P9-AQX-751

Magnetic Resonance Imaging of the Brain and Spine

SECOND EDITION

MAGNETIC RESONANCE IMAGING OF THE BRAIN AND SPINE

SECOND EDITION

EDITOR

SCOTT W. ATLAS, M.D.

Professor of Radiology
Chief of Neuroradiology and Magnetic Resonance Imaging
Neuroradiology Division
Department of Radiology
Oregon Health Sciences University
Portland, Oregon

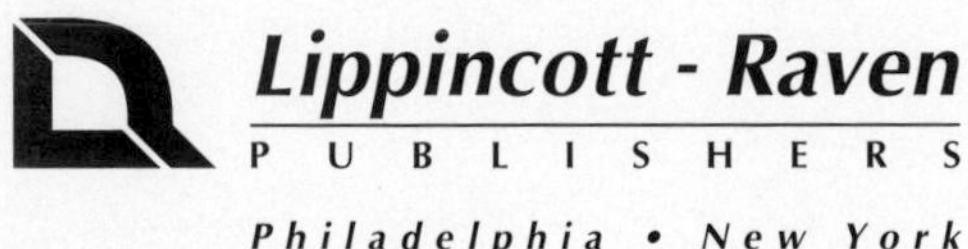

Lippincott - Raven
PUBLISHERS
Philadelphia • New York

Lippincott-Raven Publishers, 227 East Washington Square, Philadelphia, Pennsylvania 19106

Printed and bound in Japan

Library of Congress Cataloging-in-Publication Data

Magnetic resonance imaging of the brain and spine/editor, Scott W. Atlas.—2nd ed.
p. cm.
Includes bibliographical references and index.
ISBN 0-7817-0282-8
1. Central nervous system—Magnetic resonance imaging. I. Atlas, Scott W., 1955–.
[DNLM: 1. Brain Diseases—diagnosis. 2. Magnetic Resonance Imaging. 3. Spinal Diseases—diagnosis. 4. Brain—pathology. 5. Spine—pathology. 6. Spinal cord—pathology. WL 348 M196 1996]
RC349.M34M34 1996
616.8′047548—dc20
DNLM/DLC
for Library of Congress 95-6253

The material contained in this volume was submitted as previously unpublished material, except in the instances in which credit has been given to the source from which some of the illustrative material was derived.

Great care has been taken to maintain the accuracy of the information contained in the volume. However, neither Lippincott-Raven Publishers nor the editor can be held responsible for errors or for any consequences arising from the use of the information contained herein.

9 8 7 6 5 4 3 2 1

To my son,

Joseph

Contents

Contributors

Nolan R. Altman, M.D.
Clinical Associate Professor of Radiology, University of Miami School of Medicine; and Department of Radiology, Miami Children's Hospital, Miami, Florida 33136

Scott W. Atlas, M.D.
Professor of Radiology, Chief of Neuroradiology and Magnetic Resonance Imaging, Neuroradiology Division, Department of Radiology, Oregon Health Sciences University, 3181 S.W. Sam Jackson Park Road, L-340, Portland, Oregon 97201

A. James Barkovich, M.D.
Professor of Radiology, Neurology, Pediatrics, and Neurosurgery, Department of Radiology, University of California—San Francisco, 505 Parnassus Avenue, San Francisco, California 94143-0628

Laurence E. Becker, M.D., F.R.C.P.(C)
Professor, Departments of Pathology and Paediatrics, Faculty of Medicine, University of Toronto; and Pathologist-in-Chief, The Hospital for Sick Children, 555 University Avenue, Toronto, Ontario M5G 1X8 Canada

Michael D. Bell, M.D.
Clinical Assistant Professor, Department of Pathology, University of Miami School of Medicine; and Palm Beach Medical Examiner's Office, 3126 Gun Club Road, West Palm Beach, Florida 33406

Jose M. Bonnin, M.D.
Clinical Associate Professor, Indiana University, and Neuropathologist, Methodist Hospital, 1701 North Senate Boulevard, Indianapolis, Indiana 46206

Brian C. Bowen, M.D., Ph.D.
Assistant Professor, Department of Radiology, University of Miami School of Medicine, Jackson Memorial Medical Center, (R 308), 1115 N.W. 14th Street, Miami, Florida 33136

Bruce H. Braffman, M.D.
Clinical Associate Professor, Department of Radiology, University of Miami School of Medicine, Miami, Florida 33101; and Department of Radiology, Memorial Hospital, 3501 Johnson Street, Hollywood, Florida 33021

R. Nick Bryan, M.D., Ph.D.
Professor of Radiology, Neurosurgery, and Otolaryngology; Chief, Neuroradiology, Department of Radiology and Radiological Science, Johns Hopkins Medical Institutions, 600 North Wolf Street, Baltimore, Maryland 21287-2182

Sidney E. Croul, M.D.
Assistant Professor, Department of Pathology and Laboratory Medicine, Hahnemann University, Director of Neuropathology, Medical College of Pennsylvania, Broad and Vine Streets, Philadelphia, Pennsylvania 19102

Hugh D. Curtin, M.D.
Professor of Radiology and Otolaryngology, University of Pittsburgh School of Medicine, and Director, Department of Radiology, Eye and Ear Hospital, 230 Lothrop Street, Pittsburgh, Pennsylvania 15213

Leo F. Czervionke, M.D.
Associate Professor of Radiology, Department of Diagnostic Radiology, Mayo Clinic Jacksonville, 4500 San Paoblo Road, Jacksonville, Florida 32224

Mary K. Edwards-Brown, M.D.
Professor, Department of Radiology, Riley Hospital, 926 West Michigan Street, Indianapolis, Indiana 46202-5200

Adam E. Flanders, M.D.
Associate Professor, Division of Neuroradiology, Department of Radiology, Thomas Jefferson University Hospital, Suite 1072, Main Building, 10th Street and Sansom, Philadelphia, Pennsylvania 19107

Steven L. Galetta, M.D.
Associate Professor of Neurology and Ophthalmology, Department of Neurology, Hospital of the University of Pennsylvania, 3400 Spruce Street, Philadelphia, Pennsylvania 19104

Lindell R. Gentry, M.D.
Associate Professor of Radiology, Neurology, and Neurosurgery, Department of Radiology, University of Wisconsin Hospital and Clinics, 600 Highlands Avenue, Madison, Wisconsin 53792

Herbert I. Goldberg, M.D.
Professor of Radiology and Neurosurgery, Department of Radiology, Hospital of the University of Pennsylvania, 3400 Spruce Street, Philadelphia, Pennsylvania 19104

John C. Gore, Ph.D.
Professor of Diagnostic Radiology and Applied Physics, Department of Diagnostic Radiology, Yale University School of Medicine, 333 Cedar Street, New Haven, Connecticut 06510

Victor M. Haughton, M.D.
Professor of Radiology, Chief of Neuroradiology Section, Medical College of Wisconsin, 8700 West Wisconsin Avenue, Milwaukee, Wisconsin 53226

Robert W. Hurst, M.D.
Assistant Professor, Departments of Radiology, Neurosurgery, and Neurology, Hospital of the University of Pennsylvania, 3400 Spruce Street, Philadelphia, Pennsylvania 19104

Peter M. Joseph, Ph.D.
Professor, Department of Radiology, Hospital of the University of Pennsylvania, 3400 Spruce Street, Philadelphia, Pennsylvania 19104

Emanuel Kanal, M.D.
Associate Professor, University of Pittsburgh School of Medicine; and Director, MRI Department, Pittsburgh NMR Institute, Department of Radiology, University of Pittsburgh Medical Center, 200 Lothrop Street, Pittsburgh, Pennsylvania 15213

Richard P. Kennan, Ph.D.
Assistant Professor, Department of Diagnostic Radiology, Yale University School of Medicine, 333 Cedar Street, New Haven, Connecticut 06510

Walter Kucharczyk, M.D., F.R.C.P.(C)
Professor and Chair, Department of Medical Imaging, Faculty of Medicine, University of Toronto; Medical Director, Tri-Hospital Magnetic Resonance Centre, Toronto; and The Toronto Hospital, 150 College Street, Toronto, Ontario M5S 1A8 Canada

Ehud Lavi, M.D.
Assistant Professor, Division of Neuropathology, Department of Pathology and Laboratory Medicine, Hospital of the University of Pennsylvania, 3400 Spruce Street, Philadelphia, Pennsylvania 19104

Robert E. Lenkinski, Ph.D.
Professor of Radiological Science, Department of Radiology, Hospital of the University of Pennsylvania, 3400 Spruce Street, Philadelphia, Pennsylvania 19104

William M. Leue, B.A.
Corporate Research and Development Center, General Electric Company, KWC-436, P.O. Box 8, Schenectedy, New York 12309

Frank J. Lexa, M.D.
Assistant Professor, Department of Radiology, University of Pennsylvania, Hospital of the 3400 Spruce Street, Philadelphia, Pennsylvania 19104-4283

John Listerud, M.D., Ph.D.
Assistant Professor of Radiologic Sciences, Department of Radiology, Oregon Health Sciences University, 3181 SW Sam Jackson Park Road, L-340, Portland, Oregon 97201

Alexander S. Mark, M.D.
Associate Clinical Professor of Radiology and Neurosurgery, Departments of Radiology and Neurosurgery, George Washington University Medical Center; and Director of Magnetic Resonance Imaging, Department of Radiology, Washington Hospital Center, 110 Irving Street, N. West, Washington, D.C. 20010

Thomas J. Masaryk, M.D.
Head, Section of Neuroradiology, Department of Radiology, The Cleveland Clinic Foundation, 9500 Euclid Avenue, Cleveland, Ohio 44195-5001

Vincent P. Mathews, M.D.
Associate Professor, and Chief, Division of Neuroradiology, Indiana University Medical Center, University Hospital 0279, 550 N. University Blvd. Indianapolis, Indiana 46202-5253

Joseph C. McGowan, Ph.D.
Research Assistant Professor, Department of Radiology, Hospital of the University of Pennsylvania, 3400 Spruce Street, Philadelphia, Pennsylvania 19104

David G. McLone, M.D., Ph.D.
Professor of Surgery, Department of Neurosurgery, Northwestern University, Children's Memorial Hospital, 2300 Children's Plaza, Chicago, Illinois 60614

Walter J. Montanera, M.D., F.R.C.P.(C)
Assistant Professor, Department of Medical Imaging, Faculty of Medicine, University of Toronto; and Staff Neuroradiologist, The Toronto Hospital—Western Division, 399 Bathurst Street, Toronto, Ontario, M5T 2S8 Canada

Marleigh Moscatel, B.A.
Finch University of Health Sciences and The Chicago Medical School, 333 Greenberg Road, North Chicago, Illinois 60064

Frances M. Murphy, M.D., M.P.H.
Director, Environmental Agents Service, Department of Veterans Affairs; Department of Neurology, Georgetown University Medical Center; and Department of Radiologic Pathology, Armed Forces Institute of Pathology, Washington, D.C. 20306-6000

Thomas P. Naidich, M.D.
Clinical Professor of Radiology, University of Miami School of Medicine; and Director of Neuroradiology, Department of Radiology, Baptist Hospital of Miami, 8900 North Kendall Drive, Miami, Florida 33176

John Perl II, M.D.
Associate Staff, Section of Neuroradiology, Department of Radiology, The Cleveland Clinic Foundation, 9500 Euclid Avenue, Cleveland, Ohio 44195-5001

M. Judith Donovan Post, M.D.
Professor of Radiology, Neurological Surgery, and Ophthalmology; Chief, Section of Neuroradiology, Department of Diagnostic Radiology, MRI Center, University of Miami School of Medicine, Jackson Memorial Medical Center, 1115 N.W. 14th Street, Miami, Florida 33136

Charles A. Raybaud, M.D.
Professor of Radiology, Groupe Hospitalier de la Timon, Marseille, France

Bruce R. Rosen, M.D., Ph.D.
Associate Professor of Radiology, Harvard Medical School; and Co-Director, MGH-NMR Center, Department of Radiology, Massachusetts General Hospital, Building 149, 13th Street, Charlestown, Massachusetts 02129

John F. Schenck, M.D., Ph.D.
Senior Scientist, Corporate Research and Development Center, General Electric Company, Building, K1/NMR, Schenectady, New York 12309

Mitchell D. Schnall, M.D., Ph.D.
Associate Professor, Department of Radiology, Hospital of the University of Pennsylvania, 3400 Spruce Street, Philadelphia, Pennsylvania 19104

Frank G. Shellock, Ph.D.
Associate Professor, Department of Radiological Sciences, University of California—Los Angeles, School of Medicine; and Director, Research, Development, and Quality Assurance, Future Diagnostics, Inc., 6380 Wilshire Boulevard, Suite 900, Los Angeles, California 90048

James G. Smirniotopoulos, M.D.
Chairman and Professor of Radiology and Nuclear Medicine, Uniformed Services University of the Health Sciences, Bethesda, Maryland; and Department of Radiologic Pathology, Armed Forces Institute of Pathology, Washington, D.C. 20306-6000

A. Gregory Sorensen, M.D.
Instructor in Radiology, Harvard Medical School, Assistant in Radiology, Neuroradiology Section, Department of Radiology, Massachusetts General Hospital, Boston, Massachusetts 02114

Gordon Sze, M.D.
Associate Professor, Chief of Neuroradiology, Department of Diagnostic Radiology, Yale University School of Medicine, 333 Cedar Street, New Haven, Connecticut 06510

Keith R. Thulborn, M.D., Ph.D.
Associate Professor of Radiology and Psychiatry, Department of Radiology, University of Pittsburgh Medical Center, Presbyterian University Hospital, MR Research Center, B-804, 200 Lothrop Street, Pittsburgh, Pennsylvania 15213

John Q. Trojanowski, M.D., Ph.D.
Professor of Pathology and Laboratory Medicine, Division of Anatomic Pathology, Hospital of the University of Pennsylvania, 3400 Spruce Street, Philadelphia, Pennsylvania 19104-4283

Charles L. Truwit, M.D.
Associate Professor of Radiology and Neurology, and Director, Neuroradiology and Magnetic Resonance, University of Minnesota Hospital and Clinic, Box 292, 420 Delaware Street S.E., Minneapolis, Minnesota 55455

Patrick A. Turski, M.D.
Professor of Radiology, Neurology, and Neurosurgery, Chief, Section of Neuroradiology, University of Wisconsin Hospital and Clinics, 600 Highland Avenue, Madison, Wisconsin 53792

Joseph J. Wehner, M.D.
Assistant Professor of Radiology, Neuroradiology Division, Department of Radiology, University of Pittsburgh School of Medicine, 230 Lothrop Street, Pittsburgh, Pennsylvania 15213

Felix W. Wehrli, Ph.D.
Professor of Radiologic Sciences, Director of MR Education, Department of Radiology, Hospital of the University of Pennsylvania, 3400 Spruce Street, Philadelphia, Pennsylvania 19104

Michelle L. Hansman Whiteman, M.D.
Assistant Professor of Radiology and Otolaryngology, Department of Diagnostic Radiology, University of Miami School of Medicine, 1115 N.W. 14th Street, Miami, Florida 33136

Warren D. Whitlow, M.D.
Texas Neuroradiology, PA, 5430 Glen Lakes Drive, Suite 260, Dallas, Texas 75231-4362

Robert A. Zimmerman, M.D.
Professor, Department of Radiology, Children's Hospital of the University of Philadelphia, 34th Street and Civic Center Boulevard, Philadelphia, Pennsylvania 19104

Acknowledgments

The original impetus for writing the First Edition of this book can be traced to Mary Rogers, now President of Lippincott-Raven Publishers. Her support and advice has been and still is much appreciated. The publication of this Second Edition is the result of a tremendous effort under pressure by many people at Raven Press, particularly Joyce-Rachel John and Kathy Cianci. I thank them both for their availability, their admirable work ethic, and their ability to have a good time finishing this book.

Special thanks go to Krystal Vasiakin, my administrative assistant at Oregon Health Sciences University, who has worked very hard in the completion of this project. I express my appreciation to the MRI technologists and ancillary MRI staff at the Hospital of the University of Pennsylvania, where many of the images for the book were generated. I am grateful to my many friends in neuroradiology across the United States, Europe, Latin America, and Asia for sending me interesting cases and allowing me to use them here.

I am indebted to all of my past teachers in neuroradiology from whom I have had the privilege of learning, including Doctors Peter Weinberg, Kwang Kim, and Tom Naidich at Northwestern University, and Doctors Robert Grossman, Herbert Goldberg, David Hackney, Robert Zimmerman, and Larissa Bilaniuk at the Hospital of the University of Pennsylvania. Their enthusiasm for neuroradiology and their devotion to maintaining the highest level of knowledge continues to serve as an example for me. I also thank Doctor John Listerud for his unending patience with my often repetitious questioning about the physics of MRI. Any technical expertise I have about MRI is to a great extent derived from our many conversations. My appreciation also goes to all of the neuroradiology fellows and visiting radiologists who have spent time discussing cases with me. Their questions have always been an essential part of my learning process. I thank my many clinical collegues in neurology, neurosurgery, and neuropathology with whom I have had the pleasure of working, with special appreciation to Doctor Steven Galotta at the Hospital of the University of Pennsylvania and Doctor William Hoyt at the University of California at San Francisco. These clinical interactions have epitomized to me how good the interaction between clinician and neuroradiologist can be. I am certain that they have educated me more about imaging neurologic diseases than I have taught them.

I thank Doctor Lee Rogers at Northwestern University for inspiring me to pursue academic radiology and for his continued support over the years. I especially thank Doctor Robert Grossman at the Hospital of the University of Pennsylvania, who has served as mentor, friend, and advocate, since I first came to Philadelphia for my fellowship.

Finally, I thank my wife Jan for her support, for her tolerance of my time away from home, and for her direction when I need it most. And, of course, for Joey, whose smile puts it all into the appropriate perspective.

Preface to the First Edition

Although magnetic resonance imaging (MRI) has matured significantly over the past several years, it remains a changing field. There is a continuing evolution of instrumentation and software evidenced by new and developing techniques such as ultrarapid imaging and MR angiography. Both basic and clinical research continue to progress rapidly. Practically speaking, therefore, a scientifically and technically accurate book on MRI has to be completed within a short period of time, requiring a cooperative effort from all contributing authors. Needless to say, undertaking a state-of-the-art volume on this subject is a significant challenge.

Despite the rapid pace at which technological change and scientific advances proceed, the point has been reached whereby sound clinical and pathological correlations formulate a basis for the signal intensity changes seen on MRI in cerebral and spinal disease entities. MRI is presently the mainstay of imaging diagnosis for the vast majority of neurological diseases. Undoubtedly it will not only further supplant other diagnostic techniques, but functional implementation of this tool is starting to occur in clinical protocols. Morphological alterations on MRI will form only one part of the diagnostic armamentarium of the clinician, due to the integration of MR spectroscopy, flow imaging techniques, and presently unknown other implementations. This marked expansion of the use of MRI is already starting to occur and has been included at its current level in the text.

Although there are other books published on MRI of central nervous system (CNS) diseases, I believe none have truly filled the need for a comprehensive and scientifically accurate text on the subject. My concept of the scope of this endeavor entailed compiling a truly definitive work—a sophisticated, complete, and accurate book on the science that was up-to-date on the technical and clinical topics. Physicists cover physics-oriented topics, and clinicians discuss clinical applications. In an attempt to formulate the most useful rendition of complex subject matter, some chapters are co-authored by physicists and clinicians. The list of invited authors was intentionally restricted to those who possess three characteristics: (1) the highest level of knowledge in that specific area; (2) extensive background and published work in that specific field; and (3) a unique ability to teach and communicate the ideas central to that topic. I believe that each contributing author meets these requirements.

Clearly, a major strength of the modality lies in its unprecedented contrast resolution. MRI is a mirror for both gross and microscopic pathology, and it should be interpreted as such in order to glean the most information about CNS processes. Furthermore, familiarity with fundamental neuropathology and the clinical aspects of neurological disease is essential to the intelligent interpretation of MRI of the brain and spine. Several chapters in this text demonstrate a distinct tendency to stress these correlations. The chapters detailing basic aspects of nuclear relaxation, the MR imaging process, and underlying biophysicochemical alterations in disease states permit the reader to develop a fundamental understanding of current and future applications of MRI and provide an approach to the interpretation of neuroradiological MRI that is not limited to pattern recognition and rote memory.

Although a general outline of the contents of each chapter was presented to each invited contributor, a strict uniform style was not required. The compilation of differing approaches presented here is, in my opinion, refreshing to the reader. The reader will also note that from chapter to chapter some topics overlap. No rigorous attempt was made to entirely eliminate this, as differing approaches to complex topics are often beneficial to the neophyte as well as to the advanced reader. From this, one has the opportunity to more thoroughly understand basics and to learn nuances from a varied experience.

This book will be of use to neuroradiologists, neurologists, neurosurgeons, and all other clinicians who interact to discuss the results of MRI in patients with neurologic disease. It is hoped that this book will aid in this interaction by adding insight into the interpretation of scans and by promulgating a common language. Neuroradiologists and others who interpret MRI of the brain and spine will benefit from the detailed discussions concerning the basis of signal intensity derangements, whether on the fundamental level (i.e., physical or biochemical) or at the level of correlations with clinical and neuropathological findings. It is anticipated that all neuroscience personnel interested in clinical disease states and in neurological research will be able to utilize this text as a starting point and reference for proposed work utilizing MRI.

Scott W. Atlas, M.D.

Preface

At the time of the Second Edition of this book, magnetic resonance imaging (MRI) has reached a certain level of maturity. It has inarguably become the mainstay of imaging for nearly all neurologic diseases, with residual exceptions most often due to practical aspects of health care delivery in a limited resource environment, rather than because of either technical issues or medical aspects of disease. There has continued to be significant improvement in MR instrumentation as well as software. Even though economic factors impact on research, development, and the delivery side of high technology health care in the United States and throughout the world, both basic and clinical research have continued to progress. Some techniques noted as new in the First Edition (e.g., MR angiography) have improved to attain accepted clinical roles, and have the potential with slight refinement to become useful in a wider variety of cases. New and emerging techniques and a wide array of new pulse sequences for fast imaging as well as standard clinical applications are becoming incorporated into protocols. Although some functional MR techniques (e.g., MR spectroscopy) have been slow to develop defined clinical roles, new methodologies have emerged that offer a real-time display of regional brain function on a single individual in an entirely non-invasive manner. In fact, the clinical applications of MRI are on the verge of a dramatic expansion because of recent developments in the functional implementation of the technique. More than ever, a working knowledge is needed of the brain and the clinical manifestations of central nervous system (CNS) disease to exploit the available information on MRI. It is anticipated that many common diseases (e.g., psychiatric illness and learning disabilities) previously deemed inaccessible to imaging because of a lack of morphologic abnormalities will now become part of the neuroradiologist's domain. This marked expansion of the use of MRI is only beginning as the elucidation of normal brain function occurs with these techniques, which have been included at their current level in this text.

My original concept of the scope of this endeavor entailed compiling a sophisticated, complete, and accurate book on the science, as well as being up-to-date on the technical and clinical topics, such that it becomes a truly definitive work. I hope that this Second Edition moves closer toward that goal. As in the First Edition, physicists cover physics-oriented topics, and clinicians discuss clinical applications. In a further attempt to formulate the most useful rendition of complex subject matter, nearly all chapters are now co-authored by some combination of neuroradiologists, neuropathologists, physicists, neurologists, and neurosurgeons.

This volume reflects my strong belief that MRI is a mirror for both gross and microscopic pathology, and it should be interpreted as such in order to glean the most information about CNS processes. Therefore, familiarity with both the fundamentals of neuropathology and the clinical aspects of neurologic disease are essential to the optimal interpretation of MRI of the brain and spine. By virtue of improvements in spatial and contrast resolution capabilities combined with new mechanisms of eliciting MR contrast, tissue characterization by MRI has become more detailed. Extensive correlations to neuropathology, both gross and microscopic, are now found throughout the text. This ample use of color specimens is a new feature in this edition for the purpose of presenting characteristics of lesions that are or may be discernible in these advanced MR techniques. In this edition, entire chapters and selected sections of others have been considerably expanded, as a result of both increasing clinical applications from new technical developments (e.g., MR angiography) as well as more clinical experience regarding the anatomic and pathologic correlations of MR signal abnormalities (e.g., spinal trauma and spinal vascular malformations). Representative cases generously donated by colleagues around the world have improved chapters covering disorders that oftentimes are geographically limited in their occurrence. New chapters have been added to encompass not only new technology (such as functional MRI) but also new and potential clinical applications based on recently described clinicopathologic MRI correlations (e.g., diseases of the temporal bone).

MRI is not the only field in clinical neuroscience that evolved since the First Edition of this book. Recent changes in neuropathologic classifications, such as for primary brain tumors, are incorporated. Sophisticated histopathologic staining methods only recently introduced into the neuropathologist's armamentarium are presented in correlation to MRI. Changes in clinical concepts and patient management are noted and references extensively updated, so that the relevant clinical information that the radiologist needs to know to be part of the team dealing with diseases of the brain and spine is available.

The chapters detailing basic aspects of relaxation, the MR imaging process, and underlying biophysicochemical alterations in disease states are included to permit the reader to develop a fundamental understanding of current and future applications of MRI. An approach to the interpretation of neuroradiologic MRI that is not limited to pattern recognition and rote memory is provided. The basic topics have been improved by adding more text and diagrammatic discussion of *k*-space and data acquisition in an expanded coverage of both conventional and fast imaging. New contrast mechanisms and pulse sequences are also described, many of which are in the realm of clinical research but have clear potential to become integrated into clinical protocols.

As in the First Edition, a suggested list of the contents of each chapter was presented to each invited contributor, but a strict uniform style was not required. The reader will note that some topics overlap from chapter to chapter. The compilation of differing styles presented here is intentional and allows the reader to learn different approaches to complex topics. From this, one has the opportunity to more thoroughly understand the basics and to learn nuances from varied experiences.

This book is anticipated to be of most use to radiologists, neuroradiologists, neurologists, neurosurgeons, and clinicians who interact to discuss the results of MRI in patients with diseases of the brain and spine. This book will aid in this interaction by adding insight into the interpretation of scans and by promulgating a common language. While it is not possible to present complex information in a single style that is ideally suited to readers of all backgrounds, it is hoped that a varied audience can gain useful information from this text. The book is intended to be of use to the entire spectrum of potential readers, from the novice to the sophisticated, from the trainee to the experienced neuroradiologist. In this context, for example, MR physics is introduced at basic and sophisticated levels. Similarly, simplistic descriptions of signal intensity and morphologic abnormalities are noted, along with more detailed explanations of their causes. Neuroscience personnel interested in clinical disease states and in clinical neurologic research will be able to utilize this text as a starting point and as a reference for proposed work utilizing MRI.

Magnetic Resonance Imaging of the Brain and Spine

SECOND EDITION

Magnetic Resonance Imaging of the Brain and Spine, Second Edition, edited by Scott W. Atlas. Lippincott-Raven Publishers, Philadelphia © 1996.

1

Instrumentation: Magnets, Coils, and Hardware

John F. Schenck and William M. Leue

In Würtzburg, Bavaria on November 8, 1895 Wilhelm Roentgen detected a new form of radiation coming from a cathode ray tube he was studying (1). By early January in 1896 this discovery of x-rays had been reported in American newspapers and elsewhere and by the end of that month equipment already available in the MIT physics department had been used to confirm Roentgen's discovery. Clinically useful x-ray images were produced almost immediately. As an example (2), F. H. Williams presented a live demonstration of skeletal imaging to a Boston medical society in April 1896 only six months after the discovery of x-rays (2).

Compare this with the more than 40 years that elapsed between the initial description of the NMR principle and the production of the first clinically relevant MR images. The contrast between the time and effort required to develop x-ray imaging and MR imaging is a measure of the inherent complexity of whole-body MR scanners. Although the concept of nuclear magnetic resonance originated with the Dutch physicist C. J. Gorter in 1936 (3–6), NMR was not experimentally observed in bulk materials until the work of Bloch and Purcell and their associates shortly after World War II (7–11). In subsequent years, NMR was mainly used to study basic physical and chemical properties of matter—and the technique was applied mostly to test tube-sized samples or to atomic and molecular beams traveling through evacuated chambers. Between World War II and the 1970s, a few NMR studies on human or animal tissues were reported (12–16), but the key to the modern clinical uses of NMR was Lauterbur's 1973 suggestion (17) that magnetic field gradients could be used to encode position-dependent information in the NMR signal. This suggested the possibility of generating cross-sectional anatomical images. Several more years elapsed before the first images of human anatomy were produced by groups at Nottingham University in 1976 and 1977 (18–20). Several methods were suggested for converting MR signals into images—these included back projection (17), sensitive point (21), and field focusing (22–24) techniques. However, the vast majority of clinical scanning has been carried out using the Fourier techniques that were originally developed for NMR spectroscopy (25) and that were later adapted to imaging (26,27). In its most commonly used form this technique has become known under the name of spin-warp or spin-echo imaging (28).

The application of NMR to basic science engaged some of the most prominent physicists and chemists of the postwar period and it is interesting that many of these

J. F. Schenck, M.D., Ph.D., and W. M. Leue: General Electric, Corporate Research and Development Center, Schenectady, New York 12309.

leaders initially doubted the practicality of human imaging (29). To produce practical clinical scanners, it was necessary to scale the NMR apparatus up from a size designed to deal with samples in test tubes to a size capable of accepting and studying the entire human body (30,31). The development and widespread clinical utilization of MR scanners during the 1980s represented a technical tour de force. Engineering advances were combined with newly developed scientific and clinical understanding and with large financial investments to produce a completely new addition to the medical diagnostic armamentarium. During the early 1990s efforts have been aimed at improving the effectiveness and reducing the costs of conventional MR imaging and at the development of new applications to extend the range of its usefulness.

Table 1 lists some of the important scientific and technical advances crucial to the eventual development of MRI scanners along with approximate dates and the names of some of the investigators involved with them. It is, of course, not possible, in a single table, to acknowledge all of the contributors to the development of MRI. The purpose of the table is to provide orientation to the large number of basic science advances that were required before MRI could be developed, and to emphasize how recently many of these basic facts have been discovered. It is noteworthy that some elderly patients, now being scanned by a method that is based on the magnetic resonance of atomic nuclei, were born before the magnetic properties, or even the existence, of atomic nuclei were known. Magnetic resonance was the first important medical imaging modality subjected to the medical device regulations issued by the U.S. Food and Drug Administration in 1976 (32).

This chapter concentrates on topics, such as the main magnet and the gradient and rf coils, that are unique to MRI scanners. It also describes some of the computer hardware required by these devices. The chapter covers the application of MRI to proton imaging which has been by far the biggest clinical use to date. Other applications, such as spectroscopy of protons, phosphorus or other nuclei involve similar instrumental considerations except that they require even more emphasis on field homogeneity and eddy currents. A single chapter can provide only an overview of the technical aspects of MR scanners. However, recently published book-length accounts are available (33–36).

The theory of electromagnetic fields is fundamental to the description of scanner operation, and because it provides quantitatively precise descriptions of image quality and artifacts, it is of great interest to scientists and engineers concerned with scanner design and refinement. Consequently, some aspects of this theory and explanations of the mathematical expressions used in this chapter are described in an Appendix. However, advanced mathematics is *not* required to understand the basic principles of MR scanners, or to interpret clinical images, and those readers with predominantly clinical in-

TABLE 1. *Some technical and scientific milestones in MRI*

Equations governing electric and magnetic fields	Maxwell (1873)
Statistical mechanics of atoms and molecules	Maxwell (1860), Boltzmann (1872), Gibbs (1878)
Radiowaves	Hertz (1887)
Superconductivity	Onnes (1911)
Atomic structure/atomic nuclei	Rutherford (1911)
Quantum theory	Bohr, Schrödinger, and others (1913–1926)
Nuclear magnetism	Pauli (1924)
Electron spin	Uhlenbeck and Goudsmit (1926)
NMR concept	Gorter (1936)
NMR observed in atomic beams	Rabi (1939)
NMR observed in solids and liquids	Bloch, Purcell (1946)
Equations for spin relaxation (T1, T2)	Bloch (1946)
NMR relaxation mechanisms	Bloembergen, Pound, Purcell (1948)
Spin-echoes	Hahn (1950)
High field superconductors	Matthais, Kunzler (1960)
Fourier transform NMR	Ernst, Anderson (1966)
X-ray computed tomography	Oldendorf (1961), Hounsfield (1973),
Whole-body NMR for medical diagnosis	Jackson (1968), Damadian (1972), Abe (1973)
Gradient fields for imaging (zeugmatography)	Lauterbur (1973)
Selective slice excitation	Mansfield (1974), Hoult (1977)
Human imaging using gradient fields	Aberdeen, Nottingham, EMI (1976–1979)
Whole-body image using field focusing	Damadian (1978)
Human imaging using high field (1.5 T) whole-body magnets	General Electric, Oxford Instruments (1981)
Widespread clinical applications with many submodalities (multislice-multiecho spin-warp, spectroscopy, angiography, fast scanning, surface coils, etc.)	Many contributors (1980–present)

terests should feel free to skip over any unfamiliar mathematics.

THREE TYPES OF MAGNETIC FIELDS AND COILS ARE USED IN MR SCANNERS

The human body contains an enormous number of hydrogen atoms—particularly in its water (H_2O) and lipid components. It is now known that the proton at the center of each of these hydrogen atoms possesses a magnetic spin. These spins can be manipulated by applied magnetic fields and signals produced by the motion (precession) of the spins can be detected outside the body. Magnetic resonance imaging requires the application to a human patient of strong and carefully crafted magnetic fields that vary as precisely defined functions of space and time. Every MR scanner contains several sets of coils which serve as sources of the magnetic fields that are used to manipulate the magnetic spins within the patient. Scanners also contain a receiver system to detect and amplify the very weak radiofrequency (rf) field that originates within the patient once the appropriate configuration of the spins has been prepared.

In idealized terms, a scanner requires the use of three types of magnetic field: (i) there is an intense uniform (i.e., homogeneous) main field used to align (or magnetize) the spins within the patient and to drive their Larmor precession; (ii) there is a set of three orthogonal gradient fields which can be pulsed on and off and are used during the scan to give the field (and, therefore, the precessional motions) inside the patient slightly different time dependence at each position; and (iii) there is spatially a uniform but relatively low amplitude rf magnetic field oscillating near the Larmor frequency and which is pulsed on and off to produce repetitive excitation of the spins within the patient. The main magnetic field defines a direction in space which is conventionally referred to as the z-direction. The z-component of the main field at the center of the magnet is designated B_0 and is so strong that it completely dominates the effects of transverse (B_x and B_y) fields that inevitably are produced by the main magnet and the gradient coils. The transverse B_x and B_y fields are, therefore, usually inconsequential in determining the MR signal. Although small transverse static fields may ordinarily be neglected, any variations of the longitudinal field, B_z, from its central value, B_0, has a significant effect on the motion of the spin system and, therefore, also on the MR imaging process. Three separate gradient coils, one each for dB_z/dx, dB_z/dy, and dB_z/dz, are used to produce controlled variations in B_z and thereby to achieve slice selection and to encode position-dependent information in the MR signal. Ideally, the gradient coils produce longitudinal B_z fields that are precisely zero at the center of the scanner and that vary in a perfectly linear fashion, $B_z = G_x x$, $B_z = G_y y$, and $B_z = G_z z$, away from the center.

The rf excitation field is, ideally, completely uniform and at right angles to the main magnetic field. Therefore, it is a B_x or B_y field or some combination of these two components. The components are of the general form B_x or $B_y = B_1 \cos(\omega t + \phi)$ where the frequency, ω, is near the spin Larmor frequency and the amplitude, B_1, and the phase, ϕ, do not depend on position. Circularly polarized fields, produced by superimposing B_x and B_y fields with a 90° phase difference are often used because of their efficiency in both the transmit and receive modes.

To summarize, an ideal scanner would be expected to produce, over the entire region of the patient being studied, the following magnetic fields–an intense, perfectly uniform main field; $B_z = B_0$ = constant in time and place; three gradient fields each varying linearly with position and of the form $B_z = G_u u$ ($u = x, y$, or z); and an oscillating rf field perpendicular to z that is completely uniform in space. Magnetic fields are often produced by passing a current through a coil of wire which, by using a large number of turns, makes it possible to produce a strong field using only a relatively modest current. Therefore, the sources of the fields within scanners are usually referred to as coils although they are not always constructed as wire windings. It is seen that a minimum of five separate coils—one main field coil, three gradient coils, and one rf coil—each producing a distinct field pattern are required to construct an idealized MR scanner.

MAIN FIELD MAGNETS

The purpose of the main field magnet is to produce the intense static magnetic field, B_0, that is used to magnetize the nuclear spins within the patient and to drive their Larmor precession. These magnets are the key component of MR scanners and more than any other factor they determine the appearance, cost, and capabilities of these devices. The most important characteristic of these magnets is the strength of the magnetic field that they produce within the patient. Only slightly less important in the uniformity of this field strength over the desired region of imaging and the temporal stability of the field.

The official SI unit for magnetic field strength is the tesla. In addition to being officially sanctioned, the tesla is of a convenient size to measure the strengths of main magnetic fields. However, another unit of magnetic field strength, the gauss, while not an SI unit, has had a long historical usage. Also, it is still widely used by physicists and chemists and it is of convenient size to describe the smaller fields (e.g., gradient fields) associated with MR scanners. The two units have an easy to remember relationship to one another—one tesla is equivalent to 10,000 gauss—and, in this chapter, we will utilize whichever of these units is more convenient for the field under discussion. When making mathematical calculations, however, it is a good idea to express the magnetic field strength in tesla and to measure all distances in meters. It is then possible to use the equations of the standard MKS formulation of electromagnetic theory, as it is presented in modern textbooks, without need for conversion factors.

Magnetism, originating in the naturally occurring mineral magnetite (lodestone), Fe_3O_4, has been known for at least 2,500 years. In 1600 the English physician William Gilbert realized that the earth itself is a huge magnet producing what would now be described as a dipole field. Everyone on earth is, of course, continually immersed in this field, which has a strength of roughly $\frac{1}{2}$ gauss (0.05 millitesla). The fields required to create a useful NMR signal are much more intense than the earth's field. In the presence of a steady magnetic field, the magnetic spins precess around the direction of the field at a fixed rate referred to as the Larmor frequency. This frequency is linearly proportional to the magnetic field strength and is 42.576375 MHz for free protons at 1 T. Whole-body clinical MRI studies have been reported over the range from 0.02 T to 4 T (200 to 40,000 gauss) (37–38). This corresponds to a variation in Larmor frequency from 0.852 MHz to 170.3 MHz. Therefore, the range of field strengths useful for medical imaging has been demonstrated to vary by a factor of at least 200. The Larmor frequency in the earth's magnetic field is approximately 2.1 kHz. The degree of nuclear spin magnetization in such a feeble field is far too small to result in an observable NMR signal without the use of special preparation techniques and, as a result, the earth's field is not useful in clinical MRI. The NMR signal is proportional to both the degree of spin magnetization and the rate of Larmor precession. In turn, these factors are both directly proportional to the magnetic field strength, B_0. Therefore the NMR signal strength increases as the square of B_0. However, patient-generated noise increases approximately linearly with frequency. This results in a signal-to-noise ratio (SNR) that increases, in strong fields, roughly in direct proportion to B_0. This gives an intrinsic SNR advantage to higher field scanners. This advantage must be balanced, of course, with other factors in deciding on the B_0 field to use for a given scanner.

In addition to the magnitude, spatial homogeneity and temporal stability of the B_0 field, another severe requirement on the main field magnet is that it is large enough to admit the patient to the imaging region and to permit the patient to be safe and comfortable throughout the examinations which often last an hour or more. A practical consequence of this is that all scanners tend to perform better on smaller patients. At some point, roughly in the neighborhood of 250 to 300 pounds, successful scanning of patients becomes difficult. The use of larger magnets to accommodate larger patients is technically possible but, because of the cost impact, dramatic increases in scanner bore size are not likely in the near future.

All current imaging strategies require a high degree of B_0 uniformity over the region being scanned and this implies, from the basic properties of the field equations, that the patient be more or less surrounded on all sides by magnetic field sources—either electric currents or magnetic materials. Of course, compromises in source location are required to provide openings to move the patient in and out of the field and to limit claustrophobia.

There are four basic choices of magnet types available for MRI.

- Permanent magnets made from "hard" magnetic materials. These magnets do not require any external power source.
- Electromagnets (iron-core magnets) made from "soft" magnetic materials and energized by electric currents flowing in wires surrounding a portion of the magnet.
- Resistive magnets (often called air-core magnets) that utilize electric currents flowing in metallic wires or tapes wound into a series of concentric coils. The coils have a cylindrical symmetry and surround the patient.
- Superconducting magnets similar in coil geometry to the resistive magnets but which utilize zero-resistance superconducting alloys as the current conductors. These magnets are similar to permanent magnets in that they require no external power source once energized.

Magnets of all these types, along with hybrid magnets that combine more than one type of basic field source, have been used successfully for MRI. Because of their abilities to reach very strong field strengths, to maintain a high degree of temporal stability, and to achieve a very high degree of field homogeneity superconducting magnets have dominated MRI since the mid-1980s. However, scanners based on other types of magnets continue to be produced for various niches within this modality.

PERMANENT MAGNETS AND ELECTROMAGNETS

Permanent magnets and electromagnets are similar in that they both rely on magnetized materials to produce the field that is applied to the patient. The "hard" magnetic materials are difficult to magnetize but, once magnetized, they maintain their magnetization almost indefinitely without further energy input. On the other hand, the "soft" magnetic materials, used in electromagnets, can be easily magnetized by an applied current, but their magnetization vanishes if the current is switched off. Both hard and soft magnetic materials produce magnetic fields because of the alignment of microscopic, ferromagnetic (39) domains within them and both exhibit saturation. That is, once these domains are fully aligned no further increase in the magnetization can be produced. Thus, there is an upper limit to the field strengths that can be obtained from these materials.

High-carbon iron is a common hard magnetic material that has long been used to make magnetic needles for directional compasses. Many additional hard magnetic materials have been developed in modern times such as the metallic alloy, Alnico; the ceramic, barium ferrite ($BaF_{12}O_{19}$); and the rare-earth alloy, samarium cobalt ($SmCo_5$). The general features of a permanent magnet for MRI (40–41) are indicated in Fig. 1. Blocks of permanent magnet material are used to energize the device. An easily magnetized yoke of soft magnetic iron, operating on the principle of the magnetic circuit (39), is used to guide the magnetic flux from one pole of the magnet to the other. Additional soft magnetic rings can be placed next to the air gap, as indicated in the figure, to provide some shimming to improve the homogeneity. This design produces a magnetic circuit which confines most of the magnetic flux to the interior of the magnetic materials except for the air gap where the patient is to be located and, as a result, there is little problem with fringing fields. The strength of the field in the air gap is determined by the strength of the magnetization, the amount of the permanent magnet material used and by the distance between the pole faces. It is desirable to keep this air gap as small as possible to enhance the strength and homogeneity of the B_0 field. However, the gap must be large enough to accommodate the patient as well as the rf and gradient coils. If the pole faces are made from an electrically conducting material, such as iron or steel, eddy currents induced in the pole faces by the pulsed gradients will affect the scanner performance and must be taken into account in the design. The magnetization of permanent magnet materials gradually decreases with time but this usually happens so slowly that it does not affect system performance. Material limitations require that permanent magnet scanners operate at field strengths of 0.3 T or less in most cases. The combined weight of the permanent magnet and the iron yoke can be quite high and 0.3 T commercial permanent magnet scanners weigh as much as 100 tons.

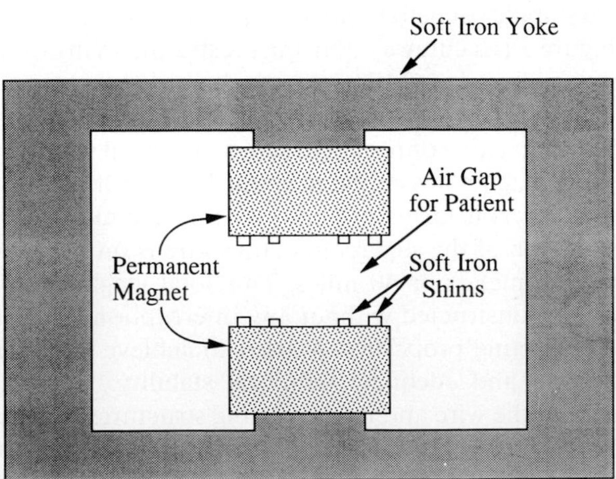

FIG. 1. Permanent magnet. A schematic cross section of a typical permanent magnet configuration. Electromagnets have similar construction but, instead of being energized by the permanent magnet material, they have current-carrying coils wound around the iron yoke. The shims are circular iron rings designed to enhance the field homogeneity in the air gap.

In 1984 a new permanent magnet material was discovered that may make it possible to construct lower weight scanners with stronger fields (42). It is an alloy of iron, neodymium, and boron with the approximate composition of $Fe_{77}Nd_{15}B_8$. Using this material, an MRI system generating 0.2 T in a 50-cm air gap and weighing 9 tons has been developed (43). A system that does not use an iron yoke has also been described (44). Although problems remain with the relatively high cost of the material and its tendency to corrode, it represents a promising approach to the issue of permanent magnet MRI systems. All permanent magnet materials are temperature sensitive. The field strength decreases as the temperature increases. For neodymium iron, a typical decrease is 1,000 ppm for a 1°C temperature rise. This undesirable temperature sensitivity is ameliorated by the large mass of the magnets which tends to reduce the fluctuations of the magnet temperature as room temperature varies.

Electromagnets are also constructed using a magnetically soft iron yoke system attached to pole faces that are designed to produce a field across a patient-containing air gap. These magnets, however, require an external power supply to energize the magnet by passing current through coils wound around the yoke. MR scanners using electromagnets are available at fields up to 0.4 T. Both electromagnet and permanent magnet systems normally produce a vertical magnet field in the direction perpendicular to the long axis of the patient's body. The magnets used in resistive and superconducting scanners, on the other hand, produce B_0 fields that are parallel to the body's long axis.

RESISTIVE MAGNETS

The first efforts to construct whole-body imaging systems in the late 1970s and early 1980s utilized, for the most part, resistive magnets that derived the magnetic field entirely from currents flowing in coils surrounding the patient and that used no magnetic materials. The systems usually used four to six coils that were wound from copper or aluminum wire or foil. The advantage of resistive magnets is that they are technically straightforward and they have a relatively low cost in comparison to superconducting systems. The chief limitations on resistive magnets result from the heat generated by the currents in the coil windings. Typical resistive magnets require 40 to 100 kilowatts from a direct current power supply continuously during operation. This necessitates the continual flow of cooling water through the coils and also through the power supply which itself dissipates many kilowatts. To avoid wasting large amounts of water, some systems use closed-cycle cooling systems which create reliability problems of their own.

The problems of heat dissipation increase rapidly with field strength and limit these magnets to approximately .15 T operation, although resistive magnets achieving somewhat higher fields have been available. Thermal expansion causes some slight motion of the coils as they are brought up to field and this can affect the field homogeneity. Once the temperature of the coils has reached a constant value the temporal stability of the magnetic field is determined by the ability of the power supply to maintain a constant current through the coils. Unlike superconducting magnets, the current-carrying coils of resistive magnets are directly accessible. This makes it possible to design magnets which have each of the coils mounted on threaded supports. Corrections to the field homogeneity can then be accomplished by adjusting the position and angular orientation of each of the coils. However, because each of the four to six coils has six degrees of freedom, the repetitive process of repositioning the coils; then measuring the resulting effect on field homogeneity; then again readjusting the coil locations; and so on can be a tedious process. Shim coils, such as are used on superconducting magnets where the main field coils are inaccessible, are not usually used on resistive magnets.

Because of the power dissipation the coil diameters are relatively small.The clear bore diameters are 60–80 cm compared to approximately 100 cm in superconducting systems. This causes resistive systems to have overall smaller openings for patients and greater difficulties in imaging heavy patients. Resistive magnets were important during the initial development of MRI but, because of substantial disadvantages relative to superconducting magnets, in the U.S. at least, they have become largely of historical interest. An exception is the work presently directed at demonstrating clinically useful applications of resistive magnets at very low field strengths on the order of .02 to .06 T.

SUPERCONDUCTING MAGNETS

As the great clinical potential of MRI became appreciated during the early 1980s reservations regarding the technical and cost challenges of utilizing whole-body superconducting magnets rapidly gave way to enthusiasm for the advantages they offered. Superconductivity has been known as an exotic property of certain metals since 1911 and over the years it has been one of the favorite topics of both theoretical and experimental solid state scientists. The key property of these materials is that they have absolutely no electrical resistance when cooled below their transition temperatures. However, this temperature is so low that liquid helium is required as a refrigerant. It is natural to try to build powerful magnets from any material with zero electrical resistance. Unfortunately, for the superconductors known before about 1950 (e.g., lead, tin and mercury), once the current density exceeds a rather low value the superconductivity vanishes and the resistance returns. Magnets made from these materials are therefore limited to producing fields of a few hundred gauss. A new class of high-field superconducting alloys (known as the type II superconductors) was discovered in the 1950s. After a great deal of metallurgical experimentation, it eventually became possible, using materials such as niobium-titanium, to build a new class of high-field magnets (45). However, except for devices designed for research laboratory purposes, there was no significant commercial application of superconductivity prior to the advent of MRI. Yet another new class of superconducting materials with very high transition temperatures was discovered in 1986. It has been hoped that these so-called high temperature superconductors would make it possible to design superconducting magnets for MRI without the requirement for refrigeration to liquid helium temperatures. However, these new materials have not yet demonstrated sufficient current carrying capability to be of use for high-field magnets.

These magnets are designed to achieve a prescribed maximum safe operating field and, in principle, they can be operated to produce any field strength up to this value. In practice, they are almost always operated at a fixed field, near the upper limit of their capabilities, which is maintained without change for months or years. Whole-body superconducting magnets are presently used in MRI scanners operating from 0.15 to 4.0 T. Typical magnet specifications would be an inhomogeneity of less than 10 ppm over a sphere 40 cm in diameter and a temporal stability of better than 0.1 ppm per hour.

Figure 2 is a cutaway drawing illustrating many of the features of modern MRI superconducting magnets. The field is produced by an intense current flowing through six coils that are connected in series. A typical superconducting magnet has a total of about 17,000 turns of wire wound on coil forms of about 0.65 meter radius. The total length of the superconducting wire is on the order of 65 kilometers or 40 miles. This total length of wire must be constructed without any interruption of its superconducting properties in order to achieve persistent operation and adequate temporal stability. The total weight of the wire and its supporting structures is on the order of 3 tons. These structures are immersed in a bath of liquid helium at 4.2°K to cool the niobium-titanium wire well below its superconducting transition temperature which is about 10°K. The transition to room temperature (298°K) is made through an intermediate liquid nitrogen stage (77°K). The spaces surrounding the liquid helium and the liquid nitrogen are both evacuated to

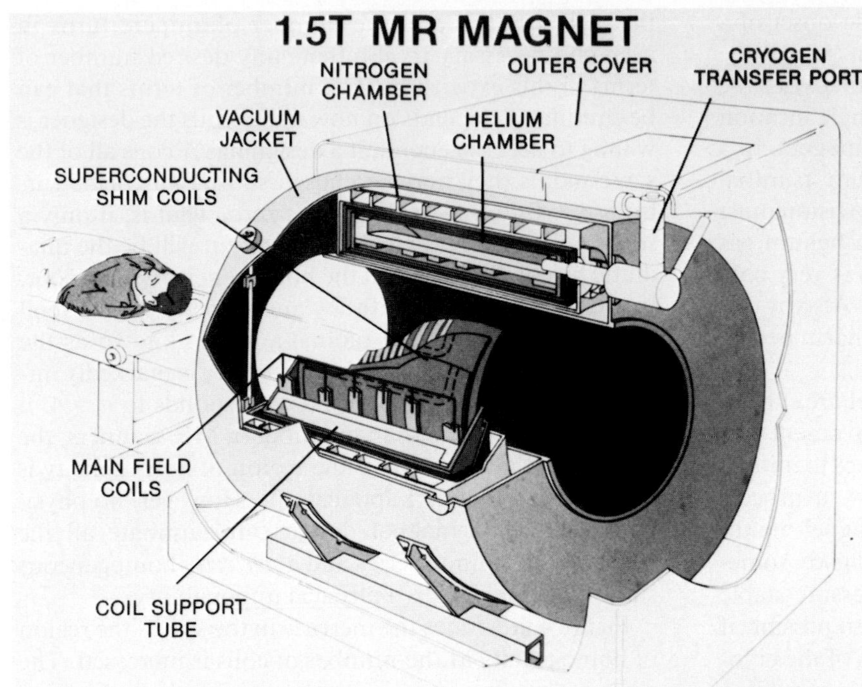

FIG. 2. Cutaway drawing of a superconducting magnet. The six main field coils and the superconducting shim coils are maintained at helium temperature. The patient table can be moved into the center of the magnet under computer control. Only in the region near the center of the cylindrical bore is the field strength and homogeneity satisfactory for MRI. (Courtesy of General Electric Medical Systems.)

minimize heat leaks into the cryogenic chambers. Nonetheless, there is an inexorable boiling of the cryogenic liquids due to thermal energy entering from the outside. This necessitates periodic refilling of the nitrogen and helium chambers. It is now common for superconducting, whole-body magnets to utilize cryogenic refrigerators that reduce or eliminate the need for refills of the cryogenic fluids. Figure 3 shows the appearance of a finished magnet.

The structure that contains the cryogenically cooled coils is called the cryostat. There are several sources of heat leaks into a cryostat—direct thermal conduction along the rods that support the weight of the coils, residual gas conduction, infrared radiation from higher to low temperatures and joule heating from eddy currents. These eddy currents are induced in metallic portions of the cryostat by pulsing of the gradient coils during imaging. The first three types of heat leak are minimized by proper cryostat design. Controlling eddy current heating, on the other hand, involves a compromise between the cryostat design and imaging performance. A 7–10 mm thick cylinder of high conductivity aluminum can be placed between the gradient coils and the main magnet coils to minimize the heat deposited in the helium temperature region. However, the use of such a shield increases the effect of eddy currents on the imaging process. For most imaging sequences now in use, however, eddy current heating is small compared to the other types of heat leak.

To maintain the superconducting state the conductor must be kept below its transition temperature. If even a small region of the wire is heated above this temperature, it begins to dissipate heat and increases still further in temperature. The result can be a self-propagating process leading to a magnet quench, wherein the entire stored energy in the magnetic field is converted into heat. This raises the temperature of the liquid helium above its boiling point and it quickly evaporates as the magnetic field

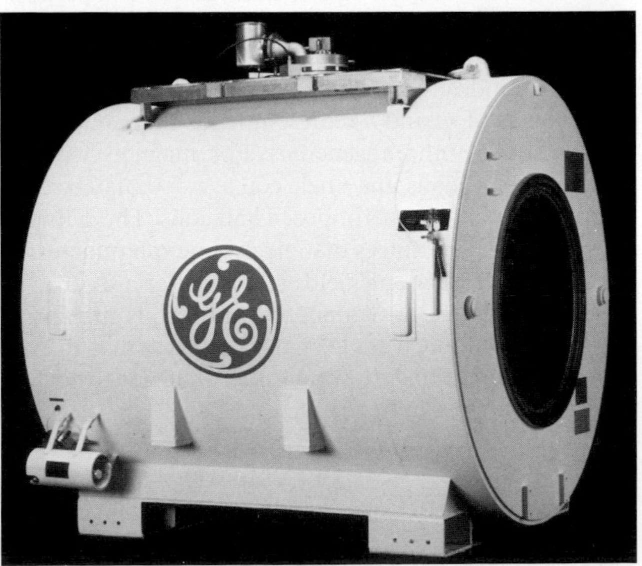

FIG. 3. A 1.5 T superconducting magnet for MRI. At the lower left is a magnetically-shielded motor. The motor is used to drive a cryogenic cooler. This device improves the thermal performance of the system and eliminates the need for liquid nitrogen in this design. (Courtesy of General Electric Medical Systems.)

collapses. Magnets are designed to sense the onset of a quench and to rapidly activate heaters that spread the energy deposition throughout the coils. Otherwise, the deposition of the total stored energy in a single location could melt the wire locally and destroy the magnet. In a controlled quench the field will decrease from its initial value to nearly zero in about one minute. Provision must be made to permit the safe removal of the helium gas that is produced during a quench. This gas is very cold and direct contact with it should be avoided. Also by displacing room oxygen it has the potential to harm people in the vicinity of a quenching magnet.

All the wires in a superconducting magnet are subject to intense forces which can cause slight movement and local frictional heating which may be sufficient to initiate a quench. This possibility is minimized by a process called training—one of the final steps in magnet manufacture—wherein the magnet is cycled to fields somewhat above its planned operating field to assure stable operation at the rated field. Quenches are also possible if a cryostat vacuum fails or if necessary refills of the cryogenic liquids are not made on time. Superconducting magnets are supplied with an emergency switch system that permits a deliberate quench in the event that someone has become trapped against or inside the magnet by a ferromagnetic object, such as an oxygen bottle.

The homogeneity of the field produced by the magnet can be analyzed in terms of the harmonic functions discussed in the appendix. The homogeneity of these designs is intrinsically good because of the cylindrical symmetry of each coil and the fact that the coils are present as identical pairs along the z axis, one or either side of the center (46–48). As described in the appendix, the static field inside the magnet can be analyzed as a superposition of independent harmonic fields which can be specified by the integers m and n. The term with $m = 0$ and $n = 0$ is the desired, perfectly homogeneous field. The other values of m and n represent fields that are present as undesirable inhomogeneities. For magnets with an odd number of coils, the single coil at $z = 0$ may be considered as a pair of superimposed half coils. The cylindrical symmetry guarantees that, neglecting manufacturing tolerances, all harmonic fields at the center are zero unless $m = 0$. The use of symmetric pairs of coils guarantees that only harmonic fields even in z, that is with n an even number, have nonzero amplitudes. The ideal field of such a coil array can be written as,

$$B_z = \sum_{\substack{n=0 \\ (n \text{ even})}}^{\infty} A_n r^n P_n^0(\cos\theta) \qquad [1]$$

The first term has $n = 0$ and $A_0 = B_0$. This term corresponds to the perfectly uniform static field that is desired. The other terms represent contaminating fields that degrade the homogeneity, particularly as r becomes large. Mathematical methods have been developed to calculate the coil positions and the number of ampere turns in each coil necessary to eliminate any desired number of terms in this expansion. The number of terms that can be eliminated depends on how many coils the designer is willing to use. In general, if a design has N coils all of the same radius they may be chosen so that all coefficients from $n = 0$ to $n = 2(N - 1)$ are zero. That is, if only a single coil is used, the first error present will be the quadratic field with $n = 2$ and the homogeneity will be poor. If two coils are used and they are properly spaced (coil separation equal to coil radius) a design known as the Helmholtz pair results, the homogeneity is markedly improved, and the first error field corresponds to $n = 4$. If six coils are used, as in many modern MR scanners, the first error is at $n = 12$ and the region of homogeneity is large enough for MRI applications. However, no physically achievable magnet design can eliminate all the terms in this infinite series and a *perfectly* homogeneous static magnetic field is a physical impossibility.

Figure 4 illustrates the increase in the size of the region of homogeneity as the number of coils is increased. The ellipses show the approximate contours where the magnitude of the total field, $B = \sqrt{B_z^2 + B_x^2 + B_y^2}$, deviates from B_0, the field at the magnet center, by 100 ppm. In a typical scanner the coil support tube diameter is about 1.3 meters and the fiberglass warm-bore tube has a diameter of about one meter. A magnet of this size that consisted of only a single coil at $z = 0$ could maintain a homogeneity of 100 ppm only over a minuscule region that is less than 1 cm in diameter. The two-coil Helmholtz pair has a substantially larger region of homogeneity and served for decades as the design of choice for scientific experiments that required homogeneous fields. However, the region of homogeneity of the Helmholtz pair is still much too small for MRI purposes. As a result, practical magnets for MRI use from 4 to 8 coils to achieve satisfactorily homogeneous fields over adequate imaging volumes.

There are inevitable imperfections in the coil locations within a manufactured magnet. These imperfections lead to the presence of harmonic error fields that would not be present in the magnet as it is ideally designed. Shimming techniques (49) are used to correct for these inevitable errors and for errors that result from the magnetization of magnetic materials in the vicinity of the magnet. Passive shimming is accomplished by placing small permanent magnets at strategic locations within the bore of the magnet to counteract field inhomogeneities once they have been mapped and characterized. This method has the advantage that no power supplies are needed to energize the permanent magnets. However, unless complete rings of iron are used (and these are difficult to manipulate inside a strong magnetic field), the individual blocks of iron produce fields that are complicated and not at all like individual harmonic fields. The correct positioning of a large number of these pieces

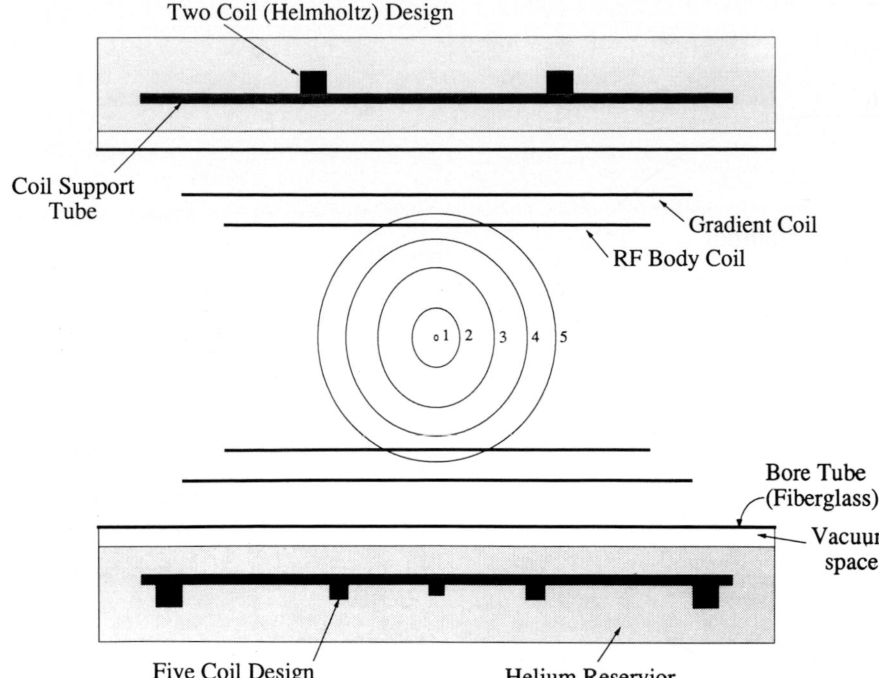

FIG. 4. Homogeneity of cylindrical bore magnets. Contours of the approximate locations where the main field inhomogeneity reaches 100 ppm are given for designs utilizing from 1 to 5 coils wound on a single cylindrical surface. For comparison, the location of some other magnet components are indicated schematically but details of the cryostat are not shown. At the top the coil locations for the two-coil (Helmholtz pair) design are indicated. These two coils are separated by a distance equal to their radius. At the bottom the location and relative strengths of the coils for the five-coil design are indicated.

of iron is time consuming. Also it may become necessary to reposition them if, for example, some magnetic material external to the magnet is moved.

Active shimming is an alternative method for improving magnet homogeneity. This method makes use of a set of specially designed coils placed within the magnet each of which is designed to produce a field which closely approximates one of the pure harmonic fields. If superconducting shim coils are used, they are located, like the main coils, within the cryostat and are maintained at liquid helium temperature. To make it possible to change the current in superconducting shim coils it is necessary to provide current leads to an external power supply. These leads can be switched from one shim coil to another and a set of currents can be built up in the array of coils to cancel out each of the harmonic fields for which a shim coil has been provided. Superconducting switches are used to restore the coil to the persistent mode once the power supply has brought each shim current to the desired value. An alternative to the use of superconducting shim coils is to provide a set of resistive shim coils which can be located within the room temperature bore of the magnet. Each of these coils also is designed to produce primarily a single harmonic field but, in this case, each coil is permanently connected to its own power supply. This makes it easy to reset the resistive shim coil currents and, therefore, shimming with these coils can be performed whenever necessary to maintain high image quality.

Many magnets are built with both resistive and superconducting shim coil sets. The more powerful superconducting shims are used to more or less permanently cancel out the major fixed inhomogeneities and the resistive shims are used for more frequent fine-tuning of the field. A scanner set may contain 10 to 15 separate coils in each set but those corresponding to low order harmonics, e.g., the B_0 shim that adjusts the main field and the gradient shims, x, y, and z, are the most crucial to image quality.

The fringing field (Fig. 5) that spreads out into the space surrounding the magnet is another important aspect of high-field superconducting magnets. At distances more than one or two meters away from the magnet, the magnitude of this fringing field is given accurately by the dipole formula

$$B(r, \theta) = \frac{\mu_0 m}{4\pi r^3} \sqrt{1 + 3\cos^2\theta} \qquad [2]$$

where m is the magnitude of the dipole moment of the magnet and is proportional to the central field, B_0. This formula shows that a given field contour extends further, by a factor of $\sqrt[3]{2} = 1.26$, along the magnet axis ($\theta = 0$). than it does transverse to the magnet ($\theta = \theta/2$). Also note that a given contour, for example the five gauss line, extends along the axis a distance that is proportional to the cube root of B_0. Therefore, if for example the central field is tripled, the position of the five gauss line only increases by $\sqrt[3]{3} = 1.44$.

For siting purposes it is often desirable to limit the extent of the fringing field by shielding the magnet (50). Active shielding is the use of additional superconducting coils with current flowing in the opposite direction to that in the main coils. These countercoils are usually much larger in diameter than the main coils or located well outside them along the z axis. They can greatly re-

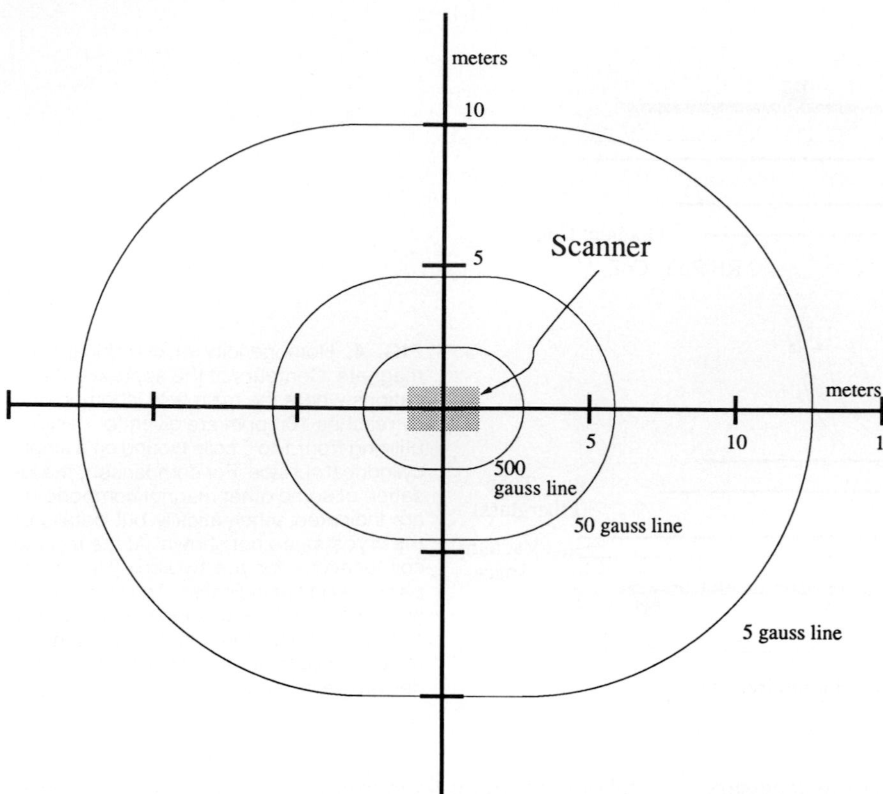

FIG. 5. Fringing field. Position of various fringing field contours for a 1.5 T whole-body magnet with a dipole moment of 5.0×10^6 ampere-m^2. For a fixed central field the dipole moment scales as the cube of the coil radius. Therefore, small-bore magnets have much less extensive fringing fields than larger magnets of the same field strength. The use of either active or passive shielding can greatly reduce the extent of the fringing field. For example, the 5 gauss line for the shielded version of this magnet is at an axial distance of 4 meters rather than at 12.5 meters as shown here.

duce the dipole moment and thereby the fringing field. Drawbacks to the use of active shielding include the substantially increased magnet size and the fact that the countercoils reduce the useful field in the center of the scanner.

Passive shielding is accomplished by using soft iron yokes external to the magnet to guide the flux from one end of the magnet to the other and thereby reducing the fringing field. The use of external iron has the agreeable property that, although it decreases the external fringing field, it increases the strength of the useful field in the center of the magnet. The disadvantages of passive shimming are that it increases the weight of the magnet and it distorts somewhat the homogeneity of the imaging field, thus putting more burden on the shim coils.

GRADIENT COILS

Three gradient coils, each with a separate power supply and each under independent computer control, are required to permit slice selection and to code position-dependent information into the NMR signal (51). Many coil shapes can be used to produce gradient fields, but in MRI using superconducting main field magnets, the most practical approach is to wind all three coils on a cylinder surrounding the patient and located inside the warm bore of the main magnet. This is the only configuration we will consider in this chapter. Coils producing the z gradient, G_z, will be considered first as they are simplest. Transverse gradient coils are more complex but a simplifying consideration is that any coil that produces a G_x field will, if rotated 90° around the z axis, produce a G_y field. Therefore, although two transverse field gradients, G_x and G_y, are needed, only one basic coil design for the transverse gradient is required. A gradient in any arbitrary direction can be generated by activating two or all three of the gradient coils simultaneously. This makes it possible to select imaging planes in any one of the principal orientations—axial, sagittal, or coronal—and also in any oblique orientation. This flexibility to select any desired scan plane electronically and without moving the patient gives MRI one of its major advantages over CT and other imaging modalities.

A z-gradient field, like the main field, may be produced by set of circular coils placed symmetrically along the z axis. The field near the center of the magnet is again given by a series of harmonics

$$B_z = \sum_{\substack{n=0 \\ (n \text{ odd})}}^{\infty} A_n r^n P_n^0(\cos\theta) \qquad [3]$$

However, the current in the coils on opposite sides of the central plane are now in opposite directions and consequently the factors A_n are all zero unless n is odd. Again, because of the cylindrical symmetry, there are no contributions to the sum unless $m = 0$. The first and most important term is for $n = 1$. This term is $B_z = A_1 r$

$\cos\theta = G_z z$, in other words a perfect z gradient. The other terms in this series represent contaminating fields that add some curvature, or nonlinearity to the field. The simplest form of gradient coil is two current loops, symmetrically placed on either side of the center and carrying current in opposite directions. Maxwell (52) showed that, if the coil radius is a, the most linear field that can be produced by this configuration places the two coils a distance $\sqrt{3}\,a$ apart. In this case the cubic contaminating field is zero and the first error term is proportional to r^5.

The remaining error terms limit the size of the region over which Maxwell pairs produce a sufficiently uniform gradient. An investigation of alternative z-gradient coils that can be wound on the surface of cylinder disclosed designs that have higher degrees of linearity, i.e., contain fewer contaminating terms, than the Maxwell pair (53). It was shown that a design current density increasing linearly with z (therefore, reversing sign at $z = 0$) produces a perfect z-gradient field throughout the inside of the cylinder. For this design, the only nonzero term in the expansion is $G_z z$—all the other coefficients are zero. This design is analogous to the infinitely long, uniformly wound solenoid which produces in its interior a perfectly uniform B_0 field. In practice, of course, it is necessary to terminate the gradient coil at some finite length. By appropriately overwinding the coil at its ends a good approximation to the ideal gradient coil can be achieved. A coil of this type, using a spiral winding which is reversed at $z = 0$ and becomes more densely wound as z increases, is shown in Fig. 6.

Transverse gradient coils may also be wound on the surface of a cylinder but the current pattern is more complex. Here the intent, ideally, is to produce a pure harmonic field proportional to H^c_{11} (as the x-gradient) or to H^s_{11} (as the y-gradient). Golay (54) invented a pattern capable of generating transverse gradient fields and designed to be placed on the surface of a cylinder (Figs. 7 and 8). This design was adapted to superconducting solenoids by Dadok (55). It can be shown that the only B_z fields generated using this four loop symmetry have n and m both odd. Furthermore, making the arcs in this

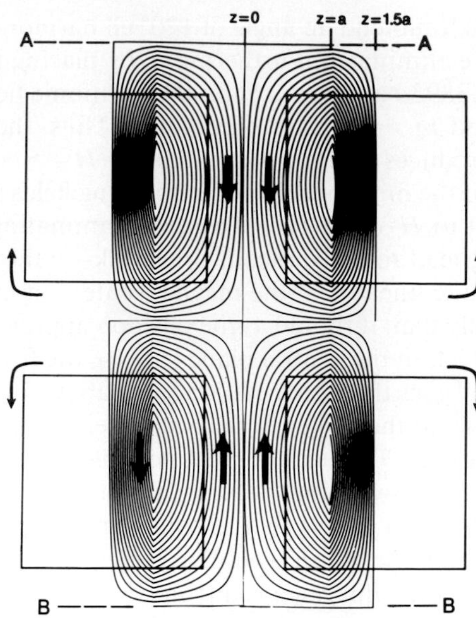

FIG. 7. Transverse gradient winding pattern. The four quadrant current pattern can be etched in copper foil and wrapped onto a cylindrical coil form so that the line AA overlaps the line BB. In this design the active current patterns extend from the center to a distance of one coil radius along the z-axis. The etching contours have a slight spiral slope to permit current to flow continuously from winding to winding. The z-location of the return currents is between 1 and 1.5 coil radii. For comparison, the rectangular overlay shows the pattern of the Golay coil design.

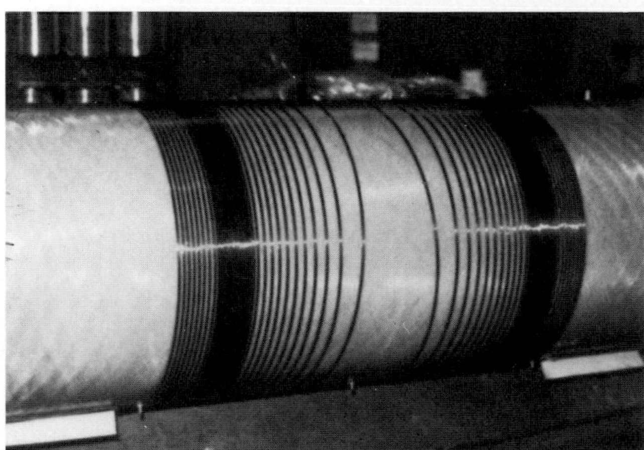

FIG. 6. z-Gradient coil. The photograph shows a coil wound on a cylindrical surface with a spiral pattern and with overwinding near the end of the coil. This pattern produces a z gradient with a high degree of linearity throughout the center of the imaging region. The overwinding begins at $z = a$ where a is the coil radius. The design shown produces a gradient field that is linear over a larger region than that of the Maxwell pair which would have coils at $z = \pm\sqrt{3}\,a/2 = \pm 0.866a$. (Courtesy of R. J. Dobberstein, General Electric Medical Systems.)

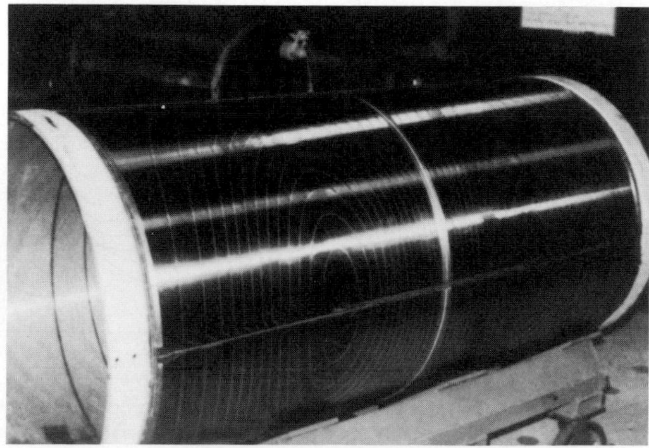

FIG. 8. Transverse gradient coil. The photograph shows the outer coil pattern of an actively shielded gradient pair. (Courtesy of R. J. Dobberstein, General Electric Medical Systems.)

design each subtend an angle of 120° all harmonics with $m = 3$ are eliminated. Furthermore, by placing the arcs at $z = \pm.3893a$ and $z = 2.569a$ the harmonic field with $n = 1$ and $m = 3$ is also eliminated. Thus, the Golay design produces a field proportional to $H^c_{11} = x$, as desired, and the first nonzero contaminating fields are proportional to H^c_{53} and H^c_{55}. These contaminating fields, however, lead to a significant drawback—although the field is quite linear near the magnet center—it increases less rapidly than it should as the position approaches the wall. In fact, in the central plane ($z = 0$), the field of the Golay coil goes through a maximum at about 70% of the distance from the center to the wall, after which it starts to decline (Fig. 9). Therefore, it is possible for two points inside the coil with the same y-value to also have the same field. This means that in spin-warp imaging these two points in the object would be projected to the same point in the image—producing a serious double exposure artifact referred to as aliasing.

A design for transverse gradient coils that overcomes the problem with aliasing has been developed (56). We take λ_ϕ and λ_z to be the two components of the surface current density on a cylinder of radius a. If a current pattern $\lambda_\phi = ca \cos \phi$ and $\lambda_z = cz \sin \phi$, where c is a constant, is established on the cylindrical surface it can be shown that the field inside the cylinder is exactly proportional to the field H^c_{11} that is desired for a transverse gradient. In practice, it is necessary to terminate the pattern at some distance along the cylinder and to provide for return current paths. However, such designs make it possible to approximate a perfect transverse gradient field as closely as desired. Although this design calls for currents with a complicated dependence on position it turns out to be possible to borrow a theorem from the hydrodynamics of nonviscous fluids—a streamline in a flow pattern may be replaced by a rigid boundary without altering the rest of the flow pattern—to show how to produce the necessary current distribution by etching an appropriate pattern into a copper sheet (57).

In practice, all gradient fields show some deviation from linearity at locations away from the center of the magnet and this leads to image distortion. However, as long as aliasing is not present, it is possible to use the exact mathematical expression for the field produced by the gradient coil to correct the image for this type of distortion.

The spin-echo imaging method relies on the application of a rapid sequence of time-varying gradient fields, on all three axes, to the patient being scanned. This requires that currents in the three gradient coils be rapidly switched by computer-controlled power supplies. The time required to switch between two current levels is one of the important factors that determines what pulse sequences can be implemented successfully on a given imager. Representative values for a common commercial scanner are that the field gradients can be switched from zero to one gauss/cm in 500 μsec. This requires that the power supply be capable of driving the coil current from zero to roughly 100 amperes in this time. This current is supplied to a gradient coil with an inductance of about 1 millihenry and a resistance of about 1 ohm. At a steady state of 100 amperes the power into each coil is 100 watts and this requires only one volt from the power supply. During the switching interval, however, a voltage, $V = L\ dI/dt = 200$ volts, is required and the instantaneous power during the ramping of the current is on the order of 20 kilowatts. For most imaging sequences the duty cycle of the gradient coils is relatively low. However, there are applications and conditions under which significant heating of these coils can occur. Some designs have in-

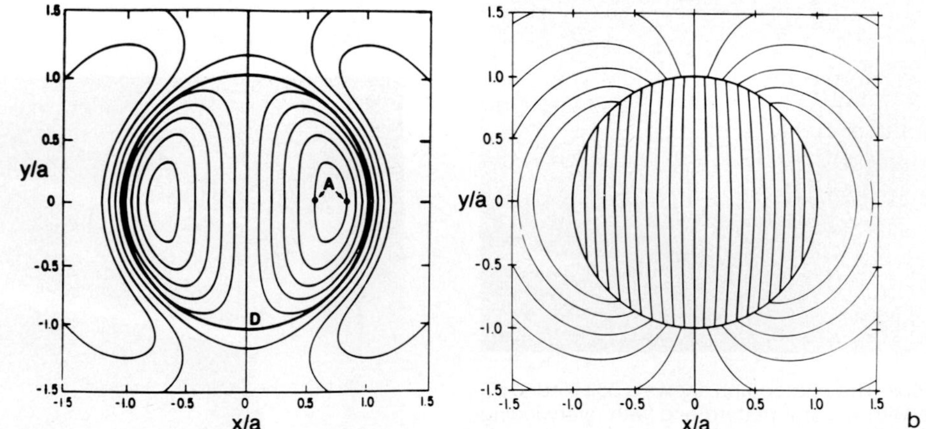

FIG. 9. Gradient field contours. The field contours in the central plane ($z = 0$) of the Golay gradient coil **(a)** and of the sinusoidally wound coil **(b)** are compared. Both designs produce a highly linear field near the axis of the coil. The field of the Golay design, however, departs significantly from linearity at points such as *D*. The aliasing artifact, which occurs when two points with the same y-value have the same gradient field, is absent in (b) but is seen in (a) where, for example, the two points A have the same transverse gradient field and, therefore, cannot be separated in a spin-warp image.

corporated water cooling of the gradient coils. This reduces the heating effects but adds additional reliability considerations to the system.

A time-dependent current is a source of electric as well as magnetic fields. When the current in a gradient coil is switched the resulting electric fields cause eddy currents to flow in any metallic conductors in the vicinity of the coil. One effect of these eddy currents, as mentioned earlier, is to provide a source of heat within the cryostat. Under most conditions a more important effect, however, is that the induced eddy currents themselves act as a source of magnetic fields that are superimposed upon the desired field produced by the gradient coil (58–60). Eddy currents are induced only during the times when the current in the gradient coils is being switched. However, once induced, the eddy currents decay relatively slowly with a complex, multiple time-constant behavior and can significantly degrade the performance of some imaging sequences.

One way to reduce the effects of eddy currents is to anticipate their actions and to tailor the wave form of the gradient current so that the *combined* magnetic field of the gradient current and the eddy current yield approximately the desired magnetic wave forms. Another approach is to build actively shielded gradient coils. These shielded gradient coils have, for each of the three primary coils, a second coil surrounding it (61–63). This second coil is in series with the main gradient coil but its current is in the opposite direction. The shielding coils are designed to largely cancel the external fields produced by the original gradient coils. As in the case of active shields for main magnets, these coils act to reduce the overall strength of the gradient field and to increase the weight of the assembly. These disadvantages are overshadowed in many cases, however, by the increase in image quality resulting from the decreased effects of eddy currents.

RADIOFREQUENCY COILS

Radiofrequency (rf) coils are required to perform two functions—transmitting and receiving signals at and near the Larmor frequency of the precessing spins (64). The term radiofrequency is applied loosely to a huge range of frequencies. Standard AM radio broadcasting used the frequency range from .54 to 1.6 MHz which is well below the proton frequency in most MR scanners. The frequency range from 3 to 26 MHz is utilized for short-wave radio broadcasting and the range from 54 to 216 MHz is used for FM radio and UHF television. To put this in perspective, note that the proton Larmor frequency at 1.5 T is 63.86 MHz. This frequency is located in the band from 60 to 66 MHz that is allocated to television broadcasting on Channel 3.

It is not surprising, therefore, that many of the electronic components in the MRI transmitter and receiver chains, such as the coaxial cables, matching and tuning networks, power amplifiers, and low level preamplifiers are similar to their counterparts in radio and TV systems. This also explains the need for careful shielding of MR scan rooms to prevent contamination of the extremely weak NMR signal, that originates inside the patient, with extraneous signals at the same frequency. Contaminating rf fields can originate either in the operation of broadcasting stations or as adventitious electromagnetic noise created during the operation of electronic equipment such as computers. It is common for MRI scanners to be surrounded by copper-mesh screened rooms so that the received NMR signal can go through at least one stage of amplification before encountering environmental electromagnetic noise. To prevent this noise from entering the scan room along electrical wiring cables, such as those used to provide current to the gradient coils, these cables are connected to electronic filters to remove high frequency noise components at the point where the cables enter the screened room.

Although the frequencies may be the same, the spatial patterns of the electromagnetic waves encountered in MRI are much different from those that are used in radio and TV broadcasting. The radio or TV signal is received at a great distance from its source and is transmitted over this distance as a traveling wave whose energy is equally divided between the electric and magnetic components. On the other hand, the electromagnetic energy of an NMR signal is almost entirely in its magnetic field and is always detected only a short distance from the precessing magnetic dipoles within the patient that are its source. In other words, the transmitting and receiving functions for NMR are carried out in the so-called near-field or standing wave zone where the source and the receiver are separated by much less than one wavelength. For example, at 1.5 T the wavelength of the proton signal is 4.5 meters which is much larger than the size of any of the coils involved in generating or detecting the NMR signal. As a consequence, except at the very highest field strengths, the wavelength of the NMR signal is not an issue in coil design. Another consequence of the differing field patterns is that entirely different receiving and transmitting antennas are required for NMR than for radio and TV. A rabbit-ear antenna can do an excellent job of receiving TV signals but it is entirely the wrong shape to use in MRI!

The initial studies of NMR were performed using continuous wave (cw) techniques. In this technique rf power is continuously supplied to the spins and the field or frequency is varied slowly through the range where the resonance occurs. However, modern MRI is almost always done using the so-called Fourier transform technique where a brief, powerful burst of rf energy (lasting at most a few milliseconds) from an rf transmitter is used to excite the spins and is followed by the detection of a signal (the free-induction-decay or FID) that lasts from roughly

10 to 1,000 milliseconds. It is possible to use the same coil for both the transmitter and receiver functions. If this is done it is necessary to protect the delicate preamplifier in the receiver chain from the brief but intense instantaneous power (.1 to 10 kilowatts) present during the transmitter pulses. This can be done by utilizing a protection circuit containing crossed diodes and coaxial cables of one-quarter wavelength (33,65). Alternatively, it is possible to use separate coils for the transmit and receive functions.

A wide range of rf coils are used for MRI. However, they all operate on similar principles and all of them can, at least theoretically, be used as transmitter coils, receiver coils, or both. It is useful to distinguish between head coils, body coils, and surface coils. Head and body coils are designed to surround the region being imaged. They are designed to produce an rf magnetic field that is essentially uniform across the region of the patient to be imaged. Body coils must be large enough to surround the patient's chest and abdomen and, often, also the table on which the patient is lying. Body coils are usually constructed on cylindrical coil forms and typically a diameter of 50 to 60 cm and a length of 70 to 80 cm. Head coils, of course, can be smaller and are typically 40 cm long and 28 cm in diameter. The term surface coil (66) is used loosely to describe a wide range of coil designs that fit closely over some specific anatomical region and provide SNR advantages for its imaging. These coils include circular (e.g., coils for the orbit and the TMJ) and rectangular coils (e.g., coils for the lumbar, spine) as well as irregular shapes designed for regions such as the cervical spine and the shoulder. A common approach to high resolution imaging is to use separate coils—a large coil (e.g., the body coil) as a transmitter and a comparatively small surface coil as the receiver. This approach takes advantage of the uniform pattern of excitation produced by the large coil and of the high sensitivity of the surface coil over local regions. The sensitivity of the surface coil, of course, is *not* uniform over its field of view, but this is balanced by the improved SNR for anatomical regions near to the coil. When separate coils are used as transmitter and receiver careful attention should be given to their interaction as both coils are tuned to the same frequency. Therefore, any current in one coil tends to excite strong currents in the other coil. This interaction can also be blocked by the appropriate use of crossed diodes and coaxial cables (67). If coil decoupling is not dealt with properly both the transmit and receive portions of the imaging sequence can be unsatisfactory.

The ideal rf field is transverse to B_0, that is in the x or y direction, and completely uniform in space. For head and body coils it can be shown that the current distribution on a cylindrical surface would produce this ideal field is a z-directed current of the form $\lambda_z = c \cos \phi$ where c is a constant. Of course, the coil has to be terminated at some finite length and return current paths must be provided. It turns out that the longer the coil is along the z axis, the more nearly the rf field approaches the desired goal of perfect uniformity. In practice, these coils have lengths that are one to two times their diameter. Shorter coils have some advantage in receiving less noise from the patient but produce a field with decreased uniformity. The simplest design for head and body coils is the saddle coil (33,64) which is essentially a four-wire approximation to the ideal current density. It is difficult, because of self-resonance effects, to build large (i.e., whole-body sized) saddle coils that will resonate properly above about 25 MHz. This limitation can be somewhat alleviated by using distributed capacitors along the length of the coil conductor.

The birdcage resonator (Fig. 10) is a coil design that is capable of resonating at higher frequencies than the saddle coil. It also possesses advantages in terms of field homogeneity and the possibility of quadrature excitation (68). This design consists of several connected loops arranged around the cylindrical surface and having series capacitances in each of the loops. A common version utilizes 16 loops to span the cylinder. A birdcage resonator has several resonant modes and frequencies but only one of these modes is useful for imaging purposes. In this mode the current in each strut of the coil varies as cos ϕ. That is, a 16-wire birdcage coil resonating in this mode provides a 16-wire approximation to the ideal current distribution and, consequently, a more uniform field than the saddle coil (Fig. 11). The multiple capacitors in the birdcage design also serve the same function as the distributed capacitors in high frequency saddle coils. Whole-body sized birdcage coils have been demonstrated to resonate readily at frequencies as high as 170 MHz.

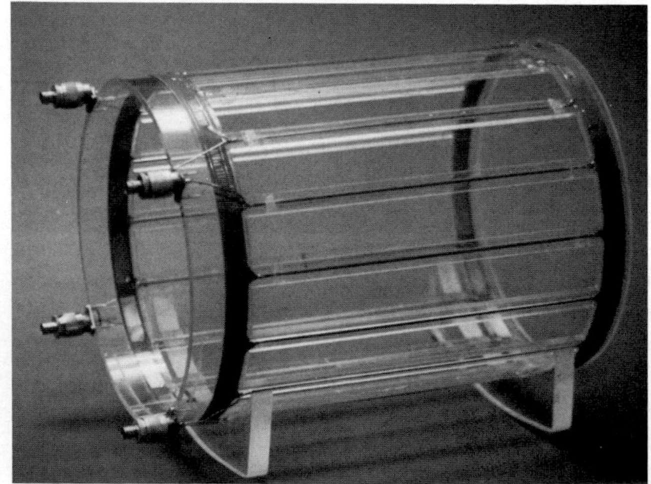

FIG. 10. Birdcage resonator. The photograph shows a head coil designed to operate at 170 MHz. Normally, only two of the four inputs would be driven. Driving two adjacent ports with equal signals 90° out of phase produces a circularly polarized field. This design has 16 struts along the z-direction while the saddle coil design has 4.

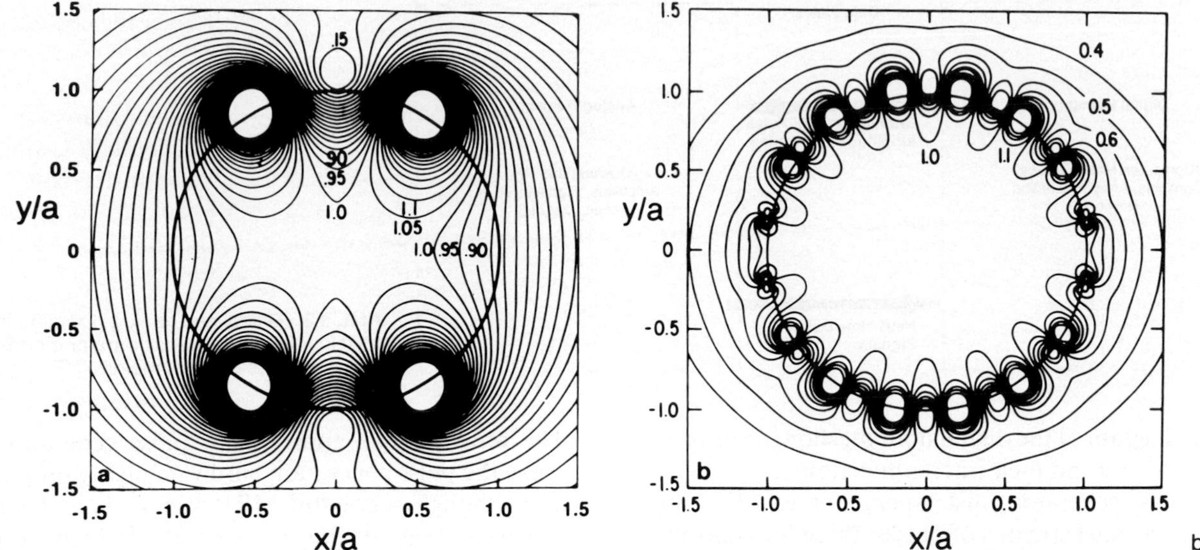

FIG. 11. Radiofrequency homogeneity patterns. If the rf field is not homogeneous across the field-of-view the nominal 90° and 180° flip angles will not be precise and will vary with position. Image shading artifacts will result. The field in the central axial plane ($z = 0$) of the saddle coil design which has its length equal to its diameter **(a)** has substantially less homogeneity than that of a 16 strut birdcage coil with length equal to 1.5 times its diameter **(b)**. (From Hayes et al., ref. 68, with permission of Academic Press.)

The birdcage design also automatically provides a second mode of oscillation, identical to the first, except that the current varies as sin ϕ rather than as cos ϕ. The first mode produces a highly uniform B_x field and the second mode produces a highly uniform B_y field. Each of these fields is linearly polarized. By using the power supply to excite both modes simultaneously, but with a 90° phase shift (called quadrature excitation), a circularly polarized rf field can be created with no additional complexity in coil design. The quadrature operation allows a saving of one half in the power required during the excitation phase and, during reception, it enhances the SNR by a factor of $\sqrt{2}$.

Although the basic problems of designing rf coils for MRI scanners have been solved, this remains an area where incremental improvements, particularly in the development of new surface coils, has the potential to significantly enhance the capabilities of this modality. An example is the recent development of surface coil arrays (69,70). Sometimes referred to as phased arrays, these designs make it possible to obtain the SNR advantages of surface coil, with the large field-of-view capabilities of head and body coils.

Patient and operation safety are crucial factors in the design of MRI scanners (71,72). For safety purposes, it should always be remembered that, during the rf transmitter pulse, large instantaneous voltages are present on the transmitter coil and cables. Care should be taken to avoid uncontrolled coupling between these voltages and other conductors—such as EKG leads and surface coil cables—in the proximity of the patient. Otherwise the possibility exists of patient injury through rf arcing (73).

DIGITAL HARDWARE

MRI was introduced as a clinical modality about ten years after computed x-ray tomography (CT) had become an established diagnostic tool. There are strong similarities in the requirements for digital hardware between MRI and CT. As a result existing implementations of the two techniques have used very similar computer hardware and software to date. Recently, the technical evolution of MRI has generated new demands on computer systems which require much greater processing power and data acquisition bandwidth. This section will discuss the basic requirements for the digital hardware and software for MRI, and describe the implications that recent developments have for current and future systems.

A useful approach to analyzing an MRI system is to divide the required functions into digital and analog domains as shown in Fig. 12. The analog functions include gradient and rf power amplifiers, the rf transceiver, probes, and the magnet itself. The digital functions include computer operations needed to exert control over the analog functions. Two principal data streams flow across the interface between these two domains: timing and amplitude information for controlling gradients and rf excitation are directed from the digital to the analog world; time-domain NMR data returns from the receiver back to the digital world for data processing. Figure 13 is

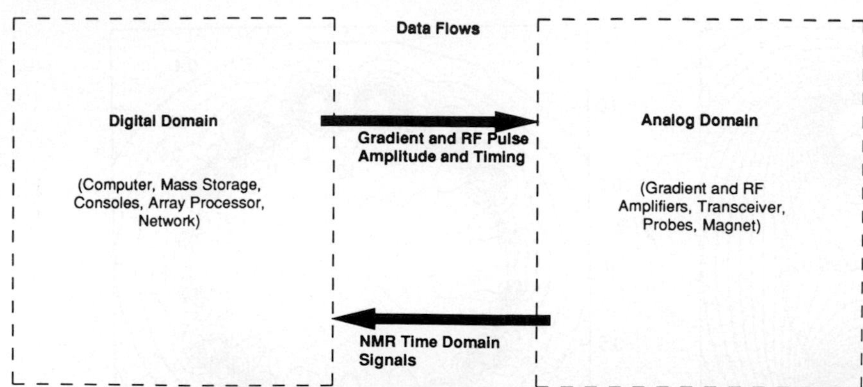

FIG. 12. Digital and analog domains for MRI. MRI involves the flow of data and commands between these two domains.

a block diagram of the digital domain showing its principal subsystems and their interconnections.

The pulse generator must generate at least four independent, parallel streams of pulses: three for controlling the gradient power supplies and one for shaping the rf transmitter output. Some implementations may also include other outputs, e.g., additional shaped waveforms for rf control, and gate outputs for utility functions. Although the spin-warp (28) technique has become the most widely used technique for MRI, there are many different pulse sequences employed for clinical and research scanning. Even within a single technique, such as two-dimensional single-plane spinwarp, several timing and amplitude parameters need to be varied to select the desired repetition rates, echo times, and field of view. The most flexible approach to pulse generation is to make the pulse generation hardware highly programmable, although successful MRI systems have been built which can generate only a few predetermined sequences.

Typical MRI pulse generators will allow adjustment of the relative timing of any pulse sequence feature in steps of 100 nanoseconds. To avoid the loss of signal and the generation of artifacts, it is necessary to generate pulses with stable and replicable timing and amplitude. For shaped pulses, sufficient dynamic range is required to avoid digitization artifacts in low-amplitude pulses. Twelve to sixteen bit digital-to-analog converters are commonly employed.

Clinical MRI systems need a number of built-in pulse sequences to handle standard scanning protocols. Rou-

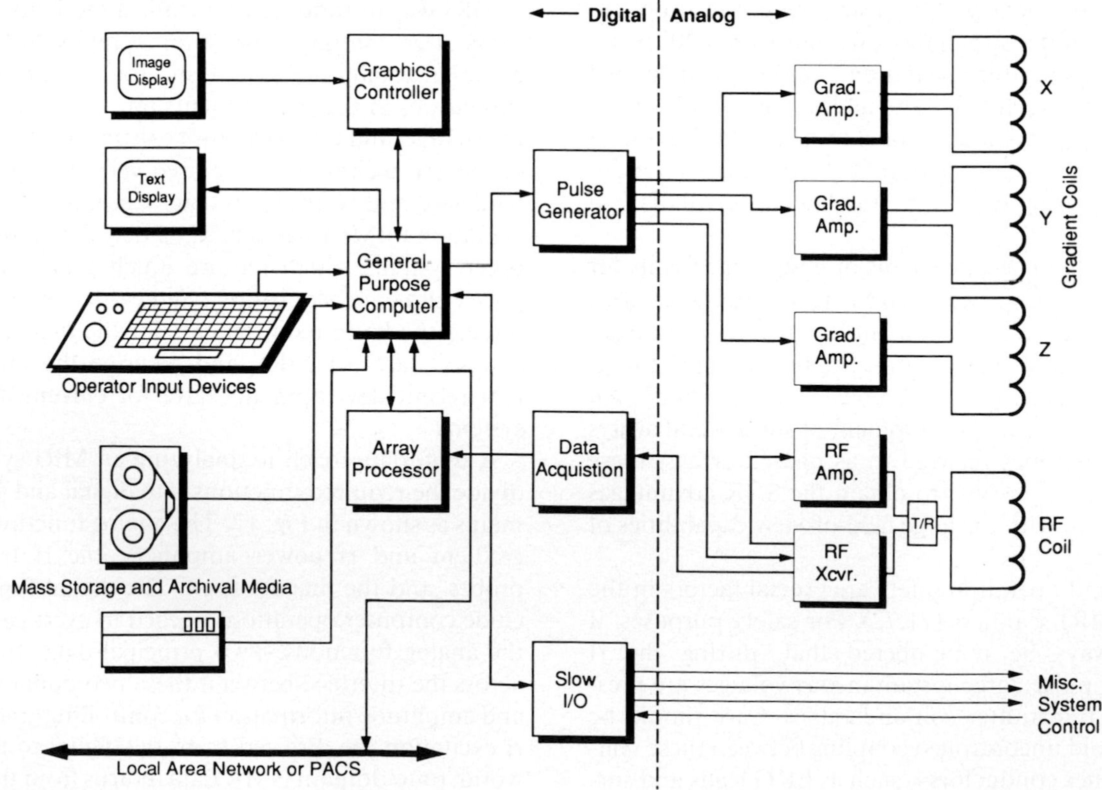

FIG. 13. Block diagram. A general purpose computer is required to generate the commands and to process the data necessary to carry out successful MRI.

tine clinical scanning usually employs a pulse sequence which acquires up to about 20 two-dimensional slices at a time in an interleaved fashion by modulating the rf waveforms. Three-dimensional sequences acquire data from an entire volume at once and generate images with a somewhat better signal-to-noise ratio, at the cost of more complicated and time-consuming data processing (74,75). Both two-dimensional and three-dimensional sequences may employ inversion recovery or multiple echoes to enhance the T1 or T2 content of the image.

Breathing, heart motion, blood flow, and other kinds of motion generate image artifacts in MRI images, principally by interfering with the phase of the acquired signal. Gating to cardiac or respiratory motion can be employed to synchronize data acquisition to reduce these distortions. Also, it is possible to record physiological information during the scan and use it during data processing to retrospectively correct phase changes (76).

The data acquisition system digitizes quadrature data at a rate sufficient to meet the Nyquist sampling criteria for the highest frequency components in the time domain data: for normal imaging, the sampling intervals are around 5 to 20 μsec per point. Some data acquisition methods, such as three-dimensional imaging, present instantaneous dynamic range demands of up to 80 Db. Analog-to-digital converters of 14 to 16 bits per channel are used to digitize the data.

The average data throughput of the data acquisition system must keep up with sustained data rates of up to about 800 kilobytes per second. For two-dimensional multislice and three-dimensional acquisition techniques, the total volume of time domain data may exceed four megabytes. Systems employing multiple parallel surface coils will multiply the data rate and data size requirements by the number of surface coils. Proposed systems would employ more than a dozen surface coils to image the spine (70), thus increasing the data handling requirements to unwieldy proportions unless specialized computational hardware is employed near the front of the signal processing chain to compress the data going to later stages.

An Array Processor (AP) is used for generating images from the time domain data. Array Processors are computers with architectures tailored for rapidly performing Fourier transforms and other algorithms related to signal processing. In some MRI systems, digitized data from the analog-to-digital converters is connected directly to a dedicated input port on the AP, thus freeing up the general-purpose computer bus for other functions.

The bulk of the signal processing for spin-warp imaging consists of multidimensional Fourier transforms. A few other operations such as anti-alias filtering, scaling, and clipping are also used. In general, the computations are easier and faster than the filtered back projection computations needed for CT data processing. Single two-dimensional images can be available for display within about 1 second after the completion of data acquisition, even using an AP of modest speed such as the single-board 15 to 20 megaflop APs available commercially. Three-dimensional image data may take much longer to process because the large data set size exceeds the data memory capacity of the AP, and so the reconstruction time is dominated by the time required to move data between a secondary storage device and the AP.

After the image data is generated, it is usually stored on a rotating magnetic disk. From there, it may be retrieved for display or transferred to an archival medium such as magnetic tape or optical disk. MR images are usually formatted as a matrix of 256×256 or 512×512 pixels, with up to 16 bits of gray scale information per pixel. The pixel data is mapped into the available contrast and brightness ranges of the display device by scaling and offsetting the pixel data. The user can continuously adjust the contrast and brightness of the image for display or filming.

Because an MRI system can acquire a large number of two-dimensional images in a short period of time, the display system may include capabilities which help to distill the large amounts of information into clinically relevant presentations. These techniques include tiled multi-image displays, the rapid sequential display of multiple images in a cine loop, multiplanar reformatting of stacks of two-dimensional images, and synthesized three-dimensional renderings of surfaces and volumes. Some of these techniques are computationally intensive and may require specialized hardware to be useful in a clinical setting (77).

Image processing that is specific to MRI includes the calculation of T1 and T2 relaxation times on a per-pixel basis (78), and correction of the brightness gradients across images caused by nonuniformities of surface coil sensitivities. Color display systems can be useful to generate functional images showing maps of relaxation times, proton density, or other physical parameters (79).

Microprocessor-based workstations that can display images and have considerable local processor power are relatively inexpensive. MRI systems can support a number of these workstations as remote image viewing stations, either directly, or as part of a hospital picture and archiving system (PACS). Several image acquisition systems (MRI, CT, and others) can also share expensive peripherals such as multiformat cameras.

In addition to acquiring data and generating pulse sequences, the computer control for an MRI system must also perform general housekeeping, hardware control, and safety monitoring. The computer can either directly control the longitudinal drive of the patient table, or merely monitor its position. The computer performs system sequencing functions during power-up and shutdown, initializes subsystems such as gradient and rf amplifiers, monitors their status, and detects anomalies. It may also monitor cryogen levels for superconducting magnets.

The operator interface to an MRI system is created and maintained by the computer. To promote greater patient throughput and reduce operator errors, the human interface for controlling the system needs to be as simple and convenient as possible. Touch-sensitive screens and special input devices such as magnetic card readers for patient data can minimize the need for using the keyboard for operator input. To increase system throughput, the computer needs to support multitasking: the ability to perform jobs such as image review, patient data entry, and archiving at the same time as patient scanning. The ability to share the computer between scanning and other functions is even more important in MRI systems than CT systems because of the long scan times.

In an MRI system, there are a number of adjustable parameters which have an impact on image quality. Some of these parameters, such as transmitter and receiver gains, may need to be adjusted for each new patient. Others, such as the rf center frequency, tend to drift out of adjustment over several hours or days. Hardware and software can be designed to automatically calibrate these parameters, or to provide the operator with feedback for manual adjustment. The computer also needs software tools to help vendor service technicians track image quality over longer periods (80). There are opportunities to employ artificial intelligence to aid in the diagnosis of difficult image quality problems. Software to analyze image artifacts and recommend adjustments or repairs can either be built into the basic software of the machine, or offered as a remote service through a modem connection to a specialized service computer.

Traditionally, CT and MRI systems have been run by an isolated computer with perhaps one or two attached consoles for image viewing. With local area networks (LANs) and wide area networks becoming inexpensive and reliable, attention is being given to using networks in a hospital environment and attaching imaging machines to these networks. Connecting an MRI system to a network provides several advantages: First, inexpensive workstations connected to the LAN can access images from the scanner from anywhere within a hospital complex. The easy electronic recreation of images can help to reduce the number of images which are photographed on film. Second, imaging systems can share expensive peripherals such as laser cameras and archival data stores. Third, administrative information used for patient record keeping can be stored in electronic data bases and logically associated with images, thus reducing costs and minimizing the loss of records and subsequent rescanning of patients. Fourth, regional health care centers can electronically exchange data with satellite clinics, saving time and reducing costs. Balancing these advantages are the high start-up costs of installing a network and concerns about the integrity and confidentiality of patient records.

The growth of PACS systems was slow in the 1970s and 1980s because of high start-up costs and a lack of universal vendor support for standard methods of image storage and transmission. However, PACS system growth appears to be poised for rapid expansion in the 1990s. Hardware costs for remote image retrieval and display stations have dropped dramatically and performance has increased, thanks to the relentless improvement in the price to performance ratio of PC-based systems. The ACR-NEMA Standards for Digital Imaging and Communication in Medicine (DICOM) (81) now enjoy widespread support from medical equipment manufacturers. The DICOM standard is compatible with computer industry standard communications protocols and hardware, which lowers the investment costs for installing a network. New image compression algorithms, such as wavelet-based imaging, permits the transmission of image data with minimal loss of quality, making teleradiology a more practical technique (82).

TRENDS IN MR INSTRUMENTATION

There are continuing efforts at many centers to improve on the capabilities of MR scanners by reducing their costs, improving image quality, shortening scan times, and increasing the number of clinically useful applications. Several areas that have been specially active in the early 1990s are discussed below.

Fast Scanning Techniques

The time required to gather the data for a conventional spin-echo image can vary over a wide range, but is usually on the order of one to ten minutes. The physical property that leads to these relatively long scan times is the long T1 relaxation time of protons in human tissues, which requires a relatively long recovery interval between successive excitation cycles. Fast scanning utilizes pulse sequences which are designed to extract more information from the spin system per unit time. Echo-planar imaging (EPI) was the first of these techniques to be proposed and has become progressively more widely used (83–85) as have a number of more recently introduced techniques (86–91). In general, fast MR images show some degradation, in terms of contrast, SNR or artifact content, relative to conventional spin-echo images. However, in many situations, these limitations are outweighed by the advantages of faster scanning such as (i) improved patient acceptance, (ii) the ability to contend with physiological motion such as respiration and cardiac activity, and (iii) the cost of performing the scan. The scan time for a single slice with the fast spin-echo (FSE) technique is on the order of 20 seconds and, in practice, this method is about two to four times faster than conventional spin-echo methods (91). The use of gradient-echo (GRASS, FLASH, etc.) techniques can reduce scan time to a few seconds per slice. EPI images of a single slice can be performed in as short a time as 40 to 60 milliseconds. The clinical relevance of the FSE approach is predominately in shortening conventional scans, while EPI and fast gradient-echo techniques permit "real-time" or "snap-shot" scanning that can partially overcome the effects of tissue motion.

Fast scan pulse sequences can usually be implemented using conventional scanner hardware. However, special gradient systems and digital hardware are required to achieve the full benefits of EPI. Provisions have been made for retrofitting some commercial scanners with specially designed EPI subsystems. In EPI the rate of data generation is increased by using stronger gradient fields and switching them more rapidly. Conventional scanners use gradient strengths of approximately 1 gauss/cm and have switching times of 500 to 1,000 milliseconds. Scanners have been developed with gradient strengths approaching 4 gauss/cm and capable of switching in 150 microseconds (89). To achieve these performance levels the gradient coils must operate at significantly higher currents and voltages. Two methods to achieve these power levels—known as the resonant and nonresonant techniques—have been developed. In the resonant approach, energy efficiency is achieved by coupling the inductance of the gradient coils with a capacitor network tuned to a desired operating frequency (84,89,92,93). The nonresonant approach uses gradient power supplies with greatly enhanced current and switching capabilities (94,95). In either case, shielded gradients are desirable to minimize eddy current effects, but the current patterns on the gradient coils do not need to be changed for these applications. There is significantly more joule heating in the gradient coils and, as a result, water cooling of these coils is usually necessary.

The enhanced strength of the readout gradients requires an increase in receiver bandwidth—to as high as 400 to 600 kHz—instead of the more standard 32 kHz. Because of the large data acquisition rate and the large number of images that can be quickly generated with EPI, it is desirable to have enhanced computer capabilities for image reconstruction. It is also desirable to have a display mechanism, such as an off-line workstation, to permit the rapid examination of a large number of images without delaying the scanning process.

The possibility of nerve or muscle stimulation by the rapidly switched gradients is of some concern in EPI (89,96). The rate of change of the magnetic field, dB/dt in tesla/second, is ordinarily used to quantify the level of this stress, although the induced electric field, E in volts/meter, is more directly relevant to tissue stimulation. The present generation of EPI scanners may be capable of a low degree of peripheral nerve stimulation and a prudent approach is certainly warranted. However, in assessing the risks and benefits of EPI it should be borne in mind that so-called magnetic stimulation in both peripheral and central nervous tissue, at dB/dt and electric field levels far beyond those present in EPI, has been widely used in clinical practice without evidence of injury (97–99).

Head-Only Scanners

Up to the present time, MR scanners have been almost universally designed to accommodate the entire human body and to be capable of imaging any anatomical region. It is an attractive idea to develop modified—presumably smaller, cheaper, and simpler—scanners dedicated to imaging only limited regions of the body, such as the head or the extremities. However, it is necessary to provide a uniform static field over the entire region to be imaged and to achieve this homogeneity it is a physical requirement that the sources of the field effectively surround this region. In other words, the anatomy to be imaged must be *inside* a powerful magnet, not simply adjacent to one. Also, it is also a physical requirement that the magnet be much larger than the desired field of view (Fig. 4). It is difficult to design a practical system which has part of a patient, such as a knee, breast, or head, inside a large magnet and the rest of the patient outside. As an example, suppose it is desired to build a small diameter, superconducting magnet to image only the human head. To provide a head-sized region of homogeneity such a magnet would be so long that its diameter would have to be at least large enough to admit the patient's shoulders. The solution to assuring an adequate region of homogeneity has usually been to make the magnet bore large enough to accommodate the entire patient even though, in any given case, only a limited region needs to be imaged. It is possible that novel, high field magnet designs will be forthcoming to permit progress in this area, but a compromise solution that utilizes conventional, large bore superconducting main magnets and smaller head-sized gradient coils provides a more immediate approach to the development of head-only scanners (100). Because of the reduced coil inductance, such scanners can have significant advantages in terms of gradient strength and switching speed.

Interventional Scanners for Image-Guided Therapy

There has recently been substantial activity to develop systems capable of performing image-guided, invasive therapeutic procedures (101). Because of its excellent ability to provide soft tissue contrast and its potential for very good positional accuracy (102), MRI has a great capability for guiding biopsies and stereotactic procedures (103,105) and in following the position of invasive devices such as endoscopes and catheters (106). MRI also has the ability to image the effects of tissue heating (107) and freezing which gives it the potential for monitoring and, eventually, controlling procedures, such as interstitial laser therapy (108–110) and focused ultrasound (111,112), that use thermal energy or cyrogenic cooling

(113) to destroy diseased tissues. To achieve the full capabilities of MRI to support image-guided therapy it is necessary to simultaneously image the tissue under treatment and provide clinical access to the patient. This access is very limited in standard MR scanners which have the patient located in the center of the imaging magnet. As a result, most of the MR-guided procedures initially reported involved scanning the patient before and/or after, but not during, the invasive procedure. Recently, a new 0.5 T system has been reported that utilizes a novel magnet design (Fig. 14). The superconducting coils are moved away from the center of the magnet and the cryostat is split into two separate, but communicating, sections. This results in a 56-cm wide zone of access at the center of the magnet. Complete access to the patient is provided by the use of divided gradient coils and the use of flexible coils for both rf transmitter and receiver functions (114). The system can continuously monitor the positions of the instruments used in the procedure by the use of optical sensors mounted on them. The clinician can operate within a sterile field and interactively control the scan plane and view near real-time images of the operative field on a field-compatible monitor located with the magnetgap. The advent of MR-guided invasive procedures has increased the need for magnetic field compatible anesthesia and patient monitoring equipment (115) as well as for field-compatible surgical instruments, catheters, and endoscopes (116).

High Field Scanners

Except for a small number of scanners operating at 2 T, most clinical MR scanners have been operated at 1.5 T or below. In the late 1980s a number of research sites began experiments with whole-body scanners operating at a 4 T (117). The early 4 T whole-body magnets were physically much larger than those of conventional clinical scanners and, because of cost and siting requirements, these systems were more suited for research than for direct clinical applications. In addition to the difficulties in constructing such powerful whole-body magnets, there are system engineering difficulties, associated with the higher rf frequency (170.3 MHz), that must be overcome to produce high quality imaging at this field strength. Conventional birdcage head coils can be operated at this frequency (64), but often there are advantages in using surface coils in both the transmitter and receiver modes. This reduces the rf power requirements, which increase substantially as the operating frequency is increased. Although, at 4 T, the T1 relaxation time for most tissues is increased by roughly 40% over that at 1.5 T, imaging techniques and pulse sequences have been developed that permit high quality head imaging at this field strength (118). A significant incentive to develop the field of high field scanning has arisen from the interest in functional brain imaging. In this case, the contrast mechanism is associated with the magnetic susceptibility difference between oxygenated and deoxygenated hemoglobin in the cerebral microvasculature, and susceptibility-based contrast is inherently greater at high field strengths (119). An important recent engineering advance has been the ability to build 3 T and 4 T magnets which are of the same physical size as conventional 1.5 T magnets. This has made it possible to develop high field scanners that have the same external appearance and operating characteristics as standard clinical scanners. Although high field systems continue to have higher costs and fringing field than standard systems, these new developments enhance the possibility of their eventual widespread clinical utilization.

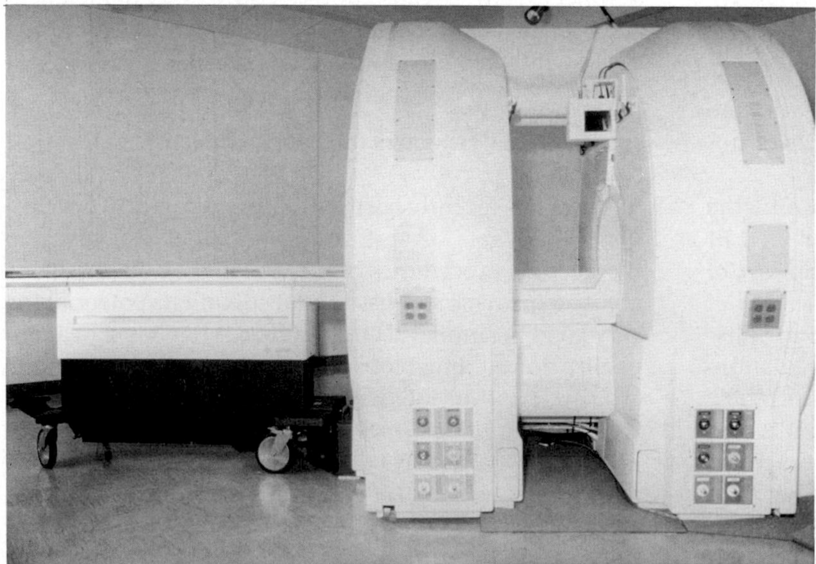

FIG. 14. System for MR-guided therapy. The superconducting open magnet configuration permits the clinician to have access to the patient, and to interactively control the scan plane. These real-time capabilities enhance the utility of MR imaging in image-guided surgery.

Appendix

ELECTROMAGNETIC THEORY AND MR SCANNERS

Electromagnetic theory (120–124) links the strength of a field at various points in space to the strength of the sources that produce it. As indicated in Table 2, all magnetic fields are produced by either electric currents or magnetized materials. In fact, atomic theory shows that the fields produced by magnetized materials also originate from electric currents, in this case microscopic currents that are internal to individual atoms and molecules. Electric fields, on the other hand, are produced by both charge accumulations and by electric currents that are changing with time. Static distributions of electric charge do not produce magnetic fields and steady currents do not produce electric fields.

The electric and magnetic effects produced by any collection of sources are described in terms of vector fields. In other words, the field at each point in space is determined only if both its strength (or magnitude) and its direction are known. A convenient method of characterizing vector fields is to specify the components of the vector along each of three preselected directions. Although other choices are often used, the most common approach is to specify components of the field along the three mutually perpendicular axes (x,y,z) of a cartesian coordinate system (125).

A magnetic field has three distinct components and each of these components usually has a different value at each point in space. Therefore, the field of a general set of sources can be very complicated to describe precisely. However, for the purposes of MRI, the desired magnetic fields have very specific and relatively simple idealized forms. It is reasonable to utilize these idealized static, gradient and rf field patterns as the framework for thinking about the magnetic fields of MRI scanners. The inevitable deviations from ideality may be analyzed, when necessary, by studying the effects of small perturbations superimposed on the basic fields.

An important property of the electromagnetic field is the principle of superposition. This states that the field produced by several sources acting simultaneously is simply the vector sum of the fields of each of the sources acting alone. In MRI the main field is applied continuously and the gradient and rf fields are activated using a programmed series of current pulses that are under computer control. The principle of superposition shows that the field at any given point within the patient, at any given instant, is the sum of the fields originating in each of these five coils. By tailoring the pulse sequence, the spins within the patient may be driven through a wide variety of motions to achieve desired imaging results.

Fortunately, modern MRI scanners are so well designed that most clinical scans can be interpreted without considering any deviations from the ideal field patterns. However, for a deeper understanding of scanner performance and limitations, deviations from these ideal patterns must be considered. For several reasons the idealized field patterns, such as a perfectly uniform static field, cannot be obtained precisely. Contending with the imperfections in magnetic field patterns represents a major portion of scanner engineering. One reason field patterns are never absolutely perfect results from the basic laws of nature as expressed in the fundamental field equations (Table 3). It is easy to show, from these equations, that no realizable source configuration can produce exactly the perfectly uniform main field and rf field and the perfectly linear gradient fields of the ideal scanner. However, in principle, it is possible to create indefinitely close approximations to these ideal fields over limited regions of space. In MR scanners the design goal is to achieve an adequate approximation to each of the ideal fields over the desired field-of-view (FOV). It is also necessary to prevent signals that originate outside this FOV from intruding on the image. Ordinarily, to achieve a higher degree of field perfection it is necessary to use a more complex coil design and this is often associated with a decrease in coil efficiency. For example, by using additional coils in the main magnet, the static field can be made more uniform. However, once this is done more current is required to achieve a given field strength. Therefore, it is necessary to make tradeoffs between coil

TABLE 2. *Fields and sources*

Types of field	Type of source	Significance to MRI
Magnetic fields	Electric currents	Main magnetic field; gradient and active shimming fields; active shielding fields.
	Magnetized matter	Main magnetic field; passive shielding and passive shimming fields; susceptibility effects.
	Electric charges	Capacitive coupling between rf coils and patients; self-resonance limitations on coil-operating frequencies.
Electric fields	Time-varying currents	Eddy currents associated with gradient pulses; inductive coupling between rf coils and patient.
	Time-varying magnetization	MR signal from precessing spins.

complexity (and cost) and the perfection of the resulting field pattern. As discussed below, deviations from the ideal field patterns associated with the basic field equations can be predicted mathematically. Therefore, they can often be significantly compensated by the use of correction formulas applied to the image before it is displayed.

Another source of imperfect field patterns is that there are inevitable limitations on the precision with which coils can be manufactured and positioned within a scanner. These manufacturing tolerances cause the field pattern of each scanner to vary somewhat from the mathematical predictions. For the static field this problem can be largely compensated by the use of shim coils as discussed earlier in this chapter. The requirements on the perfection of gradient and rf fields are not as stringent as those on the static fields and, therefore, manufacturing tolerances are less stringent for gradient and rf coils than for static field coils although they still require close attention.

All the materials located in the scanner, including the patient, have some degree of electrical conductivity and magnetic and electric susceptibility. Therefore, a third source imperfection in field patterns results from the presence of these parasitic sources. That is, even if the field patterns within the scanner were ideal, they would induce the formation of new sources (electric currents or magnetization) which would, in turn, produce secondary fields. These secondary fields would then detract from the perfection of the original fields. Three examples of induced, parasitic sources are (i) the audiofrequency eddy currents induced in metallic support structures of the scanner by the electric fields associated with the time-dependent gradient currents; (ii) the rf eddy currents induced in the patient by the electric fields associated with the rf current in the transmitter coil; and (iii) the magnetization induced in all adjacent magnetic materials (including the weak magnetization of human tissues) by the main magnetic field.

TABLE 3. *Fundamental equations relating the fields to their sources*

A) The potential fields **A** and V in terms of the sources **J**, ρ, **M**.

$$\mathbf{A} = \frac{\mu_o}{4\pi}\int\left[\frac{\mathbf{J}}{r} + \frac{\mathbf{M}\times\hat{\mathbf{r}}}{r^2}\right]dV$$

$$V = \frac{1}{4\pi\varepsilon_o}\int\frac{\rho}{r}\,dV$$

B) The fields, **B** and **E** in terms of the potentials **A** and V.

$$\mathbf{B} = \nabla\times\mathbf{A}$$

$$\mathbf{E} = \nabla V - \frac{\partial\mathbf{A}}{\partial t}$$

- The integrals are carried out over all the source positions.
- **r** and $\mathbf{r}_o$ are, respectively, the locations of the field and source points. $\hat{\mathbf{r}}$ is the unit vector from the source to the field point and r is the distance between these points.
- $\mathbf{A} = \mathbf{A}(\mathbf{r})$ is the magnetic vector potential and $V = V(\mathbf{r})$ is the electric scalar potential at the field point.
- $\rho = \rho(\mathbf{r}_o)$ is the electric charge density, $\mathbf{J} = \mathbf{J}(\mathbf{r}_o)$ is the electric current density and $\mathbf{M} = \mathbf{M}(\mathbf{r}_o)$ is the magnetization at the source point.
- $\mathbf{B} = \mathbf{B}(\mathbf{r})$ is the magnetic field and $\mathbf{E} = \mathbf{E}(\mathbf{r})$ is the electric field.
- $\varepsilon_o = 8.854 \times 10^{-12}$ farad/m is the permittivity of free space and $\mu_o = 4\pi \times 10^{-7}$ henry/m is the permeability of free space.
- At very high frequencies the retarded values of the source strengths (6) should be used to account for the finite speed of light.

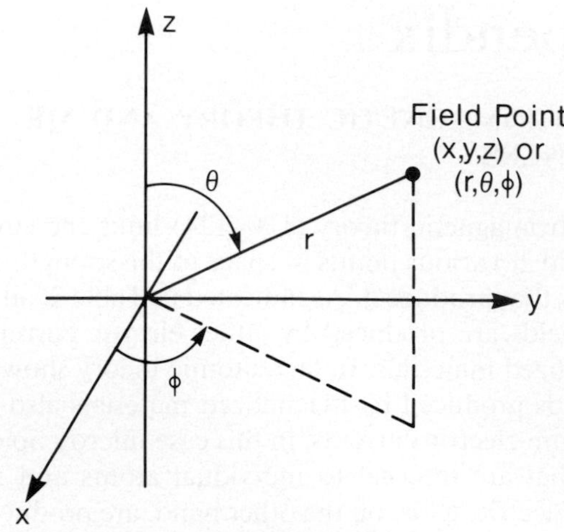

FIG. 15. Coordinate systems. The origin is usually taken as the center of the magnet. The z axis is along the direction of the B_0 field. This is along the cylinder bore in superconducting magnet systems. In this case the x direction is horizontal and the y direction is vertical. The relation between cartesian coordinates and spherical coordinates is indicated.

The coils are not designed simply to produce a given field strength at a single point but, rather, a prescribed field pattern over an extended region. Any magnetic field component can be represented over a region surrounding a given point (called the origin) as a sum of specific field patterns each of which has a characteristic, well-defined spatial variation. One version of this method, called field expansion in a series of harmonic[1] functions (120,122,126), is applicable providing that there are no sources (that is electric currents or magnetic materials) within the region where we want to represent the field and that the field is not changing too rapidly (in practice, this is true for frequencies less than 100 MHz or so) as a function of time. Ordinarily, the center of the main magnet is chosen as the origin of the coordinate system. Strictly speaking, an infinite number of terms are required to perfectly represent a magnetic field, but for most purposes only the first few terms are required. Points in the space around the origin are represented by

[1] The word harmonic is used to denote any function, $f(x,y,z)$ that satisfies Laplace's equation, $\nabla^2 f = 0$. At low frequencies and in source-free space the magnetic field components B_x, B_y, and B_z are harmonic functions.

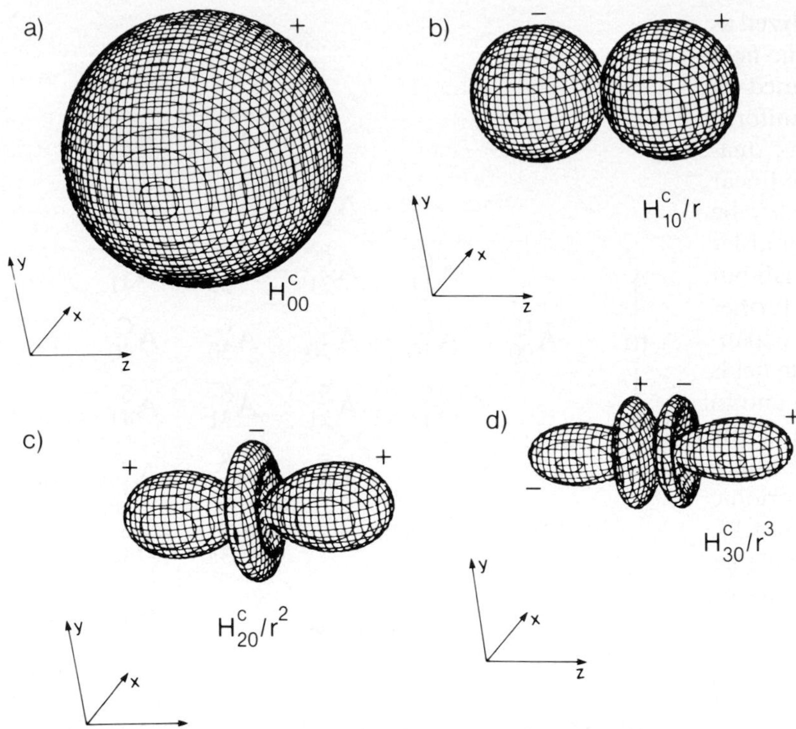

FIG. 16. Harmonic functions. These illustrations indicate how these functions vary with direction in space. The distance of the surface from the origin, R, is proportional to the absolute value of the strength of the indicated harmonic in that direction. For example, in **(b)** $R = |H^{c}_{10}|/r$. The uniform harmonic, H^{c}_{00}, is constant in all directions so the surface representing it **(a)** is a sphere. The sign of the harmonics that have multiple lobes alternates from one lobe to the next. The harmonics illustrated here all have $m = 0$. The only harmonics generated when the source has cylindrical symmetry are those with $m = 0$.

their cartesian coordinates (x,y,z), and the distance, r, of a field point from the origin is $r = \sqrt{x^2 + y^2 + z^2}$. It is often convenient to use spherical coordinates (r,θ,ϕ) as an alternative representation of the position of the field point. The relation between the cartesian and spherical coordinate representation is shown in Fig. 15.

In words, the expansion method says that at any point in the vicinity of the origin, any cartesian component

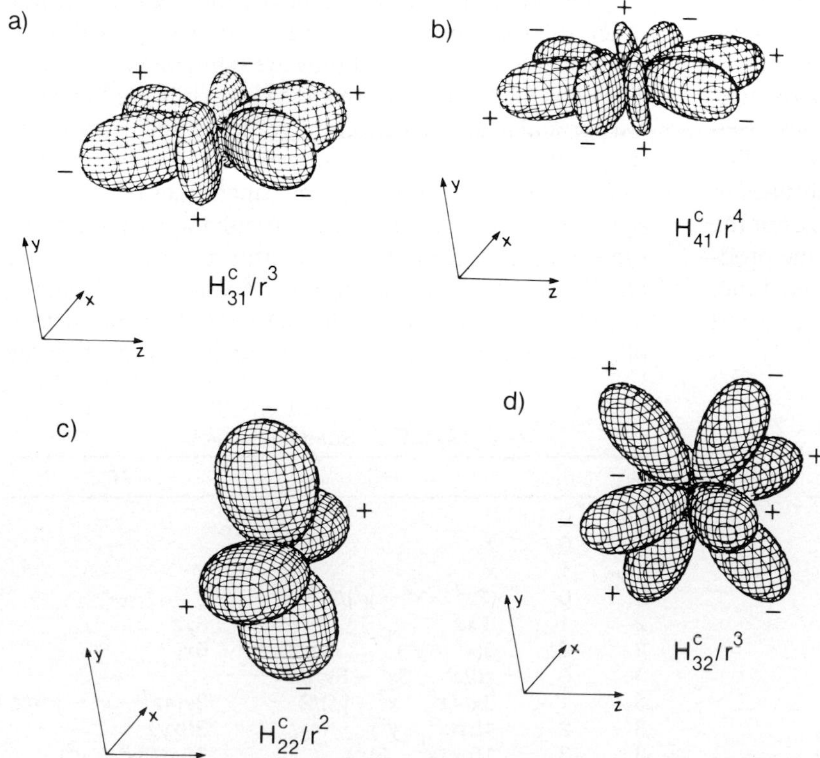

FIG. 17. Harmonic functions. As in the previous figure, the directional dependence of various harmonics are indicated. The functions illustrated here all have $m \neq 0$ and are of the type generated when the source deviates from cylindrical symmetry.

(for example, B_z) of the magnetic field can be analyzed as the superposition of an infinite number of specific field patterns each with an amplitude that is determined by the sources. This sum consists of one perfectly uniform field + three perfectly linear gradient fields + five quadratic fields + seven cubic fields and so on. The linear terms are proportional to r, the quadratic terms to r^2, the cubic terms to r^3, and so on. Therefore, the higher order fields are very small near the origin where r is small but they can become very important at locations further away from the origin. A significant merit of the expansion method is that coils can be designed to create fields corresponding to specific terms in the expansion and to eliminate or minimize undesirable terms. Each of the harmonic fields has a specific dependence on position. The way in which several of the lower order harmonic fields vary with direction is indicated in Figs. 16 and 17. For a given n, there are $2n + 1$ independent fields that vary as r^n. Mathematically a field, such as B_z, may be written as,

$$B_z = \sum_{n=0}^{\infty} \sum_{m=0}^{n} [A^c_{nm}H^c_{nm}(x, y, z) + A^s_{nm}H^s_{nm}(x, y, z)] \quad [4]$$

where n and m are integers. The functions H^c_{nm} and H^s_{nm} are known as solid harmonics. They are related to the spherical harmonics by the formulas,

$$H^c_{nm} = r^n \cos m\phi P^m_n(\cos\theta) \quad [5]$$

and

$$H^s_{nm} = r^n \sin m\phi P^m_n(\cos\theta) \quad [6]$$

The functions P^m_n (cos θ are called the associated Legendre functions. The first few of these functions are listed in Table 4. Note that H^s_{nm} is always zero if $m = 0$. In this chapter we will not go deeply into the mathematics of harmonic functions; however, they are discussed thoroughly in standard physics texts (120,122). The coefficients A^c_{nm} and A^s_{nm} (Fig. 18) are the amplitudes of the harmonics and are determined by the sources of the field. Therefore, each term in the expansion is the product of two factors—one of which, H^c_{nm} or H^s_{nm}—is a function of only the field location and one of which, A^c_{nm} and

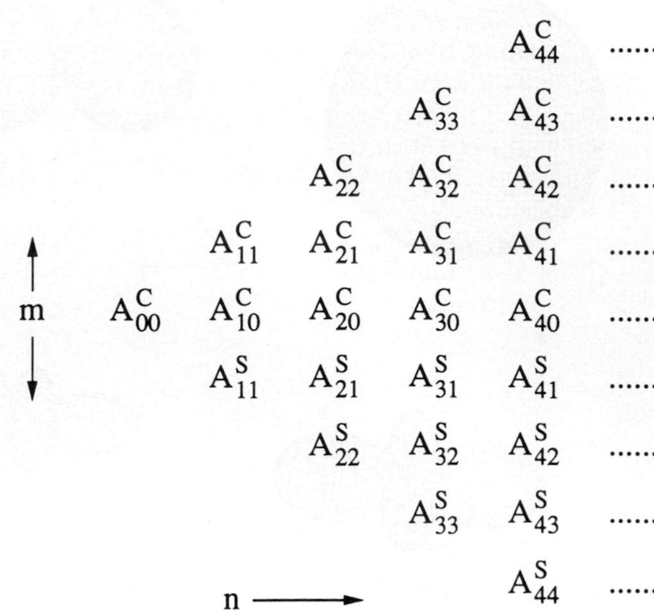

FIG. 18. Expansion coefficients. Every expansion in solid harmonics involves an array of coefficients that can be displayed as above. Generally as the order, n, increases the associated fields become less important. The symmetry of the source is important in determining the values of the coefficients. A general source will produce 25 different fields with $n \neq 4$. However, a cylindrical source will produce only the 5 fields with $m = 0$. Moreover, a cylindrical source that is symmetric about the origin will produce only the 3 fields that have both $m = 0$ and n even.

A^s_{nm} is a function only of the source properties. The lower order solid harmonics arise very frequently in discussions of MR scanners and they are tabulated in Table 5. The ideal field of each of the five basic coils used in MRI is a particular solid harmonic and the nonideal aspects of these fields result from the unwanted presence of other solid harmonics. Improving the capabilities of a coil design is often based, therefore, on enhancing the amplitude of one harmonic and eliminating or minimizing the amplitudes of all other harmonics. A very useful theorem in coil design shows that, for coils wound on the surface of a cylinder, if the angular dependence of the current

TABLE 4. *Associated Legendre functions* (n ≤ 3)

n	m	$P^m_n(\cos\theta)$
0	0	1
1	0	$\cos\theta$
1	1	$\sin\theta$
2	0	$(3\cos^2\theta - 1)/2$
2	1	$3\sin\theta\cos\theta$
2	2	$3\sin^2\theta$
3	0	$\cos\theta(5\cos^2\theta - 3)/2$
3	1	$3\sin\theta(5\cos^2\theta - 1)/2$
3	2	$15\sin^2\theta\cos\theta$
3	3	$15\sin^3\theta$

TABLE 5. *Solid harmonics*

n	m	H^c_{nm}	H^s_{nm}
0	0	1	—
1	0	z	—
1	1	x	y
2	0	$(2z^2 - x^2 - y^2)/2$	—
2	1	$3xz$	$3yz$
2	2	$3(x^2 - y^2)$	$6xy$
3	0	$z(2z^2 - 3x^2 - 3y^2)/2$	—
3	1	$3x(4z^2 - x^2 - y^2)/2$	$3y(4z^2 - x^2 - y^2)/2$
3	2	$15z(x^2 - y^2)$	$30xyz$
3	3	$15x(x^2 - 3y^2)$	$15y(3x^2 - y^2)$

density is proportional to cos $M\phi$, only magnetic field terms of the form H^c_{nm} with $m = M$ will be generated. Similarly, if the current density is proportional to sin $M\phi$ only fields of the form H^s_{nm} with $m = M$ are produced.

ACKNOWLEDGMENTS. It is a pleasure to acknowledge useful discussions and other assistance from J. Banesch, R. L. Rhodenizer, S. P. Souza, P. B. Roemer, C. L. Dumoulin, S. M. Blumenfeld, B. Johnson, R. J. Dobberstein, P. A. Bottomley, and W. A. Edelstein, and help with the preparation of the manuscript from J. A. Agresta, R. E. Argersinger, L. Macuirles, and S. M. Manell.

REFERENCES

1. Abrams HL. Radiology. In: Walton J, Beeson PB, Scott RB, eds. *The Oxford Companion to Medicine*. Oxford: Oxford University Press, 1986;1193–1198.
2. delRogato J. Francis Henry Williams. *Int J Radiat Oncol Biol Phys* 1983;9:739–749.
3. Gorter CJ. Negative result of an attempt to detect nuclear magnetic spins. *Physica* 1936;3:995–998.
4. Gorter CJ, Broer LJF. Negative result of an attempt to observe nuclear magnetic resonance in solids. *Physica* 1942;9:591–596.
5. Gorter CJ. *Paramagnetic Relaxation*. Amsterdam: Elsevier; 1947:126–127.
6. Rigden JS. *Rabi: Scientist and Citizen*. New York: Basic Books; 1987:96–120.
7. Purcell EM, Torrey HC, Pound RV. Resonance absorption by nuclear magnetic moments in a solid. *Phys Rev* 1946;69:37–38.
8. Bloch F, Hansen WW, Packard M. Nuclear induction. *Phys Rev* 1946;69:127.
9. Bloch F. Nuclear induction. *Phys Rev* 1946;70:460–474.
10. Bloch F, Hansen WW, Packard M. The nuclear induction experiment. *Phys Rev* 1946;70:474–485.
11. Bloembergen N, Purcell EM, Pound RV. Relaxation effects in nuclear magnetic resonance absorption. *Phys Rev* 1948;73:679–712.
12. Singer J. Blood flow rates by nuclear magnetic resonance measurements. *Science* 1959;130:1652–1653.
13. Bratton CB, Hopkins AL, Weinberg JW. Nuclear magnetic resonance studies of living muscles. *Science* 1965;147:738.
14. Jackson JA, Langham WH. Whole-body NMR spectrometer. *Rev Sci Instrum* 1968;39:510–513.
15. Damadian R. Tumor detection by magnetic resonance. *Science* 1971;171:1151–1153.
16. Weisman ID, Bennett LH, Maxwell LR, Woods MW, Burk D. Recognition of cancer in vivo by nuclear magnetic resonance. *Science* 1972;178:1288–1290.
17. Lauterbur PC. Image formation by induced local interactions: examples employing nuclear magnetic resonance. *Nature* 1973; 242:190–191.
18. Hinshaw WS, Bottomley PA, Holland GN. Radiologic thin-section image of the human wrist by nuclear magnetic resonance. *Nature* 1977;270:722-723.
19. Mansfield P, Maudsley AA. Medical imaging by NMR. *Br J Radiol* 1977;50:188–194.
20. Mansfield P, Pykett IL. Biological and medical imaging by NMR. *J Magn Reson* 1978;29:355–373.
21. Hinshaw WS. Image formation by nuclear magnetic resonance: the sensitive-point method. *J Appl Phys* 1976;47:3709–3721.
22. Damadian R, Minkoff L, Goldsmith M, Stanford M, Koutcher J. Field focusing nuclear magnetic resonance (FONAR): visualization of a tumor in a live animal. *Science* 1976;194:1430–1432.
23. Damadian R, Goldsmith M, Minkoff L. NMR in cancer: XVI. FONAR image of the live human body. *Physiol Chem Phys Med NMR* 1977;9:97–100,108.
24. Damadian R, Minkoff L, Goldsmith M, Koutcher JA. Field-focusing nuclear magnetic resonance (FONAR) formation of chemical scans in man. *Naturwissenschaften* 1978;65:250–252.
25. Ernst RR, Anderson WA. Application of Fourier transform spectroscopy to magnetic resonance. *Rev Sci Instrum* 1966;37:93–102.
26. Kumar A, Welti D, Ernst RR. NMR Fourier zeugmatography. *J Magn Reson* 1975;18:69–83.
27. Brunner P, Ernst RR. Sensitivity and performance time in NMR imaging. *J Magn Reson* 1979;33:82–106.
28. Edelstein WA, Hutchinson JMS, Johnson G, Redpath TW. Spin-warp NMR imaging and applications to human whole-body imaging. *Phys Med Biol* 1980;25:751–756.
29. Abragam A. *Reflections of a Physicist*. Oxford: Clarendon Press; 1986.
30. Lauterbur PC. Medical imaging by nuclear magnetic resonance zeugmatography. *IEEE Trans Nucl Sci* 1979;NS-26:2808–2809.
31. Morris PG, Mansfield P, Pykett IL, Ordidge RJ, Coupland RE. Human whole body line scan imaging by nuclear magnetic resonance. *IEEE Trans Nucl Sci* 1979;NS-26:2817–2820.
32. Makow LS. Medical device review at the Food and Drug Administration: lessons from magnetic resonance spectroscopy and biliary lithotripsy. *Stanford Law Rev* 1994;46:709–746.
33. Chen C-N, Hoult DI. *Biomedical Magnetic Resonance Technology*. Bristol: Adam Hilger; 1989.
34. Fukushima E, ed. *NMR in Biomedicine: The Physical Basis*. New York: American Institute of Physics; 1989.
35. Morris PG. *Nuclear Magnetic Resonance Imaging in Medicine and Biology*. Oxford: Clarendon Press; 1989.
36. Bronskill MJ, Sprawls P, eds. *The Physics of MRI*. Woodbury, NY: American Institute of Physics, 1993. (*Medical Physics*; vol 21).
37. Vetter J, Ries G, Reichert T. A 4-tesla superconducting whole-body magnet for MR imaging and spectroscopy. *IEEE Trans Magn* 1988;MAG-24:1285–1287.
38. Wahlund L-O, Agartz I, Almquist O, et al. The brain in healthy aged individuals: MR imaging. *Radiology* 1990;174:675–679.
39. Cullity Bd. *Introduction to Magnetic Materials*. Reading: Addison-Wesley; 1972.
40. Kaufman, L, Arakawa M, Hale J, et al. Accessible magnetic resonance imaging. *Magn Reson Q* 1989;5:283–297.
41. Battocletti JH, Myers TJ. A permanent magnet for NMR. *IEEE Trans Magn* 1989;MAG-25:3910–3912.
42. Sagawa M, Fujimura S, Togawa N, Yamamoto H, Matsuura Y. New material for permanent magnets on a base of Nd and Fe. *J Appl Phys* 1984;55:2083–2087.
43. Miyamoto T, Sakurai H, Takabayashi H, Aoki M. A development of a permanent magnet assembly for MRI devices using Nd-Fe-B material. *IEEE Trans Magn* 1989;MAG-25:3907–3909.
44. Abele MG, Chandra R, Rusinek H, Leupold HA, Potenziani E. Compensation of non-uniform magnetic properties of components of a yokeless permanent magnet. *IEEE Trans Magn* 1989;MAG-25:3904–3906.
45. Wilson MN. *Superconducting Magnets*. Oxford: Clarendon Press; 1983.
46. Garrett MW. Axially symmetric systems for generating and measuring magnetic fields, Part I. *J Appl Phys* 1951;22:1091–1107.
47. Garrett MW. Thick cylindrical coil systems for strong magnetic fields with field or gradient homogeneities of the 6th to 20th order. *J Appl Phys* 1967;38:2563–2586.
48. McKeehan LW. Gaugain-Helmholtz (?) coils for uniform magnetic fields. *Nature* 1934;133:832–833.
49. Romeo I, Hoult DI. Magnetic field profiling: analysis and correcting coil design. *Magn Reson Med* 1984;1:44–65.
50. Ishiyama A, Hondoh M, Ishida N, Onuki T. Optimal design of MRI magnets with magnetic shielding. *IEEE Trans Magn* 1989;MAG-25:1885–1888.
51. Turner R. Gradient coil design: a review of methods. *Magn Reson Imaging* 1993;11:903–920.
52. Maxwell JC. *A Treatise on Electricity and Magnetism*, 3rd ed. Oxford: Clarendon Press; 1891. Reprinted, New York: Dover; 1954. vol 2:372–373.
53. Schenck JF. Axial magnetic field gradient coil suitable for use with NMR apparatus. US patent 4,617,516:1986.

54. Golay MJE. Homogenizing coils for NMR apparatus. US patent 3,622,869:1971.
55. Dadok J. Shim coils for superconducting solenoids. *Proceedings of the Tenth Annual Conference of Experimental NMR.* Pittsburgh, PA; 1969.
56. Schenck JF, Hussain MA, Edelstein WA. Transverse gradient field coils for nuclear magnetic resonance imaging. US patent 4,646,024:1987.
57. Edelstein WA, Schenck JF. Current streamline method for coil construction. US patent 4,840,700:1989.
58. Chrissoulidis DP, Sergiadis GD, Tsiboukis TD, Kriezis EE. Pulse distortion due to eddy currents induced in a multiply excited cylindrical shell of finite length and thickness. *IEEE Trans Magn* 1989;MAG-25:4454–4461.
59. Robertson S, Hughes DG, Liu Q, Allen PS. Analysis of the temporal and spatial dependence of eddy current fields in a 40-cm bore magnet. *Magn Reson Med* 1992;25:158–166.
60. Hughes DG, Robertson S, Allen PS. Intensity artifacts in MRI caused by gradient switching in an animal-size NMR magnet. *Magn Reson Med* 1992;25:167–179.
61. Roemer PB, Hickey JS. Self shielded gradient coils for nuclear magnetic resonance imaging. US patent 4,737,716:1988.
62. Turner R. A target field approach to optimal coil design. *J Phys D* 1986;18:L147–L151.
63. Mansfield P, Chapman B. Active magnetic screening of gradient coils in MR imaging. *J Magn Reson* 1986;66:573–576.
64. Schenck JF. Radiofrequency coils: types and characteristics. In: Bronskill MJ, Sprawls P, eds. *The Physics of MRI.* Woodbury, NY: American Institute of Physics: 1993:98–134. (*Medical Physics*; vol 21.)
65. Lowe IJ, Tarr CE. A fast recovery probe and receiver for pulsed nuclear magnetic resonance spectroscopy. *J Phys E* 1968;1:320–322.
66. Schenck JF, Hart HR Jr, Foster TH, Edelstein WA, Hussain MA. High resolution magnetic resonance imaging using surface coils. In: Kressel HY, ed. *Magnetic Resonance Annual.* New York: Raven Press; 1986:123–160.
67. Edelstein WA, Hardy CJ, Mueller OM. Electronic decoupling of surface-coil receivers for NMR imaging and spectroscopy. *J Magn Reson* 1986;67:157–161.
68. Hayes CE, Edelstein WA, Schenck JF, Mueller OM, Eash M. An efficient, highly homogeneous radiofrequency coil for whole-body NMR imaging at 1.5 T. *J Magn Reson* 1985;63:622–628.
69. Requardt H, Offerman J, Erhard P. Switched array coils. *Magn Reson Med* 1990;13:385–397.
70. Roemer PB, Edelstein WA, Hayes CE, Souza SP, Mueller OM. The NMR phased array. *Magn Reson Med* 1990;16:192–225.
71. Kanal E, Shellock FG, Talagala L. Safety considerations in magnetic resonance imaging: part I an overview of current knowledge. *Radiology* 1990;176:593–606.
72. Shellock FG, Morisoli S, Kanal M. MR procedures and biomedical implants, materials and devices: 1993 update. *Radiology* 1993;189:587–599.
73. Kanal E, Shellock FG. Burns associated with clinical MR examinations. *Radiology* 1990;175:585.
74. denBoef JH, van Uijen CM, Holzcherer CD. Multiple-slice NMR imaging by three-dimensional Fourier zeugmatography. *Phys Med Biol* 1984;29:857–867.
75. Frahm J, Haase A, Matthaei D. Rapid three-dimensional MR imaging using the FLASH technique. *J Comput Assist Tomogr* 1986;10:363–368.
76. Wood ML, Henkelman RM. Suppression of respiratory motion artifacts in magnetic resonance imaging. *Med Phys* 1986;13:794–805.
77. Cline HE, Lorensen WE, Ludke S, Two algorithms for the three-dimensional reconstruction of tomograms. *Med Phys* 1988;15:320–327.
78. MacFall JR, Wehrli FW, Breger RK, Johnson GA. Methodology for the measurement and analysis of relaxation times in proton imaging. *Magn Reson Imaging* 1987;5:209–220.
79. Kamman RL, Stomp GP, Berendsen HJC, Unified multiple-feature color display for MR images. *Magn Reson Med* 1989;9:240–253.
80. Covell MM, Hearshen DO, Carson PL, Chenevert TP, Shreve P, Aisen AM, Bookstein FL, Murphy BW, Martel W. Automated analysis of multiple performance characteristics in magnetic resonance imaging systems. *Med Phys* 1986;13:815–823.
81. Bidgood WD, Horii SC. Introduction to the ACR-NEMA DICOM Standard. *Radiographics* 1992;12:345–355.
82. Lewis AS, Knowles G. Image compression using the 2-D wavelet transform. *IEEE Trans Image Processing* 1992;1:244–250.
83. Mansfield P. Multi-planar image formation using NMR spin echoes. *J Phys C: Solid State Phys* 1977;10:L55–LL58.
84. Pykett IL, Rzedzian RR. Instant images of the body by magnetic resonance. *Magn Reson Med* 1987;5:563–571.
85. Mansfield P, Ordidge RJ, Coxon R. Zonally magnified EPI in real time by NMR. *J Phys E* 1988;21:275–280.
86. Hennig J, Nauerth A, Friedburg H. RARE imaging: a fast method for clinical MR. *Magn Reson Med* 1986;3:823–833.
87. Hennig J, Friedburg H. Clinical applications and methodological developments of the RARE technique. *Magn Reson Imaging* 1988;6:391–395.
88. Wehrli FW. Fast-scan magnetic resonance: principles and applications. *Magn Reson Q* 1990;6:165–236.
89. Cohen MS, Weisskoff. Ultra-fast imaging. *Magn Reson Imaging* 1991;9:1–37.
90. Oshio K, Feinberg DA. GRASE (gradient- and spin-echo) imaging: a novel fast MRI technique. *Magn Reson Med* 1991;20:344–349.
91. Atlas SW, Hackney DB, Listerud J. Fast spin-echo imaging of the brain and spine. *Magn Reson Q* 1993;9:61–63.
92. Rzedzian RR. A method for instant whole-body MR imaging at 2.0 tesla and system design considerations in its implementation. *Abstracts of the Proceedings of the Society of Magnetic Resonance in Medicine Annual Meeting.* Berkeley, CA: Society of Magnetic Resonance in Medicine; 1987:229.
93. Harvey PR, Mansfield P. Resonant trapezoidal gradient generation for use in echo-planar imaging. *Abstracts of the Proceedings of the Society of Magnetic Resonance in Medicine Annual Meeting.* Berkeley, CA: Society of Magnetic Resonance in Medicine; 1992:588.
94. Souza SP, Roemer PB, St. Peters RL, Mueller OM, Rohling KW, Dumoulin CL, Hardy CJ. Echo planar imaging with non-resonant gradient power system. *Abstracts of the Proceedings of the Society of Magnetic Resonance in Medicine Annual Meeting.* Berkeley, CA:Society of Magnetic Resonance in Medicine; 1991:217.
95. Mueller OM, Roemer PB. Gradient speed-up circuit for NMR system. US patent 5,105,153:1992.
96. Mansfield P, Harvey PR. Limits to neural stimulation in echo-planar imaging. *Magn Reson Med* 1993;29:746–758.
97. Baker AT. An introduction to the basic principles of magnetic nerve stimulation. *J Clin Neurophysiol* 1991;8:26–37.
98. Maccabee PJ, Amassian VE, Cracco RQ, Cracco JB, Eberle L, Ruddell A. Stimulation of the human nervous system using the magnetic coil. *J Clin Neurophysiol* 1991;8:38–55.
99. Jalinous R. Technical and practical aspects of magnetic nerve stimulation. *J Clin Neurophysiol* 1991;8:10–25.
100. Roemer PB. Transverse gradient coils for imaging the head. US Patent 5,177,442:1993.
101. Jolesz FA, Stern F. The operating room of the future: report of the National Cancer Institute workshop—imaging-guided stereotactic tumor diagnosis and treatment. *Invest Radiol* 1992;27:326–328.
102. Kondziolka D, Dempsey PK, Lunsford LD, Kestle JRW, Dolan EJ, Kanal E, Tasker RW. A comparison between magnetic resonance imaging and computed tomography for stereotactic coordinate determination. *Neurosurgery* 1992;30:402–407.
103. Duckwiler G, Lufkin RB, Teresi L, Spickler E, Dion J, Vinuela F, Bentson J, Hanafee W, Head and neck lesions: MR-guided aspiration biopsy. *Radiology* 1989;170:510–522.
104. Hu X, Tan KK, Levin DN, et al. Three-dimensional magnetic resonance images of the brain: application to neurosurgical planning. *J Neurosurg* 1990;72:433–440.
105. Pitt AM, Fleckenstein JL, Greenlee RG, Burns DK, Bryan WW, Haller R. MRI-guided biopsy in inflammatory myopathy: initial results. *Magn Reson Imaging* 1993;11:1093–1099.

106. Dumoulin CL, Souza SP, Darrow RD. Real-time position monitoring of invasive devices using magnetic resonance. *Magn Reson Med* 1993;29:411–415.
107. Bleier AR, Jolesz FA, Cohen MS, Weisskoff RM, Delcanton JJ, Higuchi N, Feinberg DA, Rosen BR, McKinstry RC, Hushek SG. Real-time magnetic resonance imaging of laser heat deposition in tissue. *Magn Reson Med* 1991;21:132–137.
108. Fan M, Ascher PW, Schrottner O, Ebner F, Germann RH, Kleinert R. Interstitial 1.06 Nd:YAG laser thermotherapy in malignant gliomas under real-time monitoring of MRI: experimental studies and phase I clinical trial. *J Clin Laser Surg* 1992;10:355–361.
109. Matsumoto R, Jolesz FA, Selig AM, Carlucci VM. Interstitial Nd:YAG laser ablation in normal rabbit liver: trial to maximize the size of laser-induced lesions. *Lasers Surg Med* 1992;12:650–658.
110. Gewiese B, Beuthan J, Fobbe F, Stiller D, Mueller G, Bose-Landgraf J, Wolf K-J, Deimling M. Magnetic resonance imaging-controlled laser-induced interstitial phototherapy. *Invest Radiol* 1993;29:345–351.
111. Hynynen K, Darkazanli A, Unger E, Schenck JF. MRI-guided noninvasive ultrasound surgery. *Med Phys* 1992;20:107–116.
112. Cline HE, Schenck JF, Watkins RD, Hynynen K, Jolesz FA. Magnetic resonance-guided thermal surgery. *Magn Reson Med* 1993;30:98–106.
113. Gilbert JC, Rubinsky B, Roos MS, Wong STS, Brennan KM. MRI-monitored cyrosurgery in the rabbit brain. *Magn Reson Imaging* 1993;11:1155–1164.
114. Schenck JF, Jolesz FA, Roemer PB et al. Superconducting open configuration MRI system for image-guided therapy. *Radiology* 1995;195:[*in press*].
115. Karlik, SJ, Heatherley T, Pavan F, Stein J, Lebron F, Rutt B, Carey R, Wexler R, Gelb A. Patient anesthesia and monitoring at a 1.5-T MRI installation. *Magn Reson Med* 1988;7:210–221.
116. Schenck JF. The role of magnetic susceptibility in magnetic resonance imaging: magnetic field compatibility of the first and second kinds. 1994;[*submitted*].
117. Schenck JF, Dumoulin CL, Redington RW, Kressel HY, Elliott RT, McDougall IL. Human exposure to 4.0-Tesla magnetic fields in a whole-body scanner. *Med Phys* 1992;19:1089–1098.
118. Ugurbil K, Garwood M, Ellerman J, Hendrich K, Hinke R, Hu X, Kim S-G, Menon R, Merkle H, Ogawa S, Salmi R. Imaging at high magnetic fields: initial experiences at 4 T. *Magn Reson Q* 1993;9:259–277.
119. Ogawa S, Tank DW, Menon R, Ellermann JR, Kim S-G, Merkle H, Ugurbil K. Intrinsic signal changes accompanying sensory stimulation: functional brain mapping with magnetic resonance imaging. *Proc Natl Acad Sci U S A* 1992;89:5951–5952.
120. Ramo S, Whinnery JR, van Duzer T. *Fields and Waves in Communication Electronics*, 3rd ed. New York: Wiley; 1994.
121. Lorrain P, Carson DP, Lorrain F. *Electromagnetic Fields and Waves*. 3rd ed. New York: Freeman; 1988.
122. Jackson JD. *Classical Electrodynamics*, 2nd ed. New York: Wiley; 1975.
123. Schelkunoff SA. *Electromagnetic Waves*. New York: Van Nostrand; 1943.
124. King RWP, Smith GS, Owens M, Wu TT. *Antennas in Matter: Fundamentals, Theory and Applications*. Cambridge: MIT Press; 1981.
125. Kreyszig E. *Advanced Engineering Mathematics*, 6th ed. New York: Wiley; 1988.
126. Morse PM, Feshbach H. *Methods of Theoretical Physics*. New York: McGraw-Hill; 1953.

Magnetic Resonance Imaging of the Brain and Spine, Second Edition, edited by Scott W. Atlas. Lippincott-Raven Publishers, Philadelphia © 1996.

2

The Basis of MR Contrast

Felix W. Wehrli and Joseph C. McGowan

INNATE CONTRAST IN MAGNETIC RESONANCE

The single most distinguishing feature of (nuclear) magnetic resonance (MR), when compared to x-ray based modalities like CT, is the extraordinarily large *innate contrast* which, for two soft tissues, can be on the order of several hundred percent (Fig. 1). In x-ray imaging contrast is a consequence of differences in the attenuation coefficients for two adjacent structures and is on the order of a few percent at best. Attenuation coefficients are related to electron densities and these, of course, are roughly proportional to the atomic numbers of the elements of which the chemical constituents are composed. Therefore fat, being rich in carbon, is more "transparent" than water since oxygen has a higher atomic number than carbon. This constitutes the basis of the Hounsfield number scale.

The physical principles underlying MR are, of course, radically different from those of CT. First, MR is not a transmission technique. The signal elicited is generated by the spins themselves in response to an external perturbation. The voltage induced by the spin magnetization is proportional to the static magnetization which is proportional to the number of spins contributing to the latter. One could therefore sensibly argue that the induced signal ought to be proportional to the MR counterpart of electron density, i.e., spin density. The latter expresses the number of MR-active nuclear spins per unit volume. However, how can such a hypothesis be reconciled with the large dynamic range observed in the signal intensities when considering the relatively small differences that exist in tissue water concentration? The reason for this discrepancy is the circumstance that the MR signal commonly is acquired under *nonequilibrium conditions*. At the time of perturbation, the spins have typically not recovered from the effect of the previous perturbation, nor is the signal usually detected immediately after its creation. Spins return to equilibrium with their environment and among themselves through processes denoted *relaxation* which will be discussed in some detail below.

F. W. Wehrli, Ph.D., and J. C. McGowan, Ph.D.: Department of Radiology, Hospital of the University of Pennsylvania, Philadelphia, PA 19104.

CONTRAST AND CONTRAST-TO-NOISE

Contrast is defined as the relative signal intensity difference in an image between two adjacent anatomic structures. Assuming signal intensities S_A and S_B, contrast $C_{A,B}$ could be written as:

$$C_{A,B} = (S_A - S_B)/S_A \quad [1a]$$

or, expressed in percent:

$$C_{A,B} = 100\% \times (S_A - S_B)/S_A \quad [1b]$$

However, since the signal is always associated with

A

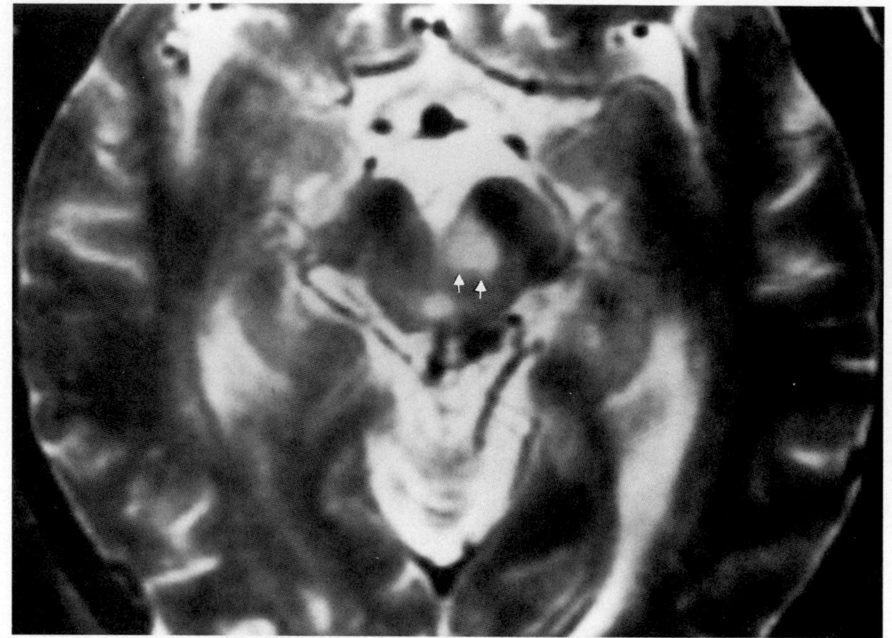

B

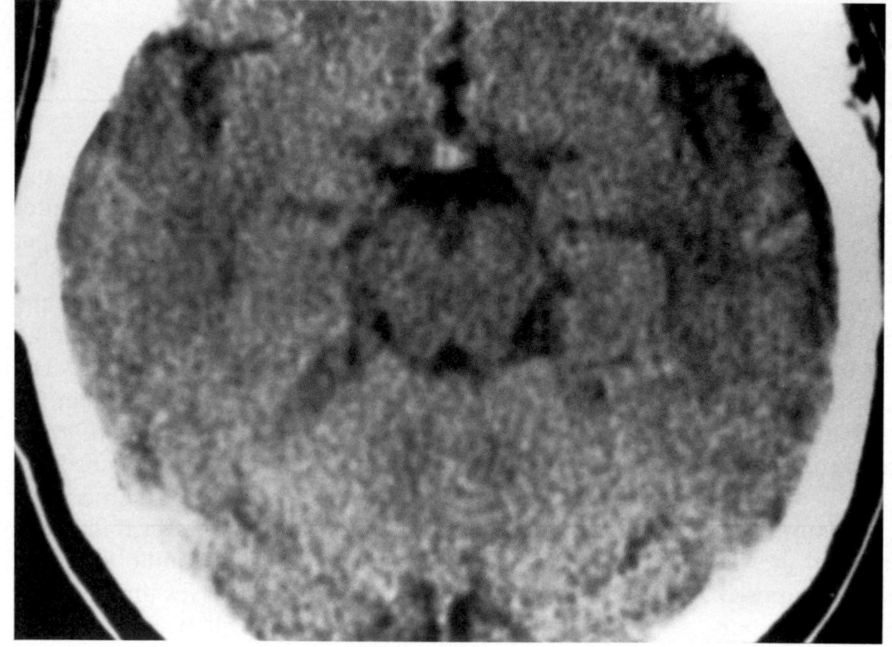

FIG. 1. The dramatically higher innate contrast of MR **(A)** relative to x-ray-based CT **(B)** is illustrated in these images where the MR scan clearly depicts a left midbrain infarction (*arrows,* **A**), but the CT scan **(B)** is normal.

noise, it is more appropriate to define a quantity which also includes the effect of noise, i.e., contrast-to-noise (CNR) (1). Therefore, instead of using the signal from one of the two tissues compared, the noise level serves as a normalization factor:

$$\mathrm{CNR}_{\mathrm{A,B}} = (S_{\mathrm{A}} - S_{\mathrm{B}})/\mathrm{Noise} \qquad [2a]$$

or

$$\mathrm{CNR}_{\mathrm{A,B}} = \mathrm{SNR}_{\mathrm{A}} - \mathrm{SNR}_{\mathrm{B}} \qquad [2b]$$

where $\mathrm{SNR}_{\mathrm{A}}$ and $\mathrm{SNR}_{\mathrm{B}}$ stand for the signal-to-noise ratios of structures A and B, respectively. If we are merely concerned with detecting a signal from background, then the background signal is zero and CNR = SNR. Figure 2 illustrates the effect of noise on visual perception. Whereas the intrinsic contrast in both images is precisely the same, CNR is not. The CNR in the image of Fig. 2a is approximately a factor of 2 lower than in Fig. 2b. We notice that it is primarily the smaller structures such as the aqueduct of Sylvius whose visualization is impaired at the lower CNR level whereas larger structures like the corpus callosum are equally well visualized in the two images. This is a fundamental finding which is well understood theoretically.

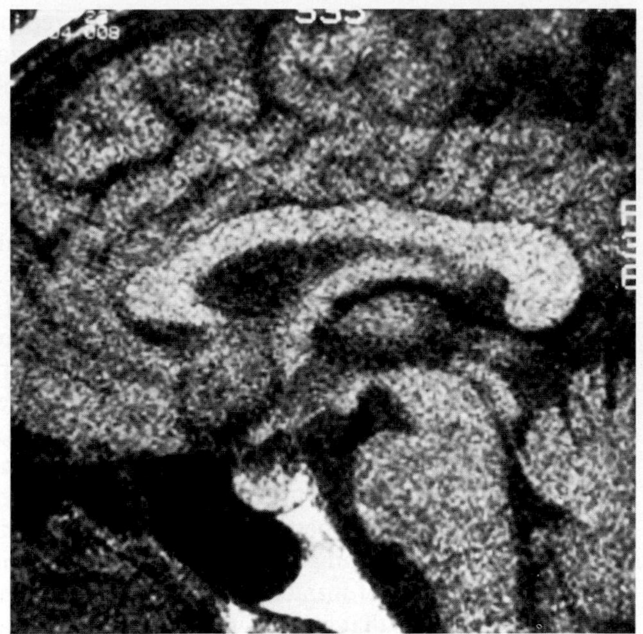

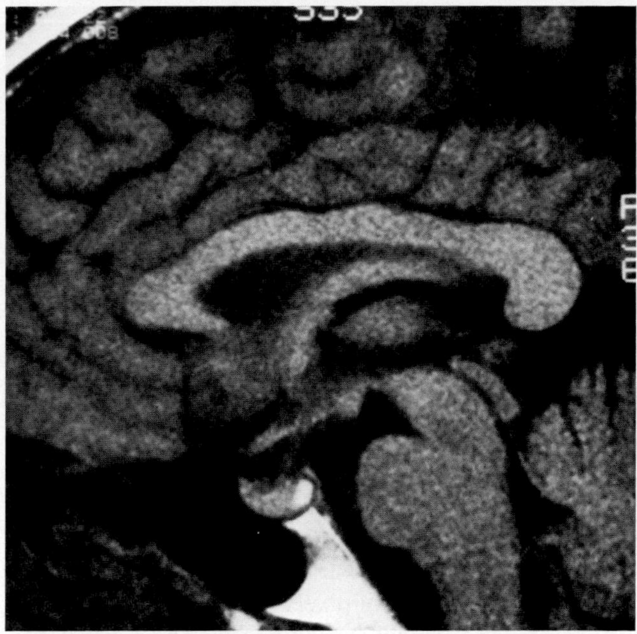

FIG. 2. Effect of noise on visual perception. Contrast in both images is the same but CNR differs. It is lower in **A** by a factor of 2. Note that the lower CNR primarily impairs visualization of small structure such as the aqueduct of Sylvius and pituitary stalk, but has little effect on visual perception of such large structures as the corpus callosum.

SIGNAL-TO-NOISE THRESHOLD

One of the fundamental questions in medical imaging is how much CNR is needed to be certain that differences between signals are real and not simply the result of noise fluctuations. This question has been addressed by Rose (2). Figure 3 shows the distribution of measured signal intensities in the presence of normally distributed (Gaussian) noise. Suppose the true value of the signal is precisely 100. However, the measured signal intensities may vary. The statistical fluctuations around the mean value can be described in terms of a probability density function for Gaussian noise:

$$p = (1/2\pi)^{1/2} \exp(-k^2/2) \qquad [3]$$

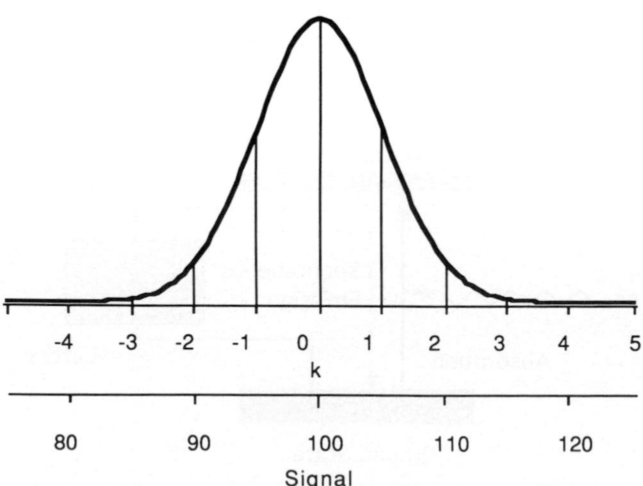

FIG. 3. Probability distribution of a signal in the presence of noise. The abscissa k is the root mean square (rms) deviation for a signal of average value 100. (Modified from Rose, ref. 2.)

In Equation 3, k corresponds to the number of standard deviations from the mean. The vertical axis of Fig. 3 thus represents the probability (p) of observing a particular value of intensity specified by the upper scale on the abscissa. The total area under the curve is unity by definition. We note that in the presence of noise the most likely value to be observed is still the mean ($\bar{X} = 100$) but a distinct probability exists that the measured value will be quite different. Hence, a legitimate question would be whether an observation of, say 110, represents a true change in signal intensity or whether it is merely due to a fluctuation of background noise. The probability for such an occurrence can be determined from the area under the probability density curve. The area under the curve between $k = 1$ and $k = 2$ is 0.13 (i.e., 13%) and represents the probability for the signal to be between 105 and 110. Likewise, the area under the curve to the right of $k = 2$ is 0.023 which means that the probability for the observation to exceed a value of 110 is 2.3%. Therefore, while a measurement greater than 110 is likely to reflect a real change in signal intensity, there still exists a finite probability that the signal is invariant (Table 1).

We can now make an assessment as to how large the signal needs to be in order not to be mistaken for noise. The signal is the brightness difference (contrast) between the spot of interest and the background. Let us assume

TABLE 1. *Probability of exceeding various values of* k

k	Probability of exceeding *k*
1	0.15
2	.023
3	1.3×10^{-3}
4	3×10^{-5}
5	3×10^{-7}
6	2×10^{-9}

for this purpose an image of 10^5 picture elements (pixels), or roughly the size of a 256 × 256 image. Hence we have 10^5 opportunities for making a mistake, i.e., mistaking a particular pixel for the signal which in actual fact might merely be a noise fluctuation. We can make this assessment by reference to Table 1 which lists the probabilities for exceeding various values of k, simply by multiplying the number of pixels by the respective probabilities. At $k = 5$ (signal exceeding noise by 5 standard deviations, i.e., SNR = 5) this probability is 3%.

If the size of the object to be discerned is larger than a single picture element, it becomes obvious that the SNR requirements are less stringent. For example, for a region of interest (ROI) of 100 pixels, the probability for a false observation (mistakenly assigning an observation to noise fluctuation) is 3% at a SNR figure of 4 ($k = 4$).

The detectability is often called the *resolving power* (not to be confused with spatial resolution). An important conclusion of the above considerations is that the contrast-to-noise requirements increase with decreasing object size. Hence, in order to detect a small abnormality or visualize a small anatomic structure, a higher level of CNR is required. This, however, is precisely what we found empirically in the images of Fig. 2. Hence, Rose's findings are universally applicable to all imaging systems but have particular significance for MR where time and thus cost considerations force us to operate in a regime only marginally above the SNR threshold needed for "safe" assessment of absence or presence of an abnormality. A more detailed discussion of this subject is provided in reference 3.

SPIN RELAXATION

We may now turn to the question regarding the mechanism of contrast in MR. We have previously seen that the extraordinary contrast seen in MR images cannot be explained in terms of differences in water concentration alone and that it is more likely due to a modulation caused by differences in the spins' ability to respond to a perturbation (e.g., a radiofrequency pulse). The return of the macroscopic spin magnetization to equilibrium is described by two independent processes, called *longitudinal and transverse relaxation*. Typically, both processes are monoexponential and thus characterized by single time constants: T1 for the longitudinal magnetization and T2 for the transverse magnetization. In the following paragraphs a cursory overview of the nature of these processes will be provided and their dependence on chemical, structural, and environmental parameters discussed.

A full appreciation of image contrast requires an understanding of the mechanisms underlying proton relaxation in biologic tissues, a subject that has been very widely researched and yet is still incompletely understood. The protons giving rise to an MR signal are mainly those in cell water and lipids (see, for example, reference 4 for a review of the subject). Protons in proteins and DNA, and those in solid structures, such as bone, usually do not contribute to the signal, mainly because their relaxation properties render them undetectable by the typical imaging system. However, it is the degree of interaction of intracellular water with macromolecular structures that governs the efficiency of water proton relaxation.

T1 Relaxation

Radiofrequency stimulation causes the nuclei to absorb energy, raising them to an excited state. The nuclei in their excited state can return to the ground state only by dissipating their excess energy to the environment, the lattice. This process is termed *spin-lattice relaxation* (Fig. 4). A direct return to the ground state by spontaneous emission of an energy quantum is a negligible process.

Return to the ground state also requires a stimulating radiofrequency field. The fields causing spin-lattice relaxation are provided by the surrounding nuclear environment, the so-called lattice. The term *lattice* refers to the highly organized network of molecules or atoms in crystalline solids. In magnetic resonance, the term has been extended to other than solid phases and describes the magnetic environment of the nuclei.

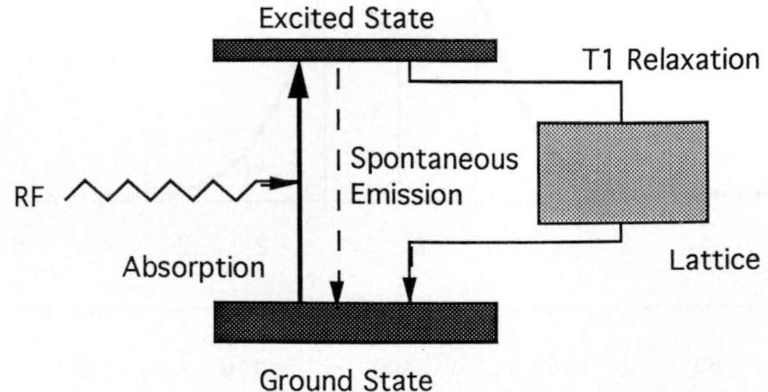

FIG. 4. Radiofrequency absorption promotes spins from the ground state to an excited state. Return to the ground state occurs through interaction with the spins' surroundings, the lattice, whereas spontaneous emission is a negligible process.

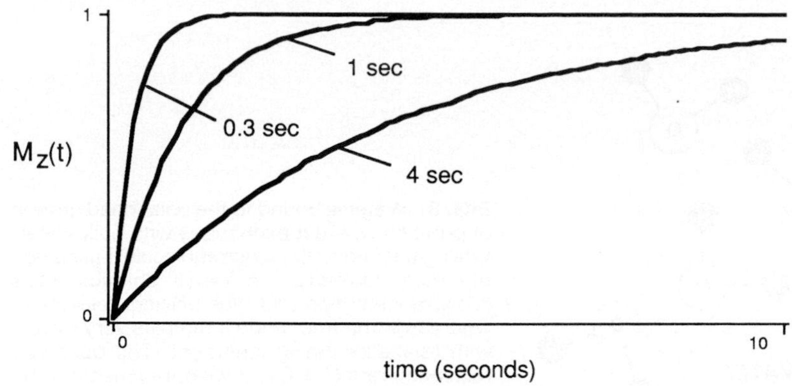

FIG. 5. Return of the longitudinal magnetization with time constants T1 typical of water protons in biological tissues.

Another, and for the purposes of understanding image contrast, more convenient definition of T1 is in terms of the return to equilibrium of the longitudinal magnetization. However, it will immediately become evident that this and the previously given definition are equivalent. Let us assume that a 90° rf pulse has been applied, converting all longitudinal to transverse magnetization. This is equivalent to equalizing the spin populations in the diagram of Fig. 5. The return to equilibrium then occurs exponentially as

$$M_z(t) = M_0\{1 - \exp(-t/\mathrm{T1})\} \qquad [4]$$

where $M_z(t)$ is the longitudinal magnetization at time t and M_0 is the magnetization in thermal equilibrium. Figure 5 plots M_z for some typical T1s found in normal biological tissues.

The lattice fields result from the presence of other magnetic nuclei, paramagnetic ions and molecules (*dipole-dipole relaxation*), and molecular magnetism, caused by fast rotation of electronic charges (spin-rotation mechanism). The most common source of lattice fields are the dipole fields produced by neighboring magnetic nuclei. For instance, in the water molecule, one of the hydrogen nuclei produces a magnetic field, thus affecting the adjacent proton (Fig. 6).

The lattice field must fluctuate to be effective in transferring energy from the excited proton to the lattice. These fluctuations must occur at a rate that matches the precessional frequency of the excited protons (Larmor frequency). In liquids, the fluctuations in the lattice field are caused by random thermal motions of molecules (*Brownian motion*), which can either be rotational or translational (Fig. 7).

Both intra- and inter-molecular relaxation processes occur. Intramolecular relaxation implies that energy is transferred between nuclei within the same molecule. Intermolecular relaxation refers to relaxation that involves nuclei in different molecules. The protons in water and lipid molecules relax primarily by the *intramolecular dipole-dipole* mechanism, which is induced by rotational rather than translational motion. The average rate at which molecules reorient (rotate or translate) is related to the size of the molecule. Small molecules (e.g., H_2O) reorient more rapidly than larger molecules (e.g., lipids). Large macromolecules (e.g., proteins or DNA) tumble very slowly due to increased frictional and inertial forces. Efficient relaxation is equivalent to short T1 relaxation times. For instance, in fat, T1 at 1.5 T field strength is of the order of about 300 milliseconds, while in pure water, it is about 3 seconds. The frequency of rotation in medium-size molecules, such as lipids, most closely matches Larmor precession at typical MR field strengths. Lipid protons, therefore, relax faster than the protons in free water molecules, which tumble at a frequency which, on the average, is much greater than the precessional frequency of the protons. Similarly, macromolecules are ineffective in causing relaxation because their tumbling rate is much lower than the precessional

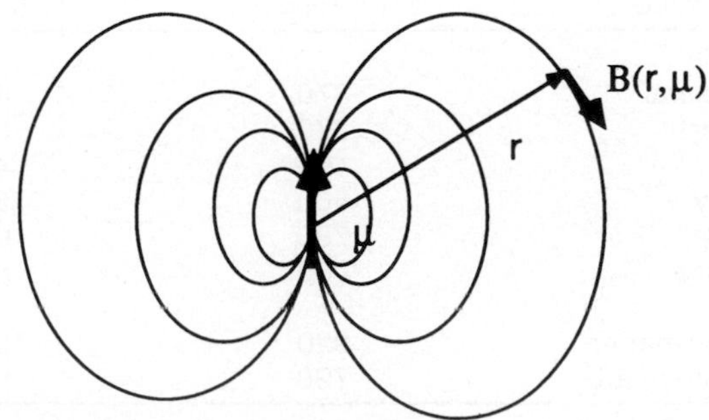

FIG. 6. Dipole field B (r, μ) generated by a nucleus of magnetic moment μ at the site of a neighboring nucleus.

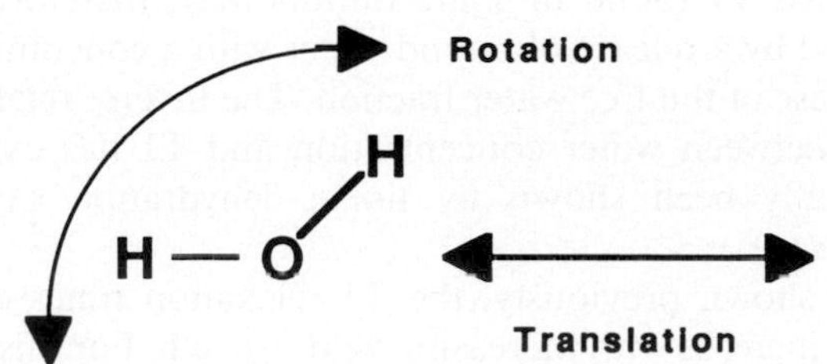

FIG. 7. Temporal modulation of magnetic field generated by nuclear dipole is caused by rotational and translational Brownian motion.

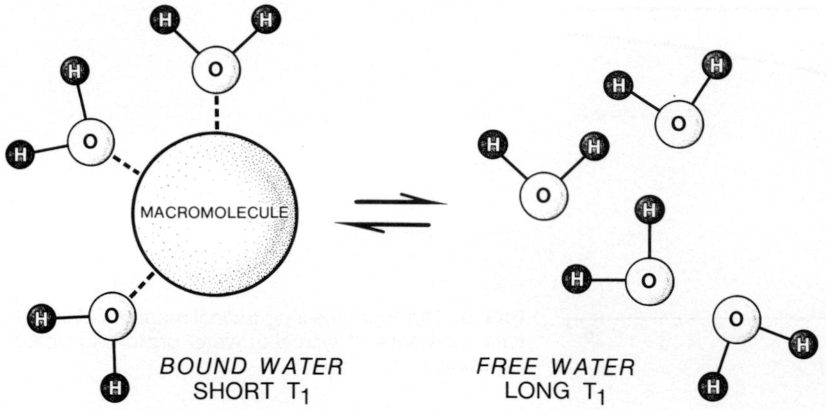

FIG. 8. Water is bound to the polar head groups of proteins where it exchanges with bulk water. While attached to the macromolecule it assumes the macromolecule's motional characteristics (slow reorientation and thus efficient relaxation) whereas in the free mode it tumbles very rapidly with relaxation being inefficient. The observed relaxation rate (1/T1) is a weighted mean of the two populations.

frequency. Since the precessional frequency is proportional to the strength of the external magnetic field, relaxation times are *field-dependent*. The relaxation rate (inverse of relaxation times) is directly related to the strength of the lattice field at the resonance frequency (ω_0). Therefore, a change in the Larmor frequency alters the relaxation in tissues. An increase in ω_0 (due to increased field strength) is, therefore, associated with decreased efficiency of relaxation (longer T1). Typically, the T1 relaxation times in biological tissue are found to increase as B^k where B is the field strength and k is an empirical parameter which was found to be on the order of 0.3–0.5 (5). In practice, this means that T1 relaxation times increase 25–40% with every doubling of the magnetic field strength.

Although free (bulk) water relaxes slowly (long relaxation time), the water in biologic tissues is found to relax much faster, typically with relaxation times of several hundred milliseconds. In order to explain this phenomenon, it was postulated that a fraction of the water in tissues is bound to the surface of proteins (4) (Fig. 8). Consequently, the motion of bound water is slowed by its proximity to the large macromolecule. The slowed molecular motion of bound water more closely matches Larmor precession and, therefore, enhances relaxation (i.e., it shortens T1). In reality, a fast equilibrium exists between free and bound water. One of the hypotheses states that this equilibrium is perturbed in certain pathologic conditions (neoplasia, abscess, demyelination). The elevated T1 found in some tumors may, therefore, be caused by a release of bound water with a concomitant increase of the free water fraction. The inverse relationship between water concentration and T1 has experimentally been shown by tissue dehydration experiments (6).

As shown previously, the T1 relaxation times gradually increase with increasing field strength. For this reason, when T1 relaxation times are reported, the field strength must be indicated. At field strengths between 0.5 and 1.5 Tesla, the T1 relaxation times in soft tissues range between about 500 msec and 1 second. Table 2 lists relaxation times in various mammalian tissues at 1.5 Tesla. Note that white matter of the corpus callosum has a shorter T1 than gray matter of the brain. This difference was correctly attributed to the lower water content of white versus gray matter, rather than the lipids in myelin. In fact, in vivo spectroscopic analysis of brain tissue afforded almost no detectable lipid peak (7). Lipids in gray and white matter exist primarily in the form of phospholipids. These molecules, however, are highly immobilized, leading to a very short spin-spin (T2) relaxation time. By contrast, lipids in the scalp and bone marrow exist in the form of mobile fatty acid triglycerides, thus accounting for the short T1 relaxation time in these tissues (Table 2).

T2 Relaxation

In the T2 relaxation process, no energy is transferred from the nuclei to the lattice. Rather, the spins exchange energy with each other, i.e., while one nucleus absorbs energy, its neighbor releases energy. The random fields generated by an ensemble of nuclei is the cause for

TABLE 2. *T1 and T2 in various mammalian tisues at 1.5 T*[a]

Tissue	T1 (msec)	T2 (msec)
Muscle		
Skeletal	870	47
Heart	870	57
Liver	490	43
Kidney	560	58
Spleen	780	62
Adipose	260	84
Brain		
Gray matter	920	101
White matter	790	92

[a] T1 was calculated using an empirical relationship for the field dependence (5); T2 values are reproduced from Table 12 of ref 5.

transverse magnetization. It is the rate of loss of the transverse magnetization that determines the T2 relaxation time. The transverse magnetization decays because the nuclear magnetic moments get out of phase (lose coherence). This loss of coherence results from the fact that all nuclear magnetic moments do not have exactly the same precessional frequency. In an ideally homogeneous external magnetic field, and in the absence of intrinsic fields, the precessional frequency of all nuclei would be the same and coherence would be sustained. However, magnetic field imperfections that lead to inhomogeneities and intrinsic fields within the tissue, cause the nuclei to precess at slightly different rates. This spread of resonance frequencies also results in a loss of phase coherence with subsequent loss of transverse magnetization. The T2 relaxation time describes the loss of transverse magnetization as a result of intrinsic fields in the sample being studied.

Figure 9 illustrates the evolution of the transverse magnetization with time as a result of transverse, T2, or spin- spin relaxation, for typical tissue proton relaxation times. This process, typically is exponential and can be described as:

$$M_{xy}(t) = M^0_{xy} \exp(-t/\mathrm{T2}) \quad [5]$$

where M^0_{xy} is the initial transverse magnetization and $M_{xy}(t)$ is the transverse magnetization at time t.

T2 is primarily related to the intrinsic field caused by protons at low and zero reorientation rate (static component of intrinsic field). T2 relaxation is, therefore, more efficient in large molecules at zero reorientational frequency than in small molecules (T2 ≤ T1). T2, therefore, is less susceptible to the magnitude of the external field. A change in resonance frequency (ω_o) will not affect the value of the intrinsic field at zero motional frequency. For this reason T2 is nearly independent of magnetic field strength (5). Nevertheless, in biological tissues there is usually a substantial correlation between T1 and T2. In normal tissue T2 is found to span a range from about 50 to 150 msec (Table 1), except in fluids like CSF or synovial fluid where T2 can be of the order of several hundred milliseconds or even seconds. As a rule we find that T2 in free water is always longer than in bound water. The prolongation of T2 observed in lesions has, therefore, again been interpreted in terms of an increase in the ratio of free to bound water.

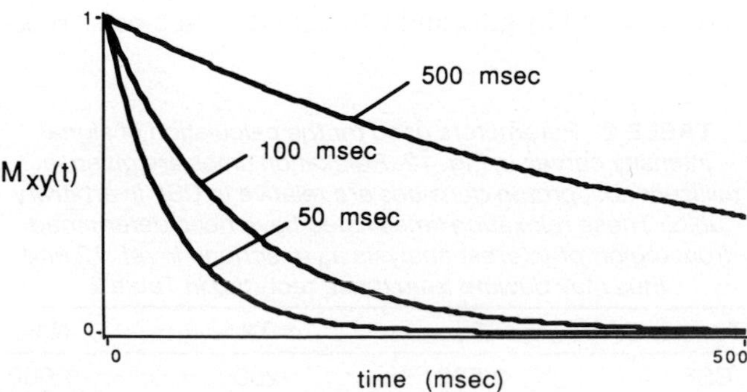

FIG. 9. Transverse magnetization as a function of time for typical proton T2 relaxation times in mammalian tissue.

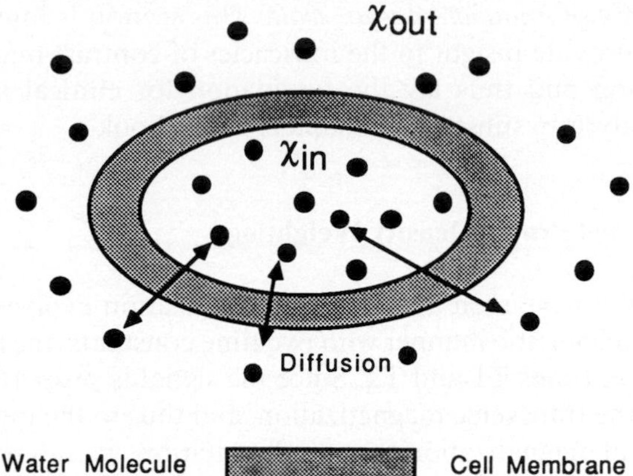

FIG. 10. Red blood cell containing paramagnetic hemoglobin (deoxy- or methemoglobin). Diffusion of water molecules along the intrinsic gradients existing between the two media is a source of effective transverse relaxation.

Susceptibility Effects

A mechanism of a very different type has its origin in local variations in magnetic susceptibility. If well defined boundaries exist between regions of different magnetic susceptibility, gradients are set up between these two regions. Spins diffusing between these two regions are dephased. Hence, this mechanism affects T2 only. The best known example is that of intact red blood cells containing either paramagnetic deoxyhemoglobin or methemoglobin as in acute or subacute hemorrhage, respectively. Very effective transverse relaxation ensues, which can lead to almost total loss in signal intensity in T2-weighted images (8,9). The mechanism of action is illustrated diagrammatically in Fig. 10, showing a red cell containing paramagnetic hemoglobin where the susceptibility inside the cell (c_{in}) is greater than outside (c_{out}). Diffusion of water molecules across the cell membrane, therefore, causes irrecoverable spin dephasing in spin-echo imaging.

CONTRAST MANIPULATION

The intriguing behavior of MR image contrast, notably the understanding and quantification of the complicated dependence on operator-selectable and intrinsic parameters, was studied extensively during the early phases of clinical magnetic resonance (10–15). The most notable distinguishing feature of MR relative to other modalities, and challenge to the newcomer, is the *ab-*

sence of a universal gray scale. This section is intended to provide insight to the intricacies of contrast manipulation and thus lay the foundation for clinical image analysis in subsequent chapters of this book.

T1 and Proton Density Weighting

We have seen above that magnetization evolves in a characteristic manner with two time constants, the relaxation times T1 and T2. Since the signal is proportional to the transverse magnetization, and thus to the longitudinal magnetization prior to rf excitation, we can predict its magnitude provided that we know the time relationship between successive rf pulses, the pulse repetition time TR, and the time between excitation and detection of the signal, the so-called echo time TE.

Let us first explore the effect of varying TR. The simplest conceivable rf pulse sequence consists of a train of equidistant 90° rf pulses which are applied every TR milliseconds (Fig. 11). The rf pulse rotates the longitudinal magnetization into the transverse plane where it is detected. Hence, the resultant signal is proportional to the longitudinal magnetization immediately before the rf pulse. Immediately after the pulse the longitudinal magnetization is zero, but it exponentially recovers during the pulse repetition time as follows:

$$M_z(\text{TR}) = M_0\{1 - \exp(-\text{TR}/\text{T1})\} \qquad [6]$$

where M_0 is the equilibrium magnetization which is assumed to be proportional to proton density. Equation 6 is equivalent to Equation 4 with t = TR.

From Equation 6 we see that the signal received is a function of both the T1 of the tissue protons as well as the TR chosen. Hence, if we know T1 for the tissues of interest, we can predict the relative signal intensities obtained from those samples for any TR. For this purpose, let us consider three common tissues: white matter (WM), gray matter (GM), and CSF, for which the relative longitudinal relaxation times follow the order: CSF ≫ GM > WM. Proton densities for the three tissues differ as follows: N(WM) < N(GM) < N(CSF). Proton density relationships are primarily apparent in signals acquired using values of TR that are long compared to T1, i.e., under conditions of nearly complete recovery of longitudinal magnetization between successive pulse sequence cycles. In Fig. 12 the signal predicted by Equation 6 is plotted using the relaxation and spin density parameters of Table 3.

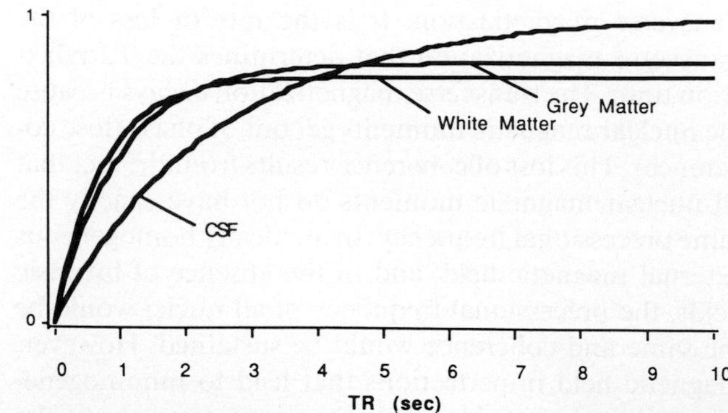

FIG. 12. MR signal calculated as a function of the pulse repetition time TR for gray matter, white matter, and CSF using the parameters of Table 3. It is assumed that 90° pulses are applied every TR sec and the signal is collected immediately thereafter. At short TR (TR < 2sec) the relative signal intensities are: WM > GM ≫ CSF and the resultant image is said to be T1-weighted, as the observed contrast primarily reflects differences in T1. At longer TR (2 sec < TR < 4 sec) the relative signal intensities are: GM > WM > CSF. Finally, at TR > 4 sec, the relative signal intensities are: CSF > GM > WM and the resultant images are said to be proton-density-weighted.

Figure 13 shows an array of axial brain images, corresponding to pulse repetition times ranging from 300 msec to 6 sec, initially in 300 msec steps of the pulse repetition time and, at longer TRs, at intervals of 600 msec. We can now follow the relative signal intensities predicted by Fig. 12. Since it is impractical to acquire such a large number of images on a single subject, the author resorted to a technique known as "image synthesis" (16,17), a discussion of which would be beyond the scope of this chapter. It suffices to state that this method permits calculation of images from a minimum of three acquired images for any desired pulse sequence parameter combination. The images shown in Fig. 13 and subsequently have virtually all the characteristics of directly acquired images.

At short TR CSF is found to be the least intense structure, followed by gray and white matter. At a pulse repe-

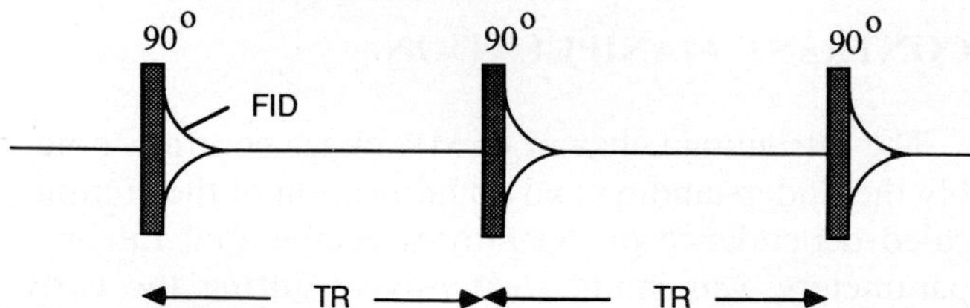

FIG. 11. Radiofrequency pulse sequence consisting of train of 90° rf pulses spaced TR milliseconds apart. Each rf pulse produces a free induction decay (FID).

TABLE 3. *Parameters used for the calculation of signal intensity curves in Fig. 12. Relaxation times are given in milliseconds, proton densities are relative to CSF in arbitrary units. These relaxation times listed have been determined from region-of-interest analysis as described in ref. 12 and thus may deviate from those reported in Table 2*

Tissue	T1	T2	N(H)
CSF	2,500	200	1.000
GM	1,000	70	0.85
WM	750	60	0.8

tition time of approximately 2 sec gray-white matter contrast vanishes, consistent with the cross-over of the signal curves for these two tissues (Fig. 12). As TR increases further, the signals pertaining to gray and white matter reach their asymptotic values, whereas the signal from CSF, by virtue of its much longer T1 continues to grow, eventually surpassing gray and white matter signal intensity. The signal evolution curves for gray matter and CSF intersect at approximately 4 sec which is consistent with the isointensity of the caudate nucleus and the anterior horns of the lateral ventricles in Fig. 13J. In all images with TR > 4 sec CSF is found to be the structure of prevailing brightness, with proton density dominating as the contrast determinant.

Inversion-Recovery

We have seen that, as the pulse repetition time increases, the signal intensity rises monotonically while contrast progresses from T1-weighted to proton density weighted. Let us now consider an alternative excitation pulse sequence where we initially perturb the spins by inverting the magnetization by means of a 180° rf pulse, followed TI milliseconds later by 90° pulse which converts the partly recovered longitudinal magnetization to transverse magnetization at which point it is detected. This process is repeated every TR milliseconds. A timing diagram for this pulse sequence which is denoted *inversion-recovery* (10, 12, 14, 18) is provided in Fig. 14. The magnetization M_z now becomes a function of both TR and the inversion delay TI (12):

$$M_z(\mathrm{TR}, \mathrm{TI}) = M_0\{1 - 2\exp(-\mathrm{TI}/\mathrm{T1}) + \exp(-\mathrm{TR}/\mathrm{T1})\} \quad [7]$$

It is readily seen that Equation 7 can assume both positive and negative values. The operator can choose to display the data with phase-sensitive reconstruction, which preserves the positive and negative values of magnetization (19). Alternatively, one may select absolute reconstruction, which displays the modulus of the magnetization, as in the following example.

We will now again plot the magnetization for the same three entities (CSF, gray and white matter) and assume again that the equilibrium magnetization is proportional to the respective proton densities. Since we have two time variables such a plot would be two-dimensional. However, we will keep TR constant at 2.5 sec and vary only the inversion delay TI (Fig. 15).

We may now attempt to correlate the predictions of Fig. 15 with images in which TI was varied systematically while holding TR constant at 2.5 seconds (Fig. 16). For reasons discussed previously the images were synthesized from the same set of acquired images as those serving as an input for the computation of the images in Fig. 13.

In spite of its superb contrast characteristics the inversion-recovery technique has so far not found widespread use in clinical imaging, the likely reason being its relative inefficiency. At a pulse repetition time of 2–3 seconds, 10–15 sections can be imaged at best in a single pass. However, it has some outstanding features which make it suited for selected applications in the CNS and body. For example, we have seen that for each T1 a value of TI exists at which the signal is exactly zero (inflection point). This permits selective suppression of undesired structures. At TR 2–3 sec, TI = 150 msec suppresses fat, which may be useful for imaging such structures as the optic nerve which is embedded in fat (20). Another, more recent application, denoted "fluid-attenuated inversion-recovery" (FLAIR) (21,22) seeks to suppress the signal from CSF by using a long inversion time in conjunction with long TE to produce heavy T2 weighting. The technique is useful in demonstrating subtle abnormalities near the spinal cord or brain–CSF interface (Fig. 17).

Recent advances in gradient-echo imaging, notably magnetization-prepared rapid gradient-echo imaging (MP-RAGE) (see Chapter 29) have led to renewed interest in inversion-recovery imaging. In this technique, a single inversion pulse, followed by a train of low flip-angle pulses, reduces scan time per section to seconds (23–25).

T2 Weighting

Spin Echo

So far we have ignored effects on signal and contrast resulting from delays in signal readout in that we have assumed that the signal is detected as soon as technically feasible following its generation. In an ideally uniform magnetic field the transverse magnetization decays with a time constant T2, the true transverse or spin-spin relaxation time. Hence, if the signal were collected some time t after its generation, it would be weakened by a factor $\exp(-t/\mathrm{T2})$. Due to spatial nonuniformities of the field, however, spins tend to get out of phase with one another faster, with a time constant T2*, the effective transverse relaxation time which is related to T2 as follows:

$$1/\mathrm{T2}^* = 1/\mathrm{T2} + \gamma\Delta B/2 \quad [8]$$

where γ is the gyromagnetic ratio and ΔB is the spread of the magnetic field across the volume of interest. Signal losses due to spatial nonuniformity may be distinguished from pure T2 effects in that they are reversible via generation of a *spin echo* which is discussed in detail in some of the standard NMR texts (26). It therefore suffices to introduce the method without detailing the underlying physical principle. Instead of directly detecting the FID

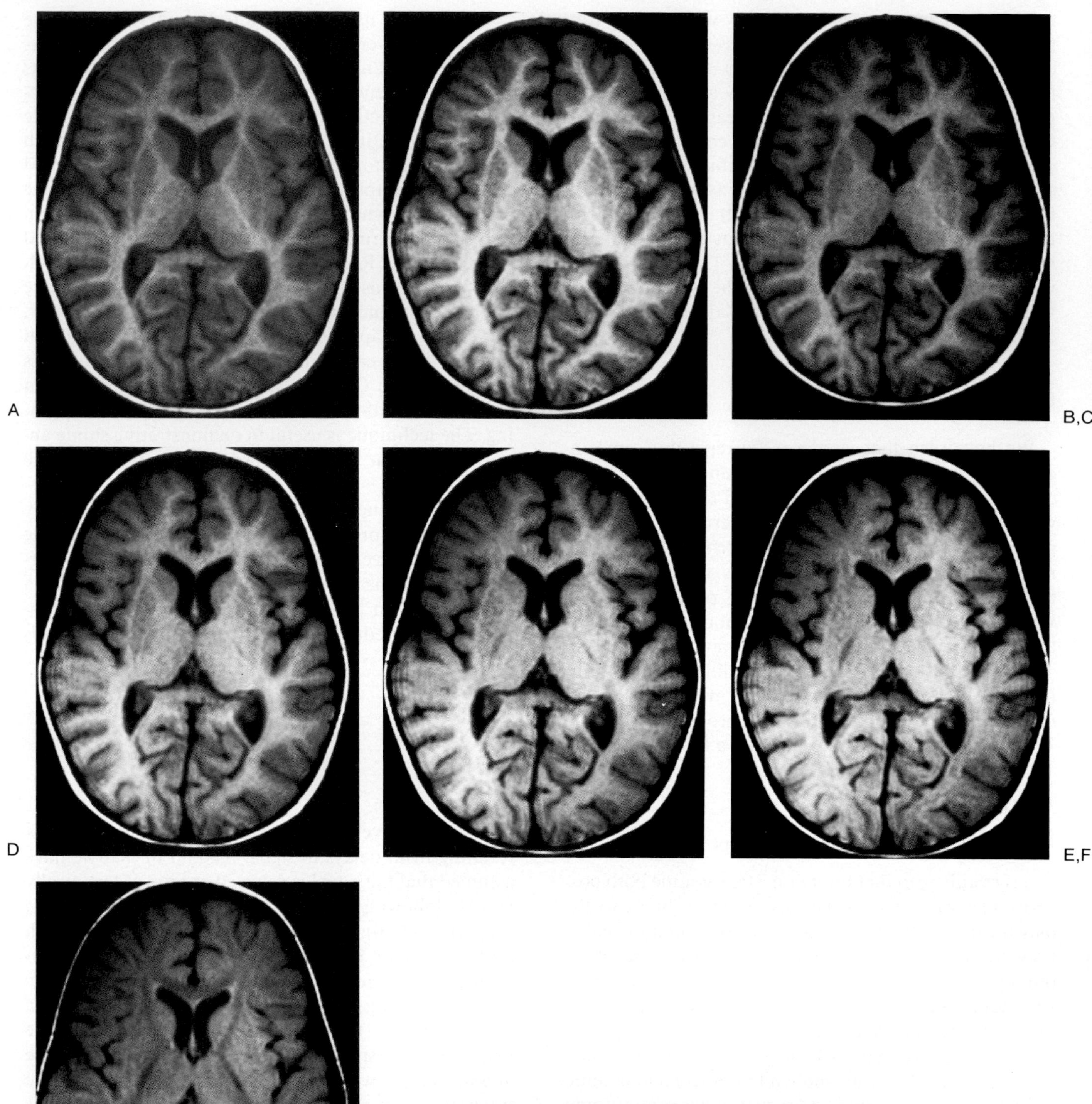

FIG. 13. Normal brain images pertaining to pulse repetition times of 300 msec (**A**), 600 msec (**B**), 900 msec (**C**), 1200 msec (**D**), 1500 msec (**E**), 1800 msec (**F**), 2400 msec (**G**), 3000 msec (**H**), 3600 msec (**I**), 4200 msec (**J**), 4800 msec (**K**), 5400 msec (**L**), and 6000 msec (**M**). Note the predicted evolution of contrast secondary to Fig. 12, notably gray-white matter contrast reversal at TR = 1800–2100 msec and gray matter–CSF contrast reversal at approximately TR = 3600 msec. All images were synthesized from basis images derived from two acquisitions as described in ref. 17 assuming an echo delay of 20 msec so as to most closely match acquired images. Further, the images have been filmed with precisely the same window width in order to avoid contrast effects from sources other than pulse timing.

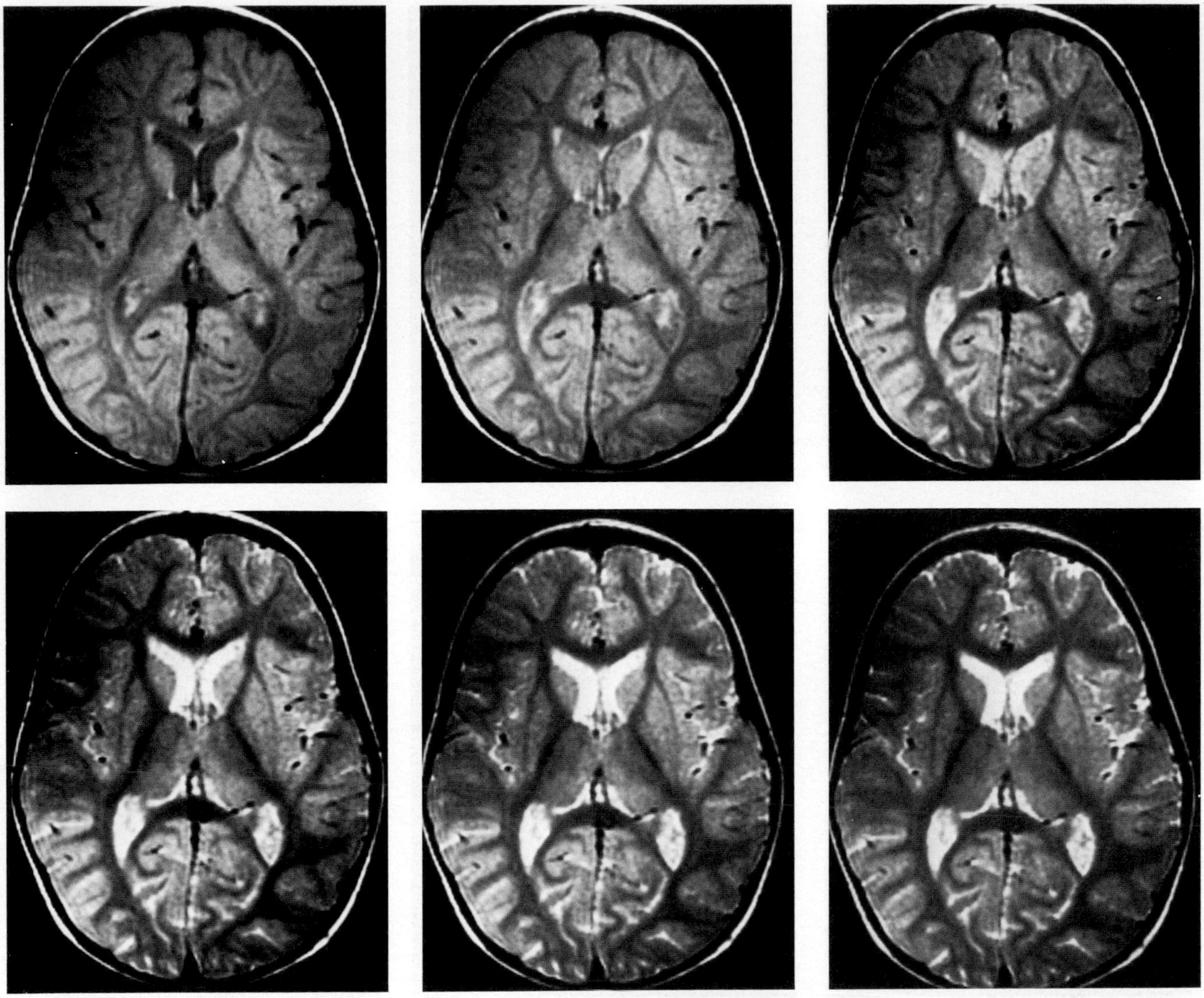

H

I,J

K

L,M

FIG. 13. *Continued.*

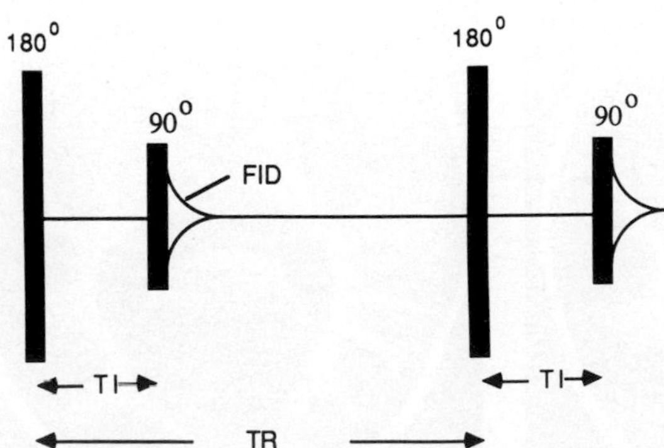

FIG. 14. Radiofrequency pulse timing diagram for the inversion-recovery pulse sequence. The initial 180° pulse inverts the magnetization, thus creating a nonequilibrium situation. During the ensuing recovery delay TI, spins partly relax and detection occurs following a 90° pulse which converts the partially recovered longitudinal to measurable transverse magnetization.

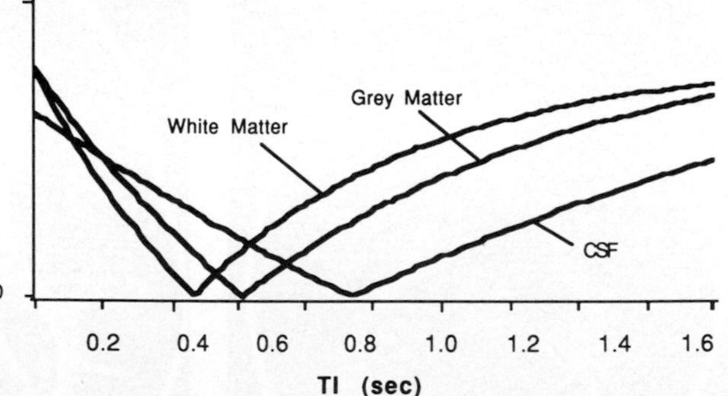

FIG. 15. MR signal calculated as a function of the inversion time TI from Equation 7 assuming a pulse repetition time TR of 2.5 sec and the parameters of Table 3 for gray matter, white matter and CSF. It is further assumed that 90° pulses are applied every TR sec and the signal is collected immediately thereafter and further that the signal represents the absolute value. Note the multiple cross-over points at which two structures are predicted to be isointense. Further, the inflection points correspond to TI values at which the signal is nulled. The relative signal intensities in the images of Fig. 16 closely match the predictions.

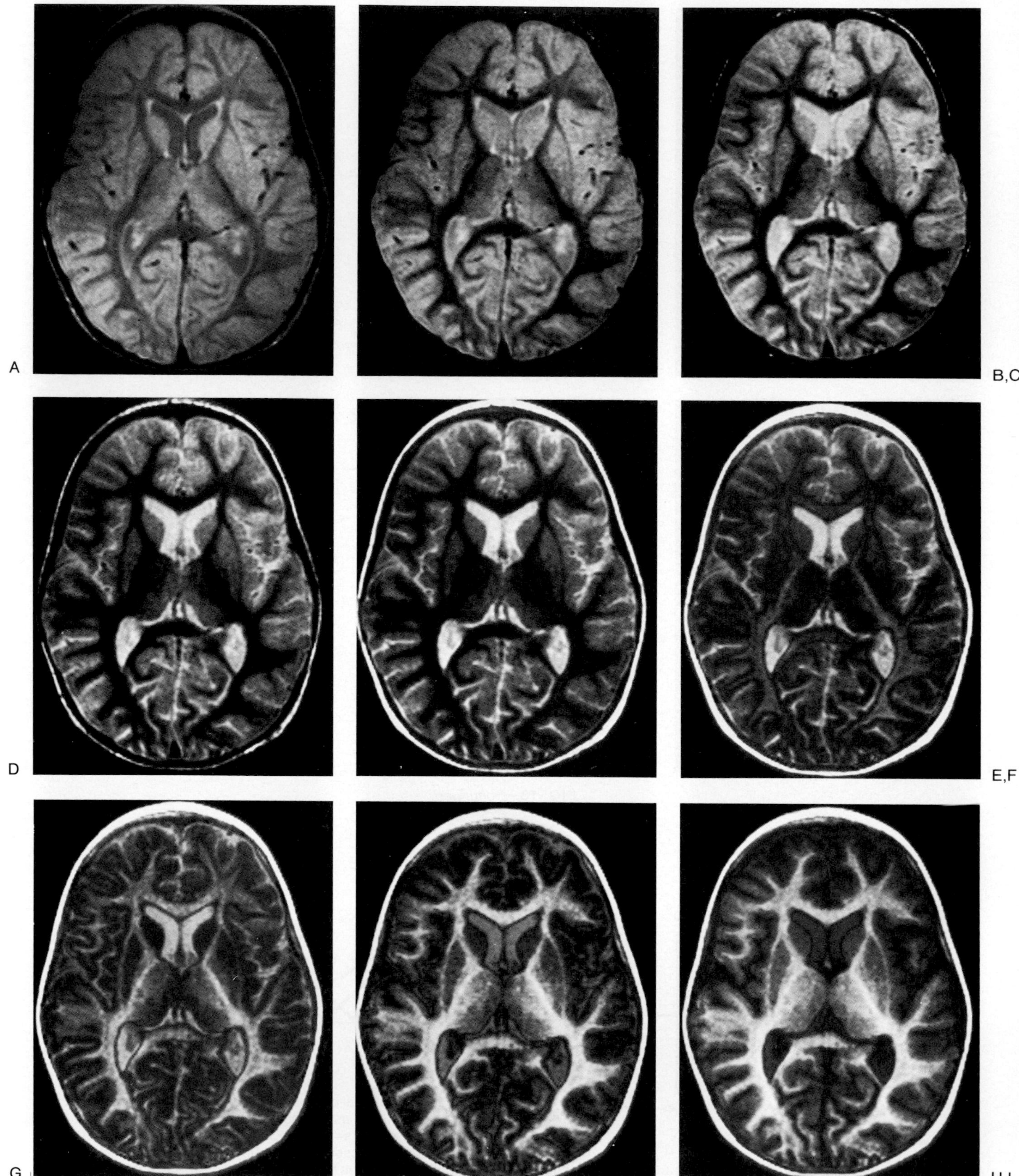

FIG. 16. Normal brain inversion-recovery images corresponding to TR = 2.5 sec and TI values of 100 msec (**A**), 200 msec (**B**), 300 msec (**C**), 400 msec (**D**), 500 msec (**E**), 600 msec (**F**), 700 msec (**G**), 800 msec (**H**), 900 msec (**I**), 1000 msec (**J**), 1200 msec (**K**). Note the complicated evolution of the relative signal intensities as TI increases. At first white matter is hypointense to gray matter (TI = 100–400 msec) whereas CSF changes from hypo to hyperintense. A second reversal of relative CSF signal intensity first occurs for white matter and subsequently also for gray matter. Finally at long TI (TI > 900 msec) the relative signal intensities follow the inverse of T1 (WM > GM > CSF).

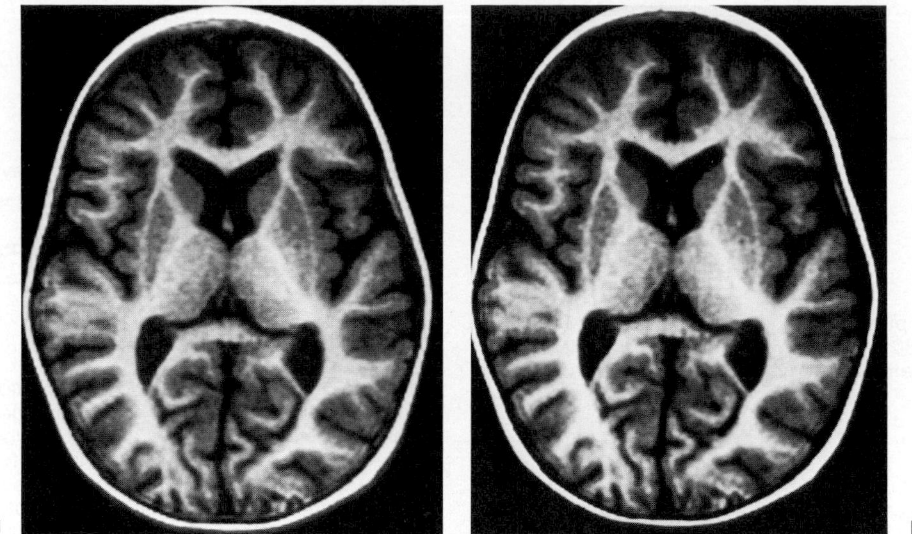

FIG. 16. *Continued.*

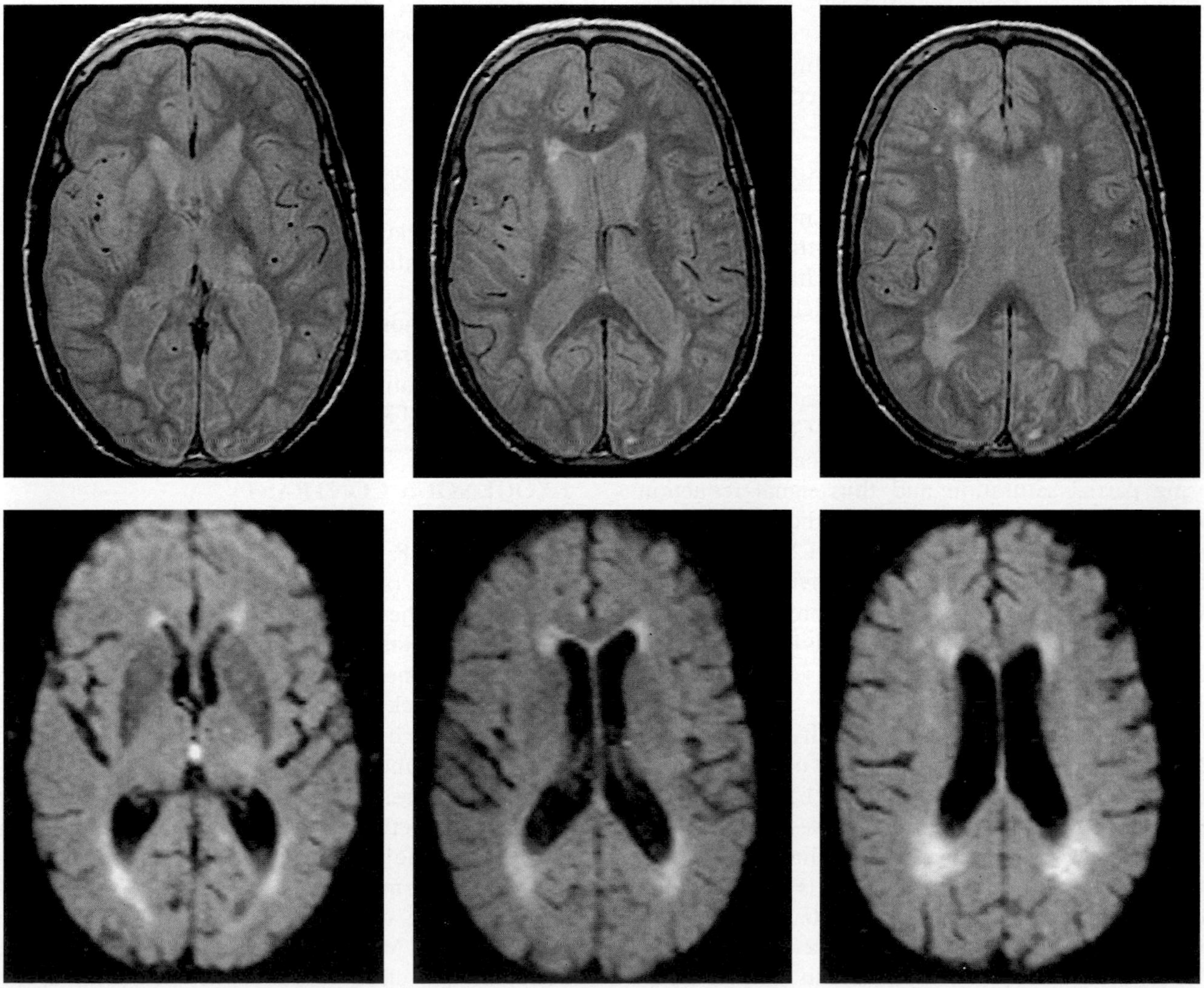

FIG. 17. FLAIR echoplanar imaging versus fast spin echo. Serial axial images show a left thalamic lesion along with multiple subcortical and deep white matter foci of high intensity on proton density—weighted fast spin echo images (**A–C**). Comparison views of EPI FLAIR (**D–F**) obtained in seconds illustrate advantage of this technique for periventricular white matter lesions.

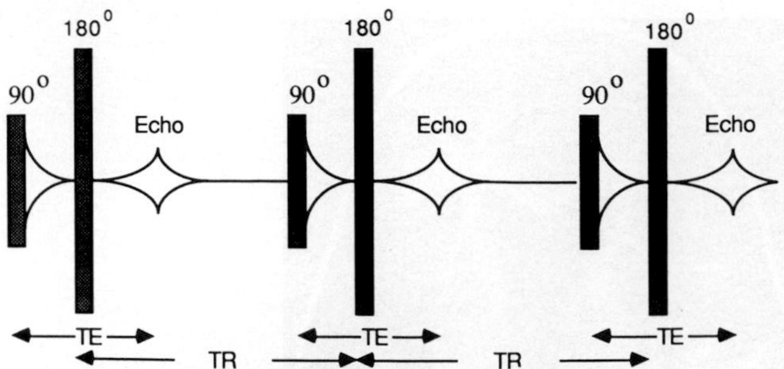

FIG. 18. Spin-echo pulse sequence: TE/2 msec after the 90° excitation pulse, a 180° phase reversal rf pulse is applied which causes the spins to refocus at time TE, creating what is denoted a "spin echo."

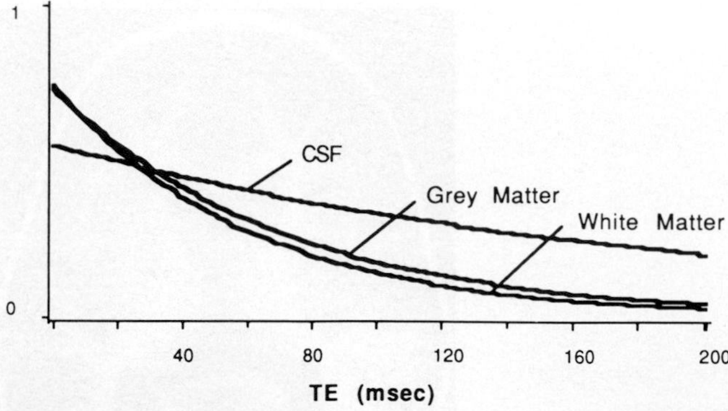

FIG. 19. MR signal calculated as a function of the echo delay TE from Equation 9 for a pulse repetition time TR of 2 sec using the parameters of Table 3 for gray matter, white matter and CSF. At short TE the relative signal intensities follow the order GM > WM > CSF with little contrast among the three tissues. The gray matter signal is highest by virtue of its proton density being higher than that of white matter. The CSF signal is suppressed due to partial saturation since at TR = 2 sec the longitudinal magnetization has only incompletely recovered. We are therefore in a mixed-weighted regime with proton density dominating for gray and white matter and T1 effects determining the relative CSF intensity. At long TR, however, the signal from CSF is predicted to prevail due its much longer T2. The resultant images are said to be T2-weighted.

signal at some delay TE following the 90° rf pulse, a 180° pulse is inserted at time t = TE/2 after the initial 90° excitation pulse. This 180° pulse can be shown to cause refocusing of the spins to form what is termed an "echo" at time t = TE, as shown schematically in the pulse sequence diagram of Fig. 18.

If we assume that 90° pulses are administered every TR seconds the amplitude of the spin echo signal is approximately given by the expression:

$$M_{xy} \approx M^0_{xy}\{1 - \exp(-\mathrm{TR}/\mathrm{T1})\} \exp(-\mathrm{TE}/\mathrm{T2}) \quad [9]$$

where M_{xy} and M^0_{xy} are the transverse magnetization at echo time and immediately following the 90° pulse, respectively, and TE is the echo delay. The longer TE the more the resultant images are T2-weighted. Figure 19 shows a plot of signal intensity as a function of the echo time TE, calculated for TR = 2 sec. We note that initially (short TE) the signal intensities for gray and white matter follow their proton densities whereas CSF is predicted to be hypointense which is a consequence of its long T1 causing partial saturation and thus signal reduction. However, as TE increases CSF is predicted to become dominant because of its much longer T2. The resultant images in this regime are called *T2-weighted.*

We will now evaluate whether these predictions can be reconciled with images in which TR was held constant at TR = 2 sec and TE was varied in 30 msec steps from 30 to 150 msec (Fig. 20).

A crucial feature of the signal intensity plot in Fig. 19 is the reversal of contrast between CSF on the one hand and gray and white matter on the other hand. Further, at the echo time where the two signal curves cross, contrast between the two anatomic entities vanishes. The echo time at which contrast reversal occurs is dictated by the pulse repetition time TR, since the initial hypointensity of CSF is caused by its long T1. Hence, increasing TR will, according to Equation 9, cause an increase in the CSF signal and, consequently, the contrast reversal point will be shifted toward shorter TEs, as shown by the signal intensity curves in Fig. 21, calculated for TR = 4 sec.

The synthesized images in Fig. 22 corroborate the predictions of Fig. 20. Note that in all six images CSF is hyperintense relative to gray and white matter. At TR = 4 sec T1 relaxation is sufficient for the protons in CSF to relax nearly completely during the TR interval thus making it the most intense structure (except at very short TE). From these experiments we see that in spin-echo imaging the relative contrast is a sensitive function of the choice of both TR and TE.

EXOGENOUS CONTRAST

As in CT, MR contrast may be enhanced through the administration of exogenous materials known as contrast agents. These materials provide MR contrast in a way fundamentally different from radiographic contrast media, acting indirectly by altering the relaxation properties of the nuclei under observation. Electron spins behave much like nuclear spins, acting as magnetic dipoles modulated by molecular motion and thus inducing relaxation (cf. Figs. 6 and 7). However, the magnetic moment of the electron is nearly three orders of magnitude greater than the proton magnetic moment. Hence the effect is greatly magnified relative to the one exerted by protons. Hence, unlike iodinated contrast agents used in x-ray imaging, MR contrast agents themselves are not detected; their effect is indirect (27). In summary, MR contrast agents contain paramagnetic ions that produce a shortening of observed T1 in water protons. The most common of these is the gadolinium ion (Gd^{3+}), a rare

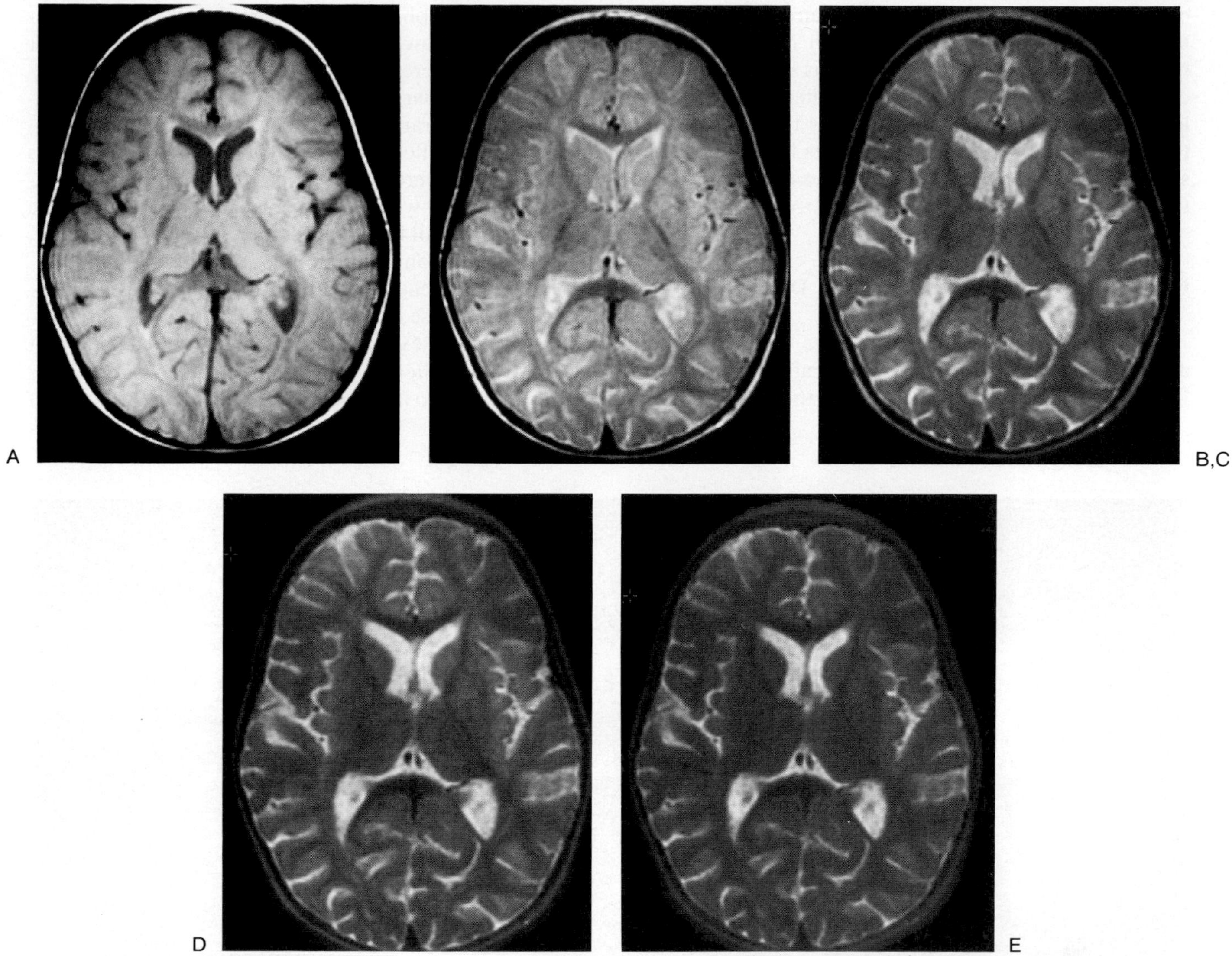

FIG. 20. Normal brain spin-echo images corresponding to TR = 2 sec with TE values of 30 msec (**A**), 60 msec (**B**), 90 msec (**C**), 120 msec (**D**), and 150 msec (**E**). The images were obtained by means of image synthesis as previously described. Note at TE = 30 msec gray–white matter contrast nearly vanishes while CSF is hypointense as predicted in Fig. 19. At TE = 60 msec, however, CSF begins to surpass the parenchymal signal to become the dominant structure as TE is further increased. Images in this regime are denoted T2-weighted since relative signal intensities now follow the order of T2 (CSF > GM > WM).

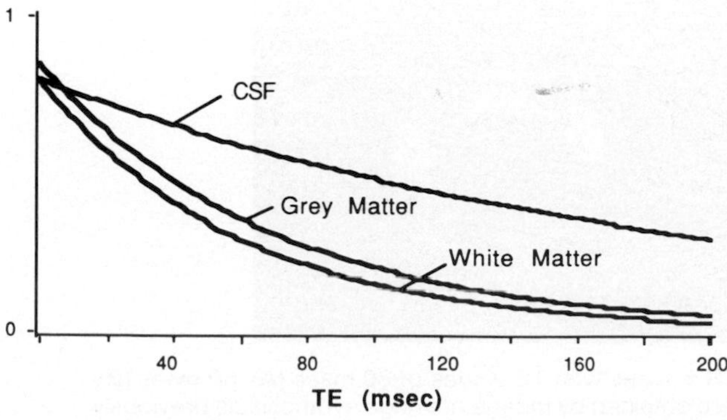

FIG. 21. Brain signal versus echo time TE, calculated for a pulse repetition time TR = 4 sec. Note that the longer TR causes an increase in the CSF signal intensity and hence a shift in the contrast reversal point between CSF on the one hand and gray and white matter, on the other hand. Hence, at short TE the images are expected to be proton-density-weighted with the signal intensity following the order CSF > GM > WM.

earth element containing seven unpaired electrons. In the presence of paramagnetic ions, T1 relaxation is enhanced and dominated by interactions between the nuclei and the unpaired electrons. The effect of this modulation in observed relaxation times is to make regions that are affected by the contrast agents hyperintense on short T1-weighted scans. The principles of action of contrast agents are discussed in Chapter 5.

CONTRAST FROM FLOW AND DIFFUSION

In addition to the relaxation times MR contrast is affected by blood and CSF flow, typically caused by inflow/outflow effects occurring during the spatial encoding process and phase shifts imparted by the imaging gradients. Blood flow imaging is treated in detail in Chapter 4. Whereas coherent flow in vessels is confined to the signal in the vascular structures themselves, diffusion of tissue water, i.e., random, incoherent motion on the molecular scale, affects the entire parenchyma and thus represents a different MR global tissue contrast mechanism. Diffusion-weighted imaging has been shown to be potentially useful for the assessment of cellular integrity, notably in the context of stroke (28,29).

Figure 23A schematically illustrates the effect of motion on the phase of spins undergoing random displacements between excitation and detection. The simplest method for achieving diffusion weighted contrast employs a spin-echo imaging technique with the addition of

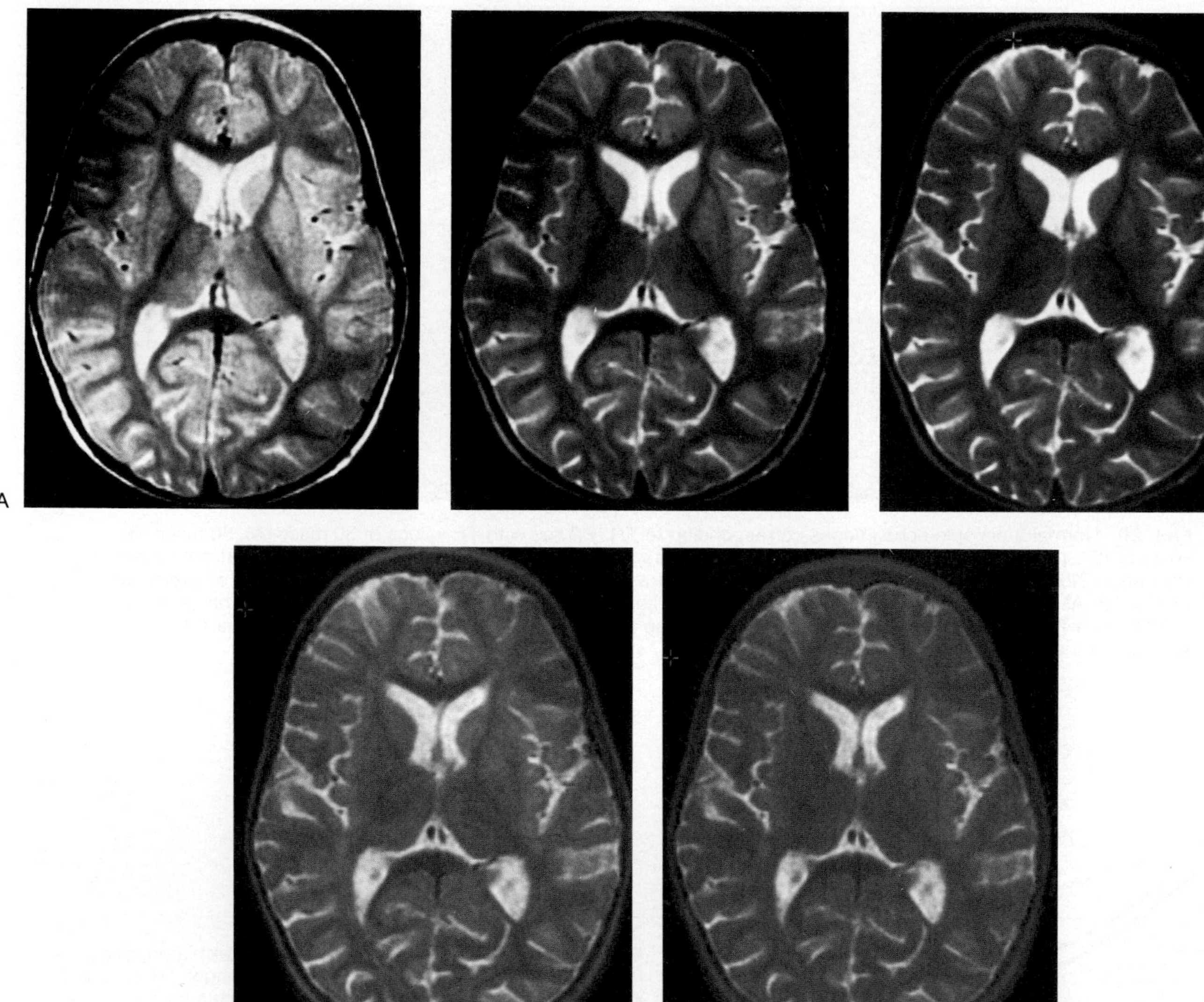

FIG. 22. Normal brain spin-echo images corresponding to TR = 4 sec with TE values of 30 msec (**A**), 60 msec (**B**), 90 msec (**C**), 120 msec (**D**), and 150 msec (**E**). The images were obtained by means of image synthesis as previously described. Note that even at the shortest TE of 30 msec CSF is the most intense structure, followed by gray and white matter. As TE is increased the images become gradually more T2-weighted.

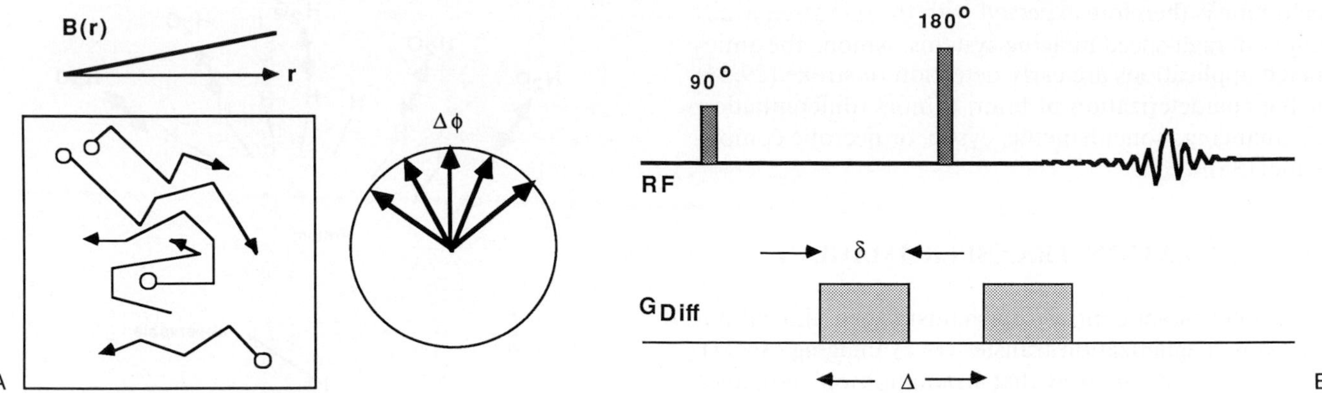

FIG. 23. A: Spins undergoing random displacements in a gradient field (*left*), accumulate random phase (*right*), thus causing an attenuation of the signal. It is obvious that faster molecular motion, such as occurs in fluids, will produce greater signal damping. **B:** The simplest pulse sequence for diffusion weighting consists of two gradient pulses of equal area, symmetric about the 180° phase reversal rf pulse. The extent of diffusion attenuation increases with increasing amplitude of the gradient, duration (δ) and spacing (Δ).

strong field balanced gradient pulses which have the effect of providing sensitivity to motion, effectively attenuating the signal amplitude by virtue of phase scrambling of the diffusing spins (30). Since the gradients are balanced, they do not spatially encode stationary protons.

For stationary spins the phase accumulated during the first gradient pulse will be exactly compensated by the second gradient. However, if the spins undergo motion, a residual phase shift remains. Further, the orientation of the field gradients determines the direction in which diffusion is measured. A most interesting finding is the anisotropy of diffusion in white matter, where it has been shown that diffusion is faster when the myelin fibers are oriented parallel to the gradient field (31–33) (Fig. 24).

Since diffusion-weighted imaging is sensitive to motion (the balanced gradients in Fig. 23B are sensitizing motion other than diffusion as well), diffusion imaging requires high-speed imaging techniques such as echoplanar imaging. More widespread clinical use of the

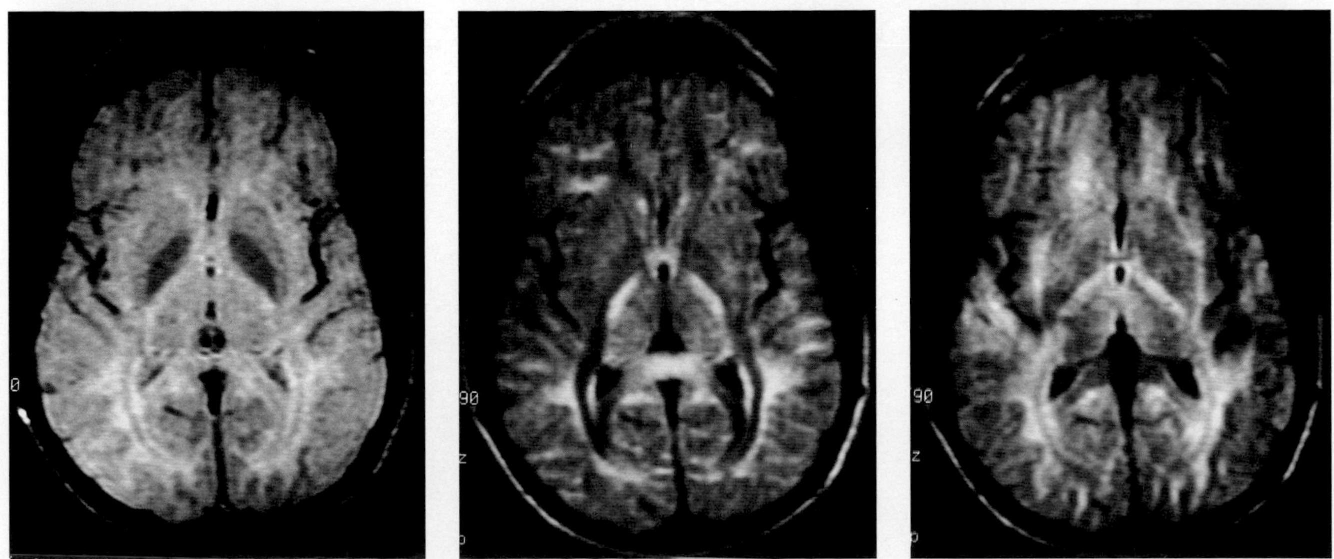

FIG. 24. Effect of anisotropic diffusion on white matter signal. The signal is attenuated whenever the white matter tracts run parallel to the diffusion-sensitizing gradients: no diffusion weighting (**A**), diffusion gradients applied in anteroposterior (**B**), and left-right (**C**) directions. Note, for example, the reduction of the signal from the corpus callosum and anterior commissure in C but not in B, owing to the transverse orientation of their fibers. Similarly, the external capsules are low intensity when the diffusion sensitivity is in the anteroposterior direction B, but high intensity in C. (Courtesy of D. Alsop, Philadelphia, PA.)

technique is therefore expected with the increased availability of high-speed imaging systems. Among the anticipated applications are early detection of stroke (29,34) or the characterization of brain tumors (differentiation of enhancing, nonenhancing, cystic, or necrotic components) (35).

MAGNETIZATION TRANSFER IMAGING

Another novel contrast mechanism with clinical potential is magnetization transfer (MT) imaging (36,37). Wolff et al. (36) showed that irradiation off resonance from the tissue water protons causes a signal reduction. They postulated the effect to arise from cross relaxation, i.e., a dipolar interaction with protons bound to macromolecules (e.g., proteins). The saturation of these protons is carried over to the observable protons via chemical exchange and other processes such as spin diffusion (Fig. 25). Therefore, in the presence of off-resonance saturation, tissue signal intensities are reduced. The extent of attenuation, however, is tissue-specific and is typically expressed in terms of the magnetization transfer ratio $r = (1 - I_S/I_0)$, where I_S and I_0 represent the signal measured with and without off-resonance irradiation. Since the efficiency of cross relaxation increases with increasing correlation time of the cross-relaxing species (de-

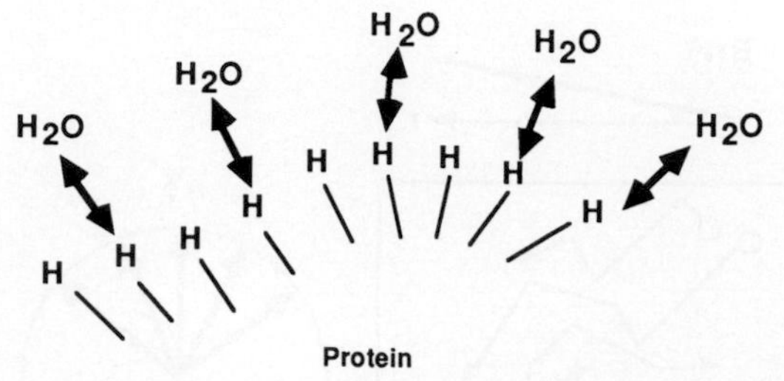

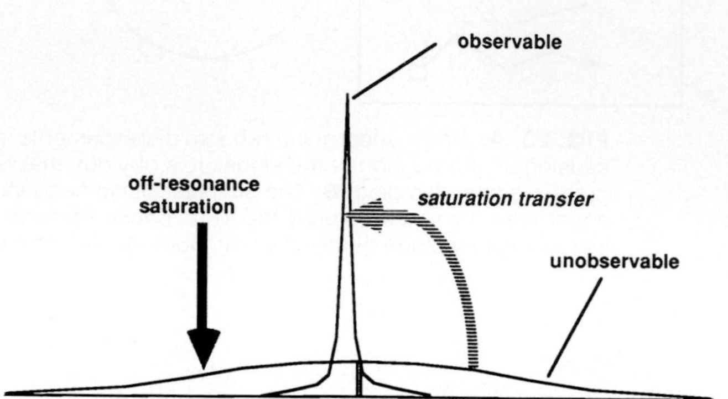

FIG. 25. Principle of magnetization transfer. **A:** Cross relaxation between (observable) water protons and nonobservable macromolecular protons. **B:** Off-resonance irradiation causes saturation of the macromolecule-bound protons. The saturation is transferred via chemical exchange or other processes to the observable protons which in turn leads to a diminution in the proton signal.

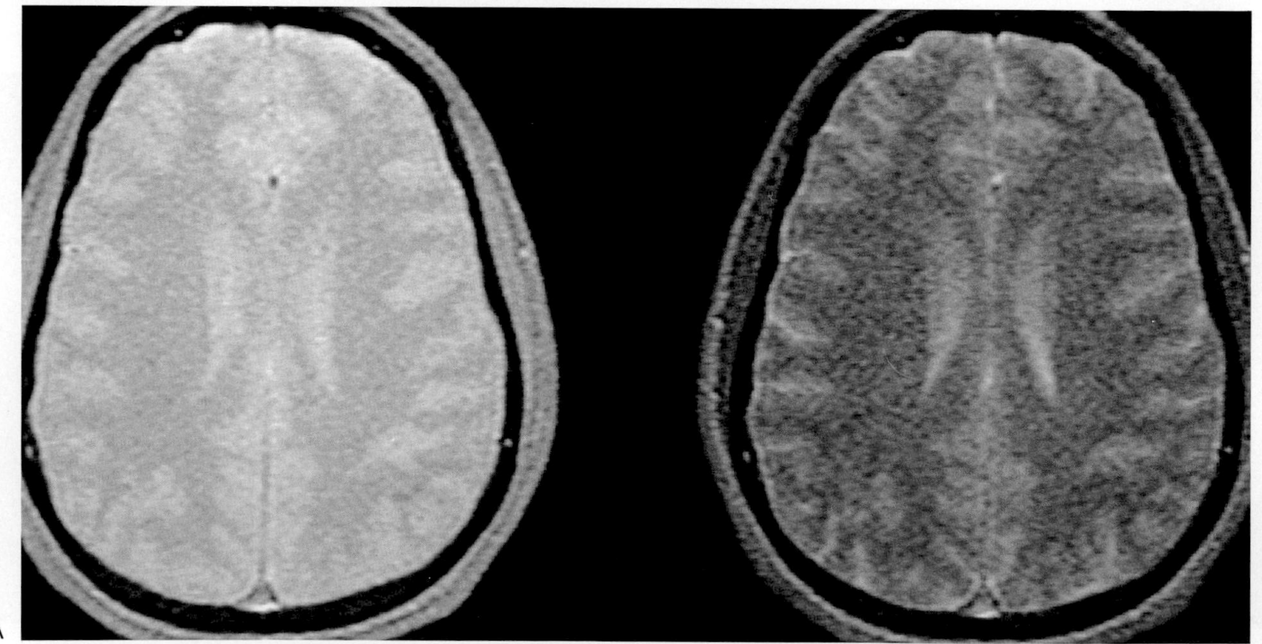

FIG. 26. Effect of off-resonance saturation on parenchymal contrast in proton-density-weighted images (TR = .100 ms, TE = 5 ms, flip angle = 7°): without **(A)** and with MT saturation **(B)**. Both images are displayed with the same window width. Note the increase in gray–white matter contrast in B, due to the greater attenuation of white matter signal intensity.

creased rate for reorientational motion), the MT ratio parallels this behavior. Dousset et al. (38) reported for normal white and gray matter r = 41.8 ± 1.3% and 38.9 ± 1.7%, as opposed to 26 ± 6% in MS lesions. The MT attenuation of parenchymal signal has been exploited in various ways, for example as a means to enhance contrast in time-of-flight angiography (see Chapter 31) (39), or for increasing the effectiveness of contrast agents (40,41). It remains to be seen whether MT provides added imaging specificity to conventional pulse sequences, or if its major role in the clinical setting will be limited to that which is based on its effectiveness as a method of background supression, as has been shown in MR angiography and in gadolinium-enhanced imaging.

In practice, MT images are obtained by applying rf excitation either through continuous-wave (36) or pulsed (38) irradiation off-resonance. Figure 26 shows a comparison of brain images of the normal human brain without and with off-resonance irradiation, obtained with the pulsed MT technique. The interpretation of contrast in MT images is complicated in that intensity variations may represent differences in exchange rates as well as relaxation times and proton densities. The development of models for a detailed quantitative understanding of the MT effect in tissues is a field of intense current research.

SUMMARY AND CONCLUSIONS

We have seen that contrast in MR is of a multiparametric nature with T1, T2, and spin density as the primary intrinsic *parameters* and TR, TE, and TI, which characterize the pulse timing relationships, as the *extrinsic parameters*. Intrinsic implies these quantities to be related to tissue chemistry while extrinsic refers to the user-selectable nature of these parameters. It has further been shown that judicious choice of the pulse sequence and timing parameters permits "weighting" of contrast toward one or the other of the intrinsic parameters. This leads to three general classes of images in which the relative signal intensities follow an established order related to a single intrinsic parameter. As a rule a data acquisition protocol should therefore be designed in such a manner that at least one set each of T1, proton density, and T2-weighted images is acquired to assure safe and reliable detection of an abnormality. Since proton density and T2-weighted images can be obtained from the same scan by producing more than one echo it usually suffices to acquire two series of images: a T1-weighted set and a proton density/T2-weighted set. Finally, contrast may be augmented through injection of paramagnetic contrast agents. New techniques such as diffusion weighting and magnetization transfer imaging increase the number of contrast parameters and provide the radiologist with an expanded set of tools.

REFERENCES

1. Edelstein WA, Bottomley PA, Hart HR, Smith LS. Signal, noise, and contrast in nuclear magnetic resonance (NMR) imaging. *J Comput Assist Tomogr* 1983;7:391–401.
2. Rose AA. Vision: *Human and Electronic*. New York: Plenum; 1973.
3. Kanal E, Wehrli FW. Signal-to-Noise Ratio, Resolution and Contrast. In: Wehrli FW, Shaw D, Kneeland JB, eds. *Biomedical Magnetic Resonance Imaging: Principles, Methodology and Applications*. New York: VCH Publishers; 1988.
4. Fullerton GD, Cameron IL. Relaxation of biological tissues. In: Wehrli FW, Shaw D, Kneeland JB, eds. *Biomedical Magnetic Resonance Imaging: Principles, Methodology and Applications*. New York: VCH Publishers; 1988.
5. Bottomley PA, Foster TH, Argersinger RE, Pfeifer LM. A review of normal tissue hydrogen NMR relaxation times and relaxation mechanisms from 1–1000 MHz. Dependence on tissue type, NMR frequency, temperature, excision and age. *Med Phys* 1984;11:425–448.
6. Fullerton GD, Potter JL, Dornbluth NC. NMR relaxation of protons in tissues and other macromolecular water solutions. *Magn Reson Imaging* 1982;1:209–228.
7. Bottomley PA, Hart HR Jr., Edelstein WA, Schenck JF, Smith LS, Leue WM, Mueller OM, Redington RW. Anatomy and metabolism of the normal human brain studied by magnetic resonance at 1.5 Tesla. *Radiology* 1984;150:441–446.
8. Thulborn KR, Brady TJ. Iron in magnetic resonance imaging of cerebral hemorrhage. *Magn Reson Q* 1989;5:23–38.
9. Gomori JM, Grossman RI, Goldberg HI, Zimmerman RA, Bilaniuk LT. Intracranial hematomas: imaging by high-field MR. *Radiology* 1985;157:87–93.
10. Bydder GM, Steiner RE, Young IR, AS Hall, Thomas DJ, Marshall J, Pallis CA, Legg NJ. Clinical NMR imaging of the brain: 140 cases. *AJR* 1982;139:215–236.
11. Crooks LE, Mills CM, Davis PL, Brant-Zawadski M, Hoenninger J. Visualization of cerebral and vascular abnormalities by NMR imaging. The effects of imaging parameters on contrast. *Radiology* 1982;144:843–852.
12. Wehrli FW, MacFall JR, Glover GH, Grigsby GN, Haughton V, Johanson J. The dependence of nuclear magnetic resonance (NMR) image contrast on intrinsic and pulse sequence timing parameters. *Magn Reson Imaging* 1984;2:3–16.
13. Hendrick RE, Nelson TR, Hendee WR. Optimizing tissue differentiation in magnetic resonance imaging. *Magn Reson Imaging* 1984;2:193–204.
14. Wehrli FW, MacFall JR, Shutts D, Breger R, Herfkens RJ. Mechanisms of Contrast in NMR Imaging. *J Comput Assist Tomogr* 1984;8:369–380.
15. Young IR. Considerations affecting signal and contrast in NMR imaging. *Br Med Bull* 1984;40:139–147.
16. Riederer SJ, Suddarth SA, Bobman SA, Lee JN, Wang HZ, MacFall JR. Automated MR image synthesis: Feasibility studies. *Radiology* 1984;153:203–206.
17. Bobman SA, Riederer SJ, Lee JN, Suddarth SA, Wang HZ, Drayer BP. Cerebral magnetic resonance image synthesis. *AJNR* 1985;6:265–269.
18. Bydder GM, Steiner RE, Blumgart LH, Khenia S, Young IR. MR imaging of the liver using short-TI inversion recovery sequences. *J Comput Assist Tomogr* 1985;9:1084–1089.
19. Young IR, Bailes DR, Bydder GM. Apparent changes of appearance of inversion-recovery images. *Magn Reson Imaging* 1985;2:81–85.
20. Atlas SW, Grossman RI, Hackney DB, et al. STIR MR imaging of the orbit. *AJNR* 1988;9:969(abst).
21. Hajnal JV, Bryant DJ, Kasuboski L, Pattany PM, De Coene B, Lewis PD, Pennock JM, Oatridge A, Young IR, Bydder GM. Use of fluid attenuated inversion recovery (FLAIR) pulse sequences in MRI of the brain. *J Comput Assist Tomogr* 1992;16:841–844.
22. White SJ, Hajnal JV, Young IR, Bydder GM. Use of fluid-

attenuated inversion-recovery pulse sequences for imaging the spinal cord. *Magn Reson Med* 1992;28(1):153–162.
23. Haase A. Snapshot FLASH MRI. Applications to T1, T2 and chemical shift imaging. *Magn Reson Med* 1990;13:77–89.
24. Mugler III JP, Brookeman JR. Three-dimensional magnetization-prepared rapid gradient-echo imaging (3D MP RAGE). *Magn Reson Med* 190;15:152–157.
25. Holsinger-Bampton A, Riederer SJ, Campeau MG, Ehman RL, Johnson CD. T1-weighted snapshot gradient-echo MR imaging of the abdomen. *Radiology* 1991;181:25–32.
26. Farrar TC, Becker ED. *Pulse and Fourier Transform Nuclear Magnetic Resonance*. New York: Academic; 1971.
27. Koutcher JA, Burt C, Lauffer RB, Brady TJ. Contrast agents and spectroscopic probes in NMR. *J Nucl Med* 1984;25:506–513.
28. Moseley ME, Kucharczyk J, Mintorovitch J, et al. Diffusion-weighted MR imaging of acute stroke: correlation with T2-weighted and magnetic susceptibility-enhanced MR imaging in cats. *AJNR* 1990;11:423–429.
29. Maeda M, Itoh S, Ide H, Matsuda T, Kobayashi H, Kubota T, Ishii Y. Acute stroke in cats: comparison of dynamic susceptibility-contrast MR imaging with T2 and diffusion-weighted imaging. *Radiology* 1993;189:227–232.
30. Le Bihan D. Molecular diffusion in nuclear magnetic resonance imaging. *Magn Reson Q* 1991;7:1–30.

Magnetic Resonance Imaging of the Brain and Spine, Second Edition, edited by Scott W. Atlas. Lippincott-Raven Publishers, Philadelphia © 1996.

3

Principles of Image Formation

Peter M. Joseph

It is readily apparent that the generation of image contrast in magnetic resonance (MR) is multifactorial and quite complex, since it depends on many operator-selected scanner inputs (e.g., pulse sequence parameters), as well as on the inherent relaxation behavior of the tissues being examined. Although one can attempt to understand images on the basis of the difference in magnetic behavior between normal tissue and areas of pathology, it is also useful to have a basic familiarity with the physics of image formation. In this chapter, the most fundamental aspects of image formation will be reviewed: the generation of the MR signal and its detection and processing to form the final image.

The source of the NMR signal is the rotation of the nuclear magnetization vector, **M**, in each voxel. As illustrated in Fig. 1, the **M** vector rotates around the magnetic field vector, $\mathbf{B}_0$, which is normally assumed to be oriented along the z axis. The direction of rotation is clockwise (from y toward x) as viewed from above, and the frequency of rotation is the Larmor frequency, f_0, given by the Larmor equation:

$$f_0 = (\gamma/2\pi)\mathrm{B}_0, \qquad [1]$$

where γ is the gyromagnetic ratio of the proton (1). The important point here is that the frequency is proportional to the field strength B_0. The unit of frequency is the Hertz, which means one cycle per second.

The actual signal appears in the form of a voltage which is induced in a specially tuned coil of wire, known as the "rf coil" (2–4). (Here "rf" stands for "radiofrequency"). The induced signal voltage will vary in a sinusoidal fashion as the **M** vector rotates, so the frequency of oscillation of the voltage will obviously be the same as the frequency of rotation of the **M** vector. Figure 2 illustrates how the rotation of the **M** vector is related to the signal voltage waveform. The angle which the vector makes with the x' axis is called the *phase* of the vector. The phase of the detected signal will depend on the angular position of the receiving coil, so that if two coils are placed at, say, 90° apart, the corresponding signal voltages will show a phase shift. This is also illustrated in Fig. 2.

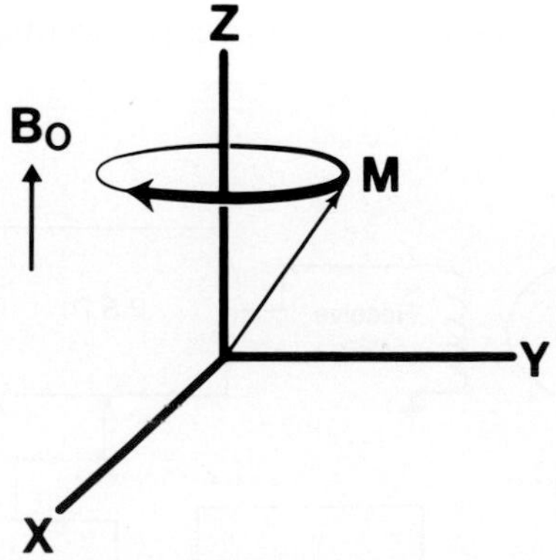

FIG. 1. The **M** vector rotates at the Larmor frequency around the $\mathbf{B}_0$ vector in the laboratory frame of reference.

P. M. Joseph, Ph.D.: Department of Radiology, Hospital of the University of Pennsylvania, Philadelphia, PA 19104.

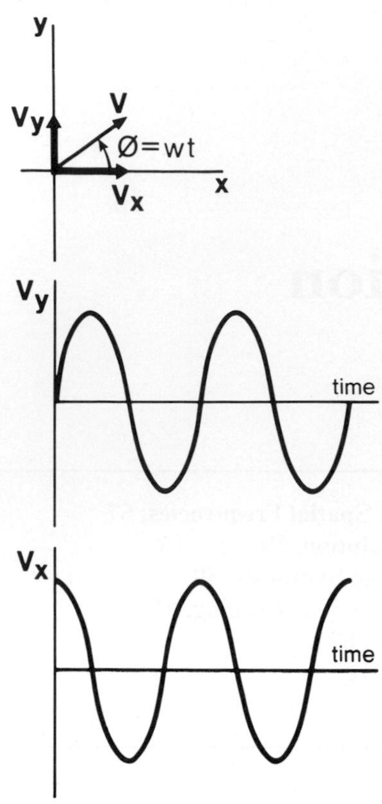

FIG. 2. In the rotating frame of reference, the **M** vector rotates at the offset frequency. The two components of voltage from the PSD, labeled V_x and V_y also oscillate at the offset frequency. Note the 90° phase shift between the V_x and V_y sine waves.

The concept of phase shift is very important in understanding many concepts in MRI and MRS. Figure 2 indicates that although the phase shift is fundamentally a shift in *time* of a sinusoidal wave, it can be thought of as a rotation in *angle* of the corresponding rotating vector. This association of phase shift with angle is so pervasive that scientists normally speak of phase shift in degrees, rather than in units of time.

THE ROTATING FRAME

In the above situation, the **M** vector is rotating very rapidly, typically millions of cycles per second, or megahertz (MHz). However, NMR most often requires that we consider very small *changes* in frequency, on the order of a few hundred or thousand cycles per second. In other words, we shall be primarily concerned with the extent to which the signal frequency *differs* from the Larmor frequency. For this purpose, it is very convenient to view the motion of the **M** vector in the *rotating frame*, which means a set of coordinate axes, x' and y', which are themselves rotating around the z axis at the Larmor frequency. In such a rotating frame, the vector **M** will appear to be stationary if it is rotating at the Larmor frequency. A good analogy to this situation is a rotating amusement park carousel which contains wooden horses on which people can ride. From the point of view of someone not on the carousel, the horses are obviously rotating around on a circular path. However, from the point of view of someone sitting on a horse, the other horses as well as himself do not appear to be rotating at all; rather, the rest of the world seems to be rotating in the opposite direction.

The rotating frame is more than a theoretical notion, however, because it relates closely to the way in which NMR signals are actually detected and processed electronically. The key component is called a phase-sensitive detector, or PSD. The purpose of the PSD is to accept the generated signal from the rf coil and produce an output which reflects the *difference* between the frequency of the received signal and that of a device called the master oscillator. As illustrated in Fig. 3, the master oscillator is also the device that generates the rf pulses which excited the spin vectors prior to reception of the signal. The function of the PSD is to produce two sine wave outputs, each of which has a frequency equal to the difference between the frequencies of the received signal and the master oscillator.

If the Larmor frequency is exactly equal to that of the master oscillator, then the PSD will produce an output of zero frequency, i.e., a static, unchanging voltage. This is analogous to the static nature of the **M** vector in the rotating frame. Furthermore, the PSD produces two outputs, and these correspond to the x' and y' components of the **M** vector in the rotating frame. Hence, from the ratio of the two PSD outputs one can easily infer the

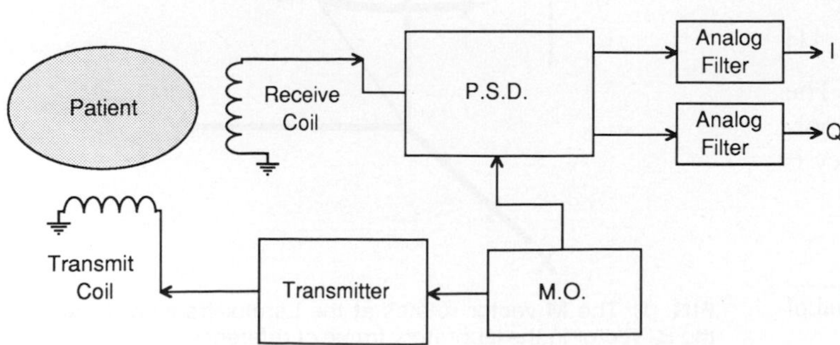

FIG. 3. Block diagram of the electronic components of an MRI system, showing how the *I* and *Q* received signal pair is obtained from the PSD. The master oscillator feeds both the transmitter coil and the receiver PSD. The *I* and *Q* signals are filtered, digitized, and fed to the system computer for further analysis. Not shown is the computer to control the pulses and the gradient coils and circuitry.

phase angle of the **M** vector in the rotating frame. The relevant equation is

$$\text{tangent (phase angle)} = V'_y/V'_x, \quad [2]$$

where V'_x and V'_y are the two voltage outputs of the PSD. Since these voltages can be digitized and measured by the system computer, the software can work with both the strength and the phase of the received signal. This ability is essential for image reconstruction.

There is no universally accepted notation for the two PSD signal components. In the engineering literature, they are called "*I*" and "*Q*," which stand for "in phase" and "quadrature." Physicists thinking of the **M** vector are likely to call them the "*x*" and "*y*" components, neglecting to use primes after the *x* and *y* because the reference to the rotating frame is understood. Mathematicians would call them the "real" and "imaginary" voltages because the two voltages can be considered to be a complex number, and complex arithmetic is essential in a detailed understanding of the Fourier transforms used in the image reconstruction process. To generate the two components, *I* and *Q*, it is necessary that the receiver be given information on the phase of the transmitter's oscillation. That is, the PSD detects the phase of the received signal with respect to the wave of the master oscillator which is also being fed into the receiver. This is illustrated in Fig. 3.

Since we shall consider the rotating frame frequency and the master oscillator radiofrequency to be the same, we can refer to either as the "rf" frequency.

FREQUENCY OFFSETS

It is impossible to understand NMR phenomena by considering only the Larmor frequency. This is because in any real system (and certainly in the human body) the magnetic field is never homogeneous but will exhibit a certain spread of values. Hence there will always be a corresponding spread of resonant frequencies, some of which are under our control and some of which are not. So, we must understand the consequences of a Larmor frequency which differs from that of the master oscillator.

If the Larmor frequency differs from the rf, the **M** vector will appear to rotate in the rf *at a frequency equal to the difference of the two frequencies*; this difference is called the *offset frequency*. Hence, the frequency of the received signal (after the PSD) will equal the offset frequency.

Obviously, the Larmor frequency could be either greater or less than the rf so, mathematically speaking, the offset frequency could be either positive or negative. The concept of negative frequency may seem puzzling at first, but it is easily understood in terms of the *direction* of motion of the **M** vector in the rotating frame. A clockwise rotation represents a positive frequency and a counterclockwise rotation represents a negative frequency. It is not possible to distinguish between these two cases if one is shown only one sine wave; only by knowing both the *I* and *Q* channel sine waves can one determine the direction of rotation. This is another illustration of the importance of PSD for NMR imaging. We shall see later that if the PSD is defective, a confusion of the positive and negative frequencies results and leads to a ghost image artifact.

USE OF GRADIENT FIELDS

A key technique in NMR imaging is the use of controlled gradients in the magnetic field (5). With this technique the homogeneity of the static magnetic field is deliberately destroyed in such a way that the *z* component of the B_0 field varies in a linear way with spatial position. This variation can be generated along either of the three directions, *x*, *y*, or *z*. In this case, the *x*, *y*, and *z* coordinates refer to the fixed, "laboratory" frame of reference and not to the rotating frame; i.e., *x*, *y*, and *z* are simply the coordinates of the pixels in the patient's body. The three gradients are called g_x, g_y, and g_z, respectively. The mathematical statement of their effect is:

$$\begin{aligned} B &= B_0 + xg_x \quad \text{for the } x \text{ gradient} \\ B &= B_0 + yg_y \quad \text{for the } y \text{ gradient} \quad [3] \\ B &= B_0 + zg_z \quad \text{for the } z \text{ gradient.} \end{aligned}$$

The meaning of a field gradient is most easily grasped in a graph of B versus either *x*, *y*, or *z*; the value of *g* is reflected in the *slope* of the line. For example, in Fig. 4 we illustrate three different examples of an *x* gradient, namely g_x positive, zero, and negative. The case of $g_x = 0$ has a horizontal line and represents a homogeneous field.

In MRI systems, the three field gradients are created by currents flowing through specially designed "gradient coils," which must not be confused with the rf coils. The strength of each gradient is proportional to the amount

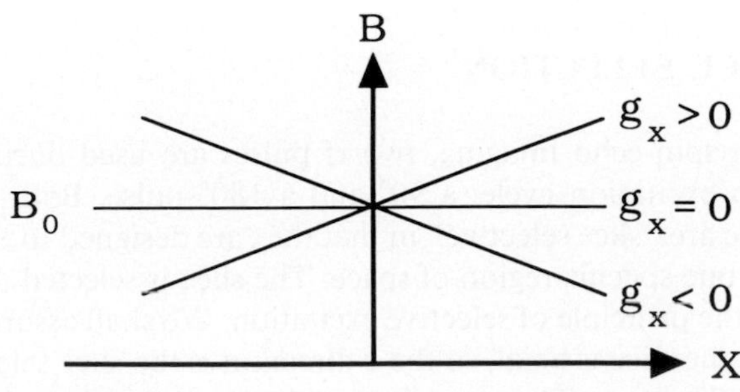

FIG. 4. Graphical illustration of various **x** gradients. The value of the gradient, g_x, is equal to the slope of the line, which can be positive, zero, or negative.

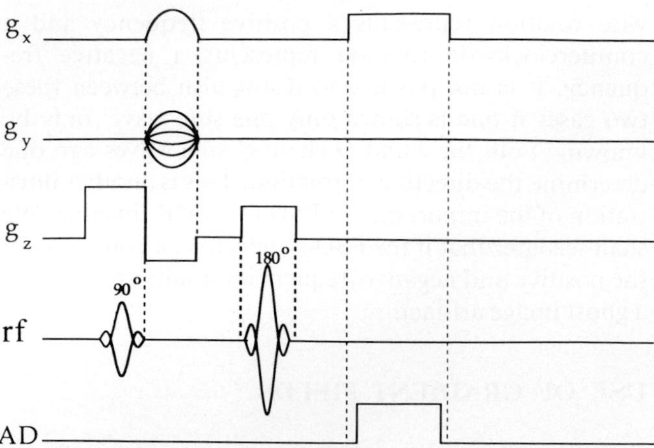

FIG. 5. The basic spin warp pulse sequence. The sequence is drawn assuming an axial scan, with *x* being the FE axis and *y* being the PE axis. In this case the exciting pulse is assumed to provide a flip angle of 90°, and a 180° pulse is used to provide a spin echo. Note that the readout gradient, g_x, is turned on during signal readout. The PE gradient, g_y, is turned on only during the time interval between excitation and readout.

of current flowing through the corresponding coil, which in turn is controlled by the system computer. The computer activates the various gradients in accordance with the requirements of the pulse sequence being used.

THE SPIN WARP PULSE SEQUENCE

To generate an image of a slice in the body requires a fairly complex pulse sequence, by which is meant a temporal sequence of pulses of radio frequency energy, gradient fields, and signal acquisition commands (6,7). Since there are three gradients operative, a graphical representation of the pulse sequence requires five lines. The fifth line, representing data acquisition, is not really a "pulse" but it is necessary to show at what times the signal is being sampled by the computer hardware.

The most commonly used pulse sequence is shown in Fig. 5. It is based on the mathematics of two-dimensional Fourier transformation, and so is often called the "2DFT" method. Another looser term for the technique is the "spin warp" method (8).

SLICE SELECTION

In spin-echo imaging, two rf pulses are used during each excitation cycle: a 90° and a 180° pulse. Both of these are "slice selective" in that they are designed to excite one specific region of space. The slice is selected using the principle of selective excitation. We shall assume that the slice is axial, so the *z* direction is the slice selection direction. The *z* gradient is turned on by the computer's pulse program at the same time as a specially shaped rf pulse. In this situation, as can be appreciated in Fig. 6, only those protons with a certain *z* position will find that their (local) Larmor frequency matches the rf frequency and so will be excited. Protons located at other positions will experience a mismatch between the Larmor and rf frequencies and will remain unexcited. More precisely, the rf pulse is specially shaped so as to contain precisely defined *range* of frequencies, and the width of this range will correspond to the slice *thickness*. Obviously, when one changes the rf frequency one will change the location of the selected slice; thus, by changing the rf frequency one "slides along" the graph of Fig. 6.

The pulse sequence shown in Fig. 5 is particularly useful because it is easily modified to allow imaging of multiple slices. Once the excitation-echo sequence (90°–180° rf pulses) are played out, which takes time TE (echo time), one then needs to wait time TR-TE for the spin vectors in the slice to recover their *z* magnetization. Since TR is usually much longer than TE, this represents a substantial fraction of the imaging time. During this recovery time interval one can apply another similar 90°–180° pulse sequence *to a different slice*. Obviously, for this method to work it is essential that the rf pulses targeted at one slice not interfere with the spins in other slices. For this reason it is essential that both the 90° and 180° pulses in Fig. 5 be *spatially selective*; i.e., both pulses are applied while the *z* gradient is energized. Each slice will have its own characteristic resonant frequency for excitation purposes, based on its position along the *z* axis when the *z* gradient is turned on. This concept is illustrated in Fig. 6 for the case of two noncontiguous slices S1 and S2, each of which has its own characteristic resonant frequency *f*1 and *f*2. Within certain limits, it is possible to image any combination of any number of slices using this technique by programming the computer to excite the volume with the appropriate radiofrequencies. Furthermore, one can easily include multiple echoes for

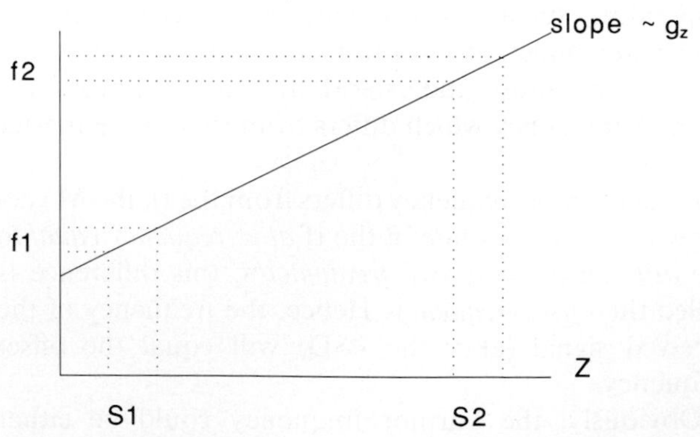

FIG. 6. Graphical representation of the principle of selective excitation. The vertical axis is frequency, which is also proportional to magnetic field. The slope of the line relating frequency to z position is proportional to g_z. With the gradient turned on, the slice S1 corresponds to frequency range *f*1 and slice S2 corresponds to frequency range *f*2.

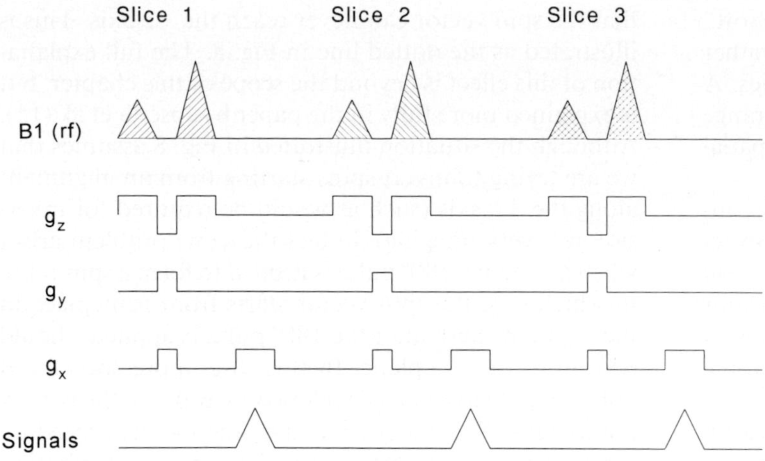

FIG. 7. Pulse sequence diagram for multiplanar spin-echo 2-D imaging. The principle is the same as shown in Fig. 5 except that different radio frequencies are used to excite and refocus the individual slices. In this diagram, the change of frequency from slice 1 to slice 2 and 3 is symbolized by the different hatch patterns under the triangular B1 wave forms. In practice, the wave forms are not triangular but are computed to provide a precisely defined slice thickness. Note that the interval between 90° pulses is this figure is *not* TR.

each slice. The obvious limit to the technique is that there must be enough time between excitations of any one slice (i.e., TR) to allow the n slices to be excited. This leads to the inherent limitation

$$\text{Number of slices} < \text{TR}/(\text{maximum TE}). \qquad [4]$$

The resulting pulse sequence is rather complex, and a block sketch of it is shown in Fig. 7. In that figure, the frequency shift between the different rf pulses is symbolized as different hatch patterns under the triangles symbolizing the 90° and 180° rf pulses. In practice, the shape of these pulses will not be triangular but will be very complex.

This picture of selective excitation, while reasonably accurate, is not entirely correct. The method described works well when the flip angles desired are not too large—up to about 90°. In any case, the flip angle is not truly constant but will vary within the slice, a fact that can upset naive calculations of relaxation times based on an assumed flip angle (9). For larger flip angles, it becomes more and more difficult to maintain a sharply defined slice profile. In particular, devising a selective pulse which achieves 180° of flip uniformly across a slice is very difficult; what tends to happen is that if the flip angle is 180° within the desired slice, then it will not be zero immediately outside the slice. In other words, the rf energy tends to spill out into adjacent slices. The best solution for this problem is to leave a *gap* between slices in the imaging protocol. Considerable effort has been devoted to finding improved pulse shapes which can more effectively provide 180° within the slice with minimal energy outside the slice (10–14).

In spectroscopy, a term often used for selective pulses is "soft," as distinguished from "hard." The distinction is based on the relative strengths and widths of the pulses used; remember that the flip angle is determined, at least on resonance, by the *product* of the B1 strength and the pulse duration ("width" on the time axis). A "hard" pulses is one which is very short in time but very strong, a "soft" pulse is the reverse. Hard pulses will tend to flip all spins by the desired flip angle more or less independent of the frequency offset. Soft pulses, on the other hand, will flip some spins more than others depending on the difference between the resonance frequency of the spins and the radiofrequency of the pulse. For slice selec-

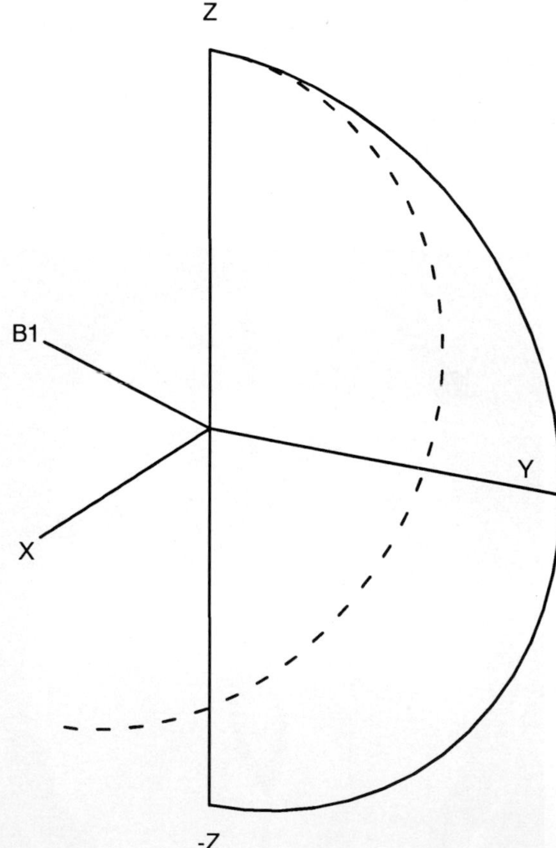

FIG. 8. Demonstration of the difficulty of achieving a 180° flip angle in the presence of magnetic field and/or frequency errors. The solid arc represents the path of the **M** vector as it rotates under the influence of a "good" B1 vector assumed to lie exactly along the x' axis in the rotating frame of reference. The dotted line represents the path of the **M** vector under the influence of a "bad" B1 rf vector which has a z component. Note that in the latter case the **M** vector can never reach the $-z$ axis.

tive purposes, all useful pulses must be considered "soft" because we only want them to be effective over a rather narrow, and well defined, range of spin frequencies. A hard pulse would tend to excite spins over a wide range of spatial positions and would produce poor spatial selectivity.

The nature of this problem can be understood by considering those protons which are *not* located at the exact center of the slice; they are, by virtue of their position and the z gradient, off resonance. Protons whose Larmor frequencies are removed from the central frequency of the slice respond in a way which is nonlinear, meaning that the flip angle achieved is not exactly proportional to the strength and time of the exciting rf pulse. The reason for this can be understood from the principle that a proton which is off resonance experiences a small magnetic field along the z direction in the rotating frame. Remember that normally, in the rotating frame on resonance, the z component of B is zero. The problem is illustrated in Fig. 8, which shows the behavior of a nominal 180° pulse applied under two conditions: on resonance and off resonance. In the on resonance case, the B1 rf field lies exactly along the x axis, so that a spin vector which is initially along the $+z$ axis will be rotated to exactly the $-z$ direction. This is shown as the solid line in Fig. 8. However, when the rf B1 field has a z component, the *spin vector will rotate around the direction of the B1 field*; the fact that the B1 vector lies out of the x-y plane implies that the spin vector can never reach the $-z$ axis. This is illustrated as the dotted line in Fig. 8. The full explanation of this effect is beyond the scope of this chapter, but is explained more fully in the paper by Joseph et al. (15). Although the situation illustrated in Fig. 8 assumes that we are trying to invert spins starting from an alignment along the $+z$ axis (such as would be required for inversion recovery imaging), in fact the same problem arises when a selective 180° pulse is needed to form a spin echo, in which case the spin vector starts from someplace in the x-y plane and, after the 180° pulse is applied, should end up in the x-y plane. In this case, more specialized pulse shapes have been developed to improve the performance (16–18). In particular, a mathematical procedure for devising "good" 180° pulses for spin-echo formation has been published by Shinnar et al. (19) and by Leroux (20). Figure 9 shows the improvement in head images using the latter type of specialized 180° rf pulses. These images of the same slice were taken with TR = 2600, TE = 30 msec, so the desired contrast should be more or less "proton density" weighted. However, in this multiplanar image set 26 slices were obtained simultaneously, so that the actual spacing between 90° excitations (irrespective of slice position) was only 100 ms. The slice thickness was 5 mm with 1-mm gaps. With perfect selective pulses, the presence of rf energy in adjacent slices should be irrelevant. However, with imperfect pulses some rf energy spills over from one slice to the

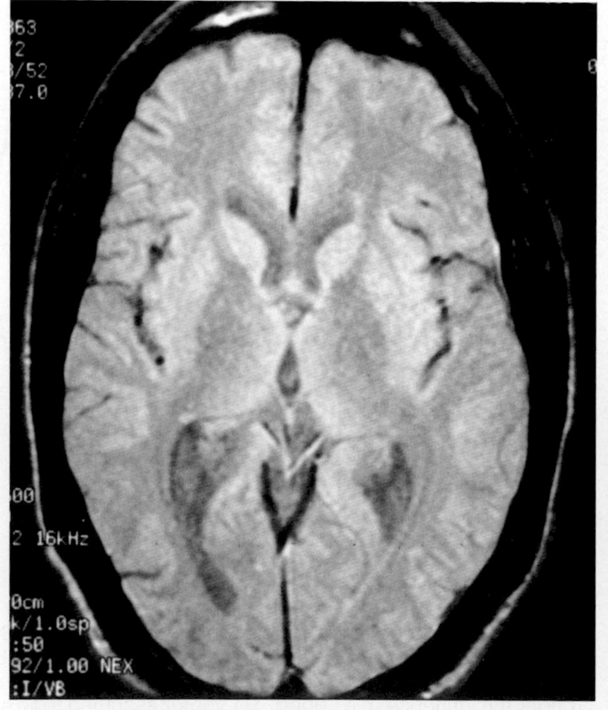

A

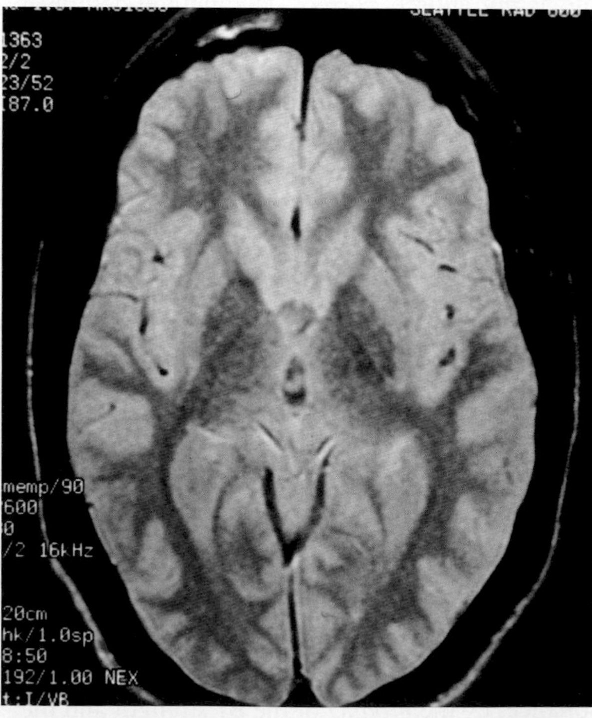

B

FIG. 9. Clinical demonstration of the value of using "good" 180° selective pulses in multiplanar spin-echo imaging. **A** was made using a "sinc" pulse which is not optimized for good slice selectivity, whereas **B** uses a pulse designed using the Shinnar-LeRoux method. Note the loss of proper gray-white contrast in A. (Images courtesy of General Electric Medical Systems, Inc.)

adjacent slices, which implies that all slices do not receive the desired TR interval between excitations. The result is a tendency to saturate the spins as if the TR were only 100 msec, so that true recovery of M_z during the TR time interval does not occur. This produces some unwanted T1 weighting of the slice in T2-weighted imaging. This effect can be seen by comparing images A and B in Fig. 9. Even with such highly optimized pulse shapes, however, it is still recommended that some gap be left between adjacent slices when acquired in the multislice mode. This effect of multislice interference from nonideal spin-echo pulses for brain imaging has been discussed in detail by Kucharczyk et al. (21).

FREQUENCY ENCODING AND RECEIVER BANDWIDTH

Ultimately, in any imaging technique it is necessary to devise some means for locating the position in space of each voxel in the imaged body. In MRI, this is done with two different techniques: frequency encoding and phase encoding. Usually, one of the image directions is frequency encoded (FE) while the other is phase encoded (PE). For the sake of discussion, we shall assume that the *x* direction is frequency encoded and the *y* direction phase encoded, although this assignment is by no means unique and many MRI machines give the user the option to alter the assignment at will.

Frequency encoding is based on the fact that the frequency of the signal, when received in the presence of a field gradient, will be a simple function of the *x* position. For example, Fig. 10A shows schematically two phantoms (P1 and P2) of water placed in the machine with the *x*-gradient turned on. In this situation the water molecules in the right-hand bottle will experience a higher Larmor frequency than will those in the left hand bottle. It must be emphasized that this is true because we are assuming that the *x* gradient is turned on *during reception of the signal*. This time interval of signal acquisition is called the "readout" period, and the corresponding FE *x* gradient is often called the "readout gradient."

Image reconstruction is based on the so-called Fourier transform (FT). This is a mathematical procedure which accepts as input the data from the received signal and produces as its output a graph or digital representation

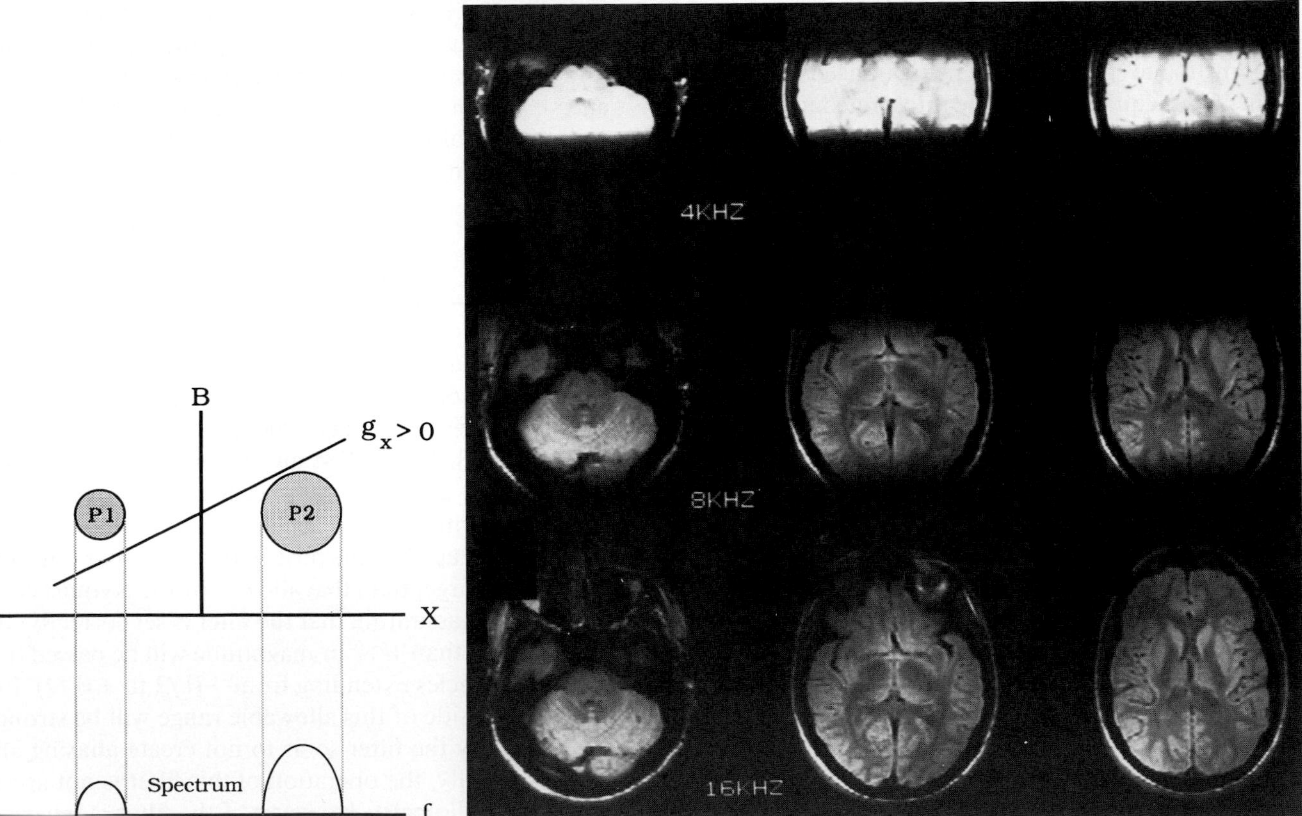

FIG. 10A: Illustration of the principle of frequency encoding of *x* position. The two phantom bottles are located at different *x* positions, and have different frequency spectra, as shown in the graph. **B:** Example of several settings of the analogue low pass filter with the FE axis vertical (anterior-posterior). Only when the setting is 16 kHz as in the lower set of images is the entire brain slice visualized. In the middle images the filter bandwidth is 8 kHz, and in the top 4 kHz. The rejection of the higher frequencies appears as a loss of signal from the outer portions of the image along the FE direction. The increased brightness of the 4 kHz images is unrelated to the narrow bandwidth.

of the frequency components of the signal. A graph of the intensity of the frequency components versus frequency is called the spectrum of the signal. Thus, the FT of the signal in Fig. 10A would consist of two bumps, as shown. From a graph of this spectrum one could easily conclude that the original object consisted of two parts, separated along the x axis as shown, with the larger being on the right. While this description of the process is obviously highly qualitative, the actual FT computer algorithm is quite quantitative, and can show in detail the quantitative distribution of frequencies in this situation. For example, if one bottle had a central portion with fewer water molecules per cubic centimeter, the resulting FT spectrum would show a dip in the middle of the corresponding bump.

An important concept in the use of frequency encoding is that of "bandwidth," which refers to the *range* of frequencies involved. As can be appreciated in Fig. 10, the range of frequencies which will enter the receiver will depend on both how far apart the two objects are as well as on the slope (i.e., strength) of the readout gradient field. Thus, for any given object whose x coordinates range from x_{min} to x_{max}, the width of the frequency range, which we shall call W, is given by:

$$W = f_{max} - f_{min} = (\gamma/2\pi)g_x(x_{max} - x_{min}). \qquad [5]$$

The quantity W would be called the *bandwidth* corresponding to the specific object being imaged.

The above equation could be interpreted to mean that the bandwidth is limited only by the gradient strength and the size of the object. However, this is not entirely correct, because there is a separate limit to the receivable bandwidth which is determined by the rate at which the computer samples the received signal. That is, even if the object and/or gradient were very large so as to imply a wide bandwidth on the received signal, there is a limit to the maximum frequency in the received signal which can be properly processed by the computer. Remember that although the signal as detected and amplified by the electronics is in analogue form, meaning that it can vary continuously as a function of time, the computer can only process discrete (called "digital") data. The digital data is obtained from the analogue data by a process called sampling, which literally means that the computer only "looks" at the received signal at certain discrete time intervals, and has no knowledge of what the signal is doing between these time intervals. This time interval, which we shall call Δt, is typically a small fraction of a millisecond. If we call N_R the number of such data acquiring samples, then obviously the duration of the data acquisition (DA) process is $N_R\ \Delta t$; i.e., shorter sample time is directly related to shorter DA time. Usually $N_R = 256$ such signal samples are obtained for each echo.

The fact that Δt is not zero implies that there is a maximum frequency which can be reliably sampled and processed. This maximum frequency is called the "Nyquist" frequency, and is equal to the inverse of the time interval, Δt:

$$W = 1/\Delta t. \qquad [6]$$

This relationship between W and Δt is easily understood if we keep in mind that to detect any wave of frequency f, one must at the minimum sample the wave twice per cycle, once when the wave is positive and once when it is negative. This implies that the maximum frequency detectable is $1/(2\Delta t)$ and the minimum frequency detectable is negative and equal to $-1/(2\Delta t)$; therefore the bandwidth, being the difference between the positive and negative frequencies, is given by Equation 6.

One easily sees that bandwidth is inversely related to the time duration of DA. This means that when the bandwidth is large, one needs less time to collect the N_R samples necessary to build an image. This in turn implies that to make the echo time as short as possible, one wants to choose as large a bandwidth as possible.

There is obviously the possibility of a conflict or contradiction between Equations 5 and 6, both of which purport to define the bandwidth of the received signal. This situation is resolved by noting that the Nyquist bandwidth (Equation 6) is the maximum *allowable* by the sampling, whereas the bandwidth given by Equation 5, corresponding to that between x_{max} and x_{min}, is the maximum *produced* by the object scanned. This latter difference is, of course, exactly what we mean by the field of view (FOV) of the imaging pulse sequence. An equivalent statement would be that the bandwidth is related to the FOV as:

$$W = (\gamma/2\pi)g_x\text{FOV}. \qquad [7]$$

If the object size exceeds the FOV, then one finds the kind of artifact known as "aliasing," which is described in another chapter.

The receiver electronics contains a circuit called a "low pass filter," which is indicated as the "analogue filter" in Fig. 3. It is called an analogue filter, as distinguished from a digital filter, because it consists of electronic components that act on the signal prior to the digitization step. The purpose of this is to filter out those frequencies larger than that allowed by the Nyquist equation. That is, assuming that the filter is set correctly, frequencies less than $W/2$ in magnitude will be passed (i.e., those frequencies extending from $-W/2$ to $+W/2$). Frequencies outside of this allowable range will be strongly attenuated by the filter so as to not create aliasing artifacts. Normally, the operation of this filter is not apparent to the radiologist. However, if the filter is set incorrectly for too low a bandwidth, then some frequencies necessary to create the image will not be passed; the result will be a sharp drop in image signal intensity beyond a certain distance from the center of the image FOV. This effect is illustrated in Fig. 10B, which shows three images of three slices of the brain. The proper frequency setting in this case would be 16 kHz. As shown, if the filter is set for 8 or 4 kHz, one loses signal at the top and bottom of the FOV. In this case the FE axis is vertical. Note there is no loss of signal in the horizontal PE direction.

In some situations, the bandwidth is of concern to the radiologist. For example, certain multiecho pulse sequences can be designed to utilize reduced bandwidth on the later echoes. This is done because the noise present with the signal can be decreased if the bandwidth is decreased, so that an image with a superior signal-to-noise ratio can be obtained (22). However, this also means that the images will differ in some ways which are unrelated to T2; for example, susceptibility and chemical shift artifacts will be significantly worse for the reduced bandwidth echo.

PHASE ENCODING

In the spin-warp method, phase encoding (PE) is used to encode the *y* position. This is accomplished by applying a brief pulse of current to the *y* gradient coil after excitation and before data readout, as shown in Fig. 5. Clearly, such a pulse will not affect either the slice-selection process nor the frequency-*x* relationship of readout. What it will do is cause a shift of phase of the spin vectors which will be proportional to their *y* position. In other words, the various spin vectors will undergo an additional (positive or negative) rotation, the angle of which will depend on where they happen to be located along the *y* axis. This is illustrated in Fig. 11.

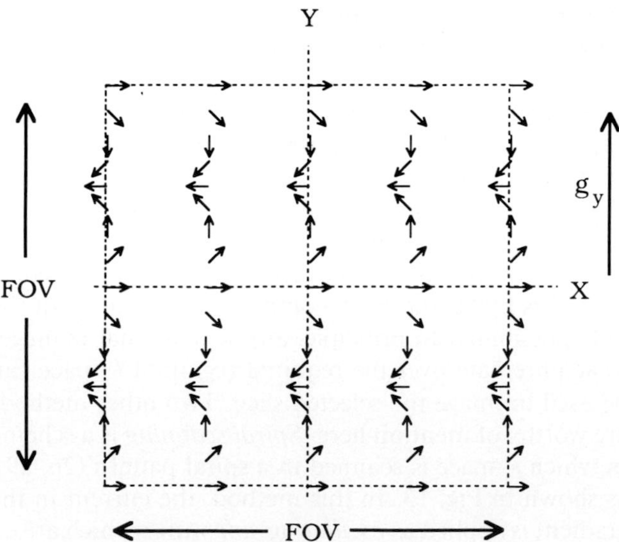

FIG. 11. Illustration of the principle of phase encoding, showing a snapshot of the phase angles of the various spin vectors within the field of view. It is assumed that a brief pulse of *y* gradient, g_y, has just been applied for a limited duration of time, resulting in the rotation of all vectors within the sample except for those at $y = 0$. Note that the angle of phase rotation varies with the *y* position, but is independent of the *x* position.

While the goal of imaging is to be able to localize each voxel in the *x-y* plane, this cannot be accomplished with just one phase encoding pulse of the type described. Rather, *it is necessary to repeat the process a large number of times using a different* y *gradient strength on each repetition.* The number of such repetitions, N_y, is normally equal to the number of *y* pixels present in the final image, although it can also be made to be a multiple of that number. As a result of this repetitive process, the total set of recorded data can be seen to be dependent on *two parameters*, namely, the PE gradient pulse that was used and the frequency of the signal within the readout window. This data is best visualized as a two-dimensional matrix, and the mathematical algorithm which processes it is called the two-dimensional FT algorithm (23).

k SPACE AND SPATIAL FREQUENCIES

Because the number of PE pulses is equal to the number of pixels, it is a common error to assume that each pixel is somehow encoded individually by each PE pulse. For example, one might think that a specific region of the body could be imaged by correspondingly restricting the range of PE gradients used. However, this is not a correct understanding of the 2DFT process. Rather, the data obtained with each pulse in the sequence is derived from the *whole* slice. To understand how the spatial encoding is achieved, it is necessary to understand the concept of spatial frequency or what physicists often call "*k*-space" (24,25).

A spatial frequency is a description of a process which is spread out in space with an sinusoidal shape. For example, a snapshot photograph of a water wave could represent a case of a spatial frequency. Spatial frequencies are measured in *cycles per unit length*, as opposed to temporal frequencies, which are measured in cycles per unit time. For example, a wave whose wavelength was 2 centimeters would be said to have a spatial frequency of $\frac{1}{2}$ cycle per centimeter. As we shall see, the maximum spatial frequency in an image is closely related to the spatial resolution and apparent sharpness of the image. In MRI, it is sometimes convenient to use the field of view (FOV) of the image as the unit of length, so that we speak of cycles per image rather than cycles per cm.

This is an important concept because *the effect of any given PE gradient pulse is to impose a definite spatial frequency on the spin vectors.* This happens by virtue of the fact the spins, whose directions are rotated through an angle that increases progressively with the *y* coordinate, end up in a situation in which their phase angles (in the rf) have a cyclic distribution in space along the *y* coordinate; hence one can see a spatial frequency in this spin pattern. This process is illustrated in Fig. 11, which shows a vertical spatial frequency of two cycles per image in the vertical direction.

Because an image is two-dimensional there can be two different directions for the spatial frequency, namely, x or y. In essence, any image can be analyzed into its spatial frequency components just as any temporal signal can be analyzed into its temporal frequency components. Physicists use the term "k-space" to describe the spatial frequency components of the images. There are two k components, namely, k_x and k_y, and they are directly proportional to the corresponding spatial frequencies. The logical way to plot these values is on a two-dimensional graph, as is shown in Fig. 12.

One very good way to understand the MRI scanning process is as a process which measures the various spatial frequency components of the image. We have seen how each PE gradient established one specific value of k_y. A similar process occurs during the readout process of frequency encoding; namely, at any given instant of time within the readout window the x spatial frequency is proportional to the time interval from the center of the spin echo within the window. The equations which describe this are simple and fairly important:

$$k_x = \gamma g_x t, \text{ and} \qquad [8]$$

$$k_y = \gamma g_y \mathrm{T}_{\mathrm{PE}},$$

where, as usual, γ is the gyromagnetic ratio of the proton, g_x and g_y are the strengths of the respective gradient fields, t is the time within the readout window, and T_{PE} is the time duration of the PE gradient pulse.

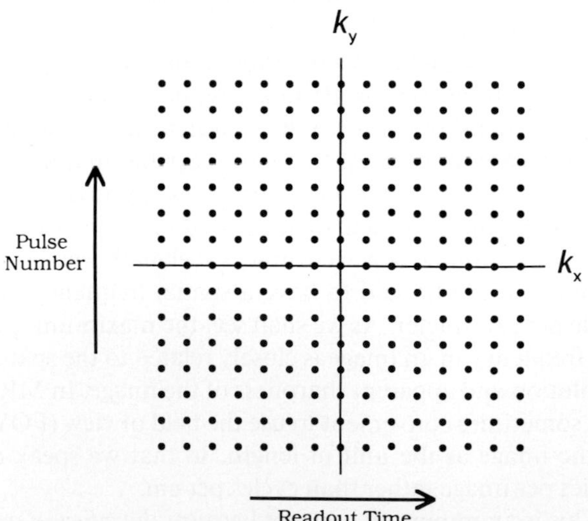

FIG. 12. Illustration of the concept of k-space. The axes are labeled k_x and k_y and represent spatial frequency, not position. To reconstruct an image it is necessary to measure the signal for a large number of points within a rectangular region in k-space. Each point in this drawing shows a single measurement made during the course of a spin warp scan. Each horizontal row of points is obtained during each readout pulse. As the pulse sequence advances the value of the PE gradient, gy, one moves sequentially up to the next row of dots.

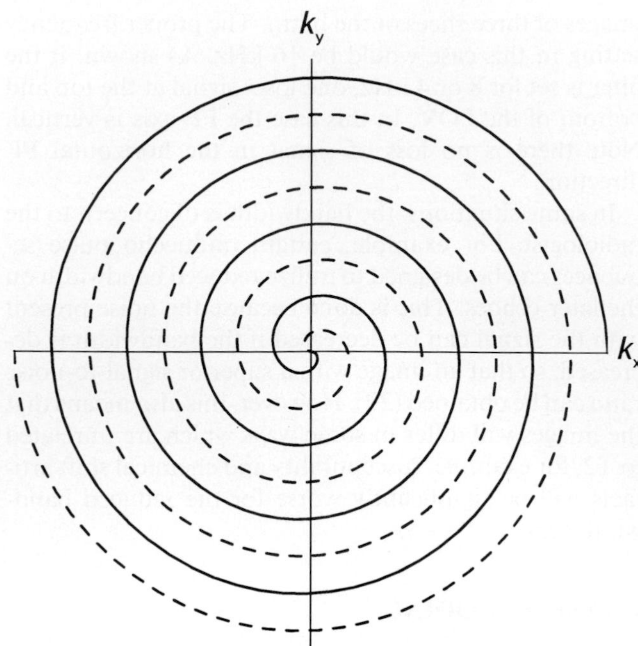

FIG. 13. Illustration of a technique for scanning k-space in a spiral pattern. In this case, two separate spiral paths are used: the solid curve starting at $k_x > 0$ and the dotted curve starting at $k_x < 0$. Either curve could be used to reconstruct the image, but by combining the curves one obtains a FOV twice as large.

The MRI scanning process can now be described by reference to the k-space diagram of Fig. 12. For any given value of PE gradient, the value of k_y is determined; this corresponds to a horizontal line in Fig. 12. The value of k_x varies from one limit to another as a function of time during the readout data acquisition window. This means that the data evolve from left to right in Fig. 12, with a different horizontal line being traced for each PE pulse. To get enough data to reconstruct an image requires that a rectangular area in Fig. 12 be traversed and the signal data obtained. To accomplish this requires that the PE gradient strength, and hence k_y, be systematically changed from pulse to pulse so that the required range from minimum to maximum is covered.

While the method of covering k-space illustrated in Fig. 12 is by far the most commonly used, it is not the only possibility. In principle, any scheme that manages to acquire data over the required region of k-space can be used to image the selected slice. Two other methods are worthy of mention here. *Spiral scanning* is a scheme in which k-space is scanned in a spiral pattern (26–29), as shown in Fig. 13. In this method, the current in the gradient is applied as *oscillating sine waves* which are either damped (starting from the outer part of k-space) or increased (starting from the center of k-space). The main advantage of this scheme over the more conventional scheme of Fig. 12 is that time is not wasted in turning the gradient currents on and off. It is impossible to actually switch the gradient currents instantaneously; this sub-

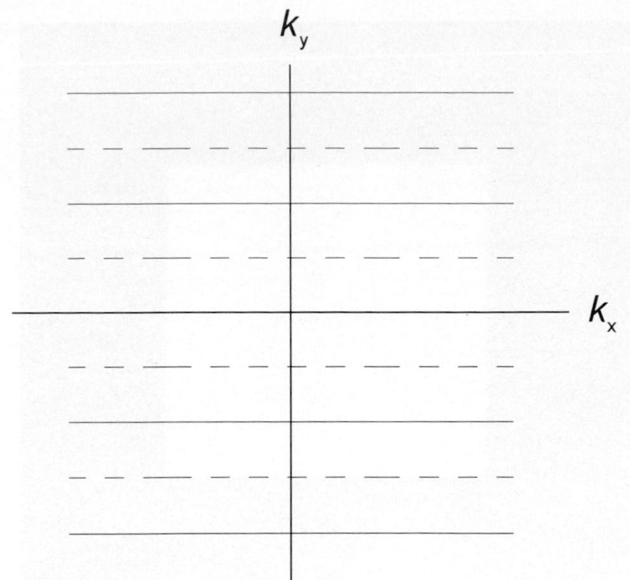

FIG. 14. Illustration of how the coverage of k-space can be accomplished by interleaving the various k_y steps. The solid horizontal lines represent k_y values obtained from one excitation, while the dotted lines represent k_y values obtained from an alternate excitation. The two sets of data are combined to provide the data needed for image reconstruction.

tlety is usually ignored when explaining the basics of imaging using diagrams like Fig. 12. Current clinical scanners need about 1 millisecond to switch the gradient currents on or off; this becomes a serious limitation when very rapid scanning is desired. The advantage of spiral scanning is that the gradients are made to oscillate continuously while the NMR data is being acquired, thus avoiding the switching time problem. The goal of this method is to rapidly cover enough k-space in a single excitation to allow a "snapshot" image to be obtained. In practice, it has not proved practical to cover all of k-space with a single spiral sweep, so several independent sweeps are used, as shown in Fig. 13.

There are various methods, known generically as *echo-planar imaging* (EPI) (30–34) which attempt to cover k-space using multiple echoes following one excitation. Ideally, this could be done in the sequential method of Fig. 12; i.e., in horizontal lines starting with k_y at its maximum negative value and increasing it sequentially with each echo until reaching the maximum positive value. However, it is usually not possible to acquire the number of phase encoding steps desired in one excitation, so multiple excitations are used. In this case, the question arises of how to organize the coverage of k-space. One successful strategy is to cover the whole range by *interleaving* the k_y values from the different excitations. This scheme, which is illustrated in Fig. 14, is widely used in techniques known under the acronyms of RARE or "fast spin echo" and is more thoroughly discussed in a later chapter in this book.

SPATIAL RESOLUTION

The spatial resolution in the image normally reflects the sharpness of the image, and can be expressed as the minimum spacing that lines need to have to be visually resolvable. Equivalently, it can be expressed as the *maximum spatial frequency in the image*. That is, to obtain a sharper image it is necessary to extend the range of k_x and k_y values covered. By reference to Equation 8, one can see that this can be accomplished either by increasing the strength of the x and y gradients, or by increasing the time intervals TE and T_{PE}. Usually, the preferred method is to increase the gradient strengths, because increasing the time intervals means both longer echo times and more sensitivity to field inhomogeneity distortions. A good demonstration of how the spin-warp process builds up a good image from a series of spatial frequencies was given by Felmlee et al. (35).

FOURIER IMAGE SYNTHESIS

The importance of the spatial frequency concept in understanding image quality problems in MRI can not be overemphasized. In most imaging methods, such as radiography, the spatial frequency concept is of secondary importance because, while it may be used in *analyzing* the images produced, it is not an essential part of the imaging process. As we have seen, in MRI the basic ("raw") data which the machine collects are measurements of the spatial frequency components (or k components) of the object. It is literally correct to describe the MRI machine itself as something that does nothing but measure spatial frequencies! The image is then created by a process of combining these components to form a recognizable digital image. This process is called *Fourier synthesis*, indicating that the computer program is a Fourier transform algorithm which adds together the various spatial waves with amplitudes determined by the MRI raw data.

In Fig. 15 we illustrate how this process works by creating two different syntheses of a square phantom. The raw data in question were not obtained with any physical MRI machine, but rather by a computer program. This means that the raw data are mathematically perfect and contains no errors of the type typically found in real machines. This was done to demonstrate the purely mathematical aspects of the synthesis process without the distracting effects of realistic physical errors.

In Fig. 15A we see the result of a synthesis using 16 spatial frequencies, i.e., the maximum frequency utilized was 16 cycles per field of view (FOV). In Fig. 15B we show the result of using four times as many spatial frequencies, up to 64 cycles per FOV. Note the obvious improvement in the sharpness of the corners of the square in the latter image. The ripples seen extending through-

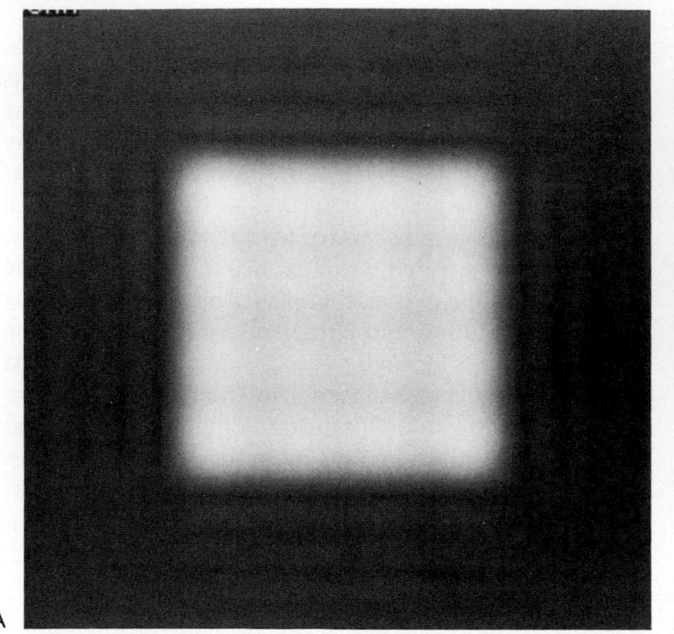

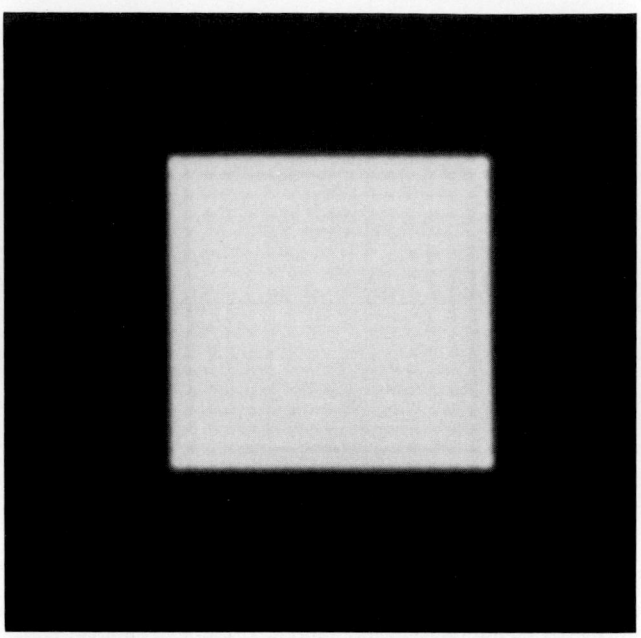

FIG. 15. Phantom images reconstructed using 16 (**A**) and 64 (**B**) cycles per field of view. The phantom is generated mathematically on a computer and represents a perfect square with no measurement or instrumental errors. Note the superior sharpness of the corners of the square in B, as well as the reduction in the Gibbs effect artifacts.

out the square are a natural consequence of the fact that we are using only a finite number of spatial waves to create our image. As is explained in the chapter on artifacts, this effect, called the "Gibbs phenomenon" or the "truncation artifact," can occasionally become significant in certain imaging situations.

A more clinical illustration of the effective contributions of different regions of k-space to the final image is shown in Fig. 16, which is taken from a review article on fast spin-echo imaging by Atlas et al. (36). In this example, two images are reconstructed from a single, complete scan of k-space. In Fig. 16A, the entire range of k_x is

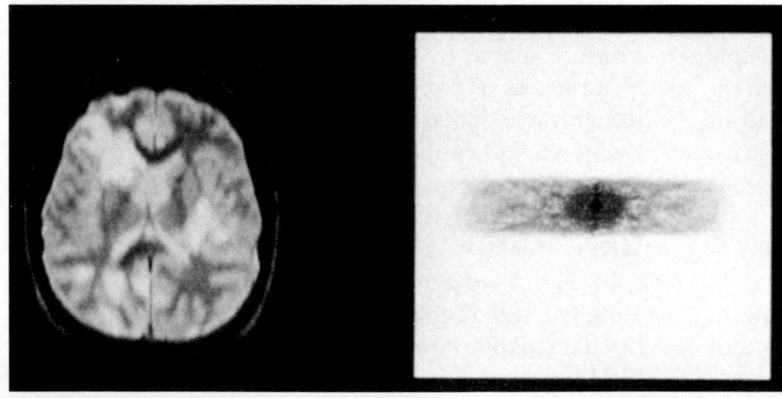
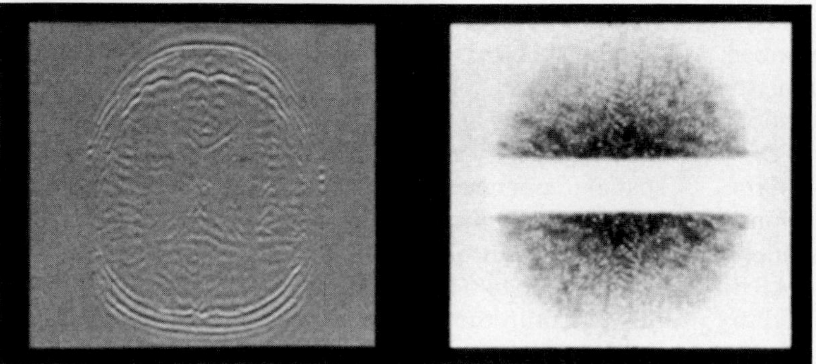

FIG. 16. Illustration of a brain image reconstructed from different parts of k-space. Image **A** shows the image reconstructed using only low (y-direction) spatial frequencies, as well as an image representation of that part of k-space used. Image **B** shows the converse, with only high k_y values used. Note that whereas image A shows normal cranial tissue contrast but with edges blurred in the vertical direction, image B shows virtually no tissue contrast but emphasizes structures with sharp edges in the y direction. (From Atlas et al., ref. 36, with permission.)

included but the contributions from large k_y are filtered out. This means that the low frequency region of k-space (that near the $k_x = k_y = 0$ origin) are properly included in the reconstructed image. Since low spatial frequencies translates into "large areas," this means that the contrast of most structures with large, homogeneous areas is reconstructed properly; this includes the ventricles and most "gross" aspects of the gray and white matter. In Fig. 16B, however, *only* the large k_y values are used. The lack of any low spatial frequency information in the image means it is not possible to distinguish most cerebral structures; i.e., they have no identifiable contrast. On the other hand, structures which have strong high k_y components, mainly surface *transitions* of high contrast which run horizontally in the image are perceivable. In this case, that includes the anterior and posterior borders between the brain and calvarium as well as the marrow and skin edges. These edges are not visible on the lateral sides of the head because those structures have high k_x, not high k_y, components.

So far we have assumed that to synthesize an image it is necessary to completely sample the symmetric region of k-space of Fig. 12, i.e., both k_x and k_y must range equally from negative to positive values. Actually, in many situations of clinical interest it is possible to obtain an image with (theoretically) one half of that data; for example, by restricting the range of k_y to be either positive or negative, but not both (37–39). This possibility lies in a particularly subtle aspect of the Fourier synthesis method; namely, it can be used to synthesize "complex" as well as "real" images. In this context, "complex" is used in the mathematical sense of having both a real and an imaginary part. The actual spin density in the patient's body is, of course, a real number, so the imaginary part of the image should be zero. Nevertheless, the method is capable of synthesizing twice as much information as we normally ask it to do, which implies that we could achieve a useful result with only one half as much data. The success of these so-called half-Fourier or half-NEX methods does *not* mean that the data in one half of k-space is zero or can be neglected. Rather, it means that it is possible to *infer* the data in the missing half from the data in the scanned half. This is based on a mathematical technique called "conjugation," which states that the data in the upper half of k-space is the mathematical complex conjugate of the data in the lower half (and vice versa). This is true only if the underlying voxel densities are strictly real numbers. In practice, the problem is somewhat more difficult because any phase shift between the upper and lower halves of k- space will create imaginary parts to the data and invalidate the method. These phase shifts could be due to such problems as patient motion or eddy currents in the gradient fields, for example. What is done in practice is to slightly overscan, i.e., scan $\frac{1}{2}$ of k-space plus a little extra into the second half. This extra information allows the computer to correct for these problems, and this technique of imaging is actually widely used in clinical practice. This factor of 2 advantage can be utilized to reduce scan time by $\frac{1}{2}$ since only $\frac{1}{2}$ the number of phase-encoding steps are required. Alternatively, when it is desired to obtain extremely short echo times, the pulse sequence can be modified so that only the right half of k-space (with $k_x > 0$) is used. In fact, in some clinical scanners this changeover is made automatically when the operator requests very short echo times in a standard 2DFT imaging method.

THREE-DIMENSIONAL IMAGING

By "three-dimensional imaging" we mean a pulse sequence in which the imaged plane is not selected using a selective excitation pulse with a z gradient as explained above. Rather, this class of imaging techniques works by *exciting the entire target volume on each excitation.* The pulse sequence for doing this is illustrated in Fig. 17. Note that the exciting radiofrequency pulse is applied in the absence of a z gradient, implying that it is not spatially selective. Obviously, some means must be used to divide up the imaged volume into the desired slices of width Δz. This is done using the principle of phase encoding; i.e., at the same time that the y phase-encoding gradient pulses are applied one also applies a set of z gradient PE pulses (40). The mathematics of phase encoding along the z axis is identical to that along the y axis. For example, the "z resolution" is equivalent to the slice thickness Δz, which is inversely proportional to the maximum z PE gradient applied. For each z phase-encoding pulse, one needs a complete set of y PE pulses, so that the total number of pulses needed is the product of N_y and N_z. This often represents a rather large number, so that

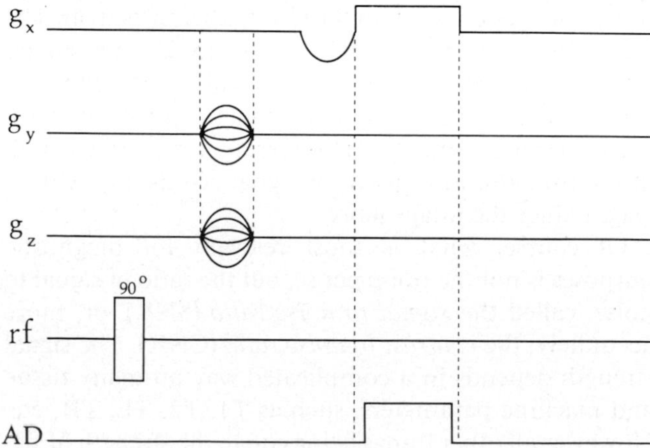

FIG. 17. Pulse sequence diagram for a simple, three-dimensional, imaging technique. In this case, the exciting rf pulse is not spatially selective, and z slice selectivity is due to the use of multiple phase encodings using the z gradient. The x and y axes are treated in a manner identical to that of 2D imaging.

such imaging techniques are usually performed using fast scan techniques with short TR (41).

IMAGE NOISE

The three main pillars of image quality are contrast, resolution, and noise. By noise we mean random variations in signal level, which appears as "mottle" in the image. Noise should be understood in two arenas: there is noise in the "raw" signal data prior to reconstruction of the image, as well as noise in the final reconstructed image. The noise in the image is due to the noise in the raw data, but may be modified by the reconstruction process. Due to the fact that the image display is controlled by the viewing window's level and width, by reducing the width one can always "push" an MRI system so that the information content is primarily limited by noise and not by spatial resolution.

The source of noise in the MR process is almost exclusively in the random motion of electrons at various stages in the system. The most important sources are the radiofrequency coil used for receiving, the first stage of rf amplification used in the receiver electronics (so-called preamplifier), and the body of the patient himself. Note that the noise does *not* depend on the random motion of the *protons* which create the NMR signal. In fact, the noise in an image is essentially unchanged if the rf transmitter is turned off entirely; the result of such an experiment will be a field of random noise uniformly distributed across the pixels of the image.

The magnitude of the image noise can be quantified as the standard deviation (SD) of the signal values measured in a strictly uniform field. This could be a basic water phantom, providing it is not so large as to show shading or other artifacts; this method is widely used to quantify computed tomography noise, for example. Alternatively, the noise could be determined as the SD of a null image generated with the rf amplifier turned off. The magnitude of the noise will be proportional to the square root of the receiver bandwidth, which, according to Equation 6, is inversely proportional to the time interval between signal samples. Therefore, increasing the length of the time duration used for signal acquisition will always reduce the image noise.

Of course, what is most relevant for diagnostic purposes is not the noise per se, but the ratio of signal to noise, called the *signal to noise ratio* (SNR), or, more accurately, the *contrast to noise ratio* (CNR). The signal strength depends in a complicated way on many tissue and machine parameters, such as T1, T2, TE, TR, etc. However, all other things being equal, the strength of signal coming from a voxel will be proportional to the number of protons in that voxel, and hence proportional to voxel volume. The voxel volume, in turn, depends on both the gradient strengths and bandwidths used. However, it turns out that the SNR depends on imaging parameters in this way:

$$\text{SNR} \propto (\text{voxel volume}) * \sqrt{(\text{signal acquisition time})} \quad [9]$$

By signal acquisition time we mean the time spent actually acquiring data. For a spin-echo technique this would be the time duration of the echo sampling. However, by increasing the number of excitations one can obviously increase this time. In fact, any technique that increases the signal acquisition time (leaving the signal strength fixed) will increase the SNR. This provides a different explanation of why a variable bandwidth technique can be useful, since bandwidth is reduced by simply increasing the time duration of the echo acceptance window in the computer's electronic programming. Similarly, *any technique that decreases voxel volume in an effort to improve spatial resolution will decrease SNR.* For example, if pixel size and slice thickness are both reduced by $\frac{1}{2}$ to improve spatial resolution, the SNR will decrease by a factor of 8; to overcome this would require increasing acquisition time by a factor of 64.

REFERENCES

1. Fukushima E, Roeder SBW. *Experimental Pulse NMR: a Nuts and Bolts Approach.* Reading, MA: Addison-Wesley; 1981:1–92.
2. Redpath TW, Selbie RD. A crossed ellipse rf coil for NMR imaging of the head and neck. *Phys Med Biol* 1984;29:739–744.
3. Arakawa M, Crooks LE, McCarten B, Hoenninger JC, Watts JC, Kaufman L. A comparison of saddle-shaped and solenoidal coils for magnetic resonance imaging. *Radiology* 1985;154:227–228.
4. Samaratunga RC, Busse LJ, Pratt RG. Resonator coils for magnetic resonance imaging at 6 MHz. *Med Phys* 1988;15:235–240.
5. Lai CM, Lauterbur PC. True three-dimensional image reconstruction by nuclear magnetic resonance zeugmatography. *Phys Med Biol* 1981;26:851–856.
6. Bottomley PA. NMR imaging techniques and applications: a review. *Rev Sci Instr* 1982;53:1319–1337.
7. Hinshaw WS, Lent AH. An introduction to NMR imaging: from the Bloch equation to the imaging equation. *Proc IEEE Trans Bio Med Eng* 1983;71:338–350.
8. Edelstein WA, Hutchison JMS, Johnson G, Redpath R. Spin warp NMR imaging and applications to human whole-body imaging. *Phys Med Biol* 1980;25:751–756.
9. Rosen BR, Pykett IL, Brady TJ. Spin lattice relaxation time measurements in two-dimensional nuclear magnetic resonance imaging: Corrections for plane selection and pulse sequence. *J Comput Assist Tomogr* 1984;8:195–199.
10. Pauly J, LeRoux P, Nishimura D, Macovski A. Parameter relations for the Shinnar-Le Roux selective excitation pulse design algorithm. *IEEE Trans Med Imaging* 1991;10:53–65.
11. Geen H, Freeman R. Band-selective radiofrequency pulses. *J Magn Reson* 1991;93:93–141.
12. Morris PG, McIntyre DJO, Rourke DE, Ngo JT. The design of practical selective pulses for magnetic resonance imaging and spectroscopy using SPINCALC. *Magn Reson Med* 1991;17:33–40.
13. Garwood M, Ke Y. Symmetric pulses to induce arbitrary flip angles with compensation for rf inhomogeneity and resonance offsets. *J Magn Reson* 1991;94:511–525.
14. Carlson JW. Exact solutions for selective excitation pulses. II. Excitation pulses with phase control. *J Magn Reson Med* 1992;97: 65–78.
15. Joseph PM, Axel L, O'Donnell M. Potential problems with selective pulses in NMR imaging systems. *Med Phys* 1984;11:772–777.
16. Murdoch JB, Lent AH, Kritzer MR. Computer-optimized narrow-

band pulses for multislice imaging. *J Magn Reson* 1987;74:226–263.
17. Runge VM, Wood ML, Kaufman DM, Silver MS. MR imaging section profile optimization: Improved contrast and detection of lesions. *Radiology* 1988;167:831–834.
18. Mao J, Mareci TH, Andrew ER. Experimental study of optimal selective 180° radiofrequency pulses. *J Magn Reson* 1988;79:1–10.
19. Shinnar M, Bolinger L, Leigh J. The synthesis of soft pulses with a specified frequency response. *Magn Reson Med* 1989;12:88–92.
20. LeRoux P. Exact synthesis of radio frequency waveforms. *Proc SMRM* 1988;7:1049–1049.
21. Kucharczyk W, Crawley AP, Kelly WM, Henkelman RM. Effect of multislice interference on image contrast in T2 and T1 weighted MR images. *AJNR* 1988;9:443–451.
22. Edelstein WA, Bottomly PA, Hart HR, Smith LS. Signal, noise, and contrast in nuclear magnetic resonance (NMR) imaging. *J Comput Assist Tomogr* 1983;7:391–401.
23. Haacke EM, Patrick JL. Reducing motion artifacts in two-dimensional fourier transform imaging. *Magn Reson Imaging* 1986;4:359–376.
24. Twieg DB. The k-trajectory formulation of the NMR imaging process with applications in analysis and synthesis of imaging methods. *Med Phys* 1983;10:610–621.
25. Cho ZH, Nalcioglu O. Methods and algorithms for fourier-transform nuclear magnetic resonance tomography. *J Opt Soc Am[A]* 1987;4:923–932.
26. Matsui S, Kohno H. NMR imaging with a rotary field gradient. *J Magn Reson* 1986;70:157–162.
27. Rand SD, Macovski A. Rapid projection MRI of short T2 species with multiple small angle excitations and oscillatory-rotary field gradients. *IEEE Trans Med Imaging* 1988;7:99–108.
28. Maeda A, Yokoyama T. Reducing chemical shift artifacts in MRI with time-varying gradients. *IEEE Trans Med Imaging* 1989;8:8–15.
29. Spielman D, Pauly J, Meyer C. Variable-density spirals for MR fluroscopy. *Proc SMRM* 1993:1261(abst).
30. Hennig J, Friedburg H, Ott D. Fast three-dimensional imaging of cerebrospinal fluid. *Magn Reson Med* 1987;5:380–383.
31. Ordidge RJ, Howseman A, Coxon R, Turner R, Chapman B, Glover P, Stehling M, Mansfield P. Snapshot imaging at 0.5 T using echo-planar techniques. *Magn Reson Med* 1989;10:227–240.
32. Stehling MK, Turner R, Mansfield P. Echo-planar imaging: magnetic resonance imaging in a fraction of a second. *Science* 1991;254:43–50.
33. Cohen MS, Weisskopf RM. Ultra-fast imaging. *Magn Reson Imaging* 1991;9:1–37.
34. Oshio K, Jolesz FA. Fast MRI by creating multiple spin echoes in a CPMG sequence. *Magn Reson Med* 1993;30:251–255.
35. Felmlee JP, Morin RL, Salutz JR, Lund GB. Magnetic resonance imaging phase encoding: a pictorial essay. *Radiographics* 1989;9:717–722.
36. Atlas SW, Hackney DB, Listerud J. Fast spin-echo imaging of the brain and spine. *Magn Reson Q* 1993;9:61–83.
37. Feinberg DA, Hale JD, Watts JC, Kaufman L, Mark A. Halving MR imaging time by conjugation: Demonstration at 3.5 kG. *Radiology* 1986;161:527–531.
38. Haacke EM, Mitchell J, Lee D. Improved contrast at 1.5 Tesla using half-Fourier imaging: application to spin-echo and angiographic imaging. *Magn Reson Imaging* 1990;8:79–90.
39. Hurst GC, Jua J, Simonetti OP, Duerk JL. Signal-to-noise, resolution, and bias function analysis of asymmetric sampling with zero-padded magnitude FT reconstruction. *Magn Reson Med* 1992;27:247–269.
40. den Boef JH, van Uijen CMJ, Holzscherer CD. Multiple-slice NMR imaging by three-dimensional Fourier zeugmatography. *Phys Med Biol* 1984;29:857–867.
41. Enzmann D, Rubin JN. Short TR, variable flip angle, gradient echo scans of the cervical spine: comparison of 2DFT and 3DFT techniques. *Neuroradiology* 1989;31:213–216.

Magnetic Resonance Imaging of the Brain and Spine, Second Edition, edited by Scott W. Atlas. Lippincott-Raven Publishers, Philadelphia © 1996.

4

Fundamentals of Flow and Hemodynamics

John Listerud and Scott W. Atlas

One of the unique characteristics of magnetic resonance imaging (MRI) is its depiction of flow, even without the administration of intravascular contrast agents. Flow-related phenomena were recognized early in the development of magnetic resonance (1,2), well before imaging techniques were even devised. The appearance of flowing fluid (e.g., blood or CSF) is important to understand for several reasons. First, it has become apparent that the signal information from flow can be exploited to provide previously unavailable physiologic information. Particularly since the initial publication by Wedeen et al. (3) showing intravascular flow as high signal intensity on in vivo magnetic resonance (MR) images, intense scientific and clinical interest has become focused upon imaging the cerebral vasculature and its pathology with MR. The various methods of imaging vascular flow and displaying it in multiple projections have been termed "MR angiography," because of the similar appearance of these images to conventional catheter angiography using iodinated contrast agents and x-rays. MR angiography (MRA) techniques are still evolving but have already improved significantly since several groups introduced the two principal techniques of data acquisition, time-of-flight and phase contrast (4–9). A strong foundation in the fundamental physical effects will certainly aid in the interpretation and rational choice between these techniques and their many permutations, most of which are operator-dependent choices (see Chapter 31). Second, the signal intensity of flowing spins is quite variable, even in normal physiologic states, so the possibility of misinterpreting normal findings as important pathologic conditions, such as vascular thrombosis or stenosis, is reduced if one has a solid conceptualization of the physical basis of flow effects. Third, signal emanating from flowing spins often generates significant artifacts which can obscure anatomy and degrade images, thereby reducing the radiologist's ability to interpret MR images and identify lesions or normal structures. The understanding of flow artifacts allows one to recognize them and implement maneuvers to eliminate or compensate for such effects (see Chapter 7).

The appearance of flowing fluid is highly dependent upon certain physical hemodynamic properties of the flow as well as specific features of the MR pulse sequence being utilized to image the region of flow. In most conditions, however, only some of these factors are operative and, in many instances, one major factor predominates over all others. The following discussion assumes a basic knowledge of the general principles of MRI and relaxation phenomena (see Chapters 2 and 3).

PHYSICAL PROPERTIES OF FLUIDS

Basic Definitions in Hemodynamics

Hemodynamics

Prior to the discussion of signal modulation based on MRI phenomena related to flowing fluid, it is important

J. Listerud, M.D., Ph.D., and S. W. Atlas, M.D.: Neuroradiology Division, Department of Radiology, Oregon Health Sciences University, Portland, OR 97201.

to have a concept of the physical nature of flow (11). The relevance of the physical properties of flowing fluids to the radiologist becomes obvious when one appreciates the most fundamental difference between MRA and catheter angiography—MRA demonstrates the physiology of flowing blood, whereas catheter angiography demonstrates the morphology of the internal lumen of vessels by virtue of filling the intravascular space with contrast agent. MRA depicts functional properties of intravascular flow, while catheter angiography depicts intraluminal anatomy.

Along with the discussion of relevant MR physics, it is useful to be fluent in the vocabulary of hemodynamics. *Dorland's Medical Dictionary* defines hemodynamics as "the study of the movements of the blood and of the forces concerned therein." As such, the subject of hemodynamics cannot be cleanly separated from the body of classical fluid mechanics. Poiseuille modeled the characteristics of blood flow through capillaries. His careful measurements of flow through small capillary tubes led him to formulate the law which now bears his name (11): the pressure drop ΔP between the two ends of a tube depends directly on laminar flow rate Q, on tube length ΔL and inversely on the fourth power of the radius r. This can be written as:

$$\Delta P = \frac{8\mu Q}{\pi r^4}\,\Delta L, \qquad [1]$$

where μ is the constant viscosity of a Newtonian fluid.

The cgs unit of viscosity is named after the discoverer of this law, the "poise." Ironically for Poiseuille, it is in the microcirculatory system where the non-Newtonian characteristics of blood are most strongly evident.

Laminar Flow, Shear Stress and Shear Strain Rate, and Viscosity

Laminar flow describes motion of fluids occurring at slow rates. Intuitively, one thinks of flow with constant velocity passing through a long rigid tube as composed of a series of concentric cylindrical sheets or laminae. As each lamina moves down the tube at a constant velocity, frictional forces from its inner and outer adjacent neighboring sheets act respectively to speed and to slow its motion (Fig. 1).

Fluid entering a tube tends to move as a plug of flow. Forward velocity is relatively constant as a function of radius until close to the lumen, where velocity quickly drops to zero. It takes time for the frictional forces slowing the outer laminae to propagate inward sufficiently to achieve the parabolic radial dependence of forward velocity characteristic of Poiseuille flow. This dependence is most easily represented mathematically in the geometrically cylindrical coordinates (r, θ, z) which are typically used to parameterize the tube lying concentrically about the z axis with inner diameter R_{lumen}. The cylindrical

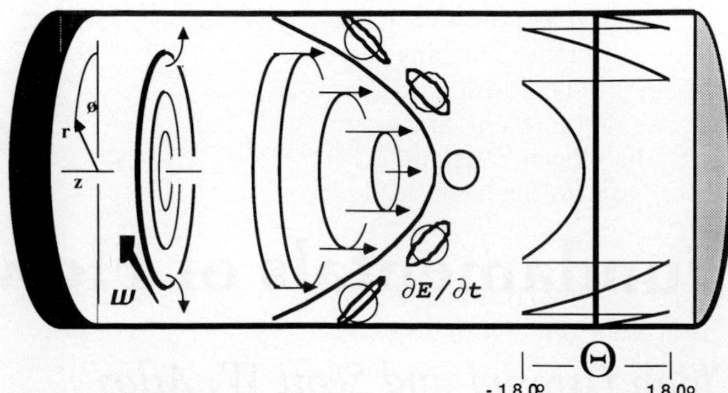

FIG. 1. With Poiseuille flow, vorticity and shear strain rate are both proportional to the radial distance. Vorticity is generated by friction with the walls, propagates inward by diffusion of momentum, and is carried downstream by convection. The interaction between fluid motion and the imaging gradients induces a phase shift which for constant flow is strictly proportional to velocity, and thus takes on the parabolic profile of fully developed laminar flow. The signal loss within a voxel element will be dependent on the range of velocities found within the voxel, and so will be more severe at the lumen.

lamina with radius r from the z axis moves as a uniform sheet with velocity v_z:

$$v_z = v_{\max}(1 - (r/R_{\text{lumen}})^2). \qquad [2]$$

Such flow is referred to as "fully developed." Conventional wisdom requires the flow to have passed a length equal to 20 diameters down a straight tube with smooth, featureless walls, before flow is admitted to be fully developed. In actual fact, the segments of the arterial tree are generally short enough that flow can be considered to be typically "plug-like" (10).

The intuitive picture of a concentric series of laminae will be useful for introducing the concept of shear stress. The shear strain rate $\partial/\partial t$ E can be thought of in two ways. In the first, it is the change in forward velocity per change in the perpendicular distance as one moves radially in a pipe or vessel, $\Delta v_z/\Delta r$. This definition is perhaps most easily associated with the picture of concentric, sliding laminae.

The second description better accounts for the name of this quantity. The definition of shear strain is borrowed from the theory of elasticity to describe the deviation in one direction per given offset in the perpendicular, in this case, a change in position along the axis per increment in the radial direction, E$\sim\Delta z/\Delta r$. Note that this is a dimensionless quantity. For an elastic material, some restoration forces described by the shear stress are proportional to the extent of deformation, as described by the shear strain. For fluid, only frictional forces are involved in resisting deformation, a fact which necessarily introduces the time rate of change of deformation into the expression for shear stress. These two definitions are the same mathematically (note that this quantity has units of (sec)$^{-1}$):

$$\Delta v_z/\Delta r = (\Delta z/\Delta t)/\Delta r = (\Delta z/\Delta r)/\Delta t. \qquad [3]$$

For example, consider flow through the common carotid, just before reaching the carotid bulb. Taking the diameter to be 5 mm, and the distance from the arch to the bulb to be 10 cm, and assuming for the sake of argument that flow is constant, then the fully developed, parabolic flow profile has a shear strain rate at the lumen of:

$$\partial/_{\partial t}\, E = \tfrac{1}{2}\, \partial/_{\partial r}\, v_z = v_{max}/R. \qquad [4]$$

(The factor of one half will be discussed further below.) For a peak velocity of 20 cm/sec and 80 cm/sec during diastole and systole, respectively, this gives shear strain rates of 40 and 160 per second, respectively.

The frictional force acting in the direction of motion per unit area of a lamina is termed shear stress Σ. Shear stress is intuitively dependent on the relative speeds of adjacent lamina, the latter being characterized by the shear strain rate. Viscosity characterizes the importance of friction in the behavior of a fluid. The fundamental definition of viscosity is as a proportionality constant between shear stress and the strain rate:

$$\Sigma = \mu\, \partial/\partial t\, E. \qquad [5]$$

Blood with a hematocrit of 40 has a viscosity of approximately 0.035 poise, which correspond to shear stresses of 1.5 and 5.6 dynes/cm, respectively, for diastole and systole. Constant flow models have demonstrated peak shear strain along the inner wall close to the flow divider of the carotid bifurcation of 3,050/sec, corresponding to shear stress of 105 dynes/cm, for flow rates corresponding to diastole (Fig. 2).

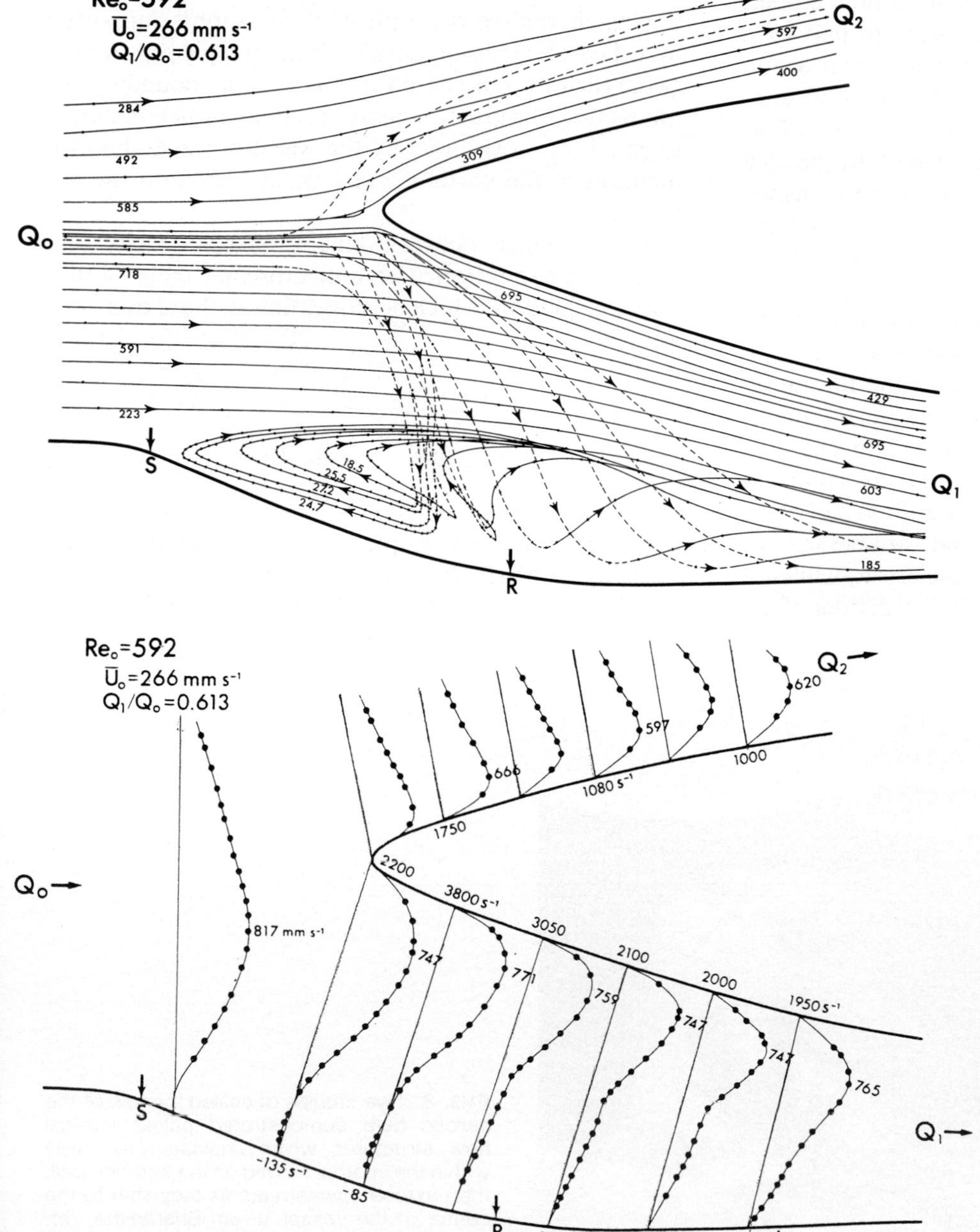

FIG. 2. This well known work demonstrates flow patterns by particle trajectory measured with high speed photography through a constant flow phantom fashioned from cadaver specimens of the human carotid artery bifurcation. (From Motomiya, ref. 12, with permission.)

The exact relation of shear stress to intimal damage has been a subject of debate for several decades. Naively, one might suppose that high shear stress would be implicated as an early contributor to the cycle of injury and healing associated with atherosclerotic plaque formation. However, the viscous stress required for endothelial cell erosion was found to occur on average for a stress of 400 dynes/cm^2, corresponding to a shear strain rate of about 11,400/sec. This strain rate probably does not occur under physiologic conditions (13,14). Furthermore, Caro argued in the late 1960s that the average location of plaque correlated with regions of very low shear stress (15). Such low stress regions were easily demonstrated at the time by an increased uptake of Evans blue dye in vivo in locations such as the outer wall of the internal carotid bulb.

The McGill and Georgia Tech constant flow models appearing approximately a decade later are part of a growing body of literature which correlate the low and oscillatory shear stress with locations of intimal thickening and early plaque in the carotid (Fig. 3) (17,18). This correlation has been implicated elsewhere in the arterial tree as well (19,20). Conversely, it is now well established that endothelial cells and the underlying connective tissue collagen will orient in vivo and in vitro with respect to a steady, unidirectional stress, with very little underlying smooth muscle, connective tissue cells, or stainable lipid (21–23). In other words, a constant shear stress in the physiologic range appears to induce the formation of a healthy vascular endothelium (Fig. 4). Furthermore, viscous stress is implicated as a controlling mechanism in related cellular functions, such as LDL receptor expression and endocytosis in cell preparations (25,26). In short, locations demonstrating low and variable viscous stress are at risk for developing atherosclerosis, while locations of high shear stress such as the flow divider of the common carotid bifurcation are spared.

Pressure and Bernoulli's Equation

The previous section described the forces which retard flow and dissipate energy. In this section, the forces of potential and kinetic energy are considered from the point of view of dimensional analysis. *Pressure* is typically defined as the force acting perpendicularly to a 2D surface, in contrast to shear stress, which acts parallel to the surface element. However, dimensional analysis of the quantity shows that it may also be written as energy per volume, or energy density.

$$\begin{aligned} \text{Pressure} &= \text{Force/Area} \\ &= \text{Force}\cdot\text{depth/Area}\cdot\text{depth} \\ &= \text{Energy/Volume} \end{aligned}$$

This alternative description of pressure is supported by a classic textbook analysis of microscopic pressurized gas particles bouncing off a macroscopic boundary. In this picture, the kinetic energy of the gas particle is shown to equal the work done by the wall to reverse the momentum of the particle and repel it back into the gas volume.

The exchange between kinetic energy density and pressure is also reflected on a macroscopic scale by Bernoulli's equation, which describes flow without frictional loss:

$$\underset{\text{Kinetic}}{\tfrac{1}{2}\rho v^2} + \underset{\text{Internal potential}}{P} + \underset{\text{Gravitational potential}}{\rho g h} = \text{Total Energy constant} \quad [6]$$

As fluid without viscosity with density ρ courses along a pathway at a macroscopic velocity v, ascending or descending to height h, its total energy remains constant and the difference is made up by the microscopic kinetic energy, described by the pressure term P.

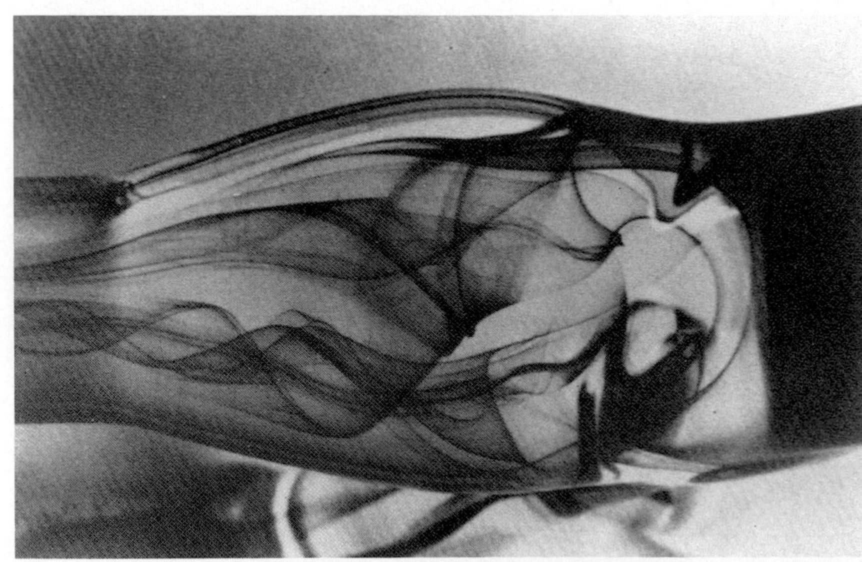

FIG. 3. Dye studies of scaled models of the carotid bulb demonstrated paired vortical flow structures which originate proximally within the internal carotid on the exterior wall, then extend downstream as they shift to the center of the vessel. (From Bharadvha, ref. 16, with permission.)

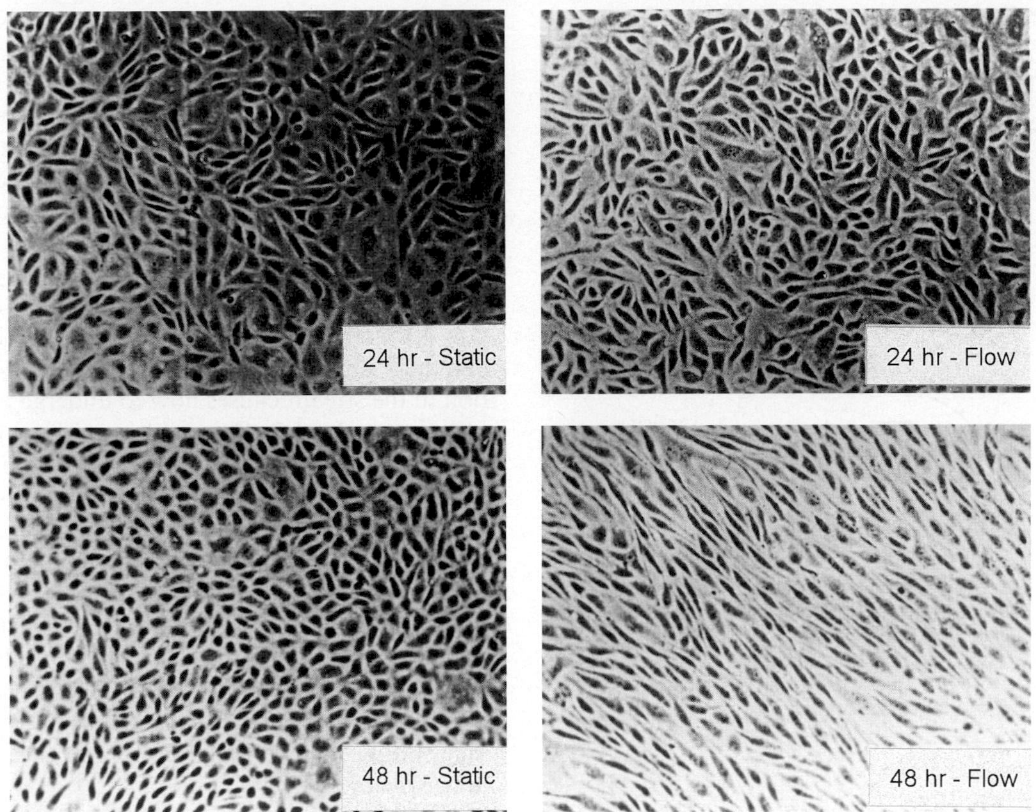

FIG. 4. Vascular endothelium cultured within a controlled flow phantom demonstrates an adaptive orientation in response to exposure to physiologic levels of shear stress. (From Dewey, ref. 24, with permission.)

Velocity Differential, Shear Strain Rate, and Vorticity

The most obvious observation one can make about a small fluid element in a flow stream during a small increment in time is a translation in the position of the element. This tells us almost nothing about the forces which are acting on the fluid element, as simple inertia is sufficient to account for translational motion. It is the relative motion of parts of the fluid element with respect to each other, as described by the velocity differential, which are needed in order to write the dynamic equations of fluid flow.

The velocity differential, by formal definition, is a matrix of quantities of partial derivatives which taken together form the vectorial derivative of the velocity vector. Intuitively it describes the time rate of distortion of a small "test" filament located at the center of the fluid element. From the formal theory of matrices, the velocity differential may be broken down into the sum of three matrix components, the diagonal, the traceless symmetric, and the anti-symmetric matrices:

Theory of Matrices

$$\underset{\substack{\text{Distortion}\\\text{of filament}}}{\overset{\substack{\text{Velocity}\\\text{differential}}}{[\partial/\partial x_i\, v_j]}} = \underset{\substack{\text{Pressure}\\\text{(gas)}}}{\overset{\substack{\text{Diagonal}\\\text{dilation}}}{(\sum \partial/\partial x_i\, v_i)I}} + \underset{\substack{\text{Shear}\\\text{strain rate}}}{\overset{\substack{\text{Symmetric}\\\text{traceless}}}{\partial/\partial t\, E}} + \underset{\substack{\text{Vorticity}\\\text{(rotation)}}}{\overset{\substack{\text{anti-symmetric}\\\text{traceless}}}{\tfrac{1}{2}[\vec{\omega}\mathbf{x}]}} \qquad [7]$$

Physical Interpretation

The physical interpretation of these quantities indicate that to first order, any distortion in a fluid element may be broken down into three kinematic quantities: a dilation, a shear strain rate, and a rotation described by a vector quantity called vorticity (Figs. 1 and 5). Dilation is a matrix operation which describes the compression or expansion of fluid filament. This action is independent of direction of the filament. In a compressible gas this term is proportional to pressure. In an incompressible fluid, this term is so small that it is neglected under all but the most extreme conditions. The shear strain rate describes the distortion of a spherical element into an ellipsoid. The effect is described by the identification of the principal axes of the ellipsoid, and the rate of distortion along each of these axes. Along these principal axes, the test filament is simply stretched or compressed in a fashion which preserves the total volume of the spheroid.

The direction of the vorticity vector defines the axis of rotation, while the rate of rotation is given by half its length. It acts on the fluid filament, as does any rotation vector, through the vector "cross-product." Obviously, a filament which is perfectly aligned with the vorticity vector is not affected by the operation of rotation. This is reflected in Thompson's theorem (27) concerning a homogeneous, nonviscous fluid. For such a fictitious fluid, a macroscopic loop formed from the connection of a series of microscopic filaments, all parallel to the vorticity

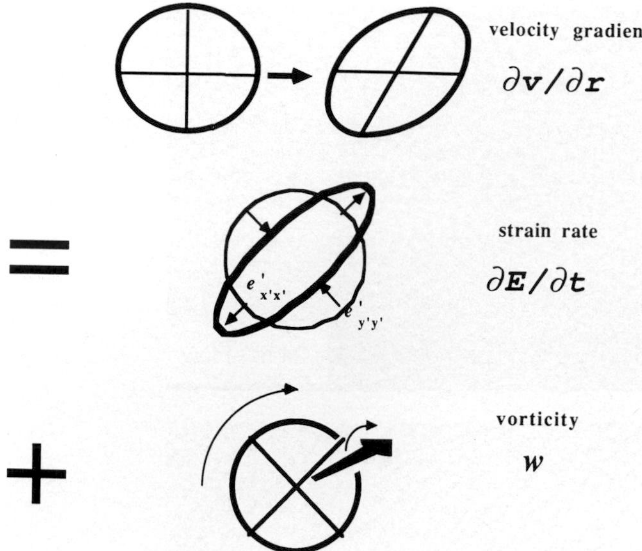

FIG. 5. To first order, the distortion of the local neighborhood by a flow pattern is given by a matrix quantity, the velocity gradient. For an incompressible fluid such as water or blood, this quantity can be further decomposed into the strain rate, which describes the tendency to distort into an oblate spheroid, and the vorticity, which describes the tendency to rotate about the local axis.

vector within their respective fluid elements, is never broken by the action of flow. In fact, for such a fluid, the entire volume may be considered to be composed of such macroscopic filaments which either close into loops which are swept downstream, or which end on boundaries.

Kinematics, Dynamics, and Turbulence

The topic of kinematics is roughly confined to the velocity vector field, or in other words, a description of flow *sans* physical forces. An important theorem from multidimensional calculus states that given any smoothly varying vector field there exists a unique flow pattern for which the velocity at any point is equal to the vector field at that point. For such a flow pattern, if one knows a particle's location at any point in time, one may predict its entire past and future trajectory. In the context of MRA, kinematics are of primary interest, as the path of a flow particle is responsible for intravoxel dephasing and for increased residence times leading to saturation.

The term "dynamics" refers to relations which describe the forces which act on fluid particles. The previous section has already introduced the relationship between the kinematic property, shear strain, and with the dynamic property, shear stress.

The term turbulence is often applied somewhat loosely to flow which exhibits complex behavior. The strict definition of turbulence requires that at any specific point within the stream, the instantaneous direction of flow is random, even though average flow is constant. To put it another way, the knowledge of the present position of a particle within a turbulent flow pattern allows only the probabilistic determination of its future and its past. Classically, flows are characterized by the Reynolds number N_R, the ratio of kinetic energy to dissipated energy per volume element. For Reynolds numbers below 2,000, flow is guaranteed to be laminar.

By gently increasing velocity, the N_R may become elevated above the critical level, while the laminar nature of flow is preserved. This is an unstable situation, however, and after some period of time, some random perturbation in the stream causes flow to undergo a transition to turbulence. At slow flow velocities, these perturbations are damped by shear strain, which "regularizes" flow and suppresses the size of the random perturbations to well below the scale of the conduit. However, once past the critical N_R, the microscopic fluid element's kinetic energy is too large for frictional forces to correct perturbations in flow direction. Turbulent flow results. The random velocity of the microscopic fluid element works against the local average velocity, and consequently frictional losses are much greater than that which is necessary simply for average transport of the fluid element downstream.

Intra-arterial flow is probably more aptly described as "disturbed," rather than either laminar or turbulent (10), since these concepts do not apply to pulsatile fluid motion. In pathologic states, such as at points distal to stenoses and in aneurysms, as well as near the normal branch-points of vessels and in curved vessels, flow patterns are known to become complicated (28,29).

Intravascular signal loss has been ascribed to intravoxel phase dispersion in in vivo imaging from complex flow characteristics due to underlying anatomy and pathophysiology. These effects have been noted primarily at vessel origins, bifurcations, and sites of focal luminal narrowing, where flow patterns are notably more complex. Note that at the center of a focally narrowed vessel, flow is accelerated, while reversal of flow occurs downstream, just distal to the site of the narrowing. Signal loss in these regions has been attributed to this combination of fluid motion with subsequent phase dispersion (30,31).

When turbulence or complex flow is present, the expected high signal intensity of flow-related enhancement, which would indicate vascular patency, may not be present, so occlusion is implied even though the vessel is patent. It remains controversial, however, whether turbulence occurs at all under normal physiologic circumstances (32). For example, the Reynolds number of the common carotid artery can be estimated at maximum velocity of 70 cm/sec and diameter of 5 mm to be approximately 100, well below critical. Although turbulence is commonly invoked as a major cause of intravoxel dephasing, the complex flow characteristics in the absence of turbulence may account for the great majority of signal loss in such techniques as MR angiography. Therefore, contrary to the situation when turbulence is present, signal loss in these regions may actually represent recoverable signal if the appropriate pulse sequence design is utilized.

The Dynamics of Flow

Stokes' Theorem and the Navier-Stokes Equation

With the vocabulary developed above, we may now consider the equation in which the forces acting on a volume of fluid are balanced. Although this necessarily involves the notions of advanced calculus, the reader is asked to bear with the notation in order that a descriptive account may be made of the main features of the "anatomy" of the equation. Two equations are relevant. The first considers the balance of forces which affect a macroscopic volume. The total rate of change of momentum, summed over the entire volume, must equal the summation of the flux of momentum across the surface, the pressure exerted perpendicularly to the surface, and the shear stresses exerted tangentially to the surface.

Force Balance Equation

Rate of Change of momentum; Momentum flux across surface; Pressure on surface; Shear stress on surface

$$\int_V \partial/\partial t \rho\vec{v}\,dV + \int_S (\vec{v}\cdot d\vec{S})\rho\vec{v} + \int_S d\vec{S}\,P = \int_S d\vec{S}\cdot\Sigma \qquad [8]$$

$$\partial/\partial t \rho\vec{v} + (\vec{v}\cdot\nabla)\rho\vec{v} + \nabla P = \mu\nabla^2\vec{v}$$

Acceleration; Convective transport of momentum; Pressure gradient; Diffusion of momentum

Navier-Stokes Equation

Historically, this equation was a great stimulus to the an important chapter in the development of vector calculus, an effort which is typified by Stokes' theorem. The intellectual question posed was the relationship between quantities which were being summed on a surface with quantities summed on the interior.

To a reader unfamiliar with this subject, a short digression on the origin of this theorem may be of interest. To condense asides contained in a footnote of Truesdell's and the preface by Spivak (33,34), the first proof of Stokes' theorem is today credited to Sir William Thompson (Lord Kelvin), and is contained in a postscript of a letter in 1850 to his close colleague, Professor Stokes of Cambridge, concerning flow confined to a two-dimensional plane. In 1854, Stokes offered it as a problem on the prestigious Smith prize, and theorem was mistakenly attributed to him by Maxwell in his opus "A Treatise on Electricity and Magnetism." By the time of his death, the theorem was universally attributed to Stokes. The importance of this theorem is difficult to overstate. Its applications include fundamental contributions to fluid flow, electromagnetism, and the Theory of General Relativity. Furthermore, its study not only stimulated the formulation of a major branch of modern mathematics, but today forms a model for the systematic development of such branches.

Stokes' theorem relates integration of a possibly multidimensional quantity over a bordering 2D surface to integration of a "derivative-like" quantity over the interior 3D volume. In the context of our discussion, the application of these ideas to the macroscopic force balance equation leads to the Navier-Stokes equation, in which related quantities are balanced on a point by point basis. In the latter equation, the accelerating force acting on a point in an interior 3D volume is related to the action of the pressure gradient, the convective transportation of momentum, and dissipation of momentum through viscous diffusion.

Reynolds Number

As flow velocity increases, the behavior of flow changes and becomes consistent with turbulence. However, high flow velocity cannot necessarily be equated with turbulence, since relatively laminar flow can be maintained at high velocity within small-diameter tubes (35). Rather, flow experiments can be uniquely characterized by a single nondimensional parameter, the Reynolds number N_R, the ratio of kinetic energy density ρV^2 stored as pressure within a volume element to the energy $\mu V/D$ dissipated by viscous losses within the element:

$$N_R = \frac{\rho V^2}{\mu V/D} = \rho VD/\mu. \qquad [9]$$

The expression relates fluid density ρ, average flow velocity V, fluid viscosity μ, and tube diameter D. For example, if the diameter is decreased in inverse proportion to an increase in the velocity, the Reynolds number remains constant.

In 1883, Reynolds discovered that past a certain flow rate corresponding to a N_R of 2,100, now known as the critical Reynolds number, the pressure drop per unit distance becomes proportional to the square of the total flow. At this point, flow is no longer parabolic. On a local macroscopic scale the flow takes on the profile of a random series of eddies which over time averages out to a "plug" profile. It now becomes inappropriate to think of flow as a layering of concentric laminae, each with its own defined speed, because flow is now random. Frictional drag, or shear stress, is no longer transmitted smoothly toward the center of the stream from vessel walls, but rather by small swirling eddies which originate at the walls and randomly migrate inward. As an approximation, therefore, the N_R can be used to predict the onset of turbulent flow; that is, if N_R is greater than 2,100, turbulent flow is likely to occur (36).

The Reynolds number makes an important appearance in the normalized Navier-Stokes equation. In this equation, all fundamental parameters of time, distance, and weight have been normalized to some "typical" value, as indicated by an overbar. For example, distance $r \rightarrow \bar{r} = r/D$. All other quantities are normalized according to appropriate combinations of the fundamental parameters, as in the velocity $\vec{v} \rightarrow \bar{\vec{v}} = \vec{v}/(D/T)$. In particular, the normalized viscosity turns out to be the inverse of the Reynolds number $\bar{\mu} = 1/N_R$.

$$\partial/\partial t \rho \vec{v} + (\vec{v} \cdot \nabla)\rho \vec{v} + \nabla P = \mu \nabla^2 \vec{v}, \quad [10]$$

$$\partial/\partial \bar{t} \bar{\rho} \bar{\vec{v}} + (\bar{\vec{v}} + (\bar{\vec{v}} \cdot \bar{\nabla})\bar{\rho}\bar{\vec{v}} + \bar{\nabla}\bar{P} = (1/N_R)\bar{\nabla}^2\bar{\vec{v}}. \quad [11]$$

This fact has important practical consequences. Often, flow patterns of interest, such as the aerodynamics of cars or planes or the hemodynamics of the carotid bulb (Fig. 5), would be difficult to study under normal conditions. Scale models with identical Reynolds numbers give identical (scaled) patterns of flow.

PHYSICS OF MOTION IN MR

The Basic Phase-Shift Effect

Gradient Moments

In all MRI sequences, controlled magnetic gradient fields are utilized to manipulate the phase and frequency of radio signals which have been elicited from the magnetic moments associated with hydrogen nuclei ("spins") by excitation with a radiofrequency transmitter. In almost all cases, several magnetic field gradient pulses are applied in carefully timed succession in order to encode the position of stationary spins in their radiofrequency signatures, phase, and frequency. The movement of a spin between pulses or during the application of a pulse is the main cause of the artifacts observed from moving spins in pulse sequences designed for stationary spins. Phase changes due to flow in the presence of field gradients are generally manifested on conventional (magnitude) images in one of three ways: signal loss from phase dispersion representing variable velocities within a given voxel, signal increase on even-numbered multiple echoes from recovery of velocity-induced phase shifts, and ghost images due to misrepresentations of phase shifts from velocity changes during the imaging sequence.

This can be understood in detail by remembering that, in the presence of any magnetic field gradient, the demodulated rf signal $\omega - \omega_{\text{Larmor}}$ of a given spin is proportional to its corresponding local magnetic field, which is equal to the product of the gradient G_z (in radians per second per centimeter), and the position z:

$$\omega - \omega_{\text{Larmor}} = G_z \cdot z. \quad [12]$$

(See Chapter 3 for definition of the Larmor frequency.) The phase change Θ that the spin's magnetization experiences can be described as (Fig. 6) (2):

$$\Theta_\tau = \int_0^\tau z_t \cdot G_z dt \quad [13]$$

As integration is a form of summation, this equation expresses an important yet simple fact which significantly aids the practical analysis of a pulse sequence: phase shifts induced by different pulses are added together. The analysis of how motion affects the MR data has been extended to define an additive series of contributing terms. For completeness, we state the analytic expressions first, then give a practical interpretation with

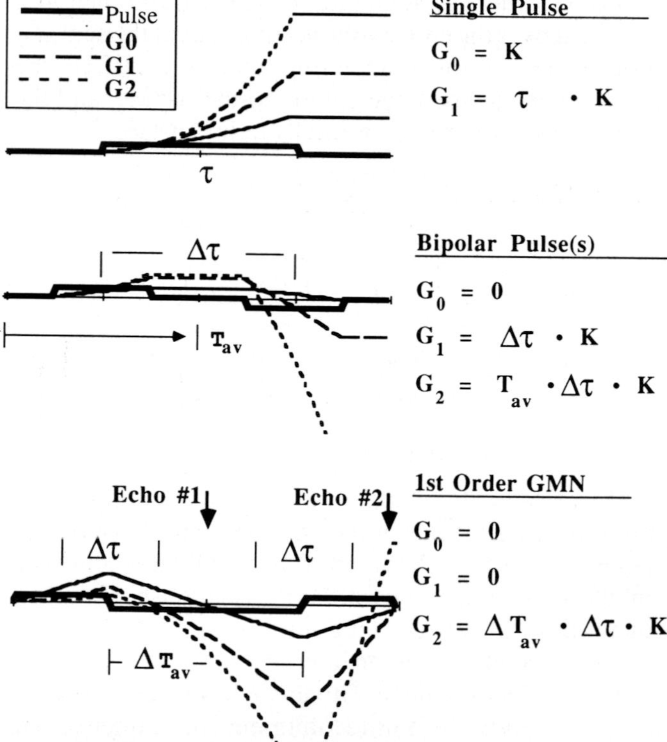

FIG. 6. Nulling of lower order gradient moments tends to extend the length of the gradient sequence. This diagram shows the 0th through 2nd order moments as functions of time for three exemplary gradient-pulse sequences: a single pulse, a bipolar pulse, and a 1st order gradient moment null (GMN) constructed from two bipolar pulses. The latter case occurs "naturally" in a dual echo sequence along the frequency-encoding axis, and its fortuitous occurrence has been dubbed the "even echo" rephasing effect. Note that at the completion of the 1st order GMN both G_0 and G_1 are zero. This can be appreciated from some simple formulas for square pulses which cover virtually all pulse sequences used in routine clinical imaging (see text).

which one may analyze the flow sensitivity of virtually any clinical imaging sequence.

The phase shift Θ is broken down into components which are associated with different types of instantaneous motion which a moving spin undergoes in the course of a pulse sequence, and each component is separately related to a *moment* of the magnetic field gradient pulse timing diagram. The prescription of the relative contributions of position z_0, velocity v_z, acceleration a_z, and so on is given by the following formal expansion, based on the Taylor series (37):

Gradient Moment Analysis of Phase Shift

$$\Theta = z_0 \cdot G_0 + v_z \cdot G_1 + a_z \cdot G_2 + d^3z/dt^3|_{t=0} \cdot G_3 + \cdots \quad [14]$$

$$z_t = z_0 \cdot 1 + v_z \cdot t + a_z \cdot \tfrac{1}{2}t^2 + d^3z/dt^3|_{t=0} \cdot \tfrac{1}{3}t^3 + \cdots \quad [15]$$

Taylor Series Expansion of Position

Here, the gradient moments are given by the general, though somewhat opaque expressions $G_i = 1/i \int t^i G_z dt$. Simpler expressions are available for the low order moments of a single pulse of strength G_{max}, of width T_{pw}, and centered at time τ. Let K be the area of the gradient pulse on a pulse timing diagram: $K = G_{max} \cdot T_{pw}$. Then the area has the dimensions of an inverse wavelength λ over which phase varies by 2π. That is to say, after this pulse, the phase of the MR signal across the object varies in the direction of the gradient, rotating a full 360° (i.e., 2π radians) in a distance λ (Fig. 1). For this single pulse, the 0th order moment is $G_0 = K$, while the first order moment is $G_1 = K \cdot \tau$.

A *bipolar pulse* is actually two gradient pulses, of equal area but opposite sense. That is, if the positive pulse caused the spin to precess clockwise, the negative pulse causes a counterclockwise phase shift. It turns out that bipolar pulses are quite commonly used in imaging, because their 0th moment obtains the condition necessary for creating a gradient echo. Consequently, the calculation of first order gradient moment of a bipolar pulse is commonly used in flow-sensitive MR imaging.

$$G_0 = K_1 - K_2 = 0, \quad [16]$$

$$G_1 = (\tau_1 - \tau_2) \cdot K = \Delta\tau/\lambda. \quad [17]$$

The second order gradient moment of a bipolar pulse pair can be expressed as the product of the average of the pulse centers and the first order gradient moment. When two bipolar pulse pairs are used to create a first order gradient moment nulling, the second order moment is easily computed from this expression (Fig. 6).

A typical application of these formulae is the calculation of the phase of a spin as it appears in the image, which turns out to be equal to the phase accumulated at the echo time, TE. On the frequency-encoding gradient axis, the dephasing gradient pulse and the portion of the readout pulse occurring before the TE have the same area. This causes the phases of all stationary spins to be equal at this time, which in turn causes their signals to interfere constructively at that moment, the very definition of the gradient-echo time. Consequently, these two gradient pulses form a "naturally occurring" bipolar pulse pair, which like all such pulse pairs imparts a velocity-dependent phase shift to the moving spin at the echo time.

In conventional imaging, the three orthogonal gradient directions are detected by distinct styles of encoding: slice-select, frequency-encoding (readout), and phase-encoding. The additive nature of the integral equation for phase shift implies that the total phase shift may be conveniently analyzed by calculating the encoding for each axis separately, then summing the results. The slice-select and frequency-encoding gradients both employ "natural" bipolar pulses, so that the net phase cumulative phase change for stationary tissue after the gradient application is zero (necessarily, the phase-encoding gradient is not bipolar and symmetrical, because the induced phase alteration is utilized for spatial encoding). Similarly, in a spin-echo sequence, the phase of the spin of stationary tissue, regardless of its position along the gradient axis, returns to zero at each multiple of TE due to the phase reversal effect of the 180° rf pulse.

Practical analysis of higher order gradient moments for all but the simplest pulse sequences requires a computer. We may make some simple observations in order to develop some intuitive understanding of gradient moments. For a single narrow gradient pulse, the gradient moment is approximately proportional to τ_n, the nth power of the pulse time. The further away from the rf excitation, the larger the time factor, especially for the higher powers.

Intravoxel Dephasing and Shear Strain Rate

Slow, straight-line flow at relatively slow rates, such as is approximated in vivo by venous blood flow, exhibits a nearly parabolic velocity profile; that is, there is a characteristic spatially dependent variation in velocity across the lumen of the vessel, where velocity is highest in the center and is zero adjacent to the vessel wall. Within individual voxels of the vessel lumen, the variation in flow velocities is greatest adjacent to the vessel wall where shear strain rate is highest, and least at the luminal center, where it is lowest (38).

Phase shift alone does not reduce signal intensity if all spins within a voxel agree in phase. Signal loss is caused, rather, by intravoxel dephasing in which spins within the same voxel acquire opposing phases, leading to destructive interference between their respective signals. It will be helpful to introduce the concept of phase dispersion, $\partial\Theta/\partial r$. Consider a voxel positioned just within the lumen of a tube through which constant Poiseuille flow is passing. At the echo time, the phase of the moving spins will be given by $\Theta = v_z \cdot G_1$, where only v_z is dependent on radial position.

Assuming Poiseuille flow of peak velocity 20 cm/sec in a tube of diameter 5 mm, then the velocity gradient $\partial v_z/\partial r$ = 80/sec. Consider sequence parameters typical for a "T1-weighted" spin-echo exam. A centered echo in a readout gradient parallel to the flow direction of strength $\frac{1}{2}$ Gauss/cm, of duration 8 msec, and separated from the dephasing gradient by 15 msec has a G_1 = 12.75 msec/mm. The phase dispersion $\delta\Theta/\delta r$ may now be calculated as

$$\partial\Theta/\partial r = \partial v_z/\partial r \cdot G_1 \qquad [18]$$

which gives 80 sec^{-1} · 12.75 msec/mm = 1.02 cycles/mm.

A pixel larger than 1 mm at the lumen of the tube contains a range of phase shifts of over 1 cycle, or 360°, ensuring significant intravoxel dephasing. This estimate accounts for the well known "black blood" artifact first noted on spin-echo imaging (39,40). In general, intravoxel dephasing can be eliminated by obeying the following condition on the phase dispersion and pixel dimension Δ:

$$\Delta\Theta \approx \partial\Theta/\partial r \cdot \Delta r \ll 2\pi. \qquad [19]$$

Intravoxel dephasing is dealt with in a variety of ways. For instance, reduction of intravoxel dephasing can be accomplished by reduction of voxel size, and by reduction of phase dispersion. Zeroing or "nulling" the first order gradient G_1 makes Θ independent of constant velocity.

First order gradient moment nulling alone does not ensure elimination of intravoxel dephasing, even for constant flow. For example, with flow around a curve, the centripetal acceleration is given by $a = v_2/R$, leading to a phase dispersion estimate of

$$\begin{aligned}\partial\Theta/\partial r &= \partial a/\partial r \cdot G_2, \\ &= 2v_z/R \cdot v_z/\partial r \cdot G_2.\end{aligned} \qquad [20]$$

These formulas indicate why the concepts of velocity gradient, strain rate, and vorticity can be expected to play an increasing role in future explanations of intra-voxel dephasing in regions of complicated flow.

Time-of-Flight Effects

Conceptually, time-of-flight effects are probably the simplest to understand. These effects include the consequences of bulk motion of spins flowing either into or out from a given imaging volume undergoing repetitive selective excitation and refocusing. Time-of-flight effects can result either in an increase in signal intensity [e.g., from more fully magnetized spins flowing into the volume (in-flow effects)], or a decrease in signal intensity [e.g., from excited spins moving out of the volume (outflow effects)].

Any volume of stationary tissue being imaged is excited once every repetition time (TR) interval. Stationary nuclei are unable to fully recover longitudinal magnetization when the TR is shorter than the T1 of the tissue, hence the repetition of the excitatory radiofrequency (rf) pulse will depress signal most significantly in structures with longer T1. This phenomenon of saturation results in signal differences between stationary spins of tissue within the slice and more fully magnetized spins flowing into the slice (1).

Note that time-of-flight effects are determined by many factors, including the velocity of flow, the slice or slab thickness of the excited volume, and the TR and the T1 relaxation time of the fluid. At the one extreme, stagnant blood acts as stationary tissue and will become saturated, emitting little signal. Spins moving into the excited volume between the 180° and the next 90° rf pulse in a traditional spin-echo sequence, however, enter in the fully relaxed state. At relatively low flow velocities, a fraction of the slice becomes filled with incoming, unsaturated spins, while the remainder of the slice is filled by spins that have not left the slice since the prior excitation, i.e., saturated spins. With increases in flow velocity, eventually the entire slice is refreshed by fully relaxed spins. Likewise, a thinner slice (or volume, if using 3DFT techniques) and a longer TR will result in a higher degree of spin replacement. The higher the proportion of relaxed (unsaturated) spins in the slice, the higher the signal intensity will be. Note that the resultant signal intensity of the incoming spins can exceed that of the stationary tissue within the slice. This signal increase related to flowing spins has been termed "flow-related enhancement" (41). Once the incoming velocity has equaled that at which there is complete replacement of spins in the slice with fresh spins, the maximum signal will be generated. This maximal flow-related enhancement occurs when velocity exceeds:

$$v_{max} = \text{slice thickness/TR} \qquad [21]$$

where v_{max} refers to the velocity at maximal signal from inflow.

As velocity continues to increase, a transition is made from the gain in intensity from inflow to a decrease in intensity due to the departure of spins from the slice during the interval between the 90° and 180° rf pulses. This corresponds to any velocity greater that the v_{max}. In spin-echo imaging, both the 90° rf and the 180° rf pulses are slice-selective, so that to emit signal, any spin would have to be within the slice for both pulses of that TR. Therefore, spins exiting the slice after the 90° rf pulse will generate no signal. In high velocity flow states, spins leaving the slice before the application of the 180° rf pulse ($\frac{1}{2}$ of the echo delay, or TE/2) will contribute no signal. Note that the longer the TE, the more spins will have left the imaging slice and will therefore yield no signal.

The type of pulse sequence will influence the impact of inflow or outflow on signal intensity. In a multislice spin-echo sequence, slices deeper within the multislice volume will have a more complicated manifestation of inflow and outflow effects which will depend on the previous excitation(s) that a spin may have received (Fig. 7). Prediction of a given spin's excitation history will depend on knowledge of inter-slice gaps, the quality of the slice profile, and the slice excitation pattern which was used (e.g., interleaved) for the purpose of reducing rf interference between adjacent slices. In gradient-echo imaging, the signal is generated by reversal of the frequency-encoding gradient, which is not a slice-selective process (as opposed to the 180° rf refocusing of spin-echo imaging). Therefore, all spins which have experienced the slice-selective (or slab-selective, as in the case of 3DFT modes) excitatory rf pulse will emit signal, even if they have moved out of the slice before refocussing has occurred (see Chapter 29). Gradient-echo imaging therefore minimizes signal loss from outflow. Gradient-echo imaging maximizes the high intensity of incoming spins (inflow effects) when these sequences are performed in a single-slice acquisition mode. Note that on gradient-echo imaging, the flip angle determines to a large extent the relative signal intensity of the incoming spins (42): the higher the flip angle, the more effective saturation of stationary spins, and, therefore, the higher the difference in signal between incoming unsaturated spins and stationary tissue.

In the discussion above, the velocity of flow was assumed to be both perpendicular to the slice and constant. In vivo, when a vessel runs oblique to the slice or even within the plane of the slice, only the component of the velocity perpendicular to the slice enters the above considerations. This implies that even relatively fast flow may exhibit high intensity from inflow effects when the course of the vessel runs parallel to the slice for a long enough distance. Furthermore, arterial (and CSF) flow has inconstant velocity because it is pulsatile. A priori, we may assume that the average velocity determines the overall signal intensity due to time-of-flight effects. However, accidental synchronization between physiologic periodicity and signal acquisition may undermine this assumption. For example, when the cardiac cycle has an R-R interval close to the TR (known as pseudogating) (43), one slice may be acquired predominantly during systole and another predominantly during diastole. Consequently, effective velocities in these slices may be dramatically different. Similarly, these effects can be obtained with intentional synchronization to the cardiac cycle. Additionally, it should be noted that time-of-flight effects are much more complex when considering intra-

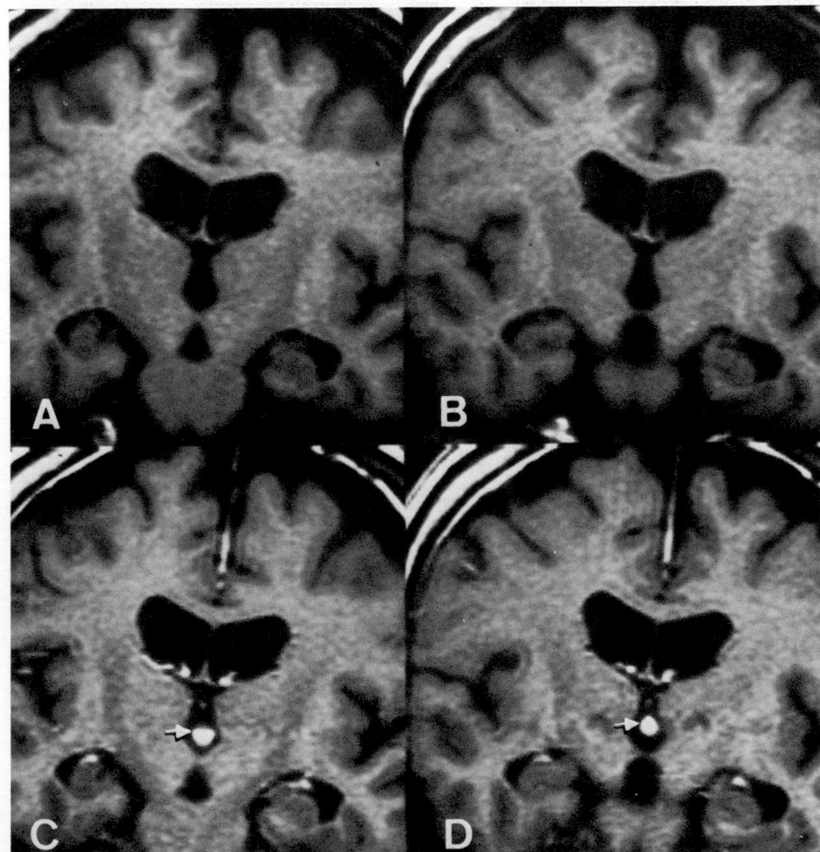

FIG. 7. Effect of rf pulse history on inflowing spins. On coronal short TR/TE spin-echo images from the middle of an imaged volume, intraventricular CSF is depicted as low signal (**A**,**B**), because of previous saturation due to interleaved slice excitation, At the same locations but in a series where these locations are the end slices of the imaged volume (**C**,**D**), note high signal intensity (*arrows,* C,D) in areas of inflowing CSF in the third ventricle.

spinal CSF flow (44,45), since spinal CSF flow is oscillatory, exhibiting varying velocity profiles as well as changing directions of flow. In the spine, CSF spins repeatedly reverse direction and are repeatedly excited as determined by TR, TE, slice thickness, interslice interval, CSF pulsation amplitude, and CSF pulsation period (44,45).

A brief comment may be made at this time in regard to the accelerated gradient systems which are imminently to be offered by the major manufacturers of MR imaging equipment. These systems make possible the use of ultra-short TR times, on the order of 4–10 msec. With current systems, there is little motivation to reduce TR times below 40 msec in most typical MRA applications, as shorter allowed TRs begin to saturate out the incoming flow signal and require several minutes for the coverage of a reasonable volume. However, as ultra-short TRs allow the acquisition of 3D volumes in significantly less than a minute, T1-shortening contrast agents may be used in effective combination with these rapid scanning methods to obtain MRA scans within the arterial bolus phase.

FLOW-RELATED ARTIFACTS

Oblique Flow Misregistration

Historically, motion effects were first described in terms of artifacts that degraded standard imaging protocols. The design of methods for overcoming artifactual signal intensities rapidly ensued and will be discussed in this section. However, the reader may find it helpful to understand that historically, the discovery and explanation not only preceded the elaboration of MR angiographic techniques, but stimulated their development.

In the presence of flow oblique to the orientation of the phase- and frequency-encoding axes, an artifactual displacement of the vascular signal relative to the location of the true vessel can occur. This vessel mismapping results from the non-simultaneous nature of spatial encoding; that is, phase-encoding and frequency-encoding are done at different time points (38). Note that vessel mismapping will only be present if the vessel generates signal intensity (either from inflow effects, or due to phase-shift compensation). In our example of a spin moving at 45° oblique to the encoding axes (Fig. 8), the y-position is encoded at the center of the phase-encoding pulse, which is often very close to the 90° rf excitation pulse. The frequency-encoded x-position is determined at the echo time TE. For a spin moving at 20 cm/sec, and a TE of 30 msec, the spin has moved 6 mm and its projection along the frequency-encoded axis has moved approximately 4 mm. Consequently, the positional encoding of the spin to the image is at a location in space that the spin did not occupy at any time. In general, a spin appears in the image at a corner of a rectangle whose diagonal is formed by connecting the positions of the spin at the phase-encoding time and the TE. The precise location (i.e., which corner of this rectangle) to which the spin will be mapped depends on the phase- and frequency-encoding directions (Fig. 8). The simplest way to reduce the degree of mismapping is to move the phase-encoding gradient pulse as close as possible to the TE.

Even-Echo Rephasing

Note that we can regain the signal loss due to constant velocity-induced phase shifts with the use of the refocusing 180° rf pulse, much as we can rephase magnetic field inhomogeneity-induced signal loss. This is an effect first noted with multiple echo imaging (46). In the case of stationary spins in the presence of an applied balanced linear gradient, phase changes linearly with time, and refocusing of the phase change imparted by gradients occurs at all echoes (assuming that no other magnetic field perturbations occur) (Fig. 6). Phase shifts associated with flow, however, are nonlinear with time and depend on many characteristics of the flow, i.e., velocity, acceleration, pulsatility, direction, linearity, or turbulence, etc.

With constant velocity flow, the phase shift is quadratic with time, which results in complete rephasing of spins at even echoes ("even-echo rephasing") (46) but incomplete rephasing of spins at odd echoes (Figs. 6 and 9). When the second echo TE does not equal the first echo TE, these velocity-induced phase shifts will not be perfectly refocused on the second echo. It should be noted that the absolute signal intensity of flow is not truly increased on even echoes. Rather, its signal is virtually identical to that of stationary fluid of the same type, except for the consequences of time-of-flight effects (inflow as well as outflow).

These observations may be explained by our expression for the phase shift of a bipolar pulse, accidentally formed for the first echo in the frequency encoding direction by the dephasing pulse, which was commonly placed just after the slice selective excitation pulse at the time, and the first half of the readout pulse.

This bipolar pulse acted to dephase signal from flowing spins destructively. A second pulse pair, with equal area and equal spacing between pulse centers, was formed by the second half and the first half of the readout gradients of the first and second echoes, respectively. However, the sense of the second bipolar pulse being opposite, it acted to cancel the dephasing caused by the first, restoring signal.

Although this effect was originally explained in terms of the spin echo sequence, it is a property of the gradient echo rather than of the rf-induced (Hahn) echo. Therefore, this principle applies equally well to gradient-echo imaging techniques. For instance, first order gradient moment nulling for constant velocity compensation es-

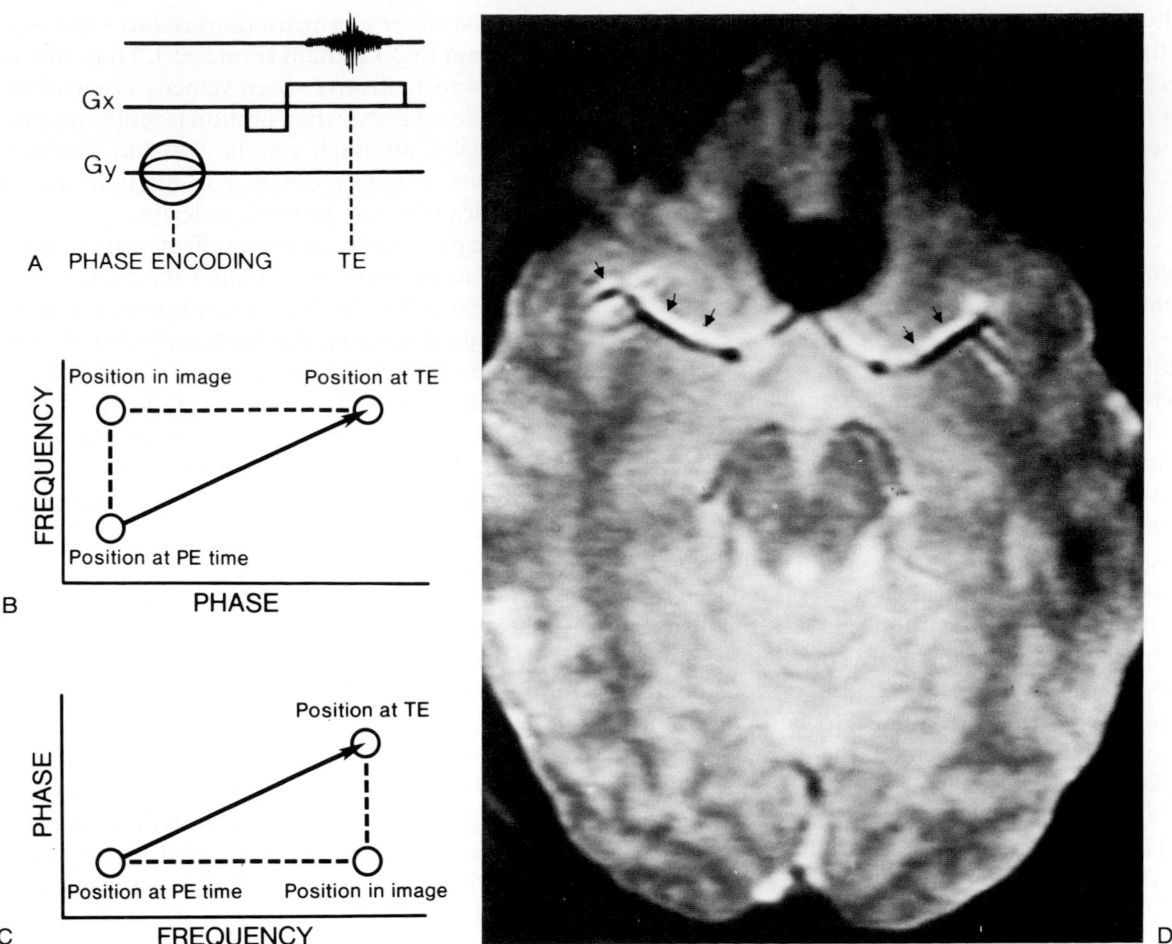

FIG. 8. Misregistration of oblique flow. The flow misregistration artifact is a consequence of the difference in time of phase encoding and frequency encoding. The phase axis is encoded at the center of the phase-encoding pulse, while frequency is encoded at the TE (**A**). If a spin moves obliquely with reference to the encoding axes during this time interval, its position is misregistered. Note that the position in the image will change if the orientation of the encoding axes is switched (**B,C**). Axial gradient-echo image (**D**) demonstrates misregistration of the high intensity from flow *(arrows)* in the middle cerebral arteries as they course obliquely.

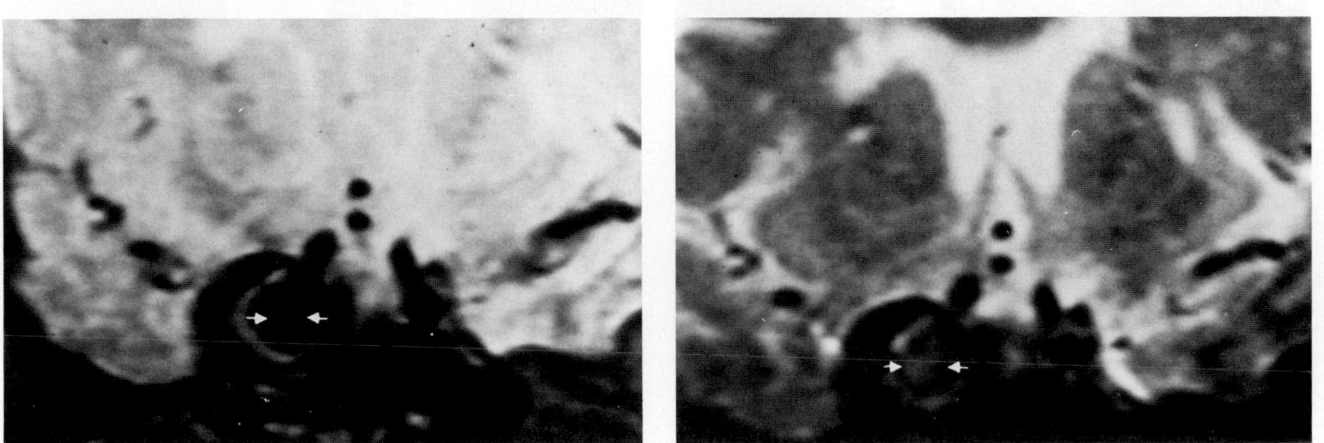

FIG. 9. Even-echo rephasing in aneurysm. Incoming flow in right cavernous carotid aneurysm (*arrows*) generates no signal on 30-msec echo (**A**), but is high intensity on 60-msec echo (**B**).

sentially amounts to the creation of an "even echo" (47) (Fig. 10). Note that the appearance of higher intensity on even echoes of a spin echo sequence, or of higher intensity on flow-compensated as compared to non-compensated sequences, can be used to imply the presence of flow.

Gradient Moment Reduction and Gradient Moment Nulling

Gradient moments of order greater than one can be nulled by additional, more complex gradient pulse waveforms. Historically, the even-echo rephasing effect is a serendipitous example of this fact. Today, most commercial systems offer gradient moment nulling by design, which can effectively be viewed as constraining the data acquisition to occur on the second echo.

The clinical utility of such sequences is reduced by the necessity of increasing the minimum TE (the higher order of moment nulling, the more complex the gradient scheme, so the longer the time required for gradient application). Furthermore, nulling of low orders of motion tends to dramatically exacerbate the higher orders. For example, a computer calculation of the second order moment of a first order-compensated sequence using a 13 msec TE generates a value of 64 radians/(mm/msec^2). Using the alternative strategy of simply offsetting the echo within the acquisition window (rather than employing first order compensation) reduces the second order moment to 2.1 radians (mm/sec^2). Thus, first order nulling is most effective when velocity is constant, but may lose effectiveness when motion is more complicated. Additionally, although systolic flow has accelerative components, second-moment contributions are usually insignificant at very short echo delays.

The most basic, and most effective method of reducing gradient moments is to reduce the area of the offending gradient pulse. There are two important examples of this in medical imaging, the fractional echo offset for the frequency-encoding gradient, and the use of 3D-volume imaging for the slice-selection gradient.

Offsetting the echo within the acquisition window toward the beginning of the frequency-encoding readout pulse reduces the area k and allows the dephasing gradient pulse to be grouped more closely to the readout gradient pulse. This is known as "asymmetric," or "partial echo" sampling. Reduction in G_1 can be proportional to the square of the offset, with one factor deriving from the decrease in area of the gradient pulse, and the other from the decrease in time interval between the centers of the dephasing gradient and the readout gradient. These maneuvers are often performed to obtain a shorter TE, and the effects of a shorter TE are occasionally confused with the effects of gradient moment reduction. However, the difference is easily demonstrated with a simple experiment in which an extended TE is used with a partial echo (Fig. 11).

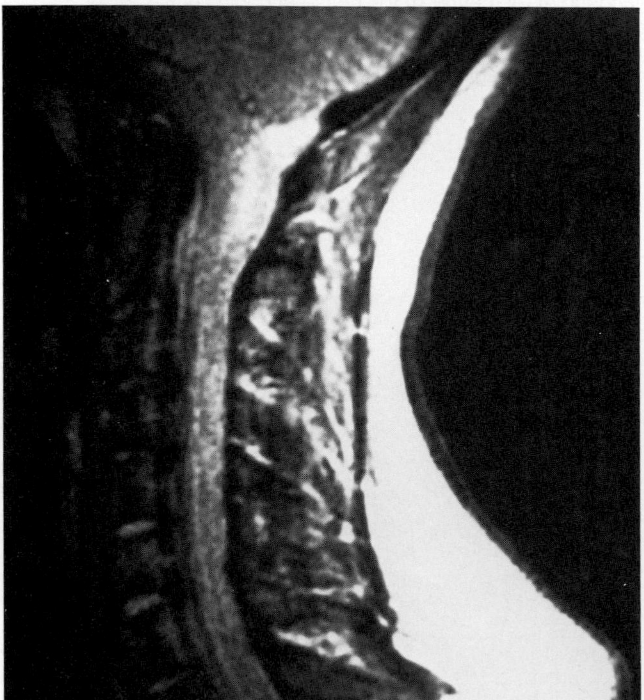

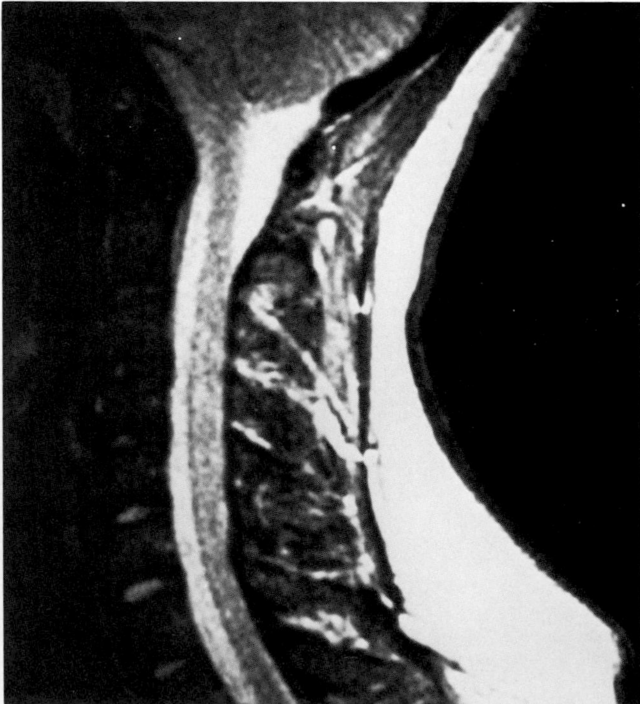

FIG. 10. First order gradient moment nulling effect on CSF flow. Long TR/long TE image of cervical spine and cord without gradient moment nulling (**A**) shows signal loss, as well as several ghost images from CSF motion, which degrade image and obscure separation of cord from CSF. Ghost images are virtually eliminated and CSF is seen as high intensity surrounding cord after gradient moment nulling (**B**).

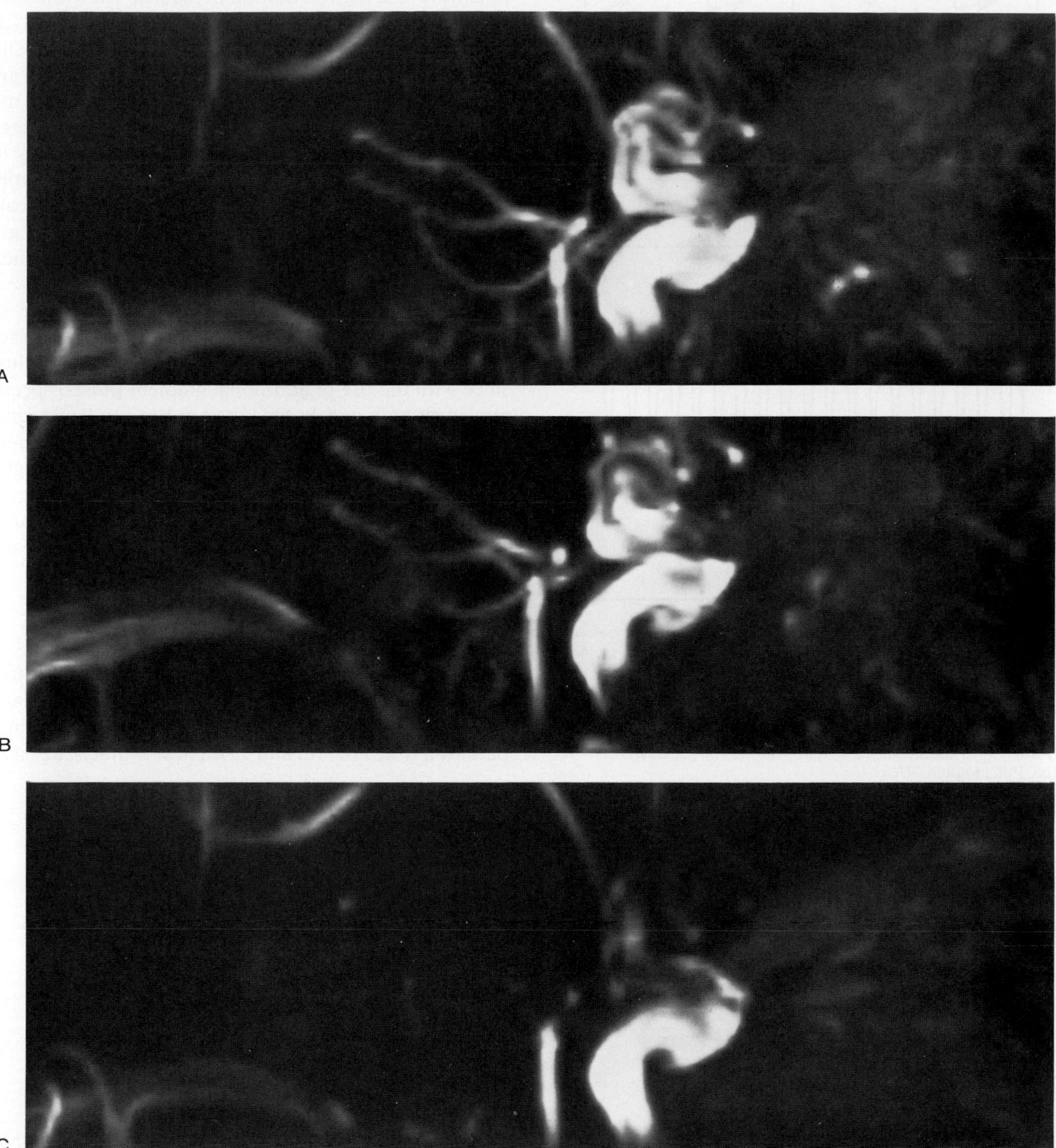

FIG. 11. Relative effects of gradient moments and TE on intravoxel phase shift-induced signal loss. **A:** MRA using TE of 6 msec with asymmetric echo sampling. **B:** MRA using TE of 12 msec with asymmetric echo sampling. **C:** MRA using TE of 12 msec with conventional symmetric echo sampling. Gradient moments play a dominant role in signal loss in MR angiography. Offset of the echo acquisition greatly reduces these moments, and is probably more important than minimizing the TE in reducing signal losses in MR angiography. On these lateral views from MR angiograms, note excellent visualization of supraclinoid carotid, anterior cerebrals, and posterior cerebral arteries using asymmetric echo sampling, regardless of TE (A,B). Using same TE as in B but with conventional echo sampling, the posterior cerebral arteries and supraclinoid carotids are not seen (C).

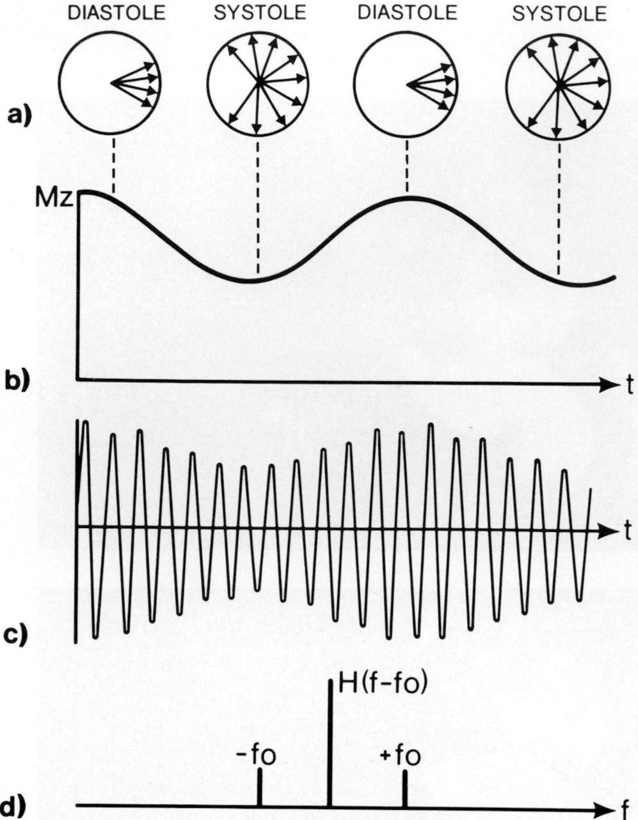

FIG. 12. Modulation of signal intensity from phase changes related to cardiac cycle. During changes in the cardiac cycle, a varying degree of phase dispersion and net phase shift occurs (**a**), causing a modulation of the longitudinal magnetization (**b**) and thus an amplitude modulation of the MR signal (**c**), which, upon Fourier transformation, results in the generation of sidebands (**d**) manifesting as displaced ghost images. (Courtesy of F. W. Wehrli, Philadelphia, PA.)

The second example highlights the fact that gradient strength for slice selection is inversely related to slice thickness. The high resolution in the slice selection direction necessary for MR angiographic techniques may be achieved by either of two extremes. The first, thin slice imaging on the order of 1.5 mm, requires maximum gradient strengths, which induce maximum gradient moments. For routine clinical use, these moments necessitate gradient moment nulling, which compensates for velocity but further extends the TE. The second, volumetric imaging, uses volumetric slab selection typically exciting slabs on the order of 30 mm. Slice-selection gradients are consequently 20 times weaker, and gradient moment nulling is virtually unnecessary.

Whatever strategy is employed, optimal pulse sequence design groups gradients together into the shortest possible total time interval. This rule is not absolute, since with the use of additional gradient pulses, specific sequences with widely separated pulses can be designed to force moments to equal zero. However, as a general rule it is quite effective, especially in reducing the higher order moments. It is anticipated that with the accelerated gradient systems now being introduced into the market by all the major manufacturers that this maneuver will enjoy a new popularity.

Ghost Images

Ghost image formation can be a troublesome artifact and commonly arises secondary to phase shifts related to periodic motion, such as respiration or cardiovascular pulsation (Figs. 10, 12, and 13). These artifacts are easily

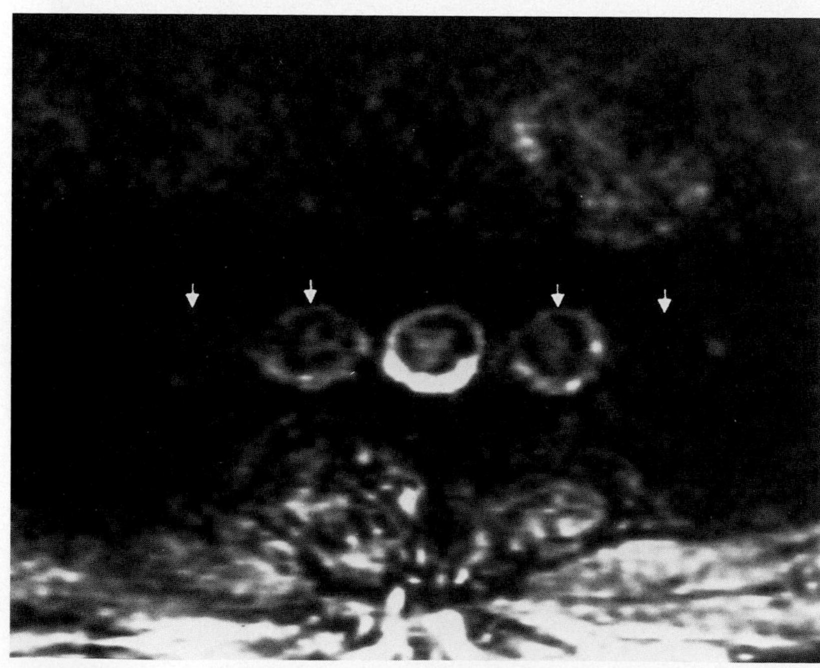

FIG. 13. Ghost images from spinal CSF motion. Ghost images *(arrows)* of high intensity CSF around spinal cord are propagated along phase-encoding axis, which is transverse in this image. Ghost images from motion of period t_p are separated by distance D, such that $D/\text{FOV} = \text{TR}/t_p$.

recognized as a series of images ("ghost images"), similar in anatomic configuration to the body part, displayed as a row of intensity along the phase-encoding axis and in line with the structure causing the artifact. The source of these motion-induced artifacts is essentially the ambiguities in the raw phase-encoding data. In the normal formation of an image, position is encoded along the phase-encoding axis by virtue of the phase-encoding gradient: the size of the phase shift imparted to the particular spin is in direct proportion to its position along the encoding gradient. During arterial pulsatile flow, for instance, the variation in flow velocity during different parts of the cardiac cycle results in displacement of spins with reference to the magnetic field gradient (phase-encoding gradient). In this situation, the phase value of a spin will be due to a combination of its phase shift corresponding to its position and that related to its movement along the gradient. The phase shift contribution due to spin movement is variable during the imaging sequence (as per the cardiac cycle), so a single, precise position of the spin will not be definable by the acquired data. Therefore, because the vector sums of these relatively narrow distributions of phase shifts still add in a coherent fashion, the signal is not attenuated, but its view-to-view variation causes mismapping of signals along the phase-encoding axis.

There are several methods of reducing the appearance of ghost image artifacts. As previously discussed, gradient waveform manipulation to null the phase shifts due to constant velocity motion can aid significantly in this endeavor, and are routinely employed in most neuroradiologic protocols (Fig. 10). Cardiac synchronization of data acquisition will effectively eliminate those artifacts related to changes in position from cardiovascular pulsation (Fig. 14), whether they are within vessels or in the CSF circulation, although it will not affect phase shift effects resulting from intravoxel velocity changes. As already noted, the degree of phase dispersion may vary between phase-encoding steps, as a direct result of variations in fluid velocity profiles during the normal cardiac cycle. As velocity increases during systole, phase dispersion increases across the voxel, whereas in diastole, the decreases in flow velocity corresponds to a reduction in the velocity spread within the voxel. View-to-view amplitude modulation of the net magnetization vector from a voxel results from this phase dispersion. The relationship of flow velocity and signal to the cardiac cycle also causes phase-related ghost images to occur. Cardiac pulsation-induced phase shifts occur when the TR is not an integral of the pulsation period (the R-R interval). According to the Fourier transformation frequency-shift theorem, the modulation that occurs in the time domain with this type of flow causes a frequency shift in the Fourier transform, so that multiple "sidebands" arise separated from the true "baseband" Fourier representation that would have been present in the absence of such motion. These sidebands are represented as phase-shift images (ghost images) whose displacement from the origin of the artifact is related to the frequency difference be-

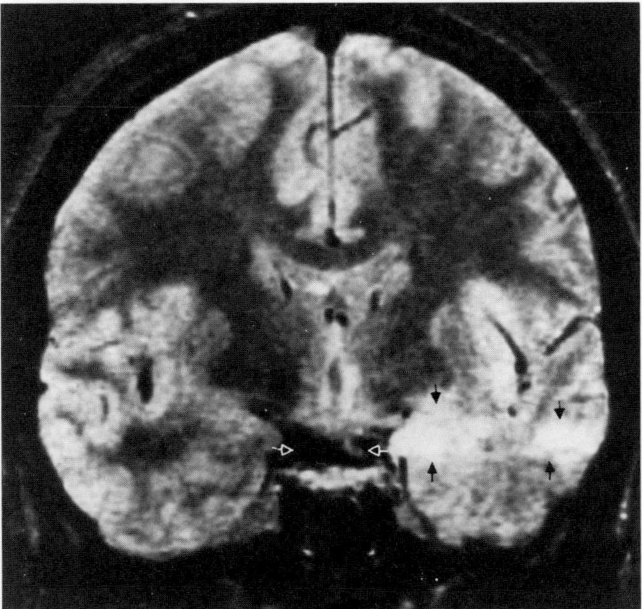
A

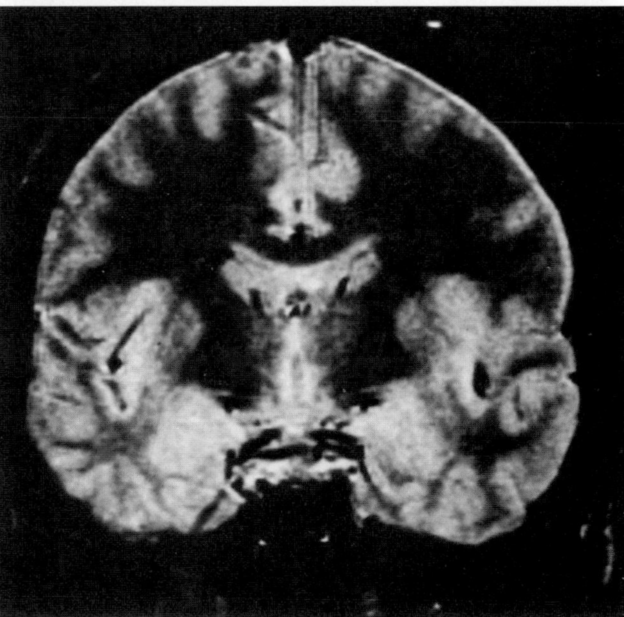
B

FIG. 14. Effectiveness of cardiac gating on image quality. Nongated coronal image through temporal lobes (**A**) shows regions of high intensity in left temporal lobe (*closed arrows,* A) and poor definition of suprasellar cistern due to signal loss (*open arrows,* A). With cardiac gating (**B**), the left temporal lobe is now normal, and the structures within the suprasellar cistern are clearly defined.

tween the heart rate (in the case of artifacts due to cardiac pulsation) and the TR (44,48) (Figs. 12 and 13).

As previously stated, gradient moment nulling will reduce the view-to-view intensity variations from phase dispersion, but it will not correct intensity changes due to inflow effects (Fig. 15). A different method of eliminating phase ghosts is based on reducing signal from the entry of unsaturated spins into the imaging volume. This method utilizes additional preparation pulses (49) to selectively saturate spins located outside the imaging volume (Fig. 16). It is applicable to the reduction of flow artifacts if one excites spins in the region where moving spins originate before they enter into the imaging volume, so that they are saturated as they flow into the slice of interest. Regardless of the degree of phase modulation, phase mismapping cannot result from flowing spins if the incoming spins generate no signal. Note that the application of these pre-saturation pulses will also eliminate (or reduce) all flow effects related to the inflow of magnetized spins, including the previously described high intensity of "flow-related enhancement." The utilization of presaturation pulses is perhaps most useful in the discrimination between slow flow and intravascular thrombus, both of which can be depicted as high signal intensity on conventional spin echo images, as well as on gradient-echo images.

FLOW DETECTION AND DIFFUSION TECHNIQUES

Time of Flight and Bolus Contrast Methods

Time-of-flight and phase-shift effects related to flow as discussed above, although initially considered only in terms of their interference with image interpretation, can be exploited, so that both qualitative and quantitative information about the state of flow can be gleaned from MRI. Although there are a wide variety of techniques which can accomplish the general goal of flow detection, all of these methods share certain methodologic features and limitations. The techniques can be simply divided along the same categories used for discussing basic flow effects: detection methods based on the detection of longitudinal magnetization and time-of-flight effects, and methods mainly concerned with the detection of phase changes due to flow.

Phase Mapping

As we have seen, a bipolar pulse imparts a phase shift to moving spins which is independent of their position by proportional to their velocity:

$$\Theta = G_1 \cdot v_z = (\Delta\tau/\lambda)v_z = v_z/V_z, \quad [22]$$

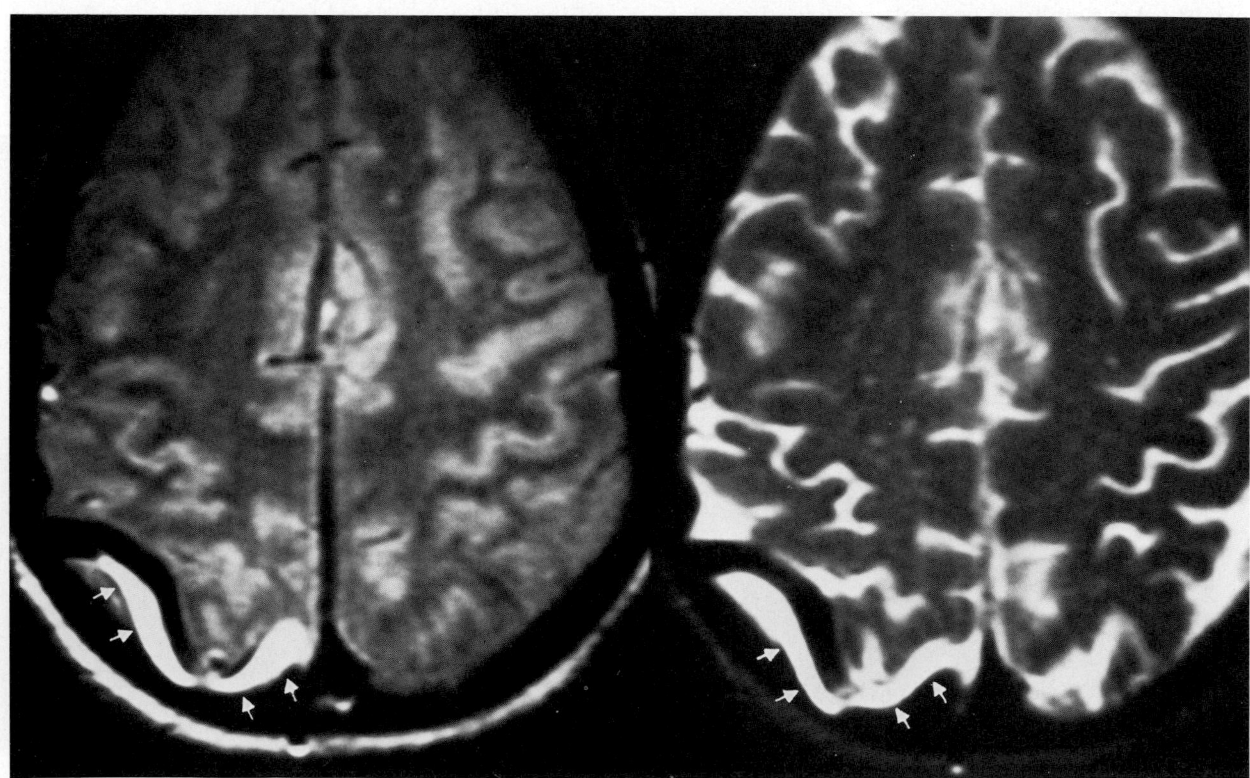

FIG. 15. First order gradient moment nulling with additional inflow effects causing high signal intensity in venous flow. Intravascular signal is high intensity in the large right parietal cortical vein (*arrows*, **A,B**) due to the combined effects of gradient moment nulling and inflow of fully magnetized spins. Also note misregistration due to obliquity of flow.

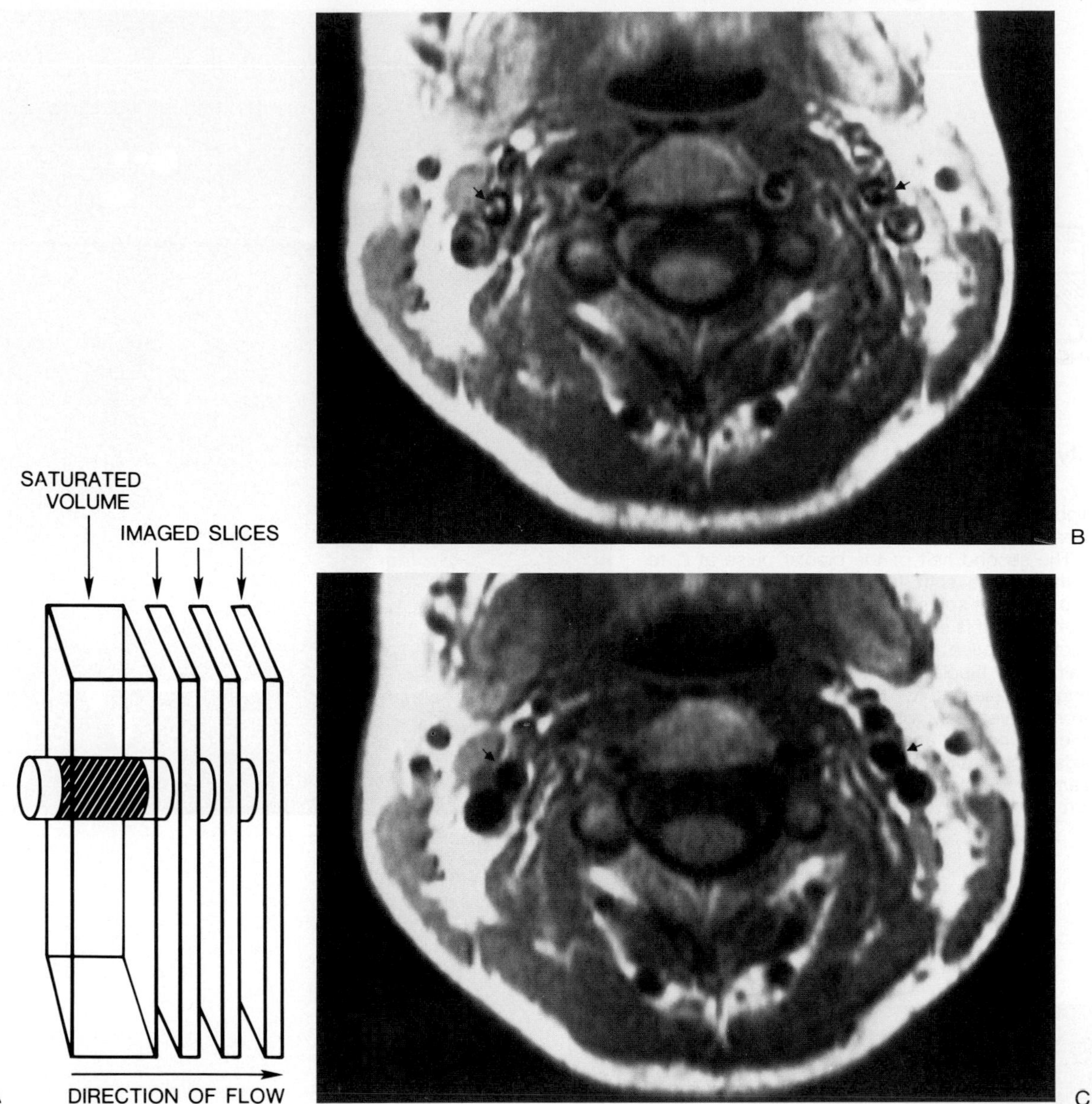

FIG. 16. A: Excitatory rf pulse is applied to volume outside region of interest and followed by a dephasing gradient pulse. Flow moving into region of interest generates no signal, since these spins are saturated. **B,C:** Axial images through neck show mixed signal in carotid arteries without saturation pulse (*arrows,* B) and absence of intraluminal signal in carotid arteries (*arrows,* C) after presaturation pulse was applied inferior to imaged volume.

where $V_z = \lambda/\Delta\tau$. Intuitively speaking, a single gradient pulse probes the position of the spin at the time center of the pulse, while two pulses of opposite sign (bipolar pulses) probe the relative motion traveled between their centers. From the Fourier point of view, phase shift can be analyzed as a new Fourier parameter pair, ν_z and $1/V_z$.

Regularly incrementing the gradient strength of the bipolar pulse pair will encode the phase proportional to velocity. A Fourier transformation will now assign intensity along a velocity axis (Fig. 17). This approach was first proposed by Moran (50) and has been implemented by several groups (3,51). This technique has potential to provide information regarding velocity distributions and to document reverse flow in the presence of antegrade flow.

Alternatively, the phase of Equation 14 may be fixed by a constant bipolar gradient pulse. As our discussion above shows, this constant phase can be used to generate a phase image calculated from the complex pixel values, which produce average velocity (7,52) (Fig. 18). Note that too large of a phase shift can result in aliasing of velocities, so that large positive velocities appear as large negative velocities. This restricts pulse sequence parameters so that the phase shift must be $-180° \leq \Theta \leq +180°$. Such a phase map can be used to quantitate total flow

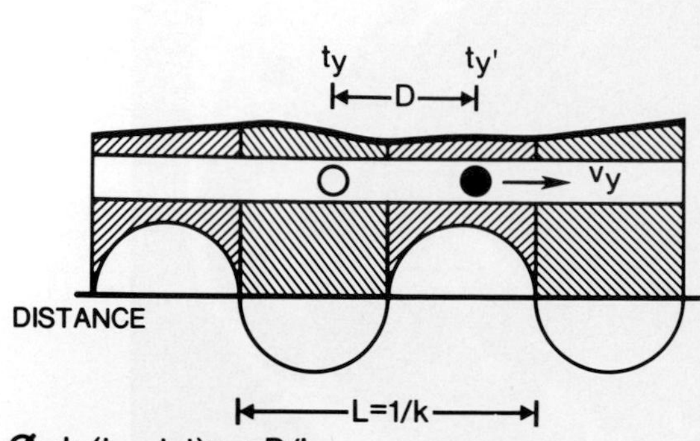

$\emptyset = k\,(ty - ty')vy = D/L$

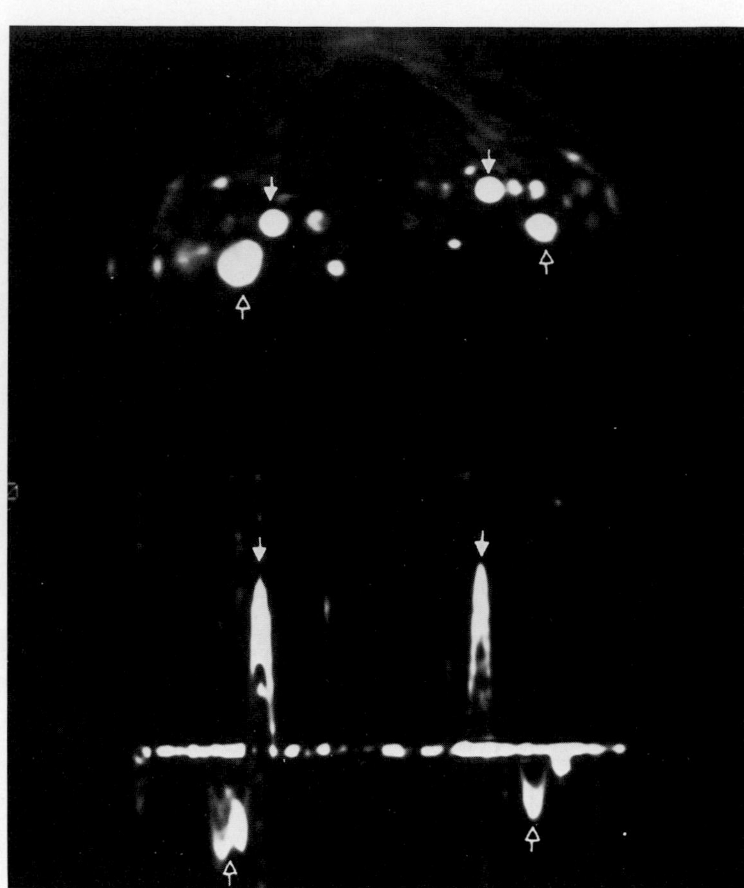

FIG. 17. Phase encoding of velocity. **A:** The first half of a bipolar gradient pulse at t_y imparts a position-dependent phase shift with a characteristic wavelength. The second half of the bipolar pulse at t'_y reverses that phase shift for stationary spins, but is unable to do so for spins that have moved with velocity v_y. The phase shift is equal to the ratio of the difference in position D relative to position at the application of each half of the bipolar gradient pulse divided by the wavelength L (see text). **B:** Velocity spectroscopy through neck vessels, with horizontal (left–right) frequency-encoding axis and vertical phase-encoding velocity axis (cephalad flow in carotid arteries indicated by *closed arrows,* caudad flow in jugular veins indicated by *open arrows*).

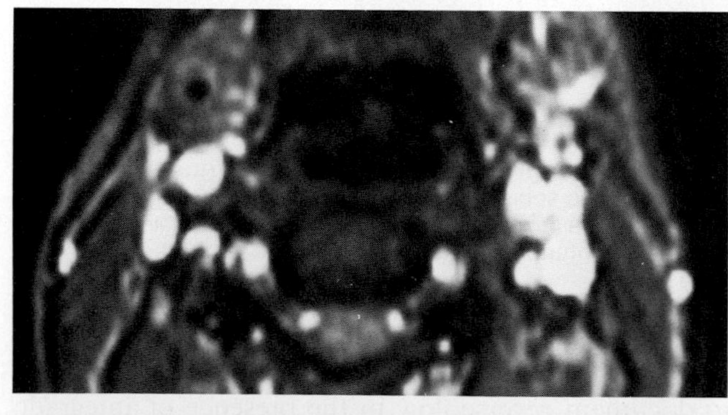

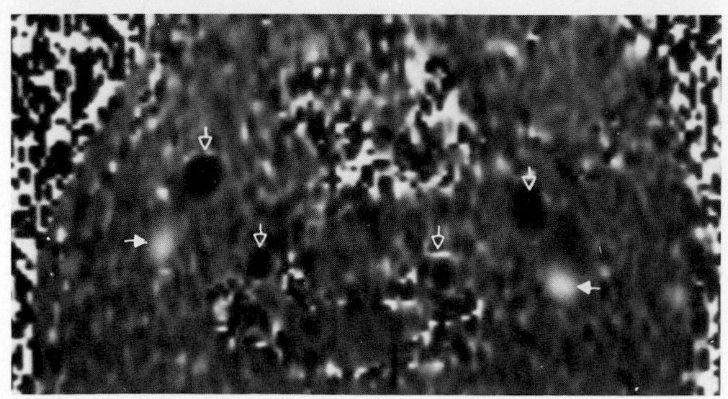

FIG. 18. Phase-contrast map of flow velocities. **A:** Gradient-echo axial image of great vessels in neck. **B:** Phase map at same slice location as **A**, where average velocity in caudal direction is proportional to signal intensity. Note signal void in carotid and vertebral arteries *(open arrows)* and high intensity in jugular veins *(closed arrows)*. (VINNIE image in B courtesy of Norbert Pelc, Sc.D.)

through a vessel by summing velocities over the cross-sectional area (52). These total flow measurements are robust, even when the angle of flow deviates from being exactly perpendicular to the slice.

Another way to detect and measure flow is by application of narrow bands of saturation to the region being imaged, prior to the actual imaging sequence. The saturated regions will appear as stationary dark stripes in regions that are stationary, including thrombi, but will be displaced or even wash out in regions of flowing blood or CSF. Such tagged regions can be created either individually with conventional selective rf pulses (53), or multiply with suitable combinations of nonselective rf pulses and gradient pulses creating spatial modulation of magnetization (SPAMM) (54,55) (Fig. 19).

Diffusion Imaging

The bipolar gradient pulse has been successfully used to detect very slow motion and even diffusion over distances as small as a few microns. In fact, the noninvasive nature of MRI makes it one of the best methods available for quantitating diffusion. In diffusion imaging, after applying an initial very large gradient pulse of area $K = 1/\lambda$ to the excited spins, which imparts a phase modulation of very small wavelength, we wait a time to allow spins to randomly diffuse away from their initial positions (56,57). After the time $\Delta\tau$ has elapsed, the reverse pulse is applied, which rephases stationary spins. However, the diffusing spins remain dephased to the extent that they have drifted in the direction of the gradient.

Classically, diffusion is described by a gaussian distribution, with variance $\sigma^2 = 2D \cdot \Delta\tau$, where the diffusion constant D for water equals 2.5×10^{-5} cm^2/sec. In the limit that each bipolar pulse is infinitely narrow, the classic expression for the loss of signal from the ideal intensity I_0 can be shown to be equal to:

$$I = I_0 \exp\{-(\sigma/\lambda)^2\}. \quad [23]$$

(The exponential term must be scaled down for gradient pulses of finite width).

For example, a spin in water has a standard deviation of 5 microns in 5 msec, 10 microns in 20 msec, and 25 microns in 125 msec. To obtain significant dephasing, we require L to be of these orders. Thus, for a gradient pulse of 50 Gauss/cm applied for 5 msec, a wavelength of 10 microns is obtained (note that conventional gradient pulses are approximately 1 Gauss/cm).

In highly ordered biological structures, such as the corpus callosum, diffusion may be restricted in one direction and not in another. Signal loss from diffusion will be greatest when the gradient is directed parallel to the orientation of the fibers (i.e., the direction of diffusion), and least when directed perpendicular. It is conceivable that cellular membranes form diffusional barriers, but the extent of these barriers varies from tissue to tissue.

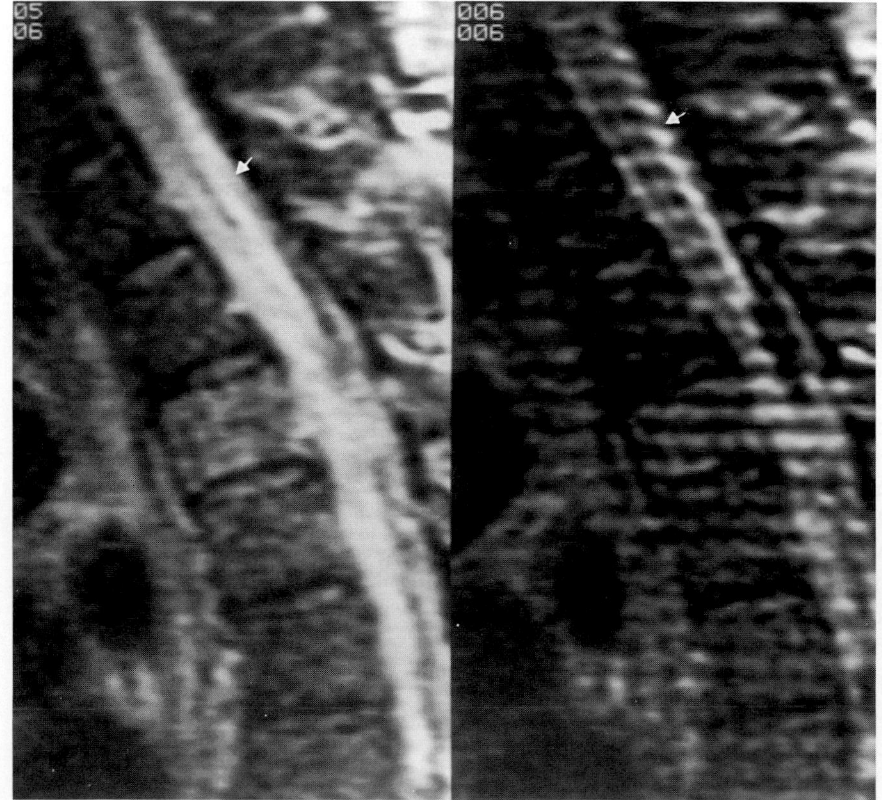

FIG. 19. SPAMM image showing CSF motion. Conventional cardiac-gated sagittal spin-echo image (**A**) of thoracic spine (2,770/70) obtained 182 msec after the R-wave shows increased intensity from CSF (*arrow,* A). Image obtained with SPAMM sequence (**B**) shows downward displacement of stripes due to motion of CSF (*arrow,* B). (From Axel and Dougherty, ref. 54.)

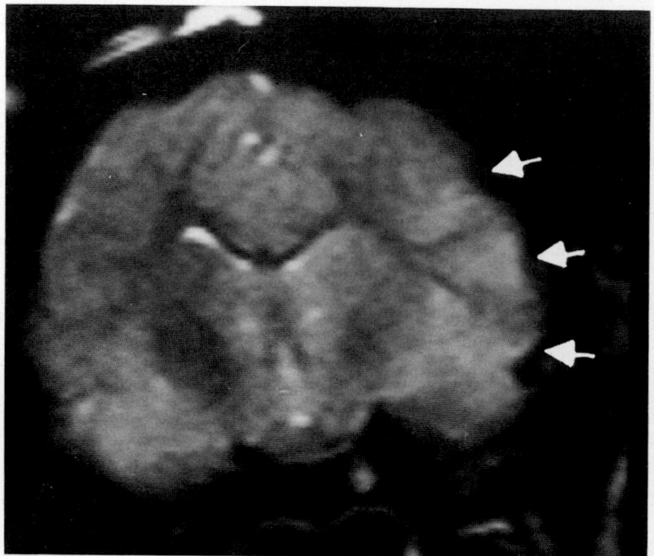

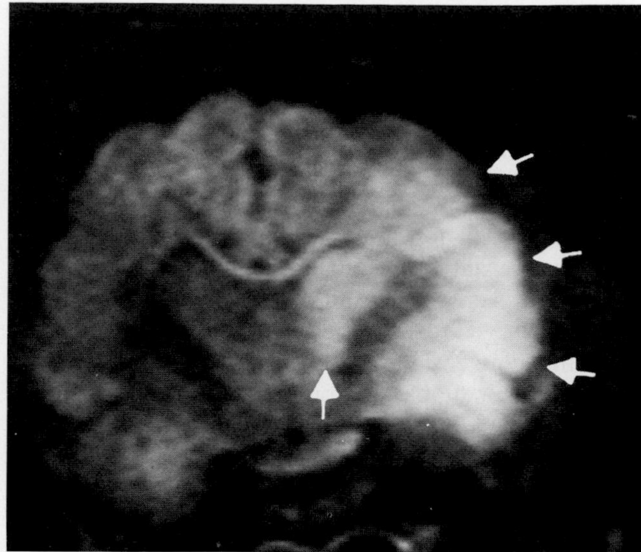

FIG. 20. Acute arterial occlusion producing perfusion deficit, "diffusion-weighted" image vs. spin-echo image. Long TR/TE spin-echo image (**A**) at 1 hour after occlusion of left middle cerebral artery has only subtle abnormal hyperintensity in distribution of occluded vessel (*arrows,* A). "Diffusion-weighted" image (**B**) shows marked hyperintensity in area of decreased perfusion at same time (*arrows,* B) possibly due to restriction of micromotion of spins in ischemic tissue. (From Moseley et al., ref. 58.)

The red blood cell membrane, for example, offers little if any impediment to the diffusion of water.

At this point in time, there is considerable controversy over whether diffusion imaging techniques are applicable to conventional imaging systems. The two major problems are limited gradient strength in whole body imaging systems and micro-motion in the living animal. Since the intensity depends on the square of the gradient pulse area, and the conventional imaging gradient is 50 times less than the above example, pulse lengths must be correspondingly longer. Diffusion imaging has been shown to be feasible in animals by Moseley (58) (Fig. 20). Future directions in diffusion imaging probably will hinge on ultra-rapid imaging techniques (59) to minimize patient-generated motion (see Chapter 29).

CONCLUSIONS

Flow phenomena on MR images present a wide variety of artifacts and represent a source of previously unavailable physiological information. Because of the increasing understanding of the basis of flow effects on MRI, techniques have been developed to overcome the majority of flow artifacts. This understanding has also led to improved pulse sequences to exploit changes related to the presence of flow. Continued software and hardware development will certainly improve flow imaging techniques, but the final clinical role of these sequences remains to be elucidated.

REFERENCES

1. Singer JR. Blood flow rates by nuclear magnetic resonance. *Science* 1959;130:1652–1653.
2. Hahn EL. Detection of sea-water motion by nuclear precession. *J Geophys Res* 1960;65:776–777.
3. Wedeen VJ, Rosen BR, Chesler D, Brady TH. MR velocity imaging by phase display. *J Comput Assist Tomogr* 1985;9:530–536.
4. Dumoulin CL, Hart HR. Magnetic resonance angiography. *Radiology* 1986;161:717–720.
5. Dumoulin CL, Souza SP, Hart HR. Rapid scan magnetic resonance angiography. *Magn Reson Imaging* 1987;5:238–245.
6. Wehrli FW, Shimakawa A, Gullberg GT, MacFall JR. Time-of-flight MR flow imaging: selective saturation recovery with gradient refocusing. *Radiology* 1986;160:781–785.
7. Nayler GL, Firmin GL, Longmore DB. Blood flow imaging by cine magnetic resonance. *J Comput Assist Tomogr* 1986;10:715.
8. Firmin DN, Nayler GL, Underwood SR, Klipstein RH, Rees SRO, Longmore DB. MR angiography, flow velocity, and acceleration measurements combined using a field even-echo rephasing (FEER) sequence. Chicago; 1986:127.
9. Masaryk TJ, Ross JS, Modic MT, Lenz GW, Haacke EM. Carotid bifurcation: MR imaging: work in progress. *Radiology* 1988;166:461–466.
10. McDonald DA. *Blood Flow in Arteries,* 2nd ed. Baltimore: Williams and Wilkins; 1974.
11. Spagnoli MV, Goldberg HI, Grossman RI, Bilaniuk LT, Gomori JM, Hackney DB, Zimmerman RA. Intracranial meningiomas: high-field MR imaging. *Radiology* 186;161:369–375.
12. Motomyia M, Karino T. Flow patterns in the human carotid artery bifurcation. *Stroke* 1984;15:50–56.
13. Elster AD, Challa VR, Gilbert TH, Richardson DN, Contento JC. Meningiomas: MR and histopathologic features. *Radiology* 1989;170:857–862.
14. Kwang SK, Rogers LF, Lee C. The dural lucent line: characteristic sign of hyperostosing meningioma en plaque. *AJR* 1983;141:1217–1221.
15. Rosenbaum AE, Rosenbloom SB. Meningiomas revisited. *Semin Roentgenol* 1984;19:8–26.

16. Bharadvha BK, Mabon RF, Giddons DP. Steady flow in a model of the human carotid bifurcation. Part I. Flow visualization. *J Biomech* 1982; 15:349–362.
17. New PFJ, Aronow S, Hesselink JR. National Cancer Institute Study: evaluation of computed tomography in the diagnosis of intracranial neoplasms. IV. Meningiomas. *Radiology* 1980; 136: 665–675.
18. Som PM, Sacher M, Strenger SW, Biller HF, Malis LI. "Benign" metastasizing meningiomas. *AJNR* 1987; 8:127–130.
19. Guidetti B, Ciappetta P, Domenicucci M. Tentorial meningiomas: surgical experience with 51 cases and long-term results. *J Neurosurg* 1988; 69:183–187.
20. Roelvink NCA, Kamphorst W, van Alphen HAM, Rao BR. Pregnancy-related primary brain and spinal tumors. *Arch Neurol* 1987; 44:209–215.
21. Dyste GN, Hitchon PW, Menezes AH, Van Gilder JC, Greene GM. Stereotaxic surgery in the treatment of multiple brain abscesses. *J Neurosurg* 1988; 69:188–194.
22. Hochberg FH, Miller DC. Primary central nervous system lymphoma. *J Neurosurg* 1988; 68:835–853.
23. Jack CR Jr, O'Neill BP, Banks PM, Reese DF. Central nervous system lymphoma: histologic types and CT appearance. *Radiology* 1988; 167:211–215.
24. Dewey CF Jr, Bussolari SR, Gimbrone MA Jr, Davies PF. The dynamic response of vascular endothelial cells to fluid shear stress. *J Biomech Eng* 1981; 103:177–185.
25. Poon T, Matoso I, Tchertkoff V, Weitzner I Jr, Gade M. CT features of primary cerebral lymphoma in AIDS and non-AIDS patients. *J Comput Assist Tomogr* 1989; 13:6–9.
26. Weingarten KL, Zimmerman RD, Leeds NE. Spontaneous regression of intracerebral lymphoma. *Radiology* 1983; 149:721–724.
27. Kerr RSC, Hughes JT, Blamires T, Teddy PJ. Lymphomatoid granulomatosis apparently confined to one temporal lobe. *J Neurosurg* 1987; 67:612–615.
28. Motomiya M, Karino T. Flow patterns in the human carotid artery. *Stroke* 1984; 15:50–56.
29. Farthing SP, Peronneau P. Flow in the thoracic aorta. *Cardiovasc Res* 1979; 13:607–620.
30. Haacke EM, Lenz GW. Improving image quality in the presence of motion by using rephasing gradients. *AJR* 1987; 148:1251–1258.
31. Lenz GW, Haacke EM, Masaryk TJ, Laub G. In plane vascular imaging: pulse sequence design and strategy. *Radiology* 1988; 166: 875–882.
32. Caro CG, Fitz-Gerald JM, Schroter RC. Observation, correlation, and proposal of a shear-dependent mass transfer mechanism of atherogenesis. *Proc R Soc London B Biol Sci* 1971; B177:109–159.
33. Kapila A, Gupta KL, Garcia JH. CT and MR of lymphomatoid granulomatosis of the CNS: report of four cases and review of the literature. *AJNR* 1988; 9:1139–1143.
34. Greco A, Jelliffe AM, Maher EJ, Leung AWL. MR imaging of lymphomas: Impact on therapy. *J Comput Assist Tomogr* 1988; 12: 785–791.
35. Bradley WG, Waluch V, Lai K, et al. Appearance of rapidly flowing blood on magnetic resonance imaging. *AJR* 1984; 143:1167–1174.
36. Bird RB, Stewart WE, Lightfoot N. *Transport Phenomena*. New York: John Wiley; 1960.
37. Sze G, Shin J, Krol G, Johnson C, Liu D, Deck MDF. Intraparenchymal brain metastases: MR imaging versus contrast-enhanced CT. *Radiology* 1988; 168:187–194.
38. von Schulthess GK, Higgins CB. Blood flow imaging with MR: Spin-phase phenomena. *Radiology* 1985; 157:687–695.
39. Russell EJ, Geremia GK, Johnson CE, et al. Multiple cerebral metastases: detectability with Gd-DTPA-enhanced MR imaging. *Radiology* 1987; 165:609–617.
40. Healy ME, Hesselink JR, Press GA, Middleton MS. Increased detection of intracranial metastases with intravenous Gd-DTPA. *Radiology* 1987; 165:619–624.
41. Bradley WG, Waluch V. Blood flow: magnetic resonance imaging. *Radiology* 1985; 154:443–450.
42. Fram EK, Dimick R, Hedlund LW, et al. Parameters determining the signal of flowing fluid in gradient refocused MR imaging: flow velocity, TR and flip angle. Montreal:1986; 84–85.
43. Haacke EM, Lenz GW, Nelson AD. Pseudo-gating: elimination of periodic motion artifacts in magnetic resonance imaging without gating. *Magn Reson Med* 1987; 4:162–174.
44. Rubin JB, Enzmann DR. Harmonic modulation of proton MR precessional phase by pulsatile motion: origin of spinal CSF flow phenomena. *AJNR* 1987; 8:307–318.
45. Rubin JB, Enzmann DR. Imaging of spinal CSF pulsation by 2DFT MR: Significance during clinical imaging. *AJNR* 1987; 8: 297–306.
46. Waluch V, Bradley WG. NMR even-echo rephasing in slow laminar flow. *J Comput Assist Tomogr* 1984; 4:594–598.
47. Pattany PM, Marino R, McNally JM. Velocity and acceleration correction in 2DFT MR imaging. *Magn Reson Imaging* 1986; 4: 154–155.
48. Bracewell RN. *The Fourier Transform and its Applications*. New York: McGraw Hill; 1978.
49. Felmlee JP, Ehman RL. Spatial presaturation: a method for suppressing flow artifacts and improving depiction of vascular anatomy in MR imaging. *Radiology* 1987; 164:559-564.
50. Moran PR. A flow velocity zeugmatographic interlace for NMR imaging in humans. *Magn Reson Imaging* 1982; 1:197–203.
51. Wehrli FW, Listerud J, Chao P, Goldberg HI. A cine bolus tracking technique for quantification of flow velocity and volume flow in arteries. Amsterdam: 1989: 100.
52. Pelc NJ, Shimakawa A, Glover GH. *Phase Contrast Cine MRI*. Amsterdam: 1989; 101.
53. Edelman RR, Mattle HP, Kleefield J, Silver MS. Quantification of blood flow with dynamic MR imaging and presaturation bolus tracking. *Radiology* 1989; 171:551–556.
54. Axel L, Dougherty L. MR imaging of motion with spatial modulation of magnetization. *Radiology* 1989; 171:841–845.
55. Axel L, Dougherty L. Heart wall motion: improved method of spatial modulation of magnetization for MR imaging. *Radiology* 1989; 172:349–350.
56. Le Bihan D, Breton E, Lallemand D, et al. MR imaging of intravoxel incoherent motions: application to diffusion and perfusion in neurologic disorders. *Radiology* 1986; 161:401–407.
57. Young IR, Hall AS, Bryant DJ, et al. Assessment of brain perfusion with MR imaging. *J Comput Assist Tomogr* 1988; 12:721–727.
58. Moseley ME, Kucharczyk J, Mintorovitch J, et al. Diffusion-weighted MR imaging of acute stroke: correlation with T2-weighted and magnetic susceptibility-enhanced MR imaging in cats. *AJNR* 1990; 11:423–429.
59. Rosen BR, Belliveau JH, Chien D. Perfusion imaging by nuclear magnetic resonance. *Magn Reson Q* 1989; 5:263–281.

Magnetic Resonance Imaging of the Brain and Spine, Second Edition, edited by Scott W. Atlas.
Lippincott-Raven Publishers, Philadelphia © 1996.

5

Contrast Agents and Relaxation Effects

John C. Gore and Richard P. Kennan

In most clinical applications of MRI the differences of intrinsic nuclear magnetic resonance properties (relaxation times or proton density) between adjacent tissues are great enough so that, by appropriate choice of pulse sequence, neighboring structures can be distinguished and the resultant image contrast is sufficient for diagnostic purposes. Contrast in NMR images arises mainly from the heterogeneous distribution of tissue relaxation times, and the lack of need for contrast materials in many important applications is one of the major advantages of MRI over x-ray techniques. There nonetheless remain other important areas in which administration of an external contrast agent is essential; to differentiate structures, to provide additional specificity in describing regions of abnormal signal, to opacify or highlight spaces, or to depict tissue vascularity and perfusion. Consequently, there has been considerable activity for many years to develop agents that, when introduced into the body, alter the NMR signals from tissues for a variety of clinical purposes, though the range and type of products approved for use in 1995 is still small. In common with other modalities, MRI contrast agents must satisfy a number of constraints, not simply that of producing a large effect in an imaging study. There are requirements that are determined by the particular clinical application. The materials must be of low or tolerable toxicity, be biocompatible, have the desirable form (e.g., for gastrointestinal use, as opposed to intravenous use), have the desired excretion pathway, and where possible be targeted with an appropriate organ specificity. These design features are all important, but will not be discussed much further in this chapter. Some have been addressed in the development of agents for other modalities, so that little new work has been done or been necessary specifically for the development of MR agents. Instead, we will concentrate solely on the underlying mechanisms of action that determine the efficacy of an agent as a contrast material in MR imaging. We will emphasize the physical principles that affect the mode of action of MR contrast agents, and consider other design factors only as they affect the fundamental efficacy of the basic interaction. That such design factors impact on the in vivo efficacy is itself a unique feature of MR contrast agents that distinguishes them from x-ray or nuclear markers. We will also illustrate how physiological and structural properties of tissue can affect the relaxation efficacy of MR contrast agents in ways that are unique to this modality and which can complicate the interpretation of MRI signals following contrast administrations. Rather than discuss a range of applications or potential agents, we will concentrate in detail on the design and reasons for the selection of the small number of materials that are in clinical use already, with special emphasis on explaining and rationalizing the choices of gadolinium-DTPA and similar compounds, and superparamagnetic iron oxide as practical agents.

In any NMR image the signal intensity at a given location depends on a combination of different factors: there may be several different proton populations present (such as fat and water) each with its own proton density M_o, relaxation times T1 and T2; there may be intrinsic variations in the magnetic susceptibility; and perhaps as-

J. C. Gore, Ph.D., and R. P. Kennan, Ph.D.: Department of Diagnostic Radiology, Yale University School of Medicine, New Haven, CT 06510.

sociated field gradients. Good contrast is obtained between different regions when these intrinsic properties vary, e.g., when T1 is longer in gray matter than white matter. In spin-echo imaging, the primary determinants of contrast are the relaxation times alone, so it is natural to design contrast agents that attempt to modify T1 or T2. Another important factor is that it is usually difficult and dangerous to significantly alter proton density, though simple liquids can be used to fill spaces in the GI tract. Thus a useful prelude to a consideration of the design of contrast agents is first to review the factors that determine T1 and T2 in tissues, which can be described using a qualitative theory of NMR relaxation.

RELAXATION THEORY IN SOLUTIONS

First, consider some underlying basic concepts of nuclear magnetization and magnetic resonance. Each hydrogen nucleus (proton) may be considered to possess spin which in turn gives rise to a magnetic dipole moment, so that it can be considered like a small bar magnet with separate poles. When a large number of such magnetic nuclei are placed in an external magnetic field they tend to align themselves in the direction of the field. Quantum theory constrains the nuclear magnetic energy states to be quantized, viz. only some energy states are permitted, analogous to the behavior of electrons orbiting the nucleus in shells. For protons in a magnetic field, this results in only two orientations of the nuclear magnet relative to the field direction being allowed, which we can naively describe as parallel and anti-parallel to the magnetic field. These two states correspond to two allowed energy levels (Fig. 1A). Since the aligned position corresponds to a lower energy level, a slightly larger number of protons populate this energy level, and they produce a net magnetization in the direction of the field.

The populations of the two energy levels in equilibrium depend on the energy difference between them, ΔE, which is proportional to $\mathbf{B}_o$, the static applied field strength. ΔE is in practice very small. For example, for protons in a magnetic field of 1 Tesla (T), ΔE is only 1.76×10^{-7} eV, which is an insignificant energy difference on the chemical or molecular scale. Since the energy difference is so small, the preference for taking one alignment rather than the other is also very weak, so that the difference in numbers of spins pointing up rather than down is very small (about 1 in a million).

NMR experiments involve inducing transitions between the two energy levels by absorption or emission of quanta with energy ΔE, which is analogous to the transitions of electrons between orbits in an atom. In the presence of not only a static field but also of an additional alternating field of frequency ω_o, where ω_o satisfies the relation

$$\Delta E = h\omega_o$$

and h = Planck's constant, the spin system absorbs energy so that the population of the upper energy level increases while that of the lower level decreases (Fig. 1B). Since only radiation of a precisely defined frequency (the Larmor frequency) is effective, the process is called a resonant process. For hydrogen nuclei in a field of 1 T, ω_o is 42.6 MHz, which is a radiofrequency field. If the energy absorbed is sufficient to equalize the populations of the two levels, saturation is said to have occurred, and no further absorption will take place. A completely or a partially saturated system will return to equilibrium because of two simultaneous processes. First, the absorbed energy will be redistributed within the spin system by processes in which every transition of a nucleus from a higher to a lower level is accompanied by a transition of a nucleus from the lower to the higher state, the process called spin-spin relaxation. Second, there will be a gradual loss of energy to the other nuclei and electrons in the material, collectively called the lattice, resulting from

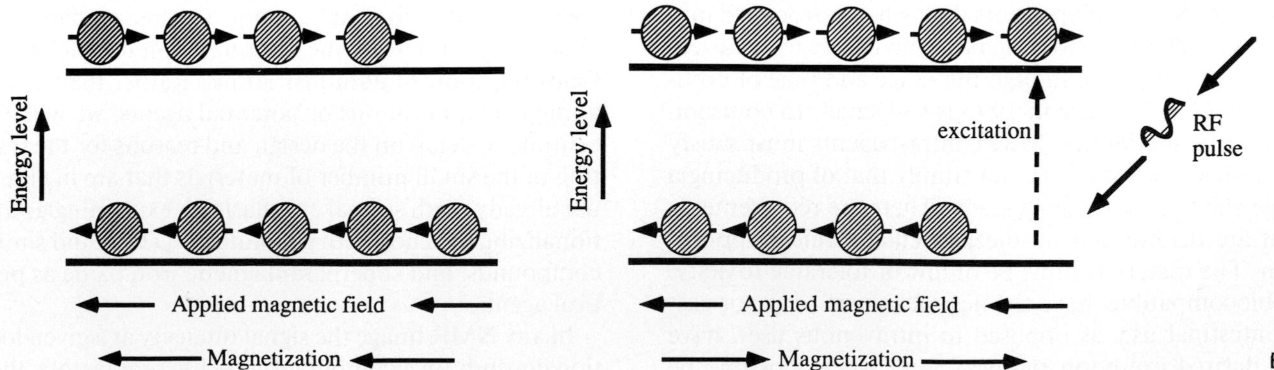

FIG. 1A: Protons are spin $\frac{1}{2}$ nuclei so that they may occupy one of only two allowed energy levels that correspond to two different orientations in the applied field. In equilibrium, the lower energy level is preferred so more nuclei align with the field than in the opposite sense. **B:** The energy difference between the two levels corresponds to a discrete transition that can be excited by absorption of a quantum of energy of precisely the right size. This corresponds in NMR to a radiofrequency excitation.

transitions of nuclei from the upper to the lower state. This second process is spin-lattice relaxation. The time constants characterizing these two processes are T2 and Tl, respectively, the spin-spin (or transverse) and spin-lattice (or longitudinal) relaxation times.

The time constants T1 and T2 yield valuable information about the local interactions experienced by nuclei. T1 describes the rate at which a nonequilibrium spin distribution exponentially approaches equilibrium following absorption of rf energy. However an excited nuclear spin does not spontaneously lose its energy but relies almost entirely on interaction with the surrounding material. Spin-lattice relaxation, where the lattice is the environment surrounding the nucleus, and includes the remainder of the host molecule as well as other solute and solvent molecules, occurs because of interactions of the excited nuclear spin dipole with the random fluctuating magnetic fields that exist on an atomic scale inside tissues. These originate from neighboring nuclei and are modulated by the motion of other surrounding dipoles in the lattice which have components fluctuating with the same frequency as the resonance frequency, ω_o. Spin-lattice relaxation is a type of stimulated recovery, in which the spins that have been excited to the upper energy level by the transmitted rf pulse are encouraged to

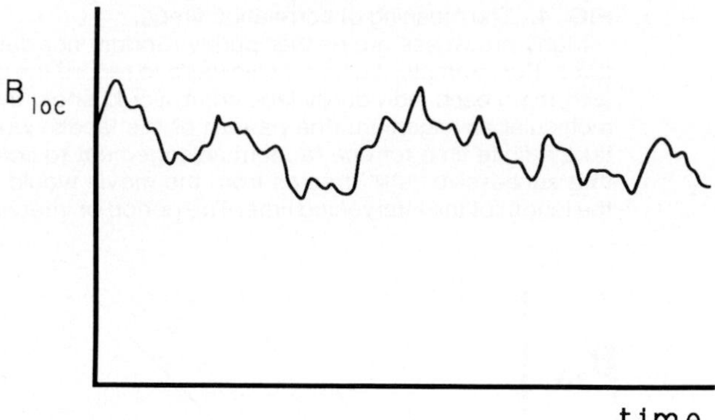

FIG. 3. The local magnetic field experienced by any proton varies as other nuclei or electrons that generate magnetic fields move past.

return to the lower level by the action of an alternating magnetic field of appropriate frequency. This stimulated recovery is very efficient when there is a local fluctuating field that can provide a magnetic perturbation at the Larmor frequency, so that there is available a quantum of energy exactly equal to the difference in levels of the nuclear spin states. A suitable source of stimulating interaction can be discovered by close inspection of the atomic environment of the protons in tissue. For example in water, each proton in a water molecule has a neighboring proton that is also a magnetic dipole which generates a magnetic field at the proton of about 5 gauss (0.5 milliTesla) (Fig. 2). This field however is constantly changing in amplitude and direction as the water molecule rotates rapidly and moves about in the liquid. It also changes as a result of intermolecular collision, translation, or chemical dissociation and exchange. The magnetic field experienced by any nucleus will fluctuate with a frequency spectrum that is dependent on the molecular tumbling due to the random thermal motion of the host and surrounding molecules (Fig. 3). The mean strength of the local field is determined by the strength of the magnetic dipoles in the medium and how close they approach to the hydrogen nuclei. Only the component of the frequency spectrum which is equal to the resonant frequency, ω_o, (or, for reasons beyond our discussion, $2\omega_o$) is effective in stimulating an energy exchange to induce transitions between nuclear spin states and lead to thermal equilibrium, i.e., T1 relaxation. In liquids the characteristic frequencies of thermal motion are of the order of 10^{11} Hz or higher, much greater than NMR frequencies of 10^7–10^8 Hz. Consequently, the component of the frequency spectrum from molecular motion that can induce T1 relaxation is small and the process is slow. As the molecular motion becomes slower, either due to lower temperature, or increased molecular size, the intensity of the fluctuations of the magnetic field at the resonance frequency increases, reaches a maximum, and then decreases again as the energy of the motion becomes increasingly concentrated in frequencies lower than the

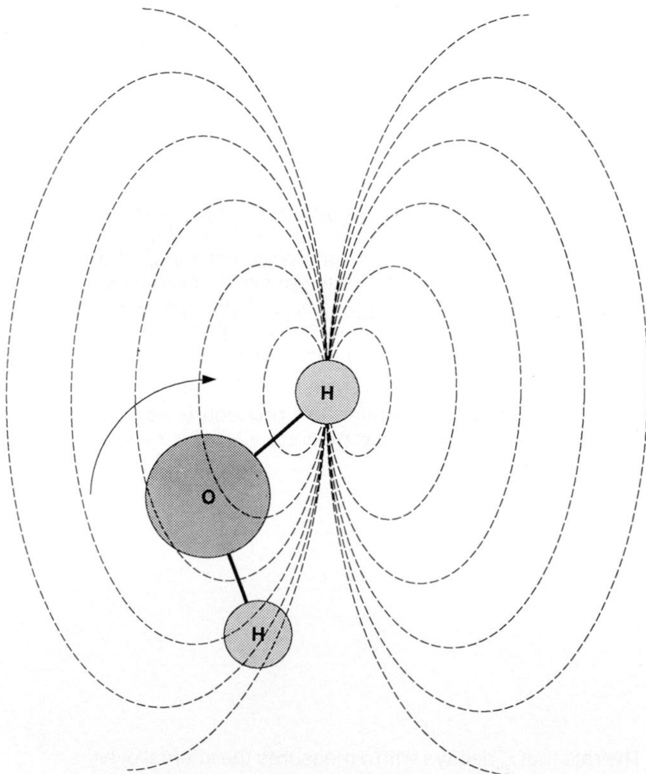

FIG. 2. A dipole can be considered as two spherical foci of magnetic flux, separated in space. The resultant field pattern is similar to that from a thin bar magnet and falls off as the inverse third power of the distance. The magnetic field around a hydrogen nucleus varies in space, and the effect on a neighboring nucleus in the same molecule changes with time if the molecule moves.

FIG. 4. The meaning of correlation times.

Many processes are neither purely random nor deterministic, but show traits both of ordered and stochastic natures. For example, if a fast movie were to record the positions of all the water molecules in a sample of liquid, starting with them each individually labeled, it would show them all moving randomly with time so that after an interval the molecular arrangement (the pattern of the labels) would bear no relation to the starting picture. However, it would take a finite time for one random arrangement to convert to another without there being an apparent evolution, so that successive "still" frames from the movie would show an apparent causal relationship that grows weaker with the length of the intervening time. The period or interval for this apparent causality to disappear is the correlation time.

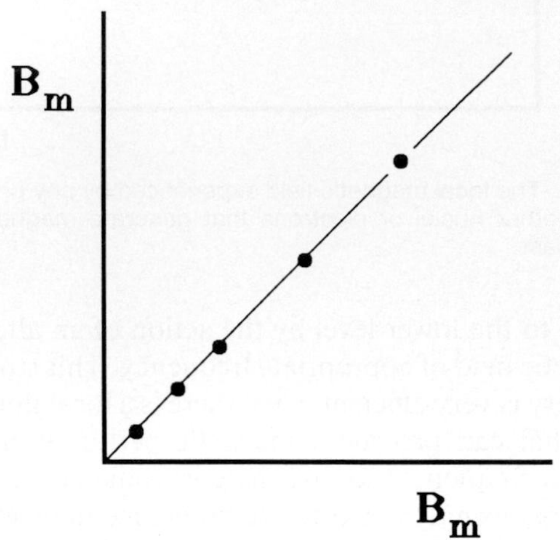

A: For the local fluctuating magnetic field experienced by a proton the correlation time can be given a precise mathematical interpretation using familiar (hopefully) statistical concepts. Consider recording the local field, $\mathbf{B}(t)$, over some time interval $0 < t < T$, by taking discrete measurements at regular sampling times $m\Delta t$, where m varies from 1 to a large number. These samples are called $\mathbf{B}_m$. If we plot the numbers $\mathbf{B}_m$ against themselves, we obviously obtain a perfect straight line relationship. The x and y variables are the same set of numbers, so they are perfectly correlated. Mathematically we can compute the correlation coefficient for the linear regression, r_0, which in this case is exactly 1.

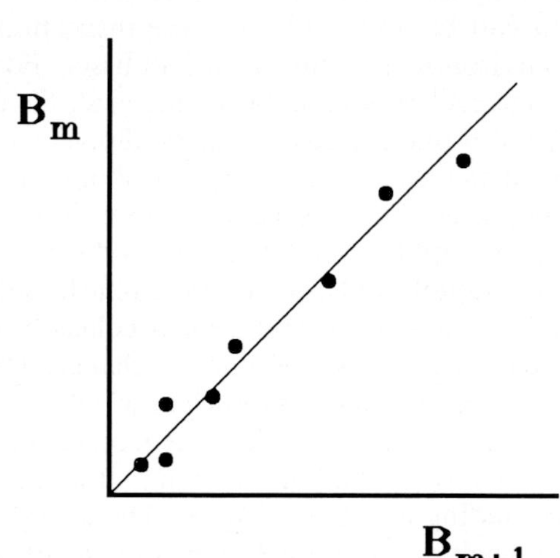

B: We can then plot a second graph, of $\mathbf{B}_m$ against $\mathbf{B}_{m+1}$, viz., the x axis variables are also $\mathbf{B}_m$ samples, but shifted 1 place in order of measurement, as though column 2 of a table had slipped one row relative to column 1. If $\mathbf{B}(t)$ does not vary too rapidly in the sample interval Δt the plot of $\mathbf{B}_m$ vs. $\mathbf{B}_{m+1}$ will be scattered about the line of regression to a degree that depends on how much change occurs.

We can then recompute the correlation coefficient, r_1, which will be less than 1. Repeating this procedure we can compute r_2 for the line $\mathbf{B}_m$ vs. $\mathbf{B}_{m+2}$ and so on. For a field modulated by random molecular motions, $r_0 > r_1 > r_2$. We can further plot the value of r_n obtained for each shift of the data, i.e., r_n vs. n.

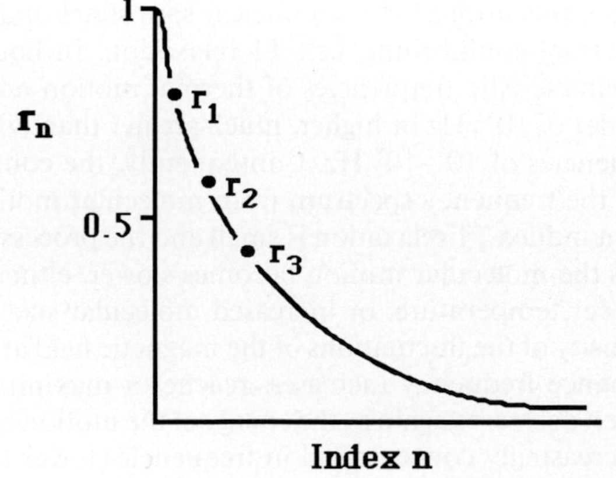

C: The rate that r_n decays with n measures the interval over which a sample of waveform of the field appears different, or unconnected, with a corresponding sample taken later. The width of the plot of r_n vs. n (which is termed the autocorrelation function) is the correlation time in units of Δt. For completely random rapidly fluctuating fields, it is short, but for systems in which it takes a relatively long time for a molecule to tumble it may be much longer (see text).

FIG. 4. *Continued.*

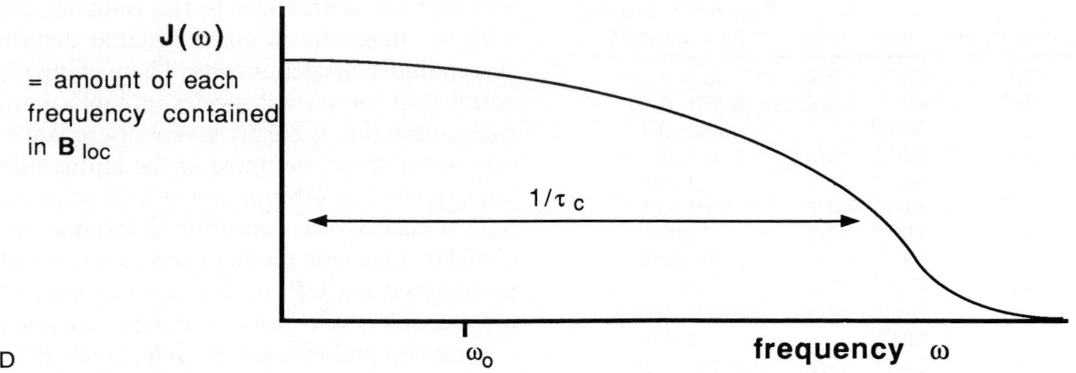

D: An alternate yet equivalent description of the fluctuating local field is the spectral density. The local field can be considered to comprise a mixture of component frequencies, a frequency spectrum. The amount at any frequency ω is denoted by $J(\omega_0)$, the spectral density. If the autocorrelation function (Fig. 4C) is of the form $\mathbf{B}^2_{loc}e^{-t/\tau_c}$, then $J(\omega)$ is of the form $\mathbf{B}^2_{loc}\,\tau_c/(1 + \omega^2\tau_c^2)$. Terms of this type may be found in the SBM equations. The width of the spectral density is $1/\tau_c$. The relaxation rate R_1 depends on $J(\omega_o)$, whereas R_2 also depends on $J(0)$.

NMR range. Thus, T1 passes through a minimum value as the molecular motion becomes slower. The effect of the molecular motion is usually expressed by a correlation time, τ_c (see below, and Fig. 4), characteristic of the time of rotation of a molecule or of the time of its translation into a neighboring position. Relaxation rates in simple liquids are affected, for example, by viscosity, temperature, and the presence of dissolved ions and molecules, which alter the correlation times of molecular motion or the amplitudes of the dipolar interactions.

PARAMAGNETIC RELAXATION

In tissue, water relaxation times are shorter than in pure water because of interactions of the water molecules with macromolecules. Proteins and other macromolecular structures exert, via protons on their surfaces, dipolar fields that fluctuate relatively slowly and which are efficient sites for relaxation. To devise external agents that reduce T1 further we need a means of affecting the amplitude and time scale of variation of the local magnetic fields experienced by water molecules. Paramagnetic agents attempt to simply do this. They are materials that on the atomic scale generate extremely strong local magnetic fields. Each agent possesses a large magnetic dipole moment compared to, say, the proton. Transition and rare earth metal ions are examples of these. The origin of their strong local fields lies in the fact that they contain unpaired electrons viz. particles with spin and electric charge (and therefore a magnetic moment) that have not been "matched" (paired off) in a chemical bond with spins of opposite character, so that there is a net residual magnetic dipole moment. The electron spin magnetic dipole is 658 times greater than the proton essentially because it has a smaller radius but the same charge, so any water molecules that approach close to an unpaired electron will experience an intense interaction that can promote relaxation. That paramagnetics have a dramatic effect on the relaxation time of protons in solution has been well understood from the earliest work in NMR. For example, Bloch (1) in his 1946 article stated that "it is recommendable to add to the substance a certain percentage of paramagnetic atoms or molecules to reduce T1," in his case in order to reduce saturation effects and speed up his observations. With the advent of NMR imaging, it was quickly realized that paramagnetic agents would likely prove useful for contrast enhancement. Lauterbur et al. (2) demonstrated the powerful effects of manganese ions in a canine model of myocardial infarction, and was able to show regional T1 effects in areas of the excised heart ex vivo. The first in vivo studies on contrast enhancement in MRI were performed by investigators from the Hammersmith Hospital, London, in the Central Research laboratories of EMI Ltd. Gore et al. (3) measured the time course of enhancement by manganese and other paramagnetic ions in rabbit tissues and demonstrated the feasibility of assessing organ uptake and excretion. The same group also performed the first human contrast studies by demonstrating the effects of oral ferrous ions on the signal from the GI tract (4).

A relatively complete theoretical description of nuclear relaxation, including a description of the effect of the dipole-dipole interaction between water molecules as well as the effects of paramagnetic ions, was given by Bloembergen, Purcell and Pound in 1948 (5). They derived a simple approximate relation, since widely quoted in the radiological literature:

$$\Delta R_1 = 12N\pi^2\gamma^2\eta\mu^2/kT \qquad [1]$$

where

ΔR_1 = increase in relaxation rate over pure solvent
N = number of ions per cm^3
μ = magnetic moment of the ion

TABLE 1. *Electron structures of elements*

	Configuration	Ion	Spin	Electron relaxation time (nanos.)
Transition	$3d^3$	Cr^{+3}	3/2	0.1–1
Metals	$3d^4$	Cr^{+2}	4/2	0.001–0.01
		Mn^{+3}		0.01–0.1
	$3d^5$	Fe^{+3}	5/2	0.1–1
		Mn^{+2}		1–10
	$3d^6$	Fe^{+2}	4/2	0.01–0.1
	$3d^7$	Co^{+2}	3/2	0.0001
	$3d^8$	Ni^{+2}	1	0.0001
	$3d^9$	Cu^{+2}	1/2	0.1
Lanthanides	$4f^7$	Eu^{+2}	7/2	0.0001–0.001
		Gd^{+3}		1–10
	$4f^9$	Dy^{+3}	5/2	0.0001–0.001
	$4f^{10}$	Ho^{+3}	4/2	0.0001–0.001
	$4f^{11}$	Er^{+3}	3/2	—

T is the temperature, γ is the gyromagnetic ratio of the proton, η the solution viscosity, and k is a physical constant.

This equation predicts that relaxation rate (the rate $R_1 = 1/T1$) should increase in direct proportion to ion concentration. The predicted linearity between rate and concentration has been observed without evidence of saturation in both simple solutions and whole tissues for a variety of paramagnetic agents. However, the slope of the line viz. the rate increase per unit concentration of material is often determined not by the paramagnetic species alone, but by the solvent and the nature of other solutes, as well as by factors within the tissue. This relationship is further discussed below, but it emphasizes a fundamental difference between contrast agents for NMR and other modalities; viz., in NMR the agent itself is not directly visualized, but rather the effect of the agent on the behavior of protons, which is not an intrinsic property of the agent alone. Equation 1 also predicts that the relaxation rate is proportional to the square of the magnetic moment. The magnetic moment is largely determined by the number of unpaired electron spins, and it is a prime factor that affects the materials' magnetic susceptibility. The electron structures for several ions of potential interest are shown in Table 1. Table 2 shows the measured relaxation rates per unit concentration for various ions, normalized to the value for copper, along with the magnetic moment squared determined from susceptibility measurements. There is obviously a good correlation for several species, notably manganese and gadolinium, but there are severe discrepancies for many others. For example, most of the lanthanide rare earth ions, typified by erbium, are at least an order of magnitude less effective as relaxation agents than would be predicted by magnetic moment considerations alone. In experiments using MRI in vivo, dysprosium and holmium, for example, have been considered as potential relaxation agents and shown to be quite ineffective at reducing T1 (6,7). This discrepancy highlights the fact that Equation 1 is an inadequate description of paramagnetic effects even in simple aqueous solution. It ignores a fundamental requirement that was introduced earlier viz. the time scale of the fluctuating magnetic field produced by the ion and experienced by the nuclei must match the frequency of the NMR transition to be affected. A more complete theoretical description was developed by Solomon (8) and by Bloembergen and Morgan (9,10). Recall that relaxation results from the action of fluctuating local magnetic fields experienced by protons, which stimulate the return to equilibrium of an excited population of spins. In water alone the dominant source of such effects is the dipole-dipole interaction between neighboring protons, mainly between hydrogen nuclei in the same water molecule. Molecular tumbling in Brownian motion causes the weak magnetic field produced by each proton to fluctuate randomly, and at the site of a neighboring proton these random alterations in the net field produce relaxation. Tl is sensitive mainly to the spectral component of such fluctuations at the Larmor frequency; T2 is sensitive also to low frequency components, as described below. The time scale characteristic of the dipolar interaction reflects molecular motion and clearly is expected to influence the efficacy of relaxation. Qualitatively, when there is a concentration of kinetic motion in the appropriate frequency range, relaxation will be efficient. We can envisage other types of motion which will be too rapid or too slow to be effective. An important

TABLE 2. *Comparison of measured relaxation rate enhancement at 20 MHz with magnetic moments, μ, both normalized to the value for copper*

Ion	$\Delta R_1/c$ (sec^{-1} mM^{-1})	$(\Delta R_1/c)_{ion}$ / $(\Delta R_1/c)_{Cu}$	$\Delta R_2/c$ (sec^{-1} mM^{-1})	$(\Delta R_2/c)_{ion}$ / $(\Delta R_2/c)_{Cu}$	$[\mu_{ion}]^2/[\mu_{Cu}]^2$
Cu^{2+}	0.83	1.00	0.98	1.00	1.00
Ni^{2+}	0.69	0.84	0.76	0.78	2.40
Cr^{3+}	4.36	5.27	10.1	10.3	3.61
Co^{2+}	0.15	0.18	0.15	0.15	6.25
Mn^{2+}	7.52	9.10	41.6	42.4	8.7
Fe^{3+}	8.37	10.1	12.8	13.1	8.7
Gd^{3+}	12.1	14.6	15.0	15.3	15.6
Er^{3+}	0.38	0.46	0.41	0.42	22.56

descriptor is the correlation time, τ_c which measures the time over which the local fluctuating field appears continuous and deterministic. It represents the time it takes on average for the field to change significantly. A more precise interpretation using simple statistical concepts is given in Fig. 4.

Paramagnetic ions accelerate relaxation by mechanisms similar to those that account for normal water relaxation. Since the relaxation rate depends on the magnetic moment squared, and the electron moment is 658 that of the proton, we expect that roughly 2.5 mmol of unpaired electrons will double the relaxation rate of water (110 molar in protons), all other factors being equal. Although in practice agents are more effective than this lower limit, it is instructive to note that such concentrations are many orders of magnitude greater than the levels typically detected in radionuclide counting experiments. This is particularly important to realize in contemplating the possibility of labeling target specific carrier molecules. Paramagnetic ions in simple solutions most effectively relax the protons in water molecules in close proximity, in the first monolayer of molecules around the ion, as discussed further below. In addition there is a weaker effect on molecules in outer spheres, which may nonetheless be effectively relaxed. If R_1 and R_2 denote the relaxation rates of protons in the coordination sphere of an aquoion, and these are rapidly exchanging position and continuously diffusing through the solvent water (intrinsic relaxation rate R_w) the overall rates will be $R'_{1,2}$

$$R'_{1,2} = (1 - u)R_w + uR_{1,2} \qquad [2]$$

where u is the fraction of time each proton spends in the coordination shell. Note that this assumes all the water has access to the inner shell of an ion. This relation will not hold when water compartments are restricted, which can be important in vivo as discussed below.

If the coordination number of the ion is q, and M and N denote the molar concentrations of the metal ion and water molecules, respectively, then:

$$u = qM/N \qquad [3]$$

$$\Delta R_{1,2} = q(R_{1,2} - R_w)/N \qquad [4]$$

where $\Delta R_{1,2}$ are the relaxivities, or increases in relaxation rates over the solvent per unit concentrations of metal. The relaxation rates $R_{1,2}$ of protons in the coordination sphere are predicted by the Solomon-Bloembergen-Morgan (SBM) equations (10):

$$R_1 = \frac{2}{15}\frac{S(S+1)g^2\beta^2 g_N^2\beta_N^2}{h^2 r^6}\left[\frac{3\tau_c}{1+\omega_I^2\tau_c^2} + \frac{7\tau_c}{1+\omega_S^2\tau_c^2}\right] + \frac{2}{3}\frac{S(S+1)a^2}{h^2}\left[\frac{\tau_e}{1+\omega_S^2\tau_e^2}\right] \qquad [5]$$

$$R_2 = \frac{1}{15}\frac{S(S+1)g^2\beta^2 g_N^2\beta_N^2}{h^2 r^6}\left[4\tau_c + \frac{3\tau_c}{1+\omega_I^2\tau_c^2} + \frac{7\tau_c}{1+\omega_S^2\tau_c^2}\right] + \frac{1}{3}\frac{S(S+1)a^2}{h^2}\left[\tau_e + \frac{\tau_e}{1+\omega_S^2\tau_e^2}\right] \qquad [6]$$

where ω_I, ω_s = Larmor frequencies for electron and proton spins, respectively.

β_N = nuclear magneton
β = Bohr magneton
g = electronic g factor
r = ion-nucleus distance
a = hyperfine coupling constant
S = electron spin quantum number
g_N = proton g factor.

At first sight these equations may appear daunting but they are actually quite simple to interpret. They state that the relaxation rates for each paramagnetic species depend on four variable quantities; first, the magnetic moment of the paramagnetic species; second, the distance between the paramagnetic center and the nucleus being relaxed; third, the frequency of the NMR measurement; and fourth, the correlation time that describes the rate of variation of the local field.

The first terms in brackets on the right-hand side describe the dipolar electron-nucleon interaction. This arises for all paramagnetics because there is a magnetic moment associated with the electron spin that has a spatial dipole dependence similar to that of the proton in Fig. 2. This is sometimes referred to as a "through space" coupling. The second terms describe a so-called scalar or contact hyperfine interaction,which is important only for some paramagnetics, and which involves spin exchange between the electron and nucleus, and is mediated by the formation of a transient chemical bond (a so-called through bond interaction). The correlation times characteristic of these two interactions are different and denoted as τ_c and τ_e, respectively. τ_c is determined by the combined effects of three processes; rotation, electron spin relaxation, and proton exchange. Rotation alters the orientation of the proton relative to the magnetic field of the electrons. The electron spin relaxation time refers to the time which elapses on average before the electron spin itself alters its orientation. Proton exchange denotes the process whereby water molecules enter and depart the hydration sphere of the paramagnetic center. Since these processes are independent their rates are additive so that

$$1/\tau_c = 1/\tau_R + 1/\tau_S + 1/\tau_M \qquad [7]$$

where τ_R, is the rotational correlation time for the ion and its hydration complex; τ_M is the exchange correlation time, the average time a proton stays in the hydration sphere of an ion; and τ_S is the electron spin relaxation time. Similarly:

$$1/\tau_e = 1/\tau_S + 1/\tau_M \qquad [8]$$

Equation 7 states that the effective correlation time is dominated by the fastest molecular process which affects it. Qualitatively, if the electron spins maintain their orientation during the course of Brownian motion and diffusion, relaxation will be primarily dependent on the rate at which water molecules randomly alter their position and orientation in the vicinity of the ions ($\tau_R \ll \tau_S$). Alternatively, if the electron spin changes its direction frequently, perhaps because of variations in its magnetic environment due to variations in the detailed atomic configuration ($\tau_S \ll \tau_R$) the magnetic field at the neighboring proton will fluctuate more rapidly and be less effective at increasing the relaxation rate. In aquo, τ_M is usually relatively long and can often be neglected, though it may be advantageous to modify the water bonding to compounds to ensure exchange is not too rapid.

The SBM description verifies that relaxation rate is proportional to the second power of magnetic moment since

$$\mu^2 \propto S(S+1) \qquad [9]$$

However, the SBM equations show a dependence on three factors in addition to magnetic moment. These are: (a) correlation time, (b) frequency, and (c) distance.

Correlation Time

The dependence on correlation time underlines the fact that the local magnetic field must fluctuate neither too slowly nor too rapidly for effective relaxation. The local field, as seen in Fig. 3, does not simply oscillate at a single frequency, but instead produces a magnetic perturbation that can be decomposed into a range of component frequencies (by the process called Fourier analysis). The constituent range of frequencies is called the power spectrum of the field, or the spectral density. NMR imaging frequencies (under 100 MHz) are relatively low compared to other atomic rates such as water molecule rotations. Materials for which the correlation time is very short spread the spectral energy over a very wide range of frequencies and consequently the amplitude in a narrow frequency range, particularly at a low NMR frequency, is actually quite low. On the other hand, agents with a longer correlation time, where the interaction is varying more slowly, tend to have more energy concentrated in the low frequency range which is relevant to the NMR frequency. So we can predict that materials with too short a correlation time will in fact be quite ineffective as relaxation agents whereas agents with a long correlation time will be more effective. Figure 5A shows this graphically and it may be seen that there is a dramatic increase in the relaxation efficiency as we increase correlation time. To produce strong relaxation effects, the paramagnetic species should have a reasonably long τ_c, and thus long τ_R and τ_S. The major discrep-

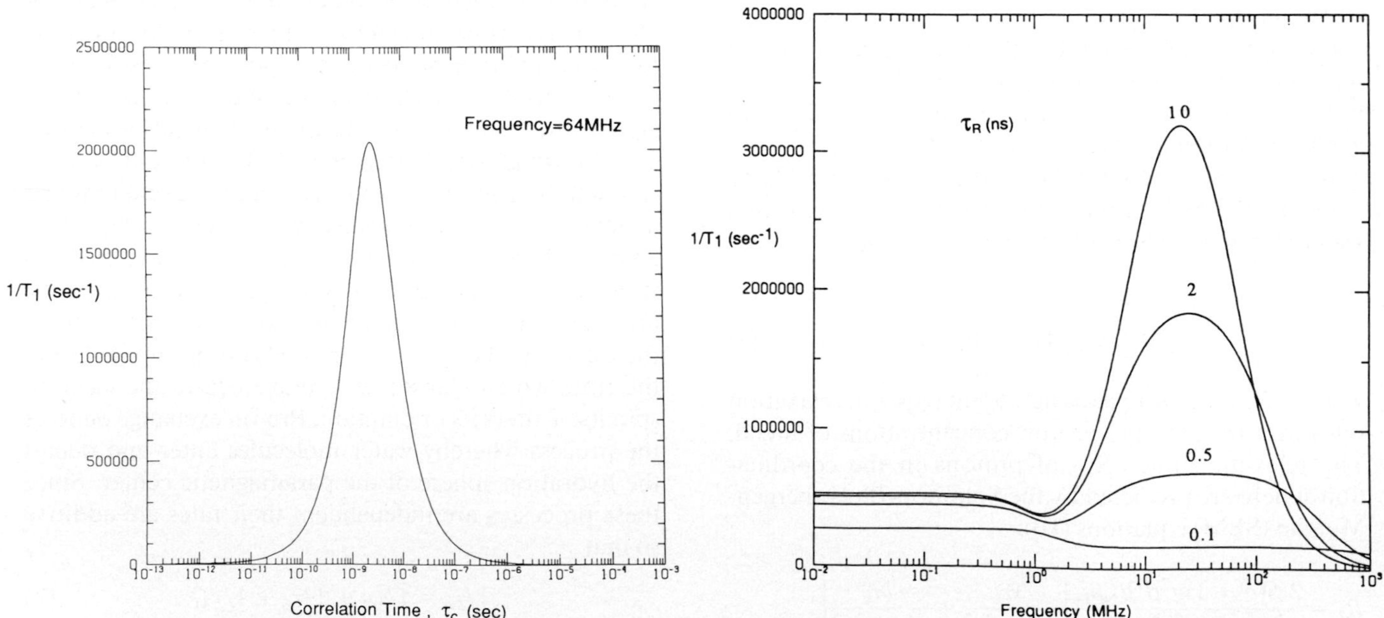

FIG. 5. The dependence of the inner sphere longitudinal relaxation rate, 1/T1, as a function of correlation time τ_c, as predicted by the Solomon-Bloembergen-Morgan equations, assuming the hyperfine contribution is negligible. This curve varies with the NMR frequency. **B:** The variation of the inner sphere longitudinal relaxation rate 1/T1 as a function of frequency (in MHz) for different values of the rotational correlation time for gadolinium, assuming $S = 7/2$, $q = 1$, $r = 3.1$ A°, $\tau_M = 3 \times 10^{-9}$ sec, $\tau_s = 10^{-10}$ sec.

ancies of the expected values of T1 in Table 1 are explicable because most of the lanthanides, cobalt, and nickel have short electron spin relaxation times ($\tau_S = 10^{-13}$ sec). Thus, the local fields they generate fluctuate too rapidly to be effective. Manganese and gadolinium have relatively long τ_S (10^{-10} sec) and thus are more effective. Furthermore, the dominant correlation time is the rotational correlation time, τ_R. This dominance imparts the characteristic that if τ_R can be lengthened, the agent will be even more effective. In particular, for the regime $\omega_I \tau_c \ll 1$, if the scalar contribution can be ignored (see below) Equation 5 reduces to:

$$R_1 = \frac{2S(S+1)g^2\beta^2 g_N^2 \beta_N^2}{15h^2 r^6}\left[3\tau_c + \frac{7\tau_c}{1+\omega_S^2\tau_c^2}\right] \quad [10]$$

and increasing τ_R ($=\tau_c$) will improve relaxivity. Such an effect may be dramatically realized when the paramagnetic species binds to a larger molecule, so that it tumbles at a slower rate or has its motion restricted; and thereby is characterized by a larger reorientation time constant. The result is a so-called proton relaxation enhancement as first described by Eisinger et al. (11). Figure 6 demonstrates the effect of free manganese binding to metal-binding sites on bovine serum albumin and γ-globulin. The amount of manganese required to shorten the solution relaxation times is much less in the presence of the macromolecules than in free solution. The behavior in the presence of the solute can be described in terms of an enhancement ratio, ε:

$$\varepsilon = \frac{R_1\,(\text{solution} + \text{ion}) - R_1\,(\text{solution})}{R_1\,(\text{solvent} + \text{ion}) - R_1\,(\text{solvent})} \quad [11]$$

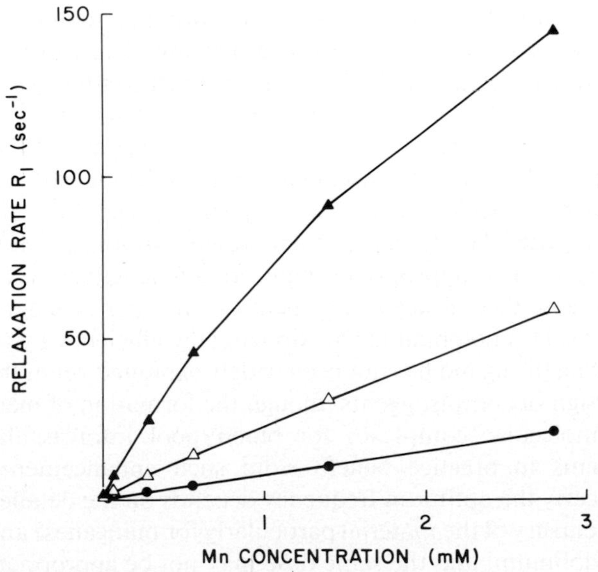

FIG. 6. Relaxation rate of Mn-doped albumin (*solid triangles*) and γ-globulin (*open triangles*) solutions at 4.5% concentration and pH 7.7 vs. Mn concentration. The rate for Mn solutions (*circles*) is also shown for comparison. (From Kang et al., ref. 12, with permission.)

For the Mn-albumin system ε is around 10 at 20 MHz, pH = 7.0 (12). For manganese introduced intravenously in whole tissues, ε is typically 5 at 20 MHz (13), showing that significant enhancements are achievable in vivo by binding effects of ions to proteins, membranes, and other high molecular weight structures. Similar properties are displayed by gadolinium. For example, Reuben (14) demonstrated enhancements of around 5 for Gd bound to BSA at 24.3 MHz, while Burton et al. (15) recorded enhancements of around 8 at 40 MHz for gadolinium bound to immunoglobulin-G, with $\tau_R = 10^{-8}$ sec. Lauffer et al. have more recently estimated enhancements of up to 10 for Gd bound via DTPA or EDTA to IgG and BSA (16).

Binding effects producing enhancements are important factors in determining the relaxation behavior of some paramagnetic species, so variations in the chemical equilibrium that may displace bound ions can have a subtle influence on proton relaxation measurements. Thus, alterations in hydrogen ion concentration (pH) or the presence of other competing ions (e.g., calcium, phosphate, or other metals) has been shown to affect the enhancement ratio and relaxation times of solutions of free metal and protein. When these competing ions are abundant, the association of the metal with the protein decreases, and bound metal ions are released to free solution, thereby becoming less effective by tumbling more rapidly (Fig. 7).

Enhancement effects are likely of major interest in the design of paramagnetic delivery methods. For example, proteins, liposomes, or monoclonal antibodies of high molecular weight can provide a suitable tumbling vehicle to lengthen the correlation time of bound gadolinium to 10^{-8} sec, and thereby provide optimal relaxivity. Furthermore, as suggested by Lauffer (17), in vivo enhancements may be obtainable by distributing agents in a tissue compartment with high microviscosity, or by forming noncovalent bonds with macromolecules in tissue. Gd-DTPA does not localize intracellularly, and exhibits much the same relaxivity in vivo as in vitro, so that it does not benefit from interacting with the more viscous cytosol.

A secondary consequence of lengthening τ_R for manganese is that such a change does not affect τ_e (Equation 8) and so does not influence the contact contribution to relaxation. It can be inferred from Table 2 and the SBM equations that the contact term accounts for much of the spin-spin relaxation of free manganese solutions, for which T1/T2 is typically 5 (in most other solutions of free ions, T1 and T2 are approximately equal). Increasing τ_R, therefore, has a less significant effect on T2 than on T1. Thus, as τ_R increases, T1/T2 decreases toward 1. The ratio T1/T2 is a sensitive index of the binding kinetics of a metal with a significant contact contribution (12).

For simple gadolinium chelates in use clinically, the in vivo correlation time is 1 to 2 orders of magnitude

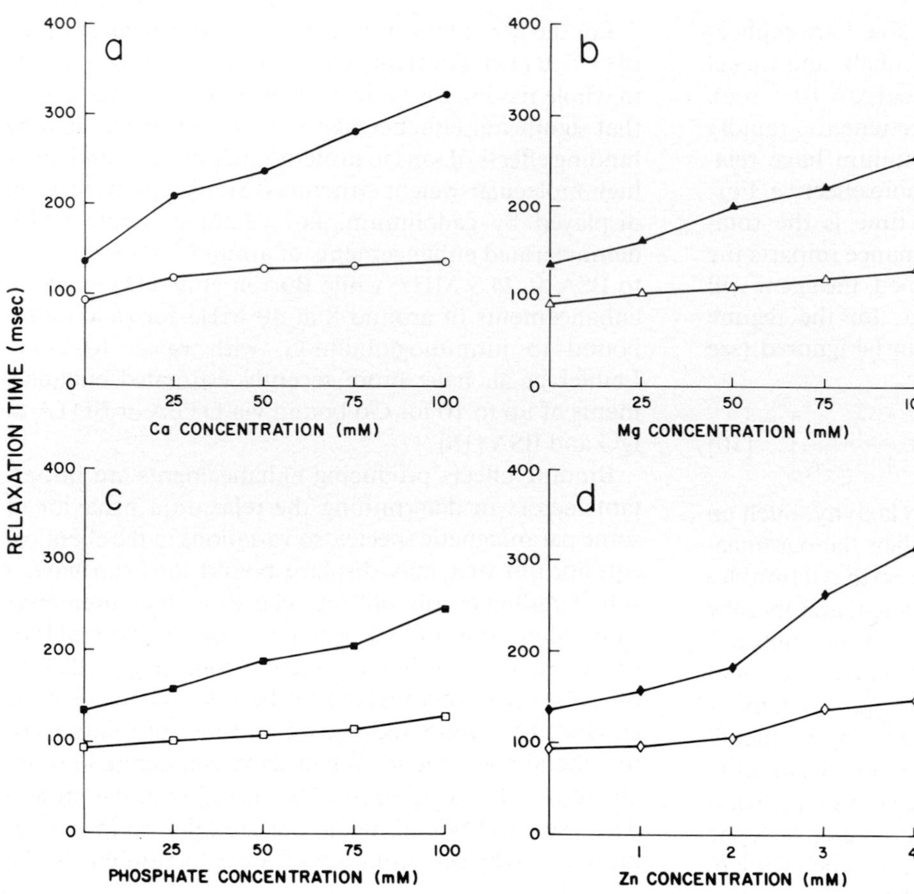

FIG. 7. Relaxation times T1 (*solid symbols*) and T2 (*open symbols*) of 4.5 g% albumin-70 μM Mn solutions at pH 7.7 titrated with Ca (**a**), Mg (**b**), phosphate (**c**), and zinc (**d**). Ionic strength was maintained at 0.3 with NaCl. (From Kang et al., ref. 12, with permission.)

shorter than the optimal that could be obtained. By attaching the metal ion by some means to a large macromolecule or complex, the rotational correlation time may become extremely long (the ion complex is essentially immobilized) and then (from Equation 7) the other correlation times become dominant. The electron spin time for gadolinium would, under such circumstances, become important, but there would then be some potential for obtaining greater relaxivity by lengthening τ_S. This could be achieved by making the metal ion complex more rigid, so that intramolecular vibrations are less effective at electron spin relaxation.

Frequency

The SBM equations predict a strong frequency dispersion of T1 and T2 in a range of frequency determined by τ_c. Frequency dispersion curves of paramagnetic complexes have been extensively studied by Koenig and coworkers (18) and are useful indicators of the dominant correlation time. The frequency dependence is illustrated graphically in Fig. 5B where the theoretical predictions of the SBM equations are plotted. There is in general a steady reduction in the relaxation efficiency as we go to higher and higher frequencies. On the other hand the SBM equations show that the frequency dependence is intimately related to the correlation time; it is the correlation time relative to the frequency that is the important factor that determines the degree of frequency dispersion. As the correlation time increases the region of maximum efficiency can be shifted to a different frequency. This may be illustrated by the work of Burton (15) on gadolinium complexed to immunoglobulin G. In this system there is a strong dispersion of Tl around a frequency of about 40 MHz. At frequencies either above or below 40 MHz more gadolinium is needed in order to achieve the same change in relaxation rate as at 40 MHz and this is a direct consequence of complexing with the macromolecule. There is a very strong dispersion for manganese bound to particular proteins around 20 MHz (18). Clearly, appropriate engineering to lengthen τ_c can increase the efficacy of an agent by an order of magnitude. This potential for maximizing the efficiency by altering the ligand has not been widely exploited yet in the design of contrast agents, though the formation of macromolecular complexes for blood pool intravascular agents in practice benefit from such enhancements. Clearly the optimum frequency depends on the detailed chemistry of the material particularly for manganese and gadolinium, and the same dose may not be appropriate at 64 MHz as at 21 MHz.

The fractional contribution to the overall relaxation time from different processes may also alter with frequency. For example, Burton et al. (15), in studies of

IgG, were able to separate the relative contributions of τ_R and τ_S to 1/T1 and 1/T2 at different frequencies. At 10 MHz, τ_R contributes only 10% to τ_c but this increases to 50% at 60 MHz. As the frequency increases from 10 MHz the contribution due to rotation increases and the contribution due to spin relaxation decreases so at 60 MHz we are actually probing a rather different chemical property of the system compared to operation at low frequency. This illustrates further the point made earlier about the difference between paramagnetic effects in NMR imaging and other sorts of contrast enhancement in radiology. In NMR the relaxation effects produced by a system are sensitive to the detailed physics and chemical composition of the surrounding material or tissue which is quite different, for example, from the behavior of iodine in CT scanning. In NMR the relaxation efficiency of a paramagnetic agent depends on exactly how it interacts with the medium as well as external effects such as the applied magnetic field strength. The frequency relation highlights the fact that paramagnetic relaxation reflects subtle molecular dynamic properties not intrinsic to the metal alone.

Distance

The sixth power inverse dependence of relaxation rate on the distance between the paramagnetic ion and the relaxing water protons means that it is particularly important to ensure that water molecules can bind directly to the ion, and the coordination number should be as high as possible. Chelating agents have been used to deliver paramagnetic materials to tissues and are favored because they reduce metal toxicity and improve solubility compared to the ion alone. There are, however, undesirable effects of using chelates on the relaxation properties of metal ions. Cage-like structures, such as EDTA and DTPA, have high association constants and they enclose metal ions and restrict access of water molecules. The word chelate is derived from the Greek word for claw, which correctly connotes the structure of the complex. Most chelated paramagnetic ions show lower relaxivities than do free ions because of the effects of restricted water access, though these can be offset by a positive enhancement effect due to the slower tumbling of the larger complex. The formation of a complex with a multidentate ligand displaces a number of water molecules from the coordination sphere. Alsaadi (19) showed the systematic decrease in relaxation rates for lanthanide complexes with ligands of increasing denticity. An important parameter is then the reduction in the number of water molecules, q, bound directly to the metal, which is approximately the number of donor atoms of the ligand. Gadolinium ions have $q = 9$ in aquo. DTPA and DOTA are both octodentate ligands, so the complex removes 8 of the 9 water sites, leaving $q = 1$.

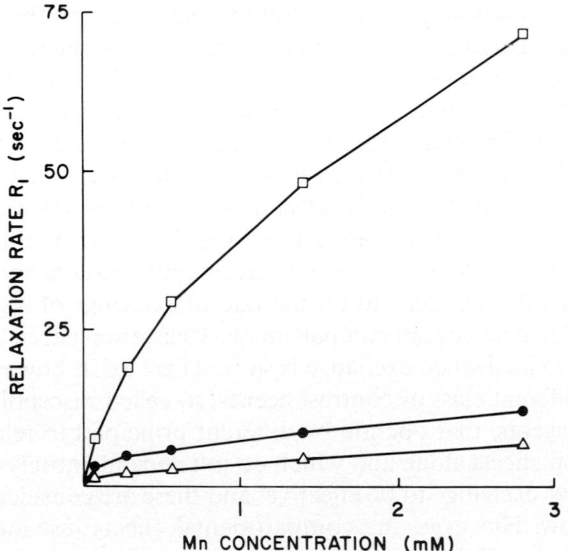

FIG. 8. Relaxation rate R_1 vs. Mn concentration of blood doped with free Mn (*squares*), Mn-EDTA (*circles*) and Mn-DTPA (*triangles*). Samples consisted of 490 μl of blood and 10 μl of $MnCl_2$. (From Kang et al., ref. 12, with permission.)

TABLE 3. *Proton relaxation enhancement factors for Mn in blood and solutions of chelates at 20 MHz*

Solution	ε
Blood	9.5
Plasma	11.5
EDTA	0.48
DTPA	0.28

From Kang et al., ref. 12, with permission.

In tissue, the chelate may prevent the type of enhancement effects described above. Figure 8 shows the different effects of manganese on the relaxation times of blood when added as free ion and chelated. It is clear, for example, that at least four times as much metal chelated with DTPA is needed to achieve the same effect as the free ion. Table 3 compares the enhancement factors for manganese in blood, in plasma and in EDTA and DTPA for a fixed amount of manganese. Whereas in blood there is a tenfold enhancement of the manganese effect, in DTPA there is a fourfold reduction in its effectiveness due to the chelation effect.

Gadolinium salts have low solubility and chelation helps prevent precipitation at tissue pH. Furthermore, chelation alters the excretion route and organ distribution, and substantially reduces toxicity, as long as the complex is stable in vivo. DTPA has proven particularly suitable for combination with gadolinium. DTPA has the highest association constant of the known aminocarboxylic acid chelates. The LD_{50} of Gd-DTPA is approximately 10 mmol/kgm in rats, about half that of common iodinated x-ray agents and 100 times the dose commonly administered in a contrast study. There remains, however, considerable interest in developing chelates that are more organ specific, stable, and reduce relaxivities to lesser extents. Of critical importance is the number of sites for water to access the inner sphere of the ion, but in general the stability of the complex and the number of sites are inversely related. In vivo, the overriding consideration is safety and stability, so that efficacy is compromised to a large extent.

There are other approaches to paramagnetic contrast enhancement in NMR. Stable free radicals offer some promise as alternatives to paramagnetic metal ions though they are in general less effective and lose their paramagnetism if they are reduced in vivo. Their paramagnetism arises from the presence of unpaired electrons in certain molecular orbitals, such as in nitroxide groups. A paramagnetic agent of special interest is molecular oxygen, which in solution is a mildly effective relaxation agent because the electron spins in the O_2 molecule are not paired off, and there is a net magnetic moment. Unfortunately, the concentration of oxygen gas in tissues is too low for this to be a major influence on tissue relaxation rates, although variations in pO_2 have been detected via the paramagnetic effects of oxygen on the fluorine-19 nucleus in perfluorocarbons, where the solubility of oxygen is much higher than in tissue water. For practical implementation in the near future, paramagnetic metal chelates are the most promising materials. By now the rationale for using Gd-DTPA and similar chelates should be clear. Although Gd does not possess the largest magnetic moment, it does exert the strongest effect on water spin lattice relaxation of all the elements. This is because its correlation time is favorable for NMR in the 10–100 MHz region. Furthermore its relaxivity can be enhanced by lengthening the rotational correlation time of the host molecule. It is not as effective at shortening transverse relaxation as manganese, but is favored because its complexes are more stable and it is more effective at shortening T1. There are several chelates, of which DTPA was the first to be used, that form extremely stable complexes with trivalent ions but which still permit reasonable access to the ion's inner sphere of influence. Improved designs for relaxation agents may be produced, but some at least will likely closely resemble Gd-DTPA in their fundamental construction and the design factors important for their effects can be understood from the theory above. The factors reviewed above describe the primary physical constraints on the design of suitable materials. The development of agents for widespread clinical use will obviously require extensive efficacy and toxicity studies as well.

EXCHANGE EFFECTS

Although there have been several other types of paramagnetic relaxation agents proposed for clinical use, to date the only materials in clinical use on a routine basis are gadolinium chelates. In most parts of the body it distributes rapidly after injection into the extracellular space, prior to excretion. In the brain however it remains intravascular in the intact organ so that it can in principle be used to detect changes in tissue vascularity. However, its effect on NMR signal may depend on compartmental effects inside tissue. For example, if there were no water exchange between the vasculature and tissue, the maximum effect on tissue NMR contrast that would be produced by such an intravascular relaxation agent is when it completely eradicates the signal from the blood (by T2 shortening), or when it so reduces the blood T1 that it does not saturate relative to host tissue. For tissue protons to experience T1 or T2 shortening by paramagnetic ions in the blood, tissue water must diffuse into the immediate hydration sphere of an ion in the time of a spin echo sequence in order to experience the local field of the ion. In a time 50 msecs, water molecules diffuse a distance of order 16 μm. Tissue water that is >16 μm from the center of a capillary will on average experience little effect, so in essence only the capillary volume and perhaps one monolayer of cells around it will show a T1 or T2 reduction, and the overall signal from the rest of the tissue may be barely effected. Under these circumstances, the maximum change in the overall signal, comparing post to pre-contrast scans, would simply be given by the fractional blood volume of that tissue, and the relaxation would no longer be adequately described by a monoexponential. If there is fast and complete exchange of the tissue water with the water in the vasculature, the resultant relaxation rate is a weighted average of the water and blood rates, and should be proportional to the ion concentration. Between these extremes, the apparent relaxation rate will depend on the diffusion radius of the water molecules in tissue, and its relationship to the average spacing of the capillaries. Similar considerations apply to agents that are targeted to particular cell types, such as the reticuloendothelial cells of the liver and spleen. The relaxation rate of much of the water in the liver may not be affected by a relaxation agent that remains in the Kupffer's cells and relies entirely on water exchange between compartments to distribute its effect. The relationship between relaxation time and concentration will then depend on the rate of exchange of water molecules between compartments. Relaxation effects are attenuated when exchange is slow. There exists however a different class of contrast agents, so-called susceptibility agents, that operate by different principles to relaxation effects alone and which do not depend entirely on water exchange to be effective, and these are considered below. However, the compartmental effects just mentioned, and their explicit dependence on the rates of water exchange between compartments, are of practical importance especially in studies involving the tracking of bolus injections of contrast materials. For example, there is widespread interest in the use of so-called first pass imaging techniques for the possible detection of perfusion deficits in myocardium, and the development of ultrafast imaging methods such as echo-planar imaging have made these possible. In principle, there is a simple relationship between the signal change seen in an imaging study and the instantaneous concentration of agent in the blood when the material remains in the vasculature. Macromolecular complexes such as polylysine or albumin labeled with gadolinium which stay in the blood have been tested for such purposes. In regions of high flow, the transit time of the material through the myocardium should be short, and the signal intensity versus time curve should reflect this (20). Visual inspection of an image during the peak of the transit of the agent might intuitively show regions of high flow as bright because the concentration of the agent is high when the fractional blood volume is large. Similarly, perfusion deficits may be expected to be relatively unrelaxed and dark because the concentration of the agent there is low. However, in addition to effects of concentration that correspond to variations in the delivery of the agent, the signal also depends on the exchange rate of water into and out of the blood, and this may not be fast. It is possible then that more water may exchange and be relaxed in regions where the flow is reduced than in regions where the flow is fast, confusing the expected relationship between concentration and signal change. Smaller molecules such as Gd-DTPA leave the blood and diffuse into the extracellular space. The situation then is even more complex, since the amount of contrast material that has time to leave by diffusion out of the capillaries may be smaller in regions of high flow than in areas of low flow. Further work is needed to clarify the inter-relationship of physical and physiological variables in different organs.

SUSCEPTIBILITY AGENTS

Agents that affect the bulk average susceptibility of tissue offer an alternative means of altering the NMR signals from tissues. In fact, all paramagnetics alter the bulk susceptibility in a measurable way, and what follows applies to Gd-DTPA to a significant extent, but there are other materials that are especially effective. Two examples of such agents are small particles of iron oxide which may be so-called superparamagnetic, and dysprosium-DTPA. The latter is a trivalent rare earth metal with 7 unpaired electrons per ion, chelated with DTPA so that the biological pharmacokinetics and distribution are closely similar to Gd-DTPA. Dysprosium-DTPA reduces the signal intensity in T2 weighted studies but shows little effect on T1-weighted scans. Dysprosium chelates can be injected intravascularly and used for first pass studies of brain perfusion and for acquiring brain blood volume maps (21). We will initially focus our discussion on the mechanisms of action of particulate susceptibility agents. However, when dysprosium or any other high susceptibility agent resides inside a blood capillary, the microvessel acts magnetically in much the same way as a small cylindrical particle, so what follows can be applied to the mode of action of intravascular agents in general (22).

Iron oxide particles have extremely high magnetic permeability (susceptibility) viz. the magnetization induced in the particle for a given applied field is extremely large. The term superparamagnetism was coined by Bean (23) to describe a type of magnetic behavior somewhat between simple paramagnetism and ferromagnetism. Paramagnetism is the phenomena already met above, for metal ions as well as for the nuclear magnetization, whereby there is a tendency for a magnetic moment to align in the same direction as an applied magnetic field. For ions such as gadolinium, the paramagnetism disappears (via relaxation) as soon as the field is removed. Iron compounds have a stronger property called ferromagnetism that arises because iron atoms have incompletely filled electron M shells. In ferromagnetics there arises a coupling (an exchange force, a force that has no adequate explanation using classical physics) between neighboring atoms such that the atoms tend to strongly align themselves even when there is no field applied. There is in effect an internal magnetic field (sometimes called the Weiss molecular field) that aligns the atoms strongly, giving rise to a large induced magnetization or ferromagnetism, characterized by its remanence after the applied external field has been removed. In polycrystalline specimens, groups of atoms that are all aligned in the same sense form discrete regions or domains, and each domain is akin to a macroscopic bar magnet with a specific magnetic axis. In a large sample of the material, there may be many such domains, each pointing in different directions until an external field is applied, which will tend to align them. The ordering may remain after the field is taken away (permanent magnetism) or until thermal agitation of the sample, perhaps accelerated by heating, destroys the alignment. As the size of the specimen decreases the number of domains decreases. When the specimen contains one or a small number of domains, the magnetization aligns with the field as it is applied, but the ferromagnetism is lost soon after the field is removed because of thermal agitation. This is then the superparamagnetism of small particles of iron oxide, characterized by possessing a strong ferromagnetism in an applied field, but with no remanence after the field has been removed. Prototype agents that have been involved in clinical trials are AMI25 and AM227, manufactured by Advanced Magnetics Inc. (Cambridge, MA). The potential for targeting very small particles using receptor-specific surface coatings has been exploited more recently by Weissleder and coworkers (24) but the mechanisms of action of all these agents rely on similar processes which are considered here.

It must be emphasized that this class of agents is intended to alter the transverse relaxation rate and not the spin-lattice relaxation, i.e., T2 (or T2*, discussed below) rather than T1. In order to properly appreciate how they operate, it is useful to first review the factors and phenomena that affect transverse relaxation. T2 describes the time for the transverse magnetization, produced in response to an rf pulse such as a 90° pulse, to decay irreversibly. The transverse component decreases whenever there is spin-lattice relaxation, i.e., T1 effects all contribute to T2, producing the well known result that T2 is always shorter than T1, since any growth of magnetization back toward equilibrium must correspond to a loss of magnetization from the nonequilibrium state produced by the rf pulses. Thus dipole-dipole interactions, and the fluctuating local fields produced by paramagnetic ions, all affect T2 at least as much as T1. There are however some other important (and sometimes dominant) processes that affect T2 only. It should always be borne in mind that the transverse magnetization is itself the residual net effect of the contributions from a large number of spins that are rotating or precessing together about the applied magnetic field direction (the z axis). They are then in phase, or coherent. The precessional Larmor frequency is proportional to the field strength. It may however be difficult to obtain magnetic fields that are extremely uniform over a sample volume, so that even in the absence of spin-spin interactions the nuclei in different parts of the specimen may experience different magnetic field strengths and therefore, the magnetization in different parts will rotate at slightly different frequencies. Immediately following a 90° pulse, the dipoles rotate together in phase in the x-y plane and produce a measureable signal, but whenever the individual dipoles rotate with slightly different frequencies, they rapidly dephase with respect to each other, viz. they "fan out" in the transverse plane, and the net precessing magnetization (and hence the signal) decreases. This signal is a free induction decay (FID) and its decay rate is conventionally denoted as 1/T2*, where

$$1/T2^* = 1/T2 + \gamma\Delta\mathbf{B}/2. \qquad [12]$$

and $\Delta\boldsymbol{B}$ denotes the range of magnetic fields experienced by the nuclei. An important point is that the transverse relaxation rate of an FID (or a gradient echo, as shown later) depends on the range of static magnetic field strengths affecting the sample.

In addition to the 90° pulse, 180° pulses, which are twice as long or have double the amplitude, are commonly used. 180° pulses rotate the direction of the magnetization in a sample so that at the end of the pulse it points in a direction that is a reflection, about an axis normal to the field direction, of where it pointed at the start of the pulse. The 90° and 180° pulses are used together in the spin echo pulse sequence. It is helpful in considering T2 relaxation processes to review how the spin echo is formed and why this technique is used in MRI. In the spin-echo sequence, a 90° pulse is first applied so that the net magnetization rotates in the x-y plane and induces in a coil a signal that decays as the spins dephase. After an interval, TE/2, a 180° pulse is applied that has the effect of collecting together the spins again at time TE. The effect is like that on a group of runners in a race who, because they move at different speeds, spread out as they get further from the start line; if they are suddenly told they are running in the wrong direction, they will all turn around and, since the farthest away are the fastest, will all arrive back at the start line together. After a time TE, therefore, the nuclei again produce a coherent arrangement that gives rise to a measureable signal or echo. If only instrumental imperfections were causing the original decay, and as long as the spins do not move, then all the dephasing effects are perfectly reversed by the 180° pulse and the echo is the same strength as the FID; but if any nonreversible changes such as those caused by molecular interactions or diffusion take place in the time TE, these are uncorrected by this technique and the echo is reduced in size. These irreversible dephasing interactions include the spin-spin couplings between nuclei. If the nuclei do not move then the rate of decay of the echo with TE does not depend on the degree of nonuniformity of the static applied field as experienced by the nuclei so the spin-echo sequence allows spin-spin interactions to be evaluated even in the presence of additional dephasing effects from nonuniformities in the magnetic field. Nonetheless, T2 dephasing effects are still induced by any apparent inhomogeneity in the static field *at the atomic level* that is not constant for time TE. Thus, whereas T1 relaxation relied on the component of the local field fluctuating at the Larmor frequency, T2 is sensitive to fluctuations at both the Larmor frequency (the "T1 contribution to T2") and at very low frequency (close to zero). In addition we can

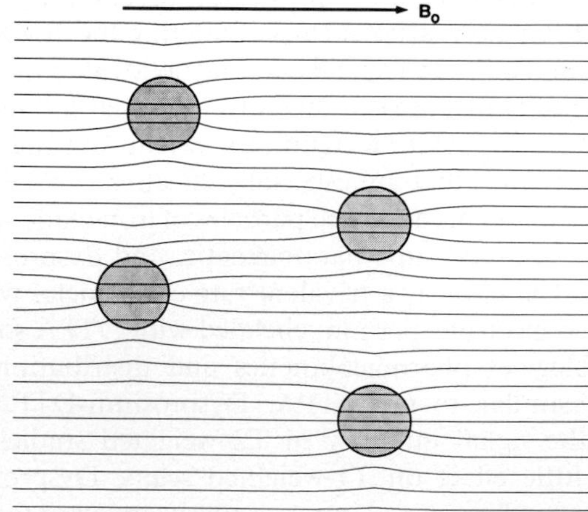

FIG. 9. Schematic representation of the variation of magnetic lines of force caused by regions of different susceptibility. The field across the sample is nonuniform, and there are regions of strong field gradient.

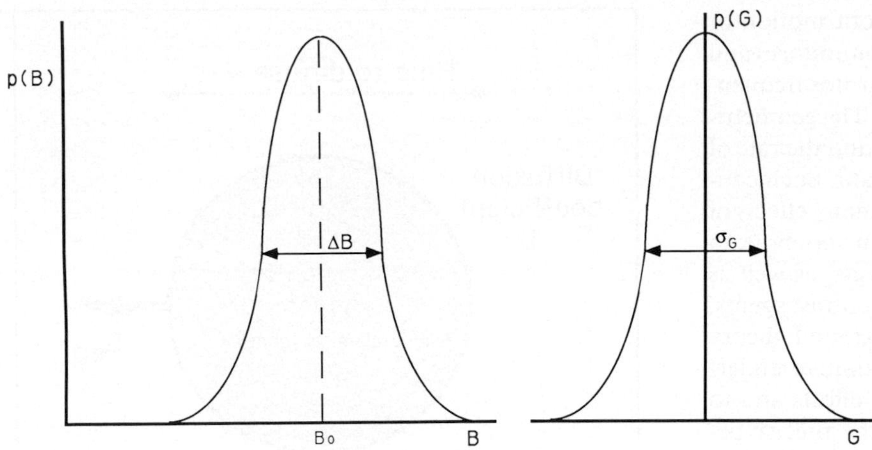

FIG. 10. In the presence of particles or regions of altered suceptibility, the field is no longer single valued. Instead there is a distribution of field values $p(\mathbf{B}) \pm \Delta\mathbf{B}$ and an associated probability $p(G) \pm \sigma_G$ that a spin at any time is in a gradient G.

predict that if molecular translational motion occurs in a nonuniform magnetic field during the time TE so that the nuclei move from one field environment to another, then the apparent transverse decay rate will increase because the frequency pattern that arises before the 180° pulse is not mirrored precisely in the interval after the 180° pulse. Any time this occurs, the 180° is not successful at reversing the dephasing effects. There can therefore occur a contribution to 1/T2 that depends on the diffusion of nuclei in a nonuniform field.

We can therefore identify various transverse relaxation processes that can be important in a medium that is magnetically inhomogeneous. Susceptibility agents may then enhance some of these processes. Figure 9 shows how, in the presence of particles that have different susceptibilities to tissue, the lines of magnetic flux within the sample are distorted and the field becomes nonuniform. The areas of altered susceptibility could be particles or blood microvessels containing a paramagnetic agent. Figure 10 shows how the field experienced by different nuclei then becomes a distribution of field values, and how the value of the field gradient experienced within each part of the sample also takes on a spread of values. A situation of special interest is illustrated in Fig. 11, which shows two examples of the distribution of a high susceptibility agent such as a lanthanide chelate within a volume element. The agent might be distributed uniformly within a voxel, as shown on the left. In this case, the agent may relax water by paramagnetic dipolar interactions (e.g., gadolinium would be more effective than dysprosium); the overall bulk susceptibility increases so there is a net shift in the NMR resonance frequency: but the region is still magnetically homogeneous and there are no intrinsic field gradients or variations. If, however, the same amount of agent is distributed in multiple small subcompartments, as shown on the right, then several other factors become important. While water inside each subcompartment may experience paramagnetic dipolar interactions, the fraction of the whole sample that is relaxed in this way depends on the water exchange across the compartment boundaries in the time of measurement. Therefore, this introduces a dependence on water diffusion and boundary permeability. A second dependence on diffusion is expected because outside the subcompartments a field perturbation is produced that is spatially nonuniform and proportional to the magnetization introduced by the agent. Random motion of the spins through these field gradients will

Uniform Distribution

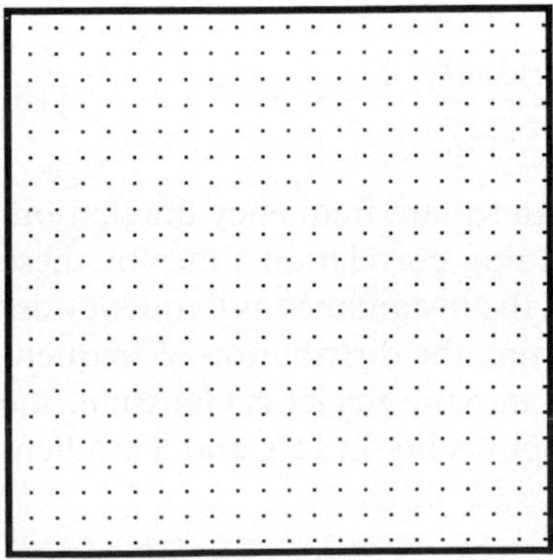

Compartmentalized

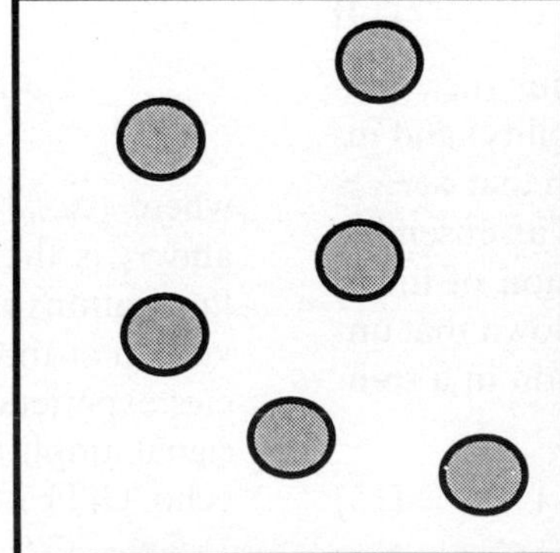

FIG. 11. Two possible distributions of a susceptibility contrast material in tissue. The left side shows the agent uniformly distributed. The magnetic field within this space is uniform. The right side shows the same amount of agent within compartments (e.g., capillaries). This introduces additional mechanisms for transverse relaxation.

contribute to spin dephasing. Even without motion or exchange of the spins the field pattern is nonuniform and thus nuclei will precess with a range of Larmor frequencies and over time the signal will dephase. The geometrical arrangement of the subcompartments and the rate of water diffusion are expected to be important. Such contributions to echo dephasing account for many effects of clinical interest, such as the signal loss from vertebrae, in hemorrhage, or in tissues with iron deposits, as well as after the administration of susceptibility contrast agents.

We now review some pertinent background theory that can be used to provide a more quantitative understanding of the behavior of susceptibility effects and to illustrate some difficulties in predicting the precise behavior of relaxation rates for different media. The loss of transverse magnetization in the presence of magnetic inhomogeneities can be separated into three regimes which are determined by the magnetic, geometric, and dynamic properties of the system. These regimes (which we shall term motionally averaged, intermediate, and static) are most easily defined in terms of the diffusive correlation time of the water molecules in the presence of the magnetic inhomogeneity, τ_D, and the characteristic variation in Larmor frequency due to the field perturbation, $\delta\omega$. For magnetic impurities that are localized τ_D is the time required for diffusion past the field perturber (a magnetic particle or a capillary), and $\delta\omega$ is the change in frequency on the surface of the magnetic inhomogeneity. For a spherical magnetic particle these quantities can be written as (22):

$$\tau_D = R^2/D \qquad [13a]$$

$$\delta\omega = \gamma B_{eq}(R), \qquad [13b]$$

where R is the radius of the sphere, and $B_{eq}(R)$ is the equatorial magnetic field evaluated on the surface of the particle (see Fig. 12).

When the diffusion rate, $1/\tau_D$, is much greater than $\delta\omega$ (i.e., $\delta\omega\tau_D \ll 1$) then diffusion is fast with respect to the spatial variations of the field perturbations and the system is said to be in a motionally narrowed regime. Gillis and Koenig (25) have shown that under these conditions the relaxation rate due to a spherical magnetic impurity may be written as:

$$R_2^{sus} = 16\tau_D(\delta\omega)^2/135, \quad \delta\omega\tau_D \ll 1 \qquad [14]$$

which varies quadratically with magnetization (i.e., quadratically with magnetic field and susceptibility) and inversely with D. When diffusion is slow, such that $\delta\omega\tau_D \gg 1$ the relaxation can be described in terms of an ensemble of spins moving through a static distribution of linear gradients. Majumdar and Gore (26) have shown that under these conditions the transverse relaxation in a spin-echo experiment is well described by:

$$R_2^{sus} = (\gamma\sigma_G \mathrm{TE})^2 D/12, \quad \delta\omega\tau_D \gg 1 \qquad [15]$$

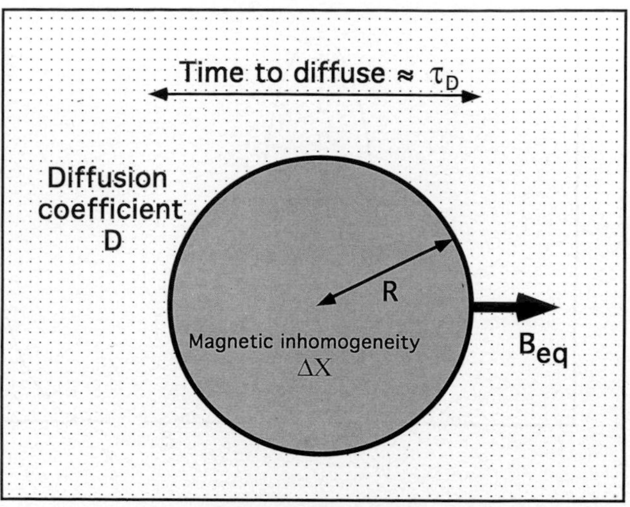

FIG. 12. A single magnetic inhomogeneity, such as a microparticle of capillary containing dysprosium, is characterized by its size (radius R) and the change in susceptibility, ΔX. This generates a field perturbation around the particle characterized by $\mathbf{B}_{eq}$, the field deviation at the surface. Nuclei around the particle take a time τ_D to diffuse a distance equal to the radius. The relative sizes of these parameters determines whether diffusion is important in increasing or decreasing the transverse decay rates.

where σ_G^2 denotes the variance of the internal gradient distribution induced by the perturbation. Under these circumstances the relaxation rate increases linearly with diffusion, and quadratically with the magnetization. When the diffusion is slow enough, such that the spin echo effectively refocuses the magnetization (also $\delta\omega\tau_D \gg 1$), there still is dephasing seen in a gradient echo due to the field inhomogeneities introduced by the perturber. Clearly the behavior differs according to the rate of diffusion, and when $\delta\omega\tau_D \approx 1$ the system is in an intermediate regime.

These different regimes, distinguished by varying correlation times, can be described approximately in terms of so-called Anderson-Weiss mean field theory (27), in which motion leads to modulations in the local field experienced by the water molecules as they move around and past different inhomogeneities. These fluctuations can again be described by a field autocorrelation function,

$$g_\omega(\tau) = \frac{\langle \Delta\omega(t)\Delta\omega(t+\tau)\rangle}{\langle \Delta\omega_0^2\rangle} = e^{-|\tau|/\tau_c} \qquad [16]$$

where $\langle \Delta\omega_0^2\rangle$ is the mean square frequency fluctuation, and τ_c is the corresponding correlation time for these fluctuations and $\Delta\omega(t)$ is the instantaneous frequency deviation at time t. Assuming the distribution of frequencies experienced by the moving nuclei is Gaussian, the signal amplitudes in a spin echo, E(TE), and a gradient echo, G(TE), are given by (27):

$$E(TE) = \exp\left[-\langle\Delta\omega_0^2\rangle\tau_c^2\left\{4\exp\left(\frac{-TE}{2\tau_c}\right) - \exp\left(\frac{-TE}{\tau_c}\right) + \frac{TE}{\tau_c} - 3\right\}\right] \quad [17a]$$

$$G(TE) = \exp\left[-\langle\Delta\omega_0^2\rangle\tau_c^2\left\{\exp\left(\frac{-TE}{\tau_c}\right) - 1 + \frac{TE}{\tau_c}\right\}\right] \quad [17b]$$

Identifying the correlation time as that due to diffusion past the field perturbation, i.e., $\tau_c = \tau_D$, the relaxation rate can be computed for different frequency fluctuations. Figure 13 shows the effective relaxation rate as a function of correlation time for a system with a mean square frequency of 400(rad/sec)^2 (corresponding to field variations of 0.75 mGauss). The relaxation time is defined as the time required for the FID and echo amplitudes to decay to e^{-1}. When the correlation time is short compared to the echo time there is little difference between the gradient echo and spin echo rates. However, as the correlation time is increased, the spin echo relaxation rate reaches a peak and then begins to decrease as refocusing becomes more effective, while the gradient echo relaxation rate approaches the static limit, R_2^*.

When diffusion is slow the correlation time is correspondingly long and the gradient echo will be far more sensitive to susceptibility effects than a spin echo. As diffusion increases the spin-echo relaxation rate also increases due to diffusion within field gradients while the gradient-echo relaxation rate begins to decrease due to motional narrowing. When diffusion is fast the gradient-echo and spin-echo rates decrease and become comparable. A similar argument can be made concerning the size of the inhomogeneity. If the perturbation is large then the field variations experienced by diffusing spins in a short time are small and the relaxation process may be considered essentially the same as in a static field. Under these conditions gradient echo relaxation is much greater than spin echo effects and is relatively insensitive to diffusion. For smaller vessels the field varies more rapidly, and the relaxation rates become sensitive to both diffusion and echo time. The correlation time varies linearly with the size of the inhomogeneity. A consequence of this is that for gradient echo sequences large vessels will always cause more efficient relaxation and hence lead to disproportionately large signal loss. It is also apparent that since the maximum spin-echo relaxation rate is determined by the ratio of the correlation time to the interpulse spacing, the behavior in single spin and multiple echo sequences will be quantitatively different even when TE is the same.

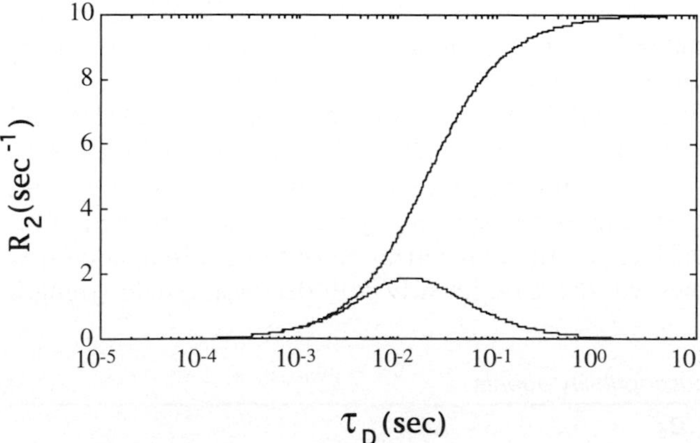

FIG. 13. A plot of Equation 17 showing spin-echo and gradient-echo relaxation rates as a function of the correlation time, for a specific set of geometric variables: capillary diameter 5 μm, TE = 50 ms, and a field deviation of 0.75 mGauss.

The magnetization M is defined as the product of the volume susceptibility and the external magnetic field $\mathbf{B}_0$. In the static regime ($\delta\omega\tau_D \gg 1$, slow diffusion or large vessels) gradient echo relaxation varies approximately linearly with M, while spin echo relaxation varies quadratically. For intermediate relaxation ($1 < \delta\omega\tau_D < 10$) the gradient-echo relaxation can vary anywhere from linear to quadratic whereas the exponent of spin-echo relaxation varies from 1.5 to 2. For fast diffusion with weak field gradients the relaxation is in a motionally narrowed regime and the relaxation varies quadratically for both spin-echo and gradient-echo measurements.

Each of the above mechanisms can be exploited and is relevant in the design of susceptibility contrast agents. Superparamagnetic iron oxide crystals and dysprosium-DTPA have been shown to be extremely effective agents at reducing T2 and T2* and there are strong indications that the change in the relaxation rate produced by such materials when they remain intravascular is significantly greater than is predicted by consideration of the blood volume fraction of the tissue alone (28). This greater efficiency is believed to be due to the fact that the susceptibility difference produced by the agents in blood capillaries sets up magnetic field gradients between the intravascular and extravascular tissue spaces. Water molecules diffusing amongst these tissue spaces experience a significant dephasing effect and consequently the apparent T2 is reduced. The effect is directly proportional to the fractional volume of tissue occupied by the blood capillaries (22) yet at the same time the effect is extended over a much greater volume of the tissue than is occupied by the capillaries themselves. Susceptibility agents therefore offer a potentially more powerful method of affecting the overall tissue signal in NMR imaging experiments. Such effects can be used to discriminate regional variations in tissue blood volume, and in conjunction with very fast imaging methods, to detect regional blood perfusion differences.

Superparamagnetic iron oxide particles are clearly effective and although the precise mechanisms by which they operate in any situation are as yet poorly documented, the relaxation rate changes produced by them

TABLE 4. *Relaxation rate change ΔR_2 (sec^{-1}) per concentration of iron (mg Fe per g medium) for AMI-25 particles in different media at 20 MHz measured by a CPMG sequence*

Medium	ΔR_2
Polyacrylamide gel	3,233
Rat liver	676
Rat spleen	305

From Majumdar and Gore, ref. 26, with permission.

are a combination of the mechanisms described earlier. The effects of AMI-25 have been shown to be field dependent (29). The measured transverse relaxation time is also dependent on the echo time TE and the specific type of pulse sequence used for the measurements, e.g., single echo and multiple echo sequences will show different degrees of reduction at the same TE values (30). Indeed, in strict analysis, the decay of the transverse magnetization cannot be completely described by a single time constant. A further important point is that the effects of susceptibility agents in any medium will depend on the detailed geometrical arrangement of the particles since this influences the pattern of the field gradients. For example, when they remain intravascular, the spacing and cross-sectional areas of capillaries will likely influence their efficacy even for the same mean concentration (22). Therefore, the proportionality constant between concentration and relaxation rate may be a variable between different tissues, or between normal and abnormal states, which will complicate the quantitation of tissue concentrations and the calibration of flow measurements. Evidence for such effects is afforded by Table 4 which shows the measured relaxation rates per unit concentration of iron oxide in different media. Furthermore, the dependence is also sensitive to the precise choice of pulse sequence.

The relative efficacies of various magnetic materials which have been shown to influence tissue contrast in magnetic resonance imaging via susceptibility effects are shown in Table 5 which lists the volume susceptibilities of the chelates of gadolinium and dysprosium, Gd-DTPA, Dy-DTPA, as well as superparamagnetic iron oxide compound, AMI-25 (25).

For a typical 70-kg person with a 5 liter blood supply, the distributed equilibrium concentration of an intravascular agent (assuming it is not removed from the circulatory system) will be 13.6*X (mM/liter), where X is the dose in millimoles per kilogram. Table 5 shows the volume susceptibilities for representative equilibrium blood concentrations of 1 mM/liter for Gd- and Dy-DTPA and AMI-25 (X = 75μmol/kg). Table 5 also shows the effect on the transverse relaxation rate and the calculated signal reduction this induces at TE = 50 ms. For intravascular agents at 1.5 T one can achieve equivalent contrast using AMI-25 at $\frac{1}{10}$ the concentration of Gd-DTPA and $\frac{1}{8}$ the concentration of Dy-DTPA. At lower field strengths the superparamagnetic species will be even more efficient than the paramagnetic agents because of saturation effects; i.e., the magnetization of the paramagnetic species will decrease linearly with decreasing field strength

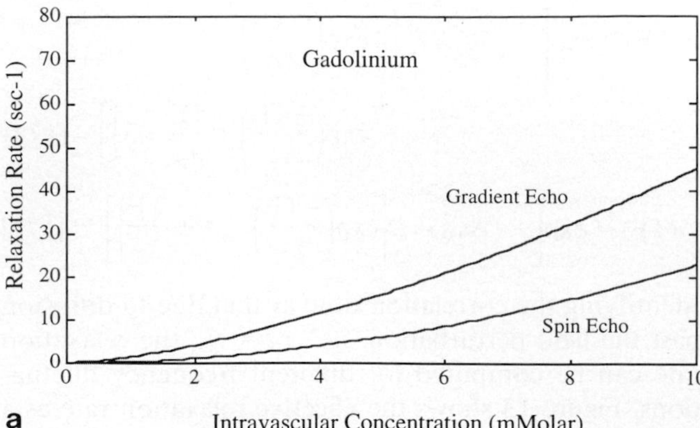

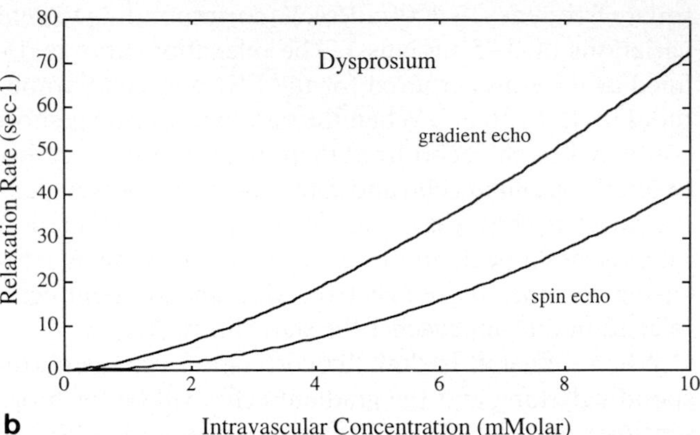

FIG. 14. Comparison of gradient-echo and spin-echo relaxation rates at TE = 50 ms calculated for gadolinium-DTPA (**a**) and dysprosium-DTPA (**b**). The capillary volume fraction was taken as 3%, $D = 0.65 \times 10^{-5}$ cm^2/s, for a collection of parallel capillaries of diameter 5 μm. (From Kennan et al., ref. 22, with permission.)

TABLE 5. *Comparison of susceptibility agents*

Material	$\Delta\chi_v$ (ppm)	$M = \Delta\chi_v \mathbf{B}_o$ ($\mathbf{B}_o$ = 2T)	ΔR_2 (sec^{-1})	S/S_0, Te = 50 ms
Gd-DTPA (1 mM)	2.55^a 10^{-2}	0.51 mGauss	1.44	0.93
Dy-DTPA (1 mM)	3.5^a 10^{-2}	0.70 mGauss	2.31	0.89
AM-I25[a] (1 mM Fe)	1.395^a	5.6 mGauss[a]	51.9[a]	0.075[a]

[a] Measured at 0.4 T. From Majumdar et al., ref. 30, with permission.

while the superparamagnetic material will remain saturated.

Figure 14 shows the calculated relaxation rate enhancement as a function of intravascular concentration for Gd-DTPA and Dy- DTPA evaluated at 85MHz. The water diffusion coefficient was taken to be $0.65*10^{-5}$ cm^2/sec, with a blood volume of 3%, and a capillary diameter of 5 μm, which is typical for brain. Figure 14A shows the spin-echo and gradient-echo relaxation rates for gadolinium while 14B shows the same information for dysprosium. In both cases we ignore dipolar relaxation mediated by exchange across the endothelial wall which is valid when the water exchange rate is slow in brain tissue. We can see that over the range of concentrations shown (0–10 mM) dysprosium is about 60% more effective in a gradient echo and 80% more effective in a spin echo. In both cases the gradient echo shows greater sensitivity to the presence of contrast agent which is characteristic of the intermediate diffusion regime.

CONCLUSIONS

In this chapter the important concepts that are invoked to explain a variety of relaxation processes in tissues are summarized. Relaxation in heterogeneous media embraces several different types of interaction, but in aqueous media such as tissue the dipole-dipole coupling dominates spin-lattice relaxation, whereas there are other effects that can be important in influencing transverse relaxation. Contrast agents for MRI can be seen as agents that employ the same physical processes as those that affect the intrinsic relaxation of tissues. The design factors for both paramagnetic relaxation agents as well as susceptibility agents can be interpreted largely in terms of the same relaxation theory that describes water behavior in heterogeneous media. In this chapter no attempt has been made to discuss methods for targeting agents, or the in vivo behavior of agents in any particular application. Whatever the method of delivery, or the circumstances of the application, the same underlying basic principles will determine the effectiveness of the agent at altering tissue relaxation times.

REFERENCES

1. Bloch F. Nuclear induction. *Phys Rev* 1946;70:460–474.
2. Lauterbur PC, Mendonca-Dias MH, Rudin AM. Augmentation of tissue water proton spin-lattice relaxation rate by in vivo addition of paramagnetic ions. In: Dutton PL, Leigh LS, Scarpa A, eds. *Frontiers of Biological Energetics,* vol 1. New York: Academic Press: 1978:752.
3. Gore JC, Doyle FH, Pennock JM. Relaxation rate enhancement observed in vivo by NMR imaging. *J Comput Assist Tomogr* 1981;304:5.
4. Gore JC. The meaning and significance of relaxation in NMR imaging. In: Witcofski RL, Karstaedt N, Partain CL, eds. *NMR Imaging.* North Carolina: Bowman Gray School of Medicine, 1981: 15–23.
5. Bloembergen N, Purcell E, Pound RV. Relaxation effects in nuclear magnetic resonance absorption. *Phys Rev* 1948;73:679–712.
6. Villringer A, Rosen RB, Belliveau JW, et al. Dynamic imaging with lanthanide chelates in normal brain: contrast due to susceptibility effects. *Magn Reson Med* 1988;6:164–174.
7. Chandra R, Pizzarello D, Keegan A, Chasen N. Study of HO^{3+} as NMR contrast agent for water proton T1 in rat tissues. *Med Phys* 1983;10:545.
8. Solomon I. Relaxation processes in a system of two spins. *Phys Rev* 1955;99:559.
9. Bloembergen N. Proton relaxation times in paramagnetic solutions. *J Chem Phys* 1957;27:572.
10. Bloembergen N, Morgan L. Proton relaxation times in paramagnetic solutions: effect of electron spin relaxation. *J Chem Phys* 1961;34:842–850.
11. Eisinger J, Shulman RG, Blumberg WE. Relaxation enhancement by paramagnetic ion binding in deoxyribonucleic acid solutions. *Nature* 1961;192:963–964.
12. Kang YS, Gore JC, Armitage IM. Studies of factors affecting the design of NMR contrast agents: manganese in blood as a model system. *Magn Reson Med* 1984;1:396–409.
13. Kang YS, Gore JC. Studies of tissue NMR relaxation enhancement by manganese: dose and time dependences. *Invest Radiol* 1984;19:399–407.
14. Reuben J. Gadolinium III as a paramagnetic probe for proton relaxation studies of biological macromolecules: binding to bovine serum albumin. *Biochemistry* 1971;10,28–34.
15. Burton DR, Forsen S, Karlstrom G, Dwek RA, McLaughlin AC, Wain Hobson S. Difficulties in determining accurate molecular motion parameters from proton relaxation enhancement measurements as illustrated by the immunoglobulin G-Gd III system. *Eur J Biochem* 1976;71:519.
16. Lauffer RB, Brady TJ. Preparation and water relaxation properties of proteins labelled with paramagnetic metal chelates. *Magn Reson Imaging* 1985;3:11–16.
17. Lauffer RB. Paramagnetic metal complexes as water proton relaxation agents for NMR imaging: theory and design. *Chem Rev* 1987;87:901–927.
18. Koenig SH, Baglin C, Brown RD III, Brewer CF. Magnetic field dependence of solvent proton relaxation induced by Gd^{3+} and Mn^{2+} complexes. *Magn Reson Med* 1984;1:496.
19. Alsaadi BM, Rossotti FJC, Williams RJP. Hydration of complexes of lanthanide cations. *J Chem Soc, Dalton Trans* 1980;2151–2154.
20. Gore JC Marjumdar S. Measurement of tissue blood flow using intravascular relaxation agents and magnetic resonance imaging. *Magn Reson Med* 1990;14:242–248.
21. Rosen BR, Belliveau JW, Aronen HJ, Kennedy D, Buchbinder BR, Fischman A, Gruber M, Glas J, Weisskoff RM, Cohen MS, Hochberg FH, Brady TJ. Susceptibility contrast imaging of cerebral blood volume: human experience. *Magn Reson Med* 1991;22: 293–299.
22. Kennan RP, Zhong J, Gore JC. Intravascular susceptibility contrast mechanisms in tissues. *Magn Reson Med* 1994;31:9–21.
23. Bean CP, Livingston JD. Superparamagnetism. *J Applied Phys* 1959;30:120S.
24. Weissleder R, Papisov M. Pharmaceutical iron oxides for MR imaging. *Rev Magn Reson Med* 1992;4:1–20.
25. Gillis P, Koenig S. Transverse relaxation of solvent protons induced by magnetized spheres: application to ferritin, erythrocytes and magnetite. *Magn Reson Med* 1987;5:323–345.
26. Majumdar S, Gore JC. Studies of diffusion in random fields produced by variations in susceptibility. *J Magn Reson* 1988;78:41.
27. Anderson PW, Weiss PR. Exchange narrowing in paramagnetic resonance. *Rev Mod Phys* 1953;25:269–276.
28. Kennan RP, Zhong J, Gore JC. On the relative importance of paramagnetic relaxation and diffusion-mediated susceptibility losses in tissues. *Magn Reson Med* 1991;22:197–203.
29. Majumdar S, Zoghbi SS, Pope CF, Gore JC. A quantitative study of relaxation rate enhancement produced by iron oxide particles in polyacrylamide gels and tissue. *Magn Reson Med* 1989;9:185–202.
30. Majumdar S, Zoghbi SS, Gore JC. The influence of pulse sequence on the relaxation effects of superparamagnetic iron oxide contrast agents. *Magn Reson Med* 1989:10:289–301.

Magnetic Resonance Imaging of the Brain and Spine, Second Edition, edited by Scott W. Atlas.
Lippincott-Raven Publishers, Philadelphia © 1996.

6

Bioeffects and Safety Considerations

Frank G. Shellock, Emanuel Kanal, and Marleigh Moscatel

During the performance of magnetic resonance imaging (MRI), the patient is exposed to three different forms of electromagnetic radiation: a static magnetic field, gradient magnetic fields, and radiofrequency (rf) electromagnetic fields. Each of these may cause significant bioeffects if applied at sufficiently high exposure levels.

Numerous investigations have been conducted to identify potentially adverse bioeffects of MRI (1–83). Although none of these have determined the presence of any significant or unexpected hazards (1–83), the data are not comprehensive enough to assume absolute safety. In addition to bioeffects related to exposure to the electromagnetic fields used for MRI, there are several areas of health concern for both the patient and health practitioner with respect to the use of clinical MRI.

This chapter will: (i) discuss the bioeffects of static, gradient, and rf electromagnetic fields with an emphasis on the data that pertains to MRI; (ii) describe and summarize the investigations that specifically apply to MRI; and (iii) provide an overview of other safety considerations and patient management aspects of this imaging technique.

F. G. Shellock, Ph.D.: Future Diagnostics, Inc. and UCLA School of Medicine, Los Angeles, CA 90048.
E. Kanal, M.D.: MRI Department, Pittsburgh NMR Institute, University of Pittsburgh, Pittsburgh, PA 15213.
M. Moscatel: Chicago, IL.

BIOEFFECTS OF STATIC MAGNETIC FIELDS

General Bioeffects of Static Magnetic Fields

There is a paucity of data concerning the effects of high-intensity static magnetic fields on humans. Some of the original investigations on human subjects exposed to static magnetic fields were performed by Vyalov (84,85), who studied workers involved in the permanent magnet industry. These subjects were exposed to static magnetic fields ranging from 0.0015 T to 0.35 T and reported feelings of headache, chest pain, fatigue, vertigo, loss of appetite, insomnia, itching, and other, more nonspecific ailments (84,85). Of note is that exposure to other potentially hazardous environmental working conditions (elevated room temperature, airborne metallic dust, chemicals, etc.) may have been partially responsible for the reported symptoms in these study subjects. Because this investigation lacked an appropriate control group, it is difficult to ascertain if there was a definite correlation between the exposure to the static magnetic field and the reported abnormalities. Subsequent studies performed with more scientific rigor have not substantiated many of the above findings (86–89).

Temperature Effects

There are conflicting statements in the literature regarding the effect of static magnetic fields on body and skin temperatures of mammals. Reports have indicated that static magnetic fields either increase or both increase and decrease tissue temperature, depending on the orientation of the organism in the static magnetic field (19,66). Other articles state that static magnetic fields have no effect on skin and body temperatures of mammals (55,61,88,90).

None of the investigators that identified a static magnetic field effect on temperatures proposed a plausible mechanism for this response, nor has this work been substantiated. In addition, studies that reported static-magnetic-field-induced skin and/or body temperature changes used either laboratory animals that are known to have labile temperatures or instrumentation that may have been affected by the static magnetic fields (19,66).

A recent investigation indicated that exposure to a 1.5 T static magnetic field does not alter skin and body temperatures in humans (61). This study was performed using a special fluoroptic thermometry system demonstrated to be unperturbed by high-intensity static magnetic fields. Therefore, skin and body temperatures of human subjects are believed to be unaffected by exposure to static magnetic fields of up to 1.5 T (55,61).

Electric Induction and Cardiac Effects

Induced biopotentials may be observed during exposure to static magnetic fields and are caused by blood, a conductive fluid, flowing through a magnetic field. The induced biopotential is exhibited by an augmentation of T-wave amplitude as well as by other, nonspecific waveform changes that are apparent on the electrocardiogram and have been observed at static magnetic field strengths as low as 0.1 T (86,91,92).

The increase in T-wave amplitude is directly related to the intensity of the static magnetic field, such that at low static magnetic field strengths the effects are not as predominant as those at higher field strengths. The most marked effect on the T-wave is felt to be caused when the blood flows through the thoracic aortic arch. This T-wave amplitude change can be significant enough to falsely trigger the rf excitation during a cardiac-gated MRI examination.

Other portions of the electrocardiogram may also be altered by the static magnetic field and this varies with the placement of the recording electrodes. Alternate lead positions can be used to attenuate the static magnetic field-induced electrocardiographic changes in order to facilitate cardiac gating studies (93). Once the patient is no longer exposed to the static magnetic field, these EKG voltage abnormalities revert to normal.

Because there are no circulatory alterations that appear to coincide with these electrocardiographic changes, no biologic risks are believed to be associated with the effects that occur in conjunction with static magnetic field strengths of up to 2.0 T (86,91,92).

Neurologic Effects

Theoretically, electrical impulse conduction in nerve tissue may be affected by exposure to static magnetic fields. However, this is an area in the bioeffects literature that contains contradictory information. Some studies have reported remarkable effects on both the function and structure of those portions of the central nervous system that were associated with exposure to static magnetic fields, whereas others have failed to show any significant changes (14,20,34,68,69,76–79,94–99). Further investigations of potential unwanted bioeffects are needed because of the relative lack of clinical studies in this field that are directly applicable to MRI. At the present time, exposure to static magnetic fields of up to 2.0 T do not appear to significantly influence bioelectric properties of neurons in humans (97–99).

In summary, there is no conclusive evidence of irreversible or hazardous biologic effects related to acute, short-term exposures of humans to static magnetic fields of strengths up to 2.0 T. However, as of 1994, there are several 3.0 and 4.0 T whole-body MR systems operating at various research sites around the world. A preliminary study has indicated that workers and volunteer subjects exposed to a 4.0 T MR system have experienced vertigo, nausea, headaches, a metallic taste in their mouths, and magnetophosphenes (which are visual flashes) (50). Therefore, considerable research is required to study the mechanisms responsible for these bioeffects and to determine possible means, if any, to counterbalance them.

Cryogen Considerations

All superconductive MR systems in clinical use today utilize liquid helium. Liquid helium, which maintains the magnet coils in their superconductive state, will achieve the gaseous state ("boil off") at approximately −268.93°C (4.22°K) (99). If the temperature within the cryostat precipitously rises, the helium will enter the gaseous state. In such a situation, the marked increase in volume of the gaseous versus the liquid cryogen (with gas-liquid volume ratios of 760 to 1 for helium and 695 to 1 for nitrogen) will dramatically increase the pressure within the cryostat (99). A pressure-sensitive carbon "pop-off" valve will give way, sometimes with a rather loud popping noise, followed by the rapid (and loud) egress of gaseous helium as it escapes from the cryostat. In normal situations this gas should be vented out of the imaging room and into the external atmosphere. It is possible, however, that during such venting some helium gas might accidentally be released into the ambient atmosphere of the imaging room.

Gaseous helium is considerably lighter than air. If any helium gas is inadvertently released into the imaging room, the dimensions of the room, its ventilation capacity, and the total amount of gas released will determine whether the helium gas will reach the patient or health practitioner who is in the lower part of the room (99). Helium vapor looks like steam and is entirely odorless and tasteless, but it may be extremely cold. Asphyxiation and frostbite are possible if a person is exposed to helium vapor for a prolonged time. In a system quench, a considerable quantity of helium gas may be released into the imaging room. This might secondarily cause difficulty in opening the room door because of the pressure differential produced. In such a circumstance, the first response should be to evacuate the area until the offending helium vapor is adequately removed from the imaging room environment and safely redirected to an outside environment away from patients, pedestrians, or temperature-sensitive material (99).

Better cryostat design and insulation have allowed the use of only liquid helium in many of the newer superconducting magnets. However, there still are a great number of magnets in clinical use that utilize liquid nitrogen as well. Liquid nitrogen within the cryostat acts as a buffer between the liquid helium and the outside atmosphere, boiling off at 77.3°K. In the event of an accidental release of liquid nitrogen into the ambient atmosphere of the imaging room, there is a potential for frostbite, similar to that encountered with gaseous helium release. Gaseous nitrogen is roughly the same density as air and is certainly much less buoyant than gaseous helium.

In the event of an inadvertent venting of nitrogen gas into the imaging room the gas could easily settle near floor level; the amount of nitrogen gas within the room would continue to increase until venting ceased. The total concentration of nitrogen gas contained within the room would be determined on the basis of the total amount of the gas released into the room, the dimensions of the room, and its ventilation capacity (the existence and size of other routes of egress, e.g., doors, windows, ventilation ducts, and fans). A pure nitrogen environment is exceptionally hazardous, and unconsciousness generally results as early as 5–10 seconds after exposure (99). It is imperative that all patients and health personnel evacuate the area as soon as it is recognized that nitrogen gas is being released into the imaging room, and they should not return until appropriate corrective measures have been taken to clear the gas from the room (99).

Dewar (cryogen storage containers) storage should also be within a well-ventilated area, lest normal boil-off rates increase the concentration of inert gas within the storage room to a dangerous level (J. E. Gray, *oral communication*, September 1989). At least one reported death has occurred in an industrial setting during the shipment of cryogens (J. E. Gray, *oral communication*, August 1989), although to our knowledge no such fatality has occurred in the medical community. There is one report of a sudden loss of consciousness of unexplained cause by an otherwise healthy technologist (with no prior or subsequent similar episodes) passing through a cryogen storage area where multiple dewars were located (A. Aisen, *oral communication*, May 1989). While there is no verification of ambient atmospheric oxygen concentration to confirm any relationship to the cryogens per se, the history is strongly suggestive of such a relationship.

Cryogens present a potential concern in clinical MR imaging despite an overwhelmingly safe record over the past 7 or more years of clinical service (99). Proper handling and storage of cryogens, as well as the appropriate behavior in the presence of possible leaks, should be emphasized at each site. An oxygen monitor with an audible alarm, situated at an appropriate height within each imaging room, should be a mandatory minimum safety measure for all sites; automatic linking to and activation of an imaging room ventilation fan system when the oxygen monitor registers below 18% or 19% should be considered at each magnet installation (99).

Electrical Considerations of a Quench

In addition to the potential for cryogen release, there is also a concern about the currents that may be induced in conductors (such as biologic tissues) near the rapidly changing magnetic field associated with a quench (5,99). In one study, physiologic monitoring of a pig and monitoring of the environment were performed during an intentional quench from 1.76 T; there seemed to be no significant effect on the blood pressure, pulse, temperature, and electroencephalographic and ECG measurements of the pig during or immediately following the quench (5).

While such a single observation does not prove safety for humans undergoing exposure to a quench, the data do suggest that the experience would indeed be similar, and that there would be no deleterious electrical effects on humans undergoing a similar experience and exposure.

BIOEFFECTS OF GRADIENT MAGNETIC FIELDS

MRI exposes the human body to rapid variations of magnetic fields due to the transient application of magnetic field gradients during the imaging sequence. Gradient magnetic fields can induce electrical fields and currents in conductive media (including biologic tissue) according to Faraday's law of induction. The potential for interaction between gradient magnetic fields and biologic tissue is inherently dependent on the fundamental field frequency, the maximum flux density, the average flux density, the presence of harmonic frequencies, the waveform characteristics of the signal, the polarity of the signal, the current distribution in the body, and the electrical properties and sensitivity of the particular cell membrane (97–99).

For animals and human subjects, the induced current is proportional to the conductivity of the biologic tissue and the rate of change of the magnetic flux density (98–101). In theory, the largest current densities will be produced in peripheral tissues (i.e., at the greatest radius) and will linearly diminish towards the body's center (98–101). The current density will be enhanced at higher frequencies and magnetic flux densities and will be further accentuated by a larger tissue radius with a greater tissue conductivity. Current paths are affected by differences in tissue types, such that tissues with low conductivity (e.g., adipose and bone) will change the pattern of the induced current.

Bioeffects of induced currents can be due either to the power deposited by the induced currents (thermal effects) or to direct effects of the current (nonthermal effects). Thermal effects due to switched gradients used in MRI are negligible and are not believed to be clinically significant (96,98,99).

Possible nonthermal effects of induced currents are stimulation of nerve or muscle cells, induction of ventricular fibrillation, increased brain mannitol space, epileptogenic potential, stimulation of visual flash sensations, and bone healing (98–103). The threshold currents required for nerve stimulation and ventricular fibrillation are known to be much higher than the estimated current densities that will be induced under routine clinical MRI conditions (96–100).

The production of magnetophosphenes is considered to be one of the most sensitive physiologic responses to gradient magnetic fields (96–99). Magnetophosphenes are supposedly caused by electrical stimulation of the retina and are completely reversible with no associated health effects (96–99). These have been elicited by current densities of roughly 17 $\mu A/cm^2$. In contrast to this level, the currents that are required for the induction of nerve action potentials is roughly 3,000 $\mu A/cm^2$ and those required for ventricular fibrillation induction of healthy cardiac tissue are calculated to be 100–1,000 $\mu A/cm^2$ (96). Although there have been no reported cases, to our knowledge, of magnetophosphenes for fields of 1.95 T or less, magnetophosphenes have been reported in volunteers working in and around a 4.0 T research system (50). In addition, a metallic taste and symptoms of vertigo seem also to be reproducible and associated with rapid motion within the static magnetic field of these 4.0 T systems (50).

Time-varying, extremely low-frequency magnetic fields have been demonstrated to be associated with multiple effects, including clustering and altered orientation of fibroblasts, as well as increased mitotic activity of fibroblast growth, altered DNA synthesis, and reduced fentanyl-induced anesthesia (49,64,99). Possible effects in multiple other organisms, including humans, have also been mentioned (99). While there have been no studies to conclusively demonstrate carcinogenic effects from exposure to time-varying magnetic fields of various intensities and durations, several reports suggest that an association between the two is still plausible (104–106).

BIOEFFECTS OF RADIOFREQUENCY ELECTROMAGNETIC FIELDS

General Bioeffects of Radiofrequency Electromagnetic Fields

Radiofrequency (rf) radiation is capable of generating heat in tissues as a result of resistive losses. Therefore, the main bioeffects associated with exposure to rf radiation are related to the thermogenic qualities of this electromagnetic field (96–99,108–116). Exposure to rf radiation may also cause athermal, field-specific alterations in biological systems that are produced without a significant increase in temperature (108–114). This topic is somewhat controversial due to assertions concerning the role of electromagnetic fields in producing cancer and developmental abnormalities, along with the concomitant ramifications of such effects (108–114). A report from the U.S. Environmental Protection Agency claimed that the existing evidence on this issue is sufficient to demonstrate a relationship between low level electromagnetic field exposures and the development of cancer (106). To this date, there have been no specific studies performed to study potential athermal bioeffects of MRI. Those interested in a thorough review of this topic, particularly as it pertains to MRI, are referred to the extensive article written by Beers (113).

Regarding rf power deposition concerns, investigators have typically quantified exposure to rf radiation by means of determining the specific absorption rate (SAR) (108–112,116–119). SAR is the mass normalized rate at which rf power is coupled to biologic tissue and is indicated in units of watts per kilogram (W/kg). Measurements or estimates of SAR are not trivial, particularly in human subjects, and there are several methods of determining this parameter for rf energy dosimetry (108–112,119).

The SAR that is produced during MRI is a complex function of numerous variables including the frequency (which, in turn, is determined by the strength of the static magnetic field), type of rf pulse (i.e., 90° or 180°), repetition time, pulse width, type of rf coil used, volume of tissue within the coil, resistivity of the tissue, configuration of the anatomical region imaged, as well as other factors (96–99). The actual increase in tissue temperature caused by exposure to rf radiation is dependent on the subject's thermoregulatory system (e.g., skin blood flow, skin surface area, sweat rate, etc.) (97–99).

The efficiency and absorption pattern of rf energy are mainly determined by the physical dimensions of the tissue in relation to the incident wavelength (108–112). Therefore, if the tissue size is large relative to the wavelength, energy is predominantly absorbed on the surface; if it is small relative to the wavelength, there is little absorption of rf power (108–112). Because of the above relationship between rf energy and physical dimensions, studies designed to investigate the effects of exposure to rf radiation during MRI that are intended to be applicable to the clinical setting require tissue volumes and anatomical shapes comparable to that of human subjects. Of additional note is that there is no laboratory animal that sufficiently mimics or simulates the thermoregulatory system or responses of man. For these reasons, results obtained in laboratory animal experiments cannot simply be "scaled" or extrapolated to human subjects (110–112,119).

MRI and Exposure to Radiofrequency Radiation

Little quantitative data has been previously available on thermoregulatory responses of humans exposed to rf radiation prior to the studies performed with MRI. The few studies that exist do not directly apply to MRI because these investigations either examine thermal sensations or therapeutic applications of diathermy, usually involving only localized regions of the body (108–110,114).

Several studies of rf power absorption during MRI have been performed recently and have yielded useful information about tissue heating in human subjects (28,58–60,62,63,65). During MRI, tissue heating results primarily from magnetic induction with a negligible contribution from the electric fields, so that ohmic heating occurs greatest at the surface of the body and approaches zero at the center of the body. Predictive calculations and measurements obtained in phantoms and human subjects exposed to MRI supports this pattern of temperature distribution (58–60,115,116).

Although one paper reported significant temperature rises in internal organs produced by MRI (65), this study was conducted on anesthetized dogs and is unlikely to be applicable to conscious adult human subjects because of factors related to the physical dimensions and dissimilar thermoregulatory systems of these two species. However, these data may have important implications for the use of MRI in pediatric patients since this patient population is typically sedated or anesthetized for MRI examinations.

An investigation using fluoroptic thermometry probes that are unperturbed by electromagnetic fields (117) demonstrated that human subjects exposed to MRI at SAR levels up to 4.0 W/kg (i.e., 10 times higher than the level currently recommended by the United States Food and Drug Administration) have no statistically significant increases in body temperatures and elevations in skin temperatures that are believed to be clinically hazardous (62). These results imply that the suggested exposure level of 0.4 W/kg for rf radiation during MRI is too conservative for individuals with normal thermoregulatory function (62). Additional studies are needed, however, to assess physiologic responses of patients with conditions that may impair thermoregulatory function (e.g., elderly patients; patients with underlying health conditions such as fever, diabetes, cardiovascular disease, or obesity; and patients taking medications that affect thermoregulation such as calcium blockers, beta blockers, diuretics, vasodilators, etc.) before subjecting them to MRI procedures that require high SARs.

Temperature-Sensitive Organs

Certain human organs that have reduced capabilities for heat dissipation, such as the testis and eye, are particularly sensitive to elevated temperatures. Therefore, these are primary sites of potential harmful effects if rf radiation exposures during MRI are excessive. Laboratory investigations have demonstrated detrimental effects on testicular function (i.e., a reduction or cessation of spermatogenesis, impaired sperm motility, degeneration of seminiferous tubules, etc.) caused by rf radiation-induced heating from exposures sufficient enough to raise scrotal and/or testicular tissue temperatures up to 38° to 42°C (118).

Scrotal skin temperatures (i.e., an index of intratesticular temperature) were measured in volunteer subjects undergoing MRI at a whole body averaged SAR of 1.1 W/kg (63). The largest change in scrotal skin temperature was 2.1°C and the highest scrotal skin temperature recorded was 34.2°C (63). These temperature changes were below the threshold known to impair testicular function. However, excessively heating the scrotum during MRI could exacerbate certain pre-existing disorders associated with increased scrotal/testicular temperatures (e.g., acute febrile illnesses, varicocele, etc.) in patients who are already oligospermic and lead to possible temporary or permanent sterility (63). Therefore, additional studies designed to investigate these issues are needed, particularly if patients are scanned at whole body averaged SARs higher than those previously evaluated.

Dissipation of heat from the eye is a slow and inefficient process due to its relative lack of vascularization. Acute near-field exposures of rf radiation to the eyes or heads of laboratory animals have been demonstrated to be cataractogenic as a result of the thermal disruption of ocular tissues if the exposure is of a sufficient intensity and duration (108,110). An investigation conducted by Sacks et al. (53) revealed that there were no discernable effects on the eyes of rats produced by MRI at exposures that far exceeded typical clinical imaging levels. However, it may not be acceptable to extrapolate this data to human subjects considering the coupling of rf radiation to the anatomy and tissue volume of the laboratory rat eyes compared to those of man.

Corneal temperatures have been measured in patients undergoing MRI of the brain using a send/receive head coil at local SARs up to 3.1 W/kg (59). The largest corneal temperature change was 1.8°C and the highest temperature measured was 34.4°C. Since the temperature threshold for rf radiation-induced cataractogenesis in animal models has been demonstrated to be between 41 to 55°C for acute, near-field exposures, it does not appear that clinical MRI using a head coil has the potential to cause thermal damage in ocular tissue (59). The effect of MRI at higher SARs and the long-term effects of MRI on ocular tissues remain to be determined.

Radiofrequency Radiation and "Hot Spots"

Theoretically, rf radiation "hot spots" caused by an uneven distribution of rf power may arise whenever current concentrations are produced in association with restrictive conductive patterns. There has been the suggestion that rf radiation "hot spots" may generate thermal "hot spots" under certain conditions during MRI. Since rf radiation is mainly absorbed by peripheral tissues, thermography has been used to study the heating pattern associated with MRI at high whole body SARs (57). This study demonstrated no evidence of surface thermal "hot spots" related to MRI of human subjects. The thermoregulatory system apparently responds to the heat challenge by distributing the thermal load, producing a "smearing" effect of the surface temperatures. However, there is a possibility that internal thermal "hot spots" may develop from MRI (65).

UNITED STATES FOOD AND DRUG ADMINISTRATION GUIDELINES FOR MR DEVICES

In 1988, MR diagnostic devices were reclassified from class III, in which premarket approval is required, to class II, which is regulated by performance standards, as long as the device(s) are within the "umbrella" of defined limits addressed below (107). Subsequent to this reclassification, new devices had only to demonstrate that they were "substantially equivalent" to any class II device that was brought to market using the premarket notification process (510[k]) or, alternatively, to any of the devices described by the 13 MR system manufacturers that had petitioned the FDA for such a reclassification.

Four areas relating to the use of MR systems have been identified for which safety guidelines have been issued by the FDA. These include the static magnetic field, the gradient magnetic fields, the rf power of the examination, and the acoustical considerations. Excerpts from the wording of the FDA Safety Parameter Action Levels are as follows (107):

Static magnetic field—Static magnetic field strengths not exceeding 2.0 T are below the level of concern for the static magnetic field. Should the static magnetic field strength exceed 2.0 T, additional evidence of safety must be provided by the sponsor.

Gradient magnetic field—Limit patient exposure to time-varying magnetic fields with strengths less than those required to produce peripheral nerve stimulation or other effects. There are three alternatives:

1. Demonstrate that the maximum dB/dt of the system is 6 T/sec or less.
2. Demonstrate that for axial gradients, $dB/dt < 20$ T/sec for $p \geqslant 120$ msec, or $dB/dt < (2{,}400/p)$ T/sec for 12 msec $< p <$ 120 psec, or $dB/dt < 200$ T/sec for $p \leqslant 12$ psec (p equals the width in microseconds of a rectangular pulse or the half period of a sinusoidal dB/dt pulse). For transverse gradients, dB/dt is considered to be below the level of concern when it is less than three times the above limits for axial gradients.
3. Demonstrate with valid scientific evidence that the rate of change of magnetic field for the system is not sufficient to cause peripheral nerve stimulation by an adequate margin of safety (at least a factor of three).

The parameter dB/dt must be lower than that either of the two levels of concern by presentation of valid scientific measurement of calculational evidence sufficient to demonstrate that the time rate of magnetic field change (*dB/dt*) is of no concern.

Radiofrequency power deposition—Options to control the risk of systemic thermal overload and local thermal injury caused by rf energy absorption are as follows:

1. If the specific absorption rate is 0.4 W/kg or less for the whole body and 8.0 W/kg or less spatial peak in any 1 g of tissue, and if the specific absorption rate is 3.2 W/kg or less averaged over the head, then it is below the level of concern.
2. If exposure to rf magnetic fields is insufficient to produce a core temperature increase of 1°C and localized heating to no greater than 38°C in the head, 39°C in the trunk, and 40°C in the extremities, then it is considered to be below the level of concern.

The parameter rf heating must be below either of the two levels of concern by presentation of valid scientific measurement or calculational evidence sufficient to demonstrate that rf heating effects are of no concern.

Acoustic noise levels—The acoustic noise levels associated with the device must be shown to be below the level of concern established by pertinent federal regulatory or other recognized standards-setting organizations. If the acoustic noise is not below the level of concern, the sponsor must recommend steps to reduce or alleviate the noise perceived by the patient (107).

MRI AND ACOUSTIC NOISE

The acoustic noise produced during MRI represents a potential risk to patients. Acoustic noise is associated with the activation and deactivation of electrical current that induces vibrations of the gradient coils. This repetitive sound is enhanced by higher gradient duty cycles and sharper pulse transitions. Acoustic noise is thus likely to increase with decreases in section thicknesses, decreased fields of view, repetition times, and echo times.

Gradient magnetic field-related noise levels measured on several commercial MR scanners were in the range of 65–95 dB, which is considered to be within the recommended safety guidelines set forth by the U.S. FDA (107). However, there have been reports that acoustic noise generated during MRI has caused patient annoyance, interference with oral communication, and reversible hearing loss in patients who did not wear ear protection (9,120). A recent study of patients undergoing MR imaging without earplugs resulted in temporary hearing loss in 43% of the subjects (9). Furthermore, the possibility exists that significant gradient coil-induced noise may produce permanent hearing impairment in certain patients who are particularly susceptible to the damaging effects of relatively loud noises (9,120).

The safest and least expensive means of preventing problems associated with acoustic noise during clinical MRI is to encourage the routine use of disposable earplugs (9,120). The use of hearing protection has been demonstrated to successfully avoid the potential temporary hearing loss that can be associated with clinical MRI examinations (9,120). MR compatible headphones that significantly muffle acoustic noise are also commercially available.

An acceptable alternative strategy for reducing sound levels during MRI is to use an "antinoise" or destructive interference technique that not only effectively reduces noise, but also permits better patient communication (122). This technique consists of a real-time Fourier analysis of the noise emitted from the MR system (122). A signal possessing the same physical characteristics but opposite phase than the sound generated by the MR system is produced. The two opposite-phase signals are then combined resulting in a cancellation of the repetitive noise, while allowing other sounds such as music and voice to be transmitted to the patient (122). A recent investigation demonstrated no significant degradation of image quality when MRI is performed with MR systems that utilize this "antinoise" method (122). While this technique has not yet found wide-spread clinical application, it has considerable potential for minimizing acoustic noise and its associated problems.

INVESTIGATIONS OF MRI BIOLOGICAL EFFECTS

Investigations performed to specifically study the potential bioeffects of MRI are summarized in Table 1 (1–83). The results of these MRI-related bioeffects studies have been predominantly negative, supporting the widely held view that there are no significant health risks associated with the use of this imaging modality. Experiments that yielded positive results either identified possible, nonspecific biological responses, determined short-term biological changes that were not considered to be deleterious, or found bioeffects that require further substantiation.

When perusing these studies, the reader should note that the dosimetric aspects of the exposure(s) to static, gradient, and/or radiofrequency electromagnetic fields were quite variable and include those that exceeded clinical exposures, simulated clinical exposures, or involved low-level, chronic exposures. In certain cases, the effects of only one of the electromagnetic fields used for MRI was evaluated. Theoretically, there is a possibility that the combination of static, gradient, and rf electromagnetic fields may produce some unusual and/or unpredictable bioeffects that are unique to MRI.

"Window" effects are often present with respect to biological changes that occur in response to electromagnetic radiation. "Window" effects are those biological

TABLE 1. *Summary of studies that investigated bioeffects of MRI*

Study description	Results	Reference
2.0 T Clinical imaging conditions Rats Studied effect of MRI on blood–brain barrier permeability	"No MRI-induced difference was detected"	Adzamil et al. (1)
1.5 T Exposure to rf radiation in excess of clinical imaging conditions Sheep Studied rf radiation-induced heating	"For exposure periods in excess of standard clinical imaging protocols the temperature increase was insufficient to cause adverse thermal effects"	Barber et al. (2)
0.5 and 1.5 T Clinical imaging conditions Human subjects Studied effect of MRI on the EEG and evaluated neuropsychological status	"No measurable influence of MRI on cognitive functions"	Bartels et al. (3)
0.04 T Clinical imaging conditions Human subjects Studied effects of MRI on cognition	"MRI did not cause any cognitive deterioration"	Besson et al. (4)
1.6 T Quenched magnet Pig Studied effect of quenching a magnet	"Our findings, which in the circumstances of this experiment, suggested that the risks are small"	Bore et al. (5)
MRI gradient-induced electric fields Dogs Studied bioeffects at high MRI gradient-induced fields	"As the strength of MRI gradient-induced fields increase, biological effects in order of increasing field and severity include stimulation of peripheral nerves, nerves of respiration and finally, the heart"	Bourland et al. (6)
0.38 T Static magnetic field only Deoxygenated erythrocytes Studied orientation of sickle erythrocytes	"Further studies are needed to assess possible hazards of MRI of sickle cell disease"	Brody et al. (7)
0.35 and 1.5 T Clinical imaging conditions Human subjects with sickle cell disease Studied effects of MRI on patients with sickle cell disease	"No change in sickle cell blood flow during MR imaging in vivo"	Brody et al. (8)
0.35 T Clinical imaging conditions Human subjects Studied effects of noise during MRI on hearing	"Noise generated by MR imaging may cause temporary hearing loss, and earplugs can prevent this"	Brummett et al. (9)
Varying gradient fields Humans Studied neural stimulation threshold with varying oscillations and gradient field strength	"The threshold decreases with the number of oscillations and increases with frequency. The repeatable threshold of 63 T/sec (1270 Hz) remains constant from 32 oscillations (25.6 msec) to 128 oscillations (102.4 msec)"	Budinger et al. (10)
0.15 T Simulated imaging conditions HL60 promyelocytic cells Studied effect of MRI of Ca^{2+}	"Results demonstrate that time-varying magnetic fields associated with MRI procedures increase Ca^{2+}"	Carson et al. (11)
Gradient magnetic fields up to 66 T/sec in dogs and 61 T/sec in humans Dogs Human subjects Studied physiologic responses to large amplitude time-varying magnetic fields	Dogs—"No motion, twitch, or ECG abnormalities" Humans—"Brief minimal muscular twitches observed on various parts of the body due to magnetic stimulation"	Cohen et al. (12)

TABLE 1. *Continued*

Study description	Results	Reference
0.5 and 1.0 T Simulated imaging conditions Cultured human blood cells Studied effect of static magnetic fields and line scan imaging on human blood cells	"Neither treatment had any significant effect on any of the parameters measured"	Cooke and Morris (13)
4.7 T Exposures to static and rf electromagnetic fields only Isolated rabbit hearts Studied effects on cardiac excitability and vulnerability	No measurable effect on strength interval relationship or ventricular vulnerability	Doherty et al. (14)
Gradient magnetic fields only Sinusoidal gradients at a frequency of 1.25 kHz with amplitudes up to 40 mT/min for a *z* coil and 25 mT/min for an *x* coil Human subjects Studied physiologic effects, physiologic responses	Observed peripheral muscle stimulation, no extrasystoles or arrhythmias	Fischer (15)
0.3, 0.5, and 1.5 T Simulated imaging conditions and static/rf and gradient fields separately Rats Studied blood–brain barrier permeability	"Increased brain mannitol associated with gradient fluid flux may reflect increased blood–brain barrier permeability or blood volume in brain"	Garber et al. (16)
2.2 to 2.7 T Simulated imaging conditions Mouse cells Studied oncogenic and genotoxic effects of MRI	"Data clearly mitigate against an association between exposure to MR imaging modalities and both carcinogenic and genotoxic effects"	Geard et al. (17)
60 T/sec Gradient magnetic fields only Human subjects Studied effects of gradient magnetic fields on cardiac and respiratory function	"No changes were observed"	Gore et al. (18)
0.1 to 1.5 T Static magnetic field only Human subjects Studied effects of static magnetic fields on temperature	Temperatures increased or decreased depending on field strength of magnet	Gremmel et al. (19)
2.11 T Static magnetic field only Isolated rat hearts Studied effect of static magnetic field on cardiac muscle contraction	"Static magnetic fields used in NMR imaging do not constitute any hazard in terms of cardiac contractility"	Gulch and Lutz (20)
2.0 T rf at 90 MHz Simulated imaging conditions Phantom Caphuchin monkey Studied temperature changes in phantom and monkey brain during high rf power exposures	"Blood flowing through the brain used the body as a heat sink"	Hammer et al. (21)
0.35 T Simulated imaging conditions Mice Studied teratogenic effects of MRI	"Prolonged midgestional exposure failed to reveal any overt embryotoxicity or teratogenicity" "Slight but significant reduction in fetal crown-rump length after prolonged exposure justifies further study of higher MRI energy levels"	Heinrichs et al. (22)
1.5 T Static magnetic field only Human subjects Studied effect of static magnetic field on somatosensory-evoked potentials	"Short-term exposure to 1.5 T static magnetic field does not affect SEPs in human subjects"	Hong and Shellock (23)

TABLE 1. *Continued*

Study description	Results	Reference
0.15 T Simulated imaging conditions Rats Studied effects on cognitive processes	"MRI procedure has no significant effect on spatial memory processes in rats"	Innis et al. (24)
2.0 T Static magnetic field only Human subjects Studied effect of static magnetic field on cardiac rhythm	Cardiac cycle length was significantly increased but this is probably harmless in normal subjects; safety in dysrrhythmic patients remains to be determined	Jehenson et al. (25)
1.5 T Simulated imaging conditions Frog embryo Studied effect of MRI on embryogenesis	"No adverse effects of MRI components on development of this vertebrate (*Xenopus laevis*)"	Kay et al. (26)
2.3, 4.7, and 10 T Static magnetic fields only Physiologic solutions (2.3 and 4.7 T) and mathematic modeling (10 T) Studied hydrostatic pressure and electrical potentials across vessels in presence of static magnetic fields	"A 10-T magnetic field changes vascular pressure in a model of the human vasculature by less than 0.2%"	Keltner et al. (27)
1.5 T Clinical imaging conditions Human subjects Studied physiologic changes during high field strength MRI	"Temperature changes and other physiologic changes . . . were small and of no clinical concern"	Kido et al. (28)
1.5 T Simulated imaging conditions Rats Studied effects of MRI on receptor-mediated activation of pineal gland indole biosynthesis	"Strong magnetic fields and/or radiofrequency pulsing used in MRI inhibited beta-adrenergic activation of the gland"	LaPorte et al. (29)
3.5 to 12 kT/sec Gradient magnetic fields only Mice Studied effect of gradient magnetic fields on pregnancy and postnatal development	"No significant difference between the litter numbers and growth rates of the exposed litters compared with controls"	McRobbie and Foster (30)
Various strong magnetic fields Gradient magnetic fields only Anesthetized rats Studied cardiac response to gradient magnetic fields	"The types of pulsed magnetic fields used in the present study did not affect the cardiac cycle of anesthetized rats"	McRobbie and Foster (31)
1.89 T Simulated imaging sequence Rats Studied taste aversion in rats to evaluate possible toxic effects of MRI	"Rats exposed to MRI did not display any aversion to the saccharin solution"	Messmer et al. (32)
1.89 T Simulated imaging sequence Mouse spleen cells Studied possible interaction between ionizing radiation and MRI on damage to normal tissue	"For the normal tissues studied, MR imaging neither increases radiation damage nor inhibits repair"	Montour et al. (33)
0 to 2.0 T Clinical imaging conditions Human subjects Studied the extent of changes of the brainstem-evoked potentials with MRI	"Routine MRI examinations do not produce pathological changes in auditory-evoked potentials"	Muller et al. (34)
1.5 T Simulated imaging conditions Human subjects Studied effect of MRI on somatosensory and brainstem auditory-evoked potentials	"It may be assumed that MRI causes no lasting changes"	Niemann et al. (35)

TABLE 1. *Continued*

Study description	Results	Reference
0.75 T Static magnetic field only Hamster cells Studied effect of static magnetic field on DNA synthesis and survival of mammalian cells irradiated with fast neutrons	"Presence of the magnetic field either during or subsequent to fast-neutron irradiation does not effect the neutron-induced radiation damage or its repair"	Ngo et al. (36)
1.89 T Static magnetic field only Mice Studied effects of long-term exposure to a static magnetic field	"No consistent differences found in gross and microscopic morphology, hematocrit and WBCs, plasma creatine phosphokinase, lactic dehydrogenase, cholesterol, triglyceride, or protein concentrations in magnet groups compared to two control groups"	Osbakken et al. (37)
0.15 T Simulated imaging conditions Rats Studied effects of MRI on behavior of rats	"Results fail to provide any evidence for short or long-term behavioral changes in animals exposed to MRI"	Ossenkopp et al. (38)
0.15 T Simulated imaging conditions Rats Studied effect of MRI on murine opiate analgesia levels	"NMRI procedure alter both day and night time responses to morphine"	Ossenkopp et al. (39)
1.0 T Static magnetic field only Mice Studied effect of static magnetic field on in vivo bone growth	"Results suggest that exposure to intense magnetic fields does not alter physiological mechanisms of bone mineralization"	Papatheofanis and Papatheofanis (40)
2.35 T Static and gradient magnetic fields only Nematodes Studied toxic effects of static and gradient magnetic fields	"Static magnetic fields have no effect on fitness of test animals" "Time-varying magnetic fields cause inhibition of growth and maturation" "Combination of pulsed magnetic field gradients in a static uniform magnetic field also has a detrimental effect on the fitness of the test animals"	Peeling et al. (41)
2.35 T Simulated imaging conditions Mice Studied the effect of MRI on tumor development	"Immune response may be enhanced following MRI exposure, as indicated by the longer latency and smaller sizes of tumors in animals receiving MRI exposure"	Prasad et al. (42)
4.5 T Simulated imaging conditions Mice Studied the effects of high-field strength MRI on mouse testes epididymes	"Little, if any, damage to male reproductive tissues from . . . high intensity MRI exposure"	Prasad et al. (43)
0.7 T Simulated imaging conditions Mouse bone marrow cells Studied the cytogenic effects of MRI	"NMR exposure causes no adverse cytogenic effects"	Prasad et al. (44)
0.15 T Simulated imaging conditions Mice Studied effects of MRI on immune system	"MR exposure has no adverse effect on the immune system, as evidenced by natural killer cell activity"	Prasad et al. (45)
2.35 T Simulated imaging conditions Human peripheral blood mononuclear cells (PBMC) Studied effect of MRI on natural killer cell toxicity of PBMC with and without interleukin-2	"In neither case was cytotoxicity affected by prior exposure to MR imaging"	Prasad et al. (46)

TABLE 1. *Continued*

Study description	Results	Reference
0.15 and 4.0 T Simulated imaging conditions Fertilized frog eggs Studied effect of MRI on developing embryos	"No adverse effect early development"	Prasad et al. (47)
0.7 T Simulated imaging conditions Frog spermatazoa, fertilized eggs, and embryos Studied effects of MRI on development	"NMR exposure, at the dose used does not cause detectable adverse effects in this amphibian"	Prasad et al. (48)
0.15 T Exposed separately to static, gradient, and rf electromagnetic fields Mice Studied separate effects of static, gradient, and rf electromagnetic fields on morphine-induced analgesia in mice	"Time-varying, and to a lesser extent, the rf fields associated with the MRI procedure inhibit morphine-induced analgesia in mice"	Prato et al. (49)
4.7 T Clinical imaging conditions Human subjects Studied bioeffects of 4.7 T scanner	"Mild vertigo" "Headaches, nausea" "Magnetophosphenes" "Metallic taste in mouth"	Redington et al. (50)
0.04 T Clinical imaging conditions Human subjects Follow-up study	"Average follow-up time was 6 months . . . none of the 35 deaths recorded was unexpected" "Using the magnetic field and radiofrequency levels currently in operation . . . we believe NMRI to be a safe, non-invasive method of whole-body imaging"	Reid et al. (51)
4.0 T rf at 8 MHz to 170 MHz No gradient magnetic fields Human subjects Studied response of human auditory system to rf pulses	"In accordance with the used rf modulation envelope three distinct chirps per sequence could be resolved" "rf induced auditory noise is usually completely masked by noise from simultaneously switched gradient fields"	Roschmann et al. (52)
2.7 T Simulated imaging conditions Rats Studied effects of MRI on ocular tissues	"There were no discernable effects on the rat eye"	Sacks et al. (53)
0.35 T Simulated imaging conditions Hamster ovary cells Studied effects of MRI on observable mutations and cytotoxicity	"NMR imaging caused no detectable genetic damage and does not affect cell viability"	Schwartz and Crooks (54)
1.5 T Static magnetic field only Human subjects Studied effect of static magnetic field on body temperature	"No effect on body temperature of normal human subjects"	Shellock et al. (55)
1.5 T Clinical imaging conditions Human subjects Studied temperature, heart rate, and blood pressure changes associated with MRI	"MR imaging . . . not associated with any temperature or hemodynamic related deleterious effects"	Shellock and Crues (56)
1.5 T Clinical imaging conditions Human subjects Studied thermal effects of MRI of the spine	"No surface 'hot spots' " "Temperature effects were well-below known thresholds for adverse effects"	Shellock et al. (57)

TABLE 1. *Continued*

Study description	Results	Reference
1.5 T Clinical imaging conditions Human subjects Studied possible hypothalamic heating produced by MRI of the head	"There was probably no direct hypothalamic heating produced by clinical MRI of the head"	Shellock et al. (58)
1.5 T Clinical imaging conditions Human subjects Studied effect of MRI on corneal temperatures	"MR imaging . . . causes relatively minor increases in corneal temperature that do not appear to pose any thermal hazard to ocular tissue"	Shellock and Crues (59)
1.5 T Clinical imaging conditions Human subjects Studied temperature changes associated with MRI of the brain	"No significant increases in average body temperature" "Observed elevations in skin temperatures were physiologically inconsequential"	Shellock and Crues (60)
1.5 T Static magnetic field only Human subjects Studied effects of static magnetic field on body and skin temperatures	"There were no statistically significant changes in body or any of the skin temperatures recorded"	Shellock et al. (61)
1.5 T Clinical imaging conditions Human subjects Studied effect of MRI performed at high SAR levels	"Recommended exposure to rf radiation during MR imaging of the body for patients with normal thermoregulatory function may be too conservative"	Shellock et al. (62)
1.5 T Clinical imaging conditions Human subjects Studied effect of MRI on scrotal skin temperature	"Absolute temperature is below threshold known to affect testicular function"	Shellock et al. (63)
0.15 T Simulated imaging conditions Anesthetized rats Studied effect of MRI on blood–brain barrier permeability	"These findings raise the possibility that exposure to clinical MRI procedures may also temporarily alter the central blood–brain permeability in human subjects"	Shivers et al. (64)
1.5 T Simulated imaging conditions Anesthetized dogs Studied effect of MRI performed at high SAR levels	"These findings argue for continued caution in the design and operation of imagers capable of high specific absorption rates"	Shuman et al. (65)
0.4 to 8.0 T Static magnetic field only Mice Studied effect of static magnetic field on temperature	"Observed a field-induced increase in temperature"	Sperber et al. (66)
0.4 to 1.0 T Static magnetic field only Human subjects Studied the effects of static magnetic fields on tissue perfusion	"Neither at the skin of the thumb nor at the forearm were the changes in local blood flow attributable to the magnetic fields applied"	Stick et al. (67)
0.4 T Static magnetic field only Human subjects Studied magnetic-field-induced changes in auditory-evoked potentials	"Strong steady magnetic fields induce changes in human auditory-evoked potentials"	Stojan et al. (68)
0.15 T Clinical imaging conditions Human subjects Studied effect of MRI on cognitive functions	"No significant effect upon cognitive functions assessed"	Sweetland et al. (69)

TABLE 1. *Continued*

Study description	Results	Reference
0.6 T/sec Gradient magnetic field only Mice Studied effect of gradient magnetic fields on the analgesic properties of specific opiate antagonists	"Results indicate that the time-varying fields associated with MRI have significant inhibitory effects on analgesic effects of specific mu-opiate-directed ligands"	Teskey et al. (70)
0.15 T Simulated imaging conditions Rats Studied effects of MRI on survivability and long-term stress reactivity levels	"Results fail to provide any evidence for changes in survivability and long-term reactivity levels in rats exposed to MRI"	Teskey et al. (71)
0.01 and 1.0 T Simulated imaging conditions and static magnetic field only *Echerichia coli* Studied effect of MRI and static magnetic field on various properties of *E. coli*	"No mutations or lethal effects observed"	Thomas and Morris (72)
1.5 T Simulated imaging conditions Mice Studied the potential effects of MRI fields on eye development	"These data suggest a potential for MRI teratogenicity in a strain of mouse predisposed to eye malformations"	Tyndall and Sulik (73)
1.5 T Simulated imaging conditions C57BL/6J mouse Studied combined effects of MRI and x-irradiation on the developing eye of the mouse	"Results . . . suggested that the MRI techniques employed for this investigation did not enhance teratogenicity of x-irradiation on eye malformations produced in the 657BL/6J mouse"	Tyndall (74)
0.35 and 1.5 T Clinical imaging conditions Human subjects Studied effects of MRI on temperature	"No significant changes in central or peripheral temperatures resulting from the application of static or dynamic radiofrequency"	Vogl et al. (75)
0.35 T Static magnetic field only Human subjects Studied effect of static magnetic field on auditory-evoked potentials	"Magnetically induced shift may be explained by changes in electric capacities of the magnetically exposed biological system"	von Klitzing (76)
0.2 T Static magnetic field only Human subjects Studied effect of static magnetic field on power intensity of EEG	"The increased control values following an inverted magnetic flux vector point to a reversible alteration of brain function induced by a static magnetic field"	von Klitzing (77)
0.2 T Static magnetic field only Human subjects studied Studied encephalomagnetic fields during exposure to static magnetic field	"Exposure to static magnetic fields as used in NMR-equipment generates a new encephalomagnetic field in human brain"	von Klitzing (78)
1.5 and 4.0 T Static magnetic fields only Rats Studied effect of magnetic field on behavior	"At 4 T . . . in 97% of the trials the rats would not enter the magnet"	Weiss et al. (79)
0.16 T Static and gradient magnetic fields only Anesthetized rats and guinea pigs Studied effects of static and gradient magnetic fields on cardiac function of rats and guinea pigs	"No change in blood pressure, heart rate, or ECG"	Willis and Brooks (80)

TABLE 1. *Continued*

Study description	Results	Reference
0.3 T Static magnetic field only Mouse sperm cell Studied effect of static magnetic field on spermatogenesis	"Acute and subacute exposure to static magnetic fields associated with diagnostic MR imaging devices is unlikely to have any significant adverse effect on spermatogenesis"	Withers et al. (81)
0.35 T Simulated imaging conditions Hamster ovary cells Studied effect of MRI on DNA and chromosomes	"The conditions used for NMR imaging do not cause genetic damage which is detectable by any of these methods"	Wolff et al. (82)
Varying gradient fields Human subjects Studied the effects of time-varying gradient fields on peripheral nerve stimulation using trapezoidal and sinusoidal pulse trains	"The thresholds of trapezoidal pulses were higher than those of sinusoidal pulses by 11% and 30%, respectively, at equivalent power level"	Yamagata et al. (83)

changes associated with a specific spectrum of electromagnetic radiation that are not observed at levels below or above this range (108,119). Both field strength and frequency "windows" have been reported in the literature (108,119). Virtually all of the experiments conducted to date on MRI biological effects have been performed at specific "windows" and the results cannot be assumed to apply to all of the various field strengths or frequencies used for clinical MRI.

A variety of different biologic systems were also used for these experiments. As previously mentioned, since the coupling of electromagnetic radiation to biologic tissues is highly dependent on organism/subject size, anatomical factors, duration of exposure, the sensitivity of the involved tissues, and a myriad of other variables, studies performed on laboratory preparations may not be extrapolated or directly applicable to human subjects nor to the clinical use of MRI. Therefore, a cautionary approach to the interpretation of the results of these studies is advisable.

ELECTRICALLY, MAGNETICALLY, OR MECHANICALLY ACTIVATED IMPLANTS AND DEVICES

The U.S. FDA requires labeling of MR systems to indicate that the device is contraindicated for patients who have electrically, magnetically, or mechanically activated implants because electromagnetic fields produced by the MR system may interfere with the operation of these devices (107). Therefore, patients with internal cardiac pacemakers, implantable cardiac defibrillators, cochlear implants, neurostimulators, bone-growth stimulators, implantable electronic drug infusion pumps, and other similar devices that could be adversely affected by the electromagnetic fields used for MRI should not be examined by this imaging technique (120,123–126). Prior ex vivo testing of certain of these implants and devices may indicate that they are, in fact, MR-compatible.

The associated risks of scanning patients with cardiac pacemakers are related to the possibility of movement, reed switch closures or damage, programming changes, inhibition, or reversion to an asynchronous mode of operation, electromagnetic interference, and induced currents in lead wires (120,123,124,126). At least one patient with a pacemaker has been scanned by MRI without incident (125). A letter to the editor recently indicated that a patient who was not pacemaker dependent underwent MRI by having his pacemaker "disabled" during the procedure (125). Although this patient sustained no apparent discomfort and the pacemaker was not damaged, it is unadvisable to routinely perform this type of maneuver on patients with pacemakers because of the potential to encounter the aforementioned hazards. Of note is the fact that there has been an MRI-related death of a patient with a pacemaker (99).

Of particular concern is the possibility that the pacemaker lead wire(s) or other similar intracardiac wire configuration could act as an antenna in which the gradient and/or rf electromagnetic fields may induce sufficient current to cause fibrillation, a burn, or other potentially dangerous events (99,120,123,124,126). Because of this theoretically deleterious and unpredicted effect, patients referred to MRI with residual external pacing wires, temporary pacing wires, Swan-Ganz thermodilution catheters, and/or any other type of internally or externally positioned conductive wire or similar device should not undergo MRI because of the possible associated risks (99,120,127).

Some types of cochlear implants employ a relatively high-field strength cobalt samarium magnet used in conjunction with an external magnet to align and retain a radiofrequency transmitter coil on the patient's head, while other types of cochlear implants are electronically activated (128). Consequently, MRI is strictly contraindicated in patients with these implants because of the possibility of injuring the patient and/or damaging or altering the operation of the cochlear implant.

Because there is a potential for affecting implants that involve magnets (e.g., dental implants, magnetic sphincters, magnetic stoma plugs, magnetic ocular implants, and other similar devices) that may necessitate surgery to replace the damaged implant, these implants should be removed from the patient prior to MRI, if possible (128–130). Otherwise, MRI should not be performed on a patient with a magnetically-activated implant or device. A patient with any other similar electrically, magnetically, or mechanically activated implant or device should be excluded from examination by MRI unless the particular implant or device has been previously demonstrated to be unaffected by the magnetic and electromagnetic fields used for MRI (120).

PATIENTS WITH METALLIC IMPLANTS, MATERIALS, AND FOREIGN BODIES

MRI is contraindicated for patients that have certain ferromagnetic implants, materials, or foreign bodies, primarily due to the possibility of movement or dislodgement of these objects (97–99). Other problems may also occur in patients with ferromagnetic implants, materials, or foreign bodies that undergo MRI including the induction of electrical current in the object, excessive heating of the object, and the misinterpretation of an artifact produced by the presence of the object as an abnormality (97,99,131–134). These latter potentially hazardous situations, however, are encountered infrequently or are insignificant in comparison with movement or dislodgement of a ferromagnetic implant or foreign body by the magnetic fields of the MR system.

Numerous investigations have evaluated the ferromagnetic qualities of a variety of metallic implants, materials, or foreign bodies by measuring deflection forces or movements associated with the static magnetic fields used by MRI (134–153). These studies were conducted in order to determine the relative risk of performing MRI on a patient with a metallic object with respect to whether or not the magnetic attraction was strong enough to produce movement or dislodgement.

A variety of factors require evaluation when establishing the relative risk of performing an MR procedure in a patient with a ferromagnetic implant, material, device, or foreign body, such as: the strength of the static and gradient magnetic fields, the relative degree of ferromagnetism of the object, the mass of the object, the geometry of the object, the location and orientation of the object in situ, and the length of time the object has been in place (98,99). Each of these should be considered before allowing a patient that has a ferromagnetic object to enter the electromagnetic environment of the MR system.

The Appendix (see pages 140–148) provides a comprehensive summary of information pertaining to biomedical implants, materials, and devices evaluated for compatibility with MR procedures. If a patient is identified to have an implant or foreign body during pre-MRI screening, this compilation of implants, materials, or foreign bodies tested for ferromagnetism should be consulted in order to determine if the object is safe (i.e., there are no or only insignificant associated deflection forces associated with the object).

Aneurysm and hemostatic clips. According to results of tests using ex vivo techniques, several aneurysm clips display ferromagnetic qualities and, therefore, are considered to be a contraindication for patients undergoing MR procedures. Unfortunately, one patient mortality has occurred as a result of a ferromagnetic aneurysm clip being displaced from its position during an MR procedure. In this incident, a 74-year-old patient with an intracranial aneurysm clip was permitted to undergo MR imaging in a 1.5-T MR system. The personnel at the site were aware that the patient had an aneurysm clip in place but it was thought to be a type that is nonferromagnetic. Only after the patient experienced a fatal intracranial hemorrhage from what appears to have been the result of motion of this aneurysm clip in the static field of the MR system was it revealed that the history provided during pre-MR screening was incorrect and that the clip was actually a ferromagnetic type.

Because of the profound safety implications related to performing an MR procedure in a patient with an aneurysm clip, we believe that each aneurysm clip, regardless of its type and known or suspected ferromagnetic qualities, should undergo ex vivo testing before implantation in a patient who may subsequently undergo an MR procedure. This ex vivo testing can take the form of subjecting the aneurysm clip to the field of a powerful, handheld permanent magnet (e.g., 3,000 G or more). If no motion or torque of the aneurysm clip is identified, the specific manufacturer, lot number, and model number of the clip should be recorded in the operative note, including the results of the evaluation of ferromagnetism. In the future, it would be easy to verify that the aneurysm clip had been tested.

If the clip is found to be ferromagnetic, it is strongly advised that it not be used for surgery. If the aneurysm clip needs to be implanted, the patient should be educated in the postoperative period and a note should be placed in the patient's chart, similar to that used to indicate a severe allergy. This will provide a warning for all further health care practitioners as well as the patient as to the possible hazards associated with MR procedures.

None of the various hemostatic vascular clips that have been evaluated were attracted by static magnetic fields up to 1.5 T. These hemostatic clips are made from nonferromagnetic materials such as tantalum and nonferromagnetic forms of stainless steel. Therefore, patients who have any of the hemostatic vascular clips listed in the table are not at risk for injury during MR procedures.

Carotid artery vascular clamps. Each of the carotid artery vascular clamps evaluated for ferromagnetism exhibited deflection forces. However, only the Poppen-Blaylock clamp was considered to be contraindicated for patients undergoing MRI because of the significant ferromagnetism shown by this object. The other carotid artery vascular clamps are believed to be safe for MRI because of the minimal deflection forces relative to their use in an in vivo application (i.e., the deflection forces are insignificant and, therefore, there is little possibility of significant movement or dislodgement of the implant).

Dental devices and materials. Various dental devices and materials have been tested for ferromagnetism. While many of them demonstrated deflection forces, only a few of these pose a possible risk to patients undergoing MRI because they are magnetically-activated devices.

Heart valves. Many of the commercially available heart valve prostheses have been tested for ferromagnetism. The majority of these displayed measurable deflection forces; however, the deflection forces were relatively insignificant compared with the force exerted by the beating heart. Therefore, patients with these heart valve prostheses may safely undergo MRI.

Intravascular coils, filters, and stents. Less than half of the different intravascular coils, filters, and stents tested were ferromagnetic (145,152). These ferromagnetic devices are usually attached firmly into the vessel wall after approximately four to six weeks following introduction (152). Therefore, it is unlikely that any of them would become dislodged by attraction from magnetic forces presently used for MRI. Patients with intravascular coils, filters, or stents in which there is a possibility that the device is not properly positioned or held firmly in place should not undergo MRI.

Ocular implants. Various ocular implants have been evaluated for ferromagnetism. Of these, the Fatio eyelid spring and retinal tack made from martensitic stainless steel displayed measurable deflection forces. While it is unlikely that the associated deflection forces would cause movement or dislodgement of these implants, it is possible that a patient with one of these implants would be uncomfortable or sustain a minor injury during MRI.

Orthopedic implants, materials, and devices. Most orthopedic implants, materials, and devices tested for ferromagnetism have been demonstrated to be made from nonferromagnetic materials. Therefore, patients with these particular orthopedic implants, materials, and devices may be imaged safely by MRI. The Perfix interference screw used for reconstruction of the anterior cruciate ligament, while composed of ferromagnetic material, does not pose a hazard to the patient undergoing MRI because of the significant force that holds it in place, in vivo. However, the resulting imaging artifact precludes diagnostic assessment of the knee using MRI.

Otologic implants. The cochlear implants evaluated for ferromagnetism are considered to be contraindicated for MRI. Besides being attracted by static magnetic fields, these implants are also electronically and/or magnetically activated. Only one of the remaining tested otologic implants has associated deflection forces. This implant, the McGee stapedectomy piston prosthesis composed of platinum and 17 Cr-4Ni stainless steel was made on a limited basis during mid-1987 and was recalled by the manufacturer. Patients with this otologic implant were issued warning cards that instruct them to not be examined by MRI.

Pellets, bullets, shrapnel, etc. Most of the pellets and bullets previously tested for ferromagnetism are composed of nonferromagnetic materials (143,145). Ammunition found to be ferromagnetic typically came from foreign countries and/or was used by the military. Shrapnel usually contains various amounts of steel and, therefore, presents a potential hazard for MRI. Furthermore, since pellets, bullets, and schrapnel may be contaminated with ferromagnetic materials, these objects represent relative contraindications for MRI. Patients with these foreign bodies should be regarded on an individual basis with respect to whether the object is positioned near a vital neural, vascular, or soft tissue structure. This may be assessed by taking a careful history and using plain film radiography to determine the location of the foreign body.

Penile implants and artificial sphincters. One of the penile implants tested for ferromagnetism displayed significant deflection forces. Although it is unlikely that this implant, the Dacomed Omniphase, would cause serious injury to a patient undergoing MRI, it would undoubtedly be uncomfortable for the patient. Therefore, this implant is regarded as a relative contraindication for MRI. Artificial sphincters that have been tested are made from nonferromagnetic materials. However, at least one artificial sphincter currently undergoing clinical trials has a magnetic component and, therefore, patients with this device should not undergo MRI.

Vascular access ports. Of the various vascular access ports tested for ferromagnetism, two showed measurable deflection forces, but the forces were felt to be insignificant relative to the in vivo application of these implants (142). Therefore, it is considered safe to perform MRI in a patient that may have one of these previously tested vascular access ports. The exception to this is any vascular access port that is "programmable" or electronically activated. Patients with this type of vascular access port should not undergo MRI.

Miscellaneous. Various types of other metallic implants, materials, and foreign bodies have also been tested for ferromagnetism. Of these, the cerebral ventricular shunt tube connector (type unknown) and tissue expander which is magnetically activated exhibited deflection forces that may pose a risk to patients during MRI. An "O-ring" washer used as a vascular marker also showed ferromagnetism, but the deflection force was determined to be minimal relative to the in vivo use of this device.

Each of the contraceptive diaphragms tested for ferromagnetism displayed significant deflection forces. However, we have performed MRI on patients with these devices who did not complain of any sensation related to movement of these objects. Therefore, scanning patients with diaphragms is not believed to be considered to be physically hazardous to patients.

According to the *Policies, Guidelines, and Recommendations for MR Imaging Safety and Patient Management* information issued by the Society for Magnetic Resonance Imaging Safety Committee (120), patients with electrically, magnetically, or mechanically activated, or electrically conductive devices should be excluded from MRI unless the particular device has been previously shown (i.e., usually by ex vivo testing procedures) to be unaffected by the electromagnetic fields used for clinical MRI and there is no possibility of injuring the patient. During the screening process for MRI, patients with these objects should be identified before their examination and prior to being exposed to the electromagnetic fields used for this imaging technique. There are implants, materials, devices, or other foreign bodies that have yet to be evaluated for MRI compatibility which may be encountered in the clinical setting. Patients that have untested objects should not be allowed to undergo MRI.

SCREENING PATIENTS WITH METALLIC FOREIGN BODIES

Patients may present to MRI with a history of metallic foreign bodies such as slivers, bullets, shrapnel, or other types of metallic fragments. The relative risk of scanning these patients is dependent upon the ferromagnetic properties of the object, the geometry and dimensions of the object, and the strength of the static and gradient magnetic fields of the MR system. Also important is the strength with which the object is fixed within the tissue and whether or not it is positioned in or adjacent to a potentially hazardous site of the body such as a vital neural, vascular, or soft tissue structure.

A patient that encounters the static magnetic field of an MR system with an intraocular metallic foreign body is at a particular risk for significant eye injury. The single reported case of a patient that experienced a vitreous hemorrhage resulting in blindness underwent MRI on a 0.35 T MR system and had an occult intraocular metal fragment that was 2.0 × 3.5 mm in size dislodge during the procedure (154). This incident emphasizes the importance of adequately screening patients with suspected intraocular metallic foreign bodies prior to MRI.

Research has demonstrated that small intraocular metallic fragments as small as 0.1 × 0.1 × 0.1 mm in size are detected using standard plain film radiographs (155). Although thin slice (i.e., ≤ 3 mm) computed tomography has been demonstrated to detect metallic foreign bodies in size down to approximately 0.15 mm, it is unlikely that a metallic fragment of this size would be dislodged during MR imaging, even with a static magnetic field up to 2.0 T (155). Metallic fragments of various sizes and dimensions ranging from 0.1 mm × 0.1 mm × 0.1 mm to 3.0 mm × 1.0 mm × 1.0 mm in size have been examined to determine if they were moved or dislodged from the eyes of laboratory animals during exposure to a 2.0 T MR system (155). Only the largest fragment (3.0 mm × 1.0 × 1.0 mm) rotated, but did not cause any discernable damage to the ocular tissue (155). Therefore, the use of plain film radiography is an acceptable technique for identifying or excluding an intraocular metallic foreign body that represents a potential hazard to the patient undergoing MRI (120). Patients with a high suspicion of having an intraocular metallic foreign body (for example, a metal worker exposed to metallic slivers with a history of an eye injury) should have a plain film radiographs of the orbits to rule-out the presence of a metallic fragment prior to exposure to the static magnetic field. If a patient with a suspected ferromagnetic intraocular foreign body has no symptoms and a plain film series of the orbits does not demonstrate a radiopaque foreign body, the risk of performing MRI is minimal (120).

Using plain film radiography to search for metallic foreign bodies is a sensitive and relatively inexpensive means of identifying patients that are unsuitable for MRI and can also be utilized to screen out patients that may have metal fragments in other potentially hazardous sites of the body (120).

Each MRI site should establish a standardized policy for screening patients with suspected foreign bodies. The policy should include guidelines as to which patients require work-up by radiographic procedures, the specific procedure to be performed (i.e., number and type of views, position of the anatomy, etc.), and each case should be considered on an individual basis. These precautions should be taken with regard to patients referred to MRI in any type of MR system regardless of the field strength, magnet type, and the presence or absence of magnetic shielding (120).

PERFORMING MRI DURING PREGNANCY

While MRI is not believed to be hazardous to the fetus, only a few investigations have examined the teratogenic potential of this imaging modality. By comparison, literally thousands of studies have been performed to examine the possible hazards of ultrasound during pregnancy and controversy still exists concerning the safe use of this nonionizing-radiation imaging technique.

Most of the earliest studies conducted to determine possible unwanted bioeffects during pregnancy showed negative results (17,22,26,31,41,47,82). More recently, one study examined the effects of MRI on mice exposed during mid-gestation (22). No gross embryotoxic effects were observed; however, there was a reduction in crown-rump length (22). In another study performed by Tyndall and Sulik (73), exposure to the electromagnetic fields used for a simulated clinical MRI examination caused eye malformations in a genetically prone mouse strain. Therefore, it appears that the electromagnetic fields used for MRI have the ability to produce developmental abnormalities.

A variety of mechanisms exist that could produce deleterious bioeffects with respect to the developing fetus and the use of electromagnetic fields during MRI (86,88,89,102,108,109,118). In addition, it is well-known that cells undergoing division, as in the case of the developing fetus during the first trimester, are highly susceptible to damage from different types of physical agents. Therefore, because of the limited data available at the present time, a cautionary approach is recommended for the use of MRI in pregnant patients.

The current guidelines of the U.S. FDA requires labeling of MRI devices to indicate that the safety of MRI when used to image the fetus and the infant "has not been established" (165). In Great Britain, the acceptable limits of exposure for clinical MRI recommended by the National Radiological Protection Board in 1983 specify that "it might be prudent to exclude pregnant women during the first three months of pregnancy" (165).

According to the Safety Committee of the Society for Magnetic Resonance Imaging (120)(this information has also been adopted recently by the American College of Radiology), MRI is indicated for use in pregnant women if other nonionizing forms of diagnostic imaging are inadequate or if the examination provides important information that would otherwise require exposure to ionizing radiation (i.e., x-ray, CT, etc.). For pregnant patients, it is recommended to inform them that, to date, there has been no indication that the use of clinical MRI during pregnancy has produced deleterious effects. However, as noted by the FDA, the safety of MRI during pregnancy has not been proved (107).

Patients who are pregnant or suspect they are pregnant must be identified prior to undergoing MRI in order to assess the risks versus the benefits of the examination. Since there is a high spontaneous abortion rate in the general population during the first trimester of pregnancy (i.e., >30%), particular care should be exercised with the use of MRI during the first trimester because of associated potential medico-legal implications relative to spontaneous abortions.

MRI AND CLAUSTROPHOBIA, ANXIETY, AND PANIC DISORDERS

Claustrophobia and a variety of other psychological reactions including anxiety and panic disorders may be encountered by as many as 5% to 10% of patients undergoing MR procedures. These sensations originate from several factors including the restrictive dimensions of the interior of the scanner, the duration of the examination, the gradient-induced noises, the ambient conditions within the bore of the scanner, etc. (156–164).

Fortunately, adverse psychological responses to MRI are usually transient. However, there has been a report of two patients with no prior history of claustrophobia who tolerated MRI with great difficulty and had persistent claustrophobia that required long-term psychiatric treatment (157). Since adverse psychologic responses to MRI typically delay or require cancellation of the examination, several techniques have been developed and may be used to avert these problems (120,156–165). These include the following:

1. Brief the patient concerning the specific aspects of the MRI examination including the level of gradient-induced noise to expect, the internal dimensions of the scanner, and the length of the examination, etc.
2. Allow an appropriately screened relative or friend to remain with the patient during the procedure.
3. Use headphones with calming music to decrease the repetitive noise created by the gradient coils.
4. Maintain physical or verbal contact with the patient throughout the examination.
5. Place the patient in a prone position. In this position, the patient is able to visualize the opening of the bore and thus alleviate the "closed-in" feeling. An alternative method to reduce claustrophobia is to place the subject feet first instead of head first into the MR system.
6. Use of scanner-mounted mirrors and mirror or prism glasses within the scanner allows the patient to see out of the scanner.
7. Use a large light at either end of the scanner to decrease the anxiety of being in a long dark enclosure.
8. Use a blindfold on the patient so that he/she is unaware of the close surroundings.
9. Use relaxation techniques such as controlled breathing and mental imagery. Also, several case reports have shown hypnotherapy to be successful in reducing MRI-related claustrophobia and anxiety.
10. Use psychological "desensitization" techniques prior to the MRI examination.

Several investigators have recently attempted to compare the effectiveness of some of the above mentioned techniques in reducing MRI-induced anxiety and/or claustrophobia (158,159,162). One such study demonstrated that providing detailed information about the MRI procedure in addition to "relaxation exercises" successfully reduced the anxiety level of a group of patients both before and during MRI. A similar anxiety reduction could not be shown in patients provided with only information or "stress reduction" counseling. Relaxation methods have also been shown to significantly decrease anxiety during other medical procedures. Certain MR system architectures employing a vertical magnetic field offer a more open design that might reduce the frequency of psychological-related problems associated with MRI procedures.

MONITORING PHYSIOLOGIC PARAMETERS DURING MRI

Because the typical MR system is constructed such that the patient is placed inside a cylindrical structure, routine observations and vital signs monitoring is not a trivial task. Conventional monitoring equipment was not designed to operate in the MRI environment where static, gradient, and rf electromagnetic fields can adversely affect the operation of these devices. Fortunately, MR-compatible monitors have been developed and are commonly used in in-patient and out-patient MRI centers (166–174).

Physiologic monitoring is required for the safe utilization of MRI in patients who are sedated, anesthetized, comatose, critically ill or unable to communicate with the MR system operator. All of the above categories of patients should be routinely monitored during MRI and, considering the current availability of MRI-compatible monitors, there is no reason to exclude these types of patients from MRI. Every physiologic parameter that can be obtained under normal circumstances in the intensive care unit or operating room can be monitored during MRI, including heart rate, systemic blood pressure, intracardiac pressure, end-tidal carbon dioxide, oxygen saturation, respiratory rate, skin blood flow, and temperature (167–174). Table 2 lists examples of MR-compatible monitors that have been successfully tested and operated at field strengths of up to 1.5 T. In addition, there are now MR-compatible ventilators for patients who require ventilatory support.

Monitors that contain ferromagnetic components (i.e., transformers, outer casings, etc.) can be strongly attracted by mid- and high-field MR systems, posing a serious hazard to patients and possible damage to the MR system. Since the intensity of standard static magnetic field falls off as the third power of the distance from the magnet, simply placing the monitor a suitable distance from the MR system is sufficient to protect the operation of the device and to help prevent it from becoming a potential projectile (171,174). If monitoring equipment is not placed in a permanently fixed position, instructions should be given to all appropriate personnel regarding the hazards of moving this equipment too close to the MR system (171,174).

In addition to being influenced by the static magnetic field, monitors may be adversely affected by electromagnetic interference from the gradient and radiofrequency pulses from the MR system (171,174). In these instances, increasing the length of the patient-monitor interface and positioning the equipment outside the rf-shielded room (e.g., the control room) will enable the monitor to operate properly. It is usually necessary to position all monitors with cathode ray tubes at a location in the magnetic fringe field such that the display is not "bent" or distorted.

Certain monitors emit spurious electromagnetic noise that can result in moderate to severe imaging artifacts (171,174). These monitors can be modified to work during MRI by adding rf-shielded cables, using fiber-optic transmission of the signals (which is becoming increasingly the method of choice in the MRI environment), or using special outer casing. Also, special filters may be added to the monitor to inhibit electromagnetic noise.

Of further concern is the fact that some monitoring equipment can be potentially harmful to patients if special precautions are not followed (171,174–177). A primary source of adverse MR system and physiologic monitor interactions has been the interface that is used between the patient and the equipment because this usually requires a conductive cable or other device. The presence of a conductive material in the immediate MR system area is a safety concern because of the potential for monitor-related burns. For example, there has been a report of an unfortunate accident involving an anesthetized patient who sustained a third- degree burn of the finger associated with using a pulse oximeter during MRI (176). Investigation of this incident revealed that the cable leading from the pulse oximeter to the finger probe may have been looped during MRI and the gradient and/or rf magnetic fields induced sufficient current to exorbitantly heat the finger probe, resulting in the finger burn (176). This problem may also occur with the use of electrocardiographic lead wires or any other cable that may be looped or form a conductive loop that contacts the patient.

Therefore, the following is recommended to prevent potential monitor-related accidents from occurring:

1. Monitoring equipment should only be utilized by trained personnel.
2. All cables and lead wires from monitoring devices that come into contact with the patient (e.g., the monitor-patient interface) should be positioned so that no conductive loops are formed.
3. Monitoring devices that do not appear to operate properly during MRI should be immediately removed from the patient and the magnetic environment.

TABLE 2. *Examples of MRI-compatible monitors and ventilators*[a]

Device and manufacturer	Function
MRI Fiber-optic Pulse Oximeter Nonin Medical Inc., Plymouth, MN	Oxygen saturation, heart rate
MR-Compatible Pulse Oximeter Magnetic Resonance Equipment Corp., Bay Shore, NY	Oxygen saturation, heart rate
MR-Compatible Pulse Oximeter Invivo Research, Inc., Orlando, FL	Oxygen saturation, heart rate
Omega 1400 Invivo Research, Inc., Orlando, FL	Blood pressure, heart rate
Omni-Trak 3100 MRI Vital Signs Monitor Invivo Research, Inc., Orlando, FL	Heart rate, EKG, oxygen saturation, respiratory rate, blood pressure
Laserflow Blood Perfusion Monitor Vasomed, Inc., St. Paul, MN	Cutaneous blood flow
Medpacific LD 5000 Laser-Doppler Perfusion Monitor Medpacific Corporation, Seattle, WA	Cutaneous blood flow
Respiratory Rate Monitor, Models 515 and 525 Biochem International, Waukesha, WI	Respiratory rate, apnea
MicroSpan Capnometer 8800 Biochem International, Waukesha, WI	Respiratory rate, end-tidal carbon dioxide, apnea
Aneuroid Chest Bellows Coulborun Instruments, Allentown, Pennsylvania	Respiratory rate
Datex CO2 Monitor Puritan-Bennett Corporation, Los Angeles, CA	Percent carbon dioxide
Wenger Precordial Stethoscope Anesthesia Medical Supplies, Santa Fe Springs, CA	Heart sounds
Fluoroptic Thermometry System, Model 3000 Luxtron, Santa Clara, CA	Temperature
Omni-Vent, Series D Columbia Medical Marketing, Topeka, KA	Ventilator
Ventilator, Models 225 and 2500 Monaghan Medical Corporation, Plattsburgh, PA	Ventilator
Anesthesia Ventilator Ohio Medical, Madison, WI	Ventilator
Infant Ventilator MVP-10 Bio-Med Devices, Inc., Madison, CN	Ventilator
Siemens-Elema Model 900C Siemens, Iselin, NJ	Ventilator

[a] Note that some of these devices may require modifications to make them MR-compatible and some of them should not be positioned closer than 8 feet from the entrance of the bore of 1.5-T MR system. Also, monitors with metallic cables, leads, or probes may cause mild-to-moderate imaging artifacts if placed near the imaging area of interest. Consult manufacturers to determine compatibility with specific MR systems.

The following is a brief description of some of the techniques for monitoring various physiologic parameters:

Monitoring blood pressure. Noninvasive blood-pressure monitors typically utilize the oscillometric technique for measuring blood pressure, using a pressure transducer connected to a pressure cuff via a pneumatically filled hose. Certain monitors (i.e., Omega 1400, Invivo Research, Orlando, FL) have adjustable audible and visual alarms as well as a strip-chart recorder.

Occasionally, the cuff inflation tends to disturb lightly sedated patients, especially pediatric patients, which may cause them to move and distort the MR image. For this reason, the noninvasive blood-pressure monitor may not represent the optimal instrument for obtaining vital signs in all patient groups. Direct pressure monitoring of systemic and/or intracardiac pressures, if necessary, can be accomplished using a fiber-optic pressure transducer made entirely of plastic.

Monitoring respiratory rate, oxygenation, and gas exchange. Monitoring of respiratory parameters during MRI of sedated or anesthetized patients is particularly important because the medications used for these procedures may produce complications of respiratory depression. Therefore, as a standard of care, a pulse oximeter, capnograph, or capnometer should always be used to monitor patients who are sedated or anesthetized during MRI.

The respiratory monitors utilized successfully on sedated pediatric or adult patients (i.e., the model 515 Respiration Monitor and model 8800 Capnometer, Biochem International, Waukesha, WI) are relatively inexpensive and can be modified for use during MR imaging by simply lengthening the plastic tubing interface to the patient so that the monitors can be placed at least 8 feet from the unshielded MR imager.

Pulse oximeters are used to record oxygen saturation and heart rate. Commercially available, modified pulse oximeters using hard wire cables have been previously used to monitor sedated and anesthetized patients during the MRI study and the recovery period with moderate success. These pulse oximeters tend to work intermittently during MRI due to interference from the gradient and/or radiofrequency electromagnetic fields. In certain instances, patients have been burned, presumably as a result of excessive current being induced in inappropriately looped conductive cables attached to the patient probes of the pulse oximeters (175–177).

Newly developed, portable fiber-optic pulse oximeters are now available for use during MR procedures (178) (see Table 2). Using fiber-optic technology to obtain and transmit physiologic signals from patients undergoing MRI has been demonstrated to be a technique that does not have any associated MRI-related electromagnetic interference. It is physically impossible for a patient to be burned using this fiber-optic monitor during MRI because there are no conductive pathways formed by any metallic materials.

Monitoring cutaneous blood flow. Cutaneous blood flow can be monitored during MRI by means of the laser-Doppler velocimetry technique. This noninvasive measurement technique uses laser light that is delivered to and detected from the region of interest by flexible, graded-index fiber-optic light wires. The Doppler-broadening of laser light scattered by moving red blood cells within the tissue is analyzed in realtime by an analogue processor that is indicative of instantaneous blood velocity and the effective blood volume and flow. A small circular probe can be attached to any available skin surface of the patient. Areas with a relatively high cutaneous blood flow (such as the hand, finger, foot, toe, or ear) yield the best results.

Hard-copy tracings obtained by laser-Doppler velocimetry can be used to determine the patient's heart rate, respiratory rate, and cutaneous blood flow. An audible signal may be activated to permit the operator to hear blood flow changes during monitoring. This technique of continuous physiological monitoring is particularly useful when there is concern about disturbing a sedated patient because it is easily tolerated.

Monitoring heart rate. Monitoring the electrocardiogram during MRI is typically required for cardiac imaging, gating to reduce imaging artifacts from the physiologic motion of cerebral spinal fluid in the brain and spine, and for determining the patient's heart rate. Artifacts caused by the static, gradient, and rf electromagnetic fields may severely distort the morphology of the electrocardiogram, making determination of cardiac rhythm during MRI extremely difficult and unreliable. Although sophisticated filtering techniques can be used to attenuate the artifacts from the gradient and rf fields, the static magnetic field produces an augmentation of the T-wave, as previously mentioned, and other nonspecific waveform changes that are in direct proportion to the strength of the field, which cannot be easily counterbalanced.

In some instances, static magnetic field-induced augmented T waves have a higher amplitude than the R waves, resulting in false triggering and an inaccurate determination of the beats per minute. Electrocardiogram artifacts can be minimized during MRI by the following: using special filters, using electrocardiogram electrodes with minimal metal, selecting lead wires with minimal metal, twisting or braiding the lead wires, and using special lead placements (173).

The previously mentioned pulse oximeters may also be used to accurately record heart rate during MRI examinations. These devices have probes that may be attached to the finger, toe, or ear lobe of the patient.

SAFETY CONSIDERATIONS OF Gd-DTPA

Although the first intravenous MRI contrast agent was only introduced into the clinical arena in mid-1988, less than six years later there are now three different contrast agents available for use. Throughout the United States, roughly one third of all MRI studies utilize contrast agents. Therefore, it is important to be familiar with the safety aspects of using these medications that are so ubiquitously present in the clinical MR environment (179–181).

The three MR imaging contrast agents approved for intravenous administration by the U.S. Food and Drug Administration (FDA) are: Magnevist (gadopentetate dimeglumine injection, Berlex Laboratories, Wayne, NJ), Omniscan (gadodiamide injection, Sanofi-Winthrop Pharmaceuticals, New York, NY; Nycomed Salutar, Oslo, Norway), and ProHance (gadoteridol injection, Bracco, Princeton, NJ). There is, in addition, another agent approved internationally named Dotarem (gadoterate meglumine, Gd-DOTA, Guebet Laboratories, Aulnay-sous-Bois, France).

All of these contrast agents are based on the element, gadolinium, and have similar mechanisms of action, biodistribution, and half-lives (180–183). Drug equilibration and physiologic biodistribution for each of the MRI contrast agents is in the extracellular fluid space, with biologic elimination half-lives roughly 1.5 hours for each of these drugs (180).

Gadolinium-based MRI contrast agents are paramagnetic substances and, therefore, develop a magnetic moment when placed in a magnetic field. The relatively large magnetic moment produced by a paramagnetic agent results in a relatively large local magnetic field that can enhance the relaxation rates of water protons in the vicinity of the MRI contrast agent. When placed in a magnetic field, gadolinium-based MRI contrast agents decrease the T1 and T2 relaxation times in tissues where it accumulates (although the T1 relaxation time is mainly affected at the dosages used in the clinical setting) with the purpose of improving image contrast between two adjacent tissue compartments, thus producing a more conspicuous abnormality, if one exists (180).

Free gadolinium ion is rather toxic, with a markedly prolonged biologic half life of several weeks. The predominant uptake and excretion of gadolinium is by the kidneys and liver. However, gadolinium ion is chelated to another structure that restricts the ion, which markedly decreases its toxicity and alters its pharmacokinetics (180). In fact, this chelation also decreases the ability of the gadolinium ion to accomplish its task of T1 shortening. The science of MRI contrast agent design and development is often a tricky act of walking the tightrope between decreasing toxicity while not overly decreasing the T1 relaxivity.

As noted above, the chelating process also alters the pharmacokinetics of the agent. For example, chelating the gadolinium ions allows for approximately a 500-fold increase in the rate of renal excretion of the substance (184,185). In each case, the chelating substance is what makes these various MRI contrast agents differ from one another.

In the case of Magnevist, the chelating agent is the DTPA molecule. In the case of Omniscan it is DTPA-BMA, and in the case of ProHance it is the HP-DO3A molecule. Magnevist has a linear structure and is an ionic compound; Omniscan has a linear structure and is nonionic; ProHance is also nonionic and possesses a macrocyclic ring structure. Despite the marked differences in these chelating molecules, their ionic versus nonionic nature, and their linear versus ring-like molecular structure, these agents appear to have remarkably similar effectiveness and safety profiles. Some differences exist—both theoretically as well as on paper—and it is these differences that we will now discuss. Multiple studies have documented the high safety index of MRI contrast agents, especially when compared to iodinated contrast media used for computed tomography (181,186–202). However, from a safety profile standpoint, it is inappropriate to compare ionic and nonionic MRI contrast agents to ionic and nonionic CT contrast agents because of the drastically different osmotic loads associated with each of these drugs.

The LD_{50} (i.e., the "fifty percent lethal dose", or LD_{50}, is the term used to denote the dose of an agent that, when administered to test animals, results in acute death of half of the population of the recipients) of these agents, as studied in rodents, is quite high: being the highest for Omniscan (>30 mmol/kg), next highest for ProHance (12 mmol/kg), and the lowest for Magnevist (6 to 7 mmol/kg). In all cases, the LD_{50} is generally in excess of roughly 300,120, and 60 times the typical diagnostic dose of 0.1 mmol/kg, respectively (180,203). There is also data to suggest that there are fewer acute cardiodepressive effects from the nonionic drugs (specifically, ProHance was used in one study) than the ionic agent, Magnevist, when injected rapidly and into a central vein (204). This may have limited clinical applicability, however, since MRI contrast agents are typically injected into peripheral veins, with only small total volumes being administered (180).

Adverse Events Related to the Use of MRI Contrast Agents

The total incidence of adverse reactions of all types for each of the MRI contrast agents ranges from approximately 2% to 4% (181,196,205). The most common reactions are nausea, emesis, hives, headaches, and local injection site symptoms, such as irritation, focal burning, or a cool sensation. With the use of Magnevist, there have also been transient elevations reported in serum bilirubin (3% to 4% of patients), and with both Magnevist and Omniscan a transient elevation in iron (15% to 30% of patients) which seem to spontaneously reverse within 24 to 48 hours (181,206). No such alterations in blood chemistry have been reported with the use of ProHance. Of special note is that here are no known contraindications for Magnevist, Ominiscan, and Prohance.

The MRI contrast agent that has had FDA approval the longest and, therefore, the one for which there is the most clinical experience and information, is Magnevist. There have been approximately 5.7 million doses administered worldwide since its approval in June of 1988. This compares to approximately 150,000 total administered doses for ProHance since its FDA approval in November, 1992 and approximately 100,000 doses for Omniscan since its FDA approval in January, 1993. There have been rare reported incidents of laryngospasm and/ or anaphylactoid-reactions (requiring interventional therapy with, e.g., epinephrine) associated with the administration of each of these agents (Dr. Reich, Associate Medical Director, Corporate Products, Sanofi Winthrop, *oral communication,* June 14, 1993) (205–214).

In consideration of the above, it may well be advisable to continue a prolonged observation period of all patients with a history of allergy or drug reaction. As stated in the package insert for Magnevist, for example: "The possibility of a reaction, including serious, fatal, anaphylactoid, or cardiovascular reactions or other idiosyncratic reactions should always be considered especially in those with a known clinical history of asthma or other allergic respiratory disorders."

Delayed reactions of hypertension, vasovagal responses, and syncope have also been reported with the use of MRI contrast agents. Accordingly, the product inserts for these drugs advise that all patients should be observed for several hours following drug administration.

Specific Adverse Events

The specific adverse events associated with the use of MRI contrast agents vary to a minor degree (205–219). It should be noted that the vast majority of these adverse events only occur at an incidence of less than 1%. Before proceeding, it might be helpful to clarify some commonly used—and misused—terminology pertaining to adverse events that occur with medications. An anaphylactoid reaction is one that involves respiratory, cardiovascular, cutaneous (and possibly gastrointestinal and/or genitourinary) manifestations (215). This is not to say that all events that have such symptoms are by definition anaphylactoid, per se. However, it does become more difficult to make the diagnosis of anaphylaxis in the absence of such symptoms, especially the classic triad of upper airway obstructive symptomatology, decreased blood pressure (or other similar severe cardiovascular symptoms), and cutaneous manifestations, such as urticaria.

As defined by the FDA, a "serious reaction" is one where an adverse experience from a drug proves fatal or life-threatening, is permanently disabling, requires inpatient hospitalization, or is an overdose (FDA Docket no. 85D-0249). A life-threatening reaction in the FDA terminology is one wherein the initial reporter (i.e., the individual initially reporting the incident) believes that the patient was at immediate risk of death from the event. In consideration of the above, one may now understand how the interpretation of an adverse event may differ from that designated by the FDA.

Magnevist

As of June 1993, there have been 13 anaphylactoid reactions with Magnevist, for an estimated anaphylactoid reaction rate of 1:450,000 (Lawrence Gifford, M.D., Director, Medical Affairs, Berlex Laboratories, *oral communication,* June, 1993). One of the patients that had an anaphylactoid reaction died and another patient suffered brain damage (at the time of this writing the patient is still in a coma) subsequent to administration of Magnevist. In each case there was a history of respiratory difficulty or allergic respiratory problem, such as asthma. As previously mentioned, the current package insert for Magnevist warns that caution should be exercised when administering this contrast agent to patients with known allergic respiratory disease.

The total reported incidence of adverse reactions to Magnevist of any kind is 2.4%, based upon a retrospective review of 15,496 patients (Lawrence Gifford, M.D., Director, Medical Affairs, Berlex Laboratories, *written communication,* June 15, 1993). Of these cases, only two reactions were labeled "serious" by FDA standards. In one of these cases, one patient being evaluated for metastatic disease died of herniation from an intracranial tumor within 24 hours of the contrast enhanced MR study. Due to the design of the present review process, this temporal association is sufficient to have the case reported as "associated" with Magnevist administration, irrespective of any perceived—or real—causal relationship. The second serious reaction in this series of patients occurred in an individual who was undergoing evaluation for vertigo and had an acute progression of vertigo following administration of Magnevist. Seizures following administration of this drug have been reported (219). In at least one case, Magnevist injection was believed to induce a seizure in a patient with a history of grand mal seizures (see product insert information for Magnevist).

There are mild elevations in serum chemistries associated with the use of Magnevist that suggest that there may be a component of mild hemolysis in some unknown manner associated with the use of this drug. However, this association is not definite and there is no evidence demonstrating increased hemolysis as a result of Magnevist being administered to patients with hemolytic anemias.

The FDA has stated concern via the package insert regarding the utilization of Magnevist, as well as the other gadolinium-based agents, in patients with sickle cell anemia. According to the package insert information for MRI contrast agents, the enhancement of magnetic moment by Magnevist, Omniscan, or ProHance may possibly potentiate sickle erythrocyte alignment. This information was based on in vitro studies that showed that deoxygenated sickle erythrocytes align perpendicular to a magnetic field and, therefore, vaso-occlusive complications may result in vivo. However, there have been no studies performed to assess the effect of the use of these MRI contrast agents in patients with sickle cell anemia and other forms of hemoglobinopathies. In addition, there has been no report of sickle crisis precipitated by the administration of any of these drugs.

Of the three MRI contrast agents, Magnevist has the highest of the osmolalities, measuring 1,960 mmol/kg of water, or roughly six to seven times that of plasma (approximately 285 mmol/kg of water) (220). Doses greater than or equal to double that used in the United States (i.e., doses of up to 0.3 mmol/kg) have already been investigated in the clinical setting (206,221–223) and have been used for quite some time in Europe, with no apparent significant deleterious effects (224).

Of note is that, since the osmolality of Magnevist is approximately six to seven times the osmolality of plasma, one might expect local irritative reactions as a possible adverse response with the use of this relatively hyperosmolar substance. Indeed, there has been at least one incident of possible phlebitis requiring hospitalization that was related temporally to the administration of an intravenous dose of Magnevist (J. LaFlore, M.D., Medical Affairs, Berlex Laboratories, *oral communication,* 1990). The mechanism(s) behind this are still unclear, although there are objective studies that have demonstrated that tissue sloughing can occur as a result of extravasation of gadolinium-dimeglumine (216,217).

There have also been several cases of erythema, swelling, and pain localized to the site of administration and proximally that were of delayed onset, typically appearing between one to four days following the intravenous administration of the gadolinium- DTPA. This typically progressed for several days, plateaued, and then resolved over several more days (218). Nevertheless, severe adverse local reactions to even considerable quantities (>10 cc) of Magnevist extravasation seem to be quite rare, at best.

Interestingly, Magnevist is the only one of the three MRI contrast agents approved in the United states that has a package insert that recommends a slow, intravenous administration at a rate not to exceed 10 ml/minute. The FDA has approved rapid bolus intravenous administration of Omniscan and ProHance. Nevertheless, studies have been performed with rapid intravenous administration of Magnevist and have indicated that there was no significant difference in the incidence of adverse effects compared with the slow, intravenous administration of this drug (194,206,218).

Omniscan

Since Omniscan is the most recently FDA approved MRI contrast agent, there is relatively little data available related to the safety aspects of this drug. Out of the estimated 100,000 doses that have been distributed, there have been 28 reports of adverse reactions of any type, of which 20 were nausea and emesis. There was a single case of laryngospasm that was successfully treated with epinephrine, as well as a single case of a patient seizing after receiving Omniscan. This patient had a history of seizure disorder. There have been no reports of patient hospitalizations or permanent disabilities related to the use of Omniscan (Dr. Lester Reich, Associate Medical Director, Corporate Products, Nicomed, *written communication*, July 1, 1993).

Omniscan has an osmolality value of 789 mmol/kg of water (220). The manufacturer of Omniscan is in the process of applying for approval of higher total dose administration for specified entities where this might be of clinical significance and benefit (Dr. Lester Reich, Associate Medical Director, Corporate Products, Nicomed, *oral communication,* June 14, 1993).

ProHance

ProHance was approved for use two months prior to the release of Omniscan, therefore, there is also a relative lack of post-market safety data concerning this MRI contrast agent. Out of the estimated 150,000 doses administered, there have been no deaths associated with the use of ProHance. Ten anaphylactoid reactions have occurred in association with the use of this MRI contrast agent, of which five required hospitalization, or ended in permanent disabilities (Rose Rogan, M.D., Director of Drug Safety, Squibb Diagnostics, *written communication,* June 15, 1993).

At this time, ProHance is the only MRI contrast agent with FDA approval to be administered for specific clinical indications up to a total dose of 0.3 mmol/kg, or a total of three times the (standard) dose for each of the other two FDA-approved MRI contrast agents. The relatively low 630 mmol/kg of water osmolality (42) of ProHance may be one of the major factors that permits use of higher doses of this MRI contrast agent to be used without significant deleterious effects on the patient. However, this is purely speculation. Here, too, total adverse effects of any type seem to total <4%, with nausea and taste disturbance each having an incidence of roughly 1.4% and all other adverse reactions being less than 1% each (A.Y. Olukotun, M.D., Vice President of Medical Affairs, Rose Rogan, M.D., Director of Drug Safety, Squibb Diagnostics, *written communication,* June, 1993).

The lower osmolality of ProHance compared to Magnevist was the subject of an investigation into the effect of extravasation of this agent versus the extravasation of Magnevist in the rat model (39). The findings indicated that extravasation of Magnevist was associated with more necrosis, hemorrhage, and edema compared to ProHance, although the authors of this report cautioned about extrapolating the results of their study to contrast agent extravasation in human subjects.

Administration of MRI Contrast Agents to Patients with Renal Failure

As previously indicated, toxicity may result from the dissociation of the gadolinium ion from its chelate. After intravenous administration of gadolinium-based contrast agents, intravascular copper and zinc (normally found in small amounts within the bloodstream), which have a competing affinity for the DTPA chelate will displace some of the gadolinium from the chelating molecule, such as DTPA, which will be released as free gadolinium ion (Gd^{+3}). Although gadolinium is a highly toxic substance, the total concentration of the released free gadolinium is very low and is cleared very rapidly, allowing for a low concentration of free ion to be maintained. In fact, in patients with normal renal function, the rate of dissociation is slower than that of clearance, thus preventing any accumulation phenomenon from occurring (185). It is also believed that the macrocyclic molecules tend to bind the gadolinium more tightly than do the linear ones (183,225).

As new physiologic sources of copper and zinc ions are "leaked" into the intravascular space in an attempt to reestablish their concentration equilibrium, they also displace more gadolinium from its chelate. This cycle continues until all the gadolinium-chelate is cleared from the body via the kidney by glomerular filtration. For this reason, there is a potential concern for the level of free gadolinium ion in cases of renal failure, as there is in patients with a decreased rate of renal clearance of all such substances from the body.

The safety of administering MRI contrast agents to patients with impaired renal function, or even overt renal failure, has not been clearly established. Although several studies suggest that it should be well-tolerated (190,206,226–229). While there is a theoretic concern that decreasing the rate of clearance of the gadolinium chelate from the body might serve to increase the concentration of free gadolinium within the body, data suggests that, for a given level of renal function, administration of lower volume doses may be safer than administering standard doses of iodine-based contrast agents to that same patient (226). Similarly, the safety of administering one of the MRI contrast agents to patients with elevated levels of copper (such as patients with Wilson's disease), or zinc has not been firmly established, and will likely depend upon factors such as the glomerular filtration rate and renal clearance rates, as well as the blood copper levels, of those patients (185). It has also been shown that Magnevist is dialyzable, with more than 95% of the administered dose being removed by the third dialysis treatment (28,52).

Chronic and Repeated Administration of MRI Contrast Agents

There is concern related to the total storage or accumulation of MRI contrast agents, or even free gadolinium ion, after multiple doses are administered throughout a patient's lifetime. The amount of detectable drug still in the liver, kidneys, and bone days after administration seems to be higher in the case of Omniscan than for Magnevist (181), and these both seem to be higher than the level for ProHance (183,225). Currently, there is no data available regarding the safety of long-term cumulative exposure to low doses of free gadolinium ion. Therefore, there may be a clinical limitation regarding the number of times a patient is scanned safely with gadolinium-based contrast drugs. As of now, however, this question remains unanswered and is a topic that warrants investigation.

Using MRI Contrast Agents During Pregnancy and Lactation

Magnevist has been shown to cross the placenta and appear within the fetal bladder only moments after intravenous administration of this drug. It is assumed that the other MRI contrast agents behave in a similar fashion and cross the blood placental barrier easily. From the fetal bladder, these contrast agents would then be excreted into the amniotic fluid and subsequently swallowed by the fetus. This will then be filtered and excreted in the urine of the fetus, with the entire cycle being repeated innumerable times.

There is no data available to assess the rate of clearance of MRI contrast agents from the amniotic fluid cycle. Therefore, it is our opinion that there is information to support the safety of the utilization of MRI contrast agents in pregnant females. Our conservative approach is to recommend against the administration of any of the MRI contrast agents to a pregnant patient until more data becomes available. Pregnant patients should only receive these drugs if the potential benefit justifies the potential risk to the fetus. In any case, should it be decided to administer MRI contrast agents to pregnant patients to facilitate MRI, the patient should be provided written informed consent that stipulates specifically that the risk associated with the use these drugs during pregnancy is presently unknown.

Magnevist has been shown to be excreted in very low concentrations (i.e., 0.011% of the total dose) in human breast milk over approximately 33 hours (231,232). The concentration of this contrast agent in breast milk peaks at approximately 4.75 hours and decreases to less than a fifth of this level (down to less than 1 μmol/liter) 22 hours after the injection (231,232). For this reason and as an extra precaution, we recommend that nursing mothers express their breasts and not breast feed for 36 to 48 hours following the administration of an MRI contrast agent to ensure that the nursing child does not receive the drug in any notable quantity by mouth. However, it should be noted that the LD_{50} of gadolinium chloride or gadolinium acetate (which easily release free gadolinium ions) when given intravenously is approximately 1,000 times lower if taken orally due to the very low absorption of gadolinium from the gastrointestinal tract (235). This supports other data which have demonstrated that 99.2% of orally administered Magnevist was fecally excreted and not absorbed (236).

REFERENCES

1. Adzamli IK, Jolesz FA, Blau M. An assessment of blood-brain barrier integrity under MRI conditions: brain uptake of radiolabeled Gd-DTPA and In-DTPA-IgG. *J Nucl Med* 1989;30:839.
2. Barber BJ, Schaefer DJ, Gordon CJ, et al. Thermal effects of MR imaging: worst-case studies in sheep. *AJR* 1990;155:1105–1110.
3. Bartels MV, Mann K, Matejcek M, et al. Magnetresonanztomographie und Sicherheit: Elektroenzephalographische und neuropsychologische Befunde vor und nach MR-Untersuchungen des Gehirns. *Fortschr Rontgenstrahlen* 1986;145(4):383–385.
4. Besson J, Foreman EI, Eastwood LM, et al. Cognitive evaluation following NMR imaging of the brain. *J Neurol Neurosurg Psychiatry* 1984;47:314–316.
5. Bore PJ, Galloway GJ, Styles P, et al. Are quenches dangerous? *Magn Reson Imaging* 1986;3:112–117.
6. Bourland JD, Nyenhuis JA, Mouchawar GA, et al. Physiologic indicators of high MRI gradient-induced fields. In: *Abstracts of the proceedings of the Society of Magnetic Resonance in Medicine.* Berkeley, CA: Society of Magnetic Resonance in Medicine; 1990: 1276.
7. Brody AS, Sorette MP, Gooding CA, et al. Induced alignment of flowing sickle erythrocytes in a magnetic field. A preliminary report. *Invest Radiol* 1985;20:560–566.
8. Brody AS, Embury SH, Mentzer WC, et al. Preservation of sickle cell blood flow patterns during MR imaging. An in vivo study. *AJR* 1988;151:139–141.
9. Brummett RE, Talbot JM, Charuhas P. Potential hearing loss resulting from MR imaging. *Radiology* 1988;169:539–540.
10. Budinger TF, Fischer H, Hentschel D, et al. Physiological effects of fast oscillating magnetic field gradients. *J Comput Assist Tomogr* 1991;15:909–914.
11. Carson JJL, Prato FS, Drost DJ, et al. Time-varying fields increase cytosolic free Ca^{2+} in HL-60 cells. *Am J Physiol* 1990;259: C687–C692.
12. Cohen MS, Weisskoff R, Rzedzian R, et al. Sensory stimulation by time-varying magnetic fields. *Magn Reson Med* 1990;14:409–414.
13. Cooke P, Morris PG. The effects of NMR exposure on living organisms. II. A genetic study of human lymphocytes. *Br J Radiol* 1981;54:622–625.
14. Doherty JU, Whitman GJR, Robinson MD, et al. Changes in cardiac excitability and vulnerability in NMR fields. *Invest Radiol* 1985;20(2):129–135.
15. Fischer H. Physiological effects of fast oscillating magnetic field gradients. *Radiology* 1989;173:(P)382.
16. Garber HJ, Oldendorf WH, Braun LD, et al. MRI gradient fields increase brain mannitol space. *Magn Reson Imaging* 1989;7: 605–610.
17. Geard CR, Osmak RS, Hall EJ, et al. Magnetic resonance and ionizing radiation: a comparative evaluation in vitro of oncongenic and genotoxic potential. *Radiology* 1984;152:199–202.
18. Gore JC, McDonnell MJ, Pennock JM, et al. An assessment of the safety of rapidly changing magnetic fields in the rabbit: implications for NMR imaging, *Magn Reson Imaging* 1982;1:191–195.
19. Gremmel H, Wendhausen H, Wunsch F. Biologische Effekte statischef Magnetfelder bei NMR-Tomographie am Menschen. Wiss, Radiologische, Klinik. Christian-Albrechts-Universitat zu Kiel; 1983.
20. Gulch RW, Lutz O. Influence of strong static magnetic fields on heart muscle contraction. *Phys Med Biol* 1986;31(7):763–769.
21. Hammer BE, Wadon S, Mirer SD, et al. In vivo measurement of rf heating in Capuchin monkey brain. *In: Abstracts of the proceedings of the Society of Magnetic Resonance in Medicine.* Berkeley, CA: Society of Magnetic Resonance in Medicine; 1278: 1991.
22. Heinrichs WL, Fong P, Flannery M, et al. Midgestational exposure of pregnant Balb/c mice to magnetic resonance imaging. *Magn Reson Imaging* 1988;6:305–313.
23. Hong CZ, Shellock FG. Short-term exposure to a 1.5 Tesla static magnetic field does not effect somato-sensory evoked potentials in man. *Magn Reson Imaging* 1989;8:65–69.
24. Innis NK, Ossenkopp KP, Prato FS, et al. Behavioral effects of exposure to nuclear magnetic resonance imaging. II. Spatial memory tests. *Magn Reson Imaging* 1986;4:281–284.
25. Jehenson P, Duboc D, Lavergne T, et al. Change in human cardiac rhythm by a 2 Tesla static magnetic field. *Radiology* 1988;166:227–230.
26. Kay HH, Herfkens RJ, Kay BK. Effect of magnetic resonance imaging on Xenopus Laevis embryogenesis. *Magn Reson Imaging* 1988;6:501–506.
27. Keltner JR, Roos MS, Brakeman PR, et al. Magnetohydrodynamics of blood flow. *Magn Reson Med* 1990;16:139–149.
28. Kido DK, Morris TW, Erickson JL, et al. Physiologic changes during high field strength MR imaging. *AJNR* 1987;8:263–266.
29. LaPorte R, Kus L, Wisniewski RA, et al. Magnetic resonance imaging (MRI) effects on rat pineal neuroendocrine function. *Brain Res* 1990;506:294–296.
30. McRobbie D, Foster MA. Cardiac response to pulsed magnetic fields with regard to safety in NMR imaging. *Phys Med Biol* 1985;30:695–702.
31. McRobbie D, Foster MA. Pulsed magnetic field exposure during pregnancy and implications for NMR foetal imaging: a study with mice. *Magn Reson Imaging* 1985;3:231–234.
32. Messmer JM, Porter JH, Fatouros P, et al. Exposure to magnetic resonance imaging does not produce taste aversion in rats. *Physiol Behav* 1987;40:259–261.
33. Montour JL, Fatouros PP, Prasad UR. Effect of MR imaging on spleen colony formation following gamma radiation. *Radiology* 1988;168:259–260.
34. Muller S, Hotz M. Human brainstem auditory evoked potentials (BAEP) before and after MR examinations. *Magn Reson Med* 1990;16:476–480.
35. Niemann G, Schroth G, Klose U, et al. Influence of magnetic resonance imaging on somatosensory potential in man. *J Neurol* 1988;235:462–465.
36. Ngo FQH, Blue JW, Roberts WK. The effects of a static magnetic field on DNA synthesis and survival of mammalian cells irradiated with fast neutrons. *Magn Reson Med* 1987;5:307–317.
37. Osbakken M, Griffith J, Taczanowsky P. A gross morphologic, histologic, hematologic, and blood chemistry study of adult and neonatal mice chronically exposed to high magnetic fields. *Magn Reson Med* 1986;3:502–517.
38. Ossenkopp KP, Kavaliers M, Prato FS, et al. Exposure to nuclear magnetic imaging procedure attenuates morphine-induced analgesia in mice. *Life Sci* 1985;37:1507–1514.
39. Ossenkopp KP, Innis NK, Prato FS, et al. Behavioral effects of exposure to nuclear magnetic resonance imaging: I. Open-field behavior and passive avoidance learning in rats. *Magn Reson Imaging* 1986;4:275–280.
40. Papatheofanis FJ, Papatheofanis BJ. Short-term effect of exposure to intense magnetic fields on hematologic indices of bone metabolism. *Invest Radiol* 1989;24:221–223.
41. Peeling J, Lewis JS, Samoiloff MR, et al. Biological effects of magnetic fields on the nemtode Panagrellus redivivus. *Magn Reson Imaging* 1988;6:655–660
42. Prasad N, Kosnik LT, Taber KH, et al. Delayed tumor onset following MR imaging exposure. In: *Abstracts of the Proceedings of the Society of Magnetic Resonance in Medicine.* Berkeley, CA: Society of Magnetic Resonance in Medicine; 1990:275.
43. Prasad N, Prasad R, Bushong SC, et al. Effects of 4.5 T MRI exposure on mouse testes and epididymes. In: *Abstracts of the Proceedings of the Society of Magnetic Resonance in Medicine.* Berkeley, CA: Society of Magnetic Resonance in Medicine; 1990: 606.
44. Prasad N, Bushong SC, Thornby JI, et al. Effect of nuclear resonance on chromosomes of mouse bone marrow cells. *Magn Reson Imaging* 1984;2:37–39.

45. Prasad N, Lotzova E, Thornby JI, et al. Effects of MR imaging on murine natural killer cell cytotoxicity. *AJR* 1987;148:415–417.
46. Prasad N, Lotzova E, Thornby JI, et al. The effect of 2.35-T MR imaging on natural killer cell cytotoxicity with and without interleukin-2. *Radiology* 1990;175:251–263.
47. Prasad N, Wright DA, Ford JJ, et al. Safety of 4-T MR imaging: a study of effects of developing frog embryos. *Radiology* 1990;174:251–253.
48. Prasad N, Wright DA, Forster JD. Effect of nuclear magnetic resonance on early stages of amphibian development. *Magn Reson Imaging* 1982;1:35–38.
49. Prato FS, Ossenkopp KP, Kavaliers M, et al. Attenuation of morphine-induced analgesia in mice by exposure to magnetic resonance imaging: Separate effects of the static, radiofrequency and time-varying magnetic fields. *Magn Reson Imaging* 1987;5:9–14.
50. Redington RW, Dumoulin CL, Schenck JL, et al. MR imaging and bio-effects in a whole body 4.0 Tesla imaging system. In: *Abstracts of the Proceedings of the Society of Magnetic Resonance in Medicine.* Berkeley, CA: Society of Magnetic Resonance in Medicine; 1988;1:20.
51. Reid A, Smith FW, Hutchison JMS. Nuclear magnetic resonance imaging and its safety implications: follow-up of 181 patients. *Br J Radiol* 1982;55:784–786.
52. Roschmann P. Human auditory system response to pulsed radiofrequency energy in rf coils for magnetic resonance at 2.4 to 170 MHz. *Magn Reson Med* 1991;21:197–215.
53. Sacks E, Worgul BV, Merriam GR, et al. The effects of nuclear magnetic resonance imaging on ocular tissues. *Arch Ophthalmol* 1986;104:890–893.
54. Schwartz JL, Crooks LE. NMR imaging produces no observable mutations or cytotoxicity in mammalian cells. *AJR* 1982;139:583–585.
55. Shellock FG, Schaefer DJ, Gordon CJ. Effect of a 1.5 T static magnetic field on body temperature of man. *Magn Reson Med* 1986;3:644–647.
56. Shellock FG, Crues JV. Temperature, heart rate, and blood pressure changes associated with clinical MR imaging at 1.5 T. *Radiology* 1987;163:259–262.
57. Shellock FG, Schaefer DJ, Grundfest W, et al. Thermal effects of high-field (1.5 Tesla) magnetic resonance imaging of the spine: clinical experience above a specific absorption rate of 0.4 W/kg. *Acta Radiol Suppl* 1986;369:514–516.
58. Shellock FG, Gordon CJ, Schaefer DJ. Thermoregulatory responses to clinical magnetic resonance imaging of the head at 1.5 Tesla: lack of evidence for direct effects on the hypothalamus. *Acta Radiol Suppl* 1986;369:512–513.
59. Shellock FG, Crues JV. Corneal temperature changes associated with high-field MR imaging using a head coil. *Radiology* 1986;167:809–811.
60. Shellock FG, Crues JV. Temperature changes caused by clinical MR imaging of the brain at 1.5 Tesla using a head coil. *AJNR* 1988;9:287–291.
61. Shellock FG, Schaefer DJ, Crues JV. Effect of a 1.5 Tesla static magnetic field on body and skin temperatures of man. *Magn Reson Med* 1989;11:371–375.
62. Shellock FG, Schaefer DJ, Crues JV. Alterations in body and skin temperatures caused by MR imaging: is the recommended exposure for radiofrequency radiation too conservative? *Br J Radiol* 1989;62:904–909.
63. Shellock FG, Rothman B, Sarti D. Heating of the scrotum by high-field-strength MR imaging. *AJR* 1990;154:1229–1232.
64. Shivers RR, Kavaliers M, Tesky CJ, et al. Magnetic resonance imaging temporarily alters blood-brain barrier permeability in the rat. *Neurosci Lett* 1987;76:25–31.
65. Shuman WP, Haynor DR, Guy AW, et al. Superficial and deep-tissue increases in anesthetized dogs during exposure to high specific absorption rates in a 1.5-T MR imager. *Radiology* 1988;167:551–554.
66. Sperber D, Oldenbourg R, Dransfeld K. Magnetic field induced temperature change in mice. *Naturwissenschaften* 1984;71:100–101.
67. Stick VC, Hinkelmann ZK, Eggert P, et al. Beeinflussen starke statische magnetfelder in der NMR-Tomographie die gewebedurchblutung? (Strong static magnetic fields of NMR: do they affect tissue perfusion?). *Fortschr Rontgenstrahlen* 1991;154(3):326–331.
68. Stojan L, Sperber D, Dransfeld K. Magnetic-field-induced changes in the human auditory evoked potentials. *Naturwissenschaften* 1988;75:622–623.
69. Sweetland J, Kertesz A, Prato FS, et al. The effect of magnetic resonance imaging on human congnition. *Magn Reson Imaging* 1987;5:129–135.
70. Teskey GC, Prato FS, Ossenkopp KP, et al. Exposure to time varying magnetic fields associated with magnetic resonance imaging reduces fentanyl-induced analgesia in mice. *Bioelectromagnetics* 1988;9:167–174.
71. Teskey GC, Ossenkopp KP, Prato FS, et al. Survivability and long-term stress reactivity levels following repeated exposure to nuclear magnetic resonance imaging procedures in rats. *Physiol Chem Phys Med NMR* 1987;19:43–49.
72. Thomas A, Morris PG. The effects of NMR exposure on living organisms. I. A microbial assay. *Br J Radiol* 1981;54:615–621.
73. Tyndall DA, Sulik KK. Effects of magnetic resonance imaging on eye development in the C57BL/6J mouse. *Teratology* 1991;43:263–275.
74. Tyndall DA. MRI effects on the tertogenicity of X-irradiation in the C57BL/6J mouse. *Magn Reson Imaging* 1990;8:423–433.
75. Vogl T, Krimmel K, Fuchs A, et al. Influence of Magnetic resonance imaging on human body core and intravascular temperature. *Med Phys* 1988;15:562–566.
76. Von Klitzing L. Do static magnetic fields of NMR influence biological signals. *Clin Physics Physiol Measure* (Bristol) 1986;7(2):157–160.
77. Von Klitzing L. Static magnetic fields increase the power intensity of EEG of man. *Brain Res* 1989;483:201–203.
78. Von Klitzing L. A new encephalomagnetic effect in human brain generated by static magnetic fields. *Brain Res* 1991;540:295–296.
79. Weiss J, Herrick RC, Taber KH, et al. Bio-effects of high magnetic fields: a study using a simple animal model. *Magn Reson Imaging* 1990;8(S1):166.
80. Willis RJ, Brooks WM. Potential hazards of NMR imaging. No evidence of the possible effects of static and changing magnetic fields on cardiac function of the rat and guinea pig. *Magn Reson Imaging* 1984;2:89–95.
81. Withers HR, Mason KA, Davis CA. MR effect on murine spermatogenesis. *Radiology* 1985;156:741–742.
82. Wolff S, Crooks LE, Brown P, et al. Tests for DNA and chromosomal damage induced by nuclear magnetic resonance imaging. *Radiology* 1980;136:707–710.
83. Yamagata H, Kuhara S, Eso Y, et al. Evaluation of dB/dt thresholds for nerve stimulation elicited by trapezoidal and sinusoidal gradient fields in echo-planar imaging. In: *Abstracts of the Proceedings of the Society of Magnetic Resonance in Medicine.* Berkeley, CA: Society of Magnetic Resonance in Medicine; 1991:1277.
84. Vyalov AM. Magnetic fields as a factor in the industrial environment. *Vestn Ross Akad Med Nauk* 1967;8:72–79.
85. Vyalov AM. Clinico-hygenic and experimental data on the effect of magnetic fields under industrial conditions. In: Kholodov Y, ed. *Influence of Magnetic Fields on Biological Objects.* Moscow: 1971. Translated by the Joint Publications Research Service. *JPRS* 1974;63-38:20–35.
86. Barnothy MF. *Biological Effects of Magnetic Fields*, vols. 1 & 2. New York: Plenum Press; 1964:1969.
87. Persson BR, Stahlberg F. *Health and Safety of Clinical NMR Examinations.* Boca Raton, FL: CRC Press; 1989.
88. Tenforde TS. *Magnetic Field Effects on Biological Systems.* New York: Plenum Press; 1979.
89. Michaelson SM, Lin JV. *Biological Effects and Health Implications of Radiofrequency Radiation.* New York: Plenum Press; 1987.
90. Tenforde TS. Thermoregulation in rodents exposed to high-intensity stationary magnetic fields. *Bioelectromagnetics* 1986;7:341–346.
91. Beischer DE, Knepton J. Influence of strong magnetic fields on the electrocardiogram of squirrel monkey (Saimiri sciures). *Aerospace Med* 1964;35:939–944.
92. Tenforde TS, Gaffey CT, Moyer BR, et al. Cardiovascular alter-

ations in Macaca monkeys exposed to stationary magnetic fields. Experimental observations and theoretical analysis. *Bioelectromagnetics* 1983;4:1–9.
93. Dimick RM, Hedlund LW, Herfkens RJ, et al. Optimizing electrocardiographic electrode placement for cardiac-gated magnetic resonance imaging. *Invest Radiol* 1987;22:17–22.
94. Abdullakhozhaeva MS, Razykov SR. Structural changes in central nervous system under the influence of a permanent magnetic field. *Bull Exper Biol Med* 1986;102:1585–1587.
95. Hong CZ. Static magnetic field influence on human nerve function. *Arch Phys Med Rehab* 1987;68:162–164.
96. Budinger TF. Nuclear magnetic resonance (NMR) in vivo studies: Known thresholds for health effects. *J Comput Assist Tomogr* 1981;5:800–811.
97. Shellock FG, Crues JV. MRI: Safety considerations in magnetic resonance imaging. *MRI Decisions* 1988;2:25–30.
98. Shellock FG. Biological effects and safety aspects of magnetic resonance imaging. *Magn Reson Q* 1989;5:243–261.
99. Kanal E, Talagala L, Shellock FG. Safety considerations in MR imaging. *Radiology* 1990;176:593–606.
100. Reilly JP. Peripheral nerve stimulation by induced electric currents: exposure to time-varying magnetic fields. *Med Biol Eng Comput* 1989;27:101–112.
101. Bernhardt J. The direct influence of electromagnetic fields on nerve and muscle and muscle cells of man within the frequency range of 1 Hz to 30 MHz. *Radiat Environ Bio Phys* 1979;16:309–323.
102. Adey WR. Tissue interactions with nonionizing electromagnetic fields. *Phys Rev* 1981;61:435–514.
103. Watson AB, Wright JS, Loughman L. Electrical thresholds for ventricular fibrillation in man. *Med J Aust* 1973;1:1179–1182.
104. Modan B. Exposure to electromagnetic fields and brain malignancy: a newly discovered menace? *Am J Ind Med* 1988;13:625–627.
105. Brown HD, Chattopadhyay SK. Electromagnetic-field exposure and cancer. *Cancer Biochem Biophys* 1988;9:295–342.
106. Pool R. Electromagnetic fields: the biological evidence. *Science* 1990;249:1378–1381.
107. F.D.A. Magnetic resonance diagnostic device; panel recommendation and report on petitions for MR reclassification. *Fed Register* 1988;53:7575–7579.
108. NCRP Report No. 86. *Biological Effects and Exposure Criteria for Radiofrequency Electromagnetic Fields.* Bethesda, MD: National Council on Radiation Protection and Measurements; 1986.
109. Erwin DN. Mechanisms of biological effects of radiofrequency electromagnetic fields: an overview. *Aviation Space Environ Med* 1988;59(Suppl 11):A21–A31.
110. Gordon CJ. Thermal physiology. In: *Biological Effects of Radiofrequency Radiation.* Washington, D.C.: EPA; 600/8-830-026A; 1984:4-1–4-28.
111. Gordon CJ. Normalizing the thermal effects of radiofrequency radiation: Body mass versus total body surface area. *Bioelectromagnetics* 1987;8:111–118.
112. Gordon CJ. Effect of radiofrequency radiation exposure on thermoregulation. *ISI Atlas Sci Plants Animals* 1988;1:245–250.
113. Beers J. Biological effects of weak electromagnetic fields from 0 Hz to 200 MHz: a survey of the literature with special emphasis on possible magnetic resonance effects. *Magn Reson Imaging* 1989;7:309–331.
114. Coulter JS, Osbourne SL. Short wave diathermy in heating of human tissues. *Arch Physical Therapy* 1936;17:679–687.
115. Bottomley PA, Edelstein WA. Power disposition in whole body NMR imaging. *Med Phys* 1981;8:510–512.
116. Bottomley PA, Redington RW, Edelstein WA, et al. Estimating radiofrequency power disposition in body NMR imaging. *Magn Reson Med* 1985;2:336–349.
117. Wickersheim KA, Sun MH. Fluoroptic thermometry. *Med Electronics* 1987;Feb:84–91.
118. Berman E. Reproductive effects. In: *Biological Effects of Radiofrequency Radiation.* Washington, D.C.: EPA; 600/8-83-026A; 1984.
119. Michaelson SM, Lin JC. *Biological Effects and Health Implications of Radiofrequency Radiation.* New York: Plenum Press; 1987.
120. Shellock FG, Kanal E. Policies, guidelines, and recommendations for MR imaging safety and patient management. *J Magn Reson Imag* 1991;1:97–101.
121. Hurwitz R, Lane SR, Bell RA, et al. Acoustic analysis of gradient-coil noise in MR imaging. *Radiology* 1989;173:545–548.
122. Goldman AM, Grossman WE, Friedlander PC. Reduction of sound levels with antinoise in MR imaging. *Radiology* 1989;173:549–550.
123. Hayes DL, Holmes DR, Gray JE. Effect of a 1.5 Tesla nuclear magnetic resonance imaging scanner on implanted permanent pacemakers. *J Am Coll Cardiol* 1987;10:782–786.
124. Gangarosa RE, Minnis JE, Nobbe J, et al. Operational safety issues in MRI. *Magn Reson Imaging* 1987;5:287–292.
125. Alagona P, Toole JC, Maniscalco BS, et al. Nuclear magnetic resonance imaging in a patient with a DDD pacemaker. *PACE* 1989;12:619.
126. Edelman RR, Shellock FG, Ahladis J. Practical MRI for the technologist and imaging specialist. In: Edelman RR, Hesselink J, eds. *Clinical Magnetic Resonance Imaging.* Philadelphia: WB Saunders; 1990.
127. ECRI. Health devices alert, a new MRI complication? May 27, 1988:1.
128. Dormer KJ, Richard GJ, Hough JVD, et al. The use of rare-earth magnet couplers in cochlear implants. *Laryngoscope* 1981;91:1812–1820.
129. Shellock FG. Ex vivo assessment of deflection forces and artifacts associated with high-field MRI of "mini-magnet" dental prostheses. *Magn Reson Imaging* 1989;7(Suppl 1):IT-03.
130. Liang MD, Narayanan K, Kanal E. Magnetic ports in tissue expanders: a caution for MRI. *Magn Reson Imaging* 1989;7:541–542.
131. Lund G, Nelson JD, Wirtschafter JD, et al. Tattooing of eyelids: magnetic imaging artifacts. *Ophthalmol Surg* 1986;17:550–553.
132. Sacco DA, Steiger DA, Bellon EM, et al. Artifacts caused by cosmetics in MR imaging of the head. *AJR* 1987;148:1001–1004.
133. Jackson JG, Acker JD. Permanent eyeliner and MR imaging. *AJR* 1987;149:1080.
134. Pusey E, Lufkin RB, Brown RKJ, et al. Magnetic resonance imaging artifacts: mechanism and clinical significance. *Radiographics* 1986;6:891–911.
135. Buchli R, Boesiger P, Meier D. Heating effects of metallic implants by MRI examinations. *Magn Reson Med* 1988;7:255–261.
136. Davis PL, Crooks L, Arakawa M, et al. Potential hazards in NMR imaging: Heating effects of changing magnetic fields and rf fields on small metallic implants. *AJR* 1981;137:857–860.
137. Shellock FG, Crues JV. High-field MR imaging of metallic biomedical implants: an in vitro evaluation of deflection forces and temperature changes induced in large prostheses. *Radiology* 1987;165:150.
138. Shellock FG, Crues JV. High-field MR imaging of metallic biomedical implants: an ex vivo evaluation of deflection forces. *AJR* 1988;151:389–392.
139. Dujovny M, Kossovsky N, Kossowsky R, et al. Aneurysm clip motion during magnetic resonance imaging: in vivo experimental study with metallurgical factor analysis. *Neurosurgery* 1985;17:543–548.
140. Shellock FG, Schatz CJ, Shelton C. et al. Ex vivo evaluation of 9 different ocular and middle-ear implants exposed to a 1.5 Tesla MR scanner. *Radiology* 1990;177(P):271.
141. Shellock FG, Schatz CJ. High-field strength MRI and otologic implants. *AJNR* 1991;12:279–281.
142. Shellock FG, Meeks T. Ex vivo evaluation of ferromagnetism and artifacts for implantable vascular access ports exposed to a 1.5 T MR scanner. *Magn Reson Imaging* 1991;1:243.
143. Teitelbaum GP, Yee CA, Van Horn DD, et al. Metallic ballistic fragments: MR imaging safety and artifacts. *Radiology* 1990;175:855–859.
144. Shellock FG. MR imaging of metallic implants and materials: a compilation of the literature. *AJR* 1988;151:811–814.
145. Shellock FG, Curtis JS. MR imaging and biomedical implants, materials, and devices: an updated review. *Radiology* 1991;180:541–550.

146. Holtas S, Olsson M, Romner B, et al. Comparison of MR imaging and CT in patients with intracranial aneurysm clips. *AJNR* 1988;9:891–897.
147. Huttenbrink KB, Grobe-Nobis W. Experimentelle Untersuchungen und theoretische Betrachtungen uber das Verhalten von Stapes-Metall-Prothesen im Magnetfeld eines Kernspintomographen. (Experiments and theoretical considerations on behaviour of metallic stapedectomy-prostheses in nuclear magnetic resonance imaging.) *Laryngorhinolootologie* 1987;66:127–130.
148. Becker R, Norfray JF, Teitelbaum GP, et al. MR imaging in patients with intracranial aneurysm clips. *AJNR* 1988;9:885–889.
149. Randall PA, Kohman LJ, Scalzetti EM, et al. Magnetic resonance imaging of prosthetic cardiac valves in vitro and in vivo. *Am J Cardiol* 1988;62:973–976.
150. Romner B, Olsson M, Ljunggren B, et al. Magnetic resonance imaging and aneurysm clips. *J Neurosurg* 1989;70:426–431.
151. Augustiny N, von Schulthess GK, Meier D, et al. MR imaging of large nonferromagnetic metallic implants at 1.5 T. *J Comput Assist Tomogr* 1987;11:678–683.
152. Teitelbaum GP, Bradley WG, Klein BD. MR imaging artifacts ferromagnetism, and magnetic torque of intravascular filters, stents, and coils. *Radiology* 1988;166:657–664.
153. Yuh WTC, Hanigan MT, Nerad JA, et al. Extrusion of a magnetic eye implant after MR examination: a potential hazard to the enucleated eye. In: *Abstracts of the Proceedings of the American Society of Neuroradiology.* American Society of Neuroradiology; 1991;97.
154. Kelly WM, Pagle PG, Pearson A, et al. Ferromagnetism of intraocular foreign body causes unilateral blindness after MR study. *AJNR* 1986;7:243–245.
155. Williams S, Char DH, Dillon WP, et al. Ferrous intraocular foreign bodies and magnetic resonance imaging. *Am J Ophthalmol* 1988;105:398–401.
156. Flaherty JA, Hoskinson K. Emotional distress during magnetic resonance imaging. *N Engl J Med* 1989;320:467–468.
157. Fishbain DA, Goldberg M, Labbe E. et al. Long-term claustrophobia following magnetic resonance imaging. *Am J Psychiatry* 1988;145:1038–1039.
158. Quirk ME, Letendre AJ, Ciottone RA. et al. Anxiety in patients undergoing MR imaging. *Radiology* 1989;170:463–466.
159. Quirk ME, Letendre AJ, Ciottone RA, et al. Evaluation of three psychological interventions to reduce anxiety during MR imaging. *Radiology* 1989;173:759–762.
160. Hricak H, Amparo EG. Body MRI: alleviation of claustrophobia by prone positioning. *Radiology* 1984;152:819.
161. Weinreb JC, Maravilla KR, Peshock R, et al. Magnetic resonance imaging: improving patient tolerance and safety. *AJR* 1984;143: 1285–1287.
162. Klonoff EA, Janata JW, Kaufman B. The use of systematic desensitization to overcome resistance to magnetic resonance imaging (MRI) scanning. *J Behav Ther Exp Psychiatry* 1986;17: 189–192.
163. Granet RB, Gelber LJ. Claustrophobia during MR imaging. *N J Med* 1990;87(6):479–482.
164. Phelps LA. MRI and claustrophobia. *Am Fam Physician* 1990;42(4):930.
165. McGuinness TP. Hypnosis in the treatment of phobias: a review of the literature. *Am J Clin Hypn* 1984;26:261–272.
166. Karlik SJ, Heatherley T, Pavan F, et al. Patient anesthesia and monitoring at a 1.5 T MRI installation. *Magn Reson Med* 1988;7: 210–221.
167. Barnett GH, Ropper AH, Johnson KA. Physiological support and monitoring of critically ill patients during magnetic resonance imaging. *J Neurosurg* 1988;68:244–250.
168. Dunn V, Coffman CE, McGowan JE, et al. Mechanical ventilation during magnetic resonance imaging. *Magn Reson Imaging* 1985;3:169–172.
169. McArdle CB, Nicholas DA, Richardson CJ, et al. Monitoring of the neonate undergoing MR imaging: technical considerations. *Radiology* 1986;159:223–226.
170. Roth JL, Nugent M, Gray JE, et al. Patient monitoring during magnetic resonance imaging. *Anesthesiology* 1985;62:80–83.
171. Shellock FG. Monitoring during MRI. An evaluation of the effect of high-field MRI on various patient monitors. *Med Electronics* 1986;Sept:93–97.
172. Shellock FG. Monitoring sedated patients during MRI [letter]. *Radiology* 1990;177:586 .
173. Wendt RE, Rokey R, Vick GW, et al. Electrocardiographic gating and monitoring during NMR imaging. *Magn Reson Imaging* 1988;6:89–95.
174. Holshouser BA, Hinshaw DB, Shellock FG. Sedation, anesthesia, and physiologic monitoring during MRI. In: Hasso AN, Stark DD, eds. *Spine and Body Magnetic Resonance Imaging.* American Roentgen Ray Society, Categorical Course Syllabus, May, 1991.
175. Kanal E, Applegate GR. Thermal injuries/incidents associated with MR imaging devices in the US: a compilation and review of the presently available data. In: *Abstracts of the Proceedings of the Society for Magnetic Resonance Imaging.* Society for Magnetic Resonance in Medicine; 1990:274.
176. Shellock FG, Slimp G. Severe burn of the finger caused by using a pulse oximeter during MRI. *AJR* 1989;153:1105.
177. Kanal E, Shellock FG. Burns associated with clinical MR examinations. *Radiology* 1990;175:585.
178. Shellock FG, Myers SM, Kimble K. Monitoring heart rate and oxygen saturation during MRI with a fiber-optic pulse oximeter. *AJR* 1992;158:663–664.
179. Runge V. Clinical application of magnetic resonance contrast media in the head. In: Runge V, ed. *Contrast Media in Magnetic Resonance Imaging: A Clinical Approach.* Philadelphia: JB Lippincott; 1992:Chap 2.
180. Oksendal A, Hals P. Biodistribution and toxicity of MR imaging contrast media. *J Magn Reson Imaging* 1993;3:157–165.
181. Harpur E, Worah D, Hals P, Holtz E, Furuhama K, Nomura H. Preclinical safety assessment and pharmacokinetics of gadodiamide injection, a new magnetic resonance imaging contrast agent. *Invest Radiol* 1993;28:S28–S43.
182. Tweedle M, Eaton S, Eckelman W, et al. Comparative chemical structure and pharmacokinetics of MRI contrast agents. *Invest Radiol* 1988;23(Suppl 1):S236–S239.
183. Tweedle M. Physiochemical properties of gadoteridol and other magnetic resonance contrast agents. *Invest Radiol* 1992;27 (Suppl 1):S2–S6.
184. Chang C. Magnetic resonance imaging contrast agents. Design and physiochemical properties of gadodiamide. *Invest Radiol* 1993;28(Suppl 1):S21–S27.
185. Cacheris W, Quay S, Rocklage S. The relationship between thermodynamics and the toxicity of gadolinium complexes. *Magn Reson Imaging* 1990;8:467–481.
186. Felix R, Schorner W. Intravenous contrast media in MRI: clinical experience with gadolinium-DTPA over four years. *Proceedings of the second annual European Congress of NMR in Medicine in Biology.* Berlin: 1988.
187. Niendorf H, Ezumi K. Magnevist (Gd-DTPA): tolerance and safety after 4 years of clinical trials in more than 7000 patients. *Proceedings of the second European Congress of NMR in Medicine in Biology.* Berlin: 1988.
188. Niendorf H, Valk J, Reiser M. First use of Gd-DTPA in pediatric MRI. *Proceedings of the second European Congress of NMR in Medicine in Biology.* Berlin: 1988.
189. Ball WJ, Nadel S, Zimmerman R, et al. Phase III multicenter clinical investigation to determine the safety and efficacy of gadoteridol in children suspected of having neurologic disease. *Radiology* 1993;186:769–774.
190. Niendorf H, Haustein J, Cornelius I, Alhassan A, Claus W. Safety of gadolinium-DTPA: extended clinical experience. *Magn Reson Med* 1991;22:222–228.
191. Sullivan M,. Goldstein H, Sansone K, Stoner S, Holyoak W, Wiggins J. Hemodynamic effects of Gd-DTPA administered via rapid bolus or slow infusion: a study in dogs. *AJNR* 1990;11:537–540.
192. Goldstein H, Kashanian F, Blumetti R, Holyoak W, Hugo F, Blumenfield D. Safety assessment of gadopentetate dimeglumine in US clinical trials. *Radiology* 1990;174;17–23.
193. Hajek P, Sartoris D, Gylys-Morin V, et al. The effect of intraarticular gadolinium-DTPA on synovial membrane and cartilage. *Invest Radiol* 1990;25:179–183.

194. Kashanian F, Goldstein H, Blumetti R, Holyoak W, Hugo F, Dolker M. Rapid bolus injection of gadopentetate dimeglumine: absence of side effects in normal volunteers. *AJNR* 1990;11:853–856.
195. Brasch R. Safety profile of gadopentetate dimeglumine. *MRI Decisions* 1989;3:13–19.
196. McLachlan S, Lucas M, DeSimone D, et al. Worldwide safety experience with gadoteridol injection (ProHance). In: *Abstracts of the Proceedings of the Society of Magnetic Resonance in Medicine.* Berkeley, CA: Society of Magnetic Resonance in Medicine; 1992:1426.
197. Berlex. A two year report on the safety and efficacy of Magnevist (gadopentetate dimeglumine) injection. In: Berlex Laboratories, Inc., 1990.
198. DeSimone D, Morris M, Rhoda C, et al. Evaluation of the safety and efficacy of gadoteridol injection (a low osmolal MR contrast agent): clinical trials report. *Invest Radiol* 1991;26(Suppl 1): S212–S216.
199. Carvlin M, DeSimone D, Meeks M. Phase II clinical trial of gadoteridol injection, a low osmolal magnetic resonance imaging contrast agent. *Invest Radiol* 1992;27:S16–S21.
200. Runge V, Bradley W, Brant-Zawadski M, et al. Clinical safety and efficacy of gadoteridol: a study in 411 patients with suspected intracranial and spinal disease. *Radiology* 1991;181:701–709.
201. McLachlan S, Eaton S, DeSimone D. Pharmacokinetic behavior of gadoteridol injection. *Invest Radiol* 1992;27(Suppl 1):S12–S15.
202. Soltys R. Summary of preclinical safety evaluation of gadoteridol injection. *Invest Radiol* 1992;27(Suppl 1):S7–S11.
203. Weinmann HJ, Gries H, Speck U. Gd-DTPA and low osmolar Gd chelates. In: Runge V, ed. *Enhanced Magnetic Resonance Imaging.* St. Louis: CV Mosby; 1989.
204. Muhler A, Saeed M, Brasch R, Higgins C. Hemodynamic effects of bolus injection of gadodiamide injection and gadopentetate dimeglumine as contrast media at MR imaging in rats. *Radiology* 1992;183:523–528.
205. LaFlore J. Goldstein H, Rogan R, Keelan T, Ewell A. A prospective evaluation of adverse experiences following the administration of Magnevist (gadopentetate dimeglumine) injection. In: *Abstracts of the Proceedings of the Society of Magnetic Resonance in Medicine.* Berkeley, CA: Society of Magnetic Resonance in Medicine; 1989:1067.
206. Niendorf H, Dinger J, Haustein J, Cornelius I, Alhassan A, Claub W. Tolerance data of Gd-DTPA: a review. *Eur J Radiol* 1991;13: 15–20.
207. Takebayashi S, Sugiyama M, Nagase M, Matsubara S. Severe adverse reaction to IV gadopentetate dimeglumine. *AJR* 1990;14: 912–913.
208. Shellock FG, Hahn P, Mink JH, Itskovich E. Adverse reaction to intravenous gadoteridol. *Radiology* 1993;189:1–2.
209. Salonen O. Case of anaphylaxis and four cases of allergic reaction following Gd-DTPA administration. *J Comput Assist Tomogr* 1990;14:912–913.
210. Tishler S, Hoffman JC. Anaphylactoid reactions to IV gadopentetate dimeglumine. *AJNR* 1990;11:1167.
211. Weiss K. Severe anaphylactoid reaction after IV Gd-DTPA. *Magn Reson Imaging* 1990;8:817–818.
212. Tardy B, Guy C, Barral G. Page Y, Ollagnier M, Bertrand C. Anaphylactic shock induced by intravenous gadopentetate dimeglumine. *Lancet* 1992;339:494.
213. Omohundro J, Elderbrook M, Ringer T. Laryngospasm after administration of gadopentetate dimeglumine. *J Magn Reson Imaging* 1992;1:729–730.
214. Chan C, Bosanko C, Wang A. Pruritis and paresthesia after IV administration of Gd-DTPA. *AJNR* 1989;10:S53.
215. American College of Radiology. *Manual on Iodinated Contrast Media.* 1991.
216. McAlister W, McAlister V, Kissane J. The effect of Gd-dimeglumine on subcutaneous tissues: a study with rats. *AJNR* 1990;11:325–327.
217. Cohan R, Elder R, A, et al. Extravascular toxicity of two magnetic resonance contrast agents: preliminary experience in the rat. *Invest Radiol* 1991;26:224–226.
218. Kanal E, Applegate G, Gillen C. Review of adverse reactions, including anaphylaxis, in 5260 cases receiving gadolinium-DTPA by bolus injection. *Radiology* 1990;177(P):159.
219. Harbury O. Generalized seizure after IV gadopentetate dimeglumine. *AJNR* 1991;12:666.
220. Watson A, Rocklage S, Carvlin M. Contrast media. In: Stark D, Bradley W, eds. *Magnetic Resonance Imaging.* St. Louis: CV Mosby; 1991.
221. Niendorf H, Haustein J, Louton T, Beck W, Laniado M. Safety and tolerance after intravenous administration of 0.3 mmol/kg Gd-DTPA. *Invest Radiol* 1991;26:S221–S223.
222. Niendorf H, Laniado M, Semmler W, Schomer W, Felix R. Dose administration of gadolinium-DTPA in MR imaging of intracranial tumors. *AJNR* 1987;8:803–815.
223. Haustein J, Bauer W, Hibertz T, et al. Double dosing of Gd-DTPA in MRI of intracranial tumors. In: *Abstracts of the Proceedings of the Society of Magnetic Resonance in Medicine.* Berkeley, CA: Society of Magnetic Resonance in Medicine; I990: 258.
224. Leander P, Allard M, Caille J, Golman K. Early effect of gadopentetate and iodinated contrast media on rabbit kidneys. *Invest Radiol* 1992;27:922–926.
225. Wedeking P, Kumar K. Tweedle M. Dissociation of gadolinium chelates in mice: relationship to chemical characteristics. *Magn Reson Imaging* 1992;10:641–648.
226. Haustein J, Niendorf H, Louton T. Renal tolerance of Gd-DTPA—A retrospective evaluation of 1,171 patients. *Magn Reson Imaging* 1990;8(S1):43.
227. Frank J, Choyke P, Girton M, Morrison P, Diggs R, Skinner M. Gadopentetate dimeglumine clearance in renal insufficiency in rabbits. *Invest Radiol* 1990;25:1212–1216.
228. Haustein J, Niendorf H, Krestin G, et al. Renal tolerance of gadolinium-DTPA/dimeglumine in patients with chronic renal failure. *Invest Radiol* 1992;27:153–156.
229. Runge V, Rocklage S, Niendorf H, et al. Discussion: gadolinium chelates. *Society of Magnetic in Resonance Imaging in Medicine workshop on Contrast Enhanced Magnetic Resonance.* Berkeley, CA; 1991:229–232.
230. Lackner K, Krahe T, Gotz R, Haustein J. The dialysability of Gd-DTPA. In: Bydder G, Felix R, Bucheler E, ed. *Contrast Media in MRI.* Bussum: Medicom Europe; 1990:321–326.
231. Schmiedl U, Maravilla K, Gerlach R, Dowling C. Excretion of gadopentetate dimeglumine in human breast milk. *AJR* 1990;154:1305–1306.
232. Rofsky N, Weinreb J, Litt A. Quantitative analysis of gadopentetate dimeglumine excreted in breast milk. *J Magn Reson Imaging* 1993;3:131–132.
235. Nell G, Rummel W. Pharmacology of intestinal permeation: In: Csaky T, ed. *Handbook of Experimental Pharmacology*, vol. 70, part II. Berlin: Springer-Verlag; 1984:489.
236. Weinmann H, Brasch R, Press W, Wesbey G. Characteristics of gadolinium-DTPA complex: a potential NMR contrast agent. *AJR* 1984;142:619–624.

Appendix

LIST OF METALLIC IMPLANTS, MATERIALS, DEVICES, AND OBJECTS TESTED FOR MOVEMENT/DEFLECTION FORCES DURING EXPOSURE TO STATIC MAGNETIC FIELDS

Metallic implant, material, device, or object	Movement/ Deflection	Highest field strength (T)	Reference
Aneurysm and hemostatic clips			
Downs multi-positional (15-7PH)	Yes	1.39	1
Drake (DR 14, DR 21) (Edward Weck, Triangle Park, NJ)	Yes	1.39	1, 2
Drake (DR 16) (Edward Weck)	Yes	0.147	1
Drake (301 SS) (Edward Weck)	Yes	1.5	2, 3
Gastrointestinal anastomosis clip, Auto Suture SGIA (SS), (United States Surgical Corp., Norwalk, CT)	No	1.5	3
Heifetz (15-7PH) (Edward Weck)	Yes	1.89	4, 5
Heifetz (Elgiloy) (Edward Weck)	No	1.89	2, 4, 5
Hemoclip, #10, (316L SS) (Edward Weck)	No	1.5	3
Hemoclip (tantalum) (Edward Weck)	No	1.5	3
Housepian	Yes	0.147	1
Kapp (405 SS) (V. Mueller)	Yes	1.89	2, 5
Kapp, curved (404 SS) (V. Mueller)	Yes	1.39	1
Kapp, straight (404 SS) (V. Mueller)	Yes	1.39	1
Ligaclip, #6, (316L SS) (Ethicon, Inc., Sommerville, NJ)	No	1.5	3
Ligaclip (tantalum) (Ethicon)	No	1.5	3
Mayfield (301 SS) (Codman, Randolph, MA)	Yes	1.5	3
Mayfield (304 SS) (Codman)	Yes	1.89	5
McFadden (301 SS) (Codman)	Yes	1.5	2, 3
Olivecrona	No	1.39	1
Pivot (17-7PH)	Yes	1.89	5
Scoville (EN58J) (Downs Surgical, Inc., Decatur, GA)	Yes	1.89	2, 5
Stevens (50-4190, silver alloy)	No	0.15	6
Sugita (Elgiloy) (Downs Surgical)	No	1.89	2, 5
Sundt-Kees (301 SS) (Downs Surgical)	Yes	1.5	2, 3
Sundt-Kees Multi-Angle (17-7PH) (Downs Surgical)	Yes	1.89	2, 5
Surgiclip, Auto Suture M-9.5 (SS) (United States Surgical Corp.)	No	1.5	3
Vari-Angle (17-7PH) (Codman)	Yes	1.89	5
Vari-Angle McFadden (MP35N) (Codman)	No	1.89	2, 5
Vari-Angle Micro (17-7PM SS) (Codman)	Yes	0.15	2, 6
Vari-Angle Spring (17-7PM SS) (Codman)	Yes	0.15	2, 6
Yasargil (316 SS) (Aesculap)	No	1.89	5
Yasargil (Phynox) (Aesculap)	No	1.89	2
Biopsy needles			
ASAP 16, Automatic 16 G Core Biopsy System, 19 cm length (304 SS) (Microvasive, Watertown, MA)	Yes	1.5	NA
Biopty-cut, biopsy needle, 14 G, 10 cm length (304 SS) (C.R. Bard, Inc., Covington, GA)	Yes	1.5	NA
Biopty-cut, biopsy needle, 16 G, 16 cm length (304 SS) (C.R. Bard, Inc.)	Yes	1.5	NA
Biopty-cut, biopsy needle, 18 G, 18 cm length (304 SS) (C.R. Bard, Inc.)	Yes	1.5	NA
Lufkin Aspiration Cytology Needle, 20 G, 5 cm length (E-Z-Em, Westbury, NY)	No	1.5	7
Ultra-Core, biopsy needle, 16 G, 16 cm length (304 SS) (Gainesville, FL)	Yes	1.5	NA
Carotid artery vascular clamps			
Crutchfield (SS) (Codman)	Yes[b]	1.5	8
Kindt (SS) (V. Mueller)	Yes[b]	1.5	8
Poppen-Blaylock (SS) (Codman)	Yes	1.5	8
Salibi (SS) (Codman)	Yes[b]	1.5	8
Selverstone (SS) (Codman)	Yes[b]	1.5	8
Dental devices and materials			
Brace band (SS) (American Dental, Missoula, MT)	Yes[b]	1.5	3
Brace wire (chrome alloy) (Ormco Corp., San Marcos, CA)	Yes[b]	1.5	3
Castable alloy (Golden Dental Products, Inc., Golden, CO)	Yes[b]	1.5	9
Cement-in keeper (Solid State Innovations, Inc., Mt. Airy, NC)	Yes[b]	1.5	9

Metallic implant, material, device, or object	Movement/ Deflection	Highest field strength (T)	Reference
Dental amalgam	No	1.39	1
Gutta Percha Points	No	1.5	NA
GDP Direct Keeper, pre-formed post, (Golden Dental Products, Inc.)	Yes[b]	1.5	9
Indian Head Real Silver Points (Union Broach Co., Inc., New York, NY)	No	1.5	NA
Keeper, pre-formed post (Parkell Products, Inc., Farmingdale, NY)	Yes[b]	1.5	1
Magna-Dent, large indirect keeper (Dental Ventures of America, Yorba Linda, CA)	Yes[b]	1.5	1
Palladium clad magnet (Parkell Products, Inc.)	Yes	1.5	10
Palladium/palladium keeper (Parkell Products, Inc.)	Yes[b]	1.5	10
Palladium/platinum casting alloy (Parkell Products, Inc.)	Yes[b]	1.5	10
Permanent crown (amalgam) (Ormco Corp.)	No	1.5	3
Stainless steel clad magnet (Parkell Products, Inc.)	Yes	1.5	10
Stainless steel keeper (Parkell Products, Inc.)	Yes[b]	1.5	10
Silver point (Union Broach Co., Inc.)	No	1.5	3
Titanium clad magnet (Parkell Products, Inc.)	Yes	1.5	10
Halo vests			
Ambulatory Halo System (AOA Co., Greenwood, SC)	Yes	1.5	11
Bremmer standard halo crown and vest (Bremmer Medical Co., Jacksonville, FL)	No	1.0	12
Bremmer halo system, MR-compatible (Bremmer Medical Co.)	No	1.0	12
EXO adjustable collar (Florida Manufacturing Co., Daytona, FL)	Yes[e]	1.0	12
Guilford cervical orthosis (Guilford & Son, Ltd., Cleveland, OH)	Yes[e]	1.0	12
Guilford cervical orthosis, modified (Guilford & Son, Ltd.)	No	1.0	12
MR-compatible halo vest and cervical orthosis (Lerman & Son Co., Beverly Hills, CA)	No	1.5	NA
Philadelphia collar (Philadelphia Collar Co., Westville, NJ)	No	1.0	12
PMT halo cervical orthosis (PMT Corp., Chanhassen, MN)	No	1.0	12
PMT halo cervical orthosis with graphite rods and halo ring (PMT Corp.)	No	1.0	12
S.O.M.I. cervical orthosis (U.S. Manufacturing Co., Pasadena, CA)	Yes[e]	1.0	12
Heart valve prostheses			
Beall (Coratomic Inc., Indiana, PA)	Yes[b]	2.35	13
Bjork-Shiley (convexo/concave) (Shiley Inc., Irvine, CA)	No	1.5	3
Bjork-Shiley (universal/spherical) (Shiley Inc.)	Yes[b]	1.5	3
Bjork-Shiley, Model MBC (Shiley Inc.)	Yes[b]	2.35	14
Bjork-Shiley, Model 22 MBRC 11030 (Shiley Inc.)	Yes[b]	2.35	14
CarboMedics Heart Valve Prosthesis Aortic, Reduced, Model R500, size 19 (CarboMedics, Austin, TX)	No	1.5	NA
CarboMedics Heart Valve Prosthesis Aortic, Reduced, Model R500, size 21 (CarboMedics)	No	1.5	NA
CarboMedics Heart Valve Prosthesis Aortic, Reduced, Model R500, size 23 (CarboMedics)	No	1.5	NA
CarboMedics Heart Valve Prosthesis Aortic, Reduced, Model R500, size 25 (CarboMedics)	No	1.5	NA
CarboMedics Heart Valve Prosthesis Aortic, Reduced, Model R500, size 27 (CarboMedics)	No	1.5	NA
CarboMedics Heart Valve Prosthesis Aortic, Reduced, Model R500, size 29 (CarboMedics)	No	1.5	NA
CarboMedics Heart Valve Prosthesis Aortic, Standard, Model 500, size 31 (CarboMedics)	No	1.5	NA
CarboMedics Heart Valve Prosthesis Mitral, Standard, Model 700, size 23 (CarboMedics)	No	1.5	NA
CarboMedics Heart Valve Prosthesis Mitral, Standard, Model 700, size 25 (CarboMedics)	No	1.5	NA
CarboMedics Heart Valve Prosthesis Mitral, Standard, Model 700, size 27 (CarboMedics)	No	1.5	NA
CarboMedics Heart Valve Prosthesis Mitral, Standard, Model 700, size 29 (CarboMedics)	No	1.5	NA
CarboMedics Heart Valve Prosthesis Mitral, Standard, Model 700, size 31 (CarboMedics)	No	1.5	NA
CarboMedics Heart Valve Prosthesis Mitral, Standard, Model 700, size 33 (CarboMedics)	No	1.5	NA
Carpentier-Edwards Model 2650 (American Edwards Laboratories, Santa Ana, CA)	Yes[b]	2.35	14

Metallic implant, material, device, or object	Movement/ Deflection	Highest field strength (T)	Reference
Carpentier-Edwards (porcine) (American Edwards Laboratories)	Yes[b]	2.35	14
Hall-Kaster, Model A7700 (Medtronic, Minneapolis, MN)	Yes[b]	1.5	3
Hancock I (porcine) (Johnson & Johnson, Anaheim, CA)	Yes[b]	1.5	3
Hancock II (porcine) (Johnson & Johnson)	Yes[b]	1.5	3
Hancock extracorporeal, Model 242R (Johnson & Johnson)	Yes[b]	2.35	14
Hancock extracorporeal, Model M 4365-33 (Johnson & Johnson)	Yes[b]	2.35	14
Hancock Vascor, Model 505 (Johnson & Johnson)	No	2.35	14
Inonescu-Shiley, Universal ISM	Yes[b]	2.35	14
Lillehi-Kaster, Model 300S (Medical Inc., Inver Grove Heights, MN)	Yes[b]	2.35	13
Lillehi-Kaster, Model 5009 (Medical Inc.)	Yes[b]	2.35	14
Medtronic Hall (Medtronic Inc., Minneapolis, MN)	Yes[b]	2.35	14
Medtronic Hall, Model A7700-D-16 (Medtronic Inc.)	Yes[b]	2.35	14
Omnicarbon, Model 35231029 (Medical Inc.)	Yes[b]	2.35	14
Omniscience, Model 6522 (Medical Inc.)	Yes[b]	2.35	14
Smeloff-Cutter (Cutter Laboratories, Berkeley, CA)	Yes[b]	2.35	3
Starr-Edwards, Model 1260 (American Edwards Laboratories)	Yes[b]	2.35	13
Starr-Edwards, Model 2320 (American Edwards Laboratories)	Yes[b]	2.35	13
Starr-Edwards, Model 2400 (American Edwards Laboratories)	No	1.5	3
Starr-Edwards, Model Pre 6000 (American Edwards Laboratories)	Yes[b]	2.35	13
Starr-Edwards, Model 6518 (American Edwards Laboratories)	Yes[b]	2.35	14
St. Jude (St. Jude Medical Inc., St. Paul, MN)	No	1.5	3
St. Jude, Model A 101 (St. Jude Medical Inc.)	Yes[b]	2.35	14
St. Jude, Model M 101 (St. Jude Medical Inc.)	Yes[b]	2.35	14
Intravascular coils, filters, and stents			
Amplatz IVC filter (Cook, Bloomington, IN)	No	4.7	15
Cook occluding spring embolization coil, MWCE-38-5-10	Yes[b,d]	1.5	NA
Cragg nitinol spiral filter	No	4.7	15
Flower embolization microcoil (platinum) (Target Therapeutics, San Jose, CA)	No	1.5	16
Gianturco embolization coil (Cook)	Yes[b,d]	1.5	15
Gianturco bird nest IVC filter (Cook)	Yes[b,d]	1.5	15, 17
Gianturco zig-zag stent (Cook)	Yes[b,d]	1.5	15
Greenfield vena cava filter, stainless steel (Medi-tech, Watertown, MA)	Yes[b,d]	1.5	15, 18
Greenfield vena cava filter, titanium alloy (Ormco, Glendora, CA)	No	1.5	15
Gunther IVC filter (William Cook, Europe)	Yes[b,d]	1.5	15
Hilal embolization microcoil (Cook, Inc., Bloomington, IN)	No	1.5	16
IVC venous clip (teflon) (Pilling Co.)	No	1.5	NA
Maas helical IVC filter (Medinvent, Lausanne, Switzerland)	No	4.7	15
Maas helical endovascular stent (Medinvent)	No	4.7	15
Mobin-Uddin IVC/umbrella filter (American Edwards, Santa Ana, CA)	No	4.7	15
New retrievable IVC filter (Thomas Jefferson University, Philadelphia, PA)	Yes[b,d]	1.5	15
Palmaz endovascular stent (Johnson & Johnson, Interventional Warren, NJ)	No	1.5	NA
Palmaz endovascular stent (Ethicon)	Yes[b,d]	1.5	15
Strecker stent (tantalum) (Medi-tech)	No	1.5	19
Ureteral stent	No	1.5	NA
Ocular implants			
Clip 50, double tantalum clip (Mira Inc.)	No	1.5	20
Clip 51, single tantalum clip (Mira Inc.)	No	1.5	20
Clip 52, single tantalum clip (Mira Inc.)	No	1.5	20
Clip 250, double tantalum clip (Mira Inc.)	No	1.5	20
Double tantaium clip (Storz Instrument Co., St. Louis, MO)	No	1.5	20
Double tantalum clip, style 250 (Storz Instrument Co.)	No	1.5	20
Fatio eyelid spring/wire	Yes	1.5	21
Gold Eyelid Spring	No	1.5	NA
Intraocular lens implants			
Binkhorst, iridocapsular lense, platinum-iridium loop	No	1.5	22
Binkhorst, iridocapsular lense, platinum-iridium loop	No	1.0	22
Binkhorst, iridocapsular lense, titanium loop	No	1.0	22
Worst, platinum clip lense	No	1.0	22
Retinal tack (303SS) (Bascom Palmer Eye Institute)	No	1.5	23
Retinal tack (titanium alloy) (Coopervision, Irvine, CA)	No	1.5	23

Metallic implant, material, device, or object	Movement/ Deflection	Highest field strength (T)	Reference
Retinal tack (303SS) (Duke)	No	1.5	23
Retinal tack (cobalt/nickel) (Grieshaber, Fallsington, PA)	No	1.5	24
Retinal tack, Norton staple (platinum/rhodium) (Norton)	No	1.5	23
Retinal tack (aluminum textraoxide) (Ruby)	No	1.5	23
Retinal tack (SS-martensitic) (Western European)	Yes	1.5	23
Single tantalum clip	No	1.5	20
Troutman magnetic ocular implant	Yes	1.5	NA
Unitech round wire eye spring	Yes	1.5	NA
Orthopedic implants, materials, and devices			
AML femoral component bipolar hip prosthesis (Zimmer, Warsaw, IN)	No	1.5	3
Cervical wire, 18 G (316L SS)	No	0.3	25
Charnley-Muller hip prosthesis Protasyl-10 alloy	No	0.3	NA
Cortical bone screw, large (titanium, Ti-6AL-4V alloy) (Zimmer)	No	1.5	26
Cortical bone screw, small (titanium, Ti-6AL-4V alloy) (Zimmer)	No	1.5	26
Cotrel rods with hooks (316L SS)	No	0.3	25
Cotrel rod (SS-ASTM, Grade 2)	No	1.5	NA
DTT, device for transverse traction (316L SS)	No	0.3	25
Drummond wire (316L SS)	No	0.3	25
Endoscopic noncannulated interference screw (titanium) (Acufex Microsurgical, Norwood, MA)	No	1.5	26
Fixation staple (cobalt chromium alloy, ASTM F 75) (Richards Medical, Memphis, TN)	No	1.5	26
Halifax clamps (American Medical Electronics, Richardson, TX)	No	1.5	NA
Harrington compression rod with hooks and nuts (316L SS)	No	0.3	25
Harrington distraction rod with hooks (316L SS)	No	0.3	25
Harris hip prosthesis (Zimmer)	No	1.5	3
Jewett nail (Zimmer)	No	1.5	3
Kirschner intermedullary rod (Kirschner Medical, Timonium, MD)	No	1.5	3
"L" Rod (cobalt-nickel) (Richards Medical Co.)	No	1.5	NA
Luque wire	No	0.3	25
Moe spinal instrumentation (Zimmer)	No	1.5	NA
Perfix interence screw (17-4 stainless steel, AL 630-Cr17) (Instrument Makar, Okemos, MI)	Yes	1.5	26
Rusch rod	No	1.5	NA
Spinal L-rod (DePuy, Warsaw, IN)	No	1.5	NA
Stainless steel plate (Zimmer)	No	1.5	3
Stainless steel screw (Zimmer)	No	1.5	3
Staple plate, large, Zimaloy (Zimmer)	No	1.5	26
Stainless steel mesh (Zimmer)	No	1.5	3
Stainless steel wire (Zimmer)	No	1.5	3
Synthes AO DCP 2, 3, 4, 5 hole plate	No	1.5	NA
Zielke rod with screw, washer and nut (316L SS)	No	0.3	25
Otologic implants			
Austin tytan piston (titanium) (Treace Medical, Nashville, TN)	No	1.5	27
Berger "V" bobbin ventilation tube (titanium) (Richards Medical Co., Memphis, TN)	No	1.5	27
Cochlear implant (3M/House)	Yes	0.6	28
Cochlear implant (3M/Vienna)	Yes	0.6	28
Cochlear implant Nucleus Mini 20-channel (Cochlear Corporation, Engelwood, CO)	Yes	1.5	29
Cody tack	No	0.6	28
Ehmke hook stapes prosthesis (platinum) (Richards Medical Co.)	No	1.5	27
Fisch piston, (Teflon, stainless steel) (Richards Medical Co.)	No	1.5	29
House single loop (ASTM-318-76 Grade 2 stainless steel) (Storz Instrument Co., St. Louis, MO)	No	1.5	27
House single loop (tantalum) (Storz Instrument Co.)	No	1.5	27
House double loop (tantalum) (Storz Instrument Co.)	No	1.5	27
House-type incus prosthesis	No	0.6	NA
House-type wire loop stapes prosthesis (276L SS) (Richards Medical Co.)	No	1.5	27, 29
House-type stainless steel piston and wire (ASTM-318-76 Grade 2 stainless steel) [Xomed-Treace Inc. (Bristol-Myers Squibb Co.)]	No	1.5	27
House wire (tantalum) (Otomed)	No	0.5	30

Metallic implant, material, device, or object	Movement/ Deflection	Highest field strength (T)	Reference
House wire (stainless steel) (Otomed)	No	0.5	30
McGee piston stapes prosthesis (316L SS) (Richards Medical Co.)	No	1.5	27, 29
McGee piston stapes prosthesis (platinum/Cr17-Ni4, SS) (Richards Medical Co.)	Yes	1.5	29
McGee Shepard's Crook stapes prosthesis (316L SS) (Richards Medical Co.)	No	1.5	27
Plasti-pore piston (316L SS/plasti-pore material) (Richards Medical Co.)	No	1.5	27, 29
Platinum ribbon loop stapes prosthesis (platinum) (Richards Medical Co.)	No	1.5	27
Reuter bobbin ventilation tube (316L SS) (Richards Medical Co.)	No	1.5	27
Richards bucket handle stapes prosthesis (316L SS) (Richards Medical Co.)	No	1.5	27, 29
Reuter drain tube	No	1.5	21
Richards Plasti-pore with Armstrong-style platinum ribbon	No	1.5	21
Richards platinum Teflon piston 0.6 mm (Teflon, platinum) (Richards Medical Co.)	No	1.5	29
Richards platinum Teflon piston 0.8 mm (Teflon, platinum) (Richards Medical Co.)	No	1.5	29
Richards piston stapes prosthesis (platinum/fluoroplastic) (Richards Medical Co.)	No	1.5	27
Richards Shepard's Crook (platinum) (Richards Medical Co.)	No	0.5	30
Richards Teflon piston (Teflon) (Richards Medical Co.)	No	1.5	29
Robinson-Moon-Lippy offset stapes prosthesis (ASTM-318-76 Grade 2 stainless steel) (Storz Instrument Co.)	No	1.5	27
Robinson-Moon offset stapes prosthesis (ASTM-318-76 Grade 2 stainless steel) (Storz Instrument Co.)	No	1.5	27
Robinson incus replacement prosthesis (ASTM-318-76 Grade 2 stainless steel) (Storz Instrument Co.)	No	1.5	27
Robinson stapes prosthesis (ASTM-318-76 Grade 2 stainless steel) (Storz Instrument Co.)	No	1.5	27
Ronis piston stapes prosthesis (316L SS/fluoroplastic) (Richards Medical Co.)	No	1.5	27
Schea cup piston stapes prosthesis (platinum/fluoroplastic) (Richards Medical Co.)	No	1.5	27, 29
Schea malleus attachment piston (Teflon) (Richards Medical Co.)	No	1.5	29
Schea stainless steel and Teflon wire prosthesis (Teflon, 316L SS) (Richards Medical Co.)	No	1.5	29
Scheer piston stapes prosthesis (316L SS/fluoroplastic) (Richards Medical Co.)	No	1.5	27
Scheer piston (Teflon, 316L SS) (Richards Medical Co.)	No	1.5	29
Schuknecht gelfoam and wire prosthesis, Armstrong style (316L SS) (Richards Medical Co.)	No	1.5	31
Schuknecht piston stapes prosthesis (316L SS/fluoroplastic) (Richards Medical Co.)	No	1.5	27
Schuknecht tef-wire incus attachment (ASTM-316-76 Grade 2 stainless steel) (Storz Instrument Co.)	No	1.5	27, 29
Schuknecht tef-wire malleus attachment (ASTM-316-76 Grade 2 stainless steel) (Storz Instrument Co.)	No	1.5	27, 29
Schuknecht teflon wire piston 0.6 mm (Teflon, 316L SS) (Richards Medical Co.)	No	1.5	29
Schuknecht teflon wire piston, 0.8 mm (Teflon, 316L SS) (Richards Medical Co.)	No	1.5	29
Sheehy incus replacement (ASTM-316-76 Grade 2 stainless steel) (Storz Instrument Co.)	No	1.5	27
Sheehy incus strut (316L SS) (Richards Medical Co.)	No	1.5	29
Sheehy-type incus replacement strut (Teflon, 316L SS) (Richards Medical Co.)	No	1.5	27
Silverstein malleus clip ventilation tube (Teflon, 316L SS) (Richards Medical Co.)	No	1.5	29
Spoon bobbin ventilation tube (316L SS) (Richards Medical Co.)	No	1.5	27
Tantalum wire loop stages prosthesis (tantalum) (Richards Medical Co.)	No	1.5	27, 29
Tef-platinum piston (platinum) [Xomed-Treace Inc. (Bristol-Myers Squibb Co.)]	No	1.5	27

Metallic implant, material, device, or object	Movement/ Deflection	Highest field strength (T)	Reference
Total ossibular replacement prosthesis (TORP) (316L SS) (Richards Medical Co.)	No	1.5	29
Trapeze ribbon loop stapes prosthesis (platinum) (Richards Medical Co.)	No	1.5	27
Williams microclip (316L SS) (Richards Medical Co.)	No	1.5	27
Xomed stapes (ASTM-318-76 Grade 2 stainless steel) [Xomed-Treace Inc. (Bristol-Myers Squibb Co.)]	No	1.5	27
Xomed ceravital partial ossicular prosthesis	No	1.5	NA
Xomed Baily stapes implant	No	1.5	21
Xomed stapes prosthesis, Robinson-style (Richard's Co., Nashville, TN)	No	1.5	21
Patent ductus arteriosus (PDA), atrial septal defect (ASD), and ventricular septal defect (VSD) occluders			
Rashkind PDA Occlusion Implant 12 mm, lot no. 07IC1391 (304 V SS) (C.R. Bard, Inc., Billerica, MA)	Yes[b]	1.5	NA
Rashkind PDA Occlusion Implant, 17 mm, lot no. 514486 (304 V SS) (C.R. Bard, Inc.)	Yes	1.5	NA
Lock Clamshell Septal Occlusion Implant 17 mm, lot no. 07BCO321 (304 V SS) (C.R. Bard, Inc.)	Yes	1.5	NA
Lock Clamshell Septal Occlusion Implant 23 mm, lot no. 07CC1903 (304 V SS) (C.R. Bard, Inc.)	Yes	1.5	NA
Lock Clamshell Septal Occlusion Implant 28 mm, lot no. 07BC1557 (304 V SS) (C.R. Bard, Inc.)	Yes	1.5	NA
Lock Clamshell Septal Occlusion Implant 33 mm, lot no. 07ACI785 (304 V SS) (C.R. Bard, Inc.)	Yes	1.5	NA
Lock Clamshell Septal Occlusion Implant 40 mm, lot no. 07ACI785 (304 V SS) (C.R. Bard, Inc.)	Yes	1.5	NA
Bard Clamshell Septal Umbrella 17 mm, lot no. 09ED1230 (MP35n) (C.R. Bard, Inc.)	No	1.5	NA
Bard Clamshell Septal Umbrella 23 mm, lot no. 09ED1232 (MP35n) (C.R. Bard, Inc.)	No	1.5	NA
Bard Clamshell Septal Umbrella 28 mm, lot no. 09ED1233 (MP35n) (C.R. Bard, Inc.)	No	1.5	NA
Bard Clamshell Septal Umbrella 33 mm, lot no. 09ED1234 (MP35n) (C.R. Bard, Inc.)	No	1.5	NA
Bard Clamshell Septal Umbrella 40 mm, lot no. 09ED1231 (MP35n) (C.R. Bard, Inc.)	No	1.5	NA
Pellets and bullets			
BBs (Daisy)	Yes	1.5	NA
BBs (Crosman)	Yes	1.5	NA
Bullet, .330 inch (copper, plastic, lead) (Glaser)	No	1.5	32
Bullet, .39 inch (Teflon, bronze) (North American Ordinance)	No	1.5	32
Bullet, 7.62 × 34 mm (copper, steel) (Norinco)	Yes	1.5	32
Bullet, .357 inch (copper, lead) (Cascade)	No	1.5	32
Bullet, .357 inch (lead) (Remington)	No	1.5	32
Bullet, .357 inch (aluminum, lead) (Winchester)	No	1.5	32
Bullet, 9 mm (copper, lead) (Remington)	No	1.5	32
Bullet, .330 inch (copper, nickel, lead) (Winchester)	Yes	1.5	32
Bullet, .357 inch (nylon, lead) (Smith & Wesson)	No	1.5	32
Bullet, .357 inch (nickel, copper, lead) (Winchester)	No	1.5	32
Bullet, .45 inch (steel, lead) (Evansville Ordinance)	Yes	1.5	32
Bullet, .357 inch (steel, lead) (Fiocchi)	No	1.5	32
Bullet, .357 inch (copper, lead) (Hornady)	No	1.5	32
Bullet, 9 mm (copper, lead) (Norma)	Yes	1.5	32
Bullet, .357 inch (bronze, plastic) (Patton-Morgan)	No	1.5	32
Bullet, .357 inch (copper, lead) (Patton-Morgan)	No	1.5	32
Bullet, .45 inch (copper, lead) (Samson)	No	1.5	32
Shot, 12 gauge, size: 00 (copper, lead) (Federal)	No	1.5	32
Shot $7\frac{1}{2}$(lead)	No	1.5	32
Shot, 4 (lead)	No	1.5	32
Shot, 00 buckshot (lead)	No	1.5	32
Penile implants			
Penile implant, AMS 700 CX Inflatable (American Medical Systems, Minnetonka; MN)	No	1.5	33

Metallic implant, material, device, or object	Movement/ Deflection	Highest field strength (T)	Reference
Penile implant, AMS Hydroflex self-contained (American Medical Systems)	No	1.5	NA
Penile implant, AMS Malleable 600 (American Medical Systems)	No	1.5	33
Penile implant, Duraphase	Yes	1.5	NA
Penile implant, Flexi-Flate (Surgitek, Medical Engineering Corp., Racine, WI)	No	1.5	33
Penile implant, Flexi-Rod (Standard) (Surgitek, Medical Engineering Corp.)	No	1.5	33
Penile implant, Osmond, external	No	1.5	NA
Penile implant, Flex-Rod II (Firm) (Surgitek, Medical Engineering Corp.)	No	1.5	33
Penile implant, Jonas (Dacomed Corp., Minneapolis, MN)	No	1.5	33
Penile implant, Mentor Flexible (Mentor Corp., Minneapolis, MN)	No	1.5	33
Penile implant, Mentor Inflatable (Mentor Corp.)	No	1.5	33
Penile implant, OmniPhase (Dacomed Corp.)	Yes	1.5	33
Penile implant, Uniflex 1000	No	1.5	NA
Vascular access ports			
Button (polysulfone polymer, silicone) (Infusaid Inc., Norwood, MA)	No	1.5	34
Dome Port (titanium) (Davol Inc./Subsidiary of C.R. Bard, Inc., Cranston, RI)	No	1.5	34
Dual MicroPort (polysulfone polymer, silicone) (Infusaid Inc.)	No	1.5	34
Dual MacroPort (polysulfone polymer, silicone) (Infusaid Inc.)	No	1.5	34
Groshung Catheter	Yes[b]	1.5	NA
Hickman Port (316L SS) (Davol Inc.)	Yes[b]	1.5	34
Hickman Port, Pediatric (titanium) (Davol Inc.)	No	1.5	34
Hickman subcutaneous port (SS, titanium, plastic components) (Davol, Inc.)	No	1.5	NA
Implantofix II (polysulfone) (Burron Medical Inc., Bethlehem, PA)	No	1.5	34
Infusaid, Model 350 (titanium) (Infusaid Inc.)	No	1.5	34
Infusaid, Model 600 (titanium) (Infusaid Inc.)	No	1.5	34
Lifeport, Model 6013 (Delrin) (Strato Medical Corp., Beverly, MA)	No	1.5	34
Lifeport, Model 1013 (titanium) (Strato Medical Corp.)	No	1.5	34
MacroPort (polysulfone polymer, silicone) (Infusaid Inc.)	No	1.5	34
Mediport (Cormed)	No	1.5	NA
MicroPort (polysulfone polymer, silicone) (Infusaid Cnc.)	No	1.5	34
MRI Port (Delrin plastic, silicone) (Davol Inc.)	No	1.5	34
Norport-AC (titanium) (Norfolk Medical, Skokie, IL)	No	1.5	34
Norport-DL (276L SS) (Norfolk Medical)	No	1.5	34
Norport-LS (titanium) (Norfolk Medical)	No	1.5	34
Norport-LS (276L SS) (Norfolk Medical)	No	1.5	34
Norport-LS (polysulfone) (Norfolk Medical)	No	1.5	34
Norport-PT (titanium) (Norfolk Medical)	No	1.5	34
Norport-SP (polysulfone, silicone rubber, Dacron) (Norfolk Medical)	No	1.5	34
PeriPort (polysulfone, titanium) (Infusaid Inc.)	No	1.5	34
Port-A-Cath, P.A.S. Port Portal (titanium) (Pharmacia Deltec, St. Paul, MN)	No	1.5	34
Port-A-Cath, Titanium Dual Lumen Portal (titanium) (Pharmacia Deltec)	No	1.5	34
Port-A-Cath, Titanium Peritoneal Portal (titanium) (Pharmacia Deltec)	No	1.5	34
Port-a-Cath, Titanium Venous Low Profile Portal (titanium) (Pharmacia Deltec)	No	1.5	34
Port-A-Cath, Titanium Venous Portal (titanium) (Pharmacia Deltec)	No	1.5	34
Port-A-Cath, Venous Portal (316L SS)	No	1.5	34
Porto-cath Pharmacin, NUTECH (Pharmacia Deltec)	No	1.5	34
Q-Port (316L SS) (Quinton Instrument Co., Seattle, WA)	Yes[b]	1.5	34
S.E.A. (titanium) (Harbor Medical Devices, Inc., Boston, MA)	No	1.5	34
Snap-Lock (titanium, polysulfone polymer, silicone) (Infusaid Inc.)	No	1.5	34
Synchromed, Model 8500-1 (titanium, thermoplastic, silicone) (Medtronic, Inc., Minneapolis, MN)	No	1.5	34
Triple Lumen Arrow	No	1.5	NA
Vasport (titanium/fluoropolymer) (Gish Biomedical, Inc., Santa Ana, CA)	No	1.5	34
Miscellaneous			
Artificial urinary sphincter, AMS 800 (American Medical Systems)	No	1.5	3
Biosearch endo-feeding tube	No	1.5	NA
Breast implant (inflatable) Inflall, 3101198 Model (Heyerschultzz)	Yes	1.5	NA

Metallic implant, material, device, or object	Movement/ Deflection	Highest field strength (T)	Reference
Cerebral ventricular shunt tube connector, Accu-Flow, straight (Codman, Randolph, MA)	No	1.5	3
Cerebral ventricular shunt tube connector, Accu-flow right angle (Codman)	No	1.5	3
Cerebral ventricular shunt tube connector, Accu-flow, T-connector (Codman)	No	1.5	3
Cerebral ventricular shunt tube connector (type unknown)	Yes	0.147	1
Contraceptive diaphragm, All Flex (Ortho pharmaceutical, Raritan, NJ)	Yes[b]	1.5	3
Contraceptive diaphragm, Flat Spring (Ortho Pharmaceutical)	Yes[b]	1.5	3
Contraceptive diaphragm, Koroflex (Young Drug Products, Piscataway, NJ)	Yes[b]	1.5	3
EEG electrodes, Pediatric E-5-GH, (gold-plated silver) (Grass Co., Quincy, MA)	No	0.3	35
EEG electrodes, Adult E-6-GH, (gold-plated silver) (Grass Co.)	No	0.3	35
Endotracheal tube with metal ring marker Trachmate	No	1.5	NA
Forceps (titanium)	No	1.39	1
Hakim valve and pump	No	1.39	1
Intraflex Feeding Tube, tungston weight, plastic	No	1.5	NA
Intrauterine contraceptive device (IUD), Copper T (Searle Pharmaceuticals, Chicago, IL)	No	1.5	36
Intrauterine contraceptive device (IUD) Lippey loop, plastic	No	1.5	NA
Intrauterine contraceptive device (IUD) Perigard (Gyne Pharmaceuticals)	No	1.5	NA
Mercury Duotube-feeding	No	1.5	NA
Mitek anchor	No	1.5	NA
Shunt valve, Holtertype (The Holter Co., Bridgeport, PA)	Yes[b]	1.5	37
Shunt valve, Holter-Hausner type (Holter-Hausner, Inc., Bridgeport, PA)	No	1.5	37
Swan-Ganz thermodilution catheter (American Edwards Laboratories, Irvine, CA)	No[c]	1.5	38
Tantalum powder	No	1.39	1
Tissue expander with magnetic port (McGhan Medical Corp., Santa Barbara, CA)	Yes	1.5	39
Vascular marker, O-ring washer (302 SS) (PIC Design, Middlebury, CT)	Yes[b]	1.5	NA
Vitallium implant	No	1.5	NA
Winged infusion set MRI compatible (E-Z-EM Inc., Westbury, NY)	No	1.5	40

Note: Manufacturer information was provided if known. SS, stainless steel; NA, not applicable. These implants, materials, devices, or objects were tested for ferromagnetism by F. Shellock or E. Kanal; however, the data have not been published.

[a] Highest field strength refers to the highest intensity of the static magnetic field that was used for the evaluation of deflection force or movement of the various metallic implants, materials, or objects tested.

[b] Denotes the metallic implants, objects, or materials that were considered to be safe for MR imaging despite being attracted by the static magnetic fields. For example, certain prosthetic heart valves were deflected by the static magnetic field but the deflection forces were considered to be less than the force exerted on the valves by the beating heart.

[c] While there is no magnetic field attraction associated with the triple-lumen thermodilution Swan-Ganz catheter, there has been a report of a catheter "melting" in patient. Therefore, this catheter would be considered a relative contraindication for MR imaging.

[d] Ferromagnetic coils, filters, and stents typically become firmly incorporated into the vessel wall several weeks following their placement, and, therefore, it is highly unlikely that they will be moved or dislodged by magnetic forces. It is recommended that coils, filters, and stents marked as [b,d] in the deflection column have a minimum 6-week wait post-placement period to assure firm implantation into vessel wall prior to an MR examination.

[e] These halo vests are known to have ferromagnetic components, however, the deflection force or amount of attraction was not determined. Refer to specific section in the chapter regarding additional information on halo vests.

REFERENCES

1. New PFJ, Rosen BR, Brady TJ, et al. Potential hazards and artifacts of ferromagnetic and nonferromagnetic surgical and dental materials and devices in nuclear magnetic resonance imaging. *Radiology* 1983;147:139–148.
2. Becker RL, Norfray JF, Teitelbaum GP, et al. MR imaging in patients with intracranial aneurysm clips. *AJR* 1988;9:885–889.
3. Shellock FG, Crues JV. High-field strength MR imaging and metallic biomedical implants: an ex vivo evaluation of deflection forces. *AJR* 1988;151:389–392.
4. Brown MA, Carden JA, Coleman RE, et al. Magnetic field effects on surgical ligation clips. *Magn Reson Imaging* 1987;5:443–453.

5. Dujovny M, Kossovsky N, Kossowsky R, et al. Aneurysm clip motion during magnetic resonance imaging: in vivo experimental study with metallurgical factor analysis. *Neurosurgery* 1985;17:543–548.
6. Barrafato D, Henkelman RM. Magnetic resonance imaging and surgical clips. *Can J Surg* 1984;27:509–512.
7. Teitelbaum GP, Lin MCW, Watanabe AT, et al. Ferromagnetism and MR imaging: safety of cartoid vascular clamps. *AJNR* 1990;11:267–272.
8. Hathout G, Lufkin RB, Jabour B, et al. MR-guided aspiration cytology in the head and neck at high field strength. *J Magn Reson Imaging* 1992;2:93–94.
9. Gegauff A, Laurell KA, Thavendrarajah A, et al. A potential MRI hazard: forces on dental magnet keepers. *J Oral Rehabil* 1990;17:403–410.
10. Shellock FG. Ex vivo assessment of deflection forces and artifacts associated with high-field strength MRI of "mini-magnet" dental prostheses. *Magn Reson Imaging* 1989;7(suppl 1):P38.
11. Shellock FG, Slimp G. Halo vest for cervical spine fixation during MR imaging. *AJR* 1990;154:631–632.
12. Clayman DA, Murakami ME, Vines FS. Compatibility of cervical spine braces with MR imaging. A study of nine nonferrous devices. *AJNR* 1990;11:385–390.
13. Soulen RL, Budinger TF, Higgins CB. Magnetic resonance imaging of prosthetic heart valves. *Radiology* 1985;154:705–707.
14. Hassler M, Le Bas JF, Wolf JE, et al. Effects of magnetic fields used in MRI on 15 prosthetic heart valves. *J Radiol* 1986;67:661–666.
15. Teitelbaum GP, Bradley WG, Klein BD. MR imaging artifacts, ferromagnetism, and magnetic torque of intravascular filters, stents, and coils. *Radiology* 1988;166:657–664.
16. Marshall MW, Teitelbaum GP, Kim HS, et al. Ferromagnetism and magnetic resonance artifacts of platinum embolization microcoils. *Cardiovasc Intervent Radiol* 1991;14:163–166.
17. Watanabe AT, Teitelbaum GP, Gomes AS, et al. MR imaging of the bird's nest filter. *Radiology* 1990;177:578–579.
18. Leibman CE, Messersmith RN, Levin DN, et al. MR imaging of inferior vena caval filter: safety and artifacts. *AJR* 1988;150:1174–1176.
19. Teitelbaum GP, Raney M, Carvlin MJ, et al. Evaluation of ferromagnetism and magnetic resonance imaging artifacts of the Strecker tantalum vascular stent. *Cardiovasc Intervent Radiol* 1989;12:125–127.
20. Shellock FG, Myers SM, Schatz CJ. Ex vivo evaluation of ferromagnetism determined for metallic scleral "buckles" exposed to a 1.5 T MR scanner. *Radiology* 1992;185(P):288–289.
21. Shellock FG, Schatz CJ, Shelton C, et al. Ex vivo evaluation of 9 different ocular and middle ear implants exposed to a 1.5 Tesla MR scanner. *Radiology* 1990;177(P):271.
22. de Keizer RJ, Te Strake L. Intraocular lens implants (pseudophakoi) and steelwire sutures: a contraindication for MRI? *Doc Ophthalmol* 1984;61:281–284.
23. Albert DW, Olson KR, Parel JM, et al. Magnetic resonance imaging and retinal tacks. *Arch Ophthalmol* 1990;108:320–321.
24. Joondeph BC, Peyman GA, Mafee MF, et al. Magnetic resonance imaging and retinal tacks [letter]. *Arch Ophthalmol* 1987;105:1479–1480.
25. Lyons CJ, Betz RR, Mesgarzadeh M, et al. The effect of magnetic resonance imaging on metal spine implants. *Spine* 1989;14:670–672.
26. Shellock FG, Mink JH, Curtin S, et al. MRI and orthopedic implants used for anterior cruciate ligament reconstruction: assessment of ferromagnetism and artifacts. *J Magn Reson Imaging* 1992;2:225–228.
27. Shellock FG, Schatz CJ. High-field strength MR imaging and metallic otologic implants. *AJNR* 1991;12:279–281.
28. Mattucci KF, Setzen M, Hyman R, et al. The effect of nuclear magnetic resonance imaging on metallic middle ear prostheses. *Otolaryngnol Head Neck Surg* 1986;94:441–443.
29. Applebaum EL, Valvassori GE. Further studies on the effects of magnetic resonance fields on middle ear implants. *Ann Otol Rhinol Laryngol* 1990;99:801–804.
30. White DW. Interaction between magnetic fields and metallic ossicular prostheses. *Am J Otol* 1987;8:290–292.
31. Leon JA, Gabriele OF. Middle ear prosthesis: significance in magnetic resonance imaging. *Magn Reson Imaging* 1987;5:405–406.
32. Teitelbaum GP, Yee CA, Van Horn DD, et al. Metallic ballistic fragments: MR imaging safety and artifacts. *Radiology* 1990;175:855–859.
33. Shellock FG, Crues JV, Sacks SA. High-field magnetic resonance imaging of penile prostheses: in vitro evaluation of deflection forces and imaging artifacts. In: *Abstracts of the Proceedings of the Society of Magnetic Resonance in Medicine.* Berkeley, CA: Society of Magnetic Resonance in Medicine; 1987:915.
34. Shellock FG, Meeks T. Ex vivo evaluation of ferromagnetism and artifacts for implantable vascular access ports exposed to a 1.5 T MR scanner. *J Magn Reson Imaging* 1991;1:243(abst).
35. Lufkin R, Jordan S, Lylcyk M. MR imaging with topographic EEG electrodes in place. *AJNR* 1988;9:953–954.
36. Mark AS, Hricak H. Intrauterine contraceptive devices: MR imaging. *Radiology* 1987;162:311–314.
37. Go KG, Kamman RL, Mooyaart EL. Interaction of metallic neurosurgical implants with magnetic resonance imaging at 1.5 Tesla as a cause of image distortion and of hazardous movement of the implant. *Clin Neurosurg* 1989;91:109–115.
38. ECRI, Health devices alert. A new MRI complication? May 27, 1988.
39. Liang MD, Narayanan K, Kanal E. Magnetic ports in tissue expanders: a caution for MRI. *Magn Reson Imaging* 1989;7:541–542.
40. To SYC, Lufkin RB, Chiu L. MR-compatible winged infusion set. *Comput Med Imaging Graph* 1989;13:469–472.

Magnetic Resonance Imaging of the Brain and Spine, Second Edition, edited by Scott W. Atlas. Lippincott-Raven Publishers, Philadelphia © 1996.

7

Artifacts

Peter M. Joseph and Scott W. Atlas

CLASSIFICATION OF ARTIFACTS

An artifact can be defined as any aspect of an image which misrepresents the anatomic and geometrical relationships within the body. Some artifacts are easily identified, such as linear streaks running across the image. Others may not be so easy to identify as artifactual, such as a subtle shift of the fat-containing tissue in a given slice, so that the radiologist must remain aware of the possibility of such a misrepresentation.

In this chapter, we will briefly discuss the appearance and physical cause of some of the more common and troublesome artifacts which appear in neurological MR images. In many cases, the effects are due to very subtle errors in the physical aspects of the scanning process, and space will permit only a brief description of the underlying mechanism producing the errors. For more detailed information the reader is referred to the bibliographic references.

P. M. Joseph, Ph.D.: Department of Radiology, Hospital of the University of Pennsylvania, Philadelphia, PA 19104.

S. W. Atlas, M.D.: Neuroradiology Division, Department of Radiology, Oregon Health Sciences University, Portland, OR 97201.

The classification used here is based on the source of the artifacts: artifacts produced by magnetic field and frequency shifts, by the finite sampling used in the scanning process, and by instrumental errors. In some cases the artifacts arise from an interaction between a patient and machine-related problem, so that a rigorous distinction between the two is not always possible (1).

ARTIFACTS DUE TO FIELD AND FREQUENCY SHIFTS

The Larmor equation for NMR states that the resonant frequency is proportional to the magnetic field present, hence any inhomogeneity in field implies an inhomogeneity of resonant frequency. Another common source of frequency differences is the chemical shift effect between fat and water. Since these are both basically frequency shift effects, the effects are similar and can be analyzed together. A very important question is whether the imaging pulse sequence uses 180° radiofrequency (rf) pulses to create a spin echo, or whether the echo is created solely using gradient pulses. The latter technique will produce, in addition to those artifacts seen in spin-echo imaging, a whole additional set of artifacts. Therefore, we will first consider those effects seen in spin-echo imaging and then examine those additional artifacts seen in gradient-echo imaging.

Frequency Errors in Spin-Echo Imaging

As we noted in Chapter 3, the method of frequency encoding of, say, the x-position coordinate, is based on the use of a controlled magnetic field gradient in the x direction to associate frequency and position in a linear way. This linear association is absolutely central to the image reconstruction process, since the Fourier transform (FT) process creates a frequency spectrum and the display system places each frequency at a specific coordinate value along the frequency encoding axis. Any process which induces a change in resonant frequency of part of an object will cause the position of that object to be shifted along the frequency-encoded direction in the reconstructed image.

The Fat-Water Chemical Shift

The water molecule, despite containing two hydrogen atoms, displays only one resonant NMR frequency. This is because the molecule rotates so rapidly that the two hydrogen atoms experience essentially the same local magnetic field. Fat, of course, is not a unique substance but appears biologically in a variety of chemical forms. Most body fats are triglycerides of fatty acids, so that the CH_2 moiety is the most common chemical component (2). The resonant frequency of the CH_2 group differs from that of water by about 3.5 parts per million (3.5 ppm) (3,4). [The unsaturated moieties −CH=CH− in some biological fat has a different chemical shift (5).] Since the magnetic field in the body in an MRI machine is approximately uniform, there will be a constant frequency shift of all such fat with respect to body water which is uniform throughout the body. For example, if the magnetic field is 1.5 Tesla, then the nominal resonant frequency for protons is 63.86 MHz, and the fat-water chemical shift is about 220 Hz.

The effect of the chemical shift is always a shift in position along the frequency-encoded (FE) axis. The reason is easily grasped from Fig. 1, which shows the frequency-position relationship for both fat and water in the presence of a gradient. The two lines are almost exactly parallel and their slope is equal to the strength of the frequency gradient, g, which could be measured in Hertz per cm. [This is directly related to the magnetic field gradient, g_x, according to $g = (\gamma/2\pi)g_x$.] Note that the two lines are displaced vertically by an amount corresponding to the frequency difference Δf, where Δf is the chemical shift frequency difference given by:

$$\Delta f\,(\text{Hz}) = 3.5 \cdot f_0\,(\text{MHz}), \qquad [1]$$

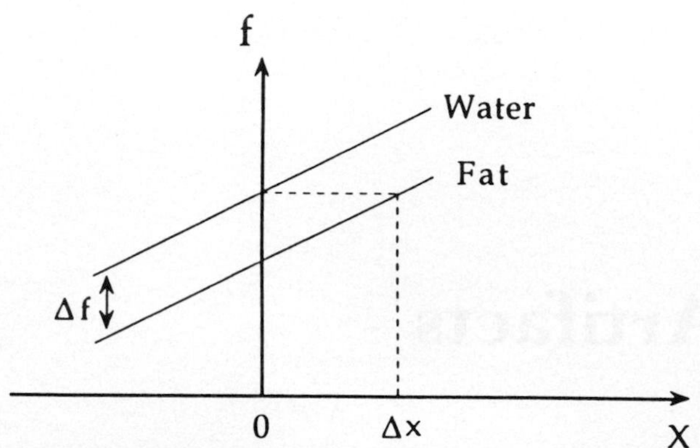

FIG. 1. Graph of frequency versus position in the presence of a gradient. Because of the chemical shift, water and fat have separate lines whose vertical separation is equal to the chemical shift frequency difference.

where f_0 is the Larmor resonance frequency (see Chapter 2). Note that Δf is proportional to f_0, and therefore to B_0, the main magnetic field. Hence high field systems will show the effect more dramatically than will lower field systems.

The reconstruction algorithm normally has no way of knowing the chemical composition of the source of the signal; i.e., it works assuming that only one substance is present (normally water). Hence an error in frequency will translate into an error in position, Δx. From inspection of Fig. 1, we see that

$$\Delta x = \Delta f/\gamma g \qquad [2]$$

(γ = gyromagnetic ratio of the proton). This equation allows an important conclusion: the amount of spatial shift in the image is inversely proportional to the strength of the applied gradient. For this reason it is not possible to specify in advance how much shift will be present in any given image, since it will depend on the strength of gradient used, which can easily vary with changes in technique. For example, in many machines, as one alters the field of view (FOV), one is really altering the strength of the readout gradient, so the size of the chemical shift will change accordingly.

The amount of shift can also be related to the bandwidth of the frequency-encoding axis. By bandwidth, in this context, we mean the range of frequency spread from one side of the image to the other. In this case the amount of shift can be calculated from a simple proportion to the bandwidth and the FOV; i.e.,

$$\Delta x = \text{FOV}\ \Delta f/W, \qquad [3]$$

where the bandwidth, W, is expressed in Hertz. Since W appears in the denominator of Equation 3, one sees that an increase in bandwidth results in a decrease in the artifactual shift; this is one reason for choosing a large bandwidth in some imaging situations. (Remember, however, that increased bandwidth also brings increased image noise; see Chapter 3.) A typical example could be a

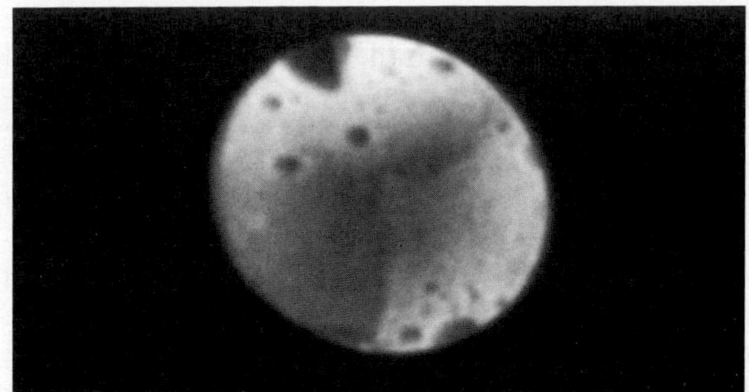

A

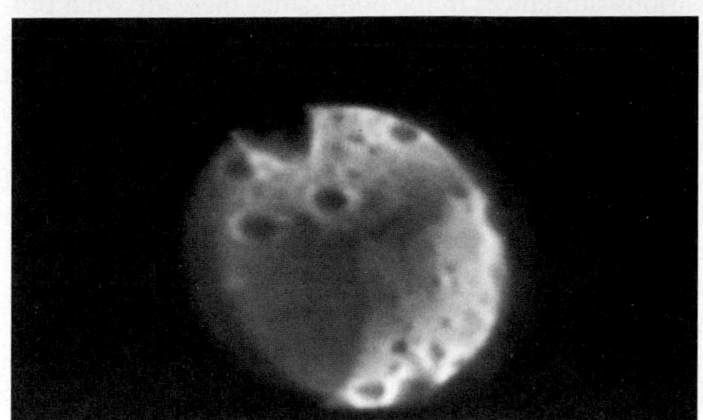

B

FIG. 2. Images of a bottle of mayonnaise. The FE axis is horizontal and the PE axis is vertical. **A** was made with a bandwidth of 11 kHz, and **B** was made with a bandwidth of 2.75 kHz. The water and fat components each produce an image with an artifactual spatial shift between them. Note the greater shift in B due to the decreased bandwidth.

bandwidth of 10,000 Hz over a FOV of 20 cm. In this case, with a main field of 1.5 T the equivalent shift would be 4.4 mm. If the image was reconstructed using 256 pixels in the FE direction, this shift corresponds to 5.6 pixels.

From the previous example it is clear that the effect is by no means negligible, and the effect can usually be seen in any part of the body in which a nonlipid organ is surrounded by fat. It will always appear as a shift of the fat with respect to the water in the FE direction, producing typically a dark region of signal void on one side of the water containing tissue. (That is, the signal that is physically present there has been shifted away). Furthermore, a region of bright signal will be found at the other end of the water-fat interface, due to the superimposition of fat and water signals.

The chemical shift effect is demonstrated for a spin-echo pulse sequence in Fig. 2, which shows a bottle of mayonnaise with a substantial fat content; the fat is dispersed throughout the volume as a suspension. Note that the fat component produces a distinctive shifted image of the bottle.

While the effect cannot be eliminated, it can be altered and mitigated in various ways so as not to interfere with diagnosis. For example, any of the various fat suppression (6–8) techniques will eliminate the effect. Another useful technique is to interchange the direction of the frequency and phase-encoding directions; this will rotate the direction of the effect by 90°, so that a critical surface of a particular organ can be visualized without the distortion that the effect produces (9).

The influence of signal bandwidth can severely degrade images and must be understood by anyone designing imaging protocols. For example, it is often desirable to use a different bandwidth on the second echo than on the first echo of a two-echo pulse sequence. This is done primarily to improve the signal-to-noise ratio of the second echo image (10). Since the second echo would be programmed to have a lower bandwidth than the first, the corresponding chemical shift effect would be worse on the second echo. This is illustrated in Figs. 2 and 3.

Figure 3 is a clinical example of the influence of receiver bandwidth on the chemical shift artifact, comparing bandwidths of 16 and 4 kHz. The improvement in signal-to-noise ratio with the lower bandwidth is evident in the brain. The chemical shift appears as a shift of the

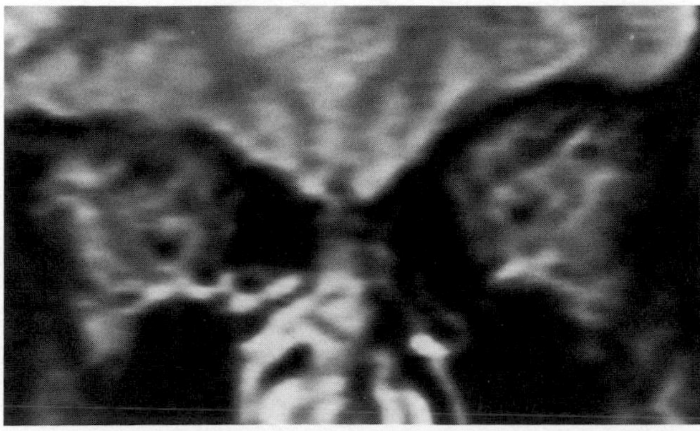

A

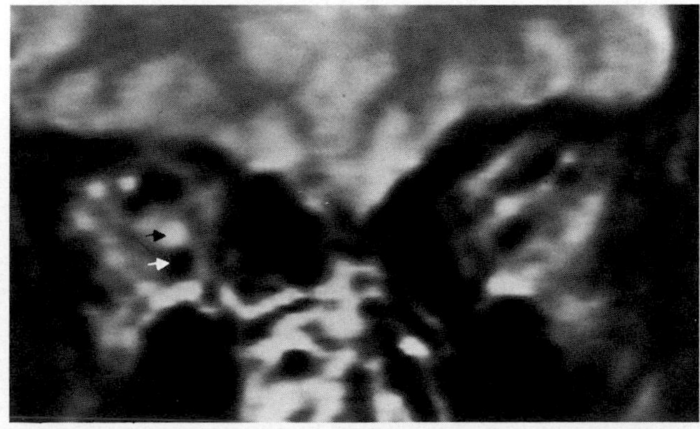

B

FIG. 3. Example of the influence of bandwidth on the chemical shift artifact. Coronal image just behind the orbits: TR = 2000, TE = 80 ms, and the frequency-encoding axis is superior-inferior. **A** used a bandwidth of 16 kHz, **B** used 4 kHz. Note the exaggerated vertical shift of the optic nerve (*black arrow*) with respect to the retro-orbital fat and the corresponding area of artifactual signal void (*white arrow*) in B.

optic nerve within the retro-orbital fat; in the 4 kHz image the shift is almost as large as the nerve itself! Even on the 16 kHz image, the shift is present but, being only one fourth as large is less apparent.

A further aspect of the chemical shift effect is a shift in the *slice-selection* direction. That is, for a given slice select gradient (g_z in our example) the z location of the fat selected will be displaced from that of the water slice by an amount given by Equations 2 and 3, except that the shift is in the z direction. This effect will not be noticed when imaging phantoms which are cylinders oriented perpendicular to the selected slice, but can be significant if the cylinder and/or the slice are at an oblique angle. Clearly, if the slice orientation is oblique to the axis of the object, the shift in the slice direction may add or subtract to the shift in the image plane. In some cases, it is possible for these two shifts to cancel, an effect which has been seen clinically in images of the female pelvis (11). In brain imaging, the nature of the chemical shift from the cranial marrow will therefore depend on the angle at which the cranium cuts through the imaging plane. Smith et al. (12) give a thorough discussion of the implications of chemical shift artifacts for brain imaging, including cases demonstrating an artifactual subdural fluid collection.

Magnetic Susceptibility

The term "magnetic susceptibility" has a technical meaning in the physics of magnetism: it refers to the universal phenomenon in which a material becomes partially magnetized when it is placed in a magnetic field. In most cases of interest to us, the magnetization, M, is proportional to the applied magnetic field, H, so a simple linear equation can describe the effect:

$$M = \chi H. \qquad [4]$$

Here χ is called the magnetic susceptibility. Substances with large χ develop a strong magnetization when placed in a magnetic field. χ can vary over many orders of magnitude, depending on the type of substance. For example, metallic iron at normal temperatures is a type of material called "ferromagnetic" and its χ value can be as high as 10,000. Certain ions, in particular iron and gadolinium, are "paramagnetic" and will show a χ value which depends on their concentration in solution and which can be on the order of 10^{-3}. All substances show an effect called "diamagnetism" in which χ is negative and of order 10^{-5}. Water and most biological substances fall into the diamagnetic class. In the case of paramagnetic and ferromagnetic materials, the diamagnetic effect is obviously overwhelmed by the positive susceptibility of the materials (see also Chapter 9).

The implications of this for MRI are rather formidable (13–15). The major effect comes not from the induced magnetization per se, but from the additional magnetic fields which are created by the magnetization. These fields are not localized to the region of the magnetized matter being considered; rather, the induced fields typically spread out for a considerable distance beyond the boundaries of the matter being magnetized (16).

First, we should note that the order of magnitude of the additional magnetic field, namely 10 ppm, while small is definitely not negligible, especially at high field strengths. (For example, it is several times larger than the fat-water chemical shift frequency difference.) Of most concern to us are the differences in magnetization of the various substances in the body, since these are what produce most of the artifacts. The worst case is one in which an object of one χ is immersed in a background of a different substance. In this case, as illustrated in Fig. 4, the magnetic field immediately surrounding the object will be highly inhomogeneous in space and the sign of the field will depend on whether the object's χ is less than or greater than that of the background. Fortunately, most soft tissues have approximately the same χ value, so useful imaging is not impossible.

One major exception to the last statement is the air-filled paranasal sinuses (17). The χ value of a substance depends somewhat on the chemical structure and is also proportional to the density of the object. Thus gases, such as air, have only about 1/1,000 the χ of most solids, so for practical purposes air can be taken as having χ = 0. In other words, an air sinus represents the equivalent of a source of negative magnetization compared to tissue, and the magnetic field immediately surrounding the sinus will be altered by amounts on the order of 10 ppm over distances comparable with the size of the sinus.

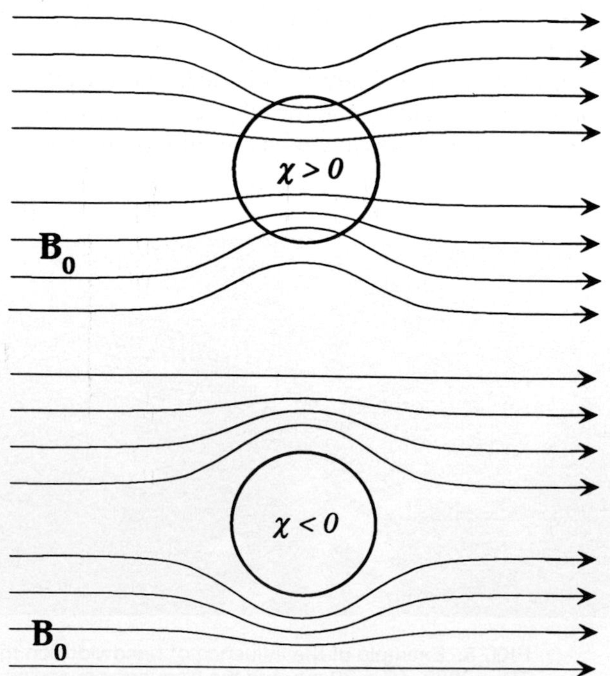

FIG. 4. Illustration of how a body of one susceptibility, when immersed in a background of differing susceptibility, distorts the magnetic field outside of the body itself.

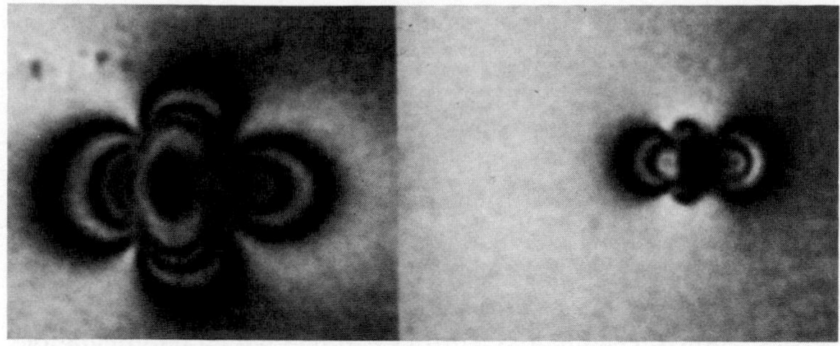

FIG. 5. Gradient-echo images of a gelatin phantom with surgical clips immersed. The $\mathbf{B}_0$ direction is from left to right in these images, as is the orientation of the magnetic moment of the magnetized clips. *Left:* stainless steel (Ethicon LS 300). *Right:* Titanium (Ethicon LT 300). With titanium the ferromagnetic effect is obviously reduced but not eliminated. (Experiment by Dr. H. L. Kundel.)

Another major source of these artifacts is the presence of material with a significant ferromagnetic susceptibility, such as residue from metallic instruments (drilling) or aneurysm clips. Many objects containing iron, such as surgical clips or mascara, can have a χ thousands of times larger than that of tissue. Furthermore, the strength of the effect is critically dependent on the detailed atomic structure of the ferromagnetic solid. For example, while iron is highly magnetic, some kinds of stainless steel are much less so. Beware, however, that even some so-called "nonmagnetic" stainless steel, while considerably less magnetic than iron, can still have a large enough χ to create serious artifacts (18). Gradient-echo images of phantoms containing surgical clips made of stainless steel and titanium are shown in Fig. 5.

In some cases the field distortion due to areas differing in χ also creates a *geometric* distortion (19). In such cases one usually finds, in addition to a region of obviously suppressed MRI signal, a thin region of increased signal which appears as a bright band. This can be understood in terms of the physics of frequency encoding. The image as viewed is really a presentation of the received signal strength per unit frequency. In the absence of significant field inhomogeneities, the FE gradient creates a linear relationship between frequency and position, so the tissue signal intensity more or less accurately reflects the density of protons in the tissue. However, as illustrated in Fig. 6, in the presence of such field distortions the field inhomogeneity can combine with the applied gradient field to create local regions in which the effective gradient is reduced. In fact, it is quite possible for protons in different spatial locations to have, under these conditions, the same frequency. The protons in these regions will all therefore appear superimposed at a given region in the image, leading to the narrow bright regions observed. Note that this "field shifting" effect has nothing to do with spin dephasing, and so will be equally important in both spin echo and gradient echo sequences. A dramatic example of this effect is shown in Fig. 7 which shows not only the large loss of signal in the occipital

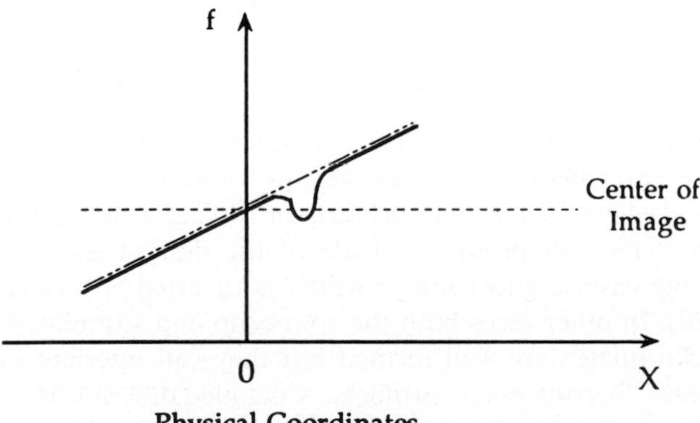

FIG. 6. Illustration of the effect of a strong local field distortion on the linearity of the frequency-encoding gradient. Because of the dip in the curve induced by some local ferromagnetic substance, there are several regions along the *x* axis which will all show no frequency offset and whose signals will all appear at the center, *x* = 0, of the image.

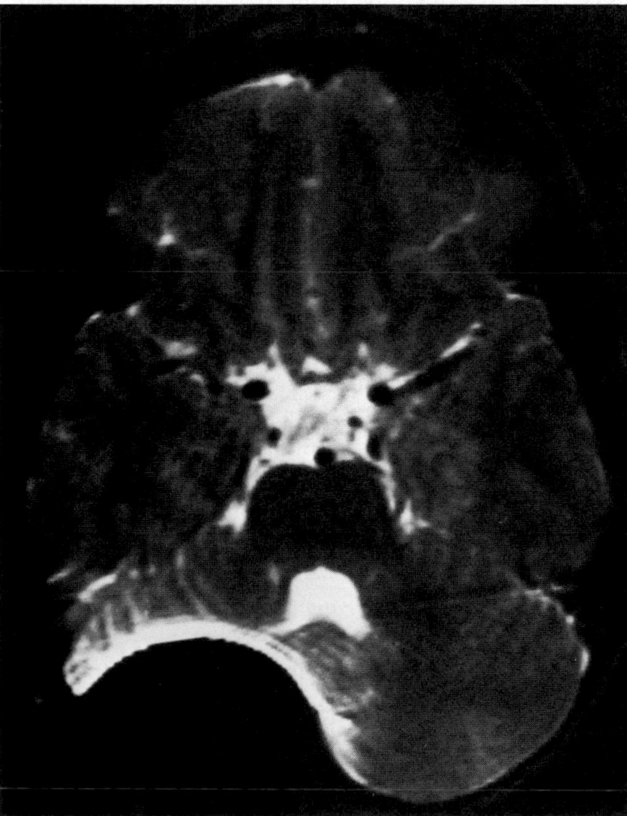

FIG. 7. Transverse spin-echo image of a patient with a ferromagnetic monitoring device in the suboccipital region. The geometric distortion is obvious; in addition note the sharp band of increased signal at the edge of the zero signal zone.

region but also the anomalous bright band immediately at the edge of the artifactual region. Obviously, in this case there are also geometric distortions in the image even in regions in which the signal strength appears to be normal. Similar effects can be seen with catheters (20) and with dental materials (21). A review of the effects of a wide range of biomedical materials and devices has been given by Shellock and Curtis (22). The influence of such susceptibility distortions has been noted in neurosurgery (23,24).

The actual influence of these susceptibility fields depends in a very subtle way on the *geometry* of the object creating the field and is often counterintuitive to people who are not expert in the behavior of magnetic fields. For example, if the object is a relatively long homogeneous cylinder then the effect inside the cylinder depends on its orientation with respect to the $\mathbf{B}_0$ field; if the cylinder axis is parallel to the $\mathbf{B}_0$ vector then there is negligible shift of magnetic *within* the cylinder. However, if the cylinder is orientated at a 90° angle with respect to $\mathbf{B}_0$ vector then one gets the maximum change in magnetic field within the cylinder. In both cases the maximum effect external to the cylinder occurs in the region where the magnetic field lines emerge from the object. Furthermore, if the object is a perfect sphere then the induced field is uniform within the object and extends beyond the object for a distance at least equal to the diameter of the object. Theoretically, the induced field extends for an infinite distance outside the object, but it decreases with increasing distance in proportion to $1/(\text{distance})^4$.

These effects were demonstrated in an experiment intended to model the apparent structural distortion of the cervical neural foramina in gradient-echo imaging (25). That experiment was concerned not with artifacts induced by foreign objects but by the susceptibility of the normal bones in the cervical spine. In a phantom, they clearly demonstrated a distortion of water immediately external to a calcium carbonate core in gradient-echo imaging. They also demonstrated similar distortion in a fresh specimen of a human cervical spine immersed in water. However, because their phantoms were not oriented in the same way as would an actual patient's spine during scanning, the quantitative aspects of their conclusions should be accepted with caution.

Eddy Currents in Nonferrous Materials

The reader should be aware that the susceptibility-induced changes in the static magnetic field are not the only source of signal loss when metallic objects are present. Another independent effect is the possible existence of eddy currents, meaning electrical currents which are induced by an oscillating magnetic field. In this case, it could be either the rf B_1 field or the changing gradient fields which induce the currents. The strength of the induced currents depends primarily on the electrical conductivity, which is quite high for all metals. However, the nature of the field perturbation depends very much on the details of the shape of the wire or metal, and in particular on whether the wire forms an open or closed loop. This means that the artifacts may appear to be variable and unpredictable. For example, Lufkin et al. (26) reported no problems with EEG electrodes made of nonferrous metals, while Teitelbaum et al. (18) reported significant signal loss from IVC filters which had negligible magnetic susceptibility.

Artifacts in Multislice Imaging

As explained in Chapter 3, multislice spin-echo imaging works by using selective B_1 rf pulse for both the 90° (exciting) and 180° pulses; the assumption is that these pulses are sufficiently selective that each one operates only on the desired slice so that the excitation of the various slices can be interleaved in time. In practice, these rf pulses (especially the 180° pulses) are imperfect and tend to irradiate protons outside of their target slices. If this effect is significant it can lead to both contrast changes (as discussed in Chapter 6) as well as noticeable artifacts.

The mechanism by which these artifacts are generated is rather subtle and is based on the physics of stimulated echoes. A stimulated echo is produced by a sequence of *three* rf pulses which are normally considered to be 90° in flip angle. The effect works by the first rf pulse rotating the **M** vector into the x-y plane, the second then rotating part of it into the z plane, and the third pulse then rotating it back into the x-y plane where it can produce the stimulated echo. The actual conditions for the echo to produce a proper image are rather complex and beyond the scope of this chapter (27–29). However, the phenomenon can be created by almost *any* sequence of three pulses applied to the same group of protons under appropriate conditions. (Of course, if the second and third pulse are exactly 180° there is only a normal spin echo, not a stimulated echo.)

The problem arises because a flip angle which is between 90° and 180° can, in effect, create both kinds of echo simultaneously. In particular, since selective pulses are never perfect, there are always some regions of the slice where the flip angle is less than 180°, as well as some irradiation of protons outside of the desired slice. In some cases a ghost image which is inverted is formed (30). In other cases both the spin-echo and stimulated-echo images are well formed but they can interfere to cause "herring bone" artifacts. A detailed description of this problem has been given by Crawley and Henkleman (31). The problem can be virtually eliminated if appropriate gradient pulses, called "crusher" or "spoiler" pulses, are applied before and after each 180° pulse (32); however, this is often not done because such gradient pulses add to the minimum echo time. Failure to include such spoiler pulses can result in either artifacts or errors in T2 estimation in multiecho pulses (33). Currently, with the development of higher quality (more selective) 180° rf pulses this artifact is rarely seen; see Chapter 3 for more details. If the problem does arise, it can usually be solved by leaving a larger gap between adjacent slices.

Frequency Errors with Gradient-Echo Imaging

The basic principle of the gradient-echo pulse sequence is illustrated in Fig. 8. As with spin-echo technique, the rf pulse, in conjunction with the *z* gradient pulse, serves to excite the spins in a particular (axial) slice. Also as with the spin-echo technique, there is a "prephasing" pulse of *x* gradient applied just after excitation which serves to temporarily dephase the spins. However, whereas a spin-echo technique would use a 180° rf pulse to refocus the spins and produce an echo, in this case that is accomplished by applying only a second *x* gradient pulse of reversed polarity. In other words, the second *x* gradient serves to reverse the dephasing introduced by the first and produces an echo at time TE, as shown.

These "gradient echoes," also called "field echoes," are in part misnamed. Like a spin echo, the signal appears to rise out of the background some time after it has apparently disappeared following excitation of the spins, i.e., after the free induction decay (FID) has decayed. However, in the case of the spin echo the decay caused by fixed field inhomogeneities is reversed, so a spin echo is relatively insensitive to the presence of fixed inhomogeneities of magnetic field. In the gradient echo the only dephasing which is reversed by the read gradient is that which was produced by the prephasing pulse! Nothing exists in the gradient-echo technique to prevent the loss of signal due to dephasing in fixed inhomogeneities, so the signal decay is most properly described by the parameter T2* rather than T2. The important conclusion is that gradient-echo imaging is equivalent to FID imaging, and the dephasing produced by all natural inhomogeneities is not reversed or compensated at all (see also Chapter 29).

One effect of any field inhomogeneity is to cause a loss of signal strength. This will occur whenever the local inhomogeneity is strong enough as to cause a significant frequency shift throughout the volume of one voxel. This situation can, especially with gradient-echo imaging, lead to large phase shifts of the various protons in the voxel, which causes the vector sum of the proton moments to be reduced; i.e., the loss of signal is due to dephasing of the protons within the voxel. This effect is, of course, more pronounced with gradient-echo imaging than with spin echo, since the SE pulse sequence, with its 180° rf pulse, tends to automatically refocus the dephased spins.

The loss of signal due to this effect is shown in the phantom images of Fig. 5. The background material was an aqueous gel designed to approximate the T1 and T2 of tissue. Embedded in each phantom was a surgical clip made of either stainless steel or titanium. The alternating bands of dark and light are due to dephasing of the water signal in regions distant from the clips. The titanium clip shows a reduced region of artifact due to its lower magnetic susceptibility. The asymmetry of the artifacts is directly attributable to the asymmetry produced by any magnetic dipole; the field is twice as strong in the longitudinal as compared with the transverse direction. The striped artifactual pattern seen in the bottom of the images is due to interference between the signal coming directly from that part of the phantom with that coming from the aliased signal on the top of the phantom. (See

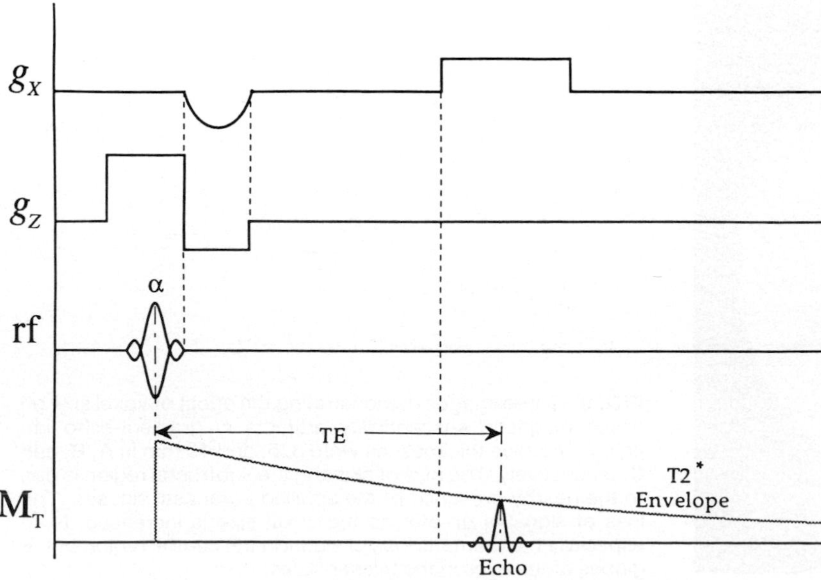

FIG. 8. Illustration of the pulse sequence for gradient-echo imaging. Slice selection is accomplished by the rf pulse and g_z gradient as with spin echo. Note the negative prephase g_x pulse followed by the positive readout g_x pulse, which is used for frequency encoding. The echo produced at time TE will be reduced due to T2* decay of the FID.

section, "Aliasing and Image Foldover"). This experiment shows rather dramatically how sensitive gradient-echo imaging is to susceptibility-induced frequency shifts.

This experiment shows how different materials can give different levels of artifact. In the real world, one may not know in an emergency situation what materials are present in patients' bodies. For example, Smith et al. (34) made a thorough survey of the artifacts created by different kinds of bullets, with results that resemble those in Fig. 5. While we are here presenting this effect as an artifact, it can also be applied to clinical diagnosis (35).

Figure 9 shows how the signal strength can be influenced by nearby differences in susceptibility. In all three images, one sees a loss of signal in the brain adjacent to the posterior ethmoid and sphenoid sinuses as well as a

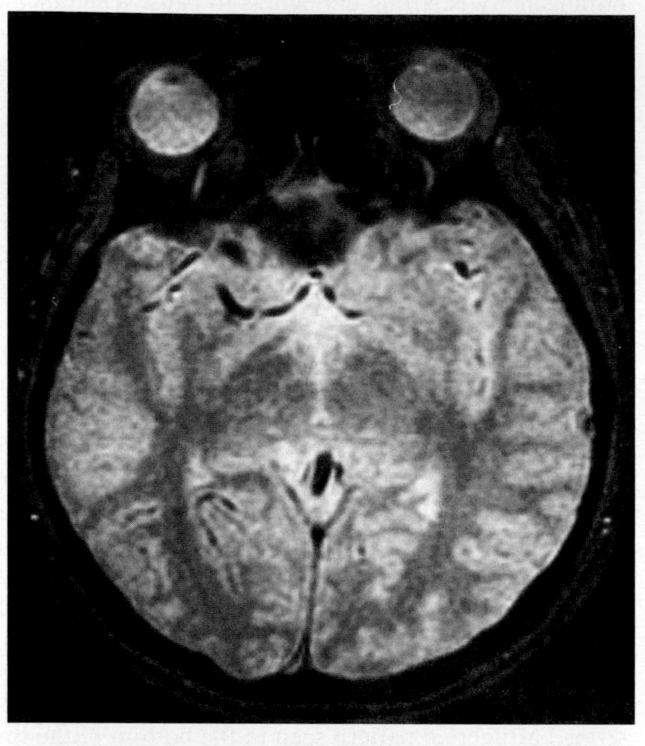

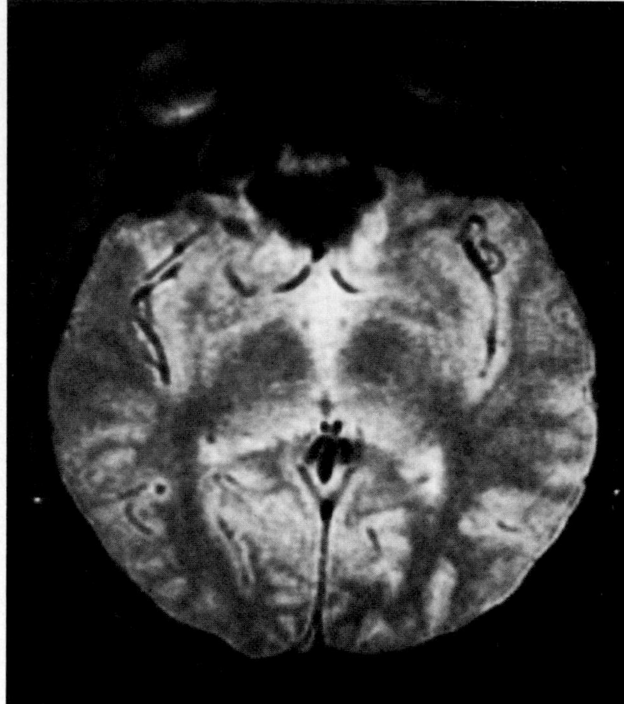

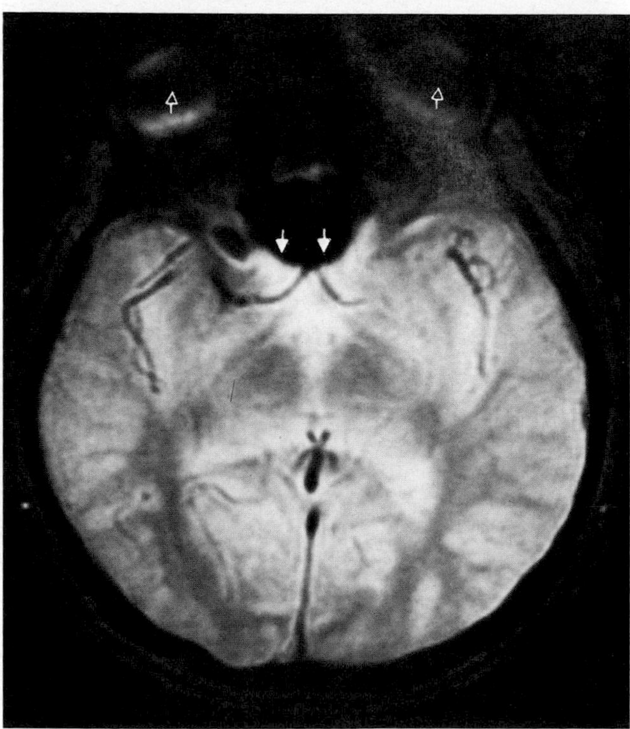

FIG. 9. Three images demonstrating the effect of voxel size on tissue magnetic susceptibility artifacts in gradient-echo imaging. The slice thicknesses were 3, 5, and 10 mm in **A**, **B**, and **C**, respectively. The loss of signal in the subfrontal region is due to the nearby presence of the air filled paranasal sinuses. The loss of signal is greater as the voxel size is increased. Note especially the dramatic loss of signal in the central region of the globes of the eyes in the thicker slices.

loss in the interior of the globe. Note that the loss increases with increasing slice thickness, being greatest for the 10 mm thick slice of Fig. 9C. (The improvement in signal-to-noise ratio with greater slice thickness is also evident in C.) Especially dramatic is the loss of signal in the center of the globe: this is the opposite behavior one would have expected from a purely linear partial volume effect.

In the clinical setting, lesions with paramagnetic substances, like hemorrhagic cavernous hemangiomas, can be associated with multiple susceptibility artifacts. These artifacts can alter the MR appearance of the lesions, so that the expected patterns of intensity are not identifiable (36).

One should understand that because the sensitivity of GE MRI is due to the magnitude of field inhomogeneity within each voxel, *the sensitivity of the effect usually increases with increasing voxel size*. Hence, one way to reduce the effect is to decrease the size of the voxels (increase image resolution), a procedure that usually involves using more time for scanning and will necessarily reduce signal-to-noise ratio. This effect is demonstrated in Fig. 9 in terms of slice thickness. On the other hand, in some cases of suspected intracranial hemorrhage, it may be desirable to enhance sensitivity to blood. This can be accomplished by using larger pixels, i.e., by deliberately "worsening" the image spatial resolution by using larger pixels (37). Since all susceptibility effects are proportional to the strength of magnetic field used, they will be less apparent at low field, and the technique of increasing voxel size is most likely to be useful under those conditions. The clinical implications of gradient-echo imaging to capitalize on enhanced sensitivity to susceptibility variations are fully discussed in Chapter 29.

We have explained why gradient-echo (GE) imaging is inherently more sensitive to induced fields than is spin echo (SE). This conclusion has been supported by several publications in the clinical radiologic literature. Watanabe et al. (38) found that SE images of the lumbar spine were superior to GE images in the evaluation of the neural foramina, epidural fat, and disk herniation, as well as in patients in whom the "bird's nest" filter had been placed in the inferior vena cava (39). Rupp et al. (40) confirmed Kundel's results (Fig. 5) that titanium fusion clips in the cervical spine gave less artifact than stainless steel. In most cases the patient is aware, or it is radiographically obvious, that a metallic foreign object is present. However, Peterman et al. (41) in an experiment using a bovine spine demonstrated that a significant source of artifact in GE images is due to microscopic residue of the steel drill bit used for surgery on the cervical spine. It appears that even using a diamond drill bit can also create such artifacts (42).

More recently implemented fast imaging techniques using "fast spin echo" have demonstrated reduced artifacts in post-operative spine cases (43).

Fat-Water Signal Cancellation

Another situation leading to a dramatic loss of image signal occurs in gradient-echo imaging whenever there is an interface between fat and water (44). The frequency difference between the two substances implies that, as a function of time after excitation, the two vectors (i.e., fat and water) will progressively diverge in phase. Indeed, this effect is the basis of a well established technique, called the "Dixon method," for distinguishing between fat and water in MRI (4).

In the case of gradient-echo imaging all echoes are offset in time. The artifact occurs for those pixels which straddle the fat-water interface. A loss of signal will occur, the magnitude of which is dependent on the fat-water phase shift which exists at the "echo" time, TE. The formula for phase shift, ϕ, is simply

$$\phi = (360°)(\Delta f)\text{TE}. \qquad [5]$$

In this formula phase shift will be in degrees if Δf is expressed in kilohertz and TE is expressed in milliseconds. The suppression of signal will depend on the exact fraction of fat and water occupying each voxel, as well as such other complicating factors as TR, the T1s of the two substances, etc. However, the effect will depend on the cosine of the phase shift angle, and maximum signal suppression will occur when ϕ is 180° or an odd multiple thereof.

A phantom example of the effect is shown in Fig. 10. This phantom contained oil and water as separated components. The echo time was adjusted so that the fat and water signals were either in phase or 180° out of phase. When the fat and water are in phase, one might (naively) expect the two signals to add together. However, the chemical shift phenomenon discussed above is still operative, so that the oil and water appear shifted relative to each other along the FE axis. Therefore, part of the oil/water interface is dark because the oil and water boundaries have been shifted in opposite directions, leaving a signal void. This phantom example illustrates the subtle way in which nature combines these two chemical shift effects: the image shift and the signal phase shift.

From Equation 5 we can conclude that the fat and water signals will be in phase with each other whenever the phase shift is a multiple of 360°, that is, whenever the echo time is equal to a multiple of $1/\Delta f$.

A clinical example of this artifact is shown in Fig. 11; again the echo times have been adjusted so that fat and water are either in phase or out of phase. Since $\Delta f = 200$ Hertz at this field, the fat and water signals will be in phase if the echo time is a multiple of 5 ms ($1/200 = 0.005$). The difference in image contrast induced by the difference in echo times is dramatic! The suppression of signal in the vertebral marrow is evident, as is the artifactual black border between the thecal sack and the epidural fat (arrows).

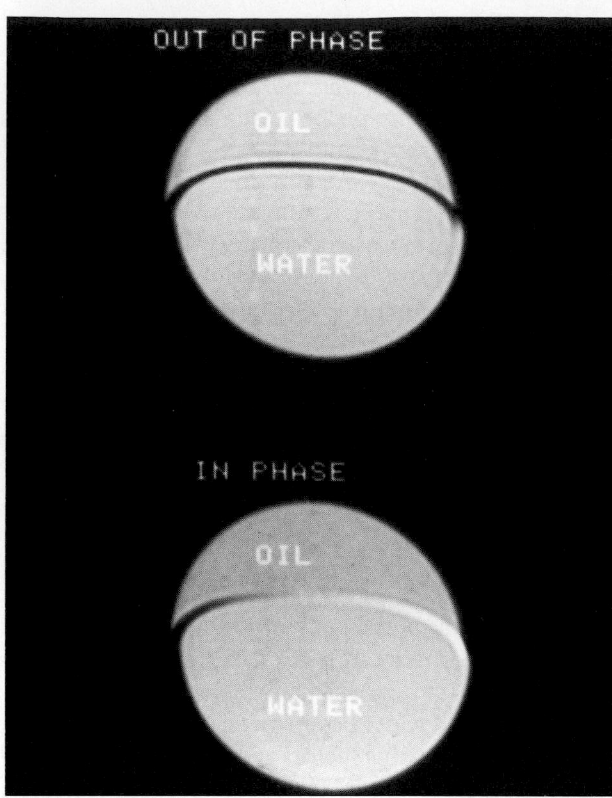

FIG. 10. Gradient-echo image of an oil-water phantom, illustrating both chemical shift and susceptibility artifacts. The echo times were adjusted so that the oil and water are in phase (bottom) and out of phase (top). The frequency-encoded axis and chemical shift direction are horizontal. The black band (top) is due to destructive interference between the oil and water signals in the region of overlap. A Gibbs artifact is also faintly visible in both the oil and water near the dark band. In the bottom image, the two signals are additive but also shifted along the FE direction.

A

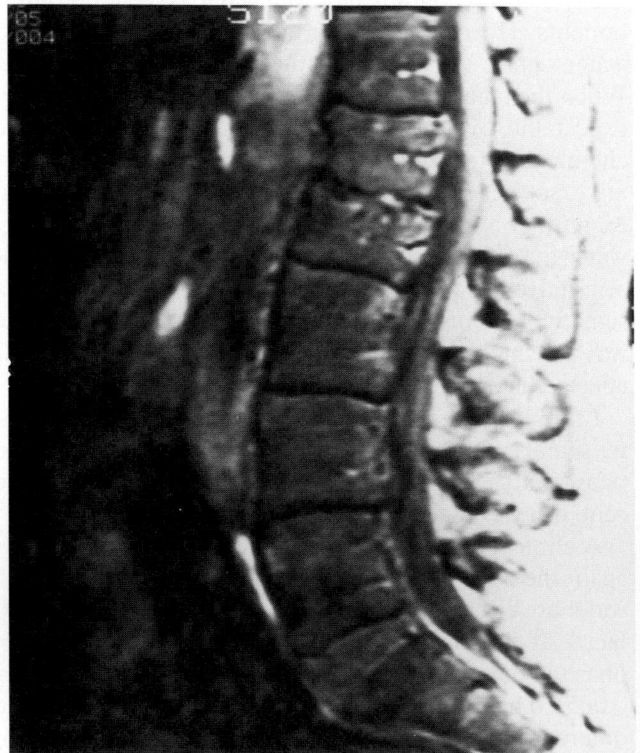

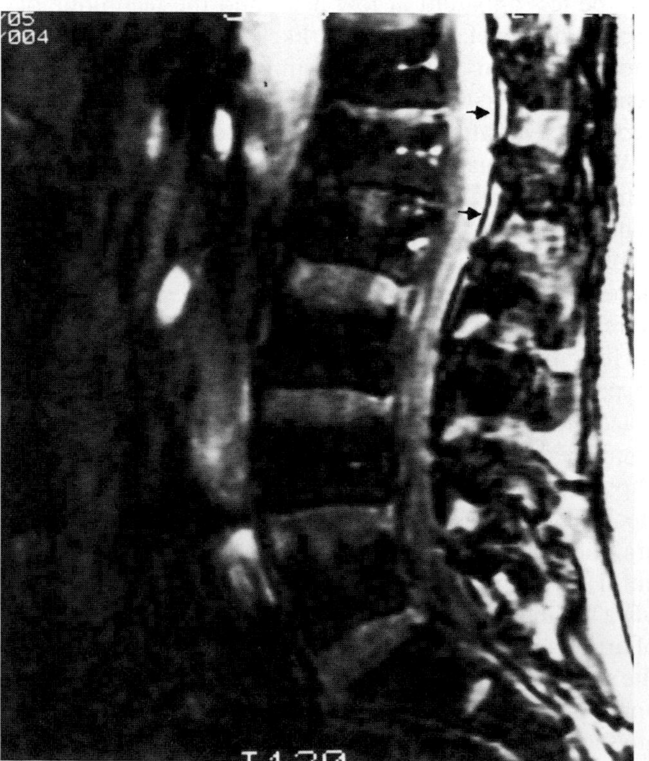

B

FIG. 11. Gradient-echo images of the lumbar spine. **A** has TE = 5 ms and **B** has TE = 8 ms. The fat and water are in phase in A and out of phase in B, creating the artifactual black band between the thecal sac and the epidural fat (*arrows*).

Chemical Shift Imaging

Obviously, the best way to eliminate artifacts caused by the chemical shift effect would be to employ a pulse sequence which explicitly separates fat and water. Ideally, one then obtains two images consisting of only fat and only water. There are a number of ways that this can be accomplished, and the literature on this subject is very large indeed (3,6). Most successful methods, however, require a high degree of magnetic field homogeneity—less than the 3.5 ppm of the fat-water shift. Some also have other disadvantages, such as increased scan time or increased image noise or incompatibility with multiplanar or multiecho imaging. In practice these techniques are only rarely used in routine neurologic imaging. The reader should note that the most widely used method, that of Dixon (4), does not provide true fat and water images, and the images produced usually closely resemble the out-of-phase gradient-echo images shown in Figs. 10 and 11.

Artifacts in Echo-Planar Imaging

By echo-planar imaging (EPI), we mean a technique in which, ideally, all of the information needed to reconstruct an image comes from multiple echoes from a single excitation; this is in contradistinction to the more usual spin-warp technique in which a separate excitation is used for each step of phase encoding (see Chapter 3). The first development of EPI was by Mansfield and Pykett (45); it was later used to obtain rapid images of the beating heart. The quality of those images was, however, rather low by today's standards. More recently this technique has been revived for the purpose of functional imaging; the goal there is to use a technique that is very sensitive to local changes in magnetic susceptibility induced by changes in blood oxygenation between venous and arterial blood (46,47). [This technique should not be confused with a similar multiecho technique called "RARE" (48) or "fast spin echo" (49) in which the various echoes are refocused using 180° rf pulses. The use of these true spin echoes will not result in increased sensitivity to magnetic susceptibility.]

Unfortunately, the increased sensitivity to magnetic susceptibility will create an increased level of image artifact (50) for the basic reason discussed earlier in this chapter. Here we want to point out two additional artifacts that will occur: a chemical shift-induced artifact in the *phase-encoded* direction as well as more subtle geometric distortions in the anatomy. These effects can cause a nonalignment between structures in the brain as visualized on conventional spin-echo and EP images.

The main task is to understand how a small frequency error, Δf, can lead to a rather large shift in the PE direction. To do this, we must examine exactly how phase encoding works in two-dimensional Fourier transform (2DFT) imaging. The magnitude of the phase-encoding gradient pulse (called g_y) is incremented by amount Δg_y between each excitation; this will increment the phase of the *n*th echo by an amount that depends on the *y* coordinate in the image. However, if for any reason there is also a frequency error Δf (such as that due to fat-water chemical shift) then there will *also* be an additional phase shift which has nothing to do with *y*. This additional phase shift will also increase in proportion to the echo time from echo to echo. Hence, the Equation for the phase of the signal on the *n*th pulse is given by the formula:

$$\phi_n = \gamma\, n\Delta g_y T_y y + nf 2\pi\Delta\text{TE}. \qquad [6]$$

Here f is the frequency offset, which is 3.5 ppm of the Larmor frequency for fat-water (200 Hz at 63 mHz), and ΔTE is the spacing between the echoes in the echo planar pulse sequence. Equation 6 shows that both the phase-encoding gradient and the frequency offset contribute to phase shift. However, the reconstruction software assumes that $f = 0$, and it will therefore determine y by looking only at the first term in Equation 6:

$$y = \phi_n/\gamma n\Delta g_y T_y. \qquad [7]$$

When $f = 0$, substituting Equation 6 into Equation 7 gives $y = y$, which is of course correct. However, when the frequency offset term is present, the result of reconstruction is to produce a different value of y gotten by substituting Equation 6 into Equation 7, namely:

$$y' = y + f\Delta\text{TE FOV} \qquad [8]$$

where FOV $= 2\phi/(\gamma\Delta g_y T_y)$ is the size of the field of view in the *y* direction. *This indicates that the true value of y is shifted by amount f ΔTE FOV in the phase-encoding direction.* This implies that fat will appear as a shifted "ghost" in the image. This is an example of the effect of the shift theorem as explained further in the section on ghosts generated by motion.

The most obvious source of such a phase shift would be the presence of fat in the imaged slice. Fat, as we have seen in Equation 5, will induce a phase shift in gradient-echo images proportional to the echo time. Such a phase shift is illustrated in the graph in Fig. 12. What is different in EPI is that we must utilize the signal from *multiple* gradient echoes, illustrated by the solid dots on the graph. Hence, fat will lead to a phase shift in the signal which increases progressively from echo to echo and is therefore indistinguishable from that which would take place if we had displaced the fat by amount given above. The result is that the fat portion of the image will be shifted along the PE direction. For comparison, Fig. 12 also shows that phase of the multiple echo signals if 180° rf pulses are used to form the echoes. In that case, due to the phase reversals that occur at the rf pulses, there is no net accumulation of phase error in the fat signal. (Of course, there will still be the chemical shift artifact in the frequency-encoded direction as discussed previously.)

By substituting numerical values for a typical case in Equation 8 we see that the shift represents a very considerable effect. For example, taking f = 200 Hz for fat-water shift at 1.5 Tesla, and ΔTE = 1 ms, we get a shift of 20% of a FOV in the phase-encoded direction. As Equation 8 shows, the magnitude of the shift is proportional to the time interval between echoes, so the actual amount would depend on what was being used in a particular scanner. Note, however, that if the echo spacing was chosen to be $\Delta TE = 1/f$ then the shift = FOV, which is equivalent to no shift at all. This is another example of the fact that if the echo spacing is set to correspond to exactly one period of the fat-water frequency difference, then water and fat are in phase at each echo and no shift artifact is created.

Echo-planar images are sometimes made utilizing one 180° rf pulse to form a spin echo (51,52). A series of gradient echoes are formed both before and after the true echo, which is usually designed for the center ($k_y = 0$) of k-space. Hence, only the single echo at $k_y = 0$ has the effects of chemical shift and inhomogeneity refocused. The rest of the echoes are essentially gradient echoes and will suffer the same sort of phase shift errors discussed above (50). In particular, the chemical shift artifact will be identical to that described by Equation 8. However, the fact that fat and water are in phase at $k = 0$ implies that, for those pixels in which they overlap, their signal intensities will add (as opposed to subtract) in the image; an example is shown in Fig. 13.

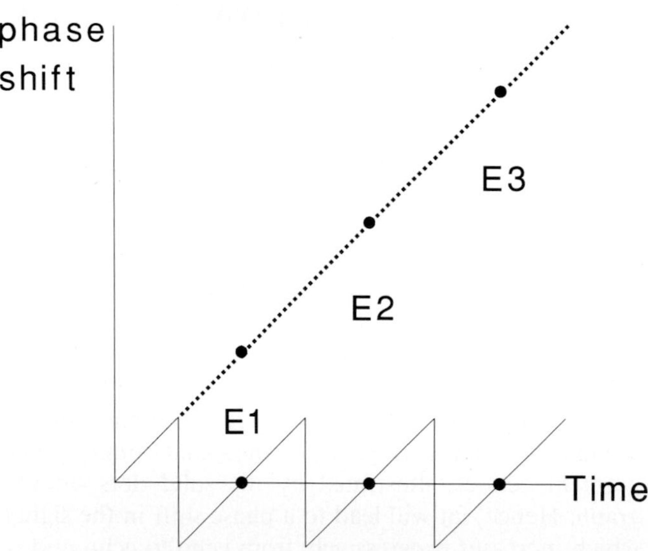

FIG. 12. Illustration of how a frequency offset error leads to phase error in echo-planar imaging. The *solid line* shows the phase of successive echo signals obtained with normal rf refocusing pulses between echoes. The *dotted line* shows the accumulation of phase error when multiple-gradient echoes are used in EPI. The time of the three echoes are indicated as E1,E2, and E3. Note that whereas the phase shift of the three rf echoes is zero, that of the three gradient echoes increases with each successive echo.

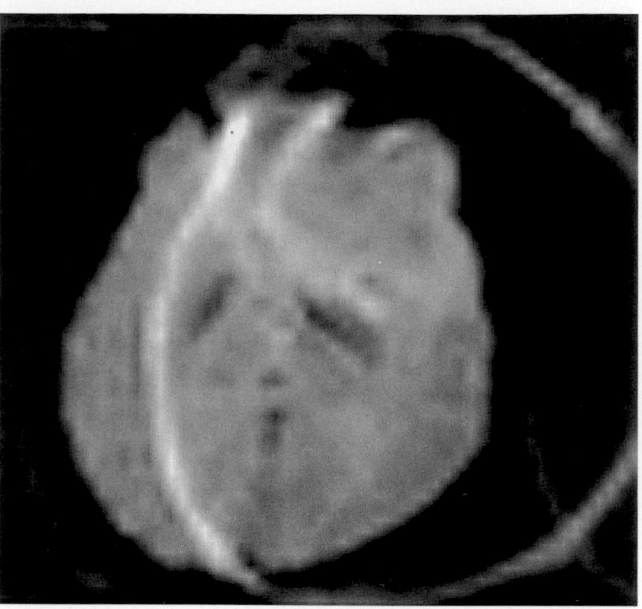

FIG. 13. Axial echo-planar 64 × 64 image through the brain using a single spin echo with TE = 100 ms. Because fat was not suppressed, the cranial marrow appears shifted by about 20% of FOV in the PE (*horizontal*) direction. In addition, a weak ghost image of the fat is visible shifted by $\frac{1}{2}$ FOV in the PE direction. The second bright artifact in the middle of the image is attributed to susceptibility effects from structures inferior to this slice.

To avoid spill-over of the cranial marrow into the brain, functional images are often made with the fat suppressed as explained elsewhere. Nevertheless, the extreme sensitivity of EPI to frequency errors means that even aqueous tissues will appear shifted if the resonant frequency is altered due to magnetic susceptibility effects. The result is an image in which the shape of the brain parenchyma is distorted.

An example is shown in Fig. 13. In this image, the phase-encoding direction is horizontal and the artifactual shift of the cranial marrow is obvious. This image also shows another more subtle artifact. It stems from the fact that EPI scans k-space in opposite directions on alternate echoes. In some cases, electronic circuits introduce a slight error due to time delay in the propagation of signals. Hence, there will be an error which alternates from even to odd echoes. This erroneous modulation of the signal creates a ghost image shifted by exactly $\frac{1}{2}$ FOV in the PE direction; this effect has been called a "time reversal ghost" (53). The weak ghost image of the cranial fat due to this effect is also faintly visible in Fig. 13.

ALIASING AND SAMPLING ERRORS

Theoretically, the Fourier transform (FT) process is capable of accurately reconstructing the image if it is given sufficient information. Specifically, the FT algorithm would require as input data measurements of all spatial frequencies, in both x and y directions. Such a data set would be literally infinite in size and is obviously impossible to obtain in a practical MRI system. Since the acquired data set is finite, we pay a price in the form of a certain ambiguity in the structure of the body being imaged, and this ambiguity causes two important artifacts.

There are two ways in which the real data set falls short of the ideal: first, the range of spatial frequencies encoded is not infinite but has definite limits, and second, even within these limits the data is obtained on a discrete grid of points in k space rather than for a continuum of k values. Both of these aspects are illustrated in Chapter 3. The artifacts created by the two processes differ considerably, however, and will be discussed separately.

The Gibbs Phenomenon and Truncation Artifacts

As we saw in Chapter 3, the use of only a finite number of spatial frequencies in synthesizing the image tends to produce an image with ripples, the spacing of which is a direct reflection of the highest spatial frequency used (54,55). The intensity of these ripples is a function of both how sharp the edges in the object are, and of the extent to which the high spatial frequencies may be attenuated by the data processing software.

To understand the dependence on object edge sharpness, recall that to reconstruct an edge sharply requires the presence of a large number of high spatial frequencies; limiting the high spatial frequency content of an image produces a blurred image. Conversely, if the object contains only edges which are not sharply defined, then the high frequencies are not needed for good reconstruction. In other words, only objects with sharp edges generate strong high frequency components.

To be more specific, the highest spatial frequency present in any reconstructed image is related to the inverse of the pixel size. This highest frequency is called the "Nyquist" frequency, and is given by the formula:

$$\nu_N = 1/(2\Delta x) \qquad [9]$$

where Δx is the pixel size. Note that if Δx has dimensions of centimeters, then the spatial frequency has dimensions of cycles per cm. In fact, the value of ν_N for any digital image is exactly $\frac{1}{2}$ cycle per pixel; this represents a wave in which alternate pixels are light and dark.

The Gibbs phenomenon refers to errors of Fourier synthesis that occur when there are strong components up to and including the Nyquist frequency. The effect is most severe when the FT reconstruction algorithm is given data which fall abruptly to zero at ν_N, as shown in Fig. 14. In such a case the reconstructed image will show strong bands or ripples of frequency ν_N. Because the artifact depends on how rapidly the frequency spectrum drops to zero, and would disappear if an infinite range of spatial frequencies were used, it can be considered to stem from the abrupt truncation of the spatial frequency spectrum and so is often called a "truncation" effect (56–58). The effect can be considerably mitigated if one is willing to process the data prior to reconstruction (59) so as to force a gradual, rather than abrupt, decrease in amplitude as ν approaches ν_N. This idea is also illustrated in Fig. 14. A variant of this technique is used on almost all MRI systems to diminish the Gibbs effect. The price paid for this is a slight blurring of the image, since the high frequency components are not present in the image in the strength that they should be. Technically speaking, such a loss of sharpness will not appear as loss of "resolution" since the maximum resolvable spatial frequency in the image has not been changed. Rather, the loss of sharpness can be quantified by using the MTF concept for image sharpness. For a discussion of this problem in the context of clinical CT image quality, see the paper by Joseph and Stockham (60).

The relevant measure of object sharpness is how rapidly the signal density changes across the length of a pixel. The effect will be strongest when either the object is sharp or when the pixels are large; i.e., the larger the pixels the more likely it is that a signal will vary rapidly across the width of one pixel. Hence the effect is usually more noticeable on larger than on smaller pixels.

The effect is most severe when the anatomy being imaged has a high contrast plane running parallel to either

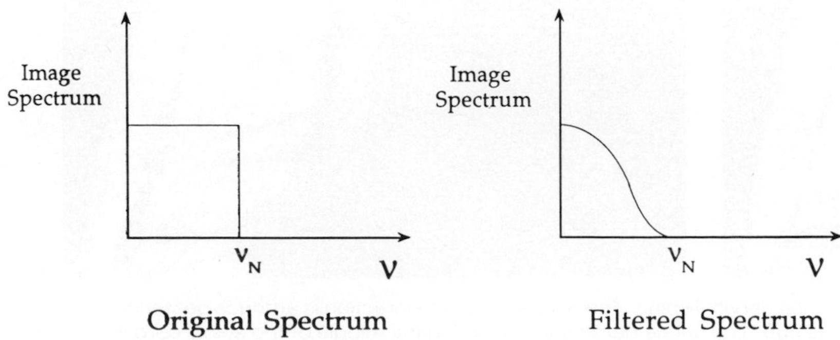

FIG. 14. Illustration of how signal filtering can reduce the strength of high spatial frequencies. **A** shows the frequency spectrum of an object with hard edges and no filtering. **B** shows how filtering can, by blurring the object, suppress spatial frequencies near the Nyquist frequency, ν_N.

the x or y axis, and the wavelength of the artifact will be equal to the length of two pixels. The effect is very commonly seen in images of the cervical spine (61) when done using only 128 pixels in the PE direction. Figure 15 demonstrates that the effect is easily seen when using 128 pixels, but is almost invisible when 256 pixels are used. This effect can occur in either the frequency- or phase-encoded directions. However, in clinical practice it is more likely to be seen in the phase-encoding direction because, to reduce scan time, fewer pixels are often used there than in the FE direction.

It has been shown that various methods of data processing or image reconstruction can mitigate the truncation artifacts with little apparent loss of resolution (62,63). Basically, these work by estimating the k-space data to beyond the limit of k_{max} by extrapolation. However, to date they have not found widespread clinical application because of the extra computing time needed for image reconstruction.

Aliasing and Image Foldover

This artifact is due to the fact that, even within the limited range of k-space covered by the scanning process, the k values are measured discretely rather than continuously, i.e., there is a minimum spacing between the various k-space values. (See Chapter 2.) The spacing between spatial frequency values, $\Delta\nu$, is inversely related to the field of view. The Equation describing this is:

$$\text{FOV} = 1/\Delta\nu. \qquad [10]$$

If $\Delta\nu$ is expressed in cycles per centimeter, then FOV will be in centimeters.

Furthermore, the Fourier synthesis mathematics implicitly assumes that the object is periodic, i.e., it assumes that the object repeats itself every FOV units of length. Of course, we know that is absurd anatomically, but this characteristic is an intrinsic aspect of Fourier analysis.

To grasp the consequences of this assumption, imagine that we start with a small object near the center of the machine. The reconstruction will of course show the object present at a corresponding position near the center of the image. Now imagine that we slowly move the object further out laterally. As it moves to the right beyond the field of view in real space, the reconstructed image will show it reappearing from the left side of the image. If we move it one full FOV laterally from the center of the machine, in the reconstructed image it will again appear to be located at the center of the FOV. The situation can be summarized as saying that any object which gives any detectable NMR signal *must* appear after reconstruction within the FOV, regardless of its true position in space. We illustrate the consequence of these

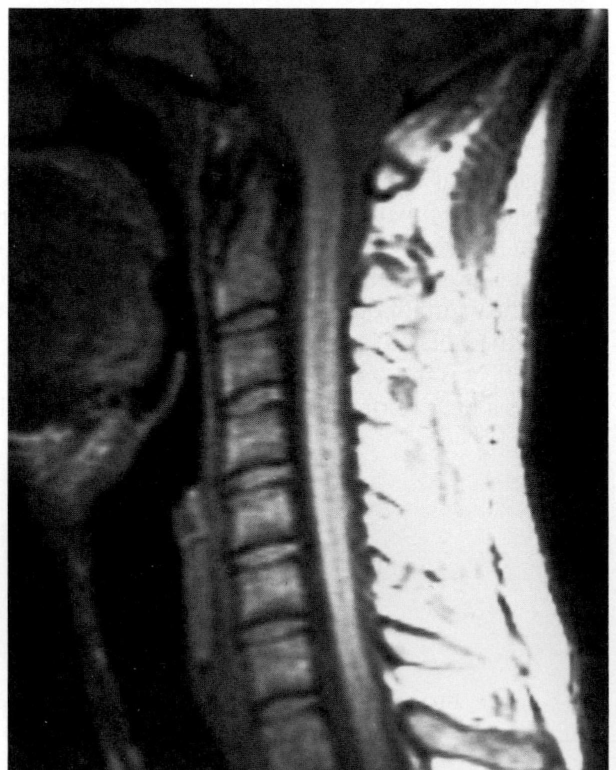
A

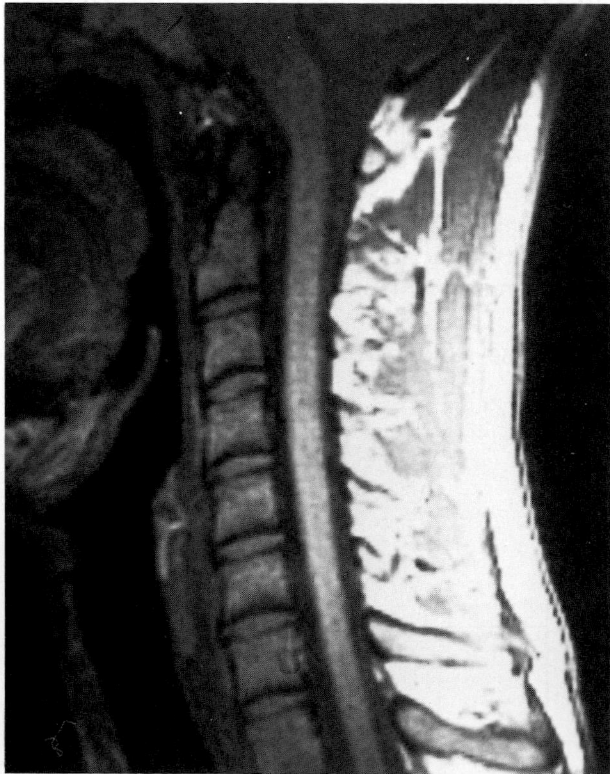
B

FIG. 15. Demonstration of the Gibbs artifact in the cervical spine. The phase-encoding direction is anterior-posterior. **A** has 128 pixels in the PE direction, while **B** has 256. The subtle dark band traversing the middle of the spinal cord in A is due to the Gibbs effect. In B the artifact is greatly reduced.

effects in Fig. 16. This phenomenon is called "aliasing" (54). In the FE direction, the result can be understood as frequency aliasing, meaning that the apparent frequency of the signal is different from its true frequency. For example, let us again consider the moving phantom example of above. In the presence of a readout gradient directed along the x axis, the resonant (temporal) frequency of the object will continue to increase as we move the object beyond the FOV. In other words, the true frequency, by definition, does not show any aliasing effect. However, the data presented to the computer is based on a finite number of samples of the signal, and these samples are spaced in time by some time interval, Δt. In this situation, the sampling process cannot properly measure frequencies higher than $f_N = 1/(2\Delta t)$, which is the temporal Nyquist frequency. (The reader must be careful not to confuse the temporal Nyquist frequency, f_N, measured in cycles per second, with the spatial Nyquist frequency, ν_N, which is characteristic of the image pixel matrix.) *Aliasing occurs when the true temporal frequency exceeds* f_N so that the apparent temporal frequency will be less than f_N. This transformation of apparent temporal frequencies due to inadequate data sampling will cause the object to appear in a different place along the x axis than it really is.

Essentially the same phenomenon occurs if we were to move the test object in the vertical, PE, direction (64). The explanation is slightly different, and can be understood by consideration of the explanation of phase encoding given in Chapter 2. The important point is that there is always some minimum value of g_y, the phase-

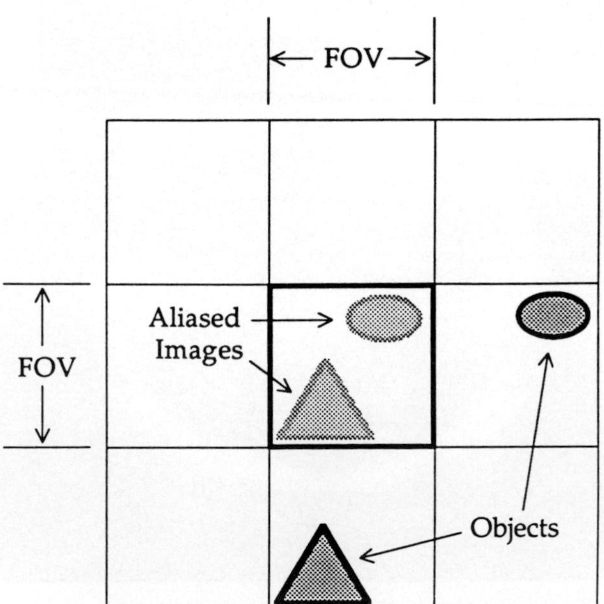

FIG. 16. Illustration of the concept of aliased field of views. Only the central (*heavy line*) FOV is intended to be imaged. The surrounding squares will alias and foldover into the central FOV. The circular object to the right and the triangle at the bottom will appear to be within the central FOV due to aliasing.

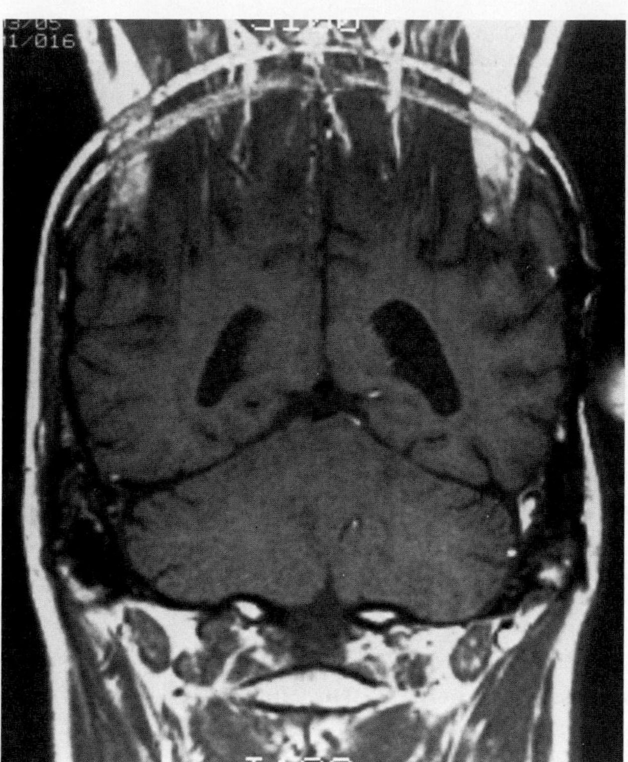

FIG. 17. Demonstration of aliasing in the phase-encoding direction. The bright signals at the top of the image are artifactual and are an aliased representation of the soft tissues of the neck lying below the FOV.

encoding gradient, in any given scan. Since the spatial frequency is directly proportional to g_y, this means a minimum y spatial frequency, ν_y. Since waves are (by definition) periodic in space, if the object is moved vertically by one spatial wavelength the signal produced will have the same phase as if it had not been moved at all. Therefore, those objects whose y position lie one FOV length away from the center of the true FOV can not be distinguished, by the phase of their NMR signal, from objects which lie at the center. The result is again a foldover of the apparent object location. This artifact is demonstrated in Fig. 17.

Filtering the FE Direction

Aliasing in the FE direction is not as troublesome as the previous discussion would suggest. The key is that it is possible to filter out the signals from objects lying outside the x FOV by electronic filtration before data sampling. This is done with a simple electronic circuit called a "low pass filter," which is analogous to the treble control on a high quality audio amplifier. This strongly attenuates the signal from any object outside the FOV on the basis of its temporal frequency and eliminates the artifact.

Unfortunately, such filtering is not possible in the PE direction, because the problem there is one of phase ambiguity and not frequency shift. If it is essential to eliminate the foldover in the PE direction, it can be done using other techniques, such as selectively forming spin echoes only for spins located within the FOV (65). Such a technique can be used, but usually is not because it is not consistent with multiplanar imaging in most cases.

Another possible solution is to restrict the sensitive region of the rf coil by applying metallic shielding to the outer parts of the body (66). This can very effectively remove the aliased portion of the body. A disadvantage of this technique is that the shielding will degrade the homogeneity of the transmitter rf field (B_1), which would mean that the flip angles would be inconsistent in areas close to the shield. This is most important in multiecho imaging, and probably least important in fast gradient-echo imaging with reduced flip angles.

In some cases, there can be a clear advantage to choosing the PE and FE directions so that the foldover effect is not troubling.

Oversampling in the PE Direction

As we have seen, it is not possible to eliminate the aliasing artifact in the PE direction by filtering. However, at the cost of increased scan time it can be eliminated by the relatively simple procedure of oversampling the PE direction. If one is willing to make twice as many PE gradient levels as is necessary to reconstruct the desired FOV, then one can obviously get enough data to reconstruct twice the desired FOV in the PE direction. For example, if a 10 cm FOV is desired with 256 pixel resolution, one could take 512 PE pulses with a FOV of 20 cm and have the same spatial resolution. However, since in this case objects would have to displaced by 20 cm from the imaged region before aliasing will occur, we have bought ourselves a factor of 2 improvement in insurance against aliasing with no loss of either spatial resolution or signal-to-noise ratio; the only price paid was a doubling of the minimum scan time. Since many clinical scans are done with multiple excitations per PE step to improve SNR, this is often not a significant disadvantage.

An alternate way to understand this technique is that one obtains a 512 pixel image and only displays the central 256 pixels; the method has a kind of built-in "digital zoom" magnification.

One possible disadvantage of this technique is increased susceptibility to phase noise artifacts (see above). In general, phase noise becomes more critical as the number of PE steps is increased. Obviously, whether this is or is not a problem will depend on the magnitude of the phase noise problems in each particular installation, since one can reduce the number of excitations accordingly.

Aliasing in Three-Dimensional Imaging

As explained in Chapter 2, three dimensional imaging is usually done using phase encoding along the z axis for slice selection rather than by selective excitation (67). This implies that the same sort of aliasing artifacts which occur in the y direction in 2D imaging can also occur in the z direction; the resulting artifacts can often be very perplexing until one realizes the nature of the problem.

As in the two-dimensional case, the relevant question is whether the "field of view" in the z direction is larger than the z dimension of the region producing signals. The z FOV is N_z times the slice thickness, Δz:

$$z\ \text{FOV} = N_z \cdot \Delta z. \qquad [11]$$

Unless the z FOV is greater than the sensitive region, aliasing and foldover will occur. The result is that the slice as viewed will contain signals emanating from other slices which are typically very far removed from the desired slice. An example is shown in Fig. 18, which is a "slice" from a 3D axial scan of the head. The bright region is the strong signal from the fat in the calvarium near the top of the head, while the presence of other tissue from the brainstem and the nasal septum is also present in the image.

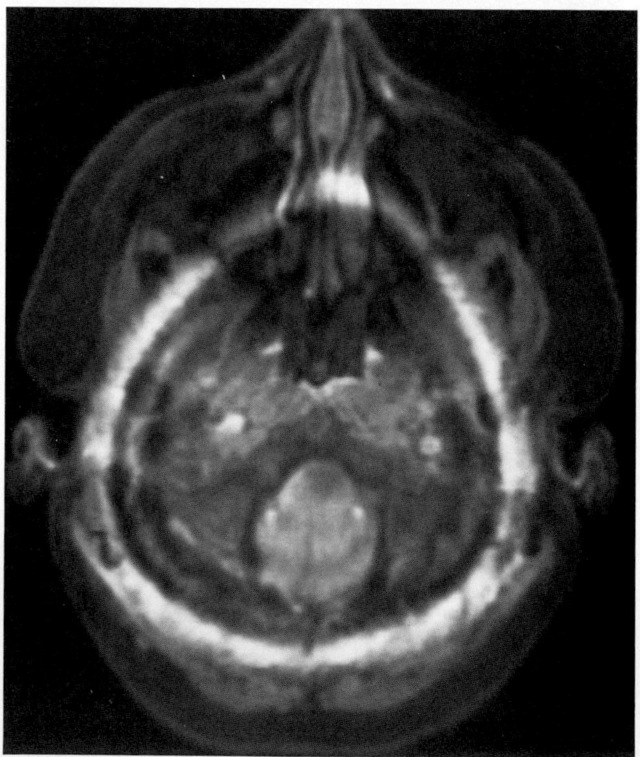

FIG. 18. Demonstration of slice aliasing in a three-dimensional, phase-encoded pulse sequence. One sees superimposed the bright fat of the upper portion of the calvarium and both neural (brainstem) and nonneural (nasal septum) signals from tissues far below the desired slice.

Since the most important way to avoid this artifact is to make sure that z FOV is larger than the thickness of the body part, this technique is most easily applied in the head to sagittal and coronal views. In those cases, one can choose z FOV so that it exceeds the AP or lateral dimensions of the head. In the case of axial 3D imaging, the problem is more difficult because it is not possible to choose z FOV to exceed the length of the entire body! In this case, the relevant body length is the length of tissue which lies within the rf receiving coil, which is usually a so-called head coil. Such a technique typically requires that the z FOV extend sufficiently far inferiorly to include the neck muscles.

An alternate way to solve the problem of axial 3D imaging is to modify the pulse sequence so that only a limited portion of the z axis is actually excited. This can be done by applying a z gradient pulse during the rf excitation process. In essence, the technique is equivalent to the selective excitation process of 2D imaging, except that the excited volume is not limited to one imaged slice but is made large enough to include the entire desired volume. In this case, it is important to make sure that the z dimension of the volume excited does not exceed the z FOV which is defined by the z phase-encoding pulse.

INSTRUMENTAL ERRORS AND ARTIFACTS

Obviously, the types of artifacts caused by instrumental failures will depend strongly on the details of the design features of each particular MRI machine. In this section we will study only those of a more universal nature, i.e., those which depend on some of the basic principles involved and are likely to be found to some degree on all machines.

Interfering Radio Signal Lines

NMR is essentially a rather weak process, and the signals produced at the terminals of the receiver rf coil are on the order of microvolts. Thus the NMR receiver is necessarily extremely sensitive. However, we live in a society in which electromagnetic fields of a wide range of frequencies are ubiquitous. Fortunately, the NMR process is also extremely selective in the frequencies used, so that only those frequencies within a few tens of kilohertz of the rf frequency are relevant. (This is always a tiny fraction of the radiofrequency used. For example, for a 1.5 T magnet the Larmor frequency is about 63 mHz.) Nevertheless, it can happen that in a given locality some radiant energy in this frequency band is present. The radiation could come from such diverse objects as computers, radio stations, television stations, arc lamps, and various sundry electronic equipment. Indeed, in some cases the most severe source of radiation in an MRI installation is the system's own computer!

If an external interfering signal is present and gets into the receiver circuitry, the result is invariably a streak running along the PE direction; i.e., the streak will lie at a certain value x along the FE direction. The reason is that the interference has a definite frequency and so the computer's Fourier analysis algorithm places the energy on the FE axis at the corresponding frequency point. This artifact is demonstrated in Fig. 19.

The only practical way to avoid this problem is to improve the shielding of the MRI room. Most installations require that the magnet room be shielded with a layer of suitable electrically conductive material, usually copper screen. Note that the shielding required is not for the static magnetic field, such as would be provided by iron plates. The most critical requirement for the rf shielding is that it be continuous, i.e., the entire room must be covered, with no breaks longer than a few centimeters. Usually the most troublesome point is the door through which patients and personnel enter the room. This must be specially designed to provide good electrical contact of the shield when the door is closed. From repeated openings, it is possible that the quality of contact could be compromised enough to allow unwanted radiation to enter the room. The problem, when seen, should respond to conventional repair measures.

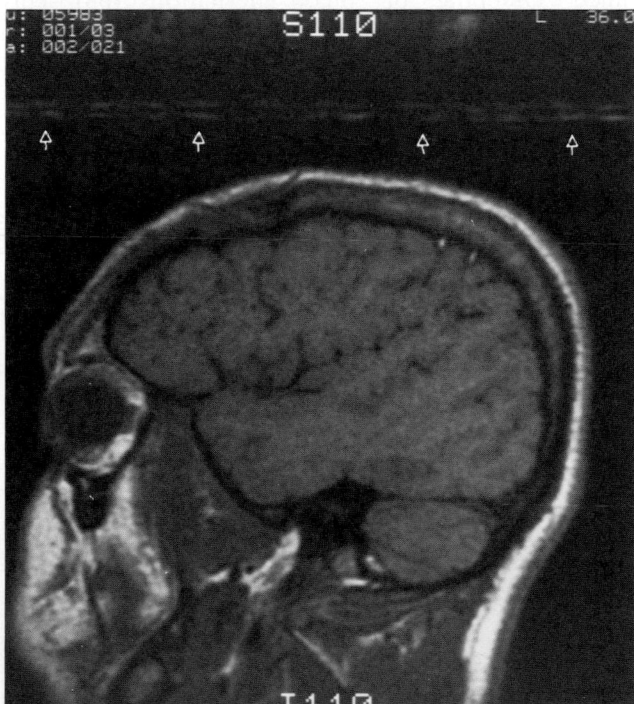

FIG. 19. Demonstration of a line artifact caused by external rf interference. The FE axis runs vertically. The horizontal line near the top of the image (*white arrows*) is due to unwanted external radiofrequency energy of a definite frequency entering into the receiver system.

Central DC Bright Spot

This artifact was rather common in the early days of this field. The effect is caused by an unwanted "DC," meaning "direct current" or zero temporal frequency, error in the receiver electronics. Ideally the receiver would produce no output when no input is present. However, it is extremely difficult to meet this condition with electronic amplifiers which must operate over a range of frequencies down to and including zero. Such amplifiers are needed after the phase sensitive detector (PSD), since the frequencies at that point are no longer in the megahertz range but depend on the difference between the Larmor frequency and the master oscillator (see Chapter 2 for discussion). Any practical amplifier will have some DC error, meaning it produces a small but constant output voltage even with no input signal present.

The result of such an error is usually a bright spot in the exact center of the image. This follows because the frequency of the erroneous voltage is zero both with respect to the FE direction and to the PE direction; essentially it means we have a "two dimensional" zero frequency error. An example is shown in Fig. 20, which is a fast image of the kidney of a rat taken without the usual protection against this artifact. The bright spot in the middle of the image is obvious.

The error is eliminated in most systems by a technique called "chopping" or "phase alternation" (68). This means that each rf exciting pulse is applied twice, each time with opposite phase. The resulting signals emerging from the PSD therefore alternate in sign. By subtracting the two signals of each pair, one cancels the DC component while the desired signal components add.

The cost of this method is obviously a doubling of the required number of pulses, which implies a doubling of the minimum scan time. If several excitations are used and averaged so as to reduce noise, this presents no problem. However, when one is interested in the fastest possible scans, the time cost is unacceptable. In that case, another technique can be used which alternates the sign of succession exciting pulses *without* doubling the total number of pulses. The computer then inverts the sign of the signal on alternate pulses to reconstruct the image properly. The effect on the DC offset is to convert it into one which changes sign with each phase-encoding pulse. The resulting artifact is then no longer a central dot but rather bright lines at the very top and bottom of the FOV. Such lines are usually irrelevant for interpreting the image and can easily be removed by software which erases those pixels from the image. For a discussion of this technique for a fast scan pulse sequence, see Bogdan and Joseph (69).

Line Frequency Noise Dots

A phenomenon closely related to the DC offset problem is caused by the presence of low frequency noise picked up from the local power lines. In the United States, power lines always have a frequency of 60 Hz, while in Europe the frequency is 50 Hz. If even a small amount of AC (alternating current) voltage from the power line is picked up by the receiver electronics, the result is an artifactual pair of dots in the image. The dots

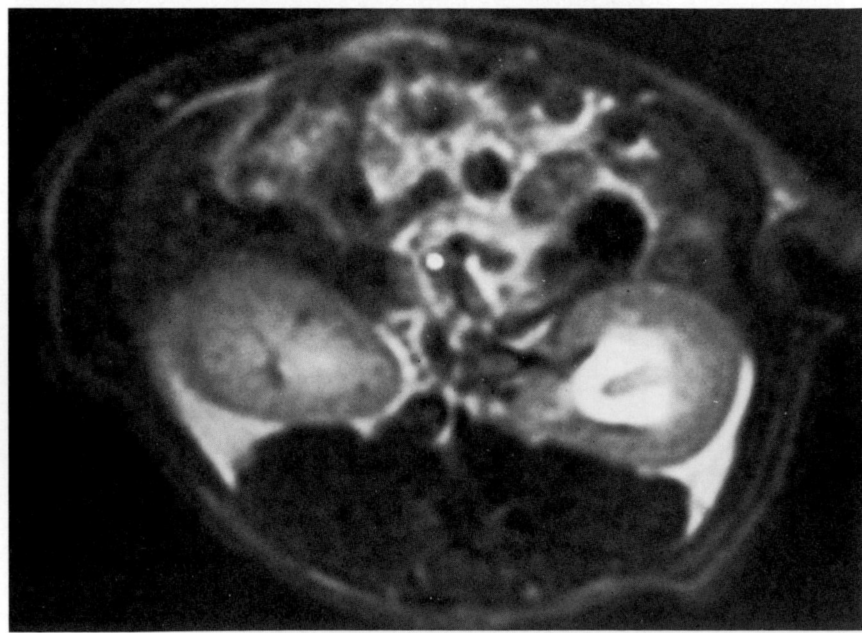

FIG. 20. Transverse slice through the kidneys of rat infused with Gd-DTPA contrast. The central bright spot is caused by a DC error in the receiver electronics. The spot is exactly centered in the original 128 × 128 pixel image, although it appears slightly above center in the figure.

will lie very close to the center of the frequency-encoding axis, since the power frequency is a small fraction of the receiver bandwidth. The reason one sees two dots is because the noise rarely appears equally in both the I and Q channels in such a way as to represent a purely rotating signal vector; i.e., it will appear to have both positive and negative frequency components. The dots will always appear symmetrically in the vertical (PE) direction. The vertical spacing of the dots is unpredictable and depends on the exact relationship between the power line and pulse repetition frequencies. In many cases, the effect can be eliminated if the TR of the pulse sequence is set to be exactly a multiple of the line frequency period. For example, with 60 Hz power lines the effect can be eliminated if the TR is exactly a multiple of 50 ms.

I/Q Imbalance Ghosts

In Chapter 3, it was explained that the MRI system needs two signals, called I and Q in engineering jargon, which should represent the components of signal along the x' and y' axes in the rotating frame. It was explained that only with both of those signals can one ascertain the direction of rotation of the **M** vector in the rotating frame. Knowledge of the direction of rotation is essential to distinguish positive from negative frequencies, hence to distinguish left from right along the FE axis.

The accurate reconstruction of positive versus negative frequencies is highly dependent on maintaining an accurate balance of the I and Q detection and amplifying systems. This is because the computer, in processing the raw data, will need to form sums and differences of the I and Q channels. Both the I and Q signals, considered separately, contain information on both positive and negative frequencies. As an extreme example of I/Q imbalance, imagine that one of the two channels was eliminated; the result would be an equal mixture of both positive and negative frequencies, and any object on one side of the FOV would appear on both sides of the image after reconstruction. A similar effect occurs in the PE direction, namely, an object in the top of the image would cast a ghost image in the bottom. The combination of these two effects is to produce a second ghost image rotated by 180° around the central point. This effect is illustrated in Fig. 21.

Of course, the MRI manufacturers take care to provide both I and Q channels to provide proper image reconstruction. However, it can happen that a very small imbalance occurs in the relative strengths of the two channels, due to drift or failure in the electronic components. In that case, the above described ghost image will occur, and its strength will be proportional to the degree of imbalance of the two channels. For example, if the two channels differ by 1% in amplification, the result will be a ghost whose MR numbers will be 1% of the true image values.

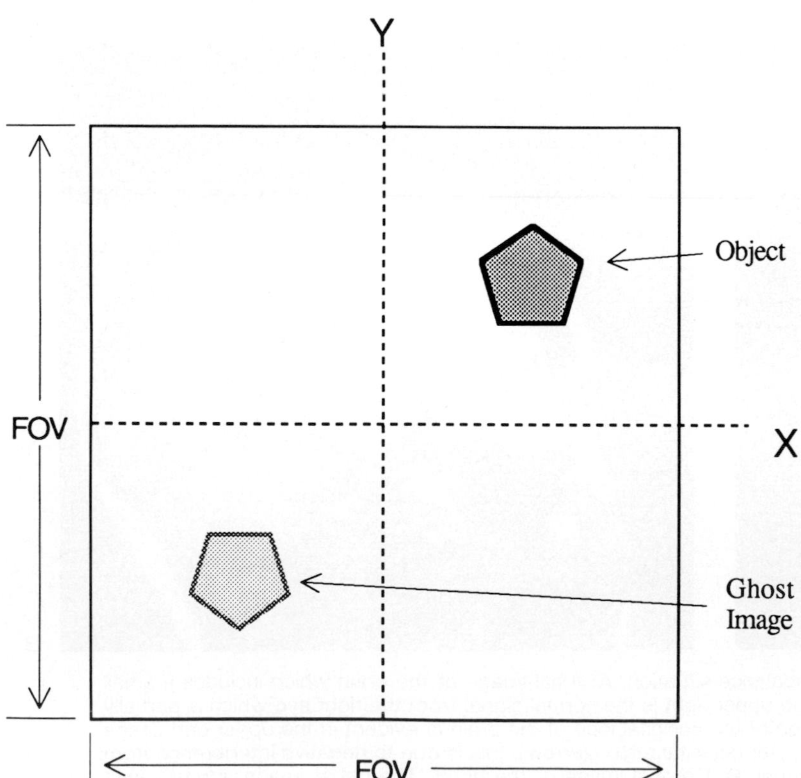

FIG. 21. Illustration of the results of receiver I/Q channel imbalance. A small imbalance creates a ghost image with both the x and y coordinates reversed. The result is a ghost image which is rotated 180° from the original.

This effect is demonstrated in Fig. 22. In part A, note the ghost image of the occipital region of the brain which appears artifactually in the upper right portion of this image. Of course, this implies that the entire image is polluted with its own ghost image artifact, so that each portion of the image contains the superimposition of both the true and ghost image. It is entirely possible that the phase of the ghost image can be reversed from that of the true image. In such a case, the ghost image signal will decrease, rather than increase, the true signal values. This effect can be seen in Fig. 22A, in the subtle dark spot seen in the occipital region. This dark spot is created by the strong orbit signal in the ghost image which is subtracting from the normal brain signal at that point.

Fig. 22B also shows this effect in a sagittal image. Again, the ghost image is rather weak and has its signal sign opposed to that of the true image; this explains the dark appearance of the ghosted scalp fat as it cuts through the cerebellum.

Since both aliasing and I/Q imbalance will cause ghost images, the reader should be careful not to confuse the two effects. I/Q imbalance causes a rotation of the image within the proper FOV, and is a purely instrumental problem which can always be corrected by appropriate repair of the equipment. The foldover produced by aliasing does not rotate the objects but rather brings into the FOV objects which are outside of it. The effect is inherent to the finite sampling used with the MRI process and is rarely due to equipment failure. A possible exception to this last statement would be a failure in the low pass analogue filter which would cause aliasing in the FE direction; this is easily correctable by proper adjustment and/or repair of the filter.

Phase Instability

This is undoubtedly one of the most common and troublesome instrumental errors, and usually results in either ghost images or a smearing of the image in the PE direction.

As explained in Chapter 2, the principle of phase encoding works by changing the PE gradient pulse amplitude in a systematic way between exciting pulses. The image is reconstructed by determining how the phase shift of the signal varies from pulse to pulse. The assumption of this method is that the only cause of phase shift between successive pulses is the changing of the PE gradient. This will be true as long as all other elements in the system, including the patient, are unchanging. If that is not true, then the phase of the signal will change in ways that have nothing to do with the value of the PE gradient, and the result will be serious errors of reconstruction as a function of position in the PE direction.

The cause of such errors could literally be anywhere in the system. However, the two most common sources are the gradient amplifiers and the rf transmitter.

The gradient amplifiers are high power, low frequency,

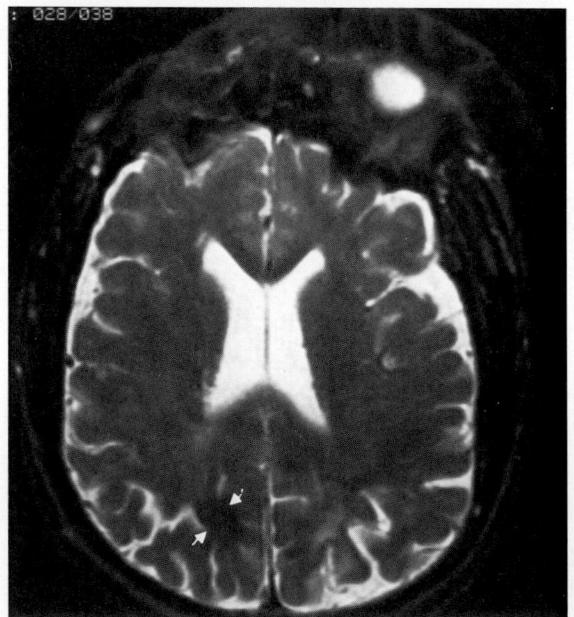

A

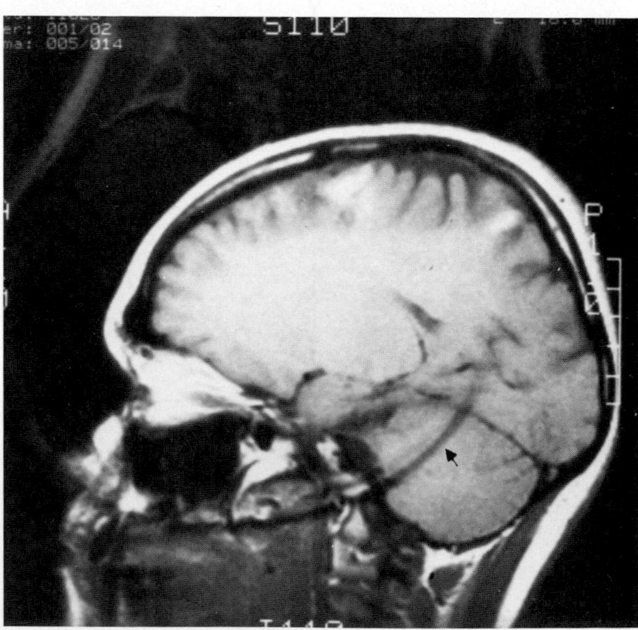

B

FIG. 22. Demonstration of a receiver I/Q imbalance situation. **A:** Axial image of the brain which includes a small portion of the right orbit. The bright spot in the upper right is the normal signal from the right eye which is partially volume averaged in this slice. The ghost image of the occipital lobe of the brain is evident in the upper part of the image. Note also the subtle dark spot in the lower occipital region (*arrow*): this is due to negative interference from the ghost component of the bright orbital signal. **B:** Coronal image of the head. The ghost image appears with reversed sign so that the scalp subcutaneous fat of the inverted ghost image appears as a dark line through the cerebellum. The neck muscles of the ghost image are faintly visible in the upper left corner of the image.

amplifiers which, under computer control, provide power to the three gradient coils. Because the coils are designed to produce a field gradient from current flowing in them, they are very sensitive to any extraneous or erroneous currents which may be applied. One source of trouble would be accidental pickup of unwanted low frequency noise. Indeed, in our highly electrified civilization we are constantly surrounded by electric and magnetic fields of frequency equal to that of the power lines (60 Hz in the United States, 50 Hz in Europe). For this reason all electronic equipment sensitive to such frequencies must be carefully shielded and decoupled from such fields. (This is often a problem in home audio systems, especially from the turntable which plays long playing records.) It must be emphasized that the gradient amplifiers in MRI systems are exquisitely sensitive to such noise, and require noise suppression at least as good as the highest quality home audio systems. Errors and noise in the gradient amplifiers can easily produce these artifacts. In fact, such errors were common in the first models of MRI machines brought to market in the early 1980s, which had inadequate digital precision in generating the PE pulses. The precision required for good quality images is roughly $1/N^2$, where N is the number of pixels across the FOV. For example, with $N = 256$ pixels, one needs a precision of about 1 part in 65,000. Such a precision, while not impossible technically, pushes the present state of electronic art to its limits. Indeed, to even verify that one's electronics are that precise requires measurement techniques considerably more sophisticated than are routinely available in electronic laboratories.

A less obvious source of phase noise is instability of the rf transmitter amplifier. This is usually a very high power device producing many kilowatts of power for use in the main "body" rf coil which surrounds the patient. In some cases, the power level is so high that water cooling is necessary. In any event, because of the high power required it is expensive and/or impractical to provide the regulation of power which would normally be provided to lower power systems. This implies that these units are susceptible to fluctuations in line voltage, such as might be produced by elevators or other electrical machinery. When this happens, the resulting variations is rf output and NMR flip angle, while fairly small, can induce significant changes in the detected signal. In this case the actual errors are probably related to rf amplitude rather than phase, but the result is still unwanted alterations in the received signal as a function of PE pulse number, so the artifacts usually appear as streaks in the PE direction.

An example of the effects of phase noise is shown in Fig. 23. The overall degeneration of image quality is obvious. Note there is significant signal level in the air outside of the head, but only in the PE direction. Since the

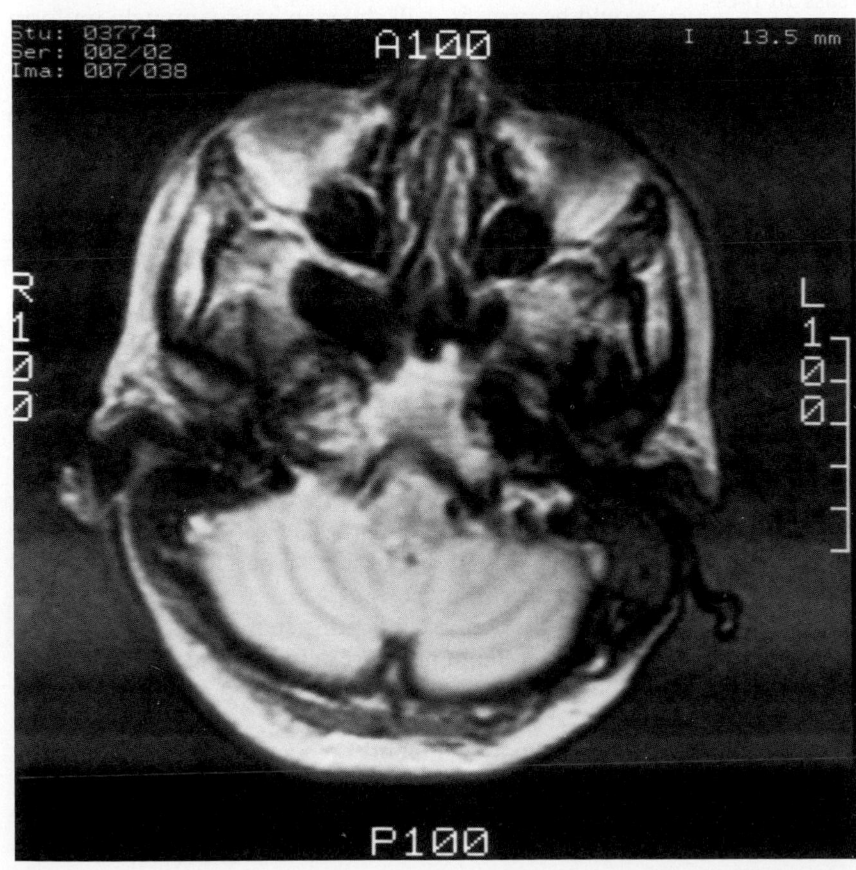

FIG. 23. Axial brain image with considerable phase noise, not due to patient motion. The PE direction is horizontal in this image. Note the considerable artifactual signal in the air outside the head in the PE direction. The dark border around the skin indicates that the ghost components have opposite phase from the true signal components in this case.

air signal is derived from the head, and not due to outside interference, we can conclude the problem is caused by phase noise. In addition to the artifactual signals, the image obviously suffers from a general degradation of sharpness and detail. Very commonly, the signal alterations due to phase noise are similar to those induced by patient motion, so that one finds a degree of blurring even when imaging static objects.

These effects are obviously highly dependent on the local environment in which the MRI machine operates. An extremely important practical question is whether the problem is caused by patient motion or by electronic instabilities. This can easily be answered by imaging an appropriate phantom, one whose spin density, T1, and T2 at least approximate those of human tissue. If artifactual signals are seen in the air surrounding the phantom, one can certainly conclude that the problem is not due to patient motion!

Receiver Overflow

Receiver overflow artifacts arise when the receiver gain, or sensitivity, is set so high that strong signals can overload the receiver electronics. Any electronic amplifier has a limited range of operation in terms of the maximum voltage level which it can properly accept and amplify. If it is given as input a voltage which exceeds this level, the result is usually a form of limiting, which means that the output voltage will not increase in proportion to the input voltage. In fact, as illustrated in Fig. 24, the output voltage quite commonly will "saturate", meaning that there is no further increase in output voltage as the input voltage is increased. Such a situation is obviously highly undesirable, and all MRI systems must provide some means of adjusting the input signal level and/or receiver gain so as to avoid this. If an error, whether human or electronic, is made, the result will be

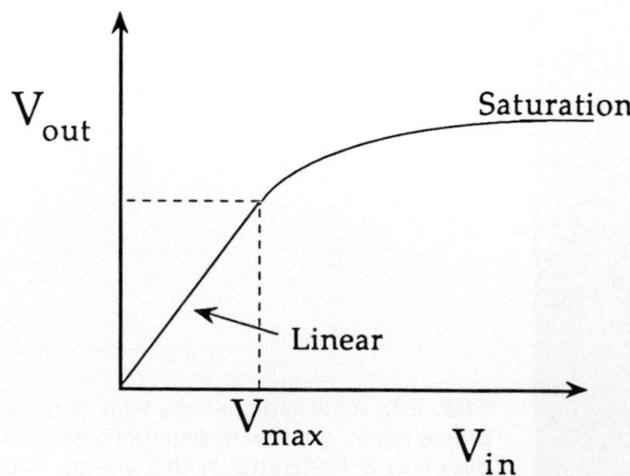

FIG. 24. Illustration of the phenomenon of receiver limitation and saturation. Ideally, the output voltage, V_{out}, would be proportional to the input voltage, V_{in}. This is true up to a certain maximum voltage, beyond which the output voltage saturates.

a class of artifacts in the image which we shall now attempt to clarify.

The problem is obviously most severe when the received signals are strongest. During the course of an imaging scan, the strength of the signals varies greatly as a function of the strength of the phase-encoding gradient. Since the purpose of the PE gradient is to dephase the spins as a function of spatial position, the signal usually gets weaker as the PE gradient strength is increased. This implies that the maximum signal will be received when the PE gradient is zero, i.e., when the system is encoding the $k_y = 0$ line in k-space (see Chapter 2). For the same reason, for a given k_y the signal is usually strongest when all of the spins are in phase with respect to the x spatial coordinate, i.e., at $k_x = 0$. In summary, at the exact center of k-space, with $k_x = k_y = 0$, the signal will have its greatest strength. Therefore, the most likely result of an overloaded receiver is to suppress the strength of this particular spatial frequency signal.

It is not difficult to understand the effect of this distortion if we remember the significance of zero spatial frequency: it represents a constant, uniform signal strength in space with no variation over the imaged plane. This means that the $k = 0$ vector represents the average strength of the signal for the entire image. If we imagine that only this $k = 0$ point is bad, the result will be an image with no obvious artifact except for an overall raising or lowering of the MRI pixel numbers. This would imply that the air background, where normally no signal would be present, will show an approximately uniform background signal level.

Unfortunately, it can happen that the receiver is adjusted so that signals other than those corresponding to the exact center of k space are also distorted. Nevertheless, it is almost always true that the k-values most likely to be affected are those of low spatial frequency, for example, 1 to 2 cycles per FOV. In this case, one will see shading artifacts which vary in a smooth way from one side of the image to another.

An example is shown in Fig. 25, which shows two coronal images which are identical except, in part B, the receiver attenuator was deliberately misset to create receiver overload. For the pulse parameters used here, the brain signal should be considerably brighter than muscle. In part B, note the halo of increased signal intensity in the air surrounding the head, as well as the artifactually low signal values in the upper part of the image and higher values in the lower. Note the absence of any geometrical distortion, indicating that the vast majority of high spatial frequencies are being received correctly.

Spatial Versus Temporal Frequency Errors

We have seen that many of the common artifacts are due to errors of a certain "frequency," either spatial or

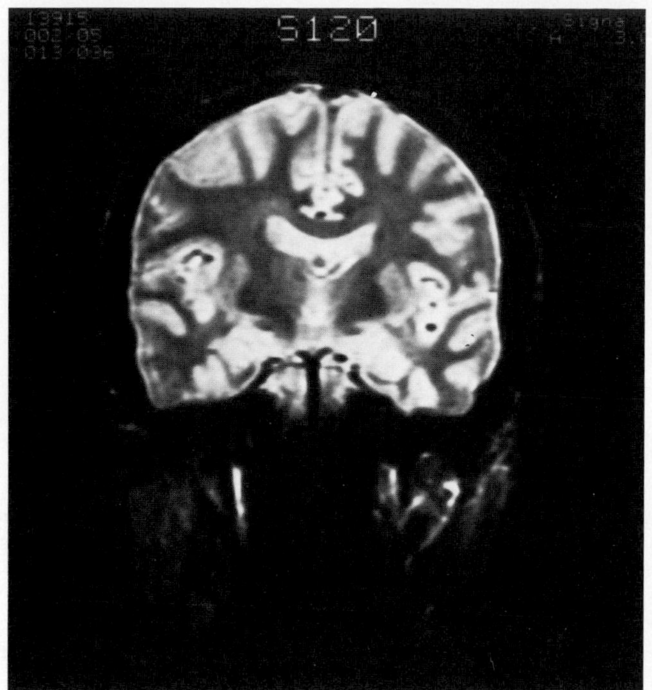

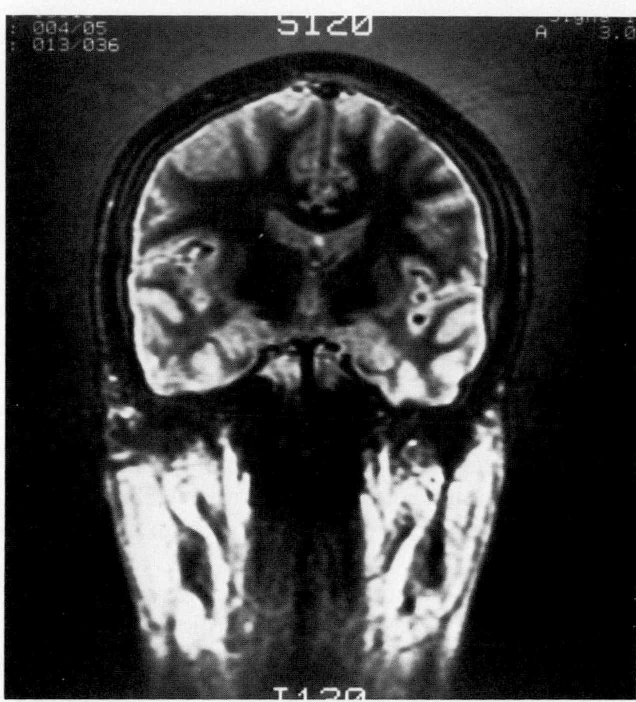

A B

FIG. 25. Demonstration of the effect of overloading the receiver. **A:** Long TR, TE coronal image of the brain made with proper receiver attenuator settings. **B:** Result of deliberate missetting of the receiver gain so as to produce saturation of the low spatial frequency signals. Note the increased signal in the air above the head ("halo"), as well as the dramatic alterations in signal strength from the top to the bottom of the image, resulting in decreased reconstructed signal from the superior cerebral structures and increased signal from the infratemporal muscles.

temporal. The distinction between these two kinds of frequency is often confusing to people who are not expert in the physics of MRI. As explained in Chapter 2, the MR signal, at any given time t, is a measure of a specific spatial frequency. The image, on the other hand, is obtained by Fourier transformation and so represents the temporal frequency distribution. For example, the DC offset error is a specific temporal frequency (zero) and so appears at a specific spot (the center) of the image. The receiver overload problem typically occurs at a specific time during the scan and so represents a specific spatial frequency (namely, $k_x = k_y = 0$); therefore its effect is seen over the entire image. If these distinctions are understood and kept in mind, many of these artifacts are easily recognized and understood.

A particularly dramatic example of an artifact at a specific spatial frequency occurs when a single "spike" of noise occurs in the receiver electronics; it will obviously affect only the spatial frequency active during the spike. The result is a "herring bone" artifact (70).

MOTION AND PULSATION ARTIFACTS

It is well known that patient motion can induce significant artifacts in MR images. Usually, this problem is much more severe in the body below the neck than in the brain, since that latter is usually firmly supported within the scanner. However, certain pulse sequences are exceptionally sensitive to even subtle motion, such as that found in major blood vessels or the CSF. It is important to understand that the nature of artifact produced by motion in MRI is completely different from what is encountered in other imaging techniques, such as radiography, ultrasound, etc. These differences stem from the fact that the MR image is not obtained directly but is reconstructed using Fourier transformation from measurements in k-space. Thus a full understanding of these artifacts involves Fourier transform mathematics which is beyond the scope of this book. However, we shall here attempt to explain the qualitative appearance of the artifacts assuming the reader has some understanding of the way in which MR images are reconstructed.

Simple Motion Blurring

If a body, or a portion of a body, is moving at velocity v for time t, then it will experience a displacement of amount

$$D = vt. \quad [12]$$

Since some MRI techniques require several minutes for scanning, it is not surprising that for some body parts D can be visually appreciable, i.e, on the order of a millimeter or more. This will necessarily appear as a blurring of magnitude D in the direction of motion. This purely kinematic argument is so basic that it applies to all imaging techniques, and is commonly called "motion blurring" in other areas of radiologic imaging. In those cases where the motion is periodic or driven by cardiac or pulmonary function, it can be reduced or eliminated by gating the data acquisition process so that the organ in question is always at the same location in space when scan data is acquired.

Certainly, motion blurring will be a part of the problem of motion artifacts in MRI, and when it is cardiac or pulmonary gating can usually mitigate it. The main problem with gating is that one loses control over the *timing* of the rf pulses, i.e., TR is determined by the patients physiologic function rather than by electronic circuits. For T1-weighted imaging or other techniques in which TR is important, this may not be an acceptable option.

Here we want to emphasize that simple motion blurring is a very minor aspect of the motion problem in MRI. The main problem comes from subtle changes in signal *phase* that are induced by the motion, and these lead to an entirely new class of artifacts, some of which can be "ghost" images.

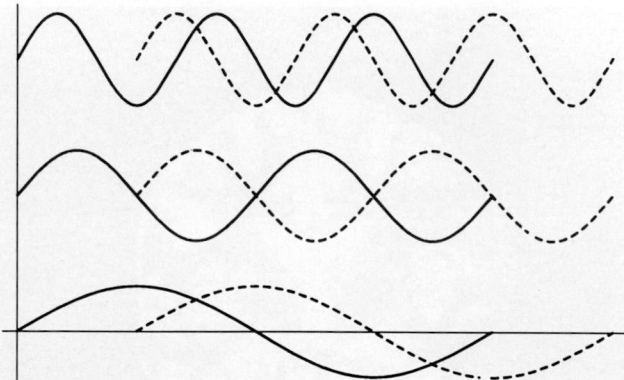

FIG. 26. Illustration of the principle of the shift theorem. Each dotted wave is shifted by the same amount from its corresponding solid wave. The frequencies of the waves are in the ratio of 1: 2:3 (*from bottom to top*). The corresponding phase shifts are 90°, 180°, and 270° for the bottom, middle, and top waves, respectively. This shows how a simple displacement results in phase shift being proportional to frequency.

Periodic Motion and Ghost Images

We saw above that many instrumental phase errors produce artifacts in the form of streaks in the phase-encoding direction. Since these errors were assumed to be random, the effects in the images are usually nonspecific. However, here we need to understand the effect of a phase error which is not random but is varying in some systematic way from one excitation to the next. The source of such motion is usually either cardiac or pulmonary function.

There are several ways to analyze this problem and they all lead to the prediction of a set of shifted or "ghost" images. The mathematical principle behind this effect stems from what is called the "shift theorem," namely, that whenever the phase shift is proportional to frequency the result is a shifted object. We shall not attempt to derive that result mathematically, but its significance is easily grasped from Fig. 26. There we see an example of six different sine waves which fall into two groups. The solid line waves all start at position $x = 0$, while the dotted line curves are all shifted by the same distance along the x axis. There are three frequencies of wave illustrated, corresponding to frequencies $f = 1$, 2, and 3 (cycles per unit length). Note that the corresponding *phase shifts* for the three sets of waves are 90°, 180°, and 270°, respectively. In other words, the phase shifts are in each case proportional to the frequency of the corresponding wave. The converse of this argument is also true, i.e., *whenever we find a phase shift proportional to frequency the result is equivalent to a net displacement of all of the waves.*

To apply this insight to the problem of MRI, we need only suppose that the phase shift is proportional to the spatial frequency, e.g., k_y. In that case, we would expect the image to appear shifted in the y (PE) direction after image reconstruction.

Actually, it rarely happens in such a simple way. More typically, some parts of the patient's body may be perfectly stationary while other parts are undergoing some sort of cyclic motion. In the case of cyclic motion, the phase shift will not simply increase with time but will oscillate in some complex manner. In this case one gets a mixture of the original, unshifted image as well as one or more ghost images.

In this context, we can focus our attention on a single (typical) voxel which spans the border between two dissimilar tissues, both of which are moving. For example in the chest the tissues might be the chest wall and edge of the lung; in the brain they might be a blood vessel and the surrounding parenchyma. Due to the pulsatile motion, the signal emitted from that voxel will vary periodically with time. Let us begin by assuming that the signal varies in accordance with a simple sine wave with frequency f; i.e., f is the frequency of physiologic motion. The signal could vary with regard to either amplitude, phase, or phase dispersion. An example of amplitude variations would be the case where the two tissue types have different signal strengths (e.g., due to T1 or T2 differences). As the two tissues move into and out of the voxel in question, its signal strength varies in a cyclic way. An example of phase variation would be the phase shift induced by flowing blood or CSF, which, as explained in Chapter 4, gives a phase shift which is velocity-dependent and so varies during the cardiac cycle. Finally, a variation in phase dispersion will occur if there is a *mix-*

ture of velocities within the voxel, as there usually is at the edges of blood vessels due to the "shear" in velocity within the vessel lumen. If the pulse sequence is not flow compensated, the result is a variation in effective signal amplitude for that voxel. (An example of this phenomenon is discussed in Chapter 4.)

The phase shifts induced by motion are always the result of motion or flow along the direction of one of the gradients used for imaging. In the normal 2DFT MR pulse sequence with a single echo, the phase shift is dependent on the velocity along any of the three gradient axes; however, the most critical are usually the slice selection or the frequency-encoding direction. The pulse sequence can be modified using the principle of gradient moment nulling (71), which is exactly the same technique used for flow compensation (FC) in flow imaging; this is discussed in more detail in Chapter 4. Other terms for this technique are "MAST" (72) and "gradient rephasing" (73). Alternatively, since the second echo is normally less sensitive to flow and velocity, it may show less motion artifact. These methods are designed to work when the motion has constant velocity, so in practice the result may not be total elimination of artifact with pulsatile motion particularly when long echo times are used. An alternate method which is effective for long echo times and is not limited to motion with constant velocity has also been published (74).

The mathematics of ghost image generation is very subtle (75,76) and we can only outline some of the more important aspects in this chapter. First, it is important to understand that regardless of the source of the signal variation, *the result is always an error propagated along the phase-encoded direction.* For example even if the motion is along the frequency-encoded direction, the ghost image(s) will be displaced along the PE direction. Furthermore, the ghost image is almost never a simple duplicate of the original image; often, only the *edges* of the structures in the original image appear (76). The reason can be understood from the following argument. Suppose one were imaging a strictly homogeneous phantom which is moving slightly. Then only those voxels near the edge of the phantom will experience any variation in signal; the central voxels will experience no signal alteration since any material lost due to motion (outflow) is automatically replaced with equivalent material flowing in. Second, *the structures experiencing variable signals will appear to be displaced in the image along the phase-encoded direction by amount:*

$$\Delta y = f \, \mathrm{TR} \, \mathrm{FOV}. \qquad [13]$$

where f = frequency of mechanical motion, and TR and FOV have their usual meanings. Notice that the distance through which the voxel appears displaced *depends on the frequency and not on the amplitude of motion.* Of course, it is intuitively obvious that large amplitude motions are in some sense worse than small amplitude motions. However, in this case the amplitude of the motion determines the *strength* of the signal as it appears in the ghost image, and not its displacement. That is, if one could somehow reduce the amplitude of motion, the result would be a weaker ghost image in the same place as with the stronger motion. If the motion amplitude is reduced to zero, the intensity of the ghost image diminishes to zero.

Equation 13 must be understood in the context of image aliasing (or "foldover") as discussed previously. For example, if the product of f and TR is exactly unity, then Δy = FOV, which really means that the ghost image reappears exactly on top of the original image (77). Expressed more prosaically, in that case one would say there is no ghost image. This is understood by noting that if f*TR = 1 then the motion and the TR pulse interval are synchronized so that the motion always places the body in the same position at the moment of NMR excitation; this is the principle of gating.

Complex Motion

Obviously, most physiologic motion is not purely sinusoidal. For one thing there is always an average value around which the signal varies. This average value is not changing with time and so determines the normal, undisplaced image. Furthermore, cardiac pulsation is not well described by a simple sine wave. However, in accordance with the basic theorem of Fourier analysis, we can always regard any *periodic* motion as composed of a "fundamental" frequency with "harmonics." (In the area of acoustics and hearing, this concept is widely understood.) We can still apply the shift theorem (Equation 13) to each component frequency. The result is an infinite set of ghost images, usually equally spaced with respect to the original, undisplaced, image. Of course, there is not room in our image display matrix for an infinite set of images, so they will "alias," or fold over, as explained previously. The result is often a confusing set of overlapping ghost images distributed along the PE direction in what appears to be a random manner.

Mitigation of Motion Artifacts

Although the basic motion blurring cannot be eliminated without some sort of gating, there are steps that can be taken to reduce the problem. The most straightforward is the use of "flow compensation" (FC), as discussed in Chapter 4. The goal of FC is to make phase shift independent of velocity. Since ghost images are partially caused by motion-induced phase errors, this will often reduce the intensity of the ghost images. However, flow compensation usually is designed to work only with motion of constant velocity, so that it cannot be completely effective with motion that is periodic. A clinical example of the effectiveness of FC for reducing ghost images can be seen in Chapter 4.

Demonstration of Ghost Images

Figure 27 shows an experiment on a moving phantom published by Joseph et al. (74). In this experiment, the phantom is moving a small amount (less than 10% of its diameter) along the frequency-encoding axis, which is horizontal in this image. In Fig. 27A, we see the image made using gating, which shows no motion-induced artifacts. When gating was disabled, as in parts B and C, one sees ghost images propagating along the phase-encoding axis. The pulse sequence used in part B is a conventional 2DFT with a rather long echo time (100 ms). Under such conditions, the signal phase is strongly influenced by motion occurring between excitation and readout. The actual amount of phase error depends on the magnitude of the motion-induced displacement and is random because the motion and NMR pulsing are not synchronized. The result is a major loss of desired signal in the true image and a group of blurred ghost images. In part C, the pulse sequence was modified in a manner similar to FC so that motion-induced phase shifts were greatly reduced. (The technique reduced phase shifts from all types of motion, not just motion with constant velocity. see ref. 74 for more details.) This virtually eliminated phase errors in the spin-echo signal; however, amplitude errors due to material at the edges of the phantom moving in and out of the voxels obviously persist. The result is blurring at the horizontal edges of the true image, as well as a "clean" set of ghost images in which only the horizontal edges are visible. This demonstrates that once phase errors are cleaned up with FC, ghost images are still possible at the borders of dissimilar materials which are in motion. That is, whereas uncontrolled phase errors occur for all regions of the phantom (Fig. 27B), magnitude errors occur only at the edges where the inflow/outflow effect takes place (Fig. 27C).

A clinical example of motion-induced ghosting is shown in Fig. 28. In this examination intravenous gadolinium contrast as well as flow compensation was used so that major blood vessels are expected to produce a strong signal. Despite the use of FC, one sees ghost images of the venous sinus projected over the cerebellum. Because of FC we can assume that phase errors are small if not negligible, so that the ghost images are being produced by the modulation of the amplitude of the signal due to normal vascular pulsation. This modulation could be due to gross movement of the blood vessel, but is more likely due to two more subtle effects. First, the degree of signal enhancement with flow is dependent on the flow

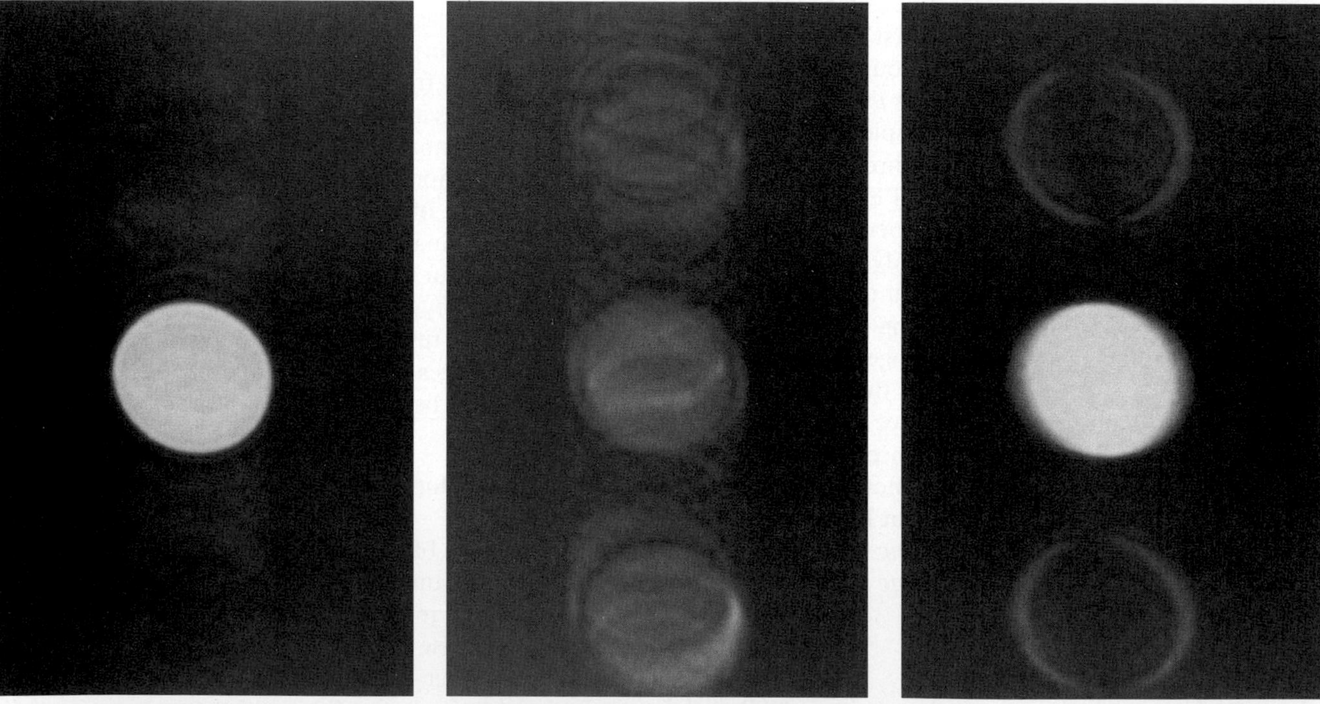

FIG. 27. Images of a simple phantom undergoing oscillatory motion in the horizontal (FE) direction. The amplitude of motion is less than 10% of the phantom's diameter. **A:** The NMR pulse sequence is gated to the motion so the image shows the phantom without artifact. **B:** With no gating, the motion induces a complex variation in signal phase due to the *x*-gradient pulses used, which diminishes the strength of the central image and creates multiple ghost images. **C:** Again without gating but using a modified *x*-gradient pulse sequence with much less motion-dependent phase shift. This greatly reduces the ghost artifacts due to phase shift, but the edges of the phantom persist in the ghosts due to amplitude variation.

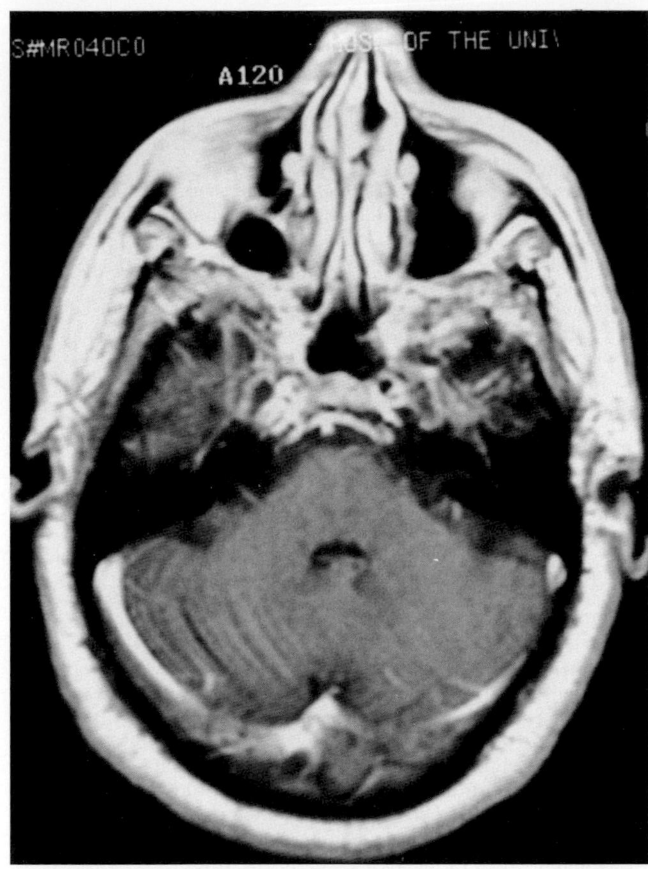

FIG. 28. Clinical image showing ghost artifacts due to the pulsation of blood within a blood vessel. This image was obtained using flow compensated spin echo with TR/TE = 750/24 ms. Despite the use of FC, artifacts are generated by the flow-induced modulation of the amplitude of signal within the lumen of the sinus. The ghost artifacts are projected over the brain parenchyma.

velocity (the so-called wash-in effect) so velocity variations will lead to signal variations within the lumen of the vessel. Second, it is possible that due to pressure variations the size of the vessel changes; this leads to major changes in signal for those pixels which straddle the edge of the lumen. In either case, the artifacts generated are associated with the *edges* of the lumen of the vessel. This is apparent in Fig. 28 since the ghost artifacts are generally much thinner than the vessel itself.

ARTIFACTS IN FAST SCANNING

By "fast scanning" here we mean any technique in which multiple excitations are used with very short TR. In this case, TR is usually significantly less than T2 for many tissues, so that the transverse component of nuclear magnetization will not decay to zero between excitations. This leads to a set of phenomena known as steady state free precession (SSFP). This presents a problem for MRI because we normally need to assume that each excitation represents a line in k-space which is independent of the preceding line; failure to achieve this will mix signals from various k values and create artifacts. The effect is especially important in three-dimensional imaging (78). Naively, one might try to suppress this effect by using "spoiler" gradient pulses between excitations, hoping that these will dephase the previously existing spins. Unfortunately, the SSFP process tends to counter this strategy. In particular, since the SSFP signal depends strongly on the phase shift, there will always be some spins whose phase shift is such as to give a stronger signal than others. For example, if there is (an inevitable) background gradient due to magnet inhomogeneity, the result will be bands of light and dark signal within the image. This effect can be mitigated by using exceptionally strong spoiler gradient pulses applied along the slice thickness axis. A better technique is to use random phases on the exciting pulses, which prevents the buildup of large SSFP magnetization. These techniques are discussed more fully in Chapter 29.

REFERENCES

1. Bellon EM, Haacke EM, Coleman PE, Sacco DC, Steiger DA, Gangarosa RE. MR artifacts: a review. *AJR* 1986;147:1271–1281.
2. Joseph PM. A spin echo chemical shift imaging technique. *J Comput Assist Tomogr* 1985;9:651–658.
3. Brateman L. Chemical shift imaging: a review. *AJR* 1986;146:971–980.
4. Dixon WT. Simple proton spectroscopic imaging. *Radiology* 1984;153:189–194.
5. Poon CS, Szumowski J, Plewes DB, Ashby P, Henkelman RM. Fat/water quantitation and differential relaxation time measurement using chemical shift imaging technique. *Magn Reson Imaging* 1989;7:369–382.
6. Joseph PM, Shetty A. A comparison of selective saturation and selective echo chemical shift imaging techniques. *Magn Reson Imaging* 1988;6:421–430.
7. Frahm J, Haase A, Hanicke W, Matthaei D, Bomsdorf H, Helzel T. Chemical shift selective MR imaging using a whole-body magnet. *Radiology* 1985;156:441–444.
8. Rosen BR, Wedeen VJ, Brady TJ. Selective saturation NMR imaging. *J Comput Assist Tomogr* 1984;8:813–818.
9. Daniels DL, Kneeland JB, Shimakawa A, Pojunas KW, Schenck JF, Hart H, Foster T, Williams AL, Haughton VM. MR imaging of the optic nerve and sheath: correcting the chemical shift misregistration effect. *AJNR* 1986;7:249–253.
10. Enzmann D, Augustyn GT. Improved MR images of the brain with use of a gated, flow-compensated, variable-bandwidth pulse sequence. *Radiology* 1989;172:777–781.
11. Smith RC, Lange RC, McCarthy SM. Chemical shift artifact: dependence on shape and orientation of the lipid-water interface. *Radiology* 1991;181:225–229.
12. Smith AS, Weinstein MA, Hurst GC, DeRemer DR, Cole RA, Duchesneau PM. Intracranial chemical-shift artifacts on MR images of the brain: observations and relation to sampling bandwidth. *AJR* 1990;154:1275–1283.
13. Luedeke KM, Roeschmann P, Tischler R. Susceptibility artifacts in NMR imaging. *Magn Reson Imaging* 1985;3:329–343.
14. Park HW, Ro YM, Cho ZH. Measurement of the magnetic susceptibility effect in high-field NMR imaging. *Phys Med Biol* 1988;33:339–349.
15. Posse S, Aue WP. Susceptibility artifacts in spin-echo and gradient-echo imaging. *J Magn Reson* 1990;88:473–492.
16. Frahm J, Merboldt KD, Hanicke W. Direct FLASH MR imaging of magnetic field inhomogeneities by gradient compensation. *Magn Reson Med* 1988;6:474–480.

17. Schick RM, Wismer GL, Davis KR. Magnetic susceptibility effects secondary to out-of-plane air in fast MR scanning. *AJNR* 1988;9:439–442.
18. Teitelbaum GP, Bradley WG, Klein BD. MR imaging artifacts, ferromagnetism, and magnetic tourque of intravascular filters, stents, and coils. *Radiology* 1988;166:657–664.
19. Bakker CJG, Moerland MA, Bhagwandien R, Beersma R. Analysis of machine-dependent and object-induced geometrical distortion in 2DFT MR imaging. *Magn Reson Imaging* 1992;10:597–608.
20. Rubin DL, Ratner AV, Young SW. Magnetic susceptibility effects and their application in the development of new ferromagnetic catheters for magnetic resonance imaging. *Invest Radiol* 1990;25:1325–1332.
21. Lissac M, Metrop D, Brugirard J, Coudert JL, Pimmel P, Briguet A, Revel D, Amiel M. Dental materials and magnetic resonance imaging. *Invest Radiol* 1991;26:40–45.
22. Shellock FG, Curtis JS. MR imaging and biomedical implants, materials, and devices: an updated review. *Radiology* 1991;180:541–550.
23. Michiels J, Bosmans H, Pelgrims P, Vandermeulen D, Gybels J, Marchal G, Suetens P. On the problem of geometric distortion in magnetic resonance images for stereotactic neurosurgery. *Magn Reson Imaging* 1994;12:749–765.
24. Bakker CJG, Bhagwandien R, Moerland MA, Ramos LMP. Simulation of susceptibility artifacts in 2D and 3D Fourier transform spin-echo and gradient-echo magnetic resonance imaging. *Magn Reson Imaging* 1994;12:767–774.
25. Tien RD, Buxton RB, Schwaighofer BW, Chu PK. Quantification of structural distortion of the cervical neural foramina in gradient-echo MR imaging. *J Magn Reson Imaging* 1991;1:683–687.
26. Lufkin R, Jordan S, Lylyck P, Vinuela F. MR imaging with topographic EEG electrodes in place. *AJNR* 1988;9:953–954.
27. Sattin W, Mareci TH, Scott KN. Exploiting the stimulated echo in nuclear magnetic resonance imaging. I. Method. *J Magn Reson* 1985;64:177–182.
28. Haase A, Frahm J. NMR imaging of spin-lattice relaxation using stimulated echoes. *J Magn Reson* 1985;65:481–490.
29. Haase A, Frahm J, Matthaei D, Haenicke W, Bomsdorf H, Kunz D, Tischler R. MR imaging using stimulated echoes (STEAM). *Radiology* 1986;160:787–790.
30. Barker GJ, Mareci TH. Suppression of artifacts in multiple-echo magnetic resonance. *J Magn Reson* 1989;83:11–28.
31. Crawley AP, Henkleman RM. A stimulated echo artifact from slice interference in magnetic resonance imaging. *Med Phys* 1987;14:842–848.
32. Crawley AP, Henkelman RM. Errors in T2 estimation using multislice multiple-echo imaging. *Magn Reson Med* 1987;4:34–47.
33. Joseph PM. Critical review:"interactions of paramagnetic contrast agents and the spin-echo pulse sequence." *Invest Radiol* 1989;24:508–509.
34. Smith AS, Hurst GC, Duerk JL, Diaz PJ. MR of ballistic materials: imaging artifacts and potential hazards. *AJNR* 1991;12:567–572.
35. Atlas SW, Grossman RI, Hackney DB, Gomori JM, Campagna N, Goldberg HI, Bilaniuk LT, Zimmerman RA. Calcified intracranial lesions: detection with gradient-echo-acquisition rapid MR imaging. *AJNR* 1988;9:253–259.
36. Kim JK, Kucharczyk W, Henkelman MR. Cavernous hemangiomas: Dipolar susceptibility artifacts at MR imaging. *Radiology* 1993;187:735–741.
37. Young IR, Cox IJ, Bryant DJ, Bydder GM. The benefits of increasing spatial resolution as a means of reducing artifacts due to field inhomogeneities. *Magn Reson Imaging* 1988;6:585–590.
38. Watanabe AT, Teitlebaum GP, Lufkin RB, Tsuruda JS, Jinkins JR, Bradley WG. Gradient-echo MR imaging of the lumbar spine: comparison with spin-echo technique. *J Comput Assist Tomogr* 1990;14:410–414.
39. Watanabe AT, Teitlebaum GP, Gomes AS, Roehm JOF. MR imaging of the bird's nest filter. *Radiology* 1990;177:578–579.
40. Rupp R, Ebraheim NA, Savolaine ER, Jackson WT. Magnetic resonance imaging evaluation of the spine with metal implants. *Spine* 1993;18:379–385.
41. Peterman SB, Hoffman JC, Malko JA. Magnetic resonance artifact in the postoperative cervical spine. *Spine* 1991;16:721–725.
42. Levitt M, Benjamin V, Kricheff II. Potential misinterpretation of cervical spondylosis with cord compression caused by metallic artifacts in magnetic resonance imaging of the post operative spine. *Neurosurgery* 1990;27:126–129.
43. Tartaglino LM, Flanders AE, Vinitski S. Metallic artifacts on MR images of the postoperative spine: reduction with fast spin-echo techniques. *Radiology* 1994;190:565–569.
44. Wehrli FW, Perkins TG, Shimakawa A, Roberts F. Chemical shift-induced amplitude modulations in images obtained with gradient refocusing. *Magn Reson Imaging* 1987;5:157–158.
45. Mansfield P, Pykett IL. Biological and medical imaging by NMR. *J Magn Reson* 1978;29:355–373.
46. Ogawa S, Lee TM, Nayak AS, Glynn P. Oxygenation-sensitive contrast in magnetic resonance image of rodent brain at high magnetic fields. *Magn Reson Med* 1990;14:68–78.
47. Menon RS, Ogawa S, Tank DW, Ugurbil K. 4 Tesla gradient recalled echo characteristics of photic stimulation-induced signal changes in the human primary visual cortex. *Magn Reson Med* 1993;30:380–386.
48. Mulkern RV, Melki PS, Jakab P, Higuchi N, Jolesz FA. Phase-encode order and its effect on contrast and artifact in single-shot RARE sequences. *Med Phys* 1991;18:1032–1037.
49. Listerud J, Einstein S, Outwater E, Kressel HY. First principles of fast spin echo. *Magn Reson Q* 1992;8:199–244.
50. Farzaneh F, Reiderer SJ, Pelc NJ. Analysis of T2 limitations and off-resonance effects on spatial resolution and artifacts in echo-planar imaging. *Magn Reson Med* 1990;14:123–139.
51. Cohen MS, Weisskopf RM. Ultra-fast imaging. *Magn Reson Imaging* 1991;9:1–37.
52. Blamire AM, Ogawa S, Ugurbil K, Rothman D, McCarthy G, Ellermann JM, Hyder F, Rattner Z, Schulman RG. Dynamic mapping of the human visual cortex by high-speed magnetic resonance imaging. *Proc Natl Acad Sci USA* 1992;89:11069–11073.
53. Feinberg DA, Turner R, Jakab PD, Kienlin Mv. Echo-planar imaging with asymmetric gradient modulation and inner-volume excitation. *Magn Reson Med* 1990;13:162–169.
54. Bracewell RN. *The Fourier Transform and Its Applications.* New York: McGraw Hill; 1978:189–215.
55. Haacke EM. The effects of finite sampling in spin-echo or field-echo magnetic resonance imaging. *Magn Reson Med* 1987;4:407–421.
56. Lufkin RB, Pusey E, Stark DD, Brown R, Leikind B, Hanafee WN. Boundary artifacts due to truncation errors in MR imaging. *AJR* 1986;147:1283–1287.
57. Levy LM, Di Chiro G, Brooks RA, Dwyer AJ, Wener L, Frank J. Spinal cord artifacts from truncation errors during MR imaging. *Radiology* 1988;166:479–483.
58. Turner DA, Rapoport MI, Erwin WD, McGould M, Silvers RI. Truncation artifact: a potential pitfall in MR imaging of the menisci of the knee. *Radiology* 1991;179:629–633.
59. Czervionke LF, Czervionke JM, Daniels DL, Haughton VM. Characteristic features of MR truncation artifacts. *AJNR* 1988;9:815–824.
60. Joseph PM, Stockham CD. The influence of modulation transfer function shape on computed tomographic image quality. *Radiology* 1982;145:179–185.
61. Bronskill MJ, McVeigh ER, Kucharczyk W, Henkelman RM. Syrinx-like artifacts on MR images of the spinal cord. *Radiology* 1988;166:485–488.
62. Amartur S, Liang ZP, Boada F, Haacke EM. Phase-constrained data extrapolation method for reduction of truncation artifacts. *J Magn Reson Imaging* 1991;1:721–724.
63. Constable RT, Henkleman RM. Data extrapolation for truncation artifact removal. *Magn Reson Med* 1991;17:108–118.
64. Pusey E, Yoon C, Anselmo ML, Lufkin RB. Aliasing artifacts in MR imaging. *Comput Med Imag Graphics* 1988;12:219–224.
65. Conturo TE, Price RR, Beth AH. Rapid local rectangular views and magnifications: Reduced phase encoding of othogonally excited spin echoes. *Magn Reson Med* 1988;6:418–429.
66. Van Hecke PE, Marchal GJ, Baert AL. Use of shielding to prevent folding in MR imaging. *Radiology* 1988;167:557–558.
67. den Boef JH, van Uijen CMJ, Holzscherer CD. Multiple-slice NMR imaging by three-dimensional Fourier zeugmatography. *Phys Med Biol* 1984;29:857–867.

68. Szumowski J, Plewes DB. Separation of lipid and water MR imaging signals by chopper averaging in the time domain. *Radiology* 1987;165:247–250.
69. Bogdan AR, Joseph PM. RASEE: a rapid spin-echo pulse sequence. *Magn Reson Imaging* 1990;8:13–19.
70. Foo TKF, Grigsby NS, Mitchell JD, Slayman BE. SNORE: Spike noise removal and detection. *IEEE Trans Med Imaging* 1994;13:133–136.
71. Pattany PM, Phillips JL, Chiu LC, Lipcamon JD, Duerk JL, McNally JM, Mohapatra SN. Motion artifact suppression technique (MAST) for MR imaging. *J Comput Assist Tomogr* 1987;11:369–377.
72. Colletti PM, Raval JK, Benson RC, Pattany PM, Zee CS, Boswell WD, Norris SL, Ralls PW, Segall HD. The motion artifact suppression technique (MAST) in magnetic resonance imaging: clinical results. *Magn Reson Imaging* 1988;6:293–299.
73. Rubin JB, Wright A, Enzmann DR. Lumbar spine: motion compensation for cerebrospinal fluid on MR imaging. *Radiology* 1988;166:225–231.
74. Joseph PM, Shetty A, Bonaroti EA. A method for reducing motion induced errors in T2-weighted magnetic resonance imaging. *Med Phys* 1987;14:608–615.
75. Wood ML, Henkelman RM. MR image artifacts from periodic motion. *Med Phys* 1985;12:143–151.
76. Haacke EM, Patrick JL. Reducing motion artifacts in two-dimensional Fourier transform imaging. *Magn Reson Imaging* 1986;4:359–376.
77. Haacke EM, Lenz GW, Nelson AD. Pseudo-gating: elimination of periodic motion artifacts in magnetic resonance imaging without gating. *Magn Reson Med* 1987;4:162–174.
78. Wood ML, Runge VM. Artifacts due to residual magnetization in three-dimensional magnetic resonance imaging. *Med Phys* 1988;15:825–831.

Magnetic Resonance Imaging of the Brain and Spine, Second Edition, edited by Scott W. Atlas. Lippincott-Raven Publishers, Philadelphia © 1996.

8

Disorders of Brain Development

Charles L. Truwit and A. James Barkovich

BRAIN DEVELOPMENT

Like all of human embryology, the brain develops in a very orderly fashion. Under normal circumstances, the neural tube closes on approximately the 24th day of gestation. After such closure, the prosencephalon, at the rostral end of the neural tube, divides into the diencephalon (future thalami, hypothalamus, and globi pallidi) and the telencephalon (future cerebral hemispheres, putamina, and caudate nuclei). Cells arising from the germinal matrix along the walls of the telencephalic ventricle will migrate away from the ependymal surface of the ventricle to form the cortical mantle (Fig. 1); cells arising in the diencephalic germinal matrix (in the wall of the future third ventricle) will give rise to the deep gray nuclei mentioned above (Fig. 2). As the cerebral hemispheres grow, they spread dorsally and laterally to cover the diencephalic structures, midbrain, and portions of the rhombencephalon in the posterior fossa.

C. L. Truwit, M.D.: Departments of Radiology and Neurology, University of Minnesota Hospital and Clinic, Minneapolis, MN 55455.

A. J. Barkovich, M.D.: Department of Radiology, University of California—San Francisco, San Francisco, CA 94143.

DISORDERS OF NEURAL TUBE CLOSURE

Cephaloceles

Cephaloceles are extracranial extensions of intracranial structures through defects in the skull and dura; that is, they are brain hernias. Under the broad category of cephalocele are meningoceles, which are herniations of leptomeninges and CSF through a skull defect, and meningoencephaloceles (abbreviated, encephalocele), which are herniations of brain tissue, leptomeninges, and CSF through a skull defect. The vast majority of cephaloceles occur in the midline, although some subtypes may occur away from the midline. In most cases, cephaloceles are detected prenatally [by obstetric ultrasound (1,2)] or at birth [by clinical presentation of a subcutaneous mass (3,4)]. In a small subset of patients, the lesions are not detected until childhood [as in obligate mouth breathers due to trans-sphenoidal cephalocele (4–6)] or until adulthood [as in occult cephaloceles of the sphenoid wing or paranasal sinuses (7,8)]. Cephaloceles may be isolated anomalies, may be seen in conjunction with other anomalies, or may be part of a syndrome, in some of which cephalocele may be the only CNS anomaly (9,10). In addition, cephaloceles are commonly seen in patients with neurofibromatosis 1.

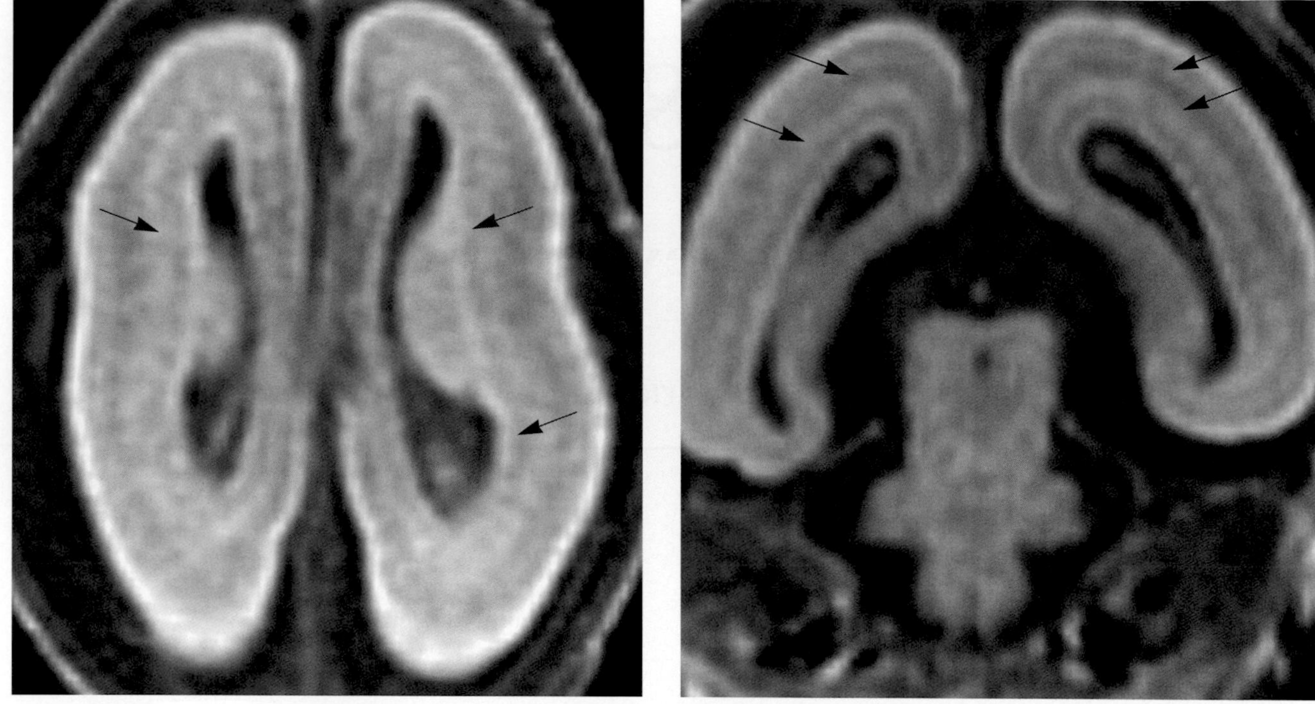

FIG. 1. Fetal brain, 14 week gestation; axial (**A**) and coronal (**B**) images from three-dimensional gradient-echo sequence obtained on fetal anatomy specimen. Images show smooth brain without sulcal development. Note germinal matrix (*arrows*, A) and normal waves of neuronal migration (*arrows*, B).

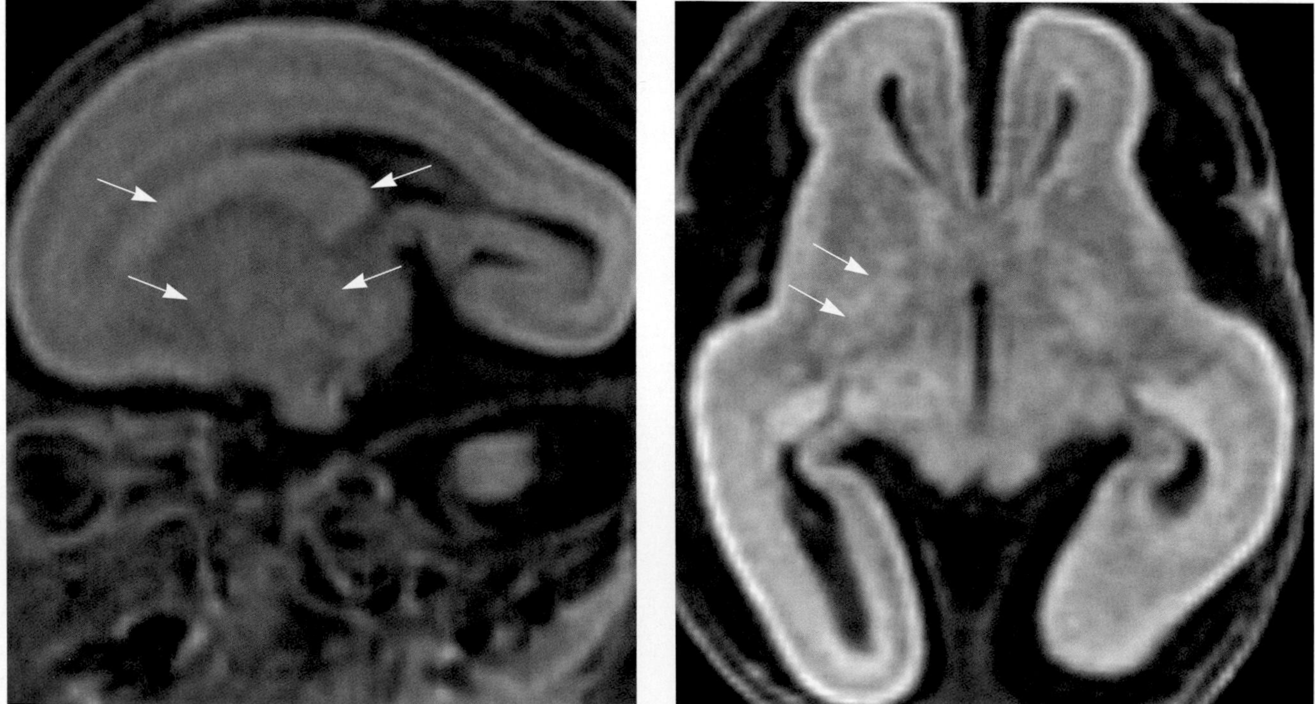

FIG. 2. Fetal brain, 14 week gestation; sagittal (**A**) and axial (**B**) images from three-dimensional gradient-echo sequence obtained on fetal anatomy specimen. Early neuronal condensations of future caudate and lenticular nuclei can be seen (*arrows*).

Cephaloceles are usually characterized by their location in the skull. Traditionally, they have been divided into four major categories: occipital, parietal, frontoethmoidal, and sphenoidal encephaloceles. With the advent of MR, however, the anatomic classification of cephaloceles has become much more specific (4). In particular, cephaloceles that involve the sphenoid bone are now subcategorized as trans-sphenoidal, transethmoidal, sphenoethmoidal, sphenomaxillary, spheno-orbital, and transalar sphenoidal. When patients with cephaloceles are scanned, the radiologist's responsibility extends beyond simple identification and description of the cephalocele-proper. The radiologist must also evaluate the subjacent dural sinuses and look for associated anomalies, such as agenesis or hypogenesis of the corpus callosum, the Dandy-Walker malformation, and subependymal heterotopic gray matter. In addition to routine multiplanar MR, cerebral MR venography may be useful in the assessment of parietal and occipital cephaloceles because the superior sagittal sinus and torcular Herophili are commonly found within the cephalocele sac. Contrast-enhanced MR sequences may also be helpful in trans-sphenoidal and post-surgical temporal cephaloceles.

The pathology of cephalocele is related to the site of involvement. Occipital cephaloceles are often large, although the contents of the sac are quite variable. Low occipital lesions may contain all or part of the cerebellum, as well as the occipital lobe(s). The cerebral hemispheres are commonly asymmetrically included. Deep brain structures tend to be more distorted than malformed, although collicular fusion and tectal deformity are often seen, and thalamic fusion and absence of the mamillary bodies may be found (11). Hydrocephalus may involve the herniated portion of the ventricle or the entire ventricular system (4). In general, the herniated brain contents have been considered dysplastic and nonfunctioning. Although this appears to be true for most cephaloceles, the concept has been questioned recently (12). In fact, at least in the case of occipital cephalocele, Oi et al. (12) have found neuronal maturation in herniated brain tissue to be complete, although they have not confirmed functional maturation of the herniated tissue. In light of their findings, they have developed a new surgical technique of intracranial transposition of the neural tissue. Since patients with occipital cephalocele often have microcephaly, due to the physiologic decompression of the cephalocele, the procedure requires two stages: in the initial phase, the cephalocele is reduced by closing the dural defect. This allows the intraventricular pulse pressure to rise and produce ventriculomegaly. With this, the cranial vault is necessarily enlarged. During the second stage, the extracranial brain is transposed into the intracranial cavity with concomitant ventricular shunting (12).

Although the issue of functioning versus nonfunctioning neural tissue may be an open question with regard to most cephaloceles, in the case of trans-sphenoidal cephaloceles, functioning brain tissue is often found within the defect. In particular, the pituitary gland and optic chiasm, although often located within the cephalocele, may function to variable degrees. Patients with neurofibromatosis 1 also have cephaloceles which can contain functioning brain tissue. The neurosurgical implications of this fact cannot be overstated. Whereas the surgical procedure on most cephaloceles involves resection of the aberrant, nonfunctioning brain, in trans-sphenoidal cephalocele, the consequences of such an approach include panhypopituitarism and blindness in a patient who preoperatively suffers little neuro-ophthalmological or neuroendocrinological deficit. The most commonly associated finding is agenesis or hypogenesis of the corpus callosum.

The plain film appearance of a cephalocele is that of a midline cranial defect with sclerotic margins. If a large amount of brain is present within the cephalocele, the craniofacial ratio will be diminished. Imaging studies will show extracranial extension of meninges, CSF, and sometimes brain through the calvarial defect (3). In general, MR is the most sensitive and accurate imaging modality for both the detection and characterization of cephaloceles. Ultrasound and CT have complimentary roles related to their convenience (US) and depiction of bony detail (CT).

Among the many features which characterize cephaloceles on MR, one of the most helpful is the general tendency of the ventricles or subarachnoid space which subtends the cephalocele to "point" toward the defect. Oftentimes, the ventricle will appear to be elongated (Fig. 3). In cases that do not involve a ventricle, generalized widening of the subarachnoid space may be seen (Fig. 4). In patients that have previously undergone surgical repair of a cephalocele, a "tract" of cerebrospinal fluid may be seen extending to deep areas of the brain from the cephalocele sac. Furthermore, the brain tissue will appear elongated and stretched toward the calvarial defect. This distortion of the brain tissue results from the fact that unmyelinated brain tissue is extremely soft and pliable and is easily deformed (13). Brain pulsations in utero presumably push this pliable unmyelinated brain outward through the defect, causing the distortion.

Although frontoethmoidal, occipital, and parietal encephaloceles are usually clinically obvious, anterior basal cephaloceles are usually clinically occult. Among such cephaloceles, the trans-sphenoidal subtype is the most important because functioning brain may be found within the sac. As noted above, patients may present toward the end of the first decade of life with nasopharyngeal obstruction (3,14). Clinical examination reveals a nasopharyngeal mass that increases in size with Val-

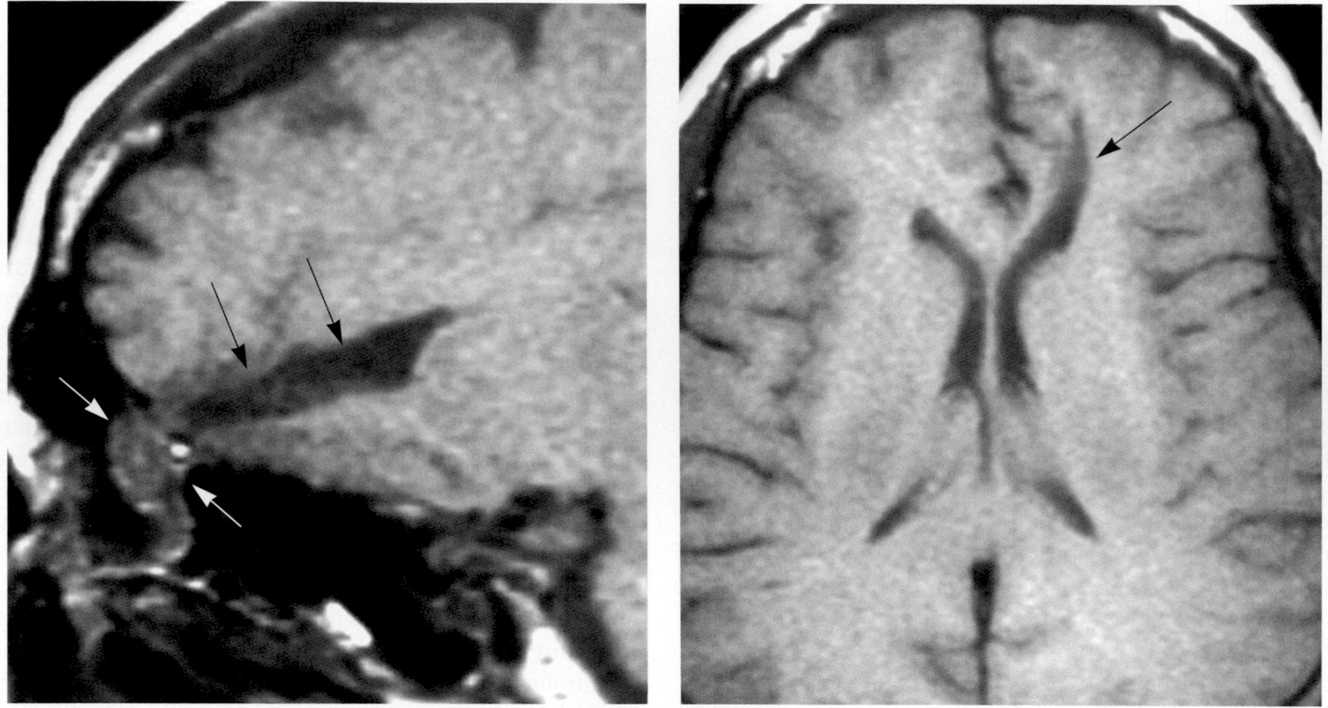

FIG. 3. Bifrontal cephaloceles. Sagittal (**A**) and axial (**B**) T1-weighted images show abnormal brain tissue (*white arrows*, A) within expected location of left ethmoid sinus. Note elongated left frontal horn (*black arrows*), typical of cephalocele. Similar findings (not shown) were apparent on right.

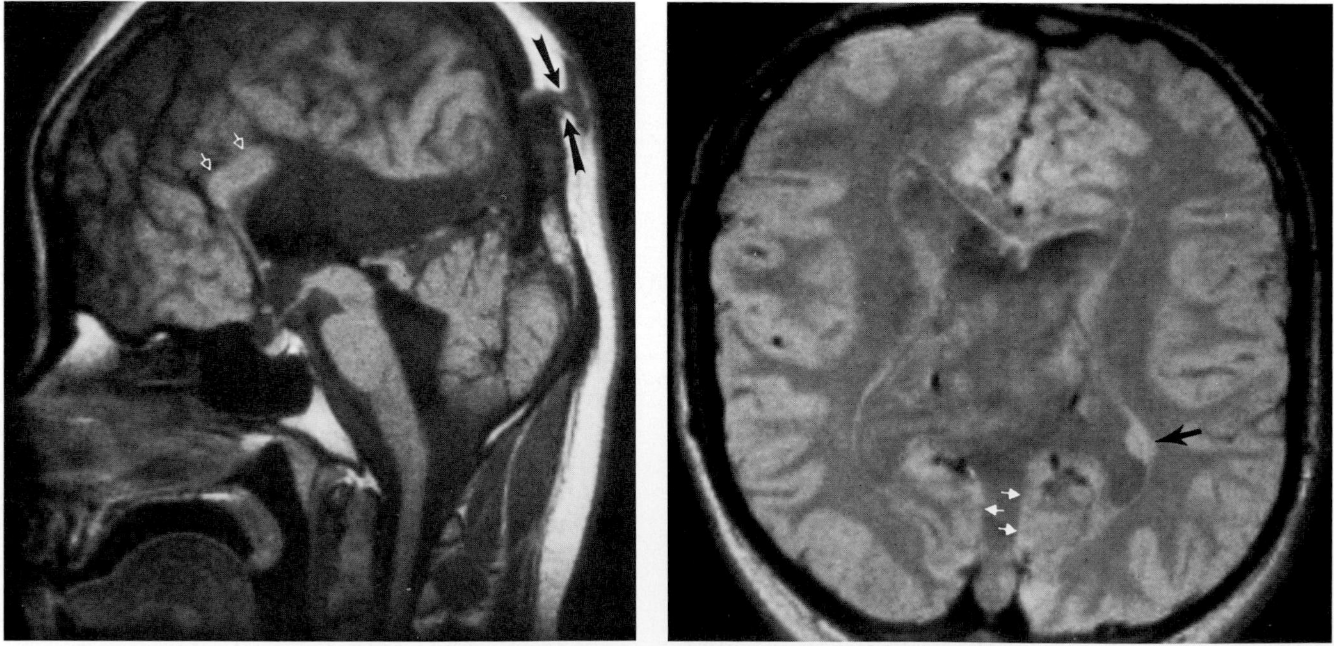

FIG. 4. Occipital encephalocele with hypogenesis of the corpus callosum and gray matter heterotopia. **A:** Sagittal SE 600/20 image shows a tract of CSF extending from the posterior incisural region dorsally to the site of the cephalocele (*arrows*). The corpus callosum (*open arrows*) is hypogenetic. The tectum and cerebellar vermis are distorted, being stretched toward the calvarial defect. Such distortion is commonly associated with encephaloceles. **B:** Axial SE 2500/30 image clearly demonstrates the tract of CSF (*white arrows*) extending from the posterior incisural space to the calvarial defect. A subependymal heterotopion is incidentally noted in the left trigone (*black arrow*).

salva's maneuver. Diminished visual acuity and hypothalamic-pituitary dysfunction almost always develop. Imaging studies reveal a variably sized defect in the sphenoid bone that, on plain films and CT, has sclerotic margins. In many cases, the defect corresponds to a persistent embryonic craniopharyngeal canal. The sac may extend through the floor of the sella into the sphenoid sinus or into the nasopharynx. In larger encephaloceles, erosion of the hard palate can be seen. Sagittal and coronal MR images will show the third ventricle, hypothalamus, pituitary gland, optic nerves, and optic chiasm elongated and stretched into the encephalocele sac (Fig. 5). Agenesis of the corpus callosum has been reported in up to 80% of these patients (14), although, with the advent of MR, more subtle cephaloceles are now discernible (Fig. 6). In such cases, associated callosal anomalies are the exception, not the rule.

Another subset of occult cephaloceles involves transalar sphenoidal cephaloceles. In such cases, patients may present in adulthood with spontaneous CSF rhinorrhea. On clinical examination, no definite abnormalities are seen. CT and MR scans reveal a small mass, often CSF-filled, within the lateral sphenoidal air cell. Associated prominence of the subjacent subarachnoid space may be seen in the medial temporal lobe (Fig. 7).

Chiari Malformations

In 1891, Chiari (15) described three malformations of the hindbrain associated with hydrocephalus. Five years later (16), he published a further study on hindbrain deformities. In that report, Chiari revised the second type of malformation described in the earlier paper as well as offered a new, fourth type of malformation. Despite countless modifications, the essence of Chiari's reports persists today.

The Chiari I malformation involves caudal displacement of the cerebellar tonsils, and sometimes the inferior vermis, through the foramen magnum into the rostral cervical spinal canal. The Chiari II malformation, also known as the Arnold-Chiari and Cleland-Chiari malformations, involves displacement of the brainstem and lower cerebellum into the cervical spinal canal. In such cases, the fourth ventricle is caudally displaced and extends below the foramen magnum. These type II abnormalities are nearly all associated with lumbar myelomeningoceles. The Chiari III malformation involves downward displacement of the medulla with herniation of the cerebellum initially through the foramen magnum, then dorsally through a cervical spina bifida, resulting in a cervical encephalocele. The Chiari IV malformation is severe cerebellar hypoplasia without displacement of brain through the foramen magnum. Since Chiari's initial descriptions, significant contributions have been made in the descriptions of the associated anomalies that are present in these disorders (17–21). In addition, numerous etiological theories have been proposed over the past century, although the definitive mechanisms remain the subject of lasting debates.

Chiari I Malformation

Chiari originally described a hindbrain malformation in association with hydrocephalus. Although it became

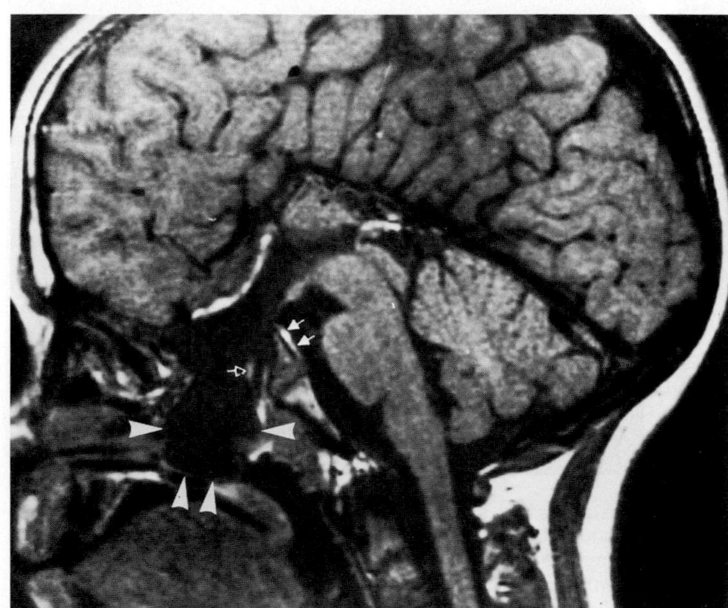
A

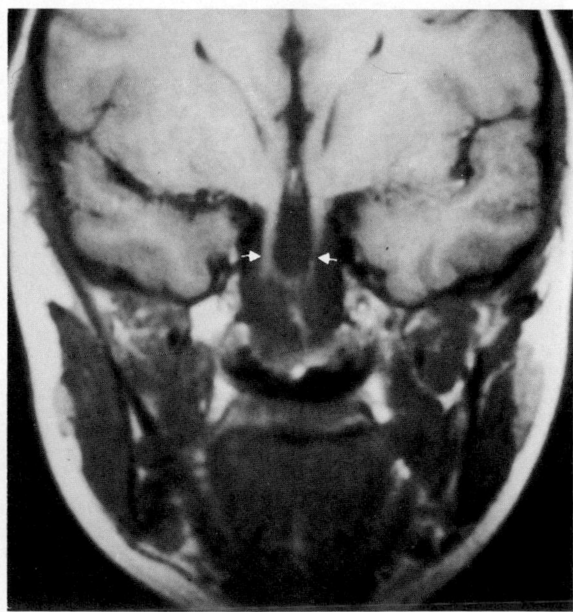
B

FIG. 5. Sphenoidal encephalocele. **A:** Sagittal SE 600/20 image shows the encephalocele extending inferiorly through the sphenoid bone into the nasopharynx (*arrowheads*). The dorsum sellae is still intact (*closed arrows*). The optic chiasm sits within the encephalocele (*open arrow*). **B:** Coronal SE 600/20 image shows the third ventricle and hypothalamus (*arrows*) sitting within the encephalocele sac.

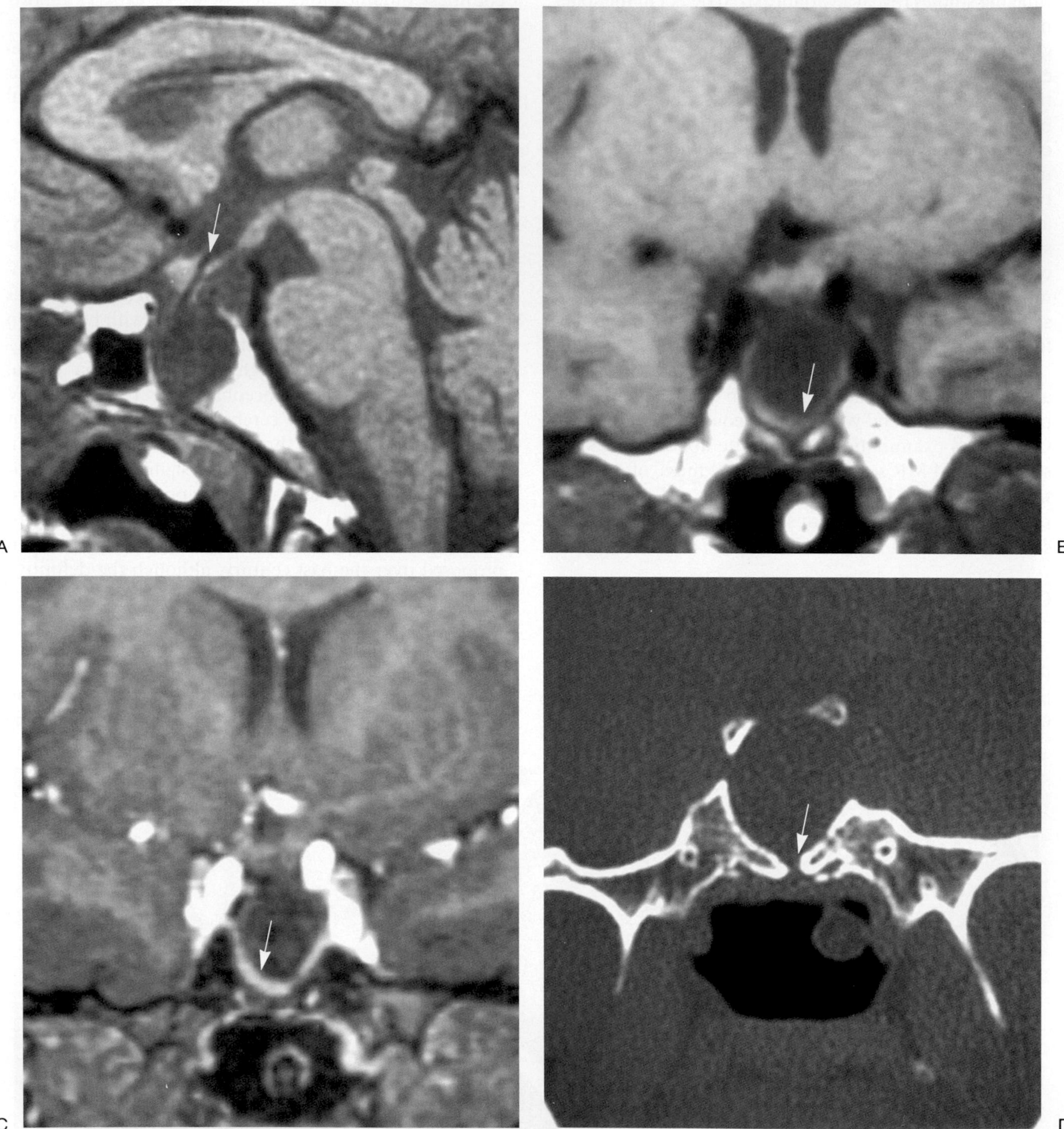

FIG. 6. Occult cephalocele in young woman with amenorrhea and short stature. Sagittal (**A**) and coronal (**B**) T1-weighted images show peculiar split infundibulum (*arrow*, A) and enlarged sella. Coronal image shows thin rim of probable pituitary tissue (*arrow*, B) along floor of sella. Unlike empty sella, infundibulum is not posteriorly displaced. Following infusion of contrast medium (**C**), normal enhancement of pituitary tissue (*arrow*, C) is seen. Coronal CT scan (**D**) shows bony defect (*arrow*, D) in floor of sella, most likely reflecting persistent craniopharyngeal canal. (From Truwit and Lempert, ref. 40, with permission.)

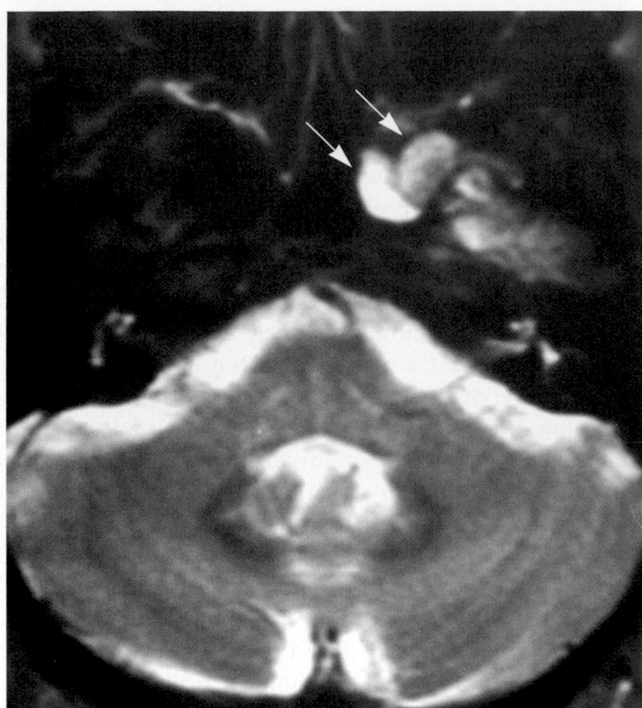

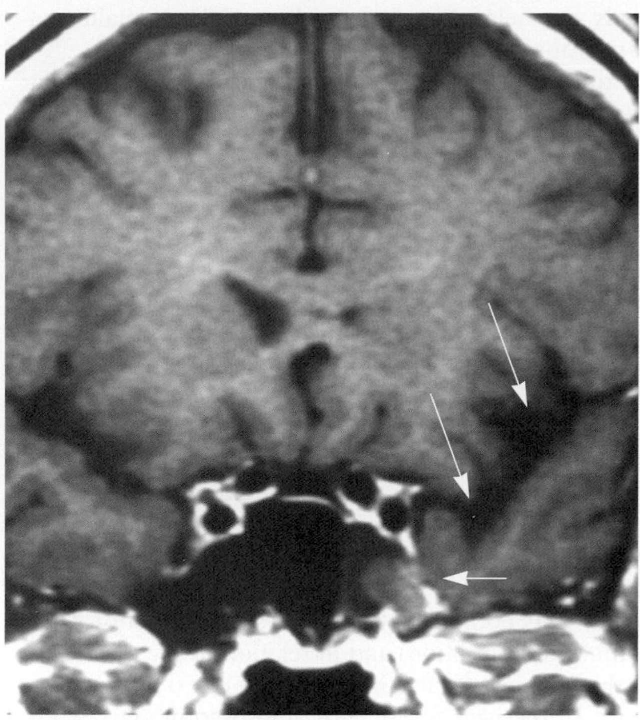

FIG. 7. Transalar cephalocele, axial T2-weighted (**A**) and contrast-enhanced coronal T1-weighted (**B**) images. Patient presented to neurosurgeon while holding paper cup beneath nose. CSF rhinorrhea in this patient was spontaneous. Cephalocele contained meninges and CSF, as well as small component of inferomesial temporal lobe (*arrows*, A). Bony defect is also apparent on coronal image (*short arrow*, B), as is generalized widening of subarachnoid space subjacent to cephalocele (*long arrows*, B). (From Truwit and Lempert, ref. 40, with permission.)

apparent that hydrocephalus is not mandatory for the diagnosis of Chiari I malformation, it is only in the past decade that the frequency of this "malformation" has become apparent. Any radiologist who reads MR scans can attest to the high frequency of encountering patients with Chiari I malformations.

The Chiari I malformation can be simply defined as inferior displacement of the cerebellar tonsils and sometimes, the inferior vermis (Fig. 8). (The Chiari I malformation has little, if anything, to do with closure of the neural tube. It is considered here only for convenience.) Traditionally, the degree of tonsillar ectopia and its relevance to the definition of the Chiari I malformation has been considered the diagnostic factor in distinguishing mild cerebellar tonsillar ectopia from a Chiari I malformation. Mild cerebellar ectopia (the caudal tips of the tonsils less than 3 mm below a line from the basion to the opisthion) has been reported to be of no clinical significance (22). In contradistinction, when the tonsils extend more than 5 mm below the foramen magnum, the incidence of clinical symptoms has been reported to rise dramatically (22). Between these limits, tonsillar ectopia of 3 or 4 mm has been considered to be of uncertain significance. The pointed morphology of the cerebellar ton-

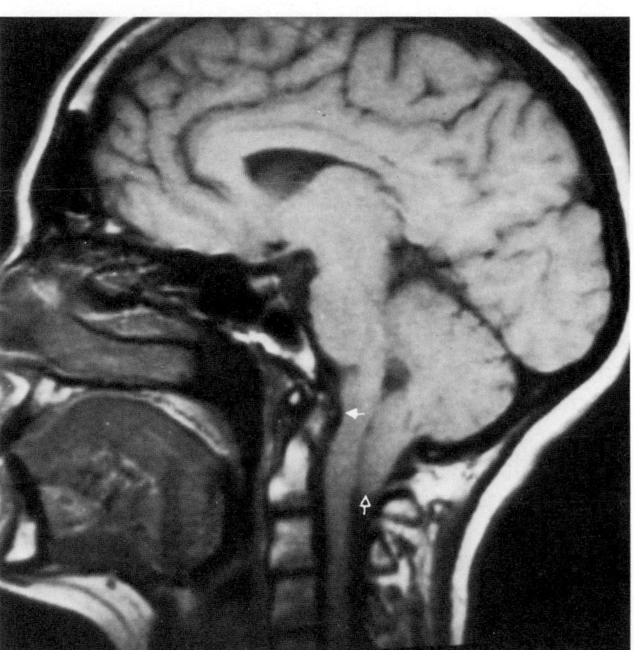

FIG. 8. Chiari I malformation. The cerebellar tonsil (*open arrow*) is enlarged and extends below the foramen magnum to the C2–C3 disc level. Moreover, there is some compression of the medulla by the odontoid process (*closed arrow*). The posterior fossa is of normal size, and the rest of the brain is unremarkable.

sils is also helpful in distinguishing Chiari I malformations from low-lying tonsils.

Probably far more relevant than the degree of tonsillar ectopia are the relative ease with which CSF passes through the foramen magnum and whether a patient with tonsillar ectopia would benefit from decompression of the foramen magnum. It is well known that patients with tonsillar ectopia of greater than 5 mm may in fact be asymptomatic if the foramen magnum is sufficient for the unimpeded dynamics of CSF flow. Moreover, such patients are likely to be at little risk of developing clinical symptoms. On the other hand, patients with milder degrees of tonsillar ectopia, if associated with altered CSF dynamics, may present—or may be at risk for presentation—with clinical symptomatology due to hydromyelia or hydrocephalus. Thus, studies of patients with Chiari I malformations in the future are likely to focus less on the static anatomic appearance of the tonsils in relation to the foramen magnum, but rather on the dynamic motion of CSF, both in relation to physiologic motion of the brain (brain pulsation) and in relation to the mechanics of the craniocervical junction (flexion, extension, rotation). In the near future, MR fluoroscopy may permit high spatial and temporal resolution imaging of the craniocervical junction in Chiari I patients with the hope of predicting which patients are likely to develop symptoms over time.

Chiari I malformations can result from a number of causes. It was originally felt that the most common cause was malformation of the craniocervical junction. The cerebellar tonsils in these patients are often abnormally large, extending down through the foramen magnum as low as the C3 or C4 level. Examination of the cervical spine in these patients may show occipitalization of the atlas, Klippel-Feil anomalies, and omovertebral bones. A second group of patients with Chiari I malformations seem to develop tonsillar ectopia as a result of (transient) intrauterine hydrocephalus; this is most likely the largest subset of patients with Chiari I malformations. What these patients have, in fact, is no more than tonsillar herniation due to their hydrocephalus. Because the tonsils are ectopic at the time of their myelination, they retain a pointed configuration and a low-lying position, even after the hydrocephalus has been treated or resolved. In conjunction with this subset are patients that develop hydrocephalus after birth. This is the subset of patients to which Chiari's original report referred. A third group of patients with ectopic cerebellar tonsils are those with acquired deformities of the foramen magnum such as platybasia and basilar invagination. A fourth group of Chiari I malformations includes patients with increased intracranial pressure not related to hydrocephalus. In this subgroup of patients, the increased pressure is usually related to intracranial mass lesions or brain swelling. Yet another subset of patients with Chiari I malformations are patients with either spinal CSF leak or spinal-peritoneal or spinal-pleural shunts (23). In these patients, decreased—not increased—intracranial pressure is the rule. Patients in any of these groups can present with cranial neuropathies as a result of brainstem compression or with pain and dissociated anesthesia of the upper extremities, resulting from associated syringohydromyelia. Lastly, a sixth group of Chiari I malformations includes those patients with myelomeningoceles and mild hindbrain malformations. Some authors prefer to classify these conditions as Chiari II malformations because of the associated myelomeningocele and the fact that such patients usually have supratentorial anomalies such as callosal hypogenesis, gyral interdigitation, and tectal beaking. We would tend to agree with this latter classification because patients in this group tend to present with hydrocephalus and myelodysplasia as opposed to brainstem compression or syringomyelia.

It should be stressed that many authors refer to "congenital" Chiari I malformations as "real Chiari I's." These patients are those of the first subset mentioned above; namely, those with Klippel-Feil deformities, etc. However, Chiari's own original description had nothing to do with such cases; he merely described tonsillar herniation due to hydrocephalus. Moreover, it is by no means clear that these are the patients that will most benefit from decompression of the foramen magnum.

The concurrence of Chiari I malformations and syringohydromyelia has been estimated to occur in up to 25% of patients with Chiari I malformations (Fig. 9). With the advent of MRI, it has become quite common to diagnose Chiari I. We believe that it is likely that the subset of patients with Chiari I and concurrent syringohydromyelia is less than 25%. Nevertheless, it is still appropriate to image the cervical spinal cord in patients discovered to have a Chiari I malformation. Conversely, patients with neuropathic deformities (Fig. 10) of the shoulder should have an MRI of the craniocervical junction to rule out a Chiari I malformation.

Unfortunately, the imaging requirements of patients with Chiari I malformations are not straightforward. In cases where the diagnosis of Chiari I malformation has already been established, the focus of MR studies should be the craniocervical junction, although at least one sequence should include the lateral ventricles to ensure that hydrocephalus is not present. Similarly, the entire cervical and upper thoracic spinal cord should be imaged in such patients, to ensure that syringohydromyelia is not present. On the other hand, most cases of Chiari I malformation are not known a priori. In such patients, it is likely that a brain MRI will be the requested study, and the Chiari I malformation will be discovered fortuitously. In such cases, it is important to follow the brain study with at least one sagittal sequence through the cervical spine to ensure that syringohydromyelia is not present. Moreover, it is not adequate to rely on the sagittal brain sequence to "clear the cervical cord." Sagittal brain

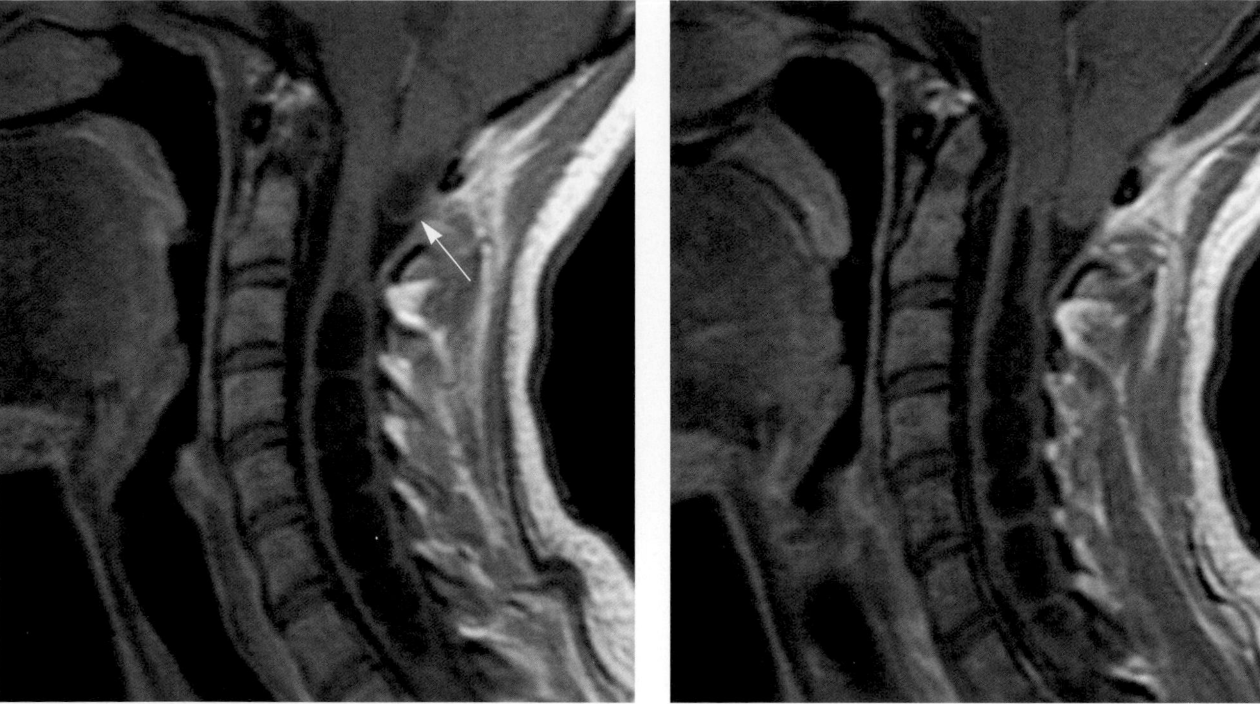

FIG. 9. Chiari I malformation with holocord syringohydromyelia. Sagittal T1-weighted images show inferiorly displaced cerebellar tonsils and syringohydromyelic cavity of entire cervical (**A**,**B**) and thoracic (not shown) cord. Note degenerated left cerebellar tonsil (*arrow*, A), due to long-standing pressure necrosis.

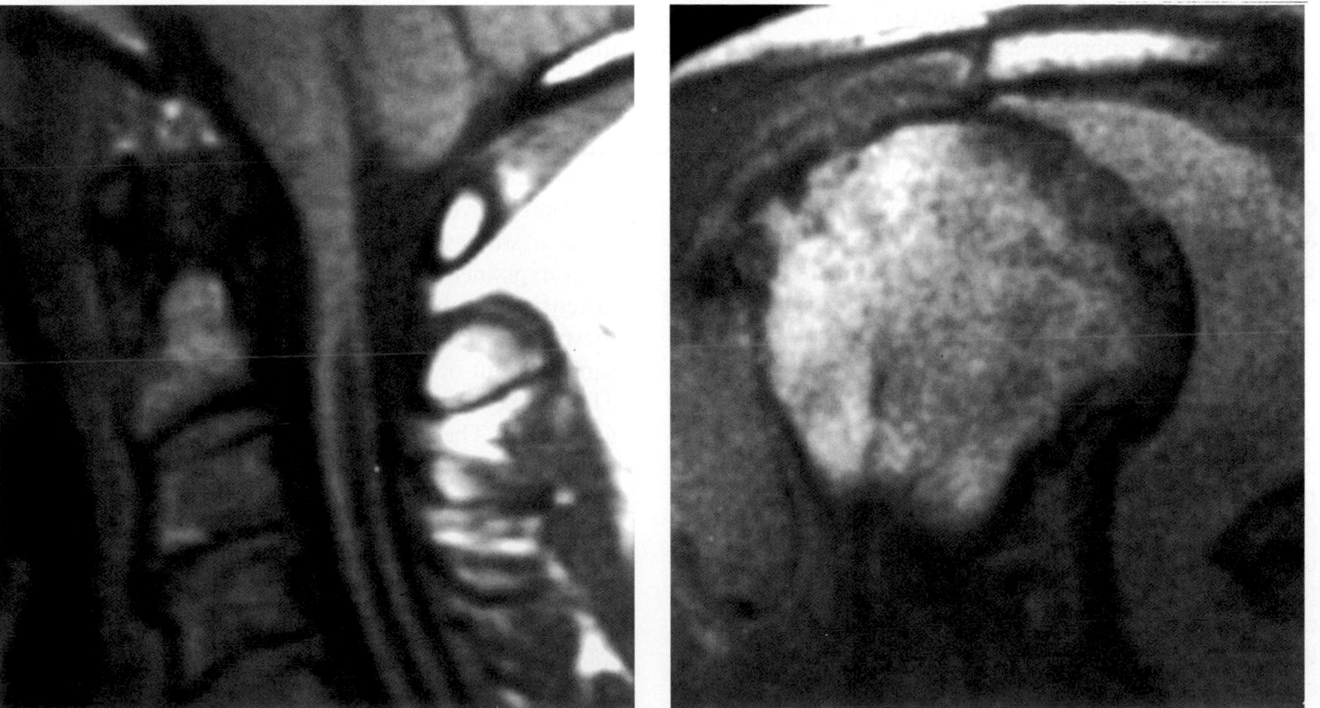

FIG. 10. Chiari I malformation with neuropathic shoulder. Sagittal (**A**) T1-weighted image shows typical features of tonsillar ectopia and syringohydromyelia. MRI of cervical spine was performed only after shoulder MRI revealed findings of neuropathic joint. Axial proton-density-weighted (**B**) image shows joint effusion and significant bone erosion.

images typically only include the upper 2 to 3 cervical segments, whereas in patients with Chiari I malformations, it is not uncommon for syringohydromyelia to involve the lower cervical and upper thoracic segments.

The surgical options available to patients with Chiari I malformations seem to evolve and recycle. Among such choices are decompression of the foramen magnum with or without duraplasty, obex plug, and a variety of shunts involving the ventricular system, the syringohydromyelic cavity, or both. At some institutions, it is currently in vogue to decompress the foramen magnum alone without breech of the dura. Plugging of the obex has been abandoned by nearly all neurosurgeons as a treatment for Chiari I malformations.

Chiari II Malformation

The Chiari II malformation is extremely complex (13,18), and its etiology remains the subject of academic debate. Even Chiari's understanding of the disorder was less than perfect and required revision in his second paper (16). Over the past century, numerous theories have been advanced to explain the etiology of the hindbrain deformity seen in Chiari II malformations. An excellent review of these theories can be found in McLone and Knepper's 1989 report (24). Briefly, the various theories can be grouped as those related to CSF dynamics, traction of the hindbrain by the tethered neural placode within the myelomeningocele, primary hindbrain dysgenesis, and primary bony dysplasia of the posterior fossa. Within the first category are Chiari, Gardner, and others. Chiari proposed simple posterior fossa herniation due to supratentorial hydrocephalus, and viewed the type 1 and 2 malformations (now known as Chiari I and II) as parts of a spectrum of disorders. Gardner, on the other hand, proposed that hydromyelia, as well as hydrocephalus, had to be involved. In his view, failure of the fourth ventricular roof to rupture (a normal event) led to pressure through the neural tube and distension and rupture, with resultant myeloschisis. In short, these theories fail to account for the small posterior fossa and associated supratentorial brain anomalies.

Traction theories seem intuitively obvious and simple: failure of normal development of the distal spinal cord and canal somehow results in tethering and consequent traction on the developing hindbrain. Beyond the surface, however, traction theories fail to explain several features. First, the caudal neural elements are not always tethered. Second, the cervicomedullary kink, a hallmark of the malformation, cannot be adequately explained by this theory. Thirdly, traction would not explain the associated supratentorial anomalies seen in Chiari II malformations. Finally, it has been shown experimentally that the forces of traction are unlikely to pass through the length of the spinal cord. Rather, they are rapidly dissipated.

The next category of theories set forth to explain the hindbrain anomaly in Chiari II malformations involves a primary malformation of the hindbrain itself. In short, proponents of such theories suggest that a failure of pontine flexure results in an elongated brainstem with both upward and downward herniation. The dysraphic state of the lower spine is not easily accounted for.

Marin-Padilla and Marin-Padilla (25) propose a primary mesodermal problem which results in a small posterior fossa. According to their theory, the posterior fossa contents are necessarily squeezed out of the small posterior fossa. This theory has received the widest support in recent years.

Lastly, McLone and Knepper (24) hypothesize that the primary defect in patients with Chiari II malformations is one of neurulation. According to their theory, such a defect results in a failure of normal rhombencephalic ventricular distention, inadequate inductive forces on the basal cranial mesoderm (i.e., small posterior fossa), and disordered formation of the cerebellum and brainstem, as well as both upward and downward herniation. In addition, the failure of fourth ventricular distention is translated to the third and lateral ventricles. Improper ventricular support for the telencephalic hemispheres ultimately results in thalamic apposition (i.e., large massa intermedia), commissural dysplasia (i.e., hypogenesis of the corpus callosum), and disordered neuronal migration (i.e., subependymal heterotopia). In short, what McLone and Knepper offer is a solution which does not invoke hydrocephalus, as suggested by Chiari and many who have followed, but a failure of normal, physiologic intrauterine hydrocephalus.

Essentially all patients with this anomaly present at birth due to obvious dorsal myelomeningocele. Surgical repair of the myelomeningocele usually occurs within the first 24 to 48 hours of life. Shortly thereafter, patients invariably develop hydrocephalus, at which point neuroimaging studies become important.

As explained, failure of rhombencephalic ventricular distension results in inadequate induction of the cranial mesoderm. Posterior fossa structures are necessarily squeezed out of the posterior fossa during their growth. The cerebellum tends to be indented superiorly by the tentorium. The tentorial insertion is often adjacent to the foramen magnum, and the dural sinuses are commonly malpositioned (26). Inferiorly, the cerebellum extends well below an invariably enlarged foramen magnum and is indented posteriorly either by the posterior arch of C1 or a "firm fibrous band" that bridges a developmental defect of the posterior arch (27). The pons is inferiorly positioned and narrow in its anteroposterior diameter. The medulla is usually positioned within the cervical spinal canal. The cervical spinal cord is also pushed inferiorly, but it is restricted in its caudal movement by the dentate ligaments that attach to the lateral aspects of the spinal cord and hold it in place, allowing a variable, but limited, amount of caudal displacement (13,18). If the medulla is pushed down further than the dentate ligaments will allow the spinal cord to move, it buckles posteriorly behind the spinal cord, forming a characteristic cervicomedullary kink (Fig. 11) (13,18). The cerebellum is squeezed not just inferiorly, but anterolaterally into the cerebellopontine and cerebellomedullary angle cisterns (Fig. 12). In severe cases, the cerebellum can wrap completely around the brainstem (13,18). The fourth ventricle is low in position, often extending through the foramen magnum into the cervical spinal canal (Figs. 12–14) its anterior-posterior diameter is narrowed (13,18). The cerebellar vermis, which is almost always herniated into the cervical spinal canal, will degenerate in areas where it is compressed by bony (or fibrous) structures. When this degeneration is severe, virtually no cerebellum may be present (Fig. 13).

Occasionally, the fourth ventricle may become isolated from the rest of the ventricular system or "trapped" as a result of aqueductal narrowing (or scarring) and diminished CSF flow through the fourth ventricular outflow foramina or basilar cisterns. To the inexperienced

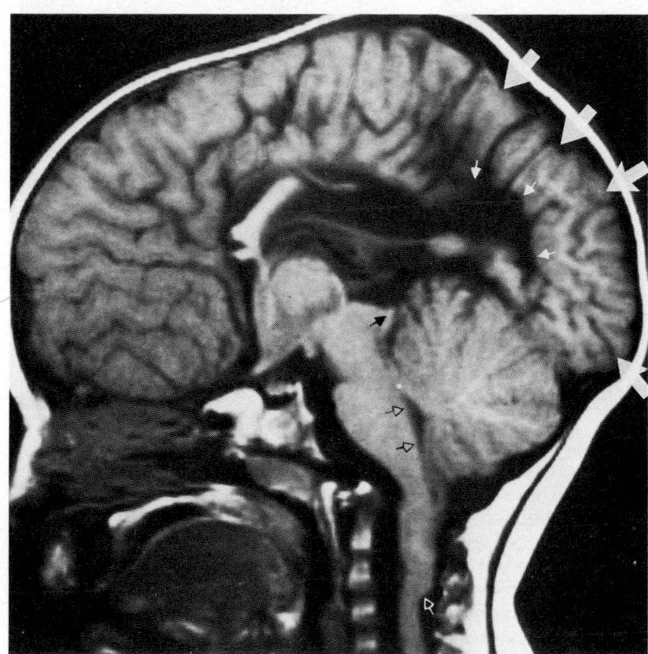

FIG. 11. Chiari II malformation. Sagittal SE 600/20 image shows several findings that are characteristic of this malformation. The pons and medulla are inferiorly displaced. The most inferior portion of the medulla extends posterior to the cervical spinal cord, forming the characteristic cervicomedullary kink (*open white arrow*). The fourth ventricle (*open black arrows*) is inferiorly displaced and narrowed in its AP diameter. The quadrigeminal plate is stretched inferiorly and posteriorly, resulting in the characteristic "beaked" shape (*closed black arrow*). There is an enlarged CSF-containing space in the posterior incisural region (*closed white arrows*), as a result of colpocephaly and shunting of the ventricles. The gyral pattern is abnormal in the posterior parietal and occipital regions (*large arrows*). This gyral configuration has been termed "stenogyria."

observer, the isolated fourth ventricle in a Chiari II malformation may look normal; indeed, in the axial plane, it may be the size of a normal fourth ventricle (Fig. 14). However, a "normal-sized" fourth ventricle in a Chiari II malformation should initiate a search for a shunt malfunction or an isolated fourth ventricle because the fourth ventricle should, in fact, be slit-like. Furthermore, when patients with Chiari II malformations have hydrocephalus or isolated fourth ventricles, the spine should be examined because of a high incidence of associated syringohydromyelia (Fig. 14C). Conversely, the development of syringohydromyelia in a myelomeningocele patient should initiate a search for shunt malfunction or an isolated fourth ventricle (18,28).

In addition to their hindbrain deformities, patients with Chiari II malformations almost always have anomalies of the supratentorial brain. The corpus callosum is abnormal in between 75% and 90% of affected patients (29); the abnormalities include hypogenesis and distortion secondary to hydrocephalus. Often, both hypogenesis and distortion are present. The callosal splenium is nearly always hypoplastic or absent. The posterior body may be normal, hypoplastic, absent, or severely attenuated due to hydrocephalus. In the more severely affected patients, the midbody, posterior body, splenium, and rostrum are absent. The caudate heads and massa intermedia are frequently enlarged in Chiari II patients. Commonly, the medial hemispheric gyri interdigitate across the interhemispheric fissure, through fenestrations of the falx cerebri (Fig. 12) (19–21). The trigones, occipital horns, and posterior temporal horns of the lateral ventricles are almost always enlarged (colpocephaly) as a result of the accompanying hypogenetic corpus callosum. After shunting, a large CSF-containing space is often present superior to the vermis, between the atria and occipital horns of the lateral ventricles (Fig. 11). This space is most likely the result of dysplastic adjacent brain and is not an enlarged suprapineal recess (19). The gyral pattern is almost always abnormal, demonstrating multiple small gyri within a cortex of normal thickness (Figs. 11 and 13). This abnormal gyral pattern, which has been termed "stenogyria," is most prominently seen over the medial aspect of the occipital lobes on sagittal MR (30). The quadrigeminal plate is almost always abnormal when viewed on the midline sagittal images. In the more severely affected cases, the inferior colliculi are markedly stretched inferiorly and posteriorly, while the superior colliculi appear hypoplastic (Figs. 10 and 11). In the less severely affected cases, the inferior colliculi are mildly prominent, and the superior colliculi appear nearly normal (Fig. 14) (13,18).

It is important to recognize that all of the findings described in the Chiari II malformations are not present in every patient. Moreover, the degree of deformity can vary widely from patient to patient. For example, the hindbrain malformation can vary from a minute poste-

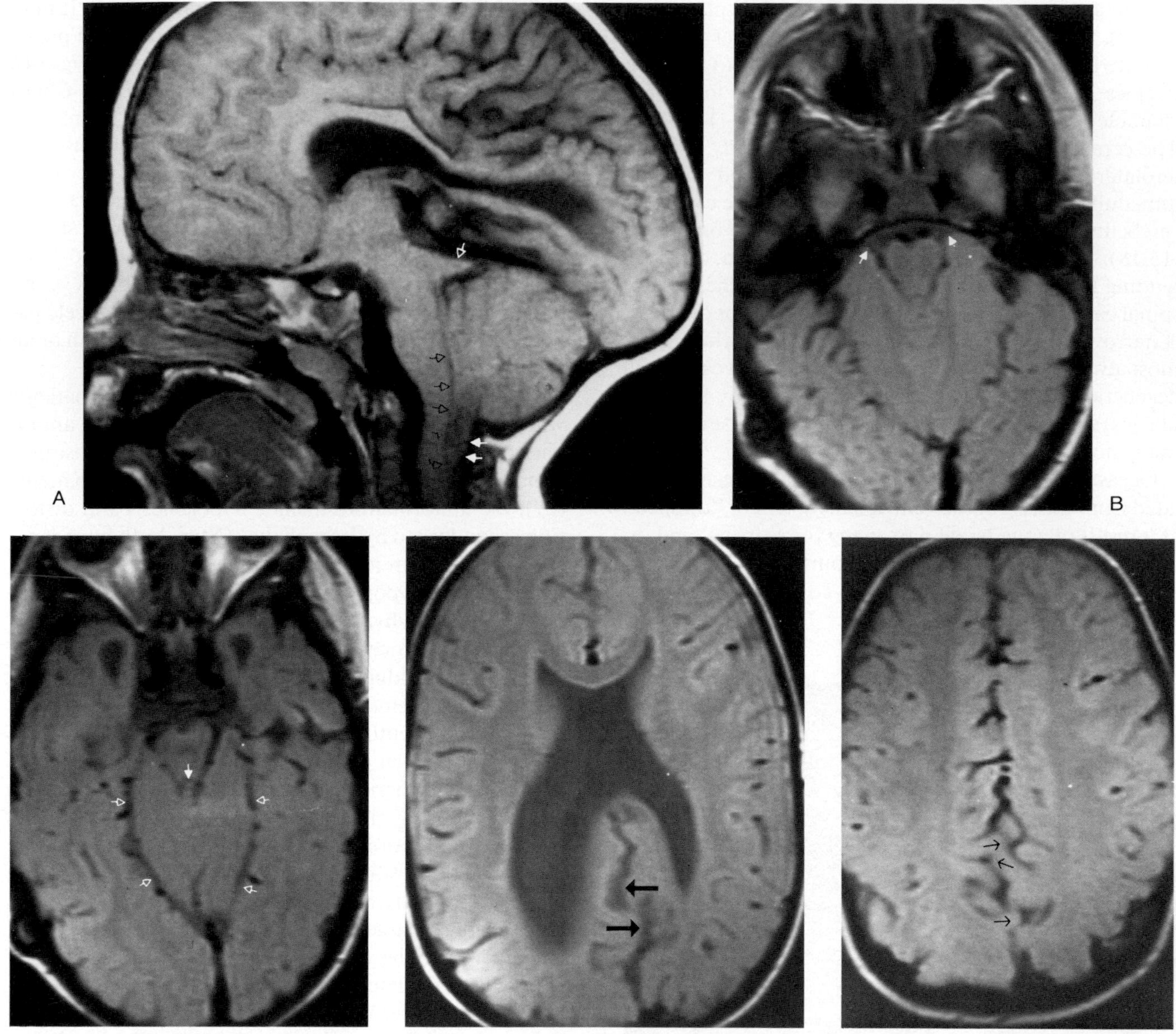

FIG. 12. Chiari II malformation. **A:** Sagittal SE 600/20 image shows an extremely low and narrow fourth ventricle (*open black arrows*) that extends below the foramen magnum. The cerebellar vermis (*closed white arrows*) is herniated into the cervical spinal canal. The corpus callosum is hypogenetic. There is pronounced "beaking" of the tectum (*open white arrow*). **B:** Axial SE 2500/30 image shows the cerebellar hemispheres extending laterally around the brainstem into the cerebellomedullary angles (*arrows*). **C:** The "beaking" of the tectum can be seen on this axial image (*closed white arrow*). The cerebellum has extended up through a widened tentorial incisura (*open white arrows*) as a result of the small posterior fossa. **D:** Axial SE 2500/30 image reveals absence of midline septum pellucidum and interdigitation of gyri across the midline (*arrows*). **E:** Axial SE 2500/30 image at the level of the centrum semiovale shows interdigitation of the gyri across the midline (*arrows*) as a result of fenestrations of the falx cerebri.

rior fossa with near total absence of the cerebellum (Fig. 13) to a relatively normal-sized posterior fossa with only cerebellar tonsillar ectopia (Fig. 11). In these milder cases, the history of a myelomeningocele repair and the associated supratentorial anomalies would indicate that these conditions should probably be classified as mild Chiari II hindbrain malformations and not as Chiari I malformations.

Chiari III Malformation

In his initial report of 1891, Chiari described a single case of caudal medullary displacement and cerebellar herniation, initially through the foramen magnum, then dorsally through a cervical spina bifida, resulting in a cervical encephalocele. Since that time, the definition of the Chiari III malformation has been expanded by some au-

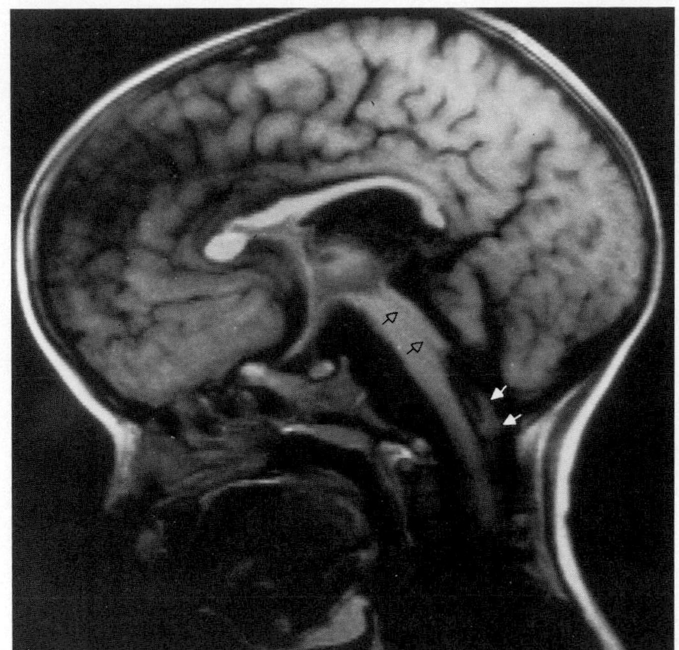

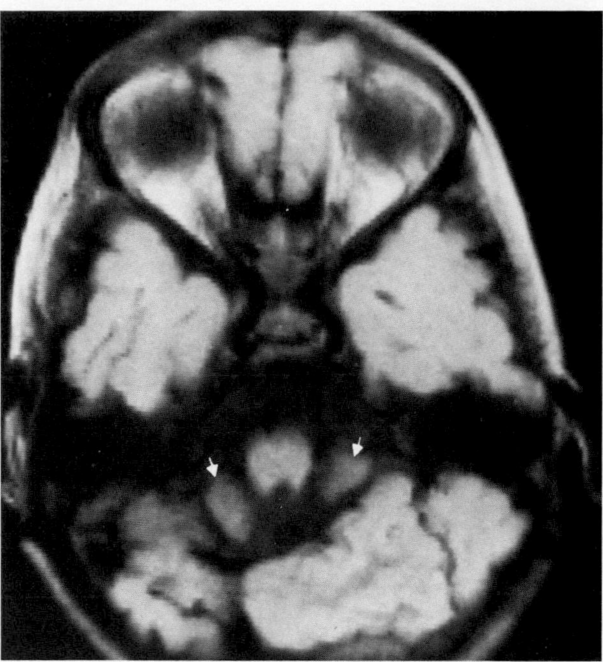

A B

FIG. 13. Chiari II malformation. **A:** Sagittal SE 500/20 image shows a hypogenetic corpus callosum. The quadrigeminal plate (*open arrows*) is extremely narrow and elongated. The brainstem is narrowed in its AP diameter and inferiorly displaced. Only a small amount of cerebellar tissue (*closed arrows*) can be identified. **B:** Axial SE 2000/30 image shows that only small remnants of the cerebellar hemispheres (*arrows*) remain. In Chiari II patients with extremely small posterior fossae, the cerebellum presumably degenerates as a result of pressure necrosis.

thors (31) to include cases of hindbrain herniation into cephaloceles which encompass both the low occipital and upper cervical regions (Fig. 15). Strictly speaking, cases that do not involve the upper cervical spinal canal should not be classified as Chiari III malformations, but simply as cephaloceles.

In general, patients with Chiari III malformations will be detected prenatally. In all cases, cerebellum herniates into the cephalocele sac (31). Variably included will be brainstem, occipital lobes, subarachnoid or ventricular CSF spaces, and dural sinuses. Deficiency of some or all of the corpus callosum is also commonly seen. Both MRI and CT will also show osseous defects involving the occiput and posterior elements of the upper cervical spine, as well as scalloping of the dorsal clivus and petrous bones, and Lükenschädel.

Chiari IV Malformation

The Chiari IV malformation (Fig. 16) is a very rare anomaly that consists of severe cerebellar hypoplasia without displacement of the posterior fossa contents through the foramen magnum.

Epidermoid/Dermoid

Epidermoid and dermoid tumors (i.e., masses) are developmental anomalies, although frequently discussed in the context of primary brain tumors (32,33). Strictly speaking, they are not neoplastic. Both lesions arise from congenital inclusions within the closing neural tube, most likely due to improper disjunction of neuroectoderm from cutaneous ectoderm within the third or fourth week of gestation. In essence, both lesions can be called ectodermal heterotopia. Both lesions are derived from tissues of epidermal origin; the primary difference between epidermoid and dermoid is that dermoids also include tissues of mesodermal origin. Both lesions may be associated with dermal sinuses and osseous defects. A very small subset of epidermoid (and possibly dermoid) tumors are not developmental in origin, but rather are the result of traumatic implantation or iatrogenic (surgical, lumbar puncture, etc.) inclusion of epidermal elements. These post-traumatic epidermoids tend to be more common in the spine, although they may occur in the head as well.

Epidermoid cysts are slightly more common than dermoids, especially in the cranial cavity. They are most fre-

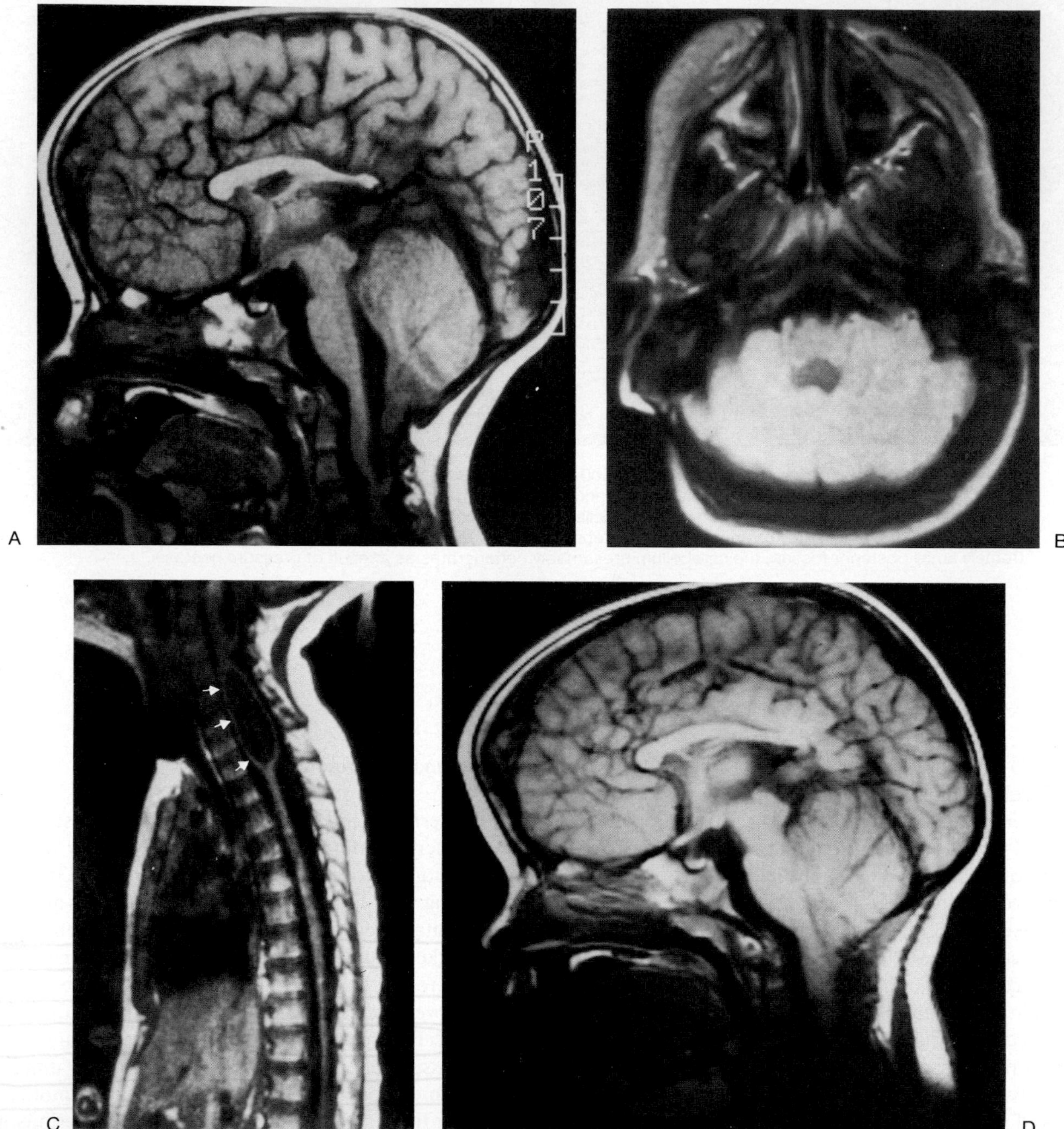

FIG. 14. Chiari II malformation with an isolated fourth ventricle. **A:** Sagittal SE 600/20 image shows a hypogenetic corpus callosum. The quadrigeminal plate is nearly normal. The fourth ventricle is too large for a patient with a Chiari II malformation. **B:** Axial SE 2500/20 image. The isolated fourth ventricle looks normal on this axial image. **C:** Sagittal SE 600/20 image through the cervical and thoracic spinal cord reveals a focal syringohydromyelia (*arrows*). Syringohydromyelia is often seen in association with an isolated fourth ventricle or nonfunctioning ventriculoperitoneal shunt in patients with a Chiari II malformation and myelomeningocele. **D:** After diversion of CSF from the fourth ventricle, the ventricle assumes a more normal (for a Chiari malformation) slit-like appearance.

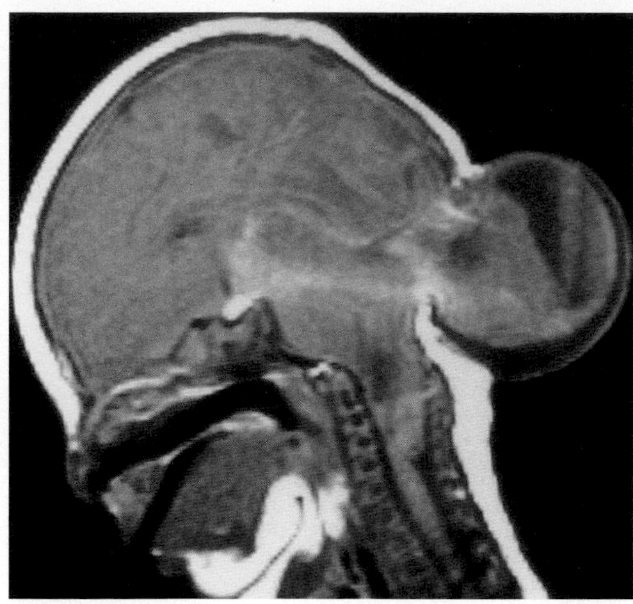

FIG. 15. Chiari III malformation. Sagittal T1-weighted image shows hindbrain malformation and herniation dorsal to upper cervical spinal cord, dysraphic posterior elements of cervical spine and suboccipital cephalocele containing malformed cerebellum. (Courtesy of Dr. Mauricio Castillo).

quently detected in mid-adulthood, owing to their very slow growth and limited symptomatology. Although they may appear anywhere in the neural axis, the majority involve the basal surface of the brain. The most common cranial sites include the cerebellopontine angle (Fig. 17) and parasellar regions. Following these sites are the rhomboid fossa (ventral to the brainstem), ventricles and choroidal fissures, and subfrontal (Fig. 18) and interhemispheric regions. Epidermoids grow locally and insinuate themselves into the subarachnoid cisterns and sulci. Symptoms related to supratentorial epidermoids include seizures and/or headaches. Patients with posterior fossa epidermoids typically present with symptoms of cranial nerve involvement and/or vertigo (34,35).

In contradistinction to epidermoid cysts, dermoids tend to show somewhat less variability in their location; they are often situated medially. Like epidermoids, they frequently involve the basal surface of the brain. Unlike epidermoids, however, dermoids tend to be somewhat more circumscribed. Although they may spread contiguously through the subarachnoid space, the more common scenario is that of rupture. When this happens, diffuse subarachnoid and intraventricular deposits are found; chemical meningitis may ensue (34,35).

On CT, epidermoids are lobulated, extra-axial masses which show low density, often similar to CSF. Their density may be slightly different than CSF, and rarely, they may be dense lesions (33,36). Intratumoral matrix is occasionally seen. Enhancement is typically not seen following intravenous or intrathecal administration of iodinated contrast medium. In contradistinction to arachnoid cysts, following intrathecal injection, contrast typically insinuates itself into the interstices of the epidermoid.

Dermoids are more straightforward on CT. The lesion usually is markedly decreased in attenuation due to the fatty nature of the tumor. Calcification may be seen in the wall of the lesion (37,38). The primary differential diagnosis is teratoma. If contrast enhancement is noted, teratoma is more likely. When a dermoid is discovered, dedicated attention should be paid to the CSF spaces, as small fatty droplets may be easily overlooked (Fig. 19). In particular, fat droplets may be seen "floating" within the frontal horns on axial or sagittal images of supine patients. These findings indicate rupture of the dermoid into the ventricular or subarachnoid space, which may be asymptomatic, but commonly evokes signs and symptoms of a chemical meningitis.

MR imaging has made the distinction between epidermoids and dermoids clear. Epidermoids commonly exhibit signal characteristics slightly different from CSF (Fig. 17), and occasionally intralesional matrix may be identified on any type of MR sequence. Particular attention should be paid to the signal intensity of the lesion on proton-density-weighted images. Most dermoids exhibit signal characteristics of fat, and chemical shift artifact is commonly seen. Occasionally, however, epidermoids may actually be hyperintense on T1-weighted images, suggesting the presence of fat—and the diagnosis of dermoid. T1 shortening of epidermoids has been attributed to "high lipid content, with mixed triglycerides containing polyunsaturated fatty acids and no cholesterol" (33) and more recently to decreased free water within inspissated, desiccated tumors (39). Like fat within dermoids, T2 shortening may be seen as well, again related to the degree of intralesional free water. Rarely, hemorrhagic epidermoids may be seen (40). In such cases, chemical shift artifact and/or fat suppressed images will help to distinguish the fatty nature of the dermoid from the similar intensities of epidermoid.

An additional diagnostic problem relates to epidermoids with signal characteristics that approximate CSF. Prior to MR imaging, such lesions were differentiated from arachnoid cysts first on the basis of morphology. Failing that, CT-cisternography would be performed, as noted above. On MRI, epidermoids that mimic arachnoid cysts are not easily discriminated. Several techniques have shown promise including gradient-echo imaging, steady-state imaging, and diffusion imaging. In the former, it is not uncommon for three-dimensional radiofrequency-spoiled gradient-recalled images to show different contrast resolution of epidermoids than spin-echo T1-weighted images. In particular, intralesional matrix, often inapparent on spin-echo images, may be revealed with gradient-echo imaging. Steady-state imaging can reveal intralesional motion, characteristic of

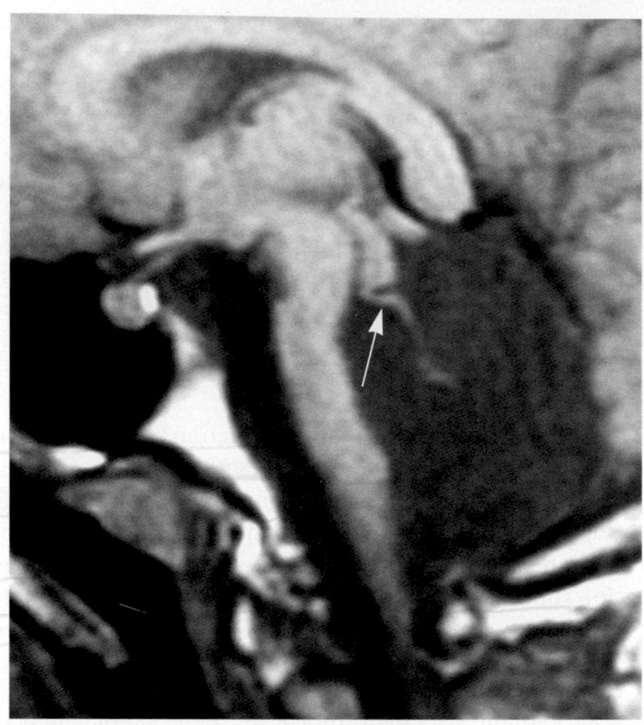

FIG. 16. Chiari IV malformation. Sagittal (**A**) and axial (**B,C**) T1-weighted images show near complete absence of the cerebellar hemispheres and vermis. Note severely hypoplastic hemispheres (*arrows*, B and C) and thin anterior medullary velum (*arrow*, A). Note the associated pontine hypoplasia. In contradistinction to Chiari II malformation, the straight sinus, torcular Herophili, and tentorium cerebelli are all in normal location. The foramen magnum appears normal.

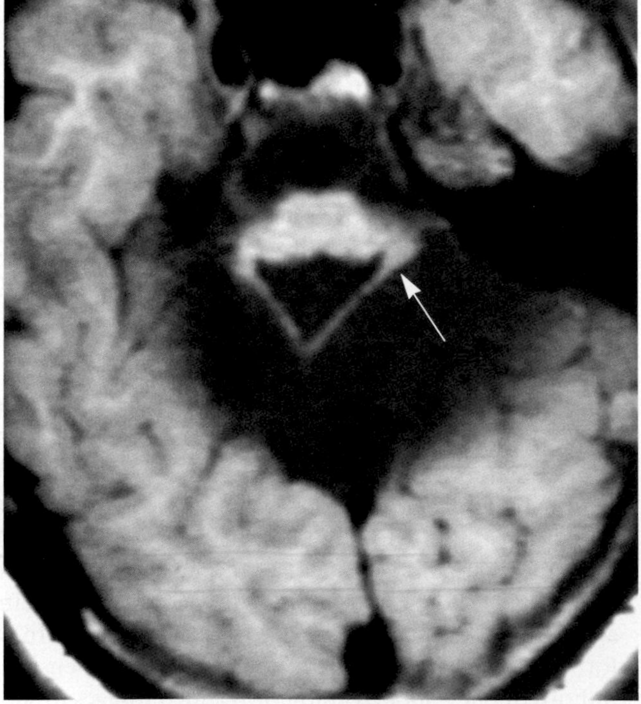

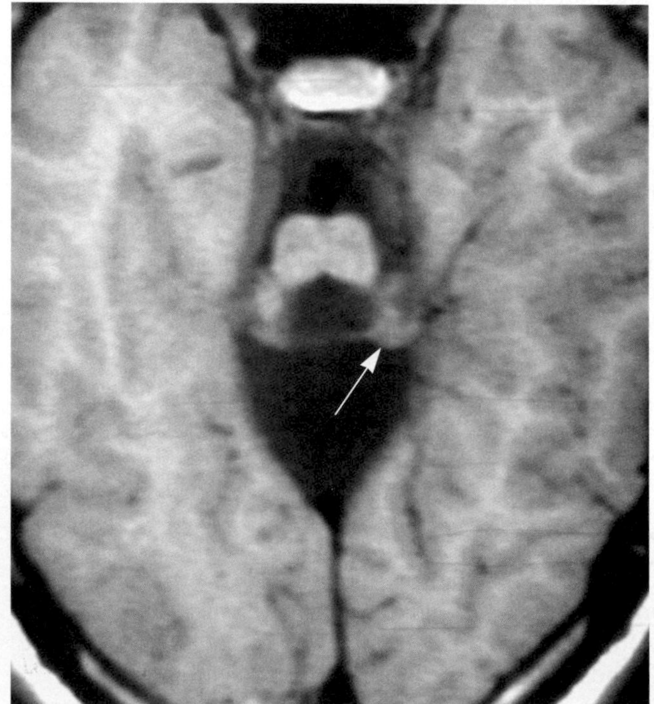

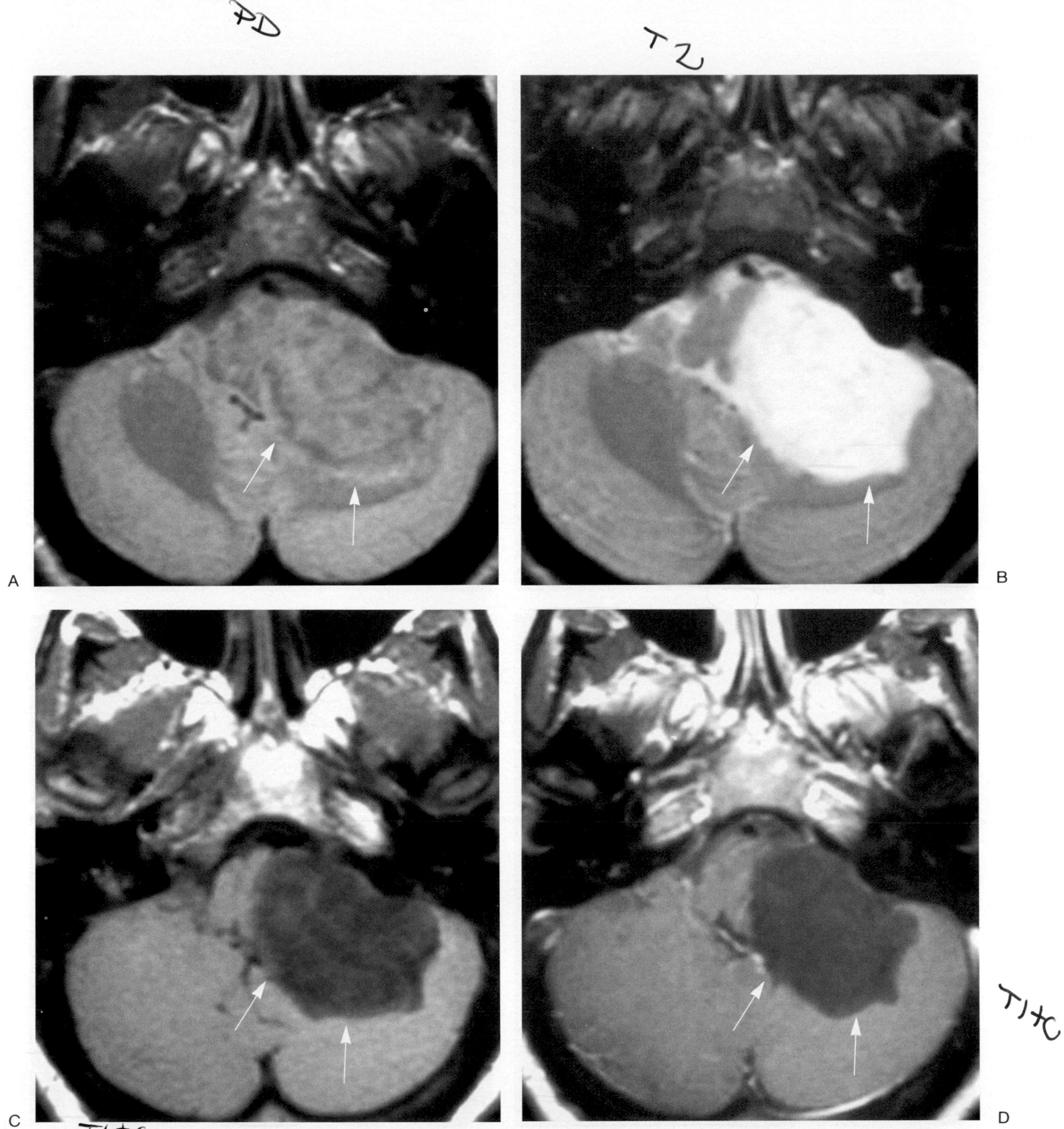

FIG. 17. Cerebellopontine angle cistern epidermoid. Axial proton-density- and T2-weighted (**A,B**) and unenhanced (**C**) and enhanced (**D**) T1-weighted images show large sharply demarcated, extra-axial mass (*arrows*) that fills the cerebellomedullary and cerebellopontine angle cisterns. Mass shows signal characteristics that are different than CSF on proton-density- and T1-weighted images. No enhancement or peritumoral edema can be seen. In addition, T1-weighted image shows intratumoral matrix, typical of epidermoid. (From Truwit and Lempert, ref. 40, with permission.)

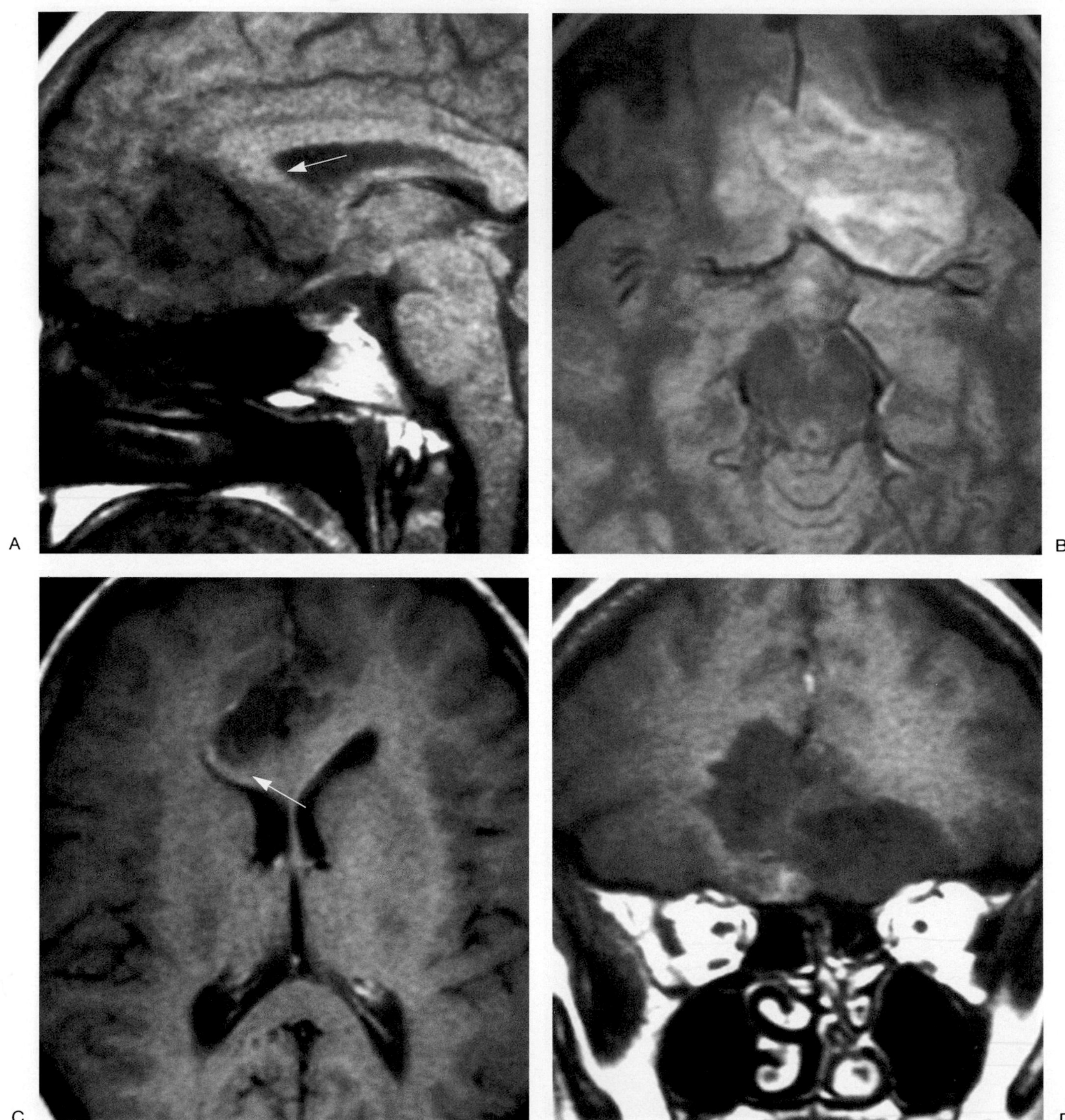

FIG. 18. Subfrontal epidermoid. Sagittal T1- (**A**), axial proton-density- (**B**), and axial (**C**) and coronal (**D**) contrast-enhanced T1-weighted images show large subfrontal mass that, at first glance, appears to cross the midline. Neither enhancement nor peritumoral edema are seen. Key feature to diagnosis is relative sparing of callosal genu (*arrows*, A,C), despite bilaterality. Tumor must be extra-axial due to callosal sparing. (From Truwit and Lempert, ref. 40, with permission.)

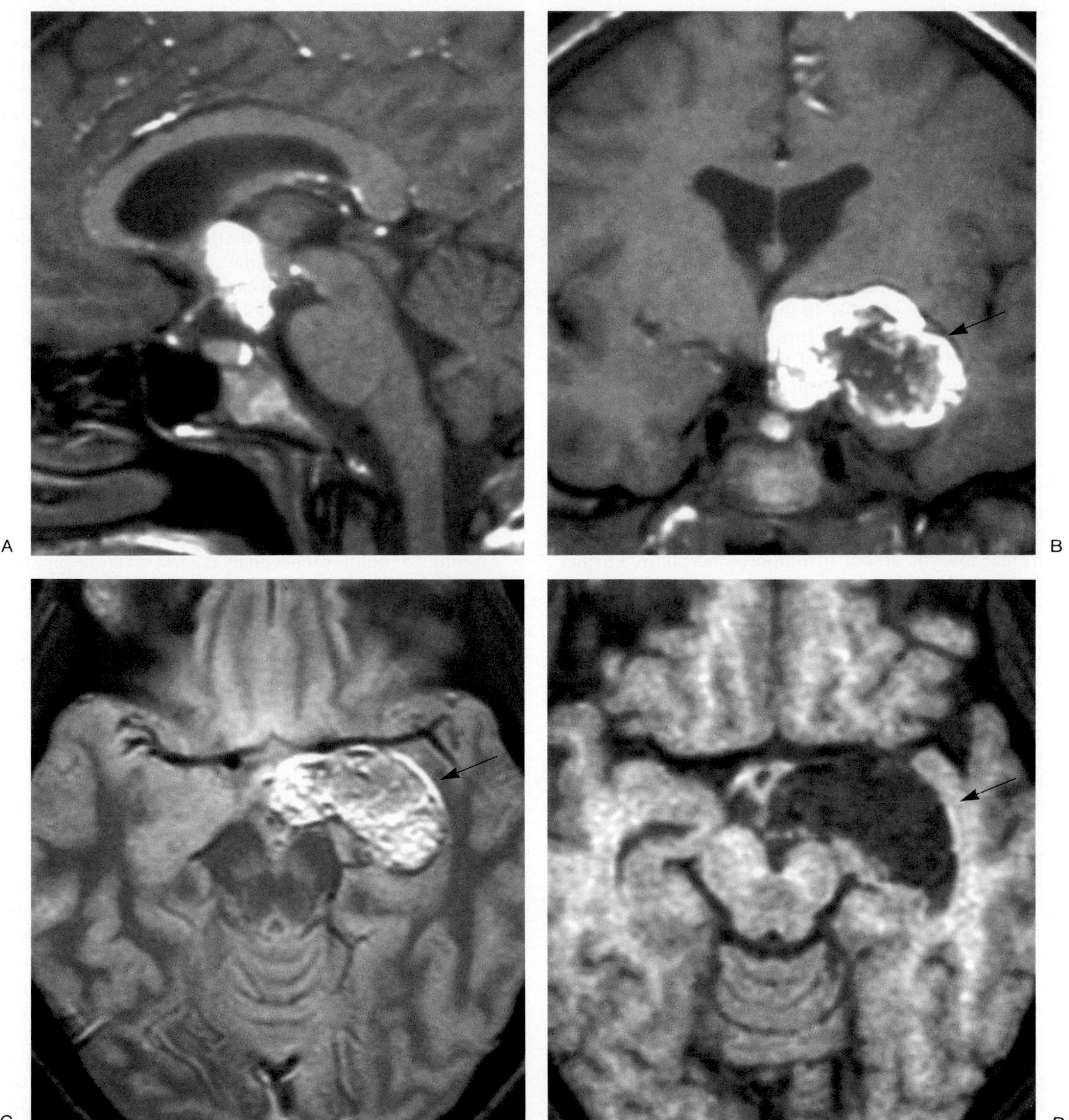

FIG. 19. Ruptured dermoid. Sagittal (**A**) and coronal (**B**) T1-weighted images show hyperintense suprasellar mass (*arrow*) that extends into and enlarges the left choroidal fissure. Hyperintensity suggest possibilities of fat, hemorrhage, and proteinaceous debris on unenhanced images. Axial proton-density-weighted image shows mild chemical shift artifact (**C**), further suggesting presence of fat. Axial T1-weighted image with fat suppression (**D**) confirms presence of fat within extra-axial lesion. T1-weighted images (A,B) also show multiple subarachnoid deposits, suggesting rupture of dermoid tumor. (From Truwit and Lempert, ref. 40, with permission.)

fluid within the arachnoid cyst. Failing that, diffusion imaging may be employed, if available. Preliminary reports have shown that the diffusion characteristics of CSF within arachnoid cysts differ considerably from the solid and semi-solid pearly matrix within epidermoids.

DISORDERS OF STRUCTURAL DEVELOPMENT

Holoprosencephaly

The holoprosencephalies are a group of disorders that are characterized by hypoplasia or aplasia of the most rostral end of the neural tube and the premaxillary segment of the face (41–44). In the past, holoprosencephaly has been considered a failure of diverticulation of the brain (failure of cleavage of the telencephalon into two cerebral hemispheres, as well as failure of cleavage of the prosencephalon into the diencephalon and telencephalon). Today, the disorder is viewed more as a global lack of forebrain induction. Indeed, Yakovlev (45) has demonstrated, in a pathoarchitectonic study of holoprosencephaly, that the prefrontal cortex ("homotypical granular cortex") that normally makes up the bulk of the frontal lobes is absent in holoprosencephaly. Furthermore, the hypothalamus, neurohypophysis, and adenohypophysis are usually hypoplastic and hypofunctional, the mamillary bodies are fused, and the olfactory system tends to be unformed (44). Associated facial anomalies, when present, result from a lack of induction of the midline segments of the face (42,44). Therefore, it may be simpler to conceptualize holoprosencephaly as a condition in which the most rostral midline sections of the brain and face are not genetically induced, and therefore, do not develop.

The severity of brain and facial deformities varies widely in holoprosencephaly. The clinical manifestations, in terms of normal development and neurologic function, vary with the amount of brain dysgenesis. Therefore, DeMeyer (41) has divided holoprosencephaly into three subcategories: alobar, semilobar, and lobar holoprosencephaly. These categories are useful for classifying holoprosencephalies of different severities. It should be noted, however, that there is no clear distinction among these different categories; in reality, they represent a spectrum of brain dysplasia, ranging from the most severe form of alobar to the nearly normal forms of lobar holoprosencephaly.

Alobar Holoprosencephaly

Alobar holoprosencephaly is the most severe form. Patients with alobar holoprosencephaly frequently have severe midline facial deformities and hypotelorism, resulting from absence or hypoplasia of the premaxillary segment of the face (41,42,44). In its most extreme form, cyclopia (fused orbits, single eyeball) and forehead proboscis are present. As the facial manifestations become slightly less severe, two severely hypoteloric orbits (cebocephaly) with proboscis between or below the orbits are seen. Examination of the brain reveals fused thalami, absence of the interhemispheric fissure and falx cerebri, a large crescent-shaped holoventricle, absence of the septum pellucidum, and, most often, a large dorsal cyst (43,44). This cyst will usually occupy more than half of the volume of the calvarium. The cerebrum is composed of a flattened mass of tissue that usually sits adjacent to the most rostral portion of the calvarium (Fig. 20). No normal structures can be appreciated grossly within the brain. Most fetuses with alobar holoprosencephaly are spontaneously (or therapeutically) aborted. They are most frequently imaged by prenatal sonography. Infants that are carried to term are stillborn or have a very short life span, and it is unusual for them to be imaged by CT or MR.

Semilobar Holoprosencephaly

Semilobar holoprosencephaly is a less severe anomaly. Patients with semilobar holoprosencephaly usually have normal facies, but they occasionally have mild facial anomalies. The interhemispheric fissure and falx cerebri are usually formed posteriorly, but are absent anteriorly (Fig. 21), where MR depicts interhemispheric continuity of cerebral cortex. The thalami are usually partially separated, resulting in a small third ventricle (Fig. 21). The hippocampal formation remains rudimentary and, as a result, the temporal horns of the lateral ventricles are large and incompletely formed. The septum pellucidum is always completely absent. A dorsal cyst may or may not be present. On sagittal images, an interhemispheric commissure that strongly resembles the posterior portions of the corpus callosum is often seen dorsal and superior to the trigones of the lateral ventricles (44,46) (Figs. 22 and 23). The anterior portions of the corpus callosum are always absent. It is debated in the developmental literature whether the "pseudosplenium" is really a corpus callosum or not (44). It should be noted, however, that, in the case of holoprosencephaly, the presence of an apparent splenium of the corpus callosum in the absence of a genu, body, and rostrum, does not imply destruction of the more anterior portions of the corpus callosum. In holoprosencephaly, the normal sequence of formation of the corpus callosum does not hold true (44,46). Rather, in holoprosencephaly one can speak of callosal dysgenesis, as opposed to hypogenesis. In addition to midline anomalies, patients with semilobar holoprosencephaly commonly have disordered neuronal migration, particularly pachygyria.

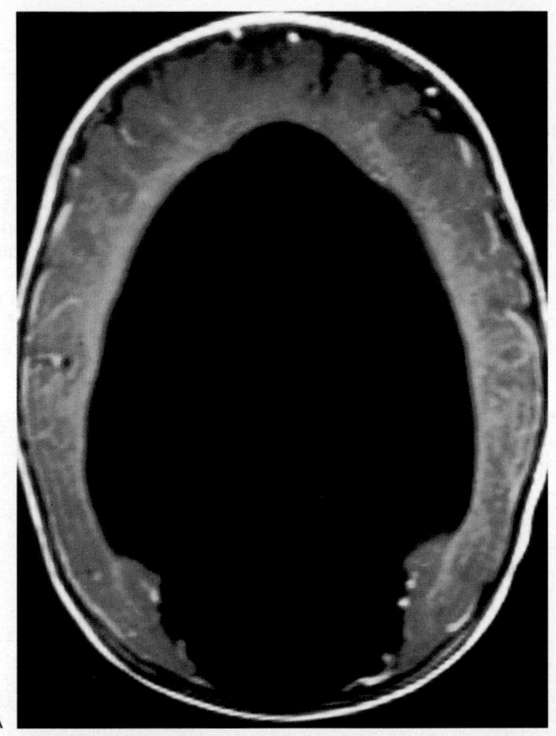

FIG. 20. A: Alobar holoprosencephaly. There is no definable interhemispheric fissure present. The falx cerebri is absent. The cerebrum is composed of a pancake-like mass of tissue situated in the rostral calvarium. A crescent-shaped holoventricle is continuous with a large dorsal cyst. **B:** Whole brain necropsy specimen viewed from above shows shallow underdeveloped interhemispheric fissure posteriorly *(arrows)* and absent interhemispheric fissure anteriorly. Note abnormal gyral pattern, with broad and smooth gyral morphology suggestive of pachygyria. **C:** Axial view of fixed specimen demonstrates monoventricle and fused thalami (*T*) with anterior continuation of gray and white matter and no interhemispheric fissure. Pachygyria is also present. (B and C from Castillo et al., ref. 199, with permission).

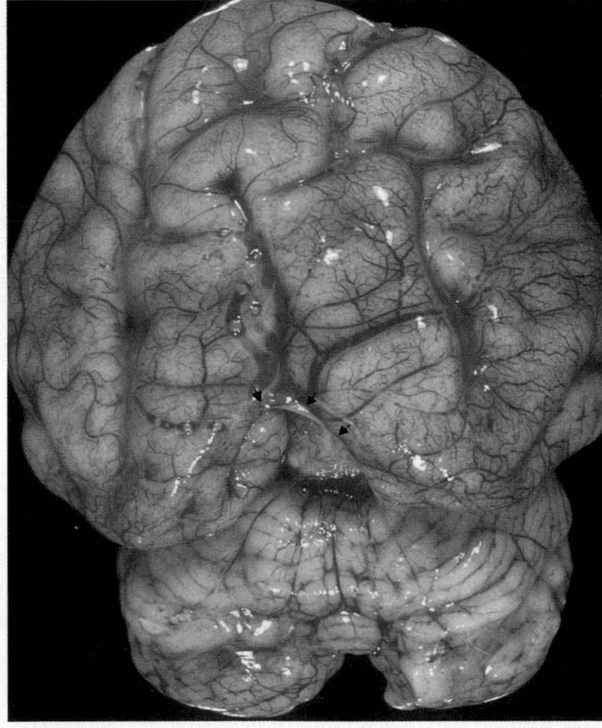

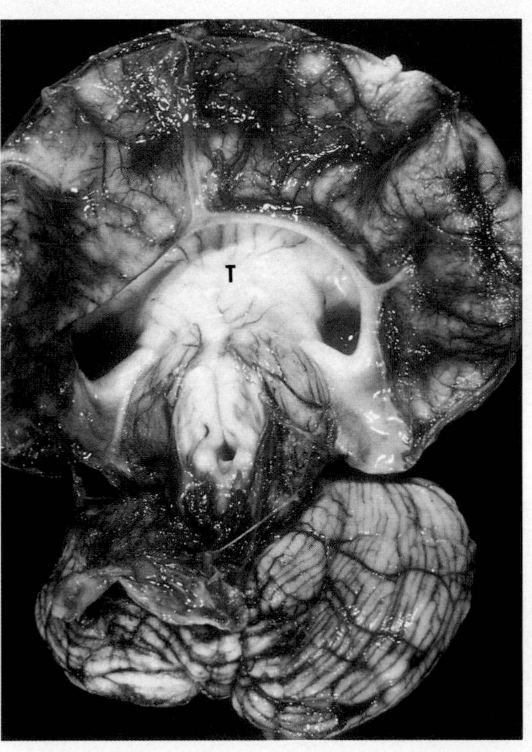

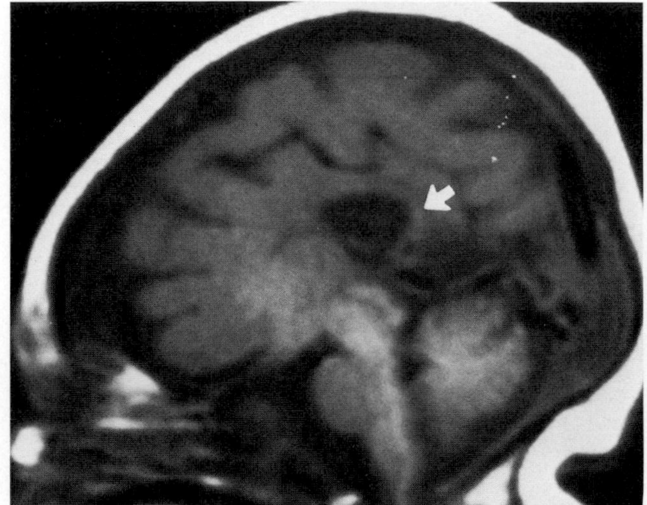

A

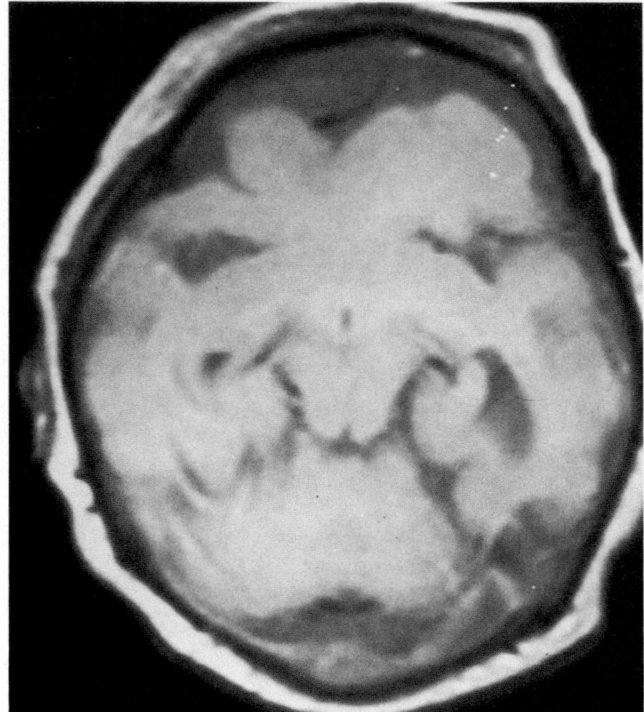

B

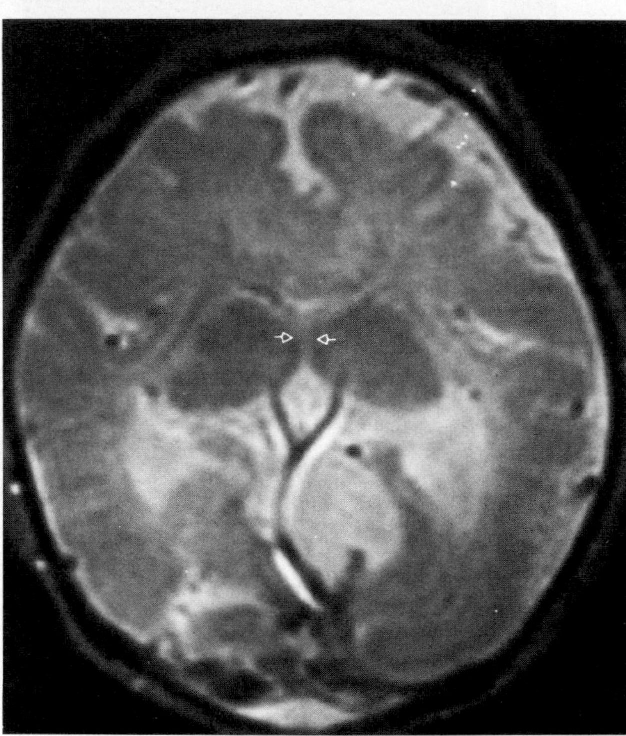

C

FIG. 21. Semilobar holoprosencephaly. **A:** Sagittal SE 600/20 image shows a markedly abnormal gyral configuration and hypoplasia of the frontal lobes. A splenium-like structure is present dorsally (*arrow*). There is debate in the developmental neuropathology literature as to whether this structure is a true splenium or a pseudosplenium. **B:** Axial SE 600/20 image reveals absence of an interhemispheric fissure and falx cerebri anteriorly. Dilatation of the temporal horns of the lateral ventricle, which results from dysplasia of the hippocampal formation. **C:** Axial SE 2800/70 image shows that the thalami are slightly separated, resulting in the formation of a rudimentary third ventricle (*arrows*).

Lobar Holoprosencephaly

The lobar form of holoprosencephaly is the most developed and least anomalous form (41,43). The interhemispheric fissure and falx cerebri extend into the frontal area of the brain, although the anterior falx is usually dysplastic (Fig. 23). The frontal horns show variable degrees of development; they may be extremely rudimentary (Figs. 22 and 23) or they may appear nearly normal. The corpus callosum shows mild dysplasia of the genu. The septum pellucidum is always absent. If a dorsal cyst is present, it is usually small. The hippocampal formations are nearly normal, and the temporal horns are well defined, appearing normal or nearly normal. Careful scrutiny will reveal some degree of hypoplasia of the frontal lobes, since the signs of lobar holoprosencephaly may be quite subtle. The olfactory bulbs, tracts, and sulci may be normal, hypogenetic, or absent.

Recently, another subset of holoprosencephaly, initially termed middle interhemispheric fusion (47), and more recently syntelencephaly (48), has been described. Perhaps the term dorsal lobar holoprosencephaly would be more consistent with the existing nomenclature of holoprosencephaly. Most cases would be classified some-

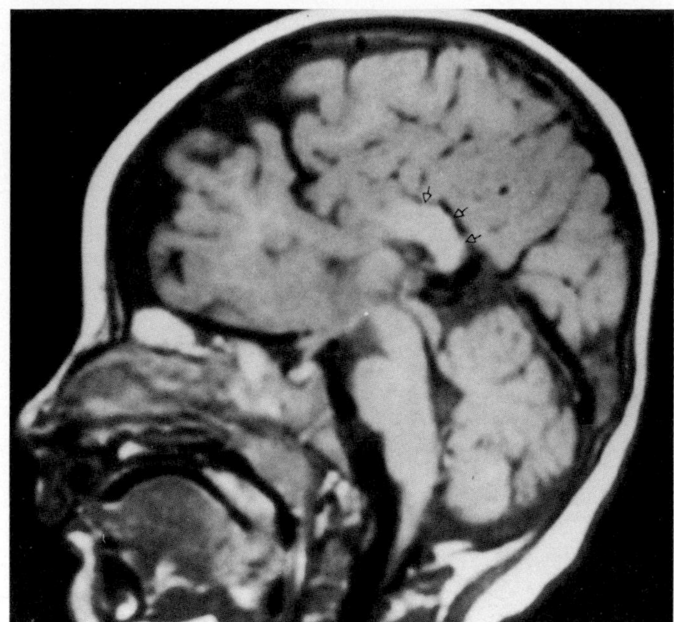

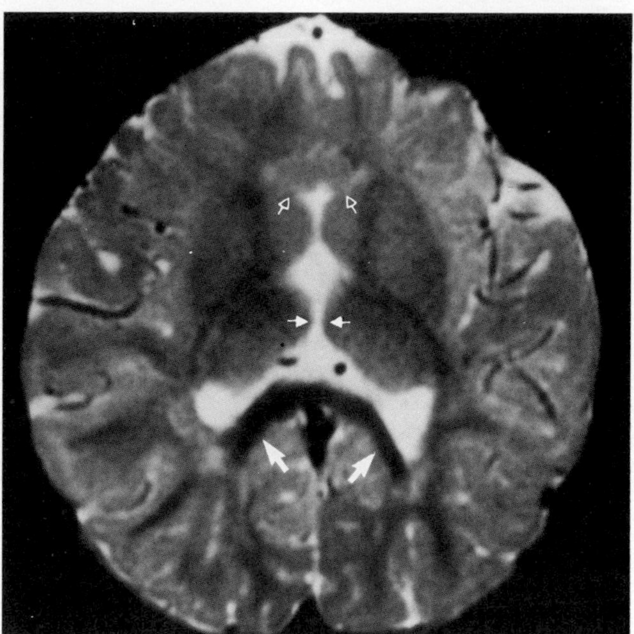

FIG. 22. Semilobar/lobar holoprosencephaly. **A:** Sagittal SE 600/20 image shows an abnormal gyral pattern and hypoplasia of the frontal lobes. A splenium-like structure is present posteriorly (*arrows*). **B:** Axial SE 2800/70 image shows fusion of the frontal lobes and slight separation of the thalami (*small closed arrows*). The dorsal interhemispheric commissure (*large closed arrows*) resembles a true splenium. Extremely rudimentary frontal horn formation is present (*small open arrows*). The presence of frontal horns would suggest that this brain should be classified as the most severe end of the spectrum of lobar holoprosencephaly. (From Barkovich, ref. 29, with permission.)

where between lobar and semilobar holoprosencephaly. Unlike semilobar holoprosencephaly, the interhemispheric fissure and falx cerebri are variably formed both posteriorly and anteriorly, with deficiency in the high frontal convexity.

In this type of holoprosencephaly, hemispheric fusion does not occur at the rostral forebrain; rather, a broad band of telencephalic fusion is seen across the frontal convexities (Fig. 24). By definition, the corpus callosum is dysgenetic, and the septum pellucidum is absent in all cases. However, rather than deficiency of the anterior corpus callosum, as in typical cases of lobar holoprosencephaly, in this variant of holoprosencephaly, it is the mid-body which is deficient. A peculiar, although not pathognomonic feature of this disorder is the presence of heterotopic gray matter "inside" the expected course of the corpus callosum (Fig. 24). The olfactory system may be deficient, as in cases of semilobar, and some cases of lobar holoprosencephaly. The face and orbits, as well as the pituitary and hypothalamus, appear normal in the few cases reported to date. The embryology of dorsal lobar holoprosencephaly is not clear since the rostro-basal forebrain appears to be less prominently involved than in the more classical forms of holoprosencephaly. It is possible that a mesenchymal failure may be related to the condition; as postulated by Barkovich and Quint (47,48), a paucity of dorsal meninx primitiva (see section, "Intracranial Lipomas") may be related to failed induction and differentiation of subjacent neural elements.

Septo-Optic Dysplasia

Septo-optic dysplasia, as described by deMorsier in 1956 (49), consists of optic nerve hypoplasia and deficiency of the septum pellucidum. In his initial report, the neuroendocrine state of his 84-year-old patient (female) was not recorded. Since that time, various clinical reports (50) have shown an association with hypothalamic-pituitary dysfunction in two-thirds of the patients (50–52). The full triad is often not seen, as the septum pellucidum may be present in up to 40% of patients (53). Visual symptoms range from nystagmus and blindness to normal vision. When hypothalamic-pituitary dysfunction is present, it is usually manifest as growth retardation secondary to diminished growth hormone and thyroid-stimulating hormone. Although the endocrine disorders have been attributed to the pituitary gland, some studies (54,55) suggest that the hypothalamus is deficient, and adenohypophyseal dysfunction is secondary. Seizures are present in half of the patients.

In addition to the triad of neuropathological changes, other features are variably present. These include schizencephaly, gray matter heterotopia, olfactory agen-

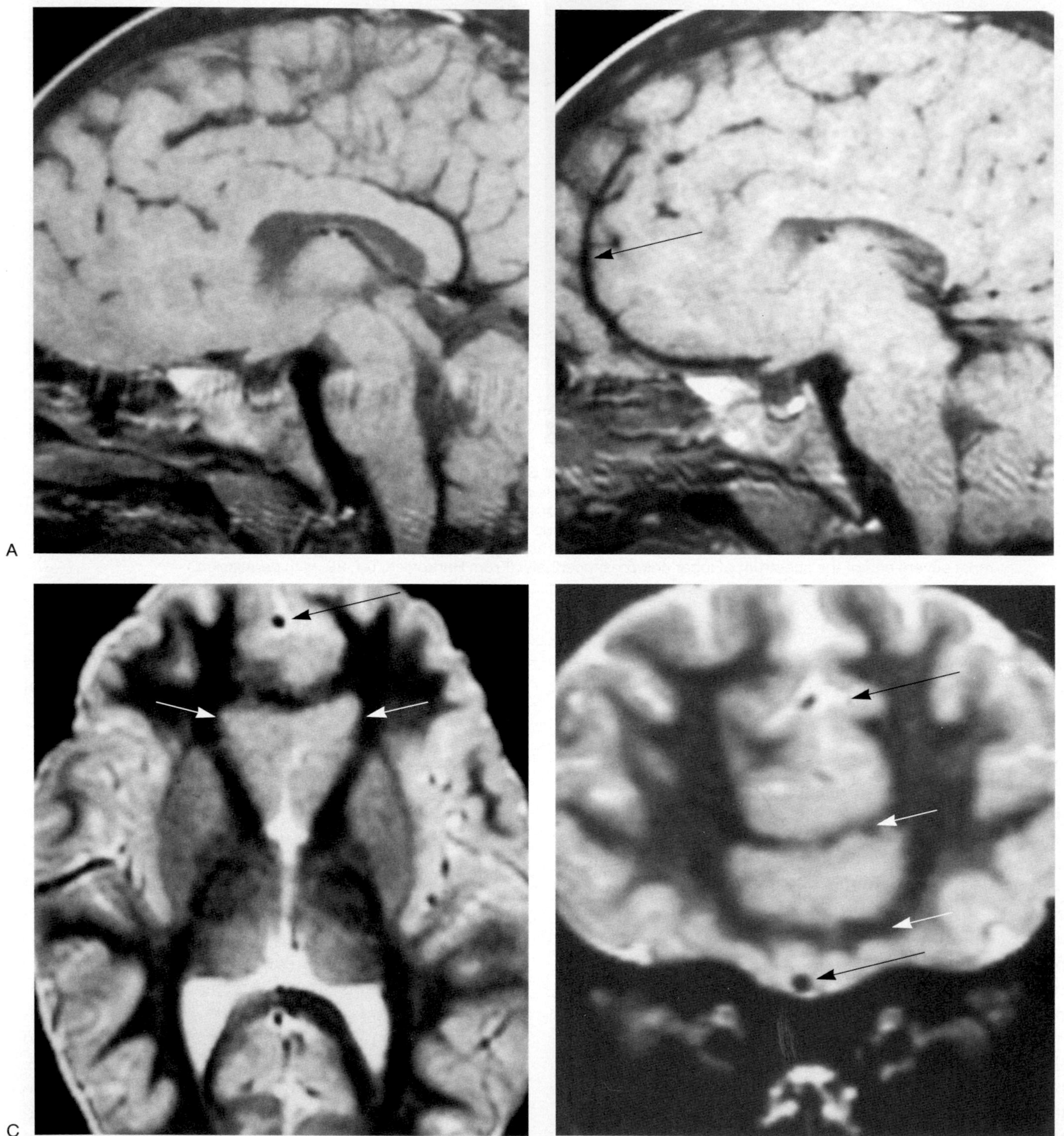

FIG. 23. Lobar holoprosencephaly. Sagittal T1-weighted images (**A,B**) show essentially normal callosal splenium and posterior body. Anterior body, genu, and rostrum, however, are not clearly visualized. This feature should prompt diagnosis of holoprosencephaly. Axial (**C**) and coronal (**D**) T2-weighted images show abnormal gray matter in place of callosal genu (*short arrows*, C), complete coaptation of frontal horns and two distinct white matter bridges of hemispheric fusion (*short arrows*, D). Note azygos anterior cerebral artery (*long arrows*), that is far more anteriorly situated than in normal patient due to hypoplastic development of interhemispheric fissure. (From Truwit and Lempert, ref. 40, with permission.)

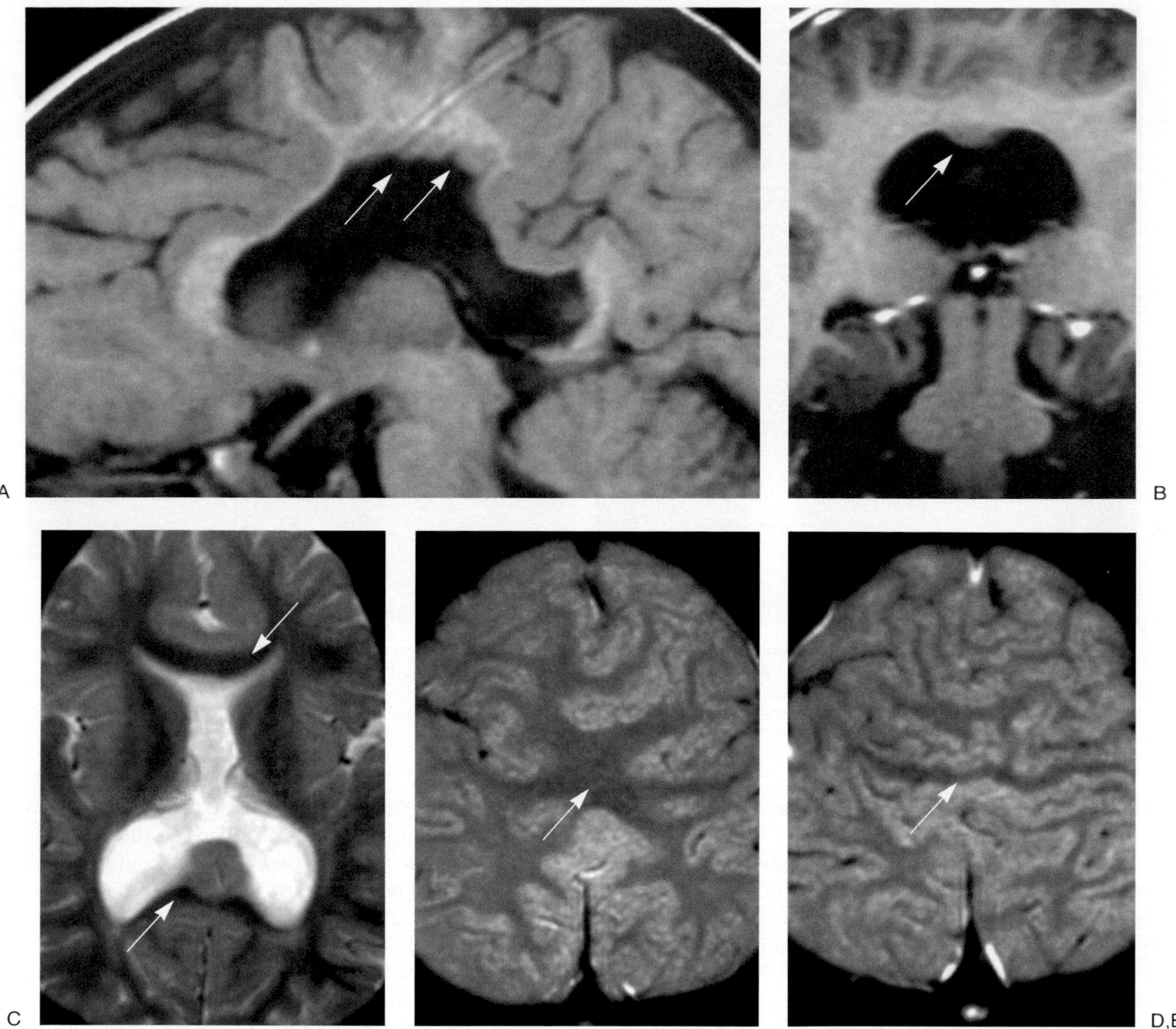

FIG. 24. Dorsal lobar holoprosencephaly. Sagittal (**A**) T1-weighted image shows marked callosal dysplasia. Although callosal genu and splenium are seen, entire callosal body is missing. (Rostrum is also hypoplastic.) Contrast-enhanced coronal (**B**) T1-weighted image shows absence of septum pellucidum and gray matter (*arrows*, A and B) beneath abnormal white matter band of hemispheric fusion. Normally, gray matter is not seen in this location. Mild hypoplasia of the temporal lobes is apparent as well. Axial T2- and proton-density-weighted images (**C–E**) show minimal distortion of callosal genu and splenium (*arrows*, C) and broad band of hemispheric fusion involving the dorsal frontal lobes (*arrows*, D,E). Because ventricles are so well formed, diagnosis is more akin to lobar, rather than semilobar, holoprosencephaly. (From Truwit and Lempert, ref. 40, with permission.)

esis or hypoplasia, and absence of the neurohypophysis (without ectopia).

The diagnosis is often suspected on the basis of ophthalmologic examination, which reveals hypoplasia of the optic discs. CT or MRI can reveal partial or complete absence of the septum pellucidum (Fig. 25), although the septum may appear normal. In addition, hypoplasia of the optic nerves and chiasm can be detected on MRI (Figs. 25 and 26) in between 50% and 80% of affected individuals. Optic nerve hypoplasia may be more apparent on MR by the use of fat suppression. MR imaging reveals concurrent schizencephaly (Fig. 25) in 50% of patients (56,57). Patients without schizencephaly commonly have diffuse white matter hypoplasia (57).

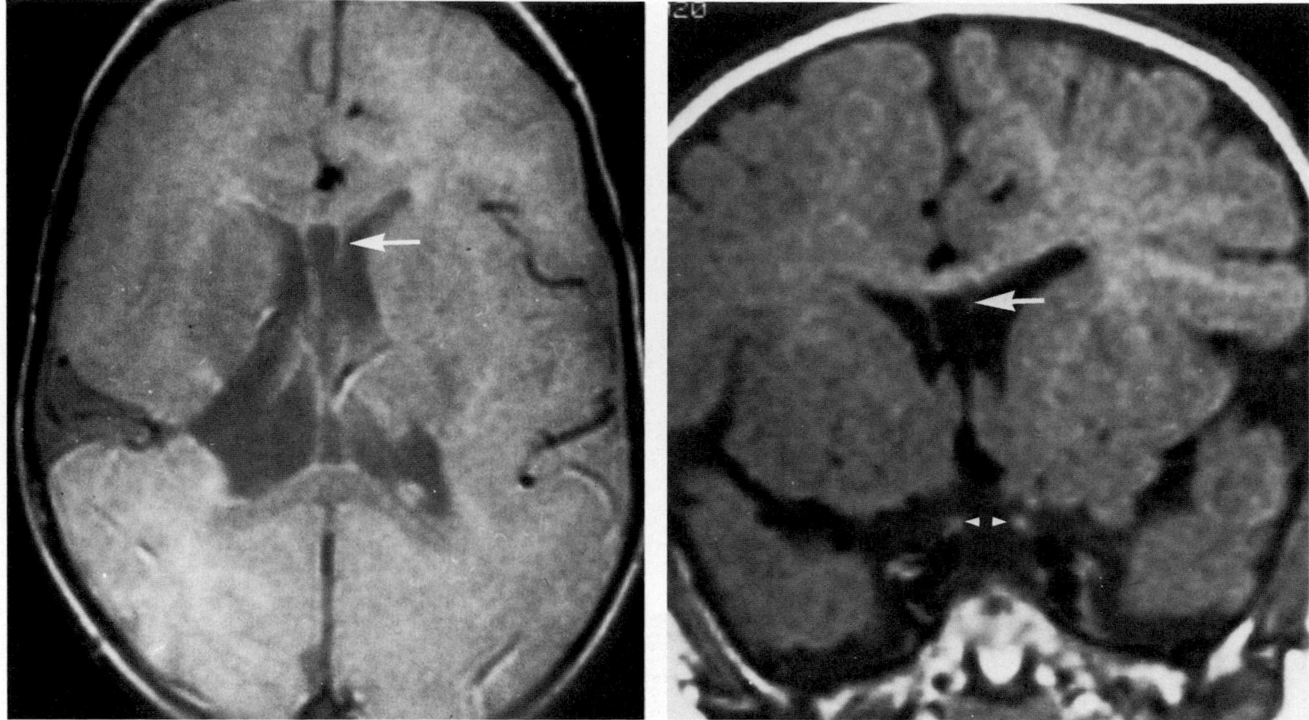

FIG. 25. Septo-optic dysplasia with schizencephaly. **A:** Axial SE 2800/30 image through the lateral ventricle reveals absence of most of the left leaf of the septum pellucidum. Only a small portion of the septum is present (*arrow*). The right leaf of the septum appears intact. A schizencephalic cleft is seen involving the posterior aspect of the right lateral ventricle. **B:** Coronal SE 600/20 image again shows the hypoplastic left septal leaf (*arrow*). The intracranial optic nerves (*arrowheads*) are hypoplastic.

Malformations of the Corpus Callosum

After closure of the anterior neuropore at about the 25th day of gestation, the rostral wall of the telencephalon is a thin layer of tissue known as the primitive lamina terminalis. During the sixth and seventh week of gestation, there is a rapid increase in the thickness of the dorsal end of the lamina terminalis near the paraphysis. This thickened, cellular region has been called the lamina reuniens (58). Axons from both hemispheres grow into this region, forming the anterior commissure, corpus callosum, and hippocampal commissure. Because the commissural plate forms in an anterior to posterior direction, the anterior commissure (the most rostral of the three) forms first, the initial fibers crossing in the rostral portion of the commissural plate at about the tenth gestational week (58). The first fibers of the hippocampal commissure begin to cross in the dorsal portion of the commissural plate at about the 11th gestational week (58). The pioneer callosal fibers then begin to cross slightly anterior to the hippocampal commissure at about the 12th gestational week (58). It is important to recognize that the entire corpus callosum does not form at the same time. In fact, the corpus callosum forms in an orderly and precise fashion. The first segment to be defined is the junction of the dorsal genu and anterior body. This is followed by the genu and anterior body, posterior body, splenium, and, lastly, the rostrum. Because of this precise sequence of development, any insult occurring to the developing brain during formation of the corpus callosum will result in the anterior portion being formed with the posterior portion absent (29). Furthermore, because the rostrum is formed last, any question of hypoplasia of the splenium can be answered by checking to see if the rostrum is present. If the rostrum is present, the splenium must be fully formed and any diminution in size will be the result of secondary atrophy and not primary hypogenesis. Moreover, a small or absent genu or body in the presence of a normal splenium and rostrum is almost certainly the result of a secondary destructive process and not primary hypogenesis. The one exception to this rule (46) is in the case of holoprosencephaly, as discussed earlier.

The commissural plate forms between approximately 8 and 16 gestational weeks, and the corpus callosum itself forms between about 12 and 20 gestational weeks (59,60). This is a time when the entire brain is developing. Therefore, it should not be surprising that anomalies of the corpus callosum are very frequently associated with other congenital brain anomalies (29,61). Some of the more common associated anomalies are the Chiari II malformation, the Dandy-Walker malformation, interhemispheric cysts, neuronal migration anomalies, cephaloceles, and midline facial anomalies (59,60). In general, these anomalies are the cause of any clinical

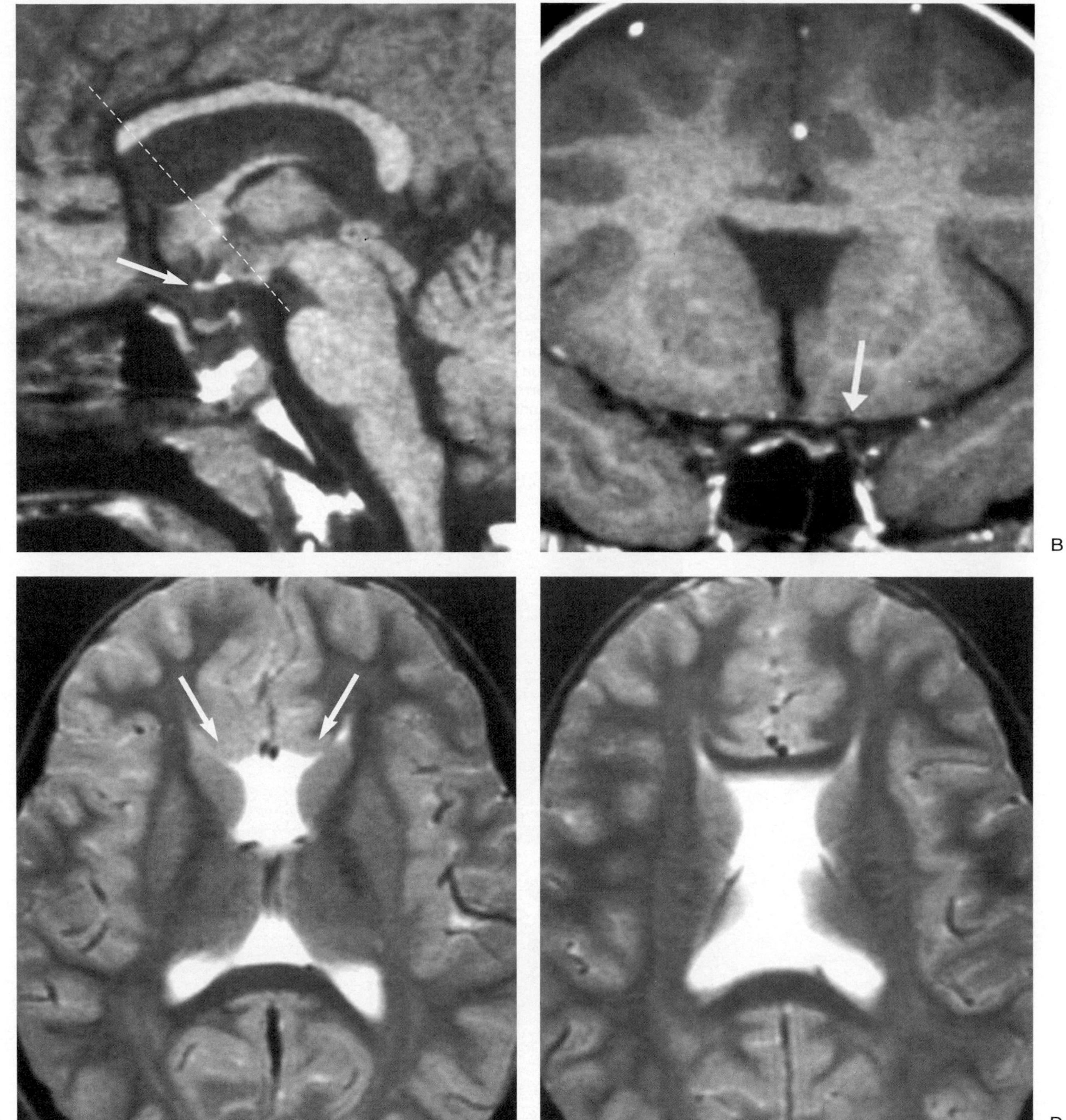

FIG. 26. Septo-optic dysplasia. Sagittal (**A**) and coronal (**B**) T1-weighted images show callosal hypoplasia involving all portions anterior to the genu-anterior body interface. Although earlier descriptions would suggest that this represents callosal dysgenesis, in fact, this appearance most likely represents an unusual form of callosal hypogenesis. If one accepts the current concept that the corpus callosum forms bidirectionally from the genu-anterior body interface, hypoplasia involving the genu and rostrum is possible, albeit unusual. The interface is defined as the callosal point along a line from the mamillary body to the corpus callosum, through the anterior commissure (*dashed line*, A). Note hypoplastic left optic nerve (*arrow*, B) and absent septum pellucidum. Chiasm also appears hypoplastic (*arrow*, A). Small lipoma of tuber cinereum is also seen. Axial proton-density-weighted images (**C,D**) show full extent of septal deficiency and frontal interhemispheric gray matter that extends all the way to the frontal horns due to hypoplasia of callosal genu (*arrows*, C). (From Truwit and Lempert, ref. 40, with permission.)

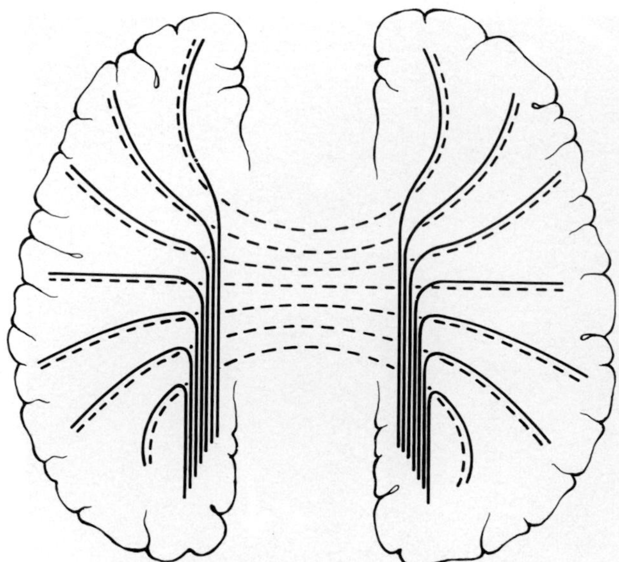

FIG. 27. The formation of the lateral callosal bundles (of Probst). As a result of a lack of normal formation of the commissural plate, axons from the cerebral hemispheres do not cross the midline. Instead, upon reaching the medial hemispheric wall, the fibers turn to course parallel to the interhemispheric fissure. The fibers run parallel to and indent the medial walls of the lateral ventricles. *Broken lines* represent normal callosal fibers. *Solid lines* represent fibers that fail to cross the midline and, instead, form the lateral callosal bundles.

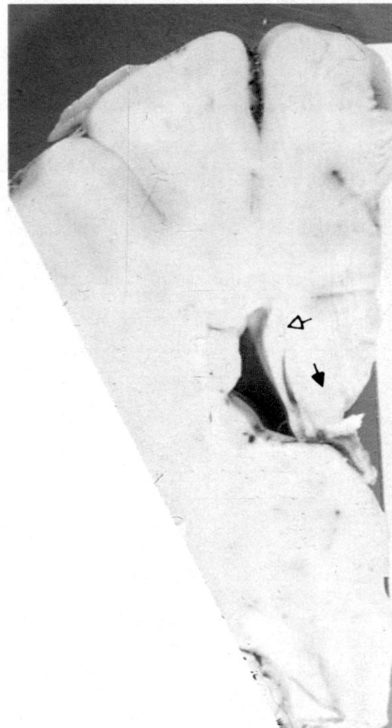

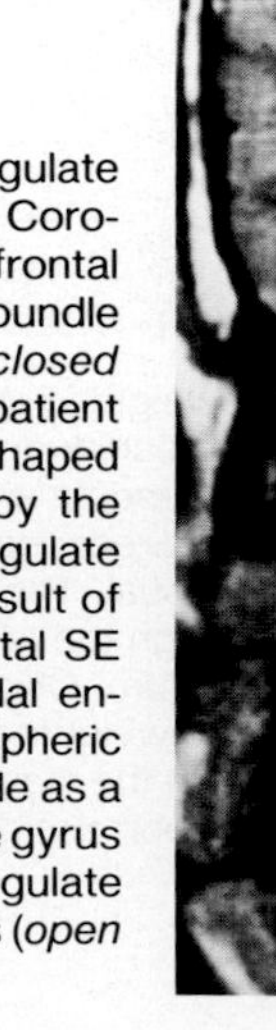

A

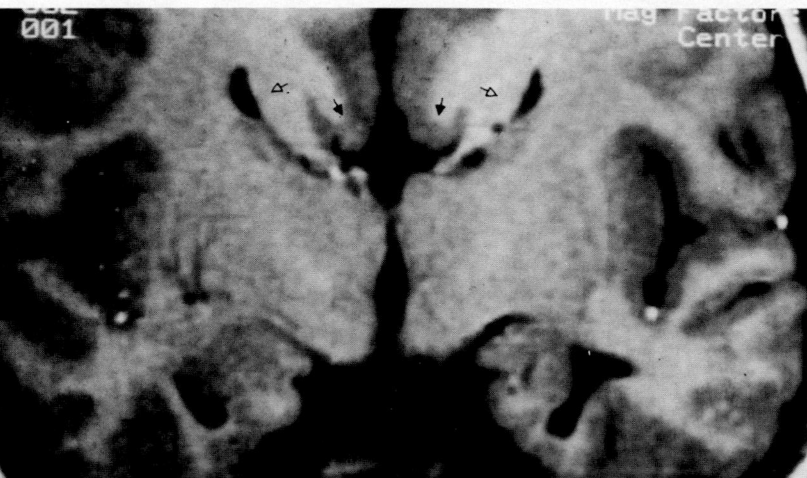

B

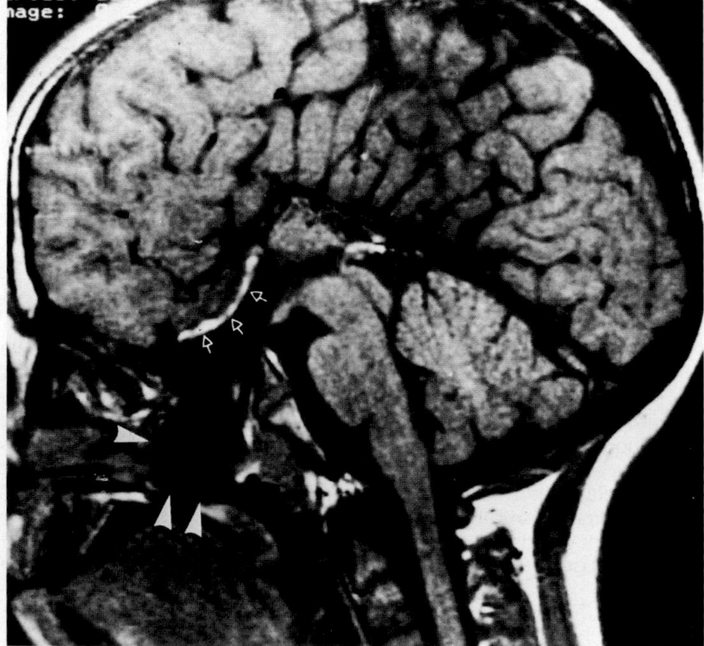

C

FIG. 28. Probst bundle and eversion of cingulate gyrus in agenesis of the corpus callosum. **A:** Coronal necropsy specimen shows concave frontal horn due to combination of Probst callosal bundle (*open arrows*) and everted cingulate gyrus (*closed arrows*). **B:** Coronal SE 600/20 image in patient with complete agenesis reveals crescent-shaped frontal horns resulting from compression by the bundles of Probst (*open arrows*). The cingulate gyri remain everted (*closed arrows*) as a result of absence of normal callosal fibers. **C:** Sagittal SE 600/20 image shows associated sphenoidal encephalocele (*arrowheads*). The mesial hemispheric sulci extend all the way into the third ventricle as a result of the lack of inversion of the cingulate gyrus and consequent lack of formation of the cingulate sulcus. Also note lipoma of lamina terminalis (*open arrows*).

symptoms; isolated agenesis of the corpus callosum is usually asymptomatic and can be detected only by sophisticated neurological testing.

Callosal agenesis results in several anatomical features that are distinct from the normal brain (29,59–61). Axons that usually cross the interhemispheric fissure within the corpus instead form fiber bundles that run medial to the medial walls of the lateral ventricles, parallel to the interhemispheric fissure (Fig. 27). These white matter fiber bundles are known as the longitudinal callosal bundles, or the bundles of Probst. The bundles of Probst invaginate the medial borders of the lateral ventricles to give them a crescentic shape when viewed in the coronal plane (Figs. 28 and 29). The third ventricle and foramina

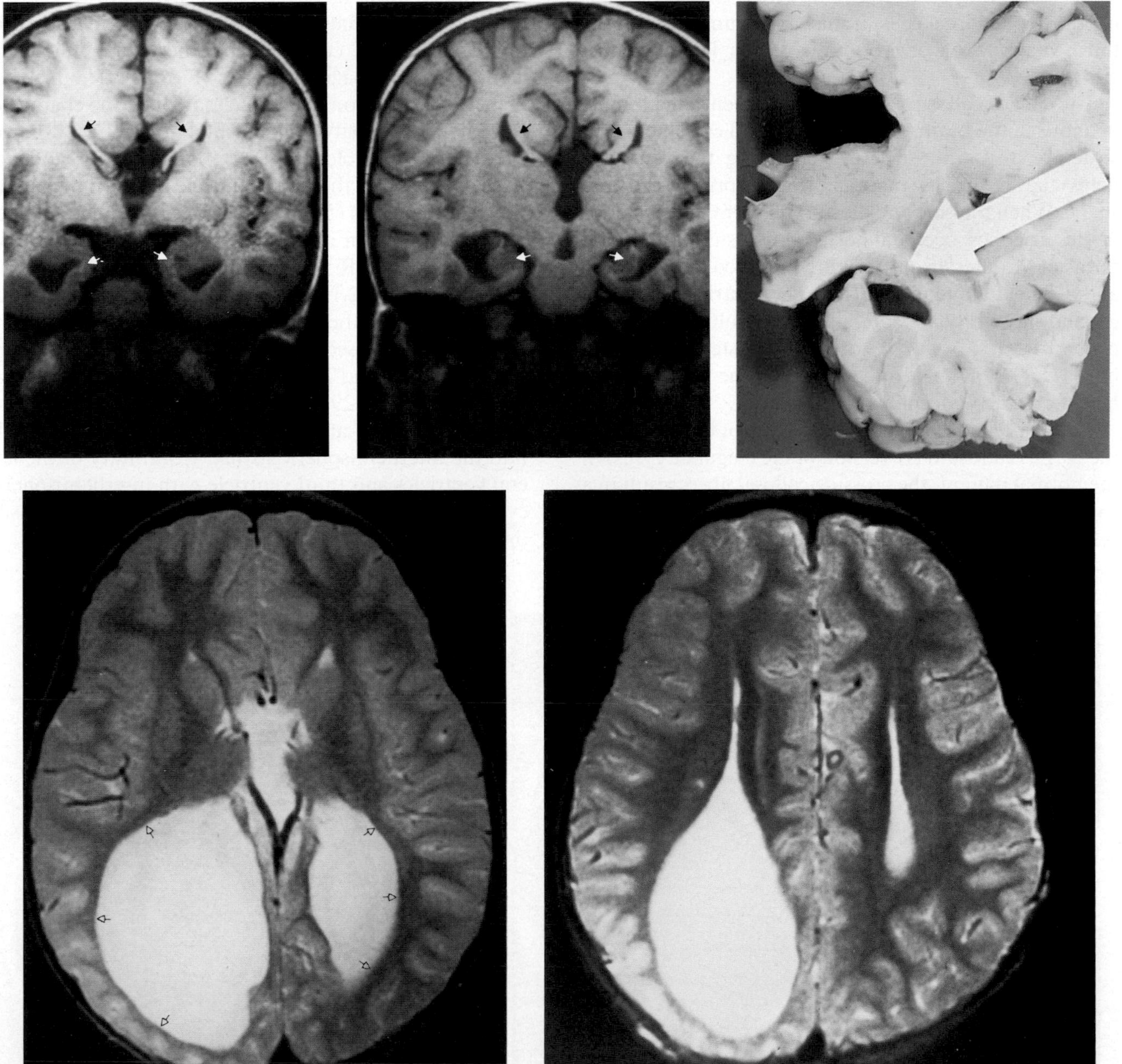

FIG. 29. Agenesis of the corpus callosum. **A,B:** Coronal SE 600/20 images reveal Probst bundles (*black arrows*) adjacent to lateral ventricles, extension of the third ventricle superiorly between the lateral ventricles, and incomplete formation and malrotation of the hippocampus (*white arrows*). **C**: Coronal necropsy specimen in callosal agenesis shows malformed hippocampus with secondarily dilated temporal horn (*arrow*). (Courtesy of Dr. Lucy Rorke, Children's Hospital of Philadelphia, Philadelphia, PA.) **D:** Axial SE 2500/70 image shows marked dilatation of the atria and occipital horns of the lateral ventricles (*arrows*). This enlargement results from disorganization of the dorsal white matter when the splenium is absent and has been termed "colpocephaly." Note paucity of posterior parietal and occipital white matter. The third ventricle extends upward between the lateral ventricles. **E:** Axial SE 2500/70 image shows that the lateral ventricles are parallel and redemonstrates deficient white matter formation posteriorly.

of Monro are usually widened in callosal agenesis; moreover, the third ventricle often extends superiorly between the bodies of the lateral ventricles (Fig. 29). Occasionally, the third ventricle extends high into the interhemispheric fissure, forming a cerebrospinal fluid (CSF) collection that is generally referred to as an interhemispheric cyst (Fig. 30). Although arachnoid cysts can occur in the interhemispheric fissure in association with agenesis of the corpus callosum, more commonly this CSF collection is lined by ependymal cells. It may communicate with the third ventricle or one or both of the lateral ventricles (59).

The corpus callosum is the most concentrated bundle of axons in the brain. As a result, it is an extremely firm structure; this firm structure bordering the ventricles helps the ventricles maintain their normal size and shape. When the corpus callosum is absent, the posterior bodies, trigones, occipital horns, and posterior temporal horns of the lateral ventricles are bordered only by loose and deficient white matter (59). The ventricles therefore expand superiorly and laterally with resultant dilatation of the trigones, occipital horns, and posterior temporal horns (Fig. 29). This configuration of the ventricles has been termed colpocephaly (60).

Another feature that is characteristic of the absence of the corpus callosum is eversion of the cingulate gyrus. In the normal patient, the crossing callosal fibers result in a superomedial displacement of the cingulate gyri, the end result being a cingulate gyrus that is oriented roughly perpendicular to the interhemispheric fissure (Fig. 31). This normal inversion of the cingulate gyrus results in the formation of the cingulate sulcus (Fig. 31). When the corpus callosum is absent, the cingulate gyri remain everted (Fig. 28), and the cingulate sulci remain unformed. As a result, the mesial hemispheric sulci course uninterrupted in a radial manner all the way into the third ventricle (Figs. 28 and 31) (29,61).

Although agenesis of the corpus callosum can be detected on axial images, such as those obtained by CT, milder degrees of callosal hypogenesis are difficult to identify without sagittal images (Fig. 32). The features that are well seen on axial images include the characteristic lateral convexity of the frontal horns (Fig. 28), parallel lateral ventricles (Fig. 29), colpocephaly, and upward extension of the third ventricle between the lateral ventricles (Fig. 29) (59). The full extent of callosal hypogenesis is well seen on midline sagittal images (Figs. 30 and 32). Other MR findings include persistent eversion of the cingulate gyri (with extension of medial hemispheric sulci into the third ventricle) (61), crescentic lateral ventricles caused by the medially located bundles of Probst (Figs. 28 and 29), hypogenesis of the hippocampal formations (Fig. 29) (61), hypoplasia of the anterior commissure (29), and extension of the third ventricle into the interhemispheric fissure. Continuity of the lateral ventricles and third ventricle with interhemispheric cysts, when present, is also appreciated much more easily on MR.

A

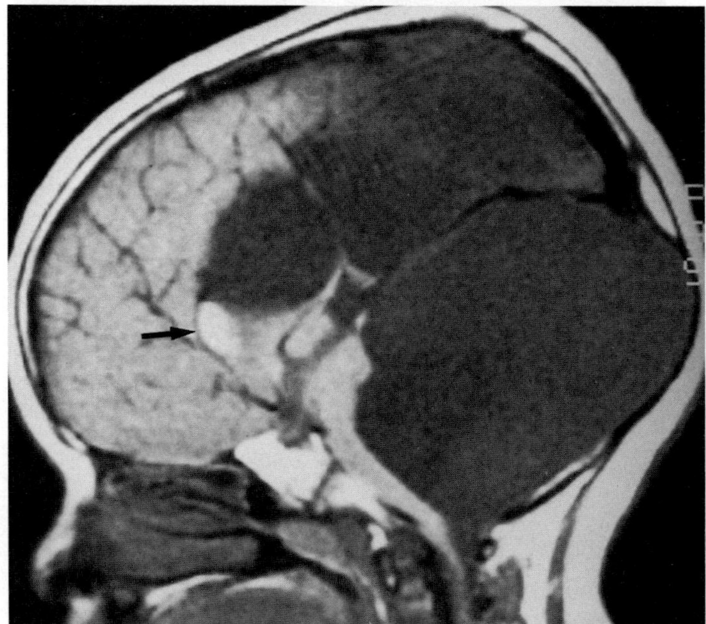

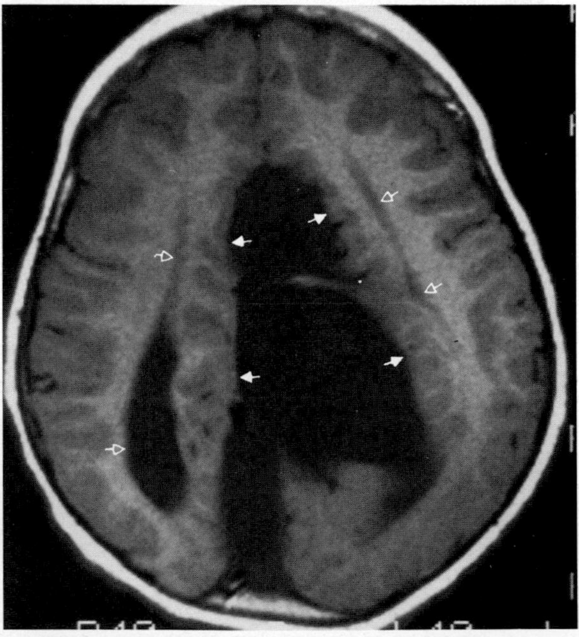

B

FIG. 30. Dandy-Walker malformation with hypogenesis of the corpus callosum and interhemispheric cyst. **A:** Sagittal SE 600/20 image shows an enlarged posterior fossa containing a huge cyst. The cerebellar vermis is absent. Only the genu of the corpus callosum (*arrow*) is present. A large CSF-intensity region is present dorsal and superior to the genu. **B:** Axial SE 600/20 image shows a large cystic midline structure (*closed arrows*) that is of CSF intensity. This left cerebral hemisphere is displaced to the left. Both lateral ventricles can be identified (*open arrows*) and are separate from the cyst.

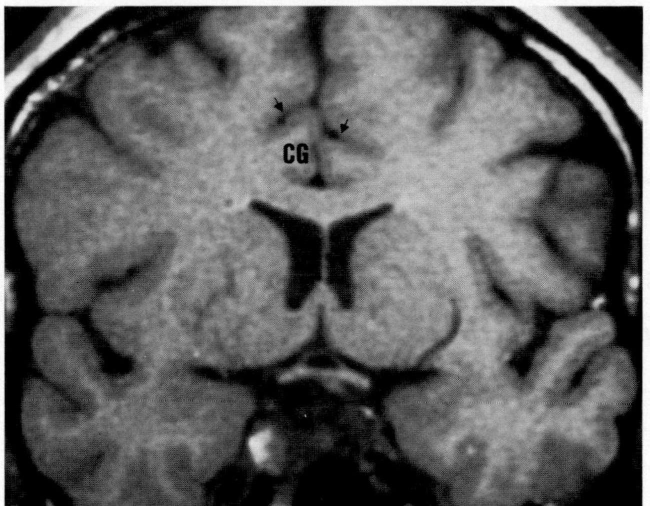

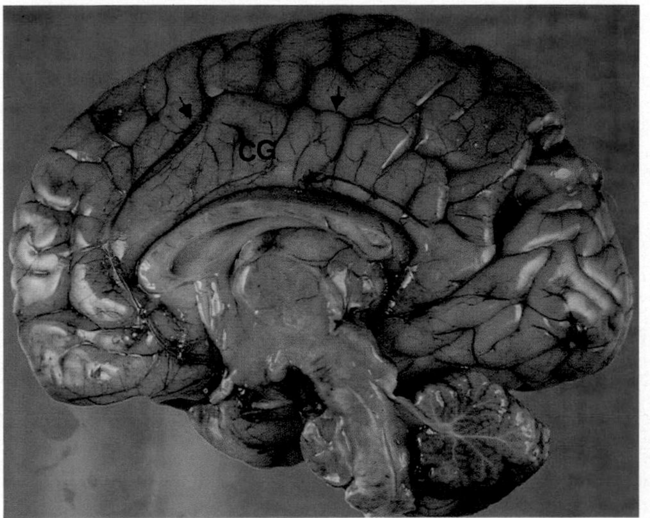

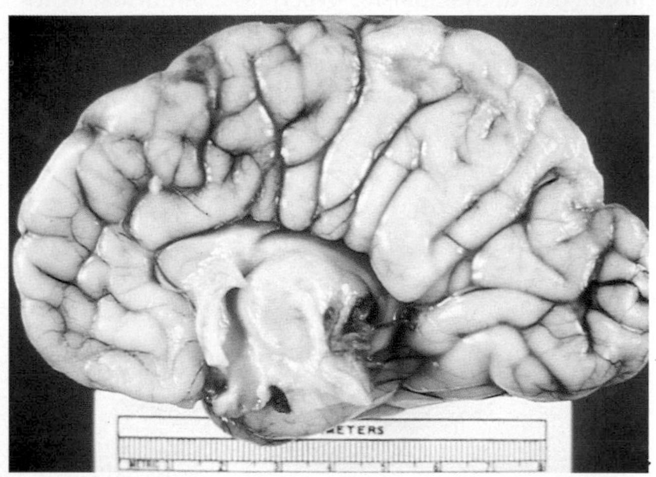

FIG. 31. Normal cingulate gyrus and cingulate sulcus formation. **A:** SE 600/20 image of normally inverted cingulate gyri. **B:** Sagittal necropsy specimen, showing normal cingulate gyrus and sulcus. **C:** Sagittal necropsy specimen in posterior agenesis of the corpus callosum. When the corpus callosum forms, one consequence of the normal crossing of the callosal fibers is inversion of the cingulate gyri (*CG* in A,B) with resultant formation of the cingulate sulci (*arrows*, A,B). In callosal agenesis (C), the lack of formation of a well-defined cingulate sulcus results in mesial hemispheric sulci radiating in an uninterrupted fashion to the roof of the third ventricle in the region of the absent corpus callosum.

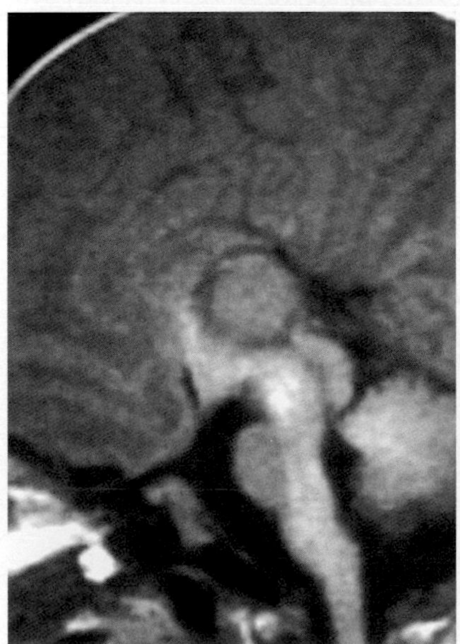

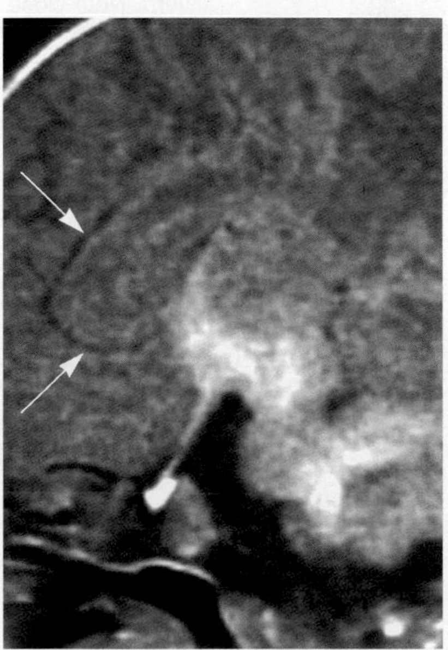

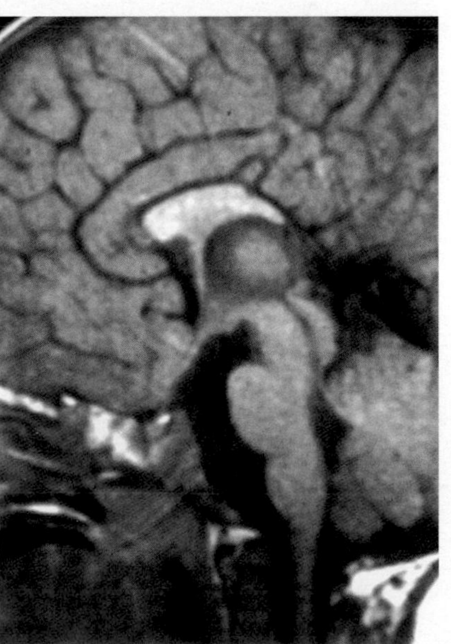

FIG. 32. Hypogenetic corpus callosum. Sagittal T1-weighted images at birth (**A,B**) and at 16 months of age show hypoplasia of corpus callosum. Early images are difficult to interpret due to absence of significant callosal myelination at birth. Presence of cingulate sulcus (*arrows*, B) is clue to diagnosis of hypogenesis, rather than agenesis. Once myelinated, full extent of callosum hypogenesis is apparent (**C**). Note absence of genu, posterior body, splenium, and rostrum. As in Fig. 27, this is not inconsistent with hypogenesis, and further supports notion of callosal development from genu-anterior body interface. (From Truwit and Lempert, ref. 40, with permission.)

Interestingly, MR has revealed a much higher incidence of callosal anomalies in patients with other brain malformations than was previously suspected (62). Therefore the corpus callosum should always be carefully scrutinized when imaging infants or children with seizures, developmental delay, or dysmorphic facial features.

Leptomeningeal Malformations

Intracranial Lipoma

Like many anomalies of the CNS, the intracranial lipoma has been the subject of abundant literature regarding its etiology, appearance, and significance. It has been proposed that lipomas are the result of mesodermal inclusion due to dysraphism, hyperplasia of normal leptomeningeal fat cells, catabolic products of neural tissue, and heterotopia of displaced dermal anlage (63). In addition, Verga (64) proposed that intracranial lipomas derive from the embryologic meninx primitiva described by Salvi (65). This latter concept failed to gain wide acceptance, primarily because it did not satisfactorily address the reason intracranial lipomas consistently occur in the same locations. This issue, however, appears now to be resolved.

The meninx primitiva is a mesodermal derivative of the neural crest. Normally, the meninx ensheaths the developing embryo; according to an orderly process, the inner meninx is resorbed leaving the subarachnoid space. For many years, it was assumed that this dissolution occurred secondary to rupture of the fourth ventricle with seepage of CSF into the extracellular matrix of the meninx primitiva. This widespread belief was based on the work of Lewis Weed (66), who cannulated both the lateral ventricle and central spinal canal of the pig embryo. Through these cannulae, he infused potassium ferrocyanide and iron-ammonium citrate, effectively replacing the CSF. Weed interpreted his findings as confirmation that CSF is initially formed by the fourth ven-

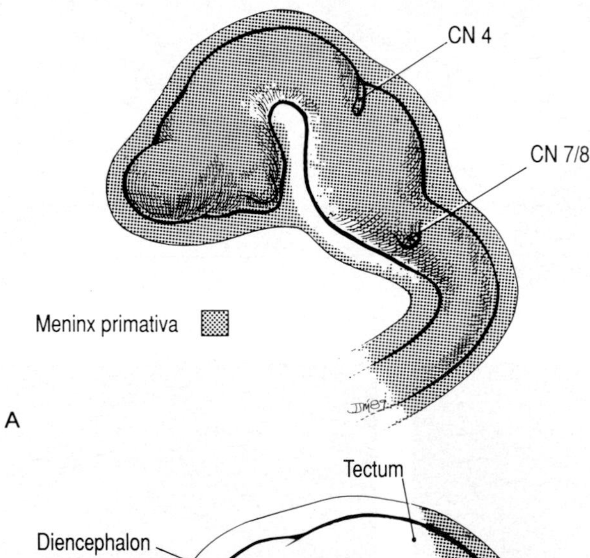

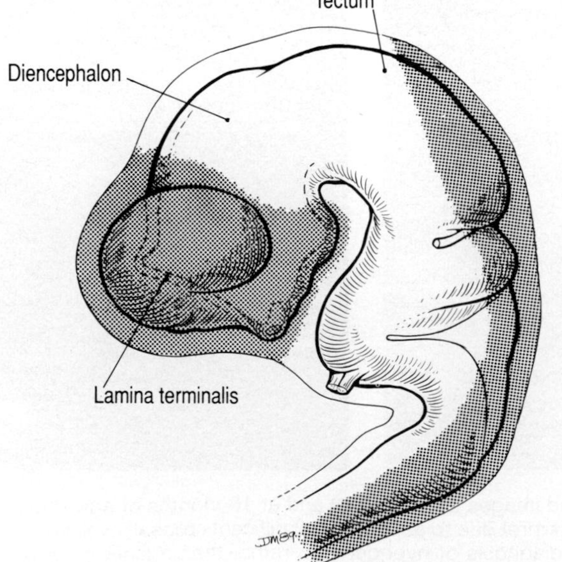

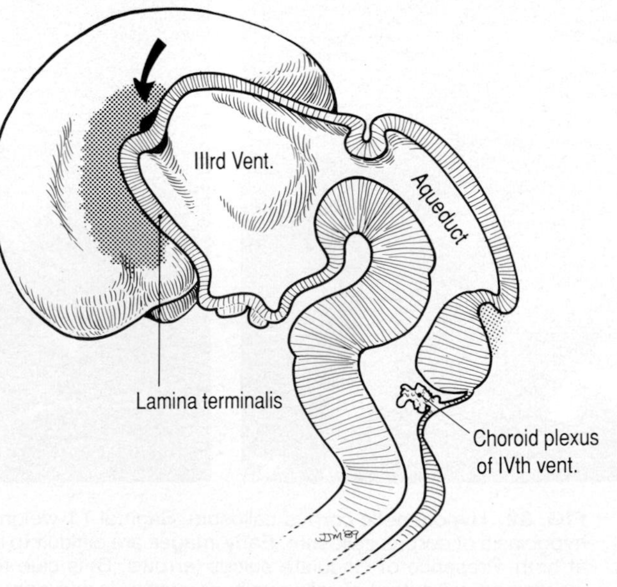

FIG. 33. **A:** Left lateral view of embryo at approximately Carnegie stage 14 (32 days, 5–7 mm) reveals earliest cavitation of meninx primitiva ventral to brainstem. *CN*, cranial nerve. **B:** At stage 18 (44 days, 13–17 mm), further dissolution of meninx has occurred; residual meninx is seen rostral to leptomeningeal septum, around (and between) telencephalic vesicles and dorsal to mes- and rhombencephali. **C:** In composite midsagittal section over stages 19–23 (48–57 days, 17–30 mm), meninx is still present rostral (dorsal) to lamina terminalis and probably within future quadrigeminal/superior cerebellar cistern. Note close proximity of choroidal fissure (*arrow*) to interhemispheric meninx, accounting for extension of lipomas into lateral ventricular choroid plexuses. *Vent.*, ventricle. (From Truwit and Barkovich, ref. 63, with permission.)

tricular choroid plexus and that with rupture of the fourth ventricular roof, CSF escapes into the extracellular space of the meninx. He showed dye initially collecting dorsal to the fourth ventricle and subsequently spreading laterally and ventrally around the brainstem. Weed concluded that the subarachnoid space must form in such a manner (66).

Unfortunately, scrutiny of Weed's methodology revealed a methodological error: he presumed that all CSF was elaborated by the choroid plexus and that only with fourth ventricular rupture could CSF escape to form the cisterns (63,67). Such a presumption is quite evident by the fact that he replaced only the intraventricular fluid. Were the subarachnoid spaces already formed or forming by the time of fourth ventricular rupture, Weed's work would have yielded the same results and in fact, this appears to be the case (63).

It was not until 1980, some 63 years after Weed's work, that Weed's results were questioned. Osaka et al. (67) showed that the cisterns develop in an orderly fashion quite different from that described by Weed. Most importantly, they showed that the prepontomedullary cisterns, not the space dorsal to the fourth ventricle, are the first subarachnoid cisterns to be created. In fact, they showed that much of the subarachnoid space has already developed at least by Carnegie stage 18 (44 days), and possibly as early as stage 14 (32 days), which is fully 4 (and possibly 16) days prior to the development of the fourth ventricular choroid plexus (Carnegie stage 19, 48 days), let alone before fourth ventricular rupture. According to the study by Osaka et al. (67), the cisterns develop first ventral to the brainstem (Fig. 33). Dissolution of the meninx then proceeds around the brainstem and over the cerebral hemispheres. The last areas to dissolve are the lamina terminalis, quadrigeminal/superior cerebellar, and suprasellar cisterns.

With this concept in mind, it was finally possible to correlate Verga's theory of maldifferentiated meninx primitiva with the formation of intracranial lipomas (63). Thus, the region with the longest window of opportunity for maldifferentiation of the meninx is the region dorsal to the lamina terminalis; hence, the relative greater frequency of pericallosal lipomas versus other intracranial lipomas. In fact, the distribution of intracranial lipomas correlates inversely, and therefore, extremely well with the pattern of cavitation and dissolution of the meninx. This concept explains essentially all intracranial lipomas as disorders of the subarachnoid space itself, rather than as neoplasms or disorders of neural tube closure.

The most common locations for intracranial lipomas are the interhemispheric fissure (pericallosal) (Figs. 34–

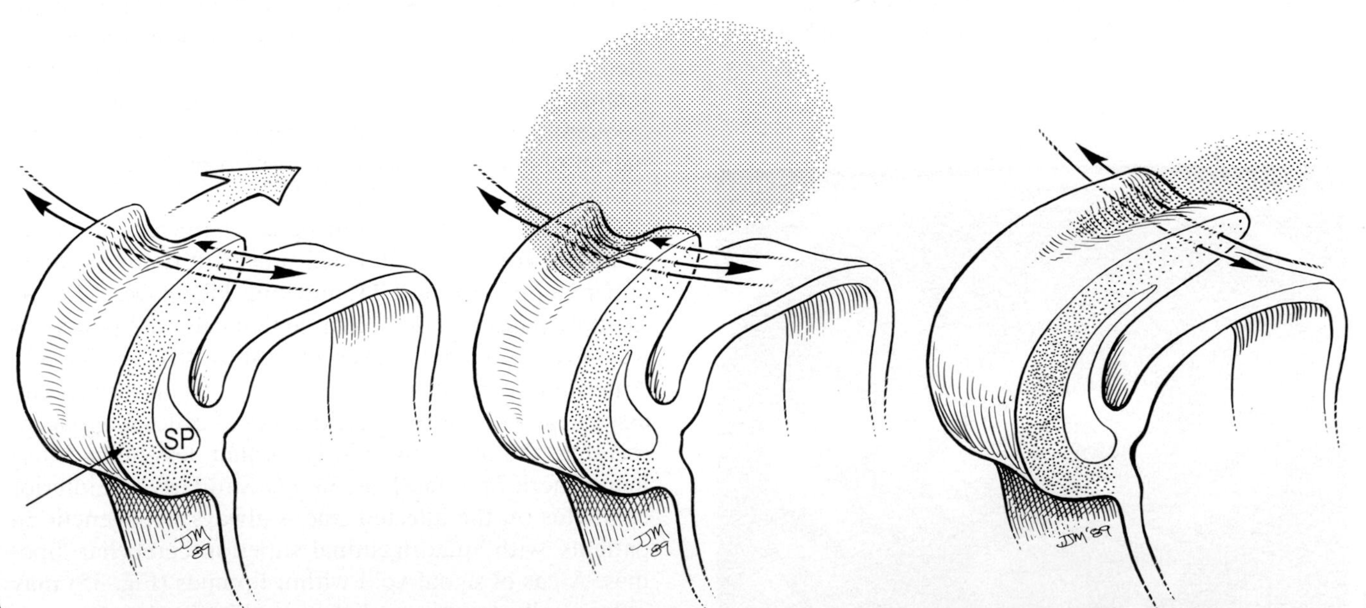

FIG. 34. A: Conceptual view of early corpus callosum shows thick commissural plate anteriorly where hemispheric transcallosal fibers have already transversed (*straight arrow*). More posteriorly, dorsal callosal groove [sulcus medianus telencephali medii (SMTM) of text] is deeper where ingrowth of fibers is still in early stage (*curved arrows*). As growth occurs, callosum thickens, meninx (not shown) dissolves, and groove fills in. SP, septum pellucidum. **B:** Interhemispheric meninx is contiguous with that of dorsal callosal groove. An insult at this early stage results in severe callosal hypoplasia; if meninx persists, a "pericallosal" lipoma may develop. **C:** At a later stage of callosal development, much of interhemispheric meninx has cavitated, leaving that of dorsal callosal groove. An insult at this stage would interfere with proper thickening of callosal body and splenium and result in dorsal ribbon lipoma or retrosplenial button. (From Truwit and Barkovich, ref. 63, with permission.)

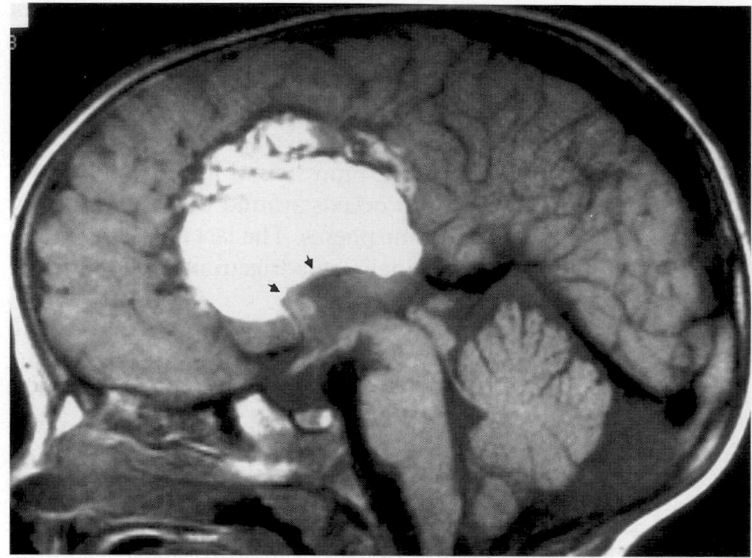

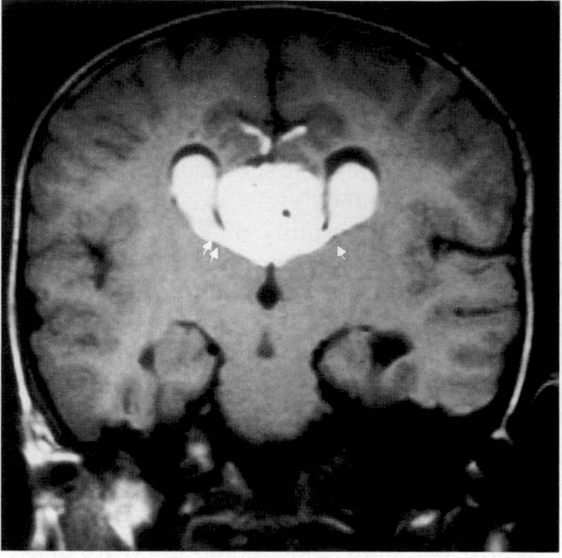

FIG. 35. Midline sagittal (**A**) and coronal (**B**) T1-weighted images, 800/20/2, at 1.5 T reveals severe callosal hypoplasia (*black arrows*) and bulky, anterior lipoma with contiguous choroidal extension (*white arrows*). Note flow void in anterior cerebral artery. (From Truwit and Barkovich, ref. 63, with permission.)

37), the suprasellar cistern (apposed to the hypothalamus or mamillary bodies) (Fig. 38), the quadrigeminal cistern (apposed to the inferior colliculi: Fig. 39), and the cerebellopontine angle (involving the seventh/eighth nerve complex: Fig. 40) (63). Uncommonly, lipomas can be seen in the sylvian fissure (Fig. 35). Because lipomas develop from the inner layers of tissue that would normally form the subarachnoid space, intracranial vessels (e.g., pericallosal arteries) and cranial nerves often course through, rather than around lipomas (63).

FIG. 36. Sagittal T1-weighted image, 500/40/1, at 0.35 T shows ribbon-like pericallosal lipoma and mild hypoplasia of dorsum of callosal body (*arrow*). (From Truwit and Barkovich, ref. 63, with permission.)

Lipomas are frequently apposed to malformed subjacent brain. For example, interhemispheric lipomas are nearly always associated with hypogenesis of the corpus callosum (Figs. 35 and 36) (63,68,69). Frontal interhemispheric lipomas are often quite bulky and may be associated with midline facial clefts and frontonasal or frontoethmoidal encephaloceles. Fat from the lipoma frequently extends into the encephalocele. This combination of anomalies has been termed midline craniofacial dysraphism (Fig. 37) (70,71).

On MRI, lipomas exhibit signal characteristics of fat (Figs. 35–40). The malformed subjacent brain is readily apparent on both short TR and long TR images. Midline sagittal images will demonstrate that callosal lipomas always extend dorsal to the corpus callosum (Figs. 34–37). Anterior interhemispheric lipomas are usually bulky and associated with more severe degrees of callosal hypogenesis than the more posteriorly located, less bulky interhemispheric lipomas (Figs. 34-37). Similarly, the inferior colliculus on the affected side is always hypogenetic in patients with quadrigeminal/superior cerebellar lipomas. Areas of signal void within lipomas (Fig. 35) may occasionally represent calcification but much more commonly represent flow void within vessels. It is important to remember that intracranial lipomas are congenital malformations and not neoplasms. As such, they enlarge only with somatic growth, not according to neoplastic growth patterns. In general, surgical management is not appropriate. Rarely, inferior collicular lipomas may be associated with hydrocephalus requiring shunt placement.

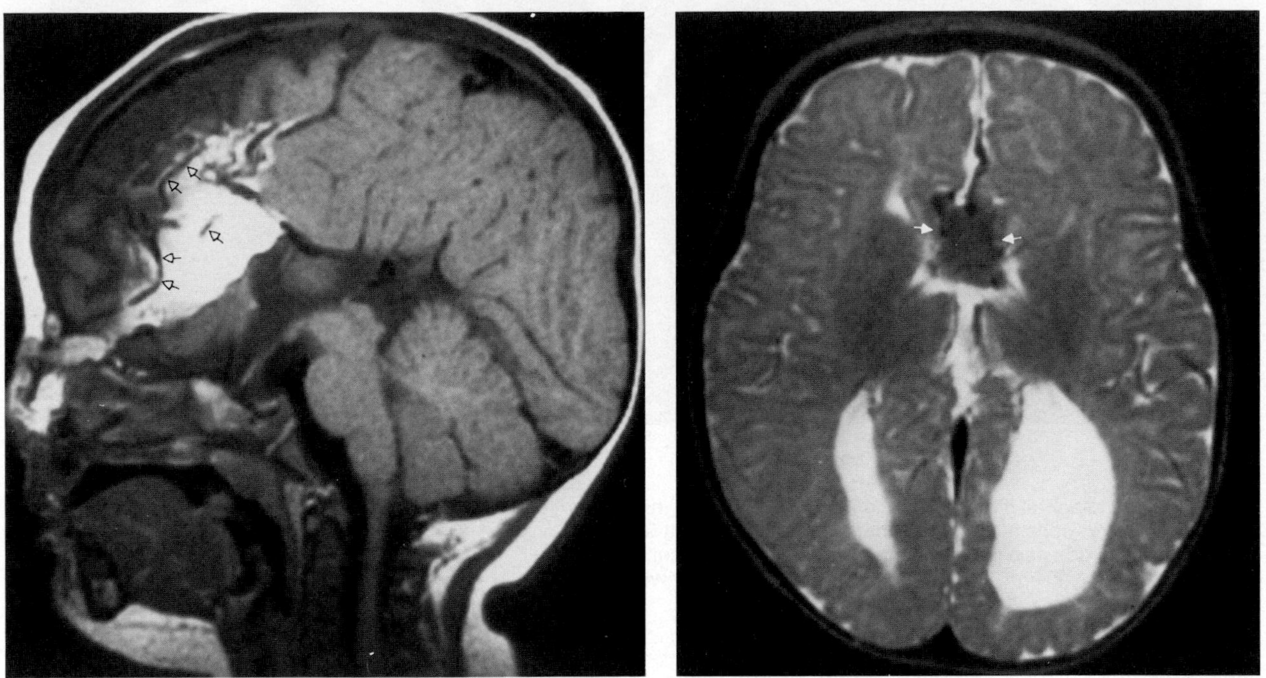

FIG. 37. Nasofrontal encephalocele in a patient with midline craniofacial dysraphism. **A:** Sagittal SE 600/20 image shows an interhemispheric lipoma extending from the midfrontal region through a defect between the frontal bones into the nasofrontal area. Note how vessels (*arrows*) course through the lipoma, which is of high signal intensity on the short TR/TE image. **B:** The lipoma (*arrows*) becomes hypointense with respect to brain on long TR/TE images.

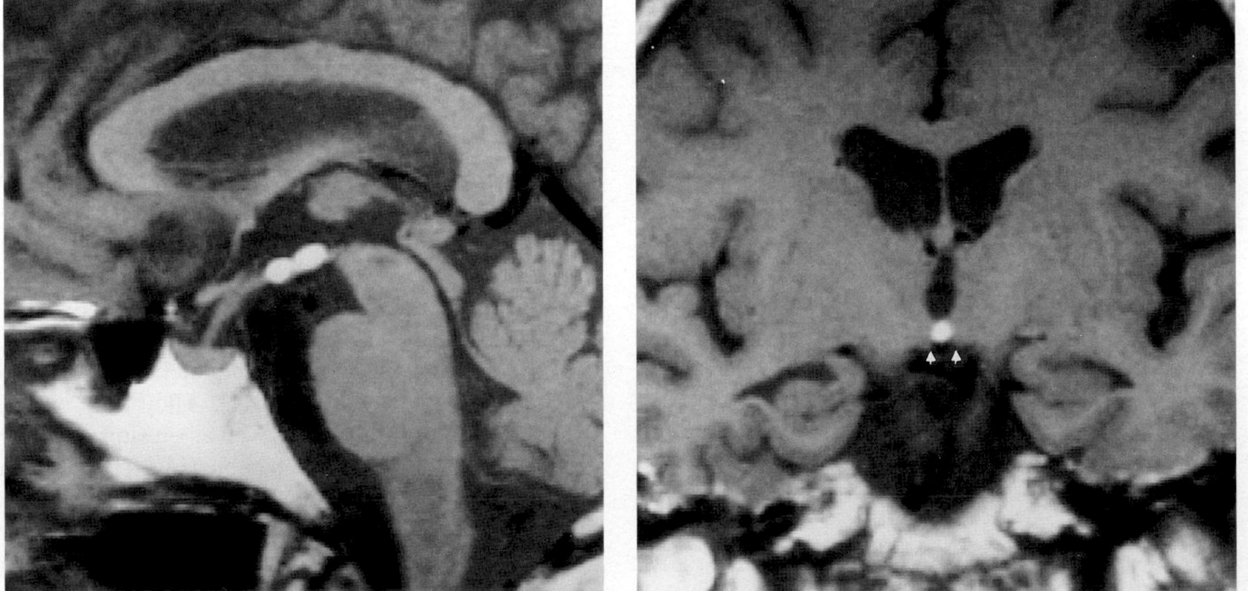

FIG. 38. Sagittal (**A**) and coronal (**B**) T-1 weighted images, 500/24/4, at 1.5 T reveal bilobed hypothalamic/mamillary body and supraseller lipoma. Mamillary bodies are hypoplastic (*arrows*). (From Truwit and Barkovich, ref. 63, with permission.)

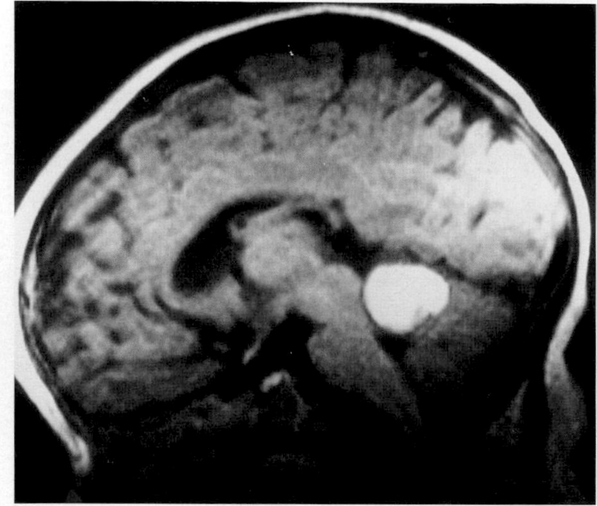

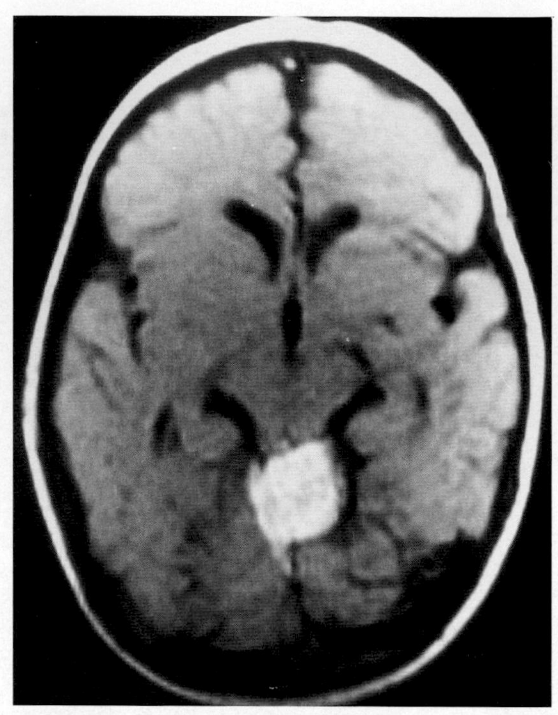

FIG. 39. Sagittal T1-weighted image, 477/30/4 (**A**), and axial proton-density-weighted image 2300/30/2 (**B**), at 0.3 T reveal hypoplasia of both left inferior colliculus and superior vermis. (From Truwit and Barkovich, ref. 63, with permission.)

Arachnoid Cyst

Intracranial arachnoid cysts are benign, developmental anomalies of the subarachnoid space. Embryologically, they derive from the meninx primitiva (see lipoma) which forms a perimedullary mesh around the developing central nervous system. With the accumulation of subarachnoid CSF, the meninx cavitates and resorbs, leaving only the subarachnoid space, subarachnoid membrane, and delicate subarachnoid trabeculae normally found throughout the subarachnoid space. During this process, it is believed that the developing arachnoid membrane splits. With time, arachnoid cells secrete fluid into the resultant cleft, and, depending on the degree of communication with the true subarachnoid space, the cleft enlarges to become a cavity, and ultimately, an arachnoid cyst (72–77).

The most common cisterns and spaces of arachnoid cysts are the cerebellopontine angle and sylvian fissure (73–76). Following these sites are the retrocerebellar area and vallecula/cisterna magna, suprasellar cistern and cerebral convexities (73–76).

On MRI, arachnoid cysts are extra-axial (Fig. 41) (72–74,78–80) (and occasionally intraventricular (Fig. 42) (81–83) fluid collections that generally exhibit signal characteristics of CSF (Fig. 41). They may exert mass effect on subjacent brain, as well as on suprajacent bone. Smooth erosion of the inner table (Fig. 41) is commonly seen in middle fossa and sylvian fissure cysts. Although vessels are typically displaced by the cyst, apparently "intracystic" vessels may be seen. In fact, such subarachnoid vessels are extracystic, but appear to be intracystic (Fig. 43), much the way a finger can be invaginated "into" a balloon, and appear to be inside. Rarely, intracystic hemorrhage (Fig. 44) may be seen (84,85).

Commonly, some difficulties arise in differentiating

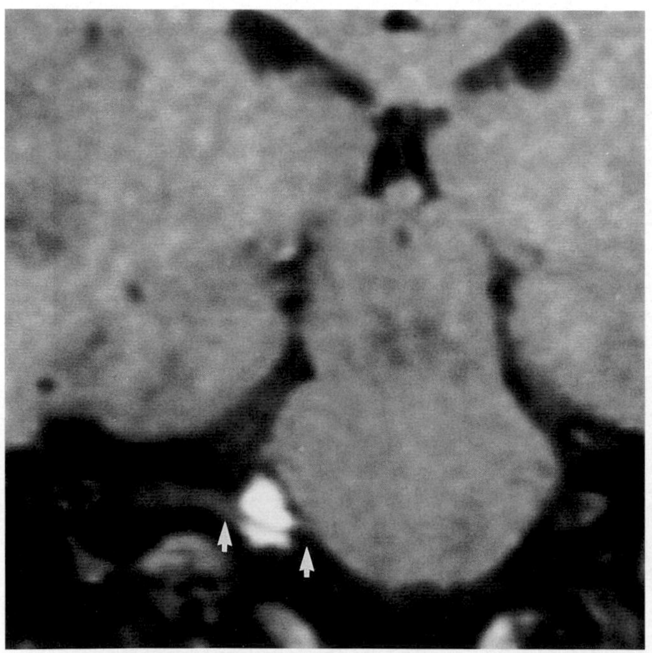

FIG. 40. Coronal T1-weighted image, 600/20/4, at 1.5 T shows seventh/eighth cranial nerve complex coursing through surgically proved right cerebellopontine angle lipoma (*arrows*). (From Truwit and Barkovich, ref. 63, with permission.)

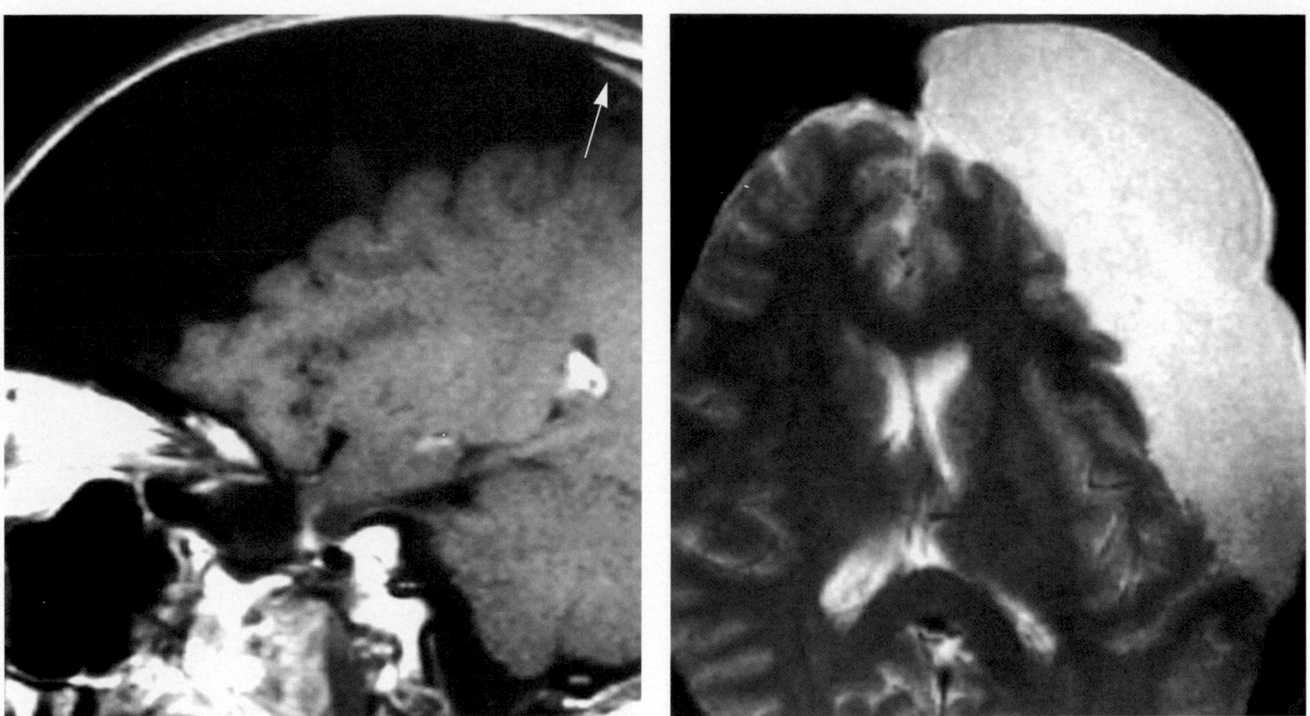

FIG. 41. Arachnoid cyst. Sagittal (**A**) contrast-enhanced T1-weighted image shows large extra-axial collection over left frontal lobe. Note smooth erosion of inner table (*arrow*), due to chronic presence of subarachnoid cyst. Axial (**B**) T2-weighted image shows marked mass effect on subjacent brain and dramatic asymmetry of hemicalvaria.

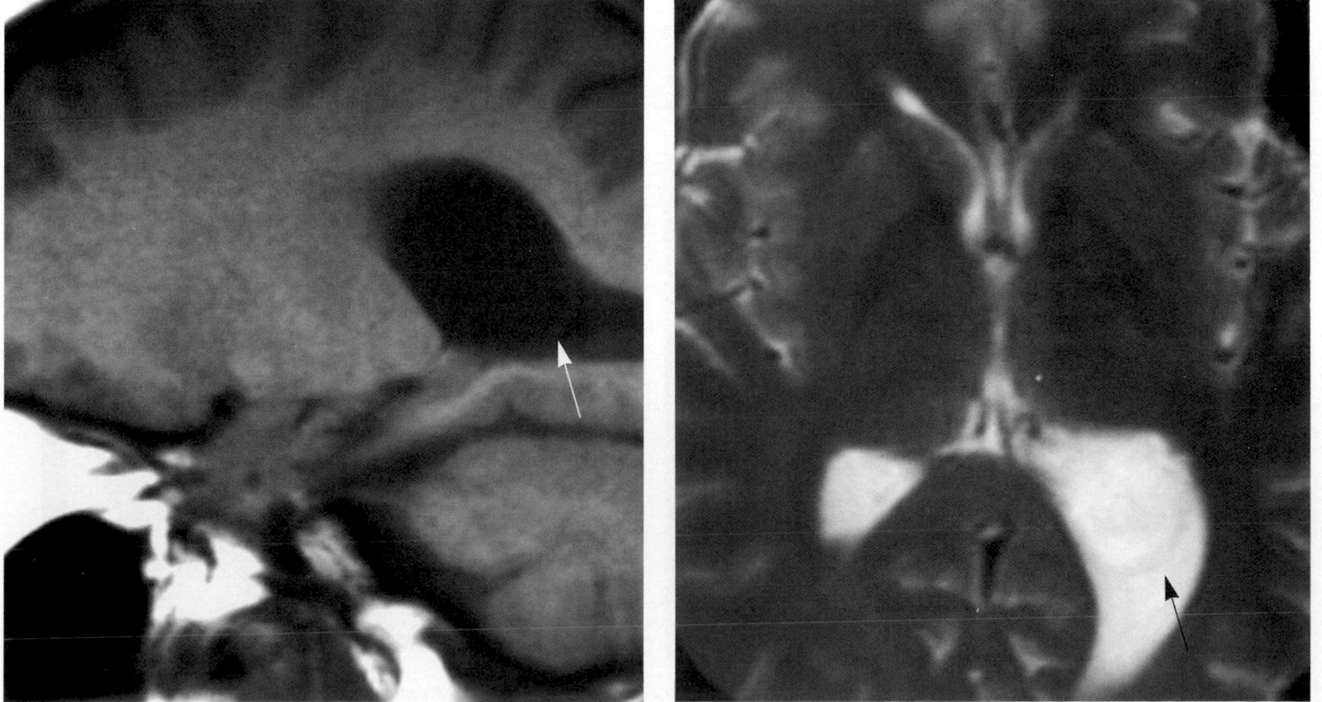

FIG. 42. Intraventricular arachnoid cyst. Sagittal (**A**) T1-weighted image shows expanded atrium of left lateral ventricle with almost imperceptible cyst membrane. Axial (**B**) T2-weighted image better shows cyst wall (*arrow*).

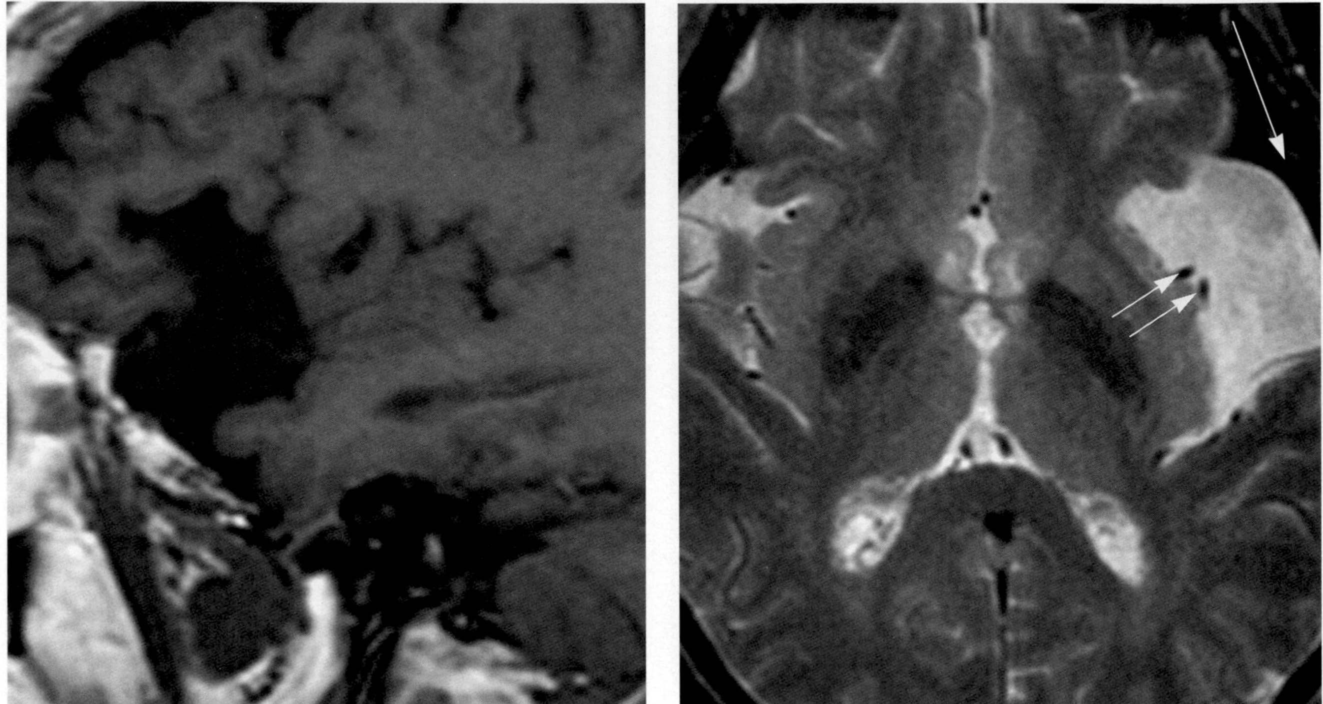

FIG. 43. Arachnoid cyst with MCA branches. Sagittal (**A**) T1- and axial (**B**) T2-weighted images show enlarged sylvian fissure with mild outward bowing of the inner table (*long arrow*, B). Signal intensities parallel those of CSF. Note middle cerebral artery branches that appear to lie within deepest portion of cyst (*short arrows*, B).

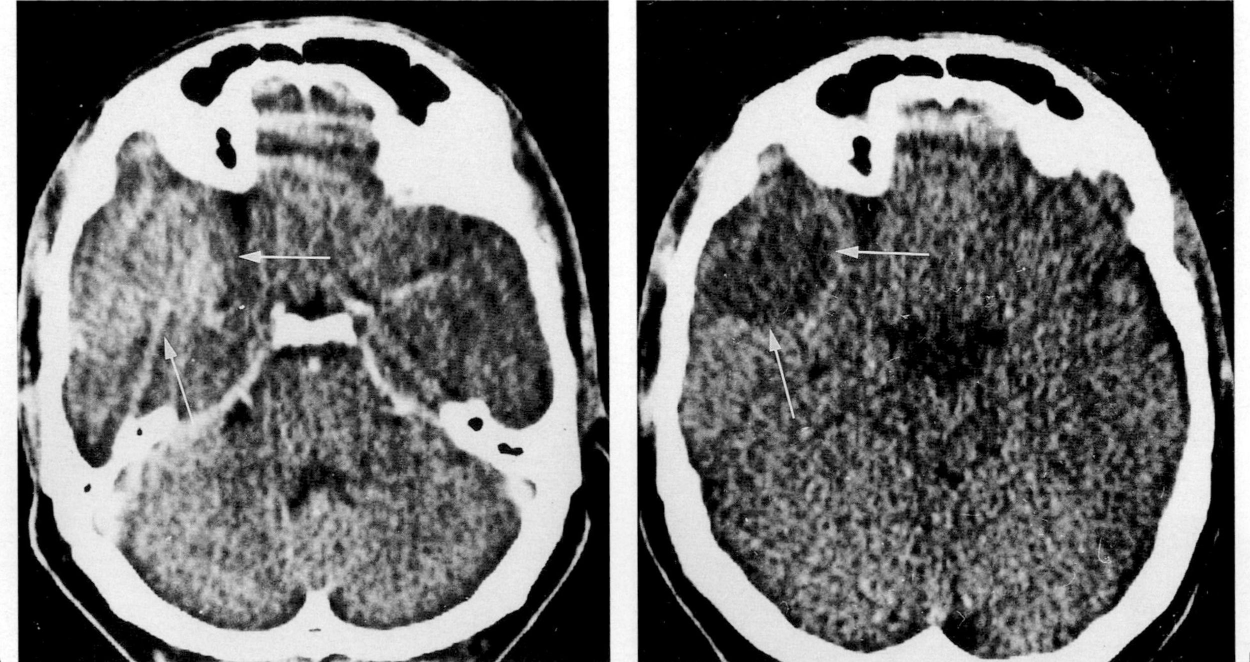

FIG. 44. Arachnoid cyst with intracystic hemorrhage. Contrast-enhanced CT (**A**) shows hyperdense mass (*arrows*, A) in right middle cranial fossa. Patient is child who suffered mild closed head injury. Follow-up non-contrast head CT (**B**) shows low attenuation arachnoid cyst (*arrows*, B) in same region. (Courtesy of Dr. Keith McMurdo.)

arachnoid cysts from epidermoid cysts. As discussed above (see epidermoid/dermoid), long TR/short TE spin-echo and spoiled gradient-echo sequences may be useful to identify intracystic matrix and slight differences in signal intensity from that of CSF, typical of epidermoid cysts and exclusive of arachnoid cysts. In addition, a common problem is the differentiation of a mega cisterna magna from an arachnoid cyst of the vallecula/cisterna magna. One often subtle clue to the diagnosis is the presence of mass effect on the subjacent vermis. This is often best seen on sagittal images as a very slight scalloping of the dorsal vermis.

Posterior Fossa Malformations

Dandy-Walker Malformations

The Dandy-Walker malformation consists of an enlarged posterior fossa with a high position of the tentorium, hypogenesis of the cerebellar vermis, and cystic dilatation of the fourth ventricle that nearly fills the posterior fossa (86–89). The cerebellar hemispheres are almost always hypoplastic. This posterior fossa malformation is best conceptualized as an intrauterine outflow obstruction of the fourth ventricle. Because of the outflow obstruction, the fourth ventricle grows upward between the developing cerebellar hemispheres, preventing their apposition and fusion in the midline. When the cerebellar hemispheres do not fuse, the vermis is not formed. Moreover, the huge fourth ventricle induces the squamous portion of the occipital bone to grow, resulting in a large posterior fossa and an apparently high tentorium.

Although fourth ventricular outflow obstruction is an easy concept to understand, it is a simplistic explanation. The Dandy-Walker malformation probably results from an in utero insult to the developing fourth ventricle and cerebellum (90). The concept of an early intrauterine insult also helps to explain the variants of the Dandy-Walker malformation, which are much more common than the classic Dandy-Walker malformation itself (90). These variants consist of hypoplasia of one or both of the cerebellar hemispheres in association with a large fourth ventricle in a normal-sized or slightly enlarged posterior fossa. They are probably the result of a less severe insult to the developing posterior fossa.

The classic Dandy-Walker malformation is associated with hydrocephalus in about 75% of patients by the age of 3 months (Fig. 45). The corpus callosum is hypogenetic in about 25% of patients (Fig. 46). Polymicrogyria or gray matter heterotopia are seen in about 10% of pa-

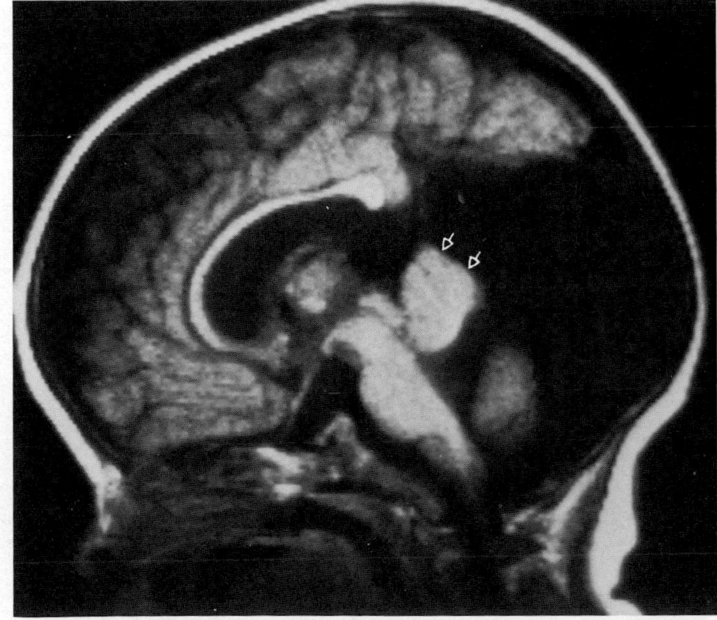

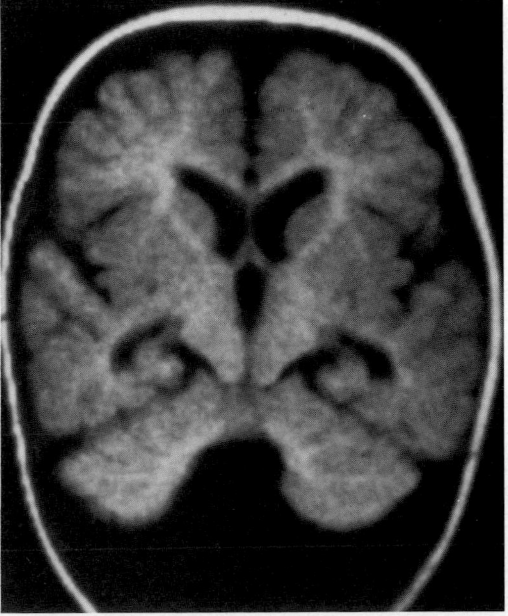

FIG. 45. Dandy-Walker malformation. **A:** Sagittal SE 500/30 image shows the classic findings of a Dandy-Walker malformation. The tentorium is elevated, and the posterior fossa is markedly enlarged. The vermis (*arrows*) is dysgenetic. The large posterior fossa is filled by an enormous fourth ventricle. **B:** Axial SE 500/30 image through the mid-fourth ventricle shows continuity of the fourth ventricle with the remainder of the CSF of the posterior fossa. The cerebellar hemispheres are slightly hypoplastic and are pushed superolaterally by the cyst. There is mild hydrocephalus.

tients, and occipital encephaloceles can be seen in 3% to 5% (88).

Associated anomalies are seen in variants of the Dandy-Walker malformation, as well, but are less common (90). This is an important concept in that it allows one to understand why developmental delay and neurological dysfunction are more common in the full-blown Dandy-Walker malformation than in the variants. Several studies have shown that, in the absence of associated supratentorial anomalies and uncontrolled hydrocephalus, patients with Dandy-Walker malformations have a good developmental prognosis (87–90). Patients with the classic Dandy-Walker malformation have a more guarded prognosis because they have a higher incidence of associated (supratentorial) anomalies.

The lack of a clear-cut differentiation between the Dandy-Walker malformation and the Dandy-Walker variants, and, for that matter, between Dandy-Walker variant and mega cisterna magna, has led to the proposal that all of the subgroups be discarded and replaced by a unifying term, that of a Dandy-Walker complex or Dandy-Walker continuum (90). The Dandy-Walker complex would include all malformations with cerebellar hypoplasia and cystic malformations of the fourth ventricle.

On imaging studies, the classic Dandy-Walker malformation is characterized by hypoplasia or absence of the cerebellar vermis, hypoplasia of the cerebellar hemispheres, a large fluid-filled fourth ventricle that extends into the cisterna magna, and a large posterior fossa with a high tentorium (Fig. 45). After shunting of the posterior fossa cyst, the cerebellar hemispheres frequently appose one another inferiorly beneath the vermis (Fig. 46).

All malformations within the Dandy-Walker complex will show some degree of cerebellar hemispheric and/or vermian hypoplasia associated with some degree of fourth ventricular dysplasia (Figs. 45 and 46). The posterior fossa may be large or normal in size. The vermis and one or both cerebellar hemispheres are hypoplastic (Figs. 45 and 46). In all patients with these malformations, it is important to look at the supratentorial structures to identify accompanying malformations. As noted above, the presence of supratentorial anomalies indicates a much more widespread insult to the developing brain, as well as a less optimistic developmental prognosis.

Joubert Syndrome

Joubert syndrome also consists of vermian hypoplasia or aplasia. In Joubert syndrome, however, no posterior fossa cyst develops, no hydrocephalus is seen, and the clinical picture is entirely different from other vermian hypoplasia syndromes. The disorder was first described in five children with periodic hyperpnea, abnormal eye

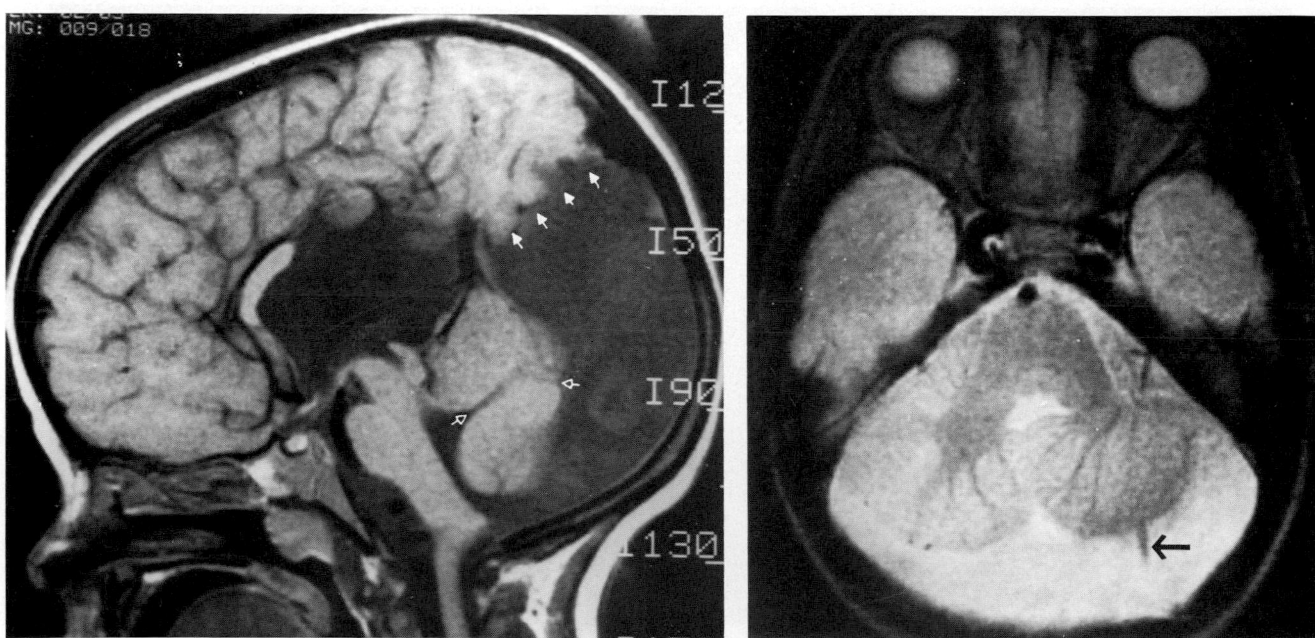

FIG. 46. Dandy-Walker malformation after shunting of the posterior fossa cyst. **A:** Sagittal SE 600/20 image shows that the corpus callosum is hypogenetic with only the genu present. The posterior fossa is enlarged as a result of the high tentorium (*closed arrows*). The vermis is rotated upward and dysgenetic. *Open arrows* mark the lower limits of the vermis. The cerebellar tissue beneath these arrows is composed of the inferior aspects of the cerebellar hemispheres, which are in apposition as a result of diversion of CSF by a shunt. **B:** Axial SE 2500/70 image at the level of the inferior fourth ventricle shows the cerebellar hemispheres in apposition without an intervening vermis. The *black arrow* points to the shunt catheter.

movements, ataxia, and mental retardation (91). Although it was reported both initially and subsequently that the vermis is agenetic, in fact, it is usually hypogenetic (26,92), as it is in most posterior fossa anomalies that involve the vermis. In addition to vermian hypoplasia, patients with Joubert syndrome have dysplastic and heterotopic cerebellar nuclei, anomalous inferior olivary nuclei, and brainstem tracts. The pyramidal decussation was absent in the lone case studied by Friede and Bolthauser (92).

MR scans of patients with Joubert syndrome reveal a peculiar pattern: subtotal aplasia of the vermis and cerebellar hemisphere disconnection. The rostral fourth ventricle is often bat-shaped (Fig. 47); the superior cerebellar peduncles are laterally splayed. Caudally, the fourth ventricle appears chalice-shaped.

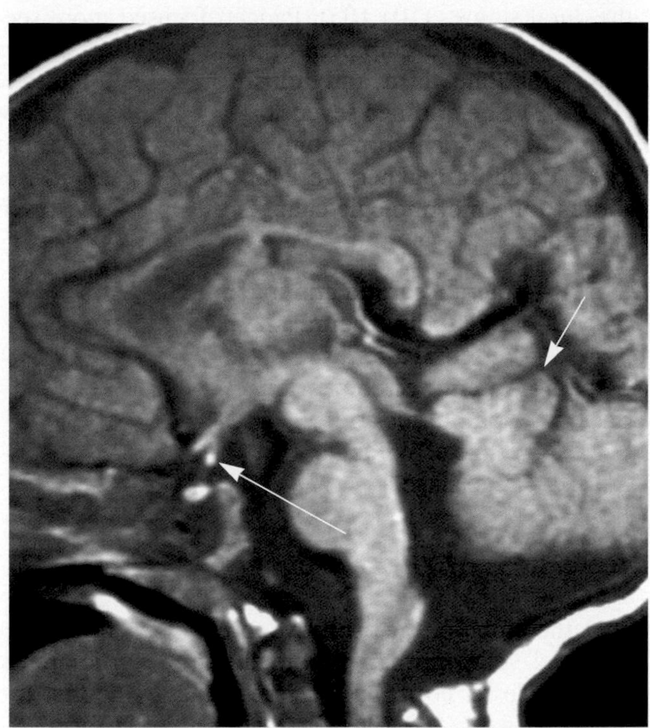

A

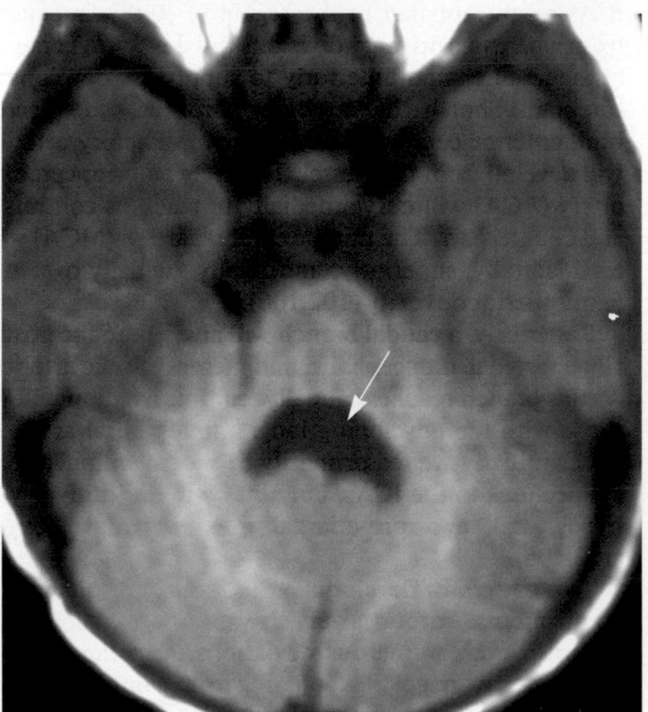

B

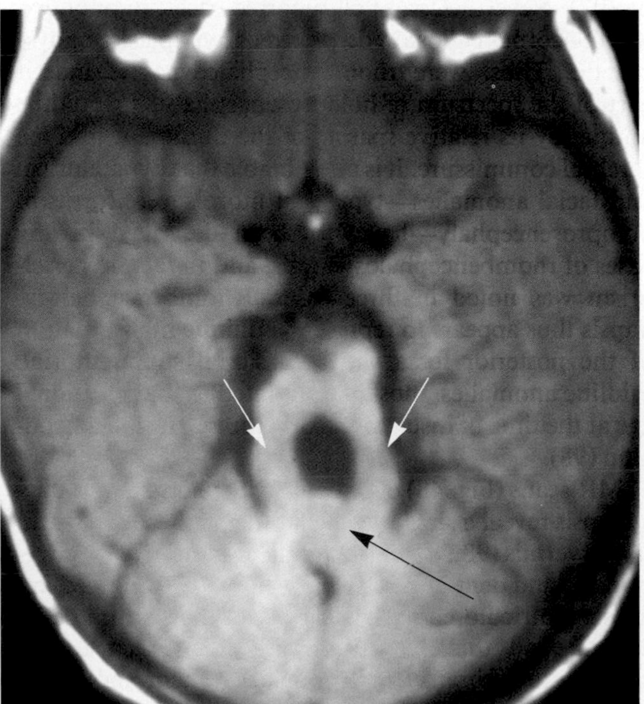

C

FIG. 47. Joubert syndrome. Sagittal (**A**) T1-weighted image shows diminutive, dysplastic superior vermis (*short arrow*, A) and enlarged fourth ventricle. Ectopic neurohypophysis (*long arrow*, A) is also seen. Axial (**B,C**) T1-weighted images show prominent, bat-shaped fourth ventricle (*arrow*, B). At level of mid-pons (B), roof of fourth ventricle should be defined by vermis, not cerebellar tonsils. More cephalad (C), elongated superior cerebellar peduncles (*short arrows*, C) and enlarged fourth ventricle are seen. Cerebellar hemispheres are essentially disconnected—hallmark of Joubert syndrome—except for small vermian remnant (*long arrow*, C). (From Truwit and Lempert, ref. 40, with permission.)

Rhombencephalosynapsis

Rhombencephalosynapsis is yet another anomaly of the cerebellar vermis. In this condition, vermian hypogenesis or agenesis is associated neither with the disconnected cerebellar hemispheres of Joubert syndrome, nor with the posterior fossa cyst of the Dandy-Walker malformation. Rather, in rhombencephalosynapsis abnormalities of cerebellar, dentate, peduncular and collicular fusion are seen, often in conjunction with supratentorial anomalies. To distinguish the disorder from that of Dandy and Blackfan (rhombocephalo-schizis), deMorsier named the disorder "rhombocephalosynapsis," which was subsequently amended by Gross to "rhombencephalosynapsis" (93,94).

The first report of rhombencephalosynapsis was described by Obersteiner in 1914. Since then, and in contrast to that case, subsequent reports have described coincident supratentorial anomalies, including deficiencies of the septum pellucidum and anterior commissure. It is easy to wonder whether rhombencephalosynapsis might be yet another subtype of holoprosencephaly. In fact, Schachenmayr described absence of the olfactory tracts and bulbs and septum pellucidum in concert with the posterior fossa malformation (95). Moreover, in reports by Gross and Kepes, rhombencephalosynapsis was associated with thalamic fusion and third ventricular deficiency (94,96). Finally, it is interesting that the hypothalamic-pituitary axis appeared normal in all case but one. In that case, the posterior pituitary lobe was absent, the septum pellucidum was absent, and the optic nerves, chiasm, and tracts were markedly hypoplastic, fulfilling the pathologic diagnosis of septo-optic dysplasia (97). Nevertheless, of all reported cases, in only two was the corpus callosum described as hypoplastic or dysgenetic. Thus, were rhombencephalosynapsis indeed part of the spectrum of holoprosencephaly, it would be unique by its relative sparing of the dominant midline cerebral commissure. It is also notable that hypotelorism and facial anomalies—typical of more severe forms of holoprosencephaly—have not been described in any cases of rhombencephalosynapsis, and in fact, hypertelorism was noted in three cases. Rhombencephalosynapsis thus appears to represent a unique malformation of the posterior fossa with occasional supratentorial, midline anomalies, most likely related to the gestational age at the time of insult to the developing rhombencephalon (98).

MR scans (Fig. 48) of patients with rhombencephalosynapsis reveal a single cerebellar hemisphere with little, if any vermis (98,99). Fusion of the middle cerebellar peduncles and dentate nuclei are seen on T2-weighted images. Ventriculomegaly, deficiency of the septum pellucidum, and thalamic fusion are often seen in the supratentorial brain (98). Anomalies of neuronal migration (Fig. 49) have been reported as well (100).

CEREBROVASCULAR ANOMALIES

Arterial Anomalies

Although considerable evolution has taken place in the nomenclature of cranial vascular development, most investigators refer to the works of Streeter and Padgett in reviewing the development of the intracranial vasculature (101–104). Streeter's work addressed the broad evolution of the intracranial vasculature, and, in particular, the dural sinuses (101,105). Padgett focused more specifically on the development of the intracranial arteries and veins (late third and fourth periods of Streeter) (102,103). She outlined seven stages of arterial development (102), which correspond to embryos of different sizes. Paraphrasing her work and relating the stages more to the morphologic changes described, the seven stages are:

Stage 1—Internal carotid and trigeminal arteries
Stage 2—Longitudinal neural and basilar arteries
Stage 3—Vertebral arteries
Stage 4—Anterior cerebral artery
Stage 5—Ophthalmic artery
Stage 6—Circle of Willis
Stage 7—Fetal stage

Carotid Agenesis/Hypogenesis

In the embryo, the primitive internal carotid arteries (ICAs) develop primarily from the third aortic arches, although lesser contributions are made by the first two arches as well (102,106). In their primitive form, the ICAs reach cephalad to the region of Rathke's pouch, from where two primary divisions will develop. A cranial branch will extend anteriorly to supply the developing forebrain. Shortly, the anterior choroidal, middle cerebral, anterior cerebral, and primitive olfactory arteries will develop from this vessel. The early anterior cerebral artery (ACA) will curve medially to reach its contralateral counterpart. The middle cerebral artery (MCA) will tend laterally, superiorly, and finally medially over the hemispheric convexity (102,106).

Posteriorly, a caudal branch will give rise to the posterior choroidal, diencephalic, and mesencephalic arteries. As this branch reaches caudally, communication will be made with the developing longitudinal neural arteries, which initially are fed primarily by the trigeminal artery connections to the ICAs, but also by the primitive otic, hypoglossal, and pro-atlantal intersegmental arteries (102,106).

This pattern of development ultimately results in the adult internal carotid artery as we know it. Along the way, however, numerous deviations from the normal adult pattern are possible, ranging from complete agenesis of the ICA(s) to segmental arterial hypoplasias and to

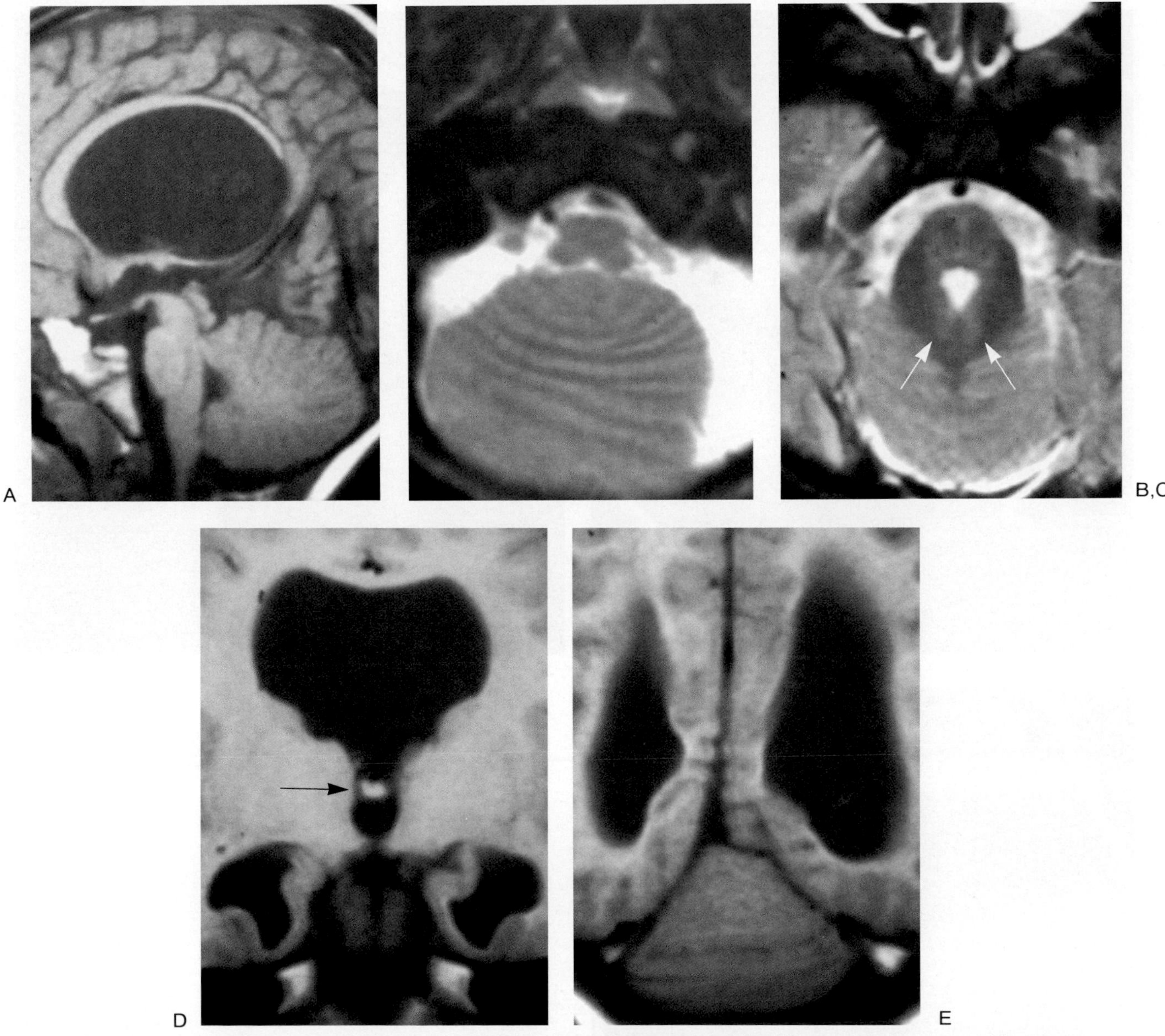

FIG. 48. **A:** Sagittal T1-weighted image, 600/15/2 (TR/TE/excitations), shows ventriculomegaly. Adjacent images (not shown) revealed contiguity of fused fornices with callosal splenium. Vermis is not seen. **B:** Axial T2-weighted image (2867/80/1) reveals hypoplastic, fused cerebellum with aberrant folial orientation and absent vermis. **C:** Slightly more cephalad, apposition or fusion of middle cerebellar peduncles and dentate fourth ventricle (*arrows*), which appears narrowed and points posteriorly. **D:** Coronal T1-weighted scan (700/15/2) shows forniceal fusion (*arrow*), ventriculomegaly with deficient septum pellucidum, and temporal lobe hypoplasia. **E:** Coronal image more posteriorly illustrates abnormal transverse orientation of cerebellar folia. (From Truwit et al., ref. 98, with permission.)

anomalous (persistent) communications with the posterior circulation or the external carotid circulation (106).

Agenesis of the ICA is an uncommon anomaly, in which there is complete absence of both the artery and the bony canal through which the artery would normally enter the cranial vault (106,107). Very rarely, the anomaly may be bilateral. Lie's thorough study of this anomaly in 1968 describes several potential outcomes, the most common of which is enlargement of the basilar artery and posterior communicating artery (PComA) to fill the MCA territory of the affected hemisphere (Fig. 50). In such cases, both ACAs fill from the normal, unaffected

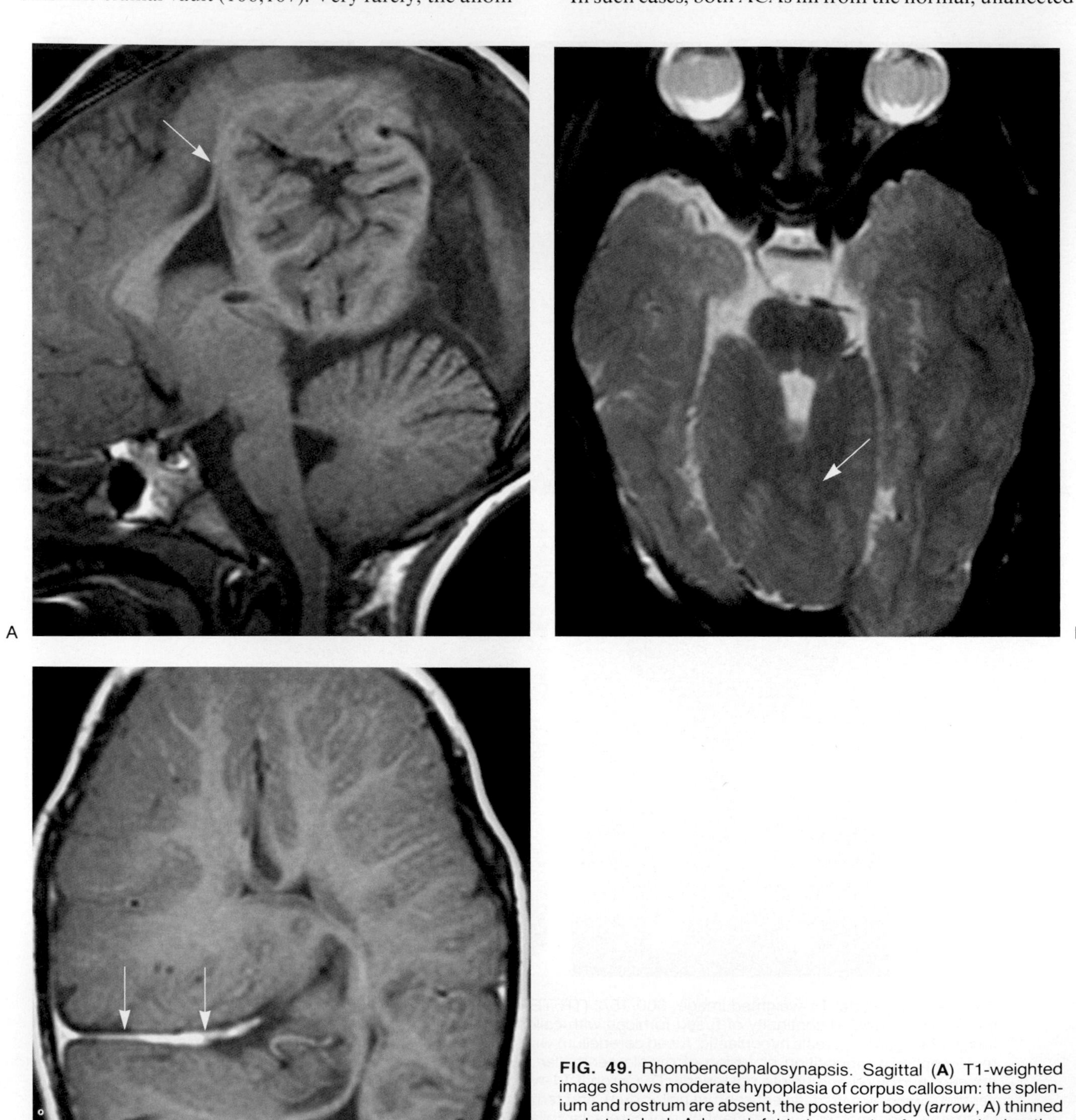

FIG. 49. Rhombencephalosynapsis. Sagittal (**A**) T1-weighted image shows moderate hypoplasia of corpus callosum: the splenium and rostrum are absent, the posterior body (*arrow*, A) thinned and stretched. A large infolded anomaly of neuronal migration is seen beneath the posterior callosal body. Within the posterior fossa, the vermis is inapparent. Axial (**B**) T2-weighted image shows typical fusion of cerebellar hemispheres. Specifically, fusion of dentate nuclei (*arrow*, B) and cerebellar white matter can be seen. Axial (**C**) T1-weighted image shows infolded cleft and enlarged venous drainage (*short arrows*, C), typical of anomaly of neuronal migration. Falcine sinus (*long arrow*, C) is also seen.

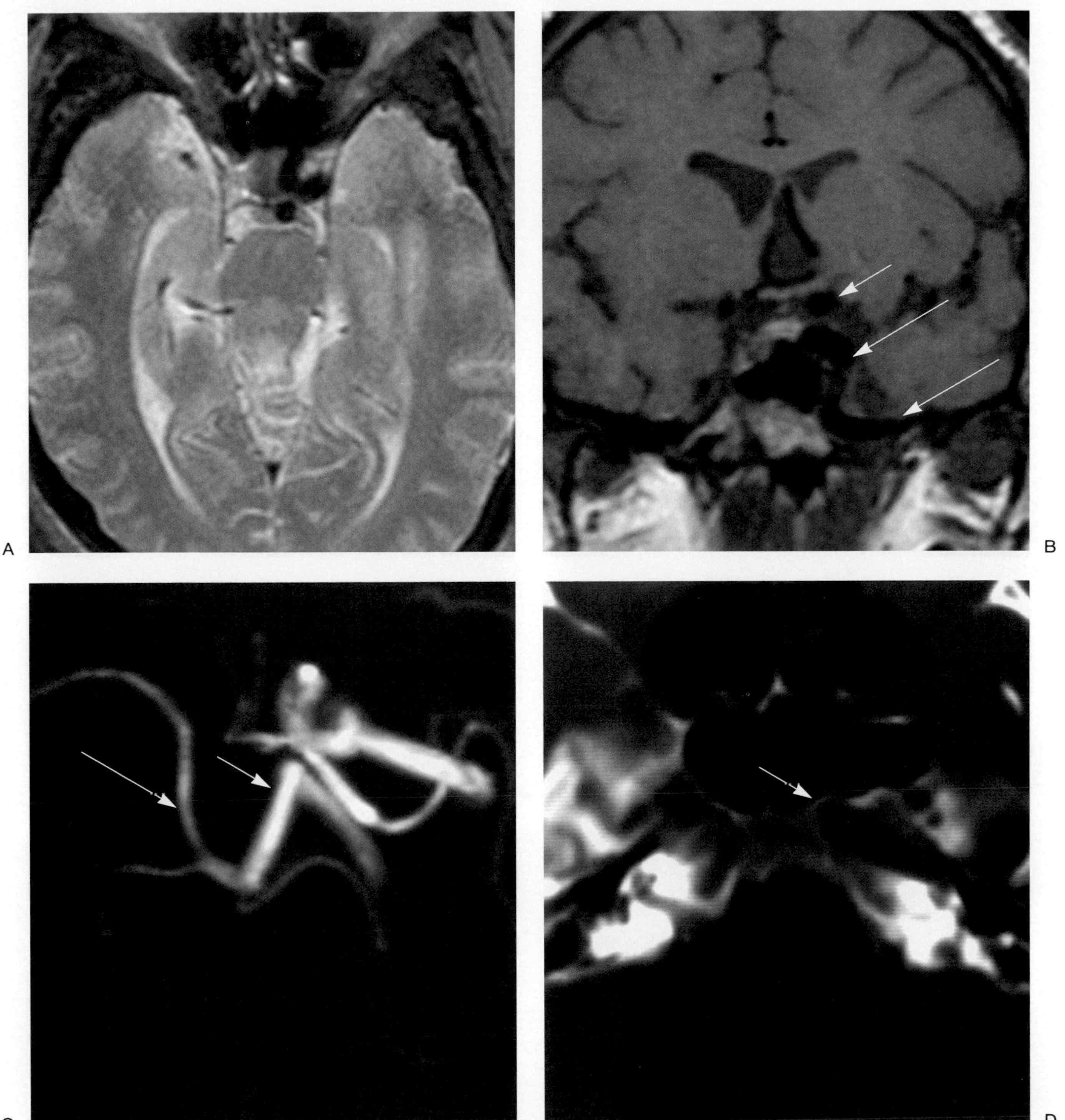

FIG. 50. Agenesis of ICA. Axial (**A**) T2-weighted and coronal (**B**) T1-weighted images show prominent flow void of left internal carotid artery (*long arrows*, B). Corresponding right internal carotid artery is not seen. Collapsed view (**C**) of three-dimensional phase contrast MR angiogram (flow velocity = 25 cm/sec) shows enlarged, tortuous basilar artery (*short double arrows*, B,C), most likely due to increased flow, as well as prominent right posterior communicating artery (*long arrow*, C). Both anterior cerebral arteries are supplied from the left. Bone detail CT (**D**) shows enlarged left carotid canal (*arrow*, D) and absence of right-sided canal. CT confirms diagnosis.

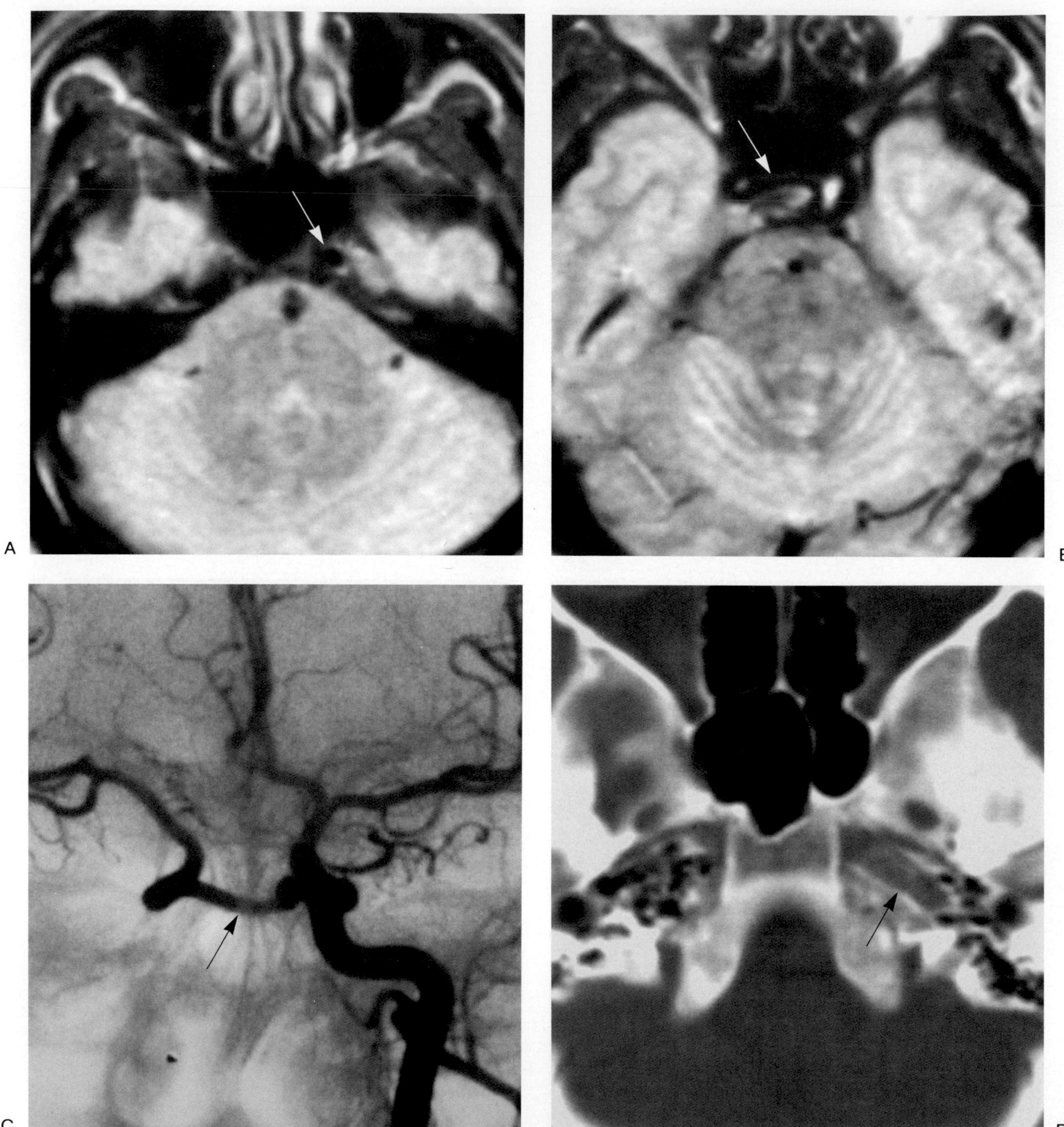

FIG. 51. Agenesis of ICA. Axial (**A,B**) proton-density-weighted images show left precavernous carotid artery (*arrow,* A), absence of normal flow void of right internal carotid artery, and abnormal trans-sellar flow void (*arrow*, B); and reconstitution of supraclinoid right internal carotid artery. Anterior posterior angiographic projection of left common carotid artery injection shows abnormal trans-sellar vessel (*arrow,* **C**). Confirmation of agenesis (versus acquired occlusion) is made by CT (**D**) which shows normal horizontal petrous carotid canal on left (*arrow*, D), but not on right. Canal would be present if disease were acquired.

carotid (106). Alternatively, persistent fetal communications through the sella turcica may provide a source of blood supply from one supraclinoid carotid artery to its contralateral counterpart (Fig. 51). The diagnosis of absent ICA may be made either by CT (absent carotid canal) or MRI (or MRA), and catheter angiography is no longer necessary. Duplex carotid ultrasound may also be helpful, although not diagnostic, by the finding of absent internal carotid flow and "externalization" of the common carotid wave forms. Less commonly, other types of connections may be detected, such as a "rete mirabile" (106,107).

In addition to agenesis, hypogenesis of the ICA may be discovered on imaging studies. This diagnosis can be suggested on MRI, but bone window CT is the definitive means of diagnosis. On CT, the bony canal will be present, but markedly hypoplastic. Angiography or MR angiography may strongly suggest the diagnosis. However, similar appearances may be seen on either catheter or MR angiography in cases of carotid dissection or moyamoya.

Trigeminal Artery and Other Variants

Once formed, the ICA offers the primary source of blood to the cerebral hemispheres and, initially, the posterior fossa. As noted above, several named branches of communication between the carotid and posterior circulation occur during vascular development. The vessels are named for their associated anatomy, such that the trigeminal artery courses in proximity to the trigeminal nerve, the hypoglossal artery through the hypoglossal canal with the nerve of the same name, and the otic through the internal auditory canal with the eighth cranial nerve. These primitive arteries present for approximately seven days in the embryo, hence accounting for their very infrequent identification in the adult. The most common of these embryonic communications is the trigeminal artery, which may be diagnosed on routine MRI (108,109). Three specific features help make the diagnosis of the trigeminal artery. First is the presence of a vessel that arises from the cavernous (or precavernous) carotid artery and courses directly posteriorly into the posterior fossa, where an abrupt medial bend is noted, and communication with the basilar artery is established. The second feature is that the basilar artery will typically be of small caliber caudal to the trigeminal artery, and the ipsilateral PComA will also be small. Although the artery is easily noted on axial images, it can be appreciated on off-midline sagittal views as well (Fig. 52). Less commonly, a variant trigeminal artery arises medially and courses through the sella and directly

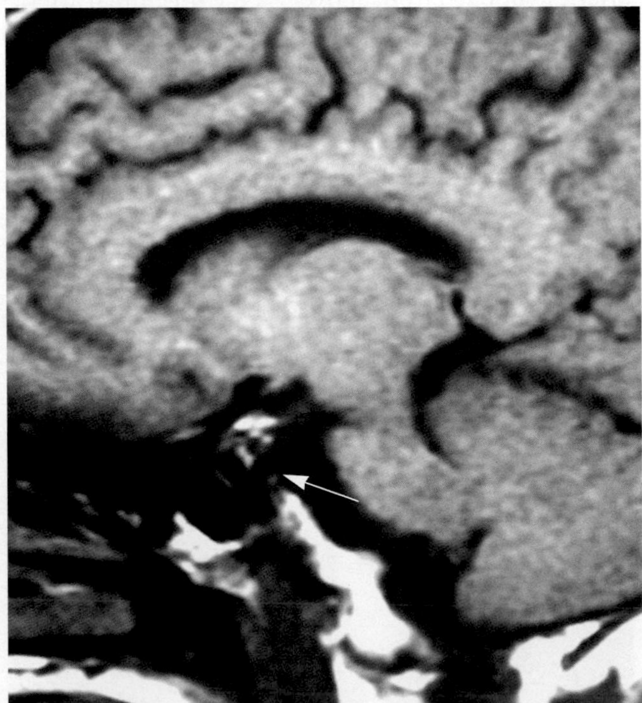

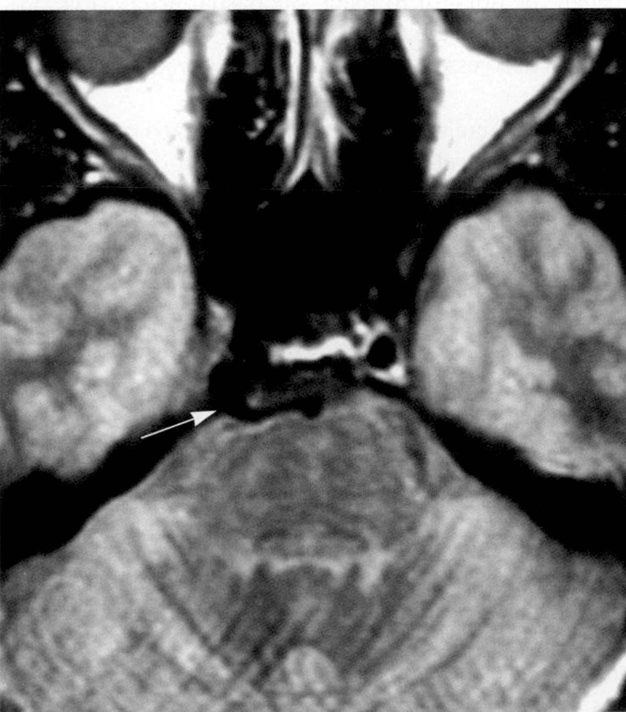

FIG. 52. Trigeminal artery. Sagittal (**A**) T1-weighted image shows an extravascular flow void (*arrow*, A) arising from the distal ascending petrous carotid artery. Axial (**B**) proton-density-weighted image shows trigeminal artery extending backward from the precavernous internal carotid artery. Note typical medial bend (*arrow*, B) as artery reaches toward the basilar artery.

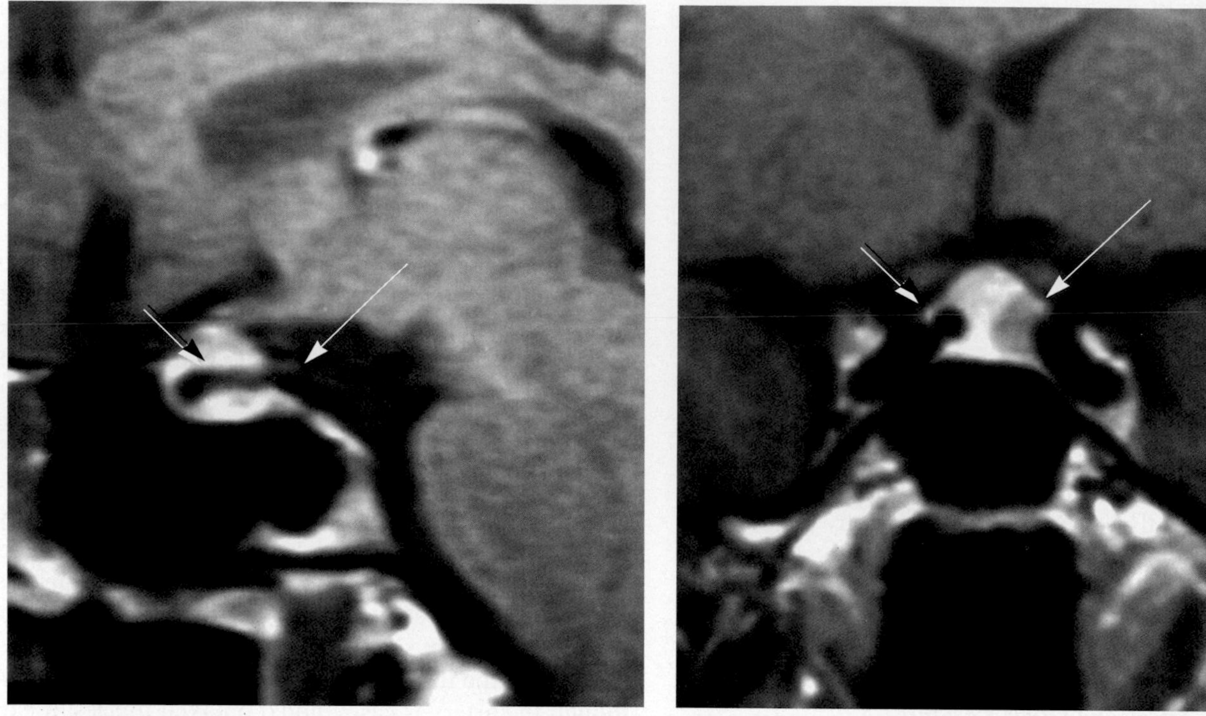

FIG. 53. Medial trigeminal artery. Sagittal (**A**) and coronal (**B**) contrast-enhanced T1-weighted images show abnormal flow void (*short arrows*, A and B) coursing through the pituitary gland and dorsum sellae (*long arrow*, A), en route to the basilar artery. Also note upwardly convex gland and microadenoma on left (*long arrow*, B). (Courtesy of Dr. William Kelly.)

through the dorsum to reach the basilar artery (Fig. 53) (108,110). Thus, the third diagnostic feature is the identification of a vessel that appears to penetrate the dorsum sellae.

The trigeminal artery is readily recognized on catheter angiography as well, and can be seen on both carotid and vertebral artery injections. Both posterior fossa embolus and vertebrobasilar insufficiency secondary to carotid bifurcation disease may be seen (110). Rarely, a trigeminal artery may be involved in the subclavian steal syndrome. In addition to such hemodynamic problems, intracranial aneurysms are reportedly more common in association with trigeminal artery, and Sturge-Weber disease has been recently described in association with trigeminal artery (111).

The other named persistent vascular communications between the carotid and posterior fossa circulation are much less common. They include the otic, hypoglossal, and pro-atlantal intersegmental arteries. There are very few reports of an otic artery (Fig. 54) (112), although its embryology is discussed by numerous authors (102, 106,113).

As noted above, during the early stages of brain development, the anterior circulation serves as the dominant intracranial vascular supply. With further growth, however, two parallel collections of primitive arterial arcades will unite along the lateral aspects of the rhombencephalon. These plexuses evolve into the longitudinal neural arteries, supplied from above, via the trigeminal arteries, and from below via the developing cervical intersegmental arteries. Depending on the growth of the posterior fossa and its complementary vascular evolution, these vascular communications between the anterior and pos-

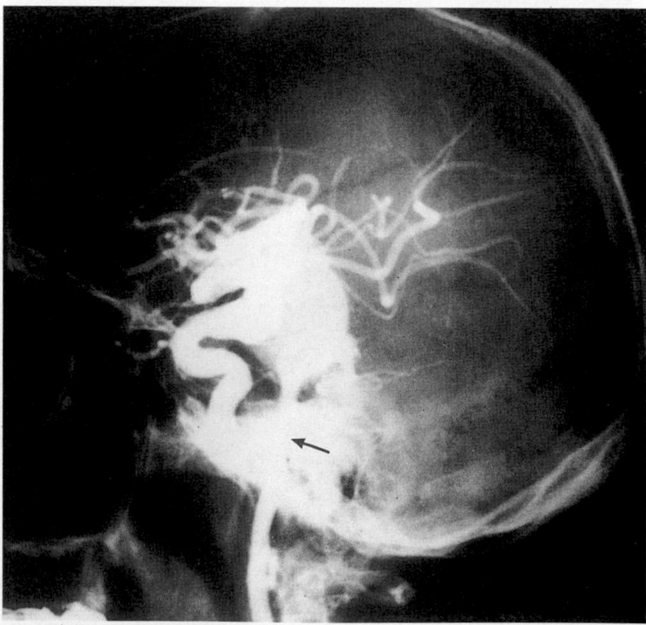

FIG. 54. Right carotid arteriogram; basilar artery, which is fed by persistent primitive acoustic artery (*arrow*). (From Franz et al., ref. 112, with permission.)

terior intracranial vasculature will recede. Ultimately, the caudal division of the ICAs, the PComAs, will supersede the trigeminal arteries as the dominant sources of collateral supply between the anterior and posterior circulation.

As the progressive development and recession of transient communications continue, the longitudinal neural arteries slowly appose and ultimately fuse in the midline, giving rise to the basilar artery. Occasionally, remnants of the prior discrete vascular channels are present in the adult and are known as basilar fenestration (Fig. 55). Continued maturation of the cervical intersegmental arteries results in the formation of two vertebral arteries, which will assume their positions as the primary sources of flow to the posterior circulation. Incomplete development of one, or rarely both, vertebral arteries will result in a hypoplastic vertebral artery with termination in the posterior inferior cerebral artery. Much more commonly, persistent embryonic communications between the vertebral and occipital arteries are seen. In fact, this is so frequently seen that it should be considered a normal variant.

Azygos Anterior Cerebral Artery

Still prior to major telencephalic hemispheric expansion, the cranial divisions of the ICAs will be dominated by the developing anterior cerebral arteries. Deep in the interhemispheric fissure an arterial plexus develops. Under normal circumstances, this plexus will evolve into the anterior communicating artery (AComA) in Padgett's stages 5 and 6 (102). Occasionally, persistence of some or all of this plexus may be noted on angiograms. Since this is the only area of the cerebral arterial vasculature that evolves such an identifiable plexus, it is not difficult to appreciate that the AComA is the most frequent location for the development of intracranial aneurysms. Incomplete resorption of any portion of this plexus could readily explain a mural weakness of the AComA, and subsequent aneurysm formation.

The ACA has been studied by several investigators (114–117). In particular, Baptista described multiple patterns of ACA development, as well as the relationship of the persistent median artery of the corpus callosum to the various adult ACA patterns (114). As noted above, the ACA evolves during stages 5 and 6. In the latter, according to Padgett, a small branch arises from the AComA, extending toward the lamina terminalis. This branch, known as the median artery of the corpus callosum, is thought to involute with the growth of the bilateral A2 segments of the ACAs. In his detailed anatomic dissections, Baptista describes an extremely high rate of persistence of the median artery of the corpus callosum in association with (i) both ACAs (i.e., triple ACAs), (ii) hypoplasia of an ACA (i.e., unilateral hemispheric supply from one ACA and contralateral hemispheric supply from the median artery of the corpus callosum), and (iii) hypoplasia or aplasia of both ACAs with dominant median artery of the corpus callosum (i.e., azygos ACA). He also describes the more common scenario of unilateral ACA hypoplasia without median artery of the corpus callosum, in which case the remaining ACA irrigates both hemispheres and simulates an azygos ACA (114). Because of this range of embryologic possibilities, radio-

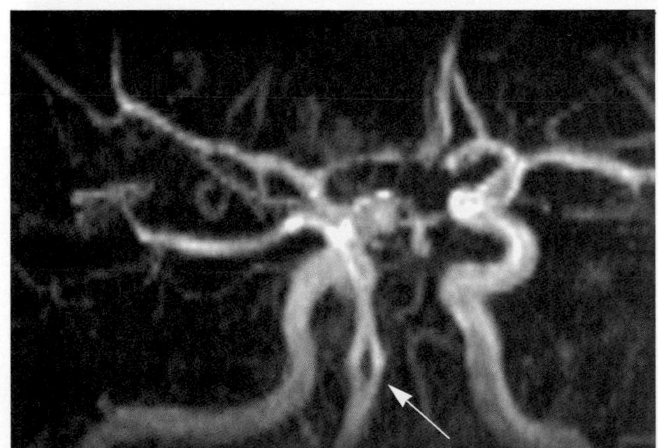

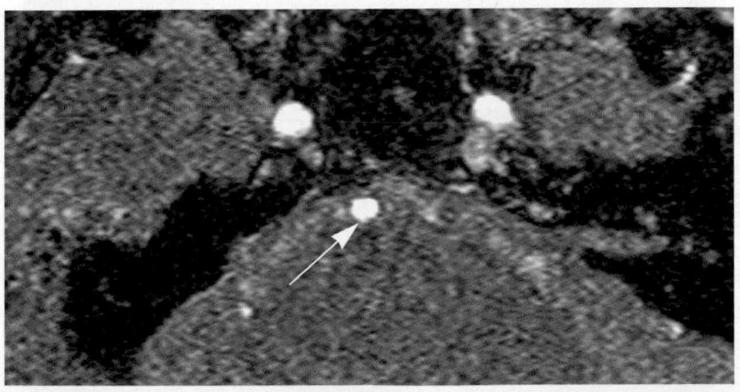

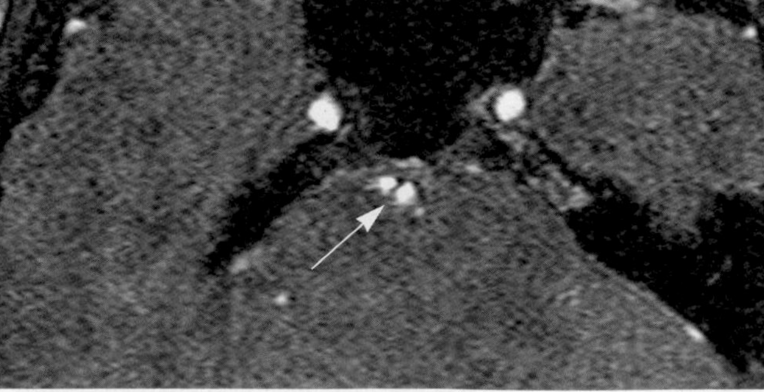

FIG. 55. Basilar artery fenestration. Shallow right anterior oblique reconstructed view from three-dimensional time-of-flight MR angiogram of intracranial vasculature shows fenestrated proximal basilar artery (*arrow*, **A**). Selected axial partitions from data set show single basilar artery (*arrow*, **B**) caudal to fenestrated artery (*arrow*, **C**).

logic definition of a true azygos ACA can be difficult (115).

The azygos (or azygous) ACA may be observed as an incidental finding, with little clinical significance, or as a feature of marked anomalous brain development, as in holoprosencephaly (Fig. 23). Uncommonly, it may be observed in association with anomalies of neuronal migration (Fig. 56). When incidental, the AComA is not

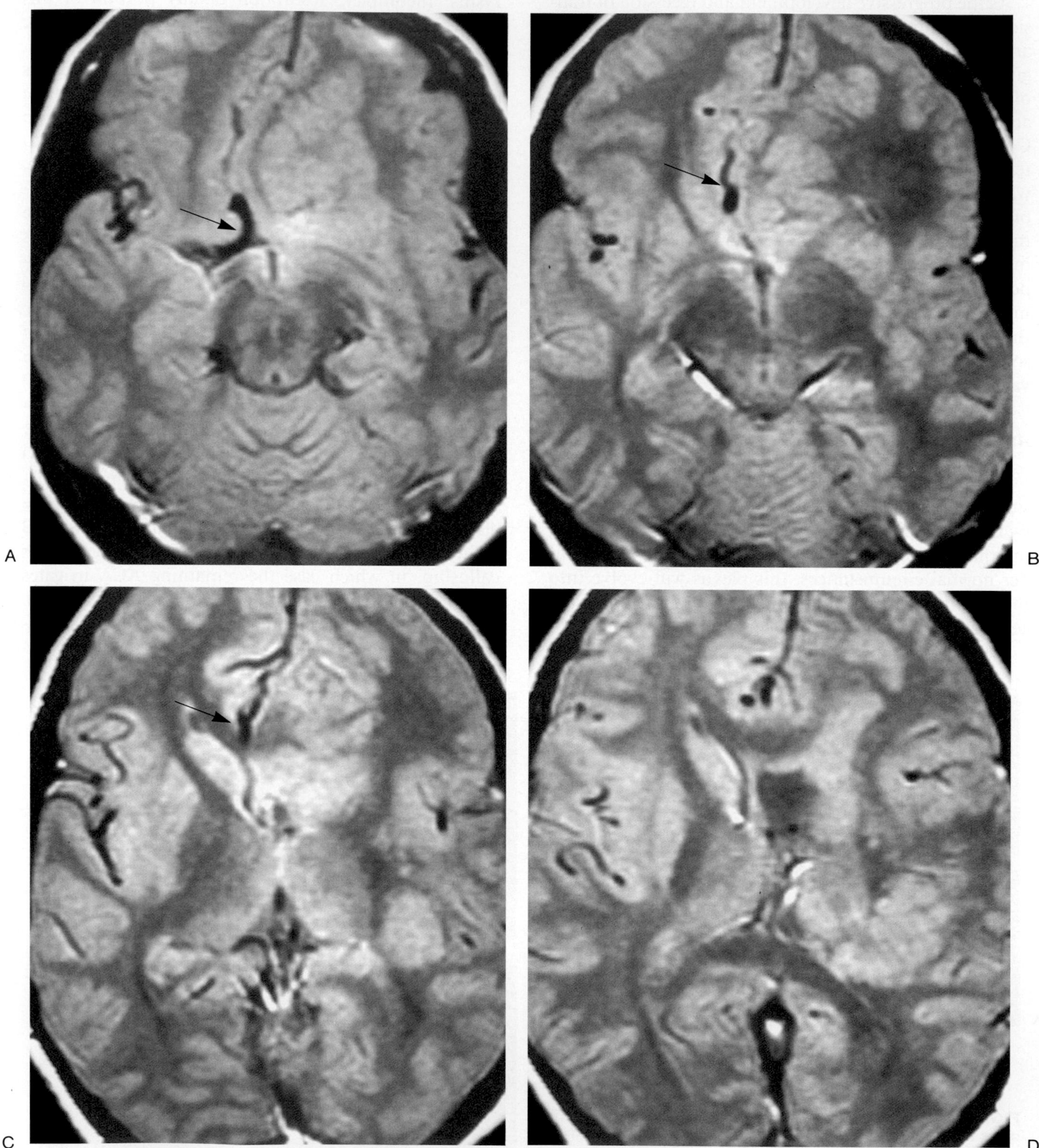

FIG. 56. Azygos anterior cerebral artery. Sequential axial (**A–D**) proton-density-weighted images show anomaly of neuronal migration. Although this case appears at first glance to represent a focal heterotopion, in fact the anomaly is a cortical dysplasia that involves the entire hemisphere; the cingulum is dysplastic and infolded into the hemisphere. Note azygos anterior cerebral artery (*arrows*). (From Truwit and Lempert, ref. 40, with permission.)

present, and the common trunk will bifurcate at the inferior margin of the falx cerebri. In this situation, the bifurcation point is susceptible to congenital and acquired aneurysm (or pseudoaneurysm) formation (Fig. 57) (118,119). Although not generally a problem on MRI, the azygos ACA may mimic an AComA aneurysm on contrast-enhanced CT (120). When associated with holoprosencephaly, the azygos ACA courses beneath, and

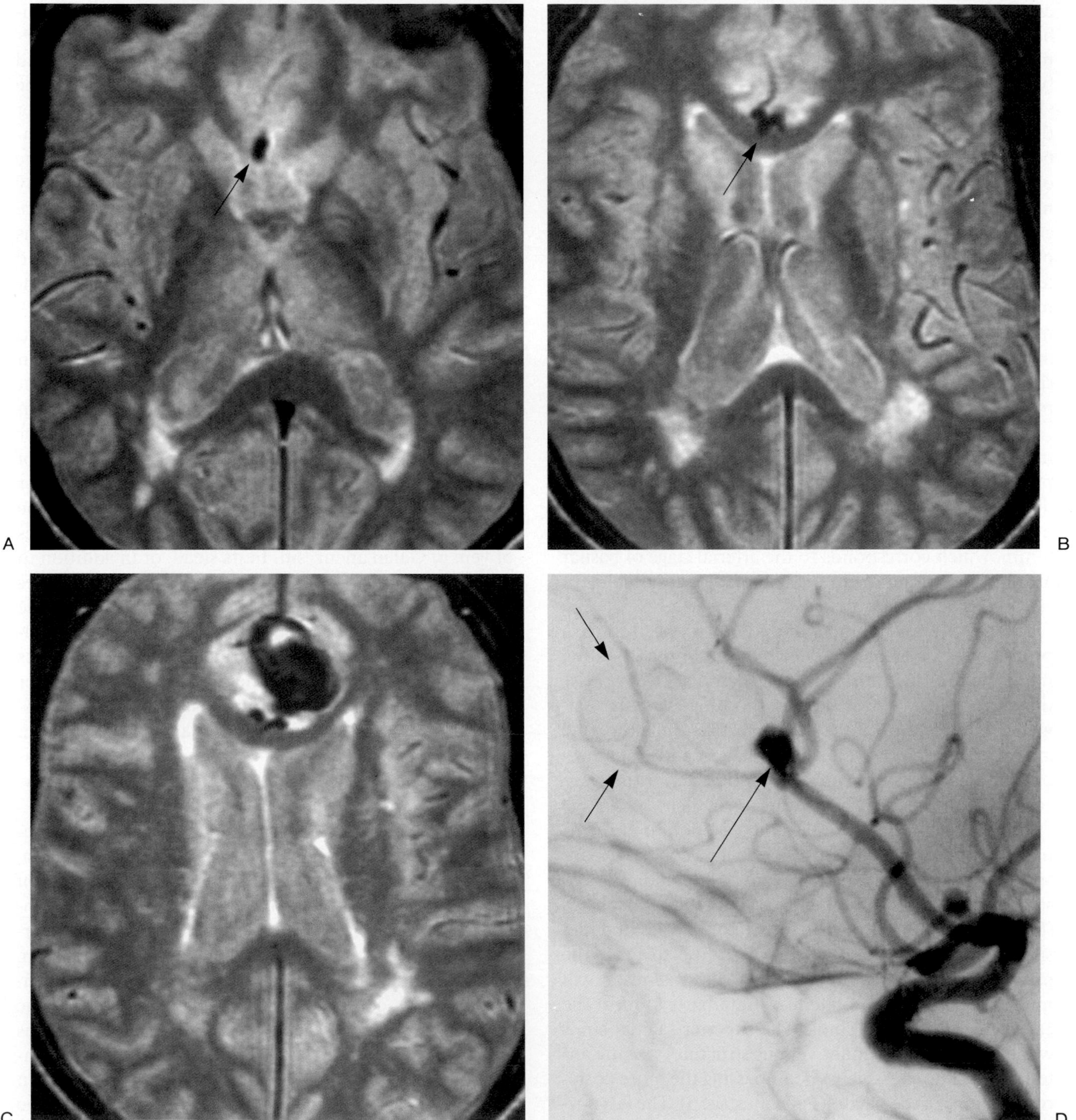

FIG. 57. Azygos anterior cerebral artery aneurysm. Axial (**A–C**) proton-density-weighted images show azygos anterior cerebral artery (*arrows*, A and B) and nearly completely thrombosed aneurysm (*arrows*, C) arising from left pericallosal artery, at point of bifurcation. Angiogram (**D**) shows small remnant of patent aneurysm (*long arrow*) and thin calcifications (*small arrows*) within wall of aneurysm. (From Truwit and Lempert, ref. 40, with permission.)

subsequently anterior to, the undivided prosencephalon, as there is neither hemispheric cleavage nor an interhemispheric fissure (117).

Venous Anomalies

The embryology of the intracranial venous pathways has also been reviewed in great detail by Padgett and others (101,103,105,121). More recently, this embryology has been reviewed by Yokota, with reference to developmental brain anomalies (122), and by Velut and Raybaud, with reference to the vein of Galen aneurysm (123,124). Although venous embryology does not follow the same chronology as that of the arteries, stages have been described which outline the course of venous development. The primary difference between arterial and venous development is that while the arterial system has essentially formed by the end of the embryonic period proper, the venous system is still evolving, with the potential for anatomic variance and anomalous development. Thus, like neuronal migration from the germinal matrix, intracranial venous development continues well into the fetal period. Not surprisingly, venous—not arterial—anomalies typically accompany anomalies of neuronal migration (125).

The first major intracranial venous structure is the primary head sinus (Padgett, stage 2), previously named the primitive rhombencephalic vessel (Sabin) and primordial hindbrain channel (Streeter) (101,103,105). At this time, the embryo is still very young, measuring only 5 to 8 mm, which corresponds to the arterial stage of basilar artery development from the bilateral longitudinal neural arteries.

Prior to the development of the primary head sinus, a primitive vascular plexus develops within the investing mesenchyme (meninx primitiva, described above). As the primary head sinus emerges, this broad vascular network organizes into three dural plexuses, including the anterior (telencephalic, diencephalic, and mesencephalic), middle (metencephalic), and posterior (myelencephalic) plexuses. They drain via their respective "stems," the anterior, middle, and posterior dural stems, into the primary head sinus. With telencephalic expansion, the anterior plexuses expand to maintain the ensheathing mesh of vascular plexus about the hemispheres (Padgett, stage 3). Along the future convexities, the mesial aspects of the bilateral plexuses fuse to form the primitive marginal sinuses. Later, these sinuses will merge with their contralateral counterparts to form the early superior sagittal sinus. The superior sagittal sinus will become the dominant venous structure, starting anteriorly and progressively encompassing the more posterior portions of the plexus (Padgett, stage 5). The last portion to resolve into a dominant structure is the supratorcular plexus. Occasionally, incomplete fusion may result in a fenestrated superior sagittal sinus (126).

Vein of Galen Aneurysm

With prosencephalic cleavage into the telencephalii, an interhemispheric cleft is formed, at the depth of which is the lamina terminalis. Further dorsally, the "telediencephalic sulcus" evaginates laterally into the telencephalic ventricles, thus forming the choroidal fissures (124). (With the development of the commissural system, the sulcus itself will mature into the interhemispheric fissure above, and the velum transversum below.) Through these bilateral fissures both meninx and primitive choroid insinuate into the ventricles. While the arterial supply will initially be dominated by the anterior choroidal arteries, the venous drainage will involve a single, transitory midline vein, the median prosencephalic vein. This embryonic and early fetal vein will ultimately recede, as development of the basal ganglia will induce formation of the true internal cerebral veins. These veins will "soon annex the venous drainage of the choroid plexus" (124). A caudal remnant of the median prosencephalic vein will become the vein of Galen.

Recently, a complex embryologic work has helped to elaborate these details and their relevance to formation of the vein of Galen aneurysm. According to Raybaud et al. (124), the venous sac of the vein of Galen aneurysm represents not a varix of the vein of Galen, but rather a varix of the persistent median prosencephalic vein (of Markowski). Persistence of this structure as an outlet for diencephalic and choroidal venous drainage obviates the need for a straight sinus; hence, its absence in many cases of vein of Galen aneurysm. In its stead, or in addition to the straight sinus, a falcine sinus is often noted in cases of vein of Galen aneurysm. This structure typifies the notion of vascular development and regression according to need. That is, as the straight sinus develops its more cephalad sister sinus, the falcine sinus, no longer dominates the deep venous drainage; hence, its regression in most cases. In the vein of Galen malformation, since venous development is arrested, it is not uncommon to see persistence of a falcine sinus with little, if any, straight sinus development (Fig. 58).

With differentiation of the telencephalii and diencephalon, lateral venous channels arise to drain the developing neural structures. Notably, the tentorial sinuses of stage 6 arises along the ventral aspect of the prosencephalon; they drain tributaries of the telencephalon (superficial and deep), as well as the ventral diencephalon. These dural channels course through the primitive tentorium. With continued prosencephalic expansion, the tentorial sinuses will recede, giving way to the basal veins (103). Another feature of stage 6 is the emergence of emissary veins, most of which will arise during stage 7. In particular, the mastoid emissary veins arise during stage 6. Although these veins typically have only a limited role in the adult, they are occasionally recruited in cases of sigmoid sinus atresia or hypoplasia. In such cases, the

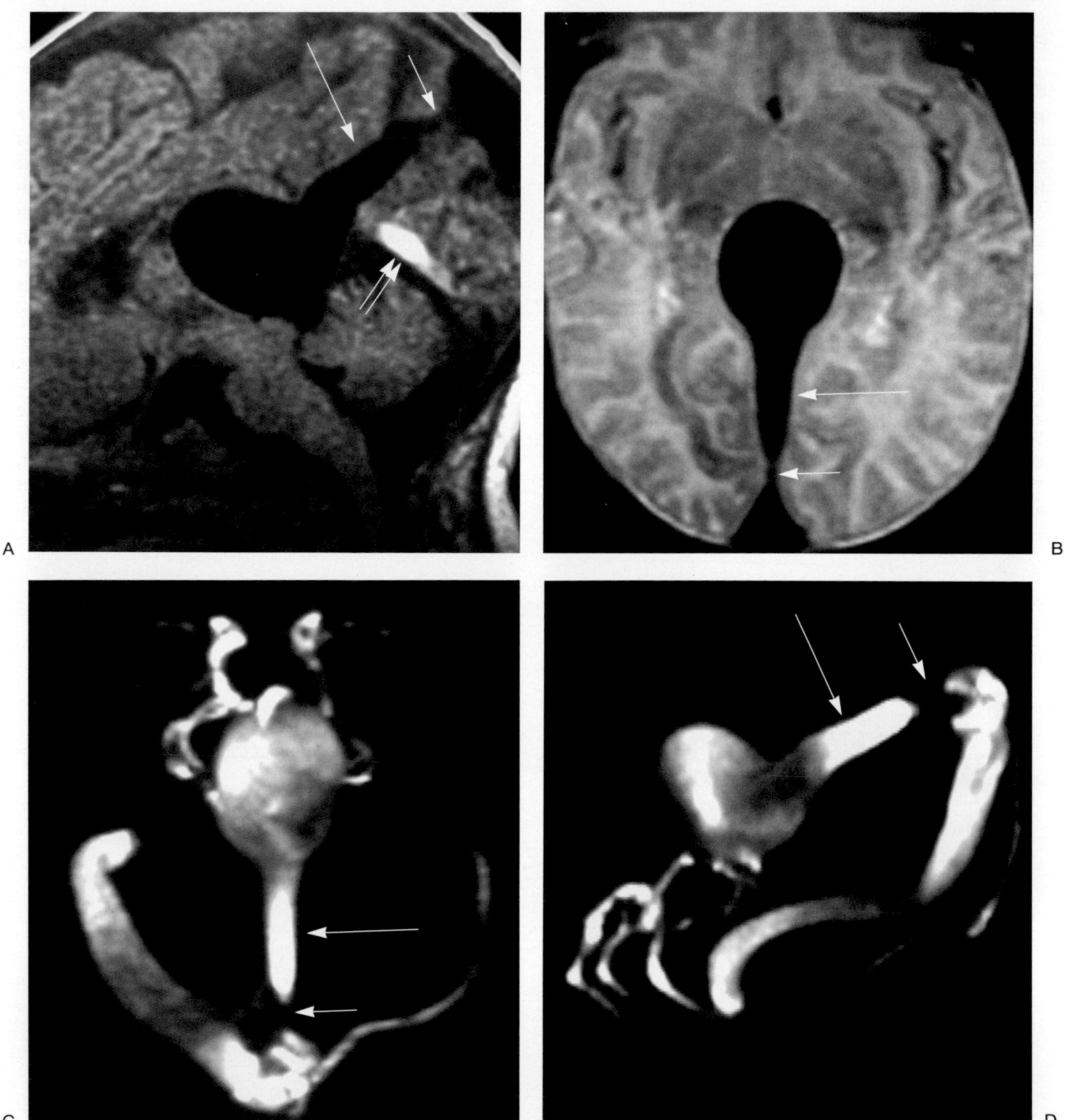

FIG. 58. Vein of Galen aneurysm with falcine sinus. Sagittal (**A**) T1- and axial (**B**) T2-weighted images show massive vein of Galen varix and enlarged falcine sinus (*long arrows*). Collapsed (**C**) and steep right anterior oblique (**D**) views from three-dimensional phase contrast MR angiogram (flow velocity = 55 cm/sec) show greater extent of malformation, as well as focal ''protective'' stenosis (*short arrows*) of falcine sinus. Because of stenosis, patient was not in congestive heart failure. Note thrombus within straight sinus (*double arrow*, A).

internal jugular veins will be hypoplastic at the skull base, only receiving inferior petrosal drainage, and large cervical muscular veins drain the majority of intracranial venous flow via the mastoid and condylar emissary veins (Fig. 59).

Growth of the posterior fossa structures also plays a determining role in the elaboration of venous sinuses. In particular, a "passive" restructuring is noted with cerebellar hemispheric growth, displacing the transverse sinuses (dural stems of the anterior/middle dural plexuses) further laterally toward their adult positions. As this occurs, a small remnant of the posterior dural plexus may persist as the occipital sinus (Fig. 60).

Venous Angioma

The final periods of intracranial venous development described by Padgett are stages 7 and 7a, referring to the "threshold of fetal period" and "fetus at the third month" (103). These periods are of particular interest since it is at this time that much of the definitive cerebral venous system appears. Moreover, many of the venous anomalies we recognize today most likely occur during the late embryonic and early fetal periods. Most notable of these anomalies is the venous angioma, more recently called a medullary venous malformation (127) and a developmental venous anomaly (128).

During Padgett's stage 7, the emergence of the superior sagittal sinus and vein of Galen were noted. In addition, however, considerable evolution of the parenchymal venous channels takes place and calvarial emissary veins are defined. With regards to the former, it is at this point that alignment of deep medullary veins and their drainage is expected. Insults to their normal development are the likely source of venous angiomas. In such cases, the medullary veins may not run parallel to each other along their course to the subependymal veins or the superficial cortical veins. Rather, a disordered "caput medusae" appearance is seen, with drainage via a dominant venous channel. This channel, known as the draining vein of a venous angioma, is typically noted in place of, rather than in addition to, the normal venous drainage of the affected brain parenchyma. Occasionally, the medullary veins may appear relatively normal; their drainage through large transcerebral veins, however, constitutes a venous anomaly essentially no different than a venous angioma. Venous angiomas may drain ei-

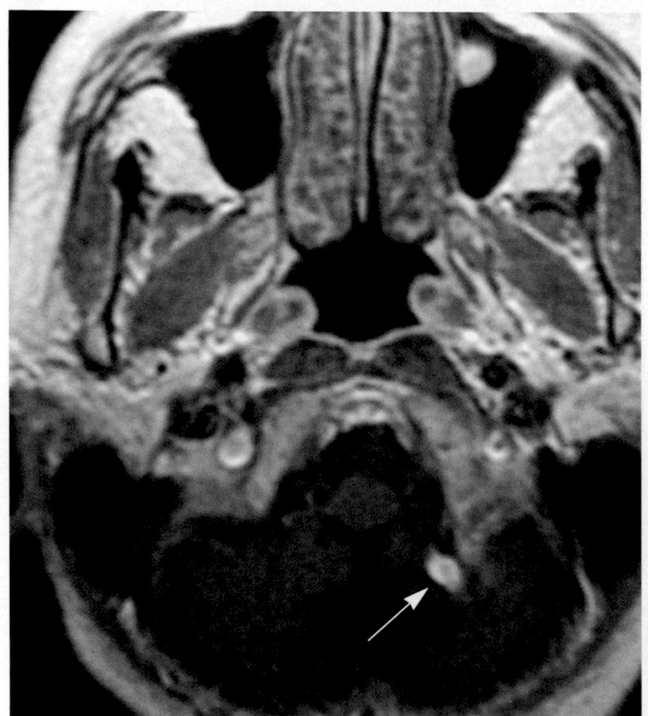

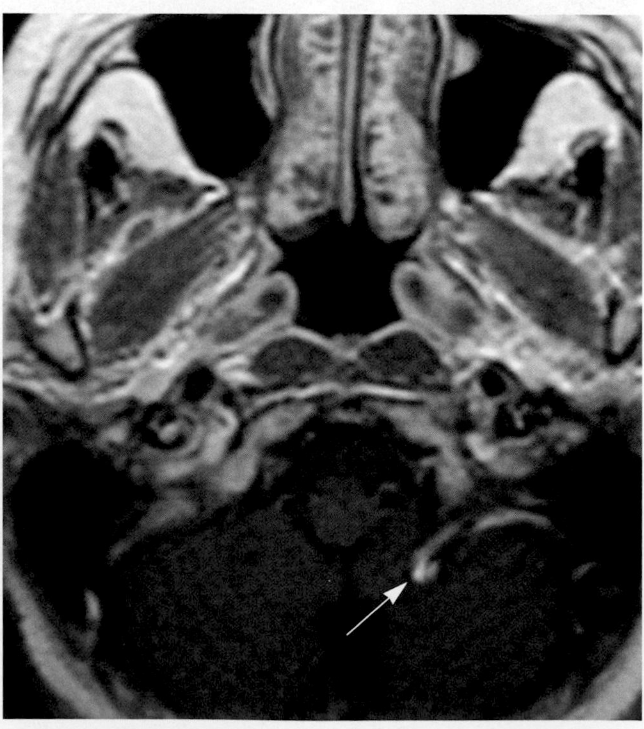

FIG. 59. Condylar emissary vein. Axial contrast-enhanced T1-weighted images show prominent vein just lateral to left cerebellar tonsil (*arrow*, **A**). Vein is about to pass through left occipital condyle. Slightly more cephalad (*arrow*, **B**), note vein extending from sigmoid sinus beneath left cerebellum. These are typical features of condylar emissary vein.

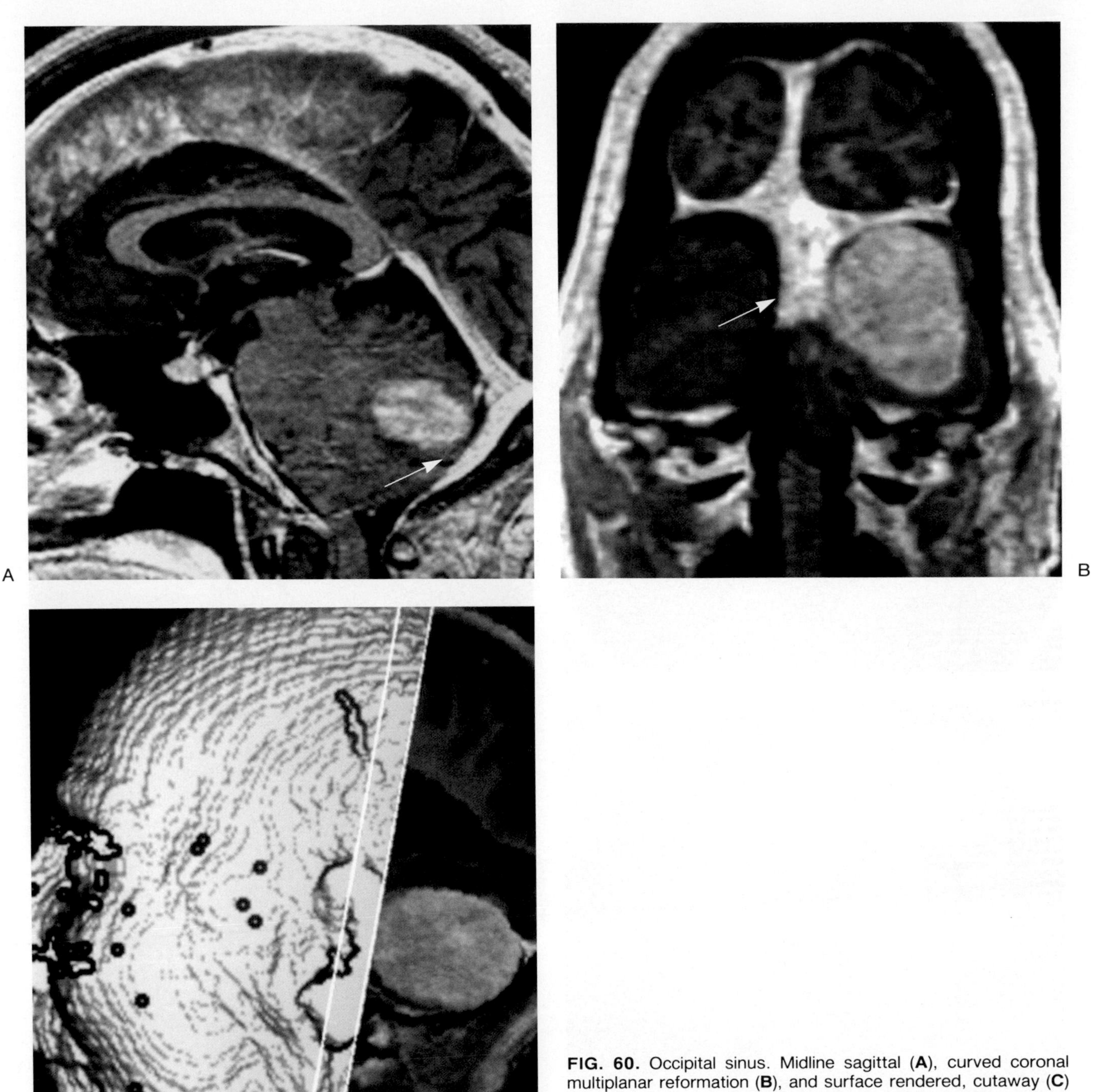

FIG. 60. Occipital sinus. Midline sagittal (**A**), curved coronal multiplanar reformation (**B**), and surface rendered, cutaway (**C**) contrast-enhanced three-dimensional gradient-echo images show enhancing posterior fossa meningioma. Note prominent occipital dural sinus (*arrows*) extending caudad from the torcular Herophili. (Courtesy of Dr. John Sherman.)

ther to the superficial or deep venous system (Figs. 61 and 62). Uncommonly, both routes of drainage are employed. Rarely, transcranial venous drainage participates; in such cases, the transcalvarial route is called sinus pericranii. Typically, this refers to a large subcutaneous, midline venous channel along the forehead with cephalad communication to the superior sagittal sinus.

The most common sites of venous angioma are the frontal lobes and the posterior fossa (Fig. 63). Usually, the caput medusae is seen within the deep white matter, although it may be seen within deep gray matter nuclei or exceptionally, within the ventricles or brainstem (129–132).

Venous anomalies may be localized aberrations of development, such as venous angioma, or they may

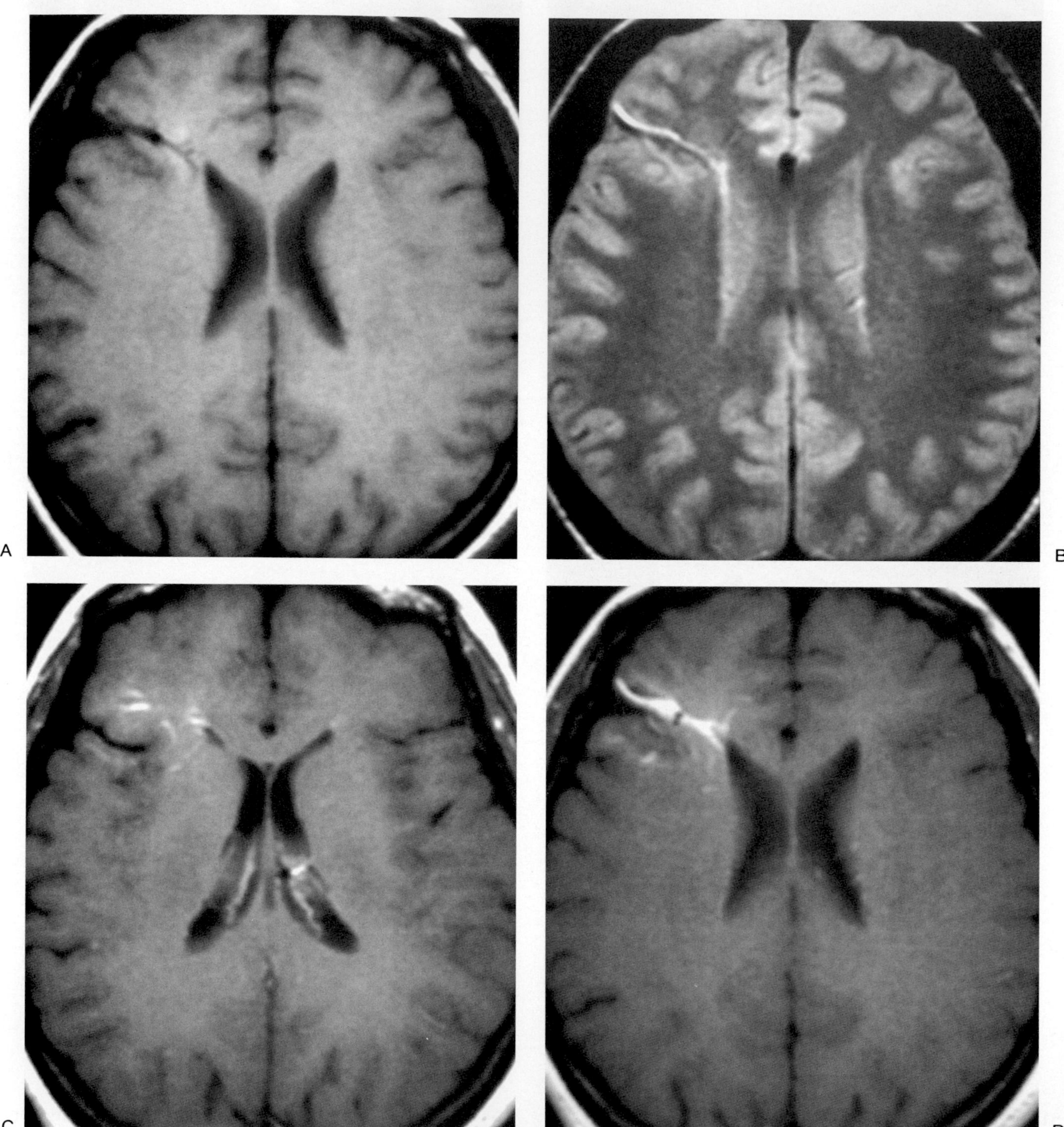

FIG. 61. Superficial venous angioma. Axial T1- (**A**), proton-density- (**B**), and contrast-enhanced (**C**,**D**) T1-weighted images show typical features of venous angioma. Note transparenchymal draining vein and few enhancing radicles of caput medusae (C). (From Truwit and Lempert, ref. 40, with permission.)

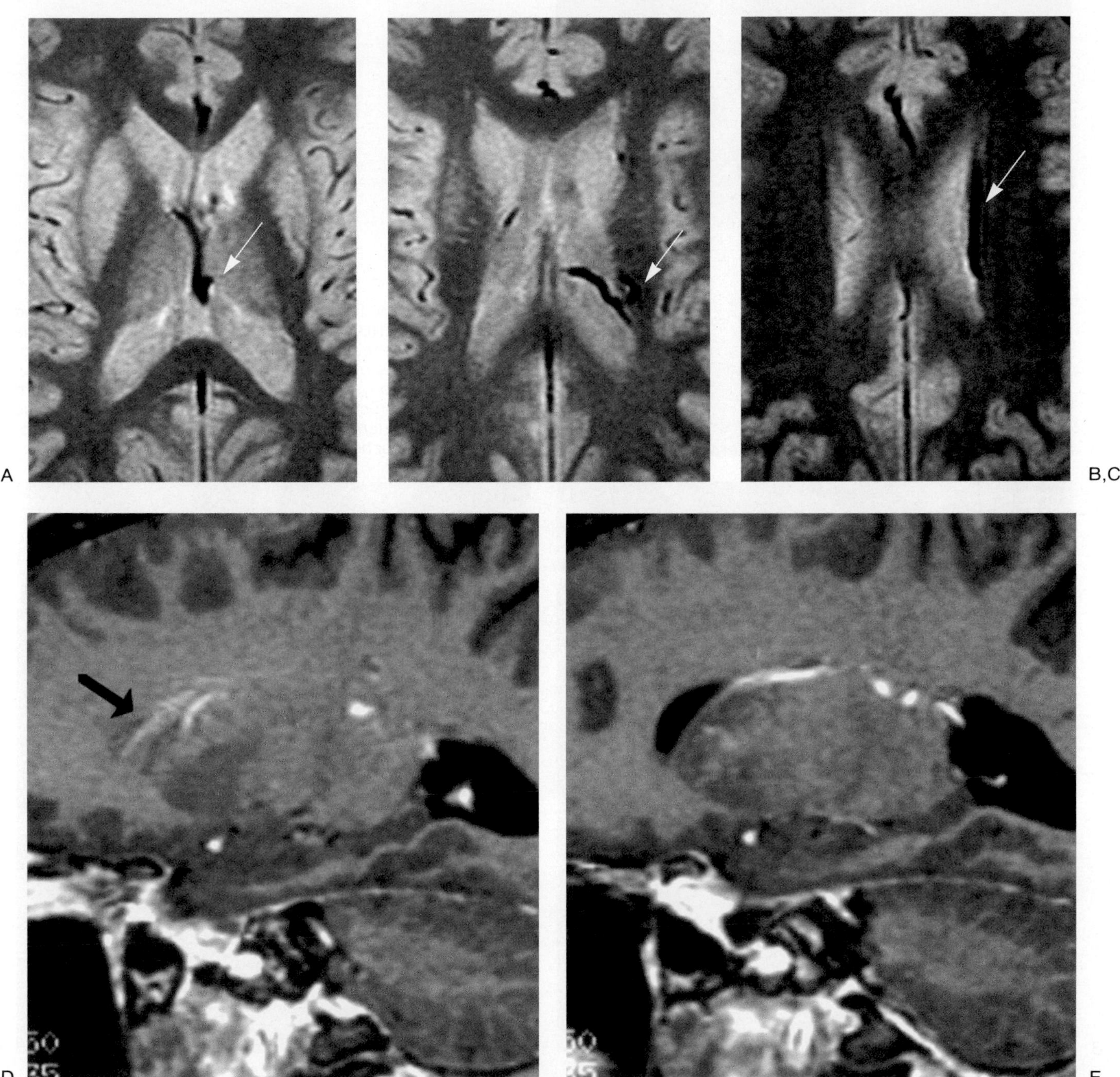

FIG. 62. Deep venous angioma. Axial (**A–C**) proton-density-weighted images through lateral ventricles show abnormal subependymal vein (*arrow*, C), that drains through the ventricle (*arrow*, B) into a shortened internal cerebral vein (*arrow*, C). Note the normal contralateral internal cerebral vein. Sagittal images (**D,E**) from contrast-enhanced three-dimensional data set show caput medusae within left caudate head (*arrow*, D) and longitudinal subependymal vein seen on axial image (C). (From Truwit, ref. 131, with permission.)

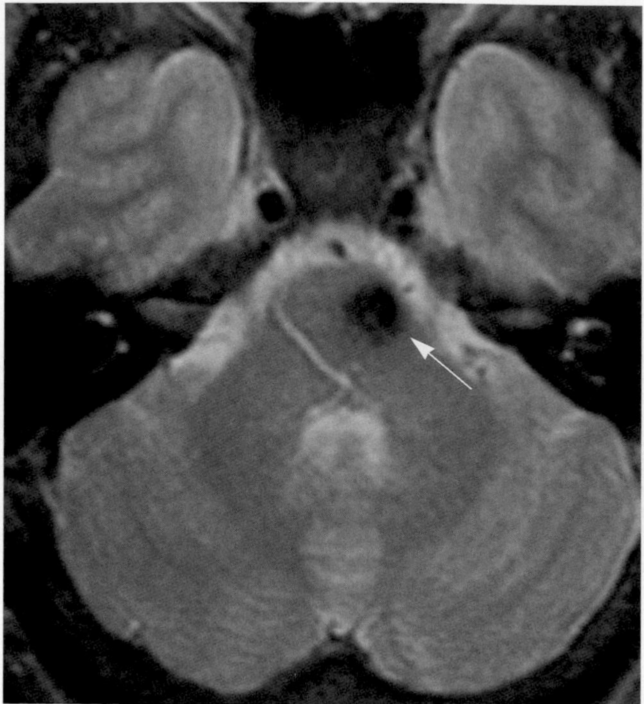

A

FIG. 63. Posterior fossa venous angioma. Axial T2- (**A**) and contrast-enhanced (**B,C**) T1-weighted images show transpontine draining vein of venous angioma. Caput medusae involves subependymal regions of floor and lateral walls of fourth ventricle. Vein drains anteriorly through the cerebellopontine angle cistern to the superior petrosal sinus (*arrows*, B and C). Note small focus of old hemorrhage (*arrow*, A) within left hemipons. This could represent either a prior hemorrhage or a cavernous angioma.

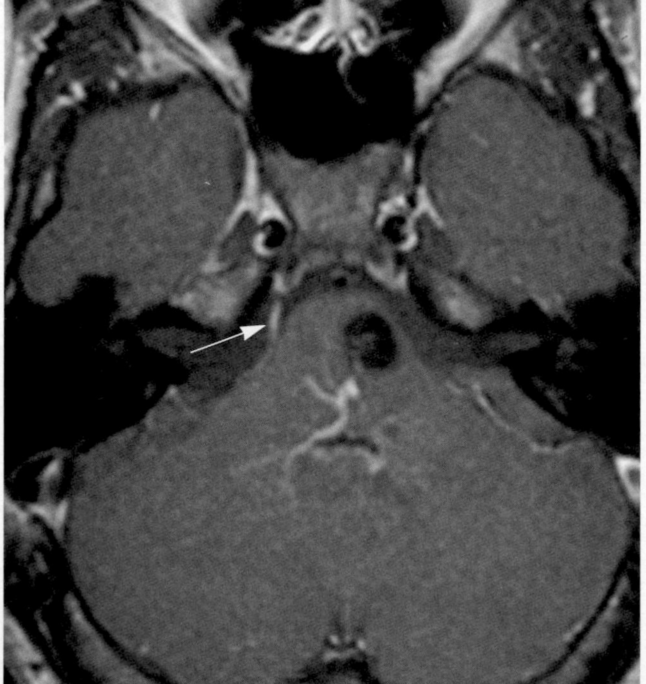

B

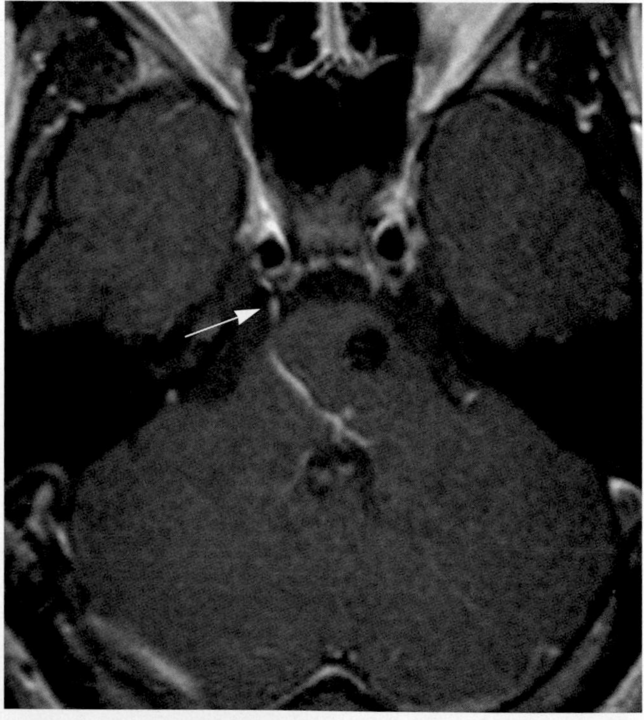

C

involve an entire brain region or hemisphere, as in the Sturge-Weber syndrome. The Klippel-Weber-Trenaunay and blue rubber bleb nevus syndromes may also involve large intracranial venous malformations.

The matter of venous angioma and associated hemorrhage continues to receive considerable attention in the neuroradiological literature. Numerous authors have attributed the hemorrhagic complications of venous angioma to associated cavernous angiomas. Although this may be true for some cases, there appear to be cases in which true arteriovenous malformations are present (Fig. 64) and account for hemorrhage as well as cases in which no associated vascular malformation can be identified. In such cases, it is possible that a component of acquired venous restrictive disease accounts for elevated venous pressure within the angioma and thus, places patients at risk for venous hemorrhage or infarction (Fig. 65).

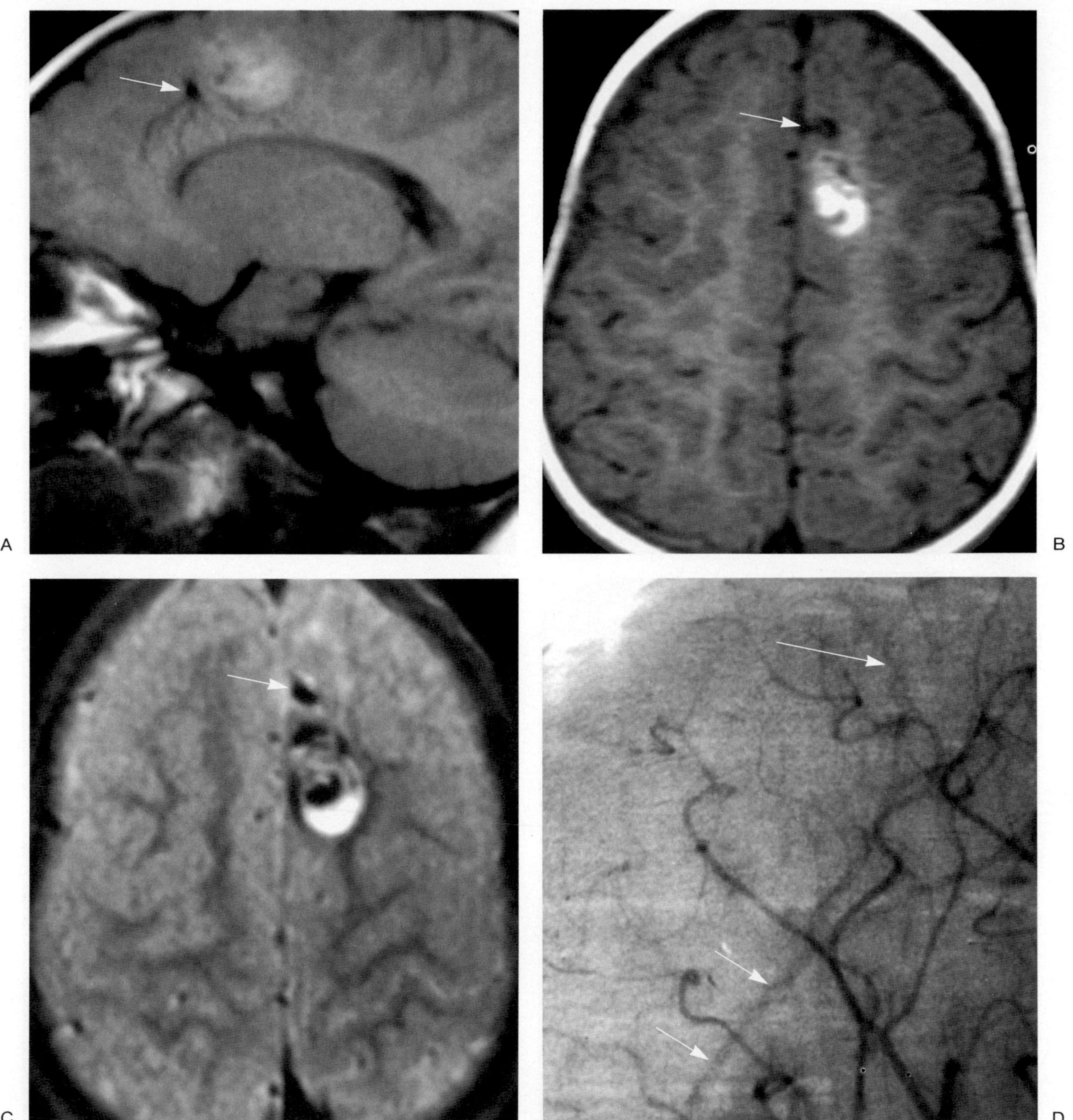

FIG. 64. Venous angioma and AVM. Sagittal (**A**) and axial T1- (**B**) and T2- (**C**) weighted images show typical caput medusae and proximal portion (*arrows*, A–C) of draining vein. Acute hemorrhage is seen within the superior frontal gyrus, just posterior to the draining vein. Magnified view of lateral projection, left internal carotid angiogram shows diminished flow through anterior cerebral artery (*short arrows*, **D**) and subtle evidence of venous flow (*long arrow*, D). Although not clearly seen on MRI or angiogram, small, true arteriovenous malformation was found at surgery. Venous angioma was identified and left intact. (From Truwit, ref. 131, with permission.)

During the late embryonic and early fetal periods, neuronal migration from the periventricular germinal matrix is actively underway. During this time, the expression of genetic disorders, as well as vascular and/or infectious insults, may result in various anomalies of neuronal migration. These range from global anomalies, such as agyria, pachygyria, or band heterotopia to more localized aberrations such as schizencephaly, cleft of polymicrogyria, or focal heterotopic gray matter. Not uncommonly associated with the arrest of neuronal mi-

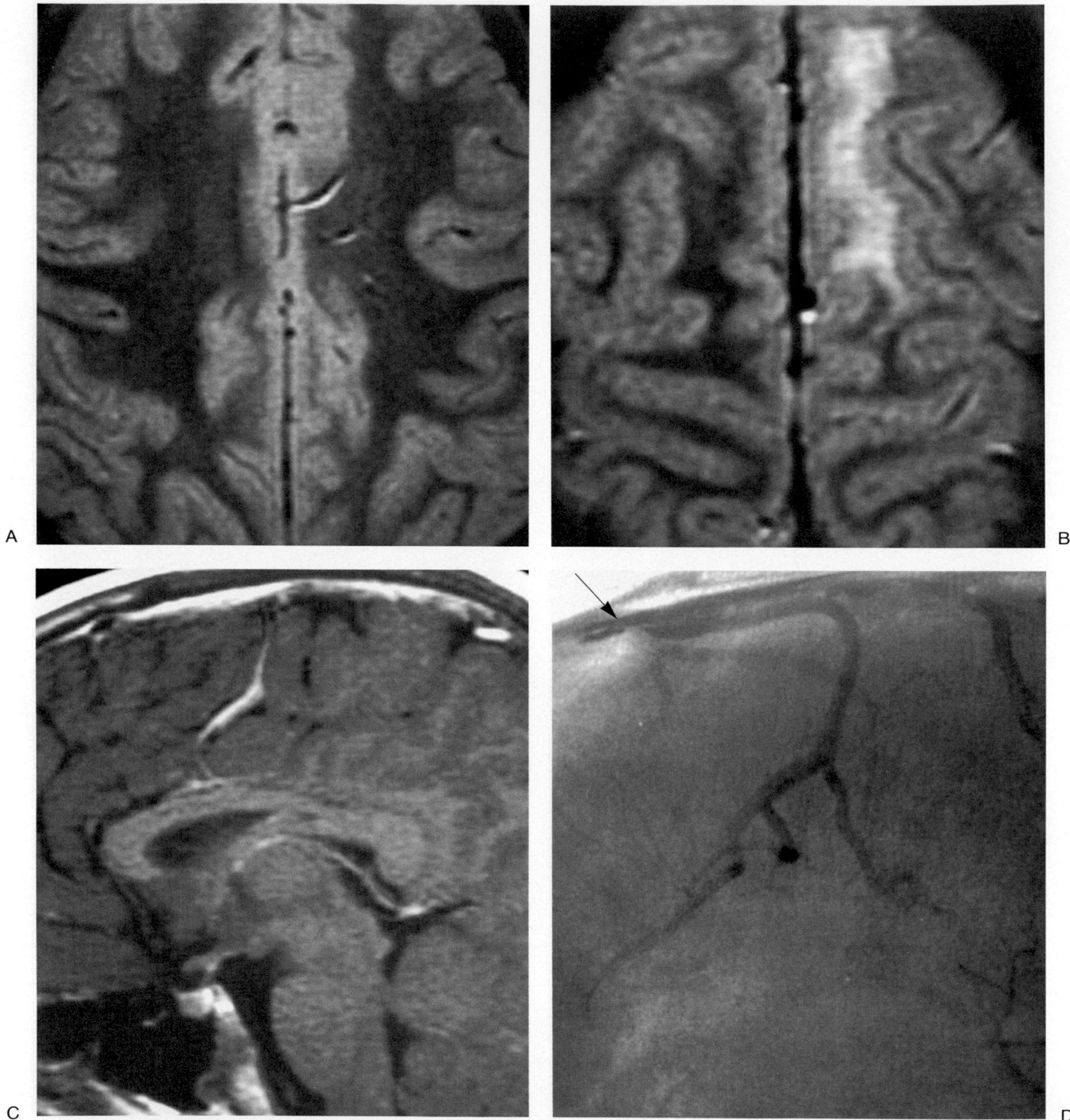

FIG. 65. Venous angioma and venous infarction. Axial (**A,B**) T2-weighted images show abnormal vascular flow voids within left cingulum and corona radiata. More cephalad, abnormal hyperintensity of subcortical white matter within left superior frontal gyrus can be seen. Features are consistent with many disorders, but venous ischemia and/or infarction must be considered. Sagittal (**C**) contrast-enhanced T1-weighted image shows prominent draining vein of venous angioma. Lateral projection (**D**) of left internal carotid artery angiogram shows large venous angioma of frontal lobe and draining vein. Note focal stenosis of venous stem (*arrow*, D) at point of entry into superior sagittal sinus. Such stenoses are typically at the junction of the venous stem and the dural sinus; the resultant elevated venous pressure is thought to be related to increased risk of venous hemorrhage, venous infarction, and possibly acquired cavernous angioma. (From Truwit, ref. 131, with permission.)

gration is an arrest of venous development (125, 133). It is likely that the venous system develops only as needed in cases of anomalous neuronal migration. With the failure of proper cortical and subcortical development is an associated failure of venous development to proceed to the next order. The result is enlarged, primitive venous channels along the course of the parenchymal anomaly. These veins are routinely identified on MRI and may simulate an arteriovenous fistula if the anomaly of neuronal migration is not appreciated (Fig. 66).

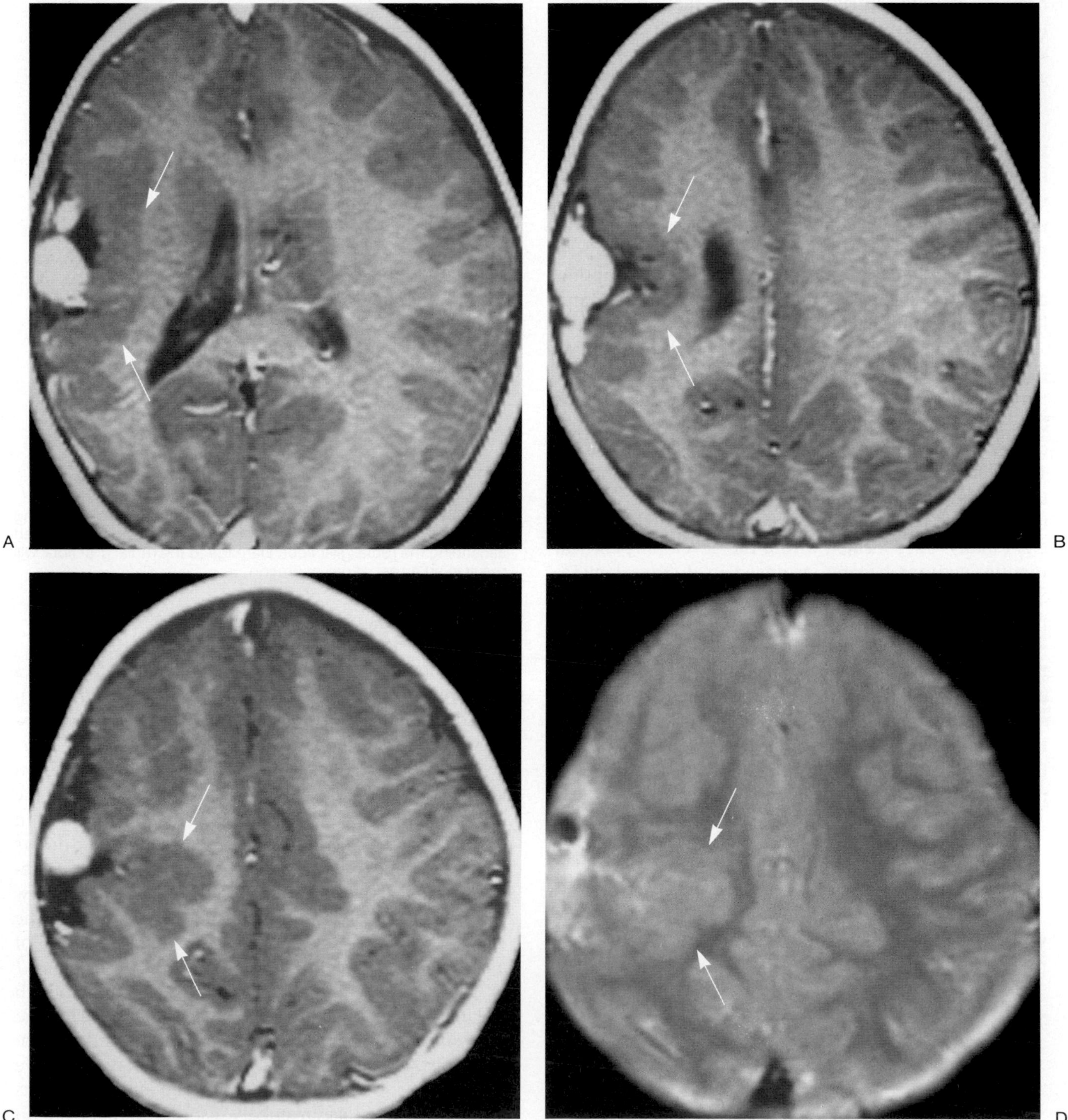

FIG. 66. Enlarged veins within polymicrogyric cleft. Axial contrast-enhanced (**A–C**) three-dimensional SPGR images of young child with seizure disorder show prominent enhancing vascular structures. Axial T2-weighted image (**D**) shows corresponding flow void. Child was referred for possible embolization of apparent arteriovenous malformation. Closer inspection of MRI, however, shows dysplastic cortex (*arrows*) underlying prominent veins. In fact, this is commonly found in cases of polymicrogyric cleft. (From Truwit, ref. 131, with permission.)

NEURONAL MIGRATION

At approximately the seventh gestational week, mitotic activity in the subependymal layer of the walls of the lateral ventricles begins (134–137). Within this area of cell proliferation, known as the germinal matrix, cells begin to migrate centrifugally to form the cerebral cortex. Initial migrations begin during the eighth gestational week. A 1:1 correlation exists between the portion of the germinal matrix in which the neurons originate and the portion of the cerebral cortex where the neurons come to rest (Fig. 67). This correlation is maintained largely by the presence of radially oriented glial fibers that span the hemisphere and act as scaffolding, along which the neurons migrate (Fig. 68). In addition, the degree of maturation of the ependyma underlying the germinal matrix may play a significant role in the degree of both neuronal migration and maturation (138). After cell migration along the radial cells is complete, these cells shrink and form the glial building blocks of the brain.

Neurons migrate away form the germinal zone according to specific patterns. Interestingly, those cells destined to reside within the deepest of the cortical layers are those cells that migrate first. These cells are followed by those destined to form the transient subplate, layer 7 (135–139). These cells actually pass through the earlier migration. Subsequent neuronal migrations also pass through the marginal layer (layer 1) to form the intervening layers. Finally, once located within the developing cortical mantle, neurons become arranged in discrete lamina. Synapses with local and distant neurons take place in a process known as cortical organization (140–142).

Migration anomalies are caused by events that inhibit normal neuronal migration. Therefore, infections, ischemia, and metabolic (genetic) derangements can all result in anomalies of neuronal migration. These anomalies are divided into several categories depending upon the severity and timing of the arrest of neuronal migration.

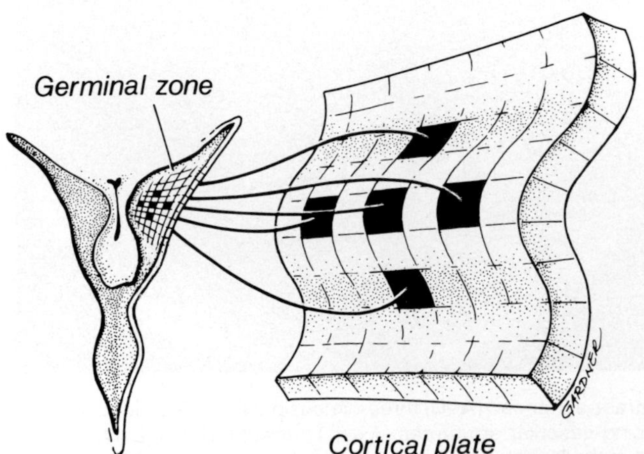

FIG. 67. Schematic drawing illustrates the relationship of the germinal matrix to the developing cortical plate. A 1:1 correspondence exists between the site of cell proliferation in the germinal zone and its eventual resting place in the cortical plate.

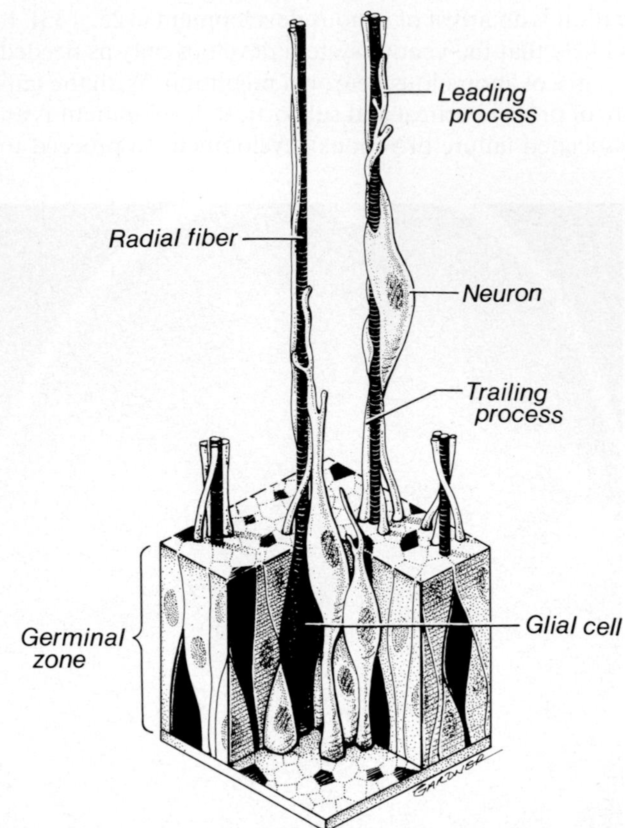

FIG. 68. Drawing demonstrates the relationship of the migrating neurons to the radial glial cells. A migrating neuron is illustrated ascending the radial glial fiber. Damage to the radial glial fiber will result in an arrest of cell migration.

Agyria and Pachygyria

The most severe of the neuronal migration anomalies is lissencephaly, which results from an abnormality in neuronal migration between about 8 and 14 weeks gestation. The lissencephalies are a group of disorders characterized by a paucity of gyral and sulcal formation known as agyria and pachygyria. Classifications of the lissencephalies have undergone considerable revision in recent years as the genetic associations of these disorders have been defined. For instance, at least two distinct subsets of classical (previously, type 1) lissencephaly are now recognized. The first subset includes patients with the Miller-Dieker syndrome; in these patients, a deletion of a lissencephaly gene known as LIS1 on chromosome 17 (17p13.3) has been identified (143,144). In children with isolated lissencephaly, on the other hand, at least two different chromosomal anomalies have been identified. In at least 40% of this subset of patients, a less extensive 17p13.3 deletion is seen. Another group of these patients have an X-linked lissencephaly disorder that appears to be related to band heterotopia (W. B. Dobyns, *personal communication*).

A second broad category of patients are those with cobblestone (formerly called type 2) lissencephaly (145–150). This group includes at least three subsets: Fukuyama muscular dystrophy, muscle-eye-brain disease, and Walker-Warburg syndrome. Yet a third broad category are those patients with lissencephaly due to intrauterine cytomegalovirus infection (151,152). These patients have a combination of pachygyria and polymicrogyria. In addition, multiple other less common categories are being recognized as part of the lissencephaly spectrum.

Patients with lissencephaly are usually microencephalic, although they may be normocephalic. Mild hypertonia and feeding problems in the newborn period are common. Profound mental retardation, generalized hypotonia with superimposed spasticity, feeding problems which often require gastrostomy, and seizures are usually seen following the newborn period.

Imaging studies show a smooth, thickened cortex with shallow, vertically oriented sylvian fissures. In more severe cases, no other sulci are present (Fig. 69). In milder cases, a few shallow sulci are seen to surround broad, flat

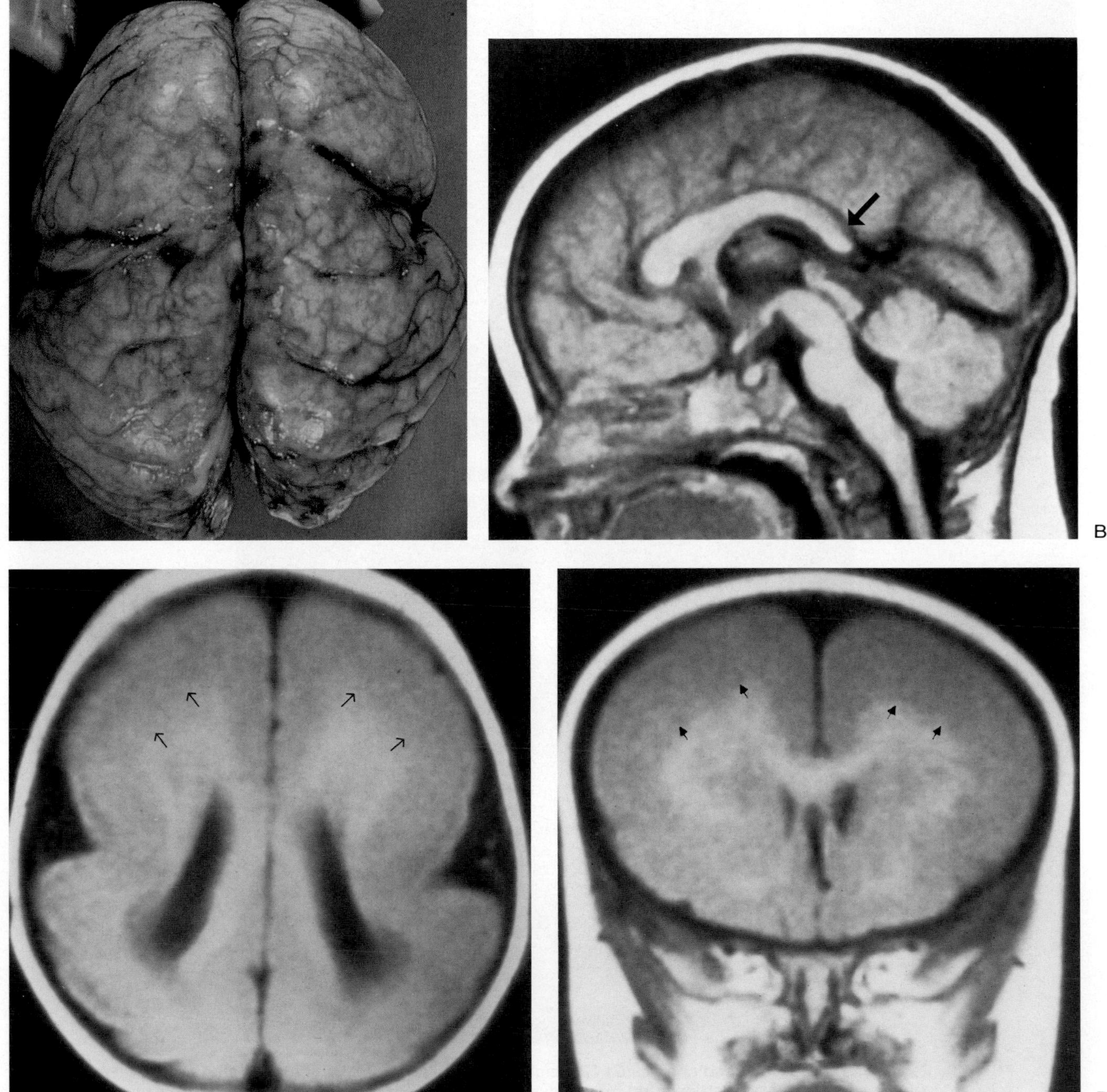

FIG. 69. Lissencephaly. **A:** Necropsy specimen shows smooth surface of hemispheres with very few sulci. **B:** Midline sagittal SE 600/25 image reveals near complete agyria. The corpus callosum is hypogenetic with a hypoplastic splenium (*arrow*) and absence of the rostrum. **C:** Axial SE 600/20 image shows a thick cortex (*arrows*) with thin underlying white matter. The shallow, vertical sylvian fissures give the brain a figure eight appearance. **D:** Coronal SE 600/20 image shows the smooth cortical surface and the thickened cortex. *Arrows* point to the gray-white junction.

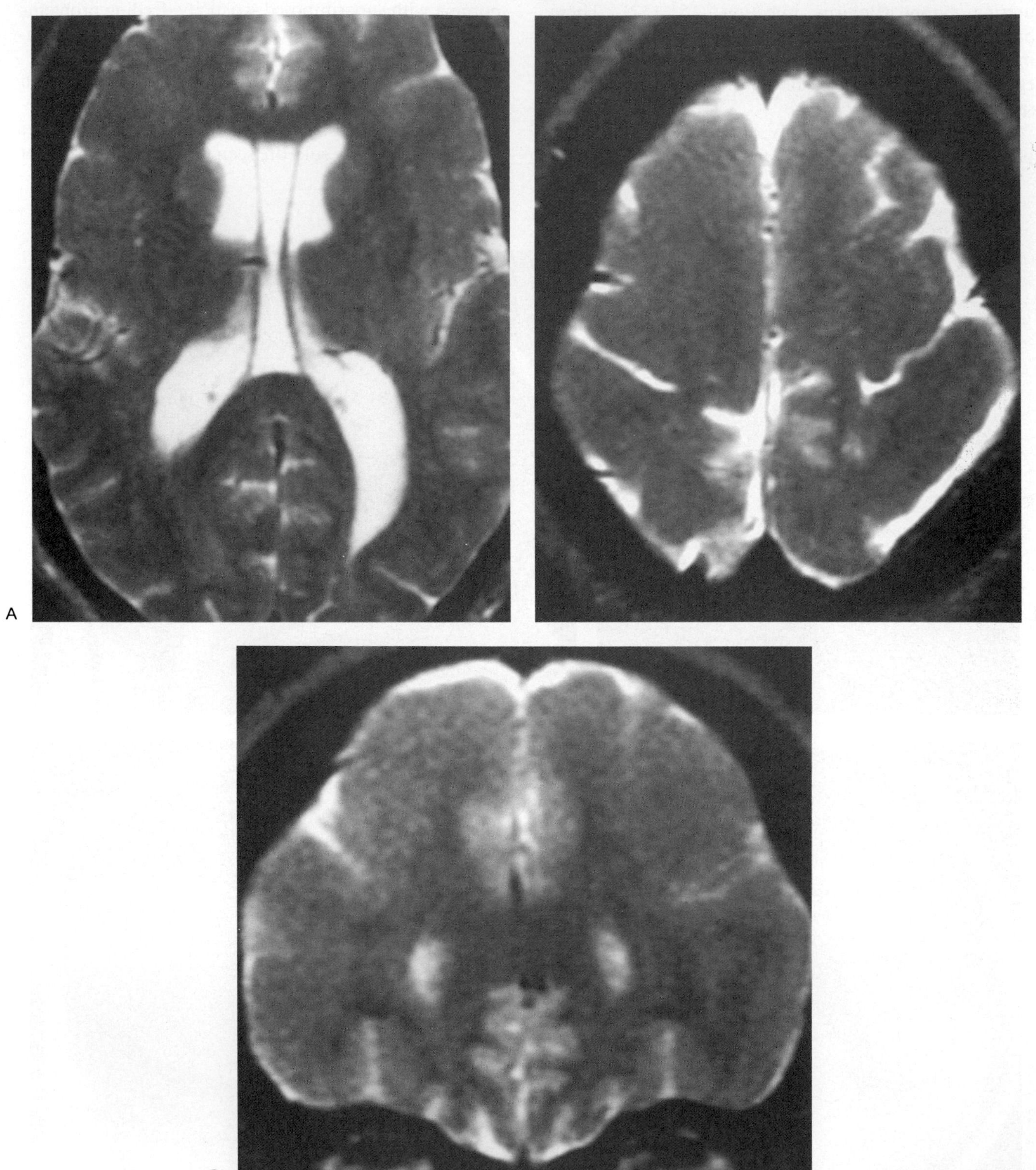

FIG. 70. Pachygyria. Axial (**A,B**) and coronal (**C**) T2-weighted images show broad, flat gyri with underdeveloped sulci. In contradistinction to polymicrogyria or cortical dysplasia, the cortex is truly thickened. (From Truwit and Lempert, ref. 40, with permission.)

gyri (Fig. 70). The cerebrum has been described as a figure eight as the result of the narrowing in the midportion by the sylvian fissures (Fig. 69). Mild callosal hypogenesis is common.

Gray Matter Heterotopia

In actuality, all anomalies of neuronal migration are heterotopia in that the primary abnormality is that normal neurons lie in abnormal locations. Heterotopia is the name given to focal collections of ectopic neurons in the cerebral hemispheres. These patients almost always present with seizure disorders. Their clinical prognosis, however, seems best to correlate with the type and degree of heterotopia. At least three broad types of heterotopia are recognized: subependymal heterotopia, focal heterotopia, and diffuse heterotopia.

MRI is far more sensitive than CT (and is clearly the study of choice) in the detection of heterotopia. On MRI, heterotopia appear as tumor-like lesions within the subependymal region or within the deep white matter. They are isointense with gray matter on all imaging sequences (153,154). Neither perilesional edema nor contrast enhancement are seen. One exception is that a heterotopic nodule might enhance either during the immediate postictal phase simply due to hyperemia or alterations of the blood–brain barrier or during the subacute post-ictal phase if the nodule infarcts consequent to the seizure. At this point, no reports of this phenomenon have been published (40).

Subependymal heterotopia may include only one or two lesions (Fig. 71) or may include nodules along the length of the lateral ventricles (Fig. 72). At least the latter appears to be X-linked in some patients (W. B. Dobyns, *personal communication*). Clinically, patients with subependymal heterotopia generally have normal development and motor skills; they present with seizures during their second or third decade of life (155).

Subependymal heterotopia are nodular lesions that appear to grow from the subependymal region into the ventricular system (Figs. 71 and 72). The differential diagnosis of this lesion is limited and includes tuberous sclerosis and ependymal metastases, especially from medulloblastoma in the pediatric population. In general, the lesions of tuberous sclerosis are iso- to hypointense to white matter, and they may or may not enhance. In addition, other manifestations of tuberous sclerosis are often present. In patients with ependymal metastases, a history of the primary tumor is usually available, and enhancement is the rule, although not without exception. In cases of medulloblastoma metastatic to the ependyma of the lateral and third ventricles, enhancement may be lacking.

Focal heterotopia tend to occur within the deep and subcortical white matter. Both small and large lesions may be seen. Patients with smaller heterotopia tend to present with seizures and often have normal motor function and development, while those with larger lesions often present with seizures, moderate or severe developmental delay, and hemiplegia (155).

On MRI focal heterotopia are readily seen as gray matter mass lesions within the hemispheric white matter. Often, subjacent subependymal heterotopia are seen as well. Ipsilateral ventricular dysmorphology may be seen. The lesions may appear to exert mass effect, although the mass effect most likely reflects a distortion of hemispheric architecture, due to the dysplasia. Uncommonly, intralesional collections of CSF and vasculature may be seen (40,155). In such cases, a careful search should be made for infolding of the adjacent cortex (Fig. 73). Such lesions are probably better classified as cortical dysplasia, rather than focal heterotopia (40,155).

The last category of heterotopia is the diffuse, or band heterotopia (also known as double cortex). Like lissencephaly, the lesion is characterized by an overlying cortex, underlying subcortical white matter, underlying band of gray matter, and an underlying band of deep white matter (Fig. 74). The cortex often appears normal, although it may appear pachygyric. Within the hemispheric white matter, a thick circumferential band of the heterotopic gray matter broadly undulates in concert with the overlying cortex, separated from the cortex by a variable amount of subcortical white matter. In general, the degree of cortical dysplasia and severity of clinical symptoms are related to the thickness of the band heterotopia; i.e., the thicker the band of heterotopic gray matter, the more anomalous (lissencephalic) the overlying cortex and the more severe the retardation (156–159). However, in contrast to findings of hypometabolism in most cortical dysplasia, (^{18}F)-fluorodeoxyglucose PET studies show glucose uptake in band heterotopia that is similar to that of normal cortex (160,161). Nevertheless, the band itself appears to be epileptogenic (162).

The deep neuronal layer of band heterotopia is essentially identical to the layer of heterotopic neurons seen in the X-linked form of classical lissencephaly (157). In both disorders, the heterotopia represent layers of neurons that have been arrested during their migration to the cortex. In reality, band heterotopia and X-linked classical lissencephaly most likely represent two ends of a spectrum. In the lissencephalic brain, few undulations of the heterotopic gray matter are seen, just as few sulci are seen. In band heterotopia, more undulations are seen, as are sulci within the overlying cortical mantle. Moreover, pedigree analyses of female patients with X-linked subcortical band heterotopia and males with X-linked classical lissencephaly have the same X-linked disorder of neuronal migration (W. B. Dobyns, *personal communication*). To date, all but one patient reported with subcortical band heterotopia are female.

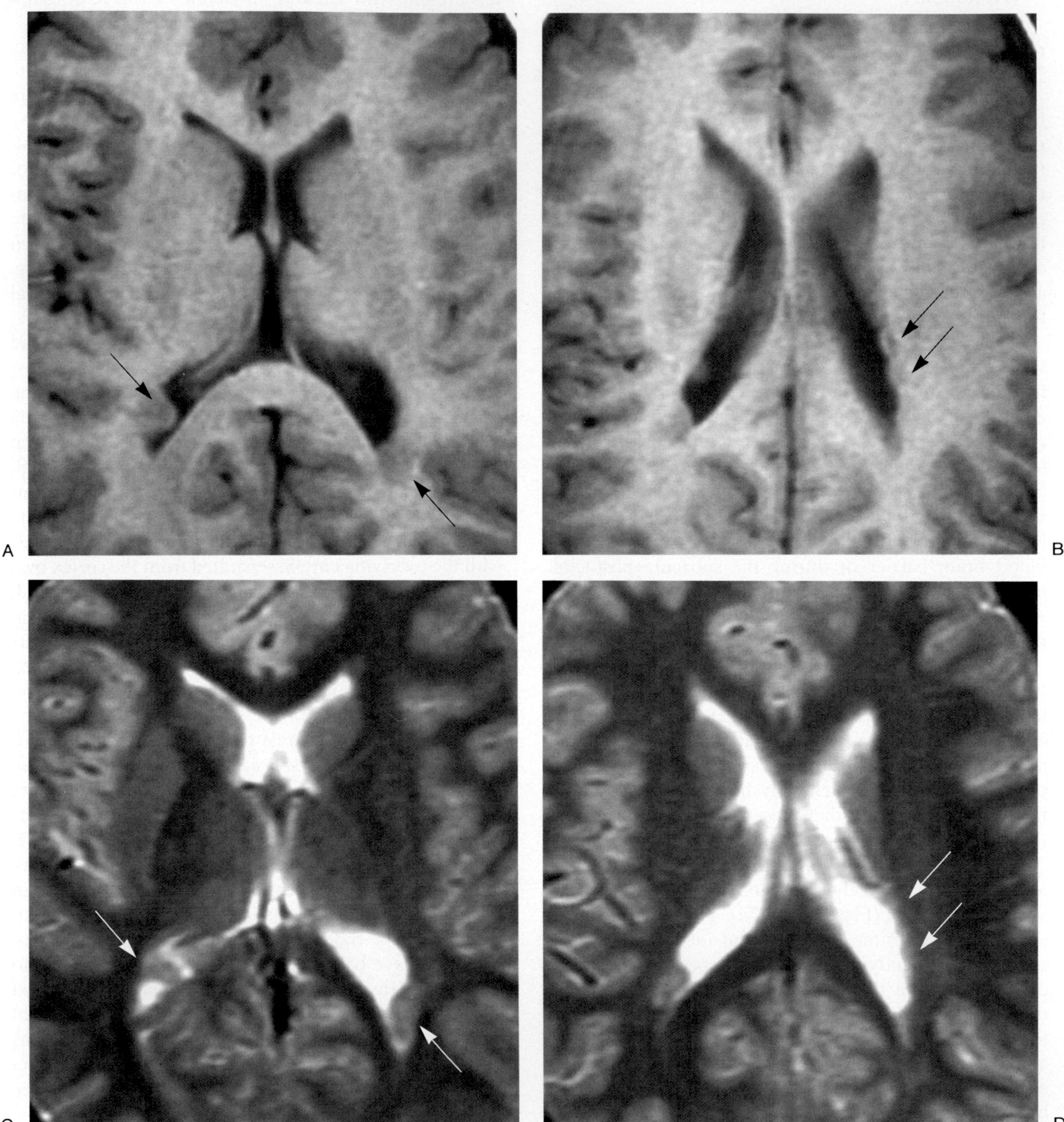

FIG. 71. Subependymal heterotopia. Axial T1- (**A**,**B**) and T2- (**C**,**D**) weighted images show multiple discrete subependymal nodules (*arrows*) whose signal intensities parallel those of gray matter. Mild dysmorphism of left lateral ventricle is seen. (From Truwit and Lempert, ref. 40, with permission.)

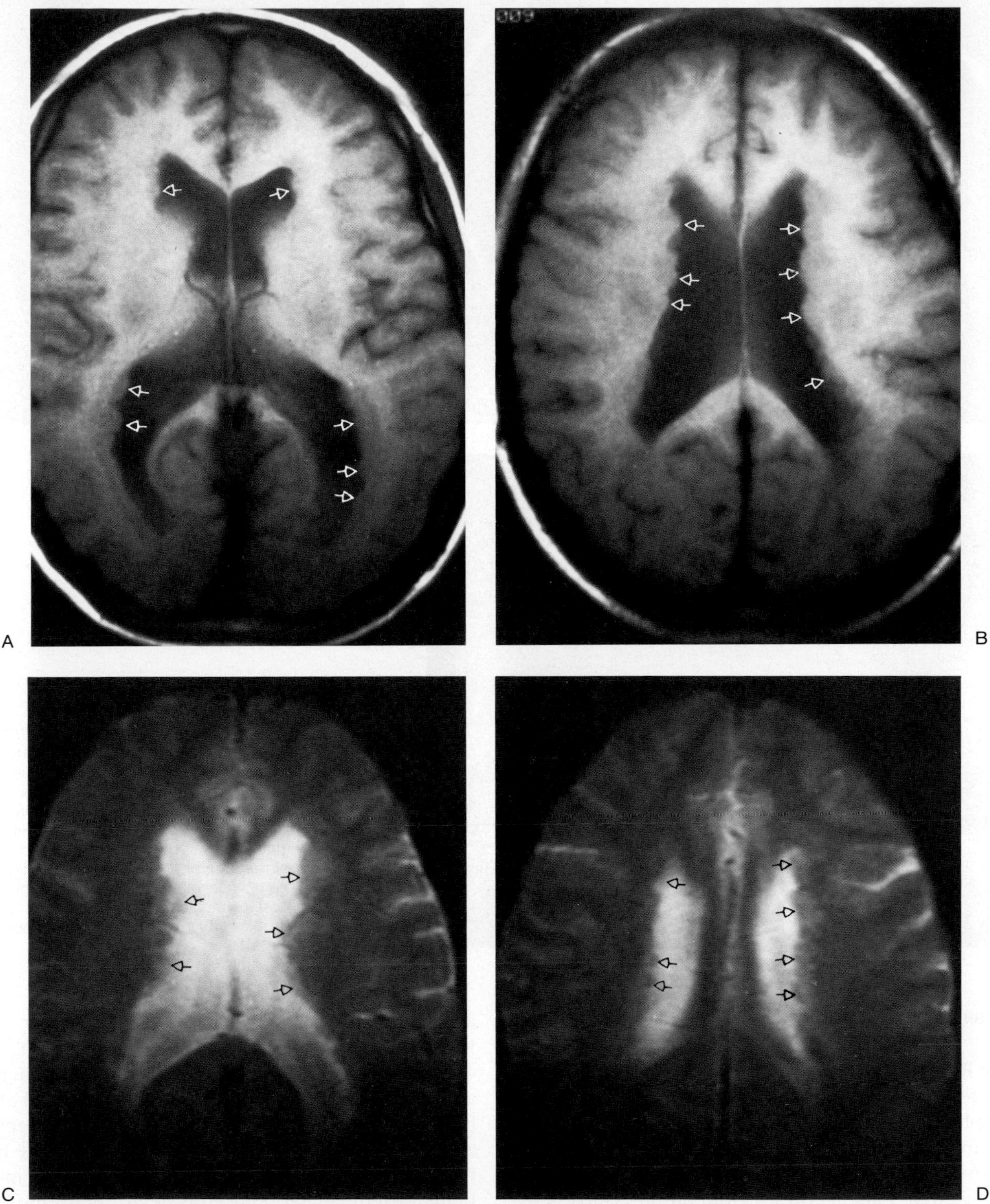

FIG. 72. Subependymal heterotopias. **A:** SE 600/20. **B:** SE 600/20. **C:** SE 2000/70. **D:** SE 2000/70. Axial SE images demonstrate multiple nodular masses lining the lateral ventricles (*open arrows*). The key to identifying these as heterotopias is their isointensity with cortical gray matter. Note that the heterotopias remain isointense with cortical gray matter on all imaging sequences.

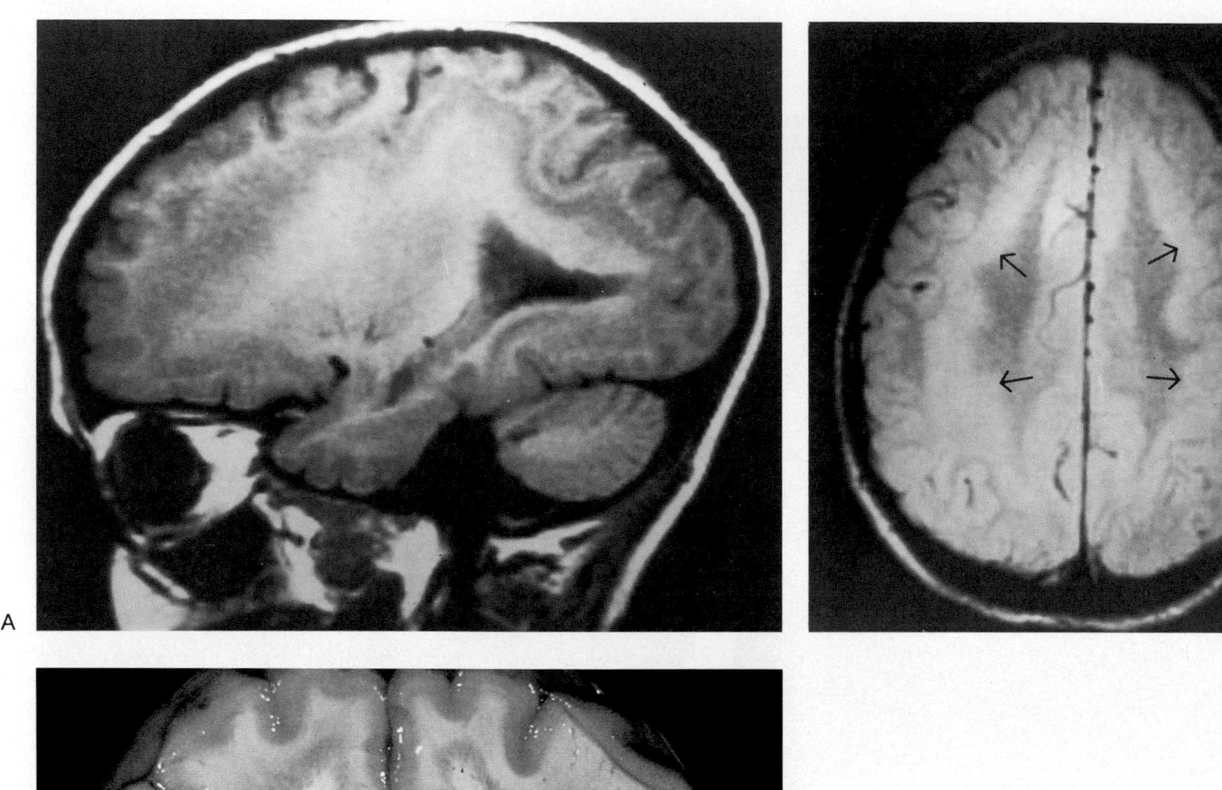

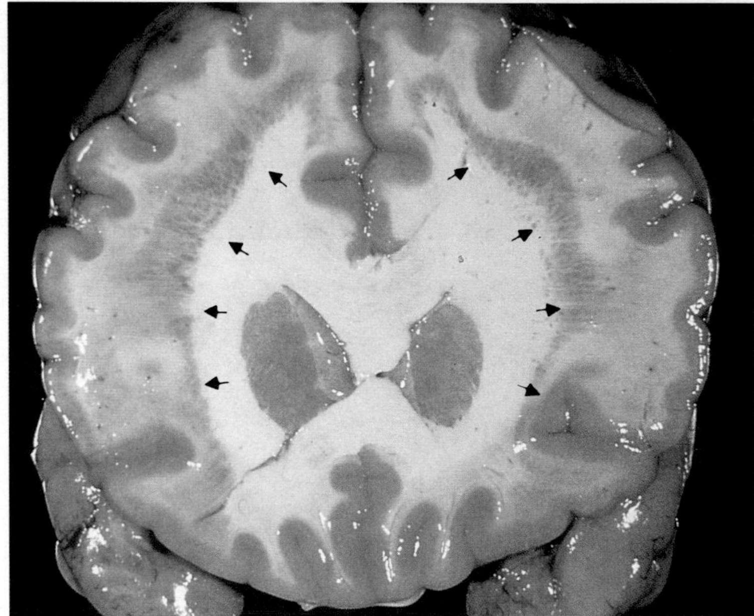

FIG. 73. Band heterotopia. **A:** Sagittal SE 600/20 image reveals a band that is isointense to gray matter running through the centrum semiovale circumferentially. A thin layer of hyperintense white matter separates a relatively normal-appearing cortex from the band. **B:** Axial SE 2800/30 image shows that the band is isointense to gray matter and separated from the cortex by a layer of hypointense white matter that interdigitates normally into the cortical gyri (*arrows* point to the band heterotopia). **C:** Coronal necropsy specimen shows band of heterotropic gray (*arrows*) between subcortical and deep white matter.

Unilateral Megalencephaly

The term unilateral megalencephaly is applied to hamartomatous overgrowth of all or part of the cerebral hemisphere (163–165). Migration anomalies are always seen in the affected portions of the hemisphere (163,164), but can be seen in the "unaffected" hemisphere as well. Patients present with an intractable seizure disorder that usually begins within the first few months of life. They are almost always hemiplegic and severely developmentally delayed (163,164). The patients usually have a large head very early in life but, possibly as a result of the intractable seizures, the head size diminishes relative to the normal curve and eventually the patients may be normocephalic or even microencephalic.

The CNS anomaly may occur in isolation or may be associated with hemihypertrophy of some or all of the body. At least one case of unilateral megalencephaly and Klippel-Weber-Trenaunay syndrome has been reported (166). The disorder may also occur in patients with the linear sebaceous nevus syndrome (167, 168), hypomelanosis of Ito (169) and neurofibromatosis 1 (170).

Imaging studies show moderate to marked enlargement of the affected cerebral hemisphere (163,171). The cortex may appear nearly normal or lissencephalic. In the more severely affected patients, the border between

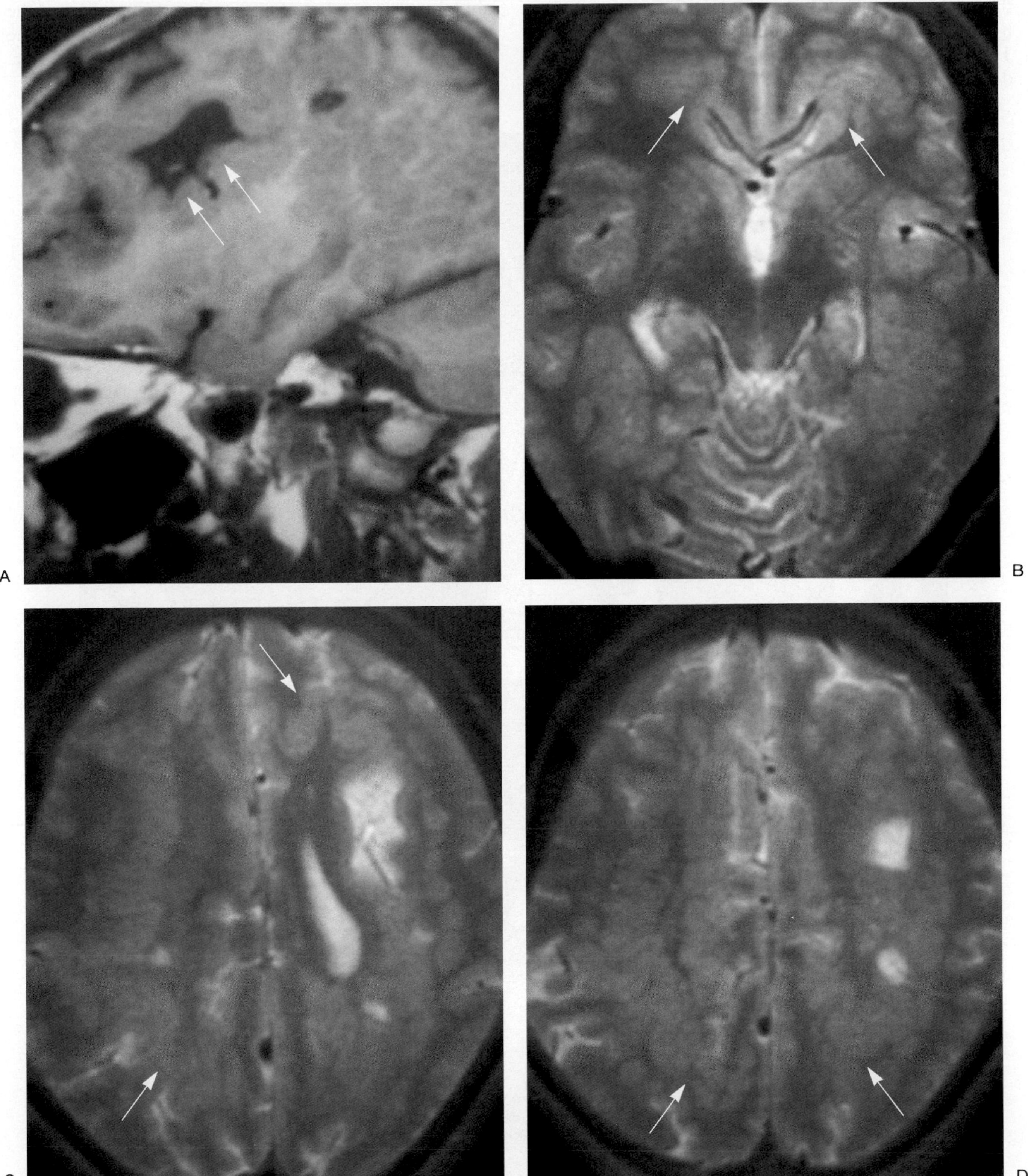

FIG. 74. Infolded cingulate gyri. Sagittal (**A**) T1-weighted image shows diffuse anomaly of neuronal migration. Large lake of CSF-intensity (*arrow*, A) is seen within migration defect. Axial T2-weighted images (**B–D**) show bilaterality of lesions and peculiar communication of heterotopic gray matter with cingulate gyri (*arrows*). CSF-lakes are actually infoldings of subarachnoid space, trapped by the infolded cingulate gyri. Multiple small foci of heterotopic gray matter are also apparent within white matter lateral to infolded cortex.

the cortex and subcortical white matter becomes indistinct (Fig. 75). Rarely, the cortex may calcify. Abnormal T1 and T2 prolongation is seen within the white matter due to heterotopia and astrocytosis. The lateral ventricle and the affected hemisphere are always enlarged, and the frontal horn often has a characteristic shape, appearing straight and pointing anteriorly and superiorly (Fig. 75) (28).

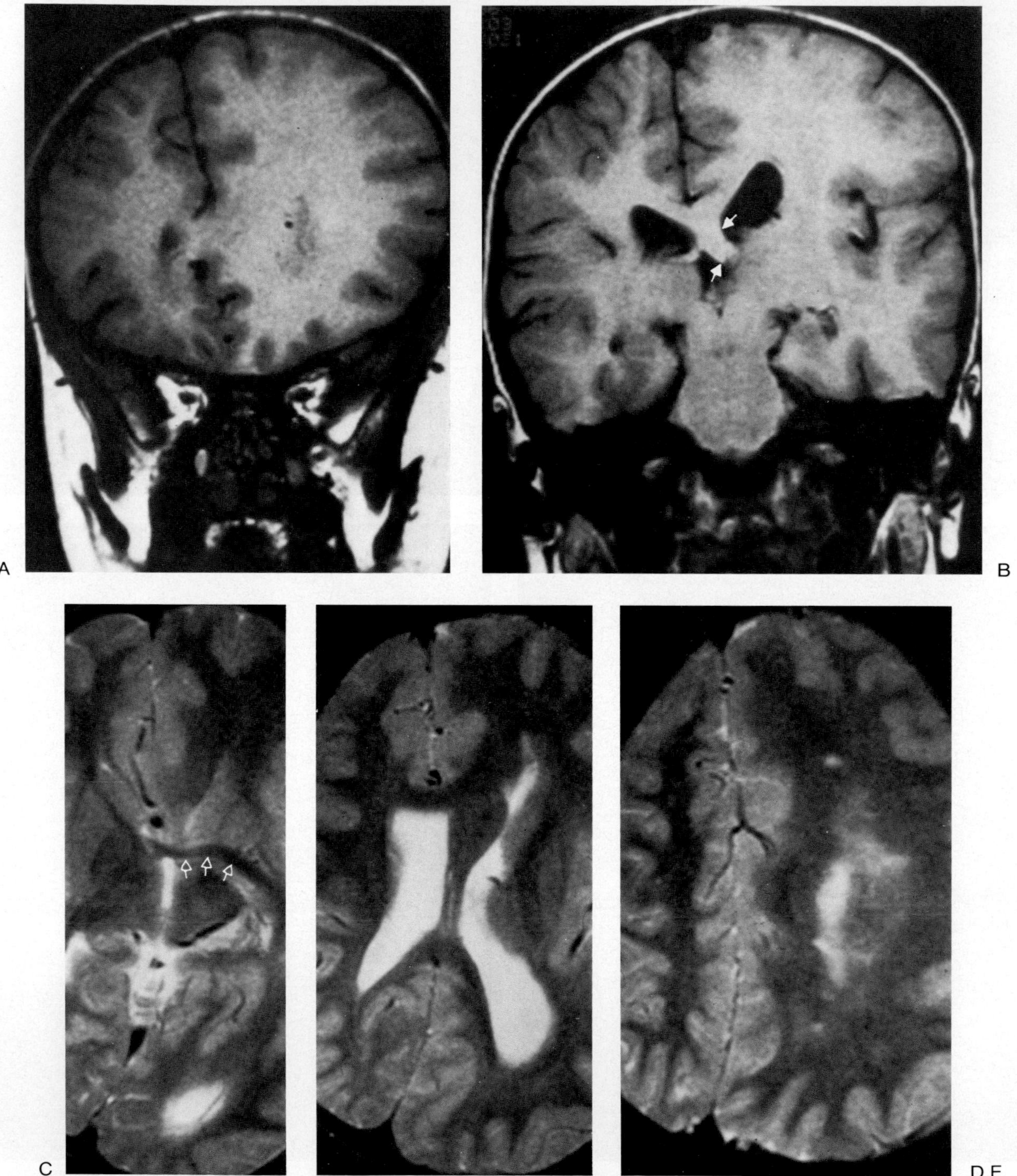

FIG. 75. Unilateral megalencephaly. **A,B:** Coronal SE 600/20 images show an enlarged left cerebral hemisphere, mainly due to marked enlargement of the left hemispheric white matter. Note enlarged left fornix and septum pellucidum (*arrows*). The left frontal cortex shows an appearance suggestive of polymicrogyria. **C–E:** Axial SE 2800/70 images show the enlarged left hemisphere, enlarged left lateral ventricle, and characteristic straightening of the left frontal horn. The left side of the anterior commissure (*open arrows*, C) and left centrum semiovale are markedly enlarged. Also note periventricular high signal intensity in the frontal region (E) resulting from heterotopia and gliosis in the white matter surrounding the enlarged ventricle.

Cortical Dysplasia

The cortical dysplasias are a group of disorders in which developing neurons complete the initial phase of neuronal migration, i.e., to the cortex, but fail to organize themselves in a normal six-layered cortical pattern (140). Cortical dysplasias thus differ from heterotopia; the former are disorders of neuronal organization,

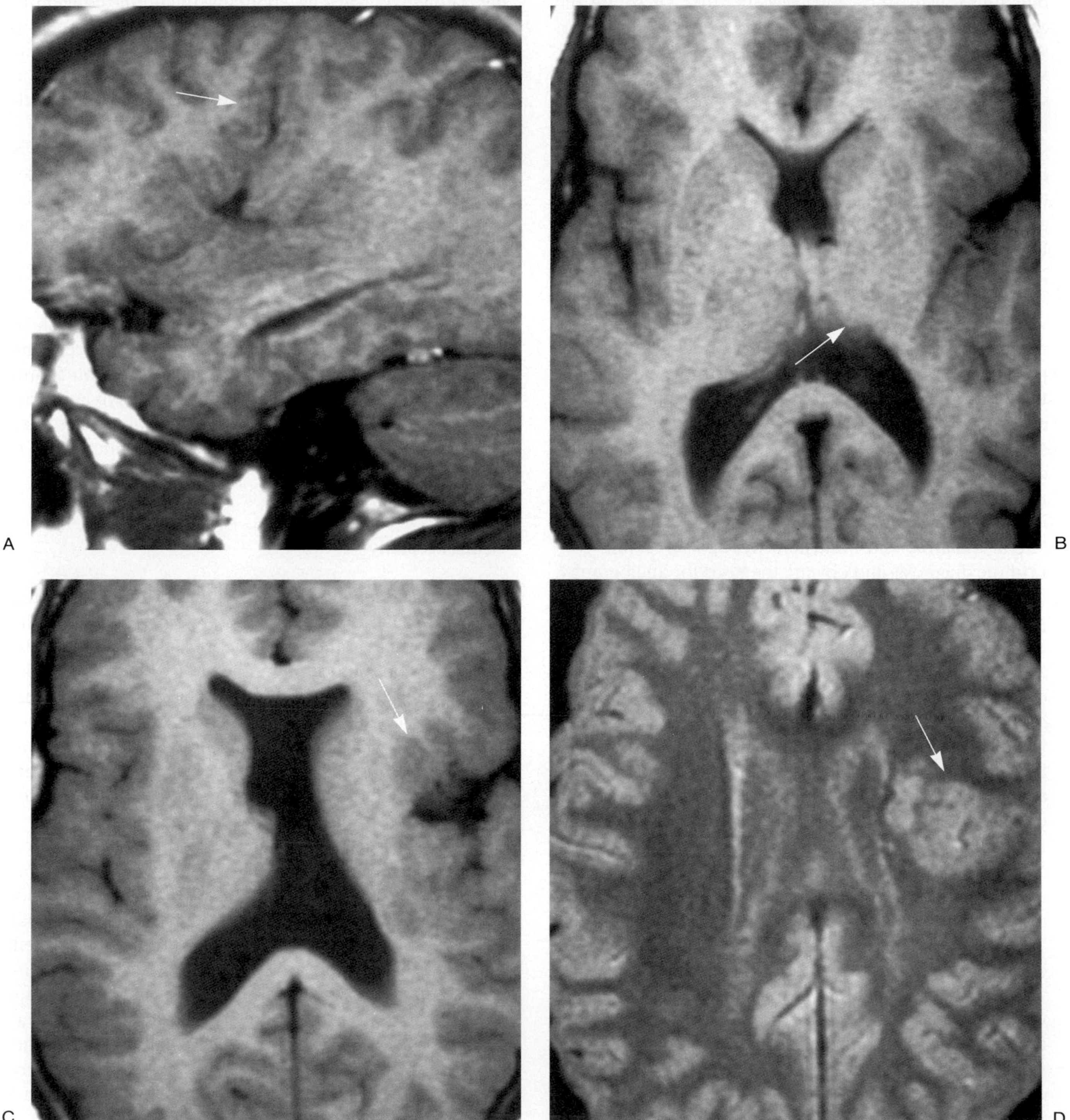

FIG. 76. Polymicrogyric cleft. Sagittal (**A**) T1-weighted image shows abnormal extension (*arrow*, A) of sylvian fissure to convexity. Note cortical dysplasia of perisylvian gray matter. In normal patient, this area is organized into long and short insular gyri. Axial T1- (**B** and **C**) and proton-density- (**D**) weighted images show thalamic hypoplasia (*arrow*, B) and cortical dysplasia (*arrows*, C,D) of infolded gyrus. Ipsilateral hypoplasia of thalamus and cerebral peduncle (not shown) are common in perisylvian cortical dysplasia. Septum pellucidum is also absent. (From Truwit and Lempert, ref. 40, with permission.)

whereas the latter are disorders of neuronal migration. Often there is overlap, with both disorders present in the same patient.

At least three types of cortical dysplasia are seen. In some cases, the dysplastic cortex is seen as a focal inward buckling toward the ventricle (Fig. 76). These are the cases that seem to be akin to a form fruste of schizencephaly and are most likely vascular in origin. Whereas schizencephaly requires a pial-ependymal seam, i.e., communication of the infolded cleft with the ventricle, clefts of polymicrogyria do not. Like schizencephaly, clefts of polymicrogyria most often occur in the posterior sylvian region, although any part of the cerebral hemisphere may be involved (Fig. 77). They are most commonly unilateral, but may be bilateral. Polymicrogyric clefts may be seen in association with a contralateral schizencephalic cleft (Fig. 78).

Nearly pathognomonic are the findings of anomalous venous drainage within the cleft and hypoplasia of the ipsilateral thalamus and cerebral peduncle. Mild hypoplasia of the corpus callosum is common. Absence of the septum pellucidum may be seen when a polymicrogyric cleft is seen in conjunction with a contralateral schizencephalic cleft. The finding of prominent vascular channels has prompted consideration of arteriovenous malformations and angiography (Fig. 66). Careful examination of the brain anomaly, and the association of ipsilateral thalamic and brainstem hypoplasia should confirm the diagnosis and obviate the need for angiography.

A second type of cortical dysplasia diffusely involves a portion of the hemisphere. It is commonly bilateral (Fig. 79), although it may be unilateral. Although it may be associated with a focal cleft of polymicrogyria at one end of the involved area, it is not generally seen with schizencephaly. The disorder is a common brain manifestation of intrauterine cytomegalovirus infection (Fig. 80). The affected cortex appears flat and congruent to the arc of normal cortex. Unlike many cases of focal polymicrogyric cleft, the ipsilateral thalamus and brainstem are not usually hypoplastic. Venous anomalies are not usually seen in this disorder unless an associated cleft is present. In a small number of patients, calcification of the affected cortex may be seen.

On MRI, the disorder may be overt or subtle. In more obvious cases, images of standard thickness will show what appears to be a thick, poorly sulcated band of cortex that simulates pachygyria. In fact, on thinner sections that overcome artifacts of volume averaging, the cortex may be relatively normal in thickness. In more subtle cases, routine 5 mm sections may not be particularly revealing. In such cases, volume acquisition gradient-echo sequences with 1.5 mm thick sections may be more helpful. Often, multiplanar assessment is required in order to detect subtle irregularities of the gray-white junction. The white matter is most commonly of normal signal intensity, although in up to 20% of cases, high intensity on T2-weighted images may be seen. This signal abnormality may represent gliosis, a feature that has not been reported in pachygyria.

The third cortical dysplasia is a newly described disorder known by various eponyms including congenital bilateral perisylvian syndrome (172), developmental Foix-Chavany-Marie syndrome (173), open opercular syndrome (174), bilateral opercular polymicrogyria (175), and bilateral central macrogyria (176), and developmental bilateral perisylvian dysplasia (177).

Clinically, congenital bilateral perisylvian syndrome is characterized by pseudobulbar palsy and moderate to severe dysarthria, both of which are present in all patients. Seizures, delayed milestones, mental retardation, and electroencephalographic abnormalities are seen in greater than 85% of patients (172). On MRI, the opercula are dysplastic and incomplete and the sylvian fissure is wide and underdeveloped. Sagittal images may show posterior extension of the sylvian fissure, exposure of the insula, and apparent thickening of the cortex on 5 mm sections. Like MRI, CT shows bilateral perisylvian cortical dysplasia, often extending to the perirolandic regions (Fig. 81). Pathologically, four-layered polymicrogyria is found (172,177).

Schizencephaly

Schizencephaly describes gray-matter-lined clefts that extend through the entire cerebral hemisphere from the lateral ventricle to the cerebral cortex (178,179). In most cases, the gray matter along the cleft is polymicrogyric; in some instances, it is more dysplastic than polymicrogyric. The clefts can be unilateral or bilateral and can appear anywhere in the brain, although they usually are perisylvian. In unilateral cases, perusal of the contralateral hemisphere is warranted, as subtle clefts of polymicrogyria are common (Fig. 78).

Presenting symptoms relate to the amount of involved brain; seizures and variable pareses are common. Patients with a narrow, unilateral cleft (Fig. 82) usually present with seizures and mild hemiparesis or visual difficulties, depending upon the location of the cleft within the hemisphere. They are otherwise developmentally normal. Patients with progressively larger clefts (Fig. 83) present with progressively larger neurological deficits because progressively more brain is missing. Patients with bilateral clefts (Fig. 84) tend to be severely retarded with early epilepsy, severe motor deficit, and blindness (28,180).

Schizencephalic clefts may be "closed," in which only a double layer of cortex (with a variable subarachnoid space and draining vein) is seen extending from the surface to the ventricle. Alternatively, they may be "open,"

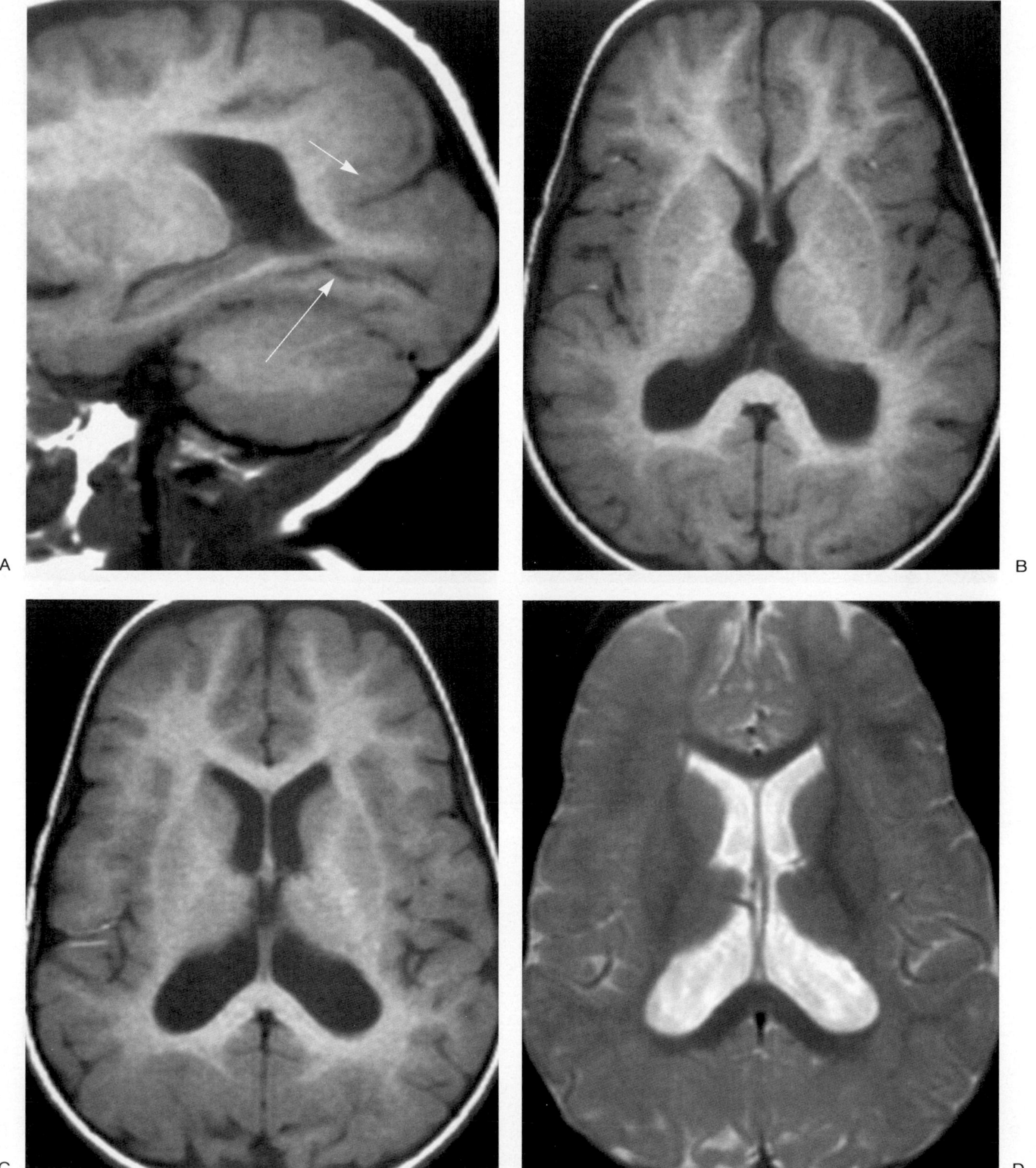

FIG. 77. Bioccipital clefts of PMG. Sagittal (**A**) T1-weighted image shows prominent cleft (*short arrow*, A) of polymicrogyria in occipitoparietal region. Axial T1- (**B,C**) and T2- (**D**) weighted images show absence of occipital horns of lateral ventricles (collateral sulcus, *long arrow;* A) and absence of subcortical white matter. Note normal fingers of peripheral white matter in frontal lobes. (From Truwit and Lempert, ref. 40, with permission.)

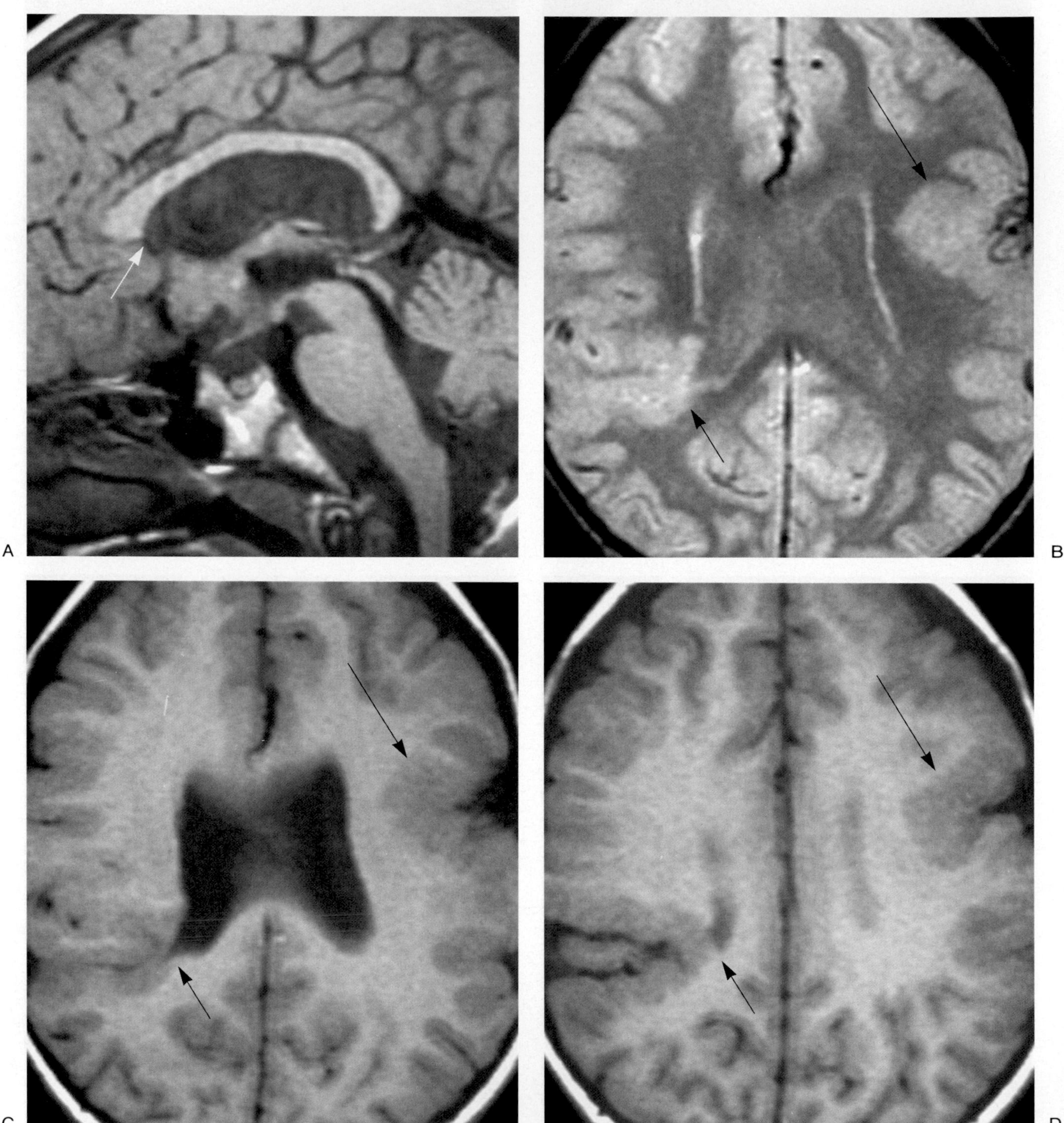

FIG. 78. Polymicrogyric cleft contralateral to schizencephalic cleft. Sagittal T1-weighted image (**A**) shows mild callosal hypoplasia. Although genu and body appear normal, splenium is mildly hypoplastic and rostrum is absent (*arrow*, A). Axial proton-density- (**B**) and T1- (**C** and **D**) weighted images show right-sided closed-lip schizencephaly with frank communication between gray matter and ventricle (*short arrow*, B–D). Careful examination of images reveals subtle cleft of polymicrogyria (*long arrow*, B–D). Septum pellucidum is also absent, and chiasm is small, consistent with septo-optic dysplasia. (From Truwit and Lempert, ref. 40, with permission.)

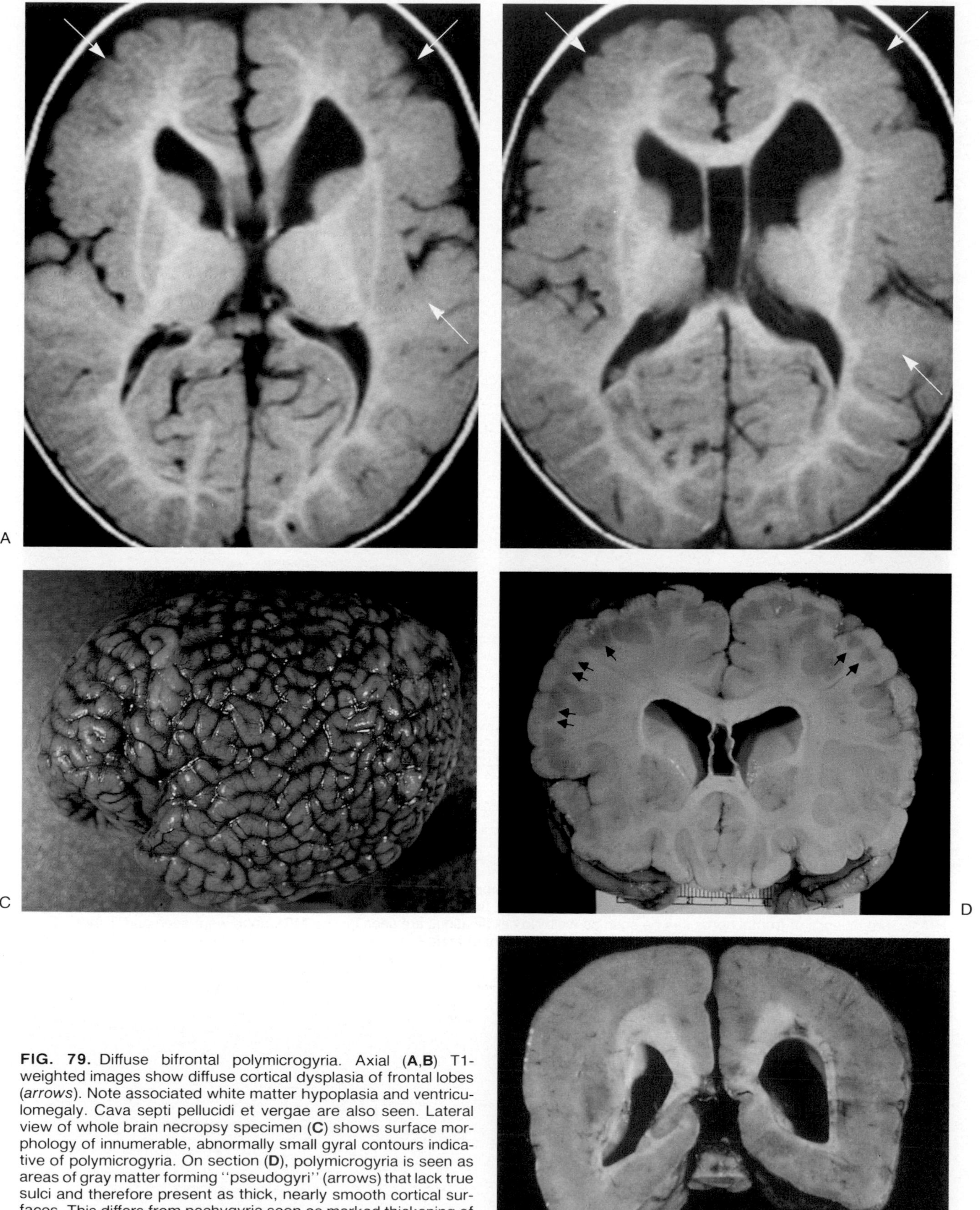

FIG. 79. Diffuse bifrontal polymicrogyria. Axial (**A**,**B**) T1-weighted images show diffuse cortical dysplasia of frontal lobes (*arrows*). Note associated white matter hypoplasia and ventriculomegaly. Cava septi pellucidi et vergae are also seen. Lateral view of whole brain necropsy specimen (**C**) shows surface morphology of innumerable, abnormally small gyral contours indicative of polymicrogyria. On section (**D**), polymicrogyria is seen as areas of gray matter forming "pseudogyri" (arrows) that lack true sulci and therefore present as thick, nearly smooth cortical surfaces. This differs from pachygyria seen as marked thickening of cortical gray matter and near absent sulcal formation on different necropsy specimen (**E**).

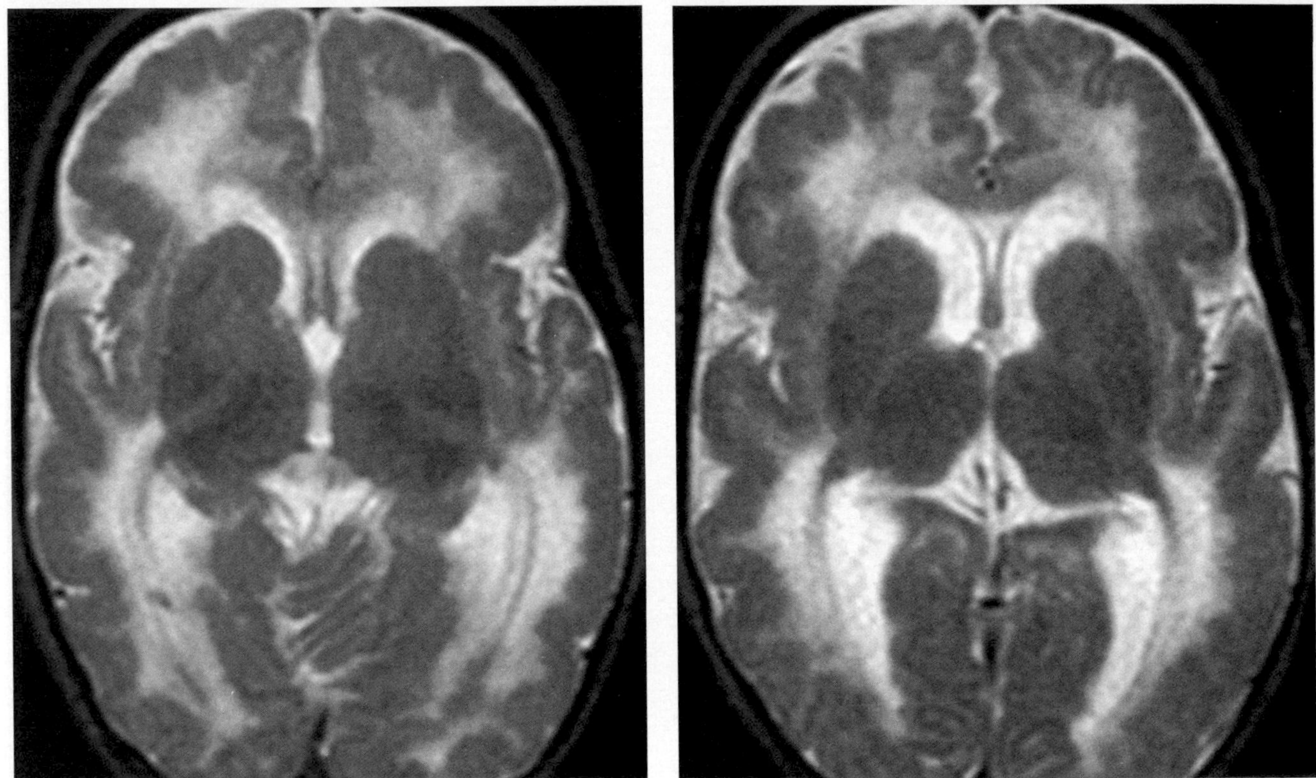

FIG. 80. Polymicrogyria secondary to intrauterine cytomegalovirus. Axial (**A**,**B**) T2-weighted images show diffuse cortical dysplasia of frontal and parietal lobes. Posterior temporal and occipital lobes appear relatively spared. Mild prominence of frontal horns can be seen as well. No calcifications are seen on the MRI; none were seen on CT (not shown). White matter is abnormally hyperintense throughout brain.

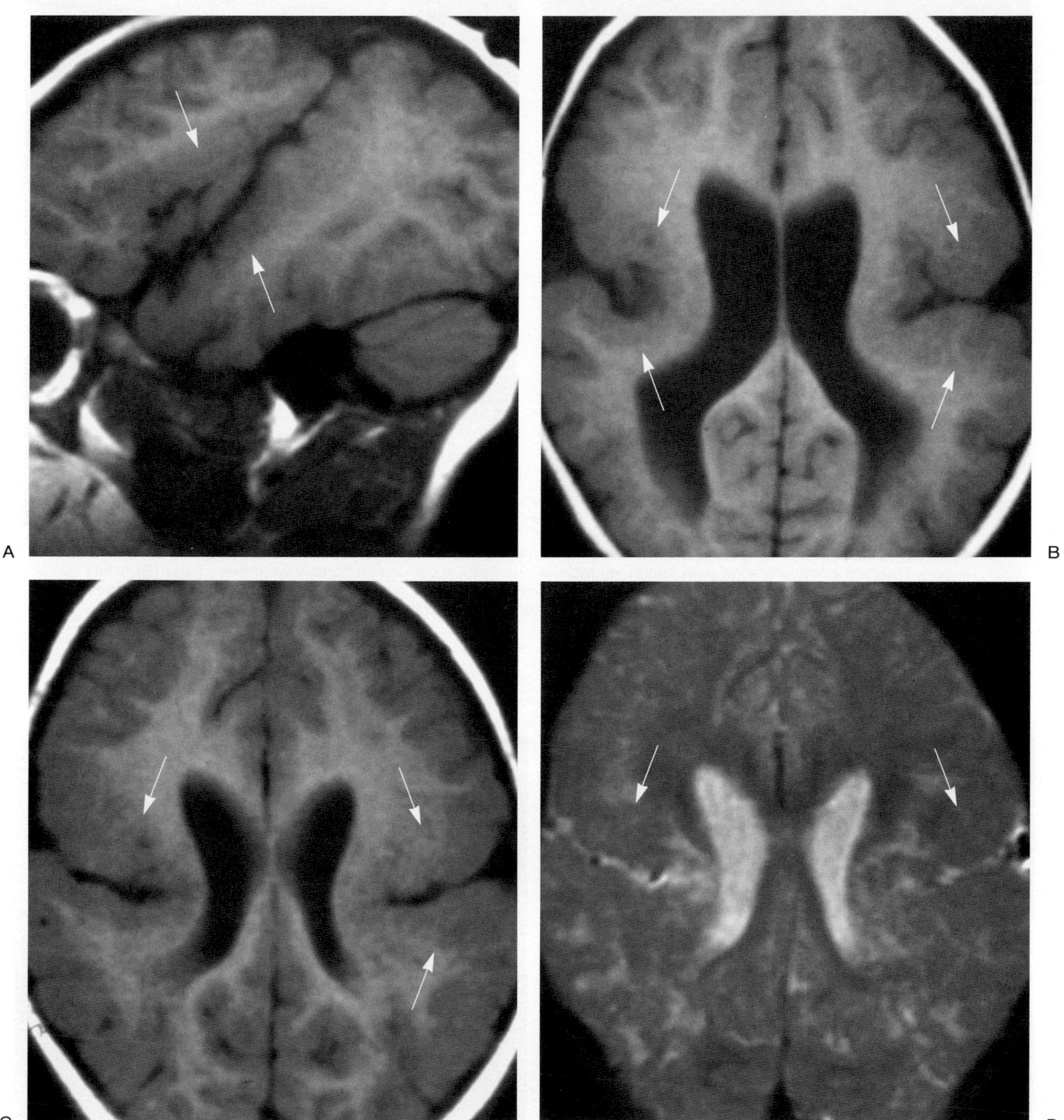

FIG. 81. Bilateral perisylvian syndrome. Sagittal (**A**) and axial (**B**,**C**) T1- and T2- (**D**) weighted images show bilateral anomalies of neuronal migration (*arrows*) overlying underdeveloped sylvian fissures. Note dorsal, perirolandic extension of sylvian fissures, typical of anomalies of neuronal migration. Bodies of lateral ventricles (C and D) show inverted appearance, typical of this disorder. (From Truwit and Lempert, ref. 40, with permission.)

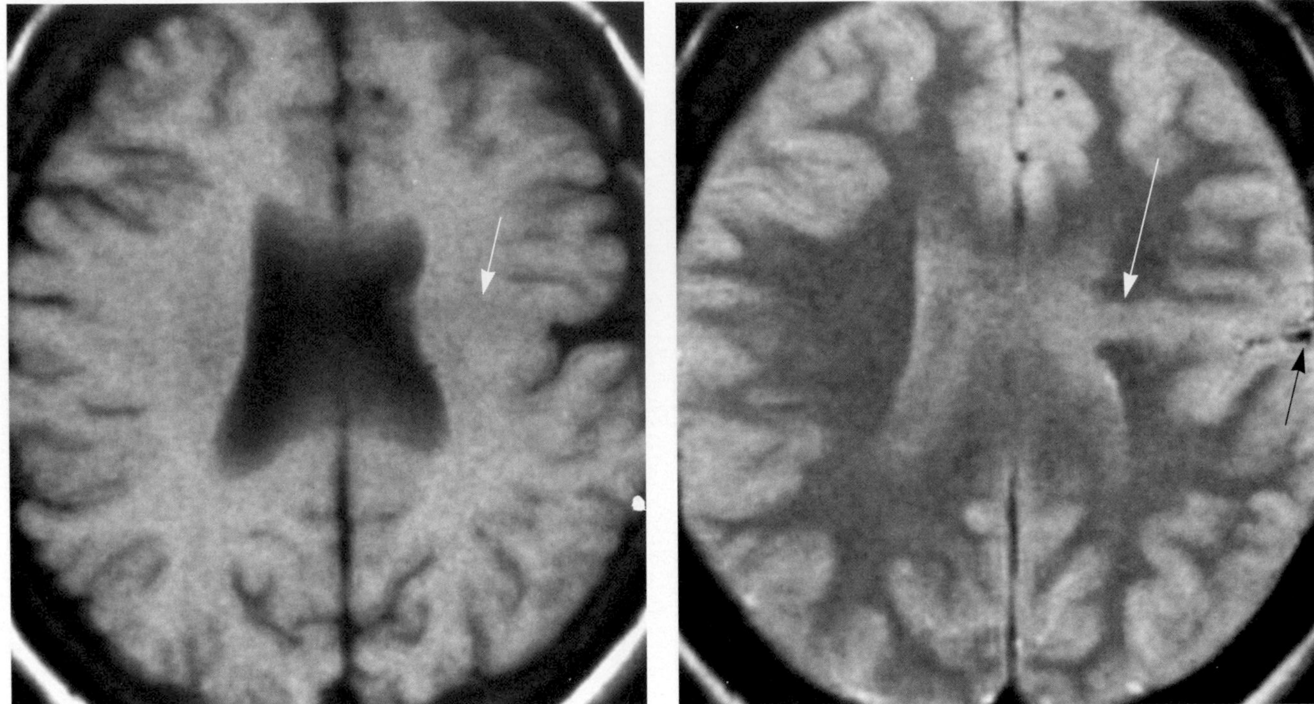

FIG. 82. Unilateral shizencephaly. Axial T1-weighted image (**A**) shows abnormal cleft along left posterior frontal region. Discrete communication with lateral ventricle is not seen. Axial proton-density-weighted image (**B**) nicely shows closed-lip schizencephaly (*long arrow*, B). Note prominent venous flow void (*short arrow*, B) within enlarged subarachnoid space over the cleft. (From Truwit and Lempert, ref. 40, with permission.)

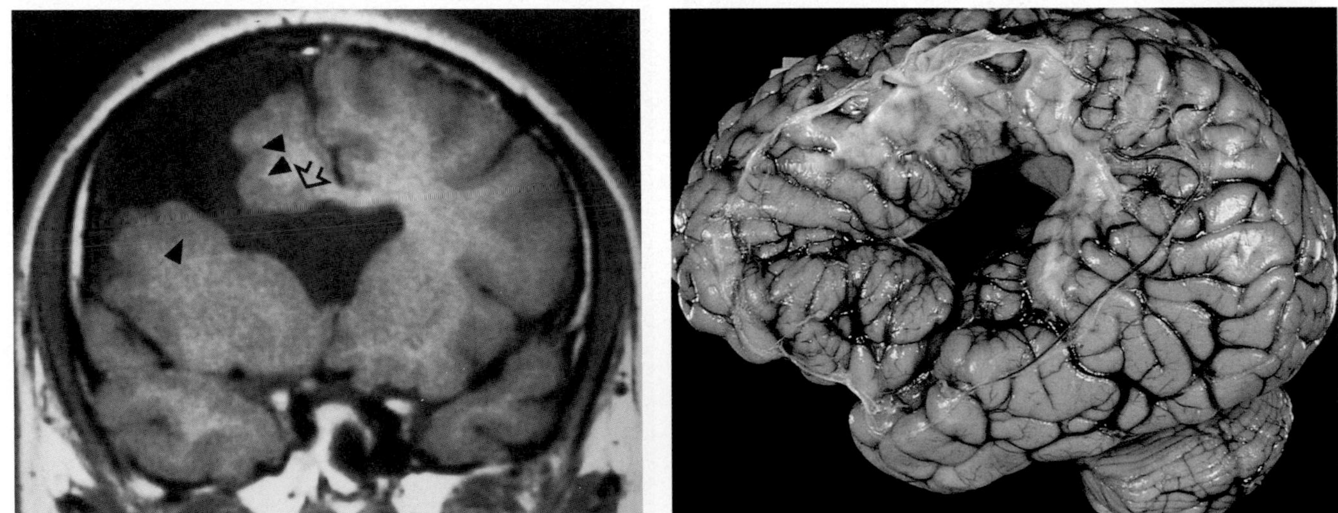

FIG. 83. A: Unilateral schizencephaly with separated lips. Coronal SE 600/20 MR image shows a large cleft in the right frontal region that extends from the inner table of the skull to the frontal horn of the lateral ventricle. The septum pellucidum is absent. Continuity of the gray matter through the cleft is clearly shown (*arrowheads*). A focus of heterotopic gray matter sits in the roof of the right lateral ventricle (*open arrow*). **B:** Lateral view of necropsy brain specimen from patient with lifelong history of seizures shows transcerebral schizencephalic cleft communicating with lateral ventricle and dysmorphic frontal gyri.

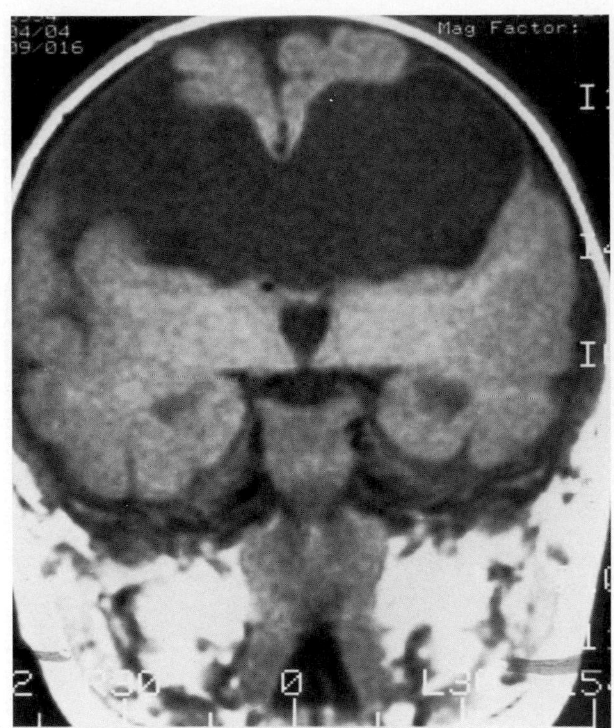

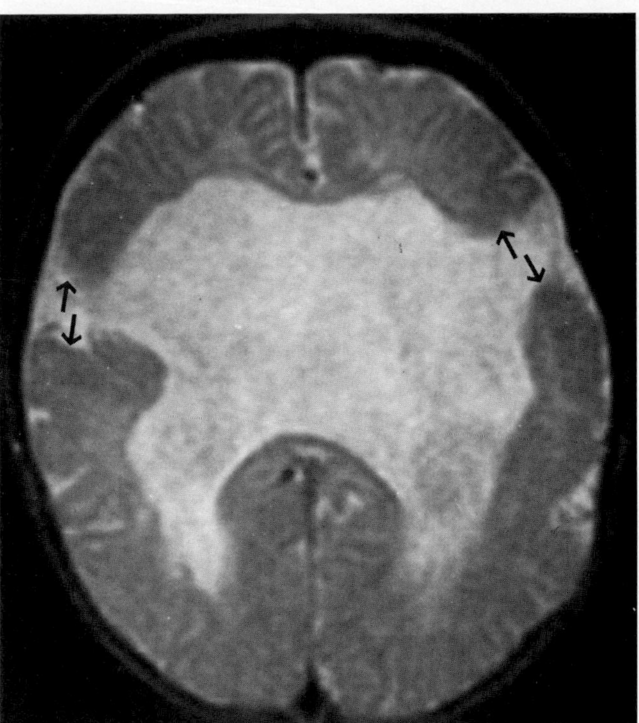

FIG. 84. Bilateral open lip schizencephaly. **A:** Coronal SE 600/20 image shows bilateral open lip schizencephalies in the posterior frontal regions. **B:** Axial SE 2800/70 image shows gray matter lining the clefts bilaterally (*arrows*). This child was severely retarded, as are all patients with bilateral open lip schizencephalies.

in which there is wide communication between the subarachnoid space and ventricle through a broad hemispheric cleft.

Imaging studies reveal transhemispheric clefts that are lined by gray matter (Figs. 78,82–85) (28,180). The cortex adjacent to the clefts almost always has an abnormal gyral pattern that can be demonstrated pathologically as polymicrogyria in most cases (26,178,179). Heterotopic gray matter lines the ventricle adjacent to the cleft in more than half of the affected patients (Fig. 83). A key feature is the presence of a ventricular dimple; this is almost always seen in cases with closed or minimally open lips. Mild hypoplasia of the corpus callosum is commonly seen. The septum pellucidum is absent or nearly completely absent in 70% to 90% of affected patients. Of those with absence of the septum pellucidum, 30% to 50% will have optic nerve hypoplasia on clinical examination. Therefore, septo-optic dysplasia is, by definition, present in 20% to 45% of patients with schizencephaly (56,57,180). The optic nerves should always be scrutinized in these patients, especially when visual symptoms are present, although optic atrophy is usually easily recognizable clinically.

In addition to the brain anomalies, in patients with open-lip schizencephaly, CSF pulsations from the lateral ventricles result in pressure effects on the inner table. In severe cases, plagiocephaly may be seen; occasionally ventriculoperitoneal shunting may be indicated for cosmetic purposes.

Kallmann Syndrome

The first association of olfactory and genital abnormalities was noted in postmortem studies by Maestre de San Juan in 1856. Weidenreich again reported the association in 1914 (181). It was not until Kallmann et al., in 1944, described eleven patients in three families with the association that a syndrome was recognized (182).

Kallmann syndrome is an inherited disorder characterized by hypogonadotropic hypogonadism and anosmia or hyposmia (181,183,184). Transmission of Kallmann syndrome can occur according to autosomal dominant, autosomal recessive, or X-linked patterns (185). In the X-linked disease, the primary disturbance has recently been linked to a failure of genetic expression of cell markers (proteins) that guide migrating neurons (186). Kallmann syndrome, therefore, is an anomaly of neuronal migration, although clearly different in its etiology and expression than the architectural and heterotopic disorders described above.

In recent years, advanced immunohistochemical studies (185,187–189) have revealed much about olfactory embryology and development. The olfactory placode in

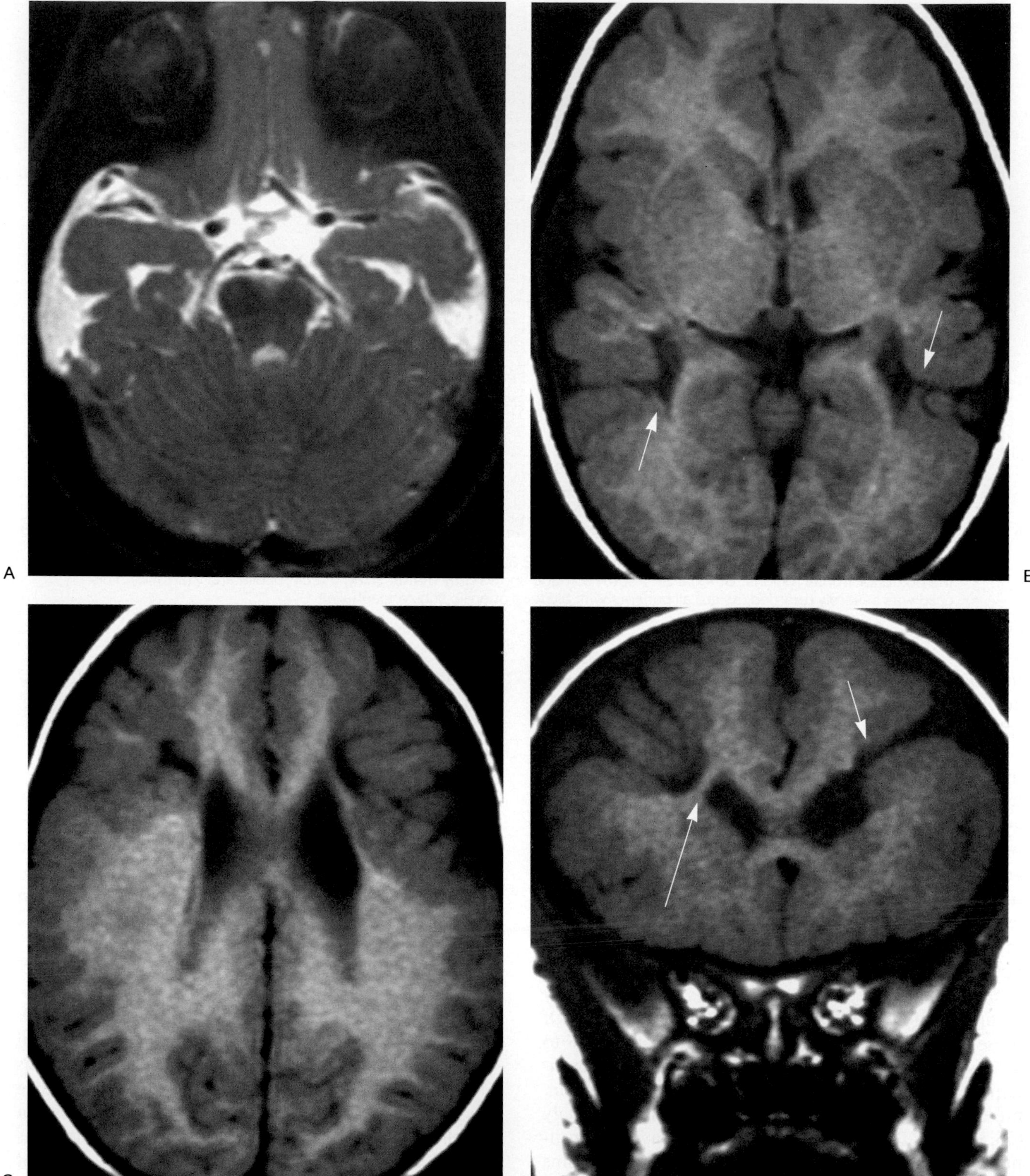

FIG. 85. Bilateral double clefts of schizencephaly and polymicrogyria. **A:** Axial T2-weighted image shows malformed temporal lobes. No white matter is seen, and cortex is dysplastic. Axial T1-weighted images (**B,C**) show bilateral closed lip schizencephalic clefts (*arrows*, B) that communicate with the posterior temporal horns. More cephalad (C), bifrontal anomalies of neuronal migration are seen. Coronal (**D**) T1-weighted image shows left side to be yet another schizencephalic cleft (*short arrow*, D). On right, however, pial-ependymal seam is not present, as small band of white matter (*long arrow*, D) can be seen separating dysplastic cortex from ventricle. (From Truwit and Lempert, ref. 40, with permission.)

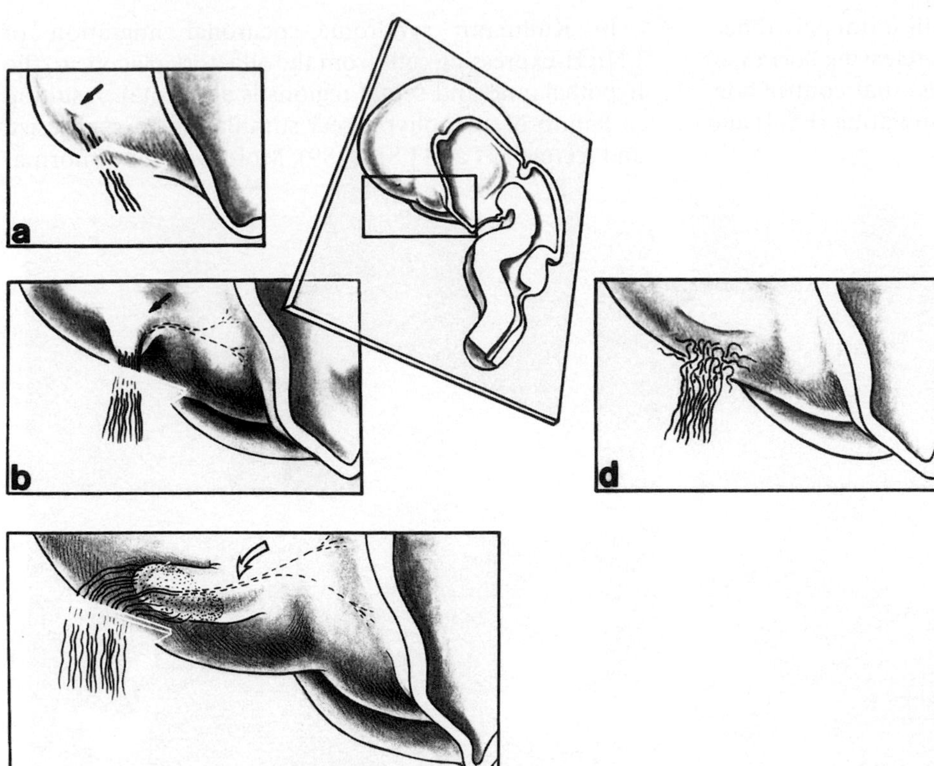

FIG. 86. Normal olfactory embryology (**A–C**) and aberrant neuronal migration (**D**) in Kallmann syndrome. Perspective (*center, unlabelled*) is from below, anterior and left looking up, posteriorly, and to the right. Early in development (A), note course of olfactory fila. With further telencephalic growth, orientation becomes more vertical (B) and, finally, posterior (C). Note terminalis nerve medial and posterior along bundle of olfactory fila and extending along primitive forebrain toward future septal and hypothalamic regions (*curved, open arrow,* C). The vomeronasal nerve is not shown. The dysplastic tangle of olfactory bulb development (*arrows,* A,B) versus failed induction of olfactory bulb (D). (Reprinted from Truwit et al., ref. 198, with permission.)

the most cephalad nasal fossa gives rise to fibers and cells which migrate anteriorly and superiorly toward the overlying telencephalic vesicles (187,190–193). From this migration, the olfactory fila will be defined. Medially, fila of the future terminalis and vomeronasal nerves accompany this olfactory fila towards the overlying brain. Once communication between the fila and the brain is established, the olfactory bulb is induced (Fig. 86). At the end of the embryonic period, the cribriform plate starts to develop and encourages the olfactory fila to aggregate into more discrete bundles, thus forming the true olfactory nerves medially, and the terminalis and vomeronasal nerves laterally.

In the normal fetus, it is along the embryologic scaffolding of the terminalis and possibly the vomeronasal nerves that cells will migrate from the nasal placode

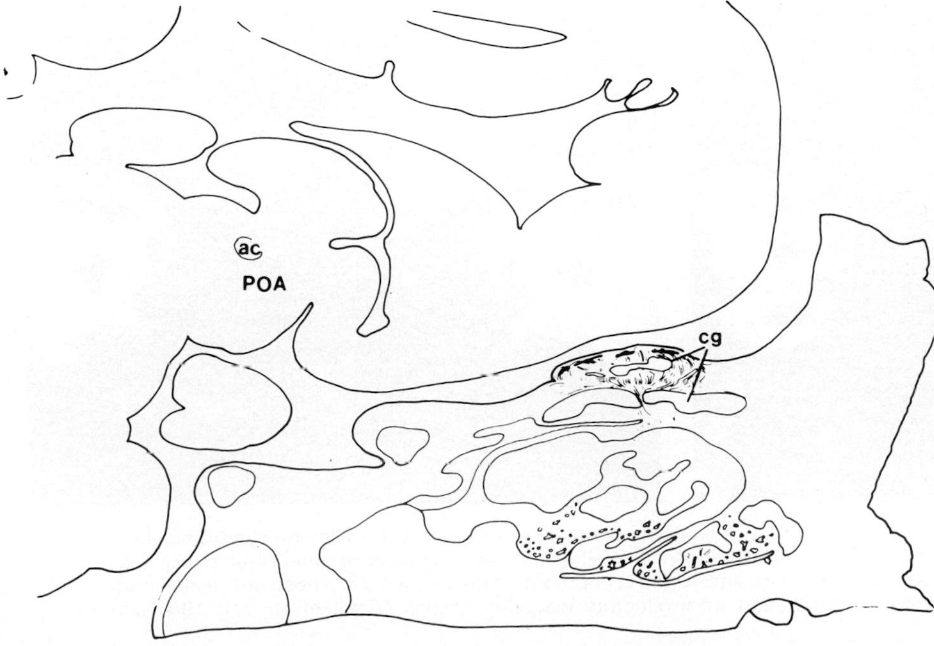

FIG. 87. Microprojection drawing of a sagittal 8-μm paraffin section through the brain and nasal cavity of a 19-week old fetus with Kallmann syndrome, showing the distribution of LHRH-expressing neurons and fibers (*thick lines* represent an LHRH fiber bundle). On the right side of the cribriform plate, lateral to midline, the tangle formed by the central processes of the olfactory nerves encompasses a part of the cartilage of the crista galli (*cg*). A few LHRH-containing nerve fibers are seen on the medial surface of this structure. LHRH-expressing cells were seen on other sections through the cribriform plate and nasal cavity (not shown), but not LHRH immunoreactivity was seen in either the median eminence of the hypothalamus or in the organum vasculosum of the lamina terminalis. *AC*, Anterior commissure; *POA*, preoptic area. (From Schwanzel-Fukuda et al., ref. 185, with permission.)

to the hypothalamus. These cells will ultimately differentiate into the luteinizing hormone-releasing hormone-releasing cells (LHRH-releasing cells) that control adenohypophyseal release of follicle stimulating (FSH) and luteinizing (LH) hormones.

In Kallmann syndrome, neuronal migration of LHRH-expressing cells from the olfactory placode to the hypothalamic and septal regions is abnormal, resulting in failure of adenohyphyseal stimulation to synthesize and secrete LH and FSH (189). Moreover, the abnormal

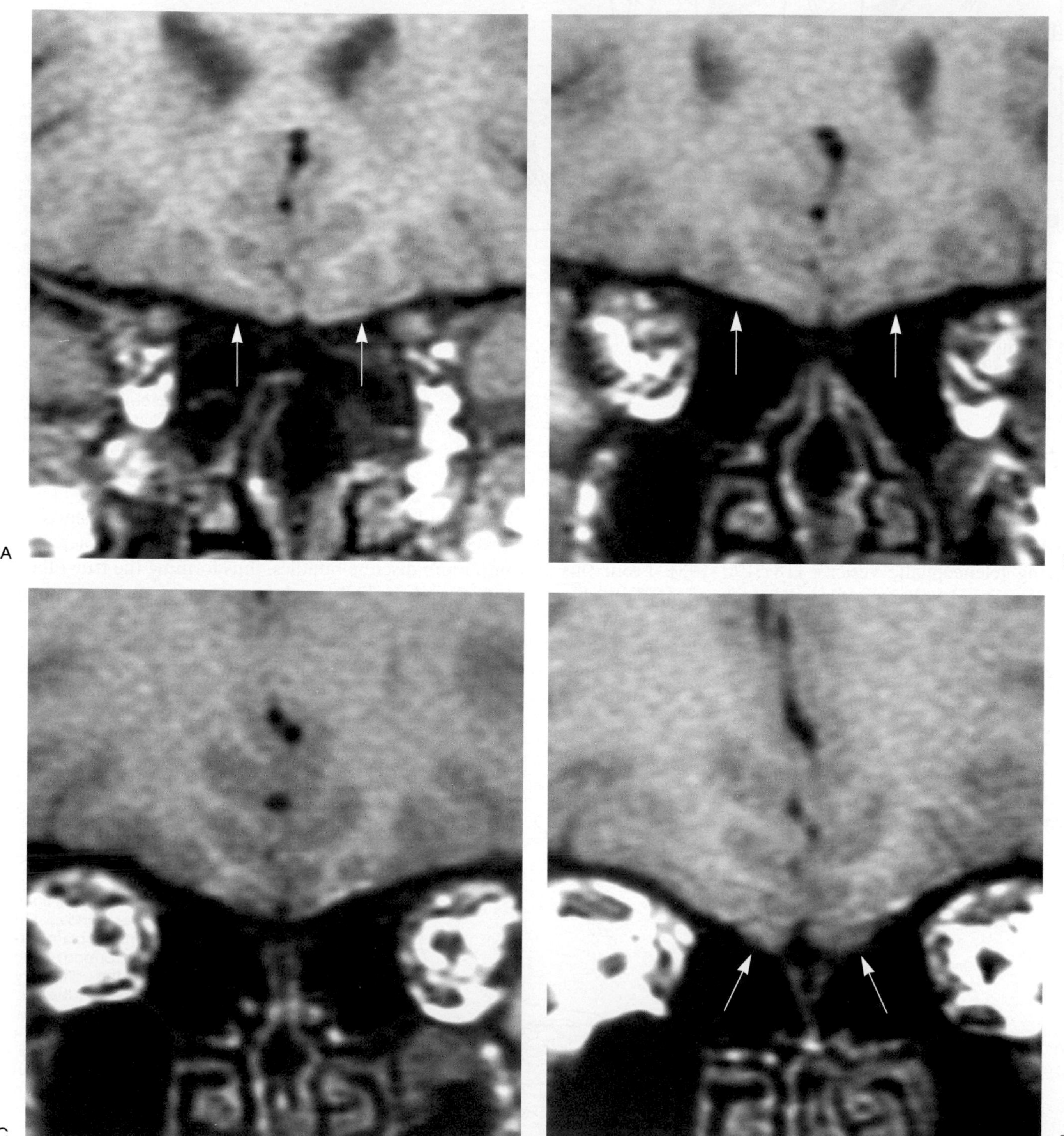

FIG. 88. Coronal T1-weighted images (600/12) from posterior to anterior in patient with Kallmann syndrome show hypoplasia of posterior olfactory sulci (*arrows*, **A,B**), absence of olfactory tracts, aplasia of anterior olfactory sulci (**C,D**), and prominent soft tissue beneath forebrain, embedded in cribriform plate (*arrows*, D). These soft-tissue nodules may represent disordered neuronal migration from olfactory placodes. (From Truwit et al., ref. 198, with permission.)

development of the olfactory placode also results in improper development of the olfactory bulbs, gyri, and sulci (Fig. 87). Clinically, these changes are manifest as hypogonadotropic hypogonadism with anosmia or hyposmia.

With the advent of MRI, Kallmann syndrome can now be detected by imaging. Initial reports showed hypoplasia of the olfactory sulci on routine axial T2-weighted images (194,195). Three subsequent reports have shown high resolution coronal T1-weighted images of the olfactory regions (196–198). In addition to the abnormalities of the olfactory bulbs, tracts, and sulci, in at least two patients of one report (198), abnormal soft tissue was present in the region between the upper nasal vault and the forebrain (Fig. 88). The authors speculated that the abnormal tissue represents the dysplastic "tangle" of disordered neuronal migration noted histopathologically by Schwanzel-Fukuda (189).

Today, high resolution, coronal, fast spin-echo T2-weighted sequences are the preferred method of morphological evaluation of the olfactory system. In patients with Kallmann syndrome, the olfactory bulbs are most likely to be absent; the tracts may be hypoplastic. The olfactory sulci may be variably present in their posterior extent; anteriorly they will be absent.

REFERENCES

1. Fleming AD, Vintzileos AM, Scorza WE. Prenatal diagnosis of occipital encephalocele with transvaginal sonography. *J Ultrasound Med* 1991;10:285.
2. Goldstein RB, LaPidus AS, Filly RA. Fetal cephaloceles: diagnosis with US. *Radiology* 1991;180:803.
3. Diebler C, Dulac O. Cephaloceles: clinical and neuroradiological appearance. *Neuroradiology* 1983;25:199–216.
4. Naidich TP, Altman NR, Braffman BH, McLone DG, Zimmerman RA. Cephaloceles and related malformations. *AJNR* 1992;13:655–690.
5. Rice JF, Eggers DM. Basal transphenoidal encephalocele: MR findings. *AJNR* 1989;10:S79.
6. Boulanger T, Mathurin P, Dooms G, Lambert M, Smellie S, Cornelis G. Sphenopharyngeal meningoencephalocele: unusual clinical and radiologic features. *AJNR* 1989;10:S80.
7. Soyer P, Dobbelaere P, Benoit S. Case report: transalar sphenoidal encephalocele. Uncommon clinical and radiological findings. *Clin Radiol* 1991;43:65.
8. Elster AD, Branch CL Jr. Transalar sphenoidal encephaloceles: clinical and radiologic findings. *Radiology* 1989;170:245–247.
9. Friede RL. Uncommon syndromes of cerebellar vermis aplasia. II: Tecto-cerebellar dysraphia with occipital encephalocele. *Dev Med Child Neurol* 1978;20:764–772.
10. Cohen MM, Lemire RJ. Syndromes with cephaloceles. *Teratology* 1982;25:161–172.
11. Karch SB, Urich H. Occipital encephalocele: a morphological study. *J Neurol Sci* 1972;15:89–112.
12. Oi S, Saito M, Tamaki N, Matsumoto S. Ventricular volume reduction technique—a new surgical concept for the intracranial transposition of encephalocele. *Neurosurgery* 1994;34:443–448.
13. Emery JL, MacKenzie N. Medullo-cervical dislocation deformity (Chiari II deformity) related to neurospinal dysraphism (myelomeningocele). *Brain* 1973;96:155–162.
14. Yakota A, Matsukado Y, Fuwa I, Moroki K, Naahiro S. Anterior basal encephalocele of the neonatal and infantile period. *Neurosurgery* 1986;19:468–478.
15. Chiari H. Über Veränderungen des Kleinhirns infolge von Hydrocephalie des Grosshirns. *Dtsch Med Wochenschr* 1891;17:1172–1175.
16. Chiari H. Über Veränderungen des Kleinhirns, des Pons unde der Medulla Oblongata infolge von congenitaler Hydrocephalie des Grosshirns. *Denkschriften der Kais Akad Wiss math-naturw* 1896;63:71–116.
17. Naidich TP. Cranial CT signs of the Chiari II malformation. *J Neuroradiol* 1981;8:207–227.
18. Naidich TP, McLone DG, Fulling KH. The Chiari II malformation: Part IV. The hindbrain deformity. *Neuroradiology* 1983;25:179–197.
19. Naidich TP, Pudlowski RM, Naidich JB. Computed tomographic signs of the Chiari II malformation: Part III. Ventricles and cisterns. *Radiology* 1980;134:657–663.
20. Naidich TP, Pudlowski RM, Naidich JB, Gornish M, Rodriguez FJ. Computed tomographic signs of the Chiari II malformation: Part I. Skull and dural partitions. *Radiology* 1980;134:64–71.
21. Naidich TP, Pudlowski RM, Naidich JB. Computed tomographic signs of the Chiari II malformation: Part II. Midbrain and cerebellum. *Radiology* 1980;134:391–398.
22. Barkovich AJ, Wippold FJ, Sherman JL, Citrin CM. Significance of cerebellar tonsillar ectopia on MR. *AJNR* 1986;7:795–799.
23. Payner TD, Pringer E, Berger TS, Crone KR. Acquired Chiari malformations: incidence, diagnosis, and management. *Neurosurgery* 1994;34:429–434.
24. McClone DG, Knepper PA. The cause of Chiari II malformation: a unified theory. *Pediatr Neurosci* 1989;15:1–12.
25. Marin-Padilla M, Marin-Padilla TM. Morphogenesis of experimentally induced Arnold-Chiari malformation. *J Neurol Sci* 1981;50:29–55.
26. Friede RL. *Developmental Neuropathology*, 2nd ed. Berlin: Springer-Verlag; 1989.
27. Blaauw G. Defect in posterior arch of atlas in myelomeningocele. *Dev Med Child Neurol* 1971;13:147–163.
28. Barkovich AJ. *Pediatric Neuroimaging*. New York: Raven Press; 1990.
29. Barkovich AJ, Norman D. Anomalies of the corpus callosum: correlation with further anomalies of the brain. *AJNR* 1988;9:493–501.
30. Wolpert SM, Anderson M, Scott RM, Kwan ES, Runge VM. The Chiari II malformation: MR imaging evaluation. *AJNR* 1987;8:783–791.
31. Castillo M, Quencer RM, Dominguez R. Chiari III malformation: imaging features. *AJNR* 1992;13:107–113.
32. Netsky MG. Epidermoid tumors: review of the literature. *Surg Neurol* 1988;29:477–483.
33. Horowitz BL, Chari MV, James R, Bryan RN. MR of intracranial epidermoid tumors: correlation of in vivo imaging with in vitro ^{13}C spectroscopy. *AJNR* 1990;11:299–302.
34. Yasargil MG, Abernathey CD, Sarioglu AC. Microneurosurgical treatment of intracranial dermoid and epidermoid tumors. *Neurosurgery* 1989;24:561–567.
35. Yamakawa K, Shitara N, Genka S, Manaka S, Takakura K. Clinical course and surgical prognosis of 33 cases of intracranial epidermoid tumors. *Neurosurgery* 1989;24:568–573.
36. Braun IF, Naidich TP, Leeds NE, Koslow M, Zimmerman HM, Chase NE. Dense intracranial epidermoid tumors. *Radiology* 1977;122:717–719.
37. Wilms G, Casselman J, Demaerel P, Plets C, De Haene I, Baert AL. CT and MRI of ruptured intracranial dermoids. *Neuroradiology* 1991;33:149–151.
38. Smith AS, Benson JE, Blaser SI, Mizushima A, Tarr RW, Bellon EM. Diagnosis of ruptured intracranial dermoid cyst: value of MR over CT. *AJNR* 1991;12:175–180.
39. Li FC, Kelly WM, Newton D, Tsuruda J, De Marco K, Kucharczyk W. Short T1/T2 epidermoids: lipid or water signal. *American Society of Neuroradiology* 1990:63.
40. Truwit CL, Lempert TE. *Pediatric Neuroimaging: A Casebook Approach*. Denver: DPS Press; 1991:264–270.
41. DeMyer W. Holoprosencephaly. In: Vinker PI, Bruyn JW, eds. *Handbook of Clinical Neurology*. Amsterdam: North Holland; 1977:431–478.
42. Cohen MM, Jirasek JE, Guzman RT, Gorlin RJ, Peterson MQ.

Holoprosencephaly and facial dysmorphia: nosology, etiology, and pathogenesis. *Birth Defects* 1971;7:125–135.
43. Fitz CR. Holoprosencephaly and related entities. *Neuroradiology* 1983;25:225–238.
44. Probst FP. *The Prosencephalies*. Berlin: Springer-Verlag; 1979.
45. Yakovlev PI. Pathoarchitectonic studies of cerebral malformation. III. Arhinencephalies (holotelencephalies). *J Neuropathol Exp Neurol* 1959;18:22–55.
46. Barkovich AJ. Apparent atypical callosal dysgenesis: analysis of MR findings in six cases and their relationship to holoprosencephaly. *AJNR* 1990;11:333–340.
47. Barkovich AJ, Quint DJ. Middle interhemispheric fusion: an unusual variant of holoprosencephaly. *AJNR* 1993;14:431–440.
48. Oba H, Barkovich AJ. Why does the callosal splenium form alone?—an analysis of holoprosencephaly. *Proceedings of the American Society of Neuroradiology*, Nashville, TN. 1994.
49. deMorsier G. Etude sur les Dysraphies crânio-encéphaliques: III. Agénésie du septum lucidum avec malformation du tractus optique. La dysplasie septo-optique. *Schweiz Arch Neurol Psychiatr* 1956;77:267–292.
50. Hoyt WF, Kaplan SL, Grumbach MM, Glaser TS. Septo-optic dysplasia and pituitary dwarfism [Letter]. *Lancet* 1970;1:893–894.
51. Morishima A, Aranoff GS. Syndrome of septo-optic pituitary dysplasia: the clinical spectrum. *Brain Dev* 1986;8:233–239.
52. Izenberg N, Rosenblum M, Parks JS. The endocrine spectrum of septo-optic dysplasia. *Clin Pediatr* 1984;23:632–636.
53. Stanhope R, Preece MA, Brook CGD. Hypoplastic optic nerves and pituitary dysfunction: a spectrum of anatomical and endocrine abnormalities. *Arch Dis Chil* 1984;59:111–114.
54. Roessmann U, Velasco ME, Small EJ, Hori A. Neuropathology of "septo-optic dysplasia" (de Morsier syndrome) with immunohistochemical studies of the hypothalamus and pituitary gland. *J Neuropath Exp Neurol* 1987;46:597–608.
55. Kam KSL, Wang C, Ma JTC, Leung SP, Yeung RTT. Hypothalamic defects in two adults patients with septo-optic dysplasia. *Acta Endocrinologica* 1986;112:305–309.
56. Chuang SH, Fitz CR, Chilton SJ, Harwood-Nash DC, Donoghue V. Schizencephaly: spectrum of CT findings in association with septo-optic dysplasia. *Abstracts of the proceedings of the annual meeting of the Radiological Society of North America*, Washington, D.C.; 1984. *Radiology* 1984;153(P):118.
57. Barkovich AJ, Fram EK, Norman D. MR of septo-optic dysplasia. *Radiology* 1989;171:189–192.
58. Rakic P, Yakovlev PI. Development of the corpus callosum and cavum septi in man. *J Comp Neurol* 1968;132:45–72.
59. Kendall BE. Dysgenesis of the corpus callosum. *Neuroradiology* 1983;25:239–257.
60. Ettlinger G. Agenesis of the corpus callosum. In: Vinker PI, Bruyn GW, eds. *Handbook of Clinical Neurology*. Amsterdam: North Holland; 1977:285–297.
61. Atlas SW, Zimmerman RA, Bilaniuk LT, et al. Corpus callosum and limbic system: neuroanatomic MR evaluation of developmental anomalies. *Radiology* 1986;160:355–362.
62. Barkovich AJ, Kjos BO, Jackson JDE, Norman D. Normal maturation of the neonatal and infant brain: MR imaging at 1.5 T. *Radiology* 1988;166:173–180.
63. Truwit CL, Barkovich AJ. Pathogenesis of intracranial lipoma: an MR study in 42 patients. *AJNR* 1990;11:665–674.
64. Verga P. Lipoma ed osteolipomi della pia madre. *Tumori* 1929;15:321–357.
65. O'Rahilly R, Müller F. The meninges in human development. *J Neuropathol Exp Neurol* 1986;45:588–608.
66. Weed LH. The development of the cerebrospinal spaces in the pig and in man. *Contrib Embryol Carnegie Institute* 1917;5:1–116.
67. Osaka K, Handa H, Matsumoto S, Yasuda M. Development of the cerebrospinal fluid pathway in the normal and abnormal human embryos. *Child's Brain* 1980;6:26–38.
68. Dean B, Drayer BP, Beresini DC, Bird CR. MR imaging of pericallosal lipoma. *AJNR* 1988;9:929–931.
69. Zettner A, Netsky MG. Lipoma of the corpus callosum. *J Neuropathol Exp Neurol* 1960;19:305–319.
70. Naidich TP, McLone DG, Bauer BS, Kernahan DA, Zaparackas ZG. Midline craniofacial dysraphism: midline cleft upper lip, basal encephalocele, callosal agenesis, and optic nerve dysplasia. *Concepts Pediatr Neurosurg* 1983;4:186–207.
71. Naidich TP, Osborn RE, Bauer B, Naidich MJ. Median cleft face syndrome: MR and CT data from 11 children. *J Comput Assist Tomogr* 1988;12:57–64.
72. Hanieh A, Simpson DA, North JB. Arachnoid cysts: a critical review of 41 cases. *Child's Nervous System* 1988;4:92–96.
73. Harsh GR IV, Edwards MSB, Wilson CB. Intracranial arachnoid cysts in children. *J Neurosurg* 1986;64:835–842.
74. Naidich TP, McLone DG, Radkowski MA. Intracranial arachnoid cysts. *Pediatr Neurosci* 1986;12:112–122.
75. Rengachary SS, Watanabe I, Brackett CE. Pathogenesis of intracranial arachnoid cysts. *Surg Neurol* 1978;9:139–144.
76. Rengachary SS, Watanabe I. Ultrastructure and pathogenesis of intracranial arachnoid cysts. *J Neuropathol Exp Neurol* 1981;40:61–83.
77. Schachenmayr W, Friede RL. Fine structure of arachnoid cysts. *Neurology* 1979;38:434–446.
78. Garcia-Bach M, Isamat F, Vila F. Intracranial arachnoid cysts in adults. *Acta Neurochir (Wien)* 1988;42(Suppl):205–209.
79. Galassi E, Tognetti F, Frank F, Fagioli L, Nasi MT, Gaist G. Infratentorial arachnoid cysts. *J Neurosurg* 1985;63:210–217.
80. Wiener SN, Pearlstein AE, Eiber A. MR imaging of intracranial arachnoid cysts. *J Comput Assist Tomogr* 1987;11:236–241.
81. Spiegel SM, Nixon B, TerBrugge K, Chiu MC, Schutz H. Arachnoid cyst of the velum interpositum. *AJNR* 1988;9:981–983.
82. Pelletier J, Milandre L, Péragut JC, Cronqvist S. Intraventricular choroid plexus "arachnoid" cyst. *Neuroradiology* 1990;32:523–525.
83. Nakase H, Hisanaga M, Hashimoto S, Imanishi M, Utsumi S. Intraventricular arachnoid cyst: report of two cases. *J Neurosurg* 1988;68:482–486.
84. Bank WO, Baleriaux D, Matos C, et al. Subarachnoid hemorrhage into preexistant arachnoid cysts: a potential pitfall in the interpretation of MRI and CT. *Proceedings of the American Society of Neuroradiology*, Washington, D.C.; 1991.
85. Eustace S, Toland J, Stack J. CT and MRI of arachnoid cyst with complicating intracystic and subdural haemorrhage. *J Comput Assist Tomogr* 1992;16:995–997.
86. Masdeu JC, Dobben GD, Azar-Kia B. Dandy-Walker syndrome studied by computed tomography and pneumoencephalography. *Radiology* 1983;147:109–114.
87. Maria BL, Zinreich SJ, Carson BC, Rosenbaum AE, Freeman JM. Dandy-Walker syndrome revisited. *Pediatr Neurosci* 1987;13:45–51.
88. Hirsch J-F, Pierre-Kahn A, Renier D, Sainte-Rose C, Hoppe-Hirsch E. The Dandy-Walker malformation: a review of 40 cases. *J Neurosurg* 1984;61:515–522.
89. Golden JA, Rorke LB, Bruce DA. Dandy-Walker syndrome and associated anomalies. *Pediatr Neurosci* 1987;13:38–44.
90. Barkovich AJ, Kjos BO, Norman D, Edwards MSB. Revised classification of posterior fossa cysts and cyst-like malformations based on results of multiplanar MR imaging. *AJNR* 1989;10:977–988.
91. Joubert M, Eisenring JJ, Robb JP, Andermann F. Familial agenesis of the cerebellar vermis. A syndrome of episodic hyperpnea, abnormal eye movements, ataxia, and retardation. *Neurology* 1969;19:813–825.
92. Friede RL, Boltshauser E. Uncommon syndromes of cerebellar aplasia. I. Joubert syndrome. *Dev Med Child Neurol* 1978;20:758–763.
93. deMorsier G. Etude sur les dysraphies crânio-encéphaliques: II. Agénésie du vermis cérébelleux. Dysraphie rhombocéphalique médiane (rhomboschizis). *Msch Psychiat Neurol* 1955;129:321–344.
94. Gross H. Die Rhombencephalosynapsis, eine systemisierte Kleinhirnfehlbildung. *Arch Psychiatr Nervenkr* 1959;199:537–552.
95. Schachenmayr W, Friede RL. Rhombencephalosynapsis: a Viennese malformation? *Dev Med Child Neurol* 1982;24:178–182.
96. Kepes JJ, Clough C, Villanueva A. Congenital fusion of the thalami (atresia of the third ventricle) and associated anomalies in a 6 month old infant. *Acta Neuropathol (Berl)* 1969;13:97–104.
97. Michaud J, Mizrahi EM, Urich H. Agenesis of the vermis with

fusion of the cerebellar hemispheres, septo-optic dysplasia and associated abnormalities. Report of a case. *Acta Neuropathol (Berl)* 1982;56:161–166.
98. Truwit CL, Barkovich AJ, Shanahan R, Maroldo TV. MR imaging of rhombencephalosynapsis: report of three cases. *AJNR* 1991;12:957–965.
99. Savolaine ER, Fadell RJ, Patel YP. Isolated rhombencephalosynapsis diagnosed by magnetic resonance imaging. *Clin Imaging* 1991;15:125–129.
100. Simmons G, Damiano TR, Truwit CL. MRI and clinical findings in rhombencephalosynapsis. *J Comput Assist Tomogr* 1993;17:211–214.
101. Streeter G. The developmental alterations in the vascular system of the brain of the human embryo. *Contrib Embryol Carnegie Inst* 1918;8:5–38.
102. Padgett DH. The development of the cranial arteries in the human embryo. *Contrib Embryol Carnegie Inst* 1948;32:205–261.
103. Padgett DH. The development of the cranial venous system in man, from the viewpoint of comparative anatomy. *Contrib Embryol Carnegie Inst* 1957;36:81–140.
104. McLone DG, Naidich TP. Embryology of the cerebral vascular system. In: Edwards MSB, Hoffman HJ, eds. *Cerebral Vascular Disease in Children and Adolescents.* Baltimore: Williams & Wilkins; 1989:1–16.
105. Streeter GL. The development of the venous sinuses of the dura mater in the human embryo. *Am J Anat* 1915;18:145–178.
106. Lie TA. Congenital anomalies of the carotid arteries. New York: Excerpta Medica Foundation, 1968.
107. Quint DJ, Silbergleit R, Young WC. Absence of the carotid canals at skull base CT. *Radiology* 1992;182:477–481.
108. Richardson DN, Elster AD, Ball MR. Intrasellar trigeminal artery. *AJNR* 1989;10:205.
109. Shintani S, Kuzuhara S, Toyokura Y. MR imaging of persistent primitive trigeminal artery. *Neuroradiology* 1990;32:79.
110. Tulsi RS, Locket NA. Persistent trigeminal artery: an anatomical study. *Aust N Z J Surg* 1985;55:397–402.
111. Loevner L, Quint D. Persistent trigeminal artery in a patient with Sturge-Weber syndrome. *AJR* 1992;158:872–874.
112. Franz M, Berlit P, Tornow K. General dysplasia of the cerebral arteries with persistent primitive acoustic artery and giant aneurysm. *Eur Arch Psychiatr Neurol Sci* 1989;238:196–198.
113. Lasjaunias PL. Craniofacial and upper cervical arteries. Baltimore: Williams & Wilkins: 1981:13–99 .
114. Baptista AG. Studies on arteries of brain. II: Anterior cerebral artery; some anatomic features and their clinical implications. *Neurology* 1963;13:825–835.
115. LeMay M, Gooding CA. The clinical significance of the azygos anterior cerebral artery. *AJR* 1966;98:602–610.
116. Szdzuy D, Lehmann R, Nickel B. Common trunk of the anterior cerebral arteries. *Neuroradiology* 1972;4:51–56.
117. Osaka K, Sato N, Yamasaki S, Fujita K, Matsumoto S, Kodama S. Dysgenesis of the deep venous system as a diagnostic criterion for holoprosencephaly. *Neuroradiology* 1977;13:231–238.
118. Niizuma H, Kwak R, Uchida K, Suzuki J. Aneurysms of the azygos anterior cerebral artery. *Surg Neurol* 1981;15:225–228.
119. Schick RM, Rumbaugh CL. Saccular aneurysm of the azygous anterior cerebral artery. *AJNR* 1989;10:S73.
120. Lightfoote JB, Grusd RS. Azygos anterior cerebral artery mimicking an anterior communicating artery aneurysm. *AJNR* 1989;10:S74.
121. Mall FP. On the development of the blood vessels of the brain in the human embryo. *Am J Anat* 1905;4:1–18.
122. Yokota A, Oota T, Matsukado Y, Okudera T. Structures and development of the venous system in congenital malformations of the brain. *Neuroradiology* 1978;16:26–30.
123. Velut S. Embryologie des veines cérébrales. *Neurochirurgie* 1987;33:258–263.
124. Raybaud CA, Strother CM, Hald JK. Aneurysms of the vein of Galen: embryonic considerations and anatomical features relating to the pathogenesis of the malformation. *Neuroradiology* 1989;31:109–128.
125. Barkovich AJ. Abnormal vascular drainage in anomalies of neuronal migration. *AJNR* 1988;9:939–942.
126. Huang YP, Okudera T, Ohta T, Robbins A. Anatomic variations of the dural venous sinuses. In: Kapp JP, Schmidek HH, eds. *The Cerebral Venous System and Its Disorders.* Orlando: Grune & Stratton; 1984:109–167.
127. Huang YP, Robbins A, Patel SC, Chaudhary MA. Cerebral venous malformations (and a new classification of cerebral vascular malformations). In: Kapp JP, Schmidek HH, eds. *The Cerebral Venous System and Its Disorders.* Orlando: Grune & Stratton; 1984:373–474.
128. Lasjaunias P, Burrows P, Planet C. Developmental venous anomalies (DVA): the so-called venous angioma. *Neurosurg Rev* 1986;9:233–244.
129. Avman N, Dinçer C. Venous malformation of the aqueduct of sylvius treated by interventriculostomy: 15 years follow-up. *Acta Neurochir (Wien)* 1980;52:219–224.
130. Tien R, Harsh GR IV, Dillon WP, Wilson CB. Unilateral hydrocephalus caused by an intraventricular venous malformation obstructing the foramen of Monro. *Neurosurgery* 1990;26:664–666.
131. Truwit CL. Venous angioma of the brain: history, significance, and imaging findings. *AJR* 1992;159:1299–1307.
132. Damiano TR, Truwit CL, Dowd CF, Symonds DL. Brainstem drainage of posterior fossa venous angiomas. *AJNR* 1994;15:643–652.
133. Watanabe M, Tanaka R, Takeda N, Ikuta F, Oyanagi K. Focal pachygyria with unusual vascular anomaly. *Neuroradiology* 1990;32:237–240.
134. McConnell S. Development and decision making in the mammalian cerebral cortex. *Brain Res Rev* 1988;13:1–23.
135. McConnell S. Fates of visual cortical neurons in the ferret after isochronic and heterochronic transplantation. *J Neurosci* 1988;8:945–974.
136. McConnell S. The generation of neuronal diversity in the central nervous system. *Annu Rev Neurosci* 1991;14:269–300.
137. Marin-Padilla M. Early ontogenesis of the human cerebral cortex. In: Peter A, Jones E, eds. *Cerebral Cortex, vol 7: Development and Maturation of the Cerebral Cortex.* New York: Plenum Press; 1988:1–34.
138. Sarnat H. Role of the human fetal ependyma. *Pediatr Neurol* 1992;8:163–178.
139. McConnell S, Kaznowski C. Cell cycle dependence of laminar determination in the developing cerebral cortex. *Science* 1991;254:282–285.
140. Barkovich A, Gressens P, Evrard P. Formation, maturation, and disorders of brain neocortex. *AJNR* 1992;13:423–446.
141. Barkovich A, Lyon G, Evrard P. Formation, maturation, and disorders of white matter. *AJNR* 1992;13:447–461.
142. Suzuki M, Choi B. Repair and reconstruction of the cortical plate following closed cryogenic injury to the neonatal rat cerebrum. *Acta Neuropathol* 1991;82:93–101.
143. Reiner O, Carrozzo R, Shen Y, et al. Isolation of a Miller-Dieker lissencephaly gene containing G protein B-subunit-like repeats. *Nature* 1993;364:717–721.
144. Dobyns WB, Reiner O, Carrozzo R, Ledbetter DH. Lissencephaly. A human brain malformation associated with deletion of the *LIS1* gene located at chromosome 17p13. *JAMA* 1993;270:2838–2842.
145. Santavuori P, Somer H, Sainio K. Muscle-eye-brain disease. *Brain Dev* 1989;11:147–153.
146. Takada K, Becker L, Takashima S. Walker-Warburg syndrome with skeletal muscle involvement: a report of three patients. *Pediatr Neurosci* 1987;13:202–209.
147. Takada K, Nakamura HTS. Cortical dysplasia in Fukuyama type congenital muscular dystrophy: a Golgi and angio architectonic analysis. *Acta Neuropathologica* 1988;76:170–178.
148. Yoshioka M, Kuroko S, Kondo T. Ocular manifestations in Fukuyama type congenital muscular dystrophy. *Brain Dev* 1990;12:423–426.
149. Yoshioka M, Saiwai S, Kuroko S, Nigami H. MR imaging of the brain in Fukuyama-type congenital muscular dystrophy. *AJNR* 1991;12:63–66.
150. Dobyns WB, Kirkpatrick JB, Hittner HM, Roberts RM, Kretzer FL. Syndromes with lissencephaly. 2: Walker, Warburg and cerebral-ocular-muscular syndromes and a new syndrome with type 2 lissencephaly. *Am J Med Genet* 1985;22:157–195.
151. Barkovich AJ, Linden C. Congenital cytomegalovirus infection

of the brain: imaging analysis and embryologic considerations. *AJNR* 1994;15:703–715.
152. Hayward JC, Titelbaum DS, Clancy RR, Zimmerman RA. Lissencephaly-pachygyria associated with congenital cytomegalovirus infection. *J Child Neurol* 1991;6:109–114.
153. Barkovich AJ, Chuang SH, Norman D. MR of neuronal migration anomalies. *AJNR* 1987;8:1009–1017.
154. Smith AS, Weinstein MA, Quencer RM, et al. Association of heterotopic gray matter with seizures: MR imaging. *Radiology* 1988;168:195–198.
155. Barkovich AJ, Kjos BO. Gray matter heterotopias: MR characteristics and correlation with developmental and neurologic manifestations. *Radiology* 1992;182:493–499.
156. Barkovich AJ, Jackson DE Jr, Boyer RS. Band heterotopias: a newly recognized neuronal migration anomaly. *Radiology* 1989;171:455–458.
157. Palmini A, Andermann F, Aicardi J, et al. Diffuse cortical dysplasia, or the "double cortex" syndrome: the clinical and epileptic spectrum in 10 patients. *Neurology* 1991;41:1656–1662.
158. Livingstone JH, Aicardi J. Unusual MRI appearance of diffuse subcortical heterotopia or "double cortex" in two children. *J Neurol Neurosurg Psychiatry* 1990;53:617–620.
159. Ianneti P, Raucci U, Basile LA, et al. Neuronal migrational disorders: diffuse cortical dysplasia or the "double cortex" syndrome. *Acta Paediatr* 1993;82:501–503.
160. Falconer J, Wada J, Martin W, Li D. PET, CT, and MRI imaging of neuronal migration anomalies in epileptic patients. *Can J Neurol Sci* 1990;17:35–39.
161. Miura K, Watanabe K, Maeda N, et al. MR imaging and positron emission tomography of band heterotopia. *Brain Dev* 1993;15:288–290.
162. Morell F, Whisler W, Hoeppner T, et al. Electrophysiology of heterotopic gray matter in the "double cortex" syndrome. *Epilepsia* 1992;33(Suppl 3):76.
163. Kalifa GL, Chiron C, Sellier N, et al. Hemimegalencephaly: MR imaging in five children. *Radiology* 1987;165:29–33.
164. King M, Stephenson J, Ziervogel M, Doyel D, Galbraith S. Hemimegalencephaly—a case for hemispherectomy? *Neuropediatrics* 1985;16:46–55.
165. Manz HJ, Phillips TM, Rowden G, McCullough DC. Unilateral megalencephaly, cerebral cortical dysplasia, neuronal hypertrophy and heterotopia: cytomorphic, fluorometric cytochemical and biochemical analyses. *Acta Neuropathol (Berl)* 1979;45:97–103.
166. Anlar B, Yalaz K, Erzen C. Klippel-Trenaunay-Weber syndrome: a case with cerebral and cerebellar hemihypertrophy. *Neuroradiology* 1988;30:360.
167. Hager B, Dyme I, Guertin S, Tyler R, Tryciecky E, Fratkin J. Linear nevus sebaceous syndrome: megalencephaly and heterotopic gray matter. *Pediatr Neurol* 1991;7:45–49.
168. Sarwar M, Schafer M. Brain malformations in livear nevus sebaceous syndrome: an MR study. *J Comput Assist Tomogr* 1988;12:338–340.
169. Peserico A, Battistella P, Bertoli P, Drigo P. Unilateral hypomelanosis of Ito with hemimegalencephaly. *Acta Paediatr Scand* 1988.
170. Cumai R, Curatolo P, Mangano S, Cheminal R, Echenne B. Hemimegalencephaly and neurofibromatosis. *Neuopediatrics* 1990;21:179–182.
171. Fitz CR, Harwood-Nash DC, Boldt DW. The radiographic features of unilateral megalencephaly. *Neuroradiology* 1978;15:145–148.
172. Kuzniecky R, Andermann F, Guerrini R, Study at CMC. Congenital bilateral perisylvian syndrome: study of 31 patients. *Lancet* 1993;341:608–612.
173. Graff-Radford NR, Bosch EP, Stears JC, Tranel D. Developmental Foix-Chavany-Marie syndrome in identical twins. *Ann Neurol* 1986;20:632–635.
174. Tatum WO, Coker SB, Ghobrial M, Abd-Allah S. The open opercular sign: diagnosis and significance. *Ann Neurol* 1989;25:196–199.
175. Becker PS, Dixon AM, Troncoso JC. Bilateral opercular polymicrogyria. *Ann Neurol* 1989;25:90–92.
176. Kuzniecky R, Andermann F, Tampieri D, Melanson D, Olivier A, Leppik I. Bilateral central macrogyria: epilepsy, pseudobulbar palsy, and mental retardation—a new recognizable neuronal migration disorder. *Ann Neurol* 1989;25:547–554.
177. Shevell MI, Carmant L, Meager-Villemure K. Developmental bilateral perisylvian dysplasia. *Pediatr Neurol* 1992;8:299–302.
178. Yakovlev PI, Wadsworth RC. Schizencephalies. A study of the congenital clefts in the cerebral mantle. I. Clefts with fused lips. *J Neuropathol Exp Neurol* 1946;5:116–130.
179. Yakovlev PI, Wadsworth RC. Schizencephalies. II. Clefts with hydrocephalus and lips separated. *J Neuropathol Exp Neurol* 1946;5:169–206.
180. Barkovich AJ, Norman D. MR imaging of schizencephaly. *AJNR* 1988;9:297–302.
181. Lightman S. Kallmann's syndrome. *J R Soc Med* 1988;81:315–316.
182. Kallmann FJ, Schoenfeld WA, Barrera SE. The genetic aspects of primary eunuchoidism. *Am J Ment Def* 1944;48:203–206.
183. Van Dop C, Burstein S, Conte FA, Grumbach MM. Isolated gonadotropin deficiency in boys: clinical characteristics and growth. *J Pediatrics* 1987;111:684–692.
184. White BJ, Rogol AD, Brown KS, Lieblich JM, Rosen SW. The syndrome of anosmia with hypogonadotropic hypogonadism: a genetic study of 18 new families and a review. *Am J Med Genet* 1983;15:417–435.
185. Schwanzel-Fukuda M, Bick D, Pfaff DW. Luteinizing hormone-releasing hormone (LHRH)-expressing cells do not migrate normally in an inherited hypogonadal (Kallmann) syndrome. *Mol Brain Res* 1989;6:311–326.
186. Franco B, Guioli S, Pragliola A, et al. A gene deleted in Kallmann's syndrome shares homology with neural cell adhesion and axonal path-finding molecules. *Nature* 1991;353:529–536.
187. Bossy J. Development of olfactory and related structures in staged human embryos. *Anat Embryol (Berl)* 1980;161:225–236.
188. Müller F, O'Rahilly R. The human brain at stage 17, including the appearance of the future olfactory bulb and the first amygdaloid nuclei. *Anat Embryol (Berl)* 1989;180:353–369.
189. Schwanzel-Fukuda M, Pfaff DW. Origin of luteinizing hormone-releasing hormone neurons. *Nature* 1989;338:161–164.
190. Pearson AA. The development of the olfactory nerve in man. *J Comp Neurol* 1941;75:199–217.
191. Pearson AA. The development of the nervus terminalis in man. *J Comp Neurol* 1941;75:39–66.
192. Humphrey T. The development of the olfactory and the accessory olfactory formations in human embryos and fetuses. *J Comp Neurol* 1940;73:431–468.
193. Humphrey T. The development of the anterior olfactory nucleus of human fetuses. *Prog Brain Res* 1963;3:170–190.
194. Klingmüller D, Dewes W, Krahe T, Brecht G, Schweikert H-U. Magnetic resonance imaging of the brain in patients with anosmia and hypothalamic hypogonadism (Kallmann's syndrome). *J Clin Endocrinol Metab* 1987;65:581–584.
195. Dewes VW, Krahe T, Klingmüller D, Harder T. MR-Tomographie beim Kallmann-Syndrom. *Fortschr Röntgenstr* 1987;147:400–402.
196. Knorr JR, Ragland RL, Brown RS, Gelber N. Kallmann syndrome: MR findings. *AJNR* 1993;14:845–851.
197. Yousem DM, Turner WJD, Li C, Snyder PJ, Doty RL. Kallmann syndrome: MR evaluation of olfactory system. *AJNR* 1993;14:839–843.
198. Truwit CL, Barkovich AJ, Grumbach MM. MR imaging of Kallmann syndrome: a genetic disorder of neuronal migration affecting the olfactory and genital systems. *AJNR* 1993;14:827–838.
199. Castillo M, Bouldin TW, Scatliff JH, Suzuki K. Alobar holoprosencephaly AJNR 1993;14:1151–1156.

Magnetic Resonance Imaging of the Brain and Spine, Second Edition, edited by Scott W. Atlas.
Lippincott-Raven Publishers, Philadelphia © 1996.

9

Intracranial Hemorrhage

Keith R. Thulborn and Scott W. Atlas

The identification of intracranial hemorrhage is essential, since its presence has important implications for clinical management and patient outcome. The MR appearance of intracranial hemorrhage can show all permutations of all possible MR signal patterns, depending on both biological variables (Table 1) and imaging parameters (Table 2). The sometimes subtle characteristics of hematoma signal intensity patterns on detailed examination provide clues to the disease processes that underlie the hemorrhagic event, thereby allowing the radiologist to make a specific diagnosis. While these complex patterns make MR image interpretation challenging, they also make hemorrhage an excellent vehicle for demonstrating the principles underlying MR contrast. This chapter aims to move beyond the simple pattern recognition style of radiological diagnosis to a more detailed description of the physics and biochemistry underlying the various MR phenomena illustrated during the evolution of cerebral hematomas. Once understood, these principles can be used to understand the signal characteristics of many other entities.

K. R. Thulborn, M.D., Ph.D.: Department of Radiology, University of Pittsburgh MR Research Center, Presbyterian University Hospital, Pittsburgh, PA 15213.
S. W. Atlas, M.D.: Neuroradiology Division, Department of Radiology, Oregon Health Sciences University, Portland, OR 97201.

The conceptual framework for understanding the MR appearance of cerebral hematoma has been summarized in multiple reviews (1–5) based on in vitro studies, animal models, and clinical observations (2,6–18). The original model (12) emphasized the roles of iron associated with hemoglobin, edema, and gross structural changes in the hematoma in determining relaxation mechanisms underlying the variable MR patterns. Iron certainly plays a major role, because of its high concentration and because its magnetic properties vary as its biochemical form, oxidation state, and spatial distribution change. Other pathophysiological processes, such as changes in integrity of the blood–brain barrier with alteration of the degree of edema or because of the presence of an underlying neoplasm, and nonparamagnetic protein concentration contribute to signal intensity patterns on these images. Recently, red blood cell volume (19), thrombus formation, and clot retraction (20) have been investigated and may be of some importance. Structural alterations, such as cavitation and hemoglobin resorption or degradation, become significant as the more acute processes of iron metabolism and edema decrease in importance during hematoma evolution.

This chapter reviews the physicochemical principles of the magnetic properties of matter and their applications to biological systems, discusses the biochemical pathways of iron metabolism and water balance in resolving

TABLE 1. *Physiologic factors influencing MR intensities of intracranial hemorrhage*

Age of hemorrhage
Site of hemorrhage
Size of hemorrhage
Local partial pressure of oxygen
Local pH
Local glucose
Hematocrit
Hemoglobin concentration
Temperature
Blood–brain-barrier integrity
Clot formation and retraction

hematomas, and presents a qualitative scheme for relating these biochemical processes to the relaxation phenomena underlying signal contrast observed in MR images of hemorrhage. Factors most important to the intensity patterns in evolving intracranial hematomas will be stressed. MR features suggestive of specific etiologies of intracranial hemorrhage will also be discussed.

MAGNETIC PROPERTIES OF MATTER

Atomic Structure

A basic understanding of the magnetic properties of matter begins with a description of fundamental atomic structure. Magnetic properties arise from the moving electric charges within individual atoms. A complete quantum mechanical description is beyond the scope of this chapter, but the nomenclature used by quantum mechanics provides a simplistic picture of the atom that is basic to understanding the origin of the magnetic properties of atoms.

An atom is composed of a positively charged nucleus containing most of the mass of the atom, and a surrounding distribution of negatively charged electrons. The sum of the electric charges of the electrons equals that of the nucleus for electrical neutrality. For ions, electrons may be lost or gained from a particular atom although the overall sum of positive and negative ions is zero. The electrons are arranged around the nucleus in an organized distribution of electronic atomic orbitals. Such orbitals are described by four quantum numbers. The derivation of these numbers is beyond the scope of this chapter, and the interested reader is referred to an excellent text (21).

The principal quantum number (n where n = 1, 2, 3, . . .) refers to the total energy of a given electron. The second quantum number (l where l = 0, 1, 2, 3, . . . , $n - 1$) refers to the total orbital angular momentum of the electron. The third quantum number (m where $m = -l \leq m \leq l$) is termed the magnetic quantum number, defining the possible values of components of the orbital angular momentum. The fourth quantum number (I where I = 0, $\frac{1}{2}$, 1, $\frac{3}{2}$,. . .) is referred to as the spin quantum number, which further defines the possible values of components of the spin angular momentum (m_I where m_I, $-I \leq m_I \leq I$).

The electronic configuration of an atom is defined by these four quantum numbers (n, l, m, I) in the following way. Electrons can be considered to occupy discrete energy levels, or shells, defined by the principle quantum number (e.g., n = 1, 2, 3, 4,. . .). Each shell is subdivided into orbitals of different total orbital angular momentum quantum numbers l = 0, 1, 2, 3, . . . , respectively, with corresponding suborbitals labeled *s, p, d, f*. . . . For example, for electronic shell n = 3, there are three orbitals given as l = 0, 1, 2. Each orbital then has discrete orbital angular momentum states given by m that are termed suborbitals. For example, for orbital l = 0, the single m = 0 suborbital is termed an s suborbital. For l = 1, there are three suborbitals, m = ≤1, 0, 1, termed p suborbitals. For l = 2, there are five suborbitals, m = −2, −1, 0, 1, 2, termed d suborbitals. The electron, with a spin quantum number $I = \frac{1}{2}$, has two states of spin angular momentum which is confined to an atom ($m_I = \pm\frac{1}{2}$). The Pauli principle states that no two electrons in an atom can have the same set of quantum numbers. This means that a maximum of two electrons are permitted to occupy each suborbital. To fill a suborbital, the two elec trons must have opposite spin ($m_I = \pm\frac{1}{2}$). Electrons fill the predicted shells beginning with the lowest energy closest to the nucleus. For orbitals of the same shell (identical energy), single electrons of equal spin momentum (i.e., identical m_I) occupy each suborbital prior to pairing with a second electron of opposite spin angular momentum. Each suborbital has a maximum of two electrons, which must have opposite spin quantum numbers ($\pm\frac{1}{2}$).

This formalized description of the electronic structure of an atom can now be applied to iron, which is of specific interest in hemorrhage. The electronic configuration of iron in the ferrous (Fe^{2+}) oxidation state (24 electrons per atom) can now be written as:

$$1s_2 2s_2 2p_6 3s_2 3p_6 3d_6$$

The volume and shape of the atomic suborbitals vary with quantum number. The s suborbital is spherical with increasing diameter as the energy of the shell increases (n = 1, 2, 3 . . . .). The p and d suborbitals show anisotropic electronic distributions that are important for

TABLE 2. *Operator-dependent factors affecting MR intensities of intracranial hemorrhage*

Magnetic field strength and homogeneity
Pulse sequence design (e.g., SE, GE, FSE, EPI)
Pulse sequence parameters (e.g., TR, TE, τ_{cpmg})

chemical-bond-forming interactions with other atoms (i.e., ligands). In the absence of ligands, the suborbitals of each shell are of equal energy (i.e., degenerate). For example, the outer five 3*d* suborbitals ($n = 3$, $l = 2$, $m = -2, -1, 0, 1, 2$) of iron are degenerate in the absence of ligands. As ligands approach the outer suborbitals, the degeneracy is removed (as shown by the energy diagram in Fig. 1). For example, the *d* suborbitals oriented directly at the approaching ligands experience electrostatic forces that increase their energy above that of the suborbitals oriented between the ligands. The energy difference between the two groups of suborbitals reflects the type of ligand, the so-called ligand field strength. As the ligands change, the energy levels of the suborbitals change within the outer shell. If the energy separation of the suborbitals increases above the energy required to pair electrons of opposite spin angular momentum ($m_l = \pm\frac{1}{2}$) within a single suborbital, then electron pairing occurs before each of the suborbitals obtains a single unpaired electron. The resultant altered electronic distribution markedly influences the magnetic properties of the atom. Figure 1 emphasizes the changes in distribution of *d* orbital energies (and therefore *d* electrons) in iron as the oxygen ligand is removed upon deoxygenation of hemoglobin (i.e., as oxyhemoglobin is converted to deoxyhemoglobin), as oxidation from ferrous (Fe^{2+}) to ferric (Fe^{3+}) iron states occurs (i.e., as deoxyhemoglobin is converted to methemoglobin), and as chelated ferric iron changes to crystalline form (chelated iron is converted to ferric oxyhydroxide).

Origin of Magnetism

A magnetic field is generated by a moving electric charge (22). The strength of the magnetic field is determined by the size of the electric charge, as well as by its momentum. The magnetic field generated by the unit charge is termed a magnetic dipole. An electron confined to an atomic orbital represents a moving charge with both orbital angular momentum and spin angular momentum. Each angular momentum of the electron (i.e., orbital and spin) generates a magnetic field. Since the nucleus also possesses an electric charge and may have nonzero spin angular momentum (spin quantum number 0, $\frac{1}{2}, \frac{3}{2}, \ldots$), it may also generate a magnetic field. However, since the magnetic moment of any charged particle is inversely proportional to its mass, and the mass of the nucleus is three orders of magnitude greater than that of the electron, the contribution of the nucleus to the magnetic properties of the atom is much less than that of the electrons. Hence, although nuclear magnetic interactions occur and nuclear magnetization is the origin of the signal used to construct the MR image, the magnetic properties of tissue are determined chiefly by the electronic configuration of the atoms and molecules.

The two major types of magnetic properties of matter most relevant to a discussion of human biological systems include the phenomena of *diamagnetism and paramagnetism.* These concepts are first reviewed in terms of the different electronic configurations of the atoms and molecules that make up the constitutive material. Other magnetic properties of matter are discussed in detail elsewhere (5) and are included herein briefly for completeness.

Diamagnetism

Most biological materials consist of elements such as carbon, oxygen, and hydrogen, in which the electrons are paired in atomic and molecular orbitals. The pairing of electrons with opposite spin angular momentum minimizes the energy state of the electrostatic and magnetic interactions of closely placed, identical charges (i.e., the electrons). In the paired condition, the net spin angular momentum of electrons is zero (i.e, there is no net magnetic moment). However, the paired electrons still have orbital angular momentum, constituting charges circulating in a confined orbital. If such a current loop is placed in an applied magnetic field, Lenz's law states that this current loop (i.e., the electrons) generates a magnetic

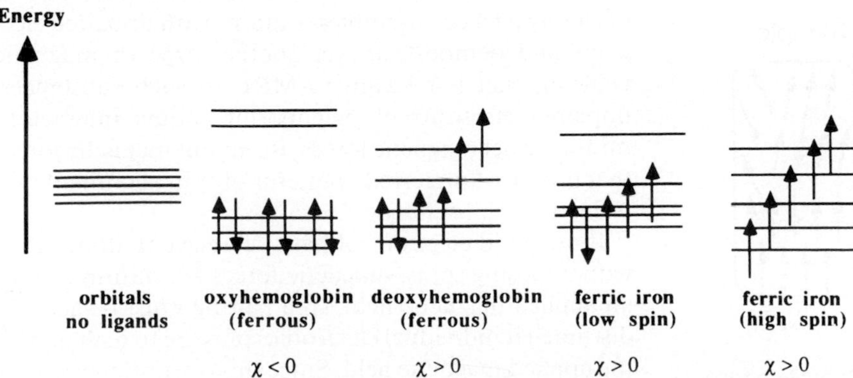

FIG. 1. Schematic representation of the electronic configuration of the five *d* suborbitals of iron in its various biochemical forms based on the relative energies of the orbitals arising from interactions with the ligands coordinated to the iron center. The number of unpaired electrons determines χ but the aggregation state of the iron determines the magnitude of the χ.

field opposing the applied magnetic field in vector direction (Fig. 2A). This reduces the magnitude of the local magnetic field within the material below that of the original applied magnetic field. Materials that reduce the magnitude of an applied magnetic field are termed *diamagnetic,* and, in fact, greater than 99% of human tissue is diamagnetic.

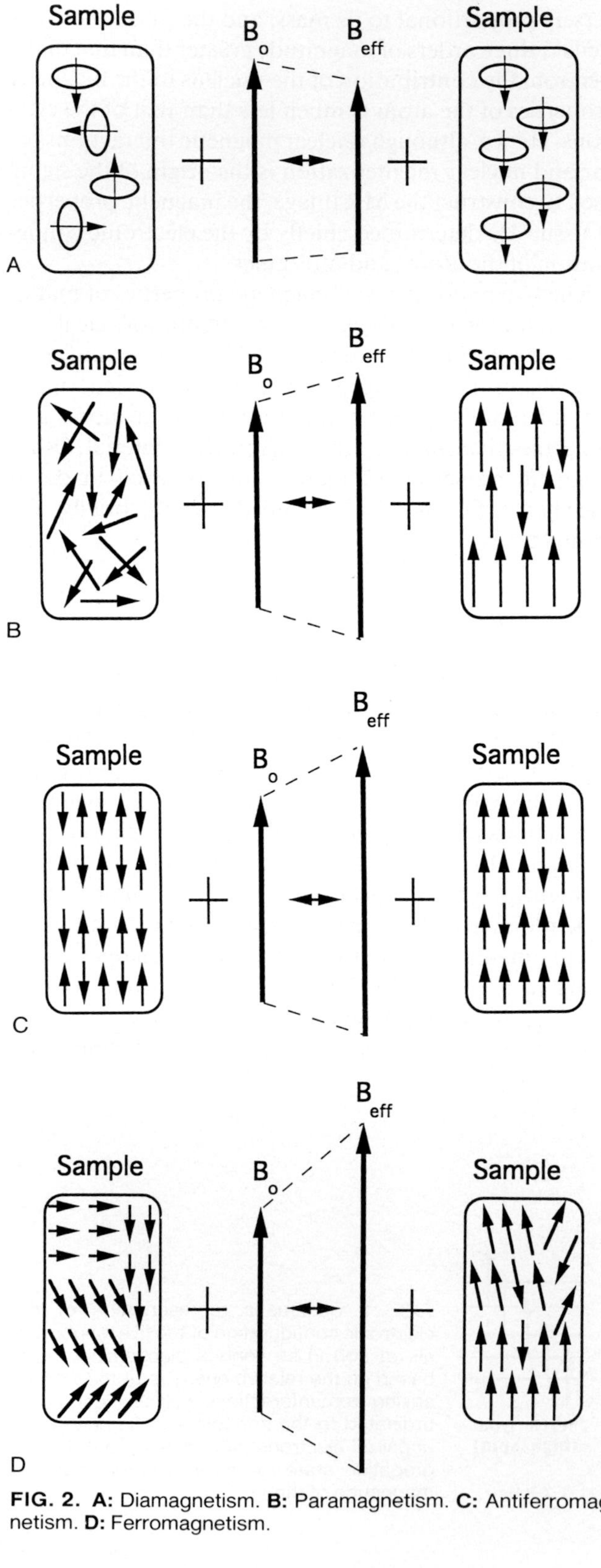

FIG. 2. **A:** Diamagnetism. **B:** Paramagnetism. **C:** Antiferromagnetism. **D:** Ferromagnetism.

Paramagnetism

Biological substances containing atomic or molecular structures with unpaired electrons have magnetic properties dominated by those unpaired electrons, due to the resultant magnetic dipole arising from the electronic spin angular momentum. Iron, in its ferrous and ferric oxidation states, is an important example of a naturally occurring substance in which the number of unpaired electrons varies with the biochemical state of the metal ion. If the magnetic dipoles of a collection of atoms or molecules are widely separated and randomly oriented in space, such that the unpaired orbital electrons on different atoms cannot interact, then the total magnetic field from that collection is zero. However, individual electronic magnetic dipoles can respond to an applied magnetic field by aligning in a parallel or antiparallel manner to that field, according to quantum mechanical requirements of the two energy state system for spin particles. The distribution of electrons between the two energy states is governed by the Boltzmann distribution. At physiological temperatures, more electrons align parallel to the applied field, resulting in an enhancement (i.e., an increase in magnitude) of that applied field (Fig. 2B). This phenomenon is analogous to the alignment of nuclear spins in the nuclear magnetic resonance (NMR) experiment. Materials that have no intrinsic magnetic field in the absence of an applied magnetic field, but augment an applied magnetic field upon exposure to it, are termed *paramagnetic.* Naturally occurring paramagnetic substances include copper, iron, and manganese.

Antiferromagnetism, Ferromagnetism, and Superparamagnetism

Some biologically important materials, such as the ferric oxyhydroxide crystalline structure of ferritin and hemosiderin (two forms of iron storage substances), consist of closely packed ensembles of atoms with unpaired electrons and demonstrate yet another type of magnetic behavior that is relevant to MRI. In such substances, unpaired electrons of neighboring atoms interact to minimize net magnetic forces. Resultant magnetic forces that produce "preferred" patterns of spin alignments are termed *exchange forces.*

If unpaired electrons of pairs of adjacent atoms align with opposing spins, magnetic forces are minimized. In an applied magnetic field, spin pairing must be actively disrupted if individual electronic spins are to realign with the applied magnetic field. Since this disruption requires energy, the overall response of the material to the applied field (i.e., the degree of augmentation of the applied field) is less than that of a paramagnetic substance. Note that the net (effective) magnetic field is still increased, in comparison with the magnitude of the original applied field (Fig. 2C). Such materials exhibiting this behavior are termed *antiferromagnetic*. The alignment pattern in antiferromagnetic substances can be disrupted if the thermal energy is increased, and initially, the response to an applied field is enhanced as the temperature is increased. Above a critical temperature, known as the Neel temperature, adjacent spin pairing is disrupted, and the antiferromagnetic substance becomes paramagnetic.

If the unpaired electrons of a group of atoms in a crystal interact to align in domains (termed *Weiss domains*), each domain has its own net magnetic field. Adjacent Weiss domains can then interact via these magnetic fields to minimize the resultant magnetic field outside the material. If that material is immersed in a high magnetic field, domains respond to both the applied field and neighboring domain fields to enhance markedly the overall field (Fig. 2D). Such materials possess a magnetic field even in the absence of an applied magnetic field and are termed *ferromagnetic*.

As the ferromagnetic crystal is reduced in size to that of a single domain, this single-domain-equivalent particle has a net magnetic dipole equivalent to that of a single domain. If a collection of such single-domain particles is free to rotate in an applied magnetic field on a time scale that is shorter than the observation time, the magnetic dipoles behave as expected for paramagnetism (discussed above). However, the larger magnetic moment of the particle (because it is a domain, or group of atoms acting as one) produces a greater enhancement of the applied magnetic field compared with paramagnetic substances. Such particles are termed *superparamagnetic* (23–25). Superparamagnetic materials do not retain their magnetic field when removed from an applied field.

If the size of the particles (which normally contain many domains) is reduced below the size of a single domain, the aligning exchange forces and disaligning thermal forces become comparable. Assuming the time scale of the observation is longer than the switching rate of the equilibrium between the aligned and disordered states, then the magnetic properties of the particles are dependent on the temperature-volume relationships, which determine the switching frequency. An aggregate of such particles behaves paramagnetically, but with a greater magnetic dipole than if no domain formed at all, and thus is termed *supermagnetic* (22).

Antiferrimagnetism and Ferrimagnetism

When a crystal lattice is composed of two different substances, the lattice symmetry can be such that the resultant structure allows exchange forces between atoms of the two substances to operate separately. This behavior resembles two separate crystals occupying the same space. The exchange forces may allow individual *opposition (antiferrimagnetism)* or group opposition *(ferrimagnetism)*.

Magnetic Susceptibility

Any material, when placed into a constant magnetic field, responds by generating its own magnetic field. The *magnetic susceptibility* of a substance (or tissue) describes this magnetic response. The induced magnetic field has two important characteristics: a magnitude and a vector direction. Materials can be categorized, based upon their induced fields (i.e., based upon their magnetic susceptibilities) (Table 3). Diamagnetic materials respond to an applied field with a very weak induced field ($\approx 10^{-6} \times$ the magnitude of the applied field), and in a vector direction that opposes that of the applied field. Paramagnetic materials have a larger induced field ($\approx 10^{-2}$ to 10^{-4} $\times$ the magnitude of the applied field), which is in the same vector direction as the applied field. Superparamagnetic and ferromagnetic materials generate a very large induced field, equal to or even greater than the applied field, and, like paramagnetic substances, the induced field is in the same vector direction as the applied field.

The tissue interaction with the static magnetic field $\mathbf{B}_0$ to produce magnetization $\mathbf{m}$, which either reduces (diamagnetism) or enhances (paramagnetism, antiferromagnetism, ferromagnetism, superparamagnetism) the effective magnetic field, $\mathbf{B}_{\text{eff}}$ within the material (note that the magnetization $\mathbf{m}$ is referring to the effects of electronic configurations, not nuclear magnetization $\mathbf{M}$, measured in the NMR experiment) can be quantified in terms of the magnetic susceptibility χ of the material where:

$$\mathbf{B}_{\text{eff}} = \mathbf{B}_0 + \mathbf{m} = \mathbf{B}_0(1 + \chi) \qquad [1]$$

where

$$\chi = \mathbf{m}/\mathbf{B}_0$$

Thus, $\chi < 0$ for diamagnetic materials, $\chi > 0$ for paramagnetic materials and $\chi = 0$ for a vacuum.

When placed into the static magnetic field of the im-

TABLE 3. *Magnetic susceptibility based upon characteristics of the induced magnetic field*

	Magnitude of **m** relative to $\mathbf{B}_0$	Effect on $\mathbf{B}_0$
Diamagnetism	10^{-6}	Opposes
Paramagnetism	10^{-2} to 10^{-4}	Augments
Superparamagnetism	> or =	Augments
Ferromagnetism	> or =	Augments

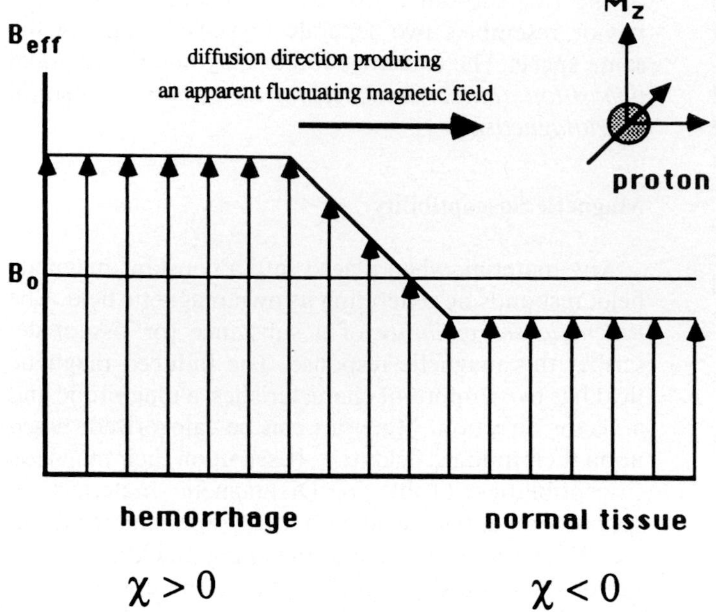

FIG. 3. The effective magnetic field $\mathbf{B}_{\text{eff}}$ is modified from the applied magnetic field $\mathbf{B}_0$ by the presence of tissue depending on whether it is diamagnetic ($\chi < 0$) or paramagnetic ($\chi > 0$). The boundary between these regions has a gradient in $\mathbf{B}_{\text{eff}}$ that functions as an apparent fluctuating magnetic field $\mathbf{b}_z$ when spins diffuse across the boundary. Thus diffusion causes $\mathbf{M}_{xy}$ relaxation characterized by T2*. As no fluctuating fields occur along $\mathbf{b}_x$ or $\mathbf{b}_y$, $\mathbf{M}_z$ and therefore T1 are unaltered.

aging magnet, therefore, tissues of different magnetic susceptibilities establish different *effective* local magnetic fields (Fig. 3). Consequently, when there are two adjacent regions of differing magnetic susceptibilities in the imaging volume, there are actually two adjacent regions of differing magnetic fields (Fig. 3). *Gradients, or differences, in magnetic susceptibility (χ) should be thought of as equivalent to magnetic field inhomogeneities.* The response of the nuclear magnetization measured in the MR image is altered dramatically by the different stages of iron metabolism found within an evolving hematoma, due to their differences in magnetic susceptibility.

MRI CONTRAST

Most clinical MR images are based on the nuclear spin system of hydrogen ($I = \frac{1}{2}$), referred to simply as protons. The proton is intrinsically the most sensitive nucleus for MRI and occurs in the highest concentration, given the abundance of water in human tissue. The protons have charge and spin and therefore behave as a magnetic dipole, as discussed for electrons above. As such, they respond to other magnetic fields such as applied external magnetic fields and to other local dipole fields produced by adjacent nuclei with nonzero spin and unpaired electrons. Image contrast is the difference in signal intensity arising from different regions of the object. If two regions have different magnetic environments, signal intensities from each region will be different and contrast will be observed. The nature of interactions between the magnetic environment and the proton spin system is discussed in terms of the MRI process.

The Nuclear Magnetic Resonance Phenomenon

The responses of a proton to the presence of an external static magnetic field $\mathbf{B}_0$, and to the perturbing influence of an oscillating magnetic field $\mathbf{B}_1$, of a radiofrequency (rf) pulse of electromagnetic energy are summarized by the Bloch equations and have been well described in many excellent texts (26–30). To be clearly distinguished from the magnetic effects of the electrons discussed above, the nuclear magnetic resonance phenomenon determining the signal measured in the MR image is based on the response of the nuclear magnetization to the surrounding magnetic environment. In the presence of $\mathbf{B}_0$, the nuclear spins realign with a net magnetization along the direction of $\mathbf{B}_0$ but with individual spins precessing about that axis at an angular frequency ω, defined by the Larmor equation:

$$\omega = \gamma \mathbf{B}_0 \quad [2]$$

where γ is the gyromagnetic ratio, a characteristic constant for the proton. The alignment of net induced nuclear magnetization, M_z, is along the direction of the static field as shown by the subscript z with no net magnetization, $\mathbf{M}_{xy}$, in the x-y plane (defined as perpendicular to the direction of the static field). The design of the receiver coils used to detect the very small currents induced by the changing magnetization of the sample is such that only transverse magnetization can be directly monitored. Therefore, the MR image is formed by generating and observing transverse magnetization M_{xy}.

This is done by application of the second magnetic field $\mathbf{B}_1$, which must oscillate at close to the Larmor precession frequency to produce the necessary torque to move $\mathbf{M}_z$, into the x-y plane (Fig. 4). The $\mathbf{B}_1$ field used is the magnetic component of electromagnetic radiation of the rf pulse. Just as the nuclear spin system gains energy, and therefore magnetization, as it is perturbed from equilibrium by $\mathbf{B}_1$, return to equilibrium when $\mathbf{B}_1$ is turned off requires dissipation of energy, and therefore magnetization, through interactions with local fluctuating magnetic fields from neighboring nuclear and electronic spin systems. These local fields can be thought of as having components $\mathbf{b}_x$, $\mathbf{b}_y$, and $\mathbf{b}_z$ along the x, y, and z axes, respectively. The process of return to equilibrium is termed relaxation and is characterized by a relaxation time or, its reciprocal, a relaxation rate.

Relaxation can be separated into two components, longitudinal and transverse relaxation, which refer to the loss of the transverse ($\mathbf{M}_{xy}$) component and reaccumulation of the longitudinal ($\mathbf{M}_z$) component of the total magnetization $\mathbf{M}$ (Fig. 4). These relaxation processes, as described by the Bloch equations, are characterized by their relaxation times, T1 and T2, respectively. Loss of transverse magnetization $\mathbf{M}_{xy}$ occurs by interaction with all three fluctuating local magnetic fields, $\mathbf{b}_x$, $\mathbf{b}_y$, and $\mathbf{b}_z$, perpendicular to the nuclear magnetization $\mathbf{M}$. In contrast, re-equilibration of longitudinal magnetization $\mathbf{M}_z$, occurs through interaction with only two local magnetic fields $\mathbf{b}_x$ and $\mathbf{b}_y$, fluctuating in the x-y plane perpendicular to $\mathbf{M}_z$. Most fluctuating fields have all three components and produce both T1 and T2 relaxation. As described below, there are mechanisms of relaxation that are highly anisotropic, in which fluctuations in $\mathbf{b}_z$ occur without fluctuations in $\mathbf{b}_x$ or $\mathbf{b}_y$ resulting in shortening of T2 but not T1. Relaxation is efficient if the magnetic interactions with other nuclear and electronic spin systems are short range, are correctly oriented for interaction, and act at or close to the Larmor frequency. The intensity of the MR signal in an image is the balance between the magnetization $\mathbf{M}_{xy}$, induced in the tissue by the rf pulse of the imaging pulse sequence and the T1 and T2 relaxation processes that return the nuclear spin system to its equilibrium state.

Relaxation Mechanisms in Hemorrhage

For diamagnetic tissues, the most important relaxation mechanism accounting for both longitudinal and transverse relaxation is attributed to proton-proton dipole-dipole interactions (24,28). Other mechanisms—scalar-spin coupling, chemical shift anisotropy, quadripolar and spin-rotational effects—are usually less important in proton MRI and are described elsewhere (27,28,30). The image contrast in hemorrhage requires discussion of two effects of nondiamagnetic substances. These are considered under *relaxivity and susceptibility* effects. A third process of *exchange* is also discussed separately.

Relaxivity Effects

The rotational and translational diffusion of water molecules in biological systems occur on a time scale that produces an isotropically fluctuating magnetic field in the range of the Larmor frequencies for protons at current imaging field strengths. If the water molecules are able to approach a paramagnetic center, then magnetic interactions between the nuclear magnetic dipoles of the water (protons) and the magnetic dipoles of the paramagnetic centers (unpaired electrons) allow efficient energy exchange to occur. This interaction results in relaxation of the water proton to its magnetic equilibrium state (31). The phenomenological equation for such intermolecular proton-electron dipole-dipole interactions

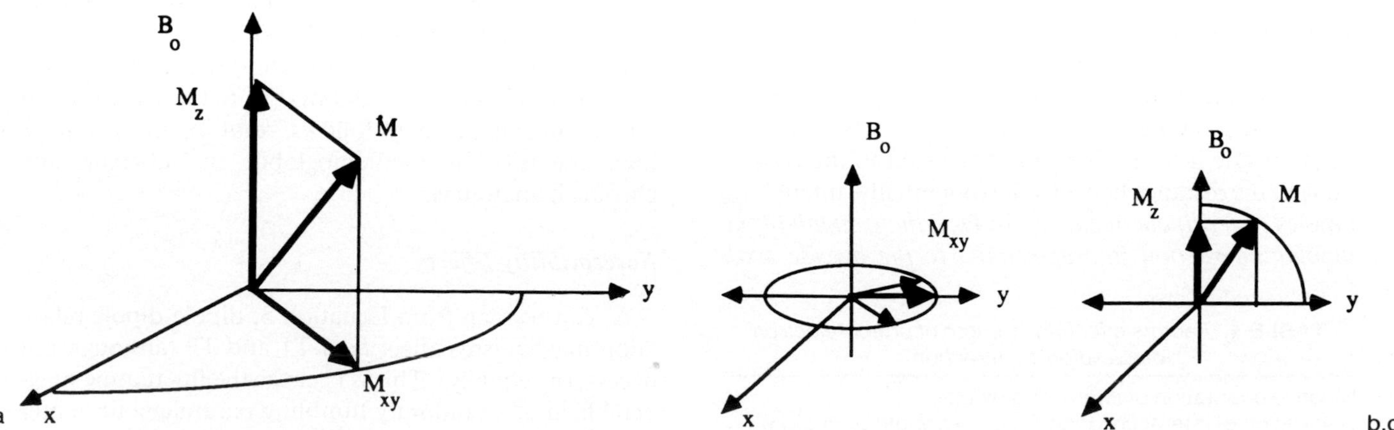

FIG. 4. Nuclear magnetization detected in the MR image is generated by rotating the equilibrium magnetization along $\mathbf{B}_0$ into the x-y plane to give $\mathbf{M}_{xy}$ (**a**), which then relaxes within the x-y plane (**b**) characterized by the transverse relaxation time T2* and along $\mathbf{B}_0$ as $\mathbf{M}_z$ (**c**) characterized by the longitudinal relaxation time T1.

with a paramagnetic agent, P, in bulk solution is given as:

$$1/T_{i(obs)} = 1/T_{i(dia)} + 1/T_{i(para)} \quad [3]$$

where

$$1/T_{i(para)} R[P] \quad [4]$$

and $i = 1, 2$; R is the relaxivity constant ($sec^{-1}\ mM^{-1}$); and $[P]$ is the concentration (mM) of the paramagnetic substance P. $1/T_{i(dia)}$ is the relaxation rate due to diamagnetic relaxation processes and $1/T_{i(para)}$ is the relaxation rate in the presence of the paramagnetic species. In the presence of a suitable paramagnetic substance, the paramagnetic term dominates over the diamagnetic term in Equation 3. The same equation applies for both longitudinal and transverse relaxation. Because T1 is generally longer than T2 in biological systems, 1/T1 is smaller than 1/T2 and so the constant term $R[P]$ contributes a greater proportion to the longitudinal relaxation rate (1/T1) than transverse relaxation rate (1/T2). The implication for MRI is that the *relaxivity effects attributed to dipole-dipole interactions with paramagnetic substances are detected with greater sensitivity on T1-weighted (short TR/TE) images than on T2-weighted (long TR/TE) images.*

The contributions of "inner-sphere" (ligand exchange in which water molecules are in the first coordination sphere of P) and "outer-sphere" (diffusion with close approach of water near, but without coordination to P) effects to paramagnetic relaxation rates can be further analyzed by the more mechanistic Solomon-Bloembergen equations, which are presented in detail elsewhere (31). It should be noted that application of Equation 3 to biological systems as complex as cerebral hematomas can only be approximate because of the heterogeneity in type and distribution of the various paramagnetic substances involved.

The strength of the dipole-dipole interaction between water and paramagnetic substances is dependent upon several factors (Table 4), including: the number of unpaired electrons in the paramagnetic material (which, in turn, determines the magnetic moment), the concentration of the paramagnetic substance, the electron spin relaxation rate, and, perhaps most relevant to the clinical images, the distance between the (potentially) interacting dipoles *(interdipole distance).* In fact, *the strength of the dipolar interaction is proportional to the inverse sixth power of the interdipole distance* (Fig. 5). The implication of this geographical restriction on the strength of relaxation enhancement is profound, when one considers the MR intensity pattern in acute hematomas. When the water proton is unable to approximate close enough to the paramagnetic center (i.e., the unpaired electrons of deoxyhemoglobin), no dipole-dipole magnetic interaction, and therefore no relaxation enhancement, occurs by relaxivity mechanisms. This failure of interaction can be ascribed to the quaternary structure of deoxyhemoglobin (Fig. 6) (32). Therefore, even though deoxyhemoglobin is clearly paramagnetic, the acute hematoma is not hyperintense on short TR/TE (T1-weighted) images. Following the acute event, when deoxyhemoglobin undergoes conversion to methemoglobin, conformational changes in the hemoglobin molecule-iron complex result in accessibility of the water proton to the unpaired electrons of iron in methemoglobin (Fig. 6) (32), and dipolar relaxation enhancement follows, resulting in the typical high intensity of methemoglobin in subacute and chronic hematomas.

TABLE 4. *Factors affecting strength of proton-electron dipole-dipole interaction*

Relative orientation of interacting dipoles
Separation of interacting dipoles, i.e., strength of PEDD α (1/interdipole distance)^6
Concentration of paramagnetic centers
Number of unpaired electrons per paramagnetic center
Electron spin relaxation rate

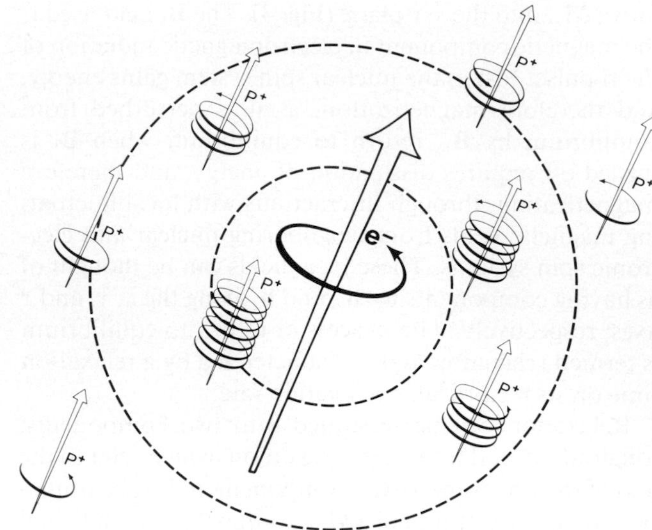

FIG. 5. Proton-electron dipole-dipole interaction schematic. The magnetic movement μ of the unpaired electron (e^-) in the paramagnetic center is much larger (~700 times) than that of the water protons (p^+), as denoted by the larger arrow of the e^-. The distance between the dipoles strongly influences the strength of the interaction (see text). The longer spirals imply stronger interactions at shorter distances between dipoles.

Susceptibility Effects

As can be seen from Equation 3, dipole-dipole relaxation mechanisms affect *both* T1 and T2 (although not necessarily equally). This is because the fluctuating magnetic field of a randomly tumbling paramagnetic center is *isotropic*, operating along the x, y, and z axes. Magnetic susceptibility-induced relaxation, in contrast, does *not* affect both T1 and T2. This *selective T2 relaxation enhancement* can be understood by considering the precise

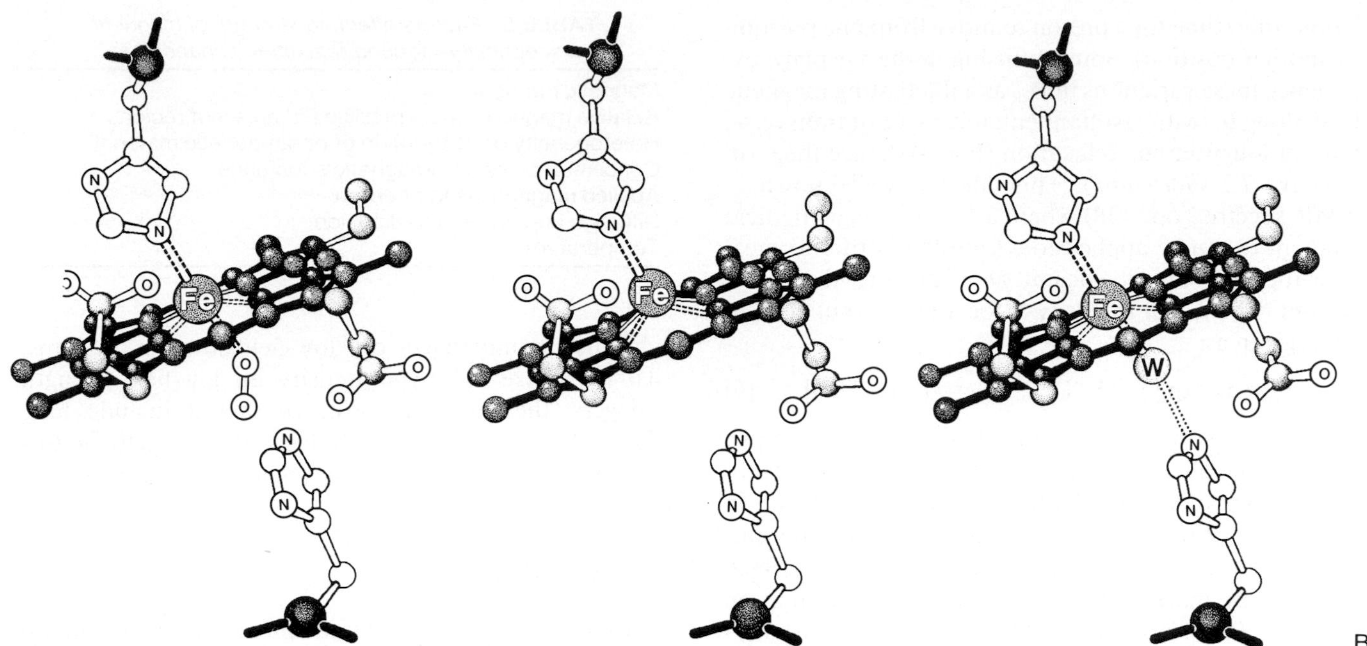

FIG. 6. Structure of hemoglobin complex in various stages of evolving hemorrhage. **A:** Oxyhemoglobin. **B:** Deoxyhemoglobin. **C:** Methemoglobin. Note that iron (Fe) is nearly within the same plane as the atoms comprising the porphyrin ring *(dark color)* in the oxyhemoglobin (A) molecule. Upon deoxygenation, there is a subtle alteration in the position of Fe to become positioned outside of the porphyrin plane (B), which prevents access to water. In the methemoglobin state (C), note that the Fe is now positioned again nearly within the plane of the porphyrin ring, allowing close approximation by water (*W*). (Courtesy of Dr. Peter Janick, Philadelphia, PA, as modified from Dickerson and Geis, ref. 32, with permission.)

mechanisms involved in generating magnetic susceptibility effects. There are two types of static magnetic fields that are highly *anisotropic,* operating only in the direction of the main field $\mathbf{B}_0$: (i) inhomogeneities in $\mathbf{B}_0$ due to magnet imperfections, and (ii) magnetic susceptibility-induced field variations $\mathbf{B}_{eff}$. If the inhomogeneities in $\mathbf{B}_{eff}$ are large over the dimensions of the voxel, the field variations produce a dispersion in frequencies within the voxel, leading to rapid loss of transverse magnetization (this has also been described as *loss of phase coherence* of spins within that voxel). The combination of this loss of transverse magnetization from $\mathbf{B}_0$ inhomogeneities with dipole-dipole relaxation mechanisms is characterized by a combined relaxation time termed T2* [note that T2* refers to total transverse relaxation, and can be described by the equation:

$$1/T2^* = 1/T2 + 1/T2' + 1/T2'' \quad [5]$$

where T2 equals the transverse relaxation induced by spin-spin interactions, T2″ equals the transverse relaxation from $\mathbf{B}_0$ inhomogeneities, and T2′ equals the transverse relaxation related to susceptibility-gradient-induced field inhomogeneities]. Spin-echo imaging minimizes the effects of static magnetic field variations (field inhomogeneities) with the use of the 180° refocusing rf pulse. In fact, this recovery of signal loss from field inhomogeneity is probably the major reason for the success of the spin-echo technique in imaging! Conversely, reversal of the readout gradient in the absence of a 180° rf pulse, which is utilized in gradient-echo imaging for generation of the echo, does not compensate for signal loss due to field inhomogeneities. As a consequence of the gradient-echo technique, gradient-echo imaging is extremely sensitive to field inhomogeneities, a feature that assumes greater importance at lower field strengths (33) (see Chapter 26).

An additional cause of phase-dispersion-induced signal loss (see also Chapter 2) distinct from that due to *static* field variations (as described above) relates to what can be considered *time-varying* magnetic field changes.

The molecular diffusion of water that occurs through regions of variable $\mathbf{B}_{eff}$ during TE (time between the 90° rf pulse and echo) produces frequency variations (Equation 2) and concomitant loss of phase coherence in the transverse plane resulting in signal loss in $\mathbf{M}_{xy}$. The local fields experienced by the moving spins over the time of diffusion, although the fields themselves are static, are analogous to a situation in which spins are stationary and the field is changing over that same period of time. In effect, then, the field itself can be considered to be varying over the time of spin diffusion. Note that this loss of signal is not recovered by the 180° rf pulse of the spin-echo sequence, so, in fact, both conventional spin-echo imaging and gradient-echo techniques are sensitive to this cause of hypointensity. This effect becomes more apparent as the echo time TE exceeds the diffusional correlation time (time for a proton to move from one position to another position). Spins diffusing in the x-y plane experience these variations in $\mathbf{B}_{eff}$ as a fluctuating magnetic field along $\mathbf{b}_z$, with resultant enhancement of transverse, but not longitudinal, relaxation (Fig. 3) (hence the term *selective T2 shortening*). This effect is well known in NMR spectroscopy (28) where a known magnetic field gradient G can be applied to a sample in order to measure the diffusion coefficient D of protons through a solvent. The signal intensity S for a Hahn spin echo at TE is given as:

$$S = S_0 \exp\left[-(\mathrm{TE}/\mathrm{T2} + \tfrac{1}{12}\cdot\gamma^2\cdot G^2\cdot D\cdot \mathrm{TE}^3)\right]. \qquad [6]$$

Differences in susceptibilities between, for example, compartmentalized paramagnetic deoxyhemoglobin within a red blood cell and diamagnetic water can result in significant T2 relaxation if sufficient diffusion is permitted to occur during the imaging sequence (Fig. 7). Such effects cause marked signal loss in acute hematomas on long TR/TE (T2-weighted) MR images without corresponding degrees of signal loss on either long TR/short TE or short TR/TE (T1-weighted) MR images. It has also been shown (34) that the use of prolonged interecho intervals (τ_{cpmg}) results in shortening of the effective T2, again by allowing more diffusion of water protons through areas of differing magnetic fields. The clinical importance of understanding this diffusion-related mechanism of T2 shortening is clear, when one considers the clinical situation of attempting to depict acute (or chronic) hemorrhage on low-field-strength systems. To maximize the hypointensity on low-field-strength imagers, the long TR protocol should include long TE with very long τ_{cpmg}. Indeed, the strength of this T2-shortening mechanism is related to several factors (Table 5).

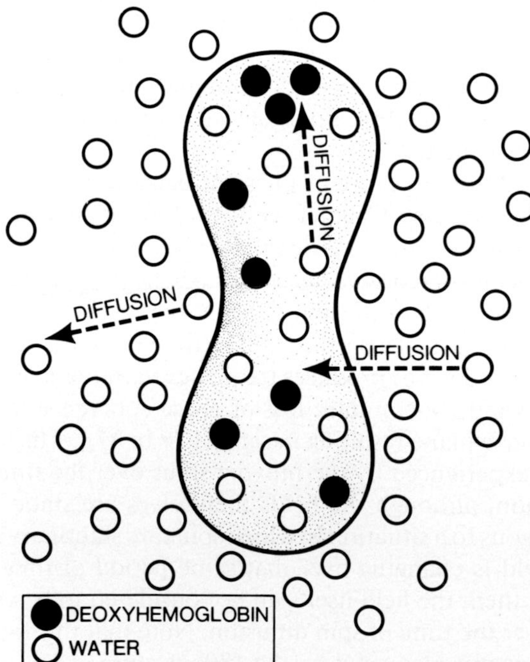

FIG. 7. Compartmentalized paramagnetic deoxyhemoglobin within regions of an intact red blood cell results in areas of different magnetic susceptibility, both within the confines of the cell as well as compared with the diamagnetic extracellular water. Therefore, as water diffuses through these regions, it experiences different magnetic fields.

TABLE 5. *Factors affecting strength of magnetic susceptibility-induced relaxation enhancement*

Magnetic moment
Relative magnetic susceptibilities of adjacent regions
Heterogeneity of distribution of paramagnetic material
Concentration of paramagnetic substance
Applied magnetic field strength
Diffusion and barriers to diffusion
Temperature

Exchange Processes

Changes in the (nonparamagnetic) protein content within the hematoma also occur as clot formation, clot contraction, and necrosis occur. From in vitro studies (35–37), increasing protein concentration would be expected to promote T1 and T2 relaxation rates. It is possible that the exchange of water between bulk phase and protein-bound (hydration layer) phases (see Chapter 2) may be a significant contributor to proton relaxation in some situations of hemorrhage, especially on low-field scanners, where paramagnetic susceptibility mechanisms are not nearly as prominent as on high-field imagers. In fact, the lack of susceptibility-induced relaxation effects accounts for the lack of marked hypointensity (and therefore, the lack of ability to detect with certainty) in most acute hematomas at low field.

Investigators (19) have demonstrated that changes in red blood cell volumes may be responsible for some of the changes in T2 relaxation rates in hematomas. With shrinkage of red blood cells due to decreases in intracellular water, it has been shown that T2 can decrease significantly in in vitro studies of blood clots. This relaxation rate increase is probably related to protein concentration-dependent changes in the correlation time (a viscosity effect) (38), but further work needs to be done to clarify the significance of this mechanism in the in vivo hematoma.

In an attempt to quantify the effects of deoxygenation, protein (hematocrit), clot formation, and clot retraction in generating signal intensity changes of acute hematomas, an investigation was performed by Clark and colleagues (20). In their study, it was apparent that the contributions of fibrin clot formation and clot retraction to T2 shortening were minimal (less than 2% combined). Furthermore, the great majority of T2 shortening was related to deoxygenation, with the remainder of change in T2 associated with hemoconcentration.

Increasing edema has also been suggested to allow increased diffusion rates by removing diffusional barriers, such as macromolecules and cell membranes, thereby promoting T2 relaxation. In areas of necrosis, diffusional barriers may not be removed to the same degree as in vasogenic edema in relatively intact tissue. The relative influences of diffusion, protein exchange, and aggregation on in vivo relaxation processes cannot be predicted as yet.

Field Strength Effects

Nuclear magnetic relaxation dispersion (NMRD) describes the variation of 1/T1 and 1/T2 with magnetic field strength. A formal mathematical treatment of NMRD has been presented elsewhere (39). The observations relevant to hemorrhage are summarized as follows. At zero magnetic field, 1/T1 = 1/T2. As field strength increases, the Larmor frequency changes according to Equation 2. The efficiency of relaxation requires matching correlation times of local fluctuating magnetic fields generated by rotational and translational diffusion to the Larmor frequency. This occurs over a wide range (10^{-10} to 10^{-11} sec) corresponding to low imaging field strengths where the effects on T1 and T2 relaxation rates are comparable. At higher fields, 1/T1 tends toward zero, but 1/T2 tends to a nonzero value termed the "secular" contribution to relaxation. This contribution to T2, but not to the T1 relaxation rate, arises from the local fluctuating fields parallel to $\mathbf{B}_0$ as described above for susceptibility-induced relaxation. Hence, higher magnetic field strengths enhance susceptibility effects. In vitro studies of deoxygenated erythrocytes show a quadratic dependence of 1/T2 on magnetic field strength over a range of 2 to 5 T (16). The importance of the imaging parameters in determining sensitivity to the susceptibility effects has been emphasized by in vitro studies of blood clots (8). Clinical experience has also indicated that higher imaging magnetic field strengths increase sensitivity of spin-echo images to susceptibility-induced relaxation mechanisms, irrespective of the source of the susceptibility variation (12,39). Note that the contrast in acute hemorrhage, for example, which is mainly based on T2 shortening from deoxyhemoglobin (12,20), may not be detected on low-field-strength systems using conventional spin-echo techniques, since the effect is approximately proportional to the square of the magnetic field (16). Therefore, the signal intensity in these lesions on low-field-strength magnets may be similar to nonparamagnetic lesions, where contrast is determined mainly by such factors as water content and the presence of macromolecules (e.g., hemoglobin and other plasma proteins, in the case of blood).

MR Imaging in Hemorrhage: Technical Considerations

MR contrast in the presence of hemorrhage is highly dependent on the mode of image acquisition (Table 2). Image acquisition protocols generally use four basic pulse sequences (Fig. 8). The spin-echo (SE) sequence uses a 90° rf pulse to convert the equilibrium longitudinal magnetization $\mathbf{M}_z$ into transverse magnetization $\mathbf{M}_{xy}$ and then a 180° rf pulse to refocus the dephasing in $\mathbf{M}_{xy}$ (due to $\mathbf{B}_0$ inhomogeneities) to generate an echo. This approach provides the time necessary for gradient switching required to perform spatial encoding. This sequence was designed to correct the otherwise deleterious effects of magnet imperfections ($\mathbf{B}_0$ inhomogeneities) that cause rapid signal loss. However, if the $\mathbf{B}_0$ inhomogeneities arise from the lesion itself, as in hematomas, the MR contrast that would have reflected this phenomenon would also be diminished. The effects of diffusion of water through the localized magnetic field gradients are not corrected unless the echo time TE is made very short rel-

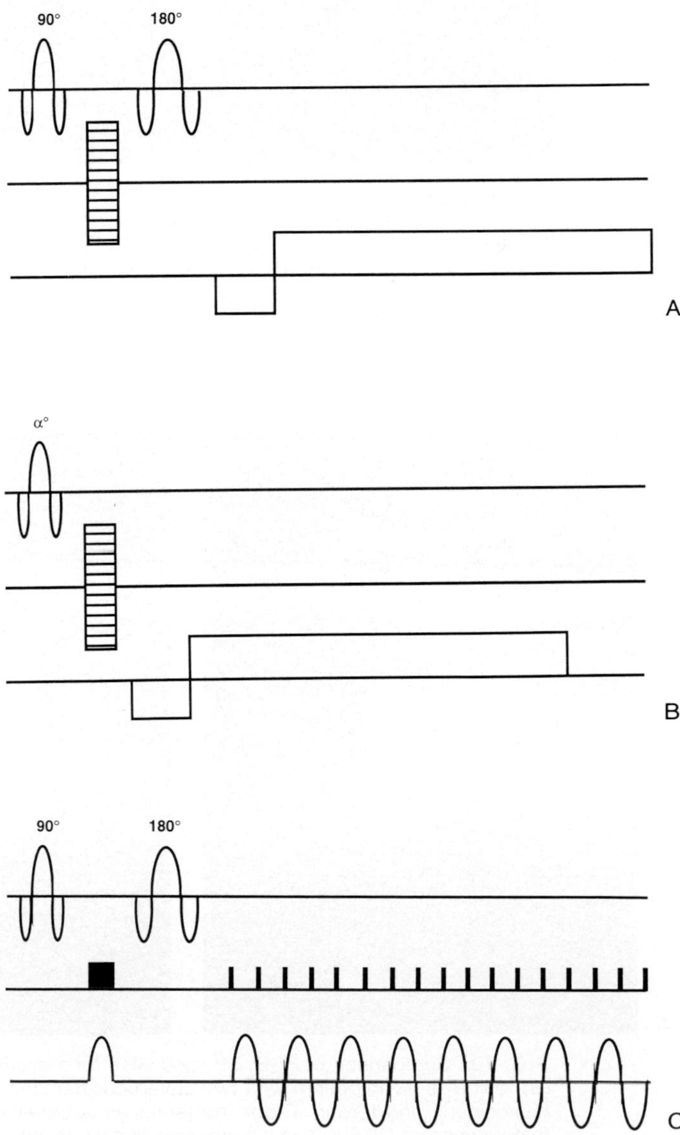

FIG. 8. Timing diagrams for spin-echo (**A**), gradient-recalled echo (**B**), and echo-planar (**C**) pulse sequences showing the rf pulses (90°, 180°, and α°) and two in-plane spatial-encoding gradients. (The slice-selection gradient is not shown as it is the same in all sequences.)

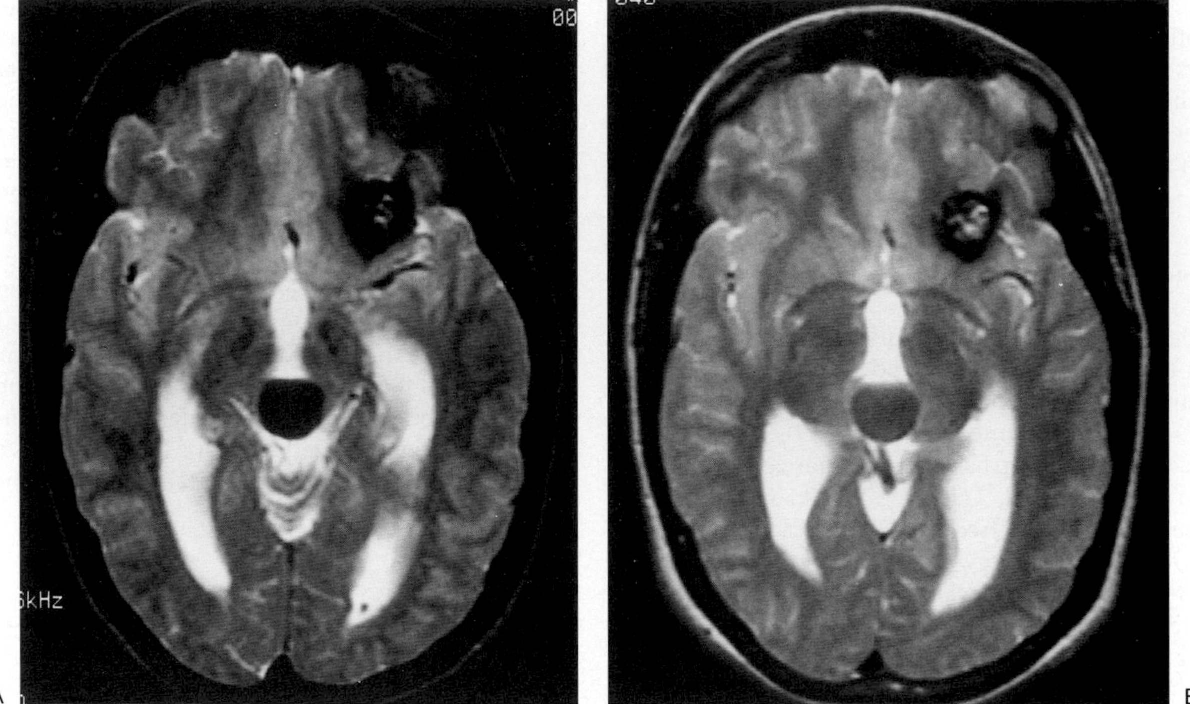

FIG. 9. Effect of interecho time τ_{cpmg}: (SE vs. FSE). Axial images obtained with the same TR and TE (or effective TE) using conventional SE (**A**) and FSE (**B**) sequences obtained in a patient with multiple cavernous hemangiomas. Note that using a long τ_{cpmg} in conventional SE (A), the acute pineal region hemorrhage is markedly hypointense, whereas using a short τ_{cpmg} in FSE (B) the lesion is less hypointense. These differences are seen despite the same TR and TE of these two images.

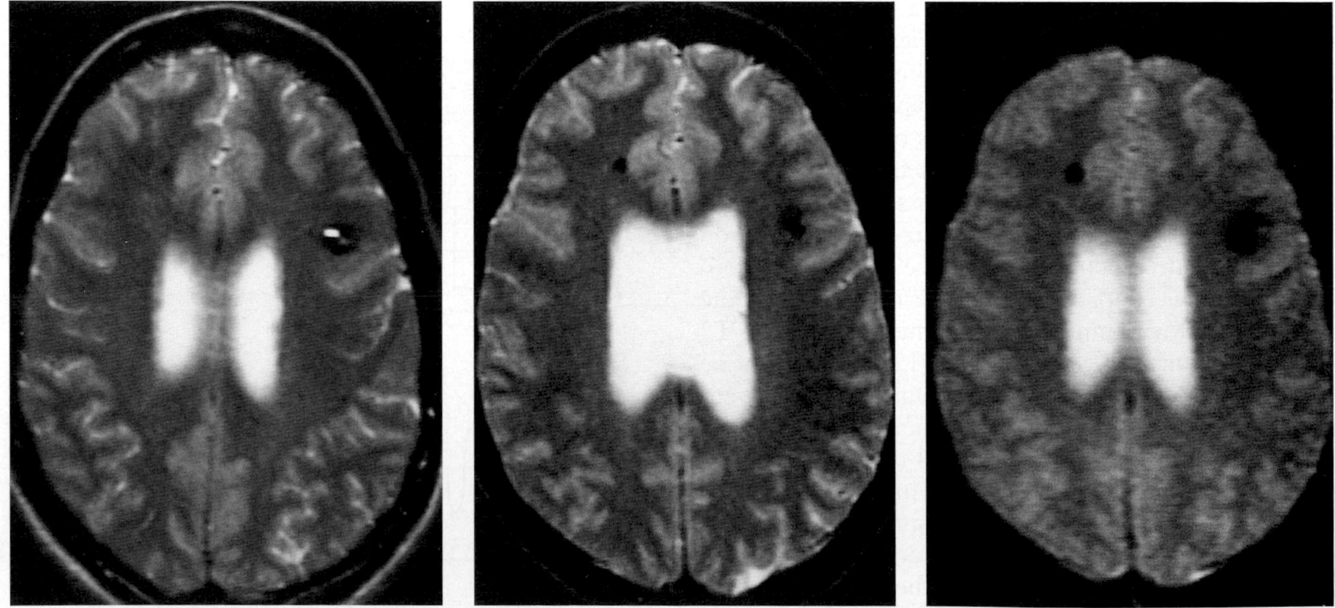

FIG. 10. Comparison of FSE, SE, and GRE for sensitivity to hemorrhage. Axial images obtained with FSE (**A**), SE (**B**), and GRE (**C**) in patient with two cavernous hemangiomas show slight differences in depiction of hypointensity of hemosiderin and ferritin. Right frontal lesion is barely visible on FSE (A), more obvious on SE (B), and markedly hypointense on GRE image (C). Internal signal pattern of left frontal lesion is only visible on FSE (A), because heightened sensitivity to susceptibility-induced signal loss on both SE (B) and GRE (C) obscures the internal architecture of the lesion.

ative to the correlation time of water diffusion. Magnet and gradient technologies have improved dramatically since SE imaging was introduced. Hence, magnet imperfections are seldom a dominant effect and values of TE are becoming much shorter without loss of image quality from artifacts generated by rapid gradient switching. These improvements have led to faster alternative and adjunctive sequences (see Chapter 29).

The gradient-recalled echo (GRE) sequence uses a rf pulse (usually less than 90°) to convert only part of the equilibrium longitudinal magnetization $\mathbf{M}_z$ into $\mathbf{M}_{xy}$ and replaces the 180° rf pulse with a gradient reversal to rephase the spins to produce the echo. Although sensitivity to paramagnetic constituents of hematomas is increased, the penalty is that normally occurring border zones of differing susceptibility (e.g., air-tissue interfaces) also produce signal loss decreasing visualization of large regions of the brain. Care must be taken to avoid mistaking artifacts for pathology in these regions particularly around the petrous bones and paranasal sinuses. Since these intravoxel dephasing effects are dependent on voxel size, various maneuvers are commonly employed to obviate problematic artifacts (see Chapter 29).

The improvement in gradient switching technology has permitted shortening of the interecho time, τ_{cpmg}, and an increase in the number of echoes per TR used in the fast spin-echo (FSE) sequence. This sequence differs from the conventional SE sequence by using a train of 180° rf pulses to generate a set of echoes which are individually spatially encoded during a single TR. This significantly shortens the total acquisition time, as several spatial encoding steps are performed in a single pulse train. The implications in the setting of cerebral hematoma are that dephasing effects in the presence of heterogeneous magnetic susceptibilities are virtually removed by the spin echoes. Moreover, the short τ_{cpmg} minimizes the signal loss effects of diffusion (Fig. 9). Hence, "T2-weighted" FSE has lower sensitivity for the hypointensity of both acute and remote hemorrhage than conventional SE images. If the clinical history suggests that hemorrhage may be present, conventional long TR/TE SE sequences or alternatively supplemental GRE scanning should be utilized (Fig. 10).

Echo-planar (EP) imaging sequences are also becoming available from all the major manufacturers. The EP sequence uses a single rf pulse train of either SE or GRE format with a complete two-dimensional spatial-encoding scheme of gradient switching ("single shot EPI"). Various ways of implementing the readout gradients are available and are outside the scope of this chapter (40). The advantage of the EP method is the very high temporal resolution, so that images of the brain can be

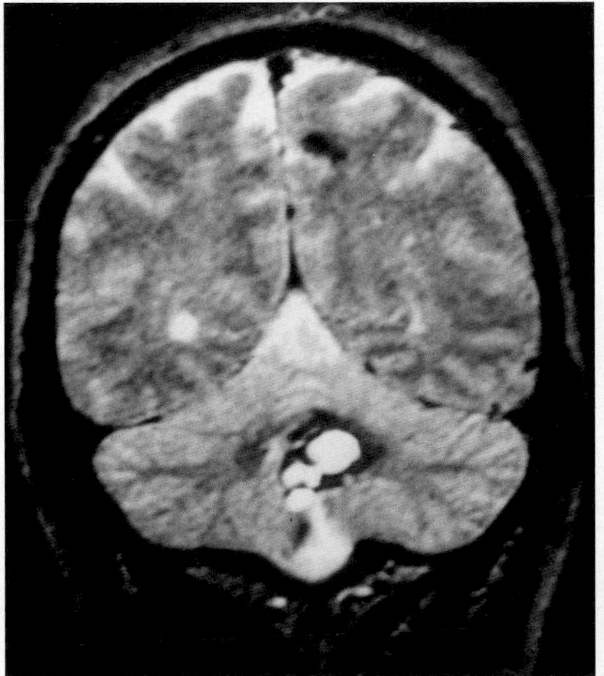
A

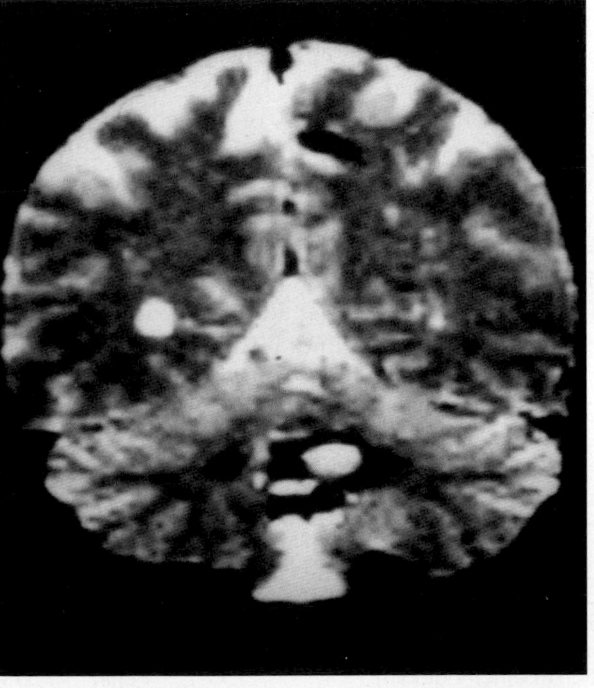
B

FIG. 11. Coronal images through the brain of a middle-aged male with multiple cavernous hemangiomas obtained using a SE sequence (**A**) (acquisition parameters: TR = 2308 msec, TE = 80 msec, matrix size = 256 × 192, 1 NEX, total acquisition time = 8:28 minute) and a EP sequence (**B**) (acquisition parameters: TR = 6000 msec, TE = 73 msec, full *k*-space, single rf pulse train, matrix size = 128 × 64, 1 NEX, total acquisition time <100 msec). The patient has multiple cavernous hemangiomas with different stages of hemorrhage, both showing increased peripheral signal loss on the EP image.

TABLE 6. *General guidelines for temporal evolution of signal intensities of hematomas on MR at 1.5 T*

Biochemical form	Approximate time of appearance	Short TR/TE[a]	Long TR/TE[a]
Oxyhemoglobin	Immediately–first several hours	≈ or ↓	↑
Deoxyhemoglobin	Hours–several days	≈ or ↓	↓↓
Intracellular methemoglobin	First several days	↑↑	↓↓
Extracellular methemoglobin	Several days–months	↑↑	↑↑
Ferritin/hemosiderin	Several days–indefinitely	≈ or ↓	↓↓

[a] Signal intensities on short and long TR/TE images are relative to normal gray matter.

obtained on the order of tens of milliseconds. EP methods are very sensitive to magnetic susceptibility effects in both the SE and GRE modes due to the nature of the variable readout gradients (note that in "spin echo" EPI, only a single 180° rf pulse is used to generate an echo at the selected TE, while many gradient reversals are used without 180° pulses; i.e., even SE EPI utilizes gradient refocusing) (Fig. 11) (see Chapters 3 and 29).

EVOLUTION OF INTRAPARENCHYMAL HEMATOMAS

Using the concepts of relaxation discussed in the preceding sections, it is possible to understand the appearance of the various stages in the biochemical evolution of intracranial hemorrhage. Although some variations can certainly occur, the vast majority of intracranial hematomas behave in a predictable fashion as they change over time (Table 6). The exact time course of biochemical changes (41) may vary, depending on the pathophysiologic state, as well as on specific imaging technical factors (Tables 1 and 2). In truth, the clinical dating of the actual hemorrhagic event is notoriously inaccurate, so the nomenclature of the temporal stages of hematomas is somewhat arbitrary. Of those factors that are intrinsic to the anatomy and pathophysiology of the lesion, those known to be most important to image interpretation include the age of the hemorrhage, the location of the bleed (i.e., intra-axial vs. extra-axial, subarachnoid vs. subdural/epidural) (42), and the presence of an underlying lesion (43,44) and its effect on the blood–brain barrier (44) and on the repair response mounted by the patient. Well-vascularized regions, for instance, would be expected to show a faster repair response than poorly vascularized regions. Such variability has been reported from biochemical studies of hemorrhage outside the central nervous system (45). Furthermore, the radiologist must be cognizant of the operator-dependent factors that potentially change the MRI appearance of hemorrhage (Table 2), including the main magnetic field strength, the exact pulse sequence parameters used (34), and the method of echo formation (i.e., SE, GRE, FSE, or EP) (6). In the following discussion, all images are spin-echo unless otherwise stated. Short TR/TE images utilized TR of 500–800 msec, and TE of 10–25 msec. Long TR images used TR of 2500–3000 msec, and TEs were either short (less than 30 msec) or long (greater than 70 msec). All images were acquired at 1.5 T.

It seems that the most important factor that determines the signal intensity of blood is related to the magnetic properties of iron in the various hemorrhage breakdown products. The magnetic properties of iron, determined by its electronic configuration, vary with its

TABLE 7. *Iron metabolic states in cerebral hemorrhage and MR relaxation effects*

Metabolic phase	Oxidation state	Distribution	Magnetic property	Relaxation process	
				Relaxivity	Susceptibility
Oxygenation (oxyhemoglobin)	Fe(II)	Within RBC	Diamagnetic	—	—
Deoxygenation (deoxyhemoglobin)	Fe(II)	Within RBC	Paramagnetic	—	+
Oxidation (methemoglobin)	Fe(III)	1) Within RBC	Paramagnetic	+	+
		2) Extracellular	Paramagnetic	+	—
Chelation/transport (transferrin, lactoferrin)	Fe(III)	Extracellular	Paramagnetic	+	+
Iron storage (ferritin, hemosiderin)	Fe(III)	Within macrophages and glial cells	Paramagnetic	—	+

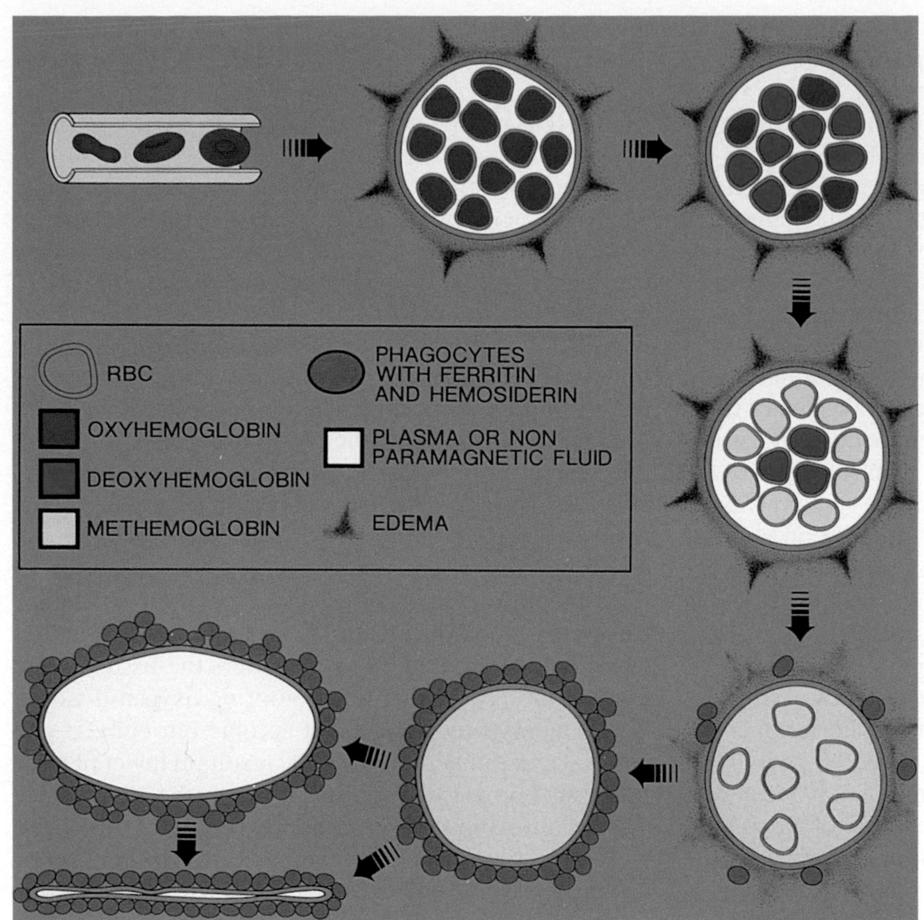

FIG. 12. Summary of biochemical evolution of resolving hematoma. Immediately after hemorrhagic event, oxyhemoglobin comprises hematoma, which is surrounded by edema. Within hours, clot retraction occurs concomitantly with deoxygenation. (Note: in the rarely seen "hyperacute hematoma," very early deoxygenation within the periphery of the hematoma can be seen.) Peripherally and subsequently throughout the hematoma, methemoglobin is formed. During the conversion to methemoglobin, red blood cell integrity is lost, edema resolves, and phagocytes accumulate iron breakdown products at the periphery of hematoma in adjacent brain parenchyma. Finally, chronic hematoma can contain nonparamagnetic fluid or is simply a collapsed cleft lined by chronic iron forms.

biochemical form, spatial distribution, and oxidation state. The changing electronic configuration is summarized in Table 7 and Fig. 12 to demonstrate how the magnetic properties of hemorrhage and hence the nuclear relaxation processes that underlie the signal contrast in the MR image depend on the biochemical pathways of iron metabolism.

Although iron is the most abundant transition metal in the human body, being vital for oxygen transport by hemoglobin in the erythrocyte of blood as well as many catalytic processes involving enzymes, free iron is toxic, as is demonstrated by toxic ingestions and iron overload states (46–48). The toxicity, believed to be due to enhanced free radical production by unchelated iron (49), requires that all iron be tightly bound in well-controlled metabolic pathways of absorption, transport, storage, and conversion into functional end products. The repair of hemorrhage requires a tightly controlled iron salvage pathway in which iron from the extravasated erythrocytes is mobilized from hemoglobin, detoxified by chelation to short-term iron transport proteins for transfer back to the reticuloendothelial system, or converted to long-term storage proteins for local deposition (47,50,51).

"Hyperacute" Hematoma

Freshly extravasated erythrocytes of arterial blood contain fully oxygenated hemoglobin. Hemoglobin is a tetramer of polypeptide chains, with each polypeptide chain having a prosthetic heme group bound within a hydrophobic cleft (32,53). Each heme group is a protoporphyrin IX, chelating a single iron in the ferrous oxidation state (6 *d* electrons). Initially, the iron is bound in octahedral geometry with six ligands. The tetrapyrrole nitrogens of the protoporphyrin constitute four ligands in a plane around the iron. The imidazole group of a histidine from the polypeptide chain is the ligand below the protoporphyrin plane, while molecular oxygen is the exchangeable ligand above the plane. The interaction of the six ligands with the metal center in *oxyhemoglobin* causes the six outer electrons in the five *d* orbitals of the ferrous ion to pair in the electronic orbitals of the lowest energy (Fig. 1). As there are no unpaired electrons in the iron (or other atoms in hemoglobin), oxygenated blood is diamagnetic ($\chi < 0$).

At the time immediately following the initial episode of bleeding, the hematoma can be considered, for practical purposes, to be composed of intact red blood cells containing oxygenated hemoglobin. Other components of blood are also present, including serum proteins, platelets, etc., but they probably contribute little to the MR image (20,52). Since there is no paramagnetic component of blood at this time, there can be no proton-electron dipole-dipole interaction, and no paramagnetic relaxation enhancement. The *"hyperacute"* hematoma would appear nearly identical to most brain lesions on MR—essentially as a high-spin-density region, with slightly shortened relaxation times (compared with water) due mainly to the macromolecular content of blood (i.e., protein content) (54). Hyperacute hematomas are extremely rare in clinical practice, since, in the great majority of patients with intracranial hemorrhage, at least several hours pass before the patient is scanned with MR. Nevertheless, this mainly theoretical lesion can rarely be seen, and would appear slightly hypointense on short TR/TE images and of high intensity on long TR/TE images (Figs. 13 and 14). Note that, in theory, the hyperacute hematoma may not be distinguishable from other intracranial mass lesions (11,55). Clues to the presence of a hyperacute hematoma may be present, however, including a rim of marked hypointensity at the periphery of the lesion on long TR/TE images (Figs. 13 and 14). This probably represents the interdigitation of blood and tissue that leads to very rapid deoxygenation of blood at the blood-tissue interface of the hematoma and a geometry that readily expresses the resultant magnetic susceptibility gradients as signal loss as discussed above. There is evidence from animal models that no iron storage products such as ferritin or hemosiderin are present at this early time (S.W. Atlas and K.R. Thulborn, *unpublished observations*).

Acute Hematoma

The role of hemoglobin is to bind oxygen in the lungs, where the partial pressure of oxygen is high enough to saturate the binding sites on the heme groups, and to transport it to the tissues, where the partial pressure of oxygen is low enough to allow dissociation. The partial pressure of oxygen in tissues undergoing aerobic respiration is lower than that required to saturate fully the oxygen-binding sites of hemoglobin, thus releasing molecular oxygen to the tissues. Within hours after bleeding, several important changes occur that dramatically affect the image of the *acute* hematoma. A cerebral hematoma causes compression of surrounding tissue, reducing perfusion and therefore oxygen delivery from fresh blood to these regions. Deoxygenation of the extravasated blood occurs due to several factors. The underperfused surrounding tissue lowers the tissue partial pressure of oxygen thereby promoting oxygen dissociation. The erythrocytes are not aerobic but convert glucose to lactate anaerobically. The resultant lower pH also promotes oxygen dissociation through the Bohr effect. The accumulation of CO_2 similarly promotes this effect.

The loss of molecular oxygen changes the coordinate geometry of the heme ferrous ion to a five-ligand system of *deoxyhemoglobin* that decreases the energy separation between the groups of higher and lower energy *d* orbitals. The six *d* electrons redistribute among the five *d* subor-

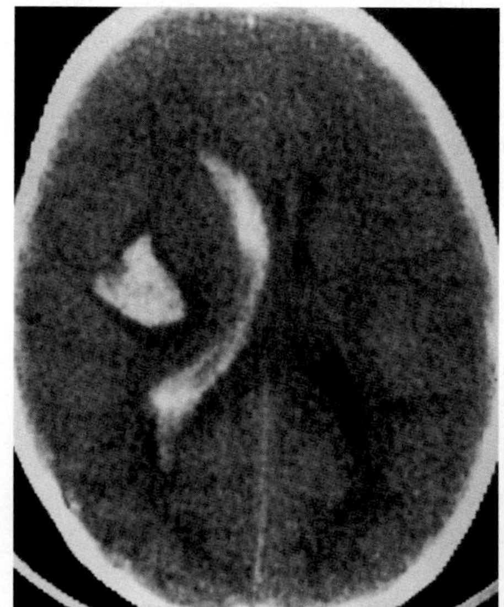
A

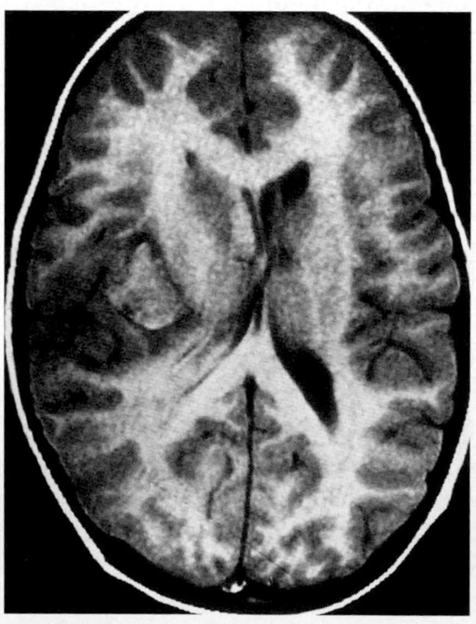

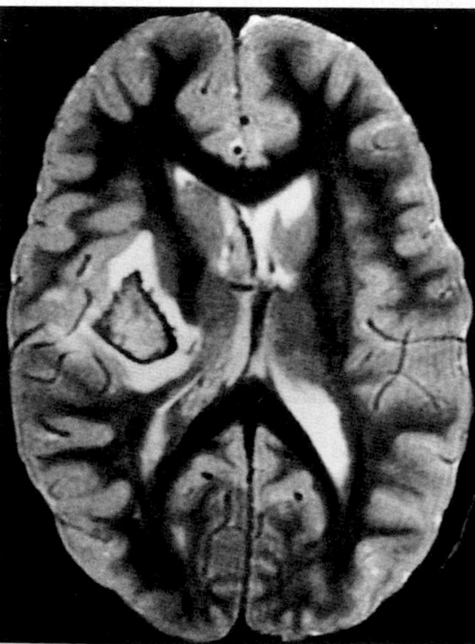
B,C

Fig. 13. A: Axial CT. **B:** Axial short TR/TE MRI. **C:** Axial long TR/TE MRI. Hyperacute hematoma in right subinsular lateral ganglionic region is hyperdense on CT (A) and has dissected into the right lateral ventricle. Hematoma is isointense to gray matter and is surrounded by low intensity from clot retraction on T1-weighted image (B). Note characteristic thin rim of marked hypointensity in periphery of hematoma on T2-weighted image (C) due to early deoxygenation. Serum and edema surrounding lesions are high intensity on T2-weighted image (C).

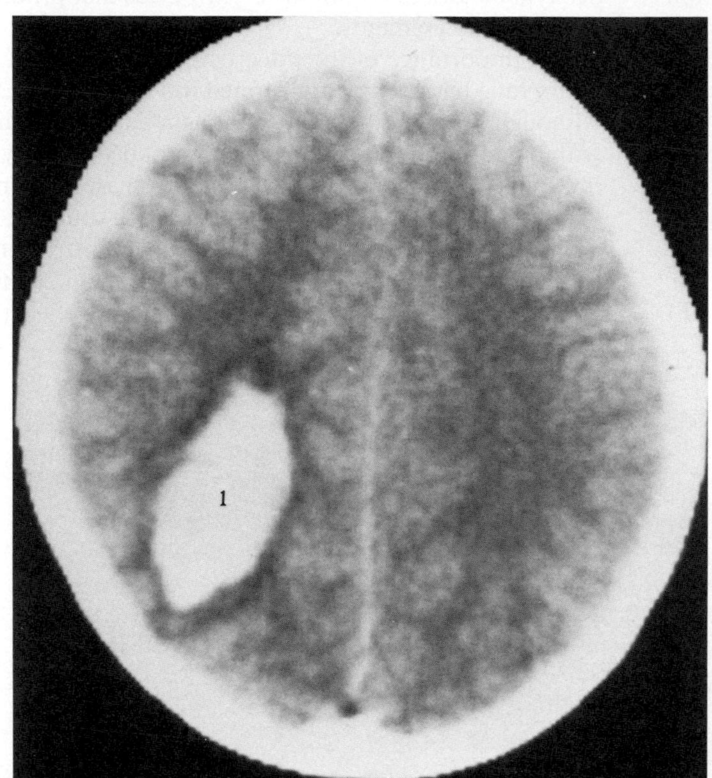

FIG. 14. Hyperacute hematoma (11 hours after ictus). **A:** CT scan. **B:** MRI scan (spoiled gradient echo; 40/5/30° to emphasize T1-based contrast). **C:** Long TR/TE MRI (3000/90). High attenuation right parietal hematoma (*1*) on CT (A) demonstrates slight hypointensity on T1-weighted image (B) and high intensity on T2- weighted image (C), consistent with diamagnetic *oxyhemoglobin.* Again, note thin rim of marked hypointensity (*closed arrows,* C) surrounding hematoma, serum adjacent to hematoma (*2*) from clot retraction, and perihematoma edema (*open arrows*, C).

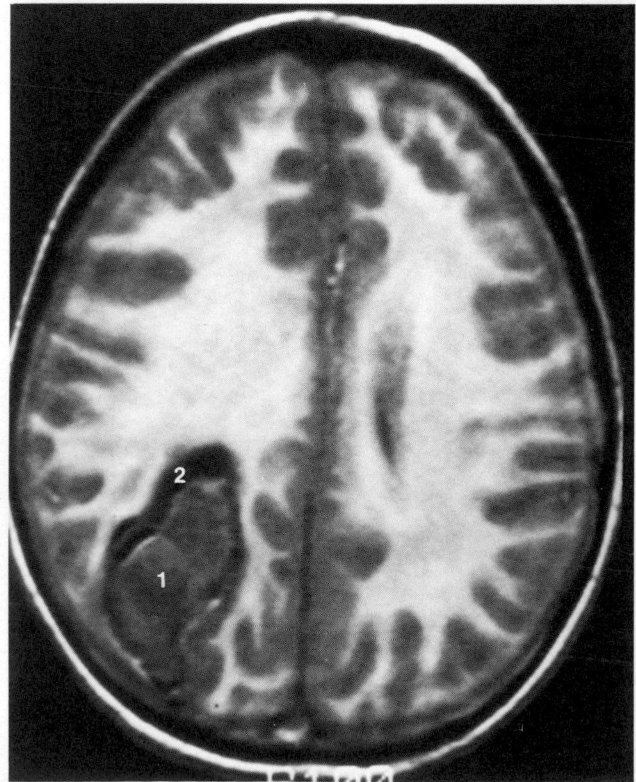

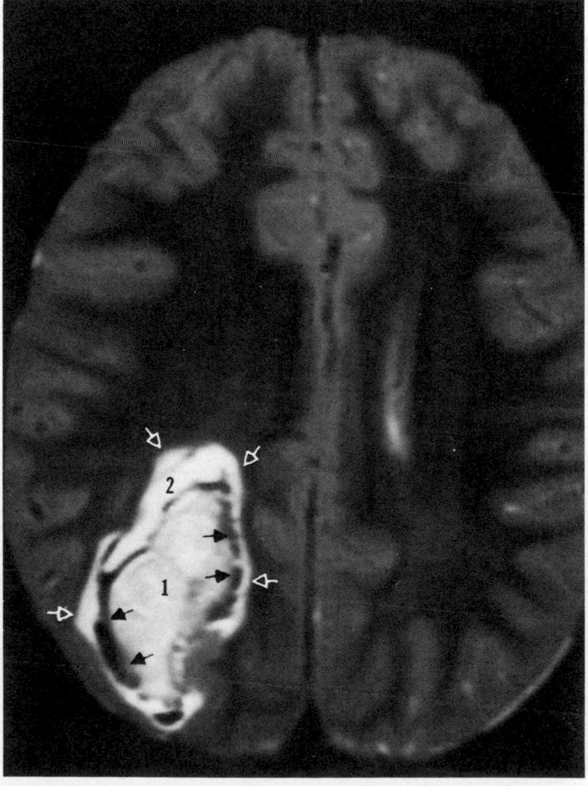

bitals, leaving four unpaired electrons of parallel spin (Fig. 1). Deoxyhemoglobin is thus paramagnetic ($\chi > 0$).

Because the paramagnetic ferrous ion is shielded from the close approach of water molecules by the hydrophobic cleft of the globin protein (Fig. 6), dipole-dipole interactions required for a relaxivity effect cannot occur. However, when deoxyhemoglobin is packaged within erythrocytes, the magnetic susceptibility of the interior of the red blood cell is different from the suspending diamagnetic environment (extracellular plasma), resulting in susceptibility variations within the hematoma. These susceptibility inhomogeneities result in T2* relaxation enhancement that is not mirrored in changes in T1 relaxation. Regardless of the precise site of the field gradients, it is the packaging of the paramagnetic deoxyhemoglobin within the erythrocytes that produces susceptibility gradients.

The importance of the integrity of the red blood cell membrane has been demonstrated in vitro (2,16,53,56). Although the actual site of the magnetic field gradient within or around the erythrocyte has not been clearly delineated, the most convincing evidence based on measurement of line widths of NMR signals for different nuclei with different intra- and extracellular distributions suggests that both intra- and extracellular magnetic field gradients are responsible for the susceptibility effect (7).

A

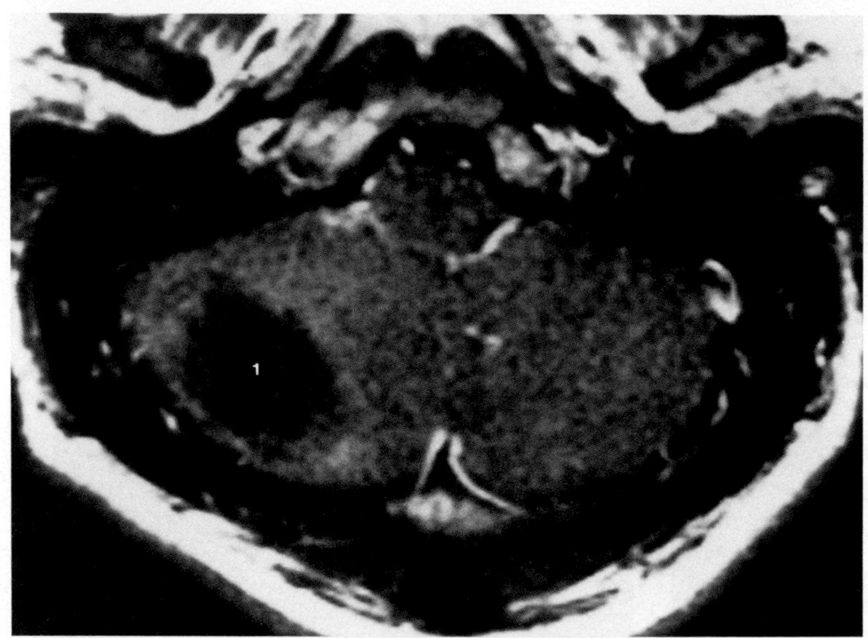

B

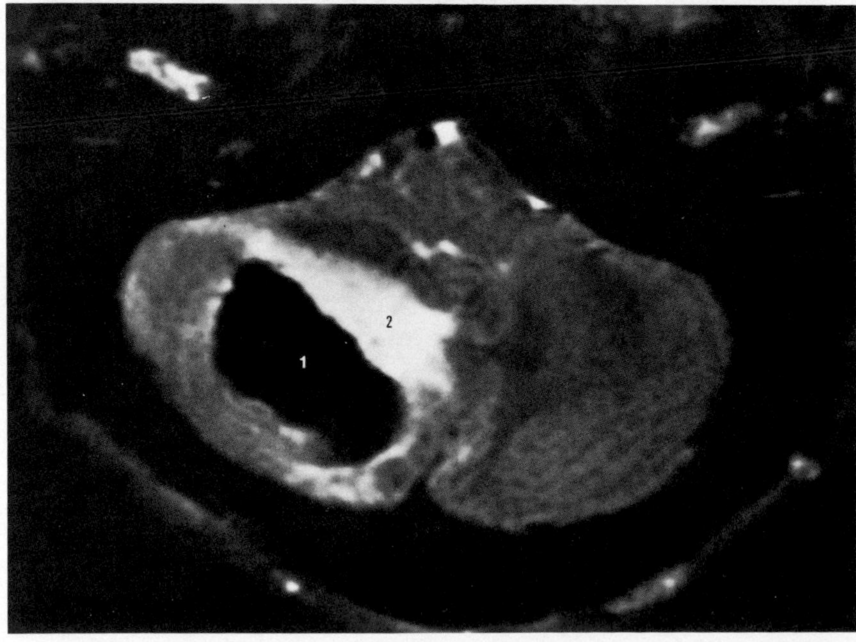

FIG. 15. Acute hematoma (less than 24 hours old). **A:** Short TR/TE MRI (600/20). **B:** Long TR/TE MRI (3000/90). Right cerebellar hematoma (*1*) containing *intracellular deoxyhemoglobin* is slightly hypointense to gray matter on short TR/TE (A) and markedly hypointense on long TR/TE image (B) with surrounding high intensity edema (2, B).

Acute hematomas, which contain intracellular deoxyhemoglobin, consequently appear as markedly hypointense on long TR/TE images (12) (Figs. 15–18). Note that the longer the TE, the more signal decay occurs (Fig. 19). Furthermore, in theory, the longer the interecho interval (the time between the 180° rf pulses, or τ_{cpmg}), the longer the time for the diffusing protons to experience differing magnetic fields, so the shorter the apparent T2 (34). It therefore follows that for the diagnosis of acute hematomas on lower field strength instruments, one should utilize a long TR, but also a very long TE and long τ_{cpmg}, to exploit as much as practically possible the diffusion-related signal decay (note that gradient-echo imaging would also be very useful on low-field systems).

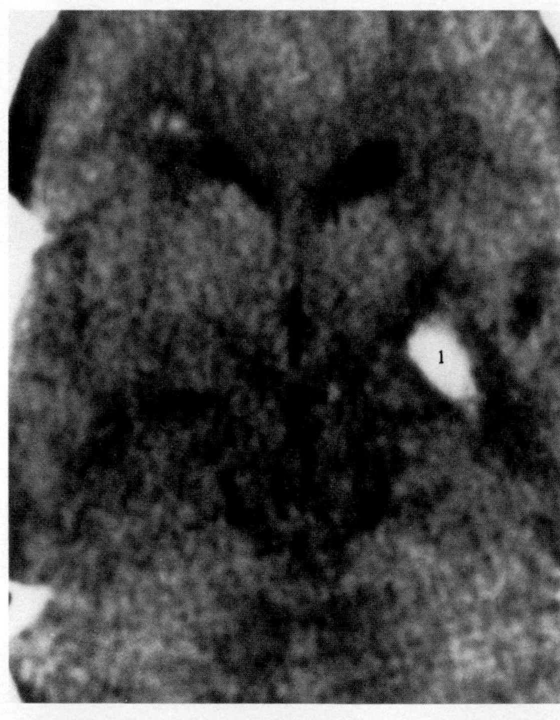

FIG. 16. Acute hematoma (less than 24 hours after trauma). **A:** CT. **B:** Short TR/TE MRI (600/20). **C:** Long TR/TE MRI (2500/80). Left ganglionic post-traumatic hematoma (*1*) (with small right frontal deep white matter hemorrhagic foci) is hyperdense on CT (A). The lesion is slightly hypointense to gray matter on short TR/TE (B) and markedly hypointense on long TR/TE (C), with surrounding edema (*arrows*, C).

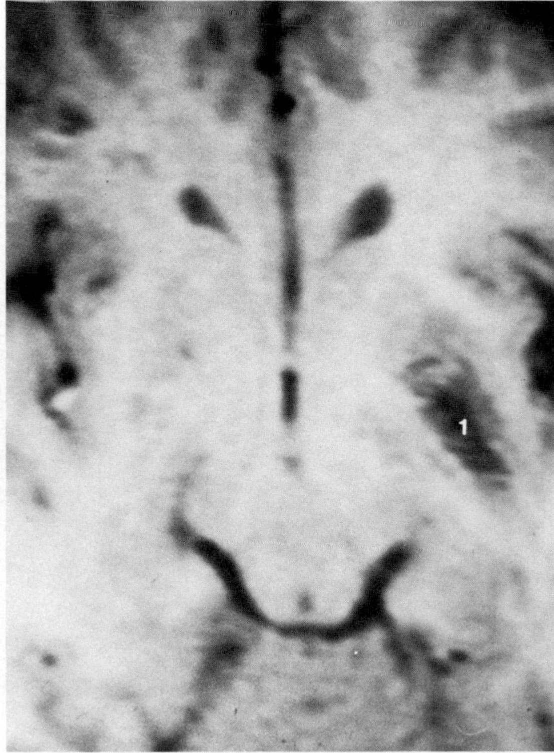

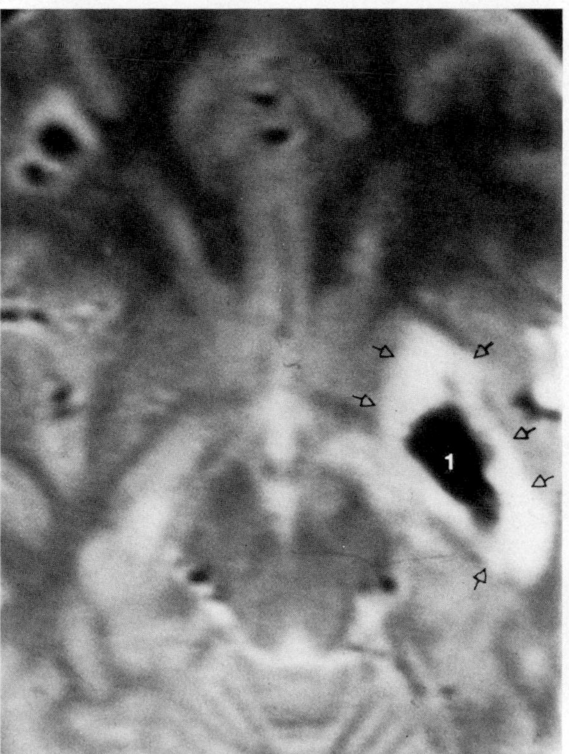

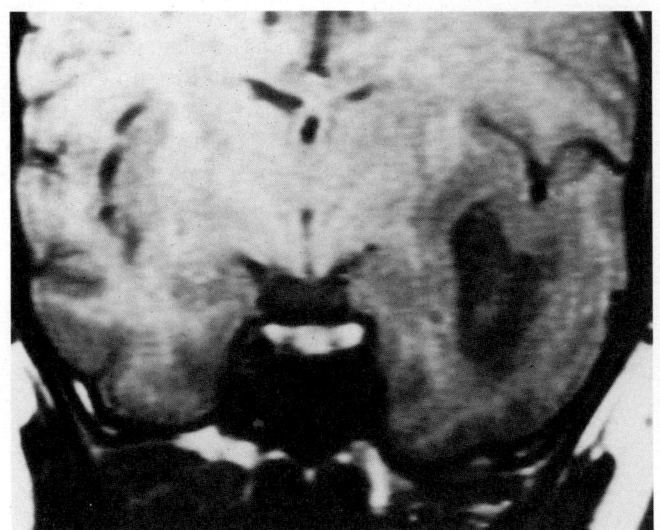
A

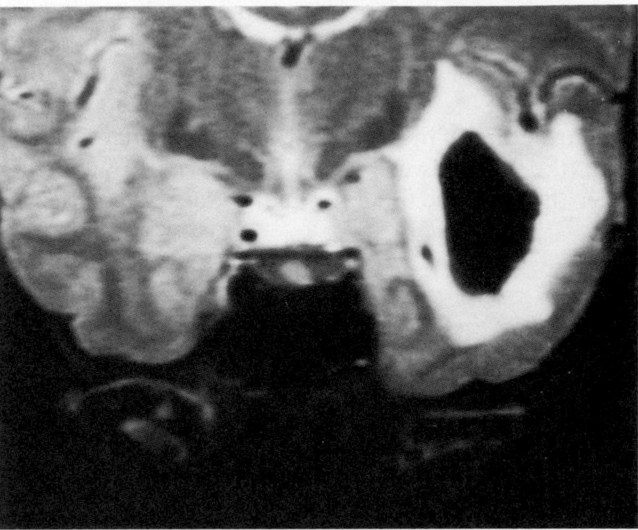
B

FIG. 17. Acute hematoma (less than 24 hours after trauma). **A:** Short TR/TE MRI (600/20). **B:** Long TR/TE MRI (2500/80). Coronal images show left temporal hematoma as hypointense on short TR/TE (A) and markedly hypointense on long TR/TE (B). The hypointensity, even on the short TR/TE image, is mainly a reflection of the very short T2 of the deoxyhemoglobin-containing clot. (From Barkovich and Atlas, ref. 1, with permission.)

Because these effects are proportional to the square of the applied magnetic field strength, very little effect is present in low-field systems (unless parameters are used to optimize visualization of T2 effects, that is, long TR and extremely long TE with a long interecho time), so that under low-field conditions using conventional spin-echo techniques, the acute hematoma is usually isointense with brain on T2-weighted images. At high field strength, low-intensity signal is seen on the long TR/TE image (Figs. 15–18). The degree of hypointensity (the amount

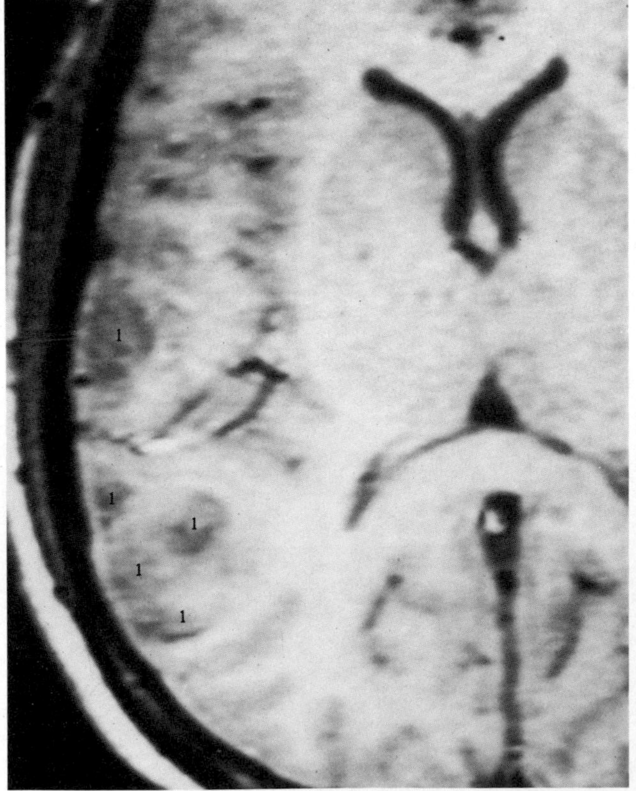

A

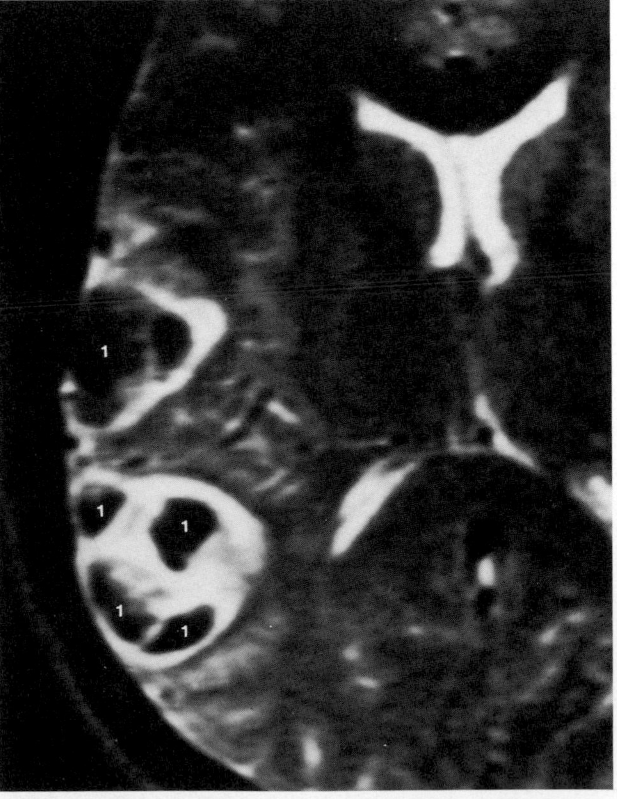

B

FIG. 18. Serial evolution of hemorrhagic contusions. **A:** Axial short TR/TE MRI (600/20), within 24 hours post-trauma. **B:** Axial long TR/TE MRI (2500/80), within 24 hours post-trauma.

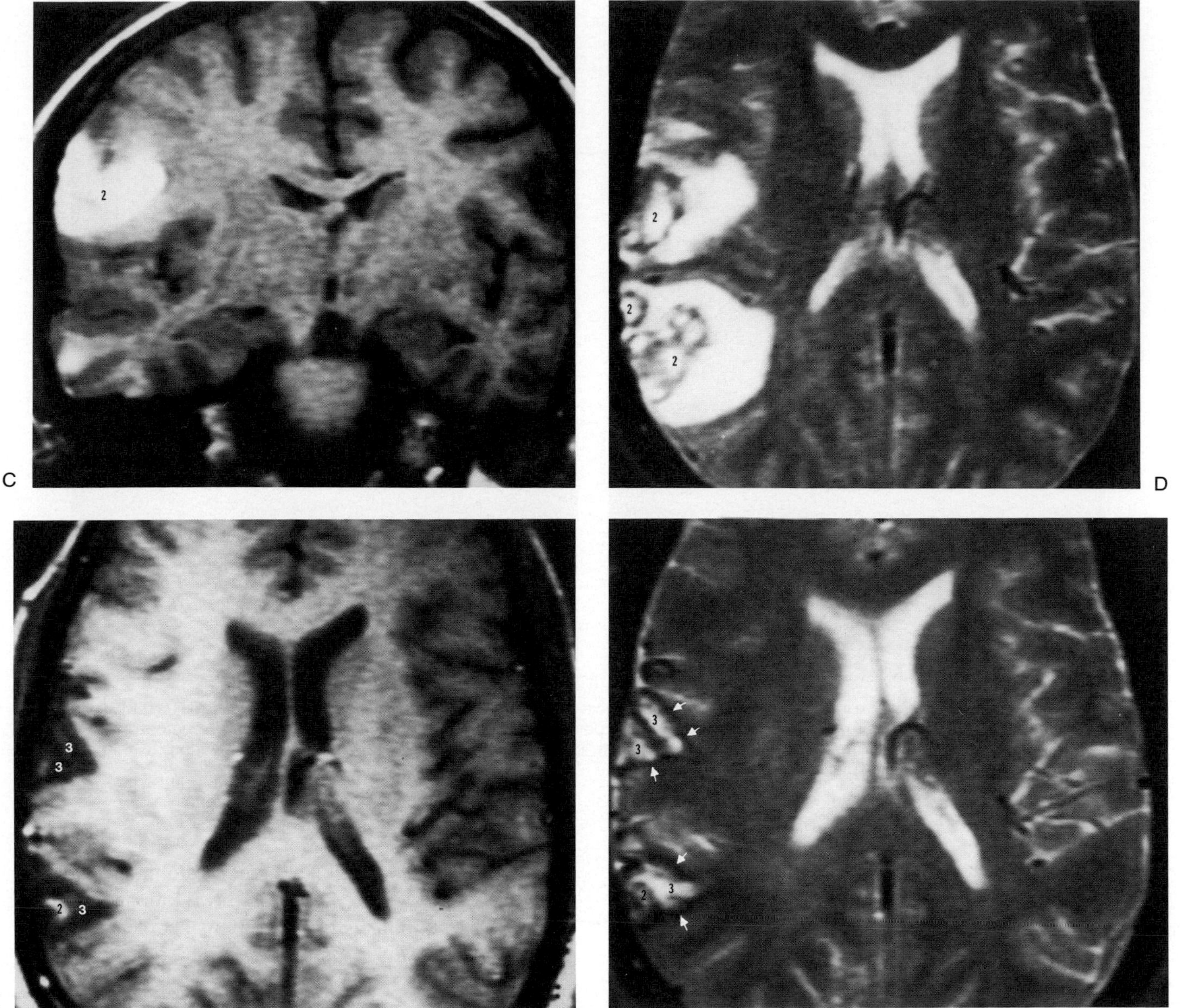

FIG. 18. (*Continued.*) **C:** Coronal short TR/TE MRI (600/20), 1 week post-trauma. **D:** Axial long TR/TE MRI (2500/80), 1 week post-trauma. **E:** Axial short TR/TE MRI (600/20), 4 months post-trauma. **F:** Axial long TR/TE MRI (2500/80), 4 months post-trauma. Acute hemorrhages (*1*) are isointense to gray matter on short TR/TE (A) and become markedly hypointense on long TR/TE (B). Subacute stage after 1 week demonstrates markedly hyperintense methemoglobin (*2*) on both short TR/TE (C) and long TR/TE images (D). Long-term follow-up (E,F) shows small subcortical areas of fluid (*3*) and methemoglobin (*2*) surrounded by marked hypointensity (*arrows*) on long TR/TE image (F). (From Barkovich and Atlas, ref. 1, with permission.)

of T2 shortening) due to intracellular deoxyhemoglobin is dependent on: the magnetic moment (which is proportional to the concentration of intracellular deoxyhemoglobin), the relative magnetic susceptibilities of the intracellular and extracellular spaces, the heterogeneity of distribution of the paramagnetic material (i.e., the deoxyhemoglobin) (57), the applied field strength, and pulse sequence parameters used in the spin-echo sequence.

During the acute hematoma stage, the retraction of clot that occurs with deoxygenation effectively raises the hematocrit. The result of increasing protein content is well known (54) and causes parallel increases in the rates of T1 and T2 relaxation (1/T1 and 1/T2). This effect is not field-dependent, would not change with oxygenation or TE, and would not be effected by the implementation of gradient refocusing (instead of rf-refocusing, as in spin-echo imaging). The signal intensity of acute hema-

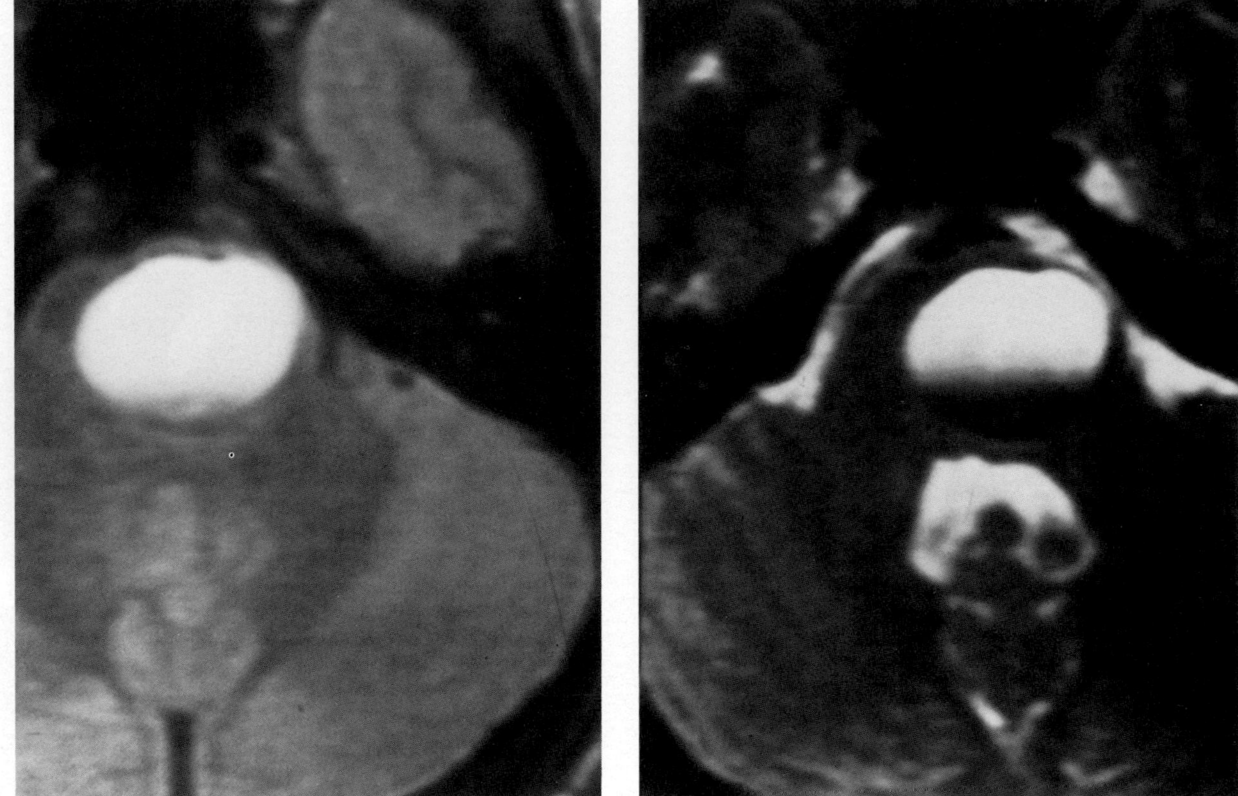

FIG. 19. Effect of change in TE on hematoma appearance. **A:** Long TR/short TE MRI (2500/30). **B:** Long TR/TE MRI (2500/120). Note the dramatic increase in degree of hypointensity in the dorsal (dependent) part of the hematoma with increasing TE. This appearance is compatible with intracellular deoxyhemoglobin layering posteriorly within cavity containing extracellular methemoglobin ventrally.

tomas is influenced only to a minor extent by the protein content (20). At this early stage of hematoma development, the surrounding edema and serum from clot retraction give a high-intensity perimeter around the hemorrhage on the long TR spin-echo images (Figs. 15–18). Fibrin clot formation and retraction have not been shown to affect significantly the in vitro appearance of the acute hematoma at 1.5 T (20).

In acute hematomas, there is no evidence of high intensity on short TR/TE images. In fact, the acute hematoma is isointense or minimally hypointense to brain on short TR/TE images (Figs. 15–18). The *lack of* hyperintensity of intracellular deoxyhemoglobin is attributed to the quaternary structure of the deoxyhemoglobin molecule, which precludes water protons from attaining the requisite proximity to the unpaired electrons of the paramagnetic deoxyhemoglobin molecule (Fig. 6). The result of the relatively large distance between water protons and the unpaired electrons of deoxyhemoglobin results in a *lack* of the dipole-dipole interaction between these substances. Therefore, no T1 shortening is observed on short TR/TE images. Note that *the hypointensity of acute hematomas on short TR/TE images is really a reflection of T2 shortening*—the signal has already decayed, due to the extremely short T2 of deoxyhemoglobin, even at the relatively short TE used on short TR/TE images. Therefore, the hypointensity on what many people call a "T1-weighted image" is actually a T2 effect!

Subacute Hematoma

The inflammatory repair response within the surrounding tissue of phagocytes, such as macrophages, infiltrates the boundaries of the hematoma to clear extravasated materials and damaged tissues. Glial cells also show phagocytic activity. Red blood cells are phagocytosed or lysed by enzymes released into the region by the inflammatory cells (41,58). As the energy status of the erythrocytes decline, the reductase enzyme systems of the RBC (NADH-cytochrome b_5 reductase, NADPH-flavin reductase) (59) used to maintain the heme iron in the ferrous oxidation state become nonfunctional. Hemoglobin is oxidized to *methemoglobin,* in which the iron, still bound to the heme moiety within the globin protein, is in the ferric state with five *d* electrons. As such, the iron is paramagnetic ($\chi > 0$). Note that if the O_2 tension is too high or too low, conversion to methemoglobin is retarded (60,61); this retardation has an effect on he-

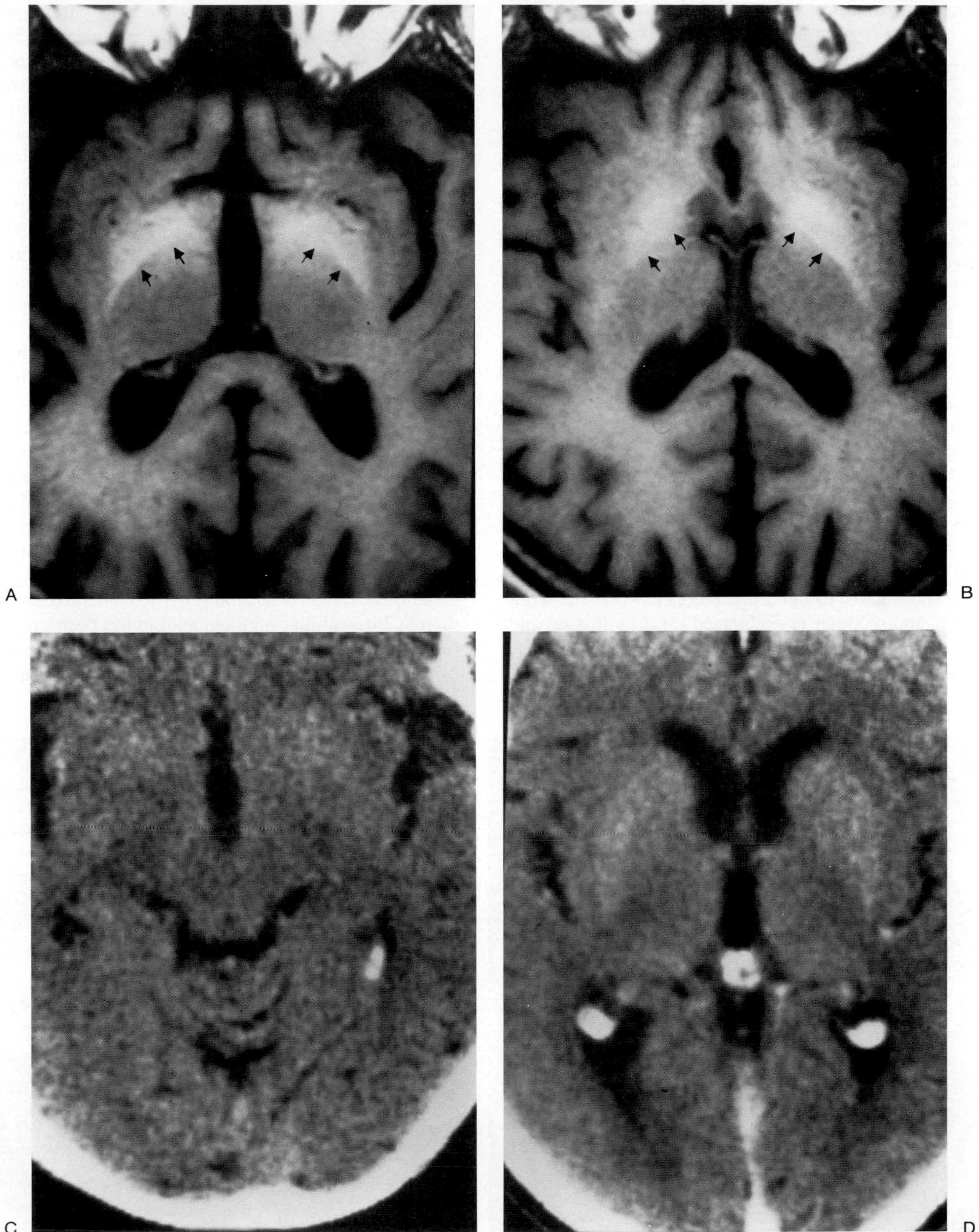

FIG. 20. Hyperintensity on short TR/TE MRI from liver disease. **A:** Short TR/TE MRI. **B:** Short TR/TE MRI. **C:** CT. **D:** CT. Short TR/TE MRI (A,B) reveals marked hyperintensity, mainly in the globus pallidus (*arrows*), bilaterally in this patient with chronic liver disease. Unremarkable CT scans (C,D) through level of basal ganglia shows no evidence of calcification or other lesion. This association may be a reflection of abnormal copper or manganese deposition.

TABLE 8. *Mimics of hemorrhage on MR—high intensity on T1-weighted images or low intensity on T2-weighted images*

Fat (biological or in oil-based contrast agents)
Very high non-paramagnetic protein concentration
Paramagnetic cations associated with hyperalimentation, liver disease, dystrophic calcification, or necrosis (iron, copper, manganese)
Calcification
Mucinous material
Intratumoral melanin
Hypermyelination
Flow effects
Normal intravascular deoxyhemoglobin (e.g., venous angioma)
Iodinated or paramagnetic contrast enhancement

matoma appearance and has been theorized as the cause of the prolonged stage of hypointensity in intratumoral bleeds (44). The globin also undergoes structural changes, ultimately irreversible, in which the ferric iron is no longer protected from the surrounding solvent (62) (Fig. 6). The electronic configuration of the iron changes from initially five unpaired electrons, one in each of the five *d* suborbitals, to one unpaired electron as the weak sixth ligand of water is exchanged for a hydroxide and then another imidazole nitrogen of a histidyl residue of the protein. These states of iron, termed *the hemichromes,* have been defined by electron paramagnetic resonance spectroscopy (63). As the paramagnetic center is now exposed to water, dipole-dipole interactions can occur to enhance relaxivity effects on T1 and T2 relaxation. For all practical purposes, high intensity is present on short TR/TE images whenever methemoglobin exists. Thus, a hematoma at this stage shows hyperintensity on short TR/TE (T1-weighted) MR images [note that there is a list of entities that can be associated with high intensity on short TR/TE images (Table 8) (Figs. 20 and 21)]. This high signal intensity of *early subacute* hematomas typically begins at the periphery of the hematoma and converges radially inward (12) (Fig. 22). Theoretically, this occurs initially at the peripheral aspect of the hematoma because the outer rim is the region with optimal conditions for the auto-oxidation of the oxyhemoglobin (12). At this early subacute stage, marked hypointensity is still present in the periphery of the hematoma on the long TR/TE spin-echo image (Fig. 22). This is the sole instance in hematomas in which both mechanisms of relaxation enhancement (i.e., proton-electron dipole-dipole interaction, and further T2 shortening from compartmentalized gradients of magnetic susceptibility) occur simultaneously (Figs. 22 and 23). The center of the hematoma remains unchanged (deoxyhemoglobin remains). Intracellular methemoglobin has been proposed to be the basis for the appearance of the MR image at this transient stage of hemorrhage (12), that is, methemoglo-

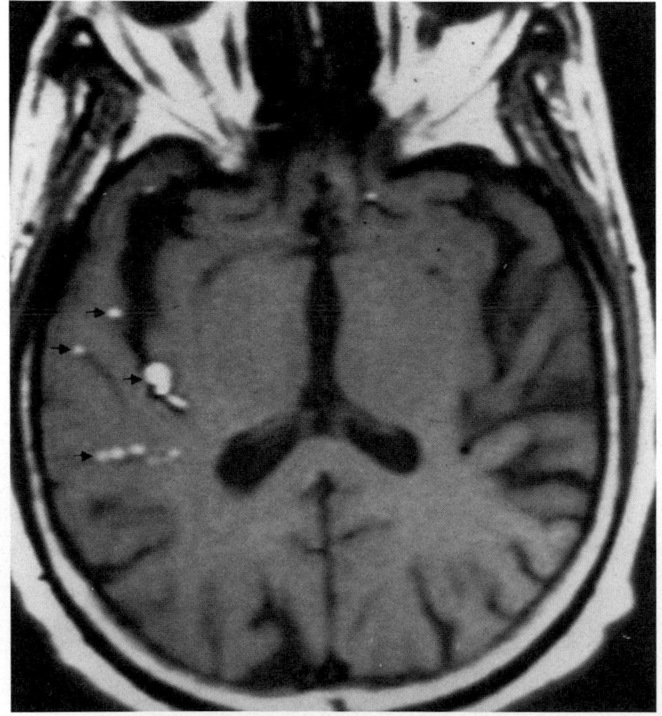
A

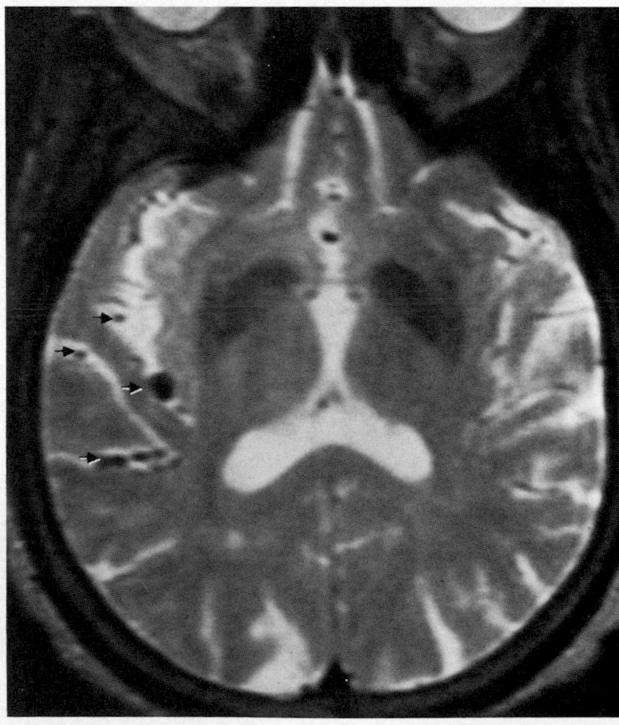
B

FIG. 21. Hyperintensity on short TR/TE due to subarachnoidal Pantopaque. **A:** Short TR/TE MRI (600/20). **B:** Long TR/TE MRI (2500/80). Small foci of hyperintensity in right sylvian fissure on short TR/TE (*arrows*, A) are hypointense on long TR/TE (B) and represent droplets of Pantopaque from prior myelogram. In this case, the signal intensity pattern resembles that of intracellular methemoglobin.

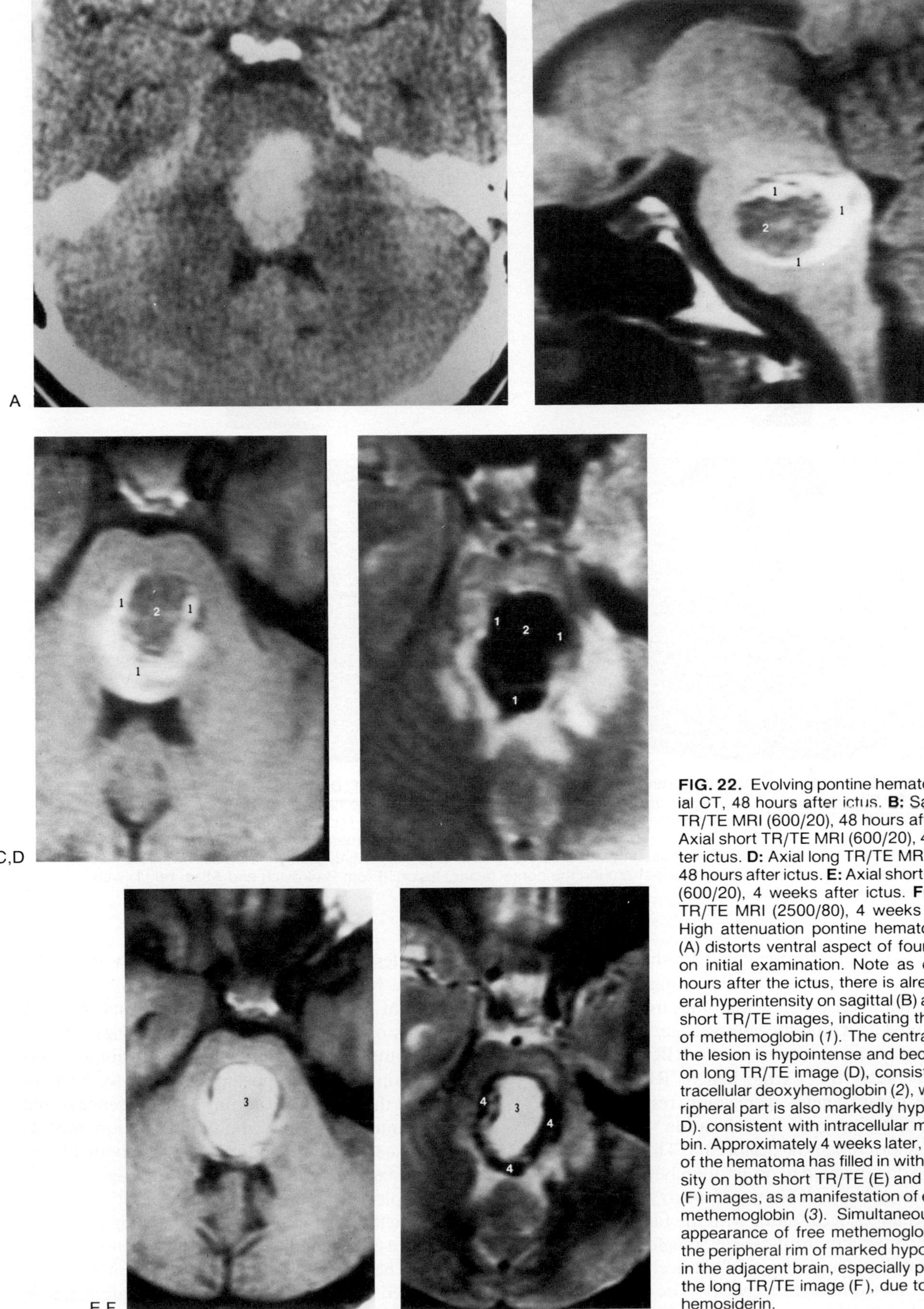

FIG. 22. Evolving pontine hematoma. **A:** Axial CT, 48 hours after ictus. **B:** Sagittal short TR/TE MRI (600/20), 48 hours after ictus. **C:** Axial short TR/TE MRI (600/20), 48 hours after ictus. **D:** Axial long TR/TE MRI (2500/80), 48 hours after ictus. **E:** Axial short TR/TE MRI (600/20), 4 weeks after ictus. **F:** Axial long TR/TE MRI (2500/80), 4 weeks after ictus. High attenuation pontine hematoma on CT (A) distorts ventral aspect of fourth ventricle on initial examination. Note as early as 48 hours after the ictus, there is already peripheral hyperintensity on sagittal (B) and axial (C) short TR/TE images, indicating the presence of methemoglobin (*1*). The central portion of the lesion is hypointense and becomes black on long TR/TE image (D), consistent with intracellular deoxyhemoglobin (*2*), while the peripheral part is also markedly hypointense (*1*, D). consistent with intracellular methemoglobin. Approximately 4 weeks later, the majority of the hematoma has filled in with hyperintensity on both short TR/TE (E) and long TR/TE (F) images, as a manifestation of extracellular methemoglobin (*3*). Simultaneous with the appearance of free methemoglobin, we see the peripheral rim of marked hypointensity (*4*) in the adjacent brain, especially prominent on the long TR/TE image (F), due to ferritin and hemosiderin.

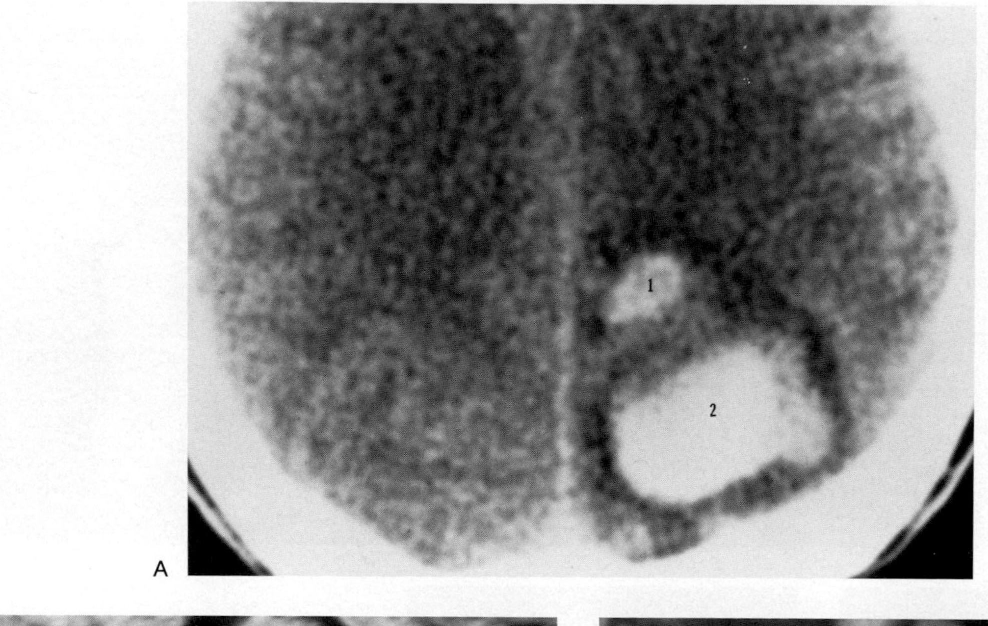

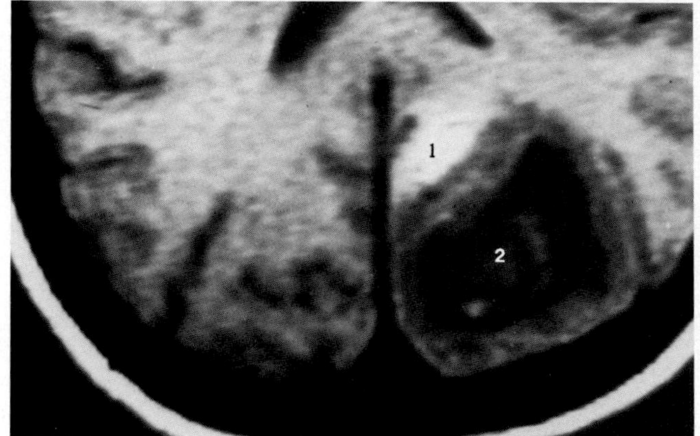

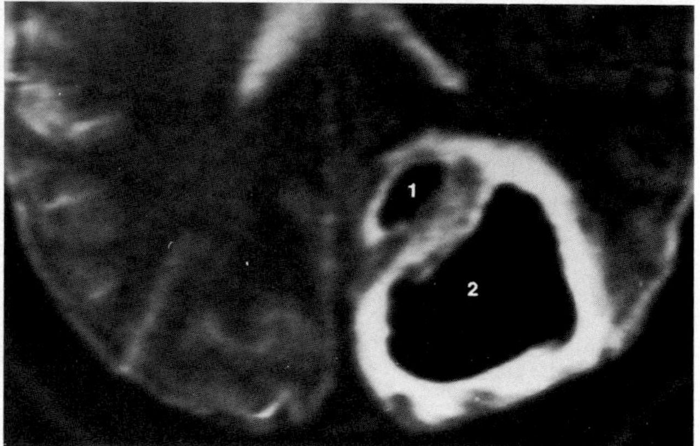

FIG. 23. Early subacute hemorrhage and acute hemorrhage, CT vs. MRI. **A:** CT. **B:** Short TR/TE MRI (600/20). **C:** Long TR/TE MRI (2500/80). Despite the fact that both left parietal lesions are high attenuation on CT (A), they represent two distinct biochemical stages of hemorrhage on MR. Ventral lesion (*1*) is hyperintense on short TR/TE (B) and markedly hypointense on long TR/TE (C), consistent with intracellular methemoglobin. Dorsal lesion (*2*) is hypointense on short TR/TE (B) and becomes black on long TR/TE (C), indicating deoxyhemoglobin within intact red blood cells. Edema is more prominent around the dorsal (acute) lesion. (From Barkovich and Atlas, ref. 1, with permission.)

bin is thought to be compartmentalized within still intact red blood cells. The approximate time range to identify these signal characteristics in hematomas usually occurs between 2 and 7 days after the hemorrhage.

The decline in energy status of the RBC causes loss of membrane integrity. As the loss of RBC integrity removes the paramagnetic aggregation responsible for the susceptibility-induced T2 relaxation process, the effective T2 shortening now disappears. This phenomenon has been documented to occur upon lysis of red cells containing deoxyhemoglobin in in vitro experiments (34). These changes occur along with the further formation of methemoglobin from deoxyhemoglobin. Hemolysis results in the accumulation of extracellular methemoglobin within the hematoma cavity. The extracellular methemoglobin further enhances T1 relaxation (34), and is manifested as high intensity on the short TR/TE images (Figs. 18, 22, and 24).

Concurrent with these changes, high signal intensity also appears on the long TR/TE images (Figs. 18, 22, and 24). A number of factors probably contribute to this seemingly contradictory appearance, since we have already stated that methemoglobin, in the absence of red blood cell integrity, allows dipolar relaxation mechanisms to ensue, which theoretically shorten both T1 and T2. At this stage of evolution, the hemorrhage is essentially a complex lesion (analogous to a solution) of paramagnetic methemoglobin and nonparamagnetic proteins, but to a great extent it is a very high proton density collection. The presence of methemoglobin shortens the T1 (compared with either a solution of nonparamagnetic protein at clinically relevant concentrations, or com-

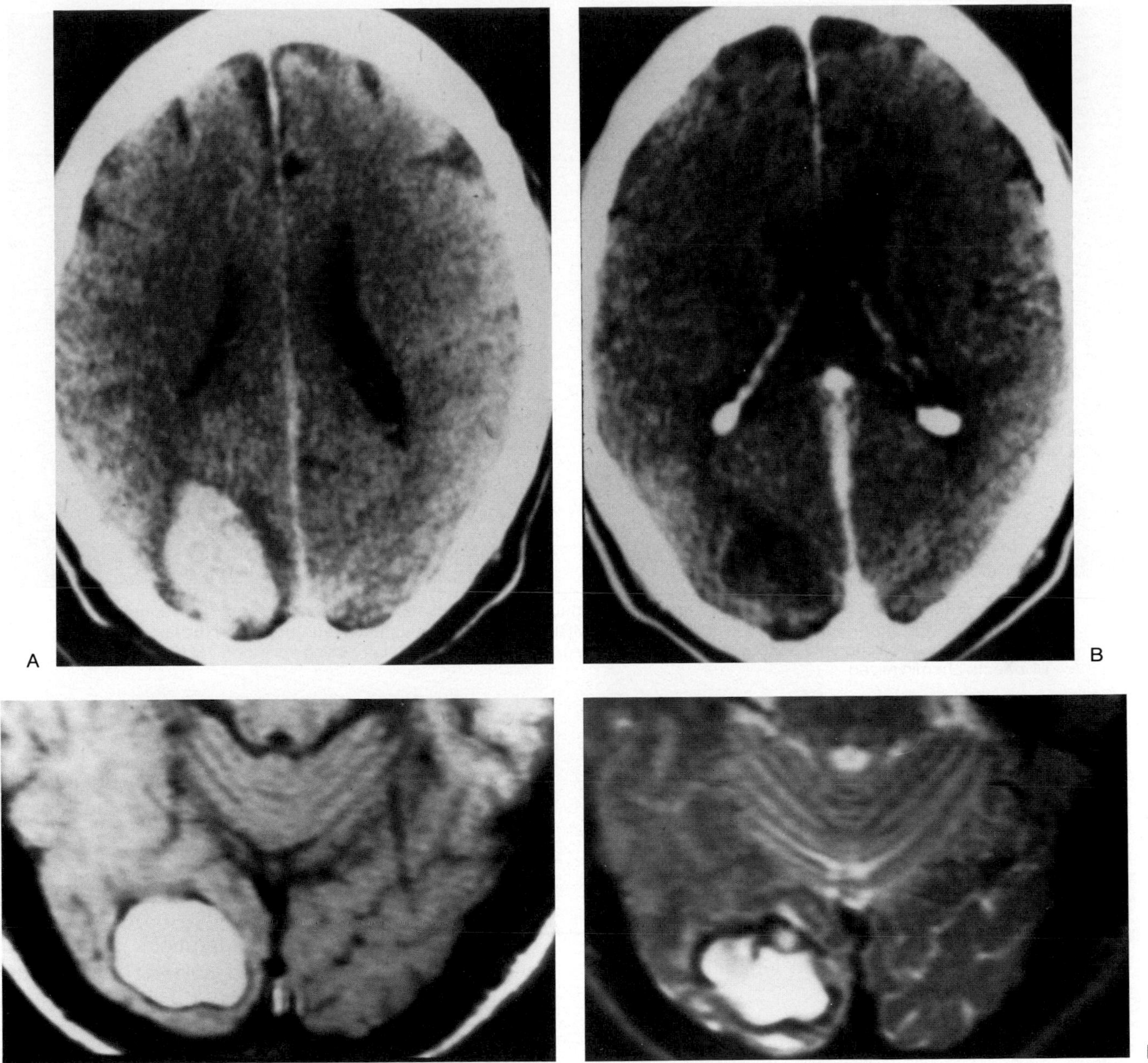

FIG. 24. Late subacute hematoma. **A:** CT on initial presentation. **B:** CT with intravenous contrast, 2-month follow-up. **C:** Short TR/TE MRI (600/20), 2-month follow-up. **D:** Long TR/TE MRI (2500/80), 2-month follow-up. Acute right parietal-occipital hematoma on initial CT (A) evolves into low attenuation mass with thin rim of enhancement on follow-up CT (B) 2 months later. Note the appearance of high intensity on both short (C) and long TR/TE (D) images with well-defined complete rim of hypointensity on long TR/TE image (D) in this late subacute hematoma. CT cannot distinguish old blood from CSF or other fluid (B), since these entities all appear as low attenuation.

pared with simple water) of this relatively high spin density (compared with brain parenchyma) lesion and causes high intensity on virtually all conventionally used spin-echo images (14). In fact, measured T1 values of subacute-to-chronic hematomas are similar to lower intensity white matter (14). Note that if one used a very long TR (e.g., >10 sec), the subacute-chronic hematoma would appear of lower intensity, since the extremely long TR would eliminate any contribution of T1 shortening to the intensity, so T2 effects would dominate the contrast (Fig. 25). After cell lysis, therefore, the *late subacute-chronic* hematoma has high intensity on long TR/TE images, which is due to T1 shortening of a high spin-density solution, as has been described by Hackney and coworkers (14). Results obtained by direct measurement by Gomori (34) and those indirectly obtained from the experiments of Bradley and Schmidt (64) and Di Chiro (11) have shown that extracellular methemoglobin causes significantly more T1 relaxation enhancement than intracellular methemoglobin. The explanation for

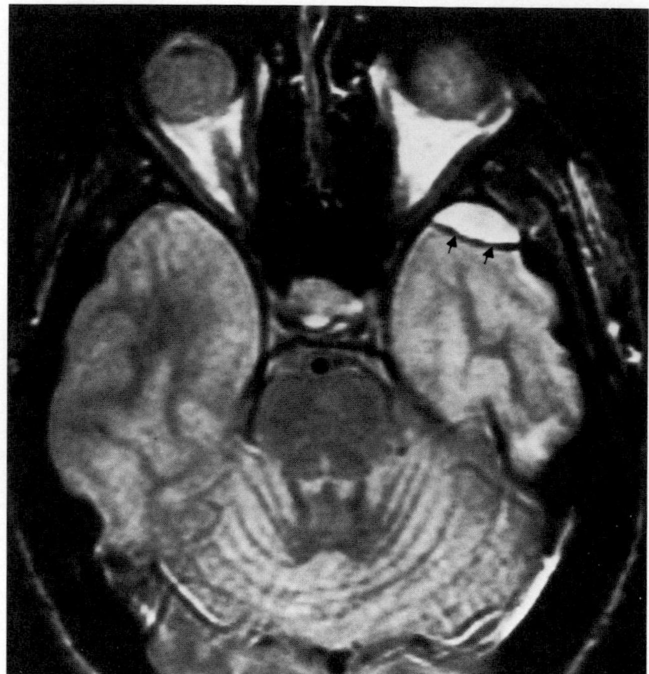

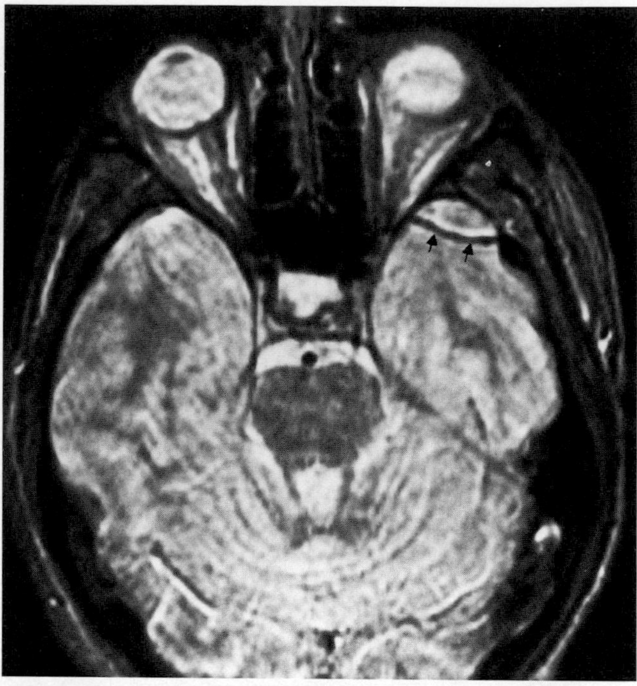

FIG. 25. Effect of very long TR on appearance of free methemoglobin in late subacute hematoma. **A:** Routine long TR/short TE MRI (3000/30). **B:** Very long TR/short TE MRI (6000/30). Although this left temporal extra-axial hematoma (*arrows*) is high intensity on routine long TR image (A), it becomes low intensity using very long TR (B), since the T1 effects are minimized.

this phenomenon, which is probably not evident on clinical images, remains obscure. Eventually, as the methemoglobin is resorbed and degraded, the amount of relaxation time enhancement declines, and the signal intensity decreases from its marked hyperintensity on short TR/TE images. Importantly, the high water content in the subacute-chronic hematoma cavity contributes significantly to the signal intensity of the chronic hematoma on both short TR and long TR spin-echo images.

Extracellular protein degradation releases iron that is detoxified by chelation to extracellular iron-binding proteins such as lactoferrin and transferrin. These binding proteins serve as detoxification and transport proteins, recycling free iron back to the reticuloendothelial system via the circulation. The chelated iron remains paramagnetic ($\chi > 0$). The iron remains accessible to water so that relaxivity effects may be expected. The specific relaxivity and susceptibility effects of ferric ions chelated to these proteins is described in vitro (36,65–67) but remains unknown for resolving in vivo hemorrhage. The concentration of these substances may be too low to have a significant role in determining signal intensity within an MR image.

Chronic Hematoma

The effects of iron storage substances on the MR characteristics of normal brain tissue have been summarized elsewhere (25,68,69). Iron from hemorrhage clearly enters and must be processed in a different manner, although the final products may be similar. Much of the intrinsic iron, and probably iron arising from hemorrhage, is as yet not biochemically characterized (25,70). After hemorrhage, heme proteins phagocytosed by macrophages and glial cells are degraded in lysosomes, with the iron being stored in the hydrophobic center of the major iron storage protein called *ferritin* (50,71). Ferritin is a water-soluble protein of about 450,000 molecular weight formed from 24 polypeptide subunits surrounding a crystalline core of ferric oxyhydroxide containing up to 4,500 ferric ions. If the quantity of available iron exceeds the capacity of the cell to synthesize apoferritin, excess iron is stored as *hemosiderin* (50). Hemosiderin is a poorly biochemically characterized, insoluble aggregation of ferric oxyhydroxide with less protein than ferritin. These storage forms with large aggregates of iron behave paramagnetically at biological temperatures ($\chi > 0$) (25,39,66,67,72), but at very low temperatures behave antiferromagnetically, and probably superparamagnetically (25). The iron in these storage forms is inaccessible to water, so relaxivity effects are not observed. Magnetic susceptibility variations are present in tissues containing such materials, with effects observed on T2*.

On MRI, along with the appearance of the extracellular methemoglobin constituting subacute-chronic hematomas, a thin rim of low signal intensity begins to appear around the hematoma in the adjacent brain parenchyma

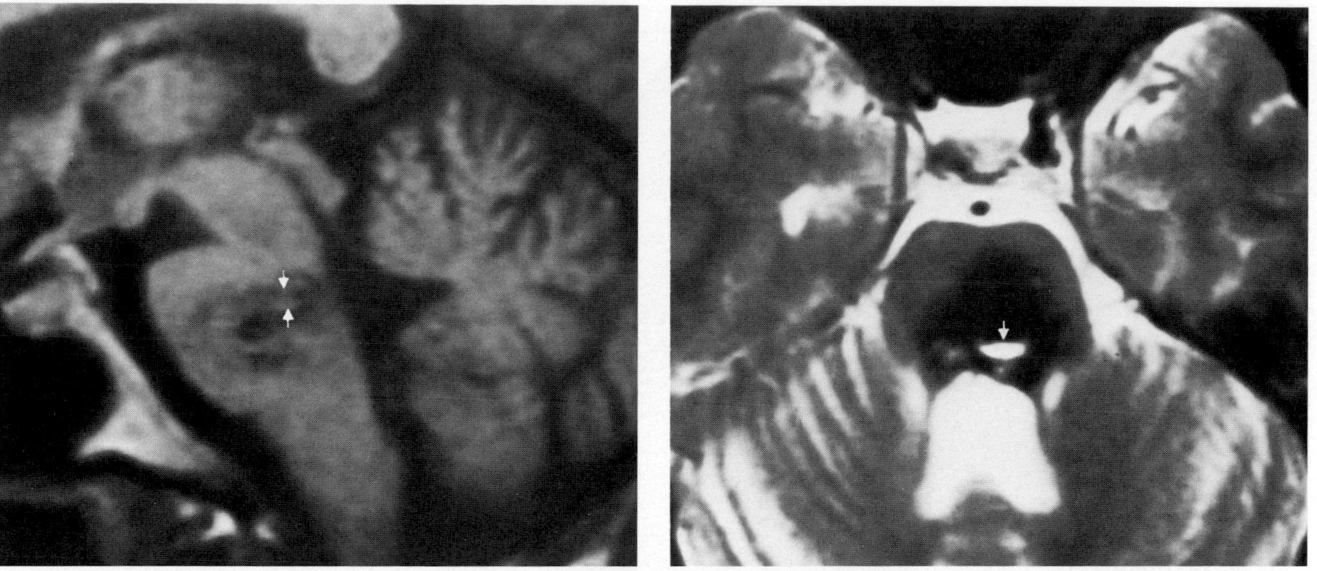

FIG. 26. Chronic hematoma with persistence of small amount of methemoglobin. **A:** Sagittal short TR/TE MRI (600/20). **B:** Axial long TR/TE MRI (3000/80). Three years after this patient's hematoma, a small amount of hyperintense methemoglobin (*arrows*, A) persists amid the dense hypointensity of ferritin/hemosiderin deposition seen on the long TR/TE image (B).

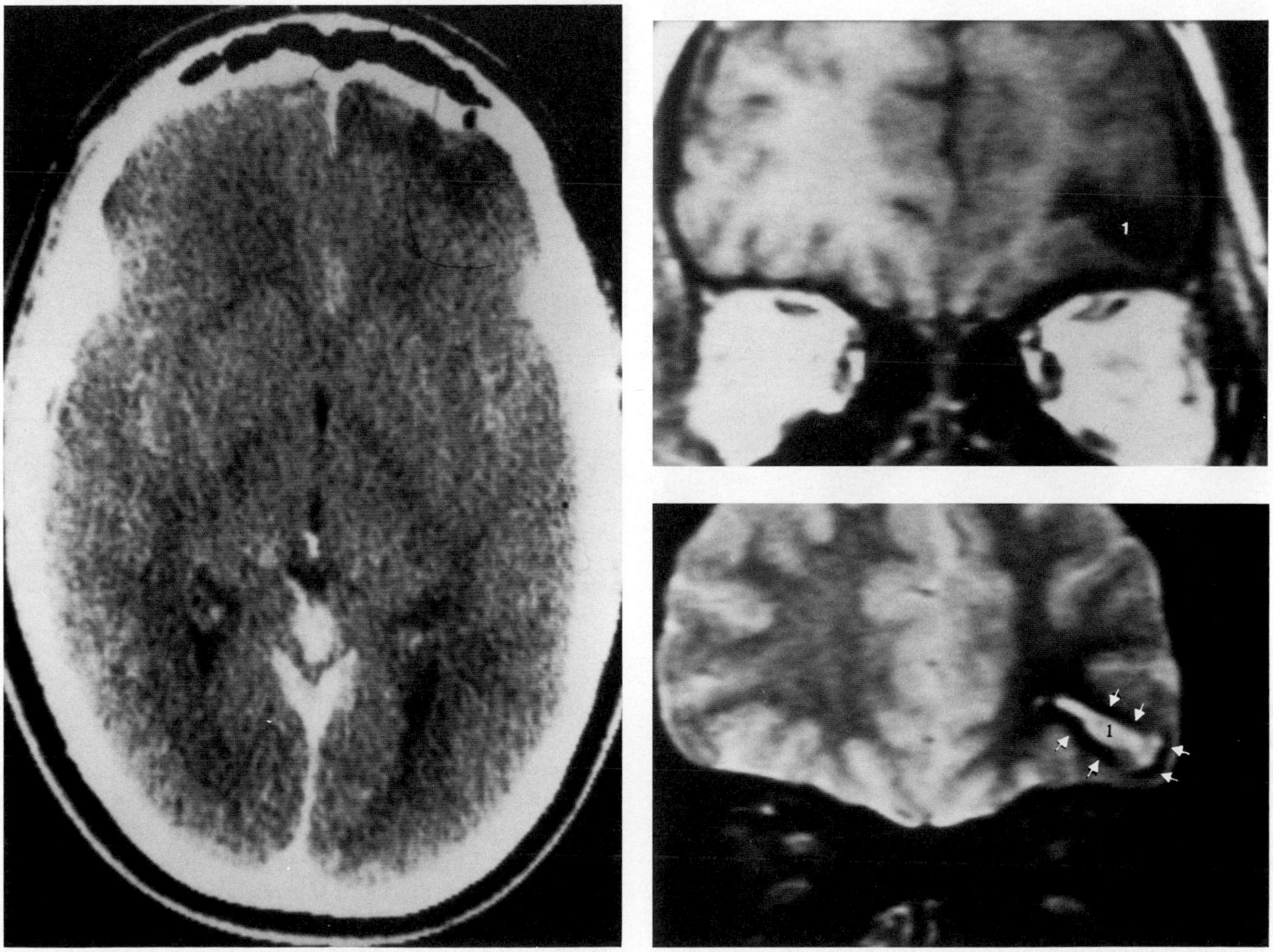

FIG. 27. Chronic hematoma with nonparamagnetic fluid centrally. **A:** Axial CT. **B:** Coronal short TR/TE MR (600/20). **C:** Coronal long TR/TE MRI (2500/80). Long-term follow-up of left frontal hematoma shows low attenuation on CT (A). Coronal MRI (B,C) reveals central CSF-like intensity (*1*) with rim of hypointensity (*arrows*).

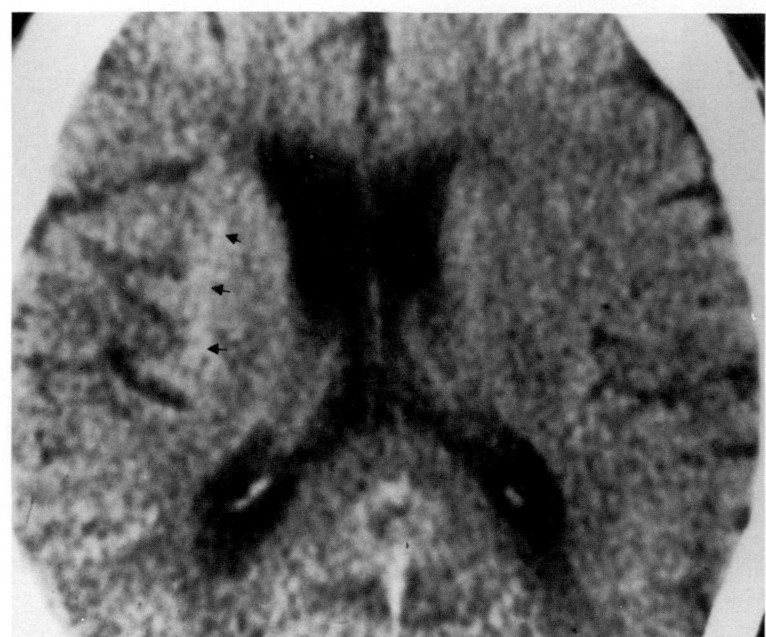

FIG. 28. Chronic hematoma with residua of slit-like cavity lined by ferritin/hemosiderin. **A:** CT scan. **B:** Short TR/TE MRI (600/20). **C:** Long TR/TE MRI (3000/90). Chronic right subinsular hematoma (*arrows*) is seen as a subtle region of slight hyperdensity on CT (A), low intensity on short TR/TE image (B), and profound hypointensity on long TR/TE image (C). No evidence of central fluid or central methemoglobin is present in this collapsed cleft, the only residua of prior hemorrhage.

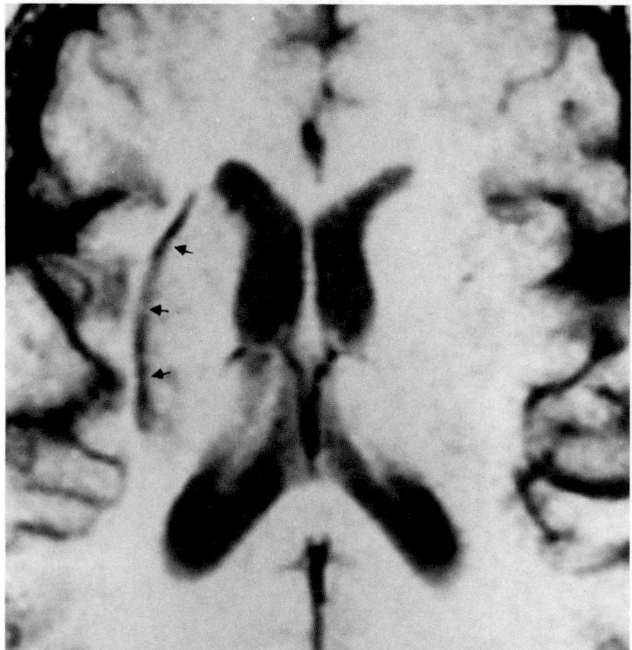

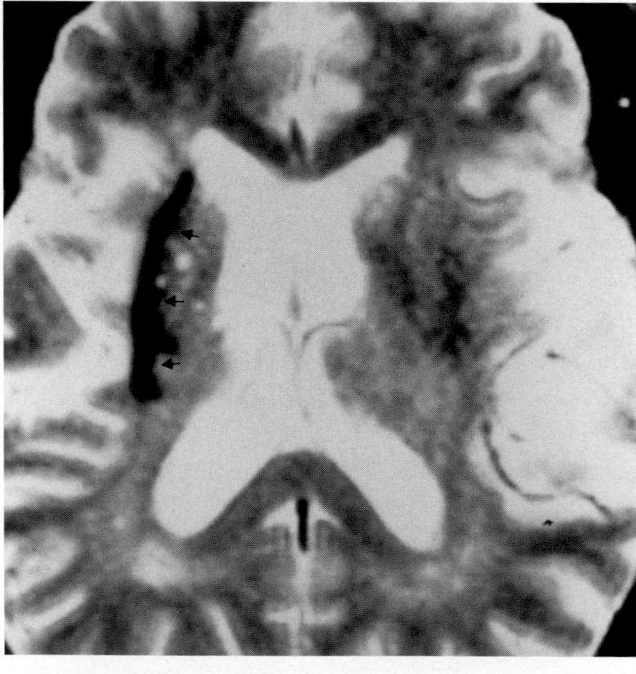

that is most marked on the long TR/TE images (12) (Figs. 18, 22, 24, and 26). This rim grows in thickness as the hematoma resolves. The source of this circumferential region of T2 shortening is the iron in the above storage forms that has been scavenged from methemoglobin breakdown products and accumulates within the lysosomes of macrophages and glial cells. An area of marked hypointensity on long TR/TE images can remain at the site of an old hemorrhage indefinitely (Figs. 26–28). This appearance is analogous to the yellow-orange staining of the brain by hemosiderin deposits seen in pathology specimens at sites of old intraparenchymal hemorrhage. The presence of the low signal intensity on long TR/TE images from old hemorrhage, when seen in association with an acute hemorrhage, can be used to imply the presence of underlying pathology related to the primary lesion (e.g., bleeding diathesis, occult cerebrovascular malformations, etc.) and is especially useful in the evaluation of suspected cases of child abuse (implying that there were multiple different episodes of bleeding). Furthermore, the absence of prominent hypointensity at the periphery of an old hematoma suggests deviation from

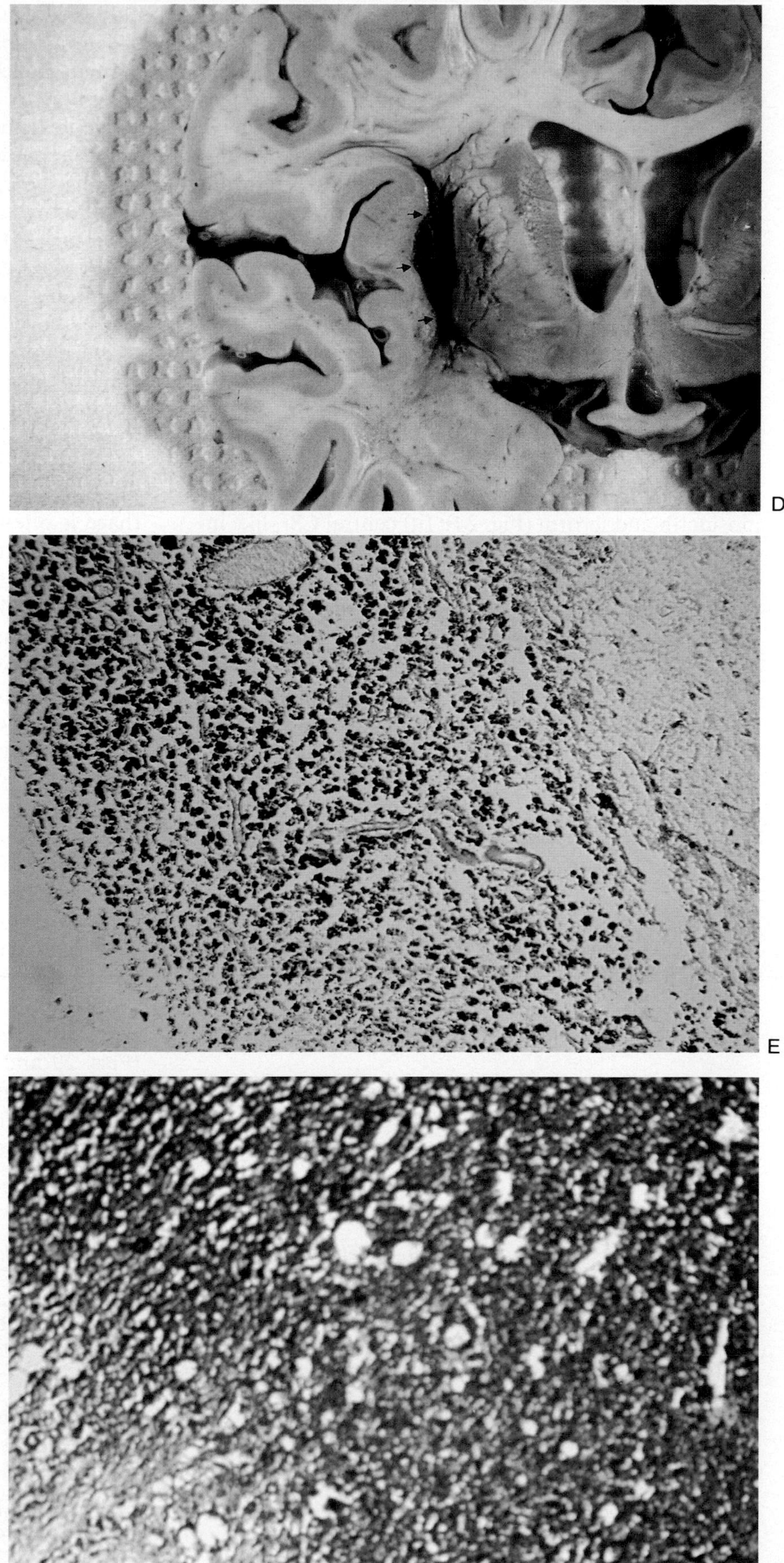

FIG. 28. (*Continued*) **D:** Necropsy specimen shows collapsed cleft in prior subinsular hematoma. **E:** Perls' stain shows positive (*dark blue*) staining indicative of hemosiderin. **F:** Immunologic stain shows positive (*dark brown*) staining for ferritin.

the normal evolution of hemorrhage and can indicate an underlying disruption of the blood–brain barrier (44).

As the methemoglobin in the cavity is slowly broken down into smaller degradation products, its T1 shortening effect is lost (63). This process can result in a slowly decreasing intensity in the cavity on short TR/TE images. These signal changes of decreasing intensity from methemoglobin degradation and resorption usually are not evident in intraparenchymal hematomas until several months after the bleed. Occasionally, methemoglobin can even persist for years (Fig. 26), although its presence after several years probably indicates either recurrent bleeding or an abnormal evolution of blood-breakdown products, one of several features of underlying tumor as the etiology of the bleed (43). Chronic hematomas may, indeed, have any of the following three appearances on spin-echo images: (i) central hyperintense methemoglobin with peripheral hypointense hemosiderin and ferritin (Fig. 24); (ii) central CSF-like intensity with peripheral hypointensity (Fig. 27); and (iii) merely a residual cleft of hypointensity (Fig. 28), whereby central methemoglobin and central fluid have been completely resorbed. Thus, by the time several months or years pass after the hemorrhagic episode, the only clue that a cavity was once hemorrhagic may be the collapsed cleft of hemosiderin in the adjacent brain. As is the case for acute hematomas, if the T2 is significantly shortened below the TE used for short TR/TE (T1-weighted) images, then the susceptibility effect will be observed on these images, and hypointensity will be seen from short T2 even on the short TR/TE image.

ATYPICAL VARIANTS OF INTRACRANIAL HEMORRHAGE

Hemorrhagic Intracranial Malignancies

Aside from the detection of brain hemorrhage, it is obviously extremely important to attempt to identify the etiology of the bleed. Hemorrhage into malignant neoplasms accounts for approximately 10% of all spontaneous intracranial hematomas (73). It occurs in up to 14% of brain metastases (74) and less than 5% of primary gliomas (75,76). Of all intracerebral metastases, those most prone to hemorrhage include melanoma, chordocarcinoma, renal cell carcinoma, bronchogenic carcinoma, and thyroid carcinoma (73,74,77). Of primary gliomas, glioblastoma multiforme, oligodendroglioma, and ependymoma (76) are most likely to demonstrate significant hemorrhage pathologically, although malignant gliomas commonly show microscopic evidence of hemorrhage. The pathogenesis of hemorrhage into intracerebral neoplasms is probably multifactorial. Factors such as high grade of malignancy, abnormal tumor vascularity, rapid tumor growth with subsequent necrosis, and vascular invasion have all been proposed as mechanisms of intratumoral bleeding (77–80). The preoperative diagnosis of tumor as the underlying etiology of intracranial hemorrhage is often extremely difficult. Computed tomography (CT) patterns of intratumoral hemorrhage are extremely variable (79). Atypical location, multiplicity of hemorrhagic lesions, and early intravenous contrast enhancement may suggest malignancy as the etiology of intracranial bleeding on CT. Cerebral angiography has also occasionally played a role in revealing underlying tumor as the cause of intracerebral hematoma. Clearly, these modalities are often of limited use in elucidating the underlying malignant lesions, as the hematoma often obliterates any evidence thereof (75).

MR signal intensity patterns of hemorrhagic intracranial malignancies differ from those of non-neoplastic intracranial hematomas (Table 9) (see also Chapter 10) and can generally be used to distinguish tumor from lesions such as occult cerebrovascular malformations (44) (see Chapter 12). In general, signal intensity patterns are more heterogeneous and markedly complex when compared with those seen from non-neoplastic hematomas (Figs. 29 and 30). In malignant lesions, multiple concomitant stages of hematoma appear, often in an atypical pattern. The complex appearance of hemorrhagic tumors is further complicated by the frequent finding of

TABLE 9. *Intratumoral hemorrhage vs. benign intracranial hematomas*

Intratumoral hemorrhage	Benign hemorrhage
Markedly heterogeneous, due to: Mixed stages of hemorrhage Debris-fluid (intracellular-extracellular blood) levels Edema + tumor + necrosis with blood	Shows expected signal intensities of acute, subacute, or chronic blood, depending on stage of hematoma
Identification of nonhemorrhagic tumor tissue	No abnormal nonhemorrhagic mass
Delayed evolution of blood-breakdown products	Follows expected orderly progression
Absent, diminished, or very irregular hypointense rim representing iron storage forms	Regular, complete peripheral hypointense rim
Persistent surrounding high intensity on long TR images (i.e., tumor/edema) and mass effect, even in late stages	Complete resolution of edema and mass effect in chronic stages

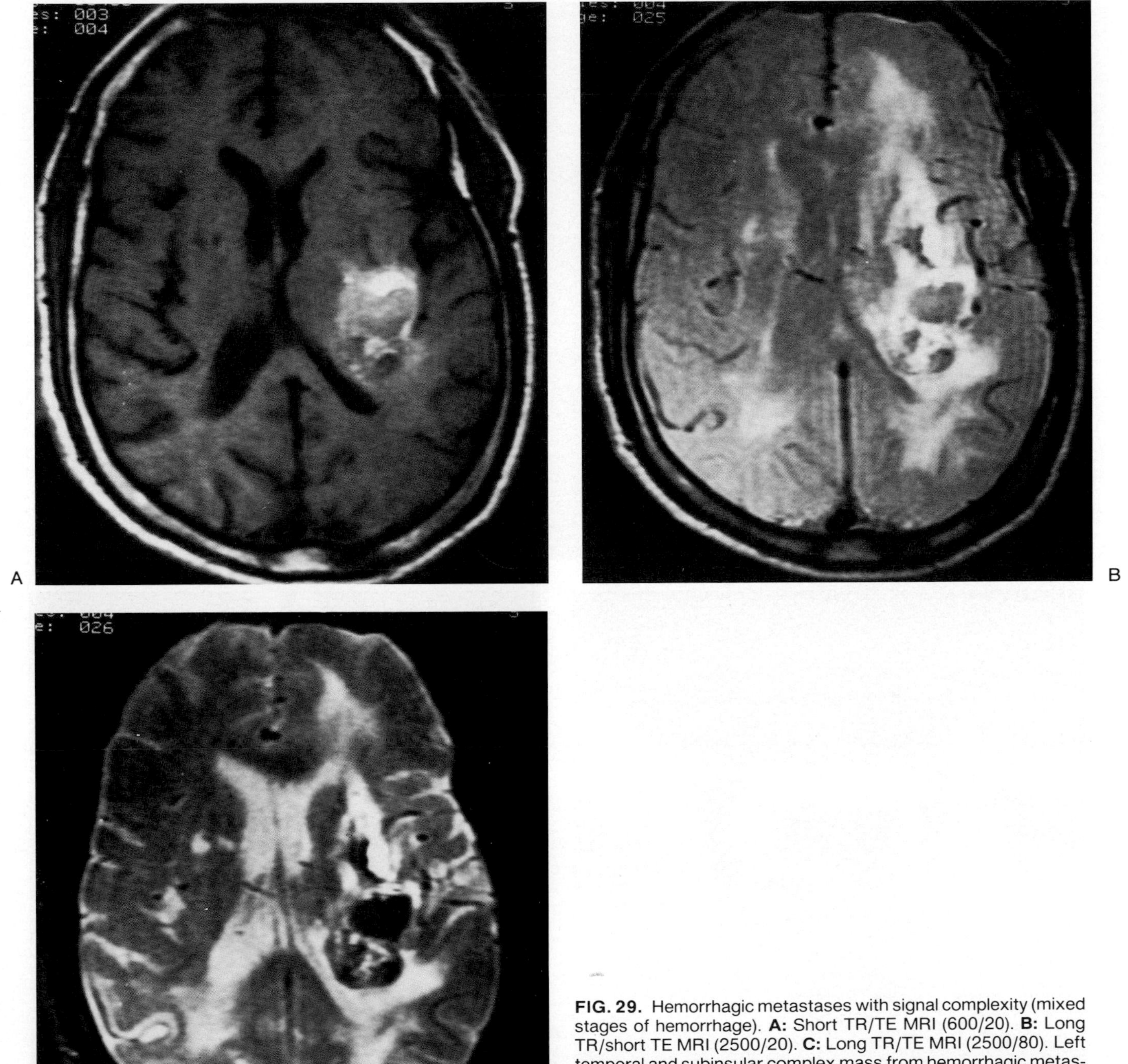

FIG. 29. Hemorrhagic metastases with signal complexity (mixed stages of hemorrhage). **A:** Short TR/TE MRI (600/20). **B:** Long TR/short TE MRI (2500/20). **C:** Long TR/TE MRI (2500/80). Left temporal and subinsular complex mass from hemorrhagic metastases shows marked signal heterogeneity, due to mixed areas of different biochemical stages of hemorrhage, including acute, early, and late subacute breakdown products, as well as nonparamagnetic high-intensity edema.

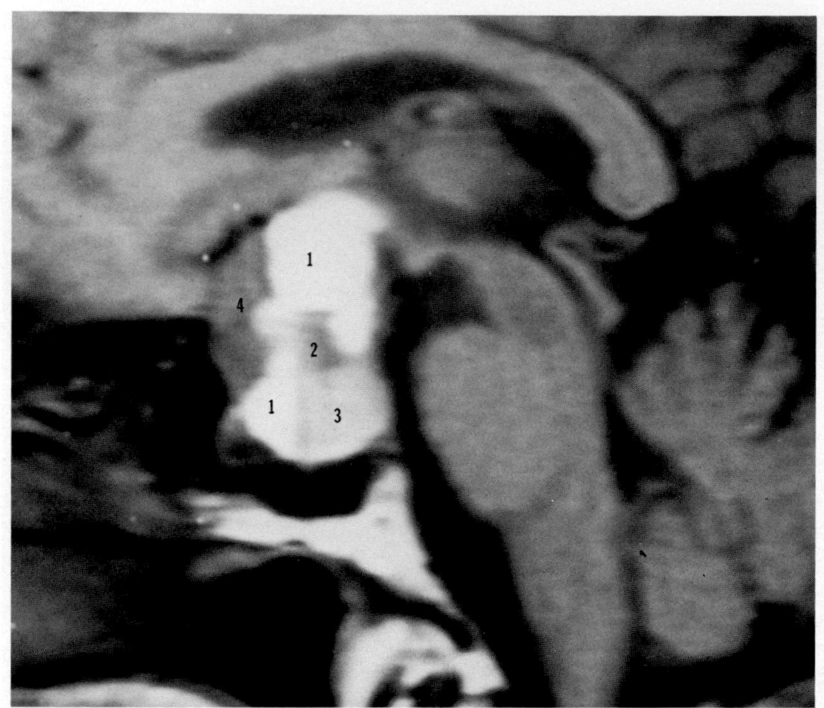

A

FIG. 30. Hemorrhagic adenoma with signal complexity (methemoglobin-deoxyhemoglobin levels). **A:** Sagittal short TR/TE MRI (600/20). **B:** Axial long TR/TE MRI (2500/80). **C:** Axial long TR/TE MRI (2500/80). Strikingly heterogeneous, hemorrhagic pituitary adenoma shows several levels, with ventral extracellular methemoglobin (*1*) and dependent intracellular deoxyhemoglobin (*2*) or intracellular methemoglobin (*3*), within areas of nonhemorrhagic tumor (*4*). Debris-fluid levels are common in hemorrhagic tumors, and represent bleeding into cystic or necrotic cavities. Also note absence of hypointensity due to iron storage products, even around areas of free methemoglobin.

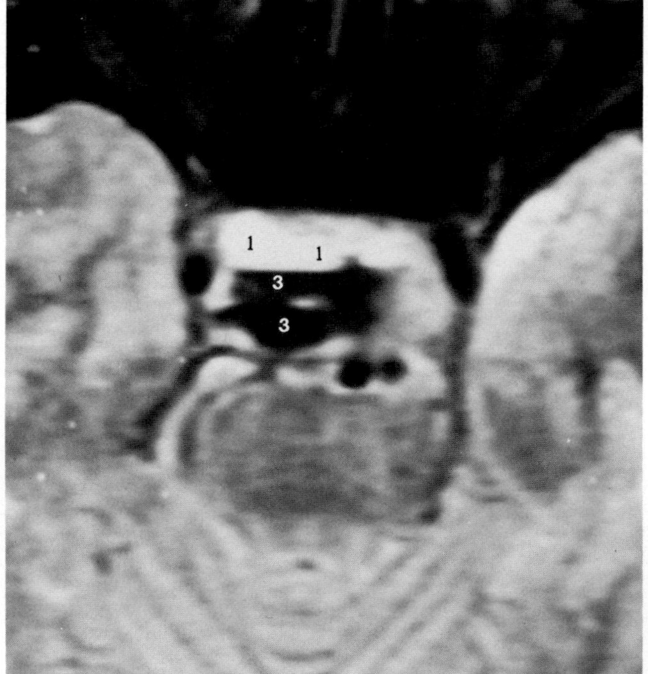

B

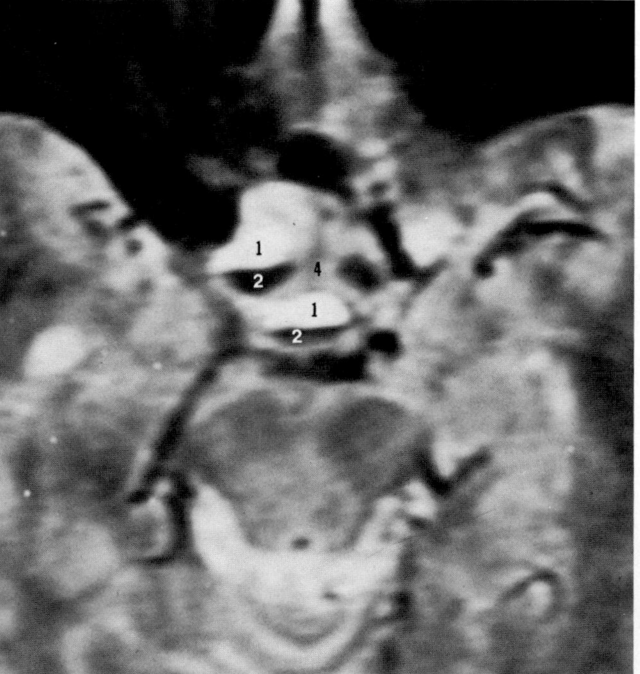

C

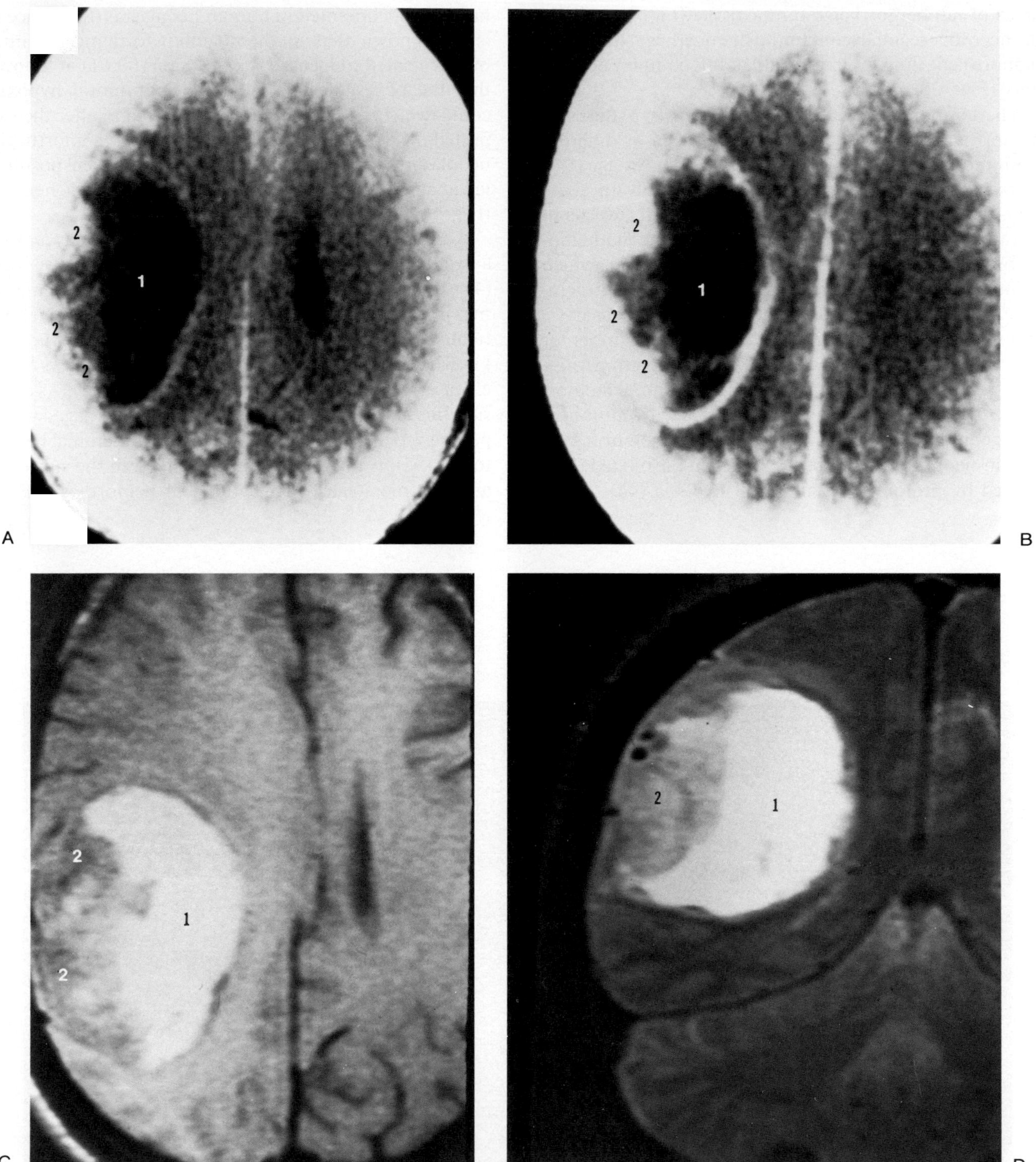

FIG. 31. Hemorrhagic glioma with nonhemorrhagic tissue and absence of hypointense rim. **A:** Axial CT, noncontrast. **B:** Axial CT, with contrast enhancement. **C:** Axial short TR/TE MRI (600/25). **D:** Coronal long TR/TE MRI (2500/80). CT (A,B) shows large right hemispheric mass with central low attenuation (*1*) and nodular enhancing masses in lateral aspect (*2*) of mass that proved to represent tumor masses projecting into hemorrhagic cavity at surgery. Note low attenuation on CT is old hemorrhage (*1*) on MR (C,D), while solid tumor (*2*) behaves as any nonparamagnetic lesion (slightly hypointense to brain on short TR/TE and hyperintense on long TR/TE). Also note absence of hypointense rim adjacent to area of old blood on long TR/TE image (D), an important sign of intratumoral hemorrhage.

areas of nonhemorrhagic tumor tissue (Fig. 31). Cystic or necrotic regions containing hemorrhage debris or hemorrhagic fluid levels also add to this complex appearance (Figs. 30 and 32).

The temporal evolution of MR intensity patterns in hemorrhagic malignancies is often delayed or different from those seen in benign intracranial hemorrhage (44). Intracellular deoxyhemoglobin is found only in acute non-neoplastic hematomas but can persist for weeks in intratumoral hemorrhage (Fig. 33). Subacute methemoglobin (high intensity on short TR/TE images), which forms initially at the periphery of nontumoral intracranial hematomas and subsequently converges over days, can remain at the periphery of hemorrhagic tumors for months. Furthermore, the lack of evolution into peripheral hemosiderin is common in intratumoral hemorrhages. This overall delay in hemorrhage evolution in malignant lesions, as compared with the evolution seen in non-neoplastic hematomas, has been postulated to be caused by profound intratumoral hypoxia (44), which has been documented in human neoplasms (81). Since it is well known that methemoglobin formation is intimately related to local oxygen tension (60,61), it follows that the persistence of marked intratumoral hypoxia could delay methemoglobin formation and alter the expected MR signal intensity patterns in hemorrhagic neoplasms. Recurrent bleeding has also been postulated as an etiology for these findings in neoplastic hemorrhages (82).

A consistent feature of hemorrhagic tumors is *lack* of a well-defined, complete, markedly hypointense rim (44), a characteristic finding in non-neoplastic hematomas in their subacute and chronic stages. It has been postulated that the persistent blood–brain barrier disruption known to occur in intracranial malignancies allows more efficient removal of iron storage products (44). As a result, this marker of prior intracranial hemorrhage, which persists indefinitely in non-neoplastic intracranial hematomas (12), is not consistently observed in the subacute and chronic stages of intratumoral hemorrhage (Figs.

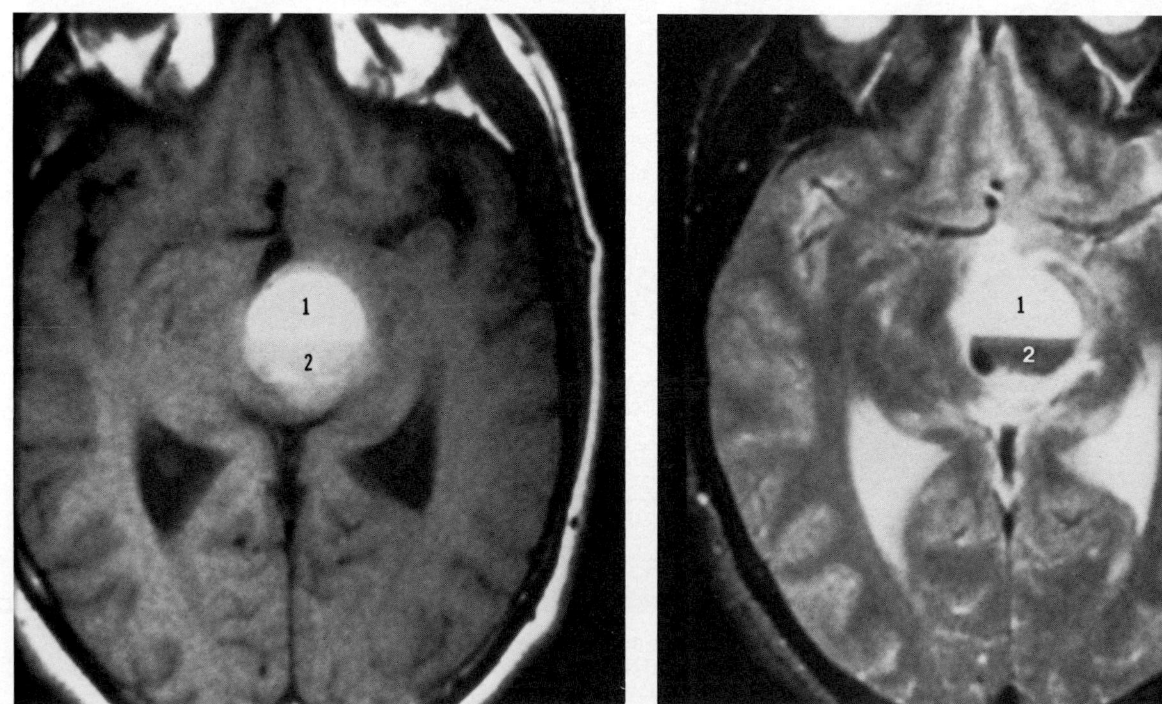

FIG. 32. Hemorrhagic astrocytoma with fluid-intracellular debris level and absence of ferritin/hemosiderin rim. **A:** Short TR/TE MRI (600/20). **B:** Long TR/TE MRI (2800/80). Left hypothalamic astrocytoma shows level of ventral extracellular methemoglobin (*1*) and dorsally layering intracellular blood (*2*) in surgically-proven hemorrhagic cystic astrocytoma. Again, there is no apparent rim of marked hypointensity around ventral methemoglobin, suggestive of tumor as underlying lesion.

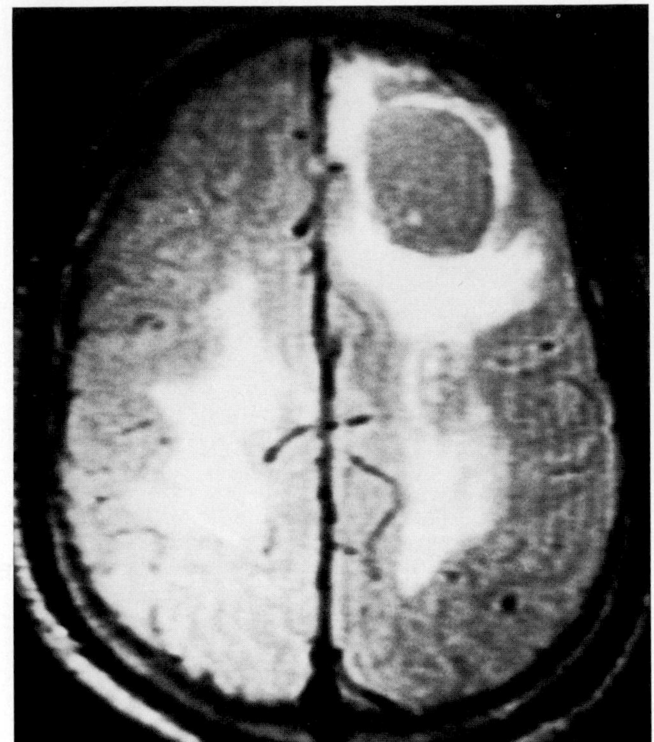
A

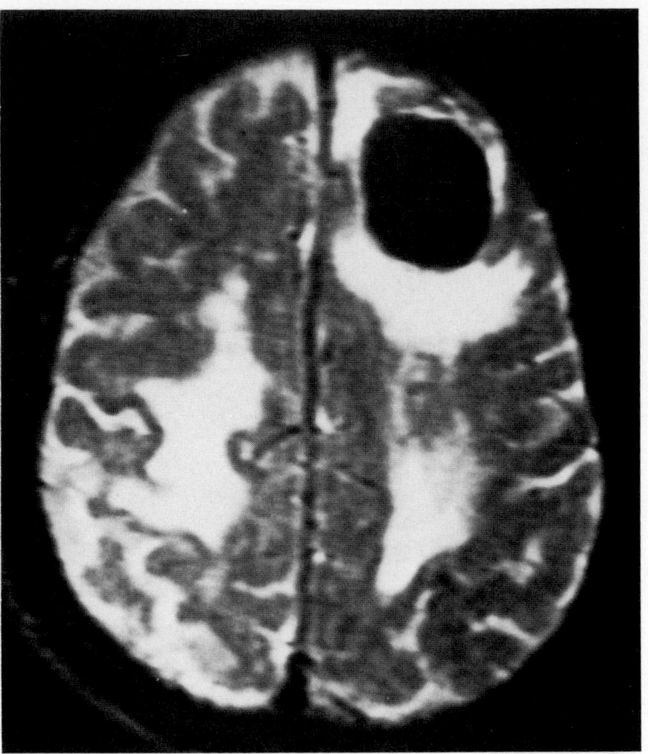
B

FIG. 33. Hemorrhagic metastasis with persistence of deoxyhemoglobin. **A:** Long TR/short TE MRI (2500/20). **B:** Long TR/TE MRI (2500/80). Large left frontal mass shows signal intensity pattern of intracellular deoxyhemoglobin in this 2- to 3-week-old hemorrhage. Note marked signal dropout on long TE image (B) as compared with short TE image (A). The persistence of deoxyhemoglobin is probably related to profound intratumoral hypoxia.

30–32). Lastly, an important finding in hemorrhagic neoplasms is the persistent and prominent perilesional high intensity (representing edema and tumor) on long TR MR images, even when the hemorrhage is in the chronic stage (Fig. 34). Edema is a well-documented, prominent feature on CT scans of intracranial metastases (83). The depiction of "edema" by MR images in the presence of an intracranial hematoma (especially when it is chronic) precludes the radiologist from confidently ascribing a benign etiology to the hemorrhage (Fig. 34).

Extra-Axial CNS Hemorrhage

While MR imaging is extremely sensitive and often specific for intracranial hemorrhage in the brain, its application in imaging extraparenchymal hemorrhage is limited in certain compartments. Subarachnoid hemorrhage, a common and often devastating event that requires immediate diagnosis and therapy, cannot be successfully imaged at present by MR techniques in the acute stage. This important pitfall in MRI of hemorrhage is well recognized (Fig. 35), and has been postulated to relate to the oxygen content of the subarachnoid space (84). The conversion of oxyhemoglobin to deoxyhemoglobin (and subsequently to methemoglobin) requires a relatively narrow range of oxygen tension (60,61). This state is rapidly achieved in isolated intracranial hematomas, resulting in characteristic marked hypointensity on long TR/TE images in the acute stage, and it is also seen in isolated clots in the subarachnoid space (Figs. 35–37). However, in acute *diffuse* subarachnoid hemorrhage, the ambient oxygen tension of the subarachnoid CSF is too high for expected evolutionary changes to occur. CT remains the imaging modality of choice for documenting acute subarachnoid blood.

After recurrent or chronic subarachnoid hemorrhage, subpial deposition of hemosiderin sometimes occurs, re-

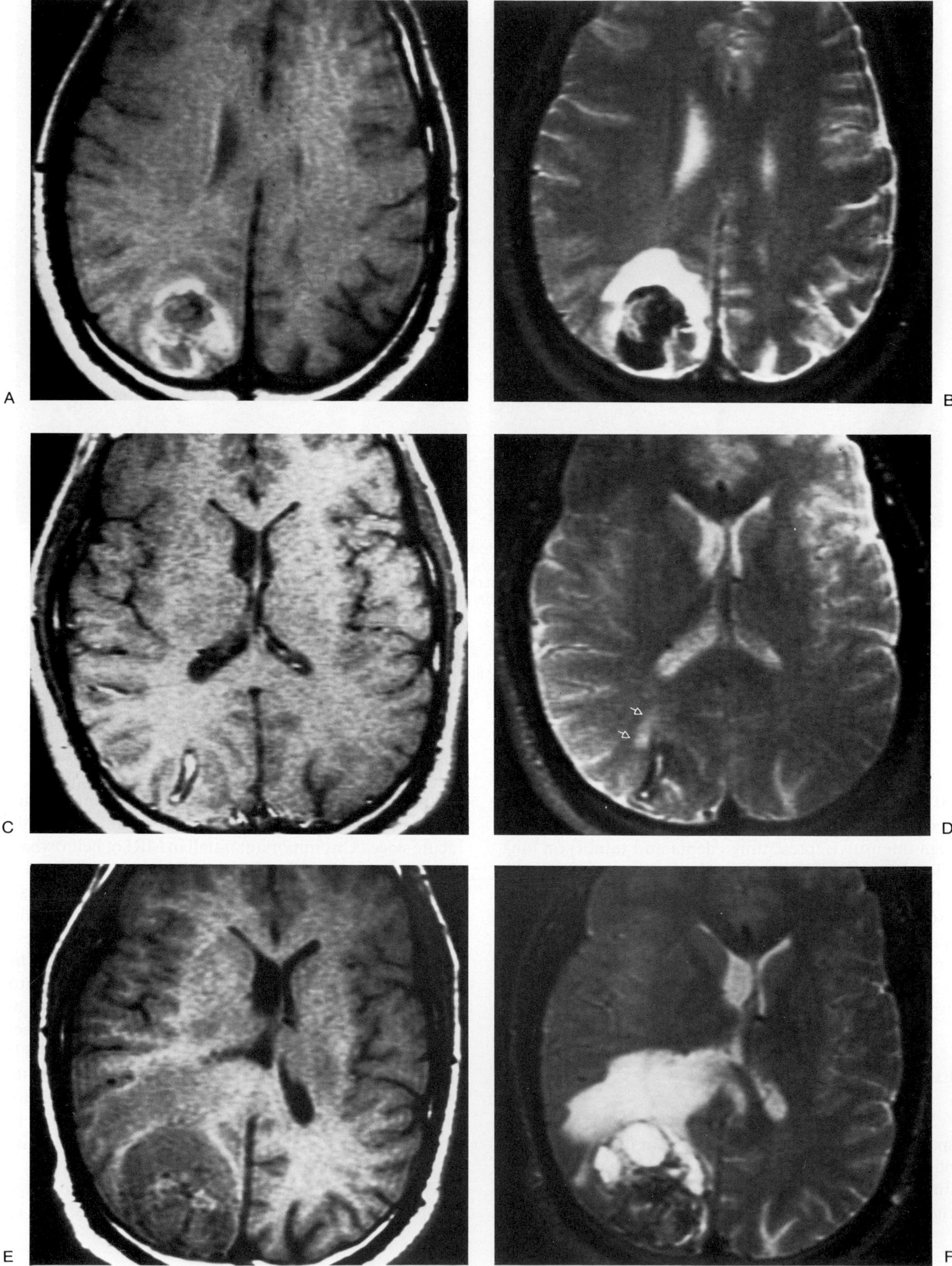
A
B
C
D
E
F

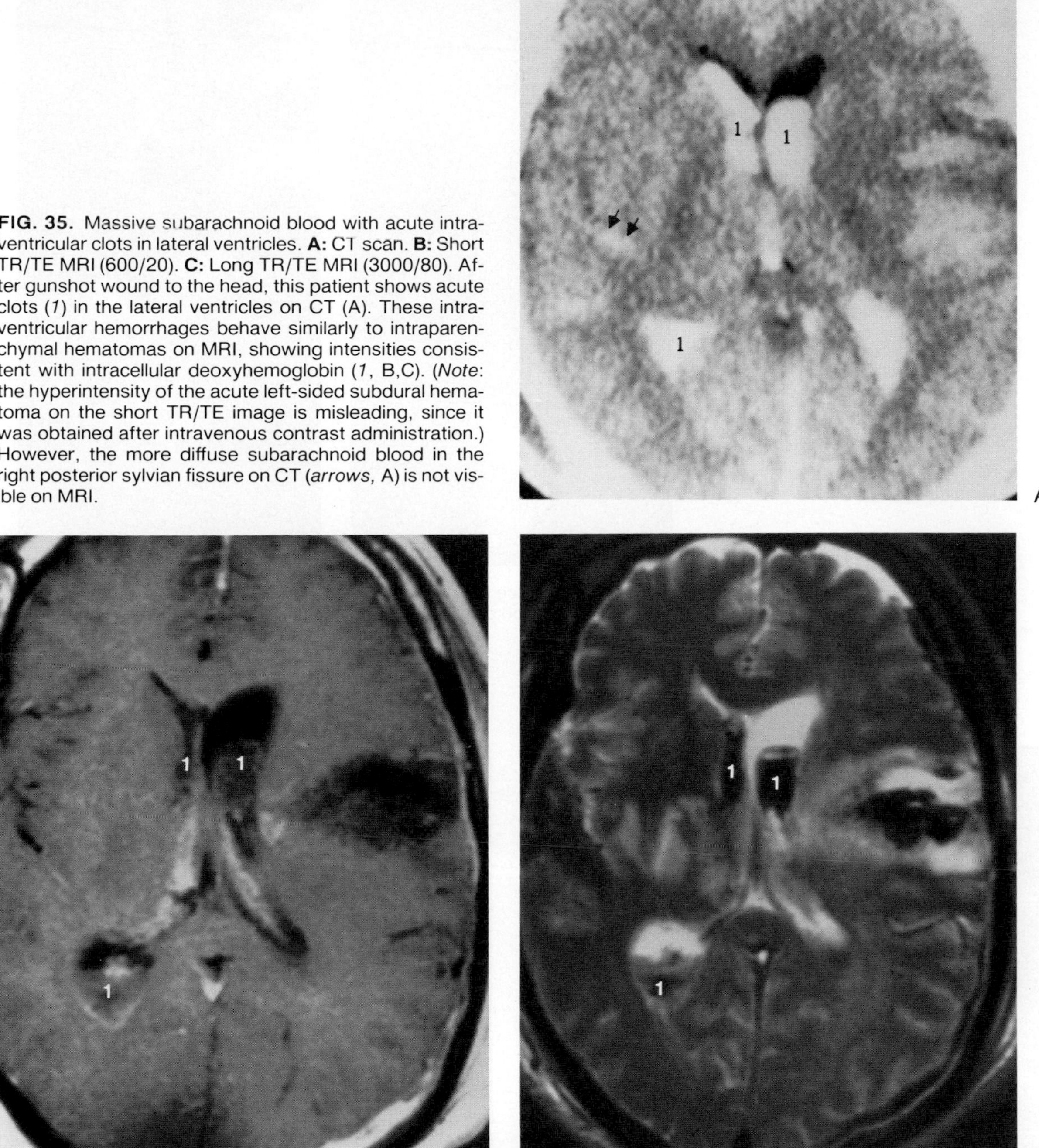

FIG. 35. Massive subarachnoid blood with acute intraventricular clots in lateral ventricles. **A:** CT scan. **B:** Short TR/TE MRI (600/20). **C:** Long TR/TE MRI (3000/80). After gunshot wound to the head, this patient shows acute clots (*1*) in the lateral ventricles on CT (A). These intraventricular hemorrhages behave similarly to intraparenchymal hematomas on MRI, showing intensities consistent with intracellular deoxyhemoglobin (*1*, B,C). (*Note*: the hyperintensity of the acute left-sided subdural hematoma on the short TR/TE image is misleading, since it was obtained after intravenous contrast administration.) However, the more diffuse subarachnoid blood in the right posterior sylvian fissure on CT (*arrows,* A) is not visible on MRI.

FIG. 34. Hemorrhagic astrocytoma, suggested by persistent peri-hematoma hyperintensity. **A:** Axial short TR/TE MRI (600/20), initial scan. **B:** Axial long TR/TE MRI (2500/80), initial scan. **C:** Coronal short TR/TE MRI (600/20), 1-month follow-up. **D:** Axial long TR/TE MRI (2500/80), 1-month follow-up. **E:** Axial short TR/TE MRI (600/20), 13-month follow-up. **F:** Axial long TR/TE MRI (2500/80), 13-month follow-up. Initial MRI (A,B) showed right parietal hemorrhage composed of central deoxyhemoglobin and peripheral methemoglobin, surrounded by high intensity on long TR image (B), a universal finding in acute/early subacute hemorrhage. One-month follow-up scan (C,D) shows evolution into appearance of chronic hematoma, with central methemoglobin, peripheral ferritin/hemosiderin, and collapse of mass with resolution of bulk of mass effect. However, the persistence of adjacent high intensity (*arrows,* D) precludes the diagnosis of benign hematoma, since there should be complete resolution of the "edema" in the chronic stage. The delayed follow-up scans (E,F) finally revealed growth of the underlying large astrocytoma, which eventually spread aggressively into both hemispheres via the corpus callosum (not shown).

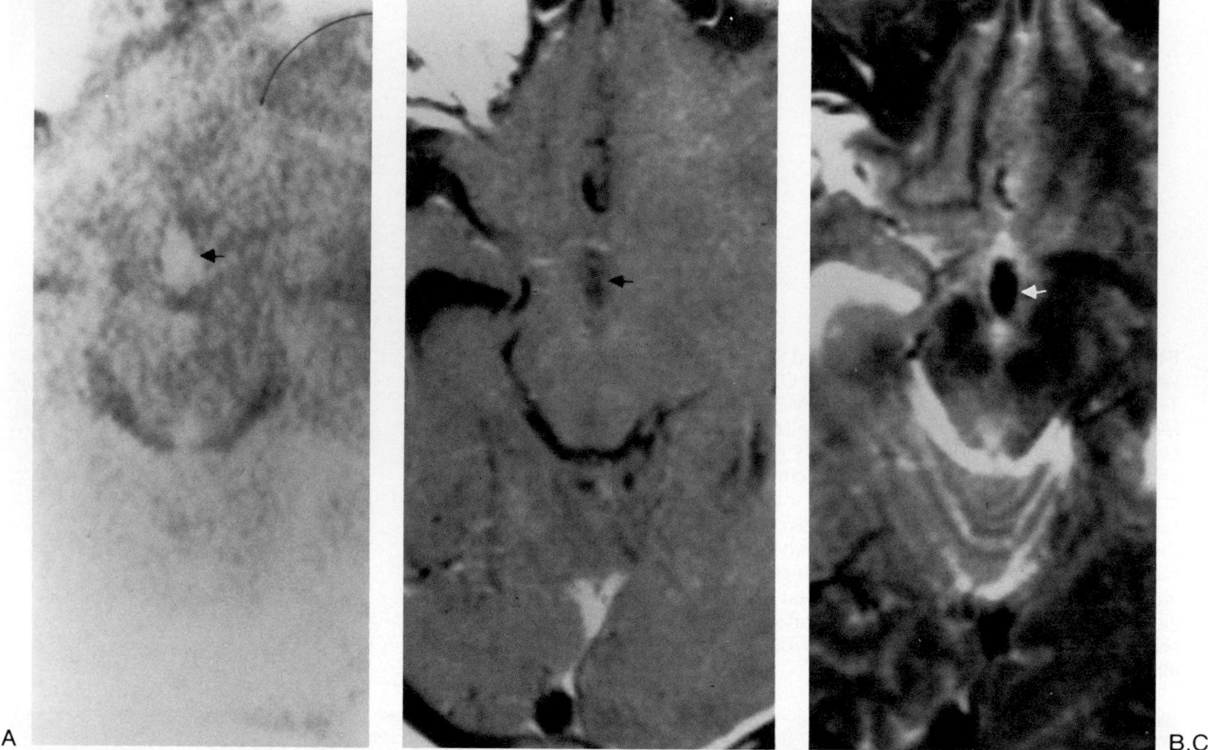

FIG. 36. Acute intraventricular clot in subarachnoid space (third ventricle). **A:** CT scan. **B:** Short TR/TE MRI (600/20). **C:** Long TR/TE MRI (3000/80). High attenuation blood on CT (A) in third ventricle (*arrow*) is seen as acute blood on short TR/TE (B) and long TR/TE (C) MR images.

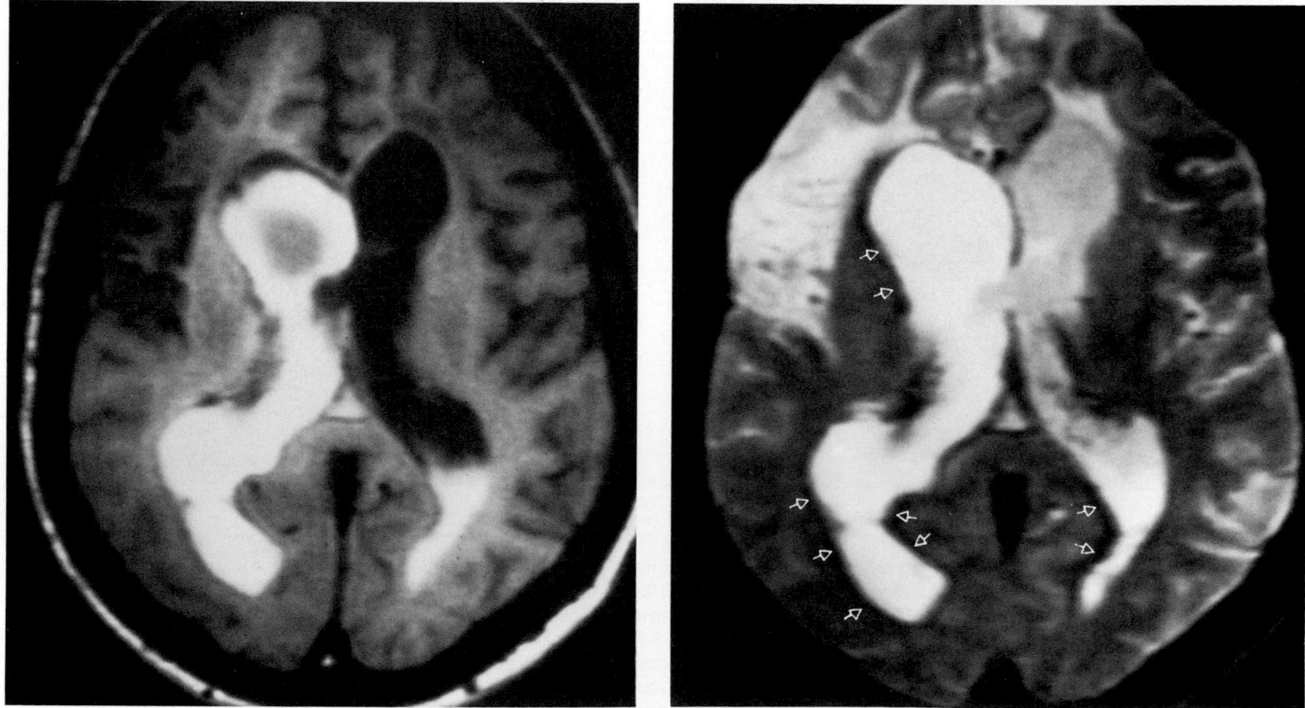

FIG. 37. Subacute clots in subarachnoid space (lateral ventricles). Massive lateral ventricle blood is hyperintense on short TR/TE (**A**) and long TR/TE (**B**) images (nearly filling right lateral ventricle), and is accompanied by subtle hypointensity along ventricular lining bilaterally (*arrows,* B), indicating ventricular siderosis in this patient with chronic intraventricular hemorrhage. Also note thickened, hypointense calvarial marrow in this patient with sickle cell disease.

sulting in superficial hemosiderosis *(superficial siderosis)* (85). This entity may be clinically incidental, but patients can demonstrate cranial nerve palsies, hearing loss, and cerebellar ataxia. Intracranial hemorrhage from tumors (Fig. 38) that continue to bleed can result in superficial hemosiderosis, which is manifested as marked hypointensity along the parenchymal surfaces on long TR/TE images. The cerebellum is a particularly common site for hemosiderin deposition in siderosis, and is typically more severely affected with hypointensity and concomitant parenchymal loss on MRI. In the absence of an intracranial cause for the siderosis, an ependymoma of the conus medullaris should be searched for as the etiology of the recurrent hemorrhage (Fig. 39). Intraventricular siderosis can also occur from neonatal intraventricular hemorrhage (86) or from intracranial vascular malformations and aneurysms (Fig. 40).

Subdural and epidural hematomas can be easily identified by SE MR images (Figs. 41 and 42). Morphologic criteria that are based on CT can also be applied to MR images for the compartmentalization of these extra-axial collections. The signal intensity patterns of evolving subdural hematomas have been reviewed (42) and appear similar to intraparenchymal hematomas in the acute and

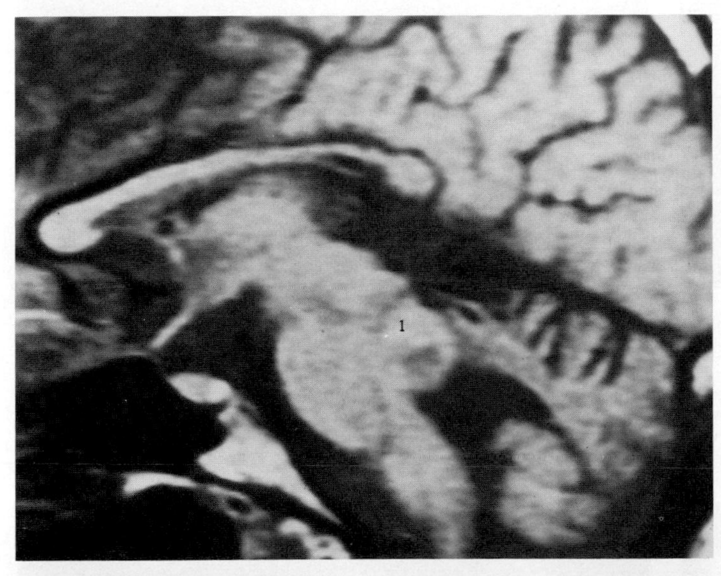

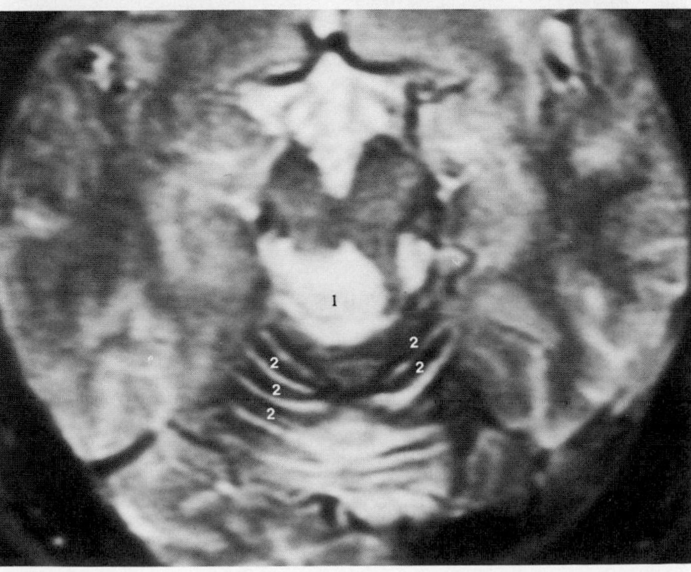

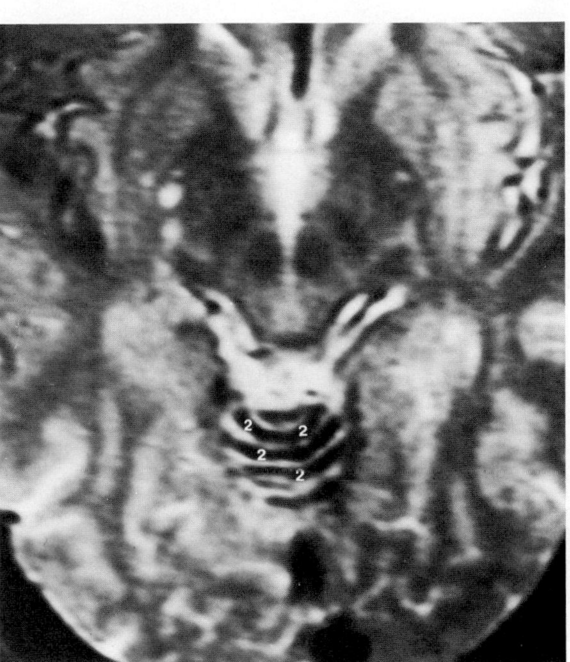

FIG. 38. Local superficial hemosiderosis from tectal glioma. **A:** Sagittal short TR/TE MRI (600/20). **B:** Axial long TR/TE MRI (2500/80). **C:** Axial long TR/TE MRI (2500/80). Note mass (*1*) involving tectum and dorsal pons with marked hypointensity on the surface of focally atrophic superior cerebellar vermis (*2*), most apparent on long TR/TE images (B,C). (From Barkovich and Atlas, ref. 1, with permission.)

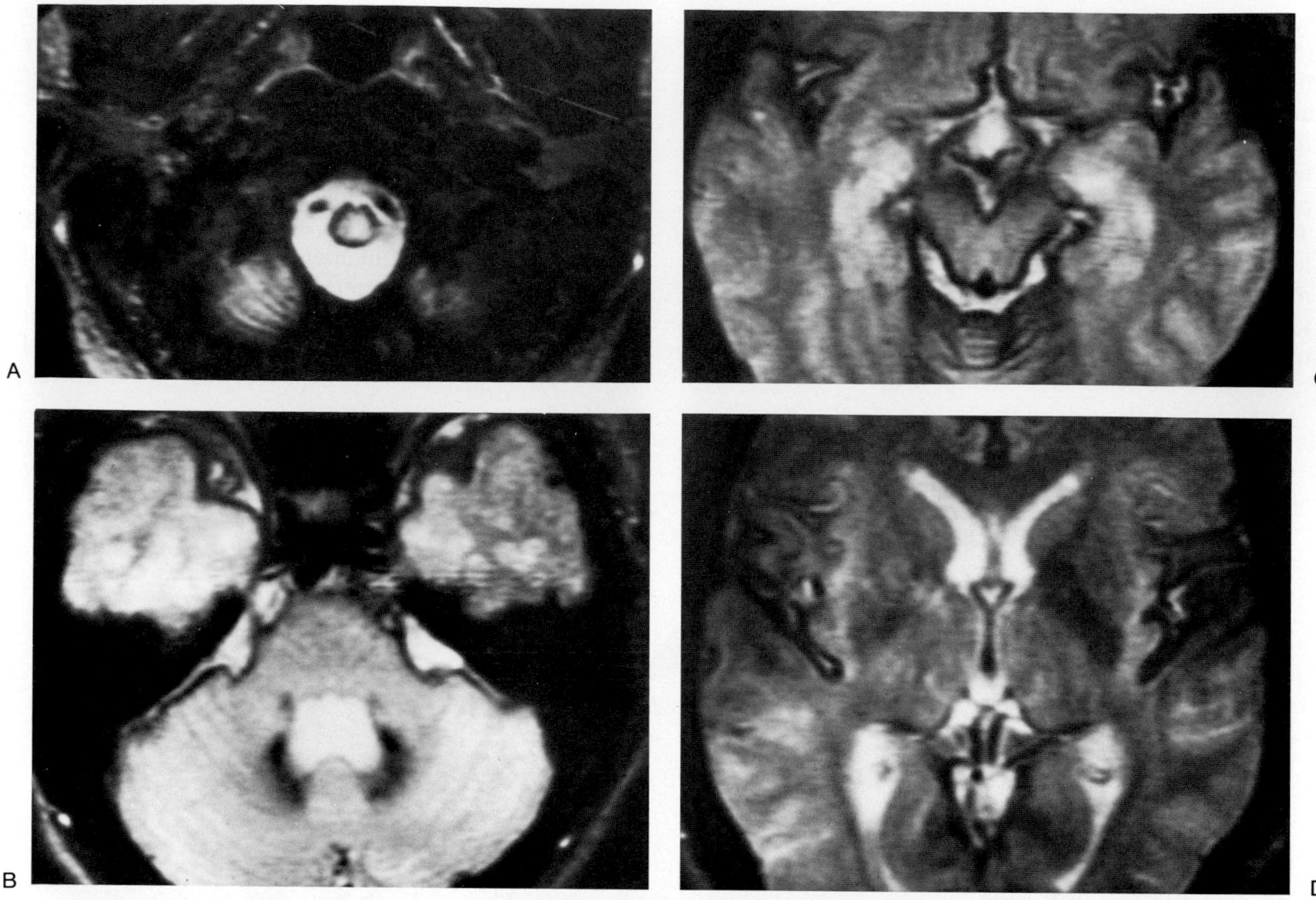

FIG. 39. Diffuse superficial hemosiderosis from spinal ependymoma. **A–D:** Serial long TR/TE MRI, inferior to superior (2500/80). Superficial marked hypointensity along surfaces of cervicomedullary junction, brainstem, and base of brain and within sylvian fissures indicates superficial hemosiderosis in this patient with filum terminate ependymoma that had repeatedly bled. This patient had sensorineural hearing loss, a fairly common clinical manifestation of this entity. (From Barkovich and Atlas, ref. 1.)

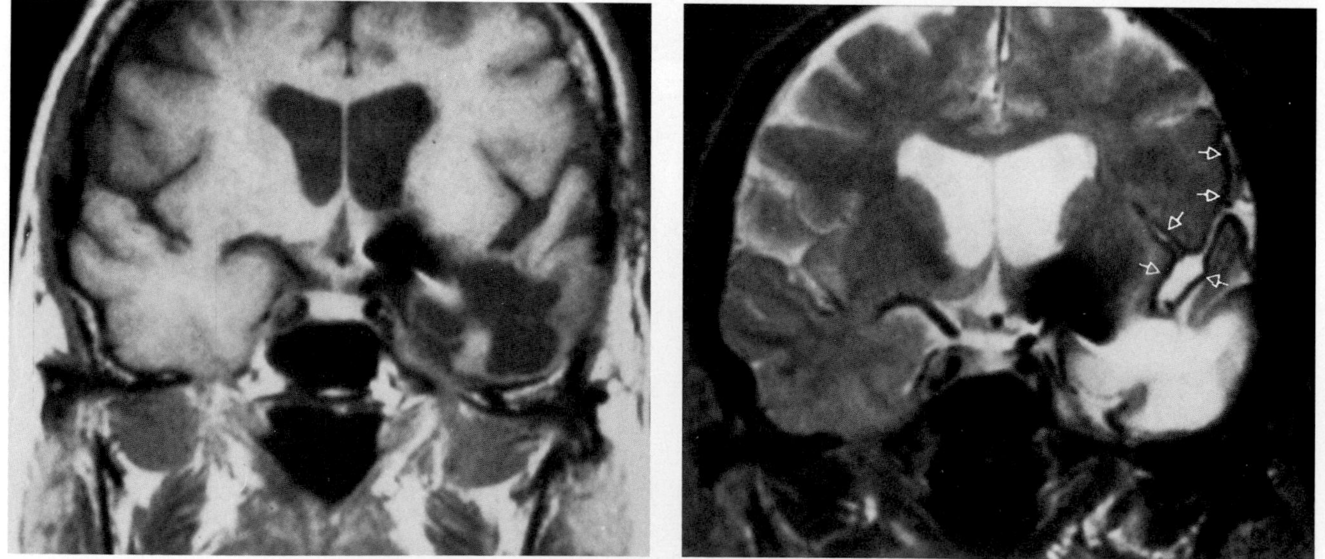

FIG. 40. Focal superficial hemosiderosis from prior aneurysmal hemorrhage. **A:** Coronal short TR/TE MRI (600/20). **B:** Coronal long TR/TE MRI (2800/80). Note thin superficial hypointensity along left sylvian fissure and opercular regions (*arrows,* B) in patient who had had prior surgical clipping of left-sided aneurysm (manifested by temporal lobe malacia and ferromagnetic clip artifact).

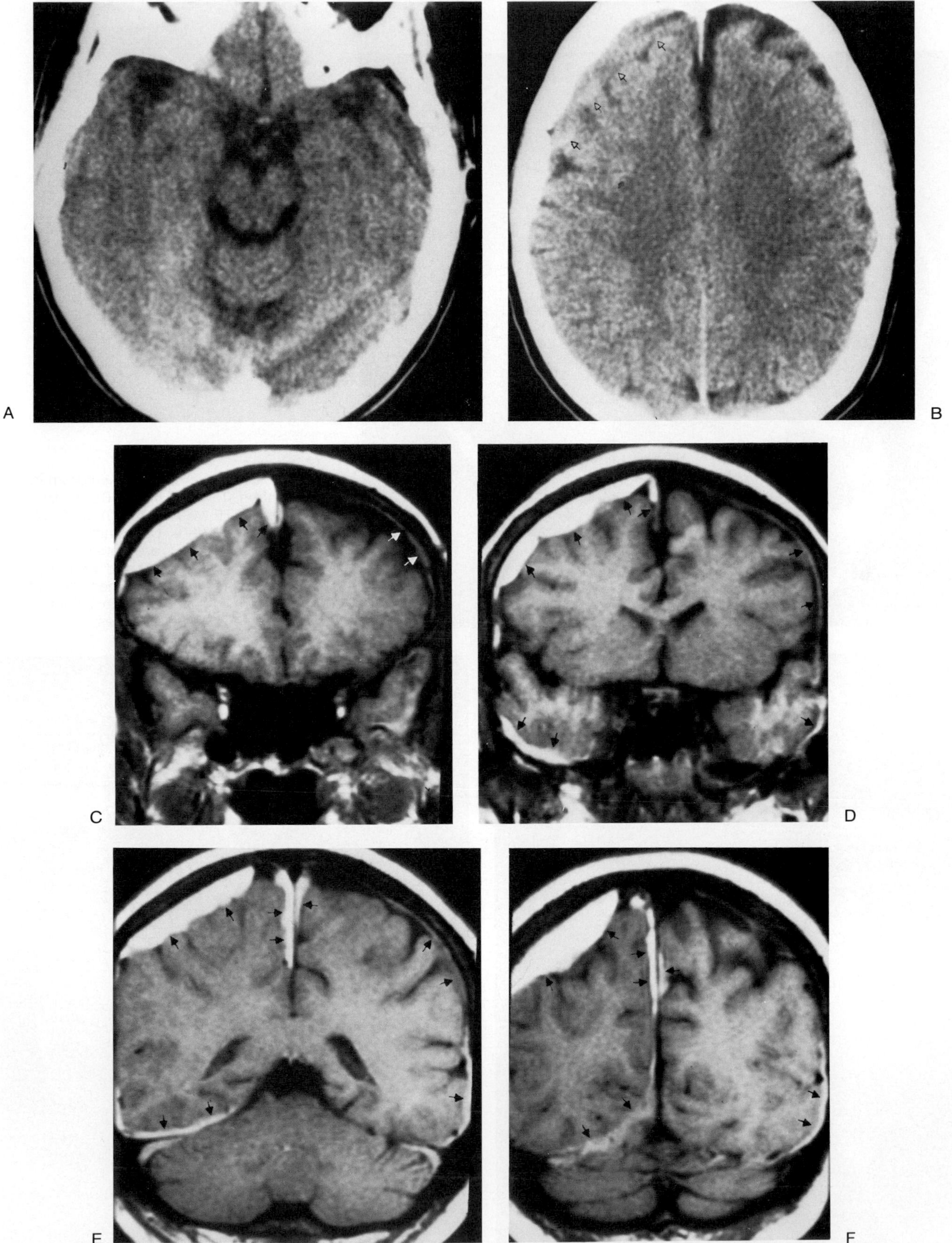

FIG. 41. Chronic subdural hematomas, CT vs. MRI. **A,B:** Axial CT scans. **C–F:** Coronal short TR/TE MRI, anterior to posterior (600/20). CT scans (A,B) only depict right frontal collection (*arrows*, B). Serial coronal MR images clearly demonstrate very extensive bilateral chronic subdural hematomas (*arrows*, C–F).

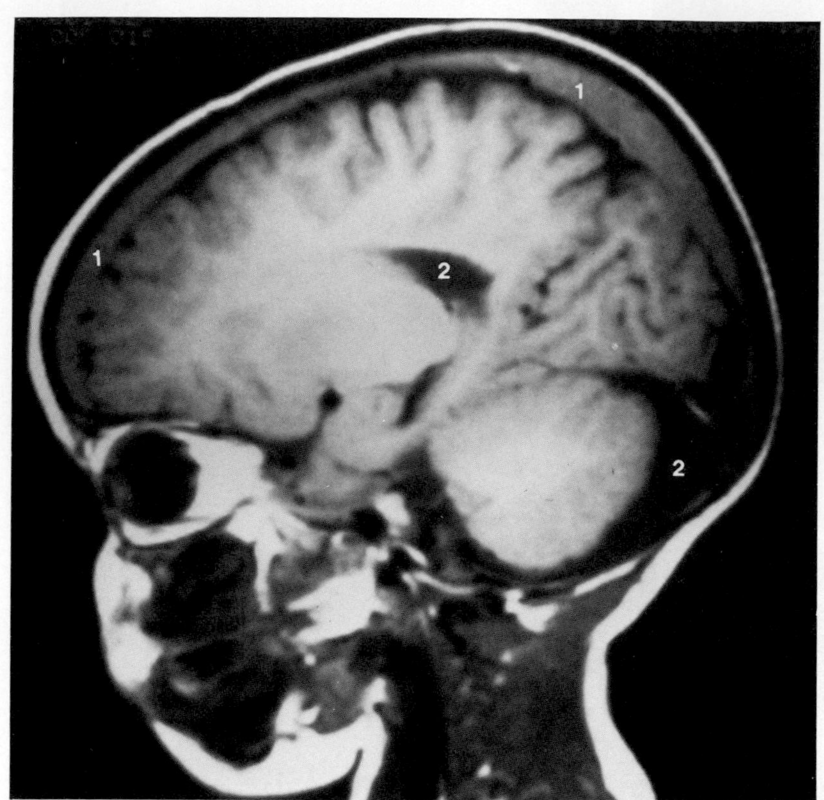

FIG. 42. Chronic subdural hematomas. **A:** Sagittal short TR/TE MRI (600/20). **B:** Axial long TR/short TE MRI (2800/30). **C:** Axial long TR/TE MRI (2800/80). Note that intensity of subdural hematomas (*1*) are higher than that of CSF (*2*) on short TR/TE (A) and long TR/short TE (B) images, distinguishing these collections from subdural hygromas, which would match the intensity of CSF on all images.

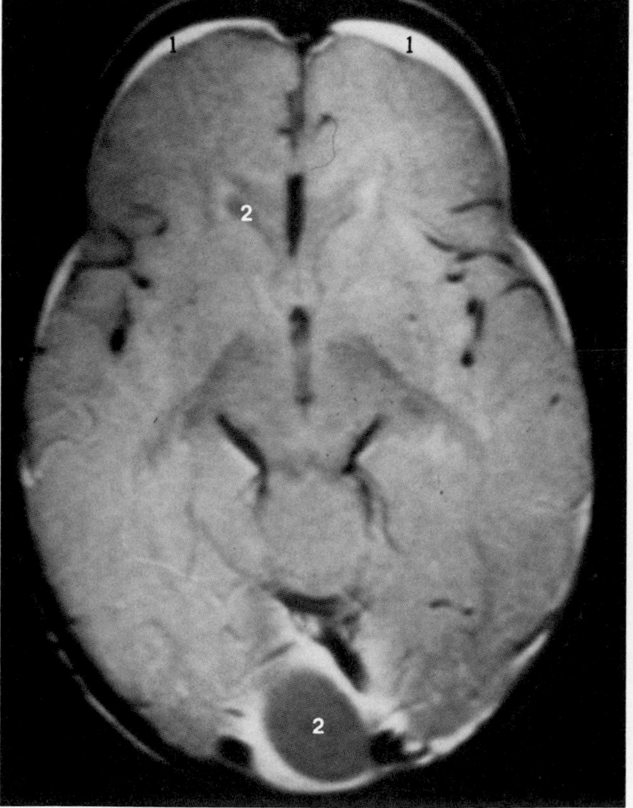

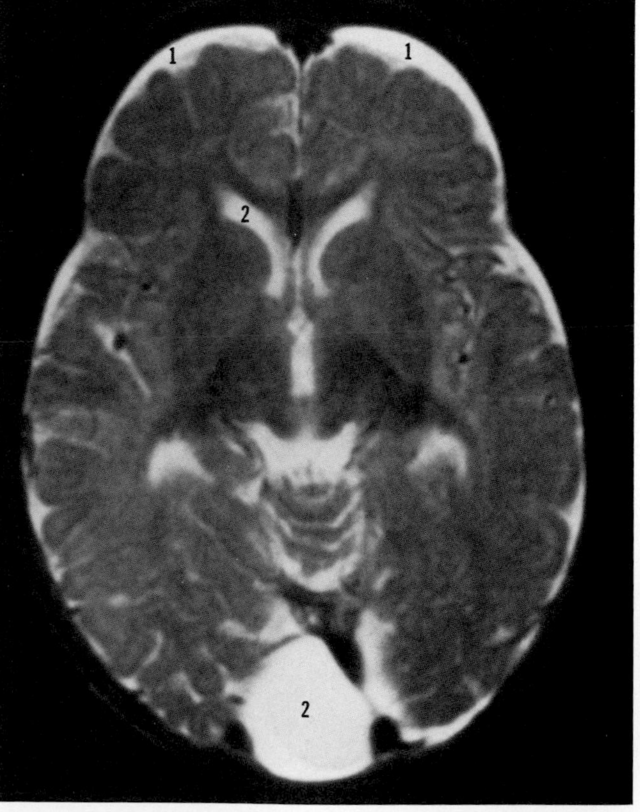

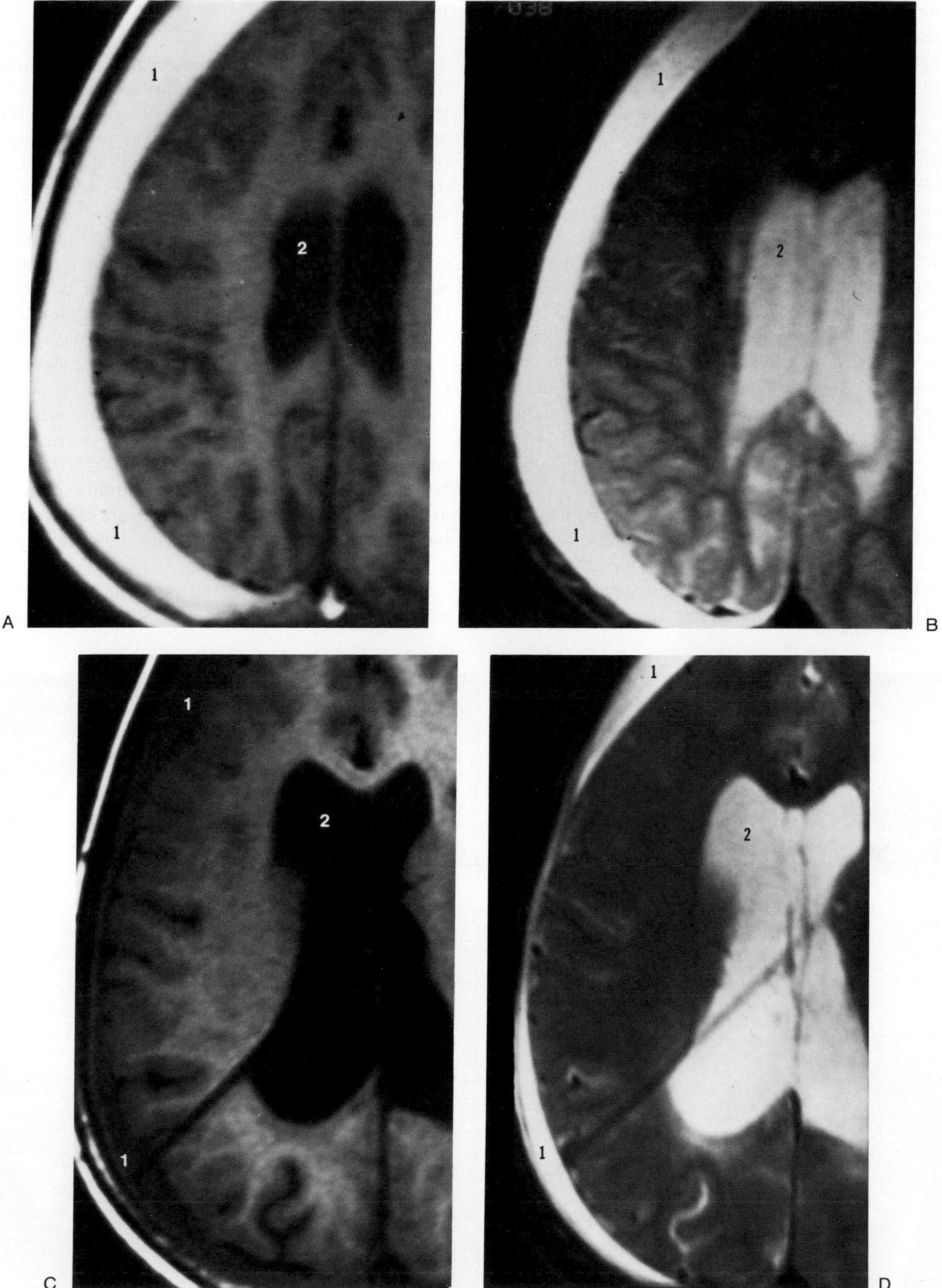

FIG. 43. Eventual decrease in intensity of chronic subdural over time. **A:** Short TR/TE MRI (600/20). **B:** Long TR/TE MRI (3000/80). **C:** Short TR/TE MRI (600/20), 2 months later. **D:** Long TR/TE MRI (3000/80), 2 months later. Chronic right-sided subdural hematoma (*1*) is markedly hyperintense on short (A) and long TR/TE (B) images. Over time, the intensity on the short TR/TE image (C) has decreased dramatically, but it still remains hyperintense to ventricular CSF (*2*). This effect is due to dilution of the concentration of methemoglobin with degradation of the hematoma.

subacute stages. Note that chronic subdural hematomas, which show low attenuation on CT scan (and thereby are indistinguishable from CSF collections), are markedly hyperintense on images because of methemoglobin content. Furthermore, as chronic subdurals evolve, progressive breakdown, resorption, and dilution effects on methemoglobin result in gradual *decrease* in intensity on short TR/TE images (Fig.43). Chronic subdurals can be only minimally hyperintense to CSF on short TR/TE MR, reflecting either a very low concentration of paramagnetic methemoglobin or a high concentration of nonparamagnetic protein (Figs. 42 and 43). Hemosiderin accumulation in the adjacent dural structures is not a consistent feature of extra-axial hemorrhage (42), presumably because of the absence of a blood–brain barrier in dura. Rebleeding into a subdural collection should be suspected if irregular hypointense membranes loculating areas of different ages of subdural are found (Fig. 44), or if there are debris-fluid levels seen within the collection (Fig. 45). An important role in MRI of extra-axial hemorrhage, with its unique ability to stage intracranial hemorrhage temporally, lies in the documentation of suspected child abuse, since the depiction of multiple sites of intracranial hemorrhage at different stages of evolution can be an important clue to this diagnosis (Fig. 46).

Pituitary Hemorrhage

Gross or microscopic hemorrhage is documented to occur in up to 27.7% of pituitary adenomas (87). Less than one-half of patients with hemorrhage into pituitary adenomas have clinical signs of true pituitary apoplexy (88). Spontaneous hemorrhage may also occur into a nontumorous pituitary but is thought to be much less common.

Pituitary apoplexy is defined by abrupt onset of headache, nausea, vomiting, photophobia, nuchal rigidity, visual disturbances, and altered levels of consciousness (89). These findings may mimic aneurysmal rupture with subarachnoid hemorrhage. Both mass effect and ischemia are thought to play roles in the development of symptomatology. Factors thought to be of etiologic importance include radiotherapy or bromocriptine therapy for existing adenoma, pregnancy, trauma, anticoagulation, lumbar puncture, and angiography (89). Note that the vast majority of pituitary hemorrhages are asymptomatic—the identification of intrapituitary blood on MR does not equate with the symptomatology of apoplexy.

The CT appearance of pituitary hemorrhage can be variable, often demonstrating only an enlarged gland

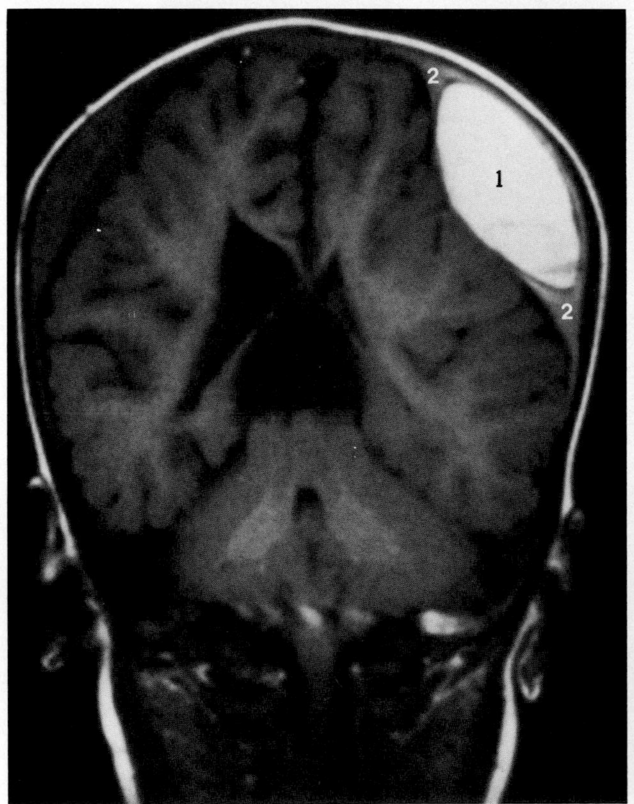

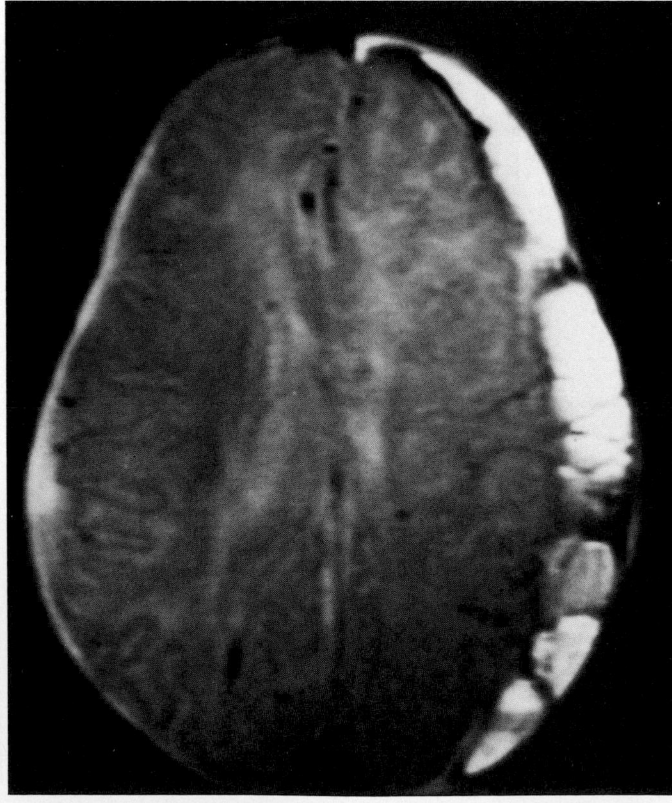

FIG. 44. Rebleed into subdural hematoma with foculated intensities and membranes. **A:** Coronal short TR/TE MRI (600/20). **B:** Axial long TR/TE MRI (2800/80). Note loculated region of high-intensity methemoglobin (*1*) within only minimally hyperintense collections (*2*) on short TR/TE image (A). The higher intensity area is more recent (it has not evolved into the lower intensity yet). Intervening hypointense membranes on long TR/TE image (B) further suggest loculations within this chronic collection.

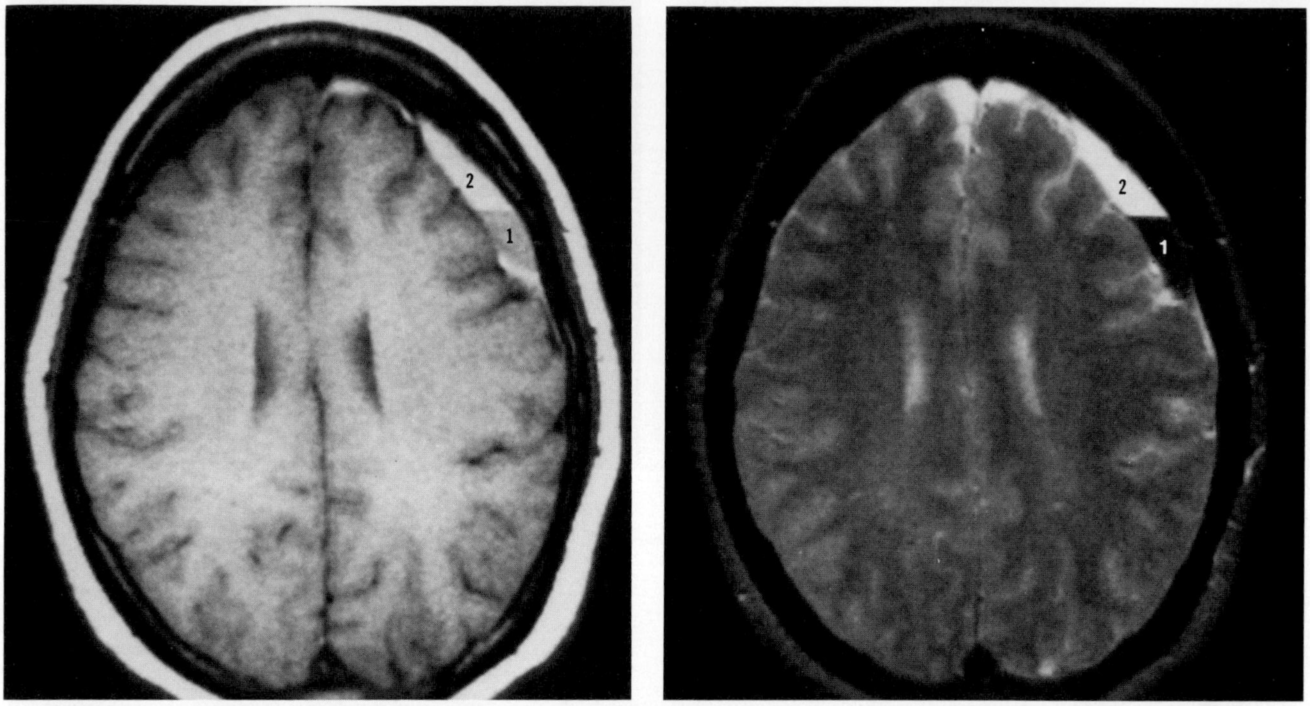

FIG. 45. Intrahematoma level suggestive of recent rebleeding. **A:** Short TR/TE MRI (600/20). **B:** Long TR/TE MRI (2800/80). Dependent intracellular deoxyhemoglobin (*1*) layers posteriorly, with anterior methemoglobin (*2*). (From Barkovich and Atlas, ref. 1, with permission.)

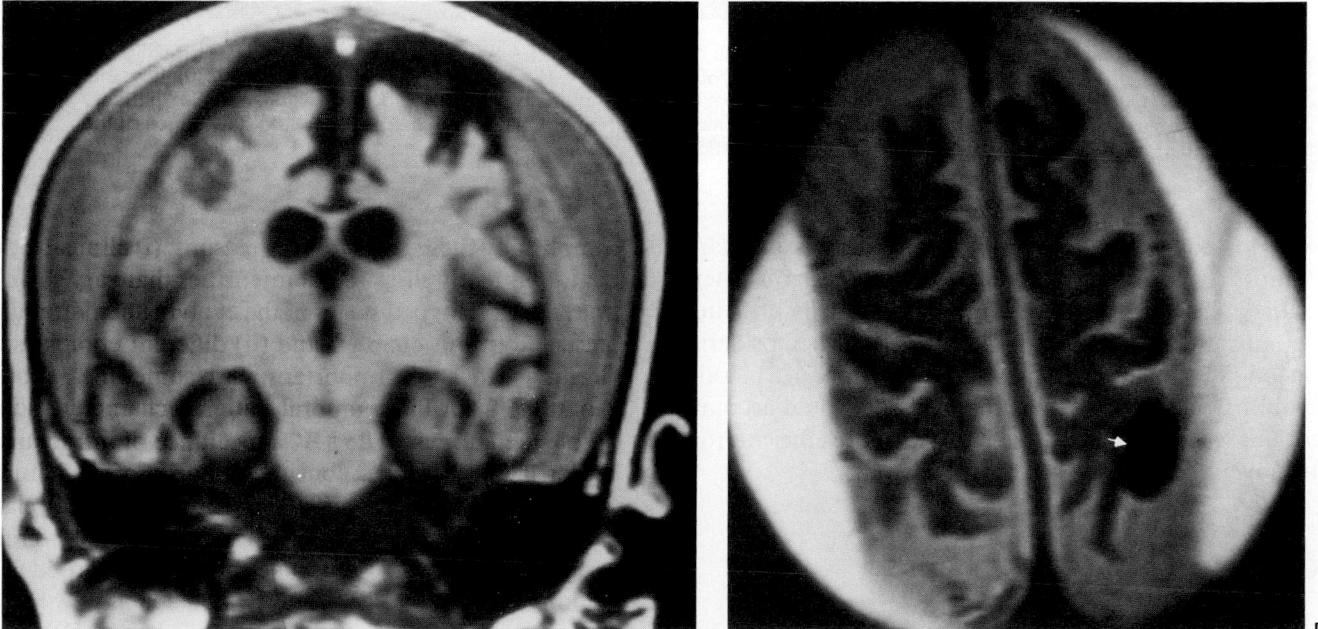

FIG. 46. Mixed ages of subdural hematomas and intraparenchymal blood, suggestive of child abuse. **A:** Coronal short TR/TE MRI (600/120). **B:** Axial long TR/TE MRI (2500/80). Membranes separating bilateral subdural hematomas of varying composition (and hence of varying ages), in combination with intraparenchymal hematoma (*arrow*, B) and marked atrophy corroborate diagnosis of multiple episodes of head trauma in this child.

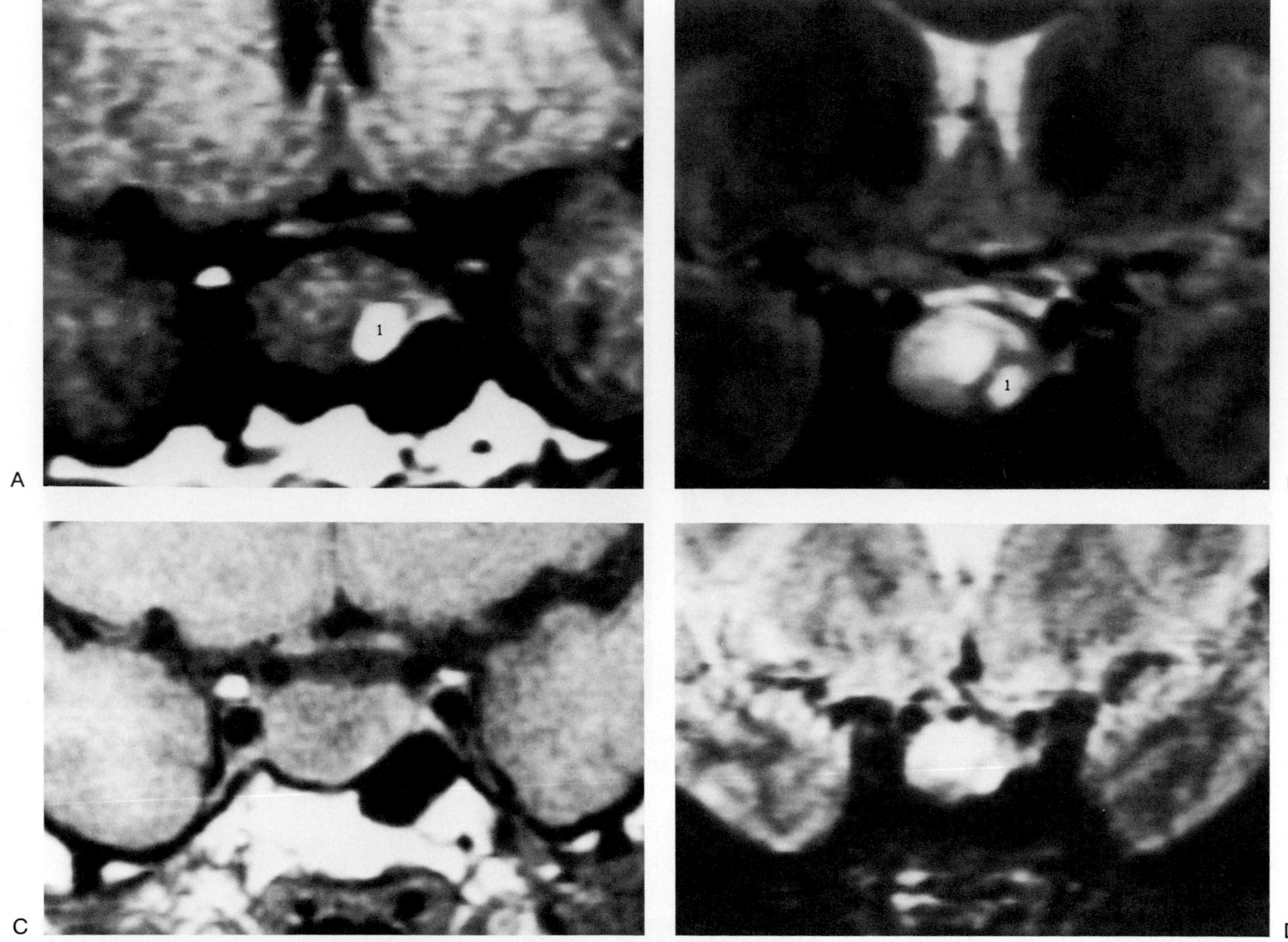

FIG. 47. Pituitary hemorrhage without iron storage hypointensity on follow-up. **A:** Coronal short TR/TE MRI (600/20), initial study. **B:** Coronal long TR/TE MRI (2500/80), initial study. **C:** Coronal short TR/TE MRI (600/20), 6 weeks later. **D:** Coronal long TR/TE MRI (2500/80), 6 weeks later. High-intensity methemoglobin (*1*) within complex pituitary adenoma is demonstrated initially (A,B). Note resolution of methemoglobin (C) 6 weeks later, without evidence of the hypointensity from iron storage forms (D). (From Barkovich and Atlas, ref. 1, with permission.)

with mixed attenuation; MRI clearly depicts pituitary hemorrhage in its various evolving states (Fig. 47). Interestingly, chronic pituitary hemorrhage usually does not demonstrate the marked hypointensity of hemosiderin on long TR/TE images (Fig. 47). The absence of a blood–brain barrier in this extracerebral tissue would account for this MR feature, because it allows more efficient iron turnover.

CONCLUSIONS

The role of the neuroradiologist in assessing MR images of patients who are suspected to have had intracranial hemorrhage is to recognize the hemorrhage and attempt to discern its etiology. Understanding the basis for the appearance of hematomas aids significantly in accomplishing these goals for two reasons: (i) clinical cases not infrequently show signal intensities that vary slightly from the stereotyped stages of the evolving hematoma as presented in this chapter; and (ii) different etiologies of bleeding can show important, but sometimes subtle, variations from the temporal patterns characteristic of simple hematomas. The MR appearance of intracranial hemorrhage is complex, but the majority of its features can be explained in terms of current concepts of relaxation, iron metabolism, and integrity of the blood–brain barrier. The presented rationale should be regarded as a working hypothesis, waiting to be updated as new information on iron biochemistry and its effects on MR relaxation phenomena become available. Image interpretation often requires correlation with the clinical history in order to interpret optimally all the features of the MR image.

REFERENCES

1. Barkovich AJ, Atlas SW. Magnetic resonance imaging of intracranial hemorrhage. *Radiol Clin North Am* 1988;26:801–820.
2. Brooks RA, Di Chiro G, Patronas N. MR imaging of cerebral hematomas at different field strengths: theory and applications. *J Comput Assist Tomogr* 1989;13:194–206.
3. Gomori JM, Grossman RI. Head and neck hemorrhage. In: Kressel HY, ed. *Magnetic Resonance Annual 1987.* New York: Raven Press, 1987;71–112.
4. Grossman RI, Gomori JM, Goldberg HI, et al. MR imaging of hemorrhage conditions of the head and neck. *Radiographics* 1988;8:441–454.
5. Thulborn KR, Brady TJ. Iron in magnetic resonance imaging of cerebral hemorrhage. *Magn Reson Q* 1989;5:23–38.
6. Atlas SW, Mark AS, Gomori JM, Grossman RI. Intracranial hemorrhage: gradient echo imaging at 1.5T. Comparison with spin-echo imaging and clinical applications. *Radiology* 1988;168:803–807.
7. Brooks RA, Brunetti A, Alger JR, Di Chiro G. On the origin of paramagnetic inhomogeneity effects in blood. *Magn Reson Med* 1989,12:241–248.
8. Bryant RG, Marill K, Blackmore C, Francis C. Magnetic relaxation in blood and blood clots. *Magn Reson Med* 1990;13:133–144.
9. Bydder GM, Pennock JM, Porteous R, Dubowitz LM, Gadian DG. MRI of intracerebral hematoma at low field (0.15 T) using T2 dependent partial saturation sequences. *Neuroradiology* 1988;30:367–371.
10. De La Paz RI, New PFJ, Buonanno FS, et al. NMR imaging of intracranial hemorrhage. *J Comput Assist Tomogr* 1984;8:599–607.
11. Di Chiro G, Brooks RA, Girton ME, et al. Sequential MR studies of intracerebral hematomas in monkeys. *AJNR* 1986;7:193–199.
12. Gomori JM, Grossman RI, Goldberg HI, Zimmerman RA, Bilaniuk LT. Intracranial hematomas: imaging by high-field MR. *Radiology* 1985;157:87–93.
13. Gomori JM, Grossman RI, Hackney DB, Goldberg HI, Zimmerman RA, Bilaniuk LT. Variable appearances of subacute intracranial hematomas on high-field spin-echo MR. *AJNR* 1987;8:1019–1026.
14. Hackney DB, Atlas SW, Grossman RI, et al. Subacute intracranial hemorrhage: contribution of spin density to appearance on spin echo MR images. *Radiology* 1987;165:199–202.
15. Sipponen JT, Sepponen RE, Sivula A. Nuclear magnetic resonance (NMR) imaging of intracranial hemorrhage in the acute and resolving phases. *J Comput Assist Tomogr* 1983;7:954–959.
16. Thulborn KR, Waterton JC, Matthews PM, Radda GK. Oxygenation dependence of the transverse relaxation time of water protons in whole blood at high field. *Biochim Biophys Acta* 1982;714:265–270.
17. Wismer GL, Buxton RB, Rosen BR, et at. Susceptibility induced magnetic resonance line broadening: applications to brain iron mapping. *J Comput Assist Tomogr* 1988;12:259–265.
18. Zimmerman RD, Heier LA, Snow RB, Liu DPC, Kelly AB, Deck MDF. Acute intracranial hemorrhage: intensity changes on sequential MR scans at 0.5T. *AJNR* 1988;9:47–57.
19. Hayman A, Chin HY, Kirkpatrick JB, Ford JJ, Taber KH. Temporal changes in RBC hydration: application to MR of blood. In: *Abstracts of the Proceedings of the American Society of Neuroradiology Annual Meeting,* Los Angeles, CA. American Society of Neuroradiology; 1990;314.
20. Clark RA, Watanabe AT, Bradley WG, Roberts JD. Acute hematomas: effects of deoxygenation, hematocrit, and fibrin-clot formation and retraction on T2 shortening. *Radiology 1990;* 175:201–206.
21. Ziock K. *Basic Quantum Mechanics.* New York: John Wiley; 1969.
22. Burke HE. *Handbook of Magnetic Phenomena.* New York: Van Nostrand Reinhold; 1986:9–57.
23. Bean CP. Hysteresis loops of mixtures of ferromagnetic micropowders. *J Appl Phys* 1955;26:1381–1383.
24. Bean CP, Livingston JD. Superparamagnetism. *J Appl Phys* 1959;30:120S–129S.
25. Schenck JF, Mueller OM, Souza SP, Dumoulin CL. Magnetic resonance imaging of brain iron using a 4 Tesla whole-body scanner. In: Frankel RB, Blakemann RP, eds. *Iron Biominerals.* New York: Plenum Press, 1990.
26. Abragam A. *Principles of Nuclear Magnetism.* Oxford: Clarendon Press, 1985.
27. Becker ED. *High Resolution NMR. Theory and Clinical Applications.* New York: Academic Press; 1980.
28. Farrar TC, Becker ED. *Pulse and Fourier Transform NMR.* New York: Academic Press; 1971:2–15.
29. Fukushima E, Roeder SBW. *Experimental Pulse NMR. A Nuts and Bolts Approach.* London: Addison-Wesley; 1981:1–25.
30. Yoder CH, Schaeffer CD Jr. *Introduction to Multinuclear NMR.* Menlo Park: Benjamin/Cummings; 1987.
31. Lauffer RB. Paramagnetic metal complexes as water proton relaxation agents for NMR imaging: theory and design. *Chem Rev* 1987;87:901–927.
32. Dickerson RE, Geis I. *Hemoglobin: Structure, Function, Evolution, and Pathology.* Menlo Park: Benjamin Cummings; 1983:1–60.
33. Edelman RR, Johnson K, Buxton R, et al. MR of hemorrhage: a new approach. *AJNR* 1986;7:751–756.
34. Gomori JM, Grossman RI, Yu-Ip C, Asakura T. NMR relaxation times of blood: dependence on field strength, oxidation state, and cell integrity. *J Comput Assist Tomogr* 1987;11:684–690.
35. Kamman RL, Go KG, Brouwer W, Berendsen HJC. Nuclear magnetic resonance relaxation in experimental brain edema: effects of water concentration, protein concentration and temperature. *Magn Reson Med* 1988;6:265–274.
36. Koenig SH, Schillinger WE. Nuclear magnetic relaxation dispersion in protein solutions. II: Transferrin. *J Biol Chem* 1969;244:6520–6526.
37. Koenig SH, Brown RD. Relaxometry of magnetic resonance imaging contrast agents. In: Kressel HY, ed. *Magnetic Resonance Annual 1987.* New York: Raven Press; 1987:263–286.
38. Koenig SH. The dynamics of water-protein interactions. Results from measurements of nuclear magnetic relaxation dispersion. In: Rowland SP, ed. *Water in Polymers.* Washington, D.C.: American Chemical Society; 1980:157–176.
39. Gillis P, Koenig SH. Transverse relaxation of solvent protons induced by magnetized spheres: application to ferritin, erythrocytes and magnetite. *Magn Reson Med* 1987;5:323–345.
40. Cohen MS, Weisskoff RM. Ultra-fast imaging. *Magn Reson Imaging* 1991;9(1):1–37.
41. Kreindler A, Marcovici G, Florescu 1. Histoenzymologic and biochemical investigations into the nervous tissue round an experimentally-induced cerebral hemorrhagic focus. *Rev Roum Neurol* 1972;9:313–319.
42. Fobben ES, Grossman RI, Atlas SW. MR characteristics of subdural hematomas and hygromas at 1.5 T. *AJNR* 1989;10:687–693.
43. Gomori JM, Grossman RI, Goldberg HI, et al. Occult cerebral vascular malformations: high field MR imaging. *Radiology* 1986;158:707–713.
44. Atlas SW, Grossman RI, Gomori JM, et al. Hemorrhagic intracranial malignant neoplasms: spin-echo MR imaging. *Radiology* 1987;164:71–77.
45. Lalonde JMA, Ghadially FN, Massey KL. Ultrastructure of intramuscular haematomas and electron-probe X-ray analysis of extracellular and intracellular iron deposits. *J Pathol* 1978;125:17–23.
46. Finch CA, Huebers HA. Iron metabolism. *Clin Physiol Biochem* 1986;4:5–10.
47. Trump BE, Valigorsky JM, Arstila AU, Mergner WJ, Kinney TD. The relationship of intracellular pathways of iron metabolism to cellular iron overload and the iron storage diseases. *Am J Pathol* 1973;72:295–324.
48. Weinberg ED. Iron, infection and neoplasia. *Clin Physiol Biochem* 1986;4:50–60.
49. Southern PA, Powis G. Free radicals in medicine. I. Chemical nature and biologic reactions. II. Involvement in human disease. *Mayo Clin Proc* 1988;63:390–408.

50. Munro HN, Linder MC. Ferritin: structure, biosynthesis and role in iron metabolism. *Physiol Rev* 1978;58:317–396.
51. Wixon RL, Prutkin L, Munro HN. Hemosiderin: nature, formation and significance. *Int Rev Exp Pathol* 1980;22:193–225.
52. Bunn HF, Forget BG. Hemoglobin structure. In: *Hemoglobin: Molecular, Genetic and Clinical Aspects.* Philadelphia: WB Saunders; 1986:13–35.
53. Cohen MD, McGuire W, Cory DA, Smith JA. MR appearance of blood and blood products: an *in vitro* study. *AJR* 1986;146:1293–1297.
54. Fullerton GD, Potter JL, Dornbluth NC. NMR relaxation of protons in tissues and other macromolecular water solutions. *Magn Reson Imaging* 1982;1:209–228.
55. Nose T, Enomoto T, Hyodo A, et al. Intracerebral hematoma developing during MR examination. *J Comput Assist Tomogr* 1987;11: 184.
56. Brindle KM, Brown FE, Campbell ID, Grathwohl C, Kuchel PW. Application of spin-echo nuclear magnetic resonance to whole cell systems: membrane transport. *Biochem J* 1979;180:37–44.
57. Majumdar S, Zoghbi SS, Gore JC. The influence of pulse sequence on the relaxation effects of superparamagnetic iron oxide contrast agents. *Magn Reson Med* 1989;10:289–301.
58. Enzmann DR, Britt RH, Lyons BE, Buxton JL, Wilson DA. Natural history of experimental intracerebral hemorrhage: sonography, computed tomography and neuropathology. *AJNR* 1981;2: 517–526.
59. Bunn HF, Forget BG. Hemoglobin structure. In: *Hemoglobin: Molecular, Genetic and Clinical Aspects.* Philadelphia: WB Saunders; 1986:634–662.
60. Neill JM. Studies on the oxidation-reduction of hemoglobin and methemoglobin. III. The formation of methemoglobin during the oxidation of autooxidizable substances. *J Exper Med* 1925;41:551.
61. Neill JM. Studies on the oxidation-reduction of hemoglobin and methemoglobin. IV. The inhibition of spontaneous methemoglobin. *J Exper Med* 1925;41:561.
62. Koenig SH, Brown RD, Lindstrom TR. Interactions of solvent with the heme region of methemoglobin and fluoro-methemoglobin. *Biophys J* 1981;34:397–408.
63. Blumberg WE. Spectroscopic properties of hemoglobins: the study of hemoglobin by electron paramagnetic resonance spectroscopy. In: Ho C, ed. *Methods in Enzymology.* New York: Academic Press; 1981:312–329.
64. Bradley WGJ, Schmidt PG. Effect of methemoglobin formation on the MR appearance of subarachnoid hemorrhage. *Radiology* 1985;156:99.
65. Aasa R, Aisen P. An electron paramagnetic resonance study of the iron and copper complexes of transferrin. *J Biol Chem* 1968;243: 2399–2404.
66. Windle JJ, Weirsema AK, Clarke JR, Feeney RE. Investigation of the iron and copper complexes of avian conalbumins and human transferrins by electron paramagnetic resonance. *Biochemistry* 1963;2:1341–1345.
67. Weir MP, Peters TJ, Gibson JF. Electron spin resonance studies of splenic ferritin and haemosiderin. *Biochim Biophys Acta* 1985; 828:298–305.
68. Cross PA, Atlas SW, Grossman RI. MR evaluation of brain iron in children with cerebral infarction. *AJNR* 1990;11:341–348.
69. Drayer B, Burger P, Darwin R, Riederer S, Herfkens R, Johnson GA. MRI of brain iron. *AJR* 1986;147:103–110.
70. Chen JC, Hardy PA, Clauberg M, et al. T2 values in the human brain: comparison with quantitative assays of iron and ferritin. *Radiology* 1989;173:521–526.
71. Harrison PM, Fischbach FA, Hoy TG, Haggis GH. Ferric oxyhydroxide core of ferritin. *Nature* 1967;216:1188–1190.
72. Boas JF, Troup GJ. Electron spin resonance and Mossbauer effect studies of ferritin. *Biochim Biophys Acta* 1971;229:68–74.
73. Scott M. Spontaneous intracerebral hematoma caused by cerebral neoplasm: report of eight verified cases. *J Neurosurg* 1975;42:338.
74. Mandybur TI. Intracranial hemorrhage caused by metastatic tumors. *Neurology* 1977;27:650.
75. Leeds NE, Elkin CM, Zimmerman RD. Gliomas of the brain. *Semin Roentgenol* 1984;19:27.
76. Russell DS, Rubinstein LJ. *Pathology of Tumors of the Nervous System,* 5th ed. Baltimore: Williams & Wilkins; 1989.
77. Davis JM, Zimmerman RA, Bilaniuk LT. Metastases to the central nervous system. *Radiol Clin North Am* 1982;20:417.
78. Little JR, Dial B, Belanger G, et al. Brain hemorrhage from intracranial tumor. *Stroke* 1979;10:283.
79. Zimmerman RA, Bilaniuk LT. Computed tomography of acute intratumoral hemorrhage. *Radiology 1980;* 135:355.
80. Zulch KJ. *Brain Tumors. Their Biology and Pathology,* 3rd ed. Berlin: Springer-Verlag; 1986.
81. Gatenby RA, Coia LR, Richter MP. Oxygen tension in human tumors: in vivo mapping using CT-guided probes. *Radiology* 1985;156:211.
82. Destian S, Sze G, Krol G, Zimmerman RD, Deck MD. MR imaging of hemorrhagic intracranial neoplasms. *AJR* 1989;152:137–144.
83. Potts DG, Abbott OF, von Sneidern JV. National Cancer Institute Study: evaluation of computed tomography in the diagnosis of intracranial neoplasms. III. Metastatic tumors. *Radiology* 1980;136: 657–664.
84. Grossman RI, Kemp SS, Yu IC, et al. The importance of oxygenation in the appearance of acute subarachnoid hemorrhage on high-field magnetic resonance imaging. *Acta Radiol* 1986;369(Suppl): 56–58.
85. Gomori JM, Grossman RI, Bilaniuk LT, et al. High-field MR imaging of superficial siderosis of the central nervous system. *J Comput Assist Tomogr* 1985;9:972–975.
86. Gomori JM, Grossman RI, Goldberg HI, et al. High-field spin-echo MR imaging of superficial and subependymal siderosis secondary to neonatal intraventricular hemorrhage. *Neuroradiology* 1987;29:339.
87. Mohanty S, Tandon PNB, Banerji AK, et al. Haemorrhage into pituitary adenomas. *J Neurol Neurosurg Psychiatry* 1977;40:987.
88. Wakai S, Fukushima T, Teramoto A, et al. Pituitary apoplexy: its incidence and clinical significance. *J Neurosurg* 1981;55:187.
89. Tindall GT, Barrow DL. *Disorders of the Pituitary.* St. Louis: CV Mosby; 1986.

Magnetic Resonance Imaging of the Brain and Spine, Second Edition, edited by Scott W. Atlas. Lippincott-Raven Publishers, Philadelphia © 1996.

10

Intra-Axial Brain Tumors

Scott W. Atlas and Ehud Lavi

The incidence of primary intracranial tumors in the United States is approximately 15,0000 new cases per year (1). While primary tumors of each of the following histopathologies can be found anywhere in the central nervous system (CNS), characteristic neuroanatomic locations can be ascertained from pathology data for many of the lesions that comprise this heterogeneous group. Although magnetic resonance imaging (MRI) has achieved remarkable sophistication in the information available from the vast array of pulse sequences, the neuroradiologist should still rely heavily upon traditional criteria, such as location in the neuraxis and the age of the patient, for specific histologic diagnoses. For instance, it has been estimated that 80% to 85% of all intracranial tumors occur in adults, the majority of which are situated in the supratentorial compartment. In the adult, the most common intra-axial supratentorial neoplasm is the glioblastoma, while metastasis is the most common intra-axial tumor of the posterior fossa. In the pediatric population, intracranial tumors are extraordinarily common amongst all tumors—the CNS is the second most common site of pediatric neoplasia. Excluding the first year of life and adolescence, the location of intracranial tumors in the pediatric age group is infratentorial in 60% to 70% of cases, of which 75% involve the cerebellum and 25% reside in the brainstem (2). Nearly all of these lesions are primary CNS tumors, but the spectrum of histologies differs remarkably from that seen in adults.

Aside from the initial recognition and characterization of these lesions (i.e., intra- versus extra-axial, neoplastic versus non-neoplastic, primary versus metastatic, cell type, and degree of malignancy), the mechanical effects and structural deformities resulting from intracranial neoplasms are also of great importance, since the cranial vault is extremely limited in its ability to accommodate increases in intracranial pressure. Therefore, the neuroradiologist must be able to appreciate the consequences resulting from the combined effects of tumors and their edema, many of which are potentially life-threatening, such as transtentorial herniation. With the advent and refinement of computed tomography (CT) and, more re-

Scott W. Atlas, M.D.: Neuroradiology Division, Department of Radiology, Oregon Health Sciences University, Portland, OR 97201.

Ehud Lavi, M.D.: Division of Neuropathology, Department of Pathology and Laboratory Medicine, Hospital of the University of Pennsylvania, Philadelphia, PA 19104.

cently, MRI, intracranial neoplasms and their effects can be more readily recognized, so that appropriate therapy can be instituted without delay and at an earlier time in their natural history. Unfortunately, it can be accurately stated that state-of-the-art imaging capabilities far exceed advances in treatment for the vast majority of brain tumors, so that in some cases, the necessity for distinction of histologic subtypes by imaging may have little practical importance at this point in time. Having said this, it is also evident that MRI has the most potential of any diagnostic method, including surgical biopsy, for allowing a complete and accurate diagnosis to be formulated in these cases. Therefore, we strongly believe that for the optimal interpretation of MRI in brain tumors, it is essential for the neuroradiologist to be particularly familiar with neuropathology in addition to the requisite mastery of neuroanatomy, since MRI abnormalities reflect pathologic findings in these lesions. Furthermore, by understanding the microscopic pathology of these lesions, the limitations of neuroimaging are often revealed just as the neuropathologist would find if he or she relied solely on gross pathology. From this deeper understanding of the current limits of MRI in CNS tumors, misinformation is less likely to be generated to the clinician primarily involved with the patient, making the radiologist more valuable in patient management. The general correlation between pathology and imaging will be stressed in this chapter.

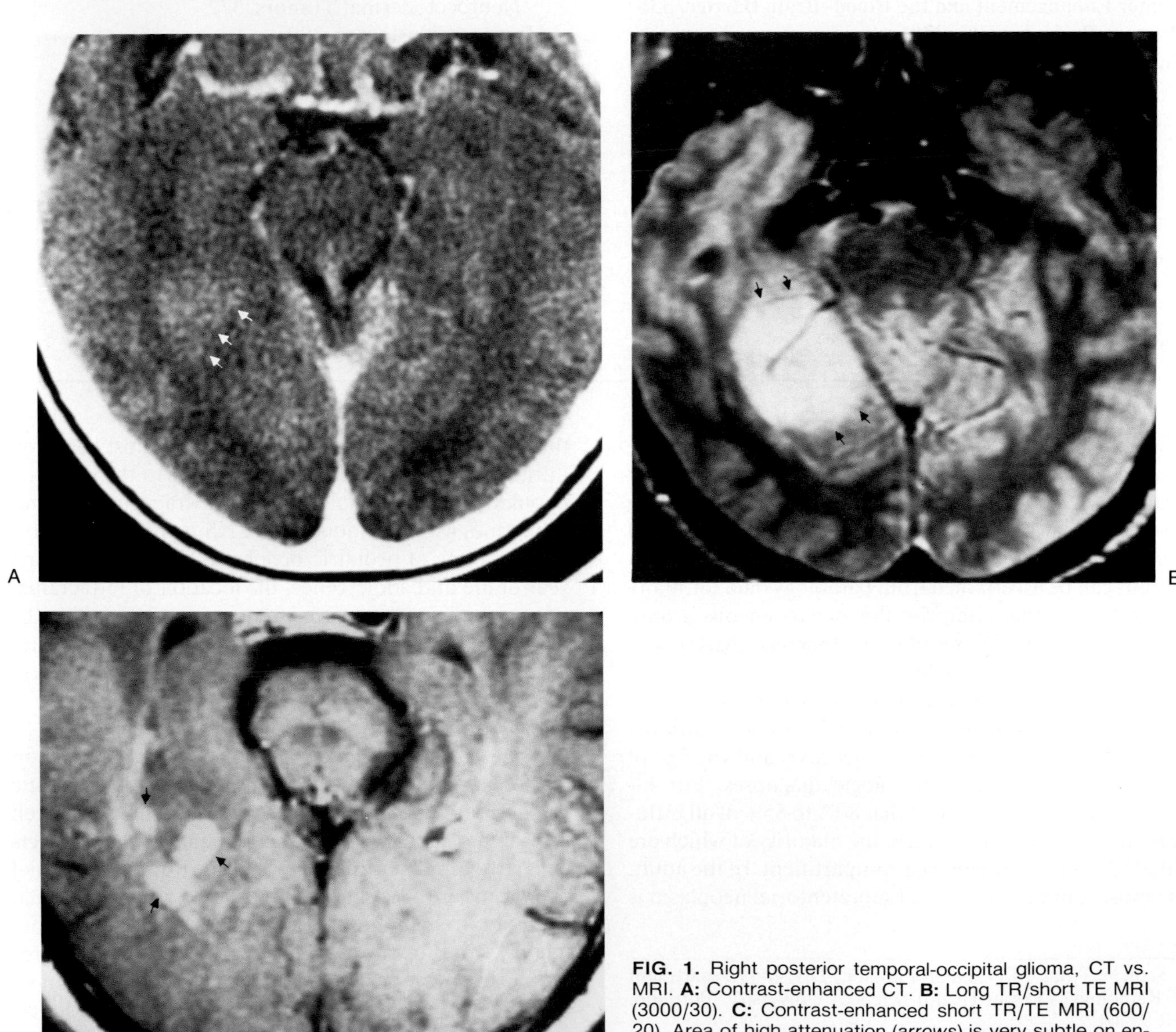

FIG. 1. Right posterior temporal-occipital glioma, CT vs. MRI. **A:** Contrast-enhanced CT. **B:** Long TR/short TE MRI (3000/30). **C:** Contrast-enhanced short TR/TE MRI (600/20). Area of high attenuation (*arrows*) is very subtle on enhanced CT (A), but stands out as high-intensity mass (*arrows*) on MRI (B) and shows definite focal nodular enhancement (*arrows*) after i.v. contrast (C).

MR IMAGING IN BRAIN TUMORS: OVERVIEW

At the time of this writing, it has become generally recognized that MR would be virtually always the imaging study of choice in the evaluation of intracerebral tumors if cost and availability were not issues. Practically speaking, of course, cost and availability are always important issues, so at virtually all medical centers, CT still plays a valuable role in the search for these lesions. MR imaging has several strengths, but despite continued refinement of hardware and software technology, some limitations remain with regard to the evaluation of intracranial tumors.

The essential reason for the enthusiasm on the part of radiologists and clinicians alike for the use of MRI in the search for brain tumors lies in the inherently high sensitivity of the technique for these lesions. Although well-controlled prospective clinical trials admittedly have never been performed, there is no question that MRI is more sensitive for brain tumors than CT, both in terms of detection (Fig. 1), as well as in showing more completely the extent of the tumor (3). This increase in sensitivity of MRI over CT also applies to metastatic disease, even when state-of-the-art CT with intravenous contrast enhancement is utilized (4,5).

The unique capability of imaging directly in multiple planes has been an important advance in imaging intracranial tumors. The major benefit of multiplanar imaging has been superior tumor localization, rather than increasing the detection rate of lesions. The decision of whether a mass is intra-axial or extra-axial is obviously important in determining the correct diagnosis, and multiplanar MRI has certainly improved our ability to make that distinction. The correct assessment of the relationship of a mass to the ventricular system is also made easier by using coronal and/or sagittal planes, in addition to the traditional axial plane of scanning (Fig. 2), which aids in differential diagnosis. The heightened sensitivity of MR combined with its ease of imaging in multiple planes are critical for treatment, as well as diagnosis. The operative approach to intracranial masses and radiotherapy portal designs are aided significantly by these capabilities. In the evaluation of the pediatric brainstem glioma, for instance, we routinely obtain sagittal long TR images for the benefit of the radiotherapist. Therefore, intracranial tumors represents one of the few entities where routine acquisition of multiple planes of imaging should be performed.

TABLE 1. *Causes of low intensity in tumors on T2-weighted MR images*

Paramagnetic effects	Iron within dystrophic calcification or necrosis
	Ferritin/hemosiderin from prior hemorrhage
	Deoxyhemoglobin in acute hemorrhage
	Intracellular methemoglobin in early subacute hemorrhage
	Melanin (or other free radicals)
Low spin density	Calcification
	Scant cytoplasm (high nucleus:cytoplasm ratio)
	Dense cellularity
	Fibrocollagenous stroma
Macromolecule content	Very high (nonparamagnetic) protein concentration
	Fibrocollagenous stroma
Intratumoral vessels	Signal void from rapid flow

TABLE 2. *Causes of high intensity in tumors on T1-weighted MR images*

Paramagnetic effects from hemorrhage	Subacute-chronic blood (methemoglobin)
Paramagnetic material without hemorrhage	Melanin
	Nautrally occurring ions associated with necrosis of calcification
	Manganese
	Iron
	Copper
Nonparamagnetic effects	Very high (nonparamagnetic) protein concentration
	Fat
	Flow-related enhancement in tumor vessels

Unfortunately, as I had written in the first edition of this chapter, the progress of MRI in the area of specificity in brain tumor evaluation still has not paralleled its gains in sensitivity and anatomic depiction. With that in mind, it is fair to say that MRI provides significantly more information about intrinsic tissue characterization, a capability which should be exploited by the neuroradiologist for determining tumor type. This ability to discriminate differences in tissue by variations in signal intensities parallels findings on gross pathology in most cases (Tables 1 and 2), and applies to several areas pertinent to tumor imaging. For instance, one of the major pathologic changes in astrocytic gliomas and one of the few prognostically significant factors on histopathology aside from general tumor cell type and overall grade, is the presence of necrosis. The identification of intratumoral necrosis is considered a poor prognostic sign found in more aggressive astrocytomas, in most cases, and should be sought by the neuroradiologist interpreting MR of brain tumors. Necrosis can be either hemorrhagic or nonhemorrhagic. The effects of necrosis on MRI are

TABLE 3. *Effects of tumor necrosis on signal intensity*

Shorten relaxation times	Hemorrhage
	Liberation of cellular iron
	Release of free radicals
	Proteinaceous debris
Prolong relaxation times	Cystic change with increased water

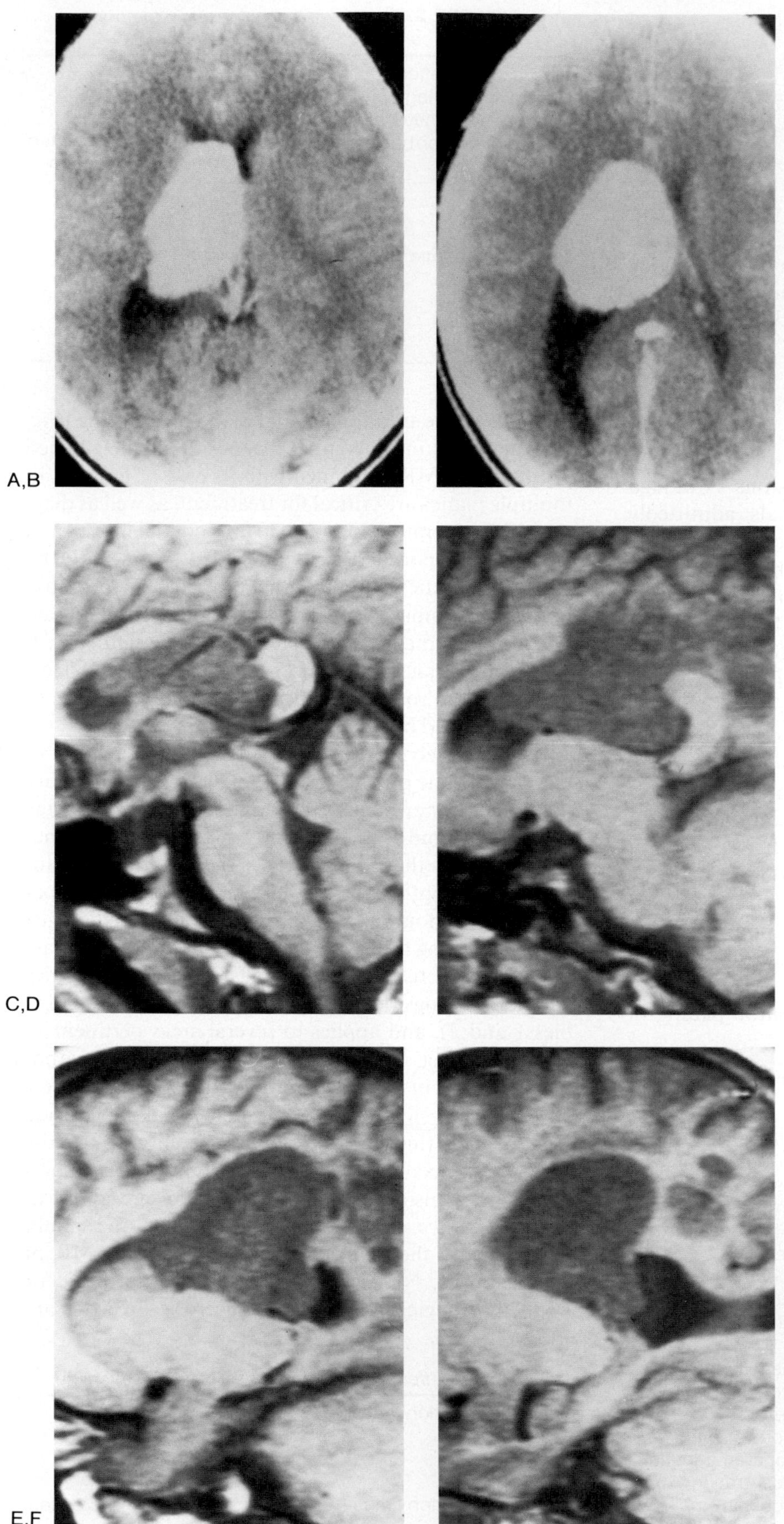

FIG. 2. Intraventricular astrocytoma, axial CT vs. sagittal MRI. **A:** Axial contrast-enhanced CT. **B:** Axial contrast-enhanced CT. **C:** Sagittal short TR/TE MRI (600/20). **D:** Sagittal short TR/TE MRI (600/20). **E:** Sagittal short TR/TE MRI (600/20). **F:** Sagittal short TR/TE MRI (600/20). Anatomic location of densely enhancing right lateral ventricular mass on CT (A,B) is more fully appreciated as originating within the ventricle, transgressing the posterior body of corpus callosum, and invading the cingulate gyrus and hemisphere on serial parasagittal MRI scans (C–F). The localization provided by MRI is valuable for surgical planning.

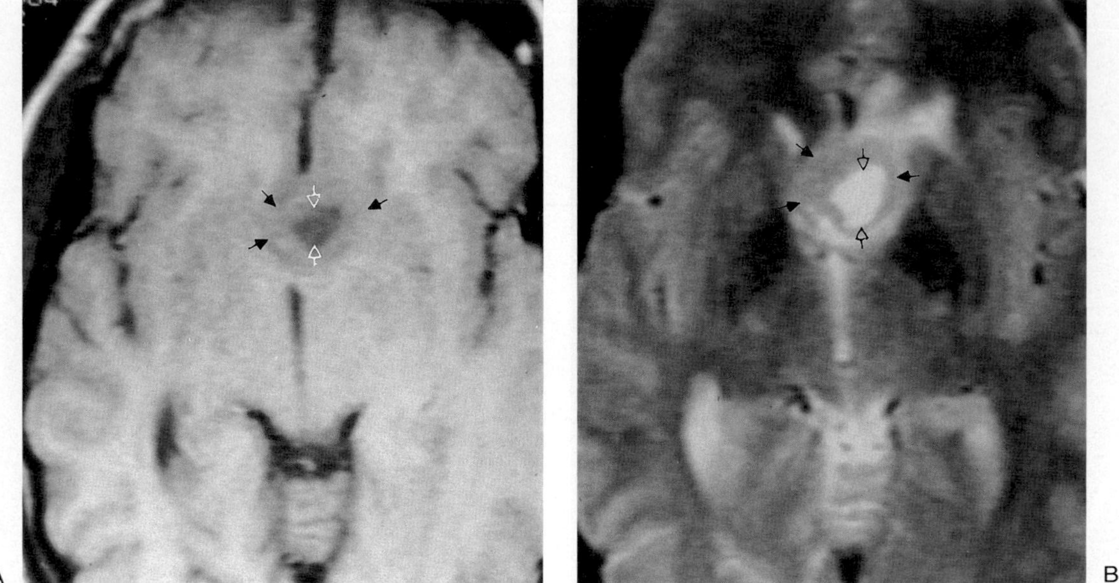

FIG. 3. Cystic necrosis in metastatic tumor. **A:** Short TR/TE MRI (600/20). **B:** Long TR/TE MRI (2500/80). Note central portion (*open arrows*) of metastasis to septum pellucidum is slightly hyperintense to CSF on short TR/TE image (A) and isointense to CSF on long TR/TE image (B) in area of cystic necrosis, while peripheral rind of non-necrotic tumor (*closed arrows*) is nearly isointense to gray matter (A,B).

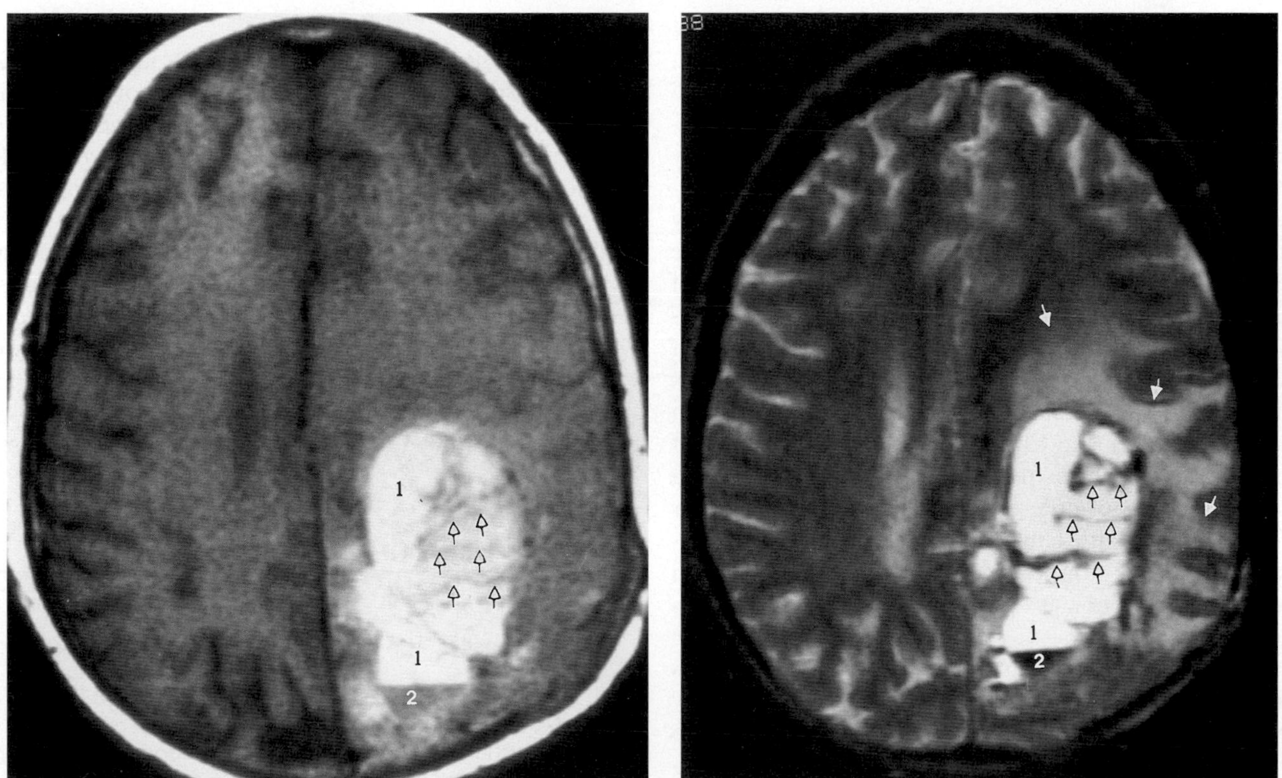

FIG. 4. Hemorrhagic necrosis in supratentorial primitive neuroectodermal tumor (PNET). **A:** Short TR/TE MRI (600/20). **B:** Long TR/TE MRI (3000/90). Intratumoral hemorrhagic necrosis displays high intensity of methemoglobin (*1*), dependent levels of intracellular deoxyhemoglobin (2), and minimal irregular strands of hypointensity (*open arrows*) within and at parts of the periphery of the lesion. The high intensity in perilesional white matter (*closed arrows*, B) represents both edema and infiltrating tumor.

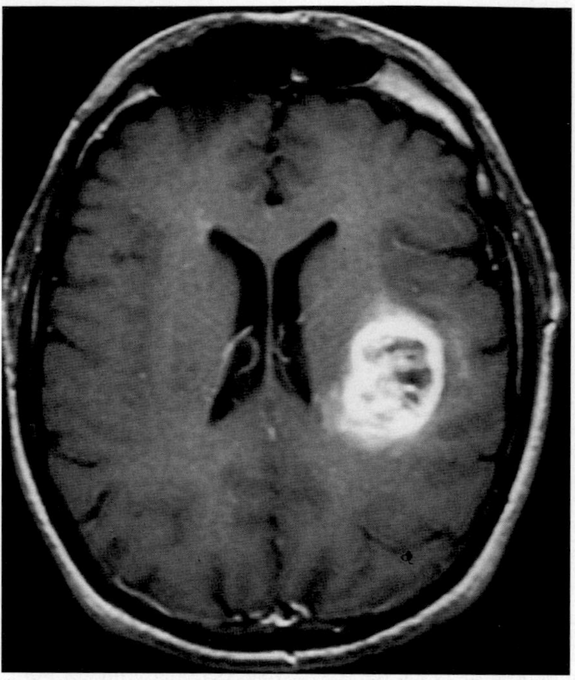

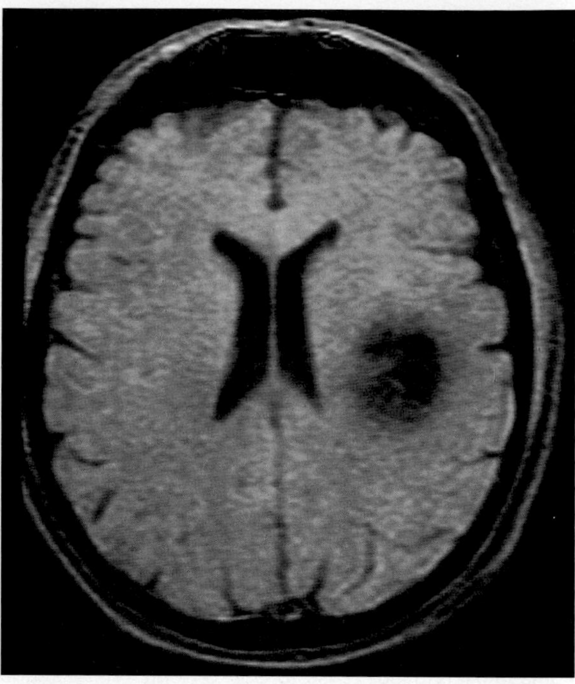

FIG. 5. Necrosis in anaplastic astrocytoma, use of magnetization transfer (MT). Gadolinium-enhanced T1-weighted MRI (**A**) shows enhancing left subinsular mass with central nonenhancing portion. MT map (**B**), where higher intensity indicates more MT effect and low intensity indicates minimal MT, shows central nonenhancing area has essentially no magnetization transfer, consistent with central cystic necrosis found at surgery.

complex and varied (Table 3), but it can often be identified with near-certainty if one uses both short TR/TE and long TR/multi-echo sequences in these cases. In general, necrosis can be either high intensity or low intensity on short TR/TE images, as well as on long TR/TE images, due to the presence of any or all of several naturally occurring paramagnetic cations and free radicals. These substances can shorten relaxation times, while regions of cystic necrosis prolong relaxation times (6). Cystic necrosis has intensities consistent with high water content (Fig. 3), and hemorrhagic necrosis parallels the complex intensities relevant to paramagnetic blood-breakdown products (Fig. 4) (see Chapter 9). The development of magnetization transfer techniques (see Chapter 2) as a potential means of differentiating populations of water protons may provide a method of detecting cystic necrosis, since protons comprising cystic necrosis should be in the "unbound" pool, as opposed to protons of intact tissue (Fig. 5).

The association of cysts with certain neoplasms has long been utilized as an aid to differential diagnosis by neuroradiologists. Preoperative cyst delineation is also helpful to the neurosurgeon when planning surgical approach. MRI is clearly superior to CT in defining cysts or cystic regions of solid masses, because of the improved sensitivity to contrast based on many different features of tissue (i.e., T1, T2, proton density). Problematically, the vast majority of neoplasms have elevated proton density, prolonged T1 and prolonged T2, just like CSF, so that most tumors are low intensity on short TR/TE images and high intensity on long TR/TE images. This does not necessarily indicate cystic structure, however. Morphology is just one of several criteria for the diagnosis of a cyst by MRI (Table 4). Cysts are generally very sharply demarcated, round or ovoid masses, but there are many exceptions to these features (7). The identification of cystic areas on MRI also requires careful scrutiny of lesion intensity relative to CSF on all of the three routinely obtained images: short TR/TE, long TR/short TE, and long TR/TE (Figs. 6 and 7). If a lesion is exactly isointense to CSF on all three of these sequences, then one can state

TABLE 4. *MRI criteria for cystic lesions*

Morphology	Sharply demarcated, round, smooth
Signal intensity	Isointense to CSF on all spin-echo images (tumor cysts can be hyperintense due to ↓ T1)
Fluid–debris levels (hemorrhage into necrotic or cystic regions)	Intracellular blood–cyst fluid Intracellular blood–extracellular blood
Motion of intralesional fluid	Lesion emanates ghost images along phase-encoding axis Intralesional signal loss (especially on steady-state sequences)

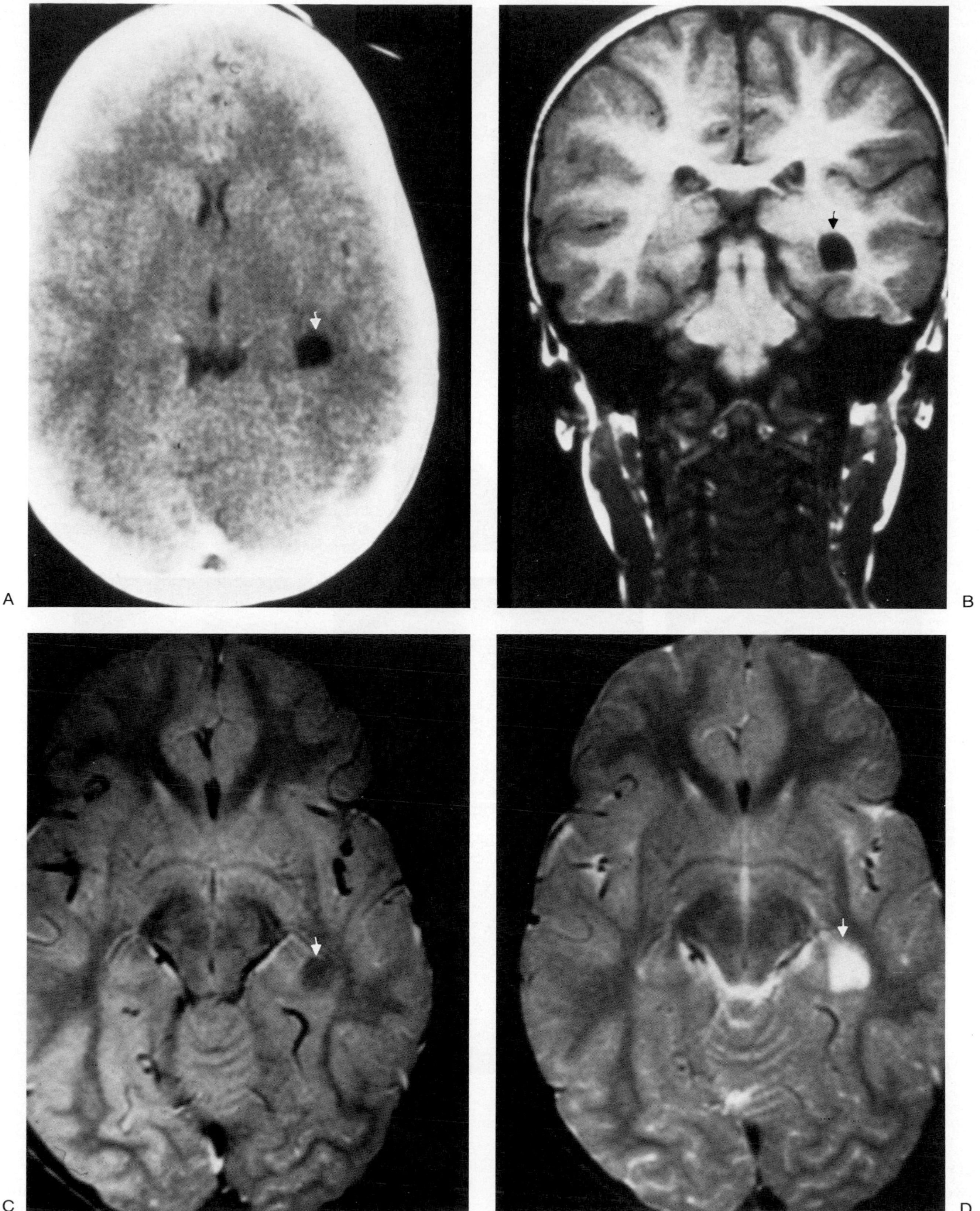

FIG. 6. Proof of cystic nature of mass by signal intensity pattern. **A:** Axial CT, glial parenchymal cyst. **B:** Coronal short TR/TE MRI (600/20). **C:** Axial long TR/short TE MRI (2800/30). **D:** Axial long TR/TE MRI (2800/80). The lesion (*arrow*, A–D) is exactly isointense to CSF on all sequences, proving its cystic nature.

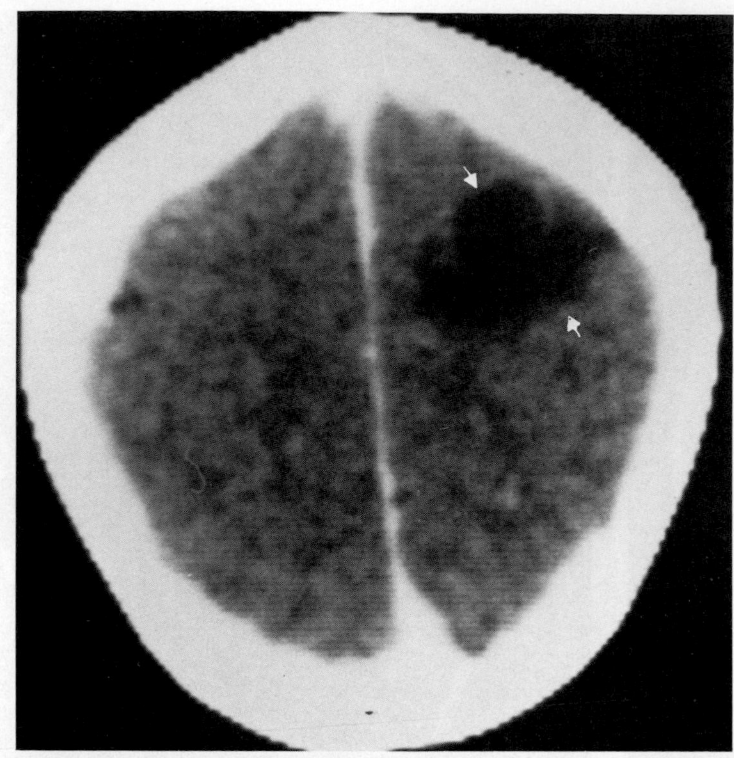

FIG. 7. Noncystic (solid) lesion by signal intensity pattern (solid ganglioglioma). **A:** Axial CT. **B:** Sagittal short TR/TE MRI (600/20). **C:** Sagittal long TR/short TE MRI (2500/20). **D:** Sagittal long TR/TE MRI (2500/80). Low-attenuation cortical mass (*arrows*) on CT (A) appears cystic. The lesion is virtually isointense to CSF on short TR/TE (B) and long TR/TE (D), but the marked hyperintensity on long TR/short TE (C) is consistent with its solid composition.

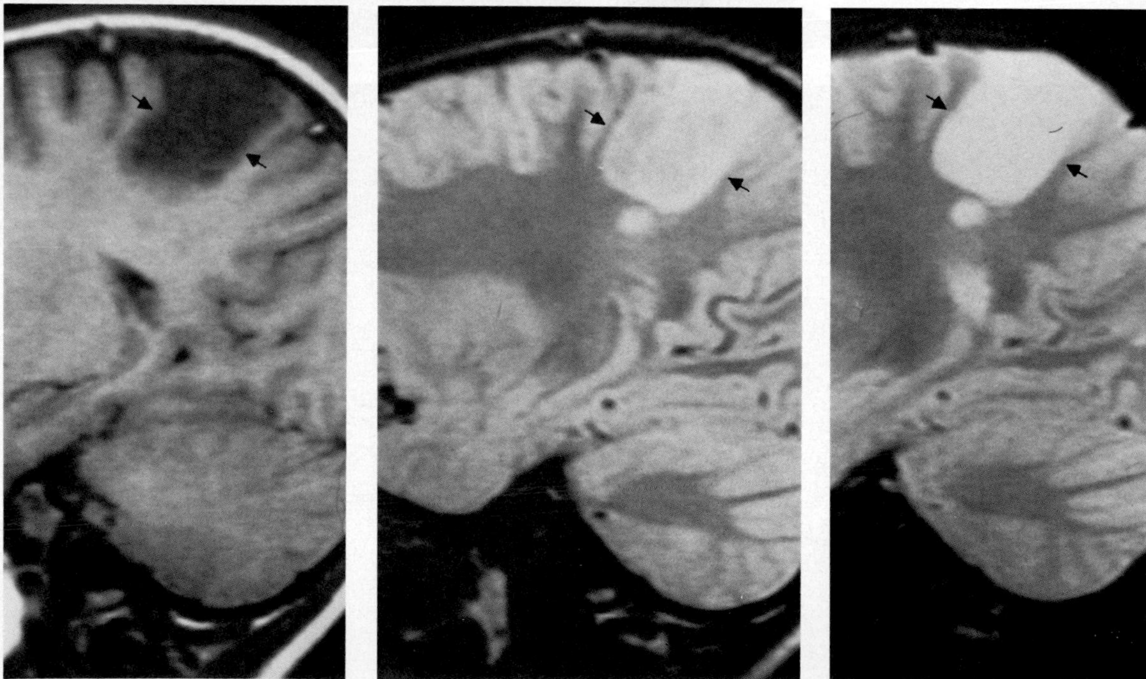

very confidently that the lesion is cystic, a pattern followed by arachnoid cysts and cysts associated with extra-axial masses. Unfortunately, it is quite common for tumor cysts (and areas of intratumoral cystic necrosis) to be of slightly higher intensity than pure CSF on short TR/TE and long TR/short TE images (Fig. 8), since highly proteinaceous debris and, more commonly, dilute concentrations of paramagnetic substances can shorten T1 enough to alter intensity on these images (8). Fluid-debris intensity levels are a pathognomonic sign of cystic tissue, and are often quite striking and frequent in cases of cystic tumors (Fig. 9). These can be found with or without intratumoral hemorrhage, and are a clear sign that a lesion is at least partly surgically drainable. An-

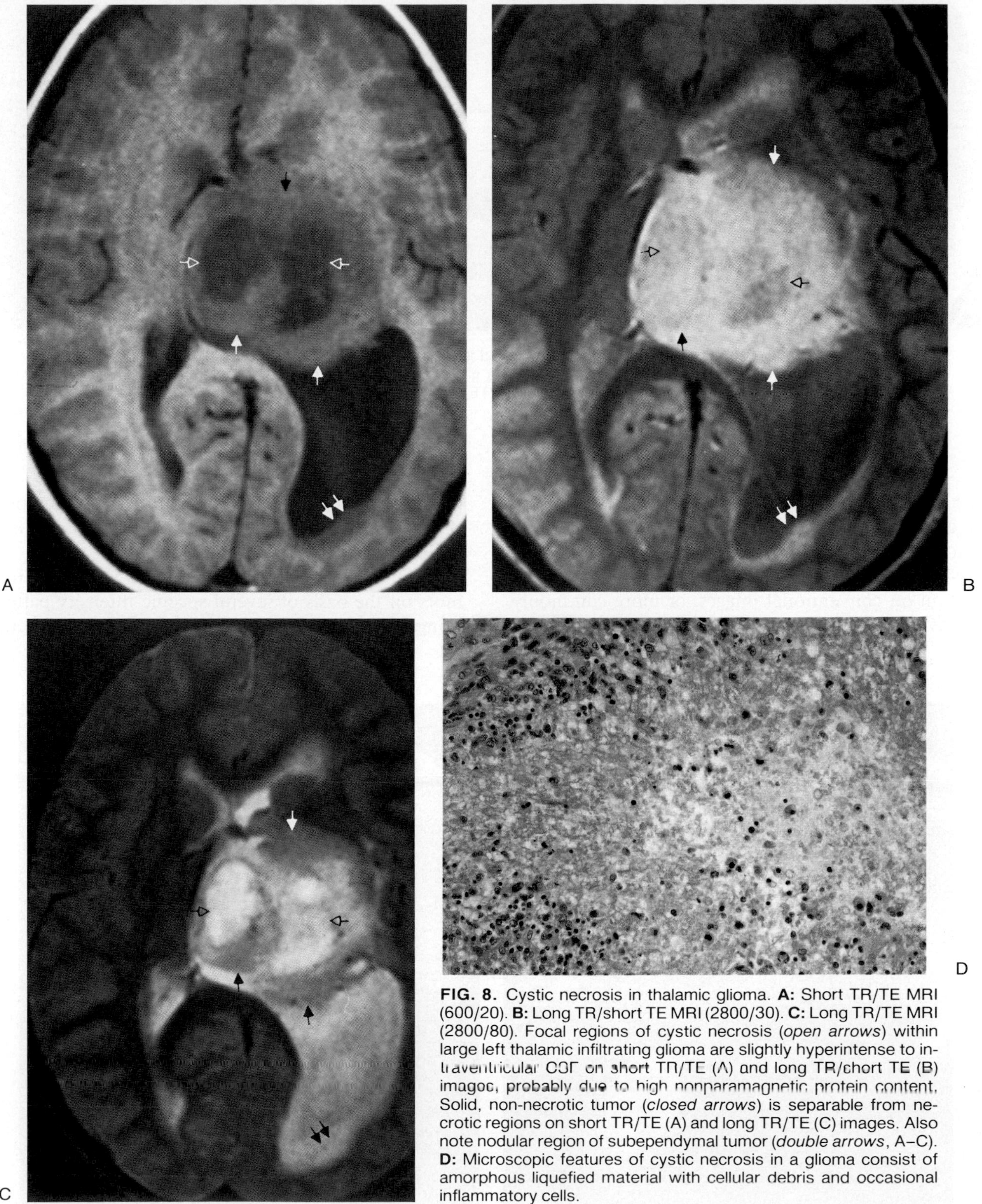

FIG. 8. Cystic necrosis in thalamic glioma. **A:** Short TR/TE MRI (600/20). **B:** Long TR/short TE MRI (2800/30). **C:** Long TR/TE MRI (2800/80). Focal regions of cystic necrosis (*open arrows*) within large left thalamic infiltrating glioma are slightly hyperintense to intraventricular CSF on short TR/TE (A) and long TR/short TE (B) images, probably due to high nonparamagnetic protein content. Solid, non-necrotic tumor (*closed arrows*) is separable from necrotic regions on short TR/TE (A) and long TR/TE (C) images. Also note nodular region of subependymal tumor (*double arrows*, A–C). **D:** Microscopic features of cystic necrosis in a glioma consist of amorphous liquefied material with cellular debris and occasional inflammatory cells.

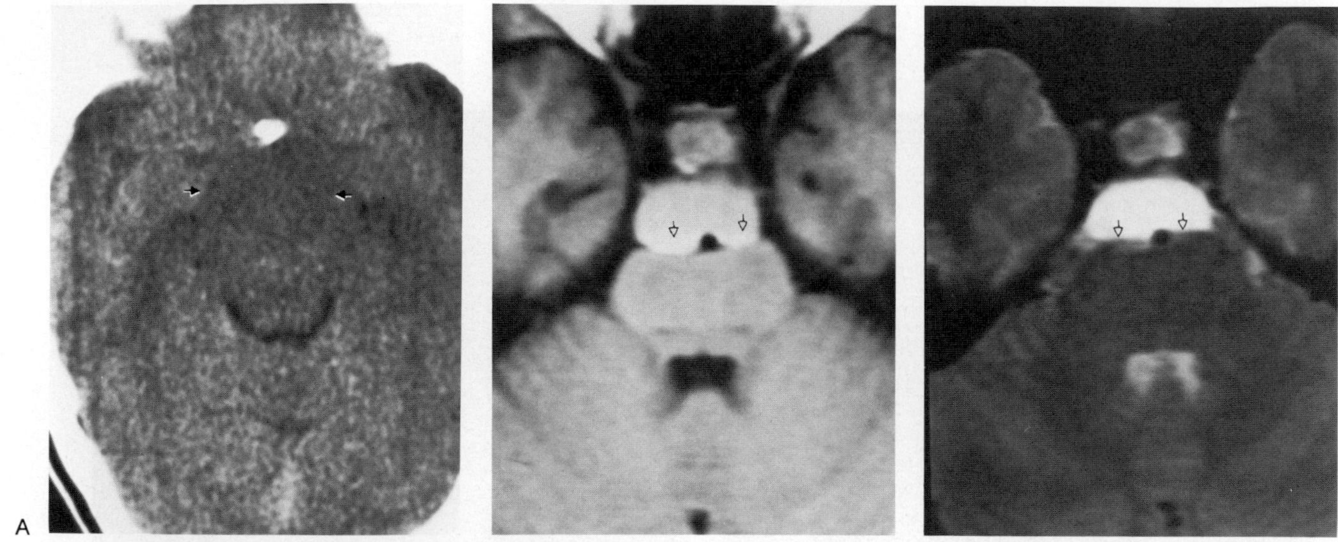

FIG. 9. Proof of cystic nature by intralesional debris-fluid level (craniopharyngioma). **A:** CT. **B:** Short TR/TE MRI (600/20). **C:** Long TR/TE MRI (2500/80). Isodense mass fills suprasellar cistern on CT (*arrows*, A). Clear level of posteriorly located, dependent, high intensity on short TR/TE *(arrows,* B) and low intensity on long TR/TE (*arrows*, C) indicates that lesion is cystic and surgically drainable.

other definite sign which, if found, reveals the cystic nature of a lesion, is the presence of artifacts due to fluid motion within the lesion. This may occasionally be seen as "ghost" images propagated along the phase-encoding direction on conventional images, or more commonly as areas of signal loss, due to dephasing. Flow-sensitive techniques (see Chapter 29) illustrate this dramatically (Fig. 10) (9), and can be useful adjuncts in evaluating tumors with MRI.

Specific diagnoses are also achieved with MRI in tumors on the basis of several specific intensity patterns, using both short TR and long TR sequences. Hemor-

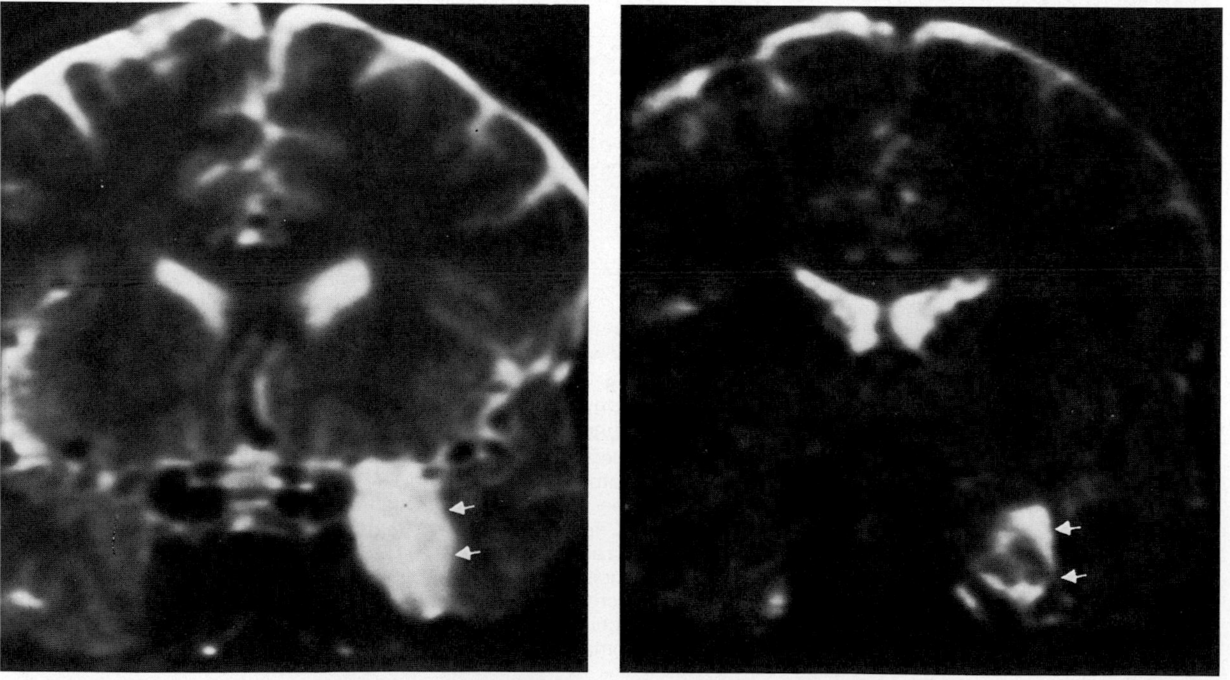

FIG. 10. Proof of cystic nature by intralesional motion artifact. **A:** Long TR/TE MRI (3000/80). **B:** 3DFT steady-state MRI (24/38/10°). CSF-intensity extra-axial mass in left middle cranial fossa on spin-echo MRI (*arrows*, A) shows marked signal drop-out on steady-state image (*arrows*, B) due to intralesional motion, proving cystic nature of mass.

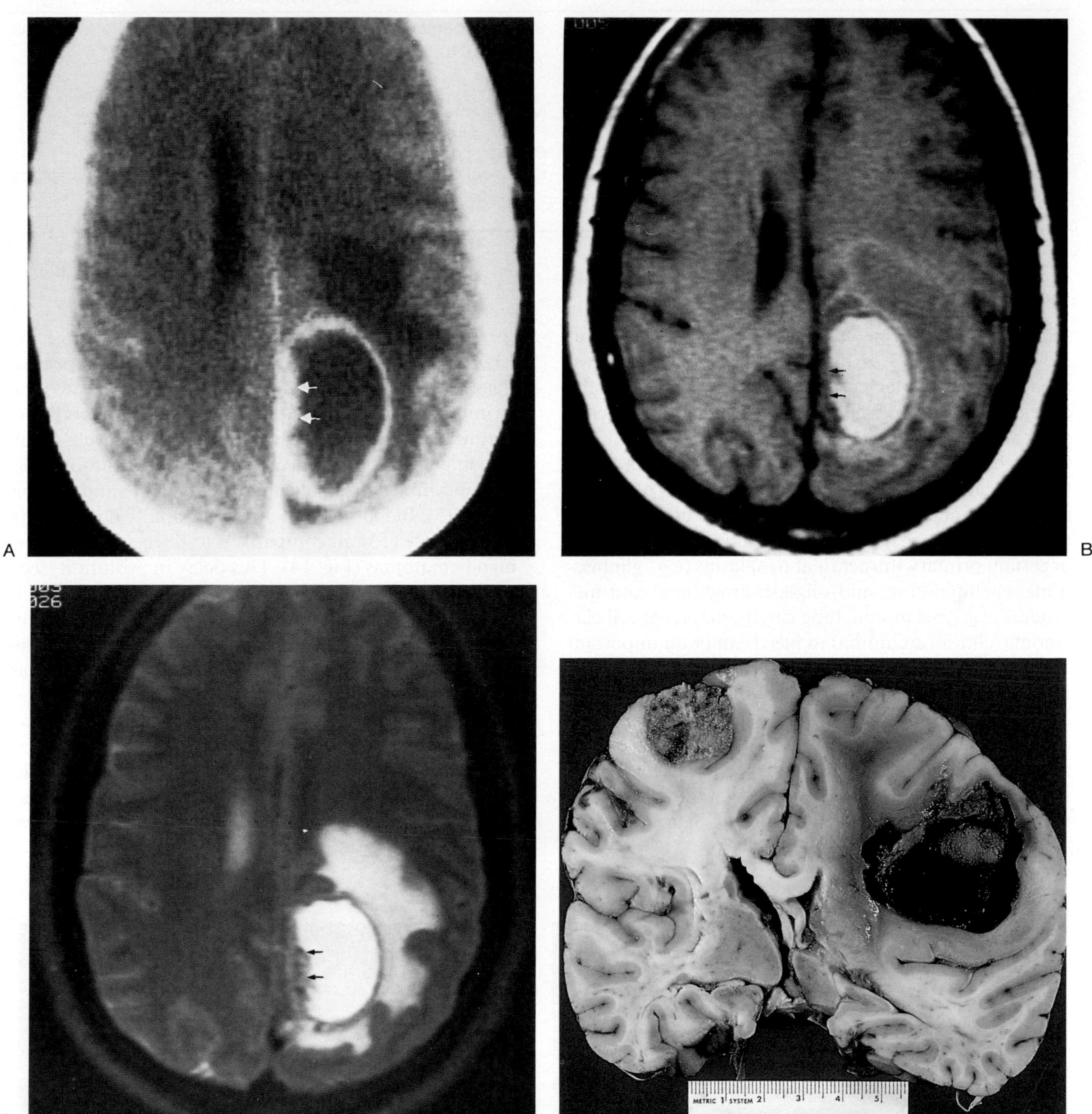

FIG. 11. Hemorrhagic metastasis, CT vs. MRI. **A:** Contrast-enhanced CT. **B:** Short TR/TE MRI (600/25). **C:** Long TR/TE MRI (2500/80). Low-attenuation mass with irregular ring enhancement and surrounding edema is present in left posterior parieto-occipital region on CT (A). The central area of low attenuation on CT is of high intensity on both short TR/TE (B) and long TR/TE (C) MRI, indicating chronic hemorrhage. Medial, irregularly enhancing portion of mass (*arrows*, A–C) represents nonhemorrhagic portion of tumor. Note absence of peripheral hemosiderin/ferritin on T2-weighted image (C), persistent edema even though hemorrhage is old, and clear nonhemorrhagic tumor tissue, all signs that differentiate between benign and tumor-associated hemorrhage. **D:** Comparable necropsy specimen shows multiple hemorrhagic metastases with solid nonhemorrhagic tumor tissue, as well as significant edema in left hemisphere, even though hematoma is old.

TABLE 5. *Intratumoral hemorrhage vs. benign intracranial hematomas*

Intratumoral hemorrhage	Benign hemorrhage
Markedly heterogeneous, related to: Mixed stages of blood Debris–fluid (intracellular–extracellular blood) levels Edema + tumor + necrosis with blood	Shows expected signal intensities of acute, subacute, or chronic blood, depending on stage of hematoma
Identification of nonhemorrhagic tumor component	No abnormal nonhemorrhagic mass
Delayed evolution of blood breakdown products	Follows expected orderly progression
Absent, diminished, or irregular ferritin/hemosiderin	Regular, complete ferritin/hemosiderin rim
Persistent surrounding high intensity on long TR images (i.e., tumor/edema) and mass effect, even in late stages	Complete resolution of edema and mass effect in chronic stages

rhage is uniquely depicted by MRI, because of the paramagnetic properties of many of the blood-breakdown products (see Chapter 9). This is simply illustrated by the appearance of chronic hemorrhage, which is low attenuation and identical to CSF on CT (Fig. 11). On MRI, old hemorrhage is easily distinguished from other fluid (like CSF), because of the paramagnetic properties of methemoglobin, one of the major constituents of chronic intracranial hemorrhage (10). The characteristic tendency of certain primary intracranial neoplasms (e.g., glioblastoma, ependymoma, and oligodendroglioma) and metastases (e.g., melanoma, lung carcinoma, renal cell carcinoma, choriocarcinoma) to bleed can be an important clue to the diagnosis (11,12), so it is desirable to be sensitive and specific for the appearance of hemorrhage.

While it is important to discover hemorrhage, it is also critical to define its etiology, and CT scanning is of limited value for this. The signal intensity pattern of intratumoral hemorrhage differs from benign intracranial hematomas (13) in several ways (Table 5). Signal intensity is extremely heterogeneous in tumor bleeds (Figs. 12 and 13), due to the combination of simultaneously appearing stages of evolving blood (from continual or repeated, intermittent bleeding), frequent intracellular blood-fluid or intracellular blood-extracellular blood levels (from bleeding into cystic or necrotic portions of tumor) (Fig. 14), and mixed areas of tumor with edema and hemorrhage (13). Blood may not evolve as rapidly if it is within tumor tissue (13), in comparison to the evolution of benign hematomas (Fig. 14). This delay in evolution (seen usually as persistent deoxyhemoglobin, which is normally found only within the first 3–5 days after hemorrhage) may be related to the well-documented intratumoral hypoxia found in human neoplasms (14), or due to repeated episodes of bleeding (15). Long after hemorrhage into tumor tissue, there is often a marked reduction or irregularity of the expected hemosiderin on long TR/TE images around the bleed (13), compared to the prominent hypointensity at the periphery of chronic benign intracranial hematomas (Figs. 15 and 16). A clear

A 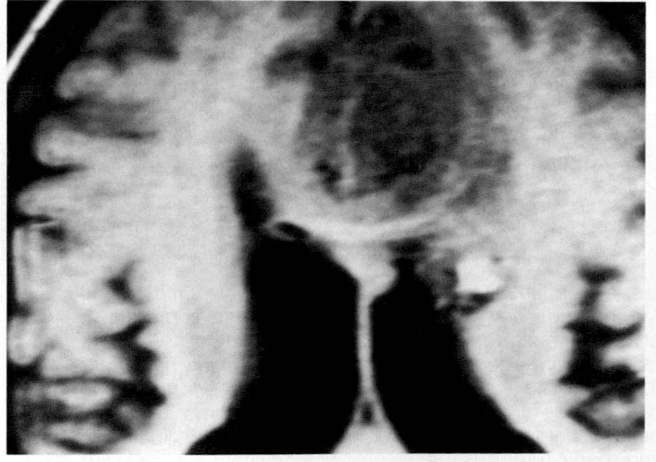

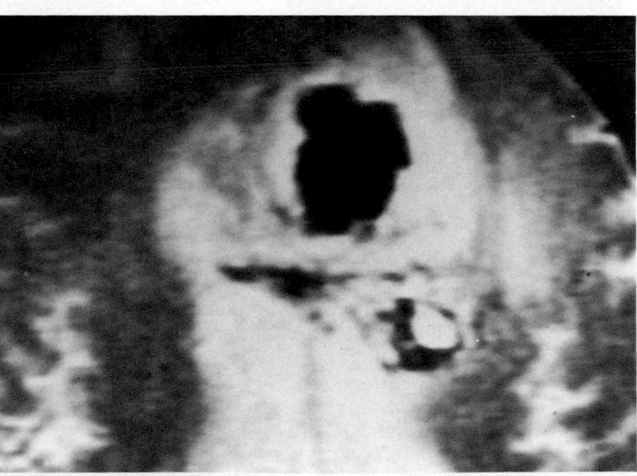 B

FIG. 12. Intratumoral hemorrhage with complex signal intensities (glioblastoma). **A:** Short TR/TE MRI (600/25). **B:** Long TR/TE MRI (2500/80). Strikingly complex, heterogeneous left frontal and callosal mass contains acute, subacute, and chronic hemorrhage, debris-fluid levels, and nonhemorrhagic tissue. This appearance is clearly different from benign hematomas and indicates intratumoral hemorrhage.

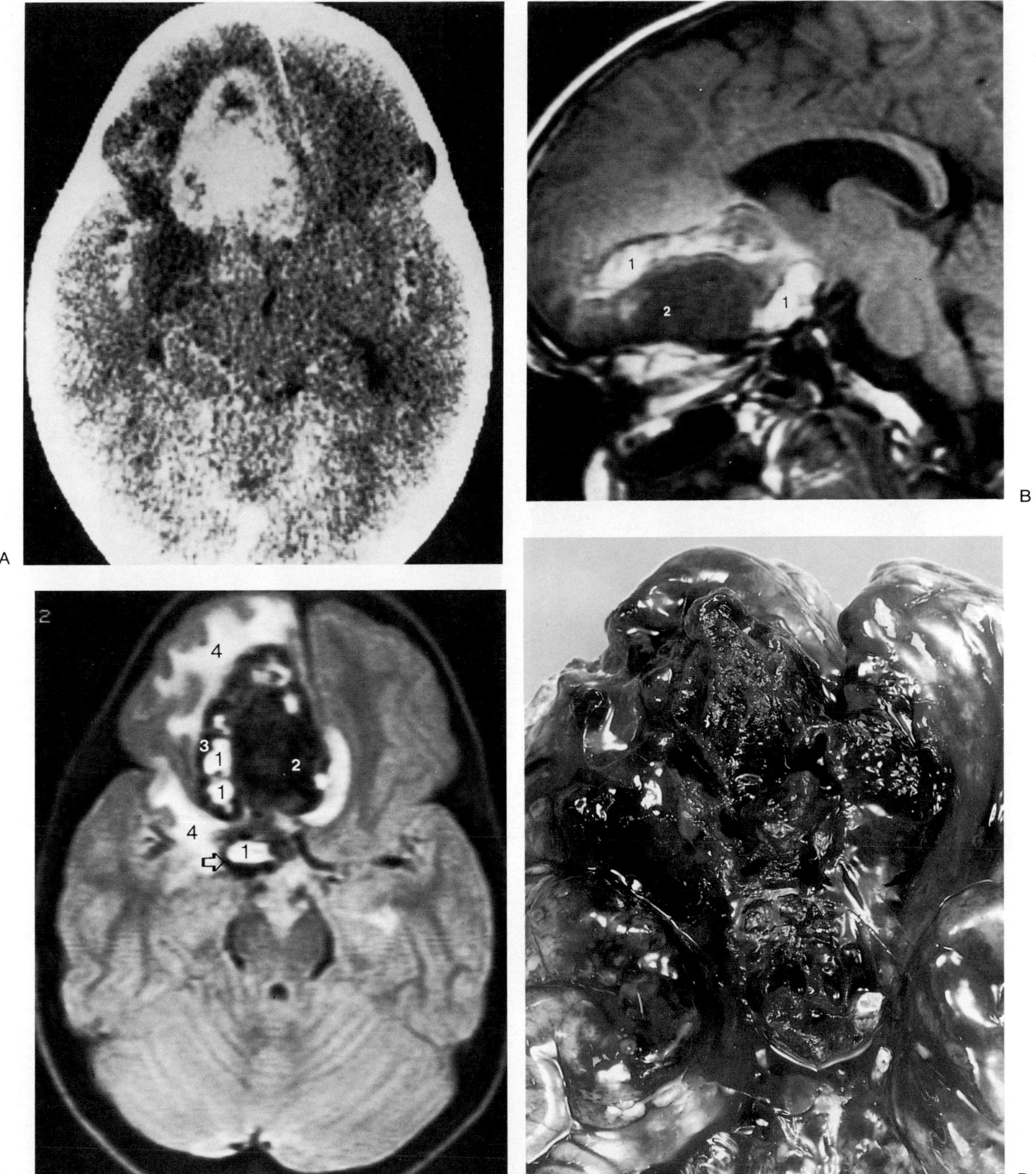

FIG. 13. Intratumoral hemorrhage with complex signal intensities (retinoblastoma metastasis). **A:** Axial CT. **B:** Sagittal short TR/TE MRI (600/25). **C:** Axial long TR/TE MRI (2500/80). **D:** Necropsy specimen. (Courtesy of Dr. Lucy Rorke, Philadelphia, PA.) Right inferior frontal hemorrhagic mass on CT (A) shows marked heterogeneity on MRI (B,C), with several different stages of hemorrhage: (*1*) methemoglobin, (*2*) deoxyhemoglobin, and (*3*) ferritin/hemosiderin. High-intensity edema (*4*, C) and fluid level (*arrow*, C) contribute to complex appearance. Tumor is grossly hemorrhagic on pathology (D).

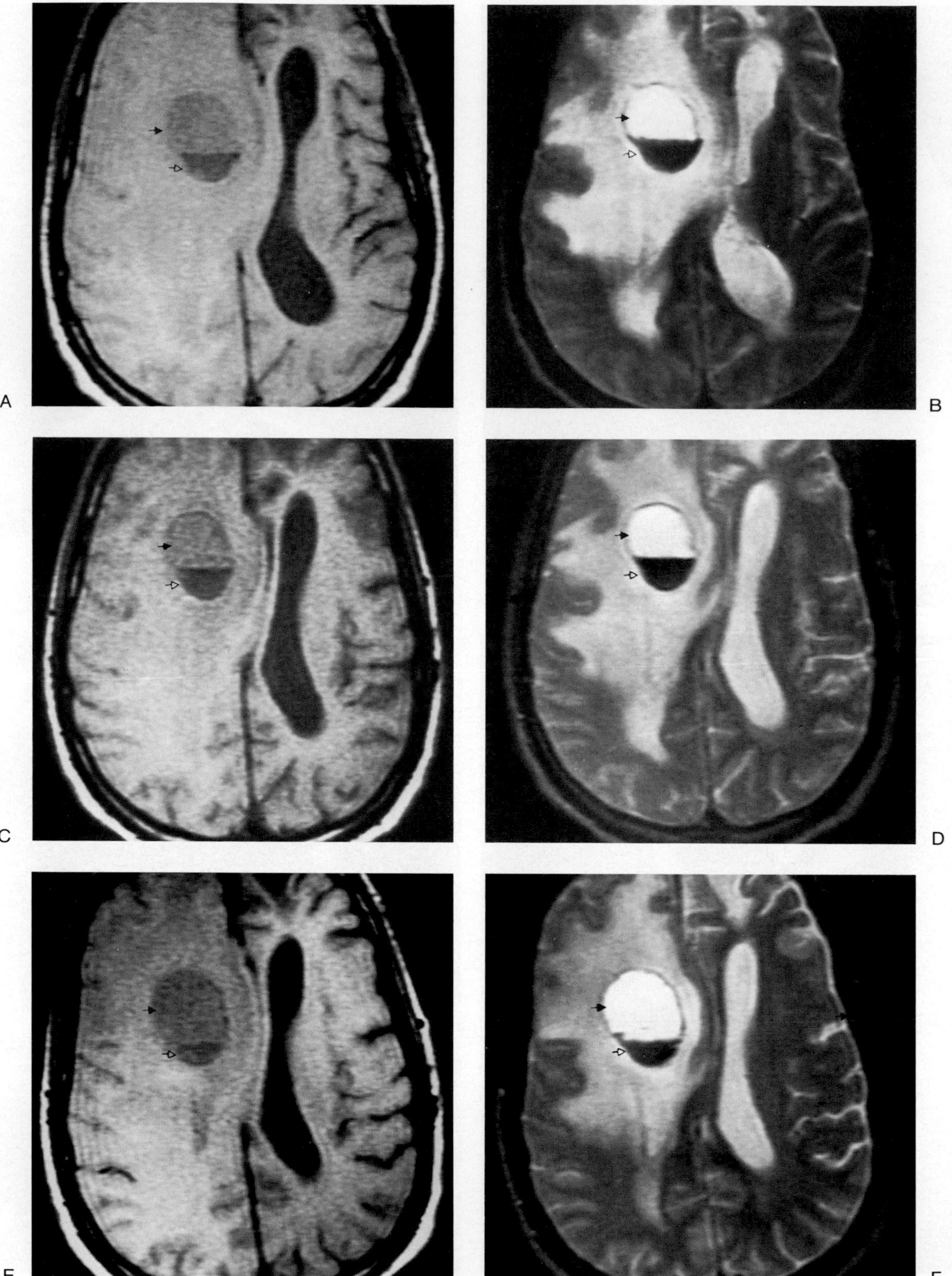

FIG. 14. Intratumoral hemorrhage with delayed evolution of blood (lung carcinoma metastasis). **A:** Short TR/TE MRI (600/20). **B:** Long TR/TE MRI (2500/80). **C:** Short TR/TE MRI (600/20), after 7 days. **D:** Long TR/TE MRI (2500/80), after 7 days. **E:** Short TR/TE MRI (600/20), after 17 days. **F:** Long TR/TE MRI (2500/80), after 17 days. Dependent layer of deoxyhemoglobin (*open arrow*) with ventral fluid (*closed arrow*) represents hemorrhage into cystic or necrotic tumor. Note persistence of deoxyhemoglobin after 17 days (normally, deoxyhemoglobin disappears by 3–5 days), indicating slowed evolution of blood-breakdown products. This is probably due to marked and persistent intratumoral hypoxia.

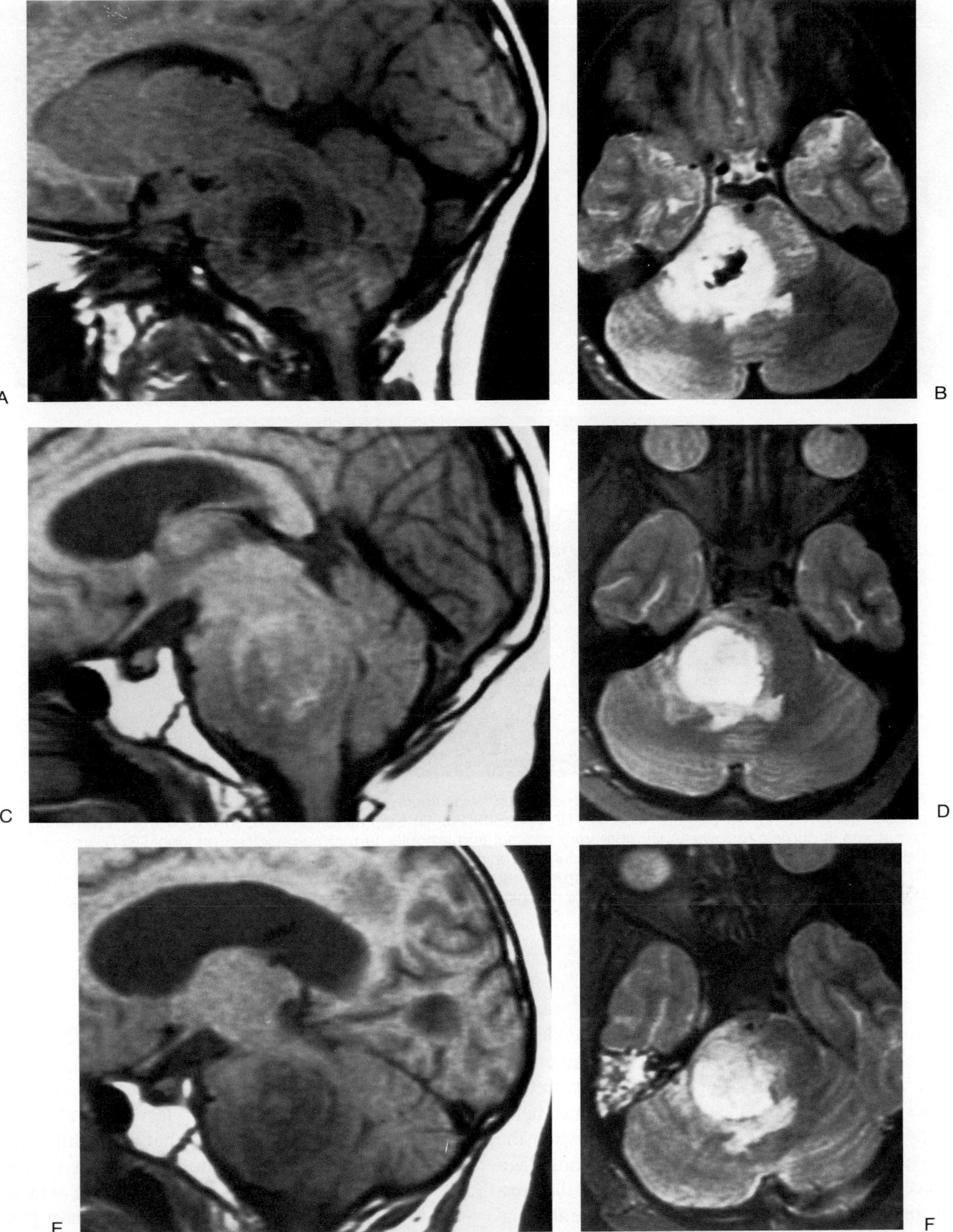

FIG. 15. Intratumoral hemorrhage with absence of ferritin/hemosiderin (brainstem astrocytoma). **A:** Sagittal short TR/TE MRI (600/20). **B:** Axial long TR/TE MRI (2500/80). **C:** Sagittal short TR/TE MRI (600/20), after 3 months. **D:** Axial long TR/TE MRI (2500/80), after 3 months. **E:** Sagittal short TR/TE MRI (600/20), after 5 months. **F:** Axial long TR/TE MRI (2500/80), after 5 months. Acute hemorrhage into center of large brainstem glioma is initially slightly hypointense on short TR/TE (A) and markedly hypointense on long TR/TE scan (B). After 3 months, hyperintense methemoglobin is seen throughout portions of tumor on short TR/TE scan (C), while virtually entire mass is of high intensity without expected significant hypointensity of hemosiderin on long TR/TE scan (D). Five months after initial bleed, methemoglobin has resolved (E), and mass is hyperintense with only minimal hypointensity on long TR/TE scan (F). The absence of ferritin/hemosiderin is thought to be a result of prolonged disruption of blood–brain barrier in tumors, which would minimize ferritin/hemosiderin accumulation.

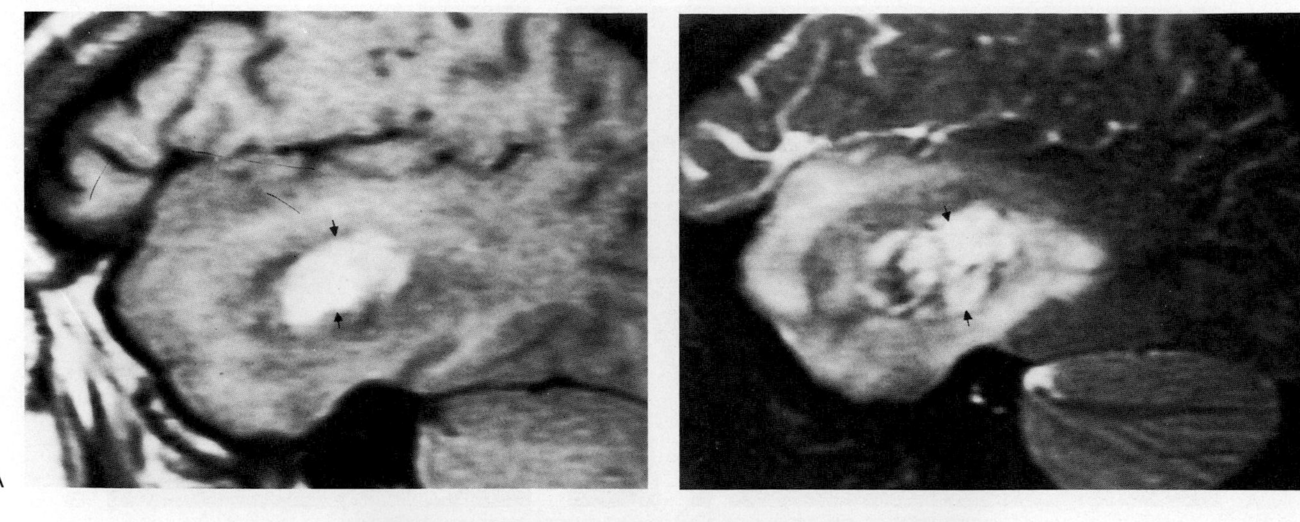

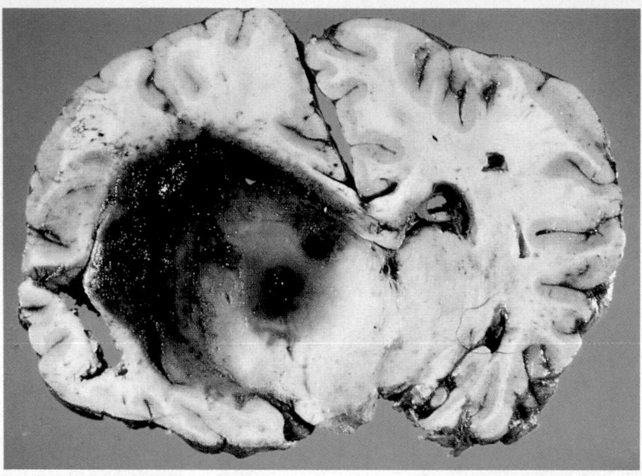

FIG. 16. Intratumoral hemorrhage with minimal ferritin/hemosiderin and persistent perihematoma high intensity (anaplastic astrocytoma). **A:** Sagittal short TR/TE MRI (600/20). **B:** Sagittal long TR/TE MRI (3000/80). Even though hematoma is chronic (*arrows*, A,B), note very minimal and irregular ferritin/hemosiderin on long TR/TE image (B). Persistent hyperintensity in temporal lobe around chronic hematoma on long TR/TE (B) indicates tumor plus edema. **C:** Brain autopsy section from anaplastic astrocytoma with hemorrhage and necrosis show persistent expansion of involved parenchyma and mass effect despite chronic nature of hemorrhage (C courtesy of Dr. N. K. Gonatas, Philadelphia, PA.)

sign of neoplasm as the underlying cause of the bleed is the identification of nonhemorrhagic tumor tissue itself (13) (Figs. 15 and 16). Lastly, the high intensity on long TR images in the parenchyma surrounding tumor hemorrhage persists and is prominent (13), even when the blood is chronic (Fig. 16), a common and ominous sign which necessitates follow-up MRI or biopsy. In the presence of any of these signs accompanying intracranial hemorrhage, one cannot ascribe the hemorrhagic event as being due to a benign cause, such as occult cerebrovascular malformation, and a work-up to exclude neoplasms must be performed.

Some components of tumors may have specific and (occasionally) pathognomonic signal intensities other than hemorrhage. Fat-containing neoplasms (e.g., teratoma, dermoid, lipoma) are easily identified on MRI, since fat is high intensity on short TR/TE and intermediate intensity on conventional long TR/TE images and parallels the intensity of subcutaneous fat (Fig. 17). The high signal of fat on newer fast spin-echo techniques makes this distinction somewhat more difficult. A more specific clue to the diagnosis of fat in tumors is the "chemical shift artifact" (see Chapter 9), which, simply put, is related to the difference in resonant frequencies between fat and water protons. This artifact is displayed as a region of signal void at fat-water interfaces and hyperintensity at water-fat interfaces, along the frequency-encoding axis (Fig. 17). Fat selective suppression methods also can play a role in the distinction of etiologies of hyperintense tumors on T1-weighted images (Fig. 18). Melanin in tumors (see section, "Metastatic Disease") is also seen as high intensity on short TR/TE and interme-

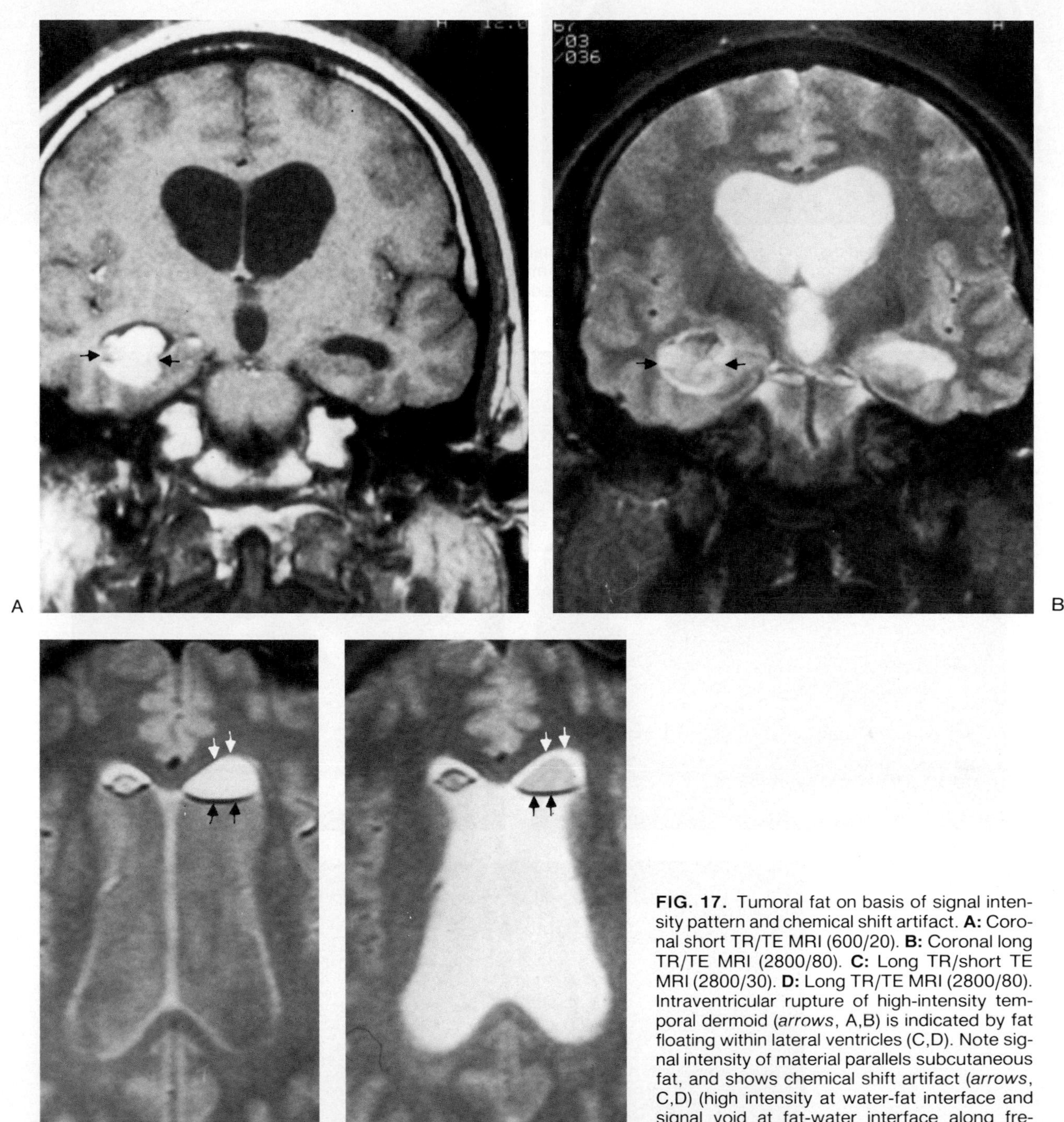

FIG. 17. Tumoral fat on basis of signal intensity pattern and chemical shift artifact. **A:** Coronal short TR/TE MRI (600/20). **B:** Coronal long TR/TE MRI (2800/80). **C:** Long TR/short TE MRI (2800/30). **D:** Long TR/TE MRI (2800/80). Intraventricular rupture of high-intensity temporal dermoid (*arrows*, A,B) is indicated by fat floating within lateral ventricles (C,D). Note signal intensity of material parallels subcutaneous fat, and shows chemical shift artifact (*arrows*, C,D) (high intensity at water-fat interface and signal void at fat-water interface along frequency-encoding gradient, which is oriented anterior-posterior).

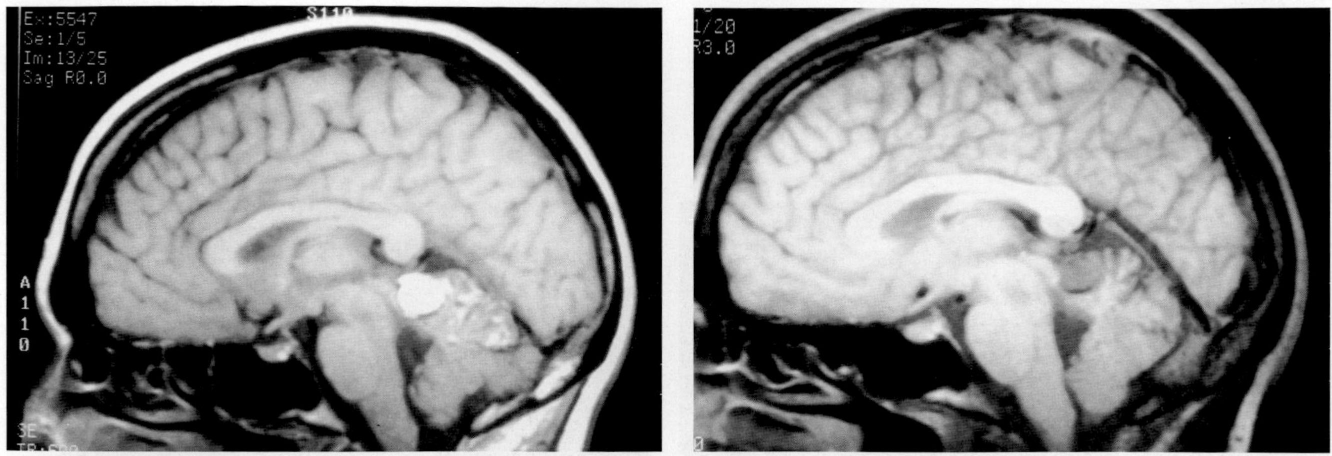

FIG. 18. Ruptured dermoid, use of fat supression. Sagittal T1-weighted MRI without (**A**) and after (**B**) fat supression shows midline superior cerebellar cistern hyperintense mass with foci of hyperintensity in vermian subarachnoid space (A) which all become low intensity after fat supression (B).

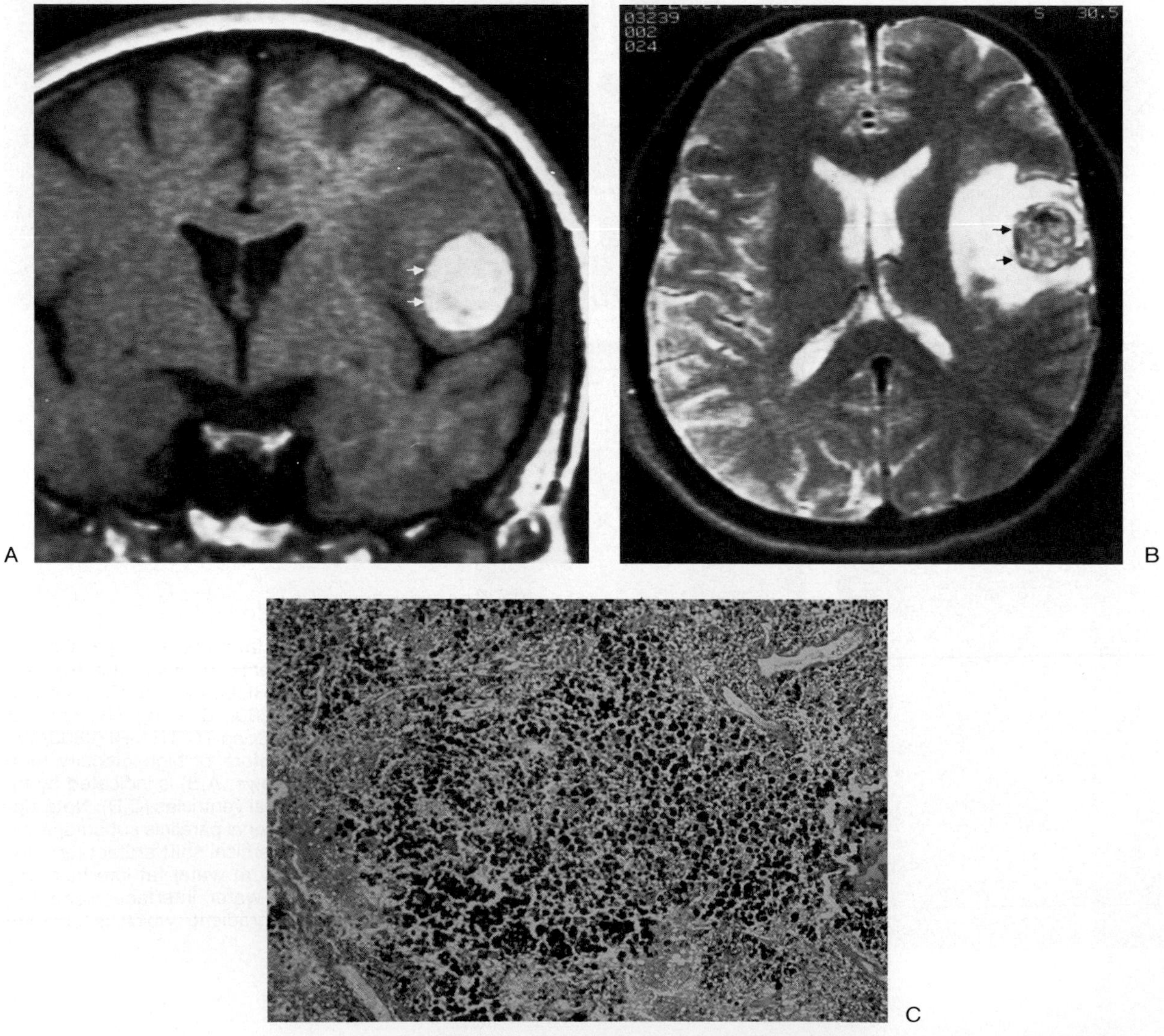

A B

C

FIG. 19. Tumoral melanin in melanoma metastasis. **A:** Coronal short TR/TE MRI (600/20). **B:** Axial long TR/TE MRI (2500/80). **C:** Histopathologic specimen (H&E, ×100). Densely melanotic, nonhemorrhagic melanoma metastasis (*arrows*, A,B) is hyperintense on short TR/TE (A) and isointense or only minimally hypointense to cortex on long TR/TE (B). This mass was densely melanotic (*dark reddish-brown staining*, C) with no evidence of iron on microscopic examination.

TABLE 6. *Intratumoral melanin vs. hemorrhage*

	Signal intensity (relative to gray matter)	
	Short TR/TE	Long TR/TE
Amelanotic tumor	↓	sl. ↑
Melanotic tumor	↑↑	= or sl. ↓
Early subacute blood (intracellular methemoglobin)	↑↑	↓↓
Late subacute blood (extracellular methemoglobin)	↑↑	↑↑

sl., slightly.

diate intensity on long TR/TE images (Fig. 19) (16), so nonhemorrhagic melanotic melanoma is distinct from amelanotic tumors and from hemorrhage based on this unique combination of signal intensities (Table 6). Unfortunately, melanoma metastases are commonly both hemorrhagic and melanotic (Fig. 20), which in many cases makes the imaging less specific. Other neoplasms that can be pigmented include medulloblastoma and melanotic neuroectodermal tumor of infancy. Profound hypervascularity associated with certain tumors can be virtually pathognomonic of hemangioblastoma or glioblastoma. These large vessels are shown on spin-echo images as linear or serpentine regions of signal void (Fig. 21) within and about neoplastic masses, and are an important sign for the diagnostician as well as for the surgeon. Intratumoral vascularity can be confirmed by using gradient-echo imaging (see Chapter 29) or MR angiography, which demonstrates these vessels as hyperintense structures. Another useful sign for differential diagnosis is seen in markedly hypercellular neoplasms, especially those with only minimal cytoplasm. These tumors are, characteristically, relatively low intensity on long TR/TE (T2-weighted) images and approximate the intensity of normal gray matter (Fig. 22). This is a characteristic MR feature of undifferentiated small round cell tumors, such as medulloblastoma, pineoblastomas, and neuroblastomas. Other tumor types also typically have low intensity on T2-weighted images, including most lymphomas, mucinous adenocarcinomas (particularly from the colon) and amelanotic melanoma metastases. Similarly, highly cellular astrocytic (generally higher grade) neoplasms have lower water content (higher solids content), which has been correlated to faster relaxation rates, although it should be noted that 1/T1 measurements are relatively insensitive to the grade of malignancy (17).

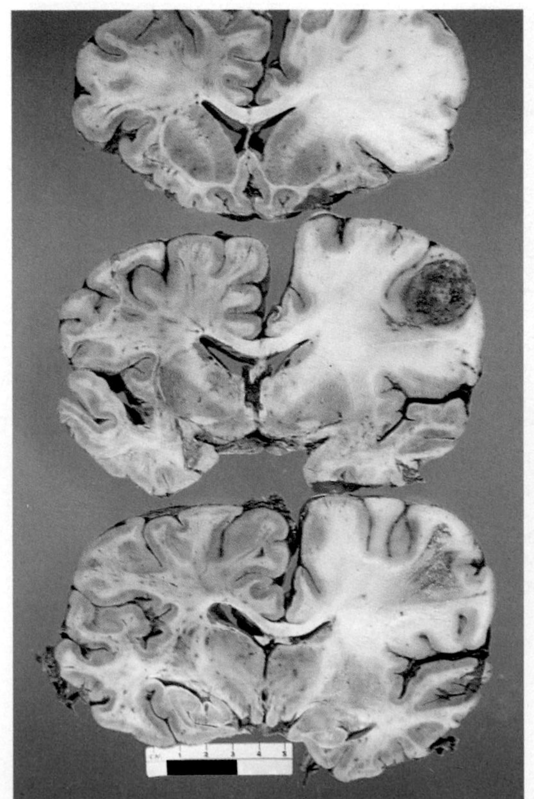

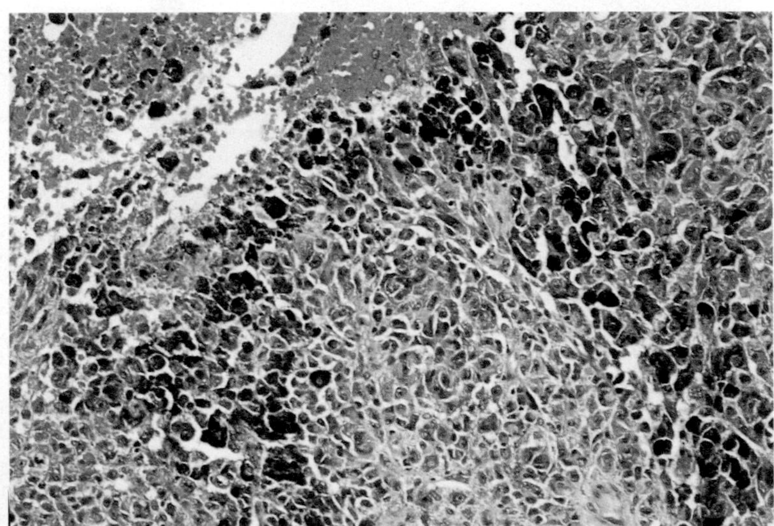

FIG. 20. Melanoma metastases with both hemorrhage and melanin content. Brain autopsy sections (**A**) show hemorrhagic melanoma metastasis in midparietal gyrus. Microscopic section from another case (**B**) exhibits nests of neoplastic cells containing melanin (fine brown pigment), in addition to hemosiderin-containing macrophages (coarse brown pigment) and fresh blood. (A courtesy of Dr. N. K. Gonatas, Philadelphia, PA.)

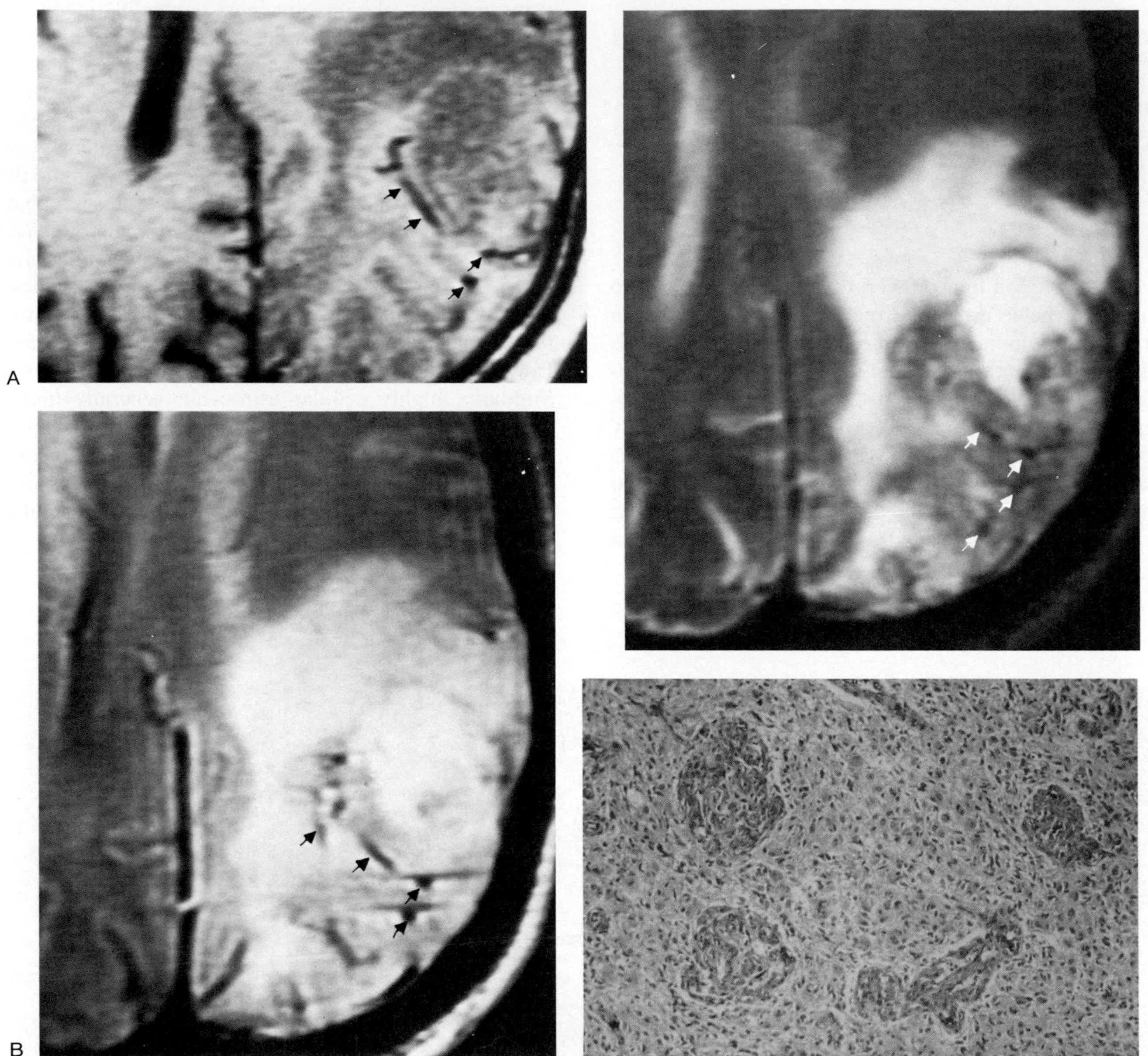

FIG. 21. Intratumoral hypervascularity as cause of hypointensity (glioblastoma). **A:** Short TR/TE MRI (600/20). **B:** Long TR/short TE MRI (2500/20). **C:** Long TR/TE MRI (2500/80). **D:** Histopathologic specimen (H&E, high-power field), different highly vascular glioma. (From Okazaki and Scheithauer, ref. 121, with permission.) Large left parietal glioblastoma shows linear and focal regions of signal void on all spin-echo images (*arrows*, A–C), indicating flow in large intratumoral vessels. Microscopic section (D) shows proliferation of angioendothelial cells (dark staining clusters of cells), indicating neovascularity induced within similar high-grade neoplasm.

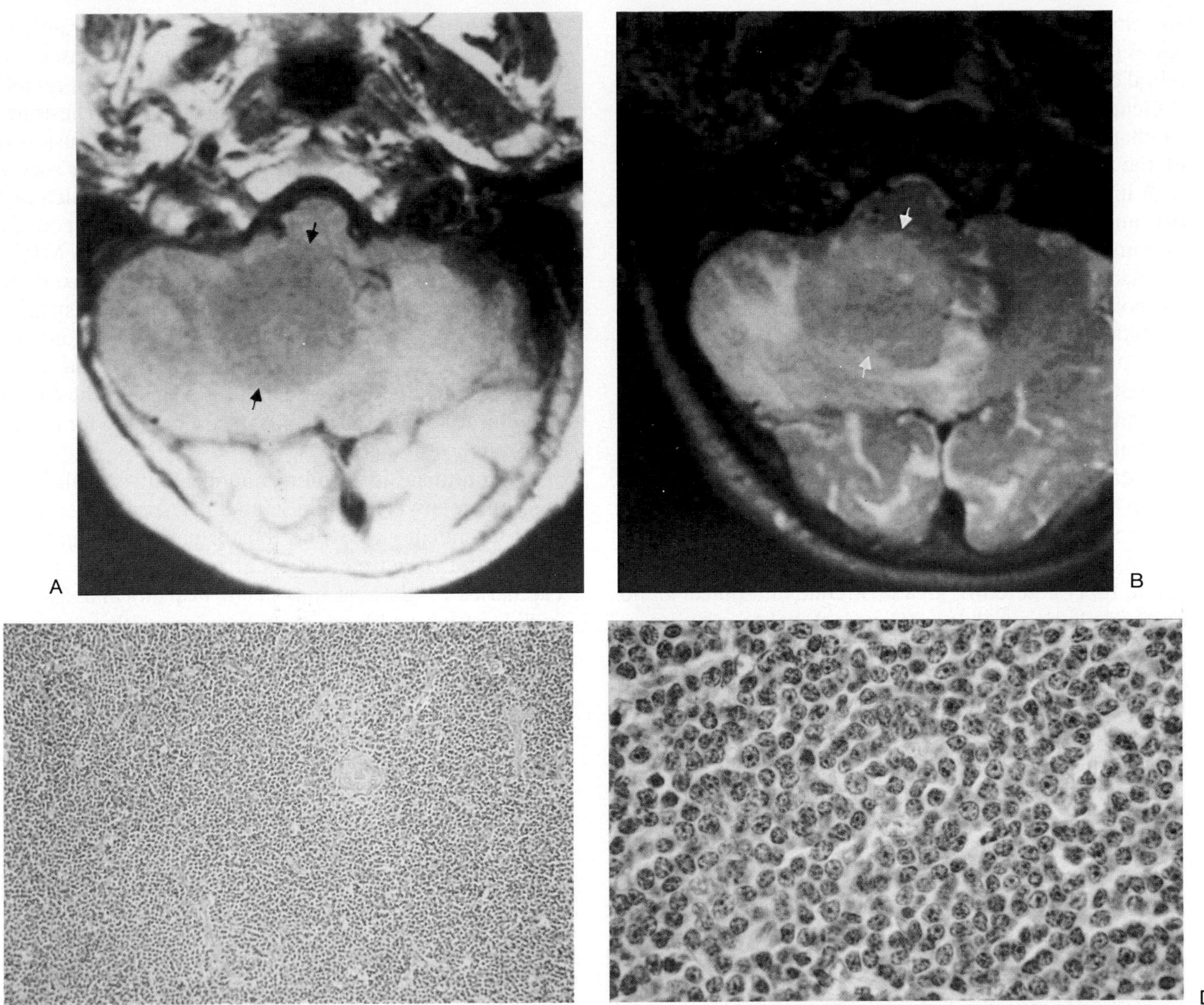

FIG. 22. Tumor with dense hypercellularity and scant cytoplasm as low intensity (lymphoma). **A:** Short TR/TE MRI (600/20). **B:** Long TR/TE MRI (2800/80). **C:** Histopathologic specimen (H&E, low-power field). **D:** Histopathologic specimen (H&E, high-power field). Right cerebellar lymphomatous mass (*arrows*, A,B) is relatively low intensity on long TR/TE image (B), consistent with its dense hypercellularity and minimal cytoplasm (high nucleus:cytoplasm ratio) revealed by microscopy (C,D).

TUMOR ENHANCEMENT AND THE BLOOD–BRAIN BARRIER

The brain is highly dependent on a constant internal milieu. This critical function is accomplished mainly by the unique endothelial cells of brain capillaries, which form a continuous wall that restricts the movement of many substances from the bloodstream to the interstitial space of the brain. These capillary cells are part of a very complex physiologic phenomenon known as the blood–brain barrier, a concept postulated first by Goldmann in 1913 (18) but not conclusively demonstrated until the 1960s by electron microscopy (19). Endothelial cells of cerebral capillaries have fused membranes, termed tight junctions, which are probably the most important feature in regulating capillary permeability in the brain. Other unique characteristics of brain capillaries include continuous basement membranes, narrow intercellular gaps, and a paucity of pinocytosis (20). All of these structures act together to function as the blood–brain barrier. Capillaries of tissues outside the nervous system typically have discontinuities in their basement membranes with wide intercellular gaps, permitting the free passage of protein molecules from the lumen of the capillary into the extravascular space (19). Aside from tight junctions between cerebral capillary endothelium, these cells are also closely surrounded by a sheath of astrocytic foot processes (Fig. 23). Their precise role of the astrocyte in cerebral capillary permeability is still not known (21).

Generally speaking, the blood–brain barrier allows the capillary endothelium layer to function as an extension of the semipermeable plasma membrane. Substances with high lipid solubility, low ionization at physiologic pH, and low plasma protein binding undergo free passage and are rapidly accommodated into cerebral extracellular space; substances with opposite characteristics are not. Water moves freely in either direction through the blood–brain barrier to maintain equal osmotic concentrations of solutes in the blood and the extracellular fluid of the brain (20). Aside from endothelial cell structure and other unique morphologic features of cerebral capillaries, there are several carrier systems and specialized enzyme-mediated systems found in these cells, which also represent part of the barrier.

Blood–brain barrier interfaces are not found in some regions of the brain, notably the choroid plexus, pituitary gland, tuber cinereum, area postrema, and pineal gland (20). Capillaries in these regions lack tight junctions, as they do in dura and pia mater. The outermost layer of arachnoid has tight junctions and acts as a barrier between CSF and brain (22). Blood–CSF barriers are also present in choroid plexus; that is, intravascular substances enter choroid extracellular space at a much faster rate than they enter CSF surrounding choroid.

In normal brain and areas of intact blood–brain barrier, the capillaries are impermeable to intravascularly injected contrast agents. Dural vessels and the aforementioned structures in which capillaries are fenestrated (e.g., pituitary, choroid plexus, etc.) allow diffusion of contrast material into their tissue's extracellular spaces. On MR images, only those regions of tissue which lack an intact blood–brain barrier enhance in the conventional sense. Note that tumor enhancement on MRI is due to accumulation of the paramagnetic contrast in the water-containing interstitial space. The contrast agent enhances the relaxation of the water protons nearby; that is, we visualize the water in the enhancing tissue as high intensity on short TR/TE images (in the case of gadolinium-containing agents) (see Chapter 5 for discussion of relaxation effects).

The rationale for tumor enhancement is multifactorial, but relatively simple. Generally speaking, tumors have a tendency to evoke the formation of capillaries within and sometimes adjacent to their tissue. Tumor capillaries in gliomas may have near-normal features with functioning blood–brain barriers, so these areas of tumor tissue will not enhance with contrast. In other, often more malignant gliomas, on the contrary, formation of capillaries is stimulated whose endothelia are fenestrated and therefore have no blood–brain barrier—these tumors should theoretically enhance (20). Metastatic lesions possess non-CNS capillaries which are similar to

A

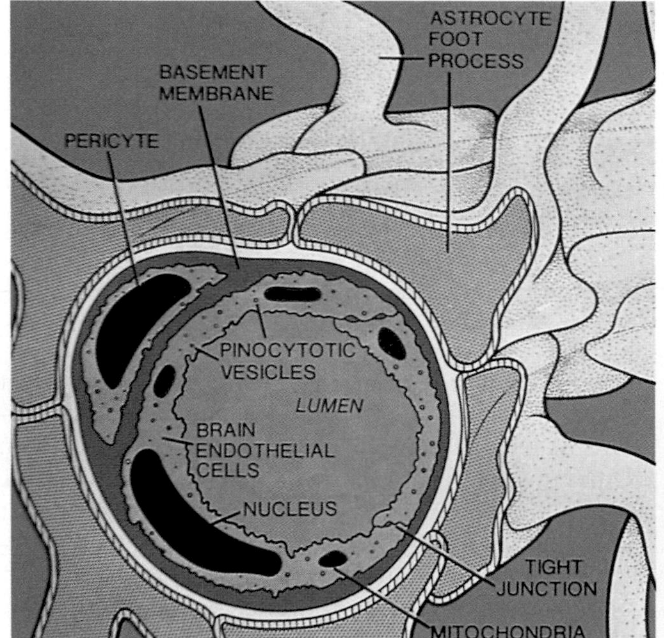

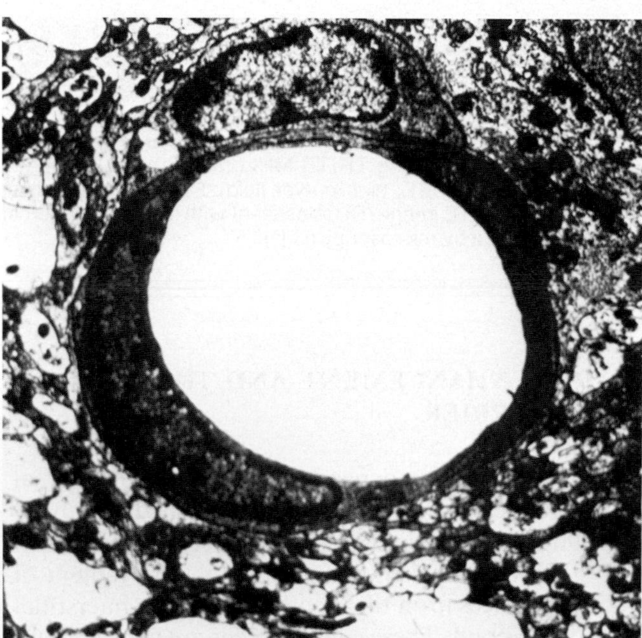

B

FIG. 23. The normal blood–brain barrier. (Modified from Goldstein and Betz, ref. 200, with permission.) **A:** Artist's conception, cerebral capillary structure. **B:** Normal cerebral capillary, electron microscopy. (Courtesy of Dr. P. Cancilla, Los Angeles, CA.) Cerebral capillaries are enveloped by astrocytic foot processes and have endothelial cells with partially fused membranes ("tight junctions," A), seen at lower right of electron micrograph (B) of normal rat brain capillary cross section.

their tissue of origin, so brain metastases virtually always enhance. Extra-axial tumors (e.g., meningiomas) arise from tissues whose capillaries lack tight junctions and, consequently, these tumors enhance. There is not usually a correlation between MRI or CT enhancement and angiographic findings of hypervascularity, although it has been suggested that the vascular pooling in angioblastic neoplasms may represent up to 20% to 30% of the noted enhancement on these studies (23). It is thought that the presence of capillary endothelia with tight junctions is the most important factor in predicting enhancement (20), but the volume of available extracellular space may also be of some relevance (23). In truth, there are several necessary precursors for contrast enhancement to occur: absence of the blood–brain barrier, adequate delivery of the contrast agent (i.e., perfusion), extracapillary interstitial space for accumulation of contrast agent, appropriate contrast agent dosage, spatial

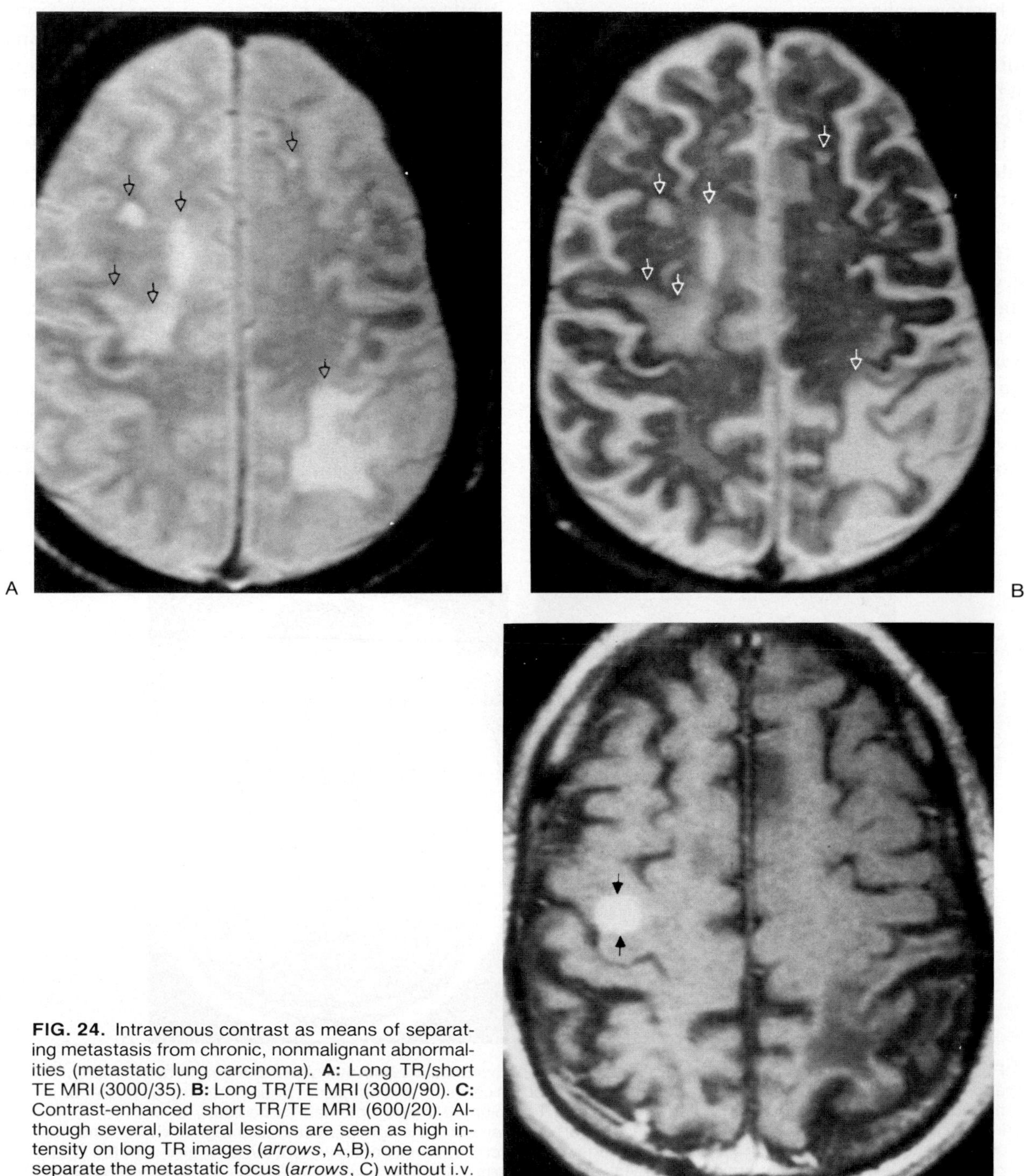

FIG. 24. Intravenous contrast as means of separating metastasis from chronic, nonmalignant abnormalities (metastatic lung carcinoma). **A:** Long TR/short TE MRI (3000/35). **B:** Long TR/TE MRI (3000/90). **C:** Contrast-enhanced short TR/TE MRI (600/20). Although several, bilateral lesions are seen as high intensity on long TR images (*arrows*, A,B), one cannot separate the metastatic focus (*arrows*, C) without i.v. gadolinium.

resolution and imaging parameters to allow its detection, and time for the contrast agent to accumulate in the region in question. Note that the formation of tumor capillaries deficient in blood–brain barrier constituents, rather than active destruction of the blood–brain barrier, is presumed to be the explanation for tumor enhancement. Moreover, the enhancement of a particular tumor may not merely be an "all or none" phenomenon; that is, the function of the blood-brain barrier should be thought of as a continuum—capillary structure (and other factors) may be aberrant to different degrees in tumors. Therefore, enhancement may be immediate or delayed, evanescent or persistent, dense and homogeneous, or minimal and irregular. Perhaps one of the most important points to remember for the radiologist is that the lack of enhancement does not necessarily signify lack of tumor. In other words, one cannot use enhancement to "separate tumor from edema" in infiltrative gliomas, since tumor clearly is often present in areas which do not enhance.

It has long been recognized that the intravenous injection of contrast agents aids in the CT delineation of many intracranial disease processes, especially neoplasia. In spite of this, the need for i.v. contrast in cranial MRI was initially debated, because it was assumed that the exquisite sensitivity of non-contrast MRI would obviate the need for contrast injection. It was also proposed that an abnormal or absent blood–brain barrier (or perhaps more appropriately, blood–tumor barrier) should also allow water (the naturally occurring contrast agent in MRI) to accumulate in the pathologic tissue. Furthermore, it was argued that many intracerebral neoplasms do not enhance on CT, so they probably would not enhance on MRI, a valid point that necessitates using long TR scanning and prohibits the reliance of the radiologist on short TR/TE images alone.

There are many situations where i.v. contrast is definitely indicated and, at times, required for complete evaluation by MRI. Distinction of nonspecific high intensity foci attributed to ischemia and aging in the deep white matter from metastases or lymphoma can be virtually impossible, unless one uses i.v. contrast. Small lesions, especially metastases to cortex, can be missed without contrast enhancement, and metastases may be indistinguishable from other chronic insults in elderly patients in the absence of contrast (Fig. 24). Patterns of contrast enhancement and relationship to mass effect often alter differential diagnosis. Leptomeningeal and subependymal metastases are certainly much better detected with i.v. contrast. These ideas will be more fully discussed in this chapter.

Aside from these instances, it has been reported that contrast enhancement can commonly occur beyond the margin of abnormality detected by unenhanced T2-weighted scans, particularly when high doses of contrast are employed (Fig. 25) (24). Owing to the exquisite sensitivity of MRI to contrast enhancement, we have also noted contrast enhancement in regions of non-tumor

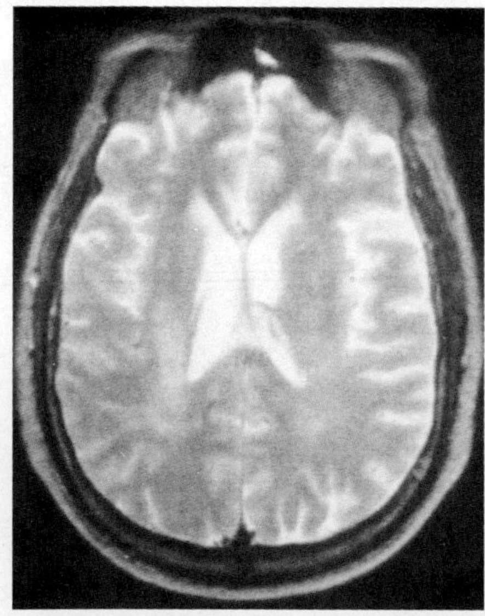

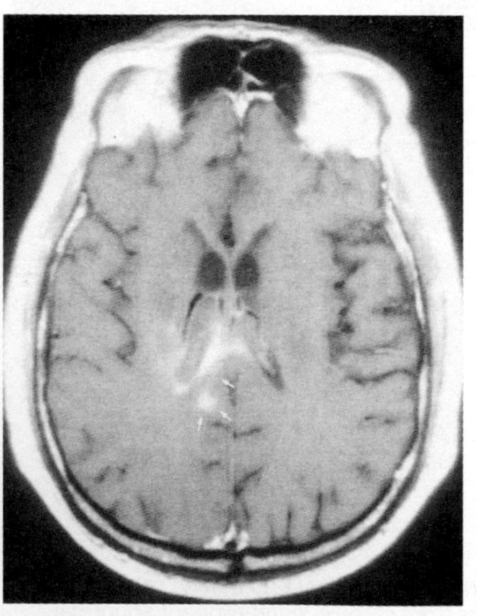

FIG. 25. A: Axial T2-weighted (2000/80) image shows a periventricular abnormal signal in the right hemisphere. No apparent abnormality was noted in the splenium of the corpus callosum and subjacent brain parenchyma posterior to the corpus callosum. **B:** Corresponding postcontrast T1-weighted image obtained immediately after intravenous injection of 0.3 mmol/kg gadoteridol, shows abnormal enhancement in the right periventricular region where abnormal signal change was observed on T2-weighted images. However, abnormal enhancement (*arrows*) also is noted in the corpus callosum and adjacent brain parenchyma along the walls of the lateral ventricles which most likely represents the spread of a tumor along the white matter tracts. (From Yuh, et al., ref. 24, with permission.)

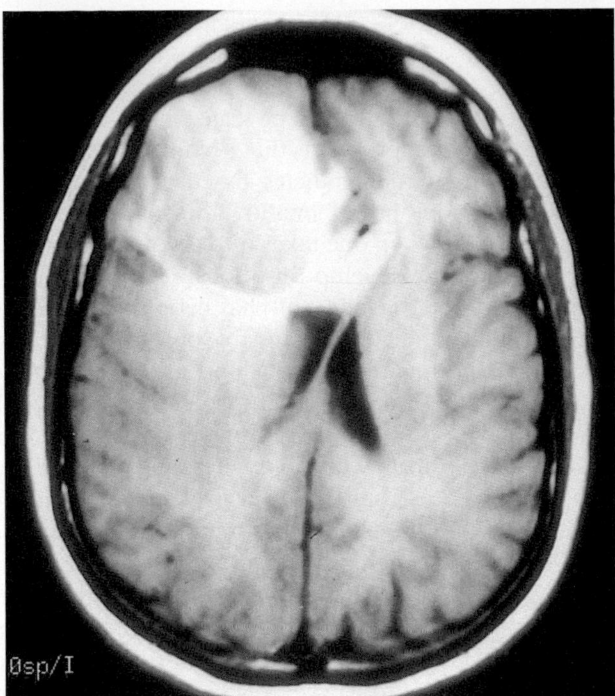

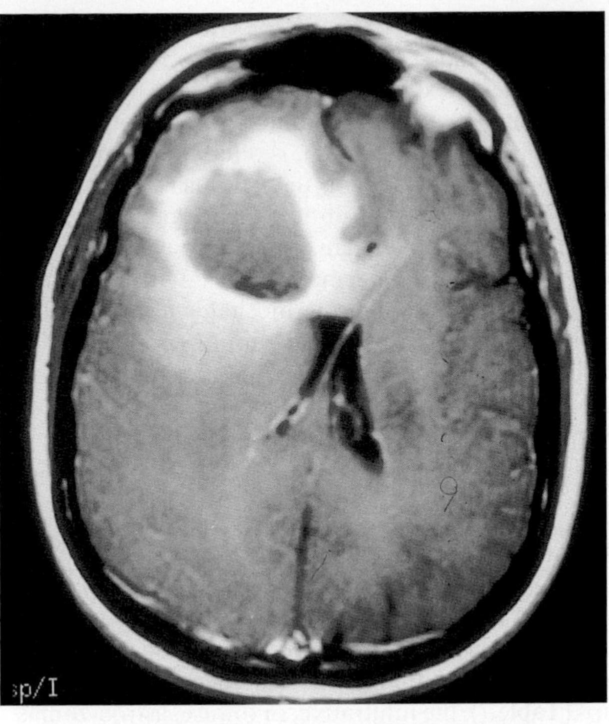

FIG. 26. Enhancement of vasogenic edema with metastasis. T1-weighted MRI shows large right frontal cystic metastasis from melanoma (**A**). After i.v. contrast (**B**), T1-weighted image shows marked enhancement of region corresponding to vasogenic edema. At pathology (not shown), no tumor cells were noted in white matter.

bearing vasogenic edema surrounding metastases (Fig. 26), a finding of uncertain significance. Heightened sensitivity to contrast enhancement has been shown by using the magnetization transfer saturation technique to suppress background parenchyma (25). Contrast agent bolus techniques in conjunction with echo-planar imaging have been advocated as a means of generating cerebral blood volume maps with MRI. Cerebral blood volume maps may aid in assessing the grade of the tumor (see Chapter 30). New applications of contrast agent usage in imaging intracranial tumors are still being explored at the time of this writing.

PRIMARY BRAIN TUMORS

Primary cerebral gliomas comprise approximately 40% to 45% of all intracranial tumors (11) and represent the largest single group. The peak incidence of gliomas occurs near the beginning of the seventh decade of life (11). The vast majority of adult gliomas are supratentorial, while 70% to 80% of these tumors in childhood are infratentorial. Although figures vary and are influenced by whether the data reflects autopsy or biopsy material, one large series (11) reports the incidence of the various histologic types as: glioblastoma 55%, astrocytoma 20.5%, ependymoma 6%, medulloblastoma 6%, oligodendroglioma 5%, and choroid plexus papilloma 2% (11). The degree of malignancy of gliomas is extremely variable and extends across the entire range of possibilities, from the low-grade, more "benign" pilocytic astrocytomas to the extremely malignant end of the spectrum, e.g., glioblastoma.

Clinical presentations are either due to focal neurologic deficits or to a generalized increase in intracranial pressure. Included in the signs and symptoms of increased intracranial pressure are increasing headache, classically most severe in the morning, nausea, vomiting, and visual symptoms. A more ominous sign of elevated intracranial pressure is obtundation and lethargy, which necessitates urgent work-up and therapy. In more malignant gliomas, these symptoms are characteristically rapidly and relentlessly progressive. A distinctly more optimistic prognosis is offered to those who initially present with focal neurologic signs or symptoms, such as seizures, an event which heralds the diagnosis in almost half of these patients (26).

As noted above, MRI appears to be more sensitive for these lesions than CT, both in terms of tumor detection and completeness of lesion delineation (3). Unfortunately, the preoperative neuroradiologic evaluation, performed with either CT or MRI, is often inconclusive regarding histologic grade of the glioma (3,27,28). In general, it appears that tumor enhancement on MRI with the use of gadopentetate dimeglumine is more sensitive than tumor enhancement on CT with iodinated contrast (29), even though the mechanism of enhancement (i.e., blood–brain barrier disruption) is identical for both agents (20,30,31). It is likely that the extreme sensitivity of MRI to contrast enhancement will not aid in distinguishing tumors of varying grades of malignancy, but will simply add sensitivity.

SUPRATENTORIAL NEOPLASMS

Tumors of Astrocytic Origin

Astrocytic brain tumors can be divided into two major groups (Table 7): the infiltrative, or diffuse, astrocytomas and the localized, non-infiltrative astrocytomas. Infiltrative astrocytomas comprise approximately 75% of astrocytic tumors of the CNS, while localized tumors make up the remainder. These two groups differ in their natural history and hence their clinical behavior and response to therapy, so this distinction is an essential one to ascertain. Many of the different histologic subtypes develop more commonly in association with neurocutaneous syndromes and in specific intracerebral locations.

Histopathologic Grading of Astrocytic Neoplasms

While it is unarguable that grading systems can be devised to categorize astrocytomas into types differing in prognosis, and that these systems are useful for the clinical management of patients harboring astrocytomas, grading these lesions "represents an attempt to establish artificial and abrupt points of division in what is actually a continuum of neoplastic evolution" (32). In fact, it is widely accepted that all such systems have significant limitations, due mainly to the intratumoral heterogeneity of these neoplasms, but also to one of the notable features of astrocytoma—the tendency to dedifferentiate into more malignant lesions over time. The process of tumor development is clearly not a static process, as documented by significant changes in degree of malignancy over time (33,34) estimated to occur in approximately 10% of cases. It should also be realized that there are several unavoidable problems that accompany any attempt to grade these malignancies based on histopathology (11). Surgical biopsy of small regions of tumor are seriously limited, when one takes into account the tendency for anaplasia to develop on a local level and the well-recognized heterogeneity of glial neoplasms. It may be the case that surgically inaccessible portions of the tumor represent the most malignant portion of the lesion. In addition to these inherent pathologic problems, grading systems do not take into account such factors as the location of the tumor, which often has significant influence on surgical accessibility and survival, and variations between different histologic interpretations.

Despite the recognized limitations of grading systems, most recent systems essentially employ a three-tiered scale. In this discussion, we have used a modification of the proposed classifications for tumors by Russell and Rubinstein (11) and Rorke (35), combined with the new three-tiered WHO classification (36) and VandenBerg's guidelines for astrocytic tumors (37). We will also employ to some extent a conventional neuroanatomic approach to the diagnosis of brain tumors that has long been used by radiologists in the interpretation of imaging studies, since it is well recognized that the clinical behavior of brain tumors can depend largely on their sites of origin. For instance, we will initially consider neoplasms of astrocytes and those of neurons according mainly to their histopathologic features. Since the majority of these lesions are far more often located in the supratentorial compartment they as such constitute the "supratentorial parenchymal tumors." Posterior fossa tumors include a variety of histologic types, but the neuroanatomic approach is well embedded in the neuroradiology literature and will be used in this chapter as well.

TABLE 7. *Classification of astrocytic brain tumors*

Diffuse (infiltrative)	Localized (circumscribed)
Astrocytoma	Pilocytic astrocytoma
Anaplastic astrocytoma	Pleomorphic xanthoastrocytoma
Glioblastoma multiforme	Subependymal giant cell astrocytoma

Infiltrative (Diffuse or Fibrillary) Astrocytic Tumors

Infiltrative astrocytomas comprise a group of neoplasms that show a wide range of tumor grade by histologic criteria. Historically, this group of tumors has been further classified and graded based on morphologic criteria in order to express differences in biological behavior, malignant potential, and survival. Early morphologic concepts introduced by Bailey and Cushing (38) included primitive, bipolar, and unipolar spongioblasts, astroblasts, and fibrillary and protoplasmic astrocytes. These terms acquired very limited use in daily clinical practice and therefore a four-tiered grading system, known as the Kernohan's classification, became popular (39). Over the years of its use, the Kernohan's classification presented several difficulties: (i) it did not separate infiltrating from non-infiltrating astrocytomas; and (ii) it presented difficulties in distinguishing grade 3 from grade 4 or grade 1 from grade 2, and therefore relied on subjective criteria which varied from interpreter to interpreter and from center to center. It therefore induced controversy and lack of uniformity when treatment modalities were compared.

As noted above, the most widely accepted approach at present to grading of infiltrating astrocytomas derives from the WHO classification of brain tumors into a three-tiered system consisting of: astrocytoma, anaplastic astrocytoma, and glioblastoma multiforme. The major criteria for this classification are: increased cell density, nuclear and/or cytoplasmic pleomorphism, mitoses, necrosis, and vascular endothelial and/or pericytic proliferation. Glioblastoma multiforme contains all of these features and typically also pseudopalisading cells around areas of necrosis and giant cell formation. Astrocytomas have none of these features, except for slight increased cellularity and minimal cellular pleomorphism. The separation between astrocytoma and anaplastic astrocytoma usually depends on the degree of cell density, cellular pleomorphism, and mitotic rate, while the distinction between anaplastic astrocytoma and glioblastoma mostly relies on the presence of necrosis and vascular endothelial proliferation. The three-tiered system is more uniform, objective, and correlates well with the biological behavior of the tumors and clinical survival rates (40–43).

Infiltrative astrocytomas can be subdivided into several types (Table 8), but most are composed of the fibrillary type of astrocyte, which is found in cerebral white matter, as opposed to the protoplasmic astrocyte found in gray matter. Mixed neoplasms are common, however. These neoplasms can occur anywhere in the CNS but are typically found in certain sites and only rarely found in others. When infiltrative astrocytomas are found in the adult population, the lesions are most often found in the cerebral hemispheres, i.e., in a supratentorial location. The infiltrative form of astrocytomas comprises approximately 75% of hemispheric astrocytomas of adults. In children, infiltrative astrocytomas are typically within the brainstem. Cerebellar hemispheric astrocytomas are only rarely of the infiltrative type, but when an adult harbors a cerebellar astrocytoma, it is more commonly infiltrative than pilocytic. In all ages, the spinal cord represents another site of origin of infiltrative astrocytomas, although it is much less common than the cerebral location (see Chapter 27).

Infiltrative astrocytomas overall have a poor prognosis, which can be traced to a significant tendency to dedifferentiate into more malignant forms and the predilection for infiltration and spread into the leptomeninges. The clinical behavior of infiltrative astrocytomas is related to the overall histopathologic grade of the lesion and, as recently described, the DNA histogram index (44), but it also varies with the age of the patient. In general, when these tumors are found in older patients, they are more aggressive, more anaplastic, and more neurologically symptomatic. On the other hand, in younger patients, infiltrative astrocytomas are usually symptomatic for a longer period of time, show slower rates of growth, and are better differentiated histologically (32). Similarly, the tendency to dedifferentiate occurs more frequently and over a shorter period of time in older patients.

Astrocytoma

Astrocytoma represents the well-differentiated subtype of infiltrative astrocytomas and comprises 25% to 30% of hemispheric gliomas in adults and approximately 30% of cerebellar gliomas found in childhood (11). The peak incidence of supratentorial astrocytomas lies between the ages of 20 and 50 years, and generally 10 years

TABLE 8. *Diffuse astrocytic brain neoplasms*

	Astrocytoma	Anaplastic astrocytoma	Glioblastoma	Gliomatosis cerebri
Typical site(s) of origin	Cerebral hemisphere (adult)	Cerebral hemisphere (adult)	Cerebral hemisphere (adult)	Cerebral hemisphere (young or middle-aged adult)
	Brainstem (child) Cerebellum (young adult)	Brainstem (child)		
Signal intensity characteristics (on long TR)	Homogeneous; high intensity	Some heterogeneity	Markedly heterogeneous; hemorrhage and necrosis common	Ill-defined; high intensity
Vascular flow voids	Not seen	Unusual	Common	Rare
Contrast enhancement	Variable; irregular	Common; irregular	Common; irregular	Uncommon
Prognosis (median survival, if available)	7–8 years	2–3 years	12 months	Estimated as months

below the age for glioblastoma (45). These tumors arise in any part of the hemisphere with relative sparing noted only of the occipital lobes (46). In the pediatric population, infiltrative fibrillary astrocytomas are mainly situated in the brainstem. When the lesions are located in deep structures, there may be bihemispheric involvement. Although astrocytoma represents the benign end of the spectrum of infiltrative astrocytomas and show a more indolent course than glioblastoma and anaplastic astrocytoma, the overall prognosis of such lesions is still grim, with median survival rates reported as approximately 7 to 8 years (47,48). Furthermore, it is recognized that about 10% of these low-grade lesions "dedifferentiate" into more malignant forms over time (11). When astrocytomas recur, progression to anaplastic astrocytoma is seen in 50% to 75% of cases (11).

These tumors pathologically are associated with the development of neuroglial fibrils and secondary to this classically develop a firm, rubbery consistency (11), but on sectioning the astrocytoma can be found to vary in texture (32). The lesions are ill-defined and expand the involved portion of brain parenchyma. They tend to blur the normally clear distinction between gray and white matter on gross examination. Degenerative microcystic formation may be encountered in these well-differentiated neoplasms, but macroscopically they are solid tumors. In distinction from the hemorrhagic cystic change in glioblastoma, the microcysts found in astrocytoma are typically filled with clear fluid (32). Calcification may be present (Fig. 27). Microscopically (Fig. 28), there is usually a clear region of hypercellularity situated within white matter, often with considerable cellular heterogeneity, even in the absence of frank anaplasia. However, the lesions can be so subtle that reactive astrocytic change is also considered. The tumor can show marked infiltration of structures without significant distortion of gross morphology. Even on microscopy, the tumor is not distinctly demarcated, consequently it is virtually impossible to completely surgically resect these lesions. Focal regions of necrosis are rare and mitotic figures are absent in astrocytoma (32) and should prompt reconsideration of the diagnosis. Dural invasion and subarachnoid and subependymal seeding are rare unless malignant degeneration has occurred.

MRI demonstrates adult astrocytomas as relatively homogeneous mass lesions of the cerebral hemisphere (Fig. 29), although heterogeneity can be seen in a proportion of cases. These lesions are usually lacking significant peritumoral "edema," which, when present, is usually confined to white matter pathways. Furthermore, the

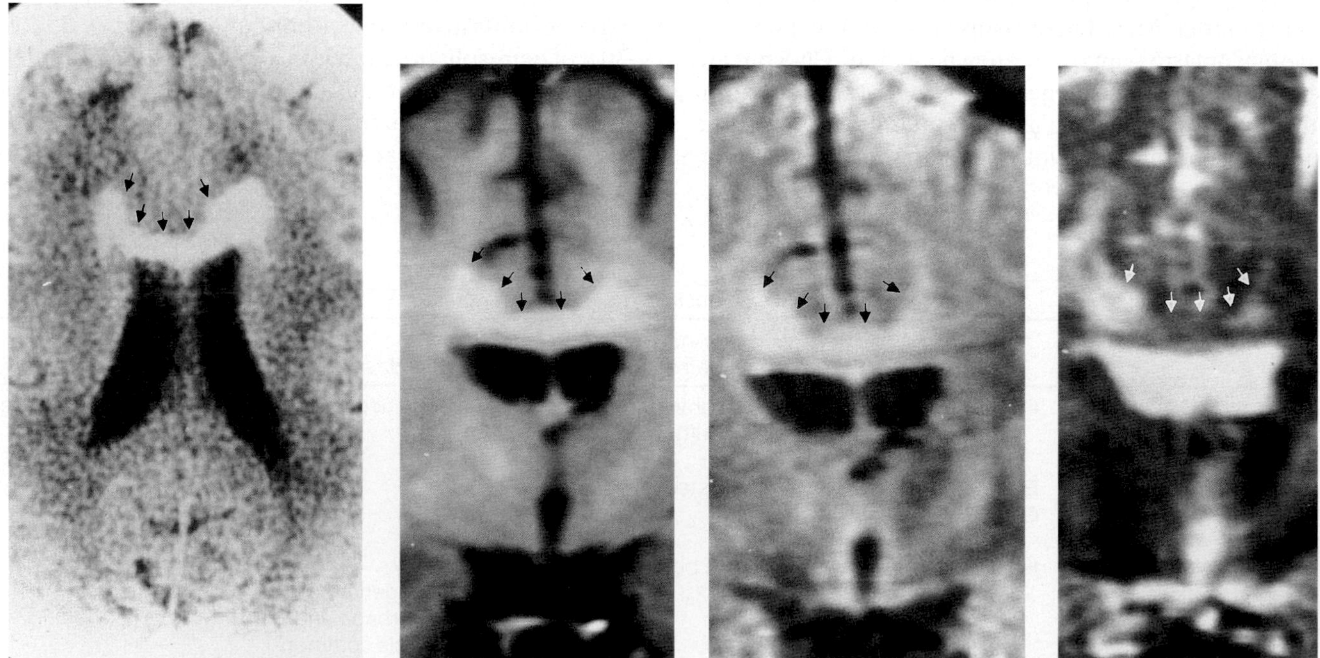

FIG. 27. Calcified astrocytoma, CT vs. MRI. **A:** Axial CT. **B:** Coronal short TR/TE MRI (600/20). **C:** Coronal long TR/short TE MRI (2500/20). **D:** Coronal long TR/TE MRI (2500/80). Area of dense calcification in corpus callosum astrocytoma (*arrows*) is of high intensity on all spin-echo MR images (B–D), probably due to associated paramagnetic cation deposition with dystrophic calcification.

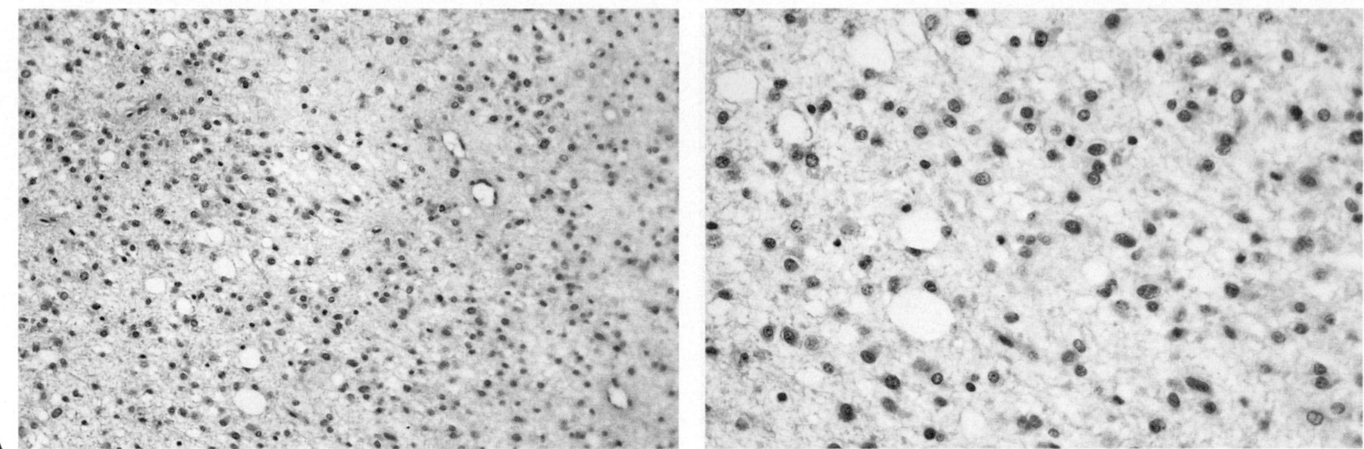

FIG. 28. Histologic features of astrocytoma. Note moderately cellular proliferation of astrocytes in a vacuolated matrix and occasional microcyst formation (**A,B**). In this low-grade astrocytoma, nuclear pleomorphism is mild, mitotic figures are rare, and no necrosis or vascular proliferation are seen. However, cell borders are ill defined and tumor cells may infiltrate beyond the grossly appearing tumor boundaries.

borders of well-differentiated astrocytomas often appear isodense to normal brain on CT. MRI, because of its higher contrast resolution, misleadingly displays these lesions as clearly defined regions of abnormal signal (Fig. 30). However, it has been documented that tumor tissue may extend beyond the confines of the imaging abnormality (49–51). Intratumoral regions suggestive of flow in vessels on MRI are not typical for astrocytoma. While focal cystic areas can occasionally be seen on imaging studies, it may not be possible to distinguish microcystic change (which is not surgically drainable) from macroscopically cystic regions of tumor on either CT or MRI. CT is estimated to identify calcification in approximately 20% of astrocytomas, a finding which is not usually evident on MRI, due to its lack of sensitivity and specificity for calcification when using spin-echo techniques (52,53). In fact, the most common glial neoplasm with calcification is the astrocytoma, in spite of the fact that oligodendrogliomas have the highest frequency of calcification.

It is not uncommon to identify cortical involvement by these tumors, which is best seen on MRI as thickening of the cortical mantle (Fig. 31), a finding which may not significantly differ from that seen in acute cortical infarction by anatomic distortion alone. Distinction can often be made if one discerns that the lesion does not obey a vascular territory, thereby indicating tumor rather than infarct. Focal parenchymal enhancement after i.v. contrast would also support a neoplastic process, since acute infarcts would not typically enhance. Occasionally, the radiologist must recommend follow-up scan in 4 to 6 weeks, in order to assess for the expected evolution (or lack thereof) of infarction.

The well-differentiated astrocytoma has a variable appearance after contrast administration, but classically astrocytoma shows no significant contrast enhancement. However, it has been reported that even up to 40% of "low grade" astrocytomas demonstrate enhancement on CT (54). Unfortunately, because of the aforementioned limitations of histopathological grading, correlations between histology and MRI are somewhat problematic. In general, contrast enhancement is not recognized as a reliable indicator of the grade of infiltrative astrocytomas.

Anaplastic Astrocytoma

The intermediate form of the infiltrative fibrillary astrocytoma is the anaplastic astrocytoma. This lesion is somewhere between the astrocytoma and the glioblastoma in its histological features and in its biological behavior. It may arise as a dedifferentiated astrocytoma, as noted above, where it is found on histopathology in over half of the cases of recurrent astrocytoma (11). It may also arise de novo (37). Clinically, the anaplastic astrocytoma is highly malignant, with median survival times of only 2 to 3 years after surgery and radiation therapy (45,55,56). These lesions generally occur in patients who are older than those with astrocytomas, but younger than those with glioblastomas. The peak incidence of anaplastic astrocytoma of the cerebral hemisphere is in the fifth decade. Anaplastic astrocytomas, when found in children, are usually centered within the pons.

On macroscopic pathology, anaplastic astrocytomas are usually more obvious mass lesions than their lower grade counterpart. They are usually easily discernible on surface examination of the involved region. On microscopic examination, the lesion shows more cellularity, nuclear pleomorphism, and mitotic figures than astrocytoma (Fig. 32). The microcystic changes often found in well-differentiated astrocytoma are lacking in the anaplastic type. As compared to glioblastoma, the necrosis

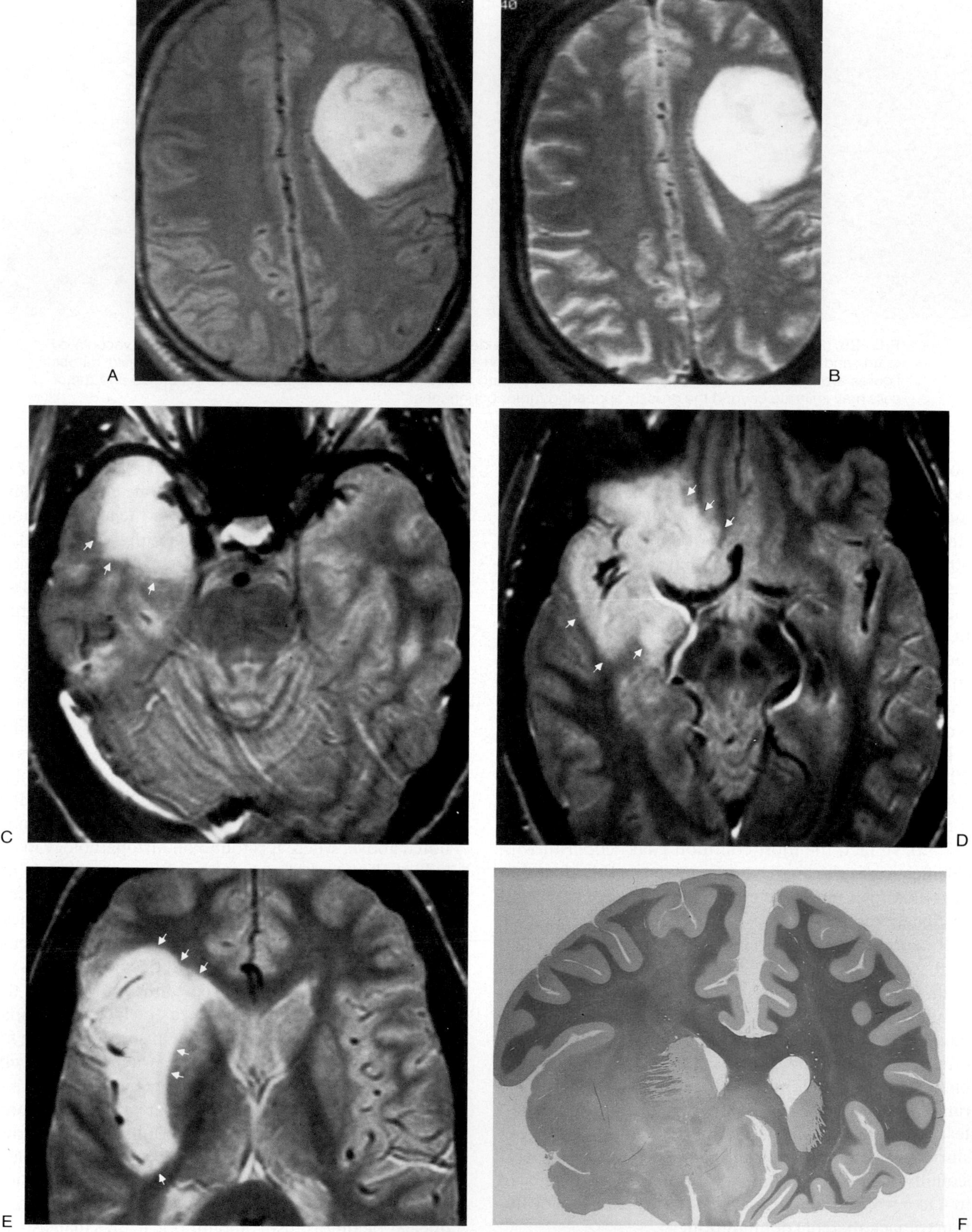
40
A
B
C
D
E
F

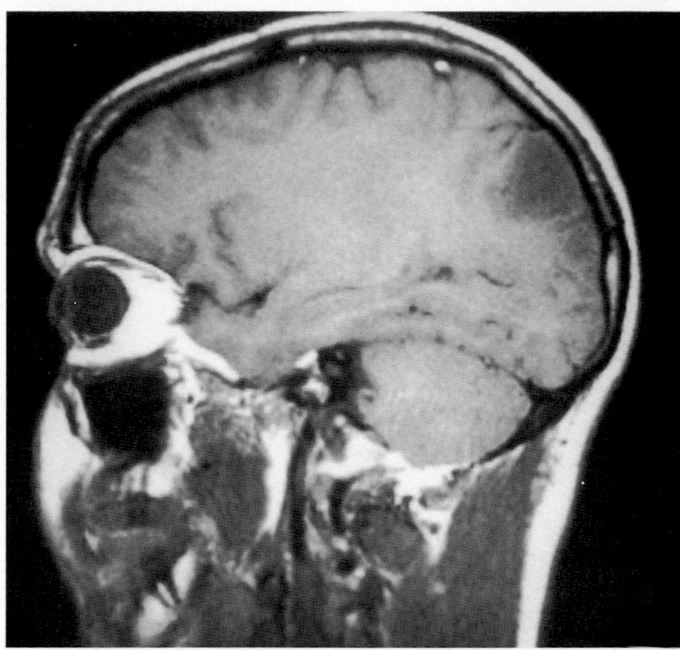

FIG. 30. Well-circumscribed appearance of proven infiltrative astrocytoma on MRI. Sagittal T1-weighted MRI (**A**) shows low-intensity mass in posterior parietal lobe. Note circumscribed appearance to lesion on proton-density (**B**) and T2-weighted (**C**) images, falsely implying non-infiltrative lesion.

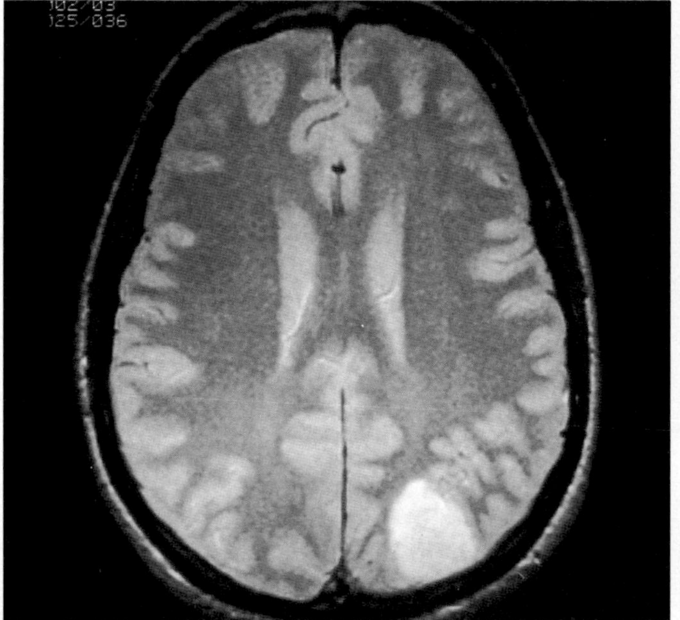

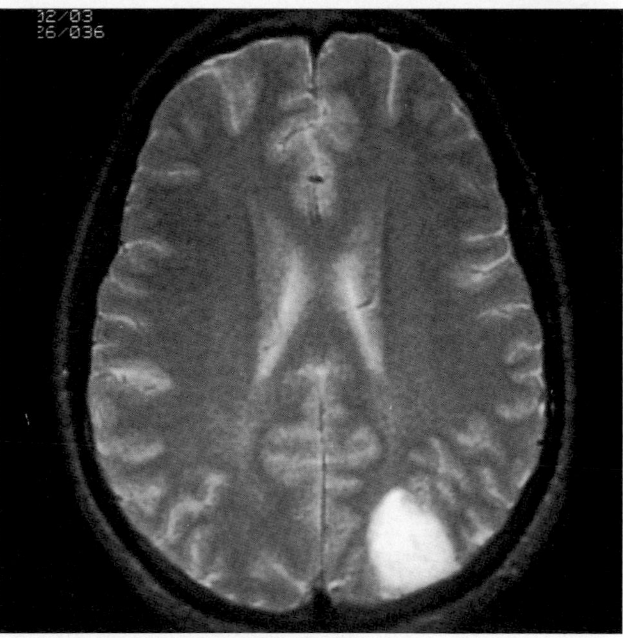

FIG. 29. Diffuse astrocytomas. **A:** Long TR/short TE MRI (2800/30), left frontal lobe astrocytoma. **B:** Long TR/TE MRI (2800/80), left frontal lobe astrocytoma. **C–E:** Long TR/short TE MRI (3000/30), right frontal temporal-insular astrocytoma (inferior to superior). **F:** Coronal necropsy specimen, myelin stain. (From Okazaki and Scheithauer, ref. 121, with permission.) High-intensity left frontal mass (A,B) is relatively homogeneous and is *not* accompanied by high signal in adjacent white matter. Similarly, high-intensity right-sided mass (*arrows*, C–E) is homogeneously hyperintense, with no evidence of hemorrhage or necrosis. Note absence of high signal in adjacent white matter. Poorly delineated nature of infiltrating astrocytoma from different patient (F) with similar lesion is seen as ill-defined, extensive region of decreased staining in right insula and deep temporal region.

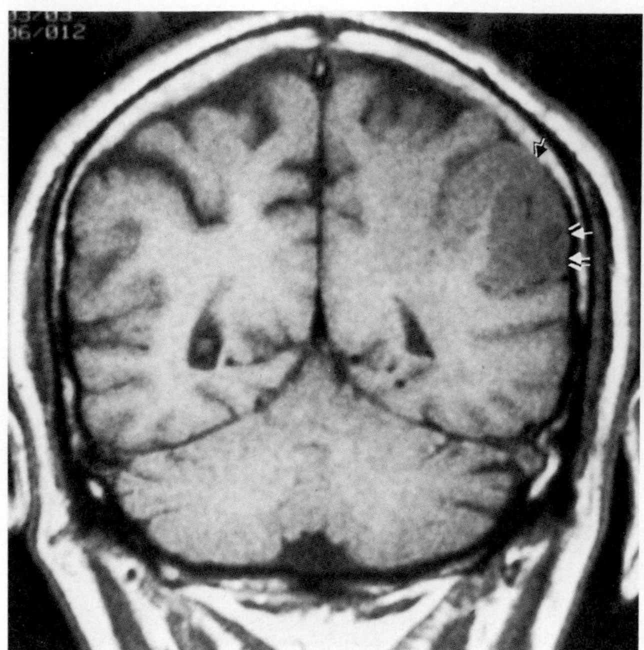

FIG. 31. Cortical astrocytoma on coronal short TR/TE MRI (600/20). Note thickening of left parietal gyrus (*arrows*), a finding that can also be seen in acute infarction.

and degree of vascular proliferation are lacking and the hypercellularity is more moderate (32). In fact, in some cases, the presence of necrosis is diagnostic of glioblastoma rather than anaplastic astrocytoma. Hemorrhage can also be seen (Fig. 33). Despite the potential confusion in differentiating anaplastic astrocytoma from glioblastoma, the treatments at this point in time are similar, so aside from prognosis the importance of such a difference is arguable.

MRI of anaplastic astrocytoma is variable, which is to be expected in a lesion that on histopathology represents a relatively large portion of the continuum of astrocytoma to glioblastoma transformation. Having said this, it can be generally stated that these lesions are typically more heterogeneous than astrocytoma, but do not show signs of frank necrosis that are highly suggestive of glioblastoma. The high intensity abnormality on T2-weighted images is commonly accompanied by an adjacent pattern consistent with vasogenic edema, as is also commonly found in glioblastoma. This "edema" pattern is a reflection of a combination of tumor and edema on histology, so the radiologist should not be misled into thinking that the tumor can be separated from the edema. Intratumoral focal regions of signal void due to prominent neovascularity can be seen (Fig. 34) but are not as common in anaplastic astrocytoma and should suggest glioblastoma.

Moreover, and perhaps even more so than for low-grade astrocytoma, contrast enhancement is extremely variable in anaplastic astrocytomas in both extent and pattern. While conventional wisdom states that higher grade astrocytomas demonstrate contrast enhancement on CT (57) and MRI (29), while lower grade astrocytomas often do not, it is important to note that there is a considerable degree of overlap. The type of enhancement is also variable and can be focal and nodular (Fig. 35), homogeneous, or ring-like. Intraventricular, subarachnoid, or subependymal spread can be seen in these lesions as well as other gliomas. The differential diagnosis on imaging studies is lengthy for these lesions, but most commonly includes other malignant lesions (i.e., solitary metastasis, mixed glioma, oligodendroglioma, and occasionally lymphoma). Non-neoplastic considerations might include abscess or cerebritis, and even (occasionally) acute or subacute infarction.

A 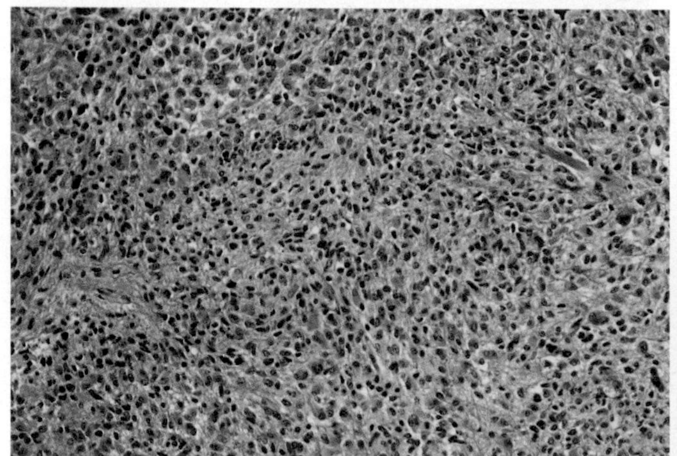

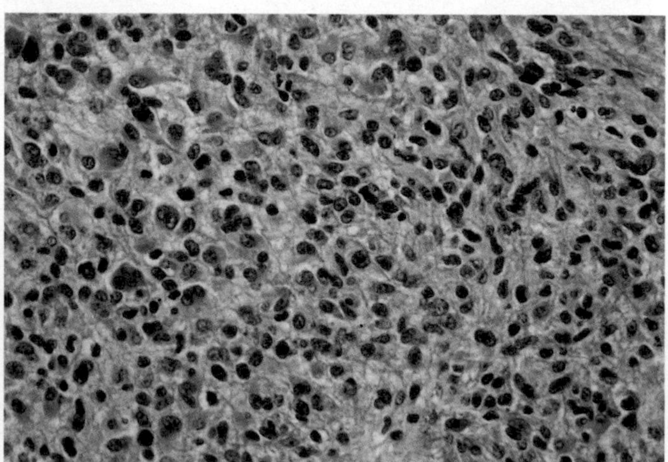 B

FIG. 32. Anaplastic astrocytoma, microscopic examination. High cellular density of pleomorphic cells in a fibrillary eosinophilic background is noted (**A**). Higher magnification (**B**) shows nuclear and cytoplasmic pleomorphism with occasional mitotic figures. Necrosis, neovascularization, and giant cell formation are not prominent features here, as they are in glioblastoma.

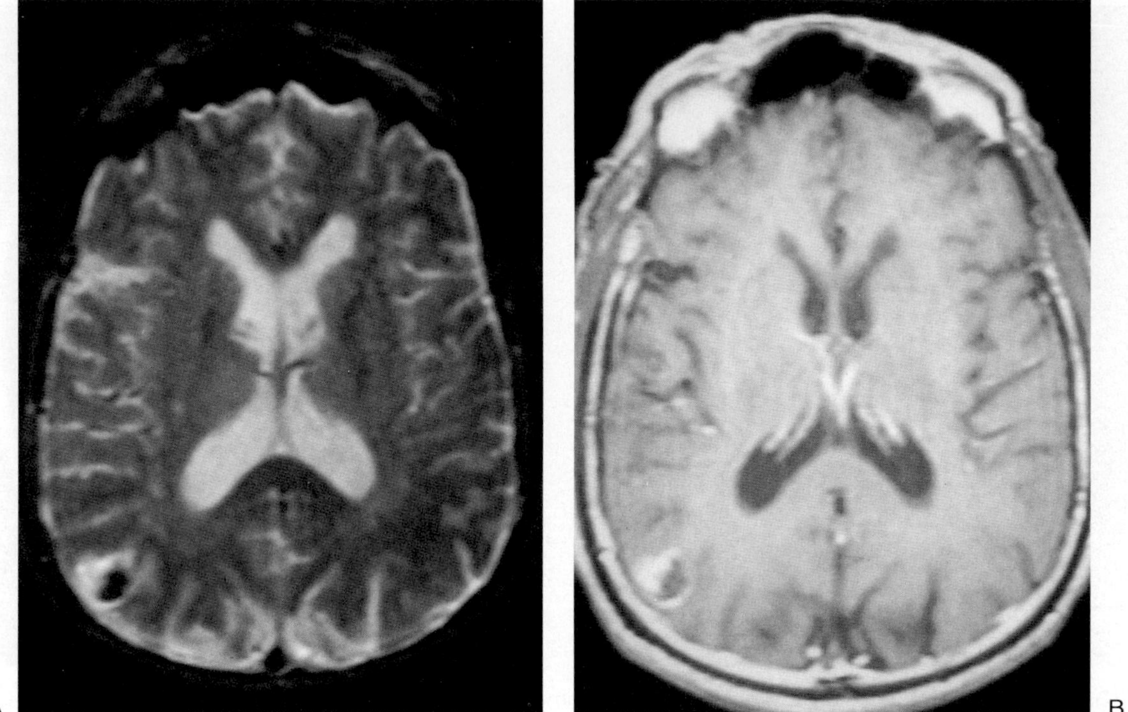

FIG. 33. Anaplastic astrocytoma with hemorrhage. T2-weighted MRI (**A**) shows right parietal subcortical hematoma. After i.v. contrast (**B**), nodular enhancement is seen in this pathologically proven anaplastic astrocytoma.

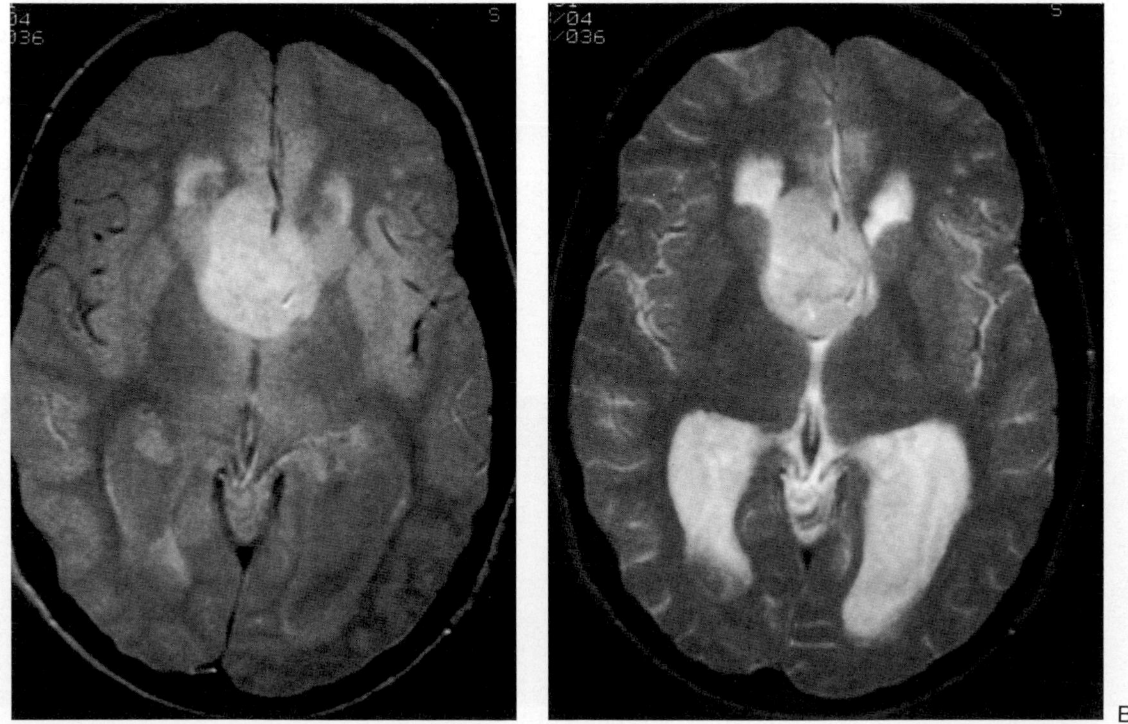

FIG. 34. Anaplastic astrocytoma with intratumoral hypervascularity. Long TR/short TE (**A**) and long TR/TE (**B**) MRI show large septum pellucidum mass which is hyperintense. Note intratumoral regions of flow due to prominent neovascularity, a more common feature of glioblastoma.

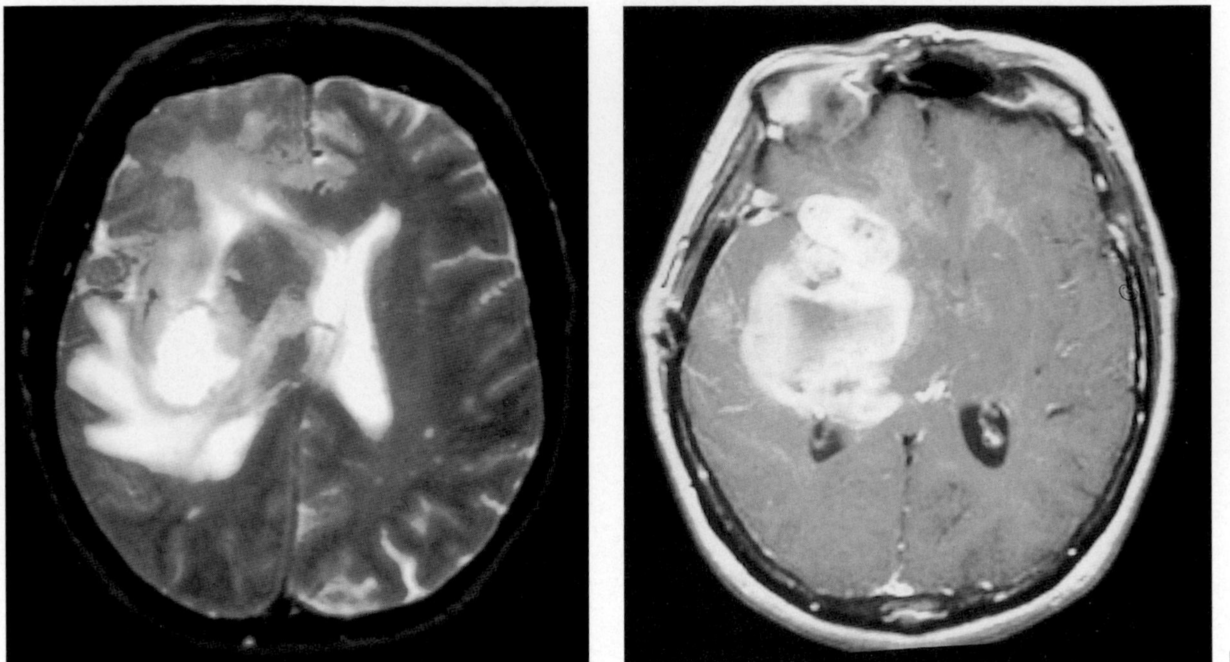

FIG. 35. Anaplastic astrocytoma with enhancement. Large heterogeneous mass with extensive "edema" (**A**) enhances prominently in an irregular fashion (**B**).

Glioblastoma

Glioblastomas, representing the most malignant end of the spectrum of neuroglial tumors, constitute approximately 15% to 20% of all intracranial tumors and nearly half of cerebral gliomas (11). The glioblastoma is the most common supratentorial neoplasm in an adult. It is thought that the majority of glioblastomas arise from an existent astrocytoma or anaplastic astrocytoma, but some arise de novo (37). According to a clinicopathologic study of 241 gliomas with necropsy data, about 7.5% of glioblastomas appear to have multicentric origin (58). Most cases are diagnosed in patients over 50 years of age, with its peak incidence in the sixth decade. Glioblastomas are rare in patients less than 30 years of age. As with gliomas in general, these lesions show a male predominance of approximately 3:2. Typically, clinical signs and symptoms of elevated intracranial pressure progress rapidly over a period often as short as one month from their initial onset. These tumors have a par-

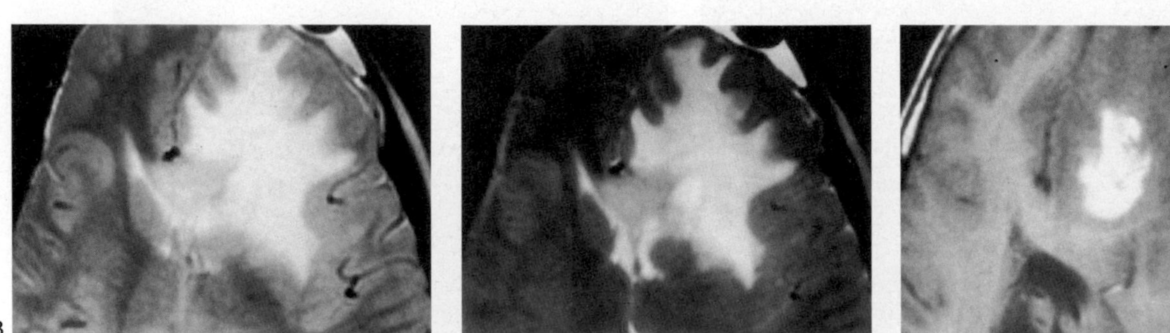

FIG. 36. Glioblastoma with extensive high intensity in white matter distribution. **A:** Axial long TR/short TE MRI (3000/35). **B:** Axial long TR/TE MRI (3000/90). **C:** Axial short TR/TE MRI (600/20), with contrast enhancement. Note mass effect and extensive high intensity, representing tumor plus edema, in white matter of left frontal lobe with extension into corpus callosum. Enhancing nodule of glioblastoma is identified on short TR/TE scan (C).

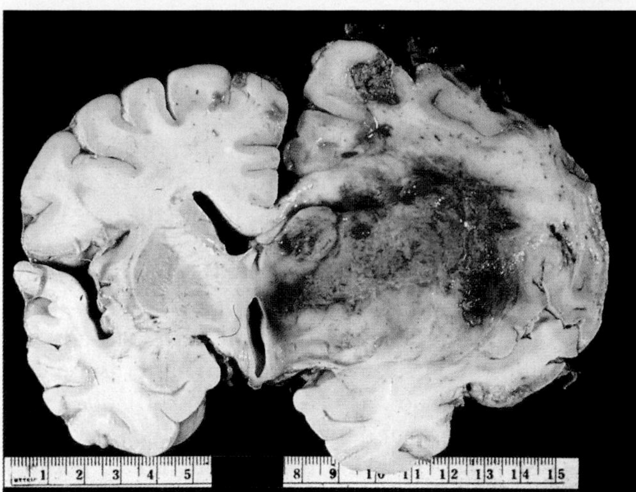

FIG. 37. Glioblastoma multiforme, gross specimen. Brain section from autopsy specimen shows nonhomogeneous cut surface with hemorrhage and necrosis (Courtesy of Dr. N. K. Gonatas, Philadelphia, PA.)

ticularly poor prognosis despite all forms of therapy, with a median survival of approximately 12 months. Factors that appear to correlate with a somewhat better prognosis (32) include younger-aged patients, development of glioblastoma as a secondary dedifferentiation rather than as the initial presentation, and surgical debulking. Recurrent glioblastomas treated with placement of interstitial radiation seeds prolongs survival by approximately one year (32).

Favored sites of localization include the frontal lobe most commonly, followed by the temporal lobe, although it is frequent that glioblastomas involve more than one lobe and can be situated in any lobe. When found in children, the most common sites are the brainstem and cerebellum. A characteristic distribution is the butterfly pattern of bihemispheric involvement with intervening corpus callosum infiltration (Fig. 36). There is a distinct tendency for malignant gliomas, especially those that are located superficially, to invade leptomeninges and dura with subsequent dissemination via the subarachnoid space. It is quite rare for these lesions to metastasize outside the CNS.

Large, irregular, but seemingly well-circumscribed mass lesions are seen on gross pathology, which typically demonstrate central necrosis, hemorrhages of varying ages, and hypervascularity, often with regions of thrombosed vessels (Fig. 37). Extensive mass effect and edematous white matter are often seen which may accompany even relatively small tumor masses (46). It should be noted that the precise mechanism of peritumoral edema formation remains poorly understood, but it is presumed to be related to the production of a vascular permeability factor known to be associated with gliomas. The histopathologic appearance of this lesion is reflected in its name of glioblastoma multiforme—the diverse nature of cell forms coupled with regions of markedly cellular tumor and focal necrosis often make the diagnosis obvious, yet the lesions are extremely variable in their appearance (32). Vascular endothelial proliferation within and adjacent to the tumor and intratumoral necrosis (Fig. 38) are highly characteristic of glioblastoma (11) and are of great prognostic significance amongst the many and varied features of these lesions on histopathology (32) (exuberant neovascularization is also a characteristic of the pilocytic astrocytoma, so in and of itself it cannot be used as a pathognomonic sign for glioblastoma). This endothelial proliferation is found not only strictly within the tumor, but it is also seen in the brain parenchyma adjacent to,

A

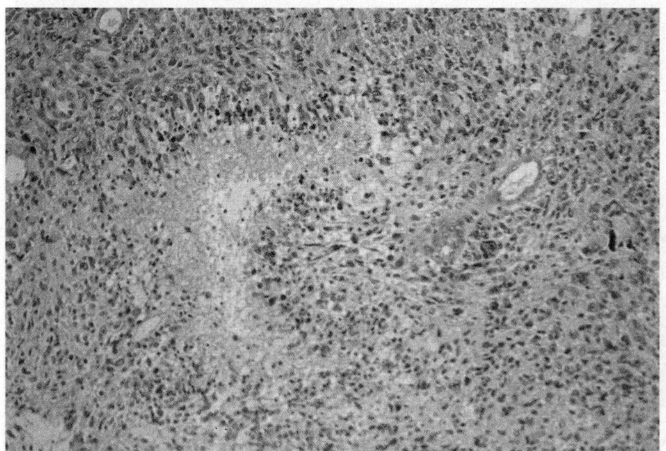

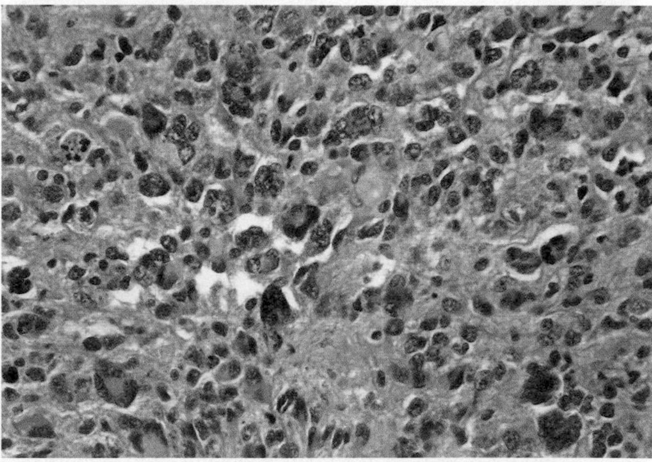

B

FIG. 38. Glioblastoma multiforme, histopathologic specimens. **A:** Note typical areas of necrosis with rim of densely arranged tumor cells (pseudopalisading) around the acellular necrotic debris. Other areas show high density of pleomorphic cells interspersed with endothelial cell-proliferating neovascularization. **B:** At higher magnification, neoplastic cells have highly pleomorphic nuclei, multinucleated giant cells, and frequent mitotic figures.

but not involved with, the infiltrating margin (37). Some pathologists separate glioblastoma from anaplastic astrocytoma on the basis of the presence of necrosis, although necrosis alone is obviously not pathognomonic of the lesion. As with all infiltrative gliomas, there is no clear margin microscopically where tumor cells stop and reactive gliosis, edema, or normal brain, in the absence of tumor, begin.

The MR imaging features of these malignancies clearly reflect the pathologic findings, and unfortunately, MRI suffers from some of the limitations seen on pathologic examination. MRI demonstrates marked tumoral heterogeneity, reflecting sites of hemorrhage, necrosis, and varying degrees of cellularity. These changes are best seen on long TR images, often showing foci of cystic necrosis and hemorrhage with debris-fluid levels (Fig. 12) and lower intensity regions in areas of hypercellularity. Linear or serpentine regions of signal void within the tumor mass on spin-echo MRI indicate the often prominent angiogenesis that characterizes glioblastomas (Fig. 21). Calcification is rare in these lesions, unless they have arisen in a lower grade lesion. Since glioblastomas, along with oligodendroglioma and ependymoma, have a tendency to bleed (11,12), it is helpful to identify any of the several features of intratumoral hemorrhage which differ from those seen in benign intracranial hematomas and suggest malignancy (13) (Table 5). These neoplasms often show significant mass effect, mainly due to fairly extensive edema which is usually apparent in the adjacent white matter (Fig. 39). To reiterate, one cannot define the "margins" of the tumor and separate tumor from edema, since this cannot even be done on microscopic pathology. In fact, what one calls "edema" is more accurately described as "tumor plus edema." The extent of the lesion is more fully delimited by MRI in comparison with CT (3), presumably due to the improved contrast resolution provided by MRI. Despite this, the radiologist should be cognizant of the fact that neoplastic tissue (i.e., microscopic tumor) extends beyond recognizable regions of abnormality, even on MR images.

The majority of glioblastomas at least partially enhance with i.v. contrast. Enhancement patterns are usually very heterogeneous (Figs. 36, 39, and 40), often with ring-like enhancement depicted as being thick, irregular and nodular, and surrounding necrotic areas, findings virtually indistinguishable from those seen in metastases and radiation necrosis. Of course, the vast majority of glioblastomas are solitary lesions (as opposed to metastases); multicentric glioblastomas are distinctly unusual (58). Multicentric malignant gliomas, whether synchronous (detected at the time of the initial presentation) or metachronous (occurring at different times, but discontinuous on pathology), cannot be differentiated from metastases without biopsy (59,60). Enhancement can often be demonstrated extending across the corpus callosum, which clearly indicates involvement by tumor (Fig. 41). Regions which enhance correlate to areas of tumor tissue on pathology (45,51), so, clearly, enhancement is helpful in guiding surgical biopsy. For the neuropathologist, it is ideal in fact for the biopsy specimen to include

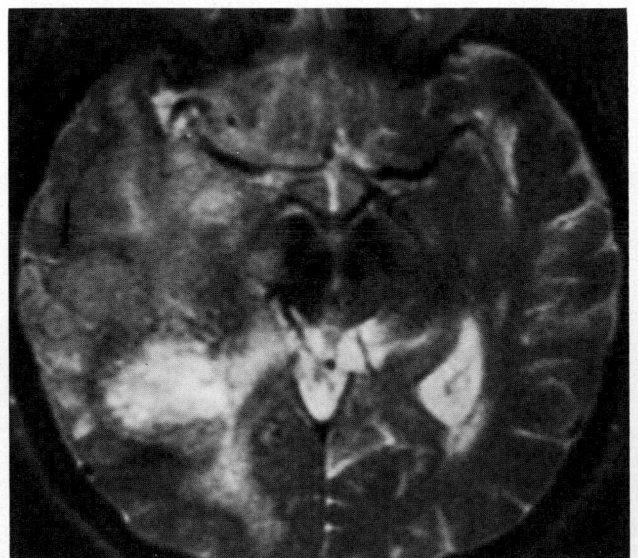

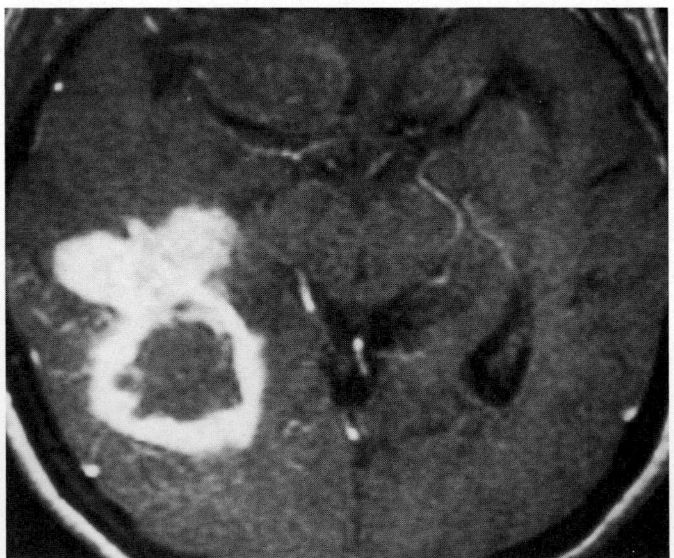

FIG. 39. Glioblastoma with thick ring of enhancement. **A:** Axial long TR/TE MRI (3000/90). **B:** Axial short TR/TE MRI (600/20), with contrast enhancement. Note extensive region of hyperintensity involving entire right frontal and temporal lobes on long TR/TE scan (A). Thick, irregular ring of enhancement (B) is highly suggestive of malignant neoplasm. Also note that only a small part of the lesion enhances, even though tumor can be found throughout the right hemisphere in this infiltrative tumor.

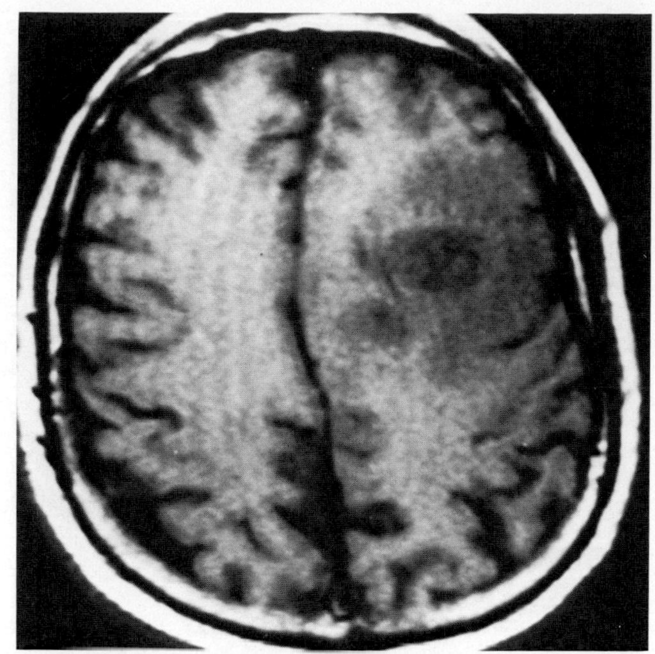
A

FIG. 40. Change in configuration of enhancing ring with time (glioblastoma). **A:** Axial short TR/TE MRI (800/20). **B:** Contrast-enhanced axial short TR/TE MRI (800/20), 5-min postinjection. **C:** Contrast-enhanced axial short TR/TE MRI (800/20), 41-min postinjection. Heterogeneous glioblastoma in left frontal lobe (A) shows thin, regular ring of enhancement (*closed arrows*) on 5-min postinjection scan (B). Note thickening of ring (*closed arrows*) with modularity on 41-min postinjection scan (C). Enhancement of tumor crossing corpus callosum (*open arrows*, B,C) also thickens with time.

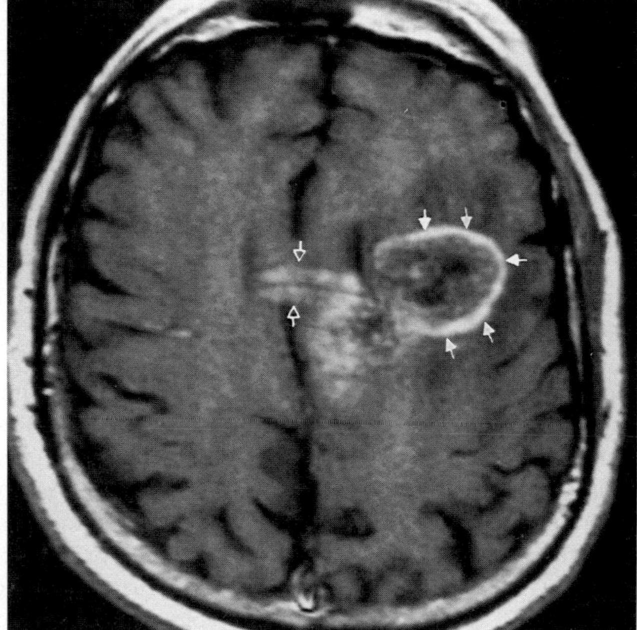
B

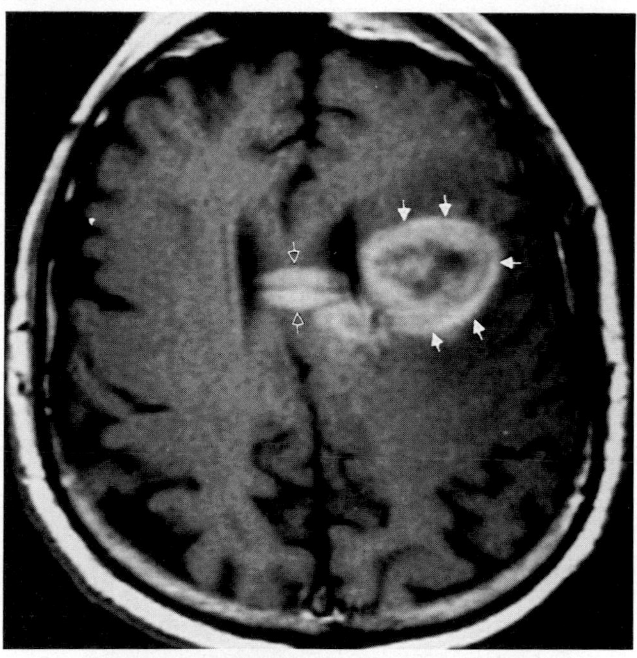
C

the enhancing ring and the adjacent necrosis, when present (32). Other indications for administering contrast include the assessment of spread of these tumors, which can occur via subependymal or subarachnoid seeding (Fig. 42), as well as, in rare cases, direct invasion of bone (61). Contrast is also useful in identifying postoperative residual or recurrent tumor. It should be realized that contrast enhancement does not correlate with the degree of hypervascularity demonstrated on angiography.

There is a differential diagnosis for the imaging appearance of glioblastoma, particularly when only some of the "classic" MRI features (intratumoral neovascularity, hemorrhage, necrosis) are identified. The differential diagnosis should include metastasis, anaplastic oligodendroglioma, and lymphoma. Radiation necrosis with the appropriate history can appear identical to glioblastoma, abscess/cerebritis with enhancement, and even cavernous angiomas with recent hemorrhage, reactive gliosis, and edema, must also be considered. Even hemangioblastoma (see later in this chapter) can appear virtually identical to glioblastoma, since intratumoral vessels, heterogeneity, enhancement, and edema can be evident in both. The large, often nonenhancing cyst of hemangioblastoma and the posterior fossa location are key to the

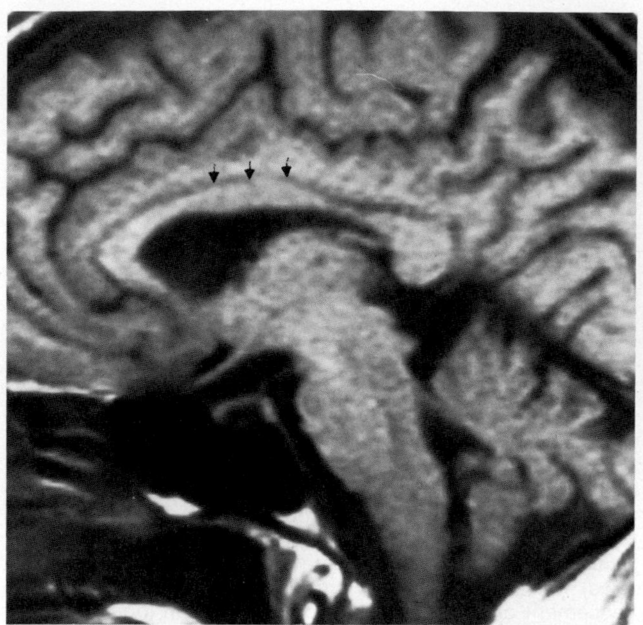

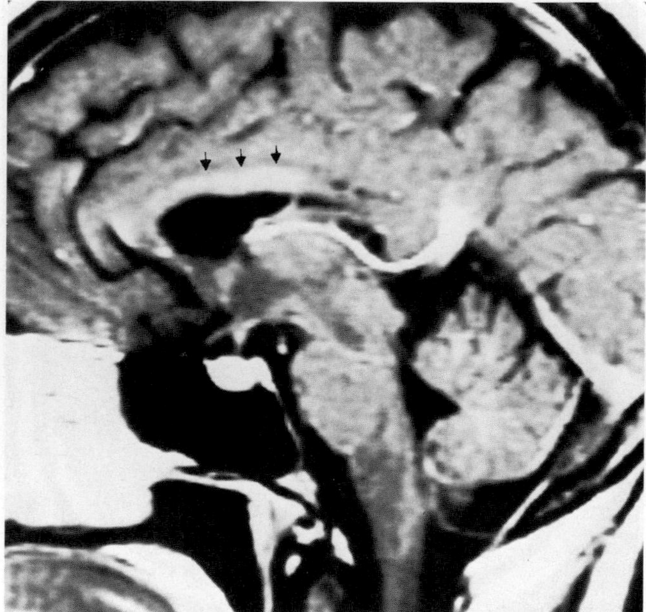

FIG. 41. Enhancement of tumor in corpus callosum (glioblastoma). **A:** Sagittal short TR/TE MRI (600/11). **B:** Sagittal short TR/TE MRI (800/26), with contrast enhancement. Slight focal expansion of body of corpus callosum (*arrows*) on precontrast scan (A) shows dense enhancement (*arrows*) after contrast injection (B).

distinction. MRI potentially narrows down this list considerably, since: (i) it is more sensitive for detecting multiple lesions, which would heavily favor lesions other than glioblastoma; (ii) the capsule of an abscess characteristically shows thin high intensity on short TR/TE and thin hypointensity on long TR/TE MR images (62), a finding not described in tumors; (iii) lymphoma most commonly is homogeneous and low intensity on T2-weighted images, a characteristic seen less commonly in glioblastoma; and (iv) hemorrhagic neoplasms usually have a relatively specific appearance (13) (Table 5), which differs in many respects from cavernous angiomas (63).

FIG. 42. Glioblastoma with subependymal spread. Post-gadolinium T1-weighted MRI shows bulky mass encasing ventricles with clear subependymal spread of tumor.

Gliomatosis Cerebri

This rare entity, known by many names but most commonly as gliomatosis cerebri (64) or diffuse cerebral gliomatosis (65), refers to a diffusely infiltrative glial neoplasia of large portions of the brain, and at times the spinal cord, with relative preservation of the underlying neural structures (64). The term is reserved for those lesions where the infiltrative extent of the tumor is out of proportion to the other histopathological features, i.e., the degree of anaplasia and the cellularity (32). Gliomatosis cerebri does not apply to all gliomas that are extremely large and should not be used by neuroradiologists in that context. An even rarer entity is leptomeningeal gliomatosis, a glioma restricted to the leptomeninges that is diagnosed only when there is no identifiable parenchymal component, although in practice the term is often applied to cases in which a small parenchymal focus is seen (32).

The clinical picture of gliomatosis cerebri is neither specific nor focal in nature, and the deficits are disproportionately mild in relation to the extent of the involvement, with personality changes and mental status disturbance the most common features (66). The disease is progressive and can last for weeks to years. The peak incidence is in the second to fourth decade (66), but all ages are affected. While its precise origins remain a subject of debate, it is considered by Russell and Rubinstein to represent the most extreme end of the spectrum of diffuse astrocytomas (11). It is still a matter of some debate whether gliomatosis cerebri is a specific pathologic entity or whether it is a term that includes a widely diverse group of astrocytic tumors that share the feature of extraordinary infiltration (32).

On pathologic studies, involved portions of the brain typically comprise nearly the extent of the cerebral hemispheres, with both gray and white matter affected, and the distinction between these regions lost. This lesion can also involve the posterior fossa, brainstem and spinal cord. On gross examination, despite the widely invasive nature of the lesion, gliomatosis cerebri may not be evident, even on lobectomy specimens (32). On microscopic examination (Fig. 43), neoplastic (usually fibrillary) astrocytes in several stages of differentiation are evident infiltrating both gray and white matter, mainly arranged in a perineuronal and perivascular distribution (66). There is concomitant thickening of the white matter and extensive demyelination in areas of neoplastic involvement, without any definite focal mass production (66). The underlying neuroanatomical architecture is often essentially preserved.

Imaging findings have been reported on both CT (67) and MRI (68). MRI shows extensive parenchymal involvement, especially of the white matter, as manifested by ill-defined regions of high intensity on long TR images (Fig. 44). Diffuse sulcal and ventricular effacement may be subtle, but if present are highly suggestive of the diagnosis. Contrast enhancement is not thought to be a common feature unless dedifferentiation has occurred. The diffuse nature of the lesion may lead to confusion with extensive demyelinating or dysmyelinating diseases, and biopsy or lobectomy is often necessary in order to make a final diagnosis. On the other hand, the pathologist is often unable to make the diagnosis on biopsy, where reactive astrocytes are seen but the diagnosis of neoplasm is not clear. Therefore, the radiologist plays an important role in the diagnosis of this rare entity.

Localized (Non-infiltrative) Astrocytic Tumors

Localized astrocytic tumors have a common tendency to be well-circumscribed and generally more differentiated than infiltrative astrocytomas, and they share a relatively favorable prognosis. The better outlook for patients harboring these lesions is due to a limited capacity for invasion and spread, and a limited tendency to progress into more malignant forms (37). This group consists of pilocytic astrocytoma, pleomorphic xanthoastrocytoma, and subependymal giant cell astrocytoma.

Pilocytic Astrocytoma

The most common form of astrocytoma in the child is the pilocytic astrocytoma, also known as the juvenile pilocytic astrocytoma (JPA). This tumor represents one of the most benign forms of glial neoplasm. The most frequent neuroanatomic location of the pilocytic astrocytoma is the cerebellar hemisphere (see section, "Posterior Fossa Neoplasms"). When supratentorial, the pilocytic astrocytoma most commonly arises in the optic nerve or diencephalon (chiasm/hypothalamus/floor of the third ventricle) (Fig. 45) (69), but it may also be found in the cerebral hemisphere, particularly in the young adult. Complete surgical resection, if anatomi-

A
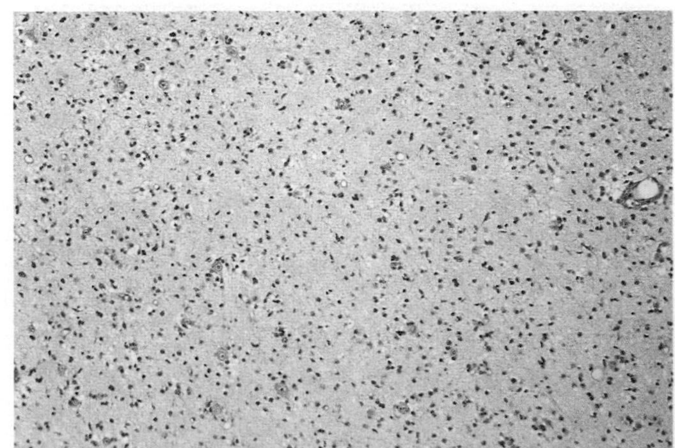
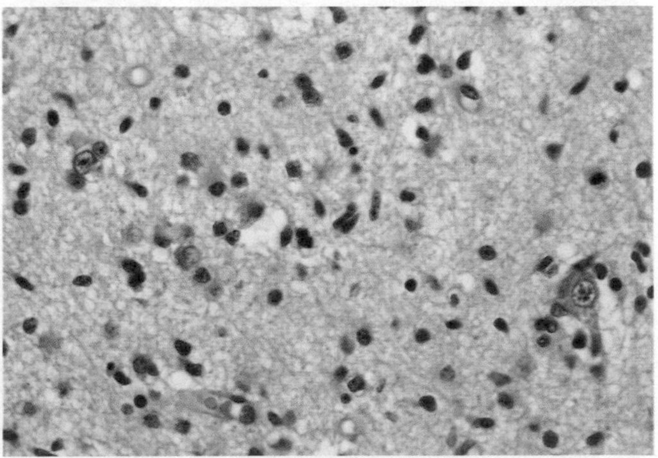
B

FIG. 43. Gliomatosis cerebri. Microscopic examination shows mild increase in cell density and diffuse astrocytic infiltration (**A**). At higher magnification (**B**), infiltration of gray matter by slightly pleomorphic astrocytes is seen, similar to infiltrating low-grade astrocytoma from which gliomatosis cannot be distinguished on a morphologic basis. A definitive diagnosis prior to autopsy can only be made by the integration of pathologic information with radiology.

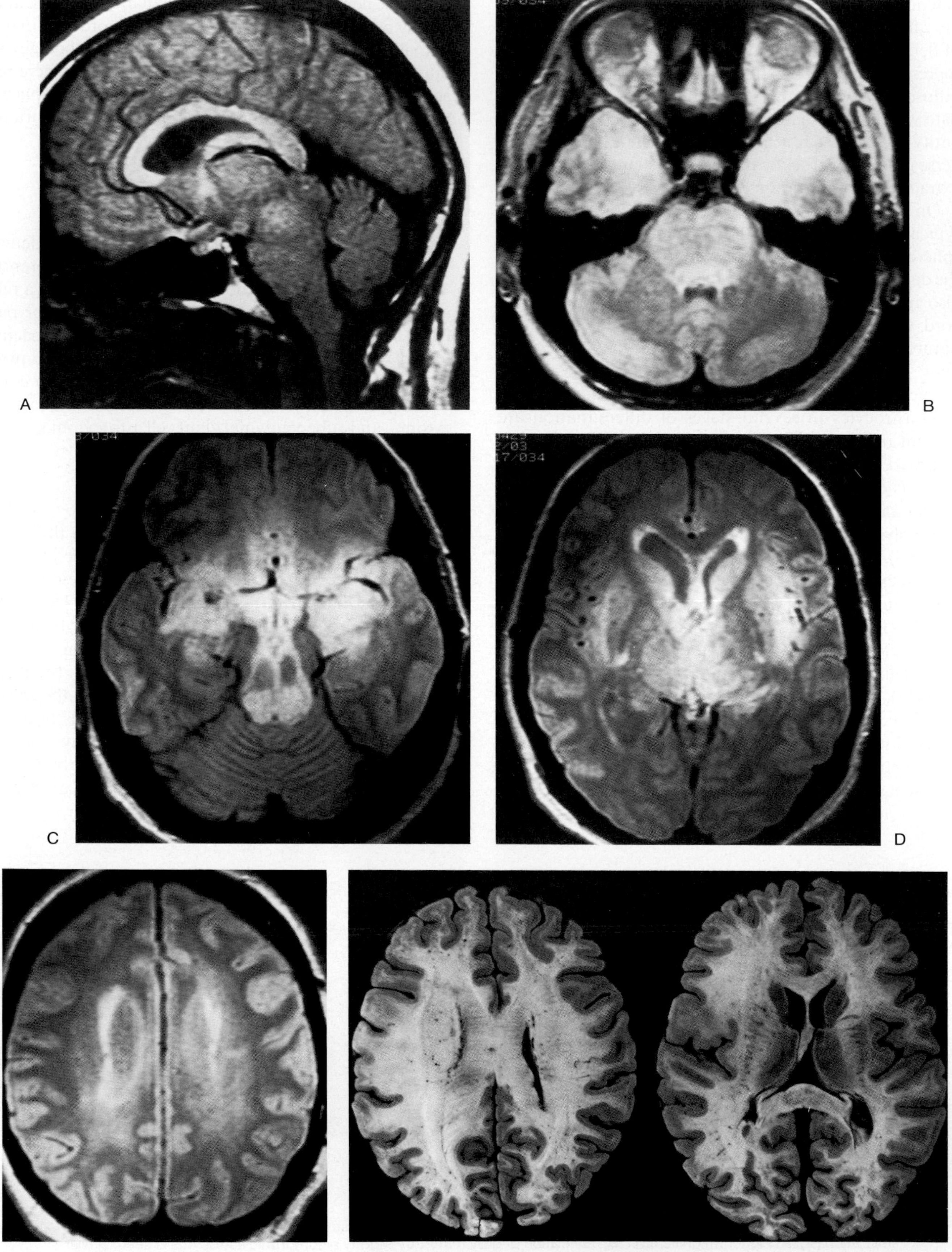
A
B
C
D
E
F

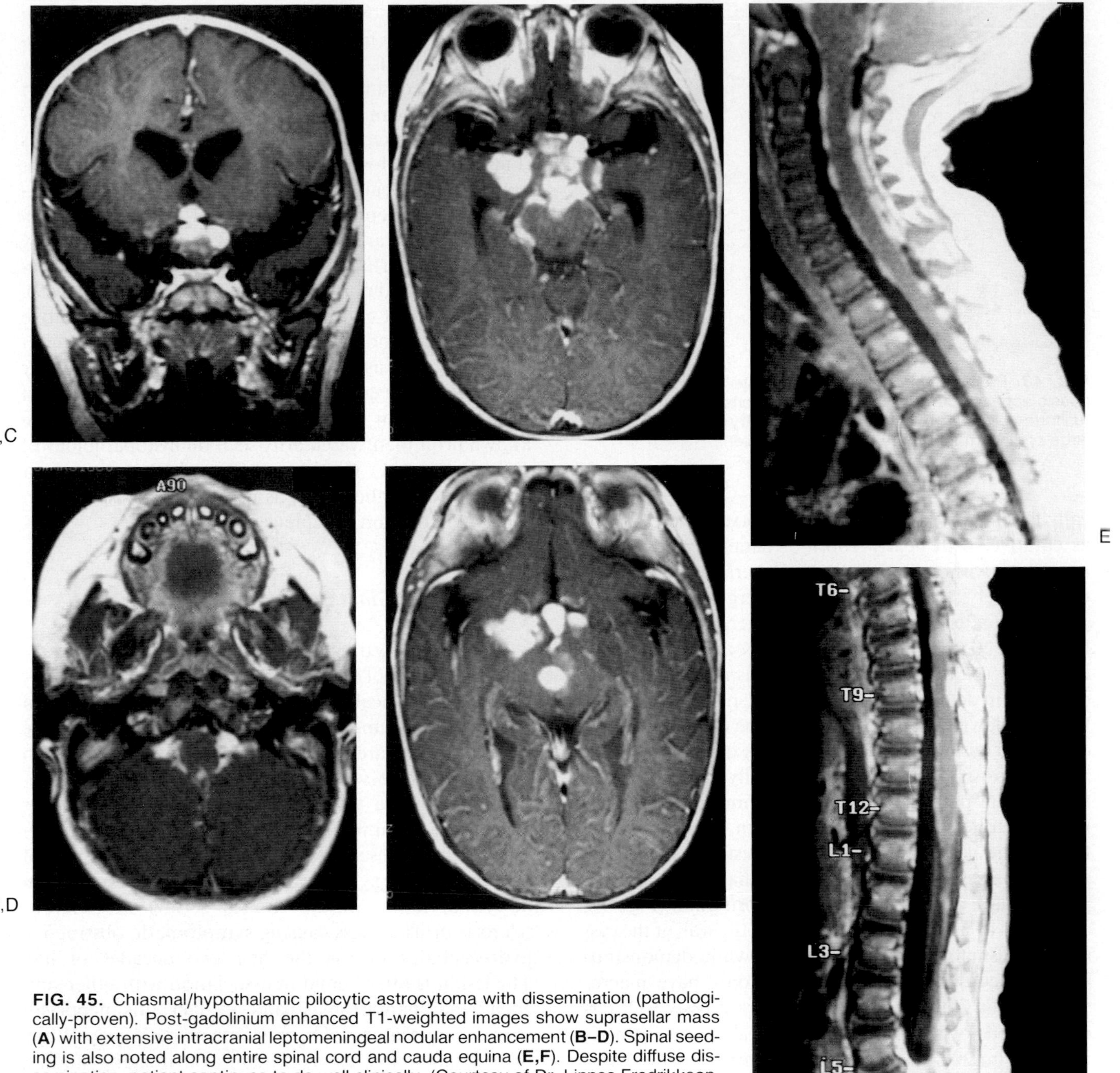

FIG. 45. Chiasmal/hypothalamic pilocytic astrocytoma with dissemination (pathologically-proven). Post-gadolinium enhanced T1-weighted images show suprasellar mass (**A**) with extensive intracranial leptomeningeal nodular enhancement (**B–D**). Spinal seeding is also noted along entire spinal cord and cauda equina (**E,F**). Despite diffuse dissemination, patient continues to do well clinically. (Courtesy of Dr. Linnea Fredrikkson, Portland, OR.)

FIG. 44. Gliomatosis cerebri. **A:** Sagittal short TR/TE MRI (600/20). **B–E:** Axial long TR/short TE MRI (2500/20), inferior to superior. **F:** Axial gross necropsy specimen from a different patient with gliomatosis cerebri. (From Okazaki and Scheithauer, ref. 121, with permission.) Extensive high intensity on long TR images (B–E) with mass effect is noted throughout brainstem, temporal lobes, bilateral insulae, and in centrum semiovale bilaterally. Presence of expansion of brainstem (A–C) helps denote tumor as etiology. Note extensive, poorly defined lesion in pathologic specimen (F), with expansion of right hemispheric white matter and loss of definition of gray-white junction.

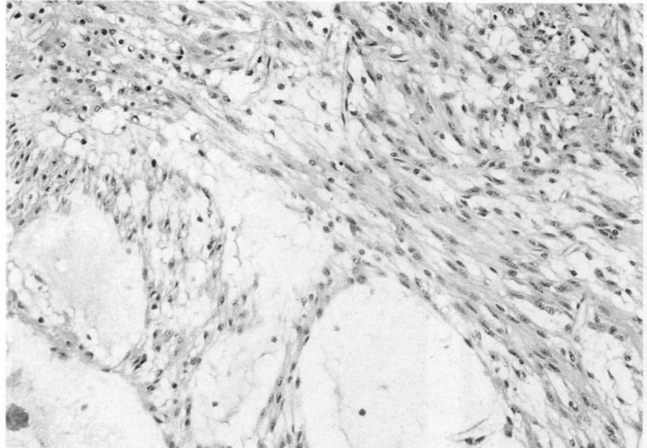

FIG. 46. Pilocytic astrocytoma, microscopic section. Note biphasic appearance with both loose and dense areas of bipolar fusiform cells with bland nuclei in a fibrillary matrix. Small and large cystic formations are typical in this lesion.

cally feasible, is the treatment of choice and is regarded as curative, with nearly 100% of patients being recurrence-free without any adjuvant therapy (70,71). Although rarely, these lesions can undergo malignant degeneration after several years (32), overall survival rates for 10 and 20 years are reported as 83% and 70%, respectively (70). (Note: optic nerve and chiasm gliomas will be discussed in detail in Chapter 22.) The peak incidence of this very slowly growing tumor is in the first two decades of life, and it is well recognized to be associated with neurofibromatosis type I, in which it usually involves the anterior visual pathway (72) and is commonly multicentric. Regardless of the site of origin, the pathologic features are nearly identical and consist of well circumscribed masses with abundant Rosenthal fibers, vascular proliferation, and conspicuous cyst formation (Fig. 46), often with a vascular tumor nodule in the wall of the cyst (11). Chiasmal/hypothalamic JPAs, while demonstrating microcystic changes, less commonly have macroscopic cysts. Although the lesions are grossly well circumscribed, overlying leptomeningeal involvement is not uncommon on pathologic examination (32); this however does not equate with potential for dissemination, a distinctly rare event (Fig. 45). As in the case of the optic nerve pilocytic astrocytoma in neurofibromatosis I (73), overlying leptomeningeal involvement is often accompanied by a prominent fibroblastic reactive change.

It is essential for the radiologist to distinguish pilocytic astrocytomas from diffuse astrocytomas, because therapy and prognosis are so distinctly different for these lesions. Usually, the MR appearance of pilocytic astrocytoma is virtually diagnostic. The highly characteristic imaging features of JPA (69) closely mirror the gross pathologic changes. The JPA is typically a sharply demarcated, lobular mass, although lesions of the diencephalon can show significant infiltrative extension on MRI (Fig. 47), a feature which often cannot be fully appreciated on CT. More than two-thirds of cases show macroscopic cyst formation (69). On MRI, the solid part of the lesion can be either isointense to brain parenchyma or markedly hyperintense on long TR images (Figs. 47–49). Most lesions have an obvious cystic component. Other features of JPA include the absence of accompanying edema or intratumoral calcification (69). Hemorrhage is rare in this lesion. These tumors virtually always show partial (usually intense) contrast enhancement of the solid portion of the tumor (Figs. 48 and 49). This is in direct contrast to most low-grade infiltrative astrocytomas, and is a feature which points out dramatically that contrast enhancement does not necessarily equate with an aggressive lesion. The significant contrast enhancement in JPAs probably correlates with the known prominent vascularity seen on histopathology of these tumors (11). Cortical-subcortical JPA may appear identical to ganglioglioma as well as pleomorphic xanthoastrocytoma on MR images.

Subependymal Giant Cell Astrocytoma

The classical setting of subependymal giant cell astrocytoma consists of a well-circumscribed lateral ventricular mass, specifically in the region of the foramen of Monro, in a young adult with tuberous sclerosis. The mass is truly a parenchymal, astrocytic neoplasm which projects into the ventricle from a subependymal location—it is not a tumor of the ependyma itself. This slowly growing tumor is very rare outside the clinical setting of tuberous sclerosis and is found in up to 10% of patients with the syndrome (74,75). It can be found as an incidental lesion in the clinical setting of tuberous sclerosis or as a mass causing symptomatic obstructive hydrocephalus during the first two decades of life. The lesion is often found in association with other subependymal hamartomas, and in fact this neoplasm shares many features of hamartoma on pathology. While these lesions have classic findings on imaging studies, their neuropathological features can be quite variable (Fig. 50). Calcification is extremely common. Although generally considered distinctly uncommon in this benign lesion (11), focal necrosis and mitoses can be identified by the pathologist and probably should not prompt aggressive therapy (76). Treatment of subependymal giant cell astrocytoma is generally restricted to surgical removal, after which long-term survival rates are excellent.

MR findings of subependymal giant cell astrocytoma hinge upon the identification of the mass in its characteristic location along with the identification of other features of tuberous sclerosis (or, of course, in a patient with the clinical diagnosis of this phakomatosis). There are

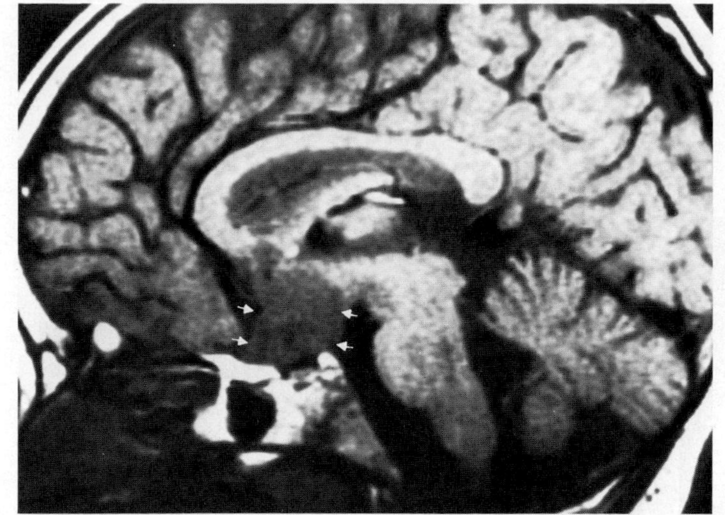

A

FIG. 47. Chiasmatic-hypothalamic pilocytic astrocytoma with infiltration. **A:** Sagittal short TR/TE MRI (600/11). **B:** Axial "spoiled" gradient-echo MRI (40/5/30°). **C:** Axial "spoiled" gradient-echo MRI (40/5/30°). **D:** Axial "spoiled" gradient-echo MRI (40/5/30°). **E:** Axial long TR/short TE MRI (3000/30). **F:** Axial long TR/short TE MRI (3000/30). **G:** Axial long TR/short TE MRI (3000/30). Suprasellar pilocytic astrocytoma (*closed arrows*) fills cistern and is homogeneous on all sequences. Note that chiasm cannot be discerned from hypothalamus, so site of origin is termed "chiasmatic-ypothalamic." Tumor infiltrates along brainstem (*open arrows*) and into medial temporal lobes and basal ganglia (B–G).

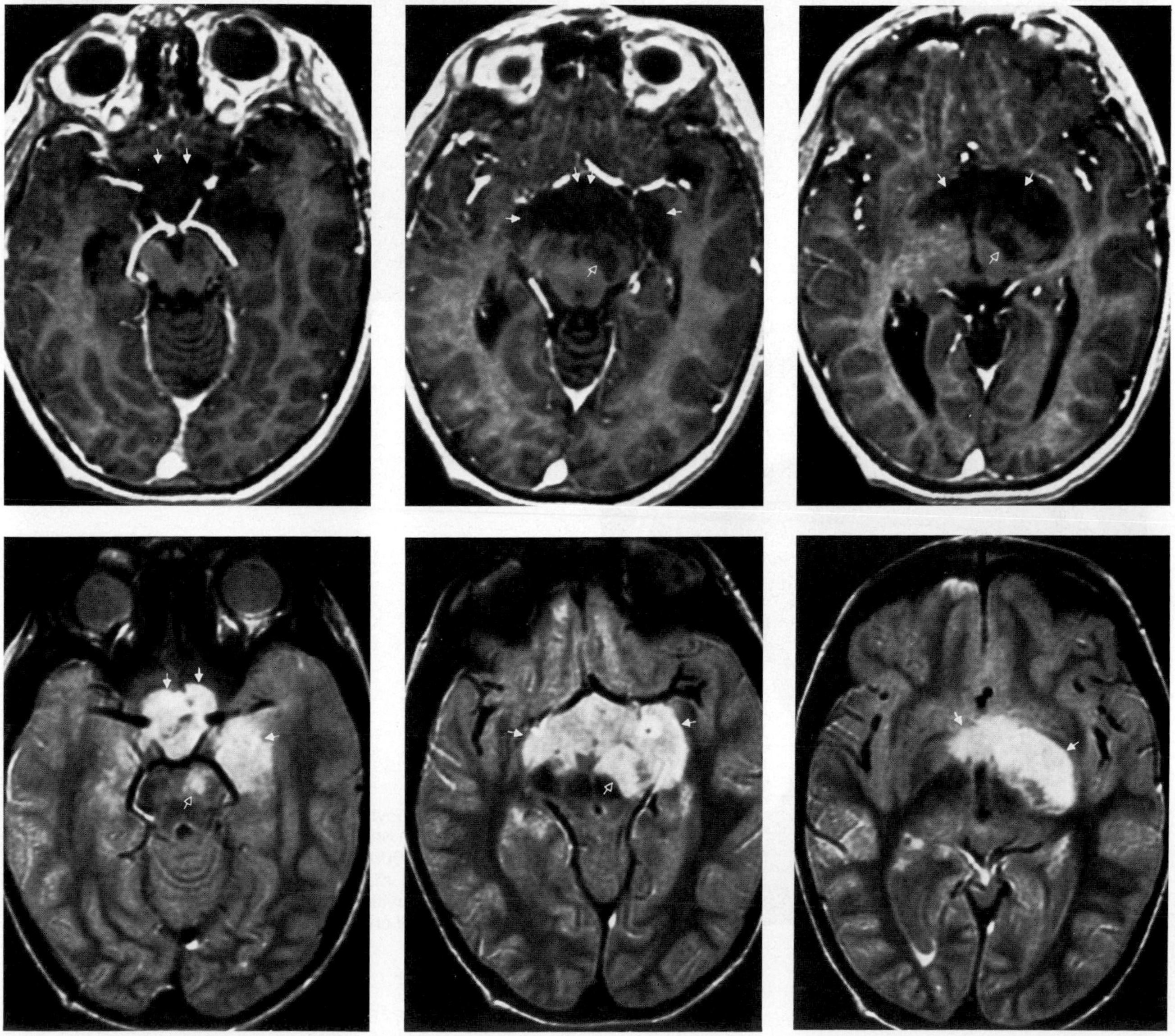

B

C,D

E

F,G

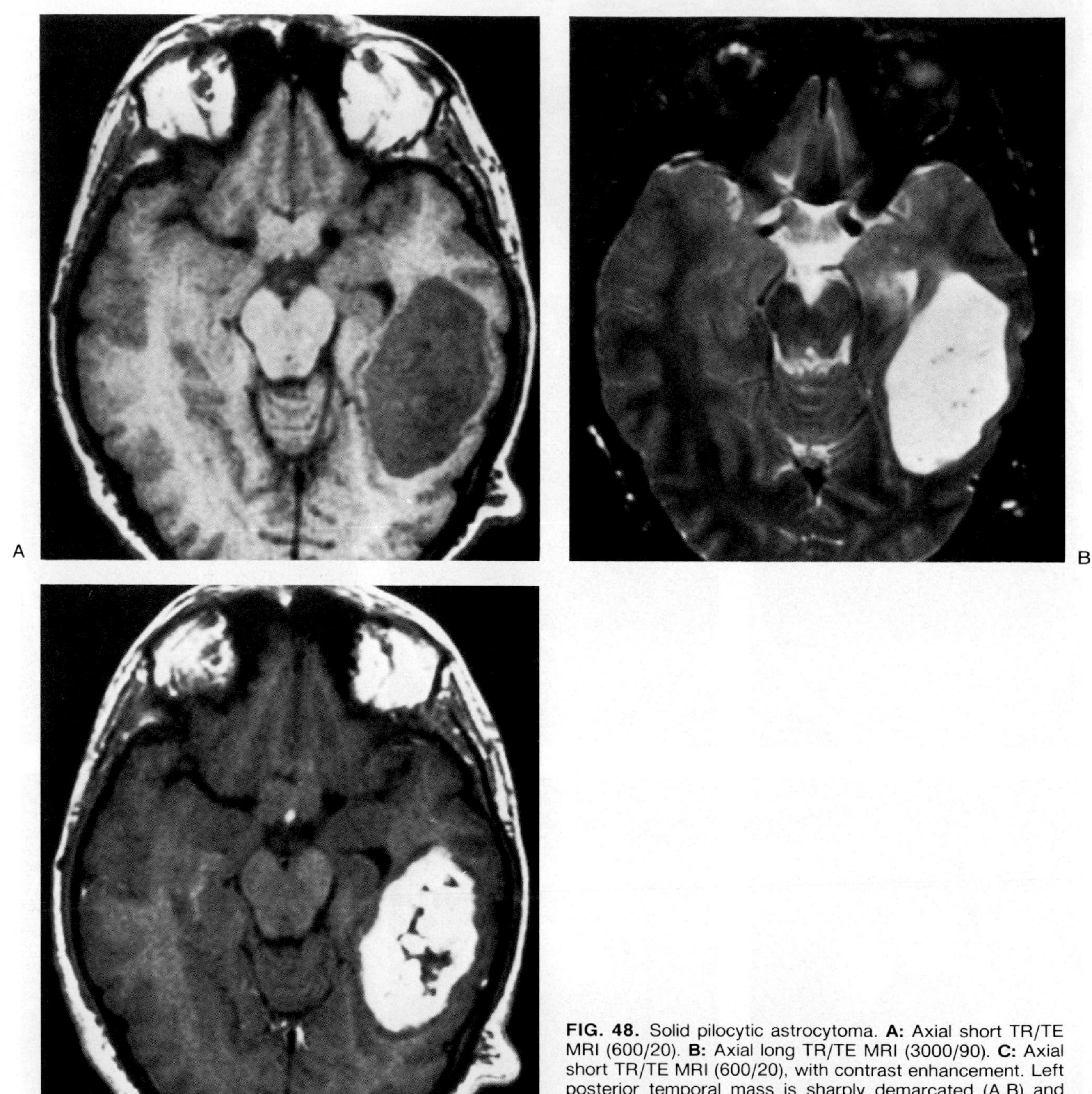

FIG. 48. Solid pilocytic astrocytoma. **A:** Axial short TR/TE MRI (600/20). **B:** Axial long TR/TE MRI (3000/90). **C:** Axial short TR/TE MRI (600/20), with contrast enhancement. Left posterior temporal mass is sharply demarcated (A,B) and densely enhances with contrast (C). Benign nature of lesion shown by its lack of change over a 5-year period.

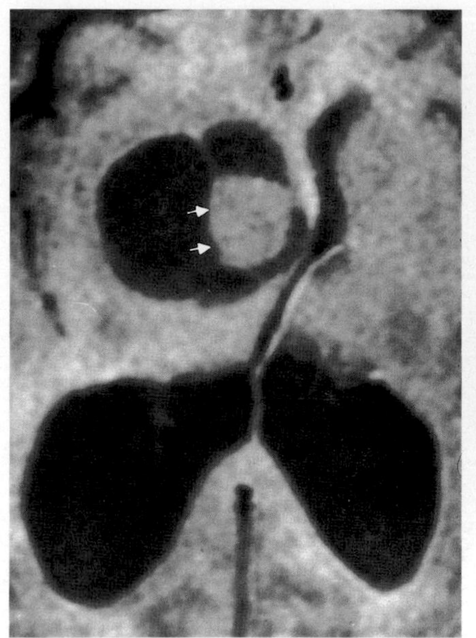

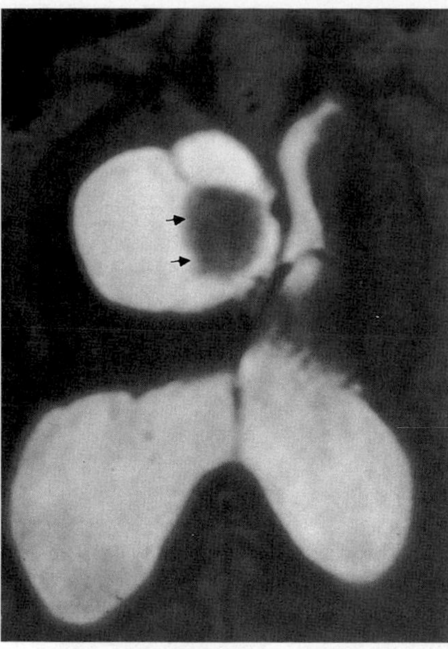

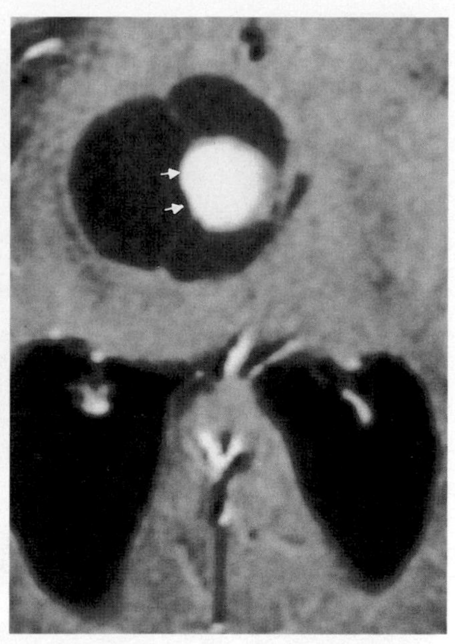

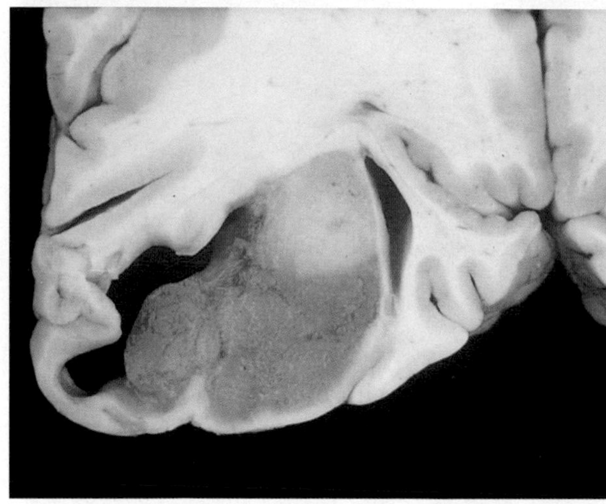

FIG. 49. Cystic pilocytic astrocytoma. **A:** Axial short TR/TE MRI (600/20). B: Axial long TR/TE MRI (3000/90). **C:** Axial short TR/TE MRI (600/20), with contrast enhancement. **D:** Coronal necropsy specimen. (From Okazaki and Scheithauer, ref. 121, with permission.) Thalamic-hypothalamic mass is partially cystic and has solid mural nodule (*arrows*, A–C), which densely enhances (C). Note typical solid nodule within partially cystic left temporal neoplasm (D) from different patient with similar lesion.

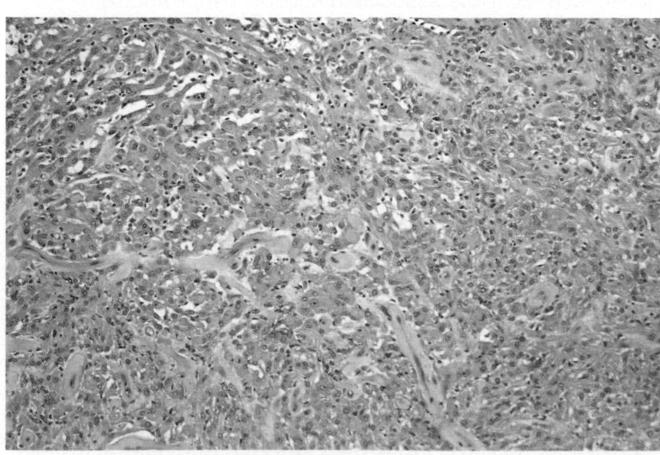

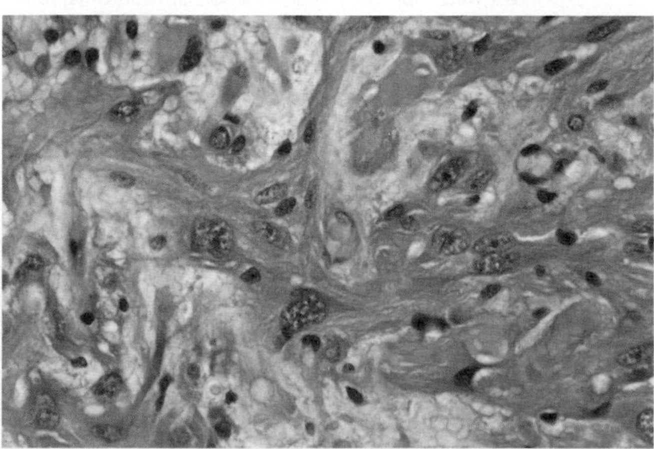

FIG. 50. Subependymal giant cell astrocytoma, microscopic sections. Features of these lesions associated with tuberous sclerosis consist of diffuse proliferation of astrocytes within a fibrillary, partially vacuolated background (**A**). At higher magnification (**B**), note heterogeneity of cells with small and very large astrocytic nuclei and abundant cytoplasm.

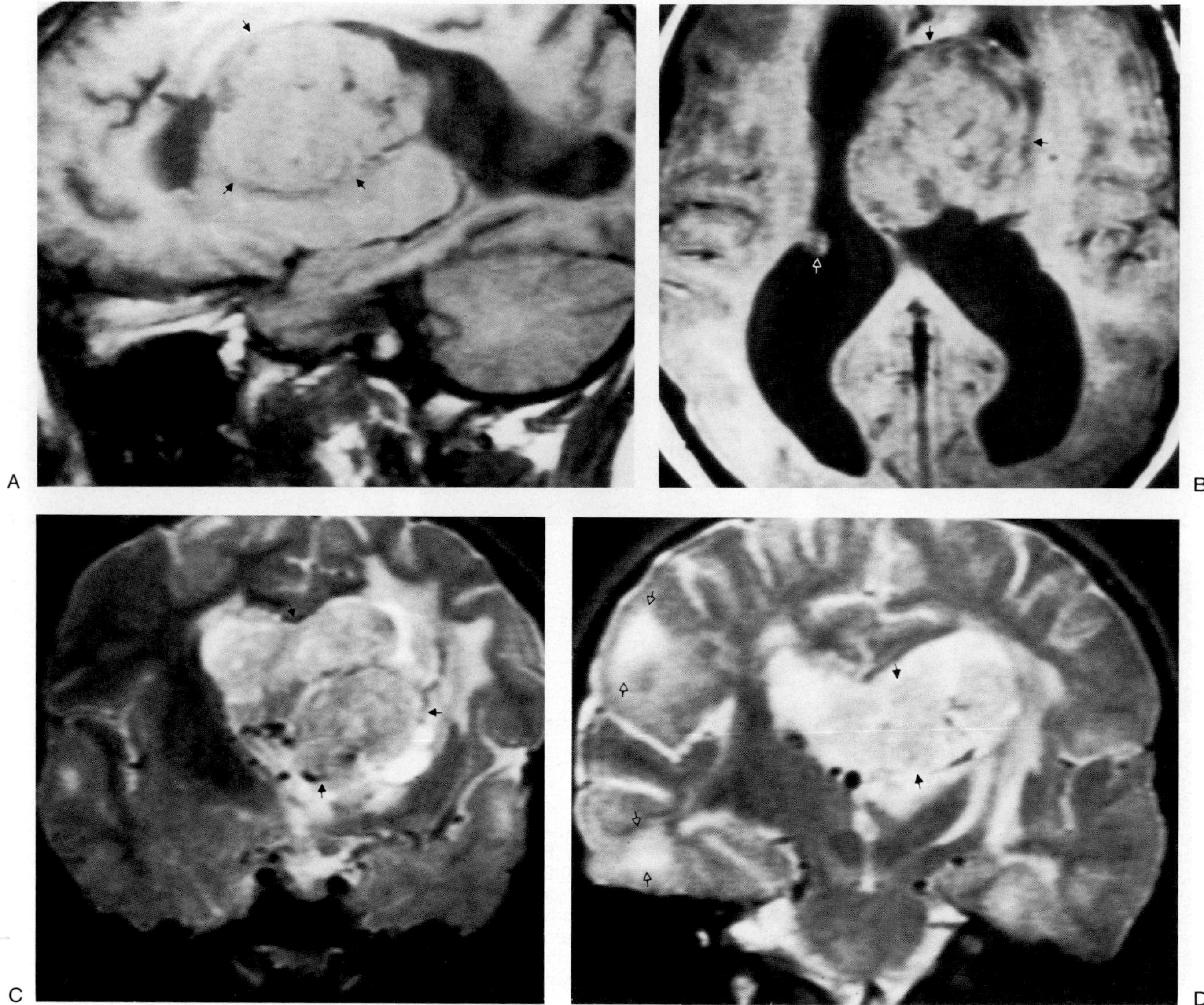

FIG. 51. Giant cell astrocytoma in patient with tuberous sclerosis. **A:** Sagittal short TR/TE MRI (600/20). **B:** Axial short TR/TE MRI (600/20). **C:** Coronal long TR/TE MRI (2500/80). **D:** Coronal long TR/TE MRI (2500/80). Intraventricular mass (*arrows*) near foramen of Monro (A) is heterogeneous (B–D). Note associated subependymal nodule (*open arrow*, B) and subcortical tubers (*open black arrows*, D).

basically four distinct intracerebral lesions seen in this syndrome (77): (i) hamartomatous cortical tubers, most commonly in the frontal lobes; (ii) radially-oriented trans-cerebral bands of heterotopic giant cells, accompanied by gliosis and dysmyelination; (iii) subependymal heterotopic nodules; and (iv) subependymal giant cell astrocytoma. Subependymal giant cell astrocytomas have been reported on MRI as hyperintense, somewhat heterogeneous masses on long TR sequences (Fig. 51) (78,79). Just as in the non-neoplastic subependymal nodules in these patients, central regions of marked hypointensity can be seen on long TR/long TE MRI and on gradient-echo images, due to susceptibility-induced signal loss from calcification and accompanying iron. Giant cell astrocytomas generally enhance with i.v. contrast (80,81), but the lack of enhancement cannot be used as exclusionary proof of this diagnosis. Moreover, the presence of enhancement in a subependymal nodule does not necessarily prove the diagnosis of giant cell astrocytoma. CT scanning is certainly more sensitive to small calcified subependymal nodules in these patients, but the spectrum of intracerebral pathology in tuberous sclerosis patients is probably more fully appreciated with MR imaging (79). Therefore, the specific diagnosis of subependymal giant cell astrocytoma is probably more definitively made with MRI (see Chapter 17).

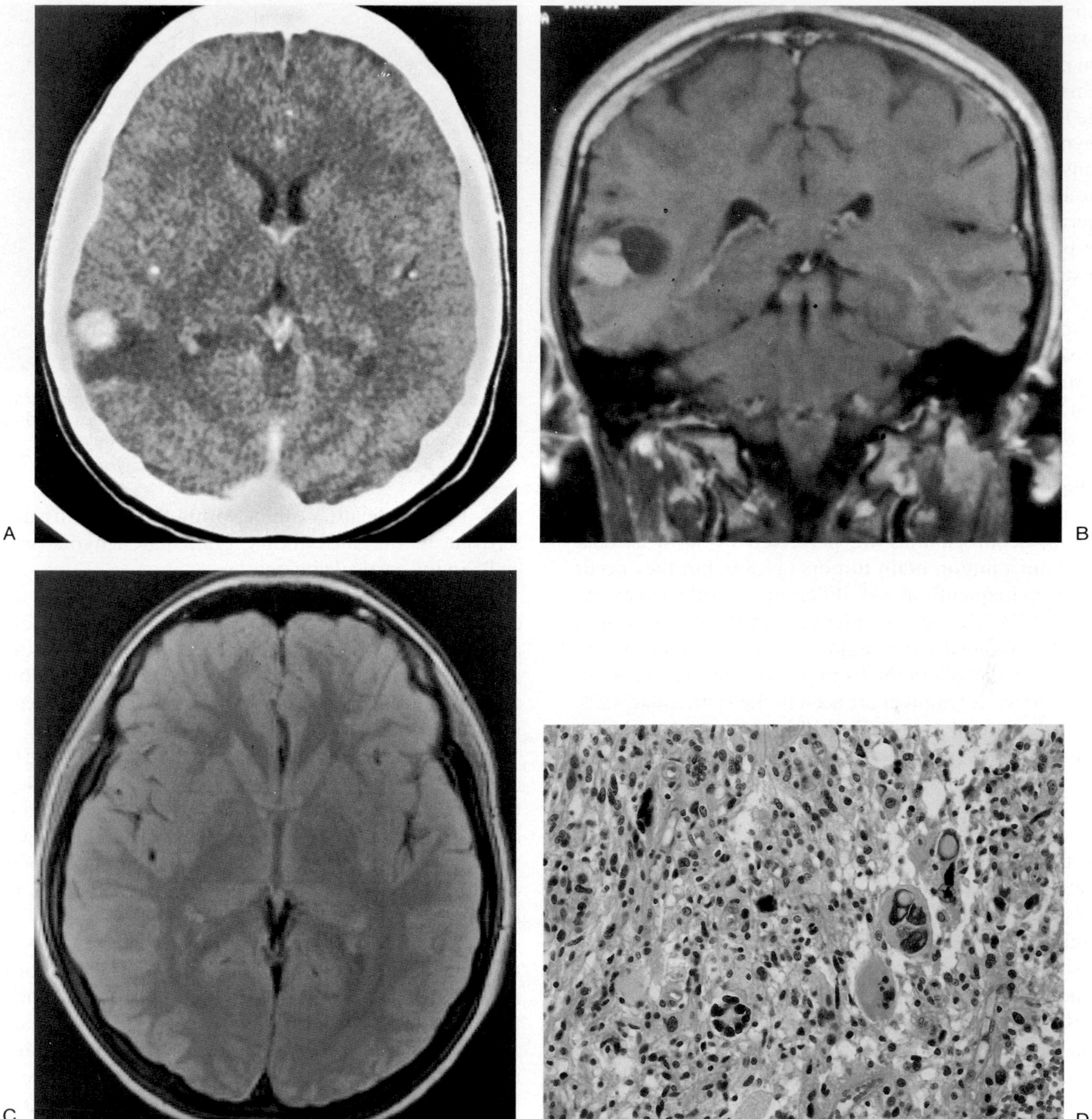

FIG. 52. Pleomorphic xanthoastrocytoma. **A:** Contrast-enhanced CT. **B:** Coronal T1-weighted MR after i.v. contrast. **C:** Axial proton density-weighted MR. **D:** Histopathologic specimen. Enhancing lesion (A,B) with subjacent cyst (B,C) is typical appearance of PXA. On pathology (D), H&E stain shows extreme nuclear and cytoplasmic pleomorphism, including large hyperchromatic nuclei and multinucleated cells as well as lymphocytic infiltrate. (From Lipper et al., ref. 82, with permission.)

Pleomorphic Xanthoastrocytoma

The pleomorphic xanthoastrocytoma (PXA) is characteristically a superficially located hemispheric neoplasm found in young adults with a long history of seizures. The temporal lobe is the most common location. The lesion is relatively rare and it is only recently recognized as a distinct entity, so it is only incompletely understood at this time. However, it is considered a much less aggressive lesion than its histologic features would suggest (32). Surgical excision alone is generally the initial treatment for this relatively benign lesion, but a significant frequency of recurrence, with malignant transformation in 10% to 25% of cases, has been noted (32). On pathology, the lesions are discrete superficial nodular masses overlying a large fluid-filled cyst. Deeper parts of the lesion may show infiltration of the subjacent parenchyma. On microscopic examination, these lesions show considerable pleomorphism and cellularity and a notable absence of mitotic figures, necrosis, and vascular proliferation (32). Imaging findings in PXA are fairly classic, despite the rarity of the lesion (82). MRI typically demonstrates a very superficial solid mass with an often large cyst immediately deep to the solid tissue (Fig. 52). On histopathology and MRI, the differential diagnosis involves pilocytic astrocytoma and ganglion cell tumor, particularly when a PXA is found with the macroscopic cyst in conjunction with a focal nodule.

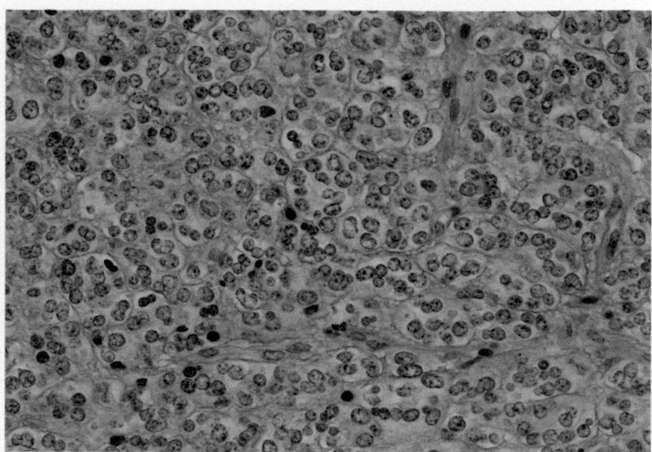

FIG. 53. Oligodendroglioma. Microscopic section demonstrates cells with regular, round nuclei and perinuclear halos ("fried egg appearance") arranged within a delicate capillary network.

Oligodendroglioma and Anaplastic Oligodendroglioma

Oligodendrogliomas are perceived by most as relatively uncommon brain tumors (11,83), but they occur nearly as frequently as well-differentiated diffuse astrocytomas (32). The peak incidence is in the fourth to fifth decades. While the vast majority of these tumors are located superficially in the frontal and frontotemporal regions, a smaller number are seen in the ventricular walls, cerebellum, and very rarely within the spinal cord (11). Although this neoplasm is regarded as having slow growth rates, as manifested by the relatively long history of symptoms (i.e., seizures or headaches) given by these patients, the postoperative survival often seems disproportionately short in comparison, with 5-year survival rates of approximately 50% and 10-year survival rates of only 10% to 30% (83), (84). However, the prognosis is considerably better than that of infiltrative astrocytomas of similar histologic grade (85). The progression of oligodendrogliomas to more anaplastic types occurs as it does in diffuse astrocytomas, but it evolves over longer periods of time (32). Traditionally, treatment has centered around surgical excision, but these lesions are infiltrative and therefore are generally not cured by surgery alone. There is evidence that the response to chemotherapy is often good, but the role of adjunctive radiotherapy continues to be debated in the literature (85–87).

Pathologically, oligodendrogliomas are solid, infiltrative lesions with poorly defined borders, like infiltrative astrocytomas (Fig. 53). They often contain cellular elements of other glial types, so are considered "mixed" in up to one-half of cases (11). These lesions are densely cellular with only minimal acellular stroma. The lesions classically exhibit extensive infiltration of cortex. Focal cystic necrosis and intratumoral hemorrhage are frequent findings, and calcification is extremely common, being associated with the walls of intrinsic blood vessels (11). The calcification can be within the tumor tissue or separate in the surrounding brain parenchyma, especially in the cortical gray matter.

Grading of oligodendrogliomas is a still unsettled area of histopathology. There is data showing that microcysts and low cellularity are favorable features, while mitoses, vascular hypertrophy, pleomorphism, and cellular atypia are unfavorable (32). However, at present there is no widely accepted grading system for these lesions.

Imaging studies of these lesions are very useful and can often suggest the specific diagnosis, based on the location, the presence of characteristic calcification, and the occasional finding of overlying calvarial change suggestive of a relatively long-standing mass lesion. Oligodendrogliomas are usually heterogeneous, but relatively low intensity (i.e., isointense to gray matter) on long TR images. These masses are typically located peripherally in the frontal lobes (88) (Fig. 54). Small cystic-appearing regions and hemorrhage are commonly found within these masses, particularly identifiable on MRI. Linear or nodular tumoral calcification on CT has been reported in 50% to 90% of oligodendrogliomas (89), which are the intracranial tumors with the highest frequency of calcification. Conventional spin-echo MRI is not sensitive to calcification itself (52), although gradient-echo imaging is highly sensitive to this finding (53) and is, therefore, a useful adjunct in imaging oligodendroglial brain tumors (Figs. 54 and 55). Furthermore, iron is often depcsited concomitantly with dystrophic calcification, and MRI is extremely sensitive to iron deposition. The extremely heterogeneous appearance of oligodendrogliomas, even on spin-echo images, can be at least in part a reflection of tumoral calcification. Edema is not usually a significant feature of lower grade oligodendrogliomas (89). Contrast enhancement has been seen in about one-half of cases (88). Calvarial erosion was demonstrated in 6/35 cases in

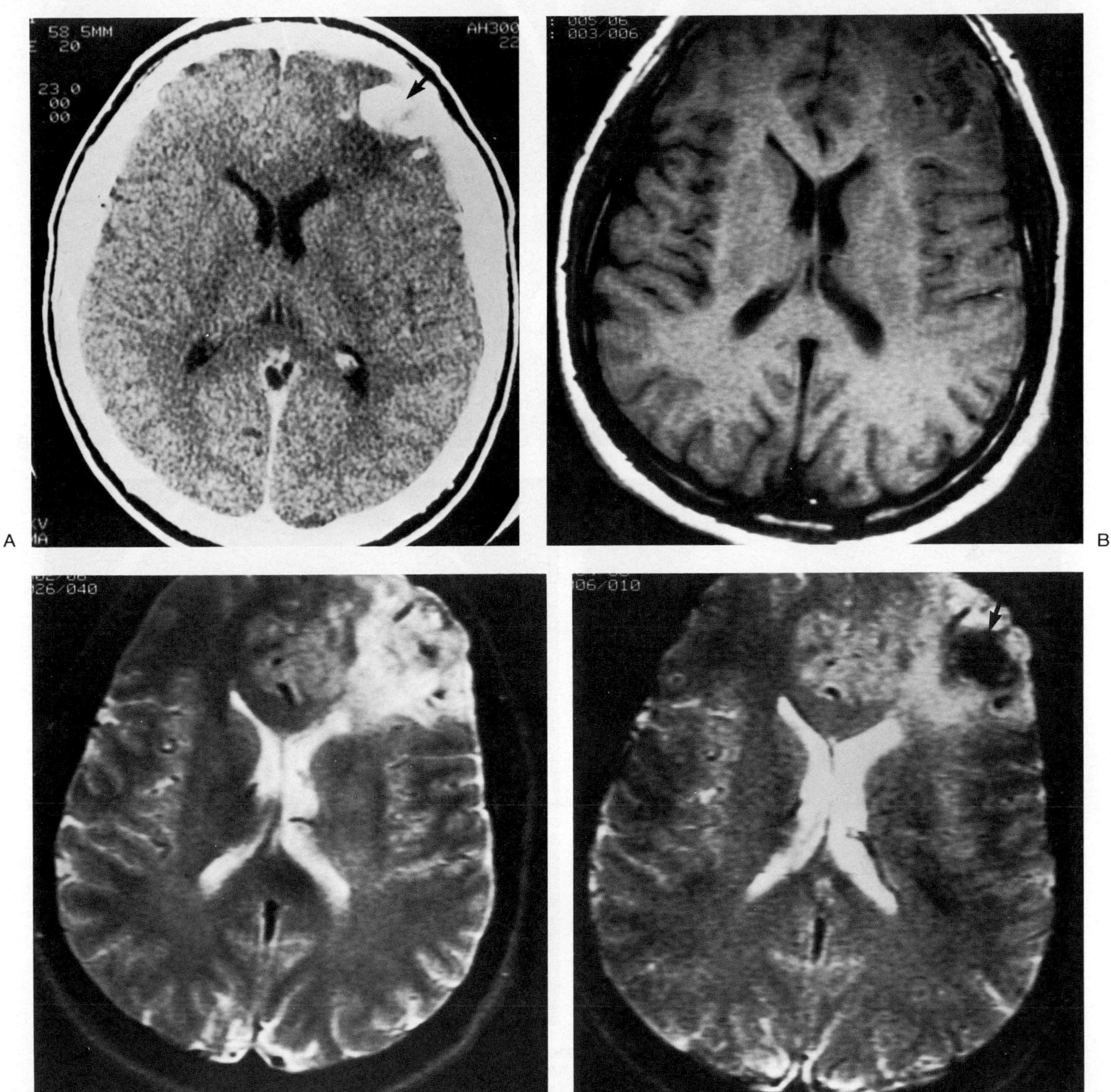

FIG. 54. Calcified oligodendroglioma, CT vs. MRI. **A:** CT. **B:** Short TR/TE MRI (600/20). **C:** Long TR/TE MRI (2500/80). **D:** Gradient-echo MRI (200/50/100). Peripheral left frontal oligodendroglioma is clearly depicted on all images, but dense calcification (*arrow*) on CT (A) is not suspected by spin-echo MRI (B,C). Gradient-echo image (D) obtained to detect magnetic susceptibility perturbations documents the entire area of calcification as marked hypointensity (*arrow*).

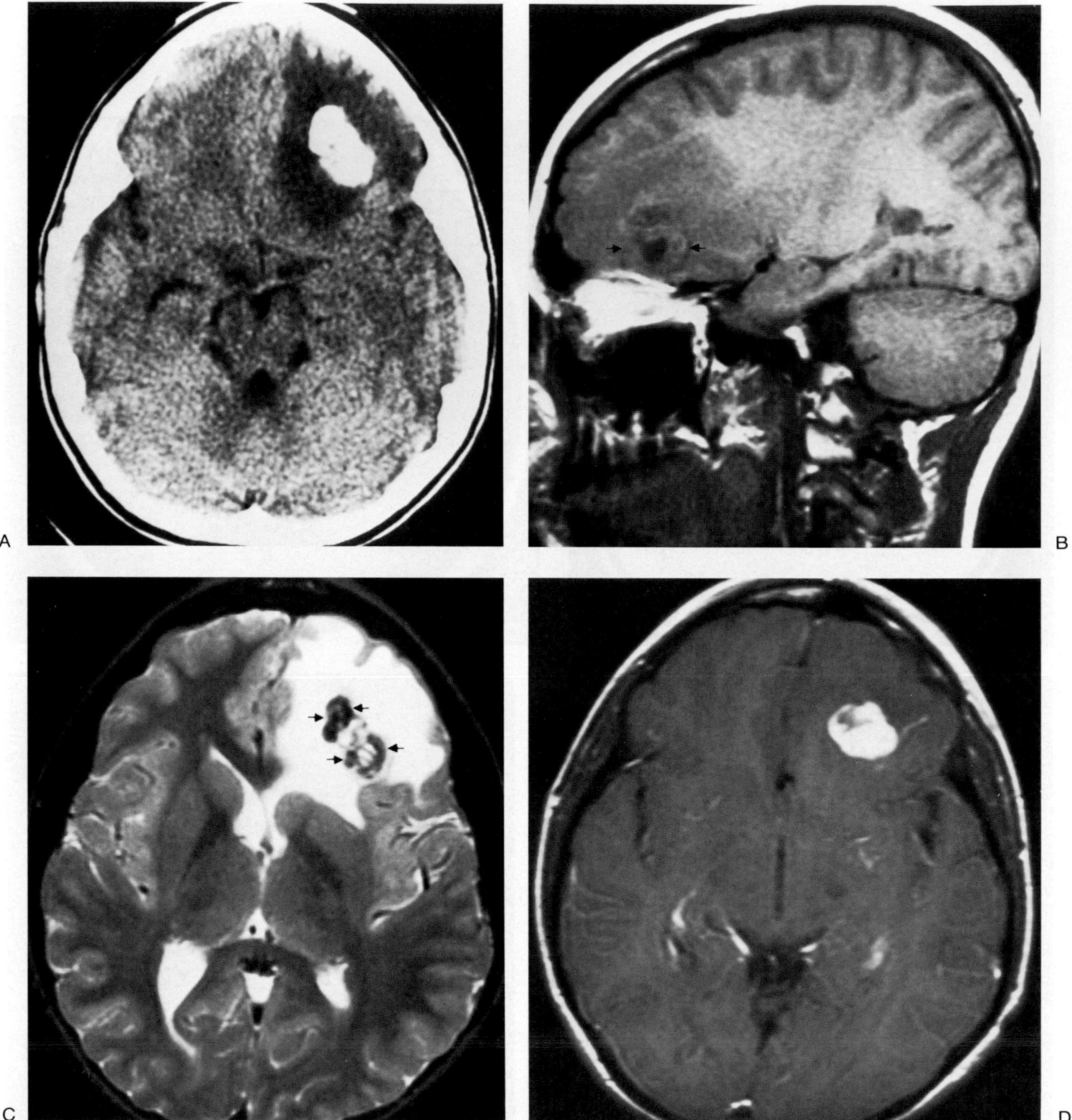

FIG. 55. Calcified oligodendroglioma with extensive "edema." **A:** Axial CT. **B:** Sagittal short TR/TE MRI (600/20). **C:** Axial long TR/TE MRI (3000/90). **D:** Axial short TR/TE MRI (800/30), with contrast enhancement. Densely calcified tumor is surrounded by low-attenuation "edema" on CT (A). Most calcification is isointense to brain on short TR/TE (*arrows*, B) and becomes markedly hypointense on long TR/TE (*arrows*, C), probably due to concomitantly deposited iron. Note extensive high-intensity "edema" on long TR/TE image (C). Calcified tumor mass enhances densely with gadolinium (D).

one study (88). On MRI, this may be a subtle finding unless significant erosion of marrow-containing medullary bone has been destroyed. The differential diagnosis of these lesions usually lies between oligodendroglioma and astrocytoma, although astrocytomas usually are more homogeneous, not as frequently calcified and often are deeper in the hemisphere. Glioblastoma, as already stated, is often quite heterogeneous and, in the case of malignant oligodendroglioma with extensive surrounding high intensity "edema" (Fig. 56), can be identical in

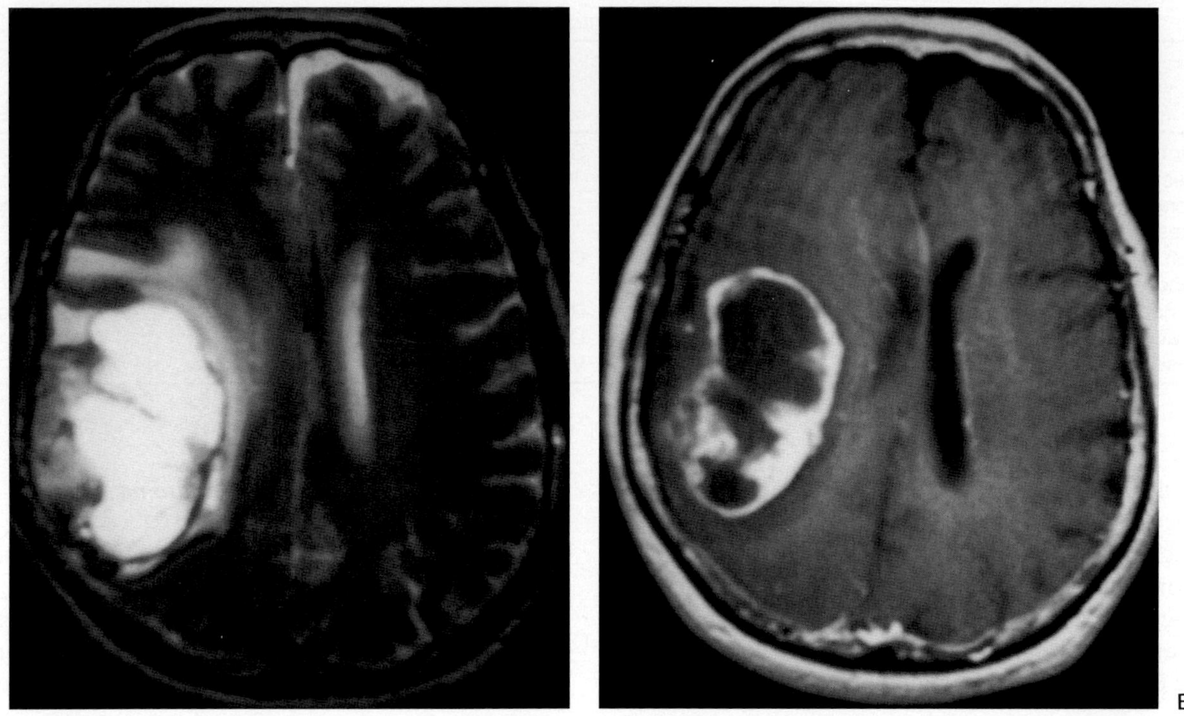

FIG. 56. Anaplastic oligodendroglioma. Heterogeneous mass on T2-weighted MRI (**A**) shows irregular ring-like enhancement (**B**).

appearance on MRI. The rare dysembryoplastic neuroepithelial tumor (DNET) of childhood and young adulthood can also look virtually identical to the oligodendroglioma, particularly when there is no significant hyperintensity of edema in association with the lesion (see below).

Tumors of Neuronal Composition

Ganglioglioma and Gangliocytoma

A distinct category of (usually) supratentorial neoplasms which illustrates the problem of mixed cell types and nomenclature of tumor classification schemes is represented by the ganglioglioma, a slowly growing tumor that mainly affects children and young adults, and is composed of both neural and glial elements (90,91). The vast majority of gangliogliomas are supratentorial (Table 9), and the temporal lobe is the predominant site (92–96), but these tumors can arise in the cerebellum, brainstem, suprasellar region, and spinal cord as well. On pathologic examination, gangliogliomas are well circumscribed tumors, typically cystic and often with focal calcification (11,94) (Fig. 57). Clinically, the slow growth and well demarcated nature of these lesions often allow surgical resection which results in an excellent prognosis in the majority of cases. Only rarely do these tumors spread via the subarachnoid space (97). Gangliocytoma is an extremely rare tumor diagnosed when the glial element is only a minor (or negligible) contributor to the overall histologic picture—a benign intraparenchymal neuronal neoplasm comprised of mature ganglion cells (11,98). The distinction between ganglioglioma and gangliocytoma is often not sharp, either histologically or on MRI, so the term ganglion cell tumor may be used. Note that despite the mature, well-differentiated histologic nature of gangliocytomas, they are still neoplasms. This entity must not be confused with neuronal heterotopia, which represents a non-neoplastic region of normal gray matter in an abnormal location. Since small biopsy specimens of heterotopia may be confused with gangliocytoma by the histopathologist on frozen section, the neuroradiologist plays an extremely important role in the differentiation of these two distinct entities.

The diagnosis of gangliogliomas on MRI centers around the delineation of a solid or partially cystic (38%) (94,96) mass lesion, preferentially located in the temporal lobe of a child or young adult. The signal intensity is nonspecific, and is usually inhomogeneously hyperintense on long TR images (Fig. 58). Most gangliogliomas show some contrast enhancement (Fig. 59) (96). Heterotopias are exactly isointense to normal gray matter (Fig. 60) on all three spin-echo images (i.e., short TR/TE, long TR/short TE, and long TR/TE), while gangliocytomas and gangliogliomas are not. The only signal aberration one might see in association with heterotopia is increased signal subjacent to the lesion, presumably indicating gli-

TABLE 9. *Pediatric supratentorial hemispheric neoplasms*

	Juvenile pilocytic astrocytoma	Ganglioglioma	Pleomorphic xanthoastrocytoma	Supratentorial PNET (cerebral neuroblastoma)	DNET
Signal intensity characteristics (on long TR images)	Sharply demarcated; commonly cystic	Sharply demarcated; commonly cystic	Sharply demarcated with subjacent cyst	Markedly heterogeneous	Sharply demarcated; heterogeneous
Contrast enhancement	Common; dense	Common; irregular	Common in solid portion	Common; irregular	Unknown
Hemorrhage	Rare	Rare	Rare	Common	Uncommon
Calcification	Uncommon	Common	Uncommon	Common	Common
Prognosis	Excellent	Excellent	Variable	Poor	Excellent

osis or dysmyelination. The main differential diagnosis on imaging studies in a child or young adult lies between ganglioglioma, JPA, and XPA, three neoplasms that all commonly show a nodular mass in association with a macroscopic cyst. CT or gradient-echo imaging to detect calcification, a more common feature of ganglioglioma, may be useful in this distinction.

Desmoplastic Infantile Ganglioglioma

Desmoplastic infantile ganglioglioma has been reported in infants less than 4 months of age. These lesions are typically massive, partially cystic tumors most often in the frontoparietal region with extensive fibrocollagenous elements, and are associated with a favorable

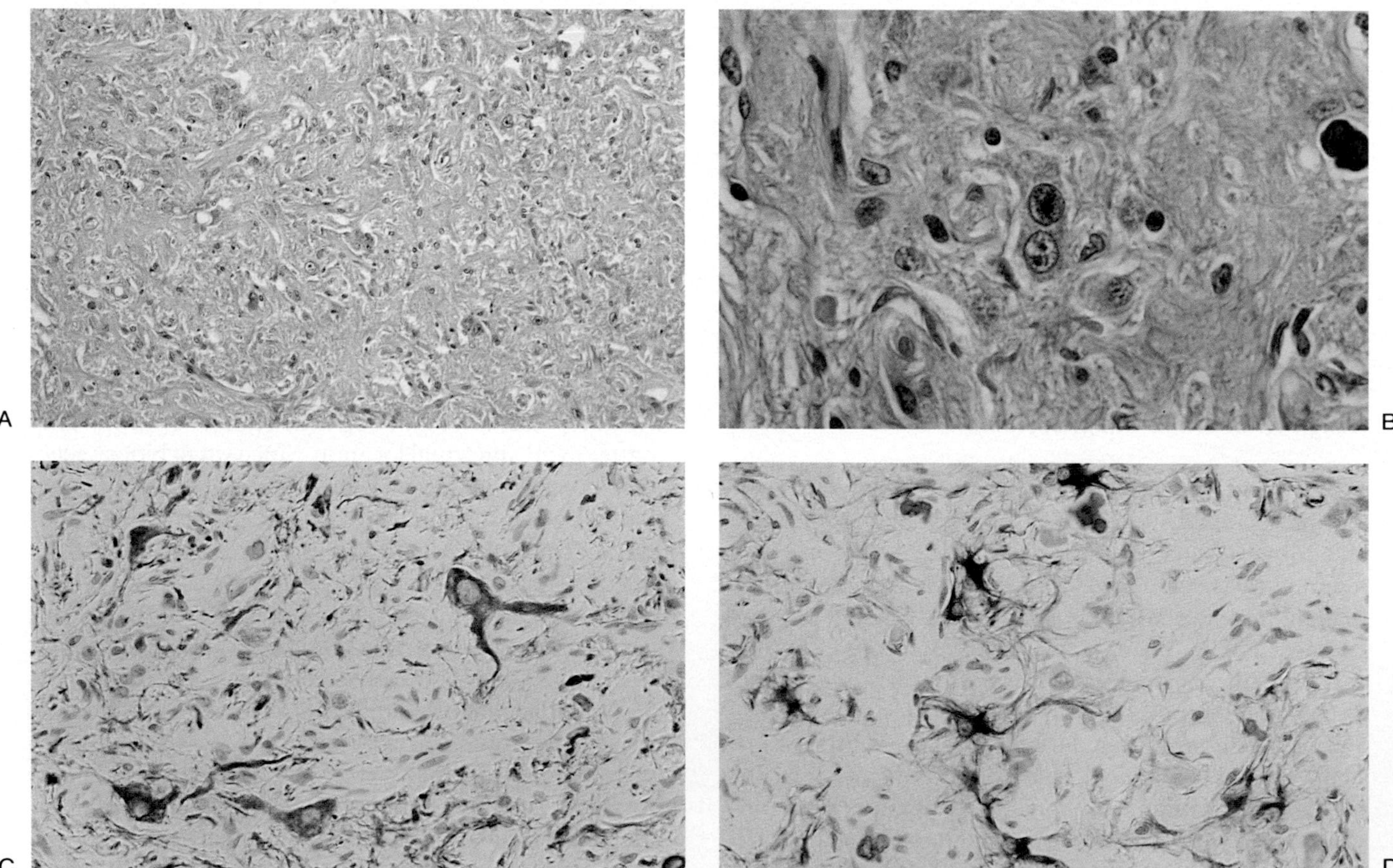

FIG. 57. Ganglioglioma, histopathologic features. Microscopic features of this slow growing tumor include a well circumscribed mass often with an extensive fibrocollagenous component (**A**). They typically contain neuronal cells with abnormal morphology, often binucleated "ganglion" cells (*center*, **B**). Neurofilament stain (**C**) is positive for cells of neuronal origin. Glial fibrillary acidic protein (GFAP)-positive astrocytes (**D**) indicates the most actively proliferating component of the tumor.

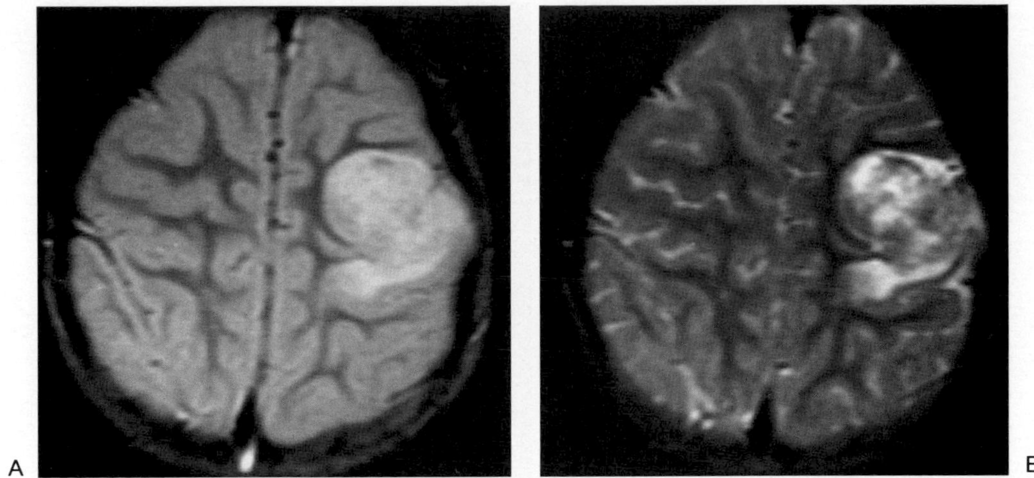

FIG. 58. Solid ganglioglioma. **A:** Long TR/short TE MRI (3000/30). **B:** Long TR/TE MRI (3000/80). Heterogeneous cortical-subcortical left frontal mass lesion is well defined and shows no associated high intensity in the adjacent white matter.

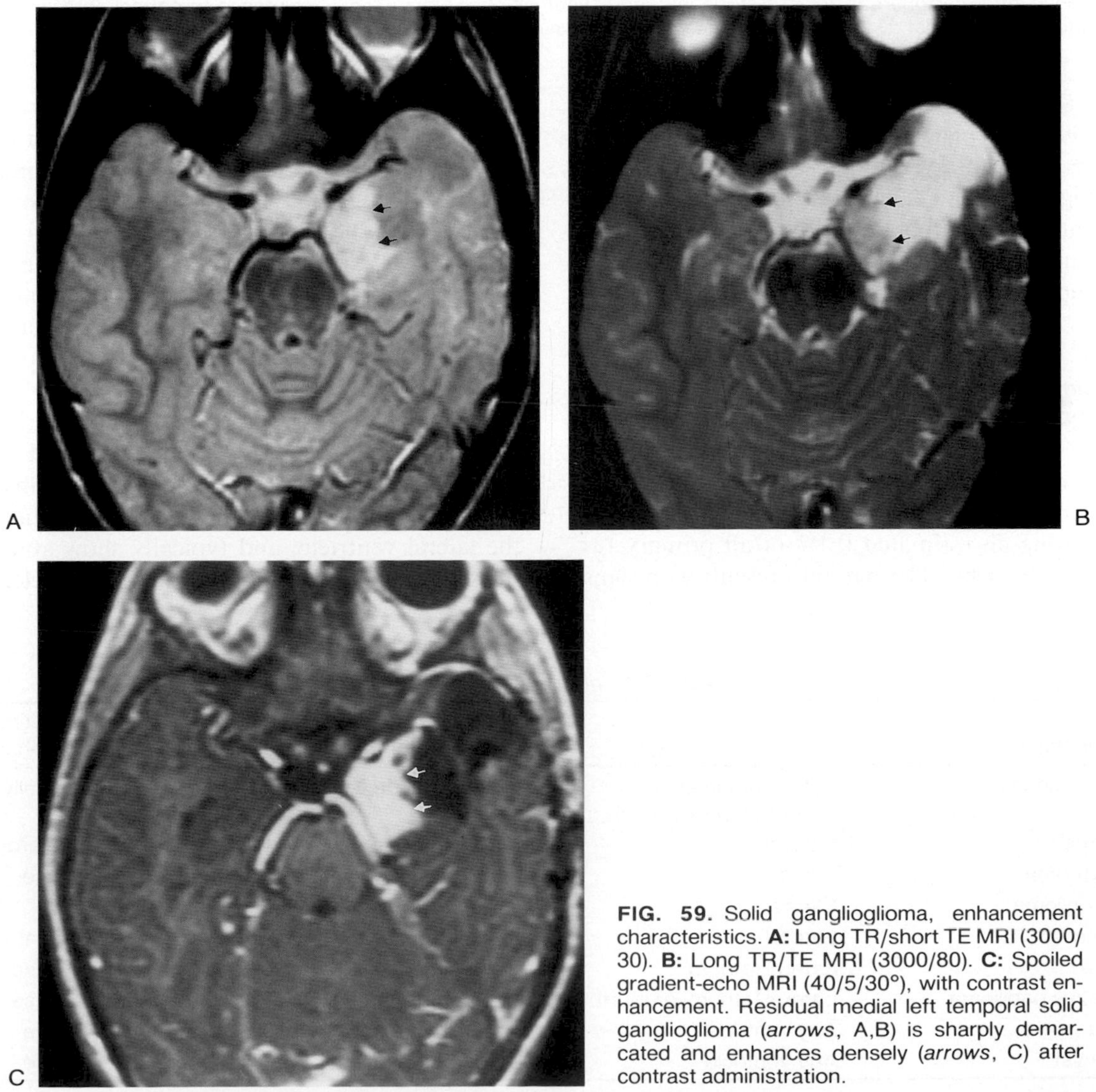

FIG. 59. Solid ganglioglioma, enhancement characteristics. **A:** Long TR/short TE MRI (3000/30). **B:** Long TR/TE MRI (3000/80). **C:** Spoiled gradient-echo MRI (40/5/30°), with contrast enhancement. Residual medial left temporal solid ganglioglioma (*arrows*, A,B) is sharply demarcated and enhances densely (*arrows*, C) after contrast administration.

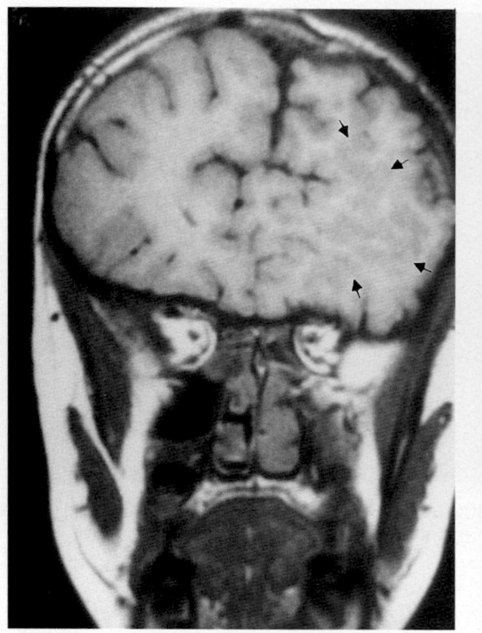

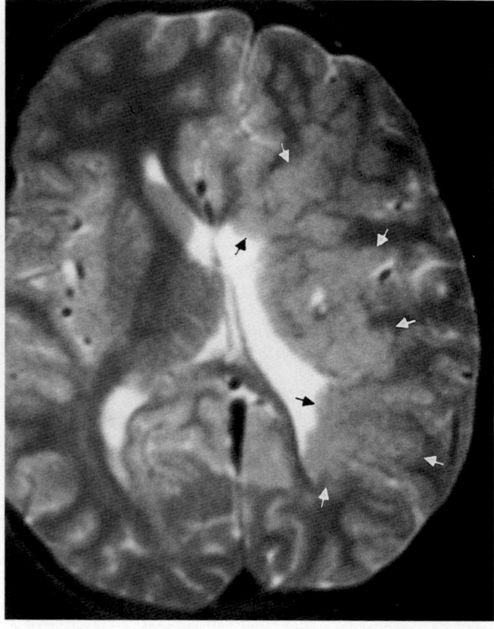

A B

FIG. 60. Heterotopia as mass lesion. **A:** Short TR/TE MRI (600/20). **B:** Long TR/TE MRI (2800/80). Apparent mass lesion in left hemisphere (*arrows*) distorts left lateral ventricle. Lesion is exactly isointense to normal cortical gray matter, a feature that distinguishes this heterotopia from a neoplasm.

prognosis (99). The collagen content and cystic nature of these lesions result in a very heterogeneous appearance on MRI (Fig. 61). The appearance may be identical to the supratentorial variant of PNET, also termed primary cerebral neuroblastoma, a tumor with a considerably worse prognosis (see PNET).

Central Neurocytoma

Central neurocytoma is a recently described relatively benign intraventricular neoplasm (Table 10) that occurs mainly in young to middle-aged adults. The lesion is rare, comprising an estimated 0.1% of all primary tumors of the CNS (100). The patient presents with signs and symptoms of hydrocephalus in the vast majority of cases. On gross pathology, central neurocytomas are well circumscribed and attached to the septum or the lateral ventricular wall. On microscopy, the tumor is made up of small well-differentiated cells with features reminiscent of neuroblastoma or oligodendroglioma. A monotonous pattern of extremely similar nuclei is notable (101). Surgery is thought to be curative in most cases, but recurrence is not uncommon (100).

Imaging studies provide a very characteristic picture that allows the diagnosis to be suspected with small differential diagnosis (100,102). These lesions are virtually always intraventricular (Fig. 62), specifically within the lateral ventricle, and typically show attachment to the septum pellucidum of the lateral ventricle. Although

TABLE 10. *Intraventricular masses*

Tumor type	Typical location	Intensity characteristics on long TR images	Contrast enhancement
Central neurocytoma	Lateal (attached to septum pellucidum)	Isointense to gray matter	Usually dense
Ependymoma	Lateral	Heterogeneous	Heterogeneous
Subependymoma	Fourth	Hyperintense to gray matter	None
Oligodendroglioma	Lateral	Heterogeneous	
Astrocytoma	Lateral	Hyperintense to gray matter	Variable; irregular
Meningioma	Lateral (atrium)	Isointense to gray matter	Dense
Choroid plexus papilloma	Lateral (atrium) or fourth	Heterogeneous	Dense
Epidermoid	Any ventricle	Sl. hyperintense to CSF	None
Arachnoid cyst	Any ventricle	Isointense to CSF	None

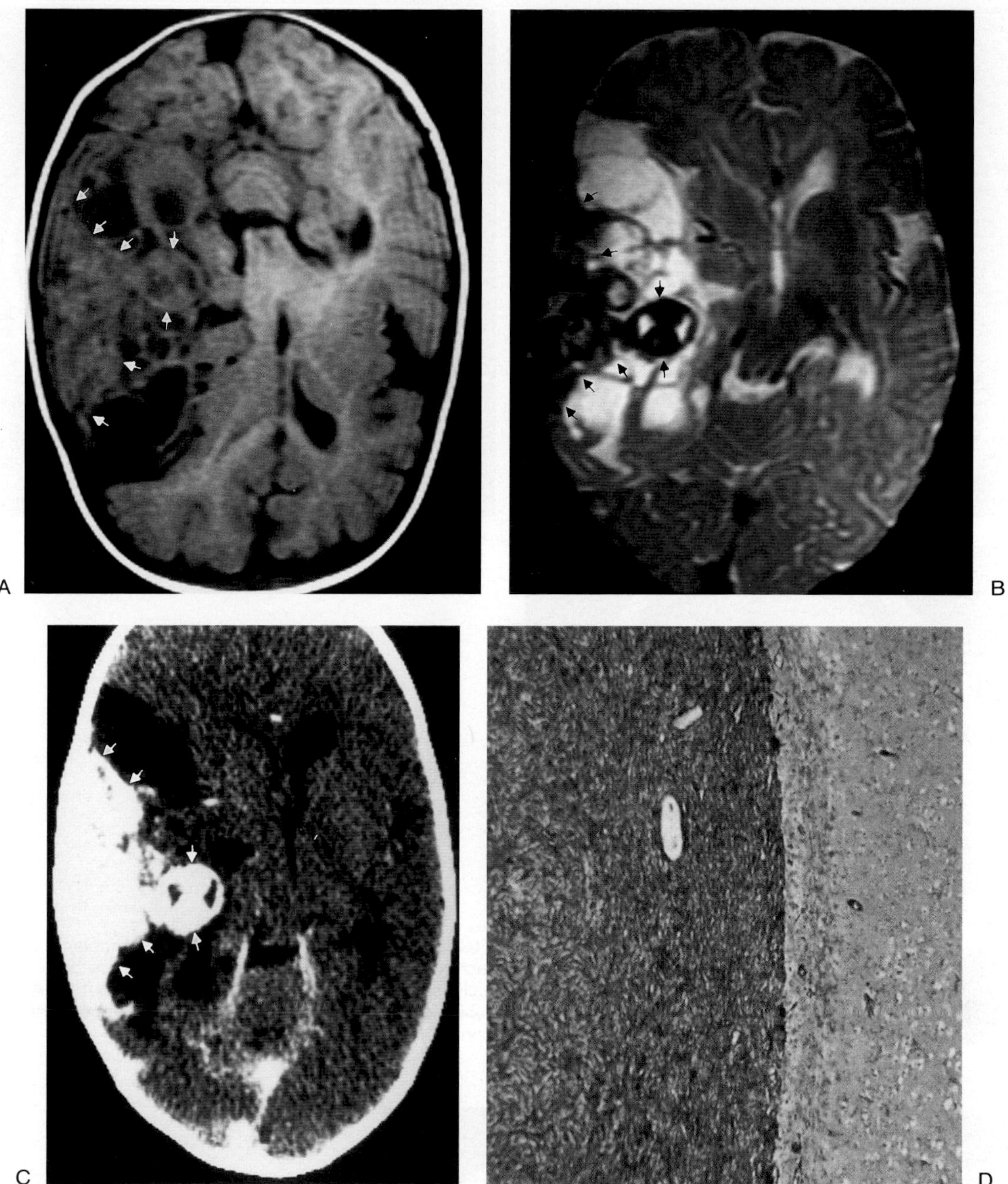

FIG. 61. Desmoplastic infantile ganglioglioma. **A:** Short TR/TE MRI (600/20). **B:** Long TR/TE MRI (3000/80). **C:** Contrast-enhanced CT. **D:** Histopathologic specimen from different patient, fibrin stain. (From Okazaki and Scheithauer, ref. 121, with permission.) Marked heterogeneity in right hemispheric mass reflects cystic areas, solid tumor, and extensive fibrocollagenous matrix (*arrows*, A,B). Fibrocollagenous region is hypointense on long TR/TE image (B). Note marked enhancement of solid and desmoplastic components of tumor (*arrows*, C). Extensive fibrocollagenous material in these lesions (*dark staining areas*, D) can masquerade as an extra-axial mass.

calcification is considered characteristic, one study showed small or large calcifications in only one-half of cases by CT (100). On MRI, these masses are nearly isointense to gray matter but more heterogeneous than heterotopias. Contrast enhancement is said to be variable, but enhancement is common (100). The differential diagnosis on MRI of this lesion is mainly ependymoma, subependymoma, and oligodendroglioma, lesions which are most often hyperintense to gray matter or more heterogeneous. Heterotopic gray matter (Fig. 63) should neither enhance nor have calcifications, and is not in contact with the septum pellucidum. Intraventricular meningiomas are usually situated more posteriorly, within the atrium of the lateral ventricle, as are choroid plexus tumors. Gangliogliomas are not typically situated within the ventricle.

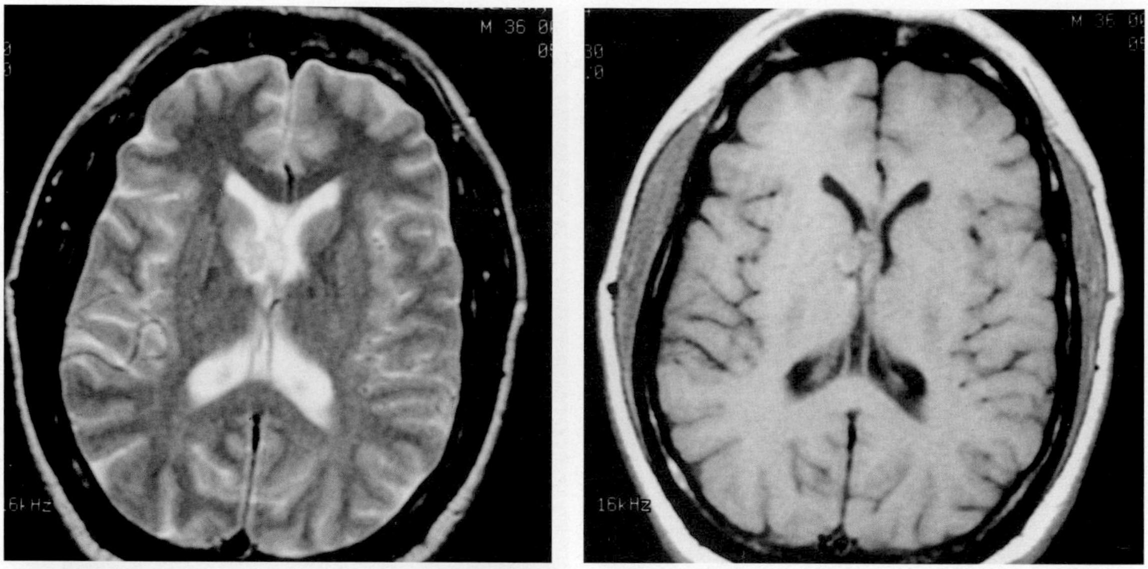

FIG. 62. Central neurocytoma. Intraventricular mass attached to septum is slightly heterogeneous but essentially isointense to gray matter on T1-weighted (**A**) and T2-weighted (**B**) images. It densely enhances after i.v. contrast (**C**).

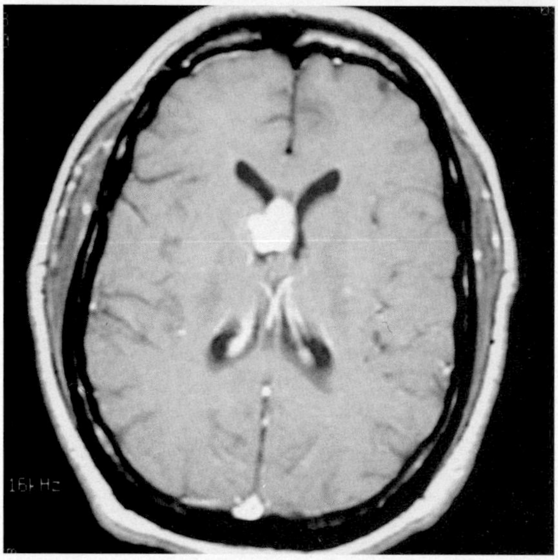

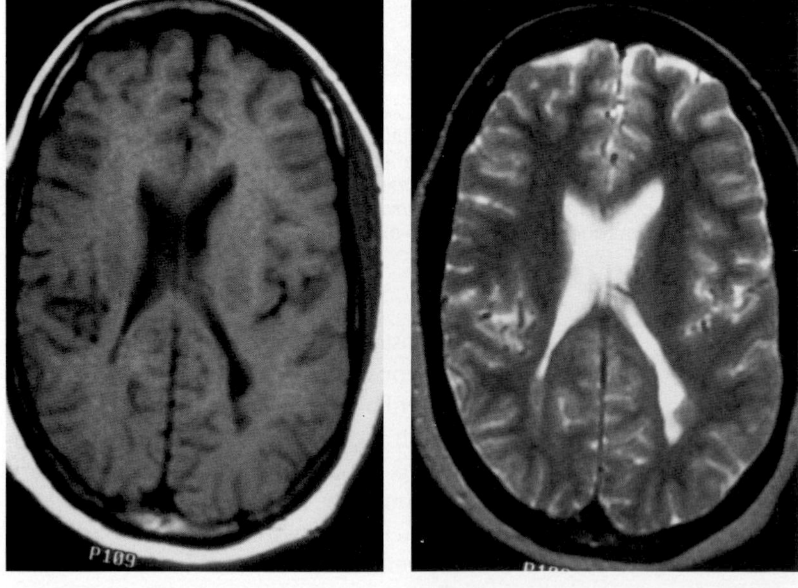

FIG. 63. Heterotopic gray matter. Mass along left lateral ventricular wall is isointense to gray matter on both T1-(**A**) and T2-(**B**) weighted images, but is in atypical location for neurocytoma.

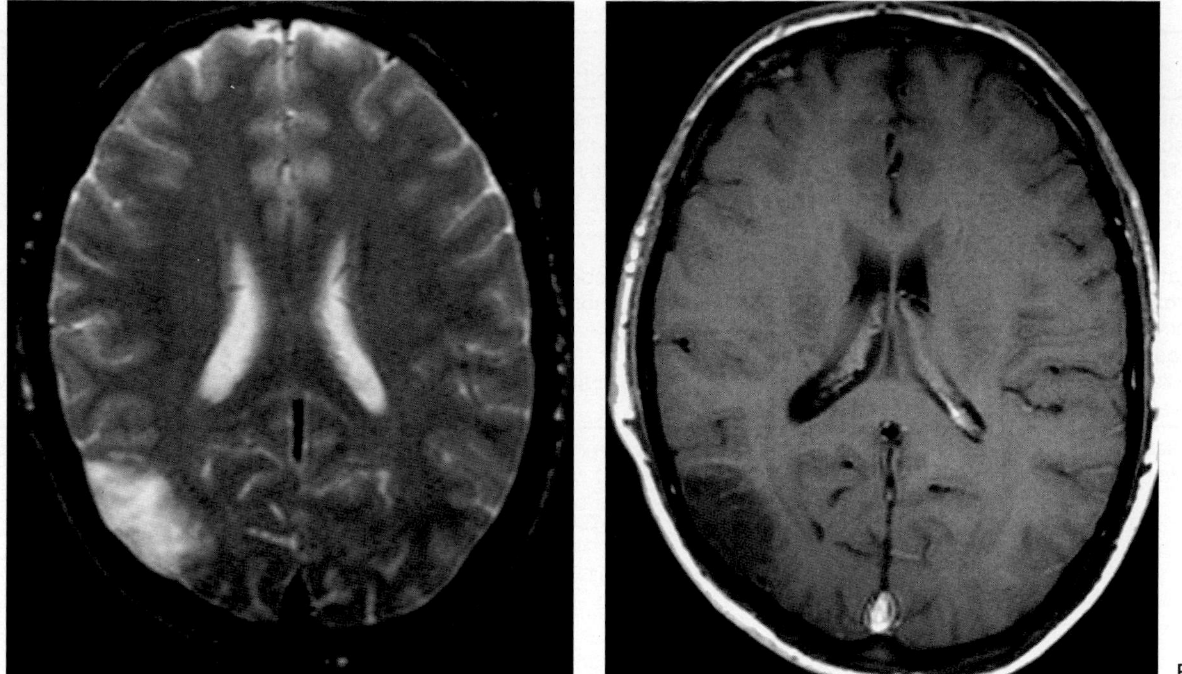

FIG. 64. DNET. DNET in a 34-year-old patient with long-standing seizures. T2-weighted image (A) shows cortical mass in posterior temporoparietal region. No enhancement is seen after gadolinium (**B**). (Courtesy of V. Mathews, M.D., Winston-Salem, NC.)

Dysembryoplastic Neuroepithelial Tumor (DNET)

The dysembryoplastic neuroepithelial tumor (DNET) is a very uncommon, extremely slow growing lesion found mainly during the first few decades of life. This cortical mass presents with long-standing seizures in virtually all reported cases. The superficial location, usually in the temporal lobe but always supratentorial in location, allows skull remodeling to occur due to the slow growing nature of the lesion. On gross pathology, gyral expansion and often small nodular elevations are seen due to the multinodular composition of the mass. Microscopic features almost always include the characteristic intracortical nodules with a wide range of size, oligodendroglial hypercellularity, and abundant mucin (101). Cortical dysplasia is also identifiable.

Imaging allows the diagnosis to be made with only few differential diagnosis considerations (Fig. 64). Since the lesions can be partially cystic and calcified, the DNET is indistinguishable from oligodendroglioma on CT and MRI when the oligodendroglioma is low grade and not associated with edema. Ganglioglioma is also a consideration, as are superficially located infiltrative astrocytomas.

POSTERIOR FOSSA NEOPLASMS

MR imaging has played an increasingly important role in the evaluation of patients suspected of harboring disease in the posterior fossa (Table 11), because of its superior, virtually artifact-free display of anatomy and pathology in this region (103–105). While the following tumors can be found outside of the confines of the posterior fossa, they are most commonly located in this region. From the radiologist's perspective, the differential diagnosis is most easily formulated using the neuroanatomical classification as a starting point, rather than any of the tumor categorizations of the neuropathologist, and subsequently using MRI for tissue characterization. Our ensuing discussion therefore, although somewhat artificial in its separation, will detail the more common neoplasms of the cerebellum and brainstem.

The posterior fossa is the most common site of primary intracranial tumors in the pediatric patient. Approximately two-thirds of intracranial tumors in children older than one year of age arise in either the brainstem or cerebellum, with cerebellar astrocytoma, primitive neuroectodermal tumor (PNET), ependymoma, and brainstem glioma the most common, in or-

TABLE 11. *Posterior fossa tumors in childhood*

	Juvenile pilocytic astrocytoma	PNET	Ependymoma	Brainstem astrocytoma[a]
Signal intensity characteristics (on long TR images)	Sharply demarcated; commonly cystic	Homogeneous; low to moderate intensity	Markedly heterogeneous	Ill-defined; high intensity
Contrast enhancement	Common in solid portion (mural nodule)	Common; dense	Common; irregular	Common (especially dorsally exophytic type)
Calcification	Uncommon	Uncommon	Common	Rare
Hemorrhage	Rare	Uncommon	Common	Uncommon
Tendency to seed CSF pathways	Extremely low	High	Low to moderate	Low
Prognosis (estimated survival)	>90% 10 yr survival	50% 5 yr survival	50% 5 yr survival	20% 5 yr survival

[a] Dorsally exophytic subgroup of brainstem astrocytoma commonly shows enhancement and has more favorable prognosis.

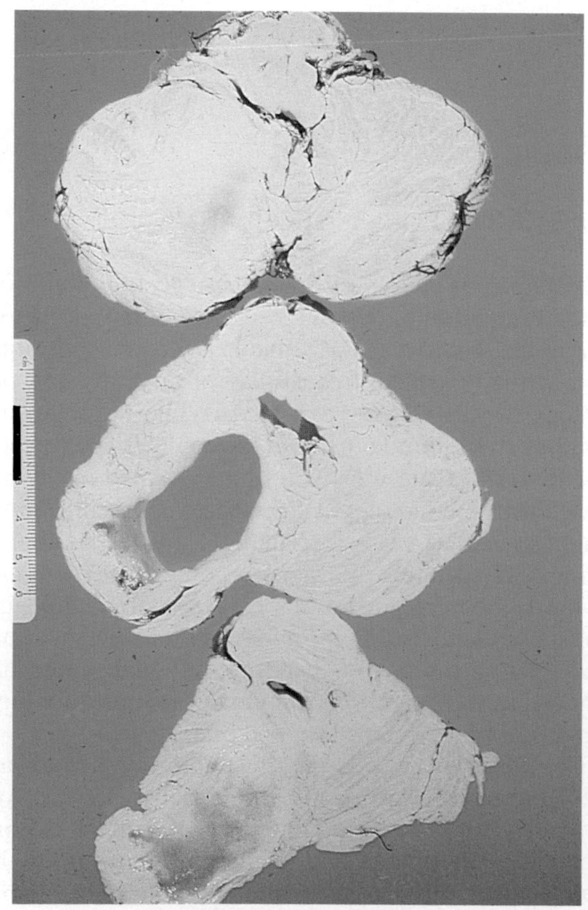

FIG. 65. Cystic cerebellar pilocytic astrocytoma on gross specimen. (Courtesy of Dr. N. K. Gonatas, Philadelphia, PA.)

der of decreasing frequency. In the neonate and young infant, infratentorial tumors are distinctly uncommon (106). Similarly, infratentorial brain tumors make up only about 15% to 20% of all intra-axial brain tumors in adults, of which the most common lesions are hemangioblastoma and metastases.

The clinical presentation of tumors in the posterior fossa, especially in the pediatric population, is essentially the same, regardless of the cell type. Signs and symptoms generally result from two pathologic conditions (107): obstruction to CSF flow causing hydrocephalus, and local neurological deficits, which depend upon whether the vermis or cerebellar hemisphere is involved.

Neuroglial, Neuronal, and Primitive Neuroectodermal Tumors

Cerebellar Astrocytoma

The cerebellar astrocytoma is the most common posterior fossa neoplasm in the child, and has long been recognized as having the highest survival rate (94% 25-year survival) (108) amongst all primary brain gliomas. The peak incidence is within the first two decades; some centers have noted a sharp peak around age four (109). The great majority (85%) of cerebellar astrocytomas are of the pilocytic variety (11) and are morphologically identical to the diencephalic or hemispheric JPA found in the supratentorial region (described earlier). These lesions are seen with a higher frequency in patients with neurofibromatosis. Interestingly, despite their benign prognosis, tumor recurrence is not uncommon and late recurrence (greater than 20 years later) has been noted (110). This peculiar violation of Collins' law regarding the period of risk for tumor recurrence (111) (nine months plus age at diagnosis) has also been reported in optic gliomas, but contrasts with the behavior of most other intracranial tumors. Grossly, the pilocytic cerebellar astrocytoma is a well circumscribed, partially cystic mass, often with a mural nodule of vascular solid tissue, situated anywhere in the cerebellum (i.e., vermis or hemisphere) (Fig. 65). The minority (approximately 15%) of cerebellar astrocytomas are of the infiltrative fibrillary type, similar to the cerebral astrocytoma of the adult. These are more frequently anaplastic microscopically and appear more infiltrative (Fig. 66). They are more apt to occur in an older age group (early adulthood) and are solid lesions, not infrequently associated with hemorrhage and necrosis.

MRI has inarguably become the clear choice for the evaluation of all posterior fossa tumors (112), and the cerebellar astrocytoma is no exception to this. The typical findings on MRI of the pilocytic type include a mass, either midline or hemispheric, comprised of a single large cyst with a nodular solid portion, often located in the wall of the cyst (Figs. 67 and 68). The clue to the specific diagnosis on MRI is the morphology of the tumor; that is, the identification of an intra-axial lesion with a large cystic component. The accurate identification of a cyst on MRI often requires careful scrutiny of signal intensity relative to CSF, as well as the use of morphologic criteria and subtle intralesional motion artifact, in order to avoid repeating the well-documented unreliability of CT (113) for this determination. The solid portion of the tumor should densely enhance with i.v. contrast, while the cyst wall may or may not enhance (Fig. 69). The nonenhancing portion of the solid part of the neoplasm probably relates to small cystic or necrotic regions within solid tumor. It should be realized that a significant proportion of these tumors are not grossly cystic, so other features are also important in the differential diagnosis. The cerebellar astrocytoma displaces and effaces, rather than fills, the fourth ventricle (Fig. 68), commonly resulting in hydrocephalus at the time of initial diagnosis. The solid portion of the tumor is often nearly isointense to normal brain on long TR images, whereas the cystic portion is either isointense to CSF or slightly hyperintense, possibly due to its higher protein content. Cerebellar astrocytomas are usually relatively homogeneous compared to ependymoma, for example, but signal heterogeneity does not preclude its diagnosis. Although calcification is not a characteristic feature of cerebellar astrocytoma, it occurs in a significant portion of these lesions (up to 20%), and therefore the use of CT for the detection of calcification has little value in the differential diagnosis.

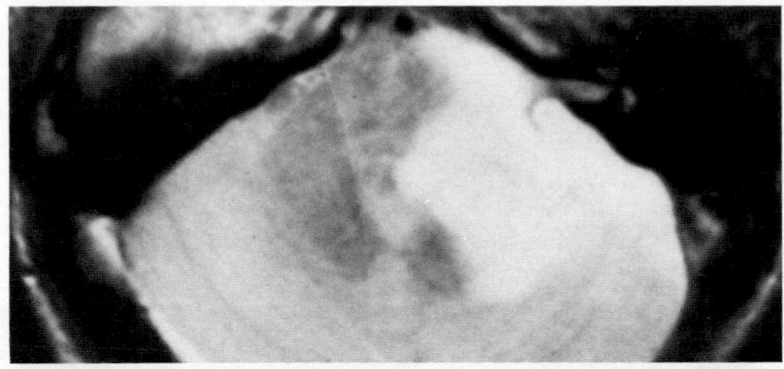

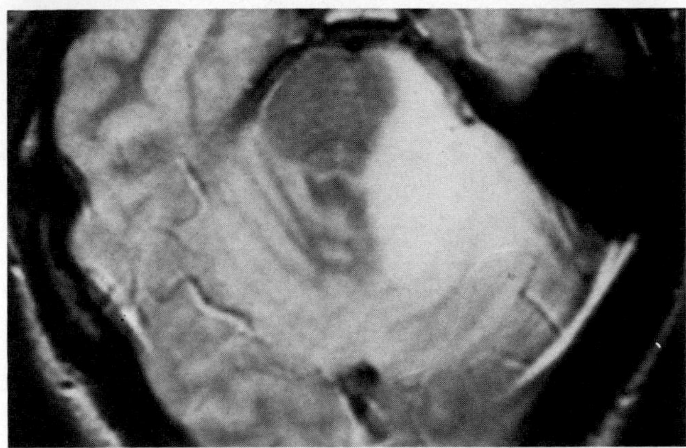

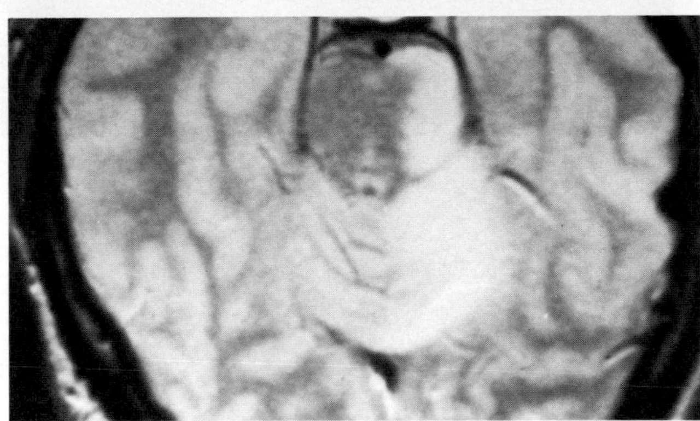

FIG. 66. Diffuse astrocytoma, left cerebellum and brainstem. **A–C:** Long TR/short TE MRI (2800/30), inferior to superior. Homogeneous high-intensity mass involves brainstem and left cerebellum and represents infiltrative, fibrillary astrocytoma, the most common type of astrocytoma in the adult posterior fossa.

Primitive Neuroectodermal Tumor (PNET)

Tumors included under the name "primitive neuroectodermal tumor" (PNET) comprise one of the most common groups of childhood CNS tumors. The designation PNET is certainly the most controversial label in brain neoplasia classification schemes amongst neuropathologists. PNET can be used to refer to a group of CNS tumors, usually of the cerebellum, thought to originate from primitive or undifferentiated neuroepithelial cells, which displays considerable histopathologic heterogene-

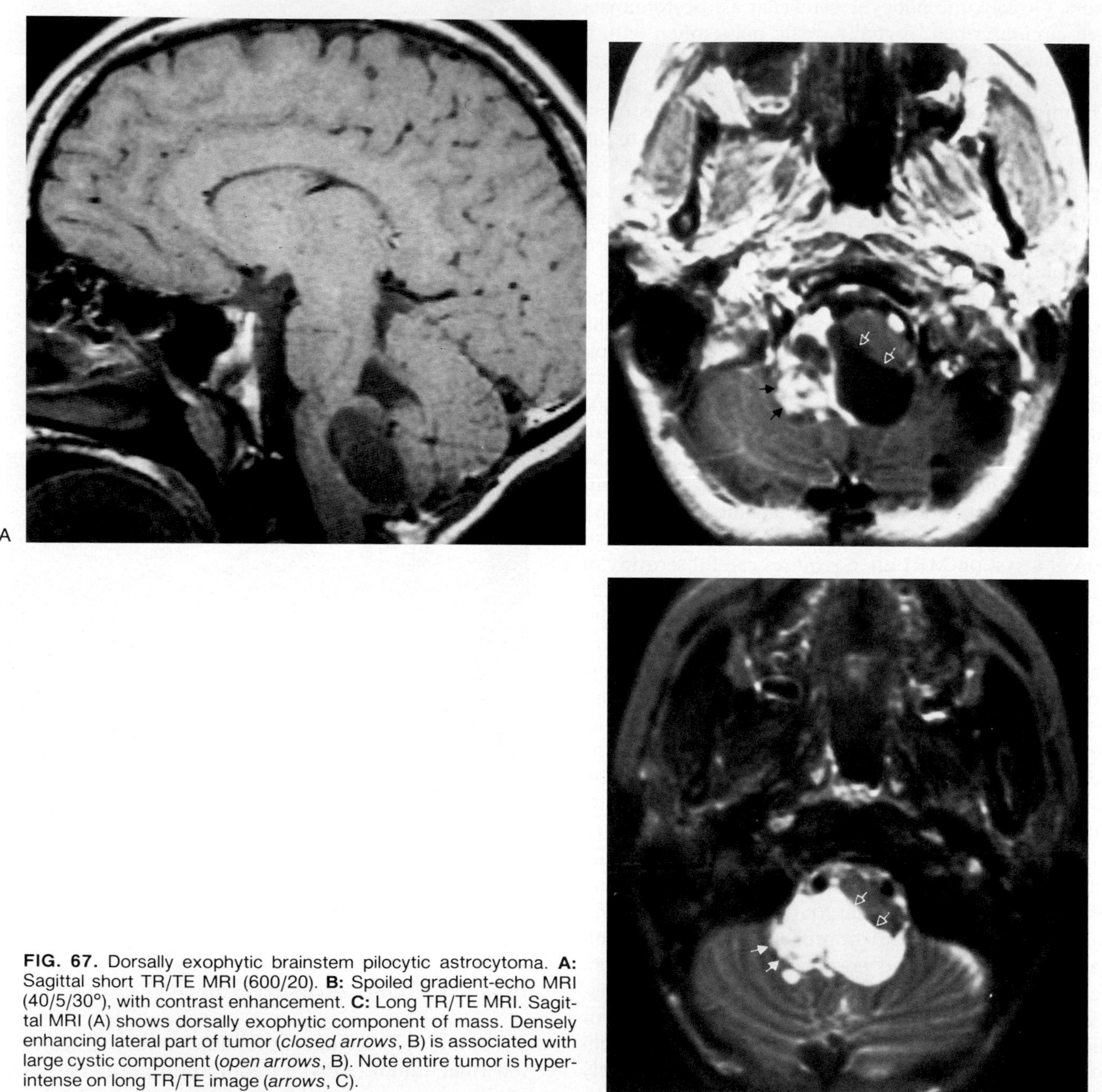

FIG. 67. Dorsally exophytic brainstem pilocytic astrocytoma. **A:** Sagittal short TR/TE MRI (600/20). **B:** Spoiled gradient-echo MRI (40/5/30°), with contrast enhancement. **C:** Long TR/TE MRI. Sagittal MRI (A) shows dorsally exophytic component of mass. Densely enhancing lateral part of tumor (*closed arrows*, B) is associated with large cystic component (*open arrows*, B). Note entire tumor is hyperintense on long TR/TE image (*arrows*, C).

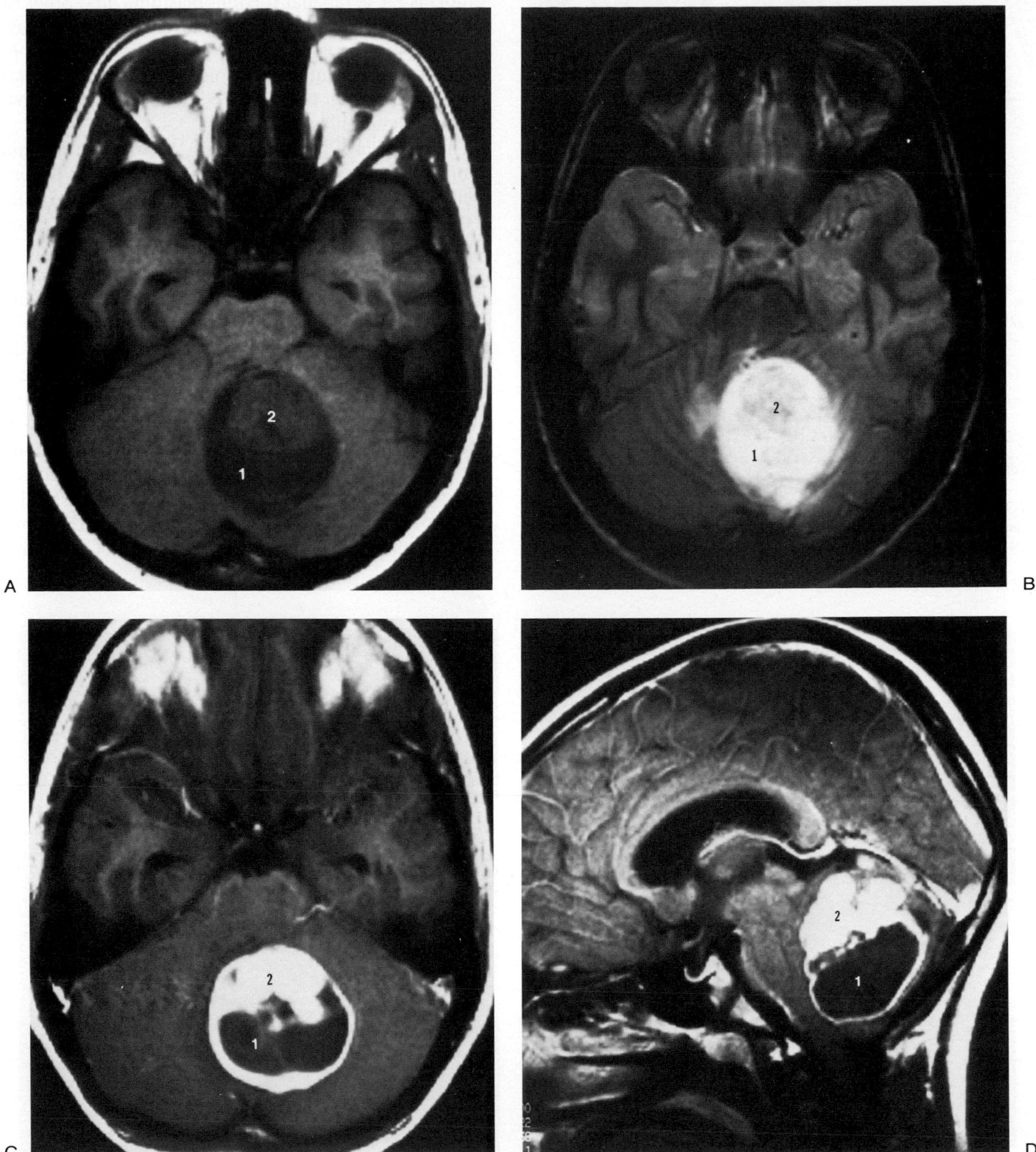

FIG. 68. Pilocytic astrocytoma, cerebellum. **A:** Axial short TR/TE MRI (600/15). **B:** Axial long TR/short TE MRI (3000/45). **C:** Axial short TR/TE MRI (600/22), with contrast enhancement. **D:** Sagittal short TR/TE (600/22), with contrast enhancement. Axial MR images (A–C) show large hemispheric mass which is partly cystic (*1*), but has mural nodule of solid tumor (*2*). Note cystic portion of tumor is higher intensity than normal CSF on long TR/short TE (B) image. Enhancement is noted in solid portion (C,D) and around wall of cyst, indicating tumoral origin of cyst.

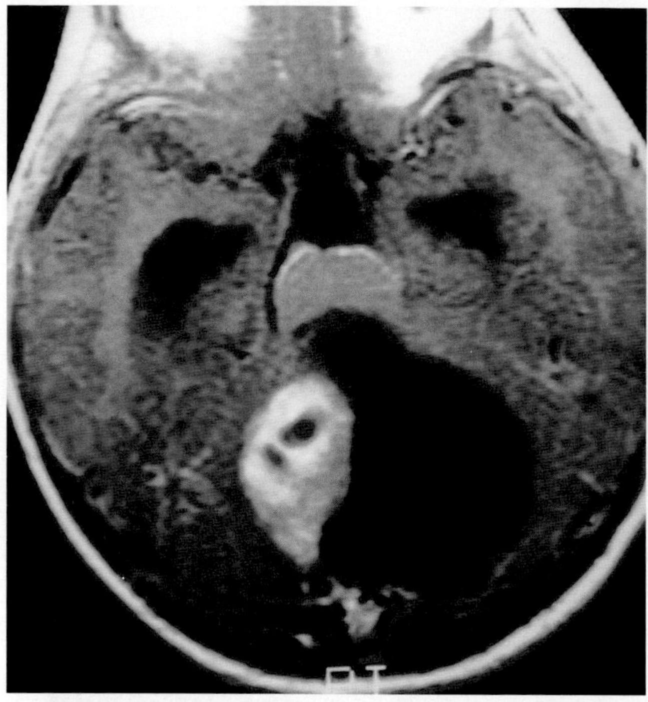

FIG. 69. Cystic pilocytic astrocytoma with nonenhancing cyst. Nodular mass in cerebellar tumor enhances but margin of large cyst does not.

ity due to the capacity of its cells to differentiate along glial or neuronal lines (11,35). The prototype of these tumors is the cerebellar medulloblastoma, and other tumors included within this designation by some authors (35) are ependymoblastoma, cerebral neuroblastoma, pineoblastoma, medulloepithelioma, and the rare variant termed melanotic vermian PNET of infancy (or pigmented medulloblastoma).

The cerebellar PNET makes up 25% of all intracranial tumors in children, second in frequency only to the cerebellar astrocytoma (11). One-half of these present in the first decade, with a peak age of between 5 and 9 years. There is a second late peak of cerebellar PNET at 20–24 years, and, in fact, up to 30% of these tumors occur in adults (11). Cerebellar PNETs can be associated with other tumors, as well as several syndromes (e.g., basal cell-nevus syndrome, Turcot syndrome, ataxia-telangiectasia). It has long been recognized that cerebellar PNET occurs most commonly in the midline, characteristically filling the fourth ventricle, but not infrequently the lesion is situated laterally, even extending into the cerebellopontine angle, in the stereotypical location of the ependymoma. Clinically, cerebellar PNET is highly malignant, with a tendency to invade the leptomeninges and disseminate throughout the CSF with a

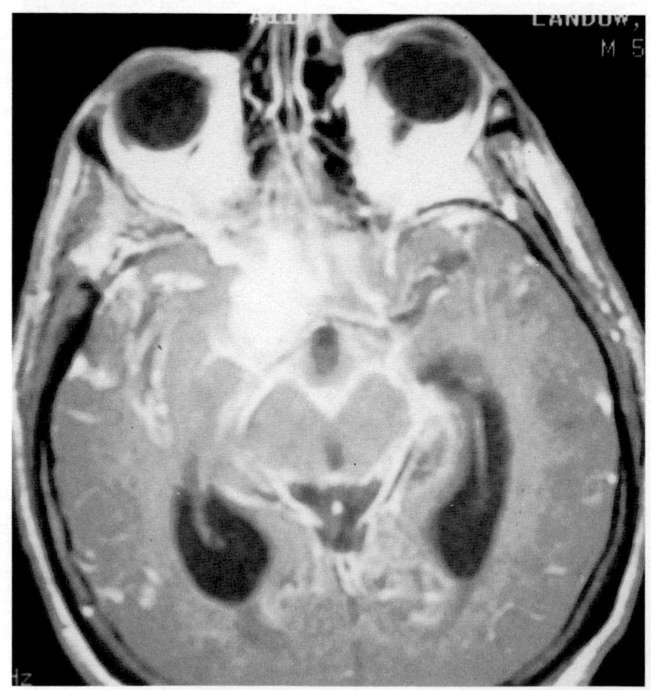

A

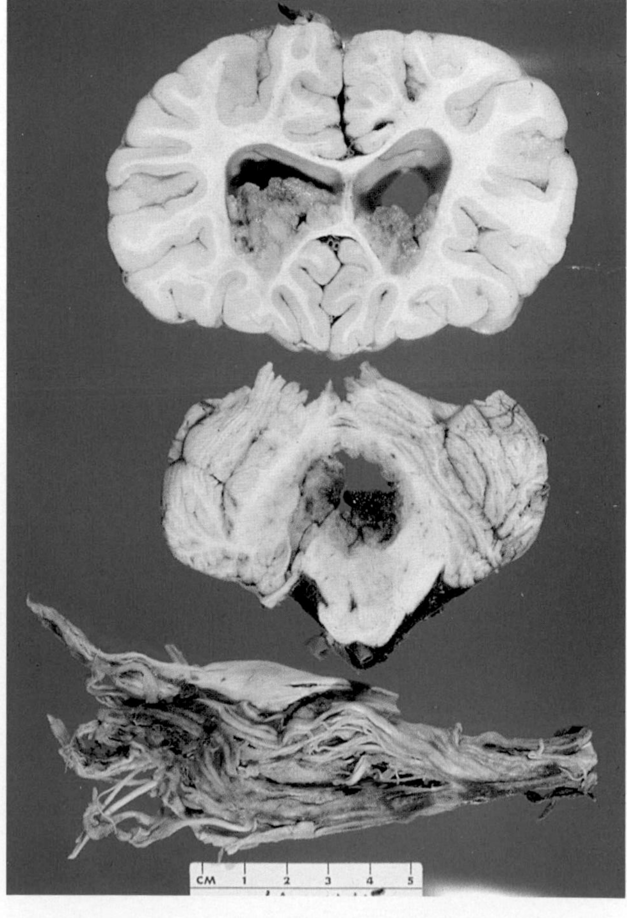

B

FIG. 70. PNET with seeding of subarachnoid space. MRI after i.v. contrast (**A**) shows extensive enhancement of basal cisterns with large subfrontal mass in disseminated PNET. Autopsy specimen of similar case (**B**) demonstrates extensive seeding of lateral and fourth ventricles with tumor, along with metastases involving the cauda equina. (Courtesy of Dr. N. K. Gonatas, Philadelphia, PA.)

remarkably high frequency (Fig. 70). The PNET is the most likely CNS tumor to metastasize outside the nervous system, most commonly to bone and at a rate approaching 5%. Survival rates have been estimated as 40% to 80% at 5 years and 40% to 50% at 10 years (114), although survival is significantly worse for patients whose tumors show necrosis (115). Brain and spinal irradiation lessens the incidence of dissemination.

Gross pathology usually shows the PNET as relatively homogeneous; although masses can show necrosis, cysts and calcification are rare (11). Laterally located masses can evoke a desmoplastic reaction from leptomeningeal invasion, causing a marked proliferation of fibrous connective tissue. The microscopic pathologic description is also pertinent to the signal intensities seen on MR images (Fig. 71). The salient features of cerebellar PNET include a monotonous, hypercellular tumor consisting mainly of small cells having only a minimal rim of cytoplasm (11). The characteristic features of cerebellar PNET on CT are well known: midline, high attenuation, densely enhancing mass with hydrocephalus (116). The MR findings are also somewhat characteristic: midline or paramedian, usually intraventricular tumor masses with relatively homogeneous signal intensity. The signal intensity of PNET on long TR images is nearly isointense to gray matter (Figs. 71 and 72); that is, these lesions are not typically markedly hyperintense. The relative low intensity of PNET can be related to several factors (Table 1), including the marked hypercellularity of the tumor, the high nucleus:cytoplasm ratio exhibited by the tumor cells, intratumoral hemorrhage with associated iron, melanin pigment, or occasionally the desmoplastic fi-

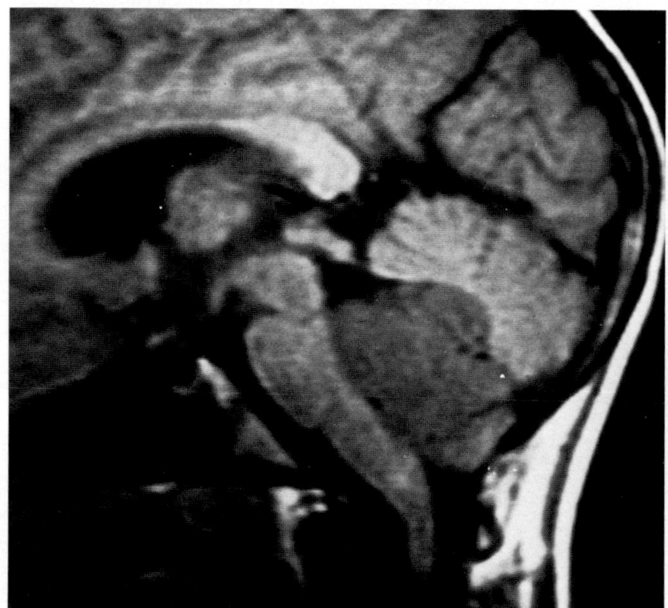
A

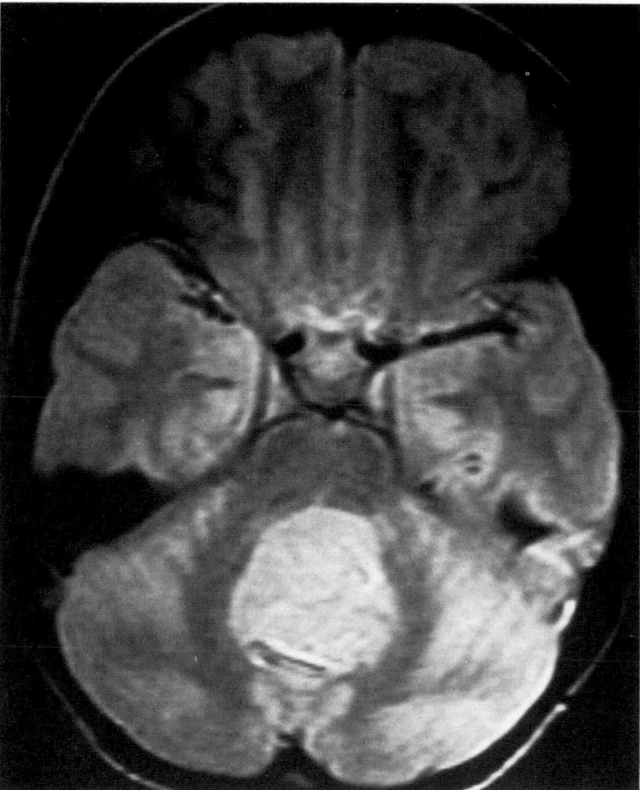
B

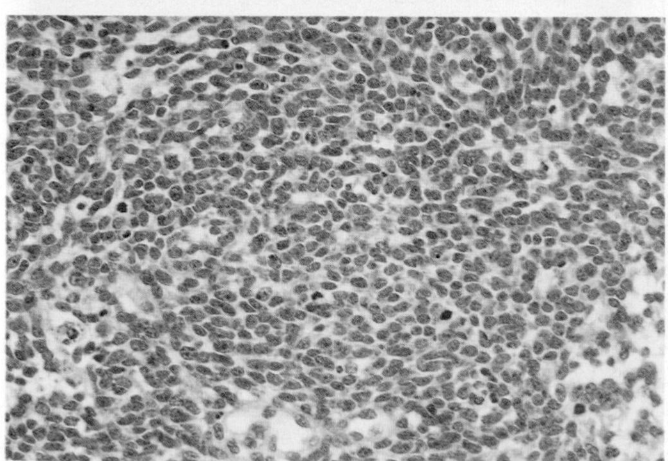
C

FIG. 71. PNET, fourth ventricle, with homogeneous signal intensity. **A:** Sagittal short TR/TE MRI (600/20). **B:** Axial long TR/short TE MRI (2500/20). Large, homogeneous mass fills fourth ventricle and displaces brainstem anteriorly (A). Note only minimal hyperintensity (relative to cortex) on long TR image (B). **C:** Microscopic section of similar PNET. Note densely cellular proliferation of sheets of cells with small dark nuclei and scarce cytoplasm, along with a high mitotic rate. There are occasional rosette formations of nuclei around an amorphous anuclear center.

brocollagenous response elicited by dural invasion. These lesions typically enhance densely after i.v. contrast. It is not uncommon for regions of heterogeneity within these tumors to be identified on MRI (117), including areas of intratumoral hemorrhage, cysts or necrosis (Fig. 72) (53). Since histologic necrosis portends a poorer prognosis, MR features of necrosis may be a useful predictor of outcome (Table 3). "Atypical" features occurred in 47% of cases in one series of CT scans on 30 untreated tumors (118), including lack of contrast enhancement, calcification, cystic or necrotic regions, or eccentric location, all present in approximately 10% of cases. These uncommon findings should also be expected when evaluating these lesions with MR imaging.

One rare supratentorial tumor considered by some as a variant of PNET is also known as cerebral neuroblastoma. These lesions occur in young children, with over 50% found within the first five years of life (11) and 10% within the first year. They are typically seated deeply within the frontoparietal hemisphere, where they are well-defined, solid masses with frequent hemorrhage, necrosis, calcification, and partial cyst formation. These tumors are densely cellular and have extensive regions of intratumoral fibrous connective tissue. Seeding of the CSF is very common. On MRI, this neoplasm is markedly heterogeneous (117,119), with focal regions of low intensity interspersed within higher intensity areas and accompanied by hemorrhagic and cystic zones (Fig. 73) (54). The MR appearance of this aggressive neoplasm in an infant is essentially identical to the rare desmoplastic infantile ganglioglioma (see the section, "Ganglioglioma"), which has a distinctly more favorable prognosis. This lesion should not be confused with the central neurocytoma on imaging, since the cerebral neuroblastoma is parenchymal while the central neurocytoma is always intraventricular.

Ependymoma

Ependymomas are common tumors in children, comprising about 10% of pediatric CNS neoplasms and 5% of all gliomas, regardless of age group (11). Intracranial ependymomas are usually found in children, while intraspinal ependymomas, the most common spinal cord tumor, are more often in adults and characteristically along the filum terminale. Two-thirds of intracranial

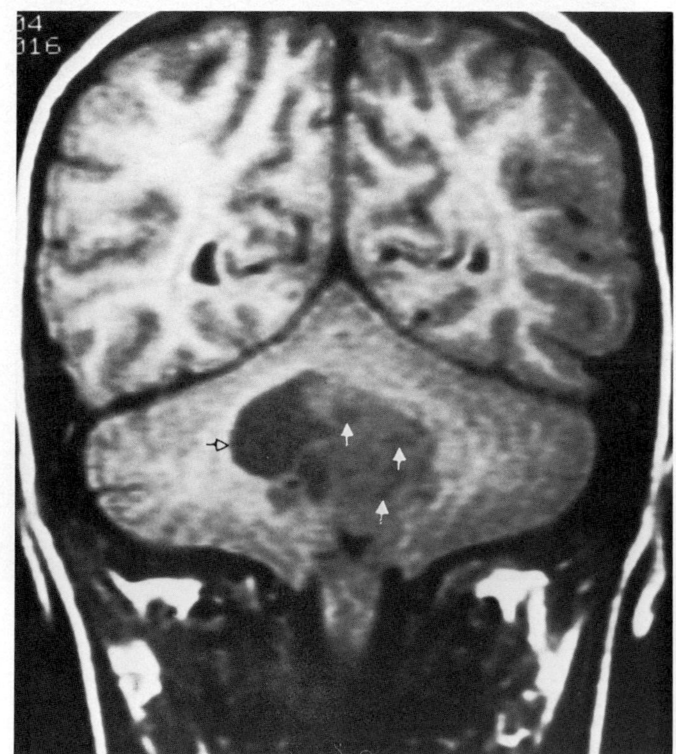

A

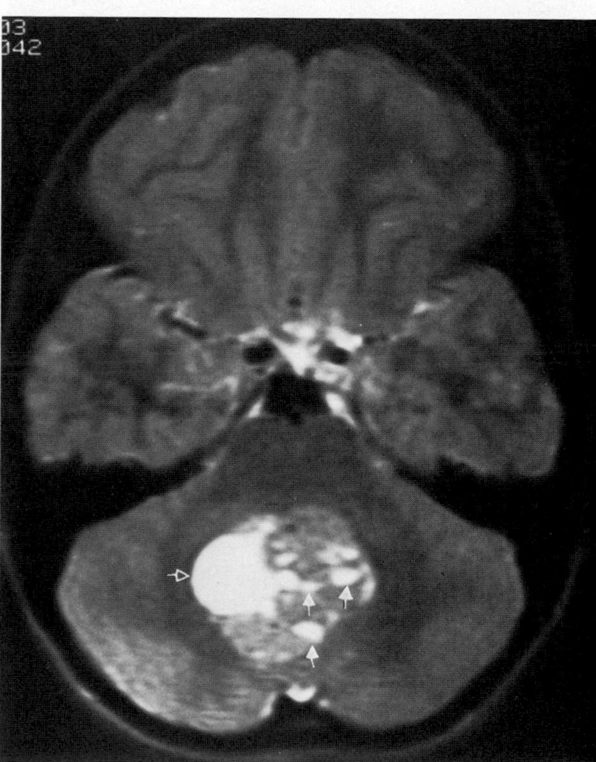

B

FIG. 72. PNET, fourth ventricle, with small areas of cystic necrosis. **A:** Coronal short TR/TE MRI (600/20). **B:** Coronal long TR/TE MRI (2500/80). Midline mass fills fourth ventricle and is associated with a trapped lateral recess of the ventricle (*open arrow*, A,B). The bulk of the mass is of low intensity on long TR/TE image (B), consistent with this tumor's high cellularity and minimal cytoplasm. Note small intratumoral areas of cystic necrosis (*closed arrows*, A,B).

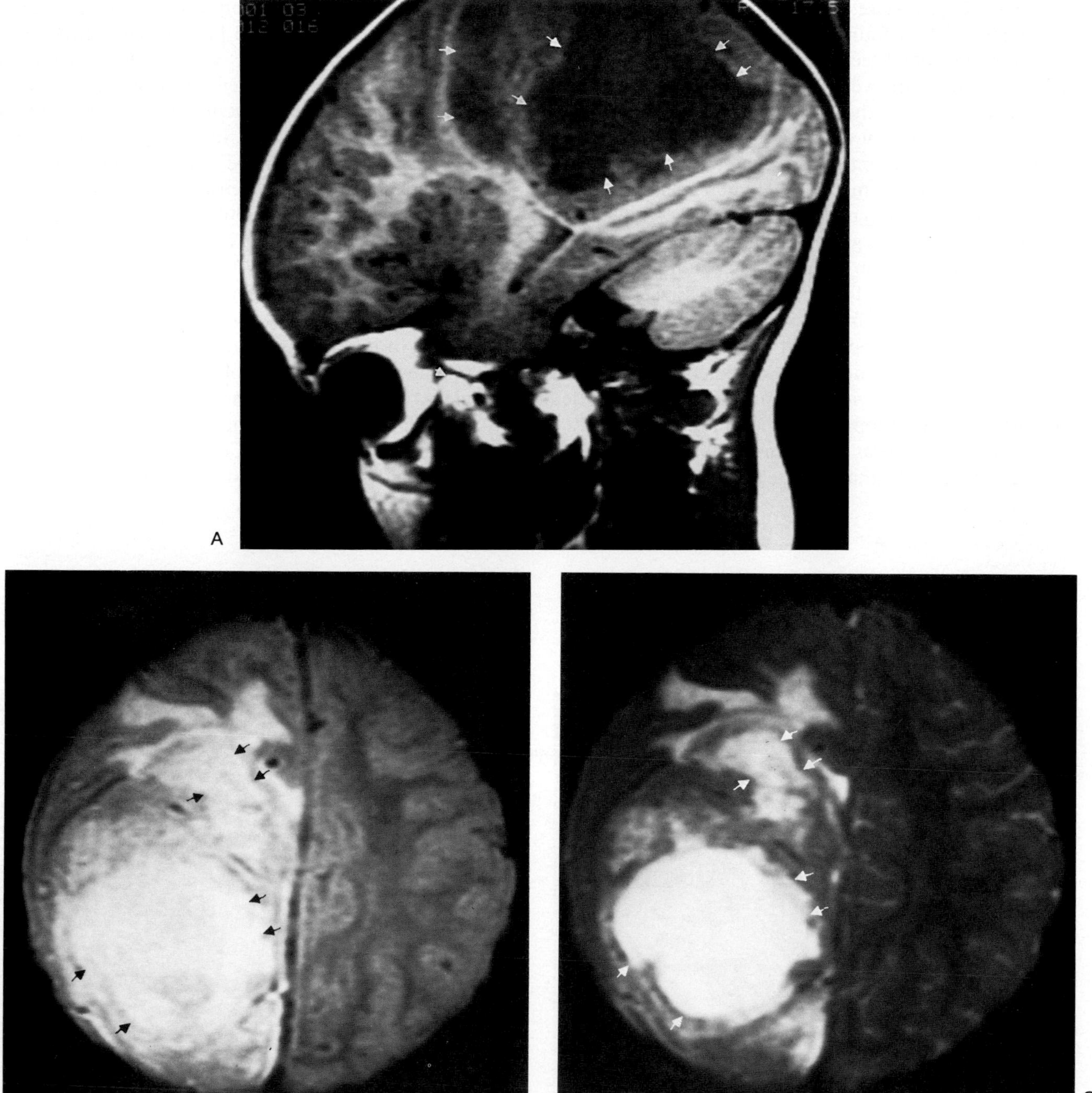

FIG. 73. Supratentorial PNET with massive cystic necrosis. **A:** Sagittal short TR/TE MRI (600/20). **B:** Axial long TR/short TE MRI (3000/30). **C:** Axial long TR/TE MRI (3000/80). Large right hemispheric mass in infant shows marked central necrosis, with necrotic portion of tumor (*arrows*) being hyperintense to CSF on long TR/short TE image (B). This common pattern of tumoral necrosis is probably due to high protein content, and reflects a shortened T1.

ependymomas are located in the infratentorial compartment (120). Their peak incidence is between 10 and 15 years of age (121). The lesions arise from the ependymal surface of the ventricular system, and are most often intimately associated with the fourth ventricle or its outlet foramina. More precisely, they characteristically arise from the floor of the fourth ventricle, tending to fill it or track along its lateral recesses into the cerebellopontine angle. After the fourth ventricle, the next most common location is the body of the lateral ventricle (Fig. 74) (57), although supratentorial ependymomas may less commonly be entirely separate from the ventricular system and center in parenchyma. Parenchymal ependymomas may arise from ependymal cell rests (122). Clinically, ependymomas are slow growing tumors, but they have a variable and often poor prognosis, depending on location and the presence of anaplasia (121). Five-year survival rates have ranged from 15% to 70% (107,121), but recent innovations in microneurosurgery have permitted some tumors to be completely excised. In light of this wide range of reported survival rates, there is still little consensus on the histopathological grading of ependymomas (Fig. 75) (29) as its features relate to prognosis (32). Burger and Scheithauer state that highly cellular lesions, especially those with vascular proliferation and mitoses, are more likely to recur, whereas necrosis within ependymomas is so common that it is of little prognostic value (32).

On gross pathologic examination (11) and on imaging studies (122–124), ependymomas are characteristically partially cystic, calcified, and hemorrhagic. MRI often shows marked heterogeneity within these neoplasms (Figs. 74, 76, and 77), as a reflection of cystic regions, areas of necrosis, acute, subacute, and chronic hemorrhage, and calcification (124). In what pathologists term "classic ependymomas," hypercellular regions are seen on MRI as relatively low intensity on T2-weighted images, as are other hypercellular neoplasms. Ependymoma, like the PNET, often is situated within the ventricle and consequently is frequently associated with hydrocephalus. Ependymomas have a particular tendency to extend through Luschka, Magendie, and then downward through foramen magnum, resulting in caudal tongue-like projections of tumor which compress dorsal and lateral aspects of the upper cervical cord (Fig. 78). This characteristic morphology has been termed the "plastic ependymoma" by Courville and Broussalian (125) and, although estimated to occur in only 10% of

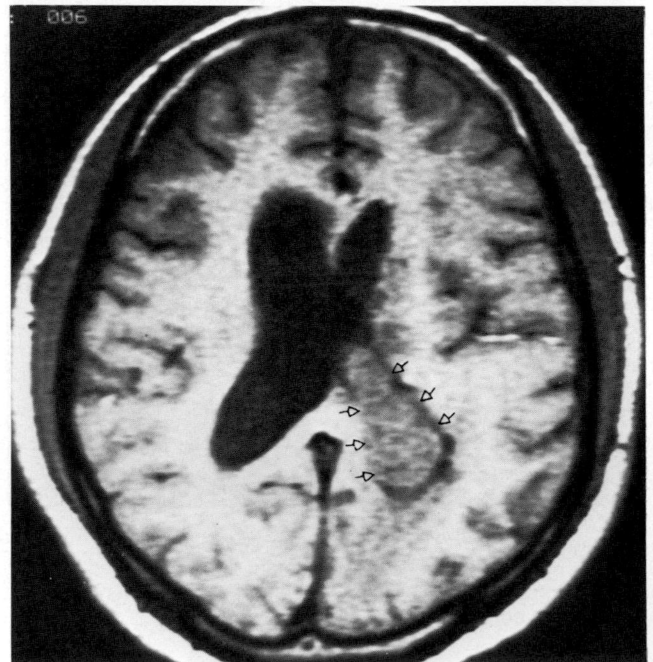

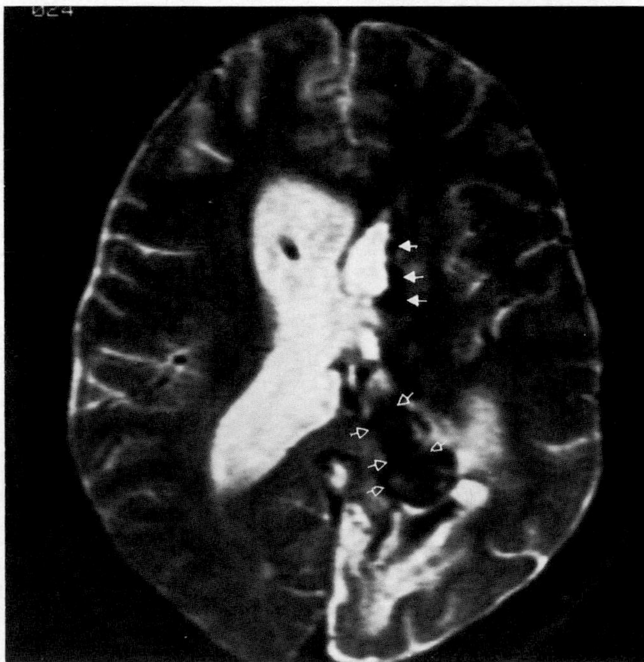

FIG. 74. Ependymoma, lateral ventricle, with hemorrhage. **A:** Short TR/TE MRI (600/20). **B:** Long TR/TE MRI (2500/80). Signal intensity in lateral ventricular ependymoma (*open arrows*) is consistent with extensive intratumoral hemorrhage. Hypointensity along left frontal horn (*closed arrows*, B) indicates ventricular hemosiderosis, due to prior hemorrhage.

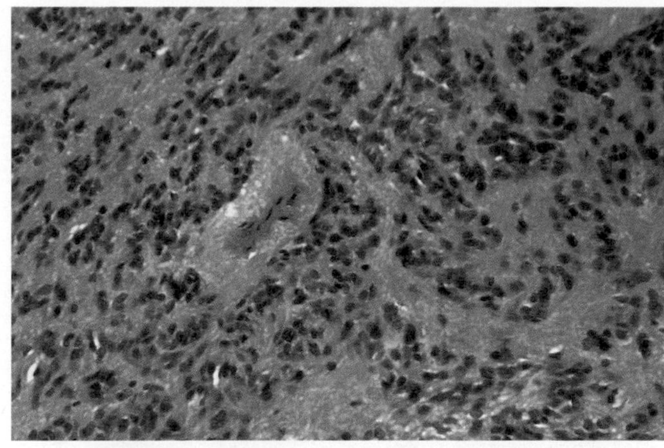

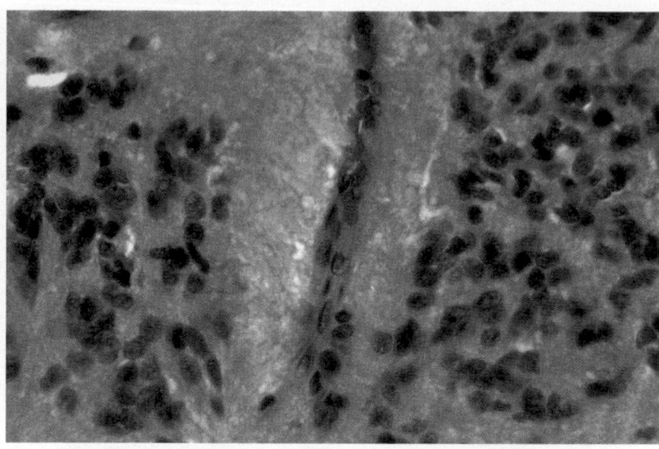

FIG. 75. Ependymoma, microscopic features. Histologic specimen shows cells with small bland nuclei and fibrillary eosinophilic matrix (**A**). Nuclear free areas, especially in perivascular regions, and tapering of fibrillary processes around blood vessels are characteristic features of ependymomas (**B**).

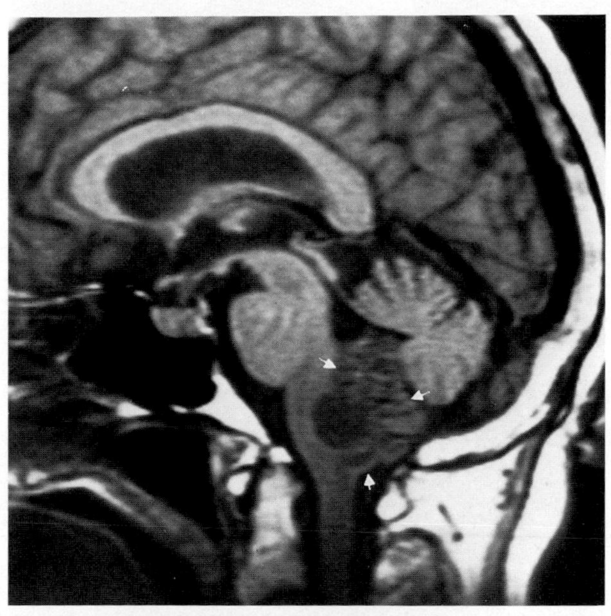

FIG. 76. Ependymoma, fourth ventricle, with marked heterogeneity. **A:** Sagittal short TR/TE MRI (600/20). **B:** Axial short TR/TE MRI (600/20). **C:** Axial long TR/TE MRI (3000/80). Mass (*arrows*) in floor of fourth ventricle shows marked signal heterogeneity, due to intratumoral hemorrhage, necrosis, and dense foci of calcification, and invades dorsal medulla.

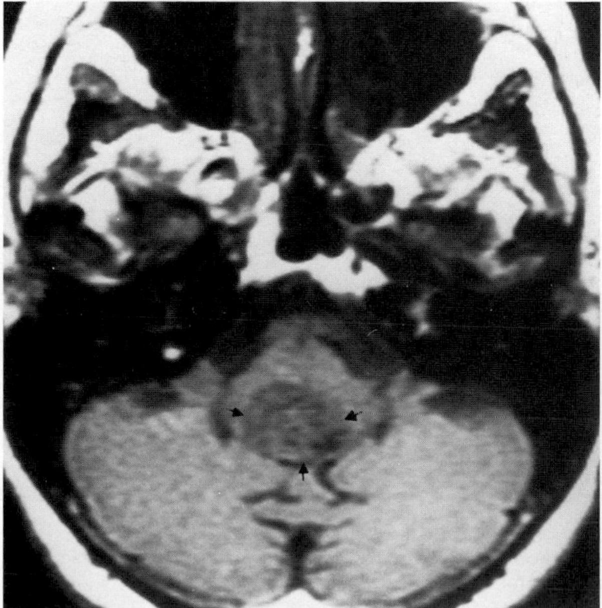

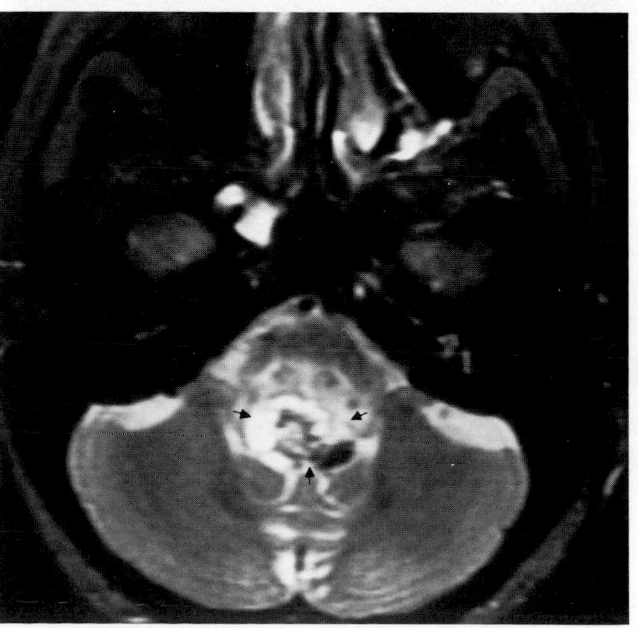

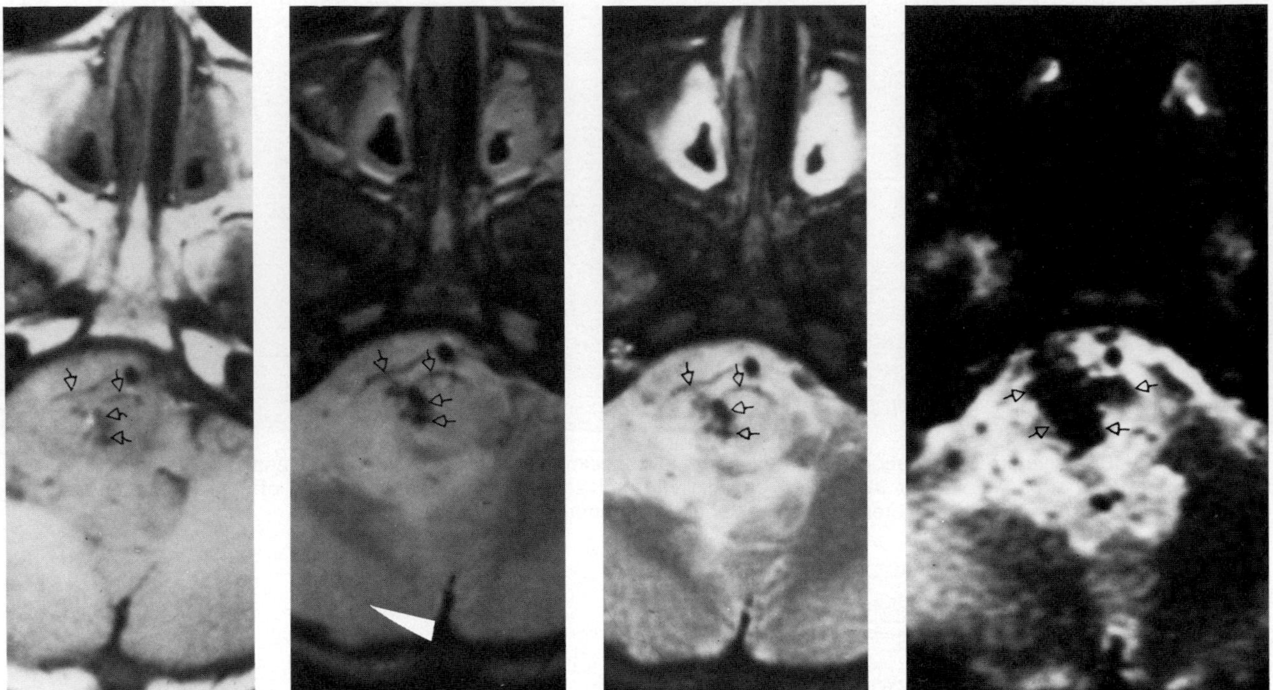

FIG. 77. Ependymoma with dense calcifications. **A:** Short TR/TE MRI (600/20). **B:** Long TR/short TE MRI (2800/30). **C:** Long TR/TE MRI (2800/80). **D:** GRASS gradient-echo MRI for detecting magnetic susceptibility gradients (200/40/10°). Right cerebellopontine angle mass has focal and linear regions of signal void (*arrows*) on spin-echo images (A–C). These regions are more prominent on GRASS scan obtained to emphasize T2*-related signal loss (*arrows*, D) and were due to dense calcification on CT (not shown).

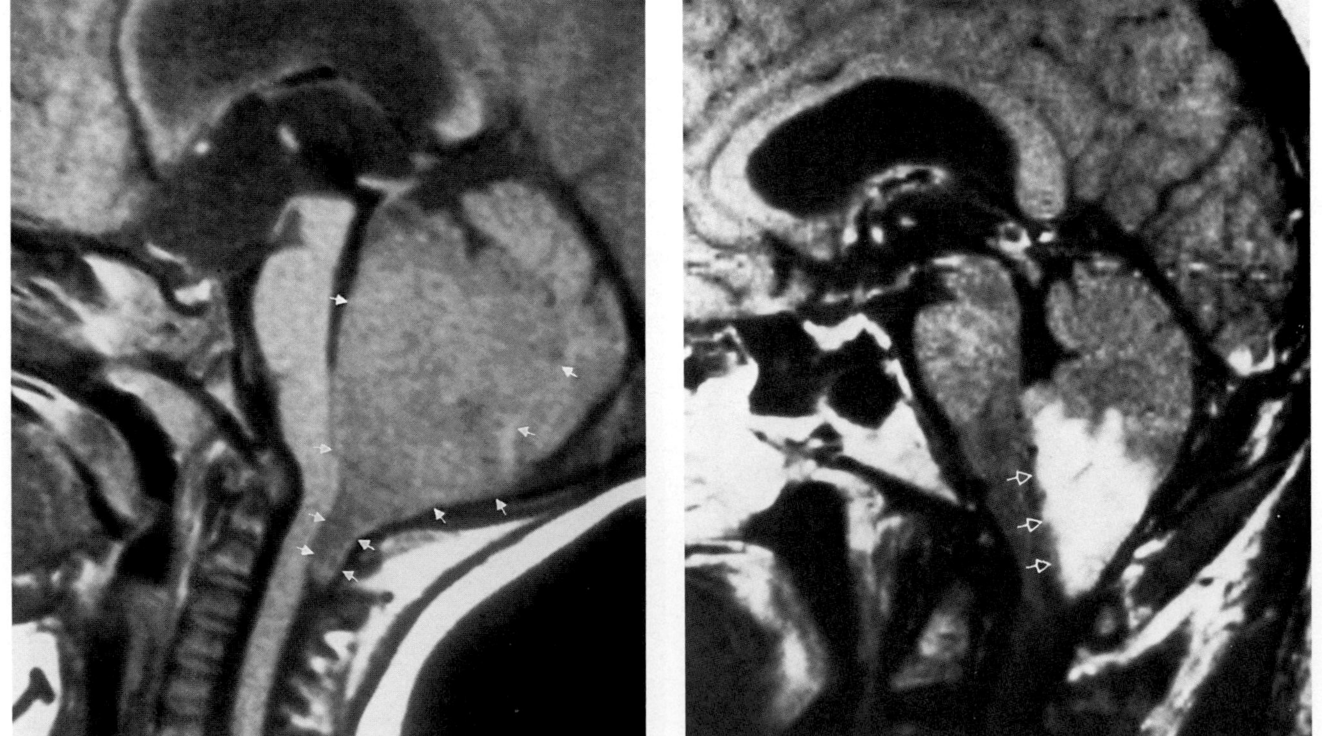

FIG. 78. "Plastic" ependymomas in two patients. **A:** Sagittal short TR/TE MRI (600/20). **B:** Sagittal short TR/TE MRI (600/20), with contrast enhancement. Masses (*arrows*) extend downward through foramen magnum and mimic tonsillar herniation. Note extensive enhancement of second patient's tumor after gadolinium (B).

cases (109), is highly suggestive of the diagnosis. This sign is not, however, specific, since cerebellar astrocytomas (particularly those arising within the vermis) can also extend inferiorly in a similar fashion (Fig. 79), although the broad-based attachment to the floor of the fourth ventricle is not present on pathologic examination (32). MRI gives an unprecedented view of the cervicomedullary junction region and can verify this finding preoperatively. It is said that ependymomas have the highest frequency of calcification of all posterior fossa tumors (45%) (109), so marked hypointensity due to calcification within these masses on gradient echo MR images (Fig. 77) (or demonstration of calcification by CT) would support the diagnosis over PNET, with the caveat that other posterior fossa neoplasms in a child, notably cerebellar astrocytoma, can have calcification. At least partial contrast enhancement occurs in virtually all ependymomas (109), but it is usually notably heterogeneous and irregular (Fig. 80), rather than densely homogeneous, as in most examples of PNET. Seeding of the CSF pathways occurs much less frequently than from PNET, with an estimated incidence of less than 5% (32), but is an important reason for the routine use of i.v. contrast when evaluating these lesions. When CSF dissemination does occur, it is usually found in conjunction with recurrence at the primary site (32). In the child, PNET and cerebellar astrocytoma should be considered in the differential diagnosis of posterior fossa ependymoma, along with choroid plexus tumor, oligodendroglioma, and even meningioma, especially in an older patient or in the presence of neurofibromatosis.

Brainstem Astrocytoma

Astrocytoma of the brainstem comprises approximately 10% of all childhood and adolescent brain tumors. They are characteristically pontine in location [64/72 cases in one series involved the pons (126)], but they also commonly extend to involve the medulla, midbrain, or cerebellum. On pathologic study, the vast majority of brainstem astrocytomas are of the diffuse (infiltrative) type, with a high tendency for anaplasia, necrosis, and hemorrhage (11). A minority (less than 20%) (11) resemble the more benign JPA on histology, particularly bulky lesions that are dorsally exophytic, which have a much better prognosis (127). Spread via the subarachnoid space is not uncommon (128). Because of their typical infiltrative nature and their neuroanatomic location, diffuse brainstem gliomas are usually not surgically resectable, so the mainstay of therapy has been irradiation. Exophytic types are often at least partially resectable. Clinically, the presentation is mainly due to either cranial nerve deficits, long tract signs, gait disturbance, or hydrocephalus (121). A sixth nerve palsy in a child is a relatively common clinical picture for this lesion and should prompt MR studies in all such cases

A 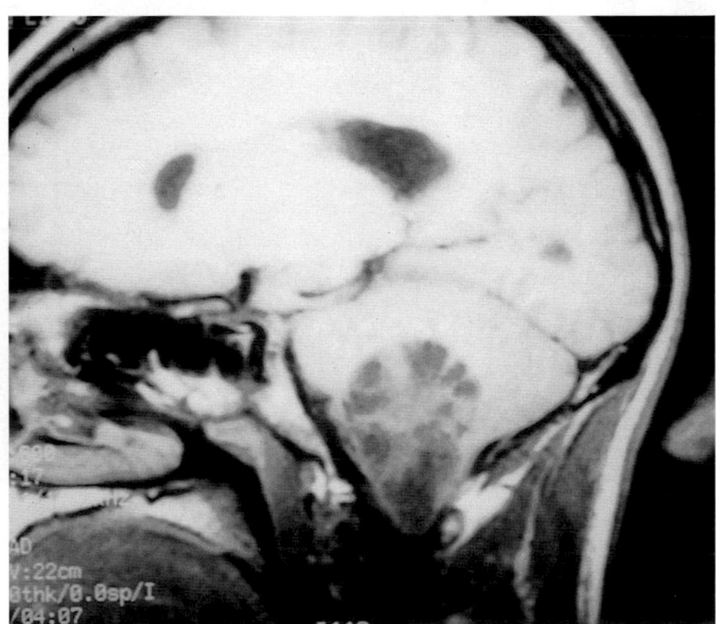

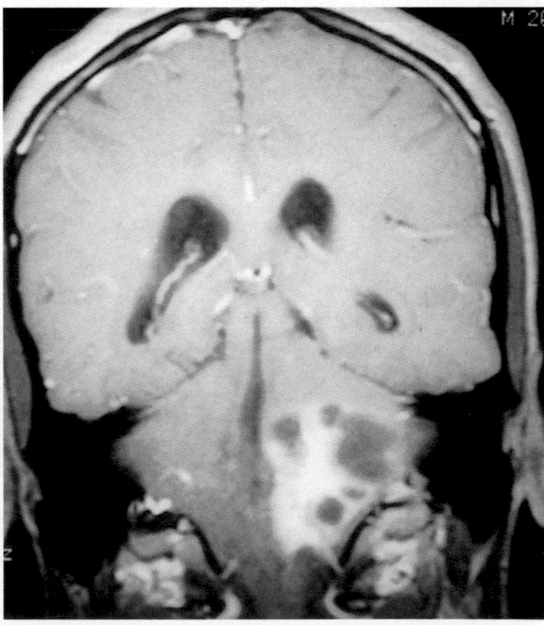 B

FIG. 79. Malignant cystic astrocytoma extending through foramen magnum. Sagittal pre-gadolinium MRI (**A**) heterogeneous, partially cystic mass involving cerebellar tonsil and extending through foramen magnum. After contrast (**B**), extensive irregular enhancement is demonstrated on coronal image.

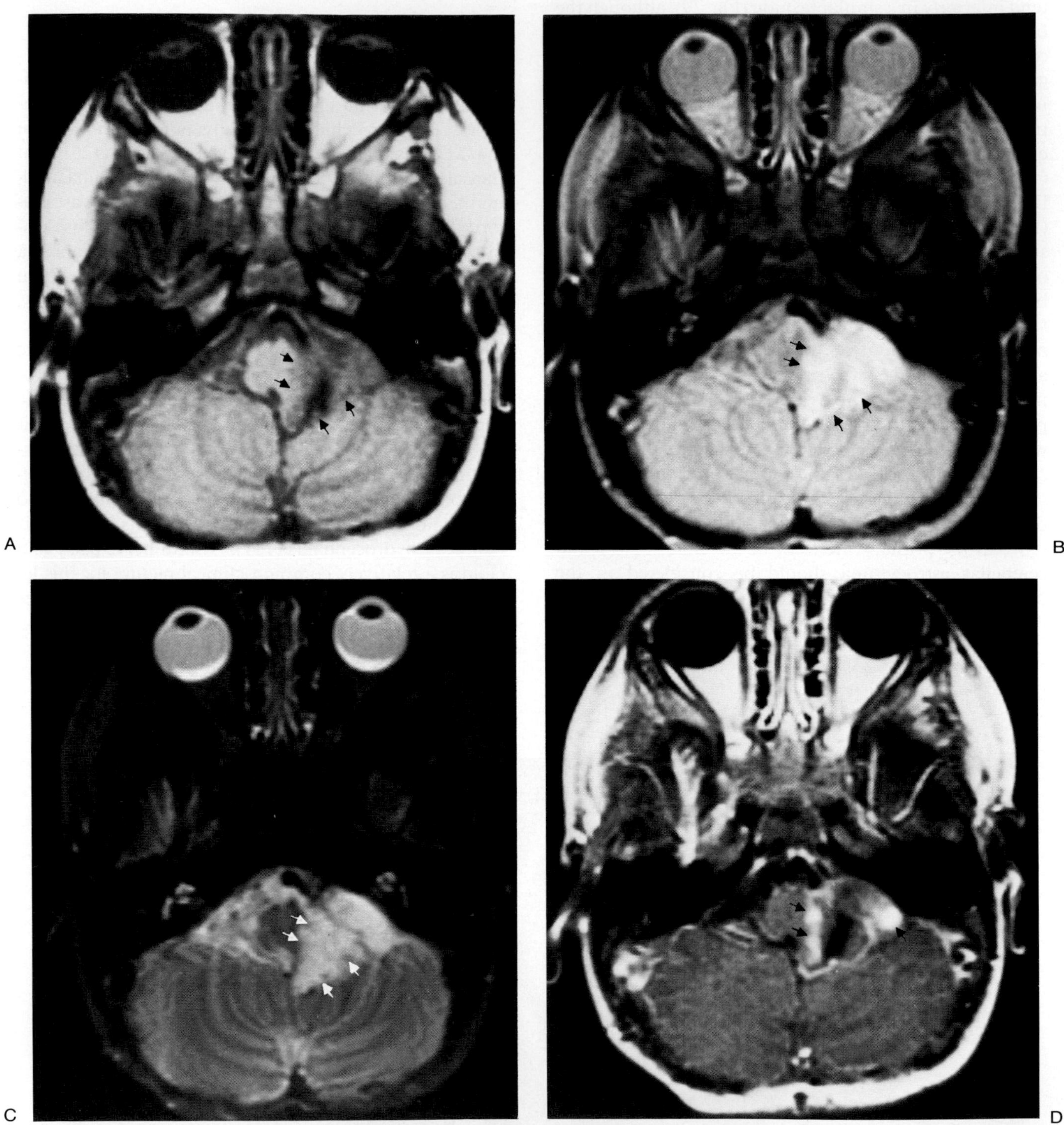

FIG. 80. Ependymoma, foramina of Luschka, with irregular enhancement. **A:** Short TR/TE MRI (600/20). **B:** Long TR/short TE MRI (3000/35). **C:** Long TR/TE MRI (3000/90). **D:** Short TR/TE MRI (800/30), with contrast enhancement. Mass lesion extends laterally out left foramina of Luschka (*arrows*, A–C) and shows partial, irregular enhancement (D) after contrast administration.

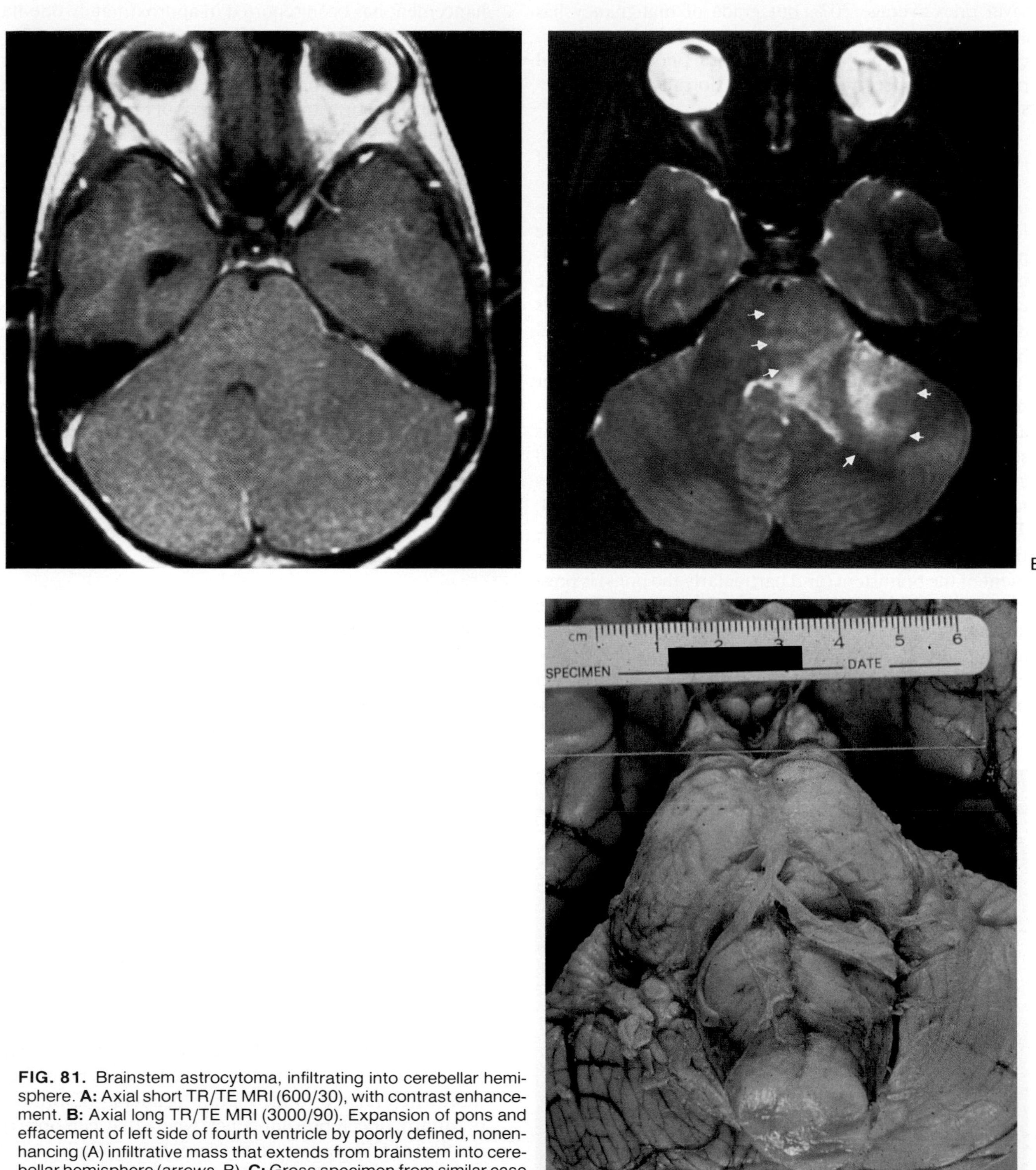

FIG. 81. Brainstem astrocytoma, infiltrating into cerebellar hemisphere. **A:** Axial short TR/TE MRI (600/30), with contrast enhancement. **B:** Axial long TR/TE MRI (3000/90). Expansion of pons and effacement of left side of fourth ventricle by poorly defined, nonenhancing (A) infiltrative mass that extends from brainstem into cerebellar hemisphere (*arrows*, B). **C:** Gross specimen from similar case shows striking enlargement of pons and lower brainstem with basilar artery "encasement." (Courtesy of Dr. N. K. Gonatas, Philadelphia, PA.)

without obvious cause. The prognosis for patients with infiltrative brainstem astrocytoma is dismal; 5-year survival rates average 20%, but grade of malignancy has some influence (126). The long-term survival rates interestingly parallel the percentage of focal pilocytic type and presumably reflect the subgroup of dorsally exophytic lesions previously mentioned (Fig. 67).

The radiographic diagnosis of this ominous lesion, prior to MRI, was often based solely on indirect signs of subtle enlargement or morphologic distortion of the pons on CT (i.e., flattening of the ventral aspect of the fourth ventricle, or a reduction in the diameter of the prepontine cistern). MRI has certainly been more sensitive for the detection of these neoplasms (105). A more complete depiction of the extent of brainstem gliomas is demonstrated on MRI, as one can clearly see intra-axial high intensity going into the cerebellum (Fig. 81) and/or upper-lower brainstem, often in the absence of clear mass effect on the prepontine cistern (Fig. 82). The overall MR imaging appearance of brainstem astrocytoma is somewhat variable, with regard to signal intensity and enhancement with i.v. contrast. Intratumoral heterogeneity is occasionally present, but cysts are not common. There is usually but not always obvious anatomic distortion of the pons morphologically. When gross enlargement of the brainstem (and particularly the pons) is present, the traditional indirect signs of pontine glioma are also seen on MRI, including invagination of the basilar artery (Figs. 81 and 83) and effacement of the prepontine cistern. An undulating ventral border of the brainstem on the sagittal image may be the initial clue to the presence of a mass lesion (Fig. 83), and, when present, significantly limits the differential diagnosis. Contrast enhancement has been reported in approximately one-half of cases (109), and is often focal and nodular (Fig. 83).

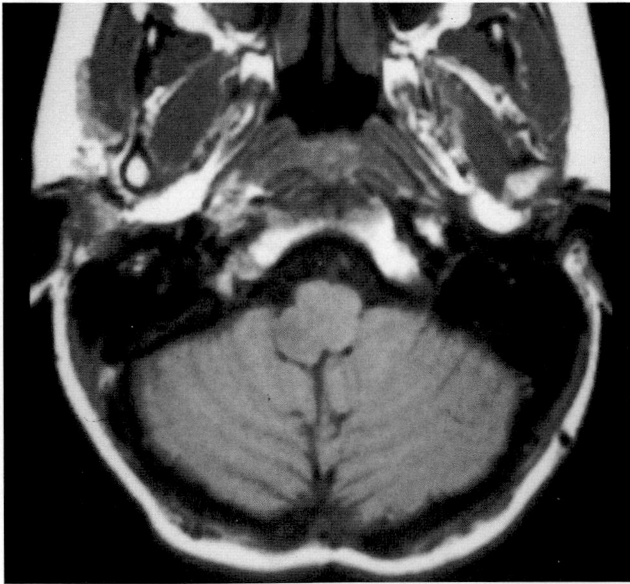

FIG. 82. Brainstem astrocytoma without prepontine cistern effacement. Note marked enlargement of right dorsolateral medulla in region of inferior cerebellar peduncle without significant ventral abnormality.

Aside from detection of the lesion, another goal of imaging is to discriminate between the diffuse astrocytoma and the pilocytic astrocytoma types of brainstem glioma. MRI displays diffuse lesions as poorly defined regions of high intensity on long TR images (Figs. 81 and 83). Pilocytic brainstem gliomas are often better circumscribed, markedly exophytic, and present as cerebellopontine angle lesions. These dorsally exophytic lesions that are often of the pilocytic variety characteristically enhance intensely and are grossly multicystic (Fig. 67). The presence of enhancement alone, however, has not correlated reliably with grade of malignancy. Depending on the geographical region of the world, the major diagnosis to be excluded is tuberculoma or other infectious mass. Other potential causes of abnormal signal intensity in the brainstem of a child or young adult include encephalitis, demyelinating disease (e.g., acute disseminated encephalomyelitis, osmotic demyelination), cavernous angioma or AVM, and rarely infarction. Clinical information often allows clear differentiation between entities on this diverse list.

Subependymoma

Subependymomas are unusual highly differentiated neoplasms which are considered variants of ependymoma, but are actually "mixed" in composition (Fig. 84), consisting of astrocytes and ependymal cells (35). These tumors are sharply demarcated, lobulated, intraventricular masses arising from beneath the ventricular lining. They are noninvasive histologically and usually very benign in clinical course. They are most frequently found at autopsy as incidental findings with no production of symptomatology, even when they are large enough to fill the fourth ventricle, their most common site of occurrence (75%) (129). Subependymomas are usually seen in males, with a mean age of 60 years. This lesion is rarely found in children. They show no tendency to undergo anaplasia or disseminate through the CSF and are one of the only glial tumors that can be truly considered benign. Symptomatic subependymomas are more often related to the septum pellucidum, foramina of Monro, or cerebral aqueduct, where they can obstruct the flow of CSF and cause hydrocephalus. While usually solid and relatively homogeneous, occasionally large subependymomas can show microcystic change, calcification, or hemorrhage. Necrosis is rarely seen on pathology.

The MR diagnosis of subependymoma hinges on its intraventricular location, with the most common site be-

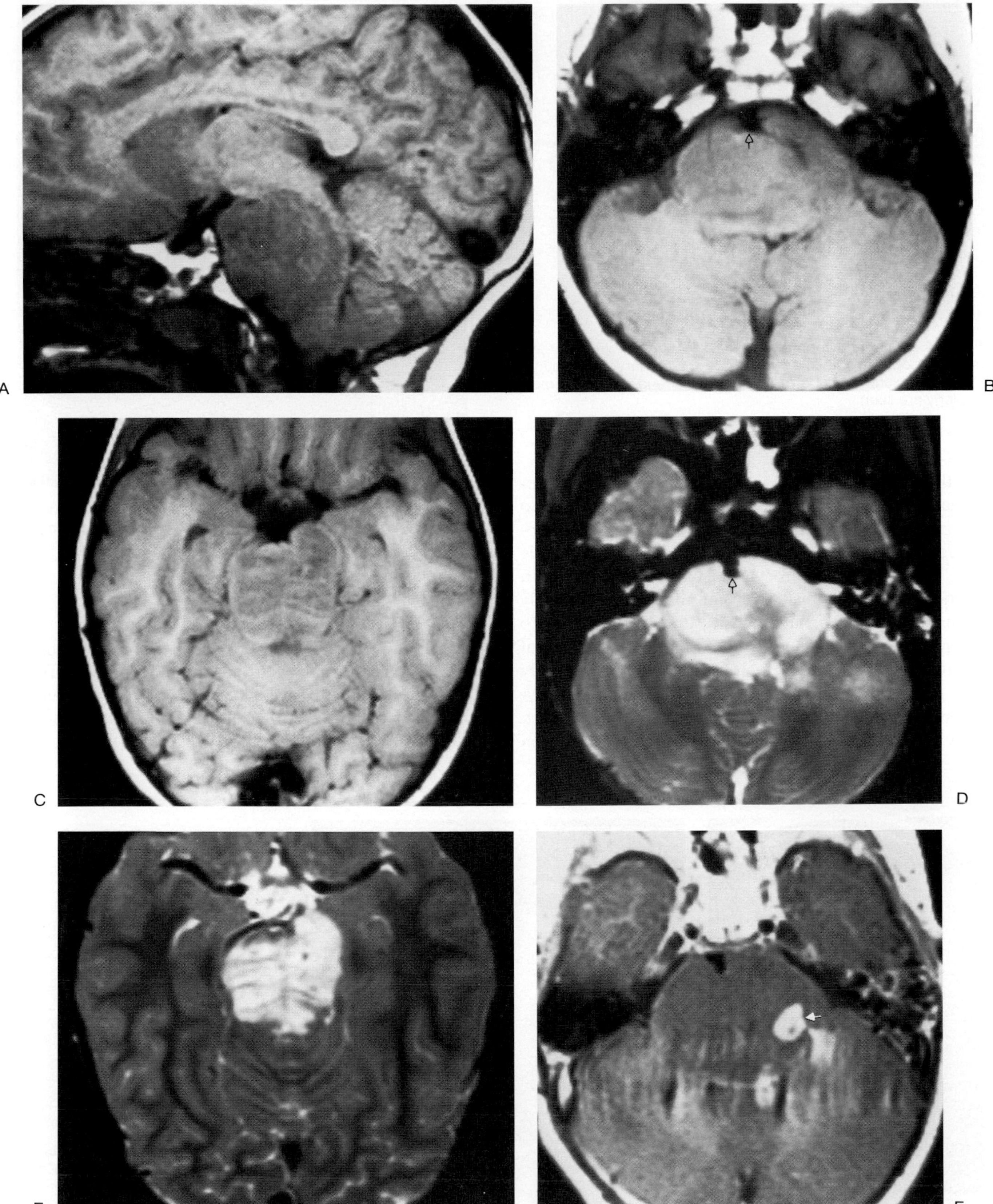

FIG. 83. Brainstem astrocytoma, massive, with nodular enhancement. **A:** Sagittal short TR/TE MRI (600/20). **B,C:** Axial short TR/TE MRI (600/20), inferior to superior. **D,E:** Axial long TR/TE MRI (3000/90), inferior to superior. **F:** Axial short TR/TE MRI (600/11), with contrast enhancement. Massive brainstem astrocytoma extends from midbrain to medulla (A–D), flattens fourth ventricle, and envelops basilar artery (*arrow*, B,D). Although tumor is extensive, only small nodular enhancement is noted after contrast administration (*arrow*, F).

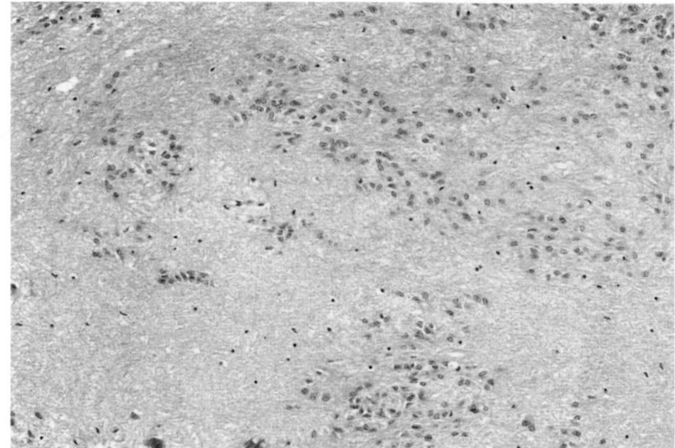

FIG. 84. Subependymoma. Histologic section shows a sparsely cellular neoplasm with low mitotic rate in a fibrillary background. Cells with bland nuclei of both ependymal and astrocytic morphology are seen.

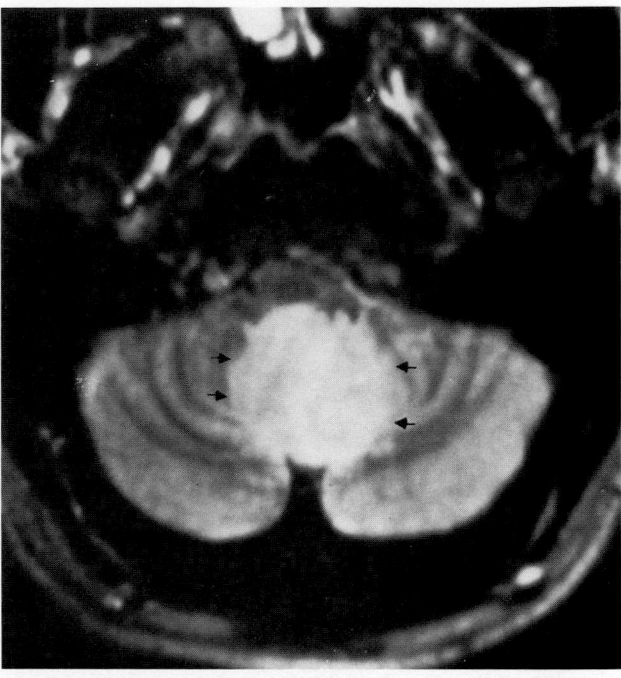

FIG. 85. Subependymoma. Long TR/short TE MRI (2800/30) shows large homogeneous mass (*arrows*) in region of floor of fourth ventricle, in patient complaining of headache. (Courtesy of Dr. Alexander Mark, Washington, D.C.)

ing the fourth ventricle (Fig. 85), typically in an asymptomatic middle-aged or elderly male. Lesions related to the lateral ventricle are usually in contact with the septum pellucidum and, therefore, may be indistinguishable on CT from central neurocytoma, particularly since both of these tumors can calcify. Small masses are relatively homogeneous in signal intensity and hyperintense to brain on long TR images (Fig. 86); large lesions reveal intensities which mirror their pathologic heterogeneity and resemble ependymoma (Fig. 87). The subependymoma typically does not enhance after i.v. contrast, which along with its hyperintensity to gray matter on long TR images, can help distinguish it from many of the other lesions that can occur in similar locations, particularly when related to the lateral ventricle. The differential diagnosis includes central neurocytoma, ependymoma, astrocytoma, oligodendroglioma, intraventricular me-

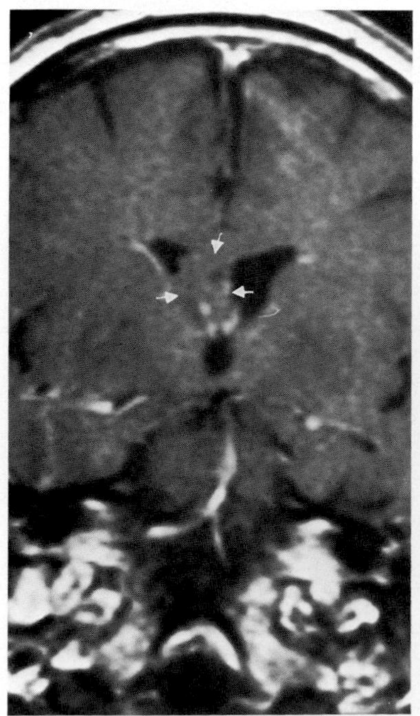

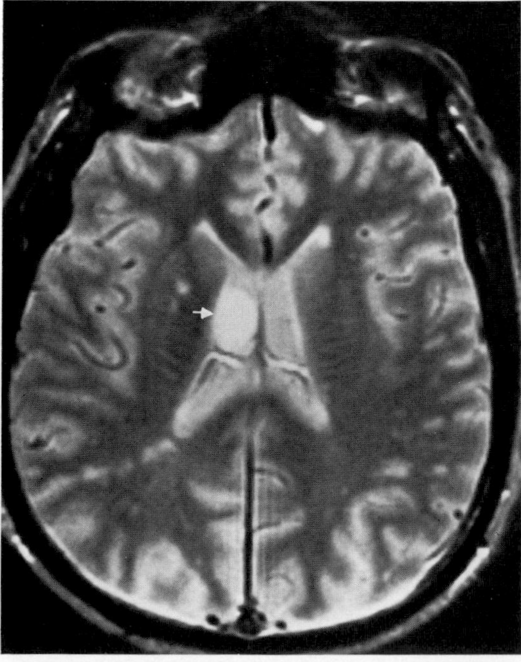

A,B

FIG. 86. Subependymoma, lateral ventricle. **A:** Coronal short TR/TE MRI (600/30), with contrast enhancement. **B:** Axial long TR/short TE MRI (3000/35). Nonenhancing, well-circumscribed mass (*arrows*) related to lateral wall of ventricle and septum pellucidum (A) is homogeneously hyperintense on long TR scan (B).

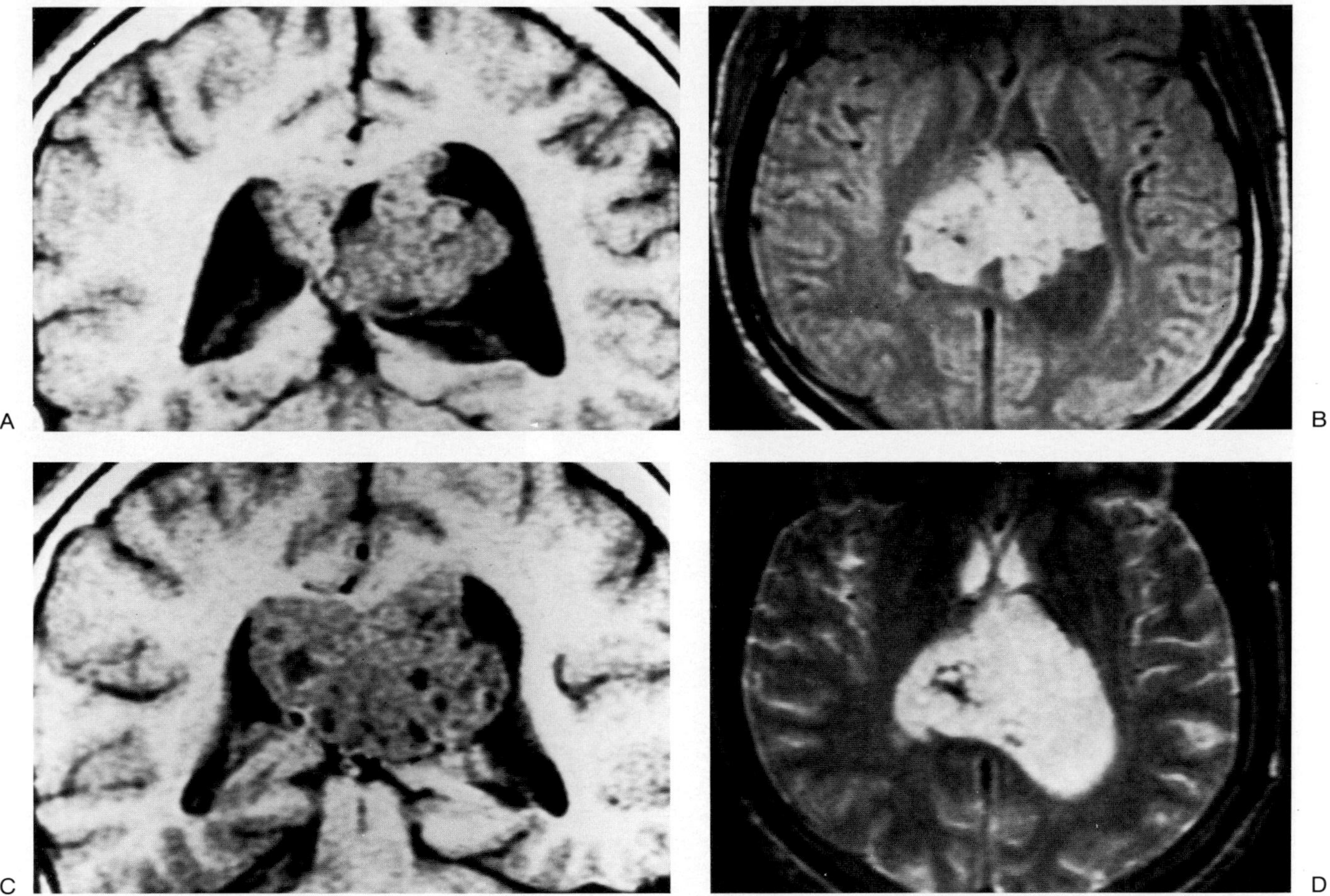

FIG. 87. Large subependymoma with marked heterogeneity. **A:** Coronal short TR/TE MRI (600/20). **B:** Coronal short TR/TE MRI (600/20). **C:** Axial long TR/short TE MRI (2500/20). **D:** Axial long TR/TE MRI (2500/80). Large heterogeneous mass involves septum pellucidum and extends into both lateral ventricles. This lesion is indistinguishable from ependymoma.

ningioma, choroid plexus tumor, as well as subependymal giant cell astrocytoma or gray matter heterotopia.

Dysplastic Cerebellar Gangliocytoma (Lhermitte-Duclos Disease)

The dysplastic gangliocytoma of the cerebellum, or Lhermitte-Duclos disease (130), is seen as a large region, often holohemispheric, of ill-demarcated mass-like thickening of cerebellar folia. It is considered a complex hamartoma or malformation, rather than a true neoplasm (121). The lesion overlaps with gangliocytoma, except that it has more of a malformative appearance than those lesions (32). Although the lesion may present in childhood, it slowly enlarges over time and is usually discovered in adults. MRI signal intensity patterns depict this extremely rare lesion as an intra-axial cerebellar mass on long TR images (131) with enlarged cerebellar folia and heterogeneous hyperintense "stripes" of dystrophic change and CSF (Fig. 88). It has not been reported to demonstrate contrast enhancement.

Hemangioblastomas

Cerebellar hemangioblastoma is a benign neoplasm of uncertain origin, which comprises approximately 7% of posterior fossa tumors in adults (11). It is the most common intra-axial neoplasm of the adult posterior fossa after metastasis. The association between hemangioblastoma and von Hippel-Lindau syndrome has been well documented. The incomplete penetrance of this inherited disease complex (autosomal dominant) makes it difficult to accurately assess the incidence of hemangioblastoma in patients with this syndrome, but it has ranged from 35% to 60% in the literature (132). Of all patients with hemangioblastoma, between 4% and 40% meet criteria for von Hippel-Lindau syndrome (133, 134). These tumors peak in incidence during the fifth and sixth decades, except in von Hippel-Lindau, where they present in younger adults (133). The cerebellum is their most frequent site, but hemangioblastoma can also be found in the area postrema of the medulla or within the spinal cord, particularly in those patients with von

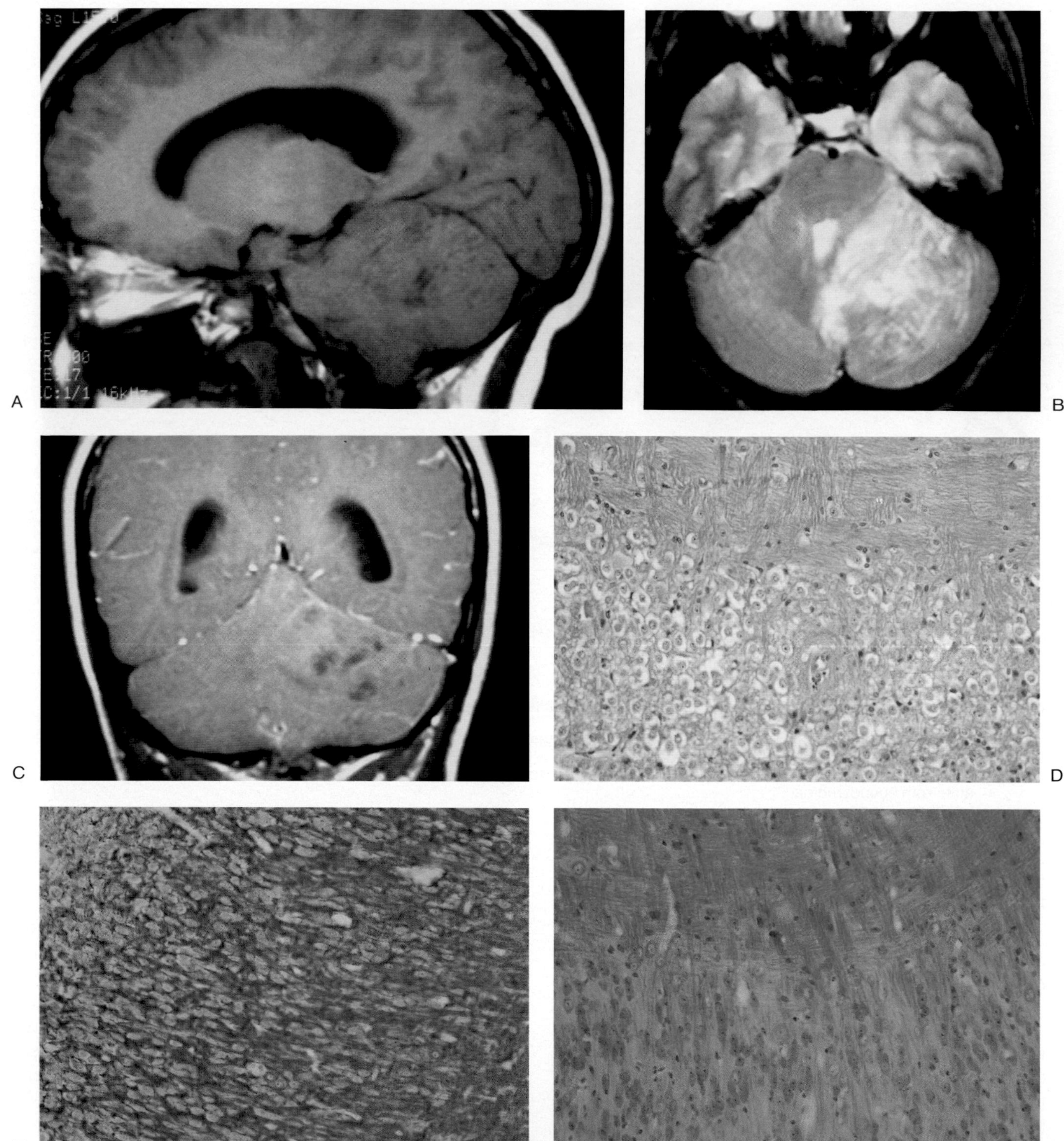

FIG. 88. Lhermitte-Duclos disease (dysplastic gangliocytoma of the cerebellum). **A:** Sagittal T1-weighted MRI. **B:** Axial T2-weighted MRI. **C:** Coronal T1-weighted MRI after i.v. contrast. **D–F:** Microscopic sections from similar case. Large expansile mass occupies most of left cerebellar hemisphere (A,B). Note irregular stripes of alternating low and high intensity (A,B), probably related to abnormal myelination pattern, and lack of enhancement (C). On microscopy, note hamartomatous hypertrophy of the granular layer neurons of cerebellum which acquire superficial resemblance to Purkinje cells (D). Hypertrophied granular cell layer cells are of neuronal origin, expressing positive immunostaining with antibodies against neurofilament (E). Abnormal myelination pattern in superficial layer of cerebellar folia is shown (F) with myelin stain (Luxol fast blue).

Hippel-Lindau. Supratentorial hemangioblastoma is exceptionally rare. Hemangioblastomas are usually solitary lesions; multiplicity is said to occur in 20% of patients with von Hippel-Lindau syndrome and only rarely in otherwise healthy patients. Multiple hemangioblastomas are also more common when they arise within the spinal cord (135).

Gross pathologic examination of hemangioblastomas reveals well-demarcated, (usually) cystic masses with highly vascularized solid nodules within the wall of the cyst (Fig. 89). Aside from the mural nodule, the cyst wall is not involved with tumor but is more often simply gliottic. The solid nidus is superficial and, in fact, virtually always abuts pia mater. Entirely solid hemangioblastomas occur in 30% to 40% of cases (136) and are the most common morphologic type if in the supratentorial compartment. Intratumoral hemorrhage can occur occasionally in association with hemangioblastoma. Microscopically, in distinction from its gross appearance, the tumor is neither encapsulated nor well circumscribed, and it can invade cerebellar parenchyma. The mural nodule is a hypervascular mass of capillaries with intervening benign-appearing neoplastic stroma. The distinction of solid hemangioblastoma from either renal cell carcinoma metastasis, another lesion of concern in von Hippel-Lindau patients, or angioblastic meningioma may at times be extremely difficult on histopathology (121).

Surgical resection is considered curative, but recurrence is common after incomplete excision of the tumor. The rate of recurrence is reduced significantly if the vascular nidus itself is removed, rather than merely the cystic portion (137). In fact, following complete surgical excision, recurrent lesions may actually represent new lesions in patients with von Hippel-Lindau. Therefore, the goals of the preoperative imaging study are severalfold: (i) to make the specific diagnosis of hemangioblastoma, (ii) to correctly identify all of the lesions, and (iii) to delineate the vascular nidus. There can be no question that MRI is the most effective noninvasive imaging modality for accomplishing these goals (134), although it has not been established whether high-resolution contrast-enhanced MRI is as sensitive as angiography for the detection of small lesions.

There are several characteristic findings on MRI (Fig. 90) which, when found in conjunction with each other, are virtually pathognomonic for this lesion and should be sought by the neuroradiologist in the presence of any intra-axial posterior fossa mass in an adult. The most important of these include: (i) the cystic nature of the mass; (ii) a peripheral, pial-based mural nodule of solid tissue which enhances markedly with i.v. contrast; and (iii) large vessels within and/or at the periphery of the mass (Fig. 90). As has been the case in the pathology literature, approximately two-thirds of cerebellar hemangioblastomas are at least partially cystic (134,138). As stated ear-

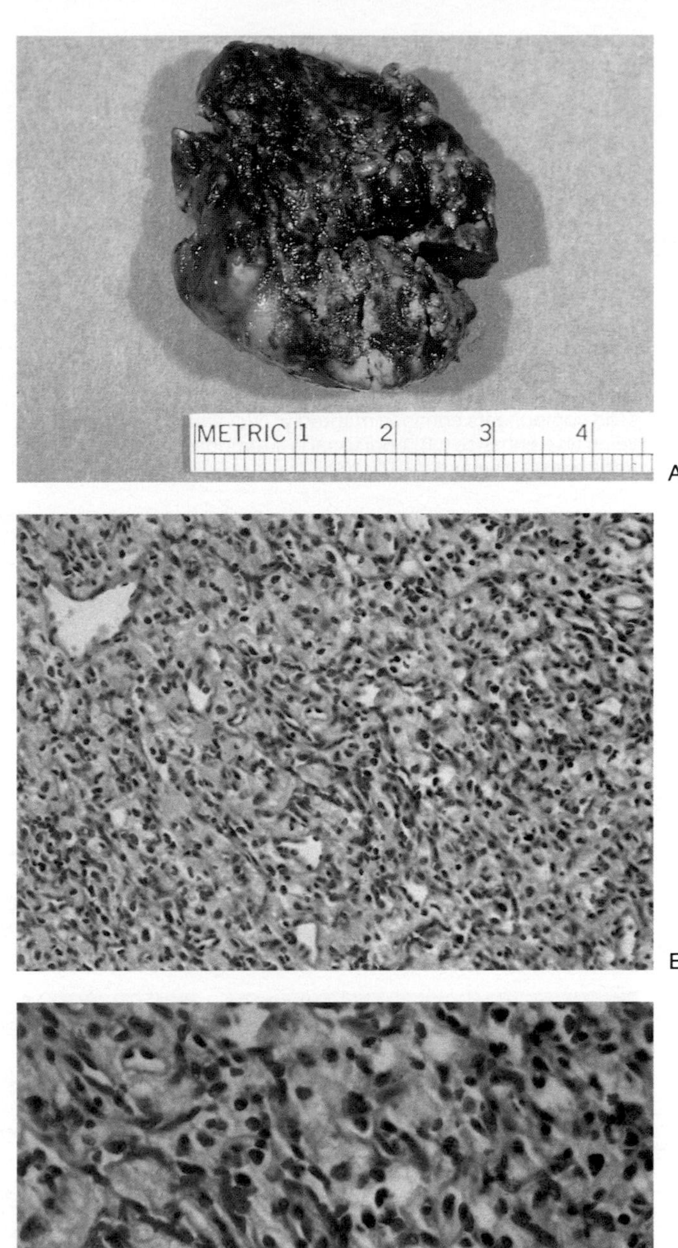

FIG. 89. Hemangioblastoma, gross and histopathologic features. Gross specimen (**A**) shows correlates of heterogeneity seen on MRI, with vascular regions admixed with solid nodular portions of tumor. Histologic examination reveals numerous vascular channels lined by plump endothelial cells. Vascular structures often form large blood-filled cysts (**B**). At higher magnification (**C**), foamy lipid-laden stromal cells with clear cytoplasm are seen admixed with endothelial cells. Red blood cells are present within the lumen of the numerous delicate vascular structures.

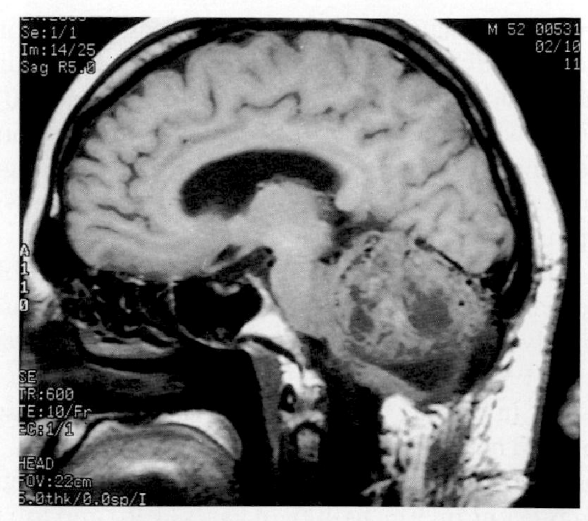

A

FIG. 90. Proteinaceous cyst in extremely vascular hemangioblastoma. Markedly heterogeneous cerebellar mass is seen on sagittal T1-weighted image (**A**), with solid, cystic, and vascular signal intensities. On proton-density-weighted (**B,C**) images, cyst is hyperintense to CSF. T2-weighted images (**D,E**) reveal heterogeneous solid component which is mainly isointense to gray matter. Note large vascular flow voids on all images at periphery of tumor and within solid portion. Edema in left uncus is noted (C,E). After i.v. contrast (**F,G**), solid components enhance markedly; cyst wall shows no enhancement. Large veins also enhance (G). Additional left temporal lobe enhancing hemangioblastoma is also clearly depicted (G).

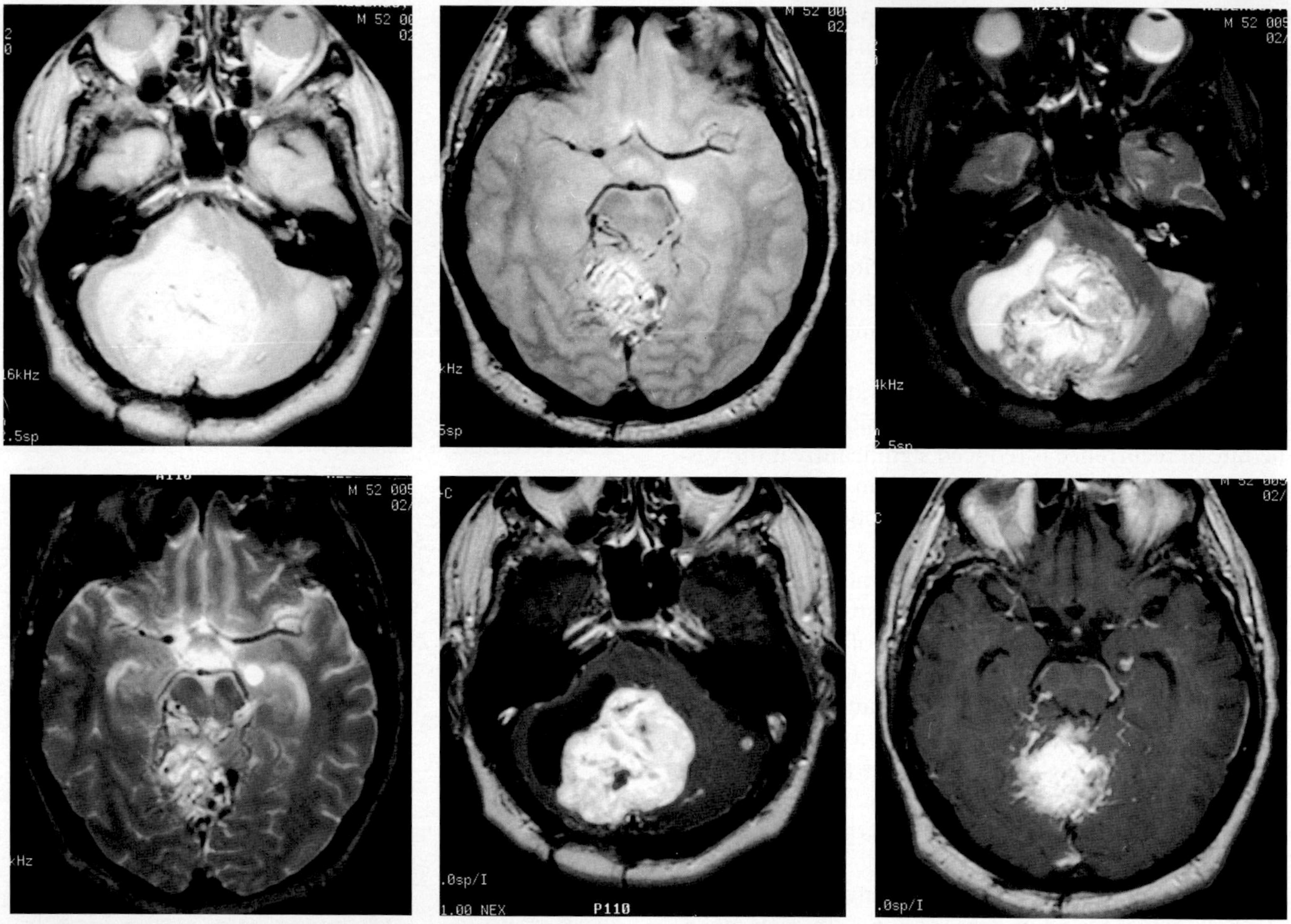

B C,D

E F,G

lier in this chapter, MRI is probably more reliable than CT in defining a cystic lesion, because there are several criteria upon which this assessment is based beyond simple morphology (Table 4). Hemangioblastoma cysts are sharply marginated and have smooth borders. The signal intensity, like all tumor cysts, is somewhat variable (134) and depends greatly on paramagnetic cations, such as those associated with hemorrhage, as well as nonparamagnetic protein concentration. Therefore, these cysts can be isointense to CSF on all spin-echo sequences (an unequivocal finding specific for cyst), but more commonly, their intensity is high relative to CSF on T1-weighted and proton-density-weighted images (Fig. 90). The mural nodule (or solid portion of the tumor) is usually only slightly hyperintense or isointense to gray matter on long TR images (134). More importantly, this portion of the hemangioblastoma always densely enhances with i.v. contrast (Fig. 90) and should abut the pia (Fig. 91). Although not typical, the cyst wall may also enhance, despite being non-neoplastic. The third feature

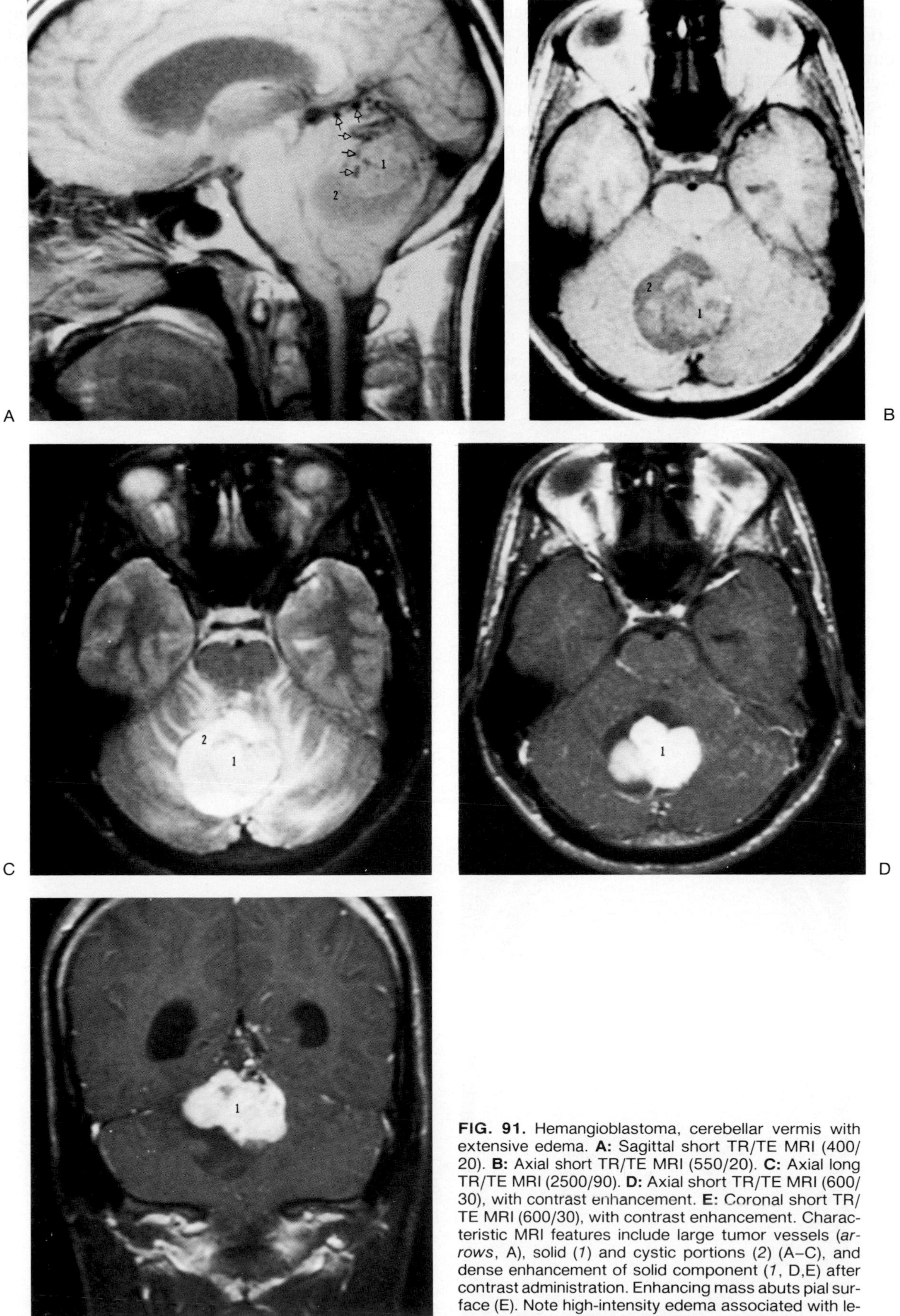

FIG. 91. Hemangioblastoma, cerebellar vermis with extensive edema. **A:** Sagittal short TR/TE MRI (400/20). **B:** Axial short TR/TE MRI (550/20). **C:** Axial long TR/TE MRI (2500/90). **D:** Axial short TR/TE MRI (600/30), with contrast enhancement. **E:** Coronal short TR/TE MRI (600/30), with contrast enhancement. Characteristic MRI features include large tumor vessels (*arrows*, A), solid (*1*) and cystic portions (*2*) (A–C), and dense enhancement of solid component (*1*, D,E) after contrast administration. Enhancing mass abuts pial surface (E). Note high-intensity edema associated with lesion (C) and tonsillar herniation from mass effect (A).

of hemangioblastomas is the presence of large associated vessels (Fig. 91), reported in 13/18 cases by spin-echo MRI, but none by CT in one study (134). Tumor vessels are depicted as serpentine or linear regions of signal void on spin-echo images. Rarely, this finding is ambiguous and gradient-echo imaging or MR angiography is helpful. Associated findings or variations may include hemorrhage (often within the cyst), additional completely solid, enhancing lesions [especially in small or supratentorial hemangioblastomas (139)] (Fig. 92), and syrinx cavities (with medullary or spinal cord lesions) (134). The constellation of MR findings can be nearly identical to that found in glioblastoma or metastases when edema is prominent or when multiple, but the posterior fossa location combined with the clinical information usually facilitate this distinction.

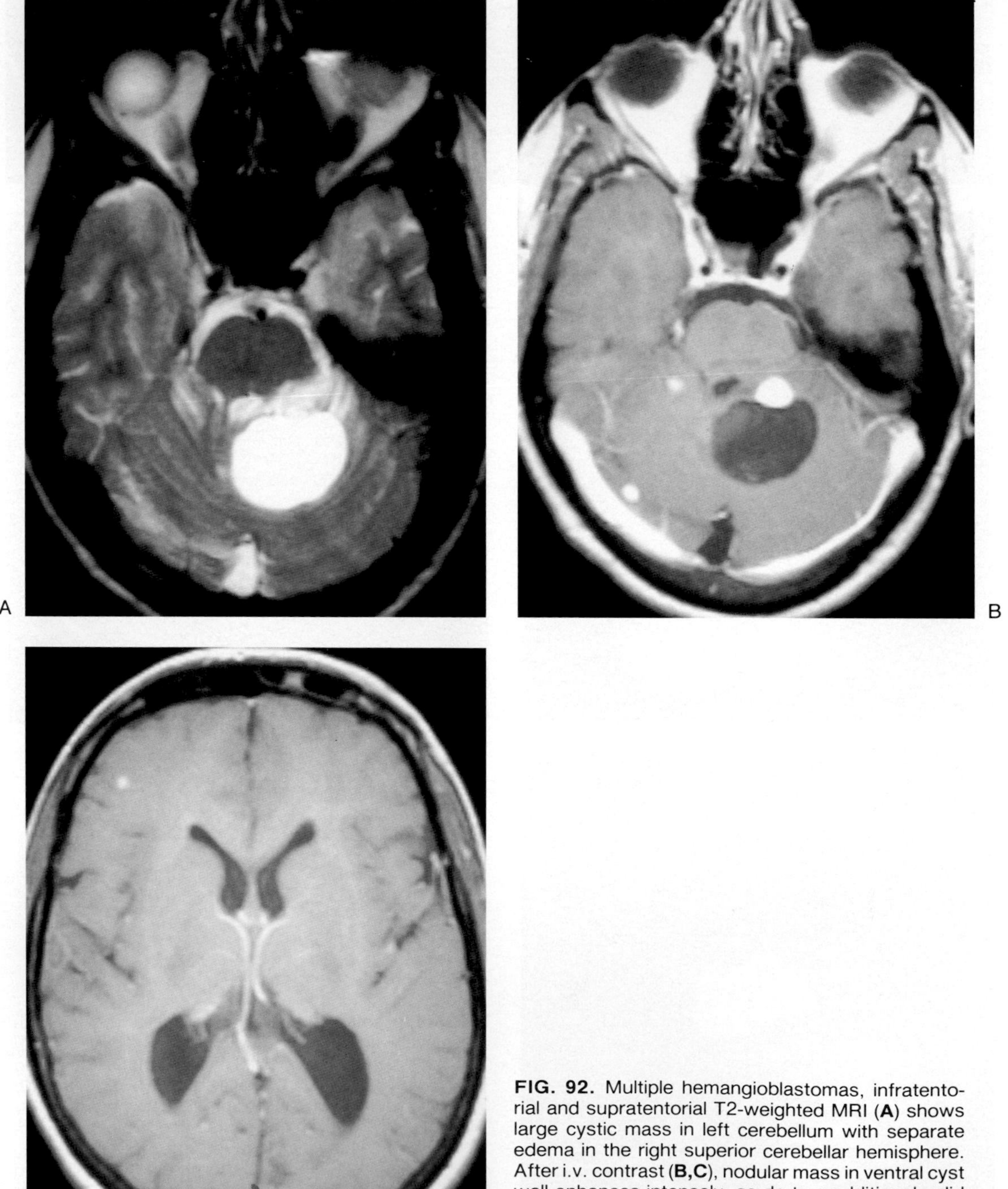

FIG. 92. Multiple hemangioblastomas, infratentorial and supratentorial T2-weighted MRI (**A**) shows large cystic mass in left cerebellum with separate edema in the right superior cerebellar hemisphere. After i.v. contrast (**B,C**), nodular mass in ventral cyst wall enhances intensely, as do two additional solid cerebellar hemangioblastomas. Typically, cyst wall does not enhance (B). Enhancing right frontal hemangioblastoma is also seen (C).

TABLE 12. *Pineal region tumors*

	Germinoma	Teratoma	Pineoblastoma	Pineocytoma	Glioma	Meningioma
Age; sex predilection	Child; male	Child; male	Child; none	Adult; none	Child; none	Adult; none
Pineal vs. parapineal	Pineal	Pineal	Pineal	Pineal	Parapineal (usually)	Parapineal (usually)
Signal intensity (heterogeneous vs. homogeneous)	Homogeneous (but often hemorrhagic)	Strikingly heterogeneous	Homogeneous (unless hemorrhagic)	Variable	Homogeneous (usually)	Homogeneous
Hemorrhage	Common	Typical	Common	Common	Rare	Rare
Calcification	Rare	Typical	Common	Common	Uncommon	Common
Brain edema or invasion	Common	Variable	Common	Uncommon	Primarily midbrain	Occasional
Tendency to metastasize	Yes	Variable	Yes	No	Variable	No
Enhancement	Dense	Variable	Dense	Dense	Variable	Dense
Prognosis	Excellent	Variable	Poor	Variable	Variable	Excellent

PINEAL REGION TUMORS

Pineal gland neoplasms are uncommon tumors, with an estimated incidence of less than 1% of all intracranial tumors (11). The clinical presentation usually develops along one of three scenarios: (i) hydrocephalus, due to aqueductal compression; (ii) Parinaud's syndrome of tectal compression (palsy of upward gaze, dissociation of light and accommodation, and failure of convergence); or (iii) endocrinologic abnormalities (e.g., precocious puberty in males with germ cell tumors) (140). Pineal cysts, on the other hand, are remarkably common as incidental findings. MR imaging has allowed a marked improvement in the preoperative delineation of benign and malignant pineal masses and in distinguishing true pineal masses from parapineal masses impinging into the region of the gland. Pineal region masses display certain imaging characteristics which correspond to their pathology and are often highly suggestive of their specific type (Table 12). Furthermore, the surgical approach of-

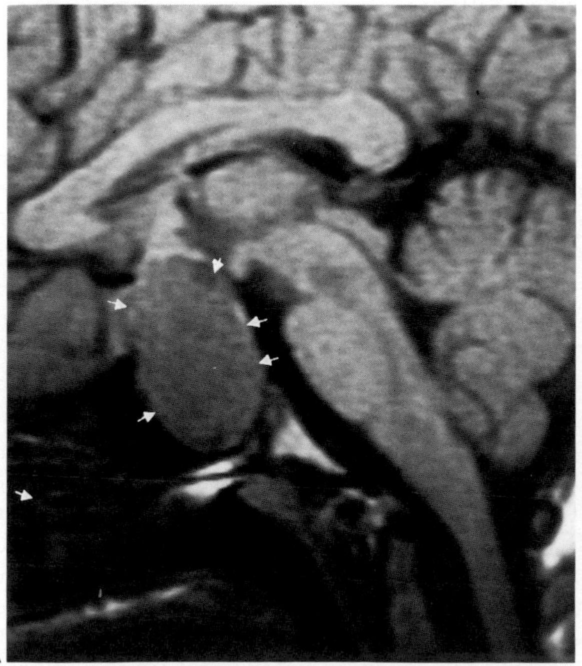

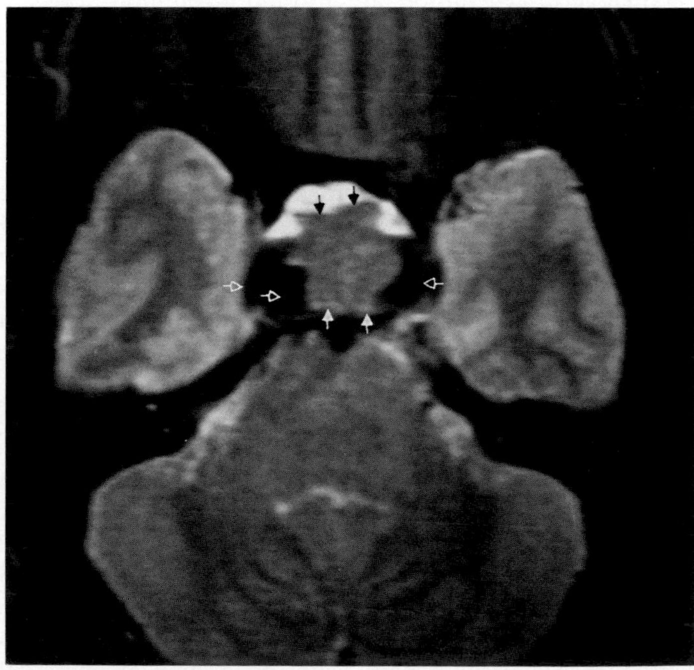

FIG. 93. Suprasellar hemorrhagic germinoma. **A:** Sagittal short TR/TE MRI (600/20). **B:** Axial long TR/TE MRI (2500/80). Intra- and suprasellar mass (*arrows*, A) elevates chiasm and hypothalamus. Note intratumoral hemorrhage on long TR/TE image, with intracellular deoxyhemoglobin (*open arrows*, B) layering posteriorly, in periphery of otherwise homogeneously low-intensity mass (*closed arrows*, B).

ten depends upon the size of the pineal mass and its precise localization relative to the tentorium (141), since the infratentorial approach is considered preferable unless there is a large component extending supratentorially (140). Therefore, neuroimaging can play a significant role in the diagnosis and management of these lesions. These tumors can be divided into two major groups: germ cell tumors, and tumors derived from pineal parenchymal cells. Pineal region glial cell tumors (e.g., astrocytomas or glioblastomas) and meningiomas usually extend from adjacent brainstem or tentorium and only rarely originate from the stroma of the pineal gland itself.

Germ Cell Tumors

Despite the somewhat problematic categorization of pineal tumors, it is well documented that the majority are of germ cell origin. There are several different tumors which constitute the family of germ cell neoplasms, including germinoma, teratoma, embryonal carcinoma, choriocarcinoma, and mixed types (11). Germ cell tumors of the CNS generally develop in the midline, most frequently in the pineal region, followed by the suprasellar area (Fig. 93) and the fourth ventricle. Laterally situated basal ganglionic germ cell tumors are less common. Germinomas are the most common type of germ cell tumor, and also are the most common pineal mass (11,141,142). There is a striking male predominance—over 90% of patients with pineal germinoma are male (11). It is not clear why this statistic does not apply to suprasellar germinomas, although other (ganglionic) intracranial germ cell tumors are also more common in males. Several studies have documented another peculiar and unexplained feature of these tumors—there is a much higher incidence in Japan. The pineal germinoma peaks in incidence at puberty, and the great majority of patients are in their first three decades of life. They are also associated with the development of precocious puberty in males (143), but the precise explanation for this remains elusive. Although these tumors are highly prone to seed the subarachnoid space and invade adjacent brain parenchyma, they are markedly radiosensitive and demonstrate good survival rates, even in the presence of widely disseminated metastases (144). Intratumoral hemorrhage is a relatively frequent pathologic finding (11). The second most common pineal germ cell tumor is a teratoma. These neoplasms have a wide variation in their degree of histologic maturity and consequently demonstrate a variable biological behavior and clinical course. They usually occur in an earlier age group than germinoma, with most seen in the first decade of life. Since these lesions are derived from all three germinal layers, they can contain hair, teeth, bone, and fat on pathologic examination (11). They are virtually always partially cystic and commonly hemorrhagic (11). Embryonal carcinoma and choriocarcinoma are much less common, have worse prognoses owing to their higher degree of malignancy, and are very frequently hemorrhagic.

The imaging features of germ cell tumors of the pineal region have been described in several reports using CT (142,145,146) and MRI (147,148). Pineal germinomas are well circumscribed, relatively homogeneous lesions which are not separable from the pineal body itself. Germinomas are typically low intensity (i.e., isointense to gray matter) on T2-weighted images (Fig. 94) (147). Intratumoral hemorrhage may be seen in these lesions, which have a propensity to invade the adjacent brain, causing edema (Fig. 94), and spread via the subarachnoid space (Fig. 95). Germinomas and their metastases enhance markedly and homogeneously after i.v. contrast administration (Fig. 94), so contrast should be given in all patients suspected of harboring these tumors. Pineal germinomas do not calcify, nor do they contain cysts, features which differ from those described for germinomas arising in the basal ganglia (149). Teratomas of the pineal are strikingly heterogeneous (Fig. 96), owing to the presence of intratumoral blood, fat, and virtually always identifiable cysts (11,146). Teratomas often have dense calcification or bone within them, as well. Enhancement of teratomas is variable. The presence of premature calcification in the pineal body itself has been stressed in the CT literature as being extraordinarily common with pineal germinomas (150), but it is not a universal finding (142) and, therefore, need not be sought with supplemental CT after the identification of the mass by MRI.

Pineal Cell Tumors

Pineoblastoma and pineocytoma are each less common than either germinoma or teratoma. These lesions do not exhibit a striking gender predilection. These tumors arise from the neuroepithelial cells of the gland itself, and although considered as very different entities, they often coexist within the same neoplasm or in a transitional form (35). Both tumors may contain melanin (151). Pineoblastoma is a highly cellular tumor composed of poorly differentiated, immature cells with very scant cytoplasm. It often shows focal hemorrhage and microscopic necrosis. This tumor is classified by Rorke as one of the primitive neuroectodermal tumors (PNET), since it appears histopathologically identical to other primitive, undifferentiated neoplasms (e.g., cerebellar medulloblastoma) and exhibits similar biological behavior. Pineoblastomas tend to disseminate early through the subarachnoid pathways, with leptomeningeal and subependymal seeding often found at the time of initial diagnosis. The prognosis in children with this

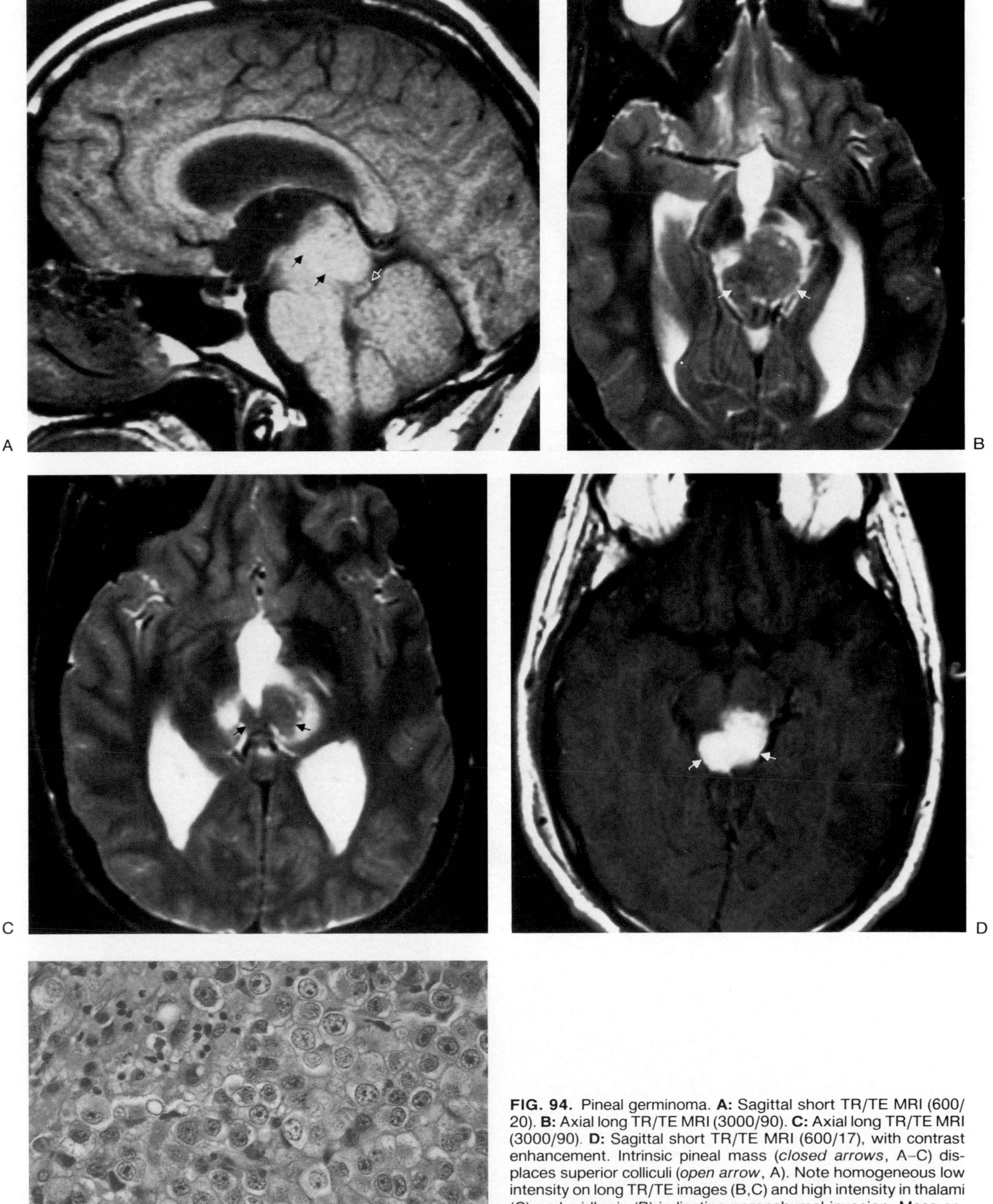

FIG. 94. Pineal germinoma. **A:** Sagittal short TR/TE MRI (600/20). **B:** Axial long TR/TE MRI (3000/90). **C:** Axial long TR/TE MRI (3000/90). **D:** Sagittal short TR/TE MRI (600/17), with contrast enhancement. Intrinsic pineal mass (*closed arrows*, A–C) displaces superior colliculi (*open arrow*, A). Note homogeneous low intensity on long TR/TE images (B,C) and high intensity in thalami (C) and midbrain (B) indicating parenchymal invasion. Mass enhances diffusely (*arrows*, D) after contrast administration. **E:** Histologic specimen of germinoma exhibits large polygonal cells with distinct boundaries and large spherical nuclei containing nucleoli, admixed with small mature lymphocytes.

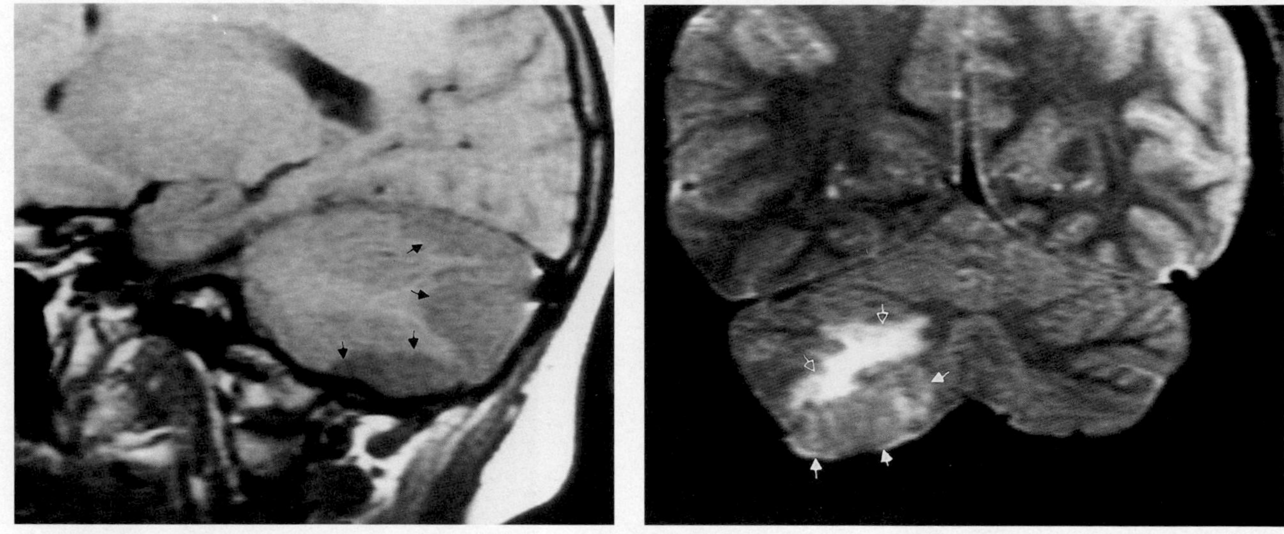

FIG. 95. Metastases from pineal germinoma. **A:** Sagittal short TR/TE MRI (600/20). **B:** Coronal long TR/TE MRI (2500/80). Large, extra-axial masses along cerebellar hemisphere (*closed arrows*, A,B) represent subarachnoidal metastases from pineal germinoma. Metastases are of low intensity on long TR/TE image (B) and are associated with high intensity in adjacent parenchyma (*open arrows*, B).

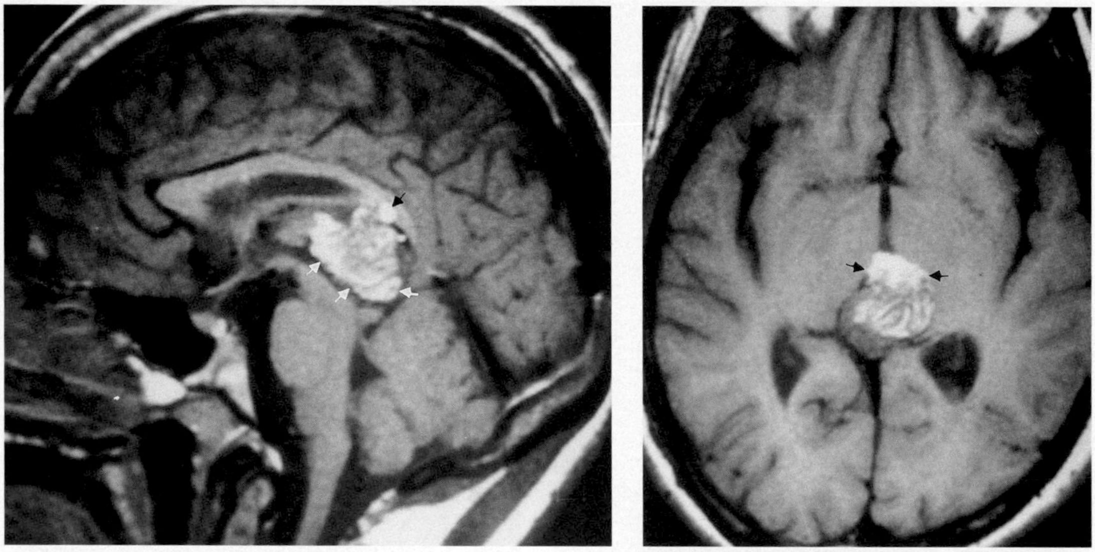

FIG. 96. Pineal teratoma. **A:** Sagittal short TR/TE MRI (600/20). **B:** Axial short TR/TE MRI (600/20). **C:** Axial long TR/TE MRI (2800/80). Inhomogeneous, partially high-intensity pineal mass (*arrows*, A,B) represents fat-containing teratoma. Fatty portion of mass parallels intensity of subcutaneous fat (A–C).

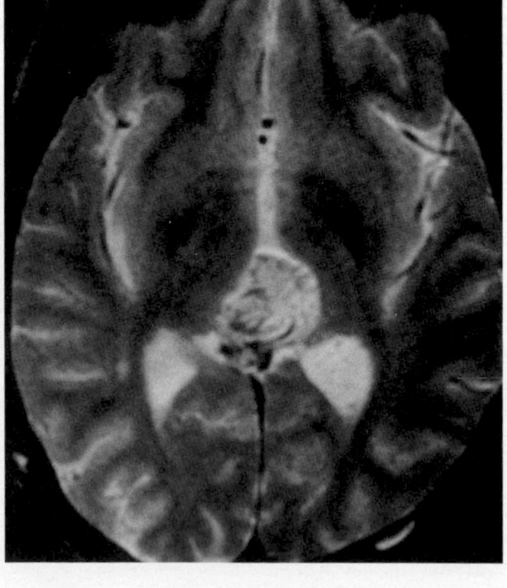

tumor is generally poor. A rare variant of pineoblastoma is the "trilateral retinoblastoma," which is the term used for a pineoblastoma in a patient with (usually) bilateral retinoblastoma (152). This is most often an inherited syndrome, and the diagnosis should be sought in any patient with bilateral retinoblastoma. Pineocytoma is more often a tumor of middle-aged and older adults. They are well-defined lesions which generally do not infiltrate brain. Pineocytomas are less cellular than pineoblastoma, and demonstrate cells with more cytoplasm (11). These are solid lesions rather than cystic on pathologic examination, so the demonstration of a cystic pineal mass should prompt the radiologist to consider simple pineal cyst rather than this neoplasm. These tumors show a slow, more benign course when they demonstrate more neuronal differentiation, but are aggressive malignancies with very poor survival rates in their less differentiated form (11).

The specific diagnosis of histopathologic type in pineal cell tumors is often not possible with MRI. However, the more important distinction is between pineal neoplasm and pineal cyst (see below). MRI depicts pineal neoplasms as lobulated, solid tumors which enhance densely with contrast. Cystic lesions should be considered as pineal cysts in the vast majority of cases. Signal intensities vary, but generally pineoblastomas are essentially isointense to gray matter on long TR/TE spin-echo images (Fig. 97), a typical pattern shared by other PNET tumors and possibly related to the known paucity of cytoplasm and overall dense cellularity (i.e., low water content) seen in these lesions. Pineal germinoma can appear identical to pineoblastoma on MRI. Pineocytomas, with a higher

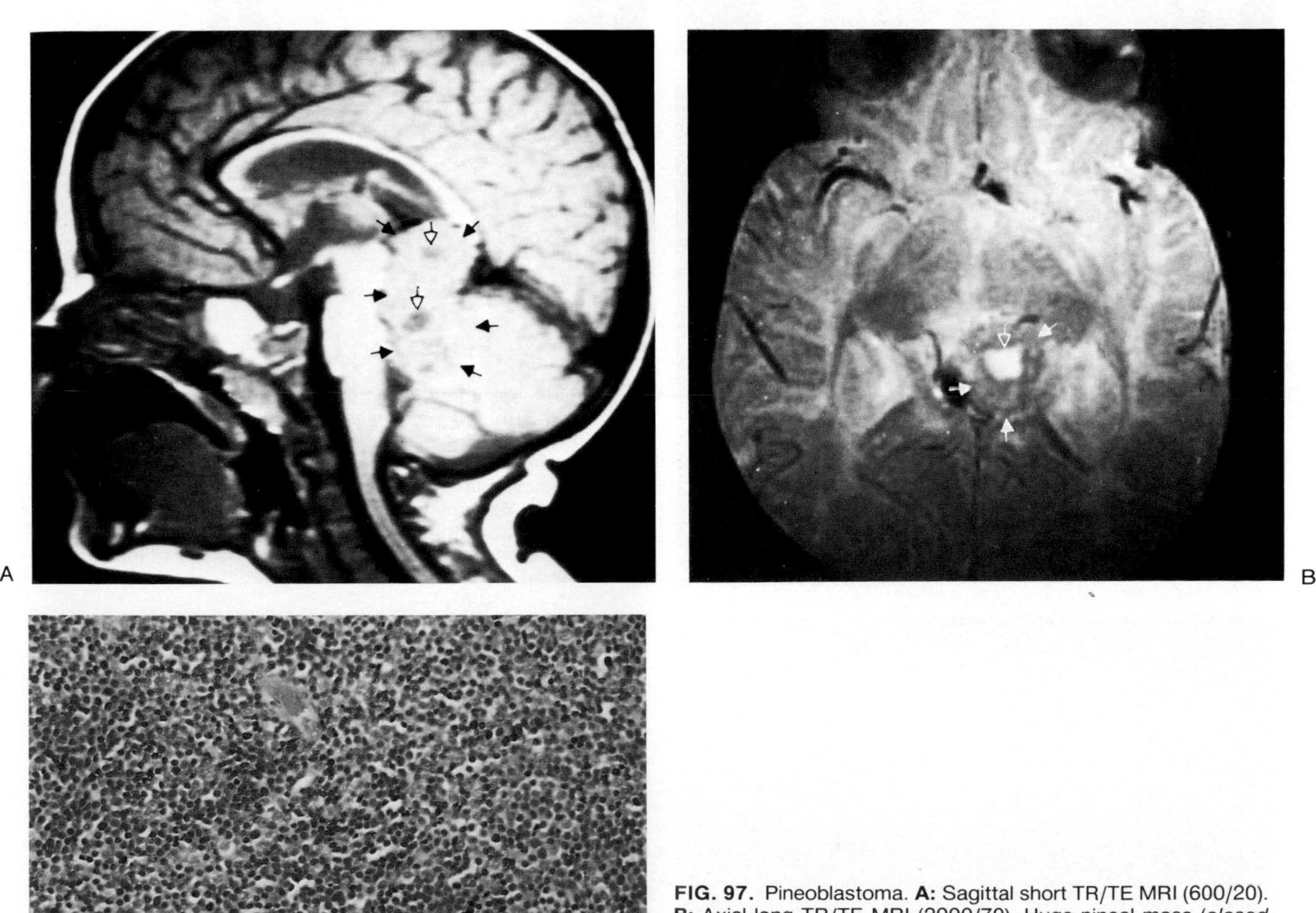

FIG. 97. Pineoblastoma. **A:** Sagittal short TR/TE MRI (600/20). **B:** Axial long TR/TE MRI (2000/70). Huge pineal mass (*closed arrows*, A,B) shows foci of cystic necrosis (*open arrows*, A,B) within otherwise low-intensity lesion on long TR/TE scan (B). **C:** Histologic specimen shows marked hypercellularity throughout tumor with infiltration by poorly differentiated cells with scant cytoplasm. (Courtesy of Dr. Alexander Mark, Washington, D.C.)

degree of cytoplasm, should have relatively higher signal intensity on long TR images (Fig. 98). Although both pineoblastoma and pineocytoma can calcify, intratumoral calcifications have been noted more commonly in pineocytoma (142,145).

Pineal Cysts

Pineal cysts are common as incidental necropsy findings, reported to be present in up to 40% of routine autopsies. These incidental lesions went virtually unno-

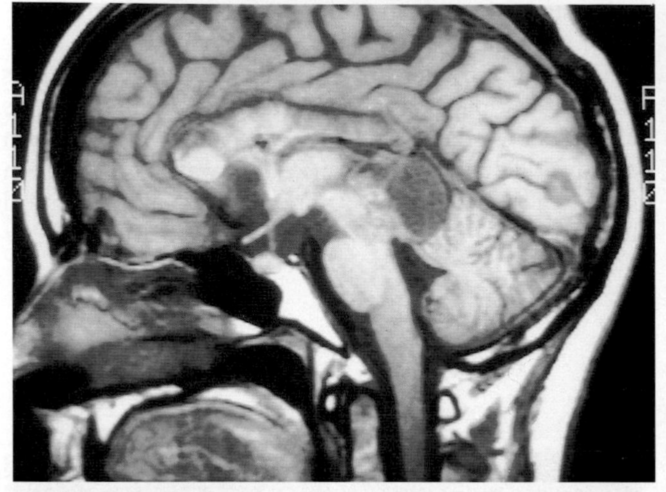

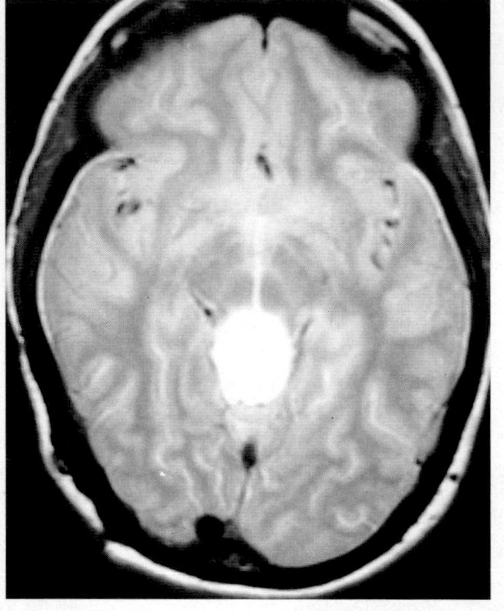

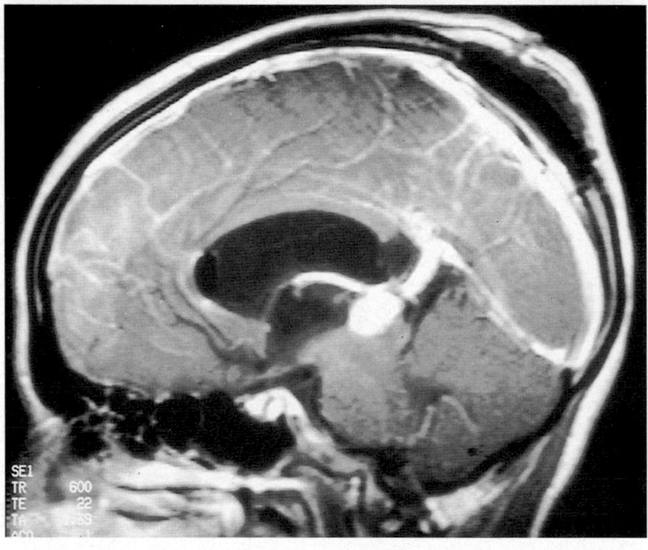

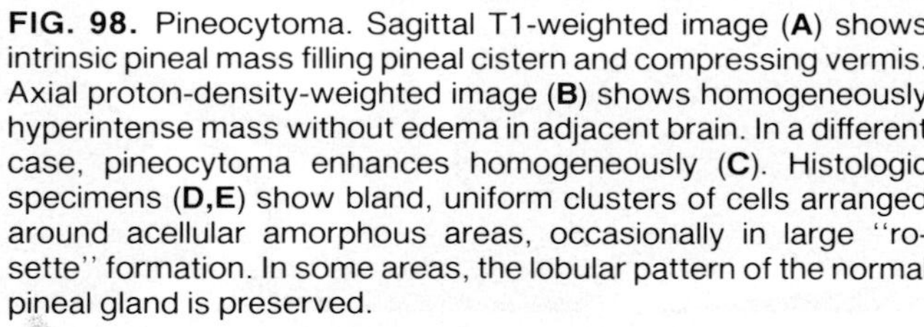

FIG. 98. Pineocytoma. Sagittal T1-weighted image (**A**) shows intrinsic pineal mass filling pineal cistern and compressing vermis. Axial proton-density-weighted image (**B**) shows homogeneously hyperintense mass without edema in adjacent brain. In a different case, pineocytoma enhances homogeneously (**C**). Histologic specimens (**D,E**) show bland, uniform clusters of cells arranged around acellular amorphous areas, occasionally in large "rosette" formation. In some areas, the lobular pattern of the normal pineal gland is preserved.

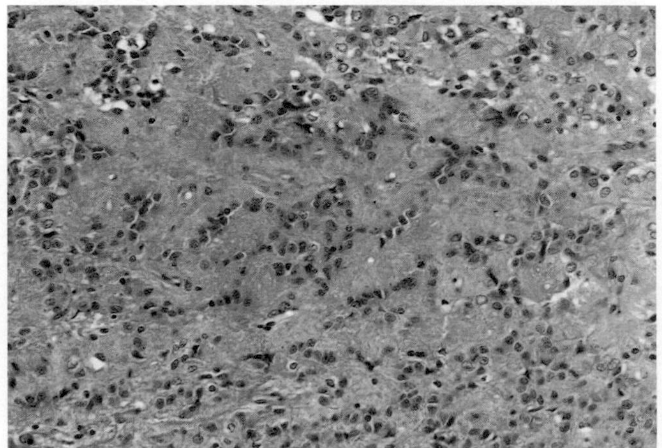

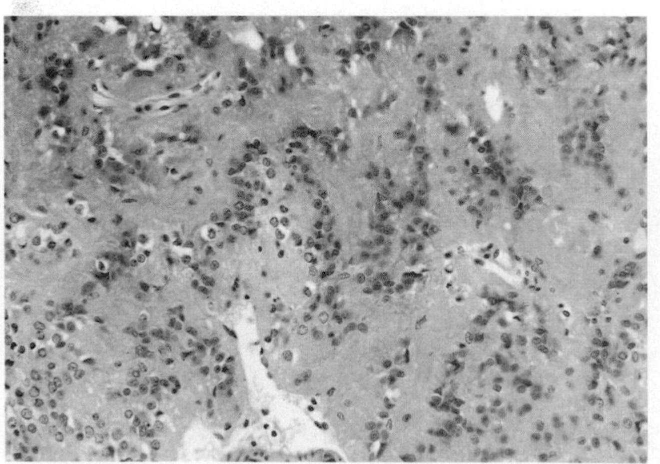

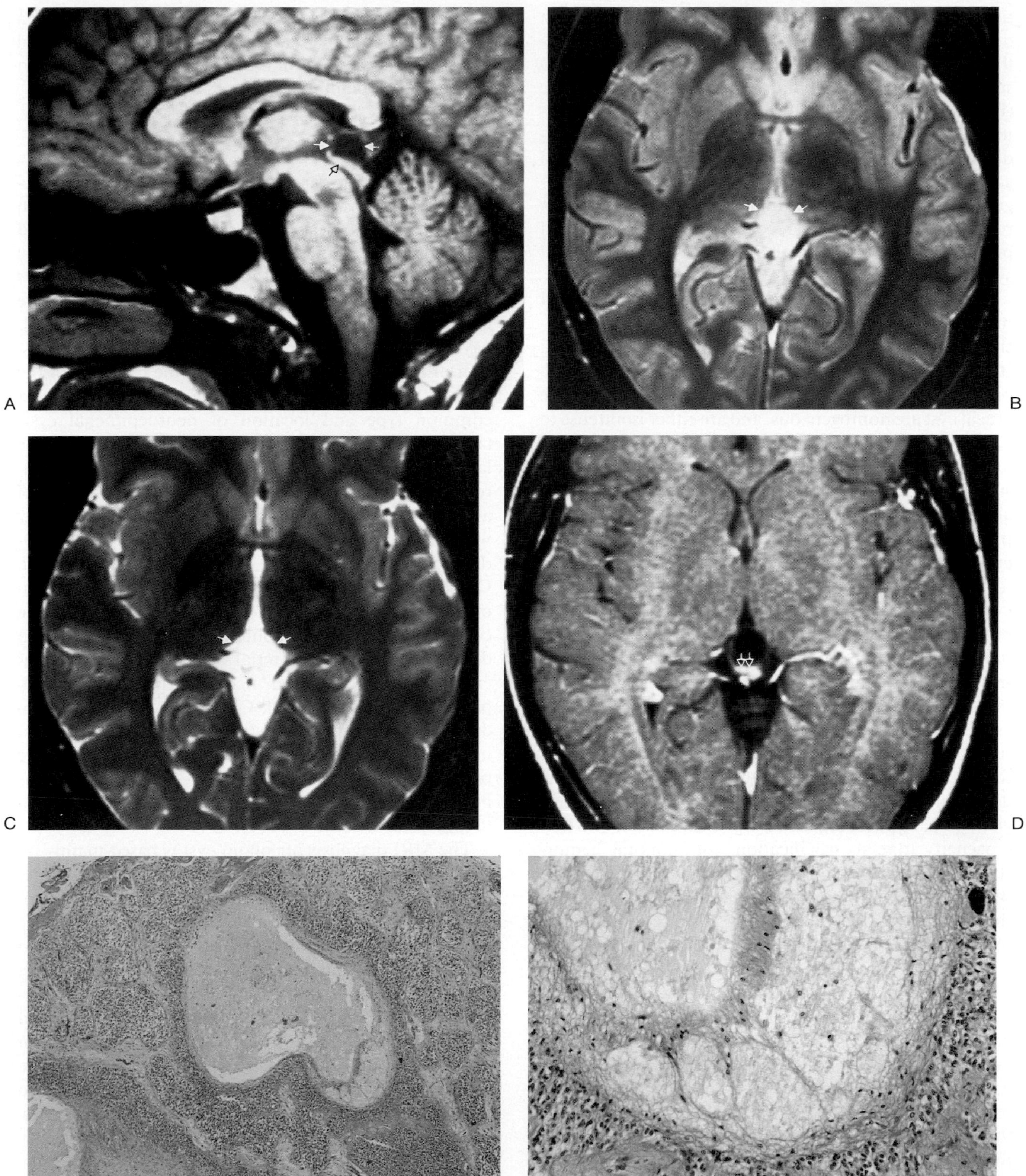

FIG. 99. Pineal cyst. **A:** Sagittal short TR/TE MRI (600/20). **B:** Axial long TR/short TE MRI (3000/35). **C:** Axial long TR/TE MRI (3000/90). **D:** Axial short TR/TE MRI (800/30), with contrast enhancement. Round, homogeneous mass in pineal (*closed arrows*, A–C) compresses superior colliculi (*open arrow*, A) in asymptomatic patient. Mass is only slightly higher in intensity than CSF on long TR/short TE image (B). Note minimal dorsal enhancement (*arrows*, D), representing either residual normal pineal parenchyma, choroid, or veins. **E,F:** Histologic specimens of small pineal glial cyst demonstrates the nature of this common finding which is derived from cystic degeneration within the glial element of the pineal gland.

ticed prior to the routine implementation of MR with direct sagittal imaging in evaluating possible brain pathology. Even large pineal cysts with apparent compression of the dorsal midbrain are usually asymptomatic (Fig. 99), but occasionally pineal cysts can bleed internally or be so large that they may be a cause of aqueductal compression with secondary hydrocephalus and gaze disorders (153, 154). The role of the neuroradiologist in this entity is to distinguish the pineal cyst from pineal neoplasm and to recognize it as a benign and probably non-contributory factor to the patient's clinical symptomatology.

The MR diagnosis of a pineal cyst is often based mainly on morphology, rather than simply signal intensity. The pineal cyst is round and smoothly marginated. It can be small and lie within a small portion of the gland, or it can replace the entire structure. The contents of the pineal cyst are homogeneous, and are either isointense to CSF or diffusely hyperintense, especially notable on the long TR/short TE image (Fig. 99). The divergence of the signal intensity from that of normal CSF should not alarm the radiologist, and in fact is the most common pattern noted (155). The relative hyperintensity of the cyst fluid may relate to factors such as isolation from flow (compared to ventricular CSF), high protein content, or even old hemorrhage, and does not signify tumor. The pineal cyst usually does not enhance intrinsically if scanning is performed immediately after injection of contrast, but surrounding residual pineal tissue will (since there is no blood–brain barrier in pineal capillaries).

In summary, there are several distinguishing MR features of pineal region tumors that should be sought when these lesions are discovered (Table 12). These include the determination of the site of origin of the mass (i.e., pineal gland or parapineal region), the presence of tumoral heterogeneity (due to calcification, intratumoral hemorrhage, fat or tumor cysts), and contrast enhancement of the lesion and any possible metastases. It is advisable, therefore, to routinely include a gradient-echo sequence for the detection of calcification (53), as well as postcontrast imaging, when evaluating pineal region masses with MR. Of course, the clinical history (e.g., age and sex, endocrinologic dysfunction) is also extremely helpful in the differential diagnosis. The relatively high percentage of radiosensitive tumors in the pineal region and the reportedly high morbidity in the past from surgical treatment has, in the past, resulted in the use of response to radiotherapy as a diagnostic test in many centers; that is, if there is dramatic tumor size reduction after 2,000 rads, therapy is completed with a total of 5,000 rads. Due to the great diversity of tumors in this region, often coupled with a less than complete tumor response, the known sensitivity of the developing brain to radiation, and significant improvements in microneurosurgical techniques, some groups now obtain histopathology in all cases before institution of therapy (141). It is clear that MR imaging with the use of i.v. contrast now provides a very sensitive and perhaps a more specific imaging tool and should be very useful in the preoperative evaluation and treatment planning of masses in this region.

COLLOID CYSTS

Colloid cysts are rare, benign epithelial-lined mass lesions related to the anterior third ventricle. Although in the past these lesions were thought to be derived from infolding of the primitive neuroepithelium (the embryologic paraphysis) (156), recent evidence suggests an origin from endoderm (157,158). These lesions are distinctive because of both their characteristic morphology and their specific location—at the anterosuperior aspect of the third ventricle, between the columns of the fornices (Figs. 100 and 101). They represent the most common type and location of neuroepithelial cysts (156), which can also occur in choroid plexus, within the lateral ventricle, subarachnoid space, and even brain parenchyma. Colloid cysts are estimated to represent 2% of all glial neoplasms (121). They become problematic only when they occlude the foramina of Monro and cause hydrocephalus, which may be intermittent and positional. One of the distinguishing features of colloid cysts from other neuroepithelial cysts, aside from location, is the composition of the cyst contents. Colloid cysts contain dense, viscid mucoid material with numerous constituents, including old blood, hemosiderin within macrophages, cholesterol crystal, CSF, and various ions (sodium, magnesium, calcium, copper, silicon, aluminum, iron, and phosphorous) (156,159), some of which are paramagnetic. Other cysts usually contain clear serous fluid, similar to CSF (differing only slightly with regard to total protein content) (160).

The MRI diagnosis of colloid cyst is based mainly on location and morphology, and although several entities may occur in this region, including choroid plexus neoplasm, meningioma, glioma, and granuloma (161), there is almost never a question about the diagnosis. Colloid cysts are remarkably varied in their signal intensity on MRI: lesions are reported as ranging from markedly hypointense (161, 162) to markedly hyperintense (161) on long TR/TE images (Figs. 100, 102, and 103). They can also be high or low intensity on T1-weighted images. This spectrum of intensities presumably relates to differences in concentration of paramagnetic substances, free water, and mucoid material. A thin wall is nearly always discernible and represents the epithelial lining. The signal intensity, as had been the experience with CT density, has not necessarily been predictive of successful and complete drainage of colloid cysts (161). Other neuroepithelial cysts appear identical in intensity to other CSF-containing lesions (e.g., arachnoid cyst)—isointense to CSF on short TR/TE, long TR/short TE, and long TR/TE images. The (nonparamagnetic) protein

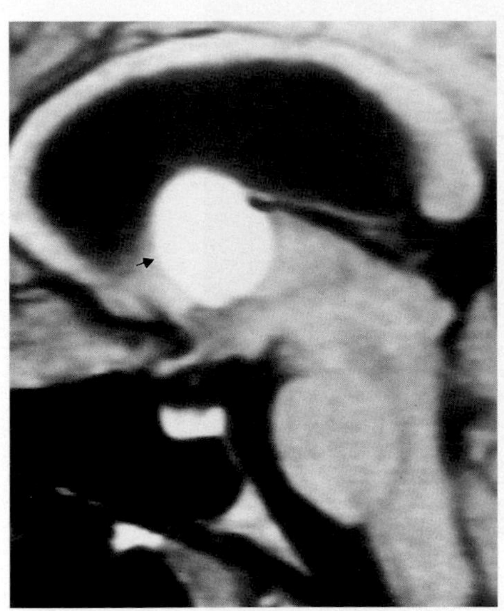
A

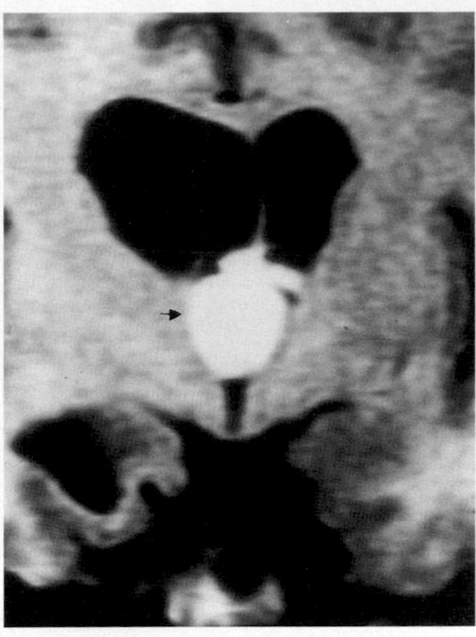

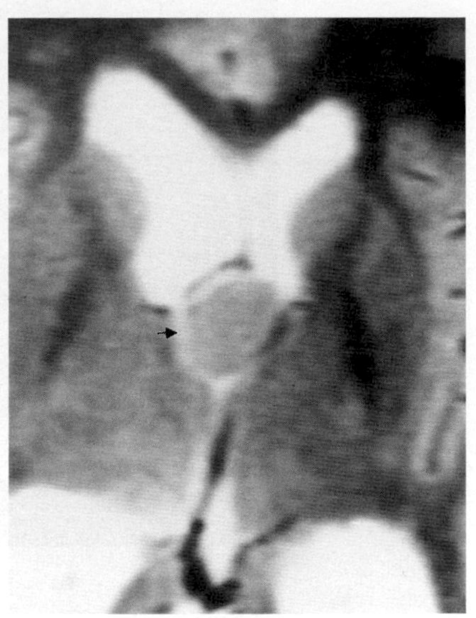

B,C

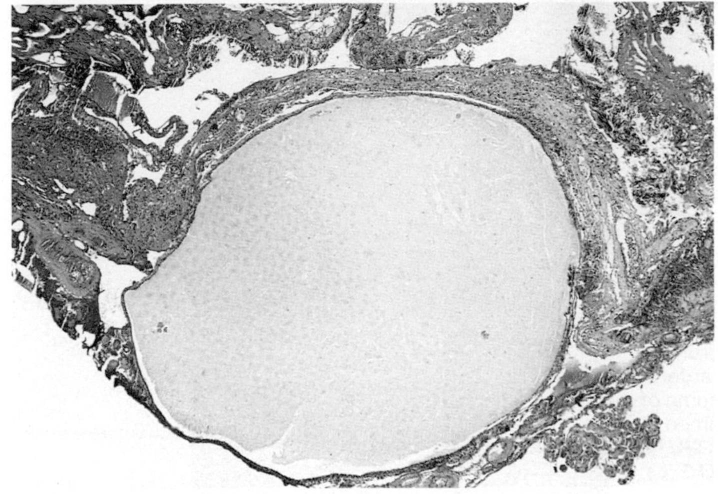
D

FIG. 100. Colloid cyst. **A:** Sagittal short TR/TE MRI (600/20). **B:** Coronal short TR/TE MRI (600/20). **C:** Axial long TR/TE MRI (2500/80). Lesion (*arrow*) is located at anterosuperior part of third ventricle, at the anterior columns of the fornices. This colloid cyst is markedly hyperintense on short TR/TE (A,B) and isointense to brain on long TR/TE image (C), similar to fat intensity (absence of chemical shift artifact implies signal not emanating from major fat peak). **D:** Histologic specimen of colloid cyst shows cystic structure lined by a single layer of flat cuboidal to low columnar, often ciliated, cells filled with PAS-positive amorphous material.

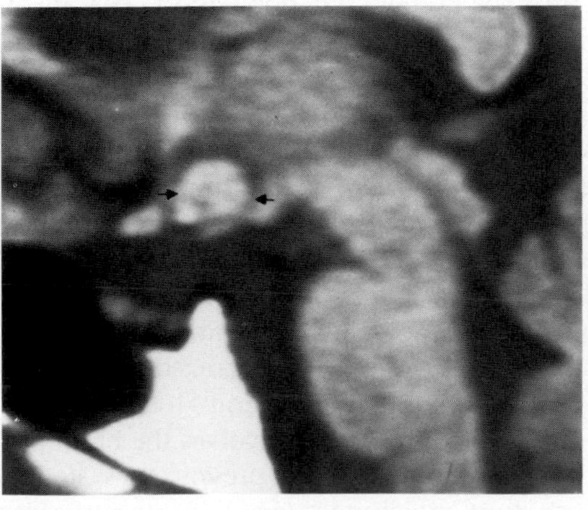

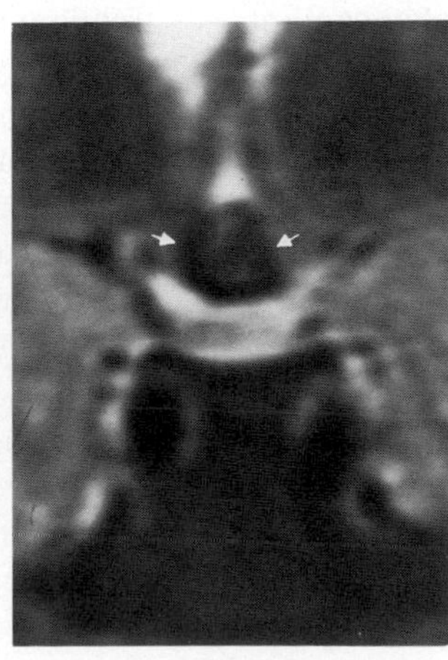
A,B

FIG. 101. Intraventricular craniopharyngioma. **A:** Sagittal short TR/TE MRI. **B:** Coronal MRI. Although intensity of craniopharyngioma can mimic colloid cyst, the differential diagnosis depends upon the location of the lesion. Note that this mass (*arrows*) is in the anteroinferior part of the third ventricle, not a site of colloid cysts (compare with Fig. 100).

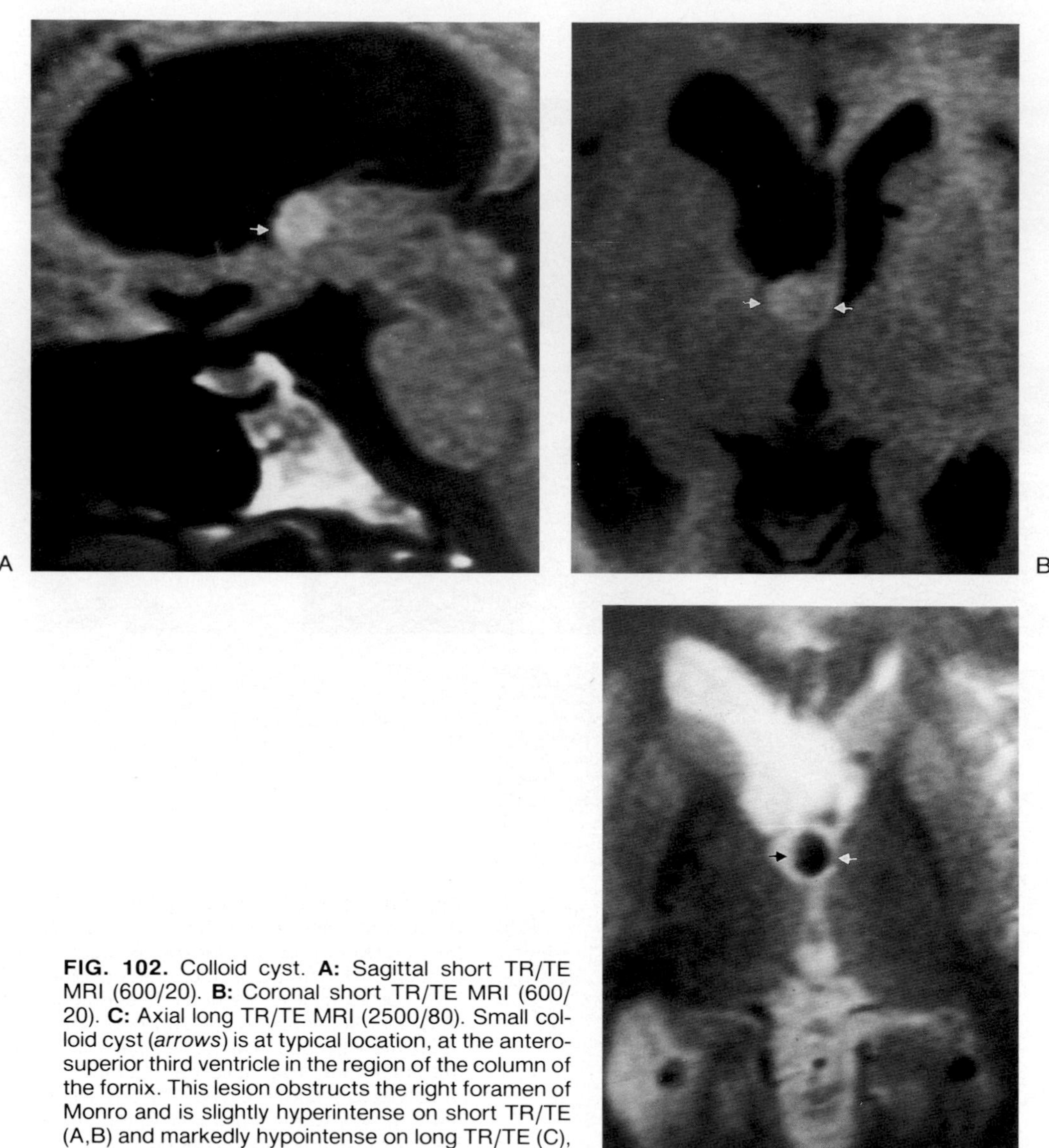

FIG. 102. Colloid cyst. **A:** Sagittal short TR/TE MRI (600/20). **B:** Coronal short TR/TE MRI (600/20). **C:** Axial long TR/TE MRI (2500/80). Small colloid cyst (*arrows*) is at typical location, at the anterosuperior third ventricle in the region of the column of the fornix. This lesion obstructs the right foramen of Monro and is slightly hyperintense on short TR/TE (A,B) and markedly hypointense on long TR/TE (C), consistent with viscous protein content.

content of cystic lesions must be extreme to cause signal intensity differences on MRI (7,8). Solid enhancement with i.v. contrast should suggest another lesion, although peripheral enhancement of colloid cysts is common and probably relates to residual pineal tissue, which inherently has no blood–brain barrier.

PRIMARY CNS LYMPHOMA

Primary lymphoma of the CNS is a rare entity with an increasing incidence, constituting approximately 1% of all primary brain tumors in the literature (163) but having a notable tripling in incidence over the past decade (164). It has been estimated that AIDS-related primary CNS lymphoma is now more common than low-grade astrocytomas and as common as meningiomas (165). Some estimates state that it has become the most common primary brain neoplasm, mainly as a result of its frequent occurrence in the AIDS population. The site of origin of primary CNS lymphoma remains controversial and unknown, since the CNS does not have endogenous lymphoid tissue nor a lymphatic circulation.

There are essentially three major groups of people at risk for developing primary CNS lymphoma: organ transplant recipients, patients with congenital immunodeficiency syndromes, and those with AIDS and other systemic diseases associated with immunodeficiency (164). The peak age of incidence in the non-AIDS population is in the sixth decade. It is recognized that nearly all primary CNS lymphoma is of the non-Hodgkin's type (11); when Hodgkin's lymphoma involves the brain parenchyma, it is almost always in the presence of systemic disease or with dural attachment (166). Focal intracerebral masses are the most common initial presentation of primary CNS lymphoma (164), whereas the subarach-

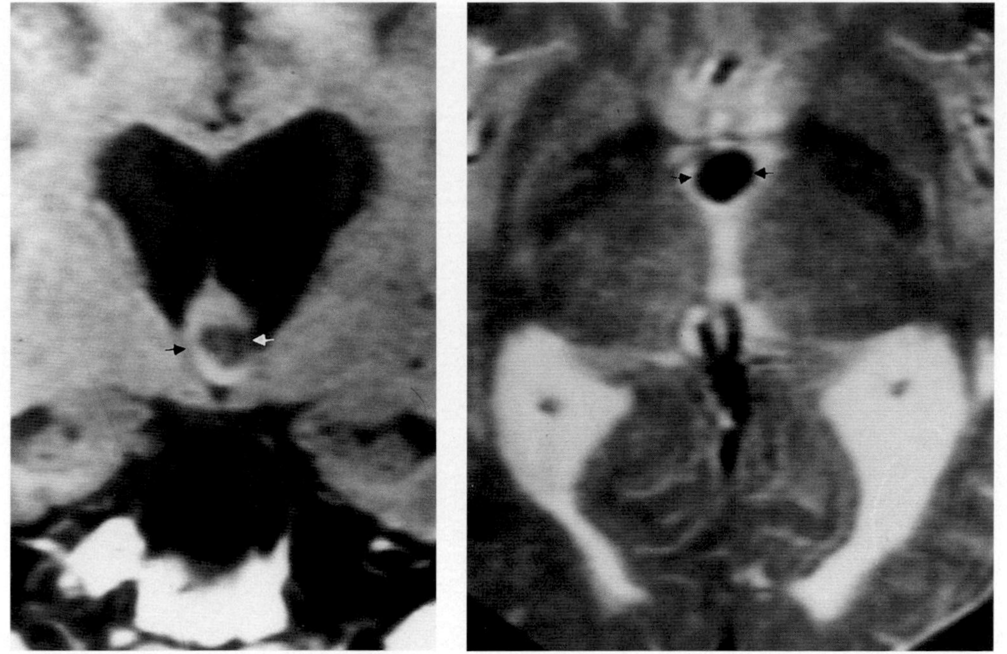

FIG. 103. Colloid cyst. **A:** Coronal short TR/TE MRI (600/20). **B:** Axial long TR/TE MRI (2500/80). Heterogeneous colloid cyst (*arrows*) has peripheral hyperintensity on short TR/TE (A) and is markedly hypointense on long TR/TE (B). Note lesion is at superior region of third ventricle (compare with Fig. 102).

noid space is an extremely common site for recurrent disease (163). The supratentorial compartment is involved in approximately 75% to 85% of patients at initial presentation (164,167). Multiplicity is very common and has been noted in up to one-half of cases. Intracranial metastases from systemic lymphoma generally fall into one of two categories: leptomeningeal (with or without parenchymal) or dural-based (11). In metastatic lymphoma of the CNS, it is exceptional for parenchymal masses to occur without leptomeningeal involvement (11).

The clinical outlook is dismal in these cases, as untreated patients survive an average of 1.5 months after diagnosis, but survival rates vary with the primary site of involvement. According to Hochberg and Miller the median survival for those with solitary parenchymal lesions was 45 months; those with multiple lesions had a median survival of nine months; those with meningeal or subependymal initial involvement survived 7.5 months (164). Steroid administration can have a dramatic effect, with CT documentation of complete regression of brain lesions reported as early as 8 hours after i.v. steroids (164). Dissemination within the CNS occurs in 60% of cases (164). In one study of AIDS-related CNS lymphoma and the role of radiotherapy, those patients who had been treated with radiation died of systemic infection, while those who had not been treated died from tumor progression (165), suggesting that early diagnosis may indeed be of value in this population.

Pathologically, parenchymal lesions are ill-defined masses with irregular borders. Microscopically, the infiltrative edges of the lesions extend along perivascular spaces and infiltrate blood vessel walls (164). Dural-based masses often spread via the Virchow-Robin perivascular spaces and directly invade the brain parenchyma.

The classical imaging findings of parenchymal lymphoma include masses which involve the deep gray matter structures, periventricular regions, and corpus callosum (167). It has been reported that up to 75% of lymphomatous masses are seen to be in contact with ependyma, meninges, or both (167). The detection of enhancement along perivascular spaces on MRI should put lymphoma at the top of the differential diagnosis, with sarcoidosis representing the only other consideration. The extent of edema on MRI is generally less than that seen in conjunction with primary gliomas or metastases of similar size (Fig. 104). Lymphomatous masses do not calcify (167) and hemorrhage is distinctly uncommon on imaging studies. MRI signal intensity patterns are extremely varied in focal intracerebral lymphoma, particularly in the AIDS population. These lesions, when deep and periventricular, are often isointense to gray matter on all spin-echo sequences, a finding shared by other small cell, hypercellular tumors (Fig. 104). However, lymphoma can also be markedly hyperintense on long TR images (Fig. 105). Enhancement after i.v. contrast occurs in the vast majority of cases and can be dense and

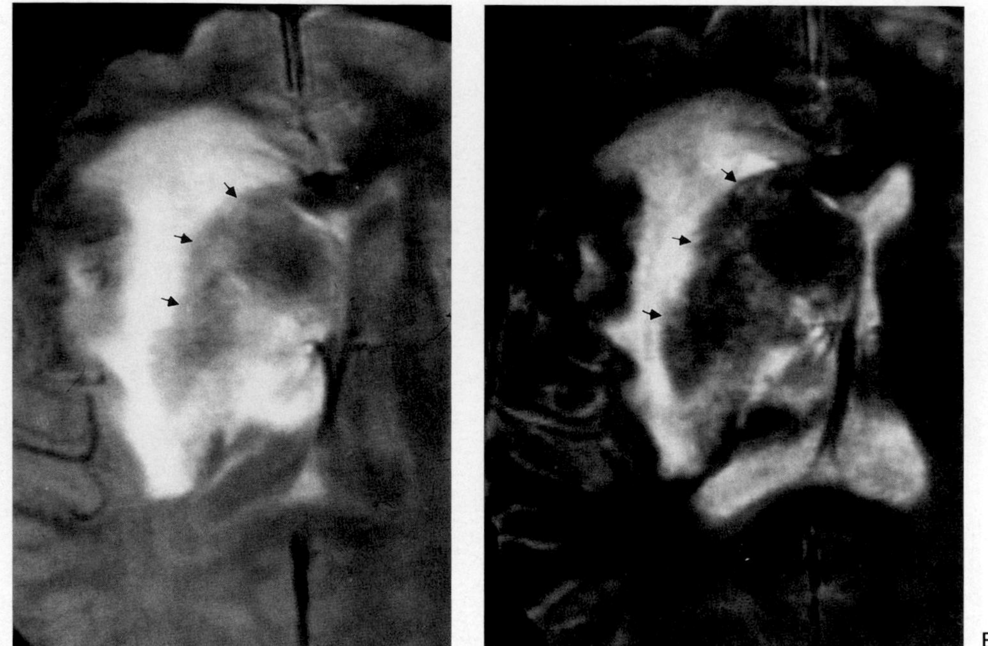

FIG. 104. Lymphoma, unifocal and of low intensity. **A:** Long TR/short TE MRI (2000/35). **B:** Long TR/TE MRI (2000/70). Right basal ganglionic mass (*arrows*) is of low intensity on long TR images (A,B) and is surrounded by only a small amount of edema, in view of the size of the lesion.

homogeneous (Fig. 106), but necrotic lesions can show ring enhancement. Reports indicate that lymphoma in AIDS patients more commonly appears as multifocal lesions (168) with ring enhancement and with more prominent edema than in the general population (169). These patients are often empirically treated with anti-toxoplasmosis agents and followed for radiographic and clinical response in the absence of tissue diagnosis. Secondary brain involvement by systemic lymphoma is indistinguishable from primary CNS lymphoma on imaging studies (170), although, as noted above, parenchymal involvement is more common in primary lymphoma. It is well recognized that leptomeningeal seeding, in the absence of parenchymal involvement, commonly escapes detection by CT scanning (171), but it appears that MRI with i.v. contrast is more sensitive to this entity (172).

The differential diagnosis of the stated imaging findings includes several entities, depending upon the appearance of the lesion. If one sees a single, deep mass having relatively homogeneous intensity similar to gray matter, dense contrast enhancement, and minimal edema, the classic description for the entity, the most likely diagnosis is lymphoma. The single most valuable

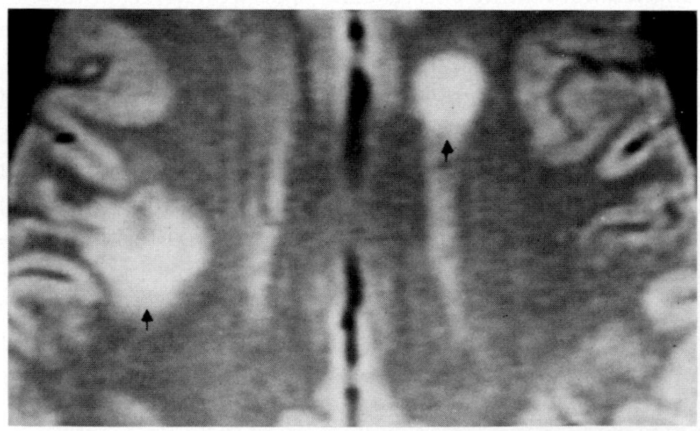

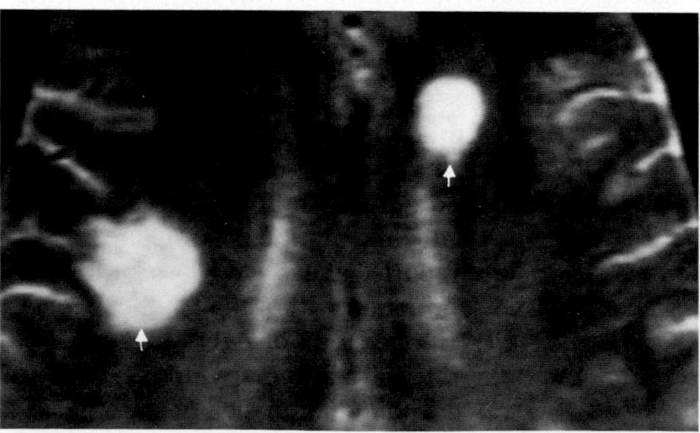

FIG. 105. Lymphoma, multifocal and of high intensity. **A:** Long TR/short TE MRI (2500/20). **B:** Long TR/TE MRI (2500/80). Two foci of marked hyperintensity in hemispheric white matter (*arrows*, A,B) illustrate variability in appearance of CNS lymphoma (compare with Fig. 104).

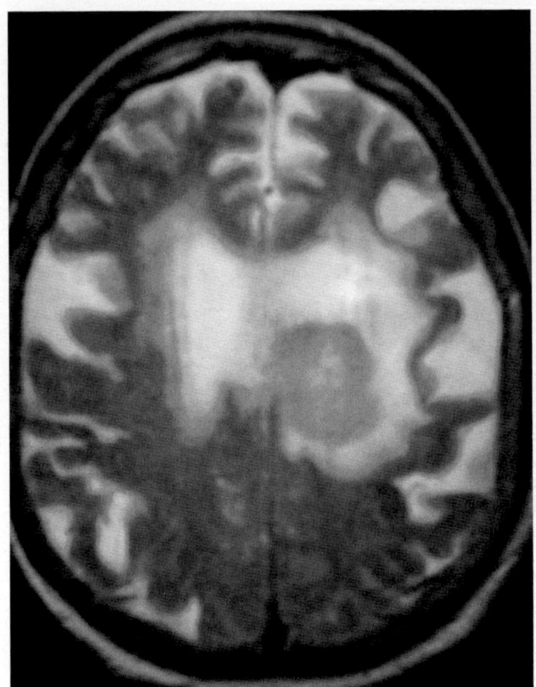

A

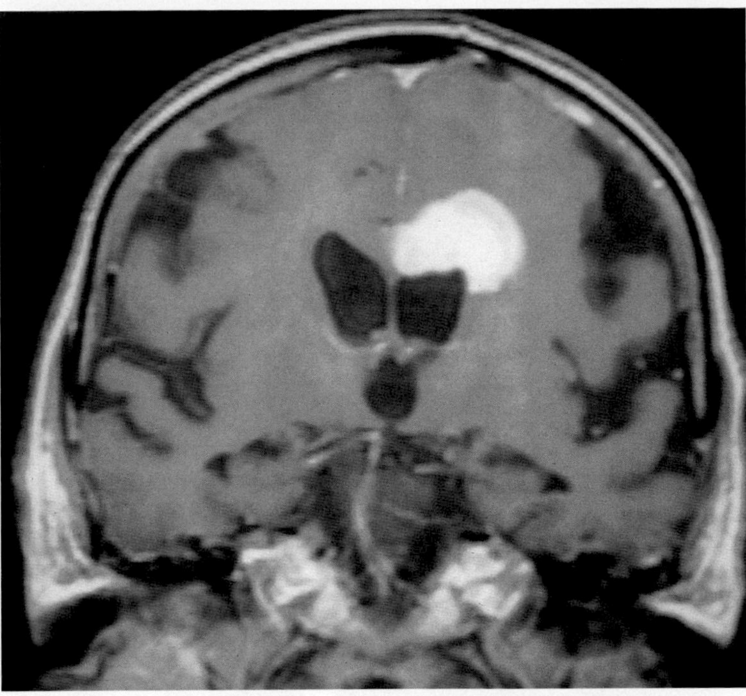

B

FIG. 106. Lymphoma with dense enhancement and "ventricular encasement." Axial T2-weighted image (**A**) shows large mass with significant edema. After i.v. contrast (**B**), note ventricular "encasement" as lesion spreads into corpus callosum, a characteristic finding in lymphoma.

MR finding in the distinction between lymphoma and toxoplasmosis in AIDS is the presence of subependymal spread (Figs. 107 and 108), which is highly suggestive of lymphoma (168). Hemorrhage is also very common in cerebral toxoplasmosis, particularly after treatment, and if present, argues against lymphoma. If a focal-enhancing parenchymal mass is accompanied by enhancement along the perivascular spaces, especially with adjacent meningeal enhancement, the only entities that should be seriously entertained are lymphoma and sarcoidosis (Fig. 109).

In the non-AIDS patient, other lesions are also in the differential diagnosis. Glioblastoma, like lymphoma, can cross the corpus callosum and enhance. Metastases are always in consideration, particularly when significant edema is noted. A hyperdense focal parenchymal mass with enhancement and minimal or no edema on CT might also describe a cavernous hemangioma, a benign lesion that has a specific appearance on unenhanced MRI (63). Parenchymal and extra-axial sarcoidosis would appear virtually identical to lymphoma. Capillary telangiectasia typically shows lace-like enhancement on MRI and is isointense to gray matter without enhancement (see Chapter 12), but this lesion should not have any mass effect. Densely enhancing dural-based lesions could implicate lymphoma, sarcoidosis, metastases (especially breast carcinoma), and meningioma (which would be the only tumor to calcify amongst these).

METASTATIC DISEASE

Metastatic spread of tumor to the brain and its coverings from extracranial sites is a relatively common occurrence which represents a frustrating therapeutic problem for the physician and an emotionally and physically debilitating event for the patient. The role of the radiologist in the search for intracranial metastases lies in detecting the lesions, making the specific diagnosis of metastases, and in localization. Approximations from literature reports concerning the incidence of metastases range from 4% to 37%, but intracranial metastases are found in up to 24% of all patients that die from cancer (173). It has also been estimated that cerebral metastases are estimated to comprise approximately 20% of all clinically detected brain tumors (174). Estimates state that 100,000 to 150,000 new cases of intracerebral metastatic disease occur each year in the United States alone (175).

While brain metastases occur in patients of all ages, the highest incidence is in patients in the fourth to seventh decade of life (176). Although brain metastases are likely to coexist with other sites of metastatic disease, the symptoms from brain metastases antedate the primary diagnosis of cancer in 45% of surgical cases (177). The neuroanatomic localization of the metastasis and its associated edema and mass effect usually determine the nature of the clinical presentation (178). These lesions may be the direct result of microscopic foci of neoplastic cells

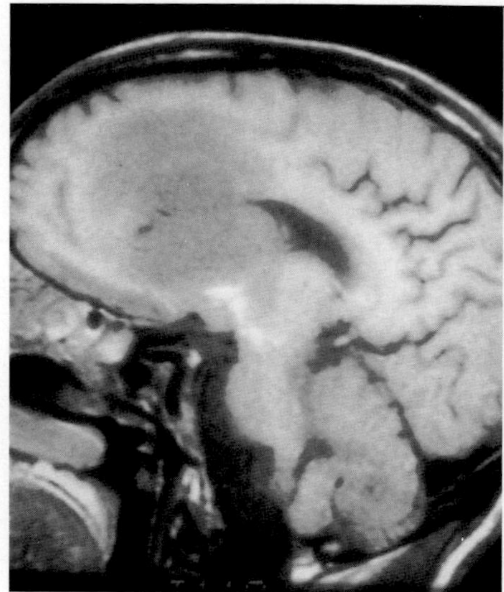

A

FIG. 107. Lymphoma in AIDS with subependymal enhancement. Bilateral ganglionic periventricular masses (**A,B**) are isointense to gray matter on T2-weighted image (B) and show extensive edema in this AIDS patient. After i.v. contrast (**C,D**), only partial enhancement is seen. Note subependymal spread along left frontal horn (C), highly suggestive of lymphoma.

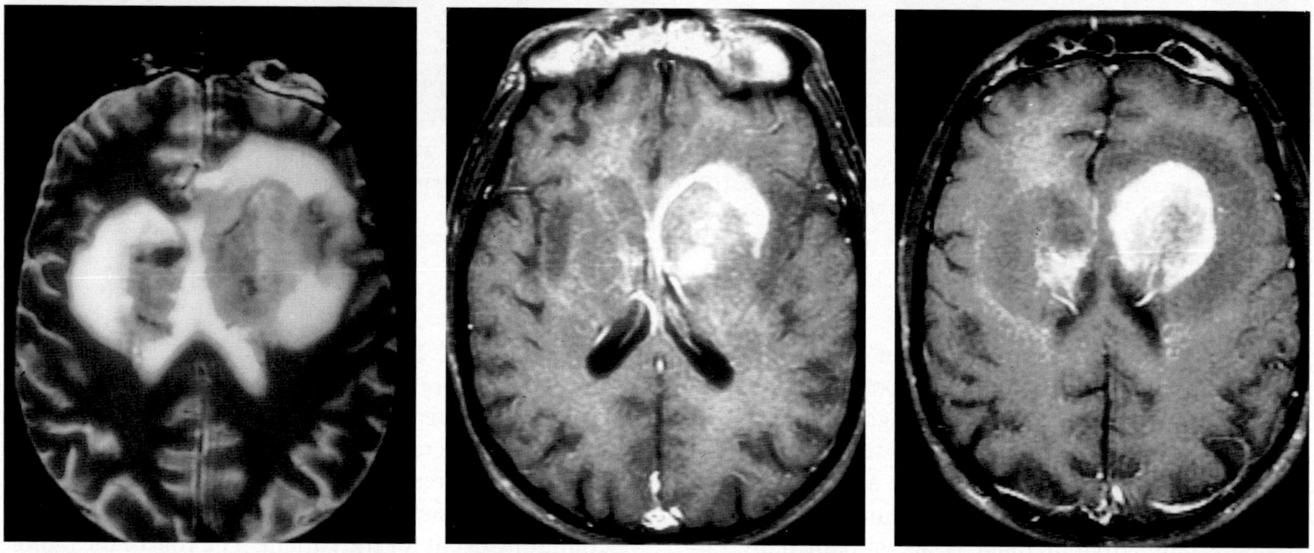

B

C,D

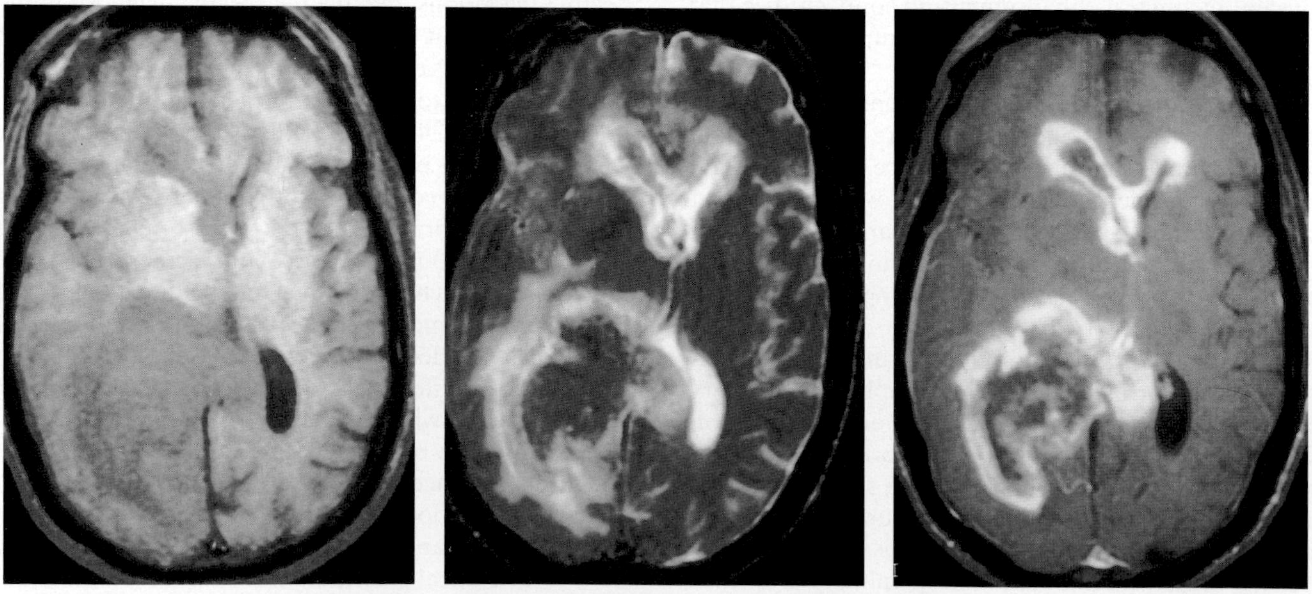

A

B,C

FIG. 108. Lymphoma in AIDS with extensive subependymal enhancement. Necrotic mass in parenchyma extends across corpus callosum on precontrast T1-weighted (**A**) and T2-weighted (**B**) images. Extensive subependymal enhancement (**C**) is noted after i.v. contrast.

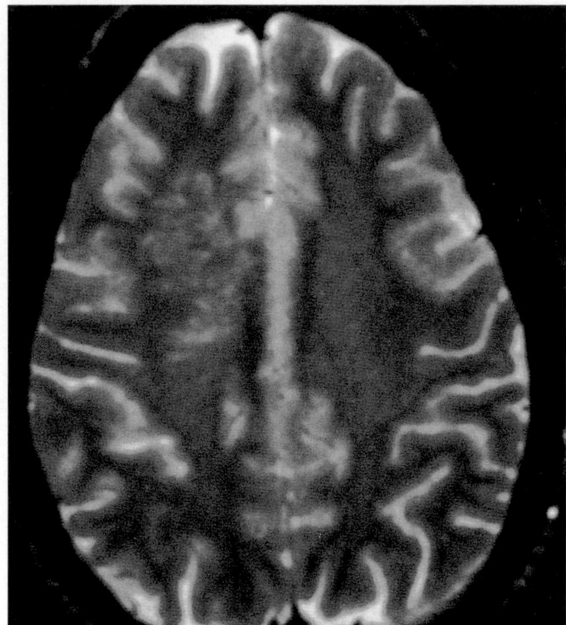

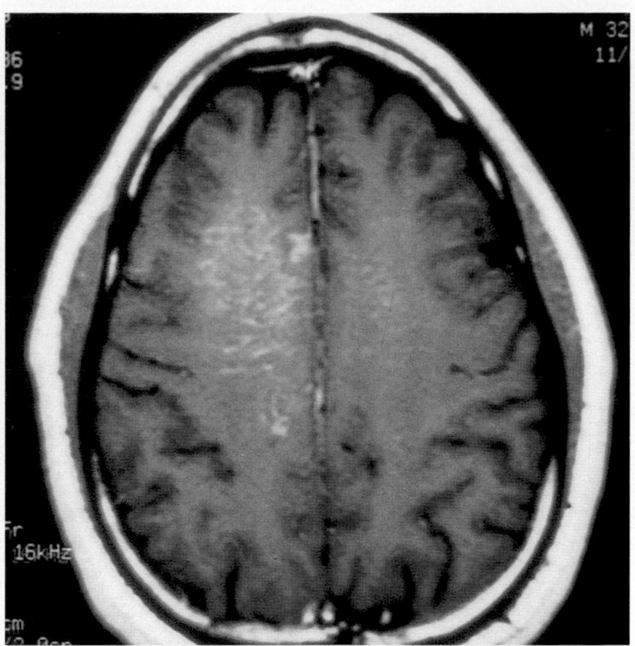

FIG. 109. Neurosarcoidosis along perivascular spaces. Subtle hyperintensity in right frontal white matter on T2-weighted image (**A**) is clarified by i.v. contrast, after which clear enhancement is noted bifrontally in a pattern indicative of infiltration along Virchow-Robin spaces (**B**) in this pathologically-proven case of sarcoidosis.

transported into the brain via the hematogenous route with subsequent growth in situ, or the metastatic deposit may be primarily to the surrounding calvarium or dural membranes and impinge upon the brain secondarily. The most common symptoms that lead to the diagnosis of brain metastasis include headaches (88%), confusion (36%), hemiparesis (35%), seizures (29%), visual problems (27%), vertigo (24%), vomiting (22%), and aphasia (17%) (177). From surgical and CT studies, roughly 80% to 85% of metastases are located in the supratentorial compartment (177,179,180). Clinically silent lesions can occur and most frequently are seen in patients with lung carcinoma [especially adenocarcinoma (40%) and oat cell carcinoma (11%)] (178) and melanoma (11%) (181). It has become apparent that the optimal screening examination for the detection of intracerebral metastases is the i.v.-enhanced MRI. A more accurate incidence of clinically unsuspected involvement of the brain by metastatic disease remains to be elucidated, now that a more sensitive method of detection exists.

Intraparenchymal metastases are the most common type of metastatic disease to affect the intracranial space. Although there are some discrepancies amongst the various reported series, it is reasonable to state that the most common sites of origin are lung, breast, skin (melanoma), gastrointestinal tract, and genitourinary tract (11,180). Furthermore, the brain is often the only site of metastases in patients with extracranial malignancy, a situation particularly common in those with bronchogenic carcinoma (182) and melanoma (181). It is generally accepted that most intracerebral metastases are multiple, regardless of the site of origin, however there is a high incidence of solitary metastasis, estimated to range from 30% to 50% and especially common in melanoma, lung, and breast carcinoma (11,183,184). Therefore, the fact that an intracerebral mass lesion is solitary does nothing to mitigate the consideration of metastasis as the diagnosis. Since surgical intervention is often indicated for solitary metastases, while radiotherapy without surgery is generally the therapy for multiple lesions, the detection of intracerebral metastases is critical to patient management.

Specific locations of intracerebral metastases generally coincide with the respective lobar volumes (11), excepting the trend of renal cell carcinoma metastases to involve the infratentorial brain (183). Early metastatic foci are commonly found at gray matter-white matter interfaces, a feature shared by all hematogenously disseminated embolic disease. This distribution has been ascribed to the dramatic narrowing of the diameter of arterioles supplying the cortex as these vessels enter the white matter (11). As noted by Henson and Urich (185), tumor emboli measuring 100–200 μm in diameter are often found lodged in the 50–150 μm lumina of arterioles. Macroscopically, intracerebral metastases are generally well circumscribed and round. Their cut surfaces are pinkish-gray and granular in appearance, but these lesions can be quite heterogeneous, owing to such factors as necrosis, liquefaction, and hemorrhage. The microscopic features can be somewhat different than those sug-

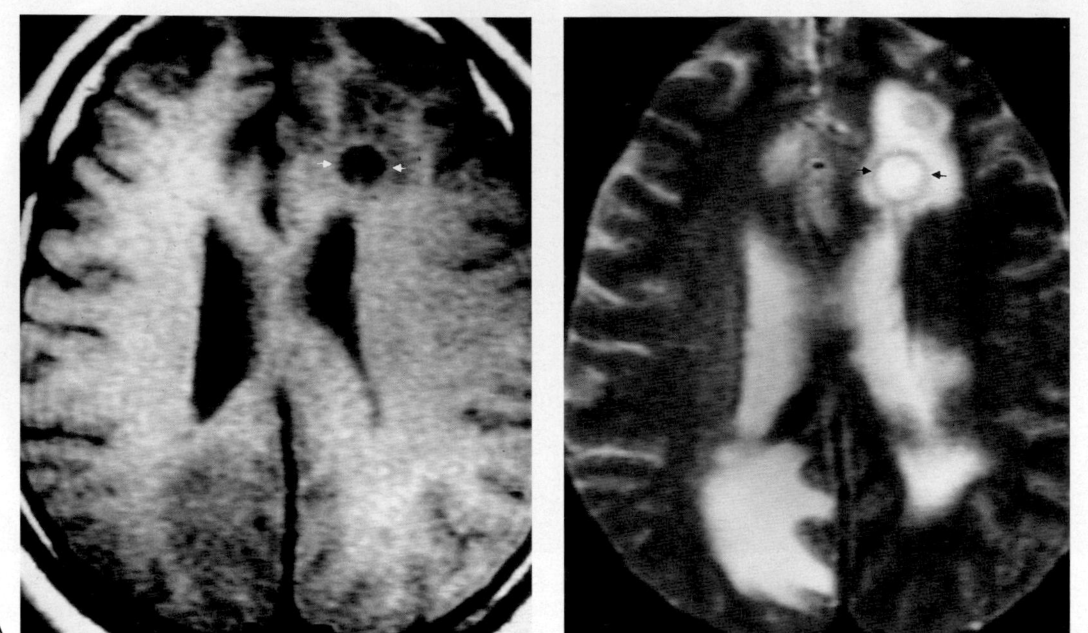

FIG. 110. Metastatic lung carcinoma, with cystic necrosis. **A:** Axial short TR/TE MRI (600/20). **B:** Axial long TR/TE MRI (2500/80). Several regions of classic edema in the white matter (i.e., vasogenic) indicate multiple metastatic foci. Left frontal lesion (*arrows*, A,B) shows central fluid-like intensity, consistent with cystic necrosis. The *absence* of a high-intensity rim on the short TR/TE image (A) differentiates this lesion from abscess.

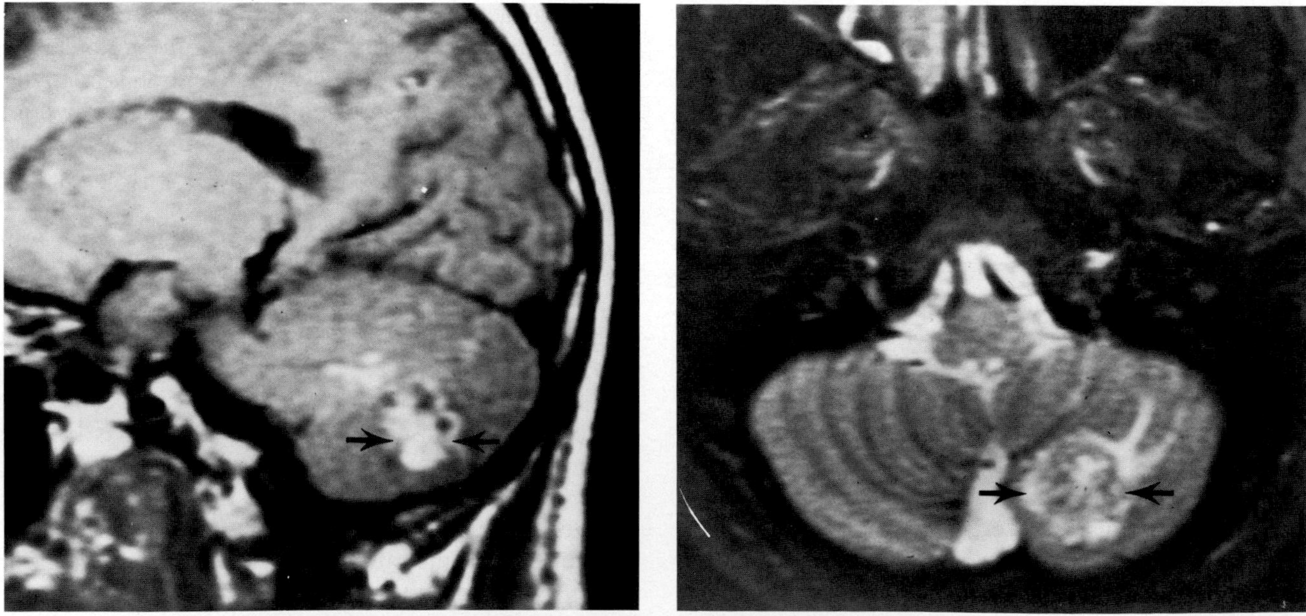

FIG. 111. Metastatic melanotic, nonhemorrhagic melanoma. **A:** Sagittal short TR/TE MRI (600/20). **B:** Axial long TR/TE MRI (2500/80). Left cerebellar hemispheric mass (*arrows*, A,B) is hyperintense on short TR/TE (A) and isointense to cortex on long TR/TE image (B), indicating melanin content. No evidence of hemorrhage is present.

gested by gross inspection, since these lesions are often less circumscribed and more infiltrative, often surrounded by reactive gliosis and perivascular invasion and extension (11). Metastases are notoriously surrounded by massive amounts of edema (Fig. 110), often extending far from the site of a relatively small metastatic focus. The edema associated with brain tumors is classified as vasogenic (186), where the major mechanism of edema formation is an underlying disturbance in vascular permeability, so that plasma proteins and other macromolecules pass freely into the perivascular space and consequently into the interstitial, extracellular space. The extent of associated edema bears no direct relationship to either the size of the metastasis, or, necessarily, to the clinical status of the patient (187).

The diagnosis of intracranial metastases has been greatly facilitated by the advent of CT scanning, especially with the use of i.v. contrast (180). Subsequently, it has been shown that MRI with i.v. contrast is more sensitive than CT for this diagnosis (4,5). Lesions are usually focal and seem to be distinguishable from their associated edema on both CT and MRI (Figs. 110 and 111). On MR, metastatic foci are generally separable from edema on long TR/TE images, as the metastasis is typically a focus of variable intensity [depending on such factors as cellularity, necrosis, hemorrhage, and (rarely) calcification] amidst a sea of high intensity edema. Intravenous contrast clearly shows the tumor focus separate from the surrounding edema. Peritumoral edema is usually prominent (180) and follows white matter boundaries, as expected from neuropathologic descriptions, which are readily identified as finger-like projections with intervening unaffected cortex (Fig. 110). The edema accompanying metastases usually does not cross the corpus callosum, nor does it involve cortex, features which often help distinguish these lesions from primary infiltrative brain malignancies. Very rarely, the vasogenic edema associated with metastases can enhance after i.v. contrast (see Fig. 26). This finding is of uncertain significance, but it presumably indicates a more marked disruption of the blood–brain barrier than that which is typically seen in metastatic disease. Edema is not a significant component of cortical metastases, however, presumably because of the paucity of interstitium in these regions. Therefore, small metastases to cortex may be missed if one relies on non-contrast, long TR scanning (Figs. 112 and 113).

Signal intensity patterns of specific metastases on MRI are usually nonspecific, in that most tumors, regardless of site of origin, appear to be extremely variable in signal, but generally prolong relaxation times (188–190). There are several specific pathologic changes in metastases which influence the MR appearance of these lesions. Areas of nonhemorrhagic cystic necrosis appear as irregular regions of CSF-like intensity surrounded by the nonnecrotic portion of the lesion (Fig. 110). Necrosis, on the other hand, has also been shown to shorten relaxation times (6), which may be due to release of intracellular naturally occurring paramagnetics (e.g., iron or copper) or to free radical peroxidation (191). Intratumoral hemorrhage, which occurs in just under 20% of metastases (192,193), is readily detected by MRI. The exquisite sensitivity for the detection of hemorrhage on MR images can give clues to the primary site of origin, since some metastases (most notably melanoma, choriocarcinoma, and renal cell carcinoma) have a particular tendency to bleed. Furthermore, detailed analysis of signal intensities in these cases can lead to the diagnosis of underlying tumor as the etiology of the intracranial hemorrhage (Fig. 11) (13) (Table 5). Specificity is also provided by MRI in the evaluation of melanoma metastases, since pathologically documented nonhemorrhagic melanotic lesions are hyperintense on short TR/TE images and isointense on long TR/TE images (16) (Figs. 19 and 111). This relaxation enhancement has been ascribed to the free radical content of melanin (194). Other lesions that can show signal patterns suggestive of their site of origin include mucinous adenocarcinomas (e.g., colon), where characteristic hypointensity is seen on T2-weighted images standing out from hyperintense edema.

While many intracerebral metastases are apparent on noncontrast scans, it has been well documented that i.v. contrast increases the sensitivity for the detection of intracerebral metastases. We believe that a normal noncontrast CT scan does little to exclude metastases (Fig. 114). It is also well recognized that the vast majority of intracerebral metastases demonstrate contrast enhancement, presumably due to deficient blood–tumor barriers in the vascular endothelium of the involved capillaries. This enhancement has been shown on both CT and MR imaging (195). It is now accepted that contrast-enhanced MRI detects many lesions which otherwise go undetected (Figs. 112 and 113) (4,5), even on high quality CT with contrast. This effect is dramatic in cortical metastases, as previously stated. Moreover, high doses of MRI contrast agents appear to allow the detection of more metastatic lesions. It has been estimated that approximately 10% of such cases alter patient management (196). Cost-benefit studies and accurate approximations of impact on patient management using high dose contrast for patients with suspected metastatic disease remain uncertain. Recent attention toward the use of stereotactic radiosurgery as an alternative to surgical resection for solitary metastases, as well as data supporting the use of adjuvant radiotherapy after surgery (175,197) makes the delineation of even small single metastases highly significant to management.

Both the morphology of the contrast enhancement and its time of occurrence may vary significantly in metastases. The patterns of enhancement on MRI can be solid and nodular, as well as ring-like in configuration. The ring enhancement of a neoplastic lesion characteris-

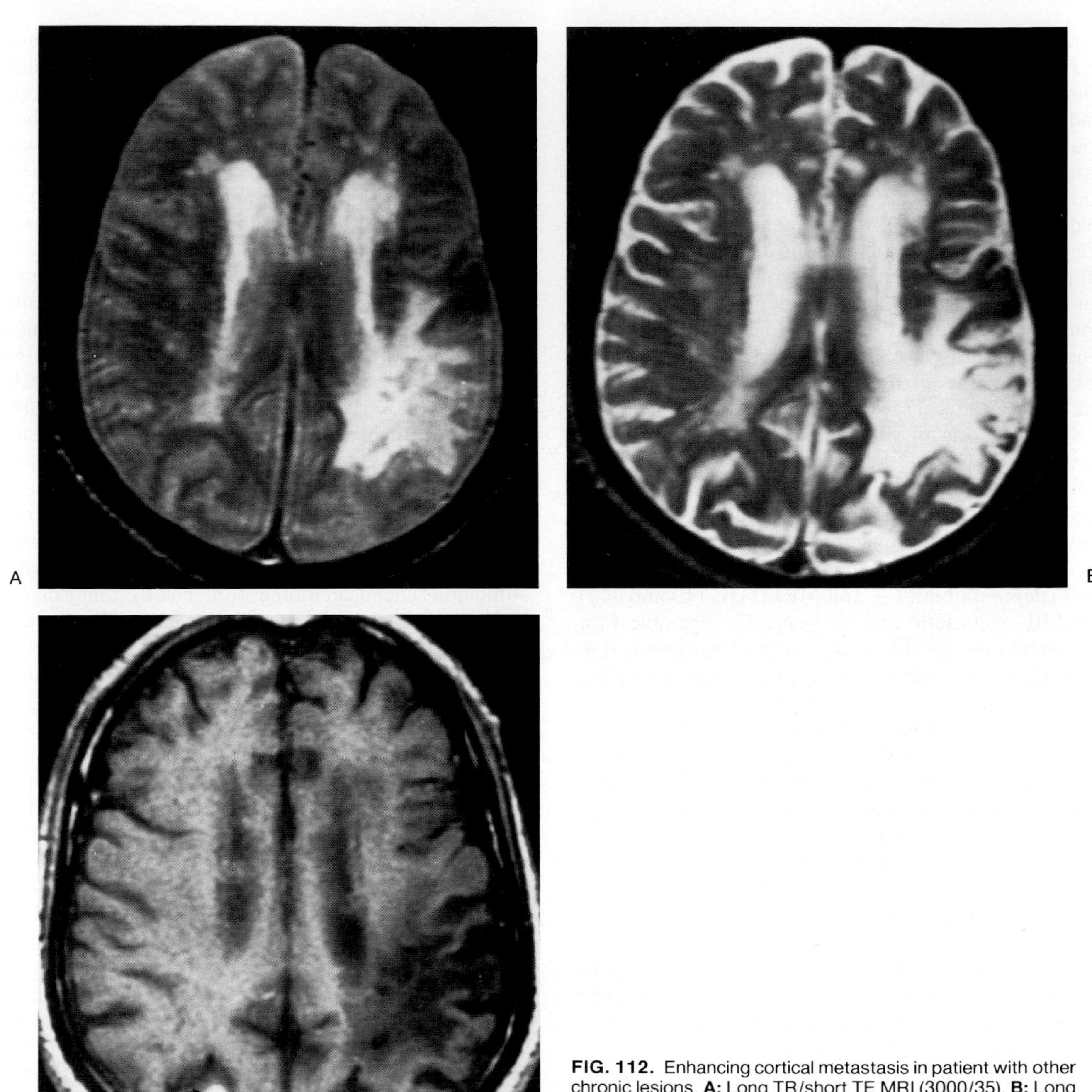

FIG. 112. Enhancing cortical metastasis in patient with other chronic lesions. **A:** Long TR/short TE MRI (3000/35). **B:** Long TR/TE MRI (3000/90). **C:** Short TR/TE MRI (600/20), with contrast enhancement. Although long TR images (A,B) show multiple areas of abnormality, postcontrast scan (C) reveals only one metastatic lesion (*arrows*, C). Note that the metastasis is not detectable on precontrast long TR/short TE image (B), due to its cortical location and consequent lack of edema.

FIG. 113. Evanescent enhancement in cortical metastases. **A:** Long TR/short TE MRI (3000/35). **B:** Long TR/TE MRI (3000/90). **C:** Contrast-enhanced CT. **D:** Short TR/TE MRI (800/20), 3 min after contrast enhancement. **E:** Short TR/TE MRI (800/20), 15 min after contrast enhancement. **F:** Short TR/TE MRI (800/20), 45 min after contrast enhancement. Precontrast long TR images (A,B) and contrast-enhanced CT (C) are normal. On initial postcontrast MRI (D), left frontal cortical metastasis is seen (*closed arrows*, D–F) and persists on 15-min postcontrast scan (E) and 45-min postcontrast scan (F). Note transient visualization of second metastasis only on 15-min scan (E) in right frontal cortex (*open arrow*, E).

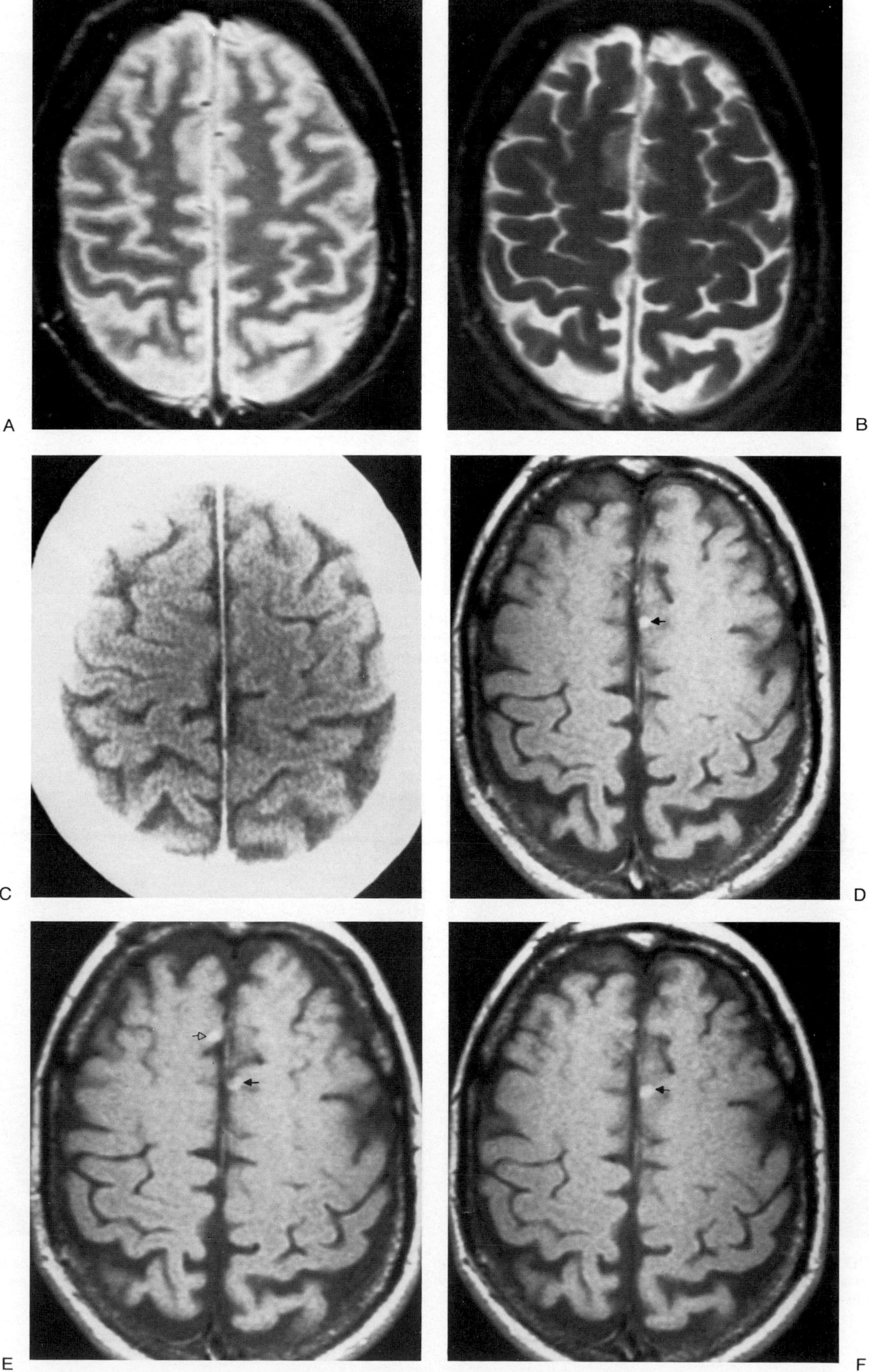
A
B
C
D
E
F

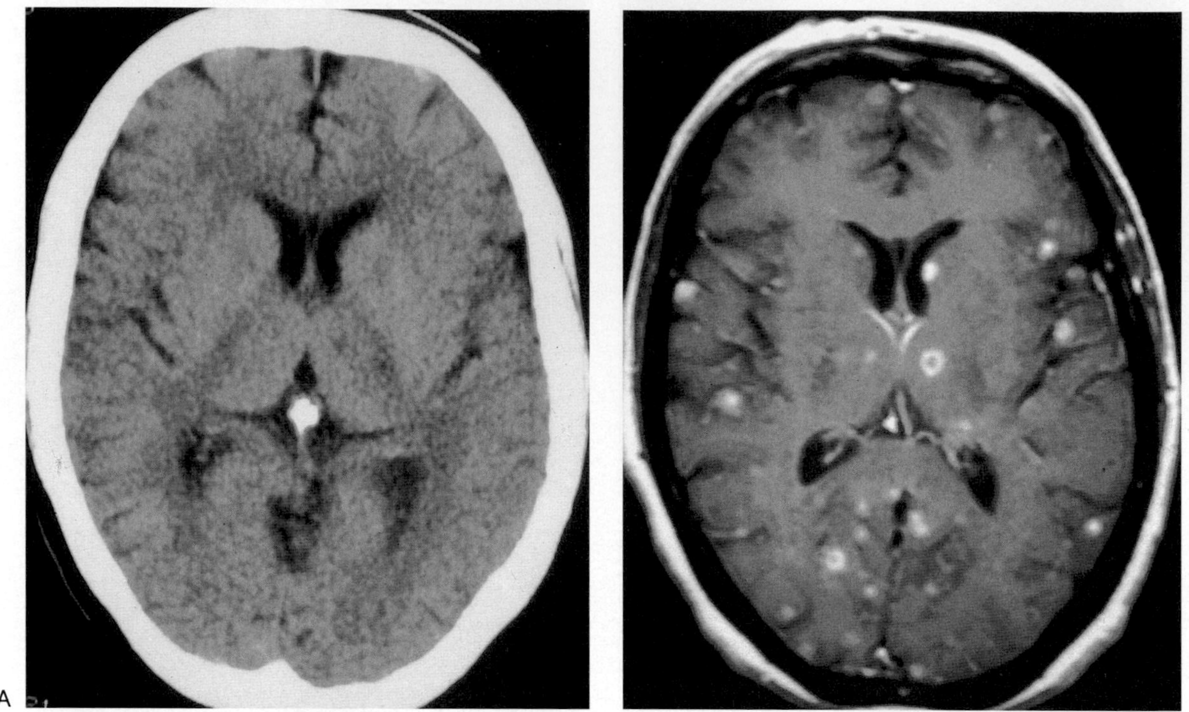

FIG. 114. Screening non-contrast CT vs. enhanced MRI for metastases. Non-contrast CT is unremarkable (**A**) except for left thalamic hypodensity. Contrast-enhanced MRI shows innumerable metastatic lesions (**B**), most of which are in gray matter and are not accompanied by significant edema.

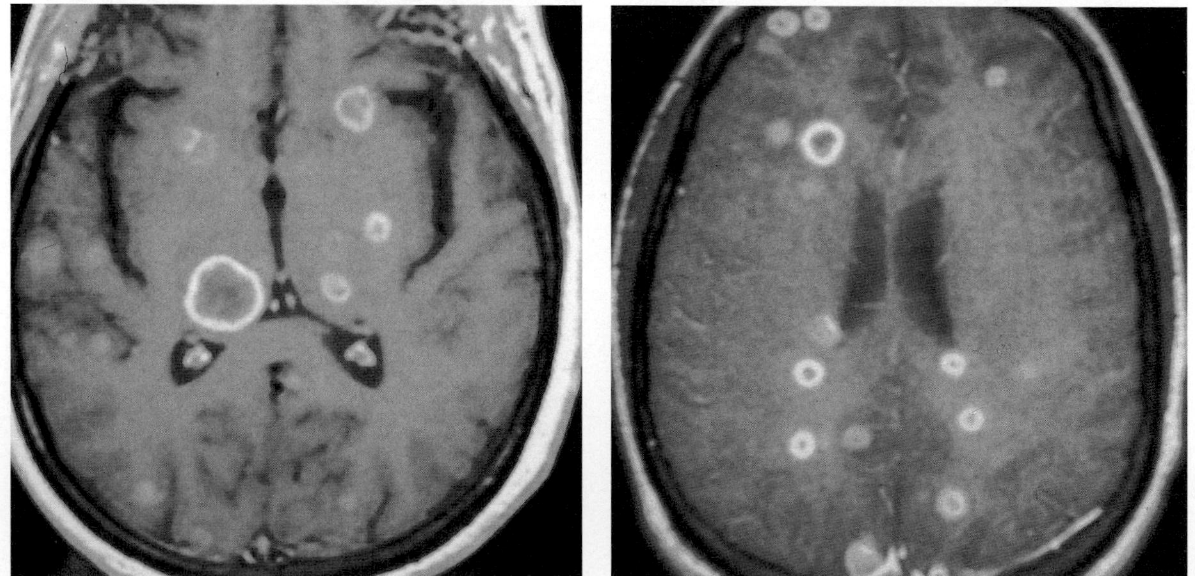

FIG. 115. Ring enhancement, metastases vs. abscesses. Although most metastases are irregular and thick-walled on enhanced studies, adenocarcinomas (**A**) and occasionally other tumors can be remarkably similar to the classic thin-walled ring-enhancing lesions of abscesses (**B**).

tically differs from the enhancement of benign conditions, such as abscess, resolving hematoma, and demyelinating disease, by its wall characteristics (180). Malignant neoplasms, but not all neoplasms, demonstrate thick, irregular, or nodular enhancement (Fig. 97), as opposed to the regular, thin, even and smooth enhancing wall of the above-mentioned benign conditions (Fig. 115).

Regarding the temporal sequence of metastatic tumoral enhancement, it appears that no uniform pattern exists. In any given patient, most metastases enhance dramatically on the immediate postcontrast scan, but other metastases in the same patient and from the same tumor may only appear on delayed scans (Fig. 113). To further complicate matters, we have observed evanescent enhancement in these lesions (Fig. 113), some of which were not visible on any unenhanced short TR or long TR scan. The general consensus amongst large centers seems to be that the immediate post-contrast scan is probably the most practical method for detecting metastases, given the fact that the radiologist will typically obtain only one postcontrast scan. Some centers inject such patients prior to entering the scanner and obtain all images postcontrast.

Regardless of the appearance of the enhancement or its time of onset, the associated findings (and clinical information) are often most helpful in making the specific diagnosis. In general, there is a greater degree of edema (and mass effect) associated with a metastatic focus when compared to the edema associated with most of the benign entities (except abscess), as well as compared to the edema associated with primary gliomas. It should be stressed that in any patient with a primary extracranial neoplasm and intracranial enhancement in a nonvascular distribution, metastases should be considered the diagnosis until proven otherwise. The major differential diagnoses of multiple enhancing lesions and edema, aside from metastases, would include abscesses, multifocal glioma, and radiation necrosis. The major differential diagnosis of a solitary, thick-walled ring-enhancing lesion in the supratentorial brain of an adult, in the absence of a history of prior irradiation, resides in primary glioblastoma versus singular metastasis, a distinction which generally cannot be made on imaging studies alone. In the solitary neoplastic posterior fossa mass of an adult which enhances, the basic differential diagnosis lies in metastasis, hemangioblastoma, or lymphoma.

RADIATION NECROSIS

Postoperative hyperintensity, hemorrhage, or malacia may persist for great lengths of time after tumor resection (Fig. 116). There are several features of recurrent tumors and radiation necrosis of which the radiologist should be cognizant. Unfortunately, microscopic recurrent or residual tumor cannot be realistically excluded with any macroscopic imaging tool, and even histopathology needs adequate tissue sample volumes and clinical correlation to make the diagnosis. Radiation necrosis for the purposes of this chapter will be confined to the delayed form, which is generally seen after treatment of malignant gliomas. Its onset is usually from 6 months to 2 years after treatment, and its occurrence is dependent on both dosage and rate of delivery. It is self-limited and is usually not problematic unless significant mass effect

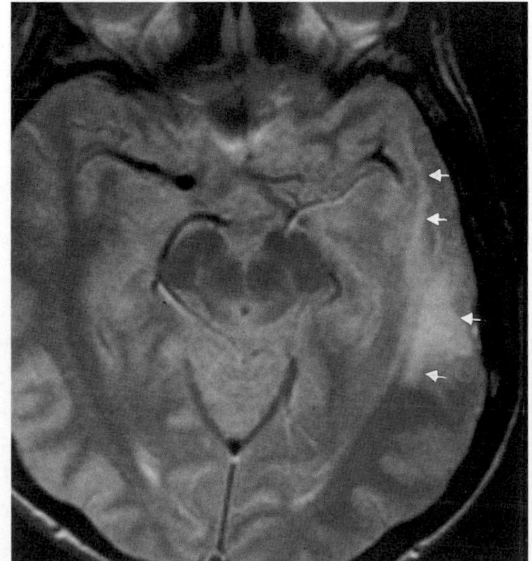

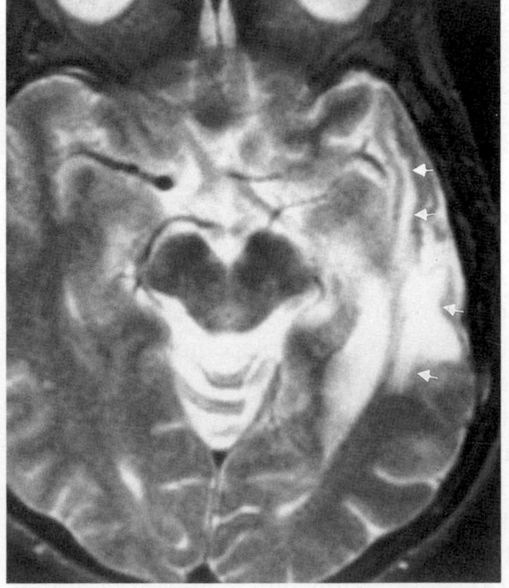

A B

FIG. 116. Difficulty distinguishing recurrent tumor from postoperative change, temporal lobe. **A:** Long TR/short TE MRI (2800/30). **B:** Long TR/TE MRI (2800/80). Persistent posterior temporal high intensity (*arrows*, A,B) is best seen on long TR/short TE (A). Malacia, reflected by enlargement of ipsilateral lateral ventricle (B) is more likely than tumor, but microscopic tumor cannot be excluded with certainty and necessitates follow-up scan.

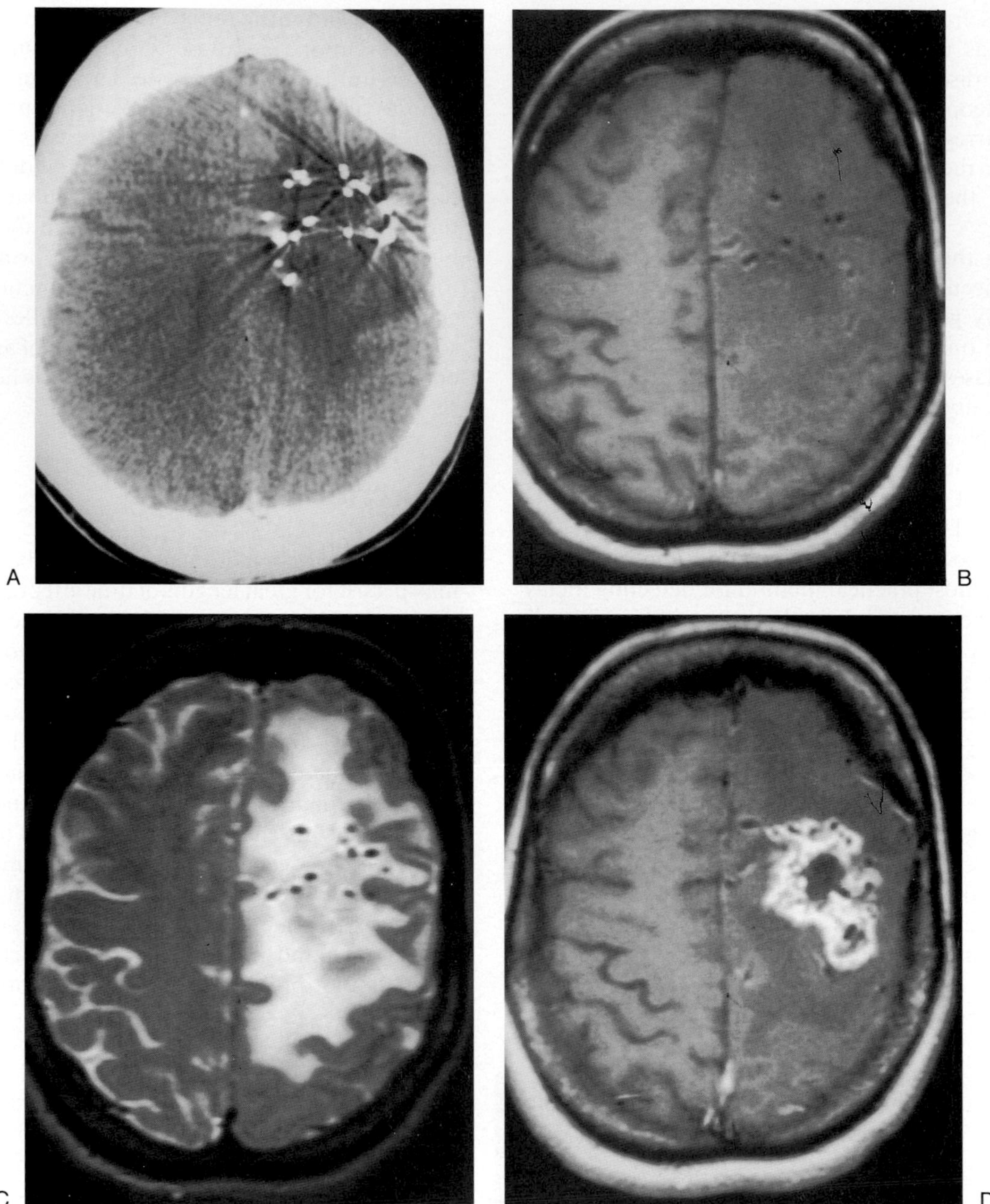

FIG. 117. Radiation necrosis after radiation seed treatment of recurrent glioblastoma. CT demonstrates radiation seed and severe edema (**A**). MRI shows extensive edema and mass effect in region of seeds (**B,C**) and thick-walled irregular enhancement (**D**) due to radiation necrosis, indistinguishable from recurrent tumor.

demands surgical decompression. It is an especially common finding after radiation seed placement (Fig. 117), from which it occurs earlier than from external beam therapy. On pathologic examination, it is a coagulative necrosis without much tissue reaction, presumably due to the ischemic nature of the event (198).

Necrosis from radiation is usually found around the original tumor bed, since that is where the radiation was directed (Fig. 118). Problematically, recurrent glioma is also typically noted in the immediate vicinity of the original lesion (55). Additionally, radiation necrosis and recurrent tumor can frequently coexist. Radiation peritumoral necrosis and vascular changes from radiation (Fig. 119) can occur sooner than the typical one-year interval (55); in fact, acute radiation encephalitis can have a disrupted blood–brain barrier and enhance dramatically on MRI. Recurrent tumor usually enhances with i.v. contrast, even if the original tumor did not. The MR assessment for recurrent tumor therefore is based on either focal mass lesion recurrence on serial scans anatomic pattern (Fig. 120), or new enhancement in or around the site of the original tumor, in comparison with the baseline postoperative scan (usually obtained 4-6 weeks after surgery). Unfortunately, one cannot differentiate radia-

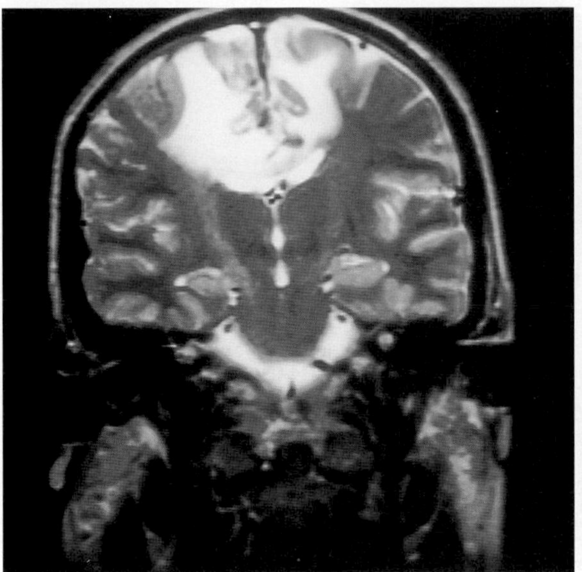

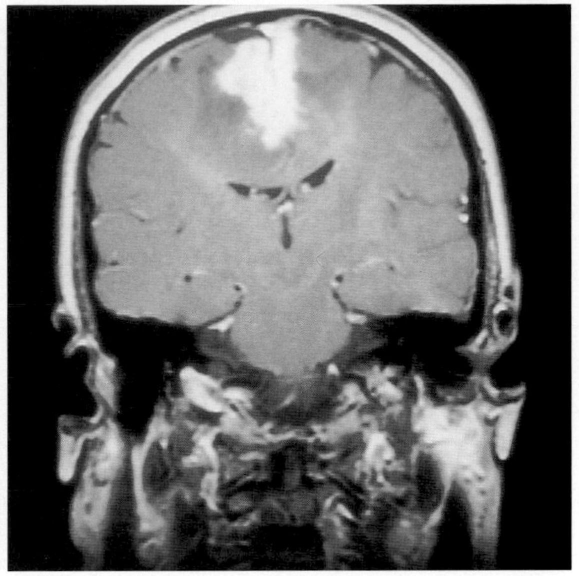

FIG. 118. Radiation necrosis after meningioma treatment. Extensive edema several months after vertex meningioma removal on T2-weighted image (**A**) is due to radiation necrosis, seen as thick cortical enhancement (**B**), rather than recurrent meningioma.

tion necrosis from recurrent tumor by MR imaging alone, but MR with MRS, MR with PET, SPECT, or functional MRI may be useful in that instance. It has been reported that thallium-201/technetium-99m HMPAO SPECT is useful in making this distinction (199). Cerebral blood volume maps from bolus injection contrast-enhanced echo-planar MRI may play a role in aiding the discrimination of recurrent tumor from radiation necrosis (see Chapter 30), since preliminary data indicates that hypometabolic regions on PET fluorodeoxyglucose studies seem to correlate with low CBV regions on MRI.

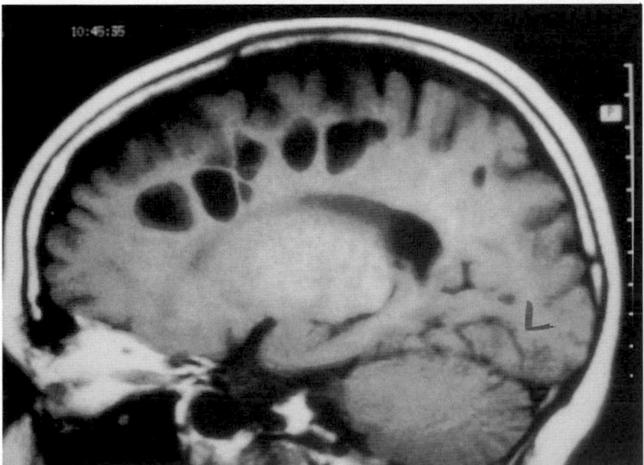

FIG. 119. Subcortical infarctions due to radiation vasculopathy seen as cystic malacia in subcortical white matter on T1-weighted image.

CONCLUSIONS

It is generally agreed at the time of this writing that all patients harboring intracranial tumors at some point along the course of diagnosis and management should undergo MR imaging. In the ideal world, the basic diagnostic work-up of intra-axial brain neoplasms, both at their initial diagnosis as well as in post-treatment follow-up, has uniformly become the role of a single imaging modality—MR with i.v. contrast. Practically speaking, this has not eliminated the utilization of CT scanning, which has its use based on availability and cost. Notwithstanding the apparent maturity of MR imaging, the technique is still evolving, with faster imaging sequences, more sophisticated hardware design, and image processing development. Having said that, spin-echo imaging remains the optimal technique for the detection and characterization of most intracranial neoplasms. High resolution, rapid imaging sequences are becoming integrated into many protocols. New types of MRI contrast agents are continually being developed, for the purposes of added safety and more effective demonstration of blood–brain barrier incompetence. Using these new developments and from comparative MR-pathologic studies, some in-roads have been made with regard to tissue characterization for specificity, but significant overlap still exists in the imaging appearance of many of these entities. Combining physiologic methods, including recently developed echo-planar techniques with contrast bolus for cerebral blood volume maps, functional MRI using task-activation studies, diffusion MRI, MR spectroscopy, and PET, with conventional anatomic MR im-

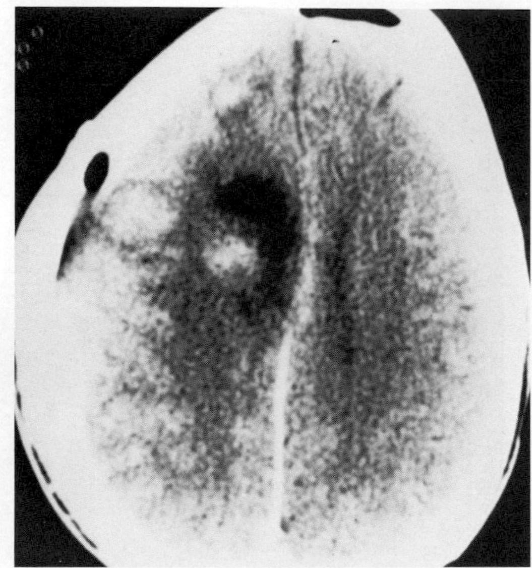

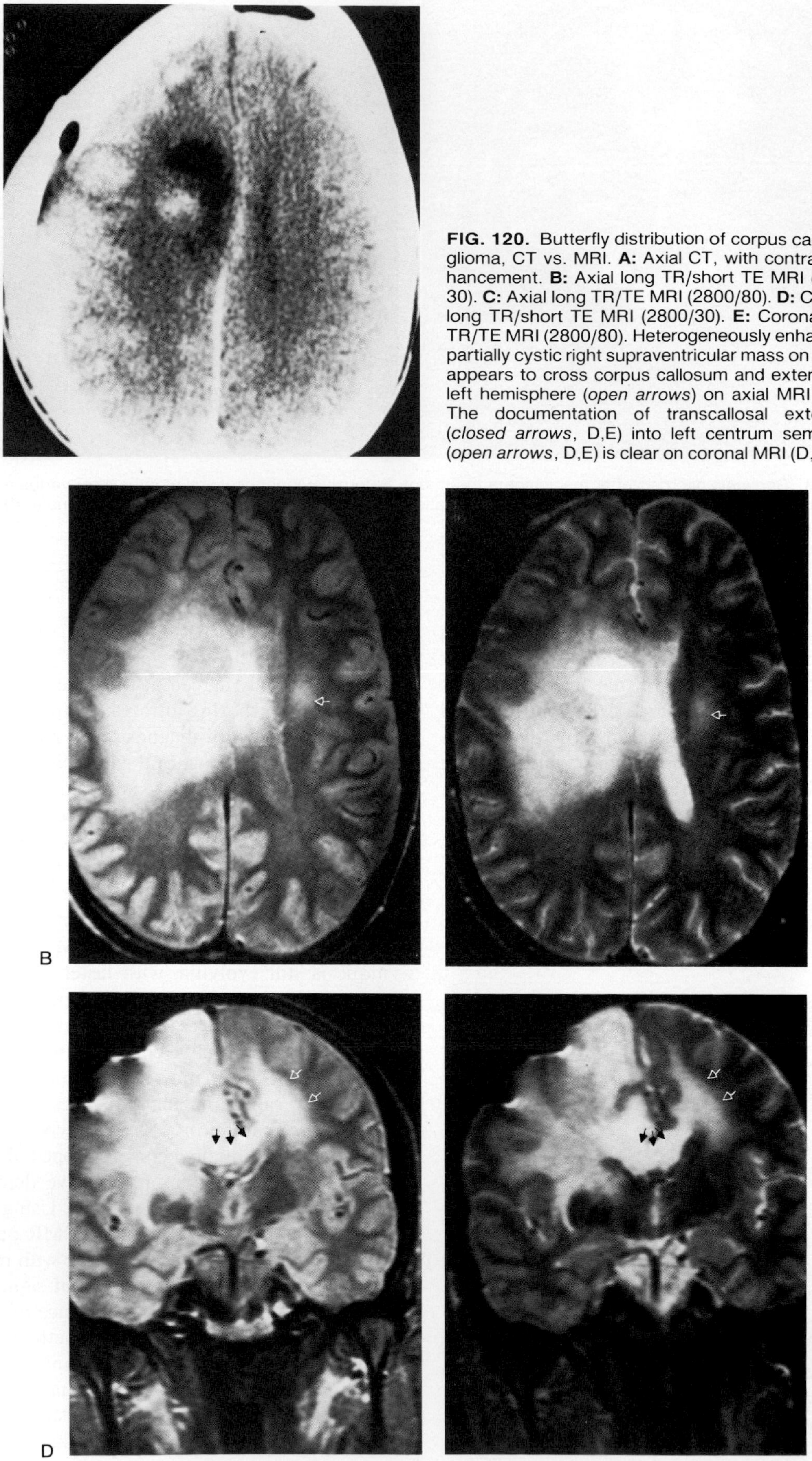

FIG. 120. Butterfly distribution of corpus callosum glioma, CT vs. MRI. **A:** Axial CT, with contrast enhancement. **B:** Axial long TR/short TE MRI (2800/30). **C:** Axial long TR/TE MRI (2800/80). **D:** Coronal long TR/short TE MRI (2800/30). **E:** Coronal long TR/TE MRI (2800/80). Heterogeneously enhancing, partially cystic right supraventricular mass on CT (A) appears to cross corpus callosum and extend into left hemisphere (*open arrows*) on axial MRI (B,C). The documentation of transcallosal extension (*closed arrows*, D,E) into left centrum semiovale (*open arrows*, D,E) is clear on coronal MRI (D,E).

aging may shed light on the natural history of these lesions and, hopefully, make an impact on patient outcome. As newer, sophisticated MR techniques have become available, it is obvious that a thorough knowledge of neuroanatomy, neuropathology, and pathophysiology is essential for the neuroradiologist to play a significant role in the diagnosis and management of these patients. It still remains to be seen whether an integrated multimodality approach to tumor imaging will provide a clinically useful tool in routine settings.

REFERENCES

1. Berens ME, Rutka JT, Rosenblum ML. Brain tumor epidemiology, growth, and invasion. *Neurosurg Clin North Am* 1990;1:1–18.
2. Farwell JR, Dohrmann GJ, Flannery JT. Central nervous system tumors in children. *Cancer* 1977;40:3123.
3. Lee BCP, Kneeland JB, Cahill PT, Deck MDF. MRI recognition of supratentorial tumors. *AJNR* 1985;6:871–878.
4. Healy ME, Hesselink JR, Press GA, Middleton MS. Increased detection of intracranial metastases with intravenous Gd-DTPA. *Radiology* 1987;165:619–624.
5. Russell EJ, Geremia GK, Johnson CE, et al. Multiple cerebral metastases: detectability with Gd-DTPA-enhanced MR imaging. *Radiology* 1987;165:609–617.
6. Kovalikova Z, Hoehn-Berlage MH, Gersonde K, Porschen R, Mittermayer C, Franke R-P. Age-dependent variation of T1 and T2 relaxation times of adenocarcinoma in mice. *Radiology* 1987;164:543–548.
7. Kjos BO, Brant-Zawadzki M, Kucharczyk W, Kelly WM, Norman D, Newton TH. Cystic intracranial lesions: magnetic resonance imaging. *Radiology* 1985;155:363–369.
8. Hackney DB, Grossman RI, Zimmerman RA, Joseph PJ, Goldberg HI, Bilaniuk LT, Spagnoli MV. Low sensitivity of clinical MR imaging to small changes in the concentration of nonparamagnetic protein. *AJNR* 1987;8:1003–1008.
9. Menick BJ, Bobman SA, Listerud J, Atlas SW. Thin section, three-dimensional Fourier transform, steady-state free precession MR imaging of the brain. *Radiology* 1992;183(2):369–377.
10. Bradley WGJ, Schmidt PG. Effect of methemoglobin formation on the MR appearance of subarachnoid hemorrhage. *Radiology* 1985;156:99–103.
11. Russell DS, Rubinstein LJ. *Pathology of Tumors of the Nervous System*, 5th ed. Baltimore: Williams & Wilkins; 1989.
12. Zimmerman H. The pathology of primary brain tumors. *Semin Roentgenol* 1984;19:129.
13. Atlas SW, Grossman RI, Gomori JM, Hackney DB, Goldberg HI, Zimmerman RA, Bilaniuk LT. Hemorrhagic intracranial malignant neoplasms: spin-echo MR imaging. *Radiology* 1987;164:71–77.
14. Gatenby RA, Coia LR, Richter MPea. Oxygen tension in human tumors: in vivo mapping using CT-guided probes. *Radiology* 1985;156:211.
15. Sze G, Krol G, Olson WL, et al. Hemorrhagic neoplasms: MRI mimics of occult vascular malformations. *Am J Radiol* 1987;149:1223–1230.
16. Atlas SW, Grossman RI, Gomori JM, et al. MR imaging of intracranial metastatic melanoma. *J Comput Assist Tomogr* 1987;11:577–582.
17. Lundbom N, Brown R, Koenig S, Lansen T, Valsamis M, Kasoff S. Magnetic field dependence of 1/T1 of human brain tumors. Correlations with histology. *Invest Radiol* 1990;25:1197–1205.
18. Goldmann EE. Vitalfarbung als zentral nervensystem. *Abh Preuss Akad Wiss Phys Klass Math Tech* 1913;1:1–60.
19. Reese TS, Karnovsky MJ. Fine structural localization of blood-brain barrier to exogenous peroxidase. *J Cell Biol* 1967;34:207–217.
20. Sage MRI. Blood-brain barrier: phenomenon of increasing importance to the imaging clinician. *AJR* 1982;138:887–898.
21. Bradbury MWB. Why a blood-brain barrier? *Trends Neurosci* 1979;2:36–38.
22. Nabeshima S, Reese TS. Barrier to proteins within the spinal meninges. *J Neuropathol Exp Neurol* 1972;31:176–177.
23. Gado MH, Phelps ME, Coleman RE. An extravascular component to contrast enhancement in cranial computed tomography. *Radiology* 1975;117:589–593.
24. Yuh W, Nguyen H, Tali E, et al. Delineation of gliomas with various doses of MRI contrast material. *AJNR* 1994;15:983–989.
25. Mathews V, Elster A. Magnetization transfer combined with gadolinium enhancement for intracranial lesions. *AJNR* 1994 [*in press*].
26. Brem H. Supratentorial astrocytomas. In: Long DM, ed. *Current Therapy in Neurological Surgery 1985–1986.* St. Louis: CV Mosby; 1985:27–29.
27. Lilja A, Bergstrom K, Spannare B, Olsson Y. Reliability of computed tomography in assessing histopathological features of malignant supratentorial gliomas. *J Comput Assist Tomogr* 1981;5:625–636.
28. Smith AS, Weinstein MA, Modic MT, et al. Magnetic resonance with marked T2-weighted images: improved demonstration of brain lesions, tumor, and edema. *AJNR* 1985;6:691–697.
29. Graif M, Bydder GM, Steiner RE, Niendorf P, Thomas DGT, Young IR. Contrast-enhanced MR imaging of malignant brain tumors. *AJNR* 1985;6:855–862.
30. Runge VM, Clanton JA, Price AC, et al. Contrast-enhanced MR imaging of the brain: experimental and clinical investigation with Gd-DTPA. *Radiology* 1984;153:145(abst).
31. Weinman HJ, Brasch RC, Press WR, Wesbey GE. Characteristics of gadolinium-DTPA complex: a potential NMR contrast agent. *AJR* 1984;142:619–624.
32. Burger PC, Scheithauer BW. Tumors of neuroglia and choroid plexus epithelium. In: *Tumors of the Central Nervous System.* Washington, D.C.: Armed Forces Institute of Pathology; 1994: 25–161.
33. Gullotta F, Kersting G, Wullenweber R. Recurrence of gliomas. A comparative clinical and morphological study with a note on the histological grading of astrocytomas. In: Kuhlendahl H, Hensall V, eds. *Modern Aspects of Neurosurgery.* Amsterdam: Excerpta Medica;1971:116–121.
34. Muller W, Afra D, Schroder R. Supratentorial recurrences of gliomas. Morphological studies in relation to time intervals with astrocytomas. *Acta Neurochir* 1977;37:75.
35. Rorke LB, Gilles FH, Davis RL, Becker LE. Revision of the World Health Organization classification of brain tumors for childhood brain tumors. *Cancer* 1985;56:1869–1886.
36. World Health Organization. *Classification of Brain Tumors.* Zurich: WHO; 1990.
37. VandenBerg SR. Current diagnostic concepts of astrocytic tumors. *J Neuropathol Exp Neurol* 1992;51:644–657.
38. Bailey P, Cushing H. *Classification of the Tumors of the Glioma Group on a Histogenetic Basis with a Correlated Study of Prognosis.* Philadelphia: J.B. Lippincott; 1926.
39. Kernohan JW, Sayre GP. Tumors of the Central Nervous System. In: *Atlas of Tumor Pathology*, section X, fascicle 35. Washington, D.C.: Armed Forces Institute of Pathology; 1952.
40. Kim T, Halliday A, Hedley-Whyte E, Convery K. Correlates of survival and the Daumas-Duport grading system for astrocytomas. *J Neurosurg* 1991;74:27–37.
41. Hoshino T, Prados M, Wilson C, Cho K, Lee K-S, Davis R. Prognosis implications of the bromodeoxyuridine labeling index of human gliomas. *J Neurosurg* 1989;71:335–341.
42. Fujimaki T, Matsutani M, Nakamura O, et al. Correlation between bromodeoxyuridine-labeling indices and patient prognosis in cerebral astrocytic tumors in adults. *Cancer* 1991;67:1629–1634.
43. Salmon I, Kiss R, Dewitte O, Gras T, Pasteels J-L, Brotchi J, Flament-Durand J. Histopathlogic grading and DNA ploidy in relation to survival among 206 adult astrocytic tumor patients. *Cancer* 1992;70:538–546.
44. Salmon I, Dewitte O, Pasteels J-L, Flament-Durand J, Brotchi J, Vereerstraeten P, Kiss R. Prognostic scoring in adult astrocytic tumors using patient age, histopathologic grade, and DNA histogram type. *J Neurosurg* 1994;80:877–883.
45. Burger PC, Vogel S, Green SB, Strike TA. Glioblastoma

multiforme and anaplastic astrocytoma. *Cancer* 1985;56:1106–1111.

46. McKeran RO, Thomas DGT. The clinical study of gliomas. In: Thomas DGT, Graham DI, eds. *Brain Tumours. Scientific Basis, Clinical Investigation and Current Therapy.* London: Butterworths; 1980:194.
47. Vertosick FJ, Selker R, Arena V. Survival of patients with well-differentiated astrocytomas diagnosed in the era of computed tomography. *Neurosurgery* 1991;28:496–501.
48. McCormack B, Miller D, Budzilovich G, Voorhees G, Ransohoff J. Treatment and survival of low grade astrocytoma in adults—1977–1988. *Neurosurgery* 1992;31:636–642.
49. Kelly P, Daumas-Duport C, Kispert D, Kall B, Scheithauer B, Illig J. Imaging-based stereotactic serial biopsies in untreated intracranial glial neoplasms. *J Neurosurg* 1987;66:865–874.
50. Greene G, Hitchon P, Schelper R, Yuh W, Dyste G. Diagnostic yield in CT-guided stereotactic biopsy of gliomas. *J Neurosurg* 1989;71:494–497.
51. Earnest F IV, Kelly PJ, Scheithauer BW, et al. Cerebral astrocytomas: histopathologic correlation of MRI and CT contrast enhancement with stereotactic biopsy. *Radiology* 1988;166:823–827.
52. Holland BA, Kucharcyzk W, Brant-Zawadzki M, Norman D, Haas DK, Harper PS. MR imaging of calcified intracranial lesions. *Radiology* 1985;157:353–356.
53. Atlas SW, Grossman RI, Hackney DB, et al. Calcified intracranial lesions: detection with gradient-echo-acquisition rapid MR imaging. *AJNR* 1988;9:253–259.
54. Marks JE, Gado M. Serial computed tomography of primary brain tumors following surgery, irradiation, and chemotherapy. *Radiology* 1977;125:119–125.
55. Burger PC. Malignant astrocytic neoplasms: classification, pathologic anatomy and response to treatment. *Semin Oncol* 1986;13:16.
56. Nelson DF, Nelson JS, Davis DR, Chang CH, Griffin TW, Pajak TF. Survival and prognosis of patients with astrocytoma with atypical or anaplastic features. *J Neurol Oncol* 1985;3:99–103.
57. Butler AR, Horli SC, Kircheff II, et al. Computed tomography in astrocytomas. A statistical analysis of the parameters of malignancy and the positive contrast-enhanced CT scan. *Radiology* 1978;129:433–439.
58. Barnard R, Geddes J. The incidence of multifocal cerebral gliomas. A histologic study of large hemispheric sections. *Cancer* 1987;60:1519–1531.
59. Kieffer SA, Salibi NA, Kim RC, et al. Multifocal glioblastoma: diagnostic implications. *Radiology* 1982;143:709–710.
60. Tassel PV, Lee Y-Y, Bruner JM. Synchronous and metachronous malignant gliomas: CT findings. *AJNR* 1988;9:725–732.
61. Woodruff WW Jr, Djang WT, Voorhees D, Heinz ER. Calvarial destruction: an unusual manifestation of glioblastoma multiforme. *AJNR* 1988;9:388–389.
62. Haimes AB, Zimmerman RD, Morgello S, et al. MR imaging of brain abscesses. *AJNR* 1989;10:279–291.
63. Gomori JM, Grossman RI, Goldberg HI, et al. Occult cerebral vascular malformations: high field MR imaging. *Radiology* 1986;158:707–713.
64. Nevin S. Gliomatosis cerebri. *Brain* 1938;61:170–191.
65. Scheinker I, Evans J. Diffuse cerebral glioblastosis. *J Neuropathol* 1943;2:178–189.
66. Couch J, Weiss S. Gliomatosis cerebri. *Neurology* 1974;24:504–511.
67. Geremia GK, Wollman R, Foust R. Computed tomography of gliomatosis cerebri. *J Comput Assist Tomogr* 1988;12:698–701.
68. Spagnoli MV, Grossman RI, Packer RJ, Hackney DB, Goldberg HI, Zimmerman RA, Bilaniuk L. Magnetic resonance imaging determination of gliomatosis cerebri. *Neuroradiology* 1987;29:15–18.
69. Lee Y, Van Tassel P, Bruner JM, Moser RP, Share JC. Juvenile pilocytic astrocytomas: CT and MRI characteristics. *AJNR* 1989;10:363–370.
70. Wallner KE, Gonzales MF, Edwards MSB, Wara WM, Shelkine GE. Treatment results of juvenile pilocytic astrocytoma. *J Neurosurg* 1988;69:171–176.
71. Forsyth P, Shaw E, Scheithauer B, O'Fallon J, Layton D, Katzmann J. 51 cases of supratentorial pilocytic astrocytomas: a clinicopathologic, prognostic, and flow cytometric study. *Cancer* 1993;72:1335–1342.
72. Alvord EC, Lofton S. Gliomas of the optic nerve or chiasm. *J Neurosurg* 1988;68:85–98.
73. Stern J, Jakobiec FA, Housepien EM. The architecture of optic nerve gliomas with and without neurofibromatosis. *Arch Ophthalmol* 1980;98:505–511.
74. De Recondo J, Haguenau M. Neuropathologic survey of the phakomatoses and allied disorders. In: Vinken PJ, Bruyn GW, eds. *Handbook of Clinical Neurology: The Phakomatoses.* Amsterdam: North Holland; 1972:19–71.
75. Frerebeau P, Benezech J, Harbi H. Intraventricular tumors in tuberous sclerosis. *Childs Nerv Syst* 1985;1:45–48.
76. Chow CW, Klug GL, Lewis EA. Subependymal giant cell astrocytoma in children. *J Neurosurg* 1988;68:880–883.
77. Bender JR, Yunis EJ. The pathology of tuberous sclerosis. *Pathol Annu* 1982;17:339–382.
78. McMurdo SK, Moore SG, Brant-Zawadzki M, et al. MR imaging of intracranial tuberous sclerosis. *AJR* 1987;148:791–796.
79. Braffman BH, Bilaniuk LT, Zimmerman RA. The central nervous system manifestations of the phakomatoses on MRI. *Radiol Clin North Am* 1988;26:773–800.
80. McLaurin RL, Towbin RB. Tuberous sclerosis: diagnostic and surgical considerations. *Pediatr Neurosci* 1985;12:43–48.
81. Tsuchida T, Kamata K, Kawamata M. Brain tumors in tuberous sclerosis. *Child's Brain* 1984;8:271–283.
82. Lipper M, Eberhard D, Phillips C, Vezina L, Cail W. Pleomorphic xanthoastrocytoma, a distinctive astroglial tumor: neuroradiologic and pathologic features. *AJNR* 1993;14:1397–1404.
83. Mork SJ, Lindegaard JF, Halvonsen TB, et al. Oligodendroglioma: incidence and biological behavior in a defined population. *J Neurosurg* 1985;63:881–889.
84. Roberts M, German WJ. A long term study of patients with oligodendrogliomas. Follow-up of 50 cases, including Dr. Harvey Cushing's series. *J Neurosurg* 1966;24:697–700.
85. Shaw EG, Scheithauer BW, O'Fallon J, Tazelaar H, Davis DH. Oligodendrogliomas: the Mayo Clinic experience. *J Neurosurg* 1992;76:428–434.
86. Wallner KE, Gonzales M, Sheline GE. Treatment of oligodendrogliomas with or without postoperative irradiation. *J Neurosurg* 1988;68:684–688.
87. Reedy DP, Bay JW, Hahn JF. Role of radiation therapy in the treatment of cerebral oligodendroglioma: an analysis of 57 cases and a literature review. *Neurosurgery* 1983;13:499–503.
88. Lee Y, Tassel PV. Intracranial oligodendrogliomas: imaging findings in 35 untreated cases. *AJNR* 1989;10:119–127.
89. Lee Y, Vonofakos D, Marcu H, Hacker H. Oligodendrogliomas: CT patterns with emphasis on features indicating malignancy. *J Comput Assist Tomogr* 1979;3:783–788.
90. Courville CB. Ganglioglioma; tumor of the central nervous system. Review of the literature and report of 2 cases. *Arch Neurol Psych* 1930;24:439.
91. Courville CB. Gangliogliomas. Further report with special reference to those occurring in the temporal lobe. *Arch Neurol Psych* 1931;25:309.
92. Zimmerman RA, Bilaniuk LT. Computed tomography of intracerebral gangliomas. *J Comput Assist Tomogr* 1979;3:24–30.
93. Denierre B, Stinchnoth FA, Hori A, Spoerri O. Intracerebral gangliogliomas. *J Neurosurg* 1986;65:177–182.
94. Dorne HL, O'Gorman MN, Melanson D. Computed tomography of intracranial gangliogliomas. *AJNR* 1986;7:281–285.
95. Johanson JH, Rekate HL, Roesmann U. Gangliogliomas: pathological and clinical correlation. *J Neurosurg* 1981;54:58–63.
96. Castillo M, Davis PC, Takei Y, Hoffman JC Jr. Intracranial ganglioglioma: MRI, CT, and clinical findings in 18 patients. *AJNR* 1990;11:109–114.
97. Wacker M, Cogen P, Etzell J, Daneshvar L, Davis R, Prados M. Diffuse leptomeningeal involvement by a ganglioglioma in a child. *J Neurosurg* 1992;77:302–306.
98. Altman NR. MRI and CT characteristics of gangliocytoma: a rare cause of epilepsy in children. *AJNR* 1988;9:917–921.
99. VandenBerg SR, May EE, Rubinstein LJ, et al. Desmoplastic supratentorial neuroepithelial tumors of infancy with divergent differentiation potential ('desmoplastic infantile ganglioglioma'). *J Neurosurg* 1987;66:58.

100. Yasargil M, von Ammon K, von Deimling A, Valavanis A, Wichmann W, Wiestler O. Central neurocytoma: histopathological variants and therapeutic approaches. *J Neurosurg* 1992;76:32–37.
101. Burger PC, Scheithauer BW. Neuronal and glio-neuronal tumors. In: *Tumors of the Central Nervous System.* Washington, D.C.: Armed Forces Institute of Pathology; 1994:163–191.
102. Kim D, Chi J, Park S, et al. Intraventricular neurocytoma: clinicopathological analysis of seven cases. *J Neurosurg* 1992;76:759–765.
103. Han JS, Bonstelle T, Kaufman B, et al. Magnetic resonance imaging in the evaluation of the brainstem. *Radiology* 1984;150:705–712.
104. Lee BCP, Kneeland JB, Deck MDF, Cahill PT. Posterior fossa lesions: magnetic resonance imaging. *Radiology* 1984;153:137–143.
105. Lee BCP, Kneeland JB, Walker RW, et al. MR imaging of brainstem tumors. *AJNR* 1985;6:159–164.
106. Radkowski MA, Naidich TP, Tomita T, Byrd SE, McLone DG. Neonatal brain tumors: CT and MRI findings. *J Comput Assist Tomogr* 1988;12:10–20.
107. McLaurin RL. Posterior fossa ependymoma. In: Long DM, ed. *Current Therapy in Neurological Surgery 1985–1986.* St. Louis: CV Mosby; 1985:40–43.
108. Gjerris F, Klinken L. Long-term prognosis in children with benign cerebellar astrocytoma. *J Neurosurg* 1978;49:179.
109. Fitz CR, Rao KCVG. Primary tumors in children. In: Lee SH, Rao KCVG, eds. *Cranial Computed Tomography and MRI.* New York: McGraw-Hill; 1987:365–412.
110. Austin EJ, Alvord EC. Recurrences of cerebellar astrocytomas: a violation of Collins' law. *J Neurosurg* 1988;68:41–47.
111. Collins VP, Loeffler RK, Tivey H. Observations on growth rates of human tumors. *AJR* 1956;76:988–1000.
112. Kucharczyk W, Brant-Zawadzki M, Sobel DF, et al. Central nervous system tumors in children: detection by magnetic resonance imaging. *Radiology* 1985;155:131–136.
113. Shillito, JJ. Cerebellar astrocytoma. In: Long DM, ed. *Current Therapy in Neurological Surgery 1985–1986.* St. Louis: CV Mosby; 1985:46–48.
114. Liebel SA, Sheline GE. Radiation therapy for neoplasms of the brain. *J Neurosurg* 1987;66:1.
115. Caputy AJ, McCullough DC, Manz HJ, Patterson K, Hammock MK. A review of the factors influencing the prognosis of medulloblastoma. The importance of cell differentiation. *J Neurosurg* 1987;66:80–87.
116. Naidich TP, Lin JP, Leeds NE, Pudlowski RM, Naidich JB. Primary tumors and other massses of the cerebellum and fourth ventricle: differential diagnosis by computed tomography. *Neuroradiology* 1977;14:153–174.
117. Figueroa RE, El Gammal T, Brooks BS, Holgate R, Miller W. MRI findings on primitive neuroectodermal tumors. *J Comput Assist Tomogr* 1989;13:773–778.
118. Zee C-S, Segall HD, Miller C, Ahmadi J, McComb JG, Han JS, Park SH. Less common CT features of medulloblastomas. *Radiology* 1982;144:97–102.
119. Davis PC, Wichman RD, Takei Y, Hoffman JCJ. Primary cerebral neuroblastoma: CT and MRI findings in 12 cases. *AJNR* 1990;11:115–120.
120. Mork SJ, Loken AC. Ependymoma. A follow-up study of 101 cases. *Cancer* 1977;40:907.
121. Okazaki H, Scheithauer B. *Atlas of Neuropathology.* New York: Gower Medical; 1988.
122. Naidich TP, Zimmerman RA. Primary brain tumors in children. *Semin Roentgenol* 1984;19:100–114.
123. Armington WG, Osborn AG, Cubberly DA, et al. Supratentorial ependymoma: CT appearance. *Radiology* 1985;157:367–372.
124. Spoto GP, Press GA, Hesselink JR, Solomon M. Intracranial ependymoma and subependymoma: MR manifestations. *AJNR* 1990;11:83–91.
125. Courville CB, Broussalian SL. Plastic ependymomas of the lateral recess. Report of eight verified cases. *J Neurosurg* 1961;18:792.
126. Jenkin RDT, Boesel C, Ertel I, et al. Brain-stem tumors in childhood: a prospective randomized trial of irradiation with and without adjuvant CCNU, VCR, and prednisone. *J Neurosurg* 1987;66:227–233.
127. Khatib Z, Heidemann R, Kovnar E, et al. Pilocytic dorsally exophytic brainstem gliomas: a distinct clinicopathologic entity. *Ann Neurol* 1992;32:458–459.
128. Packer RJ, Allen J, Nielson S, Petito C, Deck M, Jereb B. Brainstem glioma: clinical manifestations of meningeal gliomatosis. *Ann Neurol* 1983;14:177.
129. Scheithauer BW. Symptomatic subependymoma. Report of 21 cases with review of the literature. *J Neurosurg* 1978;49:689.
130. Lhermitte J, Duclos P. Sur un ganglioneuronome diffus du cortex du cervelet. *Bull Cancer (Paris)* 1920;94:99–107.
131. Smith RR, Grossman RI, Goldberg HI, et al. MR imaging of Lhermitte-Duclos disease: a case report. *AJNR* 1989;10:187.
132. Hubschmann OR, Vijayanathan T, Countee RW. Von Hippel-Lindau disease with multiple manifestations: diagnosis and management. *Neurosurgery* 1981;8:92–95.
133. Huson SM, Harper PS, Hourihan MD. Cerebellar hemangioblastoma and von Hippel-Lindau disease. *Brain* 1986;109:1297–1310.
134. Lee SR, Sanches J, Mark AS, Dillon WP, Norman D, Newton TH. Posterior fossa hemangioblastomas: MR imaging. *Radiology* 1989;171:463–468.
135. Enomoto H, Shibata T, Ito A, et al. Multiple hemangioblastomas accompanied by syringomyelia in the cerebellum and the spinal cord. Review and report of five cases. *Surg Neurol* 1984;22:197–203.
136. Okawara SH. Solid cerebellar hemangioblastoma. *J Neurosurg* 1973;39:514–518.
137. Cushing H, Bailey P. Hemangiomas of cerebellum and retina. *Arch Ophthalmol* 1928;57:447–456.
138. Elster AD, Arthur DW. Intracranial hemangioblastomas: CT and MRI findings. *J Comput Assist Tomogr* 1988;12:736–739.
139. Silbergeld J, Cohen WA, Maravilla KR, Dalley RW, Sumi M. Supratentorial and spinal cord hemangioblastomas: gadolinium enhanced MRI appearance with pathologic correlation. *J Comput Assist Tomogr* 1989;13:1048–1051.
140. Winfield JA. Pineal region tumor. In: Long DM, ed. *Current Therapy in Neurological Surgery 1985–1986.* Philadelphia: B.C. Decker; 1985:31–33.
141. Edwards MSB, Hudgins RJ, Wilson CB, Levin VA, Wara WM. Pineal region tumors in children. *J Neurosurg* 1988;68:689–697.
142. Chang T, Teng MMH, Guo W-Y, Sheng W-C. CT of pineal tumors and intracranial germ-cell tumors. *AJNR* 1989;153:1039–1044.
143. Bing JF, Globus JH, Simon H. Pubertas praecox: a survey of reported cases and their verified anatomical findings, with particular reference to tumors of the pineal body. *J Mount Sinai Hosp* 1938;4:935.
144. Borden S, Weber AL, Toch R, Wang CC. Pineal germinoma: long term survival despite hematogenous metastases. *Am J Dis Child* 1973;126:214.
145. Zimmerman RA, Bilaniuk LT, Wood JH, Bruce DA, Schut L. Computed tomography of pineal, parapineal and histologically related tumors. *Radiology* 1980;137:669–677.
146. Ganti SR, Hilal SK, Stein BM, Silver AJ, Mawad M, Sane P. CT of pineal region tumors. *AJR* 1986;146:451–458.
147. Kilgore DP, Strother CM, Strashak RJ, Haughton VM. Pineal germinoma: MR imaging. *Radiology* 1986;158:435–438.
148. Muller-Forell W, Schroth G, Egan PJ. MR imaging in tumors of the pineal region. *Neuroradiology* 1988;30:224.
149. Soejima T, Takeshita I, Yamamoto H, Tsukamoto Y, Fukui M, Matsuoka S. Computed tomography of germinomas of basal ganglia and thalamus. *Neuroradiology* 1987;29:366–370.
150. Chang CGS, Kageyama N, Kobayashi T, Yoshida J, Negoro M. Pineal tumors: clinical diagnosis with special emphasis on the significance of pineal calcification. *Neurosurgery* 1981;8:656–658.
151. Rubinstein LJ. Cytogenesis and differentiation of pineal neoplasms. *Hum Pathol* 1981;12:441–448.
152. Bader JL, Meadows AT, Zimmerman LE, Rorke LB, Voute PA, Champion LAA, Miller RW. Bilateral retinoblastoma with ectopic intracranial retinoblastoma: trilateral retinoblastoma. *Cancer Genet Cytogenet* 1982;5:203.
153. Fain J, Tomlinson F, Sheithauer B, Parisi J, Fletcher G, Kelly P, Miller G. Symptomatic glial cysts of the pineal gland. *J Neurosurg* 1994;80:454–460.

154. Wisoff J, Epstein F. Surgical management of symptomatic pineal cysts. *J Neurosurg* 1992;77:896–900.
155. Lee DH, Norman D, Newton TH. MR imaging of pineal cysts. *J Comput Assist Tomogr* 1987;11:586.
156. Shaungshoti S, Roberts MP, Netsky MG. Neuroepithelial (colloid) cysts. Pathogenesis and relation to choroid plexus and ependyma. *Arch Pathol Lab Med* 1965;80:214–224.
157. Lach B, Scheithauer B, Gregor A, Wick M. Colloid cyst of the third ventricle: a comparative immunohistochemical study of neuraxis cysts and choroid plexus epithelium. *J Neurosurg* 1993;78:101–111.
158. Inoue T, Matsusshima T, Fukui M, Iwaki T, Takeshita I, Kuromatsu C. Immunohistochemical study of intracranial cysts. *Neurosurgery* 1988;23:576–581.
159. Donaldson JO, Simon RH. Radiodense ions within a third ventricular colloid cyst. *Arch Neurol* 1980;37:246.
160. Czervionke LF, Daniels DL, Meyer GA, Pojunas KW, Williams AL, Haughton VM. Neuroepithelial cysts of the lateral ventricles: MRI appearance. *AJNR* 1987;8:609–613.
161. Waggenspack GA, Guinto FC. MRI and CT of masses of the anterosuperior third ventricle. *AJNR* 1989;10:105–110.
162. Scotti G, Scialfa G, Colombo N, Landoni L. MRI in the diagnosis of colloid cysts of the third ventricle. *AJNR* 1987;8:370–372.
163. Jellinger K, Radaszkiewicz TH, Slowik F. Primary malignant lymphomas of the central nervous system in man. *Acta Neuropathol* 1975;95.
164. Hochberg FH, Miller DC. Primary central nervous system lymphoma. *J Neurosurg* 1988;68:835–853.
165. Baumgartner J, Rachlin J, Beckstead J, Meeker T, Levy R, Wara W, Rosenblum M. Primary central nervous system lymphomas: natural history and response to radiation therapy in 55 patients with acquired immunodeficiency syndrome. *J Neurosurg* 1990;73:206–211.
166. Clark W, Callihan T, Schwartzberg L, Fontanesi J. Primary intracranial Hodgkin's lymphoma without dural attachment. *J Neurosurg* 1992;76:692–695.
167. Jack CR Jr, O'Neill BP, Banks PM, Reese DF. Central nervous system lymphoma: histologic types and CT appearance. *Radiology* 1988;167:211–215.
168. Dina T. Primary central nervous system lymphoma versus toxoplasmosis in AIDS. *Radiology* 1991;179:823–828.
169. Poon T, Matoso I, Tchertkoff V, Weitzner I Jr, Gade M. CT features of primary cerebral lymphoma in AIDS and non-AIDS patients. *J Comput Assist Tomogr* 1989;13:6–9.
170. Brant-Zawadzki M, Enzmann DR. Computed tomographic brain scanning in patients with lymphoma. *Radiology* 1978;129: 67–71.
171. Enzmann DR, Tokye KC, Hayward R. CT in leptomeningeal spread of tumor. *J Comput Assist Tomogr* 1978;2:448–455.
172. Sze G, Soletsky S, Bronen R, Krol G. MR imaging of the cranial meninges with emphasis on contrast enhancement and meningeal carcinomatosis. *AJNR* 1989;10:965–975.
173. Posner J. Management of central nervous system metastases. *Semin Oncol* 1977;4:81–91.
174. Okazaki H. *Fundamentals of Neuropathology.* New York: Igaku-Shoin; 1983.
175. Smalley S, Laws E, O'Fallon J, Shaw E, Schray M. Resection for solitary brain metastasis. Role of adjuvant radiation and prognostic variables in 229 patients. *J Neurosurg* 1992;77:531–540.
176. Vieth RG, Odom GL. Intracranial metastases and their neurosurgical treatment. *J Neurosurg* 1965;23:375–383.
177. Mahaley MS. Commentary on diagnosis and surgical management of metastatic brain. tumors. *J Neurooncol* 1987;4:191–193.
178. Tarver RD, Richmond BD, Klatte EC. Cerebral metastases from lung carcinoma: neurological and CT correlation. *Radiology* 1984;153:689–692.
179. Galicich, JH, Sundaresan N, Smith BH. Solitary intracranial metastasis. In: Long DM, ed. *Current Therapy in Neurological Surgery 1985–1986.* Philadelphia: B.C. Decker; 1985:29–31.
180. Potts DG, Abbott GF, von Sneidern JV. National Cancer Institute Study: evaluation of computed tomography in the diagnosis of intracranial neoplasms. III. Metastatic tumors. *Radiology* 1980;136:657–664.
181. Ginaldi S, Wallace S, Shalen P, Luna M, Handel S. Cranial computed tomography of malignant melanoma. *AJNR* 1980;1:531–535.
182. Rupp C. Metastatic tumors of the central nervous system; intracerebral metastases as only evidence of dissemination of visceral cancer. *Arch Neurol Psych* 1948;59:635.
183. Posner JB, Chernik NL. Intracranial metastases from systemic cancer. *Adv Neurol* 1978;19:579.
184. Meyer PC, Reah TG. Secondary neoplasms of the central nervous system and meninges. *Br J Cancer* 1953;7:438.
185. Henson RA, Urich H. *Cancer and the Nervous System. The Neurological Manifestations of Systemic Malignant Disease.* Oxford: Blackwell Scientific; 1982.
186. Klatzo I, Seitelberger F. *Brain Edema.* Vienna: Springer-Verlag; 1967.
187. Penn RD. Cerebral edema and neurological function: CT, evoked responses, and clinical examination. *Adv Neurol* 1980;28:383.
188. Damadian R, Zaner K, Hor D. Human tumors by NMR. *Physiol Chem Phys* 1973;5:381–402.
189. Komiyama M, Yagura H, Baba M, Yasui T, Hakuba A, Nishimura S, Inoue Y. MR imaging: possibility of tissue characterization of brain tumors using T1 and T2 values. *AJNR* 1987;8:65–70.
190. Rinck PA, Meindl S, Higer HP, Bieler EU, Pfannenstiel P. Brain tumors: detection and typing by use of CPMG sequences and in vivo T2 measurements. *Radiology* 1985;157:103–106.
191. Komara J, Nayini N, Bialick H, et al. Brain iron delocalization and lipid peroxidation following cardiac arrest. *Ann Emerg Med* 1986;15:384–389.
192. Mandybur TI. Intracranial hemorrhage caused by metastatic tumors. *Neurology* 1977;27:650.
193. Zimmerman RA, Bilaniuk LT. Computed tomography of acute intratumoral hemorrhage. *Radiology* 1980;135:355.
194. Atlas SW, Braffman BH, LoBrutto R, Elder D, Herlyn D. Human malignant melanomas with varying melanin content in nude mice: correlations of MRI with histopathology and electron paramagnetic resonance. *J Comput Assist Tomogr* 1990;14:547–554.
195. Claussen C, Laniado M, Schorner W, Niendorf H-P, Weinmann H-J, Fiegler W, Felix R. Gadolinium-DTPA in MR imaging of glioblastomas and intracranial metastases. *AJNR* 1985;6:669–674.
196. Yuh WT, Fisher DJ, Runge VM, et al. Phase III multicenter trial of high-dose gadoteridol MRI imaging in the evaluation of brain metastases. *AJNR* 1994;15(6):1037–1051.
197. Adler J, Cox R, Kaplan I, Martin D. Stereotactic radiosurgical treatment of brain metastases. *J Neurosurg* 1992;76:444–449.
198. Burger PC, Scheithauer BW. Reactive and inflammatory masses simulating neoplasia. In: *Tumors of the Central Nervous System.* Washington, D.C.: Armed Forces Institute of Pathology; 1994: 391–413.
199. Carvalho P, Schwartz R, Alexander E, Garada B, Zimmerman R, Loeffler J, Holman B. Detection of recurrent gliomas with quantitative thallium-201/technetium-99m HMPAO single-photon emission computerized tomography. *J Neurosurg* 1992;77:565–570.
200. Goldstein GW, Betz AL. The blood–brain barrier. *Sci Am* 1986;255:74–83.

Magnetic Resonance Imaging of the Brain and Spine, Second Edition, edited by Scott W. Atlas.
Lippincott-Raven Publishers, Philadelphia © 1996.

11

Extra-Axial Brain Tumors

Herbert I. Goldberg, Ehud Lavi, and Scott W. Atlas

The determination of a tumor's extra-axial (extracerebral) origin has significant clinical importance. The location of the mass affects treatment planning, and it is predictive of prognosis. Extra-axial masses are most frequently benign in nature.

With the advent of high-field-strength imaging, it has become apparent that in general, magnetic resonance imaging (MRI) is more informative in the visualization and complete characterization of extra-axial masses than computed tomography (CT). Not only does MRI provide pathologic information regarding histology and intrinsic tumor vascularity, but it also reveals the effects of tumors and other extra-axial masses on adjacent arterial and venous channels (encasement and invasion), which usually cannot be defined on CT study. The multiplanar imaging capability of MRI provides more complete delineation of the relationship of extra-axial masses to vital regions of surrounding brain and vascular structures. This information can be of great value to the neurosurgeon in preoperative planning.

The initial decision of the radiologist in the interpretation of MRI in the presence of an intracranial mass lesion centers around whether the mass is intra-axial or extra-axial. Several key anatomic findings strongly indicate the extra-axial location of a brain mass. Routine MRI, particularly at high field strength, will usually reveal one or more of these characteristics. MR examinations frequently will demonstrate differences between an extra-axial tumor's surface signal intensity and anatomic characteristics and that of the adjacent brain cortex. This determination by MRI permits establishment of the cardinal feature of extra-axial lesions, i.e., separation of the mass from the brain surface. In addition, MRI can identify anatomic boundary layers separating the tumor from the adjacent brain, thereby confirming its extra-axial location. These boundary layers consist of cerebral spinal fluid (CSF), pial blood vessels, and a sheet of dura, which are interposed between the tumor mass and the brain. The superior contrast resolution and multiplanar imaging capability of MRI greatly aid in defining these anatomic boundary markers. CSF clefts are recognized as crescentic bands whose intensity follows that of the spinal fluid, being of low intensity on the short TR/TE

H. I. Goldberg, M.D.: Department of Radiology, Hospital of The University of Pennsylvania, Philadelphia, PA 19104.
E. Lavi, M.D.: Division of Neuropathology, Department of Pathology and Laboratory Medicine, Hospital of the University of Pennsylvania, Philadelphia, PA 19104.
S. W. Atlas, M.D.: Neuroradiology Division, Department of Radiology, Oregon Health Sciences University, Portland, OR 97201.

(T1-weighted) images, becoming isointense on the long TR/short TE (proton-density-weighted) images, and then turning to high intensity on the long TR/TE (T2-weighted) images. CSF clefts are frequently identified only over a portion of the brain-tumor interface. Vascular clefts are recognized as rounded or curvilinear signal voids at one or more locations on the margin of the lesion on spin-echo sequences. Vascular clefts may represent either the normal arteries and veins located on that surface of the brain, or blood flow from the tumor draining into abnormally prominent veins on the brain surface.

Many extra-axial masses are situated in the posterior fossa adjacent to dense bone, which typically obscures their delineation on CT because of beam hardening artifacts. As MRI is not degraded by adjacent bony structures, MR evaluation of all masses, and in particular extra-axial lesions, in the posterior fossa is vastly superior to that of CT.

Contrast between some extra-axial masses and brain may be low on MRI. The contrast, however, is usually sufficient with most lesions not only to define the presence of the lesion and determine its extra-axial location but also to reveal signal intensity alterations, which not infrequently can correctly suggest the specific nature of the mass. Generally, it is the identification of the boundary between the lesion and the brain, rather than tissue contrast, that permits the diagnosis of the extra-axial mass.

Despite the extremely high contrast and spatial resolution capabilities of current MR techniques, there is no question that intravenous contrast agents permit the detection of many extra-axial tumors that would otherwise go undiagnosed. The enhancement of extra-axial lesions usually makes their anatomic compartmentalization obvious. Moreover, contrast enhancement is highly characteristic of many extra-axial tumors (e.g., meningiomas, metastases) and almost never found in others (epidermoid and dermoid tumors). Therefore, in most settings, we recommend the routine use of i.v. contrast in the search for extra-axial mass lesions, particularly when their detection is important to patient management. Tissue characterization of masses already noted to be situated in the extra-axial compartment is also a valuable benefit of contrast enhancement.

MENINGEAL TUMORS

Meningiomas

Meningiomas are the most common primary nonglial intracranial tumor (1). Large neurosurgical series from the United States and Europe report an incidence of from 13% to 19% of all operated brain tumors (2,3). Their occurrence is undoubtedly higher, as many asymptomatic meningiomas are found at routine autopsy (4). In a large autopsy series over a 10-year period, there was a 1.44% prevalence of meningiomas, with the cause of death being associated with only 6% of this group (5). Meningiomas mostly affect people in their middle and later decades of life. There is a strong female predilection, with a ratio of about 2:1 to males (6). Meningiomas are rare in childhood, accounting for no more than 2% of intracranial tumors (2). Childhood tumors are more apt to prove malignant than those in the older population group (7). The female prevalence does not exist in the pediatric group, and there is a frequent association with neurofibromatosis in childhood meningiomas.

Multiple meningiomas are also associated with neurofibromatosis and will be found in the younger age group of this population. A varying incidence of multiple meningiomas (1% to 8%) has been reported in the older age population. The 8% incidence of multiplicity was encountered with incidental meningiomas found in a recent autopsy series (8) and in a CT (9) study of a large number of meningiomas. This higher percent is probably therefore close to the incidence we should expect to discover with high-resolution MRI study of the brain.

Meningiomas have a distinct predilection for certain intracranial locations, although they may occur in any area where meninges exist or there are cell rests of meningeal derivation. There is a close relationship between the location of the arachnoid granulations and the prevalent sites of origin for meningiomas (10). Approximately 50% of convexity meningiomas are parasagittal or attached to the sagittal sinus. Other favorite sites include the dura adjacent to the anterior sylvian fissure region, the sphenoid wings, tuberculum sellae, perisellar region, and olfactory grooves. They may also arise from the optic nerve sheath intraorbitally or extend into the optic foramen from a tuberculum sella tumor. In the posterior fossa they frequently arise from the petrous bone in the cerebellopontine angle, the clivus, the tentorial leaf, and the tentorial free margin. Meningiomas are usually broad-based and firmly attached to the adjacent dura but can arise without any dural attachments apparently from pial meningeal cells. These pial-based meningiomas may be found in the depths of the sylvian fissure (Fig. 1) or may present intraventricularly, usually in the lateral ventricle but occasionally in the third and fourth ventricles arising from either the tela choroidea or arachnoidal cell rest within the stroma of the choroid plexus.

Initial reports on meningiomas with MRI utilizing low- and mid-field-strength units indicated poor detection and extra-axial compartmentalization of the tumors (11–13). Studies utilizing high-field-strength magnets have indicated a detection rate comparable with that of contrast CT (14,15) and an overall superiority of MRI

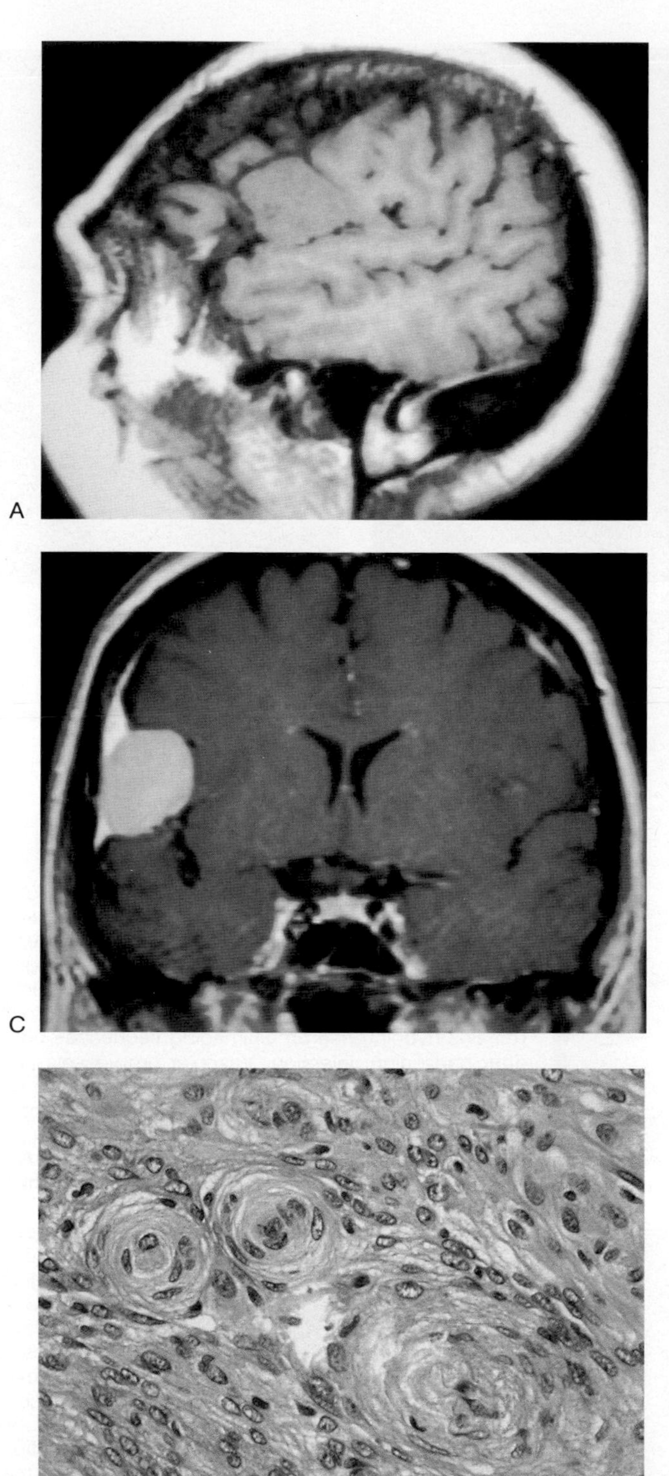

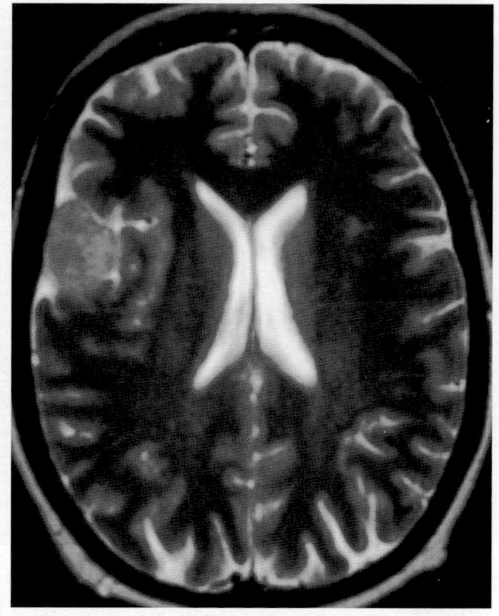

FIG. 1. Intrasylvian meningioma. Sagittal T1-weighted (**A**) and axial T2-weighted (**B**) MRI shows extra-axial intrasylvian mass nearly isointense to gray matter. After contrast (**C**), dense and homogeneous enhancement with associated dural tail is clearly seen. Multiplanar MRI is valuable here in providing precise anatomic localization prior to surgery. Histologic section (**D**) from a similar meningioma showing typical whorl formation and syncytial arrangement of cells.

in determining the tumors' extra-axial location and in defining intrinsic tumor vascularity, arterial encasement, venous sinus invasion, and marginal areas of extension. Compared with white matter, meningiomas on T1-weighted images are almost always hypointense (Fig. 2), with an occasional tumor being isointense or hyperintense. When compared with the brain cortex on T1-weighted images, a more varied intensity distribution of the tumors is present. Slightly over one-half are isointense to the cortex, with one-third being hypointense and an occasional tumor revealing hyperintensity (14). On proton-density and T2-weighted images, meningiomas

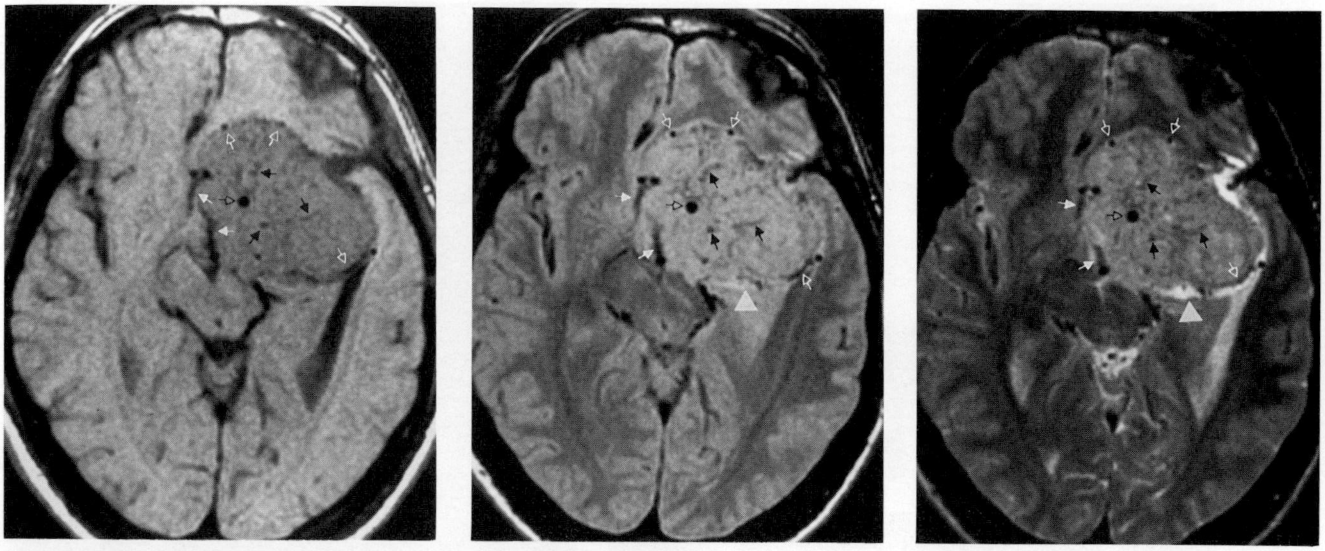

A

B,C

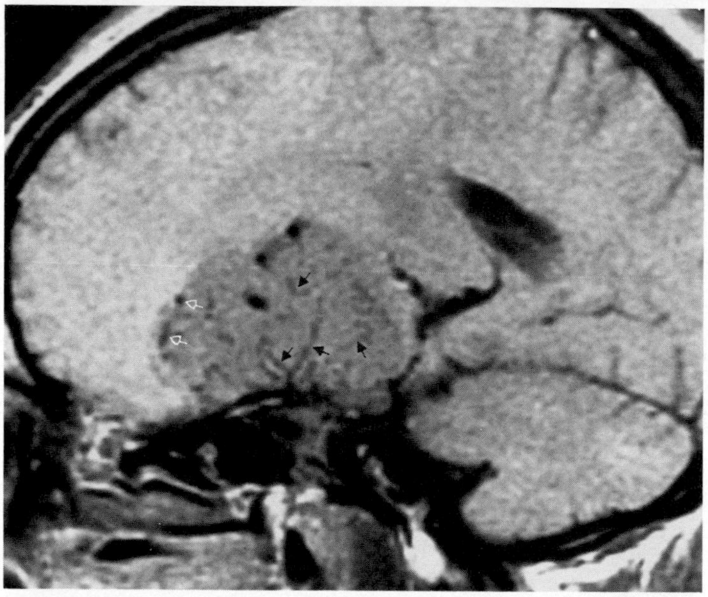

D

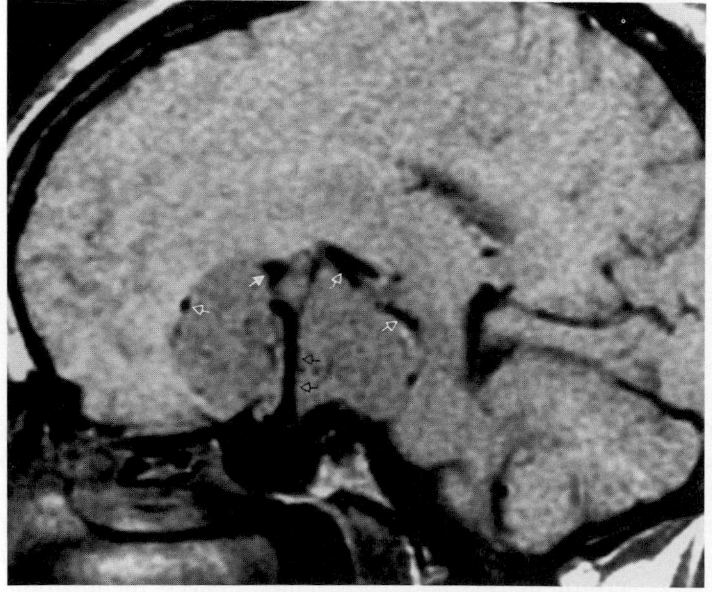

E

FIG. 2. Left sphenoid wing meningioma. A–J. Tumor vascularity (*black solid arrows*), arterial vascular rim (*white solid arrows*), venous vascular rim (*white open arrows*), entrapped internal carotid artery (*black open arrows*). **A:** Short TR/TE axial image through center of tumor that is hypointense to both white and gray matter. Tumor vascularity (also B–D,I,J) remains hypointense on all imaging sequences before and after gadolinium injection. Vascular rim vessels are small, rounded, and curvilinear signal voids at interface of tumor with brain (also B–E,I,J). Entrapped internal carotid artery remains hypointense on all imaging sequences pre- and postgadolinium administration (also B,C,E,I). **B,C:** Axial long TR/short TE (B) and long TR/TE (C) images at same level as A. Tumor is hyperintense to white matter and isointense to gray matter in both B and C and reveals inhomogeneous intensity pattern related to tumor vascularity and intrinsic mottling. CSF cleft (*white arrowhead*) containing vascular rim vessels is isointense in B and hyperintense in C. **D:** Sagittal short TR/TE image demonstrating tumor vascularity and both arterial and venous vascular rim structures. **E:** Sagittal short TR/TE image at level of carotid siphon reveals entrapped internal carotid artery and both arterial and venous vascular rim vessels. **F:** Lateral left carotid arteriogram reveals tumor vascularity, entrapped internal carotid artery, and middle cerebral artery elevated over superior margin of tumor stain. **G:** Venous phase lateral left carotid arteriogram demonstrates tumor blush and marginal venous vascular elements. **H:** Postcontrast axial CT reveals homogeneous tumor enhancement but no visualization of tumor vascularity, entrapped internal carotid artery, vascular rim, or CSF cleft. **I:** Postgadolinium axial short TR/TE image demonstrates heterogeneous tumor enhancement, rounded hypointensities of entrapped internal carotid artery, arterial vascular rim vessels, and tumor vascularity. Venous vascular rim vessels are obscured by the gadolinium. **J:** Postgadolinium coronal short TR/TE image through tumor demonstrates diffuse heterogeneous enhancement, linear hypointensities of tumor vascularity, and marginal hypointensities of elevated middle cerebral artery vascular rim elements.

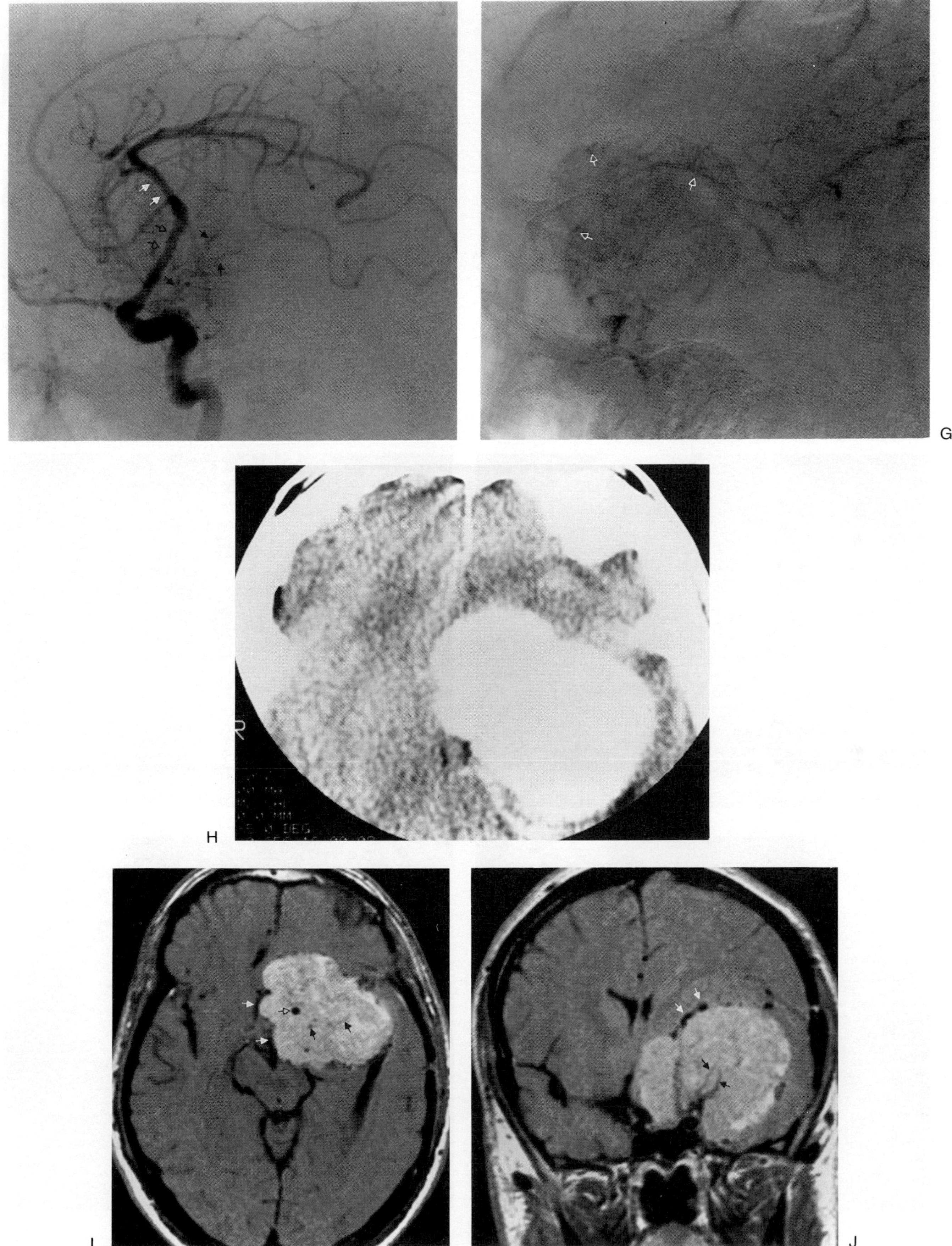
F
G
H
R
I
J

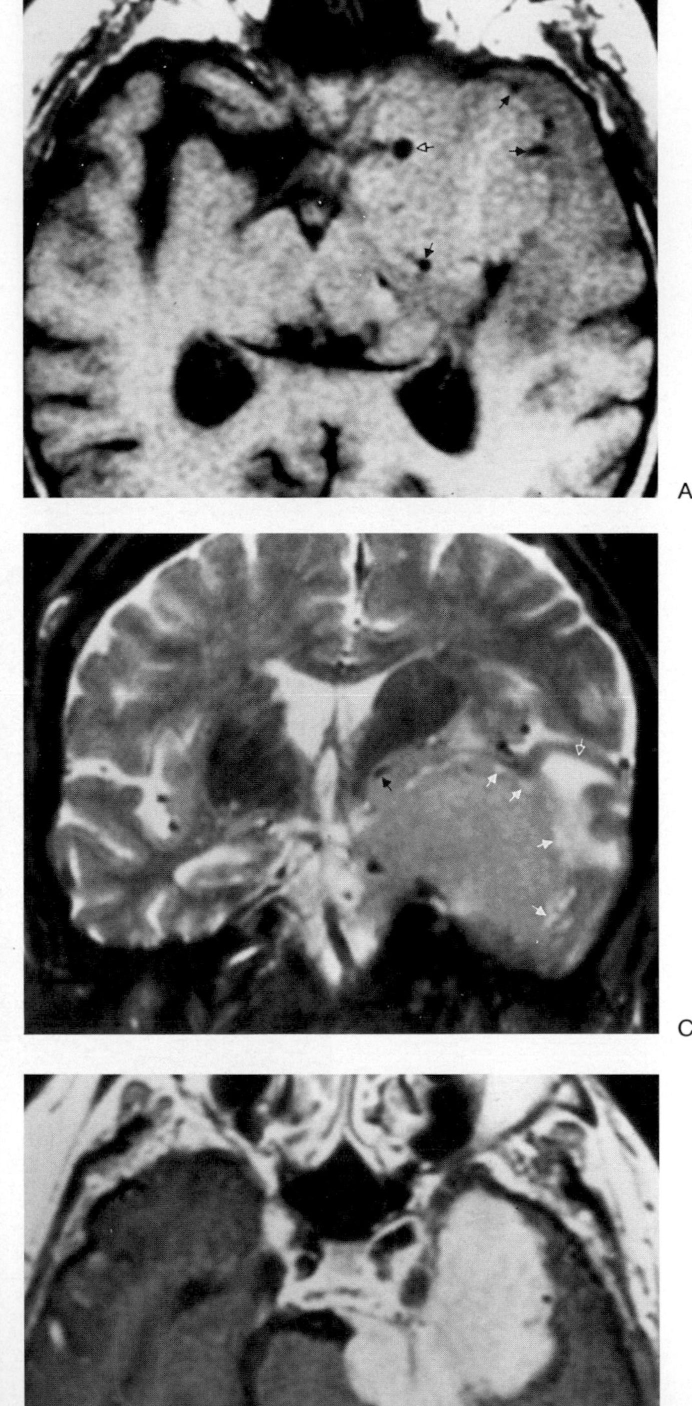

FIG. 3. Left perisellar meningioma. **A:** Axial short TR/TE image at level of optic chiasm. Tumor reveals heterogeneous intensity being both hypo- and isointense to white matter and iso- and hyperintense to gray matter. Vascular rim interface vessels (*solid arrows*) and entrapped internal carotid artery (*open arrow*) are demonstrated. **B,C:** Coronal long TR/short TE (B) and long TE (C) images through tumor. Tumor is heterogeneously hyperintense to white matter and isointense to gray matter. Only a single small vascular rim element is evident (*black arrow*), but multiple marginal curvilinear hyperintensities representing CSF clefts become apparent in C (long TR/TE image, *white arrows*). Mild temporal lobe white matter edema (*open arrow*) is evident lateral to CSF clefts. **D:** Axial short TR/TE image at level of tentorial incisura demonstrates transtentorial tumor extension onto clivus (*arrow*) and midbrain compression. **E:** Postgadolinium axial short TR/TE image at same level as D. Diffuse enhancement more sharply outlines tumor margins as well as posterior dural extension along tentorial incisura (*open arrow*).

A

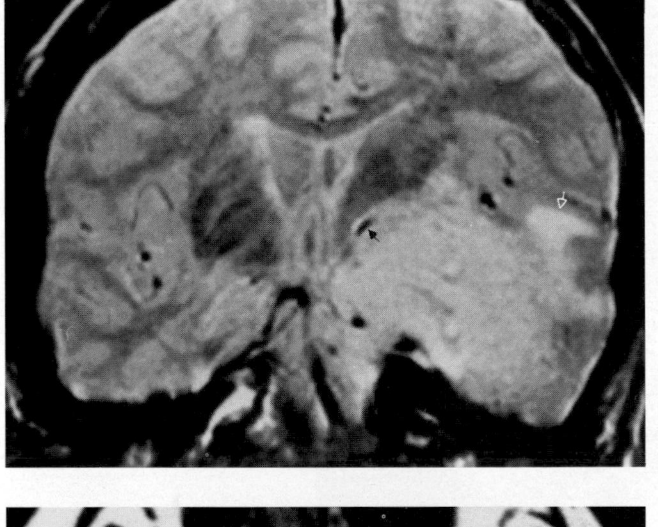

B

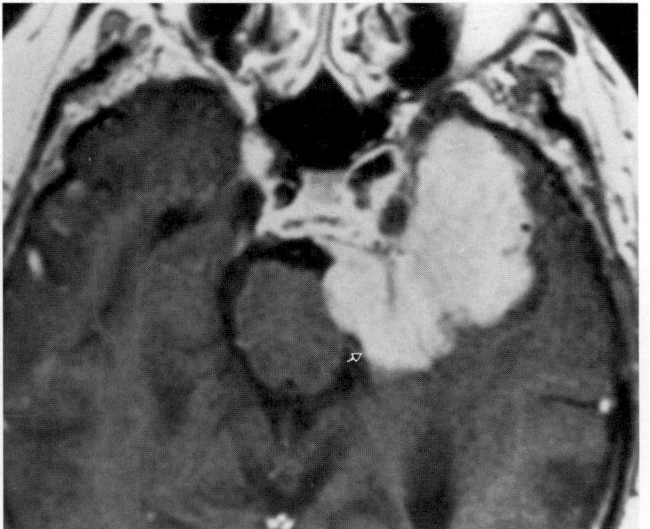

C

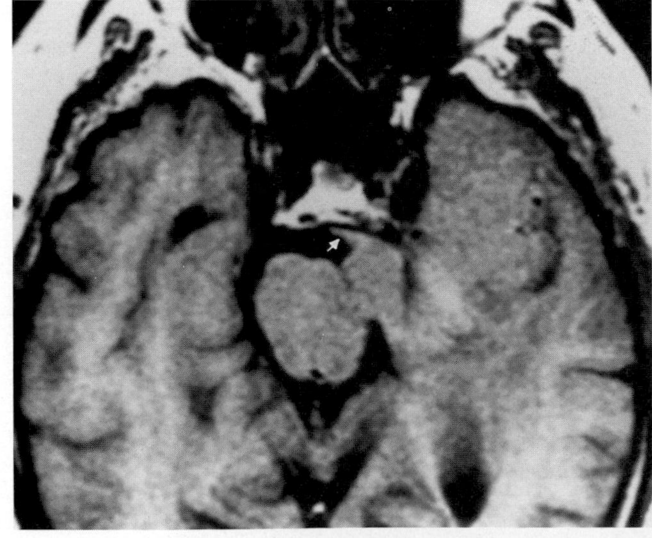

D

E

are uniformly hyperintense to the cerebral white matter in those portions (Figs. 2 and 3) that are not heavily calcified. The degree of hyperintensity is, however, widely varied on these long TR sequences. In relationship to the cerebral cortex, approximately one-half are isointense (Figs. 2 and 3) and one-half hyperintense (Fig. 4), with a rare tumor being hypointense (14). One study found a strong correlation between tumor histology and tumor intensity on T2-weighted images compared with that of the cortex (16). Almost all meningiomas that were hyperintense to the cortex were either of the syncytial or angioblastic histologic subtype. None of the fibroblastic or transitional cell type of meningiomas were hyperintense to the cortex on T2-weighted images. Transitional cell tumors were mainly isointense to the cortex as well as about one-half of the fibroblastic and some syncytial cell types. Tumors that were hypointense to the cortex on T2-weighted images (Fig. 5) were mainly in the fibroblastic or of a mixed variety with predominant fibroblastic elements.

Meningiomas may develop rare histologic variants (Fig. 6) that may have unique intensity correlates on MRI. One example is the lipoblastic (lipomatous) meningioma (17). In this unusual lesion, there is metaplastic transformation of meningioma cells into adipocytes, with the cytoplasm containing large fat droplets composed of triglycerides. This change may be present in part of or throughout the whole tumor. These meningiomas appear markedly hyperintense on T1-weighted images and become hypointense on the T2-weighted sequences (Fig. 7). A chemical shift effect may be identified at the margins of the regions of fatty transformation. This is demonstrated as a rim of hypointensity appearing at one margin of the tumor and hyperintensity at the other along the frequency-encoding axis (Fig. 7). Another fatty cell change occurring in meningiomas is of the xanthomatous type. It most frequently develops in the angioblastic variety, but may also be encountered in syncytial and fibroblastic types. This change is usually patchy within the tumor but may be more confluent. The cells with this change contain multiple small droplets composed of cholesterol and other lipids (17). Regions with xanthomatous change might be expected to demonstrate characteristic intensity patterns.

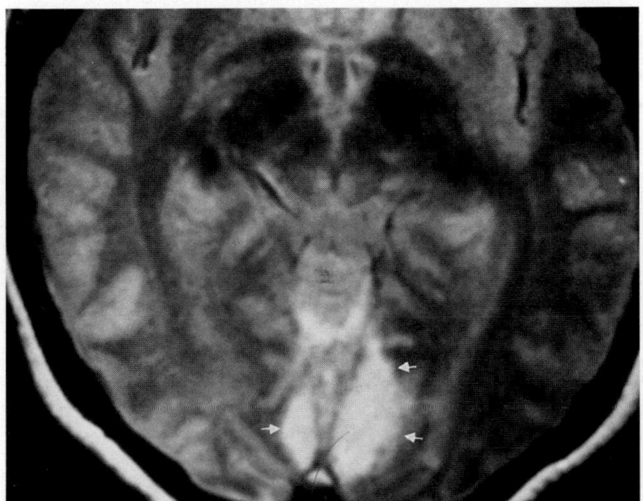

FIG. 4. Posterior inferior falx meningioma. Axial long TR/TE image. Tumor is hyperintense (*arrows*) to both white matter and gray matter and extends across the falx to opposite side.

The majority of meningiomas (84% in one series) demonstrate a heterogeneous intensity pattern that is most evident on the T2-weighted images (14). Tumor heterogeneity can be related to the presence of several factors: tumoral vascularity, cystic foci, calcifications, and an inherent speckling and mottling of uncertain etiology. In approximately one-third of meningiomas multiple factors account for signal heterogeneity. Tumor vascularity has been identified in approximately one-third of the cases and is revealed as punctate and curvilinear hypointensities within the mass on both the T1- and T2-weighted images (Fig. 2). Cystic foci develop from coalescence of cystic spaces in the microcystic and angioblastic varieties of meningioma. They appear on T1-weighted images as smooth, rounded hypointensities. On long TR/short TE images these foci are iso- to slightly hypointense. They become hyperintense on the long TR/TE images (Fig. 8). Their intensity pattern tends to follow that of CSF in the cisterns and ventricles. The cysts are usually small; however, larger cysts with the same characteristics may develop and have a tendency to be located more peripherally in the tumor. Occasionally subarachnoid cysts develop at the margins of the tumor that at times may be difficult to differentiate from the larger peripheral intratumoral cysts. Calcifications, when apparent on MRI, appear as coarse, irregular regions of hypointensity on both T1- and T2-weighted sequences (Fig. 9). Cystic foci and calcifications may be identified in approximately 20% of these tumors. The speckling and mottling pattern can be seen in approximately two-thirds of the tumors on T2-weighted images. These regions appear as fine or coarse foci, respectively, of mixed high and low signal intensity (Figs. 2, 3, and 10). This pattern is probably related to the varied cellular histology within each meningioma.

Several criteria help to establish the extracerebral localization of the meningioma, and these criteria represent the key to the diagnosis. A broad, dural-based margin is strongly suggestive, but not definitive for this localization. Bony hyperostosis and/or invasion is highly specific for an extra-axial origin (Fig. 11). However, it is infrequently present. Another highly specific characteristic for extra-axial localization is the identification of various anatomic interfaces interposed between the tumor surface and the brain surface. Three different anatomic interfaces may be identified with MRI. These consist of pial vascular structures, CSF clefts, and dural

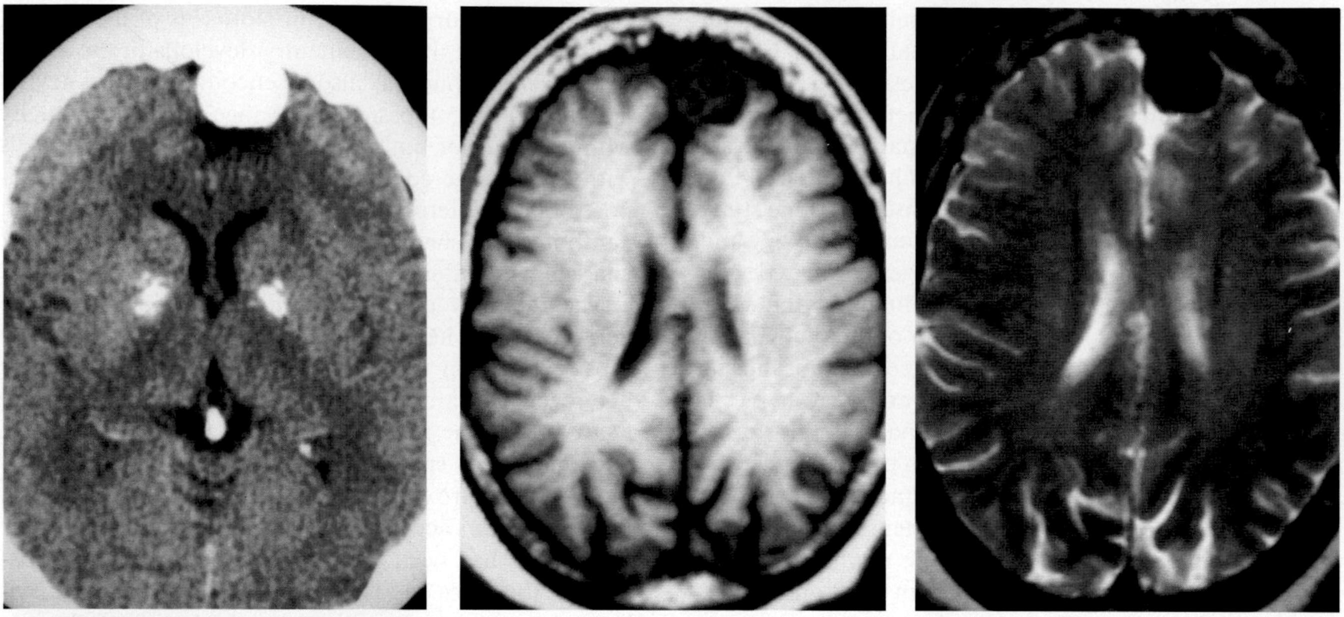

A B,C

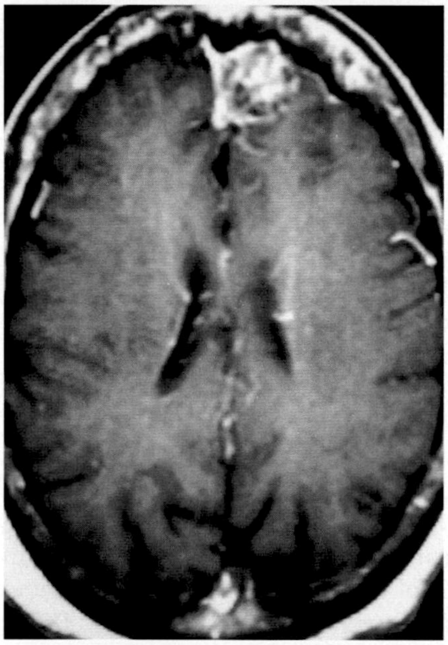

D

FIG. 5. Hypointense meningioma, densely calcified CT shows densely calcified extra-axial mass consistent with meningioma (**A**). Lesion shows marked hypointensity on MRI (**B,C**), particularly on T2-weighted image (**C**). After contrast, significant central enhancement is seen (**D**), which could not have been noted on CT due to calcific density of lesion. Histologic section of a similar meningioma (**E**) shows proliferation of cells containing bland, round to oval nuclei in a mesenchymal collagenized matrix. A characteristic feature of meningiomas is the tendency to form concentric whorls (**F**). When whorls degenerate and calcify, the result is concentric calcified structures called "psammoma bodies."

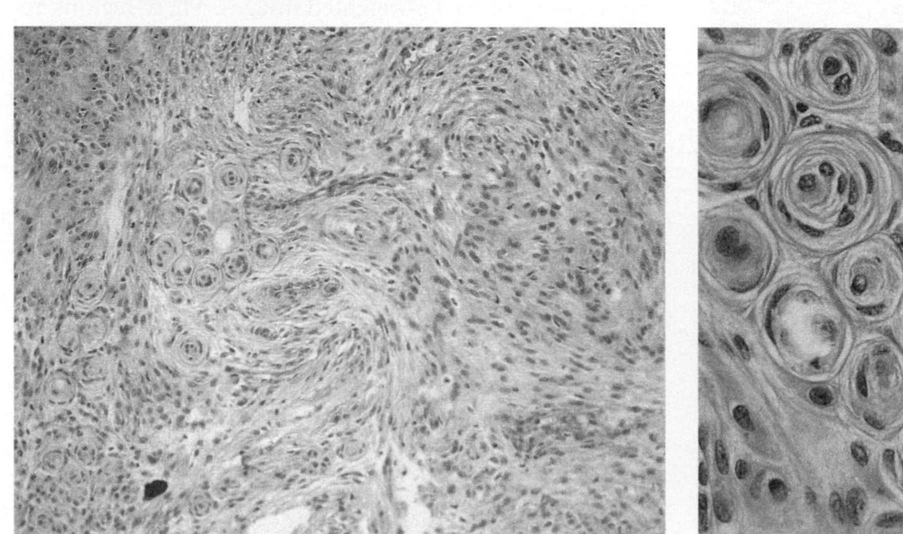

E

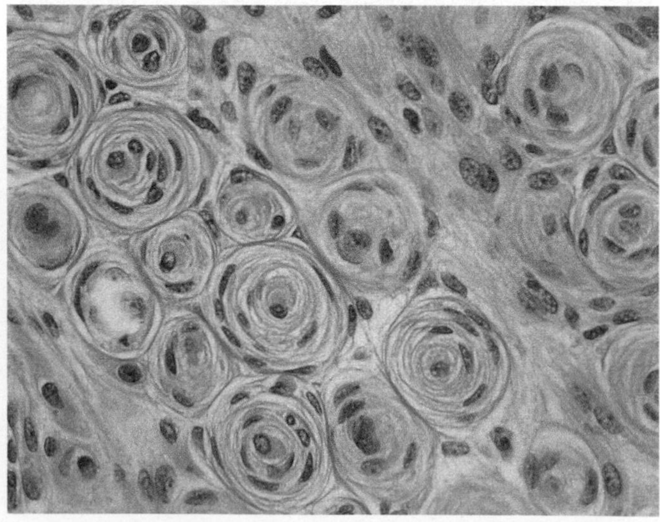

F

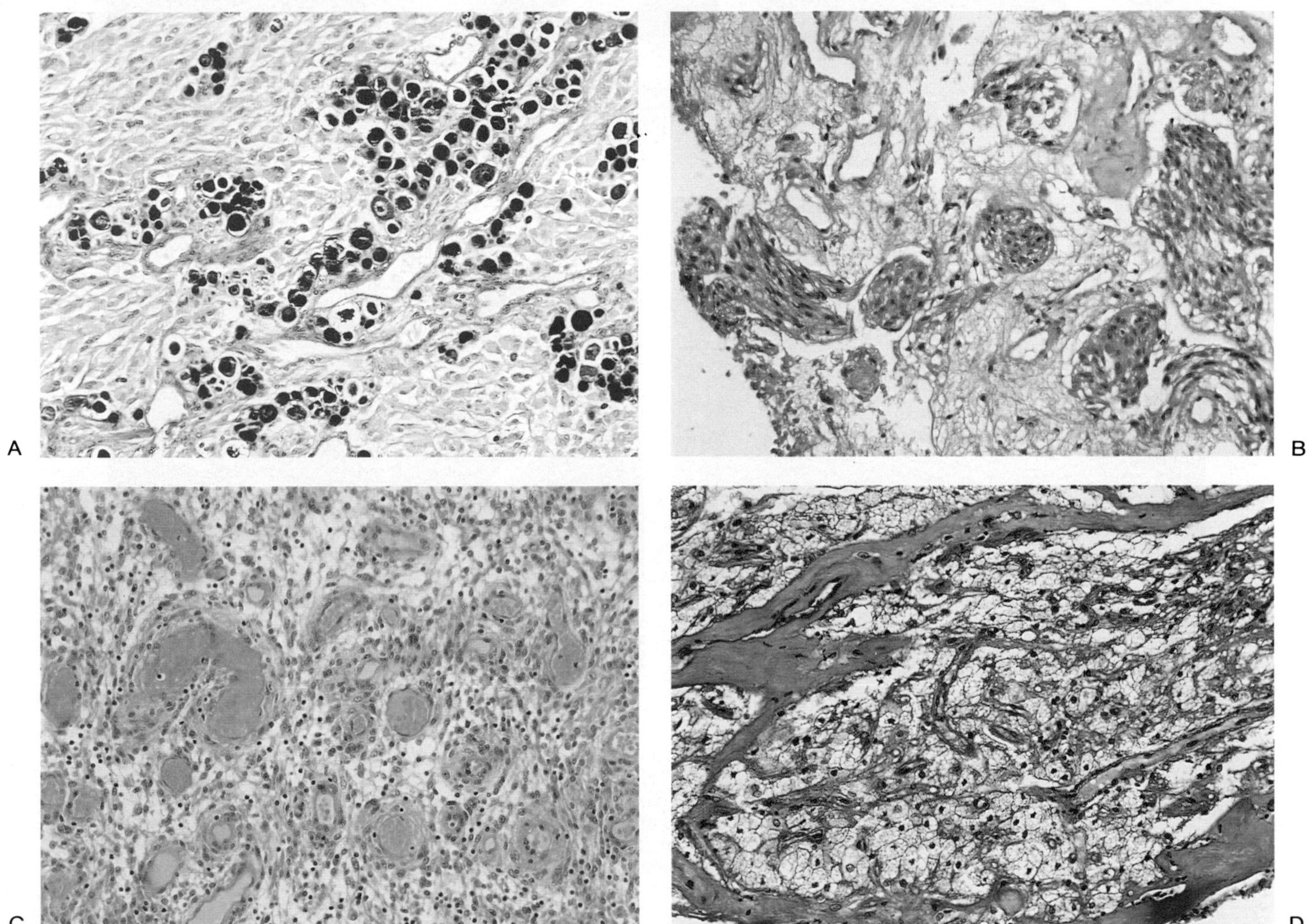

FIG. 6. Histologic variants of meningiomas which can alter MRI signal intensity. **A:** Secretory meningioma containing large PAS-positive (purple) secretory inclusions. **B:** Meningioma with myxoid degeneration. The meningothelial cells are immersed in abundant gelatinous myxoid material (blue-gray). **C:** Angiomatous meningioma. Note numerous capillary blood vessels within the tumor. **D:** Meningioma with lipomatous metaplasia. Large areas of the tumor consist of cells with vacuolated lipid-containing cytoplasm.

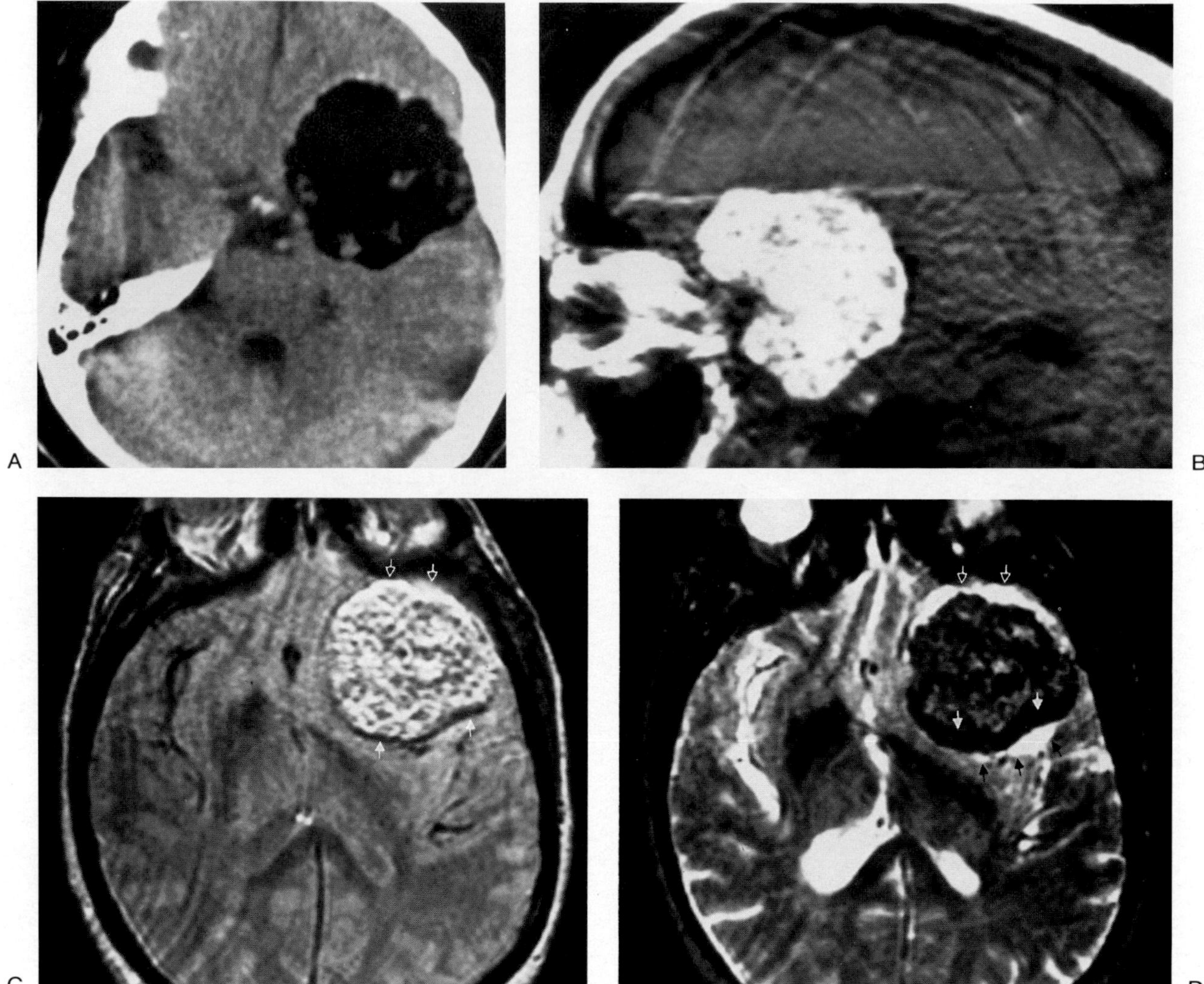

FIG. 7. Lipomatous meningioma left sphenoid wing. **A:** Axial noncontrast CT demonstrates markedly hypodense mass in left frontal temporal region containing multiple isodense irregular nodular areas. **B:** Sagittal short TR/TE image without contrast through tumor mass. Tumor is markedly hyperintense, being similar to orbital and scalp fat. It contains multiple irregular isointense foci. **C,D:** Axial long TR/short TE (C) and long TE (D) images demonstrate tumor to be heterogeneously hyperintense on long TR/short TE (C) and heterogeneously hypointense on long TR/TE image (D). A chemical shift artifact from the fat-water interface is present and demonstrated as hypointense rim in posterior portion of tumor (*solid white arrows*) and hyperintense rim at anterior margin of tumor (*open white arrows*). It is more pronounced in D due to reduced bandwidth. Note hyperintense CSF cleft evident at posterior tumor border (*black arrows*) behind hypointense chemical shift artifact in D.

FIG. 8. Right inferior temporal angioblastic meningioma. **A:** Axial noncontrast CT reveals a multicystic hyperdense right temporal lobe tumor extending to midline with evidence of brainstem compression and displacement of third ventricle to left. Mass was considered most likely intra-axial on CT. **B:** Axial short TR/TE image through temporal fossa reveals tumor to be mildly hyperintense to both gray and white matter. Multiple small and slightly larger mildly hypointense regions are present within the substance of the mass. Small rounded signal voids are evident at the anterior and posterior margins of the tumor (*white arrows*) representing vascular rim vessels. **C:** Long TR/TE axial image at level similar to B. Background intensity of tumor that was slightly hyperintense in B has become mildly hypointense. The multiple mildly hypointense foci in B become hyperintense. On the long TR/short TE image (not shown) these foci were isointense, suggesting cystic nature. Medial margin of tumor mass extends into perimesencephalic cistern and is directly compressing right cerebral peduncle (*arrows*). **D,E:** Axial short TR/TE (D) and long TR/TE (E) images through tumor at higher level than B and C. Cystic foci are larger and extend close to the tumor surface. A markedly hyperintense region is present in the posterior portion of tumor in D and remains hyperintense in E, suggesting the presence of subacute hemorrhage into a cystic focus. Rounded and curvilinear hypodensities within tumor substance in both D and E indicate prominent tumor vascularity (*black arrows*). **F:** Sagittal short TR/TE image through right temporal lobe demonstrates inferior tumor margin abutting directly on petrous ridge and sphenoid bone (*black arrows*). The hemorrhagic and multiple hypointense cystic foci are evident as well as a single marginal vascular rim vessel posteriorly (*white arrow*).

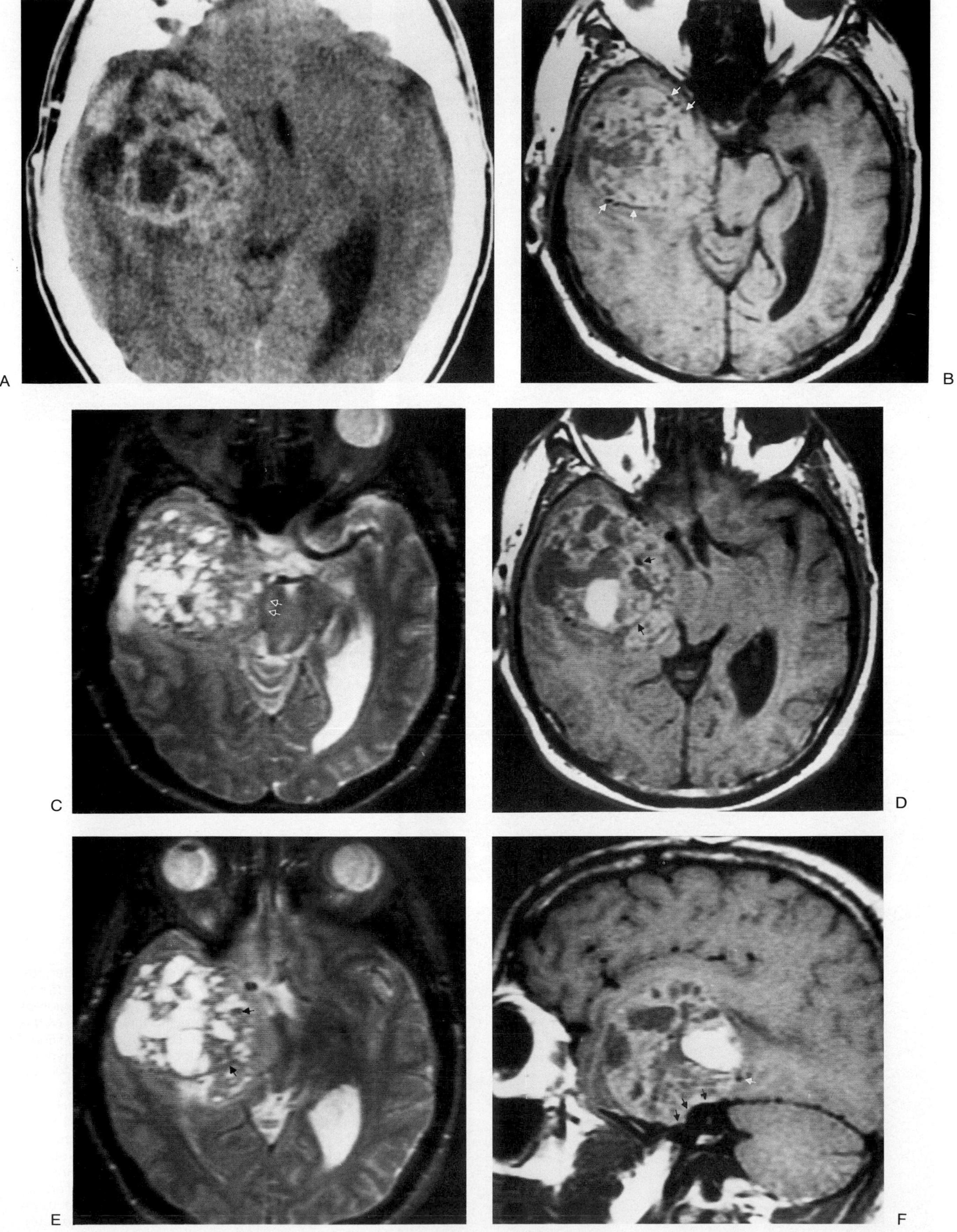
A
B
C
D
E
F

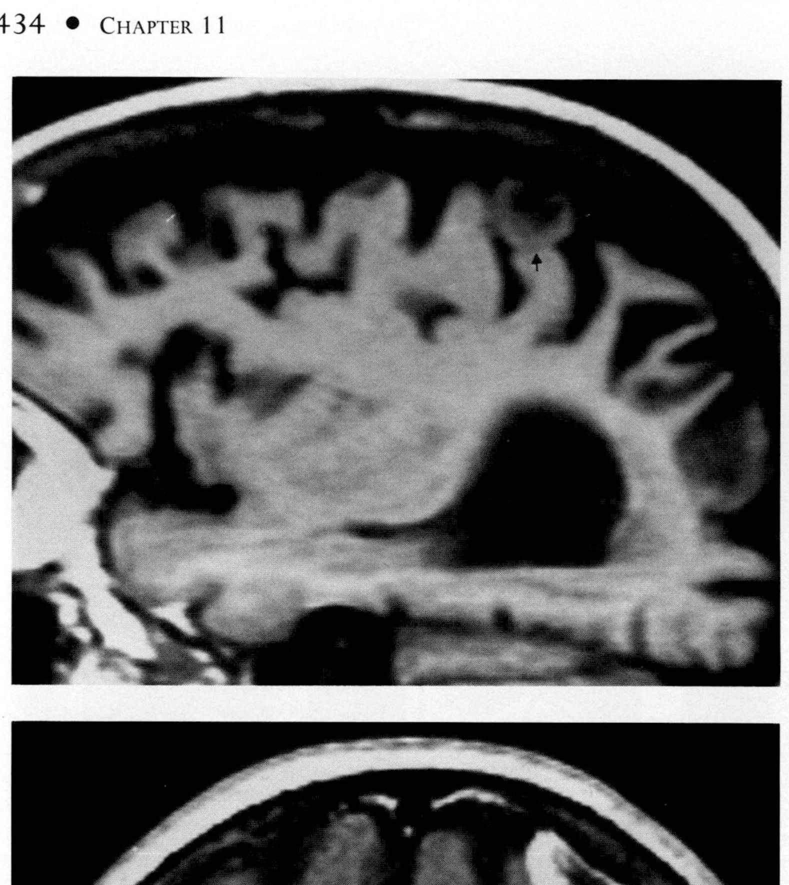

A

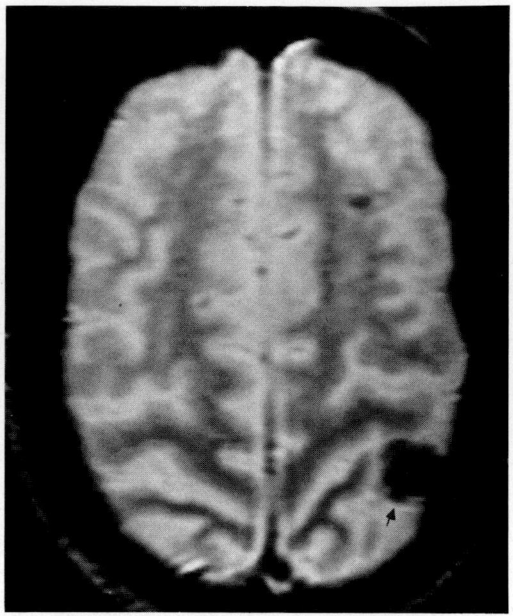

B

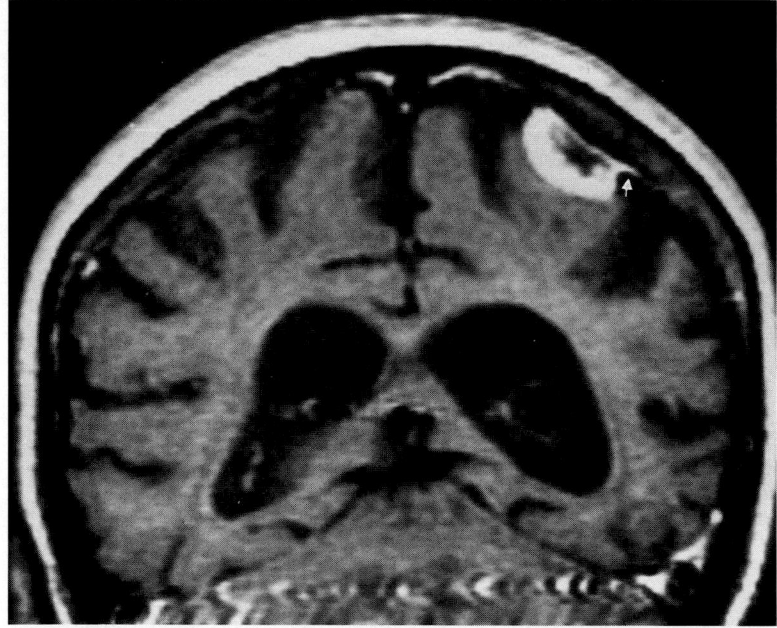

C

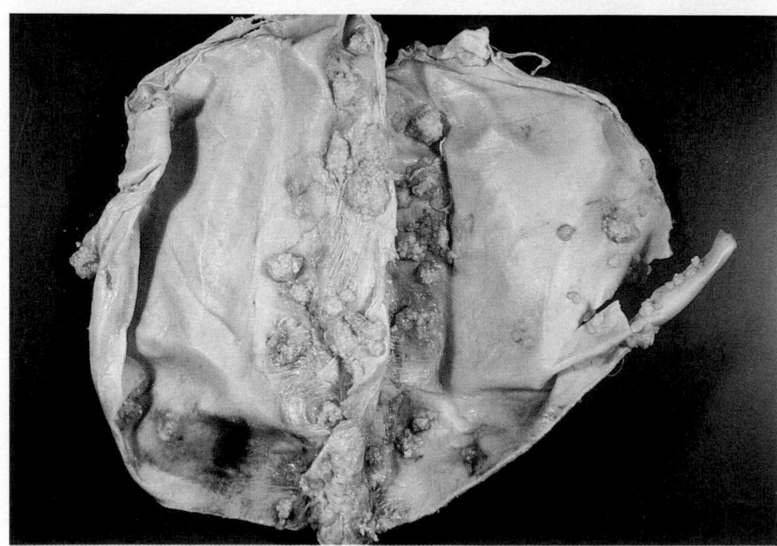

D

FIG. 9. Calcified convexity meningioma. **A:** Sagittal short TR/TE image demonstrates 1.5-cm dural-based parietal mass (*arrow*) with lobulated region of marked hypointensity occupying the majority of the central portion of the tumor. **B:** Axial long TR/TE image demonstrating similar lobulated central hypointensity within the left parietal tumor (*arrow*). Peripheral soft tissue portion of tumor obscured by high intensity of enlarged surrounding subarachnoid space. **C:** Coronal postgadolinium-enhanced short TR/TE image demonstrates peripheral enhancement of the tumor. There is a reduction in the size of the central hypointensity due to gadolinium enhancement of the outer portion of the calcified tumor region. Enhancement of a small tail of dural thickening extending inferiorly is observed (*arrow*). **D:** Dura with multiple calcified meningiomas. (Courtesy of Dr. N. K. Gonatas, Hospital of The University of Pennsylvania, Philadelphia, PA.)

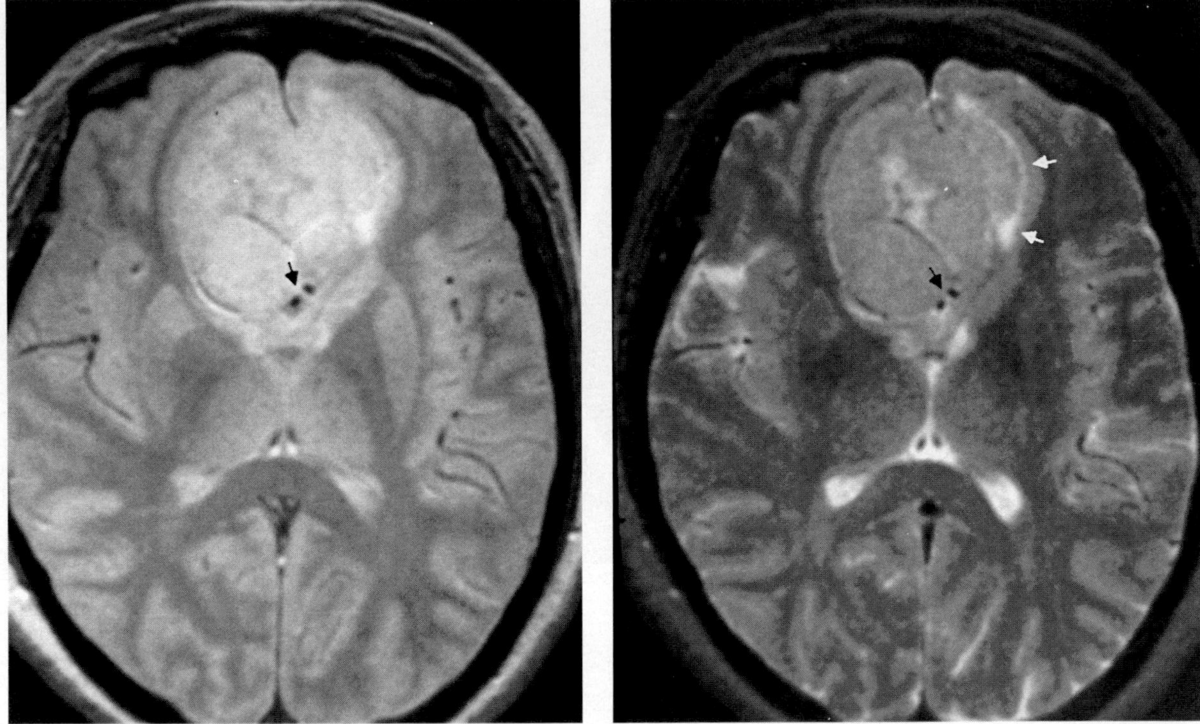

FIG. 10. Large olfactory groove meningioma. Axial long TR/short TE (**A**) and long TR/TE (**B**) multiecho images through midportion of inferior frontal tumor. Tumor demonstrates mottled hyperintensity to white matter on both the short and long echo images. On the short echo image (A) it is mildly hyperintense to gray matter but is isointense to gray matter on the second echo (B). The central portion of the tumor demonstrates a greater relative hyperintensity on the second echo, whereas on the first echo it is relatively hypointense to the rest of the tumor. An extensive CSF cleft is present around the tumor. It demonstrates curvilinear hyperintensity similar to subarachnoid and ventricular CSF on the long echo image (*white arrows*, B) and is relatively isointense on the short echo image (A). The rounded signal voids of the two anterior cerebral arteries can be observed in the midline adjacent to the posterior portion of the tumor and sitting within a small pocket of the CSF cleft (*black arrow*).

margins. With high-resolution and multiplanar MRI, one or more of these interfaces can usually be identified in essentially all cases (14). The interfaces are frequently not found along the full tumor-brain margin but in most instances are sufficient to make a highly reliable determination of extra-axial localization.

Pial blood vessel interfaces appear as punctate and curvilinear signal voids on all sequences at or along one or more margins of the tumor with the brain (Figs. 2, 8, and 10). When brain edema is present, the vascular rims may occur at the junction of the uniform high intensity of the brain edema on T2-weighted images and the more heterogeneous lower intensity of the tumor. The vascular rims may consist of either arteries or veins. For those tumors located at the base of the brain or in the proximal portions of the sylvian and interhemispheric cisterns, displaced larger brain arteries are likely to be identified at the interface (Fig. 10). Meningiomas tend to develop large marginal draining veins located at their brain surface interface. These veins are most likely the large marginal vascular structures seen with the more peripherally located meningiomas and at tumor-brain interface locations, where large arteries would not be expected to be seen (e.g., in the large basally located tumors) (Fig. 2). About 80% of the meningiomas will demonstrate a vascular marginal interface with high-resolution MRI.

CSF interfaces are also identifiable in about 80% of meningiomas on MRI. They appear as high-intensity clefts on the long TR/TE sequences and are usually isointense on the long TR/short TE images relative to the adjacent tumor and brain. On T1-weighted sequences they are low intensity (Fig. 10). CSF clefts generally follow the intensity pattern of the ventricular and subarachnoid fluid but may be of slightly higher intensity, due to the relative isolation of these thin CSF spaces from pulsation effects. They are usually separable from the high intensity of adjacent brain edema on long TR/short TE images. Also, on the long TR/TE images, a thin isointense band representing the brain cortex separates the CSF clefts from the edema. Vascular rims may be seen to lie within regions of the CSF clefts (Figs. 2 and 10). In approximately two-thirds of the meningiomas, vascular rims and CSF clefts are both present at the brain-tumor interface.

The dural margin interface is seen primarily in meningiomas of the cavernous sinus. It appears as a low-

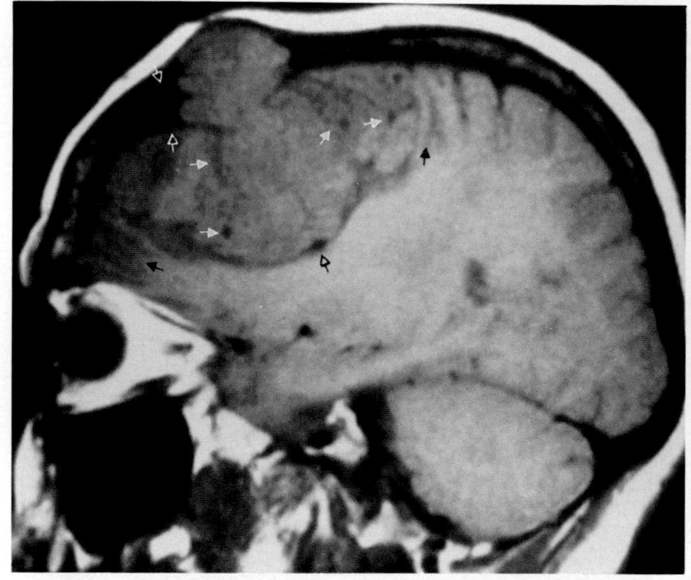

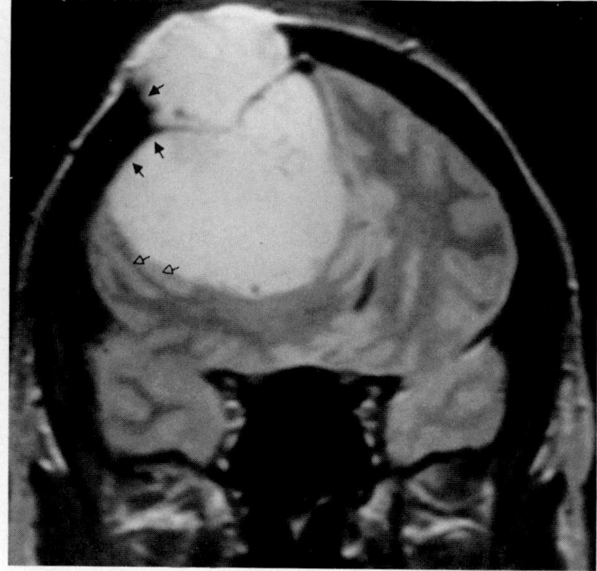

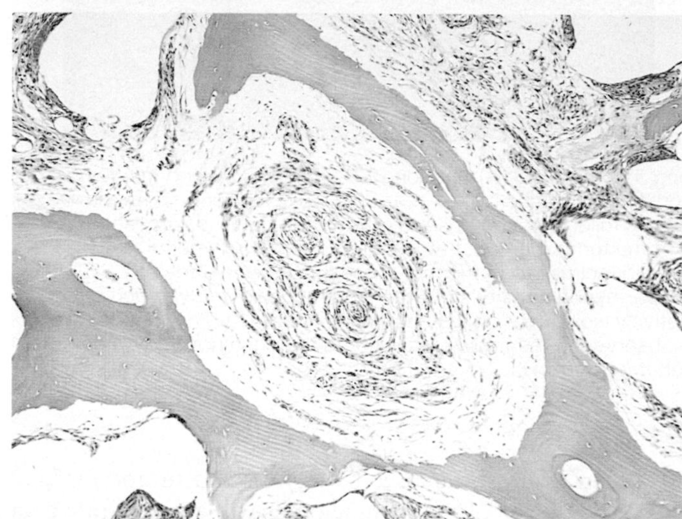

FIG. 11. Large frontal convexity meningioma growing through the calvarium with lytic and hyperostotic bony change. **A:** Sagittal short TR/TE image demonstrates large slightly hypointense frontal convexity mass with punctate and linear tumor vascularity (*solid white arrows*), a vascular rim (*open black arrow*), and accordion-like compression of marginal convolutions (*solid black arrows*). A large nodule of tumor has grown through the calvarium and presents as a scalp mass. There is a thickened signal void of the inner table at the anterior aspect of the tumor nodule that is growing through the skull (*open white arrows*). **B:** Coronal long TR/TE image demonstrates marked tumor hyperintensity. Complete destruction of the bony tables of the skull has occurred, with the tumor penetrating through into the scalp. At the lateral margin of the intracalvarial tumor there is thickening and increased hypointensity of that portion of the skull that indicates an osteoblastic hyperostotic reaction (*solid black arrows*). Again note accordion-like compression of inferior convexity cortical convolutions (*open black arrows*). **C:** Histologic section of bone trabeculae (pink bands) admixed with whorls of neoplastic meningothelial cells replacing the bone marrow. This represents meningioma invading bone rather than simply secondary hyperostotic change.

intensity rim on all imaging sequences covering the lateral margin of the tumor and separating it from the adjacent temporal lobe. Not infrequently the tumor can be seen invading through this dural margin and abutting directly on adjacent brain. Meningiomas along the falx and tentorium may also be seen invading into and through the dura to its opposite side (Fig. 12). Note that intra-axial brain tumors almost never invade dura unless there has been previous surgery. Metastatic brain tumors may occasionally grow exophytically from the brain and invade the dura. In these lesions, however, no brain-tumor interface will exist.

In comparison with CT, MRI is superior for extra-axial localization of the tumor. CT without and with contrast can define these interfaces in less than 50% of the cases in which they are identified on MRI (14). CT can identify the vascular rims only in those cases involving meningiomas at the base of the brain in which the vessels consist of the major arteries of the circle of Willis or their first order branches. CSF clefts can only be identified with CT when the tumor is adjacent to a large CSF cistern that has not been fully effaced by tumor. The high-contrast resolution on long TR MRI permits identification of very thin CSF clefts even with large tumors that are markedly compressing adjacent brain.

Another anatomic characteristic indicative of extra-axial localization of large tumors that can be recognized with MRI and less often with CT consists of arcuate bowing and compression of adjacent cortical convolutions in an onion-skin-like configuration beginning at the margin of the tumor. Large intracerebral masses located at or near the surface of the brain do not show a similar anatomic alteration (Fig. 13). Extra-axial masses compress adjacent portions of the brain together, whereas intra-

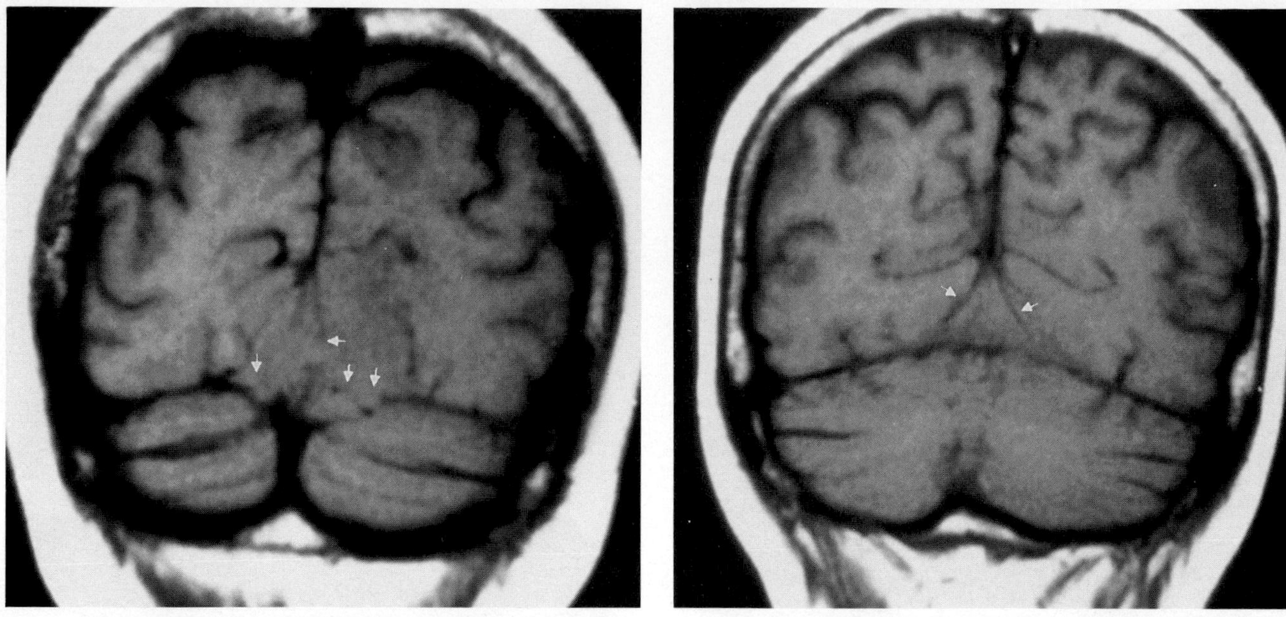

FIG. 12. Posterior falx meningioma with transfalcine, transtentorial, and straight sinus invasion. Same case as Fig. 4. **A:** Coronal short TR/TE image just anterior to the torcula demonstrates slightly hypointense tumor that is largest to the left of the midline and that has grown across the falx to the right side and inferiorly through the tentorial leafs into the posterior fossa. The hypointensity of the dura is lost where the tumor has invaded through it (*arrows*). The flow void of the straight sinus is not present, indicating obliteration by the tumor. **B:** Coronal short TR/TE image through the straight sinus anterior to the main tumor mass demonstrates isointense tissue expanding and filling the region of the proximal portion of the straight sinus (*arrows*). The dural margins of the sinus are partly destroyed by the tumor.

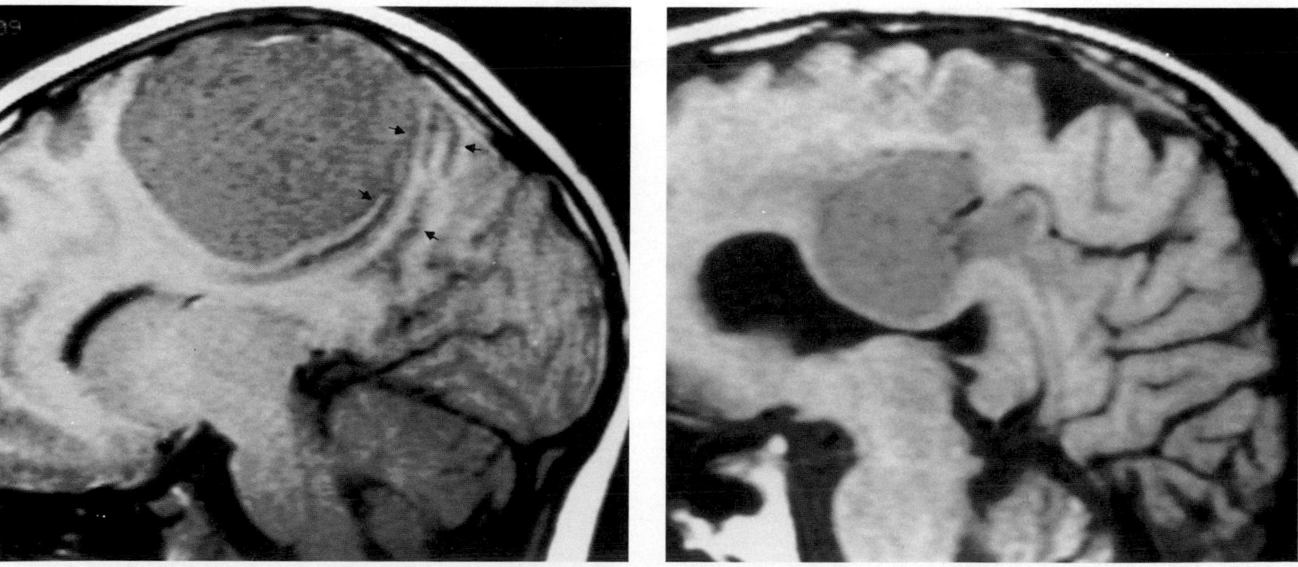

FIG. 13. A: Accordion-like compression of cortical convolutions by extra-axial tumor. Large medial parietal meningioma demonstrating arcuate bowing and accordion-like compression of cortical convolutions adjacent to the posterior margin of the tumor (*arrows*) compared with normal cortical convolutional pattern in frontal region of brain. **B:** Sagittal short TR/TE image of large medially located intra-axial metastases. Accordion-like cortical convolutional compression pattern is not present.

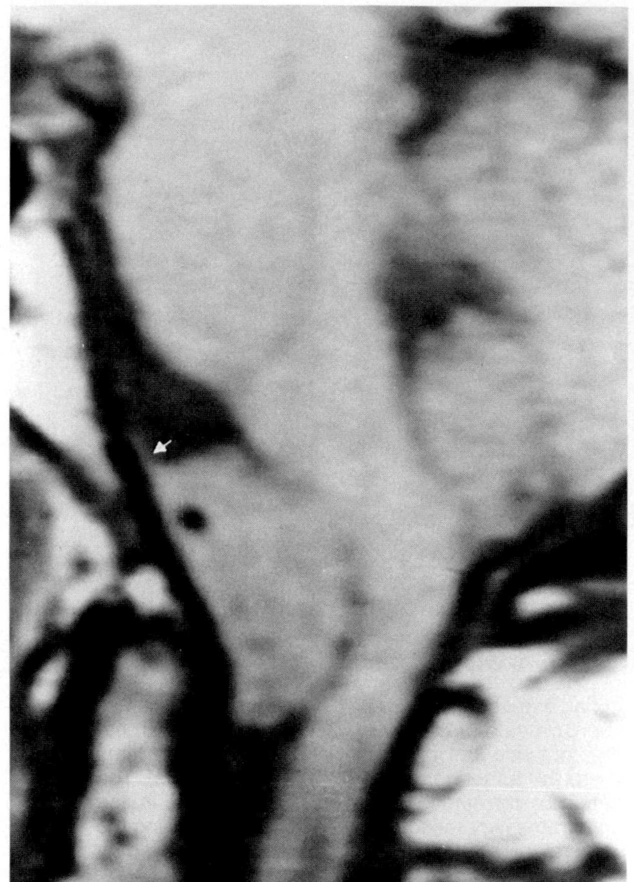

FIG. 14. Meningioma arising from inferior clivus and anterior margin of foramen magnum. Sagittal short TR/TE image demonstrates mildly hypointense tumor mass that is markedly compressing the medulla and cervical medullary junction region. It has a broad, flat attachment to the lower clivus and anterior rim of the foramen magnum. Rounded hypointensity within anterior-superior margin of tumor most likely represents entrapped vertebral artery. Small thickened dural tail can be observed extending superiorly on the clivus from the tumor margin (*arrow*).

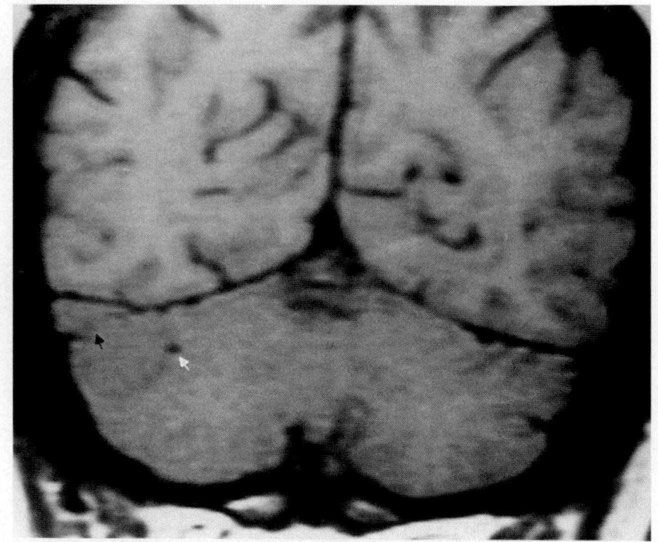

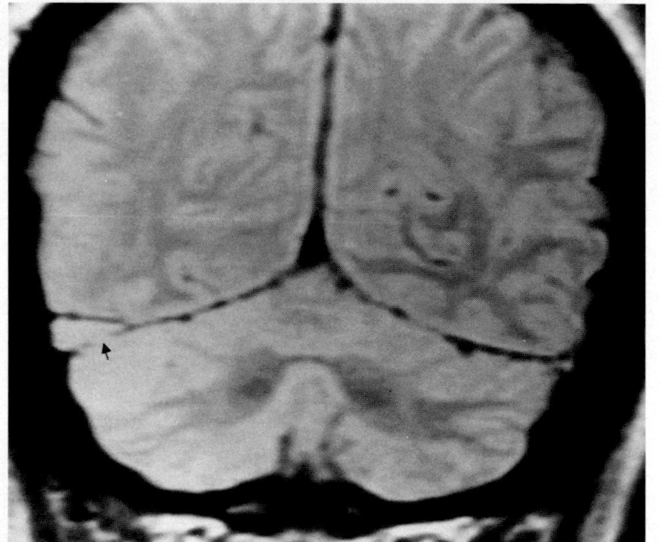

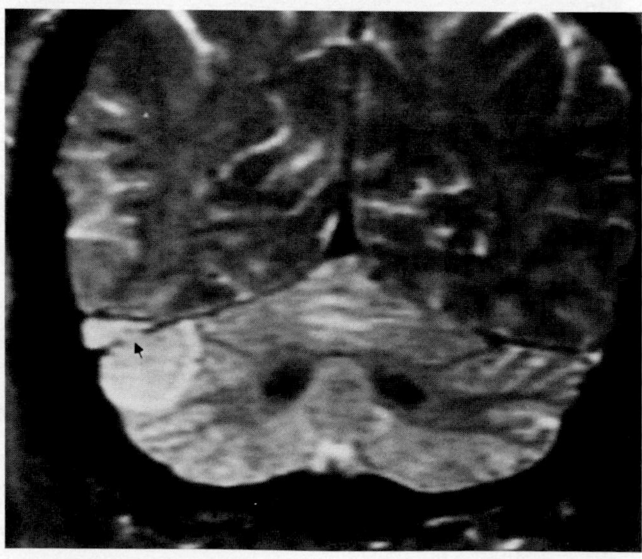

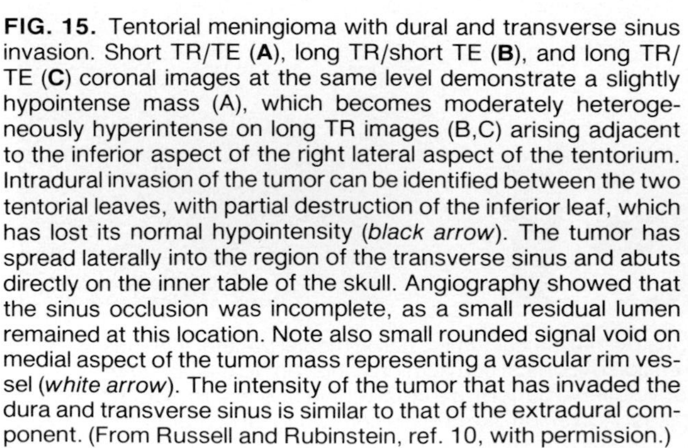

FIG. 15. Tentorial meningioma with dural and transverse sinus invasion. Short TR/TE (**A**), long TR/short TE (**B**), and long TR/TE (**C**) coronal images at the same level demonstrate a slightly hypointense mass (A), which becomes moderately heterogeneously hyperintense on long TR images (B,C) arising adjacent to the inferior aspect of the right lateral aspect of the tentorium. Intradural invasion of the tumor can be identified between the two tentorial leaves, with partial destruction of the inferior leaf, which has lost its normal hypointensity (*black arrow*). The tumor has spread laterally into the region of the transverse sinus and abuts directly on the inner table of the skull. Angiography showed that the sinus occlusion was incomplete, as a small residual lumen remained at this location. Note also small rounded signal void on medial aspect of the tumor mass representing a vascular rim vessel (*white arrow*). The intensity of the tumor that has invaded the dura and transverse sinus is similar to that of the extradural component. (From Russell and Rubinstein, ref. 10, with permission.)

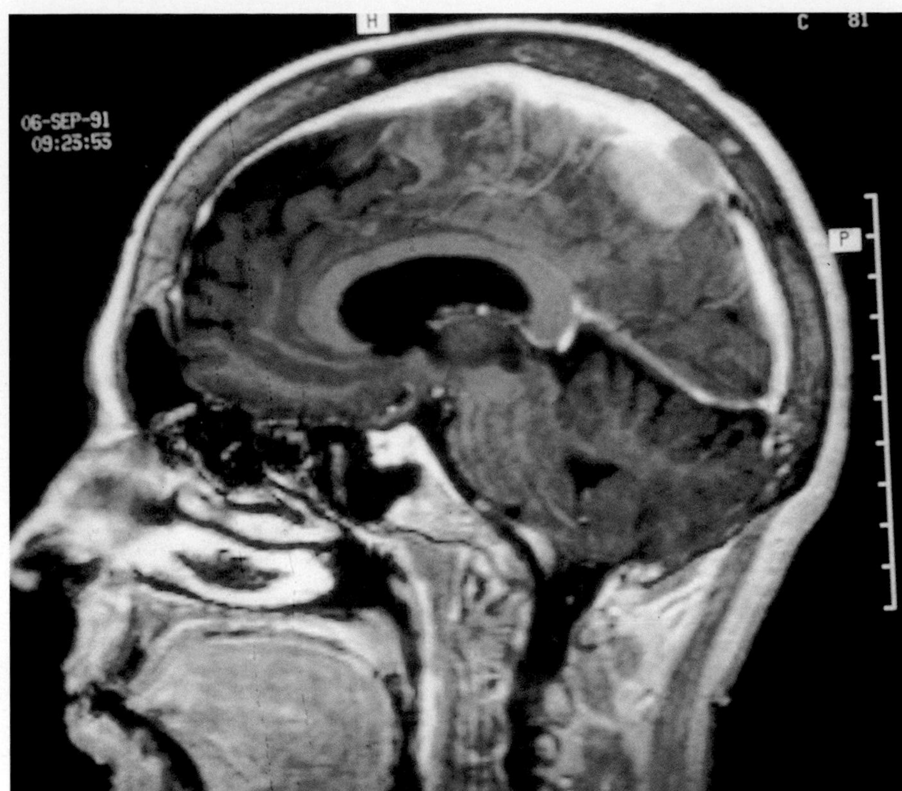

FIG. 16. Venous sinus invasion on contrast-enhanced MRI. After i.v. contrast, vertex meningioma is seen invading superior sagittal sinus, where tumor interrupts signal of enhancing venous blood in sinus.

axial masses, even when located near the surface, tend to spread parenchymal areas apart. The compression pattern on MRI from large meningiomas on the convolutions is analogous to the angiographic gyral capillary stain compression pattern often seen in association with these tumors.

MRI can depict vascular phenomena related to meningiomas much better than CT. Internal tumor vascularity (Fig. 2) and arterial encasement (Figs. 2, 3, and 14) are well demonstrated on MRI and are usually not detectable with CT (14,18), since on CT these vessels and the meningioma usually exhibit similar contrast enhancement (Fig. 2). With MRI, tumor vascularity and encased arteries with rapid flow remain hypointense on all imaging sequences even after the administration of contrast (Fig. 2). MRI is also superior to CT in demonstrating venous sinus invasion (14). Venous sinus invasion is demonstrated on MRI by the partial or complete obliteration of the sinus flow void with a soft tissue mass (Figs. 12 and 15). The intensity of the tissue within the venous sinus is usually similar to that of the adjacent tumor mass and can be appreciated on both T1- and T2-weighted sequences. CT and angiography are able to demonstrate complete sinus occlusion; however, partial sinus invasion by the meningioma usually cannot be readily detected with these imaging modalities. Sagittal and transverse sinus invasion is best demonstrated with coronal imaging (Fig. 16), whereas cavernous sinus involvement may be identified in either the coronal or axial planes. Routine T1- and T2-weighted images may not distinguish complete from near-total venous sinus obstruction. MR angiography or other MR flow techniques may improve the sensitivity of this determination.

Transdural invasion is equally well demonstrated with MRI (Figs. 12 and 15) and CT. Tumor may be demonstrated crossing from one side to the other through the tentorium cerebelli, falx cerebri, or cavernous sinus. Contrast enhancement is usually not required to demonstrate this finding with MRI. Bony hyperostosis is also equally well demonstrated with MRI (Figs. 11 and 17) and CT. Small soft-tissue components of primarily intraosseous meningiomas are frequently definable with MRI but not with CT (Fig. 18).

Meningioma calcification (Fig. 9) is less well defined with MRI than CT. Gradient-echo imaging markedly improves the sensitivity for the detection of calcifications, but specificity for this alteration will not be as great as with CT since other tissue substances such as acute or old blood products can cause a similar signal loss on gradient-echo sequences. Calcification, however, is not critical to the diagnosis in the majority of cases.

Brain edema develops in approximately 50% of meningiomas. It is more common with large lesions but may be extensive with small ones (Figs. 3, 18, and 19). Its exact cause has not been defined. Our studies have indicated its presence is significantly correlated with ei-

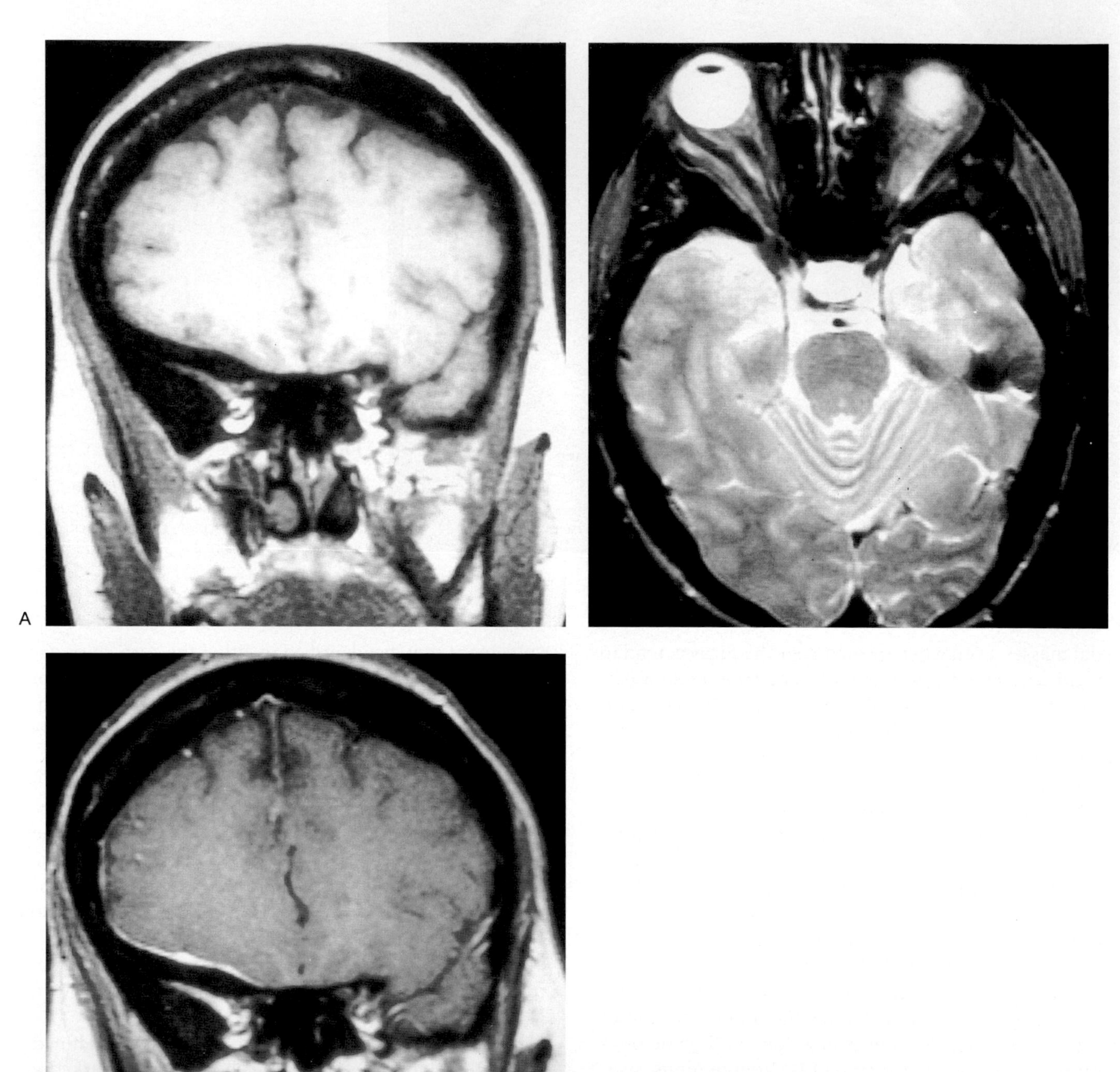

FIG. 17. Meningioma en plaque, contrast-enhancement characteristics. Coronal T1-weighted (**A**) and axial T2-weighted (**B**) images show hyperostosis of right sphenoid wing with marked hypointensity. After contrast (**C**), only thin rim of extra-axial enhancement is seen despite the extent of the lesion.

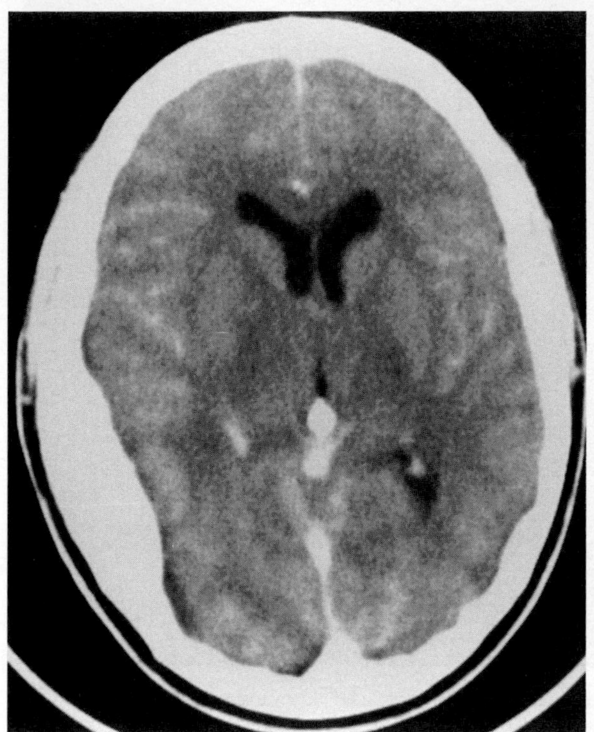
A

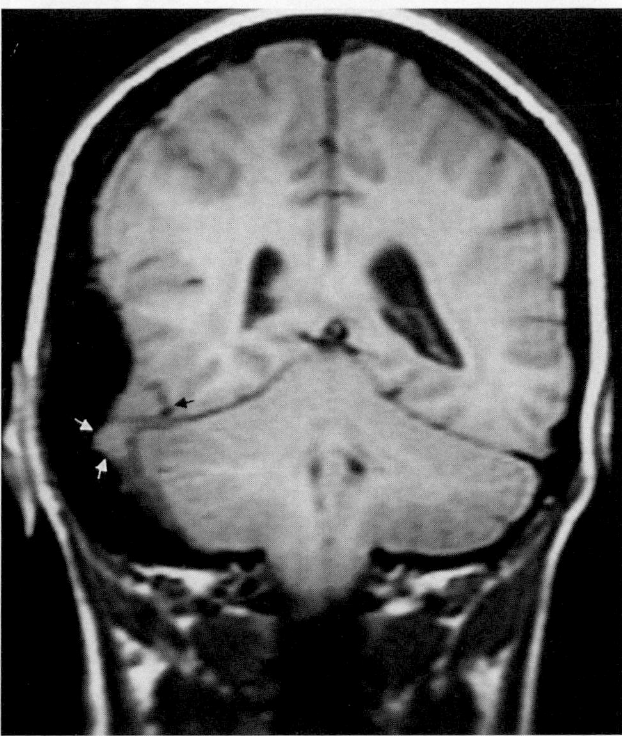
B

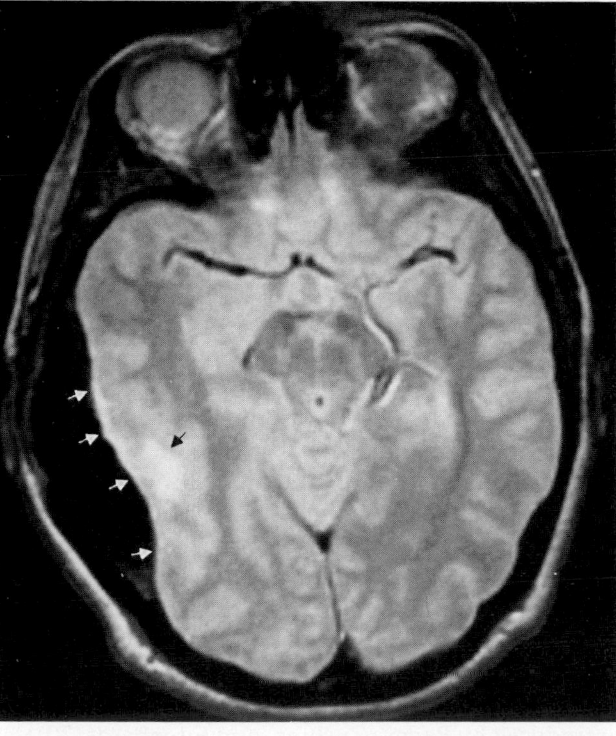
C

FIG. 18. Intraosseous meningioma with small extraosseous component. **A:** Contrast-enhanced axial CT reveals marked bony hyperostosis in right temporal parietal region without any soft tissue extraosseous component. **B:** Coronal short TR/TE image demonstrates marked hypointensity of bony hyperostosis involving the inferior temporal parietal region and extending below the tentorium into the inferior occipital bone region on the right side. A small extraosseous, extracerebral soft tissue mass that is isointense can be identified adjacent to the superior lateral leaf of the tentorium. It is marginated from the brain by a vascular rim vessel (*black arrow*). Also note the slight soft tissue thickening between the two leaves of the lateral aspect of the tentorium and the slightly higher intensity soft tissue mass in the region of the transverse sinus (*white arrows*). **C:** Axial long TR/short TE image demonstrates signal void of marked bony hyperostosis in right temporal parietal region, which appears mainly to be involving the inner table. There is a thin rim of hyperintense tissue on its inner aspect most likely representing en plaque dural tumor (*white arrows*) and a focal nodular high intensity encroaching on the lateral aspect of the right temporal lobe (*black arrow*) representing the extraosseous tumor nodule evident in B.

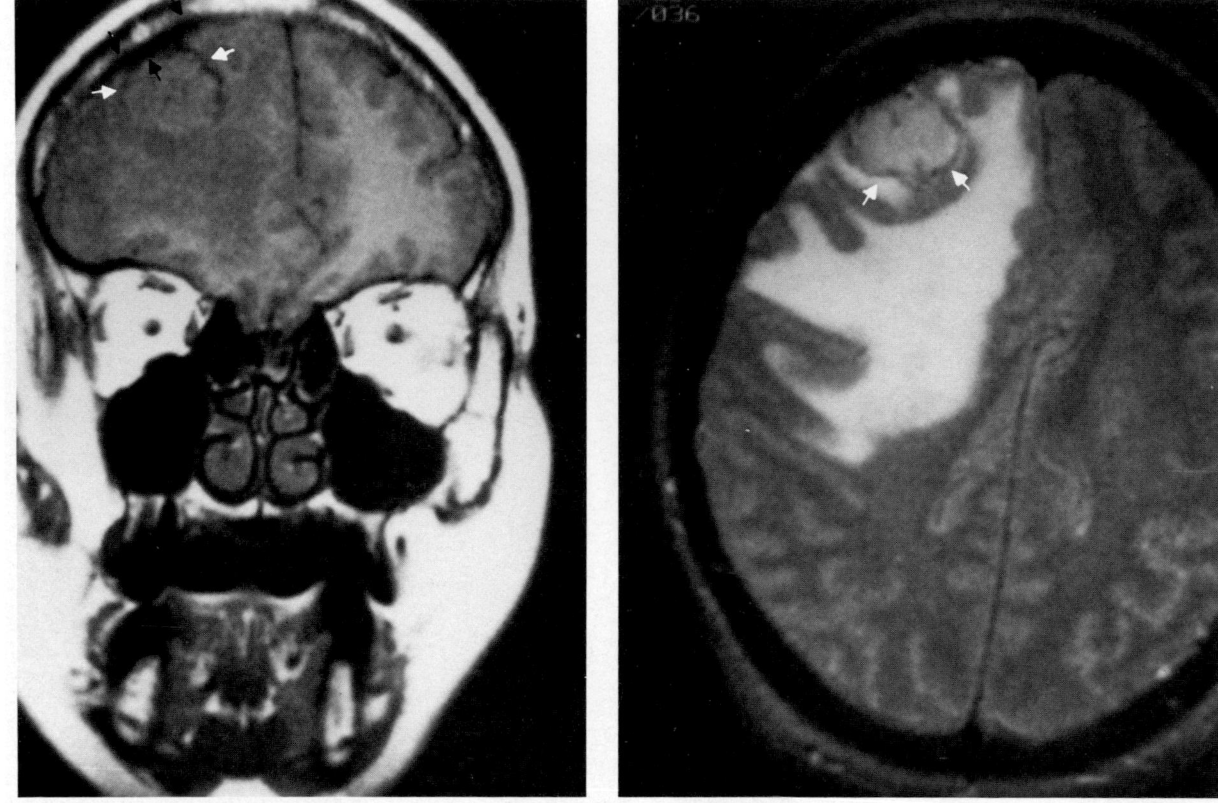

FIG. 19. Small convexity meningioma with extensive brain edema. Coronal short TR/TE image (**A**) and axial long TR/TE image (**B**) demonstrate a 2.5-cm-high convexity rounded mass outlined by vascular rim vessels (*white arrows*) from the adjacent brain. The mass abuts slightly against the inner table of the skull, which demonstrates a thickened hypointensity representing bony hyperostosis extending a short distance peripherally (*black arrows*) from the tumor base. There is extensive edema throughout the right frontal and parietal white matter.

ther the meningioma blood supply coming in some degree from cerebral pial arteries, or with its venous drainage connecting to the cortical brain veins (19). While varying amounts of edema may be present with any of the meningioma cell types, fibroblastic and transitional cell tumors have been reported to have only mild to moderate degrees of edema. Severe edema tends to be associated with meningiomas of the syncytial or angioblastic cell types (16). As indicated previously, these latter tumors also tend to be hyperintense on T2-weighted images. The degree of edema was found to be a helpful predictor of meningioma histology for meningiomas that were isointense to the cortex on T2-weighted images. Of tumors in this group that demonstrated moderately severe edema, they were mainly of the purely syncytial type or of a mixed type with significant syncytial components.

The terminology of meningiomas containing abundant vascular elements has long been the subject of debate. The concept of "angioblastic meningiomas" was first introduced by Bailey, Cushing, and Eisenhardt (20). Russell and Rubinstein (21) supported this concept and defined these tumors as a subcategory of meningiomas. They further divided angioblastic meningiomas into a hemangioblastic variant, transitional forms between hemangioblastic and classic meningiomas, and a hemangiopericytic variant. According to this classification, the hemangioblastic variant of the angiomatous meningioma is histologically identical to the cerebellar hemangioblastomas. It consists of plump endothelial cells lining multiple small capillary blood channels separated by stromal cells, often containing foamy cytoplasm rich of sudanophilic lipids. The hemangiopericytic variant is identical to hemangiopericytomas, believed to arise from the vascular wall pericytes in various organs including within the cranial and spinal cavities. These tumors are highly cellular, with a compact arrangement of polygonal cells which separate thin walled vascular spaces. Frequent mitoses and a wealth of reticulin fibers are characteristic features of hemangiopericytomas. In contradiction to Russell and Rubinstein's view, the WHO classification of nervous system tumors (22), which is widely accepted among neuropathologists, considers hemangioblastomas and hemangiopericytomas of the meninges as separate entities which should not be subclassified under meningiomas. Therefore, meningiomas which show features of increased vascular elements, or transitional forms of meningeal tumors with elements of both classic meningiomas and the other vascular tumors, are considered angiomatous (and not angioblastic) variants of meningiomas. Regardless of the classification used, angiography of all the vascular meningeal tumors generally demonstrates extensive tumor vascularity, staining, and rapid tumor circulation with enlarged early draining veins. Tumor blood supply from brain pial arteries may be a predominant feature. Cyst formation is also common, and focal and diffuse hemorrhage can occur.

MR appearance of angioblastic meningiomas may be quite varied depending on cellular and secondary changes in the tumor (Fig. 8). On T1-weighted images angioblastic meningiomas may reveal either low or high intensity depending on the degree of xanthomatous change. Those with prominent fatty accumulations will be of high intensity on T1-weighted images. On T2-weighted images these meningiomas are also usually of high intensity because of their rich capillary bed. With xanthomatous change there may be hypointensity focally or diffusely. Brain edema may be extensive. Intratumoral hemorrhage will reveal its characteristic intensities depending on the age of the hemorrhage. With cyst formation, well-demarcated foci of hypointensity are present on T1-weighted images that become markedly hyperintense on T2-weighted images.

Malignant meningiomas are rare and difficult to diagnose, because there is often considerable discrepancy between their biologic behavior (i.e., outcome) and their histologic features. The criteria for their diagnosis are therefore of somewhat limited value and a true incidence is difficult to ascertain. It has been noted that malignant meningiomas occur more frequently in males. Burger and Scheithauer (23) divide meningiomas into three groups, using both the level of histologic differentiation and the degree of aggressiveness to adjacent brain tissue: (i) typical benign meningioma; (ii) atypical meningioma, having a strong tendency to recur but lacking histologic criteria of frank anaplasia; and (iii) rare overtly malignant meningioma. These authors state that brain invasion, with deep expansile penetration of perivascular spaces with or without pial disruption, constitutes by definition a malignant meningioma. True invasion of underlying parenchyma is usually accompanied by prominent reactive gliosis. Malignant meningiomas have a distinct tendency to evoke marked brain edema. While most malignant meningiomas are only moderately anaplastic, unequivocal anaplasia on microscopy is a definite criterion for malignancy. Lastly, metastatic disease is a clear indication of malignancy. Because of problems with definitions, the recurrence rate and survival for patients harboring these lesions are difficult to assess. Generally, these lesions often result in multiple surgical procedures and radiotherapy with uncertain results. On MRI, the diagnosis of malignant meningioma is virtually impossible to make preoperatively, due to the considerable overlap of the features of these lesions with simple benign meningioma (bone destruction, brain edema), unless one detects metastatic spread.

Calvarial Invasion

Although meningiomas may cause hyperostosis of the inner table without bony invasion, many are en plaque, and some globular convexity and basal meningiomas extensively penetrate the skull, causing marked thickening of the bone along with osteoblastic reaction (Figs. 11 and 18). MRI will usually demonstrate this bony change and, in addition, the thin or thicker layer of soft tissue tumor lying adjacent to the inner table of the skull (Figs. 17 and 18). Some meningiomas arise from arachnoid cell rests in the diploic space. In these an intracranial component may not be present. Regions of soft tissue tumor within the bony thickening can be identified more readily with MRI than CT. Occasionally, bony invasion produces a lytic bony reaction (Fig. 11). The multiplanar imaging capability of MRI reveals calvarian invasion probably more frequently than does CT (14). Some tumors may extend throughout a table of the skull and present primarily as a scalp mass. Although bone destruction may appear aggressive, this finding does not correlate with malignant degeneration.

Intraventricular Meningiomas

Meningiomas may arise from arachnoid cells of the tela choroidea or from cell rests within stroma of the choroid plexi. These most commonly occur in the lateral ventricles, particularly in the region of the glomus. The MRI characteristics of these lesions are similar to meningiomas in other locations. Clinically, they are usually silent until they become large enough to block that portion of the ventricular system causing trapping and dilatation of the more distal portions. Meningiomas can usually be differentiated from choroid plexus papillomas both clinically and with MRI. Lateral ventricular choroid plexus papillomas develop mainly in young children, with meningiomas usually appearing in the middle-aged and elderly population group. Meningiomas have a smooth margin and are generally oval in configuration (Fig. 20), while papillomas frequently demonstrate very nodular, heterogeneous, irregular surfaces. Papillomas also usually present with diffuse hydrocephalus and not just dilatation of the trapped ventricular segment. This occurs either because of their overproduction of CSF or their frequent bleeding, which may cause obstructing basal arachnoiditis and/or intraventricular ependymitis. While papillomas are more frequently very heterogeneous, intraventricular meningiomas can also show sig-

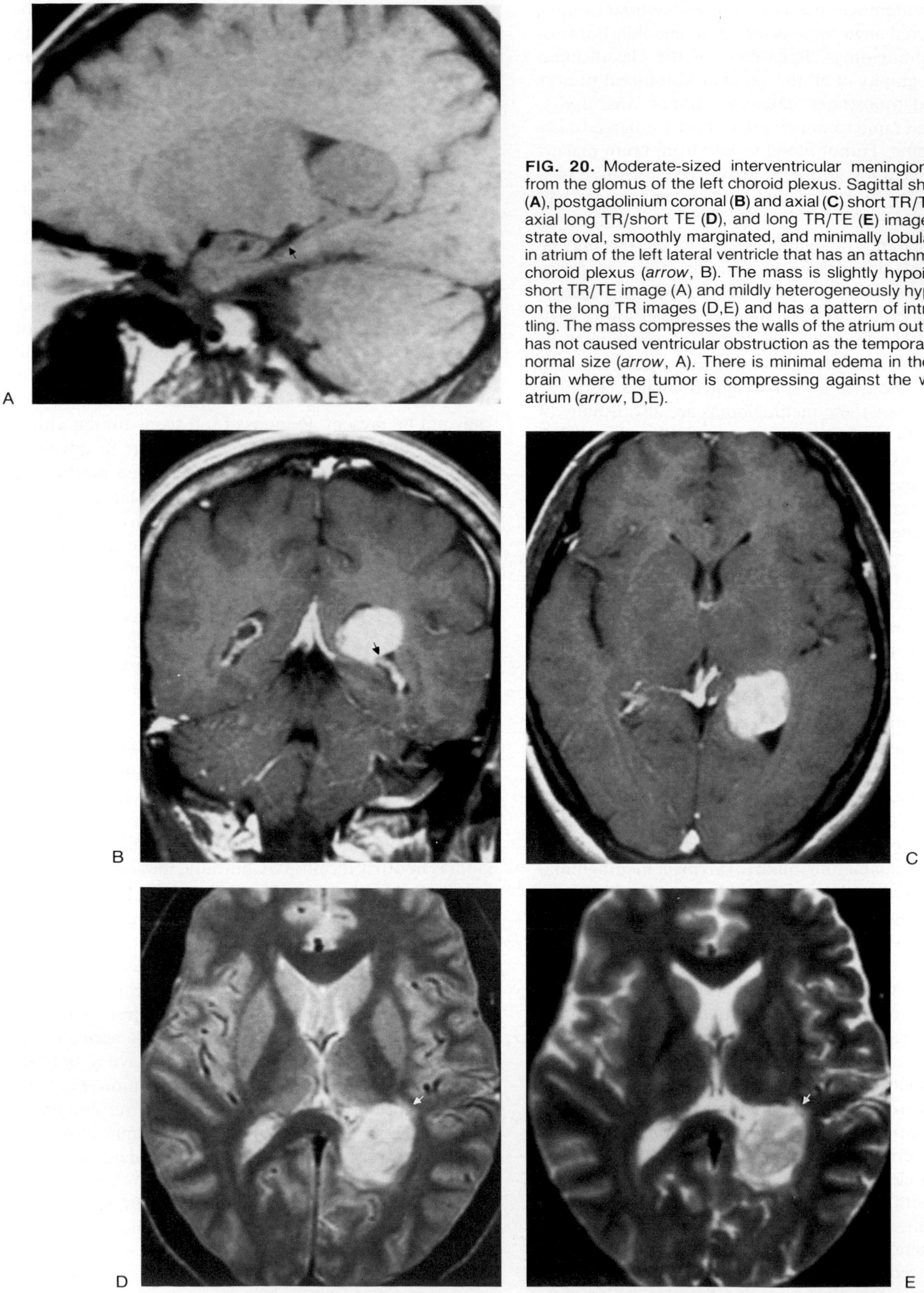

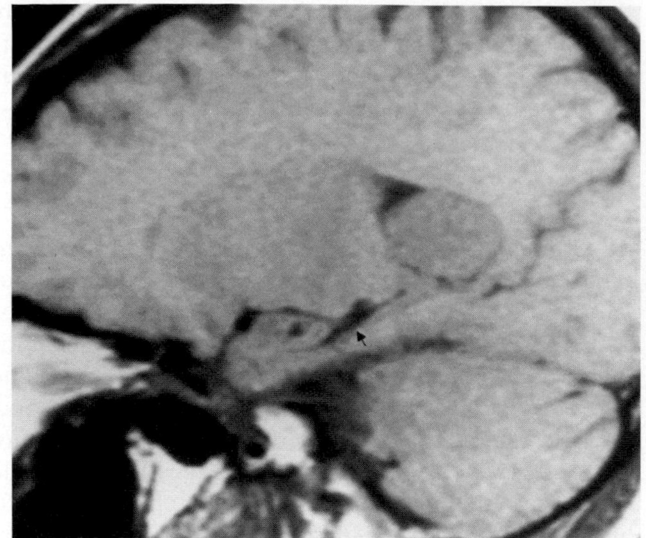

FIG. 20. Moderate-sized interventricular meningioma arising from the glomus of the left choroid plexus. Sagittal short TR/TE (**A**), postgadolinium coronal (**B**) and axial (**C**) short TR/TE images, axial long TR/short TE (**D**), and long TR/TE (**E**) images demonstrate oval, smoothly marginated, and minimally lobulated mass in atrium of the left lateral ventricle that has an attachment to the choroid plexus (*arrow*, B). The mass is slightly hypointense on short TR/TE image (A) and mildly heterogeneously hyperintense on the long TR images (D,E) and has a pattern of intrinsic mottling. The mass compresses the walls of the atrium outwardly but has not caused ventricular obstruction as the temporal horn is of normal size (*arrow*, A). There is minimal edema in the adjacent brain where the tumor is compressing against the wall of the atrium (*arrow*, D,E).

nificant heterogeneity and extensive edema (Fig. 21). Therefore, the location of the lesion and the age of the patient are the two most valuable clues to the diagnosis.

Meningiomas and Contrast Enhancement

As with radiographic contrast material, there is strong uptake of contrast by essentially all meningiomas, which usually produces marked homogeneous tumor enhancement (25–27). Contrast enhancement on MRI is almost always identifiable, even when meningiomas are densely calcified (Figs. 8 and 12). Enhancement may either be central or ring-like. This enhancement relates to the fact that meningioma capillaries have no blood–brain barrier. The degree of enhancement is usually more intense at 3 minutes after administration than at 25 or 55 min-

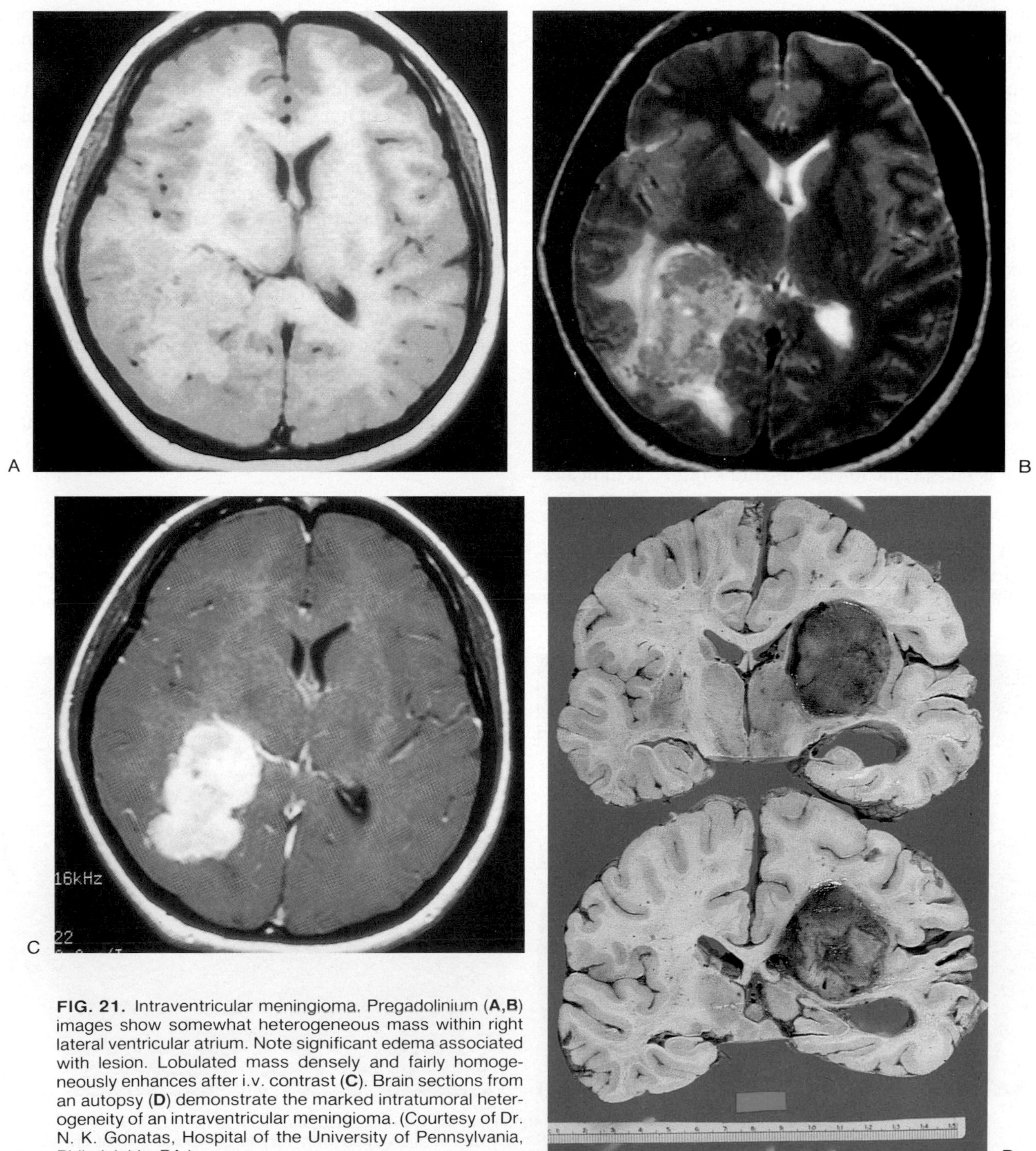

FIG. 21. Intraventricular meningioma. Pregadolinium (**A,B**) images show somewhat heterogeneous mass within right lateral ventricular atrium. Note significant edema associated with lesion. Lobulated mass densely and fairly homogeneously enhances after i.v. contrast (**C**). Brain sections from an autopsy (**D**) demonstrate the marked intratumoral heterogeneity of an intraventricular meningioma. (Courtesy of Dr. N. K. Gonatas, Hospital of the University of Pennsylvania, Philadelphia, PA.)

utes (28). Intravenous contrast is useful in demonstrating and defining the borders of symptomatic small lesions that compress or infiltrate around cortical neural structures such as the optic nerves and other cranial nerves, which may be occult on nonenhanced MRI. The anatomic boundaries of larger lesions that may be isointense to brain are clearly definable on T1-weighted enhanced scans (Figs. 2 and 3). Enhanced scans, however, may obscure some vascular rim interfaces, particularly those that are venous in nature. Slow-flowing veins will enhance with gadolinium, hiding their presence due to an intensity similar to that of the enhancing tumor (Fig. 2).

The most striking finding of contrast-enhanced MRI in meningiomas is the finding of dural enhancement adjacent to the lesion. En plaque meningiomas as well as globular convexity and basal meningiomas may infiltrate adjacent dural surfaces for several centimeters. Recognition of this infiltration can be of significant importance in surgical planning for complete tumor removal (29). Marginal dural thickening has been observed in approximately one-third of convexity meningiomas, and all gadolinium-enhanced scans have demonstrated enhancement of the dural thickening (30). Although high-resolution MRI can occasionally demonstrate marginal dural thickening without contrast (Figs. 3 and 14), gadolinium administration is clearly useful in defining the extent of dural thickening (Fig. 22) and thereby provides a valuable clue to the diagnosis (Fig. 9). Dural enhancement is *not* specific for meningioma; rather, it indicates dural involvement by any adjacent mass, whether the mass is meningioma, metastases, or invasive primary brain tumor. Meningioma dural infiltration has been surgically and histologically documented in a few cases of gadolinium-enhancing dural thickening; however, one series of cases has been recently reported that demonstrated histologically only reactive dural thickening without tumor infiltration in contrast-enhancing adjacent dura from meningioma (31).

Regardless of the precise etiology of the dural thickening and enhancement, its determination in continuity with the margins of an intracranial tumor adds another valuable MR diagnostic feature of extra-axial dural-based tumors.

Contrast administration is also extremely valuable in detecting residual and recurrent meningioma postoperatively. Tumor-brain interfaces are frequently obliterated postoperatively, and postsurgical changes in the surrounding brain further obscure evidence and definition of recurrent tumor. Although enhancing dural thickening is almost universally present after surgery, it usually appears as a thin, smooth enhancing membrane. Recurrent tumor is revealed as a lobulated thick gadolinium-enhancing mass that protrudes into the adjacent brain (Fig. 23).

Finally, contrast administration is useful in the rare instance of postradiation therapy-induced meningioma. This unusual entity should only be suspected if a new meningeal-based mass develops many years after irradiation of the primary lesion, which in most instances is a glioma. Since surgery and the original lesion have already distorted the anatomy in the region, i.v. contrast can be quite helpful in delineating these lesions (Fig. 24).

Lymphomas

Lymphomas may be primary within the central nervous system or associated with systemic involvement and present an important differential diagnosis when vis-

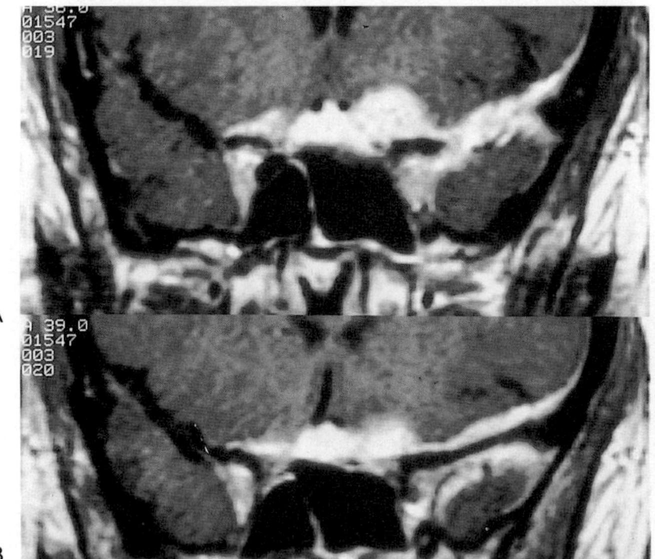

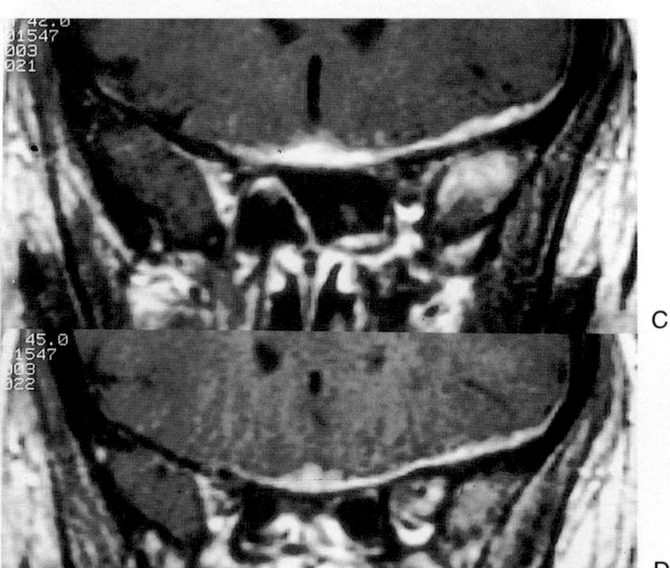

FIG. 22. Subfrontal meningioma with extensive dural enhancement. Coronal postgadolinium-enhanced MRI (**A–D**) show parasellar meningioma (A), which extends subfrontally and is associated with very large "dural tail" of enhancement (A–D).

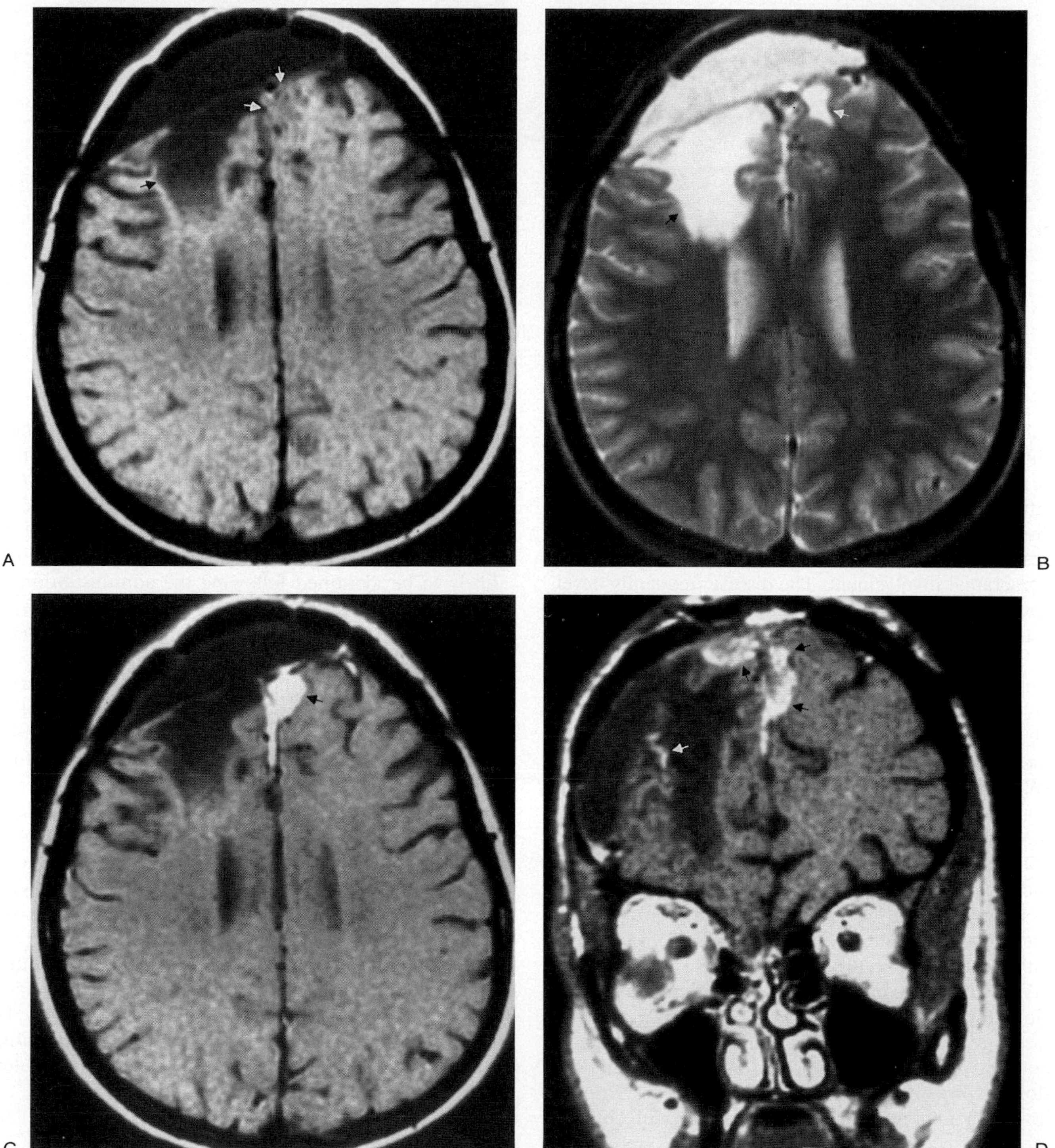

FIG. 23. Recurrent meningioma. **A,B:** Axial short TR/TE (A) and long TR/TE (B) images demonstrate what appear most likely to represent postsurgical brain changes: a bifrontal epidural hygroma, a right frontal porencephalic cavity (*black arrow*), and a left medial frontal region suggesting encephalomalacia (*white arrows*). **C,D:** Axial and coronal postgadolinium short TR/TE images demonstrate lobulated enhancing mass along the falx in the left medial frontal region with enhancing tumor extending into the right frontal parasagittal region (*black arrows*). Note also focal linear enhancement along lateral margin of right frontal porencephalic cyst (*white arrow*).

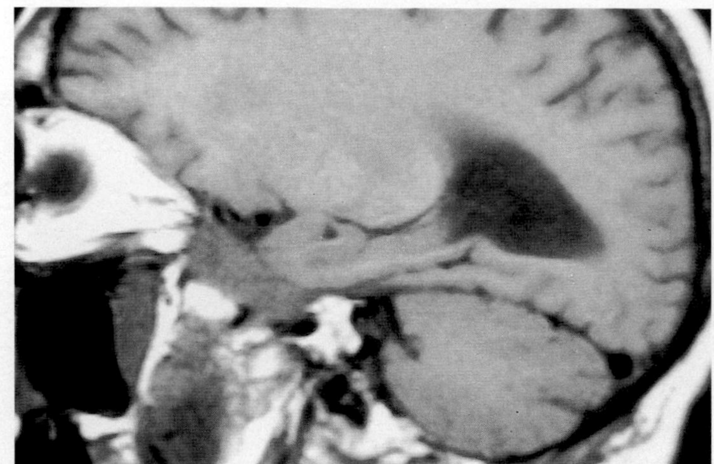

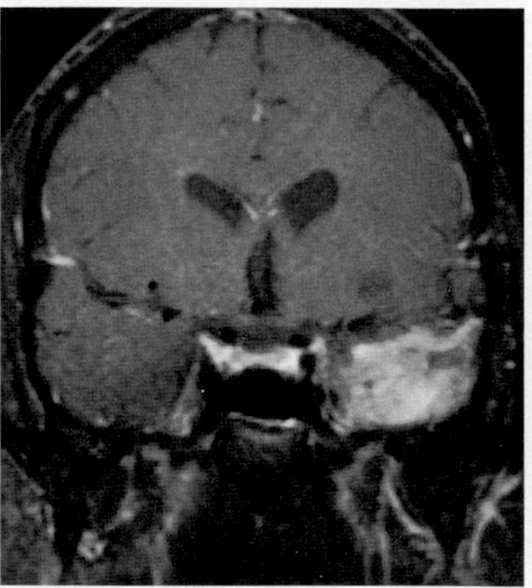

FIG. 24. Postradiation therapy meningioma. Irregular extra-axial mass (**A**) which enhances (**B**) represents radiation-induced meningioma many years following therapy for intra-axial lesion.

ualizing extra-axial brain lesions. Primary central nervous system lymphomas were previously considered to be rare lesions representing approximately only 1% of all intracranial tumors (32). All ages are affected, but the disease manifests primarily in the sixth decade. There appears to be a recent increase in the incidence of primary intracranial involvement. The disease frequently develops in immunosuppressed individuals—either transplant patients (33) with secondary iatrogenic suppression or acquired immune deficiency syndrome (AIDS) patients, in whom up to 6% of the cases may have CNS involvement (34,35). CNS involvement is frequent in individuals with systemic lymphoma. About one-third of these individuals develop secondary brain or spinal involvement (36). Multicentric foci frequently occur with both primary and secondary brain lymphomas. Although all portions of the nervous system may be involved, there is a propensity for leptomeningeal involvement, which occurs more frequently with secondary CNS lymphomas. The tumor most commonly involves the arachnoid membrane and may be present focally or diffusely throughout the CNS (37). There is frequent secondary invasion of the brain, with tumor extending along the Virchow-Robin spaces. The tumor may also locally invade the dura from the arachnoid membrane in both the primary and secondary varieties and can occasionally present as large discrete dural masses. Primary involvement of the dura also may develop with both primary and secondary cerebral lymphomas. Rarely the tumor may extend beyond the dura into the skull and extracranial compartment. When there is dural involvement the disease is frequently more extensive than in meningiomas.

Subarachnoid involvement is usually not identified with CT (38,39). It also is frequently not evident on routine MR imaging but may appear in some cases with thicker tumor plaques as high-intensity cuffing on long TR/short TE images on the surface of the brain. There may be secondary invasion into the underlying parenchyma. The lesion may be obscured on the long TR/TE sequence because of the high intensity of the adjacent CSF, which may have similar intensity to that of the tumor. Thinner plaques of subarachnoid tumor are more likely to be identified following the administration of contrast, such as gadolinium-DTPA. Thin streaks of high intensity may be identified over the surfaces of brain and along the cranial nerves (40).

Thick plaques of tumor may develop with subarachnoid and dural involvement and be evident on routine MRI. On short TR/TE images the tumor is usually isointense to the adjacent brain surface but is usually outlined by the surrounding CSF. On long TR/short TE images, the tumor may be isointense or hyperintense to the adjacent brain. On long TR/TE sequences it may be iso- or hyperintense but is frequently hypointense to the adjacent brain due to its high cellularity (Fig. 25). Following contrast administration on T1-weighted images, diffuse homogeneous enhancement develops. Contrast-enhanced images usually reveal more extensive dural spread than was evident on nonenhanced images. Differentiation from en plaque meningioma may be difficult but is suggested by its diffuse dural extension, subarachnoid extensions, hypointensity on T2-weighted images, and more frequent multicentricity.

Sarcoidosis

Intracranial involvement occurs in about 15% of people with known sarcoidosis. Primary CNS involvement may also rarely develop (41,42). Intracranial involvement manifests two patterns. Most commonly the disease appears as a granulomatous leptomeningitis but may also manifest as multiple diffuse parenchymal lesions or as a single intracerebral mass. The leptomenin-

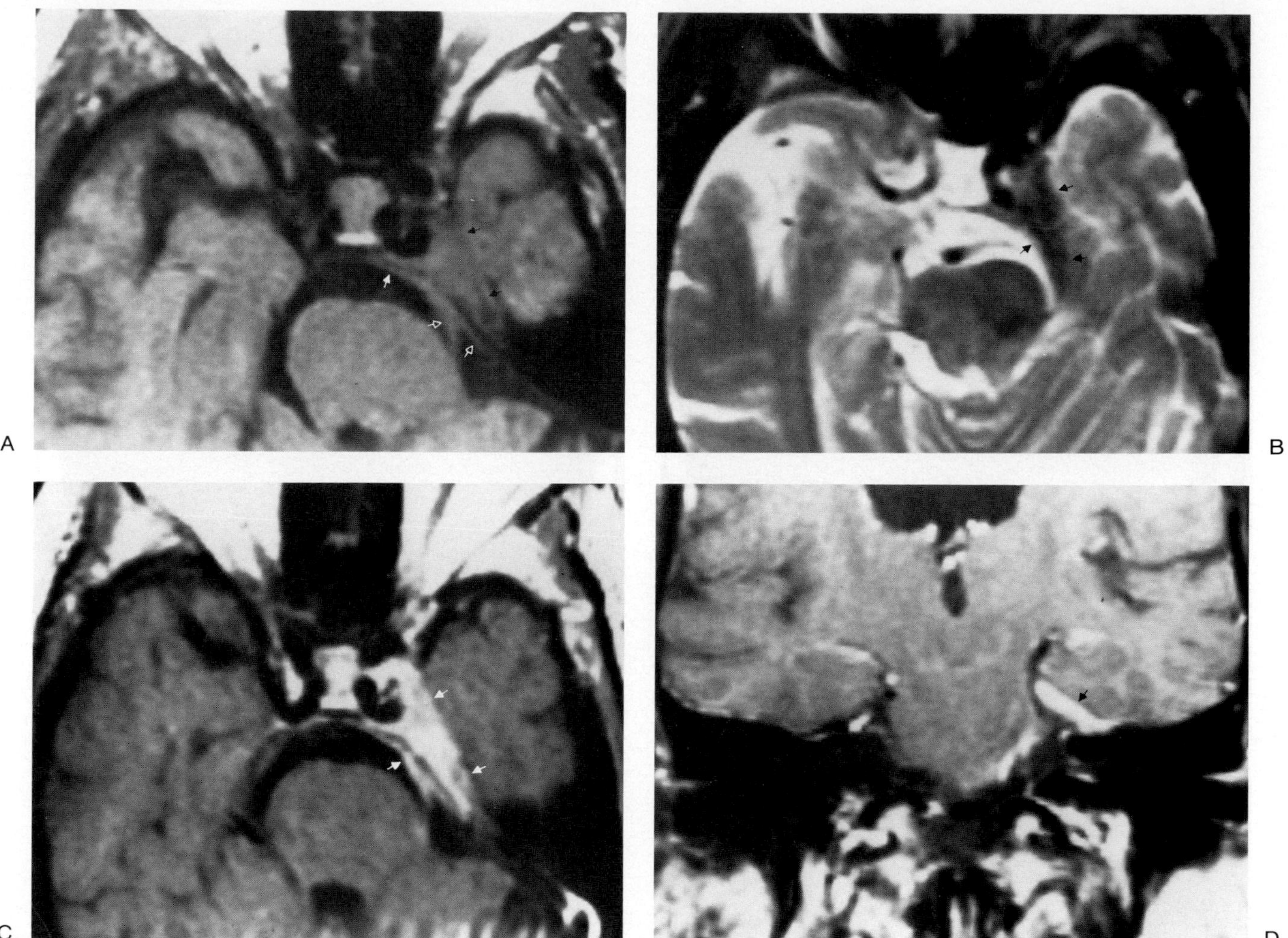

FIG. 25. Dural arachnoid lymphoma. **A:** Axial short TR/TE image demonstrates isointense soft tissue mass on medial aspect of left temporal lobe involving the lateral portion of the cavernous sinus and extending posteriorly over the petrous ridge (*black arrows*). It extends inferiorly as a thin sheet of tumor onto the left side of the clivus (*white arrow*) and laterally over the medial posterior aspect of the petrous ridge and along the fifth cranial nerve (*open white arrows*). **B:** Long TR/TE image. Tumor mass becomes moderately hypointense (*arrows*). **C:** Axial postgadolinium image demonstrates diffuse enhancement of tumor with same distribution as in A (*arrows*). **D:** Postgadolinium coronal image reveals a thick plaque of enhancement along dura on undersurface of left temporal lobe (*arrow*). On more posterior images (not shown), a thin sheet of enhancement extends over the left side of the tentorial leaf reaching almost to the occipital pole.

geal disease may secondarily involve the adjacent brain surface by infiltration along the perivascular spaces. The disease may also present as a dural-based mass.

On MR, T1-weighted images in leptomeningeal disease will frequently demonstrate isointense thickening of the subarachnoid space on the brain surface that may extend into the sulcal regions. This may be focally present in one region of the subarachnoid space or be evident diffusely throughout the brain. On T2-weighted images the lesion not infrequently appears hypointense, most likely secondary to the compact cellular nature of the granulomatous process (Fig. 26). There may be edema in the adjacent portions of the brain, which would suggest infiltration along the Virchow-Robin spaces into the parenchyma or small vessel vasculitis from the disease (Figs. 26 and 27). Following contrast administration, the subarachnoid granulomatous process demonstrates diffuse homogeneous enhancement, which more clearly outlines its extent than on noncontrast images (Figs. 26–28). The MR characteristics of the dural-based disease are similar to those of the disease in the subarachnoid space (Figs. 27 and 28). Lesions in this location may be indistinguishable from meningiomas or dural-based lymphomatous disease, so clinical correlation and biopsy (Fig. 29) is essential for accurate diagnosis.

Extra-Axial Metastases

Extra-axial intracranial metastases are common in clinical practice. In one series, 18% of autopsied patients with extracranial primary malignancies and intracranial

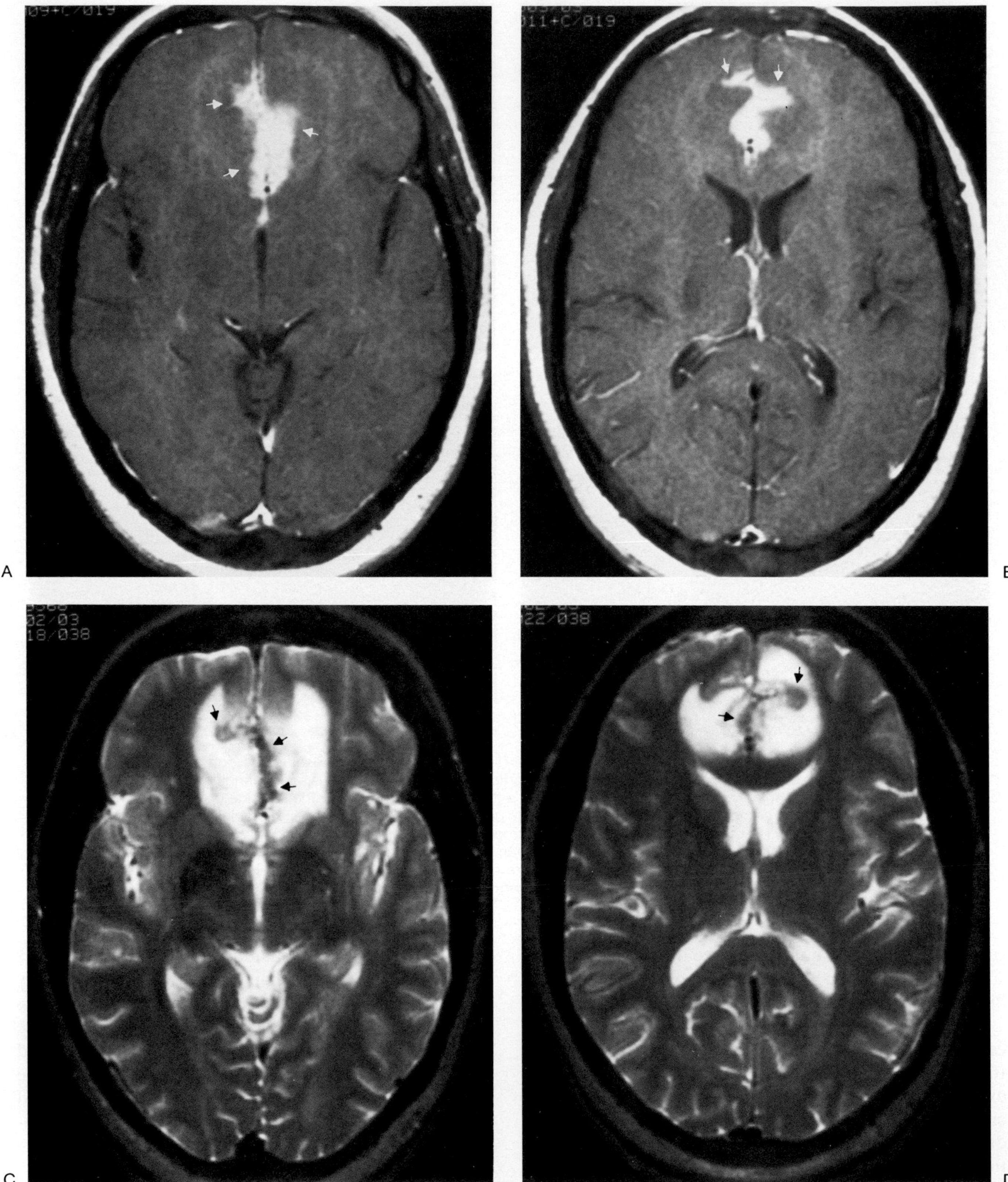

FIG. 26. Sarcoid of the pial membrane with brain invasion. **A,B:** Axial postgadolinium-enhanced short TR/TE images demonstrate thick irregular enhancement in the interhemispheric fissure with feather-like invasion into the medial cortical surfaces bilaterally (*arrows*, A) and extension into sulci (*arrows*, B). **C,D:** Long TR/TE axial images at approximately same levels as A and B, respectively. Gadolinium-enhancing tissue in A and B is slightly hypointense (*arrows*) to normal cortical tissue intensity. Hyperintensity of underlying white matter bilaterally is more extensive than enhancing tissues in A and B, suggesting the presence of secondary brain edema.

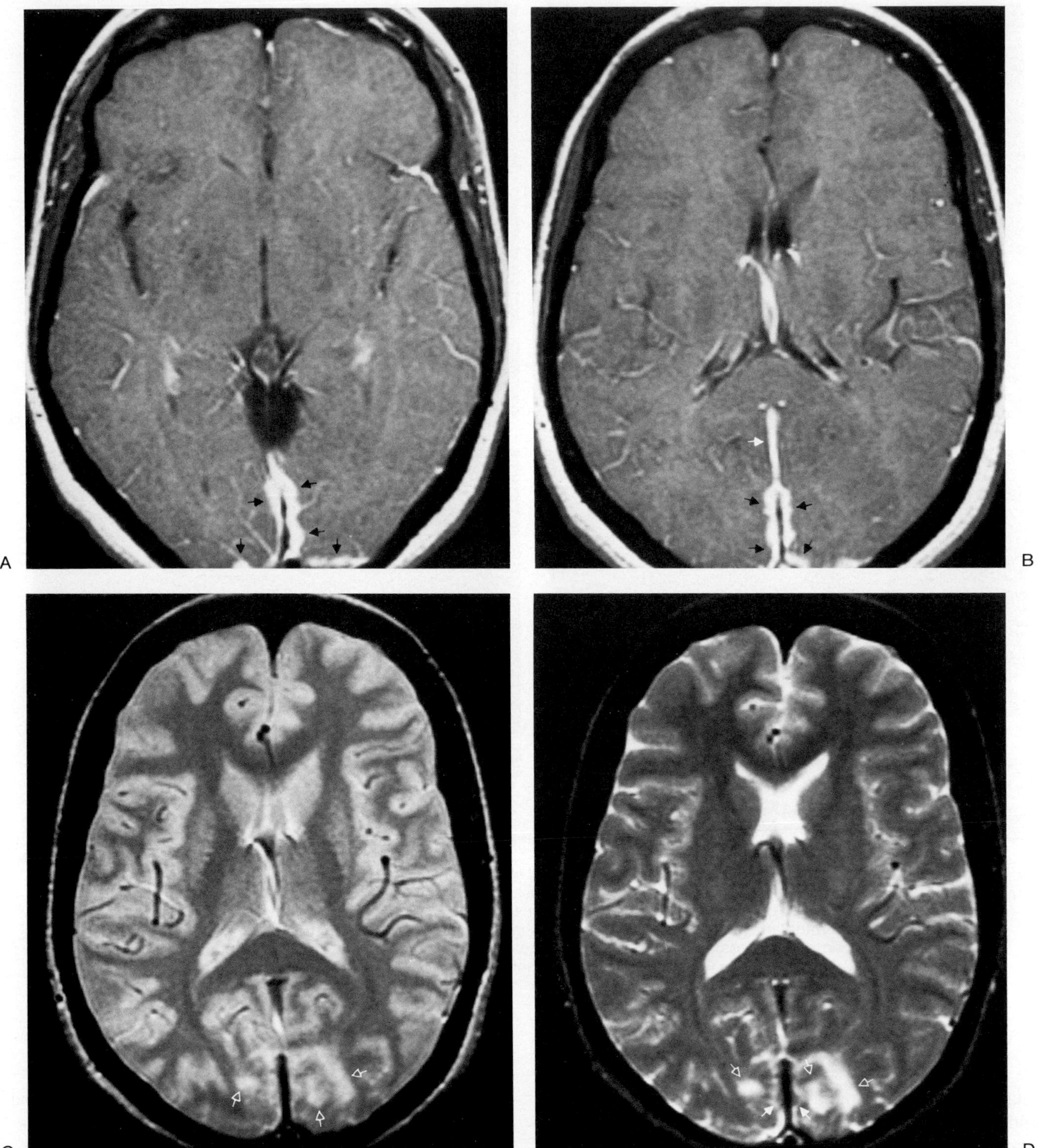

FIG. 27. Dural and leptomeningeal sarcoid. **A,B:** Postgadolinium axial short TR/TE images demonstrate lobulated enhancement on both sides of the posterior inferior aspect of the falx with extension laterally over both occipital poles (*black arrows*). Smooth linear enhancement anteriorly to inferior aspect of splenium represents a portion of the straight sinus (*white arrow*). On close inspection of B there appears to be slight enhancement within the falx in several regions. A normal falx usually does not demonstrate enhancement. **C,D:** Axial long TR/short TE (C) and long TE (D) images. In D there appears to be a subtle amount of slightly hypointense lobulated soft tissue on either side of the posterior falx, which is outlined by thin clefts of CSF (*white arrows*). This tissue is isointense in C and is less well delineated from the brain. Small regions of hyperintensity that did not enhance are present in the subjacent occipital white matter, being greater on the left than the right (*open white arrows*). This suggests transarachnoid extension with invasion into the brain along the Virchow-Robin spaces.

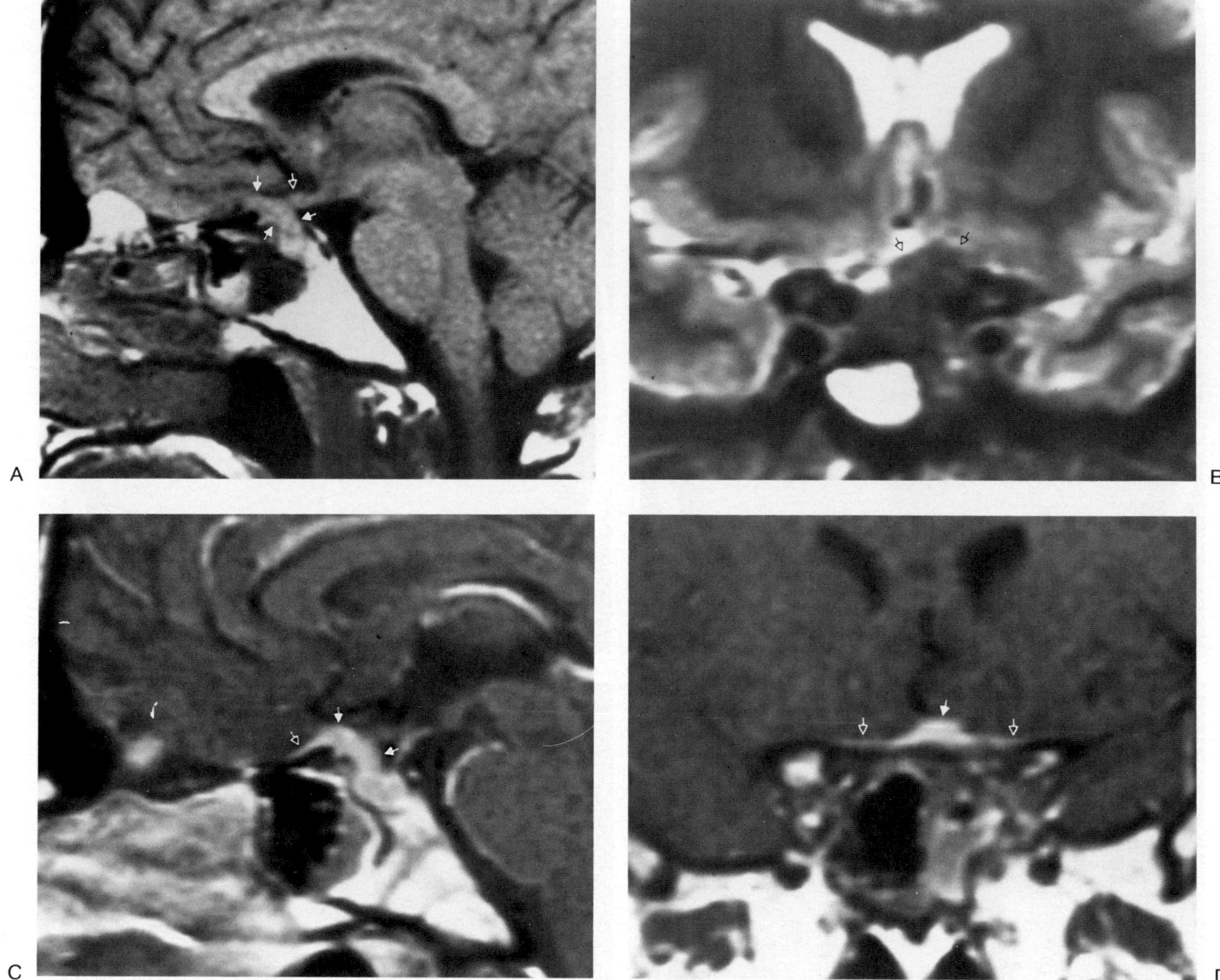

FIG. 28. Dural sarcoid of tuberculum sellae. **A,B:** Sagittal short TR/TE (A) and coronal long TR/TE (B) images demonstrate an isointense small mass in A involving the tuberculum sellae and chiasmatic groove (*solid white arrows*) that is encroaching on the left optic nerve (*open white arrow*). On the long TR/TE image (B) the mass becomes hypointense to adjacent gray matter (*arrows*). As there is no intensity change in the adjacent brain, transarachnoid invasion probably has not occurred. **C,D:** Postgadolinium short TR/TE sagittal (C) and coronal (D) images demonstrate homogeneous enhancement of the mass (*white arrows*) with thin anterior and lateral extensions of dural enhancement (*open white arrows*).

metastases had dural metastases (including both epidural and subdural) as the sole location of the metastases (43). The most common type of metastatic tumor to spread to dural sites is breast carcinoma, followed by lymphoma, prostate carcinoma, and neuroblastoma (43). Epidural metastases in adults are almost invariably secondary to metastatic tumor in the adjacent skull, and are usually associated with primary carcinomas of the breast, lung, prostate, or kidney (43–45). Pathologically, metastatic foci are focal and well-defined masses invading the dura or skull and extend to the surface of the brain, but occasionally these lesions are diffuse.

In spite of the intimate relationship of the dura to the bony calvarium and the leptomeninges to the pachymeninges, these structures present significant barriers to contiguous spread of malignant tumors. With that in mind, however, none are absolutely impenetrable, and, in fact, it is not rare to find plaques of metastatic tumor on the inner side of the dura in necropsy specimens (21). It is believed that subdural tumor implants are more likely to result from direct hematogenous seeding, rather than transgression of dura from epidural tumor (46). Although most evidence points to the arterial route as the path of transport of extracranial neoplasms to their in-

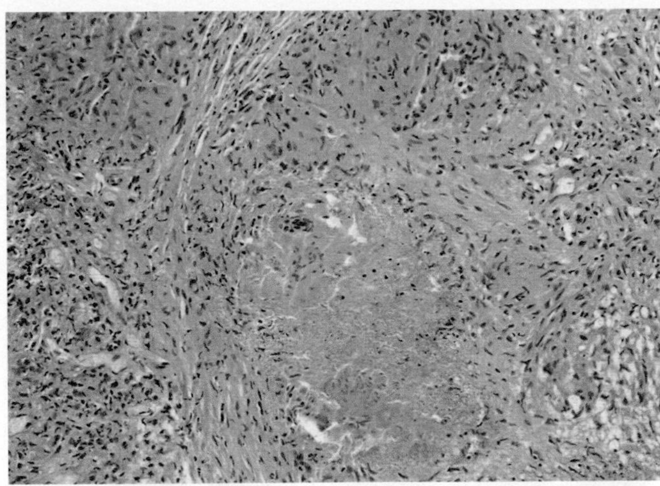
A

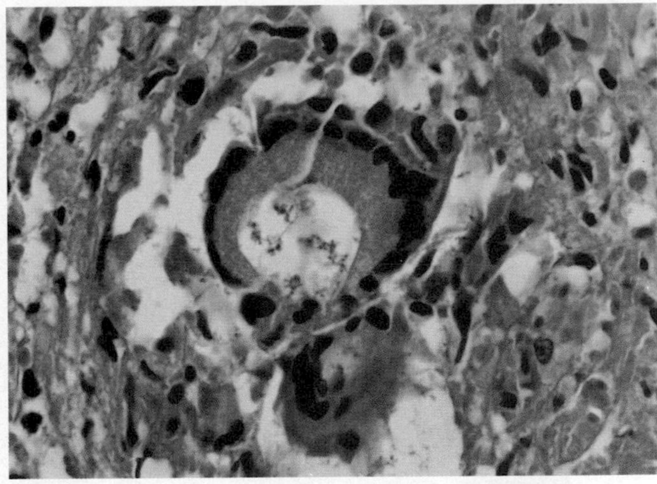
B

FIG. 29. Histologic features of sarcoidosis. The thick fibrous tissue of the dura is infiltrated by numerous small, non-caseating, occasionally necrotizing, granulomas, containing histiocytes, multinucleated giant cells and peripherally located lymphocytes (**A**). A characteristic feature of sarcoidosis is a stellate-shaped inclusion known as an asteroid body enclosed within a giant cell found in this dural granuloma (**B**).

tracranial site of spread, some authors (47) suggest that, especially in the case of subdural metastases, the epidural plexus of spinal veins plays a role in the spread of prostate carcinoma into the dural and subsequently cerebral veins, a hypothesis originally suggested by Batson (48). Symptomatology from epidural or subdural metastases are usually due to direct compressive effects of underlying brain parenchyma, so location again determines the neurologic deficit. Other less common sequelae of these lesions include venous thrombosis, which can occur either as a result of tumor invasion itself into the dural sinus, or from venous compression and stagnation. A rare consequence of dural metastases is pachymeningitis interna hemorrhagica, which entails subdural hemorrhage in association with diffuse dural metastases. Subdural hematoma due to dural metastases is usually bilateral and is most often due to breast carcinoma (21) (Fig. 30), but has been reported with many neoplasms, including prostate carcinoma and melanoma.

Leptomeningeal carcinomatosis, or carcinomatous meningitis, is an uncommon disorder which clinically is manifested by a low-grade meningitis syndrome accompanied by cranial nerve palsies, due to infiltration of the subarachnoid space and the structures around the base of the brain (49). The presence of this often elusive clinical diagnosis may also be indicated by the presence of communicating hydrocephalus. Aside from primary CNS malignancies, adenocarcinomas are the major cell type to involve the leptomeninges, particularly from lung, stomach, breast, and ovary, but melanoma is also seen in this disorder (21). It is also quite common in patients with leukemia or lymphoma (21). Grossly, examination of the brain usually demonstrates a diffuse, opaque thickening of the basal leptomeninges, with gray-white patches or yellow streaks over the surface of the brain and within sulci, obscuring superficial blood vessels (21). On microscopic examination, the subarachnoid space is filled by metastatic cellular infiltrates, which often extend along the perivascular spaces and into the brain parenchyma. The malignant infiltrate variably induces a reactive fibroblastic meningitis with inflammatory cells (21). On close inspection, most cases of leptomeningeal carcinomatosis usually are accompanied by numerous tumor deposits along the ventricular ependymal surface, which many believe represent the direct source of the diffuse subarachnoid seeding (21).

The modality of choice for the depiction of extra-axial metastases on imaging studies has, in a similar fashion to other CNS malignancies, shifted to MRI. While radionuclide bone scan still is a reasonable screening tool for bone metastases, several reports have been published which indicate that MRI may have a higher sensitivity for these lesions. Metastases to the skull are seen as focal lytic or blastic lesions of both the inner and outer tables of the calvarium on either plain films or CT. These lesions typically lack a well-defined, sclerotic border, which, if present, suggests benignity. Occasionally, metastatic lesions to skull are expansile, especially from renal cell or thyroid carcinoma. MRI depicts calvarial metastases as focal regions of abnormal low signal intensity (isointense to gray matter) on short TR/TE images, which are relatively easily seen as distinct from the high intensity of normal fatty marrow (Fig. 31). Note that these lesions can be obscured on MRI by enhancement after i.v. contrast, so precontrast images must be obtained if calvarial metastases are suspected. In addition, benign intradiploic epidermoid may be indistinguishable from calvarial metastasis.

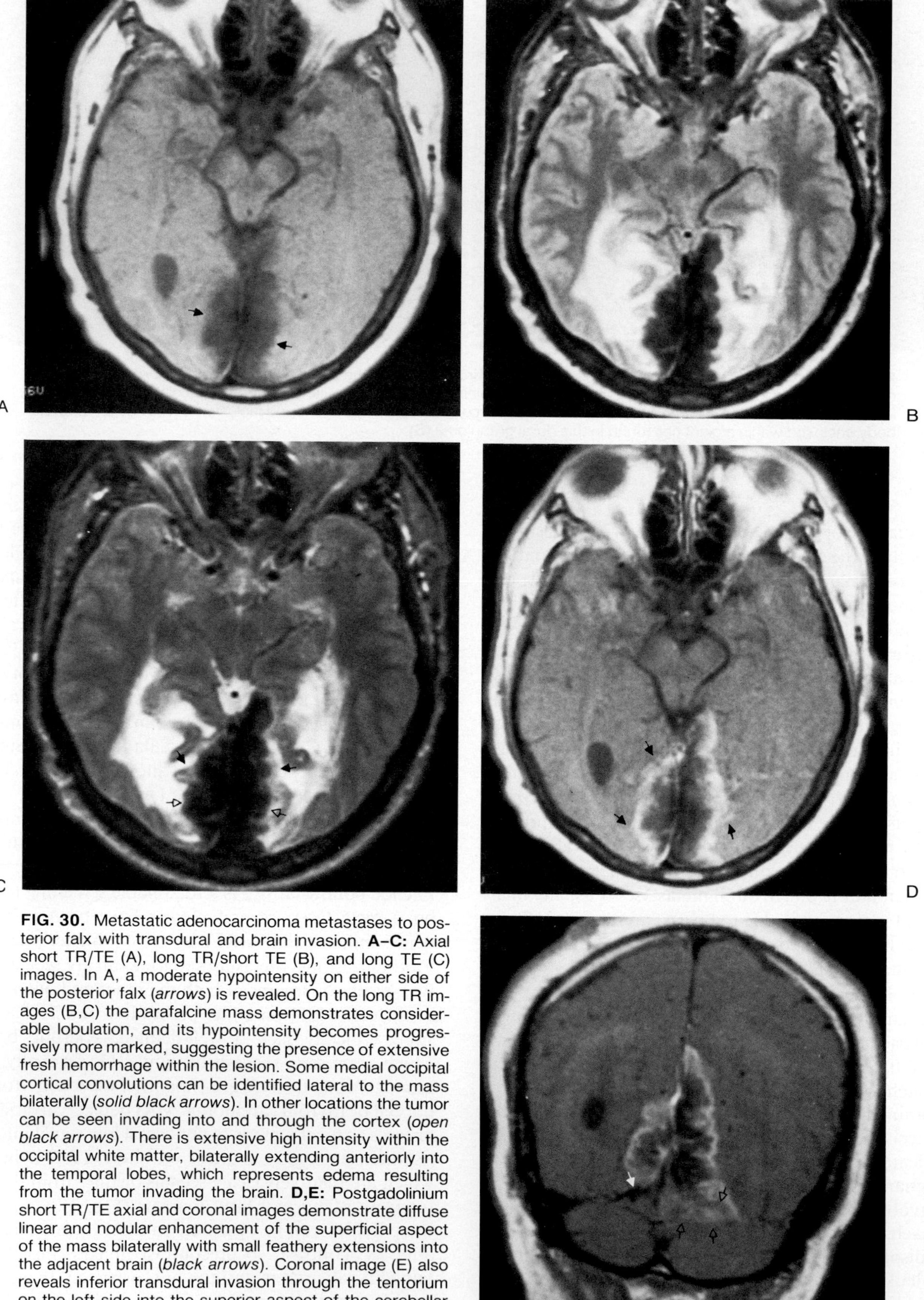

FIG. 30. Metastatic adenocarcinoma metastases to posterior falx with transdural and brain invasion. **A–C:** Axial short TR/TE (A), long TR/short TE (B), and long TE (C) images. In A, a moderate hypointensity on either side of the posterior falx (*arrows*) is revealed. On the long TR images (B,C) the parafalcine mass demonstrates considerable lobulation, and its hypointensity becomes progressively more marked, suggesting the presence of extensive fresh hemorrhage within the lesion. Some medial occipital cortical convolutions can be identified lateral to the mass bilaterally (*solid black arrows*). In other locations the tumor can be seen invading into and through the cortex (*open black arrows*). There is extensive high intensity within the occipital white matter, bilaterally extending anteriorly into the temporal lobes, which represents edema resulting from the tumor invading the brain. **D,E:** Postgadolinium short TR/TE axial and coronal images demonstrate diffuse linear and nodular enhancement of the superficial aspect of the mass bilaterally with small feathery extensions into the adjacent brain (*black arrows*). Coronal image (E) also reveals inferior transdural invasion through the tentorium on the left side into the superior aspect of the cerebellar (*open arrows*). Note normal position of right tentorium (*white arrow*).

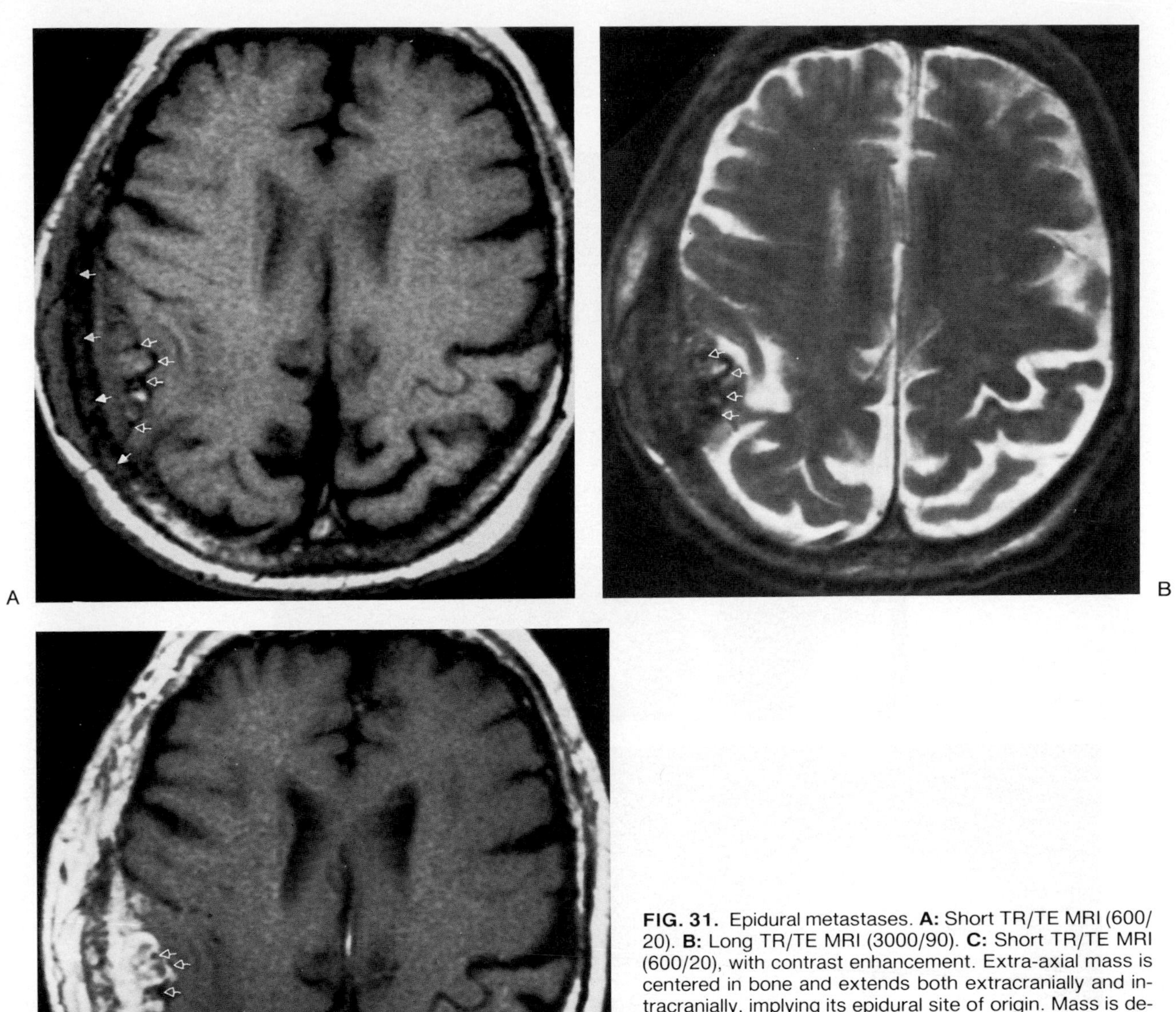

FIG. 31. Epidural metastases. **A:** Short TR/TE MRI (600/20). **B:** Long TR/TE MRI (3000/90). **C:** Short TR/TE MRI (600/20), with contrast enhancement. Extra-axial mass is centered in bone and extends both extracranially and intracranially, implying its epidural site of origin. Mass is delineated by vascular cleft (open arrows, A–C) between lesion and brain. Also note intervening cortex interposed between mass and underlying, high-intensity edematous white matter on long TR/TE image (B), proving extra-axial location. Involvement of diploic fatty marrow is seen as replacement of normal high-intensity on precontrast short TR/TE by low-intensity tumor (closed arrows, A). Note that the distinction between tumor, normal marrow, and subcutaneous fat is obscured after contrast administration.

The intracranial epidural extent of skull metastases and the presence of subdural disease is well documented by both CT and MRI, although subtle dural-based tumor is probably better seen on MRI, since CT scans are often limited by artifacts emanating from bone (e.g., in the regions of the inferior frontal and temporal lobes and at the vertex). The role of the radiologist in these cases is mainly to correctly discern extra-axial disease from superficial cortical, intra-axial lesions. It can also be helpful to distinguish epidural from subdural masses. Both modalities usually demonstrate epidural tumor as the characteristic biconvex mass which displaces brain parenchyma away from the inner table (Fig. 31). Subdural metastatic lesions, in contrast to subdural fluid collections (e.g., hematoma, hygroma), often appear very similar in intensity and shape to epidural metastases. These lesions are solid masses of neoplastic tissue and do not necessarily have the typical crescentic appearance of subdural hematomas, since they do not merely passively fill the potential space of the subdural compartment. The major feature of epidural disease which allows distinction from subdural tumor is the neoplastic involvement of overlying calvarium (Fig. 31), a nearly universal finding in epidural metastases. Recent implementations of

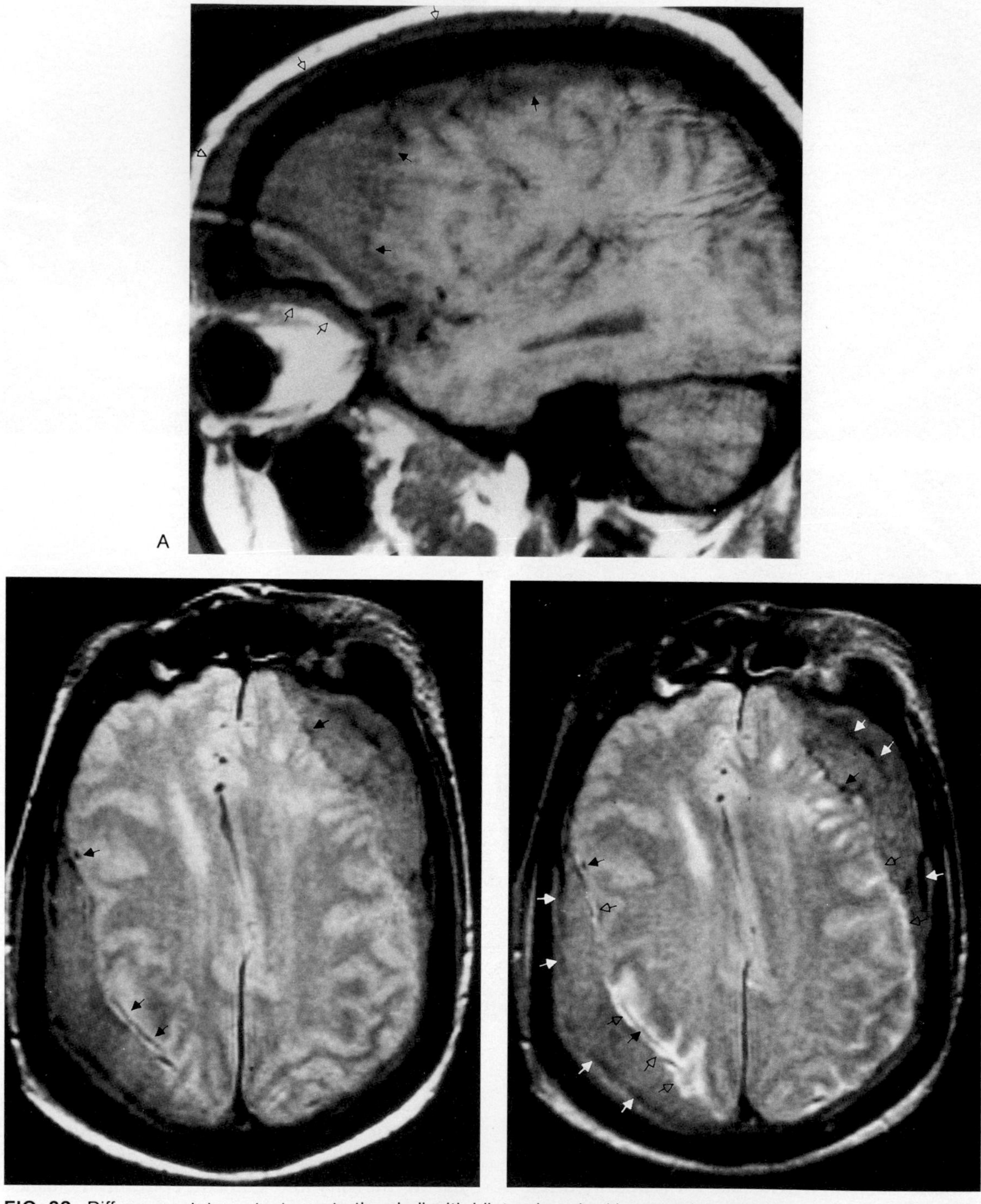

FIG. 32. Diffuse prostate metastases to the skull with bilateral marked intracranial extension. **A:** Sagittal short TR/TE image through left side of brain reveals loss of the normal high signal intensity from the fatty marrow within the diploic space. There is a large frontal slightly hypointense mass that is compressing the underlying brain surface (*solid black arrows*). There are smaller masses in the subgaleal space extracranially and in the roof of the orbit (*open black arrows*). **B,C:** Axial long TR/short TE (B) and long TE (C) images demonstrate large mildly hypointense intracranial masses in the left frontal parietal and right parietal occipital regions. Hypointensities from surface brain vessels (*solid black arrows*) and a CSF cleft (open black arrows, C) separates the tumor from the brain. There is a fragmented linear hypointensity that roughly parallels the inner table of the skull running through the outer portion of both extracerebral masses (*white arrows*). These most likely represent the elevated dura invaded from calvarial tumor. There is hyperintensity of the gyri in the right posterior parietal and left anterior frontal regions that may represent edema from either tumor invasion of the brain or blood flow compromise in the leptomeningeal arteries and veins in these regions by the tumor (*white arrows*).

fast spin-echo MR techniques, unfortunately, results in intradiploic tumor deposits and normal marrow becoming isointense on "T2-weighted" images. Therefore, fat-suppressed postcontrast imaging should be performed in these cases. Subcutaneous (subgaleal) extension of metastatic tumor centered in the skull is easily depicted by both CT and MRI. MRI also allows better definition of the dura itself. Note that displaced gray matter (i.e., cortex) is identifiable between the mass and subcortical white matter (Fig. 31) when an extra-axial lesion is present. MRI is superior at depicting several signs and structures which are not only pathognomonic of extra-axial disease, but also allow specific identification of the involved compartment (Fig. 31): (i) the identification of a CSF or vascular cleft between the lesion and normal brain, (ii) direct visualization of the displaced dura and its relationship to the mass (especially after i.v. contrast), and (iii) the documentation of displaced cortical veins, which lie between the extra-axial lesion and the brain.

Signal intensity patterns on MRI are usually not specific in the evaluation of types of extra-axial tumor, since most metastases are slightly hypointense to cortex on short TR/TE images and are slightly hyperintense on long TR/TE images. This does differ somewhat from the most typical pattern described in meningiomas, which are classically nearly isointense to cortex on all sequences (50). Unfortunately, some metastatic lesions, particularly those of small cell primary neoplasms (Fig. 32), are

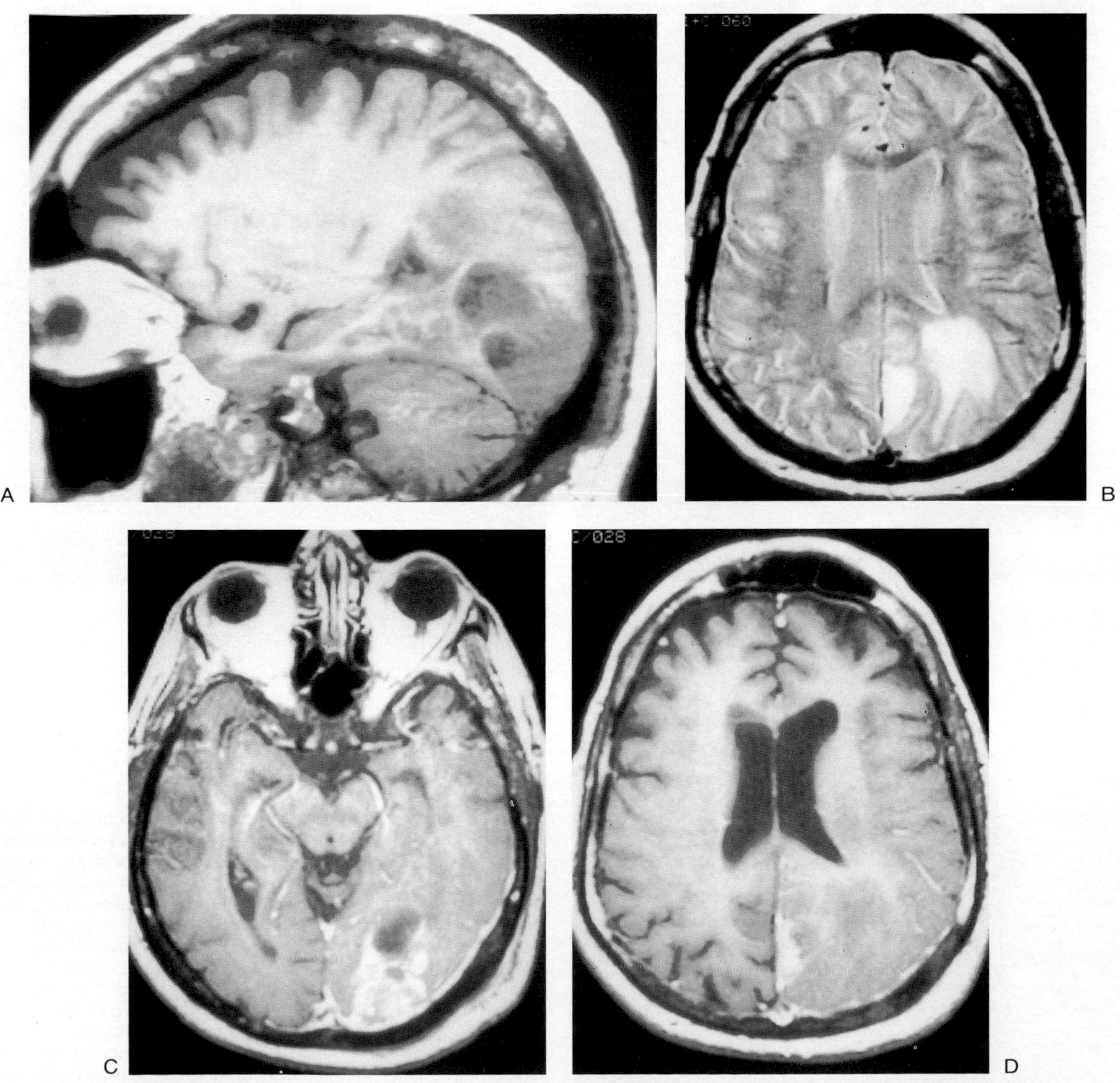

FIG. 33. Intraparenchymal and subdural metastases, prostate carcinoma. Extensive edema and heterogeneous signal on T1-weighted (**A**) and proton-density-weighted (**B**) images is due to subdural metastases with parenchymal invasion, as clarified by i.v. contrast (**C,D**). Parenchymal metastases with secondary involvement of dura cannot be excluded.

isointense to gray matter on MRI. It is not uncommon for subdural metastases to invade brain parenchyma (Fig. 33). Obviously clinical information is the most helpful evidence of metastatic disease. Other non-neoplastic lesions, such as sarcoidosis or empyema, can appear identically to metastases on MR studies. Signal intensity patterns are helpful, however, in separating extra-axial hemorrhage from tumor, since the various stages of extra-axial hemorrhage have relatively specific intensities (51). Intravenous contrast agents might increase the detection of neoplastic causes of extra-axial hemorrhage. Bone invasion would indicate a neoplastic etiology of the mass. It is likely that the sensitivity of MRI increases with the use of contrast agents for small extra-axial metastases, as is the case for other extra-axial lesions.

It is well known that contrast-enhanced CT is relatively insensitive for the detection of leptomeningeal metastatic disease (52,53), especially from leukemia or lymphoma. It has also become apparent that MRI without i.v. contrast is strikingly inadequate for documenting this entity (54). Several reports have shown that i.v. contrast-enhanced MRI, however, is extremely sensitive for the detection of leptomeningeal diseases (55). It appears that leptomeningeal carcinomatosis is most readily detected, short of cytologic examination of CSF, with

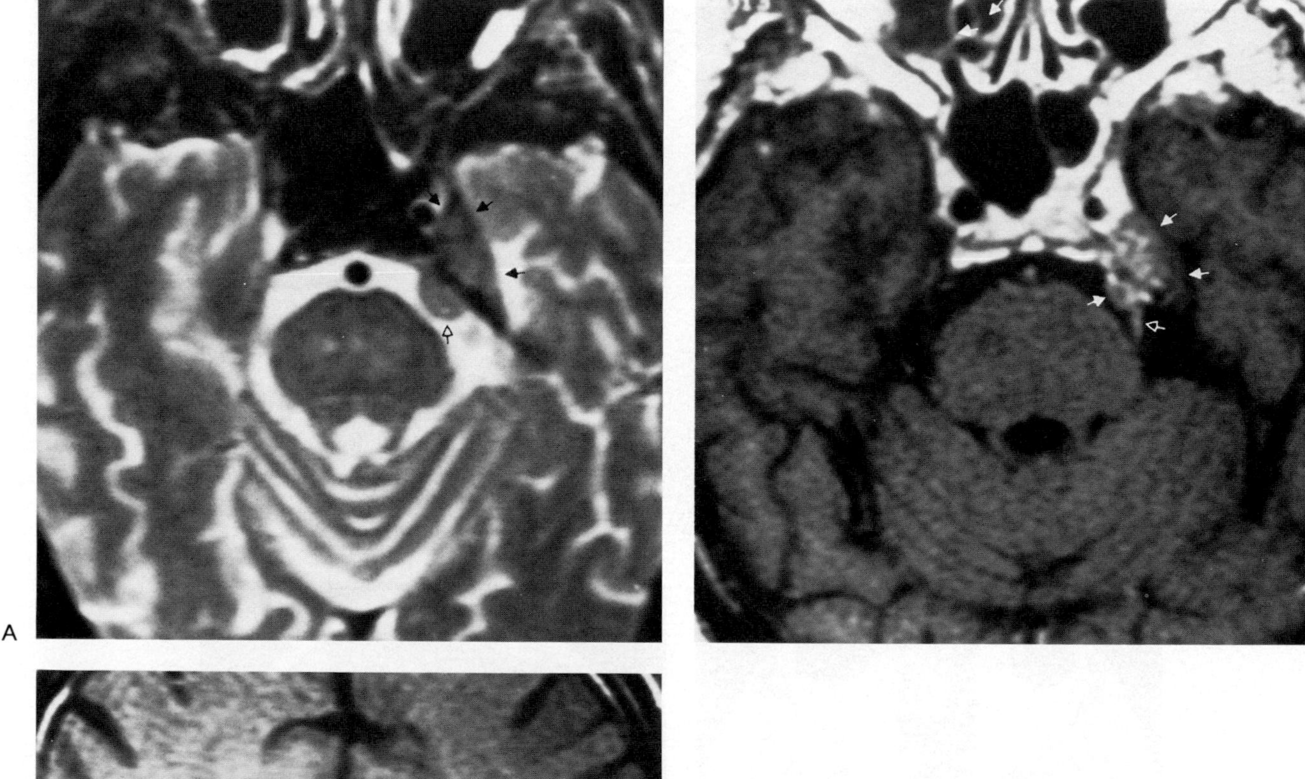

FIG. 34. Arachnoid metastases most likely secondary to seeding from superficial brain metastases in a patient with esophageal carcinoma. **A:** Axial long TR/TE image demonstrates hypointense mass expanding Meckel's cave on the left side (*solid black arrows*) with a small hemisphere-shaped extension of the tumor posteriorly into the pontine cistern (*open black arrow*). **B:** Postgadolinium-enhanced axial short TR/TE scan reveals mild heterogeneous enhancement of the tumor identified in A (*solid white arrows*). In addition, there is enhancement noted along the proximal portion of the left fifth nerve (*open white arrow*). **C:** Postgadolinium coronal short TR/TE image reveals multiple cortical and subcortical enhancing nodules within the cerebellum (*arrows*). One of these lesions could be the source of the arachnoid metastases identified in A and B. Alternatively, these lesions could be the result of secondary brain invasion from hematogenous leptomeningeal metastases. The former is probably more likely.

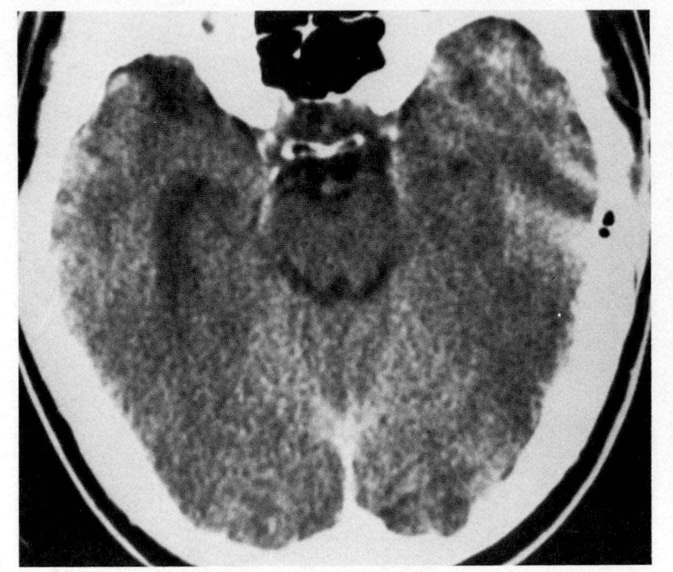
A

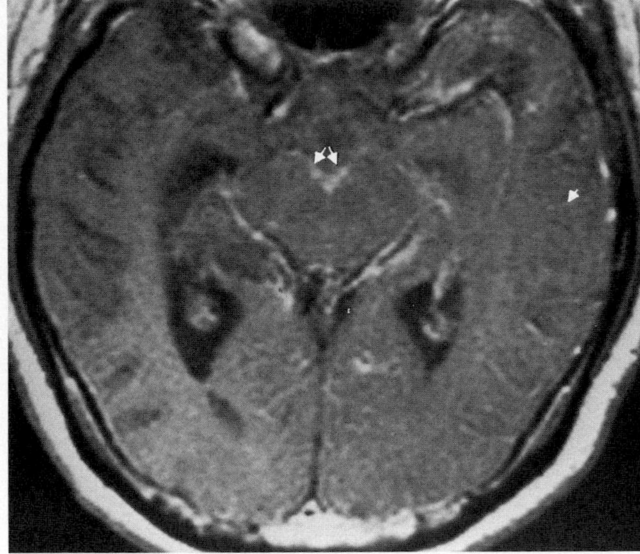
B

FIG. 35. Subarachnoid seeding by tumor (glioblastoma), CT vs. MRI. **A:** CT, with contrast enhancement. **B:** Short TR/TE MRI (600/20), with contrast enhancement. In spite of normal enhanced CT (A), subtle enhancement of interpeduncular fossa is seen on MRI (arrows, B) in patient with proven seeding of glioblastoma.

MRI and i.v. contrast (40,56). On both CT and MRI, this disorder, when demonstrated, is seen as prominent enhancement of the leptomeninges (Figs. 34 and 35) and, at times, ependymal surfaces. Leptomeningeal involvement with tumor (Fig. 36) usually cannot be differentiated from other diffuse meningeal conditions, such as infectious meningitis. Although MR is most certainly the most sensitive imaging method to date, subependymal/ependymal tumor seeding does not necessarily enhance on MRI in all cases, so it can be inferred that subtle cases will be missed. As with CT, even if the MRI demonstrates only hydrocephalus in a patient with a known extracranial malignancy, the diagnosis of leptomeningeal carcinomatosis should be suspected and examination of CSF for cytologic evidence of malignancy should be recommended.

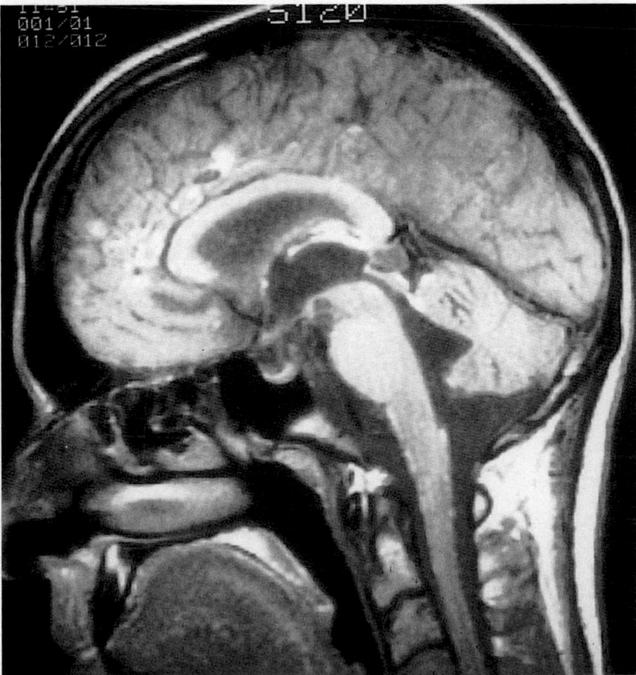

A

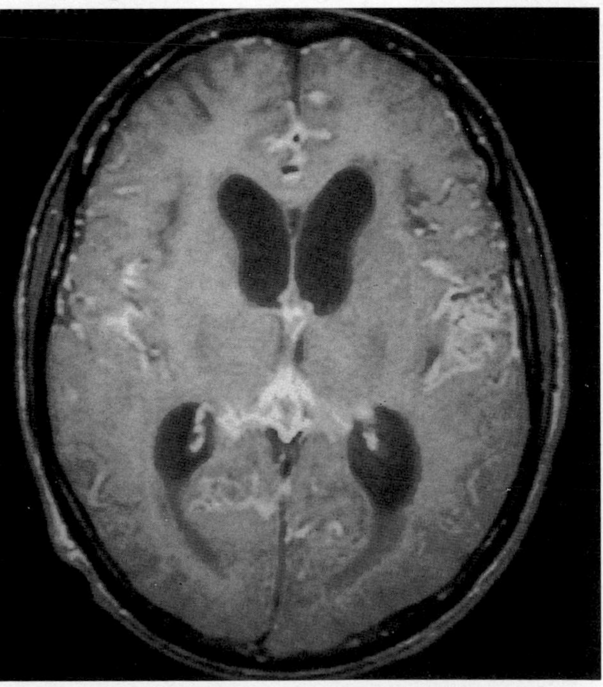
B

FIG. 36. Primary leptomeningeal melanosis. Sagittal precontrast T1-weighted image (**A**) shows subtle hyperintensity along surfaces of lower brainstem and cervical spinal cord, the clue to this rare diagnosis. Note extensive enhancement of leptomeninges after contrast (**B**).

FIG. 37. Clival chordoma. **A:** Sagittal short TR/TE image reveals slightly hypointense large mass destroying the greater part of the clivus and extending markedly both into the nasopharynx anteriorly (*solid black arrows*) and backwards into the posterior fossa, where it is markedly compressing the pons and medulla oblongata (*open black arrows*). A tongue-like extension of tumor extends inferiorly into the upper cervical canal (*solid white arrow*). Curvilinear, rounded, and corkscrew-like hypointensities are extensively present within the mass, most likely representing tumor vascularity (*open white arrows*). **B,C:** Axial long TR/short TE (B) and long TE (C) images demonstrate the mass to be heterogeneously hyperintense (*white arrows*). The rounded and irregular curvilinear vascular hypointensities can be noted again (*open black arrows*). Larger patchy, irregular, less hypointense foci, which are more pronounced on the long TE image (*solid black arrows*, C), suggests regions of histologic variation probably representing more compact cellular tissue. Other considerations might include partially calcified regions or multiple small acute hemorrhages. **D:** Histologic section of a clivus chordoma showing cells arranged in "chords" or bands within a fibro-myxoid matrix. **E:** Higher magnification of chordoma cells exhibiting resemblance to the physaliphorous notochord origin with small hyperchromatic nuclei, and eosinophilic vacuolated cytoplasm.

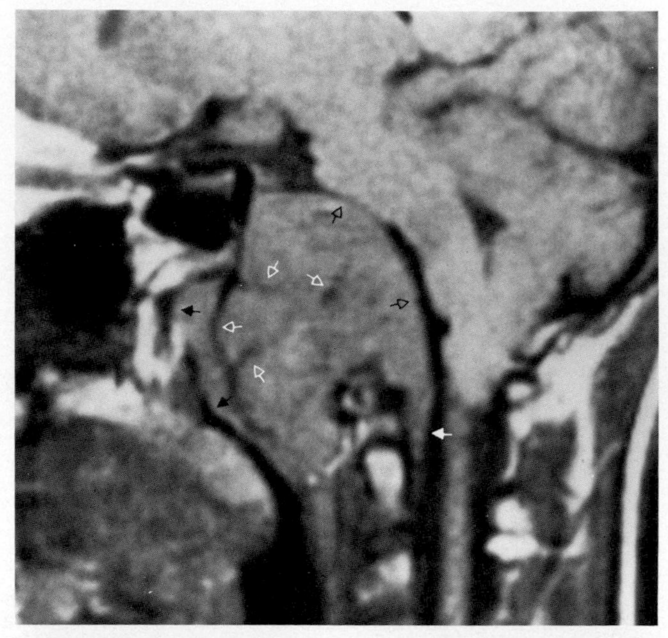
A

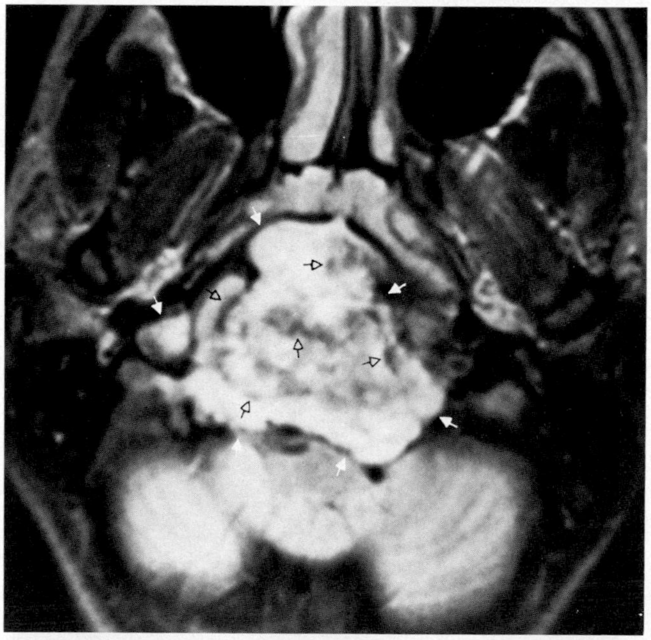

B

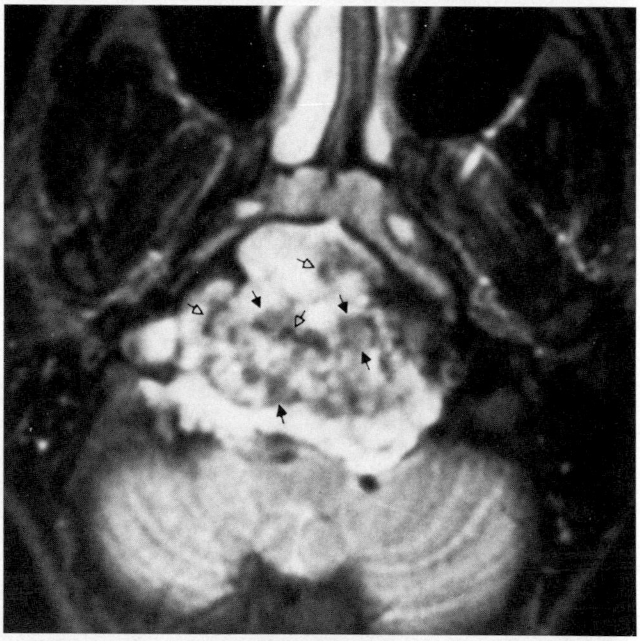

C

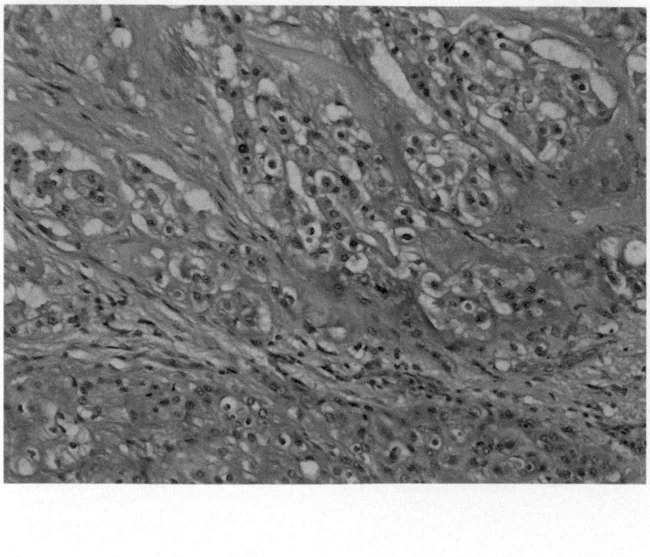

D

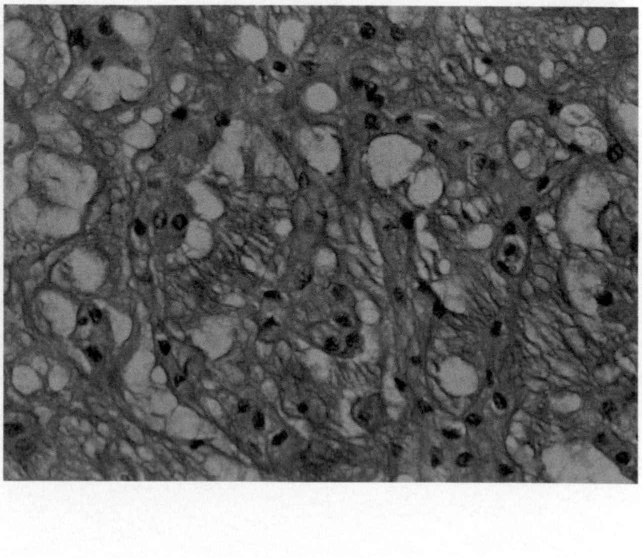

E

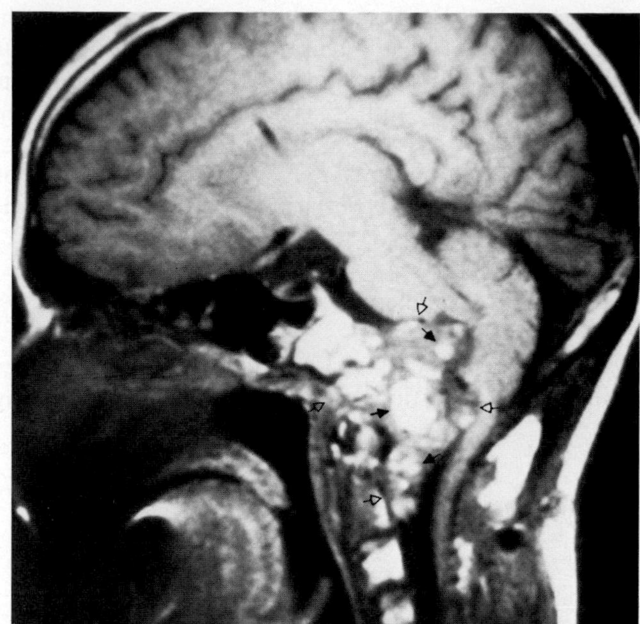

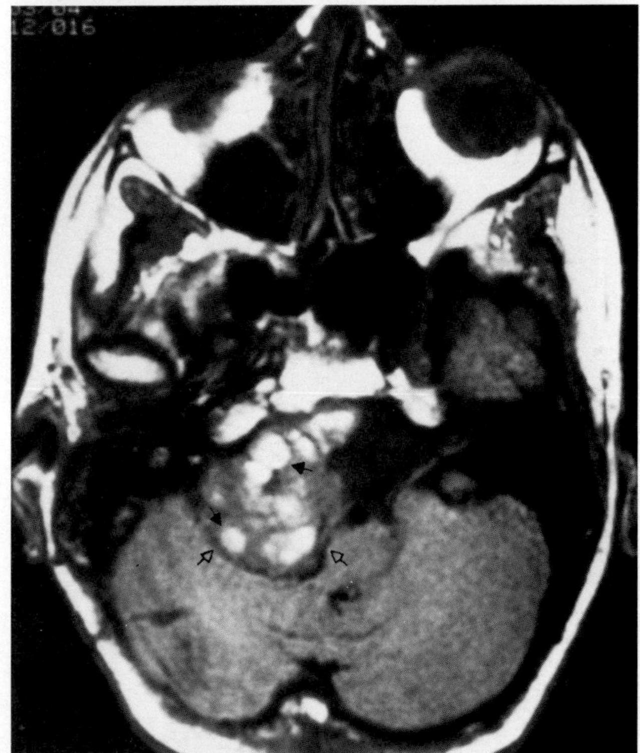

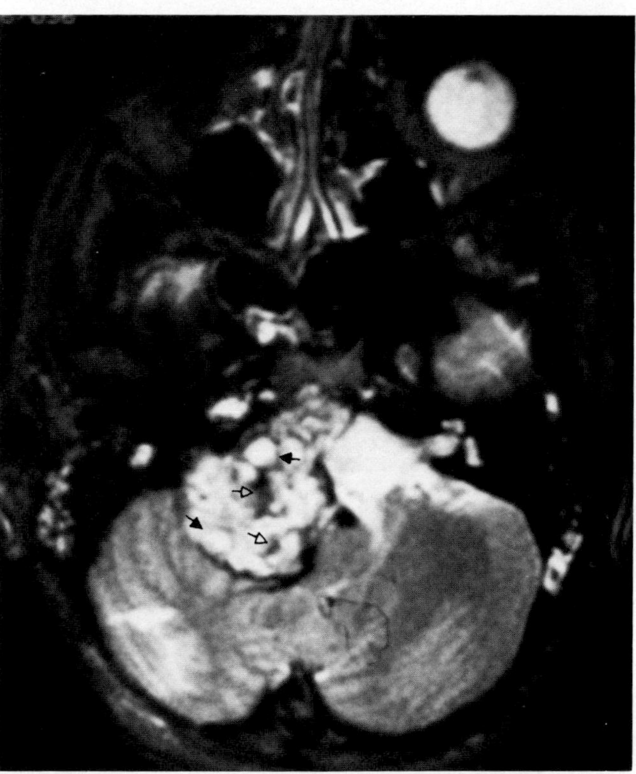

FIG. 38. Hemorrhagic clival chordoma. **A,B:** Short TR/TE sagittal (A) and axial (B) images demonstrate extensive destruction of the lower half of the clivus by a large tumor that extends into the posterior fossa and upper cervical canal (*open black arrows*). There is marked compression of the medulla oblongata and upper cervical cord. Multiple, various-sized, rounded, and lobular well-defined foci of marked hyperintensity are evident (*black arrows*). **C:** Axial long TR/TE image at a level close to that of B. The focal rounded and lobular areas of hyperintensity in B remain hyperintense in C (*solid black arrows*), strongly suggesting the presence of subacute hemorrhage. Isointense regions of the tumor in B become markedly hyperintense in C. Some small, rounded, and linear hypointensities in B remain similar in C (*open black arrows*), suggesting either tumor vascularity or areas of calcification.

BONE TUMORS

Chordomas

Chordomas are tumors of notochordal tissue remnants that most frequently affect the sacrum but not uncommonly involve the clivus. Intracranial chordomas usually become bulky masses that spread through the dura into the middle or posterior cranial fossae compressing the brain, brainstem, and cerebellum. They are very prone to invade anteriorly into the nasopharyngeal region. Besides invading the dura they may extend into the subarachnoid space but rarely invade the brain directly. Brain involvement may be the result of myelomalacia as a result of compression of cerebral tissue or from entrapment and occlusion of leptomeningeal and dural arteries and veins. The peak age at which clival chordomas appear is between 20 and 40 years of age, with a male predominance of 2:1. These tumors are usually highly vascular and frequently develop focal calcifications. On MRI, sagittal short TR/TE images demonstrate the tumor best. It is manifested by a moderately hypointense lesion that replaces the hyperintense clival fatty marrow. On long TR/TE images, it is usually hyperintense, with considerable heterogeneity (Fig. 37). The inhomogeneous intensity pattern may be related to focal areas of calcification, tumor vascularity, variations in cellular histology (Fig. 37), and a tumoral hemorrhage (Fig. 38). Occasionally, chordomas can be completely homogeneous on MRI. These lesions typically still enhance with i.v. contrast; rarely enhancement is not seen (Fig. 39). The diagnosis in these cases hinges upon the identification of relationship to the clivus, usually with bone changes, but the differential diagnosis should include epidermoid tumor as well. CT should be performed in these cases to detect subtle calcifications.

Other clival tumors may mimic chordomas on MRI. These include primarily metastatic disease and chondrosarcomas.

Eosinophilic Granuloma

This disease is part of a wide spectrum of pathologically similar conditions ranging from a diffuse malignant

FIG. 39. Homogeneous nonenhancing chordoma on MRI. Irregular mass in prepontine cistern on all sagittal (**A**) and axial images (**B,C**) extends into right cavernous sinus and partially destroys clivus and dorsum sella. No enhancement is seen in **D**. Similar signal intensities and lobulation can be seen with epidermoid tumor.

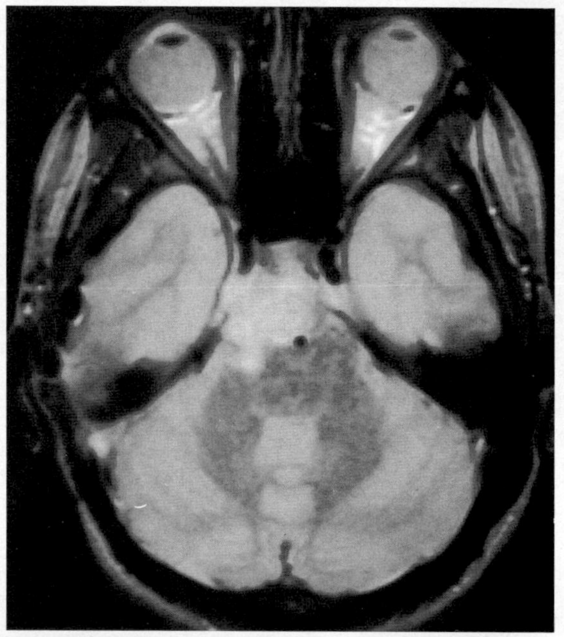

B

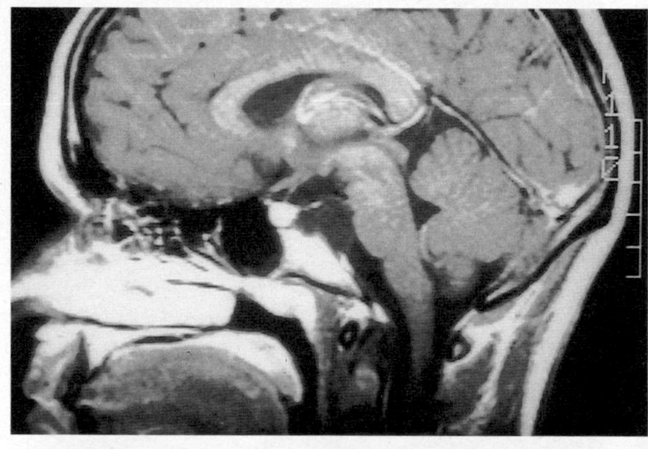

A

C

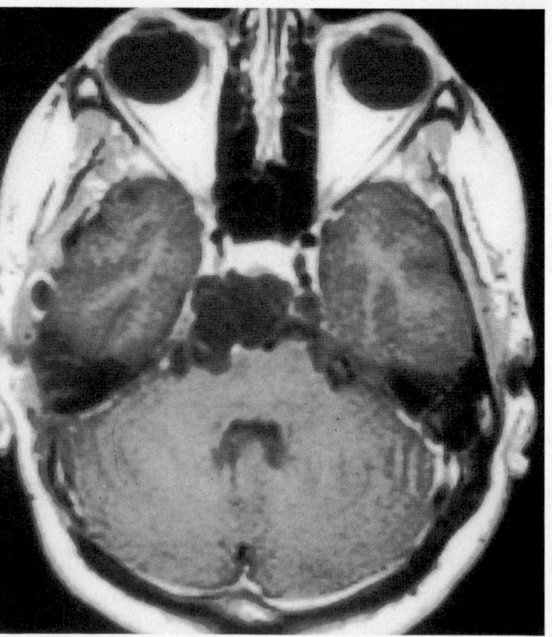

D

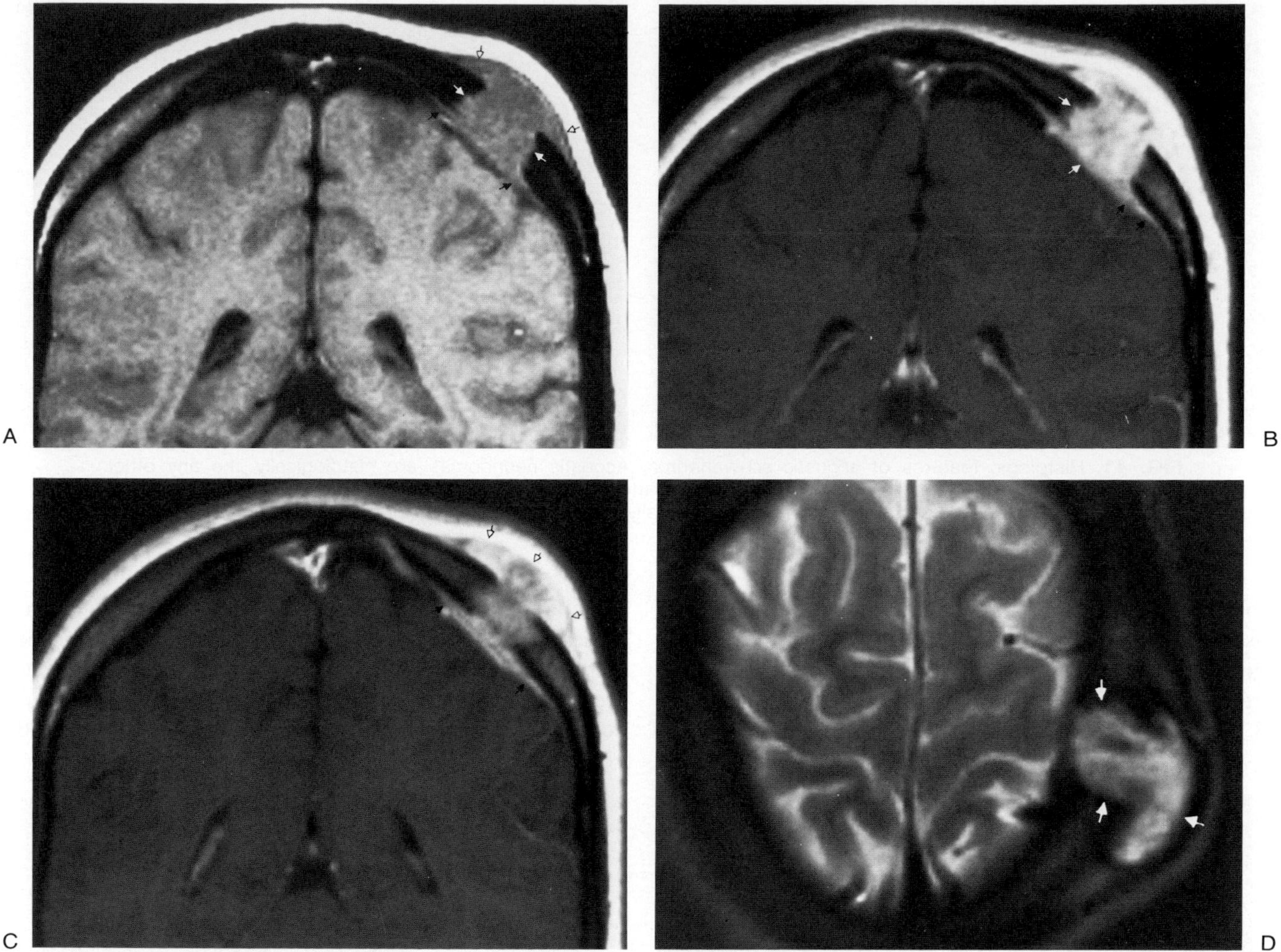

FIG. 40. Eosinophilic granuloma of the skull. **A–C:** Coronal short TR/TE pregadolinium (A) and postgadolinium (B,C) images demonstrate a slightly hypointense inhomogeneous calvarial soft tissue mass (*white arrows*) that is completely destroying all three tables (loss of signal void from bone) and not causing secondary reactive bony thickening. The mass extends peripherally from the region of its penetration onto the dura (*black arrows*). A larger soft tissue component is present subgaleally that has a collar-button-like appearance (*open black arrows*). **D:** Axial long TR/TE image demonstrates mild inhomogeneous hyperintensity of the lesion (*arrows*). (Courtesy of Dr. David S. Titelbaum.)

systemic form affecting primarily children (Letterer-Siwe disease) to the benign eosinophilic granuloma of adults. The disease may affect the brain or the skull. With skull involvement there may be epidural and epicranial extension. MRI will demonstrate a destructive lesion of the bone with soft tissue tumor in the epidural and subgaleal spaces. The lesion may be seen as a hypointense mass on short TR/TE images and a hyperintense lesion on long TR/TE sequences (Fig. 40). The specific diagnosis rests upon clinical and pathologic findings.

NERVE SHEATH TUMORS

Acoustic Schwannoma

Acoustic schwannomas constitute approximately 7% to 8% of all primary intracranial neoplasms. They most frequently arise from the vestibular portion of the eighth cranial nerve. They are frequently seen in association with neurofibromatosis type II disease, in which they are typically bilateral. The tumors will generally involve the intracanalicular portion of the nerve and in most instances also demonstrate a mass in the cerebellopontine angle.

Histologically, acoustic schwannomas are circumscribed encapsulated tumors that may be lobulated but are frequently ovoid or tubular in shape. Histologically, many of the lesions are composed of two distinct types of tissue (Fig. 41) (57). Antoni type A tissue has a compact texture composed of interwoven bundles of bipolar spindle cells. There are numerous fine fibers within the stroma paralleling the axis of the cells. Mature collagen fibers may be present. The cellular elements may be arranged in bundles and whorls, which can vary in size and

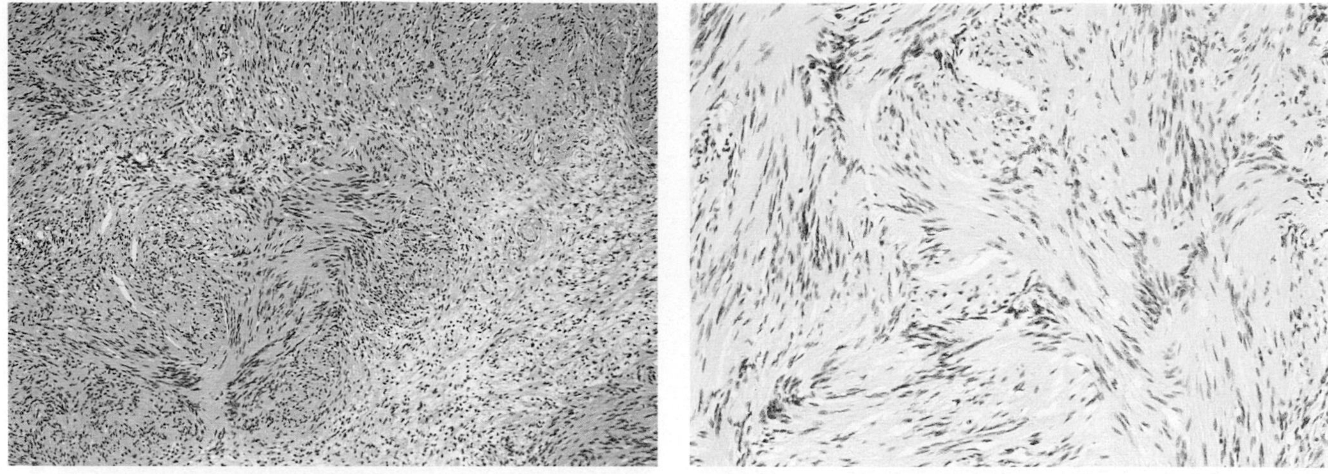

FIG. 41. Histologic features of acoustic schwannoma. Acoustic neurinomas are histologically like any other schwannoma of the peripheral nerves. Note a biphasic pattern of growth with "Antoni A" dense areas and "Antoni B" loose areas (**A**). The cells are spindly and occasionally are lined around a nuclear-free area, called "Verocay body" (**B**).

compactness. Antoni type B is intermingled with type A tissue and is usually well demarcated from it. Type B tissue has a loose texture containing tumor cells. There is frequently mucinous and microcystic change in the type B tissue. Large cysts may develop from confluence of smaller cystic areas. Other histologic variants may occur. These consist of extensive fibroblastic change in the stroma with dense hyalinized collagen bands as well as regions of focal calcification and fatty xanthomatous change. There is often prominent tumor vascularity, and

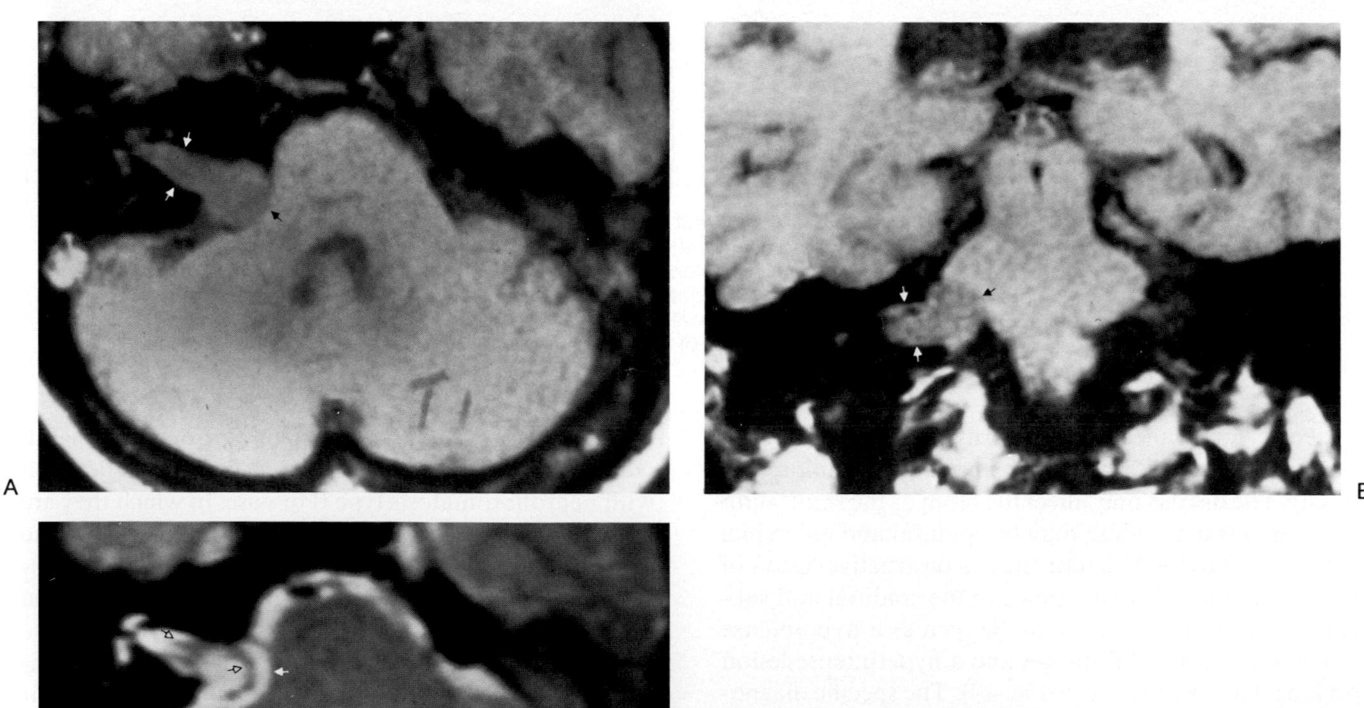

FIG. 42. Cerebellopontine angle and intracanalicular acoustic schwannoma. **A,B:** Short TR/TE axial (A) and coronal (B) images at the level of the internal auditory canals reveal a slightly hypointense soft tissue mass expanding the right internal auditory canal (*white arrows*) and extending into the cerebellopontine angle cistern, where it mildly compresses the posterior lateral aspect of the pons (*black arrow*). **C:** Axial long TR/TE image at same level as A reveals inhomogeneous hyperintensity of the tumor. Within a high-intensity tumor background there are linear and curvilinear bands of slight hypointensity (*open black arrows*). The outer rim of tumor has a hyperintensity similar to that of CSF, from which it is not significantly demarcated (*solid white arrows*).

blood vessels may show regions of focal sinusoidal dilatation or telangiectatic changes. Intratumoral thrombosis of vessels may occur as well as areas of focal hemorrhage.

On MRI, thin-section (3 mm) axial short TR/TE images will reveal most tumors, which are generally larger than 3 mm in size (58,59). The tumors are usually well demarcated from adjacent CSF on these images and reveal mild hypointensity (Fig. 42). On long TR images the tumors are usually heterogeneously hyperintense (59) and are better defined on the short echo. On the long-echo image the hyperintensity of the CSF may obscure the lesion because of similarities in intensity (Fig. 42). The heterogeneous pattern is more frequently appreciated on long TR images but may also be present on short TR images. The heterogeneous pattern on the short TR sequence may consist of patchy, ill-defined regions of mild hypo- and isointensity (Fig. 43) probably represent-

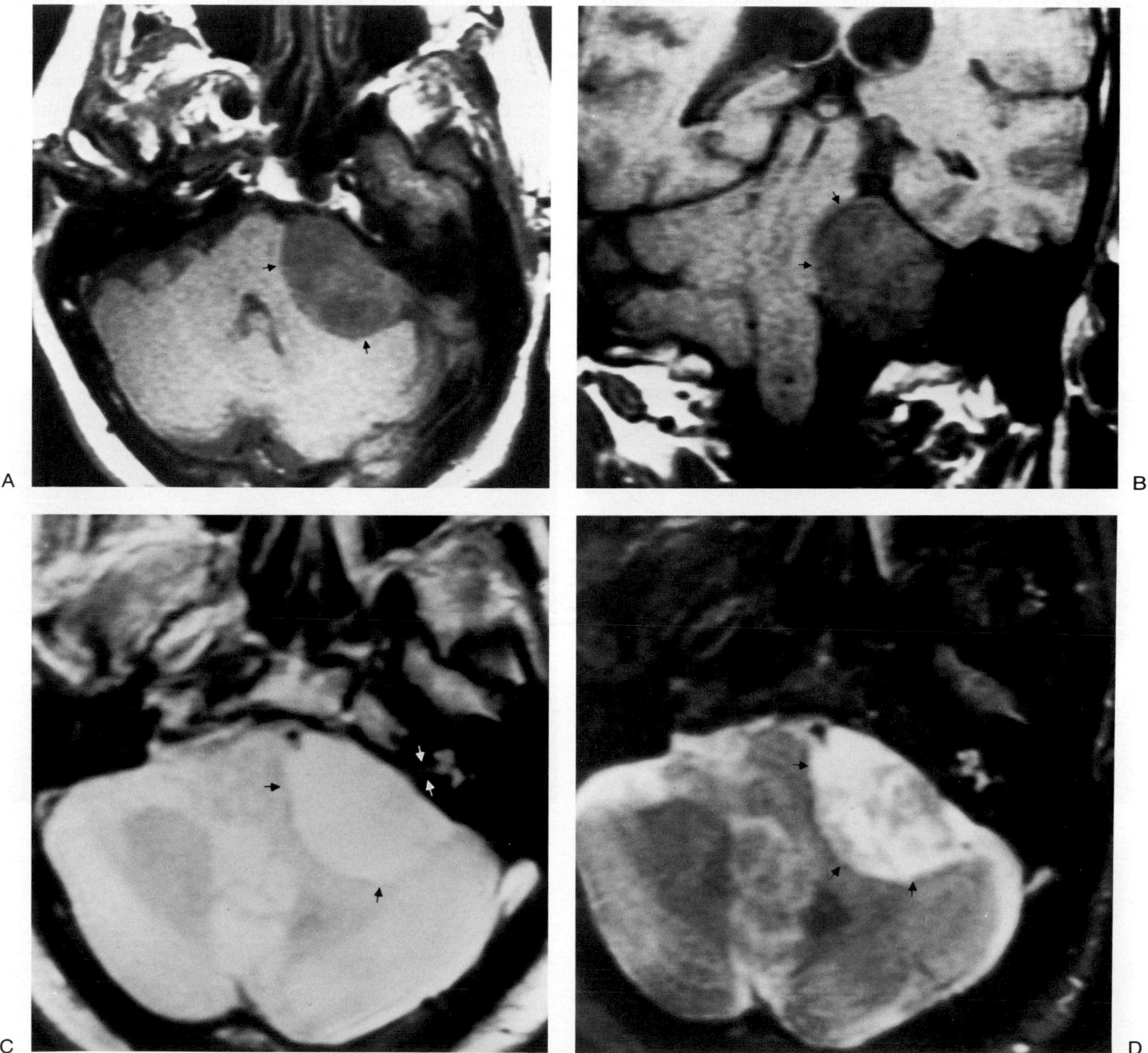

FIG. 43. Large heterogeneous left cerebellopontine angle acoustic schwannoma with no intracanalicular extension. **A,B:** Short TR/TE axial (A) and coronal (B) images demonstrate a large heterogeneously hypointense mass in the left cerebellopontine angle that is markedly compressing the pons and anterior lateral aspect of the cerebellum (*black arrows*). The tumor is broad-based against the posterior surface of the petrous ridge and does not extend into the internal auditory canal. Its internal architecture consists of large, patchy mildly hypointense and isointense regions. **C,D:** Axial long TR/short TE (C) and long TE (D) images demonstrate the broad base of the large hyperintense mass (*black arrows*) on the posterior petrous surface and no tumor extension into the internal auditory canal, which is of normal size (*white arrows*). The mass is heterogeneously hyperintense, seen best at window settings in D consisting of patchy isointense regions (which were also the isointense regions in A and B) within a diffuse background of tumor hyperintensity.

ing areas of different cellular histology (Antoni type A and type B tissue), well-defined oval regions of hypointensity similar to that of CSF, which probably represent cystic change (Fig. 44), and well-defined small oval and curvilinear regions most likely representing conspicuous tumor vascularity (Fig. 45). On long TR images the hyperintensity of the tumor background may contain linear and curvilinear bands of mild hypointensity as well as larger areas of iso- and hyperintensity representing the MRI appearance of Antoni A and B tissue regions (Figs. 42 and 43). The cystic change will demonstrate well-demarcated focal areas of hyperintensity that may be very similar to that of the adjacent CSF (Fig. 44). Tumors with marked vascularity or focal nodular calcifications will reveal similar hypointensity on both long TR and short TR series (Fig. 45). It should be noted that significant heterogeneity with cystic and/or hemorrhagic regions on MRI is more typical of acoustic schwannoma than meningioma.

These tumors can usually be demonstrated within the internal auditory canal without the use of contrast enhancement in most instances (59,60). A soft tissue density obscuring the individual seventh and eighth nerves should be observed in lesions that are 5 mm or greater in size. Contrast enhancement will demonstrate smaller intracanalicular tumors that may not be otherwise fully defined even on high-resolution routine series (Figs. 46 and 47). The widening of the internal auditory canal will usually be appreciated best on axial images, which will demonstrate the entire length of the canal on a single slice, in contrast to the coronal image (Fig. 42), which will generally not reveal the entire length of the canal on a single section (59). Also erosion of the posterior wall of the canal will be best appreciated in the axial view on the short TR sequence. Contrast enhancement may show extension of cisternal tumor into the canal in the absence of canal expansion (Fig. 46). The contrast enhancement of the tumor may be homogeneous (Fig. 46) but is fre-

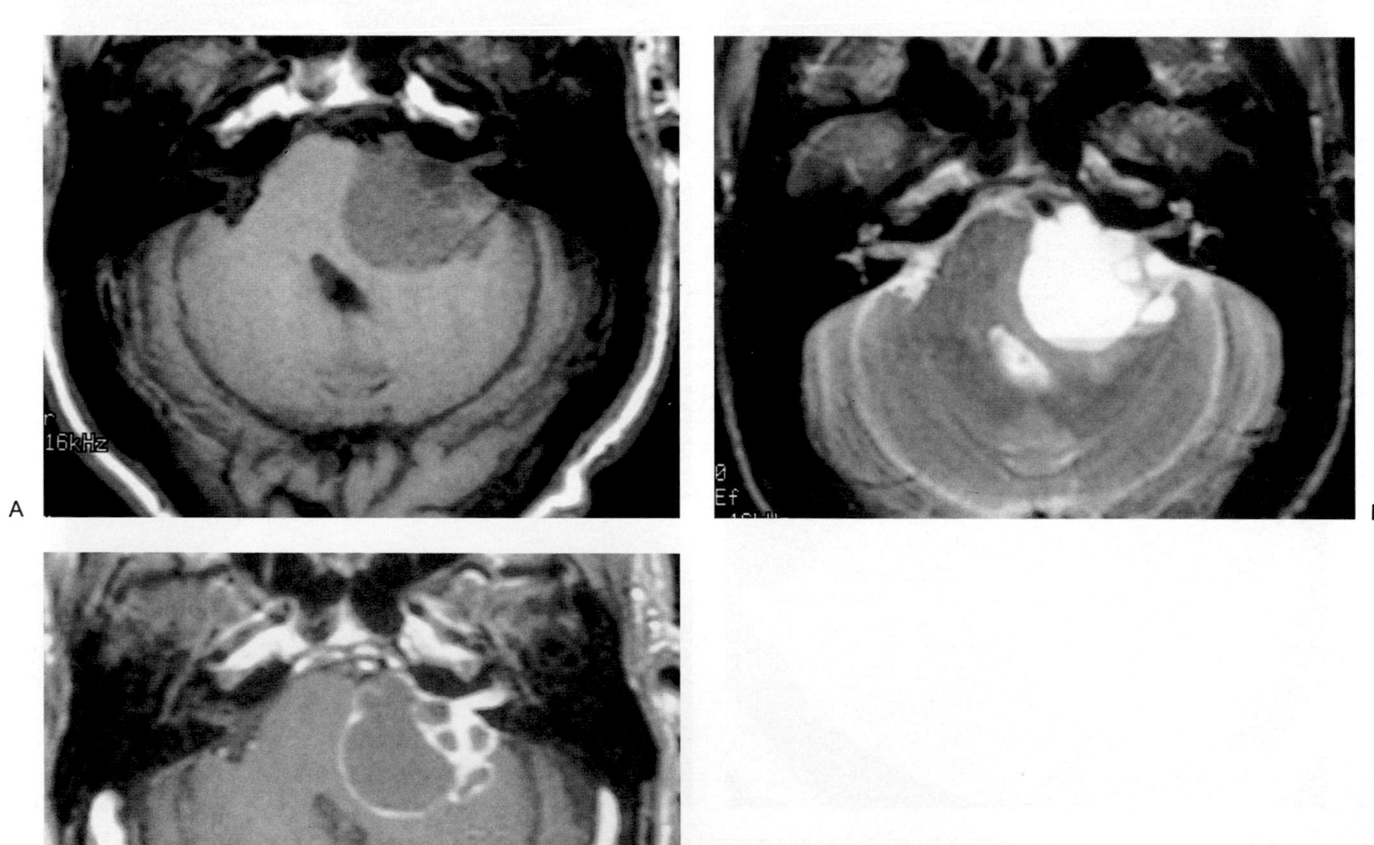

FIG. 44. Acoustic schwannoma with cystic changes. Unenhanced T1-weighted and T2-weighted images **(A,B)** reveals large cerebellopontine angle mass with associated cysts. After contrast **(C)**, the vast majority of the mass that extends far into the internal auditory canal is noted to be cystic.

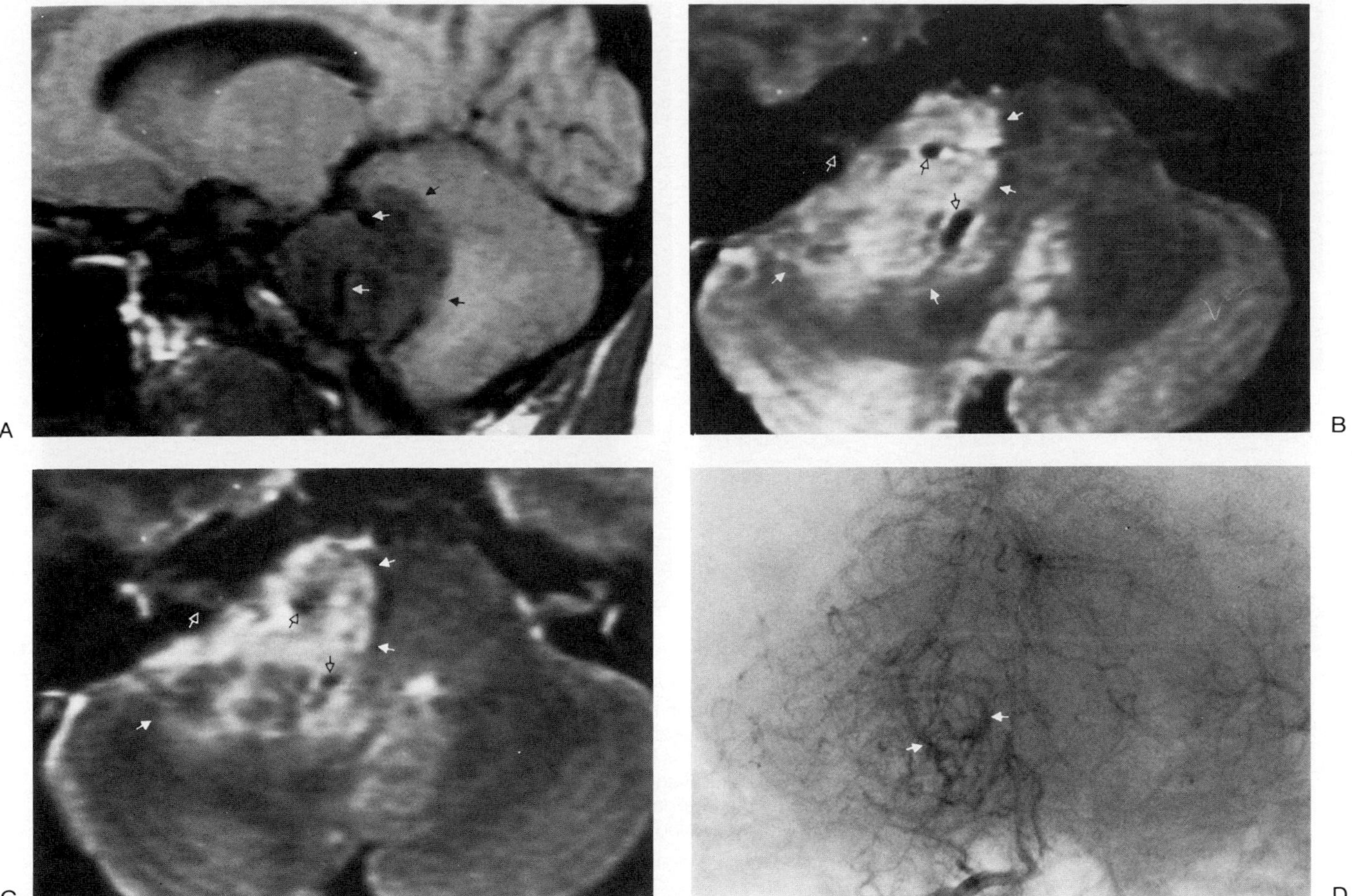

FIG. 45. Vascular acoustic schwannoma. **A:** Sagittal short TR/TE image through right side of cerebellum demonstrates a large heterogeneously hypointense mass anteriorly in the posterior fossa (*black arrows*). The mass consists of ill-defined patchy and nodular regions of moderate hypointensity and well-defined oval and curvilinear tubular-like structures of marked hypointensity (*white arrows*). These latter hypointense regions represent vascular channels within the tumor. **B,C:** Axial long TR/short TE (B) and long TE (C) images at the level of the internal auditory canals. Hyperintense mass with marked heterogeneity (*white arrows*) is present behind the right petrous ridge. The mass does not involve the right internal auditory canal (*open white arrow*). The mass is poorly separated from the cerebellum. Within the mass there are several well-defined rounded regions of marked hypointensity, similar in both images (*open black arrows*), which represent the large tumor blood vessels. **D:** Frontal projection, right vertebral arteriogram, late capillary–early venous phase, reveals vascular tumor stain behind the right petrous bone consisting of many small blood vessels and dilated irregular veins (*white arrows*). These vessels correspond to the well-defined regions of marked hypointensity in A–C.

quently inhomogeneous, presenting a pattern similar to what may be evident on long TR images (Fig. 48).

In the acoustic schwannoma there is usually an intracanalicular portion of the tumor associated with a cisternal mass. About 20% of acoustic schwannomas, however, have no intracanalicular component or only a very small knuckle of tumor extending into the canal (Fig. 43). These tumors are usually oval to hemispheric in shape and may present as a broad-based mass against the petrous ridge. Lesions with this configuration and without intracanalicular extension cannot usually be differentiated from meningiomas in the cerebellopontine angle. Their tissue intensity also will be quite similar to their anatomic configuration. A vascular rim and/or a CSF cleft can usually be identified between the tumor and the adjacent pontocerebellar tissue. There is frequent compression of the posterior lateral aspect of the pons and middle cerebellar peduncle by tumor masses that are 1 cm or greater in diameter.

Trigeminal Nerve Schwannoma

Schwannomas may occur on other cranial nerves, with those on the trigeminal nerve next in frequency to eighth nerve tumors. The tumors of the fifth cranial

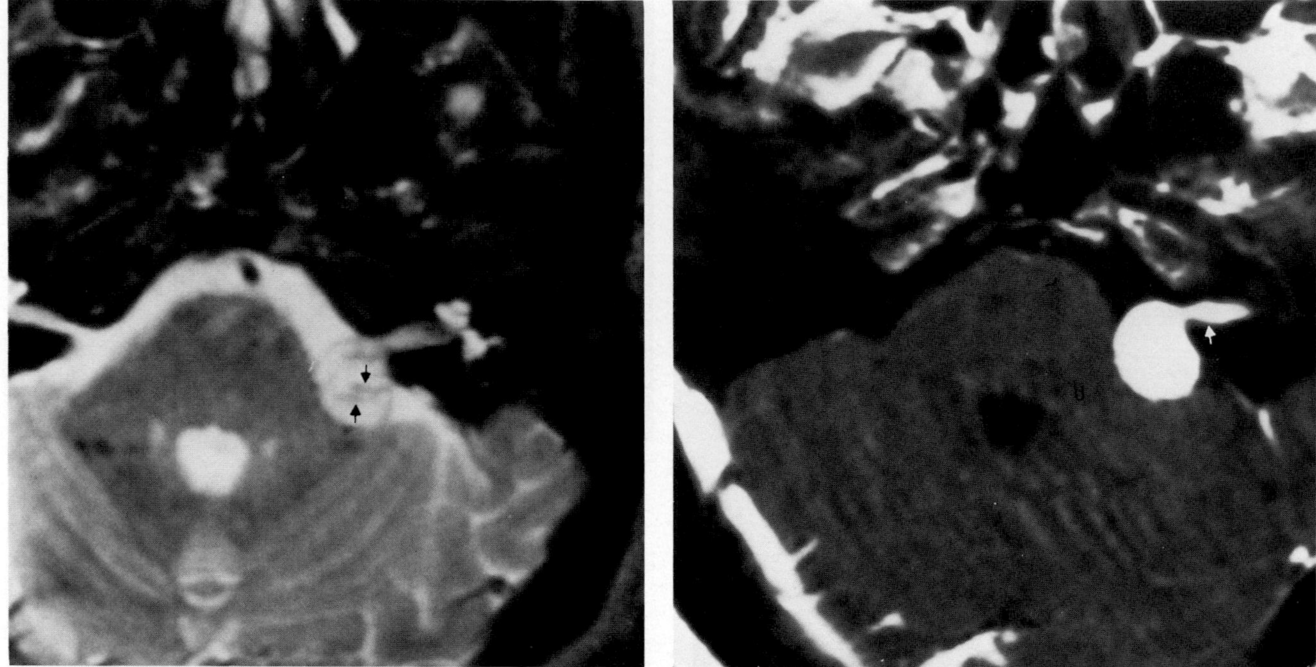

FIG. 46. Left acoustic schwannoma with gadolinium enhancement. **A:** Axial long TR/TE image at level of internal auditory canal reveals a 1-cm diameter hyperintense mass in the left cerebellopontine angle cistern containing several incomplete horizontal isointense bands (*black arrows*). The anterior medial and posterior lateral margins of the tumor are demarcated from the CSF by curvilinear isointense bands also. There is minimal asymmetry of the internal auditory canals, with the left side being slightly larger, but tumor tissue within the canal cannot be definitely defined. **B:** Postgadolinium axial short TR/TE image at the level of the internal auditory canal demonstrates uniform enhancement of the cisternal tumor with a band of enhancing tumor extending to the lateral aspect of the internal auditory canal (*white arrow*).

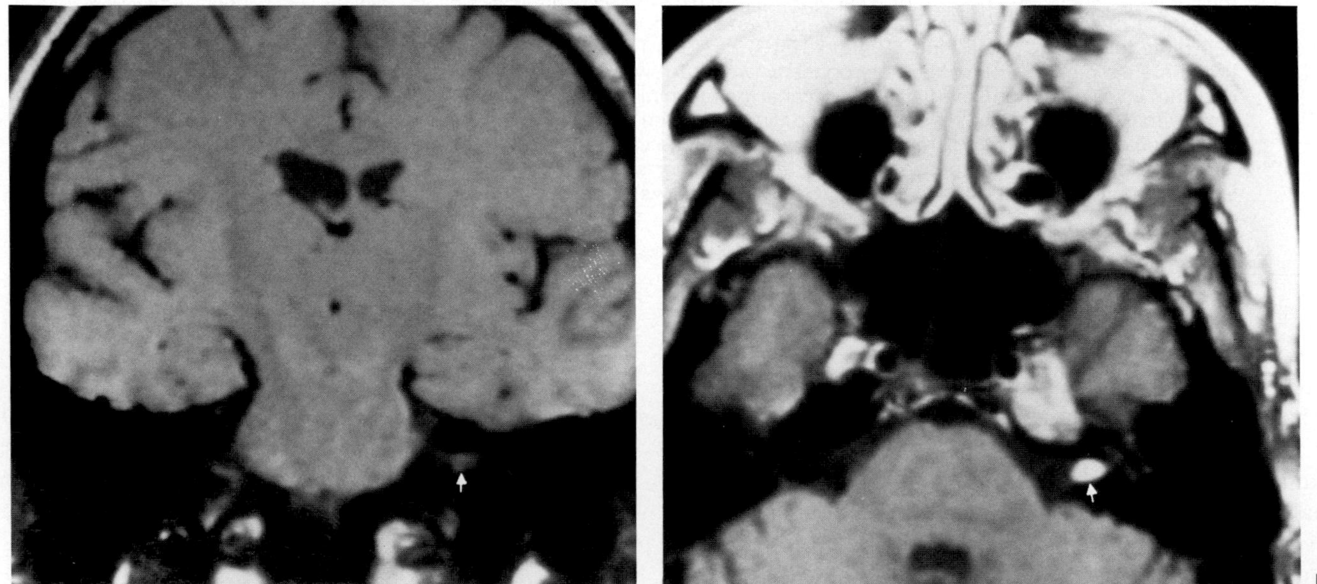

FIG. 47. Intracanalicular acoustic schwannoma. **A:** Coronal short TR/TE image through level of left internal auditory canal demonstrates minimal isointense tissue within medial aspect of left internal auditory canal (*white arrow*). Left internal auditory canal is not enlarged in this projection. **B:** Postgadolinium axial short TR/TE image through level of internal auditory canals demonstrates oval enhancing mass within left internal auditory canal that is mildly expanded in this projection (*white arrow*).

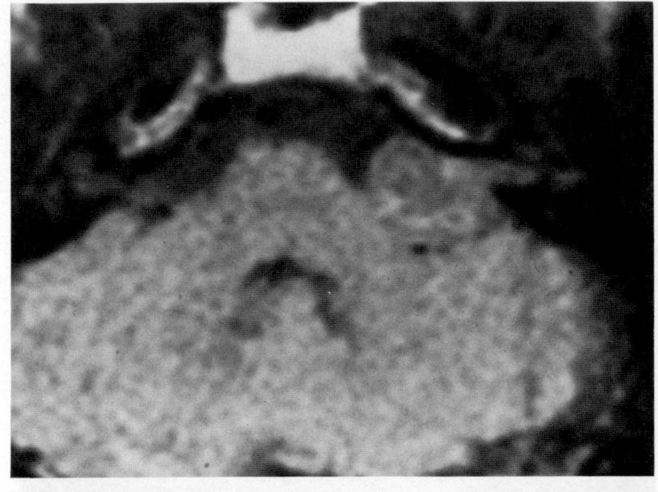

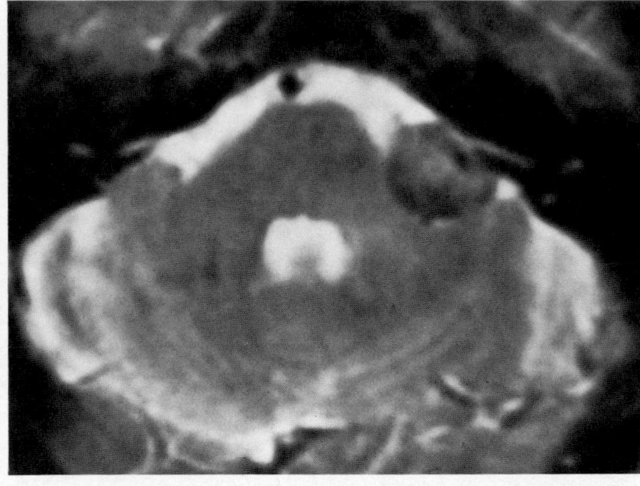

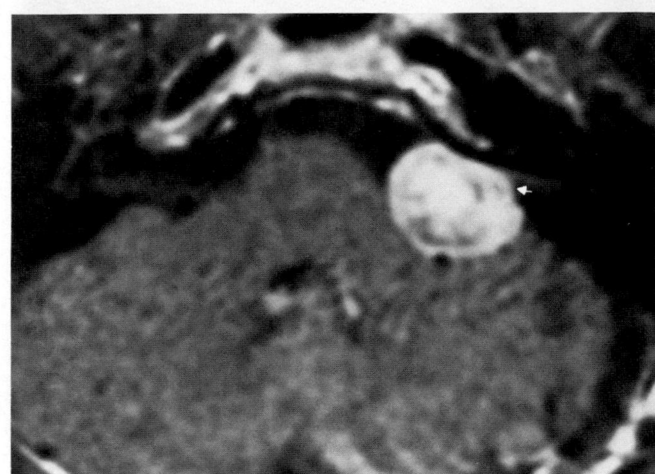

FIG. 48. Left acoustic schwannoma with heterogeneous intensity pattern and heterogeneous gadolinium enhancement. **A:** Axial short TR/TE image at level of internal auditory canal shows moderate-sized left cerebellopontine angle cistern mass with heterogeneous intensity pattern. The central region of the tumor shows an irregular-shaped large region of mild hypointensity surrounded by a nodular band of isointense tumor tissue. Inferiorly in the tumor peripheral to the zone of isointensity, there is a thin layer of tumor tissue that is mildly hypointense. **B:** Axial long TR/TE image at a level slightly superior to A. The tumor tissue shows approximately reversed intensities to that in A. The tissue in A that was slightly hypointense is mildly hyperintense in B, and the tissue that was isointense in A is hypointense in B. **C:** Postgadolinium axial short TR/TE image at a level almost identical to that of A. There is heterogeneous enhancement of the tumor with the nonenhancing portion located in the region of the isointense tissue in A and hypointense tissue in B. The internal auditory canal is not enlarged, and only a small knuckle of tumor extends into its medial aspect (*white arrow*).

nerve will be seen along the course of the nerve, involving its pontine cisternal segment and/or its extension into Meckel's cave at the petrous apex and the cavernous sinus (Fig. 49). Schwannomas of the fifth nerve will demonstrate intensity characteristics similar to those of acoustic schwannomas. The key to this diagnosis is the neuroanatomic localization of the fifth nerve pathway, often best appreciated on coronal images.

EXOPHYTIC BRAIN TUMORS IN THE CEREBELLOPONTINE ANGLE CISTERN

Ependymomas of the fourth ventricle and its lateral recess not infrequently extend into the cerebellopontine angle as an exophytic mass. These tumors will demonstrate mild hypointensity on short TR images and may have a very irregular lobulated surface. They not infrequently will encase the basilar and vertebral arteries (Fig. 50). A mass within the fourth ventricle may occasionally be demonstrated, although at times it is minimal in size. The lesion may arise in the lateral recess of the fourth ventricle and not be defined as arising from the ventricular surface. On the long TR series invasion of the tumor into the subependymal area or into the pontomedullary and cerebellar parenchyma may be demonstrated (Fig. 50) in a portion of these exophytic masses. They otherwise strongly mimic the appearance of an acoustic schwannoma, which is only located in the cerebellopontine angle cistern and does not extend into the internal auditory canal. Ependymomas have no specific intensity pattern on MRI, but they very commonly show marked heterogeneity, intratumoral hemorrhage and necrosis, and irregular contrast enhancement (see Chapter 10).

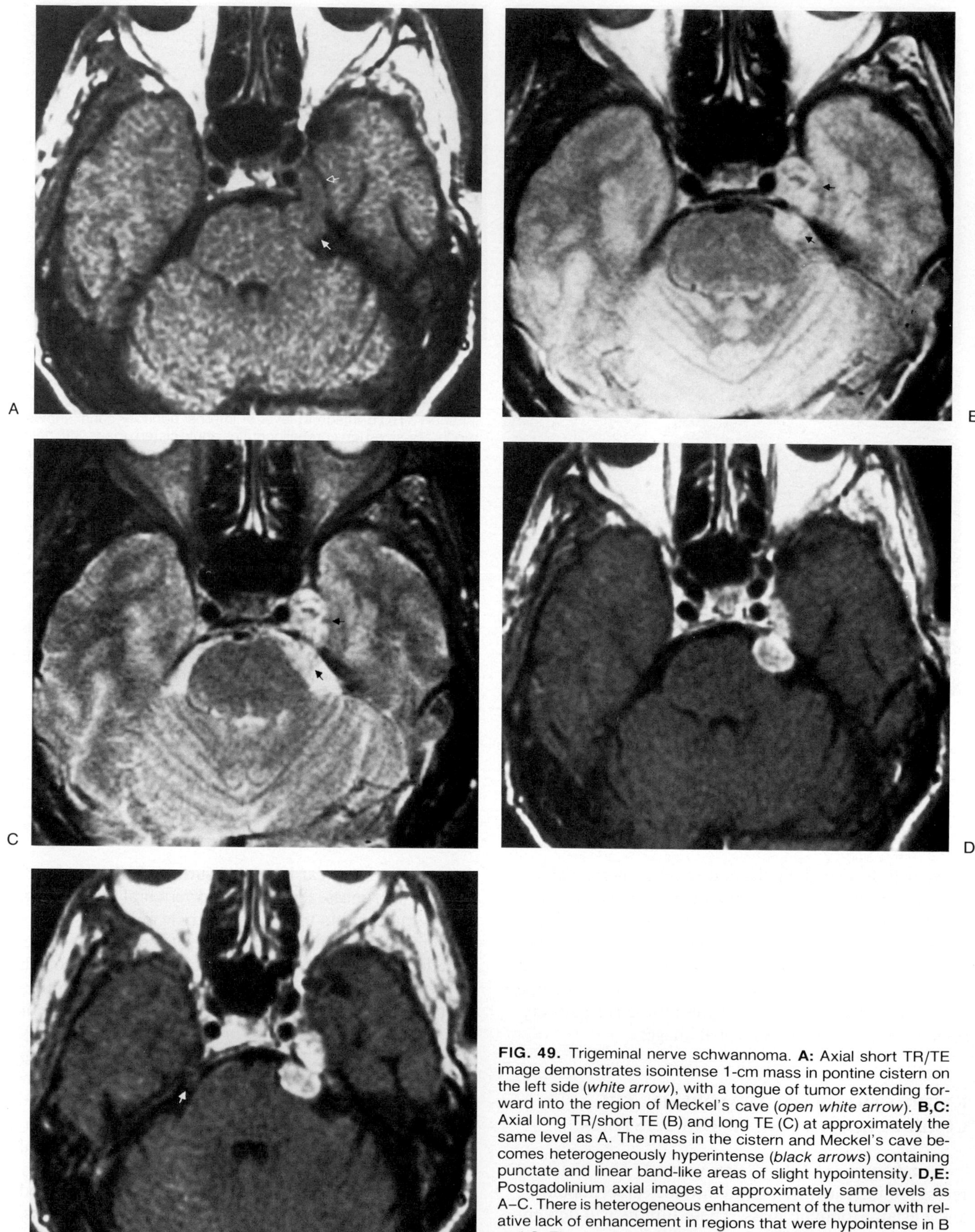

FIG. 49. Trigeminal nerve schwannoma. **A:** Axial short TR/TE image demonstrates isointense 1-cm mass in pontine cistern on the left side (*white arrow*), with a tongue of tumor extending forward into the region of Meckel's cave (*open white arrow*). **B,C:** Axial long TR/short TE (B) and long TE (C) at approximately the same level as A. The mass in the cistern and Meckel's cave becomes heterogeneously hyperintense (*black arrows*) containing punctate and linear band-like areas of slight hypointensity. **D,E:** Postgadolinium axial images at approximately same levels as A–C. There is heterogeneous enhancement of the tumor with relative lack of enhancement in regions that were hypointense in B and C. The mass in the cistern is occupying the position of the fifth cranial nerve with the normal fifth nerve seen on the right side (*white arrow*, E).

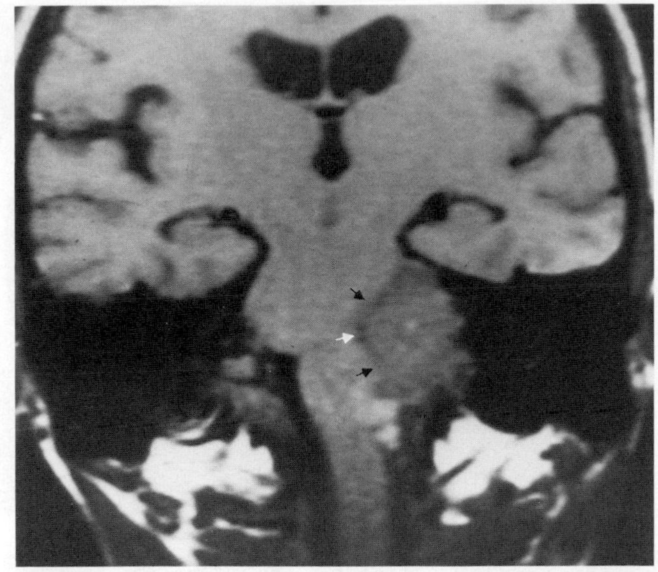

A

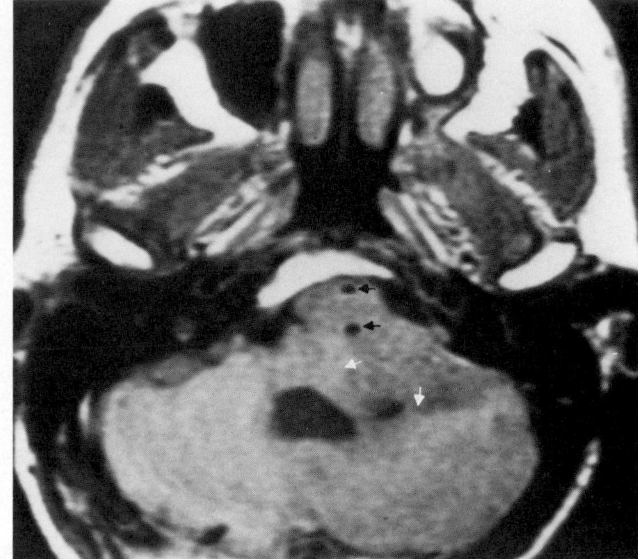

B

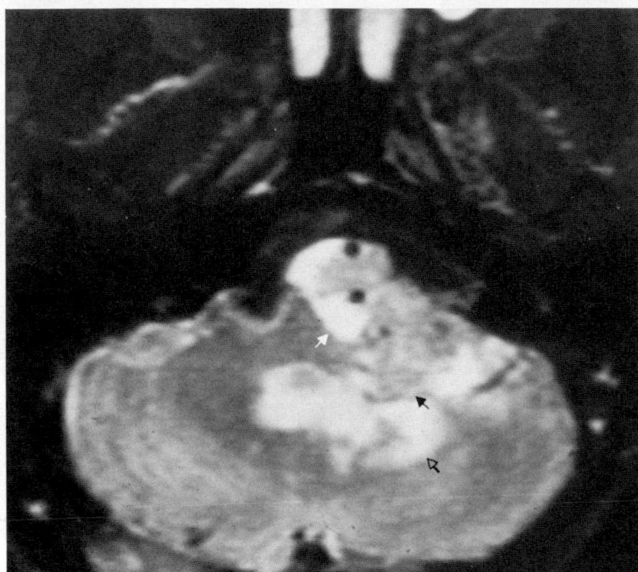

C

FIG. 50. Exophytic ependymoma of the fourth ventricle. **A:** Coronal short TR/TE image at pontomedullary junction region demonstrates lobulated slightly hypointense mass on the left side (*black arrows*). Two small vascular rim vessels (*white arrow*) are seen at the tumor pontine junction indicating the extra-axial position of the mass at this location. **B:** Axial short TR/TE image at level of fourth ventricle demonstrates slightly hypointense mass behind left petrous ridge and clivus. The mass encases the vertebral arteries (*black arrows*) and distorts the pontomedullary junction and anterior cerebellum on the left side (*white arrows*). **C:** Axial long TR/TE image at level of fourth ventricle demonstrates mass to be hyper- and isointense in moderate-sized areas. In A, a hyperintense focus appears to be invading into the pontomedullary junction (*white arrow*). An isointense region of the tumor extends back to the left anterior lateral margin of the fourth ventricle and appears to be invading into the adjacent middle cerebellar peduncle (*black arrow*). There is hyperintensity, most likely representing cerebellar edema alongside the left posterior lateral aspect of the fourth ventricle (*open black arrow*).

MALDEVELOPMENTAL CYSTS AND TUMORS

Arachnoid Cysts

There are many possible etiologies for the development of arachnoidal cysts. Some are acquired secondary to an inflammatory reaction in the subarachnoid space related to an episode of leptomeningitis, head trauma, or primary subarachnoid hemorrhage, or associated with brain tumors that are extra-axial or on its surface. A large number, however, are the result of congenital abnormality in the development of the arachnoid membrane (61,62). These arachnoid cysts represents approximately 1% of intracranial masses, with about one-half to two-thirds occurring in the middle cranial fossa (63). Other locations include the frontal convexity region and cisterns in the suprasellar, quadrigeminal, and foramen magnum region. They can also be within the ventricular system (Fig. 51). They are frequently asymptomatic but become symptomatic when they compress the brain sufficiently to cause headache and obstruction of the CSF pathways, resulting in hydrocephalus. The arachnoid cysts in the middle cranial fossa are frequently associated with what is believed to be primary hypogenesis of the temporal lobe (64). Arachnoid cysts frequently cause erosion and expansion of the overlying portion of the calvarium (Fig. 52). They do not develop calcifications in

A

FIG. 51. Arachnoid cyst. Intraventricular mass enlarges right lateral ventricle (**A**). Note lesion is isointense to CSF on T1-weighted (A), proton-density-weighted (**B**), and T2-weighted (**C**) images, except for minimal differences attributed to insulation from the normal CSF flow dynamics found within the ventricle. No contrast enhancement is seen in **D**.

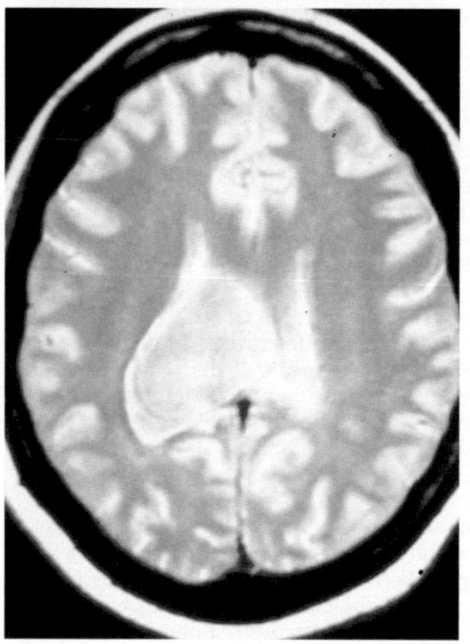

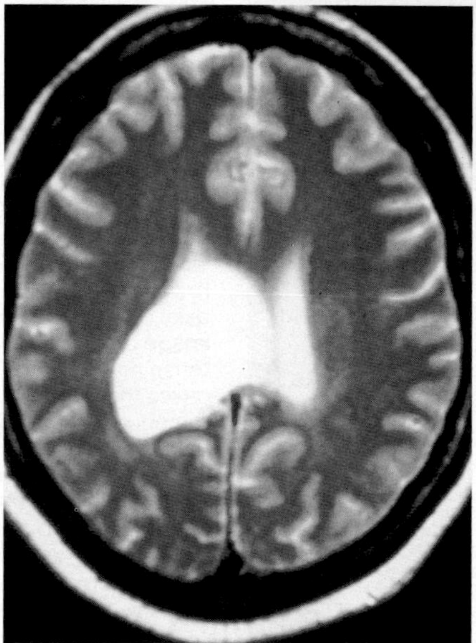

B,C

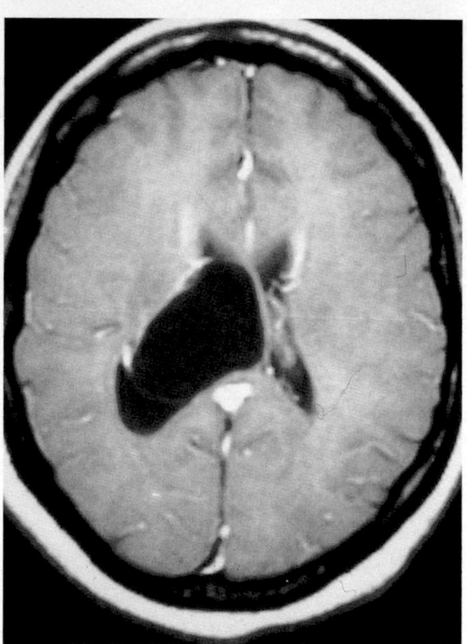

D

their walls and demonstrate no contrast enhancement (65). The superficial brain vasculature is displaced inward and may be outlined against the inner cyst wall (Fig. 52). Intensity will usually follow almost exactly that of CSF (64,66)—low intensity on short TR/TE images, isointensity on long TR/short TE images, and hyperintensity on long TR/TE images (Figs. 52 and 53). Pulsation artifacts may occasionally be seen within the larger cysts and are revealed as focal streaks of hypointensity on the long TR series.

Epidermoid Cysts

Intradural epidermoid cysts are congenital lesions of ectodermal origin. They most likely result from incomplete cleavage of the neural from the cutaneous ectoderm at the time of closure of the neural to between 3 and 5 weeks of gestation, with the retention of ectopic ectodermal cells in the neural groove (67). Histologically they are composed of an internal layer of stratified squamous epithelium covered by an external fibrous capsule. The cysts grow by progressive desquamation of epithelial cells with their conversion to keratin and cholesterol crystals (68). The tumor grows slowly, is soft and very pliable, conforming to the shape of the adjacent brain and cerebral spinal fluid spaces in which it is growing. The cysts frequently referred to as "pearly tumors" because of their gross external appearance account for approximately 0.2% to 1.8% of brain tumors. Although congenital in nature, they usually do not present clinically until the third or fourth decades. The cysts may be extradural or intradural in location. The intradural lesions are frequently located in the cisterns of the cere-

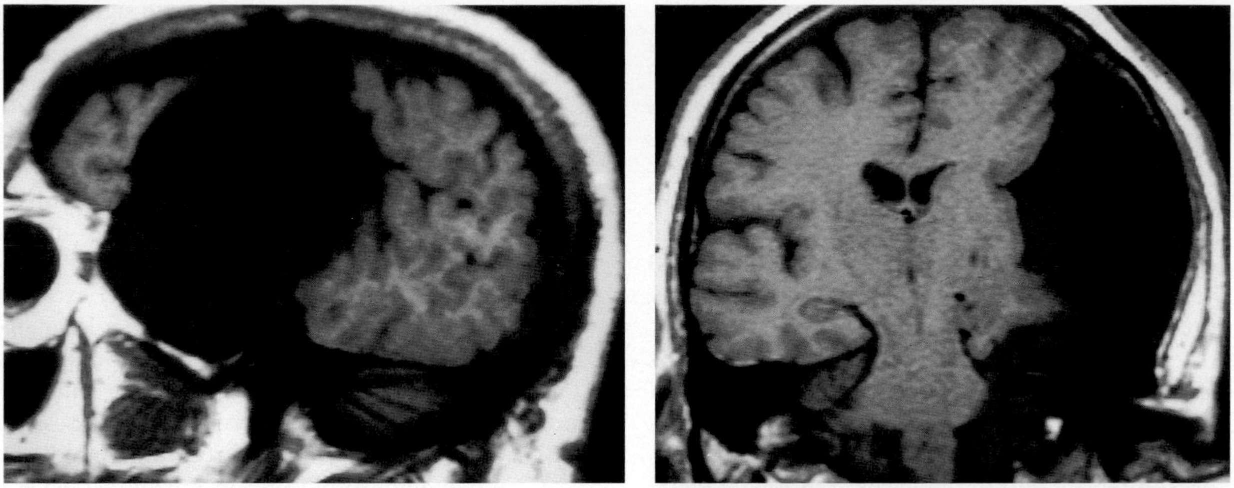

FIG. 52. Arachnoid cyst with skull remodeling and signal heterogeneity due to fluid motion. Sagittal **(A)** and coronal **(B)** T1-weighted images show a huge extraaxial mass with enlarged, remodeled middle cranial fossa (B) that extends into the posterior fossa. Intralesional heterogeneity on T1- and T2-weighted images **(C)** is due to motion of the fluid within the arachnoid cyst.

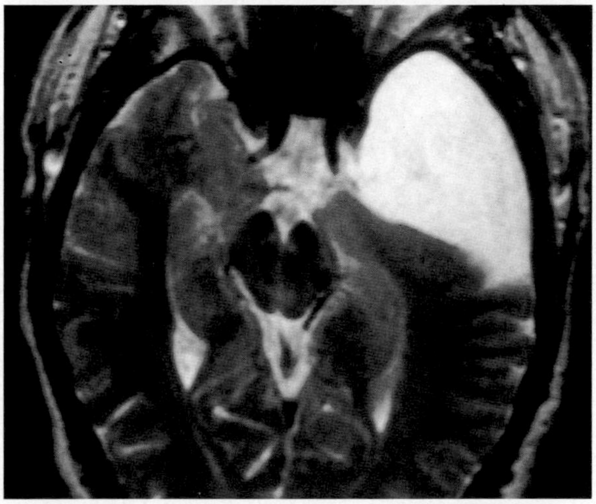

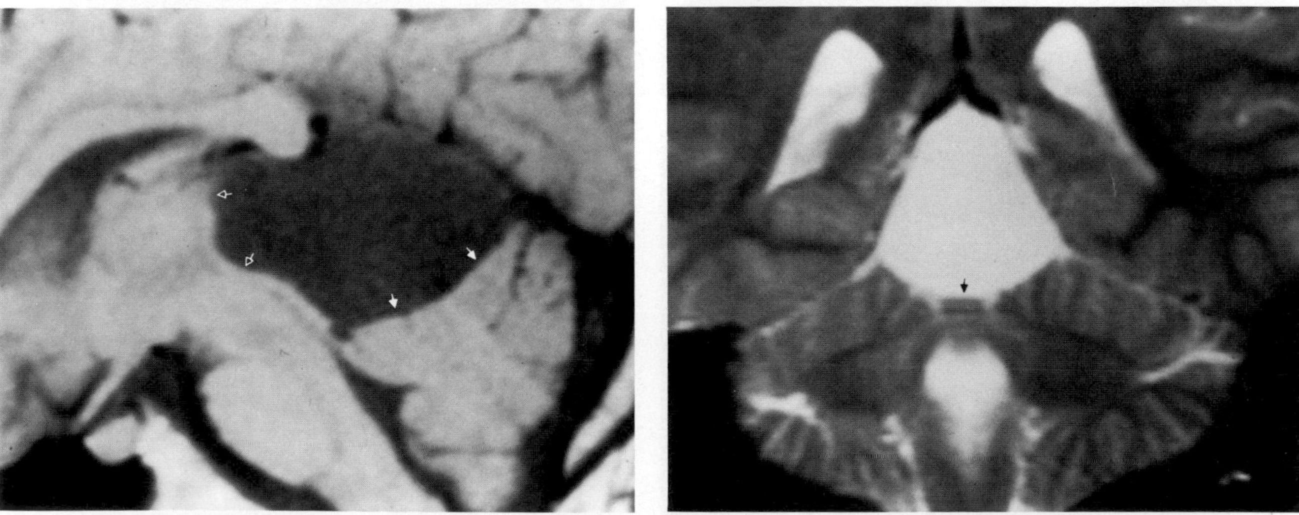

FIG. 53. Arachnoid cyst of quadrigeminal cistern. **A,B:** Sagittal short TR/TE (A) and coronal long TR/TE (B) images demonstrate a large extracerebral collection in the region of the quadrigeminal cistern that has similar intensity to that of ventricular fluid, being hypointense in A and hyperintense in B. The mass compresses the superior vermis inferiorly (*white arrows*, A; *black arrow*, B) and the posterior third ventricle and upper aqueduct (*open white arrows* in A), which, however, remain patent as no hydrocephalus is present.

bellopontine angle, supra- and parasellar regions (Fig. 54), and middle cranial fossa, as well as the cisterna magna. Tumors may also develop in the tela choroidea, usually in the temporal horn of the lateral ventricle but occasionally in the fourth ventricle. On CT the lesions are hypodense and do not enhance with contrast material (69). They are difficult to differentiate from arachnoid cysts based on their density; however, their external surface is usually lobulated in configuration compared with the smooth surface of an arachnoid cyst. There may occasionally be focal calcifications in their walls.

On short TR/TE MR images, epidermoid tumors demonstrate mild hypointensity, usually between that of the CSF and the brain parenchyma. There is usually mild inhomogeneity of low intensity, with some patchy regions of isointensity within the lesion. On long TR/TE sequences the tumors show marked hyperintensity similar to or greater than that of CSF, with significant heterogeneity of the signal intensity (70–72). The low-intensity signals within the tumor hyperintense pattern are probably the result of the cellular debris and solid cholesterol crystals within the cysts (Fig. 55). A high-intensity rim may surround the portion of the cyst on long TR/TE sequences that probably represents a CSF cleft. The tumors may be dumbbell-shaped in configuration and extend from the middle cranial fossa into the posterior fossa. They may have a smooth external surface but in most instances demonstrate a lobulated appearance. No free fatty acids have been found in epidermoid cysts that are low intensity on the short TR/TE sequences (73). In the vast majority of cases, epidermoids are distinctly different from arachnoid cysts on MRI, in that epidermoid tumors are almost never isointense to CSF on long TR/short TE images.

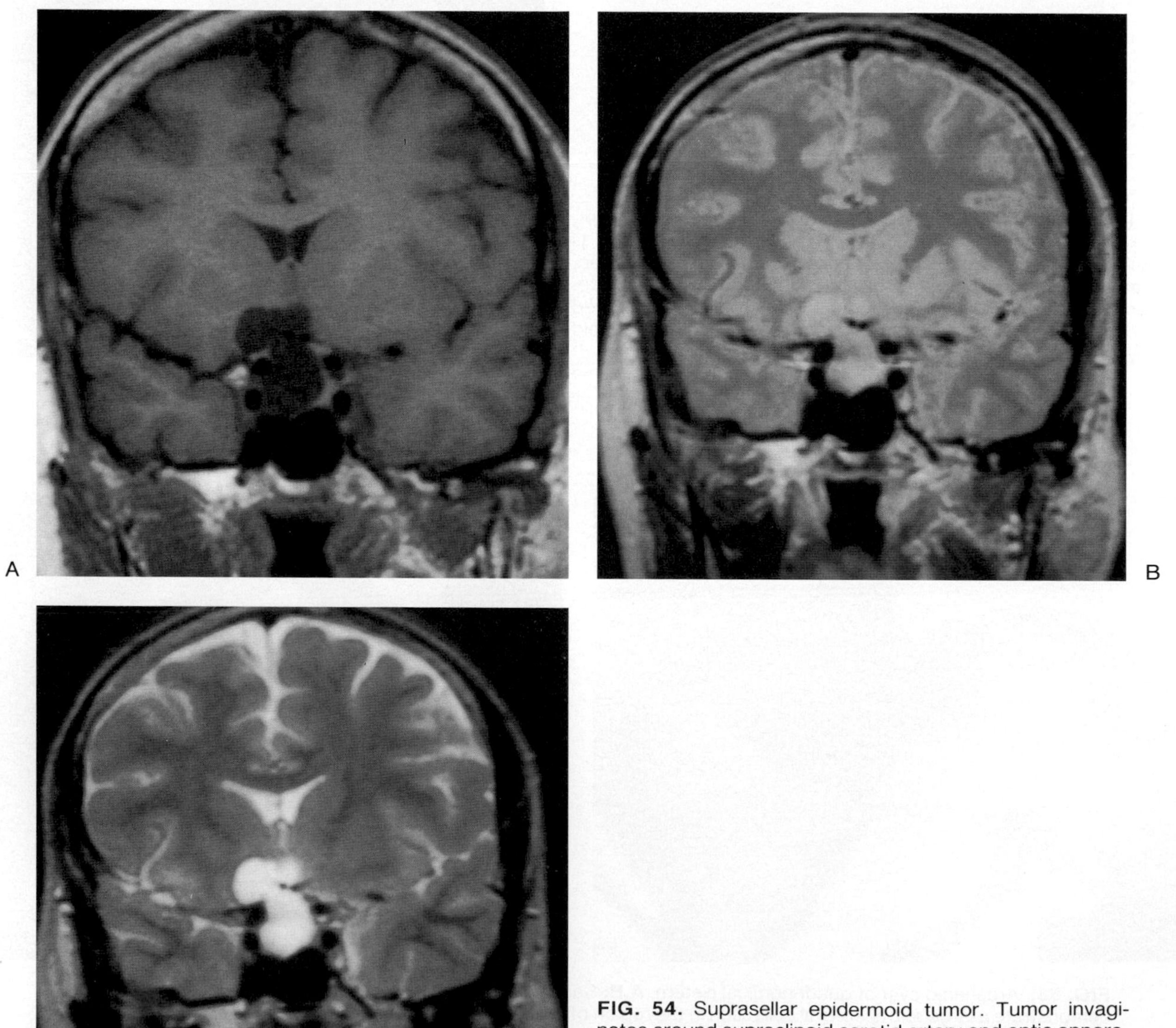

FIG. 54. Suprasellar epidermoid tumor. Tumor invaginates around supraclinoid carotid artery and optic apparatus (**A–C**). Note lesion is minimally different from CSF intensity on proton-density-weighted image (B).

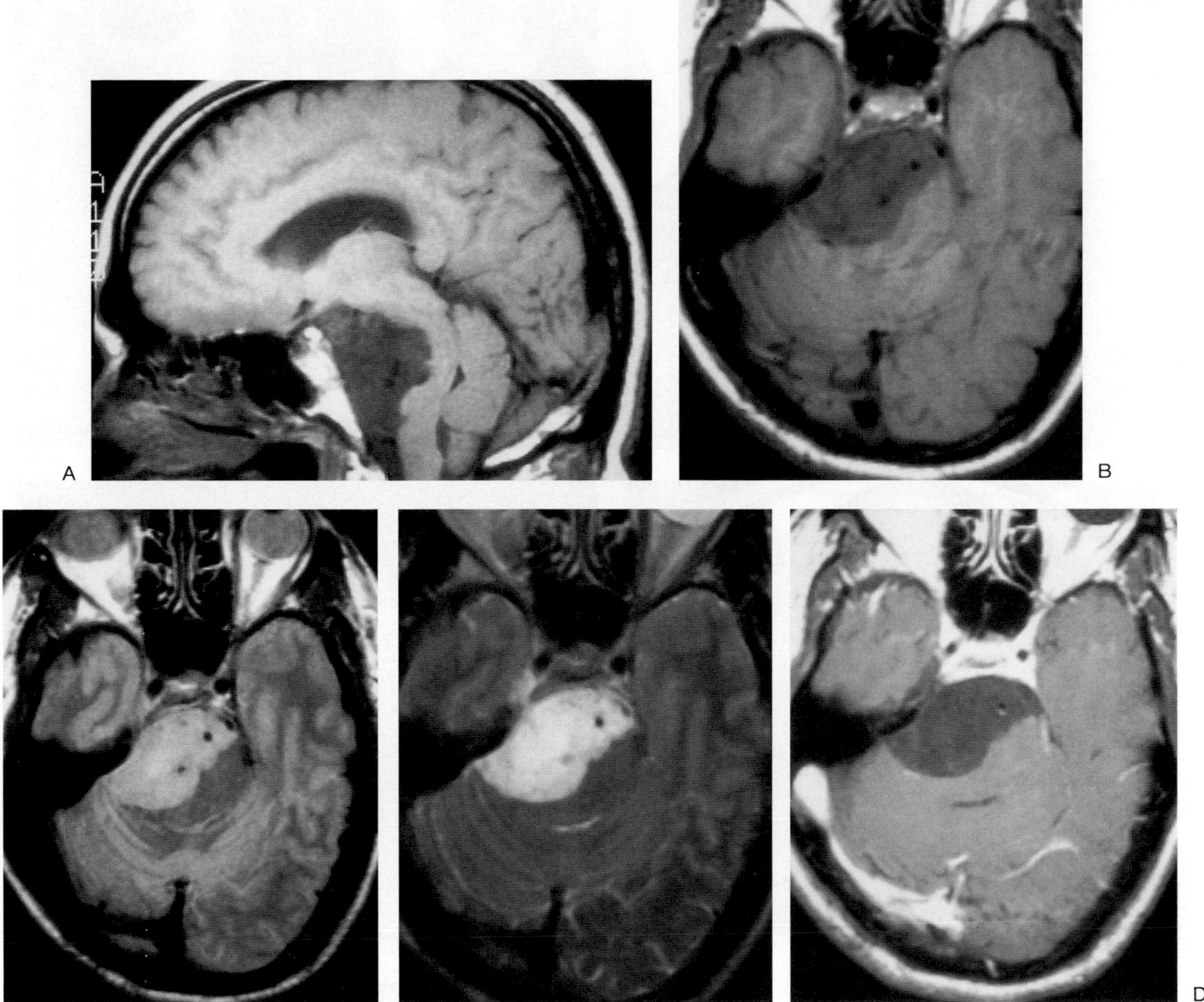

FIG. 55. Epidermoid tumor, cerebellopontine angel cistern. Irregular, lobulated morphology on sagittal T1-weighted **(A)** and heterogenous signal intensity on axial images **(B–D)** without enhancement **(E)** make diagnosis of the epidermoid tumor virtually certain. Note the typical encasement of the basilar artery, rather than the displacement that would be seen if the lesion was an arachnoid cyst (B–E).

Dermoid Cysts

Intracranially these are rarer tumors than epidermoid cysts. As with epidermoid cysts, they arise from inclusion of ectodermoid elements in the neural groove at its time of closure. Not uncommonly there is a persistent defect in the overlying skin, with a sinus tract extending into the intracranial portion. Clinically, they usually present in the third decade and are most commonly located in the posterior fossa in the midline but may occur in the cisterns about the sella turcica and elsewhere. They may also have an intraventricular location arising within the cisterns of the tela choroidea in the lateral, third, or fourth ventricular regions. Microscopically, these cysts may contain elements from all layers of the skin. Much of the wall of the cysts may be lined (as in epidermoid tumors) by stratified squamous epithelium supported by an outer collagen layer. More solid portions of the tumor may contain hair follicles along with sebaceous, sweat, and apocrine glands. Calcification may develop in the portion of the walls, and there may be bone and cartilage within some of the cysts (74).

Dermoid cysts typically demonstrate marked hyperintensity on short TR/TE MR images (75) (Fig. 56) due to their fatty content, which consists of triglycerides and unsaturated fatty acids (73). On long TR images, the

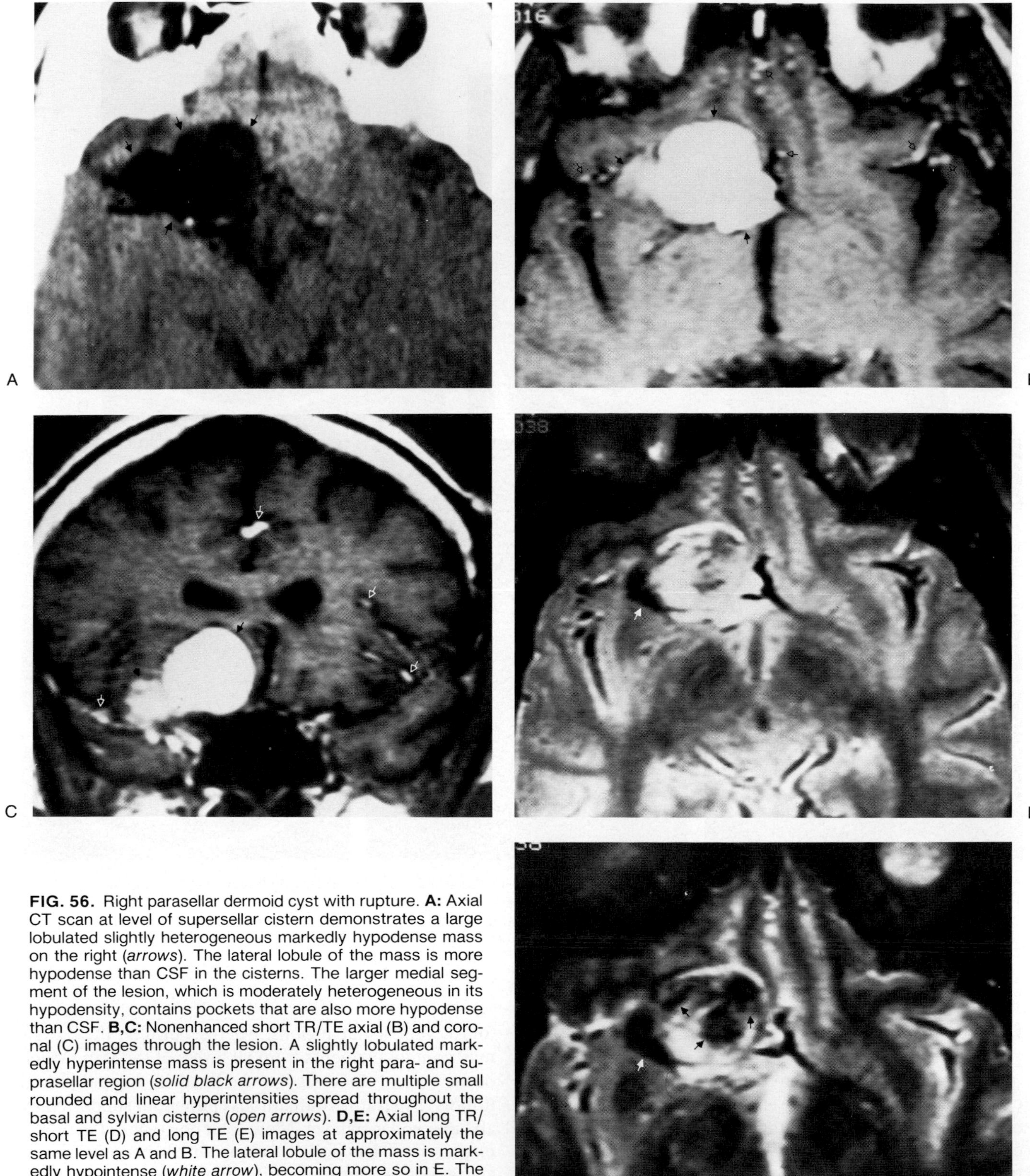

FIG. 56. Right parasellar dermoid cyst with rupture. **A:** Axial CT scan at level of supersellar cistern demonstrates a large lobulated slightly heterogeneous markedly hypodense mass on the right (*arrows*). The lateral lobule of the mass is more hypodense than CSF in the cisterns. The larger medial segment of the lesion, which is moderately heterogeneous in its hypodensity, contains pockets that are also more hypodense than CSF. **B,C:** Nonenhanced short TR/TE axial (B) and coronal (C) images through the lesion. A slightly lobulated markedly hyperintense mass is present in the right para- and suprasellar region (*solid black arrows*). There are multiple small rounded and linear hyperintensities spread throughout the basal and sylvian cisterns (*open arrows*). **D,E:** Axial long TR/short TE (D) and long TE (E) images at approximately the same level as A and B. The lateral lobule of the mass is markedly hypointense (*white arrow*), becoming more so in E. The larger medial lobule demonstrates considerable heterogeneity of its intensity. There is a background of hyperintensity containing smaller and larger foci of marked hypointensities, which become more pronounced in E (*black arrows*).

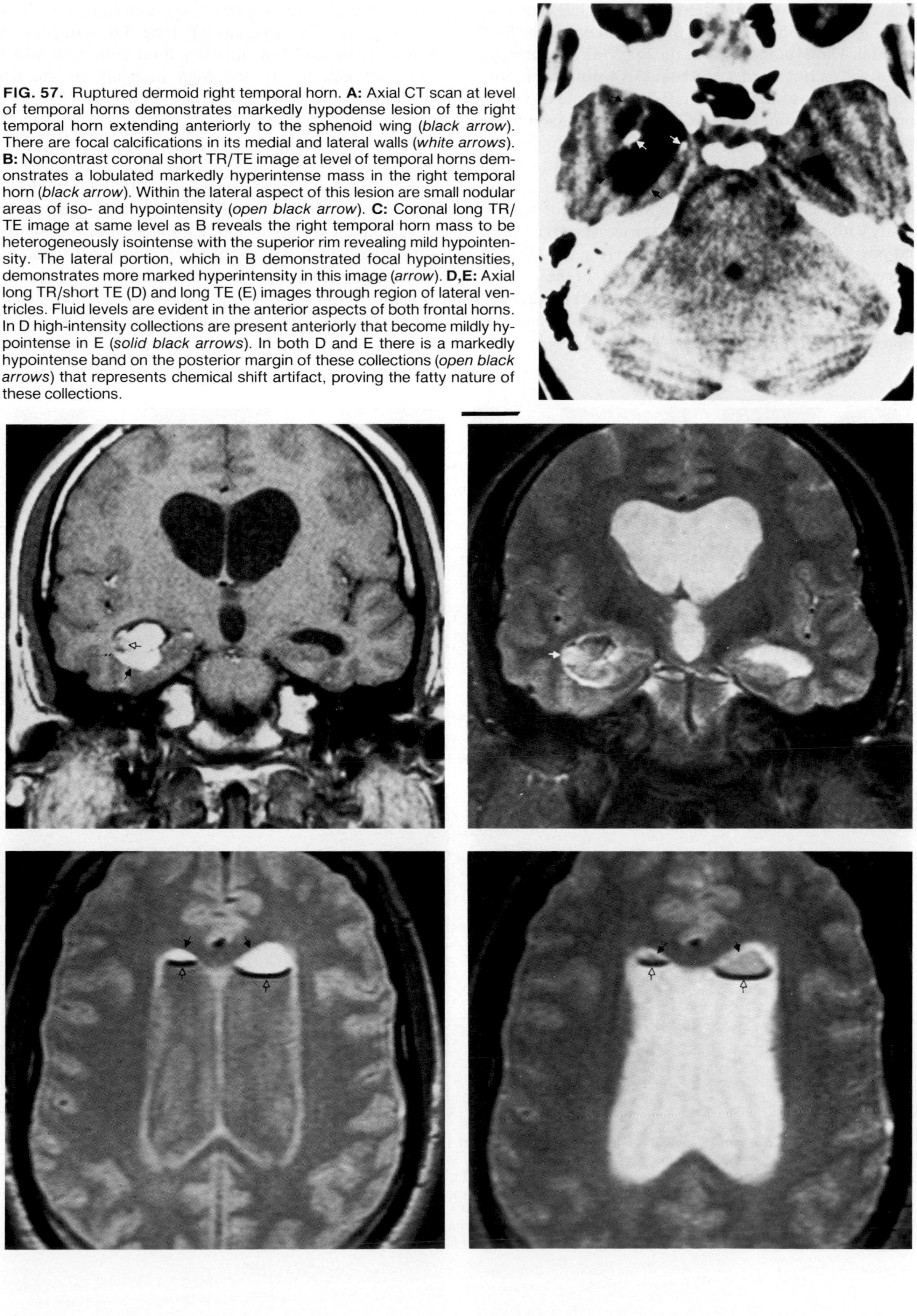

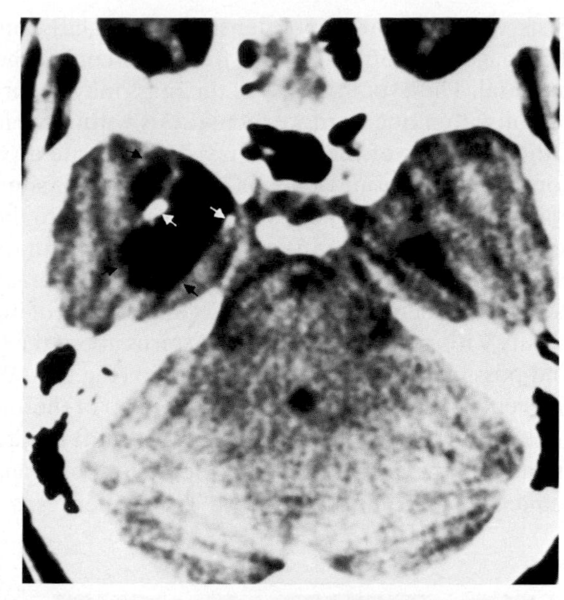

FIG. 57. Ruptured dermoid right temporal horn. **A:** Axial CT scan at level of temporal horns demonstrates markedly hypodense lesion of the right temporal horn extending anteriorly to the sphenoid wing (*black arrow*). There are focal calcifications in its medial and lateral walls (*white arrows*). **B:** Noncontrast coronal short TR/TE image at level of temporal horns demonstrates a lobulated markedly hyperintense mass in the right temporal horn (*black arrow*). Within the lateral aspect of this lesion are small nodular areas of iso- and hypointensity (*open black arrow*). **C:** Coronal long TR/TE image at same level as B reveals the right temporal horn mass to be heterogeneously isointense with the superior rim revealing mild hypointensity. The lateral portion, which in B demonstrated focal hypointensities, demonstrates more marked hyperintensity in this image (*arrow*). **D,E:** Axial long TR/short TE (D) and long TE (E) images through region of lateral ventricles. Fluid levels are evident in the anterior aspects of both frontal horns. In D high-intensity collections are present anteriorly that become mildly hypointense in E (*solid black arrows*). In both D and E there is a markedly hypointense band on the posterior margin of these collections (*open black arrows*) that represents chemical shift artifact, proving the fatty nature of these collections.

A

B

C

D

E

cysts usually show hypointensity, particularly on long TE images (Fig. 56), again due to the presence of the fatty material. The hypointensity of the mass may be throughout or within one or more loculations within the lesion. Other portions of the cysts may demonstrate a pattern consisting of inhomogeneous hyperintensity, similar to epidermoid tumors. The cysts may rupture into the subarachnoid space (Fig. 56) or, for those arising in the tela choroidea, intraventricularly (Fig. 57). Subarachnoid rupture will demonstrate droplets and streaks of high intensity within the subarachnoid cisterns about the tumor and possibly more distally in the brain (Fig. 56). Within the ventricles a fat-fluid level will develop in the anterior superior portions (Fig. 57). A chemical shift artifact will frequently be projected into the lesion on long TR sequences (Fig. 57). On short TR sequences a high-intensity fluid level will be present anterior to the hypointensity of CSF, whereas on long TR sequences an intermediate and low-intensity fluid collection will be observed anterior to the high intensity of the CSF (Fig. 57).

Subarachnoid Lipomas

These lesions arise from a congenital abnormality of the leptomeningeal membranes. Normal embryologic development results in the reabsorption of the meninx primitiva, which is the primitive meningeal tissue initially formed. This results in the subarachnoid cisterns. If reabsorption of this tissue is incomplete, there may be differentiation of the cells into lipomatous tissue. These tumors are usually located in the subarachnoid space

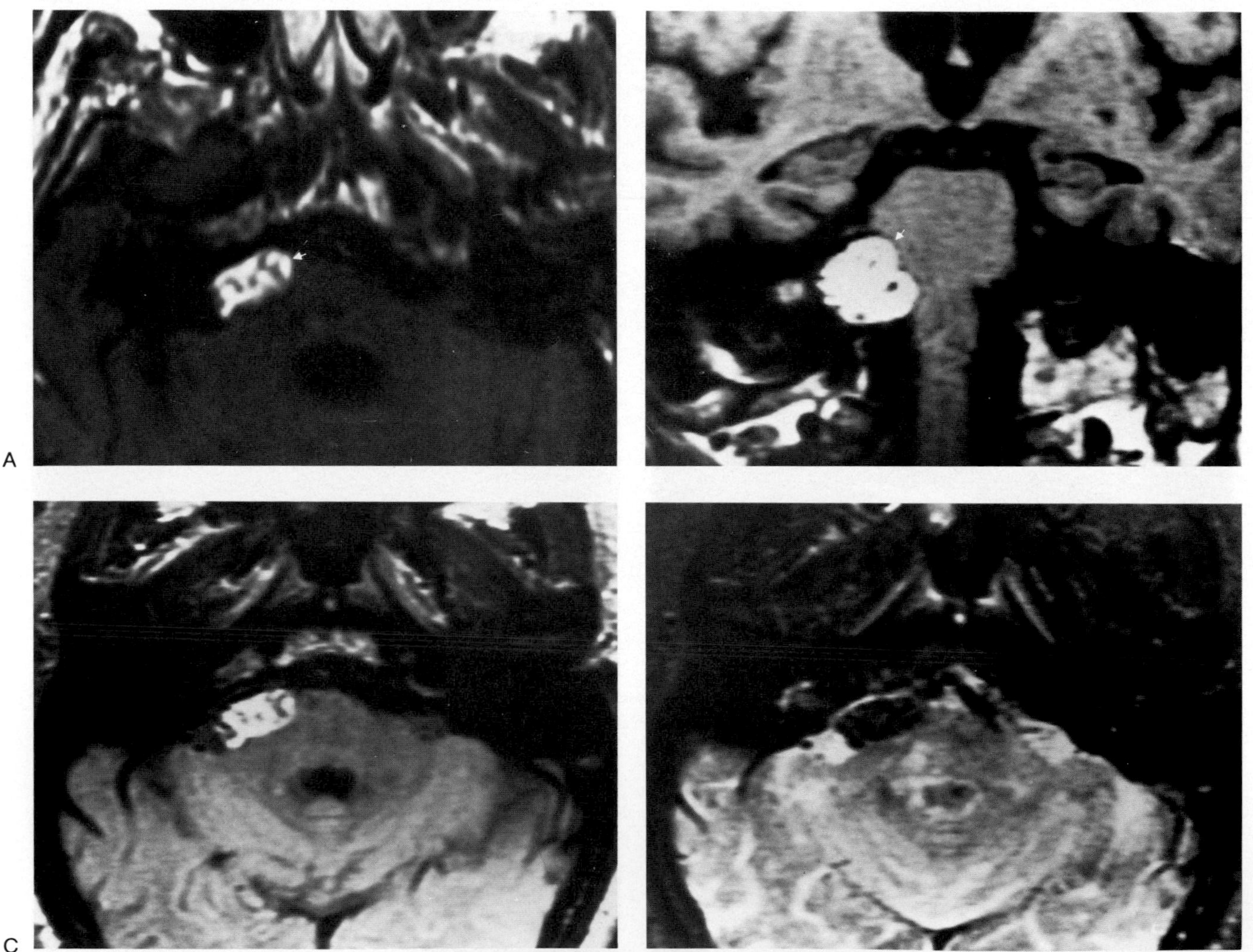

FIG. 58. Right cerebellopontine angle lipoma. **A,B:** Short TR/TE axial (A) coronal (B) images without contrast at the level of the cerebellopontine angles. There is a slightly lobulated hyperintense mass containing irregular internal strands of hypointensity situated in the medial aspect of the right cerebellopontine angle cistern (*arrow*). **C,D:** Axial long TR/short TE (C) and long TE (D) images at approximately the same level as A. On the short TE image (C), the lesion characteristics are similar to that in A, while in the long TE image (D), the background intensity of the lesion becomes moderately hypointense and the band-like densities become even more hypointense relative to brain parenchyma. These intensity changes suggest the presence of fibrous bands within a lipomatous mass.

and are most frequently found in the pericallosal cistern; large lesions in this location are known as corpus callosum lipomas (76). They may also be found in the quadrigeminal, chiasmatic, perimesencephalic, cerebellopontine angle, and sylvian cisterns (77). The lesions are frequently incidental and asymptomatic but may cause compression of the brain with obstructive hydrocephalus when enlarged or may infiltrate around the cranial nerves, producing focal symptoms. When there is pericallosal cistern involvement there is frequent corpus callosum hypogenesis or agenesis. Microscopically the lesion contains adipose cells and a variable amount of collagen fibers in an uneven distribution (78). The tumor may infiltrate around neural tissues and around small blood vessels. Some tumors may contain neuronal ganglion cells and islands of fibrillary neuroglia. Some lesions may also contain a prominent vascular pattern, giving rise to an angiolipomatous variant.

On MR the lesion will be hyperintense on short TR/TE images either uniformly or containing isointense nodules and bands representing the nonlipomatous elements within the lesion (79). On long TR/TE sequences the lesion becomes hypointense and frequently more heterogeneous (Fig. 58). There may be a pathognomonic chemical shift artifact evident.

Hypothalamic Hamartomas

This lesion consists of mature neuronal ganglionic tissue projecting from the hypothalamus down into the retrosellar cistern. It is usually attached to the tuber cinereum or mamillary bodies. These lesions are commonly associated with precocious puberty. They usually measure 1 to 2 cm in diameter. In addition to mature ganglionic cells, the lesion consists of myelinated and unmyelinated fibers, which in places form compact bundles, as

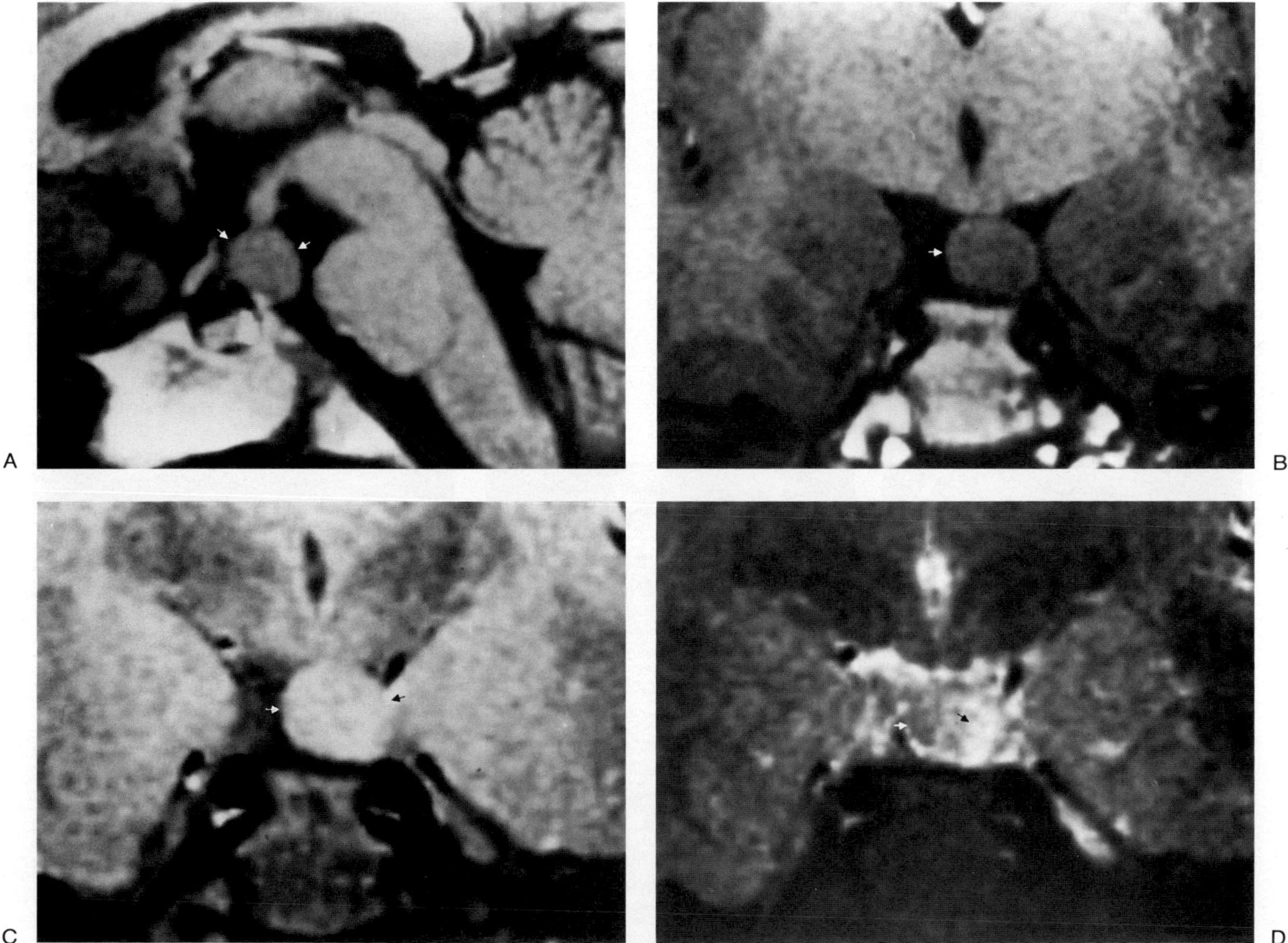

FIG. 59. Hypothalamic hamartoma in 6-year-old girl. **A,B:** Short TR/TE sagittal (A) and coronal (B) images at the level of the hypothalamus. A 1-cm mass is present in the retrosellar region abutting against the floor of the third ventricle superiorly (*white arrow*). The mass is isointense to gray matter. **C,D:** Coronal long TR/short TE (C) and long TE (D) images at the same level as B. The mass (*white arrow*) remains isointense to gray matter but contains a band of slightly more hyperintense tissue on its left side (*black arrow*).

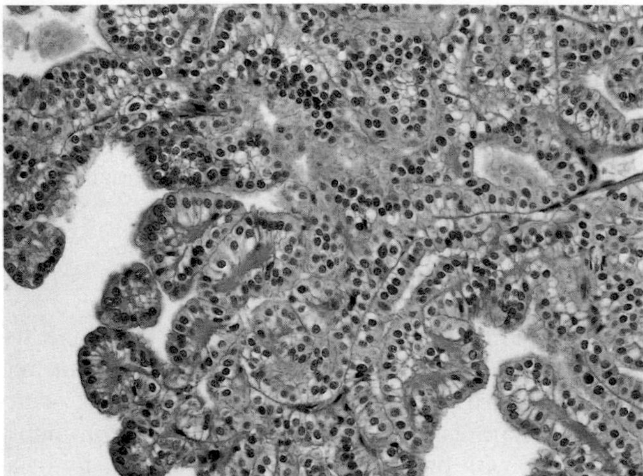

FIG. 60. Choroid plexus papilloma, histopathology. Histologic section of a choroid plexus papilloma exhibiting finger-like papillae lined by epithelial cells, surrounding a fibrovascular core.

well as various types of glial cells with a variable amount of fibrillary gliosis within the lesion.

On MRI, short TR/TE sequences demonstrate a slightly hypointense mass approximately 1 to 2 cm in diameter in the retrosellar cistern, which abuts against the floor of the hypothalamus. The mass will generally be isointense to adjacent gray matter. Long TR images demonstrate that the mass in general remains nearly isointense to adjacent gray matter and may contain patchy regions of slightly higher intensity (Fig. 59). The higher intensity areas may represent the gliotic regions seen histologically.

CHOROID PLEXUS PAPILLOMAS

These tumors can be mistaken for other ventricular tumors such as meningiomas and ependymomas. Papillomas of the choroid plexus that arise from its surface epithelium constitute approximately 0.5% of all intracranial tumors (80). Approximately 40% occur in the fourth ventricle (usually in adults), 10% in the third ventricle, and 43% in one of the lateral ventricles (81). About 10% of the cases involve the choroid plexus, which projects into the cerebellopontine angle cistern. There may be a multifocal origin of these tumors in approximately 4% of the cases. In children choroid plexus papillomas constitute a more frequently intracranial tumor, accounting for 1.5% to 6.4% (82,83) of all intracranial pediatric neoplasms. In children 80% of the papillomas arise in the lateral ventricle, 16% in the fourth ventricle, and 4% in the third ventricle (83). Of pediatric tumors that presented within the first 60 days of life, 42% were reported to be choroid plexus papillomas (84).

Microscopically, papillomas are very irregularly lobulated masses projecting into the ventricular cavity from the region of the choroid plexus (Fig. 60). Large tumors locally expand the ventricle in which they are growing and may cause trapping, with dilation of its more peripherally draining segments. The tumors may show regions of heavy calcification with bone formation. Their stroma consists of highly vascularized connective tissue supporting a papilla composed of a single layer of columnar or epithelial cells. Hemorrhage and cystic regions may develop within the tumor (Fig. 61). Hydrocephalus frequently occurs with choroid plexus papillomas as a result

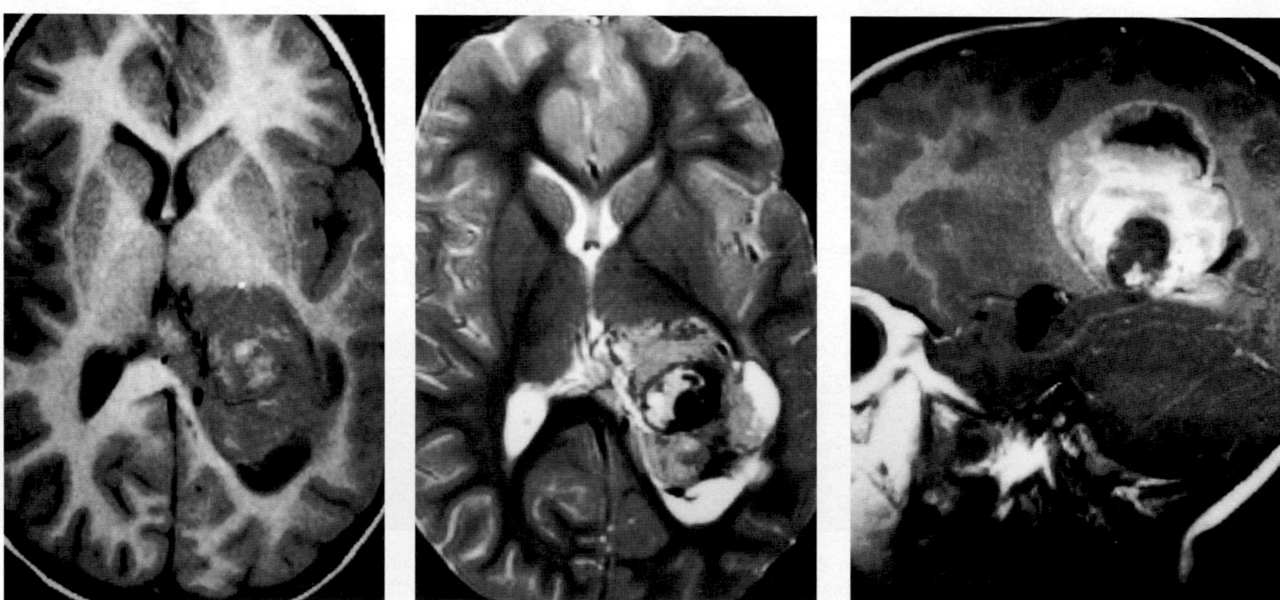

FIG. 61. Choroid plexus papilloma with intratumoral necrosis. Large heterogeneous intraventricular mass with hemorrhage and necrosis (**A,B**) enhances irregularly (**C**). Despite heterogeneity, lesion is benign.

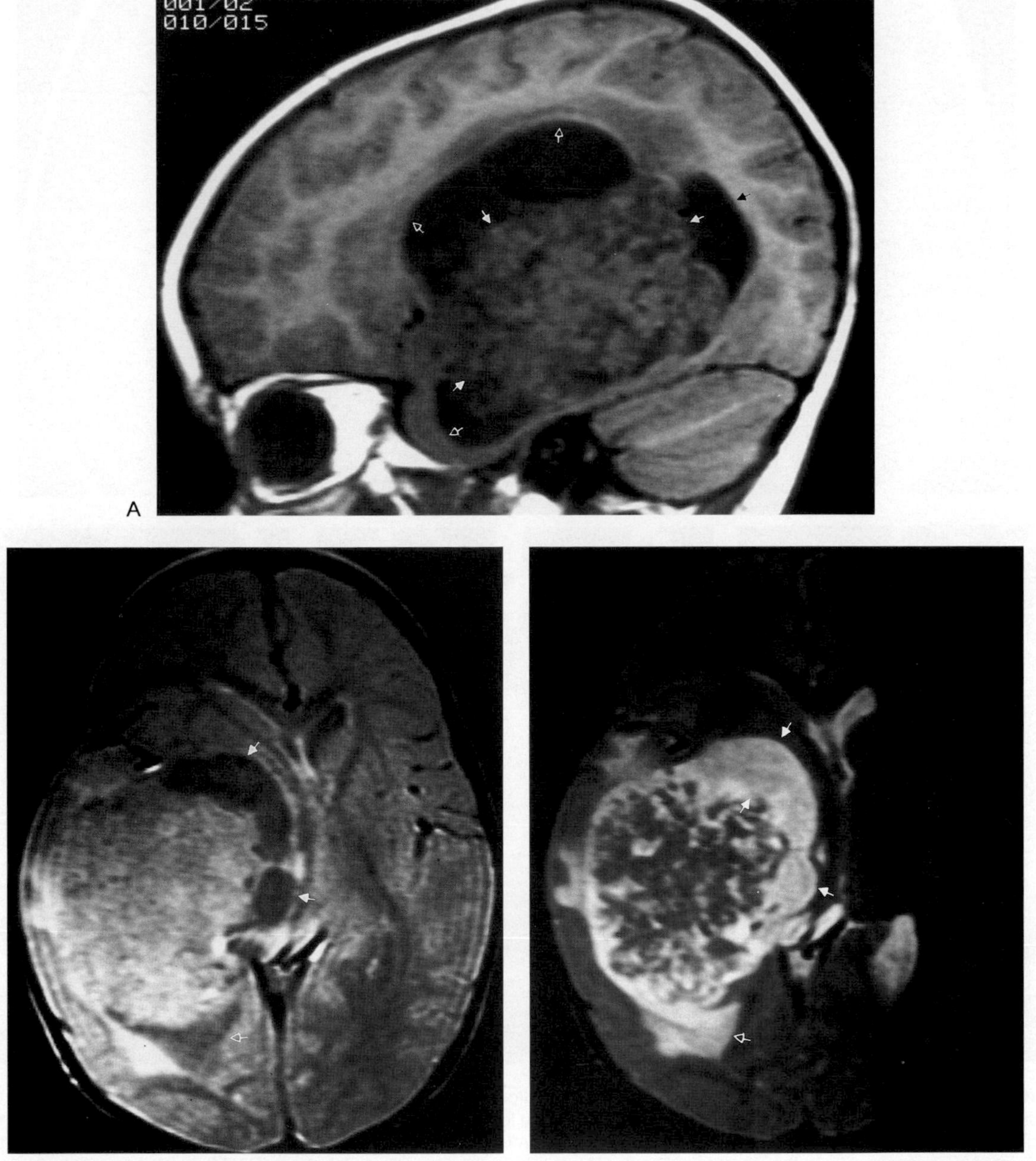

FIG. 62. Choroid plexus papilloma, right lateral ventricle, in a 1-month-old infant. **A:** Sagittal short TR/TE image at level of right temporal horn. There is a very large irregularly lobulated mass within the right temporal horn and atrial region that is isointense to gray matter (*white arrows*). It contains multiple punctate, linear, and patchy regions of more marked hypointensity. There is marked dilatation of the temporal horn (*open white arrows*) and occipital horn (*black arrow*) due to trapping by the tumor. **B,C:** Axial long TR/short TE (B) and long TE (C) images at level of the atrium demonstrate the large right temporal-atrial mass to be mainly isointense to gray matter but containing large patchy areas of mild hyperintensity on the short TE image (B). On the long TE image (C), very irregular hypointensities become apparent throughout the tumor. Only the trapped right temporal horn (*solid white arrows*) and occipital horn (*open black arrow*) are dilated. The left lateral ventricle is normal in size, and there is marked compression of the right frontal horn and third ventricle.

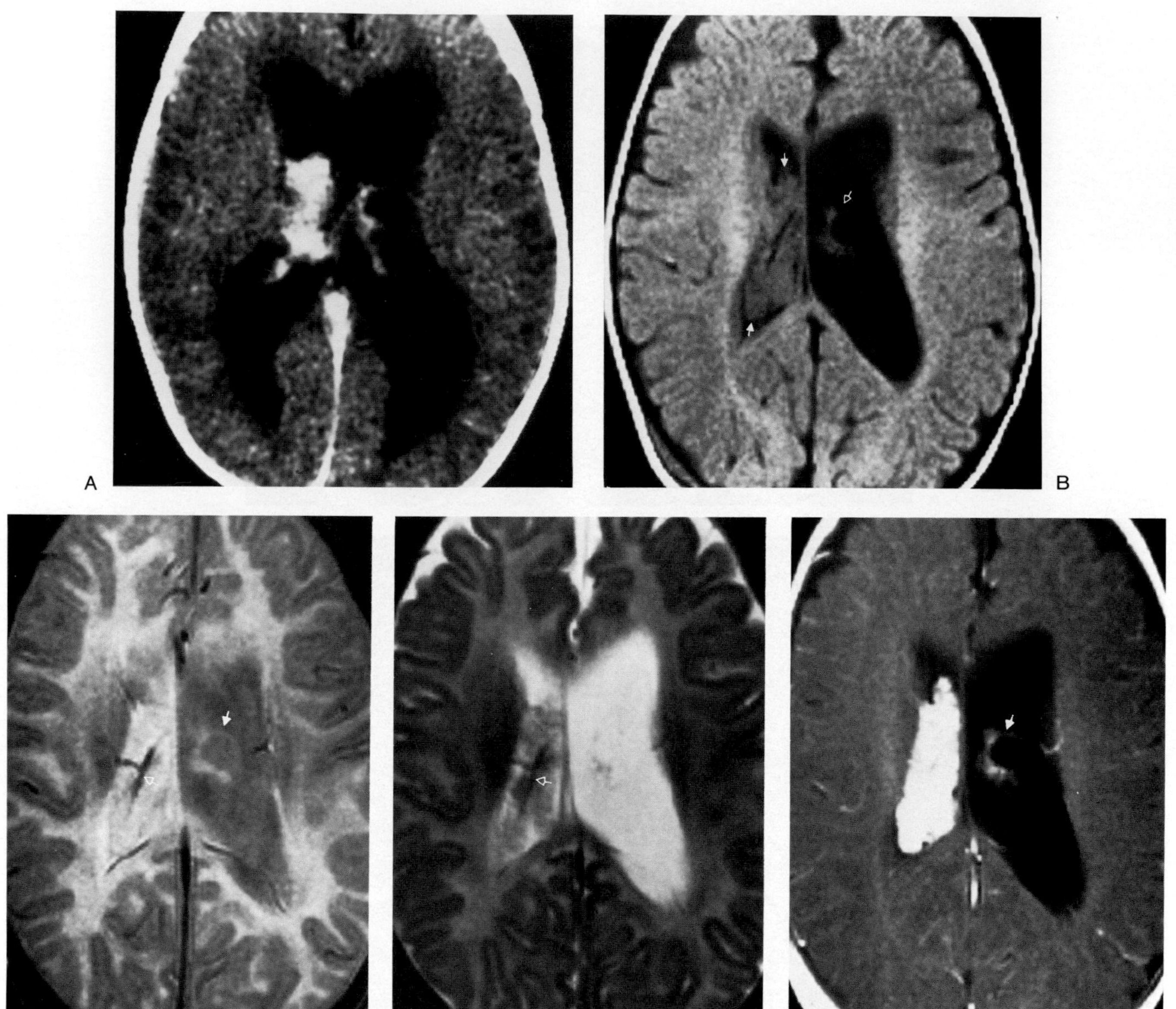

FIG. 63. Bilateral choroid plexus lateral ventricular papillomas with hydrocephalus. **A:** Axial contrast-enhanced CT scan at level of lateral ventricles reveals a very irregularly lobulated contrast-enhancing mass within the body of the right lateral ventricle. There is also slightly increased prominence of the enhancing choroid plexus in the body of the left lateral ventricle. Marked bilateral ventricular dilatation is present. **B:** Axial short TR/TE image at level of lateral ventricle postshunting of right lateral ventricle. Compared with A, the right lateral ventricle has decreased markedly in size. A very irregularly lobulated mass isointense to gray matter fills the body of the right lateral ventricle (*arrows*). In the body of the left lateral ventricle there is an irregular band of isointense tissue that appears to contain a low-intensity cyst-like region in its lateral aspect (*open arrow*). **C,D:** Axial long TR/short TE (C) and long TE (D) images at level of lateral ventricles. The mass in the right lateral ventricle becomes mildly hyperintense in C and moderately hypointense in D. Linear hypointensities within the mass most likely represent enlarged choroidal veins (*open arrow*). The cystic nature of the lesion in the body of the left lateral ventricle can be best appreciated in C (*arrow*) as the lesion is obscured on the long TE image (D) by the hyperintensity of the surrounding CSF. **E:** Postgadolinium axial short TR/TE image at level of lateral ventricles demonstrates diffuse moderately homogeneous enhancement of the tumor in the right lateral ventricle, showing its irregular lobulated shape. The smaller tumor in the body of the left lateral ventricle is more clearly outlined and its cystic nature confirmed (*arrow*).

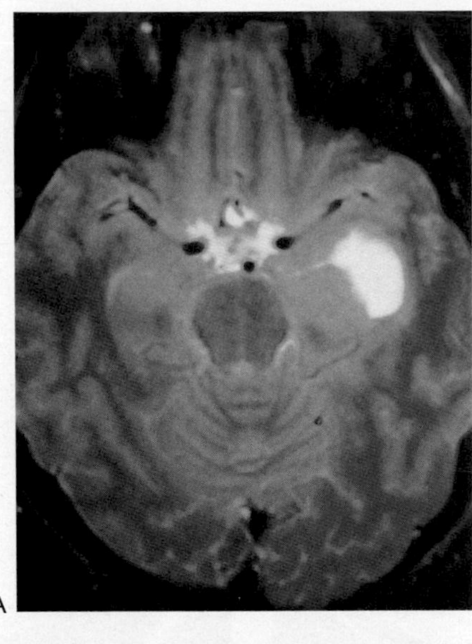

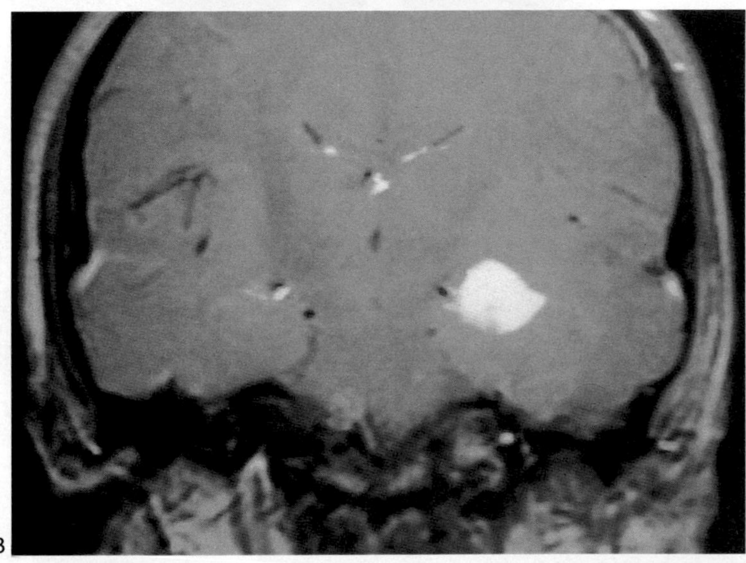

FIG. 64. Homogeneous choroid plexus papilloma in temporal horn (**A**) enhances densely (**B**) and is indistinguishable from other intraventricular lesions.

of either the overproduction of cerebral spinal fluid and/or the occurrence of blockage in the subarachnoid cisterns or interventricular pathways from adhesions resulting from tumor hemorrhage (83,85).

On MR, short TR/TE images demonstrate that the tumor usually has a very lobulated margin and is iso- to slightly hypointense to gray matter (Fig. 62). It may contain multiple punctate linear and patchy regions of more marked hypointensity resulting from tumor calcification and vascularity (86,87) (Fig. 62). On long TR/TE sequences the tumors may show a very heterogeneous hyperintensity as a result of similar factors, as well as from the presence of iron from old hemorrhages in the tumor (Fig. 62). Cyst-like changes may be present within the lesion, and bilateral hydrocephalus may be evident without evidence of obstruction in the CSF pathways (Fig. 63). Enlarged blood vessels within the tumor may be seen as punctate and curvilinear regions of hypointensity on both short and long TR sequences (Fig. 63). Multicentric tumors may be present (Fig. 63). Gadolinium administration will demonstrate enhancement throughout the tumor (Figs. 63 and 64) that may be heterogeneous in its pattern depending on the degree of tumor calcification, vascularity, and cystic change present. Certain tumors may be heavily calcified (Fig. 65). Contrast administration will demonstrate enhancement outside the calcified hypointense regions and also within the calcified area (Fig. 65). Lesions located in the third ventricle will generally produce hydrocephalus because of obstruction at the foramen of Monro. In some tumors the long TR/TE images demonstrate mild hypointensity of the lesion (Fig. 66). Tumors situated in the fourth ventricle may

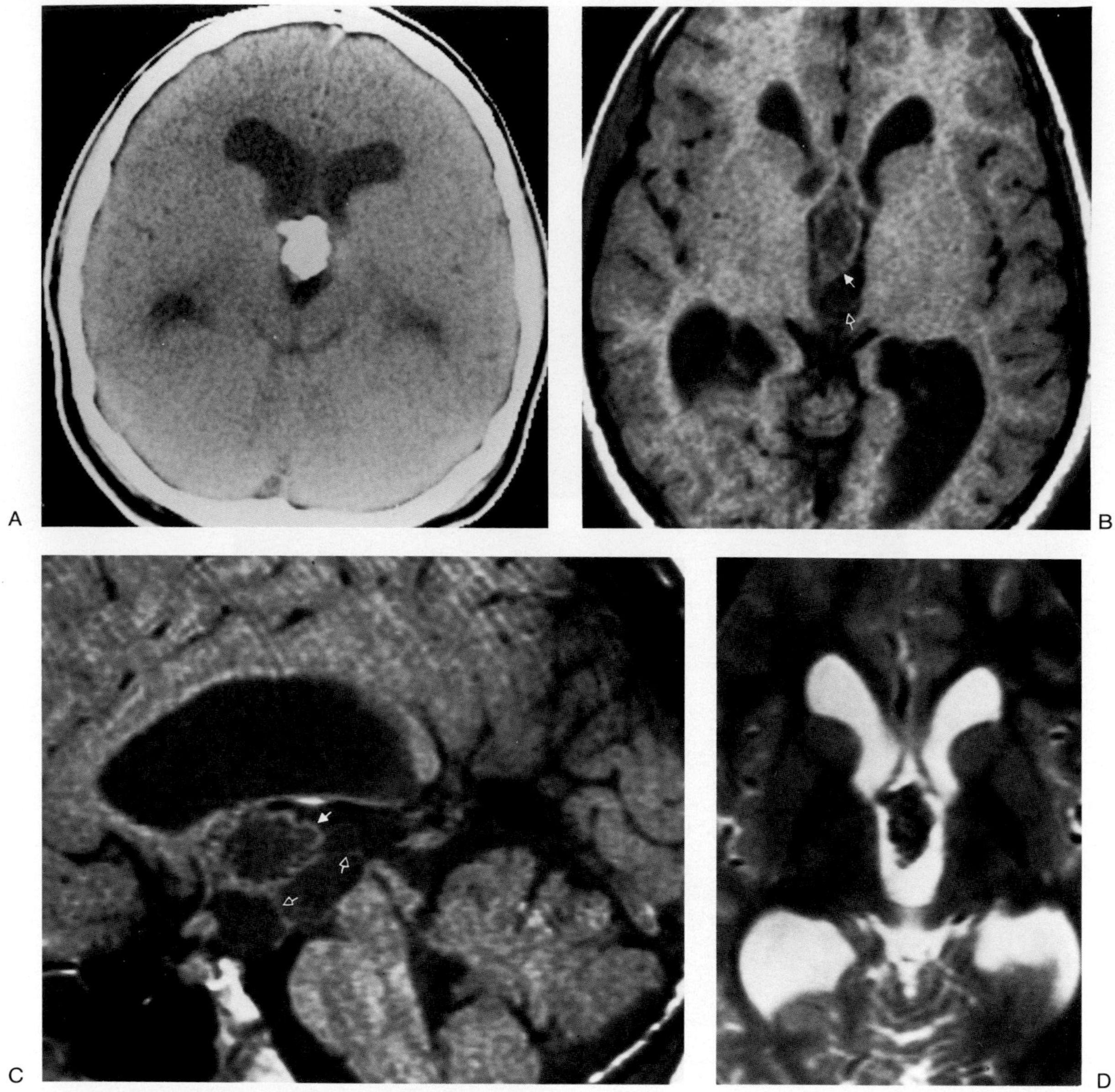

A

B

C

D

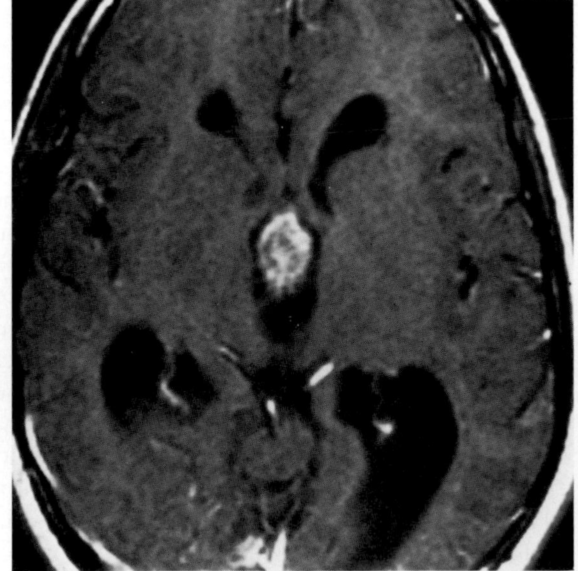

E

FIG. 65. Calcified cystic choroid plexus papilloma of third ventricle. **A:** Noncontrast axial CT scan demonstrates irregularly lobulated high-density mass in anterior third ventricle with dilatation of the lateral ventricles. **B,C:** Short TR/TE axial (B) and sagittal (C) images demonstrate a lobulated rim of isointense soft tissue surrounding a relatively hypointense portion of the mass (representing the area of calcification in A) in the anterior superior aspect of the third ventricle (*white arrow*). Multiple septa extend peripherally from this portion of the mass (*open white arrows*), creating several moderate-sized cystic pockets that expand the anterior and inferior aspect of the third ventricle. These collections are slightly less hypointense than surrounding CSF. The lateral ventricular dilatation is most likely related to tumor obstruction of the third ventricle. The aqueduct and the fourth ventricle are normal in size, as demonstrated in C. **D:** Long TR/TE axial image demonstrates marked hypointensity of the calcified portion of the lesion but contains within it several patchy areas of isointensity. **E:** Postgadolinium axial short TR/TE image demonstrates intense enhancement in the peripheral portion of the third ventricular tumor and some milder patchy enhancement in the central calcified region.

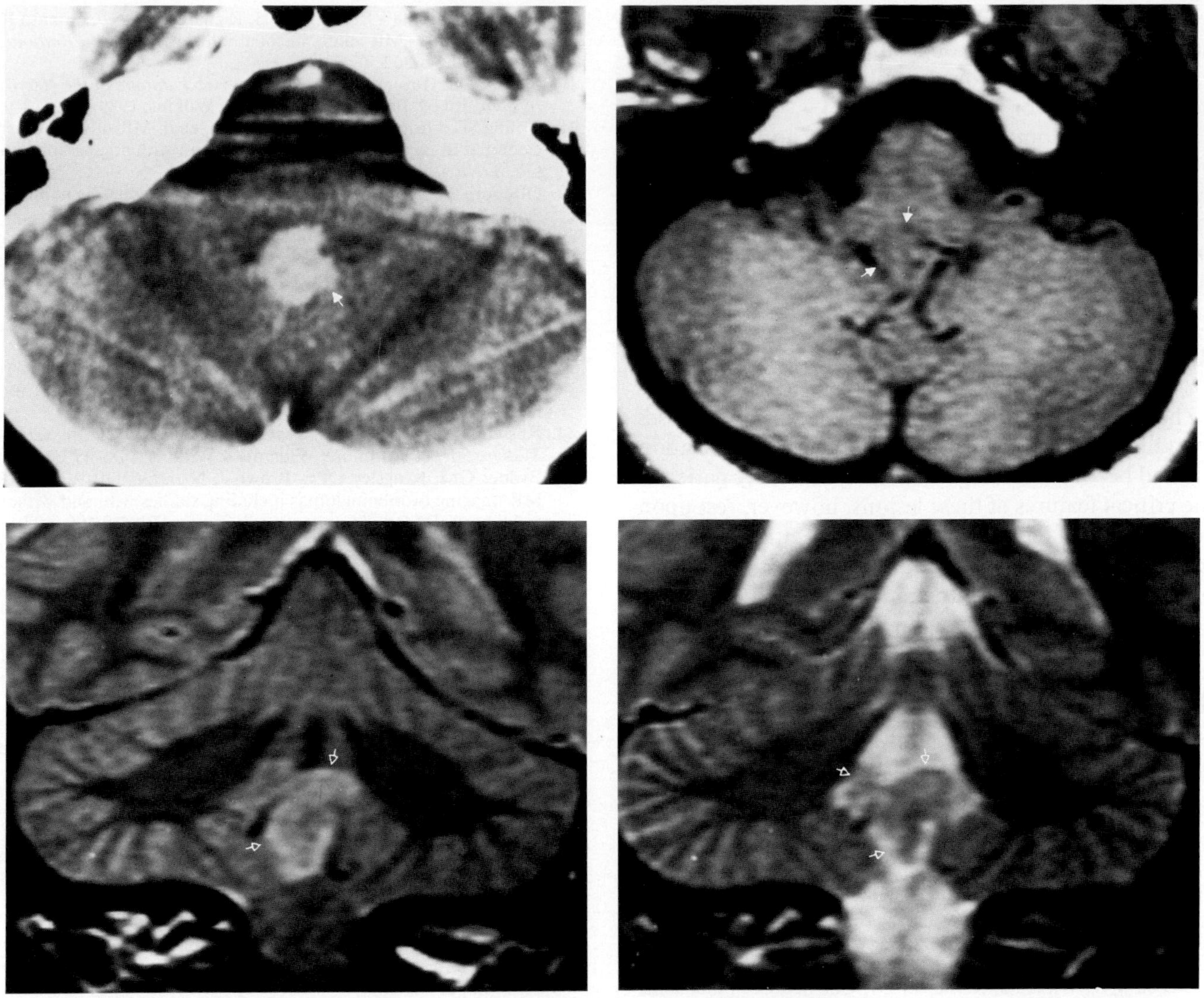

FIG. 66. Fourth ventricular choroid plexus papilloma. **A:** Contrast-enhanced axial CT scan at level of fourth ventricle demonstrates irregularly lobulated mass within the fourth ventricle (*arrow*). **B:** Short TR/TE axial image through lower fourth ventricle demonstrates isointense tissue within inferior fourth ventricle and foramen of Magendie (*arrows*). **C,D:** Coronal long TR/short TE (C) and long TE (D) images through fourth ventricle demonstrate irregularly lobulated mass within the fourth ventricle extending slightly through the foramen of Magendie. The tumor is heterogeneous and mildly hyperintense in C and heterogeneous and mildly hypointense in D (*arrows*).

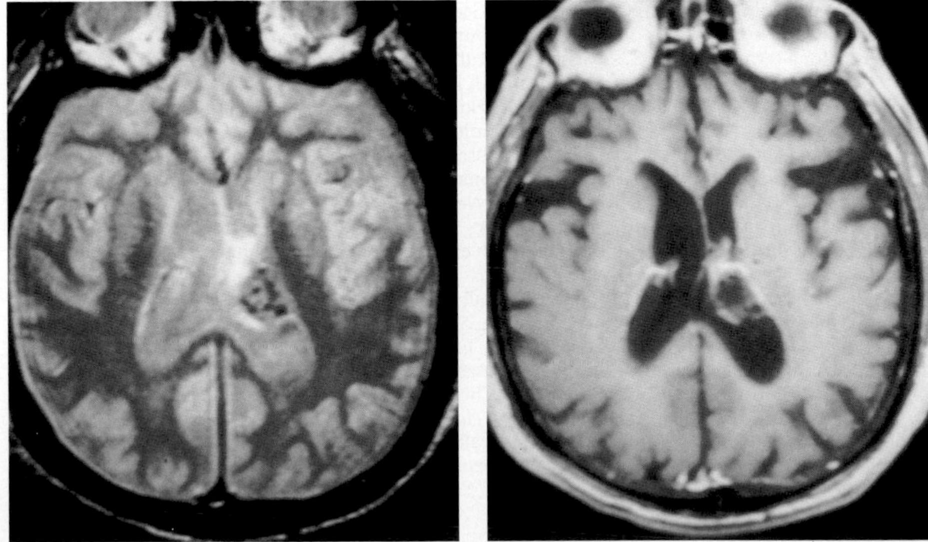

FIG. 67. Xanthogranulomatous change in choroid plexus. Heterogeneous, partially cystic signal in enlarged left lateral ventricular choroid plexus (**A**), which partially enhances (**B**) is benign xanthogranulomatous degeneration in this case.

reveal a moderately lobulated mass within the ventricle that does not invade through the ventricular wall but may extend out of the fourth ventricle through the foramen of Magendie or Luschka (Fig. 66).

Xanthogranulomatous change in the choroid plexus is a benign degenerative phenomenon most commonly seen bilaterally in lateral ventricle choroid. This dystrophic change is usually not mistaken for neoplastic involvement, but occasional cases are difficult to distinguish from other masses (Fig. 67).

CONCLUSIONS

The evaluation of intracranial extra-axial brain masses is readily made with MRI, and in fact some correlation is found between histology and signal intensity patterns. The critical features of these lesions, however, rest upon identification of the extra-axial site of origin. Boundaries between brain parenchyma and the mass should be sought when assessing intracranial tumors, since treatment and prognosis hinge upon this diagnosis.

REFERENCES

1. Hardman JM. Non-glial tumors of the nervous system. In: Schochet SS Jr, ed. *Neuropathology*, vol 3 of Rosenberg RN, ed. *The Clinical Neurosciences.* New York: Churchill Livingstone; 1983: 119.
2. Cushing H, Eisenhardt L. *Meningiomas. Their Classification, Regional Behaviour, Life History and Surgical End Results.* Springfield, IL: Charles C Thomas: 1938:69.
3. Grant FG. A study of the results of surgical treatment in 2,326 consecutive patients with brain tumor. *J Neurosurg* 1956;13:479–488.
4. Wood MW, White RJ, Kernohan JW. One hundred intracranial meningiomas found incidentally at necropsy. *J Neuropathol Exp Neurol* 1957;16:337–340.
5. Rausing A, Ybo W, Stenflo J. Intracranial meningioma—a population study of ten years. *Acta Neurol Scand* 1970;46:102–110.
6. Kepes JJ. *Meningiomas. Biology, Pathology and Differential Diagnosis.* New York: Masson; 1982:17.
7. Deen HG Jr, Scheithauer BW, Ebersold MJ. Clinical and pathological study of meningiomas of the first two decades of life. *J Neurosurg* 1982;56:317.
8. Nakasu S, Hirano A, Shimura T, Llena JF. Incidental meningiomas in autopsy study. *Surg Neurol* 1987;27:319.
9. Sheehy JP, Crockard HA. Multiple meningiomas: a long-term review. *J Neurosurg* 1983;59:1–5.
10. Russell DS, Rubinstein LJ. *Pathology of Tumours of the Nervous System*, 5th ed. Baltimore: Williams & Wilkins; 1989:455.
11. Brant-Zawadzki M, Norman D, Newton TH, et al. Magnetic resonance of the brain: the optimal screening technique. *Radiology* 1984;152:71–77.
12. Bradley WG Jr, Waluch V, Yadley RA, Wycoff RR. Comparison of CT and MR in 400 patients with suspected disease of the brain and cervical spinal cord. *Radiology* 1984;152:695–702.
13. Zimmerman RD, Fleming CA, Saint-Louis LA, Lee BC, Manning JJ, Deck MD. Magnetic resonance imaging of meningiomas. *AJNR* 1985;6:149–157.
14. Spagnoli MV, Goldberg HI, Grossman RI, et al. Intracranial meningiomas: high-field MR imaging. *Radiology* 1986;161:369–375.
15. Yeakley JW, Kulkarni MV, McArdle CB, Haar FL, Tang RA. High-resolution MR imaging of juxtasellar meningiomas with CT and angiographic correlation. *AJNR* 1988;9:279–285.
16. Elster AD, Challa VR, Gilbert TH, Richardson DN, Contento JC. Meningiomas: MR and histopathologic features. *Radiology* 1989;170:857–862.
17. Russell DS, Rubinstein LJ. *Pathology of Tumours of the Nervous System*, 5th ed. Baltimore: Williams & Wilkins; 1989:470.
18. Young SC, Grossman RI, Goldberg HI, et al. MR of vascular encasement in parasellar masses: comparison with angiography and CT. *AJNR* 1988;9:35–38.
19. O'Moore PV, Goldberg HI, Gonatas N. Factors relating to meningioma brain edema. *AJNR* 1983;4:1138.
20. Bailey P, Cushing H, Eisenhardt L. Angioblastic meningiomas. *Arch Pathol* 1928;6:953.
21. Russell DS, Rubinstein LJ. *Pathology of Tumors of the Nervous System*, 5th ed. Baltimore: Williams and Wilkins; 1989.
22. World Health Organization. Classification of Brain Tumors. Zurich: WHO; March, 1990.
23. Burger PC, Scheithauer BW. Tumors of Meningothelial Cells. In: *Tumors of the Central Nervous System.* Washington, D.C.: Armed Forces Institute of Pathology; 1994:259–286.
24. Russell DS, Rubinstein LJ. *Pathology of Tumours of the Nervous System*, 5th ed. Baltimore: Williams & Wilkins; 1989:473.
25. Bydder GM, Kingsley DPE, Brown J, Niendorf HP, Young IR. MR imaging of meningiomas including studies with and without gadolinium-DTPA. *J Comput Assist Tomogr* 1985;9:690–697.
26. Felix R, Schorner W, Laniado M, et al. Brain tumors: MR imaging with gadolinium-DTPA. *Radiology* 1985;156:681–688.
27. Berry I, Brant-Zawadzki M, Osaki L, Brasch R, Murovic J, Newton TH. Gd-DTPA in clinical MR of the brain. *AJNR* 1986;7:789–798.
28. Breger RK, Papke RA, Pojunas KW, Haughton VM, Williams AL, Daniels DL. Benign extra-axial tumors: contrast enhancement with Gd-DTPA. *Radiology* 1987;163:427–429.
29. Borovich B, Doron Y. Recurrence of intracranial meningiomas: the role played by regional multicentricity. *J Neurosurg* 1986;64: 58–63.
30. Wilms G, Lammens M, Marchal G, et al. Thickening of dura surrounding meningiomas: MR features. *J Comput Assist Tomogr* 1989;13:763–768.
31. Tokumaru A, O'uchi T, Eguchi T, et al. Prominent meningeal enhancement adjacent to meningioma on Gd-DTPA-enhanced MR images: histopathologic correlation. *Radiology* 1990;175:431–433.
32. Jellinger K, Radszkiewicz T, Slowk F. Primary malignant lymphomas of the central nervous system in man. *Acta Neuropathol* 1975;(Suppl vi):95.
33. Helle TL, Britt RH, Colby TV. Primary lymphoma of the central nervous system. Clinicopathological study of experience at Stanford. *J Neurosurg* 1984;60:94.
34. Gill PS, Levine AM, Meyer PR, et al. Primary central nervous system lymphoma in homosexual men. Clinical, immunologic, and pathologic features. *Am J Med* 1985;78:742.
35. So YT, Beckstead JH, Davis RL. Primary central nervous system lymphoma in acquired immune deficiency syndrome: a clinical and pathological study. *Ann Neurol* 1986;20:266.
36. Barnard RO, Scott T. Patterns of proliferation in cerebral lymphoreticular tumours. *Acta Neuropathol* 1977;(Suppl vi):125.
37. Russell DS, Rubinstein LJ. *Pathology of Tumours of the Nervous System*, 5th ed. Baltimore: Williams & Wilkins; 1989:605–611.
38. Brant-Zawadzki M, Enzmann DR. Computed tomographic brain scanning in patients with lymphoma. *Radiology* 1978;129:67–71.
39. Pagani JJ, Libschit HI, Wallace S, Hayman LA. Central nervous system leukemia and lymphoma: computed tomographic manifestations. *Am J Neuroradiol* 1982;2:397–404.
40. Sze G, Soletsky S, Bronen R, Krol G. MR imaging of the cranial meninges with emphasis on contrast enhancement and meningeal carcinomatosis. *AJNR* 1989;10:965–975.
41. Cahill DW, Salcuman M. Neurosarcoidosis—a review of the rare manifestation. *Surg Neurol* 1981;15:204–211.
42. Silverstein A, Feuer MM, Siltzbach LE. Neurologic sarcoidosis: study of 18 cases. *Arch Neurol* 1965;12:1–11.
43. Posner JB, Chernik NL. Intracranial metastases from systemic cancer. *Adv Neurol* 1978;19:579.
44. Meyer PC, Reah TG. Secondary neoplasms of the central nervous system and meninges. *Br J Cancer* 1953;7:438.

45. Tsukada Y, Fouad A, Pickren JW, Lane WW. Central nervous system metastasis from breast carcinoma. Autopsy study. *Cancer* 1983;52:2349–2354.
46. Willis RA. *The Spread of Tumours of the Human Body.* 3rd ed. London: Butterworths; 1973.
47. Castaldo JE, Bernat JL, Meier FA, Schned AR. Intracranial metastases due to prostatic carcinoma. *Cancer* 1983;52:1739.
48. Batson OV. Function of vertebral veins and their role in the spread of metastases. *Ann Surg* 1940;112:138.
49. Henson RA, Urich H. *Cancer and the Nervous System. The Neurological Manifestations of Systemic Malignant Disease.* Oxford: Blackwell Scientific; 1982.
50. Spagnoli MV, Goldberg HI, Grossman RI, Bilaniuk LT, Gomori JM, Hackney DB, Zimmerman RA. Intracranial meningiomas: high-field MR imaging. *Radiology* 1986;161:369–375.
51. Fobben ES, Grossman RI, Atlas SW, et al. MR characteristics of subdural hematomas and hygromas at 1.5T. *AJNR* 1989;10:687–693.
52. Lee Y-Y, Glass JP, Geoffray A, Wallace S. Cranial computed tomographic abnormalities in leptomeningeal metastasis. *AJR* 1984; 143:1035–1039.
53. Enzmann DR, Tokye KC, Hayward R. CT in leptomeningeal spread of tumor. *J Comput Assist Tomogr* 1978;2:448–455.
54. Davis PC, Friedman NC, Fry SM, Malko JA, Hoffmann JC Jr, Braun IF. Leptomeningeal metastasis: MR imaging. *Radiology* 1987;163:449–454.
55. Mathews VP, Kuharik MA, Edwards MK, et al. Gd-DTPA enhanced MR imaging of experimental bacterial meningitis: evaluation and comparison with CT. *AJNR* 1988;9:1045–1050.
56. Frank JA, Girton M, Dwyer AJ, Wright DC, Cohen PJ, Doppman JL. Meningeal carcinomatosis in the VX2 rabbit tumor model: detection with Gd-DTPA-enhanced MR imaging. *Radiology* 1988;167:825–829.
57. Russell DS, Rubinstein LJ. *Pathology of Tumours of the Nervous System*, 5th ed. Baltimore: Williams & Wilkins; 1989:541.
58. Goldberg HI, Spagnoli MV, Grossman RI, Hackney DB, Zimmerman RA, Bilaniuk LT. High field MRI evaluation of acoustic neuroma. *Acta Radiol Suppl* 1986;369:173–175.
59. Press GA, Hesselink JR. MR imaging of cerebellopontine angle and internal auditory canal lesions at 1.5T. *AJNR* 1988;9:241–251.
60. Daniels DL, Millen SJ, Meyer GA, et al. MR detection of tumor in the internal auditory canal. *AJNR* 1987;8:249–252.
61. Shaw CM, Alvord EC. Congenital arachnoid cysts and their differential diagnosis. In: Vinken PJ, Bruyn GW, eds. *Handbook of Clinical Neurology. Congenital Malformations of Brain and Skull, Part II.* Amsterdam: North Holland; 1977:75–135.
62. Starkman SP, Brown TC, Linell SA. Cerebral arachnoid cysts. *J Neuropathol Exp Neurol* 1958;17:484–500.
63. Galassi E, Giancarlo P, Gaist G, et al. Arachnoid cysts of the middle cranial fossa: a clinical and radiological study of 25 cases treated surgically. *Surg Neurol* 1980;14:211–219.
64. Robertson SJ, Wolpert SM, Runge VM. MR imaging of middle cranial fossa arachnoid cysts: temporal lobe agenesis syndrome revisited. *AJNR* 1989;10:1007–1010.
65. Sato K, Shimosi T, Yaguchi K, et al. Middle fossa arachnoid cyst: clinical neuroradiological and surgical features. *Childs Brain* 1983;10:301–316.
66. Gandy SE, Heier LA. Clinical and magnetic resonance features of primary intracranial arachnoid cysts. *Ann Neurol* 1987;21:342–348.
67. Burger PC, Fogel FS. *Surgical Pathology of the Central Nervous System and its Coverings.* New York: John Wiley; 1982:117–123.
68. Russell, DS, Rubinstein LJ. *Pathology of Tumours of the Nervous System*, 5th ed. Baltimore: Williams & Wilkins; 1989:695.
69. Davis KR, Roberson GH, Taveras JM, New PF, Trevor R. Diagnosis of epidermoid tumor by computed tomography. Analysis and evaluation of findings. *Radiology* 1976;119:347–353.
70. Steffey DJ, De Filipp GJ, Spera T, Gabrielsen TO. MR imaging of primary epidermoid tumors. *J Comp Assist Tomogr* 1988;12:438–440.
71. Tampieri D, Melanson D, Ethier R. MR imaging of epidermoid cysts. *AJNR* 1989;10:351–356.
72. Yuh William TC, Barloon TJ, Jacoby CG, Schultz DH. MR of fourth-ventricular epidermoid tumors. *AJNR* 1988;9:794–796.
73. Horowitz BL, Chari MV, James R, Bryan RN. MR of intracranial epidermoid tumors: correlation of in vivo imaging with in vitro ^{13}C spectroscopy. *AJNR* 1990;11:299–302.
74. Russell DS, Rubinstein LJ. *Pathology of Tumours of the Nervous System*, 5th ed. Baltimore: Williams & Wilkins; 1989:692.
75. Newton DR, Larson TC III, Dillon WP, Newton TH. Magnetic resonance characteristics of cranial epidermoid and teratomatous tumors. *AJNR* 1987;8:945.
76. Zettner A, Netsky MG. Lipoma of the corpus callosum. *J Neuropathol Exp Neurol* 1960;19:305–319.
77. Kazner E, Stochdorph O, Wende S, Grumme T. Intracranial lipoma. *J Neurosurg* 1980;52:234–245.
78. Russell DS, Rubinstein LJ. *Pathology of Tumours of the Nervous System*, 5th ed. Baltimore: Williams & Wilkins; 1989:706.
79. Truwit CL, Williams RG, Armstrong EA, Marlin AE. MR imaging of choroid plexus lipomas. *AJNR* 1990;11:202–204.
80. Bohm E, Strong R. Choroid plexus papillomas. *J Neurosurg* 1961;18:493–500.
81. Rovit R, Schechter M, Chodroff P. Choroid plexus papillomas: observations on radiographic diagnosis. *AJR* 1970;110:608–617.
82. Heiskanen D. Intracranial tumors in children. *Child's Brain* 1977;3:69–79.
83. Pascual-Castroviejo I, Villarejo F, Perez-Higueras A, Morales C, Pascual-Pascual S. Childhood choroid plexus neoplasms: a study of 14 cases less than 2 years old. *Eur J Pediatr* 1983;140:51–56.
84. Radkowski MA, Naidich TP, Tomita T, Byrd SE, McLone DG. Neonatal brain tumors: CT and MR findings. *J Comput Assist Tomogr* 1988;12:10–20.
85. Milhorat TH, Hammock MK, Davis DA, Fenstermacher JD. Choroid plexus papilloma. I. Proof of cerebrospinal fluid overproduction. *Childs Brain* 1976;2:273–289.
86. Hooper KD, Foley LC, Nieves NL, Smirniotopoulos JG. The intraventricular extension of choroid plexus papillomas. *AJNR* 1987;8:469–472.
87. Coates TL, Hinshaw DB, Peckman N, et al. Pediatric choroid plexus neoplasms: MR, CT, and pathologic correlation. *Radiology* 1989;173:81–88.

Magnetic Resonance Imaging of the Brain and Spine, Second Edition, edited by Scott W. Atlas.
Lippincott-Raven Publishers, Philadelphia © 1996.

12

Intracranial Vascular Malformations and Aneurysms

Scott W. Atlas and Robert W. Hurst

Along with the maturation of conventional magnetic resonance (MR) imaging over the past few years, many technical advances in MR software and hardware have developed that are particularly well suited to the depiction of lesions of the cerebral vasculature. These innovations have allowed an exquisitely detailed, noninvasive characterization of most intracranial vascular pathologic conditions using what have now become standard techniques. It is well established now that MR imaging is the most specific and sensitive noninvasive modality for the detection of intracranial vascular malformations of all types, whether angiographically demonstrable or angiographically occult. Moreover, aside from subarachnoid hemorrhage (1), MR is more sensitive to the documentation of the sequelae of these lesions and complications of their treatment than computed tomography (CT) scanning. In fact, MR has virtually replaced CT as the screening modality of choice for intracranial vascular malformations and their complications in all clinical settings except in the search for acute subarachnoid blood (2).

In certain clinical settings and pathologies, it has even become apparent that the complete preoperative assessment of some types of vascular malformations (generally those without arterial components), as well as all secondarily related intracerebral pathology, can be made with MR alone. The continued refinement and development of newer pulse sequences, such as a variety of improvements to MR angiography (MRA), promise even more sensitive and sophisticated methods for detecting and specifically defining these lesions based on anatomic and pathophysiologic criteria as well as temporal evolution. Most recently, MR techniques have evolved that can demonstrate dynamic physiology rather than strictly anatomic derangement (i.e., "functional" MRI; fMRI) (see Chapter 30). These functional MRI techniques are beginning to be explored in the clinical setting and seem to be well suited to the regional mapping of brain functions in the presence of vascular malformations that occupy "eloquent" cortex (3). The ultimate role of fMRI in the study of vascular malformations, both for preoperative mapping as well as for more detailed investigations of anomalous development of cortical representations in the presence of congenital space-occupying lesions like AVMs, remains to be fully defined.

Although we recognize that MRI has now become part of the standard work-up of patients suspected (or known) to harbor these lesions, catheter angiography continues to be the definitive modality for the study of many of these lesions and is still the mainstay of diagnosis in the pre- and postoperative evaluation of arteriovenous malformations (AVMs) as well as aneurysms. It should be emphasized that, despite all the improvements in both

S. W. Atlas, M.D.: Neuroradiology Division, Department of Radiology, Oregon Health Sciences University, Portland, OR 97201.

R. W. Hurst, M.D.: Departments of Radiology, Neurosurgery, and Neurology, Hospital of the University of Pennsylvania, Philadelphia, PA 19104.

conventional MRI and sophisticated MRA techniques, intracranial aneurysms in particular still cannot be definitively excluded by any noninvasive modality, leaving conventional intra-arterial catheter angiography as the gold standard at this juncture for aneurysm diagnosis.

VASCULAR MALFORMATIONS

Vascular malformations of the brain have been classified by McCormick (4) and Russell and Rubinstein (5) into four major pathologic types: (a) AVM; (b) cavernous angioma; (c) capillary telangiectasia; and (d) venous angioma. The basis for these classifications is the fact that each of these entities has its own distinct pathologic abnormalities. In addition, each has its unique clinical presentation, treatment, and in most cases MRI characteristics. Although not typical, clinical imaging studies andnecropsy specimens have demonstrated that mixed vascular malformations, having pathologic characteristics of two or more of the major types, may also occur (6–10).

Aside from these congenital (developmental) lesions, a distinct entity is the dural AVM. The dural AVM (or fistula) represents an acquired vascular lesion, characterized by arteriovenous (AV) shunting involving vessels within the dural venous sinuses and coverings of the brain. Estimates of the overall incidence of vascular malformations involving the brain range from 0.1% to 4%.

Arteriovenous Malformations

The most common clinically symptomatic cerebrovascular malformation is the AVM. AVMs have an estimated incidence of about one seventh that of intracranial aneurysms (11), which corresponds to approximately 0.14% of the population. AVMs represent congenital anomalies of blood vessel development and result from preservation of direct communication between arterial and venous channels without an intervening capillary network (12).

The focus of all therapy in the management of the patient harboring an AVM is the tangle of abnormal vessels representing the site of this primitive communication—the *nidus*—which replaces the normal arterioles and capillaries with a low resistance, high flow vascular bed (Fig. 1). The nidus permits increased flow through the arterial feeding vessels to the AVM and delivers increased blood volume under relatively high pressure into the cerebral venous system. Therefore, it is of paramount importance in pretherapy imaging to delineate this vascular nidus.

Clinical Features

Although congenital, AVMs most commonly are not clinically apparent until the second through the fourth decades of life, with most having become symptomatic by the time the patient reaches age 40 years (13). In

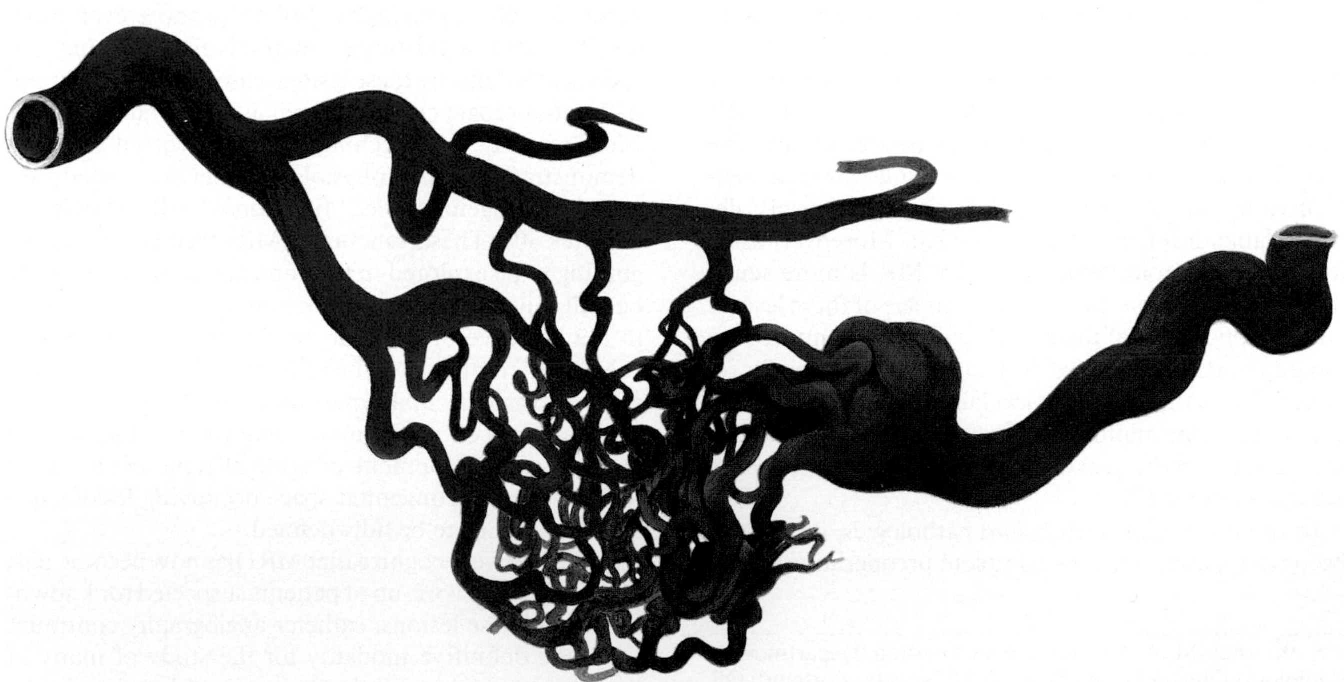

FIG. 1. AVM, artist's depiction. Tangle of vascular nidus receives supply from multiple enlarged, tortuous arteries. Markedly enlarged proximal draining veins carry arterialized blood.

adults, the most common initial symptom is related to acute intracranial hemorrhage, although larger AVMs are more likely to present with seizures rather than acute hemorrhage (14). Seizures and progressive neurologic deficits follow hemorrhage in frequency, and other less common clinical manifestations may also occur. In those cases where the AVM becomes apparent in the pediatric age group, hemorrhage is more likely than seizures to be the initial clinical event (15).

Intracranial hemorrhage heralds the existence of the AVM in 30% to 55% of patients and most often occurs during the second or third decade (16–18). More than 70% of patients who become symptomatic due to acute intracranial hemorrhage do so before age 40 years. Intracranial hemorrhage associated with AVMs is most often intraparenchymal, with the presumed site of bleeding being the nidus or proximal arterialized venous drainage. Intraventricular and subarachnoid hemorrhage may also occur, although AVMs represent the etiology of only a small minority of nontraumatic subarachnoid hemorrhages. On the other hand, the occurrence of nontraumatic isolated intraventricular hemorrhage (i.e., without subarachnoid hemorrhage) in an adult should always suggest the presence of an underlying AVM.

The rate of bleeding from AVMs has received much attention in the clinical literature. Until quite recently, it was generally thought that the incidence of bleeding from cerebral AVMs was much lower than that of intracranial (saccular) aneurysms. Current data, however, suggest a rate of hemorrhage in the range of 2% to 4% per year. It appears that the rate of hemorrhage from an AVM is at least as high (19) and probably exceeds that of aneurysmal hemorrhage from long-term follow-up studies (17,18).

Each occurrence of hemorrhage from an AVM is associated with a mortality of 10% to 15%, with an overall annual mortality rate in the range of 1%. In addition, permanent neurologic deficit associated with hemorrhage is estimated to be approximately twice the risk of death, that is, 20% to 30% per episode of hemorrhage, for an annual incidence in the range of 2%. The risk of rebleeding after the initial hemorrhage from cerebral AVM is estimated to be 6% during the first year (20). After the first year, the rebleeding rate decreases to that of the rate of initial hemorrhage in patients with symptomatic AVMs who had no clinical history of bleeding, estimated to be 2% to 4% per year (11,16). No significant increase in the risk of AVM hemorrhage has been associated with hypertension or specific situations, such as physical activity, pain, or trauma (11,16,21).

A high incidence of underlying AVM has been reported by many investigators in patients presenting with intracranial hemorrhage after cocaine abuse (22,23), so the diagnosis must be aggressively pursued in that specific clinical setting.

Seizures are also a common clinical manifestation of intracranial AVMs, reported as an initial symptom in from 20% to 60% of cases in several large series (11,14,20,24). More often associated with AVMs situated in the temporal and frontal regions, seizures will affect more than half of AVM patients younger than 30 years.

Acute or progressive neurologic deficits may result from the presence of an intracranial AVM. Although acute neurologic deficits have been reported to accompany 90% of AVM-associated intraparenchymal hemorrhages, neurologic deficits may arise in the absence of bleeding. In fact, the risk of significant morbidity and mortality is high in AVMs, whether or not the lesion has ruptured. Crawford et al. (17) followed 217 patients who had conservative management of their AVMs for a mean period of more than 10 years. They estimated that aside from the risk of hemorrhage, the risk of seizure disorder was 18%, and the risk of neurologic dysfunction was 27% during the 20-year follow-up in conservatively treated patients. In Anderson's study (25), there was a 25% risk of a patient becoming disabled because of intellectual impairment, even without hemorrhage.

Progressive and transient deficits have been ascribed to a number of potential pathophysiologic mechanisms. Among those proposed include "steal" of blood flow from adjacent normal regions of brain into the low resistance, high flow vessels feeding the AVM. Dilation of arterial supply to the AVM or enlarged draining veins may result in mass effect with resultant compression and neurologic dysfunction. Hydrocephalus may develop, either as a result of prior hemorrhage or by compression of adjacent CSF pathways. Venous hypertension represents an additional cause of neurologic dysfunction that may affect brain adjacent to or at a distance from the AVM nidus.

Headache is another frequently described clinical manifestation of intracranial AVMs that affects more than half of patients at some time during their clinical course (26). Although no characteristic headache pattern is consistently observed in AVM patients, a number of authors have reported atypical migraine-like pain with associated visual complaints. The incidence of true migraine, however, appears no higher in patients with AVMs than in the general population. AVMs with arterial supply from dural arteries may cause headache as a result of involvement of the pain-sensitive dura. Other mechanisms of pain include increased intracranial pressure, hemorrhage, hydrocephalus, or mass effect.

Additional clinical associations of AVMs include subjective bruit, which was noted in nearly 30% of patients in one series (16). Objective cranial bruit is an infrequent finding in adult patients with AVMs. Compression of cranial nerves is a rare symptom, most often reflected in atypical facial pain from involvement of cranial nerve V.

Hemifacial spasm and glossopharyngeal neuralgia due to involvement of the VIIth and IXth nerves have also been described (26).

Pathologic Findings

Although AVMs can be found throughout the central nervous system (CNS), intracranial AVMs are located in the supratentorial compartment in approximately 80% to 93% of cases. Supratentorial AVMs usually arise over the convexities and involve the distribution of the middle cerebral artery (MCA), typically visible over the surface of the cerebral hemisphere. However, deep-seated lesions are not uncommon. When AVMs are situated within deep structures, their venous drainage typically enlarges the deep venous system; in children, this may result in a massive enlargement of the vein of Galen ("vein of Galen aneurysm"). AVMs are most often solitary lesions, but they can be multiple when part of certain syndromes (27), including hereditary hemorrhagic telangiectasia (Rendu-Osler-Weber disease) and mesencephalo-oculo-facial angiomatosis (Wyburn-Mason syndrome).

On direct inspection, the gross pathologic appearance of an AVM is a tangled cluster of irregularly dilated vessels with varying wall thicknesses and luminal sizes (Fig. 2). Classically, AVMs appear as wedge-shaped clusters of vessels, with the apex of the wedge directed toward the ventricular surface and the base located at the cortical margin. Intervening brain parenchyma is not found within the vascular nidus itself, but feeding and draining vessels are separated by parenchyma when examining the malformation in its entirety (28).

Typically, neither displacement nor mass effect on adjacent structures is present unless either hemorrhage has occurred, or there has been development of large venous varices involved in the drainage of the lesion. With time, feeding arteries of the AVM gradually enlarge with increased flow, and venous drainage pathways undergo progressive dilatation and tortuosity. Approximately 10% of AVMs have associated arterial aneurysms, the vast majority of which occur on arteries hemodynamically related to the lesion (29,30). In one recent series, more than 98% of aneurysms originated from arteries hemodynamically or anatomically related to the AVM (30).

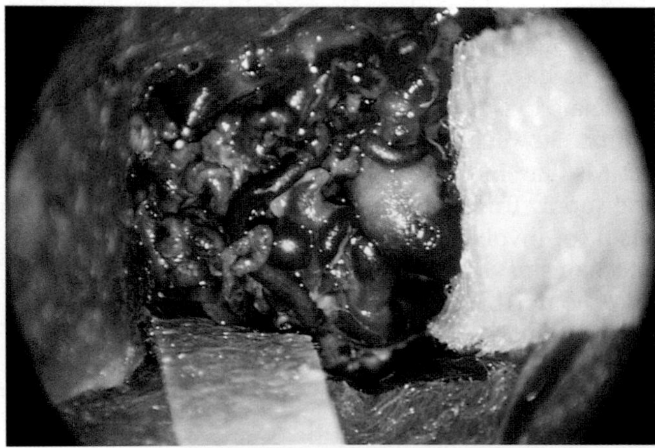

FIG. 2. AVM, intraoperative photograph. (Courtesy of Dr. E. Flamm, Philadelphia, PA.) Note well-circumscribed AVM with vessels of varying caliber and states of thrombosis.

On histopathologic examination, arterial channels in AVMs usually show well-defined elastic laminae, a feature absent in the venous channels. Wall thickening of both arterial and venous channels is often present with hyperplasia of smooth muscle cells, fibroblasts, and connective tissue. In many cases, focal areas of wall thinning may be found, representing sites of possible hemorrhage. Regions of thrombosis and recanalization are often present. Intervening and adjacent brain parenchyma frequently exhibit degenerative changes, seen as mild or extensive gliosis and demyelination (Fig. 3), often with concomitant parenchymal atrophy (28,31). Evidence of prior hemorrhage is also frequently present, as evidenced by ferritin, hemosiderin, and other iron-storage forms. Calcification may involve not only vessel walls but also adjacent brain parenchyma.

Pretreatment Grading of AVMs

Grading systems have been developed in an effort to rank individual AVMs into groups predictive of the difficulty associated with a specific treatment and the probable response to that treatment. Ideally, such a system should be sufficiently simple for easy application, yet comprehensive enough to permit grading of all AVMs. It should therefore encompass all features of the lesion that influence risks of the specific treatment modality, and it should accurately predict the degree of risk associated with the treatment. Although such an ideal grading system does not exist, a number of systems have been proposed.

Surgical grading scales are based on clinical, anatomic, and/or physiologic characteristics of the AVM and the patient. Features studied have included the age and sex of the patient, the presence of neurologic deficits, and the occurrence of prior hemorrhage. The number and location of feeding arteries, site and size of the AVM nidus, and pattern of venous drainage have also been included in various grading systems (32–36).

A relatively simple and widely used AVM grading system is that proposed by Spetzler and Martin (35). This system assigns a numerical grade to the AVM, with higher grades indicating more surgically difficult lesions. It requires evaluation of three features: (a) the size of the nidus, (b) the location of the nidus, and (c) the venous

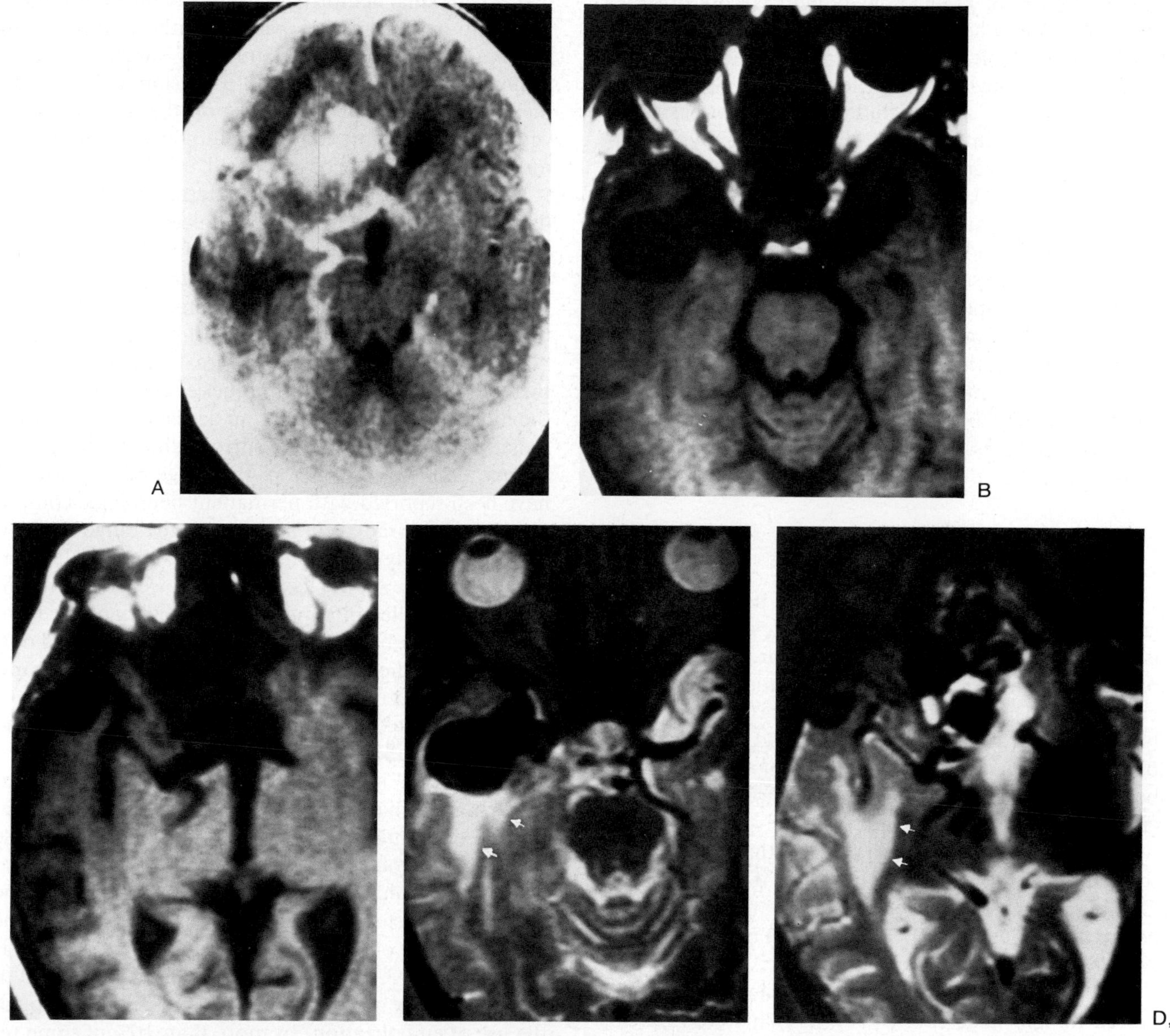

FIG. 3. Right hemispheric AVM, CT vs. MR. **A:** CT after contrast administration. **B:** Short TR/TE MR (600/20). **C:** Short TR/TE MR (600/20). **D:** Long TR/TE MR (3000/80). **E:** Long TR/TE MR (3000/80). CT (A) shows right frontal enhancing mass lesion with punctate calcification, which was originally interpreted as neoplasm. Large regions of signal void on MR (B–E) denote AVM with venous aneurysm, while surrounding high intensity on long TR/TE image (*arrows*, D,E) represents gliosis in adjacent parenchyma.

drainage pattern. The nidus size is scored as small (<3 cm), medium (3–6 cm), or large (<6 cm), with 1, 2, or 3 points given, respectively. Venous drainage is categorized as either superficial (score of 0), if drainage is entirely into the cortical venous system, or deep (score of 1), if any or all drainage enters the deep system. The location of the nidus is determined to be within either "eloquent" (score of 1) or "noneloquent" (score of 0) regions of brain, where "eloquent" areas are those with readily identifiable neurologic function and resultant disabling neurologic deficit when injured. By this definition, "eloquent" areas include sensorimotor, visual, or language cortex; internal capsule; thalamus; hypothalamus; brainstem; cerebellar peduncles; and deep cerebellar nuclei (Table 1).

The numerical score from these features are added to give the overall grade of the AVM. For instance, a Grade I lesion would be small, located in noneloquent cortex, and have only superficial venous drainage. A Grade V AVM would be large, involve eloquent cortex, and have deep drainage. In this system, large or diffuse AVMs encompassing the entirety of critical structures are classified as Grade VI because surgical resection of such lesions would be associated with unavoidable disabling neurologic deficit or death.

Therapy

Since AVMs have a grim prognosis if untreated, the goal of management (in the appropriate clinical setting) is complete obliteration of the nidus for cure. A variety of therapeutic arms are available for patients with intracranial AVMs, including surgery, intravascular embolotherapy, and radiotherapy, often used in some combined approach. Traditional treatment for AVMs has been surgical excision of the nidus. Complete surgical excision can be achieved in approximately 80% of AVMs with mortality and morbidity better than that arising from the natural history of the lesion if left untreated. Combined operative morbidity and mortality rates equals approximately 10% when taking into account all AVMs, regardless of grade (19).

Most postoperative morbidity in Heros' series occurred in very large AVMs, AVMs that were immediately adjacent to critical anatomy, and AVMs with deep venous drainage (i.e., those that would be classified as Spetzler Grade V). If one only considered AVMs of Grades I through IV, morbidity and mortality was only 4.5% in Heros' series. Because the rates of immediate rebleeding and mortality and morbidity associated with hemorrhage from AVMs are lower than those associated with aneurysmal hemorrhage, acute or emergent surgical intervention is limited to patients with life-threatening intracranial hemorrhage. Timing of surgery is determined by the characteristics of the lesion and the judgment of the surgeon. Depending on the risk associated with surgical treatment alone, adjunctive or alternative forms of therapy may be employed.

Radiosurgery or stereotactic external beam radiation therapy uses focused irradiation directed at the AVM nidus. Radiosurgery is usually pursued in those cases considered unsuitable for resection, because of either location of the AVM nidus or overall operative risk. Generally, the size of the nidus must be <3.5 cm for the AVM to be considered suitable for treatment by these methods. Radiotherapy techniques cause obliteration of the nidus secondary to radiation damage, with minimal radiation exposure of the surrounding brain parenchyma. Obliteration rates in the range of 75% to 90% have been reported with permanent neurologic complications (due to radiation necrosis) in the range of 3% to 10% (37–40). Significant controversy over the role of radiotherapy for AVMs continues, however, as recent studies have called into question the efficacy of any form of radiotherapy based on apparently worse reported outcomes from radiotherapy as compared to those from microsurgery in some hands (41).

Interventional neuroradiologic techniques can also contribute significantly to the management of the patient with an AVM. Embolization of AVMs using endovascular techniques has been found extremely useful in presurgical devascularization of the nidus and to decrease blood flow through the lesion. Embolization has also been shown to have a role in decreasing the size of the AVM nidus before radiosurgical therapy. Because the maximum size of the target diameter in radiosurgery is in the range of 3.5 cm, larger AVMs may be reduced in size and thereby made amenable to radiosurgery through the use of embolization. In more than 10% of some reported series, complete obliteration of AVMs has been achieved by embolization, making further therapy unnecessary (42). In most instances, however, embolization is used as part of a combined therapeutic approach to the lesion, most often before surgical resection.

TABLE 1. *"Eloquent" areas of brain*[a]

Primary sensory, motor, visual cortex
Speech areas of dominant hemisphere
Deep gray matter nuclei, internal capsule, thalami
Brainstem
Cerebellar nuclei

[a] The term "eloquent" is probably misleading here because it can be argued that all cerebral cortex is eloquent, particularly when noting recent functional brain imaging studies.

MR Imaging

Complete imaging evaluation of an AVM requires the acquisition of sufficient information upon which to select, plan, and carry out therapy. Features of the lesion to be evaluated include (a) the number, location, and specific identification of arterial supplies to the AVM (including collateral circulation to the AVM and vascular steal from adjacent normal brain); (b) associated vascular lesions (e.g., aneurysms); (c) the presence of hemorrhage (acute or chronic); (d) the location, size, and flow characteristics of the nidus; (e) venous drainage of both the AVM and the normal brain, including the presence of venous thrombosis, outflow restriction, or mass effect; and (f) follow-up of any prior therapy (35,43).

Although cerebral angiography clearly remains the definitive method of fully characterizing the vascular supply and venous drainage of intracranial AVMs, recent advances with MRI allow specific diagnosis of these lesions in the vast majority of cases. It has been recognized that improved anatomic delineation of the AVM nidus, its relationship to vital cerebral structures, and improved definition of the lesion in three-dimensional space with the use of MRI (Fig. 4) has contributed significantly to optimizing surgical approach (44) and has allowed treatment of some lesions that previously would have been thought to be inoperable (19).

Associated hemorrhage and other parenchymal changes, as well as post-therapy follow-up are best evaluated with the use of MRI in conjunction with supplemental MRA. MR information derived from these types of studies is complementary to the angiographic evaluation and clearly contributes significantly to accurate diagnosis and optimal therapeutic decisions (Fig. 5).

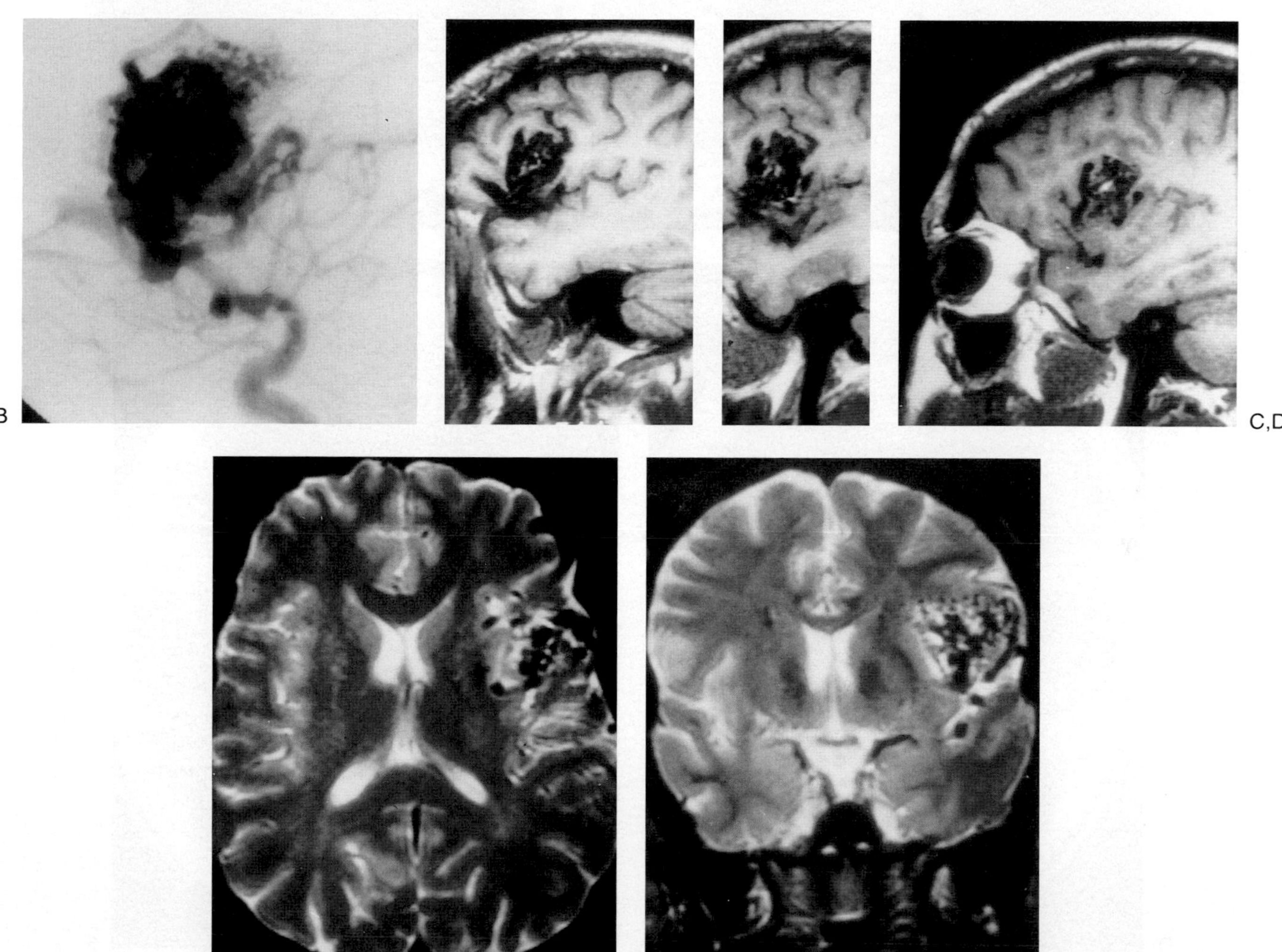

FIG. 4. AVM, complete anatomic delineation by MR. **A:** Arteriogram, oblique lateral view. **B–D:** Short TR/TE MRI, lateral to medial. **E:** Axial long TR/TE MRI. **F:** Coronal long TR/TE MRI. Although left frontal AVM is clearly defined by arteriography (A), the relationship of the lesion to sylvian fissure and its precise localization within inferior frontal gyrus (B–F) are fully defined in 3D space by multiplanar MRI. Signal void in lesion is evidence for high flow state in this frontal AVM.

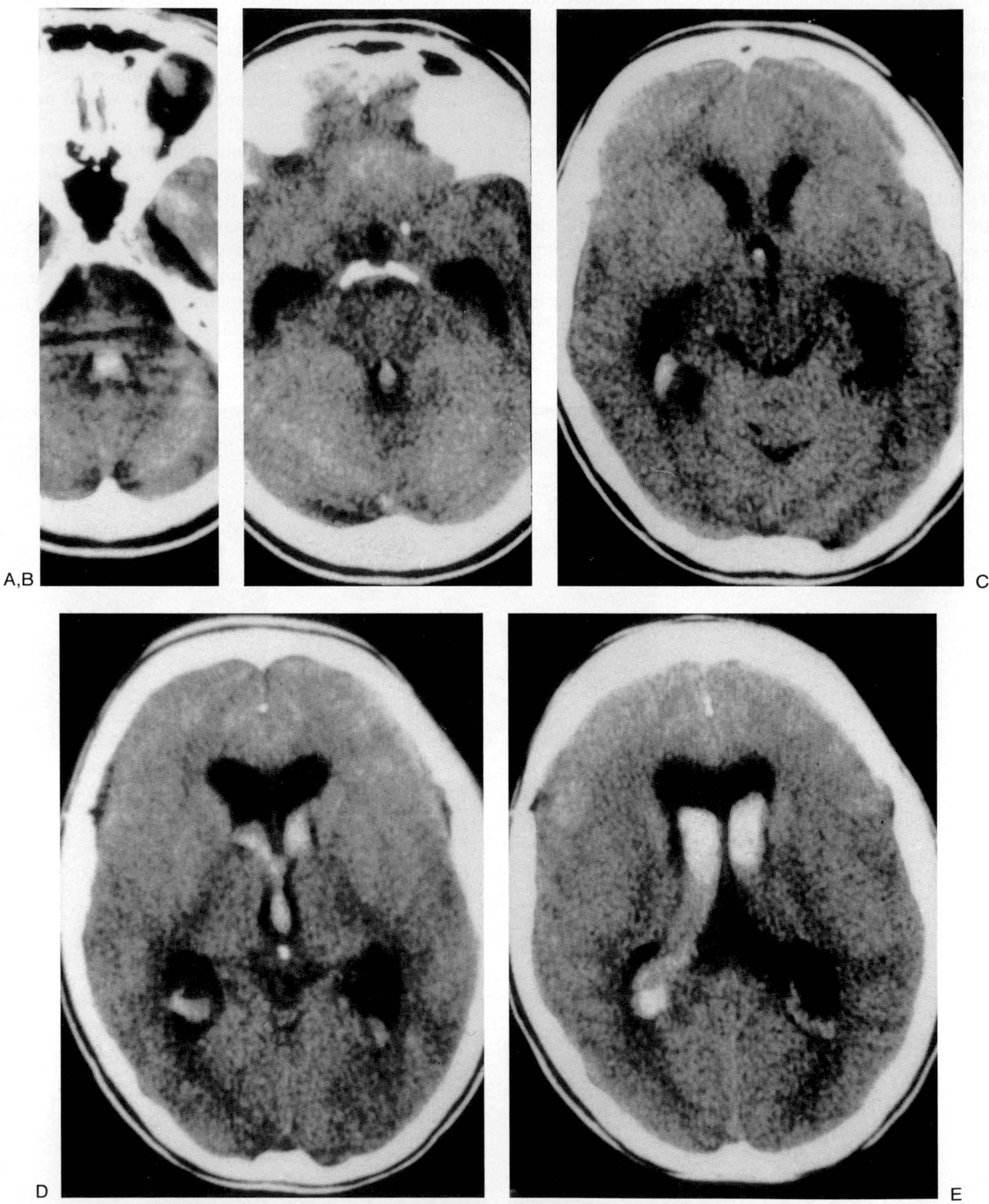

FIG. 5. AVM preoperative localization by MR. **A–E:** Axial CT, inferior to superior. **F–H:** Sagittal short TR/TE MRI. **I,J:** Axial long TR/TE MRI. The underlying cause of the acute intraventricular hemorrhage with hydrocephalus on CT (A–E) and MRI (F–J) is revealed as vascular flow voids of AVM nidus situated within atrium of left lateral ventricle on sagittal (F,G) and axial (I,J) MRI. Intraventricular localization altered the surgical approach in this case.

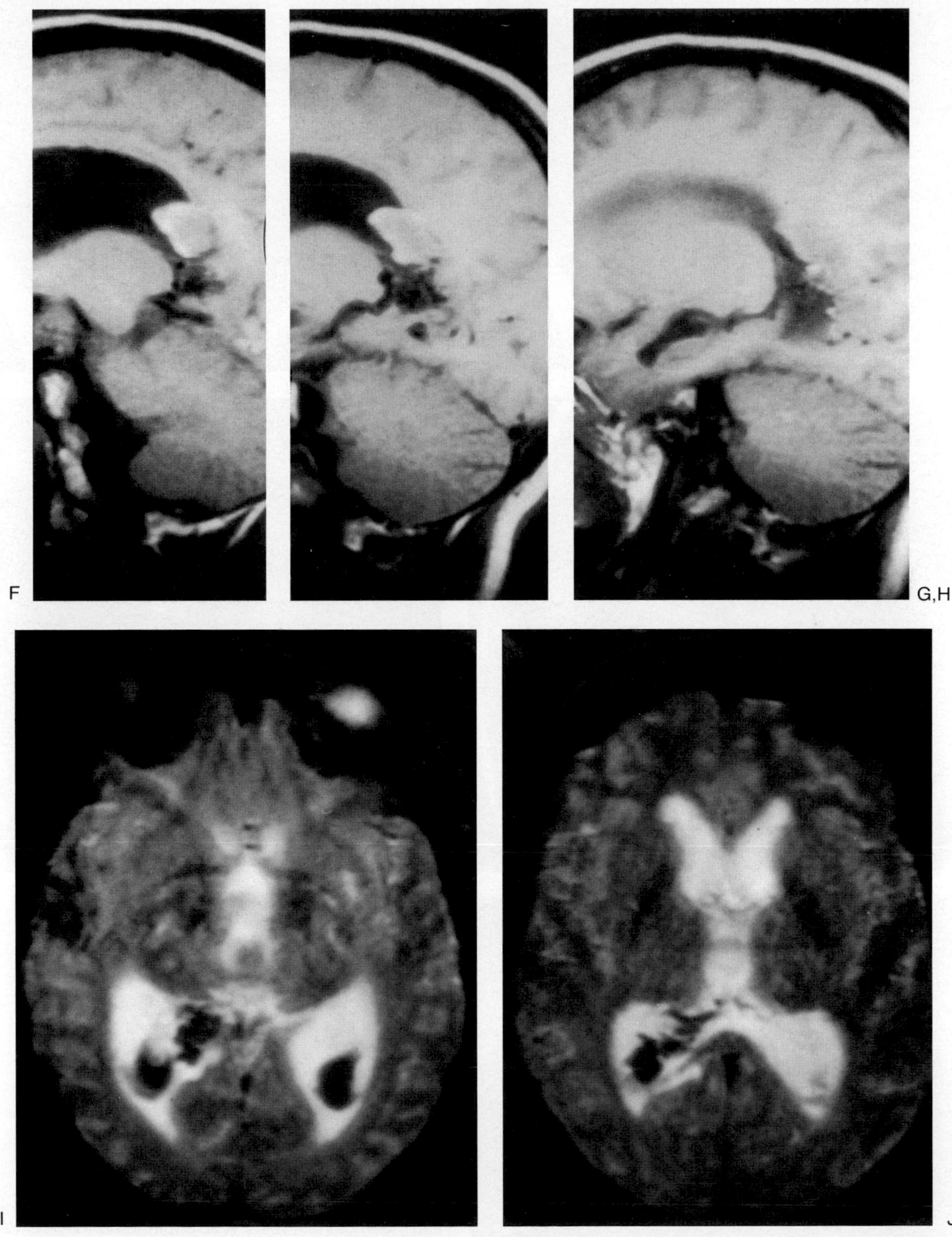

FIG. 5. *Continued.*

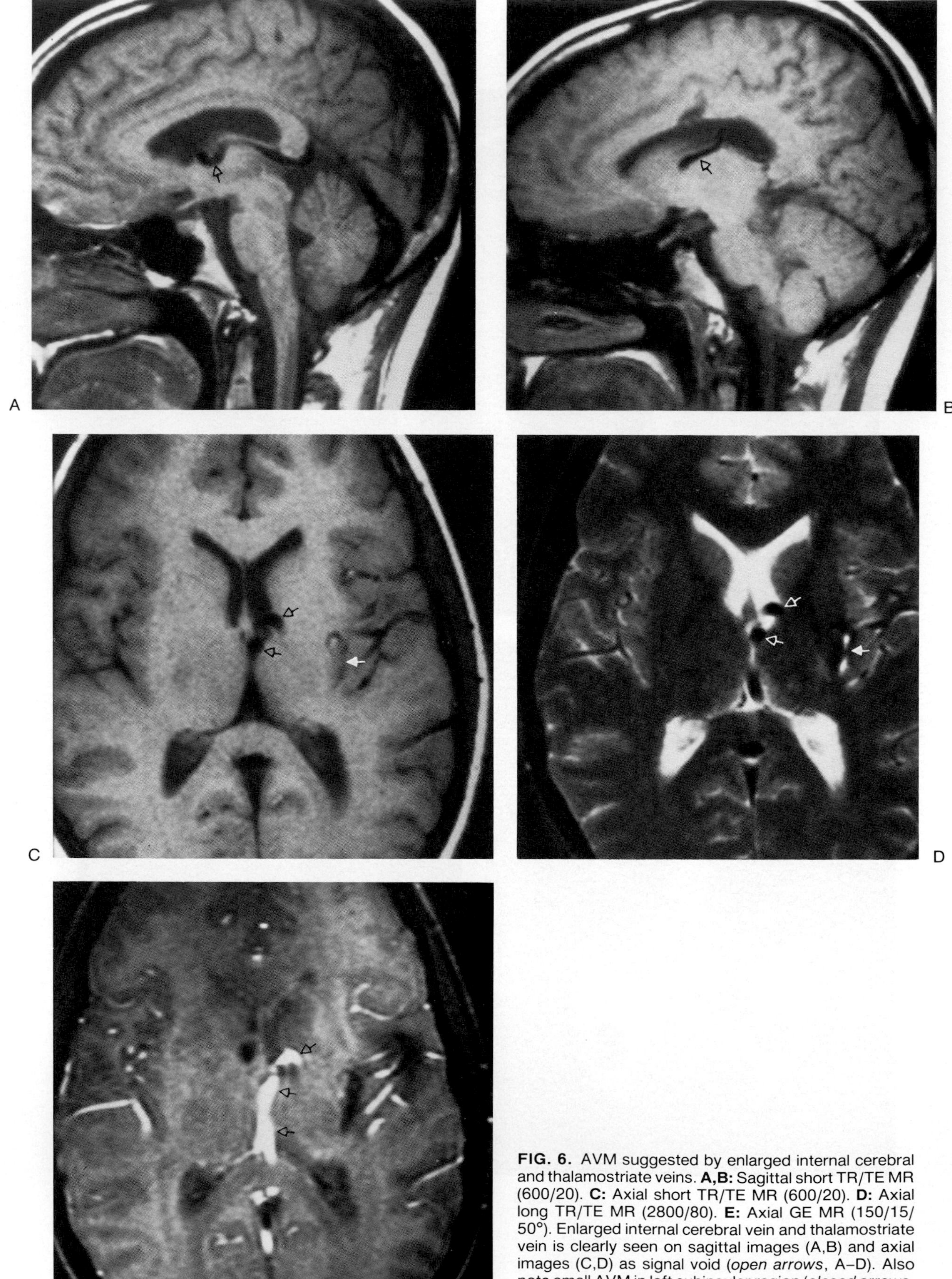

FIG. 6. AVM suggested by enlarged internal cerebral and thalamostriate veins. **A,B:** Sagittal short TR/TE MR (600/20). **C:** Axial short TR/TE MR (600/20). **D:** Axial long TR/TE MR (2800/80). **E:** Axial GE MR (150/15/50°). Enlarged internal cerebral vein and thalamostriate vein is clearly seen on sagittal images (A,B) and axial images (C,D) as signal void (*open arrows*, A–D). Also note small AVM in left subinsular region (*closed arrows*, C,D). Enlarged veins are high intensity on GE image (E).

The typical AVM on spin-echo (SE) MR is depicted as a cluster of focal round, linear, or serpentine areas of signal void (see Figs. 3–5), representing dilated vascular channels containing relatively rapidly flowing blood (45).

Although large high flow AVMs are usually obvious diagnoses on MR imaging, subtle enlargement of deep veins occasionally may be the only clue to the diagnosis of these high flow lesions (Fig. 6). Note that certain MR sequences can result in high intensity in areas of flowing blood (Figs. 6 and 7), because of either flow-related enhancement or even echo rephasing (46) or because of the now routine incorporation of gradient moment nulling into SE imaging. High intensity from these phenomena is generally a reflection of slower flow. Gadolinium enhancement of the enlarged vessels also occurs in those vessels with relatively slow flow, that is, mainly the venous side of the lesion. AVM niduses can partially enhance after gadolinium (Fig. 8), but the rapidly flowing blood within arterial feeding vessels generally does not enhance. Despite the traditional teaching stating that intraparenchymal AVMs demonstrate little or no mass effect on imaging studies unless hemorrhage has occurred, enlargement of draining veins can result in fairly significant mass effect (Figs. 9), even in the absence of hemorrhage, in up to one third of cases (16).

Aside from the features of the intracranial AVM itself, associated findings on MRI may provide further insight into the natural history of these lesions and aid in predicting the development of secondary clinical deficits in individual patients. The presence and age of any associated intraparenchymal hemorrhage and its resultant mass effects are clearly seen on MR. Associated intraparenchymal hemorrhage can be aged on the basis of signal intensity patterns (see Chapter 9). Staining of adjacent brain by iron-storage products can suggest prior subclinical hemorrhage from a clinically asymptomatic AVM. Intraventricular or superficial cortical hemosiderosis from prior (or recurrent) subarachnoid hemorrhages is a frequent accompaniment to vascular malformations. This entity, not usually seen on CT, is often an incidental MR finding, but patients can develop cranial nerve palsies, most commonly sensorineural hearing loss, or extraventricular obstructive hydrocephalus. Long TR/TE (T2-weighted) SE and gradient-echo (GE) images demonstrate marked hypointensity along the surface of the brain parenchyma or along the ependymal surface of the

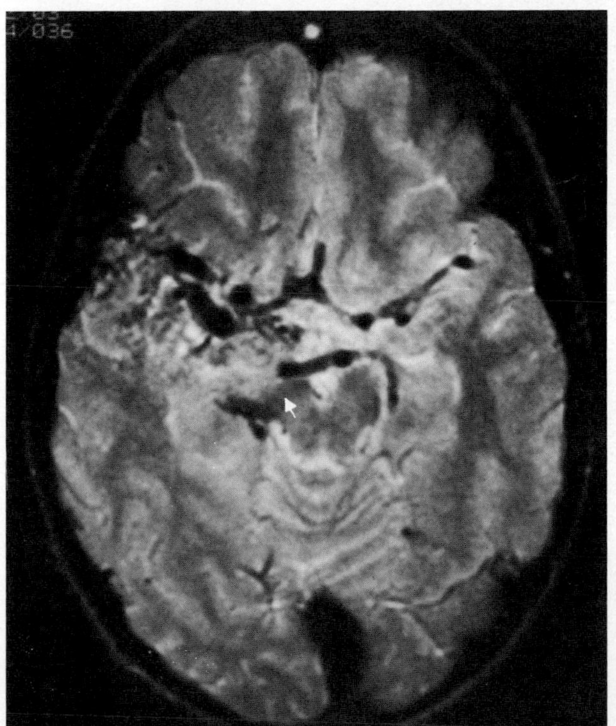

A

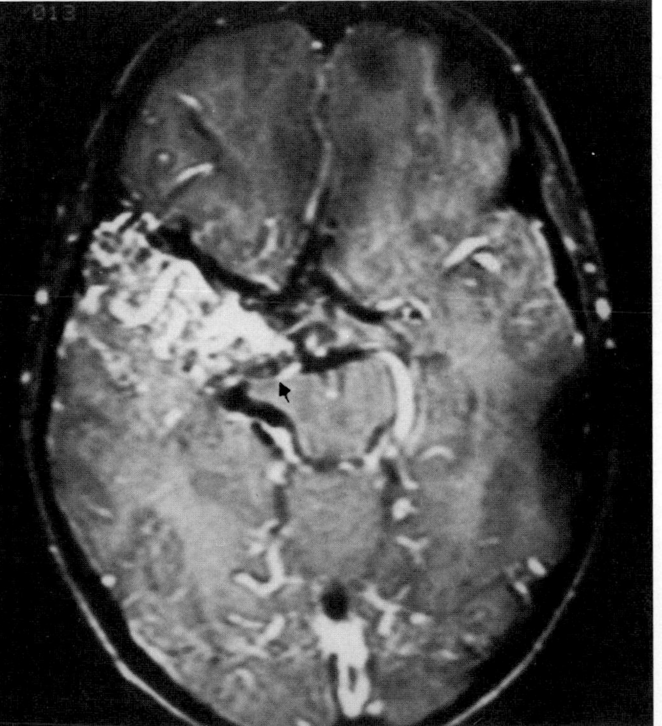

B

FIG. 7. Right frontotemporal AVM, SE vs. GE characteristics. **A:** Long TR/TE SE MR (2800/80). **B:** GE MR (150/15/50°). Note the typical appearance of wedge-shaped cluster of vessels in right frontotemporal region, seen as linear and round areas of signal void on SE image (A). The AVM is high intensity on GE image (B), and is apparently larger than suspected from SE image alone, because of clearer depiction of regions of slow flow, which were isointense to brain on long TR/TE SE image (A). Mass effect is seen on right cerebral peduncle (*open arrow*). (From Atlas, ref. 163, with permission.)

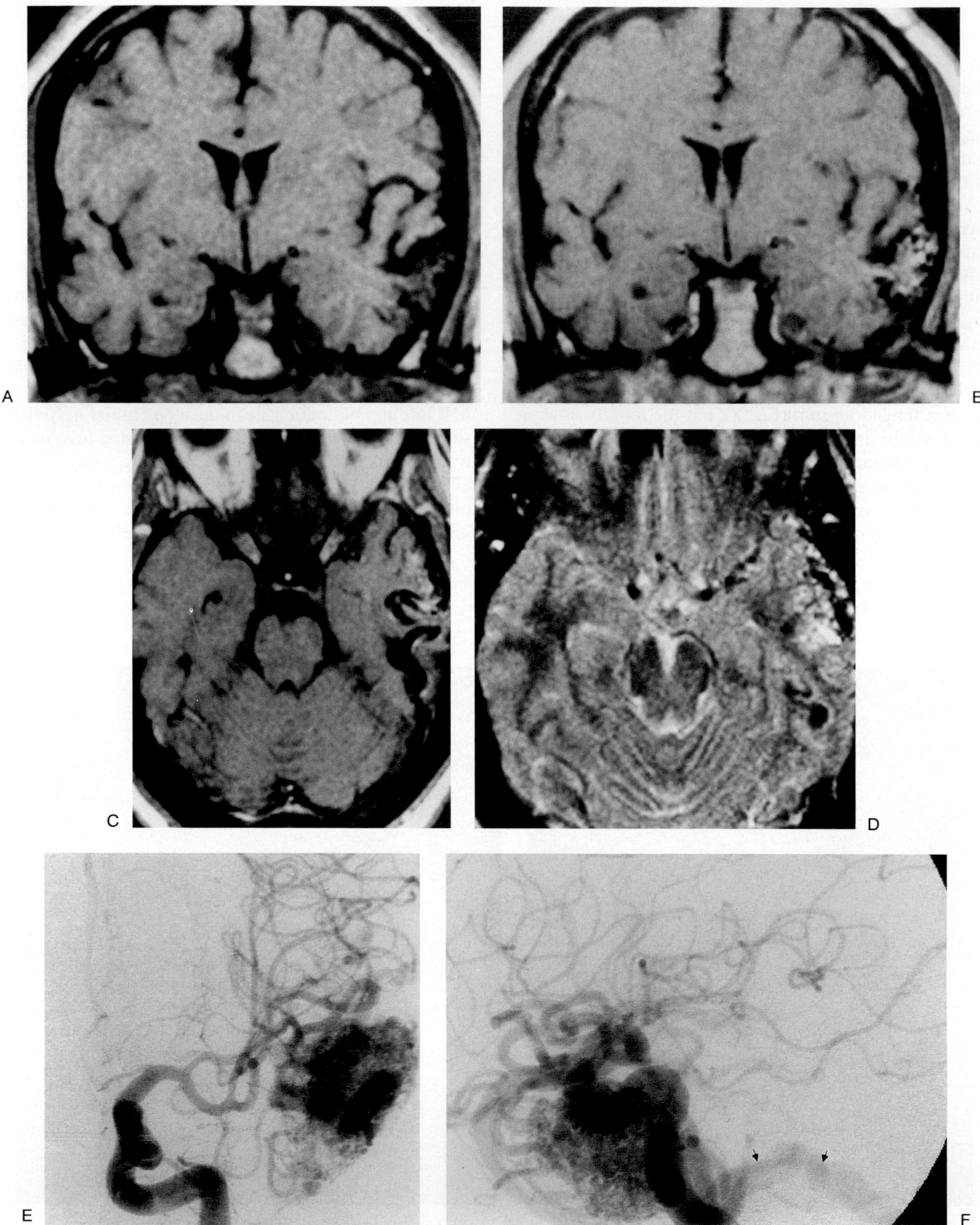

FIG. 8. AVM with enhancing nidus. Coronal unenhanced (**A**) and enhanced **(B)** T1-weighted images (650/25) demonstrate multiple areas of signal void within atrophic left temporal gyrus. Heterogeneous enhancement of nidus is present. Axial enhanced T1- (**C**) and (**D**) T2-(3000/100) weighted images show heterogeneous signal within nidus and enlarged draining vein (*arrows*). **E:** AP and lateral (**F**) views of left ICA injection demonstrate AVM nidus with enlarged early draining vein (*arrows*).

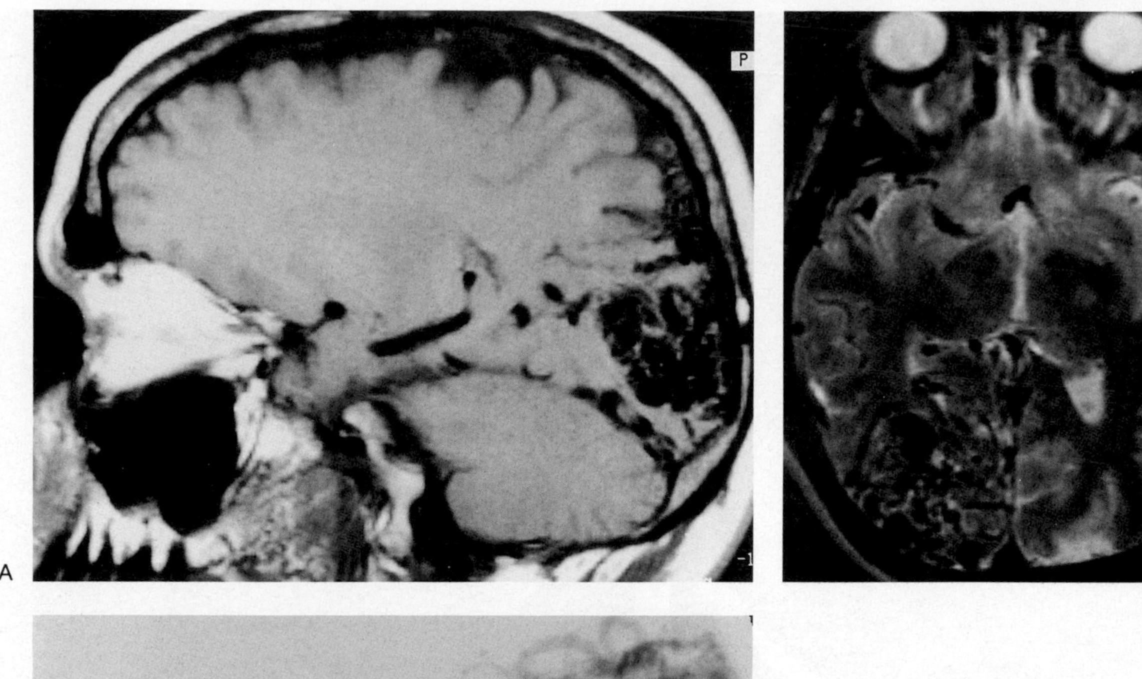

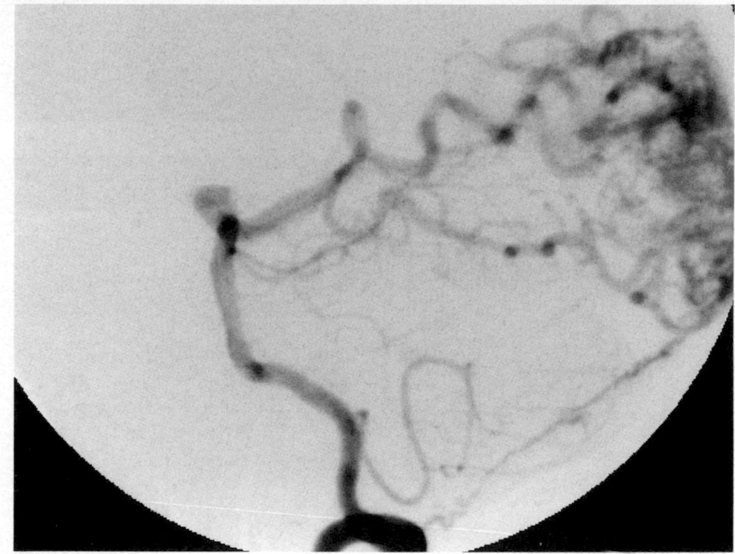

FIG. 9. AVM with mass effect in the absence of hemorrhage. Wedge-shaped nidus of occipital AVM (**A,B**) fed by dural and pial vessels (**C**) has mass effect on atrium of left lateral ventricle and effaces sulci (A,B) despite lack of hemorrhage.

ventricle (Fig. 10) (47) in this entity. Venous occlusive disease, probably an important pathophysiologic feature of many AVMs, should be searched for on MR. This can be suggested by massively dilated vessels (nearly always representing veins) of either the deep or superficial venous system. Enlargement of the medullary veins, even in the contralateral hemisphere from the site of the AVM, is an important clue to venous occlusive disease (particularly in dural AV fistulae—see below). Signal intensity alterations representing gliosis and/or secondary demyelination in the vicinity of the AVM are easily demonstrated as well and implies chronic vascular ischemia, perhaps because of "steal" from adjacent brain.

To determine the precise role of MRI in the diagnostic work-up of intracerebral AVMs, several investigators have studied patients with these lesions and compared MRI findings to those of other imaging modalities (44,48,49). MRI has been shown to be superior to both CT and catheter angiography for demonstrating the neuroanatomic location of the nidus and the relationship of its supplying and draining vessels to deep ganglionic structures, the ventricular system (Figs. 5 and 11), and the corpus callosum (Fig. 12). This information is critical to treatment planning, whether surgical, endovascular, or radiosurgical (50).

MR is more accurate than CT in determining the overall size of the nidus, probably because of the ease of imaging in multiple planes with MR (see Fig. 4). The size of the AVM nidus is important for many reasons, including an overall increase in operative grade (and risk) with increasing nidus size, and the potential for normal perfusion pressure breakthrough after a large nidus is re-

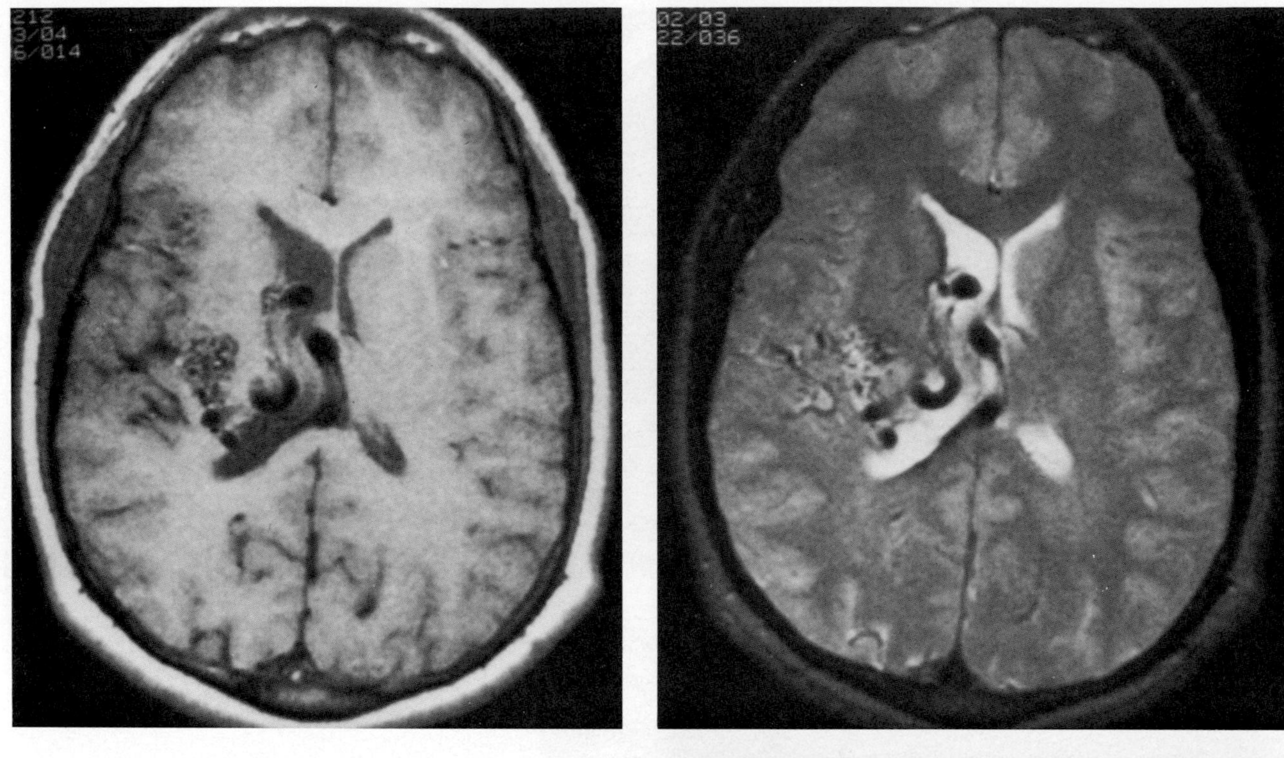

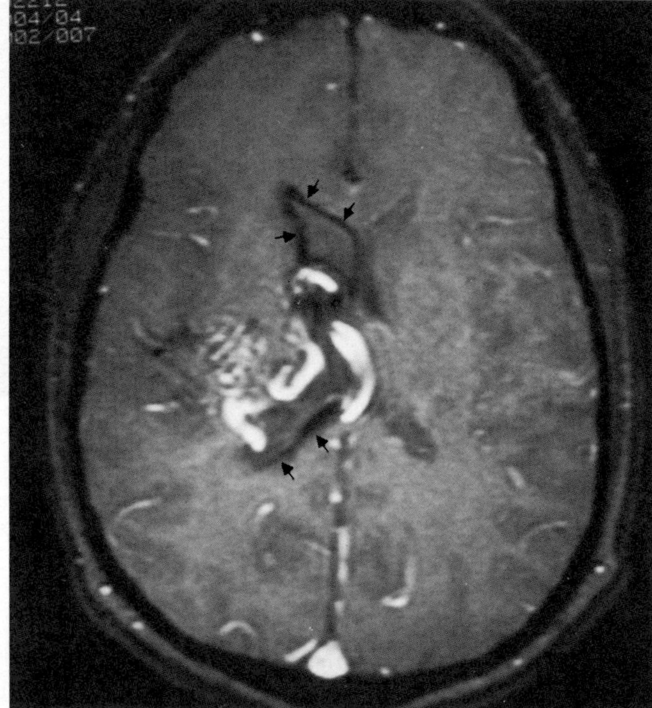

FIG. 10. Intraventricular AVM with intraventricular siderosis. **A:** Short TR/TE MR (600/20). **B:** Long TR/TE MR (2800/80). **C:** GE MR (150/15/50°). Right ganglionic and intraventricular AVM is unambiguously depicted as round and serpentine regions of signal void on SE images (A,B) and as high intensity on GE image (C). Note marked hypointensity lining right lateral ventricle (*arrows,* C), more obvious on GE image (C), indicating prior intraventricular hemorrhage. (From Atlas et al., ref. 76, with permission.)

FIG. 11. AVM adjacent to blood-filled lateral ventricle. Axial T1-weighted (**A**) and T2-weighted FSE (**B**) images demonstrate increased signal of subacute hemorrhage in the right mid-temporal lobe with interventricular extension. Adjacent areas of signal void are present. Interventricular hemorrhage within the third and fourth ventricles is present on sagittal T1-weighted image (**C**). Frontal projection compressed view MRA (**D**) (phase contrast 90 cm/sec VENC) outlines portion of nidus and enlarged early draining vein. Enlarged feeding arteries from MCA (*arrows*) and PCA (*open arrows*) are seen. AP right ICA (**E**) and right vertebral artery (**F**) injections illustrate enlarged arterial feeding vessels from MCA (*arrows*) and PCA (*open arrows*) as well as early filling vein.

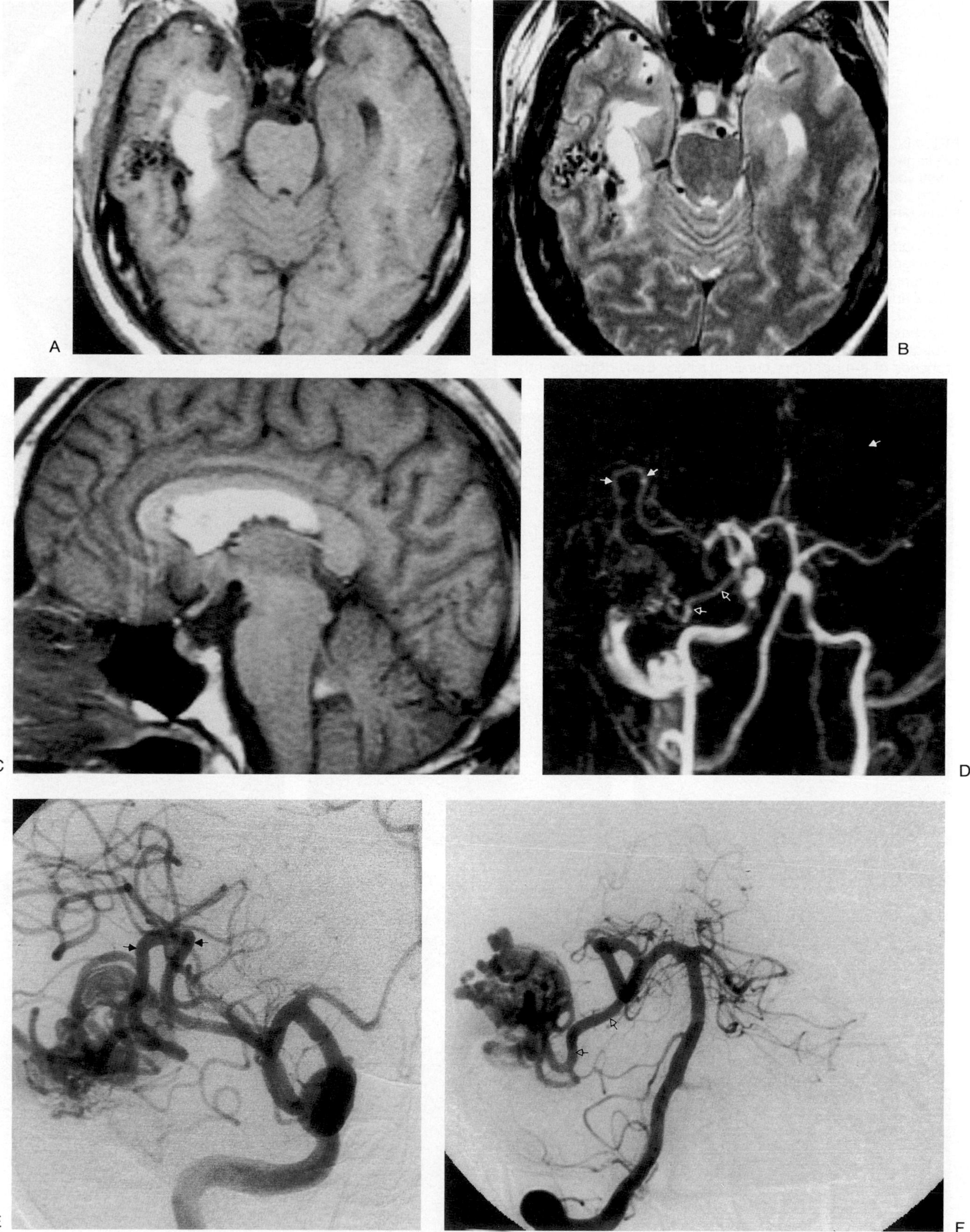
A
B
C
D
E
F

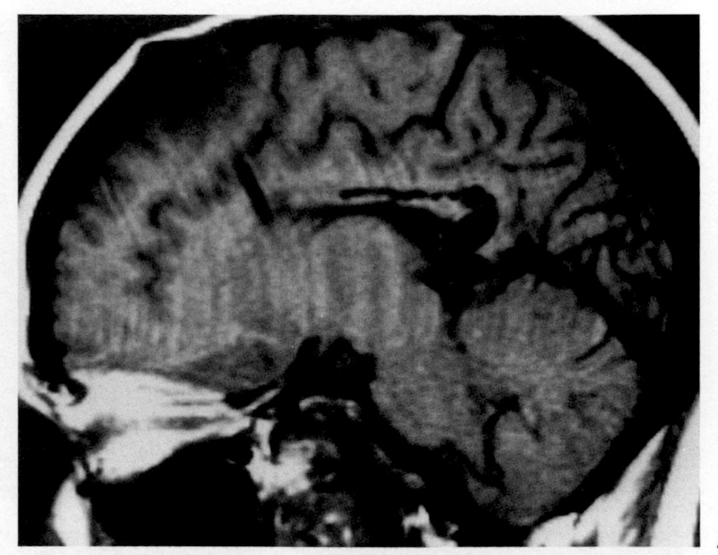

FIG. 12. AVM involving corpus callosum. T1-weighted (500/16) sagittal (**A**) and axial (**B**) images demonstrate serpentine signal voids within posterior body and splenium of corpus callosum. Splenium adjacent to the nidus shows decreased signal (shunt had been placed following interventricular hemorrhage 10 years earlier). Following administration of gadolinium, partial enhancement of the nidus occurs (**C**). Axial T2-weighted (2350/90) image (**D**) shows flow voids within splenium and adjacent decreased signal of iron-storage products. Early (**E**) and late (**F**) phase of right ICA injection shows filling of AVM nidus via distal anterior cerebral artery branches. Enlarged posterior communicating artery fills nidus through posterior choroidal and posterior pericallosal branches of the posterior cerebral artery. Early drainage into the deep venous system is present (*arrows*).

A

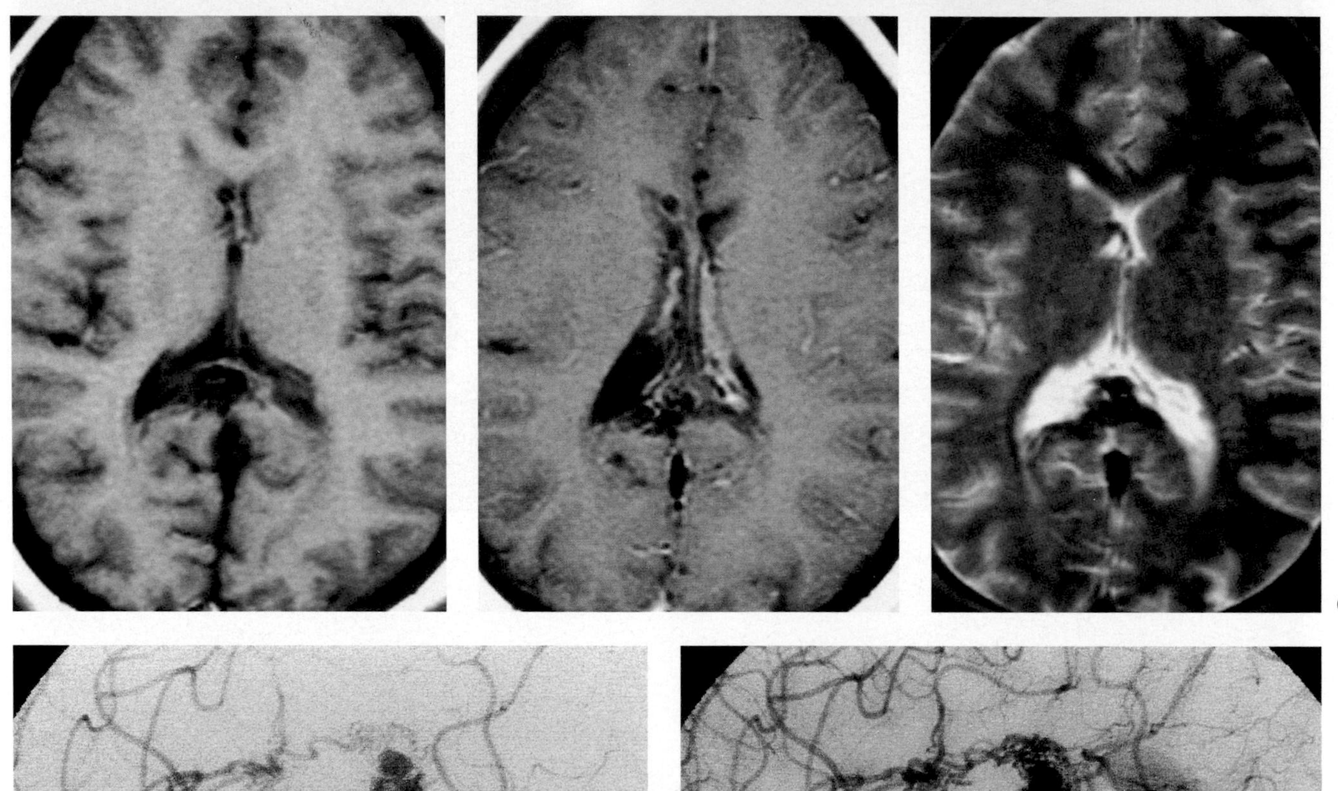

B C,D

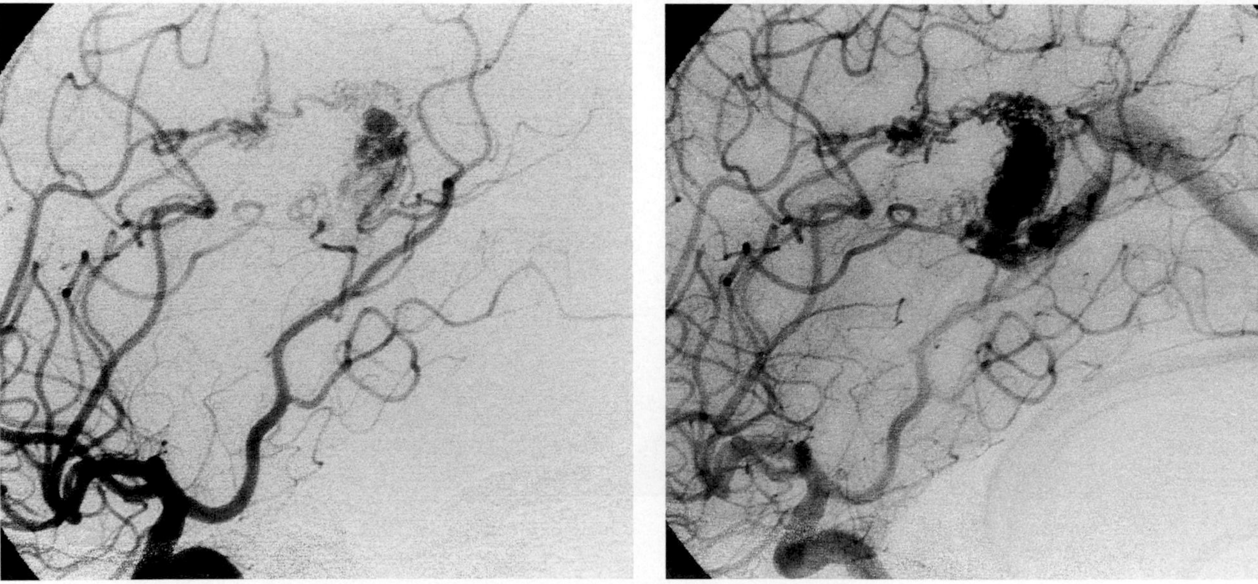

E F

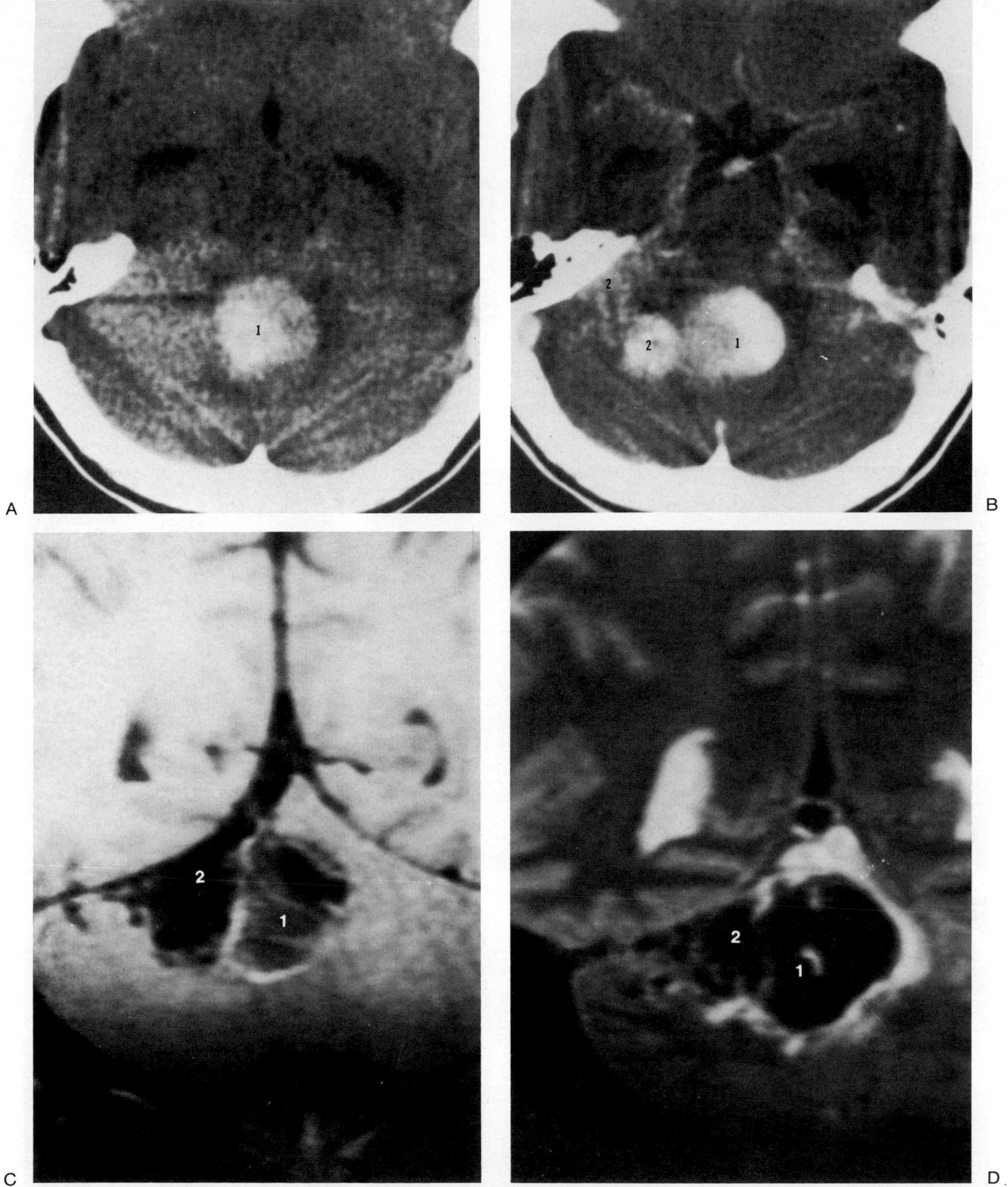

FIG. 13. Acute cerebellar hematoma with AVM. **A:** Axial CT. **B:** Axial CT with contrast enhancement. **C:** Coronal short TR/TE MR (600/20). **D:** Coronal long TR/TE MR (2500/80). Vermian hematoma (*1*) is identified on all images. Note enhancement along right side (*2*, B), which represents nidus and enlarged draining veins, seen on MR (*2*, C,D) as signal void. (From Atlas, ref. 163, with permission.)

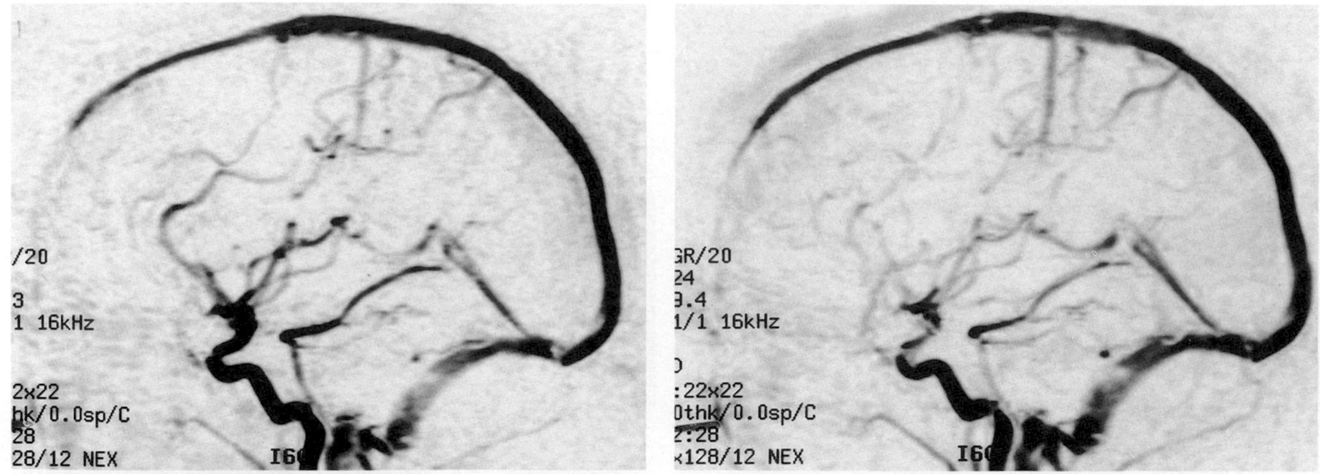

FIG. 14. AVM characterization using velocity-encoded MRA. **A:** 2D phase-contrast MRA using high velocity sensitivity. **B:** 2D phase-contrast MRA using low velocity sensitivity. At high velocity encoding values (VENCs), high flow vessels (arterial feeders, nidus) are particularly well seen (A). At low VENC, the venous side of the lesion is better seen (B).

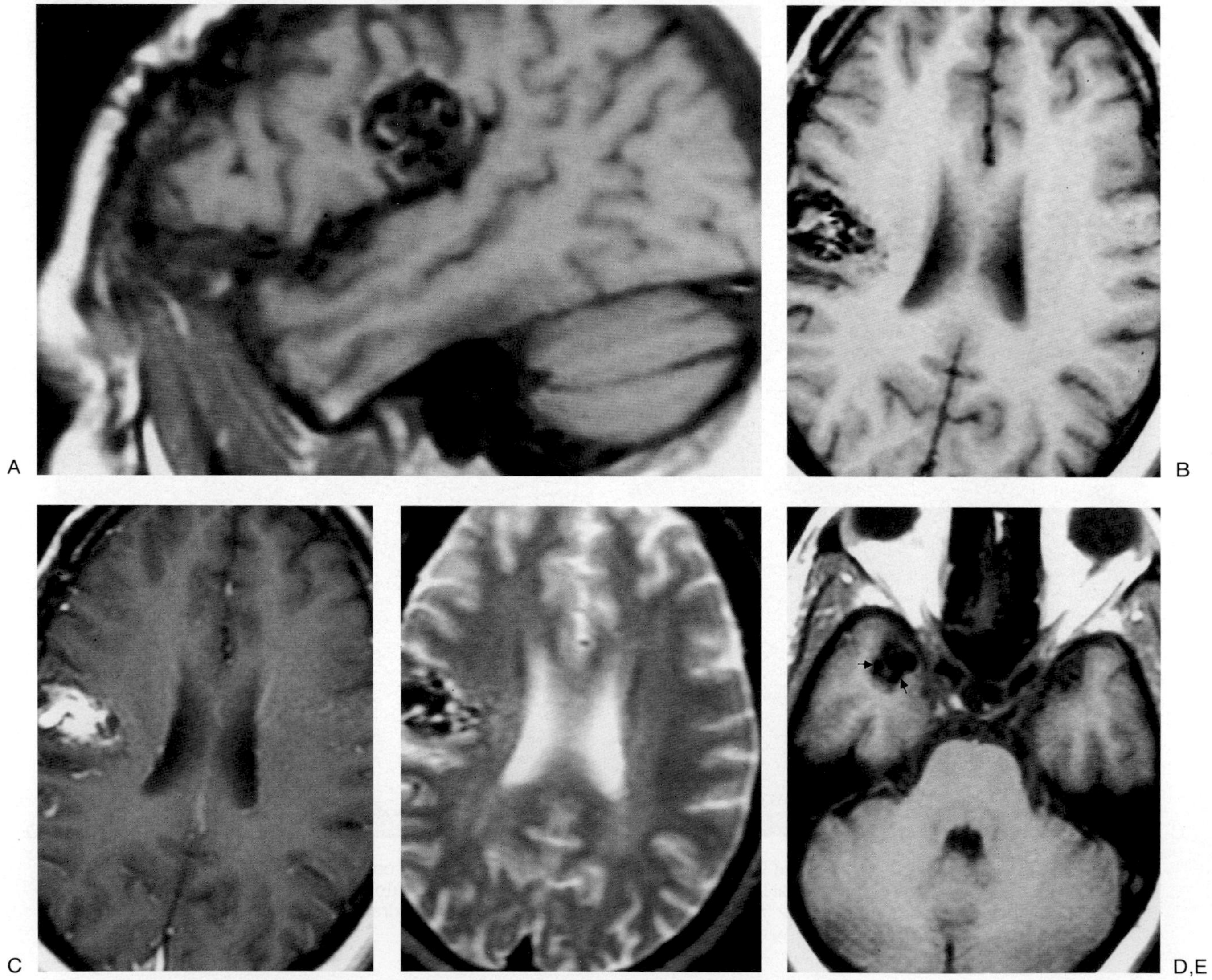

A B

C D,E

FIG. 15. AVM with aneurysm on feeding artery (A–G). Sagittal (**A**) and axial (**B**) T1-weighted (549/27) images demonstrate an area of heterogeneous signal and flow voids, which enhances heterogeneously following gadolinium (**C**). Axial T2-weighted (2500/90) image (**D**) shows flow voids of nidus. Axial T1-weighted image (**E**) demonstrates focal area of MCA enlargement representing an aneurysm at the MCA bifurcation (*arrows*).

sected (51). The potential for hemorrhage is also related to AVM size, where smaller AVMs tend to present more often with hemorrhage than larger AVMs (52). MR is also superior to CT for demonstrating the degree of nidus obliteration after intra-arterial embolization. In such cases, MRI often allows clear depiction of the thrombosed portion of the lesion and accurate differentiation of patent from thrombosed vessels, a distinction that even conventional arteriography may not be able to make with certainty because of the many physiologic changes in flow after endovascular therapy (44). MR is more sensitive than either CT or angiography at delineating hemorrhagic complications of AVMs, especially those that are subacute or chronic (Figs. 10,12, and 13).

Conventional catheter angiography remains superior to MR in depicting the specific arterial supply and venous drainage of the AVM. Even thin section, high resolution MRI can only implicate abnormal veins or arteries in an AVM on the basis of enlargement, a feature that may not be present in all involved vessels. Similarly, MRA is a nonselective technique that cannot define with certainty the specific feeding arteries and draining veins, although approaches to selective MRA are being developed (Fig. 14) (see Chapter 31). Moreover, one must detect and characterize aneurysms that are associated with the AVM because certain types are reported to have an extremely high risk of rupture (53). Obliteration of symptomatic aneurysms is now considered a part of the surgical management of AVMs (30), so these lesions must be defined on imaging studies (Fig. 15). If MRA is performed in these patients, then the region of interest is not limited to the AVM itself and must include the circle of Willis and feeding arteries into the nidus.

Differential Diagnosis

Because AVMs are frequently associated with intracranial hemorrhage, the question of the diagnosis is often raised when the patient presents after an episode of intracranial hemorrhage. In the presence of any intracerebral hematoma, the radiologist must search for evidence of large vessels to suggest AVM (Figs. 13 and 16). It is important to realize that the failure to identify large vessels on MRI in the presence of an acute hematoma does not entirely exclude an AVM as the cause of the hemorrhage (Fig. 17). Small AVMs can occasionally even be angiographically occult because of a variety of factors, including compression of the lesion by adjacent hematoma, vasospasm, extremely slow flow, and thrombosis. These lesions are often referred to as "cryptic" AVMs.

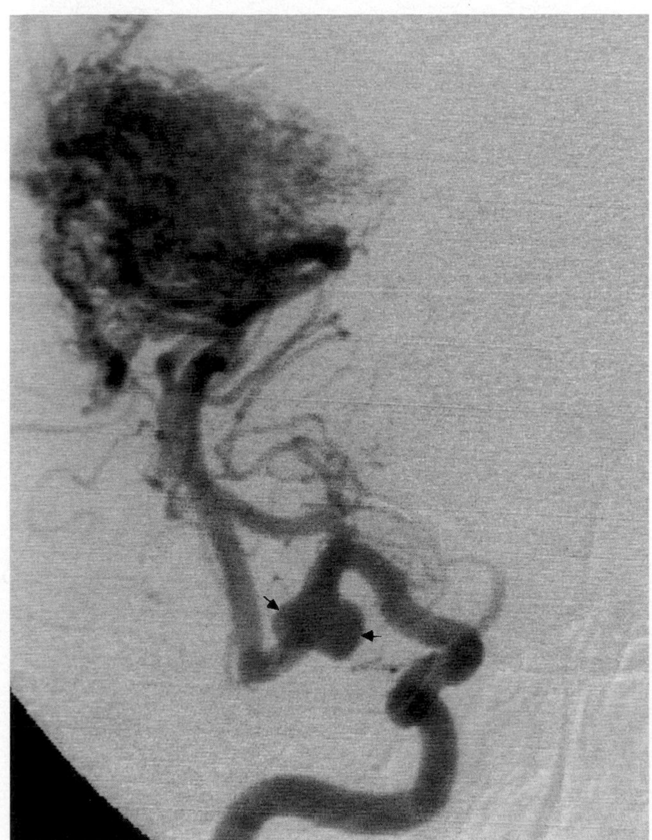
F

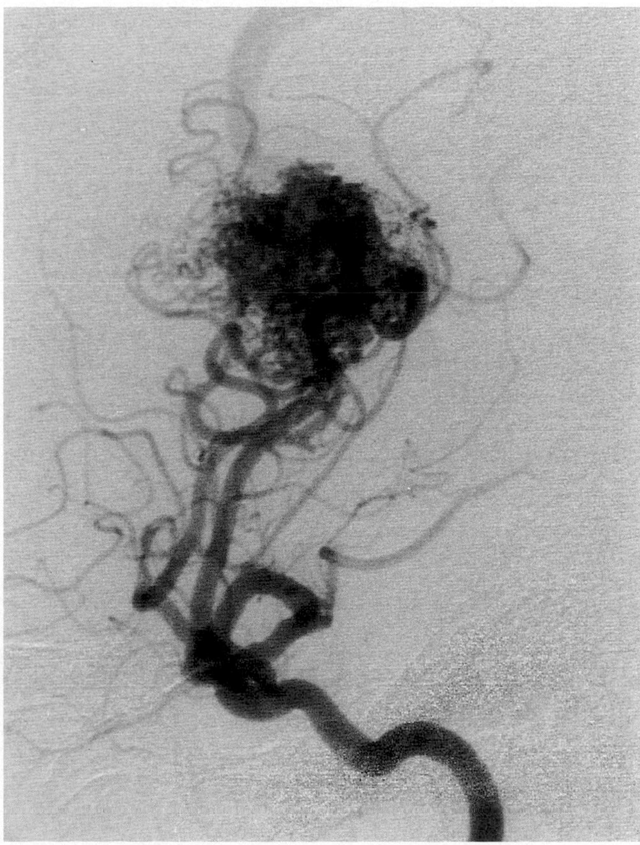
G

FIG. 15. *(Continued.)* AP (**F**) and lateral (**G**) left ICA injection demonstrating MCA aneurysm (*arrows*), AVM, and early vein draining superiorly.

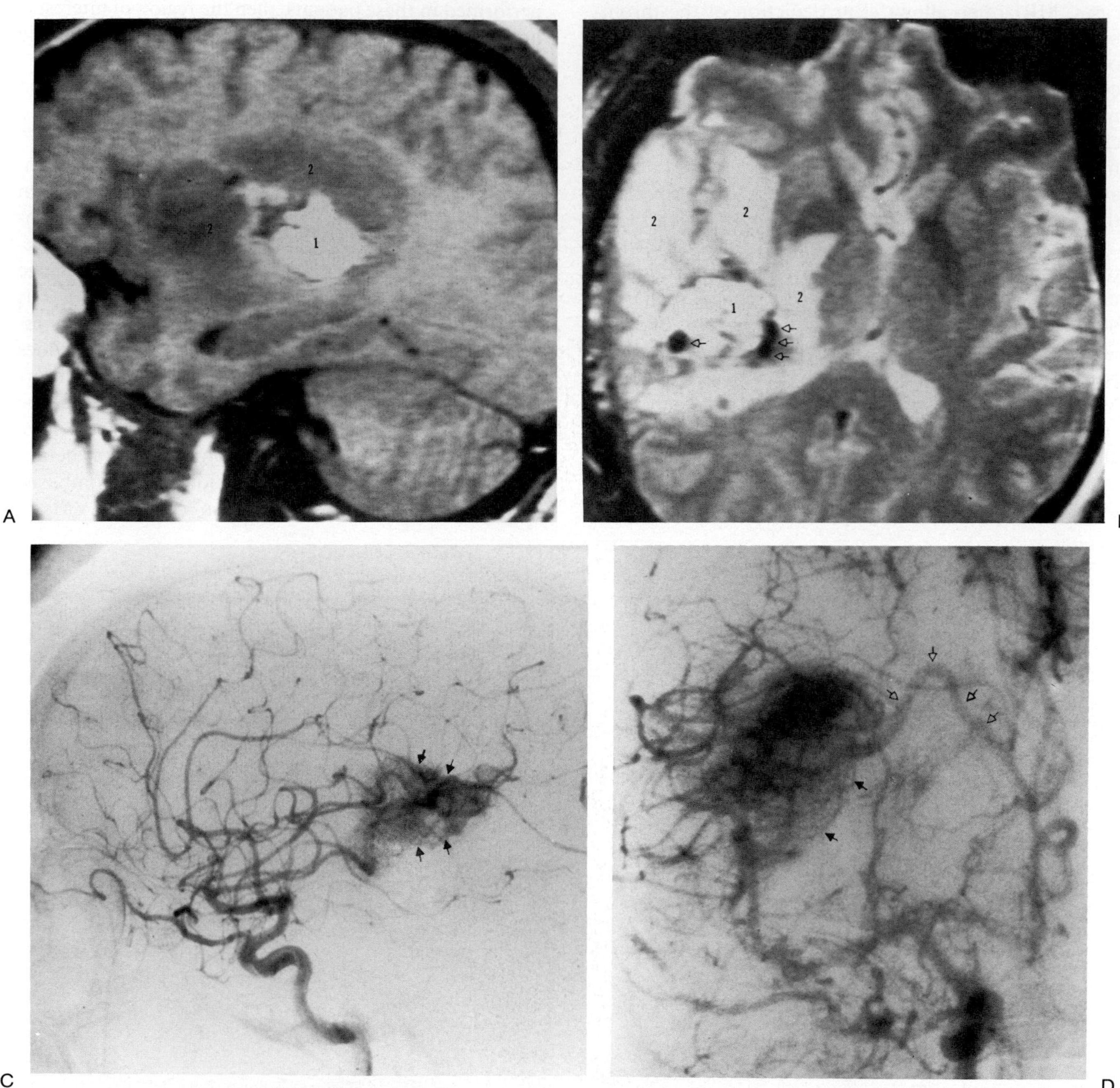

FIG. 16. Subacute posterior sylvian hematoma with AVM. **A:** Sagittal short TR/TE MR (600/20). **B:** Axial long TR/TE MR (2500/80). **C:** Arteriogram, lateral view. **D:** Arteriogram, AP view. Posterior sylvian hematoma (*1*) is identified on MR images (A,B) with surrounding edema (*2*). Note AVM nidus (*arrows*, C,D) with enlarged draining vein (*open arrow*, D), suggested by MR (*open arrow*, B) as signal void.

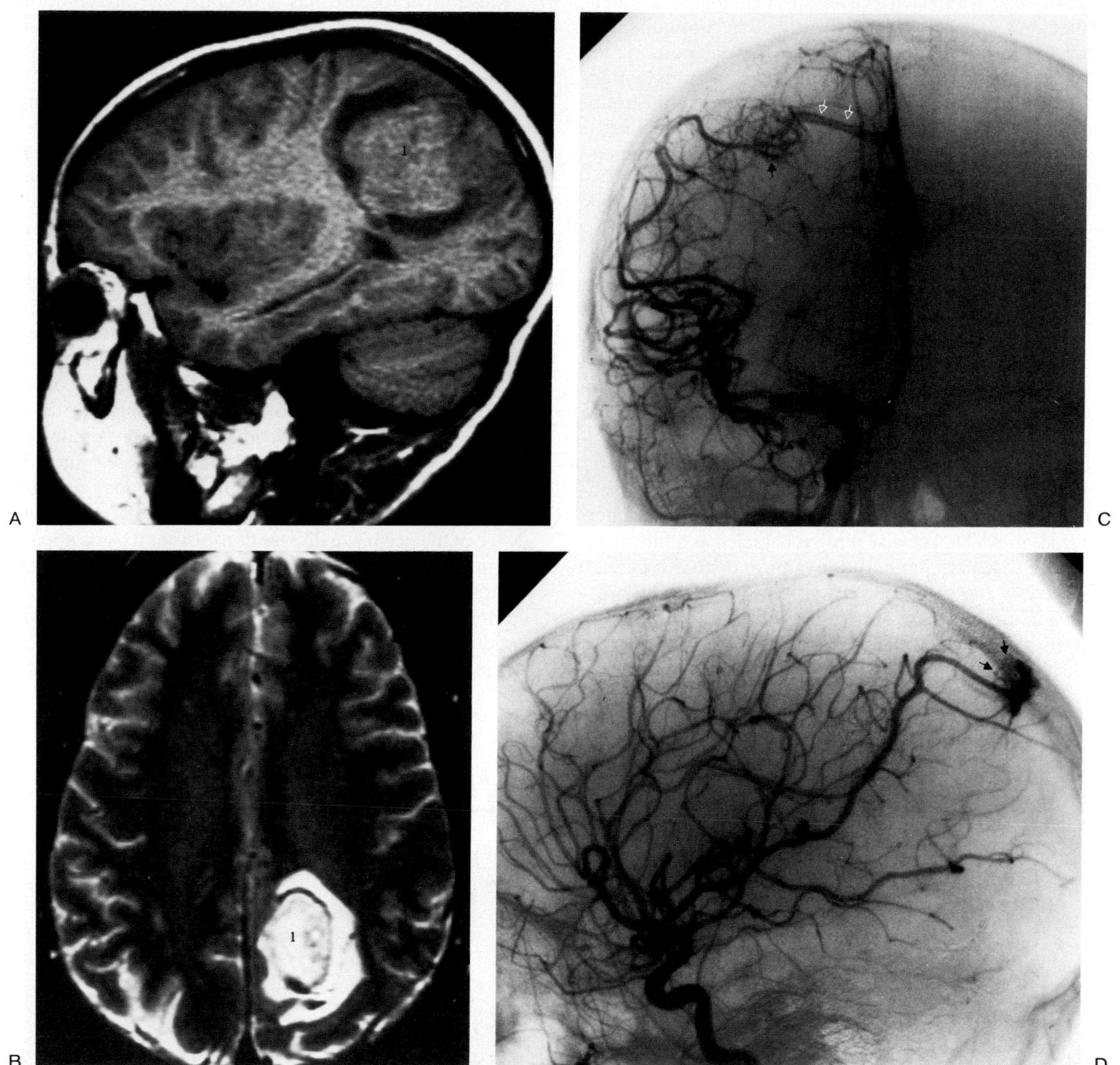

FIG. 17. Hyperacute hematoma with cryptic AVM. **A:** Sagittal short TR/TE MR (600/11). **B:** Axial long TR/TE MR (3000/80). **C:** Lateral view, arterial phase, angiogram. **D:** AP view, arterial phase, angiogram. Parietal mass (*1*, A,B) represents hyperacute hematoma (see Chapter 9), with no definite evidence of AVM on MRI. Arteriogram shows posterior parietal AVM with small nidus (*closed arrows*, C,D) and draining vein (*open arrows*, D).

A major part of the role of the radiologist once the identification of an intracerebral hemorrhage has been made on MRI is the search for any associated enlarged vessels, because the diagnosis of an underlying AVM is of paramount importance in these cases. A point of confusion may arise when a cavernous hemangioma is identified, but vascular channels are noted in contiguity with the lesion (Fig. 18). The keys to the diagnosis of the "mixed malformation," comprised of cavernous hemangioma plus venous angioma (discussed later in this chapter), are the recognition of two features of the associated vessels: (a) the characteristic "spoke-wheel" morphology of the enlarged vessels (Fig. 18), or (b) the very slow flow through these vessels (shown by either SE intensities or with gadolinium enhancement) (Fig. 19).

Occasionally, a hypervascular neoplasm with markedly enlarged vessels will manifest as an acute hematoma. The only potential source of confusion with AVM might be a hemangioblastoma, which can certainly be associated with markedly enlarged vascular channels and intraparenchymal hematoma. The typical macrocystic component and the identification of the enhancing mural nodule of hemangioblastoma will separate this entity from AVM in the vast majority of cases.

Although the diagnosis of AVM is usually unambiguous on MR, one other lesion can superficially masquerade as an AVM, because it too is depicted as abnormally dilated vascular channels. Moyamoya disease is characterized by the occurrence of progressive symmetric occlusion involving the bifurcations of the internal carotid arteries (ICAs), as well as the proximal anterior and middle cerebral arteries. The occlusive process stimulates the development of an extensive network of enlarged basal, transcortical, and transdural collateral vessels (Fig. 20). The angiographic appearance of the innumerable tiny collateral vessels, termed "puff of smoke" or "moyamoya" in Japanese, gives the condition its name.

Moyamoya disease has a bimodal age presentation with the first peak occurring in the first decade of life, associated with cerebral infarction as progressive carotid occlusion develops. Adult patients most often present in the fourth decade with intracranial hemorrhage arising from the rupture of the delicate network of collateral vessels. Hemorrhage from moyamoya is intraparenchymal in 60% of cases, with intraventricular hemorrhage accounting for nearly all the rest (54,55). Occasionally, isolated subarachnoid hemorrhage is the initial manifestation of the disease.

Characteristically, flow voids representing large collaterals and the markedly enlarged striate vessels are seen on MRI amid the deep ganglionic structures (56,57) (Fig. 20). Absence of the expected flow void within the cavernous and supraclinoid portions of the ICAs is a consequence of narrowing and ultimately occlusion of these vessels. Changes resulting from ischemia or rupture of the fragile enlarged network of collateral vessels, including regions of infarction or hemorrhage, may also be seen. This diagnosis is clearly defined by MRI when evidence of the occlusive disease of the distal ICAs is apparent in conjunction with the flow voids representing the enlarged striate vessels.

Most often the underlying occlusive process is idiopathic and is more commonly seen in Oriental patients. An identical picture may result from progressive distal

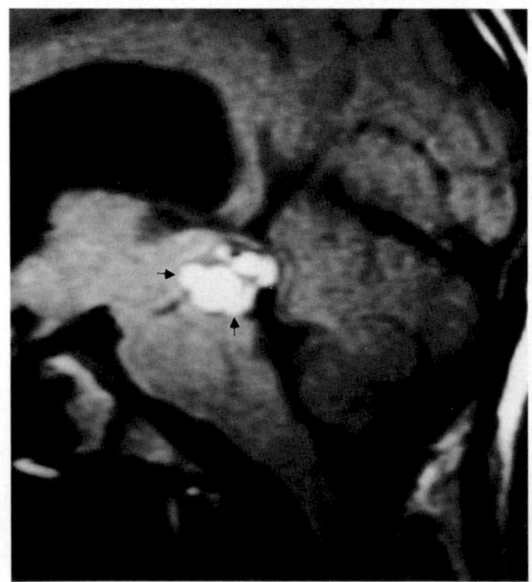
A

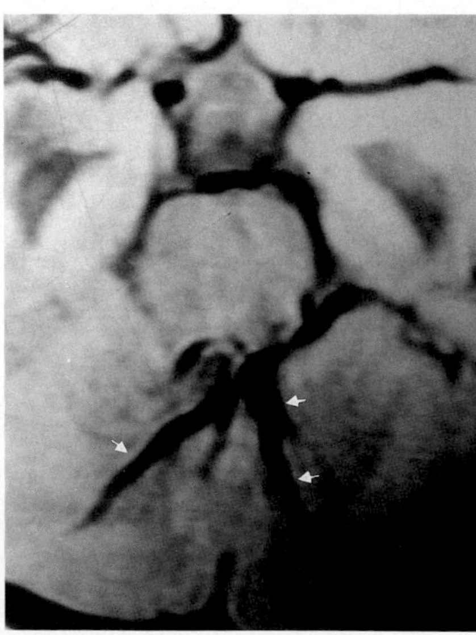

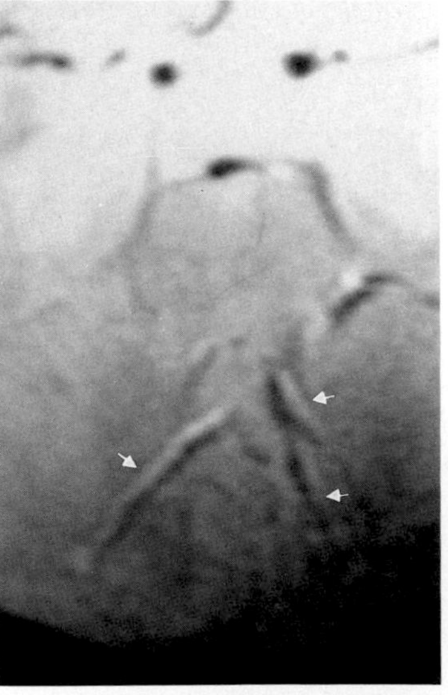
B,C

FIG. 18. Venous angioma in association with a cavernous hemangioma. **A:** Sagittal short TR/TE MR (600/20). **B:** Axial long TR/short TE MR (2000/30). **C:** Axial long TR/TE MR (2000/60). Hemorrhagic tectal mass (*arrows*, A) represents cavernous hemangioma in association with venous angioma (*arrows*, B,C). Note even echo rephasing in slowly flowing venous malformation (B,C). (From Atlas, ref. 166, with permission.)

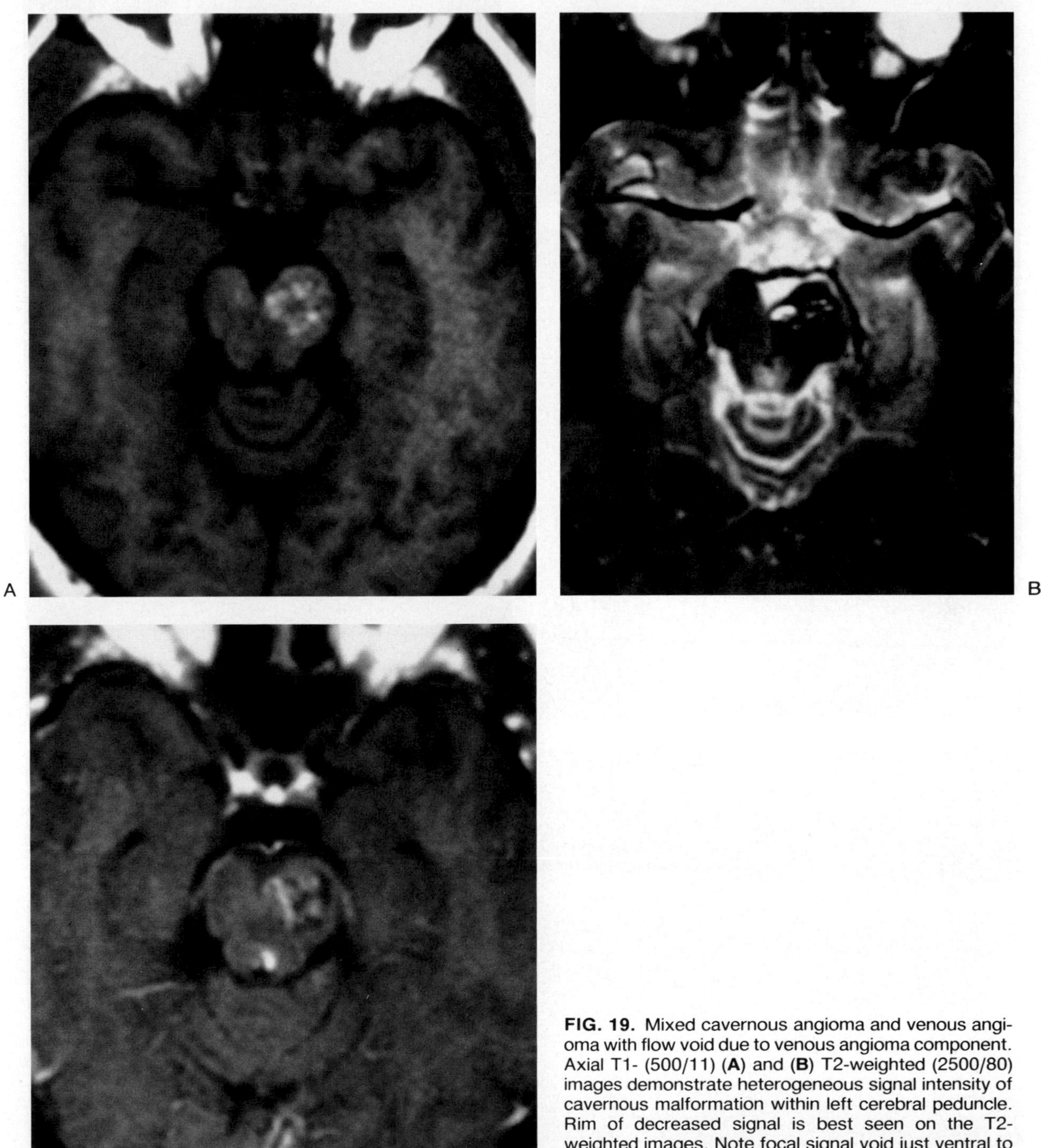

FIG. 19. Mixed cavernous angioma and venous angioma with flow void due to venous angioma component. Axial T1- (500/11) (**A**) and (**B**) T2-weighted (2500/80) images demonstrate heterogeneous signal intensity of cavernous malformation within left cerebral peduncle. Rim of decreased signal is best seen on the T2-weighted images. Note focal signal void just ventral to aqueduct. Enhanced T1-weighted image (**C**) shows enhancement of slow flow within venous angioma component.

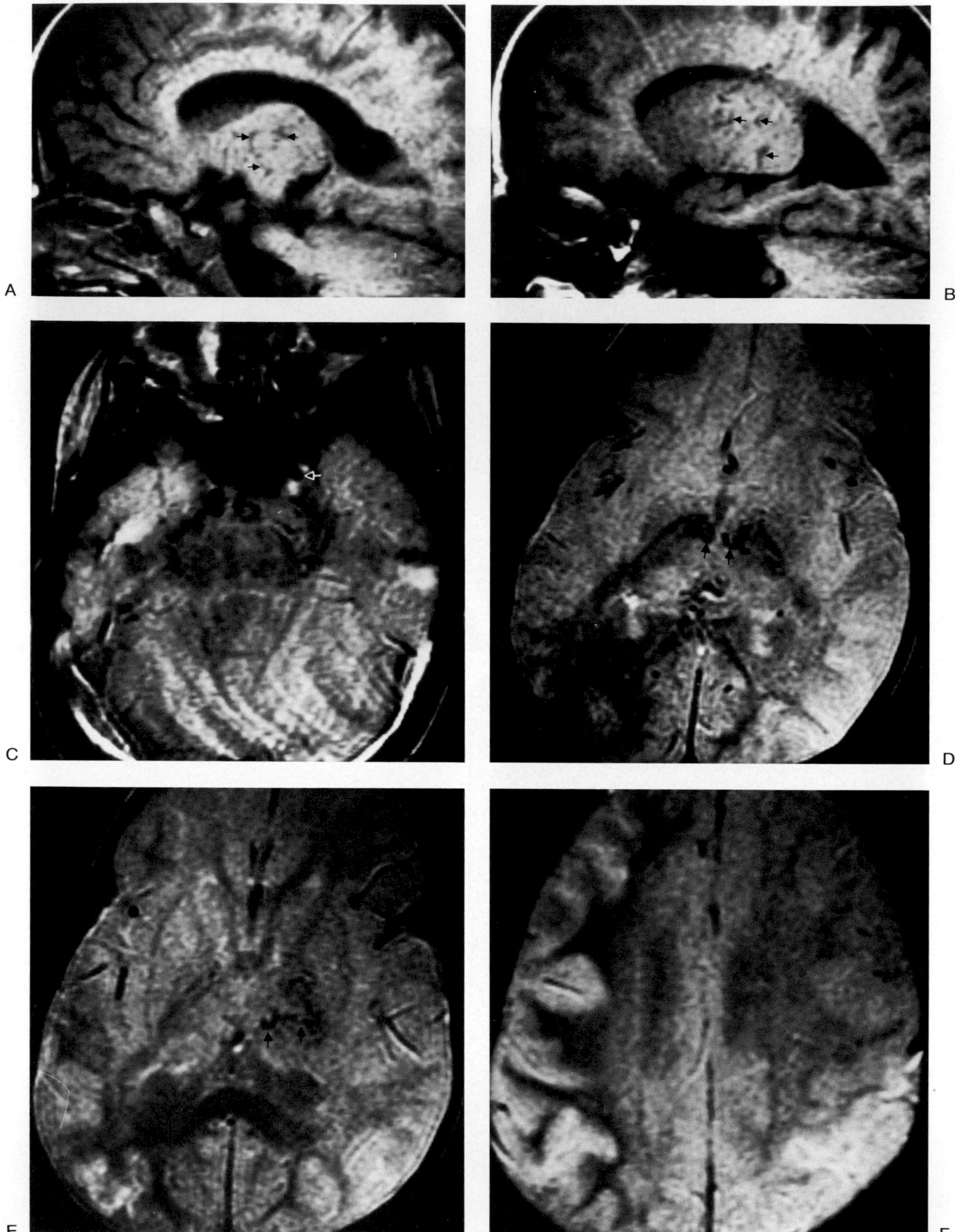

FIG. 20. Enlarged striate vessels due to "moyamoya" collateral enlargement from carotid occlusion. **A,B:** Sagittal short TR/TE MR (600/20). **C–F:** Axial long TR/short TE MR (3000/30), inferior to superior. Enlarged striate vessels course through basal ganglionic regions bilaterally (*arrows*, A–E). Note narrowed left cavernous carotid (*open arrow*, C) and extensive bilateral cortical infarctions (D–F).

internal carotid occlusion arising from any other etiology that is accompanied by collateral development. Such causes include neurofibromatosis, sickle cell disease, and as a delayed effect of radiation therapy to the suprasellar region. An increased incidence of moyamoya changes may also be present in patients with Down syndrome. On close inspection, the MRI changes associated with moyamoya are usually quite characteristic and should not be confused with the findings of an AVM.

Post-Therapy MRI

In addition to the initial pretreatment evaluation of the patient harboring an intracranial AVM, MRI has gained increasing importance in the assessment of these patients after treatment has been completed. Several investigators have studied the effects of radiosurgery on intraparenchymal AVMs, based on imaging (58–60). Expected pathologic changes after therapy include deposition of collagen within the subendothelial space of the nidus, resulting in gradual narrowing and thrombosis of the lesion. A significant reduction in nidus size after therapy is usually clearly recognized on MRI, even without MRA. This is depicted as a decrease in previously recognizable flow void with increased signal intensity on T2-weighted images and persistent contrast enhancement in the area of the nidus. Significant evidence of reductions in AVM flow generally do not occur until at least 12 months after the initial treatment (50) (Fig. 21). It should be noted that CT is inaccurate in evaluating residual AVM nidus size after radiosurgery because persistent contrast enhancement is demonstrated even after complete obliteration.

Complications of this treatment may also be monitored by MR. Changes in the surrounding parenchyma have been noted as early as 3 months after treatment and include transient vasogenic edema and radiation necrosis. Most often asymptomatic, vasogenic edema is a frequent finding in these patients and is characterized by hyperintensity on T2-weighted images in white matter surrounding the nidus. Symptomatic radiation necrosis occurs in an estimated 3% to 4% of patients and is seen as high intensity with mass effect and irregular enhancement (Fig. 22). Hemorrhage can be concomitant with radiation necrosis.

Specialized MR Techniques in AVMs

MR Angiography

Since the initial publication by Wedeen et al. (61) showing intravascular flow as high signal intensity on in vivo MR images, intense scientific and clinical interest has become focused on imaging the cerebral vasculature and its pathology with MR. The various methods of imaging vascular flow and displaying it in multiple projections have been termed "MR angiography", because of the similar appearance of these images to conventional catheter angiography using iodinated contrast agents and x-rays. MRA techniques are clearly still evolving but have already improved significantly since several groups introduced the two principle techniques of data acquisition, time-of-flight (TOF) and phase contrast (PC) (62–67).

The major impetus for the development of MRA as a potential replacement for catheter angiography in the

A

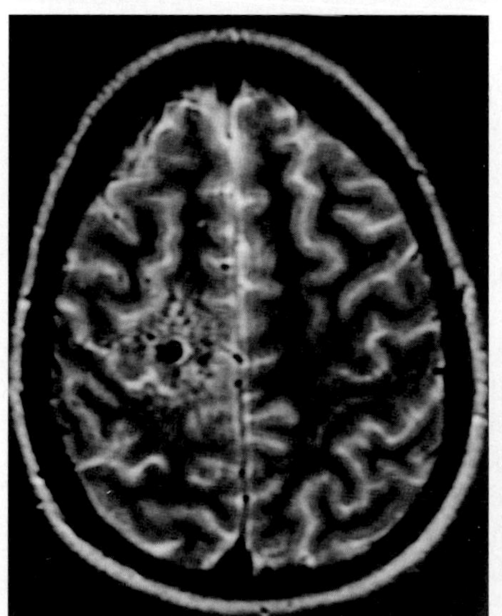

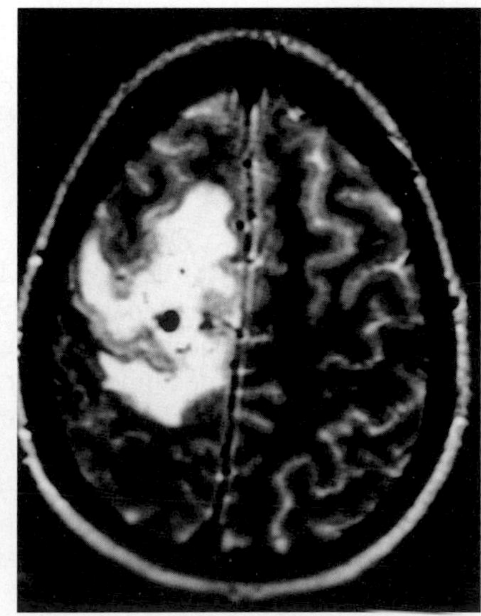

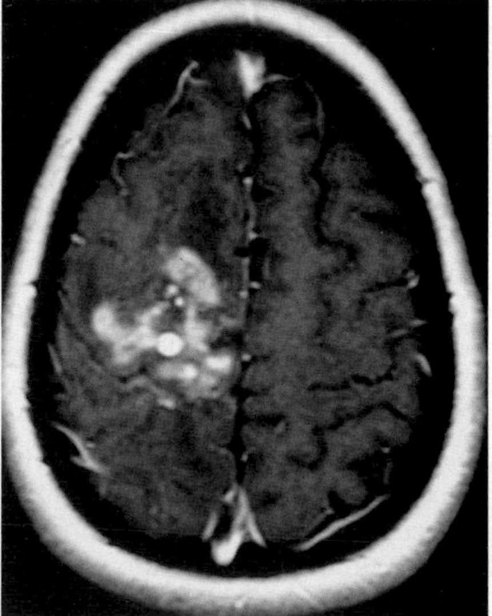

B,C

FIG. 21. AVM with extensive radiation necrosis after treatment. **A:** Pretherapy MRI. Supraventricular AVM is clearly seen as signal voids in patient without neurologic deficit. **B,C:** Post-therapy MRI. Severe edema (B) with marked contrast enhancement (C) indicates extensive radiation necrosis in patient who developed hemiparesis.

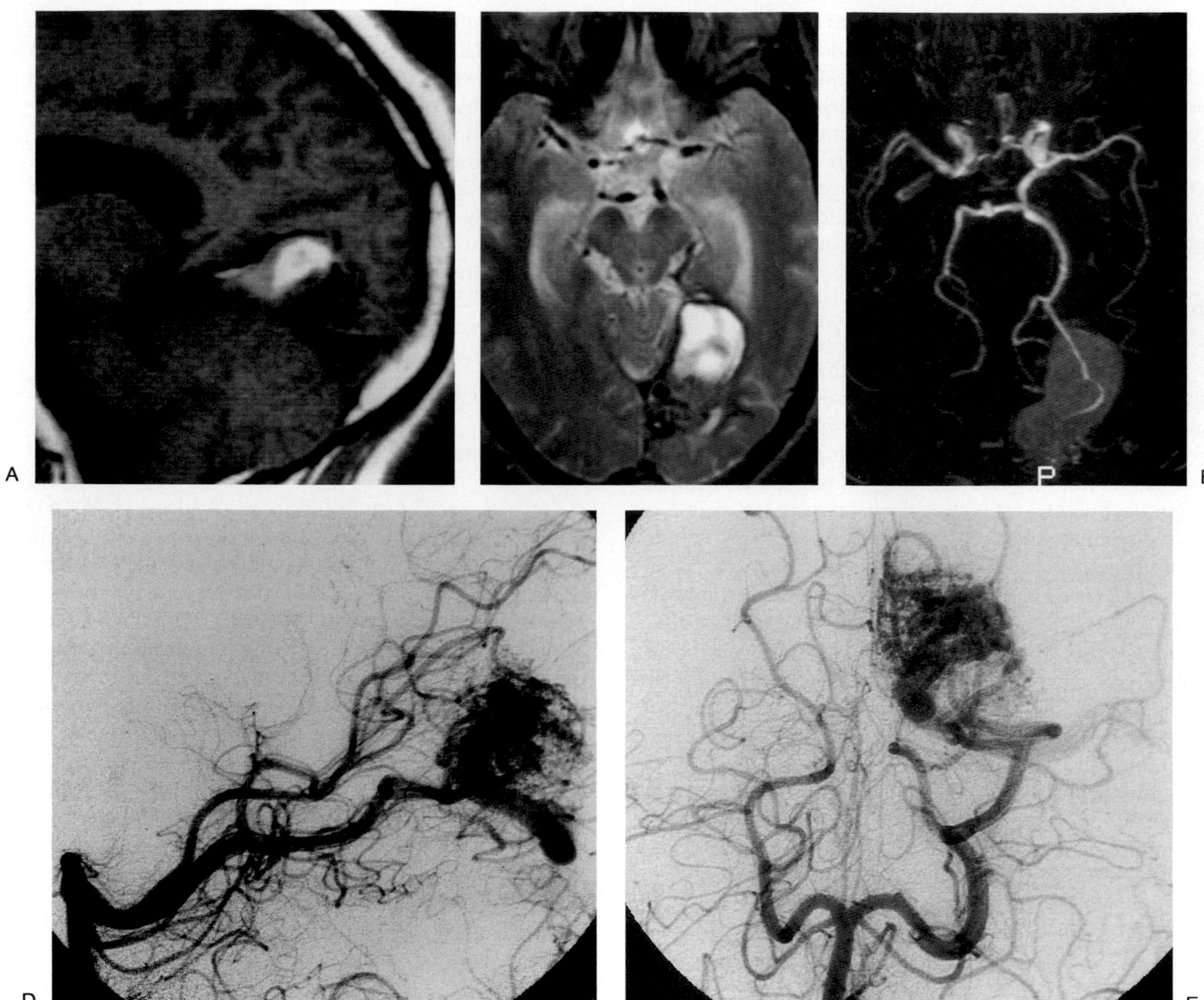

FIG. 22. AVM with adjacent hematoma, MRI vs. TOF MRA. Sagittal T1-(700/12) (**A**) and axial T2-(2300/80) weighted (**B**) images demonstrate intraparenchymal hemorrhage with adjacent areas of signal void. 3D TOF MRA (**C**) shows feeding vessels originating from left PCA as well as their relationship to the area of high signal hematoma. Lateral (**D**) and AP (**E**) vertebral artery injection showing arterial supply, nidus, and superficially draining vein.

diagnosis of neurologic diseases is the morbidity and mortality of cerebral catheter angiography. According to a recent review (68), aside from local complications due at the puncture site itself, there is approximately a 4% incidence of neurologic event, a 1% fixed neurologic deficit incidence, and a small but definable (<0.1%) incidence of death from these procedures. It should be recognized, however, that in competent and well trained hands, cerebral angiography is certainly well documented to be a safe procedure and has, in fact, become much safer with the improvement in equipment, contrast agents, and techniques (69). The second motivation for developing MRA for the work-up of neurologic disease, particularly in the United States in the current health care climate, is the hospital cost of catheter angiography, a factor that varies widely and is too complex a subject for this review.

More specific characterization of regions of signal void on SE images as regions of blood flow, rather than from dense calcification or hemorrhage, can be obtained by using gradient refocused, limited flip angle techniques (64,70). These techniques form the basis of TOF and PC MRA (see Chapter 31). On these sequences, regions of flowing blood are most often demonstrated as high signal intensity (see Fig. 7). These techniques can be relatively rapid methods of clarifying ambiguous regions of signal intensity on SE images as flowing blood (such as subependymal vessels or vessels near cortical margins). The presence of major venous sinus occlusion accompanying the AVM can also be clarified with MRA techniques. It is clear that at least some familiarity of the physics of flow is essential to the appropriate design and implementation of these techniques (71) (see Chapters 4 and 29).

The fundamental role for such flow imaging techniques as MRA in the diagnostic work-up of the patient with an AVM is controversial at this point in the evolution of these techniques (72).

Although no one doubts that MRA can demonstrate the vascular nature of a high flow AVM, the importance of simply showing the tangle of vessels on an image is arguable, because the mere identification of the lesion is usually accomplished even with conventional SE MRI (see Fig. 11). In fact, the AVM can sometimes be even more clearly separated from adjacent hematoma by MRI rather than MRA (see Fig. 22). MRA in those AVMs that are fed by enlarged dural vessels is a valuable tool because dural feeding arteries are often not seen well on conventional SE MRI because of their intrinsic signal void superimposed against the background of signal void of skull base and calvarium. The search for dural vessels involved in AVMs is a clear indication for supplemental MRA rather than MRI alone (see "Dural AV Fistulae," below).

One could make a strong argument that the assessment of AVM nidus size might be an appropriate indication for MRA of these lesions, whether pretreatment or post-treatment, for several reasons. First, many neurosurgeons classify AVMs at least in part based on nidus size, in terms of prognosis (35,52). Second, it is common practice to evaluate these patients after radiotherapy and/or embolization to determine the residual nidus, particularly if one desires to avoid exposing these patients to invasive catheter angiograms multiple times. Third, most institutions that treat some AVMs with a form of radiotherapy triage these lesions based on the size of the nidus, where lesions less than 3.5 cm are candidates for such therapy (37–40).

MRA does represent a potentially effective way to demonstrate a quantifiable nidus size in three-dimensional space (Fig. 23). Unfortunately, it can be difficult to separate nidus vascularity from draining veins in many cases. Moreover, it is a subject of ongoing debate in the neurosurgical literature whether any form of radiotherapy is indicated in any AVM, based on worse reported outcomes of radiotherapy as compared to those from microsurgery (41). Quantification of intravascular flow in AVMs may be a future indication for MRA, as an adjunct to the multifaceted treatment plan and follow-up of patients harboring these lesions by using phase-contrast MRA techniques (73).

A further indication for MRA in AVM patients is the search for associated aneurysms. The sensitivity and specificity of MRA for aneurysms is still not clear, but indications are that more than 90% of circle of Willis aneurysms larger than 3 mm are detected by intracranial MRA if state-of-the-art acquisition and postprocessing methodology are used (74) (see the section "Intracranial Aneurysms," below).

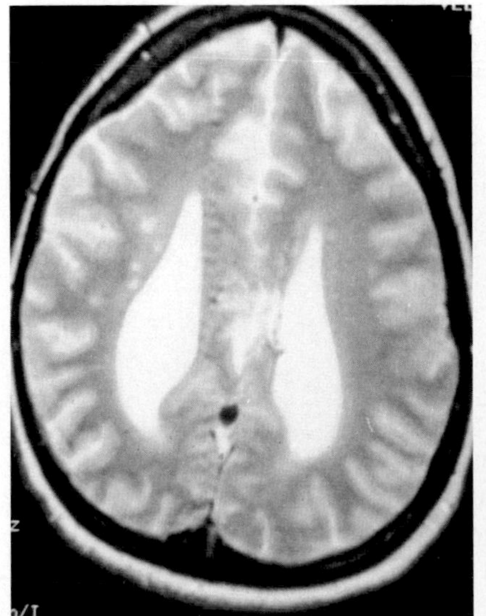
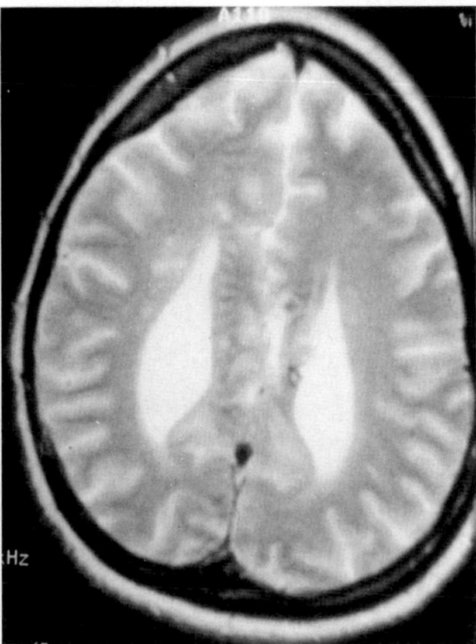
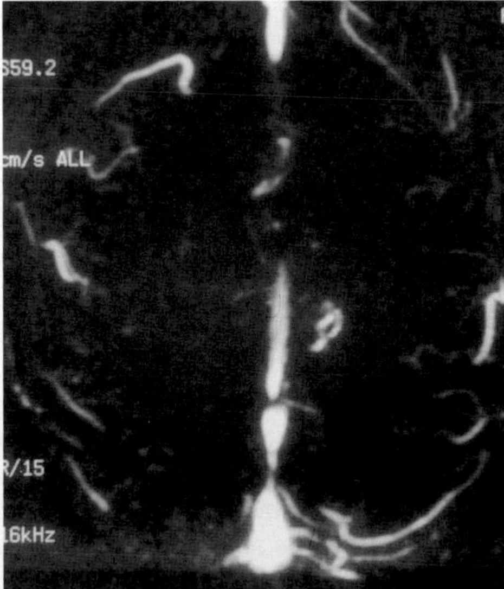

A,B C

FIG. 23. MRA in assessment of residual nidus after radiotherapy. Axial T2-weighted MRI (A,B) shows abnormal signal in left mesial hemisphere, but it is difficult to clearly define residual lesion. **C:** 3DPC MRA defines residual vascularity.

Important pitfalls in using MRA for documenting flow must be recognized by the radiologist. If flow is turbulent (75), as is often the case in high flow AVMs (76), in-plane, or extremely slow (71), flowing blood may be manifest as low intensity on all "white blood" MRA methods. Furthermore, subacute-chronic intravascular clot is often difficult or impossible to distinguish from intravascular flowing blood on the GE images (76) that comprise TOF MRA (see Fig. 22). Other MRA methods have been used with more success in differentiating flowing blood from clot, including most importantly both two-dimensional (2D) and three-dimensional (3D) PC MRA techniques. In the clinical setting of an intracranial hematoma and, in fact, in any search for the source of an intracranial hemorrhage, the major advantage of PC MRA is its specificity for flow because this technique is based on differences in phase between moving and stationary spins, rather than simply the T1 differences that characterize TOF methods. PC MRA, however, has its own unique limitations and artifacts (see Chapters 4 and 31). Therefore, we believe that, in the hunt for intracranial AVMs, MRA techniques should be used only in conjunction with conventional SE imaging (as an adjunctive MR method), rather than as the sole pulse sequence (76). Generally speaking, although MRI better delineates AVM nidus localization, and conventional arteriography is clearly superior in depicting overall angioarchitecture, the potential usefulness and the noninvasiveness of MRA should encourage its use in cases of suspected intracranial AVMs.

Functional MRI in AVMs

Blood oxygen level–dependent contrast (BOLD) imaging (77) is a noninvasive functional MRI (fMRI) technique for localizing regional brain signal intensity changes in response to task performance. This technique uses no intravenous contrast agents and depends mainly on regional changes in endogenous intravascular paramagnetic deoxyhemoglobin. Signal intensity changes in BOLD fMRI are attributed to the documented mismatch between increases in regional cerebral blood flow and cerebral blood volume and to the much less profound increase in oxygen extraction in response to regional activation (78,79).

As opposed to contrast bolus MRI techniques (80) and positron emission tomography (PET), the performance of BOLD fMRI measurements are not limited by contrast agent dose or radiation limits, so several activation experiments can be performed without these considerations. The use of fMRI for the localization of definable cortical functions in relation to the site of AVM nidus as an aid to operative planning has been explored (81). We have also demonstrated that aberrant mapping of cortical functions can occur in the presence of an AVM that is situated in the expected location of primary sensorimotor cortex (81) (Fig. 24), implying neural plasticity. The precise clinical role of such imaging in the setting of intracranial AVMs is promising but as of yet undefined (see Chapter 30).

Cavernous Angioma

Cavernous angiomas (or *cavernomas*) account for approximately 8% to 16% of all cerebrovascular malformations from post-mortem studies. It is estimated that 4% of the population harbors this lesion. They represent a distinct pathologic subtype of vascular malformation, typically appearing as discrete, compact honeycomb-like masses of endothelial-lined sinusoidal vascular spaces, which contain essentially thrombosed blood (28,31). This lesion is believed to be congenital, although the peak incidence of symptom onset is between the third and fifth decades of life. Cavernous angiomas may occur in either the brain or spinal cord. Intracranial lesions affect males and females equally, whereas those in the spine show a female predominance. Most cavernous angiomas occur in the cerebral hemispheres, in either a superficial or subcortical location, but a superficial location with proximity to either the subarachnoid space (SAS) or ventricle is particularly common. Involvement of the deep cerebral structures, including basal ganglia, thalamus, and internal capsule, occurs in only 10% of cases. Roughly one quarter of the lesions involve the infratentorial compartment, with the cerebellum and brainstem equally affected. The pons is the most common brainstem location. Extra-axial locations have been described infrequently, including lesions arising from leptomeninges (82,83) or cranial nerves. The lesions are frequently multiple (approximately 20–30% of cases), with a familial pattern in 10% to 15% of patients, suggesting that a genetic basis may be present in some cases (84–86). When familial, the lesions have a very strong tendency to be multiple (87). MRI has also documented that cavernous angiomas change in size, morphology, and composition over time. Moreover, the de novo development of these lesions has also been described in patients with the familial type (87).

Clinical Features

The increased sensitivity of MRI (86) for the detection of cavernous angiomas has highlighted the relatively high number of lesions that are asymptomatic. In fact, these lesions are not uncommonly found incidentally at post-mortem (28). In one study of familial cavernous angiomas, 61% of patients were symptomatic, but it can be inferred that a higher percentage of lesions evoke no symptoms (87). If symptoms do occur, the clinical presentation may include seizures, hemorrhage, or progres-

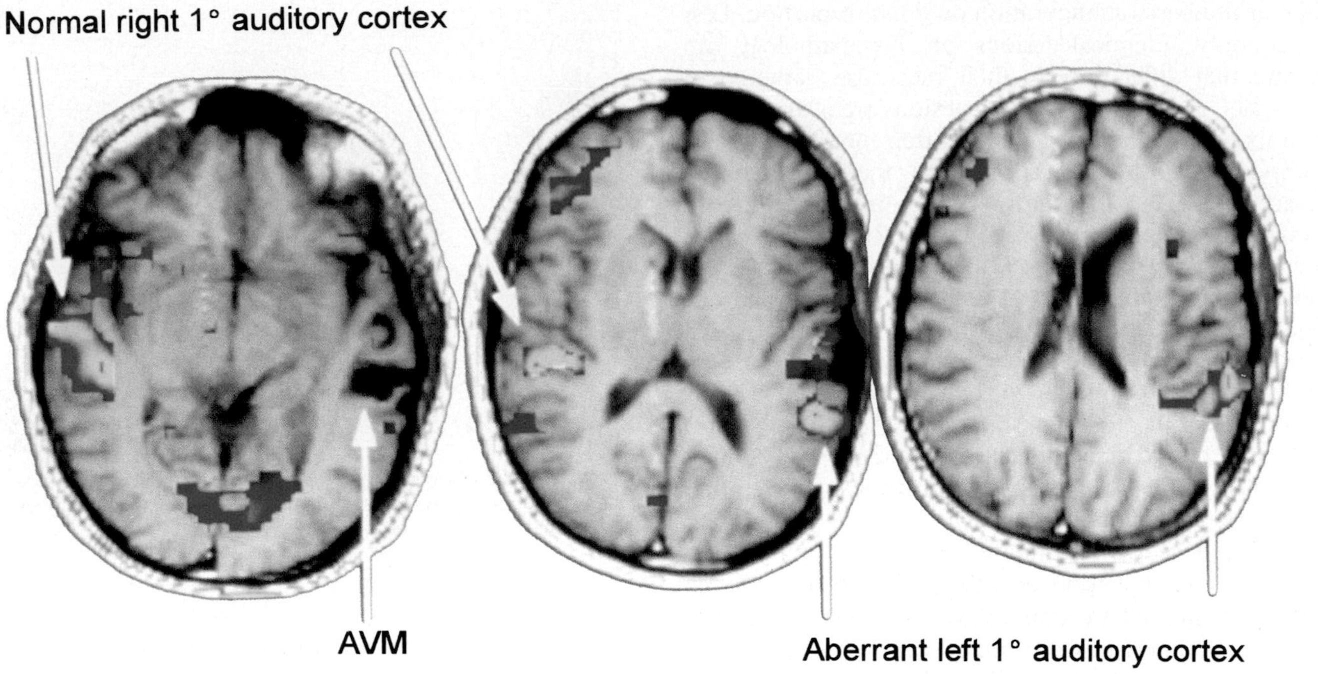

FIG. 24. Functional MRI in AVM, patient without neurologic deficit (color slide, three images). Activation is seen posterior and superior to left temporal lobe AVM nidus when patient is presented with auditory stimulus (**A–C**). Aberrant mapping of auditory cortex (posterior and superior to expected location) implies plasticity of developing brain.

sive neurologic deficit. Cavernous angiomas represent the second most common type of vascular malformation to be symptomatic. Seizures are the most common symptom associated with cavernous angiomas, occurring in 40% to 60% of those patients with symptoms, and are the most frequent manifestation of those lesions that are situated in the supratentorial compartment. Patients may have a long-standing seizure disorder and relate no acute episode to indicate hemorrhage in the past. Seizures associated with cavernous angiomas are most often focal and are believed to arise from the irritative effects of hemosiderin, gliosis, and compression on adjacent cortex. The lesions vary considerably in their responsiveness to medical management, and refractory seizures are a rather common indication for surgical excision.

Clinically evident hemorrhage is the most concerning consequence of cavernous angiomas. Like other symptoms of these lesions, hemorrhage occurs with the highest incidence in the second and third decades of life and affects males and females equally. Limitations in the imaging of these lesions in the pre-MRI era made it difficult to estimate accurately the frequency of hemorrhage associated with their presence. It is now clear that subclinical hemorrhage is a common occurrence, but the size of the hemorrhage is usually small and most often not accompanied by the devastating effects of AVM-associated hemorrhage (28). Recent studies using MRI suggest that clinically significant hemorrhage occurs in 10% to 13% of patients. Several investigators have estimated that the risk of hemorrhage from a cavernous angioma is in the range of 0.1% to 1.1% per year for each lesion (88–90). Hemorrhage may be associated with seizures or with the acute development of neurologic deficits. Most often intraparenchymal hemorrhage occurs with similar frequencies, regardless of the location of the lesion. Clinical consequences vary, so that small hemorrhages in critical locations (e.g., brainstem) are more likely to produce symptoms. Extension of hemorrhage into subarachnoid or intraventricular space is not common. Repeat hemorrhages, each with clinically evident sequelae, are not infrequent, and some evidence suggests that cavernous angiomas become more aggressive after an episode of bleeding (89).

Progressive neurologic deficit is an uncommon manifestation of supratentorial cavernous angiomas, but occur more often with those in the infratentorial space. Although sometimes arising from an episode of frank hemorrhage, progressive deficits are more likely to be caused by slow enlargement of the malformation secondary to chronic or recurrent extravasation of blood, thrombosis, or other poorly understood mechanisms.

Pathologic Findings

Pathologically identical regardless of their location in the CNS, cavernous angiomas are typically dark blue, well circumscribed, lobulated mass lesions with a grape-like or mulberry configuration on gross inspection. Less commonly, identical lesions on histopathology are found that differ only in their racemose, rather than compact, appearance (28). The lesions are nearly always intraparenchymal, and they are often found in either a subpial location, protruding into the subarachnoid space, or adjacent to a ventricle. Leptomeningeal sites of origin have been reported (Fig. 25). Rarely, cavernous angiomas are extradural, with most reported cases of such lesions involving intraspinal sites (91,92). The vast majority range in diameter from a few millimeters to a few centimeters. Within the lesion is subacute to chronic clotted blood. Although virtually always well demarcated by a rim of gliotic brain stained by hemosiderin pigment from prior hemorrhages (Fig. 26) or diffusion of red cell pigment from prior intracavernous sequestration (4), the lesions are not encapsulated.

On microscopic examination, a honeycomb of multiple, partially collagenized endothelial-lined sinusoidal vascular channels are seen that vary in caliber. The walls of these channels may be thin, irregularly thickened and hyalinized, or partially calcified. Even when thickened, no muscularis or elastica is present in vessel walls, differentiating the vessels of cavernous angioma from those of AVM. Another distinguishing feature of the vessels found in cavernous angiomas is their close apposition within the substance of the lesion, reflecting the absence of interposed brain tissue (Fig. 27). Intraluminal thrombosis of varying stages is frequently identified, reflecting the extremely slow flow or stagnation through the lesions in vivo. Staining of the lesions and adjacent parenchyma with hemosiderin and iron-storage products within macrophages and astrocytes (28) provides evidence of chronic low grade seepage of blood in virtually all cases. Adjacent parenchymal atrophy and gliosis may also be found. In some cases, mixed forms of vascular malformations have been identified that share features of both cavernous angioma and capillary telangiectasia (10,93). Additionally, the co-existence of cavernous angioma and venous angioma (developmental venous anomaly) can be seen (6,7,9).

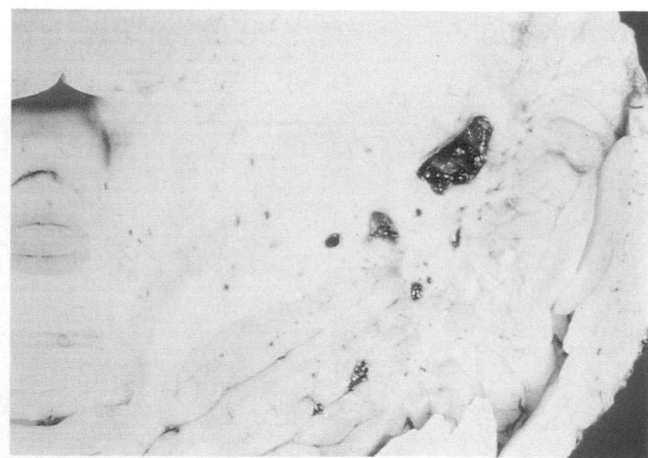

FIG. 26. Cavernous angiomas with surrounding hemosiderin, necropsy specimen. Gross examination reveals classic staining of adjacent brain by hemosiderin.

Imaging Characteristics

These lesions are typically angiographically occult, hence they have also been called "occult cerebrovascular malformations," or OCVMs as a reflection of the normal cerebral angiogram seen in the vast majority of cases ex-

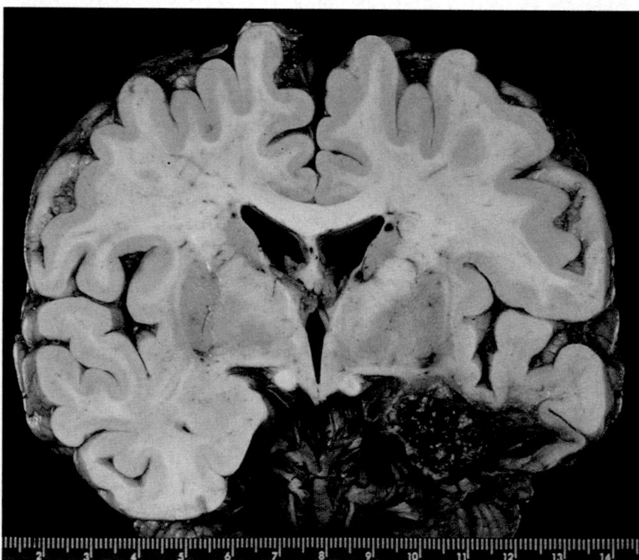

FIG. 25. Extra-axial origin of cavernous angioma. (Courtesy of Dr. P. Burger, Charlottesville, VA.) Infratemporal cavernous angioma arises from meninges and elevates temporal lobe.

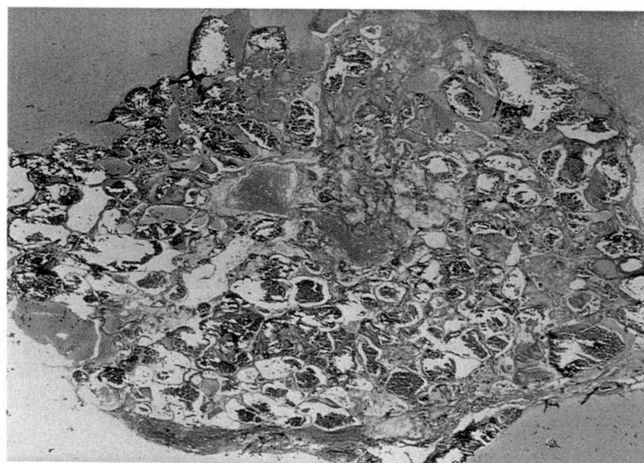

FIG. 27. Cavernous angioma, low power section. Thrombosed vascular spaces in superficial subpial location without intervening brain parenchyma characterize the cavernous angioma. (From Okazaki and Scheithauer, ref. 8, with permission.)

cepting mass effect if acute hematoma is present. Occasionally, a late, minimal contrast stain is seen, but AV shunting is never a feature of cavernous hemangioma.

CT demonstrates these lesions as focal, high-attenuation masses with variably present calcification (Fig. 28), in the absence of edema or mass effect (94). Enhancement is typically mild on CT, but may not be identifiable. Rigamonti et al. (86) studied nine relatives harboring pathologically proven cavernous angiomas using both CT and MRI. CT allowed the detection of 11 lesions, whereas MRI showed 38 lesions, illustrating the increased sensitivity of MRI for the detection of cavernous angiomas.

MRI features of cavernous angiomas are characteristic and are considered diagnostic of these lesions (95), obviating angiography in the vast majority of cases

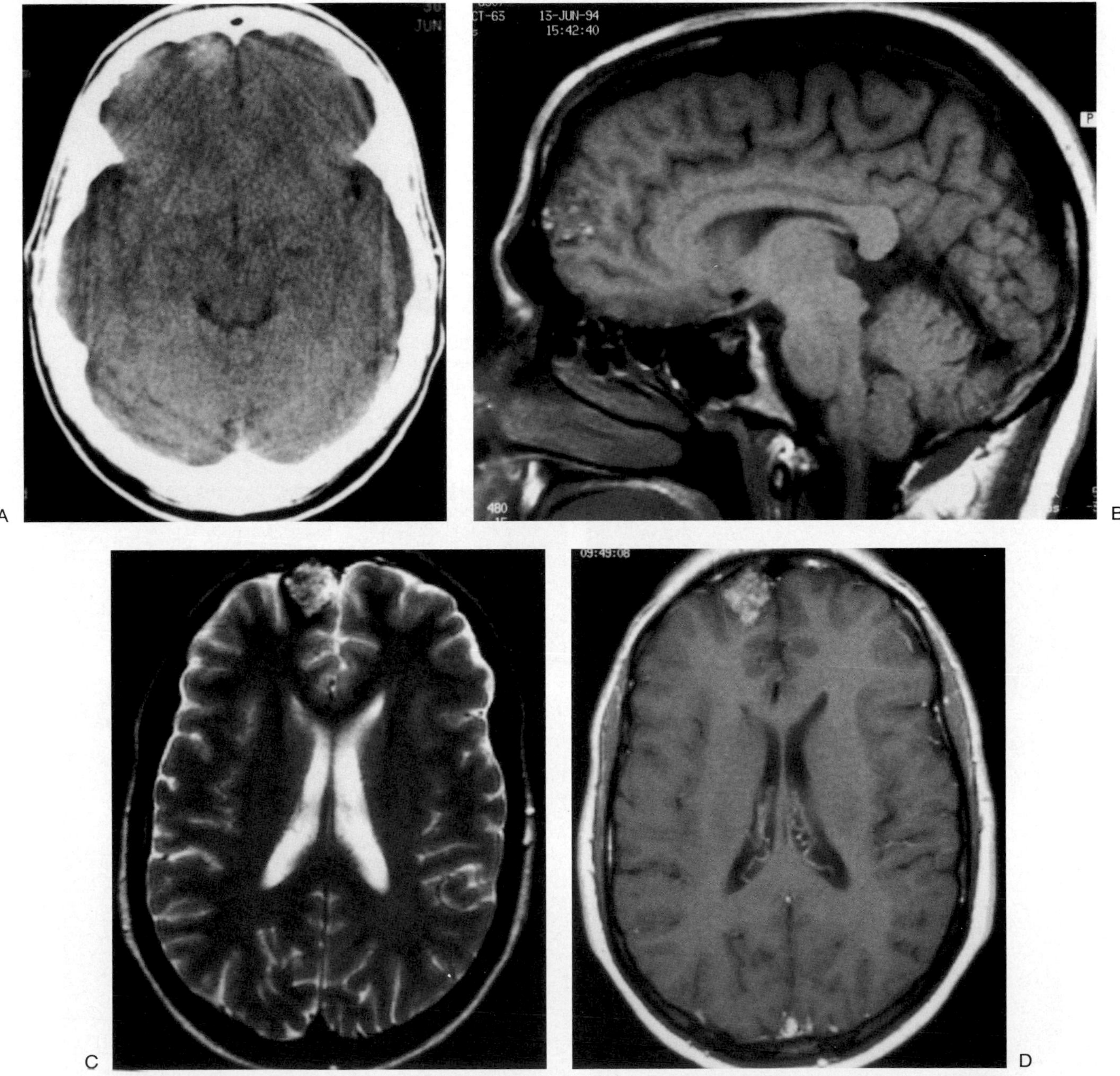

FIG. 28. Cavernous angioma, CT and MR appearance. **A:** Axial CT. **B:** Sagittal short TR/TE MR. **C:** Axial long TR/TE MR. **D:** Axial postcontrast short TR/TE MR. CT (A) shows hyperdense superficial mass in frontal lobe. Subpial mass with round collections of hyperintense methemoglobin (B,C) surrounded by dense, complete rim of hypointensity on T2-weighted image (C) characterize this lesion with high degree of specificity. Enhancement is also typical (D).

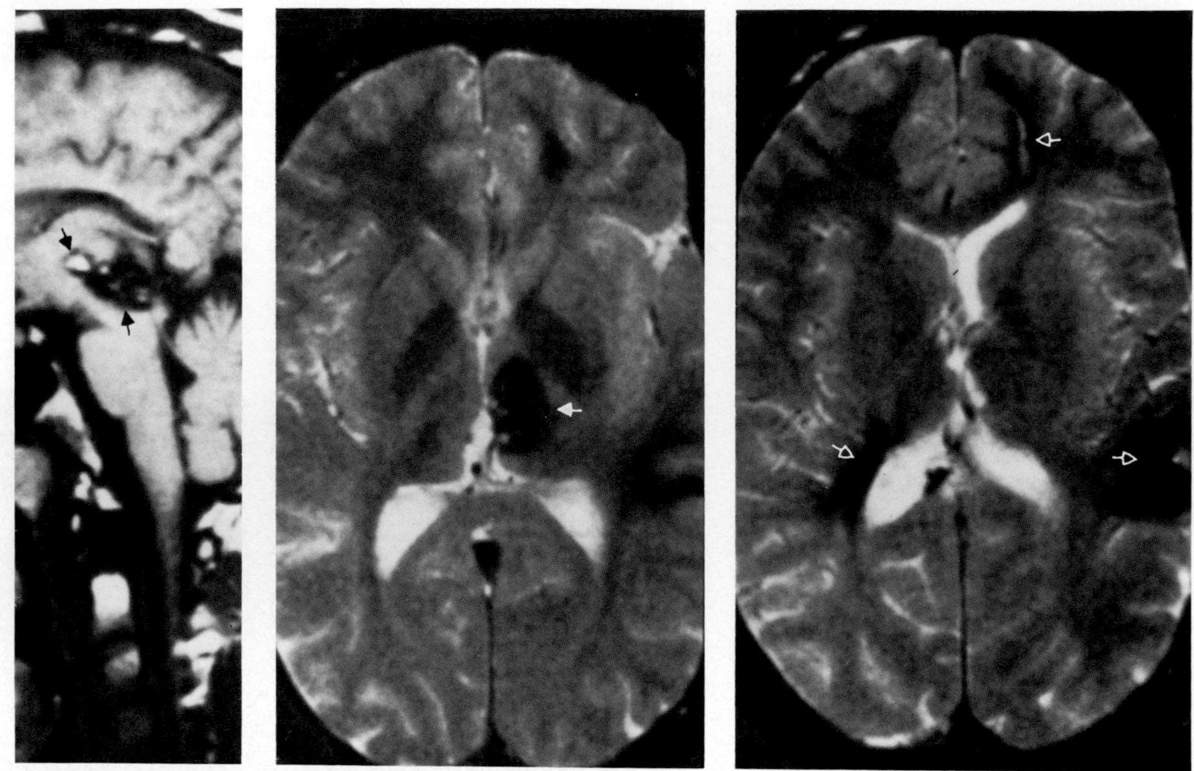

FIG. 29. Multiple cavernous angiomas. **A:** Sagittal short TR/TE MR (600/20). **B:** Axial long TR/TE MR (2800/80). **C:** Axial long TR/TE MR (2800/80). Dorsal thalamic-hypothalamic hemorrhagic lesion (*closed arrows*, A,B) has typical features of this lesion. Note multiple other cavernous angiomas (*open arrows*) on long TR/TE images (B,C).

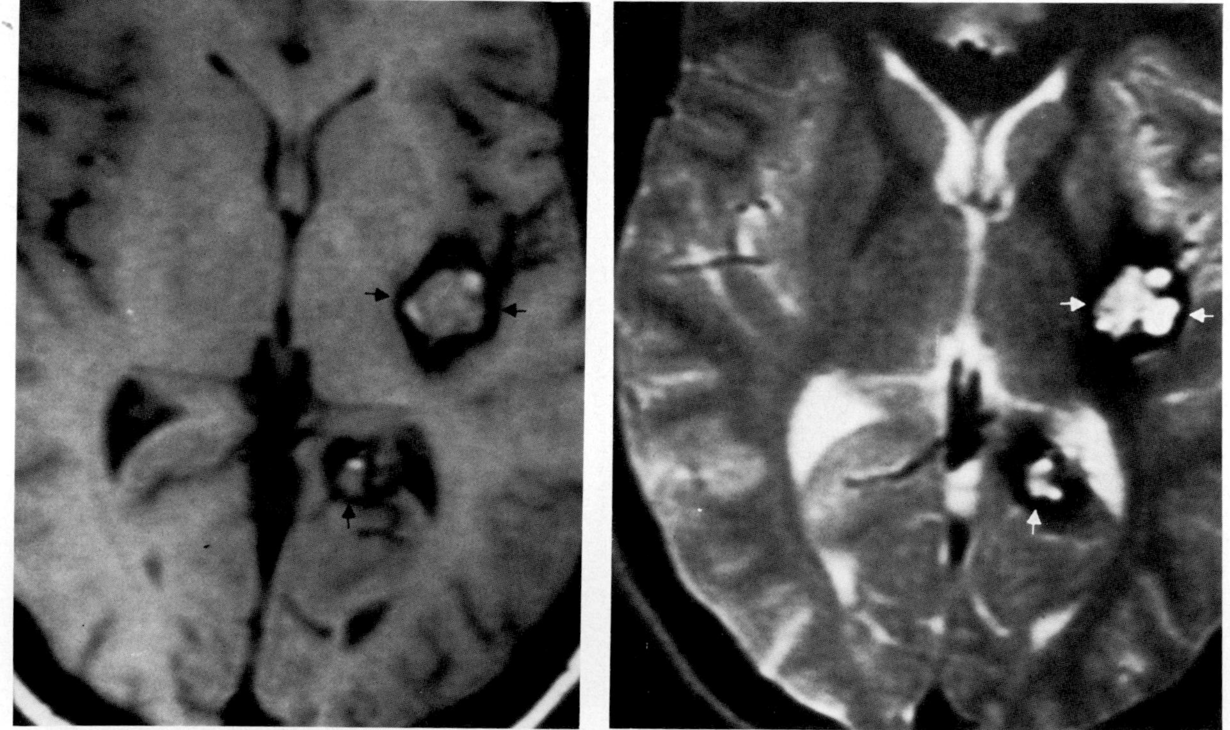

FIG. 30. Multiple cavernous angiomas. **A:** Short TR/TE MR (600/20). **B:** Long TR/TE MR (2500/80). Left subinsular and periatrial hemorrhagic lesions (*arrows*, A, B) have typical features of OCVM, with focal methemoglobin, complete rim of markedly hypointense iron-storage products, and no edema. (From Atlas, ref. 163, with permission.)

(Figs. 28–30). These key features include (a) focal central heterogeneity containing areas corresponding to subacute-chronic hemorrhage (methemoglobin), (b) circumferential, complete rings of markedly hypointense iron-storage forms around these high intensity central areas, (c) no mass effect or edema, and (d) no demonstrable feeding arteries or draining veins can be associated with developmental venous anomalies (venous angiomas) (see Fig. 17), which may lessen the specificity of MRI (7). The presence of remote blood-breakdown products within and around these lesions is often demonstrable in patients who relate no history of clinical hemorrhagic event, supporting the idea that this appearance is more often due to seepage of blood pigments from intracavernous sequestration rather than from frank hemorrhage. On MRI, cavernous hemangiomas typically show contrast enhancement (Figs. 31 and 32).

Aside from the potential confusion from the associated venous anomaly, other pitfalls occur in the interpretation of MRI when a cavernous angioma is suspected (see Table 2). The distinction of cavernous angioma from hemorrhagic neoplasm on MR images may be difficult if a relatively recent hemorrhage has occurred, but the absence of edema, the absence of identifiable nonhemorrhagic tumor tissue, complete rings of extensive ferritin/hemosiderin in the adjacent parenchyma, and the presence of expected temporal evolution of the hematoma on serial MR scans usually allow confident differentiation from neoplasm (96) (also see Chapters 9 and 10). Focal hypointensity on T2-weighted images in isolation can be due to a variety of pathologic conditions, including cavernous angioma, residua of remote hypertensive hemorrhage, treated toxoplasmosis, prior radiation therapy, disseminated intravascular coagulopathy (Fig. 33) and amyloid angiopathy (Fig. 34). The utilization of GE imaging (see Chapter 29) for its heightened sensitivity to hemorrhage and therefore cavernous angiomas occasionally presents two problems in diagnosing this entity. First, the hypointensity arising from the heterogeneity of magnetic susceptibilities when the lesion is present can mask all intrinsic signal characteristics, thereby precluding the specific diagnosis. Second, focal susceptibility artifacts from any cause may uncommonly appear as peripheral rings of hypointensity with central artifactual hyperintensity (97), thereby mimicking the characteristic appearance.

Capillary Telangiectasia

Capillary telangiectasias (sometimes called *capillary angiomas*) are usually small, solitary lesions that most commonly occur in the pons. These represent a collec-

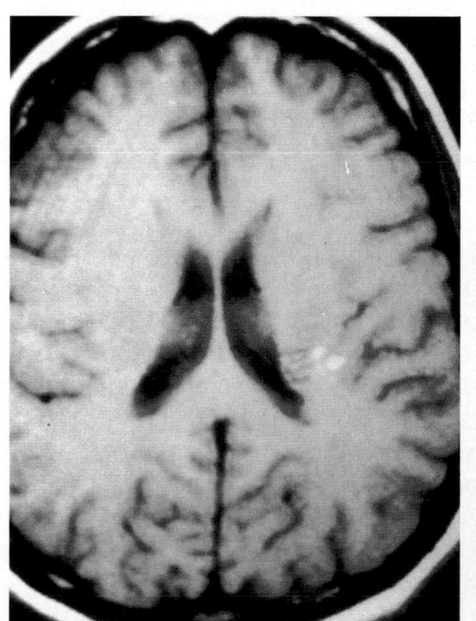
A

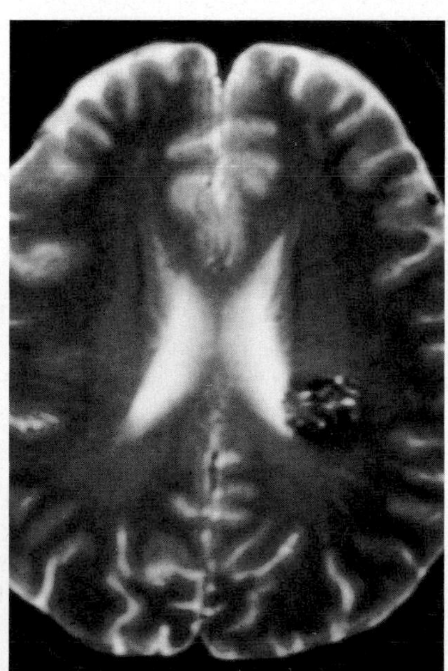

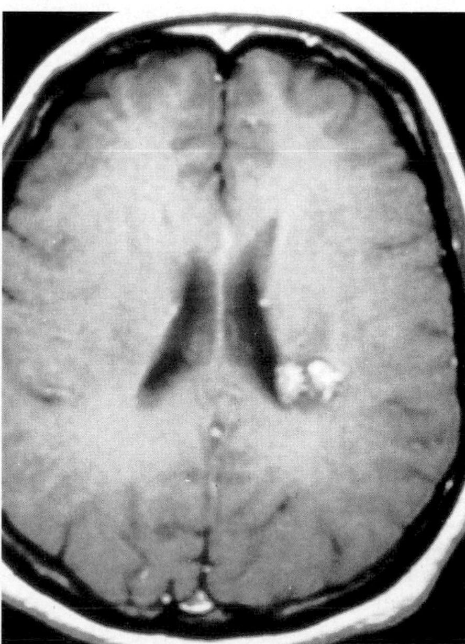
B,C

FIG. 31. Cavernous angioma, enhancement characteristics on MR. **A:** T1-weighted MR. **B:** Axial T2-weighted MR. **C:** Axial postcontrast T1-weighted MRI. Classical appearance on unenhanced (A,B) images enhances slightly after gadolinium (C).

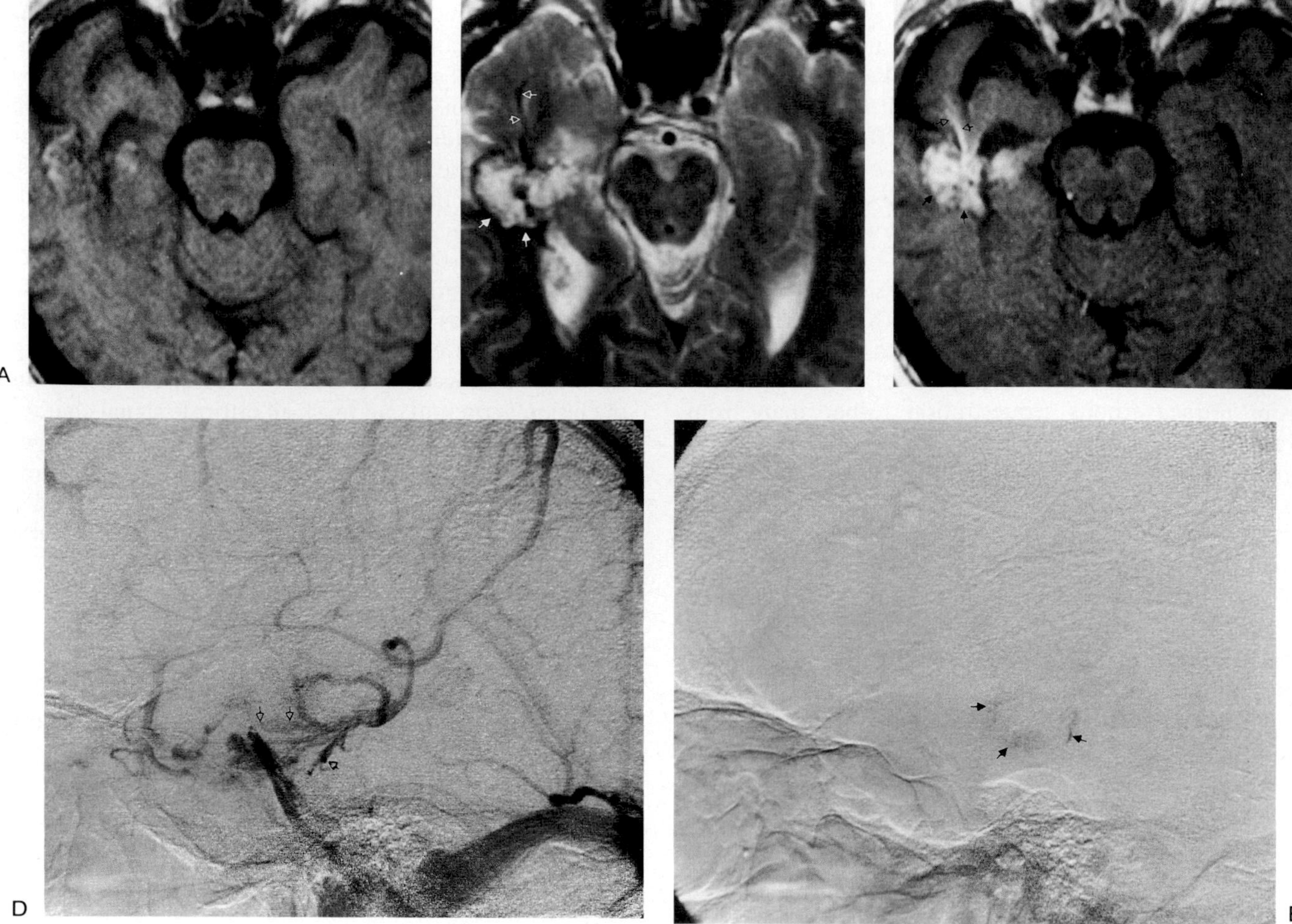

FIG. 32. Cavernous malformation with associated venous angioma. Unenhanced axial T1-(**A**) (700/20) and T2-(**B**) (3500/93) weighted images demonstrate heterogeneous signal intensity adjacent to the right temporal horn without associated mass effect. Rim of decreased signal intensity surrounding cavernous malformation is best seen on the T2-weighted images (*arrows*), as are linear areas of decreased signal (venous angioma) within the temporal lobe (*open arrows*). **C:** Enhanced T1-weighted image (700/20) with diffuse enhancement of the cavernous malformation (*arrows*) and improved visualization of linear vascular structures of the venous angioma (*open arrows*). **D:** Venous phase of right internal carotid injection demonstrates venous angioma (*open arrows*), whereas **E:** very late (>20 sec) phase shows contrast stagnation within the cavernous malformation (*arrows*).

tion of pathologically dilated capillaries, which on histologic examination reveal aneurysmal enlargement with marked variability within a delicate network of these vessels. Intervening brain parenchyma is identifiable within the lesion (in distinction from cavernous hemangiomas)

TABLE 2. *Differential diagnosis of cavernous angioma*

Cavernous angioma
Subacute to chronic isolated intraparenchymal hematoma
Amyloid angiopathy
Radiation therapy–associated hemorrhage
Hemorrhagic metastasis
Melanotic melanoma metastasis
Infection (esp. treated toxoplasmosis)

(28,31). In the vast majority of cases, the intervening and adjacent brain tissue is normal on pathologic examination, without gliosis or residua of prior hemorrhage (28).

Although most of these lesions are clinically silent and therefore incidental findings on both imaging and necropsy, they occasionally can be associated with hemorrhage and can also be found in concert with other vascular malformations (as can cavernous hemangiomas) (7).

It can be difficult to differentiate cavernous angiomas from capillary telangiectasias when the lesion is in the pons and is an incidental finding if hemorrhage has occurred (although the fact that hemorrhage has indeed occurred implies the diagnosis of cavernous angioma rather than capillary telangiectasia). Therefore, as noted above, an often-used term for this group of entities for

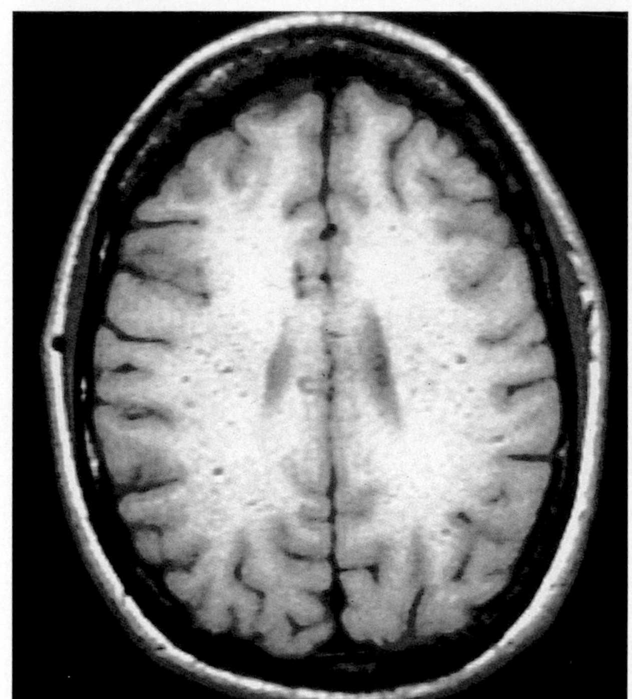

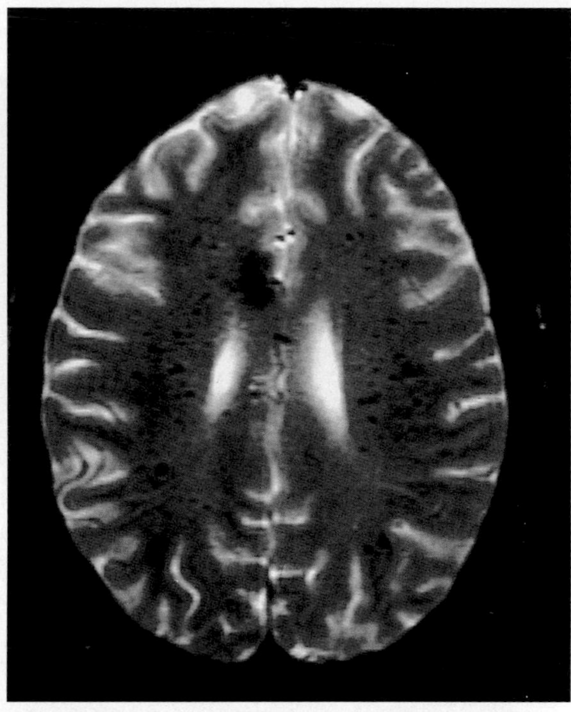

FIG. 33. DIC as multiple focal hypointensities in T2-weighted MRI. **A:** Short TR/TE MR. **B:** Long TR/TE MR. Multiple punctate foci of marked hypointensity in subcortical and deep white matter are seen best on T2-weighted image (B). Absence of any hyperintensity on T1-weighted image (A) and location of lesions make cavernous angiomas less likely.

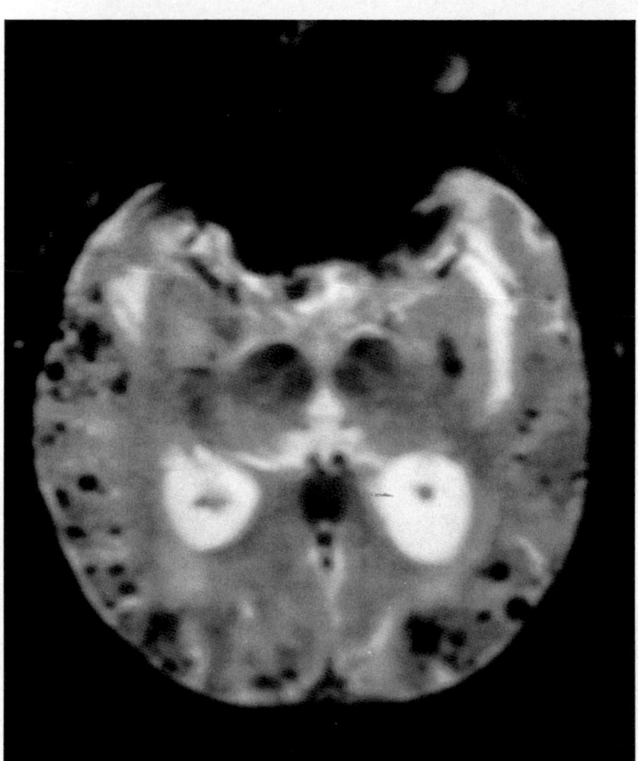

FIG. 34. Amyloid angiopathy as subcortical focal hypointensities. Numerous focal hypointensities in subcortical white matter in elderly patient can occasionally be the manifestation of amyloid angiopathy and can be confused with multiple cavernous angiomas.

clinicians that is more descriptive is OCVM because these lesions are usually angiographically occult (98).

More importantly, cavernous angioma and capillary telangiectasia typically have different clinical manifestations (cavernous angiomas commonly declare themselves with seizures or intracranial hemorrhage, whereas capillary telangiectasias are most often clinically silent), and therefore different management issues. Therefore, it is important to recognize those instances when the MRI findings are specific for capillary telangiectasia. The capillary telangiectasia should be suspected when there is a lace-like region of stippled contrast enhancement with no (or only subtle) abnormality on unenhanced SE images (Figs. 35 and 36). There occasionally may be a minimal hypointensity associated with the lesion, presumably representing residua of subclinical bleeding. This may be detected only with highly sensitive GE techniques (see Fig. 36). The diagnosis can be confidently made when the lesion demonstrates all these features, is asymptomatic, and particularly when it is situated in its classic location, that is, the pons. It should be noted that capillary telangiectasias are occasionally found in the cerebral hemispheres (Fig. 37) and other locations (see Fig. 35). The key to distinguishing the enhancement of capillary telangiectasia from other similar enhancing lesions, notably lymphoma when periventricular, is the absence of any signal abnormality on the unenhanced images. The associated findings of other portions of a mixed vas-

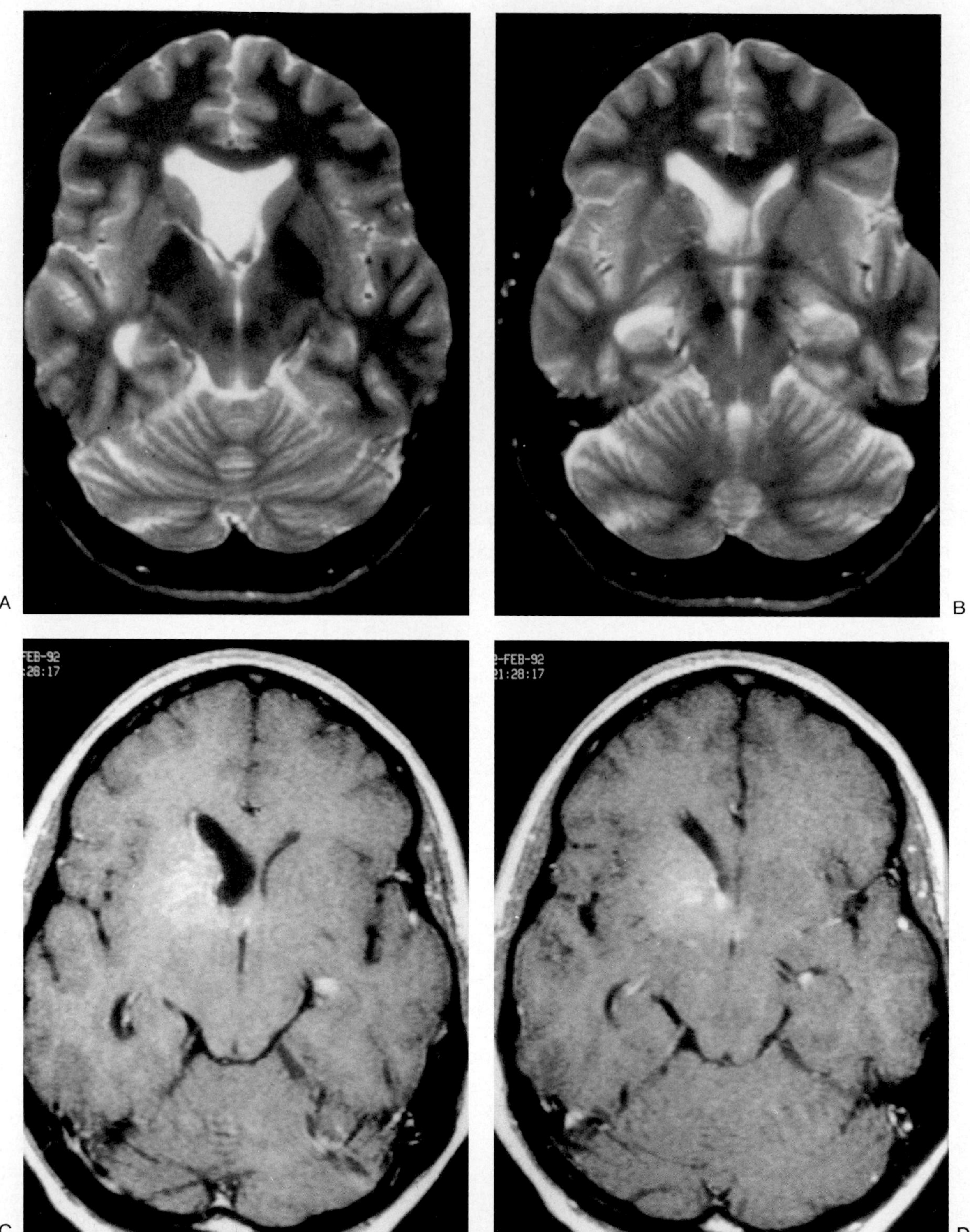

FIG. 35. Capillary telangiectasia, basal ganglia. **A,B:** Long TR/TE MR. **C,D:** Short TR/TE MR after intravenous contrast. Dilated right frontal horn and only subtle signal change in right basal ganglia can be seen on unenhanced MR (A,B). After gadolinium (C,D), lace-like enhancement is seen in right caudate head, right putamen, and anterior limb of internal capsule in this asymptomatic patient. The pattern of enhancement in an essentially normal noncontrast region is typical of this lesion.

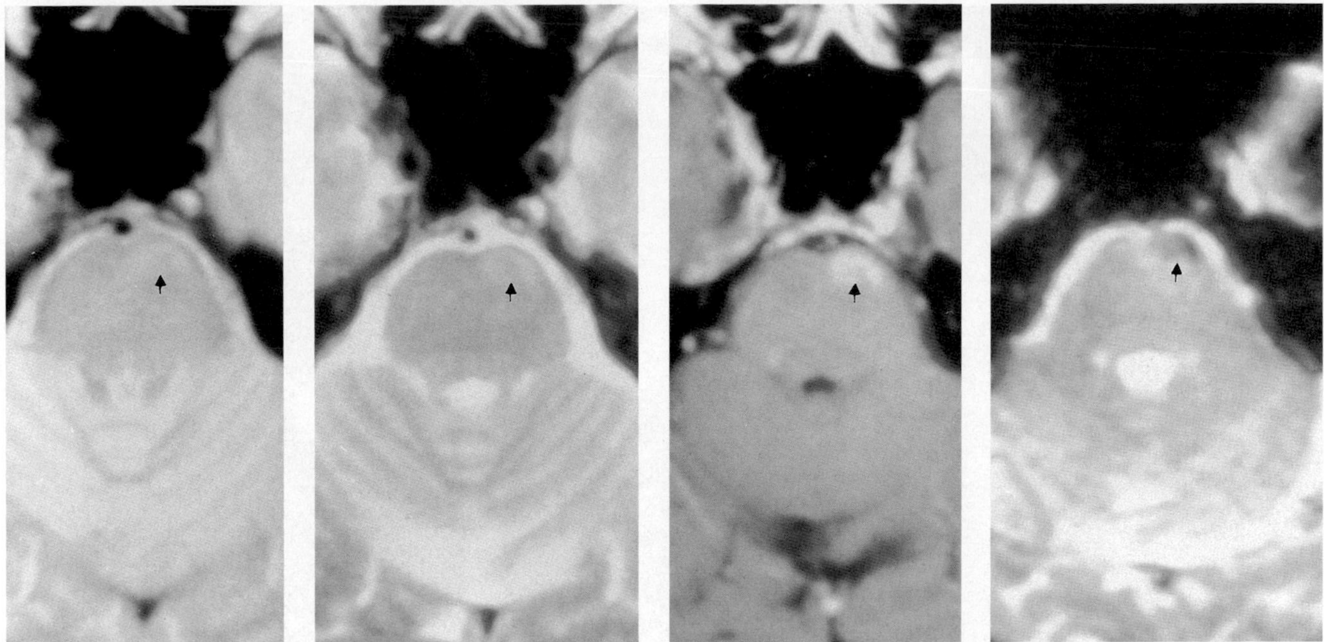

FIG. 36. Capillary telangiectasia, pons. **A:** Long TR/short TE MR. **B:** Long TR/long TE MR. **C:** Short TR/TE MR after intravenous contrast. **D:** GE MR (T2* weighted). Minimal signal abnormality in right ventrolateral aspect of pons can be seen on unenhanced MR (*arrow*, A,B). After gadolinium (C), lace-like enhancement is seen in region (*arrow*). Note subtle hypointensity (*arrow*) throughout lesion on GE image (D), presumably indicating residua of prior subclinical hemorrhage in this asymptomatic patient.

cular malformation are also helpful, when present (Fig. 38).

Venous Angioma

Venous angiomas (also known as *developmental venous anomalies* or *venous malformations*) are considered by most to be incidental malformations of venous drainage patterns. There is no arterial component in this entity. Intervening brain tissue is present between the veins comprising the lesion, and this brain tissue is usually normal without evidence of hemosiderin staining or gliosis (28). Venous angiomas may represent the most common cerebrovascular malformation, accounting for 63% of vascular malformations in one large autopsy study, with an overall incidence of 2% (99). They are generally thought to be clinically silent, although there is some controversy regarding their possible association with hemorrhage (100).

Venous angiomas occur throughout the cerebrum and cerebellum; Burger and Scheithauer state that they can also involve the spinal cord (28). This lesion consists of a tuft of abnormally enlarged medullary venous channels that are radially arranged around, and drain into, a central venous trunk (Fig. 39). The common trunk drains intracerebrally into the deep or superficial venous system (101). In the spinal cord, the enlarged draining veins associated with a venous angioma must be considered in a differential diagnosis with normally prominent veins seen along the dorsal aspect of the lumbar cord and enlarged draining veins of a dural spinal AVM (28) (see Chapter 28).

Because they represent anatomically variant but physiologically competent venous drainage pathways of a normally functioning region of brain, only rarely have

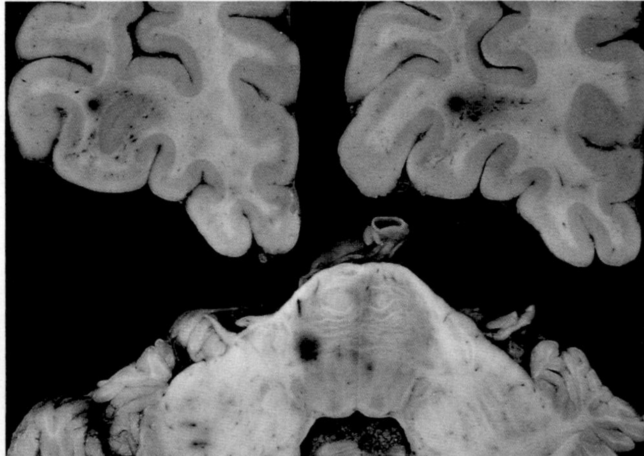

FIG. 37. Capillary telangiectasia, necropsy specimen. Axial section from necropsy specimen shows typical morphology of capillary telangiectasias, with abnormally ectatic vessels and interposed brain parenchyma in lesions involving brainstem and cerebral hemisphere. (From Okazaki and Scheithauer, ref. 8, with permission.)

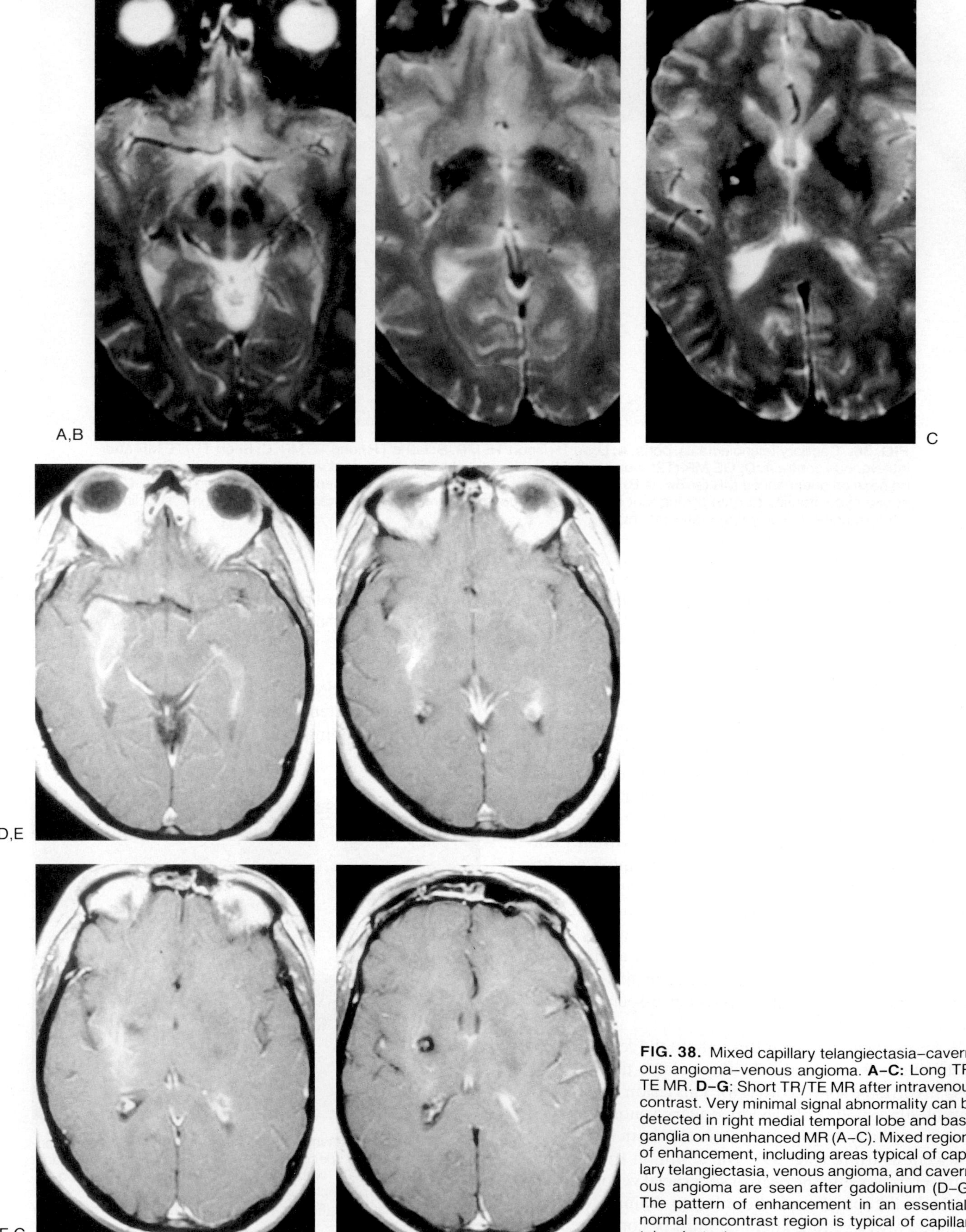

FIG. 38. Mixed capillary telangiectasia–cavernous angioma–venous angioma. **A–C:** Long TR/TE MR. **D–G**: Short TR/TE MR after intravenous contrast. Very minimal signal abnormality can be detected in right medial temporal lobe and basal ganglia on unenhanced MR (A–C). Mixed regions of enhancement, including areas typical of capillary telangiectasia, venous angioma, and cavernous angioma are seen after gadolinium (D–G). The pattern of enhancement in an essentially normal noncontrast region is typical of capillary telangiectasia.

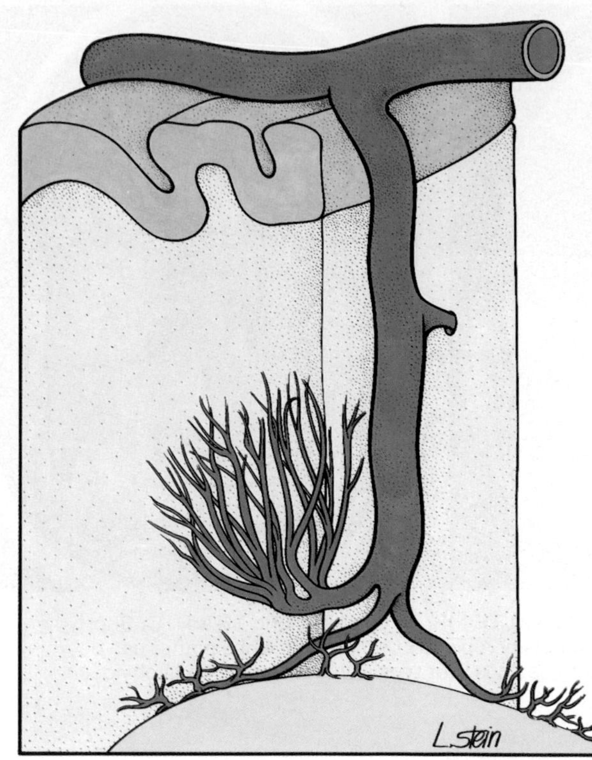

FIG. 39. Venous angioma, artist's depiction. Radially arranged veins along roof of lateral ventricle drain into enlarged cortical vein in the pattern characteristic of this anomaly.

neurologic symptoms been attributed to venous angiomas. Nonetheless, clinical symptomatology, particularly intracranial hemorrhage, has been reported in patients with venous angiomas (102). Although the potential may exist for the increased blood flow through the normally tiny medullary veins to cause rupture, the vast majority of cases are thought to remain asymptomatic throughout life. Most cases of symptoms associated with venous angiomas have been found in patients who also harbor cavernous malformations in contiguity with the venous angioma, that is, mixed vascular malformations (103). The link between venous angioma and clinical symptoms remains controversial. It has been noted that venous angiomas occur frequently with solitary cavernous angiomas, yet only very rarely when multiple cavernous angiomas are present (Shibata, 1995 ASNR, paper 99).

Angiography, contrast-enhanced CT, and contrast-enhanced MRI delineate typical curvilinear vascular channels receiving drainage from a "spoke-wheel"–appearing collection of small tapering veins arranged in a radial pattern (Figs. 17, 40, and 41). The larger central draining vein empties into a large cortical vein, a dural sinus, or a subependymal ventricular vein. Angiographic characteristics also include normal arterial and capillary phases, with opacification of the lesion usually occurring during normal venous phase and remaining opacified through the late venous phase. Venous angiomas may be overlooked on first pass on unenhanced MRI (see Fig. 40), where sometimes only the large central vein is obvious as a linear flow void. The venous nature of the vascular channel is implied on unenhanced long TR MRI when the venous slow flow is high intensity because of gradient moment nulling techniques (often misregistered because of oblique flow) (see Fig. 41), and on close inspection the radially arranged veins are also revealed. An anatomic clue to the diagnosis is the location of the venous angioma, typically intimately associated with the lateral ventricle (Figs. 40 and 42) and draining into a subependymal vein. As already stated, venous angiomas can co-exist with other OCVMs, an association that should be actively sought with GE techniques in symptomatic patients. GE MR imaging allows rapid confirmation of flowing blood within these incidentally discovered malformations when necessary, although they have a characteristic appearance on conventional SE images (104). GE imaging can occasionally show marked hypointensity within venous angiomas. This should not be mistaken for hemorrhage, but it is simply a reflection of the paramagnetic deoxyhemoglobin within venous blood (see Fig. 42). MRA is unnecessary in the vast majority of cases.

Dural Arteriovenous Malformations

Dural AVMs (or AV fistulae) are vascular malformations that have different angioarchitecture, clinical presentation, natural history, imaging features, and therapy

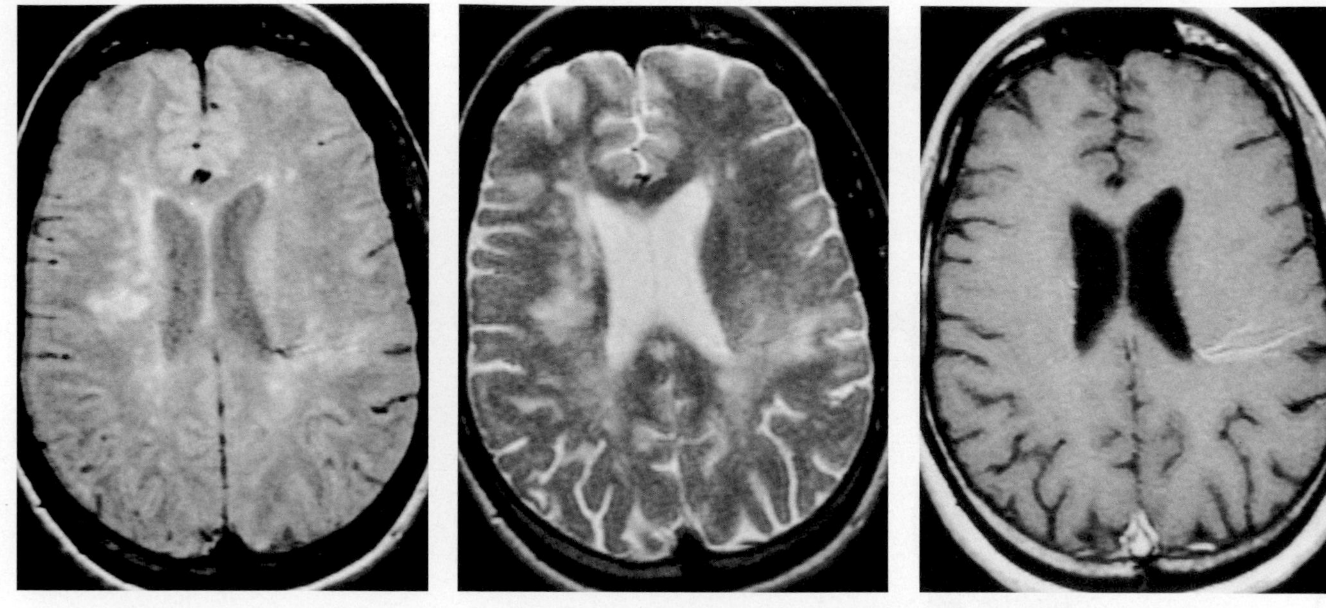
A B,C

FIG. 40. Venous angioma, pre- vs. postcontrast MR. **A:** Long TR/short TE MR. **B:** Long TR/long TE MR. **C:** Short TR/TE MR after contrast enhancement. Suggestion of linear low intensity regions in left parietal white matter can be noted on unenhanced MR (A,B) in patient with multiple white matter lesions, but typical venous angioma is obvious after intravenous contrast (C).

from parenchymal AVMs of the brain. Dural AVMs (DAVMs) comprise about 10% to 15% of all intracranial vascular malformations (105). Approximately 35% of posterior fossa AVMs are purely dural in supply; more than half of DAVMs are in the posterior fossa. They represent AV shunts located within the dura or tentorium, most often involving the walls of the large dural venous sinuses (Fig. 43). Arterial supply is primarily via meningeal branches of the external carotid artery, internal carotid artery (ICA), or vertebral artery. DAVM drainage is into the dural venous sinuses or other dural or leptomeningeal venous channels. Thrombosis or obstruction of the involved venous sinus has frequently been associated with DAVMs. Retrograde filling of the involved ve-

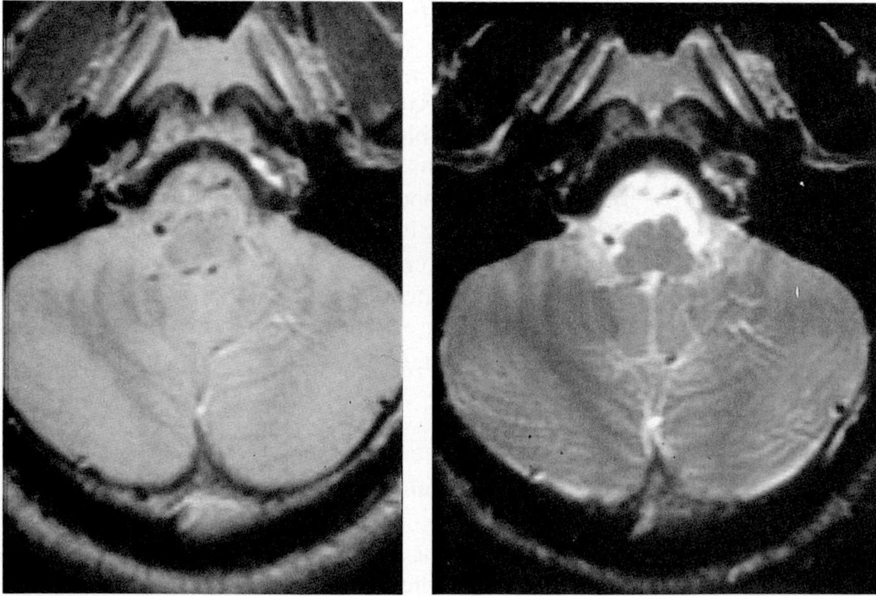
A,B

FIG. 41. Venous angioma as high intensity with gradient moment nulling. **A:** Long TR/short TE MR. **B:** Long TR/long TE MR. Flow-compensated images (A,B) show slightly misregistered hyperintensity in cerebellar venous angioma because of oblique orientation of vessels.

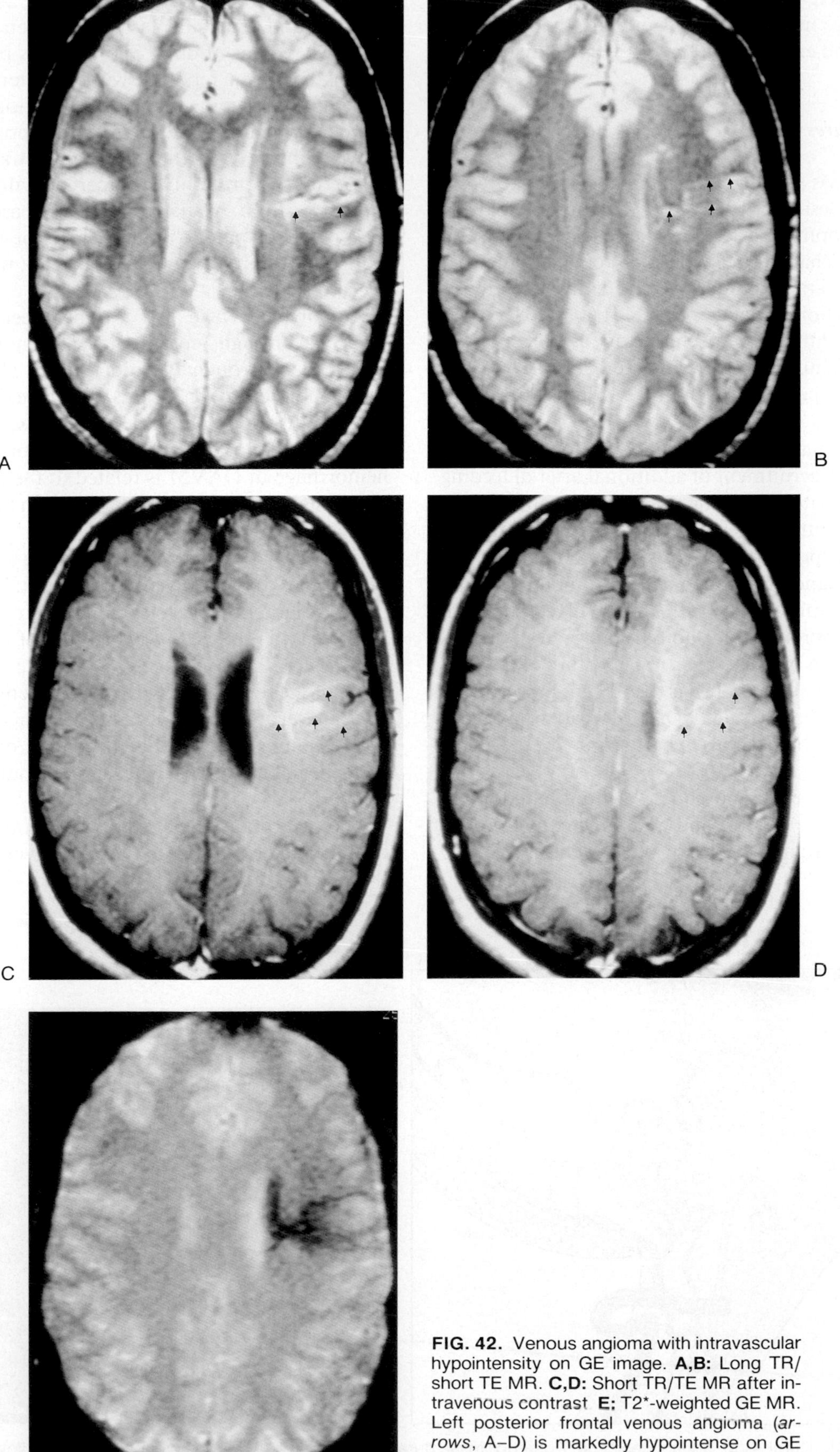

FIG. 42. Venous angioma with intravascular hypointensity on GE image. **A,B:** Long TR/short TE MR. **C,D:** Short TR/TE MR after intravenous contrast. **E:** T2*-weighted GE MR. Left posterior frontal venous angioma (*arrows*, A–D) is markedly hypointense on GE image (E), more likely because of deoxyhemoglobin in venous blood, than hemorrhage.

nous sinus and reflux into pial veins may also be present. When drainage into pial veins is present, the veins may be tortuous and enlarged, often with variceal dilatation.

Clinical Features

Most DAVMs present later in life and are believed to be acquired lesions (106). The pathophysiology of DAVM development as well as the temporal course of vasculopathic changes in the lesions remain somewhat controversial. Trauma, surgery, and sinus thrombosis are potential etiologic factors (Fig. 44) (107,108). It has been postulated that veno-occlusive disease affecting the dural venous sinus results in enlargement of normally present microscopic AV shunts within the sinus wall (109).

Initially, drainage from the shunts is into the involved venous sinus. Recruitment of additional arterial feeding vessels occurs with increasing AV shunting and venous hypertension within the sinus. In some cases, the increased venous pressure and sinus obstruction favor retrograde filling and enlargement of leptomeningeal and pial veins communicating with the involved sinus. In such cases, compromise of venous drainage from regions of involved brain may occur, as may rupture of the delicate, enlarged pial veins. It has also been shown in an animal model that acquired DAVMs can occur after chronic intracerebral venous hypertension, even without veno-occlusive disease (110).

The natural history and clinical symptomatology of DAVMs is highly variable and to a large extent dependent on the location of the lesion and its venous drainage pathways (108). Cranial bruit, tinnitus, and headache are frequent and reflect increased flow, often involving pain-sensitive regions of dura. Spontaneous regression of the lesions has been reported without intervention. Many patients do not come to medical attention because of the frequently benign clinical course. In approximately 15% of cases, however, patients sustain intracranial hemorrhage, most commonly intraparenchymal or subarachnoid in location. A smaller number of cases are identified as a result of parenchymal deficits or seizures arising from venous infarction or impairment of venous drainage and ischemia.

Hemorrhage from DAVMs has been demonstrated to occur through leptomeningeal venous connections rather than through the nidus itself. Hemorrhage has been reported only in lesions with reflux into leptomeningeal veins and not in those cases whose drainage is confined to the dural sinuses. Consequently, the risk of hemorrhage in DAVM is related to the presence of leptomeningeal venous drainage, which in turn is a factor of the location of the lesion (111).

DAVMs may be classified according to the dural sinus or region of dura involved by the shunt. DAVMs involving the sigmoid-transverse sinuses are the most common, making up nearly two thirds of cases in Awad's review of 377 reported cases in the literature (112). Because of the tendency for drainage to remain confined to the transverse and sigmoid sinuses, reflux into leptomeningeal veins is rare in this location. Consequently, the incidence of hemorrhage in sigmoid-transverse DAVMs is low.

The cavernous sinus is the second most common location, with nearly 12% of DAVMs involving this region.

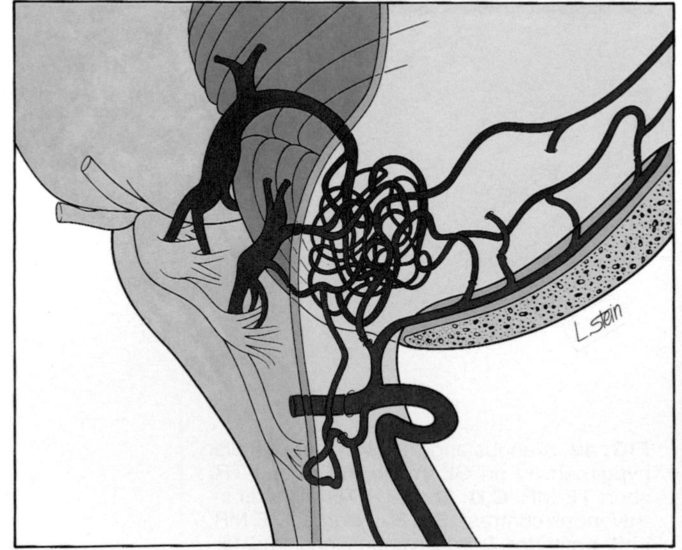

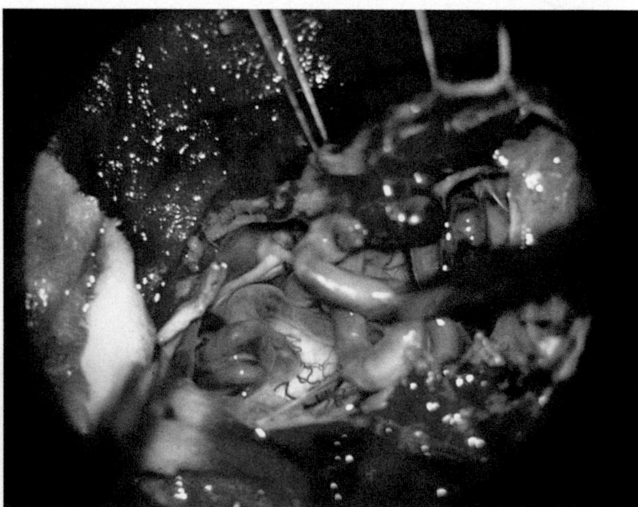

FIG. 43. Dural AVM, artist's depiction. Posterior fossa dural AVM has enlarged vessels because of high flow shunt within dural margin at skull base.

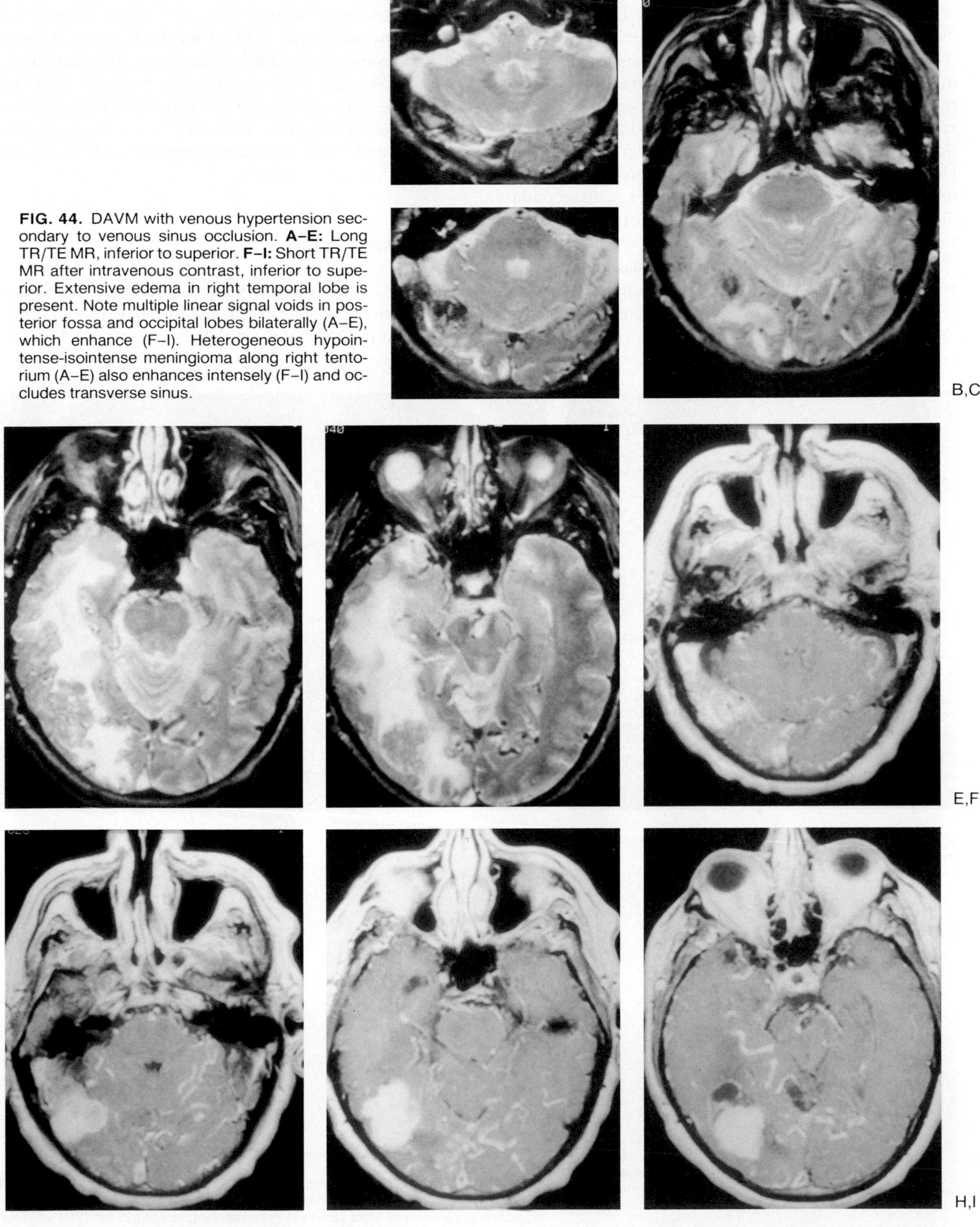

FIG. 44. DAVM with venous hypertension secondary to venous sinus occlusion. **A–E:** Long TR/TE MR, inferior to superior. **F–I:** Short TR/TE MR after intravenous contrast, inferior to superior. Extensive edema in right temporal lobe is present. Note multiple linear signal voids in posterior fossa and occipital lobes bilaterally (A–E), which enhance (F–I). Heterogeneous hypointense-isointense meningioma along right tentorium (A–E) also enhances intensely (F–I) and occludes transverse sinus.

DAVMs of the cavernous sinus comprise a unique group of intracranial vascular malformations. These lesions are usually found in middle-aged women, often with hypertension. Leptomeningeal venous drainage is uncommon in this location, and consequently intracranial hemorrhage from this lesion is rare. In cavernous DAVM, symptoms are highly suggestive of the diagnosis, a situation distinctly different from noncavernous DAVMs. Drainage into the cavernous sinus often results in compromise of cranial nerves III, IV, and VI, with secondary diplopia. Drainage into the ophthalmic veins is extremely common in DAVMs of the cavernous sinus, and red eye with proptosis secondary to engorgement of the veins of the orbit is a frequent complaint (113). Secondary glaucoma from impairment of venous drainage from the globe may also occur.

DAVMs of the tentorial-incisural region, anterior fossa, convexity–sagittal sinus, and sylvian–middle fossa represent additional DAVM locations (114). Although these lesions are much less common, the incidence of leptomeningeal venous drainage is very high with DAVMs in these regions. Consequently, the vast majority of lesions in these locations have a very aggressive course and most commonly present with intracranial hemorrhage (Figs. 45–47).

MR Characteristics

The role of MRI in DAVMs has been discussed in the literature (115). The actual site of the fistulous communication in DAVM is virtually never seen on MRI. The

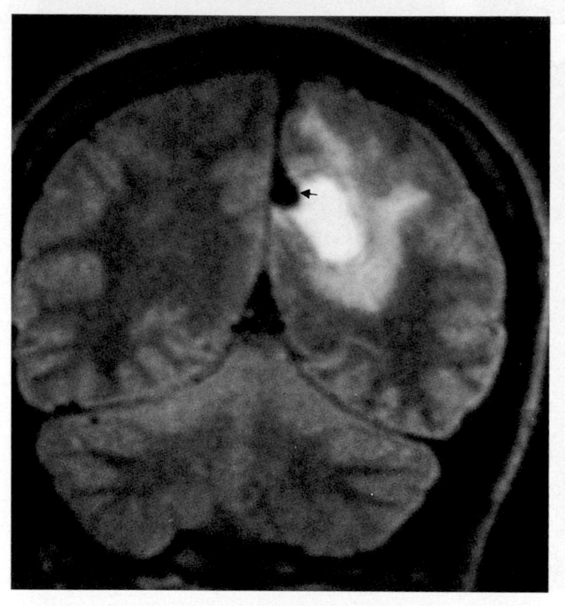

A

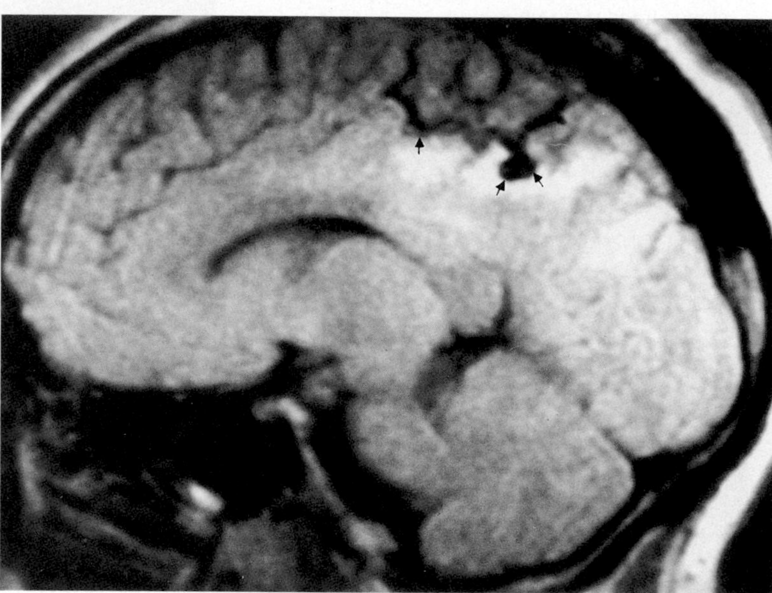

B

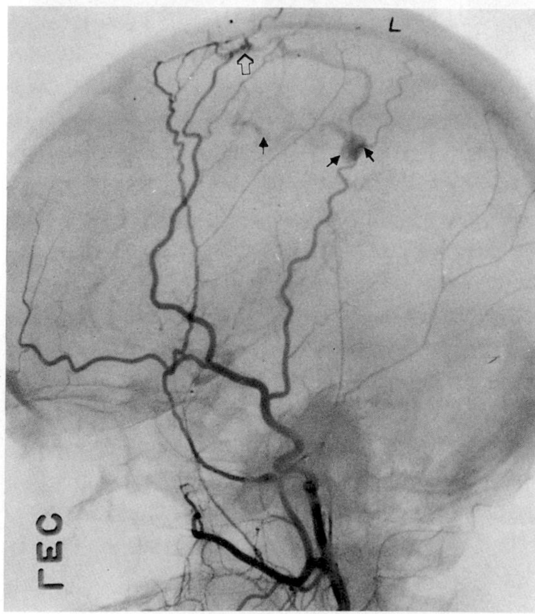

C

FIG. 45. DAVM of superior sagittal sinus. **A:** Coronal T2- (2000/80) and (**B**) sagittal T1- (800/20) weighted images showing left parietal hematoma with adjacent area of flow void (*arrows*) representing enlarged cortical vein with area of ectasia. **C:** Lateral view of left external carotid artery injection showing DAVM of superior sagittal sinus region (*open arrow*) with filling of enlarged cortical vein (*arrows*).

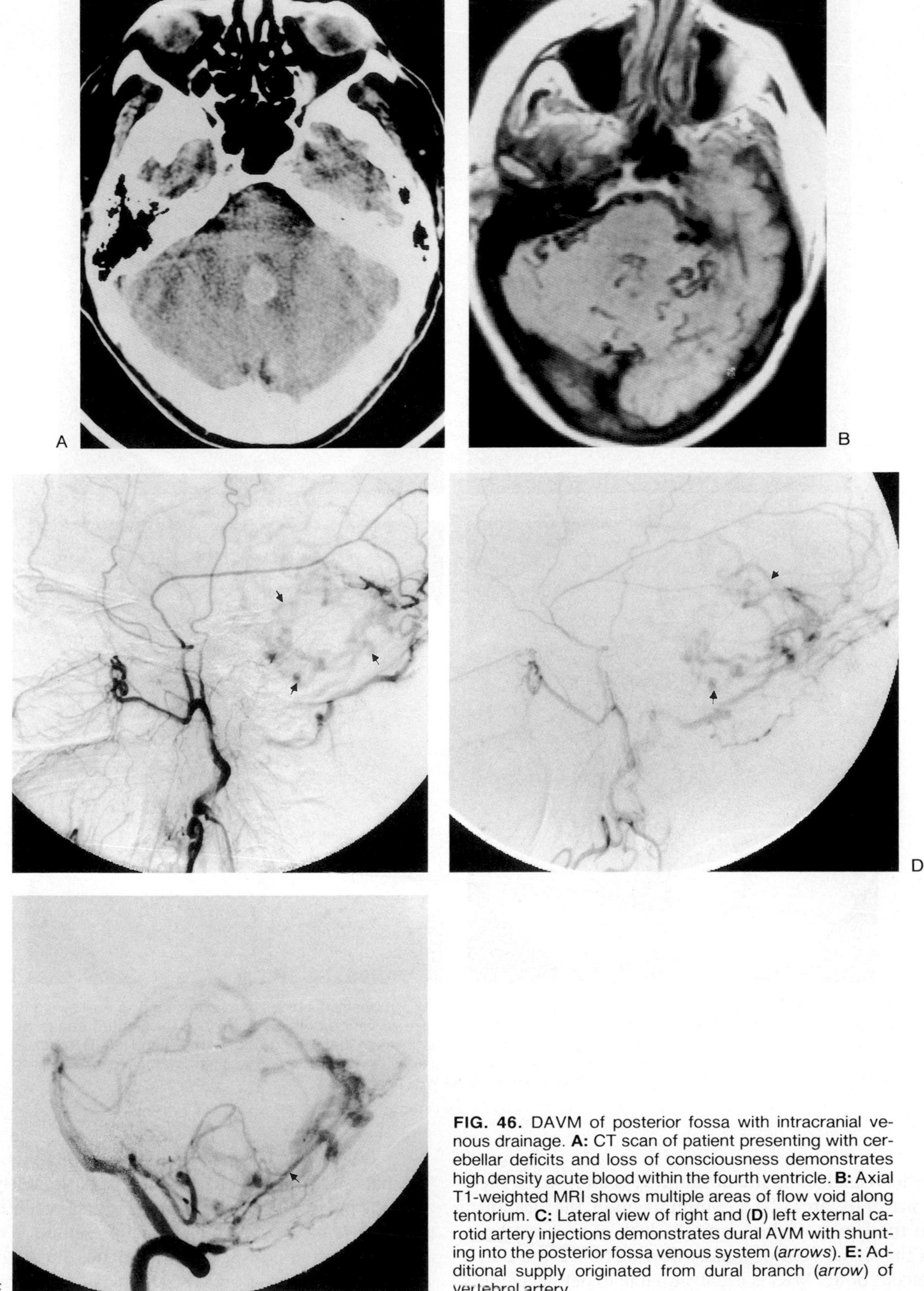

FIG. 46. DAVM of posterior fossa with intracranial venous drainage. **A:** CT scan of patient presenting with cerebellar deficits and loss of consciousness demonstrates high density acute blood within the fourth ventricle. **B:** Axial T1-weighted MRI shows multiple areas of flow void along tentorium. **C:** Lateral view of right and (**D**) left external carotid artery injections demonstrates dural AVM with shunting into the posterior fossa venous system (*arrows*). **E:** Additional supply originated from dural branch (*arrow*) of vertebral artery.

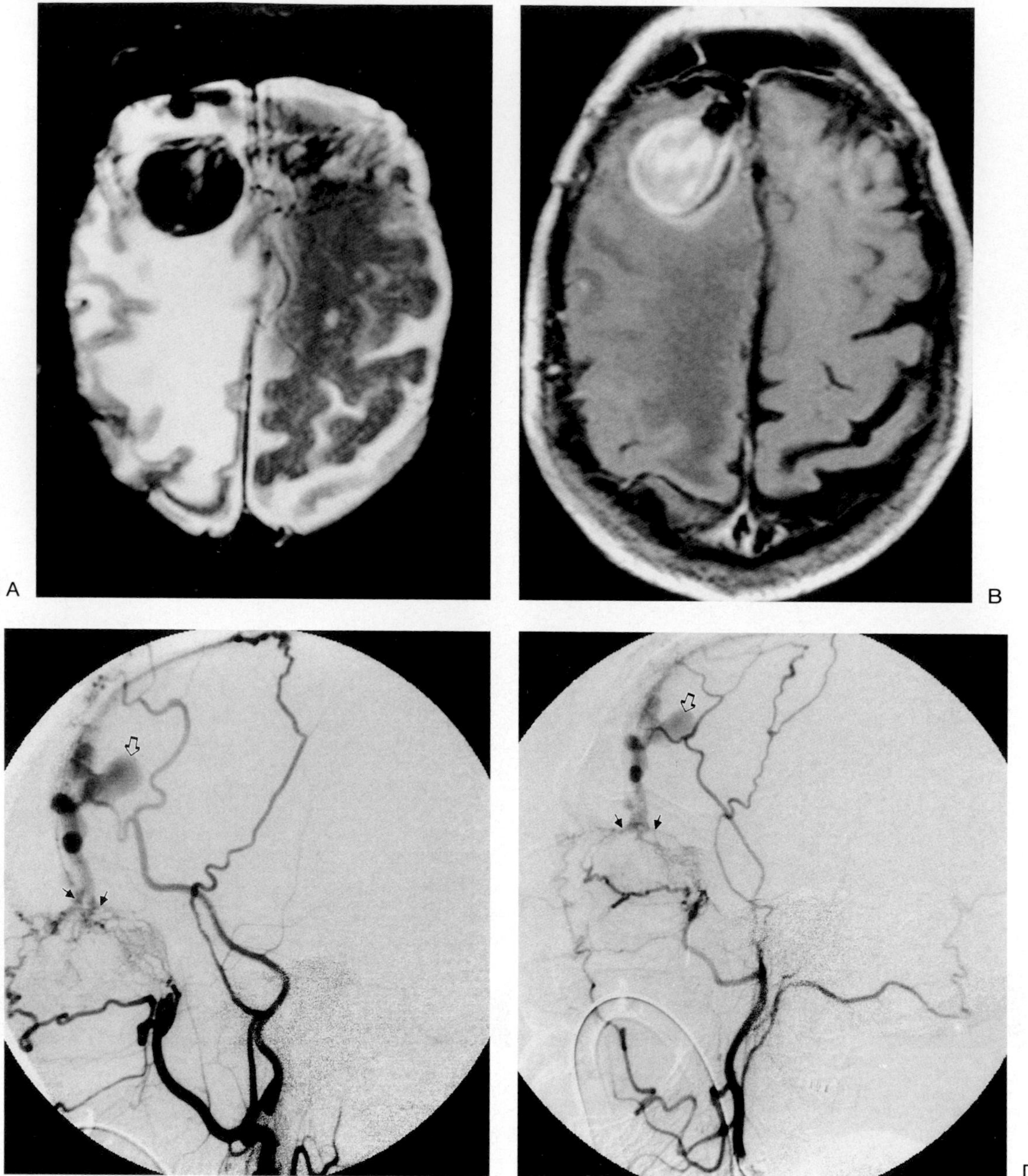

FIG. 47. DAVM of anterior fossa. Axial T2-weighted image (**A**) demonstrates mass with signal void as well as signal abnormality affecting entire right hemisphere from compromise of venous drainage. Axial T1-weighted image (**B**) shows spherical lesion enhances following administration of gadolinium. Lateral views of right (**C**) and left (**D**) external carotid artery injections demonstrate DAVM of anterior fossa (*arrows*) with drainage into intracranial veins and filling of large venous varix (*open arrow*). No supply from the ICAs was present.

failure to visualize the site of shunting is ascribed to the small size of the area of AV communication, the location within the leaves of dura, and the lack of contrast between the signal void of rapidly flowing blood and that of adjacent bone. MRI is usually unable to delineate the arterial supply to DAVMs (Fig. 48), again because of the relatively small size of meningeal feeding arteries. Nevertheless, MRI is extremely useful in the evaluation of the patient with DAVM (Table 3), particularly those with the potential for an aggressive course because of pial venous drainage. Since the clinical presentation of these patients is often nonspecific and vague, the often subtle clues to the diagnosis on MRI can play an extremely important role in the management of these patients.

DAVM should be suspected when large draining veins and feeding vessels are found exclusively in superficial,

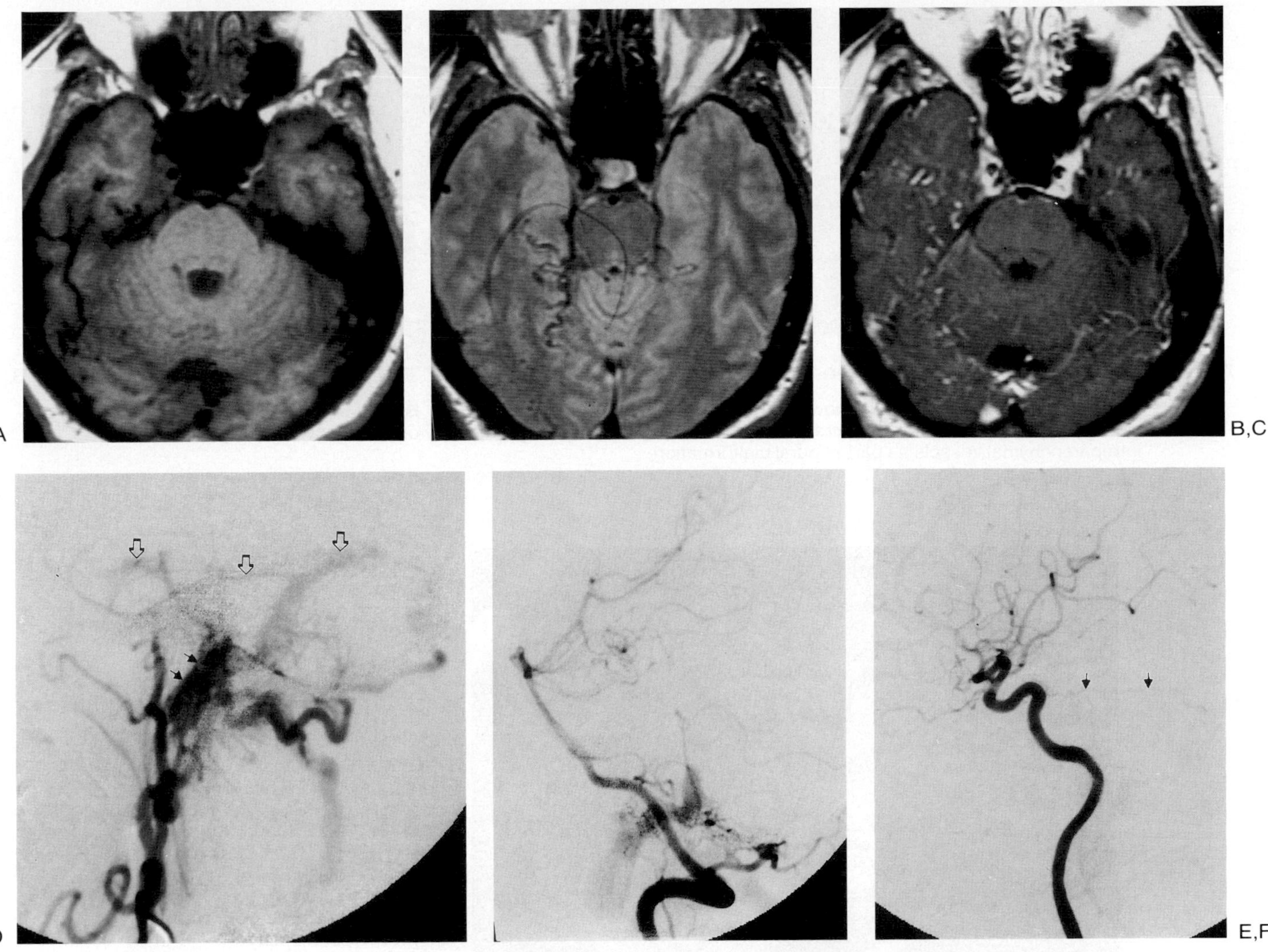

FIG. 48. DAVM of jugular region with intracranial drainage. **A:** Axial T1 (650/11) unenhanced and (**B**) density-weighted MRI showing serpentine flow voids along inferior temporal lobe representing intracranial venous drainage from DAVM in right jugular fossa. **C:** Enhanced T1-weighted image with areas of slow flow enhancement within the intracranial venous drainage. **D:** Lateral right external carotid artery injection shows filling of DAVM (*arrows*) with intracranial drainage retrograde into transverse sinus, petrosal sinuses, and cavernous sinus (*open arrows*). Later film showed filling of cortical veins. **E:** Lateral view of left vertebral artery injection showing additional supply from dural branches of vertebral artery. **F:** Lateral right ICA injection showing enlarged tentorial branch of cavernous ICA (artery of Bernasconi and Cassanari) (*arrows*) also feeding the lesion.

dural-based locations (Figs. 49 and 50). Dilatation of cortical veins in the absence of visualization of a parenchymal vascular nidus should suggest the diagnosis of DAVM. In one study (115), MRI was able to define accurately all cases of cortical vein dilatation associated with veno-occlusive disease that were seen at catheter angiography. A highly suggestive, if not specific, MRI sign of DAVM with veno-occlusive disease is the finding of prominent medullary veins (Hurst and Atlas, *unpublished data*).

TABLE 3. *MRI findings in dural AVMs*

Enlarged superficial cortical veins
Venous sinus occlusion
Enlarged deep medullary veins (2° to venous hypertension)
Edema
Venous infarction
Subcortical hematoma

AVM, arteriovenous malformation.

The enlarged medullary veins are frequently found in both hemispheres, and often in supratentorial as well as infratentorial locations (see Fig. 44). This sign is more obvious on postcontrast MRI and is a reflection of the venous hypertension that frequently accompanies these lesions. The enlarged medullary veins are often seen in conjunction with edema, presumably reflecting venous congestion (113). We believe that the demonstration of medullary vein enlargement on MRI is a specific sign of venous hypertension due to DAVM with venous outflow

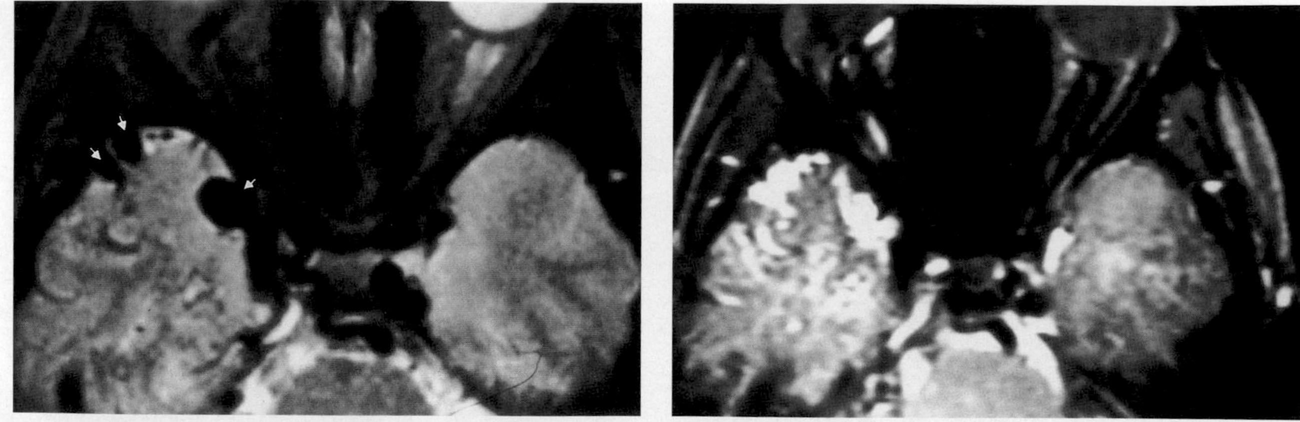

FIG. 49. DAVM with venous outflow obstruction. **A:** Long TR/TE MR (2800/80). **B:** GE MR (150/15/50°). Note large superficial vessels in right middle cranial fossa (*arrows*, A), seen as high intensity on GE image (B) along with smaller intraparenchymal vessels as part of dural malformation.

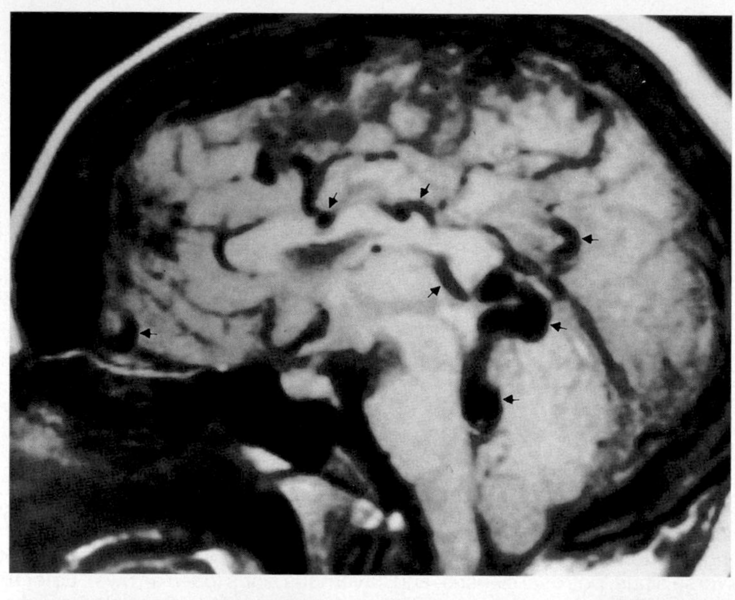

FIG. 50. DAVM with evidence of venous hypertension. **A:** Sagittal short TR/TE MR (600/20). **B:** Axial short TR/TE MR (600/20). **C:** Axial GE MR (150/15/50°). Note extensive evidence of enlarged venous structures as regions of signal void (*arrows*, A,B), which fill in with hyperintensity on GE image (*arrows*, C). The diffuse nature of the enlarged deep and superficial venous system implies venous hypertension, consistent with venous sinus occlusions.

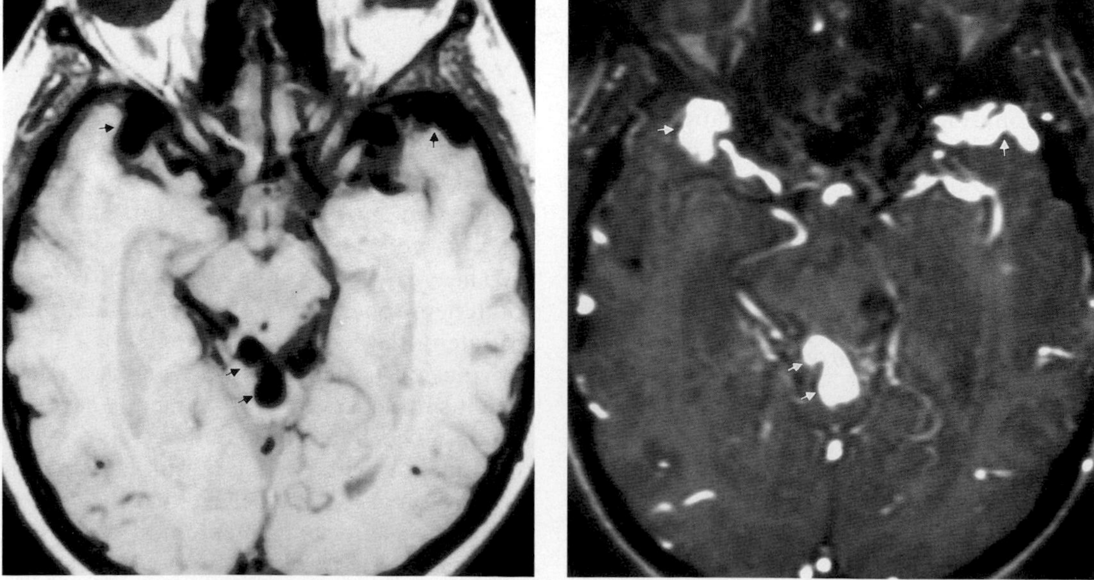

obstruction. It is an indication of significant venous hypertension and may correspond to clinically apparent encephalopathy in these patients. The documentation of thrombosis of the major dural sinuses is usually clear on conventional SE images, but MRA can play an adjunctive role. Parenchymal changes secondary to venous hypertension (venous infarction and parenchymal hemorrhage) are also well evaluated by MRI. One study has shown that nearly 80% of DAVM cases with MRI evidence of abnormal venous drainage had parenchymal complications.

MRA has been of use in demonstrating AV shunting in DAVMs in a variety of intracranial locations. This has been particularly true in cases with extensive involvement of the sigmoid-transverse sinuses, which may be characterized by large areas of visible nidus and relatively high flow. MRA may be useful in DAVMs near the skull base, where MR even with gadolinium is often unremarkable (Fig. 51). Although the diagnosis of DAVMs of the cavernous sinus has also been documented by the finding of abnormal drainage patterns into the orbit or across the intercavernous sinuses, the nidus in cavernous DAVMs is small and usually not visualized directly, even on MRA. Although MR cannot delineate the small vessels supplying these lesions, depiction of cavernous sinus or superior ophthalmic vein thrombosis is exquisite on MR images (117) (see Chapter 22). Thrombosis of cavernous DAVMs can occur spontaneously and may be precipitated by diagnostic angiography.

Since direct visualization of the shunt in DAVMs is generally not possible on MR, the technique cannot definitively exclude DAVMs, particularly those without cortical venous drainage. The role of MRI in DAVMs is (a) to document parenchymal complications of these lesions, (b) to suggest veno-occlusive disease by defining abnormal cortical venous drainage, (c) to indicate venous hypertension and thereby implicate DAVM with venous outflow obstruction by delineating enlarged deep medullary veins, and (d) to exclude other causes of venous dilatation (e.g., parenchymal AVM, isolated dural sinus thrombosis).

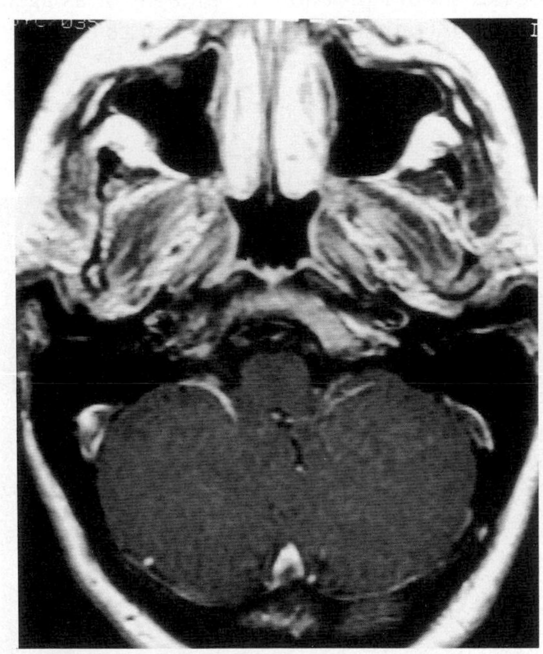
A

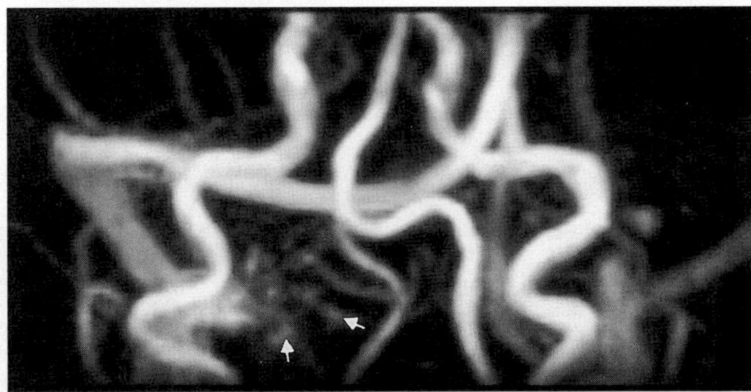
B

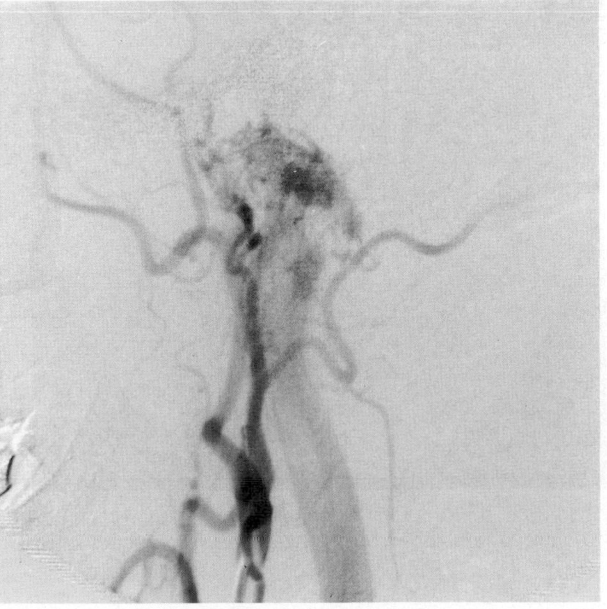
C

FIG. 51. DAVM of jugular region, MRA vs. MRI. MR imaging, including contrast-enhanced axial T1-weighted images (**A**), show no abnormality. Phase-contrast MRA sequence (**B**) demonstrates increased vascularity in the region of the right jugular fossa (*arrows*). **C:** Lateral angiographic injection of right external carotid artery shows DAVM in the jugular region with AV shunting into the right jugular vein. No intracranial venous drainage was present.

INTRACRANIAL ANEURYSMS

Cerebral aneurysms are found in 1% to 14% of the population (118), suggesting that approximately 11 million people in the United States harbor this lesion. Intracranial aneurysms represent the most common atraumatic cause of subarachnoid hemorrhage (SAH) and, indeed, SAH is the most frequent presenting manifestation of intracranial aneurysm (118). Unruptured aneurysms are most often asymptomatic. Assuming a maximum prevalence of unruptured aneurysms of 0.5% and an incidence of SAH of 10/100,000 per year, an annual risk of aneurysm rupture of 2% has been calculated. Operation on incidentally discovered, unruptured aneurysms is recommended because of the serious morbidity (20–25%) and mortality (50–60%) of SAH, and because the morbidity and mortality of surgery for unruptured aneurysms is low (119,120), with the best outcomes being for those less than 25 mm, that is, nongiant aneurysms. The specific timing of aneurysm surgery for ruptured aneurysms remains somewhat controversial, but there is convincing evidence and little controversy that early operation offers the best hope for good outcome. In a randomized, prospective study to investigate this question, Ohman (121) found that at 3 months post-SAH, 92% of the acutely operated (0–3 days) group were functionally independent, whereas only 79% of the 4- to 7-day group and 80% of the 8-day or later group were considered independent.

Saccular Aneurysms

Aneurysms may be classified based on a number of features, including morphology (saccular, fusiform), size, location (intradural, extradural), and etiology (congenital, traumatic, neoplastic, dissecting, mycotic, atherosclerotic). Overlap of many characteristics and uncertainty regarding etiology, however, often makes a rigid separation into categories unsatisfactory, controversial, or impossible. Nevertheless, we will use the term "saccular aneurysm" to include all arterial outpouchings of unknown origin that are not associated with inflammation or tumor (122).

The vast majority of intracranial aneurysms are saccular aneurysms. Most saccular aneurysms are isolated lesions without any underlying predisposing factor (genetic predisposition, collagen-vascular disease, AVM). According to Stehbens, there is no sound scientific evidence of a congenital, developmental, or inherited weakness in the parent vessel wall (123). Currently, hemodynamic stresses are thought to represent the most likely cause of aneurysms. Hypertension and collagen-vascular diseases should probably be thought of as aggravating conditions, rather than primary causes of these lesions

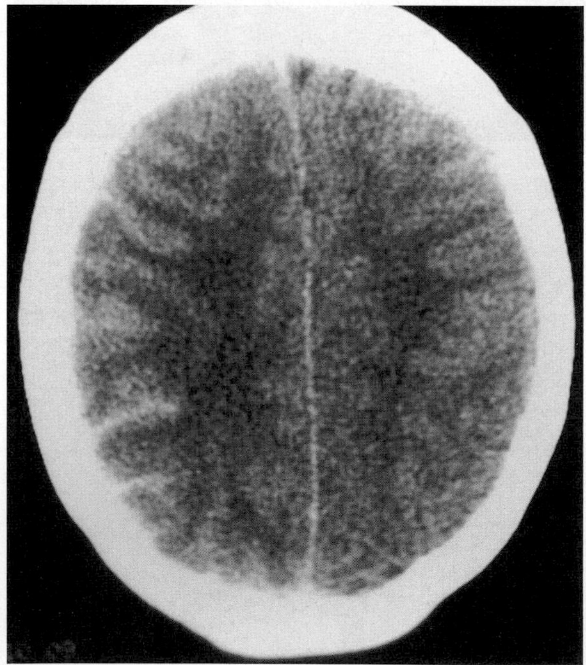

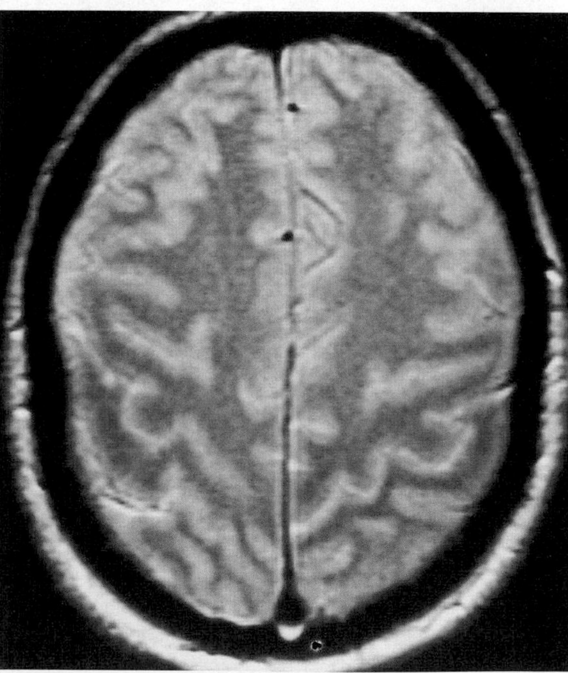

FIG. 52. Acute SAH, CT vs. MR. **A:** Noncontrast CT. **B:** Long TR/short TE MR. Obvious acute subarachnoid blood in right parietal region on CT (A) is difficult to discern among many regions of slight hyperintensity along sulci bilaterally on MR (B).

(124). In less than 5% of cases, aneurysms are associated with septic emboli, head trauma, or neoplasia. In these instances, aneurysms are typically at peripheral sites or in regions other than branch points.

Saccular aneurysms usually occur at vessel bifurcations, typically on the convexity of a curve in the parent vessel, and point in the direction that flow would have continued had the curve not been present. Larger arteries in the region of the circle of Willis are most frequently involved. More than 90% of saccular aneurysms originate at one of the following five locations: the junction of the anterior cerebral and the anterior communicating artery, the ICA at the origin of the posterior communicating artery, the bifurcation of the MCA, the tip of the basilar artery, and the bifurcation of the ICA (125). In approximately 20% to 25% of cases, aneurysms are multiple.

Traditional methods of identifying the origin of subarachnoid hemorrhage in a patient with multiple aneurysms have rested on either CT correlation of the site of the hemorrhage (126,127) or angiographic morphologic changes in ruptured aneurysms. For instance, anterior interhemispheric blood correlates to ruptured anterior communicating aneurysms, whereas sylvian fissure hemorrhage typically indicates MCA bifurcation aneurysm rupture. Angiographic demonstration of bleeding site has rested on features such as size, luminal irregularity, and associated spasm (128).

The current diagnostic work-up for a patient with suspected aneurysm should be tailored to the clinician's index of suspicion for aneurysmal rupture but, generally speaking, this lesion must be detected with accuracy and in the shortest period of time to optimize therapy. Therefore, conventional catheter angiography remains the modality of choice for its diagnosis. The cardinal diagnostic sign of ruptured aneurysm is a severe headache of sudden onset, and CT scan remains the most sensitive imaging method for the detection of acute subarachnoid blood.

The usefulness of MRI in the diagnosis of acute SAH has been a subject of considerable interest, largely because of the prognostic importance of its identification. In fact, MRI is notoriously poor for documenting this entity (Figs. 52 and 53), unless the SAH is massive (Fig. 54). It has been proposed that the lack of visualization of diffuse subarachnoid blood on SE MR images is related to the relatively high pO_2 in the CSF, which thereby prevents paramagnetic deoxyhemoglobin from forming (129). Several studies have attempted to evaluate the ability of MRI to depict acute SAH (130,131). No convincing data have yet been published to indicate a role for MRI in the initial diagnosis of acute SAH (1). On the other hand, isolated acute clot in the SAS can be routinely detected on MR images (see Chapter 9).

Nonruptured aneurysms are usually asymptomatic, but there are several instances in which compression of

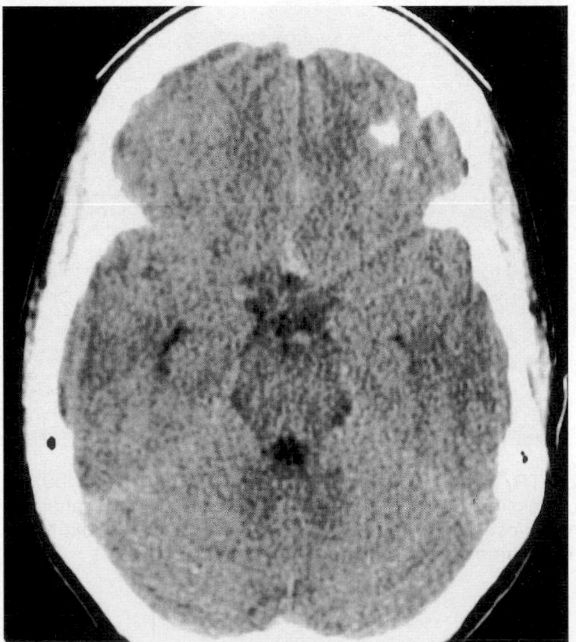

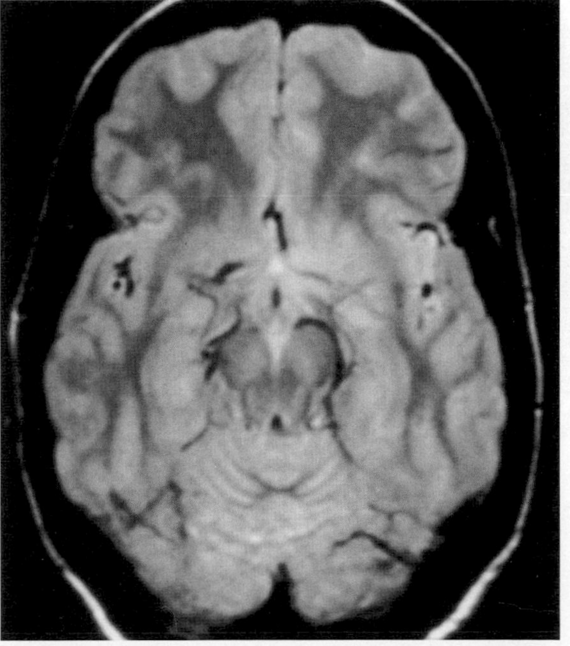

FIG. 53. Acute SAH, CT vs. MR. **A:** Noncontrast CT. **B:** Long TR/short TE MR. Clearly depicted acute subarachnoid blood in cistern of lamina terminalis and within anterior interhemispheric fissure on CT (A) is impossible to distinguish from normal CSF in sylvian fissures and interpeduncular fossa on MR (B), even though long TR/short TE techniques were used, i.e., those purported to be the most sensitive to acute subarachnoid blood.

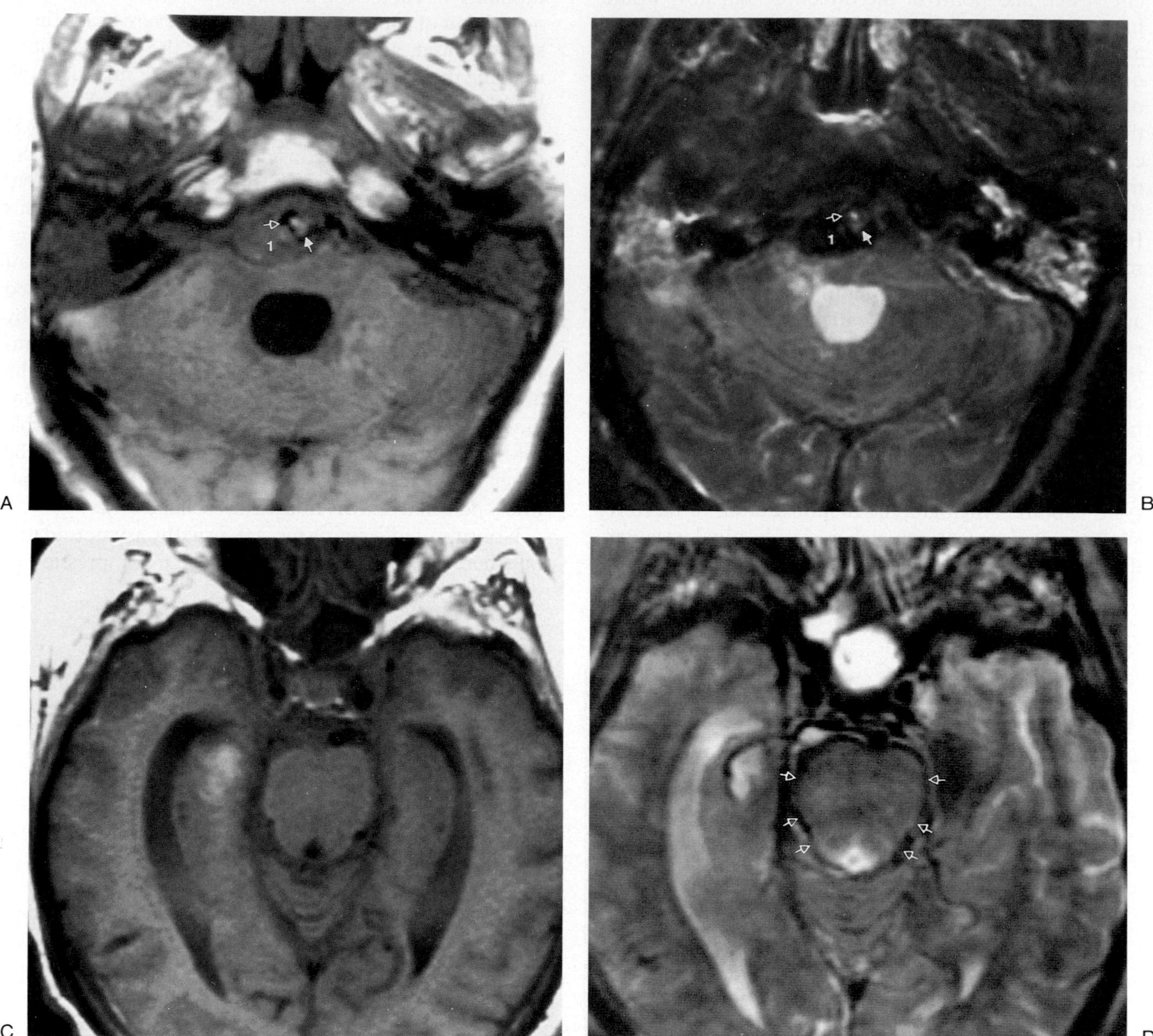

FIG. 54. Massive acute SAH from PICA aneurysm. **A:** Short TR/TE MR (600/20). **B:** Long TR/TE MR (3000/80). **C:** Short TR/TE MR (600/20). **D:** Long TR/TE MR (3000/80). Massive, acute SAH (*1*) surrounds right vertebral artery (*open arrows*, A,B) with adherent perianeurysmal hematoma (*closed white arrows*, A,B). Acute subarachnoid blood is noted surrounding brainstem (C,D), depicted as marked hypointensity on long TR/TE image (*arrows*, D).

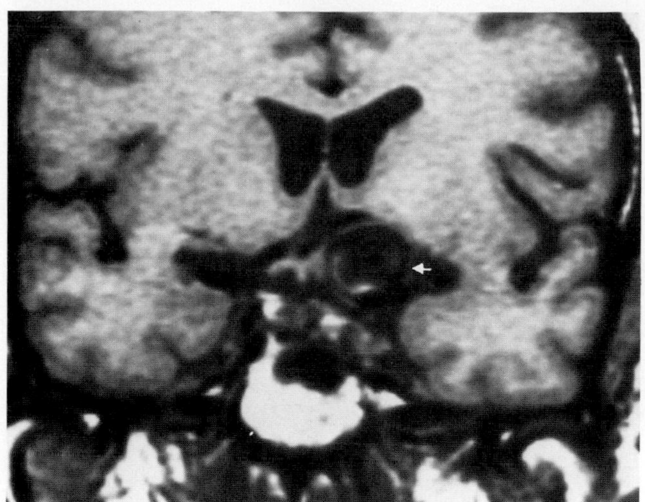

FIG. 55. Compression of optic chiasm and tract by aneurysm in patient with right homonymous hemianopsia. Coronal short TR/TE image demonstrates large aneurysm (*arrow*) compressing left side of optic chiasm and origin of left optic tract in this patient with complete, homonymous field defect.

adjacent structures by aneurysmal masses causes symptoms. Aneurysms can compress optic nerve or chiasm (Fig. 55), cranial nerves III to VI, hypothalamus, or brainstem, depending on their size and location. An isolated and complete third nerve palsy (ptosis, diplopia, pupillary dilatation, strabismus) is a classic finding in patients with aneurysm (posterior communicating or basilar tip), and when this finding is appreciated by the clinician, the search for aneurysm should be prompted. Any adult with a painful, complete third nerve palsy must be given the diagnosis of aneurysm until proven otherwise because in such patients a high percentage have unruptured posterior communicating-ICA aneurysm (118). Isolated third nerve palsy can also be a sign of microvascular disease, particularly common in diabetes. The third nerve palsy of diabetes (or any etiology of infarction) characteristically spares the pupil (pupillary fibers run in the peripheral portion of the nerve, and infarctions characteristically involve the central nerve) and often recovers completely over several weeks. Other masses of the third nerve can present as third nerve palsies as well (Fig. 56).

After aneurysmal clipping, MRI is probably the most useful noninvasive imaging modality in the postoperative assessment of these patients (132), although the assessment of rebleeding into the SAS is essentially not visible on MR. Although some ferromagnetic artifacts emanate from these devices, significantly less obscuration of brain is seen as compared to that on CT scans. Virtually all aneurysm clips in current use are composed primarily of nonferromagnetic material, which generally shows no movement in a magnetic field. Although Phynox and Sugita Elgiloy contain ferromagnetic material, they usually do not demonstrate movement when introduced into MR scanners at currently used field strengths.

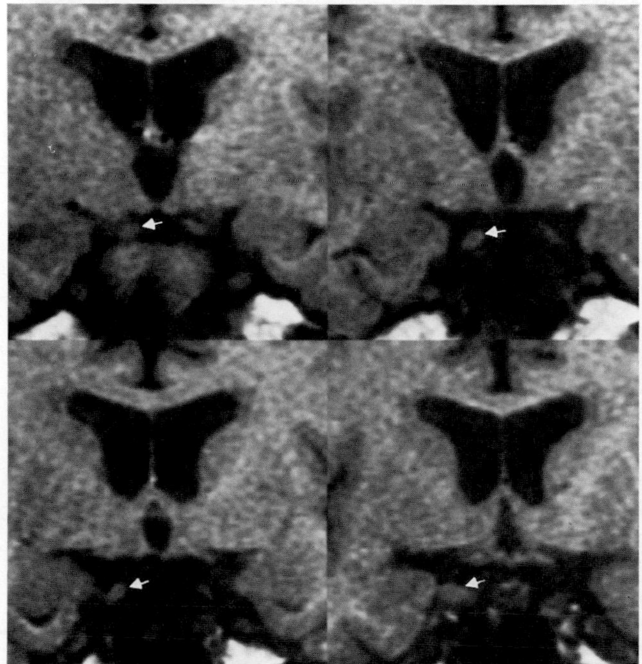

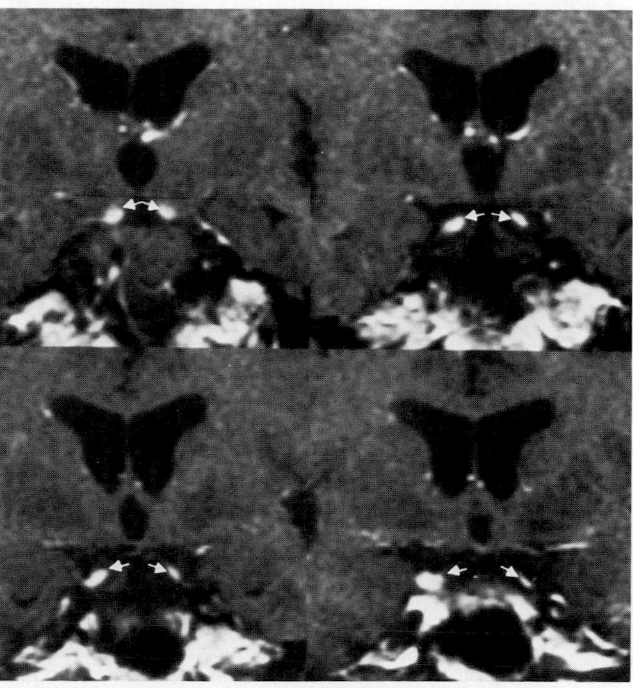

FIG. 56. Third nerve palsy due to intrinsic oculomotor nerve lesion. **A:** Serial coronal short TR/TE MR, posterior to anterior (600/11). **B:** Serial coronal short TR/TE MR, posterior to anterior (600/11), with contrast enhancement. Thin section images show marked enlargement of right third nerve (*arrows*, A). Both third nerves intrinsically enhance after contrast administration (*arrows*, B) in this patient with probable lymphoma and right third nerve palsy.

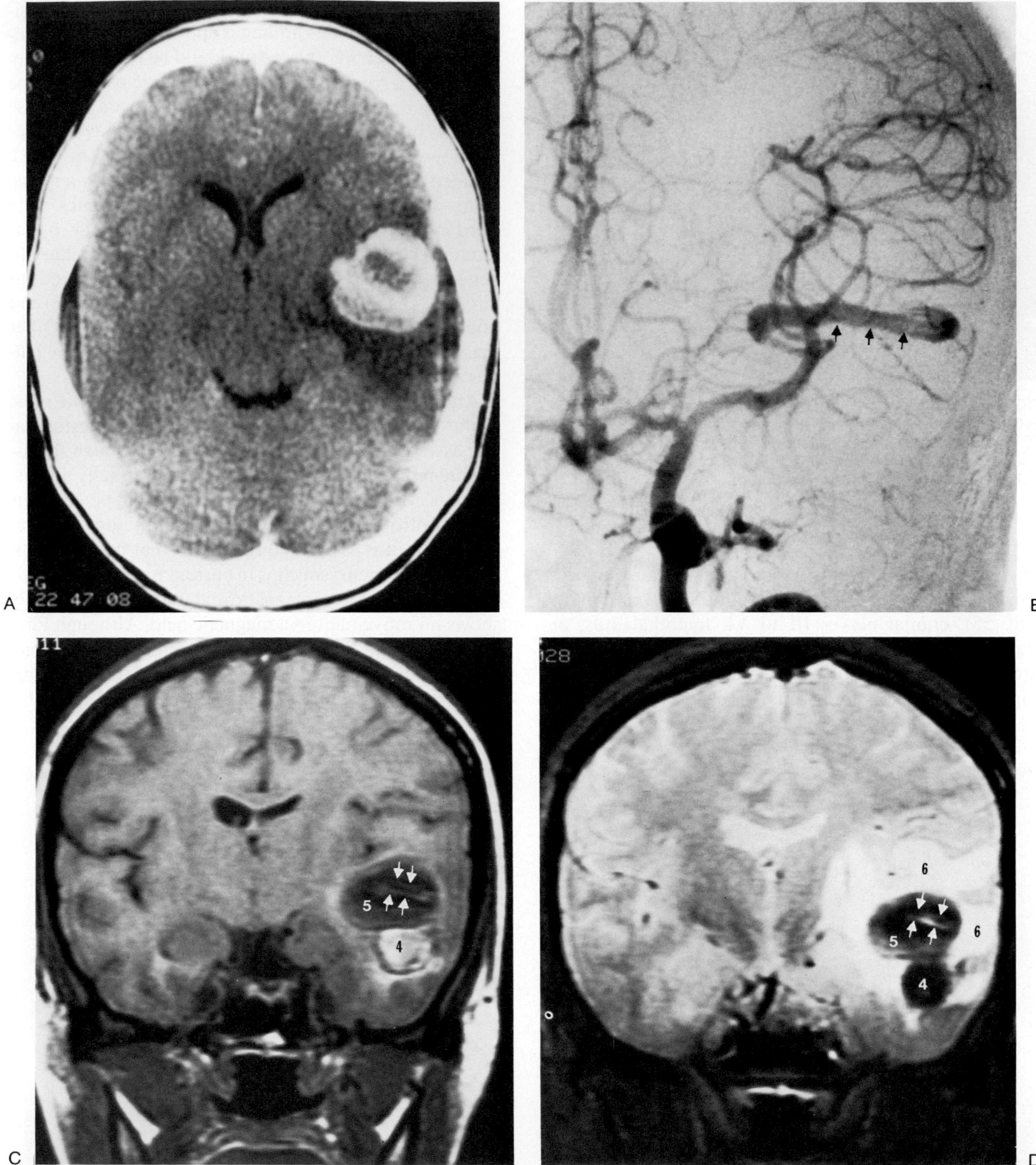

FIG. 57. Partially thrombosed MCA giant aneurysm. **A:** Axial CT. **B:** Arteriogram, AP view. **C:** Coronal short TR/TE MR (600/20). **D:** Coronal long TR/TE MR (2500/80). CT (A) shows nonspecific middle cranial fossa hematoma. Arteriogram (B) documents left middle cranial fossa mass, with deviation and elevation of sylvian vessels, and thin, horizontally oriented residual patent lumen (*arrows*, B) of giant aneurysm. MR (C,D) shows horizontally oriented patent lumen surrounded by stripes of hyperintensity (*arrows*, C,D), representing either methemoglobin or very slow flow. Note extraluminal hematoma (*4*), thrombosed part of lumen with various intensities (*5*), and edema (*6*). (From Atlas, ref. 163, with permission.)

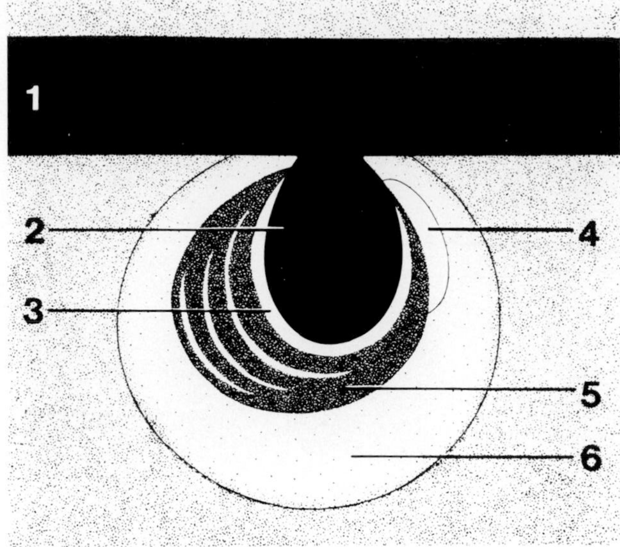

FIG. 58. Partially thrombosed giant aneurysm, artist's conception. Note several features that often allow differentiation of this lesion from simple hematoma and allow a specific diagnosis to be made. *1*, parent vessel; *2*, patent lumen of aneurysm; *3*, periluminal hyperintensity; *4*, extra-aneurysmal hemorrhage; *5*, thrombosed portion of lumen with layered stages of clot; *6*, associated edema. (From Atlas, ref. 163, with permission.)

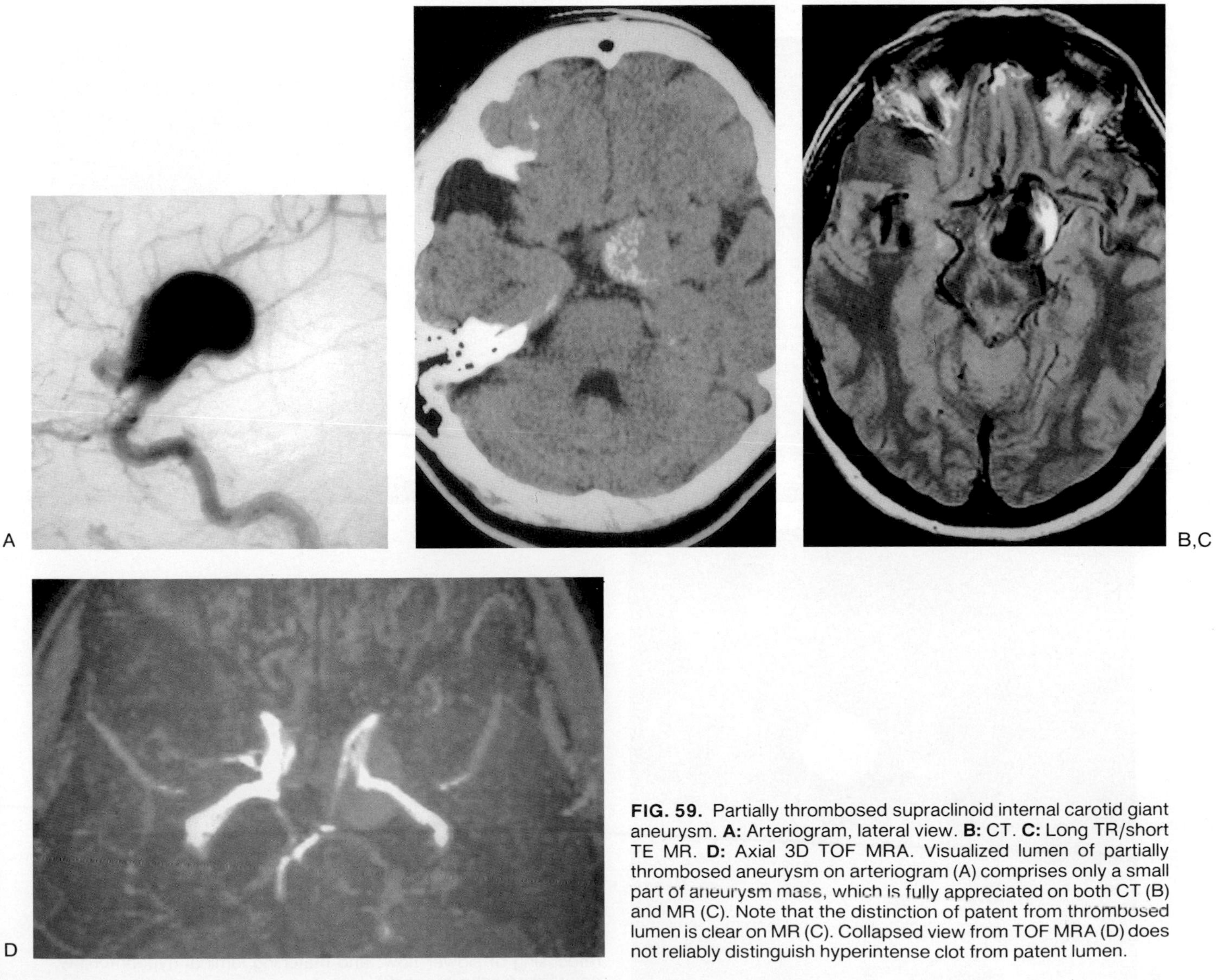

A

B,C

D

FIG. 59. Partially thrombosed supraclinoid internal carotid giant aneurysm. **A:** Arteriogram, lateral view. **B:** CT. **C:** Long TR/short TE MR. **D:** Axial 3D TOF MRA. Visualized lumen of partially thrombosed aneurysm on arteriogram (A) comprises only a small part of aneurysm mass, which is fully appreciated on both CT (B) and MR (C). Note that the distinction of patent from thrombosed lumen is clear on MR (C). Collapsed view from TOF MRA (D) does not reliably distinguish hyperintense clot from patent lumen.

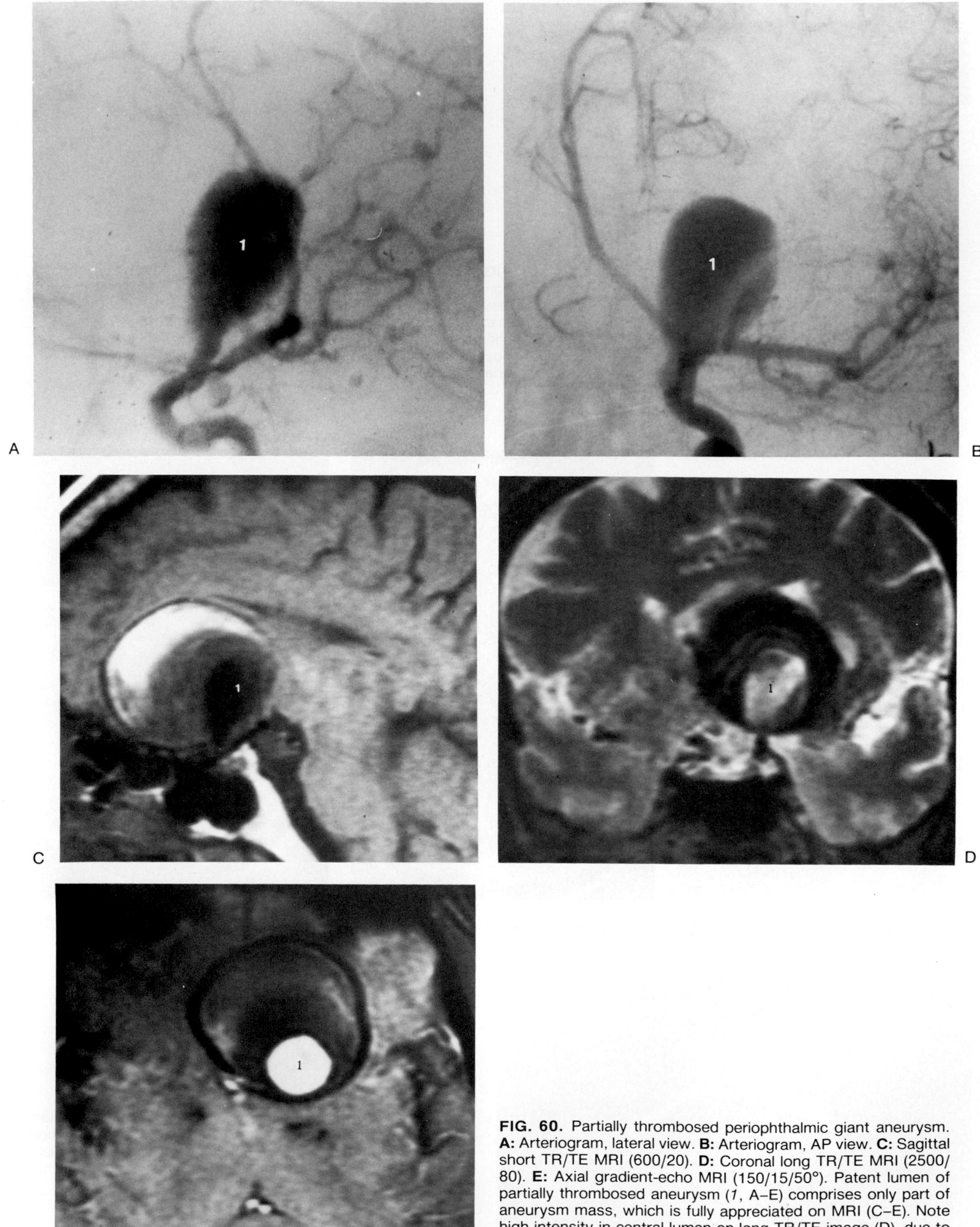

FIG. 60. Partially thrombosed periophthalmic giant aneurysm. **A:** Arteriogram, lateral view. **B:** Arteriogram, AP view. **C:** Sagittal short TR/TE MRI (600/20). **D:** Coronal long TR/TE MRI (2500/80). **E:** Axial gradient-echo MRI (150/15/50°). Patent lumen of partially thrombosed aneurysm (*1*, A–E) comprises only part of aneurysm mass, which is fully appreciated on MRI (C–E). Note high intensity in central lumen on long TR/TE image (D), due to refocusing of slower flow, and matching luminal hyperintensity on gradient-echo image (E).

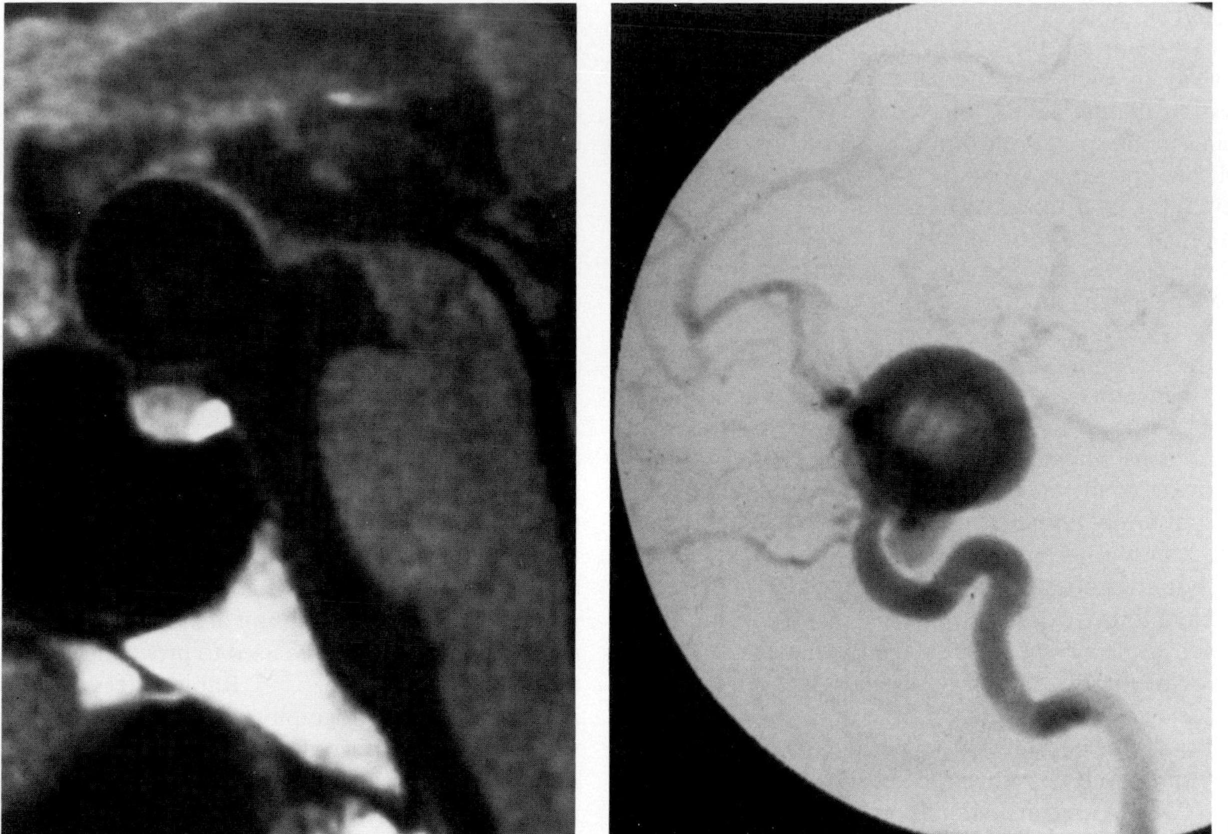

FIG. 61. SE flow characteristics in giant cavernous aneurysm. **A:** Short TR/TE MR (600/20). **B:** Long TR/TE MR (2500/80). Left cavernous carotid aneurysm shows slight signal in central portion of lumen (*1*) on short TR/TE (A) and hyperintensity on long TR/TE (B), because of slower flow centrally and signal void in peripheral area of more rapid flow.

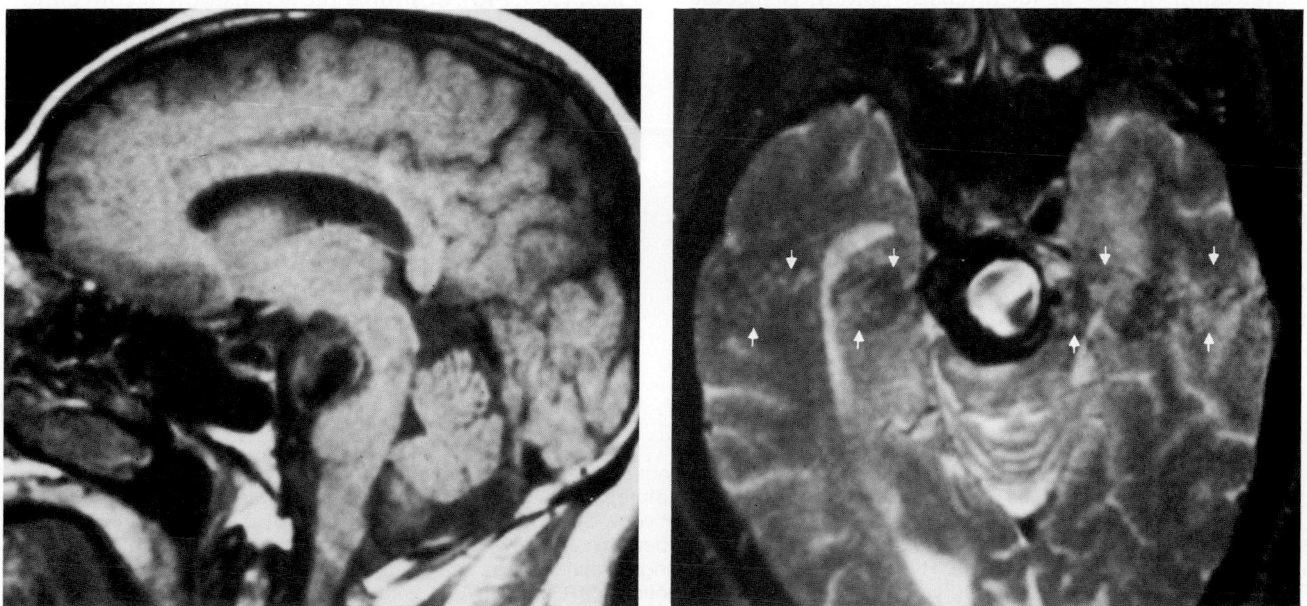

FIG. 62. Intraluminal high intensity in aneurysm on long TR/TE image with ghost artifacts. **A:** Sagittal short TR/TE MR (600/20). **B:** Axial long TR/TE MR (2800/80). Giant basilar aneurysm shows signal void on short TR/TE image (A) and compresses brainstem. Note intraluminal high intensity due to refocusing of slow flow by gradient moment nulling on long TR/TE image (B). Ghost images (*arrows*, B) along phase-encoding axis prove vascular nature of mass. (From Atlas, ref. 163, with permission.)

It should be noted that recent reports (see Chapter 6) have cast doubt on the notion that aneurysm clips are consistent in their response to large magnetic fields. Moreover, many patients have undergone aneurysm clipping in the past with ferromagnetic clips, some of which may move on exposure to magnetic fields. The potential for fatal intracranial hemorrhage after movement of a ferromagnetic aneurysm clip in an MRI unit (133) emphasizes the necessity for identifying the exact type of aneurysm clip used (see table in Chapter 6).

Giant Aneurysms

Aneurysms whose greatest diameter exceeds 2.5 cm are termed "giant aneurysms" (134). These lesions are most commonly found in middle-aged women and usually present with signs more indicative of a mass lesion (134), but SAH does occur (135). Most giant aneurysms are related to the extradural internal carotid within the cavernous sinus or MCA, but a high percentage occur at the apex of the basilar artery. Basilar giant aneurysms are associated with particularly poor outcomes. The CT identification of partially thrombosed giant intracranial aneurysms is well described (136), and angiography, although directly imaging patent portions of the lumen in these lesions, clearly is insufficient to define the entire extent of this lesion (see Figs. 59 and 60).

Because of their dual component nature (thrombosed portion with layered clot and patent portion with flowing blood), partially thrombosed giant aneurysms have a characteristic appearance on MR images (137), and identification of this signal intensity pattern is specific for this lesion (Figs. 57–60). The MR signs of partially thrombosed giant intracranial aneurysms are (a) a well-circumscribed mass lesion containing mixed signal intensities representing various stages of clot in the thrombosed portion of the lumen, (b) evidence of flow (signal void or other flow phenomena) within the patent portion of the residual lumen, (c) (usually) periluminal hyperintensity around the patent residual lumen, reflecting either slow flow or methemoglobin, and (d) flow void in the parent vessel anatomically related to the aneurysm. Perianeurysmal hemorrhage and intraparenchymal edema may also be seen in the surrounding brain, outside the confines of the partially thrombosed aneurysm mass. SAH will generally not be clearly definable on MRI.

The important clue to the diagnosis of a partially thrombosed giant aneurysm is the recognition of flowing blood within the mass, which is pathognomonic of the entity. Rapidly flowing blood through the patent portion of the lumen appears as an area of signal void on SE images, because these spins do not remain within the same slice for both the 90° and 180° pulses (which are slice selective), and therefore no SE is produced (45). Other mechanisms, such as spin-phase dispersion (138), may also contribute to signal void. It must be appreciated that the patent portion of the lumen can be seen as high intensity on certain pulse sequences, due to either flow-related enhancement, or rephasing phenomena (Fig. 61) (46), or gradient moment nulling. Flow phenomena, especially ghost image pulsation artifacts, arising from the intraluminal signal can be used to prove the vascular nature of these lesions (Fig. 62). Rapid MRI with GE techniques and MR angiography (see Chapters 29 and Chapter 31) can quickly confirm the patency of the residual lumen in aneurysms (76). It should be noted that MRA, particularly when implemented with 3D TOF volume acquisitions, can fail to demonstrate giant aneurysms by virtue of saturation of the slow intraluminal flow that characterizes these aneurysms. Intravenous contrast (Fig. 63), alternative or modified MRA acquisition techniques with superior background suppression (see Chapter 31), postprocessing methods more sensitive to slow flow (139,140), or simply the acquisition of conventional SE images are all methods by which the slow flow within the residual patent lumen of these lesions can be demonstrated.

In summary, the presence of three specific SE MR characteristics allows differentiation of partially thrombosed giant aneurysms from isolated intracerebral hematomas: (a) flow phenomena with the patent portion of the lumen (usually flow void), (b) laminated thrombus of mixed stages in the clotted portion of the lumen, and (c) recognition of the anatomic relationship of signal

FIG. 63. MRA of slowly filling giant aneurysm, pre- and postcontrast enhancement. **A:** Axial short TR/TE MR (800/30). **B:** Axial long TR/TE MR (2500/80). **C:** Axial view, compressed 3D TOF MRA image. **D:** Axial view, compressed 3D TOF MRA image, after contrast enhancement. **E:** AP view, 3D TOF MRA image of left carotid. **F:** AP view, 3D TOF MRA image of left carotid, after contrast enhancement. **G:** AP view, conventional angiographic image of left carotid, early arterial phase. **H:** AP view, conventional angiographic image of left carotid, later arterial phase. Supraclinoid carotid giant aneurysm is clearly seen on conventional MR images (A,B), with central high intensity implying slower flow centrally. Compressed stack of slices from MRA series before intravenous contrast (C) fails to reveal giant aneurysm. Similar projection image after contrast administration (D) shows high intensity (*arrows*, D) from enhancement of slowly filling lumen. Three-dimensional projection MRA image of left carotid artery before contrast administration (E) shows only the peripheral portion of the aneurysm (*open arrows*, E). After intravenous contrast (F), entire aneurysm is visualized. Arteriography (G,H) reveals peripheral early filling of aneurysm (*open arrows*, G) and finally entire lumen is visualized (H).

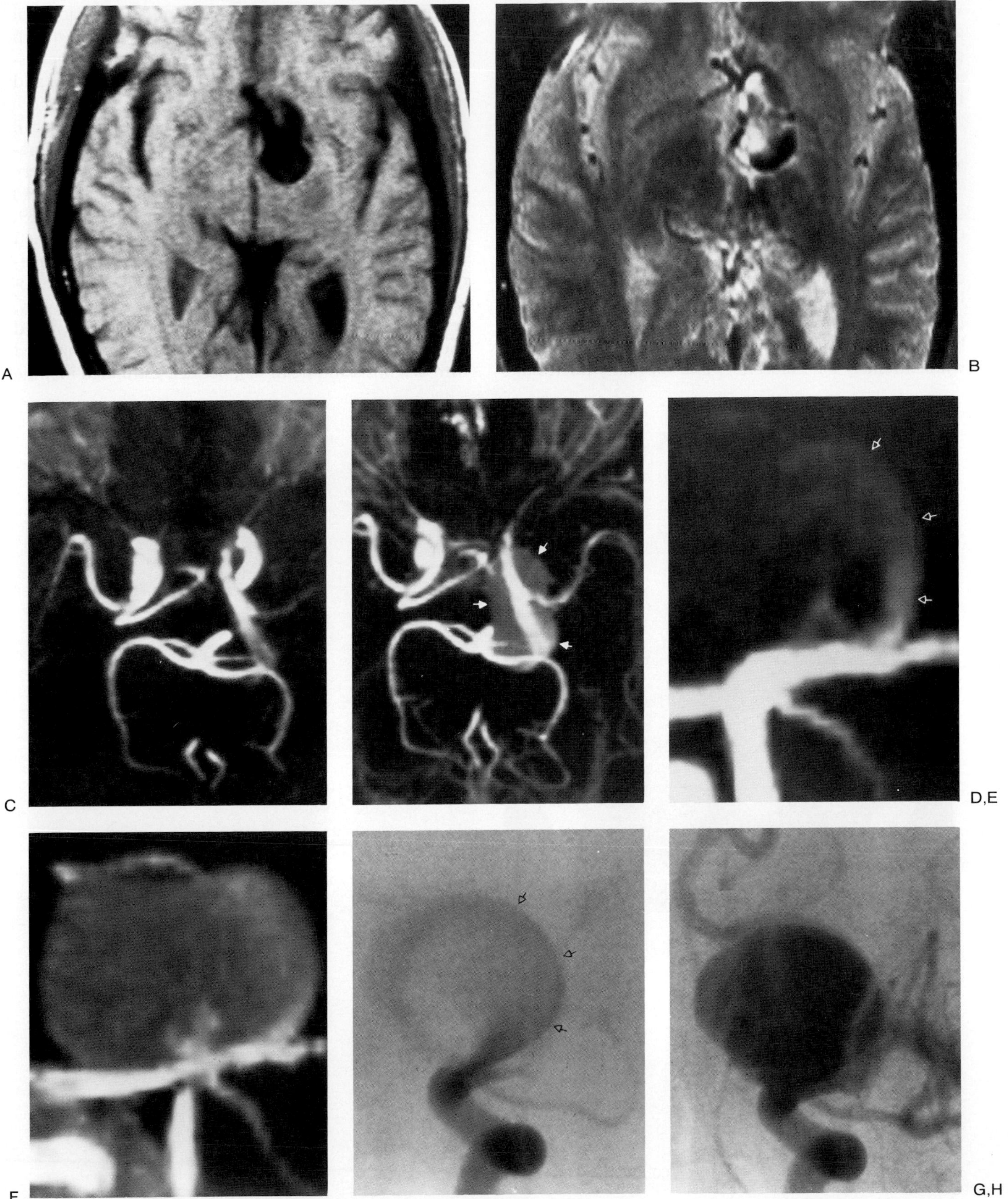
A
B
C
D,E
F
G,H

void in the parent vessel. It is clear that more complete and specific characterization of the giant aneurysm components and associated extra-aneurysmal parenchymal abnormalities is possible with MRI as compared to either CT or angiography.

MR Angiography in the Search for Aneurysms

The question frequently arises as to the practical role of MRI and MRA in the evaluation of patients suspected of harboring an intracranial aneurysm. Aneurysms most commonly present as acute SAH and as such are a medical emergency, in that, beyond the high mortality reflected by those patients who do not survive the initial bleed, a ruptured aneurysm represents a treatable disease with extremely high morbidity and mortality if left untreated (118). Furthermore, unruptured intracranial aneurysms represent a major, growing public health problem, with a tremendous cost in terms of diagnostic work-up, hospitalization, morbidity, mortality, and treatment (141).

The value of having an imaging technique that can function reliably as a screening examination for intracranial aneurysms is irrefutable, because of the known very low morbidity (4%) and mortality (approaching 0%) when an unruptured aneurysm is operated on (119, 120,124). Moreover, an effective screening method would permit the early detection of intracranial aneurysms in patients and family members with a higher potential incidence of aneurysms and allow early surgery, before aneurysm rupture. The detection of unruptured aneurysms would significantly reduce costs associated with diagnosis and treatment because estimated lifetime

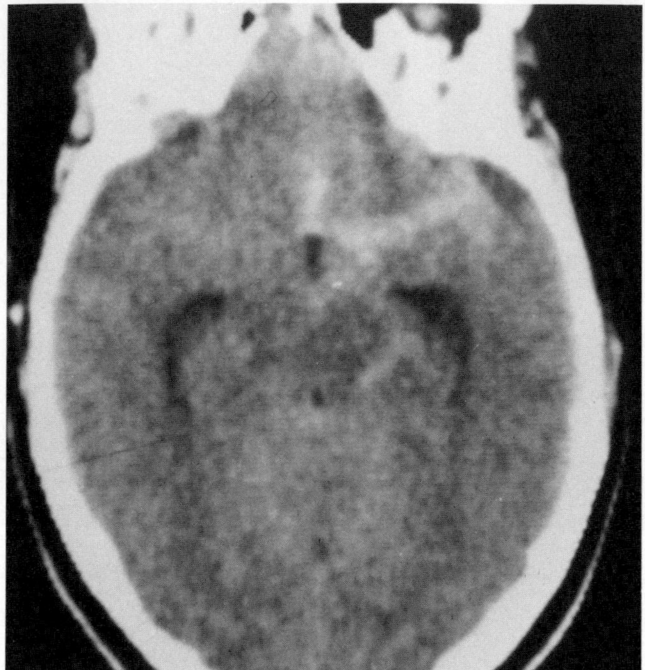
A

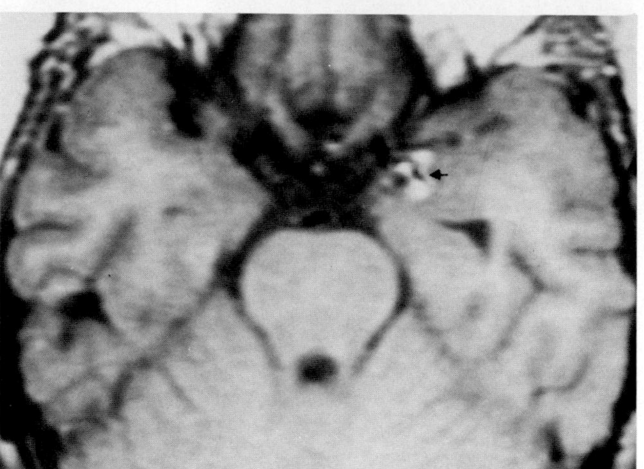
B

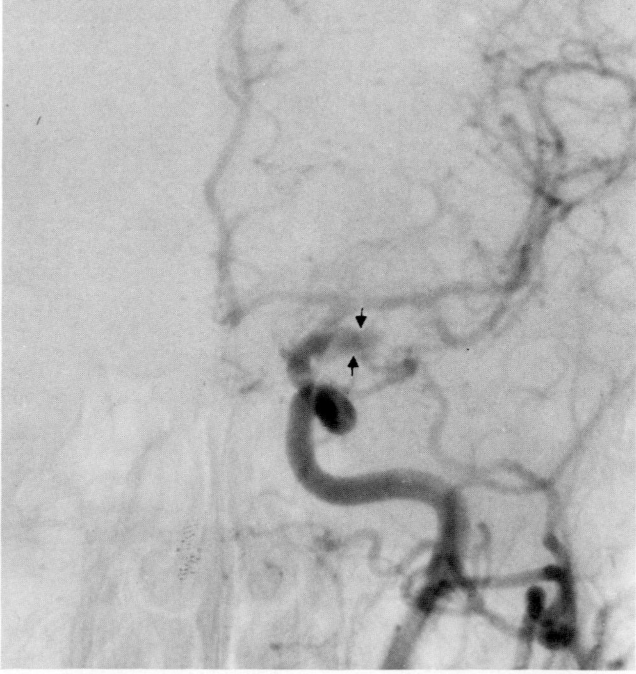
C

FIG. 64. Detection of perianeurysmal hemorrhage, indicating origin of bleed. **A:** CT. **B:** Short TR/TE MR (600/20). **C:** Arteriogram, AP view. CT scan shows left-sided SAH. MR reveals high intensity hemorrhage adjacent to left posterior communicating aneurysm (*arrows*, B), confirmed by arteriogram (*arrows*, C). (From Atlas, ref. 163, with permission.)

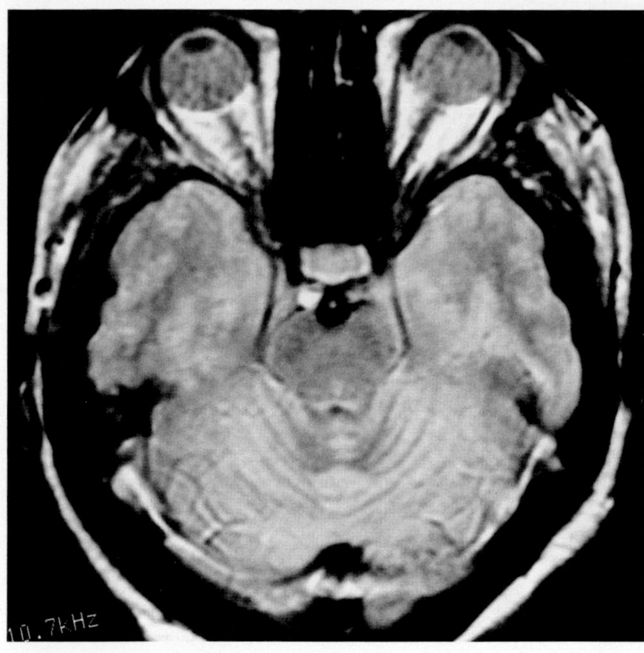

FIG. 65. Perianeurysmal hemorrhage on MR. Long TR/short TE MR shows blood clot alongside basilar aneurysm in prepontine cistern.

costs of unruptured aneurysms are dramatically lower than those of ruptured aneurysms. On the other hand, it should be stressed that any attempt to replace catheter arteriography for aneurysms with another imaging test must take into account the extremely high (60–70%) fatality rate in untreated ruptured aneurysms. In other words, it must be clearly understood that a missed (undetected) aneurysm is a life-threatening circumstance, because this is a treatable disease with a tragic outcome likely if left untreated.

Aneurysms may be diagnosed on MRI, mainly based on the identification of regions of flow void in an area morphologically consistent with a saccular aneurysm. In selected cases, MRI may also provide information regarding the bleeding site in patients with multiple aneurysms (142) by the identification of hemorrhage adjacent to the aneurysm (Figs. 64 and 65). MRI may also aid in guiding the work-up for subacute SAH (Fig. 66). It is clear, though, that the difficulties in discerning intracranial aneurysms with intraluminal signal void from dense

A

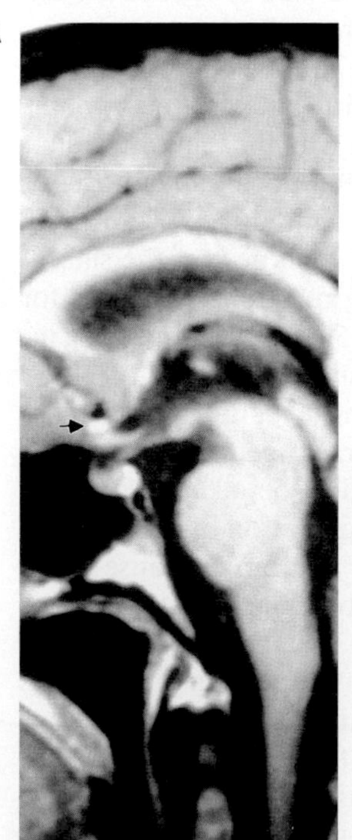

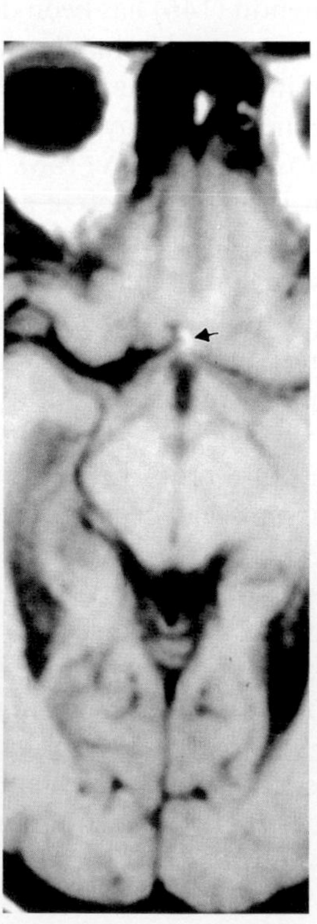

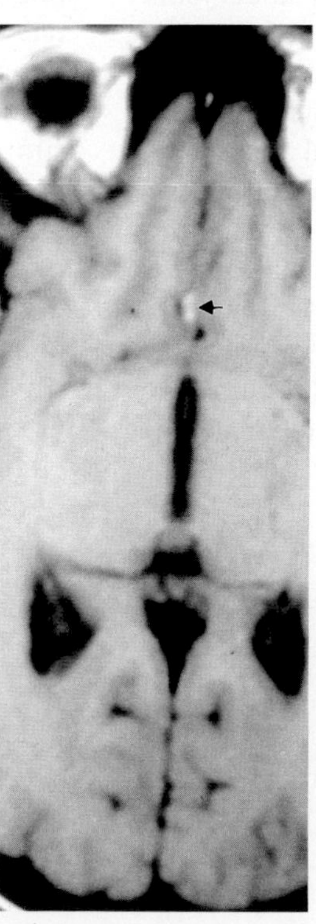

B,C

FIG. 66. MRI as an aid to site of origin of SAH. Sagittal (**A**) and axial (**B,C**) short TR/TE MR images show hyperintense subacute SAH (*arrows*) in anterior interhemispheric fissure and cistern of lamina terminalis, making the diagnosis of anterior communicating artery rupture likely as a source of bleeding in this patient with a normal angiogram (not shown).

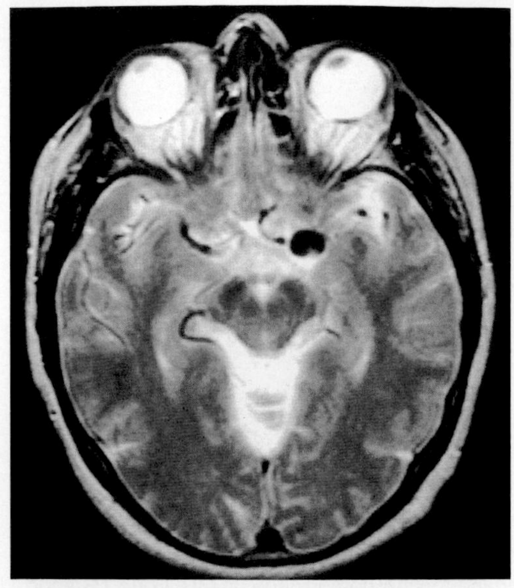

A

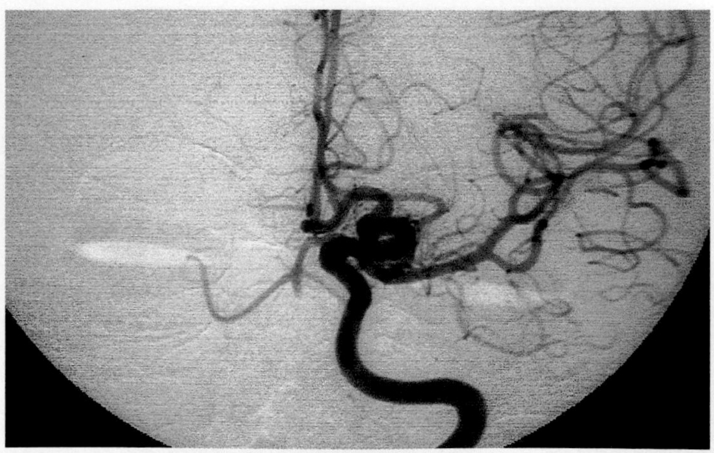

B

FIG. 67. Signal void of looping vessel masquerading as aneurysm. **A:** Axial long TR/TE MR. **B:** Arteriogram, ICA injection. Rounded signal void on MR (A) appears to indicate carotid bifurcation aneurysm, but arteriogram (B) shows marked tortuosity and redundancy but no aneurysm.

bone of the anterior clinoid process, for instance, or from normal looping MCA, preclude relying on standard axial images for this diagnosis (Fig. 67). In the investigation with MR of patients suspected of harboring intracranial aneurysms, it is absolutely essential to (a) use high resolution 3D imaging with thin slices, and (b) generate projection images from postprocessing of the 2D data (see Chapter 31).

A number of studies have evaluated the role of MRA in the identification of intracranial aneurysms (74,143–145). The best data suggest that approximately 90% of angiographically confirmed intracranial aneurysms more than 3 mm in diameter may be identified through the use of MRA when state-of-the-art postprocessing is used. MRA may be of use in screening asymptomatic populations at increased risk for intracranial aneurysms (Table 4). Limitations remain, however, including the depiction of complex and small aneurysms, accurate definition of aneurysm morphology (a key indicator of prior rupture) and in particular the reliable identification of lesions with turbulent intraluminal flow. As is the case with SAH, however, it is clear that MRI/MRA cannot be used to exclude definitively the presence of an aneurysm (72) and currently has no role in the initial evaluation of patients with either acute SAH or acute third nerve palsy, situations in which catheter angiography is required.

TABLE 4. *Populations that may be at higher risk for intracranial aneurysms*

Polycystic kidney disease
Coarctation of the aorta
Fibromuscular dysplasia
Family history of saccular aneurysm
Marfan's syndrome
Ehlers-Danlos syndrome

Several methods of increasing the intravascular signal-to-background ratio have been studied to reduce the problem of insensitivity of intracranial MRA (particularly 3D TOF) to slow flow, as in large aneurysms (see Chapter 31). These technical improvements can be divided into two main groups, based on their approach to this problem: (a) minimizing background signal, and (b) reducing flow saturation. The use of an off-resonance saturation pulse to elicit the magnetization transfer (MT) phenomenon (146) has been described to reduce the signal of brain parenchyma (background) while sparing the signal of intravascular blood (147).

A second major way of reducing background signal is simply to use PC MRA (148), in which background suppression is highly effective and clinically advantageous (139,149). Spin saturation has been reduced by a variety of ways, including reducing the thickness of the slab in 3D acquisitions and combining multiple thin slabs for anatomic coverage (MOTSA) (150–152), by injecting intravascular contrast agents to shorten the T1 of blood (153–155) (Fig. 68), and by using a spatially varying excitation pulse (156–158). Contrast agent use for MRA of aneurysms has been reported to be of limited value, because along with its reduced saturation of slow arterial flow comes obscuration of other anatomy because of enhancement of basilar venous structures (154). Perhaps the most important advance in data acquisition for intracranial MRA lies in high resolution techniques (157,159). Voxel sizes approaching 0.1 mm^3 are now attainable, and appear promising for improving the delineation of small vessels and presumably small aneurysms. Great promise is also seen with recent improvements in

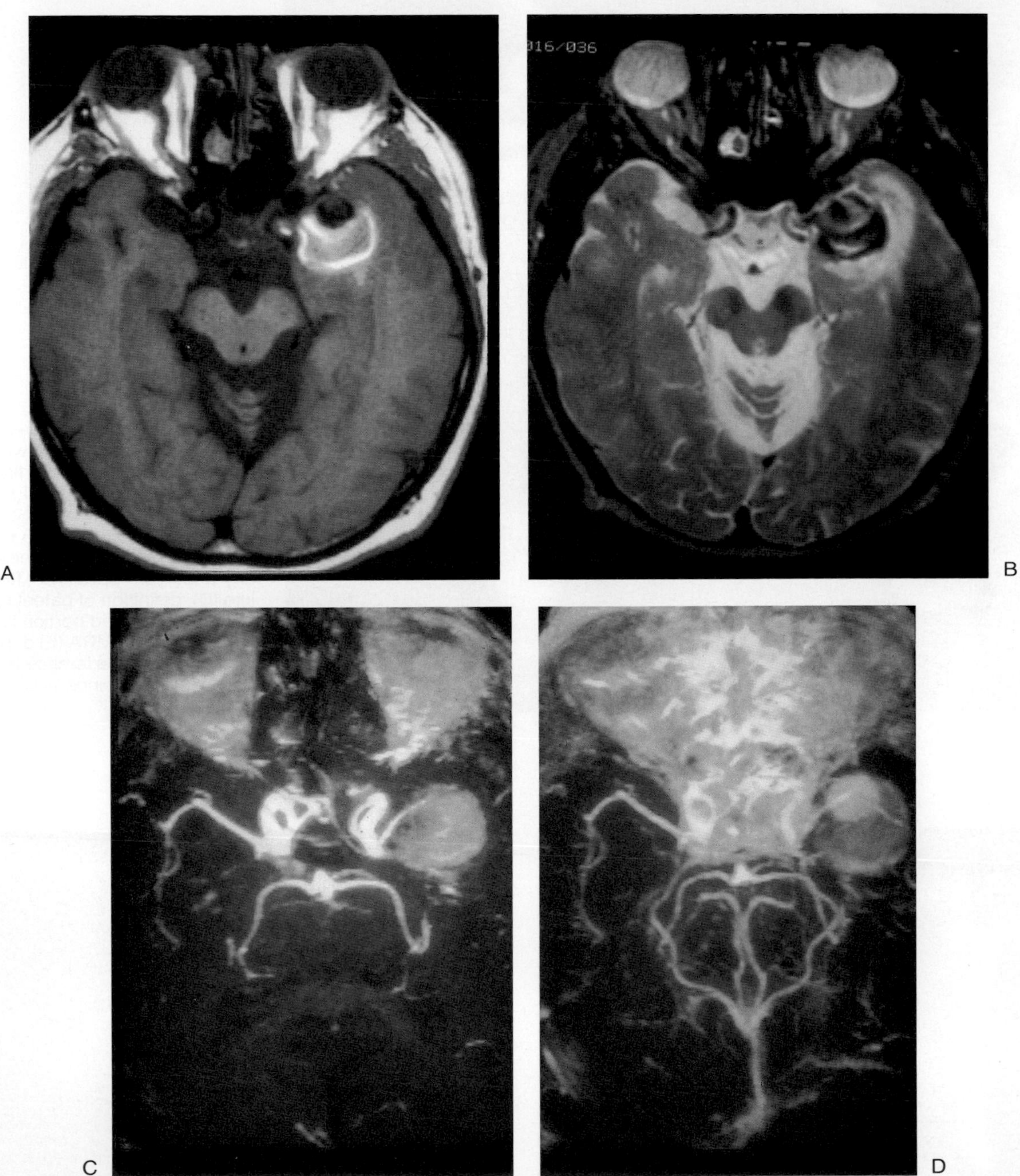

FIG. 68. MRA in partially thrombosed giant aneurysm, pre- vs. postgadolinium (A–H). **A:** Short TR/TE MR. **B:** Long TR/TE MR. **C:** 3D TOF MRA precontrast, collapsed view. **D:** 3D TOF MRA after intravenous contrast, collapsed view.

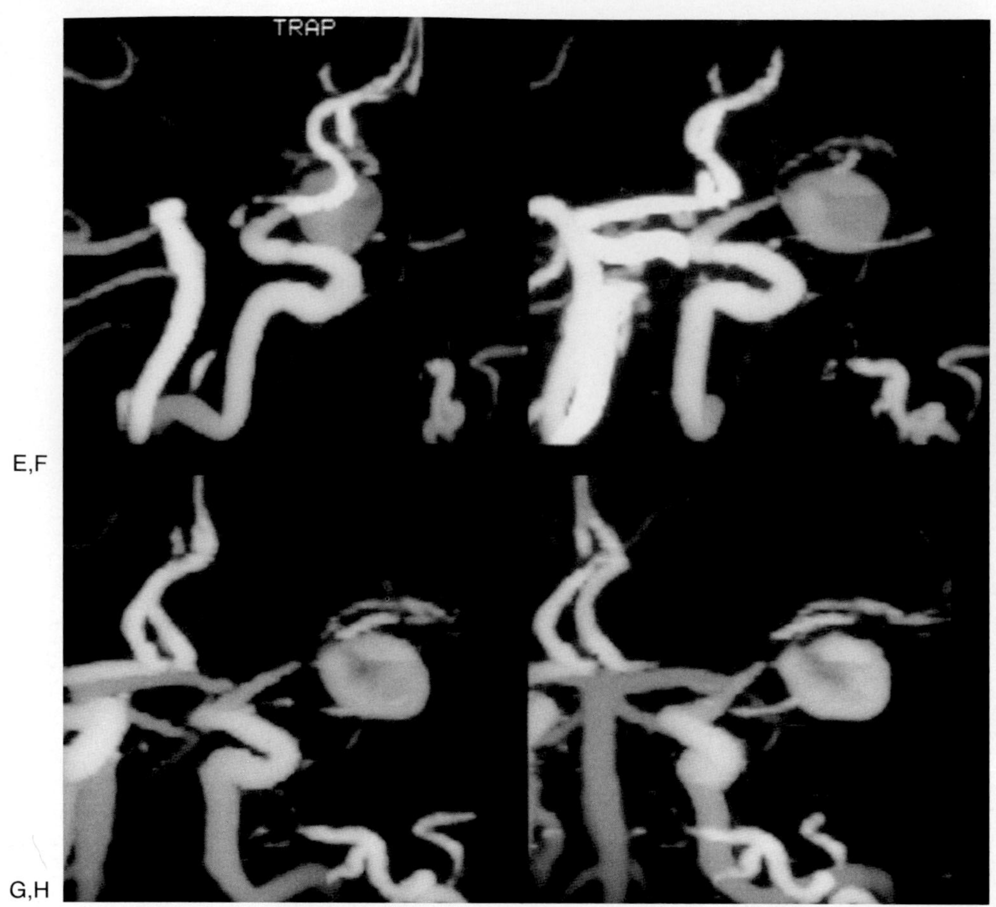

FIG. 68. (*Continued*) **E–H:** 3D PC MRA precontrast, four views about the cephalocaudad axis. Partially thrombosed middle cerebral bifurcation aneurysm is clearly seen on SE MR (A,B). Precontrast TOF MRA (C) shows high intensity from clot, but it does not show any aneurysm patency. After gadolinium (D), definition of patent lumen ventral to thrombosed portion is obtained. Phase-contrast MRA (E) depicts aneurysm without interference from thrombosed portion, since it is specific for flow.

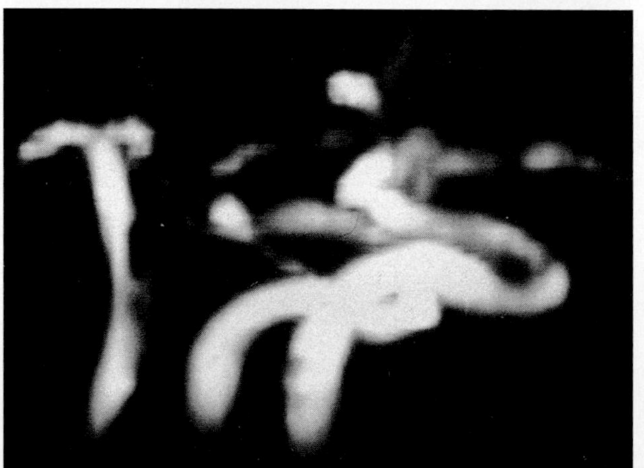

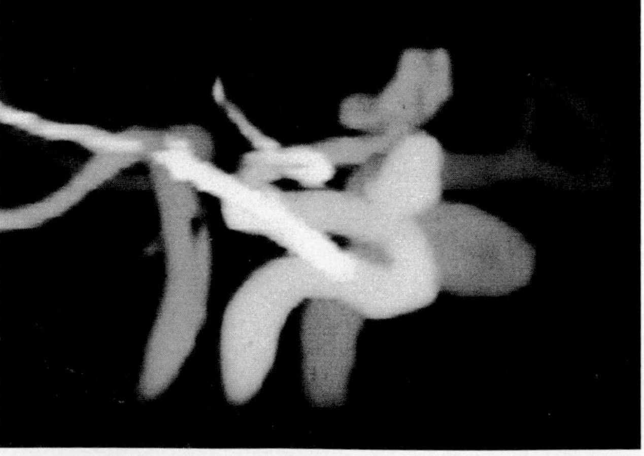

FIG. 69. MRA using advanced postprocessing for aneurysm characterization. **A:** Conventional MIP postprocessing of MRA, oblique view. **B:** Advanced (STANDOUT) postprocessing of MRA, oblique view. Although conventional MIP (A) does not clearly identify aneurysm, the STANDOUT image of the same MRA data (B) fully defines periophthalmic aneurysm.

post-processing (160–162) techniques (Fig. 69). Although MRA techniques have significantly improved with a number of recent innovative techniques (see Chapter 31 for a more complete discussion), we have yet to eliminate the need for conventional arteriography for intracranial aneurysms.

REFERENCES

1. Atlas SW. MR imaging is highly sensitive to acute subarachnoid hemorrhage . . . not! *Radiology* 1993;186:319.
2. Atlas SW. Imaging vascular intracranial disease: current status. *Curr Opin Radiol* 1990;2:18–25.
3. Howard RS, Maldjian J, Alsop D, et al. Functional MRI in the assessment of cerebral gliomas and AVMs prior to surgical or endovascular therapy. SMR Annual Meeting Book of Abstracts, San Francisco, 1994.
4. McCormick WF. The pathology of vascular ("arteriovenous") malformations. *J Neurosurg* 1966;24:807–816.
5. Russell DS, Rubinstein LJ. *Pathology of Tumors of the Nervous System,* 5th ed. Baltimore: Williams and Wilkins; 1989.
6. Takamiya Y, Takayama H, Kobayashi K, Mine T, Suzuki K. Familial occurrence of multiple vascular malformations of the brain. *Neurol Med Chir* (*Tokyo*) 1984;24:271–277.
7. Rigamonti D, Spetzler RF. The association of venous and cavernous malformations. Report of four cases and discussion of the pathophysiological, diagnostic, and therapeutic implications. *Acta Neurochir* 1988;92:100–105.
8. Okazaki H, Scheithauer B. *Atlas of Neuropathology*. New York: Gower Medical Publishing; 1988.
9. Goulao A, Alvarez H, Monaco RG, Pruvost P, Lasjaunias P. Venous anomalies and abnormalities of the posterior fossa. *Neuroradiology* 1990;31:476–482.
10. Awad I, Robinson J, Mohanty S, Estes M. Mixed vascular malformations of the brain: clinical and pathologenetic considerations. *Neurosurgery* 1993;33:179–188.
11. Perret G, Nishioka H. Arteriovenous malformations. An analysis of 545 cases for craniocerebral arteriovenous malformations and fistulae reported to the cooperative study. *J Neurosurg* 1966;25: 467–490.
12. Kaplan HA, et al. Vascular malformations of the brain. An anatomical study. *J Neurosurg* 1961;27:630.
13. Wilkins RH, Rengachary SS. Vascular malformations. In: *Neurosurgery*. New York: McGraw-Hill; 1985:1448–1473.
14. Waltimo O. The relationship of size, density and localization of intracranial arteriovenous malformations to the type of the initial symptom. *J Neurol Sci* 1973;19:13–19.
15. Gerosa MA, Cappellotto P, Licata C, et al. Cerebral arteriovenous malformations in children (56 cases). *Childs Brain* 1981;8:356–371.
16. Brown RDJ, Wiebers DO, Forbes G, et al. The natural history of unruptured intracranial arteriovenous malformations. *J Neurosurg* 1988;68:352–357.
17. Crawford PM, West CR, Chadwick DW, Shaw MDM. Arteriovenous malformations of the brain: natural history in unoperated patients. *J Neurol Neurosurg Psychiatry* 1986;49:1–10.
18. Ondra S, Troupp H, George E, Schwab K. The natural history of symptomatic arteriovenous malformations of the brain. *J Neurosurg* 1990;73:387–391.
19. Heros RC, Korosue K. Arteriovenous malformations of the brain. *Curr Opin Neurol Neurosurg* 1990;3:63–67.
20. Graf CJ, Perret GE, Torner JC. Bleeding from cerebral arteriovenous malformations as part of their natural history. *J Neurosurg* 1983;58:331–337.
21. Szabo M, Crosby G, Sundaram P, et al. Hypertension does not cause spontaneous hemorrhage of intracranial arteriovenous malformations. *Anesthesiology* 1989;70:761–763.
22. Brust JCM, Richtor RW. Stroke associated with cocaine abuse—? *NY State J Med* 1977;77:1473–1475.
23. Lichtenfeld PJ, Rubin DB, Feldman RS. Subarachnoid hemorrhage precipitated by cocaine snorting. *Arch Neurol* 1984;41: 223–224.
24. Mendalow A, Erfurth A, Grossary K, et al. Do cerebral arteriovenous malformations increase in size? *J Neurol Neurosurg Psychiatry* 1987;50:980–987.
25. Anderson EB, Petersen J, Mortensen EL, Udesen H. Conservatively treated patients with cerebral arteriovenous malformation: mental and physical outcome. *J Neurol Neurosurg Psychiatry* 1988;51:1208–1212.
26. Woodard E, Barrow D. Clinical presentation of intracranial arteriovenous malformations. In: Barrow D, ed. *Intracranial Vascular Malformations*. Park Ridge, Ill: AANS; 1990:53–61.
27. Willinsky RA, Lasjaunias P, Terbrugge K, Burrows WP. Multiple cerebral arteriovenous malformations (AVMs). Review of our experience from 203 patients with cerebral vascular lesions. *Neuroradiology* 1990;32:207–210.
28. Burger PC, Scheithauer BW. Vascular tumors and tumor-like lesions. In: *Tumors of the Central Nervous System*. Washington, D.C.: Armed Forces Institute of Pathology; 1994:287–299.
29. Miyasaka K, Wolpert SM, Prager RJ. The association of cerebral aneurysms, infundibula and intracranial arteriovenous malformations. *Stroke* 1982;13:196–203.
30. Cunha e Sa MJ, Stein BM, Solomon RA, McCormick PC. The treatment of associated intracranial aneurysms and arteriovenous malformations. *J Neurosurg* 1992;77:853–859.
31. Okazaki H. *Fundamentals of Neuropathology*. New York: Igaku-Shoin; 1983.
32. Luessenhop A, Gennarelli T. Anatomical grading of supratentorial arteriovenous malformations for determining operability. *Neurosurgery* 1977;1:30–35.
33. Pellitieri L, Carlsson C, Grevsten S, et al. Surgical versus conservative treatment of intracranial arteriovenous malformations: a study in surgical decision making. *Acta Neurochir* (*Wien*) 1979;29(Suppl):1–86.
34. Luessenhop A, Rosa L. Cerebral arteriovenous malformations. *J Neurosurg* 1984;60:14–22.
35. Spetzler RF, Martin NA. A proposed scheme for grading intracranial arteriovenous malformations. *J Neurosurg* 1986;65:476–483.
36. Steinmeier R, Schramm J, Muller H, Fahlbush R. Evaluation of prognostic factors in cerebral arteriovenous malformations. *Neurosurgery* 1989;24:193–200.
37. Steiner L. Radiosurgery in cerebral arteriovenous malformations. In: Flamm E, ed. *Cerebrovascular Surgery*. New York: Springer-Verlag; 1986.
38. Steiner L, Lindquist C, Adler JR, et al. Clinical outcome of radiosurgery for cerebral arteriovenous malformations. *J Neurosurg* 1992;77:1–8.
39. Lunsford L, Kondziolka D, Bissonette D, Maitz A, Flickinger J. Stereotactic radiosurgery of brain vascular malformations. *Neurosurg Clin North Am* 1992;3:79–98.
40. Fabrikant J, Levy R, Steinberg G, et al. Charged particle radiosurgery for intracranial vascular malformations. *Neurosurg Clin North Am* 1992;3:99–139.
41. Sisti MB, Kader A, Stein BM. Microsurgery for 67 intracranial arteriovenous malformations less than 3 cm in diameter. *J Neurosurg* 1993;79:653–660.
42. Berenstein A, Lasjaunias P. *Surgical Neuroangiography*. New York: Springer-Verlag; 1992.
43. Shi YQ, Chen XC. A proposed scheme for grading intracranial arteriovenous malformations. *J Neurosurg* 1986;65:484–489.
44. Smith HJ, Strother CM, Kikuchi Y, et al. MR imaging in the management of supratentorial intracranial AVMs. *AJNR* 1988;9: 225–235.
45. Axel L. Blood flow effects in magnetic resonance imaging. *AJR* 1984;143:1157–1166.
46. Bradley WG, Waluch V. Blood flow: magnetic resonance imaging. *Radiology* 1985;154:443–450.
47. Gomori JM, Grossman RI, Bilaniuk LT, et al. High-field MR imaging of superficial siderosis of the central nervous system. *J Comput Assist Tomogr* 1985;9:972–975.
48. Valavanis A, Schubiger O, Wichmann W. Classification of brain arteriovenous malformation nidus by magnetic resonance imaging. *Acta Radiol Suppl* (*Stockholm*) 1986;369:86–89.

49. Nussel F, Wegmuller H, Huber P. Comparison of magnetic resonance angiography, magnetic resonance imaging, and conventional angiography in cerebral arteriovenous malformations. *Neuroradiology* 1991;33:56–61.
50. Kjellberg RN, Hanamura T, Davis KR, et al. Bragg-peak proton beam therapy for arteriovenous malformations of the brain. *N Engl J Med* 1983;309:269–274.
51. Spetzler RF, Wilson CB, Weinstein P, et al. Normal perfusion pressure breakthrough theory. *Clin Neurosurg* 1978;25:651–672.
52. Spetzler RF, Harggraves RW, McCormick PW, Zabramski JM, Flom RA, Zimmerman RS. Relationship of perfusion pressure and size to risk of hemorrhage from arteriovenous malformation. *J Neurosurg* 1992;76:918–923.
53. Perata HJ, Tomsick TA, Tew JM Jr. Feeding artery pedicle aneurysms: association with parenchymal hemorrhage and arteriovenous malformation in the brain. *J Neurosurg* 1994;80:631–634.
54. Suzuki J, Kodama N. Moyamoya disease: a review. *Stroke* 1983;14:104–109.
55. Yonakawa Y, Handa J, Okuno T. Moyamoya disease: diagnosis, treatment, and recent achievement. In: Barnett HJ, Stein BM, Mohr JP, Yatsu FM, eds. *Stroke: Pathophysiology, Diagnosis, and Management*, 2nd ed. New York: Churchill, 1985:805–831.
56. Hasuo K, Tamura S, Kudo S, et al. Moyamoya disease: the use of digital subtraction angiography in its diagnosis. *Radiology* 1985;157:107–111.
57. Fujisawa I, Asato R, Nishimura K, et al. Moyamoya disease: MR imaging. *Radiology* 1987;164:103–105.
58. Marks MP, DeLapaz RL, Fabrikant JI, et al. Intracranial vascular malformations: Imaging of charged-particle radiosurgery. Part I. Results of therapy. *Radiology* 1988;168:447–455.
59. Marks MP, DeLapaz RL, Fabrikant JI, et al. Intracranial vascular malformations: imaging of charged-particle radiosurgery. Part II. Complications. *Radiology* 1988;168:457–462.
60. Lunsford L, Flickinger J, Coffey R. Stereotactic gamma knife radiosurgery: initial North American experience in 207 patients. *Arch Neurol* 1990;7:169–175.
61. Wedeen VJ, Rosen BR, Chesler D, Brady TH. MR velocity imaging by phase display. *J Comput Assist Tomogr* 1985;9:530–536.
62. Dumoulin CL, Hart HR. Magnetic resonance angiography. *Radiology* 1986;161:717–720.
63. Dumoulin CL, Souza SP, Hart HR. Rapid scan magnetic resonance angiography. *Magn Reson Imag* 1987;5:238–245.
64. Wehrli FW, Shimakawa A, Gullberg GT, MacFall JR. Time-of-flight MR flow imaging: selective saturation recovery with gradient refocusing. *Radiology* 1986;160:781–785.
65. Nayler GL, Firmin GL, Longmore DB. Blood flow imaging by cine magnetic resonance. *J Comput Assist Tomogr* 1986;10:715.
66. Firmin DN, Nayler GL, Underwood SR, Klipstein RH, Rees SRO, Longmore DB. MR angiography, flow velocity, and acceleration measurements combined using a field even-echo rephasing (FEER) sequence. Chicago: 1986;127.
67. Masaryk TJ, Ross JS, Modic MT, Lenz GW, Haacke EM. Carotid bifurcation: MR imaging: work in progress. *Radiology* 1988;166: 461–466.
68. Hankey GJ, Warlow CP, Sellar RJ. Cerebral angiographic risk in mild cerebrovascular disease. *Stroke* 1990;21:209–222.
69. Grzyska V, Freitag J, Zeumer H. Selective arterial intracerebral DSA: complication rate and control of risk factors. *Neuroradiology* 1990;32:296–299.
70. Haase A, Frahm J, Matthaei D, et al. Rapid NMR imaging using low flip-angle pulses. *J Magnet Reson* 1986;67:258–266.
71. Fram EK, Dimick R, Hedlund LW, et al. Parameters determining the signal of flowing fluid in gradient refocused MR imaging: flow velocity, TR and flip angle. *Book of Abstracts*, Fifth Annual Meeting, SMRM, 1986:84–85.
72. Atlas SW. MR angiography in neurological disease: state of the art. *Radiology* 1994;193:1–16.
73. Marks MP, Pelc NJ, Ross MR, Enzmann DR. Determination of cerebral blood flow with a phase-contrast cine MR imaging technique: evaluation of normal subjects and patients with arteriovenous malformations. *Radiology* 1992;182:467–476.
74. Sheppard L, Listerud J, Goldberg HI, Hurst RW, Flamm E, Atlas SW. MR angiography of intracranial aneurysms using a sophisticated multifeature extraction post-processing method. *1994 RSNA Book of Abtracts*, 1994 (*in press*).
75. Evans AJ, Blinder RA, Herfkens RJ, et al. Effects of turbulence on signal intensity in gradient echo images. *Invest Radiol* 1988;23:512–518.
76. Atlas SW, Fram EK, Mark AS, Grossman RI. Vascular intracranial lesions: applications of fast scanning. *Radiology* 1988;169: 455–461.
77. Ogawa S, Lee TM, Kay AR, Tank DW. Brain magnetic resonance imaging with contrast dependent on blood oxygenation. *Proc Natl Acad Sci* 1990;87:9868–9872.
78. Fox PT, Raichle ME. Focal physiological uncoupling of cerebral blood flow and oxidative metabolism during somatosensory stimulation in human subjects. *Proc Natl Acad Sci* (*USA*) 1986;83: 1140–1144.
79. Fox PT, Raichle ME, Mintun MA, Dence C. Nonoxidative glucose consumption during focal physiologic neural activity. *Science* 1988;241:462–464.
80. Belliveau J, Kennedy D, McKinstry R, et al. Functional mapping of the human visual cortex by magnetic resonance imaging. *Science* 1991;254:716–719.
81. Maldjian J, Howard R, Alsop DA, et al. Functional MRI in AVMs prior to surgical or endovascular therapy. *Book of Abstracts, Annual Meeting of the RSNA, 1994.*
82. Simard JM, Garcia-Bengochea F, Ballinger WEJ, Mickle JP, Quisling RG. Cavernous angioma: a review of 126 collected and 12 new clinical cases. *Neurosurgery* 1986;18:162–172.
83. Scott RM, Barnes P, Kupsky W, Adelman LS. Cavernous angiomas of the central nervous system in children. *J Neurosurg* 1992;76:38–46.
84. Bicknell J, Carlow T, Kornfield M, Stovring J, Turner P. Familial cavernous angiomas. *Arch Neurol* 1978;35:746–749.
85. Cosgrove R, Bertrand G, Fontaine S, Robitaille Y, Melanson D. Cavernous angiomas of the spinal cord. *J Neurosurg* 1988;68:31–36.
86. Rigamonti D, Hadley MN, Drayer BP, et al. Cerebral cavernous malformations. Incidence and familial occurrence. *N Engl J Med* 1988;319:343–347.
87. Zambramski JM, Wascher TM, Spetzler RF, et al. The natural history of familial cavernous malformations: results of an ongoing study. *J Neurosurg* 1994;80:422–432.
88. Curling O, Kelly D. The natural history of intracranial cavernous and venous malformations. *Persp Neurol Surg* 1990;1:19–39.
89. Robinson J, Awad I, Little J. Natural history of the cavernous angioma. *J Neurosurg* 1991;75:709–714.
90. Barrow D, Krisht A. Cavernous malformations and hemorrhage. In: Awad I, Barrow D, eds. *Cavernous Malformations*. Park Ridge, Ill: AANS; 1993: 65–80.
91. Enomoto H, Goto H. Spinal epidural cavernous angioma. *Neuroradiology* 1991;33:462–465.
92. Goldwyn D, Cardenas C, Murtagh F, Balis G, Klein J. MRI of cervical extradural cavernous hemangioma. *Neuroradiology* 1992;34:68–69.
93. Tomlinson FH, Howser OW, Scheithauer BW, Sundt T, Okasaki H, Parisi JE. Cavernous angioma. Angiographically occult vascular malformations: a correlative MR imaging and histological study. *J Neurosurg* 1993;78:328.
94. Kucharczyk W, Lemme-Pleghos L, Uske A, et al. Intracranial vascular malformations: MR and CT imaging. *Radiology* 1985;156:383–389.
95. Gomori JM, Grossman RI, Goldberg HI, et al. Occult cerebral vascular malformations: high field MR imaging. *Radiology* 1986;158:707–713.
96. Atlas SW, Grossman RI, Gomori JM, Hackney DB, Goldberg HI, Zimmerman RA, Bilaniuk LT. Hemorrhagic intracranial malignant neoplasms: spin-echo MR imaging. *Radiology* 1987; 164:71–77.
97. Kim J, Kucharczyk W, Henkelman R. Cavernous hemangiomas: dipolar susceptibility artifacts at MR imaging. *Radiology* 1993;187:735–741.
98. Cohen HCM, Tucker WS, Humphreys RP, et al. Angiographically cryptic histologically verified cerebrovascular malformations. *Neurosurgery* 1982;10:704–714.

99. Sarwar M, McCormick W. Intracerebral venous angioma: case report and review. *Arch Neurol* 1978;35:323–325.
100. Latchaw RE, Truwit CL, Heros RC. Venous angioma, cavernous angioma, and hemorrhage. *AJNR* 1994;15:1255–1257.
101. Lasjaunias P, Berenstein A. *Functional Vascular Anatomy of Brain, Spinal Cord, and Spine*. Berlin, Heidelberg, New York: Springer-Verlag; 1990.
102. Malik GM, Morgan JK, Boulos RS, Ausman JI. Venous angiomas: an underestimated cause of intracranial hemorrhage. *Surg Neurol* 1988;30:350–358.
103. McCormick P, Michelson W. Management of cavernous and venous malformations. In: Barrow D, ed. *Intracranial Vascular Malformations*. Park Ridge, Ill: AANS; 1990:197–217.
104. Augustyn G, Scott J, Olson E, Gilmore R, Edwards M. Cerebral venous angiomas: MR imaging. *Radiology* 1985;156:391–395.
105. Vinuela F, Fox AJ, Pelz DM, Drake CG. Unusual clinical manifestations of dural arteriovenous malformations. *J Neurosurg* 1986;64:554–558.
106. Chaudhary MY, Sachdev VP, Cho SH, Weitzner IJ, et al. Dural arteriovenous malformations of the major venous sinuses: an acquired lesion. *AJNR* 1982;3:13–19.
107. Houser O, Baker HJ, Rhoton AJ, et al. Intracranial dural arteriovenous malformations. *Radiology* 1972;163:55–64.
108. Houser O, Campbell J, Campbell R, Sundt T. Arteriovenous malformation affecting the transverse dural venous sinus: an acquired lesion. *Mayo Clin Proc* 1979;54:651–661.
109. Halbach VV, Higashida RT, Heishima GB, Mehringer CM, Hardin CW. Transvenous embolization of dural fistulas involving the transverse and sigmoid sinuses. *AJNR* 1989;10:385–392
110. Terada T, Higashida R, Halbach VV, et al. Development of acquired arteriovenous fistulas in rats due to venous hypertension. *J Neurosurg* 1994;80:884–889.
111. Lasjaunias P, Chue M, TerBrugge K. Neurological manifestations of intracranial dural arteriovenous malformations. *J Neurosurg* 1986;64:724–730.
112. Awad I, Little J. Dural arteriovenous malformations. In: Barrow D, ed. *Intracranial Vascular Malformations*. Park Ridge, Ill: AANS; 1990:219–226.
113. Taniguchi RM, Goree JA, Odom GL. Spontaneous carotid cavernous shunts presenting diagnostic problems. *J Neurosurg* 1971;35:384–391.
114. Martin N, King W, Wilson C, et al. Management of dural arteriovenous malformations of the anterior cranial fossa. *J Neurosurg* 1990;72:692–697.
115. De Marco JK, Dillon WP, Halbach VV, Tsuruda JS. Dural arteriovenous fistulas: evaluation with MR imaging. *Radiology* 1990;175:193–199.
116. Willinsky R, Terbrugge K, Montanera W, Mikulis D, Wallace MC. Venous congestion: an MR finding in dural arteriovenous malformations with cortical venous drainage. *AJNR* 1994;15: 1501–1507.
117. Savino PJ, Grossman RI, Schatz NJ, et al. High-field magnetic resonance imaging in the diagnosis of cavernous sinus thrombosis. *Arch Neurol* 1986;43:1081–1082.
118. Sahs AL, Perret GE, Locksley HB, et al. *Intracranial Aneurysms and Subarachnoid Hemorrhage: A Cooperative Study*. Philadelphia: JB Lippincott; 1969.
119. Rosenorn J, Eskesen V, Schmidt K. Unruptured intracranial aneurysms: an assessment of the annual risk of rupture based on epidemiological and clinical data. *Br J Neurosurg* 1988;2:369–378.
120. Solomon RA, Fink ME, Pile-Spellman J. Surgical management of unruptured intracranial aneurysms. *J Neurosurg* 1994;80: 440–446.
121. Ohman J, Heiskanen O. Timing of operation for ruptured supratentorial aneurysms: a prospective randomized study. *J Neurosurg* 1989;70:55–60.
122. Mohr J, Kistler J, Zambranski J, Spetzler R, Barnett H. Intracranial aneurysms. In: Barnett H, Mohr J, Stein B, Yatsu F, eds. *Stroke: Pathophysiology, Diagnosis, and Management*. New York, Edinburgh, London, Melbourne: Churchill Livingstone; 1986:643–677.
123. Stehbens WE. Etiology of intracranial berry aneurysms. *J Neurosurg* 1989;70:823–831.
124. Weir BKA. Intracranial aneurysms. *Curr Opin Neurol Neurosurg* 1990;3:55–62.
125. Rhoton A. Anatomy of saccular aneurysms. *Surg Neurol* 1980; 14:59–66.
126. Scotti G, Ethier R, Melancon D, et al. Computed tomography in the evaluation of intracranial aneurysms and subarachnoid hemorrhage. *Radiology* 1977;123:85–90.
127. Aalmaani WS, Richardson AE. Multiple intracranial aneurysms: identifying the ruptured lesion. *Surg Neurol* 1978;9:303–305.
128. Wood EH. Angiographic identification of the ruptured lesion in patients with multiple cerebral aneurysms. *J Neurosurg* 1964;21: 182–198.
129. Grossman RI, Kemp SS, Yu IC, et al. The importance of oxygenation in the appearance of acute subarachnoid hemorrhage on high-field magnetic resonance imaging. *Acta Radiol (Suppl)* 1986;369:56–58.
130. Jenkins A, Hadley DM, Teasdale GM, Condon B, Macpherson P, Patterson J. Magnetic resonance imaging of acute subarachnoid hemorrhage. *J Neurosurg* 1988;68:731–736.
131. Ogawa T, Inugami A, Shimosegawa E, et al. Subarachnoid hemorrhage: evaluation with MR imaging. *Radiology* 1993;186:345.
132. Holtas S, Olsson M, Romner B, Larsson E, Saveland H, Brandt L. Comparison of MR imaging and CT in patients with intracranial aneurysm clips. *AJNR* 1988;9:891–897.
133. Klucznik R, Carrier D, Pyka R, Haid R. Placement of a ferromagnetic intracerebral aneurysm clip in a magnetic field with a fatal outcome. *Radiology* 1993;187:612–614.
134. Bull J. Massive aneurysms at the base of the brain. *Brain* 1969;92: 535–570.
135. Drake CG. Giant intracranial aneurysms: experience with surgical treatment in 174 patients. *Clin Neurol* 1979;26:12–95.
136. O'Neill M, Hope T, Thompson G. Giant intracranial aneurysms: diagnosis with special reference to computerized tomography. *Clin Radiol* 1980;31:27–39.
137. Atlas SW, Grossman RI, Goldberg HI, et al. Partially thrombosed giant intracranial aneurysms: correlation of MR and pathologic findings. *Radiology* 1987;162:111–114.
138. von Schulthess GK, Higgins CB. Blood flow imaging with MR: spin-phase phenomena. *Radiology* 1985;157:687–695.
139. Atlas SW, Listerud J, Goldberg HI. MR angiography of the circle of Willis: three dimensional Fourier transform time-of-flight versus three dimensional Fourier transform phase contrast imaging. *RSNA Book of Abstracts* 1991;1:119.
140. Atlas SW, Listerud J, Chung W, Flamm E. Intracranial aneurysms: depiction on MR angiograms with a multifeature extraction post-processing algorithm. *Radiology* 1994;192:129–139.
141. Wiebers DO, Torner JC, Meissner I. Impact of unruptured intracranial aneurysms on public health in the United States. *Stroke* 1992;23:1416–1419.
142. Hackney DB, Lesnick JE, Zimmerman RA, et al. MR identification of bleeding site in subarachnoid hemorrhage with multiple intracranial aneurysms. *J Comput Assist Tomogr* 1986;10:878–880.
143. Ross JS, Masaryk TJ, Modic MT, Ruggieri PM, Haacke EM, Selman WR. Intracranial aneurysms: evaluation by MR angiography. *AJNR* 1990;11:449–456.
144. Schuierer G, Huk WJ, Laub G. Magnetic resonance angiography of intracranial aneurysms. *Neuroradiology* 1992;35:50–54.
145. Gouliamos A, Gotsis E, Vlahos L, et al. Magnetic resonance angiography compared to intra-arterial digital subtraction angiography in patients with subarachnoid hemorrhage. *Neuroradiology* 1992;35:46–49.
146. Eng J, Ceckler TL, Balaban RS. Quantitative 1H magnetization transfer imaging in vivo. *Magn Reson Med* 1991;17:304–314.
147. Edelman RR, Ahn SS, Chien D, et al. Improved time-of-flight MR angiography of the brain with magnetization transfer contrast. *Radiology* 1992;184:395–399.
148. Dumoulin CL, Souza SP, Walker MF, et al. Three-dimensional phase contrast angiography. *Magn Reson Med* 1989;9:139–149.
149. Huston J, Rufenacht DA, Ehman RL, Wiebers DO. Intracranial aneurysms and vascular malformations: comparison of time-of-flight and phase-contrast MR angiography. *Radiology* 1991;181: 721–730.
150. Blatter DD, Parker DL, Robison RO. Cerebral MR angiography

with multiple overlapping thin slab acquisistion. Part I. Quantitiative analysis of vessel visibility. *Radiology* 1991;179:805–811.
151. Blatter DD, Parker DL, Ahn SS, et al. Cerebral MR angiography with multiple overlapping thin slab acquisition. Part II. Early clinical experience. *Radiology* 1992;183:379–389.
152. Parker DL, Yuan C, Blatter DD. MR angiography by multiple thin slab 3D acquisition. *Magn Reson Med* 1991;17:434–451.
153. Creasy J, Price RR, Presbrey T, Goins D, Partain CL, Kessler RM. Gadolinium-enhanced MR angiography. *Radiology* 1990; 175:280–283.
154. Chung W, Atlas SW, Listerud J. Contrast material-enhanced MR angiography for intracranial aneurysms with 3D time-of-flight and 3D phase contrast techniques. *RSNA Book of Abstracts* 1992;121.
155. Bradley WG, Widoff BE, Yan K, Song SJ, Brown SM, Nissenbaum MA, et al. Comparison of routine and gadodiamide-enhanced 3D time-of-flight MR angiography in the brain. *RSNA Book of Abstracts* 1992;122.
156. Purdy DE, Cadena G, Laub G. The design of variable tip angle slab selection (TONE) pulses for improved 3D MR angiography. *SMRM Book of Abstracts* 1992;882.
157. Ross JA, Ruggieri PM, Tkach JA, Masaryk TJ, Modic MT. High resolution, magnetization transfer saturation, variable flip angle, time-of-flight MR angiography of the intracranial vasculature. *RSNA Book of Abstracts* 1992;720.
158. Hiehle J, Chung W, Atlas SW, Listerud J, Goldberg HI, Schneider E. Ramped excitation magnetization transfer 3D Fourier transform time-of-flight MR angiography in the intracranial circulation: comparison with 3D Fourier transform phase contrast imaging. *RSNA Book of Abstracts* 1993;14.
159. Lewin JS, Laub G. Intracranial MR angiography: direct comparison of three time-of-flight techniques. *AJNR* 1991;12:1133–1139.
160. Hu X, Alperin N, Levin DN, Tan KK, Mengeot M. Visualization of MR angiographic data with segmentation and volume-rendering techniques. *J Magn Reson Imag* 1991;1:539–546.
161. Listerud J, Atlas SW, McGowan JC, Butler N. TRAP: traced ray by array processor. *SMRM Book of Abstracts* 1991;757.
162. Lin W, Haacke EM, Smith AS, Clampitt ME. Gadolinium-enhanced high resolution MR angiography with adaptive vessel tracking: preliminary results in the intracranial circulation. *J Magn Reson Imag* 1992;2:277–284.
163. Atlas SW. Intracranial vascular malformations and aneurysms: current imaging applications. *Radiol Clin North Am* 1988;26: 821–837.

Magnetic Resonance Imaging of the Brain and Spine, Second Edition, edited by Scott W. Atlas. Lippincott-Raven Publishers, Philadelphia © 1996.

13

Cerebral Ischemia and Infarction

Vincent P. Mathews, Warren D. Whitlow, and R. Nick Bryan

Stroke is a commonly used but imprecise term that describes a clinical event—sudden onset of neurologic deficit secondary to cerebrovascular disease. The symptomatology of stroke has three main etiologies: cerebral infarction, intraparenchymal hemorrhage, and subarachnoid hemorrhage. Stroke patients have been extensively studied by numerous imaging techniques (1–3), but no routine imaging examination currently allows for the precise diagnosis and delineation of the most common form of stroke—cerebral infarction—nor its usual precursor, ischemia. Currently, the diagnosis of acute infarction is based primarily on the clinical observation of an acute neurologic deficit and the exclusion of other diagnostic possibilities by x-ray computed tomography (CT) scanning and metabolic tests (4). CT is often normal in the first 24 to 48 hours (5), and therefore may not establish a definitive diagnosis. Stable xenon CT and single positron emission CT (SPECT) with newer blood flow radiopharmaceuticals may be sensitive to ischemia, but are temporally nonspecific and of low anatomic resolution. Other imaging tests, such as positron emission tomography (PET) (6,7), are often neither available nor practical. A significant consequence of the resultant imprecise diagnosis of early cerebral ischemia may be ineffectual management. This possibility is of increasing importance as new therapies for acute infarction evolve and become a routine part of patient care. Magnetic resonance (MR), with its improved soft tissue contrast and new physiologic imaging capabilities, offers new opportunities for the early detection and delineation of ischemia and infarction that will hopefully improve our understanding of the disease and lead to improved patient outcome.

V. P. Mathews, M.D. : Department of Radiology, Bowman Gray School of Medicine, Wake Forest University, North Carolina Baptist Hospital, Winston-Salem, NC 27157.

W. D. Whitlow, M.D.: Texas Neuroradiology, P.A., 5430 Glen Lakes Drive, Suite 260, Dallas, TX 75231.

R. N. Bryan, M.D., Ph.D.: Department of Radiology and Radiological Science, Johns Hopkins Medical Institutions, Baltimore, MD 21287.

PATHOPHYSIOLOGY OF CEREBRAL ISCHEMIA

For nervous tissue to function properly and maintain its morphologic integrity, there must be a continuous and steady supply of critical metabolites such as oxygen and glucose as well as a continually operating system for removal of metabolic by-products such as CO_2. Simplistically, cerebral blood flow (CBF) is responsible for this continuous replenishment of metabolic requirements and removal of by-products. While cerebral blood flow is physiologically quite complex, the final demands placed on it are relatively straightforward. Normal CBF implies normal delivery of blood to the brain with an adequate concentration of oxygen and glucose.

The word "ischemia" is often loosely used to cover all abnormalities of CBF, but, by definition, ischemia is disruption of the entire blood flow. Oligemia indicates a reduction in blood flow. Anoxemia and hypoxemia indicate absent or reduced oxygen in the blood whereas anoxia or hypoxia connote absent or reduced oxygen in the pulmonary alveoli. A reduced level of blood glucose is hypoglycemia. Therefore, abnormalities of CBF can be broken down into three main categories (8):

1. Ischemic or oligemic—diminished blood supply.
2. Anoxemic or hypoxemic—decreased blood oxygen. This may be due to:
   a. Ischemia
   b. Anoxia or hypoxia—condition of tissue-insufficient oxygen tension in the alveoli
   c. Anemia—inadequate hemoglobin for O_2 transfer.
3. Hypoglycemia—decreased blood glucose.

It is obvious then that regions of cerebral ischemia not only have abnormal blood flow but also lack adequate levels of oxygen and glucose. On the other hand, the brain may be hypoxic from respiratory dysfunction but not ischemic or hypoglycemic. The multiple permutations of these factors are obvious, but it must be remembered that clinically it is relatively unusual to see any factor independently altered. For instance, respiratory dysfunction with hypoxia sufficient to produce cerebral infarction seldom occurs without significant cardiovascular dysfunction with associated ischemia.

Clinically, ischemia is far more common than the other types of CBF abnormalities and will be the main topic covered in this chapter. In addition, we will primarily discuss alterations in CBF that produce at least the risk of permanent functional and morphologic alterations of the brain, i.e., infarction.

In general, if ischemia, regardless of the physiologic type, is sufficient to produce a permanent effect, the brain responds in a pathologically stereotyped fashion. When nervous tissue is not supplied with adequate metabolites for functional and morphologic integrity, the tissue dies in a similar fashion, regardless of etiology. Infarcted brain, whether produced by ischemia, anoxia, anemia, or hypoglycemia, is remarkably similar in pathologic appearance.

PATHOLOGY OF CEREBRAL INFARCTION

Acute Stage

The neuron is the cell most sensitive to ischemia (followed by the astrocyte, oligodendroglia, and microglia). Because of this, the earliest cytologic changes occur within the neuron and may be seen as quickly as 20 minutes after complete ischemia. The neurons show microvacuolation which, by electron microscopy, consists of swollen, disorganized mitochondria. This may be the only change for 6 hours. The remainder of the nervous tissue is normal both macroscopically and microscopically. More obvious ischemic cell changes are seen at 4 to 6 hours, at which time the neurons begin to shrink, the nuclei stain more intensely, and the cytoplasm becomes eosinophilic. Electron micrographs reveal additional disruption of mitochondria, aggregation of ribosomes and swollen endoplasmic reticulum, and Golgi complex. At this time, perivascular spaces enlarge with associated expansion of astrocytic end feet. Subsequently, synaptic "encrustations" appear on the surface of the neurons that continue to shrink and lose their subcellular integrity. At the end of 24 hours, most of these acute necrotic changes are complete (9).

Macroscopically, the infarction becomes evident as "softening" of the brain with loss of the border between cortex and white matter and development of focal swelling with effacement of adjacent gyri (9). This focal swelling is at a maximum between 24 to 48 hours and is probably initially due to intracellular cytotoxic edema. Later there is an associated or superimposed extracellular vascular edema (10). One must remember that these earliest effects of cerebral infarction are relatively subtle, even at the microscopic level. The very earliest pathologic changes are evident, at best, within one-half to one hour after the insult. Functionally, permanent damage may be accomplished within 5 to 10 minutes.

Subacute Stage

Beginning at approximately 24 to 48 hours, the reparative processes of necrotic resorption begin (9). This is characterized by an ingrowth of microglial cells that begin to phagocytize the necrotic tissue. In addition, there is proliferation of astrocytes and endothelial cells with new capillaries. These resorptive and reparative processes are most marked at the periphery of the infarction and proceed toward the center. As the necrotic tissue is removed via macrophages and new blood vessels, there are remnant cavities and cysts occupying the previous nervous tissue spaces with intervening and surrounding glial scar tissue. If the infarction is of sufficient size, there may be an overall volume loss of brain tissue. This replaces the earlier cerebral swelling. In large infarcts, complete resorption of necrotic tissue may not take place and regions of central coagulation necrosis may persist.

Chronic Stage

In the late stages of cerebral infarction, the resorption of necrotic tissue is complete and one is left with glial scar, encephalomalacic cysts and, if of sufficient size, shrunken gyri, enlarged sulci, and adjacent ventricular dilation (9). This final pathologic state of the infarction is usually reached by the second to fourth week, although in some instances active resorption of tissue may persist for months. These general pathophysiologic changes occur in nearly all types of ischemic insults to the nervous system if infarction occurs. However, the specific appearances of an infarction will vary not only in location and size, but also in pattern, which is somewhat dependent on the specific etiology.

This pathologic description of infarction applies to "bland" infarcts. These are infarcts without a hemorrhagic component. However, many infarcts will have associated hemorrhage. In a hemorrhagic infarction, there is more disruption of the vasculature than in the bland infarction. Endothelial breaks allow diapedesis of red blood cells out of the vessels with subsequent small petechial hemorrhages (9). Occasionally, frank disruption of vessels occurs, resulting in intraparenchymal hematomas. Hemorrhagic infarction is thought to occur most commonly when ischemically damaged endothelium is reperfused. For instance, in embolic disease, the emboli initially lodge in more proximal vessels producing the ischemic insult. Subsequently, as the emboli are lysed, circulation is restored to the ischemic area, resulting in secondary hemorrhage. In venous infarction, the venous obstruction blocks the normal blood efflux. However, the distal arterial and capillary bed are still exposed to systemic blood pressure, which may disrupt the ischemic vessels. Hemorrhagic components of infarcts are secondary and, therefore, are generally not present during the very early stages of infarction. It is also noteworthy that most hemorrhagic infarcts from thromboembolic disease predominantly affect the gray matter, whereas venous hemorrhagic infarcts predominantly affect the white matter (11).

In addition to these classic pathologic changes, there are several additional factors to keep in mind. First, it is unclear which, if any, of the very early histologic changes of the brain in response to ischemia are reversible. This is an important scientific topic and is of increasing importance to the clinical radiologist as our imaging techniques become more sensitive and acute stroke therapies are developed.

In addition to the morphologic changes of the neuralglial tissue itself, ischemia alters the morphology and function of the cerebral vasculature. During the acute phase, prominence of perivascular spaces is noted, which may be due to swollen astrocytic end feet or direct damage to the endothelium. During the subacute stage, increased endothelial pinocytosis is present as well as disruption of some of the tight junctions between endothelial cells. These two histologic changes are related to the functional breakdown of the blood–brain barrier (BBB), which allows leakage of intravascular elements into the adjacent brain parenchyma. The abnormal endothelium and BBB is present not only in original blood vessels, but also is present in the new blood vessels that form around the periphery of the infarction and grow inward during the reparative process. After a period of weeks, the endothelium usually recovers to a more normal state with reestablishment of the integrity of the BBB (12). Along with these morphologic changes of blood vessels, there are physiologic changes including loss of autoregulation of adjacent blood vessels. Although cerebral infarction is generally associated with decreased CBF and cerebral blood volume, there may be areas of increased CBF and cerebral blood volume ("luxury perfusion") in ischemic areas around the margins of the lesion (13).

MR OF ISCHEMIC INFARCTION

Conventional Spin-Echo and Gradient-Echo MRI

For routine evaluation of stroke, MR imaging (MRI) examinations should include spin density–weighted (SDW), T2-weighted (T2-weighted) (3–3,500/22–35, and 3–3,500/80–120), and T1-weighted (T1-weighted) (5–600/20–35) spin-echo (SE) sequences. Scans generally consist of 5-mm thick slices with a 0-mm to 2.5-mm gap, 128 to 256 × 256 matrix, 20-cm to 24-cm field of view (FOV), one acquisition for 1.0 and 1.5 T (Tesla) double-echo sequences, and two acquisitions for 0.5-T systems. For T1-weighted sequences, two acquisitions are used at 0.5 T, one at 1.0, and 1.5 T. Gradient-echo (GE) scans are also obtained to evaluate T2-weighted effects to increase the sensitivity for blood products. In some cases, T1-weighted images performed after the intravenous injection of gadolinium may help to define areas of BBB breakdown and to visualize flow abnormalities within the larger vessels.

Acute infarctions are more frequently visible on MR than on CT scans. In the first 24 hours, approximately 80% of MR scans are positive compared to 60% percent of CT scans (14). On follow-up scans, approximately 90% of both CT and MR scans are positive.

On MRI, regions of increased signal intensity (SI) due to acute infarctions are usually observed on both SDW and T2-weighted images. The SDW changes often are more conspicuous (Fig. 1A). This is particularly evident for lesions involving cortical gray matter. In addition, when structures such as the internal and external capsules, thalamus, and basal ganglia are involved, better anatomic delineation is seen with the SDW image. When a lesion is near a ventricle or subarachnoid space, the presence of cerebrospinal fluid (CSF) may make it difficult to identify the lesion on T2-weighted images because both CSF and the lesion may have similar signal intensities.

The earliest SI changes usually involve the gray matter, where the increased SI is associated with very

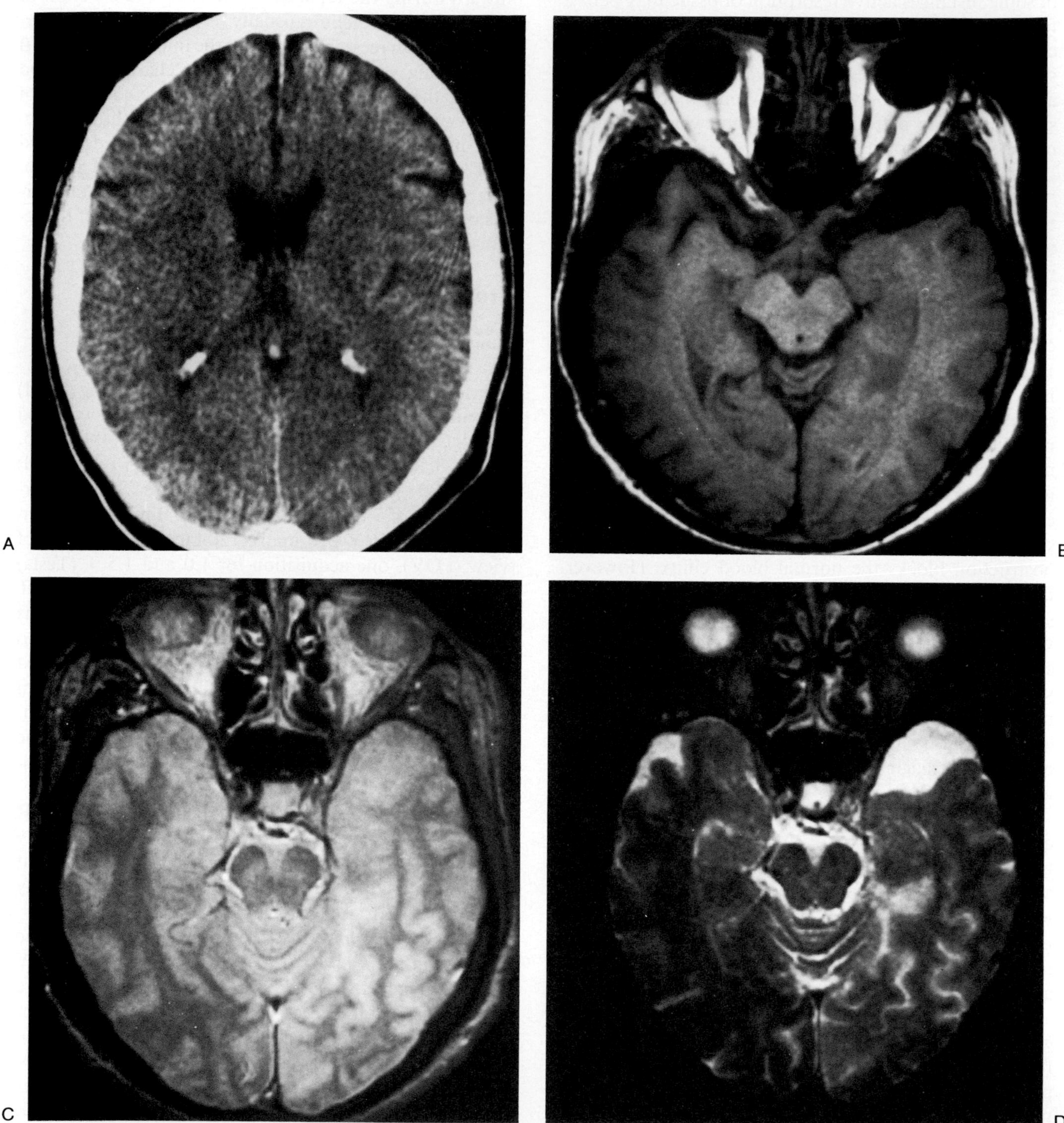

FIG. 1. A–H. Left occipital and posterior temporal lobe infarction with hemorrhagic evolution. **A:** CT scan shows subtle sulcal effacement left occipital lobe. **B:** T1-weighted image shows swollen gyri. SDW (**C**) and T2-weighted (**D**) images show increased SI of gyri in left posterior temporal and occipital lobes.

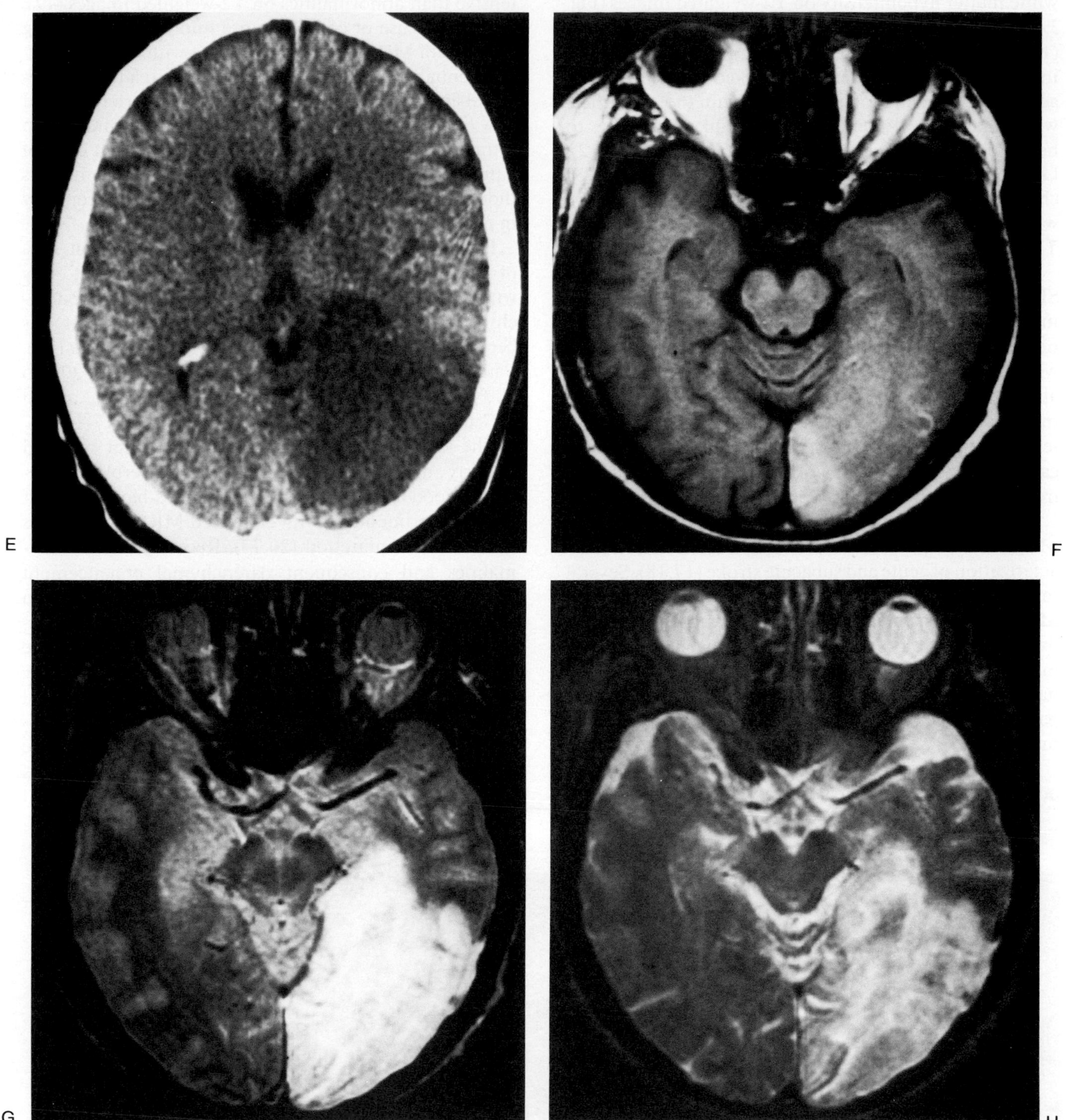

FIG. 1. (*Continued.*) **E:** CT scan 2 weeks later shows better defined infarction. **F:** T1-weighted image shows increased SI consistent with hemorrhage. SD (**G**) and T2-weighted (**H**) images show better defined infarction with additional white matter edema. (From Bryan, et al., ref. 15, with permission.)

subtle gyral swelling of a vascular territory. In typical cases, the white matter appears normal in the first 24 hours. However, not infrequently, there is subcortical white matter hypointensity on T2-weighted images (Fig. 3A). This has been ascribed to iron and/or free radicals (14), but it is of uncertain etiology at the time of this writing. It should be noted that this marked hypointensity in acute cortical infarction is located within the subcortical white matter, and therefore is most likely not due to hemorrhage, which occurs in the affected cortex (Fig. 2). On both initial and follow-up scans, T1-weighted SI changes are the least sensitive for detection of stroke (15), which is not unexpected because of the negative mix of T1 and SD contrast (16).

In the typical *subacute infarction*, the relatively subtle SI changes seen initially are more obvious with further increase in SDW and T2-weighted SI (see Fig. 1B). Gray matter, especially gyral, swelling is more obvious and white matter abnormalities are now seen. The accentuated gray matter changes in combination with white matter changes result in much more obvious lesions, often with more mass effect. In approximately 20% of cases, there will be regions of increased T1-weighted SI indicating hemorrhagic component.

Recently, the use of paramagnetic contrast agents in MRI has been shown to improve the detection and characterization of acute and subacute stroke (17,18). Several investigations have described gadolinium-enhanced MRI of infarction (17–24). Four types of contrast enhancement have been described on T1-weighted images in patients with cerebral infarction: a) intravascular enhancement, b) meningeal enhancement, c) mixed compartment enhancement, and d) parenchymal enhancement (17).

Intravascular and meningeal enhancement typically occur earlier than parenchymal enhancement and have peak incidences on the second day after infarction (Figs. 3 and 4). Intravascular enhancement is seen in 75% of strokes in the first week and can precede or be more extensive than abnormalities on T2-weighted images (17), making the use of contrast more important in imaging stroke with MR than it is in imaging with CT. Intravascular enhancement on MRI has been correlated with cerebral arteriography and is related to slow arterial blood flow (25). Meningeal enhancement is less common than intravascular enhancement, being identified in 35% of patients in the first week. Meningeal enhancement is thought to be due to meningeal irritation and is seen only in peripheral infarctions (17).

During the fourth to seventh days after infarction, 35% of patients will demonstrate enhancement not only within vessels and meninges but also within the parenchyma. This mixed compartment enhancement has been termed the *transitional stage of enhancement* (17). Parenchymal enhancement has been observed in 20% to 40% of patients studied less than 6 days after ictus and in 90% to 100% of patients studied after 1 week (17,21).

The infrequent parenchymal enhancement reported in early infarction in clinical studies is perplexing because blood–brain barrier abnormalities have been detected experimentally with enhanced MRI within hours after cerebral infarction (26,27). Recently, BBB abnormalities and consequent parenchymal enhancement have been detected during the first week of infarction in 100% of patients when magnetization transfer (MT) imaging or high doses of paramagnetic contrast agents are used (Fig. 4). Utilization of delayed MRI, MT imaging, and high-dose gadolinium administration also increased the frequency of detection of meningeal and intravascular enhancement (28). The increased sensitivity of these techniques, however, makes these enhancement patterns less useful in the dating of cerebral infarction as discussed

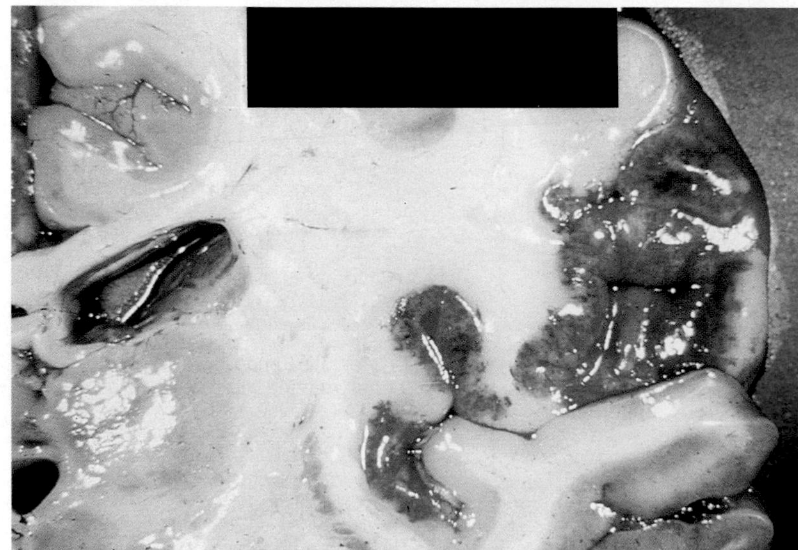

FIG. 2. Cortical hemorrhage, gross specimen. Note typical cortical location of hemorrhage associated with embolic infarction. (Courtesy of H. Goldberg, M.D., Philadelphia, PA).

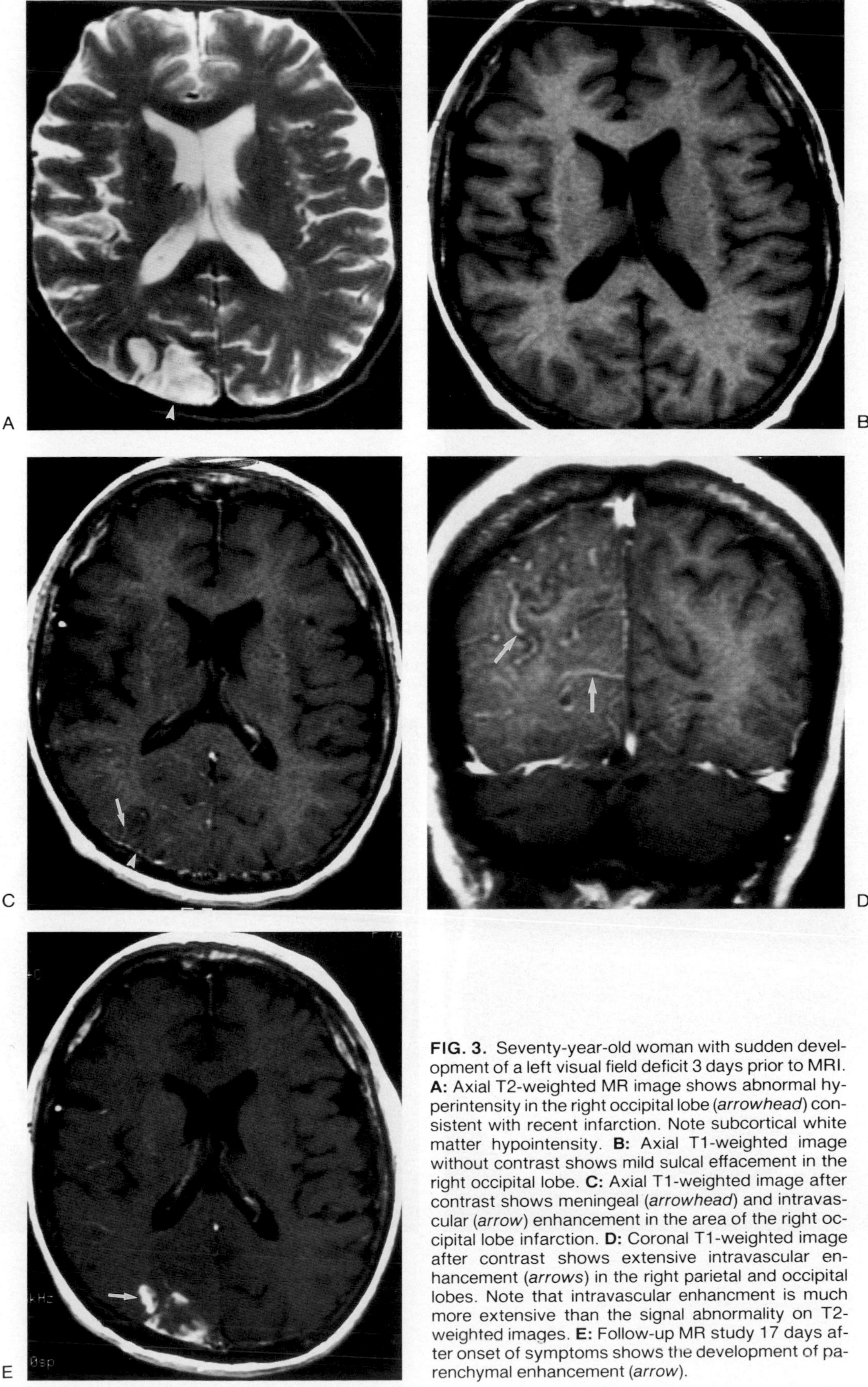

FIG. 3. Seventy-year-old woman with sudden development of a left visual field deficit 3 days prior to MRI. **A:** Axial T2-weighted MR image shows abnormal hyperintensity in the right occipital lobe (*arrowhead*) consistent with recent infarction. Note subcortical white matter hypointensity. **B:** Axial T1-weighted image without contrast shows mild sulcal effacement in the right occipital lobe. **C:** Axial T1-weighted image after contrast shows meningeal (*arrowhead*) and intravascular (*arrow*) enhancement in the area of the right occipital lobe infarction. **D:** Coronal T1-weighted image after contrast shows extensive intravascular enhancement (*arrows*) in the right parietal and occipital lobes. Note that intravascular enhancment is much more extensive than the signal abnormality on T2-weighted images. **E:** Follow-up MR study 17 days after onset of symptoms shows the development of parenchymal enhancement (*arrow*).

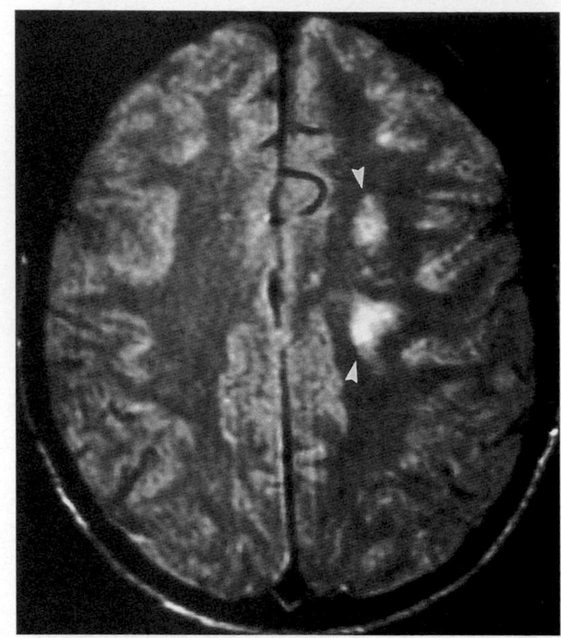

A

FIG. 4. Sixty-five-year-old male with a 7-day history of right arm weakness. **A:** Axial proton-density–weighted MR image shows abnormal hyperintensity (*arrowheads*) due to a left hemispheric infarction. **B:** Axial T1-weighted image after contrast administration shows no abnormal enhancement. **C:** Axial T1-weighted image after contrast with magnetization transfer saturation shows extensive enhancement (*arrows*) in the left hemisphere. This exam was performed approximately 15 min after B and shows the abnormality to be much more extensive than was indicated by the proton-density–weighted image.

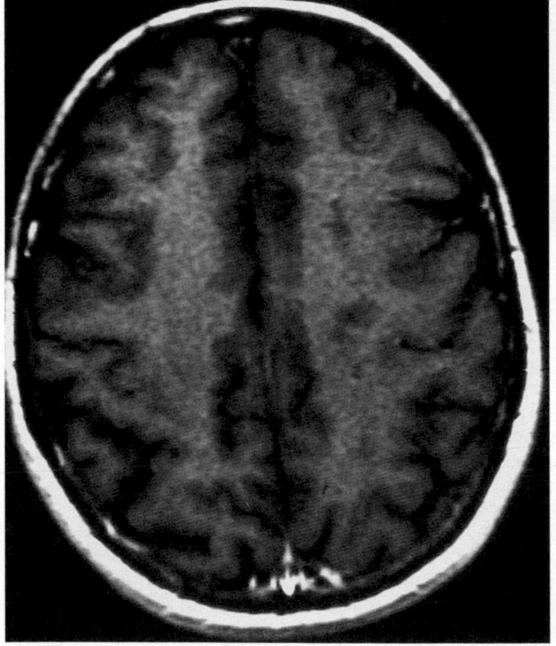

B

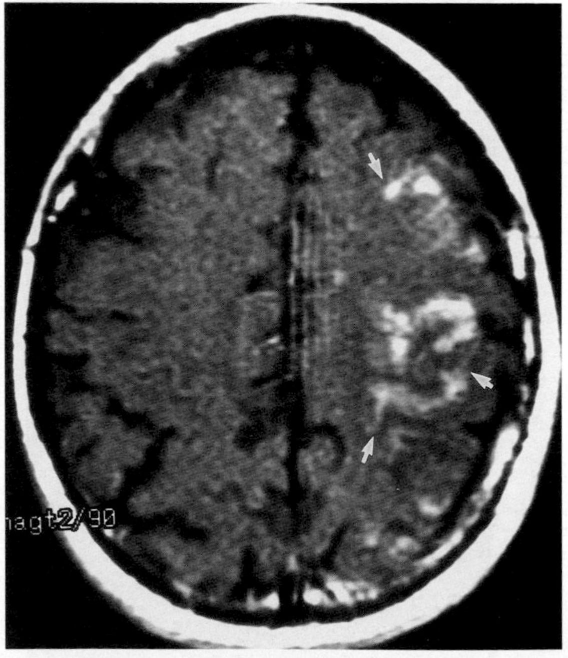

C

above (17). However, the overall improvement in the detection of enhancement may be helpful in identifying infarctions when images without contrast are normal, as in the hyperacute stage (18) as well as in the subacute phase when "fogging" may occur (29,30). Contrast enhancement may also be useful when numerous stroke-like lesions are present on T2-weighted images, the ages of which cannot be determined clinically or radiologically without contrast (31).

The *chronic stage* of cerebral infarction is usually considered to begin when the integrity of the BBB is restored, edema has resolved, and most of the resorption of necrotic tissue is complete. This takes longer with larger infarctions, both pathologically and by MR, but is usually accomplished by 3 to 4 weeks. The MR of chronic infarctions is characterized by a smaller, better defined zone of altered SI than seen on earlier scans. In addition, the SDW and T2-weighted SI is greater. Contrast enhancement does not usually occur. The increased SI is due to greater water content secondary to the cystic cavitation making up the bulk of the residual tissue. There is a net loss of tissue volume and hence focal atrophy is present with dilatation of the adjacent sulci and ventricles. As time progresses, the lesions continue to shrink, with the atrophic changes becoming more obvious and the infarction itself less obvious. Rarely, in very small infarctions, the parenchymal lesion may become undetectable by MR and only the atrophic changes indicate the previous insult.

Clinical results suggest that in the setting of acute stroke, MRI signal changes of increased SD and T2 (and probably T1) are generally irreversible and associated with cell death and infarction. We have seen few cases of acute stroke in which a region of abnormal MRI SI reverted to normal (Fig. 5). Thus, MRI signal changes may actually be indicators of "cell death." This is not to imply that increased SD and T2 are associated with cell death in general; clearly, this is not true. Rather, in certain cases in which the clinical picture is of acute stroke and there is a MR "pattern" of acute stroke with primary involvement of gray matter in a vascular pattern, the SI changes may be relatively specific for cell death. This finding could be important in planning the initial management of stroke patients and for the evaluation of therapies.

Another critical factor in the diagnosis and current management of acute stroke is determination of the presence of a hemorrhagic component. In cases of obvious acute hematoma, both CT and MR show typical changes of increased radiodensity and decreased SI on T2 and GE

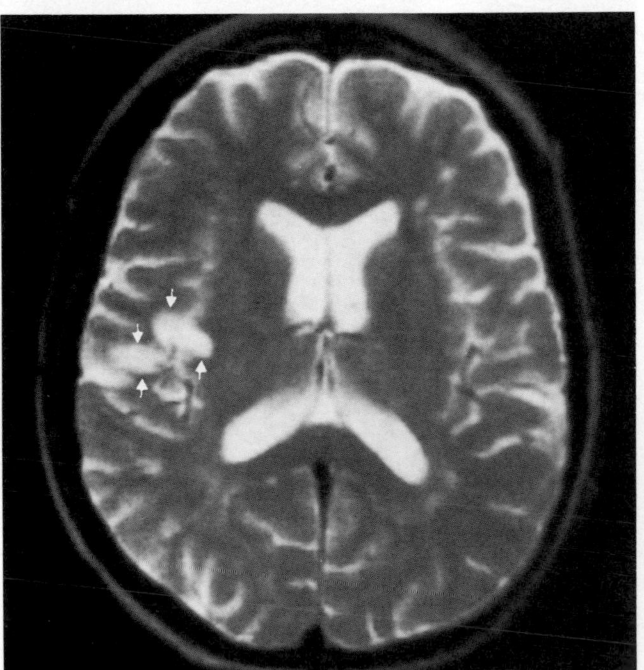
A

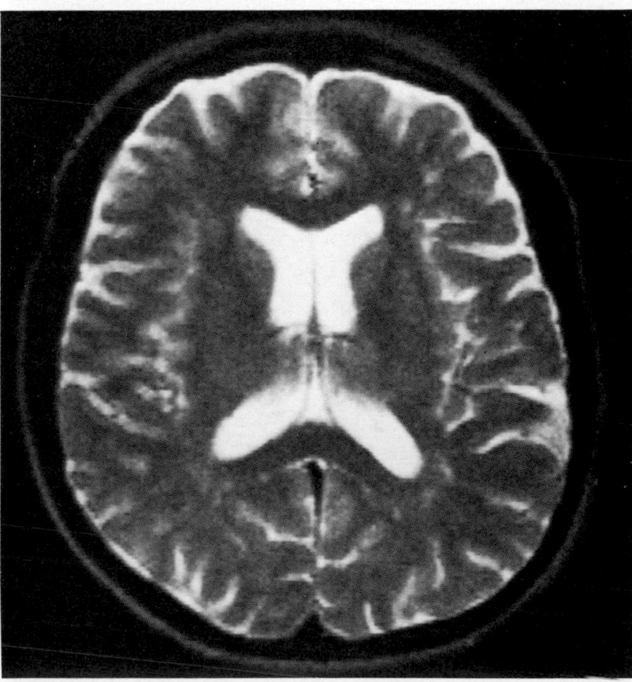
B

FIG. 5. Apparent resolution of right sylvian cortical "infarction." **A:** Initial T2-weighted image shows increased SI right sylvian cortex. **B:** On follow-up day 7, T2-weighted image shows resolution of signal abnormalities.

MR scans (Fig 6). However, there are reports indicating that acute hemorrhage may not be obvious on MRI, particularly if GE scans are not performed (32). Theoretically, early hemorrhagic lesions might not have adequate time for the fluid resorption, hemoglobin concentration, clot formation, and/or accumulation of high concentrations of deoxyhemoglobin that contribute to the typical appearance of hemorrhage on MRI (33,34). However, we believe that the combination of SE and GE generally obviates the need for such studies as CT to detect intracerebral hemorrhage. This is not true for subarachnoid hemorrhage, which is not well detected by MRI.

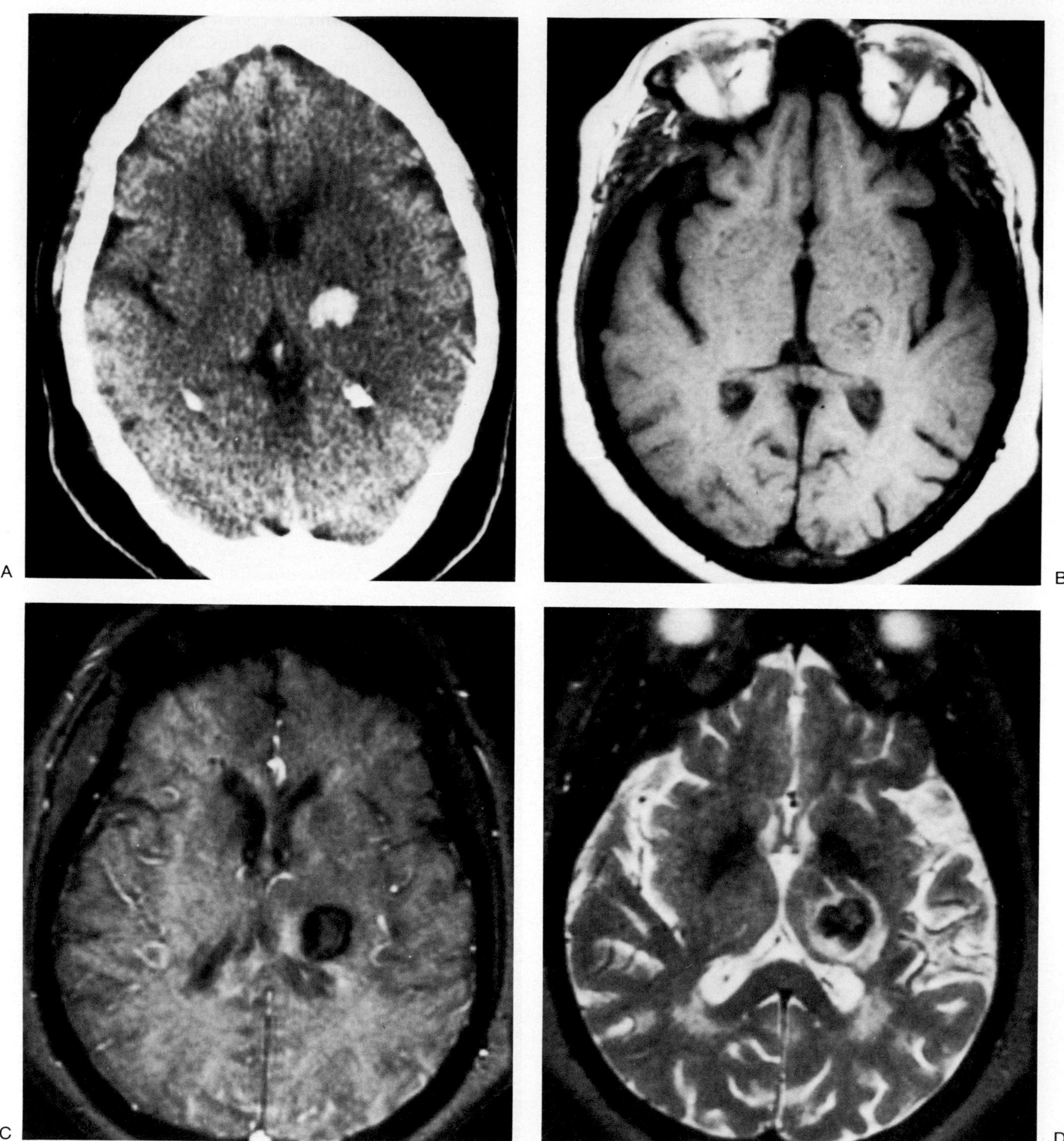

FIG. 6. Acute left thalamic hematoma. **A:** CT scan shows increased density left thalamus. **B:** T1-weighted image shows isotense to decreased SI. **C,D:** GE and T2-weighted images show decreased SI.

An important point relative to hemorrhage in stroke is its comparative frequency, as reflected by increased SI on T1-weighted images (Figs. 1A and 7). This "hemorrhagic" pattern differs from the usual hematoma. In particular, it may not be associated with decreased SI on T2-weighted images; nor are T2* effects reflected by decreased SI on GE images. Furthermore, the presence of "methemoglobin" signal in the first day of ischemia is not in keeping with the usual 3- to 4-day time course of oxidation of hemoglobin to methemoglobin. The most likely explanation is that these lesions are not frank hematomas, but "ischemic petechial infarctions." The early formation of methemoglobin in these lesions might be explained by the exposure of oxy- and deoxyhemoglo-

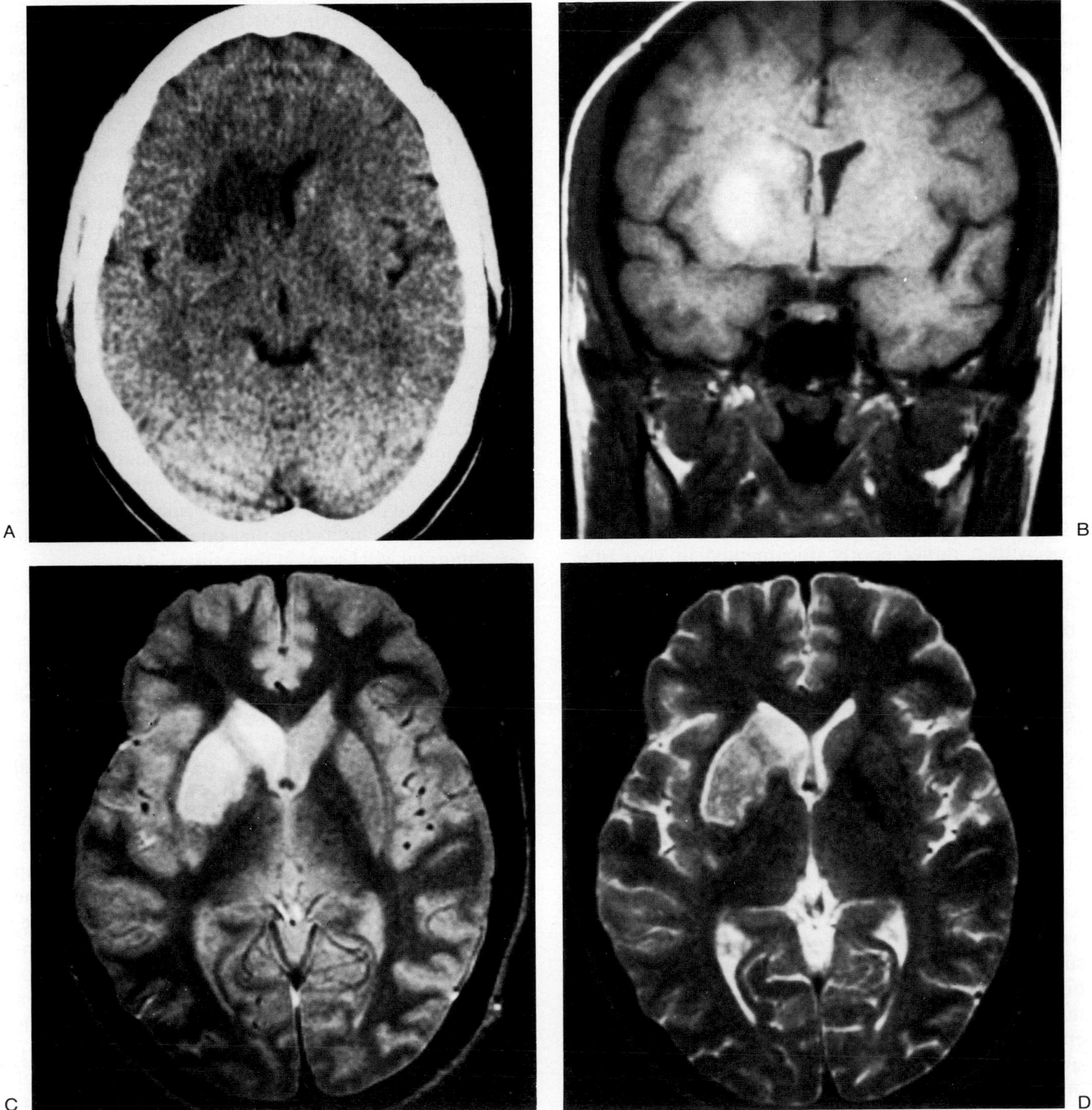

FIG. 7. Acute petechial hemorrhagic infarction right basal ganglia. **A:** CT shows decreased density right basal ganglia without evidence of hemorrhage. **B:** T1-weighted image shows increased SI consistent with early methemoglobin formation. **C,D:** SD and T2-weighted images show relatively nonspecific increased SI.

bin to free radicals in the ischemic area. Free radicals are known to accelerate the oxidation of hemoglobin to methemoglobin (35). Ischemic areas with reperfusion have been experimentally shown to have increased free radical formation, which could lead to accelerated methemoglobin formation. Such methemoglobin conversion could occur in red blood cells (RBCs) in stagnant capillaries or in small petechiae in the ischemic area. However, the lack of signal loss in GE imaging suggests that there is little magnetic susceptibility heterogeneity in these lesions. Although we have no proven explanation for the lack of magnetic susceptibility heterogeneity in these ischemic lesions, it is possible that the heterogeneity accounting for susceptibility effects within the usual hematoma is not only due to heterogeneity from RBC membrane partition, but from other aspects of the lesion, such as clot matrix. Because these hemorrhagic infarctions are not frank hematomas, they do not have clot formation and associated heterogeneity. At the present time, we have not seen progressive hemorrhage in these lesions and do not believe that anticoagulation is contraindicated.

MR OF AREAS AT RISK OF INFARCTION

We believe MR is the most sensitive, accurate, and practical means of imaging acute infarction. However, the significance of the observed signal changes as well as their relationship to the pathophysiology of acute stroke needs to be clarified. Stroke is a temporally dynamic disease with a rather poorly documented in vivo time course that begins with regions of tissue at risk of infarction. These at-risk areas may or may not proceed to irreversible infarction. Initially, inadequate tissue perfusion leads to depletion of intracellular energy stores, a decrease in oxidative phosphorylation, increased glycolysis, and early cellular injury (36). This sequence is followed by a series of biochemical events culminating in cell death—the so-called ischemic cascade (37), with loss of high energy metabolites and finally cell death (38). These primary events may be accompanied or followed by secondary phenomena such as edema, mass effect, and endothelial damage.

It is postulated that the initial signal changes observed with conventional MRI reflect changes in intracellular water arising from loss of normal energy homeostasis, subsequent membrane dysfunction (particularly Na/K pumps), increased intracellular H_2O, diminished binding of water to macromolecules, and consequent increases in T1 and T2 (39,40). According to this hypothesis, cells (neurons and/or glia) will maintain reasonable intracellular water biophysics, including water concentration and relaxation times, until a lethal level of ischemia (approximately 12 mL/100 g per min) is reached. It has been shown that intracellular sodium, and probably potassium, become affected at these lower ischemic levels (41). Because there is an intimate relationship between intracellular water and intracellular sodium and potassium, this level of insult may be required to change the proton MRI signals, in which case they would be relatively irreversible. However, more carefully controlled experiments, in which CBF and tissue metabolic parameters such as adenosine triphosphate (ATP), lactate, and intracellular Na are monitored, are required to document these ideas.

Although conventional MRI may be accurate at delineating infarcted tissue, it is clear that it does not detect areas at risk of infarction. For instance, acute infarctions show a progression of size in 30% of cases, an important finding (15). In addition, 5% of lesions "appear" after the first 24 hours (Fig. 8). Thus, despite the sensitivity of MRI to early infarction, dynamic events occur after the first 24 hours, leading to additional tissue infarction. The significance of this finding is the implication of a larger tissue area "at risk" of infarction that is not currently identified by routine MRI scans.

These human clinical findings are in keeping with previous reports on the MRI appearance of acute infarction (42) in animal experiments. Numerous animal experiments indicate that conventional MRI signal changes do not occur until 2 to 4 hours after the onset of ischemia (43). During the early postictal period there are clearly tissues at risk of infarction that are not identified by this technique. There are also increasing numbers of reports of normal patient MRI scans performed earlier than 6 hours postictus, indicating that one may not expect to see abnormal MRI scans at these times (44).

At least two mechanisms might account for this progression of disease. There may be a core of immediate infarction, where blood flow is lowest, surrounded by the "penumbra" or area at risk of infarction (45), where blood flow is diminished, but not lethal in the first 24 hours. Because of an ischemia/time interdependency related to cell death, there may be a progressive infarction of the penumbra as the metabolic reserves of more distal cells become inadequate.

Another mechanism relates to proximal thromboemboli that produce proximal end vessel occlusion and central infarction (46,47). Subsequently, lysis and breakup of the proximal thromboemboli occurs and results in the lodging of smaller emboli in more distal vessels. This sequence results in secondary peripheral end vessel infarction. This pathophysiologic mechanism should apply only to thromboembolic strokes. The general pattern observed with the progressive MR changes in stroke is proximal disease initially (in terms of arterial anatomy), followed by more peripheral extension that is consistent with either mechanism. Other factors could also influence infarction progression such as vascular spasm or reperfusion. With the advent of effective therapies for acute ischemia, it will become increasingly important to

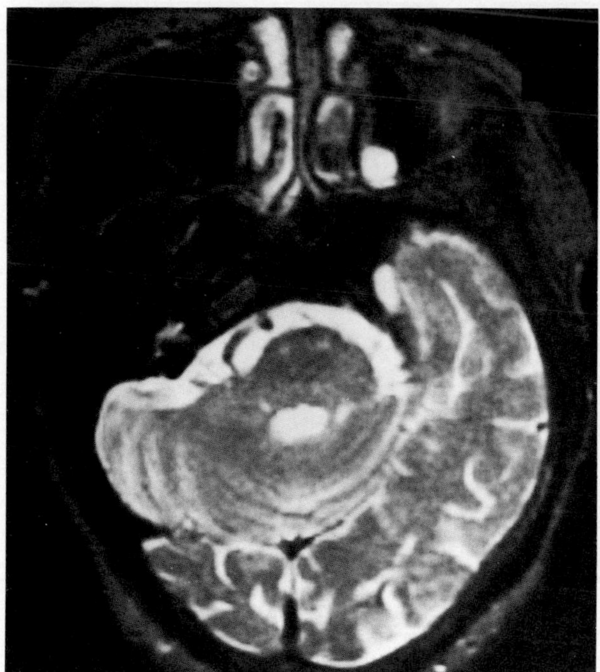
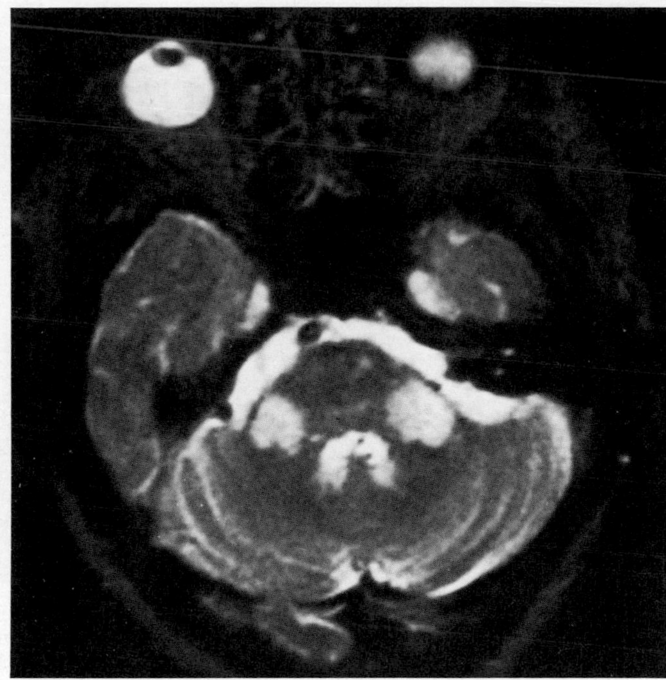

A B

FIG. 8. Brainstem infarctions in patient with basilar artery thrombosis syndrome. **A:** Initial T2-weighted image does not show lesion. **B:** Follow-up T2-weighted image shows bilateral brainstem infarctions.

identify areas at risk of infarction, in addition to already infarcted tissue. Fortunately, these ischemic areas at risk can now be detected with new MR methods, including MR angiography, perfusion/diffusion MRI, and MR spectroscopy.

MR Angiography

Since arterial occlusion is the most significant cause of cerebral ischemia, the assessment of the blood supply to the brain is important in the evaluation of stroke patients. Even though MRI has improved the detection of the parenchymal changes associated with acute stroke, it can only indirectly assess patency of intracranial vessels by demonstrating the presence or absence of intraluminal flow void. Accurate determination of the patency of the internal carotid artery is difficult with conventional MRI because the presence of a flow void in the internal carotid artery siphon does not exclude significant stenosis in the proximal extracranial internal carotid artery (48,49) and the presence of isointense signal within the arterial lumen may be due either to occlusion or high grade stenosis causing very slow flow (48). MR angiography (MRA) has been developed to optimize the evaluation of blood flow with MR techniques. A number of clinical studies have investigated the use of MRA in cerebrovascular disease, focusing their evaluations primarily either on the carotid bifurcation or the intracranial circulation.

Most clinical MRA studies of the extracranial carotid have used time-of-flight (TOF) techniques (50–58), although both two-dimensional (2D) (59) and three-dimensional (3-D) (60) phase contrast (PC) MRA have demonstrated carotid stenosis. Two-dimensional TOF MRA has particular utility in the neck because it is fast, can be used to cover a large area, and is sensitive to a wide range of flow velocities (Fig. 9). Errors in lumen definition, however, are a problem with TOF MRA. These errors may be due to: a) dephasing of blood due to higher order motion, b) shortcomings of image reconstruction techniques, c) signal loss due to T2* dephasing, d) misregistration artifacts, e) vessel wall motion, and f) partial volume averaging (61).

Despite these limitations, 2D TOF MRA has been shown to correlate significantly with conventional angiography in the grading of carotid bifurcation stenoses (51,52,55). Using a variety of grading classifications, exact agreement between MRA and conventional angiography in classifying stenoses into mild, moderate, severe, and occluded categories has ranged from 44% to 93% (50,52,54–56). Because of the sources of inaccuracy in defining vessel lumen diameter described above, the most frequent error of MRA is overestimation of stenosis (50,52,54–57), usually by one grade (52,55). Since the overestimation is not directly proportional to the actual degree of stenosis, useful correction factors have not been developed (57). Nevertheless, both 2D and 3D TOF have high sensitivity (94% to 100%) and specificity (93% to 97%) for detecting hemodynamically significant stenosis (>70% lumen diameter narrowing) (51,56,62). Preliminary studies (62) have demonstrated that the overestimation of stenosis can be overcome with a sup-

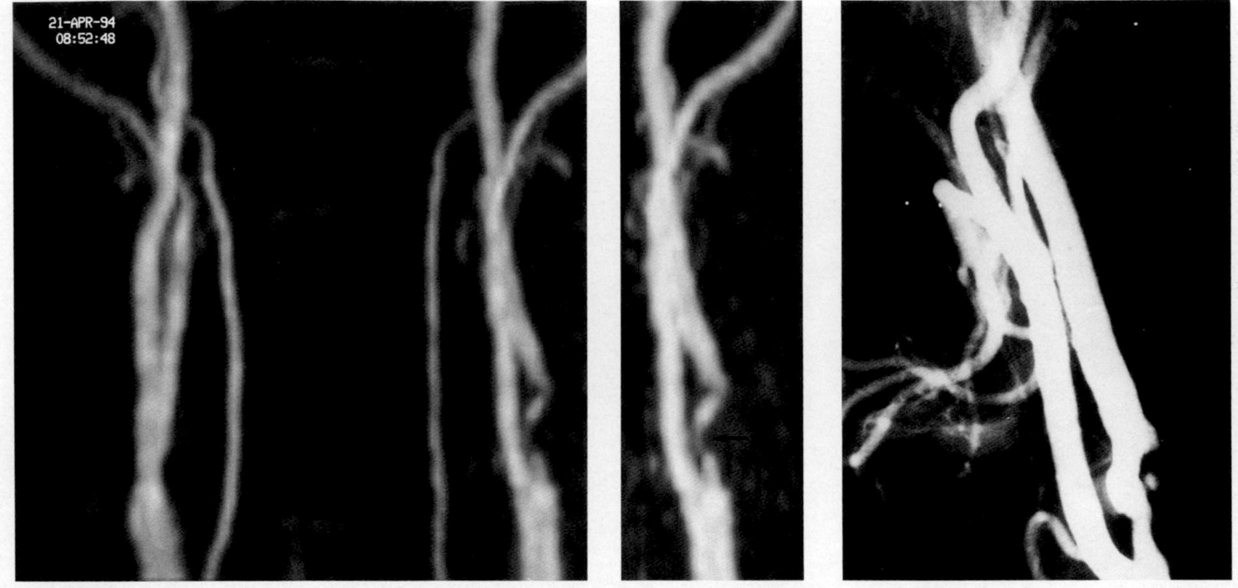

FIG. 9. **A:** AP, MIP MRA image showing both carotid and vertebral arteries. **B:** Detail 2D TOF MRA of left carotid artery (from A) shows irregular narrowing at the origin of the left internal carotid artery (*arrow*). **C:** RPO view from left common carotid angiogram shows irregular atherosclerotic narrowing at the origin of the left internal carotid artery corresponding to the MRA findings. Note the overestimation of the stenosis and nonvisualization of the small ulcer on MRA.

plemental high resolution 3D TOF technique (Fig. 10), which minimizes intravoxel dephasing. Since such methods are more prone to saturation effects (which might falsely show slow flow as occlusion), 2D TOF scanning is still considered an important part of the carotid MRA protocol.

A particular problem with overestimation of lumen narrowing is complete signal loss in a stenosed area with preserved distal flow. This precludes calculation of percent stenosis. Studies (57,62) have shown that this focal signal void on 2D MRA corresponded to ≥70% diameter stenosis on catheter angiography in most but not all pa-

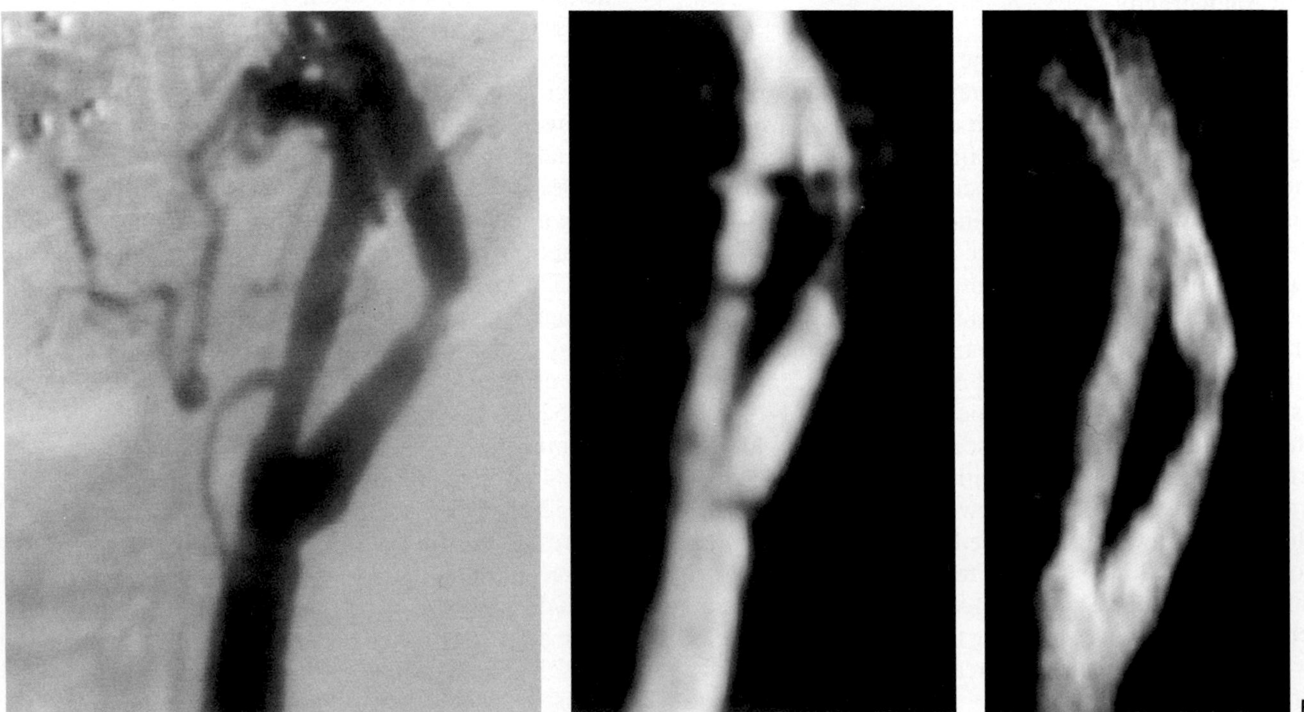

FIG. 10. Depiction of carotid stenosis, 2D TOF vs. 3D TOF MRA. Catheter arteriogram (**A**), 2D TOF MRA (**B**), 3D TOF high resolution MRA (**C**). By arteriography (A), proximal internal carotid stenosis measures approximately 40%. 2D TOF (**B**) falsely implies high-grade stenosis, while 3D TOF (**C**) more accurately defines lumen diameter.

compensatory vasodilatation that occurs until collateral circulation becomes insufficient (89). Perfusion imaging can also show the effectiveness of reestablishing blood flow on tissue perfusion (90). In the first clinical study of dynamic contrast-enhanced T2-weighted MRI, decreased blood volume in the area of infarction was detected in 57% of patients during the first 48 hours after onset of symptoms. This initial technique did not reliably detect infarctions smaller than 2 cm or less than 10 hours old. One major shortcoming of this study that used GE perfusion imaging techniques was the inability to image the entire brain (91). However, echo-planar techniques overcome this problem and have greater sensitivity in detecting perfusion deficits in stroke (92).

As mentioned above, diffusion imaging utilizes pulse sequences sensitive to small scale motions of water molecules that reflect both tissue perfusion and diffusion. These motions result in a random or pseudo-random distribution of phase shifts, which reduce signal amplitude. A diffusion coefficient can be measured by comparing images that have different sensitivities to diffusion (84). A calculated diffusion image can be obtained by subtracting an image performed with normal gradient pulses from an image generated by a pulse sequence that differs from the first only by the addition of gradient pulses. These gradient pulses increase the effect of spin motion on the SI. Thus, the effects of SD, T1, and T2 are removed, and the SI of the calculated image depends on intravoxel incoherent motions only (93).

Experimental studies of diffusion imaging using very strong field gradients have demonstrated abnormalities related to cerebral ischemia within 1 hour of ischemic onset whereas T2-weighted images on the same animals demonstrated abnormalities only after 2 to 3 hours (94–97). However, diffusion abnormalities may not be detected this early if standard field gradients are used (88). Decreased diffusion has been reported during the initial hours of experimental ischemia (88–90,96–99). Although several potential mechanisms have been proposed for this observed diminished diffusion, the most plausible explanations are that reduced cell membrane permeability or the development of cytotoxic edema account for the experimental findings (98). In one study areas of restricted diffusion after 30 to 180 minutes of permanent MCA occlusion corresponded closely with infarction size by pathologic analysis at 24 hours (96). Diffusion abnormalities have been reported to reverse if reperfusion occurs within 2 hours (97,100), although reversible lesions had less intense diffusion abnormalities than irreversible areas of restricted diffusion (97). In the subacute stage of infarction, as vasogenic edema progresses, diffusion increases. Further increases in diffusion have been reported as infarction evolves to the chronic phase. Areas of gliosis demonstrate faster diffusion than edema, and regions of cyst formation show even faster diffusion than gliotic areas (101).

Clinical studies using standard field gradients have confirmed the experimental results by finding diffusion abnormalities before the development of lesions on T2-weighted images (102) and observing an initial reduction of diffusion in acute infarction that was followed by increasing diffusion as infarction evolved (Fig. 13) (102–105). However, the results of clinical studies have been less consistent and dramatic than those of experimental studies, probably because of technological limitations. Echo-planar imaging, which uses stronger field gradients and is less affected by patient motion, promises to improve the clinical use of diffusion imaging.

By combining diffusion and perfusion MRI, recent experimental studies have demonstrated ischemic penumbrae, or areas at risk for infarction, at the periphery of acute infarctions (89,99). One study (99) of middle cerebral artery occlusion demonstrated a core of absent perfusion that was surrounded by a zone of reduced perfusion. Only the core of severely impaired perfusion had restricted diffusion within 1 hour. Within 24 hours, however, the entire area destined to infarction demonstrated restricted diffusion. This report suggests that brain tissue with decreased perfusion but normal diffusion is at risk for infarction, but that tissue with restricted diffusion is not viable. Preliminary observations of a core of infarction and a surrounding area of partial ischemia has been reported in humans as well (92). Future studies will need to determine in patients whether the outcome of the MR perfusion/diffusion-defined ischemic penumbrae can be affected by therapeutic interventions.

MR Spectroscopy

MR spectroscopy (MRS) has been employed as one of the most powerful and widely used analytical techniques in chemistry for several decades. More recently, it was discovered that it was possible to obtain MR spectra from living tissue (106). Interest in in vivo MRS is generated by its ability to monitor, noninvasively, metabolic processes in situ. Since most clinical high-field (1.5 T) MR imagers can be upgraded to perform MRS at fairly low cost, the potential exists for the extensive use of MRS as a diagnostic and prognostic tool. Even though any nucleus with a nonzero nuclear spin can generate a MR signal, in vivo MRS studies of cerebral ischemia have been almost solely confined to the ^{1}H and ^{31}P nuclei because of their intrinsically higher sensitivity relative to other nuclear species.

Phosphorus MRS can detect signals from ATP, phosphocreatine (PCr), inorganic phosphate (Pi), and various phosphomonoesters and phosphodiesters. In addition, the chemical shift of Pi is sensitive to pH (107), allowing the estimation of intracellular pH. Experimental studies have extensively utilized ^{31}P in the study of cerebral ischemia. Within minutes of cerebral ischemia, ^{31}P MRS has

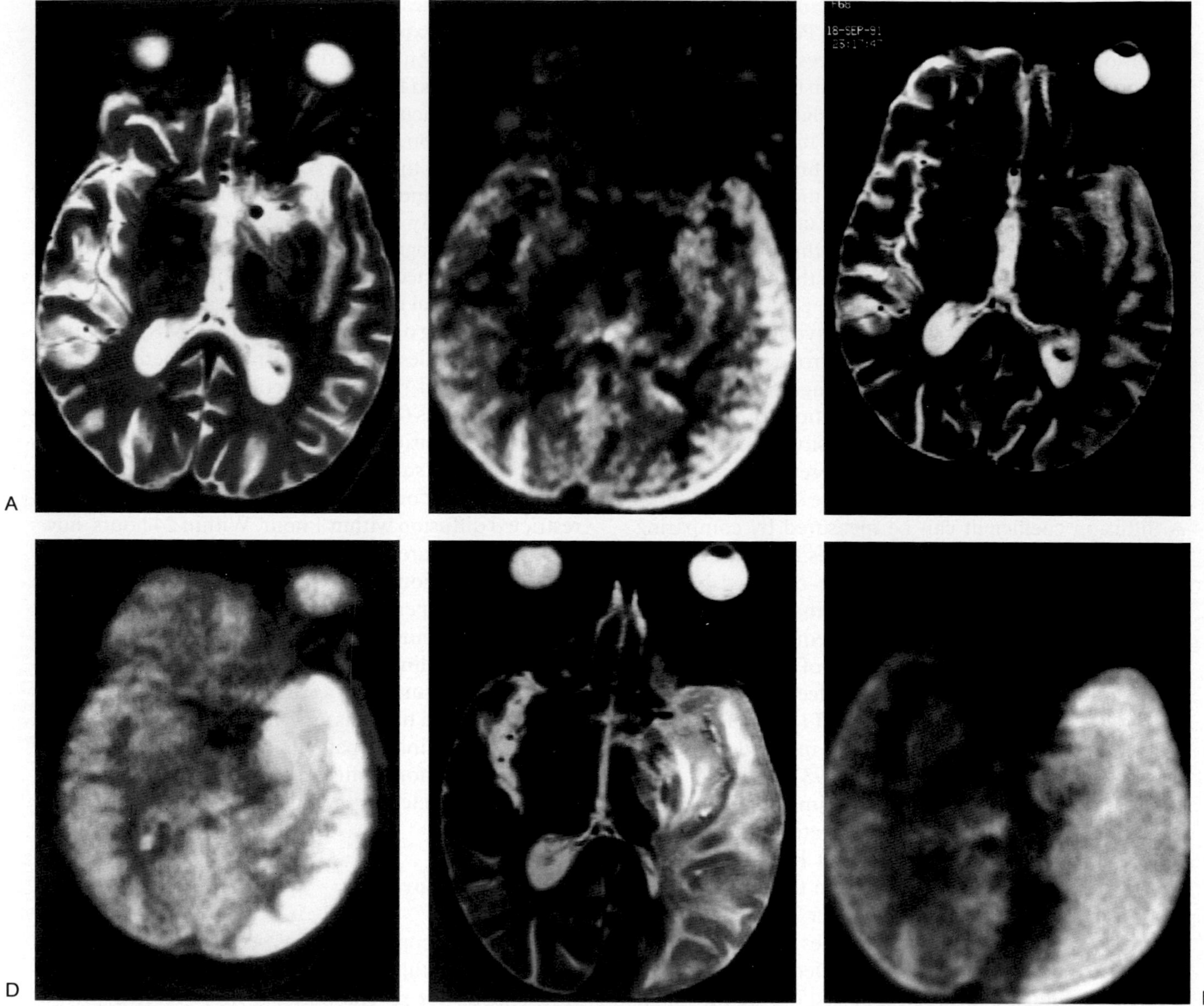

FIG. 13. Diffusion-weighted imaging demonstrates lesions before SE imaging. T2-weighted images and diffusion-weighted images from a 68-year-old woman 105 minutes, 13 hours, and 9 days after she suffered a sudden onset of global aphasia, right-sided hemiplegia, and right homonymous hemianopia from which she never recovered. MRA (*not shown*) demonstrated absence of flow throughout the intracranial portion of the left internal carotid artery. (Parameters of diffusion-weighted images are given in the text of ref. 102). **A:** T2-weighted image at 105 min shows no parenchymal lesion in the left hemisphere. **B:** Diffusion-weighted image at 105 min demonstrates hyperintensity in the cerebral cortex of the left hemisphere relative to the right. Relative apparent diffusion coefficient (ADC) was 0.60. **C:** T2-weighted image at 13 hours shows early changes (increased signal) of evolving parenchymal lesion in the left hemisphere. **D:** Diffusion-weighted image at 13 hours demonstrates greater degree of hyperintensity in the area of evolving infarct. Relative ADC was 0.40. Study at 34 hours (*not shown*) demonstrated mass effect on T2-weighted image and relative ADC of 0.36. **E:** T2-weighted image at 9 days shows the fully evolved infarct. **F:** Diffusion-weighted image at 9 days demonstrates a matching area of hyperintensity. Relative ADC was 0.60. (From Warach et al, ref. 102, with permission.)

demonstrated depletion of high energy phosphates, reduction of PCr/Pi ratio, and decreases in the intracellular pH (108). The degree of metabolic changes detected by ^{31}P MRS correlate with the severity of stroke based on electroencephalogram (EEG) abnormalities (109). Recent MRS clinical studies have evaluated stroke in the acute, as well as subacute and chronic, phases. During the first 48 hours of clinical cerebral ischemia ^{31}P MRS detects cerebral acidosis, significant reduction of ATP, and significant increases in Pi. Serial studies show a transition from early acidosis to later alkalosis during the first 3 weeks after infarction (110). Others have also have demonstrated increased pH (111) as well as reduced metabolite concentrations (112,113) in patients with strokes several weeks old. The clinical significance of pH changes as infarction evolves is unclear because neurologic status does not appear to correlate with the degree of acidosis or alkalosis (110). Unfortunately, ^{31}P MRS sensitivity is relatively low, resulting in fairly large voxels of 9 cm^3, which significantly limits clinical studies of stroke.

The higher sensitivity of ^{1}H MRS permits the recording of spectra from voxels as small as 1 cm^3 in the human brain (114). ^{1}H spectra of the brain contain major resonances from choline (Ch)-containing compounds, total creatine (Cr), which includes creatine and phosphocreatine, and *N*-acetyl aspartate (NAA). The peak typically designated as NAA may also contain contributions from other *N*-acetyl groups (115). Signals from lactate protons are not normally observed above noise in vivo but may be observed in pathologic conditions, particularly ischemia (Fig. 14). The presence of the large water signal (cerebral water proton concentration is approximately 80 mol, whereas the metabolites in the proton spectrum are 10 mmol or less) has limited the development of ^{1}H MRS. However, efficient water suppression techniques have been developed that allow the application of ^{1}H MRS to clinical studies.

^{1}H MRS has detected abnormal lactate accumulation within minutes of cerebral ischemia in animal experiments (116,117). Cerebral ischemia and infarction also cause reduction of the NAA peak amplitude, presumably due to neuronal loss. A lactate threshold for lethal cerebral injury has been suggested by Plum, who postulated that infarction occurs as brain lactate concentration exceeds 17 mmol/g (118). This threshold may relate to tissue pH, but other studies have shown independent changes in lactate concentration and intracellular pH indicating that lactate is not the only determinant of intracellular pH (119,120). Changes in CBF have an important effect on metabolite concentrations as measured by ^{1}H MRS. Specifically, one study showed that lactate concentration increased when CBF fell below 20 ml/100 g per min (121). MRS can also be used to study the effects that pharmacologic interventions have on ischemic injury (122).

The first clinical ^{1}H MRS studies of stroke included patients examined a few days to years after infarctions (123–125). One of these studies proposed that neuronal injury could be represented by a spectral pattern of normal Ch with concomitant decreases in NAA and Cr (123). However, significant decreases in Ch as well as Cr and NAA in areas of chronic infarction have also been reported (125).

More recent ^{1}H MRS studies of acute and chronic infarction have focused their discussions on the detection of lactate and NAA. NAA is associated with the presence of neurons (126). Reduction of NAA in both acute and chronic infarction has been attributed to loss of viable neurons (127–130). The concept of a penumbra of tissue at risk surrounding a central core of infarction has been supported by MRS observations. One study showed that NAA concentrations were lower at the center of infarctions than at the margins of the lesions (129). Another

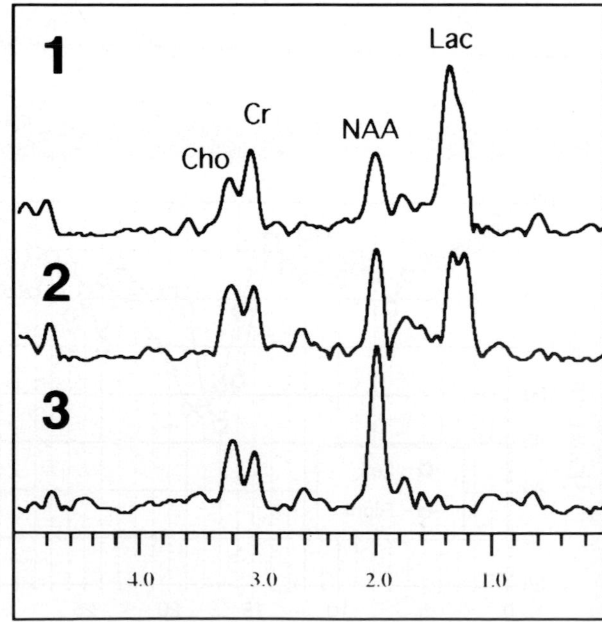

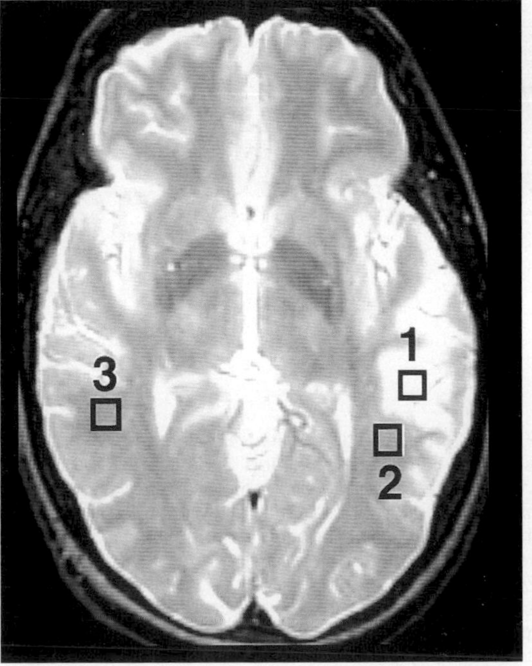

FIG. 14. Magnetic resonance spectroscopy. Selected voxel (1) from 2D chemical shift imaging (CSI) MRS shows increased lactate and decreased NAA in infarcted tissue seen on T2-weighted MRI. Ischemic region with normal T2-weighted SI is characterized by less lactate and greater NAA (2). Normal control spectra (3).

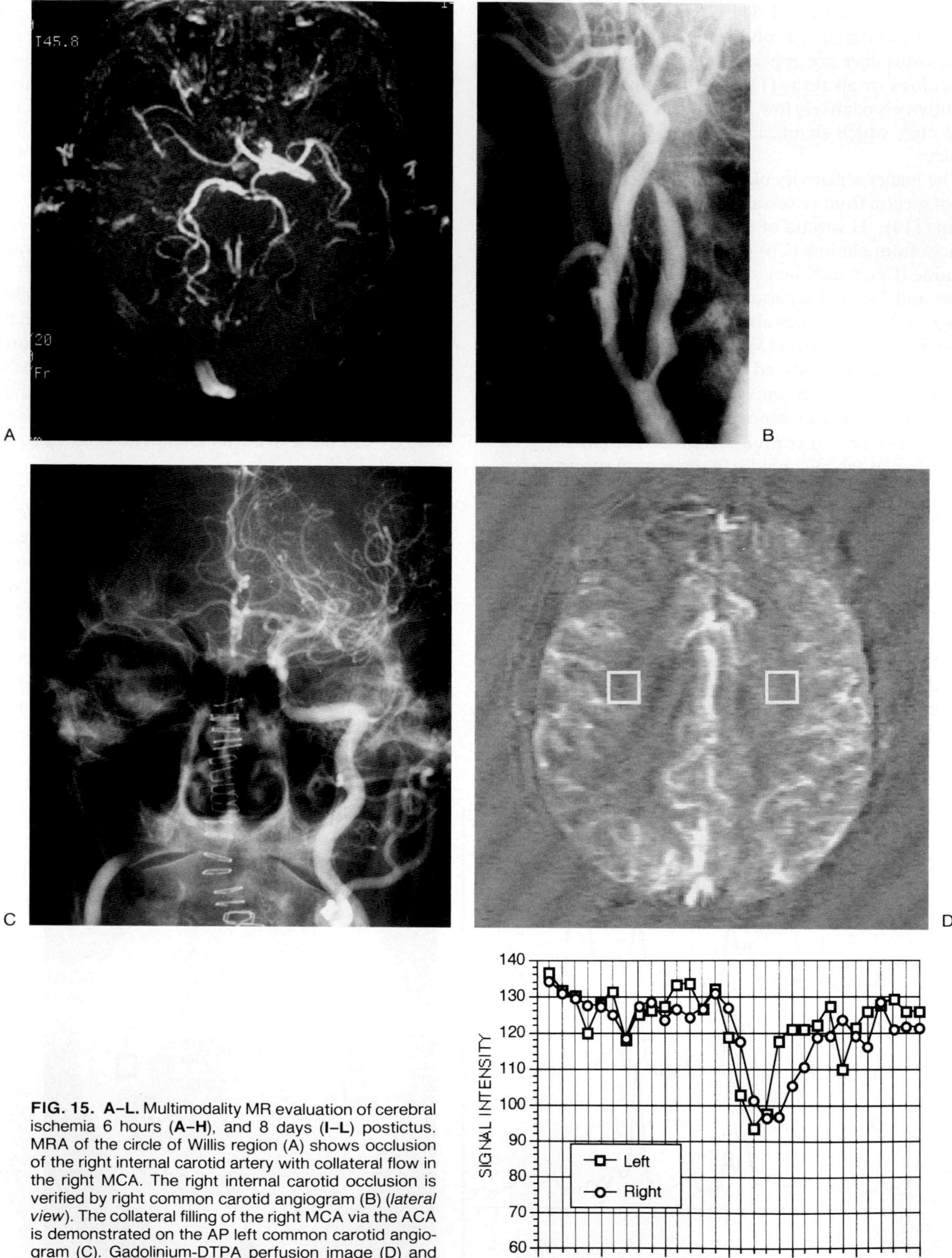

FIG. 15. A–L. Multimodality MR evaluation of cerebral ischemia 6 hours (**A–H**), and 8 days (**I–L**) postictus. MRA of the circle of Willis region (A) shows occlusion of the right internal carotid artery with collateral flow in the right MCA. The right internal carotid occlusion is verified by right common carotid angiogram (B) (*lateral view*). The collateral filling of the right MCA via the ACA is demonstrated on the AP left common carotid angiogram (C). Gadolinium-DTPA perfusion image (D) and time intensity curve (E) reveal a relative delay in signal loss in the right hemisphere.

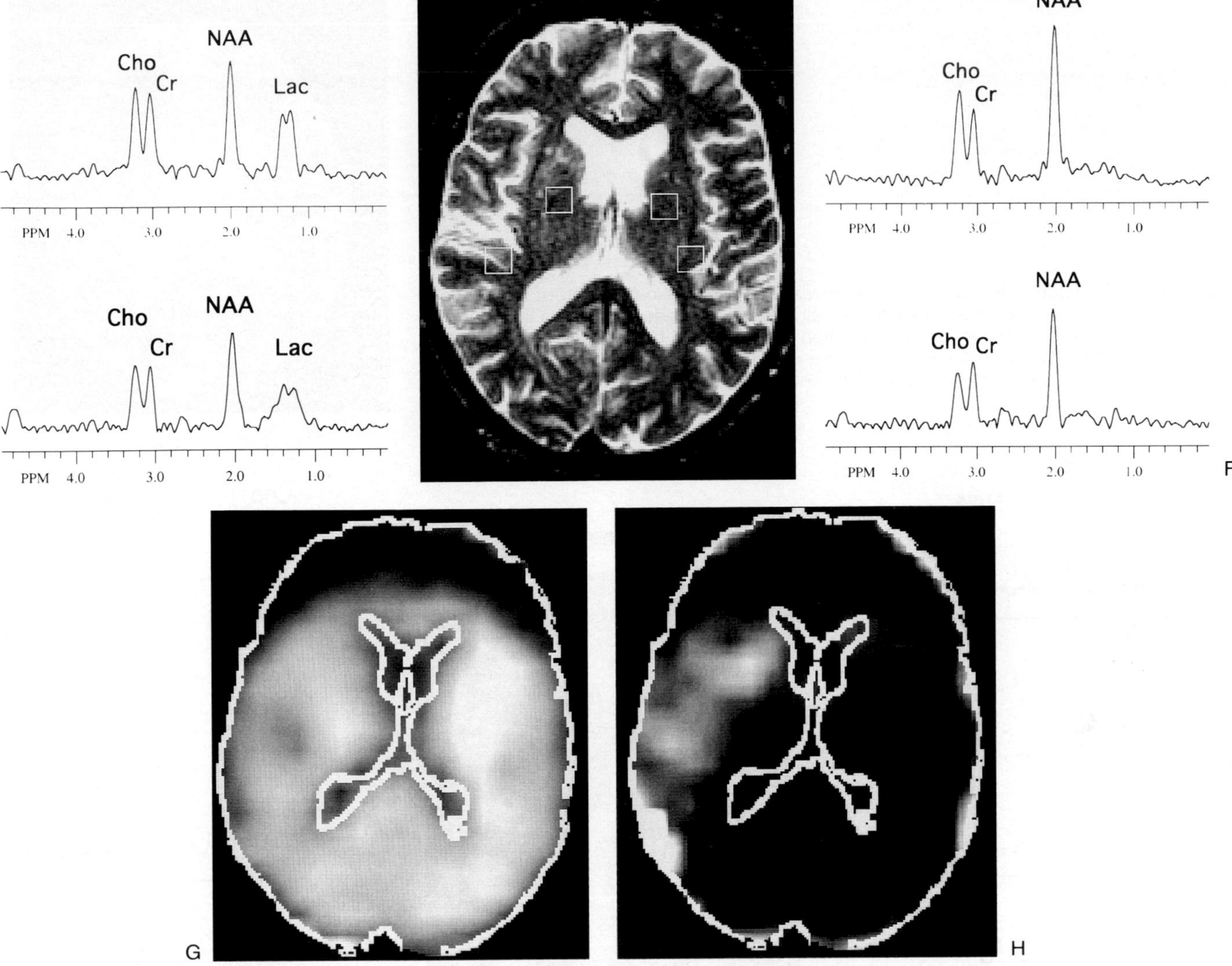

FIG. 15. (*Continued.*) T2-weighted MRI scan (F) is normal whereas selected voxels from 2D CSI MRS reveal ischemia in the right hemisphere reflected by increased lactate. Corresponding 2D CSI NAA (G) and lactate (H) images.

study observed progressive declines in NAA during the first 2 weeks of infarction suggesting loss of viable neurons (130).

Lactate is produced by the acutely ischemic brain through anaerobic metabolism. In the subacute and chronic stages of infarction, brain macrophages may contribute to detectable lactate concentrations (131). Consistent with experimental work, lactate was uniformly present during the initial hours of clinical infarction or ischemia (128–130). Lactate concentrations were highest in the first 2 to 3 days and declined over the next several days in uncomplicated stroke (130–132). Lactate levels were greatest in the center of an infarction where NAA is lowest, further supporting the idea of heterogeneous injury in cerebral infarction (133). Even though lactate has been reported to decline to nearly undetectable levels after 2 to 4 weeks, lactate has been identified in some chronic infarctions (123,125,127).

Multimodality MR of Acute Ischemia and Infarction

With the availability of these new MR techniques it is now possible to extensively evaluate and define not only regions of cerebral infarction but regions at risk of infarction (133). We have recently applied conventional MRI, MRA, perfusion MRI, and MRS to acute stroke victims and successfully delineated infarctions, major vessel occlusions, regions of hypoperfusion, and metabolically compromised tissue (Figs. 15 and 16). This multi-MR modality approach to acute cerebral ischemia offers great potential for the precise diagnosis of cerebral

FIG. 15. (*Continued.*) Follow-up studies reveal an infarction in the head of the caudate nucleus on T2-weighted image (I) with a small amount of residual lactate in the infarcted area only (J). 2D CSI image reveals infarction characterized by decreased NAA (K) and residual lactate (L) in the infarction. This series of examinations reveals the ability of MRA, gadolinium perfusion imaging, and MRS to identify regions at risk of infarction as well as infarcted tissue.

I

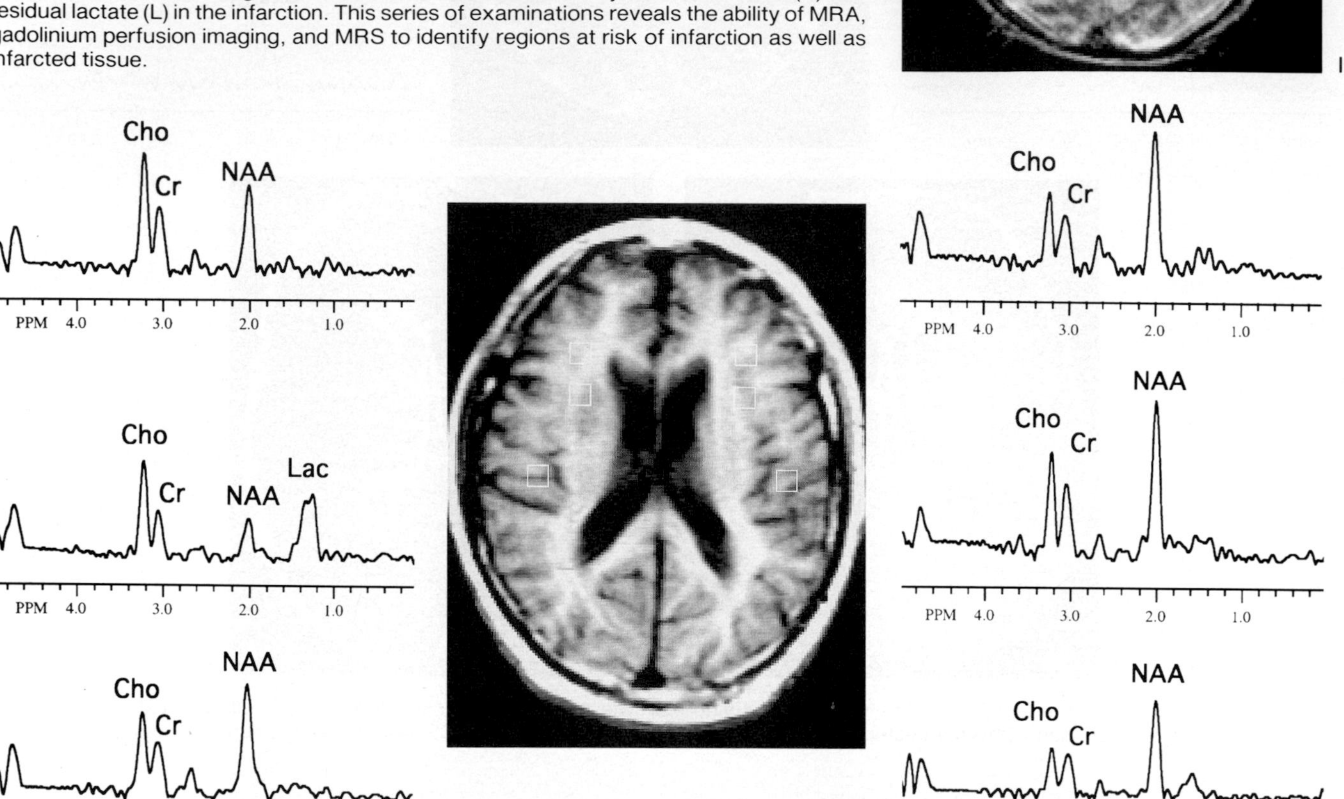

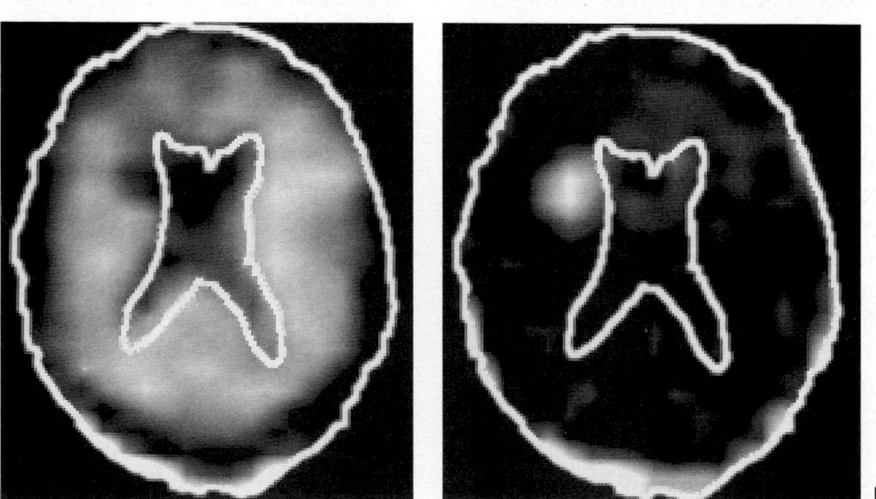

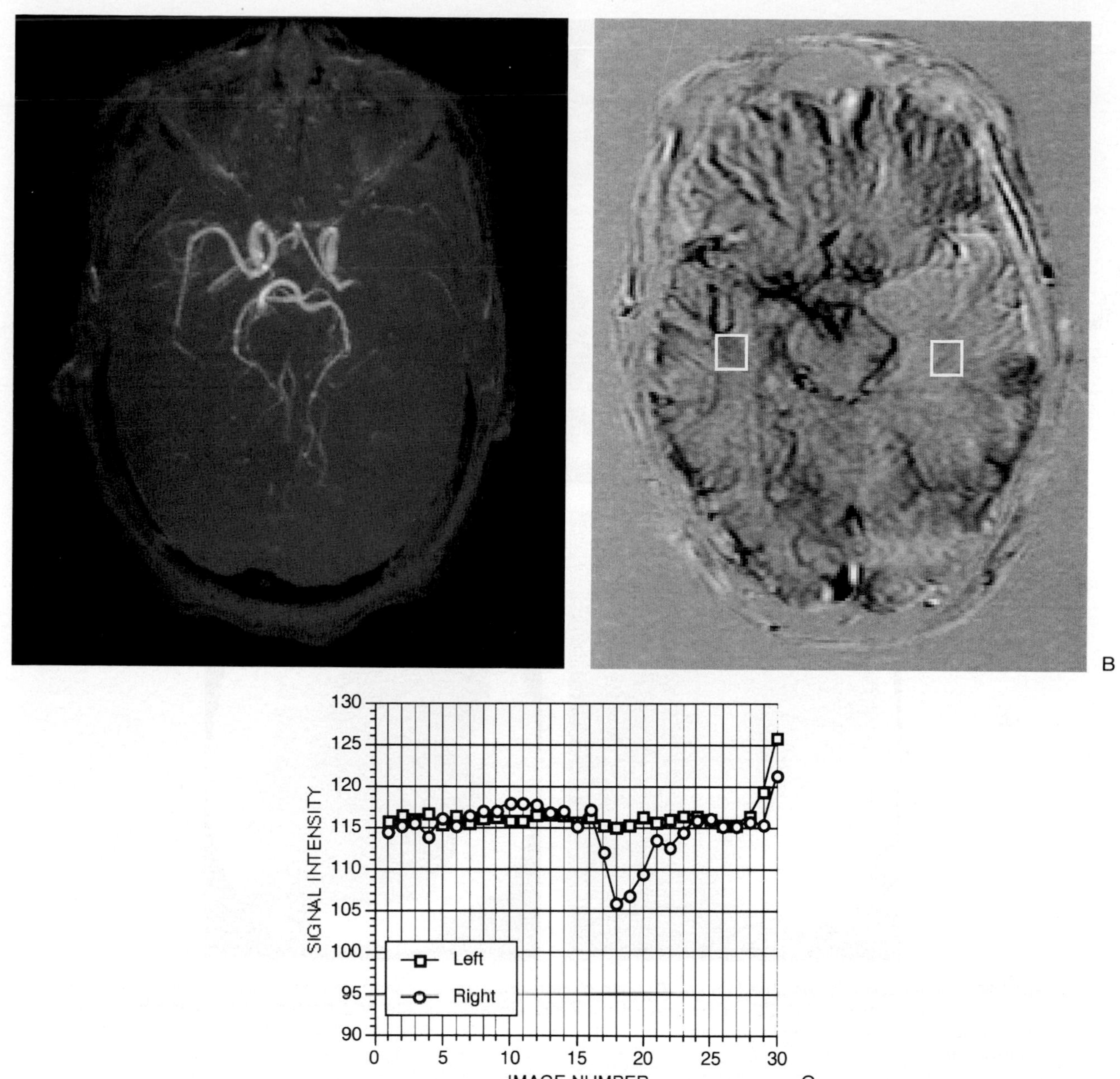

FIG. 16. A–F. Multimodality MR evaluation of cerebral ischemia 4 hours postictus. **A:** MRA of circle of Willis reveals occlusion of the left middle cerebral artery. Gadolinium-DTPA perfusion subtraction image (**B**) and time/intensity curve (**C**) reveals no signal loss in the left MCA territory.

ischemia and its sequela, which may be critical for patient management.

SPECIFIC APPEARANCES OF ISCHEMIC LESIONS

Large Vessel Arterial Occlusive Disease

Thromboembolism is the most common etiology of infarction secondary to arterial occlusive disease. The MR appearance is dependent on the site or sites of occlusion, the duration and degree of occlusion, and the adequacy of collateral circulation. The pattern of cerebral infarction resulting from occlusion of a blood vessel is largely dependent on vascular anatomy. A good working knowledge of major vascular territories is a prerequisite to the proper interpretation of the MR exam, especially in the evaluation of thromboembolic infarction. Collateral support of the major vascular territories will modify the extent of infarction following occlusion. This may, in

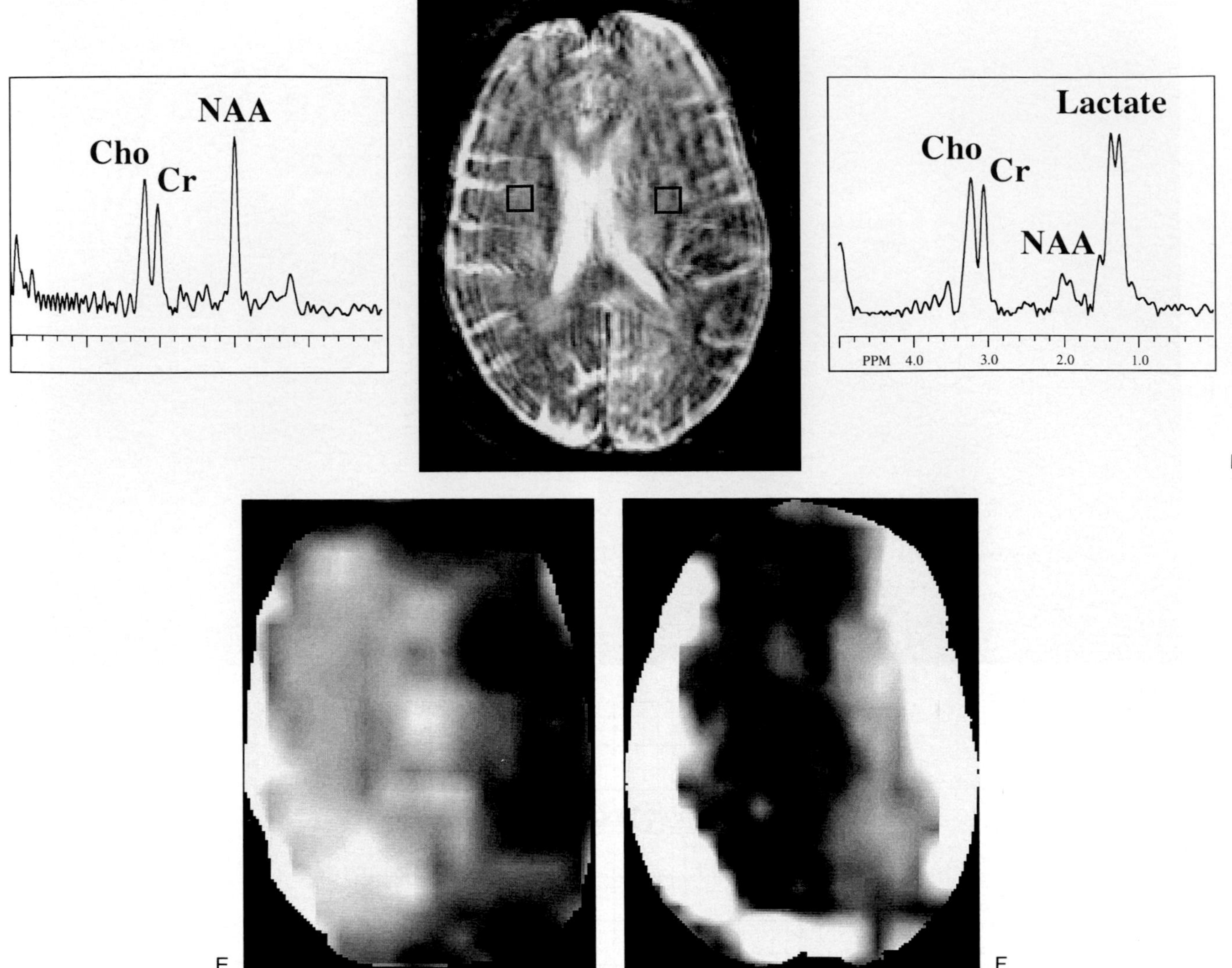

FIG. 16. (*Continued.*) T2-weighted image (**D**) (with motion artifacts) demonstrates only subtle swelling in the left hemisphere, but selected 2D CSI voxels reveal markedly elevated lactate and decreased NAA throughout the left hemisphere. 2D CSI NAA (**E**) and lactate (**F**) image show changes of typical acute infarction throughout the left hemisphere.

part, explain the variable clinical course and MR appearance of many ischemic infarctions. Recanalization of occluded vessels also modifies infarction (134). In the case of single intracranial major vessel occlusions, the extent of SI changes found on MR may closely follow the vascular anatomic distributions to be discussed below (Fig. 17A,B). Conversely, in the case of proximal disease or pancerebral hypoperfusion, the anastomotic border zones or so-called watershed zones between the major territories are often the most severely involved, reflecting the vulnerability of this most distal perfusion bed (Fig. 17C).

Occlusion of the internal carotid artery is usually preceded by stenosis permitting the development of collateral pathways assuming no significant embolism. The stenosis or occlusion produces a wide spectrum of clinical and pathologic findings, from normal to extensive infarction (135). The determining factor is, of course, the adequacy or inadequacy of collaterals. When collaterals are inadequate the infarction often occurs in the border

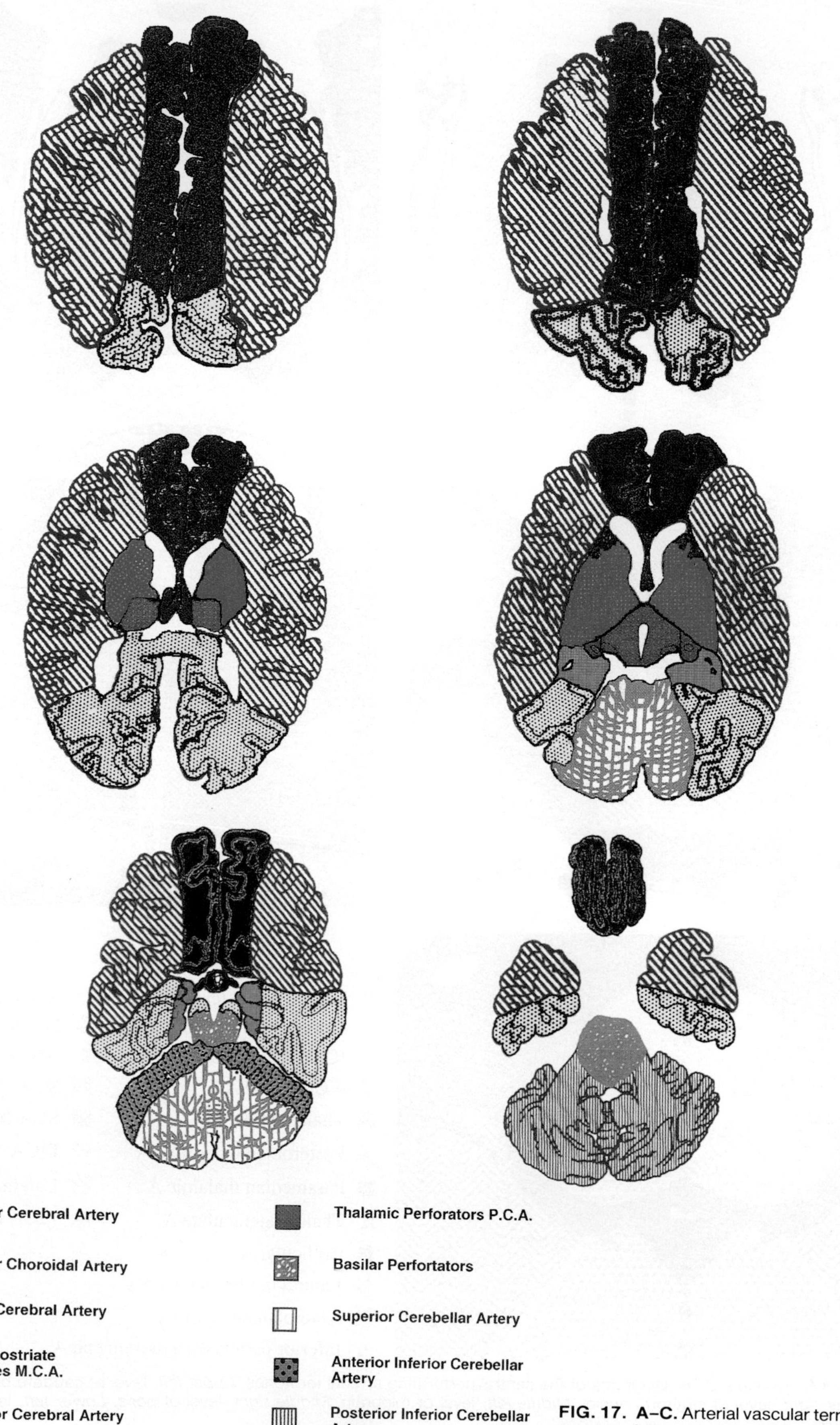

FIG. 17. A–C. Arterial vascular territories. **A:** Diagrams of the major arterial territories.

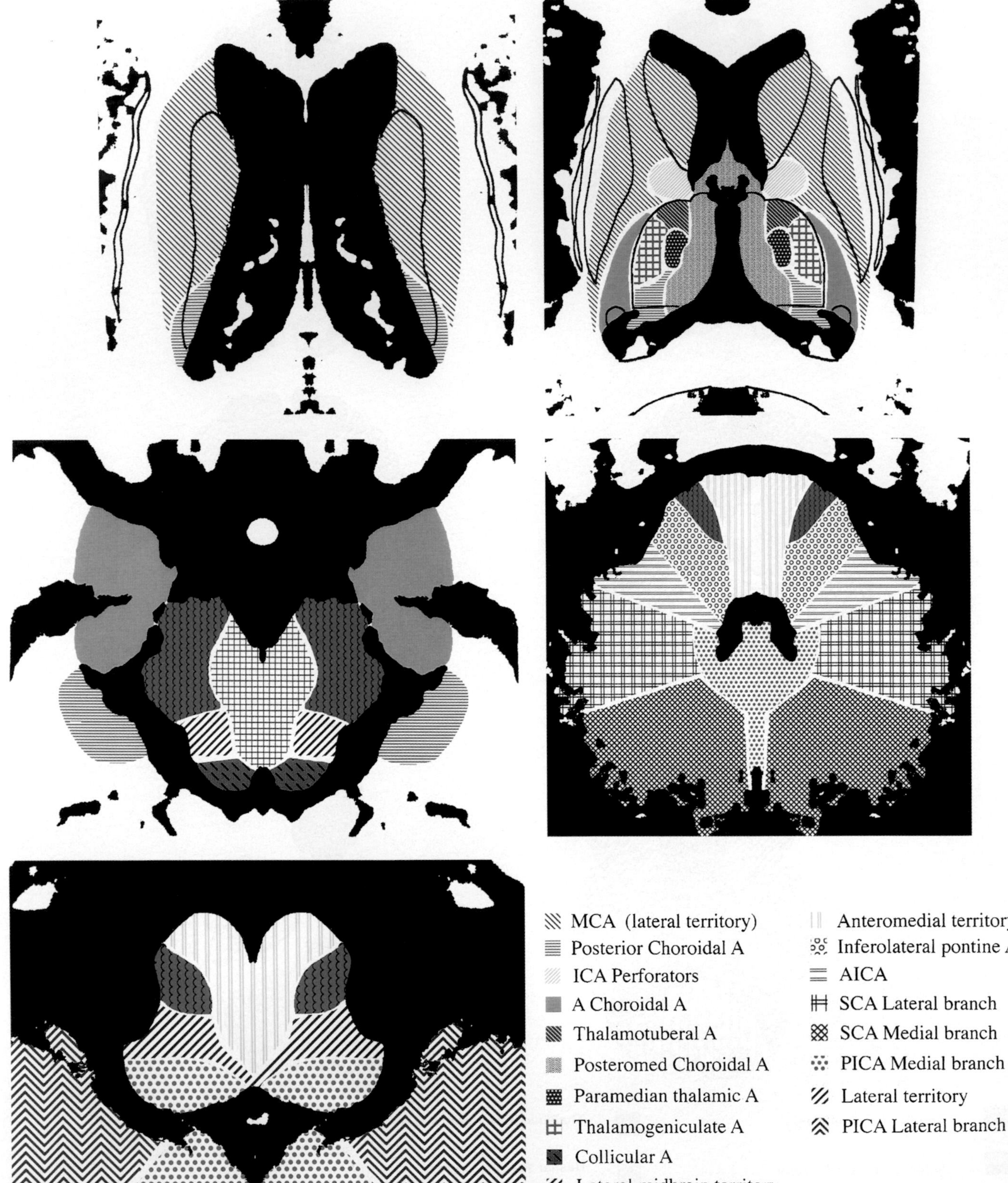

FIG. 17. (*Continued.*) **B:** Diagrams of the central perforating arterial territories. *Upper left,* level of caudate bodies. *Upper right,* level of lentiform nuclei. *Middle left,* level of midbrain. *Middle right,* level of pons. *Lower left,* level of medulla.

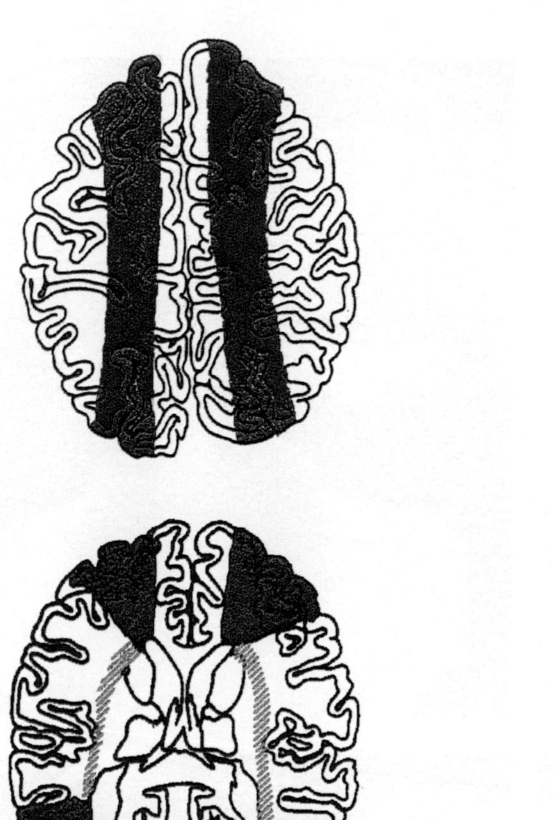

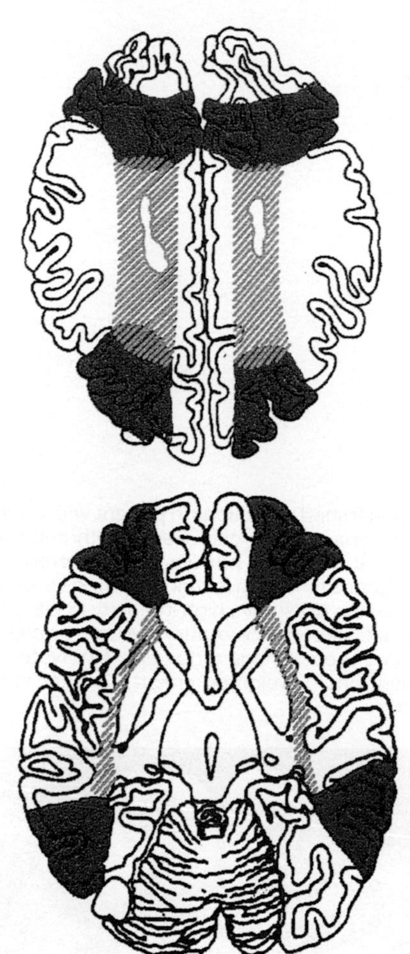

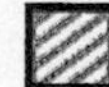

FIG. 17. (*Continued.*) **C:** Diagrams of the arterial border zones.

zone between major vascular territories (Fig. 18). Since the anterior cerebral circulation is frequently adequately supplied via the anterior communicating artery, the middle cerebral territory often bears the brunt of such an ischemic insult. Should the thrombosis involve the anterior cerebral artery as well, infarction of the hemisphere excluding the posterior cerebral territory may occur (Fig. 19). Rarely, an incomplete circle of Willis results in an internal carotid artery, which supplies all three major supratentorial vessels. Occlusion of such a vessel can result in massive infarction because collateral circulation is minimal. Such extensive infarction may be accompanied by significant brain swelling and may result in herniation, further vascular compromise, and even death.

Intracranially, the cerebral hemispheres are supplied almost entirely by three major arteries: the anterior, middle, and posterior cerebral arteries. Each of these give rise to two types of branches: deep ganglionic and peripheral

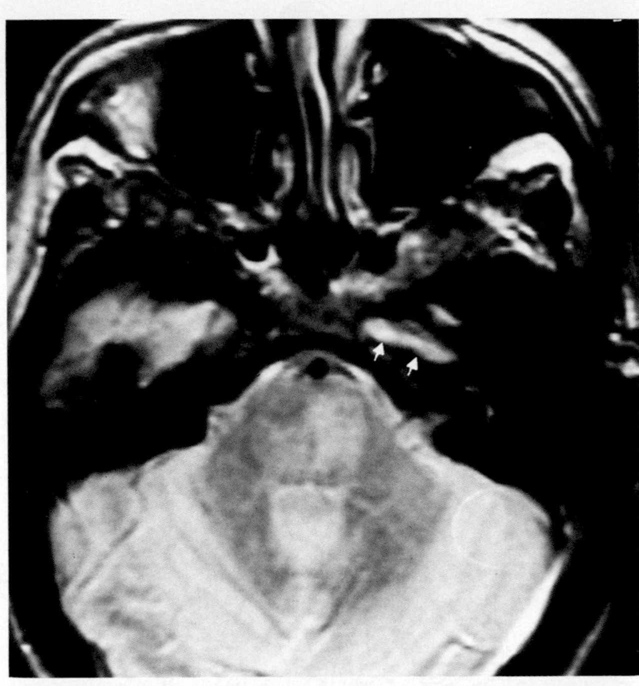

FIG. 18. Watershed infarctions in patient with proximal ICA occlusion from basal meningitis. Sections through skull base show abnormal intensity in petrous carotid (*arrows*) on SDW image (**A**), consistent with either thrombosis or stagnant flow. SDW image (**B**) shows high intensity in watershed distribution in left deep white matter (*closed arrows*, B) with small region of hemorrhage (*open arrows*). Note extensive enhancement on T1-weighted image (**C**) after intravenous gadolinium.

A

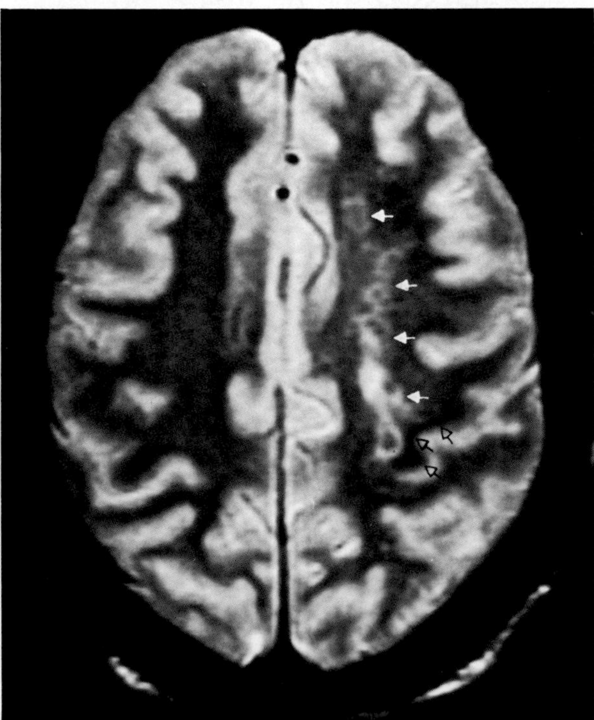

B

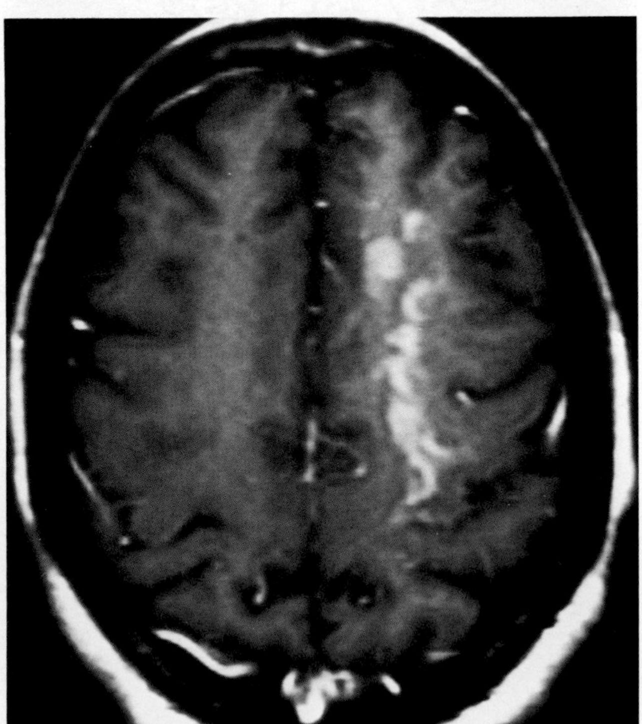

C

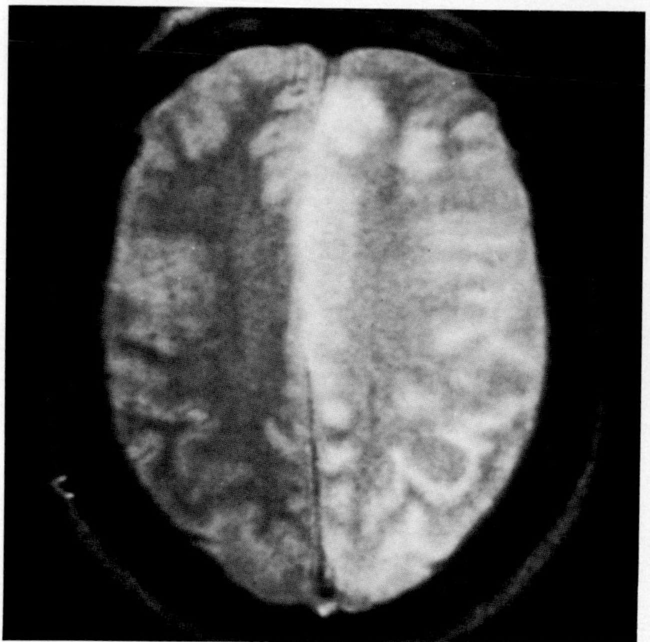

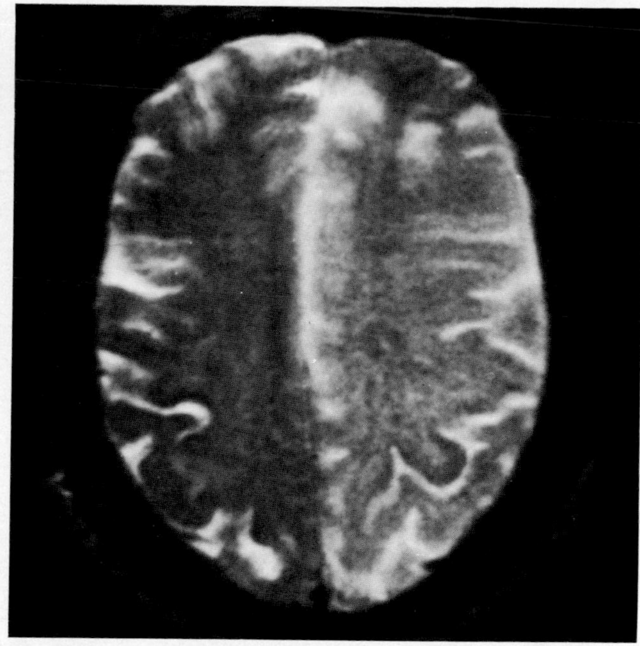

FIG. 19. Anterior and middle cerebral artery infarction secondary to ICA occlusion with increased SI in both arterial distributions on SDW (**A**) and T2-weighted (**B**) images.

or cortical. The deep ganglionic branches arise from the proximal portions of the vessels and the associated communicating arteries that make up the anastomotic circle of Willis. Along with the anterior choroidal artery, these ganglionic branches provide the vascular supply to the deep central portion of the telencephalon and diencephalon. The distal or cortical branches ramify over the infoldings of the cerebrum to supply the cortex and underlying white matter of the cerebral hemispheres. These two types of branches have distinct perfusion territories and distinct clinical and radiographic pictures in the case of occlusion. In humans there are poor anastomoses between various components of the deep circulations and strong anastomoses between the peripheral cortical branches of the three major arteries (136). There are poor anastomoses between the deep and superficial circulations. A brief summary of cerebral vascular anatomy as it relates to patterns of infarction follows, but no attempt is made to describe in detail the anatomic course and relationships of intracranial arteries as they have been extensively covered in previous publications (137–139).

The anterior cerebral artery is the smaller of the distal two branches of the internal carotid artery and gives rise first to one or more medial striate arteries, including the recurrent artery of Huebner, which enter the anterior perforated substance to supply the anterior and medial portions of the caudate nucleus and adjacent portions of the internal capsule. Occlusion of this branch presents a characteristic wedge-shaped or sickle-shaped infarction lateral to the frontal horn of the lateral ventricle. The anterior cerebral artery subsequently gives rise to orbital, frontal polar, callosal marginal, and pericallosal cortical branches that supply the inferior and medial surfaces of the frontal lobe, the genu and anterior two-thirds of the body of the corpus callosum and fornix, as well as the septum pellucidum (Fig. 20) (140).

The middle cerebral artery is the largest branch of the internal carotid artery and gives rise to numerous lenticulostriate arteries, which supply the anterior perforated substance. These supply the anterior two-thirds of the internal capsule and portions of the globus pallidus and putamen, as well as the bulk of the caudate nucleus. The peripheral cortical branches of the middle cerebral artery supply the anterolateral portions of the temporal lobes as well as the entire lateral convexity of the frontal, temporal, and parietal lobes. Major middle cerebral territory infarctions may involve the deep ganglionic and/or peripheral cortical distributions (Fig. 21).

The anterior choroidal artery is a small branch of the supraclinoid carotid artery that courses posteriorly to enter the choroidal fissure. It supplies the optic tract anteriorly, the choroid plexus posteriorly, and several branches to the hippocampal formation, lateral thalamus, and a large portion of the posterior limb of the internal capsule. Despite the theoretical vulnerability of this artery, demonstration of isolated infarctions of its territory are unusual in clinical practice.

The posterior cerebral arteries may originate from the basilar tip or the internal carotid artery. In either case, there are deep and superficial branches. The deep ganglionic branches include the thalamoperforate, thalamogeniculate, and posterior choroidal arteries. In addition,

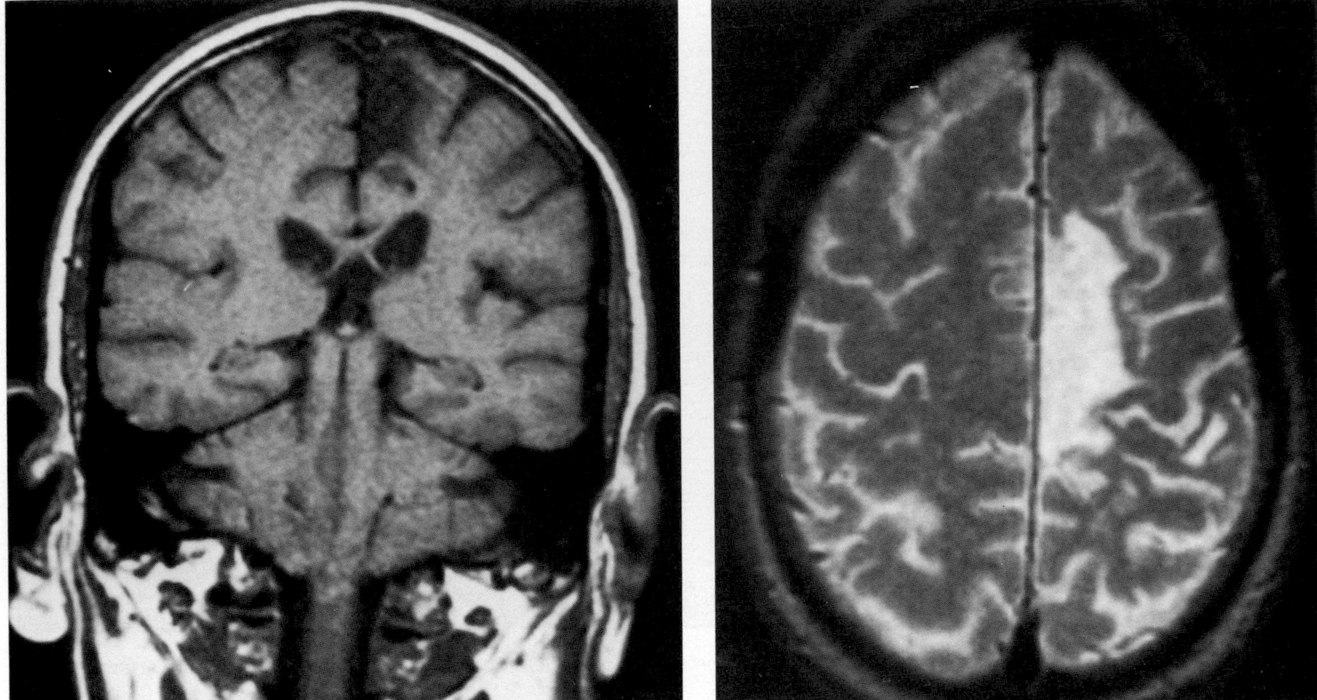

FIG. 20. Chronic anterior cerebral infarction. T1- and T2-weighted images show well-defined left anterior cerebral infarction with fluid-like SI on T2-weighted image.

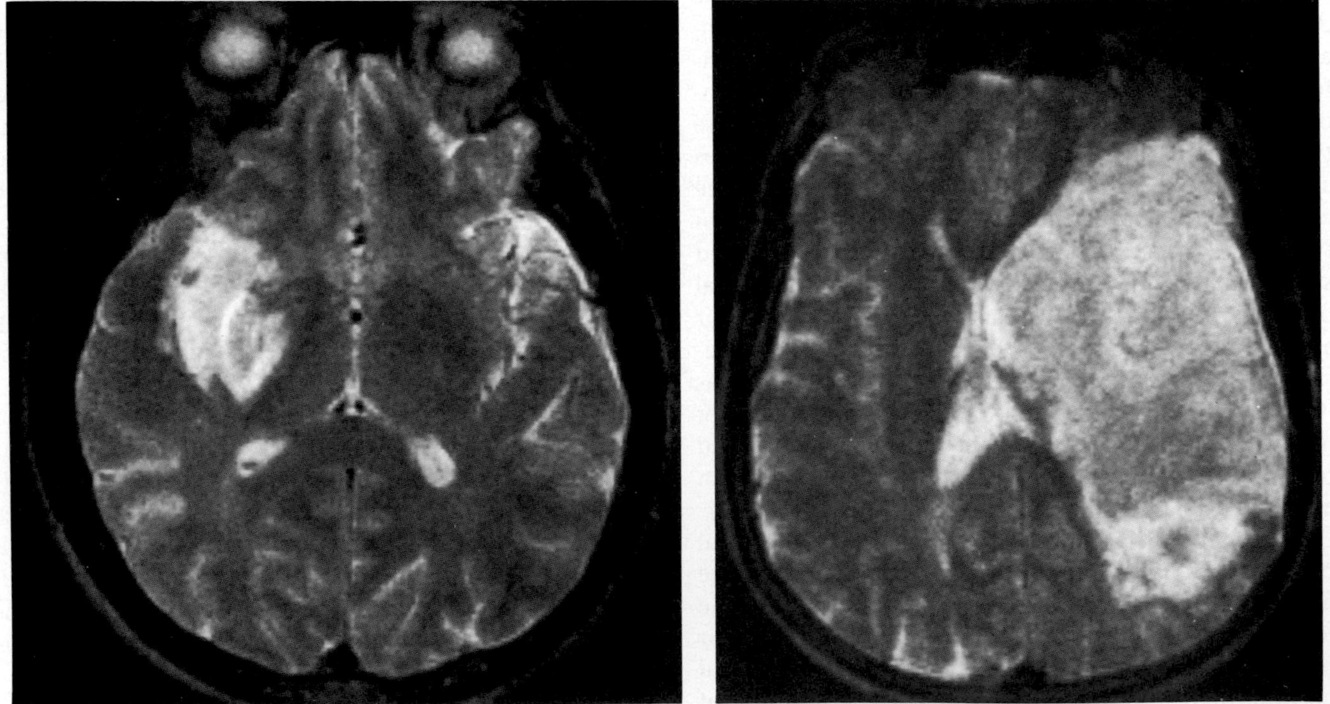

FIG. 21. Middle cerebral artery infarctions. **A:** Middle cerebral artery infarction with involvement of ganglionic perforator, T2-weighted image. **B:** Involvement of both ganglionic perforator and peripheral cortical region, T2-weighted image.

a number of small direct perforator branches enter the ventral surface of the midbrain. The peripheral branches of the posterior cerebral arteries include the posterior temporal, occipital, and parieto-occipital arteries, which supply the posterior-inferior temporal lobe, most of the occipital lobe, and the medial portion of the parietal lobe. Not infrequently there is distal basilar occlusive disease, with the occluded segment involving the origin of a posterior cerebral artery and perforating vessels. This results in ischemia in the distribution of both ganglionic and peripheral territories (Fig. 22). One particular variation in the posterior circulation can be a source of confusion when infarction of its territory has occurred. This vessel has been called the paramedian thalamic artery or the "artery of Percheron" (141), a variable branch (or branches) usually emanating from the proximal posterior cerebral artery, between the division of the terminal basilar artery and the posterior communicating artery. Infarctions due to occlusion of these vessels are extremely variable in extent (142), but classically involve both paramedian thalami. Infarctions of the artery of Percheron therefore are typically bilateral (Fig. 23), and represent a unique circumstance in which bilateral lesions can be traced to a single arterial occlusion.

The blood supply to the posterior fossa can be divided conveniently into four territories: the posterior inferior cerebellar artery, the anterior inferior cerebellar artery, the superior cerebellar artery, and the vertebrobasilar perforators. Variations in the pattern of the major branches of the distal vertebral and basilar arteries are extensive. This is especially true with the supply to the mesencephalon, where branches of the anterior choroidal, posterior cerebral, superior cerebellar, and perforating branches of the posterior communicator and basilar arteries are involved. The following is a brief summary of the classical distribution of the vessels supplying the posterior fossa (139,143).

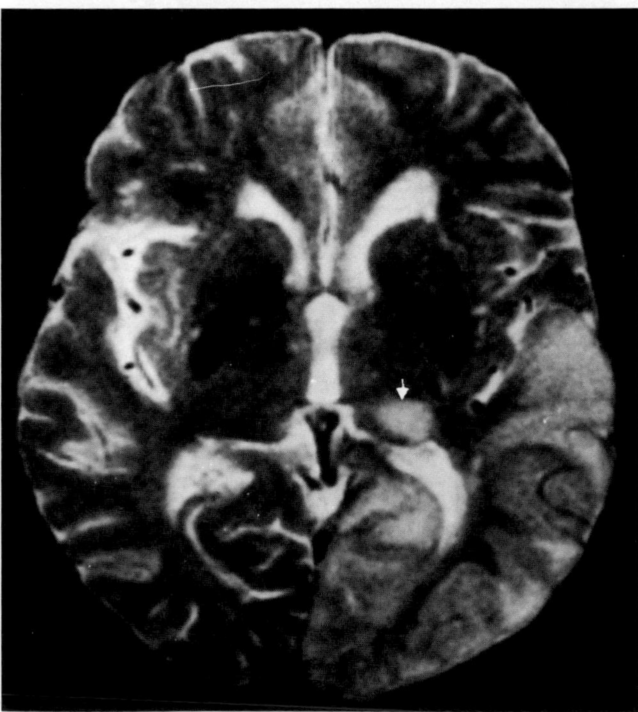

FIG. 22. Left posterior occipital artery distribution infarction including thalamogeniculate territory (*arrow*), T2-weighted image.

The posterior inferior cerebellar artery arises from the distal vertebral artery and supplies perforators to the retro-olivary portion of the medulla, the inferior vermis, cerebellar tonsil, and inferolateral surface of the cerebellar hemisphere. The anterior inferior cerebellar artery arises from the midbasilar artery and supplies some circumferential branches to the dorsal medulla as well as the anterior cerebellum. It overlaps considerably and variably with the territory of the posterior inferior cerebellar artery. The superior cerebellar artery supplies branches to the mesencephalon including the quadrigeminal plate, superior medullary velum, superior vermis, and cerebellar hemispheres. Vermian branches anastomose with posterior inferior communicating artery (PICA) branches, and hemispheric branches with those of the anterior inferior cerebellar artery (AICA). Anastomotic interconnections between distal branches of the PICA, AICA, and superior cerebellar artery (SCA) serve to limit infarction in the cerebellum; however, collateral supply to the brainstem is generally poor.

Infarctions of the cerebellum and brainstem are frequently seen with MRI, which is far superior to CT studies, which are limited because of artifacts emanating from the skull base. However, many patients with posterior fossa infarctions are neurologically devastated and poor candidates for good MR exams as motion artifacts are increased. Infarctions in the brainstem are small in relation to the extent of clinical damage produced. The small lesion combined with the technical problems cited above may serve to render some of these lesions undetectable by routine clinical MR. In general, however, MRI is superior to CT in detecting posterior fossa infarctions (Fig. 24).

Approximately two thirds of cerebral emboli are from atherosclerotic disease. Other sources of emboli include the heart in patients with valvular disease, cardiac thrombi, and atrial myxomas (144,145). Peripheral venous thrombi may reach the brain through the pulmonary circulation and cardiac shunts. Septic emboli may originate from the lung, fat emboli from major fractures, and air embolism from surgical procedures or hyperbaric accidents. Most of these embolic situations result in numerous small emboli and infarctions. The vessels most frequently involved in embolic disease are the middle cerebral artery, followed by the posterior cerebral artery. Regardless of etiology, these emboli produce a sudden complete focal or regional ischemia allowing little or no

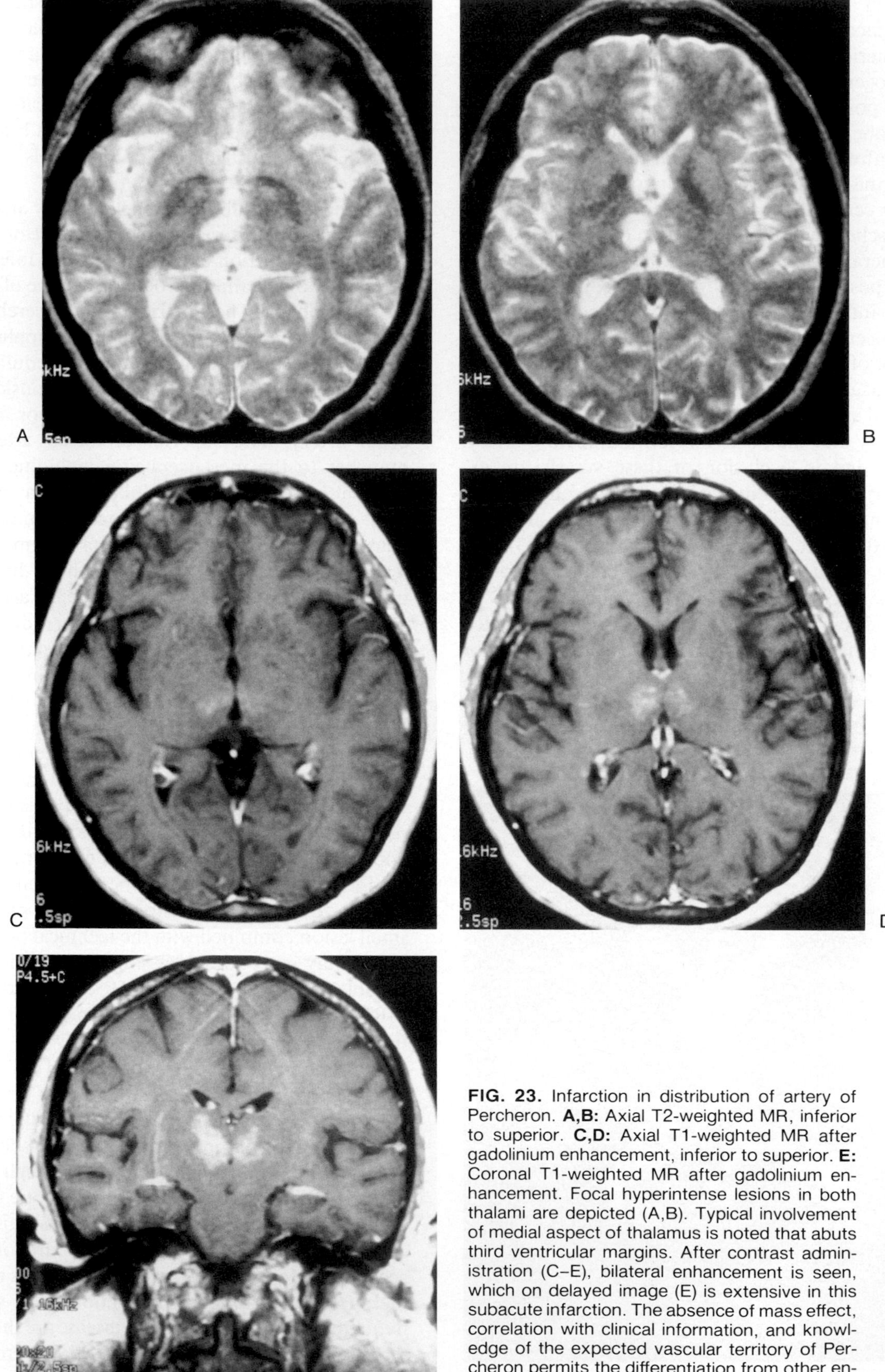

FIG. 23. Infarction in distribution of artery of Percheron. **A,B:** Axial T2-weighted MR, inferior to superior. **C,D:** Axial T1-weighted MR after gadolinium enhancement, inferior to superior. **E:** Coronal T1-weighted MR after gadolinium enhancement. Focal hyperintense lesions in both thalami are depicted (A,B). Typical involvement of medial aspect of thalamus is noted that abuts third ventricular margins. After contrast administration (C–E), bilateral enhancement is seen, which on delayed image (E) is extensive in this subacute infarction. The absence of mass effect, correlation with clinical information, and knowledge of the expected vascular territory of Percheron permits the differentiation from other entities, such as lymphoma or glioma.

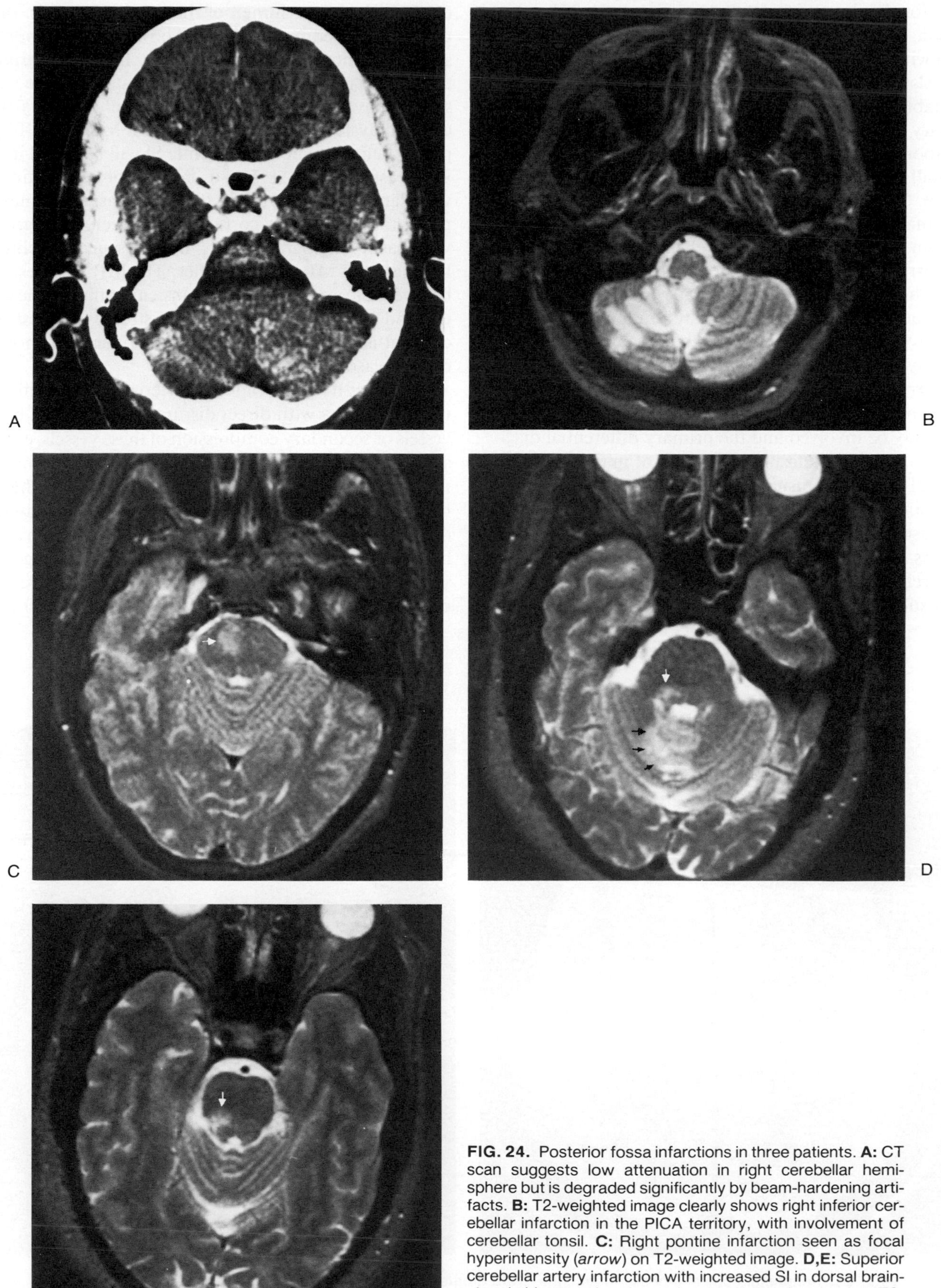

FIG. 24. Posterior fossa infarctions in three patients. **A:** CT scan suggests low attenuation in right cerebellar hemisphere but is degraded significantly by beam-hardening artifacts. **B:** T2-weighted image clearly shows right inferior cerebellar infarction in the PICA territory, with involvement of cerebellar tonsil. **C:** Right pontine infarction seen as focal hyperintensity (*arrow*) on T2-weighted image. **D,E:** Superior cerebellar artery infarction with increased SI in dorsal brainstem (*white arrow*) and superior vermis (*black arrows*) on T2-weighted images.

time for development of collateral circulation. For this reason, smaller, more peripheral infarctions are often seen with these diseases (Fig. 25). Many of these emboli are relatively quickly lysed and blood vessel circulation reestablished. There may or may not be associated secondary hemorrhage of the infarction. The hemorrhagic component of an embolic infarction may occupy only a small portion of the lesion or, occasionally, the entire lesion. The hemorrhagic component is confined predominantly to the gray matter whereas the white matter seldom exhibits hemorrhagic change. Small areas of hemorrhagic infarction are frequently missed by x-ray CT examination because of partial volume effects with radiolucent nonhemorrhagic infarction, but MR is very sensitive to the T_1 shortening of hemorrhage and, consequently, is much more sensitive than CT in diagnosing hemorrhagic infarction (Fig 26).

If emboli are multiple, more than one vascular territory may be involved and the primary differential diagnosis is cerebral metastasis. The lack of mass effect and clinical correlation usually resolves this question. If not, then simply repeating the scan in approximately 7 days will usually show the evolutionary nature of embolic lesions.

Cerebral ischemia secondary to vasospasm is common after subarachnoid hemorrhage (146). Although there is constriction of the lumen of the involved vessels, there usually is not complete vascular obstruction. Minor vasospasm is not associated with any clinical abnormalities, nor change on MR scans. Moderate to severe vasospasm may produce significant cerebral ischemia with cerebral dysfunction and an abnormal MR scan. If so, a poorly defined region of ischemic SI will be noted in the vasospastic region, which usually involves a definable vascular bed (Fig. 27) (147). If severe, mass effect may be present. There is good correlation between the degree of vasospasm angiographically, the presence of clinical findings, and MR abnormalities. The MR changes may be reversible and, in fact, the transient nature of the clinical and MR abnormalities would strongly suggest that cerebral ischemia does not produce infarction in most cases of vasospasm.

Other less frequent causes of arterial occlusive disease include trauma with direct disruption of cerebral blood vessels or secondary compression of these vessels, extrinsic compression of cerebral blood vessels by large masses, moyamoya disease (vascular occlusive disease of the distal internal carotid artery in children), fibromuscular dysplasia, clotting disorders [particularly hypercoagulable states with thrombosis (148,149)], and congenital vascular anomalies. Migraine may also produce significant ischemia presumably due to vasospasm (150,151).

A 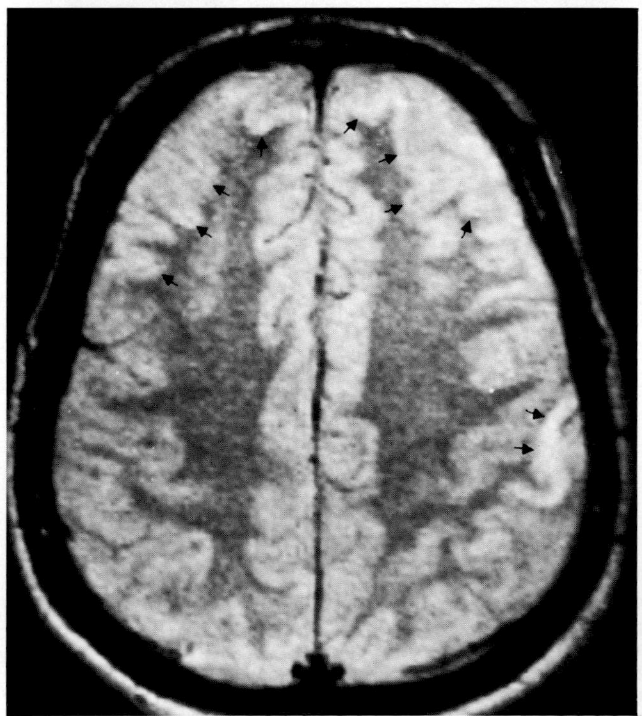

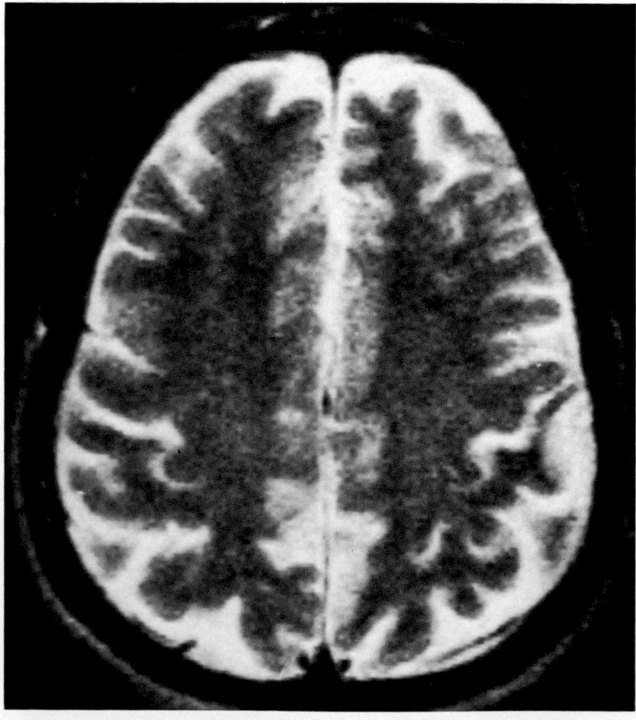 B

FIG. 25. Peripheral cortical embolic infarctions. Note greater conspicuity of these bilateral peripheral infarctions *(arrows)* on SDW image (**A**) compared to T2-weighted image (**B**).

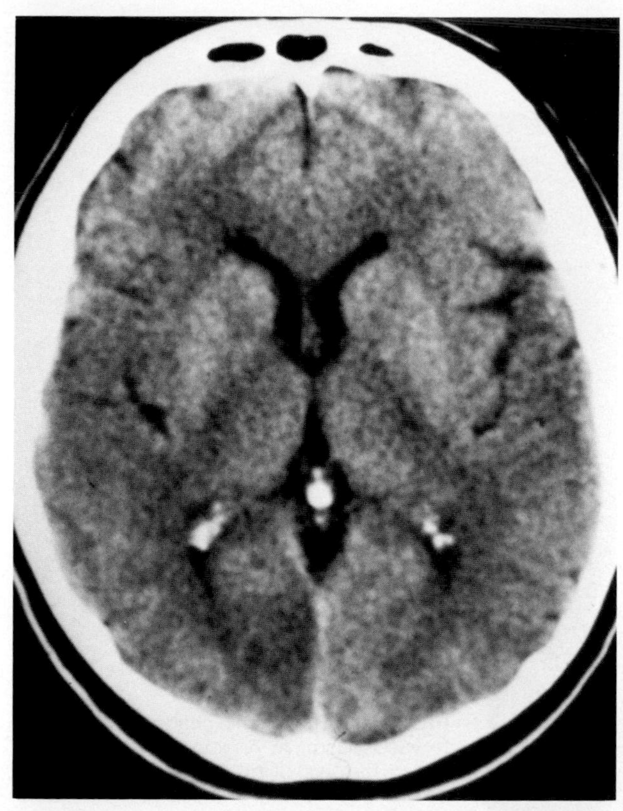

A

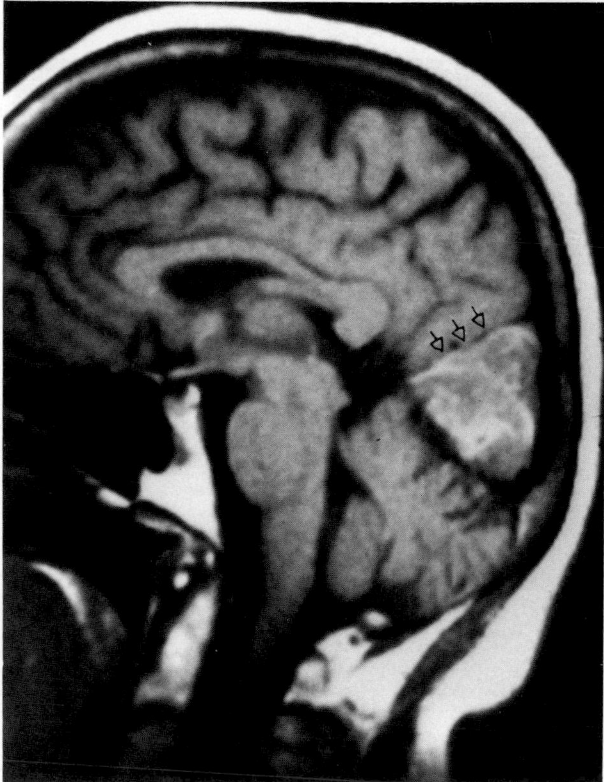

B

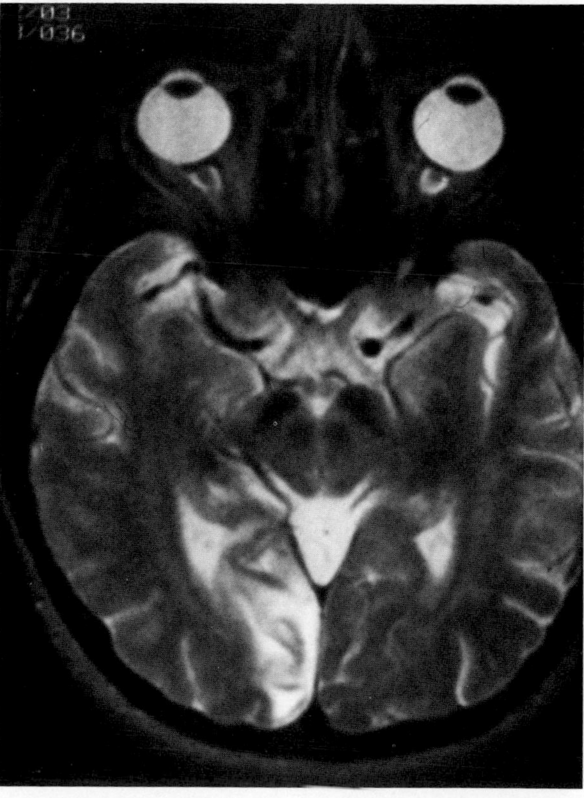

C

FIG. 26. Hemorrhagic infarction, CT vs. MRI. **A:** Axial CT. **B:** Sagittal T1-weighted image. **C:** Axial T2-weighted image. A shows subtle hypodensity in right occipital lobe with no evidence of hemorrhagic component. Note hyperintensity in occipital lobe on sagittal T1-weighted image (B), nicely demarcated anatomically by parieto-occipital sulcus above (*open arrows*). Infarction is also obvious on T2-weighted image (C).

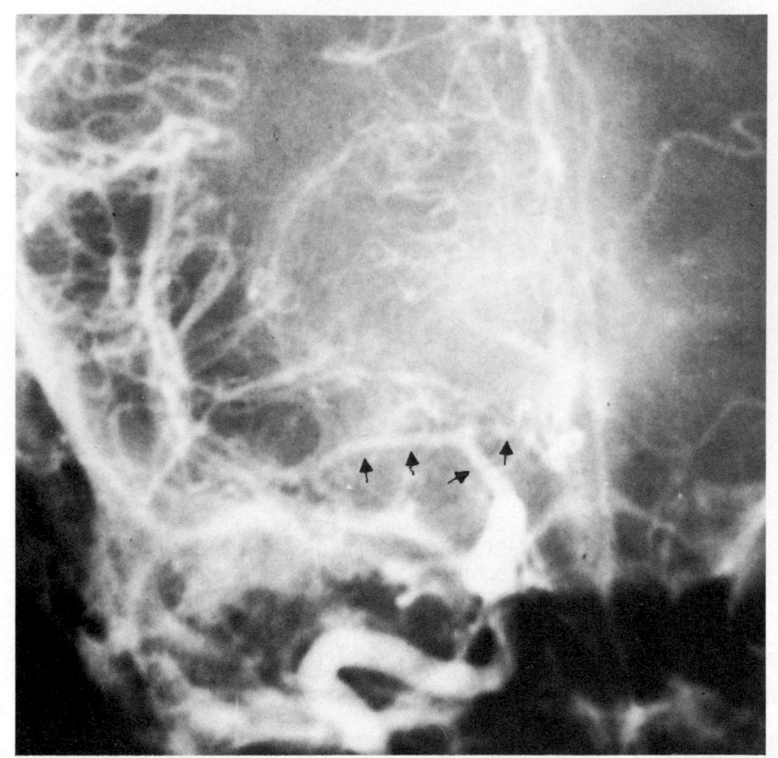

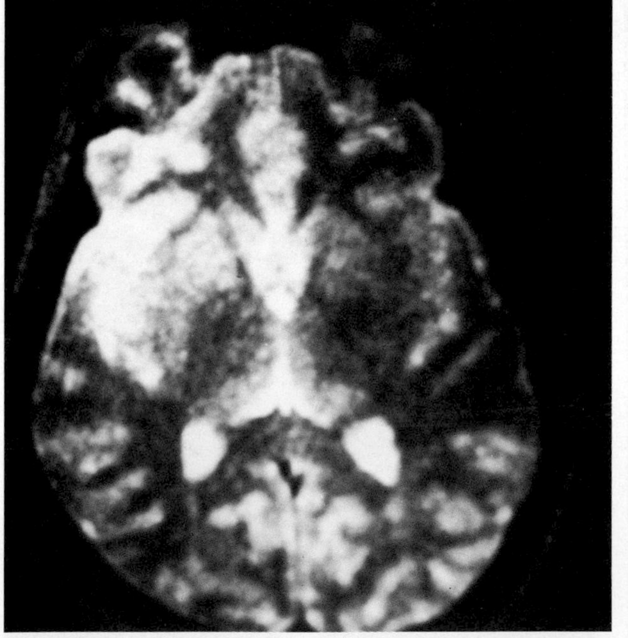

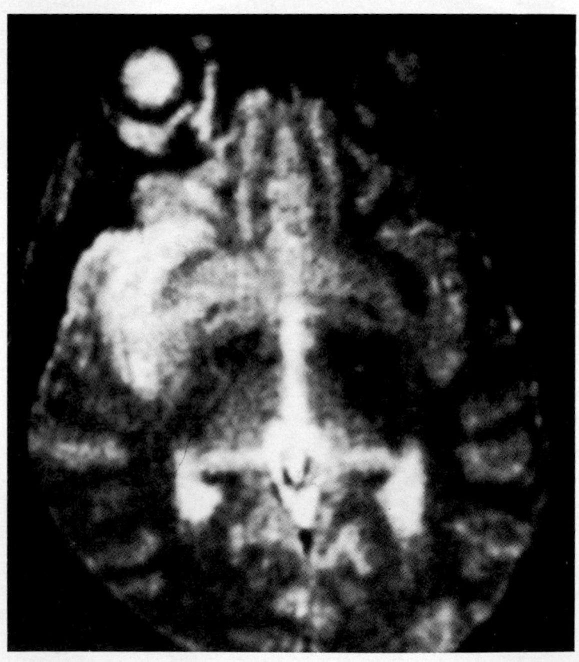

FIG. 27. MR ischemic changes secondary to vasospasm. **A:** Angiogram shows vasospasm (*arrows*) of internal carotid artery and its branches. **B,C:** Increased SI right middle cerebral artery distribution, T2-weighted images.

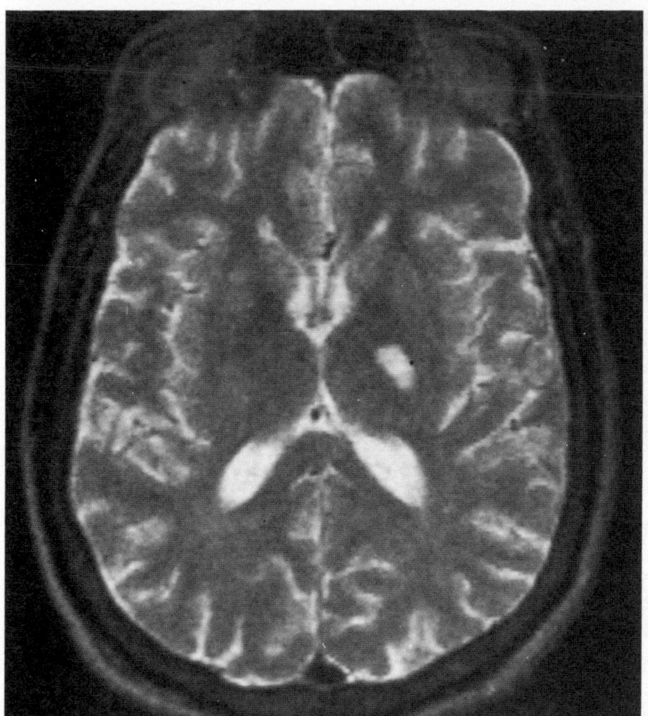

FIG. 28. Lacunar infarction left posterior limb internal capsule, T2-weighted image. (From Mathews, et al, ref. 184, with permission.)

Regardless of etiology, the final insult to the brain is infarction that accounts for the MR abnormalities that provide only indirect information as to the underlying etiology.

Small Vessel Arterial Occlusive Disease

Although small peripheral cerebral infarctions are usually not secondary to primary atherosclerotic cerebral vascular disease, small deep infarctions in the capsular and ganglionic as well as deep white matter regions are usually secondary to primary cerebral vascular disease, although the specific etiology remains somewhat controversial. These lesions have been attributed either to arteriosclerosis, hypertension, or microaneurysms (152). Regardless of specific etiology, these small "lacunar" infarctions may be difficult to see during the first 24 hours, but will become distinguishable as small high-signal lesions by the second or third day (153). The lesions most frequently involve the lenticulostriate territory but not the entire distribution of these vessels, which would suggest major occlusion of the middle cerebral artery. The MR abnormalities mostly involve the gray matter in this region, the lentiform nuclei, thalamus, caudate, and pons. This is secondary to the greater effect ischemic changes have on gray matter and not necessarily to lack of involvement of adjacent white matter. Most lacunar infarctions are generally considered clinically "silent," although this is being increasingly questioned. In contrast, the internal capsules are frequently involved in clinically apparent acute lacunar infarction (Fig. 28). During the chronic stage, these small infarctions resolve to very small (<1 cm) ovoid lesions in the ganglionic region. Since lacunar infarctions are due to diffuse small vessel disease, they are often multiple—30% in one series (154) (Fig. 29).

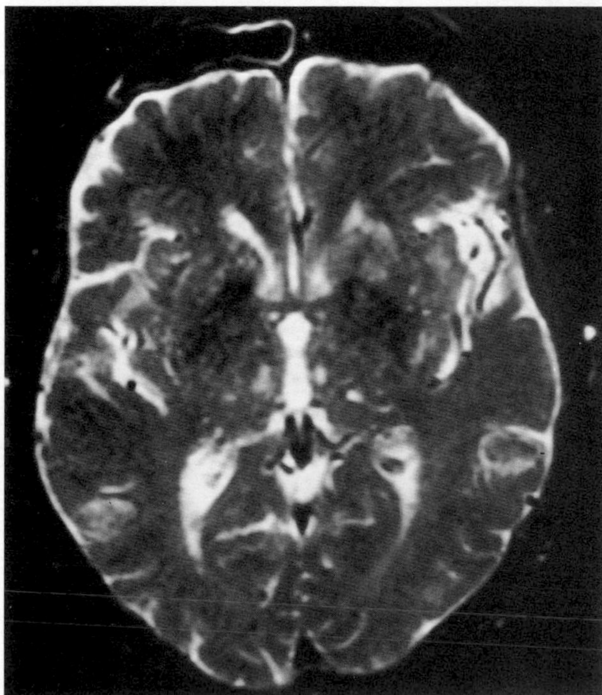

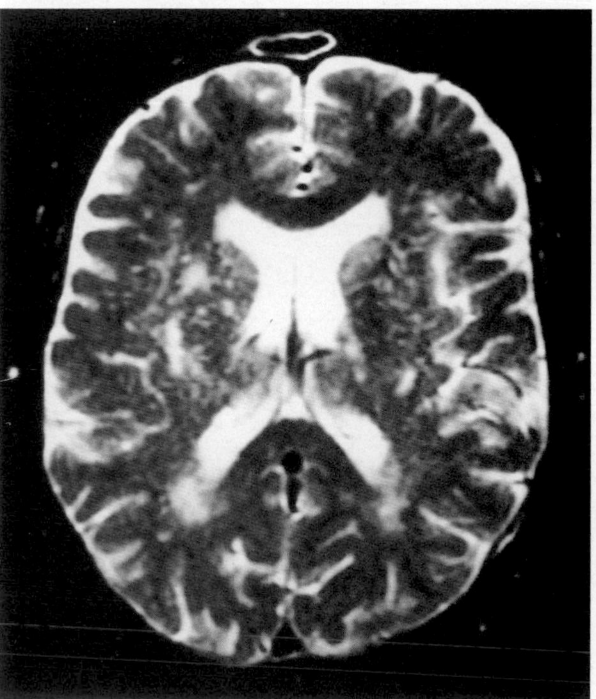

FIG. 29. T2-weighted MRI scans show many small (<10 mm) lesions in the basal ganglia and thalamus.

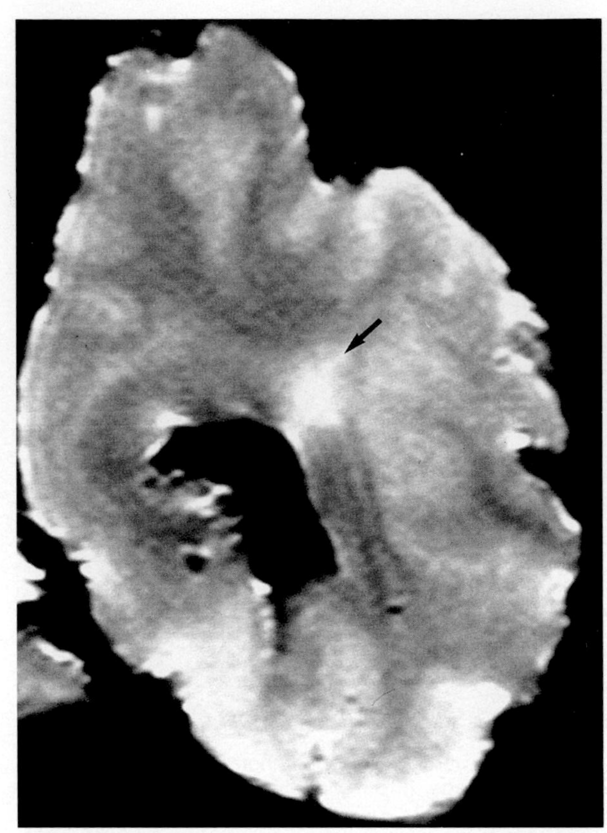

A

FIG. 30. A: MRI (TR = 2600 msec, TE = 20 msec) of a 1-cm thick brain slice cut at a coronal oblique angle (toward the mammillary bodies) through the occipital area of the brain of an 88-year-old woman. She had Alzheimer's disease with dementia, senile plaques in the cortex, and neurofibrillary tangles. This MR image shows a large, confluent area of leuko-araiosis (*arrow*) lateral and superior to the atrium of the left lateral ventricle. **B:** Demyelination (*pale area*) in the periventricular leuko-araiosis lesion, which is shown in the occipital brain slice in A. Kultschitsky's myelin stain; 100 mm-thick celloidin section. Original magnification 2.5×. **C:** Tortuous arteriole entering the area of leuko-araiosis shown in A and B. Brain surface is toward reader's right. This arteriole arises from a pial artery at the surface border zone (watershed), an area already imperiled with a tenuous blood supply. The tortuosity increases the length of the vessel and there are kinetic energy losses associated with each abrupt change in direction: both decrease perfusion pressure. 100 mm-thick celloidin section stained for the enzyme alkaline phosphatase, which remains functional in the endothelium of the arterioles and capillaries after ethanol fixation. Original magnification, 5×. (A, Courtesy of D. Moody and W. Brown, Winston-Salem, NC.)

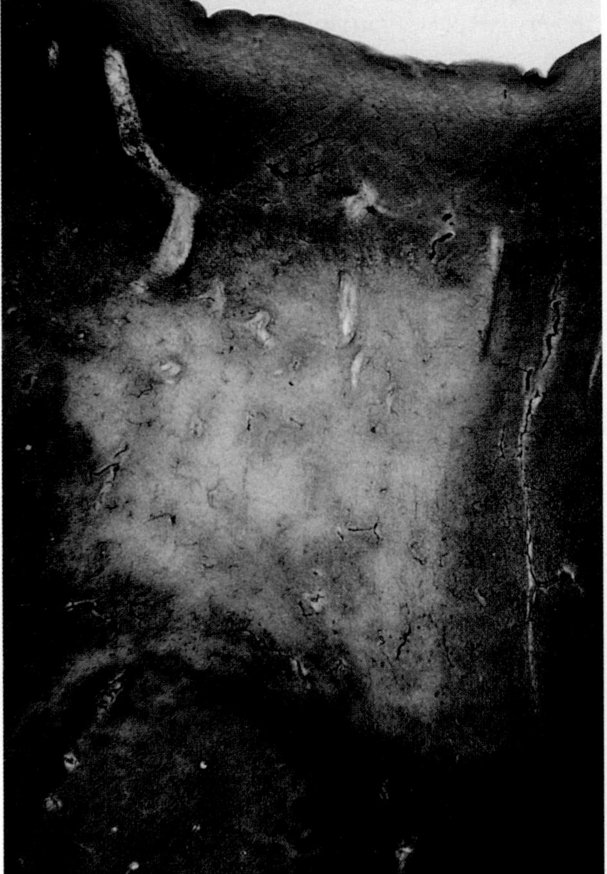

B

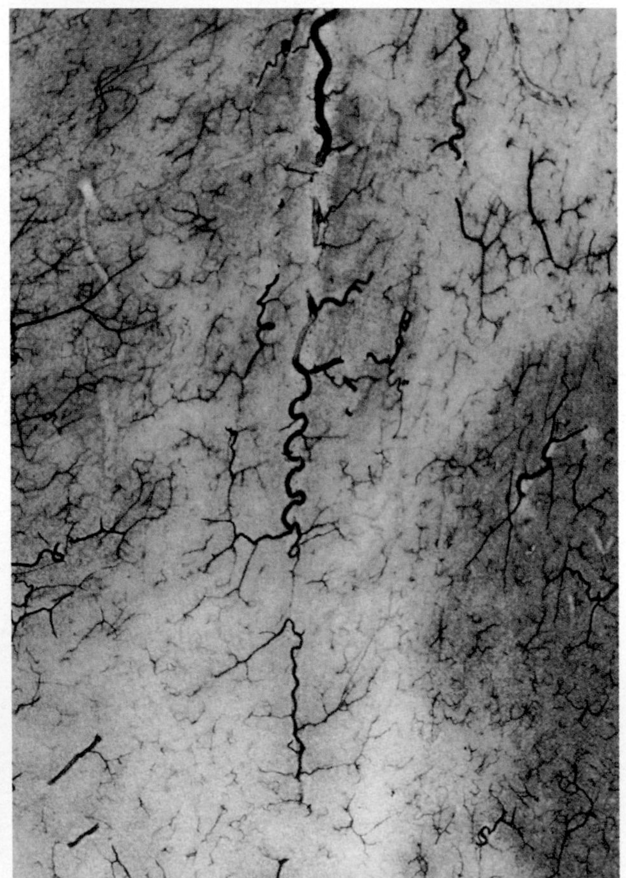

C

MRI is very sensitive to white matter disease in vivo. Deep white matter hyperintensity on MRI is now known to be a common finding, particularly in elderly people. Most of these lesions are now thought to be ischemic in origin. They may be focal or diffuse but predominate in the periventricular or deep white matter. Hachinski et al. (155) proposed that these white matter foci be called "leuko-araiosis," literally meaning "white rarefaction." This definition is based on the CT finding of decreased density in the white matter. Even though these white matter foci can be detected by CT, MRI is much more sensitive. In a comparative study of CT and MRI, only 11 of 155 hyperintense areas on MRI were identified on CT (156). True leuko-araiosis must be distinguished from normal areas of hyperintensity on MRI. These normal areas include areas of late myelination adjacent to the atria of the lateral ventricles (157); focal breakdown of the ependymal lining resulting in increased periependymal extracellular fluid anterolateral to the frontal horns (158); decreased myelination in the parietopontine tracts in the region of the posterior internal capsules bilaterally (159); and perivascular spaces accompanying penetrating vessels at the base of the brain or high convexities (160). True leuko-araiosis is seen as areas of hyperintensity on proton density and T2-weighted images within the deep or subcortical white matter. No mass effect is present and little if any abnormality is present on T1-weighted images (Fig. 30). Various brain regions differ in their susceptibility to developing white matter abnormalities because of their differing blood supplies. The centrum semiovale is particularly susceptible because it is supplied by long arteries and arterioles, (161) whereas the corpus callosum is relatively resistent because it is supplied by short to intermediate length arteries and arterioles (162). Various conditions such as aging, diabetes mellitus, and atherosclerosis can intensify the development of leuko-araiosis by compromising brain microcirculation. However, it is now becoming increasingly clear that hypertension is the main etiologic culprit (Fig. 31). Generally, these hypertensive/ischemic white matter changes are chronic in nature, although the classic acute hypertensive encephalopathy of Binswanger can produce acute and even reversible white matter signal changes (163). Several studies have correlated imaging findings with pathology (164–169). The spectrum of pathology reported ranges from perivascular atrophic demyelination to gliosis to frank infarction.

Cerebral infarction is clinically typified by focal neurologic deficits with acute onset. However, multiple scattered infarctions may result in the more obscure condition of multi-infarction dementia (MID) (170). After Alzheimer's disease, this is thought to be the most common etiology of dementia. Clinically, it is characterized by a more discretely stepwise progression than Alzheimer's disease. Often there are transient focal neurologic deficits due to the most recent infarction. In most cases, some focal neurologic deficit will persist to contrast this disease with Alzheimer's, although these may be relatively subtle clinical findings. Although MID may be secondary to single or a few large infarctions, the disease is usually due to multiple small infarctions, none of which involve an entire major vessel territory. The etiology is usually arteriosclerosis with or without associated hypertension. Obviously, a variety of other diffuse ischemic or hypoxic insults with infarction can result in dementia, but there are usually additional clinical abnormalities and these patients are not usually included in the MID group.

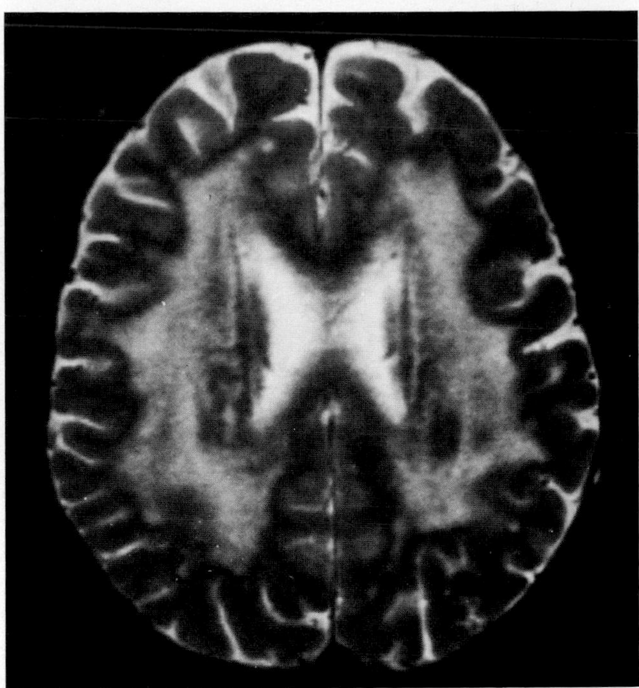

FIG. 31. Patient with chronic hypertension and diffuse increased SI in the subcortical white matter (T2-weighted image).

In contrast to the other clinical conditions involving cerebral infarction, MID is not dominated by the acute and subacute phases. Rather, it is the chronic aspect of this disease that brings the patient to the physician for clinical evaluation and the initial MR. Therefore, it is unusual in these patients to observe the acute and subacute phases of cerebral infarction. Rather, one sees the effects of multiple or diffuse chronic ischemia. In most cases, there will be diffuse cerebral atrophy characterized by lateral ventricular and sulcal dilatation plus focal lesions with atrophy and/or abnormal parenchymal SI (171,172) (Fig. 32).

To differentiate these patients from those with Alzheimer's disease, some focality must be demonstrable by

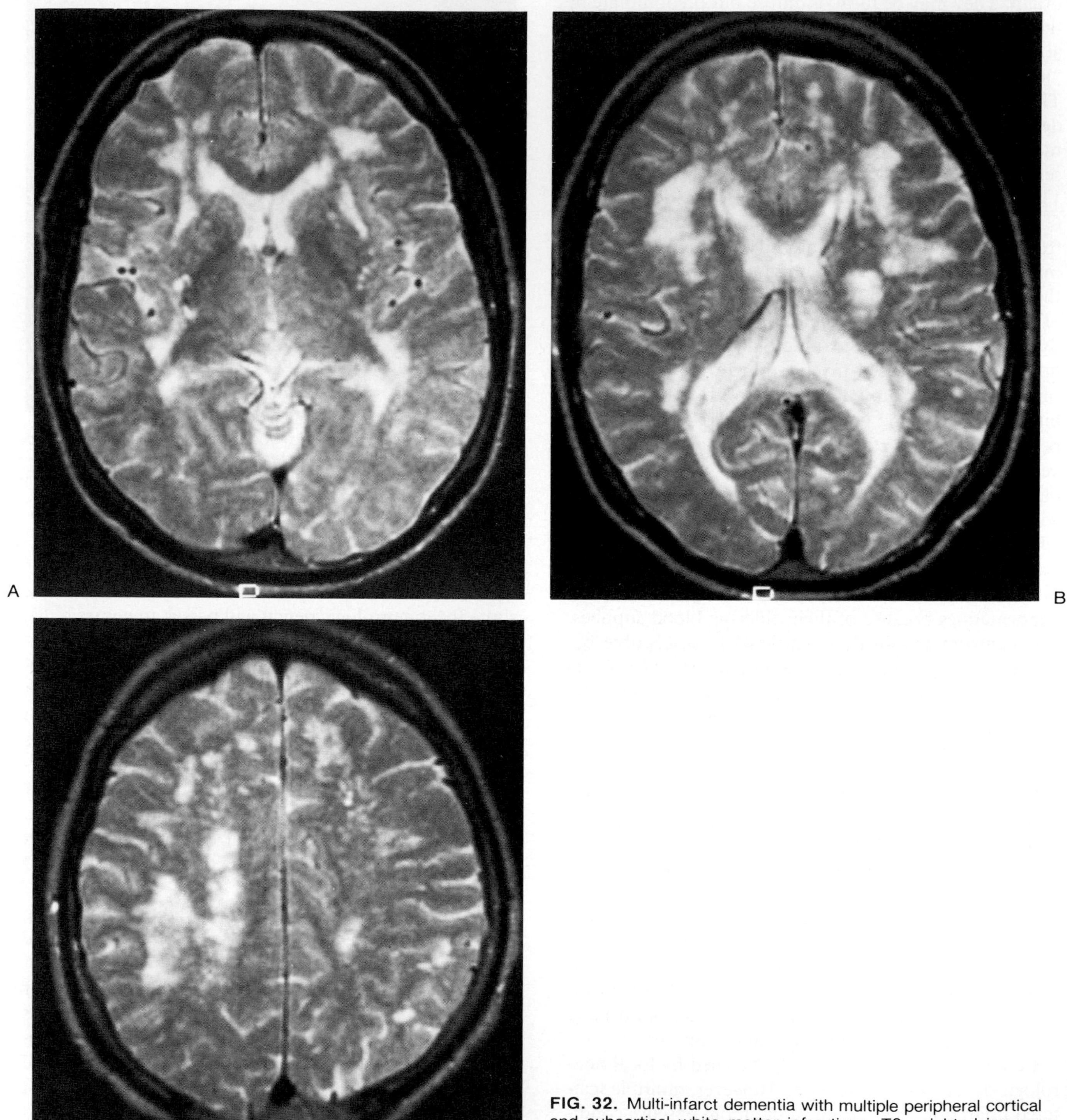

FIG. 32. Multi-infarct dementia with multiple peripheral cortical and subcortical white matter infarctions, T2-weighted images **(A–C)**.

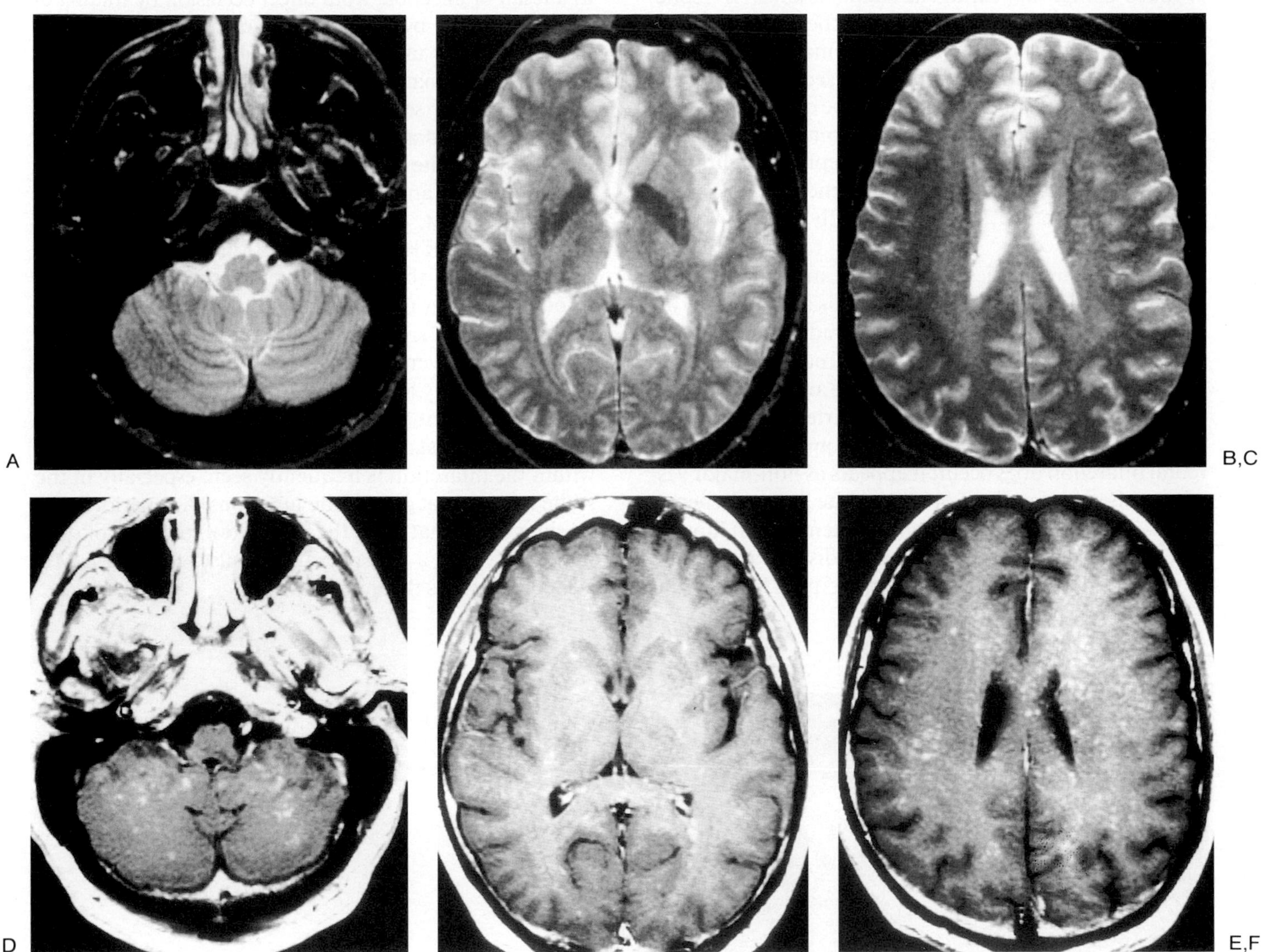

FIG. 33. Granulomatous angiitis, pathologically proven. **A–C:** Axial T2-weighted images, inferior to superior. **D–F:** Axial T1-weighted images after gadolinium enhancement, inferior to superior. T2-weighted images (A–C) are nearly normal, with only a few scattered foci of hyperintensity in the white matter. After contrast, multiple tiny foci of enhancement are clearly seen throughout infratentorial and supratentorial brain parenchyma, mainly located in white matter, presumably due to inflammatory necrosis of vascular endothelium.

MR. In a few cases, patients with clinically or pathologically established multi-infarct dementia may have lesions so small, peripheral, and scattered that they are not individually noticeable. This will result in an atrophic pattern identical to that of Alzheimer's disease or even "normal" atrophy secondary to aging.

A variety of less common small vessel occlusive diseases, including arteritis, either septic or nonseptic, may produce similar-appearing ischemic lesions. If septic, there may be secondary invasion of the vessel wall and environs. In this case, the infarction may be due to the initial intraluminal occlusion or the secondary arteritis with destruction of the vessel. This type of septic vascular occlusion may present as a typical small peripheral infarction or a larger proximal insult. Septic vasculitis secondary to meningitis or meningoencephalitis has a different appearance and is frequently due to venous occlusion.

Nonseptic arteritidies includes the autoimmune diseases, particularly lupus erythematosus and polyarteritis nodosa, granulomatous angiitis, and radiation or chemical arteritis. Many forms of arteritis remain quite difficult to diagnose by any means because arteriography and even biopsy can be normal. In these arteritides, focal cerebral infarction is not particularly common. When cerebral infarction does occur, it appears as non-major vessel peripheral infarctions or deep white matter ischemic disease (Fig. 33). Central nervous system (CNS) lupus is reflected as subcortical white matter disease and diffuse atrophy in most cases, although there may be acute infarctions, even hemorrhagic, in 20% of cases (172) (Fig. 34). Clinical and laboratory information is usually necessary for the specific diagnosis of these lesions.

Venous Occlusive Disease

Occlusion of the venous drainage of the CNS may occur as a result of infection, from direct occlusion by trauma or surgery, invasion by tumor such as meningioma, or pathologic thrombosis usually seen with hypercoagulable states such as disseminated intravascular coagulation, primary polycythemia, or secondary polycythemia due to hypovolemia from dehydration or blood loss (173).

There are quite extensive venous collateral channels from the brain and if the occlusive process is slow, or limited in extent, no symptoms may be produced. On the other hand, if large (i.e., occlusion of the major dural sinus) or abrupt, the stasis will diminish or obstruct flow through the arterial-capillary bed and produce cerebral ischemia and infarction (Fig. 35). These infarctions will tend to involve venous territories that are quite different and anatomically less consistent than arterial territories. Hence, a different geographic pattern is seen on MR, often being bilateral and subcortical (Fig. 36). Hemorrhage within the infarction is frequently seen, especially in the white matter or at gray-white junctions. A superior sagittal sinus (SSS) that lacks the usual flow void and/or does not opacify with a flow refocusing pulse sequence is MR evidence of sinus thrombosis.

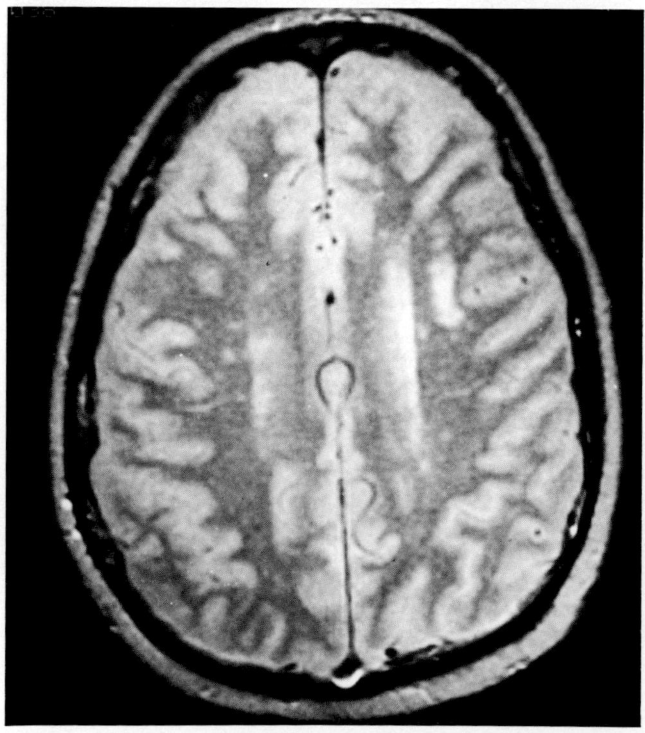

FIG. 34. Lupus cerebritis with multiple small subcortical white matter infarctions, SDW image.

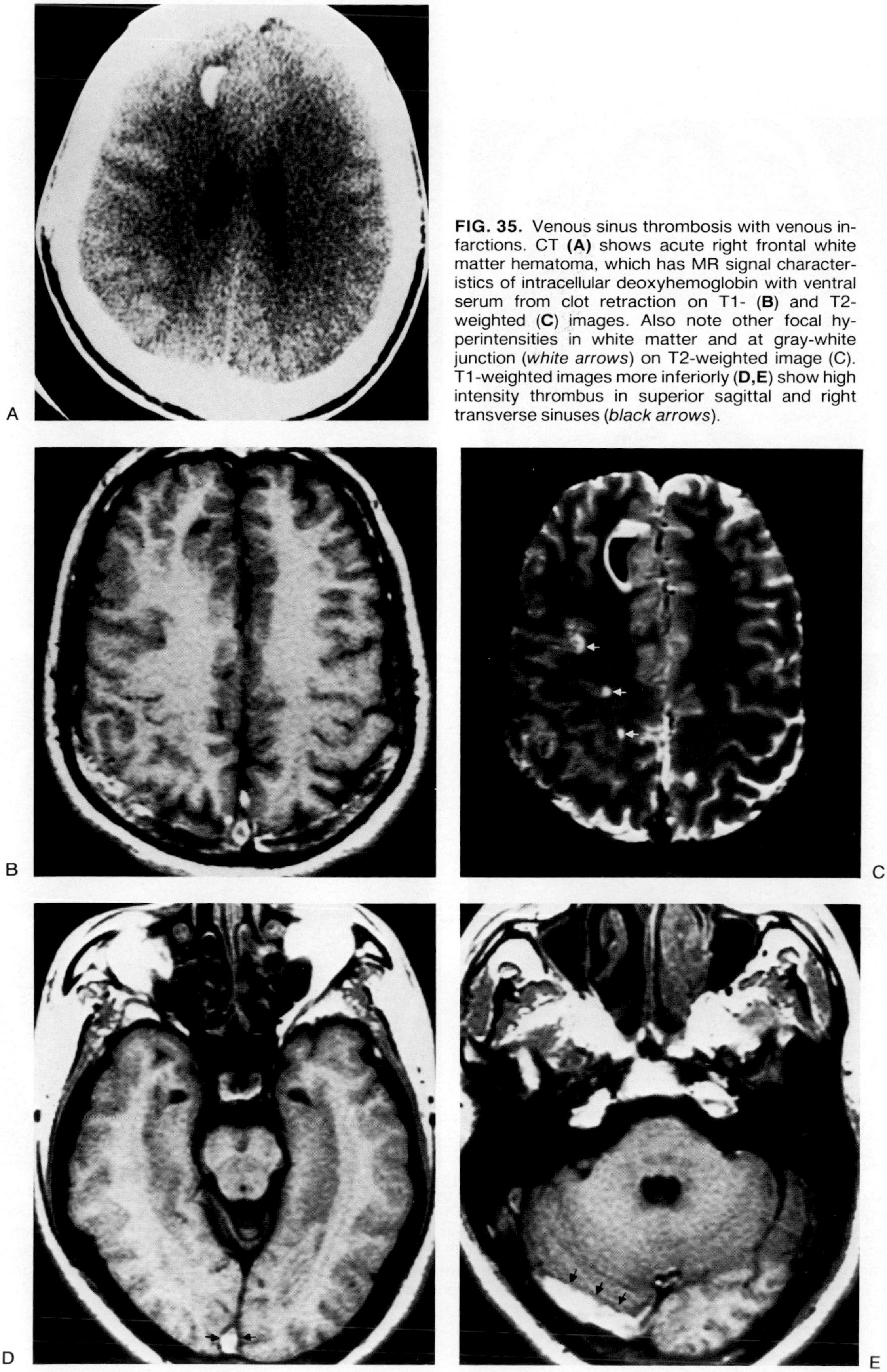

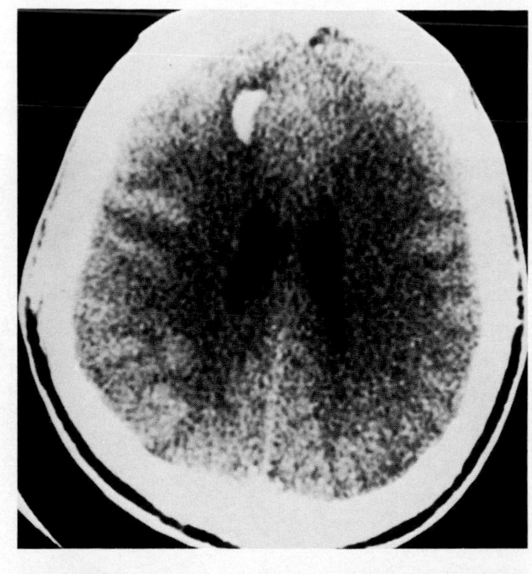

A

FIG. 35. Venous sinus thrombosis with venous infarctions. CT **(A)** shows acute right frontal white matter hematoma, which has MR signal characteristics of intracellular deoxyhemoglobin with ventral serum from clot retraction on T1- (**B**) and T2-weighted (**C**) images. Also note other focal hyperintensities in white matter and at gray-white junction (*white arrows*) on T2-weighted image (C). T1-weighted images more inferiorly (**D,E**) show high intensity thrombus in superior sagittal and right transverse sinuses (*black arrows*).

B

C

D

E

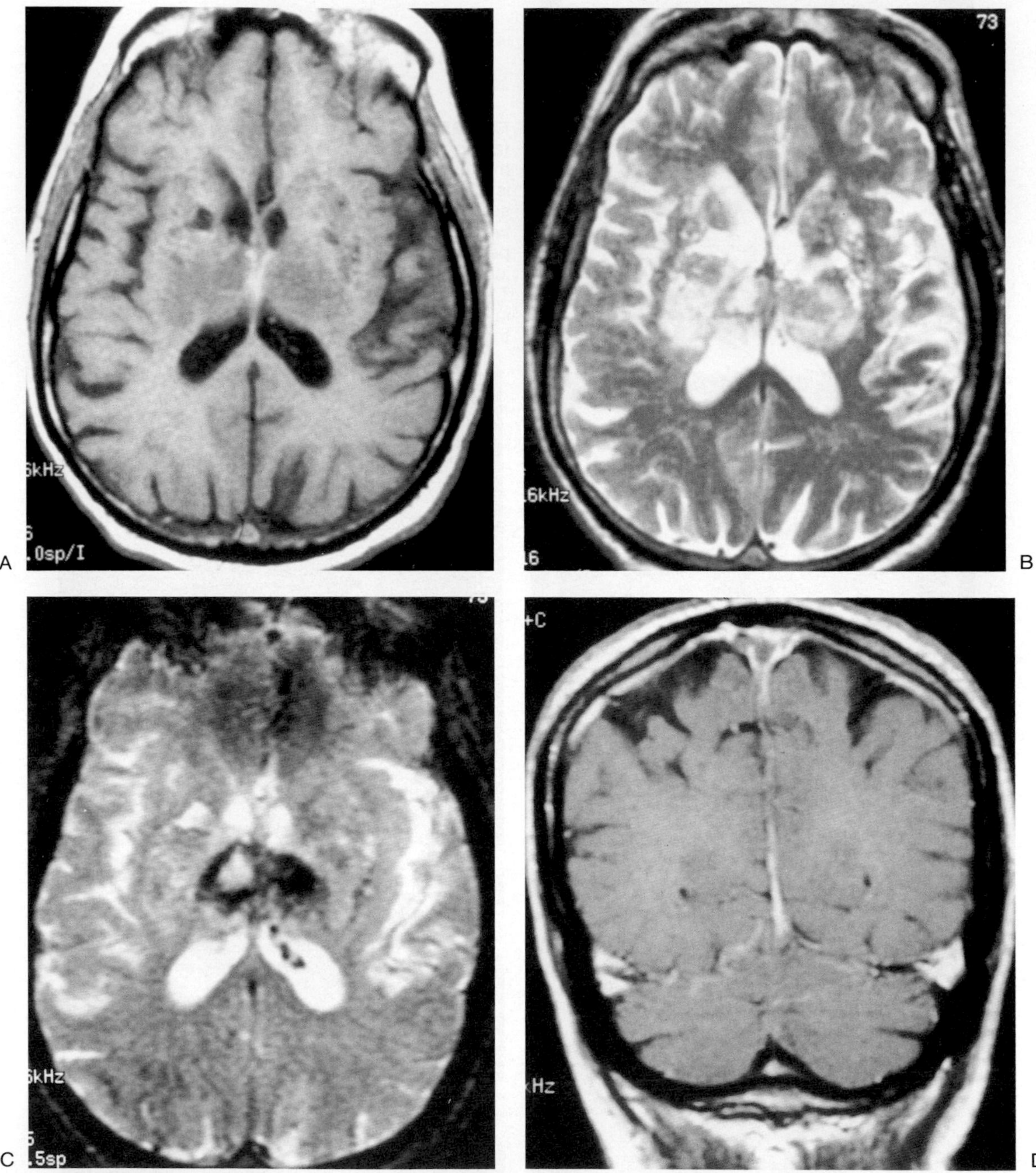

FIG. 36. Bilateral venous infarctions due to deep venous system thrombosis. **A:** Axial T1-weighted MR. **B:** Axial T2-weighted MR. **C:** Axial T2-weighted GE MR. **D:** Coronal T1-weighted MR after contrast enhancement. Bilateral thalamic and ganglionic infarctions are noted (A,B). Diagnosis is made by detection of hyperintense thrombus within internal cerebral veins and superior sagittal sinus (A). GE MR (C) allows detection of hemorrhagic components, a common finding in venous infarctions. After intravenous gadolinium, coronal MR (D) shows equivalent of "delta sign," i.e., enhancement around isointense thrombus within superior sagittal sinus.

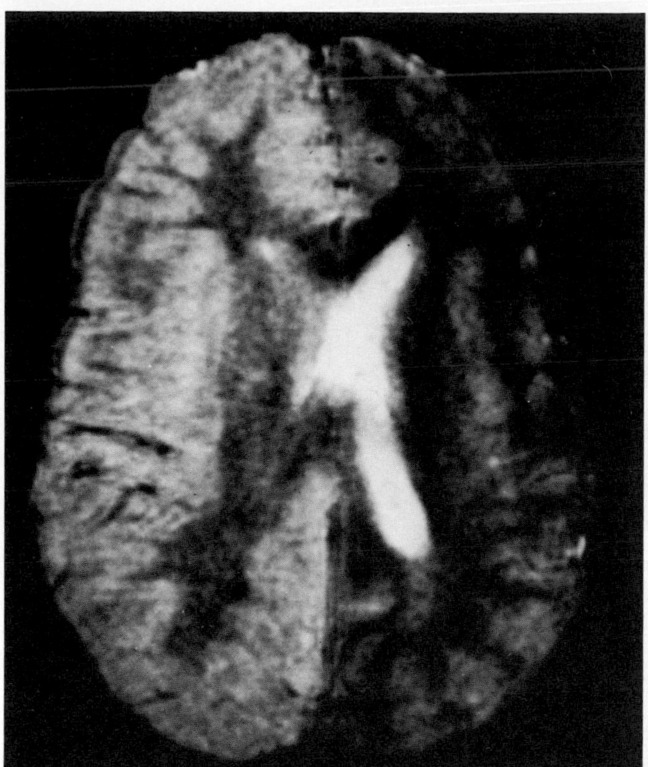

FIG. 37. Eight-year-old child with meningoencephalitis and acute stroke syndrome, T2-weighted image. Note striking gyral swelling.

Septic venous vasculitis occurs more commonly than arterial disease with meningitis and meningoencephalitis. It may produce cortical necrosis. This is particularly common in children with *Hemophilus influenza* meningitis. Rather than small focal lesions, there are usually diffuse irregular serpiginous lesions involving the cerebral gyri (174). In the acute phase of this condition, the scans may be relatively unremarkable or show diffuse swelling and subtle SDW and T2-weighted changes. In the subacute stage there is often quite striking gyral enlargement with or without underlying edema (Fig. 37). During the chronic stage, there may be marked sulcal dilatation and loss of the cortical gray matter secondary to diffuse necrosis.

Nonocclusive Infarction

Cerebral infarction in the absence of vascular occlusion is physiologic in origin (rather than anatomic) and may be secondary to cerebral hypoxemia, hypotension, anemia, hypoglycemia, or metabolic enzymatic deficiencies such as the mitochondrial encephalopathies.

Hypoxic-ischemic encephalopathy (HIE) results when there is a global rather than focal reduction in bloodflow, oxygen, or glucose supply. The pattern of brain tissue damage depends on the duration of the insult as well as individual variables such as patient age and collateral circulation.

In premature infants HIE results in selective damage to the periventricular white matter, which, in the developing fetus, is the vascular watershed zone and has a relatively high metabolic demand (175). This ischemic insult results in periventricular leukomalacia (PVL), which manifests on MRI as loss of white matter volume, hyperintensity of periventricular white matter on long TR images due to gliosis and/or cyst formation, and ventriculomegaly (176–179) (Fig. 38). In some cases, the loss of white matter is so dramatic that the ventricular margins are wavy and follow the contour of the cortical gray matter. In these cases the sulci are deep and in close proximity to the ventricles (179). The loss of white matter also is evident on sagittal images, which reveal a gracile corpus callosum.

When the hypoxic insult occurs late in the third trimester or in the perinatal or neonatal period of a full-term infant, the lesions are typically located in the gray matter, both deep gray matter nuclei and cortex, as well as the subcortical white matter. Acutely, these lesions may be difficult to see on MR, particularly on T2-weighted images (Fig. 39). Chronically, on long TR images, there often is hyperintensity due to gliosis and/or cyst formation within the gray matter structures, most commonly involving the putamen and thalami (180). Acute cortical laminar necrosis may result in hypointensity of the cortical ribbon on long TR images, although contrast enhancement may be the most obvious finding on MR (Fig. 40) (181). When hypoxia is severe or prolonged in full-term neonates or infants, there may be dramatic loss of supratentorial brain tissue resulting in cystic encephalomalacia of the cerebral hemispheres but relative preservation of cerebellum, brainstem, and diencephalic structures. Cystic encephalomalacia can be seen on imaging studies as multiseptated fluid collections replacing brain parenchyma. In addition to these ischemic lesions, hemorrhagic lesions, particularly in the basal ganglia, commonly occur in full-term infants with HIE (177).

HIE in older children and adults typically results in watershed infarctions in the zones between the anterior, middle, and posterior cerebral artery territories as described elsewhere. Since neurons are the elements most sensitive to hypoxic-ischemic injury, gray matter structures show great sensitivity to this type of injury. In particular, the hippocampus, cerebral cortex, Purkinje cells of the cerebellum, caudate, and putamen are highly sensitive to hypoxia. Imaging findings may be very subtle in these areas in cases of mild hypoxia-ischemia, but high resolution images may show hyperintensity on long TR images.

The classic toxic, hypoxic infarction is that secondary to carbon monoxide poisoning. Interestingly enough, this disease most profoundly affects the capsular white

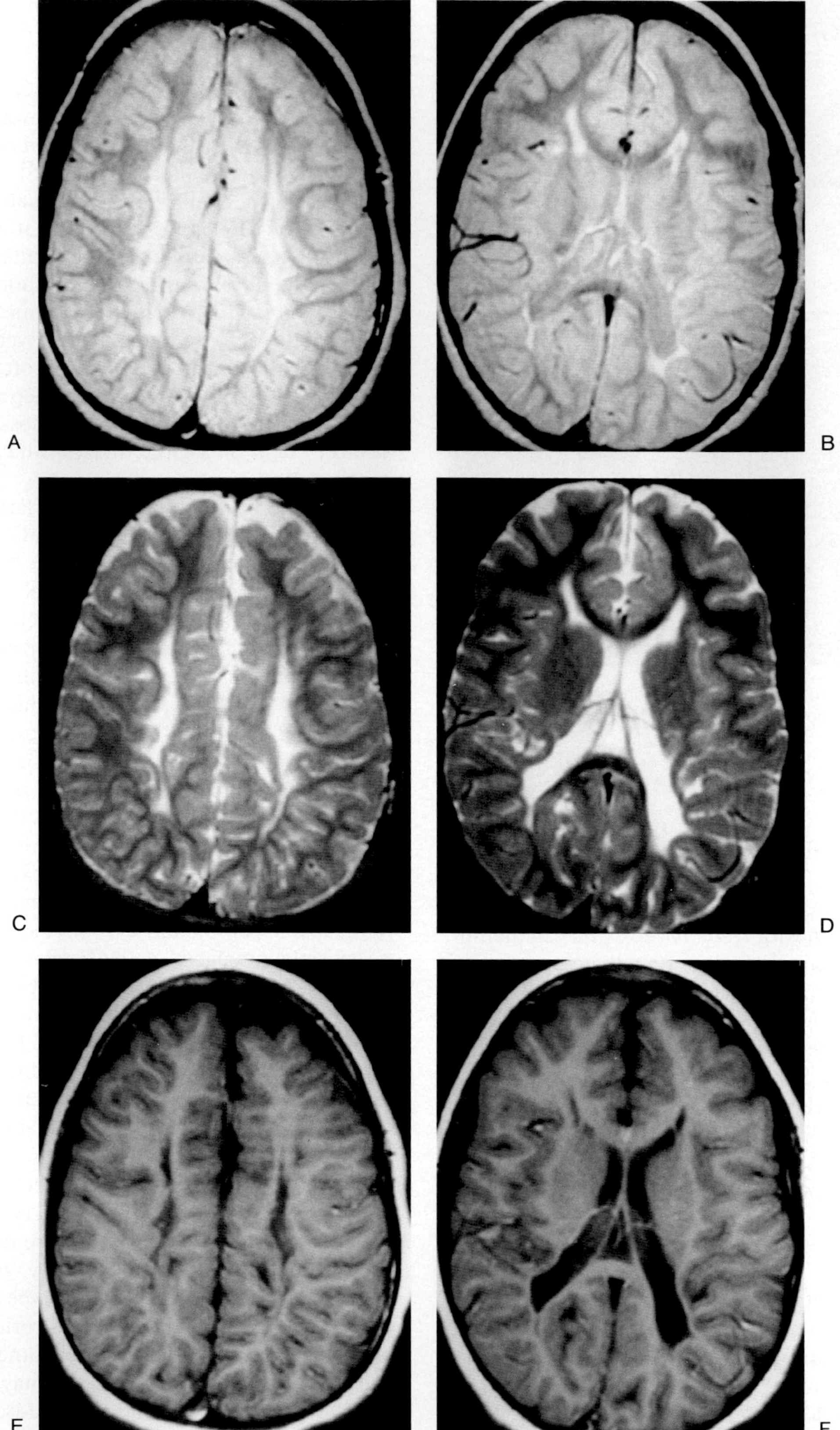

FIG. 38. Periventricular leukomalacia. Six-year-old child who was born at 30 weeks' gestational age. SD (**A,B**), T2-weighted (**C,D**), and T1-weighted (**E,F**) images show periventricular gliosis, loss of white matter, and undulating margins of the lateral ventricles.

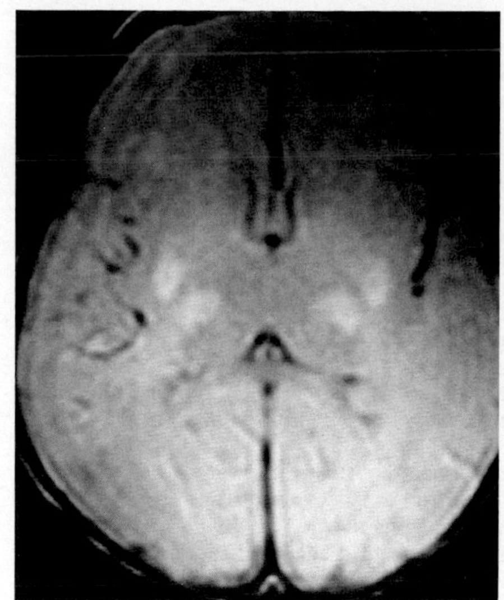
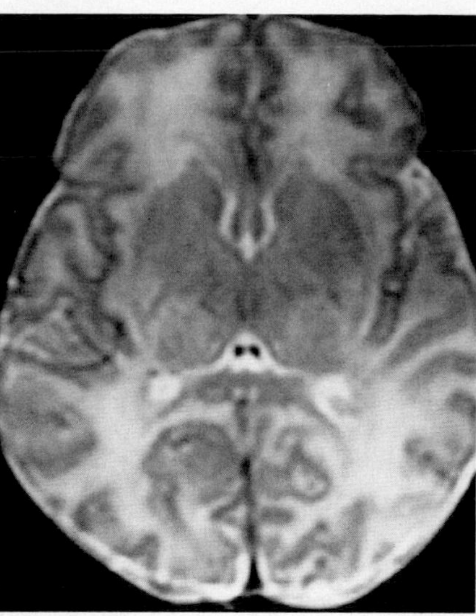
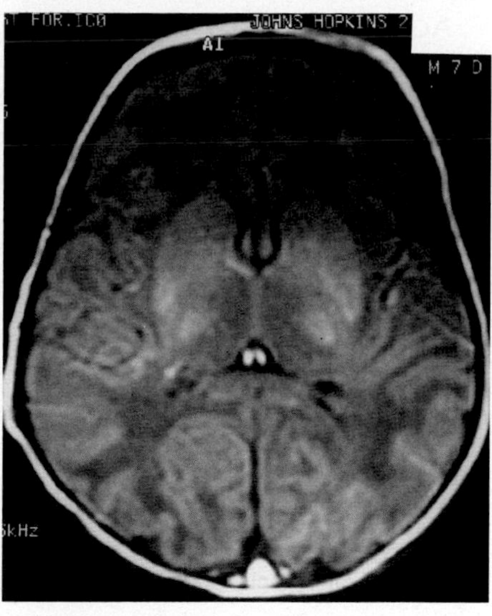

A B,C

FIG. 39. Acute basal ganglia infarction in 7-day-old, term baby who experienced an hypoxic episode. SDW (**A**) and T1-weighted (**C**) images show increased SI in lentiform nucleus and thalamus. T2-weighted (**B**) image is relatively normal, probably due to high water content and long T2 of neonatal brain.

matter and globus pallidus. Cerebral infarction secondary to hypoglycemia alone is rare, although it can occur (182). In contrast to anemic hypoxic infarction, hypoglycemic infarction predominantly involves the peripheral gray matter.

Cerebral ischemia secondary to "steal" may occur in occlusive disease such as subclavian stenosis, or secondary to high-flow arteriovenous malformations that shunt blood away from normal brain. This seldom results in acute infarction, but may produce a chronic functional and morphologic loss of neural tissue with secondary cerebral atrophy (183). On MR, the atrophic changes may be noted but, in addition, demonstration of the vascular lesion itself is usually seen.

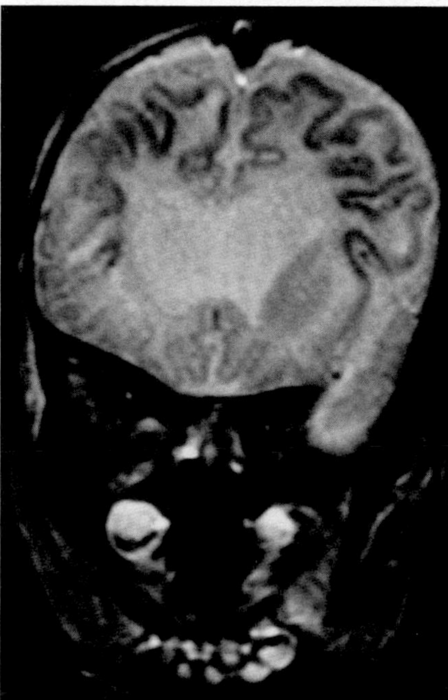
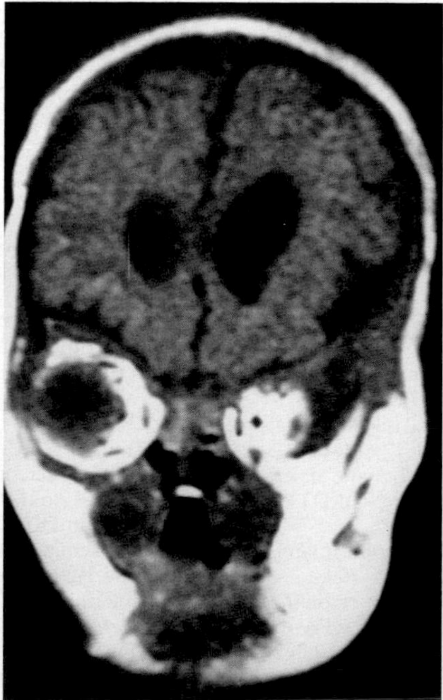
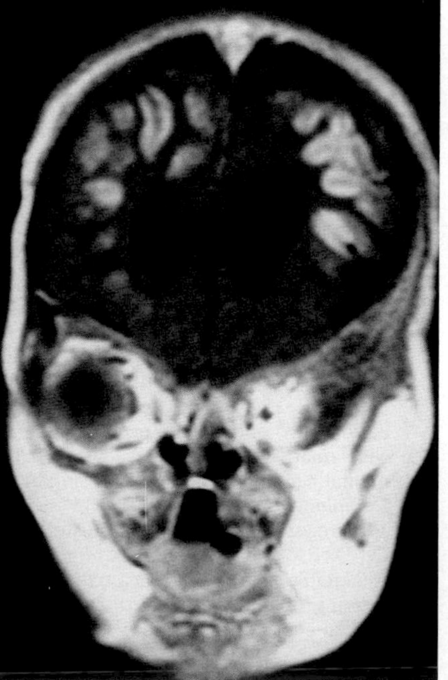

A B,C

FIG. 40. Acute cortical necrosis in premature infant with anoxic episode. Coronal T2-weighted image (**A**) shows subtle hypointensity in cortex whereas T1-weighted image (**B**) shows slight cortical hyperintensity. Postcontrast T1-weighted image (**C**) shows dramatic contrast enhancement.

ACKNOWLEDGMENTS. We thank Douglas Price for his assistance in the preparation of the manuscript, and Errol Candy, M.D., for his generous contribution of the pediatric case material.

REFERENCES

1. Brant-Zawadski M, Weinstein P, Bartkowski H, Moseley M. MRI and spectroscopy in clinical and experimental cerebral ischemia: a review. *AJR* 1987;148:579–588.
2. Kricheff IJ. Arteriosclerotic ischemic cerebrovascular disease. *Radiology* 1987;162:101–109.
3. Welch KMA, Levine SR, Ewing JM. Viewing stroke pathophysiology: an analysis of contemporary methods. *Stroke* 1986;17(6): 1071–1077.
4. Hachinski V, Norris JW. *The Acute Stroke*. Philadelphia: F.A. Daus Co., 1985.
5. Hakim AV, Rynder-Cooke A, Melanson D. Sequential computerized tomographic appearance of strokes. *Stroke* 1983;14:893–897.
6. Bushnell DL, Gupta S, Mlcoch AG, Romyn A, Barnes WE, Kaplan E. Demonstration of focal hyperemia in acute cerebral infarction with iodine-123 iodoamphetamine. *J Nucl Med* 1987; 28:1920–1923.
7. Wise RJS, Rhodes CG, Gibbs JM, Hatazawa J, Palmer T, Frackowiak RSJ, Jones T. Disturbance of oxidative metabolism of glucose in recent human cerebral infarcts. *Ann Neurol* 1983;14:627–637.
8. Brierley JB. Cerebral hypoxia. In: Blackwood W, Corsellis JAN, eds. *Greenfield's Neuropathology*. Chicago: Year Book Medical Pubishers; 1976;43–85.
9. Einsiedel-Lechtape H, Kleihues P. Pathology of cerebral vascular insufficiency. In: Newton TH, Potts DG, eds. *Radiology of the Skull and Brain: Anatomy and Pathology*. St. Louis: The C.V. Mosby Co; 1977;3173–3196.
10. Katzman R, Clasen R, Klatzo I, Meyer JS, Pappius HM, Ealtz AG. Report of joint committee for stroke resources. IV. Brain edema in stroke. *Stroke* 1977;8:512–540.
11. Zulch KJ. Hemorrhage, thrombosis, embolism. In: Minckler J, ed. *Pathology of the Nervous System*, vol. 2. New York: McGraw-Hill; 1968;1499–1536.
12. Klatzo I. Pathophysiologic aspects of cerebral ischemia. In: Tower DB, ed. *The Nervous System, Vol. 1: The Basic Neurosciences*. New York: Raven Press; 1975;313–322.
13. Heiss WD, Hayakawa T, Waltz AG. Patterns of changes of blood flow and relationships to infarction in experimental cerebral ischemia. *Stroke* 1976;7:454–459.
14. Ida M, Mizunuma K, Hata Y, Tada S. Subcortical low intensity in early cortical ischemia. *AJNR* 1994;15:1387–1393.
15. Bryan RN, Levy LM, Whitlow WD, Killian JM, Preziosi TJ, Rosario JA. Diagnosis of acute cerebral infarction: comparison of CT and MRI. *AJNR* 1991;12:611–620.
16. Bryan RN, Weathers SW, Blackwell RD. CNS magnetic resonance imaging. *Curr Neurol* 1988;8:251–294.
17. Elster AD, Moody DM. Early cerebral infarction: gadopentetate dimeglumine enhancement. *Radiology* 1990;177:627–632.
18. Crain MR, Yuh WTC, Greene GM, et al. Cerebral ischemia: evaluation with contrast enhanced MRI. *AJNR* 1991;12:631–639.
19. McNamara MT, Brant-Zawadzki M, Berry I, et al. Acute experimental cerebral ischemia: MR enhancement using Gd-DTPA. *Radiology* 1986;158:701–705.
20. Virapongse C, Mancuso A, Quisling R. Human brain infarcts: Gd-DTPA–enhanced MRI. *Radiology* 1986;161:785–794.
21. Imakita S, Nishimura T, Yamada N, et al. Magnetic resonance imaging of cerebral infarction: time course of Gd-DTPA enhancement and CT comparison. *Neuroradiology* 1988;30:372–378.
22. Miyashita K, Naritomi H, Sawada T, et al. Identification of recent lacunar lesions in cases of multiple small infarctions by magnetic resonance imaging. *Stroke* 1988;19:834–839.
23. Elster AD. MR contrast enhancement in brainstem and deep cerebral infarction. *AJNR* 1991;12:631–639.
24. Sato A, Takahashi S, Soma Y, et al. Cerebral infarction: early detection by means of contrast-enhanced cerebral arteries at MRI. *Radiology* 1991;178:433–439.
25. Meuller DP, Yuh WTC, Fisher DJ, Chandran KB, Crain MR, Kim Y-H. Arterial enhancement in acute cerebral ischemia: clinical and angiographic correlation. *AJNR* 1993;14:661–668.
26. Mathews VP, Monsein LH, Pardo CA, Bryan RN. Histologic abnormalities associated with gadolinium enhancement on MR images in the initial hours of experimental cerebral infarction. *AJNR* 1994;15:573–579.
27. Lanens D, Spanoghe M, Van Audekerke J, Van der Linden A, Domisse R. Complementary use of T2- and postcontrast T1-weighted NMR images for the sequential monitoring of focal ischemic lesions in the rat brain. *Magn Reson Imag* 1993;11:675–683.
28. Mathews VP, King JC, Elster AD, Hamilton CA. Cerebral infarction: effects of dose and magnetization transfer saturation at gadolinium-enhanced imaging. *Radiology* 1994;190:547–552.
29. Uchino A, Miyoshi T, Ohno M. Fogging effect and MRI: a case report of pontine infarction. *Radiat Med* 1990;8:99–102.
30. Asato R, Okumura R, Konishi J. Fogging effect in MR of cerebral infarct. *J Comput Assist Tomogr* 1991;15:160–162.
31. Miyashita K, Naritomi H, Sawada T, et al. Identification of recent lacunar lesions in cases of multiple small infarctions by magnetic resonance imaging. *Stroke* 1988;19:834–839.
32. Bryan RN, Weathers SW, Blackwell RD. CNS magnetic resonance imaging. *Curr Neurol* 1988;8:251–294.
33. Edelman RR, Johnson K, Buxton R, et al. MR of hemorrhage: a new aproach. *AJNR* 1986;7:751–756.
34. Miyashita K, Naritomi H, Sawada T, et al. Identification of recent lacunar lesions in cases of multiple small infarctions by magnetic resonance imaging. *Stroke* 1988;19:834–839.
35. Grotta JC. Can raising CBF improve outcome after acute cerebral infarction? *Stroke* 1987;18:264–267.
36. Erecinska M, Silver IA. ATP and brain function. *J Cereb Blood Flow* 1989;9:2–19.
37. Siesjo BK, Agardh C-D, Bengisson F. Free radicals and brain damage. *Cerebrovasc Brain Metab Rev* 1989;1:165–211.
38. Symon L, Wang A, Momma F. Aspects of cerebral ischemia in humans: clinical correlates of primate thresholds. In: Cervos-Navarro J, Ferszt R, eds. *Stroke and Microcirculation*. New York: Raven Press; 1987;1–4.
39. Bose B, Jones SC, Lorig R, Friel HT, Weinstein M, Little JR. Evolving focal cerebral ischemia in cats: spatial correlation of nuclear magnetic resonance imaging, CBF, tetrazolium staining, and histopathology. *Stroke* 1988;19:28–37.
40. Mano I, Levy RM, Crooks LE, Hosobuchi Y. Proton nuclear magnetic resonance imaging of acute experimental cerebral ischemia. *Invest Radiol* 1983;17:345–351.
41. Eleff SM, Maruki Y, Monsein LH, Traystman RJ, Bryan RN, Koehler RC. Sodium, ATP, and intracellular pH transients during reversible complete ischemia of dog cerebrum. *Stroke* 1991; 22:233–241.
42. Brant-Zawadzki M, Pereira B, Weinstein P, et al. MRI of acute experimental ischemia in cats. *AJNR* 1986;7:7–11.
43. Dewitt LD, Kistler JP, Miller DC, Richardson EP, Buonanno FS. NMR-neuropathologic correlation in stroke. *Stroke* 1987;18(2): 342–351.
44. Yuh WTC, Crain MR, Loes DJ, Greene GM, Ryals TJ, Sato Y. MRI of cerebral ischemia: findings in the first 24 hours. *AJNR* 1991;12:621–629.
45. Gadian DG, Frackowiak SJ, Crockard HA, et al. Acute cerebral ischaemia: concurrent changes in CBF, energy metabolites, pH, and lactate measured with hydrogen clearance and ^{31}P and ^{1}H nuclear magnetic resonance spectroscopy. I. Methodology. *J Cereb Blood Flow Metab* 1987;7(2):199–206.
46. Figols J, Cervos-Navarro J, Sampaolo S, Ferszt R. Microthrombi in the development of ischemic irreversible brain infarct. In: Cervos-Navarro J, Ferszt R, eds. *Stroke and Microcirculation*. New York: Raven Press; 1987;69–74.
47. Price TR. Progressing ischemic stroke. In: Barnett JM, Mohr JP,

Stein BM, Yatsu FM, eds. *Stroke*. New York: Churchill Livingstone; 1986; 1059–1068.
48. Brant-Zawadzki M. Routine MRI of the internal carotid artery siphon: angiographic correlation with cervical carotid lesions. *AJNR* 1990; 11:467–471.
49. Lane JI, Flanders AE, Doan HT, Bell RD. Assessment of carotid artery patency on routine spin-echo MRI of the brain. *AJNR* 1991; 12:819–826.
50. Litt AW, Eidelman EM, Pinto RS, et al. Diagnosis of carotid artery stenosis: comparison of 2DFT TOF MRA with contrast angiography in 50 patients. *AJNR* 1991; 12:149–154.
51. Masaryk AM, Ross JS, DiCello MC, et al. 3DFT MRA of the carotid bifurcation: potential and limitations as a screening examination. *Radiology* 1991; 179:797–804.
52. Pan XM, Anderson CM, Reilly LM, et al. Magnetic resonance angiography of the carotid artery combining two- and three-dimensional acquisitions. *J Vasc Surg* 1992; 16:609–618.
53. Polak JF, Bajakian RL, O'Leary DH, et al. Detection of internal carotid artery stenosis: comparison of MRA, color doppler sonography, and arteriography. *Radiology* 1992; 182:35–40.
54. Riles TS, Eidelman EM, Litt AW, et al. Comparison of magnetic resonance angiography, conventional angiography, and duplex scanning. *Stroke* 1992; 23:341–346.
55. Heiserman JE, Drayer BP, Fram EK, et al. Carotid artery stenosis: clinical efficacy of two-dimensional TOF MRA. *Radiology* 1992; 182:761–768.
56. Laster RE, Acker JD, Halford HH, et al. Assessment of MRA versus arteriography for evaluation of cervical carotid bifurcation disease. *AJNR* 1993; 14:681–688.
57. Huston J, Lewis BD, Wiebers DO, et al. Carotid artery: prospective blinded comparison of two-dimensional TOF MRA with conventional angiography and duplex US. *Radiology* 1993; 186: 339–344.
58. Polak JF, Kalina P, Donaldson MC, et al. Carotid endarterectomy: preoperative evaluation of candidates with combined doppler sonography and MRA. *Radiology* 1993; 186:333–338.
59. Kido DK, Barsotti JB, Rice LZ, et al. Evaluation of the carotid artery bifurcation: comparison of magnetic resonance angiography and digital subtraction arch aortography. *Neuroradiology* 1991; 33:48–51.
60. Pernicone JR, Siebert JE, Potchen EJ, et al. Three-dimensional phase-contrast MRA in the head and neck: preliminary report. *AJNR* 1990; 11:457–466.
61. Lin W, Haache EM, Smith AS. Lumen definition in MRA. *J Magn Reson Imag* 1991; 1:327–336.
62. Mittl R, Broderick M, Xarpenter J, et al. Blinded reader comparison of magnetic resonance angiography and duplex ultrasonography for carotid artery bifurcation stenosis. *Stroke* 1994; 25:4–10.
63. Masaryk TJ, Modic MT, Ross JS, et al. Intracranial circulation: preliminary clinical results with three-dimensional (volume) MRA. *Radiology* 1989; 171:793–799.
64. Creasy JL, Price RR, Presbrey T, Goins D, Partain CL, Kessler RM. Gadolinium-enhanced MRA. *Radiology* 1990; 175:280–283.
65. Marchal G, Michiels J, Bosmans H, et al. Contrast-enhanced MRA of the brain. *J Comput Assist Tomogr* 1992; 16(1):25–29.
66. Lin W, Tkach JA, Haache EM, et al. Intracranial MRA: application of magnetization transfer contrast and fat saturation to short gradient-echo velocity-compensated sequences. *Radiology* 1993; 186:753–761.
67. Pike GB, Hu BS, Glover GH, et al. Magnetization transfer TOF magnetic resonance angiography. *Magn Reson Med* 1992; 25: 372–379.
68. Edelman RR, Ahn SS, Chien D, et al. Improved TOF MRA of the brain with magnetization transfer contrast. *Radiology* 1992; 184: 395–399.
69. Blatter DD, Parker DL, Robison RO. Cerebral MRA with multiple overlapping thin slab acquisition. Part I. Qualitative analysis of vessel visibility. *Radiology* 1991; 179:805–811.
70. Davis WL, Warnock SH, Harnsberger R, et al. Intracranial MRA: single volume vs. multiple thin slab 3D TOF acquisition. *J Comput Assist Tomogr* 1993; 17(1):15–21.
71. Heiserman JE, Drayer BP, Keller PJ. Intracranial vascular stenosis and occlusion: evaluation with three-dimensional time-of-flight MRA. *Radiology* 1992; 185:667–673.
72. Rither J, Wentz K, Rautenberg W, et al. Magnetic resonance angiography in vertebrobasilar ischemia. *Stroke* 1993; 24(9):1310–1315.
73. Wentz KU, Rither J, Schwartz A, et al. Intracranial vertebrobasilar system: MRA. *Radiology* 1994; 190:105–110.
74. Fujita N, Hirabuki N, Fujii K, et al. MRI of middle cerebral artery stenosis and occlusion: value of MRA. *AJNR* 1994; 15:335–341.
75. Blatter DD, Parker DL, Ahn SS, et al. Cerebral MRA with multiple overlapping thin slab acquisition. Part II. Early clinical experience. *Radiology* 1992; 183:379–389.
76. Ross MR, Pelc NJ, Enzmann DR. Qualitative phase contrast MRA in the normal and abnormal circle of Willis. *AJNR* 1993; 14:19–25.
77. First G, Steinmetz H, Fischer H. Selective MRA and intracranial collateral blood flow. *J Comput Assist Tomogr* 1993; 17(2):178–183.
78. Edelman RR, Mattle HP, O'Reilly GV, et al. Magnetic resonance imaging of flow dynamics in the circle of Willis. *Stroke* 1990; 21(1):56–65.
79. Mattle H, Edelman RR, Wentz KU, et al. Middle cerebral artery: determination of flow velocities with MRA. *Radiology* 1991; 181: 527–530.
80. Marks MP, Pelc NJ, Ross MR, Enzmann DR. Determination of CBF with a phase-contrast cine MRI technique: evaluation of normal subjects and patients with arteriovenous malformations. *Radiology* 1992; 182:467–476.
81. Warach S, Li W, Ronthal M, et al. Acute cerebral ischemia: evaluation with dynamic contrast-enhanced MRI and MRA. *Radiology* 1992; 182:41–47.
82. Garcia JH, Anderson ML. Physiopathology of cerebral ischemia. *CRC Crit Rev Neurobiol* 1989; 4(4):303–324.
83. Raichle ME. The pathophysiology of brain ischemia. *Ann Neurol* 1983; 13(1):2–10.
84. Rosen BR, Belliveau JW, Chien D, Cohen MS, Weisskopf RM. MR perfusion imaging. In: Kressel HY, Modic MT, Murphy WA, eds. *MR 1990.* Chicago: Radiological Society of North America, Inc; 1990:69–84.
85. Edelman RR, Mattle HP, Atkinson DJ, et al. CBF: assessment with dynamic contrast-enhanced T2-weighted MRI at 1.5T. *Radiology* 1990; 176:211–20.
86. Villringer A, Rosenm BR, Belliveau JW, et al. Dynamic imaging with lanthanide chelates in normal brain: contrast due to magnetic susceptibility effects. *Magn Reson Med* 1988; 6:164–174.
87. Belliveau JW, Rosen BR, Kantor HL, et al. Functional cerebral imaging by susceptibility-contrast NMR. *Magn Reson Med* 1990; 14:538–546.
88. Finelli DA, Hopkins AL, Selman WR, Crumrine RC, Bhatti SU, Lust WD. Evaluation of experimental early acute cerebral ischemia before the development of edema: use of dynamic, contrast-enhanced and diffusion-weighted MR scanning. *Magn Reson Med* 1992; 27:189–197.
89. Maeda M, Itoh S, Ide H, Acute stroke in cats: comparison of dynamic susceptibility-contrast MRI with T2- and diffusion-weighted MRI. *Radiology* 1993; 189:227–232.
90. Kucharczyk J, Vexler ZS, Roberts TP, et al. Echo-planar perfusion-sensitive MRI of acute cerebral ischemia. *Radiology* 1993; 188:711–717.
91. Warach S, Li W, Ronthal M, Edelman RR. Acute cerebral ischemia: evaluation with dynamic contrast enhanced MRI and MRA. *Radiology* 1992; 182:41–47.
92. Warach S, Wielopolski P, Edelman RR. Identification and characterization of the ischemic penumbra of acute human stroke using echo planar diffusion and perfusion imaging. In: *Abstracts of the Proceedings of the Society of Magnetic Resonance in Medicine.* Berkeley, CA: Society of Magnetic Resonance in Medicine; 1993:249.
93. LeBihan D, Breton E, Lallemand D, Grenier P, Cabanis E, Laval-Jeantet M. MRI of intravoxel incoherent motions: applications to diffusion and perfusion in neurologic disorders. *Radiology* 1986; 161:401–407.

94. Moseley ME, Kucharczyk J, Mintorovitich J, et al. Diffusion-weighted MRI of acute stroke: correlation with T2-weighted and magnetic susceptibility-enhanced MRI in cats. *AJNR* 1990;11: 423–429.
95. Moseley ME, Kucharczyk J, Mintorovitich J, et al. Early detection of regional cerebral ischemia in cats: comparison of diffusion and T2-weighted MRI and spectroscopy. *Magn Reson Med* 1990;14:330–346.
96. Minematsu K, Li L, Fisher M, Sotak CH, Davis MA, Fiandaca MS. Diffusion-weighted magnetic resonance imaging: rapid and quantitative detection of focal brain ischemia. *Neurology* 1992; 42:235–240.
97. Minematsu K, Li L, Sotak CH, Davis MA, Fisher M. Reversible focal ischemic injury demonstrated by diffusion-weighted magnetic resonance imaging in rats. *Stroke* 1992;23:1304–1311.
98. Dardzinski BJ, Sotak CH, Fisher M, Hasegawa Y, Li L, Minematsu K. Apparent diffusion coefficient mapping of experimental focal cerebral ischemia using diffusion-weighted echo-planar imaging. *Magn Reson Med* 1993;30:318–325.
99. Quast MJ, Huang NC, Hillman GR, Kent TA. The evolution of acute stroke recorded by multimodal magnetic resonance imaging. *Magn Reson Imaging* 1993;11:465–471.
100. Mintorovitch J, Moseley ME, Chileuitt L, Shimizu H, Cohen Y, Weinstein PR. Comparison of diffusion- and T2-weighted MRI for the early detection of cerebral ischemia and reperfusion in rats. *Magn Reson Med* 1991;18:39–50.
101. Takahashi M, Fritz-Zieroth B, Chikugo T, Ogawa H. Differentiation of chronic lesions after stroke in stroke-prone spontaneously hypertensive rats using diffusion weighted MRI. *Magn Reson Med* 1993;30:485–488.
102. Warach S, Chien D, Li W, Ronthal M, Edelman RR. Fast magnetic resonance diffusion-weighted imaging of acute human stroke. *Neurology* 1992;42:1717–1723.
103. Chien D, Kwong KK, Gress DR, Buonanno FS, Buxton RB, Rosen BR. MR diffusion imaging of cerebral infarction in humans. *AJNR* 1992;13:1097–1102.
104. LeBihan D, Breton E, Hallemand D, et al. Separation of diffusion and perfusion in intravoxel incoherent motion MRI. *Radiology* 1988;168:497–505.
105. Young IR, Hall AS, Bryant DJ, et al. Assessment of brain perfusion with MRI. *J Comput Assist Tomogr* 1988;12:721–727.
106. Hoult D, Busby S, Gadian D, et al. Observation of tissue metabolites using ^{31}P nuclear magnetic resonance. *Nature* 1974;252: 285–287.
107. Petroff O, Prichard J, Alger J, den Hollander J, Shulman R. Cerebral Intracellular pH by ^{31}P nuclear magnetic resonance spectroscopy. *Neurology* 1985;35:781–788.
108. Hope PL, Cady EB, Chu A, Delpy DT, Gardiner RM, Reynolds EOR. Brain metabolism and intracellular pH during ischemia and hypoxia: an in vivo ^{31}P and ^{1}H nuclear magnetic resonance study in the lamb. *J Neurochem* 1987;49:75–82.
109. Komatsumoto S, Mioka S, Greenberg JH, Koshizaki K, Subramanian VH, Chance B, Reivich M. Cerebral energy metabolism measured in vivo by ^{31}P-NMR in middle cerebral artery occlusion in the cat—relation to severity of stroke. *J Cereb Blood Flow Metab* 1987;7:557–562.
110. Levine SR, Helpern JA, Welch KMA, et al. Human focal cerebral ischemia: evaluation of brain pH and energy metabolism with ^{31}P NMR spectroscopy. *Radiology* 1992;185:537–544.
111. Sappey-Marinier D, Hubesch B, Matson GB, Weiner MW. Decreased phosphorus metabolite concentrations and alkalosis in chronic cerebral infarction. *Radiology* 1992;182:29–34.
112. Welch KMA, Helpern JA, Robertson WM, Ewing JR. ^{31}P topical magnetic resonance measurement of high energy phosphates in normal and infarcted brain. *Stroke* 1985;16:151.
113. Bottomley PA, Drayer BP, Smith LS. Chronic adult cerebral infarction studied by phosphorus NMR spectroscopy. *Radiology* 1986;160:763–766.
114. Hanstock CC, Rothman, Prichard JW, Jue T, Shulman RG. Spatially localized ^{1}H NMR spectra of metabolites in the human brain. *Proc Natl Acad Sci USA* 1988;85:1821–1825.
115. Frahm J, Michaelis T, Merboldt K-D, et al. On the N-acetyl methyl resonance in localized ^{1}H NMR spectra of the human brain. *In Vivo NMR Biomed* 1991;4:201–204.
116. Petroff OAC, Prichard JW, Ogino T, Shulman RG. Proton magnetic resonance spectroscopic studies of agonal carbohydrate metabolism in rabbit brain. *Neurology* 1988;38:1569–1574.
117. Monsein LH, Mathews VP, Barker PB, et al. Irreversible regional cerebral ischemia: serial MRI and proton MR spectroscopy in a non-human primate model. *AJNR* 1993;14:963–970.
118. Plum F. What causes infarction in ischemic brain? *Neurology* 1993;33:222–233.
119. Nakada T, Houkin D, Hida K, Kwee IL. Rebound alkalosis and persistent lactate: multinuclear (^{1}H, ^{13}C, ^{31}P) NMR spectroscopic sudies in rats. *Magn Reson Med* 1991;18:9–14.
120. Lotito S, Blondet P, Francois A, et al. Correlation between intracellular pH and lactate levels in the rat brain during potassium cyanide induced metabolism blockade: a combined ^{31}P-^{1}H in vivo nuclear magnetic spectroscopic study. *Neurosci Lett* 1989; 97:91–96.
121. Crockard HA, Gadian DG, Frackowiak, et al. Acute cerebral ischaemia: concurrent changes in CBF, energy metabolites, pH, and lactate measured with hydrogen clearance and ^{31}P and ^{1}H nuclear magnetic resonance spectroscopy. II. Changes dring ischaemia. *J Cereb Blood Flow Metab* 1987;7:394–402.
122. Kucharczyk J, Mintorovitch J, Moseley M, et al. Ischemic brain damage: reduction by sodium-calcium ion channel modulator RS-87476. *Radiology* 1991;179:221–227.
123. Fenstermacher MJ, Narayana PA. Serial proton magnetic resonance spectroscopy of ischemic brain injury in humans. *Invest Radiol* 1990;25:1034–1039.
124. Bruhn H, Frahm J, Gyngell ML, Merboldt KD, Hanicke W, Sauter R. Cerebral metabolism in man after acute stroke: new observations using localized proton NMR spectroscopy. *Magn Reson Med* 1989;9:126–131.
125. Duijn JH, Matson GB, Maudsley AA, Hugg JW, Weiner MW. Human brain infarction: proton MR spectroscopy. *Radiology* 1992;183:711–718.
126. Birken D, Olendorf WH. N-acetyl aspartatic acid: a literature review of a compound prominent in 1H-NMR spectroscopic studies of the brain. *Neurosci Biobehav Rev* 1989;13:23–31.
127. Ford CC, Griffey RH, Matwiyoff NA, Rosenberg GA. Multivoxel ^{1}H-MRS of stroke. *Neurology* 1992;42:1408–1412.
128. Felber SR, Aichner FT, Sauter R, Gerstenbrand F. Combined magnetic resonance imaging and proton magnetic resonance spectroscopy of patients with acute stroke. *Stroke* 1992;23:1106–1110.
129. Gideon P, Henricksen O, Sperling B, Christiansen P, Olsen TK, Jfrgensen HS, Arlien-Sfborg P. Early time course of N-acetylaspartate, creatine and phosphocreatine, and compounds containing choline in the brain after acute stroke. A proton magnetic resonance spectroscopy study. *Stroke* 1992;23:1566–1572.
130. Graham GD, Blamire AM, Rothman DL, et al. Early temporal variation of cerebral metabolites after human stroke. A proton magnetic resonance spectroscopy study. *Stroke* 1993;24:1891–1896.
131. Petroff OAC, Graham GD, Blamire AM, et al. Spectroscopic imaging of stroke in humans: histopathology correlates of spectral changes. *Neurology* 1992;42:1349–1354.
132. Henriksen O, Gideon P, Sperling B, Olsen TK, Jfrgensen HS, Arlien-Sfborg P. Cerebral lactate production and blood flow in acute stroke. *J Magn Reson Imag* 1992;2:511–517.
133. Barker PB, Gillard JH, vanZijl PCM, et al. Acute stroke: evaluation with serial proton MR spectroscopic imaging. *Radiology* 1994;192:723–732.
134. Irino T. Review of the clinical reports about recanalization of occluded cerebral artery (author's translation). *Brain Nerve* 1978; 30:135–151.
135. Radue EW, Moseley IF. Carotid artery occlusion and computed tomography. *Neuroradiology* 1978;17:7–12.
136. Scharrer E. The functional significance of the capillary bed in the brain of the opossum. *Anat Rec* 1939;75:319–322.
137. Hilal SK. Arterial occlusive disease in infants and children. In: Newton TH, Potts DG, eds. *Radiology of the Skull and Brain: Angiography: Specific Disease Processes,* vol. 2, book 4. St. Louis: CV Mosby Co: 1974;2286–2309.
138. Kilgore BB, Fields WS. Arterial occlusive disease in adults. In: Newton TH, Potts DG, eds. *Radiology of the Skull and Brain:*

Angiography: Specific Disease Processes, vol. 2, book 4. St. Louis: CV Mosby Co: 1974;2310–2343.
139. Tedeschi GS. *Neuropathology: Methods and Diagnosis.* Boston: Little, Brown; 1970.
140. Berman SA, Hayman LA, Hinck VC. Correlation of CT cerebral vascular territories with function: anterior cerebral artery. *AJNR* 1980;1:259–263.
141. Percheron G. The anatomy of the arterial supply of the human thalmus and its use for the interpretation of the thalmic vascular pathology. *Z Neurol* 1973;205:1–13.
142. Castaigne P, Lhermitte F, Buge A, Escourolle R, Hauw JJ, Lyon-Caen O. Paramedian thalmic and midbrain infarcts: clinical and neuropathologic study. *Ann Neurol* 1981;10:127–148.
143. Carpenter MB. *Human Neuroanatomy,* 7th ed. (formerly *Strong and Elwyn's Human Neuroanatomy*). Baltimore: Williams and Wilkins; 1976.
144. Lieberman A, Haas WK, Pinto R, et al. Intracranial hemorrhage and infarction in anticoagulated patients with prosthetic heart valves. *Stroke* 1978;9:18–24.
145. Poeck K, Ringelstien EB, Hacke W. *New Trends in Diagnosis and Management of Stroke.* Berlin: Springer–Verlag; 1987.
146. Saito I, Shigeno T, Aritake K, Tanishima T, Sano K. Vasospasm assessed by angiography and computerized tomography. *J Neurosurg* 1979;51:466–475.
147. Adams HP, Love BB. Medical management of aneurysmal subarachnoid hemorrhage. In: Barnett JM, Mohr JP, Stein BM, Yatsu FM, eds. *Stroke.* New York: Churchill Livingstone; 1992: 1029–1055.
148. Amit M, Camfield PR. Neonatal polycythemia causing multiple cerebral infarcts. *Arch Neurol* 1980;37:109–110.
149. Buonanno FS, Cooper MR, Moody DM, Laster DW, Ball MR, Toole JF. Neuroradiologic aspects of cerebral disseminated intravascular coagulation. *AJNR* 1980;1:245–250.
150. Bousser MG, Baron JC, Iba-Zizen MT, Comar D, Cabanis E, Castaigne P. Migrainous cerebral infarction: a tomographic study of CBF and oxygen extraction fraction with the oxygen-15 inhalation technique. *Stroke* 1980;11:145–153.
151. Dorfman LJ, Marshall WH, Enzmann DR. Cerebral infarction and migraine: clinical and radiologic correlations. *Neurology* 1979;29:317.
152. Fisher CM. Capsular infarcts: the underlying vascular lesions. *Arch Neurol* 1979;36:65–73.
153. Nelson RF, Pullicino P, Kendall BE, Marshall J. Computed tomography in patients presenting with lacunar syndromes. *Stroke* 1980;11:256–261.
154. Brown JJ, Hesselink JR, Rothrock JF. MR and CT of lacunar infarcts. *AJR* 1988;151:367–372.
155. Hachinski VC, Potter P, Merskey H. Leuko-araiosis. *Arch Neurol* 1987;44:21–23.
156. Lechner H, Schmidt R, Bertha G, Justich E, Offenbacher H, Schneider G. Nuclear magnetic resonance image white matter lesions and risk factors for stroke. *Stroke* 1988;19:263–265.
157. Barkovich AJ, Kjos BO, Jackson DE. Normal maturation of the neonatal and infant brain: MRI at 1.5T. *Radiology* 1988;166: 173–180.
158. Sze G, DeArmond SJ, Brandt-Zawadski M, et al. Foci of MRI signal (pseudolesions) anterior to the frontal horns: histologic correlations of a normal finding. *AJNR* 1986;7:381–387.
159. Mirowitz S, Sartov K, Gado MG, et al. Focal SI variations in the posterior internal capsule: normal MR findings and distinction from pathologic findings. *Radiology* 1989;172:535–539.
160. Jungreis CA, Kanal E, Hirsch WL, et al. Normal perivascular spaces mimicking lacunar infarction: MRI. *Radiology* 1988;169: 101–104.
161. Moody DM, Bell MA, Challa VR. The corpus callosum, a unique white matter tract: anatomic features that may explain sparing in Binswanger's disease and resistance to flow of fluid masses. *AJNR* 1988;9:1051–1059.
162. Moody DM, Bell MA, Challa VR. Features of the cerebral vascular pattern that predict vulnerability to perfusion or oxygenation deficiency: an anatomic study. *AJNR* 1990;11:431–439.
163. Zeumer H, Schonsky B, Sturm KW. Predominant white matter involvement in subcortical arteriosclerotic encephalopathy (Binswanger disease). *J Comput Assist Tomogr* 1980;4:14–19.
164. Awad IA, Johnson PC, Spetzler RF, et al. Incidental subcortical lesions identified on magnetic resonance imaging in the elderly. II. Post-mortem pathologic correlations. *Stroke* 1986;17:1090–1097.
165. Brun P, Englund E. A white matter disorder in dementia of the Alzheimer's type: a pathoanatomical study. *Ann Neurol* 1986;26: 873–887.
166. Kirkpatrick JB, Hayman LA. White matter lesions of the clinically healthy brains of elderly subjects: possible pathologic basis. *Radiology* 1987;162:509–511.
167. Braffman BH, Zimmerman RA, Trojanowski JQ, et al. Brain MR: pathologic correlation with gross and histopathology. 2. Hyperintense white matter foci in the elderly. *AJNR* 1988;9:629–636.
168. Grafton ST, Sumi SM, Stimac GK, Alvord EC Jr, Shaw C-M, Nochlin D. Comparison of postmortem magnetic resonance imaging and neuropathologic findings in the cerebral white matter. *Arch Neurol* 1991;48:293–298.
169. Munoz DG, Hastak SM, Harper B, Lee D, Hachinski VC. Pathologic correlates of increased signals of the centrum ovale on magnetic resonance imaging. *Arch Neurol* 1993;50:492–497.
170. Hachinski VC, Lassen NA, Marshall J. Multi-infarct dementia: a cause of mental deterioration in the elderly. *Lancet* 1974;2:207–210.
171. Hershey LA, Modic MT, Greenbough PG, Jaffe DF. Magnetic resonance imaging in vascular dementia. *Neurology* 1987;37:29–36.
172. Gonzalez-Scarano F, Lisak RP, Bilaniuk LT, Zimmerman RA, Atkins PC, Sweimann B. Cranial computed tomography in the diagnosis of systemic lupus erythematosus. *Ann Neurol* 1979;5: 158–165.
173. Lavin PJM, Bone I, Lamb JT, Swinburne LM. Intracranial venous thrombosis in the first trimester of pregnancy. *J Neurol Neurosurg* 1978;41:726–729.
174. Palal PM, Palal KP. Cerebrovascular manifestations of infectuous disease. In: *Handbook of Clinical Neurology,* vol. 55. Amsterdam: Elsevier Science Publications; 1989:441–442.
175. Volpe JJ. Neonatal hypoxic-ischemic brain injury. *Pediatr Clin North Am* 1976;23:383–397.
176. McArdle CB, Richardson CJ, Hayden CK, Nicholas DA, Amparo EG. Abnormalities of the neonatal brain: MRI. Part II. Hypoxic-ischemic brain injury. *Radiology* 1987;163:395–403.
177. Keeney SE, Adcock EW, McArdle CB. Prospective observations of 100 high-risk neonates by high-field (1.5 T) magnetic resonance imaging of the CNS. II. Lesions associated with hypoxic-ischemic encephalopathy. *Pediatrics* 1991;87:431–438.
178. Wilson DA, Steiner RE. Periventricular leukomalacia: evaluation with MRI. *Radiology* 1986;160:507–511.
179. Flodmark O, Lupton B, Li D, et al. MRI of periventricular leukomalacia in childhood. *AJNR* 1989;10:111–118.
180. Truwit CL, Barkovich AJ, Kock TK, Ferriero DM. Cerebral palsy: MR findings in 40 patients. *AJNR* 1992;13:67–78.
181. van der Knaap MS, Smit LS, Nauta JJP, Lafeber HN, Valk J. Cortical laminar abnormalities—occurrence and clinical significance. *Neuropediatrics* 1993;24:143–148.
182. Hezgason CM. Blood glucose and stroke. *Stroke* 1988;19(8): 1049–1053.
183. Mohr JP, Hilal SK, Stein BM. AVMs and other vascular anomalies. In: Barnett JM, Mohr JP, Stein BM, Yatsu FM, eds. *Stroke.* New York: Churchill Livingstone; 1992;645–670.
184. Mathews VP, Barker PB, Bryan RN. Magnetic resonance evaluation of stroke. *MRQ* 1992;8(4):245–263.

Magnetic Resonance Imaging of the Brain and Spine, Second Edition, edited by Scott W. Atlas.
Lippincott-Raven Publishers, Philadelphia © 1996.

14

Head Trauma

Lindell R. Gentry

Trauma constitutes one of the most important causes of morbidity and mortality in the modern world (1,2). Thus far, preventive measures have had little impact on the incidence of trauma and are unlikely to do so in the near future (1,2). For this reason, concerted efforts must be made to improve the clinical outcome of each individual patient with head injury. This can only be accomplished if we can more accurately define the true extent of initial brain injury, achieve a better understanding of the different types of traumatic lesions (3–7), and develop more focused and effective means of treatment and rehabilitation.

It is also essential that we expand our abilities to accurately predict final outcome from head injury. In the past we have almost exclusively relied on clinical indicators of injury to provide prognostic information. Diagnostic tests, such as computed tomography (CT), have been of limited value in predicting eventual outcome (8–12). The most widely used clinical indicator of head injury is the Glasgow Coma Scale (GCS) score (13). This score provides an index of injury severity by assessing three aspects of neurologic function: (a) eye opening to external stimuli, (b) motor response to stimuli, and (c) verbal response. An important limitation of this scale is that different types of traumatic lesions can produce similarly low GCS scores (14,15). For example, low GCS scores may be seen with subdural hematomas, epidural hematomas, cortical contusions, intracerebral hematomas, and diffuse axonal injury. Although these patients may have similar GCS scores, their neurologic outcomes may be quite different (14,15).

Until recently, imaging played a small role in efforts to predict the final outcome from head injury. This was primarily due to the low sensitivity of prior diagnostic tests to many types of traumatic lesions (7,15–17). This limitation was significantly diminished, however, with the development of magnetic resonance imaging (MRI) (2–7). More accurate prediction of neurologic outcome is now achievable with a combination of clinical and imaging information than was possible with clinical indicators alone (5–7).

In this chapter I will review the current role of MRI and magnetic resonance angiography (MRA) in evaluating patients with head injury. The capabilities and limitations of CT, MRI, and MRA for imaging these patients will be addressed. The classification, mechanisms, and pertinent clinical features of different types of traumatic lesions will also be reviewed. Important imaging signs that can assist in predicting outcome from head injury will be discussed.

EPIDEMIOLOGY OF HEAD INJURY

The most common cause of death and permanent disability in the first few decades of life is trauma (1,2). The

L. R. Gentry, M.D.: Department of Radiology, Section of Neuroradiology, University of Wisconsin Hospital and Clinics, Madison, WI 53792.

neurologic components of trauma are responsible for the vast majority of these deaths and disabilities. Recent reports have estimated the annual incidence of head injury to be from 0.2 % to 0.3% of the total population per year (2). The incidence of head injury peaks at 550 per 100,000 population for the ages of 15–24 (2). The incidence then declines slightly until the age of 50, when it again starts to increase (2). About 500,000 cases of head injury can be expected to occur in the United States each year (2). Up to 10% of the new cases will be fatal and 20% to 40% will be of at least moderate severity (2). As many as 5% to 10% of those that survive the initial trauma will experience some degree of residual neurologic deficit (2,7).

Head injury mortality rates are estimated at 25 per 100,000 population each year (2,7). Fatal head injuries are four times more common in males than females (2,7). Traffic-related injuries account for 20% to 50% of head injury deaths (2,7). Gunshot wounds to the head are responsible for 20% to 40% of deaths. Falls and nonfirearm assaults account for the majority of the remaining deaths (2,7). Falls typically account for a higher percentage of injuries at both extremes of life. Seventy-five percent of head injuries in preschool children are secondary to falls (2,7). Falls are also responsible for a greater proportion of head injuries in the elderly population. Regrettably, two thirds of all head injury deaths occur prior to hospitalization (2,7). Measures designed to reduce mortality from head injury, therefore, will be unproductive unless preventative actions are also incorporated (7).

RELATIVE ROLES OF IMAGING STUDIES FOR HEAD TRAUMA IMAGING

Remarkable advances have occurred in the past few decades in the management of patients with head injury. CT spearheaded these advances by providing, for the first time, a rapid method for detecting most treatable forms of head injury (18–30). Modern CT scanners can assess a head injury patient in less than 5 minutes, allowing prompt diagnosis of expanding intracranial hematomas and thereby facilitating early surgical intervention (7). The fast examination time, wide availability, lack of contraindications, and high accuracy for detecting hemorrhage have made CT the diagnostic study of choice for initial evaluation of head injury patients (Table 1) (7). This is likely to be true for the immediate future, although MRI is now beginning to contend for this role (3–7,31–59). Factors that limit the more widespread use of MRI as the primary diagnostic study for evaluation of trauma patients are greater cost, lesser availability, slightly longer examination time, greater difficulty of patient monitoring, lower accuracy for detecting fractures, and physician unfamiliarity with the MRI appearance of traumatic lesions (31–47). These limitations have been greatly reduced during the last few years and now offer little impediment to the current use of MRI for evaluating head injury patients (3–6,31–59).

The slightly longer exam time for MRI is currently less of a limitation than it has been in the past (7). While many first generation magnetic resonance (MR) scan-

TABLE 1. *Diagnostic flow chart for evaluation of acute head injury patients*

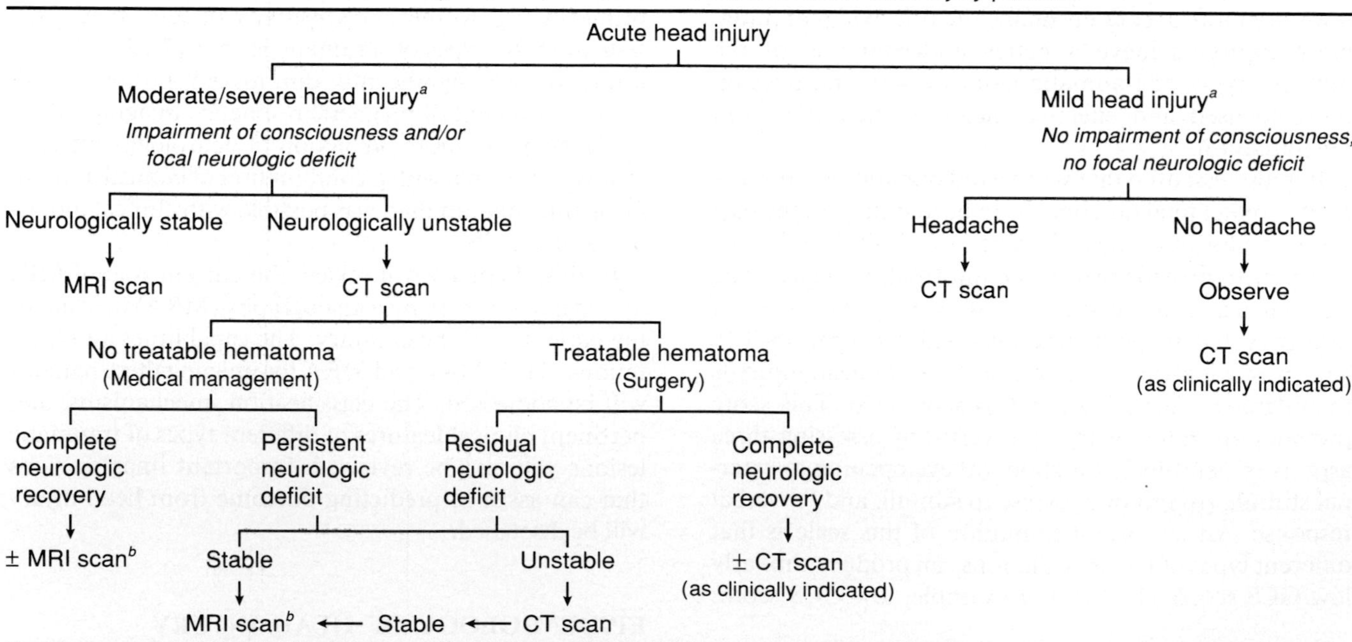

[a] Mild = GCS 13–15; moderate = GCS 8–12; severe = GCS <8.
[b] Within 2 weeks of injury.

ners required at least 10 minutes to acquire even the shortest diagnostic scans, this limitation has been largely overcome by a variety of fast imaging techniques (see Chapter 29). It is currently possible to obtain high quality T1-weighted scans in 2 to 3 minutes using standard short TR/TE spin-echo (SE) techniques (7). Sufficient quality T1-weighted images can be obtained in even less time using gradient-recalled echoes (GRE) (7,51–57). In the proper clinical setting, T1-weighted scans alone are adequate for detecting virtually all significant intracranial hematomas (3,7). Recently, fast spin-echo (FSE) pulse sequences have been developed that allow true proton-density (PD-weighted) and T2-weighted scans to be obtained in 2–3 minutes (Figs. 1 and 2) (7,47). Conventional long TR/TE SE scans of diagnostic quality still require 8–10 minutes to obtain. T2*-weighted GRE scans (Fig. 3) that have an adjunctive role in the evaluation of both acute and chronic trauma can be acquired in less than 2 minutes (48,49). Recently available echoplanar hardware and pulse sequences have made it possible to obtain T2-weighted scans within seconds. Notably, most currently available MR scanners can complete a thorough study of head injury patients in 15 minutes or less (7).

Another major drawback to the use of MRI has been the logistic difficulty of safely imaging severely injured patients in the MRI environment (3–7,45,46). These difficulties have been substantially overcome with the development of self-shielded magnets, wider and more accessible scanning gantries, and a wide range of nonferromagnetic life-support and monitoring devices that are compatible with the MRI environment. The latter has greatly facilitated the evaluation of these critically ill patients (46). Nowadays, every physiologic parameter that might need to be monitored in these patients can be safely monitored (7,46). Sensors for monitoring respiratory rate and effort, invasive or noninvasive blood pressure, arterial oxygen saturation (pulse oximetry), heart rate and rhythm, end-expiratory CO_2 levels, electrocardiographic (ECG) activity, temperature, and intracranial pressure are available (46). Several types of respirators and ventilators that are MRI compatible are also available (46). A complete discussion of this topic is beyond the scope of this article. Kanal and Shellock have recently summarized many important concerns, principles, and techniques regarding patient monitoring in the MRI environment (46).

Now that both CT and MRI are viable diagnostic options, one is faced with a decision as to which examination should be used for the initial evaluation of head injury patients. Although it is best to use an approach tailored to each individual patient, several general guidelines can be provided (Table 1) (7). Neurotrauma patients are usually categorized into three clinical groups,

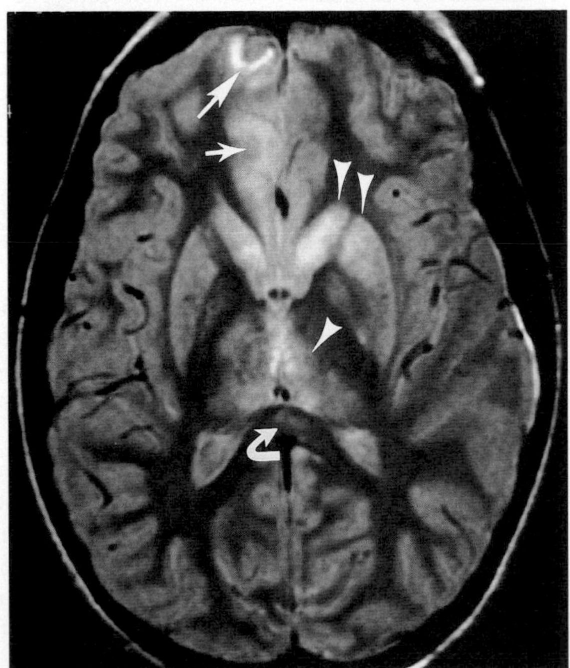

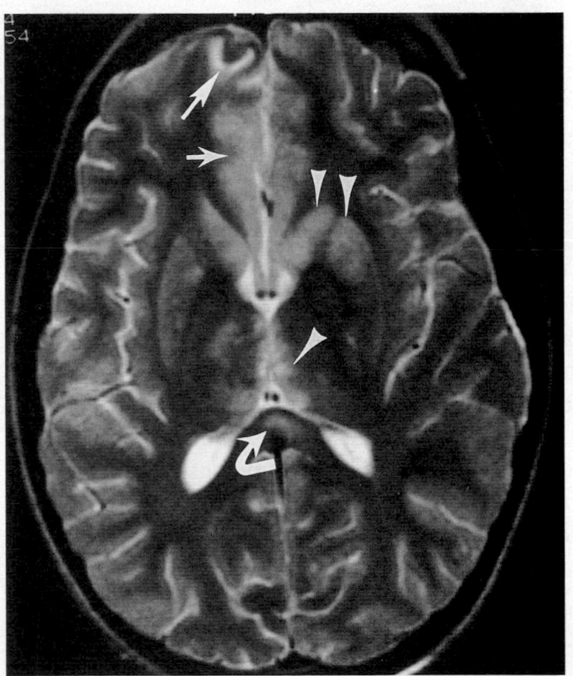

FIG. 1. DAI, anoxic brain injury, anterior cerebral artery infarction. Axial FSE scans in a 25-year-old man obtained 3 days after severe head injury that was accompanied by a period of anoxia. **A:** PD-weighted (TR/TE$_{eff}$ = 2500/18) and **(B)** T2-weighted (TR/TE$_{eff}$ = 2500/90) FSE scans acquired with a scan time of 4.2 minutes reveal areas of DAI in the corpus callosum (*curved arrows*) and frontal white matter (*large arrows*). Also present are widespread areas of anoxic injury (*arrowheads*) in deep gray matter nuclei (caudate, putamen, thalami), as well as bilateral anterior cerebral artery distribution infarctions (*small arrows*).

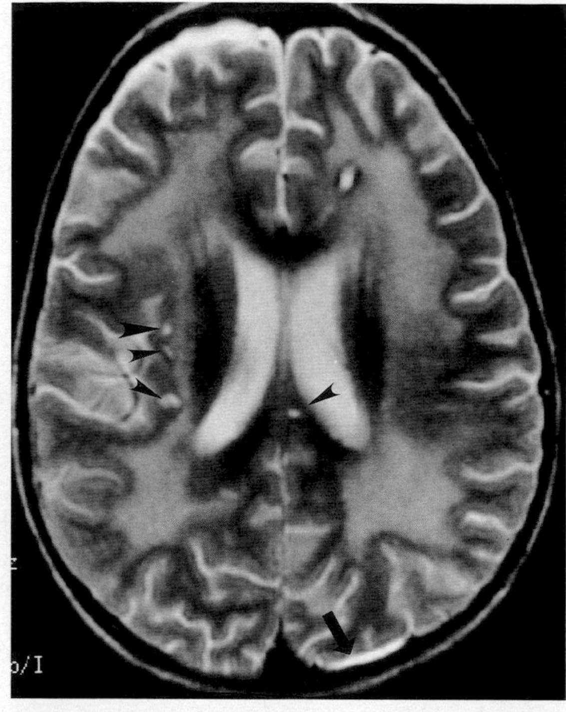

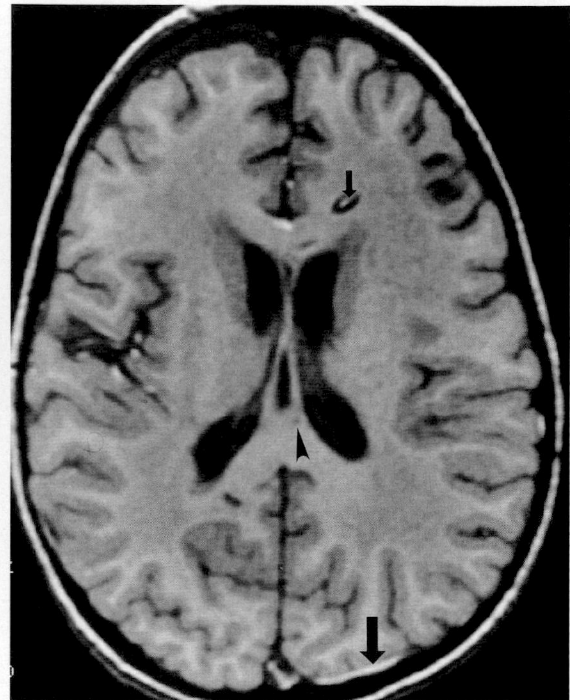

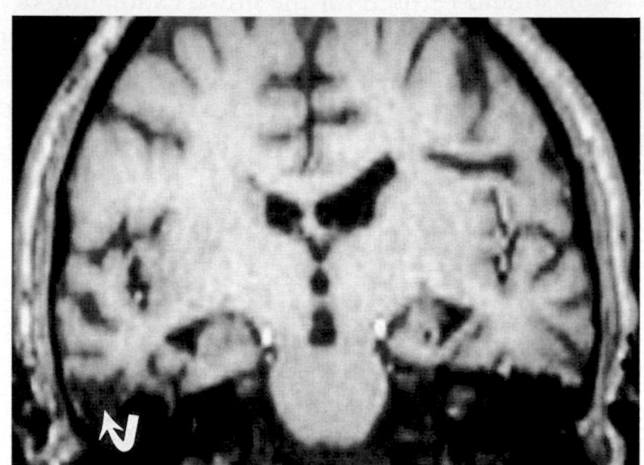

FIG. 2. DAI, cortical contusion, subdural hematoma, posttraumatic hydrocephalus. **A:** Axial T2-weighted (TR/TE_{eff} = 3000/100) FSE. **B:** 3D-volume acquisition SPGR (29/14/35°; 128 partitions, 1.3 mm partition thickness, 11 minute scan time) MR scans obtained on an 18-year-old man 3 weeks after severe head injury. **C:** Coronal reformatted image obtained from the SPGR scan data in B. Numerous small focal DAI lesions (*arrowheads,* A,B) are seen in the corpus callosum and extreme capsule. A small subacute subdural hematoma (*large arrows,* A,B), temporal lobe contusion (*curved arrow*, C), and diffuse white matter edema from posttraumatic hydrocephalus are also present. Also note the high signal intensity of flowing fluid, seen on the flow-sensitive SPGR pulse sequence (B,C), within numerous branches of the middle and posterior cerebral arteries and within a patent shunt catheter (*small arrow*, A).

depending on the degree of impairment of the admission GCS score: 1. mild (GCS = 13–15), 2. moderate (GCS = 8–12), and 3. severe (GCS <8) (7,28–30).

Mild acute head injury patients generally present after head trauma with headaches, slight transient disorientation, or confusion (30). By definition, these patients have little or no persistent impairment of consciousness (30). Some clinicians maintain that mild head injury patients can be safely managed by clinical observation alone without initially obtaining any imaging study (28). Others, however, strongly advocate early diagnostic evaluation (29). Statistically speaking, this group has a low incidence of significant pathology on diagnostic studies (28,29). Specific patients, however, may have traumatic lesions, especially skull fractures and extraparenchymal hematomas (30). They are less likely than those with more severe degrees of injury, however, to have significant intraparenchymal lesions. CT is the most efficacious method for evaluating the lesions most commonly found in this group of patients (Table 1) (7). Skull fractures, extraaxial hematomas, and intracerebral hematomas are accurately detected by CT. Although MRI is slightly more accurate than CT for detecting extraaxial hematomas, those that are missed by CT are usually small and are typically managed in a conservative fashion (7). Small nonhemorrhagic intraaxial lesions [diffuse axonal injury (DAI), contusions] will undoubtedly be missed by CT but these rarely alter the clinical management or outcome of mild head injury patients (28,30).

The moderate and severe head injury categories share many clinical features and management concerns (7). These two groups, therefore, will be considered together. Neurologically unstable patients in these two categories should be initially studied with CT (7). These patients,

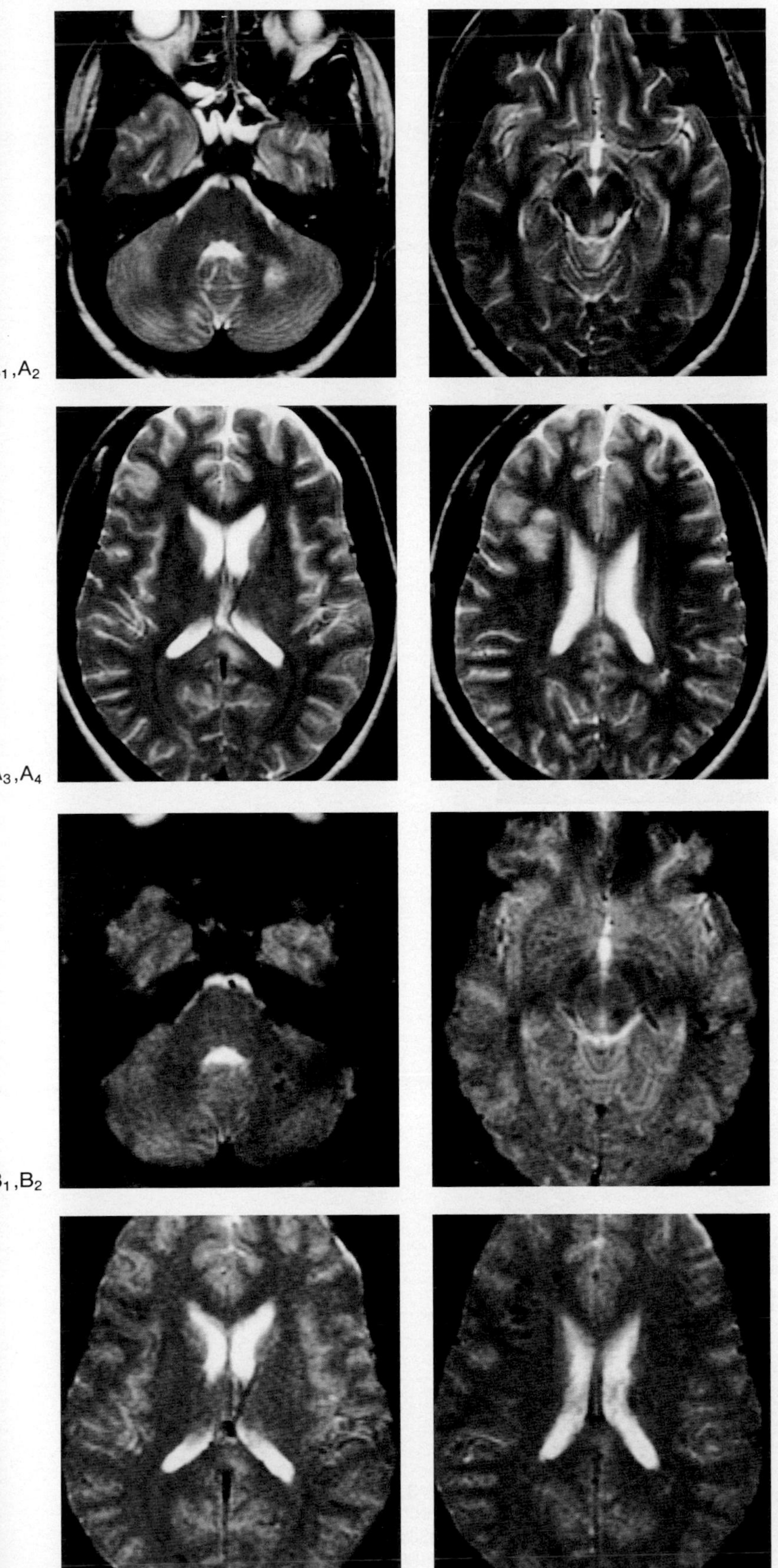

FIG. 3. Extensive DAI with hemorrhage, comparisons of MRI techniques. Acute head trauma, fast spin echo **(A)** versus gradient echo **(B)**. Focal lesions of diffuse axonal injury are clear on fast spin-echo images (A) in deep white matter of left cerebellum, dorsolateral rostral midbrain, splenium of corpus callosum, and deep and subcortical supratentorial white matter. Note demonstration of hypointense hemorrhages in most of these sites as well as in other subcortical (gray-white junction) locations on gradient echo images (B).

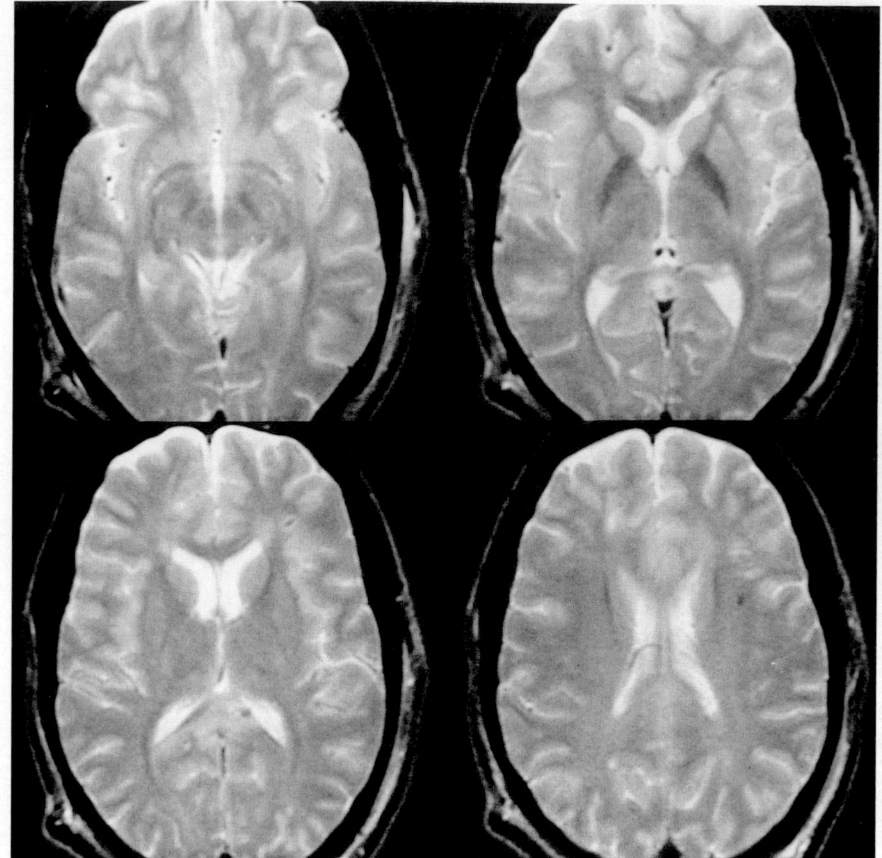
C

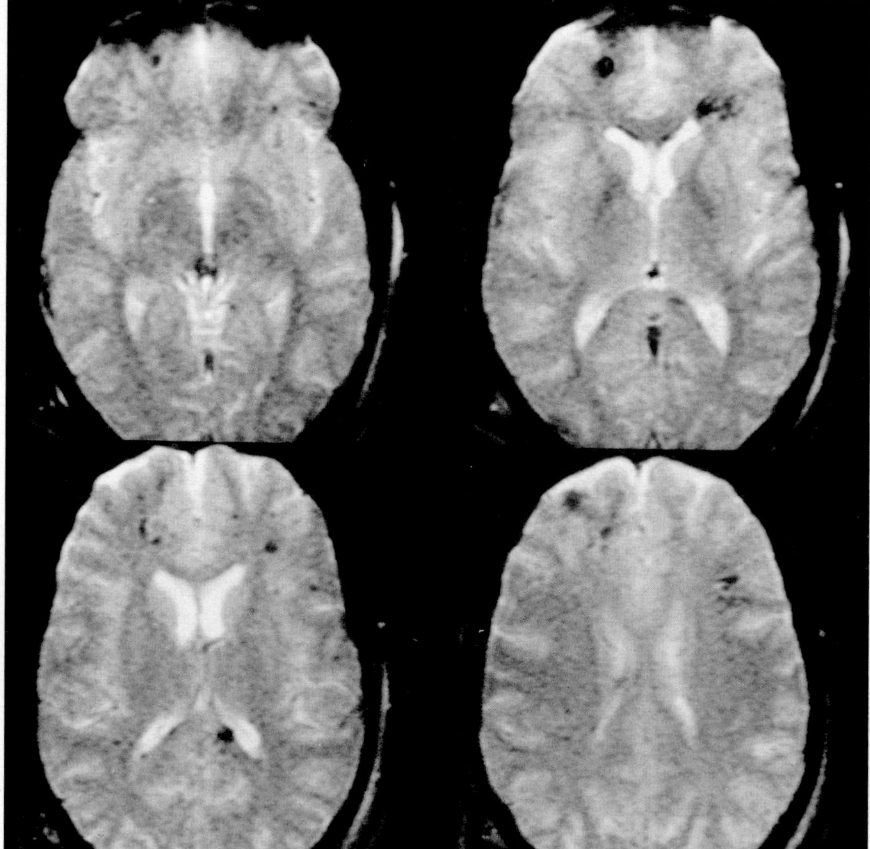
D

FIG. 3. (*Continued.*) Acute head trauma, spin echo **(C)** versus gradient echo **(D)**. High intensity lesions of DAI are seen in typical sites (gray-white junctions, corpus callosum) on spin-echo images (C). Extensive hemorrhages are seen to better advantage on gradient echo images (D).

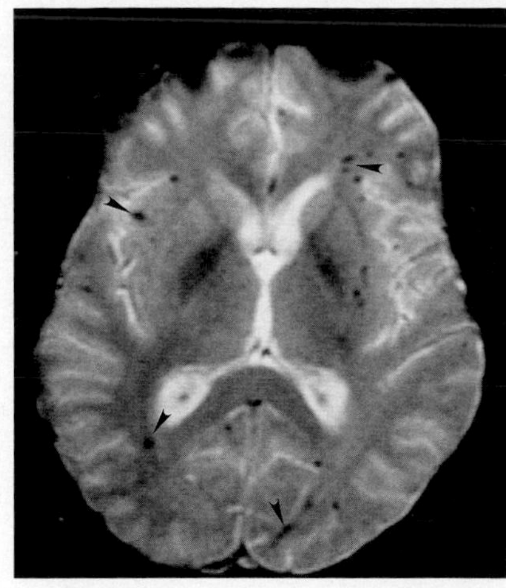

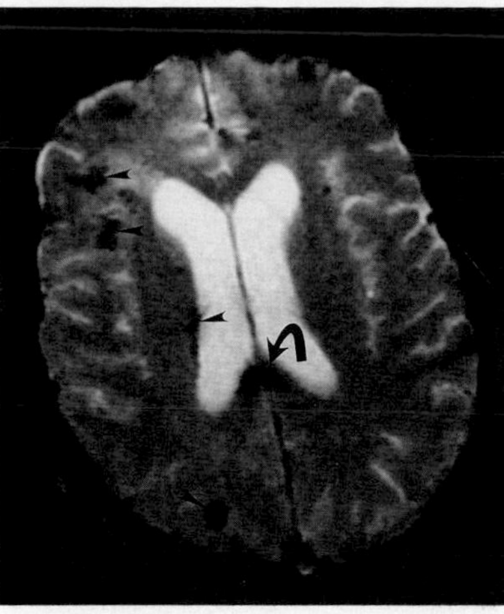

E,F

FIG. 3. (*Continued.*) Remote head trauma (**E,F**). Axial T2*-weighted gradient echo (400/40/10°) scans obtained 3 months after severe head injury demonstrate typical remote sequelae of DAI. Numerous small focal areas of hemosiderin deposition are seen in the splenium of the corpus callosum (*curved arrow*) and deep cerebral white matter (*arrowheads*) at sites of prior shearing injury. Once edema associated with the acute injury has resolved, DAI lesions may be quite indistinct on conventional SE pulses sequences, even at high field strength. T2*-weighted scans, therefore, are essential for evaluating patients with a remote history of head injury.

by definition, already have significant impairment of consciousness and focal neurologic deficits that are deteriorating. The most critical issue in this situation is to rapidly detect potentially treatable hematomas or other surgically correctable lesions (7). Although CT may miss several important types of injuries, it is still the most efficient means of rapidly excluding these lesions (7). Moderate and severe head injury patients who are initially stable can be primarily evaluated by MR (3–7,45). It is advantageous to use MR in these patients, if possible, since it is considerably more sensitive for detecting most traumatic parenchymal and extraparenchymal lesions (3–7,45).

In the opinion of this author all moderate to severe head injury patients should be evaluated with MR at some point in time during the first 2 weeks after injury (Table 1). The full extent of traumatic brain injury will not be fully determined if only CT is used to evaluate this group of patients (3–7,17). MRI is clearly more valuable than CT for assessing the full magnitude of injury (3–7). It also provides more accurate information regarding the expected degree of final neurologic recovery (17). The MRI study can be done as the initial exam in stable patients (3–7,45). In unstable patients, however, it is best to initially study the patients with CT scanning and postpone the MRI exam until they can be safely imaged (7). It is advisable to obtain the MRI study within the first 2 weeks after injury, if possible, since most parenchymal lesions are more visible during this time period. Edema and axoplasmic leakage around areas of neuronal disruption will be maximal during the first 2 weeks, rendering lesions more conspicuous. Smaller lesions will be more difficult to detect over the ensuing weeks as intra- and extracellular edema gradually subsides (7). After the edema does resolve, many traumatic intraaxial lesions may be quite indistinct on CT and standard SE MRI scans (7).

A CT scan is also the study of choice for evaluation of neurologically or hemodynamically unstable patients who have significant impairment of consciousness (Table 1) (7). The most critical issue in this situation is rapid detection of potentially treatable hematomas or other surgically correctable lesions. Although CT may miss several important types of injuries, it is still the most efficient means of excluding treatable hematomas (7). In unstable patients it is unwise to spend even a few extra minutes to obtain MR scans when a CT scan can more quickly and safely answer the urgent questions. Similarly, CT is always the study of choice for evaluation of patients with rapid changes of neurologic status at any point in time after acute head injury (Table 1).

MAGNETIC RESONANCE IMAGING STRATEGIES AND TECHNIQUES

Although seemingly counterintuitive, there are some definite advantages of low- and ultra-low-field systems for examining patients with acute head injury (45). These systems typically offer improved patient access, facilitate better physiologic monitoring, require less modification of existing monitoring and life-support equipment, and reduce the danger associated with bringing ferromagnetic equipment into the scanning room (7,45). Despite these low-field advantages, there are also many benefits of high-field systems for evaluating head injury patients (7). At higher field strength, signal-to-noise (SNR) and contrast-to-noise (CNR) ratios are usually greater for comparable scan times (7). With low-field systems, maintaining a short exam time requires the sacrifice of one or more of the following: SNR, spatial resolution, contrast resolution, slice thickness, and number of scans acquired (7). High-field MR also offers superior detection and characterization of hemorrhage, especially in the acute (deoxyhemoglobin) and chronic (hemosiderin-ferritin) phases (39,48), as well as more specificity in the hyperacute stage (S. W. Atlas, *unpublished data*) (see Chapter 9). Additionally, high-field systems usually provide more homogeneous static magnetic fields and furnish steeper magnetic gradients. These two features help to improve the quality of scans acquired with "fast" GRE pulse sequences without undue magnetic susceptibility artifacts (Figs. 2 and 3) (7,50–57).

The best MR protocol for a specific acute head injury patient will vary, depending upon individual circumstances. The patient's clinical condition must always be of principal concern (7). It may be necessary to delay the MR exam or substitute a CT scan in some patients if they are neurologically unstable (Table 1) (7). When the MR study is performed, it is best to obtain the MR images as rapidly as possible. Generally speaking, however, MR image and exam qualities are inversely related to pulse sequence acquisition time and total MR study time, respectively (7). A judgment must often be made as to how much time can be safely permitted for answering all of the critical questions. An abbreviated exam, tailored to address the most crucial questions in the shortest time possible, may be necessary in some cases (7).

With the above-mentioned considerations in mind, the MR study should be structured so that it can detect all intracranial hematomas, identify nonhemorrhagic forms of injury, provide sufficient anatomic information to classify lesions, guide surgical treatment, and provide an estimation of long-term prognosis (3–7,17). The primary emphasis should be directed at maximizing the sensitivity of the examination since these objectives can only be met if all traumatic lesions are accurately identified. Most traumatic lesions can usually be identified if images are obtained in at least two imaging planes using T1-weighted, PD-weighted, T2-weighted, and T2*-weighted sequences (3–7).

Multiple imaging planes are very beneficial for detection and characterization of traumatic lesions (3–7). For example, superficial lesions are most reliably detected when the imaging plane is perpendicular to the cortical base of the lesion (3). Multiplanar imaging is also helpful for detection of small lesions (e.g., traumatic brainstem lesions) since they may be missed because of partial volume effects or an interslice gap (6). Multiple planes are also essential for determining the exact location of traumatic lesions. Precise localization is necessary for accurate classification of lesions, which, in turn, has great impact on defining the long-term prognosis (17). For example, it can be quite difficult with only one plane of imaging to determine whether a small lesion close to the cortical surface of the brain is a cortical contusion or a peripheral DAI lesion. Only when the imaging plane is perpendicular to the adjacent calvarium can this be reliably established. It is desirable to have both T1-weighted and T2-weighted scans in at least two perpendicular planes for precisely localizing and classifying traumatic lesions. Since this is rarely possible because of time constraints, a reasonable compromise is a study composed of T2-weighted scans in one plane (axial or coronal) and T1-weighted scans in two planes. It is usually best to obtain the T1-weighted scans both perpendicular to and in the same plane as the T2-weighted scans (2–7).

The visibility of a lesion on a particular pulse sequence is influenced by a number of factors: lesion size and location, presence and age of hemorrhage, presence of edema, and MR acquisition parameters (3). The most important factor that affects lesion visibility is the MR pulse sequence that is utilized (3). Overall, PD-weighted and T2-weighted SE scans are most sensitive for detecting traumatic lesions across the whole time course of injury (3–7). This is especially true for nonhemorrhagic lesions. In several double-blind studies, T2-weighted scans (2000–2300/80–100) were found to be most effective for initial detection of both hemorrhagic and nonhemorrhagic lesions (3–6,45). In one study, T2-weighted SE scans detected 93% of nonhemorrhagic and 93% of hemorrhagic lesions as compared with T1-weighted scans (68% and 87%) and CT scans (18% and 90%), respectively (3). PD-weighted and T2-weighted conventional SE images, therefore, are sufficient for detection and categorization of most traumatic nonhemorrhagic intraaxial lesions.

More recently it has become possible to obtain T2-weighted and PD-weighted scans using recently developed rapid spin-echo techniques, such as FSE (Figs. 1 and 2) (7,47). The FSE pulse sequence allows images with true proton-density and T2 weighting to be obtained in a fraction of the time required for conventional SE techniques and can be implemented on conventional scanners (7,47) (see Chapter 29) Since FSE utilizes rf refocusing pulses to generate echoes, true T2 contrast is maintained (7,47). The FSE sequence, therefore, is less prone to magnetic susceptibility-induced artifacts when compared with T2*-weighted GRE sequences that use gradient-refocusing to generate echoes (7,47). This can be disadvantageous in the case of traumatic brain injury, however, where it is desirable to identify hematomas by their distinctive areas of susceptibility-induced hypointensity arising from paramagnetic iron (Fig. 3) (7,47).

Accurate detection of hemorrhage also constitutes an important aspect of trauma imaging. MR was initially thought to be insensitive for detection of some hematomas. As more experience was gained with the MR appearance of hemorrhage, however, it became apparent that MR was extremely sensitive to hemorrhage throughout all stages of its evolution (3,39). The sensitivity of different MR pulse sequences to hemorrhage does vary with the age of the hematoma and the specific biochemical nature of the hemoglobin (39), as well as a variety of intrinsic and operator-dependent factors. The reader is referred to Chapter 9, where the temporal MR appearance of hemorrhage is discussed in greater detail.

Briefly, however, hyperacute hematomas less than 4–6 hours of age will, for simplicity's sake, be considered to be primarily composed of hemoglobin that is in a fully oxygenated state (oxyhemoglobin) (39). Oxyhemoglobin is diamagnetic and therefore (unlike deoxyhemoglobin, methemoglobin, and chronic iron storage forms such as hemosiderin) does not produce significant shortening of the T1, T2, or T2* relaxation times (39). Hyperacute hematomas, therefore, may have signal intensities that are quite similar to that of adjacent brain parenchyma or any nonparamagnetic lesion on all MR pulse sequences (39). It was initially thought that MRI might not be able to detect these relatively isointense lesions. It is now clear that few significant hyperacute hematomas will be overlooked if MR images are acquired with T1-weighted, T2-weighted, PD-weighted, and T2*-weighted sequences (3,7). Invariably there is enough anatomic distortion, perifocal edema, and MR signal intensity difference between hyperacute hematomas and brain parenchyma to allow their recognition (3,7). Moreover, it appears that hyperacute hematomas on high-field MR have a characteristic rim of marked hypointensity on T2-weighted images, which has been postulated to represent marginal hematoma deoxygenation (S. W. Atlas, *unpublished data*).

The acute stage of a hematoma begins with the conversion of oxyhemoglobin to deoxyhemoglobin (39). This usually begins at 4 to 6 hours after the bleed and last for 3 to 7 days, depending on the size of the hematoma (3,7,39). The most efficacious MR pulse sequences for detection of hematomas in the deoxyhemoglobin stage are those that are strongly T2-weighted (3,7,39). At high field strength, many radiologists believe that T2-weighted SE scans are satisfactory for this purpose (7,39,48), although T2*-weighted GRE scans do offer higher sensitivity for acute and remote hemorrhage, even at high field (Fig. 3). The conspicuity of susceptibility-induced hypointensity on T2-weighted spin-echo scans, however, is significantly less at lower field strength (39). T2* relaxation effects are known to be inversely related to the square of the strength of the main magnetic field (39). It is especially important, therefore, to augment conventional T2-weighted SE scans with T2*-weighted GRE scans when imaging trauma patients with a low or ultra-low field strength MR system (7,39,48).

Subacute hematomas result when the deoxyhemoglobin is further metabolized (oxidized) into methemoglobin (3,7,39). Methemoglobin typically begins to appear at the periphery of a hematoma at 2 to 3 days postinjury (39). It then gradually fills in the remainder of the hematoma over the next few days (39). Some methemoglobin usually persists within a hematoma for at least 2 to 3 months after trauma, especially in larger lesions (39). Methemoglobin-containing hematomas will have a very high signal intensity on T1-weighted MR pulse sequences. Either conventional spin-echo, inversion recovery, or GRE techniques can be used to provide strongly T1-weighted images (7), which are the most sensitive for detection of these subacute hematomas (Fig. 2) (3). The relative advantages and disadvantages of each of these pulse sequences for imaging trauma patients have been previously discussed by Gentry (7) and will be summarized later in this chapter.

Chronic hematomas arise several months after injury as the methemoglobin within the lesion is further metabolized and partially converted into hemosiderin (39). Iron storage forms, including hemosiderin and ferritin, are then engulfed by phagocytic cells at the periphery of the resolving hematoma (39). This results in a variably sized, primarily cystic central cleft with a peripheral rim composed of iron-laden phagocytic cells (39). The disappearance of methemoglobin from the hematoma coincides with a loss of hyperintensity on T1-weighted pulse sequences (39). At this point, strongly T2-weighted or T2*-weighted pulse sequences again become most sensitive for detecting the blood products (7,48–50). Conventional T2-weighted SE scans at high field strength will often reveal these foci of hemosiderin deposition as faint areas of susceptibility-induced signal loss (39). Hemosiderin may be much less apparent or even invisible on T2-weighted SE images at low field strength, however (39). The sensitivity of conventional T2-weighted SE scans to hemosiderin can be improved by using relatively long TR (>3500) and TE (>100) times at both high- and low-field strengths (39). T2*-weighted GRE scans are even more helpful for detecting areas of hemosiderin deposition (Fig. 3) (7,48–50). These scans are considerably more sensitive than T2-weighted SE scans for detecting areas of remote hemorrhage at high field and are important for detecting hemosiderin at low- to intermediate-field (<0.5 Tesla) strength (7,48–50).

Importantly, MRI is much more sensitive and specific than CT for detecting and characterizing traumatic hemorrhage that is more than 2 weeks of age. Although the hyperdensity of the blood will disappear on CT scans after 1 to 2 weeks, the specificity of MR for blood products will persist for a much longer period of time (7). Methemoglobin is usually visible on T1-weighted scans for several months after a bleed and hemosiderin staining may be detectable on T2*-weighted scans for several years (3–6,39,48). This can be particularly important when evaluating nonaccidental injury in children since MRI will be more specific for a much longer time after trauma than will CT (7,58–59).

T1-weighted images obtained with a short TR, short TE conventional SE pulse sequence are usually sufficient for evaluation of most pathologic processes in the central nervous system. This author has found that strongly T1-weighted images, however, are especially useful for evaluation of patients with head injury (2–7). They are particularly beneficial for detection of traumatic lesions in the corpus callosum, deep cerebral white matter, and brainstem (5–7). The conspicuity of nonhemorrhagic lesions in these areas is often much better on strongly T1-weighted scans than on T2-weighted scans (2–7). Improved T1 contrast also provides better visualization of paramagnetic forms of iron (methemoglobin) that shorten T1 relaxation. Images with enhanced T1 contrast can be obtained with either inversion recovery (IR) (TR/TI/TE = 2100/600/30) or strongly T1-weighted GRE (MP-RAGE, FLASH, SPGR) pulse sequences (Fig. 2) (7). Inversion recovery has been effectively used for this purpose at some centers (3–7).

Superb T1 contrast can also be achieved on many MR systems with relatively short imaging times using T1-weighted GRE (7,51–54). The various manufacturers use different acronyms to describe comparable pulse sequences based on quite similar principles (SPGR, FLASH, RF-FAST, etc.) (Fig. 2). In general, these pulse sequences combine extremely short TR intervals (TR <10–30) and echo formation using GRE techniques (7,51–54). This combination, in turn, makes it practical to acquire the scan data as a three-dimensional (3D) volume set. This is advantageous in that SNR is markedly improved over two-dimensional (2D) techniques, smaller section thicknesses are possible, and the 3D data can be retrospectively reformatted in any plane; provided that small partition thicknesses are utilized (7,51–54). A very short TE interval serves to reduce T2 relaxation effects and improves T1 tissue contrast. The short TE also helps to minimize magnetic susceptibility artifacts (7,51–54). The resultant T1 contrast obtainable with these images is superior to that possible with conventional SE techniques and is quite comparable to that found with IR, but images are acquired in much shorter scan times. Excessive patient motion can seriously impair image quality when using 3D acquisitions because of the relatively longer scan times inherently accompanying these sequences (7). As would be expected, this can be a significant drawback in uncooperative patients.

Magnetization-prepared rapid gradient-echo (e.g., MP-RAGE) imaging is a recently introduced method for rapidly achieving superb T1 contrast resolution (7,55–57). The MP-RAGE sequence utilizes a preparatory 180° rf pulse to invert the spins in a manner quite similar to an IR sequence (7,55–57). Small flip angles and gradient-refocused echoes allow for the use of much shorter TR (TR <8–10 msec) and TE times than can be used with conventional IR. The short TR time, in turn, makes it feasible to utilize 3D volume acquisitions. The MP-RAGE sequence is very similar to the SPGR sequence with regard to its benefits, limitations, and image characteristics (7) (these and other GRE pulse sequences are more fully described Chapter 29).

MRA has become another important diagnostic tool for the evaluation of vascular pathologies of the central nervous system (see Chapter 31). The current role of MRA for evaluation of traumatic vascular injury, however, will be covered later in this chapter.

GENERAL MECHANISMS OF INJURY

Holbourn's early pioneering work concerning the mechanisms of head injury has served as a fundamental basis for understanding the means by which traumatic stresses produce cerebral injury (Fig. 4) (60,61). Using a gelatin model of the brain, he concluded that injury to the brain occurred through two major mechanisms: (a) direct injuries due to skull distortion (contact phenomenon) and (b) indirect injuries that arise irrespective of skull deformation. The former is produced by localized fracture or inbending of the skull with direct injury to adjacent brain parenchyma. Neural damage, therefore, is typically superficial and localized to the immediate vicinity of the calvarial injury. Examples of lesions caused by this mechanism are cortical lacerations due to depressed fracture fragments and epidural hematomas secondary to lacerations of meningeal arteries.

The second mechanism operates irrespective of skull deformation and, in fact, may produce extensive neural damage, even in the absence of a direct blow to the head. Holbourn (60,61) emphasized that neural injuries by indirect mechanisms could be produced only through two types of structural deformations. *Compression-rarefaction strain* is characterized by a change in cell volume without a change in shape and is of minimal importance in the production of cerebral injury. Neurons are highly resistant to injury by compression-rarefaction strain due to their innate noncompressibility. Injuries due to compression-rarefaction strain have been postulated by some authors, but, as Holbourn points out, the magnitude of force required to injure the brain through deformations of this type greatly exceeds that generated by even the most severe blows. For this reason, the terms *coup* and *contracoup* injuries are quite misleading and should be discarded since they incorrectly imply injury by compression-rarefaction strain (60,61).

Shear-strain deformation is characterized by a change in shape without a change in volume and is responsible for the vast majority of mechanically induced lesions. Because of their inherently low rigidity, neurons are extremely susceptible to shear-strain deformations. These shear-strains develop because of differential movements of one portion of the brain with respect to another. Shear-strain forces are greatest at the junction of tissues of different density and rigidity (cerebrospinal fluid [CSF]/brain, gray/white matter, brain/pia-arachnoid, pia-arachnoid/dura, skull/dura). As Holbourn points out (60,61), only four possible types of forces can produce shear-strain deformation (linear/rotational acceleration, centrifugal/Coriolis forces). Of these four, only linear and rotational acceleration are of sufficient magnitude to produce neuronal injury. Furthermore, rotational acceleration plays a much more important role than linear acceleration in the production of cerebral in-

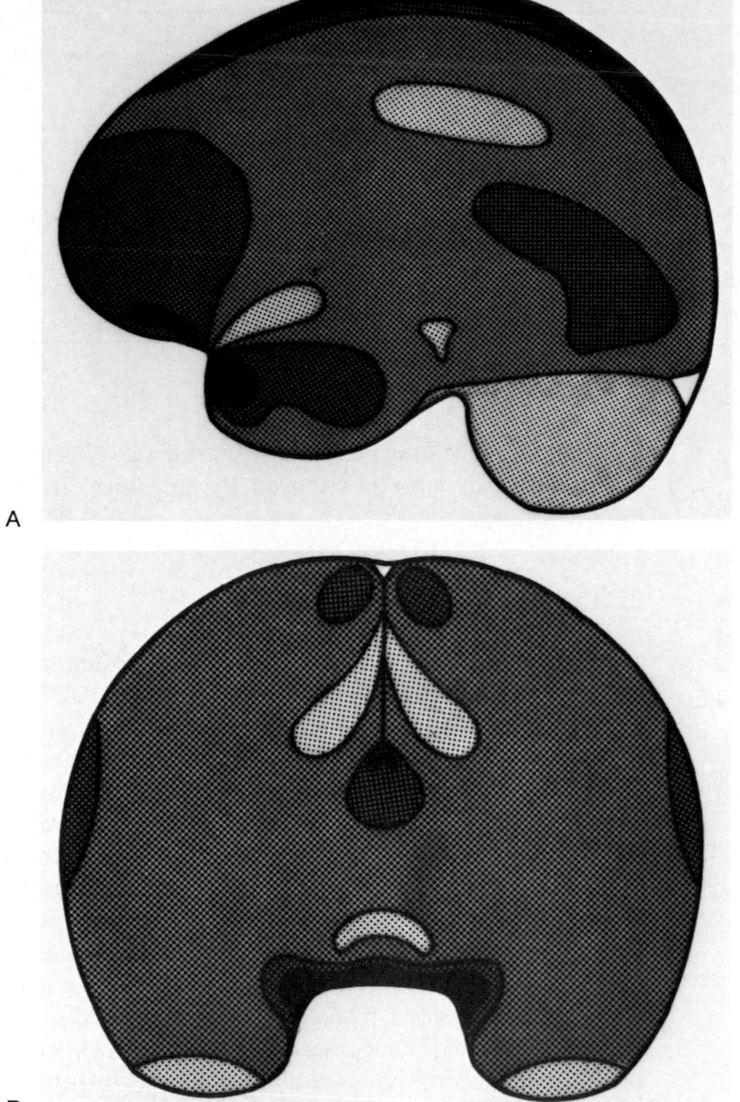

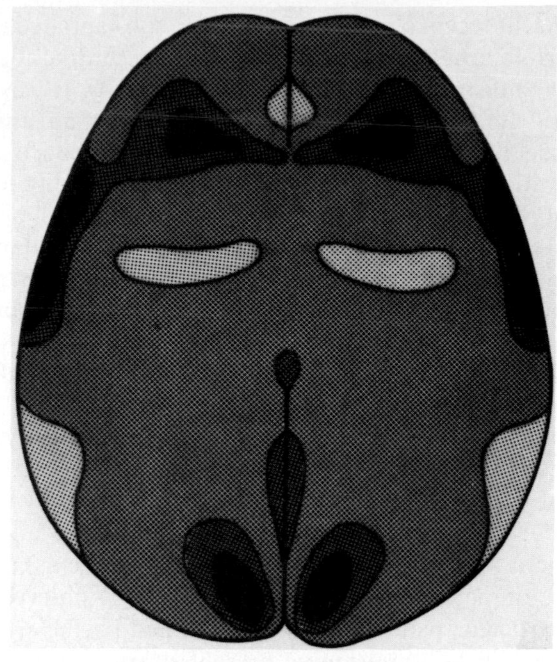

FIG. 4. Theoretical distribution of shear-strain forces during rotational acceleration of the head. Holbourn has experimentally mapped the locations of maximum shear-strain force during rotational acceleration of the head in the **(A)** sagittal, **(B)** coronal, and **(C)** axial planes (60). A greater frequency of rotationally induced traumatic lesions is to be anticipated in the more highly susceptible, darkly shaded regions. (Adapted from Holbourn, ref. 60, and reprinted from Gentry et al., ref. 4, with permission.)

juries. Lesions from the latter tend to be limited to subdural hematomas and small superficial contusions (60,61).

Unlike traumatic lesions from contact phenomenon, rotationally induced shear-strain lesions are typically widespread (bilateral and multiple), can occur remote from the site of impact, and may be either superficially or deeply situated (Figs. 3–7) (60,61). The location of lesions produced by this mechanism, as would be expected, closely corresponds to the locations of maximum shear-strains that develop during rotational acceleration of the head. The expected anatomic distribution has been experimentally mapped by Holbourn (60,61) for the three orthogonal planes of rotation using a gelatin brain model (Fig. 4). Despite the limitations of this model, the distribution of traumatic lesions in fatal head injuries and animal trauma models has generally followed Holbourn's theoretical predictions. The *location* of rotationally induced shear-strain lesions is primarily *dependent* on the plane of rotation and is *independent* of the direction of rotation within a given plane. The *location* of maximum shear-strain is also *independent* of the distance from the center of rotation, the arc of rotation, and the duration and intensity of the force. The *magnitude* of shear-strain deformation is *dependent* upon these factors, however. Figure 4 illustrates the location of maximum shear-strain for all three orthogonal planes of rotation (60,61).

For a number of years Holbourn's classic work went ignored. Strich was the first to recognize the significance of Holbourn's observations with the publication of a pathologic description of shearing injuries of the white matter (62,63). Most of Holbourn's observations have also been supported by other postmortem studies (64–

70). Our recent clinical series has also substantiated most of Holbourn's theoretical predictions regarding the expected distribution of traumatic lesions (4). It was not until Gennarelli et al. (71,72) developed an animal model of cranial trauma, however, that Holbourn's observations were experimentally confirmed. In an important series of experiments using a primate model of cranial trauma, these authors have confirmed that all of the major types of traumatic lesions can be reproduced by nonimpact inertial loading of the head in an appropriate manner (71,72). The exact nature of the resulting injury will depend upon the type (angular, linear), rate, duration, and plane of head acceleration.

Rotationally induced shear-strain injury typically produces lesions at one of four topographical levels: (a) cortical surface of brain (contusions), (b) cerebral white matter (diffuse axonal injury), (c) brainstem, and (d) penetrating blood vessels (arteries or veins). The predominate types of lesions that will be observed in a particular patient will be determined by the specific mechanical circumstances present during trauma. Although neurons are the most susceptible tissue to rotationally induced shear-strain deformations, nonneuronal tissues (penetrating blood vessels, bridging veins, pia-arachnoid) may also be injured by this mechanism (60,61).

TABLE 2. *Classification of traumatic intracranial lesions*[a]

- A. Primary lesions
  - 1. Primary neuronal injuries
    - a. Diffuse axonal injury
    - b. Cortical contusion
    - c. Subcortical gray matter injury
    - d. Primary brainstem injury
  - 2. Primary hemorrhages
    - a. Epidural hematoma
      - Arterial origin
      - Venous origin
    - b. Subdural hematoma
    - c. Intracerebral hematoma
    - d. Intraventricular hemorrhage
    - e. Subarachnoid hemorrhage
  - 3. Primary vascular injuries
    - a. Carotid-cavernous fistula
    - b. Arterial pseudoaneurysm
    - c. Arterial dissection/laceration/occlusion
    - d. Carotid sheath hematoma
    - e. Dural sinus laceration/occlusion
  - 4. Traumatic pia-arachnoid injuries
    - a. Post-traumatic arachnoid cyst
    - b. Subdural hygromas
  - 5. Cranial nerve injuries
- B. Secondary lesions
  - 1. Territorial arterial infarction
  - 2. Boundary and terminal zone infarction
  - 3. Diffuse hypoxic injury
  - 4. Diffuse brain swelling/edema
  - 5. Pressure necrosis (due to brain displacement and herniation)
  - 6. Secondary brainstem injury
  - 7. Secondary hemorrhage
  - 8. Other (e.g., fatty embolism, infection)

[a] Modified from Gentry et al, ref. 4.

TABLE 3. *Classification of traumatic brainstem injury*[a]

- I. Primary brainstem injury
  - A. Direct superficial laceration or contusion
  - B. Diffuse axonal injury
  - C. Multiple primary petechial hemorrhages
  - D. Pontomedullary rent or separation
- II. Secondary brainstem injury
  - A. Secondary (Duret) hemorrhages
  - B. Focal brainstem infarcts from vascular compromise
  - C. Compression, displacement, and deformity
  - D. Pressure necrosis from transtentorial herniation
  - E. Diffuse hypoxic/anoxic/ischemic injury
- III. Combined primary and secondary brainstem injury

[a] Modified from Gentry et al., ref. 6.

CLASSIFICATION

A variety of classification systems for head injury have been proposed (Tables 2 and 3) (4–7,15,60,61,64–72). Despite some differences, most authors are in agreement that two basic types of traumatic lesions exist. *Primary lesions* are those that arise as a direct result of the initial traumatic force. *Secondary lesions* are those that develop subsequent to initial impact. The latter either arise from sequelae of primary lesions or from the neurologic effects of systemic injuries. The distinction between primary and secondary lesions is not merely an academic one but one that has great therapeutic ramifications (4–7,17,64–70). Secondary lesions, by definition, are potentially preventable, provided that causative factors are quickly recognized and appropriate treatment promptly instituted. The neurologic effects of primary lesions, however, may or may not be treatable, depending on the type of lesion. Extraaxial hematomas often show dramatic response to treatment while intraaxial lesions generally are not reversible.

Over the last three decades there have been significant improvements in the mortality and morbidity rates for patients with traumatic brain injury. These advances can be traced to a simultaneous refinement in our ability to accurately distinguish between different types of lesions and to provide specific treatment for each type. The development and widespread use of CT (8–16,18–30) and MRI (3–6,17,31–59) has led to earlier detection and treatment of curable lesions and more focused therapy in patients with nonreversible lesions to minimize the development of secondary lesions. The evolution of uniform, reproducible classification systems has greatly facilitated improvements in patient care (Tables 2 and 3).

Virtually all primary traumatic intraaxial lesions arise as a result of shear-strain deformation of either neurons or blood vessels produced by rotational acceleration of the head (60,61). Since most primary neuronal lesions are produced by the same type of deformation and differ only by their location, it seems most valid to base their classification on the latter point (Tables 2 and 3) (4,17). Primary intraaxial lesions clearly fit into four anatomically well-defined categories: (a) diffuse axonal injury, (b) cortical contusion, (c) subcortical gray matter injury, and (d) brainstem injury (3–7,17). This method of classification is applicable to both radiologic imaging and pathologic analysis and avoids imprecise nomenclature (e.g., coup/contrecoup, gliding contusion, etc.).

CT has never been particularly useful for classification and staging of injury (4–17,65,71). Its low sensitivity for nonhemorrhagic lesions and the difficulty of obtaining multiplanar images has severely limited its usefulness (3–6,17). MRI offers distinct advantages over CT for classification of traumatic cerebral lesions. Firstly, more lesions can be classified with MRI than with CT because of its much higher sensitivity (3–6,17,35–38,40–44). Also, the ability of MRI to obtain images in multiple planes is particularly beneficial since this allows more reliable localization and classification of the lesions (4).

There is little difficulty using the classification scheme in Tables 2 and 3 in separating the various types of primary lesions, since the anatomic location of each type of lesion is distinctive (4). One may encounter some difficulty in distinguishing primary and secondary lesions, since both types are often found in the same locations (3–6). This problem, however, is not unique to MRI since it is not always possible to make this distinction, even at autopsy (60–70). Despite these problems, MRI distinction between primary and secondary lesions can generally be made on the basis of lesion size, shape, location, and distribution, and in conjunction with the timing of when the lesions first appeared.

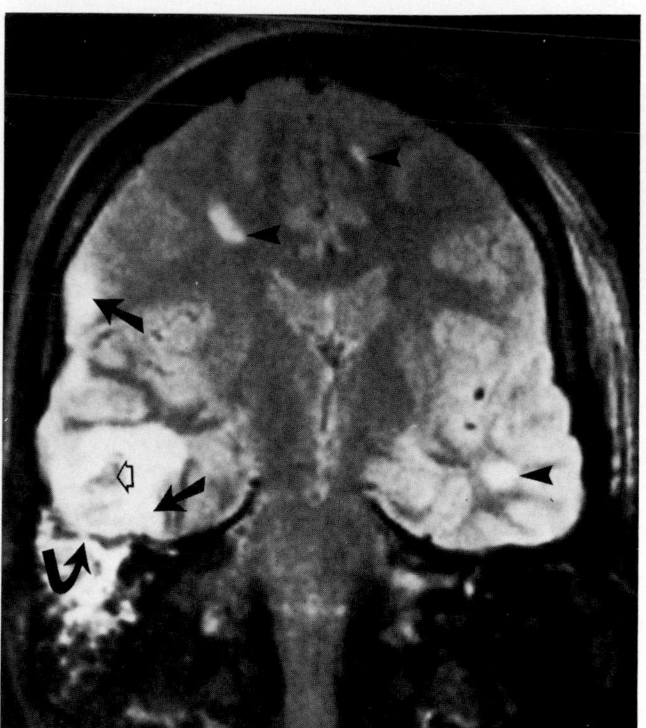

FIG. 5. DAI and cortical contusion. A coronal T2-weighted (2300/80) image reveals the typical MR appearances of deep white matter DAI and cortical contusion. Cortical contusions (*arrows*), by definition, primarily affect cortical gray matter and always extend to the surface of the brain. Areas of hemorrhage (*open arrow*) can often be seen within larger nonhemorrhagic zones of contusion. Lobar white matter DAI lesions (*arrowheads*), on the other hand, always spare the overlying cortex. They are often found in the deep white matter of the frontal and temporal lobes, especially at the corticomedullary junction. DAI lesions are usually nonhemorrhagic and tend to be ovoid in shape. Note the fracture of the tegmen antri of the temporal bone (*curved arrow*), which was responsible for CSF otorrhea. (From Gentry et al., ref. 4, with permission.)

Diffuse Axonal Injury

Diffuse axonal injury is one of the most common types of primary injury found in patients with severe head trauma (3–6,41,62–72). DAI constituted approximately 48% of all primary lesions in our earlier trauma series (3–4). DAI is characterized by multiple, small, focal traumatic lesions scattered throughout the white matter (Figs. 3, 5, and 6). Most lesions spare the overlying cortex, frequently being located at the gray-white matter interface. Occasionally, the cortex may be secondarily involved by larger lesions. DAI lesions are usually (80%) nonhemorrhagic in nature. Lesions range in size from 5 to 15 mm, with peripheral lesions tending to be smaller than more central ones. Lesions are usually ovoid to elliptical in shape, with the long axis parallel to the direction of the axonal tracts that are involved. When present, DAI lesions tend to be multiple, with as many as 15–20 lesions found in some severely injured patients. Autopsy and histopathologic studies have shown that the extent of axonal injury always exceeds that visualized macroscopically (62–72). It is likely that all current imaging modalities, including MRI, greatly underestimate the true extent of DAI. In all probability, MRI detects only those regions of DAI where axonal disruption is confluent enough to allow visualization.

Classically, patients with DAI present with severe loss of consciousness starting at the moment of impact (64–72). Patients with DAI usually have significantly greater impairment of consciousness than do patients with many other primary lesions, such as cortical contusions, intracerebral hematomas, and extraaxial hematomas (3–6,17,64–72).

DAI tends to occur in three fundamental anatomical areas: (a) lobar white matter, (b) corpus callosum, and (c) the dorsolateral aspect of the upper brainstem (Figs. 1–3 and 5–9) (3–7,60–72). Adams et al. have emphasized that DAI tends to occur in these three areas in successive stages, with the involvement becoming sequen-

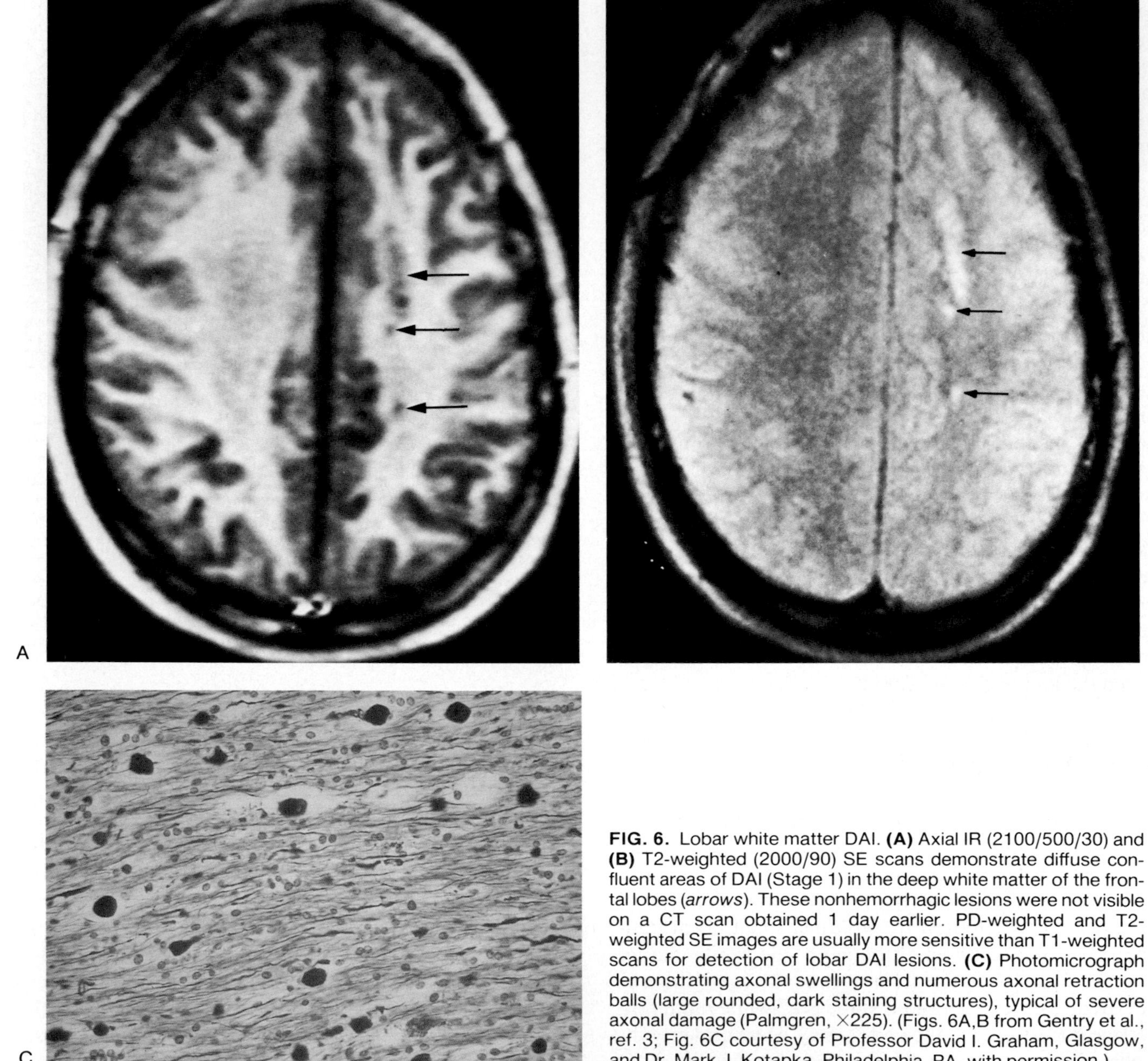

FIG. 6. Lobar white matter DAI. **(A)** Axial IR (2100/500/30) and **(B)** T2-weighted (2000/90) SE scans demonstrate diffuse confluent areas of DAI (Stage 1) in the deep white matter of the frontal lobes (*arrows*). These nonhemorrhagic lesions were not visible on a CT scan obtained 1 day earlier. PD-weighted and T2-weighted SE images are usually more sensitive than T1-weighted scans for detection of lobar DAI lesions. **(C)** Photomicrograph demonstrating axonal swellings and numerous axonal retraction balls (large rounded, dark staining structures), typical of severe axonal damage (Palmgren, ×225). (Figs. 6A,B from Gentry et al., ref. 3; Fig. 6C courtesy of Professor David I. Graham, Glasgow, and Dr. Mark J. Kotapka, Philadelphia, PA, with permission.)

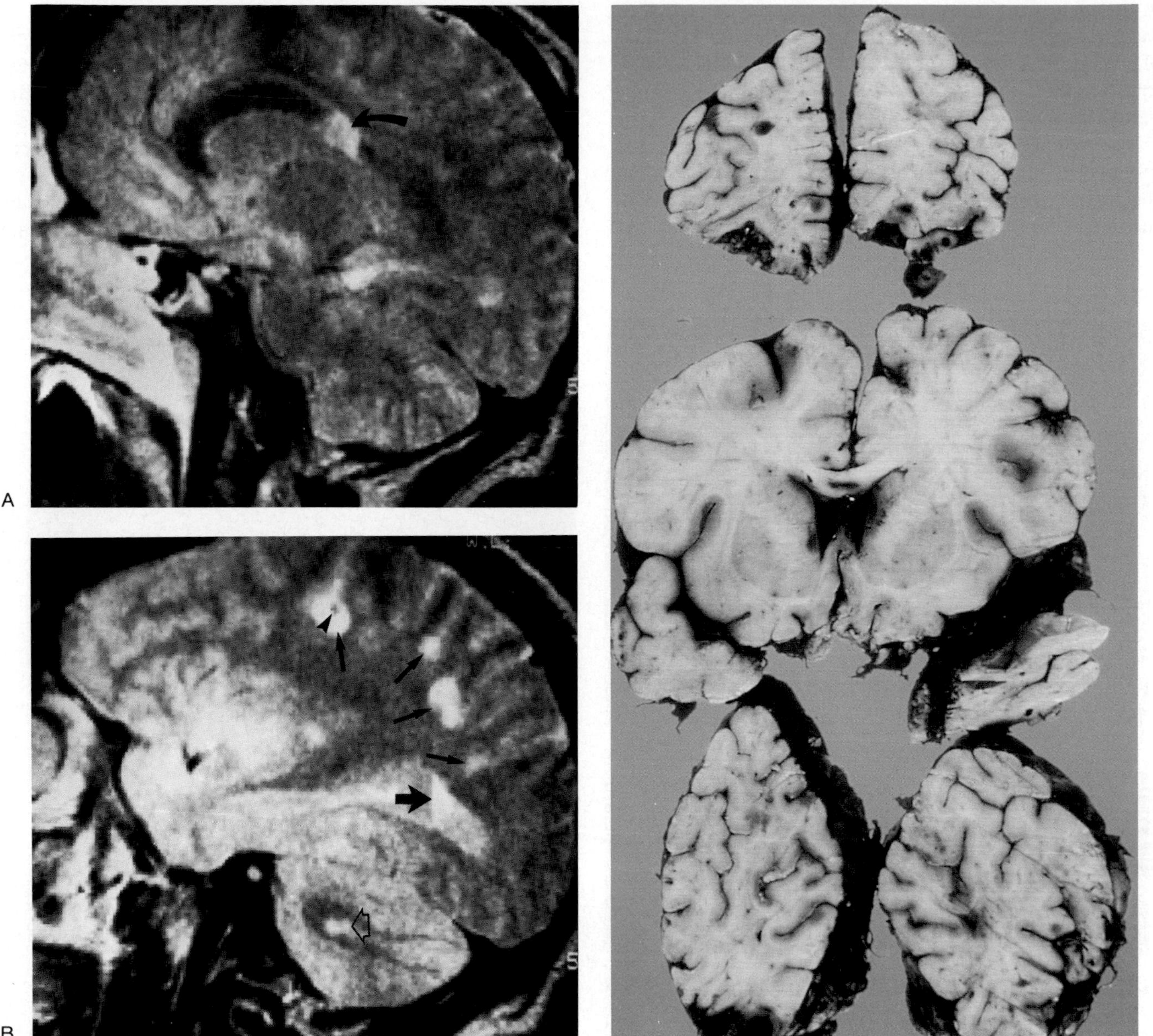

FIG. 7. Extensive DAI, intraventricular hemorrhage. **(A,B)** Sagittal T2-weighted SE MR scans of a patient with DAI of the lobar white matter (*small arrows*), body of the corpus callosum (*curved arrow*), and brainstem (brachium pontis; *open arrow*). The involvement of these three anatomic areas by DAI has been called *Stage 3 DAI*. The majority of the visualized DAI lesions are nonhemorrhagic, although a small petechial hemorrhage (*arrowhead*) is present in one lesion. A CSF/blood sedimentation level in the lateral ventricle (*large arrow*) indicates IVH. Intraventricular hemorrhage is found in the vast majority of patients with DAI of the corpus callosum and most likely arises from "shearing" injury of nearby subependymal veins. **(C)** Serial coronal sections show subcortical hemorrhagic shearing injury in the right parieto-occipital lobe, cortical hemorrhagic contusions, corpus callosal lesion, and massive intraventricular and subarachnoid hemorrhage (C courtesy of Dr. Nicholas Gonatas, Philadelphia, PA.)

tially deeper with increasing severity of trauma (64–67,72). In patients with mild head trauma, DAI lesions may be confined to the white matter of the frontal and temporal lobes (Stage 1) (Figs. 5 and 6). Patients with more severe rotational acceleration may develop lesions in the lobar white matter as well as the posterior half of the corpus callosum (Stage 2) (Figs. 1–3). If the trauma is of even greater severity, DAI lesions will additionally be found in the dorsolateral aspect of the midbrain and upper pons (Stage 3) (Figs. 7–9).

The majority (67%) of DAI lesions will be found in the lobar white matter (4,64–72). Most of these are found at the gray-white matter junction with a smaller number in the deep central white matter (corona radiata) (Figs. 3–6). Stage 1 DAI typically involves the parasagittal regions of the frontal lobes and the periventricular regions of the temporal lobes. Occasionally, DAI lesions will occur in the parietal and occipital lobes. About 8% of DAI lesions involve the internal and external capsules, while only 4% of lesions are found in the cerebellum (4).

The corpus callosum is the second most common area involved with DAI (21% of DAI lesions) (4). DAI of the corpus callosum invariably occurs in conjunction with DAI of the lobar white matter (Stage 2 DAI). The vast majority of callosal lesions (72%) occur in the posterior body and splenium (Figs. 1–3 and 7–9) (4,5,67,73–75). When DAI lesions are found in more rostral areas of the corpus callosum, they are usually found in conjunction

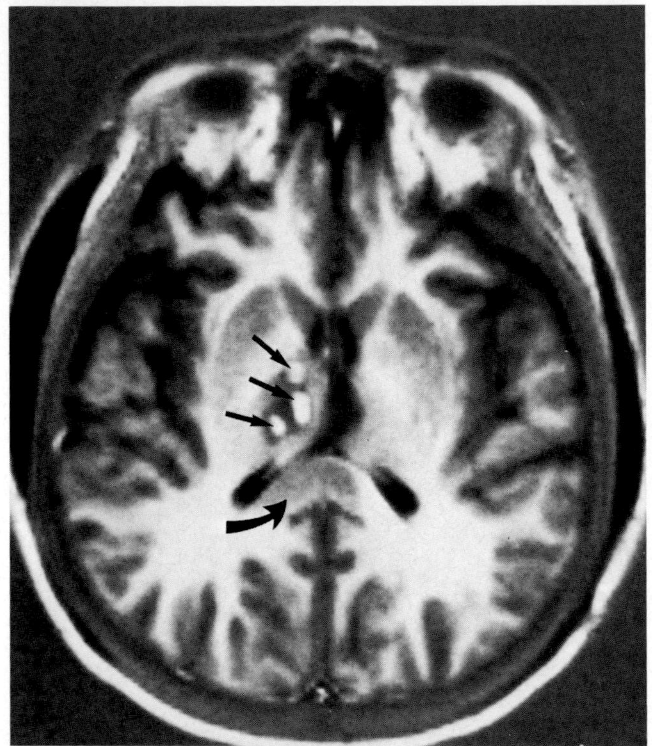

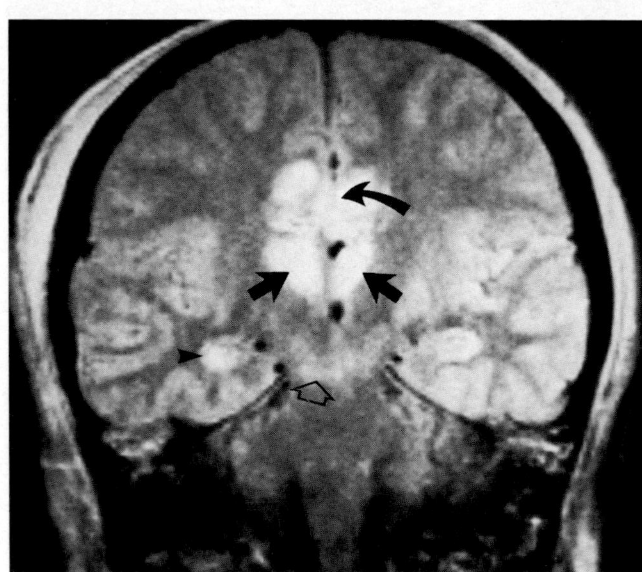

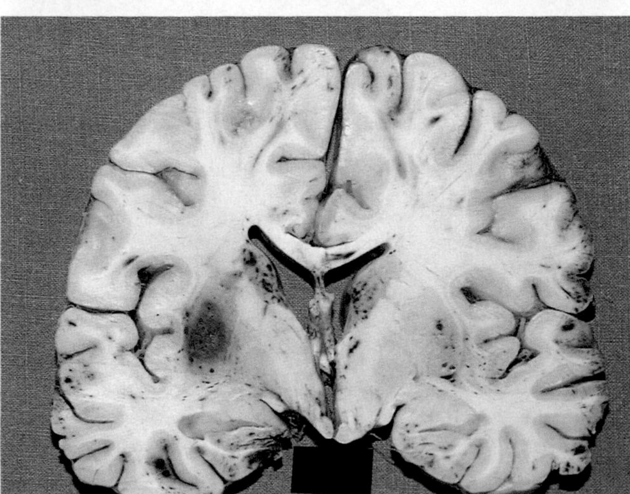

FIG. 8. DAI of the corpus callosum and brainstem, subcortical gray matter injury. **(A)** Axial IR (2100/500/30) and **(B)** coronal T2-weighted (2000/90) SE scans of a 21-year-old female who presented with severe instantaneous loss of consciousness following head trauma. Numerous DAI lesions are present in the splenium of the corpus callosum (*curved arrows*), upper brainstem (*open arrow*), and white matter of the frontal and temporal lobes (not shown). Since DAI lesions of the corpus callosum are usually quite large and easily visible, they often herald the presence of more subtle DAI lesions elsewhere (e.g., lobar white matter, dorsolateral brainstem). Multiple subcortical gray matter hemorrhages (*small arrows*) and infarcts (*large arrows*) are present in the thalami. These lesions are most likely due to shear-strain induced injury of the thalamoperforating arteries. **(C)** Coronal section at the level of the internal capsule and basal ganglia demonstrates hemorrhage in the midportion of corpus callosum, small contusions (see hippocampus), and deep ganglionic/deep white matter hematoma. (C courtesy of Professor David I. Graham, Glasgow, and Dr. Mark J. Kotapka, Philadelphia, PA.)

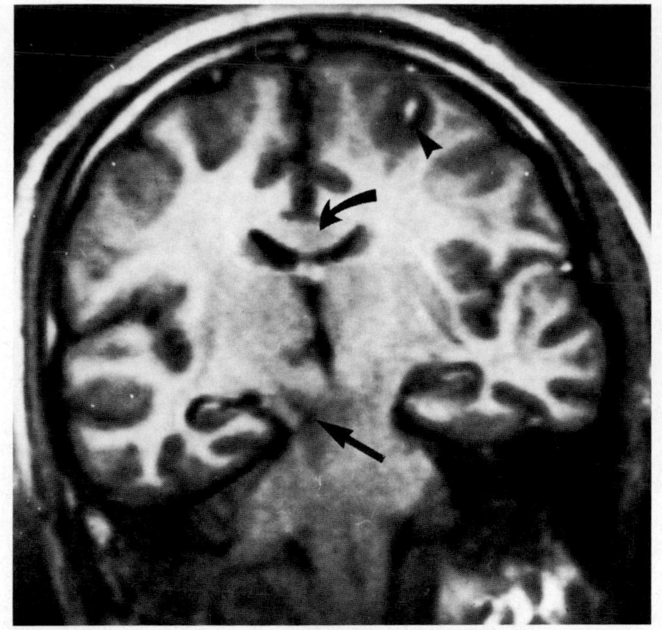

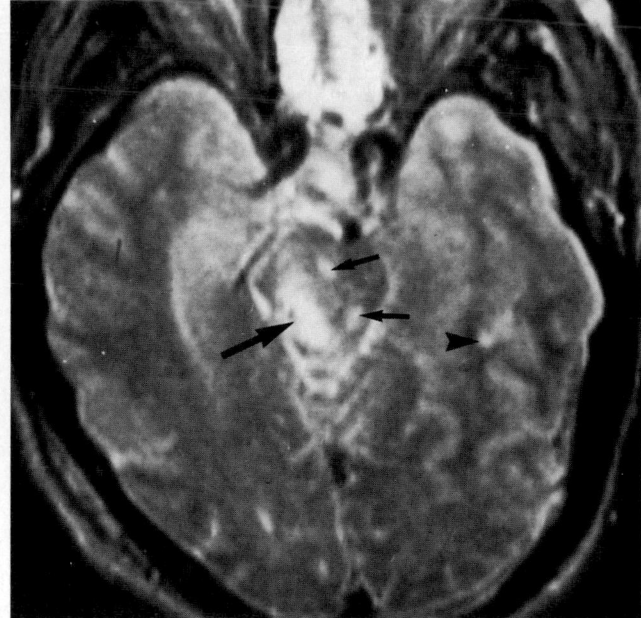

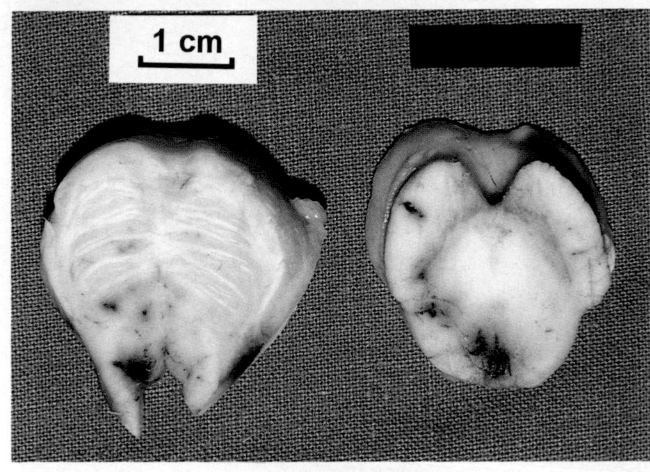

FIG. 9. Primary BSI. **(A)** Coronal IR (2000/500/30) and **(B)** axial T2-weighted (2000/100) SE MR scans of a 43-year-old man with clinical evidence of primary BSI. There is extensive signal abnormality in the right dorsolateral aspect of the upper brainstem from severe DAI (*large arrows*). Smaller DAI lesions are present in the left midbrain (*small arrows*). Primary brainstem DAI is invariably accompanied by similar lesions in the corpus callosum (*curved arrow*) and deep lobar white matter (*arrowheads*; Stage 3 DAI). (From Gentry et al., ref. 6, with permission.) **(C)** Gross specimen shows primary hemorrhagic lesion in dorsolateral quadrant of rostral brainstem typical of DAI involving midbrain. (C courtesy of Professor David I. Graham, Glasgow, and Dr. Mark J. Kotapka, Philadelphia, PA.)

with lesions of the splenium. Callosal DAI lesions may be quite large and occasionally may involve the entire corpus callosum. These lesions are usually unilateral and slightly eccentric to the midline, but may also be bilateral and symmetric (4,5).

The mechanism for production of traumatic corpus callosum injury was originally thought to be due to traumatic laceration of the corpus callosum by the free edge of the falx (76). It is now generally accepted that this mechanism is implausible and that corpus callosum injury is mediated by rotationally induced shear-strain forces (5,71–72). Gennarelli et al. (72) have shown in primate experiments that nonimpact rotational acceleration of the head in the lateral or oblique-lateral direction will uniformly produce shearing injury of the corpus callosum. Although the falx does not play a direct role in callosal injury, it may play an indirect one. Tensile and shear-strain forces do not develop between tissues of the same density if they are free to move together as a unit (5). With lateral or oblique-lateral movements of the head, the rigid falx prevents the cerebral hemispheres from moving across the midline. Shear-strains, therefore, develop across the connecting point (corpus callosum) of the two hemispheres. The shape of the falx does play an important role in the location of traumatic lesions in the corpus callosum (5). Anteriorly, less strain develops in the corpus callosum, since the falx is shorter and can allow transient displacement of portions of the brain across the midline. Posteriorly, the falx is longer and effectively prevents this displacement, allowing greater shearing and tensile strains to develop within the fibers of the corpus callosum. This seems to be the most plausible explanation for the selective vulnerability of the posterior half of the corpus callosum that most authors have observed (5).

DAI of the brainstem is the third area that is frequently involved with DAI (Stage 3 DAI) but this will be discussed as a separate topic.

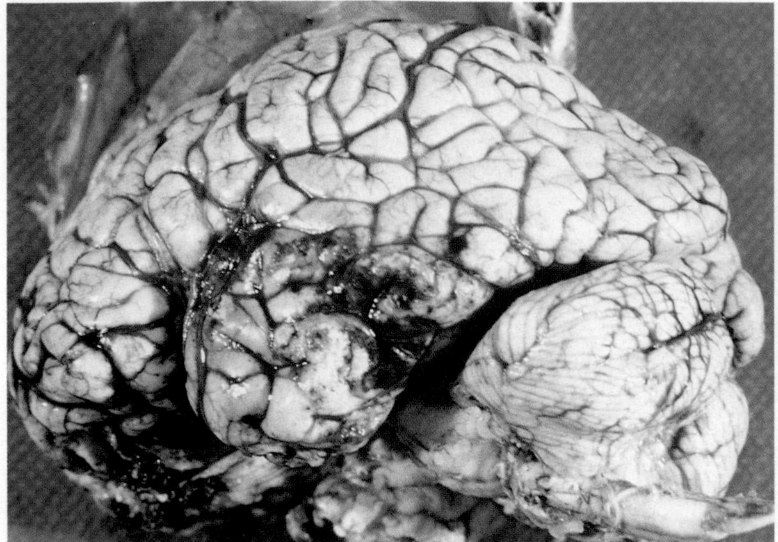

A

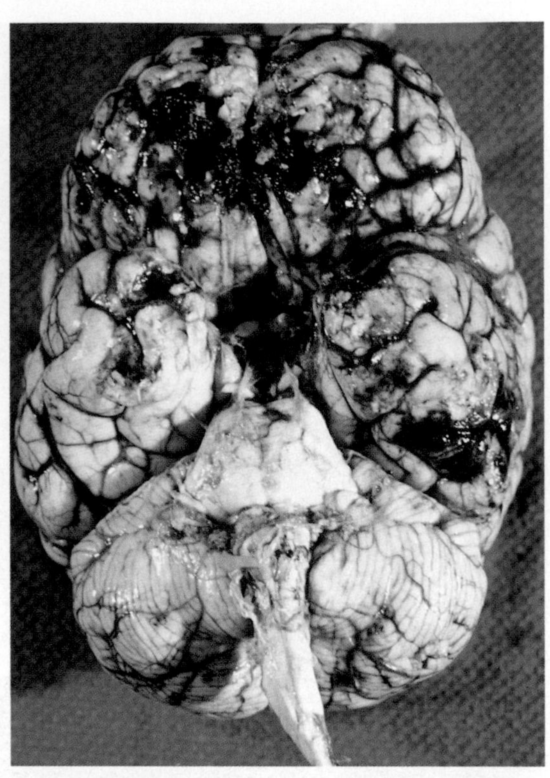

B

FIG. 10. Cortical contusions. **(A)** Lateral and **(B)** inferior views of the brain of a patient who died from head trauma demonstrate the typical appearance and distribution of traumatic cortical contusions. Contusions are often hemorrhagic, superficially located, and typically involve the inferior, lateral, and anterior surfaces of the frontal and temporal lobes.

A

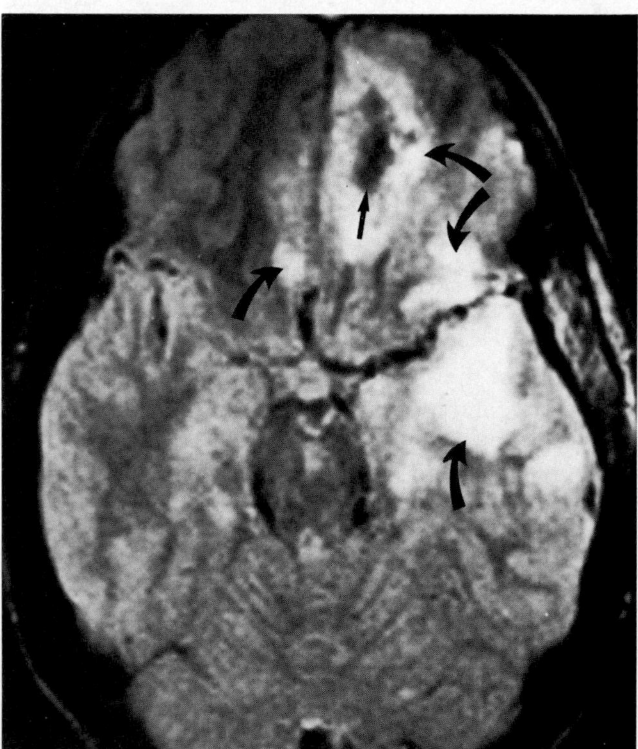

B

FIG. 11. Multiple cortical contusions. **(A,B)** Axial T2-weighted (2300/80) SE scans obtained 5 days after trauma. There are multiple hemorrhagic and nonhemorrhagic contusions (*curved arrows*) in the inferior frontal and anterior and medial temporal lobes. The lesion distribution is consistent with that expected from Holbourn's observations (60,61). Contusions often contain small focal areas of petechial hemorrhage (*arrows*) surrounded by larger zones of nonhemorrhagic injury. This patient experienced a good neurologic recovery despite the extensive nature of the contusions. Patients with contusions usually have a good neurologic outcome or are only mildly disabled unless the lesions are very large or are accompanied by other more ominous lesions, severe mass effect, or secondary BSI (17). (From Gentry et al., ref. 4, with permission.)

Cortical Contusions

Cortical contusions are the second frequently encountered group of primary intraaxial lesions. They comprised about 44% of intraaxial lesions in our own recent series (3,4). Cortical contusions, by definition, must primarily involve the superficial gray matter of the brain (Figs. 5 and 10–13) (4,67,76–79). The underlying white matter is usually spared unless the contusion is extremely large (67). Because gray matter is much more vascular than white matter, contusions are much more likely to be hemorrhagic than are DAI lesions (52% vs. 19%) (Fig. 10) (3,4). The hemorrhagic foci may vary in size from small petechia scattered throughout a much larger nonhemorrhagic zone of injury to multiple large confluent regions of hemorrhage occupying most of an entire lobe (Figs. 12 and 13). Contusions, when present, tend to be multiple and bilateral (Figs. 10 and 11) (4,67).

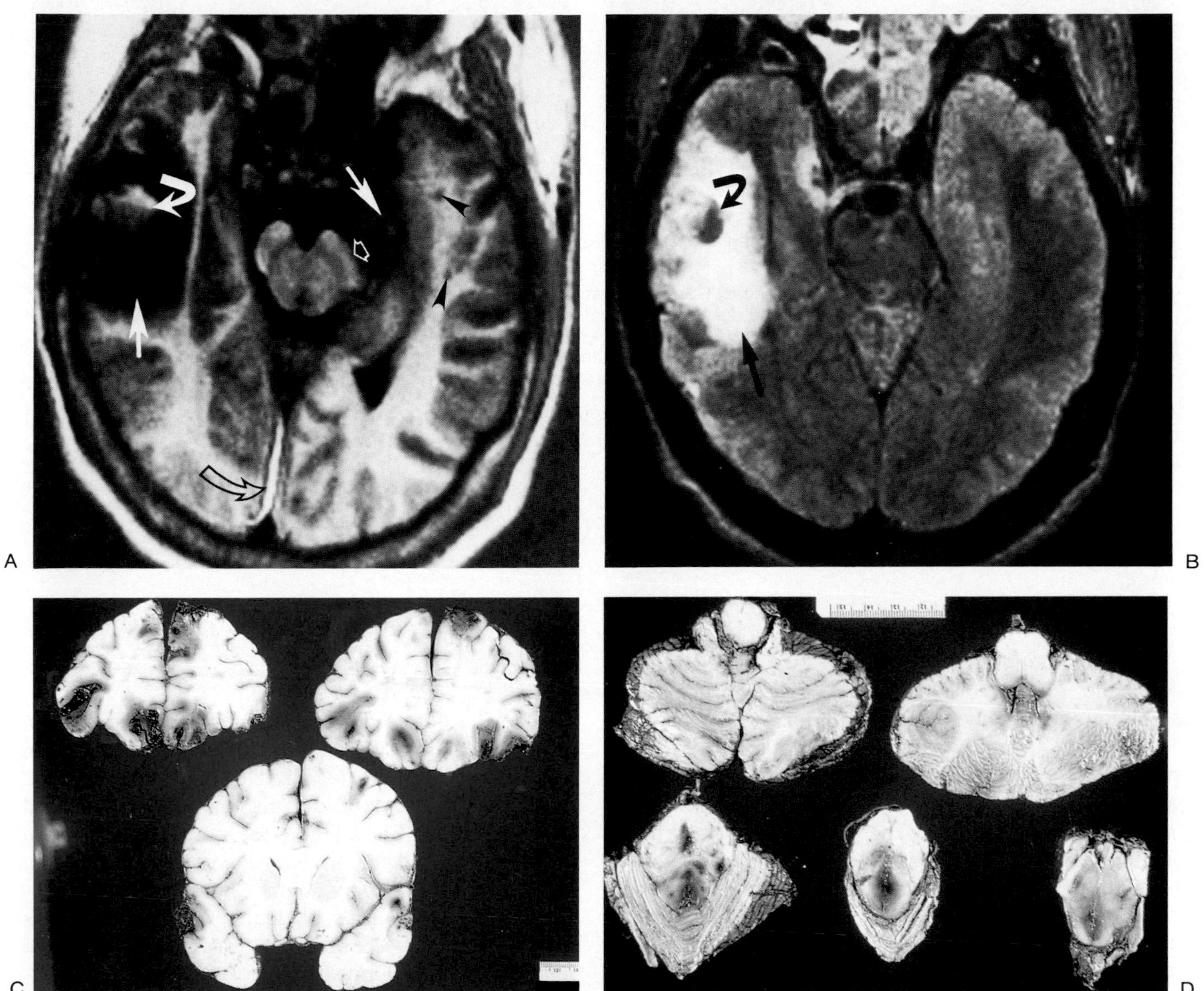

FIG. 12. Bilateral temporal lobe contusions with brainstem displacement. Axial **(A)** IR (2100/600/30) and **(B)** T2-weighted (2300/80) SE MR scans in a head injury patient with a new left third nerve palsy and acute brainstem dysfunction. There are bilateral temporal lobe contusions (*arrows*) with a large area of hemorrhage in one lesion (*curved arrows*). The left temporal lobe uncus is medially herniated and produces compression, displacement, and rotation of the brainstem (*open arrow*). Although the ventrolateral aspect of the midbrain is compressed, no focal intrinsic brainstem lesions are seen. The patient responded well to treatment and had a good final outcome. Brainstem dysfunction due to deformity and displacement from transtentorial herniation may have a good outcome if no focal intrinsic secondary lesions are seen in the brainstem (17). Also noted are several temporal lobe DAI lesions (*arrowheads*) and an interhemispheric SDH (*curved open arrow*). (From Gentry et al., ref. 6, with permission.) Serial sections through supratentorial brain **(C)** show extensive cortical contusions. In sections through posterior fossa **(D)**, note "coning" deformity of brainstem due to descending transtentorial herniation with secondary brainstem Duret hemorrhages. (C and D courtesy of Dr. Nicholas Gonatas, Philadelphia, PA.)

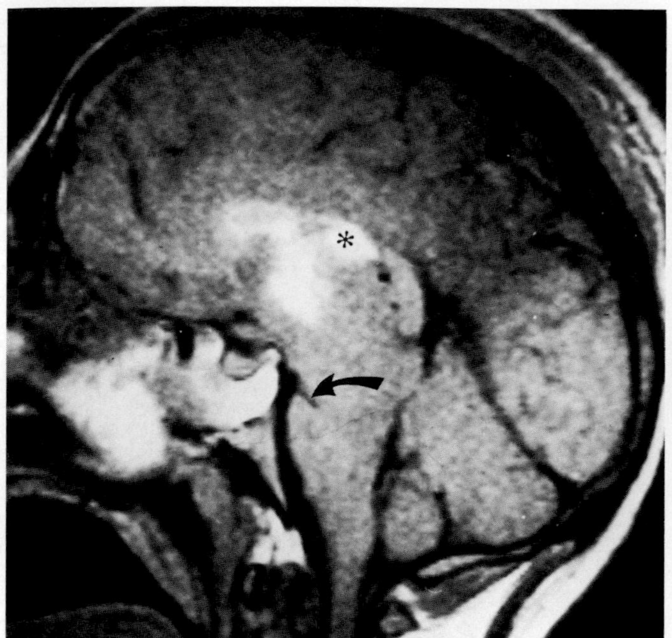

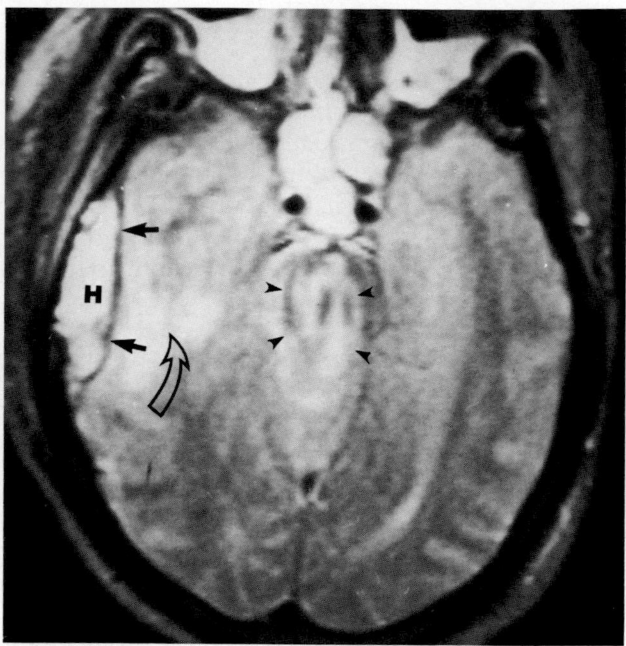

FIG. 13. Epidural hematoma and secondary BSI due to transtentorial herniation. **(A)** Sagittal T1-weighted (400/26) and **(B)** axial T2-weighted (2300/80) SE scans of a patient with new signs of secondary BSI 10 days after initial trauma and conservative management of an EDH (H). The EDH can be easily differentiated from SDH by characteristic displacement of dura mater (*arrows*) away from the calvarium. Note the signs of transtentorial herniation with marked compression of the perimesencephalic cisterns, caudal displacement of the midbrain, and obliteration of the interpeduncular cistern (*curved arrow*). There is severe midbrain deformity (*arrowheads*) and extensive areas of signal abnormality within the midbrain due to intrinsic secondary BSI. Also note the IVH, temporal contusion (*curved open arrow*), and hemorrhagic corpus callosum DAI (*asterisk*). (From Gentry et al., ref. 6, with permission.)

Contusions most commonly involve the temporal (46%) and frontal (31%) lobes (4,60,61,67). Particularly prone to injury are the inferior, anterior, and lateral aspects of these lobes (Fig. 10) (4). Temporal lobe lesions are most likely to occur just above the petrous bone or posterior to the greater sphenoid wing. Frontal lobe lesions tend to lie just above the cribriform plate, orbit, planum sphenoidale, and lesser sphenoid wing (Figs. 10 and 11). The parietal and occipital lobes are implicated much less frequently (13%). Cerebellar contusions constitute approximately 10% of contusions and are typically found in the superior vermis, tonsils, and inferior hemispheres (4).

In our series of trauma patients, cortical contusions were much less likely to be associated with severe initial impairment of consciousness as compared with DAI (3–6,17). Severe impairment of consciousness typically only occurred when the contusions were either very large, multiple, bilateral, or associated with DAI or secondary brainstem injury.

Subcortical Gray Matter Injury

Adams et al. (65,67) have described an uncommon diffuse type of injury characterized by multiple petechial hemorrhages primarily localized to the upper brainstem, basal ganglia, thalamus, and regions around the third ventricle (Fig. 8). These lesions are most commonly seen in severely injured patients who die shortly after trauma. It has been postulated by Adams et al. (65–67), and consistent with Holbourn's predictions (60,61), that this form of injury is secondary to disruption of multiple small perforating blood vessels.

We have also encountered a few patients with similar types of traumatic lesions. These lesions constituted only about 5% of all primary intraaxial lesions in our study (4). The majority of lesions were found in the thalamus and putamen, although some were seen in the caudate nucleus and globus pallidus. A much higher percentage of these lesions are hemorrhagic than for any other type of primary intraaxial lesion (4). This is most likely due to the high vascularity of the basal ganglia and thalamus that are supplied by a rich network of perforating vessels. Head injury patients who have this type of injury as the dominant abnormality usually have very profound neurologic deficits and very low initial Glasgow Coma Scale scores (4,17). Patients with multiple lesions of this type also generally have a very poor prognosis (17).

Primary and Secondary Brainstem Injury

Brainstem injury (BSI) can be separated into primary and secondary forms, depending on when the injury occurs (Table 3) (6,11,25, 26,70,80–92). Primary lesions are those that result from the initial traumatic force, while secondary ones are those that develop subsequent to initial trauma. Much of the current knowledge regarding the imaging appearance of primary and secondary BSI has arisen from autopsy studies (62–72,80–82), because CT has never been sensitive enough to allow detection and characterization of most types of BSI (3,6,25–26,87). MRI now makes it possible to effectively evaluate and characterize BSI in nonfatally injured patients (6).

Primary BSI can be classified into four major types (Table 3) (6). One type is due to direct forces (6,84), while the other three are due to indirect ones (6,64–67). The first type of primary BSI is thought to be quite rare. With severe displacement of the brain, the dorsolateral aspect of the upper brainstem may strike the free edge of the tentorium, producing a superficial contusion or laceration (84). The colliculi, superior cerebellar peduncles, and lateral aspect of the cerebral peduncles are most susceptible to this uncommon form of injury. Individual susceptibility to BSI by this mechanism is highly influenced by considerable variation in size and shape of the tentorial incisura (93). Unlike brainstem DAI, this type of injury is not necessarily associated with involvement of the cerebral white matter and corpus callosum.

Indirect forces are responsible for the vast majority of cases of primary BSI (6,64–67,71,72). The most common type, by far, is that associated with widespread DAI (Figs. 7–9) (71–72). Brainstem DAI, according to Adams (64–67), rarely occurs without the presence of histologically similar lesions in the corpus callosum and deep cerebral white matter (Figs. 7–9). DAI lesions in these three locations form a frequently associated triad that has been previously described by Adams (64–67). We also found this highly significant association in our own group of patients (3–6,17). All of our patients with primary BSI, with one exception, had multiple DAI lesions in the frontotemporal white matter, and the vast majority also had lesions in the corpus callosum. Unless the brainstem lesions are accompanied by lesions in other portions of the brain, the diagnosis of primary brainstem DAI should be made with extreme caution (64–67). In addition, the diagnosis cannot be confidently made in the presence of transtentorial herniation, cisternal compression, or posterior fossa mass effect, which may produce secondary BSI (64–67).

Brainstem DAI lesions are characteristically located in the dorsolateral quadrants of the rostral brainstem (midbrain and upper pons) (Fig. 9) (6,62–72). The ventral aspect of the pons and midbrain and the entire medulla are typically spared (6,64–67). There is a strong predilection for injury to specific fiber tracts, such as the superior cerebellar peduncles and medial lemnisci (64–67). Less commonly, lesions may involve the lateral aspect of the midbrain and cerebral peduncle (6). Since the lesions are usually nonhemorrhagic, they may be difficult to visualize with CT (3,6).

A third type of primary BSI has been described by Tomlinson (82) and Adams (64–67). This type consists of multiple petechial hemorrhages that are scattered throughout the brain but are particularly prominent in the deep central white matter, hypothalamus, thalamus, and periaqueductal regions of the rostral brainstem. Although the location is similar to that of brainstem DAI, there is no specific association with lesions of the lobar white matter, corpus callosum, or superior cerebellar peduncles (64–67). The distribution of these petechial hemorrhages is also quite different from secondary (Duret) hemorrhages that are described later in this chapter. Histologically these lesions are characterized by multiple, primarily microscopic, perivascular collections of blood (64–67,82). This type of injury is usually associated with a grim prognosis (64–67) and may represent shear-strain injury to numerous small penetrating blood vessels in the brainstem (6,17).

A fourth type of primary BSI is the pontomedullary separation or rent (64–67,85–86). Unlike brainstem DAI, this lesion may occur in the absence of more widespread cerebral damage (64–67). It is characterized by a hyperextension induced tear of the ventral surface of the brainstem at the junction of the pons with the medulla (64–67,85,86). This may range from an incomplete tear to complete brainstem avulsion. This type of injury is typically (86) but not invariably (85) fatal.

Secondary BSI can arise from two general mechanisms: (a) systemic factors (anoxia, hypotension, ischemia), and (b) severe mechanical compression or displacement of the upper brainstem (Table 3) (6,11,64–70,80–92). Diffuse hypoxic or ischemic BSI usually occurs in conjunction with supratentorial ischemic injury. Brainstem involvement with diffuse hypoxia is usually a late or terminal event. The brainstem is usually spared until just before death (6).

Mechanical compression is invariably secondary to transtentorial herniation caused by increased intracranial pressure, intracranial hematomas, multiple contusions, or diffuse edema (Figs. 12–15) (6,11,64–70,80–92). Mechanical compression may initially cause only distortion and displacement of the brainstem (Fig. 12) (6). Clinical signs and symptoms of brainstem dysfunction may be potentially reversible (17,83,90–92), especially if the only radiographic findings of BSI are displacement or compression of the brainstem (Fig. 12) (6,17). If mechanical compression is prolonged, however, there is often development of focal intrinsic secondary lesions within the brainstem that are unlikely to be completely reversible (Figs. 13–15) (6,17). In our prior MR series of patients with traumatic brainstem injury, we identified two main types of abnormalities in patients with clinical evidence of secondary BSI: (a) indirect signs from associated mass effect and (b) focal intrinsic lesions within the brainstem (6,17).

Indirect signs of BSI were present in all our patients with clinical manifestations of secondary BSI, as well as in a few patients without clinical evidence of BSI (6). Rotation, angulation, ovoid compression, and craniocaudal shortening of the upper brainstem were some of the more commonly observed indirect signs of secondary BSI (Figs. 12–15) (6). Other common but less specific indirect signs include compression of the fourth ventricle and basal cisterns, herniation of the parahippocampal gyrus into the tentorial incisura, and posterior cerebral artery distribution infarcts (Figs. 12–15) (6).

In our prior series of BSI patients studied with MRI, indirect signs of secondary BSI were usually but not invariably accompanied by focal intrinsic lesions within the brainstem (6). We found the topographical distribution of intrinsic secondary BSI lesions to be significantly different ($p < 0.02$) when compared with the location of lesions seen in patients with primary BSI (6). The majority of primary lesions (60%) were located in the dorsal and dorsolateral aspects of the upper brainstem, while intrinsic secondary lesions were typically (87%) found in the ventral and ventrolateral aspects (6).

Several types of intrinsic secondary lesions may be seen within the brainstem (Table 3) (6). Secondary (Duret) hemorrhages consist of centrally placed, generally midline, collections of blood in the tegmentum of the rostral pons and midbrain (6,64–67,80,82,88,89). These hemorrhages may vary from numerous petechia to massive central tegmental hemorrhages involving the entire upper brainstem. They are usually located in the ventral and paramedian aspects of the midbrain and upper pons, with relative sparing of the dorsolateral aspects of the brainstem (6,64–67). Duret hemorrhages are not limited to head injury patients but also occur following transtentorial herniation from other causes. Most authors believe that secondary brainstem hemorrhages result from stretching or tearing of the penetrating arteries as the upper brainstem is caudally displaced during transtentorial herniation (6,69,82,88,89). Focal brain-

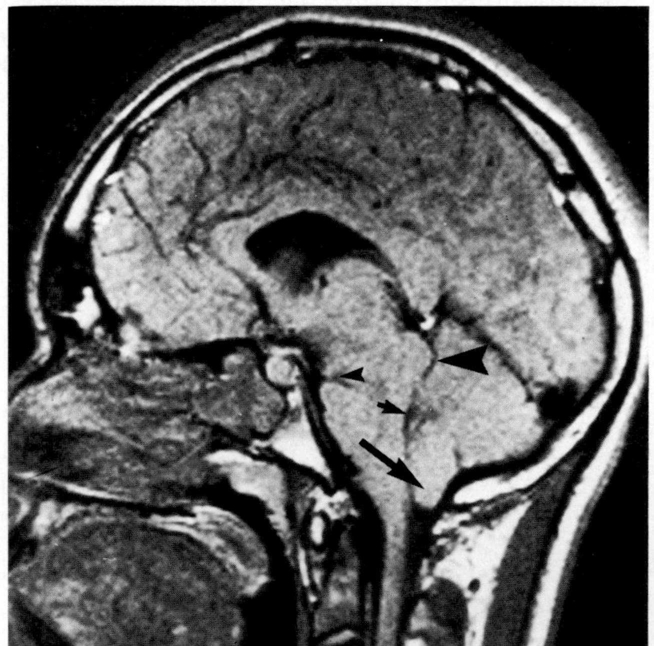

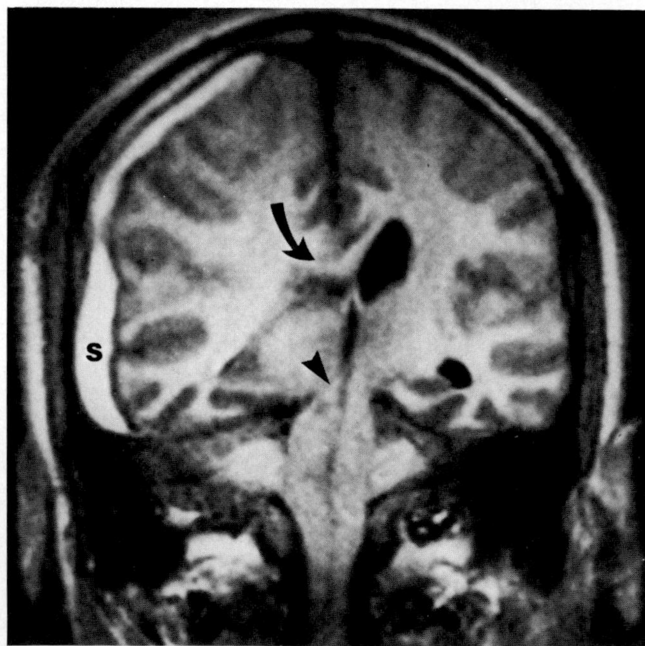

FIG. 14. Subacute subdural hematoma: tonsillar, subfalcine, and transtentorial herniation. **(A)** Sagittal T1-weighted (600/20) SE and **(B)** coronal IR (2100/500/30) MR scans demonstrate a large crescent-shaped subacute SDH (S), which is comprised of hemoglobin in the methemoglobin state. There is anatomic evidence of tonsillar (*large arrow*) and subfalcine (*curved arrow*) herniation. Also present are specific signs of transtentorial herniation, including fourth ventricular compression (*small arrow*), midbrain deformity (*large arrowhead*), and compression of the interpeduncular cistern (*small arrowhead*). Multiplanar MR is very helpful for revealing the size and shape of SDHs as well as demonstrating associated displacement, compression, and anatomic distortion of the brainstem.

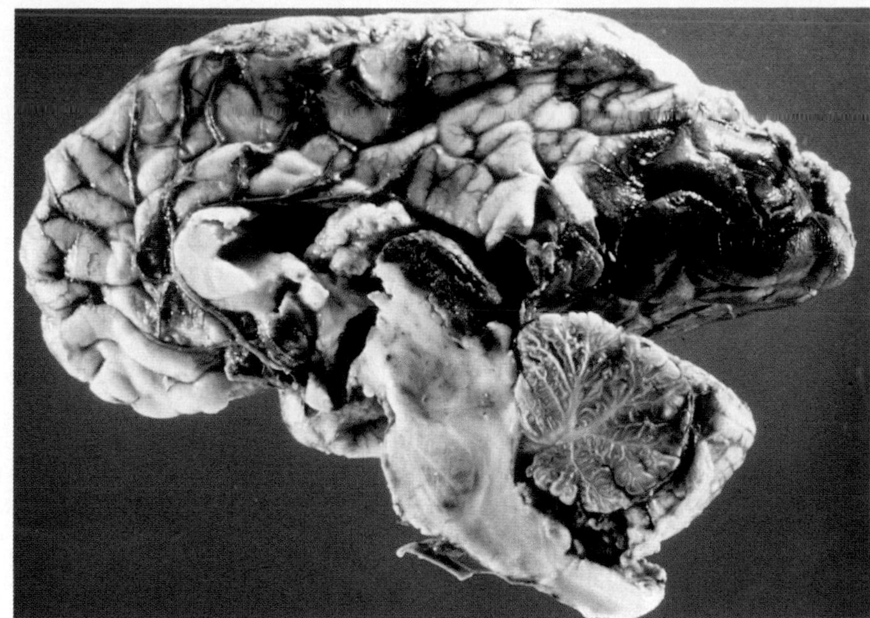

FIG. 15. Fatal secondary brainstem injury due to transtentorial herniation. Thirty-seven-year-old man with fatal head injury from bilateral SDHs. The specimen reveals the typical autopsy changes of secondary brainstem injury due to transtentorial herniation. Marked craniocaudal shortening, kinking, and deformity of the brainstem as well as severe compression of the fourth ventricle are present. Pressure necrosis and hemorrhagic infarction are seen within the midbrain. The most prominent abnormalities, however, are extensive areas of hemorrhagic infarction in the posterior thalamus and medial parieto-occipital lobes from posterior cerebral artery occlusion. The latter is due to injury of this vessel as it is compressed between the herniated medial temporal lobe and the edge of the tentorium. (From Gentry et al., ref. 4, with permission.)

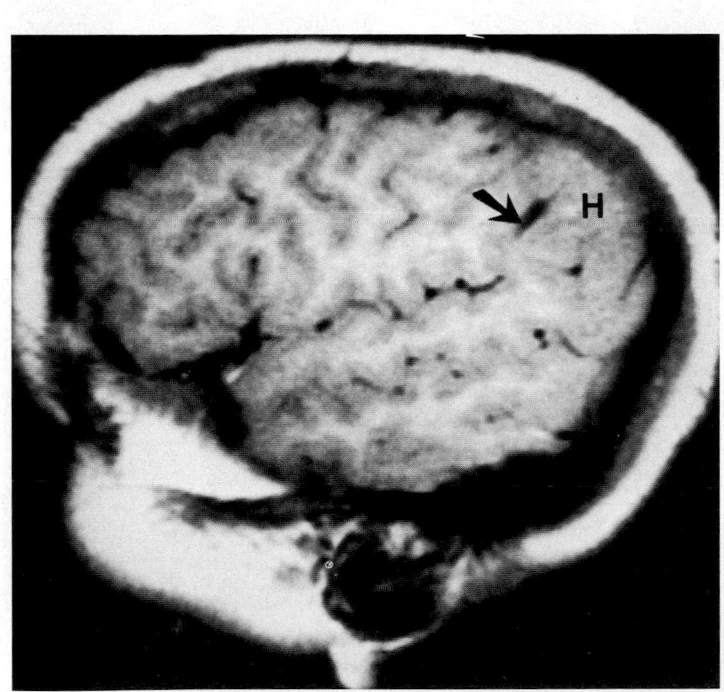

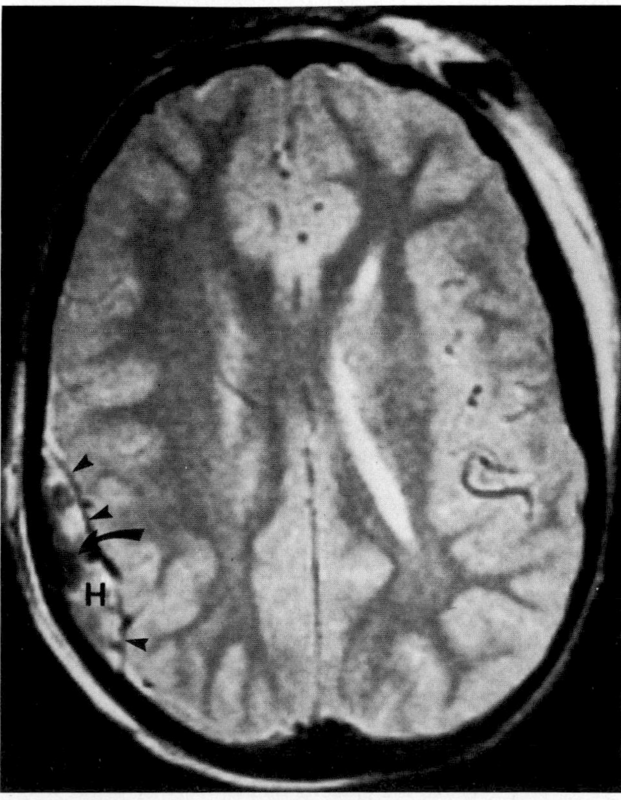

FIG. 16. Acute epidural hematoma. **(A)** Sagittal T1-weighted (600/20) and **(B)** axial T2-weighted (2000/90) SE scans reveal a hyperacute (6-hour-old) right parietal EDH (H). (A) The EDH is isointense to gray matter on the T1-weighted SE scan, being recognizable only by displacement of adjacent cortical veins (*arrow*). (B) A thin, low intensity line, representing displaced dura (*arrowheads*), aids in recognition of the nearly isointense hematoma. Although the majority of the hematoma has a signal intensity that is consistent with oxyhemoglobin, a small area of low intensity deoxyhemoglobin is noted on the long TR/TE images (*curved arrow*).

stem infarcts may also occur through the same mechanism (6,70,82). Although differentiation of brainstem infarcts from DAI lesions can be difficult, the location of infarcts is typically in the central tegmentum of the pons and midbrain, while DAI usually involves the dorsolateral midbrain (6). Severe pressure necrosis involving the entire upper brainstem is commonly seen in individuals who eventually die from prolonged brainstem compression due to transtentorial herniation (Figs. 13 and 15) (6,68,80,82).

Primary Hemorrhages

Traumatic hemorrhage can result from injury to any of the cerebral vessels (meningeal, pial; artery, vein, capillary). The site, shape, and anatomic pattern of the resulting hemorrhage will be determined by the exact location and type of vessels that are injured (Table 3). The anatomic features of different types of primary hemorrhages on MR scans are identical to those seen on CT studies. The temporal MR appearance of hemorrhage has been previously described in this chapter. The MR appearance will vary with the age of the lesion and the specific parameters that are used to acquire the MR images (39).

Epidural hematomas are most commonly of arterial origin (94–99). They usually arise from direct laceration or tearing of meningeal arteries (typically the middle meningeal artery) by skull fractures (94–99). A fracture is present in 85% to 95% of cases (94–99). Occasionally (9%) they may occur from stretching and tearing of meningeal arteries in the absence of fractures (94). The latter is particularly common in children and is usually due to transient deformation and depression of the calvarial vault (94). Arterial epidurals typically occur in the temporal or temporoparietal region (Figs. 13, 16, and 17). A fracture can often be seen on the MR scan due to hemorrhage or fluid that often extends between the fracture margins (3,6). The dura can often be seen to be displaced away from the inner table of the skull (Figs. 13, 16, and 17) (3,6). It is visualized as a thin line of low signal intensity between the brain and the lenticular-shaped hema-

A

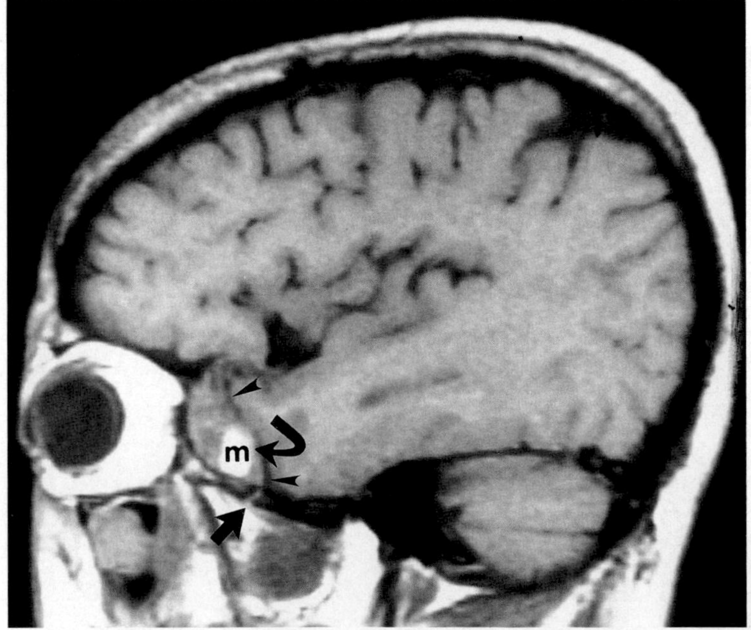

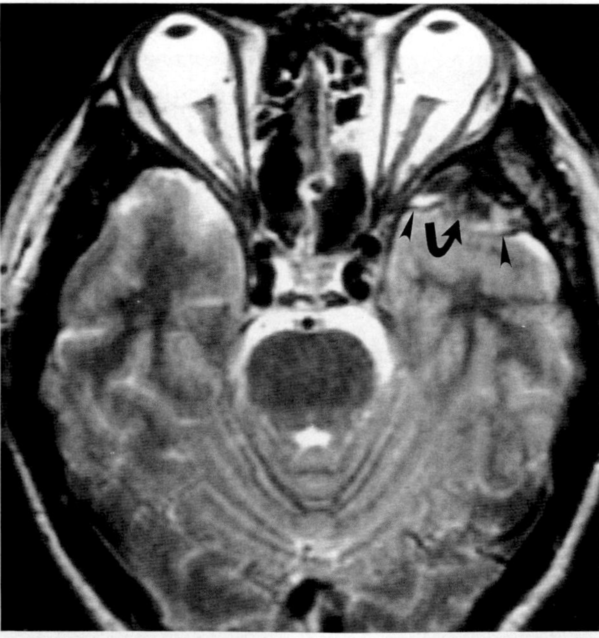

B

FIG. 17. Epidural hematoma. **(A)** Sagittal T1-weighted (600/20) and **(B)** axial T2-weighted (2500/90) SE scans reveal a 3-day-old middle cranial fossa EDH (*curved arrows*). Despite its small size, the hematoma is clearly seen to lie within the epidural space, displacing the dura mater (*arrowheads*) away from the calvarium. This acute EDH is hypointense to gray matter on the T2-weighted scan due to the presence of deoxyhemoglobin and intracellular methemoglobin. MR signal hyperintensity from methemoglobin (m) is noted in a portion of the EDH on the T1-weighted scan. A skull fracture (*arrow*) is faintly seen. The location of this EDH, just posterior to the lesser sphenoid wing, would raise the possibility of a venous origin.

toma. Visualization of the dura on MR scans allows one to be absolutely certain of the diagnosis of an epidural hematoma. With CT one cannot always differentiate small epidurals from subdurals since the former may not have the classic lenticular shape and may not be associated with a fracture (7).

Venous epidural hematomas are much less common than those of arterial origin (94–99) and are usually due to laceration of a dural sinus by occipital, parietal, or sphenoid bone fractures (99). The most common locations of venous epidurals are (a) the posterior fossa from laceration of the transverse or sigmoid sinus (Fig. 18); (b) the middle fossa from injury to the sphenoparietal sinus (Fig. 17); and (c) the parasagittal area from a tear of the superior sagittal sinus. Differentiation of arterial and venous epidural hematomas is often possible with MRI and may have some therapeutic and prognostic significance (99). Venous epidurals are more variable in shape than those of arterial origin (94,99). All, however, are invariably separated from adjacent brain by displaced dura matter that is easily seen on PD-weighted and T2-weighted scans. Another characteristic feature of venous epidurals is that they always lie adjacent to a dural sinus that is transgressed by a fracture line (94,100–102). Frequently, the injured dural sinus will be stripped away from the adjacent calvarium by the expanding hematoma (Fig. 18) and, occasionally, the sinus will be occluded by the fracture-induced intimal tear (98). MRI can often be quite helpful for differentiating arterial and venous epidurals, and determining whether the dural sinus is occluded. Patency of the sinus can usually be established by MRI or MRA without the necessity of performing a conventional arteriogram. A venous epidural, unlike a subdural hematoma, will often lie both above and below the tentorium. The lower pressure of the injured vein also means that these lesions may expand more slowly than arterial lesions and, therefore, may be delayed in onset (94,100,101). Posterior fossa epidurals are much less frequent (2% to 29%) than supratentorial lesions (94,100,101), more likely (85%) to be of venous origin (94,100,101), and more likely to be associated with a poor outcome (100,101).

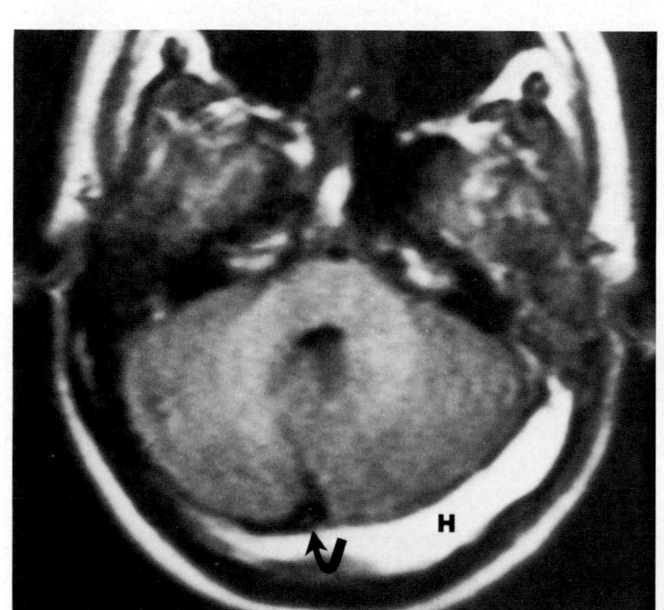

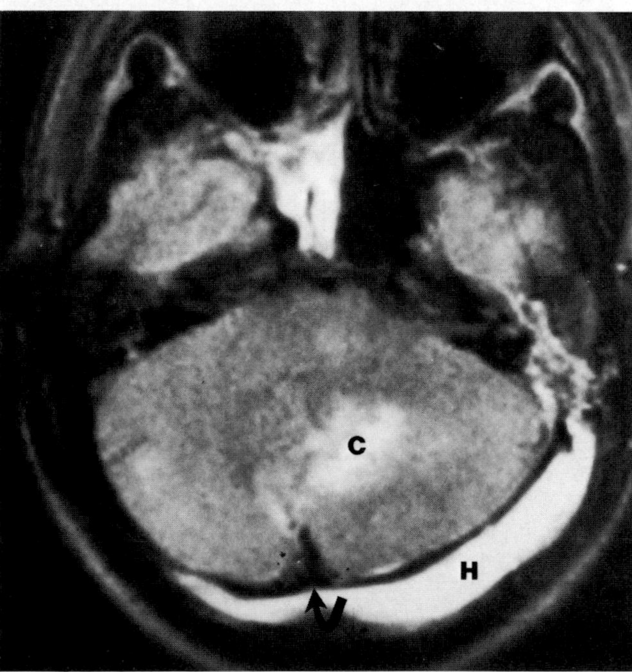

FIG. 18. Posterior fossa venous epidural hematoma and cerebellar contusion. Axial **(A)** IR (2100/600/30) and **(B)** T2-weighted (2000/90) MR scans reveal a large subacute posterior fossa venous EDH (H). The EDH displaces the venous confluence (*curved arrows*), transverse sinus, and dura mater away from the occipital bone. The EDH is noted to extend across the midline, posterior to the venous confluence, clearly differentiating it from a SDH. The patent venous confluence and transverse sinus are identified by their high-velocity flow void. An extensive cerebellar contusion (c) is also present.

Subdural hematomas (SDH) are typically caused by stretching and tearing of bridging veins (Fig. 19) that traverse the subdural space as they leave the cortical surface of the brain to drain into the dural sinuses (64,67,71,72,76,102). These veins are quite susceptible to shear-strain injury when the relatively mobile brain moves in relationship to the fixed dural sinuses (60,61). Subdural hematomas may be produced by either rotational or linear acceleration (60,61,71,72). Symptoms of isolated SDH are quite variable (asymptomatic, headache, unconscious) (9,15,102,103). Generally, patients with SDH do not have as severe impairment of consciousness as those who have primary neuronal injuries unless there is severe mass effect or other associated lesions (65,67,103). The outcome from SDH continues to be poor (35% to 90% mortality), primarily because of secondary forms of injury and associated underlying brain injury (102,103). Survival is significantly better if large subdurals with mass effect are evacuated within 4 hours of injury (103).

Although most SDH are usually found along the supratentorial convexity (Figs. 14, 19, and 20), some will

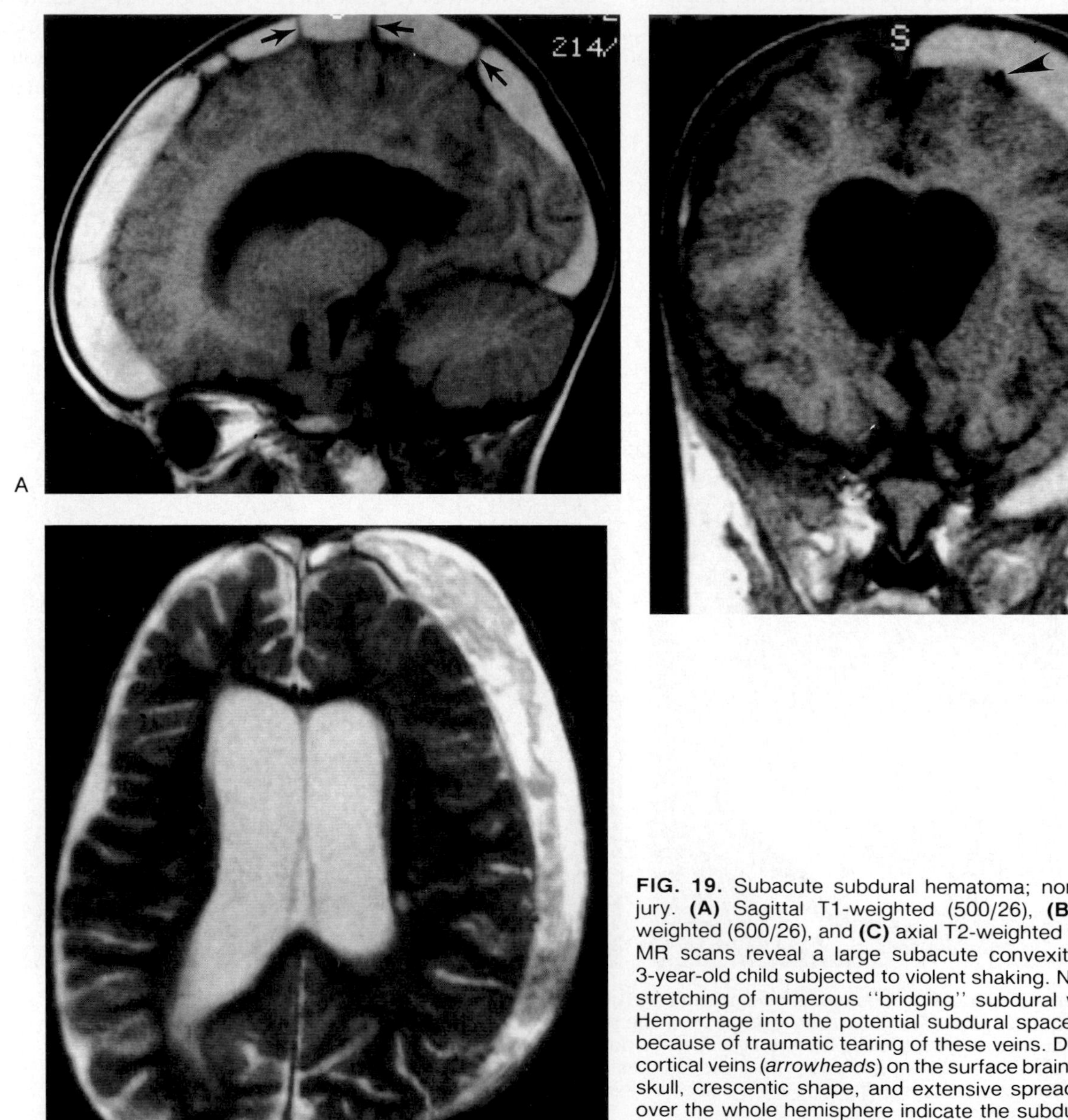

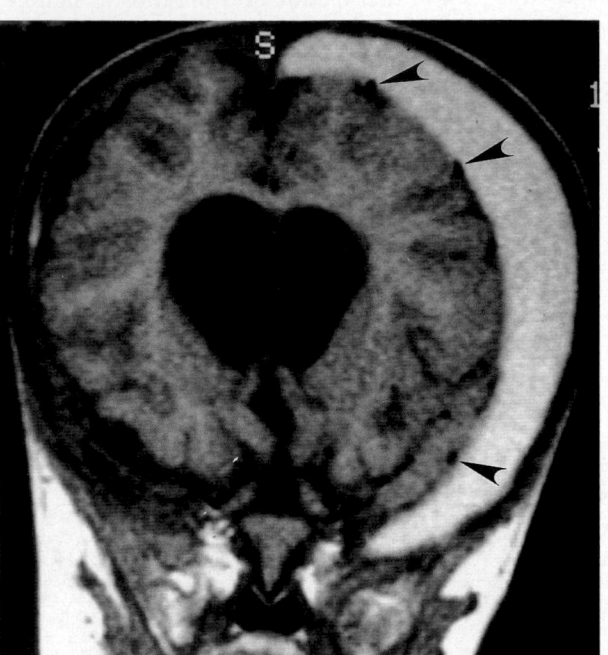

FIG. 19. Subacute subdural hematoma; nonaccidental injury. **(A)** Sagittal T1-weighted (500/26), **(B)** coronal T1-weighted (600/26), and **(C)** axial T2-weighted (2300/100) SE MR scans reveal a large subacute convexity SDH in this 3-year-old child subjected to violent shaking. Note the severe stretching of numerous "bridging" subdural veins (*arrows*). Hemorrhage into the potential subdural space has occurred because of traumatic tearing of these veins. Displacement of cortical veins (*arrowheads*) on the surface brain away from the skull, crescentic shape, and extensive spread of the lesion over the whole hemisphere indicate the subdural location of the hematoma. Numerous fibrous septations are noted within the SDH on the T2-weighted scan, suggesting multiple compartments to the lesion.

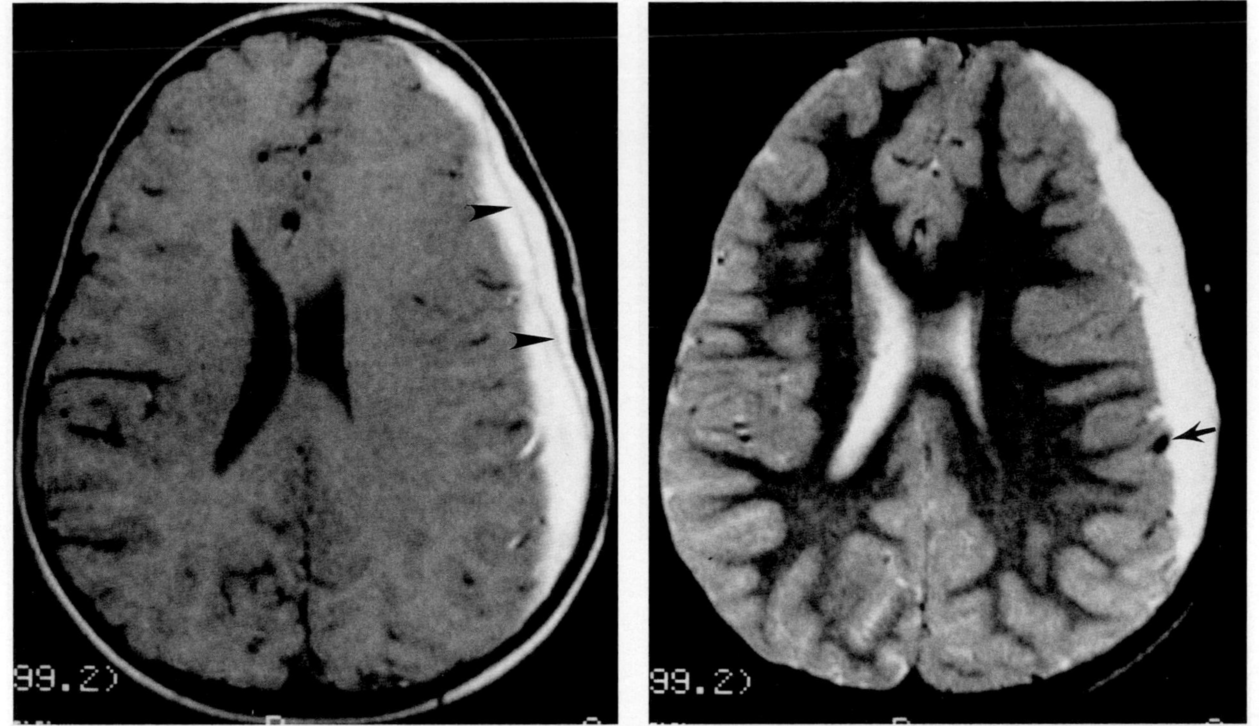

FIG. 20. Subacute subdural hematoma. **(A)** T1-weighted (600/26) and **(B)** T2-weighted (2300/100) SE scans reveal a large 12-day-old subacute convexity SDH. The cortical veins (*arrow*) on the surface brain are markedly separated from the skull by the extensive crescentic-shaped SDH. There is compression and displacement of the left lateral ventricle and septum pellucidum. The SDH is primarily composed of hemoglobin in the methemoglobin state, as demonstrated by the short T1 of the lesion on the T1-weighted image. A faint secondary subdural membrane (*arrowheads*) suggests multiple episodes of hemorrhage. MR is usually more helpful than CT for identifying the multicompartmental nature of SDH and guiding drainage.

be located in the posterior fossa (Fig. 21), along the falx (Fig. 12), and adjacent to the tentorium (Fig. 21) (102,103). The latter two locations are especially common in children (104,105). Interhemispheric and tentorial leaf subdural hematomas are commonly found in children who are victims of nonaccidental injury (58,59,104,105) by means of violent shaking (shaken-baby syndrome) (Fig. 21). Although these hematomas are not completely specific for child abuse, their presence should always alert one to the possibility of this syndrome.

MR scans in patients with SDH reveal the typical crescentic collection of blood between the brain and the falx, tentorium, or inner table of the skull (3–7,58,59,104,105). The MR signal appearance of the SDH will vary with the age of the lesion, as described earlier in this chapter. Subdurals will be visualized on all MRI pulse sequences as crescentic areas that have a signal intensity that is always higher than that of the adjacent cortical bone (3–6). There are many advantages of MRI over CT when evaluating patients with SDH. First of all, MRI has been shown to be considerably more sensitive than CT for detection of SDH (3). In our own series of acute to subacute SDH, CT detected only 53% of lesions as compared with T1-weighted and T2-weighted MR scans, which detected 70% and 95% of lesions, respectively (3). The wide difference in the contrast between the hematoma and signal void of cortical bone is responsible for the exquisite sensitivity of MRI to these lesions. Those subdurals that are missed with CT, however, are almost always only 1–2 mm in thickness and of no clinical significance (3). Secondly, MRI can be quite helpful for evaluation of patients with CT-suspected bilateral isodense SDH (3,6,38). Unlike CT scanning, these lesions are quite conspicuous on MR scans. CT isodense SDH will have a high intensity signal on all MR pulse sequences since they are typically composed of free methemoglobin in solution (3). Contrast-enhanced CT scans are no longer necessary for confirmation of these lesions. A third advantage of MRI for evaluation of SDH is the ability to image the lesions in more than one plane. This is often helpful in determining the severity of the mass effect and whether the hematoma should be managed conservatively or operatively (17). Lastly, in contradistinction to CT, MR more clearly reveals the multicompartmental nature of some subacute to chronic SDH (Figs. 19 and 20). This information may be helpful for surgical drainage of these complex lesions (7).

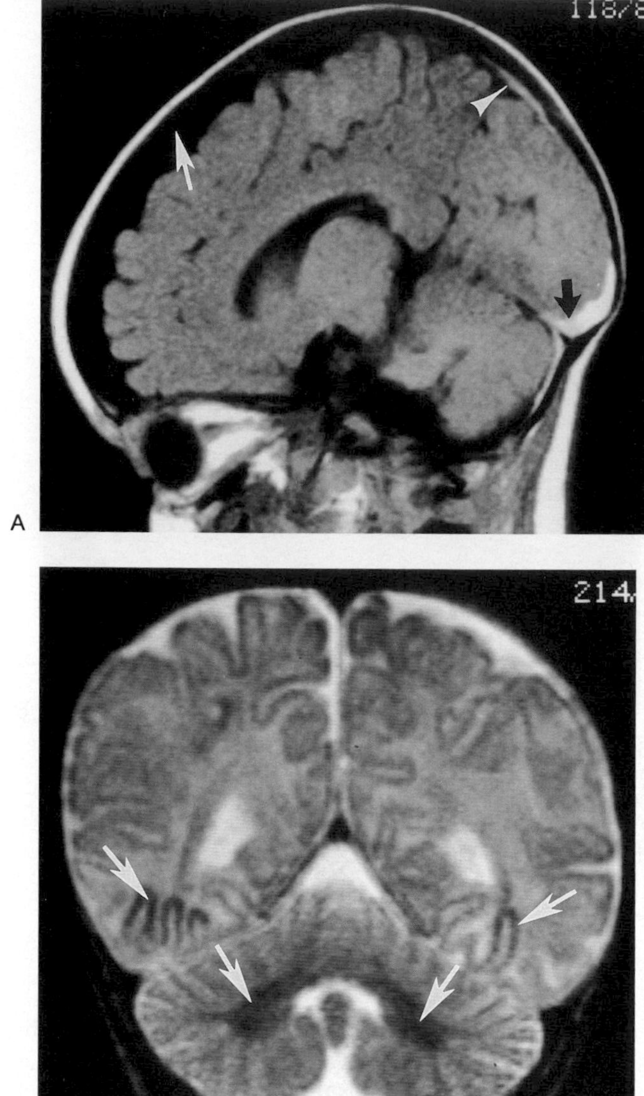

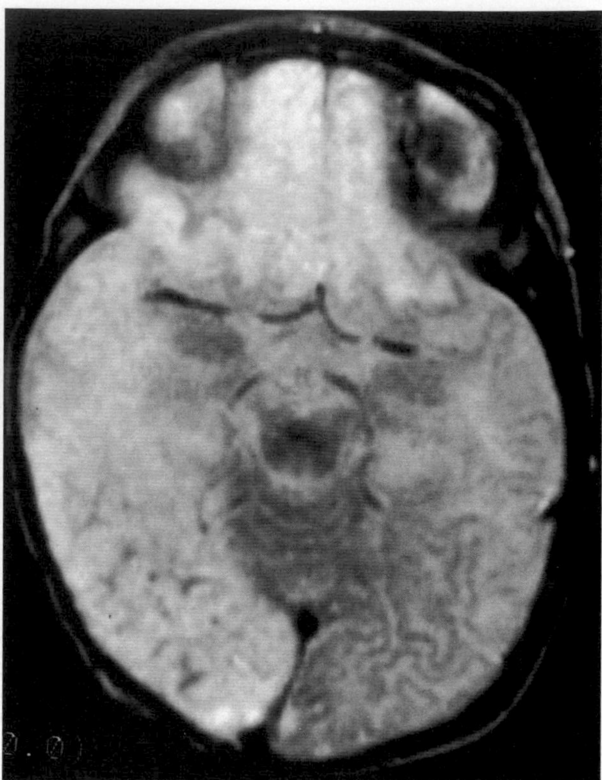

FIG. 21. Nonaccidental injury; subdural hematoma; ischemic infarction. **(A)** Sagittal T1-weighted (600/26), **(B)** axial PD-weighted (2300/30), and **(C)** coronal T2-weighted (2300/90) SE MR scans in a child who sustained multiple episodes of nonaccidental head trauma with possible strangulation. (A) Multiple SDHs of different ages are present, including chronic convexity (*white arrow*), subacute peritentorial (*arrow*), and subacute convexity (*arrowhead*) lesions. (B) Extensive MR signal hyperintensity from diffuse cerebral swelling and extensive ischemic infarction is present in both hemispheres but most severe in the right middle, right posterior, and bilateral anterior cerebral artery distributions. (C) Note the loss of normal gray-white matter differentiation on this strongly T2-weighted scan. Normal MR signal intensity and better gray-white differentiation is noted in the less involved portions (*arrows*) of the cerebellum and inferior temporal lobes.

Traumatic *intracerebral hematomas* are focal collections of blood that most commonly arise from rotationally induced shear-strain injury to intraparenchymal arteries or veins (Fig. 22) (7,60,61,102,106–108). They may occasionally result from penetrating injury to a vessel (102). Intracerebral hematomas (ICH) may vary from a few millimeters to several centimeters in size and occur in 2% to 16% of trauma victims (102,106–108). Differentiation from hemorrhagic contusions or DAI is often difficult (102,106–108). The distinction rests primarily with the fact that ICH primarily expand between relatively normal neurons, while the hemorrhage within contusions is interspersed in areas of simultaneously injured and edematous brain (7,102). The published variability in outcome from these lesions is likely the result of a failure to make this distinction (17,67,102,106–108). Prognosis of an isolated ICH is often quite good (108) unless it causes marked mass effect, is associated with DAI, or is associated with multiple shear-strain related basal ganglia hemorrhages (17,67,102,106,107).

Intracerebral hematomas are usually (80% to 90%) located in the frontotemporal white matter (Fig. 22) (95) or basal ganglia (102,106–108). These lesions are frequently associated with other primary neuronal lesions and calvarial fractures (102,107). Unlike patients with cortical contusions, DAI, or primary BSI, however, these patients may not lose consciousness and often (30% to 50%) remain lucid throughout the duration of their injury (102). Signs, symptoms, and clinical course are variable but similar to those seen with extraaxial hematomas. Temporal lobe hematomas are especially unpredictable, however, in that even small lesions may produce secondary BSI due to focal medial temporal lobe herniation (17,102). Delayed ICH should always be

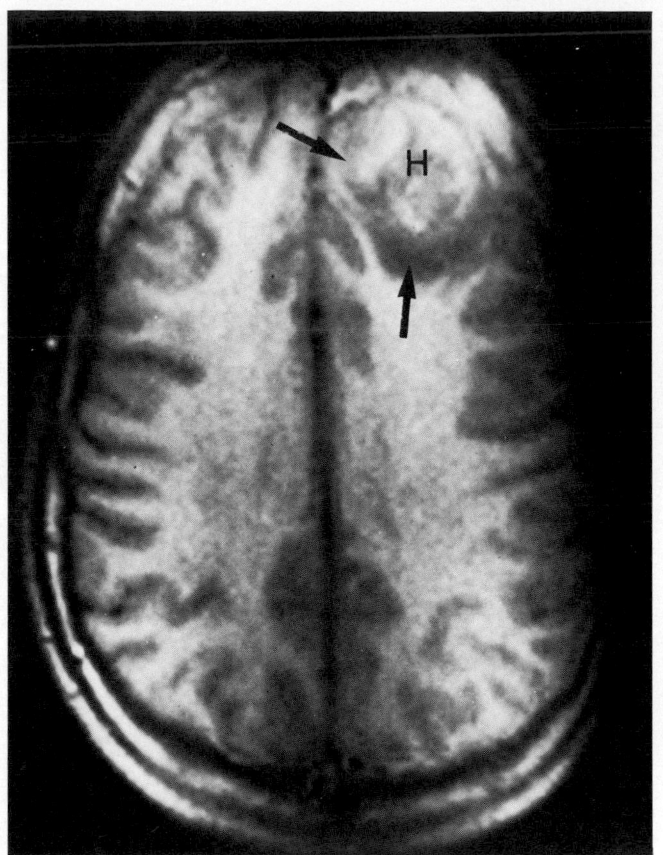

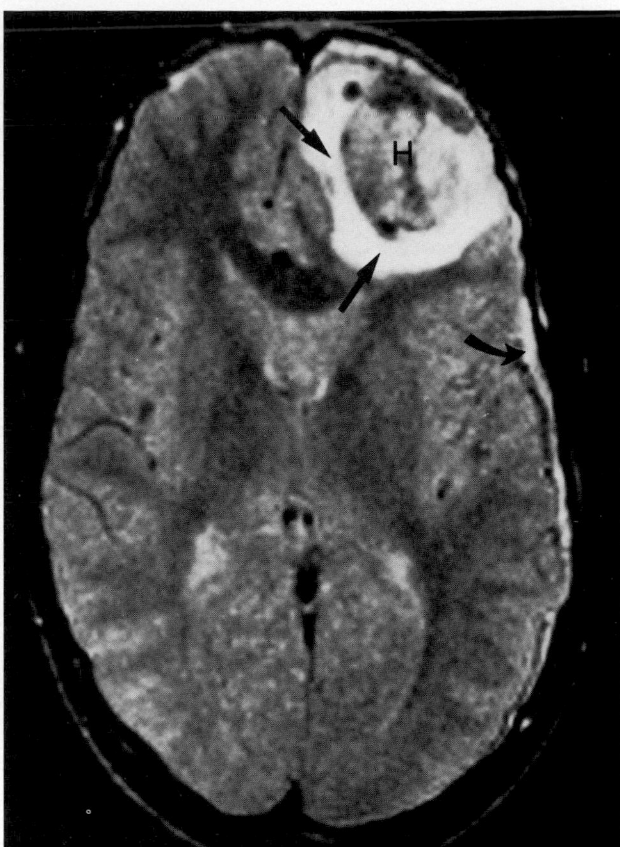

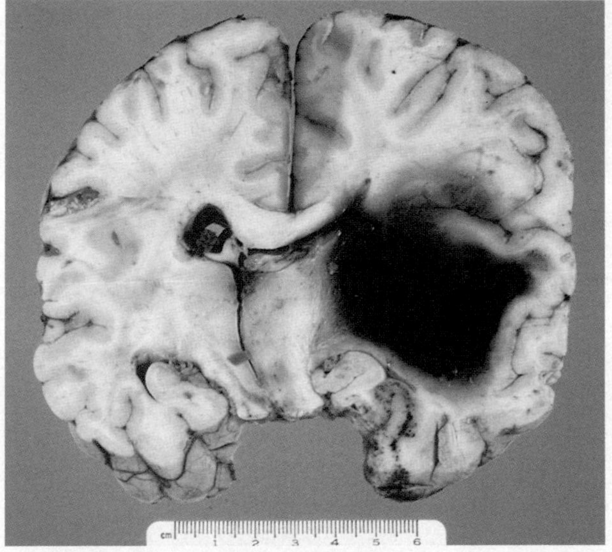

FIG. 22. Hyperacute intracerebral hematoma. **(A)** IR (2100/500/30) and **(B)** T2-weighted (2300/80) SE low field MR scans reveal a large hyperacute frontal ICH (H). Despite the isointense appearance of this 6-hour-old oxyhemoglobin-containing ICH, it is clearly visible with MR because of perifocal edema (*arrows*), mass effect, and anatomic distortion. An acute SDH (*curved arrow*) is also seen. **(C)** Coronal pathologic section from another patient with a huge acute ICH. Also present are midline displacement from subfalcine herniation, hemispheric swelling, and medial temporal lobe pressure necrosis and contusion from transtentorial herniation. ICH tend to separate and displace the adjacent neural tissue. Hemorrhagic contusions, on the other hand, tend to have the areas of hemorrhage interspersed with the injured brain tissue.

considered in patients who have a deterioration of their level of consciousness since they may occur in 2% to 8% of all patients with severe head injury (102).

Intraventricular hemorrhage (IVH) is quite common in patients with head injury, varying in incidence from 3% to 35% of cases, depending upon the severity of trauma (Fig. 7) (3–5,102). Intraventricular hemorrhage may be caused by a variety of traumatic lesions (DAI, intracerebral hematoma, large contusions) (3–5,102). The etiology of IVH in most cases, however, appears to be due to rotationally induced tearing of subependymal veins on the ventral surface of the corpus callosum and along the fornix and septum pellucidum (5). These veins are often disrupted by the same force that causes DAI of the corpus callosum (Fig. 7). In our published series of trauma victims (5), we found that IVH occurred in 60% of patients with DAI of the corpus callosum but in only 12% of patients without callosal injury ($p < 0.002$). IVH

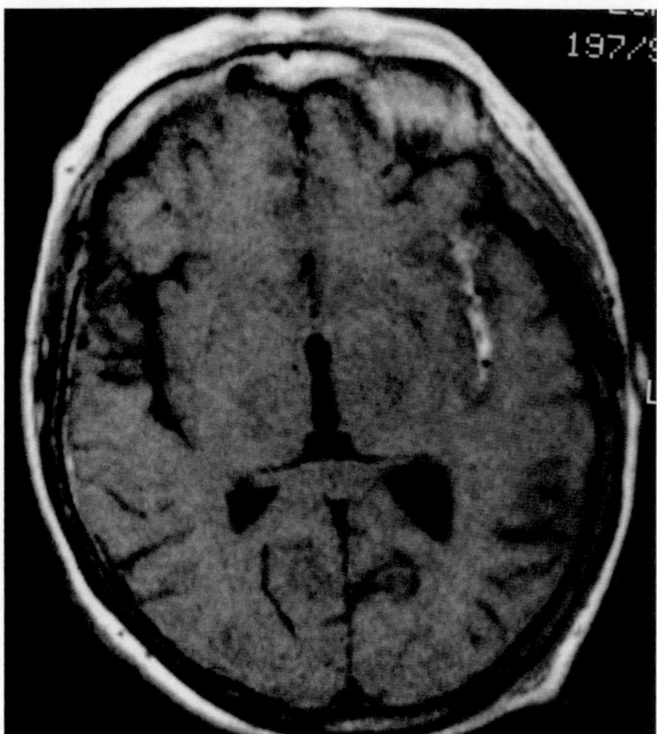

FIG. 23. Traumatic subarachnoid hemorrhage. Axial T1-weighted (500/20) MR scan reveals a considerable amount of blood within the left Sylvian fissure. SAH can occasionally be seen on MR scans, especially in the subacute phase and when the clot is large. SAH, however, tends to evolve and disappear more rapidly than hemorrhage in other locations.

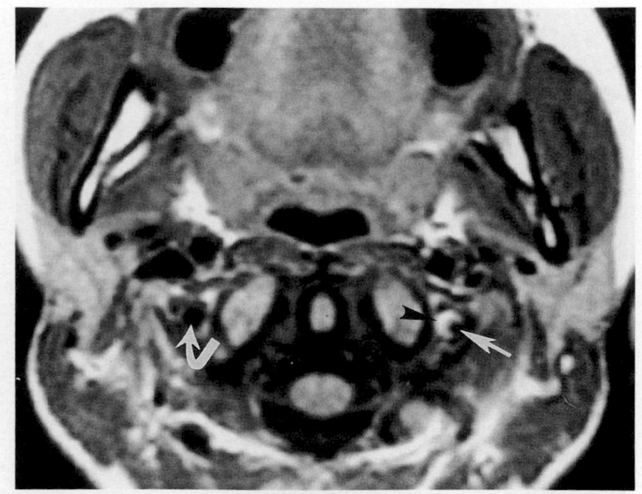

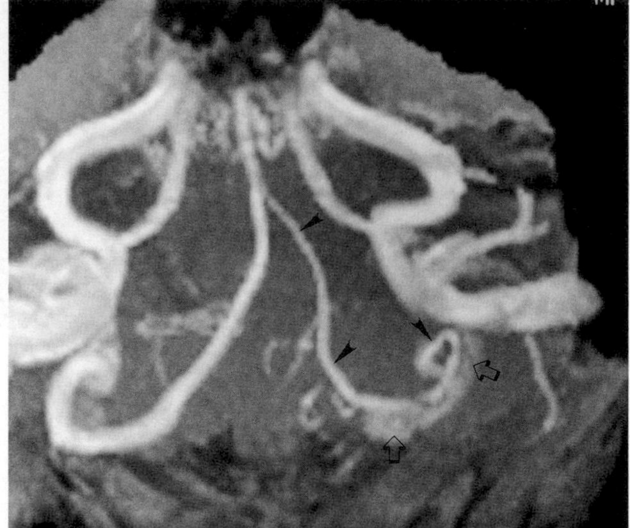

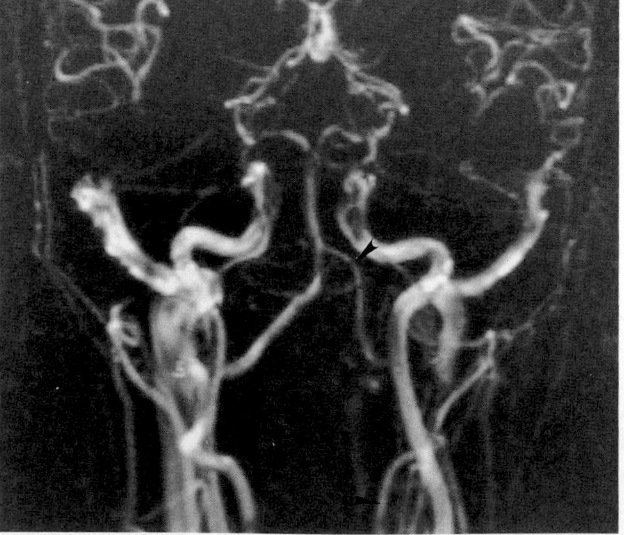

FIG. 24. Traumatic vertebral artery dissection with intramural hematoma. Thirty-six-year-old female presenting with diplopia and nystagmus after striking her head and neck while skiing. **(A)** Axial T1-weighted (549/19) SE scan reveals the right vertebral artery (*curved arrow*) to have a normal flow void, indicating patency of this vessel. There is a marked reduction of the normal flow void in the left vertebral artery (*arrow*), however, due to the presence of a dissecting intramural hematoma (*arrowhead*) containing high signal intensity methemoglobin. **(B)** 3D TOF (maximum intensity pixel projection) and **(C)** 2D phase contrast MRA images confirm the patency of the right vertebral artery (*arrowheads*) but demonstrate marked irregularity and a reduction in the caliber of the vessel lumen. Note that the intramural hematoma (*open arrows*) is visible on the TOF image because of the very short T1 of methemoglobin but is not visible on the phase contrast study since the later excludes stationary spins.

in patients without callosal injury were invariably due to dissection of large ICH into the ventricular system. The MR appearance of IVH will vary depending on its age, presence or absence of clotting, and whether or not erythrocyte lysis has occurred (3–6). The blood is invariably hyperintense to CSF on short TR/TE scans, however, easily allowing detection (3–6).

Subarachnoid hemorrhage (SAH) is considerably more difficult to detect with MRI than with CT (3,109,110). In our own series of trauma victims who had CT-documented SAH, the hemorrhage was seen in only 15% of cases with MRI (3). SAH is typically visualized with MRI only when there are large focal clots (Fig. 23). It may be seen more optimally with either T1-weighted or T2-weighted scans, depending on the age of the hemorrhage (3). It is usually detected more easily in the subacute phase as areas of T1 shortening in the subarachnoid space (Fig. 23) (3). Bradley and Schmidt (109) and Chakeres and Bryan (110) have comprehensively reviewed the theoretical considerations regarding visibility of SAH of various ages on different MRI pulse sequences, but it should be clearly understood that MRI is not sensitive to the presence of acute subarachnoid hemorrhage.

Primary Vascular Injuries

Traumatic vascular injuries are likely to be much more prevalent than have been previously reported in the literature (7,111–120). Asymptomatic vascular lesions may escape detection in the initial stages because of a low index of suspicion (7,111–112). In many instances, there may be a significant delay between the time of trauma and the onset of symptoms (Figs. 24–26)

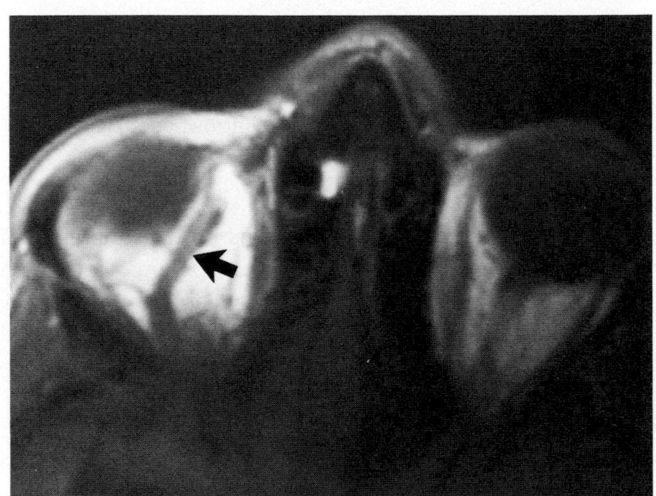

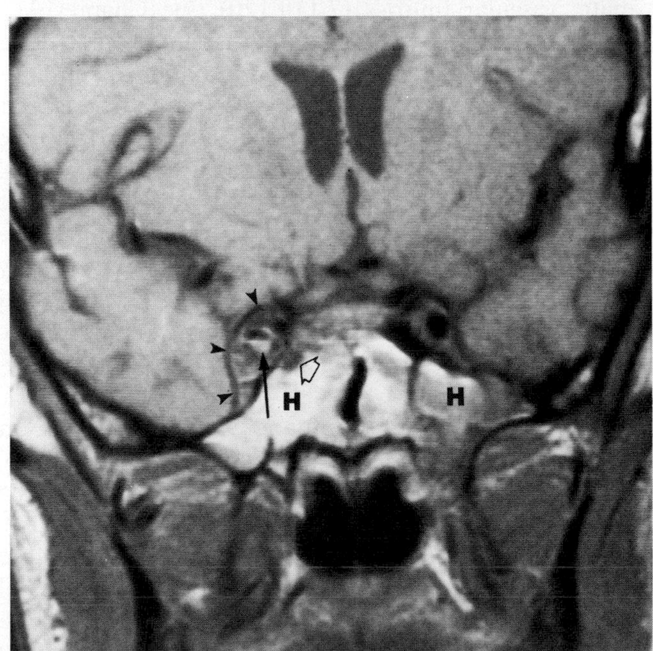

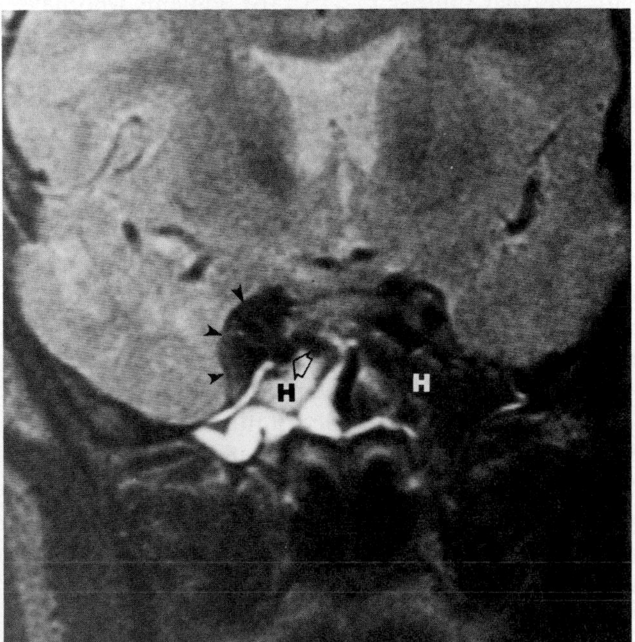

FIG. 25. Traumatic carotid artery laceration, dissection, and pseudoaneurysm; partially thrombosed carotid-cavernous fistula. **(A)** Axial T1-weighted (600/20) MR image reveals a markedly dilated superior ophthalmic vein (*arrow*). A flow void was not observed in this vein on multiple different MR pulse sequences, indicating thrombosis. Coronal **(B)** PD-weighted (2000/20) and **(C)** T2-weighted (2000/90) scans through the cavernous sinus reveal fluid and hemorrhage (*H*) of different ages in the sphenoid sinus. The right cavernous sinus (*arrowheads*) is enlarged due to the fistula. The internal carotid artery lumen is markedly compressed by an intramural hematoma (*arrow*) secondary to traumatic carotid dissection. Also visualized is a small angiographically proven pseudoaneurysm (*open arrows*) that was responsible for an episode of severe epistaxis one day prior to the MR scan. (From Gentry et al., ref. 115, with permission.)

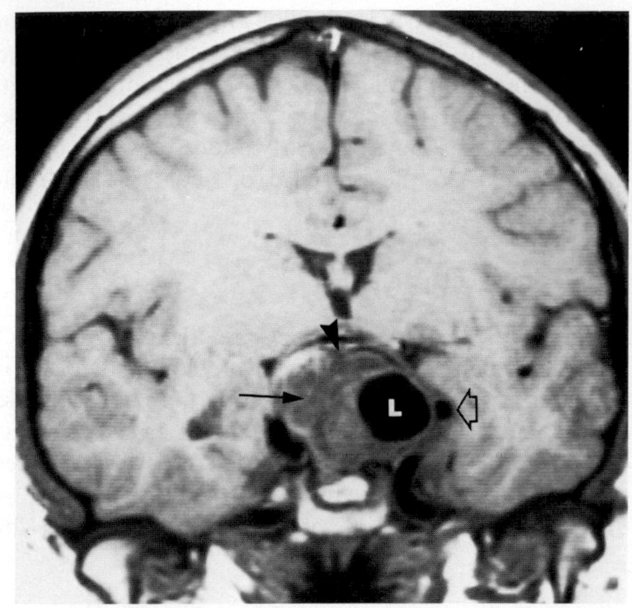

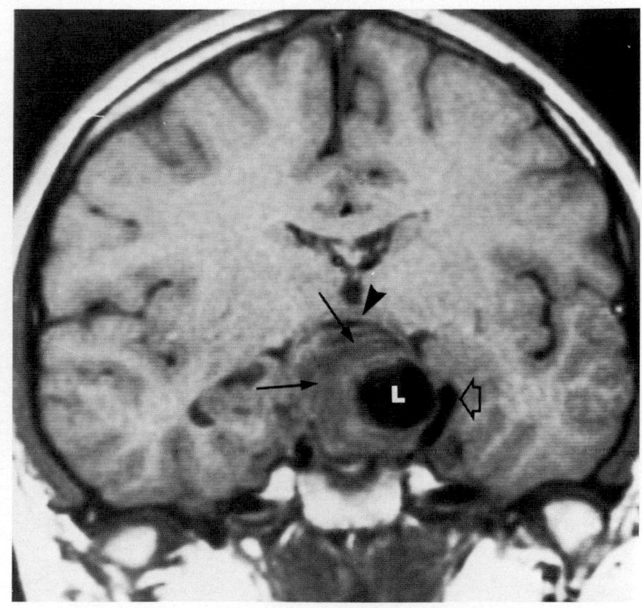

FIG. 26. Posttraumatic internal carotid artery pseudoaneurysm. **(A,B)** Coronal T1-weighted (600/20) scans reveal a traumatic pseudoaneurysm completely filling the suprasellar cistern. The thrombosed peripheral portion of the aneurysm is characterized by concentric laminated regions of intermediate to high signal intensity (*arrows*), while the central unclotted lumen (*L*) has a high-velocity signal void due to rapidly flowing arterial blood. The pseudoaneurysm is seen to be closely related to the patent left internal carotid artery (*open arrows*). The optic chiasm (*arrowheads*) is markedly displaced and compressed by the aneurysm. (From Gentry et al., ref. 115, with permission.)

(115,116). Many symptomatic lesions also go unrecognized in the acutely injured patient because they are masked by other intra- or extracranial injuries (7,111–112,115). Often the clinical symptoms and imaging findings arising from primary traumatic vascular injuries are attributed to other traumatic parenchymal injuries (e.g., contusions, SDH, ICH) (111,112).

CT scanning is very helpful in some respects in identifying those patients who are at increased risk for traumatic vascular injuries (7,115,116). Patients who have basal skull fractures that extend across the carotid canal, sphenoid bone (especially body, greater/lesser wings), petrous pyramid, and occipital bones have a much higher incidence of symptomatic and asymptomatic vascular injuries (7,115,116). Although CT scanning does accurately reveal these fractures, many patients with fractures do not have vascular injuries. Additionally, the exact nature of the vascular injury is not usually apparent with CT (115,116). CT is a good screening test, therefore, for identifying many of the patients who are at increased risk of traumatic vascular injury (115). It is a poor diagnostic test, however, for definitive documentation of the presence or absence of injury and for characterization of the exact nature of the injury.

MRI is slightly less accurate than CT for detection of basal skull fractures but is considerably more sensitive and specific for detection and characterization of the vascular injuries themselves (7,45,115). MRI provides the ability to directly visualize the vessel lumen and its contents, vessel wall, perivascular tissues, and adjacent bone (7,115). MRI itself can usually confirm patency of a vessel if multiple different pulse sequences are used (115,118,119). The nature of an occlusion or the severity of vessel narrowing can often be appreciated on sectional MR images if close attention is paid to the vascular structures (6,115,118). MRI, for this reason, can be considered an effective screening test for vascular injuries (115).

MRA offers a more definitive but noninvasive way to assess patients with symptomatic or asymptomatic traumatic vascular injuries (7,119,120) (see Chapter 31). MRA is especially valuable in that it can be obtained at the same setting as the MRI scan in patients who have MR findings that are suspicious for traumatic vascular injuries (7). MRA cannot yet be considered as definitive a diagnostic study as conventional arteriography (7). Generally, however, it can accurately reveal most types of traumatic vascular injuries in a rapid noninvasive manner (7,119,120). Conventional arteriography may be necessary for definitive diagnosis of subtle lesions and for endovascular treatment of several types of traumatic vascular injuries (severe hemorrhage, epistaxis, carotid-cavernous fistulae) (7).

The appearance of traumatic vascular injuries on MRI/MRA scans will vary, depending on the severity, location, and exact nature of the lesion. Spasm may be the only finding with minimal arterial injury (111,112), and this is not usually directly visible with MRI. More extensive laceration of the vessel may produce an intimal flap or damage to the vasa vasorum with subsequent development of a dissection and intramural hematoma

(Figs. 24 and 25) (7,111,112,118). These hematomas may significantly compromise the arterial lumen and impair flow (7). Slow arterial flow may be manifest on standard SE images by a diminution or disappearance of the normal "flow void" (Figs. 24 and 25) (7,115,118,119). A narrowed but patent vessel can be differentiated from an occluded one through the use of flow-sensitive pulse sequences (Fig. 2) or MRA (Fig. 24).

Arterial dissection, laceration, and occlusion can occur through a variety of mechanisms: laceration by skull fractures, penetrating injuries, blunt trauma, and stretching of the artery (7,111,112,115,117–120). Fractures of the skull base are one of the most common causes of arterial injury (7,111,112). These typically result from displaced fracture fragments that lacerate the vessel (115,116). The exact pathology will depend on the precise location and severity of arterial injury (Table 3) (Figs. 23–27) (7,111–120).

The internal carotid arteries are most vulnerable to fracture related dissections and occlusions in the area near the anterior clinoid process and clinocarotid canal (Fig. 25) (111–116). Patients with fractures in this area should be carefully screened for the possibility of a vascular injury. Thin-section short TR/TE MR scans can often provide a definitive diagnosis of vessel occlusion or dissection, obviating the necessity of arteriography (Fig.

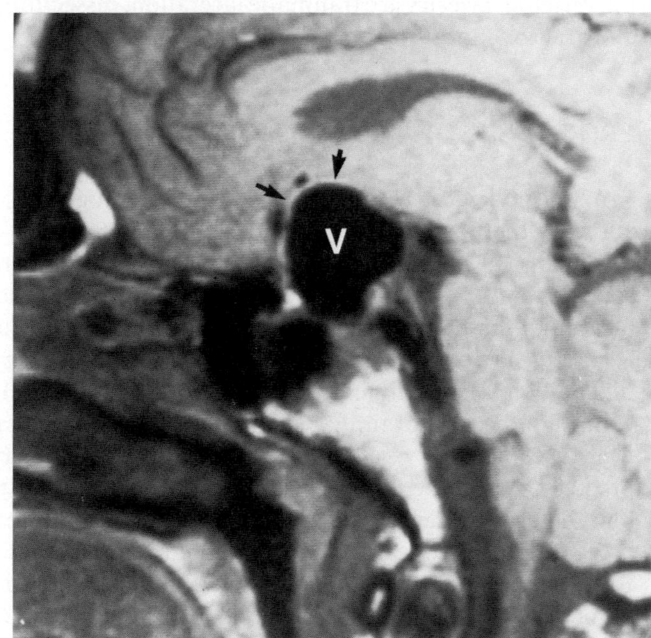

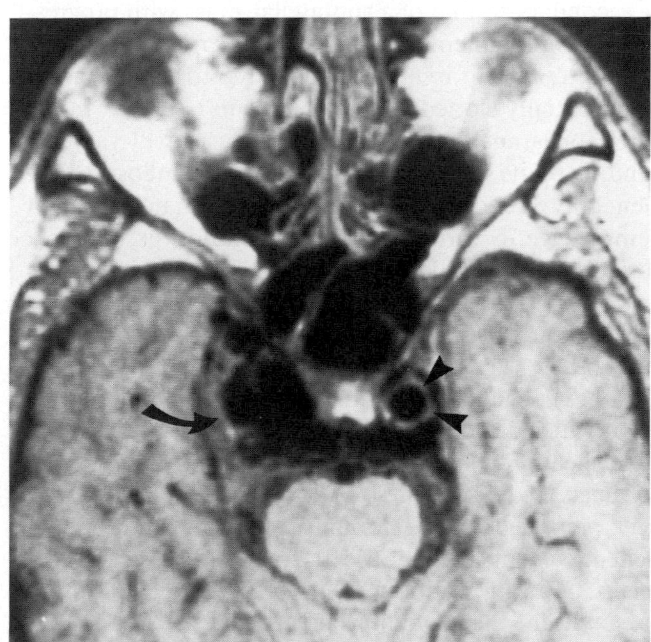

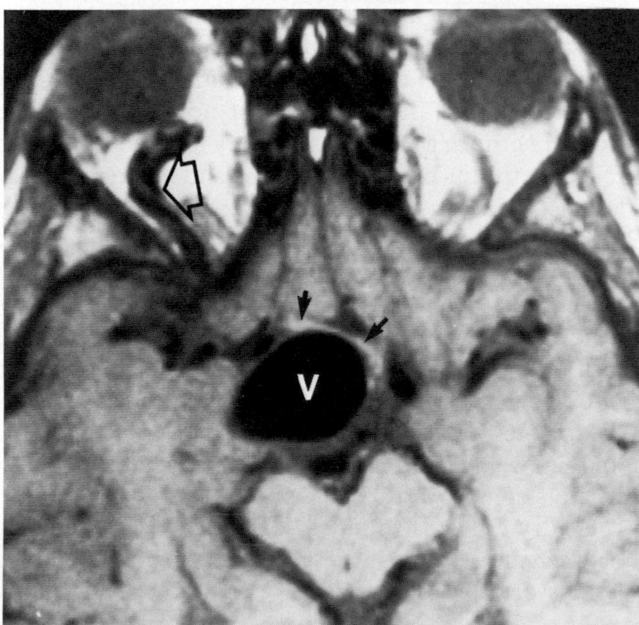

FIG. 27. Carotid-cavernous fistula with optic chiasm compression. **(A)** Sagittal and **(B,C)** axial T1-weighted (600/20) scans reveal a markedly enlarged superior ophthalmic vein (*open arrow*) and cavernous sinus (*curved arrows*) with evidence of high-velocity flow void characteristic of a carotid-cavernous fistula. The wall of the contralateral internal carotid artery (*arrowheads*) is well visualized, but the ipsilateral wall is not visible, presumably due to extensive arterial disruption. The optic chiasm and nerves (*short arrows*) are markedly displaced and compressed by a venous diverticulum (*V*) from the enlarged cavernous sinus.

25) (115). In fact, MRI may provide even more information than angiography in some cases, since the intramural hematoma is never directly visualized at angiography (7,115,118). Carotid lacerations in this region are often accompanied by simultaneous optic nerve injuries (Figs. 26 and 27) and, conversely, there is a much higher incidence of traumatic vascular injuries in patients who present with traumatic optic neuropathy (7,115). The combination of MRI and MRA should be strongly considered in any patient who presents with either of these two diagnoses (115).

Occasionally, the adventitial layer will be left intact and a pseudoaneurysm (Fig. 26) will develop (111–117,120). These false aneurysms can develop over a period of a few weeks to a few years. Symptoms will usually be secondary to that of a suprasellar mass with progressive bitemporal hemianopia, palsies of cranial nerves 3–6, or intermittent ischemic events due to embolization from partially clotted pseudoaneurysms (111–115). The MRI appearance of the pseudoaneurysm will vary depending on its size, age, and extent of thrombosis (115). Generally there will be concentric, laminated rings of hemorrhage in various stages of evolution as well as a variably sized patent lumen that can be recognized by its flow void (115).

When the full thickness of the arterial wall is torn, several other types of vascular lesions may develop (111,112). The precise nature of the lesion will depend upon which segment of the carotid artery is torn. A carotid sheath hematoma may be seen if rupture occurs in the neck (111,112). These patients usually present with neck pain, neck mass, Horner's syndrome, and cerebral ischemic events (111,112,119). A carotid-cavernous fistula (CCF) will result if a full-thickness arterial tear occurs within the cavernous sinus (Figs. 25 and 27) (111,112, 115–117,119). The MRI appearance of the CCF will depend upon the size and type of arterial tear and the pattern of venous drainage. The fistula may be "high flow" if a large tear is present (111,112), and there will be marked enlargement of the superior ophthalmic vein, cavernous sinus, and petrosal sinuses (Figs. 25 and 27). There will be MRI evidence of rapid flow (flow void) in these venous structures (115,119). There may be moderate proptosis, enlargement of extraocular muscles, and swelling of the preseptal soft tissues of the orbit. There may be bilateral enlargement of the superior ophthalmic veins when there is free communication of the fistula through the cavernous plexus of veins (111,112). If the drainage of the fistula is predominately via the inferior petrosal sinus, the superior ophthalmic vein may not be significantly enlarged. Less commonly, only a small intracavernous branch of the internal carotid artery will be avulsed and the fistula may be of a "low-flow" variety (111,112). The MR scan findings may be much less obvious in these cases. Finally, massive SAH will occur if the carotid laceration is intradural and of full thickness (Fig. 23).

Rarely, a skull fracture will lacerate the middle meningeal artery and its associated vena comitantes. When this occurs the patient may not develop the expected epidural hematoma since it may be "self-evacuating" through a dural (meningeal artery–meningeal vein) fistula (112). These may be completely asymptomatic or they may produce tinnitus because of increased flow through the petrosal sinuses and internal jugular vein. The MRI findings in these cases are usually limited to venous distention. Injuries of the vertebral arteries are also quite common, producing a wide spectrum of pathologies that closely correspond to those seen with injuries of the carotid arteries (111,112). The most common injuries of the vertebral arteries are traumatic laceration, dissection, and arteriovenous fistula (Fig. 24) (111,112).

PROGNOSIS OF HEAD INJURY

A full review of the many and varied demographic, clinical, therapeutic, and radiographic factors (13–17,27,80,95,96,121,122) that must be considered when assessing and predicting clinical outcome to traumatic head injury is beyond the scope of this chapter. Only a few MR imaging factors that have been shown to be significantly related to final prognosis will be covered (17). Clinical indicators of injury, such as the Glasgow Coma Scale, although very valuable, are not always reliable at predicting outcome (14,17,121). For example, similarly low Glasgow coma scores can occur from many different types of traumatic lesions, but the outcome from these various lesions may be quite different. Prior to the development of MRI, diagnostic studies had been of minimal value in predicting outcome (3–6,17). A number of reports have found an unsatisfactory correlation between CT scan findings and eventual outcome (8–10,17). The primary reason for the poor correlation has been the low sensitivity of CT for detection of nonhemorrhagic lesions (17). Since MRI is significantly more sensitive than CT for detecting both hemorrhagic and nonhemorrhagic lesions, MR scan findings have more closely paralleled final clinical outcome (17).

Gentry et al. (17) have attempted to identify MR scan findings that could be used to predict long-term neurologic outcome. They correlated the initial MR scan findings, initial Glasgow Coma Scale scores, and clinical data in 62 patients with moderately severe head injury with the long-term Glasgow outcome (17). Certain MR scan findings were found to closely parallel acute clinical indicators of injury (GCS scores).

Gentry (3–6,15) found a strong inverse relationship between mean initial GCS scores and the number of DAI lesions detected by MRI ($p < 0.001$). The higher the number of DAI lesions that were detected per patient, the lower was the mean admission GCS score. Low initial GCS scores were also significantly related to the presence of traumatic DAI lesions in the corpus callosum ($p < 0.001$) and primary DAI lesions of the upper brainstem ($p < 0.001$). Only a negligible correlation, however, was found between mean admission GCS scores and the presence of cortical contusions, epidural hematomas, and subdural hematomas.

Certain MR scan findings were also found to strongly correlate with long-term prognosis (17). The number of DAI lesions detected on the initial posttraumatic MRI study showed a strong inverse relationship ($p < 0.001$) with long-term Glasgow outcome. While 80% of patients without DAI lesions had a good recovery, only 27% of those with more than 10 lesions had a good outcome. Patients with MRI evidence of primary BSI also had a more dismal prognosis ($p < 0.005$) than those without injury. Additionally, MRI evidence of DAI of the corpus callosum was significantly associated with a poor prognosis ($p < 0.001$). It is unlikely, however, that the poor outcome in these patients is directly related to callosal injury but to the presence of more widespread DAI in the brainstem and deep white matter. Traumatic callosal injury appears to serve as a "marker" of DAI in more critical areas of the brain.

The mean number of cortical contusions was not found to be significantly related to final clinical outcome (17) unless there was definite MRI evidence of mass effect (transtentorial herniation, midbrain deformity, intrinsic secondary BSI). Also, no significant correlation was found between Glasgow outcome and the presence of isolated subdural or epidural hematomas unless they were large enough to produce transtentorial herniation. Small isolated subdural hematomas without mass effect had a prognosis that was uniformly good. Even those patients with transtentorial herniation and mild brainstem compression due to subdural hematomas did well if the hematoma was promptly evacuated and no intrinsic secondary BSI lesions were seen on MR scans (17). The prognosis of patients with subdural or epidural hematomas was only ominous when there was MRI evidence of marked transtentorial herniation, severe brainstem deformity, and intrinsic secondary brainstem lesions (17).

Although the number of their cases was very small, patients who had MRI signs of both brainstem compression and intrinsic secondary lesions within the brainstem had a much more dismal prognosis than if only brainstem deformity was present (17). The dysfunction of a compressed and deformed brainstem appears to be more reversible than one in which the deformity is also accompanied by focal intrinsic secondary lesions. This is consistent with the report by Seelig et al. (90) and others (89–92) that acute brainstem dysfunction may be reversible in some cases with rapid and appropriate treatment.

REFERENCES

1. Kraus JF. Epidemiology of head injury. In: Cooper PR, ed. *Head Injury*. 2nd ed. Baltimore, MD: Williams and Wilkins, 1987:1–19.
2. Frankowski RF, Annegers JF, Whitman S. Epidemiological and descriptive studies. Part 1: The descriptive epidemiology of head trauma in the United States. In: Becker DP, Polishock J, eds. *Central Nervous System Trauma Status Report*. Bethesda, MD: National Institute Neurological and Communicative Disorders and Stroke, National Institutes of Health, 1985;33–51.
3. Gentry LR, Godersky JC, Thompson B, Dunn VD. Prospective comparative study of intermediate-field MR and CT in the evaluation of closed head trauma. *AJNR* 1988;9:91–100; *AJR* 1988;150:673–682.
4. Gentry LR, Godersky JC, Thompson B. MR imaging of head trauma: review of the distribution and radiopathologic features of traumatic lesions. *AJNR* 1988;9:101–110; *AJR* 1988;150:663–672.
5. Gentry LR, Thompson B, Godersky JC. Trauma to the corpus callosum: MR features. *AJNR* 1988;9:1129–1138.
6. Gentry LR, Godersky JC, Thompson BH. Traumatic brainstem injury: MR imaging. *Radiology* 1989;171:177–187.
7. Gentry LR. Imaging of closed head injury. *Radiology* 1994;191:1–17.
8. French BN, Dublin AB. The value of computerized tomography in the management of 1000 consecutive head injuries. *Surg Neurol* 1977;7:171–183.
9. Lanksch W, Grumme T, Kazner E. Correlations between clinical symptoms and computerized tomography findings in closed head injuries. In: Frowein RS, Wilcke D, Karimi-Nejad A, Brock M, Klinger M, eds. *Advances in Neurosurgery: Head Injuries—Tumors of the Cerebellar Region*, Vol. 5. Berlin: Springer-Verlag, 1978:27–29.
10. Snoek J, Jennett B, Adams JH, Graham DI, Doyle D. Computerized tomography after recent severe head injury in patients without acute intracranial hematoma. *J Neurol Neurosurg Psychiat* 1979;42:215–225.
11. Cooper PR, Maravilla K, Kirkpatrick J, et al. Traumatically induced brainstem hemorrhage and the computerized tomographic scan: clinical, pathological and experimental observations. *Neurosurgery* 1979;4:115–124.
12. Clifton GL, Grossman RG, Makela ME, Miner ME, Handel S, Sadhu V. Neurological course and correlated computerized tomography findings after severe closed head injury. *J Neurosurg* 80;52:611–624.
13. Teasdale G, Jennett B. Assessment of coma and impaired consciousness: A practical scale. *Lancet* 1974;2:81–84.
14. Eisenberg HM. Outcome after head injury: General considerations and neurobehavioral recovery. Part I: General considerations. In: Becker DP, Polishock J, eds. *Central Nervous System Trauma Status Report*. Bethesda, MD: National Institute Neurological and Communicative Disorders and Stroke, National Institutes of Health, 1985:271–280.
15. Lobato RD, Cordobes F, Rivas JJ, et al. Outcome from severe head injury related to the type of intracranial lesion: a computerized tomography study. *J Neurosurg* 1983;59:762–774.
16. Cooper PR, Maravilla K, Moody S, Clark WK. Serial CT scanning and the prognosis of severe head injury. *Neurosurgery* 1979;5:566–569.
17. Gentry LR, Godersky JC, Thompson BH. Prognosis after severe head injury: MRI correlation with Glasgow outcome scale. [*Submitted*.]
18. Moseley IF, Zilkha E. The role of computerized axial tomography (EMI-scanning) in the diagnosis and management of craniocerebral trauma. *J Neuroradiol* 1976;3:277–296.
19. Dublin AB, French BN, Rennick JM. Computed tomography in head trauma. *Radiology* 1977;122:365–369.
20. Koo AH, LaRoque RL. Evaluation of head trauma by computed tomography. *Radiology* 1977;123:345–350.
21. Zimmerman RA, Bilaniuk LT, Gennarelli T. Computed tomography of shearing injuries of the cerebral white matter. *Radiology* 1978;127:393–396.

22. Tsai FY, Huprich JE, Gardner FC, Segar HD, Teal JS. Diagnostic and prognostic implications of computed tomography of head trauma. *J Comput Assist Tomogr* 1978;2:323–331.
23. Sweet RC, Miller JD, Lipper M, Kishore PRS, Becker DP. Significance of bilateral abnormalities on the CT scan in patients with severe head injury. *Neurosurgery* 1978;3:16–21.
24. Tsai FY, Teal JS, Itabashi HH, Huprich JE, Hieshima GB, Segall HD. CT of posterior fossa trauma. *J Comput Assist Tomogr* 1980;4:291–305.
25. Tsai FY, Teal JS, Quinn MF, et al. CT of brainstem injury. *AJNR* 1980;1:23–29; *AJR* 1980;134:717–723.
26. George B, Thurel C, Pierron D, Ragueneau JL. Frequency of primary brainstem lesions after head injuries: a CT analysis from 186 cases of severe head trauma. *Acta Neurochir (Wien)* 1981;59:35–43.
27. Lipper MH, Kishore PRS, Enas GG, Domingues da Silva AA, Choi SC, Becker DP. Computed tomography in the prediction of outcome in head injury. *AJNR* 1985;6:7–10, *AJR* 1985;144:483–486.
28. Mohanty SK, Thompson W, Rakower S. Are CT scans for head injury patients always necessary? *J Trauma* 1991;31:801–805.
29. Stein SC, Ross SE. The value of computed tomographic scans in patients with low-risk head injuries. *Neurosurgery* 1990;26:638–640.
30. Williams DH, Levin HS, Eisenberg HM. Mild head injury classification. *Neurosurgery* 1990;27:422–428.
31. Sipponen JT, Sepponen RE, Sivula A. Nuclear magnetic resonance (NMR) imaging of intracerebral hemorrhage in the acute and resolving phases. *J Comput Assist Tomogr* 1983;7:954–959.
32. Sipponen JT, Sepponen RE, Sivula A. Chronic subdural hematoma: demonstration by magnetic resonance. *Radiology* 1984;150:79–85.
33. Gandy SE, Snow RB, Zimmerman RD, Deck MDF. Cranial nuclear magnetic resonance imaging in head trauma. *Ann Neurol* 1984;16:254–257.
34. Moon KL Jr, Brant-Zawadzki M, Pitts LH, Mills CM. Nuclear magnetic resonance imaging of CT-isodense subdural hematomas. *AJNR* 1984;5:319–322.
35. Hans JS, Kaufman B, Alfidi RJ. Head trauma evaluated by magnetic resonance and computed tomography: A comparison. *Radiology* 1984;150:71–77.
36. DeLaPaz RL, New PFJ, Buonanno FS, et al. NMR imaging of intracranial hemorrhage. *J Comput Assist Tomogr* 1984;8:599–607.
37. Levin HS, Handel SF, Goldman AM, Eisenberg HM, Guinto FC. Magnetic resonance imaging after "diffuse" nonmissile head injury. *Arch Neurol* 1985;42:963–968.
38. Zimmerman RA, Bilaniuk LT, Grossman RI et al. Resistive NMR of intracranial hematomas. *Neuroradiology* 1985;27:16–20.
39. Gomori JM, Grossman RI, Goldberg HI, Zimmerman RA, Bilaniuk LT. Intracranial hematomas: imaging by high field MR. *Radiology* 1985;157:87–93.
40. Snow RB, Zimmerman RD, Gandy SE, Deck MDF. Comparison of magnetic resonance imaging and computed tomography in the evaluation of head injury. *Neurosurgery* 1986;18:45–52.
41. Zimmerman RA, Bilaniuk LT, Hackney DB, Golberg HI, Grossman RI. Head injury: early results comparing CT and high-field MR. *AJNR* 1986;7:757–764, *AJR* 1986;147:1215–1222.
42. Dooms GC, Uske A, Brant-Zawadzki M, et al. Spin-echo MR imaging of intracranial hemorrhage. *Neuroradiology* 1986;28:132–138.
43. Wilberger JE, Deeb Z, Rothfus W. Magnetic resonance imaging in cases of severe head injury. *Neurosurgery* 1987;20:571–576.
44. Groswasser Z, Reider-Groswasser I, Soroker N, Machtey Y. Magnetic resonance imaging in head injury patients with normal late computed tomography scans. *Surg Neurol* 1987;27:331–337.
45. Orrison WW, Gentry LR, Stimac GK, Tarrel RM, Espinosa MC, Cobb LC. Blinded comparison of cranial CT and MR in closed head injury. *AJNR* 1994;15:351–356.
46. Kanal E, Shellock FG. Patient monitoring during clinical MR imaging. *Radiology* 1992;185:623–629.
47. Jones KM, Mulkern RV, Schwartz RB, Oship K, Barnes PD, Jolesz FA. Fast spin-echo MR imaging of the brain and spine: current concepts. *AJR* 1992;158:1313–1320.
48. Atlas SW, Mark AS, Grossman RI, Gomori JM. Intracranial hemorrhage: gradient-echo MR imaging at 1.5 T: comparison with spin-echo imaging and clinical application. *Radiology* 1988;168:803–807.
49. Unger EC, Cohen MS, Brown TR. Gradient-echo imaging of hemorrhage at 1.5 Tesla. *Magn Reson Imaging* 1989;7:163–172.
50. Seidenwurm D, Tze-Kong M, Kowalski K, Weinreb JC, Kricheff II. Intracranial hemorrhagic lesions: evaluated with spin-echo and gradient-refocused MR images at 0.5 and 1.5 T. *Radiology* 1989;172:189–194.
51. Hennig J, Naureth A, Friedburg H. RARE imaging: a fast imaging method for clinical MR. *Magn Reson Med* 1986;3:823–833.
52. Shogry ME, Elster AD. Cerebrovascular enhancement in spoiled GRASS (SPGR) images: comparison with spin-echo technique. *J Comput Assist Tomogr* 1992;16:48–53.
53. Dean BL, Lee C, Kirch JE, Runge VM, Dempsey RM, Pettigrew LC. Cerebral hemodynamics and cerebral blood volume: MR assessment using gadolinium contrast agents and T1-weighted Turbo-FLASH imaging. *AJNR* 1992;13:39–48.
54. Lee C, Dean BL, Kirsch JE, et al. Cerebral infarction: assessment of patterns using ultra-fast MR contrast imaging. *AJNR* 1992;13:277–279.
55. Brant-Zawadzki M, Gillian GD, Nitz WR. MP-RAGE: a three-dimensional, T1-weighted, gradient-echo sequence—initial experience in the brain. *Radiology* 1992;182:769–775.
56. Mugler III JP, Brookeman JR. Rapid three-dimensional T1-weighted MR imaging with the MP-RAGE sequence. *J Magn Reson Imaging* 1991;1:561–567.
57. Runge VM, Kirsch JE, Thomas GS, Mugler JP III. Clinical comparison of three dimensional MP-RAGE and FLASH techniques for MR imaging of the head. *J Magn Reson Imaging* 1991;1:493–500.
58. Sato Y, Yuh WTC, Smith WL, Alexander RC, Kao SCS, Ellerbroek CJ. Head injury in child abuse: evaluation with MR imaging. *Radiology* 1989;173:653–657.
59. Bruce DA, Zimmerman RA. Shaken impact syndrome. *Pediatr Ann* 1989;18:482–494.
60. Holbourn AHS. Mechanics of head injuries. *Lancet* 1943;2:438–441.
61. Holbourn AHS. The mechanics of brain injuries. *Br Med Bull* 1945;3:147–149.
62. Strich SJ. Diffuse degeneration of the cerebral white matter in severe dementia following head injury. *J Neurol Neurosurg Psychiatry* 1956;19:163–185.
63. Strich JS. Shearing of nerve fibers as a cause of brain damage due to head injury, a pathological study of twenty cases. *Lancet* 1961;2:443–448.
64. Adams JH, Mitchell DE, Graham DI, Doyle D. Diffuse brain damage of immediate impact type: relationship to primary brainstem damage in head injury. *Brain* 1977;100:489–502.
65. Adams JH, Graham DI, Scott G, Parker LS, Doyle D. Brain damage in fatal non-missile head injury. *J Clin Pathol* 1980;33:1132–1145.
66. Adams JH, Graham DI, Murray LS, Scott G. Diffuse axonal injury due to nonmissile head injury in humans: an analysis of 45 cases. *Ann Neurol* 1982;12:557–563.
67. Adams JH. Head injury. In: Adams JH, Corsellis JAN, Duchen LW, eds. *Greenfield's Neuropathology*. 4th ed. New York: John Wiley and Sons, 1984:85–124.
68. Clifton GL, McCormick WF, Grossman RG. Neuropathology of early and late deaths after head injury. *Neurosurgery* 1981;8:309–314.
69. Hardman JM. The pathology of traumatic brain injuries. In: Thompson RA, Green JR, eds. *Complications of Nervous System Trauma. Advances in Neurology*, Vol 22. New York: Raven Press, 1979:15–50.
70. Jellinger K, Seitelberger F. Protracted post-traumatic encephalopathy: pathology, pathogenesis, and clinical implications. *J Neurol Sci* 1970;10:51–94.
71. Gennarelli TA, Spielman GM, Langfitt TW, et al. Influence of the type of intracranial lesion on outcome from severe head injury. *J Neurosurg* 1982;56:26–32.
72. Gennarelli TA, Thibault LE, Adams JH, Graham DI, Thompson

CJ, Marcincin RP. Diffuse axonal injury and traumatic coma in the primate: In: Dacey RG Jr, Winn HR, Rimel RW, Jane JA, eds. *Trauma of the Central Nervous System*. New York: Raven Press, 1985:169–193.
73. Lindenberg R, Fisher RS, Durlacher SH, Lovitt WV Jr, Freytag E. Lesions of the corpus callosum following blunt mechanical trauma to the head. *Am J Pathol* 1955;31:297–317.
74. Komatsu S, Sato T, Kagawa S, Mori T, Namiki T. Traumatic lesions of the corpus callosum. *Neurosurgery* 1979;5:32–35.
75. Shigemori M, Kojyo N, Yuge T, Tokutomi H, Nakashima H, Kuramoto S. Massive traumatic hematoma of the corpus callosum. *Acta Neurochir* 1986;81:36–39.
76. Rowbotham GF. The mechanisms of injuries of the head. In: *Acute Injuries of the Head*. 3rd ed. Edinburgh: Churchill Livingstone, 1949:1–37.
77. Lindenberg R, Freytag E. The mechanism of cerebral contusions: A pathologic-anatomic study. *Arch Pathol* 1960;69:440–469.
78. Ommaya AK, Gennarelli TA. Cerebral concussion and traumatic unconsciousness. Correlation of experimental and clinical observations on blunt head injuries. *Brain* 1974;97:633–654.
79. Gurdjian ES, Webster JE, Lissner HR. Observations on the mechanism of brain concussion, contusion, and laceration. *Surg Gynecol Obstet* 1955;101:680–690.
80. Rosenblum WI, Greenberg RP, Seelig JM, Becker DP. Midbrain lesions: frequent and significant prognostic feature in closed head injury. *Neurosurgery* 1981;9:613–620.
81. Crompton MR. Brainstem lesions due to closed head injury. *Lancet* 1971;1:669–673.
82. Tomlinson BE. Brainstem lesions after head injury. *J Clin Pathol (Suppl) (R Coll Pathol)* 1970;4:154–165.
83. Turazzi S, Alaxandre A, Bricolo A. Incidence and significance of clinical signs of brainstem traumatic lesions: study of 2600 head injury patients. *J Neurosurg Sci* 1975;19:215–222.
84. Saeki N, Ito C, Ishige N, Oka N. Traumatic brainstem contusion due to direct injury by tentorium cerebelli. *Neurol Med Chir (Tokyo)* 1985;25:939–944.
85. Pilz P. Survival after ponto-medullary junction trauma. *Acta Neurochir (Suppl)* 1983;32:75–78.
86. Britt RH, Herrick MK, Mason RT, Dorfman LJ. Traumatic lesions of the pontomedullary junction. *Neurosurgery* 1980;6:623–631.
87. Zuccarello M, Fiore DL, Trincia G, De Caro R, Pardatscher K, Andrioli GC. Traumatic primary brainstem haemorrhage: a clinical and experimental study. *Acta Neurochir (Wien)* 1983;67:103–113.
88. Friede RL, Roessmann U. The pathogenesis of secondary midbrain hemorrhages. *Neurology* 1966;16:1210–1216.
89. Caplan LR, Zervas NT. Survival with permanent midbrain dysfunction after surgical treatment of traumatic subdural hematoma: the clinical picture of a Duret hemorrhage. *Ann Neurol* 1977;1:587–589.
90. Seelig JM, Greenberg RP, Becker DP, Miller JD, Choi SC. Reversible brain-stem dysfunction following acute traumatic subdural hematoma. *J Neurosurg* 1981;55:516–523.
91. Gruszkiewicz J, Doron Y, Peyser E. Recovery from severe craniocerebral injury with brainstem lesions in childhood. *Surg Neurol* 1973;1:197–201.
92. Gyori E. Prolonged survival without neurological deficit following traumatic dorsolateral brainstem injury. *Clin Neuropathol* 1985;4:121–126.
93. Sunderland S. The tentorial notch and complications produced by herniations of the brain through that aperture. *Br J Surg* 1958;45:422–438.
94. Zimmerman RA, Bilaniuk LT. Computed tomography staging of traumatic epidural bleeding. *Radiology* 1982;144:809–812.
95. Baykaner K, Alp H, Ceviker N, Keskil S, Seckin Z. Observation of 95 patients with extradural hematomas and review of the literature. *Surg Neurol* 1988;30:339–341.
96. Lobato RD, Rivas JJ, Cordobes F, et al. Acute epidural hematoma: analysis of factors influencing outcome of patients undergoing surgery in coma. *J Neurosurg* 1988;68:48–57.
97. Bricolo A, Pasut ML. Extradural hematoma toward zero mortality. A prospective study. *Neurosurgery* 1984;14:8–12.
98. Servadei F, Faccani G, Roccella A, et al. Asymptomatic extradural haematomas: results of a multicenter study of 158 cases in minor head injury. *Acta Neurochir (Wien)* 1989;96:39–45.
99. Knuckey NW, Gelbard S, Epstein MH. The management of "asymptomatic" epidural hematomas: a prospective study. *J Neurosurg* 1989;70:392–396.
100. Milo R, Razon N, Schiffer J. Delayed epidural hematoma: a review. *Acta Neurochir (Wien)* 1987;84:13–23.
101. Pozzati E, Tognetti F, Cavallo M, Acciarri N. Extradural hematomas of the posterior cranial fossa: observations on a series of 32 consecutive cases treated after the introduction of computed tomographic scanning. *Surg Neurol* 1989;32:300–303.
102. Cooper PR. Post-traumatic intracranial mass lesions. In: Cooper PR, ed. *Head Injury*, 2nd ed. Baltimore, MD: Williams and Wilkins, 1987:238–284.
103. Seelig JM, Becker DP, Miller JD, Greenberg RP, Ward JD, Choi SC. Traumatic acute subdural hematoma. Major mortality reduction in comatose patients treated within four hours. *N Engl J Med* 1981;304:1511–1518.
104. Zimmerman RA, Bilaniuk LT, Bruce D, Schut L, Uzzell B, Goldberg HI. Computed tomography staging of craniocerebral injury in the abused child. *Neuroradiology* 1979;130:687–690.
105. Cohen RA, Kaufman RA, Myers PA, Towbin RB. Cranial computed tomography in the abused child with head injury. *AJNR* 1985;6:883–888; *AJR* 1986;146:97–102.
106. Jayakumar PN, Sastry Kolluri VR, Basavakumar DG, Arya BYT, Das BS. Prognosis in traumatic basal ganglia haematoma. *Acta Neurochir (Wien)* 1989;97:114–116.
107. Colquhoun IR, Rawlinson J. The significance of haematomas of the basal ganglia in closed head injury. *Clin Radiol* 1989;40:619–621.
108. Katz DI, Alexander MP, Seliger GM, Bellas DN. Traumatic basal ganglia hemorrhage: clinicopathologic features and outcome. *Neurology* 1989;39:897–904.
109. Bradley WG Jr, Schmidt PG. Effect of methemoglobin formation on the MR appearance of subarachnoid hemorrhage. *Radiology* 1985;156:99–103.
110. Chakeres DW, Bryan RN. Acute subarachnoid hemorrhage: in vitro comparison of magnetic resonance and computed tomography. *AJNR* 1986;7:223–228.
111. Davis JM, Zimmerman RA. Injury of the carotid and vertebral arteries: review article. *Neuroradiology* 1983;25:55–69.
112. Kassell NF, Boarini DJ, Adams HP Jr. Intracranial and cervical vascular injuries. In: Cooper PR, ed. *Head Injury*, 2nd ed. Baltimore, MD: Williams and Wilkins, 1987:327–354.
113. Barr HWK, Blackwood W, Meadows SP. Intracavernous carotid aneurysms: a clinical-pathological report. *Brain* 1971;94:607–622.
114. Mokri B, Piepgras DG, Sundt TM Jr, Pearson BW. Extracranial internal carotid artery aneurysms. *Mayo Clin Proc* 1982;57:310–321.
115. Gentry LR. Facial trauma and associated damage. *Radiol Clin North Am* 1989;27:435–466.
116. Gentry LR. Diagnostic evaluation of facial trauma. *Radiology Rep* 1989;2:41–58.
117. Komiyama M, Hakuba A, Yasui T, Yagura H, Fu T, Baba M, Nishimura S. Magnetic resonance imaging of intracavernous pathology. *Neurol Med Chir (Tokyo)* 1989;29:573–578.
118. Goldberg HI, Grossman RI, Gomori JM, Asbury AK, Bilaniuk LT, Zimmerman RA. Cervical internal carotid artery dissecting hemorrhage: diagnosis using MR. *Radiology* 1986;158: 157–161.
119. Magnetic resonance applications in cerebral injury. Sklar EM, Quencer RM, Bowen BC, Altman N, Villanueva PA. *Radiol Clin North Am* 1992;30:353–366.
120. Edwards JD, Sapienza P, Lefkowitz DM, Thorpe PE, McGregor PE, Agrawal DK, Samocha MS. Posttraumatic innominate artery aneurysm with occlusion of the common carotid artery at its origin by an intimal flap. *Ann Vascular Surg* 1993;7:368–373.
121. Giannotta SL, Weiner JM, Karnaze D. Prognosis and outcome in severe head injury. In: Cooper PR, ed. *Head Injury*, 2nd ed. Baltimore, MD: Williams and Wilkins, 1987:464–487.
122. Jennett B, Bond M. Assessment of outcome after severe brain damage: A practical scale. *Lancet* 1975;1:480–484.

Magnetic Resonance Imaging of the Brain and Spine, Second Edition, edited by Scott W. Atlas. Lippincott-Raven Publishers, Philadelphia © 1996.

15

White Matter Diseases

Mary K. Edwards-Brown and Jose M. Bonnin

The visualization of disorders of the cerebral white matter is unquestionably one of the major areas in neurological disease where magnetic resonance imaging (MRI) has become the standard and, in many instances, the only acceptable imaging modality. This can be traced to the inarguable advance in the sensitivity of the technique for detecting pathology of the white matter. There is a wide variety of causes of white matter lesions on MRI, and MRI, though highly sensitive, is only rarely specific for their etiology. Histologic and pathologic examination are far more specific, notwithstanding the lack of known causes for the majority of these entities. The purpose of this chapter is to discuss the MRI findings in white matter diseases and relate them to the underlying pathophysiologic processes. Knowledge of the pathologic basis for demyelination and dysmyelination improves our understanding of the MRI findings in these disease states and thereby improves the specificity of our diagnoses. Furthermore, it is becoming clear that MRI is the most sensitive indicator of white matter disease among all diagnostic methods, including bedside examination. MRI has therefore evolved beyond its adjunctive role in most diseases of the CNS to become an essential component of the work-up of all patients suspected of harboring such pathology.

There is no question that MRI is far superior to computed tomography (CT) in detecting and demonstrating the extent of intracerebral white matter diseases (Fig. 1) (1–3). Moreover, lesions affecting extracerebral sites, such as the optic nerves and spinal cord, are frequently seen on MRI, but have only rarely been reported by CT. This high sensitivity of MRI, when coupled with its lack of specificity, unfortunately results in the depiction of similar appearing but clinically diverse white matter processes. This discrepancy between sensitivity and specificity can actually limit the clinical relevance of MRI findings of white matter lesions in many patients, particularly when MRI is interpreted without input from the clinician. To maximize the interpretation of MR images in white matter diseases, it is essential to acquire an adequate clinical history, to recognize the various disease patterns that correspond to pathology, and to understand the variability in the appearances of these diseases on different pulse sequences (4) as well as variation simply due to the natural history of the disease. New developments in MRI, including spectroscopy, diffusion-weighted imaging, and magnetization transfer tech-

M. K. Edwards-Brown, M.D.: Department of Radiology, Riley Hospital, Indianapolis, IN 46202-5200.
J. M. Bonnin, M.D.: Department of Pathology and Laboratory Medicine, Methodist Hospital, Indianapolis, IN 46206.

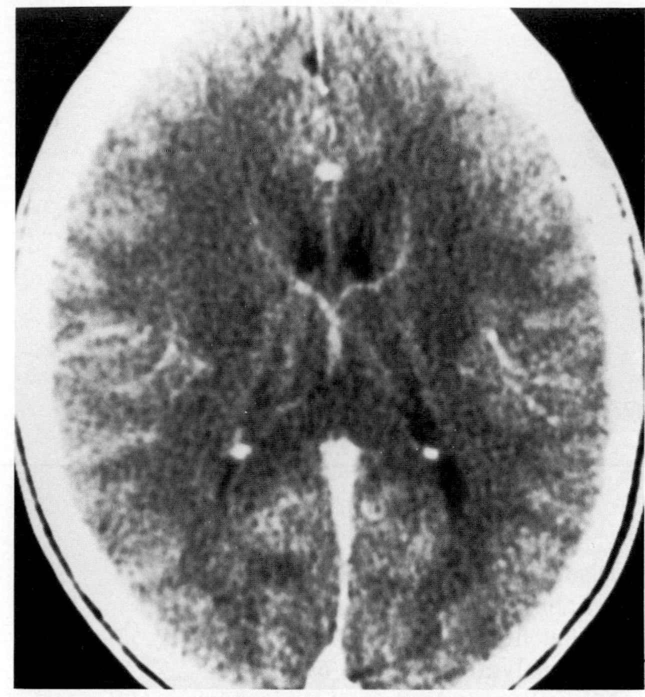

A

FIG. 1. Acute MS, enhanced CT vs. MRI. **A:** Contrast-enhanced CT is normal. **B:** Long TR/short TE MRI (3000/30) shows obvious large area of high intensity in periatrial right occipital white matter. **C:** Contrast-enhanced T1-weighted MR (600/20) image demonstrates clear enhancement in portions of the large white matter lesion (*arrows*).

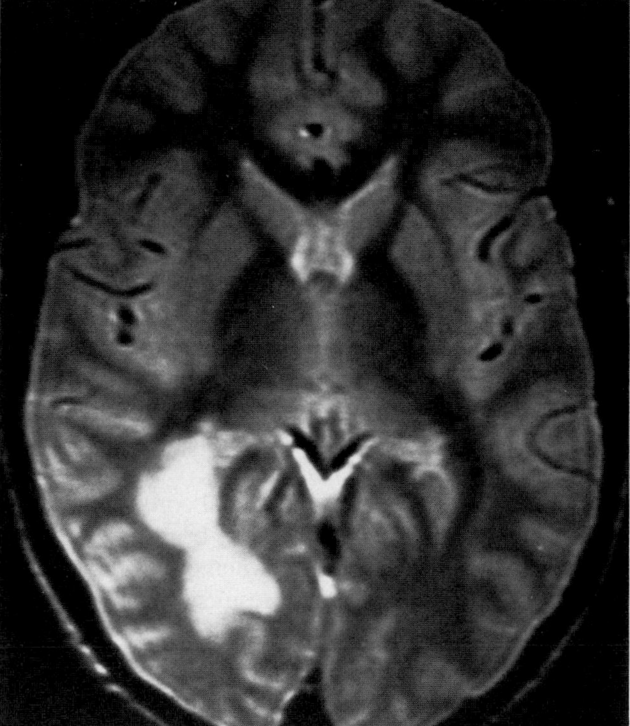

B

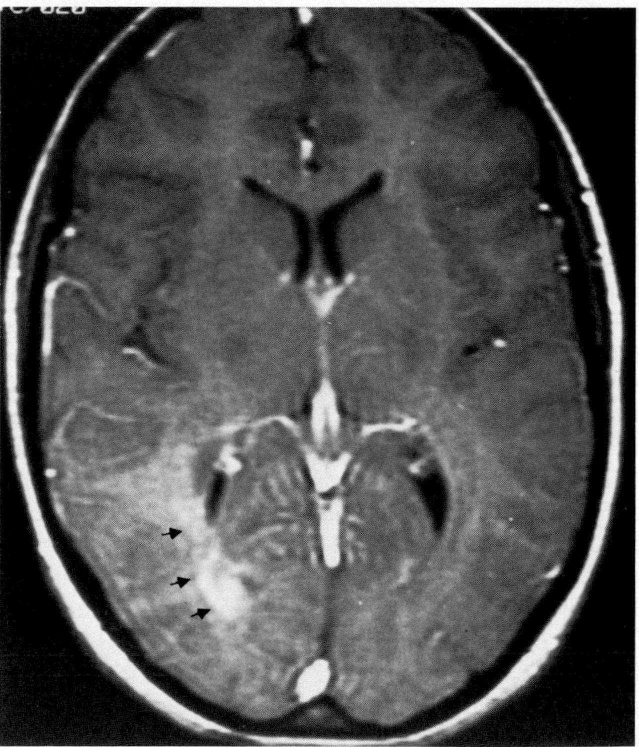

C

niques appear promising as methods to further our understanding of white matter diseases by potentially offering both improved sensitivity and possibly specificity for defining underlying histopathological alterations. Precise experimental methodology, long-term clinical follow-up, and detailed histopathologic correlations are required to ascertain the veracity of these newer techniques, the development of which provide continuing challenges to the radiologist.

WHITE MATTER STRUCTURE AND DEVELOPMENT

White and gray matter are normally composed of slightly different amounts of water and have different macromolecular components, notably lipid. Myelinated white matter contains 12% less water than gray matter. White matter also differs in organizational structure from most other tissues in that it is comprised of bundles

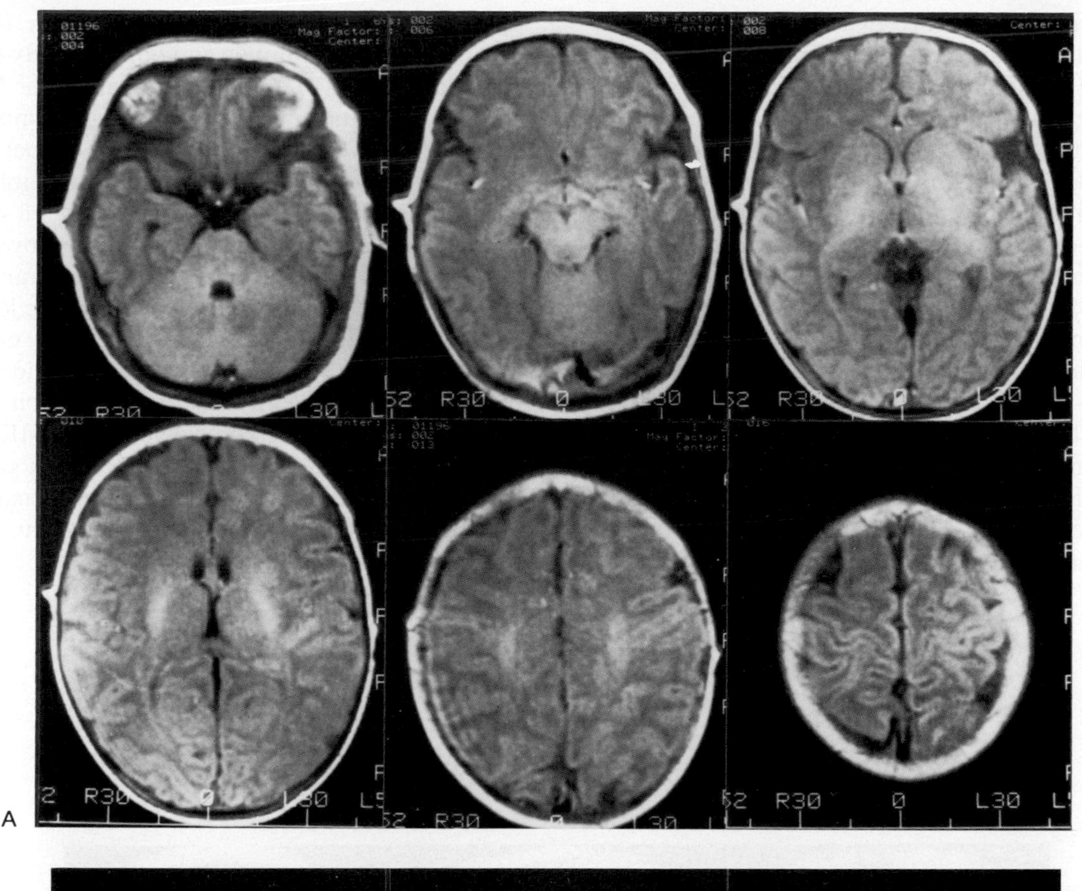

A

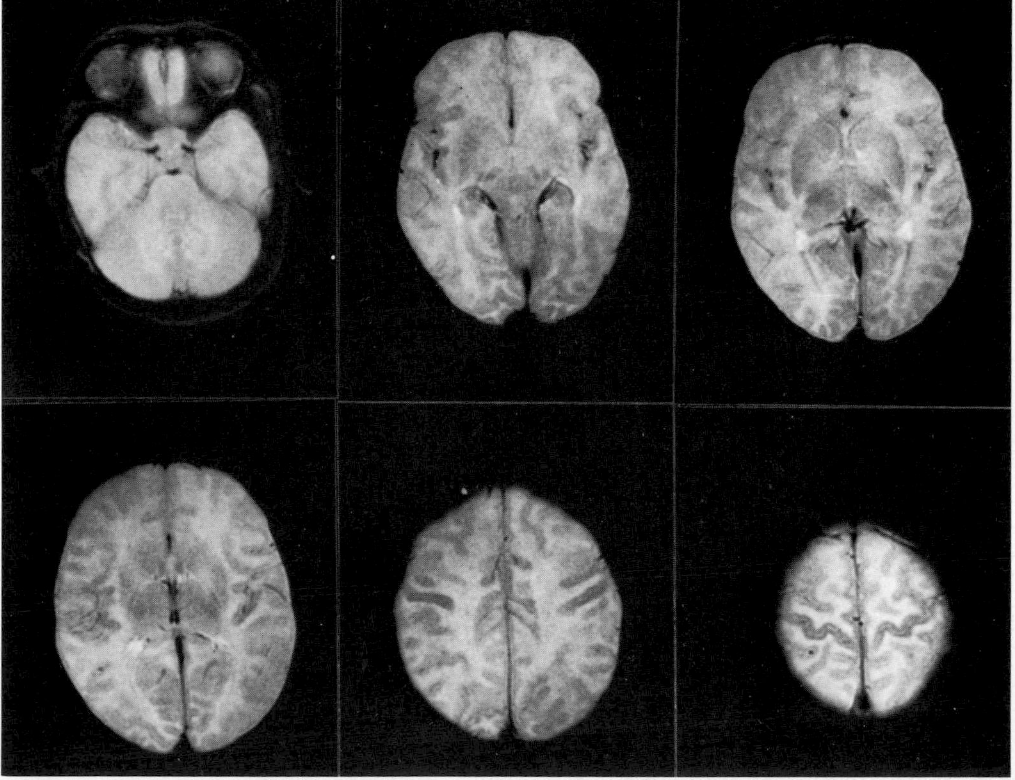

B

FIG. 2. Cranial MR image of a 2-week-old infant. **A:** SE 600/20 images show high intensity in the dorsal brainstem, the decussation of the superior cerebellar peduncles, the optic tracts, the posterior limbs of the internal capsules, the optic radiations, and the central corona radiata. Increased intensity is also present in the rolandic and prerolandic gyri, corresponding to known myelination of the white matter within these structures shortly after birth. **B:** SE 2500/70 images reveal low intensity in the dorsal brainstem, posterior aspect of the posterior limb of the internal capsule, ventral lateral thalamus, and perirolandic gyri. The decreasing signal intensity on T2-weighted images corresponds more closely to the temporal sequence of brain myelination as demonstrated with histochemical staining techniques.

of axons, which are bounded by a phospholipid plasma membrane surrounding the innermost layer of a myelin sheath. Since the quantity of tissue water and the interactions between tissue water and macromolecules that affect water mobility are responsible to a large degree for proton relaxation behavior and MRI signal intensities, it is assumed that these water content differences and the unique lipid content of white matter are responsible for differences in the appearance of white matter and gray matter on MR scanning. Mature white matter differs from gray matter in cholesterol, galactocerebroside, sphingomyelin, and total phospholipid content (5). These lipids account for the stability and strength of the myelin membrane. Any process, including metabolic injury or ischemia, that changes the chemical composition of myelin will result in a less stable structure that is more susceptible to injury (6). Although myelin contains large numbers of hydrogen protons, the hydrogen atoms of lipids do not contribute appreciably to the MR signal, because they are immobile and bound tightly to the long chain fatty acids (7). Lipid protons affect the MR image by communication with the surrounding mobile water protons, either by chemical exchange or magnetization transfer (or both) by way of transiently immobilized water protons. Cholesterol and sphingomyelin are known to alter the relaxation rates of lipid protons by shortening T1 relaxation times and by magnetization transfer effects even more than would be predicted by the lesser water content of white matter (7–9). However, a more recent in vitro study by Kucharczyk et al. (5) provides evidence that although sphingomyelin, cholesterol, phosphatidylcholine, and galactocerebroside all affect MR relaxivity and magnetization transfer, it is likely that galactocerebroside is the major cause of the shorter relaxation times and stronger magnetization transfer effects of normal myelinated white matter.

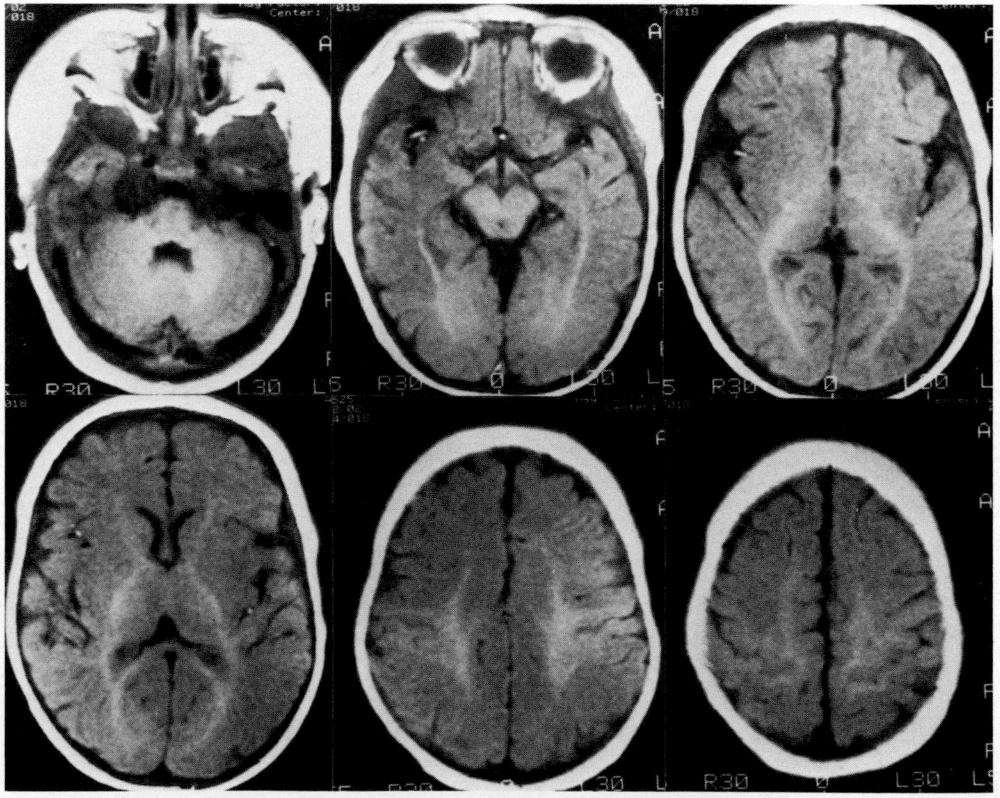

FIG. 3. Cranial MR image of a 3-month-old infant. SE 600/20 images show high intensity in the middle cerebellar peduncles and in the ventral aspect of the brainstem. High intensity is now seen in the anterior limbs of the internal capsule and in the optic radiations all the way to the striate cortex. High signal extends through the centrum semiovale to the subcortical white matter in the pre- and postcentral gyri. The cortical gray matter and subcortical white matter are essentially isointense at this age, making structural abnormalities difficult to detect on T1-weighted images. T2-weighted images are helpful in the detection of structural abnormalities at this age.

The process of myelination of the brain occurs in a progressive and systematic fashion which has been clearly described both from histologic studies and from review of MRI examinations (6,10). The process of progressive myelination of the brain is affected by certain diseases. When interpreting MRI examinations of children less than one year of age it is important to compare the myelination seen to that of published normals (Figs. 2–11). Table 1 lists the milestones of normal myelination seen on MR imaging at 1.5 Tesla. As illustrated in the table, different rates of myelination are implied by T1-weighted images and T2-weighted images of the brain. Although the exact mechanisms are not fully understood at the time of this writing, it is known that the changes on T1-weighted MRI parallel increases in certain lipids that occur during the formation of myelin from oligodendrocytes (6). The changes on T2-weighted MRI occur during the period of maturation of the myelin sheath seen histologically as tightening of the spiral of myelin around the axon (6).

DEMYELINATING DISEASES

Demyelinating diseases, also known as myelinoclastic diseases, are diseases in which normally formed myelin is later destroyed. The pathologic hallmark of all demyelinating disease is the destruction of myelin with relative sparing of axons, which differentiates demyelinating diseases from conditions with breakdown of myelin as a secondary phenomenon of neuronal destruction. MRI to date cannot distinguish lesions of myelin versus those involving axons with secondary myelin breakdown. *Primary* demyelinating diseases are those where the demyelination is the sole disease process, occurring in the absence of systemic disease (11) (see Table 2).

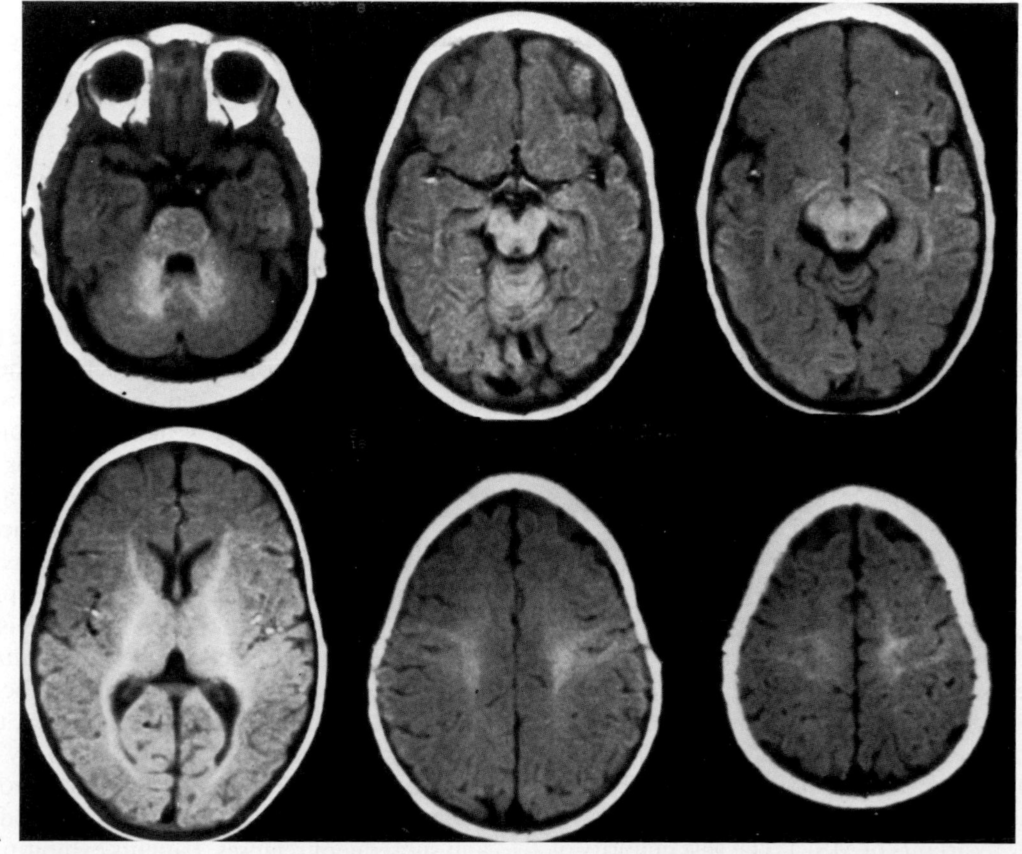

FIG. 4. Cranial MR image of a 4-month-old infant. **A:** SE 600/20 images show a significant increase in the myelination of the anterior limbs of the internal capsule. The splenium of the corpus callosum is now of high intensity. Notice that the cortical gray matter and subcortical white matter are isointense, resulting in difficulty detecting structural abnormalities.

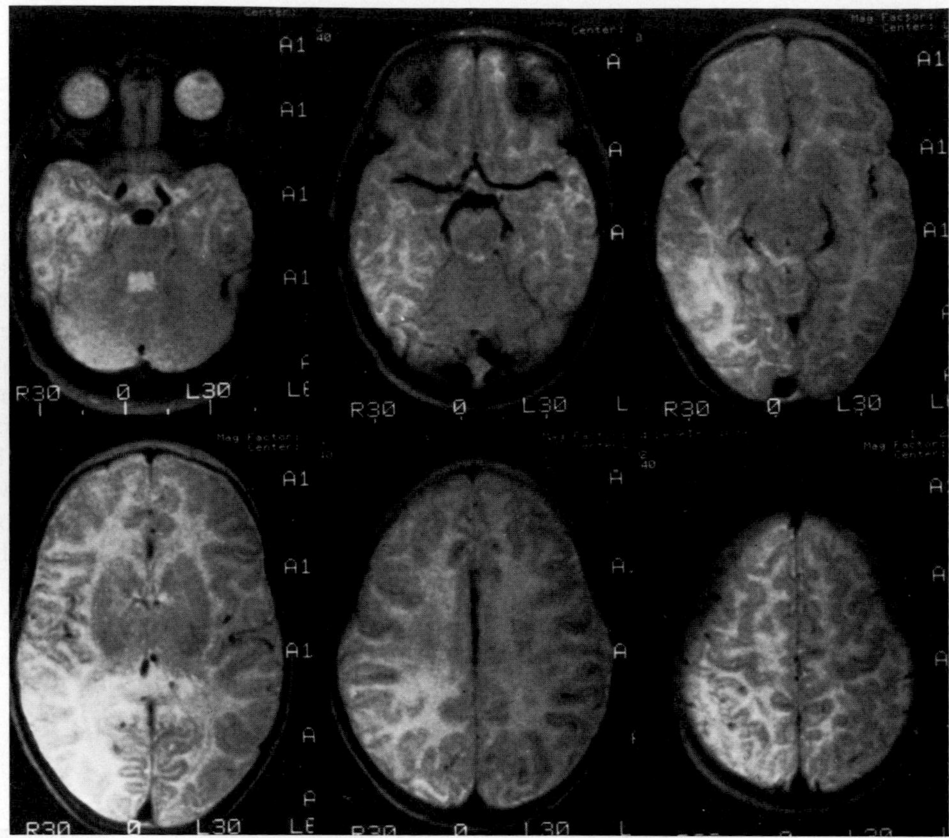

FIG. 4. (*Continued.*) **B:** The SE 2500/70 image is essentially unchanged from the infant demonstrated in Fig. 1.

With a few exceptions, the causes of myelinoclastic diseases are unknown. The known pathogenic agents and mechanisms in either human diseases or animal models include viral infection, post-infectious or post-immunization immune responses, and toxic chemical agents.

Multiple Sclerosis

Clinical Features

Multiple sclerosis (MS) is the most common and most extensively studied of all the demyelinating diseases, yet the etiology of MS is still poorly understood. There are several different disease patterns of white matter that are generally considered different forms of MS (see Table 2 and the section, "Variants of MS"). The vast majority of MS cases are categorized into the *classic* form, or Charcot type. Although most patients initially present in the third and fourth decades, 15% come to attention before the age of 20 and 10% after 50 years of age (12). Females are slightly more commonly afflicted. The first clinical symptom is often impaired or double vision. The patients may complain of weakness, numbness, tingling, and gait disturbances. As the disease progresses, loss of sphincter control, blindness, paralysis, and dementia may develop. Patients rarely experience pain with multiple sclerosis, except that which is associated with eye movement in those patients with an episode of optic neuritis. The clinical course of classic MS is variable, but most patients experience a *relapsing-remitting* course of exacerbations and remissions of multifocal neurologic deficits. Early in the course of the disease, recovery after relapse is often complete, but the majority of these cases show a protracted course with progression of deficits. Other cases are progressive without episodic remissions and subsequent relapses. Patients exhibiting the *chronic-progressive* pattern typically have more severe spinal cord involvement. Late in the classic form of the disease, severe neurologic disability with cognitive impairment

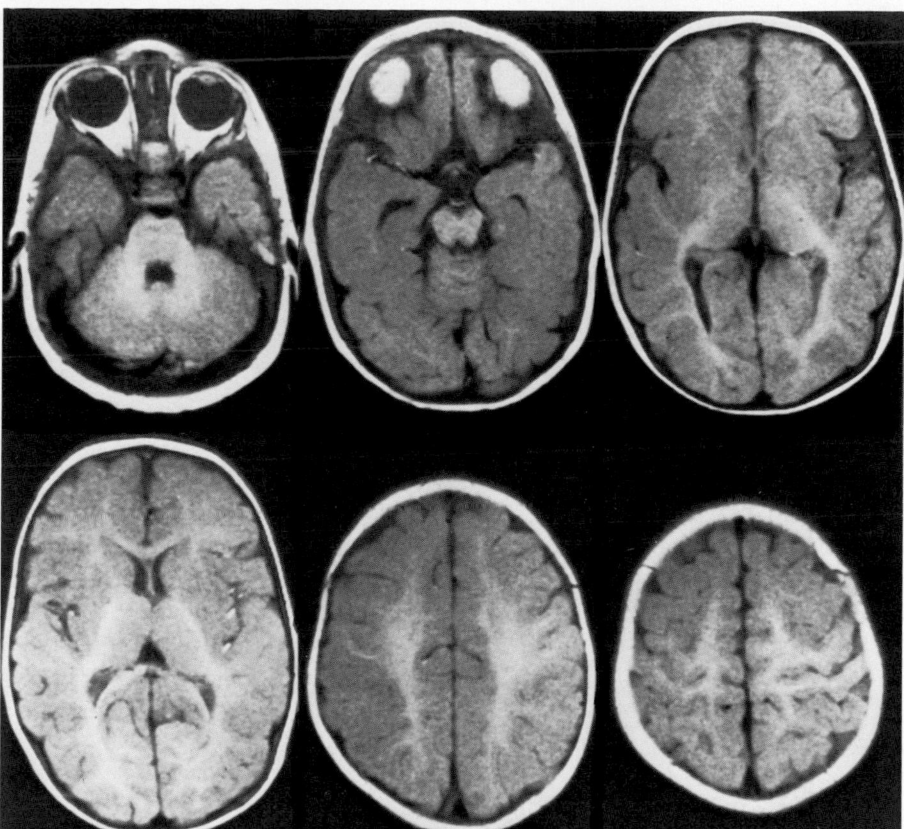

FIG. 5. Cranial MR image of a 6-month-old infant. **A:** SE 600/20 images show the splenium and genu of the corpus callosum to be of high signal intensity. There has been significant progression of the maturation of the centrum semiovale. The subcortical white matter, most notably in the occipital and paracentral regions, is now hyperintense with respect to the overlying cortex. **B:** SE 2500/70 images reveal a mild diminution of signal intensity within the central centrum semiovale. The basal ganglia are now of very low signal intensity with respect to the surrounding brain. The splenium of the corpus callosum is of low intensity.

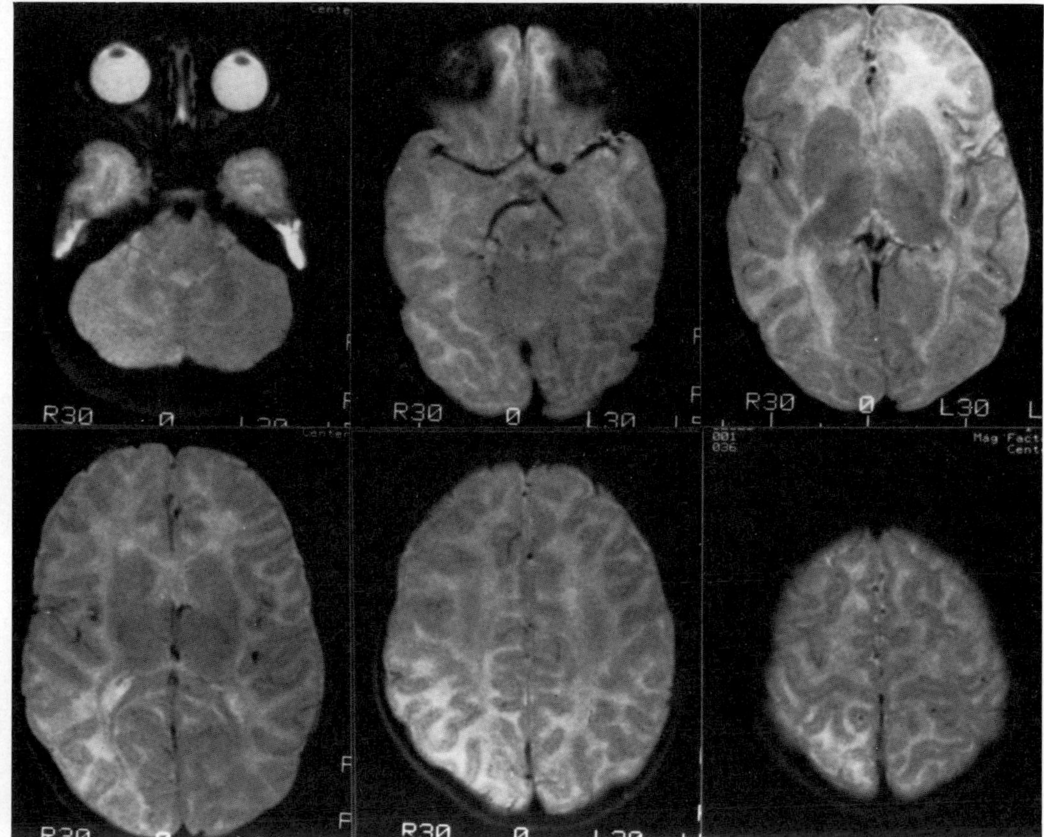

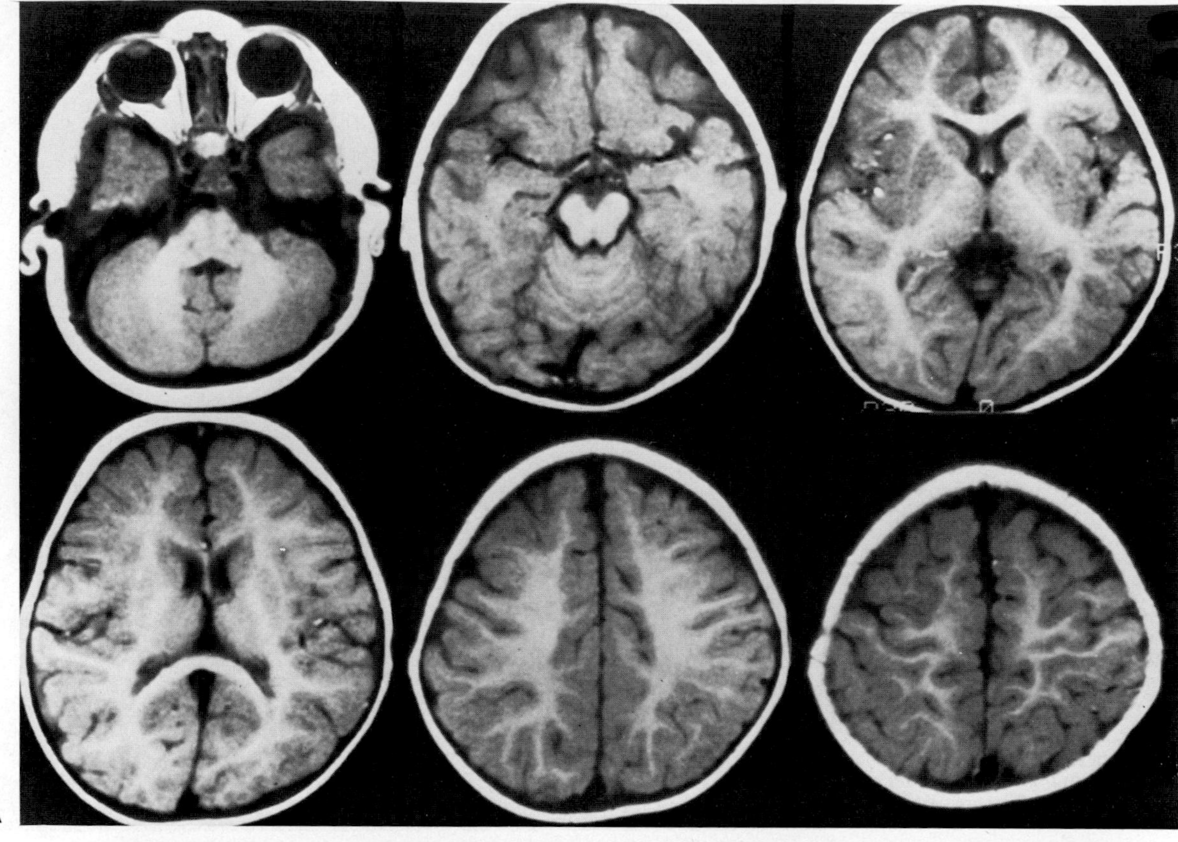

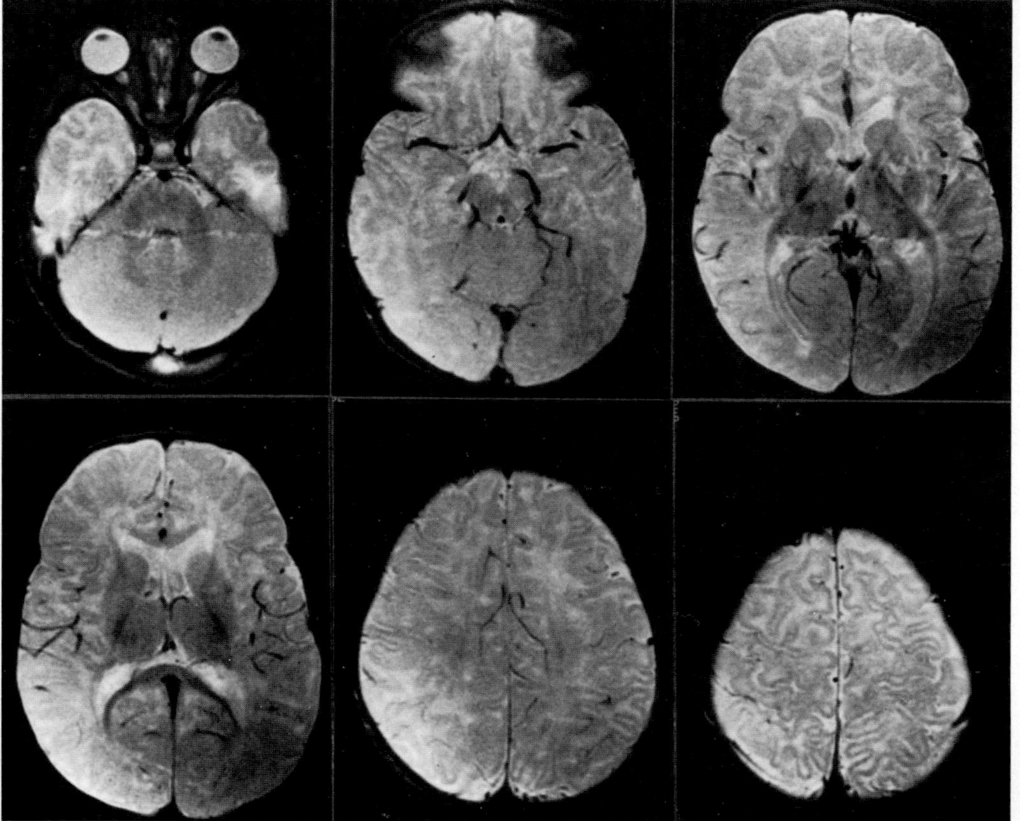

FIG. 6. Cranial MR image of an 8-month-old infant. **A:** SE 600/20 images show myelination of all deep white matter. The subcortical white matter is of high intensity in the paracentral and occipital regions but has not quite matured in the frontal and posterior temporal/parietal areas. **B:** SE 2500/70 images show diminished signal intensity in the anterior limbs of the internal capsule. Both the splenium and genu of the corpus callosum are of low intensity. The hemispheric white matter is becoming isointense with cortex.

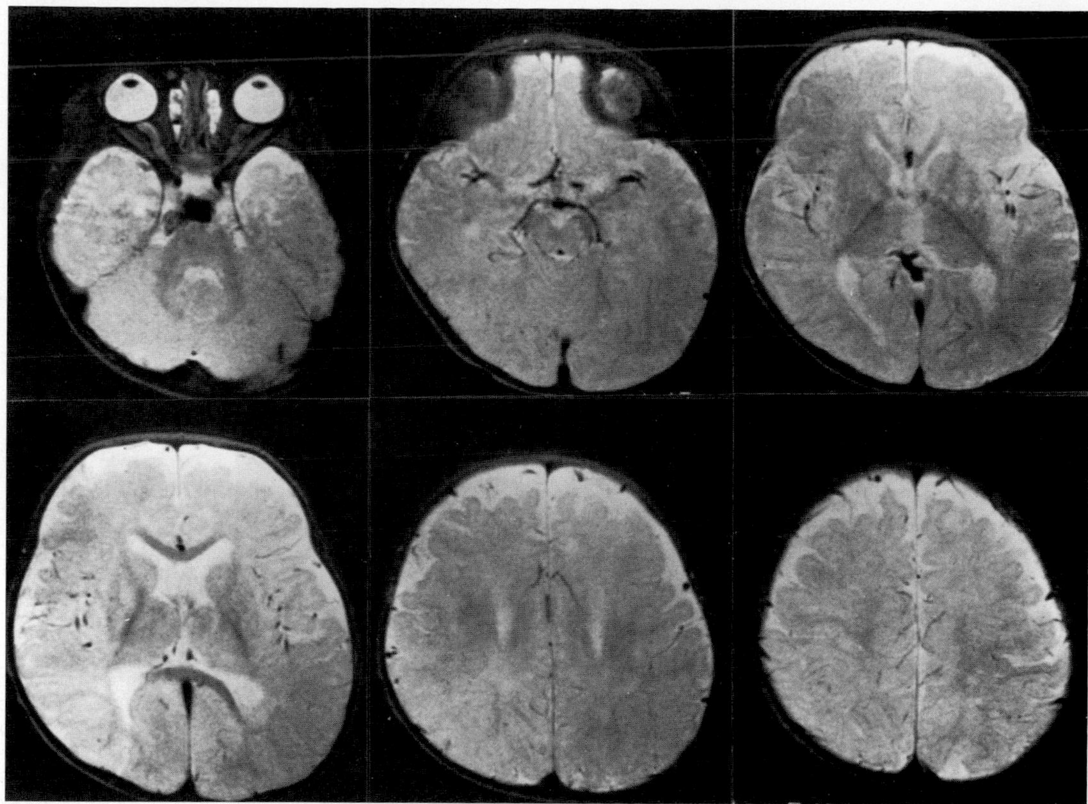

FIG. 7. Cranial MR image of a 10-month-old infant. SE 2500/70 images reveal diminished intensity of the white matter diffusely throughout the brain. This results in a near isointensity of the deep nuclei, white matter, and cortex. For this reason, structural abnormalities of the brain are best identified on short TR/TE images at this age.

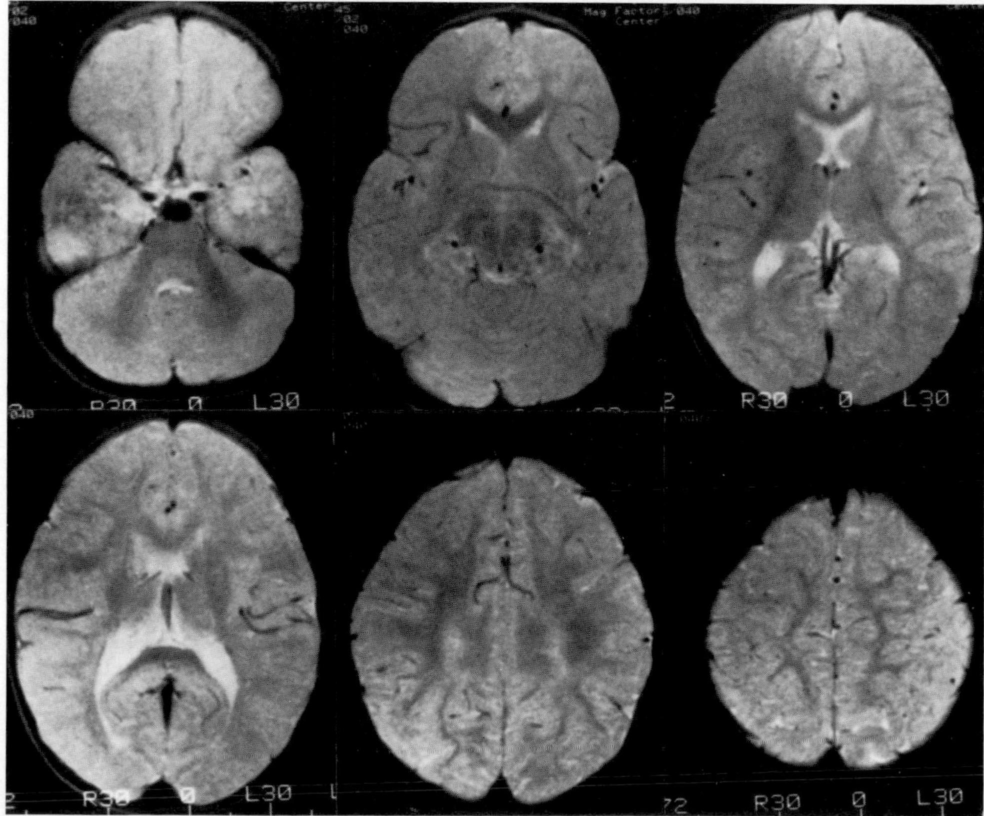

FIG. 8. Cranial MR image of a 15-month-old infant. The maturation of the deep white matter has progressed significantly since the 10-month-old stage. The subcortical white matter is now hypointense in the paracentral and calcarine regions. Maturation is slowest in the frontal and posterior parietal/temporal regions.

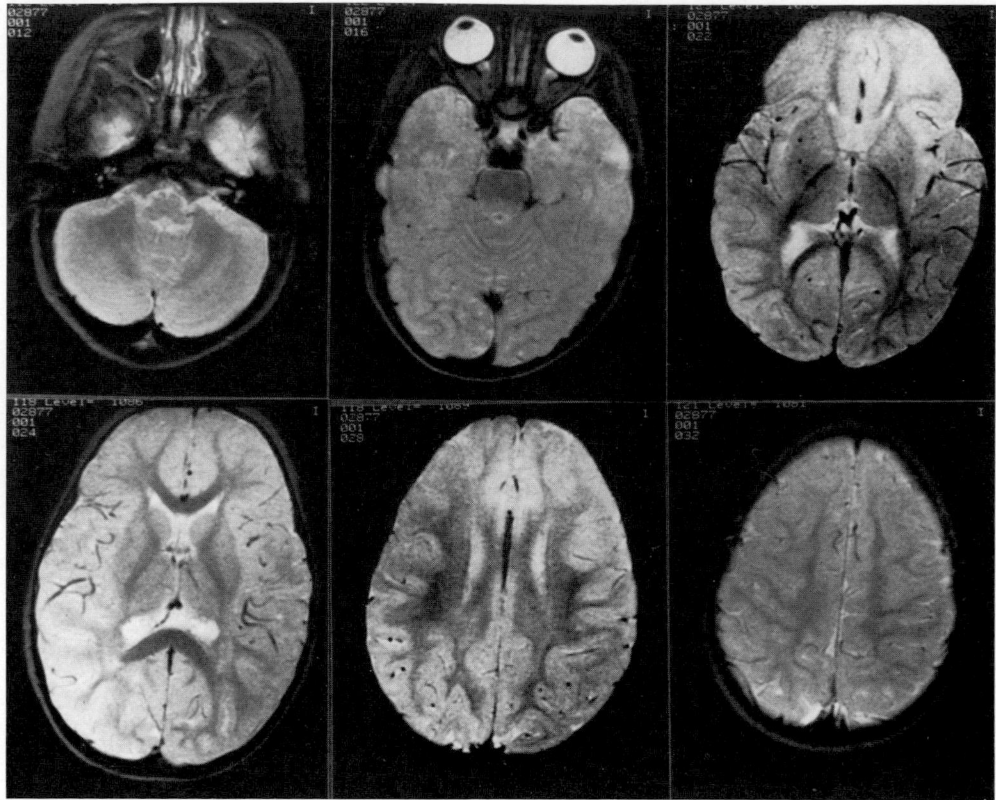

FIG. 9. Cranial MR image of an 18-month-old child. White matter maturation is complete except for the subcortical white matter in the frontal and posterior parietal regions and some patchy areas dorsal to the trigones.

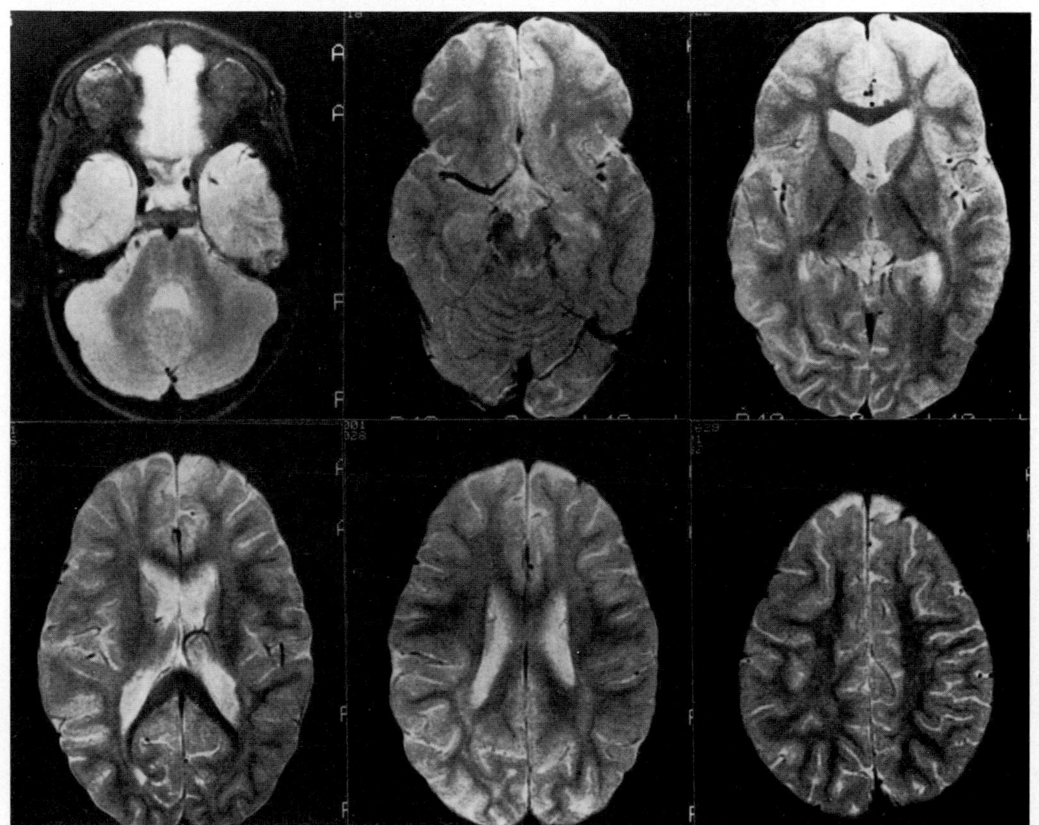

FIG. 10. Cranial MR image of a 24-month-old child. The appearance of the brain is mature except for some patchy high signals dorsal to the trigones of the lateral ventricles.

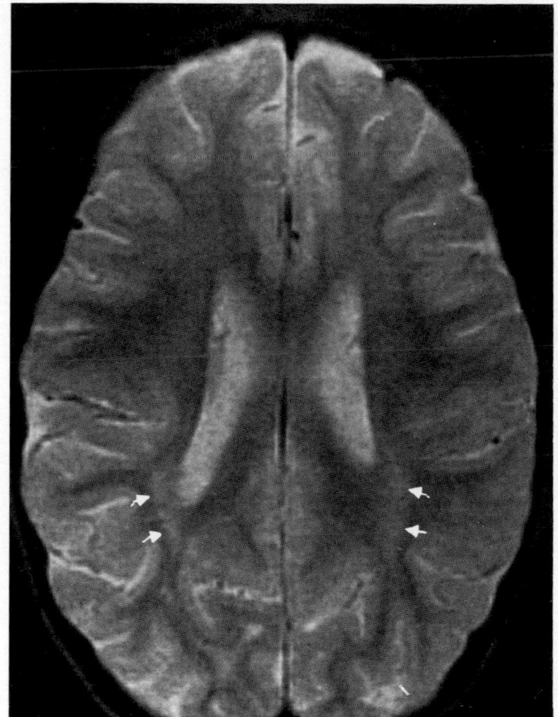

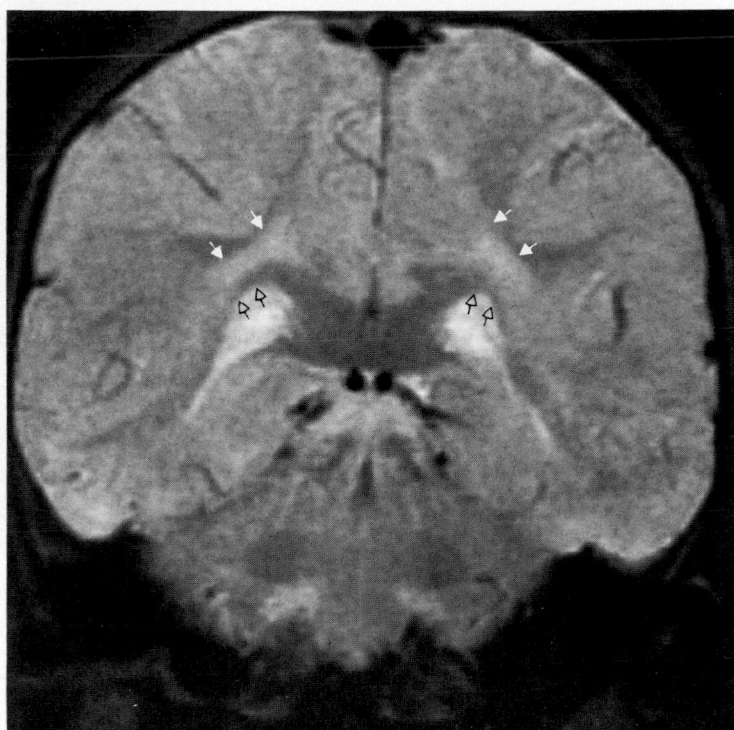

FIG. 11. Axial **(A)** and coronal **(B)** SE 2500/70 images show persistent increased intensity superior and posterior to the trigones of the lateral ventricles (*arrows*). These areas are believed to represent regions of slow myelination within the brain. The layer of myelinated white matter (*open arrows*) between the ventricular wall and the patchy area of high signal intensity, and the normal distance between the border of the ventricle and the cortical gyri are important in differentiating this normal finding from periventricular leukomalacia.

is common, regardless of the overall time course of the progression (13).

While MS has been extensively studied for many years, its cause is still unknown. It is likely that exogenous factors acting on a substrate of an inherited susceptibility are responsible for MS. Hypotheses concerning the identity of the agents responsible for the disease cover a wide spectrum of possibilities and include those based on infection, autoimmune mechanisms, some combination of infection and autoimmune reaction, and toxic-metabolic causes. While straightforward mendelian inheritance has been excluded, there is strong evidence for a genetic predisposition to develop the disease (14). At this point in time, there is a significant body of information suggesting a viral etiology in genetically susceptible individuals (12).

The Diagnosis of MS

MRI has fundamentally changed the clinical evaluation of patients with MS. It has become generally accepted that the sensitivity of MRI to MS lesions far exceeds that of the clinical examination as well as any other imaging modality, i.e., CT scanning (15,16). This basic fact is in agreement with studies that have shown significant pathologic evidence of MS in optic nerves of asymptomatic patients (17) and reports of unexpectedly discovered MS lesions on necropsy examination of brains and spinal cords (11). On the other hand, while MRI has increased the sensitivity to lesions of MS, the diagnosis may still be missed in up to 25% of patients with a proven clinical diagnosis (15). It is widely accepted that MRI is unfortunately not specific for the diagnosis of MS, in that many white matter lesions that mimic those of MS may be detected in both normal volunteers and patients harboring other pathologic conditions, although some MRI studies report very high degrees of specificity (18). For these reasons, MRI data cannot be the sole criterion for the diagnosis of MS, but must be included with clinical and laboratory findings to establish the diagnosis.

Because the diagnosis of MS can be difficult to make with confidence, elaborate criteria have been developed to establish the degree of certainty of the diagnosis, including sets of findings described in the literature based on Schumacher criteria, Poser criteria, and Bartel criteria. Prior to the development of MRI scanning, criteria based purely on the clinical picture were employed, but have largely been replaced by others that include the information from imaging studies and CSF analysis. The Bartel criteria, used at our institution, establish the diagnosis as "possible," "probable," or "definite" (19). Using

TABLE 1. *Chronology of white matter intensity changes*

Anatomic region	Age region appears bright on T1-weighted image (short TR/TE)	Age region appears dark on T2-weighted image (long TR/TE)
Infratentorial space		
Dorsal medulla	Birth	Birth
Dorsal midbrain	Birth	Birth
Inferior cerebellar peduncle	Birth	Birth
Superior cerebellar peduncle	Birth	Birth
Middle cerebellar peduncle	Birth–1 month	3–6 months
Cerebellar deep white matter	1–3 months	8–18 months (deep to peripheral)
Supratentorial space		
Corticospinal tract	Birth	
Posterior limb internal capsule to central portion of centrum semiovale		
Posterior limb internal capsule to cerebral peduncle		Birth
Ventrolateral thalamus	Birth	
Internal capule		
Anterior limb	3 months	7–11 months
Posterior limb	Birth	Birth–7 months (posterior to anterior)
Pre- and postcentral gyrus	1 month	9–12 months
Centrum semiovale		2–4 months
Optic nerve, chiasm, tract	Birth	Birth–1 month
Optic radiation		3 months
Calcarine subcortical white matter		4 months
Subcortical white matter (except frontal and posterior parietal)	3 months 8 months	
Subcortical white matter (occipital lobe)		9–18 months (deep to peripheral)
Adult pattern	12 months	24 months
Corpus callosum		
Splenium	3–4 months	6 months
Body	4–6 months	6–8 months
Genu	6 months	8 months

TABLE 2. *Demyelinating diseases*

Primary Demyelinating Diseases
Acute disseminated encephalomyelitis
- Classic (postinfectious, postimmunization, idiopathic)
- Acute hemorrhagic leukoencephalitis (hyperacute type)

Multiple sclerosis
- Classic (Charcot type)
- Acute (Marburg type)
- Diffuse cerebral sclerosis (Schilder type)
- Concentric sclerosis (Balo type)
- Neuromyelitis optica (Devic type)

Demyelinating Disorders Associated with Systemic Disease
- Central pontine myelinolysis (osmotic demyelination)
- Progressive multifocal leukoencephalopathy
- Marchiafava-Bignami disease

Modified from Allen and Kirk, ref. 11.

the Bartel method (19), three criteria must be met before the diagnosis of multiple sclerosis can be considered "definite": (i) history of neurologic symptoms with relapse and remission; (ii) evidence of two or more anatomically separate lesions in the central nervous system obtained by clinical examination, electrophysiologic tests, or imaging techniques; and (iii) evidence of immunologic disturbance involving the central nervous system revealed by a demyelinative spinal fluid profile. Diagnosis of multiple sclerosis may be considered "probable" when there is evidence of two separate lesions in the central nervous system and when the patient satisfies only one of the two remaining essential criteria. Finally, patients with evidence of a single lesion or clinical deficit, but satisfying one or both of the remaining essential criteria, would be diagnosed as "possible" multiple sclerosis

(19). Many patients may present with only one neurologic deficit but have several demyelinating lesions in neurologically silent areas in the brain. Detecting these lesions is important in establishing the certainty of the diagnosis of multiple sclerosis. MRI provides an excellent method for evaluating the nerve axis for clinically silent multifocal disease (Fig. 12). Visual, auditory, and somatosensory-evoked responses may also be used to help establish the multifocality of disease (20). The greatest limitation of evoked responses, though, is the narrow scope of the studies, which measure only a fraction of the potentially affected pathways. Spinal fluid analysis, with attention to oligocolonal bands, myelin basic protein, and immunoglobulin G, is also an important contributor in establishing the diagnosis of multiple sclerosis (21).

Pathologic Findings

While it is widely recognized that there is a characteristic pattern of distribution of plaques in brains affected by MS, considerable variation is noted from patient to patient. In the chronic stage, plaques often involve large areas of the hemispheric white matter. For still unknown reasons, there is a distinct propensity for involvement of certain regions of white matter, most notably the periventricular white matter, optic nerves, brainstem, and spinal cord. The characteristic susceptibility of the periventricular regions to MS plaques is not uniform; however, most plaques are seen with particular frequency at

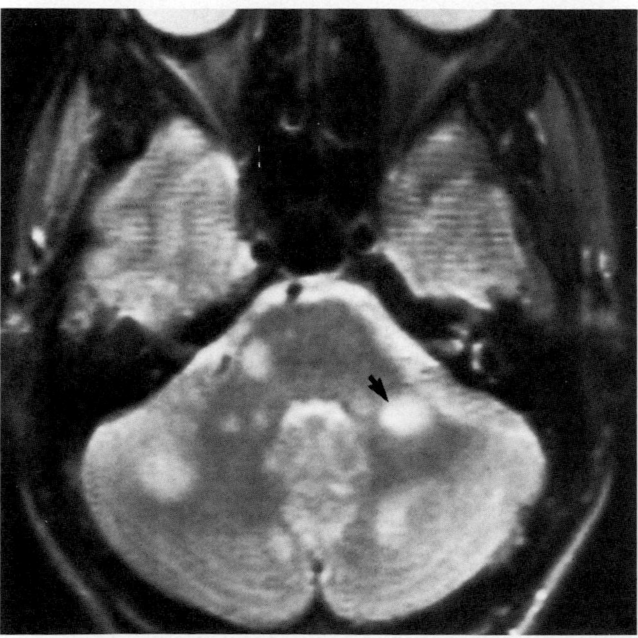

FIG. 12. Multiple sclerosis. Axial T2-weighted image (2000/80) shows multiple hyperintense abnormalities consistent with white matter demyelination. The brachium pontis lesion is common in MS (*arrow*). Note that many of these lesions are clinically silent.

specific sites and seem to be anatomically related to subependymal veins (11). About 50% occur in a periventricular distribution, predominantly near the angles of the lateral ventricles (Fig. 13). The periaqueductal region and the floor of the fourth ventricle are also frequently involved (Fig. 14). Although MS plaques are typically situated within white matter, gray matter lesions are not uncommon on pathologic examination. In one study, 74% of plaques involved deep white matter, while 17% were entirely within gray matter (22).

The morphologic features of the foci of demyelination or MS "plaques" vary considerably on pathology, from the acute to the chronic phase. Grossly, the acute lesions vary in their appearance according to the severity of the lesions. It should also be noted that different neuropathologists stress different features in their descriptions of early lesions in MS and have somewhat contrasting views as to what pathologic findings constitute the early lesion (11). Moreover, it is recognized that the definitive neuropathologic aging of MS lesions is often not possible. Most early lesions have a swollen, wet texture, and a pink-gray color. Histologically, the early (acute) lesions are characterized by fragmentation of the myelin with "myelin ball" formation and relative preservation of the axons (Fig. 15). Acute lesions also show microglial infiltration. Perivascular lymphocytic cuffing may or may not be observed (Fig. 16). Oligodendrocytes are recognizable in the acute phase, but disappear within a few weeks in the subacute phase. At that stage, neutral fat may be detected in the extracellular space and in the cytoplasm of macrophages. Plaques that occur in the gray matter are usually associated with preservation of neurons. In the chronic phase, months after the initial event, fibrillary gliosis appears, and atrophy and cavitation may develop (Fig. 17). At this stage the myelin sheaths are interrupted at the edge of the plaque of demyelination, where glial cells persist, indicating an active cellular margin even in old plaques (23). Remyelination can also be noted. Histopathologically "active" lesions, therefore, are those that typically show demyelination, myelin fragmentation, intact axons, microglial infiltration, and reactive astrocytes, with variable degrees of perivascular inflammation. Lesions that can be termed "inactive" by histopathological criteria generally show gliosis with hypocellularity, usually complete demyelination with abrupt borders, little or no perivascular inflammation, absence of myelin breakdown products, few lipid-laden macrophages, and often a slight reduction in axonal number as a secondary finding (11,24).

Some plaques demonstrate incomplete myelin loss and ill-defined margins and are often referred to as "shadow plaques" (11). Features of shadow plaques have been at least in part attributed to the phenomenon of remyelination. Remyelination has been clearly documented to occur, although incompletely, in acute le-

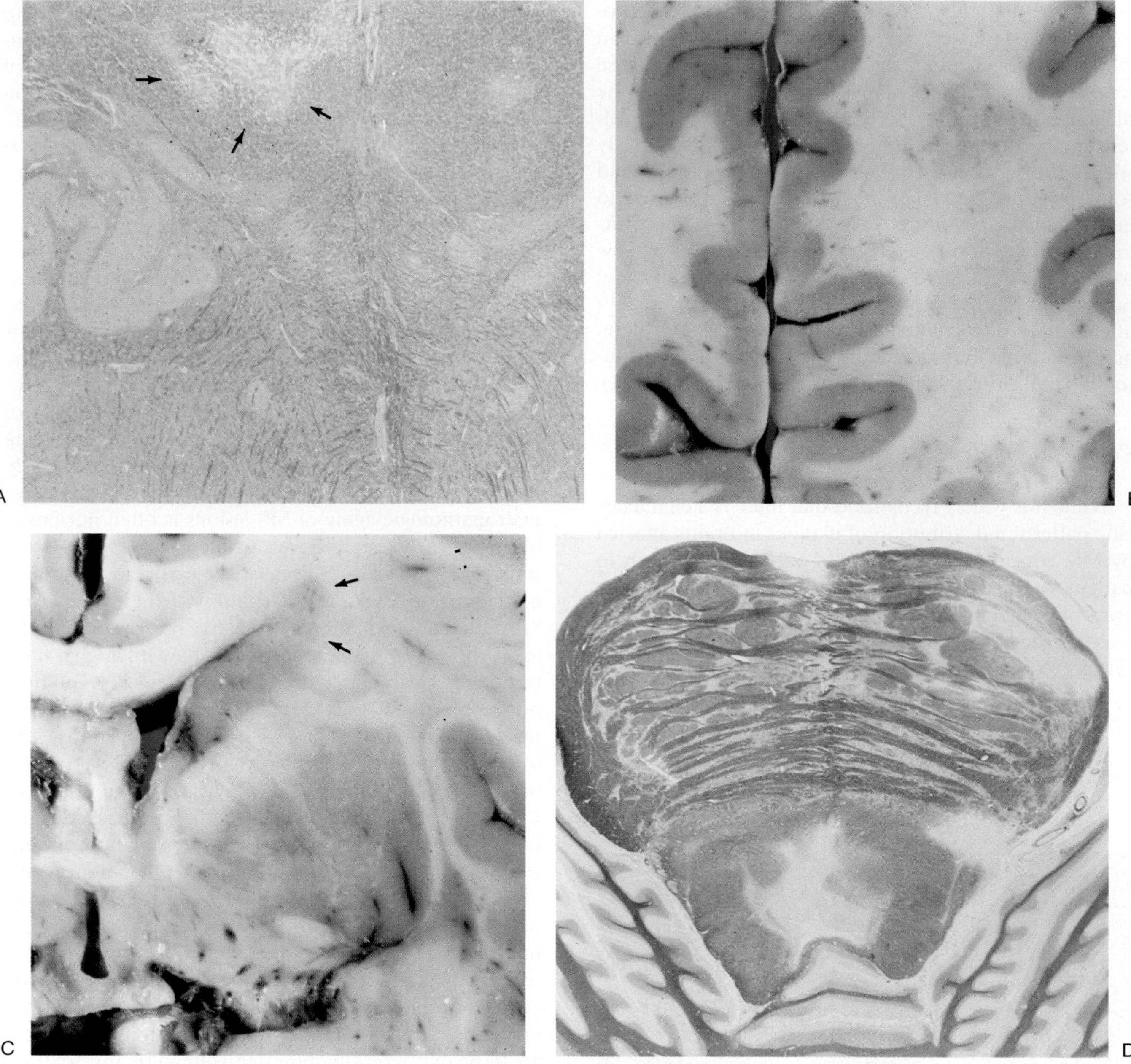

FIG. 13. Chronic MS. **A:** Multiple sclerosis plaque in the corticospinal tract (*arrows*) in medulla oblongata. Note a small plaque in the contralateral tract. (Luxol fast blue—H&E, ×40.) **B:** Plaque of demyelination in the hemispheric white matter of the frontal lobe in a patient with the classical (Charcot) type of multiple sclerosis. **C:** Multiple sclerosis plaque in the angle of the lateral ventricle, just above the body of the caudate nucleus. Note also the severe demyelination of the dorsal portion of the optic chiasm and optic tracts. **D:** Upper pons with periventricular, tegmental, and base multiple sclerosis plaques. (Myelin stain, ×45.)

sions. In chronic shadow plaques, it is thought that simultaneous demyelination and remyelination are occurring (11).

Aside from these focal findings in MS, it is also known that diffuse abnormalities can be found in the CNS. Very mild histologic abnormalities have been described in macroscopically normal white matter in brains of established MS cases (25), including diffuse gliosis, perivascular inflammation, lipofuscin deposition, collagenized veins, and small foci of demyelination. These findings have also been demonstrated in spinal cases (26), and suggest that a diffuse involvement of mild abnormality can occur without focal plaque formation (11). In association with this diffuse type of lesion, the meninges can also rarely be involved with inflammatory cells identified in the subarachnoid space (27).

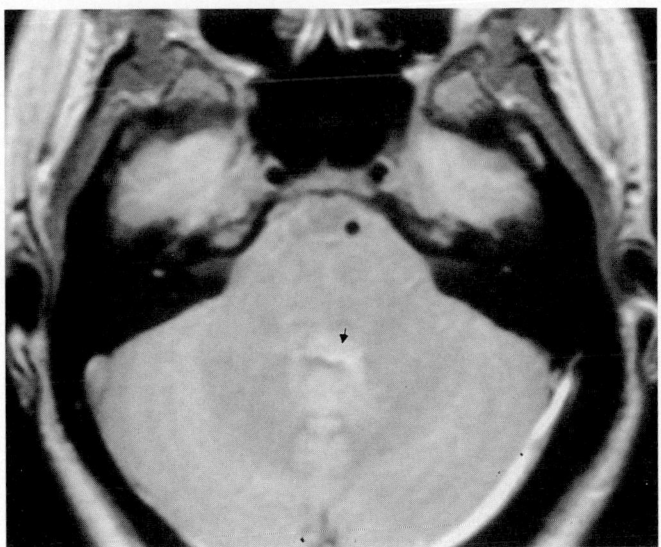
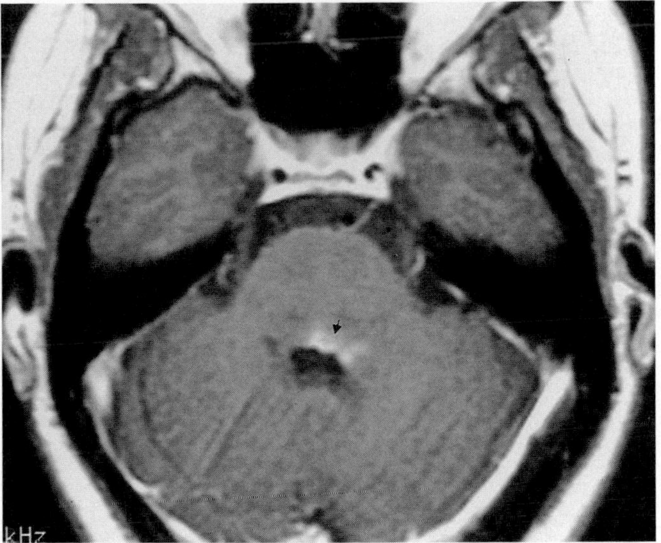

FIG. 14. MS in patient with ocular motility disorder. **A:** Proton-density-weighted MRI. **B:** T1-weighted MRI post-gadolinium. Ill-defined hyperintensity near floor of fourth ventricle in left facial colliculus (*arrow*, A) shows enhancement after intravenous contrast (*arrow*, B) in patient with new diplopia.

Variants of MS

Less common variants of MS are occasionally seen and differ from classic MS in their clinical presentation and course as well as histopathologic findings (see Table 2) (11). *Acute MS (Marburg type)* occurs as an infrequent variety of MS, most commonly in younger patients. It is often preceded by fever and typically has inexorable, rapid progression to death within months. This fulminant form of MS has also been seen as a terminal event in classic MS. Pathologic findings of extensive myelin destruction, severe axonal loss, and early edema are seen. Treatment is directed at reducing the inflammation. Although acute fulminant MS is associated with high morbidity and mortality, it may respond to aggressive immunosuppressive therapy (28). *Neuromyelitis optica (Devic type)* is a syndrome of acute onset of severe optic nerve and spinal cord demyelination that appear at approximately the same time and dominate the clinical picture. Often, the symptoms and signs are not in complete isolation, but are part of a more generalized disorder. About one-half of these patients die within several months. It is

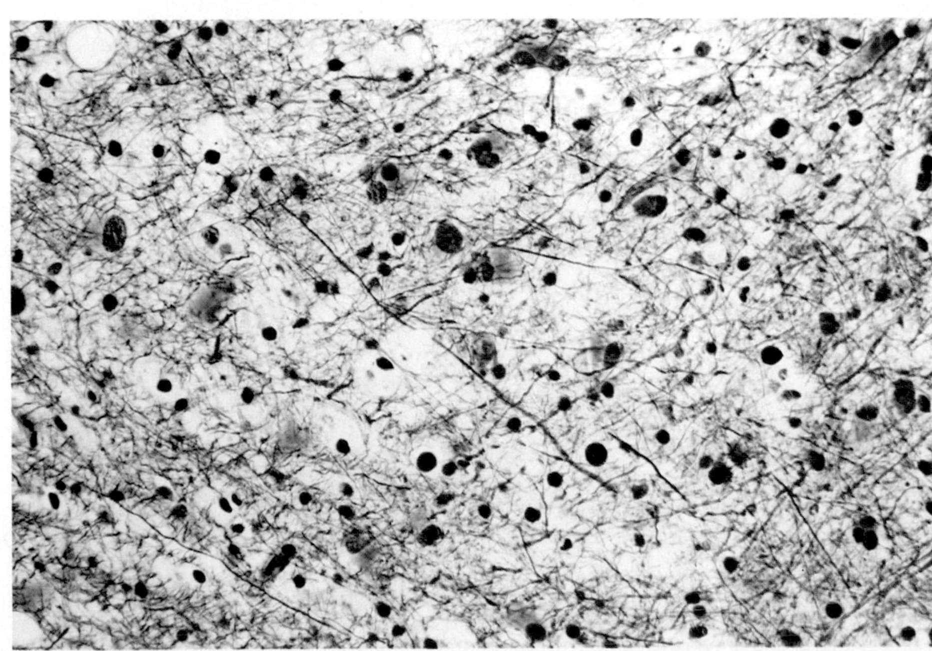

FIG. 15. Subacute MS. Partial preservation of axons in an old plaque of demyelination (Silver impregnation for nerve fibers, ×100).

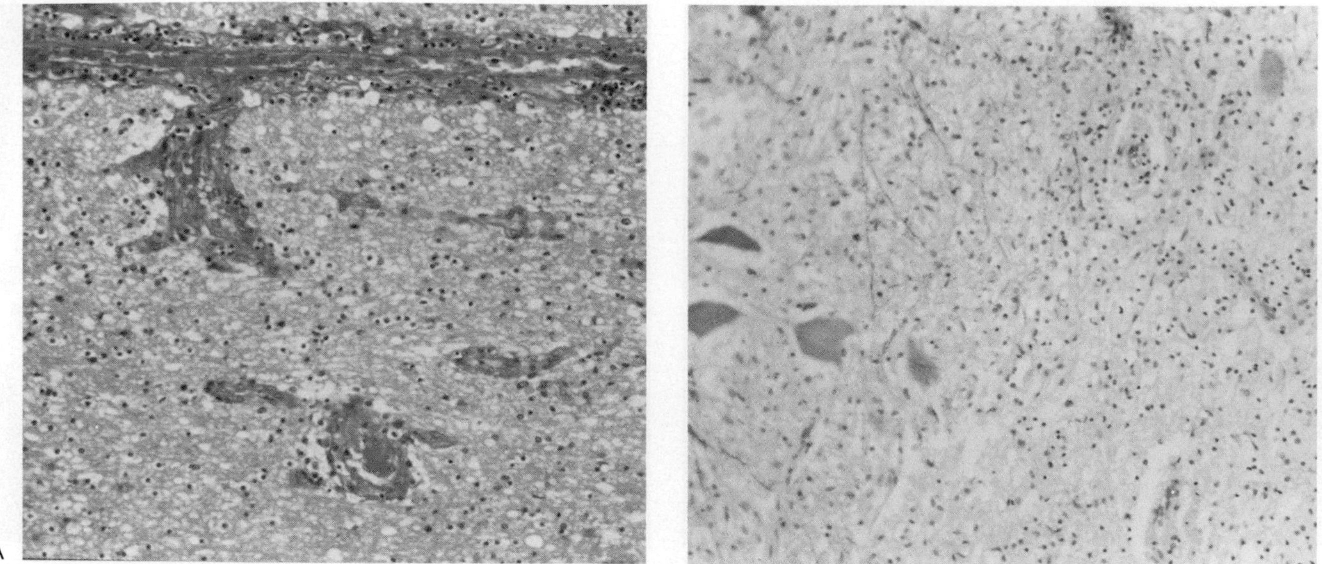

FIG. 16. Acute MS. **A:** Focus of demyelination with marked expansion of perivascular spaces by foamy macrophages, lymphocytes, and plasma cells. (H&E, ×100.) **B:** Multiple sclerosis plaque in subcortical white matter with intense infiltration with microglial cells and sparing of neurons. (Luxol fast blue—H&E, ×100.)

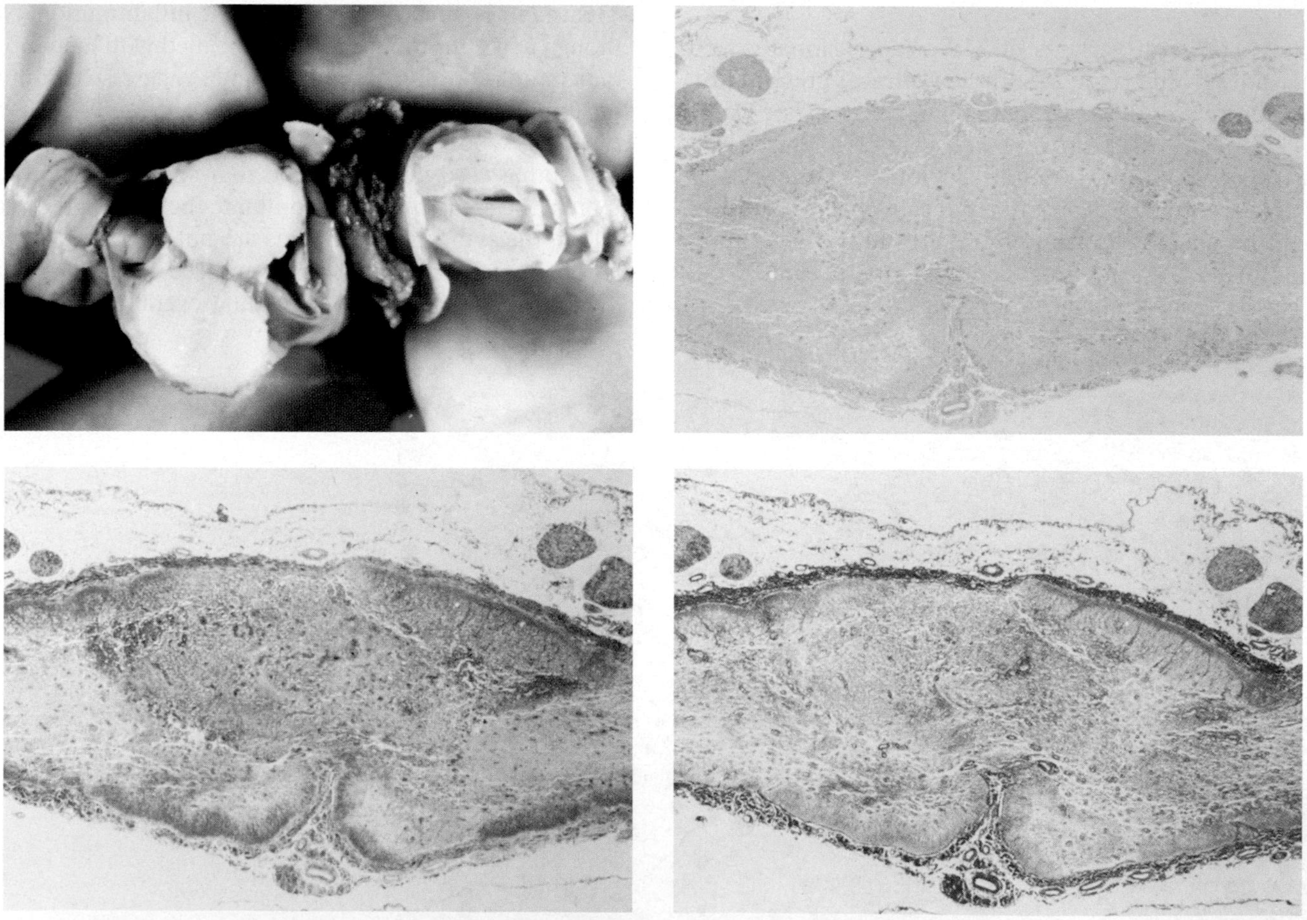

FIG. 17. Spinal cord MS. **A:** Spinal cord in a patient with chronic multiple sclerosis (*right*) and in a normal, age-matched control patient (*left*). **B:** Marked shrinkage of the cord in its AP diameter and almost complete loss of myelin sheaths. Note the preservation of the myelin sheaths in the dorsal roots (stained dark blue). (Luxol fast blue—H&E, ×20.) **C:** Partial preservation of axons in lateral and anterior columns. (Silver impregnation for nerve fibers, ×20.) **D:** Marked fibrillary gliosis. (Holzer's stain for glial fibrils, ×20.)

clear that several entities can produce this clinical syndrome, but the term is reserved for those without other underlying diseases. The relationship of Devic syndrome to MS is still controversial. *Schilder type,* or *diffuse sclerosis,* refers to an entity consisting of extensive, confluent, asymmetric demyelination of both cerebral hemispheres with involvement of the brainstem and cerebellum. Late in the disease, wallerian degeneration and cavitation can be seen. *Concentric sclerosis (Balo type)* is a very rare type of demyelinating disease in which large regions with alternating zones of demyelinated and myelinated white matter are found. The myelinated regions may reflect remyelination, rather than spared normal myelin. This progressive disease is more often found in young patients and is more common in the Philippines. When encountered, Balo concentric sclerosis has a pathognomonic appearance on both pathology and MRI (Fig. 18) (29).

MRI Findings in MS

The MR appearance of MS generally reflects the histologic findings. Acute inflammation appears as a rounded area of high signal intensity on T2-weighted sequences (where the repetition time, TR, is long, i.e., greater than 2 seconds) (Figs. 19 and 20). Gadolinium enhancement and even significant mass effect may be seen during the acute phase (23,28) (Figs. 21–23). Acute MS (Marburg type) may also present as areas of clearly defined rings within or surrounding plaques of demyelination (30) (Fig. 24). These rings have signal characteristics on T1-weighted images consistent with the presence of paramagnetic material, with slight increase in signal intensity. Enhancement is typically seen in the region of these rings. This appearance most likely represents the presence of free radicals in the macrophage layer forming the margin of an acute plaque (30). Plaques of Balo concentric sclerosis are striking in their unique concentric rings of alternating destroyed and intact myelin (Fig. 18).

In classic MS, the area of inflammation decreases in size with time and leaves a smaller residual plaque of high intensity, often more linear or punctate in appearance than the initial lesion. Treatment with steroids may also be associated with a marked reduction in lesion enhancement and morphology (Fig. 25). High intensity lesions in MS do not necessarily indicate demyelination, but rather might merely reflect transient inflammation. Occasionally the plaque will contain a cavity large enough to present as a fluid-containing cyst. With progression of disease, atrophy is apparent, and increased iron deposition is concomitantly found in the basal ganglia (31) (Fig. 26). Plaques are commonly situated in the periventricular location, internal capsule, corpus callosum, pons (Fig. 27), and brachium pontis but may appear throughout the myelinated white matter and not uncommonly in the gray matter (Fig. 28). When the plaques are located in the immediate periventricular region they may not be apparent on long TR/TE images (where CSF is high intensity) and "proton-density-weighted" (long TR/short TE) images will better define the MS lesions as bright signal adjacent to darker CSF (Fig. 29). Note that the anatomic distribution of the lesions should *not* be considered key to the diagnosis, since "exceptional" locations are in fact quite commonly encountered.

The corpus callosum is a region that is especially sensitive to demyelination with multiple sclerosis, possibly due to its intimate neuroanatomic relationship to the lateral ventricular roofs and its relationship to small penetrating vessels. Sagittal MR imaging has been advocated for the depiction of the majority of the corpus callosal lesions, although many can be clearly identified on conventional axial images, particularly using proton-density-weighted parameters. In up to 93% of MS patients, focal lesions can be identified in the inferior aspect of the corpus callosum on sagittal views (32,33) (Fig. 30). Long TR images typically show focal corpus callosal lesions to best advantage (Fig. 30), but the anatomic distortion with focal thinning in the inferior aspect of the corpus callosum may be easily appreciated on T1-weighted lesions in many cases (Fig. 30). While it has been advocated that the appearance of the corpus callosum involvement on MRI may be specific for MS (32), there is no question that ischemic lesions can be noted to have a virtually identical appearance. We believe that there is no single pathognomonic sign of MS on brain MRI.

Intracranial involvement with MS may appear quite similar to many other white matter diseases on MRI, with scattered foci of high intensity in the white matter on T2-weighted spin-echo images. Contrast enhancement may be used to add specificity to the finding of multiple hyperintensities on T2-weighted images, since the finding of enhancing along with nonenhancing lesions is quite common in MS (Figs. 21, 22, and 31) but makes many other diagnoses unlikely. Similarly, the temporal changes in enhancing and nonenhancing lesions common in MS cases is very different from other entities. Periventricular lesions of MS commonly appear as linear abnormalities oriented perpendicular to the lateral ventricle, due to the propensity of MS plaques to occur in a periventricular location. Although this is common, the appearance of an MS lesion on MRI is highly variable and certainly not specific. MS can also appear as very subtle, diffuse hyperintensity in the white matter. Moreover, it has been shown by several studies that quantitative analysis of relaxation times in "normal appearing" white matter in MS patients differs from that of normal volunteers (34–39). These nonvisual findings of quantitative differences in proton relaxation times may

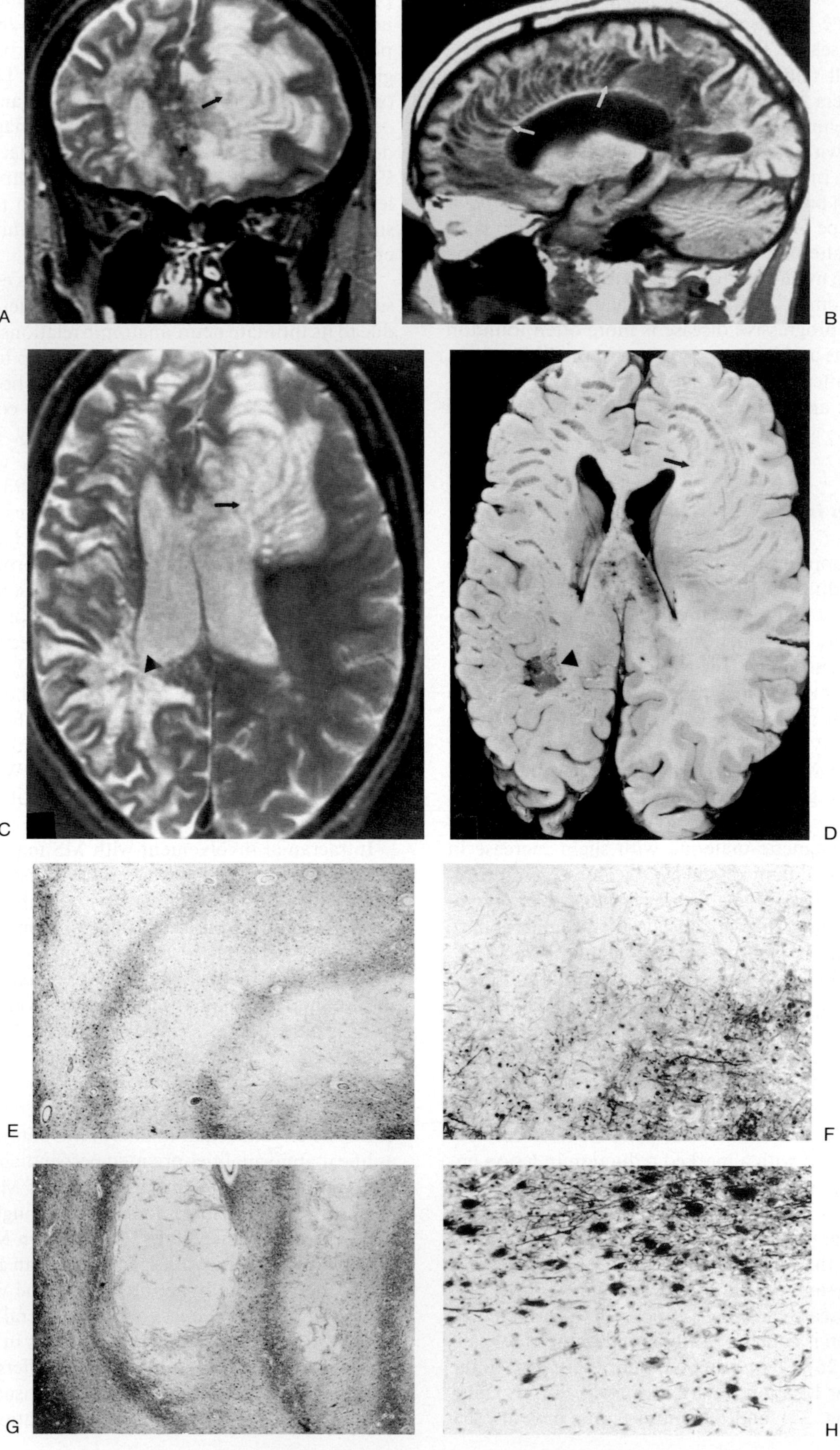
A
B
C
D
E
F
G
H

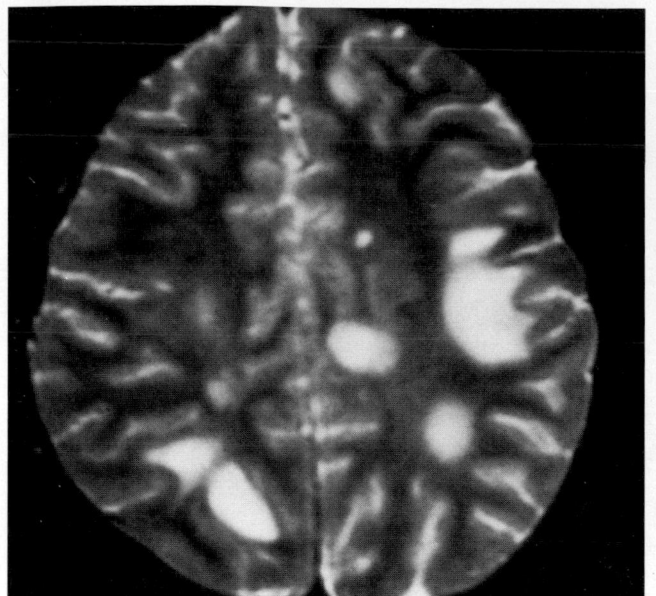
A

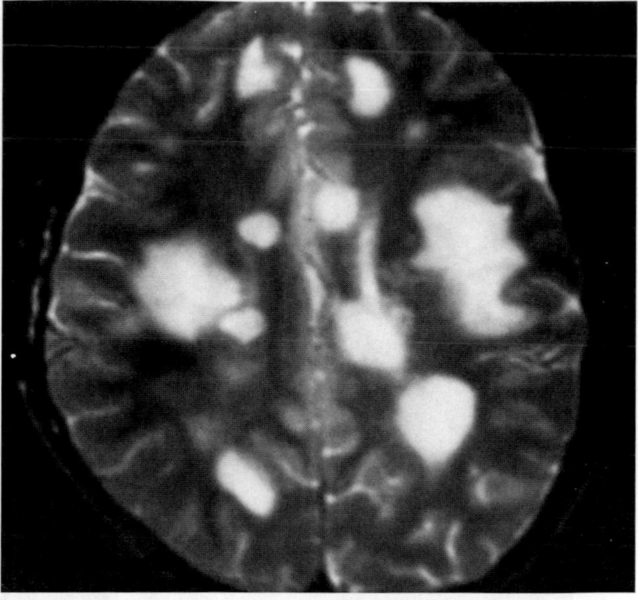
B

FIG. 19. Appearance of new lesions in acute MS. **A:** Baseline T2-weighted MRI (3000/90) shows several focal regions of hyperintensity in subcortical white matter. **B:** T2-weighted MRI (3000/90) 9 days later, after progression of symptoms, reveals multiple new areas of hyperintensity due to acute disease.

be a reflection of the subtle histologic changes reported by pathology studies found in the absence of focal plaques or macroscopic lesions in brains known to be affected by MS (25). Finally, it has even been reported that meningeal enhancement after intravenous contrast agent administration has been seen in association with MS (40).

Proton MR spectroscopy has been studied by several investigators in MS and related animal models of demyelinating disease. The development of and continued research with spectroscopy in MS is driven mainly by the lack of specificity of standard MRI techniques in this disease, notwithstanding the relative correlation between "active" disease and contrast enhancement reported in some studies (24,41). While still purely a research tool at the time of this writing, this technique shows promise in defining the precise biochemical nature of the intracerebral lesions, and in separating early edematous lesions from those areas that contain demyelination and/or incomplete remyelination (42,43). Decreased levels of *N*-acetylaspartate (NAA) have been reported in chronic plaques of MS (44) as well as in normal appearing white matter (45,46). The reduction of NAA, the putative neuronal marker, has been interpreted as an indicator of secondary neuronal loss following prior demyelination, and consequently a potential marker of irreversible damage. Other investigators have reported abnormal hydrogen spectra in MS consistent with the presence of free lipids or cholesterol breakdown products (47,48), which correspond to degradation products of myelin. Proton spectra of enhancing lesions have suggested the presence of lipids and other myelin breakdown products (49) or amino acids (42). These findings suggest that spectroscopy will be of use in staging the histopathologic changes, thereby providing a window to observe the natural history of the disease, and potentially in monitoring the response to therapies (see Chapter 32).

Additional methods of MRI investigation continue to

FIG. 18. Balo concentric sclerosis **A:** Sagittal T1-weighted MRI (600/12). **B:** Coronal T2-weighted MRI (2500/90). **C:** Axial T2-weighted MRI (2500/90). **D:** Axial gross necropsy specimen. **E,F:** Photomicrographs (original magnification ×12, Luxol fast blue stain). **G:** Photomicrograph (original magnification ×80, Bielschowsky stain). **H:** Photomicrograph (original magnification ×120, Luxol fast blue stain). Striking lamellated pattern of alternating bands of demyelination and relatively normal white matter, reflecting either spared or remyelinated regions, is clear on both T1- and T2-weighted MRI (A,B, *straight arrow*, C) and gross specimen (*straight arrow*, D). Cavitary appearance in parts of lesion is also demonstrated (*straight arrows*, A,B). Prior biopsy site is indicated in right parietal lobe (*curved arrow*, C,D). Photomicrographs of cerebral white matter (E–H) show extent of lamellated tissue abnormality, where pale areas represent demyelination with persistence of cellular background (E) and areas of cystic necrosis (F). Axonal preservation is seen in area of myelin loss (upper part of G). Demyelination margin is seen in H. Large cell bodies are astrocytes. (From Gharagazloo et al., ref. 29, with permission.)

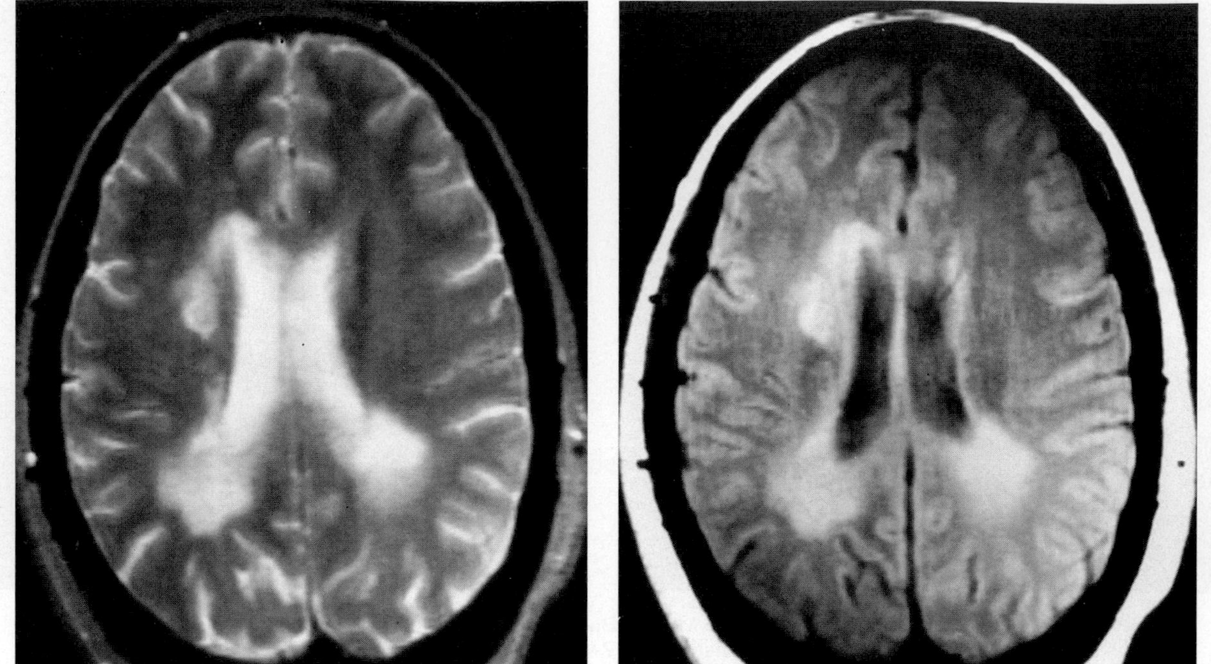

FIG. 20. Acute MS. **A:** Large, ill-defined areas of bright signal on T2-weighted images (2000/80) are typical of lesions seen in patients with acute symptoms. **B:** Proton-density images (2000/20) show the lesions with better contrast compared to the lateral ventricles.

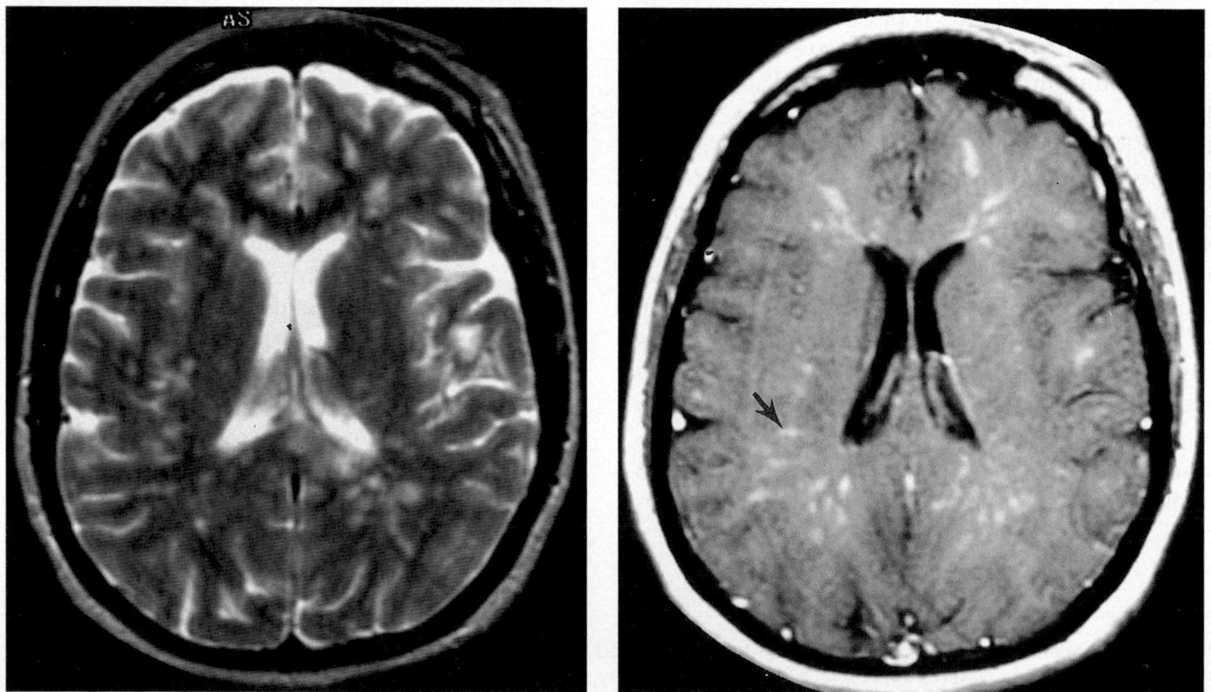

FIG. 21. Enhancing and nonenhancing lesions in acute MS. **A:** Multiple hyperintense lesions present of axial T2-weighted image (2000/80). **B:** Gadolinium-enhancement on T1-weighted image shows enhancement of acute plaques (*arrow*).

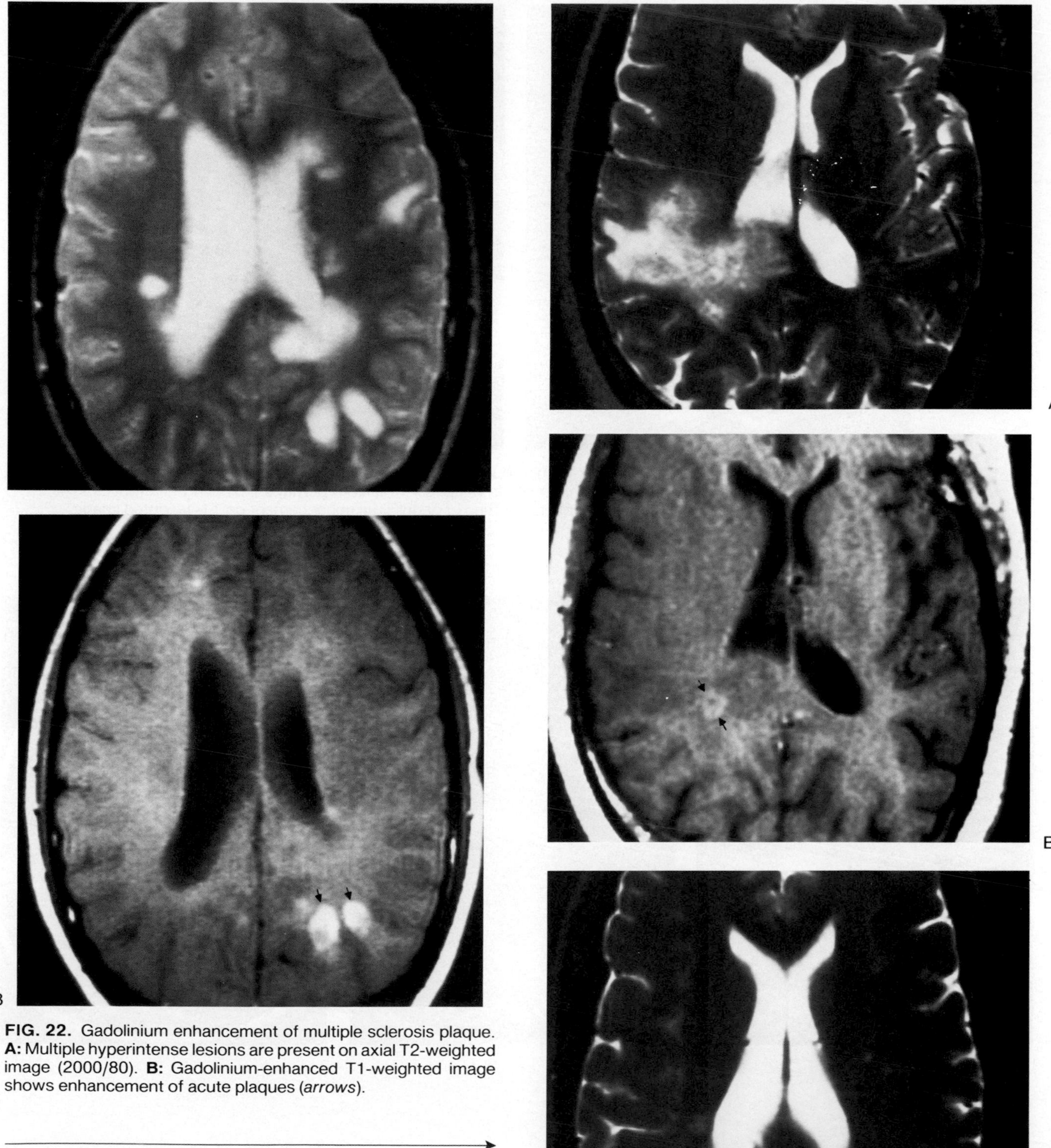

FIG. 22. Gadolinium enhancement of multiple sclerosis plaque. **A:** Multiple hyperintense lesions are present on axial T2-weighted image (2000/80). **B:** Gadolinium-enhanced T1-weighted image shows enhancement of acute plaques (*arrows*).

FIG. 23. Acute MS appearing as mass lesion. **A:** T2-weighted MRI (3000/80) shows large mass lesion in right temporoparietal lobe white matter, extending into splenium of corpus callosum and effacing right lateral ventricle. **B:** Contrast-enhanced T1-weighted image (600/20) shows small ring lesion of enhancement (*arrows*). **C:** Several months later, lesion has almost completely resolved on T2-weighted MRI (3000/90).

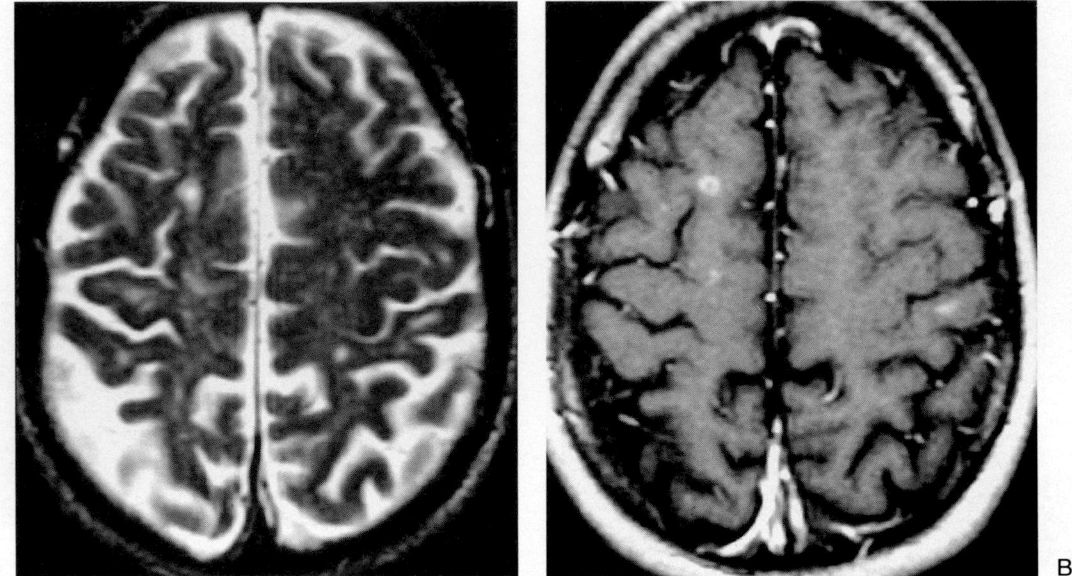

FIG. 24. Ring enhancement in acute MS. **A:** T2-weighted image (2000/80) shows "target lesion" with markedly hyperintense signal in the center and slight hyperintensity in periphery of lesion, perhaps indicating differences in degree of demyelination centrally compared to periphery. **B:** Ring of gadolinium enhancement on T1-weighted image (600/20).

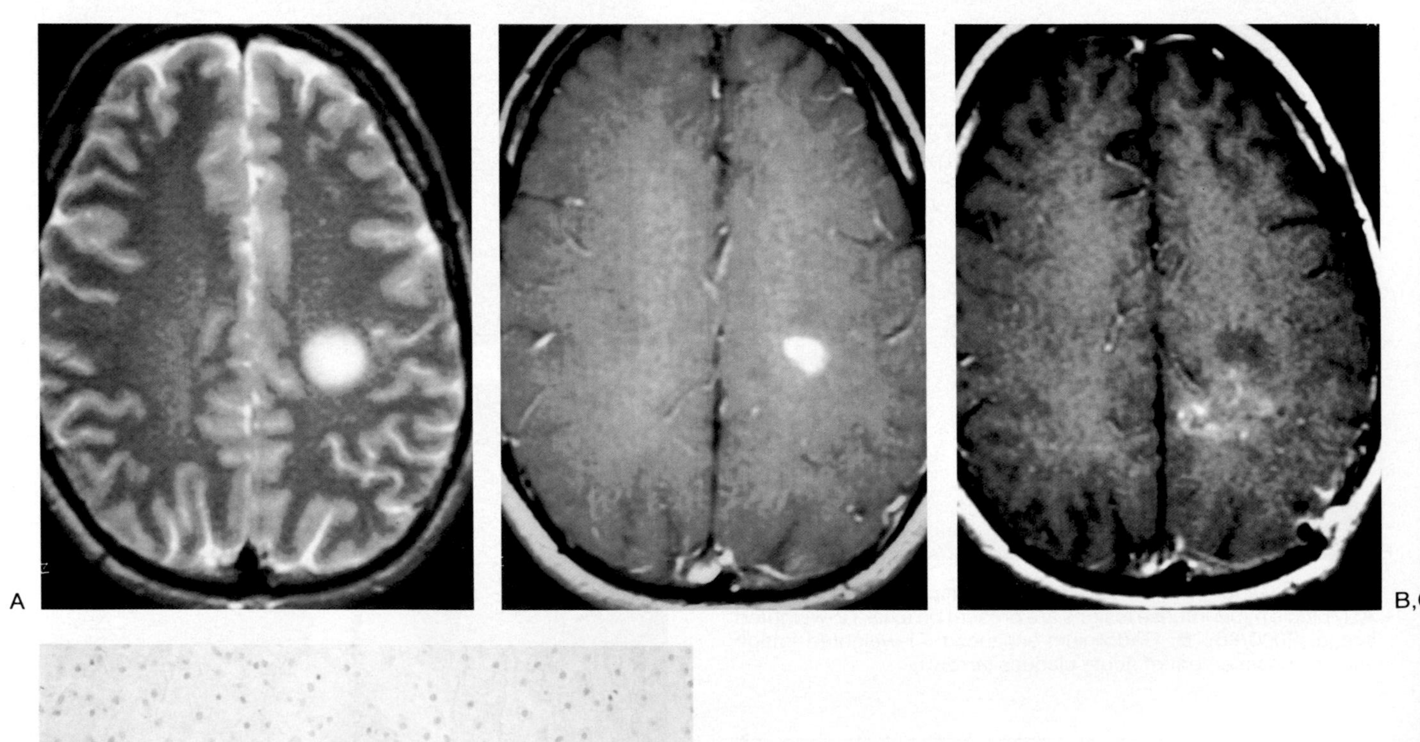

FIG. 25. Change in MS lesion appearance after steroid therapy. **A:** T2-weighted MRI. **B:** T1-weighted MRI after gadolinium. **C:** T1-weighted MRI after steroid treatment. **D:** Biopsy specimen, stain for lymphocytes. Note large lesion in left centrum semiovale during acute presentation (A), which enhances markedly (B). After steroids (C), dramatic reduction in enhancement is seen. Biopsy prior to steroids showed classic perivascular lymphocytes (D).

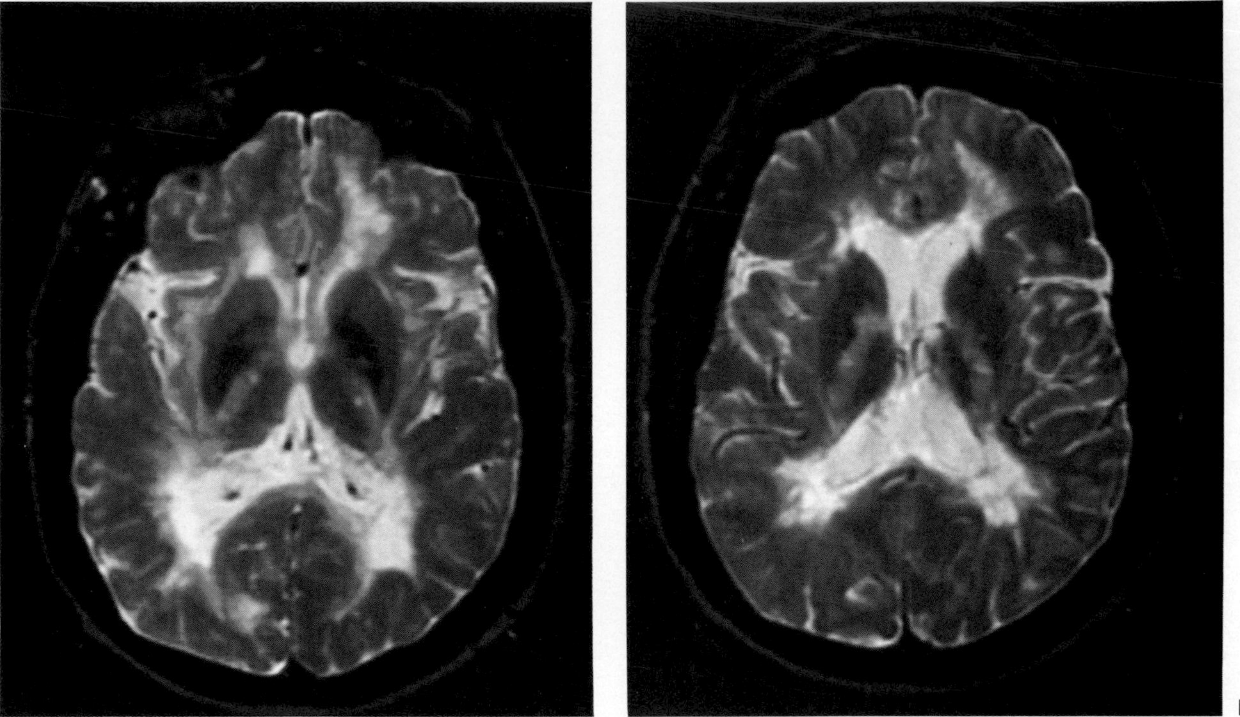

FIG. 26. Patient with longstanding MS has extensive white matter disease, involving periventricular and capsular white matter on T2-weighted images (**A,B**). Note concomitant abnormal hypointensity throughout basal ganglia and thalami bilaterally.

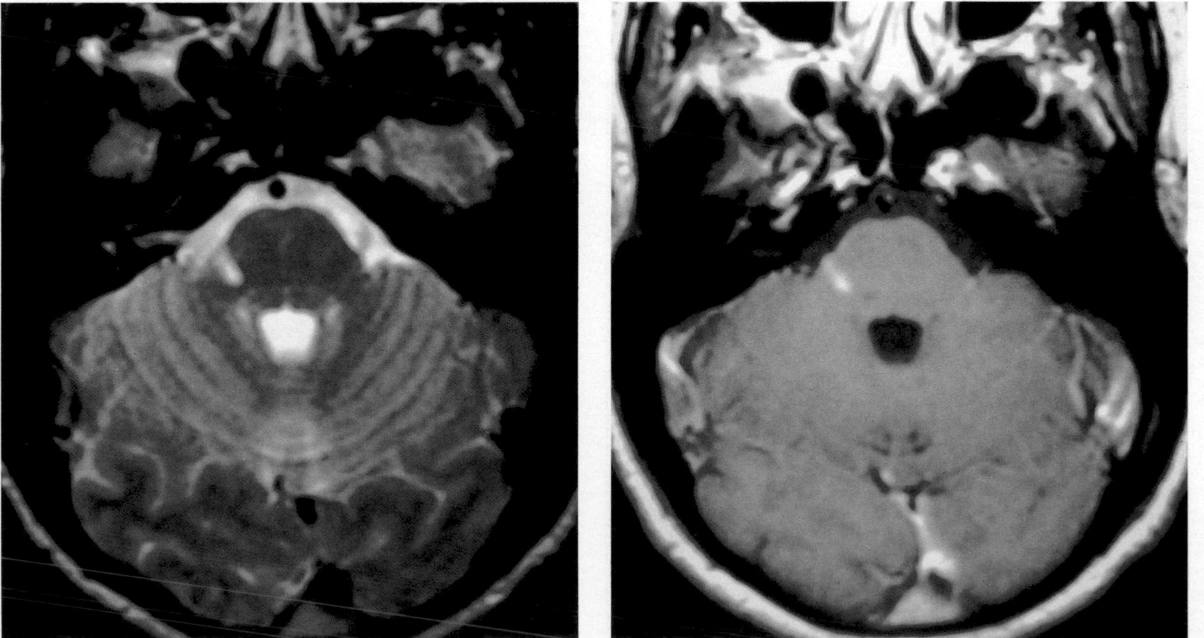

FIG. 27. Pontine lesion in patient with right paresthesias and MS. **A:** T2-weighted MRI. **B:** T1-weighted MRI after gadolinium. Focal lesion in right pons (A) enhances (B) and is situated in pathway of fibers of cranial nerve V in a patient with V_1 distribution sensory disturbance.

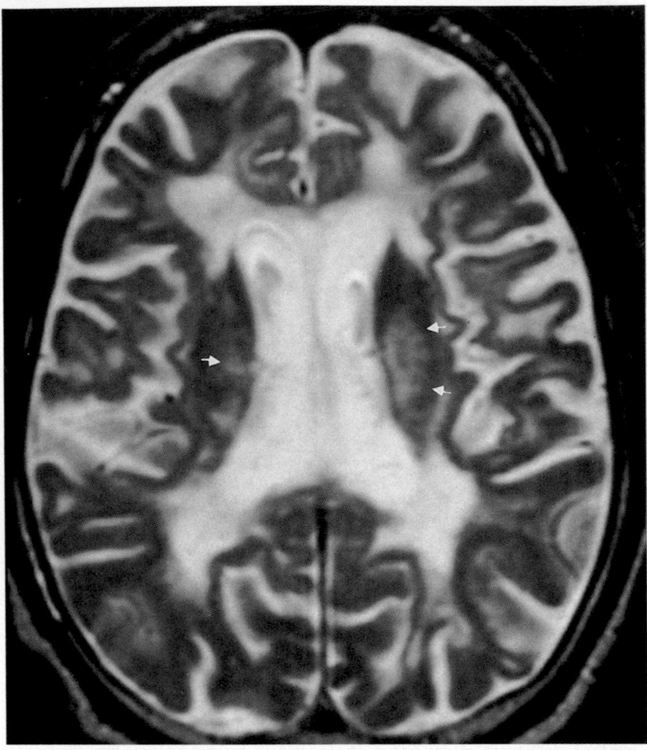

FIG. 28. Extensive white matter and ganglionic hyperintensity in MS. Extensive hyperintensity is present throughout most of the periventricular white matter on T2-weighted images (2800/80). Note sparing of the subcortical U-fibers and involvement of superior aspects of lentiform nuclei bilaterally (*arrows*).

be developed that may have applications in the evaluation of MS and other white matter diseases. Magnetization transfer techniques have been applied to brain MRI in an attempt to characterize MS lesions (50). This pulse sequence technique, which can be implemented on a conventional scanner, exploits differences in relaxation between immobilized water transiently bound to macromolecules and water protons not associated with macromolecules. The hypothesis underlying these investigations is that demyelination results in more free water, i.e., a reduction in the "bound" fraction of water, as compared to myelinated white matter or intact but edematous tissue. Selective suppression of immobilized water is accomplished by the application of an off-resonance saturation pulse, which saturates the broad resonance of protons bound to macromolecules. Transiently bound protons exchange with free water protons by diffusion (see Chapter 2). Magnetization transfer (MT) ratios have been calculated in a simple experimental design that compares relative degrees of saturation transfer in different regions of brain. Using this experimental design, it has been shown in some studies that MT ratios are higher (i.e., there is more signal reduction due to the saturation pulse) in normal mature (myelinated) white matter as compared to gray matter. In experimentally-produced early edematous experimental allergic encephalomyelitis (EAE) lesions, little MT change was noted from normal white matter; significant

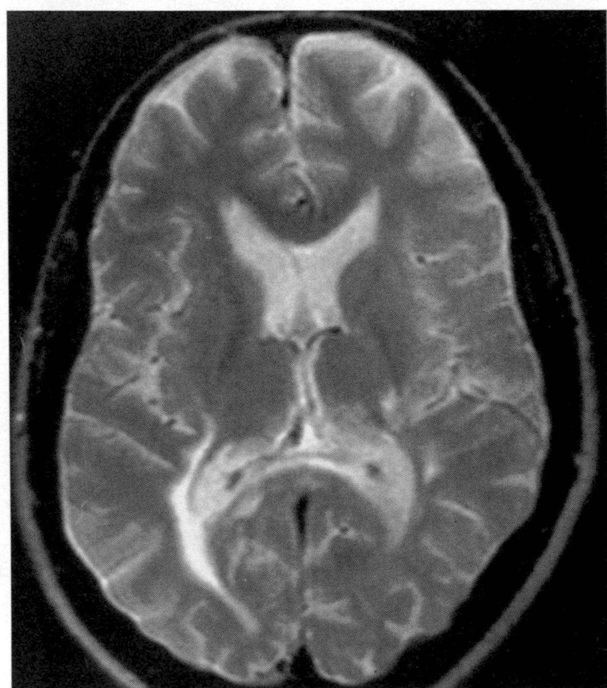

A

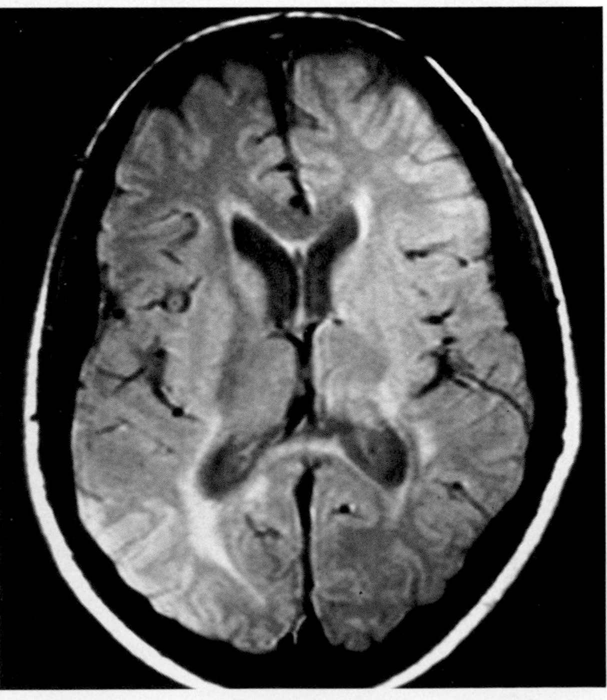

B

FIG. 29. MS with more extensive disease on proton-density-weighted image. **A:** Periventricular disease is subtle in the frontal horn region on T2-weighted sequence (2000/80). **B:** Proton-density-weighted image (2000/20) better defines the extent of the periventricular disease.

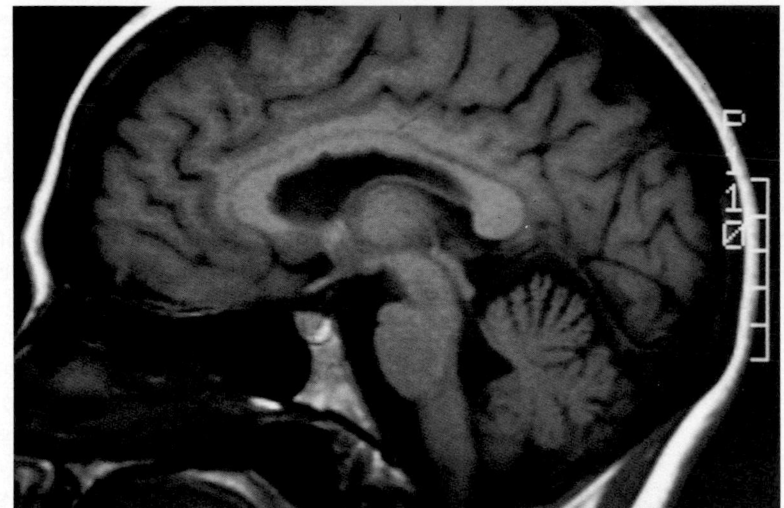

A

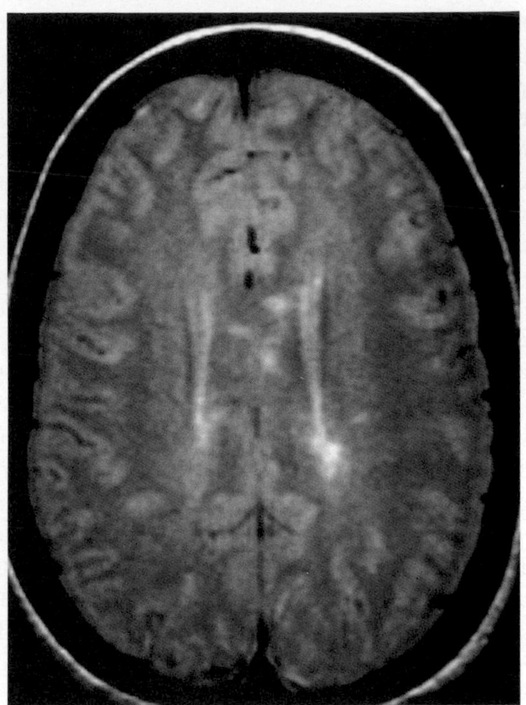

B

FIG. 30. Corpus callosal lesions in MS. Sagittal T1-weighted image **(A)** shows marked irregularity of inferior surface of corpus callosum. Axial proton-density-weighted image **(B)** shows hyperintense foci within corpus callosum and periventricular regions.

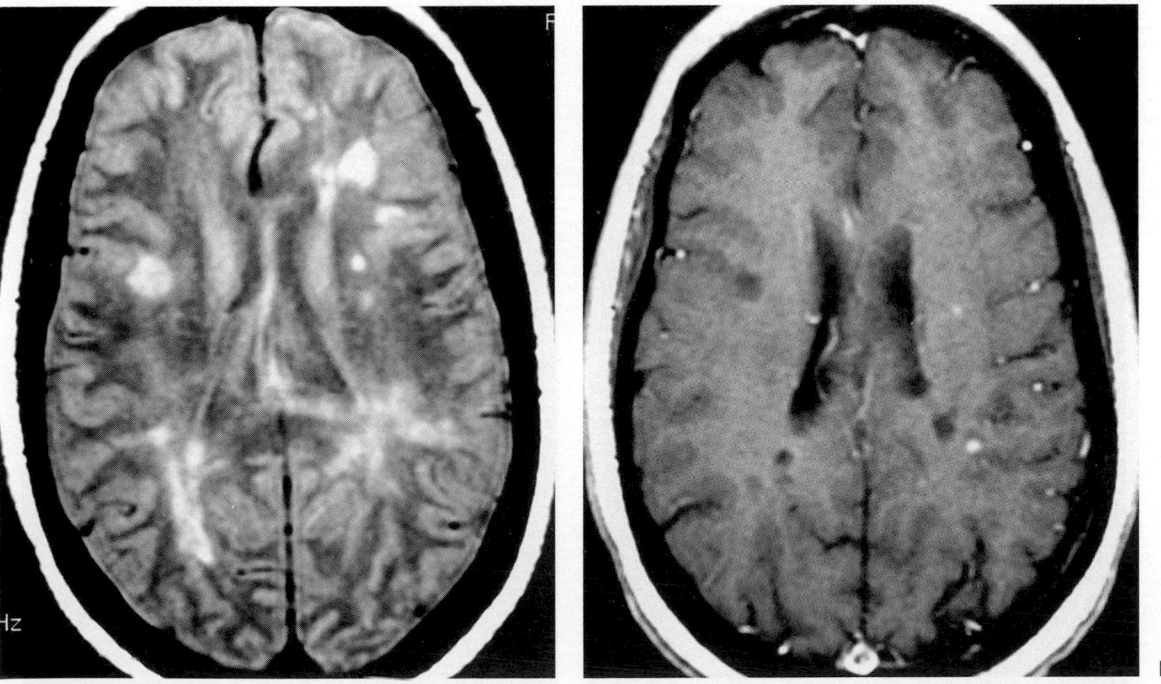

A B

FIG. 31. Acute and chronic MS. **A:** Proton-density-weighted images (2000/20) reveal multiple lesions in periventricular white matter. **B:** Gadolinium-enhanced T1-weighted image (600/20) shows single enhancing lesion, but several chronic, nonenhancing cavities.

reduction in MT in MS plaques in humans was reported (50). In one study of a small number of gadolinium-enhancing MS lesions, the MT effect was more reduced from normal as compared to the MT effect in nonenhancing lesions (51). This reduction in MT corresponded to the presence of abnormal proton MR spectroscopy resonances that were consistent with active demyelination. Interestingly, in that study (51), the normal appearing white matter in the MS patients showed similar MT ratios to those of white matter in normal volunteers, raising the possibility that the overall sensitivity of the MT technique to changes may not actually be higher than that of calculated T1- and T2-relaxation times. Clearly, the data regarding MT and demyelinating diseases is preliminary at the time of this writing.

Another recent development is diffusion-weighted MR imaging. The basis of contrast in diffusion imaging is that translational molecular motion of water causes a loss of spin coherence and hence a loss of signal intensity, when imaged with an appropriately sensitive technique in the presence of strong magnetic fields generated by the application of "diffusion gradients." The unique organizational structure of mature (myelinated) white matter has been postulated to cause anisotropy of diffusion, i.e., a directional restriction of water diffusion, as compared to gray matter (52) (Fig. 32). While it is not clear whether the myelin itself is the source of the anisotropy, it has been reported that focal demyelinating lesions in the white matter lose their anisotropy. In one primate study of EAE, white matter lesions were seen on diffusion-weighted MRI earlier than on spin-echo MRI (53). Moreover, diffusion imaging has been utilized in imaging the developing white matter in young children, where evidence of diffusion-related signal changes do not occur to a significant degree until changes compatible with myelination are seen on spin-echo MRI (54). Preliminary evidence suggests that diffusion-weighted imaging might differentiate acute from chronic MS plaques (55). This technique generally requires modified scanner hardware and is best accomplished with the use of strong gradient systems with fast switching times. It is presently in limited use at this time. There are several limitations to diffusion-weighted imaging, including the requirement for total absence of subject motion, since the technique derives its signal from its exquisite sensitivity to differences in motion on the molecular level. Most of

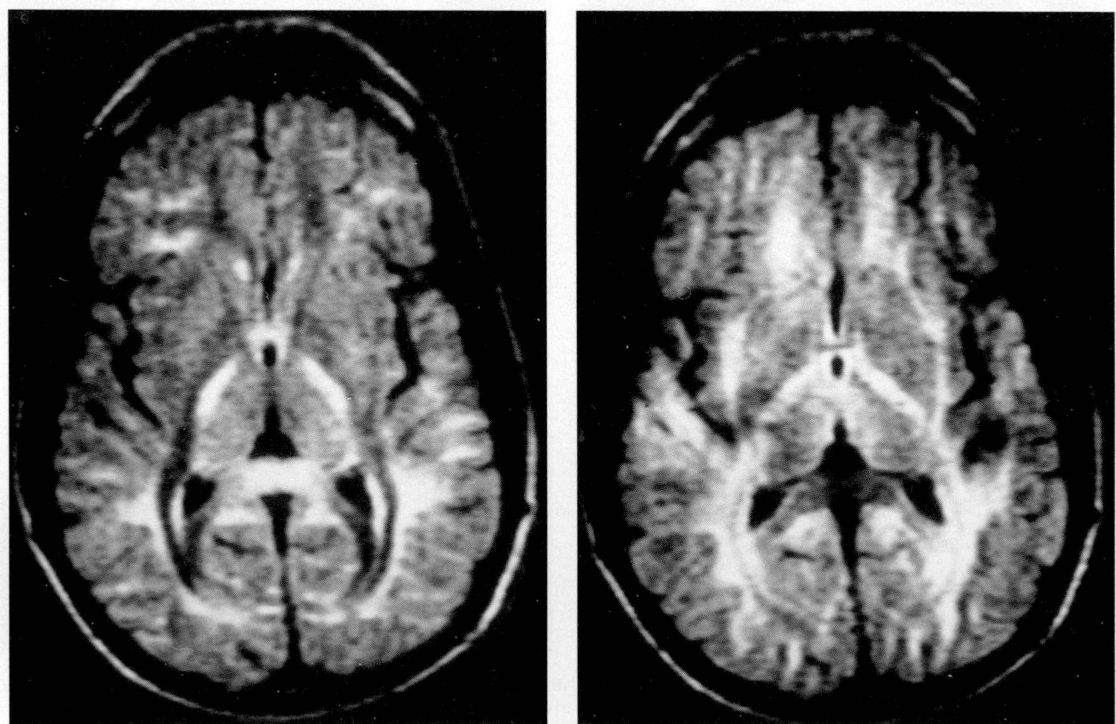

FIG. 32. Diffusion-weighted MRI showing anisotropy of white matter. High intensity is seen in white matter with fibers oriented perpendicular to direction of diffusion-sensitive gradient, since selective signal loss in diffusion-sensitive direction occurs. Therefore, note change in signal of corpus callosum and anterior commissure when diffusion direction is changed from anterior-posterior **(A)** to left-right **(B)**. (Images courtesy of D. Alsop, Philadelphia, PA.)

these problems are solved when echo planar imaging is utilized (see Chapter 30).

Extracerebral Lesions in MS

Spinal cord plaques are also often demonstrated on MRI, but MRI may not be as sensitive in the detection of spinal cord lesions as it is for brain lesions. If a patient is shown to have an intramedullary lesion that is suspected to represent spinal cord MS, it is probably most reasonable to perform a head MRI to screen for asymptomatic multifocal disease in addition to scanning the spinal cord (56), with the caveat that a normal brain MRI in no way excludes MS as the diagnosis. Most lesions detected within the spinal cord are found in the cervical region, perhaps due to the improved ability of the current MR scanners to image the cervical cord compared with the thoracic, rather than any predisposition of the cervical spinal cord to MS (Fig. 33), although some necropsy evidence shows the cervical region to be most commonly affected. Gradient-echo images, typically used for rapid imaging of the spine in the search for degenerative disc disease, should probably not be used for screening for MS plaques in the spinal cord, since it is generally believed that this technique is less sensitive than spin-echo MRI to typical intraparenchymal lesions (Fig. 34). Routine use of rapid spin-echo techniques has become standard in the search for the intramedullary lesions of MS in the spinal cord. Gadolinium contrast administration will occasionally demonstrate enhancement of the acute spinal lesions of MS (Fig. 35), depending on the nature of the blood–cord barrier at the time of the scan. Enhancing MS plaques can be virtually indistinguishable from neoplastic lesions and other inflammatory lesions of the spinal cord (see Chapters 25 and 27), particularly when the spinal cord is enlarged due to edema. Therefore, clinical correlation and often serial follow-up scanning is necessary to formulate a specific diagnosis, especially in those cases where MRI of the brain is normal.

Optic nerve involvement in MS is quite common clinically and at autopsy (17), but routine spin-echo sequences, even with high resolution, often fail to detect optic nerve involvement in clinically affected individuals. Other pulse sequences, including short tau inversion recovery (STIR) and fat suppressed fast spin echo, show promise in detecting optic neuritis with a high degree of sensitivity (57). In these techniques, optic neuritis appears as abnormal high signal intensity within the affected nerves (Fig. 36). The parameters we use at our institution for the STIR sequence are: TR = 2000, TE = 150, and TE = 30. More recently, it has become clear that high resolution T2-weighted fast spin-echo MRI with fat suppression, as well as high resolution post-contrast enhanced T1-weighted images also can often detect intraneural signal abnormalities (see Chapter 22). It should be realized by the radiologist that it is unclear whether it is significant to detect optic neuritis on imaging studies in patients with clinically evident optic neuritis (see Chapter 22). There is strong evidence that optic neuritis is often the first evidence of MS, being the initial manifestation in about 20% of cases and occurring

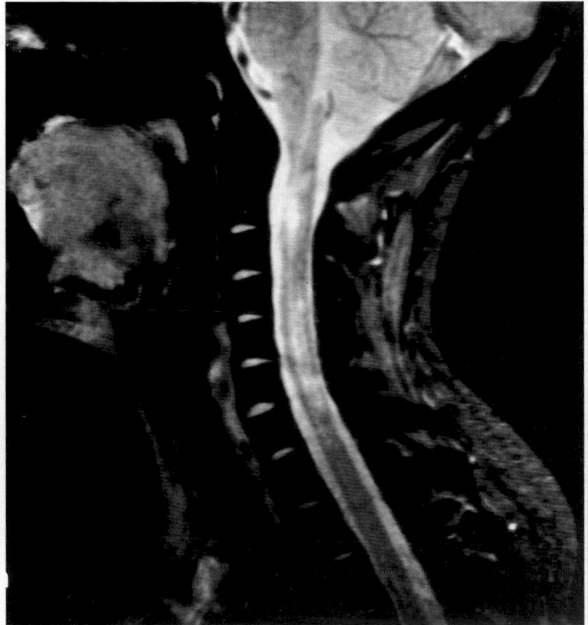

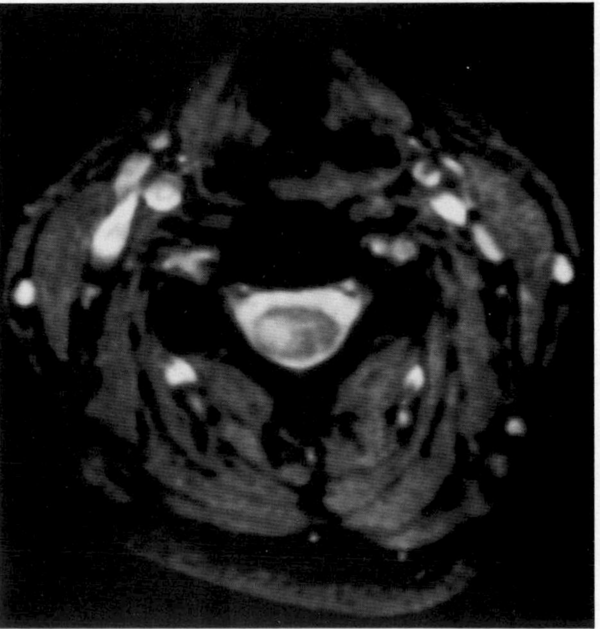

FIG. 33. Extensive cervical spinal cord lesions with MS. **A:** Sagittal T2-weighted image (2000/80) shows extensive irregular high signal within the cord substance. **B:** Axial T2-weighted image shows typical peripheral location of MS plaque.

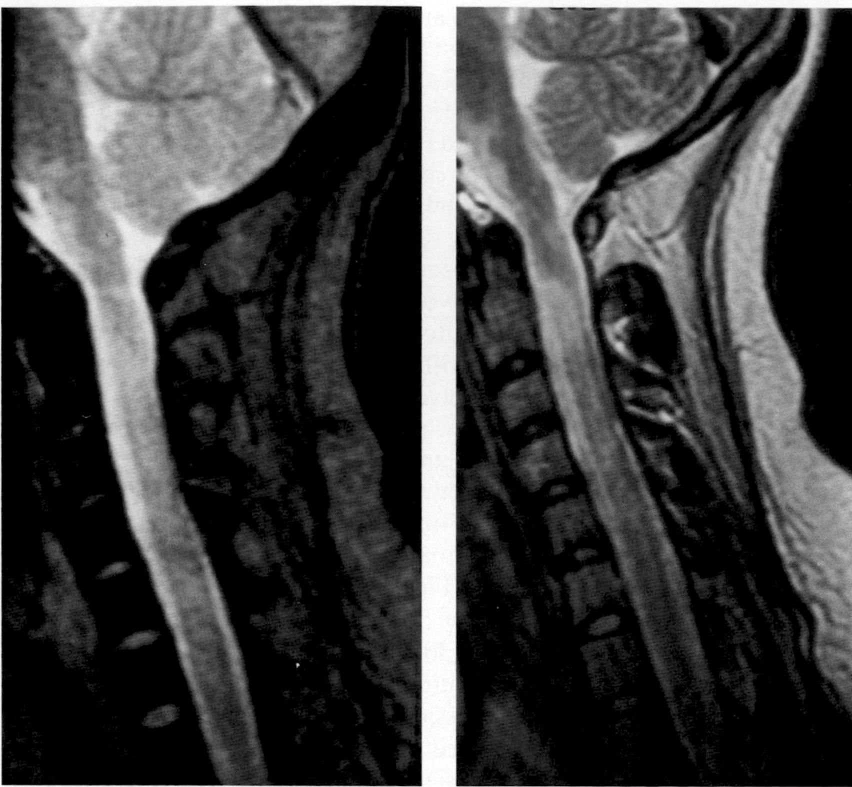

FIG. 34. Cervical spinal cord MS, gradient echo vs. spin echo. **A:** Lesion in spinal cord is poorly seen on sagittal gradient-echo T2-weighted image (600/18, Flip angle 25°). **B:** Sagittal spin-echo T2-weighted image is much more sensitive to disease.

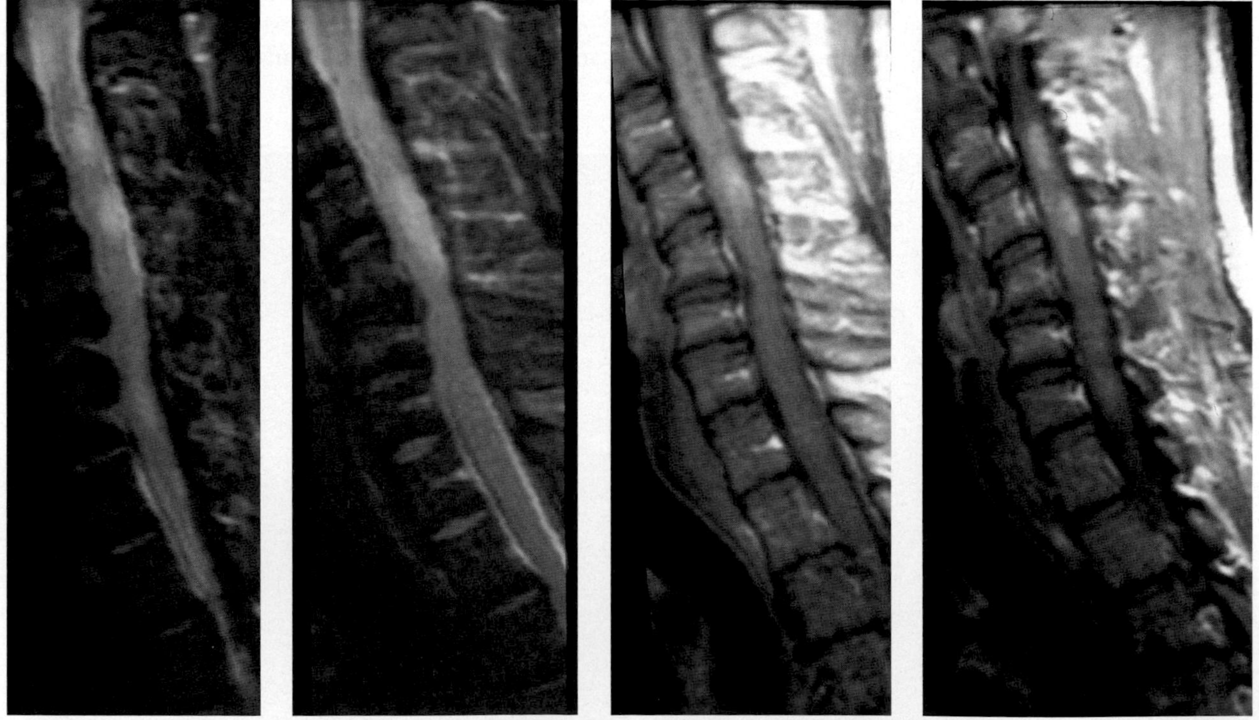

FIG. 35. MS in cervical spinal cord with enhancement. **A,B:** Sagittal T2-weighted MRI. **C,D:** Sagittal T1-weighted MRI after gadolinium. Focal intramedullary lesions (A) show partial enhancement (B) in this MS patient with new symptoms.

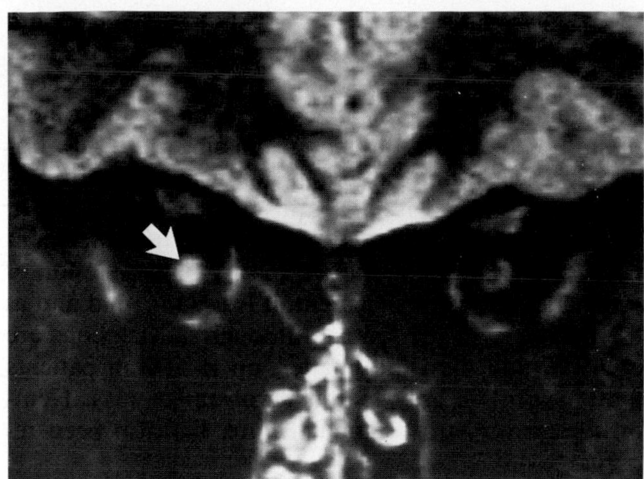

FIG. 36. Multiple sclerosis with optic neuritis. Coronal image through the optic nerves on a STIR sequence (2000/150/30) shows the right optic nerve to be bright compared with the left (*arrow*).

during the course of the disease in 50% of cases. It is also estimated that 45% to 80% of patients with isolated optic neuritis go on to develop MS at some point during the next 15 years, although most who do develop MS do so within the first 5 years. In patients with clinically diagnosed optic neuritis, many clinicians feel that the role of MRI is twofold (58): (i) to exclude the rarely found alternative cause of the clinical symptomatology aside from optic neuritis, and (ii) to detect the presence of intracerebral lesions. Recent data from the Optic Neuritis Treatment Trial at 2-year follow-up showed that steroid treatment of acute optic neuritis reduced the risk of developing MS from 36% to 16% *only in those patients with abnormal focal lesions on brain MRI* at the time of the acute presentation (59). Therefore, although it may not be important to detect the optic nerve lesion in optic neuritis, MRI appears to be important in prognosis and in guiding therapy for patients with optic neuritis.

Virally-Induced Demyelination

Many viruses cause encephalitis or myelitis by infecting and destroying the nervous tissue in the brain and spinal cord (see also Chapters 16 and 25), but some have a peculiar tropism for the white matter. Potential mechanisms of demyelination attributed to viruses include (i) direct infection of oligodendrocytes, (ii) immune-induced oligodendrocytes or myelin destruction by immune reactions against viral antigens, (iii) secondary damage from immune complex formation, and (iv) antimyelin autoimmune reactions (11).

Progressive multifocal leukoencephalopathy (PML) is probably the best known virally induced demyelinating disease. It is caused by reactivation of a latent papovavirus (the JC virus) infection. This disorder affects immune-compromised patients, and in years prior to the acquired immune deficiency syndrome (AIDS), PML was found primarily in leukemia or lymphoma patients. The non-AIDS population affected by PML is generally middle-aged and either harbors an underlying disease affecting immunocompetence, such as leukemia, lymphoma, sarcoidosis, malignancy, or tuberculosis, or is receiving immunosuppressive therapy. Rarely, patients with PML have neither an underlying systemic disease nor an immunodeficiency (60). More recently, the majority of cases of PML have occurred as a complication of AIDS. PML typically presents with an insidious onset of dementia and variable neurologic deficits, including visual loss, weakness, and ataxia. The disease progresses to profound neurologic deficits and death usually within 6 months (61).

PML is characterized pathologically by focal or confluent areas of demyelination, mainly distributed throughout the cerebral white matter (Fig. 37). The gray matter may also be affected, but the lesions are often less conspicuous. The foci of demyelination can have a resemblance to those of multiple sclerosis, but occasionally they are large and confluent, mimicking foci of ischemic necrosis or cystic degeneration. The ultimate diagnosis of PML is finalized by the microscopic pathologic features demonstrated by a variety of staining techniques. Striking cytologic features include large, highly atypical astrocytes with bizarre appearing nuclei and intranuclear inclusions in oligodendrocytes (Fig. 38). Since the virus is found within oligodendrocytes, it is concluded that the lesion of PML is a result of failure of infected oligodendrocytes to maintain myelination. Rare inflammatory cells, usually lymphocytes, may also be present (62).

Classically, PML appears on MRI as asymmetric, bi-

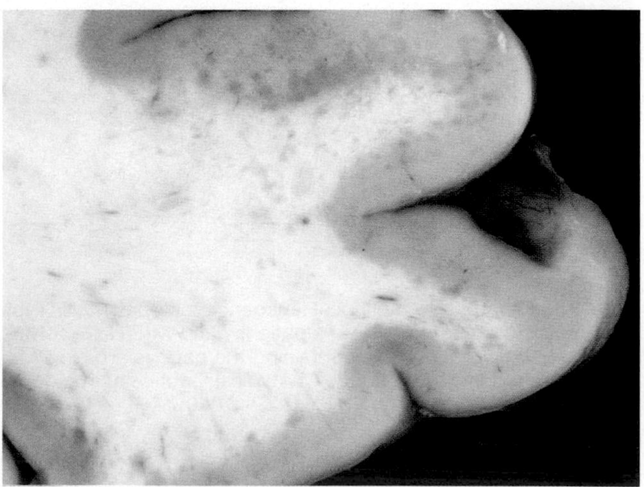

FIG. 37. Progressive multifocal leukoencephalopathy. Multiple small foci of demyelination in subcortical white matter are noted, along with small lesions in cortex, in this necropsy specimen from patient with PML and AIDS.

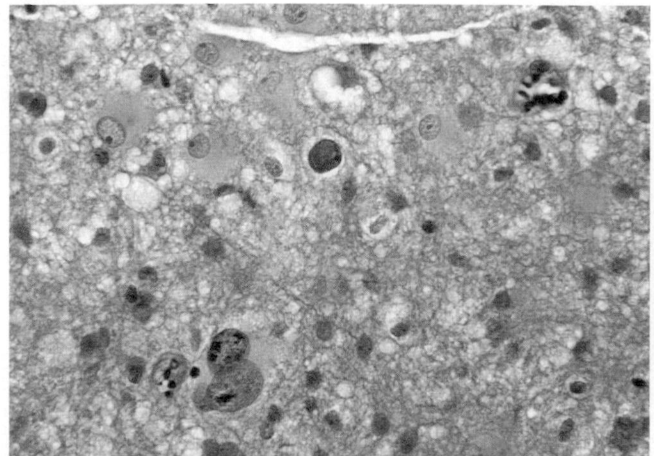
A

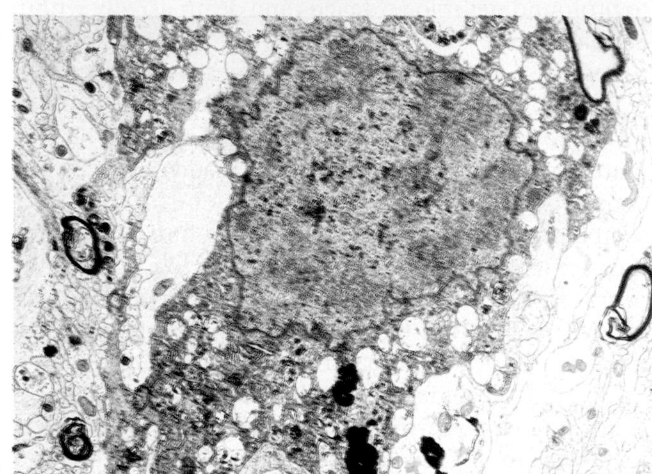
B

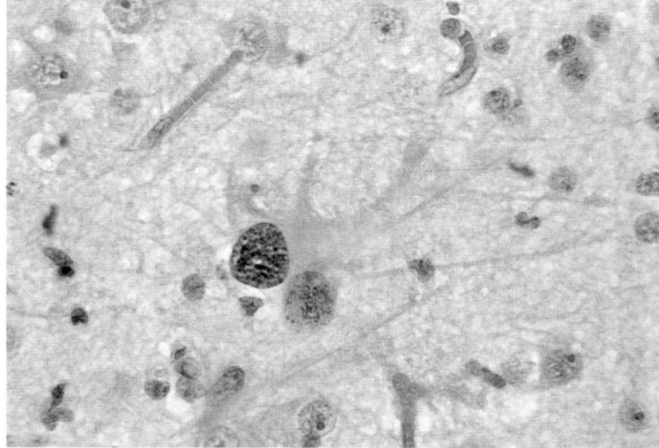
C

FIG. 38. Progressive multifocal leukoencephalopathy. **A:** Typical oligodendroglial inclusion in a patient with PML (H&E, ×400). **B:** Oligodendroglial nucleus containing the papovavirus in PML. Electron micrograph (×10,000). **C:** Atypical reactive astrocytes in a focus of demyelination in PML (H&E, ×1000).

lateral, patchy areas of demyelination with a preference initially for the subcortical white matter and a slight preference for the parietal region (30,63) (Fig. 39). Early in the course of the disease, single lesions are common in PML. The disease progresses quickly to involve greater amounts of white matter becoming confluent in the later stages (Figs. 40 and 41). Some degrees of mass effect can be noted, and in these cases, differentiation from neoplasm (i.e., glioma) may not be possible (Fig. 40). Enhancement is usually absent on MRI, possibly attributable to the paucity of perivenous inflammation (61). In the literature, however, isolated cases of enhancement with PML have been reported (64). When the lesion of PML does show enhancement, it is usually mild and at the periphery of the lesion. Although most lesions are clearly within the white matter, up to 50% of patients may have some gray matter involvement (61). Hemorrhage, a very uncommon feature, has also been reported (61).

In patients with AIDS, many other disease processes may affect the white matter and mimic PML. These include diseases with multifocal involvement predominantly of white matter, most notably encephalitides, including cytomegalovirus, toxoplasmosis, or encephalitis from the AIDS virus, HIV-1 (Fig. 42) (see Chapter 16 for a complete discussion). Mass effect is more common with lymphoma and toxoplasmosis, but as noted can occasionally be present in PML (61).

Subacute sclerosing panencephalitis (SSPE) is now a very rare disease resulting from a slow infection reactivated after an episode of measles. Probably because of widespread measles immunization in this country, there

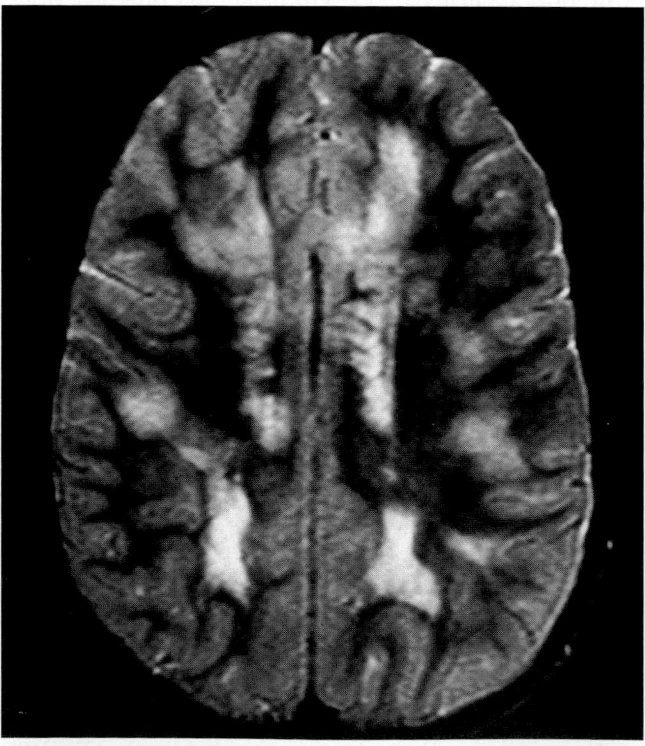

FIG. 39. PML in patient with AIDS. Extensive white matter lesions seen on T2-weighted image (2000/80), with predilection for subcortical white matter.

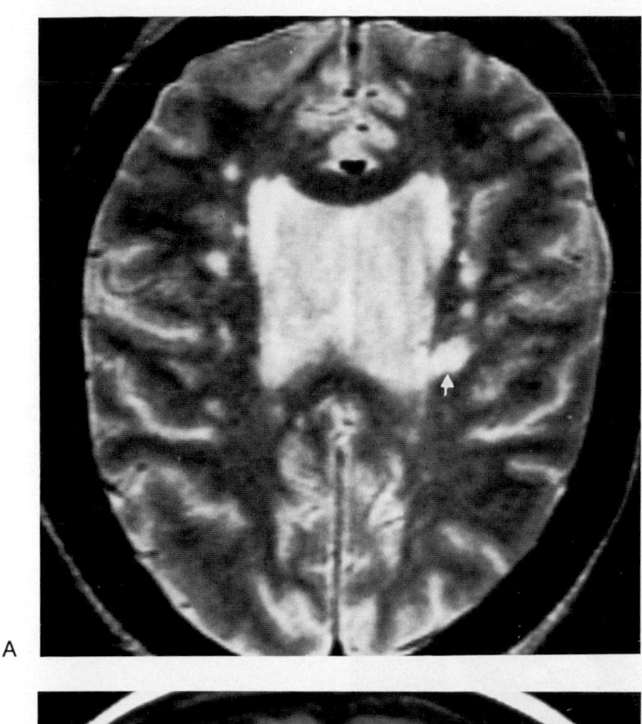

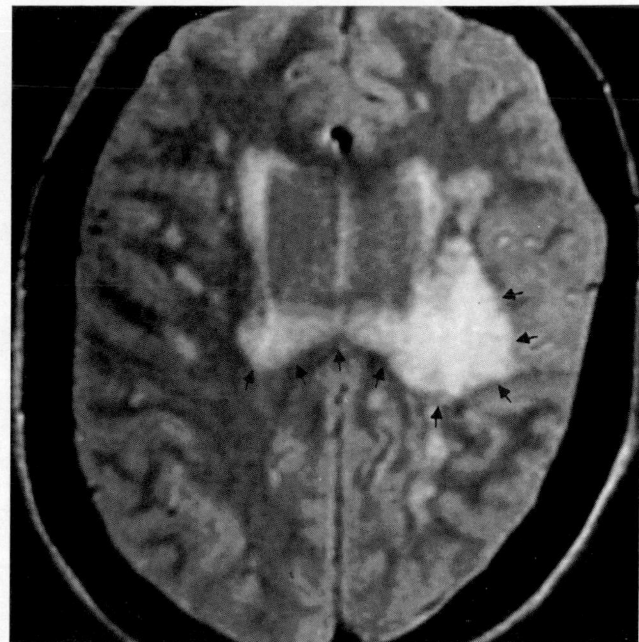

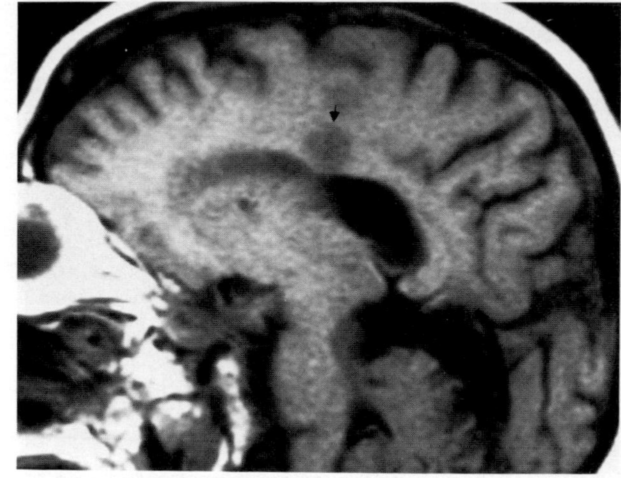

FIG. 40. PML with mass effect, pathologically proven. **A:** Axial long TR/short TE (3500/30), initial scan. **B:** Axial long TR/short TE (3000/30), 1 month after initial scan. **C:** Sagittal T1-weighted image (600/11), 1 month after initial scan. Initial MRI (A) shows scattered nonspecific white matter focal hyperintensities, with a slightly larger lesion in left parietal white matter (*arrow*, A). Progressive worsening of symptoms led to follow-up MRI 1 month later (B,C), which showed marked enlargement of lesion (*arrows*, B) that now crossed corpus callosum (B). Note focal mass effect (*arrow*, C), which led to erroneous MRI diagnosis of glioma.

has been a marked decrease in incidence (65). While this is essentially a disease of the pediatric age group, a latency of several years may be present, with the age of onset of SSPE between 3–20 years. Clinical features include initially behavioral changes with progressive myoclonus, ataxia, and seizures. MR and CT findings are of edematous periventricular white matter lesions with significant mass effect, initially compressing the ventricles, followed by an end-stage appearance of marked cerebral atrophy. SSPE usually progresses to death in 6 months to 6 years. While many theories have been espoused to explain the long latency of the infection and the temporal course of the disease, none are completely accepted.

A rare entity of progressive encephalitis has been reported to follow congenital and other rubella infections. This "progressive rubella panencephalitis" (66) should at least be considered in the differential diagnosis of SSPE.

Immune-Mediated White Matter Diseases

Occasionally, following a viral illness, a patient will develop an autoimmune response to white matter, with variable and usually reversible demyelination. Guillain-Barré syndrome and acute disseminated encephalomyelitis (ADEM) are examples of virally induced, immune-mediated white matter diseases. ADEM in its most common form usually presents as a monophasic, self-limited illness within weeks following a viral infection. Analysis of CSF in ADEM usually shows either only mild signs of inflammation or it is normal. The most common virus associated with ADEM is measles, followed by rubella, chickenpox, Epstein-Barr, mumps, and pertussis. Seizures and focal neurologic deficits commonly present 5 days to 2 weeks after a viral illness or immunization. The neurologic deficits usually resolve

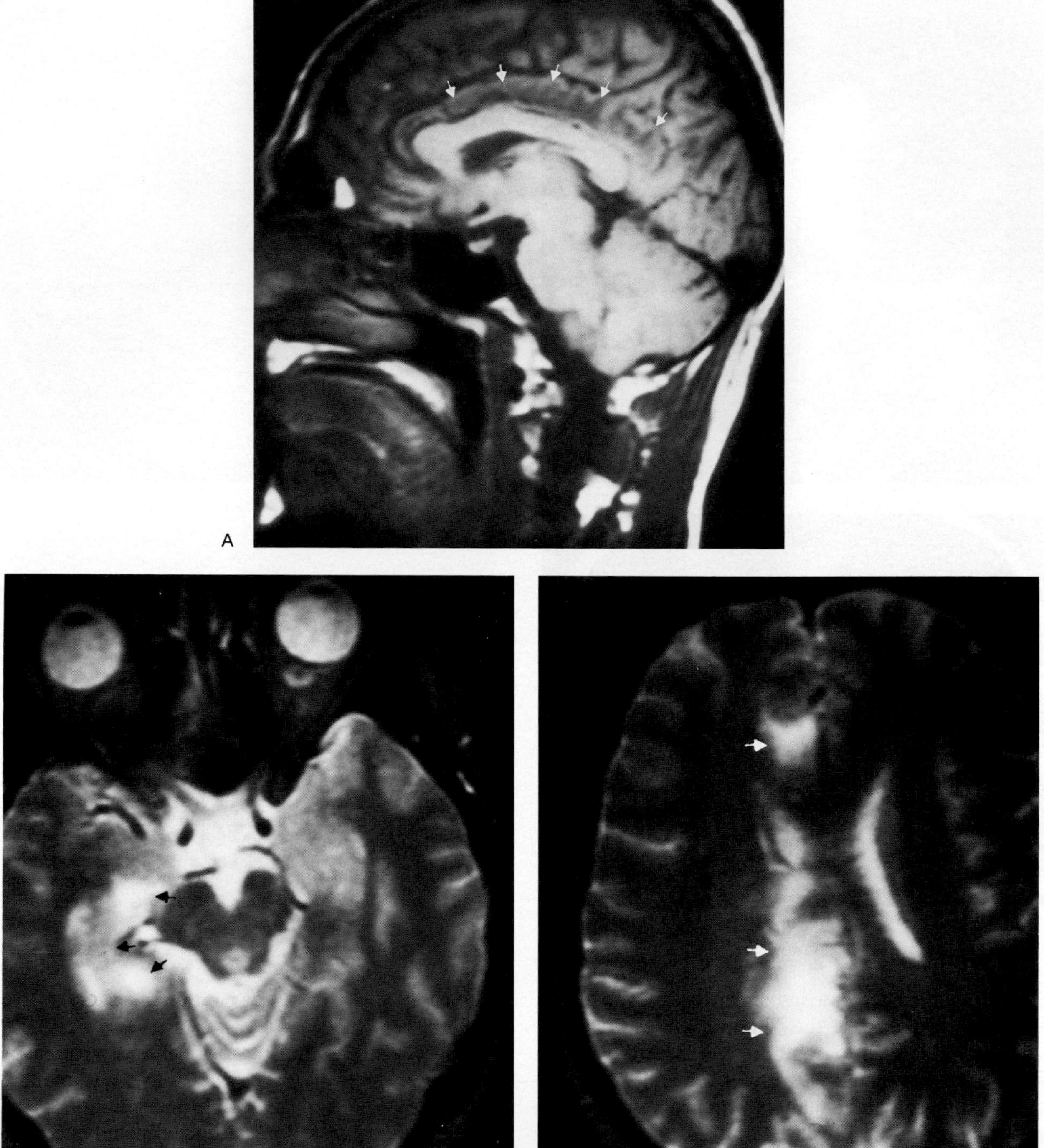

FIG. 41. PML involving gray and white matter of limbic system. **A:** Sagittal T1-weighted (600/20) MRI shows low-intensity lesion extending throughout right cingulate gyrus (*arrows*). **B,C:** Axial T2-weighted images (2800/80) show high signal intensity in right uncus and parahippocampal gyrus (*arrows*, B) and in subcortical white matter and cortex of right cingulate gyrus (*arrows*, C).

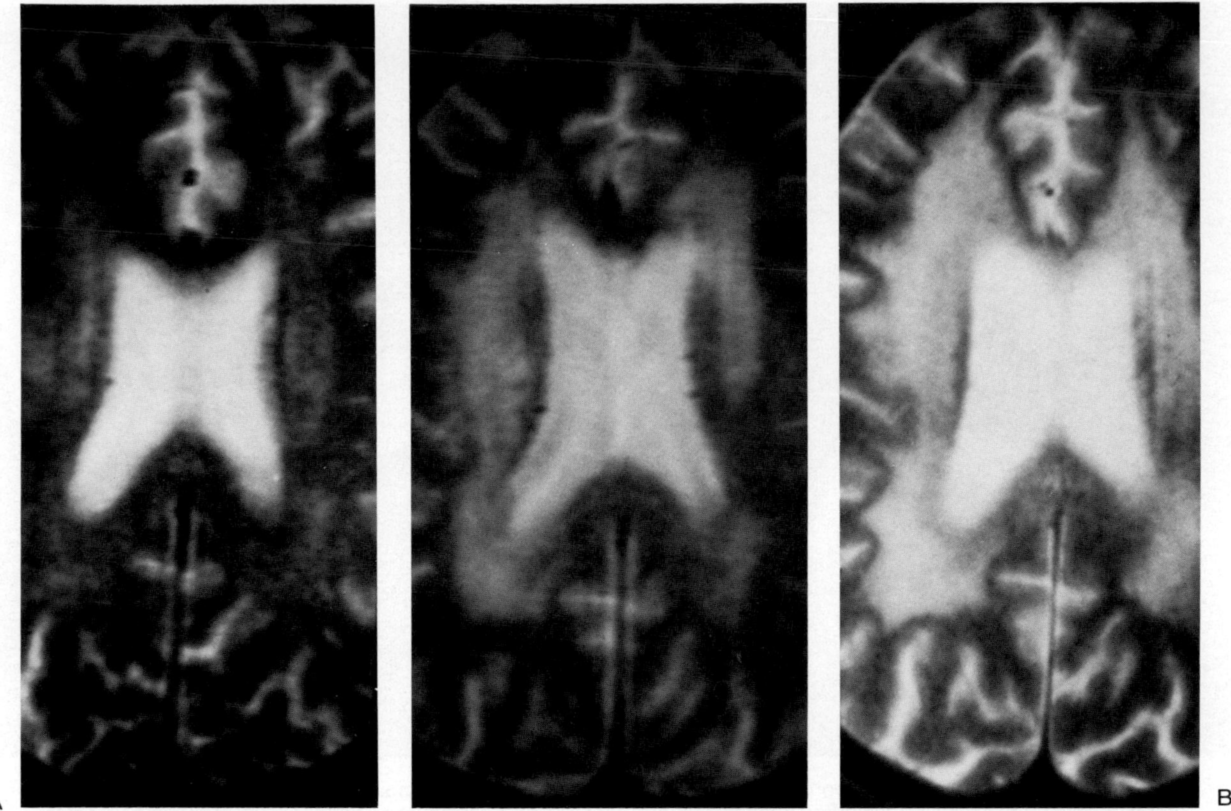

FIG. 42. Progressive white matter involvement with HIV encephalitis. **A:** Baseline T2-weighted image (2500/70). **B:** T2-weighted image (2800/80) 9 months later. **C:** T2-weighted image (2800/80) 13 months after baseline. Note progressive and extensive white matter abnormality in patient with AIDS and HIV encephalitis over time.

spontaneously within 1 month, although permanent sequelae occur in 10% to 20% of cases (67,68). The residual complications of ADEM are most commonly related to frequent seizures. A few children have a progressive downhill course, with severe paresis, neurologic dysfunction, and death.

A perivenous inflammatory process is seen on pathologic examination with confluent areas of demyelination. In distinction from viral encephalitides, virus is generally not found on examination of brain tissue in this disorder. The histologic appearance of ADEM is similar to that of experimental allergic encephalomyelitis (particularly the chronic form), supporting the hypothesis that ADEM results from an autoimmune response to a CNS antigen triggered by viral infections.

The lesions of ADEM appear virtually identical to most MS lesions on MRI studies, and some patients, initially diagnosed as ADEM, develop exacerbations of their neurologic symptoms. Some of these cases eventually become reclassified as MS. Most ADEM lesions are located in the subcortical white matter, with asymmetric involvement of both hemispheres, with or without brainstem disease (Fig. 43). There is predominant involvement of the white matter, but lesions may involve gray matter as well (Fig. 44). Lesions may be large but charac-

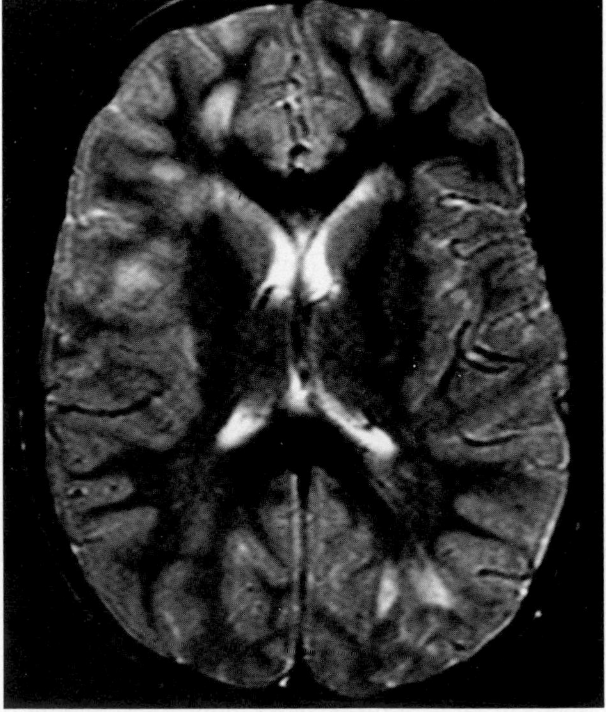

FIG. 43. ADEM. Scattered white matter lesions are seen in the subcortical region on T2-weighted axial image (2000/80).

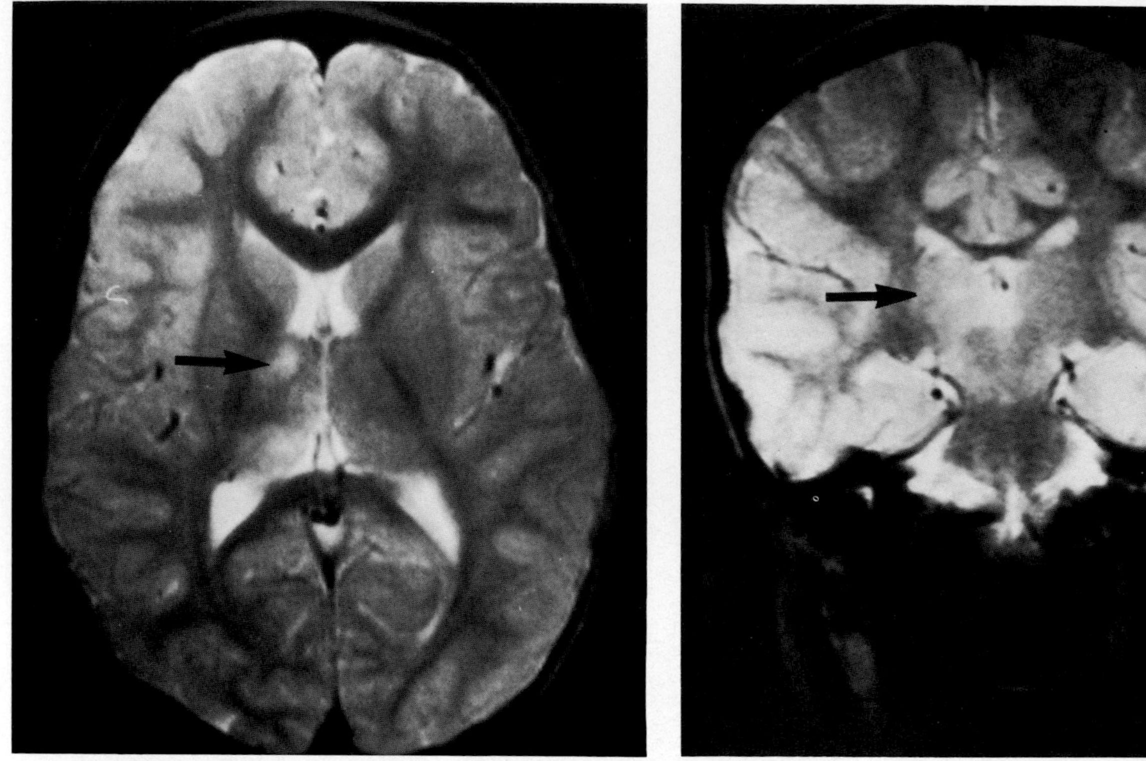

FIG. 44. Acute disseminated encephalomyelitis. **A:** Gray matter involvement is seen as increased signal in the thalamus (*arrow*) on this axial T2-weighted image (2000/80). **B:** Coronal T2-weighted sequence (2000/80) shows extensive gray matter lesion (*arrow*).

teristically show only mild mass effect as compared to that expected with the size of the lesions (Figs. 45 and 46) and typically show prompt regression in response to steroid therapy (28,67). While enhancement can be seen with ADEM, the absence of enhancement does not lessen the likelihood of the diagnosis. Involvement of the spinal cord is common (Fig. 47).

Acute hemorrhagic leukoencephalopathy is considered a rare hyperacute form of ADEM, which is a fulminant form of the disease. This entity is typically seen in young patients who have an abrupt onset of progressive neurologic deficits and often go on to death. Acute hemorrhagic leukoencephalopathy has been reported following viral respiratory infections and sepsis, as well as in association with a variety of diseases presumed to have allergic etiologies, including ulcerative colitis and asthma (69). Histopathologically, vessel wall necrosis, perivascular edema, inflammatory cells, perivascular demyelination, and hemorrhages surrounding thrombosed capillaries are identified (11). White matter lesions can be confluent and usually contain small foci of hemorrhage (70) (Fig. 48), although occasionally large hemorrhages are seen. The pathophysiology of the disease is thought to be a result of deposition of circulating immune complexes secondary to a circulating antibody response (11).

Central Pontine and Extrapontine Myelinolysis (Osmotic Demyelination)

Central pontine myelinolysis is a demyelinating disorder found commonly in alcoholics, but the disorder is also found in association with many systemic disorders with electrolyte abnormalities (71,72), including chronic pulmonary disease, liver and kidney diseases, and neoplasia. Because of the common association with rapidly corrected hyponatremia, the term "osmotic demyelination syndrome" has been proposed (73). The symptoms of central pontine myelinolysis are quadriparesis, pseudobulbar palsy, and changing levels of consciousness, including coma and death (74). A state of pseudocoma (locked-in syndrome) may precede death by a few days. Many patients progress to death, but with the improved detection of the disease with MRI, many more cases have been described with survival accompanied by varying degrees of residual neurologic deficits. Histologically, the area of myelin breakdown is sharply demarcated and displays extensive loss of oligodendrocytes, infiltration with foamy macrophages, and reactive astrocytosis. A significant number of neurons and axis cylinders are spared (75).

The MR findings are of high intensity on T2-weighted sequences corresponding to the regions of demyelination

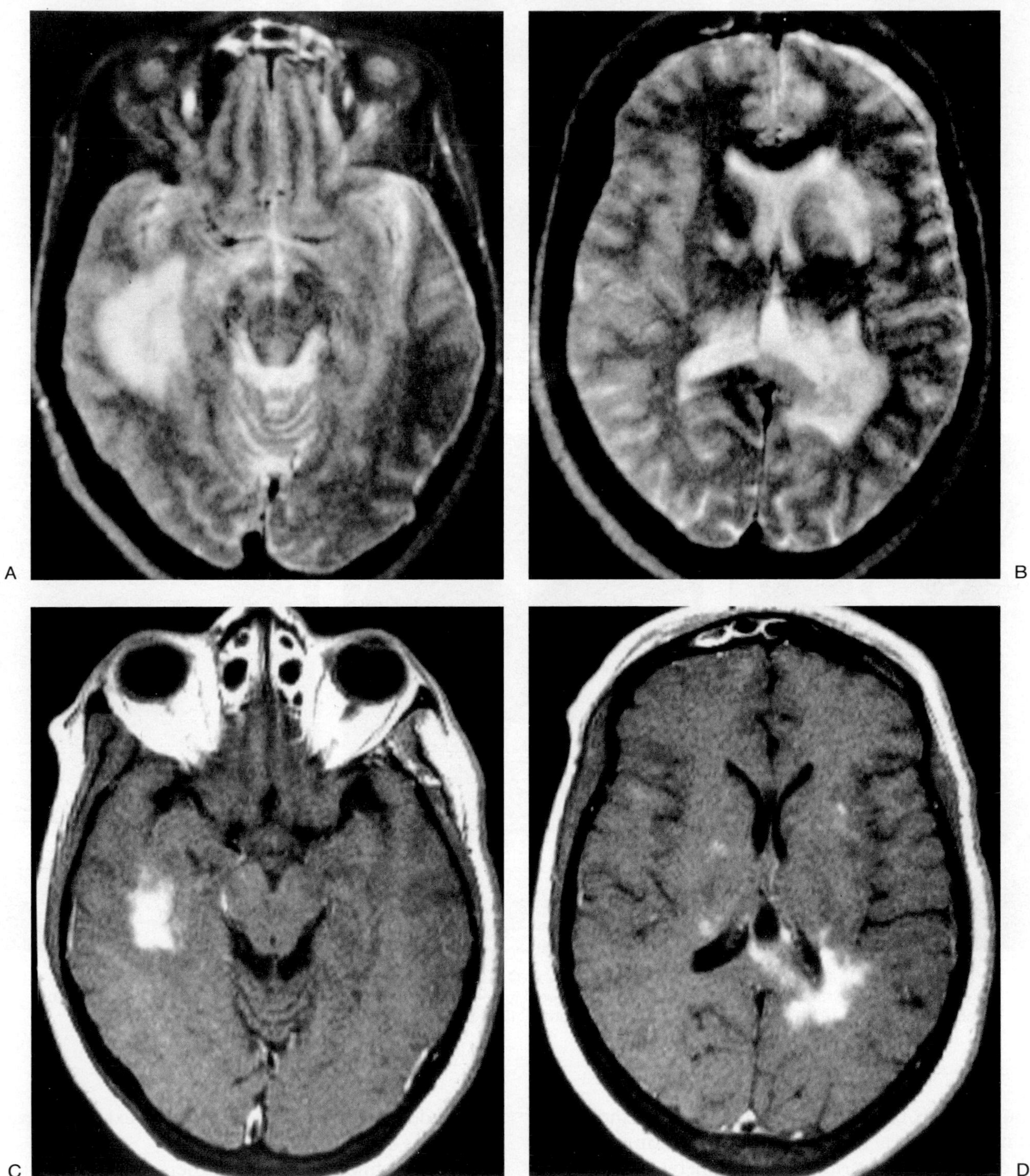

FIG. 45. ADEM with mass-like appearance and dense enhancement (biopsy proven). **A,B:** T2-weighted MRI. **C,D:** T1-weighted MRI after gadolinium. Multiple large lesions involve both white and gray matter and extend into corpus callosum (A,B). Note absence of significant mass effect in light of size of lesions. Dense enhancement of portions of lesions is seen (C,D), including corpus callosum lesion.

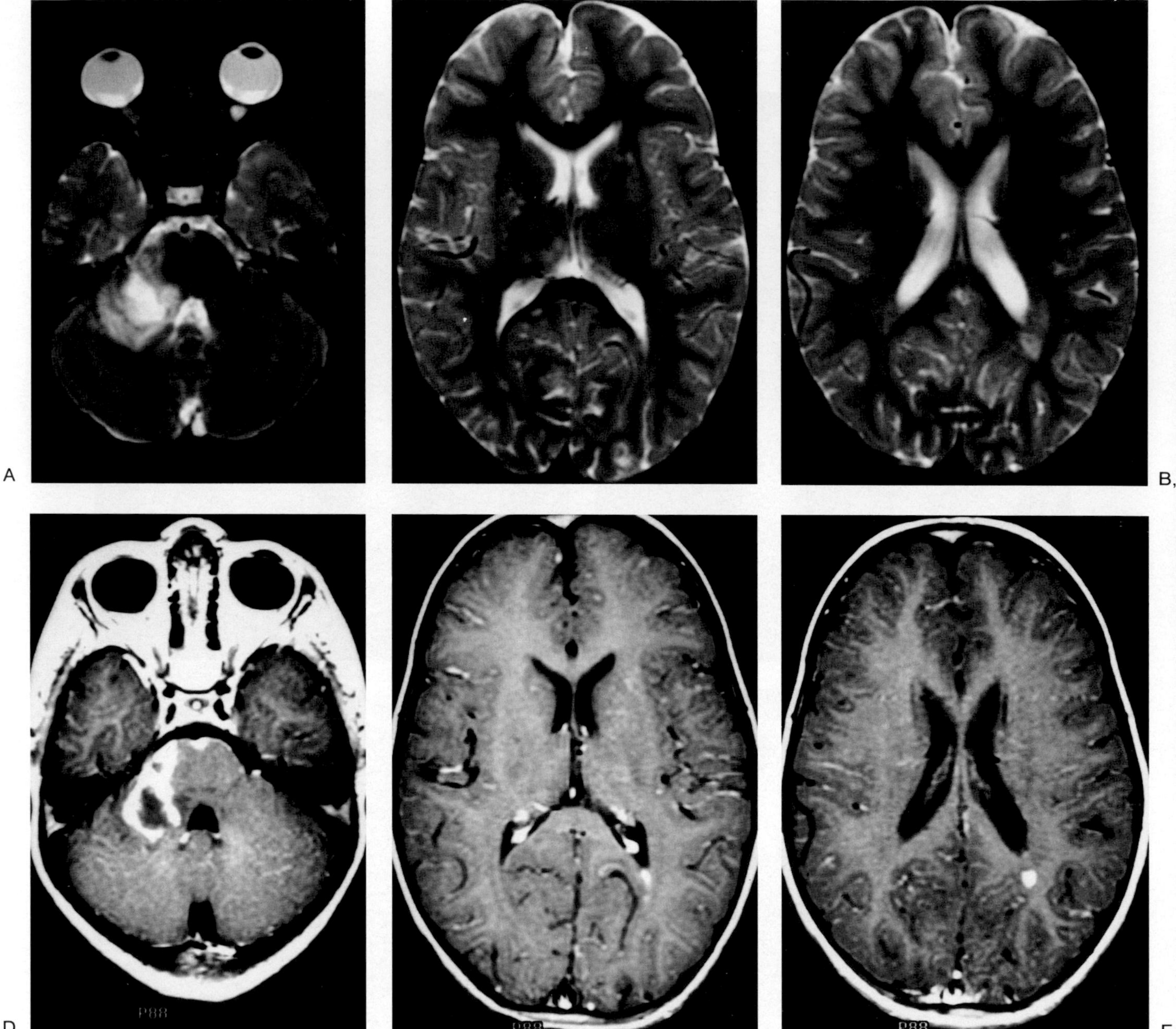

FIG. 46. ADEM as multiple masses (biopsy proven). **A–C:** T2-weighted MRI. **D–F:** T1-weighted MRI after gadolinium. Child after viral illness presented with ataxia. Focal lesions with some mass effect (A–C) involve both gray (B) and white matter (A,C). Significant irregular enhancement (D–F) is also seen.

throughout the brain, but most prominent in the upper and middle pons (71–74). The pontine lesion is central, with characteristic sparing of the peripheral pial and ventricular surface rim of tissue (Fig. 49). Gadolinium contrast enhancement is occasionally seen at the periphery of the area of acute pontine myelinolysis (Fig. 50). Extrapontine sites of myelinolysis may also occur in association with electrolyte disturbance and its rapid correction (77). These abnormalities may be seen even without significant pontine abnormality, and characteristically involve deep white matter, particularly external capsules, as well as deep gray matter (Fig. 51).

The MR findings of osmotic demyelination, although often characteristically located, must be interpreted in light of the clinical setting. Unfortunately, the clinical diagnosis can be difficult to ascertain, so the recognition of the pattern of abnormalities by the astute radiologist often prompts a thorough search of the electrolyte results. Particularly when white matter lesions are seen beyond the pons, many entities can be considered in the differ-

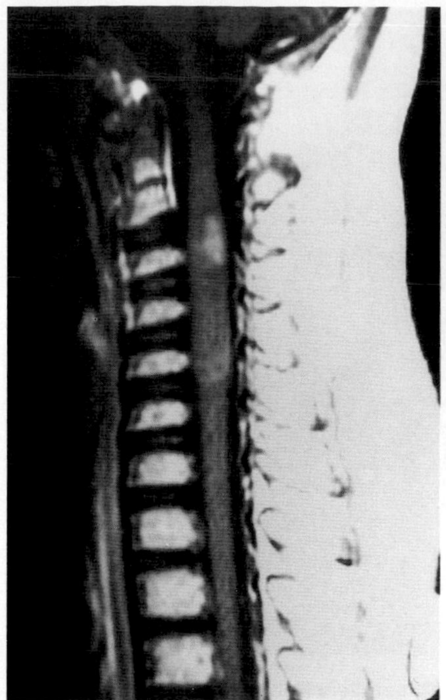

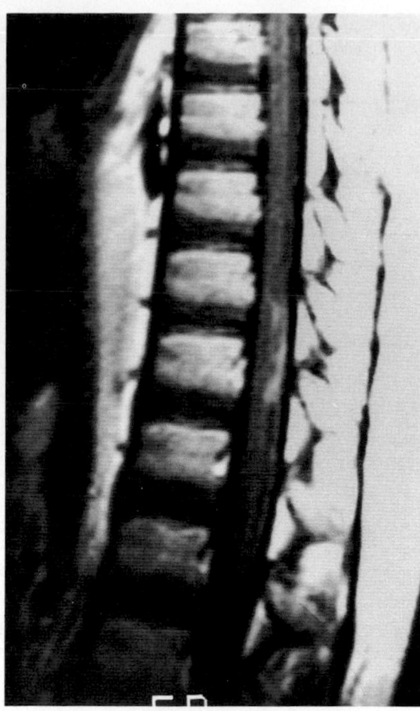

A,B

FIG. 47. Enhancement of spinal cord lesions in ADEM. Abnormal enhancement is present in the cervical **(A)** and thoracic **(B)** spinal cord.

ential diagnosis, including ischemia, multiple sclerosis, encephalitis, toxic exposures, and radiation therapy effects. Even brainstem gliomas may present with central increased signal on T2-weighted images in a pattern quite similar to central pontine myelinolysis, and should be considered in those patients with a more insidious onset of neurologic dysfunction. Therefore, while the spectrum of findings in pontine and extrapontine myelinolysis is diverse, the key to the MRI diagnosis is the bilateral involvement of the deep and capsular white matter, often accompanied by abnormalities in the thalami and basal ganglia.

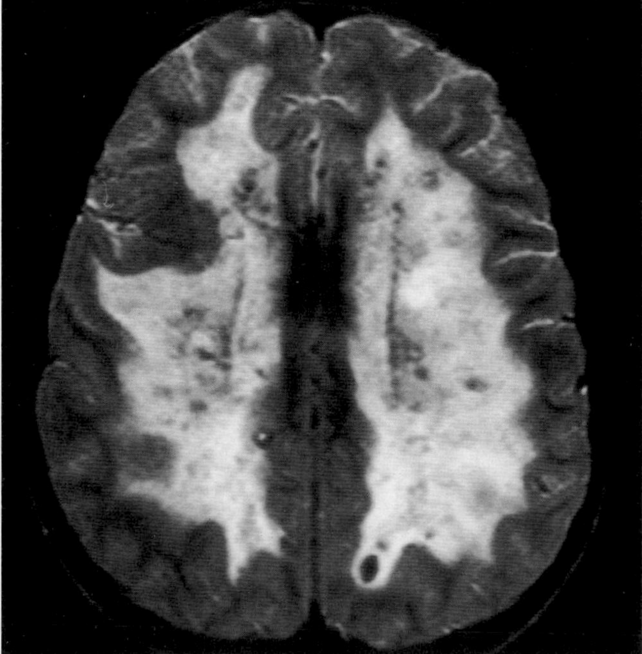

FIG. 48. Hemorrhagic leukoencephalopathy. Extensive abnormal signal involving the supraventricular white matter is present, with acute hemorrhage present as foci of marked hypointensity within the white matter lesions.

LEUKODYSTROPHIES

In the leukodystrophies, also known as dysmyelinating diseases, an enzyme deficiency prevents normal formation of maintenance of white matter. This group of diseases is characterized by progressive destruction of the myelin of the white matter. The exact nature of the enzymatic defect is not equally clear in each of the disease processes. The destruction of myelin is due to deficient catabolism of portions of the complex proteins in the myelin sheaths, resulting in accumulation of different catabolites in the various diseases of this group. The clinical picture is one of progressive mental deterioration. Patients present with mental retardation, weakness, and long track signs as well as visual, auditory, and somatosensory-evoked potentials (78). The diseases progress to frank dementia, spasticity, and unresponsiveness. In most patients the disease is evident early in the first decade. The common leukodystrophies (metachromatic leukodystrophy, Krabbe's and Canavan's diseases) are transmitted by an autosomal recessive pattern of inheritance. Adrenal leukodystrophy in the classic form and Pelizaeus-Merzbacher disease, found only in boys, are inherited as a sex-linked recessive disorder.

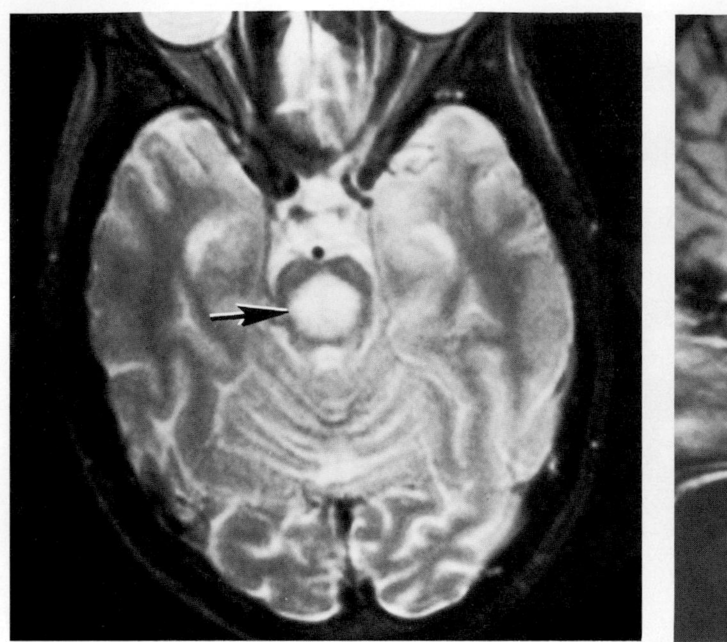

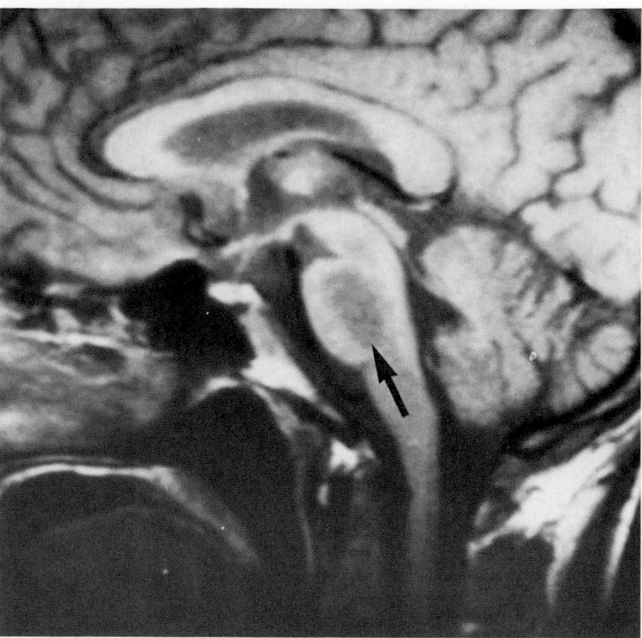

FIG. 49. Central pontine myelinolysis. **A:** T2-weighted axial image (2000/80) shows characteristic bright lesion most prominently within the midpons (*arrow*), with surrounding rim of normal-appearing pontine parenchyma. **B:** Sagittal T1-weighted image (800/26) demonstrates a low-signal lesion within the pons and medulla (*arrow*). (From Edwards, ref. 76, with permission.)

The MR picture is that of progressive white matter lesions eventually resulting in diffuse cerebral atrophy. Although the disease pattern on MRI is similar for all of the leukodystrophies in the later stages, there are some distinguishing features early in the disease course (79–81).

Sudanophilic Leukodystrophies

The sudanophilic leukodystrophies include several poorly defined diseases that cause an accumulation of sudanophilic droplets containing cholesterol and triglycerides in the white matter. Pelizaeus-Merzbacher disease

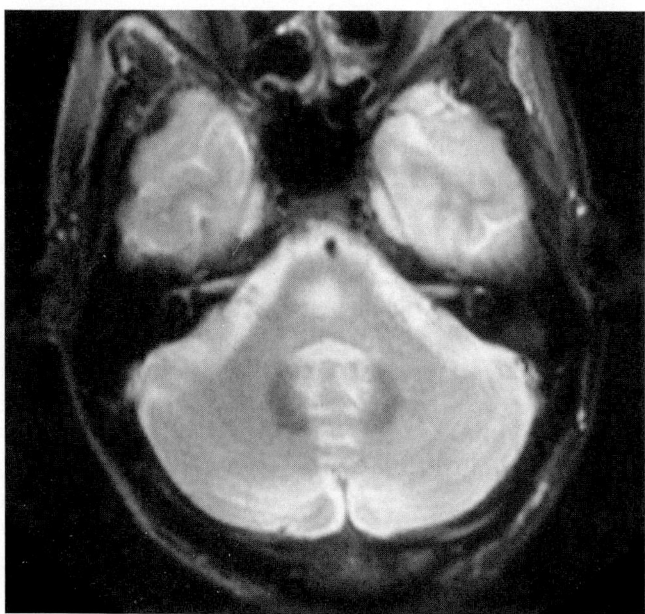

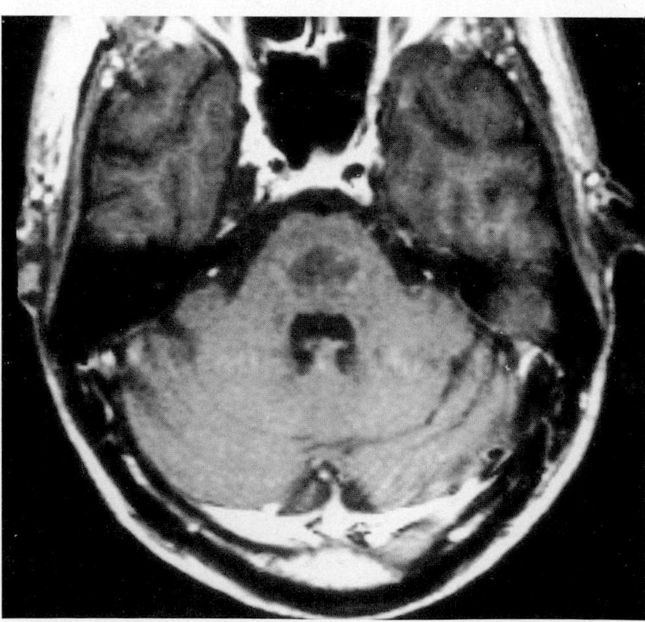

FIG. 50. Central pontine myelinolysis. **A:** T2-weighted axial image (2000/80) shows lesion within the midpons, with surrounding rim of normal-appearing pontine parenchyma. **B:** Contrast-enhanced T1-weighted image (600/26) demonstrates faint enhancement at the margins of the pontine lesion.

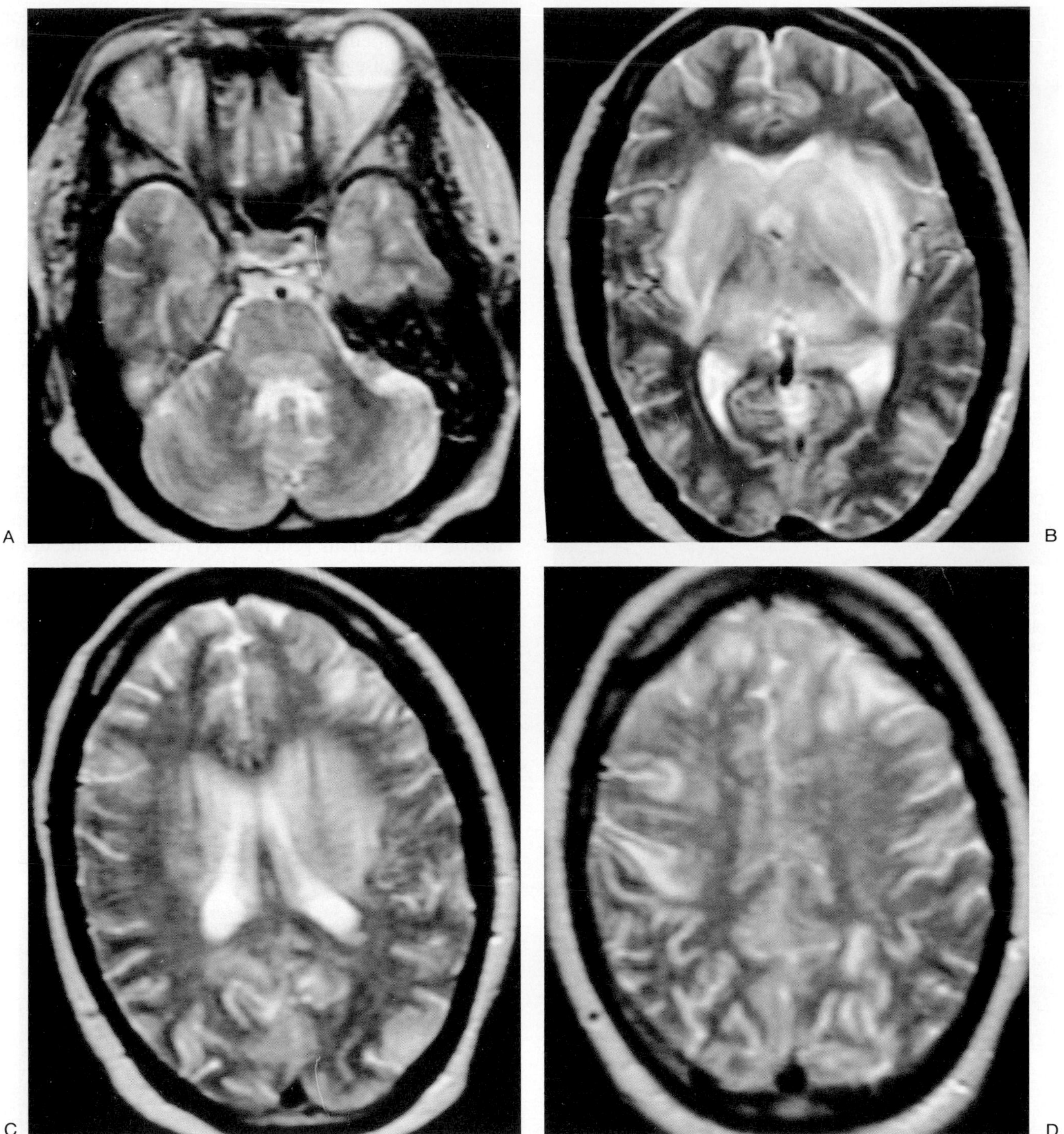

FIG. 51. Extrapontine myelinolysis. Serial T2-weighted MRI from inferior to superior (**A–D**) show extensive patchy abnormality particularly in basal ganglia, thalami, and external capsules. Lesions are also seen in deep and subcortical white matter with minimal abnormality in pons.

and Cockayne's syndrome are the two best known sudanophilic leukodystrophies (65). The clinical presentation of all of the sudanophilic leukodystrophies is that of neurologic dysfunction, presenting early in childhood. In Pelizaeus-Merzbacher disease, symptoms are usually observed within the neonatal period; in Cockayne's syndrome, children may be normal until late in infancy. Typically, abnormal eye movements are observed, and patients have head shaking, ataxia, and slow development. Progressive dysfunction evolves rapidly to spasticity and encephalopathy. Children with Pelizaeus-Merzbacher usually die in childhood, but those with

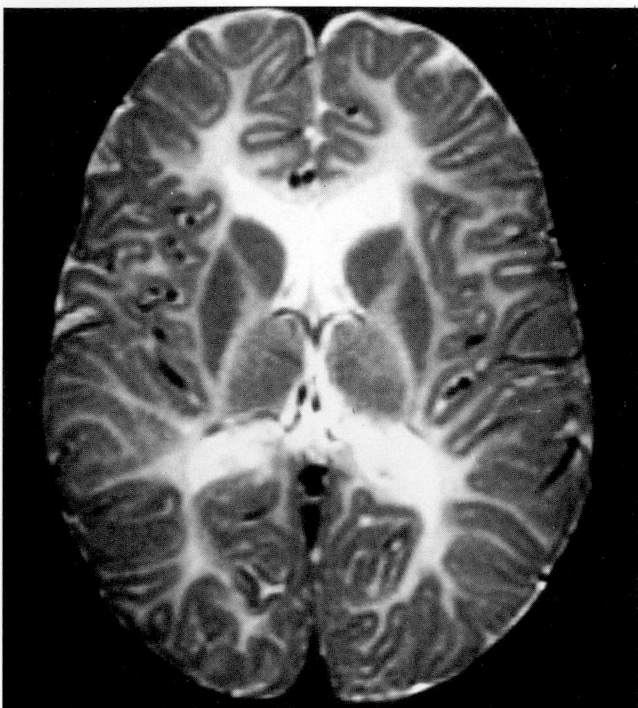

FIG. 52. Pelizaeus-Merzbacher disease. Extensive lesions in the white matter with atrophy and secondary abnormal iron deposition in the basal ganglia are seen on this T2-weighted axial image (2000/80).

Cockayne's syndrome may live long enough to develop dwarfism. Patients with the classic form of Pelizaeus-Merzbacher disease usually develop marked brain atrophy, which is particularly severe in the posterior fossa (cerebellum and brainstem). Histologically, the demyelination appears widespread, but "islands" of myelin preservation are scattered throughout the white matter "tigroid" pattern. An intense reactive proliferation of astrocytes is also present. As in other types of myelin diseases, the axis cylinders tend to be preserved. Cockayne's syndrome is also characterized by patchy preservation of myelin without sparing of U-fibers and also by granular mineralization of the capillaries, capillary neural parenchyma, cerebral cortex, and basal ganglia. Patients with Cockayne's syndrome may also have segmental demyelination in peripheral nerves (79).

On both CT and MRI the late phase of the disease is characterized by widespread white matter lesions and atrophy (Fig. 52). The tigroid appearance seen histologically is only rarely demonstrated on MR imaging (Fig. 53). Increased signal on T2-weighted images in a symmetric distribution, progressively replacing the entire white matter, characterizes the appearance of both of these diseases (Fig. 54) (80). Variable degrees of calcification may be observed in the basal ganglia and cerebellum, usually more extensive in Cockayne's syndrome.

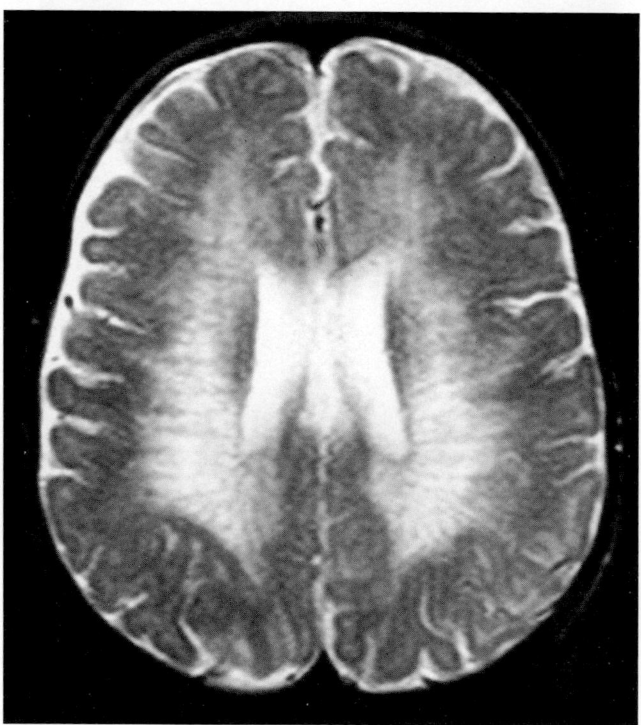

FIG. 53. Pelizaeus-Merzbacher disease with unusual tigroid appearance on T2-weighted image (2000/80).

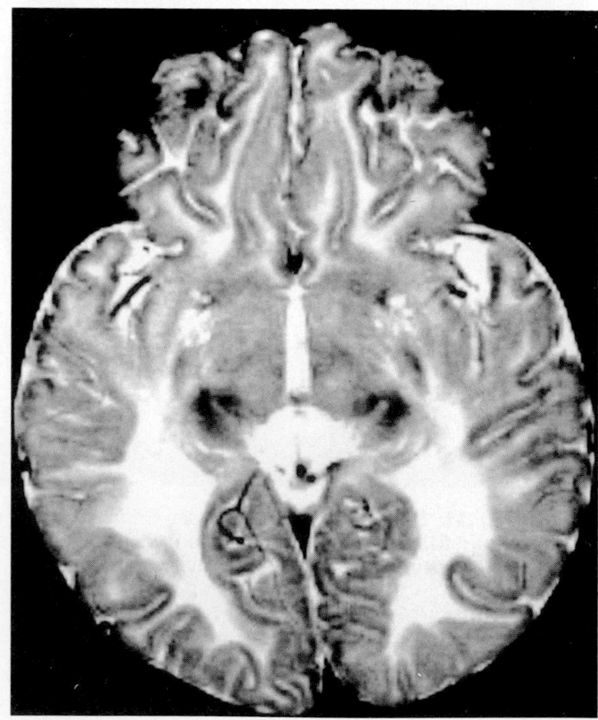

FIG. 54. Cockayne's disease. Bilaterally symmetric lesions are present throughout the white matter on axial T2-weighted image (2000/80).

Canavan's Disease

Canavan's disease is also known as van Bogaert-Canavan disease or spongy degeneration of the cerebral white matter. It is inherited as an autosomal recessive disease found predominantly in children of Ashkenazi Jewish decent. The diagnosis depends on brain biopsy confirmation. Histologically, there is a fine network of cysts, which give the characteristic spongy appearance. The distribution is most prominent in the subcortical white matter, with relative sparing of the internal capsule (65).

At pathologic examination the brain is abnormally enlarged in Canavan's disease. The deeper cortex and subcortical white matter are edematous and soft (81). During the first two years of life the ventricles are usually narrowed. As the child ages the ventricles gradually increase in size as a result of loss of tissue. The histologic appearance is that of cortical and subcortical vacuolation, giving a spongy appearance. During the early stage of Canavan's disease there is relative sparing of the deep areas of white matter, but after two years there is a more diffuse pattern of myelin destruction (81).

The MR appearance of Canavan's disease is that of diffuse increased signal throughout the white matter symmetrically on T2-weighted images, with relative sparing of the internal capsules. The demyelination in Canavan's disease is known to begin in the subcortical arcuate fibers. The putamen tends to retain a dark signal, with the globus pallidus more commonly affected (81) (Figs. 55 and 56). Cerebral atrophy is a later finding in Canavan's disease.

Krabbe's Disease

Children with Krabbe's disease experience a predictable neurologic deterioration that is less variable than the other leukodystrophies. Three distinct phases of the disease are seen clinically. Following an initial healthy and normal first few months of life, the child by six months of age presents with spasticity and irritability. Fever, without signs of infection, may occur. The child fails to progress in development, and neurologic regression begins. The second phase is characterized by rapid deterioration in motor function, with chronic opisthotonos and myoclonic jerking, accompanied by hyperpyrexia, hypersalivation, and hypersecretion from the lungs. In the third phase the child appears to be decerebrate, with no discernable mental activity. The intense muscular tone of the second phase is replaced by flaccid paralysis. The child dies quickly, by infection, aspiration, or neurologic deterioration (82).

In Krabbe's disease the histologic finding is that of large macrophages containing myelin breakdown products, called globoid cells (65). The CT appearance is one of increased density within the thalami, caudate, and corona radiata. The MR findings are of increased signal in-

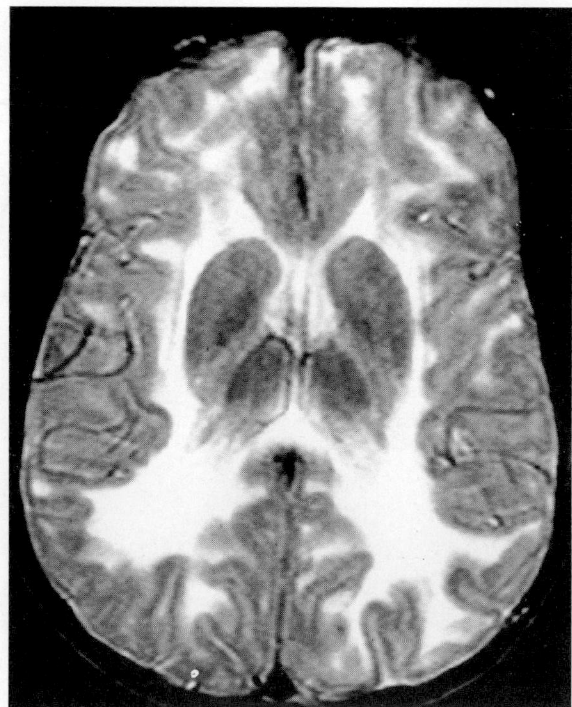

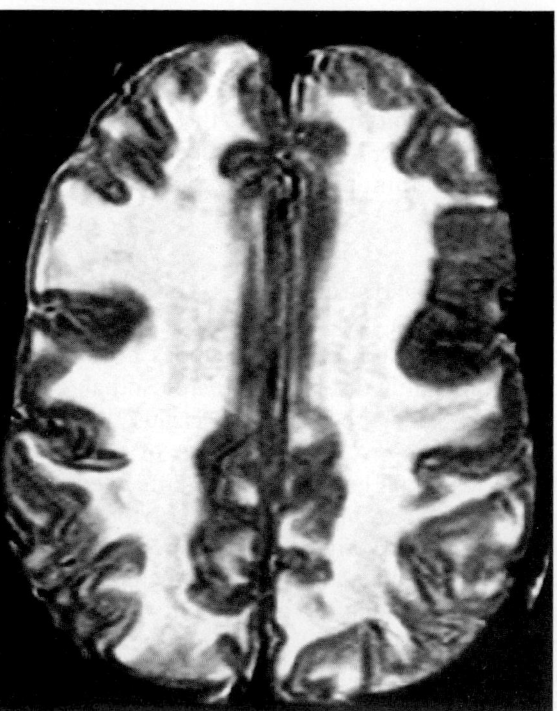

FIG. 55. Canavan's disease. T2-weighted images (**A,B**) in child with macrocephaly shows diffuse high-signal abnormality in supratentorial white matter, with relative sparing of internal capsules bilaterally.

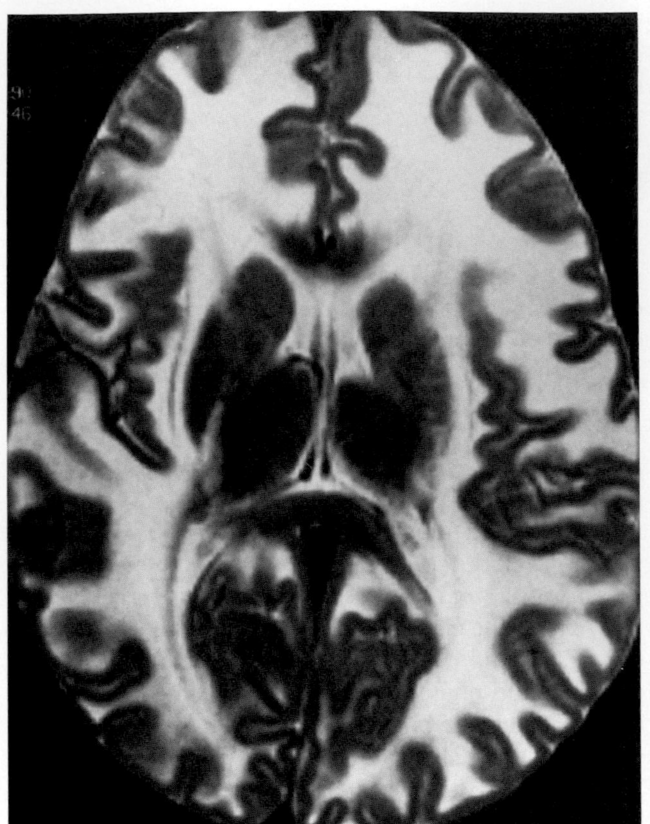

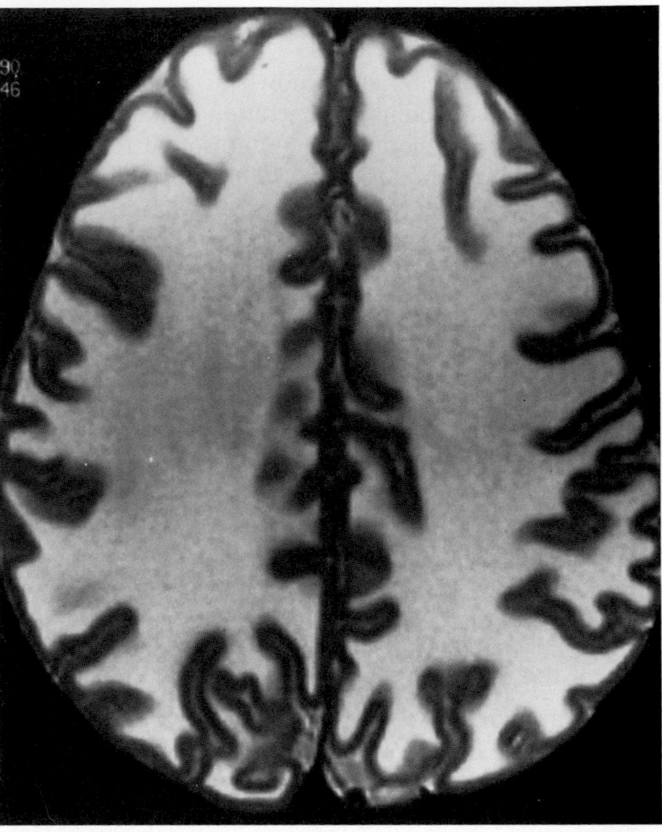

FIG. 56. Canavan's disease. T2-weighted images (**A,B**) in child with macrocephaly denote near-complete high-signal abnormality in supratentorial white matter, which is enlarged in relative volume. Note relative sparing of internal capsules bilaterally.

tensity in the periventricular white matter, with an initial predilection for the optic radiations and splenium of the corpus callosum (82) (Fig. 57). Lesions are generally symmetric and commonly involve the basal ganglia and centrum semiovale. With progressive loss of white matter, atrophy is common late in the course.

Metachromatic Leukodystrophy

Metachromatic leukodystrophy includes a group of progressive white matter disorders with autosomal recessive inheritance (82). These disorders are caused by a deficiency of arylsulfatase A. The diagnosis of metachromatic leukodystrophy is based on the finding of enzyme activity of arylsulfatase A in the urine and peripheral leukocytes (82). If enzyme activity in the urine and peripheral leukocytes is normal additional tests including measurement of urinary sulfatide, assessment of fibroblast sulfatide catabolism, and sural nerve biopsy are usually diagnostic (82). The prenatal diagnosis can be made by culturing amniotic fluid cells from which enzyme activity can be determined. A heterozygote carrier for the disease can be detected by measuring enzyme activity in leukocytes, aiding genetic counseling (82).

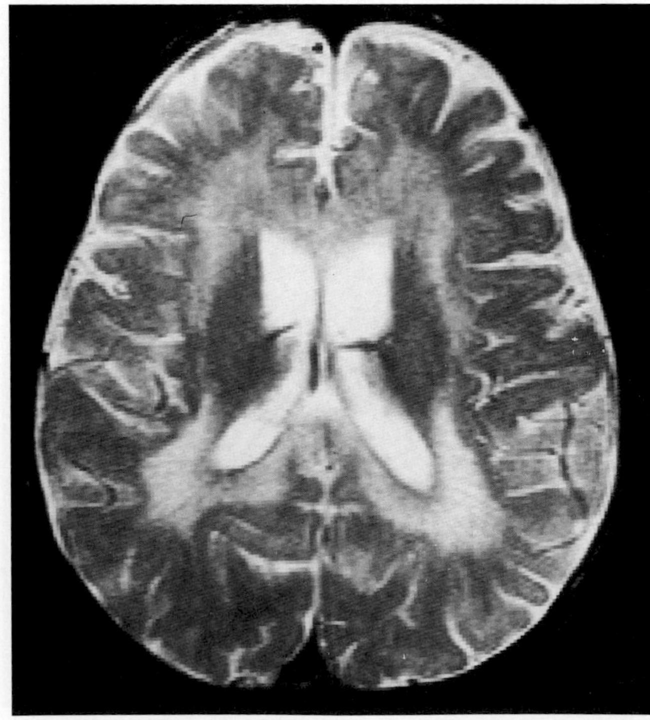

FIG. 57. Krabbe's disease. Symmetric lesions in the periventricular white matter on the T2-weighted sequence (2000/80). Note preference for posterior white matter.

There are four principal forms of the disease, congenital, late infantile (presenting at age 2–3 years), juvenile (presenting at 4–6 years), and the adult variant (65). In one family only one variant of metachromatic leukodystrophy occurs. The congenital form is rare, presents with seizures at birth, and is followed by death within a few days or weeks. The late infantile form is the most common. The child presents with difficulty in walking, marked by frequent falls within the second and third year of life (65,82). The disease progresses quickly with poor speech, mental deterioration, and hypertonia, which evolve to decerebrate and decorticate posture within 3–6 months. Seizures are common. In the less common juvenile form, symptoms usually do not develop until 4 years. The clinical picture is similar to the late infantile form, except that the child is old enough to manifest behavioral disturbances as well.

Pathologic examination of the brain initially reveals involvement of the white matter in a patchy distribution, but with time the entire white matter is affected, often in a symmetric fashion, resulting in a butterfly configuration (82). There is relative preservation of the arcuate U-fibers noted histologically (Fig 58). In cases of severe or longstanding metachromatic leukodystrophy, the white matter is reduced to a narrow strip 1 to 2 cm in diameter with compensatory enlargement of the ventricles. Demyelination is present predominantly in the cerebral hemispheres, and to a lesser extent in the cerebellum, brainstem, and spinal cord. Microscopic examination reveals

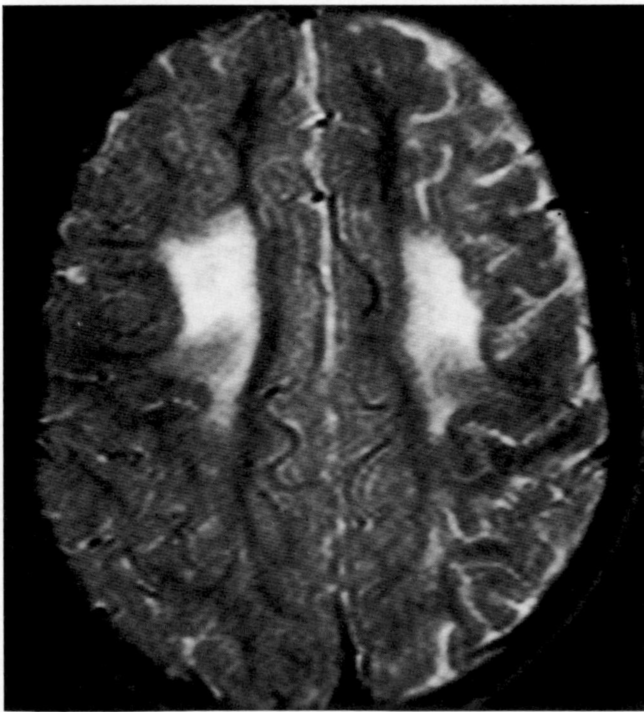

FIG. 58. Metachromatic leukodystrophy. Note the severe demyelination and the partial preservation of the subcortical fibers (U-fibers).

loss of myelin followed by axonal degeneration (82). Numerous macrophages containing metachromatic sulfatides are scattered throughout the white matter (83). Fibrous gliosis is found within the lesions. Oligodendroglia are missing from areas of demyelination and are reduced in number even in areas where the myelin is still intact (82). There are no inflammatory cells within areas of demyelination.

MRI of metachromatic leukodystrophy reveals extensive white matter lesions usually beginning in the frontal region, and showing posterior progression (Fig. 59), unlike findings in most of the other leukodystrophies. The pattern is usually completely symmetric, confluent, and sparing the subcortical U-fibers and myelin of the basal ganglia (84). The white matter tracks that myelinate during the latter part of infancy show greatest involvement, accounting for the frontal predominance. Cerebellar lesions are found frequently in metachromatic leukodystrophy, and may help differentiate this disease from the other leukodystrophies. Enhancement has not been reported. Atrophy is present late in the disease.

Adrenoleukodystrophy

Adrenoleukodystrophy is an X-linked recessive disorder involving the white matter of the brain and spinal cord as well as the adrenal cortex. Even in patients without prior diagnosis of adrenoleukodystrophy, there is often a history of men on the mother's side of the family having died of Addison's disease or of an unknown neurologic illness, perhaps diagnosed as Schilder's disease (82). Typically a boy presents with neurologic symptoms in late childhood, between the ages of 5 and 9. A boy, in previous good health, may develop behavior problems, decreasing mental function, and visual and hearing disorders (65). The disease progresses to motor signs and ataxia. Symptoms of Addison's disease commonly appear before the neurologic symptoms, but may follow mental deterioration, and occasionally may never present. The disease is progressive, but the rate of deterioration is variable. In the final stages, the patient suffers with severe seizures, spastic quadriplegia, and decorticate posturing (82). Patients are blind, deaf, and mute. Within a few years of onset most boys have died.

Pathologic examination of the brain in adrenoleukodystrophy reveals atrophy with cystic cavitation of the central white matter. The cerebral cortex and gray matter are of normal thickness. There is enlargement of the ventricles. Histologic examination reveals confluent demyelination in a symmetric fashion, usually bilaterally in the occipital regions, with extension across the splenium of the corpus callosum. The demyelination progresses forward and outward from the occipital lesion until most or all of white matter is involved. There is usually relative sparing of the subcortical U-fibers. Cerebellar involvement is common.

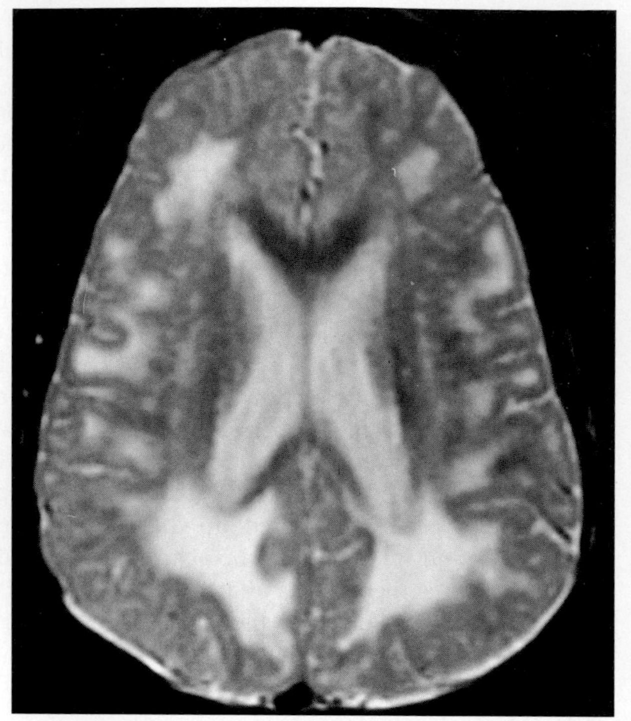

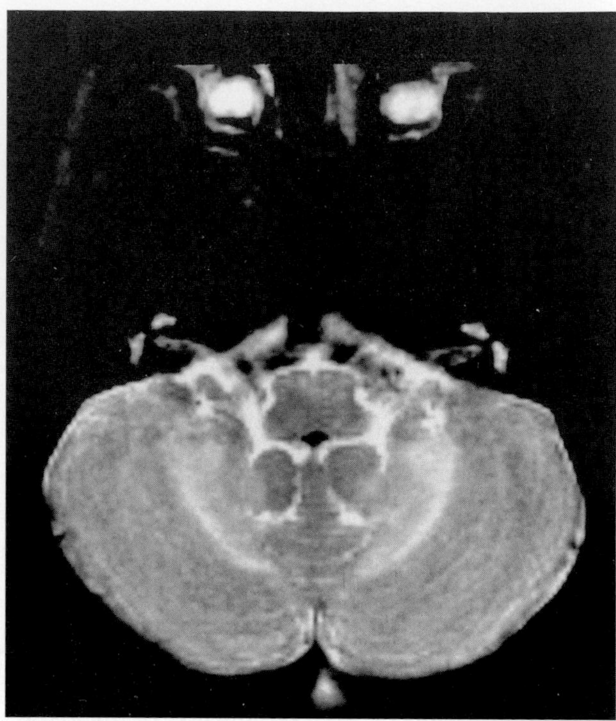

FIG. 59. Metachromatic leukodystrophy. **A:** Extensive disease throughout white matter on T2-weighted image (2000/80). **B:** Cerebellar involvement is common, as seen on axial T2-weighted sequence (2000/80).

The histologic findings reflect the zones of activity seen on imaging studies. The central portion of the lesion reveals absent myelin sheaths and oligodendroglia. Glial stranding and scattered astrocytes with no evidence of active disease are present. The next zone of involvement shows evidence of active inflammation with many macrophages filled with lipid. Intact axons are identified both with and without myelin sheaths. In the outer zone, there is active myelin destruction, but more axonal sparing.

The enzymatic defect, related to oxidation of long-chain fatty acids, results in characteristic cytoplasmic inclusions in the skin, adrenal gland, and conjunctiva, sites where biopsies are often specific (85).

The CT and MR appearance of adrenoleukodystrophy is somewhat specific, with symmetric areas of white matter abnormality surrounding the atria of the lateral ventricles, spanning the splenium of the corpus callosum (78). Although the periatrial location is far more common, frontal predominance and holohemispheric patterns have been described (86). At the lateral margin of the zones of demyelination, contrast enhancement appears, corresponding to areas of active demyelination accompanied by inflammation (Schaumberg's zones 1 and 2) (Figs. 60–62). As in all white matter diseases, MRI has been found to be more sensitive than CT in the detection of the acute demyelinating lesions of adrenoleukodystrophy (84), with the exception of the detection of calcification, an uncommonly reported finding in the parieto-occipital region (86). Proton spectroscopy shows promise in the evaluation of adrenoleukodystrophy (87). The spectra appear characteristic enough to suggest use of MR spectroscopy as a noninvasive diagnostic technique with potential for prognostic assessment of adrenoleukodystrophy (87).

Adrenomyeloneuropathy probably represents a phenotypic adult variant of adrenoleukodystrophy (82). Adrenomyeloneuropathy may occur in either sex, but males with the disease have symptoms of adrenal insufficiency. Adrenomyeloneuropathy is similar in clinical presentation and MR appearance to adrenoleukodystrophy, but the disease progresses more slowly.

Alexander's Disease

Alexander's disease, a rare disorder, is unusual for leukodystrophies in that it occurs sporadically without a familial incidence. There are three forms of the disease, infantile, juvenile, and adult. The infantile form is the most common. The diagnosis is usually made within the first year of life when the infant presents with developmental delay, macrocephaly, spasticity, and seizures (78,88). Progressive deterioration of intellectual functioning and spasticity are followed by death in early childhood. The duration of the illness is usually about 3 years.

Pathologic examination reveals an enlarged brain. The histologic examination is distinctive in the extensive demyelination with a large number of Rosenthal fibers

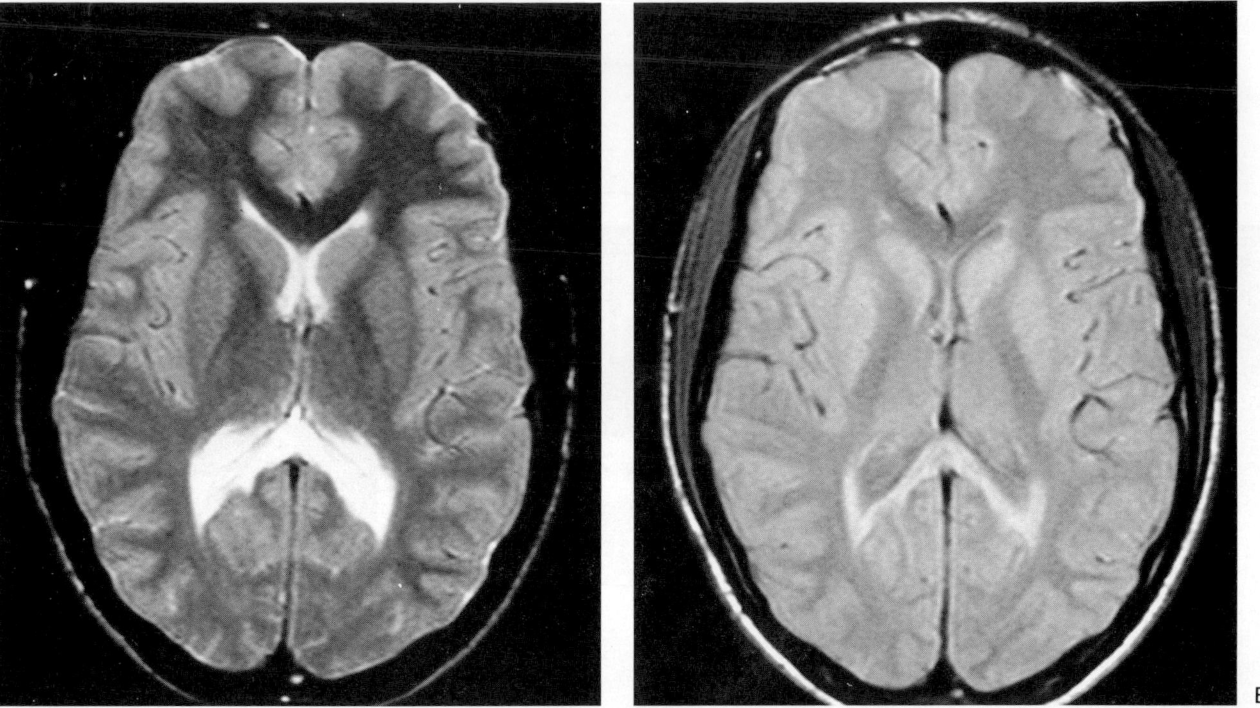

FIG. 60. Adrenoleukodystrophy. Early involvement with disease is seen only in the splenium of the corpus callosum on T2-weighted image (2000/80) **(A)** and proton-density-weighted image (2000/20) **(B)**.

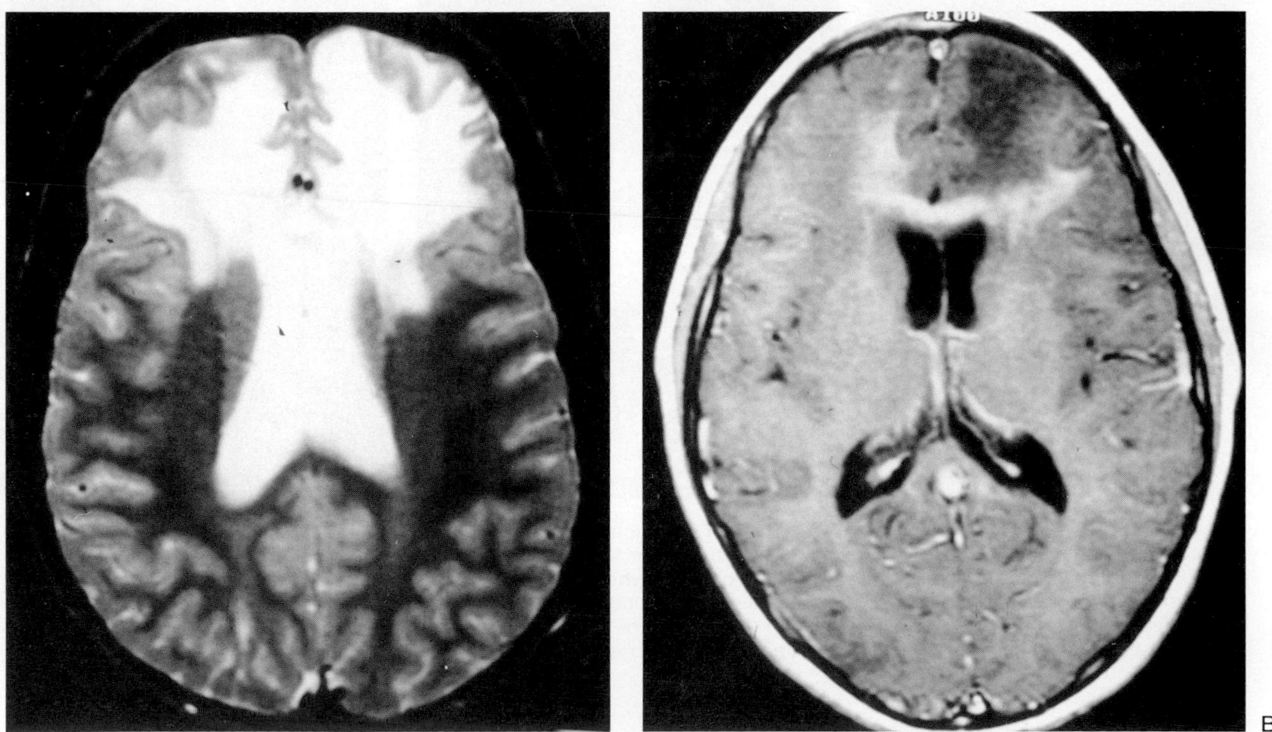

FIG. 61. Advanced adrenoleukodystrophy with unusual feature of frontal involvement. **A:** Bright signal is present spanning the genu of the corpus callosum on axial T2-weighted image (2000/80). **B:** Gadolinium-contrast enhancement is present at the leading edge of the demyelination.

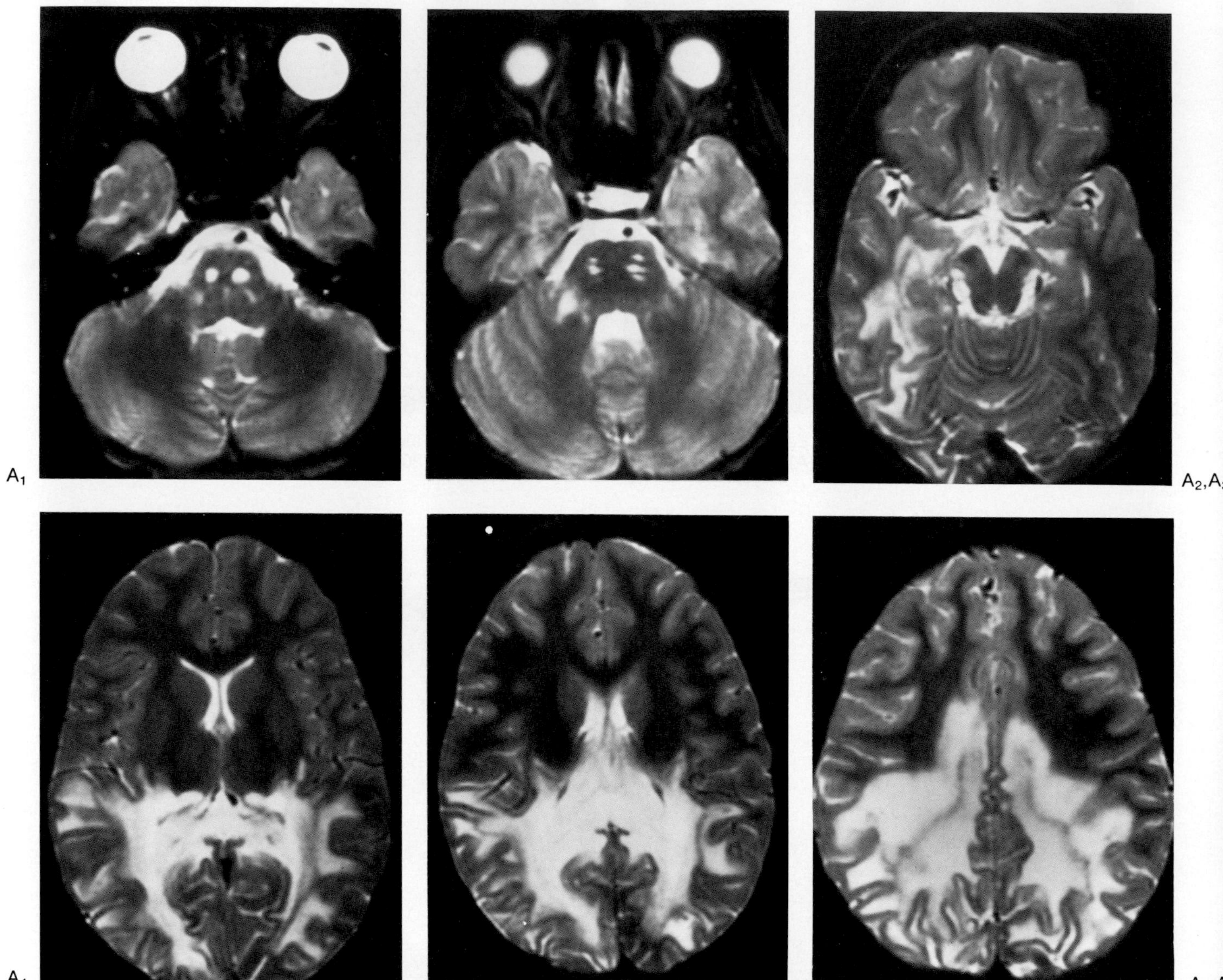

FIG. 62. Adrenoleukodystrophy. **A_1–A_6**: Serial T2-weighted images (3000/90), inferior to superior. **B_1–B_6**: Serial contrast-enhanced T1-weighted images (600/20), inferior to superior. Note extensive high intensity abnormality on T2-weighted images (A) in bilateral parietal and occipital white matter through corpus callosum, extending into lateral geniculate bodies and pulvinar of the thalami down corticopontine tracts inferiorly into pyramids of medulla. Post-contrast images (B) show enhancement of leading edges of these areas, including occipital optic radiations into geniculate bodies, and descending corticopontine tracts bilaterally.

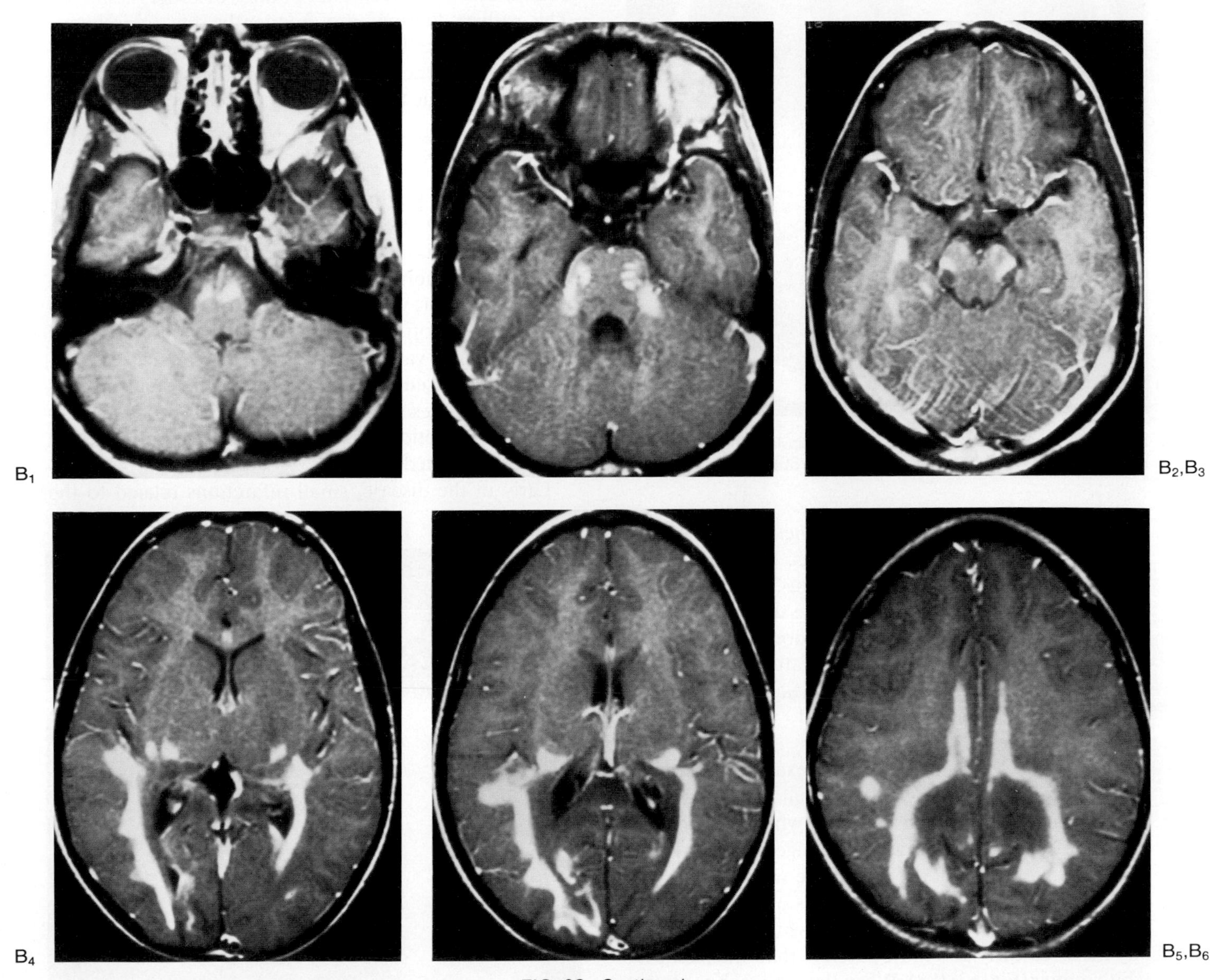

FIG. 62. *Continued.*

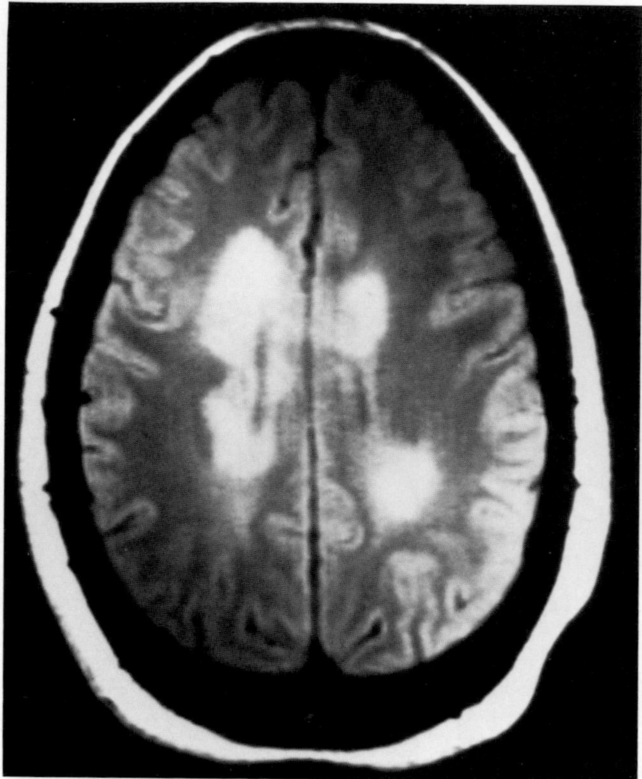

FIG. 63. Alexander's disease. Periventricular bright signal is present on T2-weighted axial image (2000/80).

(degenerated astrocytic processes). The Rosenthal fibers are found in the perivascular spaces, subpial regions, subependymal white matter, thalamus, and basal ganglia. The basal ganglia and cortex are usually relatively well preserved. There is a frontal predominance. Extensive demyelination is typical. Cavitation is common, and there is *no* sparing of the subcortical U-fibers. The cerebellum is less often affected than in other leukodystrophies.

The CT and MR appearance of Alexander's disease is that of an evolving course with normal appearing brain progressing to generalized gray and white matter atrophy. The MR picture is that of prolonged T1 and T2 relaxation involving any portion of the white matter, including the internal capsule (which is usually spared in Canavan's disease) (88). The frontal white matter is usually involved early and more severely than the periatrial white matter (Fig. 63) (88). When the entire white matter is involved in a patient with macrocephaly, the differential diagnosis is mainly between Canavan's and Alexander's diseases.

DISORDERS OF LIPID METABOLISM

This group of disorders includes a number of inherited diseases characterized by an abnormal sphingolipid metabolism, which in most instances leads to the intracellular deposition of lipid within the brain (78). These disorders have a relentless, progressive course that cannot be altered and vary only in the rate of intellectual and visual deterioration. These include Tay-Sachs disease, Gaucher's disease, Niemann-Pick disease, Fabry's disease, and ceroid lipofuscinosis. These disorders are uncommon, and MR experience is limited. In many cases, there are no abnormalities on MRI until late in the course. The MR appearance of these disorders is similar. The earliest findings are frequently due to ischemic changes in the basal ganglia. Bright signal on T2-weighted sequences is seen within areas of infarction, and hemorrhagic lesions may be present (82).

Fabry's Disease

This is a rare sex-linked systemic disorder with symptoms appearing late in childhood, but occasionally not recognized until the second or third decade of life. The first manifestation is usually a punctate angiectatic skin rash; later, fever, weight loss, and pain in the joints and abdomen develop (78). The neurologic manifestations of periventricular vascular disease are a relatively late development. Vascular disease involving the small arteries and arterioles results in premature periventricular ischemia and infarction (Fig. 64). Cerebral hemorrhage has also been reported.

Early in the disease, small infarctions related to the

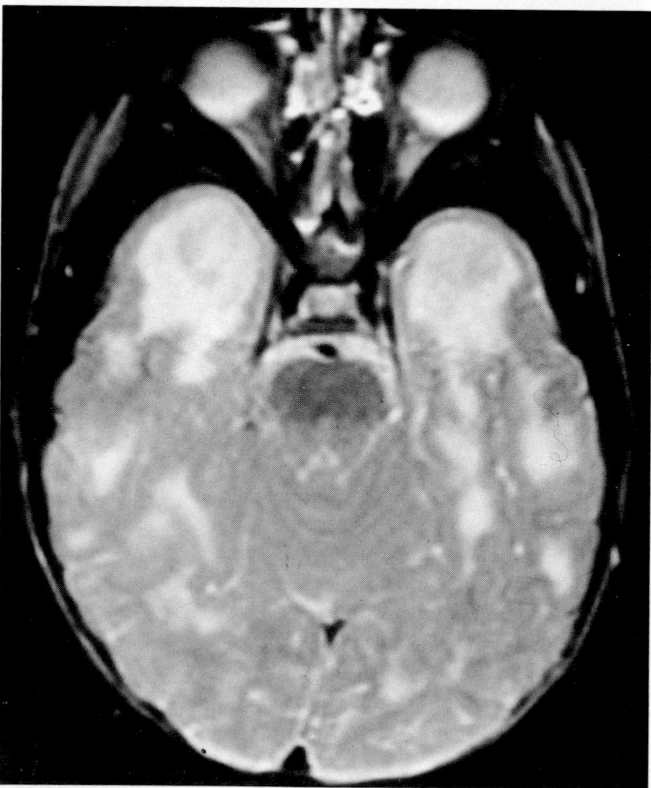

FIG. 64. Fabry's disease. Extensive white matter disease late in course on T2-weighted image (2000/80).

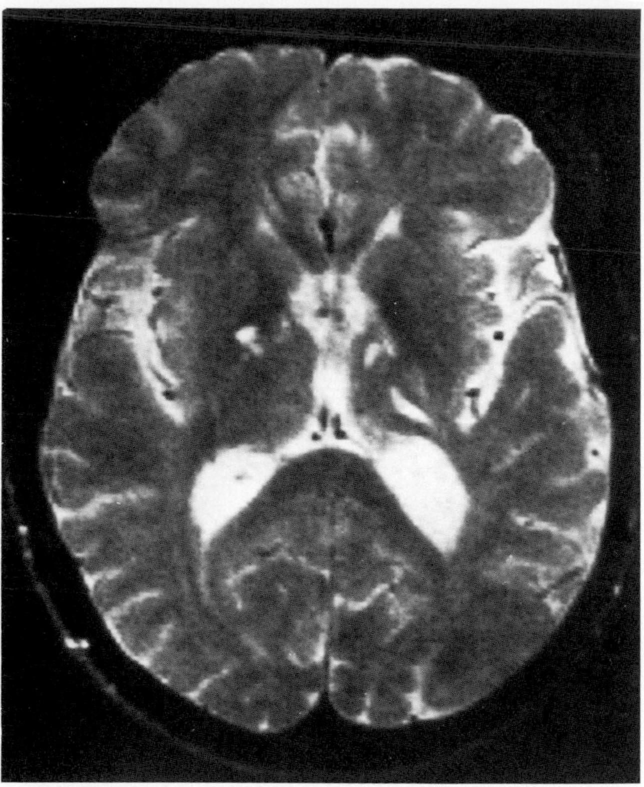

FIG. 65. Fabry's disease. Punctate perivascular lesions are present in the basal ganglia and thalamus on T2-weighted sequence.

vascular disease appear as small, focal bright lesions on long TR/TE sequences. The basal ganglia are the most common location for small lacunar infarcts in Fabry's disease (Fig. 65) (90).

Gaucher's Disease

Gaucher's disease includes several autosomal recessive lipid storage diseases in which there is a deficiency of glucocerebroside (78). Several forms are recognized, with varying severity of the enzyme deficiency. The diagnosis is made by the clinical picture, by the presence of Gaucher's cells in the bone marrow, and by finding reduced glucocerebroside beta-glucosidase in the cultured skin, fibroblasts, or blood leukocytes (78). The clinical presentation is that of splenomegaly, hepatomegaly, thrombocytopenia, lesions of the long bones, and variable neurologic signs. The adult form of Gaucher's disease, which may be found even in children, does not have neurologic manifestations. Neurologic symptoms include seizures, developmental regression, spasticity, mental deficiency, incoordination, and tics.

MR and CT findings are similar to those of Fabry's disease, with atrophy, infarction, and occasional hemorrhage (Fig. 66) (80).

MUCOPOLYSACCHARIDOSES

Mucopolysaccharidoses include a group of inherited metabolic diseases in which there is an enzyme deficiency resulting in the inability of lysosomes to degrade mucopolysaccharides (65). Hunter's disease is inherited by sex-linked transmission; all of the other mucopolysaccharidoses are inherited by autosomal recessive transmission. The clinical picture is that of variable skeletal, visceral, and central nervous system involvement. Morquio's disease, and far less common Scheie's and Difer-

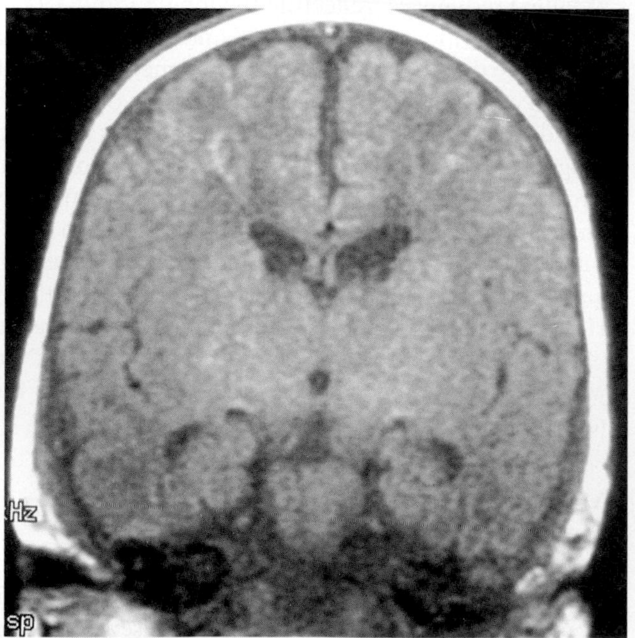

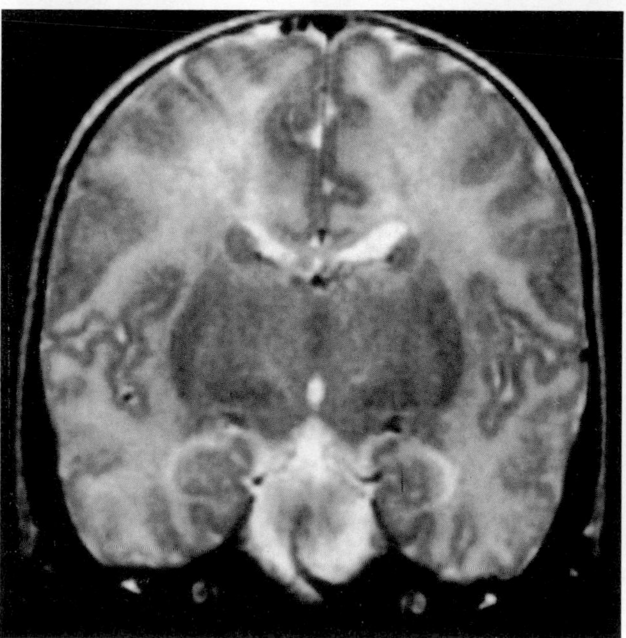

FIG. 66. Gaucher's disease. **A:** T1-weighted sequence (800/20) demonstrates subacute blood in the centrum semiovale. **B:** T2-weighted sequence (2000/80) shows widespread white matter lesions.

TABLE 3. *Classification of the mucopolysaccharidoses*

		Sites of involvement		
Type	Eponym	Bone	Viscera	CNS
IH	Hurler	+	+	+
IS	Scheie	+	+	−
I H/S	Hurler-Scheie	+	+	+
II	Hunter	+	+	+
III A–D	Sanfilippo	−	−	+
IV A, B	Morquio	+	−	−
VI	Maroteaux-Lamy	+	−	+
VII	Sly	+	+	+
VIII	Diferrante	+	−	−

rante's diseases, are the only mucopolysaccharidoses in which the patients are not mentally retarded or severely delayed in development (65). A gargoyle-like face and dwarfism are characteristic manifestations of the mucopolysaccharidoses (91). Spinal cord compression is common, especially at the upper cervical level and foramen magnum. The cord compression results from skeletal narrowing and dural thickening from mucopolysaccharide deposits. Spinal cord compression may also be due to atlantoaxial subluxation or thoracic gibbus. The classification of the mucopolysaccharidoses is presented in Table 3 (65).

MR findings are quite variable. In some patients there may be no intracranial abnormalities on either MRI or CT (91). In cases with mild involvement, thickening of the skull and slight ventricular enlargement may be the only findings. When the disease is advanced, findings include hydrocephalus, dural thickening, and periventricular white matter lesions (Fig. 67) (94). The periventricular lesions may be seen as multiple small areas of bright signal on T2-weighted sequences, and dark areas on T1-weighted sequences, reflecting the long T1 and T2 characteristics of the lesions (Figs. 68 and 69). The punctate lesions are due to perivascular involvement with the disease, in which there is a large accumulation of vacuolated cells distended with mucopolysaccharide. As the disease progresses, the lesions become more widespread and larger, reflecting the development of infarcts in demyelination (91). Bone marrow transplant has been used as a method of therapy in the mucopolysaccharidoses. MRI has been used to follow the progression of patients with Hurler's syndrome treated with bone marrow transplant (92). Improvement in myelination and improved gray white differentiation has been reported following bone marrow transplant (92).

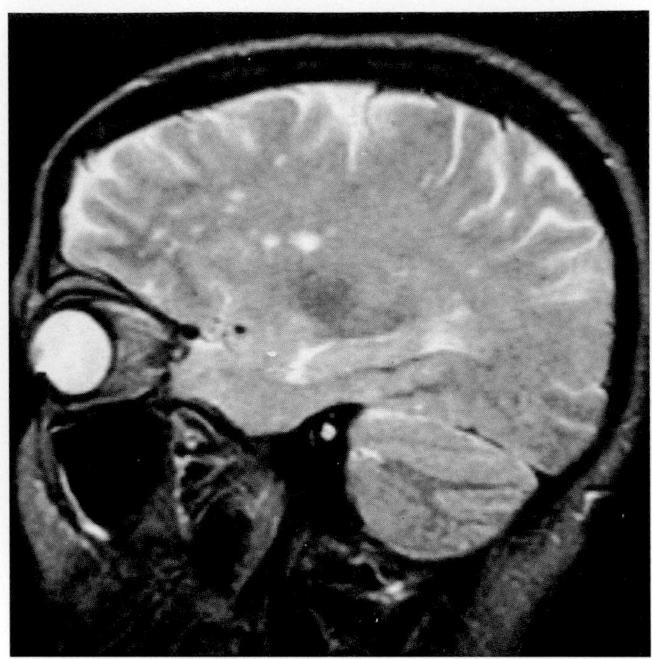

FIG. 68. Mucopolysaccharidosis II, Hunter's disease. Abnormal bright signal in the periventricular region on T2-weighted image (2000/80) reflects the perivascular involvement.

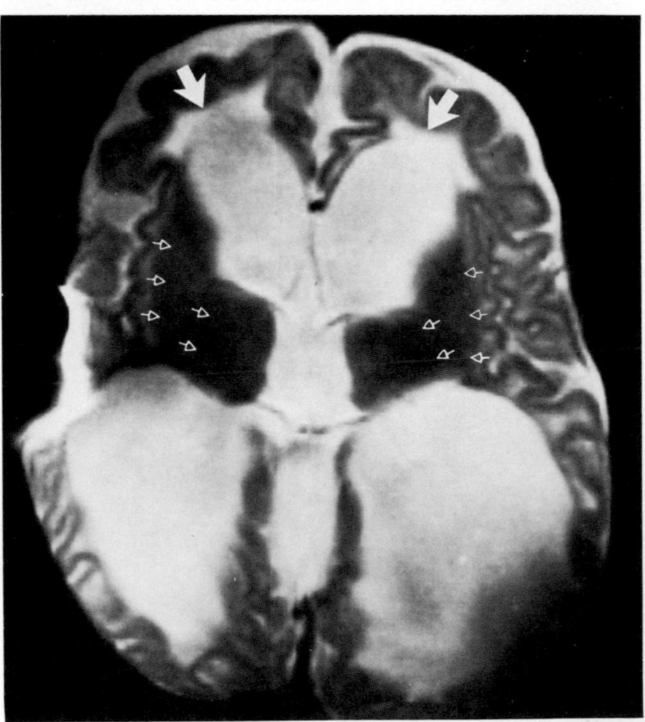

FIG. 67. Hurler's disease. Hydrocephalus, white matter thinning, and periventricular lesions of abnormal bright signal (*large arrows*) on T2-weighted axial image (2000/80) are characteristic of advanced mucopolysaccharidoses. Also note abnormally prominent iron deposition in the thalamic and basal ganglia (*open arrows*), which is a nonspecific reflection of cerebral pathology.

MISCELLANEOUS LESIONS OF WHITE MATTER

White matter lesions may be the primary MR finding in many disease processes considered elsewhere in this text. Tumor, trauma, and even normal aging (Fig. 70) may present with MR findings isolated to the white

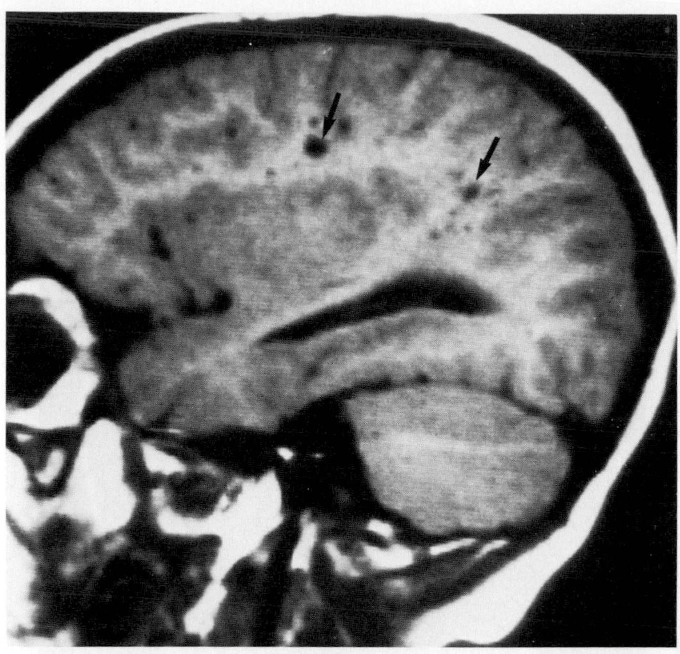

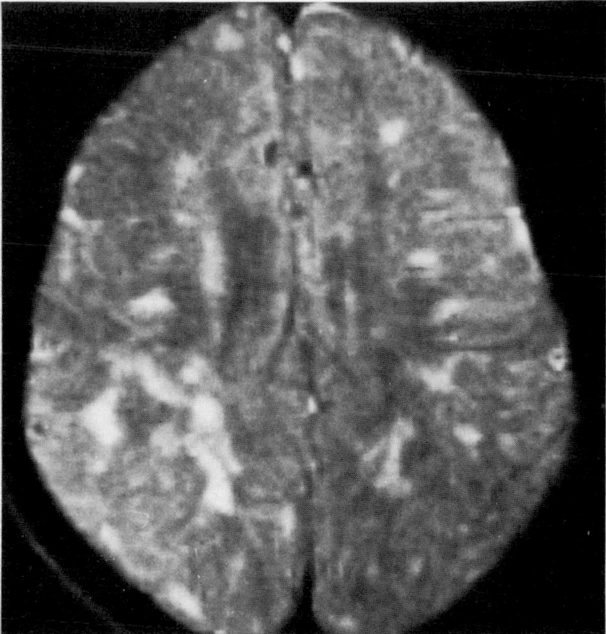

FIG. 69. Mucopolysaccharidosis VI. **A:** Unusual punctate cavitary lesions are seen within the white matter on axial T1-weighted sequence (800/26) (*arrows*). **B:** Axial T2-weighted sequence shows punctate periventricular bright signal reflecting predilection of disease for perivascular involvement.

matter. Inherited diseases or syndromes such as neurofibromatosis (Fig. 71) may have hamartomas involving white matter that appear as small areas of bright signal on T2-weighted images. Small collections of normal gray matter, the result of a disturbance in migration, appear as islands of abnormal tissue intermixed with white matter (Fig. 72). Although innumerable entities have white matter manifestations, the following are diseases that most commonly may be confused with MS and the other primary white matter diseases.

FIG. 70. Senescent white matter change. A single focus of bright signal is present in the posterior periatrial region in this asymptomatic 66-year-old man.

Ischemia and Arteritis

The most common lesion that may mimic the demyelinating or dysmyelinating disorders of small vessel ischemic disease is in the periventricular location. Periventricular ischemic disease is characteristic of elderly, hypertensive, and diabetic hypertensive patients (93,94). The lesions are bright on T2-weighted sequences that are usually patchy and multifocal (Fig. 73) (93). The deep white matter of the centrum semiovale and optic radiations are the most commonly affected areas. Basal ganglia lesions, when present, may help differentiate ischemia from MS. Especially in the elderly, small white matter lesions are common, and may not correlate with any neurologic deficits. When the lesions are extensive, there does appear to be some correlation between white matter ischemic disease and dementia; clinical correlation is always necessary, however, to make the diagnosis of subcortical arterial sclerotic encephalopathy (SAE). In younger patients, ischemia may be the result of embolic disease, hypoxia, dissection, arteritis, and migraine. Hypoxia in the infant and child commonly causes periventricular lesions that may mimic the leukodystrophies

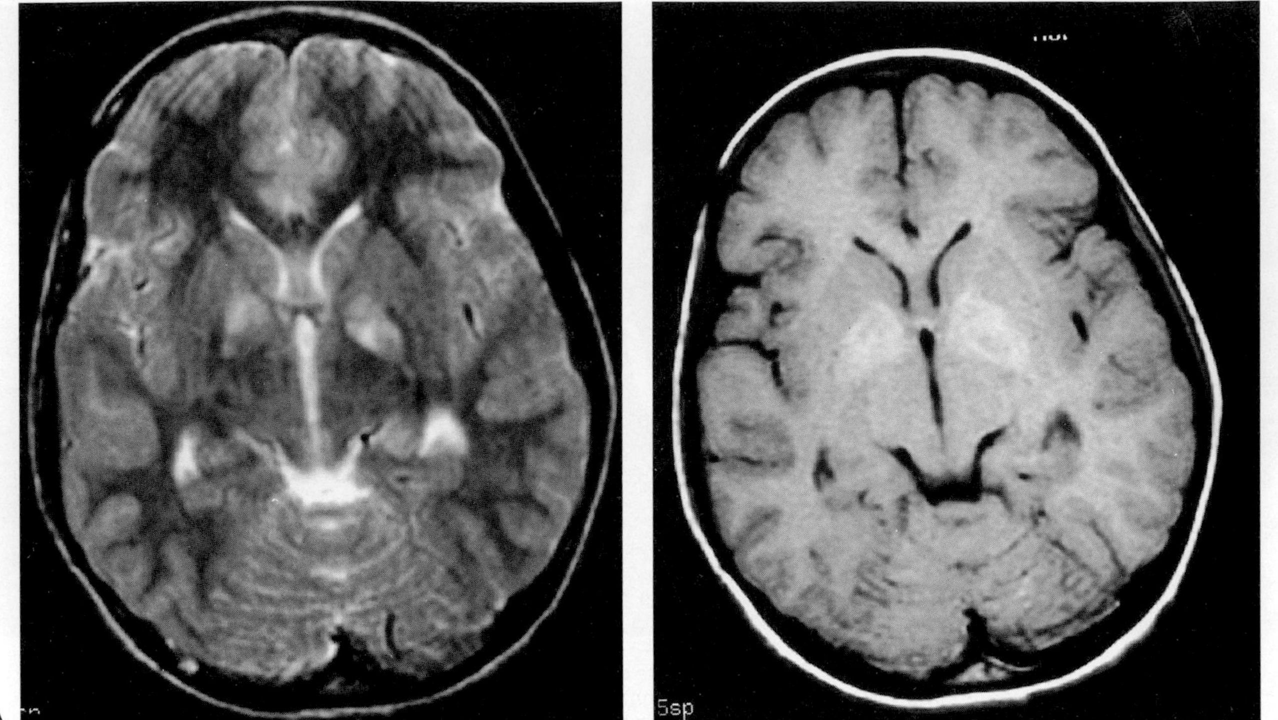

FIG. 71. Neurofibromatosis. **A:** Small hyperintense lesions involving basal ganglia and internal capsules on T2-weighted image (2000/80) could mimic demyelination. **B:** Lesions may also appear bright on T1-weighted image (600/20), but this finding is more common in children.

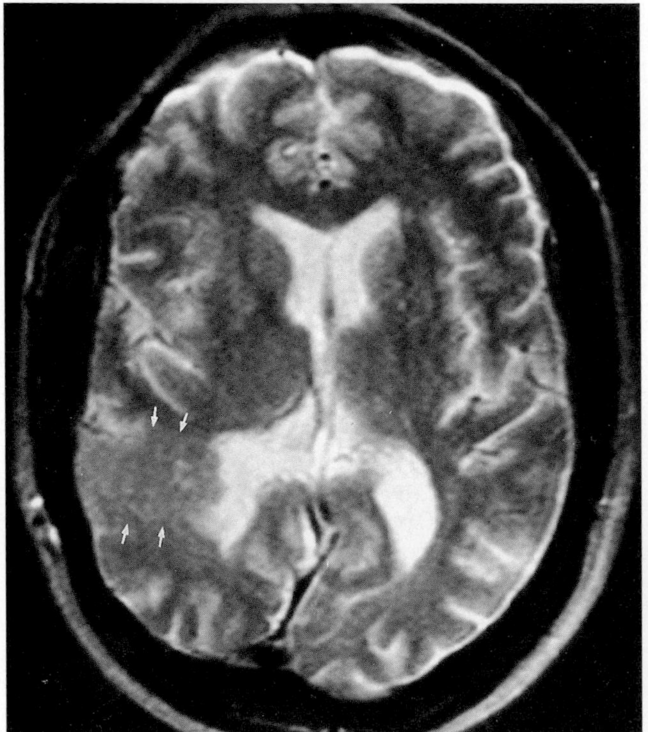

FIG. 72. Heterotopias. Islands of tissue isointense to normal gray matter situated within the white matter (*arrows*) create characteristic appearance of disorders of migration on axial T2-weighted image (2000/80).

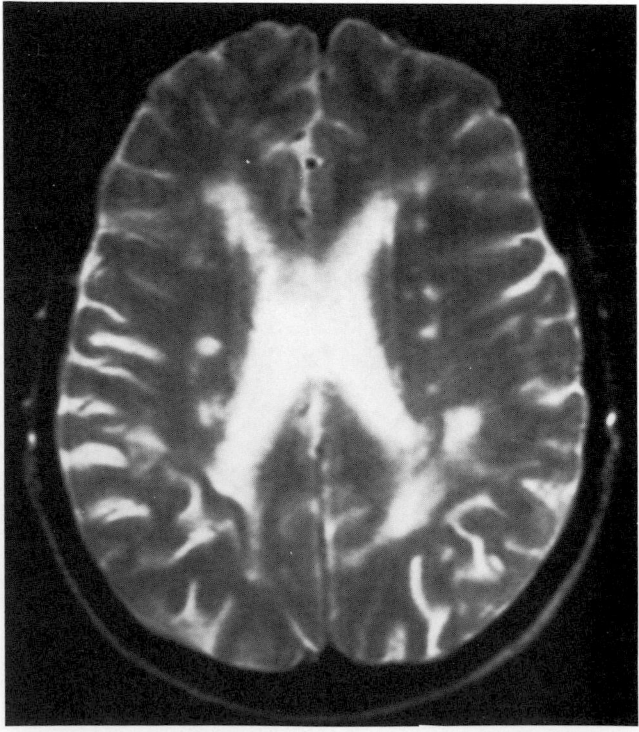

FIG. 73. Ischemia, adult. Widespread periventricular ischemia with patchy bright signal in white matter appears quite similar to MS and other white matter lesions on T2-weighted sequence.

(Figs. 74 and 75). Complicated migraine may appear on MRI as irregular areas of potentially reversible ischemia predominantly within the white matter. Patchy white matter lesions can be seen throughout the white matter in addition to the classic globus pallidus lesions following acute carbon monoxide intoxication (96).

The differentiation between systemic lupus erythematosus (SLE) and MS may be particularly difficult both clinically and on MRI (Fig. 76). Overt cortical infarctions are certainly more typical of SLE than MS, but most cases are not, in fact, easily distinguished. Areas of arteritis appear similar to other ischemic lesions, except that foci of arteritis tend to be more patchy, bilateral, and widespread than with other ischemic processes (Fig. 77). Arteritis is sometimes reversible and responsive to steroid therapy. As with other causes of hypoxic injury, hemorrhage is a common sequelae to arteritis, and this is distinctly uncommon in MS.

Sarcoidosis

Sarcoidosis is a systemic granulomatous disease with neurologic involvement in up to 10% of patients (97–99). Most patients are affected between the ages of 20–40. There is a slight predilection for females and blacks. It may present with multifocal white matter lesions iden-

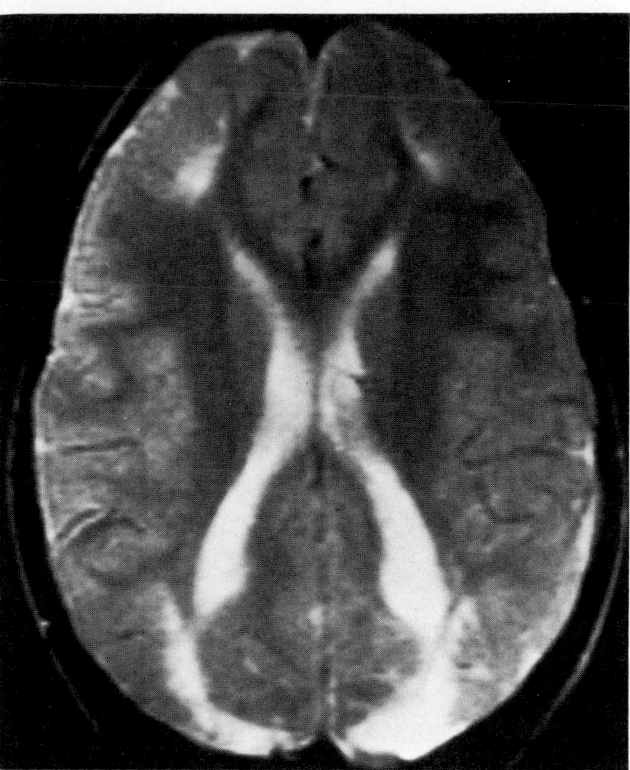

FIG. 75. Ischemia, child. Severe hypoxic damage at age 2 years created symmetric white matter lesions on T2-weighted sequence.

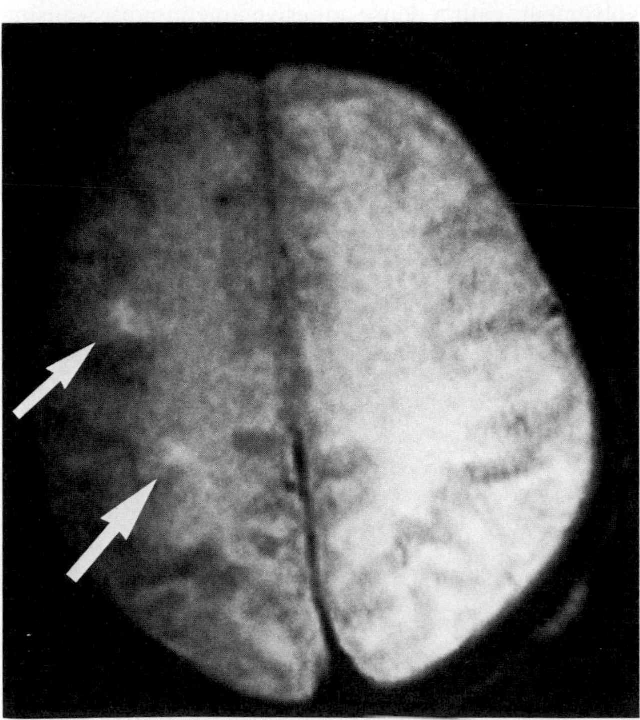

FIG. 74. Ischemia, infant. Two giant, focal bright lesions at the gray-white matter junction (*arrows*) are the only MR findings in a 1-month-old child with severe hypoxic injury on T2-weighted sequence (3000/120). Undermyelinated white matter with increased water content makes detection and differentiation of white matter lesions difficult.

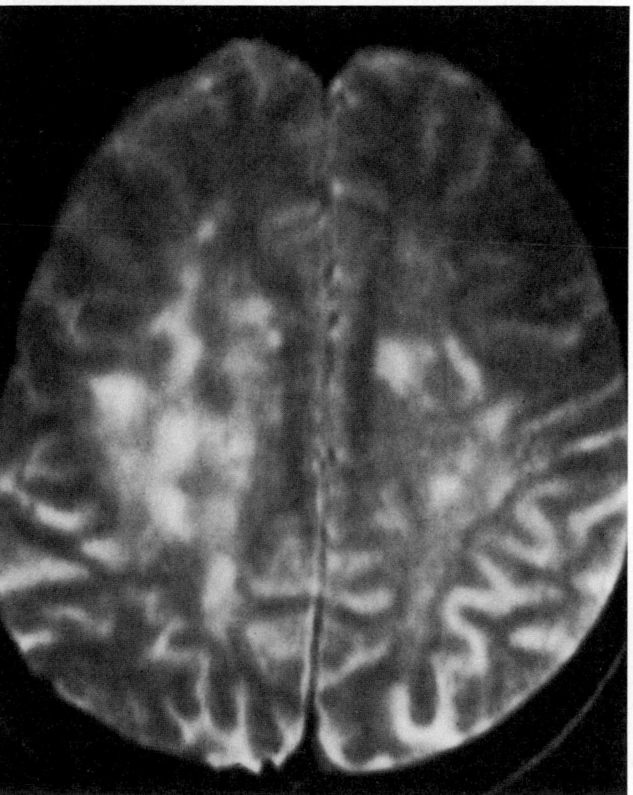

FIG. 76. Arteritis. Scattered bright lesions predominantly within white matter in the centrum semiovale are present in this patient with lupus arteritis on T2-weighted sequence (2000/80).

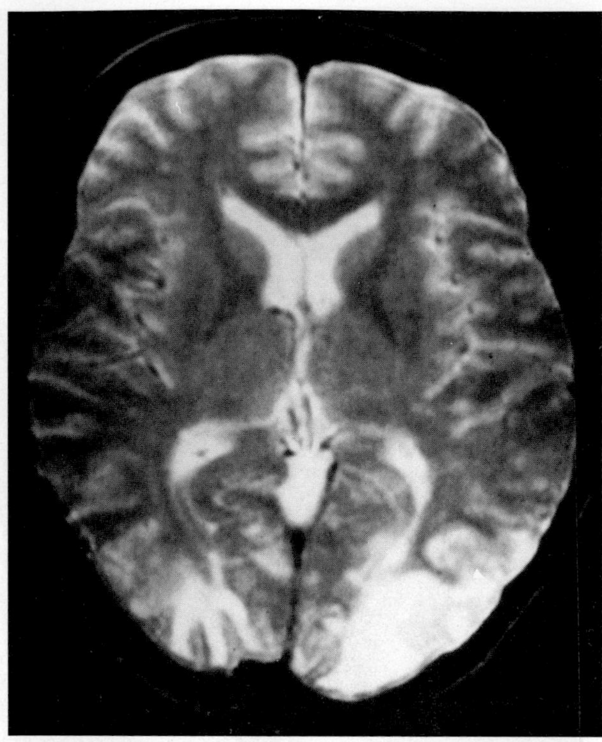

A

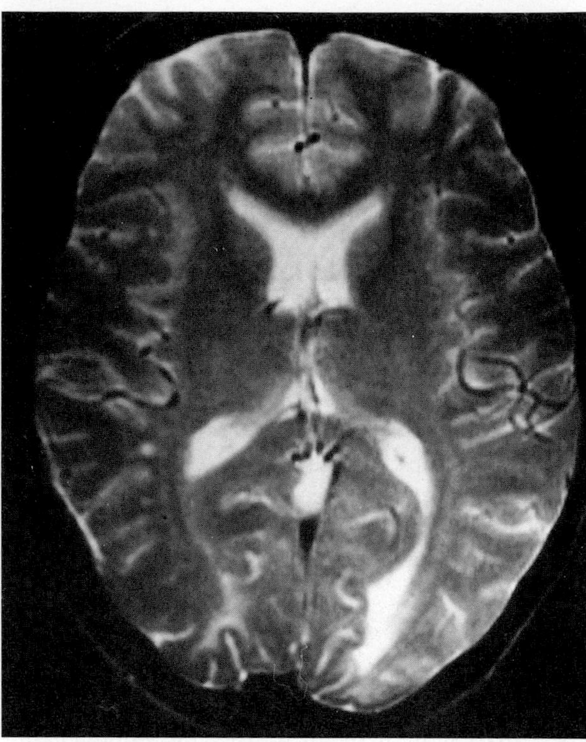

B

FIG. 77. Lupus vasculopathy. **A:** Scattered bright lesions predominantly within occipital lobes are present in this patient with lupus vasculopathy on T2-weighted image (2000/80). **B:** Marked improvement in lesions with steroid therapy, but residual abnormality persists (2000/80).

tical in appearance to both SLE and MS (98). The clinical diagnosis may be characteristic if the patient has hilar adenopathy, anergy, hypercalcemia, uveitis, and a positive Kveim test (99). There are some patients with neurosarcoidosis, however, who have no systemic manifestations of disease.

Intracranial findings include meningovascular involvement, with a dense adhesive arachnoiditis causing cranial nerve deficits and inflammation of the pituitary gland and hypothalamus. On MRI, meningitis may be seen as abnormal enhancement of the meninges on T1-weighted images. Parenchymal involvement is usually

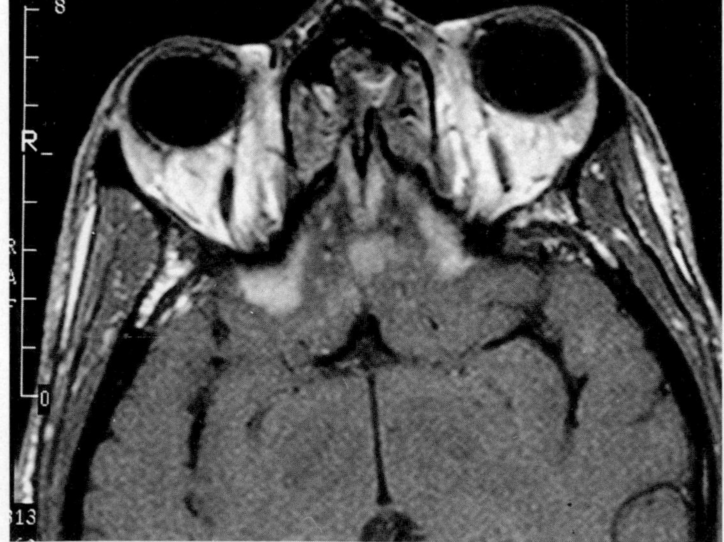

A

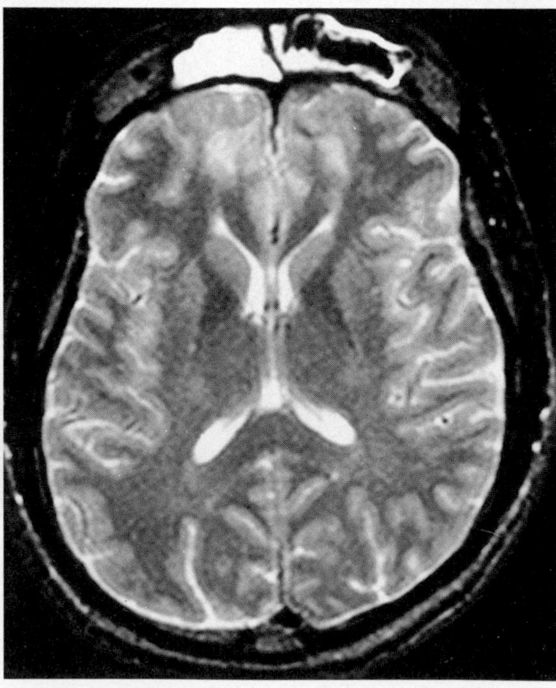

B

FIG. 78. Sarcoidosis with white matter abnormality. **A:** Gadolinium-enhanced T1-weighted image shows high intensity along surfaces of orbitofrontal region bilaterally. **B:** Bifrontal high intensity is present in the subcortical white matter on T2-weighted sequence.

peripheral within the gray matter and subcortical white matter (Fig. 78). Disease in the subependymal region is not uncommon, and may be the predominant lesion (99). Neurosarcoidosis is commonly found in the periaqueductal region and may involve the pineal gland (99).

Radiation and Chemotherapy Effects

Arteritis and secondary ischemic lesions of brain may result from chemotherapy and radiation therapy. Determining whether the patient's symptoms are due to an exacerbation of the neoplasm or to the effects of therapy can be a confusing clinical question. Symptoms of radiation- or chemotherapy-induced arteritis are similar to those of an intracranial mass: seizures, headaches, confusion, and focal neurologic deficits. MRI can be of great value in differentiating primary from secondary neurologic dysfunction. Most recurrent or residual tumors appear as focal areas of enhancement with surrounding edema. The white matter lesions caused by radiation-induced arteritis may be transient or permanent (Figs. 79 and 80) (102). The initial changes of transient white matter edema are of little clinical consequence. The chronic changes can be marked, with devastating clinical sequelae. These include radiation necrosis, widespread leukomalacia, calcifying microangiopathy, and

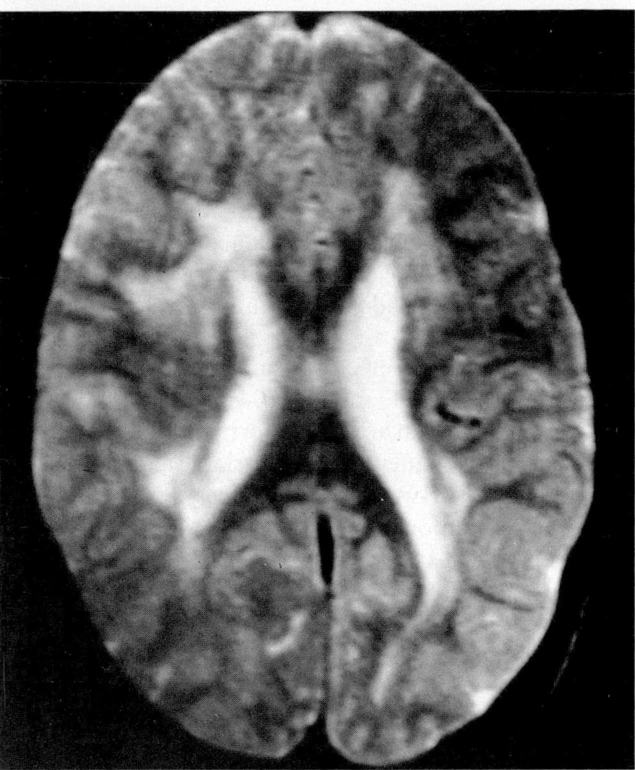

FIG. 79. Radiation-related ischemic change. Bright signal reflects radiation therapy effects in the periventricular regions on T2-weighted sequence (2000/80).

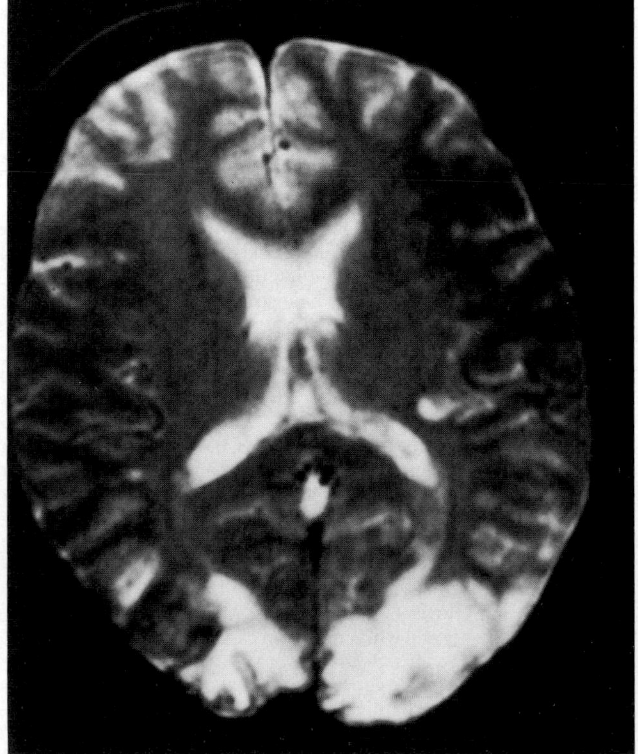

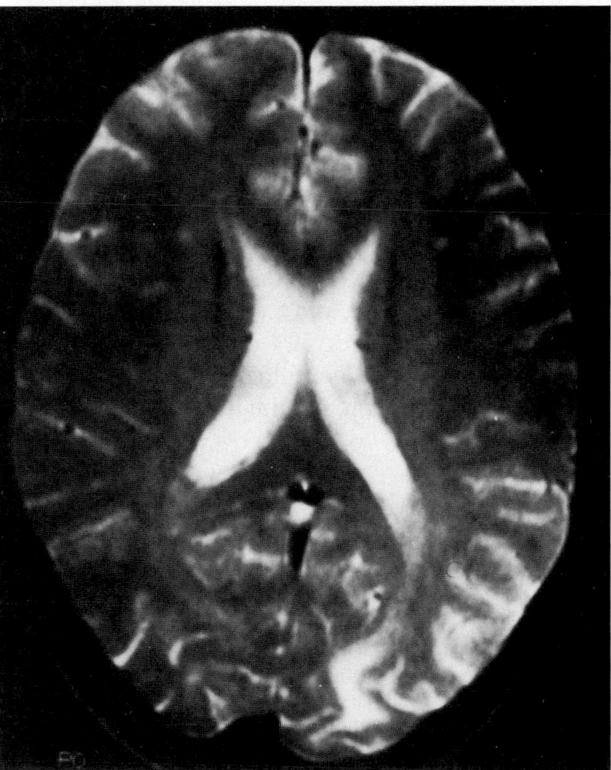

FIG. 80. Arteritis in patient with both radiation therapy and experimental chemotherapy for breast cancer. **A:** Marked bilateral occipital lesions are present on this T2-weighted sequence (2000/80), involving both gray and white matter. **B:** Following cessation of chemotherapy and administration of steroids, the lesions are largely resolved.

atrophy (102). Focal atrophy of any portion of the central nervous system can occur, including the optic nerves, resulting in optic atrophy, and the pituitary gland, resulting in panhypopituitarism. In children, the younger the patient at the time of radiation therapy, the more devastating the result. In combination with chemotherapy, the effects of radiation may be even more severe (Fig. 80). A subacute leukoencephalopathy can be seen as a consequence of the combination of intrathecal methotrexate and irradiation of the central nervous system (103).

Areas of radiation necrosis can be focal or disseminated within the white matter (104). Radiation necrosis appears acutely as an area of abnormal signal brightness on T2-weighted sequences, with variable gadolinium enhancement on T1-weighted sequences. Mass effect and edema are common findings in radiation necrosis and the lesion may, based on imaging findings alone, be indistinguishable from neoplasm. Later in the course, ventricular enlargement and atrophic changes predominate. The diffuse changes of radiation therapy on MRI appear as extensive, confluent white matter lesions, scalloped laterally, adjacent to the cortical gray matter, due to arcuate, U-fiber damage (102). The corpus callosum is usually spared.

L-Asparaginase, an enzyme used in treating acute leukemia, has been associated with intracranial sinus thrombosis in 1–2% of children (105). Hemorrhagic infarcts, the result of sinus thrombosis, present as seizures, obtundation, headache, or hemiparesis. MRI has been of great value in detecting thrombosis early in children treated with L-asparaginase, and in documenting subcortical white matter changes, many of which are transient after cessation of therapy.

Bone marrow transplantation is another source of treatment-related changes in the white matter. This modality has become one of the mainstays in the treatment of recurrent leukemia and other disseminated cancers, as well as for aplastic anemia, and a variety of inborn errors of metabolism. In one series, 59% of pediatric bone marrow recipients developed neurologic complications, including cerebral infarction, meningitis, and meningoencephalitis (106).

REFERENCES

1. Jackson JA, Leake DR, Schneiders NJ, et al. Magnetic resonance imaging in multiple sclerosis: results in 32 cases. *AJNR* 1985;6:171–176.
2. Jacobs I, Kinkel WR, Polachini I, et al. Correlations of nuclear magnetic resonance imaging, computerized tomography, and clinical profiles in multiple sclerosis. *Neurology* 1986;36:27–34.
3. Scotti G, Scialfa G, Biondi A, et al. Magnetic resonance in multiple sclerosis. *Neuroradiology* 1986;28:319–323.
4. Runge VM, Price A, Kirshner HS, et al. Magnetic resonance imaging of multiple sclerosis: a study of pulse-technique efficacy. *AJR* 1984;143:1015–1026.
5. Kucharczyk W, Macdonald PM, Stanisz GJ, Henkelman RM. Relaxivity and magnetization transfer of white matter lipids at MR imaging: importance of cerebrosides and pH. *Radiology* 1994;192:521–529.
6. Barkovich AJ, Lyon G, Evrard P. Formation, maturation, and disorders of white matter. *AJNR* 1992;13:447–461.
7. Koenig SH, Brown RD, Spiller M, Lundbom, N. Relaxometry of brain: why white matter appears bright in MRI. *Magn Reson Med* 1990;14:482–490.
8. Koenig SH. Cholesterol of myelin is the determinant of gray-white matter contrast in MRI of the brain. *Magn Reson Med* 1991;20:285–296.
9. Fralix TA, Ceckler TL, Wolff SD, Simon SA, Balaban RS. Lipid bilayer and water proton magnetization transfer: effect of cholesterol. *Magn Reson Med* 1991;18:214–223.
10. Staudt M, Schropp C, Staudt F, Obletter N, Bise K, Breit A. Myelination of the brain in MRI: a staging system. *Pediatr Radiol* 1993;23:169–176.
11. Allen IV, Kirk J. Demyelinating diseases. In: Adams JH, Duchen LW, eds. *Greenfield's Neuropathology.* New York: Oxford University Press; 1992:447–520.
12. Batchelor JR. Histocompatibility antigens and their relevance to multiple sclerosis. *Br Med Bull* 1977;33:72.
13. Heaton RK, Nelson LM, Thompson DS, et al. Neuropsychiatric findings in relapsing-remitting and chronic-progressive multiple sclerosis. *J Consult Clin Psychol* 1985;53:103–110.
14. McAlpine D. Some aspects of the natural history. In: McAlpine D, Lumsden CE, Acheson ED, eds. *Multiple Sclerosis. A Reappraisal.* Edinburgh: Churchill Livingstone; 1972:83–98.
15. Mushlin AI, Detsky AS, Phelps CE, et al. The accuracy of magnetic resonance imaging in patients with suspected multiple sclerosis. *JAMA* 1993;269:3146–3151.
16. Paty DW, Oger JJF, Kastrukoff LF, Hashimoto SA, Hooge JP, Eisen AA. MRI in the diagnosis of MS: a prospective study with comparison of clinical evaluation, evoked potentials, oligoclonal banding, and CT. *Neurology* 1988;38:180–185.
17. Ulrich J, Groebke-Lorenz W. The optic nerve in multiple sclerosis. A morphological study with retrospective clinicopathological correlations. *J Neuroophthalmol* 1983;3:149–159.
18. Yetkin FZ, Haughton VM, Papke RA, Fischer ME, Rao SM. Multiple sclerosis: specificity of MR for diagnosis. *Radiology* 1991;178:447–451.
19. Bartel DR, Markand ON, Kolar OJ. The diagnosis and classification of multiple sclerosis: evoked responses and spinal fluid electrophoresis. *Neurology* 1983;33:592–601.
20. Cutler JR, Aminoff MJ, Brant-Zawadzki M. Evaluation of patients with multiple sclerosis by evoked potentials and magnetic resonance imaging: a comparative study. *Ann Neurol* 1986;20:645–648.
21. Farlow MR, Markand ON, Edwards MK, et al. Multiple sclerosis: magnetic resonance imaging, evoked responses, and spinal fluid electrophoresis. *Neurology* 1986;36:828–831.
22. Brownell B, Hughes JT. The distribution of plaques in the cerebrum in multiple sclerosis. *J Neurol Neurosurg Psychiatry* 1962;25:315–320.
23. Grossman RI, Gonzalez-Scarano F, Atlas SW, Galetta S, Silberberg DH. Multiple sclerosis: gadolinium enhancement in MR imaging. *Radiology* 1986;161:721–725.
24. Nesbit GM, Forbes GS, Scheithauer BW, Okazaki H, Rodriguez M. Multiple sclerosis: histopathologic and MR and/or CT correlation in 37 cases at biopsy and three cases at autopsy. *Radiology* 1991;180:467–474.
25. Allen IV, McKeown SR. A histological, histochemical, and biochemical study of the macroscopically normal white matter in multiple sclerosis. *J Neurol Sci* 1979;41:81–91.
26. Allen IV, Glover G, Anderson R. Abnormalities in the macroscopically normal white matter in cases of mild or spinal multiple sclerosis (MS). *Acta Neuropathol* 1981;(Suppl VII):176–178.
27. Adams CWM. The general pathology of multiple sclerosis: morphological and chemical aspects of the lesions. In: Hallpike JF, Adams CWM, Tourtellotte WW, eds. *Multiple Sclerosis: Pathology, Diagnosis, and Management.* Baltimore: Williams & Wilkins; 1983: 203–240.
28. Niebler G, Harris T, Davis T, Roos K. Fulminant multiple sclerosis. *AJNR* 1992;13:1547–1551.

29. Gharagozloo AM, Poe LB, Collins GH. Antemortem diagnosis of Balo concentric sclerosis: correlative MR imaging and pathologic features. *Radiology* 1994; 191:817–819.
30. Powell T, Sussman JG, Davies-Jones GAB. MR imaging in acute multiple sclerosis: ringlike appearance in plaques suggesting the presence of paramagnetic free radicals. *AJNR* 1992; 13:1544–1546.
31. Drayer B, Burger P, Darwin R, Riederer S, Herfkens R, Johnson GA. MRI of brain iron. *AJR* 1986; 147:103–110.
32. Gean-Marton AD, Venzina LG, Marton KI, Stimac GK, Peyster RG, Taveras JM, Davis KR. Abnormal corpus callosum: A sensitive and specific indicator of multiple sclerosis. *Radiology* 1991; 180:215–221.
33. Wilms G, Marchal G, Kersschot E, Vanhoenacker P, Demaerel P, Bosmans H, Carton H, Baert AL. Axial vs sagittal T2-weighted brain MR images in the evaluation of multiple sclerosis. *J Comput Assist Tomogr* 1991; 15:359–364.
34. Lacomis D, Osbakken M, Gross G. Spin lattice relaxation (T1) times of cerebral white matter in multiple sclerosis. *Magn Reson Med* 1986; 3:194–202.
35. Brainin M, Neuhold A, Resiner T, Maida E, Lang S, Deecke L. Changes within the "normal" cerebral white matter of multiple sclerosis patients during acute attacks and during high dose cortisone therapy assessed by means of quantitative MRI. *J Neurol Neurosurg Psychiatry* 1989; 52:1355–1359.
36. Miller DH, Johnson G, Tofts PS, MacManus D, McDonald WI. Precise relaxation time measurements of normal-appearing white matter in inflammatory central nervous system disease. *Magn Reson Med* 1989; 11:331–336.
37. Armspach JP, Gounot D, Rumbach L, Chambron J. In vivo determination of multiexponential T2 relaxation times in the brain of patients with multiple sclerosis. *Magn Reson Imaging* 1991; 9: 107–113.
38. Haughton VM, Yetkin FZ, Rao SM, et al. Quantitative MR in the diagnosis of multiple sclerosis. *Magn Reson Med* 1992; 26:71–78.
39. Barbosa S, Blumhardt LD, Roberts N, Lock T, Edwards RHT. Magnetic resonance relaxation time mapping in multiple sclerosis: normal appearing white matter and the "invisible" lesion load. *Magn Reson Imaging* 1994; 12:33–42.
40. Barkhof F, Valk J, Hommes OR, Scheltens P. Meningeal Gd-DTPA enhancement in multiple sclerosis. *AJNR* 1992; 13:397–400.
41. Grossman RI, Gonzalez-Scarano F, Atlas SW, Galetta S, Silberberg DH. Multiple sclerosis: gadolinium enhancement in MR imaging. *Radiology* 1986; 161:721–725.
42. Grossman RI, Lenkinski RE, Ramer KN, Gonzalez-Scarano F, Cohen JA. MR proton spectroscopy in multiple sclerosis. *AJNR* 1992; 13:1535–1543.
43. Richards TL. Proton MR spectroscopy in multiple sclerosis: value in establishing diagnosis, monitoring progression, and evaluating therapy. *AJR* 1991; 157:1073–1078.
44. Arnold DL, Matthews PM, Francis G, Antel J. Proton magnetic resonance spectroscopy of human brain in vivo in the evaluation of multiple sclerosis: assessment of the load of the disease. *Magn Reson Med* 1990; 14:154–159.
45. van Hecke P, Marchal G, Johannik K, Demaerel D, Wilms G, Carton H, Baert AL. Human brain proton localized NMR spectroscopy in multiple sclerosis. *Magn Reson Med* 1991; 18:199–206.
46. Miller DH, Austin SJ, Connelly A, Youl BD, Gadian DG, McDonald WI. Proton magnetic resonance spectroscopy of an acute and chronic lesion in multiple sclerosis. *Lancet* 1991; 337:58–59.
47. Larsson HBW, Christiansen P, Jensen M, Frederiksen J, Heltberg A, Olesen J, Henriksen O. Localized in vivo proton spectroscopy in the brain of patients with multiple sclerosis. *Magn Reson Med* 1991; 22:23–31.
48. Wolinsky JS, Narayana PA, Fenstermacher MJ. Proton magnetic resonance spectroscopy in multiple sclerosis. *Neurology* 1990; 40: 1764–1769.
49. Narayana PA, Wolinsky JS, Jackson EF, McCarthy M. Proton MR spectroscopy of gadolinium-enhancing multiple sclerosis plaques. *J Magn Reson Imaging* 1992; 2:263–270.
50. Dousset V, Grossman RI, Ramer KN, Schnall MD, Young LH, Gonzalez-Scarano F, Lavi E, Cohen JA. Experimental allergic encephalomyelitis and multiple sclerosis: lesion characterization with magnetization transfer imaging. *Radiology* 1992; 182:483–491.
51. Hiehle JF, Lenkinski RE, Grossman RI, et al. Correlation of spectroscopy and magnetization transfer imaging in the evaluation of demyelinating lesions and normal appearing white matter in multiple sclerosis. *Magn Reson Med* 1994; 32:285–293.
52. Moseley ME, Kucharczyk J, Mintorovitch J, et al. Diffusion-weighted MR imaging of acute stroke: correlation with T2-weighted and magnetic susceptibility-enhanced MR imaging in cats. *AJNR* 1990; 11:423–429.
53. Heide AC, Richards TL, Alvord EC, Peterson J, Rose LM. Diffusion imaging of experimental allergic encephalomyelitis. *Magn Reson Med* 1993; 29:478–484.
54. Sakuma H, Nomura Y, Takeda K, et al. Adult and neonatal human brain: diffusional anisotropy and myelination with diffusion-weighted MR imaging. *Radiology* 1991; 180:229–233.
55. Larsson H, Tomsen C, Frederiksen J, Stubgaard M, Henriksen O. In vivo magnetic resonance diffusion measurement in the brain of patients with multiple sclerosis. *Magn Reson Imaging* 1992; 10: 7–12.
56. Edwards MK, Farlow MR, Stevens JC. Cranial MR in spinal cord MS: diagnosing patients with isolated spinal cord symptoms. *AJNR* 1986; 7:1003–1005.
57. Smith RR, Edwards MK, Farlow MR, et al. Imaging of optic neuritis using STIR MR. *AJNR* 1989; 10:905(abst).
58. Brodsky MC, Beck RW. The changing role of MR imaging in the evaluation of acute optic neuritis. *Radiology* 1994; 192:22–23.
59. Beck RW, Cleary PA, Trobe JD, et al. The effect of corticosteroids for acute optic neuritis on the subsequent development of multiple sclerosis. *N Engl J Med* 1993; 329:1764–1769.
60. Walker DL. Progressive multifocal leukoencephalopathy: an opportunistic viral infection of the central nervous system. In: Vinken PJ, Bruyn GW, eds. *Infections of the Nervous System*, vol 43. Amsterdam: Elsevier/North-Holland; 1978;43: 307–341.
61. Mark AS, Atlas SW. Progressive multifocal leukoencephalopathy in patients with AIDS: appearance on MR images. *Radiology* 1989; 173:517–521.
62. Richardson EP Jr. Progressive multifocal leukoencephalopathy. *N Engl J Med* 1961; 265:815–823.
63. Levy JD, Cottingham KL, Campbell RJ, et al. Progressive multifocal leukomalacia and magnetic resonance imaging. *Ann Neurol* 1986; 19:399–401.
64. Heinz ER, Drayer BP, Haenggeli CA, et al. CT in white matter disease. *Radiology* 1979; 130:370–378.
65. Diebler C, Dulac O. *Pediatric Neurology and Neuroradiology*. Berlin: Springer-Verlag; 1987.
66. Esiri M, Kennedy P. Virus diseases. In: Adams JH, Duchen LW, eds. *Greenfield's Neuropathology*. New York: Oxford University Press; 1992:335–399.
67. Saito H, Endo M, Takase S, et al. Acute disseminated encephalomyelitis after influenza vaccination. *Arch Neurol* 1980; 37:564–566.
68. Shoji H, Kusuhara T, Honda Y, Hino H, Kojima K, Abe T, Watanabe M. Relapsing acute disseminated encephalomyelitis associated with chronic Epstein-Barr virus infection: MRI findings. *Neuroradiology* 1992; 34:340–342.
69. Graham DI, Behan PO, More IAR. Brain damage complicating septic shock. Acute hemorrhagic leucoencephalitis as a complication of the generalised Schwartzman reaction. *J Neurol Neurosurg Psychiatry* 1979; 42:19–28.
70. Dangond F, Lacomis D, Schwartz RB, Wen PY, Samuels M. Acute disseminated encephalomyelitis progressing to hemorrhagic encephalitis. *Neurology* 1991; 41:1697.
71. Rippe DJ, Edwards MK, D'Amour PG, Holden RW, Roos KL. MR imaging of central pontine myelinolysis. *J Comput Assist Tomogr* 1987; 111:724–726.
72. Mascalchi M, Cincotta M, Piazzini M. Case report: MRI demonstration of pontine and thalamic myelinolysis in a normonatremic alcoholic. *Clin Radiol* 1993; 47:137–138.
73. Gerard D, Healy ME, Hesselink JR. MR demonstration of mesencephalic lesions in osmotic demyelination syndrome (central pontine myelinolysis). *Neuroradiology* 1987; 29:582–584.

74. Miller GM, Baker HL, Okazaki H, Whisnant JP. Central pontine myelinolysis and its imitators: MR findings. *Radiology* 1988; 168: 795–802.
75. Endo Y, Oda M, Hara M. Central pontine myelinolysis. A study of 37 cases in 1,000 consecutive autopsies. *Acta Neuropathol (Berl)* 1981;53:145–153.
76. Edwards MK, Smith RR. White matter diseases. *Top Magn Reson Imaging* 1989;2(1):41–48.
77. Dickoff DJ, Raps M, Yahr MD. Striatal syndrome following hyponatremia and its rapid correction. A manifestation of extrapontine myelinolysis confirmed by magnetic resonance imaging. *Arch Neurol* 1988;4:112–114.
78. Menkes JH. Metabolic diseases of the central nervous system. In: Menkes JH, ed. *Textbook of Child Neurology,* 3rd ed. Philadelphia: Lea & Febiger; 1985:1–122.
79. Friede RI. *Developmental Neuropathology,* 2nd ed. Berlin: Springer-Verlag; 1989.
80. Mirowitz SA, Sartor K, Prensky AJ, Gado M, Hodges FJ III. Neurodegenerative diseases of childhood: MR and CT evaluation. *J Comput Assist Tomogr* 1991;15:210–222.
81. Hatten HP Jr. Dysmyelinating leukodystrophies: "LACK proper myelin." *Pediatr Radiol* 1991;21:477–482.
82. Valk J, van der Knapp MS. *Magnetic Resonance of Myelin, Myelination, and Myelin Disorders.* Berlin: Springer-Verlag; 1989.
83. Lake BD. Lysosomal enzyme deficiencies. In: Adams JH, Corsellis JAN, Duche IW, eds. *Greenfields's Neuropathology,* 4th ed. New York: John Wiley; 1984:526–530.
84. Demaerel P, Faubert C, Wilms G, Casaer P, Piepgras U, Baert AL. MR findings in leukodystrophy. *Neuroradiology* 1991;33: 368–371.
85. Moser HW, Moser AE, Singh I, et al. Adrenoleukodystrophy: survey of 303 cases: biochemistry, diagnosis, and therapy. *Ann Neurol* 1984;16:628–641.
86. Hong-Mango ET, Muraki AS, Huttenlocher PR. Atypical CT scans in adrenoleukodystrophy. *J Comput Assist Tomogr* 1987; 11:333–336.
87. Tzika AA, Ball WS Jr, Vigneron DB, Dunn RS, Nelson SJ, Kirks DR. Childhood adrenoleukodystrophy: assessment with proton MR spectroscopy. *Radiology* 1993;189:467–480.
88. Schuster V, Horwitz AE, Kreth HW. Alexander's disease: cranial MRI and ultrasound findings. *Pediatr Radiol* 1991;21:133–134.
89. Nelson MD Jr, Wolff JA, Cross CA, Donnell GN, Kaufman FR. Galactosemia: evaluation with MR imaging. *Radiology* 1992; 184:255–261.
90. Boothman BR, Bamford JM, Parsons MR. Magnetic resonance imaging in Fabry's disease. *J Neurol Neurosurg Psychiatry* 1988; 51:1240–1241.
91. Murata R, Nakajima S, Tanaka A, et al. MR imaging of the brain in patients with mucopolysaccharidosis. *AJNR* 1989;10:1165–1170.
92. Johnson MA, Desai S, Hugh-Jones K, Starer F. Magnetic resonance imaging of the brain in Hurler syndrome. *AJNR* 1984;5: 816–819.
93. George AE, de Leon MJ, Kalnin A, et al. Leukoencephalopathy in normal and pathologic aging. 2. MR of brain lucencies. *AJNR* 1986;7:567–570.
94. Takahashi S, Higano S, Ishii K, Matsumoto K, Sakamoto K, Iwasaki Y, Suzuki M. Hypoxic brain damage: cortical laminar necrosis and delayed changes in white matter at sequential MR imaging. *Radiology* 1993;189:449–456.
95. Schouman-Claeys E, Henry-Feugeas M-C, Roset F, Larroche J-C, Hassine D, Sadik J-C, Frija G, Gabilan JC. Periventricular leukomalacia: correlation between MR imaging and autopsy findings during the first 2 months of life. *Radiology* 1993;189:59–64.
96. Chang KH, Han MH, Kim HS, Wie BA, Han MC. Delayed encephalopathy after acute carbon monoxide intoxication: MR imaging features and distribution of cerebral white matter lesions. *Radiology* 1992;184:117–122.
97. Delaney P. Neurologic manifestations in sarcoidosis. Review of the literature, with a report of 23 cases. *Ann Intern Med* 1977;87: 336–345.
98. Smith AS, Meisler DM, Tomsak RL, et al. High signal periventricular lesions in patients with sarcoidosis: neurosarcoidosis or multiple sclerosis? *AJNR* 1989;10:898–891.
99. Hayes WS, Sherman JL, Stern BJ, et al. MR and CT evaluation of intracranial sarcoidosis. *AJNR* 1987;8:841–845.
100. Hausegger DA, Millner MM, Fluckiger F, Justich E. Mitochondrial encephalomyopathy—two years follow-up by MRI. *Pediatr Radiol* 1991;21:231–233.
101. Johns DR, Stein AG, Wityk R. MELAS syndrome masquerading as herpes simplex encephalitis. *Neurology* 1993;43:2471–2473.
102. Hecht-Leavitt C, Grossman RI, Curran SJ, et al. MR of brain radiation injury: experimental studies in cats. *AJNR* 1987;8:427–431.
103. Peylan-Ramu N, Poplack DG, Pizzo PA, et al. Abnormal CT scans in asymptomatic children with acute lymphocytic leukemia after prophylactic treatment of the central nervous system with radiation and intrathecal chemotherapy. *N Engl J Med* 1978;298: 815–818.
104. Robain O, Dulac O, Dommergues JP, et al. Necrotizing leukoencephalopathy complicating treatment of childhood leukaemia. *J Neurol Neurosurg Psychiatry* 1984;47:65–72.
105. Priest JR, Ramsay NKC, Steinberz PG, et al. A syndrome of thrombosis and hemorrhage complicating L-asparaginase therapy for childhood acute lymphoblastic leukemia. *J Pediatr* 1982;100:984–989.
106. Wiznitzer M, Packer RJ, August CS, Burkey ED. Neurological complications of bone marrow transplantation in childhood. *Ann Neurol* 1984;16:569–576.

Magnetic Resonance Imaging of the Brain and Spine, Second Edition, edited by Scott W. Atlas. Lippincott-Raven Publishers, Philadelphia © 1996.

16

Intracranial Infection

Michelle L. Hansman Whiteman, Brian C. Bowen, M. Judith Donovan Post, and Michael D. Bell

The incidence of central nervous system (CNS) infection has increased dramatically in the United States and elsewhere over the past decade, despite advances in antibiotic therapy. This is primarily due to the high incidence of CNS infection in patients with AIDS and the increasing numbers of individuals with HIV-related disease. Prompt detection and accurate diagnosis of CNS infection is critical as most of these disorders are readily treatable.

Computed tomography (CT) and magnetic resonance (MR) imaging often provide complementary information concerning many pathologic processes, but it is clear that MR imaging is most often the procedure of choice because of better inherent contrast resolution, multiplanar imaging, and the lack of artifact from compact bone. This is particularly true for the imaging of the posterior fossa, white matter disease, and small lesions without appreciable mass effect. MR is clearly superior to CT in the detection of remote hemorrhage as well as early ischemia and infarction. Postcontrast MR imaging is also more sensitive to meningeal pathology than contrast CT.

In general, long TR/long TE (T2-weighted) images have more contrast resolution and greater sensitivity to pathologic changes, whereas short TR/short TE (T1-weighted) images have better anatomic resolution and better delineate morphology. For the purposes of this chapter, long TR/long TE (T2-weighted) images refer to spin echo MR with a TR of 1500 to 3000 msec and a TE of 80 to 120 msec. Short TR/short TE (T1-weighted) images refer to a TR of 300 to 700 msec with a TE of 10 to 30 msec. Proton-density images refer to a TR of 1500

M. L. Hansman Whiteman, M.D.: Department of Diagnostic Radiology, University of Miami School of Medicine, Miami, FL 33136.

B. C. Bowen, M.D., Ph.D.: Department of Radiology, University of Miami School of Medicine, Miami, FL 33136.

M. J. Donovan Post, M.D.: Section of Neuroradiology, Department of Radiology, University of Miami School of Medicine, Miami, FL 33136.

M. D. Bell, M.D.: Department of Pathology, University of Miami School of Medicine; Palm Beach Medical Examiner's Office, West Palm Beach, FL 33406.

to 3000 msec and a TE of 20 to 40 msec. Both the signal characteristics and enhancement pattern must be considered in the evaluation of any infectious process involving the CNS.

VIRAL INFECTIONS

Viral Infection

Intracranial viral infection is usually a multifocal or diffuse inflammatory process, i.e., an encephalitis, that often involves the meninges as well (1). The disease process may result from acute or latent infection of the CNS. In the United States, acute viral encephalitis is most often due to arthropod-borne viruses ("arboviruses," an epidemiologic designation rather than a taxonomic classification). Of these "arboviruses," two families of viruses, togaviruses (alphaviruses and flavaviruses) and bunyaviruses (California group) are responsible for the majority of cases (2,3).

In the general population, aseptic meningitis is most often due to enteroviruses (especially coxsackieviruses and echoviruses) and less frequently due to herpes simplex viruses (HSV) or mumps virus (3). Viruses that may result in a meningitis in the acquired immunodeficiency syndrome (AIDS) population include human immunodeficiency virus (HIV) and the herpes viruses, especially cytomegalovirus (CMV) and occasionally herpes simplex virus type 1 and 2 (HSV-1 and HSV-2).

Pathologically, the primary features of viral encephalitis include neuronal degeneration and inflammation. Gross histopathologic findings range from unremarkable to diffuse brain congestion and edema with hemorrhage and necrosis (as in HSV-1, HSV-2, and some arboviral encephalitis). There is often some degree of cerebral edema as well as congestion of meningeal vessels.

On MR, the pathologic changes that result from viral encephalitis appear as scattered or confluent areas of hyperintensity on T2-weighted images and are isointense or hypointense on T1-weighted images, with variable mass effect (4–6). Foci of subacute hemorrhage (extracellular methemoglobin) demonstrate increased signal intensity on both long TR and short TR images (7). Localized or generalized atrophy, resulting from chronic or prior infection, may appear more prominent on short TR images. Although these general features apply to most of the viral encephalitides, certain infections demonstrate particular features that may be characteristic and are thus helpful in the differential diagnosis. These are described in the ensuing pages.

Herpes Viruses

The herpes viruses are a large group of double-stranded DNA viruses including HSV-1, HSV-2, CMV, Epstein-Barr virus (EBV), varicella-zoster virus (VZV), B virus, herpes virus 6, and herpes virus 7 (8). All have a similar molecular structure with a double-stranded DNA core and an envelope comprised of variable glycoproteins (9). These differing glycoproteins engender distinct differences among the viruses within the family (9). CNS infection by the herpes virus family may be either via a hematogenous route or via neuronal transmission of an extracerebral focus of infection (10).

After initial acquisition of the virus by the host, there is a primary viremia and seeding of the CNS may occur. The virus gains access to neuronal tissue either by diffusion through the blood-brain barrier or by infecting endothelial cells within intracranial blood vessels. This is the mechanism of infection in CMV, HSV-2, EBV, HSV 6, HSV 7, and neonatal cases of HSV-1. In nonneonatal HSV-1, VZV, and B virus, the infection originates in a peripheral neuron and is transported centrally within the axon to the brain (8).

Initial infection can result in clinical expression but more frequently the virus persists in an inactive form and is later reactivated by some stimulus (11). Clinical expression is proportionate to the degree of viral replication within neuronal tissue (8). Symptoms may vary from an aseptic meningitis to a severe encephalitis, with headache, fever, altered mental status, and focal or diffuse neurologic deficit (9).

Pathologically, the herpes virus family results in perivascular cuffing and an inflammatory infiltrate (9). Hemorrhage and necrosis may be seen in the more aggressive infections, HSV-1, HSV-2, and B virus (12). Inclusion bodies within individual cells may also be identified (9).

Herpes Simplex Virus Type 1

Herpes simplex virus type 1 (HSV-1) is the causative agent in 95% of herpetic encephalitis and is the most common cause of fatal sporadic encephalitis (13–15). Mortality from HSV encephalitis ranges from 50% to 70%. In adults, this infection usually arises in those individuals with pre-existing antibodies and thus represents viral reactivation. In children, HSV-1 acquisition is usually postnatal and in neonates HSV-2 is much more frequent than HSV-1, accounting for 80% to 90% of neonatal herpes virus infections and almost all the congenital herpes virus infections (16).

Clinical symptoms in the adult population include a nonspecific alteration in mental status, a diminished level of consciousness, focal neurologic deficit, and fever (8). Cerebrospinal fluid (CSF) findings are nonspecific and isolation of HSV from the CSF is rare (9). Electroencephalography (EEG) demonstrates activity localized to the temporal lobes (8). Definitive diagnosis is on the basis of brain biopsy (17). Polymerase chain reaction (PCR), a DNA amplification technique, may prove useful in obtaining a more accessible and rapid diagnosis from the CSF.

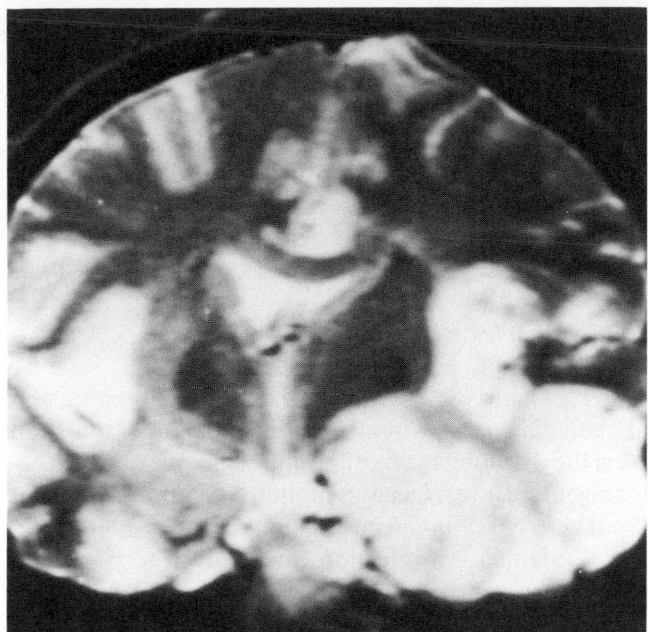

FIG. 1. Herpes simplex (type 1) encephalitis in a child. Coronal long TR/long TE (2500/80) MRI shows bilateral temporal lobe hyperintensity with mass effect. Note bilateral insular cortex involvement, left cingulate gyrus abnormality, and sparing of the putamen.

In non-AIDS patients, HSV-1 may result in a necrotizing encephalitis of the temporal lobes and the orbital surfaces of the frontal lobes (18). The insular cortex, cerebral convexity, and posterior occipital cortex may become involved (18). Disease is usually bilateral, with sparing of the basal ganglia (19). The cingulate gyrus may also become involved later in the course of the disease (20).

In adults, HSV-1 encephalitis is thought to result from reactivation of a latent HSV-1 infection in the trigeminal ganglion with intracellular spread of virus along the branches of cranial nerve V that innervate the meninges of the anterior and middle cranial fossae (21). Rhombencephalitis (pontine infection) may occur and may be related to retrograde viral transmission along the cisternal portion of cranial nerve V to the brainstem (22).

CT demonstrates hypodense lesions in the temporal lobes with or without involvement of the frontal lobes. Enhancement and hemorrhage are infrequent (23). Correlation of CT, MR, EEG, and CSF studies reveals the greater sensitivity of MR over CT (24). MR demonstrates the early edematous changes of herpes encephalitis, with increased signal seen in the temporal and inferior frontal lobes on T2-weighted images (25,26) (Figs. 1 and 2). This hyperintense signal involves both cortex and white matter, and may be seen as early as 48 hours following the onset of signs and symptoms (5), compared to 3 to 5 days for evidence on pre- and postcontrast CT (27,28), and 4 to 11 days for single photon emission computed tomography (SPECT) brain scans using either ^{123}I-iodoamphetamine (IMP) or ^{99m}Tc-hexamethylpropyleneamine oxime (HMPAO) (29). MR is thus considered the study of choice in imaging HSV encephalitis (8).

As areas of involvement enlarge and coalesce, there is associated mass effect. Extension from the temporal lobes across the sylvian fissure to the isle of Reil is well seen, as is frequent sparing of the putamen (30). MR will

A

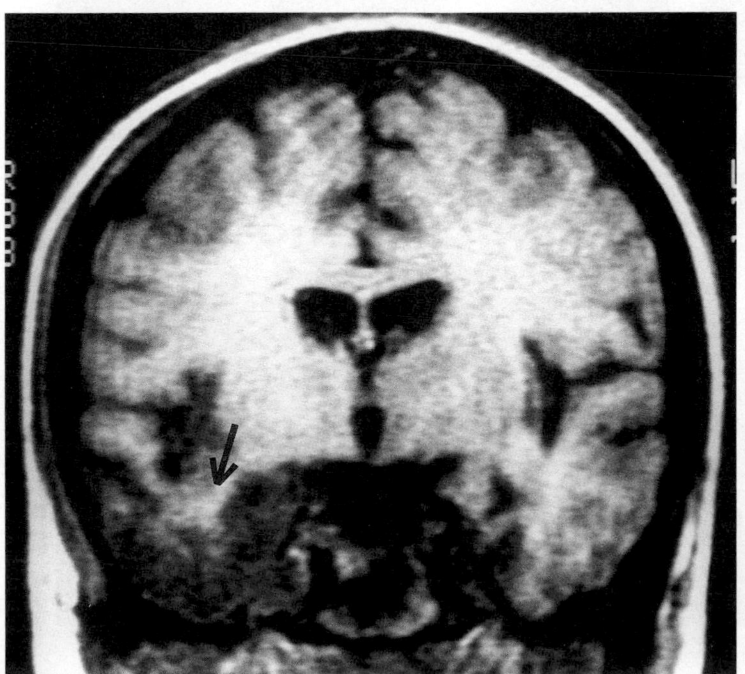

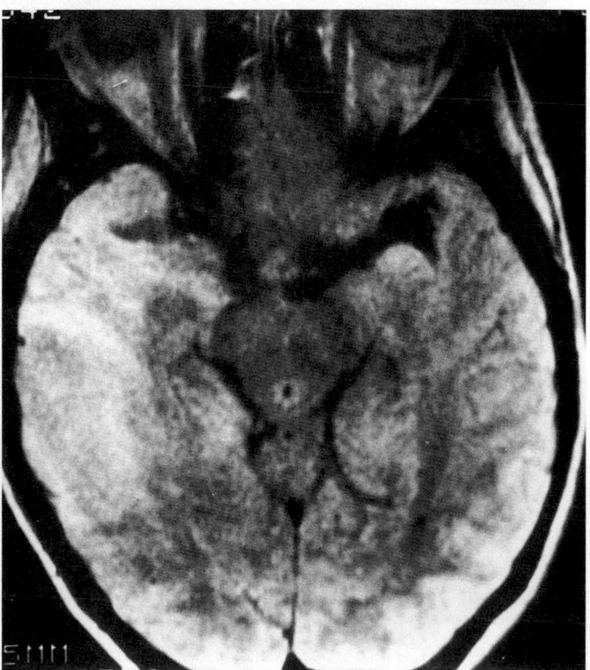

B

FIG. 2. Herpes simplex encephalitis (HSV-I). **A:** T1-weighted coronal MR image (600/20) reveals hypointense signal involving the gray and white matter of the right temporal lobe (*arrow*) in a 26-year-old female technician who worked in a virology lab. **B:** Proton-density axial MR image (1999/56) of the same patient reveals increased signal in the right temporal lobe with loss of the gray-white junction.

often demonstrate bitemporal involvement when CT shows only unilateral infection (4,5). Enhancement is often absent in the early stages, but gyriform enhancement may be seen with disease progression. Focal hemorrhage is consistently present at autopsy, yet is often not detected or is less apparent on CT. Acute hemorrhage on MR may appear as a focus of moderate to marked hypointensity on gradient-echo images (31) or on T2-weighted images (6,7) and nearly isointense on T1-weighted images. MR is more sensitive than CT to the presence of subacute hemorrhage, which is apparent as hyperintense signal on both T1-weighted and T2-weighted images (7) (Fig. 3). MR may also be used to monitor response to treatment with acyclovir (32). A late sequela is atrophy, which is well seen on multiplanar, spin echo MR, particularly on T1-weighted images. Mortality from HSV encephalitis ranges from 50% to 70%.

Infection with HSV-1 and HSV-2 has been reported in AIDS patients (20,33), but is an infrequent complication of AIDS, occurring in 2% of AIDS autopsy cases (34). In AIDS patients, HSV often results in diffuse rather than localized temporal/frontal involvement (20). Mild to severe forms of both HSV-1 and HSV-2 encephalitis have been reported (35) and may coexist with other infections (34–36). Typical pathologic findings of necrotizing encephalitis may be absent in the AIDS patient, even when HSV-1 or HSV-2 is cultured from the brain tissue (33). In these immune-compromised patients, there appears to be an inverse relationship between the degree of immunodeficiency and the severity of the inflammation induced by the herpes viruses (37) as well as the rapidity of disease progression. CT scanning in AIDS patients with HSV infection is most often either normal or may reveal atrophy only (33).

Herpes Simplex Virus Type 2

Herpes simplex virus type 2 (HSV-2) is a major cause of neonatal encephalitis. The primary route of infection is via the maternal birth canal, although infrequently, hematogenous transplacental in utero infection can occur (8). The CNS is involved in approximately 30% of infected infants (38). Infection can result in seizures, microcephaly, microphthalmia, ventriculomegaly, multicystic encephalomalacia, and death (8).

Pathologic examination demonstrates acute and chronic parenchymal and leptomeningeal inflammation (8). In contrast to the temporal/frontal predilection seen in adults, HSV neonatal infection is diffuse and may therefore result in widespread brain destruction (39).

Early CT findings include subtle hypodensity of the periventricular white matter with relative sparing of the

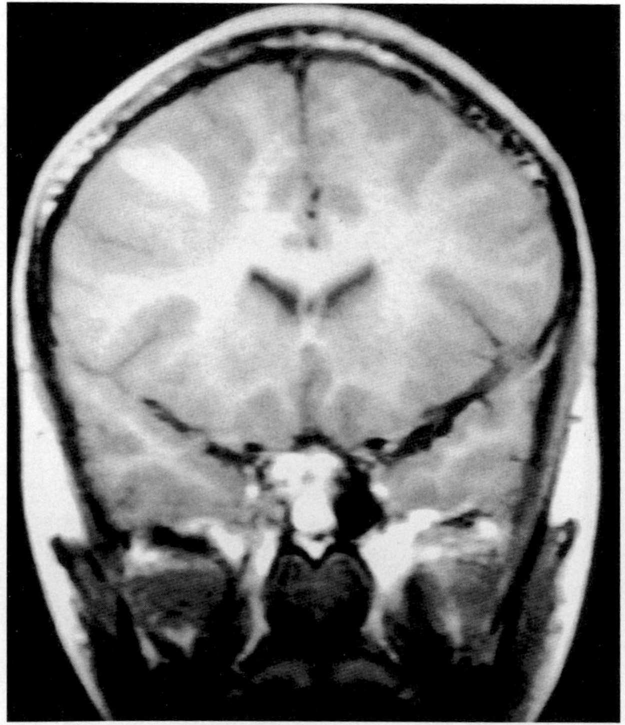

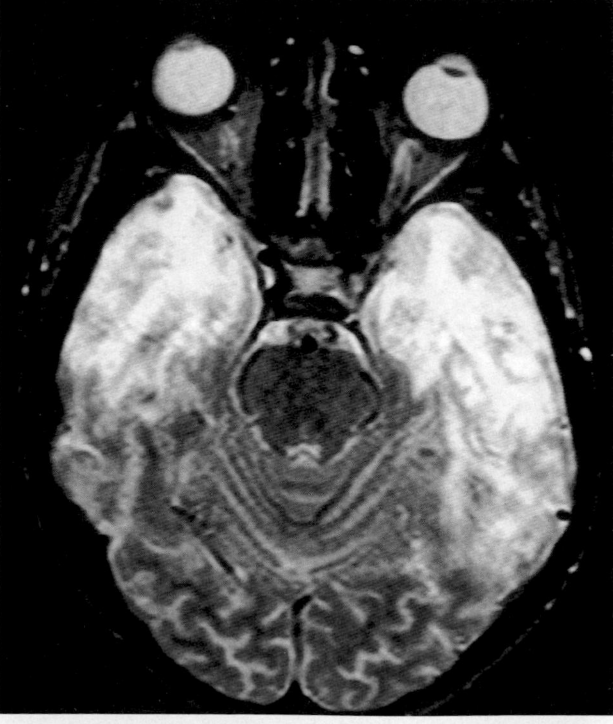

FIG. 3. Herpes simplex encephalitis. **A:** Coronal T1-weighted MR image without contrast (600/20) reveals a focus of subacute hemorrhage in the right frontal lobe, not apparent on a CT scan performed earlier the same day. This patient was a 10-year-old boy presenting with confusion, who rapidly progressed to become encephalopathic. **B:** T2-weighted axial image (2433/80) in the same patient reveals bilateral hyperintense signal in both temporal lobes, involving both gray and white matter.

central gray matter and posterior fossa (8). This may progress to increased white matter lucency and a finger-like increase in density of the cortex (40). This increased density is thought to result from an increase in cortical blood flow as a consequence of cortical infection (40). With disease progression, CT may show focal hemorrhagic necrosis, parenchymal calcification, and cystic encephalomalacia (18).

On MR, early findings include a loss of distinction at the gray/white matter interface. Edema may be difficult to distinguish from surrounding unmyelinated immature white matter because both have increased signal on T2-weighted images (8).

Varicella-Zoster Virus

Varicella-zoster virus (VZV) is the cause of two distinct clinical disorders: varicella (chicken pox) and herpes zoster infection (shingles) (8). Both disorders result in similar histopathologic changes in the skin (9). CNS infection may be seen in both entities and can result in hemorrhagic necrosis with intranuclear inclusions (9).

Varicella (chicken pox) is highly contagious with a generalized skin eruption occurring primarily in children, and usually of no serious consequence in those who are healthy (8). Encephalitis, however, may result in the immunocompromised patient (8). Varicella CNS infection may result in transverse myelitis, meningoencephalitis, cerebellar ataxia, and aseptic meningitis (8,9). Neurologic complications of varicella are seen in less than 1% of infected patients (8,41). Symptoms of cerebellar ataxia are often concurrent with the skin eruptions (8).

Neuroimaging is often negative in patients with cerebellar ataxia, which is usually self-limited (9). Meningoencephalitis is an uncommon CNS complication of varicella, which is of greater severity with fever, headache, vomiting, seizures, and alteration in mental status occurring 11 days to several weeks following the onset of the rash (42,43). CSF reveals a mild to moderate lymphocytic pleocytosis and elevated protein. EEG may also be diffusely abnormal (8). On MR, multifocal areas of increased signal in the cortex have been observed on T2-weighted images. In immunocompetent patients, mortality is low, with complete or near complete recovery as the usual outcome (8).

Zoster CNS infection may present as an encephalitis, neuritis, myelitis, and/or herpes ophthalmicus (8). These rarely complicate the clinical course in healthy adults with shingles, but in immunodeficient patients, there is an increased risk of CNS involvement (8). In immunocompetent patients, cranial and peripheral nerve palsies are the most common neurologic disorders seen in zoster infection (44), whereas diffuse encephalitis is the most frequent manifestation seen in AIDS patients and other immunosuppressed patients (45). Latent virus residing in the ganglia of cranial nerves (especially cranial nerves V and VII) can reactivate and spread retrograde to the brainstem, resulting in encephalitis (46). Fever, meningismus, and altered mental status in a patient with shingles should suggest the diagnosis (8). CSF is nonspecific, with a mild lymphocytic pleocytosis, a slightly elevated protein, and a normal glucose (8). MR may demonstrate increased signal in the brainstem and supratentorial gray matter on T2-weighted images (8), and may reveal brainstem enlargement (4) despite a negative CT (4,47) (Fig. 4).

Diffuse encephalitis associated with VZV infection is rare. It is usually seen in immunocompromised patients (1), and the white matter may be more involved than the gray matter. The involved areas appear hyperintense on T2-weighted images and may be a result of direct infection and/or an immune-mediated reaction. Vasculitis may also occur (46).

Cranial and peripheral nerve palsies are the most common neurologic manifestations of herpes zoster. The palsies occur in dermatomes involved by the characteristic skin lesions (44). Involvement of cranial nerve V results in pain in the distribution of the trigeminal nerve associated with headache and sometimes a change in the corneal reflex (8). The first division of cranial nerve V is the branch most frequently affected (Herpes zoster ophthalmicus) and presents with pain and a vesicular eruption in the distribution of the ophthalmic division of cranial nerve V. Fat-suppressed MR imaging with gadolinium may demonstrate enhancement of the intraorbital portion of the trigeminal nerve (48). A contralateral hemiplegia may develop and is usually preceded by the herpes ophthalmicus by several weeks to months (49). The immunodeficient patient is at increased risk for this complication (50). The pathogenesis of the hemiplegia is thought to result from viral infection of the larger intracranial arteries, resulting in cerebral angiitis and formation of mycotic aneurysms (50). CT and MR may reveal cerebral infarction (50). Angiography may demonstrate segmental constrictions or occlusions, which are often unilateral and involve the proximal ipsilateral middle cerebral artery (MCA), anterior communicating artery (ACA), or carotid siphon (49). The prognosis for this complication of herpes zoster ophthalmicus is variable, but can be fatal (51).

Epstein-Barr Virus

Epstein-Barr virus (EBV) is the etiologic agent in infectious mononucleosis. EBV is associated with a number of CNS disorders including Guillain-Barré syndrome, meningoencephalitis, transverse myelitis, and chronic fatigue syndrome (52,53). These may occur in the presence or absence of infectious mononucleosis (54). CNS complications are seen in approximately 5%

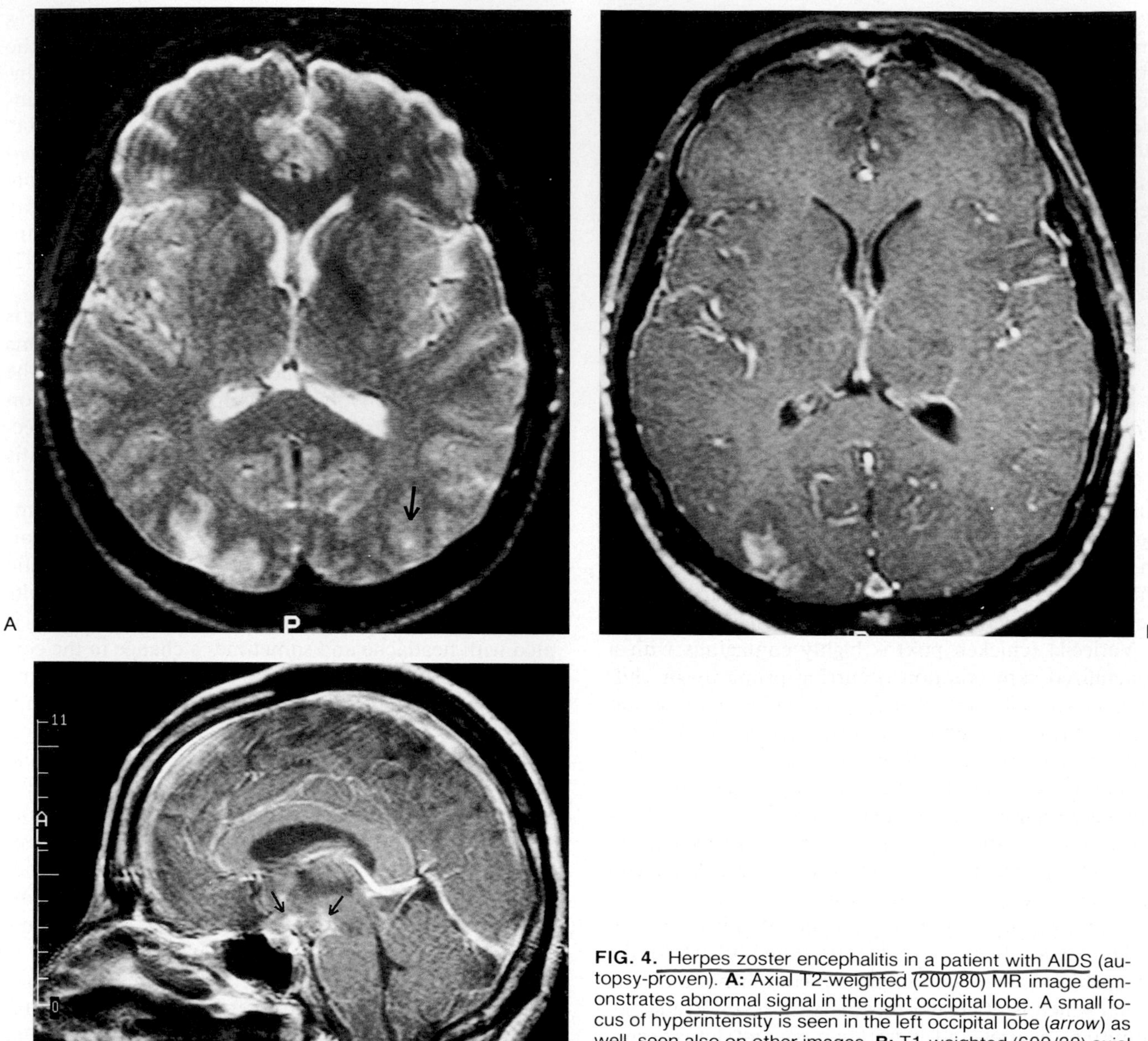

FIG. 4. Herpes zoster encephalitis in a patient with AIDS (autopsy-proven). **A:** Axial T2-weighted (200/80) MR image demonstrates abnormal signal in the right occipital lobe. A small focus of hyperintensity is seen in the left occipital lobe (*arrow*) as well, seen also on other images. **B:** T1-weighted (600/30) axial MR from the same patient reveals focal enhancement in the right occipital region, primarily involving gray matter. **C:** Midline sagittal T1-weighted (600/30) image demonstrates enhancement in the suprasellar and interpeduncular cisterns (*arrows*).

of patients with infectious mononucleosis (55). A diffuse encephalitis is seen in less than 1% of patients with infectious mononucleosis (55) with a short but severe clinical course and a good prognosis for recovery (54). MR may reveal multifocal areas of hyperintensity on T2-weighted images in gray matter or at the gray-white junction (54).

Cytomegalovirus

In adults, cytomegalovirus (CMV) is a frequent pathogen in the AIDS population and in other immunocompromised patients, occurring not only in the CNS, but throughout the body. CMV more often presents outside the CNS, involving the respiratory tract, liver, gastrointestinal tract, genitourinary tract, and/or hematopoietic system (33). This virus exists in a latent form in the vast majority of the population, with nearly 90% of adults having antibodies to CMV (1). Reactivation usually results in a subclinical or mild infection, mimicking mononucleosis (56,57). However, in a minority of immunodeficient patients, reactivation results in disseminated infection and/or severe necrotizing meningoencephalitis (58) and ependymitis (58). CMV may involve the central and/or peripheral nervous system (59,60).

Neurologic manifestations of CMV thus include acute or chronic meningoencephalitis, cranial neuropathy, vasculitis, retinitis, myelitis, brachial plexus neuropathy, and peripheral neuropathy (61–64).

In AIDS patients, CMV may coexist with other lesions, including toxoplasmosis and cryptococcosis, and may be clinically silent (58). Approximately 15% to 30% of adult AIDS patients demonstrate CMV on neuropathologic examination (34,59).

The pathologic hallmark of CMV is the "owl's eye," an enlarged cell with a distended nucleus containing eosinophilic viral inclusions, surrounded by a halo, resulting in the characteristic appearance (58). The "owl's eye" appearance can be seen in ependymal cells, subependymal astrocytes, oligodendroglia, endothelial cells, and neurons. Ependymal involvement is quite common. Infrequently, CMV infection may result in extensive destruction of gray and white matter (33). Other typical histopathologic findings in the CNS include well circumscribed microglial nodules (34), and CMV intranuclear inclusions may also be found in the spinal cord, spinal nerves, and retina (65).

CMV meningoencephalitis may be seen in HIV-seropositive patients as well as in otherwise healthy adults. This may be subclinical in immunocompetent and in immunocompromised patients (34,59,66) Less often, subacute symptoms develop over days to months with fever, confusion, altered mental status, memory loss, and progressive dementia (58). CMV meningoencephalitis is most commonly seen in transplant patients (67) and in patients with AIDS. Brain involvement may be diffuse or limited to the subependymal regions (1,68). CSF findings and complement fixation blood titers are nonspecific, and thus the clinical diagnosis can be difficult (61).

CT is frequently insensitive in the imaging of CMV encephalitis (58). The most frequent manifestation on CT is atrophy (61,69). Infrequently, white matter hypodensity may be apparent (69,70). Ring-enhancing lesions have also been described (68). CT grossly underestimates the degree of involvement by CMV (33). In addition to atrophy and white matter hypodensity, periventricular and subependymal enhancement may be seen (33) and is best visualized with a double dose-delayed technique (70).

MR has far greater sensitivity than CT in the detection of CNS CMV infection (58). In addition to atrophy, MR may demonstrate increased signal on T2-weighted images in the periventricular white matter (70), which may be patchy and is less often confluent (6,71) (Fig. 5). In-

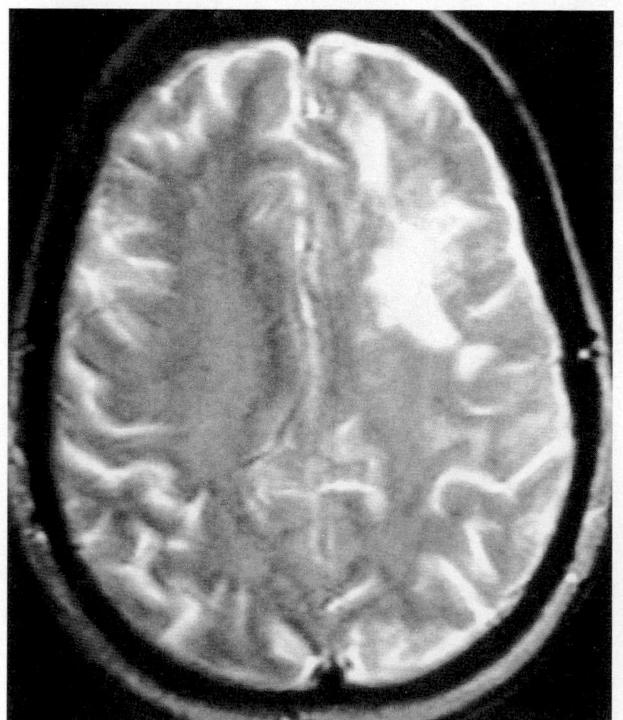

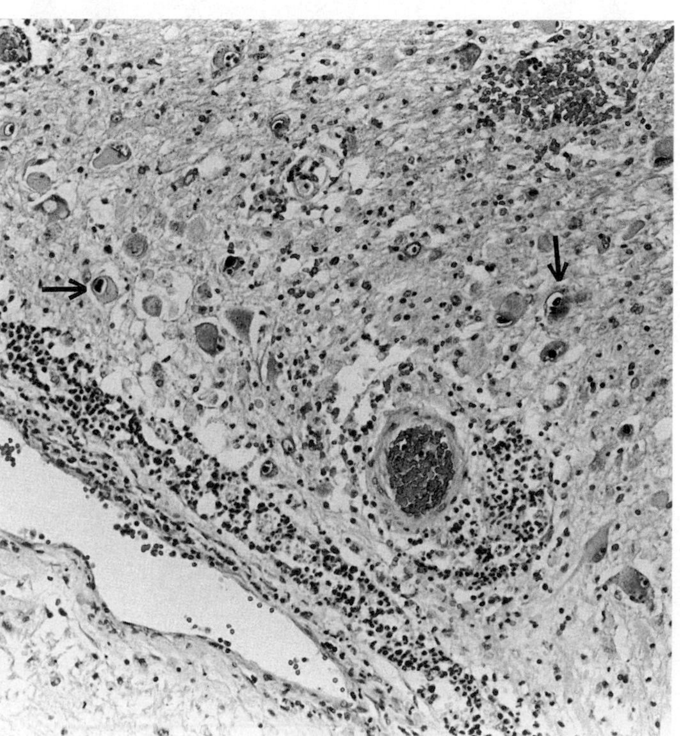

FIG. 5. Cytomegalovirus. **A:** T2-weighted (2400/80) axial MR scan reveals a large patchy area of increased signal in the frontal white matter, without mass effect, in this renal transplant patient on immunosuppressive therapy. **B:** Subependymal neurons with intranuclear inclusions surrounded by clear halos or "owl's eyes" (*arrows*) and perivascular involvement is characteristic of CMV infection (H & E, original magnification ×20). (From Whiteman et al., ref. 77, with permission.)

frequently, subependymal enhancement is evident and, if present, is a valuable diagnostic clue (58) (Fig. 6). Fat-suppressed MR with gadolinium may reveal a thickened and enhanced choroid/retina in patients with CMV retinitis (72), a hemorrhagic retinitis seen frequently in the AIDS population.

CMV is often seen in the pediatric population and is the most common cause of serious fetal and neonatal encephalitis (73). CMV infection acquired in utero is a result of transplacental transmission from primary maternal infection. Thirty to 40% of cases of maternal primary infection result in fetal infection (74). Infected infants are often born prematurely (75). Only 10% of infants with congenital CMV are symptomatic at birth, with evidence of jaundice, thrombocytopenia, chorioretinitis, and hepatosplenomegaly (8,75). Fifty to 75% have microcephaly (76). In utero acquisition of CMV may result in intracranial parenchymal necrosis and hydrocephalus (1). Seizures, optic atrophy, sensorineural hearing loss, and mental retardation may become evident (16). CT demonstrates atrophy, encephalomalacia, ventricular enlargement, periventricular calcification, and por-

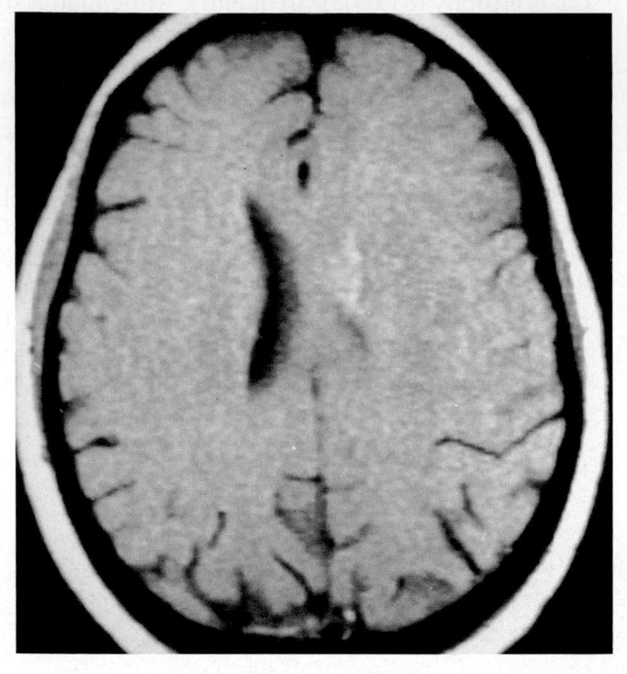
A

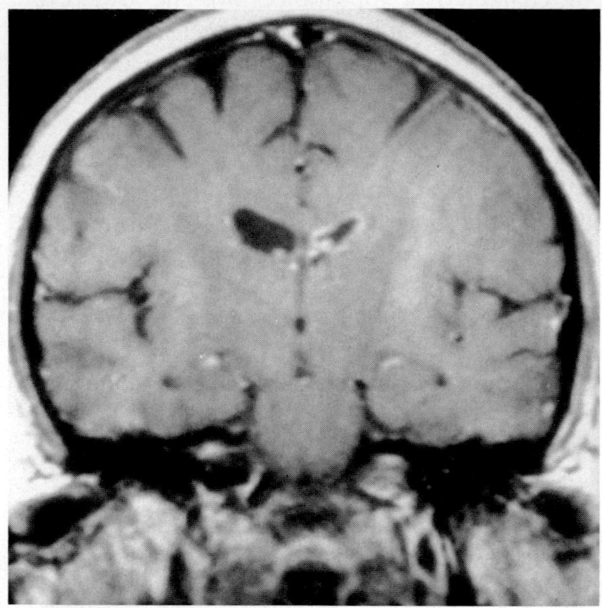
B

C

FIG. 6. Cytomegalovirus. **A:** Axial T1-weighted (900/20) MR image obtained after gadolinium administration (0.1 mm/Kg) reveals periventricular/subependymal enhancement along the left lateral ventricle. **B:** Coronal T1-weighted (900/20) postcontrast image of the same patient again demonstrates smooth subependymal/periventricular enhancement. **C:** "Shaggy" appearance of the frontal horns due to CMV ventriculitis.

encephaly (77). Periventricular calcification (mineralizing microangiopathy) and cystic encephalomalacia are also seen in other TORCH (toxoplasmosis, rubella, CMV, and herpes simplex) infections and are easily detected by neuroimaging (78,79). Calcification of the cortex and basal ganglia are present less commonly, but can also be seen in congenital CMV infection (77).

An important advantage of MR over CT is the demonstration of migrational abnormalities that can result from the teratogenic effect of CMV infection. The migrational abnormalities are often associated with other evidence of congenital CMV infection and include the lissencephaly-pachygyria spectrum (80,81).

Human Retroviruses

The human retroviruses that may cause neurologic disease include HIV and the human T-cell lymphotropic virus type I (HTLV-1). HIV, a lentivirus, has two subtypes: HIV-1 (formerly known as HTLV-III) and HIV-2 (82,83). Although HIV-1 is present on all continents, HIV-2 has been found mainly in West Africa (84,85). HTLV-I infection, which is endemic in Southern Japan, the Caribbean, and parts of Africa and South America, is uncommon in North America, although its prevalence appears to be on the rise (83).

The neurologic manifestations of HIV infection in the absence of superimposed opportunistic infection or neoplasm include encephalopathy, myelopathy, peripheral neuropathy, and myopathy (35,86–89). The presence of HIV-1, an RNA virus, within the CNS has been documented in 73% of adults and children with AIDS (90). In the brain, replicating HIV is most frequently associated with multinucleated giant cells and macrophages (87). These cells appear to be the chief targets of infection by HIV and are related to the progressive encephalopathy seen in AIDS (91–93). Polymorphic microglia are also frequently infected. Oligodendrocytes and astrocytes are infrequently infected, and neurons are only rarely infected by HIV (91–93).

The most common neurologic complication seen in AIDS patients is subacute encephalitis (35,61,69,86). This subacute encephalitis is present in 28% of adult AIDS autopsies (34). Clinical presentation includes a progressive dementia associated with motor and/or behavioral dysfunction (86). Early difficulties with memory and concentration are often followed by apparent apathy and social withdrawal and may be mistaken for symptoms of depression (94). Headache is also a frequent complaint, and seizures are seen in approximately 10% of cases (95). The subacute encephalitis has been attributed to CMV in some cases (96,97), although HIV itself appears to be the etiologic agent in the vast majority of cases (86,93,97). The pathologic correlate of HIV encephalopathy is found to be myelin pallor associated with HIV-infected multinucleated giant cells (33), microglial nodules, gliosis, and vacuolar degeneration (90). Clinicopathologic correlation in patients with AIDS dementia complex (ADC) suggests the primary pathologic substrate is subacute encephalitis with multinucleated giant cells rather than microglial nodules (66). Electron microscopy reveals retrovirus particles within these multinucleated giant cells, and their presence strongly correlates with ADC (66). There are sparse infiltrates of lipid-laden macrophages, gemistocytic astrocytes, and lymphocytes (34). The multinucleated giant cells may be present within the cortex, basal ganglia, and/or white matter (87). Diffuse atrophy is usually present. Gross examination often reveals only atrophy (98).

Initially, lesions are present in the white matter and extend to the basal ganglia and cortex with disease progression (66). In some patients the white matter lesions predominate, whereas in others, the gray matter is more severely affected (71). Lesions may also be located in the brainstem, cerebellum, and spinal cord (66).

Although foci of demyelination are present, this is a secondary and comparatively late finding. Small, ill-defined foci of demyelination are interspersed in a general pattern of myelin pallor (99). There is little edema and a paucity of inflammatory cells. Milder cases may demonstrate reactive astrocytosis and myelin pallor in the absence of multinucleated giant cells, inflammation, or atrophy (100).

HIV may also directly result in acute encephalitis (101) as well as acute or chronic meningitis (90,102). The viral meningitis usually presents with fever, headache, and meningeal signs and usually remits spontaneously, but can recur (71). Neuroimaging is usually negative (35,68).

In patients with subacute encephalitis, CT is often negative or reveals atrophy only. White matter lesions are infrequently detected by CT in patients with HIV encephalopathy (35,86). In some cases, although MR has shown diffuse white matter disease and HIV has been cultured from brain tissue, the CT has been negative (92). In general, the clinical diagnosis of HIV encephalitis significantly antedates the radiographic evidence of disease (98,103).

The effects of cerebral HIV infection are clearly more evident on MR than CT (86,100). Cortical atrophy is the most frequent MR finding and is usually the only early alteration (98,104). Both cortical and central atrophy progress on serial MR examination (98,104). T2-weighted images reveal hyperintense lesions without mass effect in the periventricular white matter and centrum semiovale that correspond to foci of demyelination and vacuolation. Lesions do not enhance. Lesions may vary from scattered, isolated, unilateral foci to confluent bilateral involvement, and may be symmetric or asymmetric (Fig. 7). The extent of disease roughly parallels the clinical neurologic deterioration (98). Although MR may demonstrate these signal changes in the white matter, it cannot detect the microglial nodules and multinucleated giant cells seen at histopathology. It has been argued that a diffuse pattern of periventricular white matter hyperintensity suggests HIV encephalitis (103, 104), in contradistinction to the multifocal pattern produced by progressive multifocal leukoencephalopathy (PML) (103). However, the variability in size, extent, and distribution of lesions in both HIV-related demyelination and PML, especially early in the course of disease, precludes a definitive diagnosis based on the MR appearance alone. Clinical correlation, however, is extremely helpful as HIV encephalitis often presents with encephalopathy whereas PML is usually associated with a focal neurologic deficit.

A multicenter AIDS cohort study found sulcal enlargement and multifocal signal abnormalities on T2-weighted images in 63% of asymptomatic HIV-seropositive homosexual males compared to 48% of HIV-seronegative homosexual males (105). MR abnor-

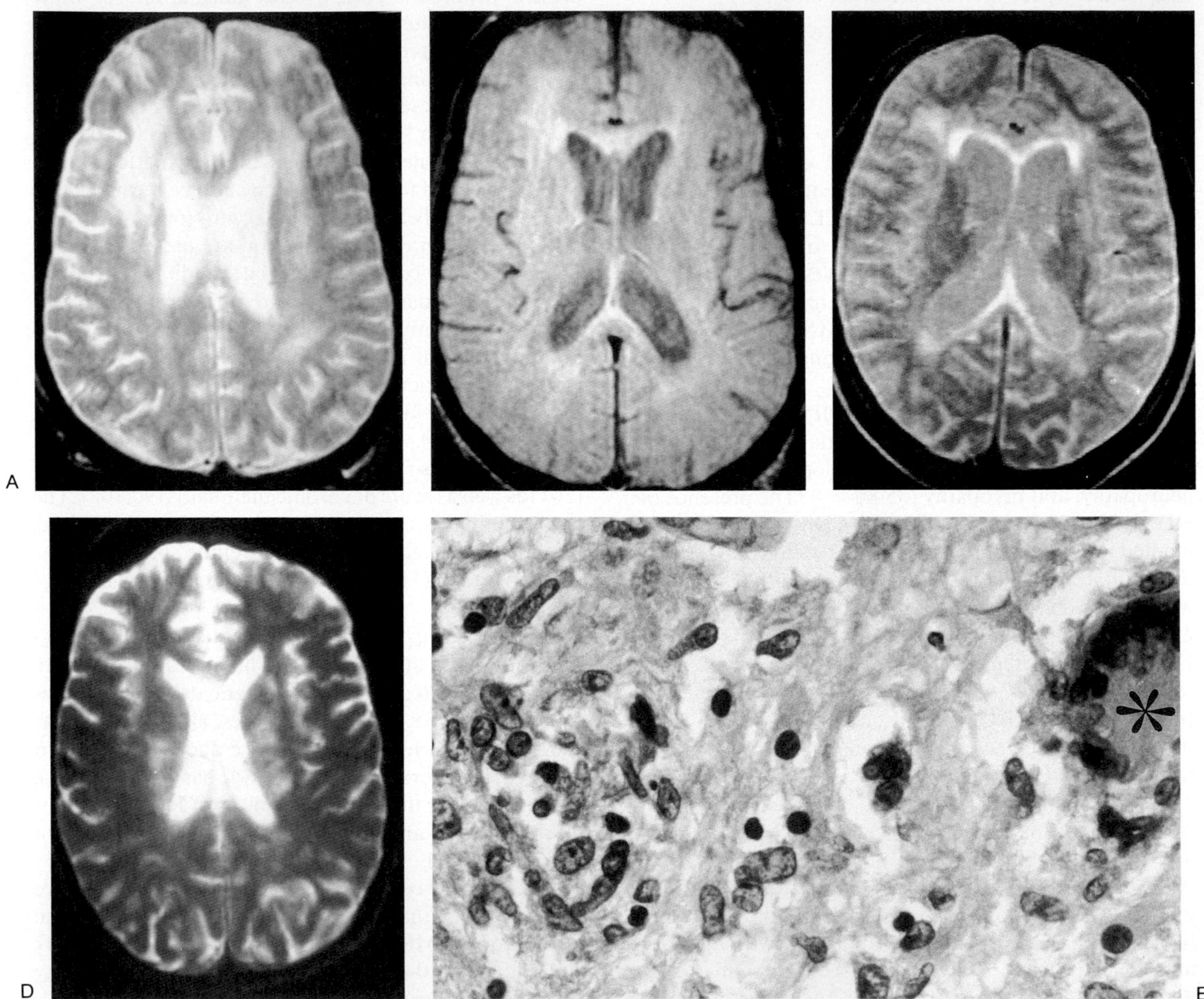

FIG. 7. HIV encephalitis. **A:** Axial T2-weighted image (2400/80) reveals patchy, asymmetric areas of increased signal involving the periventricular and, to a lesser degree, the subcortical white matter, without mass effect. Also note the presence of atrophy. Autopsy-proven HIV encephalitis. **B:** Axial proton-density image (2400/40) of same patient seen in A. Again note asymmetric areas of increased signal within the white matter. There is also involvement of the corpus callosum. **C:** Proton-density axial MR scan (2200/80) of a different patient reveals predominantly periventricular white matter disease, with some asymmetric involvement of the subcortical white matter. **D:** Another example of HIV encephalitis in a 34-year-old AIDS patient with a progressive encephalopathy. Again note periventricular areas of hyperintensity. **E:** Microglial nodules are seen in HIV encephalitis containing macrophages, microglia, astrocytes, and multinucleated giant cells (*asterisk*) (mucicarmine, original magnification ×80).

malities have been reported in approximately 50% of patients with AIDS-related complex (ARC) and 69% of patients with AIDS (106). These abnormalities included sulcal and ventricular enlargement, as well as patchy areas of hyperintensity on T2-weighted images without mass effect. These patchy areas become more diffuse, homogeneous, and confluent with clinical progression from subtle cognitive dysfunction to gross dementia (106).

Other authors have found abnormal MR exams in 13% of asymptomatic HIV-seropositive patients and 46% of symptomatic HIV-seropositive patients (107). Again, increasing cerebral atrophy and white matter disease were found to parallel the development of clinically evident neurologic disease (107).

Another study obtained initial MR exams on asymptomatic HIV-seropositive patients, with repeat studies performed at 2 to 4 years (108). Eighty percent of these exams were found to be normal and remain normal. Twenty percent had minor abnormalities that were static and stable. Serial examination of patients with mild neurologic symptoms revealed 50% of MR scans were mildly abnormal, but remained stable (108). The MR findings of minor abnormalities in asymptomatic HIV-seropositive patients may not be clinically significant as they apparently remain stable. Zidovudine (ZDV) therapy has shown partial regression of HIV-related white matter disease on MR imaging associated with improvement in cognitive function (103).

Proton MR spectroscopy has been found to detect cerebral abnormalities in HIV-infected patients. One study (109) found the NAA/Cr (*N*-acetyl aspartate/creatine) ratio to be significantly reduced in the patient group compared to the control group and was also lower in symptomatic compared to asymptomatic patients. The mean Cho/Cr (choline/creatine) ratio was significantly elevated in the patient population compared to the control group. All control spectra were found to be normal by "blinded" readers, whereas 80% of patient spectra were determined to be abnormal. MR imaging studies of these same individuals did not reveal significant differences in the white matter of the patient group versus the control group. Thus, it appears MR proton spectroscopy may reveal abnormalities before standard imaging techniques and holds a promise of early diagnosis of biochemical alterations in HIV-infected patients. Further research is necessary to determine the reliability of these findings as well as their clinical utility.

Another study (110) also found significant reductions in NAA/choline and NAA/Cr ratios in HIV-seropositive patients with neurologic dysfunction. NAA is a putative neuronal marker and thus the reduced ratios would support a theory of neuronal loss (and/or dysfunction) as a contributing factor to ADC. These reduced ratios correlated with the presence of diffuse abnormalities on MR imaging but did not correlate well with focal lesions. Cho/Cr was also elevated in patients with low CD4 counts and abnormal MR exams (110). A number of patients in this study had normal MR images but abnormal spectra (11/103) whereas another group had normal spectra but abnormal imaging (22/103). Thus, the information provided by both techniques appears to be complementary.

Pediatric HIV

In the United States, approximately 2% of AIDS patients are children, and 5% to 25% of AIDS cases worldwide occur in children (111). Seventy percent of pediatric AIDS is secondary to congenital infection via maternal transmission (112). Pediatric HIV infection may result in a progressive encephalopathy with loss of intellectual capability, motor milestones, and the development of weakness and pyramidal tract signs (113,114). This progressive encephalopathy is estimated to occur in 30% to 50% of HIV-seropositive children (115). The subacute encephalitis is likely due directly to the HIV infection (116,117). Other pediatric manifestations of direct HIV infection include microcephaly, cognitive defects, spasticity, seizures, and ataxia.

Pathologic examination reveals large multinucleated cells infected with HIV present in the brains of these children, along with inflammatory cell infiltrates and extensive calcific vasopathy, primarily involving small vessels in the basal ganglia, but also seen in the pons and cerebral white matter (87,116,117). It is postulated that during the acute phase of HIV infection, there is damage to the vascular wall of small and medium-sized arteries with secondary calcium deposition in the walls and adjacent brain (116,117). Reduced brain volume is likely related to myelin loss or diminished myelination because neuronal loss is uncommon (71).

CT most often reveals atrophy and ventricular enlargement (112,114–116). White matter hypodensity is seen infrequently. Basal ganglia calcification is often present and usually bilateral. Enhancement of the basal ganglia has also been reported (114–116). Calcifications may also be seen in the white matter of the frontal lobes (115). Serial CT scans obtained on patients treated with 3'-azido-3'deoxythymidine (zidovudine, ZDV, or AZT, Burroughs Wellcome Co., Research Triangle Park, NC) has shown improvement of the atrophic changes (112).

On MR, patchy areas of white matter disease are evident as hyperintense lesions on T2-weighted images. There is no mass effect and no enhancement. Serial MR studies reveal progression of white matter involvement, which correlates well with the progression of dementia.

Although CMV, toxoplasmosis, and PML have all been described in the pediatric AIDS population (113,114,118,119), opportunistic infections are far less common in children as compared to HIV-infected adults (113,114,117). This is partly due to a lack of exposure,

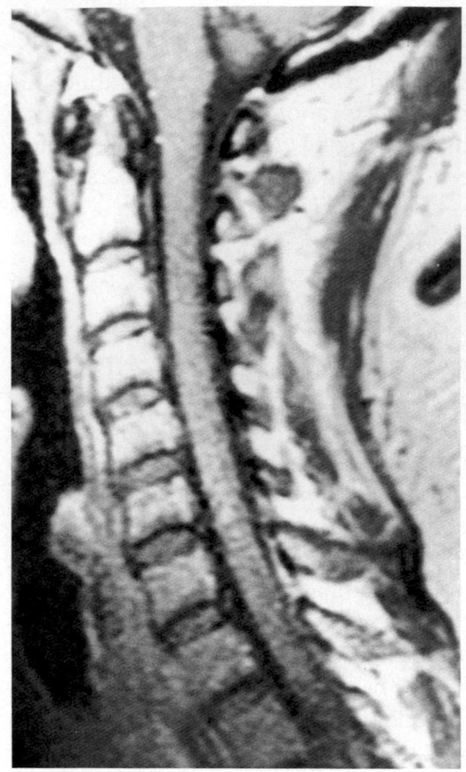

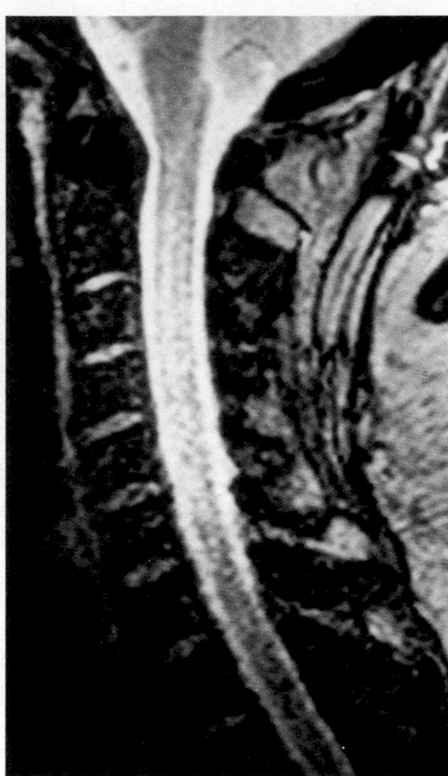

A,B

FIG. 8. Tropical spastic paraparesis. **A:** T1-weighted postcontrast sagittal MR image (600/20) of a patient with a progressive paraparesis and seropositive for HTLV-I. There is no enhancement. **B:** Gradient-echo (600/18) sagittal image of the same patient reveals abnormal increased signal throughout most of the cervical cord, without expansion.

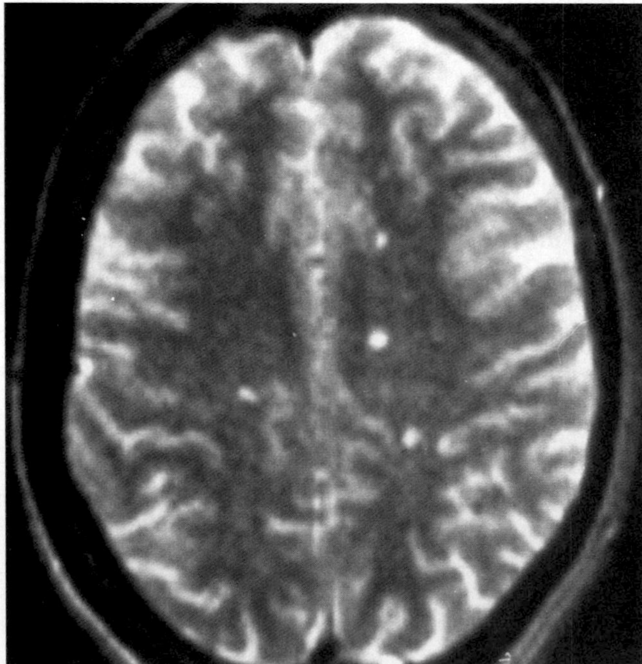

FIG. 9. Tropical spastic paraparesis (TSP). A 36-year-old woman with a 5-year history of a spastic, progressive paraparesis had markedly elevated levels of serum antibodies to HTLV-I antigen. T2-weighted (2400/100) scan reveals multiple, bilateral, punctate nodular hypointense foci, without mass effect, in the periventricular and subcortical white matter. Similar foci were present in the pons and cerebellar white matter (*not shown*).

as many of these infections are a result of reactivation. Approximately 15% of neuroimaging studies of pediatric AIDS patients reveal a focal lesion as a result of opportunistic infection or CNS lymphoma (87,115).

HTLV-1

HTLV-1 is a human retrovirus that is totally distinct from HIV in natural history and cellular effects (120). HTLV-1 has been linked to adult T-cell leukemia/lymphoma (121,122) and is considered the etiologic agent in tropical spastic paraparesis (TSP) and HTLV-1-associated myelopathy (HAM) (123,124). Although clinically similar to certain forms of multiple sclerosis (MS) (125), TSP is a distinct entity based on epidemiologic studies and serologic tests (120,126). HAM and TSP are characterized by a slowly progressive paraparesis, mild sensory disturbance, and urinary incontinence.

Autopsy studies have shown both HAM and TSP to involve the spinal cord primarily, especially the thoracic cord, where inflammatory changes, demyelination, and axonal loss may be seen (124,127) (Fig. 8). A more widespread chronic meningoencephalomyelitis is also present, with inflammatory changes involving the meninges, brainstem, and both supratentorial and infratentorial white matter. Thickening of the media and adventitia of blood vessels in the subarachnoid space, the spinal cord, and the brain suggests a vasculitis as well (127). Although HTLV-1 has been isolated from CSF lymphocytes of a patient with HAM (128), it is uncertain whether the neuropathologic changes are due to HTLV-1-infected lymphocytes or to direct neurotropism of the retrovirus (120).

T2-weighted MR imaging of the brain reveals punctate and nodular discrete hyperintense foci, without mass effect, in the periventricular and subcortical white matter in approximately 50% of patients (129,130) (Fig. 9). Lesions are most often discrete but may be confluent (131). The appearance is nonspecific and must be differentiated from other white matter lesions such as MS, Lyme disease, HIV-related demyelination, ischemia, and vasculitis. The white matter lesions do not enhance (132). Serial studies reveal an increase in number of these white matter lesions in affected patients (132).

Progressive Multifocal Leukoencephalopathy

Progressive multifocal leukoencephalopathy (PML) is a progressive demyelinating disorder arising from CNS infection with a papovavirus. The etiologic agent is a human polyomavirus, the JC virus, which belongs to the papova family of CNS viruses (*pa*pilloma, *po*lyoma, *vac*uolating virus) (133).

PML was first described by Astrom et al. in 1958 (134). In 1965, electron microscopy revealed innumerable virus-like particles within inclusion bodies of oligodendrocytic nuclei (135,136). In 1971, the virus was isolated from the post-mortem brain of a patient with PML (137). The initials of this donor patient were JC, and thus the virus was termed the JC virus. The target of the JC virus is the oligodendrocyte, which forms and maintains the myelin sheath (138). Infection of the oligodendrocyte causes cytolytic destruction and thus results in myelin loss (139). The axon is usually spared. Electron microscopy can identify intranuclear inclusions within the oligodendrocyte consisting of JC virus particles (136,140). Enlarged, abnormal astrocytes are also a pathologic feature of PML. These astrocytes are multinucleated with numerous large processes (141) (Fig. 10). Microscopic foci of scattered demyelination enlarge over time and co-

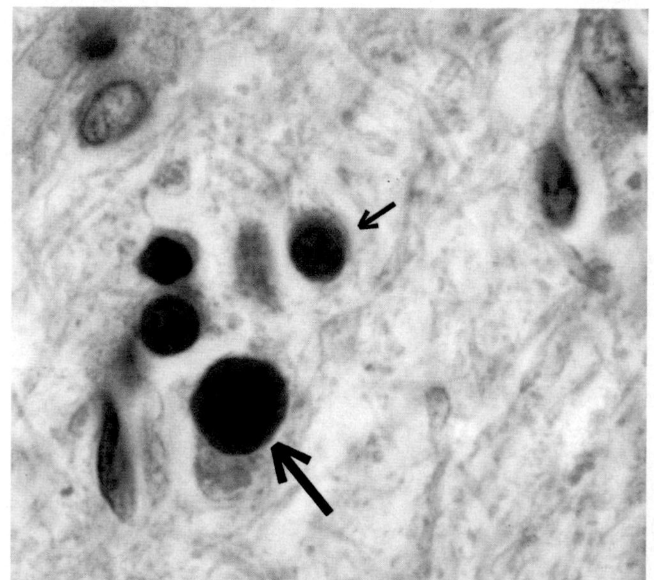
A

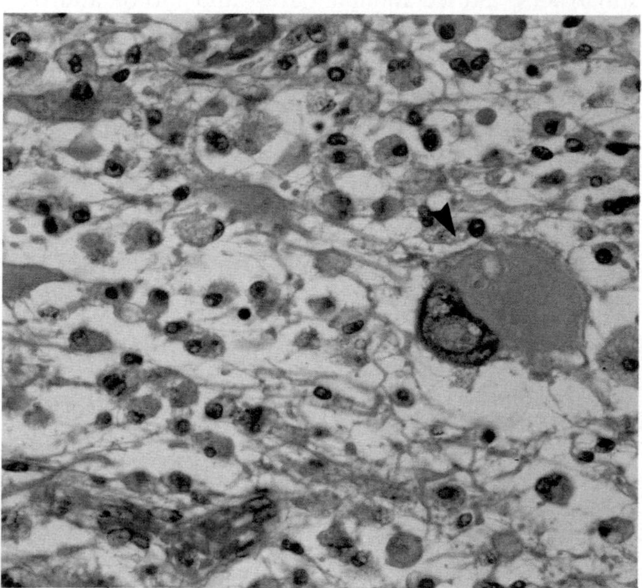
B

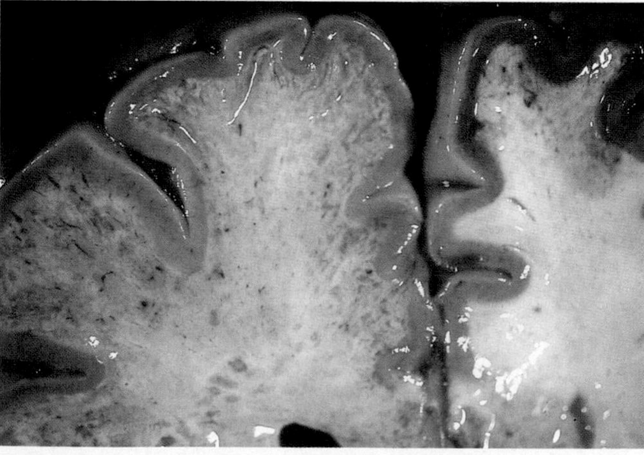
C

FIG. 10. Progressive multifocal leukoencephalopathy. **A:** High power photomicrograph reveals an oligodendrocyte in the center of the field, packed tightly with intranuclear inclusions (*large arrow*). For comparison, an uninfected oligodendrocyte (*small arrow*) is also indicated (H & E stain, original magnification ×200). **B:** Gemistocytic astrocytosis (*arrow*) from same case seen in A (H & E stain; original magnification ×120). (From Whiteman et al., ref. 119, with permission.) **C:** Gross specimen reveals brownish discoloration of the white matter on the right, due to the loss of myelin in PML.

alesce (139). Gross examination of the brain reveals a gray or brownish discoloration of the white matter as a result of the myelin loss (119).

Seroepidemiologic studies indicate the JC virus infects 80% of the human population before adulthood without producing overt illness (141). Antibodies to the JC virus are nearly ubiquitous among the adult population worldwide (119,142). The virus typically remains latent unless there is reactivation due to immunodeficiency (142). Before the era of AIDS, PML was primarily associated with other immunodeficient disorders, including renal transplantation, autoimmune disease, tuberculosis, sarcoidosis, Whipple's disease, nontropical sprue, and lymphoproliferative disorders (134). Patients treated with chemotherapy are also at increased risk for PML. Currently, PML appears to have a stronger association with AIDS than with any other immunosuppressive disorder (143) and 55% to 85% of recent PML cases are attributable to AIDS (102,144). PML is present in approximately 5% of AIDS patients at autopsy (119).

Clinical presentation of PML includes memory loss, visual deficit, personality change, cognitive and speech disturbances, altered mental status, and motor and/or sensory abnormalities with a progressive neurologic decline (134,145). Less frequent signs and symptoms include vertigo, seizures, headache, and aphasia (102,134). There is relentless progression of disease, with death often occurring within 9 months of the onset of symptoms (134). The most common symptoms of PML are hemiparesis, visual impairment, and altered mentation (102,119); patients with lesions of the posterior fossa exhibit ataxia, dysarthria, and dysmetria (146,147). Homonomous hemianopsia is the most frequent visual deficit. Spinal cord involvement is rare (1,148).

On CT, PML appears as a focal hypodensity within the white matter, usually without significant mass effect and usually without enhancement. Most often lesions are present in both periventricular and subcortical white matter, although involvement may be isolated to either the subcortical or periventricular white matter (119). CT may be negative in early lesions (149). Patchy enhancement is seen occasionally (119). Serial scans demonstrate progressive disease.

MR demonstrates far greater sensitivity than CT in the imaging of PML, in defining both the extent and number of lesions (119,138). MR is thus the procedure of choice in imaging of PML (138). On T2-weighted images, lesions demonstrate increased signal intensity in the periventricular and/or subcortical white matter (Fig. 11). Lesions may be initially small, but usually progress to larger areas of involvement (Fig. 12). A multifocal distribution pattern is seen, which may be unilateral but is more often bilateral and asymmetric (119). There is an absence of mass effect and lesions rarely enhance. When enhancement is present, it is faint and peripheral (119) (Fig. 13). The subcortical lesions follow the gray-white interface, resulting in a "scalloped" appearance because of involvement of subcortical U-fibers (119) (Fig. 14). On T1-

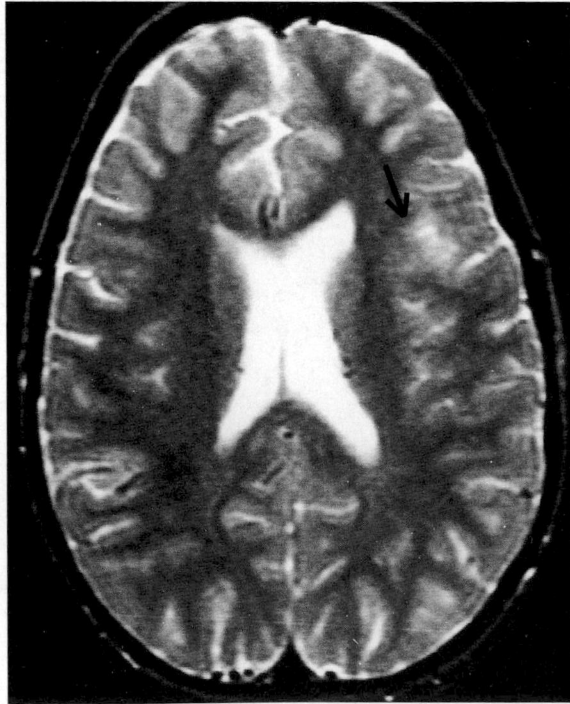

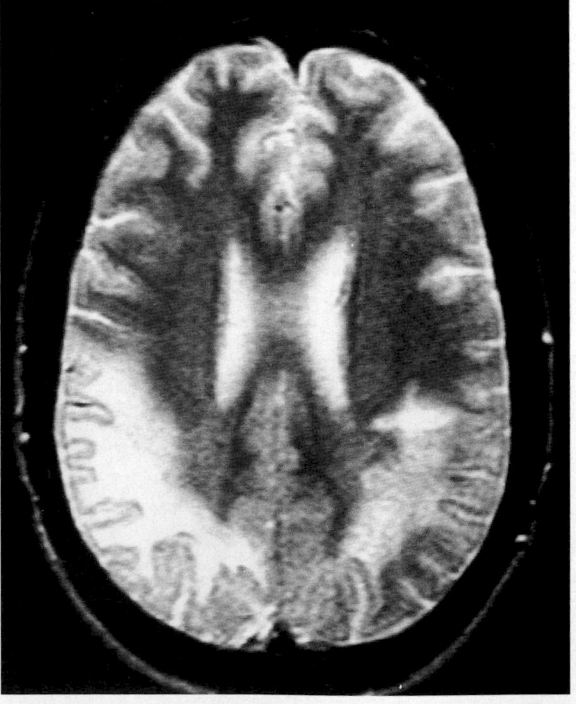

FIG. 11. Progressive multifocal leukoencephalopathy (autopsy-proven). **A:** Subtle disease is noted in the left frontal subcortical region (*arrow*) on this T2-weighted (2400/80) MR image. **B:** Florid, bilateral parieto-occipital involvement is noted in a different patient, also with PML. T2-weighted (2200/80) axial MR reveals hyperintensity of the parieto-occipital white matter, without mass effect.

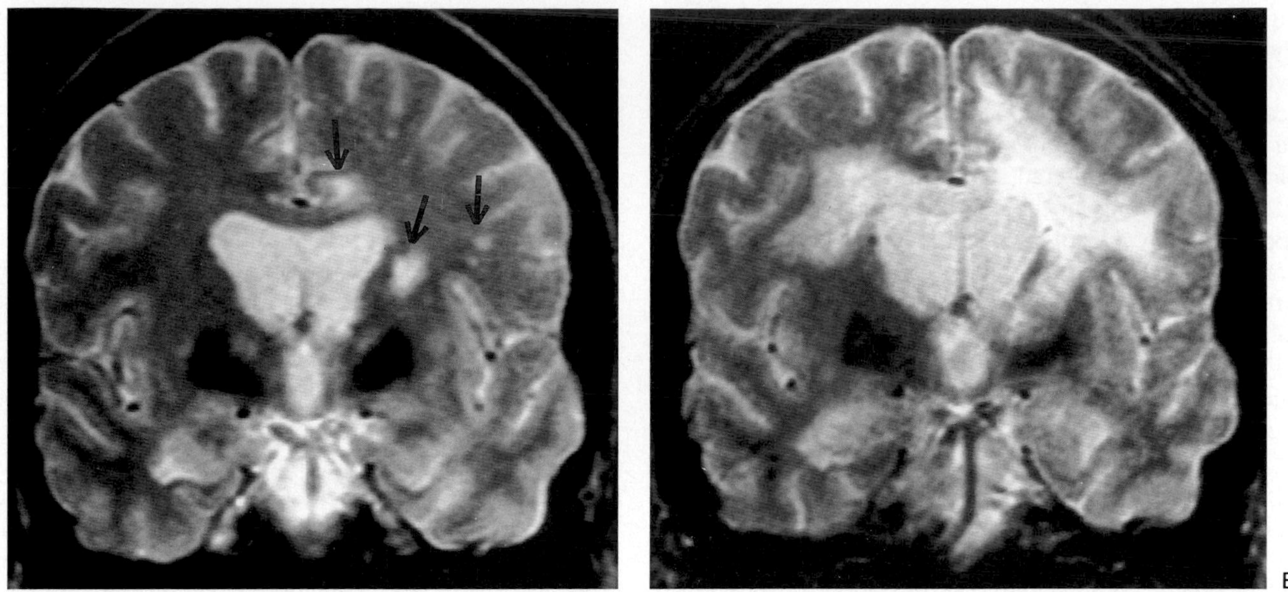

FIG. 12. Progressive multifocal leukoencephalopathy (biopsy and autopsy proven). **A:** Initial T2-weighted (2400/80) coronal MR scan demonstrates small foci of disease (*arrows*). **B:** This scan, obtained 3 months later on the same patient as in A, reveals marked progression of disease that is now bilateral and also involves the corpus callosum and basal ganglia.

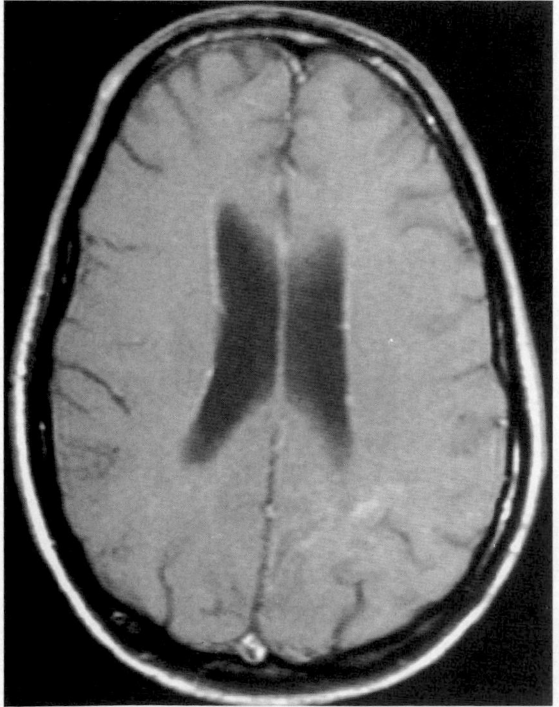

FIG. 13. Progressive multifocal leukoencephalopathy (autopsy- and biopsy-proven). T1-weighted (600/20) postgadolinium MR image of a patient with pathologically proven PML reveals faint enhancement along the edge of a lesion.

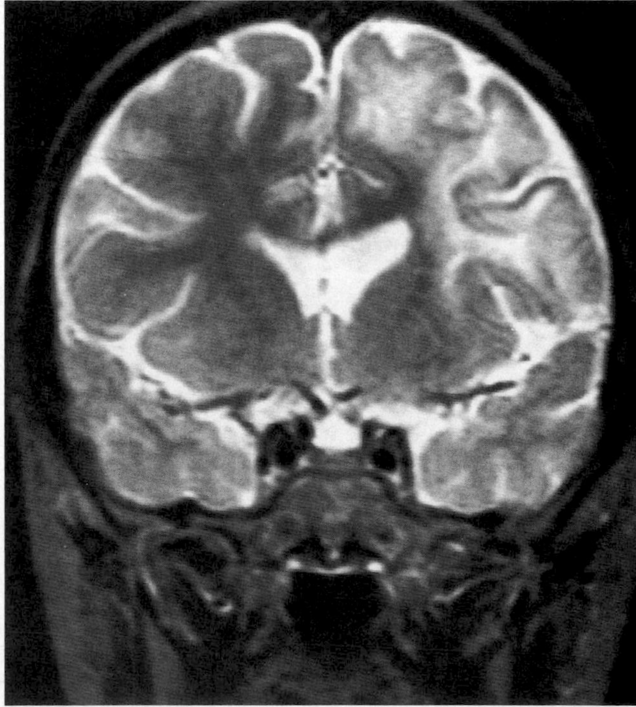

FIG. 14. Progressive multifocal leukoencephalopathy (pathologically-proven). T2-weighted (1750/80) axial MR scan of a child with PML who became HIV positive following liver transplantation for biliary atresia. Note "scalloping" of the white matter.

weighted images, the lesions are usually hypointense to parenchyma, although early lesions may be isointense (Fig. 15). By contrast, HIV-related demyelination is usually isointense on T1-weighted images. Any lobe may be involved by PML, but the frontal and parieto-occipital locations are most common and thus correlate well with the symptoms of homonomous hemianopsia, focal neurologic deficit, and altered mentation.

PML commonly affects the posterior fossa (Fig. 16). Approximately 1/3 of PML cases have some involvement of the posterior fossa (119). There are often synchronous supratentorial lesions, although PML may be isolated to the infratentorial region in about 10% of cases (71). PML may also appear to involve the deep gray structures because of involvement of small myelinated fibers which course through the basal ganglia and adjacent parenchyma (119).

In AIDS patients, PML may be difficult to distinguish radiographically from HIV-related demyelination. PML is more often multifocal, asymmetric, with "scalloping" and a greater predilection for the subcortical white matter. HIV encephalitis is more often diffuse, symmetric, and periventricular in location. Clinical correlation is essential, as mentioned earlier, because HIV encephalitis most often presents with global disturbance and dementia whereas PML presents with focal motor or sensory deficit and dementia is infrequent (77).

Effective treatment remains elusive. Future investigation must be directed toward therapy that specifically targets the JC virus (139).

Subacute Sclerosing Panencephalitis

A slow, progressive infection by a measles virus (morbillivirus genus) causes the often fatal condition known as subacute sclerosing panencephalitis (SSPE). Typically, children between the ages of 5 and 12 years old who had clinical measles before the age of 3 years are affected (150). Four clinical stages have been described progressing from initial mental or behavioral abnormalities (Stage I) to loss of cerebral cortical function (Stage IV) over a period of 1 to 3 years (151). Death usually occurs within 2 to 6 years. The diagnosis is established by the presence of elevated titers of measles antibodies in the CSF and serum, abnormal complexes on EEG, and clinical manifestations. Estimated yearly incidence is approximately one case per million population (75). Pathologically, the primary abnormalities involve white matter, especially the centrum semiovale, where variable

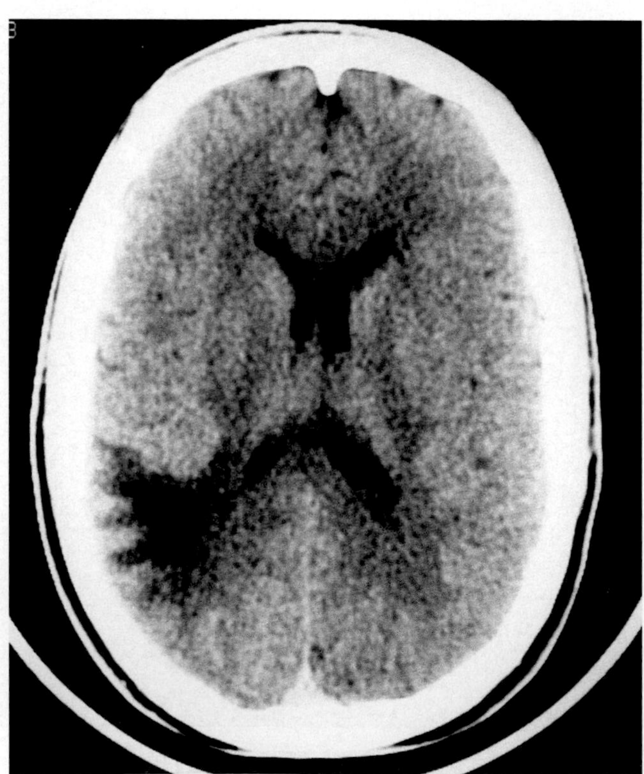
A

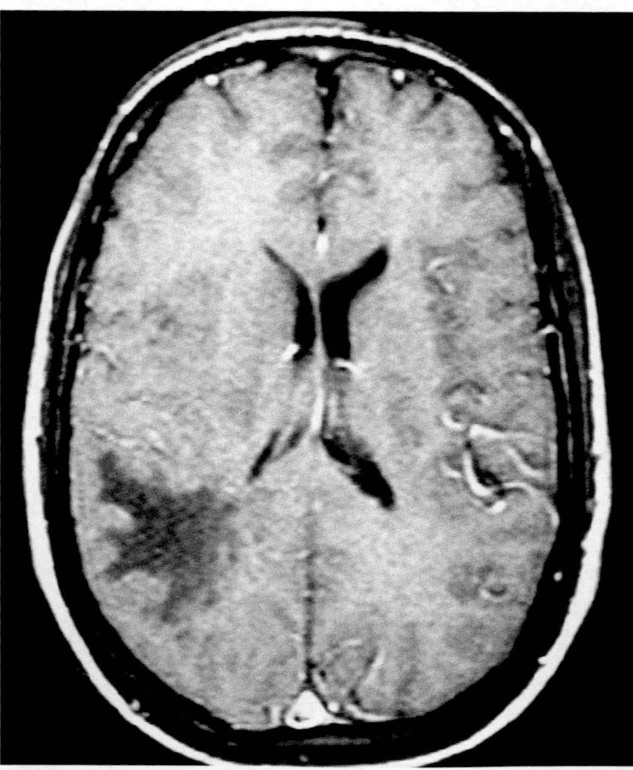
B

FIG. 15. Progressive multifocal leukoencephalopathy (autopsy-proven). **A:** Axial postcontrast CT reveals hypodense lesion on the right, without enhancement. **B:** Postgadolinium (0.1 mm/Kg) T1-weighted MR of the same patient reveals marked hypointensity of the lesion, without significant enhancement.

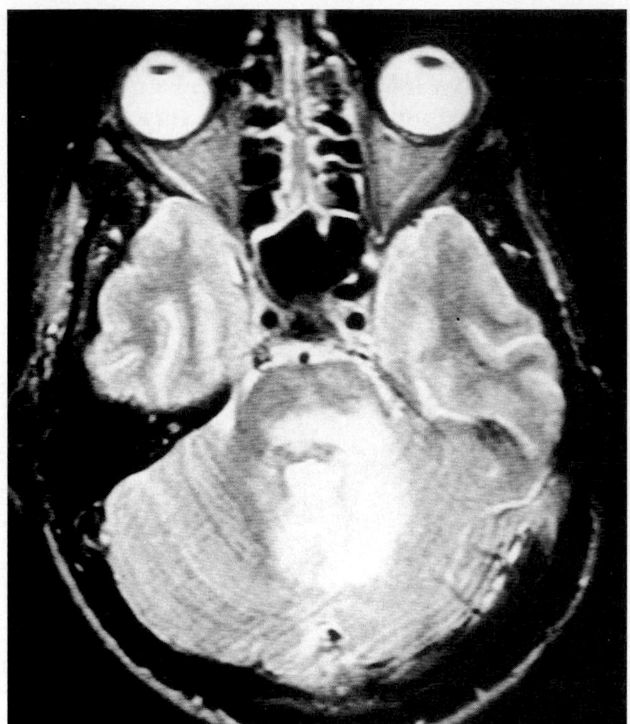

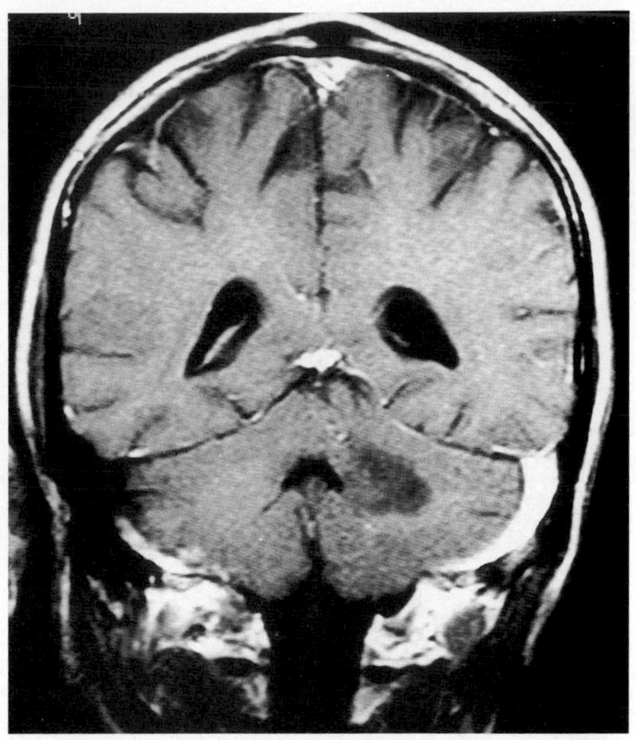

FIG. 16. Progressive multifocal leukoencephalopathy (biopsy-proven). **A:** T2-weighted (2650/80) axial MR of a patient with AIDS reveals hyperintense signal bilaterally in the cerebellum, the pons, and the cerebellar peduncles, without mass effect on the fourth ventricle. **B:** Coronal postgadolinium (0.1 mm/Kg) T1-weighted scan reveals hypointense signal in the posterior fossa on the left, without appreciable enhancement or mass effect.

degrees of patchy (Stages I and II) to diffuse (Stages III and IV) demyelination and gliosis are found (1). Inflammation is usually minimal. Neuronal loss and gliosis occur in the gray matter, and pathologic changes may also be found in the basal ganglia, pons and thalamus.

MR demonstrates the periventricular white matter lesions, as well as those in the basal ganglia, which are only infrequently detected by CT (150,152). Patients with Stage III and IV disease have diffuse bilateral periventricular white matter signal abnormalities because of prolonged relaxation times and increased water content (150,152). There is no mass effect. Frontal and/or occipital white matter involvement may be more extensive (150). Focal, well-circumscribed areas of hyperintensity on T2-weighted images can be seen in the basal ganglia, especially the putamen (153). These lesions are usually bilateral, and may be either symmetric (153) or asymmetric (150). T2-weighted images may demonstrate hyperintense lesions, undetected by CT, in the cerebellar white matter and pons. These areas of abnormal signal are thought to correspond to the demyelination and gliosis that are seen on pathologic examination (154,155). Atrophy may be the only finding in very slowly progressive cases of SSPE (156).

Another paramyxovirus, mumps virus, can cause lesions of the basal ganglia similar to those described for SSPE, as well as scattered hyperintense foci in the cerebral and cerebellar white matter, thalami, and brainstem on T2-weighted images (157,158). These findings, however, occur in the setting of an acute encephalitis (159).

Creutzfeldt-Jakob Disease

Creutzfeldt-Jakob disease (CJD) results in an uncommon, rapidly progressive dementia that may be difficult to distinguish clinically from other forms of dementia (160). This fatal disease of the CNS was first described by Creutzfeldt in 1920 and by Jakob in 1921 (161,162). Like kuru and scrapie, CJD is thought to be caused by an "unconventional virus" known as a prion (163). Prions are small proteinaceous infectious particles that differ from standard viruses in that they contain little or no nucleic acid and do not evoke an immune response during infection (163). The specific mechanism by which this prion causes CNS degeneration is unknown. Most cases are sporadic (163), 10% to 15% of cases are familial (1). A few cases have been linked to corneal transplantation, injection of growth hormone, and implantation of cerebral electrodes (163). Incidence is estimated at 0.25 to 2 cases per million population per year worldwide (164).

Clinical presentation is classically that of a rapidly progressive dementia associated with upper motor neuron dysfunction and myoclonic jerks. Most patients are between the ages of 40 and 80 years (160). The clinical symptoms of CJD are diverse. Some patients present with sensory abnormalities, confusion, and/or inappropriate behavior, or with cerebellar ataxia (165). A number of clinical subtypes have been identified, which include the myoclonus type, Heidenhain's syndrome, dyskinetic type, intermediate type, amyotrophic type, ataxic form, Alpers' disease, and the Gerstmann-Straussler syndrome (166). The prognosis is poor, with a mean

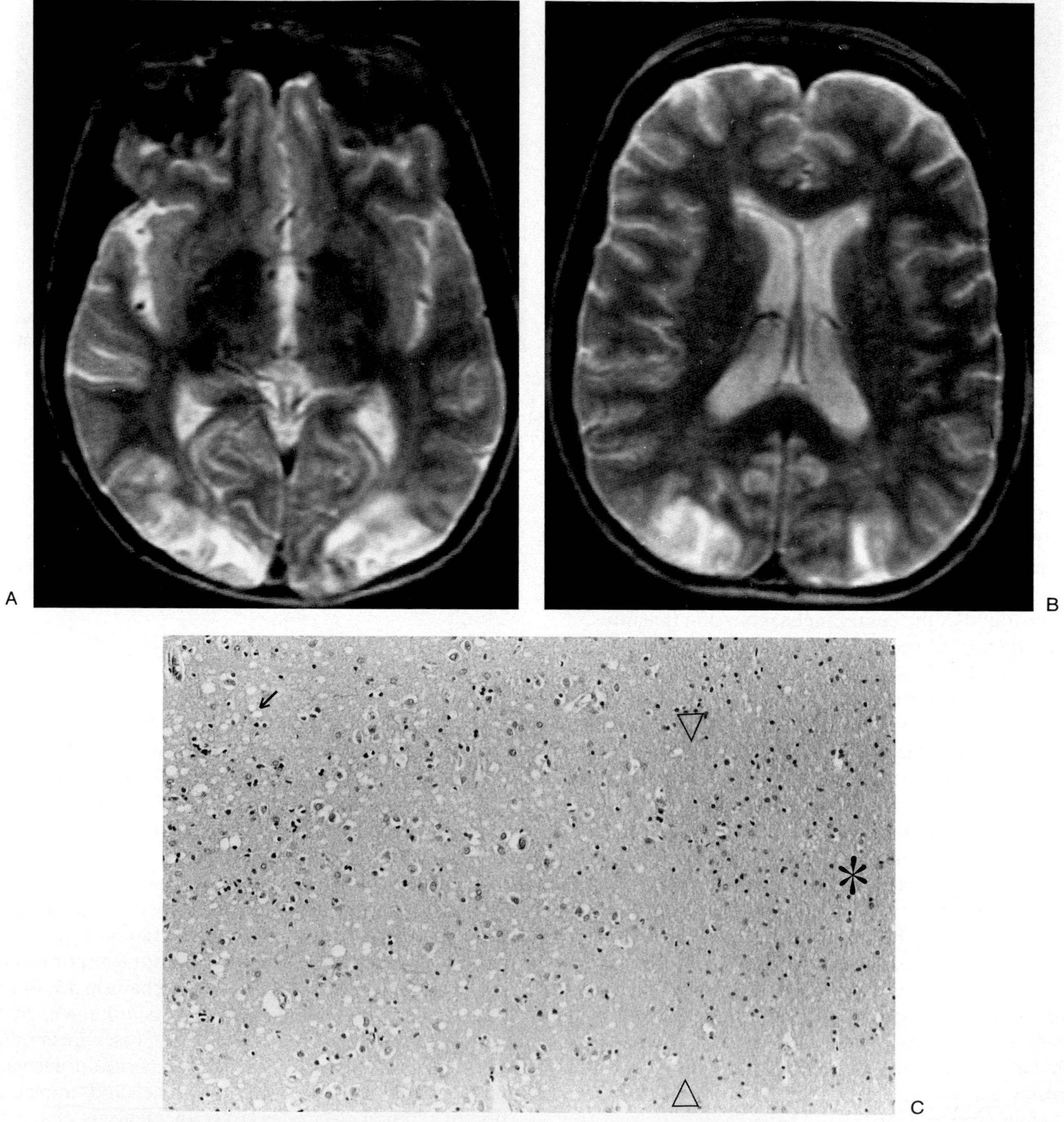

FIG. 17. Creutzfeldt-Jakob disease (pathologically proven). **A,B:** T2-weighted (2400/80) axial MR images reveal hyperintense signal involving cortical and subcortical regions of both occipital lobes. These findings are compatible with the occipitoparietal pathologic subtype (vide supra). **C:** Pathologic specimen of a different patient demonstrates numerous vacuoles (*small arrow*) within the cerebral cortex, sparing the white matter (*asterisk*) (H & E, original magnification ×20). *Arrowheads* denote cortex/white matter interface.

survival of less than 1 year from the onset of symptoms and only 10% surviving for more than 2 years (167). EEG reveals diffuse slowing with superimposed bursts of sharp waves (160). CSF is usually normal, but may show a slightly elevated protein content (1).

Microscopically, CJD is characterized by spongiform change in the cortical as well as subcortical gray matter, with loss of neurons and replacement gliosis. White matter is usually spared, except for secondary wallerian degeneration (168,169). There is, however, considerable topographic variation. Atrophy may occur diffusely or may be predominantly confined to cortex, cerebellum, thalamus, basal ganglia, or specific tracts (1). Inflammatory changes are absent (170). CJD may be divided into three main pathologic variants: frontopyramidal (33%), occipitoparietal (18%), and diffuse cortical/basal ganglia type (49%). Any of these variants may also reveal lesions of the thalamus, midbrain, cerebellum, or spinal cord (171).

CT of patients with CJD is most often normal but may reveal atrophy in approximately 20% of cases (172). Initial CT studies that are normal may progress to atrophy on follow-up examinations (169,173). Hypodense lesions of the occipital lobes have been reported (160). In patients with CJD, CT is most useful in excluding focal lesions that may contribute to the clinical symptoms (169).

MR has been shown to be more sensitive than CT in the detection of abnormalities in CJD (Fig. 17) (160). MR may only reveal atrophy in some cases (160). T2-weighted images have shown symmetric increased signal in other patients in the caudate nuclei (174), corpus striatum, thalamus and cortex (175), basal ganglia (176), periventricular white matter (177), and occipital lobes (160). Lesions do not enhance and do not demonstrate mass effect.

Acute Disseminated Encephalomyelitis

In acute disseminated encephalomyelitis (ADEM), neurologic signs and symptoms typically begin 5 days to 2 weeks following a viral illness (especially varicella, measles, and rubella) or vaccination, and resemble signs and symptoms associated with primary viral encephalitis, toxic encephalopathy, or acute multiple sclerosis (MS) (178,179). Headaches, fever, and drowsiness may be the initial symptoms (180). Thereafter, there is rapid progression to seizure or focal neurologic deficit that can further progress to coma and death (181). Thus, antemortem diagnosis of ADEM is made infrequently. The pathologic hallmark of this disease is multifocal perivenous demyelination, thought to be a consequence of complement-mediated endothelial damage, with absence of recoverable virus from the brain (178,182).

MR demonstrates patchy areas of increased signal intensity on T2-weighted images in the deep and subcortical white matter of the cerebral hemispheres, as well as in the cerebellar white matter and brainstem (Fig. 18) (179,183). The spinal cord may be involved. Characteristically, there are few lesions, with an asymmetric distribution and an absence of hemorrhage. The location of the lesions on MR often correlates with the clinical signs and symptoms. Thus, MR is the study of choice, as CT is either normal or reveals abnormalities that correlate poorly with neurologic deficits (184).

The lesions in ADEM usually exhibit no mass effect, although enlargement of the medulla has been described in one case (179). Although multiple lesions may demonstrate enhancement, not all lesions necessarily enhance (180,181). Treatment is with high-dose steroids, resulting in clinical improvement as well as progressive resolution of the MR signal abnormalities.

The differential diagnosis for this MR appearance includes embolic infarction (which should conform to a vascular distribution, involving both gray and white matter), vasculitis (which may also involve both gray and white matter), acute hemorrhagic leukoencephalopathy (which would demonstrate evidence of hemorrhage), and MS. MS and ADEM may be indistinguishable by plain and contrast MR, although a greater number of enhancing lesions can be seen with ADEM. The clinical course of the disease will often distinguish one entity from the other. Typical MR findings in combination with the appropriate clinical presentation may suggest the diagnosis of ADEM and MR may be used, as well, to follow response to therapy (179).

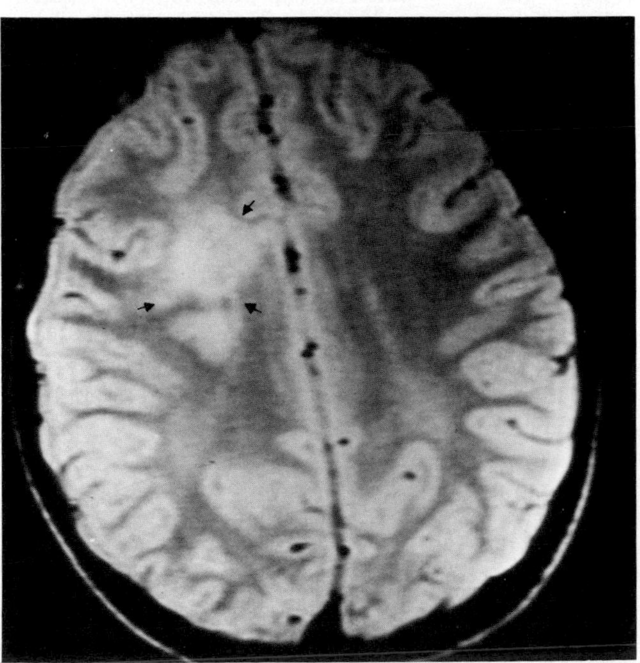

FIG. 18. Acute disseminated encephalomyelitis. Proton-density axial MR image reveals focal regions of hyperintensity (*arrows*) within the white matter. Clinical correlation is essential to making a diagnosis of ADEM.

Rasmussen's Encephalitis

Rasmussen's encephalitis, first described in 1958 (185), is a childhood disorder of severe epilepsy and progressive neurologic deficits with frequent episodes of epilepsia partialis continua and, less often, generalized status epilepticus (186). The seizures are intractable, and resistant to medical therapy. Partial motor seizures predominate, although a mixture of seizure types may occur. Permanent motor deficits result, associated with mental deterioration (186). The brain damage may be so insidious in onset and gradual in course that the clinical diagnosis may not be readily apparent. The intractable seizures may necessitate hemispherectomy because medical treatment is often ineffective (186).

The specific cause of Rasmussen's encephalitis is unknown, although pathologic findings suggest a chronic viral encephalitis. The disease tends to affect one hemisphere, although bilateral involvement at initial presentation has also been reported (187). Microscopic features include perivascular lymphocytic cuffing of round cells, microglial proliferation, and scattered glial nodules (186). With disease progression, cortical atrophy, spongy degeneration, and neuronal loss is seen without evidence of active inflammation.

CT obtained early in the course of the disease is often normal. Chronic cases demonstrate focal and progressive atrophy of the affected hemisphere, which correlates well with EEG abnormalities (186). Initial MR exams may also be normal. Serial scans demonstrate focal or hemispheric atrophy, and T2-weighted images may reveal areas of increased signal in the white matter and/or putamen (186). Xenon CT cerebral blood flow studies reveal decreased flow to the affected hemisphere (186). Similarly, ^{18}F-fluorodeoxyglucose (FDG) PET scans demonstrate decreased tracer uptake at involved sites (186).

BACTERIAL INFECTIONS

Pyogenic Bacteria

The most commonly encountered forms of pyogenic bacterial infection of the CNS are focal cerebritis, abscess, meningitis, and extra-axial (subdural or epidural) empyema.

Cerebritis Abscess

Pathologically, cerebritis is described as a localized yet poorly demarcated area of parenchymal softening with scattered necrosis, edema, vascular congestion, petechial hemorrhage, and perivascular inflammatory infiltrates (188,189). Commonly, cerebritis results from direct spread of infection, either otorhinologic infection or meningitis (including retrograde septic thrombophlebitis), or from hematogenous spread from an extracranial focus of infection.

T2-weighted spin-echo MR images demonstrate early cerebritis as an area of increased signal intensity indistinguishable from, or slightly hypointense to, surrounding edema (6). The inherent sensitivity of proton-density and T2-weighted images to alterations in tissue water enables earlier detection of cerebritis compared to CT (30). On T1-weighted images, cerebritis appears isointense to slightly hypointense to adjacent normal brain parenchyma, with associated mass effect, manifested by sulcal effacement or ventricular compression. T1-weighted images also reveal foci of subacute hemorrhage as hyperintense relative to normal and edematous brain. Contrast enhancement is minimal and inhomogeneous.

A focus of cerebritis progresses to abscess when the central zone of necrosis within the area of cerebritis becomes liquefied, better defined and encircled by a collagen capsule, which itself is surrounded by a prominent zone of gliosis (188,189). The evolution to abscess has been characterized by four stages: early cerebritis, late cerebritis, early capsule formation, and late capsule formation (188–190). In the final stage, the collagen capsule is complete and the surrounding area of cerebritis extends only minimally beyond the capsule, which is less well developed on its ventricular side than on its cortical side, probably related to slight differences in perfusion. Daughter abscesses become apparent during this stage.

The length of time required to form a mature abscess varies from 2 weeks to several months (188,191). In adults, abscesses arising from hematogeneous spread are most often caused by anaerobic bacteria or a mixture of anaerobes and aerobes (191,192). In children, staphylococci, streptococci, and pneumococci are the most common pathogens (188,191). In patients with a history of trauma or prior neurosurgical procedure, abscesses are usually due to *Staphylococcus aureus* (188,191).

Most patients present in the late cerebritis or mature abscess stages (6). In more than 50% of cases of hematogenously disseminated infection, a solitary abscess is found that is usually located at the gray-white matter junction in the distribution of the anterior or middle cerebral arteries, i.e., most commonly in the frontal and parietal lobes (188). Cerebellar abscesses constitute 2% to 14% of all brain abscesses (193,194).

Pyogenic abscesses possess characteristic MR features, which are frequently sufficient to make an accurate diagnosis (195). In the usual case of a mature abscess with central liquefactive necrosis, the center of the cavity is slightly hyperintense to CSF whereas the surrounding edematous brain is slightly hypointense to normal brain parenchyma on T1-weighted images (30,195) (Fig. 19). On T2-weighted images the signal intensities are quite variable depending on the TE chosen and the protein

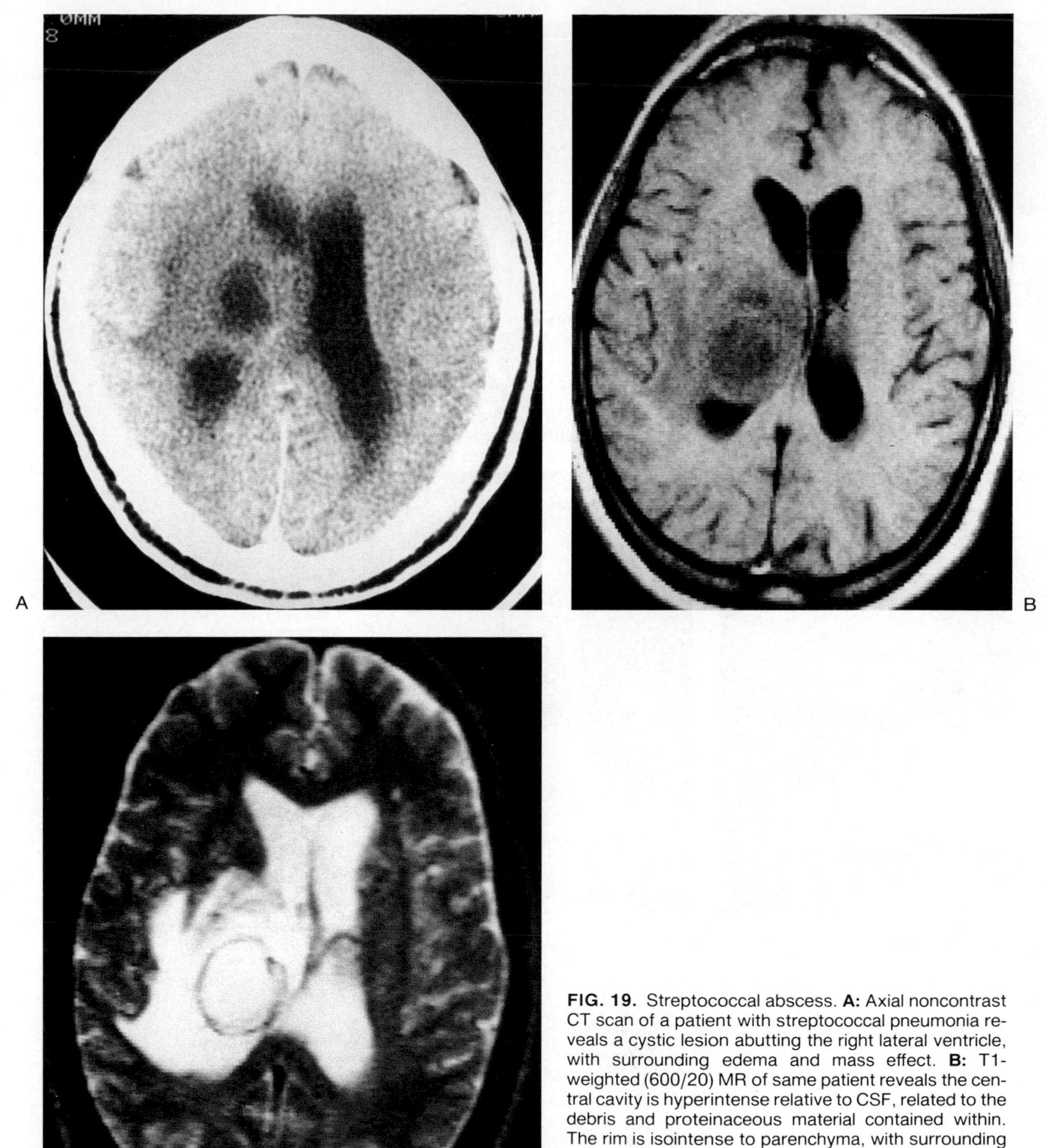

FIG. 19. Streptococcal abscess. **A:** Axial noncontrast CT scan of a patient with streptococcal pneumonia reveals a cystic lesion abutting the right lateral ventricle, with surrounding edema and mass effect. **B:** T1-weighted (600/20) MR of same patient reveals the central cavity is hyperintense relative to CSF, related to the debris and proteinaceous material contained within. The rim is isointense to parenchyma, with surrounding hypointense edema and mass effect, with midline shift. **C:** T2-weighted (2000/80) MR of same case reveals marked hypointensity of the abscess rim. The central cavity and edema both appear isointense to CSF.

composition and fluidity of the material in the central cavity. With a long TE (>100 msec) the differences in intensity between CSF, cavity fluid, and edema usually diminish. This is because the contribution of T2 relaxation to the signal intensity on long TR images is maximized. The T1 contribution to contrast is significant at short and intermediate TE, and it is this contribution to contrast that gives the central proteinaceous fluid and the brain edema a higher signal intensity than CSF. Without protein and other macromolecular components that shorten T1 (196), the cavity fluid would be nearly equal to CSF in signal intensity.

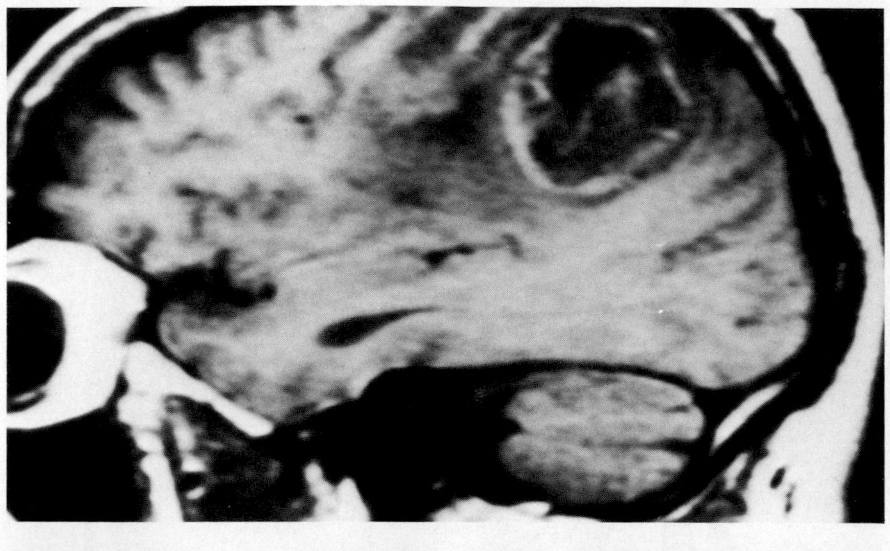

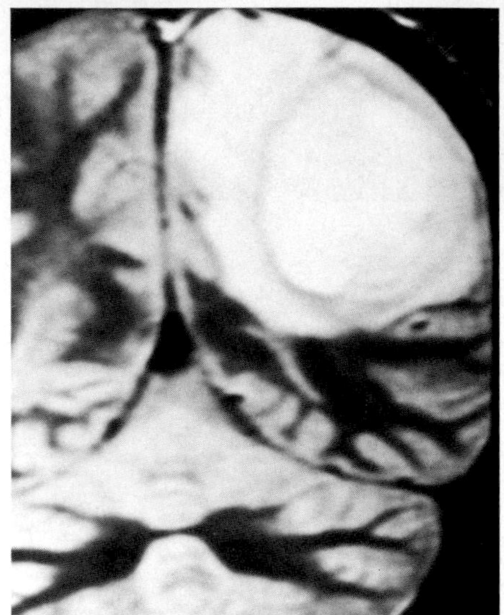
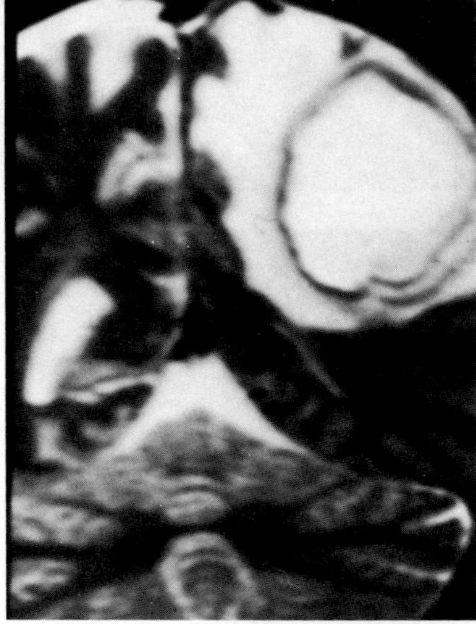

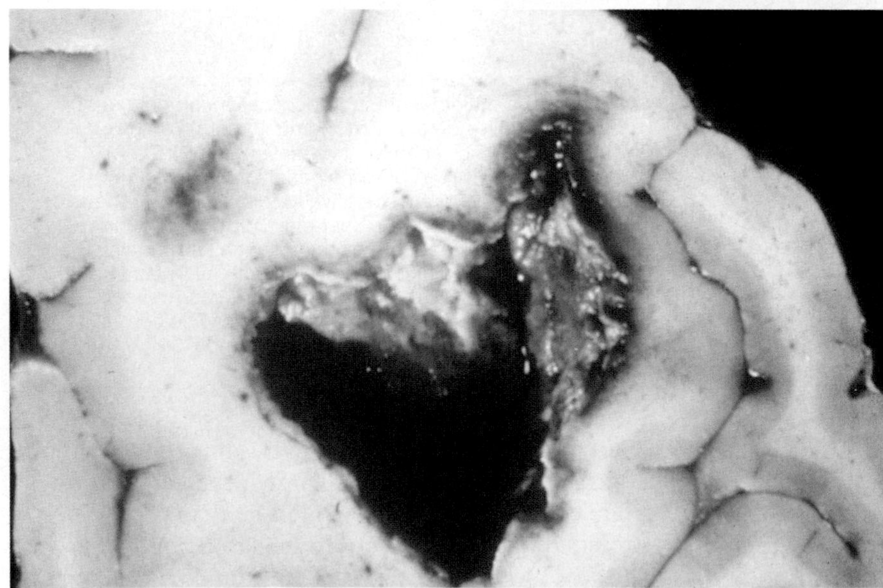

FIG. 20. MR characteristics of pyogenic bacterial abscess. **A:** Sagittal T1-weighted (600/20) MR (noncontrast) reveals a thin rim of hyperintensity at the periphery of the lesion. **B:** Proton-density (2500/20) and **C**, T2-weighted (2500/80) coronal images demonstrate hypointensity of the same peripheral rim. The etiology of this hypointense rim has been ascribed to both hemorrhage and free radical formation in the abscess capsule (*see text*). Central cavity is necrotic and amenable to surgical drainage. **D:** Gross specimen from a different patient demonstrating the necrotic cavity of a bacterial abscess.

On unenhanced MR images, the mature abscess often has a rim with distinctive features (6,195) (Fig. 20). The rim is isointense to slightly hyperintense to white matter on TW1 and is hypointense on T2-weighted images. The rim reportedly does not show the mesial thinning seen with the collagen capsule, nor is the rim identical to the ring enhancement seen on contrast studies (6). The signal properties of the rim seen on MR have been attributed to collagen, hemorrhage, or paramagnetic free radicals within phagocytosing macrophages, which are heterogeneously distributed in the periphery of the abscess (6,30,195). In the latter hypothesis, localized shortening of T1 and T2 relaxation times accounts for the signal properties. Support for this hypothesis is based on the fact that a similar hypointense rim on T2-weighted images has been observed for granulomas, which are not notably hemorrhagic and for some metastases, which have no pathologic evidence of iron deposition or hemorrhage, but do have abundant macrophages (6). To complicate matters further, however, it is well established that free radicals promote the formation of methemoglobin so, in fact, both hemorrhage and free radicals may play a role in the generation of the described signal characteristics. The hypointense rim resolves within successful surgical and/or medical treatment of the abscess with a reduction in phagocytic activity. Thus, the rim may be a better indicator of response to treatment than residual enhancement, which can persist on contrast studies for months after completion of therapy (6,197). Other lesions that may have a hypointense rim on T2-weighted images include evolving hematomas and infrequently metastases.

The ring enhancement of an abscess capsule on postgadolinium MR images parallels the enhancement seen on postcontrast CT images (Fig. 21) (195,198). By CT, the ring is usually smooth and thin walled ($\approx$5 mm thick), and is often thinner along the medial margin, possibly because of variation in perfusion of gray and white matter. Less often nodular or solid enhancement, incomplete thin rings, or thick and irregular rings may be observed. Daughter abscesses appear as adjacent smaller enhancing rings, often along the medial margin of the parent abscess.

Edema surrounding an abscess may be greater in volume than the abscess itself, and causes much of the associated mass effect. If an abscess ruptures into the ventricular system and ependymitis develops, there is enhancement of the ventricular margin in addition to the ring enhancement of the abscess, which heralds a poor prognosis (199). Purulent material within the CSF may show increased signal intensity on both T1- and T2-weighted images (30).

In studies on experimentally produced brain abscesses, Grossman and colleagues have shown that nonenhanced T2-weighted images are very sensitive in identifying parenchymal areas of abnormality, whereas T1-weighted images with enhancement add specificity by demonstrating the "ring enhancement" characteristic of certain lesions (198). In addition, gadolinium-enhanced MR is better than contrast-enhanced CT in detecting small abscesses with necrotic centers and in showing ring-enhancing lesions long after these lesions have evolved to nodular enhancement by CT. The differential diagnosis for a ring-enhancing lesion includes primary brain tumor (high-grade astrocytoma), metastasis, infarction (bland or septic), resolving hematoma, thrombosed aneurysm, arteriovenous malformation, radiation necrosis, AIDS-related lymphoma, and other inflammatory conditions (e.g., demyelinating disease, granulomata, etc.) (200–202). Helpful radiographic clues that may differentiate one lesion from another include the pattern of enhancement, the presence of "daughter" rings, time course, location, ependymal and/or meningeal enhancement, and extra-axial collections (197, 199,200). Also, an abscess will often exhibit mesial thinning of the ring (thought to be related to differences in white vs. gray matter perfusion) and, of course, the clinical scenario. The false-negative rate for the diagnosis of abscess is low (reported to be $\leq$1% for CT) (203,204). However, patients receiving steroid therapy or antibiotic treatment may show a significant reduction in the degree of ring enhancement associated with an abscess (197,199).

The standard treatment of mature brain abscess is surgical drainage and/or excision, whereas cerebritis and some cases of abscess may be managed with antibiotics (197). Mortality has decreased from 40% to 50% to less than 5% (211). In cases with daughter abscess formation, intraoperative ultrasound guidance is recommended to ensure that all abscesses are identified and drained. After successful surgical and/or medical treatment, serial MR scans reveal a decrease in the edema, mass effect, and degree of enhancement associated with the abscess. A small focus of enhancement may persist even after a full course of antibiotics, yet the lesion usually resolves within the succeeding 3 to 4 months (197,205). With healing, an area of gliosis, and occasionally focal calcification is all that remains. Postoperatively, the MR appearance of resolving abscess may be complicated by the presence of subacute or chronic hemorrhage.

Septic Emboli

Patients with a history of intravenous drug abuse, bacterial endocarditis, or cyanotic heart disease are at risk for the development of septic embolism leading to cerebrovascular occlusions. Depending on the size of the emboli (188), the MR findings may vary from major arterial branch infarction to multiple small abscesses located at the gray-white matter junction, secondary to occlusion of small arteries and arterioles. Multiple small abscesses

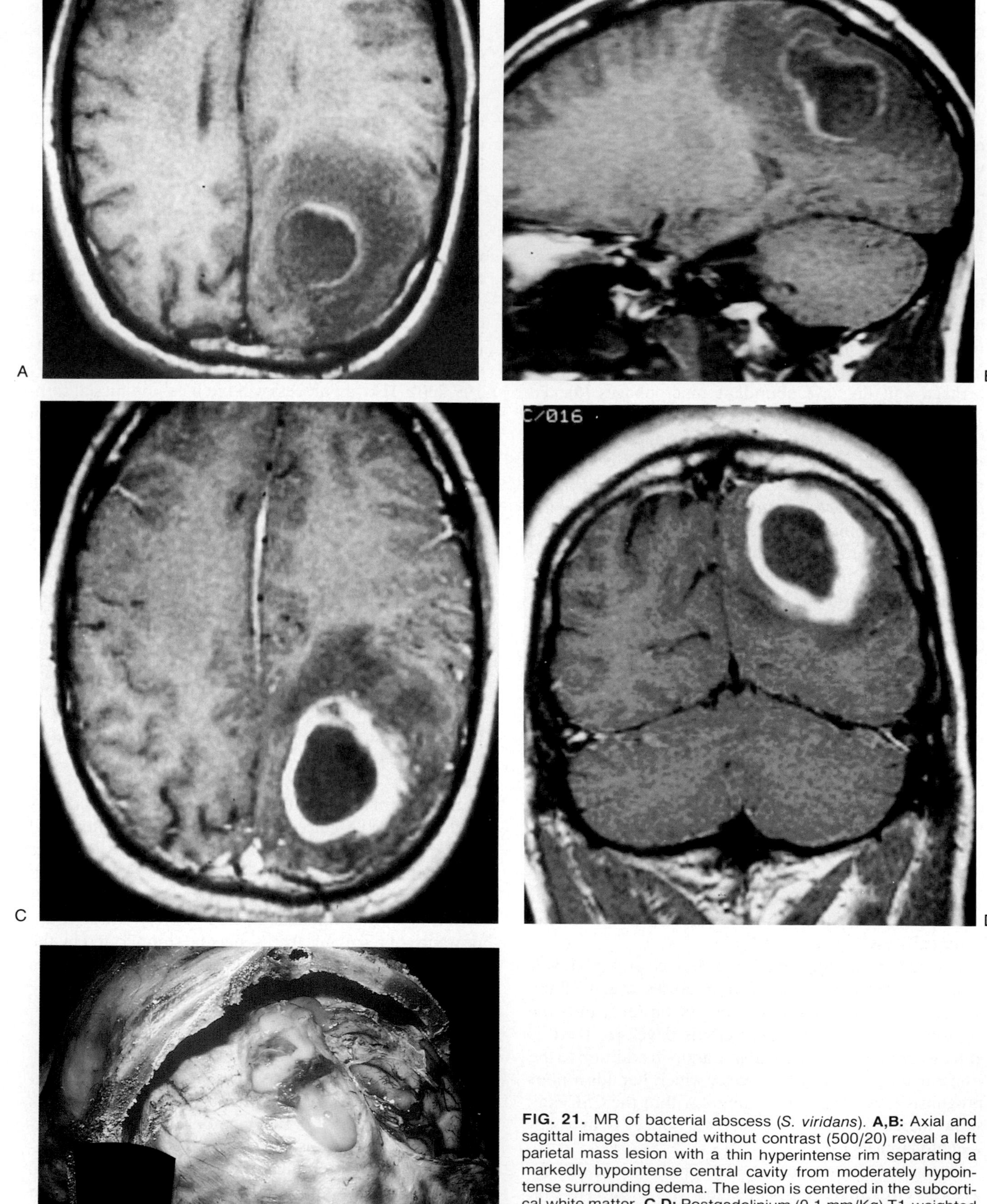

FIG. 21. MR of bacterial abscess (*S. viridans*). **A,B:** Axial and sagittal images obtained without contrast (500/20) reveal a left parietal mass lesion with a thin hyperintense rim separating a markedly hypointense central cavity from moderately hypointense surrounding edema. The lesion is centered in the subcortical white matter. **C,D:** Postgadolinium (0.1 mm/Kg) T1-weighted scans (500/20) show thick ring enhancement, with mesial thinning. **E:** Gross specimen from another patient reveals a superficial brain abscess with overlying empyema.

may mimic toxoplasma encephalitis and should be considered in the differential diagnosis when enhancing intracranial lesions are seen in an AIDS patient with a history of intravenous drug use. The small abscesses are accompanied by surrounding edema and mass effect, which is well demonstrated on MR (Fig. 22).

Mycotic aneurysms, which can occur as a result of septic embolism, involve intermediate to small cerebral ar-

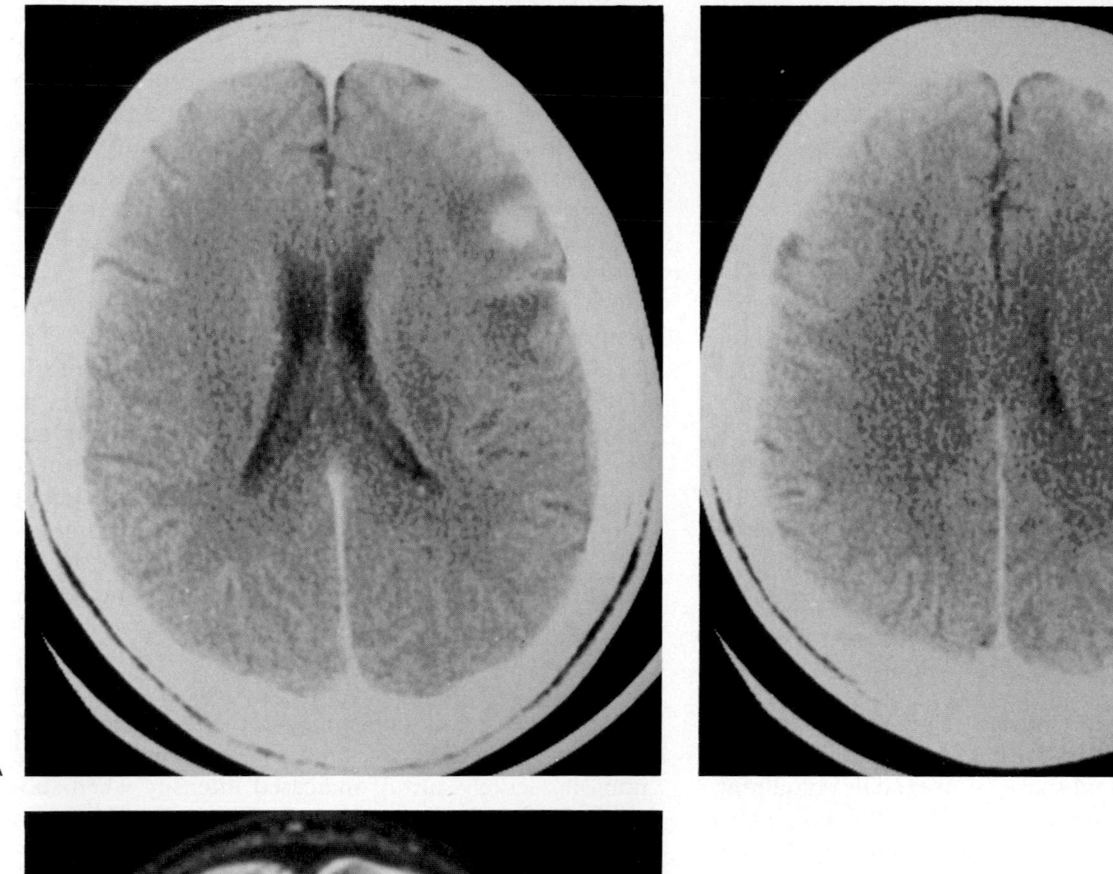

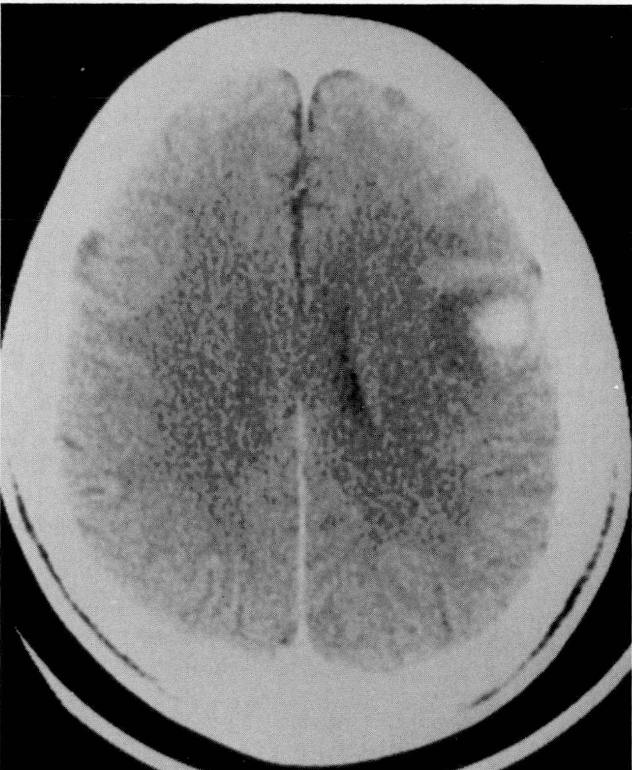

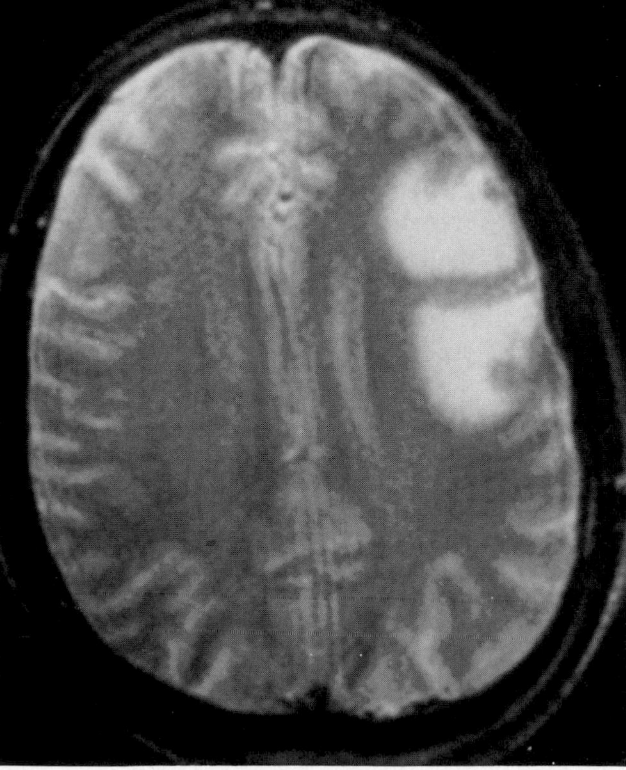

FIG. 22. Autopsy-proven septic emboli with abscess formation (*S. aureus*) in a 29-year-old man with AIDS and a history of intravenous drug abuse. **A,B**: Postcontrast CT scans demonstrate nodular foci of enhancement at the gray-white matter junction in the left frontal and frontoparietal regions. **C**: T2-weighted (2400/80) MR of the same patient reveals areas of hyperintensity with slight mass effect. The patient failed to respond to initial treatment for presumed toxoplasmosis.

teries, and thus are usually located in more peripheral arterial branches than congenital aneurysms (206,207). Although mycotic aneurysms are usually small and thus difficult to detect, the degree of suspicion should be high when reading MR scans of patients at risk. Mycotic aneurysm should be suspected in a patient with a history of infection and evidence of parenchymal or subarachnoid hemorrhage. MR angiography may be helpful in this regard, but catheter angiography should be performed for definitive diagnosis because these aneurysms must be recognized early for prompt initiation of therapy.

Meningitis

Pyogenic organisms may reach the leptomeninges and produce a meningitis via several different routes. These include hematogenous spread (the most frequent source of infection), direct spread from an adjacent (e.g., otorhinologic) focus of infection, or penetrating injury with direct inoculation (the least common source of infection). In the general population, *Streptococcus pneumoniae, Neisseria meningitidis*, or *Hemophilus influenzae* account for most cases of acute suppurative meningitis due to hematogenous spread, whereas in neonates, gram-negative rods (*Escherichia coli, Citrobacter,* etc.) and group B Streptococci are the principle pathogens (188,200).

Pathologically, acute leptomeningitis results in congestion and hyperemia of the pia-arachnoid and distention of the subarachnoid space by an exudate containing polymorphonuclear neutrophils (188). Subsequent to the initial infection, several complications may develop in the ensuing days to weeks. These complications are seen in approximately 50% of adult patients with bacterial meningitis. Blood vessels exposed to the inflammatory exudate may undergo spasm and/or thrombosis, resulting in arterial or venous infarction. Cerebrovascular disorders are the most frequent complication of bacterial meningitis in adults. Cortical infarction results in disruption of the pia, which normally acts as a barrier to the spread of infection. This facilitates the development of cerebritis/abscess in the subpial cortex and adjacent white matter. Parenchymal involvement, with edema and mass effect, may be localized or diffuse. Infection and necrosis of the arachnoid permits formation of a subdural collection, which may become infected (empyema). As a result of the subarachnoid inflammatory exudate, CSF pathways may become obstructed, producing hydrocephalus. Involvement of the ependymal lining of the ventricles, i.e., ventriculitis, may occur, but it is a relatively uncommon complication of leptomeningitis.

Unenhanced MR scans of patients with uncomplicated acute bacterial meningitis may be unremarkable (6,156). Postgadolinium MR studies can demonstrate leptomeningeal enhancement analogous to that seen on contrast CT. However, this enhancement is often better demonstrated by MR, with its multiplanar capability. In experimental studies performed on dogs with *S. aureus* meningitis, T1-weighted MR images with gadolinium demonstrated abnormal leptomeningeal enhancement that more closely approximated the extent of inflammatory cell infiltration than CT (208). Multiplanar MR is better than CT in demonstrating the distention of the subarachnoid space (with widening of the interhemispheric fissure), which is reported to be an early finding in severe meningitis (30). Plain and contrast MR also detects better the complications of meningitis described above such as infarction, cerebritis/abscess, empyema/effusion, hydrocephalus and ventriculitis (208).

Cortical and subcortical ischemic infarctions are evident as areas of increased signal intensity on T2-weighted images and are seen earlier by MR than CT (209). Occlusion of small perforating arteries results in focal infarcts of the basal ganglia, whereas spasm of anterior or middle cerebral arteries may lead to massive infarctions. Cortical venous occlusions, with or without dural venous thrombosis, result in hyperintense areas in the subpial cortex and underlying white matter, which do not conform to an expected arterial distribution. A favored site for this complication is near the vertex, secondary to superior sagittal sinus thrombosis (210). Hemorrhagic infarctions have a characteristic appearance on T2-weighted images, depending on the age of the infarct, with areas of hemorrhage appearing decreased in signal intensity acutely and of increased intensity when subacute. On T1-weighted images, the hemorrhage increases in signal intensity with evolution from the acute to subacute phase (7,209). For subacute infarcts, the pattern of enhancement on MR mimics the gyriform pattern seen on contrast CT. Vascular narrowing or occlusion may be documented by spin-echo or gradient-echo MR sequences or by MR angiography (212).

Cerebritis and edema also appear as areas of increased signal intensity on T2-weighted MR images. Differentiation of cerebritis from infarction should become apparent with time because cerebritis typically evolves to a well formed abscess, whereas the signal changes present in arterial infarction will conform to a distinct vascular distribution. However, these entities can be difficult to distinguish.

Subdural collections are detected sooner and their extent is better demonstrated by MR than CT because of the multiplanar capability of MR and the lack of artifact from bone. On MR, subdural effusions can often be distinguished from empyema because effusions are isointense to CSF signal, whereas empyema, with a higher protein content, are often of greater signal intensity than CSF on T1-weighted images and proton-density images. Subdural effusions, such as those that occur in association with *H. influenzae* meningitis in children, may be bilateral and are usually crescentic collections adjacent to the frontal and parietal lobes (213). Calcification of the margins of an effusion is an uncommon late sequela (214). Postgadolinium images should show an enhancing membrane associated with an empyema but not with a simple effusion (215). The presence of signal alterations in the cortex subjacent to an extra-axial collection more likely indicates empyema, with associated cortical inflammatory changes, than a simple effusion.

Hydrocephalus may be either communicating or obstructive, and is a complication seen more frequently in children than in adults (200). Obstructive hydrocephalus is demonstrated by both CT and MR, however T1-weighted images in the sagittal and coronal planes permit direct evaluation of midline structures (such as the cerebral aqueduct) and better delineate the site of obstruction. CSF dynamics can be displayed cinematographically (216). Periventricular CSF accumulation ("transependymal migration") secondary to ventricular obstruction is seen on proton-density and T2-weighted images as areas of hyperintense signal surrounding the ventricular system. Similar periventricular hyperintensity may be seen in cases of ependymitis without hydrocephalus; however, in those cases contrast MR would demonstrate ependymal enhancement. One sequela of ependymitis is the "trapped" fourth ventricle, which has an appearance of an expanding posterior fossa cystic mass (217) with resulting obstructive hydrocephalus.

Empyema

Purulent collections in the subdural and/or epidural space are uncommon, occurring one fourth (218,219) to one half (220) as often as intracerebral abscesses. In 65% to 90% of cases, the empyema is secondary to otorhinologic infection, which has spread by direct invasion of the extra-axial space and/or by retrograde thrombophlebitis via bridging emissary veins (219,220). The remaining cases of empyema are related to previous head trauma (penetrating injury, infected subdural hematoma) or neurosurgical procedure and, less often, as a complication of bacteremia or meningitis (219).

Subdural empyema (SDE) should be considered a neurosurgical emergency, and neuroimaging is essential to early diagnosis. When empyema results from sinusitis or mastoiditis it is often associated with seizures, focal deficits, and rapid neurologic deterioration, progressing from obtundation to coma (6,215). Empyemas that occur secondary to prior trauma or surgery are usually more indolent clinically. Mortality associated with subdural empyema now approaches 10% (6), compared with approximately 40% in the pre-CT era (214,215).

The value of CT in the early diagnosis of SDE has been controversial (221,222). Currently, MR is the study of choice as the presence and extent of extra-axial collections are better defined by MR (218). The increased sensitivity and specificity of MR are due to direct multiplanar imaging, increased contrast resolution, and the absence of artifact from bone. Although SDE may be lentiform or crescentic in shape, epidural empyema (EDE) is typically lentiform. It is possible to differentiate SDE from EDE when the latter is continuous across the midline and/or when there is a hypointense rim on both T1 and T2-weighted images, representing medially displaced dura, seen at the interface between a collection and the brain (218).

SDE is most commonly located over the cerebral convexity and is frequently bilateral, based on the results of CT studies (215). A paratentorial location is the least common (199). On T1-weighted images convexity and interhemispheric SDE appear hypointense relative to brain and hyperintense to CSF. On proton-density and T2-weighted images the collections are hyperintense to brain and isointense to hyperintense relative to CSF. These signal characteristics are typical of proteinaceous fluid with T1 and T2 values intermediate between gray matter/white matter and CSF. The signal intensity of the collection may not be markedly different from underlying brain if there is significant edema secondary to ischemia and/or early cerebritis.

In the early stages of SDE, T2-weighted images can demonstrate a thin hyperintense convexity and interhemispheric collection not visible by CT (6). Paratentorial and subtemporal extension is well demonstrated on coronal MR images. MR demonstrates sulcal effacement and associated parenchymal abnormalities better than CT (218). T2-weighted images, which are very sensitive to abnormal tissue-water distribution, may show cortical hyperintensities that are reversible and are thought to represent edema related to transient ischemia produced by inflammatory vasospasm and venous stasis (6,218). Gradient-echo and spin-echo MR can demonstrate cortical vein and/or dural sinus thrombosis (31,223) and also demonstrate the characteristic signal properties of acute and subacute hemorrhagic infarctions.

Prominent enhancement of the margin of an empyema is an important diagnostic feature on CT and is due to formation of a membrane of granulomatous tissue on the leptomeninges and inflammation in the subjacent cerebral cortex (215,219). The marked degree of enhancement seen on CT with an empyema rarely occurs with subdural hematoma (SDH), although a thin rim of enhancement is not uncommon for chronic SDH. On MR, however, even noninfected SDH enhances markedly on postgadolinium images. SDE may be differentiated from subacute/chronic SDH (weeks to months old) when the latter is hyperintense on T1- and T2-weighted images because of the presence of extracellular methemoglobin and other iron forms (7).

As the source of the infection may be otorhinologic, MR is quite sensitive in detecting inflammatory changes in the paranasal sinuses and mastoid air cells, usually as areas of increased signal intensity on T2-weighted images. Enhancement is usually prominent and peripheral. Mucopyocele may have decreased signal on T2-weighted images related to chronic inspissated secretions.

Spirochetes

The two primary spirochetal infections to be discussed include Lyme disease and syphilis. The tick-transmitted spirochete *Borrelia burgdorferi* is responsible for a multisystem disease, lyme borreliosis, which occurs worldwide (224,225). *B. burgdorferi* is found in deer, mice, raccoons, and birds worldwide, with transmission to humans by infected ixodid ticks (226–228). There has been a tenfold increase in reported cases in the United States over the past decade (227). The disease usually manifests clinically in several stages and the skin, joints, heart, and nervous system are primarily affected (226). Neurologic abnormalities develop in only about 11% of patients with the characteristic initial skin lesions (erythema chronicum migrans). However, CNS involvement may occur without a history of skin manifestations (229,230). In stage I Lyme disease the characteristic rash may be accompanied by headache, stiff neck, myalgia, or neuralgia (231,232). Neurologic manifestations typically occur months to years after the initial tick bite, i.e., during stage 2 (disseminated) or stage 3 (persistent) infection (225). Aseptic meningitis, cranial neuritis, (especially Bell's palsy), and cerebellar ataxia and cardiac abnormalities are among the manifestations of stage 2, whereas encephalitis, which may be acute or chronic, mild or severe, is usually manifested in stage 3 (225,233), often accompanied by arthritis (231).

Meningitis results from direct spirochetal invasion of the CSF (224,230). In the past, based on clinical, laboratory, and imaging findings (229,233), an immune complex mechanism has been proposed to explain parenchymal involvement. More recently, brain biopsies of patients with Lyme disease and encephalitis have revealed a small number of spirochetes within the brain parenchyma, accompanied by only a minimal inflammatory response (230). While CNS involvement is reminiscent of tertiary stage syphilis, neuropathologic findings equivalent to meningovascular syphilis, gumma, and tabes dorsalis have not been demonstrated in Lyme disease (230).

In many cases, MR scans have been normal, which is not unexpected if the patient is clinically stage 1 or 2. In other cases, multiple bilateral periventricular and/or subcortical hyperintense lesions have been identified on T2-weighted images without mass effect (230,234) (Fig. 23). The lesions are said to resemble MS plaques (230), although the differential diagnosis must also include vascular etiologies as well as other infectious demyelinating processes. Lesions may be seen in the basal ganglia. The brainstem may be involved (230,234). MR is more sensitive than CT in detecting the lesions of Lyme disease. Multifocal parenchymal enhancement as well as meningeal enhancement has been reported (235). Dilated Virchow-Robin spaces may also be evident. Treatment is with antibiotics.

Neurosyphilis is a chronic infection with three well-characterized stages. The causative agent is *Treponema pallidum,* a spirochete. Between 1986 and 1989, the incidence of syphilis rose sharply in both men and women, largely as a consequence of AIDS (236). Without therapy, 5% to 10% of patients develop clinical evidence of neurosyphilis. Approximately 1% to 3% of HIV-infected patients demonstrate evidence of neurosyphilis.

Neurosyphilis is most often asymptomatic. CNS involvement may occur at almost any stage of systemic infection (236). Neurosyphilis may occur weeks to decades after the initial infection and occurs in one third of patients who progress to the late stages of syphilis (236). There are two major clinical categories of symptomatic neurosyphilis: meningovascular and parenchymatous. Mixed features are common, and the parenchymatous manifestations include general paresis and tabes dorsalis. The usual interval of infection to symptom onset in the general population is 5 to 10 years for meningovascular syphilis, 20 years for general paresis, and 25 to 30 years for tabes dorsalis, although this time course appears to be accelerated in HIV-infected patients (237).

Meningeal neurosyphilis may present as an acute meningitis and may result in hydrocephalus, cranial neuritis, and/or formation of gummas (236). There is widespread thickening of the meninges, meningeal lymphocytic infiltrates, and perivascular lymphocytic infiltrates (188). Cranial nerve involvement is most commonly with cranial nerves II and VIII.

Vascular neurosyphilis is usually characterized by headache and focal neurologic deficit related to a vascular event, with abnormal CSF findings. Two types of vascular involvement have been described in neurosyphilis: Heubner's endarteritis and Nissl's endarteritis. The Heubner type of arteritis is more commonly encountered, affecting large and medium-sized arteries with resultant irregular luminal narrowing and ectasia. Less frequently, the Nissl-Alzheimer type of arteritis is present, primarily involving small vessels in which a luminal narrowing occurs as a consequence of intense proliferation of endothelial and adventitial cells. Both types of arteritis may result in vascular occlusion.

Syphilitic gummas are circumscribed masses of granulation tissue surrounded by mononuclear epithelial and fibroblastic cells with occasional giant cells and perivas-

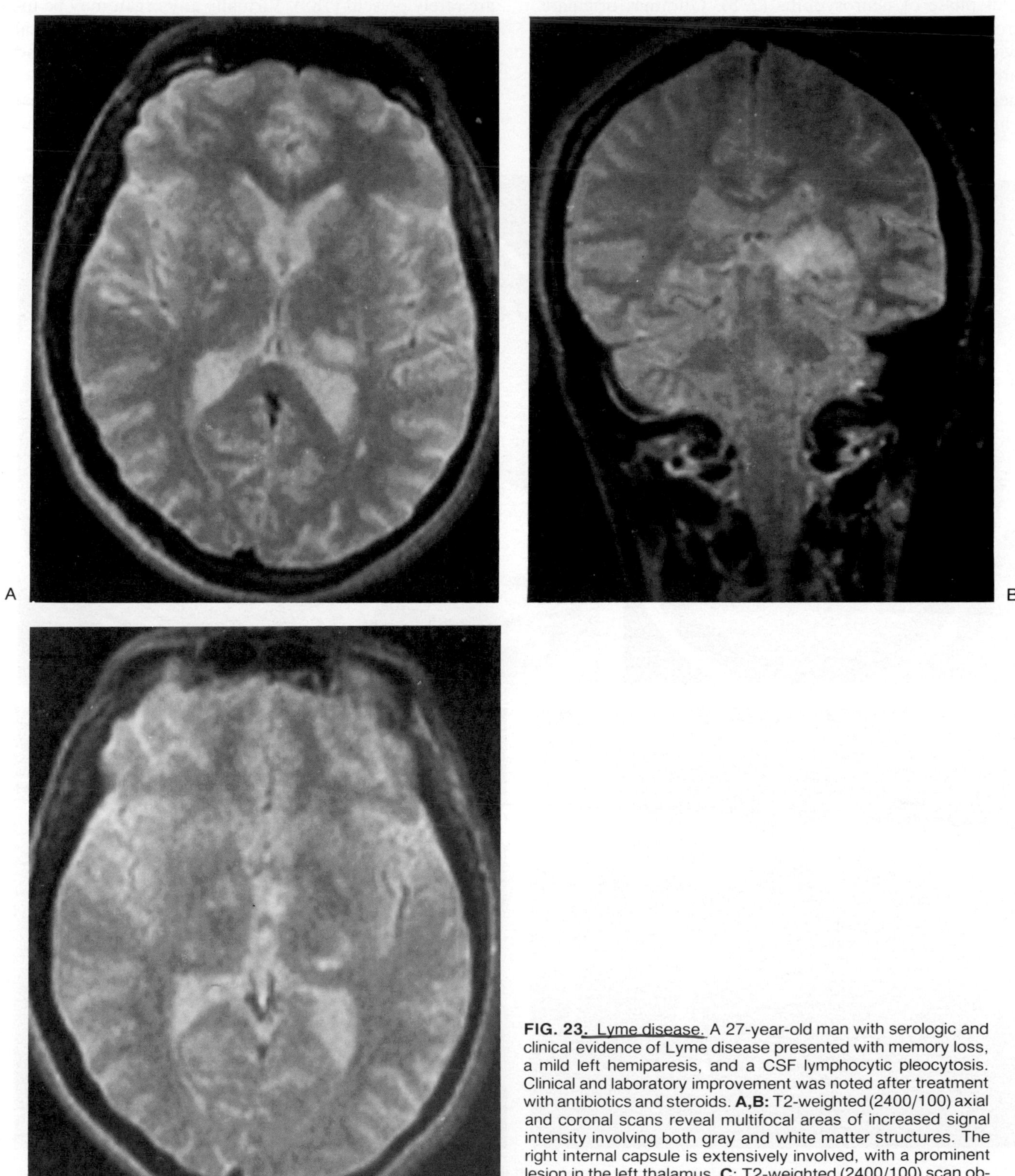

FIG. 23. Lyme disease. A 27-year-old man with serologic and clinical evidence of Lyme disease presented with memory loss, a mild left hemiparesis, and a CSF lymphocytic pleocytosis. Clinical and laboratory improvement was noted after treatment with antibiotics and steroids. **A,B:** T2-weighted (2400/100) axial and coronal scans reveal multifocal areas of increased signal intensity involving both gray and white matter structures. The right internal capsule is extensively involved, with a prominent lesion in the left thalamus. **C:** T2-weighted (2400/100) scan obtained 2 months later reveals a decrease in size of the left thalamic lesion.

culitis. Gummas are created by an intense localized leptomeningeal inflammatory reaction early in the meningeal phase of neurosyphilis (238). Gummas originate from the meningeal connective tissue and blood vessels with spread to the adjacent parenchyma. The gummas are usually seen overlying the cerebral convexities, adherent to both dura and brain parenchyma. The lesions vary in size from 1 mm to 4 cm (188) and may be multiple, but are most often solitary. There may be central caseous necrosis within the lesion, but spirochetes are rarely present (188). Virtually any organ may be involved, with the most common sites being skin, skeletal system, mouth, upper respiratory tract, larynx, liver, and stomach. CNS gummas are seen infrequently.

General paresis is a reflection of diffuse parenchymal damage and may result in alterations of personality and

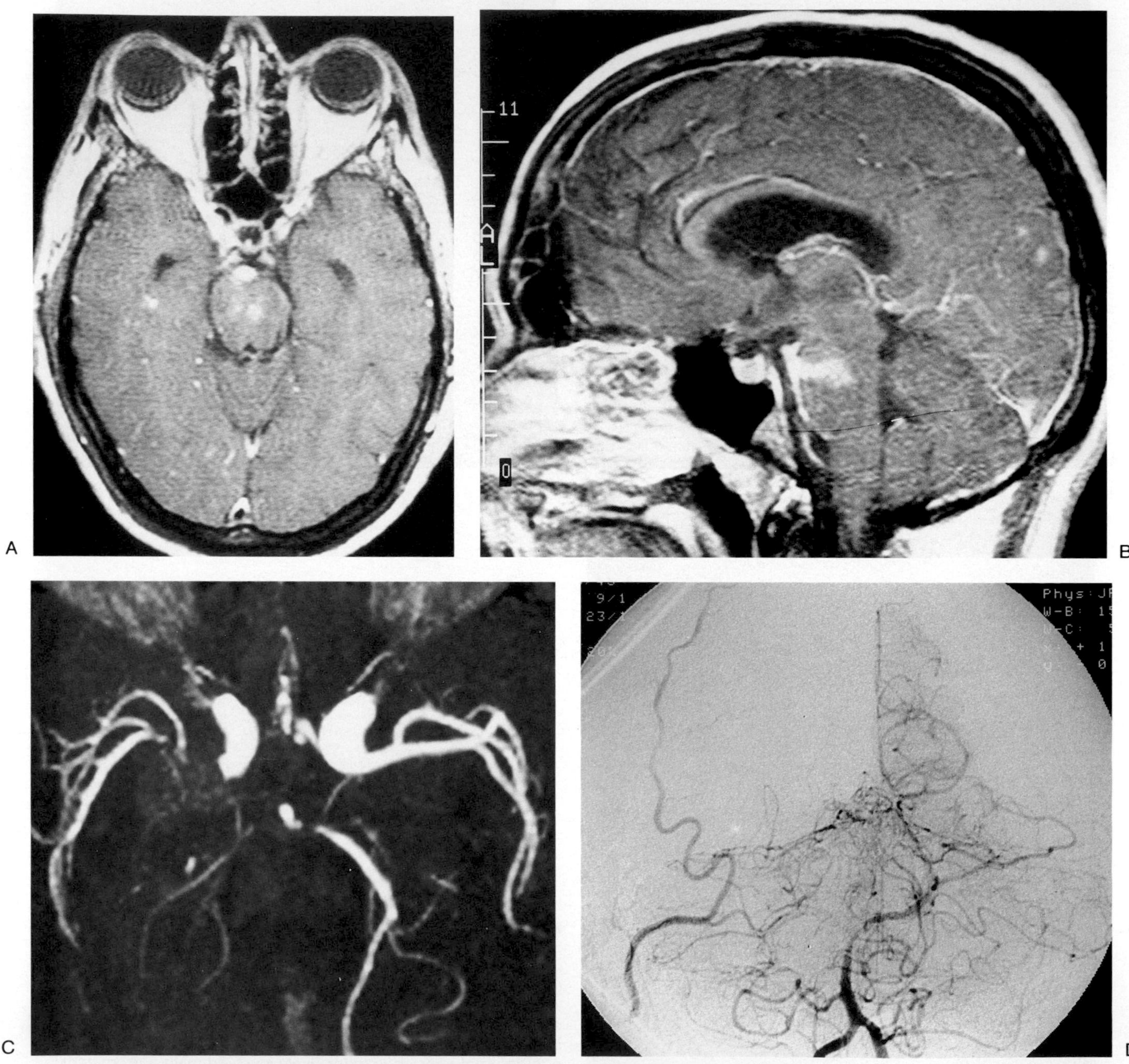

FIG. 24. Meningovascular syphilis. **A,B:** Axial and sagittal postcontrast T1-weighted images (600/20) reveal enhancement within the brainstem due to subacute ischemia/infarction. There is also abnormal meningeal enhancement surrounding the basilar artery. A focus of enhancement is also seen in the right temporal lobe. **C:** Image from a 3-D TOF MR angiogram (48/8,20°) demonstrates occlusion of the right posterior cerebral artery, and focal narrowing of the proximal left posterior cerebral artery (P_1 segment). **D:** Conventional angiogram, vertebral injection, reveals occluded right posterior cerebral artery with marked narrowing of the distal basilar artery and proximal left posterior cerebral artery (P_1 segment).

affect, illusions, delusions, hallucinations, memory loss, loss of judgement and insight associated with speech disturbances, hyperactive reflexes, and the Argyll-Robertson pupil. General paresis is associated with chronic meningoencephalitis. Neuropathologic examination reveals cortical atrophy and ependymitis on gross examination (188). Microscopic evaluation reveals degenerative neuronal changes with gliosis and scattered microglia (188). Spirochetes may be found in the cortical gray matter (188).

Tabes dorsalis is a myelopathy associated with atrophic, degenerated, and demyelinated dorsal nerve roots and posterior spinal columns. A triad of symptoms (lightning pains, dysuria, and ataxia) and a triad of signs (Argyll-Robertson pupil, areflexia, and loss of proprioception) are the characteristics of this disorder (239). The Argyll-Robertson pupil, seen in both tabes dorsalis and general paresis, is a small, irregular pupil that accommodates but does not react to light (240).

Diagnostic confirmation of neurosyphilis is based on

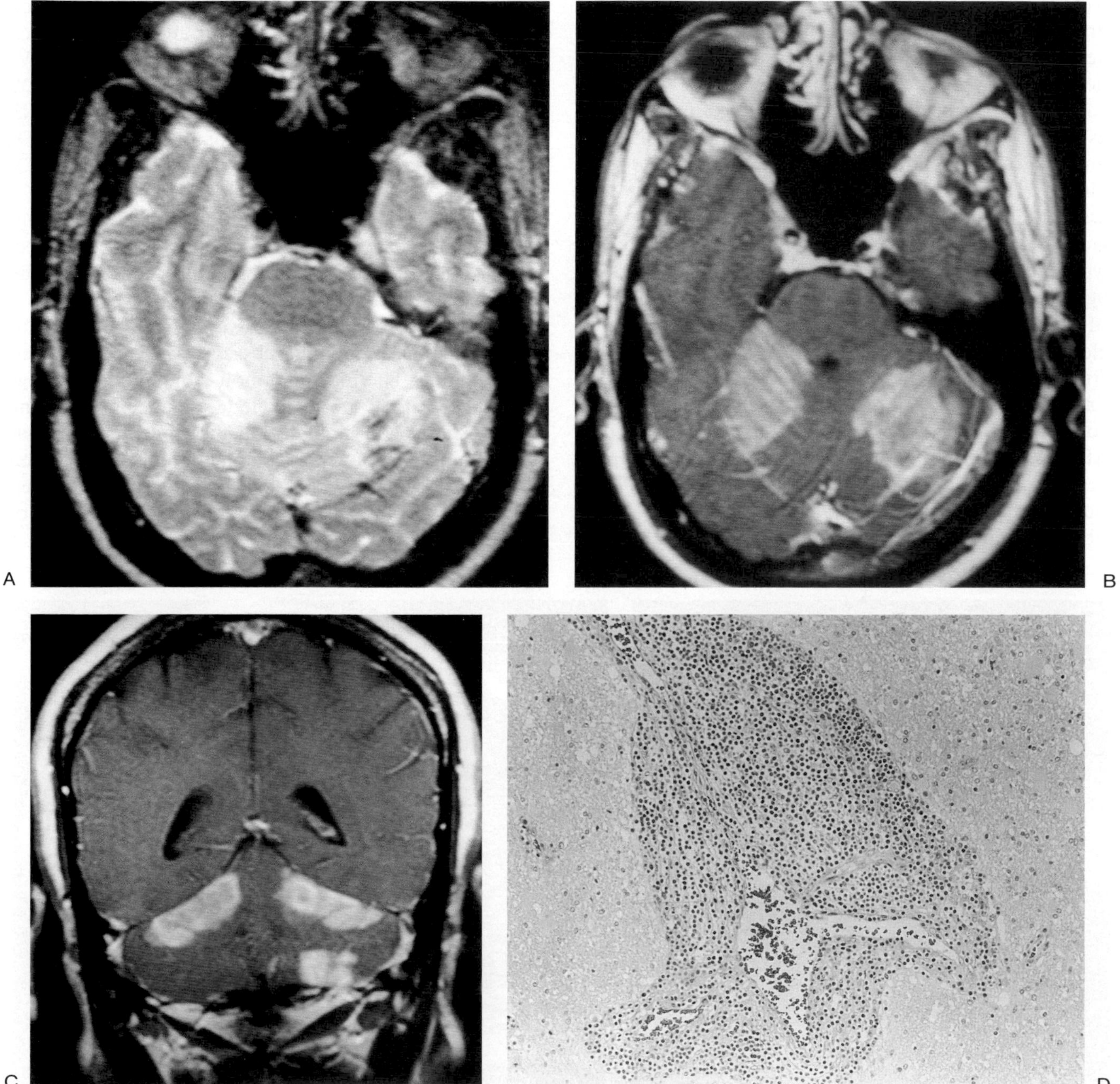

FIG. 25. Meningovascular syphilis. **A:** Bilateral regions of hyperintense signal are seen in the cerebellum on this T2-weighted (2400/80) image. **B,C:** Multiple, bilateral areas of enhancement are seen on these postgadolinium (0.1 mm/Kg) images, which conform to multiple arterial distributions. **D:** Perivascular infiltration by lymphocytes and plasma cells is typical of meningovascular syphilis (H & E, original magnification ×20).

a positive serum fluorescent treponemal antibody absorption test (FTA), CSF pleocytosis, elevated CSF protein levels, and a positive CSF Venereal Disease Research Laboratory (VDRL) test. A positive CSF VDRL is highly specific for active neurosyphilis but the test is negative in approximately 50% of patients with neurosyphilis (236). Serum VDRL is negative in one third to one half of all cases (236,241,242). Specific criteria pertaining to elevated CSF white blood cell counts and elevated protein levels permit a diagnosis of neurosyphilis in those patients with a negative CSF VDRL but a positive serum FTA. Meningovascular syphilis responds promptly to treatment with penicillin G (240). Treatment of general paresis and tabes dorsalis is far less successful.

Just as the histopathologic appearance of neurosyphilis is quite varied, so too are the radiographic manifestations. On CT, one third of studies are negative and one third reveal only cerebral atrophy (243,244). Small infarcts or foci of ischemia secondary to the vasculitis may be apparent on both CT and MR. On MR, multiple focal hyperintensities are seen on T2-weighted images involving both gray and white matter in cortical and subcortical locations (Fig. 24). Multiple arterial distributions are affected, involving both supratentorial and infratentorial structures with a predilection for the basal ganglia. MR is superior to CT in demonstration of these ischemic regions (245) (Fig. 25). When CT reveals a solitary focus, MR can demonstrate multiple infarcts in the same patient, suggesting the possibility of a vasculitis (245). Postgadolinium images may reveal enhancement in areas of subacute infarction (243,245), and meningeal enhancement may also be present, again seen to better advantage on MR than CT (Fig. 26). Gummas appear as mass lesions, with nodular or ring enhancement, at the brain surface. Adjacent meningeal enhancement may be present (Fig. 27).

Mycobacterium Tuberculosis

In the United States, there has been a rise in the number of TB cases since 1986 (246,247) as well as an increase in extrapulmonary manifestations (248) that may be attributed to the AIDS epidemic. Information derived from clinic-based studies in Miami and San Francisco suggests 28% to 31% of patients with TB are HIV-seropositive (249,250). Conversely, 5% to 9% of AIDS patients have tuberculosis (all sites included) (246). CNS tuberculosis occurs in 2% to 5% of all patients with TB (251,252) and in 10% of those with AIDS-related TB (251,253).

Adult TB is most often a postprimary infection, whereas most cases in children are due to primary infection (254). Ten to 30% of current adult TB cases are due to primary infection (255,256).

CNS tuberculosis may take a variety of forms, including tuberculous meningitis, abscess, focal cerebritis, and tuberculoma. The most common radiographic findings associated with CNS TB include enhancement of the basal cisterns, granulomata, calcifications, hydrocephalus, meningeal enhancement, and infarction, most often of the basal ganglia. Coexistent pulmonary TB is often present (257,258), seen in 25% to 83% of cases of CNS TB.

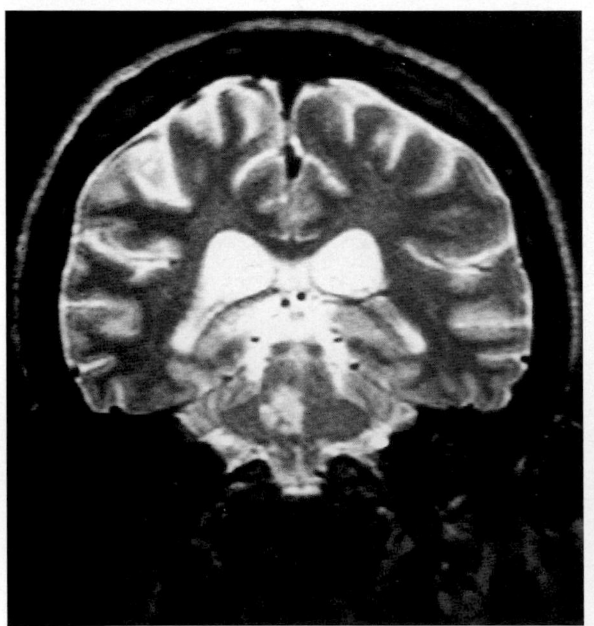

A

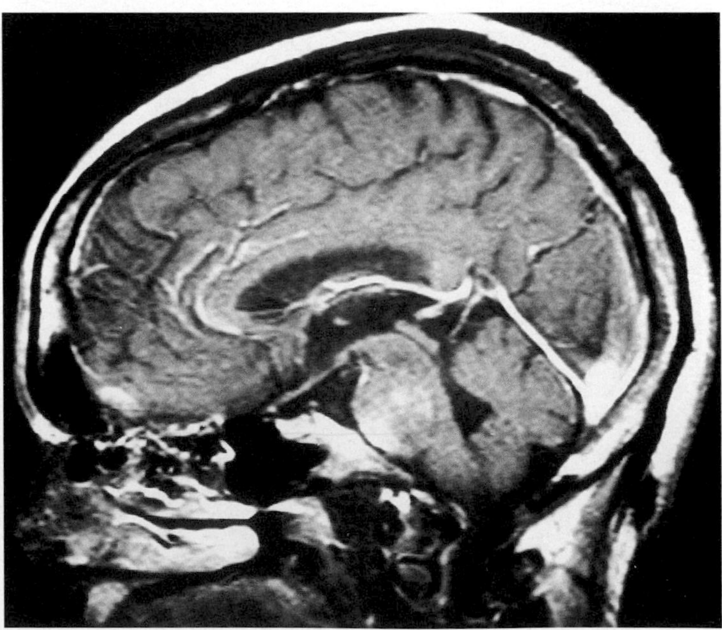

B

FIG. 26. Meningovascular syphilis. **A:** Subacute infarction is seen as an area of increased signal in the brainstem on this T2-weighted (2550/80) coronal image. **B:** Postgadolinium scan demonstrates prominent enhancement of the pons.

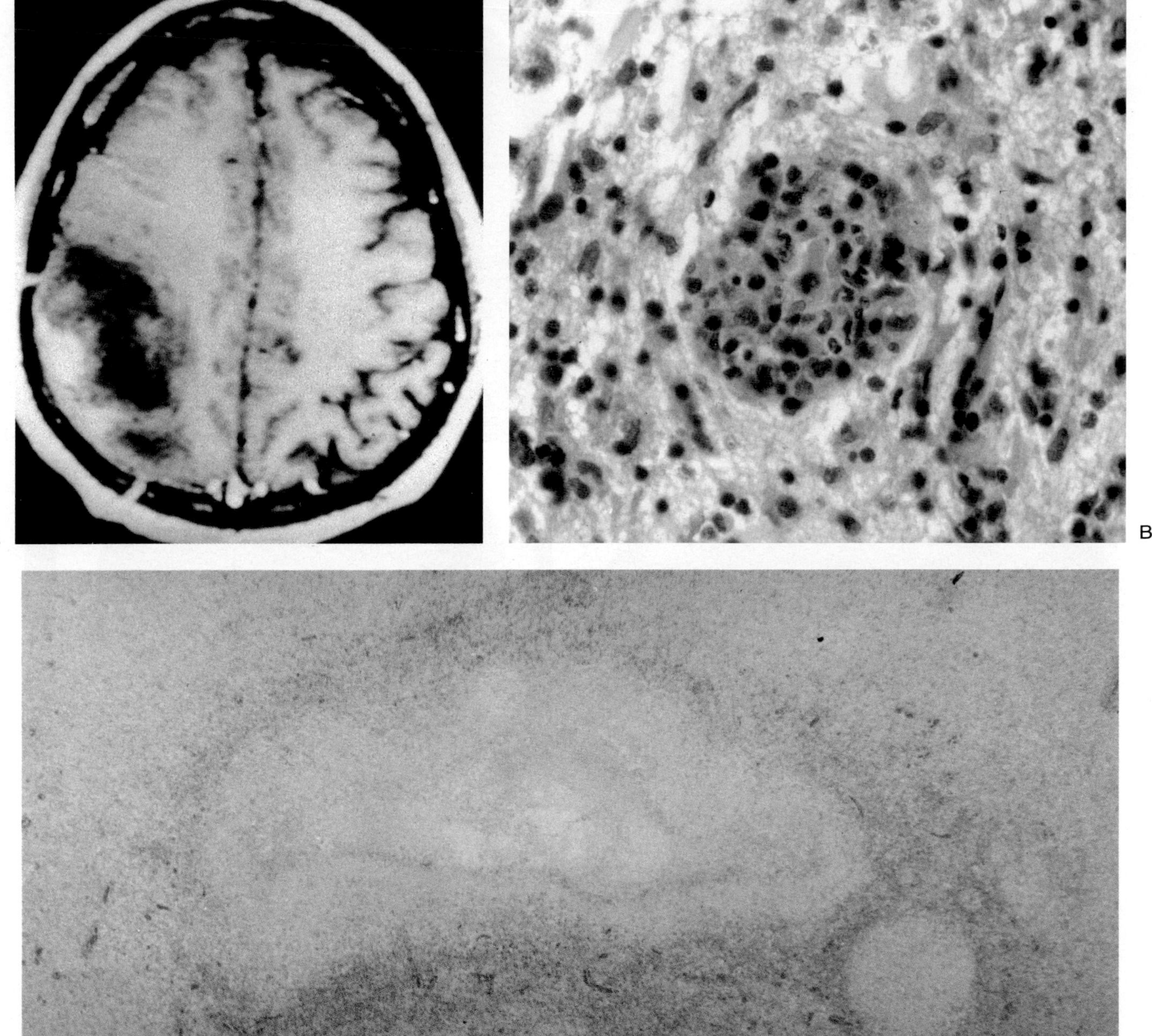

FIG. 27. Syphilitic gumma (pathologically proven). **A:** Postcontrast MR scan reveals peripheral enhancement in the right parietal region with surrounding edema and mass effect. There is overlying meningeal enhancement as well. **B:** Biopsy specimen of patient A reveals a syphilitic gumma with parenchymal infiltration of lymphocytes and plasma cells (H & E, original magnification ×150). (From Berger et al., *Neurology* 1992;42:1282–1287, with permission.) **C:** This syphilitic gumma from another patient consists of central coagulative necrosis surrounded by inflammatory cells including macrophages, lymphocytes, and plasma cells (H & E, original magnification ×2).

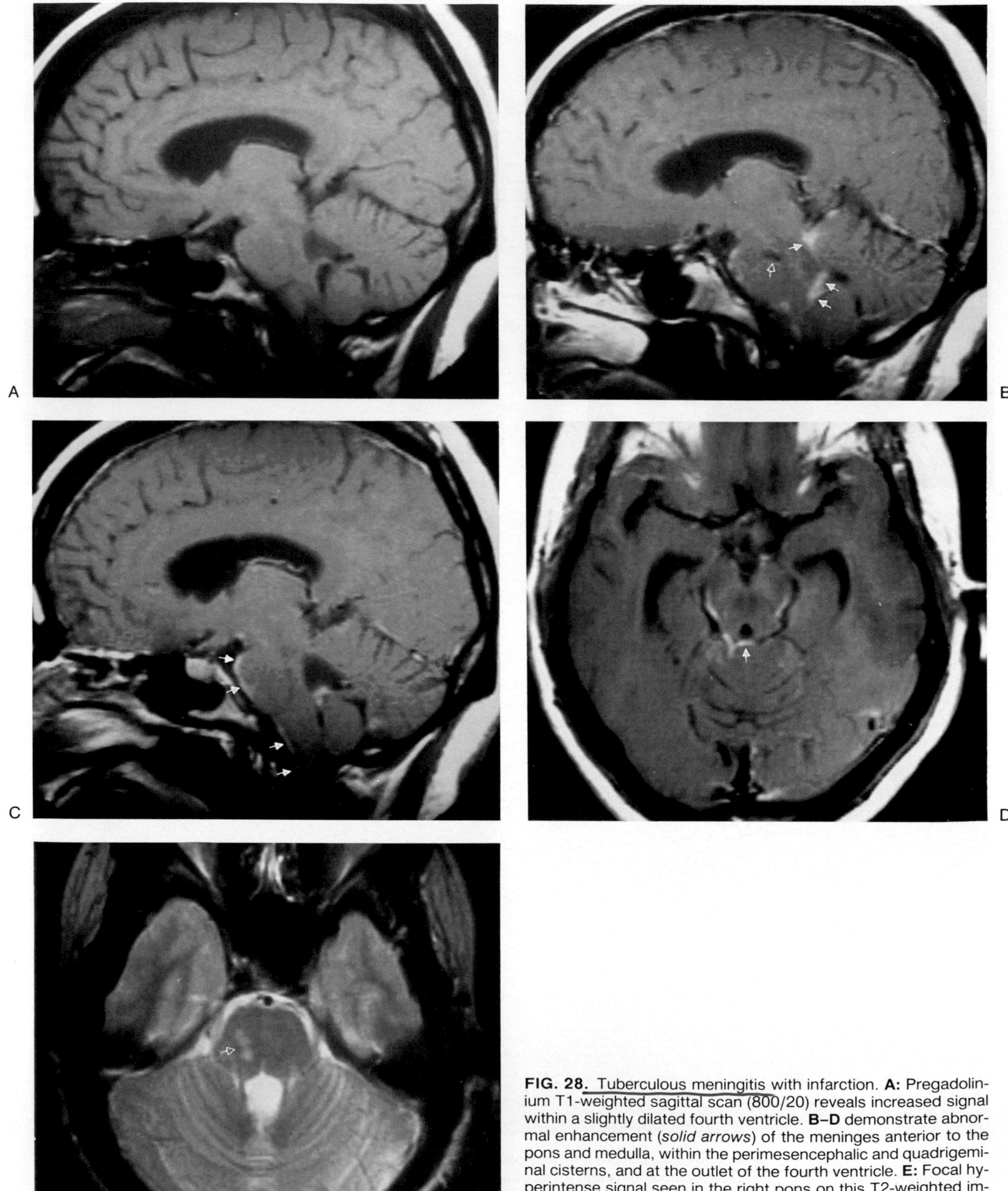

FIG. 28. Tuberculous meningitis with infarction. **A:** Pregadolinium T1-weighted sagittal scan (800/20) reveals increased signal within a slightly dilated fourth ventricle. **B–D** demonstrate abnormal enhancement (*solid arrows*) of the meninges anterior to the pons and medulla, within the perimesencephalic and quadrigeminal cisterns, and at the outlet of the fourth ventricle. **E:** Focal hyperintense signal seen in the right pons on this T2-weighted image (2400/80) represents an area of infarction (*open arrow*). It can also be seen in scan B as an area of well-defined hypointense signal (*open arrow*) without enhancement.

Leptomeningitis due to CNS tuberculosis most often presents with fever, headache, altered mental status, and meningeal signs. Two different mechanisms are proposed for the pathogenesis of TB meningitis (6,30,259). The first mechanism suggests rupture of subependymal or subpial granulomata into the CSF. The second proposed pathogenesis involves penetration of the walls of meningeal vessels by hematogenous spread, usually from a gastrointestinal or pulmonary source. By either mechanism, the basal meninges are involved early in the course of infection and, characteristically, a thick gelatinous exudate is found in the basal cisterns (259). Arteries that course through this exudate can become directly involved by the inflammatory infiltrate, indirectly by reactive endarteritis obliterans, or by both processes, with consequent spasm and intimal changes resulting in thrombosis and infarction. Arteritis is present in approximately 28% to 41% of cases with basilar meningitis (260). Infarctions are even more common in children (261). The middle cerebral artery and its branches are most often affected, especially the small perforating branches supplying the basal ganglia (200,259). These infarcts are commonly bilateral. Although both CT and MR can demonstrate these infarctions, there is earlier detection with MR (209).

Both CT and MR can also document communicating hydrocephalus, a common sequela of tuberculous meningitis (262). Cisternal enhancement is often quite striking and may be seen well on both CT and MR. Meningeal enhancement is far better demonstrated by postgadolinium MR than CT (Fig. 28). The hydrocephalus encountered in TB is usually of the communicating type, secondary to blockage of the basal cisterns by the inflammatory exudate, but occasionally may be of the obstructive type, secondary to a focal parenchymal lesion with mass effect or due to entrapment of a ventricle by granulomatous ependymitis (30,188,259).

CSF studies typically reveal a pleocytosis with a low glucose and slightly elevated protein. Elevated adenosine deaminase (ADA) levels (>9 μ/L CSF) in the CSF may be helpful in establishing an early diagnosis, as cultures take several weeks and may delay urgent therapy resulting in irreversible damage (263). Polymerase chain reaction (PCR) can also be used to establish a diagnose, usually within 1 to 2 days.

Overall mortality for tuberculous meningitis is more than 25% and even higher in children, with pediatric mortality rates reported between 17% and 71.9% (6,264). Those who survive are frequently left with a significant deficit. Long-term morbidity among patients with TB meningitis is 66% (264). These sequelae include mental retardation, paralysis, rigidity, cranial nerve palsy, seizures, and speech or visual deficits (264). These complications result from infarction, hydrocephalus, and/or tuberculous involvement of the brain parenchyma and cranial nerves (264).

The most common parenchymal form of CNS TB is tuberculous granuloma (tuberculoma). Granulomata may be secondary to hematogenous spread of systemic disease or may evolve from extension of CSF infection into the adjacent parenchyma via cortical veins or small penetrating arteries (188). Pathologically, the granuloma is composed of a central zone of solid caseation necrosis, surrounded by a capsule of collagenous tissue, epithelioid cells, multinucleated giant cells, and mononuclear inflammatory cells. Few tubercle bacilli are seen on smears (265,266), but may be demonstrated in the necrotic center and throughout the capsule (267). Outside the capsule, there is parenchymal edema and astrocytic proliferation (267). Tuberculomas may be found in the cerebrum, cerebellum, subarachnoid space, or subdural or epidural space. Parenchymal disease most often involves the corticomedullary junction and periventricular regions, as expected for hematogenous dissemination. Most tuberculomas are supratentorial (258,268). Parenchymal disease can occur with or without coexistent meningitis (156).

On CT, tuberculomas are seen in only a minority of patients with TB meningitis (259). Of these patients with parenchymal tuberculomas, 10% to 34% have multiple lesions (6,269). Contrast CT demonstrates a small ring-enhancing lesion that correlates with the pathologic findings of central necrosis and peripheral organization (270). One third of patients may demonstrate the "target sign" that appears as a central calcification or punctate enhancement surrounded by a region of hypodensity with surrounding rim enhancement (271). This sign is suggestive of TB, but not pathognomonic.

On noncontrast MR studies, granulomata appear isointense to gray matter on T1-weighted images and may have a slightly hyperintense rim (possibly secondary to the presence of paramagnetic species, which shorten the T1 relaxation time) (272). On T2-weighted images, the tuberculomas exhibit variable signal. They are often isointense or hypointense to brain parenchyma and it is postulated that this relative hypointensity is related to T2 shortening by paramagnetic free radicals produced by macrophages, which are heterogeneously distributed throughout the caseous granuloma (6). Alternatively, the diminished signal on T2-weighted images may be attributed to the mature tuberculoma being of greater cellular density than brain (272). Granulomas may also be hyperintense to brain on T2-weighted images; this is likely due to a greater degree of central liquefactive necrosis in these lesions. There is usually associated mass effect. Surrounding edema may be minimal in small lesions and, in general, there is less edema than that surrounding a pyogenic abscess of comparable size, based on CT studies (199,273). Edema surrounding tuberculomata is relatively more prominent in the early stages of granuloma formation (272).

Postgadolinium images of TB granulomas demon-

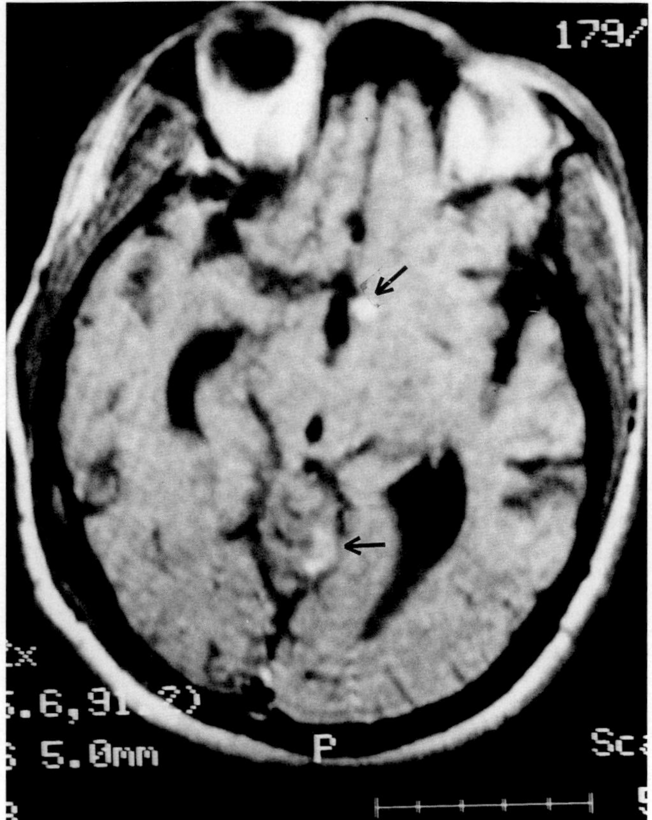

FIG. 29. Tuberculous granulomata in an AIDS patient (pathologically proven). T1-weighted MR (500/20) obtained after contrast reveals focal, nodular areas of enhancement (*arrows*) without significant edema or mass effect.

strate intense nodular and ring-like enhancement (Fig. 29). Healed tuberculomas may calcify in up to 23% of cases and these are usually more evident on CT than MR (269). On MR images, the calcifications are more evident on gradient-echo than on spin-echo imaging. Atrophy is frequently a long-term sequela of tuberculous CNS infection. Full resolution of cerebral tuberculoma requires months to years of medical therapy. The length of time required is related more to the size of the original lesion than to any other single factor (269).

Tuberculous abscess is a rare complication (259). In contrast to the solid caseation seen in the granuloma (with few tubercle bacilli present), the abscess is formed by semiliquid pus that is teeming with tubercle bacilli (265,266). The wall of a tuberculous abscess lacks the giant cell epithelioid granulomatous reaction of a TB granuloma (274). It is postulated that the abscess may be due to liquefactive breakdown of a more typical caseated tuberculoma (274). TB abscesses are larger than tuberculomas and have a more accelerated clinical course (275). The appearance is similar to that of bacterial abscess, although it is often multiloculated (149,251). On CT, the tuberculous abscess is hypodense with surrounding edema and mass effect. Postcontrast images demonstrate ring enhancement that is usually thin and uniform, but less often may be somewhat irregular and thick. The appearance is related to the central zone of liquefactive necrosis with pus and surrounding inflammation. This central area is thus of increased signal on T2-weighted images (6). The enhancement pattern on MR is similar to that on CT.

Comparison studies of HIV-seropositive and HIV-seronegative patients with tuberculous meningitis have shown hydrocephalus to occur with similar frequency in the two groups (249). Nonenhancing lesions (presumably infarcts) are seen more frequently in the HIV-seropositive group as compared to the HIV-seronegative group. Meningeal disease is also more prominent in the HIV-seropositive group. Enhancing parenchymal lesions are more common as well in the HIV-seropositive patients (249). Thus, infarction, meningeal enhancement, and parenchymal disease appear to be more common in patients with TB who are also HIV-infected. This is supported by the results of another comparative study that found mass lesions on imaging studies in 60% of HIV-infected patients with TB meningitis but in only 14% of the non–HIV-infected patients with TB meningitis (276).

Approximately 16% of both HIV-seronegative and HIV-seropositive patients demonstrate resistance to at least one of the drugs (isoniazid, rifampin, streptomycin, ethambutol) commonly used to treat TB (277). This often results from transmission of resistant organisms from TB patients who have received inadequate or inappropriate therapy (278).

FUNGAL INFECTIONS

CNS infection by certain fungi, namely the systemic or deep mycoses, results in a granulomatous reaction, with variable degrees of suppuration (188). Intracranial blood vessels, leptomeninges, and/or brain parenchyma may become involved, producing MR (and CT) findings that are often indistinguishable from those of TB (6,279). Focal parenchymal lesions can mimic pyogenic abscesses or tumors (279). CT underestimates the extent of pathology in patients with fungal disease (280). Although MR is certainly a more sensitive technique, it may be unable to distinguish among the various types of fungal disease.

Despite this general lack of diagnostic specificity, certain findings are more commonly associated with particular fungal pathogens. The most frequently encountered systemic mycoses may be divided into those genera that usually infect only immunocompromised patients (Aspergillus, Candida, Mucor) and those that also infect the immunocompetent (Cryptococcus, Coccidioides, Histoplasma, and Blastomyces) (279). Aspergillus, Candida, Mucor, and Cryptococcus are ubiquitous, whereas the remaining fungi are endemic to certain geographic regions of the world (281). In addition, the pathophysiology of mycotic lesions in the CNS varies with the type of fungal form (188). Fungi that grow in infected tissue as yeast cells (Cryptococcus, Histoplasma) are spread hematogenously, reach the microvasculature of the meninges, penetrate the vessel walls, and result in an acute or chronic leptomeningitis. Less frequently, parenchymal lesions such as granulomas and/or abscesses are encountered (Fig. 30).

Fungi that grow in infected tissue as hyphae only (Aspergillus, Mucor) or as pseudohypha (Candida) tend to involve the parenchyma rather than the meninges, as these larger hyphae forms have limited access to the meningeal microcirculation (188). Hyphae form mycelial colonies capable of invading and obstructing large, medium, and small arteries leading to infarction as well as cerebritis. Pseudohyphae, which represent adherent yeast cells and their progeny, are larger than individual cells but smaller than true hyphae. Thus, CNS infection with Candida species often results in scattered parenchymal granulomatous microabscesses secondary to small

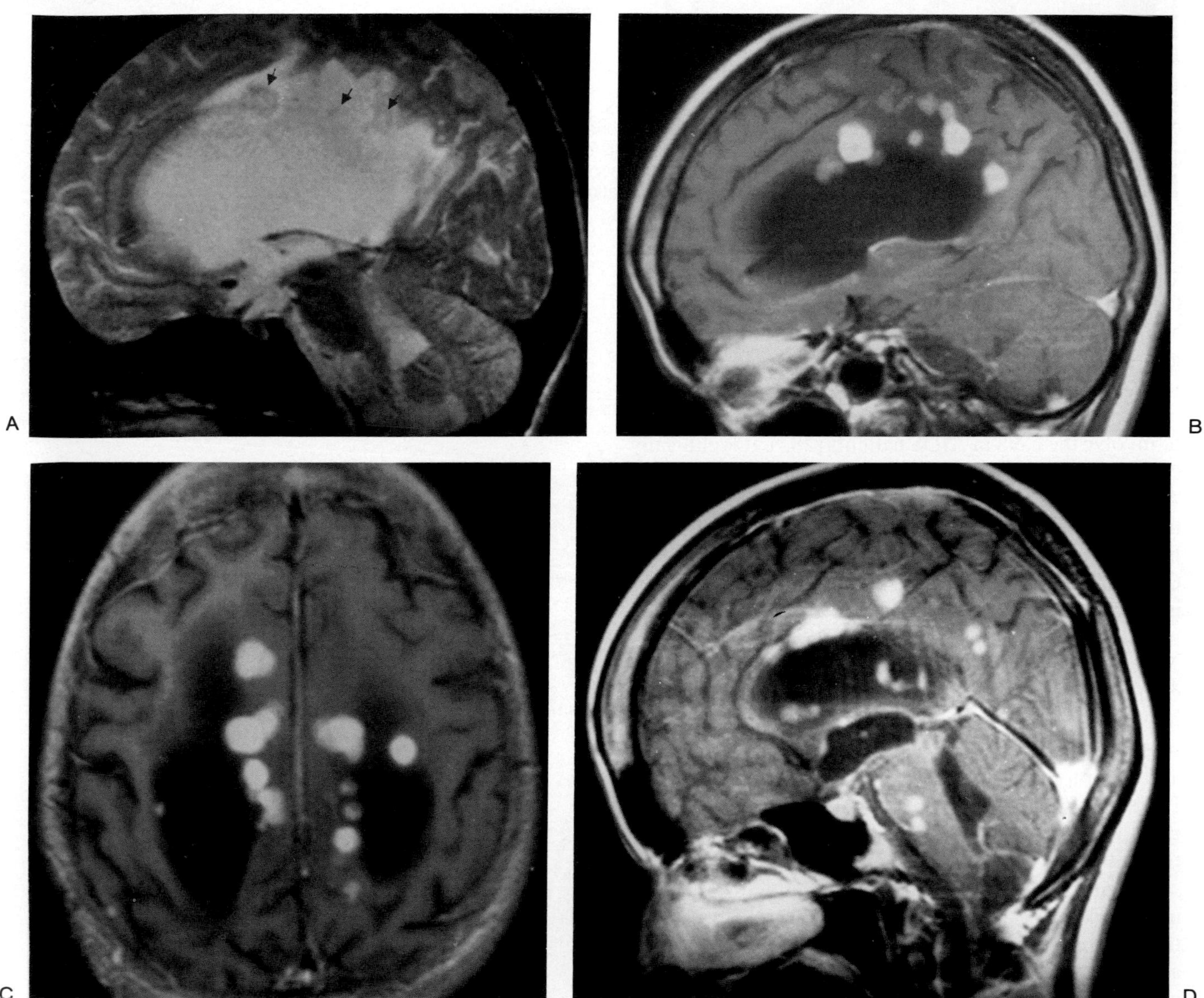

FIG. 30. A–F. Histoplasmosis with parenchymal granulomas, meningitis, and hydrocephalus. **A:** T2-weighted left parasagittal (2000/80) scan shows subependymal nodules (*arrows*) that are nearly isointense to brain parenchyma. **B:** Corresponding postgadolinium T1-weighted (700/20) parasagittal image reveals marked enhancement of the nodules. **C,D:** Postgadolinium T1-weighted (700/20) axial and midsagittal scans demonstrate not only the subependymal and periventricular granulomas, but several pontine granulomata as well.

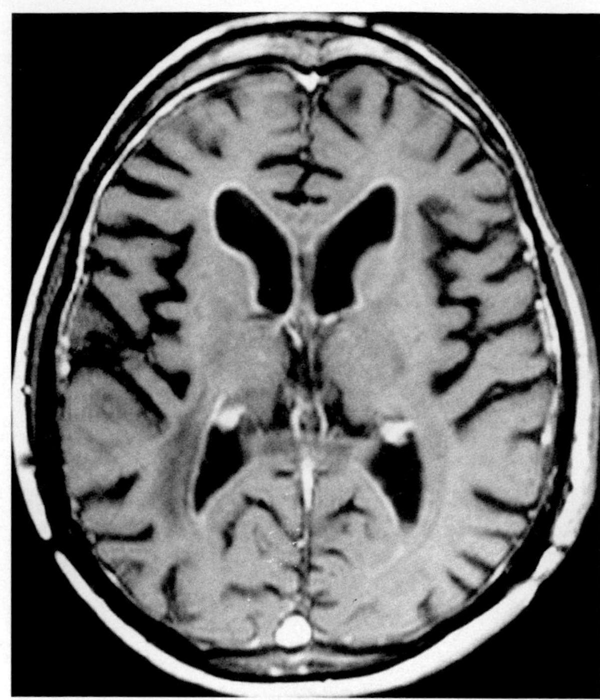

E

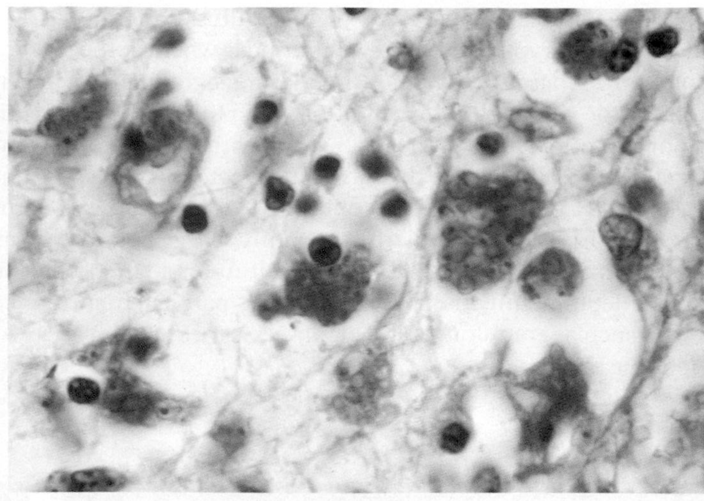

F

FIG. 30. (*Continued.*) **E:** After treatment, residual meningeal and subependymal enhancement persists. **F:** The 2- to 4-μ PAS-positive yeast cells of histoplasma capsulatum are seen in the macrophages of this brain with histoplasma encephalitis (periodic-acid Schiff, original magnification ×200).

vessel (arteriole) occlusion and tissue breakdown (30). Clinically, meningitis is also associated with candidiasis, and presumably results from penetration of the meningeal microvasculature by individual or small groups of yeast cells.

Cryptococcus neoformans is the most common fungus to involve the CNS in AIDS patients (282). It is clinically evident in 6% to 7% of AIDS patients (283). In 45% of all AIDS patients with cryptococcosis, that infection is the first manifestation of their immunodeficiency (283). Inhalation is the usual mode of infection. Cryptococcal CNS infection results in a basilar meningitis (282). This is usually a subacute meningitis with headache as the most common and sometimes the sole symptom (35). In one study of 35 patients with CNS cryptococcosis, 66% complained of headache, altered mental status was seen in 29%, and fever was present in 26% (284). Clinical presentation may also include neck stiffness (284), seizures, and symptoms of increased intracranial pressure (61). Diagnosis is made via India ink preparation, detection of cryptococcal antigen in the CSF, or fungal culture of the CSF.

Imaging findings in cryptococcal meningitis are often unremarkable. CT is frequently negative (69,149). Positive CT findings are often nonspecific, including atrophy and communicating hydrocephalus (68,149,285). Meningeal enhancement can be seen, but is uncommon (149,286) (Fig. 31). Although MR may also be negative, it is far more sensitive than CT (165). Gadolinium-enhanced studies reveal meningeal enhancement that is inapparent on noncontrast images (287).

Spread of infection to the parenchyma occurs via hematogenous dissemination or via direct spread of meningeal infection to the cortex. Parenchymal disease in cryptococcal CNS infection may take a variety of forms, and the literature is somewhat confusing on this topic. Four patterns may be encountered: (a) parenchymal mass lesions, also known as cryptococcomas,

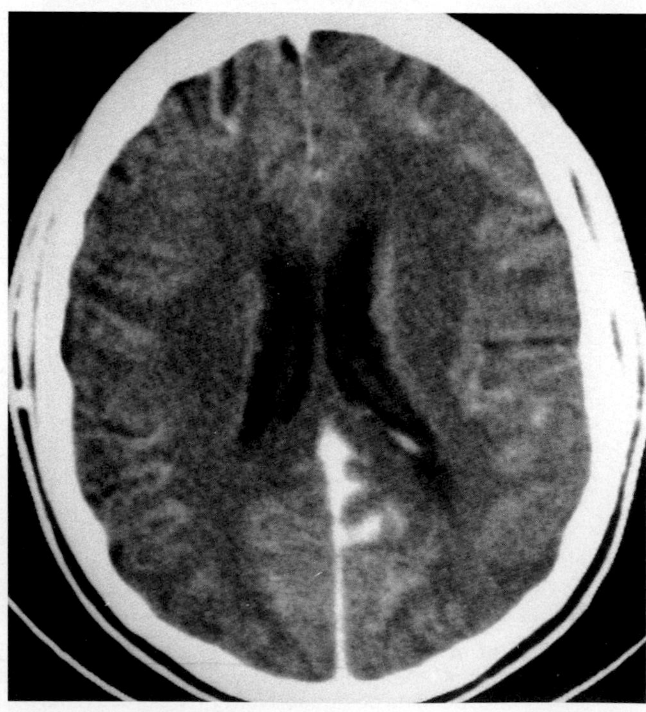

FIG. 31. Cryptococcal meningitis. Postcontrast axial CT scan demonstrates thick meningeal enhancement in this AIDS patient with evidence of cryptococcal antigen in the CSF.

(b) dilated Virchow-Robin spaces, (c) parenchymal/leptomeningeal nodules, and (d) a mixed pattern. Cryptococcomas represent a collection of organisms, inflammatory cells, and gelatinous mucoid material (288). The relative amount of each constituent may vary, and can result in an imaging appearance that has been termed "gelatinous pseudocyst." Alternatively, the constituents may differ in relative concentration, and can thus appear as an isodense or isointense mass lesion on imaging studies. Pathologic examination, however, reveals pseudocystic areas filled with mucoid material in both these types of lesions (288).

In AIDS patients with CNS cryptococcosis, the symptoms and pathologic findings are often muted, perhaps because of the inability to mount a significant cell-mediated immune response (71). This may also account for the paucity of radiographic findings in many cases (71). The cryptococcomas seen in AIDS patients thus rarely demonstrate enhancement, although the lesions seen in immunocompetent patients may enhance.

Dilated Virchow-Robin spaces are perivascular spaces that become distended with fungus and mucoid material (288). As the vessels extend from the basal cisterns to the brain substance, fungal invasion results in the production of voluminous mucoid material, which promotes enlargement of the perivascular spaces. This is most evident in the basal ganglia and midbrain but may be seen throughout the brain (288). In such cases, the infectious agent is outside the parenchyma and therefore does not incite a significant inflammatory response. The parenchymal/leptomeningeal nodules represent small cortical granulomas (71).

The imaging findings in cryptococcal infection may vary with the host population. In the immunocompromised population with CNS cryptococcosis, hydrocephalus is seen in approximately 9% (284). In contrast, among non-AIDS patients with CNS cryptococcal infection, hydrocephalus is present in approximately 25% (289). Thus, hydrocephalus is less common in the immunodeficient patient, and abnormal enhancement is also less frequent. The lower frequency of hydrocephalus may be attributed to the lack of inflammatory leptomeningeal reaction in the immunosuppressed patient and the paucity of resulting adhesions within the basal cisterns.

A number of imaging findings may be encountered in CNS cryptococcosis. Focal hypodensities (>3 mm) are often seen within the basal ganglia, which do not enhance. Those represent the dilated Virchow-Robin spaces described above, distended by cryptococcal organisms and mucinous material. Parenchymal cryptococcomas vary in appearance. Larger cystic masses with septations may be seen in the basal ganglia (Fig. 32). These gelatinous pseudocysts do not demonstrate significant enhancement, especially when present in AIDS

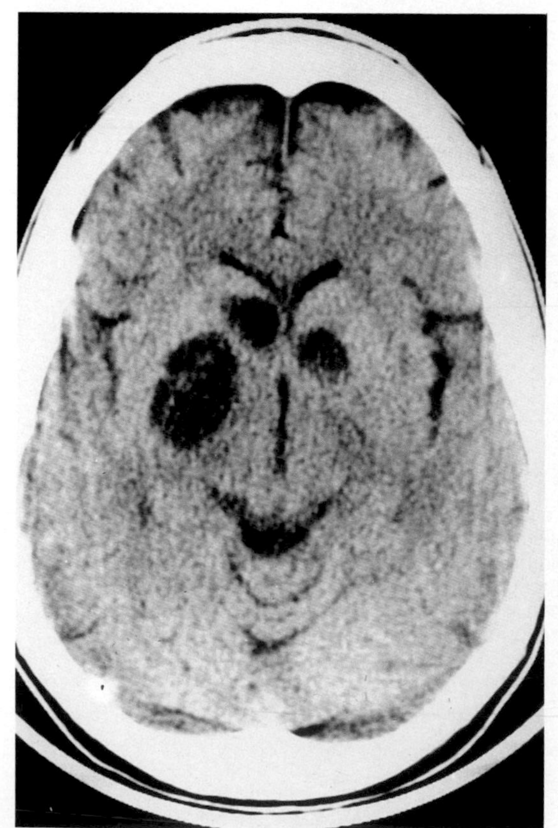

A

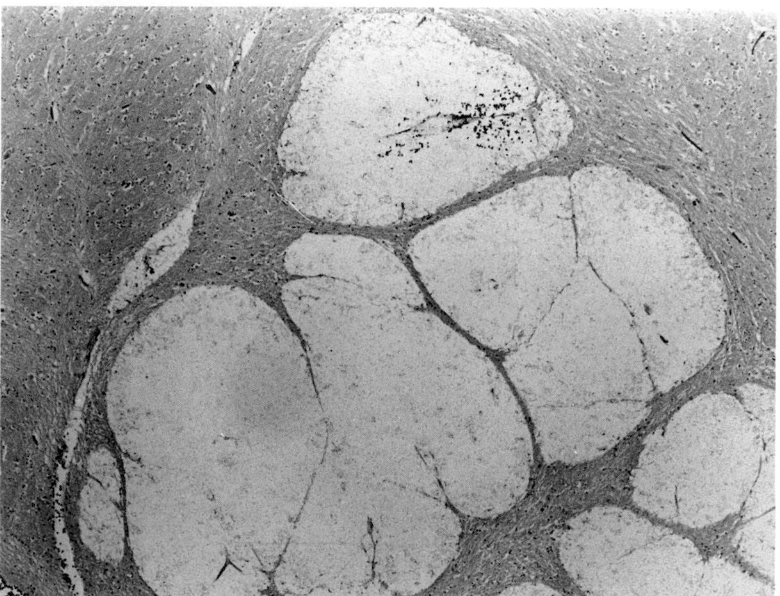

B

FIG. 32. Gelatinous pseudocysts (cryptococcomas). **A:** Noncontrast CT of a patient with documented cryptococcal meningitis reveals cystic mass lesions in both basal ganglia with mild mass effect. On contrast scans, the lesions did not enhance. **B:** Low power photomicrograph of cryptococcoma. The clear areas are filled with mucoid material (H & E, original magnification ×8).

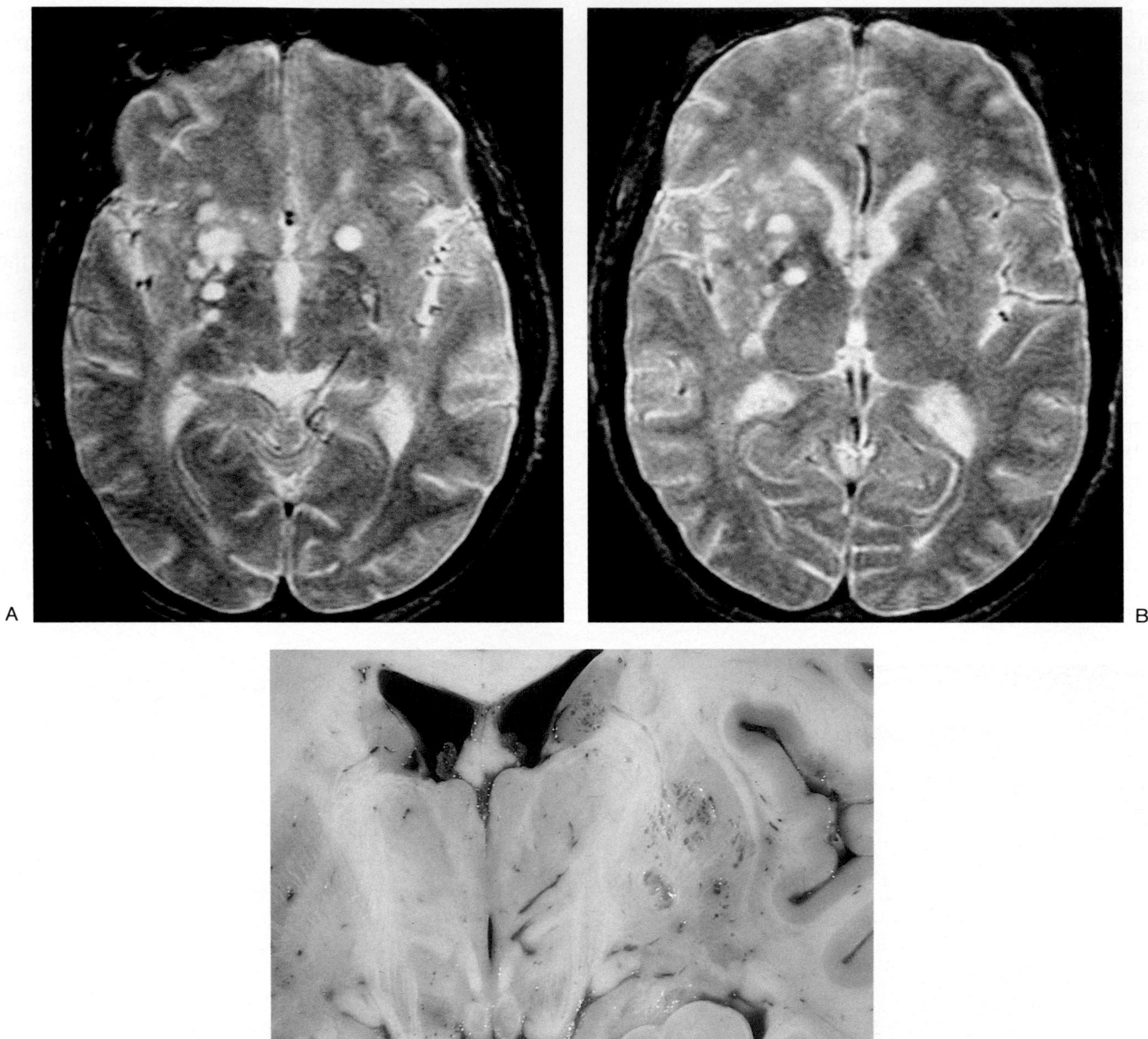

FIG. 33. Cryptococcosis. **A,B:** Axial T2-weighted images (2650/80) of a patient with cryptococcal infection demonstrate foci of increased signal in the basal ganglia, bilaterally, without mass effect. These lesions did not enhance on contrast images. While the majority of these lesions represent dilated Virchow-Robin spaces filled with cryptococcal fungi and mucoid material, the larger lesions likely represent small cryptococcomas. These are difficult to distinguish radiographically but are apparent pathologically. **C:** Autopsy specimen of another case demonstrating dilated Virchow-Robin spaces in the caudate nuclei and in the globus pallidus and putamina, bilaterally.

patients. The lesions may have mild mass effect but there is no surrounding edema. In general, parenchymal disease in cryptococcosis is less widely distributed and incites less edema than toxoplasma encephalitis (290). CT may also demonstrate hypodense or isodense lesions with ring or solid enhancement, particularly in the basal ganglia and cerebral hemispheres (291). Intraventricular cryptococcocomas have been reported (284). Lastly, peripheral small enhancing nodules may be present consistent with cortical granulomas. Noncontrast CT may reveal calcification of these miliary lesions (291).

MR demonstrates punctate clustered foci of signal abnormality that are isointense to CSF on all sequences, compatible with dilated Virchow-Robin spaces (291). These are primarily located in the basal ganglia, are bilateral, and are often symmetric (Fig. 33). Similar findings may be present in the midbrain (291). These foci do not enhance with gadolinium and are not associated with edema or mass effect. Mass lesions (cryptococcomas) again have a variable appearance, depending on the relative constituents of the particular lesions. Gelatinous pseudocysts are isointense to CSF on T1-weighted and T2-weighted images and do not demonstrate edema or enhancement, although there may be mass effect depending on the size of the lesion. These are primarily seen in the basal ganglia, and may be bilateral. These vary in size from <3 mm to several centimeters. Thus, foci of signal abnormality <3 mm on MR may represent either small cryptococcomas or dilated Virchow-Robin spaces (288). MR is far more sensitive than CT in detecting these lesions (288). Cryptococcomas may also appear as mass lesions in the basal ganglia and/or cerebral hemispheres and may be associated with edema, mass effect, and enhancement. In contrast to the gelatinous pseudocysts, these lesions are not isointense to CSF on all sequences. Another pattern of cryptococcal involvement of the CNS has been reported as multiple miliary enhancing parenchymal and/or leptomeningeal nodules (291), suggestive of granulomata.

The MR findings in *Candiasis* are nonspecific. On T2-weighted images the candida abscess appears as an area of well demarcated, hypointense signal surrounded by a larger area of high signal intensity, representing edema (6,33). Some have termed this a "target appearance" (282). Rarely, CNS candida may also present as meningitis (282), meningoencephalitis (35), and granulomata (282).

Aspergillus and mucormycosis involve the CNS by direct extension from nasal cavity/paranasal sinus infection or by hematogenous dissemination. CNS aspergillus (usually *A. fumigatus* infection) is more commonly due to hematogenous dissemination (188). When there is direct extension, vascular invasion is observed, which may involve the cavernous sinus and Circle of Willis, resulting in angiitis, thrombosis, and infarction. Extension to the subarachnoid space may result in meningitis and meningoencephalitis (30,200).

When there is hematogenous spread, usually from a pulmonary focus, aspergillus hyphae lodge in cerebral vessels, cause occlusion, and grow through the vessel walls, producing hemorrhagic infarction. This converts to septic infarction with associated cerebritis and abscess formation, usually in the distribution of the anterior and middle cerebral arteries. Those lesions do not usually reveal granulomatous inflammation histologically (188). On MR, lesions may be well demarcated with ring enhancement typical of an abscess, or lesions may be poorly circumscribed areas of prolonged T1 and T2 relaxation time, with or without mass effect and enhancement (Fig. 34).

CNS mucormycosis is a phycomycosis due to the genus *Mucor*. It occurs in the uncontrolled diabetic or immunocompromised patient, although it is rarely seen in AIDS patients. CNS mucormycosis is most often of the rhinocerebral (craniofacial) type, with spread of infection along perivascular and perineural channels through the cribriform plate into the frontal lobe or through the orbital apex into the cavernous sinus (Fig. 35). Paranasal involvement appears as mucosal thickening, usually without air-fluid levels, and bone destruction, if present, is a late finding (292,293). Intracranial mucormycosis causes either infarction or fungal abscess, and usually involves the base of the brain and cerebellum following invasion of the infratemporal fossa or orbit (293). Infarction or abscess may occur at a site remote from the primary focus of infection, because of vascular dissemination. Direct invasion or vascular dissemination in mucormycosis may result in a basal meningitis.

MR is superior to CT in evaluation of skull base lesions and in evaluation of vascular occlusive disease, and is thus the study of choice in imaging these fungal infections. MR demonstrates both hemorrhagic and nonhemorrhagic infarction. Sinus inflammation is usually hyperintense on T2-weighted images, although aspergillosis is often markedly hypointense on both T1-weighted and T2-weighted images and may demonstrate peripheral enhancement with gadolinium (294). Direct intracranial extension is well demonstrated on multiplanar T2-weighted images as areas of hyperintensity and on post-gadolinium T1-weighted images as abnormal meningeal or parenchymal enhancement (Fig. 36).

CNS infection with *Coccidioides immitis* results from hematogenous spread of endospores from a pulmonary infection. The 2- to 5-mm diameter endospores likely infect the meninges the same way as the individual yeast cells of cryptococcus or histoplasma (188,281). Typically, there is meningeal inflammation with infectious purulent and caseous granulomas, particularly at the base of the brain (188,199). The most common MR and CT findings are (a) abnormal enhancement of the

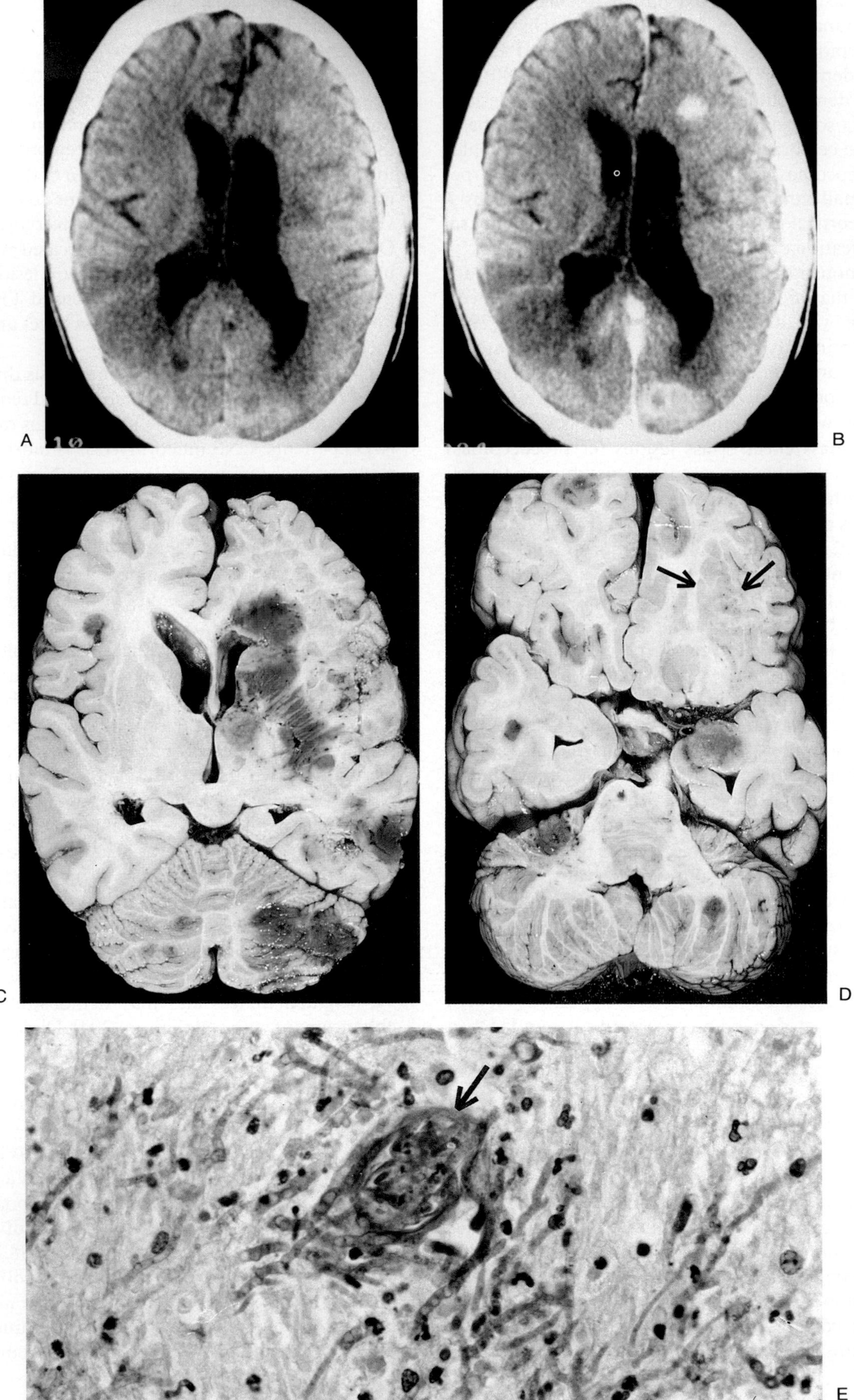
A
B
C
D
E

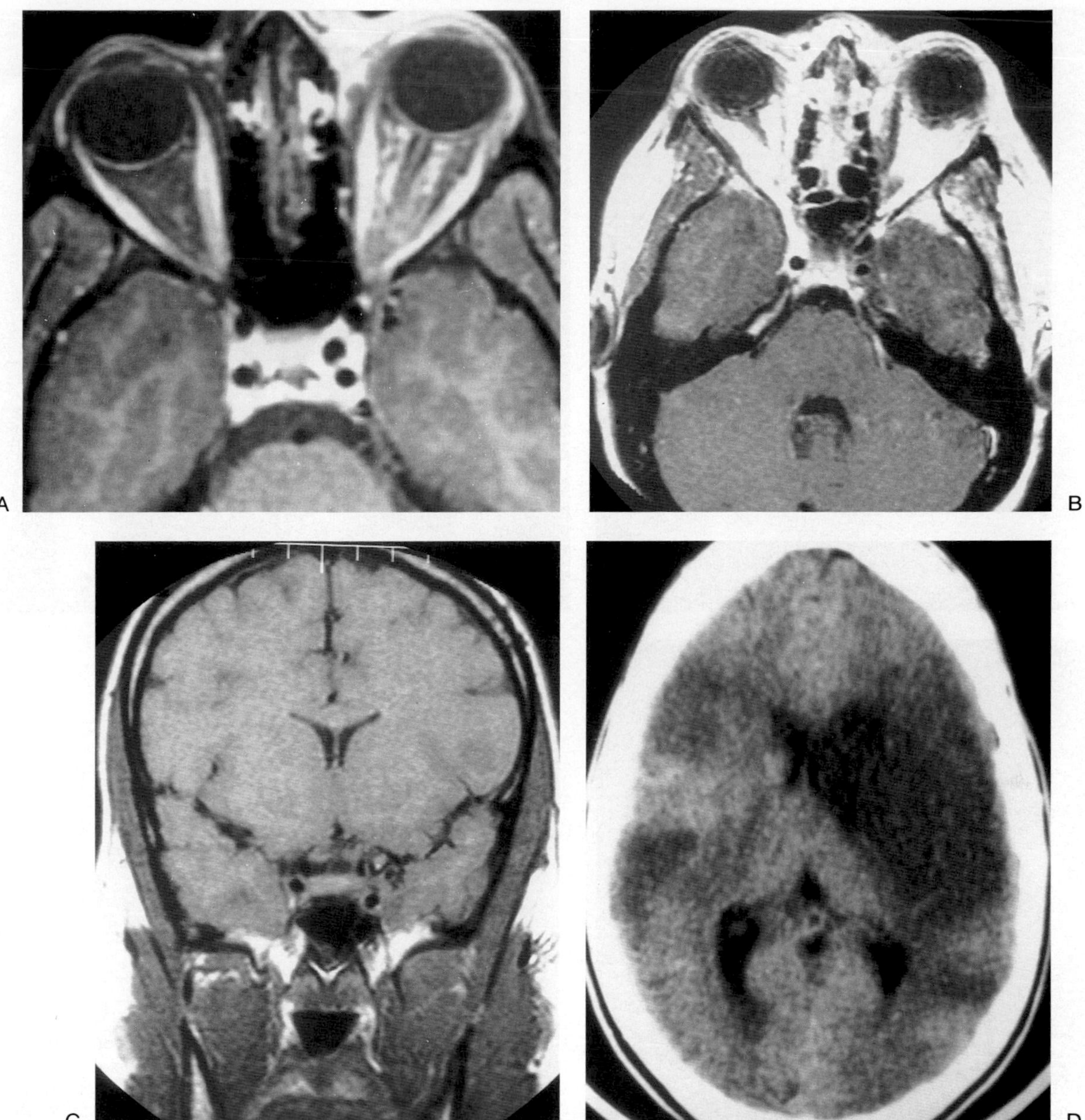

FIG. 35. *Rhizopus* (species of Mucormycosis). **A:** An 18-year-old diabetic woman presented with complaints of left eye pain. T1-weighted axial image of the orbits with fat suppression demonstrates abnormal enhancement throughout the retrobulbar fat on the left. Note also the presence of sinus inflammatory changes. **B:** Axial T1-weighted MR (600/20) postgadolinium performed 24 hours after A reveals a mass in the cavernous sinus and slight narrowing of the left cavernous carotid artery. The cavernous sinus mass represents fungal invasion of the cavernous sinus by *Rhizopus* (a species of mucormycosis), which was obtained from the biopsy of the paranasal sinuses. **C:** Coronal T1-weighted (600/20) image without contrast demonstrates bulging of the left cavernous sinus with loss of the lateral dural margin and inferior displacement of the cavernous carotid artery. **D:** Noncontrast axial CT of this patient obtained soon after the MR demonstrates multiple areas of acute infarction due to vascular occlusion by fungal invasion. Despite aggressive medical therapy, the patient died several days later.

FIG. 34. Aspergillosis (autopsy proven). **A:** Noncontrast CT demonstrates slightly increased density in the left frontal and left occipital regions, compatible with petechial hemorrhage. Abnormal wedge-shaped hypodensity is seen on the right, adjacent to the right lateral ventricle with mass effect, consistent with infarction. **B:** Contrast CT reveals enhancement of the left frontal and occipital lesions. There is nodular enhancement of the frontal lesion and thick ring enhancement of the occipital lesion. At autopsy, these were small abscesses, with vascular invasion and hemorrhage. **C:** Autopsy specimen of same case as in A and B. Numerous hemorrhagic foci are evident, due to vascular invasion and hemorrhagic infarction. **D:** Autopsy specimen, same case. Again note multiple hemorrhagic areas of involvement. Incidentally noted at autopsy was an area of bulk heterotopia in the left frontal region (*arrows*) with tissue characteristics similar to cortical gray matter. **E:** Branching, septate hyphae are seen in this pathologic specimen (same patient, A–E). Invasion of blood vessels (*arrow*) is a hallmark of aspergillus infection (periodic-acid Schiff, original magnification ×80).

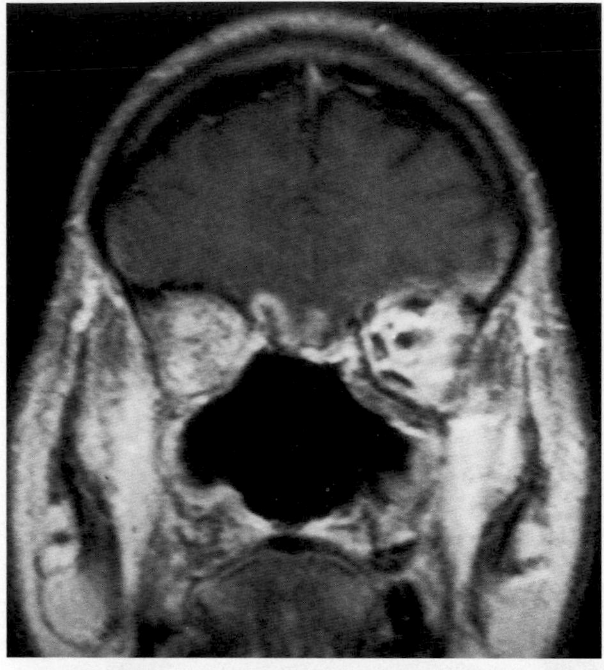

A

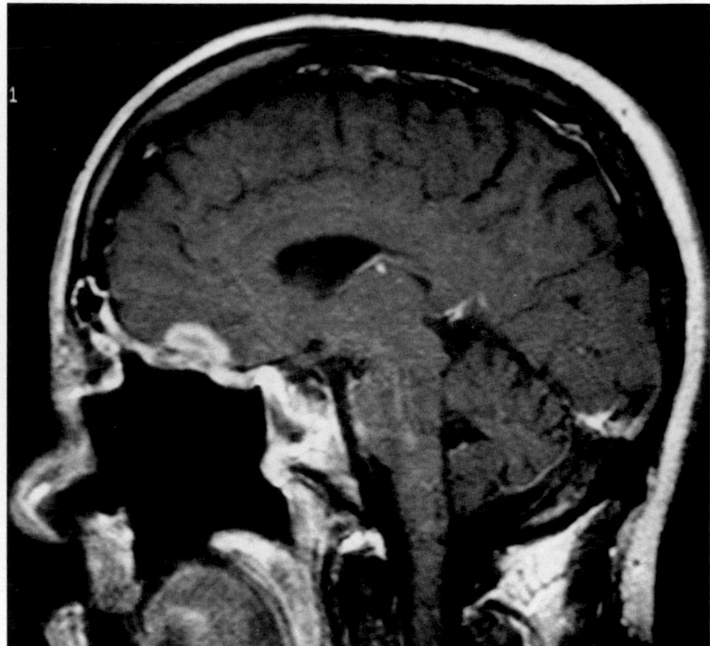

B

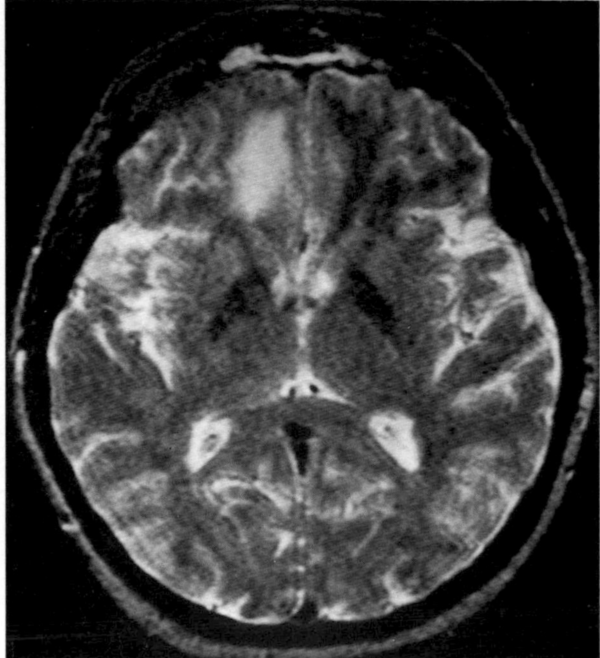

C

FIG. 36. Mucormycosis. **A,B:** This patient was found to have facial mucormycosis and was treated aggressively with surgery and medical therapy. An extensive maxillectomy was performed along with a right orbital exenteration. Coronal and sagittal images obtained after gadolinium administration demonstrate ring enhancement in the gyrus rectus, due to fungal infection, along with enhancement along the surgical margins. Also note postoperative changes in the right orbit. **C:** T2-weighted (2400/80) axial MR demonstrates increased signal at the site of intracranial involvement. The frontal lobe abscess improved on vigorous medical treatment with a good clinical result.

meningeal surfaces over the convexities and in the basal cisterns, which may be obliterated or distorted, (b) communicating hydrocephalus, and (c) entrapment of the fourth ventricle, or a portion of the third or lateral ventricles, secondary to ependymitis with resulting obstructive hydrocephalus (295,296) (Fig. 37). Less commonly, focal white matter or deep gray matter enhancing lesions are identified, representing granulomas (295,296). Although vasculitis may occur in coccidiomycosis, vascular occlusion is rare (296,297).

Neurosarcoidosis, which occurs in approximately 5% of patients with sarcoid, may have MR findings that mimic those of TB and fungal infection. Meningitis and vasculitis occur more often than parenchymal disease (298,299). Typically, there is basal or diffuse granulomatous leptomeningitis with secondary involvement of the optic chiasm, hypothalamus, floor of the third ventricle, and pituitary gland (300). These findings are best seen on multiplanar postgadolinium T1-weighted images (Fig. 38). Ischemia or infarction, as a result of vasculitis, may be seen as focal hyperintense foci in the white matter and basal ganglia on T2-weighted images (6,298).

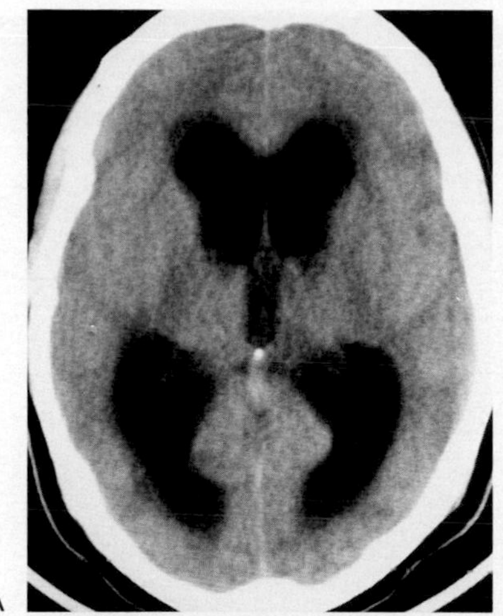

A

FIG. 37. Coccidiomycosis. This patient had a history of extensive, chronic coccidiomycosis infection, involving both brain and spine. **A:** Noncontrast CT demonstrates communicating hydrocephalus due to chronic meningitis. **B:** Sagittal T1-weighted (600/20) MR of the cervical spine reveals a syrinx cavity containing proteinaceous fluid, higher in signal than the CSF. Note also marked enlargement of the fourth ventricle with brainstem compression. **C:** Postgadolinium sagittal scan of the C-spine reveals meningeal enhancement along the cord surface with a large central syrinx. **D:** Postgadolinium sagittal T1-weighted (700/20) scan of the lumbar and lower thoracic region reveals the syrinx extends the entire length of the spinal cord. The syrinx collapsed after shunting of the intracranial hydrocephalus. (From Sklar et al., ref. 347, with permission.) **E:** Coccidiomycosis meningitis reveals the various stages of the coccidioides immitis sporangia from early sporangia (*arrowhead*) to mature sporangium (*large arrow*) to ruptured sporangium with its numerous sporangiospores (*small arrow*). It is the latter structures that elicit the pyogenic reaction or meningitis (H & E, original magnification ×80).

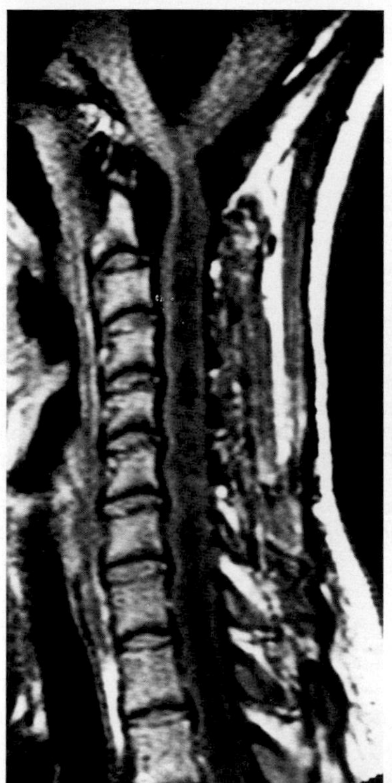

B

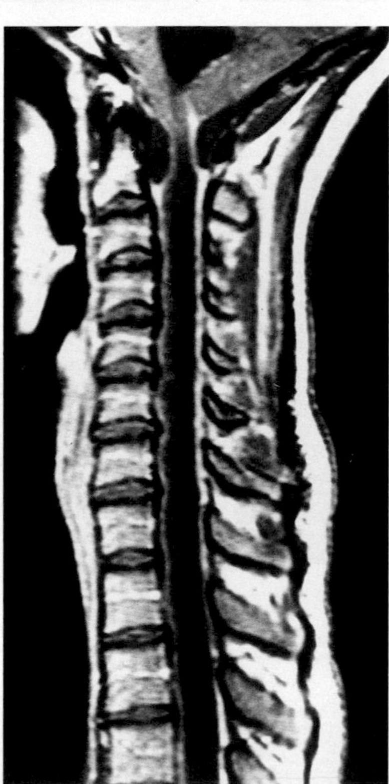

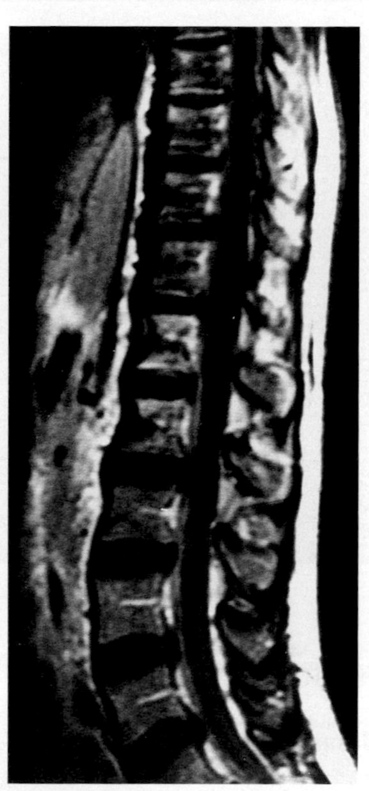

C,D

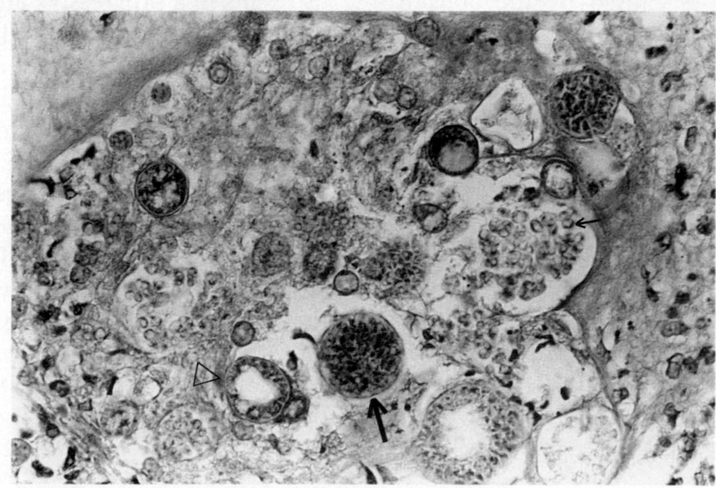

E

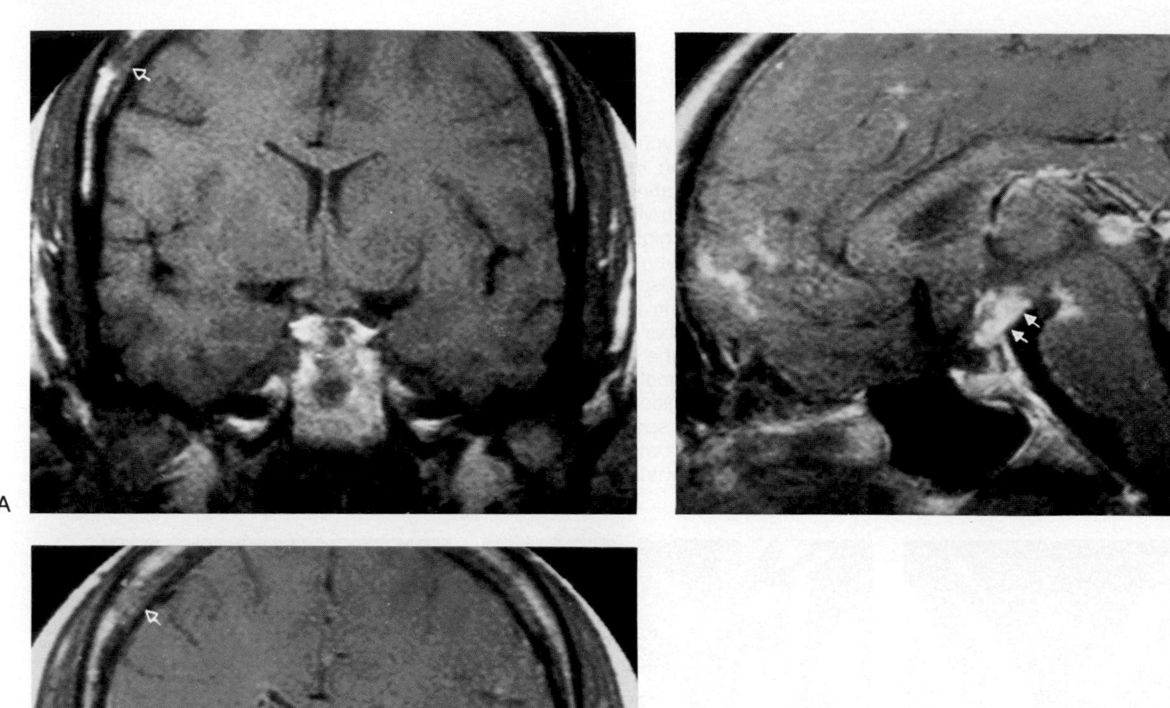

FIG. 38. Neurosarcoidosis in a 30-year-old woman with biopsy-proven sarcoidosis and chronic meningitis. **A:** Noncontrast coronal T1-weighted (700/20) MR. **B:** Postgadolinium coronal and sagittal **(C)** scans (700/20) demonstrate enlargement and enhancement of the optic chiasm and hypothalamus (*solid arrows*). There is also abnormal enhancement of the basal cisterns and cerebellar folia. Note also the focal hypointense signal seen in the right frontal bone on scans (**A,B**) (*open arrow*), which is due to calvarial involvement by sarcoidosis.

PARASITIC INFECTIONS

Toxoplasma Encephalitis

Toxoplasma encephalitis is caused by the obligate intracellular protozoan *Toxoplasma gondii* with a worldwide distribution. Seropositivity for adults in the Unites States ranges from 20% to 70% (35,188). In the immunocompetent patient, infection may be subclinical or may result in a benign course with self-limiting adenopathy, with or without fever (188,301). Before the era of AIDS, fulminant necrotizing encephalitis as a result of toxoplasma infection occurred only in those patients with significant immunodeficiency such as collagen vascular disease, underlying malignancy, organ transplantation, and patients maintained on steroids or undergoing chemotherapy or radiation treatment (301–303). The major transmission of toxoplasma is via raw meat (36,280). Transmission is also possible via bodily secretions, raw milk, transfusions, organ transplantation, contaminated needles, cat feces, and via in utero exposure (36).

In patients with HIV infection, toxoplasma encephalitis results in a progressive and often fatal encephalitis if untreated (35,61,304). The clinical course includes headache, fever, altered mental status, confusion, lethargy, seizure, and focal neurologic deficit (35,61,304). Toxoplasma encephalitis is the most common opportunistic brain infection seen in AIDS patients presenting with altered mental status, fever, seizure, and/or focal neurologic deficit (282,285,286,304). It is present in approximately 10% of adult AIDS autopsies (34). Since seropositivity for toxoplasmosis is so widespread, a positive titer alone is nondiagnostic, only indicating past or recent exposure. A negative titer, however, in a patient with a mass lesion of the CNS should arouse suspicion of other possible etiologies. It should be noted, however, that up to 22% of AIDS patients with toxoplasma encephalitis may not have detectable antitoxoplasma IgG antibodies (305). CSF findings in this infection are nonspecific.

Pathologically, parenchymal toxoplasma lesions have three distinct zones: (a) a central zone, which is avascular, contains few organisms, and demonstrates coagulative necrosis, (b) an intermediate zone, which is engorged with blood vessels, contains numerous free extracellular and intracellular tachyzoites (with very few encysted organisms), and has fewer areas of necrosis, and (c) a peripheral zone, with few vascular changes, more encysted organisms (bradyzoites), and fewer tachyzoites, with little necrosis (304). Inflammatory reaction is most intense in the intermediate zone. There is endothelial cell swelling and proliferation with cuffing of venules by lymphocytes, plasma cells, and macrophages. Toxoplasma lesions do not have capsules. When leptomeningitis is present, it involves only the meninges directly adjacent to the areas of encephalitis. Although small vessel thrombosis and necrosis are characteristically associated with the lesions, arteritis of large vessels is absent.

Pathologic diagnosis is made on hematoxylin and eosin (H & E) stains. In more difficult cases, electron microscopy of formalin-fixed material may be utilized, or standard, immunoperoxidase procedures may be employed in diagnostic evaluation (304).

Early imaging of patients with acute neurologic deterioration is imperative as the results will often dictate clinical management and appropriate therapy can be promptly instituted. On CT, toxoplasma encephalitis characteristically appears as multiple areas of isodensity or hypodensity. There is a predilection for the basal ganglia (in 75–88%) and the corticomedullary junction (36,304). Lesions may involve the posterior fossa (149). Hemorrhage has been reported (92,123), although it is uncommon. The lesions vary in size from less than 1 cm to over 3 cm (304). There is surrounding mass effect and edema, of variable degree (149).

Postcontrast CT demonstrates ring or nodular enhancement. Ring enhancement is more common, with central hypodensity. The rings are usually thin and smooth but may be thick and irregular (304), especially in the larger lesions. Double-dose delayed (DDD) technique (78 g of iodine by bolus/drip infusion with delayed scanning at 1 hour) has been found to be extremely effective in detecting these lesions (35,138,149,304). DDD technique permits maximal enhancement. The central portion of ring lesions of toxoplasma may fill in on delayed scans (149).

The radiologic appearance correlates well with the pathologic findings, with the central hypodensity corresponding to the region of avascular coagulative necrosis. The enhancing ring corresponds to the region of intense inflammation and the peripheral zone may appear as edema on neuroimaging studies (304). Pathologic-radiologic correlation has revealed that the pathologic extent of these lesions is often greater than the area of contrast enhancement seen on CT (304).

Toxoplasma encephalitis is effectively treated with pyramethamine and sulfadiazine with dramatic clinical improvement (35,61,68,149). Serial scans obtained while the patient is on therapy demonstrate a decrease in the number and size of the lesions, with a reduction in edema and mass effect. These changes usually occur within 2 to 4 weeks after initiation of treatment (68,149,286), but may take up to 6 months to completely resolve (35,36). Treated lesions have a variable appearance on CT. Sites of prior disease may appear normal, may demonstrate encephalomalacia and focal atrophy, or may calcify (149). The larger, more complex lesions tend to resolve more slowly and often may result in encephalomalacia. Despite radiographic resolution, in the presence of a persistent cellular immunodeficiency, toxoplasma encephalitis will frequently recur if therapy is discontinued, and thus life-long maintenance medication is required (35,149).

Spin-echo MR imaging without and with gadolinium is more sensitive to both new and old lesions of toxoplasma encephalitis than pre- and postcontrast CT (35,36,138) (Fig. 39). On T2-weighted images, active lesions may vary in signal intensity (Fig. 40). Lesions may be hyperintense to parenchyma and thus indistinguishable from surrounding high intensity edema. Lesions may also be isointense or hypointense centrally surrounded by high signal edema (71,138). This latter appearance has been called a "target" sign (138) and is nonspecific.

On T1-weighted images the lesions are isointense to hypointense on noncontrast images. Postgadolinium (0.1 mm/Kg) studies reveal ring or nodular enhancement in active lesions, clearly distinguishable from surrounding high intensity edema. The enhancement pattern is similar to that seen on CT (149). Hemorrhage in toxoplasma lesions is uncommon.

MR has a greater sensitivity than CT, particularly for small lesions at the corticomedullary junction. Toxoplasma is commonly seen in the basal ganglia and lesions are often multiple. As a result of greater sensitivity, MR is capable of detecting more lesions than CT. MR may also be positive in cases in which the CT is completely negative (35,36). On postgadolinium MR imaging, only 14% of patients with toxoplasma encephalitis will demonstrate a solitary lesion (305) whereas the vast majority will have multiple sites of involvement (305) (Fig. 41). Thus, the lack of multiplicity on a high quality MR study should prompt suspicion of other possible pathology.

Treated lesions may become mineralized ("calcified") and thus show small foci of decreased signal on T1-weighted and T2-weighted images, which may be more prominent on gradient-echo studies. In some cases, de-

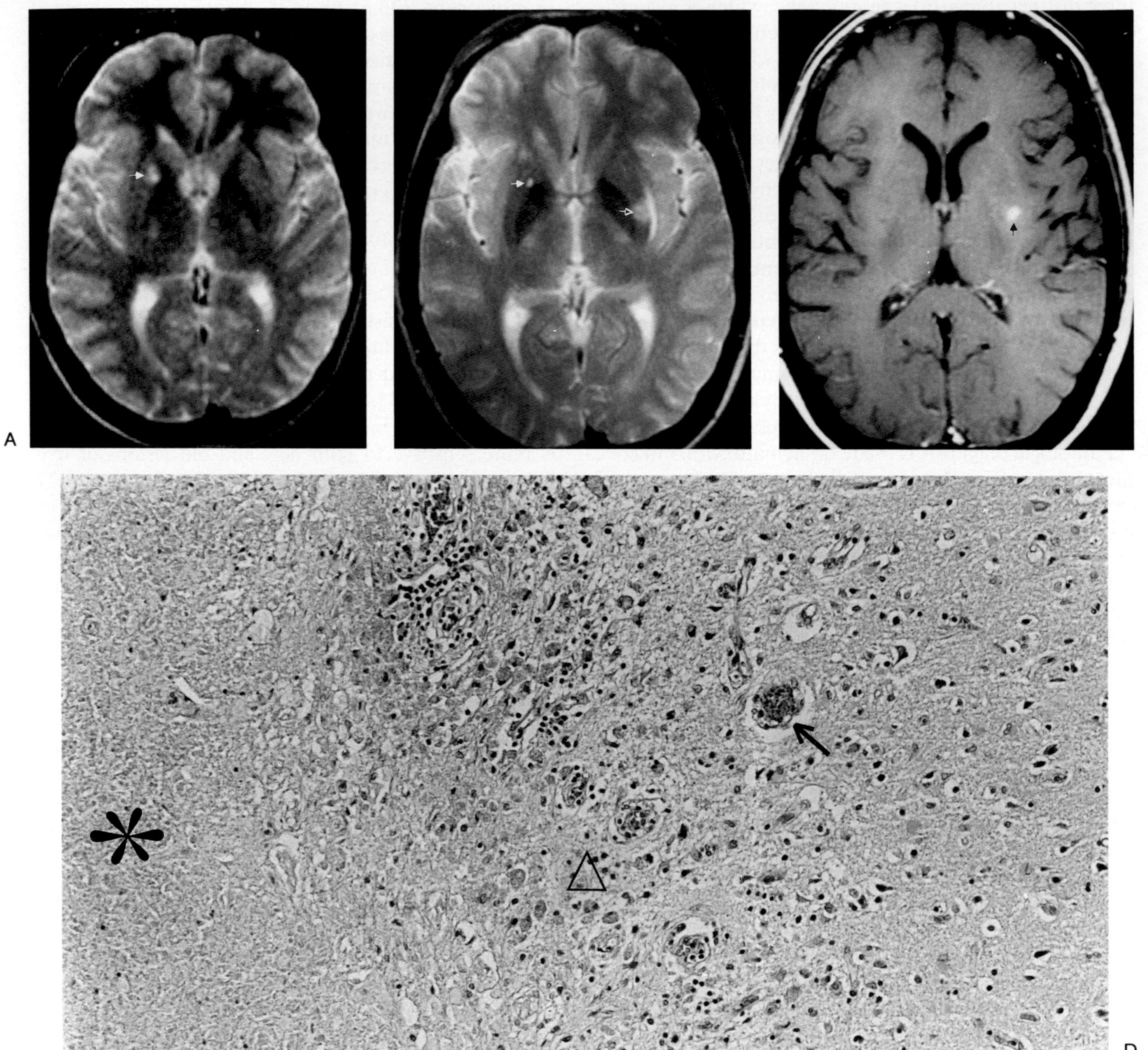

FIG. 39. Toxoplasma encephalitis (new and old lesions). **A:** Initial T2-weighted scan (2400/100) demonstrates focal hyperintense signal in the right basal ganglia (*white arrow*). The patient was treated with antitoxoplasma medication. The patient was noncompliant, however, and returned 3 months later with recurrent seizures. **B:** Subsequent study reveals the right-sided lesion has diminished in size (*white arrow*). However, a new lesion has appeared on the left (*open arrow*), with edema involving the external capsule. **C:** Postgadolinium T1-weighted (800/20) image demonstrates nodular enhancement of the new left-sided lesion (*arrow*) without appreciable enhancement of the old, right-sided lesion. **D:** Typical pathologic findings seen in toxoplasma include an area of central coagulative necrosis (*asterisk*), an adjacent region of neovascularization with engorged blood vessels (*arrowhead*), and a relatively unaffected neuropil with toxoplasma cysts (*large arrow*) (H & E, original magnification ×20).

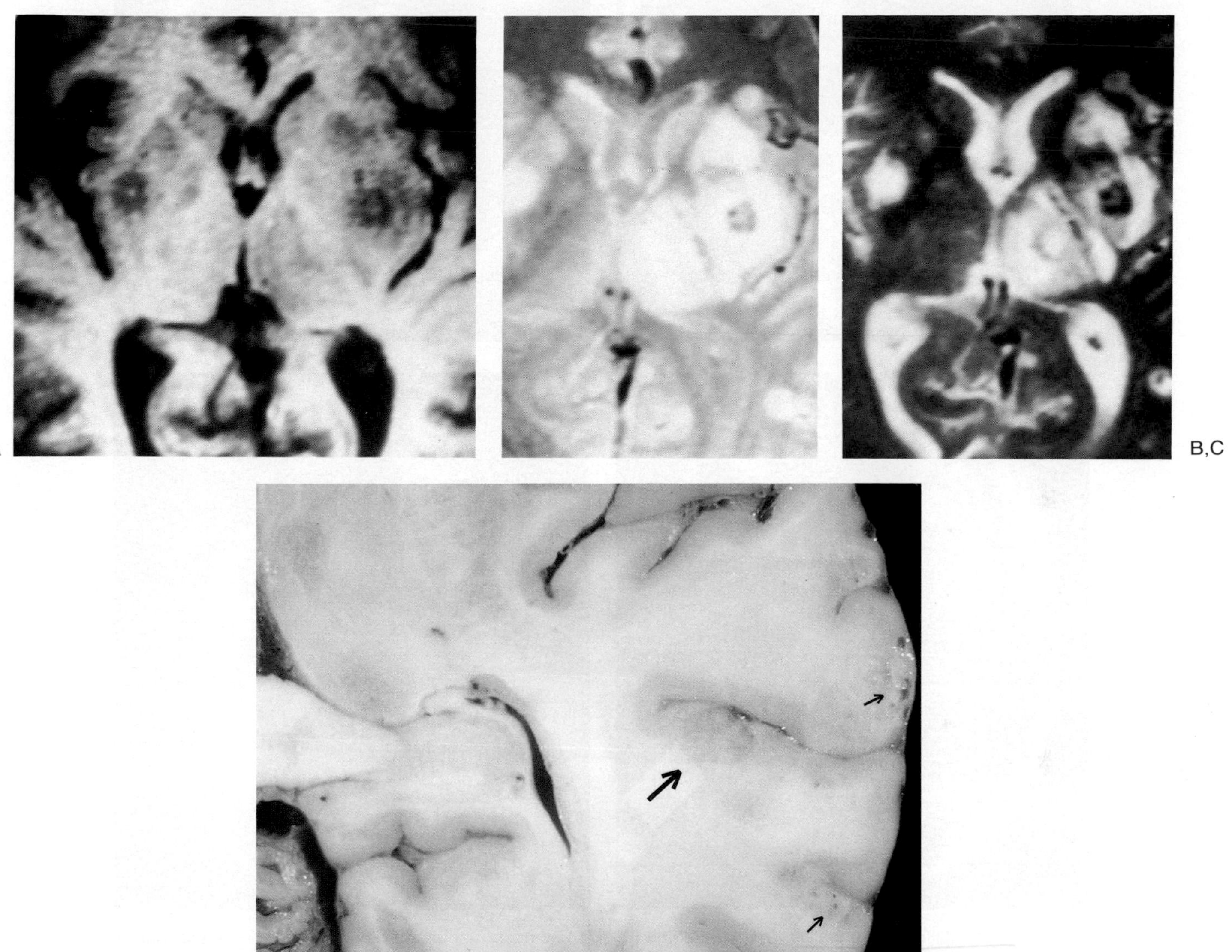

FIG. 40. Toxoplasma encephalitis. **A,** T1-weighted, **B,** proton-density and **C,** T2-weighted images were obtained before initiation of medical therapy. Bilateral foci with heterogeneous signal are noted to involve the deep gray structures, with mass effect and edema. **D:** Pathologic gross specimen of another patient with toxoplasma reveals the small foci of coagulative necrosis (*small arrows*), typical of toxoplasma encephalitis. The largest lesion (*large arrow*) has a reddish rim due to neovascularization.

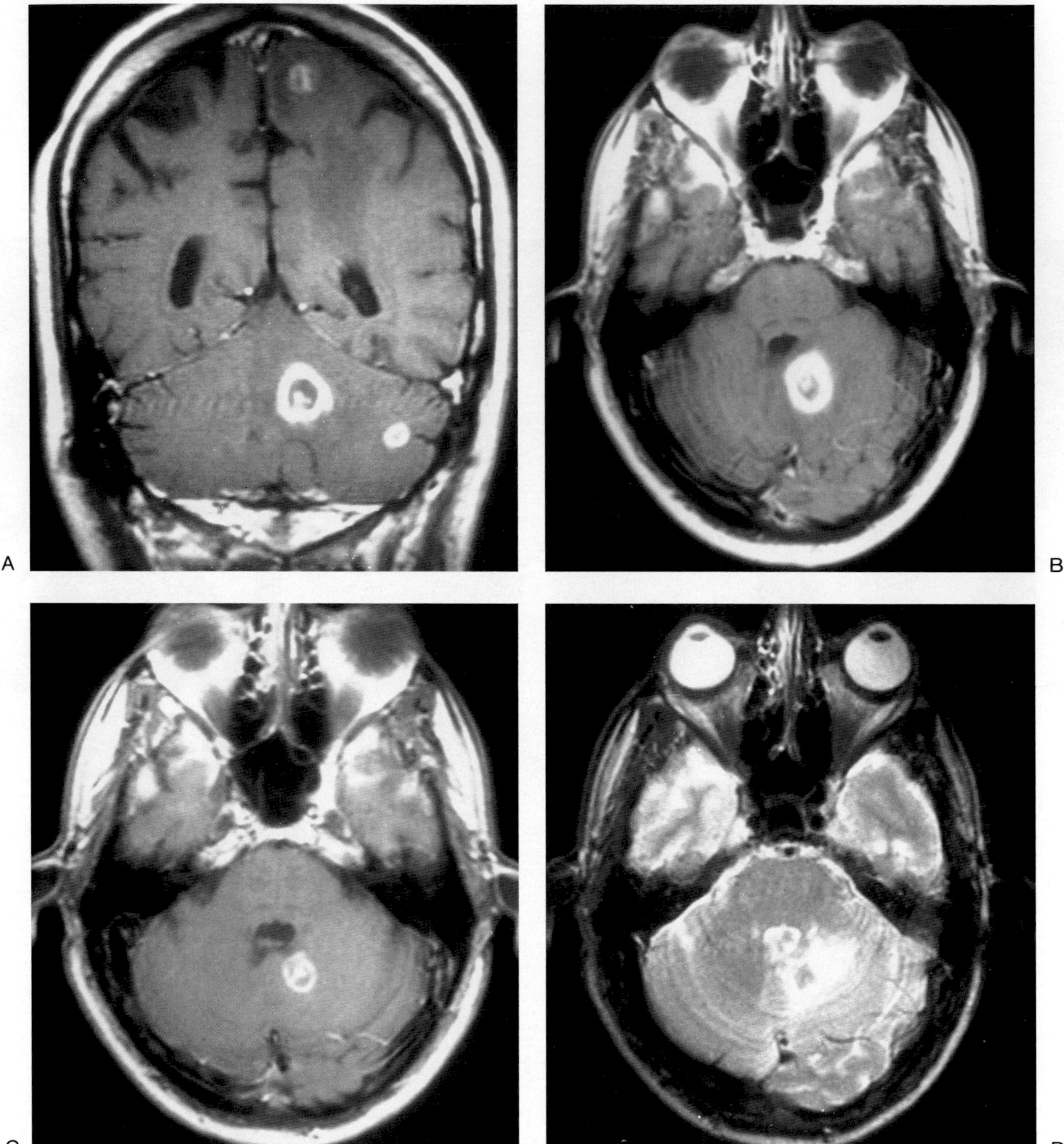

FIG. 41. Toxoplasma encephalitis. **A:** T1-weighted (800/20) postcontrast image demonstrates ring-enhancing lesions in the left parietal lobe at the corticomedullary junction and in the posterior fossa as well. **B:** Axial scan through the posterior fossa again shows a ring-enhancing lesion adjacent to the fourth ventricle with mass effect. **C:** Repeat study obtained after 2 weeks of medical therapy (pyrimethamine/sulfadiazine) reveals a decrease in the size and degree of enhancement. **D:** T2-weighted image (2400/80) obtained at the same time as C shows an isointense lesion surrounded by edema with minimal mass effect.

tection of these mineralized lesions is better on CT (306). Some treated lesions may reveal bright signals on T1-weighted and T2-weighted MR images, possibly due to mineralization with paramagnetic species (i.e., manganese, iron, copper, etc.) (306) (Fig. 42). Thus, the mineralized lesions may have foci of increased or decreased signal on MR. High intensity areas may also represent variation in the deposition of calcium hydroxyapatite or subacute hemorrhage (7).

In the past, early biopsy of these enhancing lesions had been advocated to establish promptly the diagnosis in order to institute appropriate therapy (35,68,304). For the last several years, these cases have been handled more conservatively. Since toxoplasmosis is fairly common in AIDS patients, those who present with typical clinical and radiographic findings are placed on appropriate medical therapy and follow-up scans are obtained in 10 days to 2 weeks. Consistent improvement on serial stud-

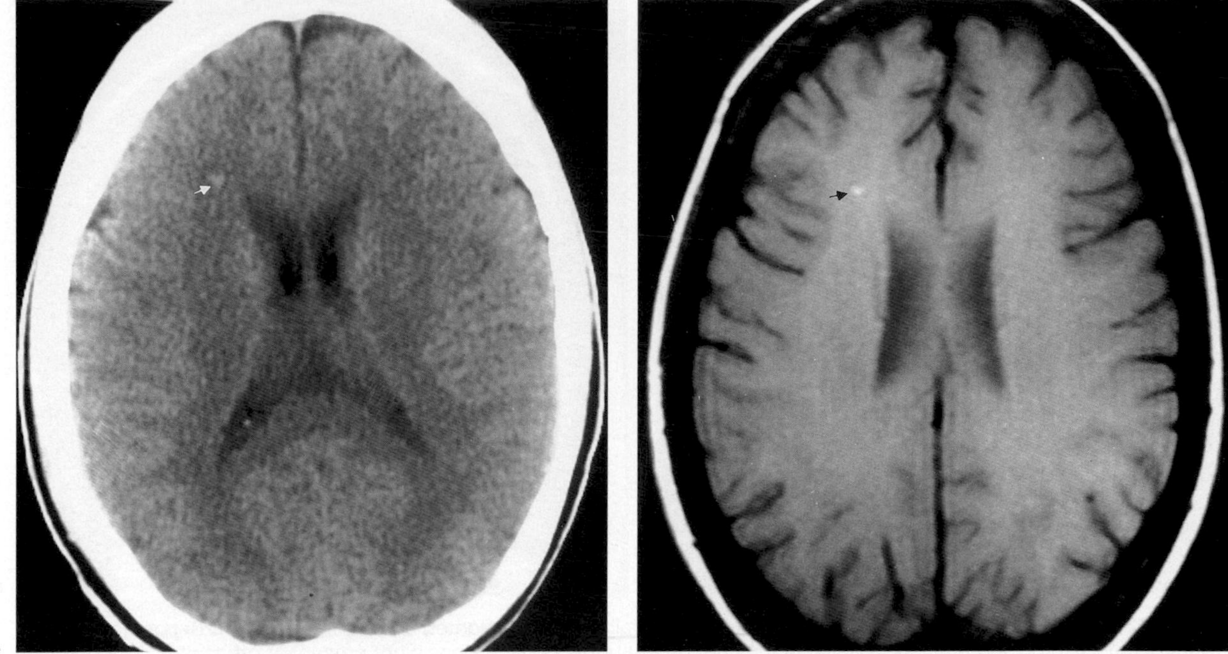

FIG. 42. Treated toxoplasma encephalitis. **A:** Noncontrast CT shows a focal hyperdensity in the right frontal white matter (*arrow*). **B:** T1-weighted noncontrast MR (800/20) obtained 4 months after the CT reveals a hyperintense focus in the same location. Although most treated toxoplasma lesions that calcify are hypointense, some may appear as hyperintense foci because of mineralization with paramagnetic species (i.e., manganese, iron, copper, etc.).

ies is presumptive evidence of toxoplasma encephalitis. An important caveat, however, is that *all* lesions need to be followed to resolution, as multiple pathologies may coexist in any one patient. Lack of considerable improvement should prompt biopsy because a focal enhancing mass lesion may represent primary CNS lymphoma or possibly another type of infection. A second caveat is that it is impossible to assess lesion activity accurately if the patient is on steroid treatment. Steroids will reduce the degree of enhancement and diminish the associated edema and mass effect and it is therefore impossible to determine if there has been a true response to antitoxoplasma therapy.

Primary CNS lymphoma is often difficult to distinguish from toxoplasma encephalitis on CT and MR imaging. Whereas toxoplasma is often multicentric but may be solitary, primary CNS lymphoma is often solitary but may be multicentric as well (Fig. 43). Since treatment of these lesions is completely different, it becomes necessary for the radiologist and the clinician to distinguish between these two entities. Thallium-201 brain SPECT has become invaluable in enabling this distinction. Metabolically active tissue, such as tumor, will demonstrate increased uptake relative to the surrounding parenchyma (307), whereas infectious lesions do not. While Thallium-201 brain SPECT is nonspecific, and will be positive for other types of tumor, a positive study in an HIV-seropositive patient is highly indicative of a primary CNS lymphoma (307) (Fig. 44). This study can be obtained quickly after clinical presentation and may preclude the need for 10 to 14 days of therapy with reevaluation. AIDS patients presenting with intracranial mass lesions are begun on antitoxoplasma therapy and sent for nuclear imaging with thallium-201 brain SPECT. Positive scans are suggestive of CNS lymphoma, and biopsy is urged. Negative studies are presumed to be due to an infectious agent, and the patient is continued on medical therapy for toxoplasma encephalitis with follow-up scans obtained in 10 to 14 days. The sensitivity of the thallium scan is limited by resolution and tumors less than 6 to 8 mm in size may not be detected (307). Lymphomatous lesions limited to the subependymal region may also go undetected.

Toxoplasmosis is also a common cause of congenital CNS infection, second only to CMV. Toxoplasmosis involves 1/1,000 to 1/10,000 pregnancies in the United States per year (75).

Clinically significant findings occur when the fetus is infected before 26 weeks of gestational age (308). Signs and symptoms may be subclinical initially, with development of seizures. Chorioretinitis may be present bilaterally. Severely affected infants have microcephaly. Neuroimaging studies reveal hydrocephalus and intracranial calcifications, most commonly in the cortex and basal ganglia, and these calcifications are located more diffusely than those seen in CMV. Ependymitis results is aqueductal stenosis and thus hydrocephalus (301).

Cysticercosis

Cysticercosis is the most common parasitic infection of the human CNS, worldwide (309). It is seen in both

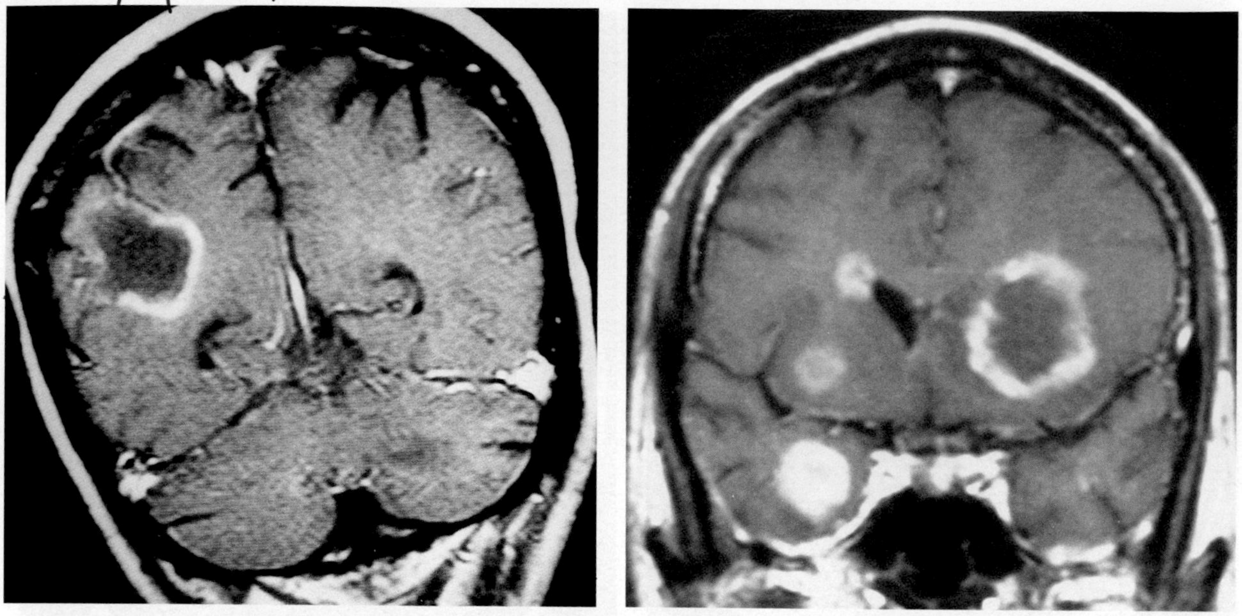

lymphoma Toxo

A B

FIG. 43. Primary CNS lymphoma vs. toxoplasma encephalitis. **A:** T1-weighted coronal image (600/20) postgadolinium reveals a large ring-enhancing lesion in the right parietal lobe. Other lesions were present at other sites, including the left cerebellum (note edema). This patient had biopsy-proven toxoplasma encephalitis. **B:** T1-weighted coronal MR (600/20) in a different patient reveals solid and ring-enhancing lesions as well as periventricular enhancement surrounding the right frontal horn. This patient had biopsy-proven CNS lymphoma. The CNS lymphoma seen in AIDS patients is often necrotic centrally and thus appears as a ring-enhancing lesion, quite similar to toxoplasma encephalitis. Both toxoplasma and lymphoma may be either uni- or multifocal. Thus, there can be difficulty in distinguishing between these entities radiographically. The distinction is essential, however, because of the marked difference in treatment of these diseases.

immunosuppressed and immunocompetent individuals from endemic regions. Neurocysticercosis is endemic in Mexico, Central and South America, India, and China (309). Cases have been reported from Eastern Europe, Africa, Asia, and Portugal (309). Immigration to the United States has resulted in an increased prevalence of this disease in the United States (309).

The causative agent in cysticercosis is the pork tapeworm, *Taenia solium.* Humans may be either the definitive host in the life cycle (infected with a tapeworm), or may be the intermediate host (infected with the cysticercus) (309).

When humans ingest insufficiently cooked pork that contains the viable larvae of *T. solium* (cysticerci), they become the definitive host for the tapeworm (309). Humans are the only definitive host for this cestode (309). Following ingestion, the cysticercus larva develops in the small intestine into a tapeworm, 1 to 8 m long. This tapeworm is usually asymptomatic but does release eggs that pass into the stool (309). If these ova contaminate food or water that is then eaten by the pig, the life cycle continues in the pig as the intermediate host.

Humans may also become the intermediate host after ingestion of contaminated food or water. Within the stomach, gastric juices dissolve the thick outer shell of the ova to release the oncospheres (309). These oncosphores, the primary larvae, penetrate the stomach and intestinal mucosa and enter the blood stream. They may deposit in any tissue, but show a predilection for the brain (309). Other sites include the retina, skeletal muscle, heart, and subcutaneous tissues (309).

Intracranially, the oncospheres may burrow into brain parenchyma, meninges, ependyma, and choroid plexus. Spinal cord involvement can occur, but is rare (310). There are four patterns of neurocysticercosis: parenchymal, subarachnoid, intraventricular, and mixed (311). The parenchymal type is probably the most common (295).

Initial cerebral infection by the larva is usually asymptomatic and results in a small edematous lesion (312). The secondary larvae or cysticerci then develop into cysts. Mature parenchymal cysts are present 2 to 3 months after the original host ingestion of ova (309). This stage is often asymptomatic but may result in seizures.

Each cyst measures 3 to 18 mm in diameter and contains a scolex (313). When alive, the cyst provokes minimal surrounding inflammation and remains viable for 2 to 6 years after infestation (309). As the cyst dies, antigens and metabolic products leak from the wall into the surrounding brain, inciting an intense inflammatory reaction in the adjacent parenchyma, with edema and mass effect. The patient may become symptomatic with seizures or focal neurologic signs. The clear cyst fluid becomes turbid and gelatinous (313). The cyst then collapses, degenerates, and often calcifies (309).

If oncospheres lodge in the meninges or choroid plexus, the infection may involve the ventricular system and/or subarachnoid space (309). The subarachnoid

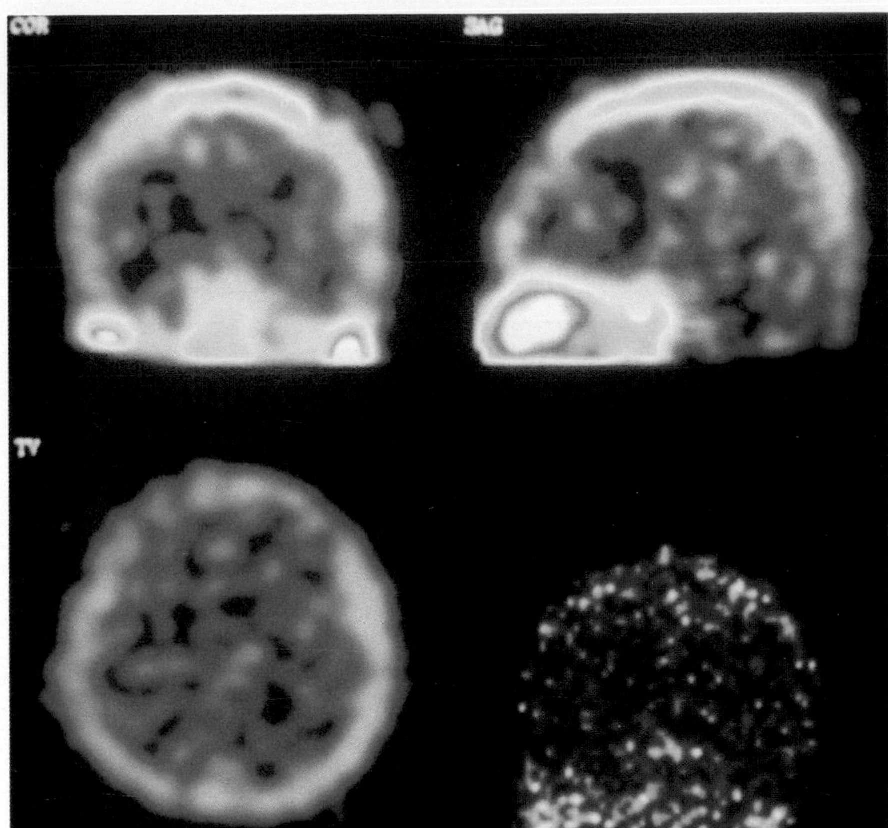

A

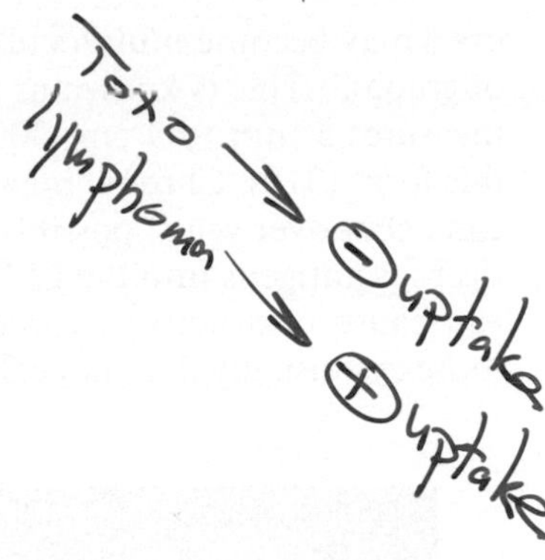

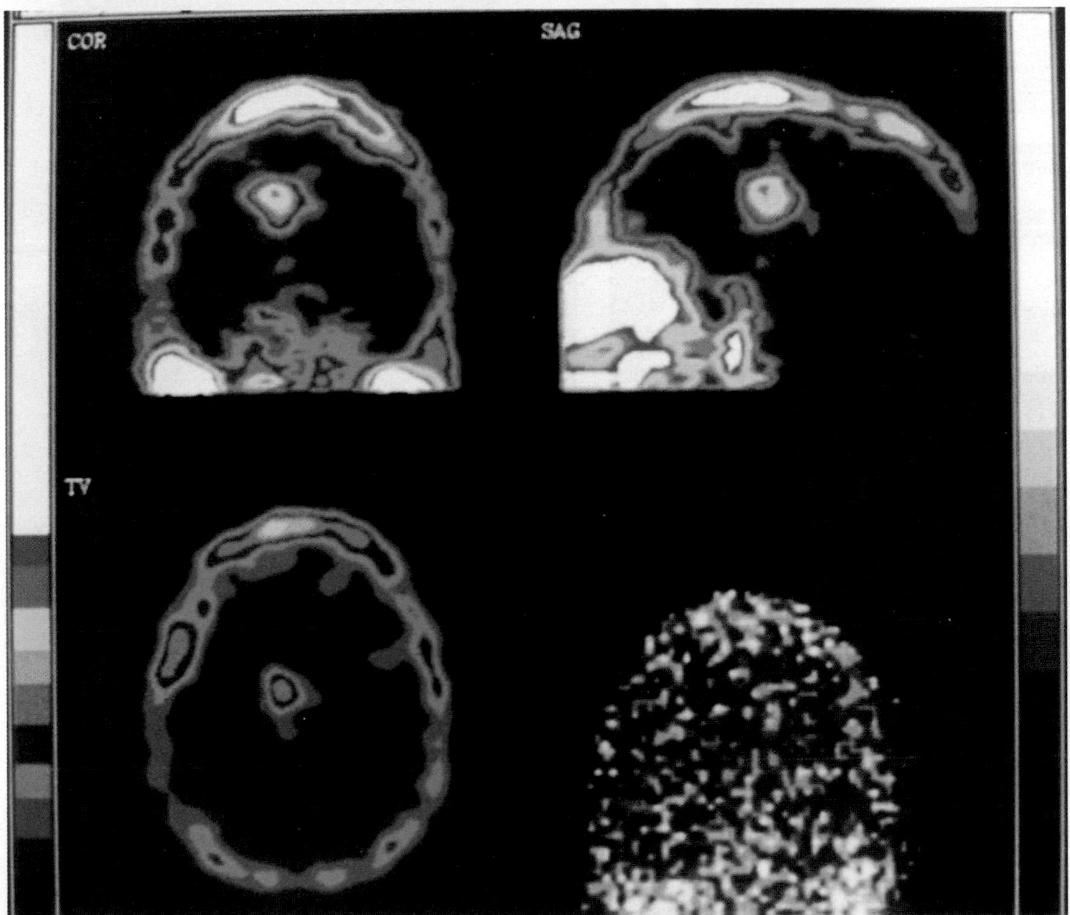

B

FIG. 44. Primary CNS lymphoma vs. toxoplasma encephalitis by Thallium-201 brain SPECT. **A:** Coronal, sagittal, transverse, and planar images from Thallium-201 Brain SPECT of an AIDS patient with multifocal enhancing lesions by CT. No focal uptake is identified. Brain biopsy confirmed toxoplasma encephalitis. The patient responded well to medical therapy. **B:** Coronal, sagittal, transverse, and planar images from Thallium-201 Brain SPECT of an AIDS patient with a ring-enhancing lesion in the pericallosal region. Note focal uptake in the same region of abnormality, consistent with neoplasm. Brain biopsy confirmed primary CNS lymphoma.

cysts may become multiloculated, resembling a "cluster of grapes." This is known as the racemose form, which measures 5 mm to 9 cm (309). The scolex is absent in this form (310). Chronic meningitis and/or ventriculitis can occur over years, possibly because of leakage of cysticercus antigens into the CSF (309). The racemose cyst can cause obstructive hydrocephalus (314). The racemose cyst usually does not calcify after degeneration.

In endemic regions, there may be recurrent ingestion of ova and thus the intracranial cysts are found in different stages of evolution. Additionally, some lesions resolve more slowly than others, also accounting for different stages of disease within an individual patient. In the untreated host, the entire process of resolution of a single lesion will take 2 to 10 years (309).

CSF is abnormal in about 50% of cases (309). Opening

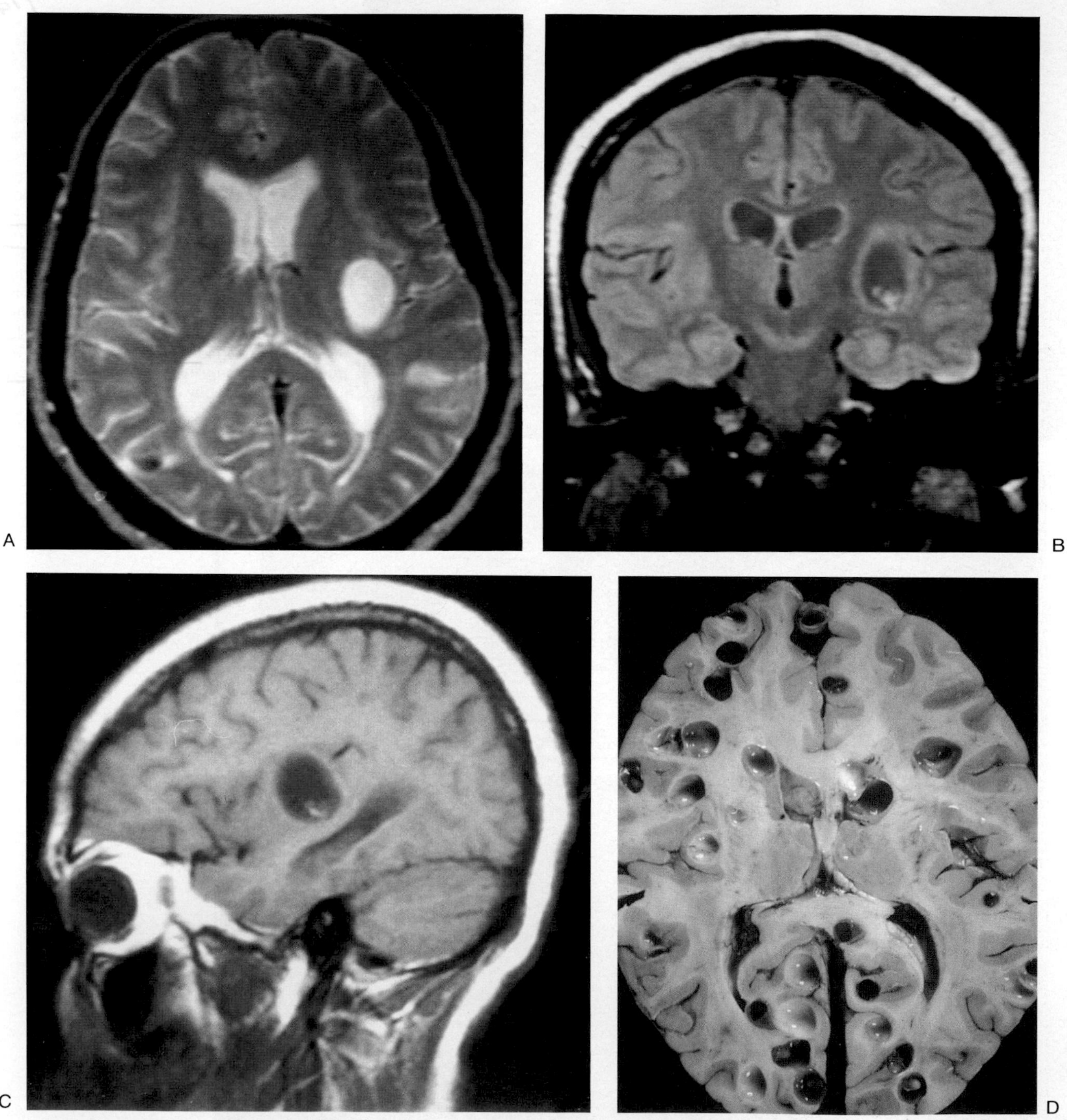

FIG. 45. Cysticercosis. **A:** T2-weighted (2550/80) axial image demonstrates a large cystic lesion in the left basal ganglia without edema or mass effect. **B:** Proton-density coronal image (2550/20) demonstrates the cyst to be isointense to CSF with a hyperintense mural nodule that is seen best on the intermediate weighted images. **C:** Sagittal T1-weighted scan (600/20) without contrast reveals the cystic lesion with a well-defined mural nodule, minimal if any mass effect, and no surrounding edema. The cyst wall is thin and smooth. **D:** Autopsy specimen of another patient with innumerable cysts of cysticercosis. Note the paucity of mass effect despite the number of lesions.

pressures may be elevated in 40% of cases. A lymphocytic pleocytosis may be present in the CSF (315).

Imaging findings in neurocysticercosis are quite often characteristic. The initial infection results in a small edematous lesion that is hypodense on CT and hyperintense on T2-weighted MR images. These usually do not enhance (316), although some peripheral or punctate enhancement may be seen. Nodules may then appear that do show some enhancement (316). These represent protoscoleces, which are within cysticerci but without cyst fluid. The mature cysts are readily apparent on CT and MR, measuring 5 to 20 mm (317). This is the vesicular stage (Fig. 45). Cysts may be near the gray-white junction but are also seen in the basal ganglia, cerebellum, and brainstem. There is little, if any, edema. The cyst wall is thin and smooth. The protoscolex can be identified as a focal nodule within the cyst, and is better demonstrated by MR than CT, although it may be seen on both studies. Because of the bright signal of the CSF on T2-weighted images that may obscure the scolex, the mural nodule is best seen on proton-density images (317,318) (Fig. 46). The cyst wall only occasionally enhances at this stage

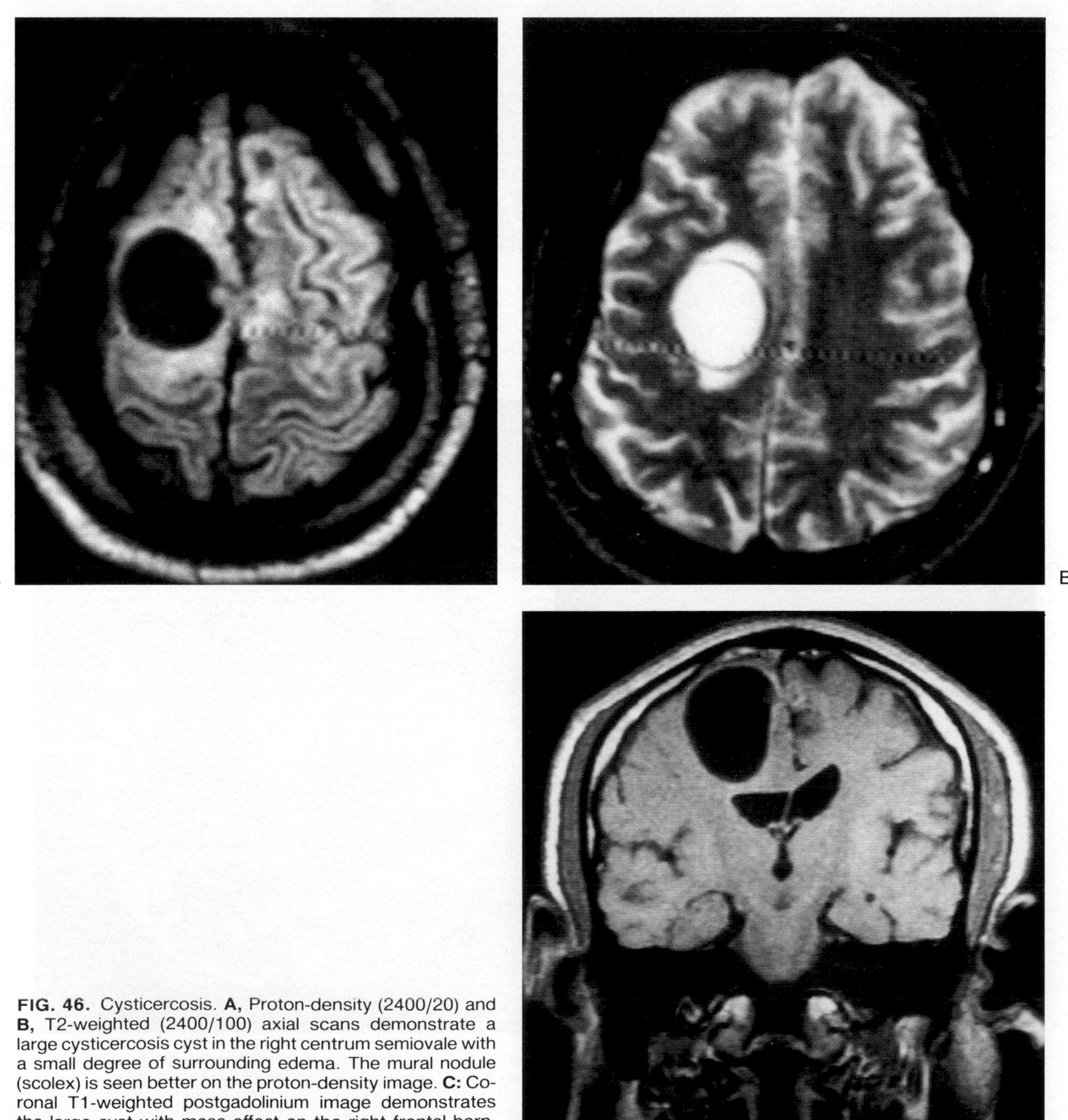

FIG. 46. Cysticercosis. **A,** Proton-density (2400/20) and **B,** T2-weighted (2400/100) axial scans demonstrate a large cysticercosis cyst in the right centrum semiovale with a small degree of surrounding edema. The mural nodule (scolex) is seen better on the proton-density image. **C:** Coronal T1-weighted postgadolinium image demonstrates the large cyst with mass effect on the right frontal horn. Note faint enhancement along the medial edge of the lesion, near the mural nodule.

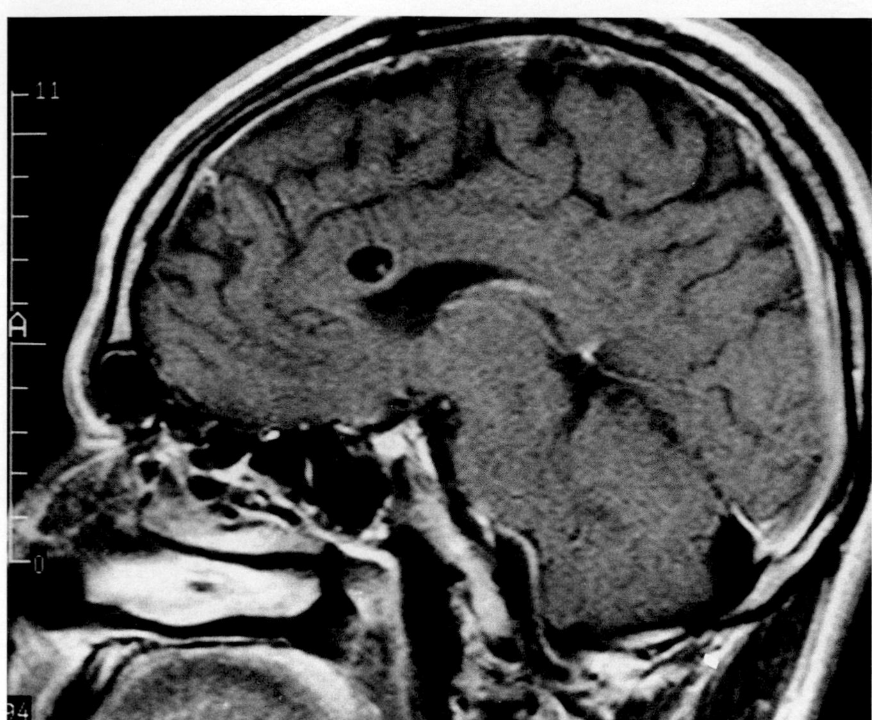

FIG. 47. Cysticercosis T1-weighted (600/20) sagittal image, postgadolinium, demonstrates a cyst in the corpus callosum with an enhancing scolex and faint enhancement along the inferior aspect of the cyst. This patient was asymptomatic, and was scanned because of head trauma. He had recently come to the United States from Mexico.

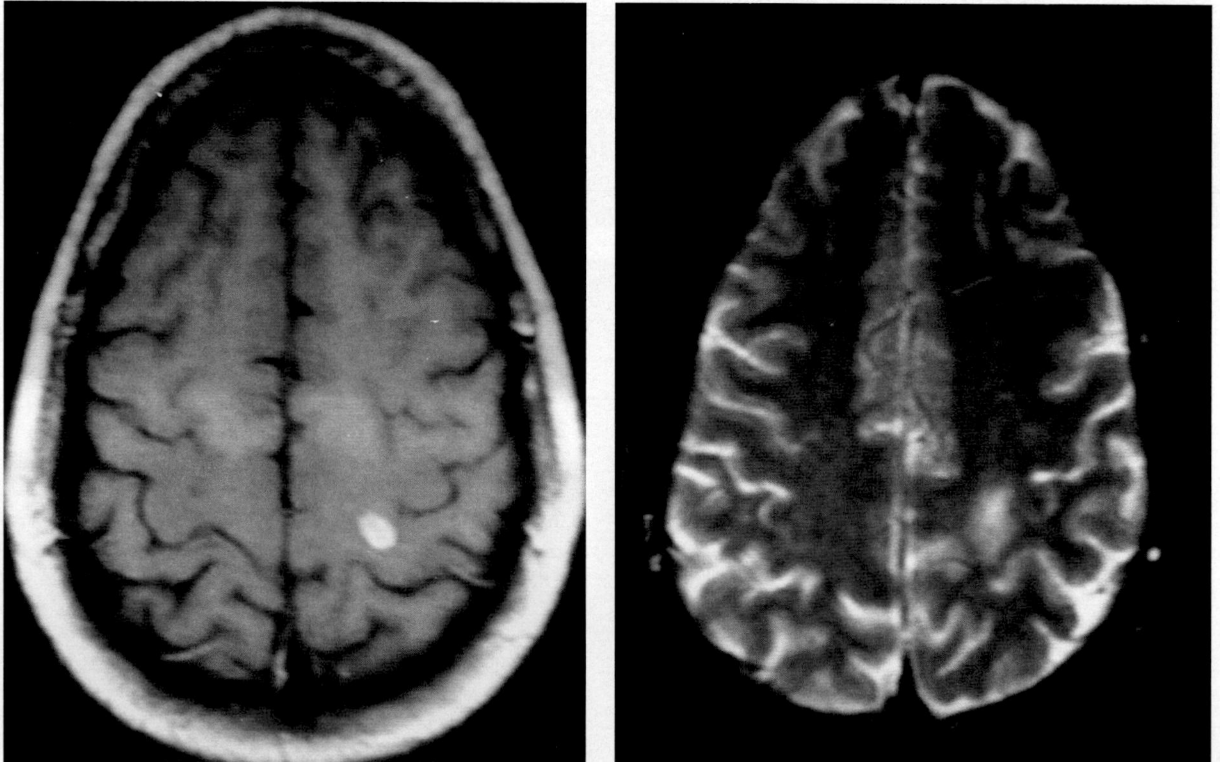

FIG. 48. Cysticercosis. **A:** This degenerating cyst has retracted and demonstrates enhancement on this T1-weighted (750/20) axial scan. **B:** Focal edema is seen on the T2-weighted image (2200/80) at the site of the cyst degeneration.

(Fig. 47). The cysts are isointense to CSF on all MR sequences and of fluid density on CT. MR often reveals a greater number of viable lesions compared with CT.

As the larva dies, the host inflammatory response results in formation of a fibrous capsule that often demonstrates ring enhancement on CT and MR. Degenerating cysts may be hyperintense on both T1- and T2-weighted images because of the proteinaceous fluid and debris accumulated within the cyst (319). This is the colloidal vesicular stage. Degenerating cysts incite surrounding edema, which is evident on MR as increased signal on T2-weighted images and on CT as surrounding hypodensity. In the granular nodular stage the cyst retracts and forms a granulomatous nodule, which may show ring or solid enhancement (320) (Fig. 48).

In the final nodular calcified stage, the lesion becomes mineralized. The granulomatous nodules are replaced by gliosis and eventually calcification (320) (Fig. 49). Calcified lesions may be easier to identify on CT but can be seen as small foci of hypointense signal on spin-echo T2-weighted images, and may be more apparent on gradient-echo imaging.

On CT, the intraventricular and subarachnoid cysts are often difficult to identify as they are isodense to CSF and the subarachnoid lesions do not enhance (310). The intraventricular cysts may enhance. These lesions are better demonstrated by MR, particularly because the fourth ventricle is the most common site for intraventricular cysticercosis (317,318) (Fig. 50). Hydrocephalus is often present. Within the subarachnoid space, the cerebellopontine angle and suprasellar cisterns are the most common locations. These racemose ("grape-like") subarachnoid cysts can sometimes be difficult to delineate, even with MR. The clue to their presence may be the focal widening of a CSF space or an inflammatory response in the adjacent parenchyma. Infection of the subarachnoid space may result in communicating hydrocephalus because of the chronic meningitis and MR may show enhancement of the basal cisterns. Cysts have also been reported within the spinal cord (Fig. 51). Plain films of the extremities may reveal calcification within skeletal muscle, suggestive of cysticercosis (310).

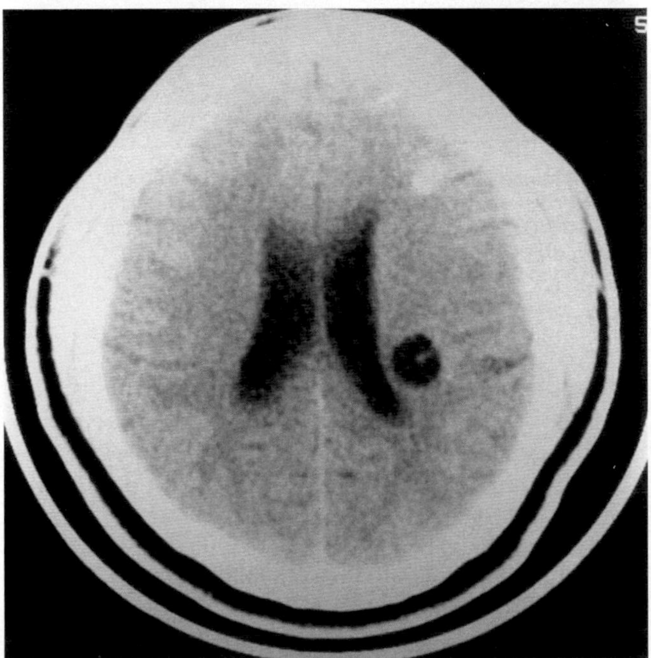

FIG. 49. Cysticercosis. Axial noncontrast CT demonstrates a left frontal calcification at the site of a prior cyst. A lesion in the vesicular stage is seen adjacent to the left lateral ventricle.

The diagnosis of cysticercosis is based on clinical, radiographic, and serologic indicators. Treatment is most often with praziquantel. Intraventricular cysts may not respond as well as parenchymal cysts, and may require surgical treatment if ventricular obstruction is present.

Amoeba

Several amebic organisms may involve the CNS. These infections are rare, with *Entamoeba histolytica, Naegleria fowleri* and *Acanthamoeba* being the most frequently encountered.

Entamoeba histolytica is the etiologic agent in cerebral amebiasis. It is an intestinal parasite endemic to the southern Unites States, South America, Latin America, Southeast Asia, and Africa (321). The route of infection is via ingestion of cysts. Most patients thus infected are asymptomatic or have a mild colitis (322). CNS infection occurs in patients who have had intestinal infestation, and the mode of spread is likely hematogenous (323,324). Many of these patients also harbor liver abscesses (324,325).

Patients with cerebral amebiasis are usually between the ages of 20 and 40 years, with men affected 10 times as often as women (323,325). Symptoms are nonspecific, including headache, vomiting, lethargy, seizures, meningeal signs, and stupor (321). Concomitant gastrointestinal or pulmonary symptoms may be present, and may provide the clue to the diagnosis (321). Antiamebic antibodies are usually present in the serum (326). CSF findings are nondiagnostic (324). Prognosis is extremely poor, as cerebral infection is usually fatal (323,325). Early treatment with metronidazole and prompt surgical intervention may improve the outcome (321).

Pathologically, multiple lesions are often seen, varying in size from 2 to 60 mm, with central necrosis. The lesions are commonly hemorrhagic (324). Focal or generalized meningitis may be seen (324). Amebae are present, but can be missed.

Imaging findings have been described in isolated case reports. CT has revealed single or multiple ring enhancing lesions (327,328). Multiple enhancing lesions have also been seen on MR (327). The diagnosis should be considered in patients from (or travellers to) endemic regions with multiple brain and liver abscesses (321).

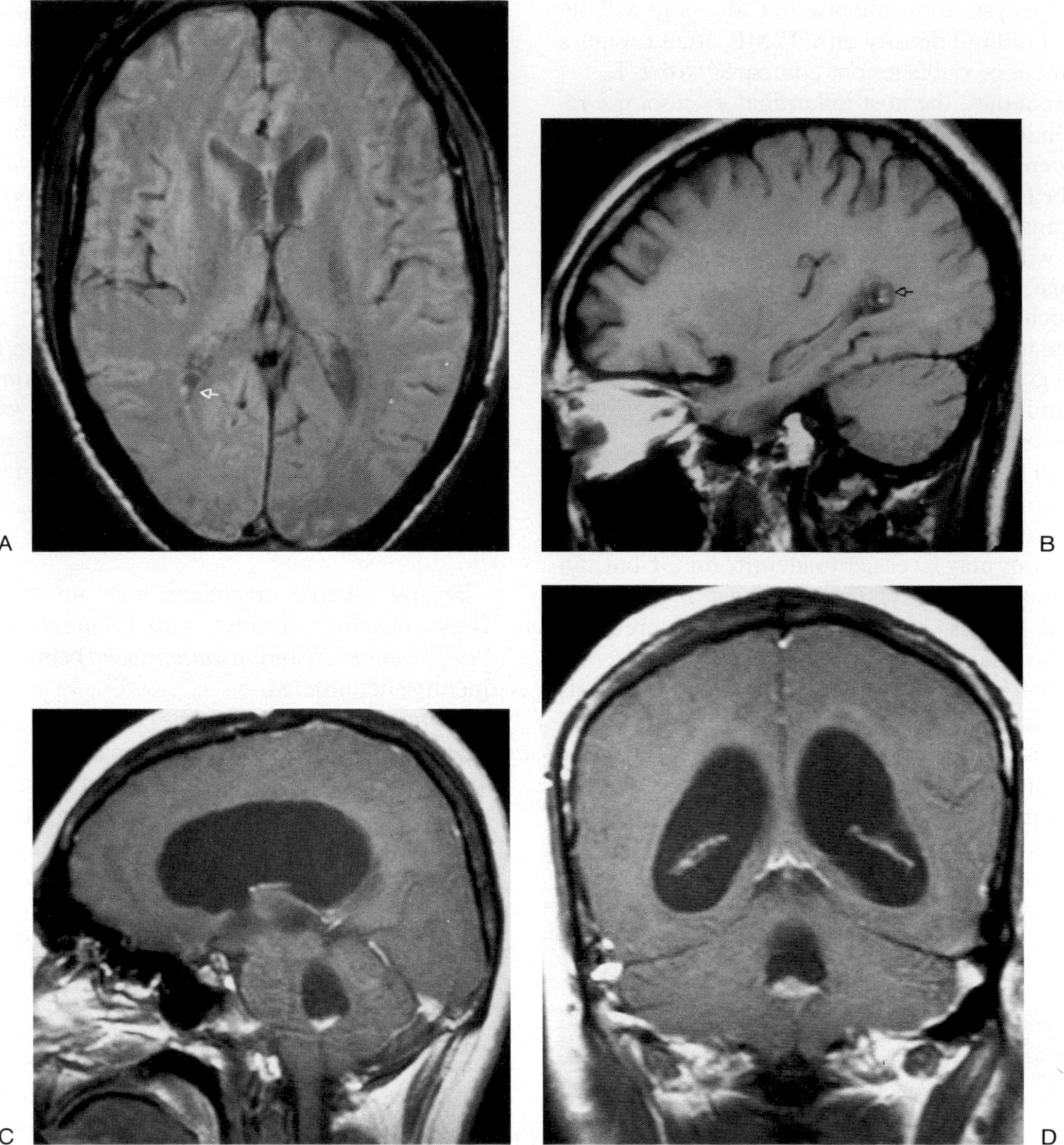

FIG. 50. Intraventricular cysticercosis. **A:** Proton-density (2400/20) image reveals a small cyst in the right atrium (*arrow*) that is isointense to CSF with a hyperintense mural nodule. A scolex may be seen in the intraventricular cysts, although it is absent in the subarachnoid form. **B:** Sagittal T1-weighted (600/20) scan again shows the intraventricular cyst (*arrow*) with a prominent mural nodule. **C,D:** T1-weighted (600/30) postgadolinium scans of a different patient with an enhancing lesion at the outlet of the fourth ventricle, resulting in hydrocephalus. At surgery, the mass was found to be a cysticercosis cyst with some inflammatory reaction.

N. fowleri is the pathogen that causes primary amebic meningoencephalitis (PAM) in humans (329). *N. fowleri* is a protozoan found in lakes, ponds, and soil (329,330). This is a rare but fatal infection (331), with males affected twice as often as females (332). Infection usually occurs in an immunocompetent host, and children are primarily affected (329).

Infection occurs while the host is swimming in infected waters. The organism enters the nasal cavity and then invades the anterior cranial fossa across the cribriform plate (333,334). The organisms can then spread directly into the brain or may spread along vascular channels.

Clinical presentation is similar to that of bacterial meningitis, with headache, seizure, fever, photophobia, and progression to stupor or coma (321). Death often occurs within several days. No effective or optimal drug regimen has been established (321).

A diffuse purulent exudate is often seen in patients with PAM, most prominent in the region of the olfactory bulbs, the site of organism entry (321). Brain necrosis may result, with the frontal and temporal lobes most severely affected. There is hyperemia of the meninges with evidence of superficial hemorrhage (333). CT may reveal cisternal and meningeal enhancement (335). MR findings have not been reported.

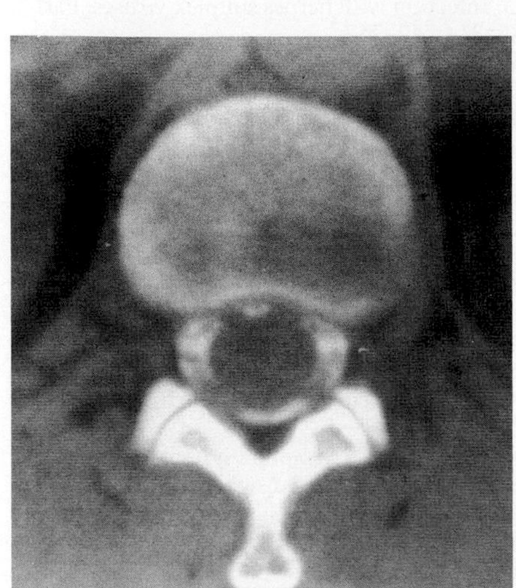
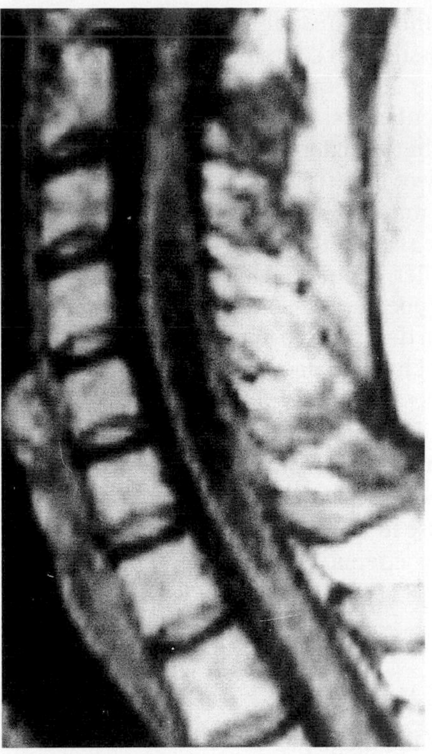
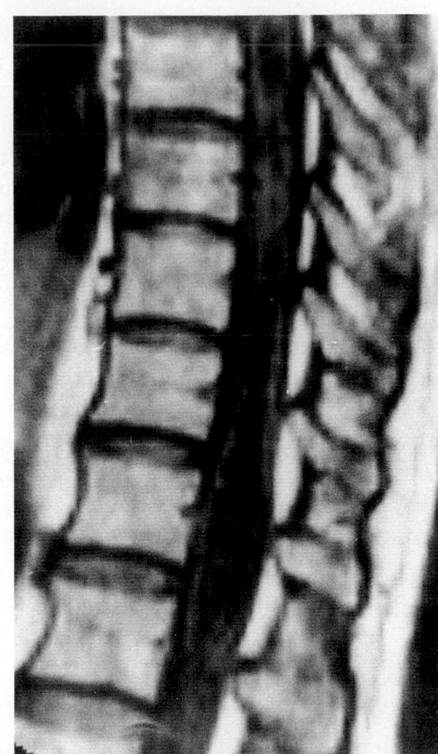

A B,C

FIG. 51. Intramedullary cysticercosis. **A:** Postmetrizamide CT at the T12–L1 level shows symmetric enlargement of the cord. **B:** Sagittal T1-weighted (700/26) image reveals an intramedullary cyst with cord expansion extending from C3 to C7. **C:** T1-weighted sagittal image shows CSF intensity signal within the thoracic cord with an expansile intramedullary cyst at the conus medullaris. Myelotomy of the conus medullaris revealed a cysticercus cyst. (From Castillo, ref. 348, with permission.)

Acanthamoeba infection results in granulomatous amebic encephalitis (GAE) (336). These protozoa are found worldwide in warm, moist climates. Those affected are usually immunocompromised (332). Males are affected five times more often than females (332).

CNS spread can occur via direct invasion to the meninges or via a hematogenous route. The clinical course of GAE is more insidious compared to PAM. Over a 2- to 4-week period, patients complain of headache, low grade fever, and may have focal neurologic signs. CSF analysis is nondiagnostic. The infection is usually fatal within 2 to 4 weeks, although survivors have been reported (337,338). There is no proven effective therapy (321).

Gross pathology reveals single or multiple focal inflammatory masses or brain abscesses. Microscopically, there is granulomatous inflammation (329,339). Vascular invasion may occur, resulting in a necrotizing vasculitis (329) or mycotic aneurysm formation (339).

CT may reveal ring-enhancing lesions (340) or gyriform enhancement (341). MR has been reported to show areas of increased signal on T2-weighted images at involved sites (340).

Hydatid Disease

The pathogen responsible for CNS hydatid disease is Echinococcus, and specifically *E. granulosus.* Echinococcus is endemic to the Middle East, South America, Australia, and countries in proximity to the Mediterranean Sea. Even in endemic regions, hydatid disease of the CNS is unusual, accounting for only 2% of intracranial space-occupying lesions (342). Echinococcus is a tapeworm that lives in the gastrointestinal tract of mammals. The intermediate host is usually sheep, but humans may also become intermediate hosts (321). The life cycle continues with passage of eggs into the feces of the definitive host. These are ingested by the intermediate host. The organism penetrates the wall of the intestine and spreads along venous channels and lymphatics (343). The agent is most often deposited in liver and/or lung, although the brain may also act as an end organ. The parasite then forms a slowly enlarging cyst. *E. multilocularis* may also infest the brain, forming clusters of smaller grape-like cysts termed "alveoli" (321).

Clinical presentation is due to mass effect by the cyst. Because of their slow growth, the lesions may be asymptomatic until they are quite large. Signs and symptoms include nausea, headache, vomiting, seizures, papilledema, hemiparesis, and cranial nerve palsies.

Pathologic examination of the cysts produced by *E. granulosus* reveals two layers. The internal layer, the endocyst, is formed by the organism. This endocyst is composed of a laminated membrane of mucopolysaccharide, which is lined inside by a germinal layer of cells. The outer layer, the ectocysts, is formed by the host reaction to the lesion, and is composed of glial tissue (321). Cysts enlarge by 1 to 5 mm/year (321).

CT most commonly reveals a unilocular cyst that is CSF equivalent, with local mass effect but no edema or enhancement. Because of the chronicity of these lesions, cysts near the inner table of the skull may cause bone erosion (344,345). Calcification may be seen in the cyst wall or in an internal septation. Smaller multilocular cysts may be seen, with a "grape-like" appearance. Contrast enhancement and edema have been described in association with the multiloculated form of hydatid disease (344,346). A recent MR report of a pathologically proven hydatid cyst revealed a 1-cm unilocular cyst that was slightly hyperintense to gray matter on proton-density images and CSF equivalent on T2-weighted images. The cyst was slightly hyperintense to CSF on T1-weighted images, without surrounding edema or enhancement. Mild mass effect was noted (321).

CONCLUSIONS

Neuroimaging plays a critical role in the diagnosis of intracranial infection. Many types of CNS infection are now seen more commonly, as a result of AIDS. Clinical findings are frequently nonspecific and thus imaging studies are often instrumental in the diagnosis and management of these patients. Although MR is an exquisitely sensitive technique, and is thus the study of choice in imaging these patients, specificity may lag behind sensitivity. Thus, correlation with other imaging studies (CT, thallium-201 brain SPECT, proton spectroscopy, etc.) is needed, as is clinical and laboratory correlation for definitive diagnosis.

REFERENCES

1. Leestma JE. Viral infections of the nervous system. In: Davis RL, Robertson DM, eds. *Textbook of Neuropathology*. Baltimore: Williams & Wilkins; 1985;704–787.
2. Rennels MB. Arthropod-borne virus infections of the central nervous system. *Neurol Clin* 1984;26:241–254.
3. Jubelt B. Enterovirus and mumps virus infections of the nervous system. *Neurol Clin* 1984;2:187–207.
4. Davidson HD, Steiner RE. Magnetic resonance imaging of infections of the central nervous system. *AJNR* 1985;6:499–504.
5. Schroth G, Kretzschmar K, Gawehn J, Voight K. Advantages of magnetic resonance imaging in the diagnosis of cerebral infections. *Neuroradiology* 1987;29:120–126.
6. Sze G, Zimmerman RD. The magnetic resonance imaging of infections and inflammatory diseases. *Radiol Clin North Am* 1988;26:839–859.
7. Barkovich AJ, Atlas SW. Magnetic resonance of intracranial hemorrhage. *Radiol Clin North Am* 1988;26:801–820.
8. Tien RD, Feldberg GJ, Osumi AK. Herpes virus infections of the CNS: MR findings. *AJR* 1993;161:167–176.
9. Whitley RJ, Schlitt M. Encephalitis caused by herpes viruses, including B virus. In: Scheld WM, Whitley RJ, Durach DT, eds. *Infection of the Central Nervous System*. New York: Raven Press; 1991;41–86.
10. Johnson RP, Mims CA. Pathogenesis of virus infection of the nervous system. *N Engl J Med* 1968;278:23–30.
11. Roizman B, Sears A. Inquiring into mechanisms of herpes simplex virus latency. *Annu Rev Microbiol* 1988;41:543–555.
12. Booss J, Esiri MM. Sporadic encephalitis: 1. In: *Viral Encephalitis: Pathology, Diagnosis and Management*. Boston: Blackwell Scientific; 1986;55–93.
13. Corey L, Spear PG. Infection with herpes simplex viruses. Part 1. *N Engl J Med* 1986: 314:686–691.
14. Corey L, Spear PG. Infection with herpes simplex viruses. Part 2. *N Engl J Med* 1986; 314:749–757.
15. Weiner LP, Fleming JO. Viral infections of the nervous system. *J Neurosurg* 1984; 61:207–224.
16. Shaw DWW, Cohen WA. Viral infection of the CNS in children: imaging features. *AJR* 1993;160:125–133.
17. Morawetz RB, Whitley RJ, Murphy DM. Experience with brain biopsy for suspected herpes encephalitis: review of forty consecutive cases. *Neurosurgery* 1983;12:654–657.
18. Kissane JM. *Anderson's Pathology*, Vol. 2, 9th ed. St. Louis: CV Mosby; 1990:2160–2161.
19. Schroth G, Gawehn J, Thron A, Vallbracht A, Voigt K. Early diagnosis of herpes simplex encephalitis by MRI. *Neurology* 1987;37:179–183.
20. Jordan J, Enzmann DR. Encephalitis. *Neuroimag Clin North Am* 1991;1:17–38.
21. Damasio AR, Van Hoesen GW. The limbic system and the localization of herpes simplex encephalitis. *J Neurol Neurosurg* Psychiatry 1985;48:297–301.
22. Soo MS, Tien RD, Gray L, Andrews PI, Friedman H. Mesenrhombencephalitis: MR findings in nine patients. *AJR* 1993;160: 1089–1093.
23. Hindmarsh T, Lindquist M, Olding-Stenkvist E, et al. Accuracy of computed tomography in the diagnosis of herpes simplex encephalitis. *Acta Radiol* 1986;369:192–196.
24. Gasecki AP, Steg RE. Correlation of early MRI with CT scan, EEG and CSF: analysis in a case of biopsy proven herpes simplex encephalitis. *Eur Neurol* 1991;31:372–375.
25. Bale JF, Anderson RD, Grose C. Magnetic resonance imaging of the brain in childhood herpes virus infections. *Pediatr Infect Dis J* 1987;6:644–647.
26. Neils EW, Lukin R, Tomsick TA, Tew JM. Magnetic resonance imaging and computerized tomography scanning of herpes simplex encephalitis; report of two cases. *J Neurosurg* 1987;67:592–594.
27. Zimmerman RD, Russell EJ, Leeds NE, Kaufman D. CT in the early diagnosis of herpes simplex encephalitis. *AJR* 1980;134:61–66.
28. Davis JM, Davis KR, Kleinman GN, et al. Computed tomography of herpes simplex encephalitis with clinico-pathological correlation. *Radiology* 1978;129:409–416.
29. Launes J, Nikkinen P, Lindroth L, et al. Diagnosis of acute herpes simplex encephalitis by brain perfusion single photon emission computed tomography. *Lancet* 1988;1:1188–1191.
30. Zimmerman RA, Bilaniuk LT, Sze G. Intracranial infection. In: Brant-Zawadzki M, Norman D, eds. *Magnetic Resonance Imaging of the Central Nervous System*. New York: Raven Press; 1987;235–257.
31. Atlas SW, Mark AS, Fram EK, Grossman RI. Vascular intracranial lesions: applications of gradient-echo MR imaging. *Radiology* 1988;169:455–461.
32. Lester JW, Carter MP, Reynolds TL. Herpes encephalitis: MR monitoring of response to acyclovir therapy. *J Comput Assist Tomogr* 1988;12:941–943.
33. Post MJD, Berger JR, Hensley GT. The radiology of central nervous system disease in the acquired immunodeficiency syndrome. In: Taveras JM, Ferrucci JT, eds. *Radiology: Diagnosis-Imaging-Intervention*, Vol 3. Philadelphia: JB Lippincott; 1988;1–26.
34. Petito CK, Cho E-S, Lemann W, Navia BA, Price RW. Neuropathology of acquired immunodeficiency syndrome (AIDS): an autopsy review. *J Neuropath Exp Neurol* 1986;45:635–646.
35. Levy RM, Bredesen DE, Rosenblum ML. Neurological manifestations of the acquired immunodeficiency syndrome (AIDS): ex-

perience at UCSF and review of the literature. *J Neurosurg* 1985;62:475–495.
36. Levy RM, Rosenbloom S, Perrett LV. Neuroradiological findings in the acquired immunodeficiency syndrome (AIDS): a review of 200 cases. *AJNR* 1986;7:833–839.
37. Price R, Chernik NL, Horta-Barbosa L, Posner JB. Herpes simplex encephalitis in an anergic patient. *Am J Med* 1973;54:222–228.
38. Osborn RE, Byrd SE. Congenital infections of the brain. *Neuroimag Clin North Am* 1991;1:105–118.
39. Herman TE, Cleveland RH, Kushman DC, Taveras JM. CT of neonatal herpes encephalitis. *AJNR* 1985;6:773–775.
40. Enzmann D, Chang Y, Augustyn G. MR findings in neonatal herpes simplex encephalitis type II. *J Comput Assist Tomogr* 1990;14:453–457.
41. Applebaum E, Rachelson MH, Dolgopol VB. Varicella encephalitis. *Am J Med* 1953; 15:223–230.
42. Johnson R, Milbourn PE. Central nervous system manifestations of chicken pox. *Can Med Assoc J* 1970;102:831–834.
43. McKendall RR, Klawans HL. Nervous system complications of varicella-zoster virus. In: Vinker PJ, Bruyn GW, eds. *Handbook of Clinical Neurology*, Vol. 34. Amsterdam: North-Holland 1978;161–183.
44. Gershon A, Steinberg S, Greenberg S, et al. Varicella-zoster associated encephalitis: detection of specific antibody in cerebrospinal fluid. *J Clin Microbiol* 1980;12:764–767.
45. Reichman RC. Neurological complications of varicella-zoster infection. In: Dolin R, ed. Herpes-zoster varicella infections. *Ann Intern Med* 1978;89:375–388.
46. Tenser RB. Herpes simplex and herpes zoster. Nervous system involvement. *Neurol Clin* 1984;2:215–240.
47. Furman JM, Brownstone PK, Balch RW. Atypical brainstem encephalitis: magnetic resonance imaging and oculographic features. *Neuroradiology* 1985;35:438–440.
48. Tien RD, Hesselink JR, Szumowski J. MR fat suppression combined with Gd-DTPA enhancement in optic neuritis and perineuritis. *J Comput Assist Tomogr* 1991;15:223–227.
49. Eidelberg D, Sotrel A, Horoupian DS, Neumann PE, Pumarola-Sune T, Price R. Thrombotic cerebral vasculopathy associated with herpes zoster. *Ann Neurol* 1986; 19:7–14.
50. O'Donohue JM, Enzmann DR. Mycotic aneurysm in angiitis associated with herpes zoster ophthalmicus. *AJNR* 1987;8:615–619.
51. Doyle PW, Gibson G, Dolman CL. Herpes zoster ophthalmicus with contralateral hemiplegia: identification of cause. *Ann Neurol* 1983;14:84–85.
52. Bernstein TC, Wolff HG. Involvement of the nervous system in infectious mononucleosis. *Ann Intern Med*1950;33:1120.
53. McKee KT, Wright PE, Kilroy AW, et al. Herpes encephalitis after infectious mononucleosis. *South Med J* 1981;74:238.
54. Tolly TL, Wells RG, Sty JR. MR features of fleeting CNS lesions associated with Epstein-Barr infection. *J Comput Assist Tomogr* 1989;13:665–668.
55. Silverstein A, Steinberg G, Nathanson M. Nervous system involvement in infectious mononucleosis: the heralding and/or major manifestation. *Arch Neurol* 1972;26:353–358.
56. Boyd JF. Adult cytomegalic inclusion disease. *Scott Med J* 1980;25:266–269.
57. Wong T-W, Warner NE. Cytomegalic inclusion disease in adults. Report of 14 cases with review of literature. *Arch Pathol Lab Med* 1962;74:403–422.
58. Post MJD, Hensley GT, Moskowitz LB, Fischl M. Cytomegalic inclusion virus encephalitis in patients with AIDS: CT, clinical and pathologic correlation. *AJR* 1986; 146:1229–1234.
59. Ball JF Jr. Human cytomegalovirus infection and disorders of the nervous system of patients with the acquired immune deficiency syndrome. *Arch Neurol* 1984;41:310–320.
60. Wiley CA, Nelson JA. Role of human immunodeficiency virus and cytomegalovirus in AIDS encephalitis. *Am J Pathol* 1988;133:73–81.
61. Britton CB, Miller JR. Neurologic complications of acquired immunodeficiency syndrome (AIDS). *Neurol Clin* 1984;2:315–339.
62. Dorfman LJ. Cytomegalovirus encephalitis in adults. *Neurology* 1973;23:136–144.
63. Duchowny M, Caplan L, Siber G. Cytomegalovirus infection of the adult nervous system. *Ann Neurol* 1979;5:458–461.
64. Rosen PP. Cytomegalovirus infection in cancer patients. *Pathol Ann* 1978;131:175–208.
65. Post MJD, Sheldon JJ, Hensley GT, et al. Central nervous system disease in acquired immunodeficiency syndrome: prospective correlation using CT, MR imaging and pathologic studies. *Radiology* 1986;158:141–148.
66. Navia BA, Cho E-S, Petito CK, Price RW. The AIDS dementia complex: II. Neuropathology. *Ann Neurol* 1986;19:525–535.
67. Schneck SA. Neuropathological features of human organ transplantation. Survey of 31 cases. *Lancet* 1973;1:962–967.
68. Levy RM, Pons VG, Rosenblum ML. Central nervous system mass lesions in the acquired immunodeficiency syndrome (AIDS). *J Neurosurg* 1984;61:9–16.
69. Snider WD, Simpson DM, Nielsen S, et al. Neurological complications of acquired immune deficiency syndrome: analysis of 50 patients. *Ann Neurol* 1983;14:403–418.
70. Ramsey RG, Geremia GK. CNS complications of AIDS: CT and MR findings. *AJR* 1988;151:449–454.
71. Sze G, Brant-Zawadzki MN, Norman D, Newton HT. The neuroradiology of AIDS. *Semin Roentgenol* 1987;22:42–53.
72. Tien RD, Chu PK, Hesselink JR, Szumowski J. Intra- and paraorbital lesions: value of fat suppression MR imaging with paramagnetic contrast enhancement. *AJNR* 1991; 12:245–247.
73. Hanshaw JB. Congenital cytometalovirus infection. *N Engl J Med* 1973;288:1406–1407.
74. Pass RF, Stagno S, Myers GJ, Alford CA. Outcome of symptomatic congenital cytomegalovirus infection: results of long term longitudinal follow-up. *Pediatrics* 1980; 66:758–782.
75. Fitz CR. Inflammatory diseases of the brain in childhood. *AJNR* 1992;13:551–567.
76. Whitley RJ, Stagno S. Perinatal virus infection. In: Scheld WM, Whitley RJ, Durack DT, eds. *Infection of the Central Nervous System*. New York: Raven Press; 1991;167–200.
77. Whiteman MLH, Post MJD, Bowen BC, Bell MD. AIDS-related white matter diseases. *Neuroimag Clin North Am* 1993;3:331–359.
78. Bale JF Jr, Bray PF, Bell WE. Neuroradiologic abnormalities in congenital cytomegalovirus infection. *Pediatr Neurol* 1985;1:42–47.
79. Boesch C, Issakainen J, Kewitz G, Kikinis R, et al. Magnetic resonance imaging of the brain in congenital cytomegalovirus infection. *Pediatr Radiol* 1989;19:91–93.
80. Hayward JC, Titelbaum DS, Clancy RR, Zimmerman RA. Lissencephaly-pachygyria associated with congenital cytomegalovirus infection. *J Child Neurol* 1991;6:109–114.
81. Sugita K, Ando M, Makino M, Takanashi J, Fujimoto N, Niimi H. Magnetic resonance imaging of the brain in congenital rubella virus and cytomegalovirus infections. *Neuroradiology* 1991;33:239–242.
82. Gallo RC, Salahuddin SZ, Popovic M, et al. Frequent detection and isolation of cytopathic retroviruses (HTLV-III) from patients with AIDS and at risk for AIDS. *Science* 1984;224:500–503.
83. Rosenblatt JD, Chen ISY, Wachsman W. Infection with HTLV-I and HTLV-II: evolving concepts. *Semin Hematol* 1988;25:230–246.
84. Curran JW, Morgan WM, Hardy AM, et al. The epidemiology of AIDS: current status and future prospects. *Science* 1985;229:1352–1357.
85. Clavel F, Mansinho K, Chamaret S, et al. Human immunodeficiency virus type 2 infection associated with AIDS in West Africa. *N Engl J Med* 1987;316:1181–1185.
86. Navia BA, Jordan BD, Price RW. The AIDS dementia complex: I clinical features. *Ann Neurol* 1986;19:517–524.
87. Petito CK. Review of central nervous system pathology in human immunodeficiency virus infection. *Ann Neurol* 1988;23(suppl):S54–S57.
88. Bailey R, Baltch A, Venkatish R, et al. Sensory motor neuropathy associated with AIDS. *Neurology* 1988;38:886–891.
89. Simpson DM, Bender AN. Human immunodeficiency virus-associated myopathy: analysis of 11 patients. *Ann Neurol* 1988;24:78–84.
90. Ho DD, Rota TR, Schooler RT. Isolation of HTVL-III from ce-

rebrospinal fluid and neuronal tissue of patients with neurologic syndromes related to the acquired immunodeficiency syndrome. *N Engl J Med* 1985;313:1493–1497.

91. Gaburda DH, Ho DD, de la Monte SM, et al. Immunohistochemical identification of HLTV—II antigen in brains of patients with AIDS. *Ann Neurol* 1986;20:289–295.
92. Gartner S, Markovits P, Markovits DM, et al. Virus isolation from and identification of HTLV-III/LAV-producing cells in brain tissue from a patient with AIDS. *JAMA* 1986 256:2365–2371.
93. Sharer LR, Cho E-S, Epstein LG. Multinucleated giant cells and HTLV-III in AIDS encephalopathy. *Hum Pathol* 1985;16:760.
94. Ho DD, Bredesen DE, Vinters HV, et al. The acquired immunodeficiency syndrome (AIDS) dementia complex. *Ann Intern Med* 1989;111:400.
95. Levy RM, Bredesen DE, Rosenblum ML et al. Central nervous system disorders in AIDS. In: Levy JA, ed. *AIDS Pathogenesis and Treatment*. New York: Dekker; 1988:371.
96. Nielsen SL, Petito CK, Urmacher CD, Posner JB. Subacute encephalitis in acquired immunedeficiency syndrome: a postmortem study. *Am J Clin Pathol* 1984;82:678–682.
97. Shaw GM, Harper ME, Hahn BH, et al. HTLV-III infection in brains of children and adults with AIDS encephalopathy. *Science* 1985;227:177–181.
98. Post MJD, Tate LG, Quencer RM, et al. CT, MR and pathology in HIV encephalitis and meningitis. *AJNR* 1988;9:469–476.
99. Price RW, Navia BA, Cho E-S. AIDS encephalopathy. *Neurol Clin* 1986;4:285–301.
100. McArthur JC, Becker PS, Parisi JE, et al. Neuropathological changes in early HIV-I dementia. *Ann Neurol* 1989;26:681–684.
101. Carne CA, Tedder RS, Smith A, et al. Acute encephalopathy coincident with seroconversion for anti-HTLV-III. *Lancet* 1985;2:1206–1208.
102. Berger JR, Kaszowitz B, Post MJD, Dickinson G. Progressive multifocal leukoencephalopathy associated with human immunodeficiency virus infection. A review of the literature with a report of sixteen cases. *Ann Intern Med* 1987;78–87.
103. Olsen WL, Longo FM, Mills CM, Norman D. White matter disease in AIDS: findings at MR imaging. *Radiology* 1988;169:445–448.
104. Chrysikopoulous HS, Press GA, Grafe MR, et al. Encephalitis caused by human immunodeficiency virus: CT and MR imaging manifestations with clinical and pathologic correlation. *Radiology* 1990;175:185–191.
105. McArthur JC, Cohen BA, Selnes OA, et al. Low prevalence of neurological and neuropsychological abnormalities in otherwise healthy HIV-infected individuals: results from the multicenter AIDS cohort study. *Ann Neurol* 1989;26:601–611.
106. Grant I, Atkinson JH, Hesselink JR, et al. Evidence for early central nervous system involvement in the acquired immunodeficiency syndrome (AIDS) and the human immunodeficiency virus (HIV) infections. *Ann Intern Med* 1987;107:828–836.
107. Post MJD, Levin BE, Berger JR, et al. Sequential cranial MR findings of asymptomatic and neurologically symptomatic HIV positive subjects. *AJNR* 1992;13:359–370.
108. Post MJD, Berger JR, Duncan R, Quencer RM, Pall L, Winfield D. Asymptomatic and neurologically symptomatic HIV-seropositive subjects: results of long-term MR imaging and clinical follow-up. *Radiology* 1993;188:727–733.
109. Jarvik JG, Lenkinski RE, Grossman RI, et al. Proton MR spectroscopy of HIV-infected patients: characterization of abnormalities with imaging and clinical correlation. *Radiology* 1993;186:739–744.
110. Chong WK, Sweeney B, Wilkinson I, et al. Proton spectroscopy of the brain in HIV infection: correlation with clinical, immunologic, and MR imaging findings. *Radiology* 1993;188:119–124.
111. Wood BP. Children with acquired immune deficiency syndrome. *Invest Radiol* 1992; 27:964–970.
112. Curless RG. Congenital AIDS: review of neurologic problems. *Child Nerv Syst* 1987;5:9–11.
113. Belman AL, Novick B, Ultmanm MH, et al. Neurological complication in children with acquired immune deficiency syndrome. *Ann Neurol* 1984;16:414.
114. Epstein LG, Sharer LR, Joshi VV. Progressive encephalopathy in children with acquired immune deficiency syndrome. *Ann Neurol* 1985;17:488–496.
115. Epstein LG, Sharer LR, Goudsmit J. Neurological and neuropathological features of human immunodeficiency virus infection in children. *Ann Neurol* 1988;23(suppl 6):S19–S23.
116. Belman AL, Ultmann MH, Horoupian D, et al. Neurological complications of infants and children with acquired immunedeficiency syndrome. *Ann Neurol* 1985;18:560–566.
117. Sharer LR, Epstein LG, Joshi VV, Rankin LF. Neuropathological observations in children with AIDS and HTLV-III infection of brain. *J Neuropathol Exp Neurol* 1985;44:350.
118. Post MJD, Curless RG, Gregorios JB, et al. Reactivation of congenital cytomegalic inclusion disease in an infant with HTLV-III associated immunodeficiency: a CT-pathologic correlation. *J Comput Assist Tomogr* 1986;10:533–536.
119. Whiteman MLH, Post MJD, Berger JR, et al. Progressive multifocal leukoencephalopathy in 47 HIV-seropositive patients: neuroimaging with clinical and pathologic correlation. *Radiology* 1993;187:233–240.
120. Editorial—HTLV-I comes of age. *Lancet* 1988;1:217–219.
121. Poiesz BJ, Ruscetti FW, Gazdar AF, et al. Detection and isolation of type-C retrovirus particles from fresh and cultured lymphocytes of a patient with cutaneous T-cell lymphoma. *Proc Natl Acad Sci* USA 1980;77:7415–7419.
122. Yoshida M, Miyoshi I, Hinuma Y. Isolation and characterization of retrovirus from cell lines of human adult T-cell leukemia and its implication in the disease. *Proc Natl Acad Sci USA* 1982;79:2031–2035.
123. Osame M, Igata A, Matsumoto M, et al. HTLV-I associated myelopathy: a report of 85 cases. *Ann Neurol* 1987;22:116.
124. Piccardo P, Ceroni M, Rodgers-Johnson P, et al. Pathological and immunological observations on tropical spastic paraparesis in patients from Jamaica. *Ann Neurol* 1988;23(suppl):S156–S160.
125. Koprowski H, DeFreitas EC, Harper ME, et al. Multiple sclerosis and human T-cell lymphotropic retroviruses. *Nature* 1985;318:154–160.
126. Rodgers-Johnson P, Morgan O StC, Mora C, et al. The role of HTLV-I in tropical spastic paraparesis in Jamaica. *Ann Neurol* 1988;23(suppl):S121–S126.
127. Akizuki S, Nakazato O, Higuichi Y, et al. Necropsy findings in HTLV-I associated myelopathy. *Lancet* 1987;1:156–157.
128. Hirose S, Uemura Y, Fujishita M, et al. Isolation of HTLV-I from cerebrospinal fluid of a patient with myelopathy. *Lancet* 1986;2:237–398.
129. Tournier-Lasserve E, Gout O, Gessain A, et al. HTLV-I brain abnormalities on magnetic resonance imaging, and relation with multiple sclerosis. *Lancet* 1987;2:49–50.
130. Mattson DH, McFarlin DE, Mora C, Zaninovic V. Central nervous system lesions detected by magnetic resonance imaging in an HTLV-I antibody positive symptomless individual. *Lancet* 1987;2:49.
131. Hara Y, Takahashi M, Ueno S, Yoshikawa H, Yorifuji S, Tarui S. MR imaging of the brain in myelopathy associated with human T-cell lymphotropic virus type I. *J Comput Assist Tomgr* 1988;12:750–754.
132. Kira J, Fujihara K, Itoyama Y, Goto I, Hasuo K. Leukoencephalopathy in HTLV-I-associated myelopathy/tropical spastic paraparesis: MRI analysis and a two year follow-up study after corticosteroid therapy. *J Neurol Sci* 1991;106:41–49.
133. Richardson EP Jr. Progressive multifocal leukoencephalopathy 30 years later. *N Engl J Med* 1988;318:315–317.
134. Brooks BR, Walker DL. Progressive multifocal leukoencephalopathy. *Neurol Clin* 1984;2:299–313.
135. Silverman L, Rubinstein LJ. Electron microscopic observation on a case of progressive multifocal leukoencephalopathy. *Acta Neuropathol* (Berlin) 1965;5:215–224.
136. ZuRhein GM, Chou E-S. Particles resembling papovaviruses in human cerebral demyelinating disease. *Science* 1965;148:1477–1479.
137. Padget BL, Walker DL, ZuRhein GM, et al. Cultivation of papova-like virus from human brain with progressive multifocal leukoencephalopathy. *Lancet* 1971;1257–1260.
138. Post MJD, Sheldon JJ, Hensley GT, et al. Central nervous system disease in acquired immunodeficiency syndrome: prospective

correlation using CT, MR imaging and pathologic studies. *Radiology* 1986;158:141–148.
139. Major EO, Amemiya K, Tornatore CS, et al. Pathogenesis and molecular biology of progressive multifocal leukoencephalopathy, the JC virus-induced demyelinating disease of the human brain. *Clin Micro Rev* 1992;5:49–73.
140. Mazlo M, Tariska I. Morphological demonstration of the first phase of polyomavirus replication in oligodendroglia cells of human brain in progressive multifocal leukoencephalopathy (PML). *Neuropathology* 1980;49:133–143.
141. Greenfield JG. *Greenfield's Neuropathology*, 4th ed. New York: Wiley & Sons; 1984:261–288.
142. Walker DL. Progressive multifocal leukoencephalopathy. In: Vinken PJ, Bruyn GW, Klawans HL, eds. *Handbook of Clinical Neurology, Vol. 47. Demyelinating Diseases.* Amsterdam: Elsevier Science Publishers; 1985:503–524.
143. Stoner G, Ryschkewitsch CF, Walker DL, Webster HD. JC papovavirus large tumor (T)-antigen expression in brain tissue of acquired immune deficiency syndrome (AIDS) and non-AIDS patients with progressive multifocal leukoencephalopathy. *Proc Natl Acad Sci USA* 1986;23:2271–2275.
144. Krupp LB, Lipton RB, Swerdlow ML, et al. Progressive multifocal leukoencephalopathy: clinical and radiographic features. *Ann Neurol* 1985;17:344–349.
145. Blum LW, Chambers RA, Schwartzman RJ, Streletz LJ. Progressive multifocal leukoencephalopathy in acquired immune deficiency syndrome. *Arch Neurol* 1985;42:137–139.
146. Jones HR, Hedley-Whyte T, Friedberg SR, et al. Primary cerebellopontine progressive multifocal leukoencephalopathy diagnosed premortem by cerebellar biopsy. *Ann Neurol* 1982;11:199–202.
147. Parr J, Horoupian DC, Winkelman C. Cerebellar form of progressive multifocal leukoencephalopathy (PML). *Can J Neurol Sci* 1979;6:123–128.
148. Bauer W, Chamberlain W, Horenstein S. Spinal demyelination in progressive multifocal leukoencephalopathy. *Neurology* 1987;19:287.
149. Post MJD, Kursunoglu SJ, Hensley GT, et al. Cranial CT in acquired immunodeficiency syndrome: spectrum of diseases and optimal contrast enhancement technique. *AJNR* 1985;6:743–754.
150. Tsuchiya K, Yamauchi T, Furui S, et al. MR imaging vs CT in subacute sclerosing panencephalitis. *AJNR* 1988;9:943–946.
151. Jabbour JT, Garcia JH, Lemmi H, et al. SSPE: a multidisciplinary study of eight cases *JAMA* 1969;207:2248–2254.
152. Takemoto K, Koizumi Y, Kogame S, et al. Magnetic resonance imaging of subacute sclerosing panencephalitis. *Jpn Clin Radiol* 1986;31:999–1004.
153. Woodard KG, Weinberg PE, Lipton HL. Basal ganglia involvement in subacute sclerosing panencephalitis: CT and MR demonstration. *J Comput Assist Tomogr* 1988;12:489–491.
154. Duda EE, Huttenlocker PR, Patronas NJ. CT of subacute sclerosing panencephalitis. *AJNR* 1980;1:35–38.
155. Schoeman JF, Bezing K-LV, Hewlitt RH. Correlative clinical, neuroradiological and pathological findings in subacute sclerosing panencephalitis. A report of 5 cases. *S Afr Med J* 1982;62:447–450.
156. Sze G. Infections and inflammatory diseases. In: Stake DD, Bradley WG Jr, eds. *Magnetic Resonance Imaging.* St. Louis: CV Mosby; 1988:316–343.
157. Goutiere F, Alcardi J. Acute neurological dysfunction associated with destructive lesions of the basal ganglia in children. *Ann Neurol* 1982;12:328–332.
158. Tarr RW, Edwards KM, Kessler RM, Kulkarni MV. MRI of mumps encephalitis: comparison with CT evaluation. *Pediatr Radiol* 1987;17:59–62.
159. Donohue WL, Playfair FD, Whitaker L. Mumps encephalitis: pathology and pathogenesis. *J Pediatr* 1955;47:395–412.
160. Falcone S, Quencer RM, Bowen BC, Bruce JH, Naidich TP. Creutzfeldt-Jakob disease: focal symmetrical cortical involvement demonstrated by MR imaging. *AJNR* 1992;13:403–406.
161. Kirschbaum WR. *Jakob-Creutzfeldt disease.* New York: American Elsevier Publishing Co; 1968.
162. Gajdusek DC. Unconventional viruses and the origin and disappearance of Kuru. *Science* 1977;197:943–960.
163. Prusiner SB. Prions and neurodegenerative diseases. *N Engl J Med* 1987;317:1571–1581.
164. Masters CL, Harris JO, Gajdusek DC, Gibbs CJ Jr, Bernoulli C, Asher DM. Creutzfeldt-Jakob disease: patterns of worldwide occurence and the significance of familial and sporadic clustering. *Ann Neurol* 1979;5:177–188.
165. Asher DM. Slow viral infections of the human nervous system. In: Scheld MW, Whitley RJ, Durack DT, eds. *Infections of the Central Nervous System.* New York: Raven Press; 1991.
166. Webb RM, Leech RW, Brumback RA. Spongiform encephalopathies: the physician's responsibility. *South Med J* 1990;83:141–145.
167. Brown P, Rodgers-Johnson P, Cathala F, Gibbs CJ Jr, Gajdusek DC. Creutzfeldt-Jakob disease of long duration: clinipathological characteristics, transmitability, and differential diagnosis. *Ann Neurol* 1984;16:295–304.
168. Park TS, Kleinman GM, Richardson EP. Creutzfeldt-Jakob disease with extensive degeneration of white matter. *Acta Neuropathol* (Berlin) 1980;52:239–342.
169. Kovanen J, Erkinjuntti T, Iivanainen M, et al. Cerebral MR and CT imaging in Creutzfeldt-Jakob disease. *J Comput Assist Tomogr* 1985;9:125–128.
170. Beck E, Daniel PM, Matthews WB, et al. Creutzfeldt-Jakob disease, the neuropathology of a transmission experiment. *Brain* 1969;92:699–716.
171. Kirschbaum WR. Comments on the tabulated cases and compilation of the data. In: *Jakob-Creutzfeldt Disease.* New York: American Elsevier Publishing; 1968:114–129.
172. Galvez S, Cartier L. Computed tomography findings in 15 cases of Creutzfeldt-Jakob disease with histological verification. *J Neurol Neurosurg Psychiatry* 1984;47:1244–1246.
173. Kitagawa Y, Gotoh F, Koto A, et al. Creutzfeldt-Jakob disease: a case with extensive white matter degeneration and optic atrophy. *J Neurol* 1983;229:97–101.
174. Pearl GS, Anderson RE. Creutzfeldt-Jakob disease: high caudate signal on magnetic resonance imaging. *South Med J* 1989;82:1187–1190.
175. Gertz HJ, Henkes H, Cervos-Navarro J. Creutzfeldt-Jakob disease: correlation of MRI and neuropathologic findings. *Neurology* 1988;38:1481–1482.
176. Milton WJ, Atlas SW, Lavi E, Mollman JE. Magnetic resonance imaging of Creutzfeld-Jakob disease. *Ann Neurol* 1991;29:439–440.
177. Kruger H, Meesmann C, Rohrbach E, Muller J, Mertens HG. Panencephalopathic type of Creutzfeldt-Jakob disease with primary extensive involvement of white matter. *Eur Neurol* 1990;30:115–119.
178. Alford EC. Acute disseminated encephalomyelitis and "allergic" neuroencephalopathies In: Vinken PJ, Bruyn GW, eds. *Handbook of Clinical Neurology*, Vol. 9. New York: American Elsevier; 1980:501–571.
179. Atlas SW, Grossman RI, Goldberg HI, et al. MR diagnosis of acute disseminated encephalomyelitis. *J Comput Assist Tomogr* 1986;10:798–801.
180. Caldemeyer KS, Harris TM, Smith RR, Edwards MK. Gadolinium enhancement in acute disseminated encephalomyelitis. *J Comput Assist Tomogr* 1991;15:673–675.
181. Broich K, Horwich D, Alavi A. HMPAO-SPECT and MRI in acute disseminated encephalomyelitis. *J Nucl Med* 1991;32:1897–1900.
182. Hart MN, Earle KM. Hemorrhagic and perivenous encephalitis: a clinical-pathological review of 38 cases. *J Neurol Neurosurg Psychiatry* 1975;38:585–591.
183. Dunn V, Ball FJ Jr, Zimmerman RA, et al. MRI in children with postinfectious disseminated encephalomyelitis. *Magn Reson Imaging* 1986;4:25–32.
184. Lukes SA, Norman D. Computed tomography in acute disseminated encephalitis. *Ann Neurol* 1983;13:567–572.
185. Rasmussen T, Olszweski J, Lloyd-Smith D. Focal seizures due to chronic localized encephalitis. *Neurology* 1958;8:435–455.
186. Tien RD, Ashdown BC, Lewis DV Jr, Atkins MR, Burger PC.

Rasmussen's encephalitis: neuroimaging findings in four patients. *AJR* 1992;158:1329–1332.

187. Rasmussen T, Andermann F. Update on the syndrome of "chronic encephalitis" and epilepsy. *Cleve Clin J Med* 1989; 56(suppl):S181–S184.
188. Parker JC Jr, Dyer MC. Neurologic infections due to bacteria fungi, and parasites. In: Doris RL, Robertson DM, eds. *Textbook of Neuropathology*. Baltimore: Williams & Wilkins; 1985:632–703.
189. Enzmann DR, Britt RH, Yeager AS. Experimental brain abscess evolution: computed tomographic and neuropathologic correlation. *Radiology* 1979;133:113–122.
190. Enzmann DR, Britt RD, Placone R. Staging of human brain abscess by computed tomography. *Radiology* 1983;146:703–708.
191. Alvord EC Jr, Shaw CM. Infectious anergic and demyelinating diseases of the nervous system. In: Newton TH, Potts DG, eds. *Radiology of the Skull and Brain: Anatomy and Pathology*, Vol. 3. St. Louis: CV Mosby; 1977:3088–3172.
192. Heineman HS, Braude AI. Anaerobic infection of the brain: observations on 18 consecutive cases of brain abscess. *Am J Med* 1963;35:682–697.
193. Morgan H, Wood MW. Cerebellar abscesses: a review of 7 cases. *Surg Neurol* 1975;3:93–96.
194. VanDellen JR, Bullock R, Postma MH. Cerebellar abscess: the impact of computed tomographic scanning. *Neurosurgery* 1987;21:547–550.
195. Haimes AB, Zimmerman RD, Morgello S, et al. MR imaging of brain abscesses. *AJR* 1989;152:1073–1085.
196. Som PM, Dillon WP, Fullerton GD, et al. Chronically obstructed sinonasal secretions: observations on T1 and T2 shortening. *Radiology* 1989;172:515–520.
197. Whelan MA, Hilal SK. Computed tomography as a guide in the diagnosis and follow-up of brain abscesses. *Radiology* 1980;135: 633–671.
198. Grossman RI, Joseph PM, Wolf G, et al. Experimental intracranial septic infarction: magnetic resonance enhancement. *Radiology* 1985;155:649–653.
199. Lee SH. Infectious diseases. In: Lee SH, Rao KCVG, eds. *Cranial Computed Tomography*. New York: McGraw-Hill Book Co; 1983:505–546.
200. Post MJD, Hoffman TA. Cerebral inflammatory disease. In: Rosenberg RN, ed. *The Clinical Neurosciences. Neuroradiology*, vol. 4. New York: Churchill Livingstone; 1984:525–594.
201. Coularu CM, Seshul M, Donaldson J. Intracranial ring lesions: can we differentiate by computed tomography? *Invest Radiol* 1980;15:103–112.
202. Dobkin JF, Healton EB, Dickson PC, Brust JC. Nonspecificity of ring enhancement in "medically cured" brain abscess. *Neurology* 1984;34:139–144.
203. Shaw MDM, Russell JA. Value of computed tomography in the diagnosis of intracranial abscess. *J Neurol Neurosurg Psychiatry* 1977;40:214–220.
204. Price H, Danziger A. The role of computed tomography in the diagnosis and management of intracranial abscess. *Clin Radiol* 1978;29:571–577.
205. Robertheram EB, Kessler LA. Use of computerized tomography in nonsurgical management of brain abscess. *Arch Neurol* 1979;36:25–26.
206. Frazee JG, Cahan LD, Winter J. Bacterial intracranial aneurysms. *J Neurosurg* 1980;53:633–641.
207. Bohmfalk GL, Story JL, Wissinger JP, et al. Bacterial intracranial aneurysm. *J Neurosurg* 1978;48:369–382.
208. Mathews VP, Kuharik MA, Edwards MK, et al. Gd-DTPA-enhanced MR imaging of experimental bacterial meningitis: evaluation and comparison with CT. *AJNR* 1988;9:1045–1050.
209. Brandt-Zawadzki M, Kucharczyk W. Vascular disease: ischemia. In: Brandt-Zawadzki M, Norman A, eds. *Magnetic Resonance Imaging of the Central Nervous System*. New York: Raven Press; 1987:221–234.
210. Goldberg HI. Stroke. In: Lee SH, Rao KCVG, eds. *Cranial Computed Tomography*. New York: McGraw-Hill Book Co; 1983: 631–640.
211. Zimmerman RD, Weingarten K. Neuroimaging of cerebral abscesses. *Neuroimag Clin North Am* 1991;1:1–16.
212. Bradley WG Jr, Waluch V. Blood flow: magnetic resonance imaging. *Radiology* 1985;154:443–450.
213. Cockrill HH Jr, Dreisbach J, Lowe B, et al. Computed tomography in leptomeningeal infection. *AJR* 1978;130:511–515.
214. Nelson JD, Watts CC. Calcified subdural effusion following bacterial meningitis. *Am J Dis Child* 1969;117:730–733.
215. Zimmerman RD, Leeds NE, Danziger A. Subdural empyema: CT findings. *Radiology* 1984;150:417–422.
216. Quencer RM, Hinks RS, Post MJD, Calabro G. Intracranial flow of cerebrospinal fluid: qualitative and quantitative evaluation with cine MR imaging. *Radiology* 1989;173:115.
217. Zimmerman RA, Bilaniuk LT, Gallo E. CT of the trapped fourth ventricle. *AJR* 1978; 130:503–506.
218. Weingarten K, Zimmerman RD, Becker RD, et al. Subdural and epidural empyemas: MR imaging. *AJNR* 1989;152:615–621.
219. Moseley IF, Kendall BE. Radiology of intracranial empyemas, with special reference to computed tomography. *Neuroradiology* 1984;26:333–345.
220. Blaquiere RM. The computed tomographic appearances of intra- and extracerebral abscesses. *Br J Radiol* 1983;56:171–181.
221. Luben MG, Whelan MA. Recent diagnostic experience with subdural empyema. *J Neurosurg* 1980;52:764–771.
222. Sadhu VK, Handel SF, Pinto RS, Glass TF. Neuroradiologic diagnosis of subdural empyema and CT limitations. *AJNR* 1980;1: 39–44.
223. Macchi PH, Grossman RI, Gomori JM, et al. High field MR imaging of cerebral venous thrombosis. *J Comput Assist Tomogr* 1986;10:10–15.
224. Steere AC, Grodzicki RL, Kornblatt AN, et al. The spirochetal etiology of Lyme disease. *N Engl J Med* 1983;308:733–740.
225. Steere AC. Lyme disease. *N Engl J Med* 1989;321:586–596.
226. Pachner AR. Spirochetal diseases of the CNS. *Neurol Clin* 1986;4:207–222.
227. Wickelgren I. At the drop of a tick. *Sci News* 1989;135:76–82.
228. Steere AC, Malawista SE, Syndman DR, et al. Lyme arthritis: an epidemic of oligoarthritis in children and adults in three Connecticut communities. *Arthritis Rheum* 1977;20:7–17.
229. Steere AC, Broderick TF, Malawista SE. Erythroma chronicum migrans and Lyme arthritis: epidemiologic evidence for a tick vector. *Am J Epidemiol* 1978;108:312–321.
230. Pachner AR, Duray P, Steere AC. Central nervous system manifestations of Lyme disease. *Arch Neurol* 1989;46:790–795.
231. Steere AC, Malawista SE, Nardin JA, Ruddy S, Askenase PW, Andiman WA. Erythema chronicum migrans and Lyme arthritis: the enlarging clinical spectrum. *Ann Intern Med* 1977;86:685–698.
232. Steere AC, Bartenhagen NH, Craft JE. The early clinical manifestations of Lyme disease. *Ann Intern Med* 1983;99:76–82.
233. Reik L Jr., Smith L, Khan A, Nelson W. Demyelinating encephalopathy in Lyme disease. *Neurology* 1985;35:267–269.
234. Fernandez RE, Rothberg M, Ferencz G, Wujack D. Lyme disease of the CNS: MR imaging findings in 14 cases. *AJNR* 1990;11: 479–481.
235. Rafto SE, Milton WJ, Galetta SL, Grossman RI. Biopsy-confirmed CNS Lyme disease: MR appearance at 1.5T. *AJNR* 1990;11:482–484.
236. Tien RD, Gean-Marton AD, Mark AS. Neurosyphilis in HIV carriers: MR findings in six patients. *AJR* 1992;158:1325–1328.
237. Katz DA, Berger JR, Duncan RC. Neurosyphilis. A comparative study of the effects of infection with human immunodeficiency virus. *Arch Neurol* 1993;50:243–249.
238. Kaplan JG, Sterman AB, Horoupian D, et al. Leutic meningitis with gumma: clinical, radiographic, and neuropathologic features. *Neurology* 1981;31:464–467.
239. Merrit HH. The early clinical and laboratory manifestations of syphilis of the central nervous system. *N Engl J Med* 1990;223: 446–450.
240. Holmes KK. Syphilis. In: Isselbacher KJ, Adams RD, Braunwald E, Petersdorf RG, Wilson JD, eds. *Harrison's Principles of Internal Medicine*, 9th ed. New York: McGraw-Hill Book Co; 1980: 716–726.
241. Fujimara NJ. Human immunodeficiency virus infection and syphilis. *J Am Acad Dermatol* 1989;21:141–142.
242. Simon RP. Neurosyphilis. *Arch Neurol* 1985;42:606–613.

243. Godt P, Stoeppler L, Wischer U, Schroeder HH. The value of computed tomography in cerebral syphilis. *Neuroradiology* 1979;18:197–200.
244. Ihmeidan IH, Post MJD, Katz D, et al. Radiographic findings in HIV+ patients with neurosyphilis. *AJNR* 1989;10.896.
245. Holland BA, Perrett LV, Mills CM. Meningovascular syphilis: CT and MR findings *Radiology* 1986;158:439–442.
246. Centers for Disease Control. Tuberculosis and acquired immunodeficiency syndrome—New York City. *MMWR* 1987;36:785–795.
247. Reider HL, Cauthen GM, Kelly GD, et al. Tuberculosis in the United States. *JAMA* 1989;262:385–389.
248. Mehta JB, Dutt A, Harvill L, et al. Epidemiology of extrapulmonary tuberculosis. A comparative analysis with pre-AIDS era. *Chest* 1991;99:1134–1138.
249. Pitchenik AE, Burr J, Suarez M, Fertel D, et al. Human T-cell lymophotropic virus-III (HTLV-III) seropositivity and related disease among 71 consecutive patients in whom tuberculosis was diagnosed: a prospective study. *Am Rev Respir Dis* 1987;135: 875–879.
250. Theuer CP, Hopewell PC, Elias D, Schecter GF, et al. Human immune deficiency virus infection in tuberculosis patients. *J Infect Dis* 1990;162:8–12.
251. Berenguer J, Moreno S, Laguna F, Vicente T, et al. Tuberculous meningitis in patients infected with the human immunodeficiency virus. *N Engl J Med* 1992;326:668–672.
252. Curless RG, Mitchell CD. Central nervous system tuberculosis in children. *Pediatr Neurol* 1991;7:270–274.
253. Bishburg E, Sunderam G, Reichman LB, Kapila R. Central nervous system tuberculosis with the acquired immunodeficiency syndrome and its related complex. *Ann Intern Med* 1986;105: 210–213.
254. Starke JR. Modern approach to the diagnosis and treatment of tuberculosis in children. *Pediatr Clin North Am* 1988;35(3):441–464.
255. Khan MA, Kovnat DM, Bachus B, et al. Clinical and roentgenographic spectrum of pulmonary tuberculosis in the adult. *Am J Med* 1977;62:31–38.
256. Woodring JH, Vandiviere HM, Fried AM, et al. Update: the radiographic fetures of pulmonary tuberculosis. *AJR* 1986;146: 497–506.
257. Bagga A, Kalra V, Ghai OP. Intracranial tuberculoma. *Clin Pediatr* 1988;27:487–490.
258. Draouat S, Abdenabi B, Ghanem M, Bourjat P. Computed tomography of cerebral tuberculosis. *J Comput Assist Tomogr* 1987;11:594–597.
259. Sheller JR, DesPrez RM. CNS tuberculosis. *Neurol Clin* 1986;4: 143–158.
260. Leiguarda R, Berthier M, Starkstein S, et al. Ischemic infarction in 25 children with tuberculous meningitis. *Stroke* 1988;19:200–204.
261. Schoeman J, Hewlett R, Donald P. MR of childhood tuberculous meningitis. *Neuroradiology* 1988;30:473–477.
262. Chang K-H, Han M-H, Roh JK, et al. Gd-DTPA–enhanced MR imaging in intracranial tuberculosis. *Neuroradiology* 1990;32: 19–25.
263. Ribera E, Martinez-Vasquez JM, Ocana I, et al. Activity of adenosine deaminase in cerebrospinal fluid for the diagnosis and follow-up of tuberculous meningitis in adults. *J Infect Dis* 1987;155:603–607.
264. Thomas MD, Chopra JS, Walia BNS. Tuberculous meningitis (TBM). *J Assoc Phys Ind* 1977;25:633–639.
265. Tyson G, Newman P, Strachen WE. Tuberculous brain abscess. *Surg Neurol* 1978;10:323–325.
266. Whitener DR. Tuberculous brain abscess: report of a case and review of the literature. *Arch Neurol* 1978;35:148–155.
267. Dastur DK. Neurotuberculosis. In: Minckler J, ed. *Pathology of the Nervous System*, vol. 3. New York: McGraw Hill Book Co; 1972:2412–2422.
268. Villoria MF, de la Torre J, Munoz L, et al. Intracranial tuberculosis in AIDS: CT and MRI findings. *Neuroradiology* 1992;34: 11–14.
269. Jinkins JR. Computed tomography of intracranial tuberculosis. *Neuroradiology* 1991; 33:126–135.
270. Gupta RK, Jena A, Sharma DK, et al. MR imaging of intracranial tuberculomas. *J Comput Assist Tomogr* 1988;12:280– 285.
271. Van Dyk A. CT of intracranial tuberculosis with specific reference to the "target sign." *Neuroradiology* 1988;30:329–336.
272. Gupta RK, Jena A, Sharma DK, et al. MR imaging of intracranial tuberculomas. *J Comput Assist Tomogr* 1988;12:280– 285.
273. Newton TH, Norman D, Alvord EC, et al. The CT scan in infectious diseases of the CNS: In: Norman D, Korobkin M, Newton TH, eds. *Computed Tomography*. San Francisco: University of California Press; 1977:719–740.
274. Wouters EFM, Hupperts RMM, Vreeling FW, et al. Successful treatment of tuberculous brain abscess. *J Neurol* 1985;23:118–119.
275. Yang PJ, Reger KM, Seeger JF, et al. Brain abscess: an atypical CT appearance of CNS tuberculosis. *AJNR* 1987;8:919–920.
276. Dube MP, Holtom PD, Larsen RA. Tuberculous meningitis in patients with and without human immunodeficiency virus infection. *Am J Med* 1992;93:520–524.
277. Shafer RW, Chirgwin KD, Glatt AE, et al. HIV prevalence, immunosupression and drug resistance in patients with tuberculosis in an area endemic for AIDS. *AIDS* 1991;5:399–405.
278. Centers for Disease Control. Primary resistance to antituberculous drugs—United States. *MMWR* 1983;32:521–523.
279. Lyons RW, Andriole VT. Fungal infections of the CNS. *Neurol Clin* 1986;159–170.
280. Enzmann DR, Brant-Zawadzki M, Britt RH. CT of central nervous system infections in immunosuppressed patients. *AJNR* 1980;1:239–243.
281. Kobayashi GS. Fungi. In: Davis BD, Dulbecco R, Eisen HN, Ginsbert HS, eds. *Microbiology*. New York: Harper and Row; 1980:817–850.
282. DeLaPaz, RL, Enzmann D. Neuroradiology of acquired immunodeficiency syndrome. In: Rosenblum ML, et al., eds. *AIDS and the Nervous System*. New York: Raven Press; 1988:121–153.
283. Davenport C, Dillon WP, Sze G. Neuroradiology of the immunosuppressed state. *Radiol Clin North Am* 1992;30:611–637.
284. Popovich MJ, Arthur RH, Helmer E. CT of intracranial cryptococcosis. *AJNR* 1990;11:139–142.
285. Whelan MA, Kricheff II, Handler M, et al. Acquired immunodeficiency syndrome: cerebral computed tomographic manifestations. *Radiology* 1983;149:477–484.
286. Kelly WM, Brant-Zawadzki M. Acquired immunodeficiency syndrome: neuroradiologic findings. *Radiology* 1983;149:485–491.
287. Riccio TJ, Hesselink JR. Gd-DTPA enhanced MR of multiple cryptococcal brain abscesses. *AJNR* 1989;10:565–566.
288. Mathews VP, Alo PL, Glass JD, Kumar AJ, McArthur JC. AIDS-related CNS cryptococcosis: Radiologic-pathologic correlation. *AJNR* 1992;13:1477–1486.
289. Tan CT, Kuan BB. Cryptococcus meningitis, clinical-CT scan considerations. *Neuroradiology* 1987;29:43–46.
290. Balakrishnnen J, Becker PS, Kumar AJ, et al. Acquired immunodeficiency syndrome: correlation of radiologic and pathologic findings in the brain. *Radiographics* 1990;10:201–216.
291. Tien RD, Chu PK, Hesselink JR, et al. Intracranial cryptococcosis in immunocompromised patients: CT and MR findings in 29 cases. *AJNR* 1991;12:283–289.
292. Centeno AS, Bentson Jr, Mancuso AA. CT scanning in rhinocerebral mucormycosis and aspergillosis. *Radiology* 1981;140:383–389.
293. Gamba JL, Woodruff WW, Djang WT, Yeates AE. Craniofacial mucormycosis: assessment with CT. *Radiology* 1986;160:207–212.
294. Shapiro MD, Som PM. MRI of the paranasal sinuses and nasal cavity. *Radiol Clin North Am* 1989;27:447–475.
295. Rodriguez-Carbajal J, Palacios E, Naidich TA. Infections and parasitic disorders—supratentorial. In: Taveras JM, Ferrucci JT, eds. *Radiology: Diagnosis-Imaging-Intervention*, Vol. 3. Philadelphia: JB Lippincott; 1986:1–22.
296. Dublin AB, Phillips HE. Computed tomography of disseminated cerebral coccidioidomycosis. *Radiology* 1980;135:361–368.
297. Kobayaski RM, Coel M, Niwayama G, et al. Cerebral vasculitis in coccidioidal meningitis. *Ann Neurol* 1977;1:281–284.

298. Stern BJ, Krumholz A, Johns C, et al. Sarcoidosis and its neurological manifestations. *Arch Neurol* 1985;42:909–917.
299. Leeds NE, Zimmerman RD, Elkin CM, et al. Neurosarcoidosis of the brain and meninges. *Semin Roentgenol* 1985;20:387–392.
300. Kumpe DA, Rao KCVG, Garcia JH, Heck AF. Intracranial neurosarcoidosis. *J Comput Assist Tomogr* 1979;3:324–330.
301. Carey RM, Kimball AC, Armstrong D, Lieberman PH. Toxoplasmosis. Clinical experiences in a cancer hospital. *Am J Med* 1973;54:30–38.
302. Remington JS. Toxoplasmosis in the adult. *Bull NY Acad Med* 1978;50:211–227.
303. Vietzke WM, Gelderman AH, Grimley PM, Vaslamis MP. Toxoplasmosis complicating malignancy. Experience at the National Cancer Institute. *Cancer* 1968;21:816–827.
304. Post MJD, Chan JC, Hensley GT, et al. Toxoplasma encephalitis in Haitian adults with acquired immunodeficiency syndrome: a clinical-pathologic-CT correlation. *AJR* 1983;140:861–868.
305. Porter SB, Sande MA. Toxoplasmosis of the central nervous system in the acquired immunodeficiency syndrome. *N Engl J Med* 1993;2:1643–1648.
306. Atlas SW, Grossman RI, Hackney DB, et al. Calcified intracranial lesions: detection with gradient echo acquisition rapid MR imaging. *AJNR* 1988;253–259.
307. Ruiz A, Ganz WI, Post MJD, et al. Use of Thallium-201 brain SPECT to differentiate cerebral lymphoma from toxoplasma encephalitis in AIDS patients. Presented at the 26th Annual Conference of the American Society of Neuroradiology, Vancouver, Canada, May 13–16, 1993.
308. Becker LE. Infections of the developing brain. *AJNR* 1992;13:537–549.
309. Davis LE, Kornfeld M. Neurocysticercosis: neurologic, pathogenic, diagnostic and therapeutic aspects. *Eur Neurol* 1991;31:229–240.
310. McCormick GF. Cysticercosis: review of 230 patients. *Bull Clin Neurosci* 1985;50:76–101.
311. Carbajal JR, Palacios E, Azar-Kia B, et al. Radiology of cysticercosis of the central nervous system including computed tomography. *Radiology* 1977;125:127–131.
312. Lopes-Hernandez A. Clinical manifestations and sequential computed tomographic scans of cerebral cysticercosis in childhood. *Brain Dev* 1983;5:269–277.
313. Escobar A. The pathology of neurocysticercosis. In: Palacios E, Rodriguez-Carbajal J, Taveras JM, eds. *Cysticercosis of the Central Nervous System*. Springfield: Charles C Thomas; 1983:27–59.
314. Lobato RD, Lamas E, Portillo JM, et al. Hydrocephalus in cerebral cysticercosis. *J Neurosurg* 1981;55:786–793.
315. Scharf D. Neurocysticercosis. *Arch Neurol* 1988;45:777–780.
316. Kramer LD, Locke GE, Byrd SE, et al. Cerebral cysticercosis: documentation of natural history with CT. *Radiology* 1989;171:459–462.
317. Lotz J, Hewlett R, Alheit B, Bowen R. Neurocysticercosis: correlative pathomorphology and MR imaging. *Neuroradiology* 1988;30:35–41.
318. Suss RA, Maravilla KR, Thompson J. MR imaging of intracranial cysticercosis: comparison with CT and anatomopathologic features. *AJNR* 1986;7:235–242.
319. Spickler EM, Lufkin RB, Teresi L, Lanman T, Leveque M, Benston JR. High signal intraventricular cysticercosis on T1 weighted MR imaging. *AJNR* 1989;10:S64.
320. Chang K-H, Lee JH, Han MH, Han MC. The role of contrast-enhanced MR imaging in the diagnosis of neurocysticercosis. *AJNR* 1991;128:509–512.
321. Falcone S, Quencer RM, Post MJD. Magnetic resonance imaging of unusual intracranial infections. *Topics Magn Reson Imag* 1994;6:41–52.
322. Walsh JA. Problems in recognition and diagnosis of amebiasis; estimation of the global magnitude of morbidity and mortality. *Rev Infect Dis* 1986;8:228–238.
323. Orbison JA, Reeves N, Leedham CL, Blumber JM. Amebic brain abscess. Review of the literature and report of five additional cases. *Medicine* 1951;30:247–282.
324. Banerjee AK, Bhatnagar RK, Bhusnurmath SR. Secondary cerebral amebiasis. *Trop Geogr Med* 1983;35:333–336.
325. Lombardo L, Alonso P, Arroyo LS, Brandt H, Mateos JH. Cerebral amebiasis. Report of 17 cases. *J Neurosurg* 1964;21:704–709.
326. Martinez-Paloma A, Ruiz-Palacios G. Amebiasis. In: Warren KS, Mahmoud AAF, eds. *Tropical and Geographic Medicine*, 2nd ed. New York: McGraw Hill; 1990.
327. Dietz R, Schanen G, Kramann B, Erpelding J. Intracranial amebic abscesses: CT and MR findings. *J Comput Assist Tomogr* 1991;15:168–170.
328. Tikly M, Denath FM, Hodkinson HJ, Saffer D. Computed tomographic findings in amoebic brain abscess. *S Afr Med J* 1988;73:258–259.
329. Martinez AJ. *Free Living Amebas: Natural History, Prevention, Diagnosis, Pathology and Treatment of Disease*. Boca Raton: CRC Press; 1985.
330. Franke ED, MacKiewicz JS. Isolation of Acanthamoeba and Naegleria from the intestinal contents of fresh water fishes and their potential pathogenicity. *J Parasitol* 1982;68:164–166.
331. Fowler M, Carter RF. Acute pyogenic meningitis probably due to Acanthamoeba sp.: a preliminary report. *Br Med J* 1965;2:740–742.
332. Duma RJ. Primary amebic meningoencephalitis. In: Warren KS, Mahmoud AAF, eds. *Tropical and Geographic Medicine*, 2nd ed. New York: McGraw Hill; 1990.
333. John DT. Primary amebic meningoencephalitis and the biology of Naegleria fowleri. *Annu Rev Microbiol* 1982;36:101–123.
334. Martinez AJ, Duma RJ, Nelson EL, Moretta E. Experimental Naegleria meningo-encephalitis in mice. Penetration of the olfactory mucosal epithelium by Naegleria and pathologic changes produced: a light and electron microscope study. *Lab Invest* 1973;29:121–133.
335. Lam AH, de Silva M, Procopis P, Kan A. Primary amoebic (Naegleria) meningo-encephalitis. *J Comput Assist Tomogr* 1982;6:620–623.
336. Martinez AJ. Is Acanthamoeba encephalitis an opportunistic infection? *Neurology* 1980;30:567–574.
337. Kwame Ofori-Kwakye S, Sidebottom DG, Herbert H, Fischer EG, Visvesvara GS. Granulomatous brain tumor caused by Acanthamoeba (*abstr*). *J Neurosurg* 1986; 64:505–509.
338. Callicott JH Jr, Nelson C, Jobes MM, et al. Meningoencephalitis due to pathogenic free living amoebae. Report of two cases. *JAMA* 1989;206:579–582.
339. Martinez AJ, Sotelo-Aveila C, Alcala H, Willaert E. Granulomatous encephalitis intracranial arteritis and mycotic aneurysm due to a free living ameba. *Acta Neuropathol* 1980;49:7–12.
340. Matson DO, Rovah E, Lee D, Armstrong RT, Parke JT, Baker CJ. Acanthemoeba meningoencephalitis masquerading as neurocysticercosis. *Pediatr Infect Dis J* 1988;7:121–124.
341. Wessel HB, Hubbard J, Martinez AJ, Willaert E. Granulomatous amebic encephalitis (GAE) with prolonged clinical course, CT scan findings, diagnosis by brain biopsy and effect of treatment (*abstr*). *Neurology* 1980;30:442.
342. Dew KHR. *Hydatid Disease. Its Pathology, Diagnosis, and Treatment*. Sydney: Australian Medical Publishing; 1928.
343. Schantz PM, Okelo GBA. Echinococcus (hydatidosis). In: Warren KS, Mahmoud AAF, eds. *Tropical and Geographic Medicine*, 2nd ed. New York: McGraw Hill; 1990.
344. Demir K, Karsli AF, Kaya T, Devrimci E, Alkan K. Cerebral hydatid cysts: CT findings. *Neurology* 1991;33:22–24.
345. Baassiri A, Hadded F. Primary extradural intracranial hydatid disease: CT appearance. *AJNR* 1984;5:474–475.
346. Hamza R, Touibi S, Jamoussim M, Bardi-Bellogha I, Chtioui R. Intracranial and orbital hydatid cysts. *Neuroradiology* 1982;22:211–214.

Magnetic Resonance Imaging of the Brain and Spine, Second Edition, edited by Scott W. Atlas.
Lippincott-Raven Publishers, Philadelphia © 1996.

17

Central Nervous System Manifestations of the Phakomatoses and Other Inherited Syndromes

James G. Smirniotopoulos and Frances M. Murphy

There are many commonly encountered central nervous system lesions that are manifestations of inherited syndromes. The most common and extensively studied of these syndromes are the "neurocutaneous" syndromes. Also called the "phakomatoses," these disorders have variable patterns of inheritance, and some appear to be congenital malformations without hereditary genetic defects. These diseases are very common, and neuroimaging plays a central role in the diagnosis and management of patients with these diseases. Neuroimaging studies are important for three reasons. First, these diseases have prominent and often pathognomonic imaging findings. The diagnosis can often be made entirely on the basis of a magnetic resonance (MR) or computed tomography (CT) scan; in other cases a clinical impression can be confirmed using imaging studies. Less commonly, an unsuspected case may be identified when imaging is obtained for unrelated reasons, for example, after trauma or for nonspecific symptoms and signs such as headaches or seizures. Second, once a proband-affected individual is recognized, all the first-degree relatives (parents, siblings, children) should be screened to determine whether they are also affected. Third, all individuals who are identified with these syndromes should undergo routine periodic surveillance, using both clinical examinations and neuroimaging studies, to monitor the progression of existing lesions and/or the development of new manifestations. Clinical management is thus dependent on serial neuroimaging studies. In addition, genetic testing and appropriate counseling should be provided for affected family members.

GENERAL CONCEPTS

The terms "neurocutaneous" and "phakomatosis" both colloquially imply that the described condition affects both the skin and the central nervous system (CNS). There are more than thirty so-called neurocutaneous syndromes described in the literature. The most frequent and important are:

J. G. Smirniotopoulos, M.D.: Department of Radiologic Pathology, Armed Forces Institute of Pathology, Washington, DC 20306-6000.

F. M. Murphy, M.D.: Department of Neurology, Georgetown University Medical Center, Washington, DC 20007.

Descriptive Name	*Common Eponym*
Neurofibromatosis Type 1 (NF1)	von Recklinghausen disease
Neurofibromatosis Type 2 (NF2)	Bilateral VIIIth nerve schwannoma
Tuberous sclerosis (TS)	Bourneville disease
Encephalotrigeminal angiomatosis	Sturge-Weber (SW) syndrome
Cerebelloretinal hemangiomatosis	von Hippel-Lindau (VHL) syndrome
Ataxia-telangiectasia (AT)	Louis-Barr syndrome

Although grouped together as "neurocutaneous," even some of the more commonly known syndromes, for example, von Hippel-Lindau disease, do not affect the skin at all. The word "phakoma" was coined by the Dutch ophthalmologist van der Hoeve to describe the ocular/retinal findings of von Recklinghausen neurofibromatosis (NF1) and tuberous sclerosis (TS). He thought that these ocular lesions were similar benign hamartomatous conditions and that these inherited disorders were, therefore, also interrelated. However, TS and NF1 are two completely distinct conditions that have only the most superficial similarities to one another. The "phakoma" of NF1 is a patch of myelinated nerve fibers (neurons) and the ocular mass in TS is a benign glial proliferation of astrocytes. van der Hoeve subsequently added Sturge-Weber syndrome and von Hippel-Lindau syndrome to his grouping of phakomatoses.

NEUROFIBROMATOSIS TYPE 1

The NIH, through its consensus panels, has defined two distinct inherited nerve-sheath disorders that are called "neurofibromatosis type 1" and "neurofibromatosis type 2" (1,2). Alternatively, Riccardi has suggested that there may be as many as eight different versions of "neurofibromatosis" (3). NF1 is the classic von Recklinghausen or "peripheral" disease. It is far more common than NF2, and NF1 has very prominent clinically evident external lesions, including superficial tumors (neurofibromas) and macular hyperpigmentation (café-au-lait spots, or CAL), that facilitate clinical recognition. NF1 is "true" neurofibromatosis, characterized by an inherited predisposition for the development of benign peripheral nerve sheath tumors (neurofibromas), and significant CNS abnormalities that include true neoplasms (usually optic nerve gliomas) as well as dysplastic and hamartomatous/heterotopic lesions. Many of the more common manifestations, as well as the NIH (2) diagnostic criteria (in italics) are summarized in Table 1. Of historical interest, Joseph Merrick (the original "Elephant Man") did not have neurofibromatosis, but another phakomatosis called Proteus syndrome (4,5).

TABLE 1. *Common findings in von Recklinghausen/Type 1 neurofibromatosis*[a]

Brain/orbit/ocular
Lisch nodules (iris hamartomas)
Eyelid plexiform neurofibroma
Optic nerve glioma
Retinal patch of myelinated nerves
Pulsatile exophthalmos (sphenoid dysplasia)
Multifocal T2-weighted hyperintensities
Basal ganglia T1-weighted hyperintensities
Chiasmatic and other gliomas
Moya-Moya, aneurysms, and/or multiple infarcts
Macrocephaly (>97th percentile)
Cutaneous/subcutaneous
Café-au-lait spots (CAL) (>6, 5 mm in children, 15 mm in adults)
Axillary and intertriginous freckling (can be smaller than CAL)
Cutaneous/subcutaneous neurofibroma (2 or more)
Plexiform neurofibroma (only 1 needed)
Elephantiasis neuromatosa
Skeletal/spinal
Acute cervical kyphoscoliosis
Simple scoliosis
Lateral thoracic meningocele
Pseudoarthrosis (especially congenital)
Sphenoid dysplasia/hypoplasia
Ribbon ribs
Lambdoid suture defect
Focal gigantism
Spinal root/dumbbell neurofibroma (2 or more)
Dysplastic enlargement of spinal foramina
Dysplastic enlargement of optic and auditory canals
Vascular/visceral/endocrine
Pheochromocytoma
Parathyroid adenoma
Renal artery stenosis
Medullary carcinoma of thyroid

[a] NIH (2) criteria for diagnosis in italics—two or more features needed.

NF1 is an autosomal dominant disorder without racial or sexual predilection. The incidence is estimated at 1 in 2,000 to 1 in 3,000 births, and the prevalence is documented at about 1 in 4,000 in North America (6). NF1 is an extremely pleomorphic disorder, and, although we may dwell on those individuals with classic stigmata, who suffer significant morbidity and mortality from symptomatic lesions, many patients are asymptomatic, with few obvious findings, and enjoy a normal lifespan. This latter group of patients may not be diagnosed until an autopsy or diagnostic testing for an unrelated disease reveals the characteristic features. However, in most individuals the diagnosis is commonly made on the basis of the prominent cutaneous findings, or is detected while screening first-degree relatives of an affected individual.

Less than half the patients with NF1 will have a positive family history that suggests a high rate of spontaneous mutation. Historic accounts, in the older literature, of spontaneous and/or sporadic cases should be viewed with some skepticism, however, because the clinical features of NF1 are extremely variable. It is difficult to exclude familial cases of von Recklinghausen neurofibromatosis in the absence of a thorough evaluation, which should include a physical examination, neuroimaging of the brain (and probably the spine), slit-lamp examination of the eyes, or genetic testing. Genetic linkage analyses have shown that the gene responsible for NF1 is on the long arm of chromosome 17 (7,8). The normal gene appears to function as a tumor-suppressor oncogene, and, with only a single copy of the gene, tumorigenesis is suppressed. However, if both copies of the gene are absent, a variety of neoplasms and non-neoplastic lesions are likely to develop. This NF1 oncogene concept follows the two-hit theory that is used to explain inherited retinoblastoma. The first "hit" removes one copy of the gene from the germ cell line and therefore affects every somatic cell in the body. The affected individual is now "primed" for the second "hit" required for tumorigenesis. The loss of the only remaining protective gene probably occurs during periods of rapid cell division, for example, during embryonic and fetal growth, and with the rapid growth spurt that occurs with puberty. The second hit then affects a subpopulation of somatic cells producing the characteristic neoplastic and dysplastic manifestations. Although the major effects of the abnormal chromosome 17 gene are on the nervous system [both peripheral (PNS) and central (CNS)] and the skin, virtually all organ systems and tissues of the body are affected.

In some series, more than half of all patients with probable NF1 have abnormal neuroimaging of the brain and/or orbit (9). Both hamartomatous and neoplastic lesions occur, including optic nerve and parenchymal gliomas as well as multifocal signal changes (bright foci on T2-weighted MR) in the brainstem, cerebellar white matter, dentate nucleus, basal ganglia, periventricular white matter, optic nerve, and optic pathways (10–14) (Figs. 1–5). In most of these published series, there has not been histologic verification of these lesions. Although the T2 hyperintensities should be followed using serial examinations, they most probably represent either abnormal myelination or some hamartomatous change (10,11,15). The radiologic criteria for distinguishing these lesions as "hamartomas" (rather than more ominous neoplasms) are absence of mass effect, absence of a spreading (vasogenic) pattern of edema, and absence of contrast enhancement or hemorrhage. One exception to these rules is the lesion in the globus pallidus; these demonstrate abnormally high signal intensity on T1-weighted images in more than half the patients who have them, and are often associated with mild mass effect (10,16). These T1-weighted hyperintensities could be produced by increased myelination (and increased lipid?) from heterotopic Schwann cells, or perhaps from ectopic melanin (16). Both Schwann cells and melanocytes are derived from the neural crest, but are not normally present within the brain parenchyma. Although there has been no large-scale confirmation of these heterotopic Schwann cells as the cause of the T1-weighted hyperintensities, heterotopic Schwann cells have been seen histologically, in patients with and without neurofibromatosis (15). Ferner et al. reported that there is no association between the presence of the globus pallidus abnormalities and detectable cognitive impairment (17).

Optic nerve gliomas (ONGs), especially those that present in childhood, are an important and often diagnostic feature of NF1 (Figs. 6 and 7). In childhood, both the sporadic ONGs and especially those associated with NF1 are almost invariably juvenile pilocytic astrocytomas (JPAs) (Fig. 8). These are low grade (WHO I) astrocytomas and are histologically identical to those occurring in the pediatric cerebellum as the "cystic cerebellar astrocytoma" (18). Approximately 2% to 5% of all brain tumors in childhood are ONGs, and about 70% of the patients with ONGs will have NF1 (19). Although almost 50% of all cases of childhood JPA (with and without NF1) present in the optic chiasm and hypothalamus, less than 3% of them are limited to the intraorbital portions of the optic tract (Figs. 9 and 10). Conversely, 5% to 40% of patients with NF1 will develop ONGs, and these typically present under the age of 10 years (mean of 6 years) (6,10,11,14). Surveillance is extremely important for these young patients, since up to 80% with their ONGs are asymptomatic at the time of diagnosis. The primary findings of ONG include abnormal optic nerve thickening and abnormal enhancement (10,20). In ONG, the optic nerves may also appear beaded, and become elongated and tortuous—often "kinking" within the orbit. However, dural ectasia of the optic nerve sheath, without a neoplasm, can mimic the enlargement and beaded configuration of an optic glioma (Fig. 11). The presence of bilateral ONGs is considered specific for NF1 (21).

Serial studies may reveal the development, progressive growth, and even the regression of untreated ONG in patients with NF1, continuing the controversy about the management of these patients (21,22). Hoyt and Baghadassarian suggested that ONG behaves in an indolent fashion, more like a hamartoma than a true neoplasm, and they recommended conservative management (23). In many institutions definitive resection is postponed as long as there is useful vision remaining in the eye, unless the ONG is causing hydrocephalus, or other structures are compressed from mass effect (24,25), whereas other authors recommend a biopsy for confirmation, surgical resection, and radiation treatment (26–28). Furthermore, the use of radiation, either alone or as an adjunct to surgery, is also questioned. Irradiation of tissues that are prone to tumorigenesis (such as in patients with inherited retinoblastoma and in the phakomatoses) is relatively contraindicated because it may stimulate the development of additional new neoplasms.

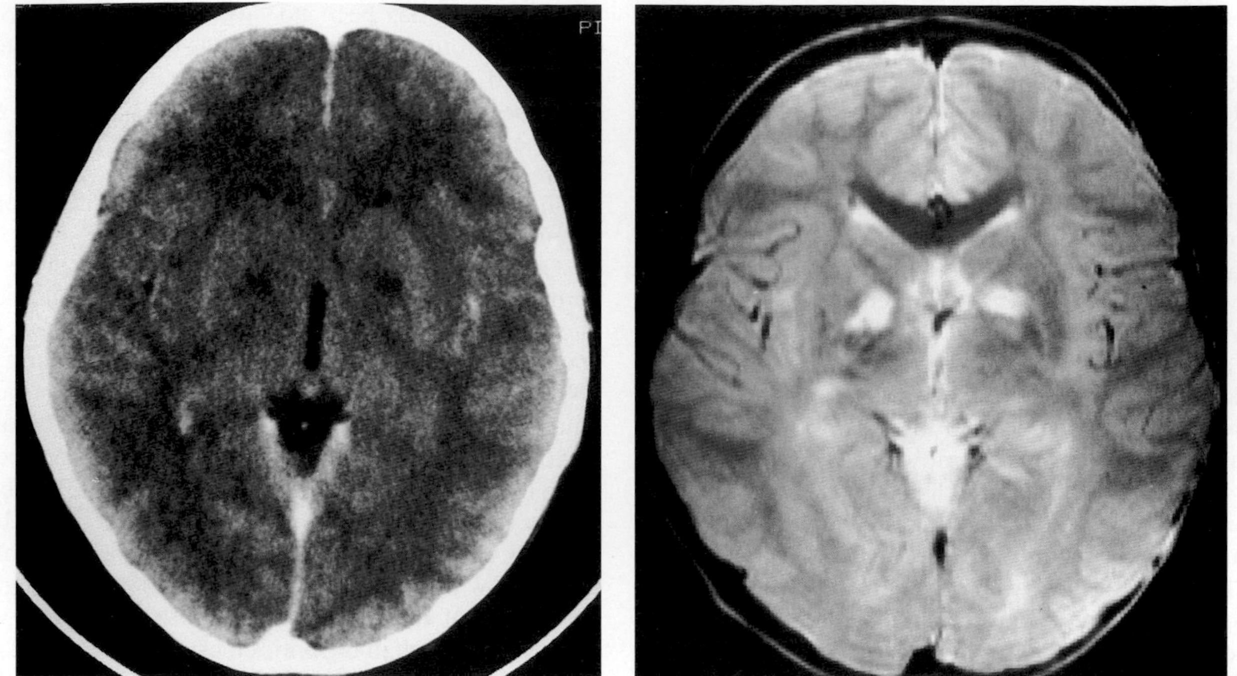

FIG. 1. NF1. Globus pallidus lesion. **A:** Contrast-enhanced CT scan demonstrates bilateral abnormal lucency in the globus pallidus region of the lenticular nuclei. There is no evidence of mass effect or edema, nor is there any contrast enhancement. The remainder of the brain is normal. **B:** T2-weighted axial MR in the same patient demonstrates bilateral abnormal signal hyperintensity in the globus pallidi. There is no mass effect or vasogenic edema.

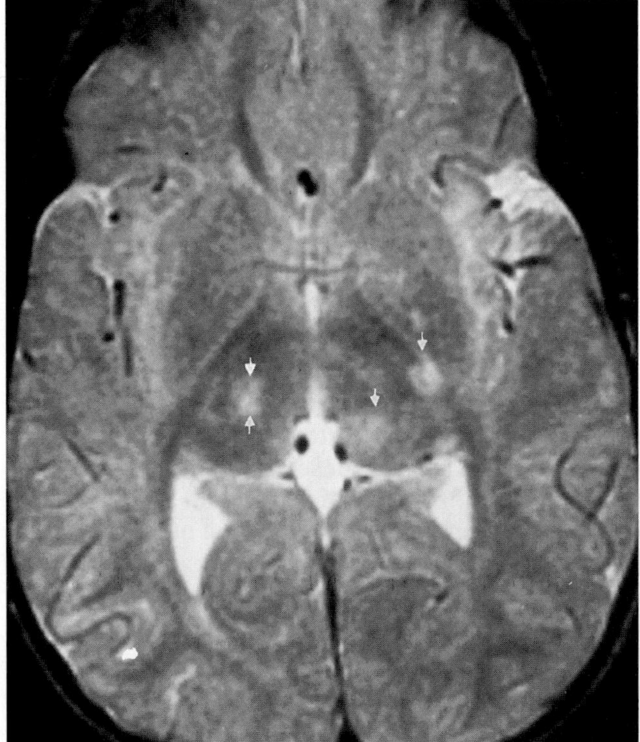

FIG. 2. Small foci of hyperintensity on long TR/TE image of NF1 patient with bithalamic lesions (*arrows*).

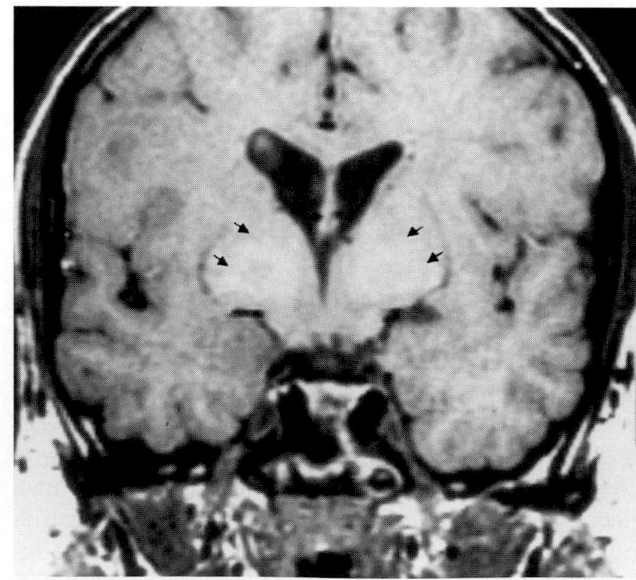

FIG. 3. Marked high intensity in basal ganglia on short TR/TE MR (*arrows*) may correlate with pigment deposition (*see text*).

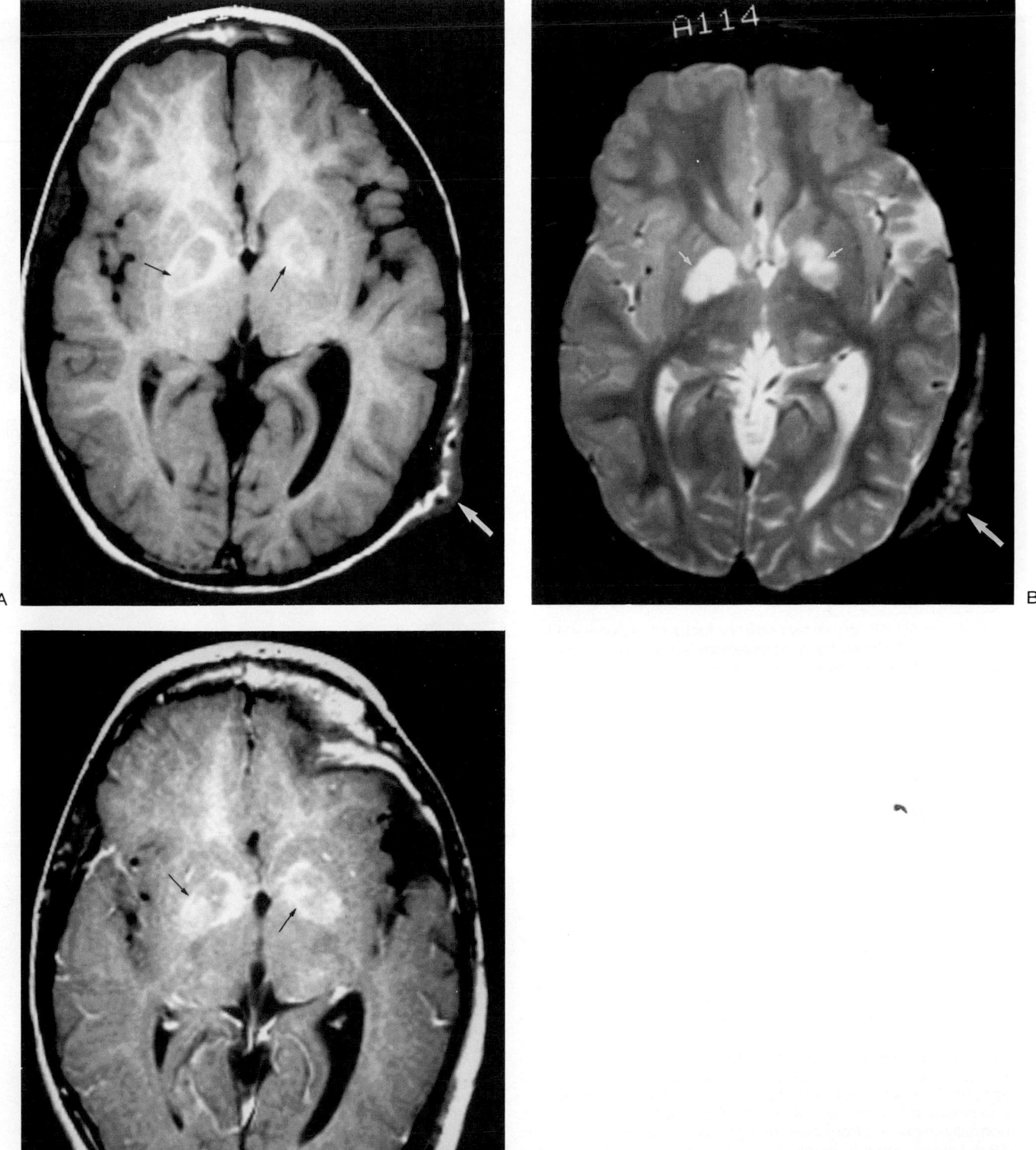

FIG. 4. NF1 patient with areas of hyperintensity involving both globus pallidi (*small arrows*) and left temporal scalp neurofibroma (*large arrow*) on both short TR/TE (**A**) and long TR/TE (**B**) images. Note enhancement of pallidus lesions bilaterally (**C**) on postcontrast scan.

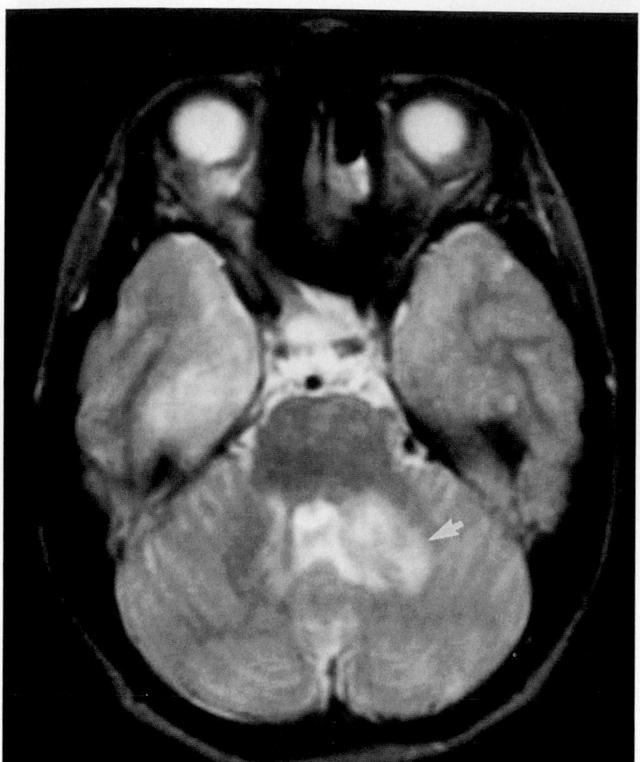

FIG. 5. Long TR/TE MR shows solitary focus of hyperintensity in white matter of left cerebellar hemisphere (*arrow*). The suggestion of mass effect demands close follow-up.

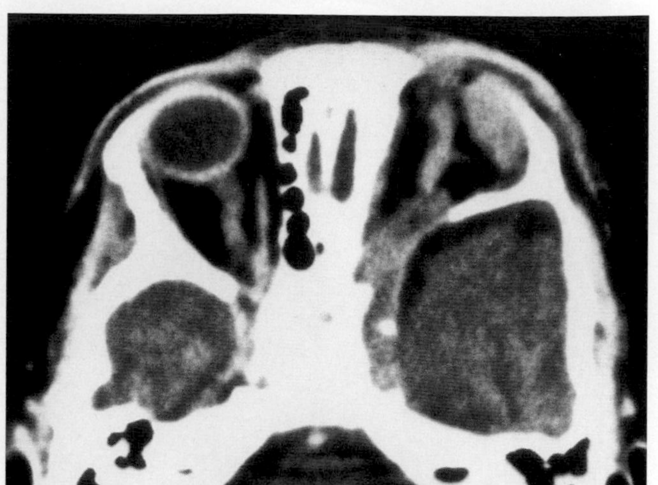

A

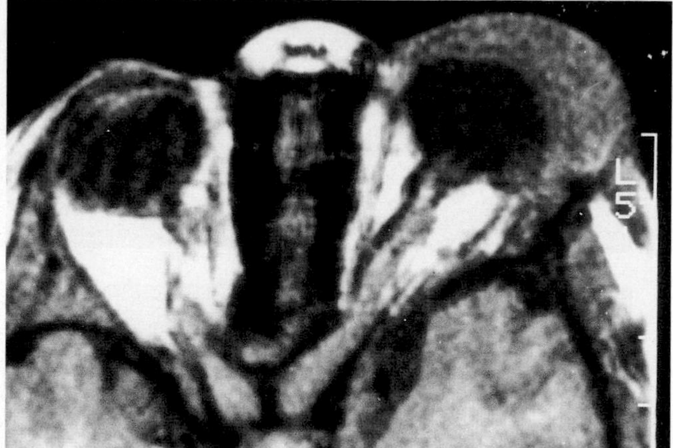

B

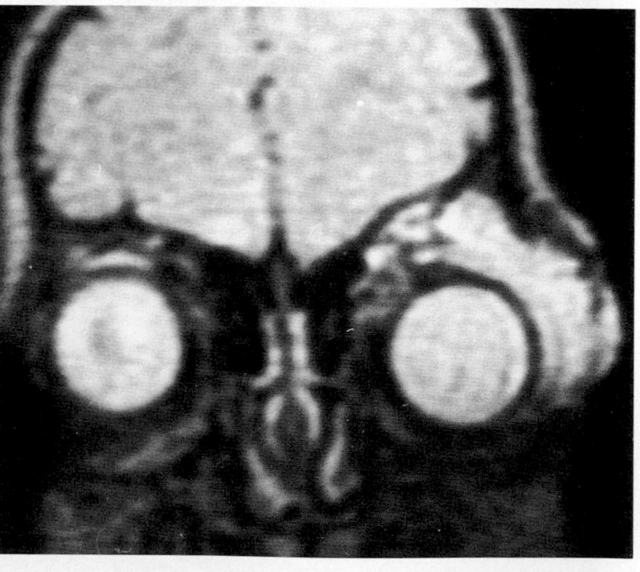

C

FIG. 6. NF1 with sphenoid hypoplasia. **A:** This enhanced CT scan demonstrates enlargement of the left middle fossa with secondary encroachment on the left orbit. The left sphenoid is hypoplastic and associated with a wide open superior orbital fissure. The soft tissue density in the outer aspect of the left orbit is an extraconal plexiform neurofibroma. **B:** T1-weighted MR in the same patient demonstrates anterior displacement of the left temporal tip, causing secondary proptosis. Also visualized is abnormal thickening of the left eyelid produced by a diffuse subcutaneous plexiform neurofibroma. Both optic nerves are abnormally thickened from bilateral optic nerve gliomas. **C:** On the T2-weighted coronal image, the subcutaneous plexiform neurofibroma is almost uniformly hyperintense. Note the inferior displacement of both the left globe and the surrounding intraconal orbital fat.

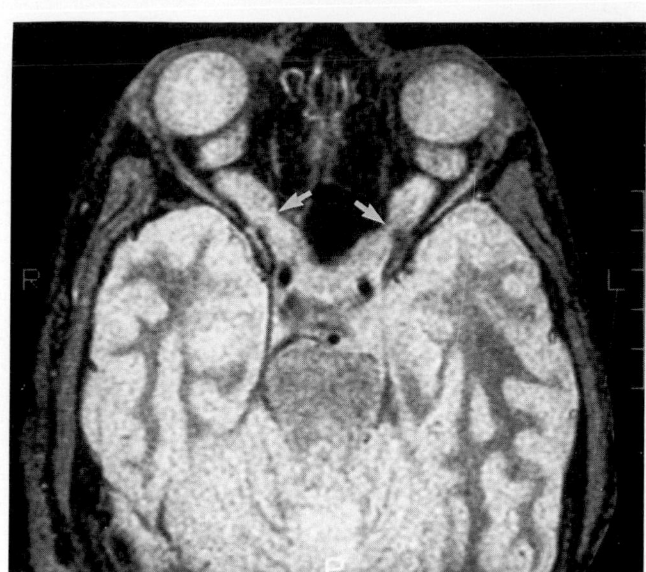

FIG. 7. Bilateral optic nerve gliomas in patient with NF1 show fusiform enlargement (*arrows*) on STIR inversion recovery MR image.

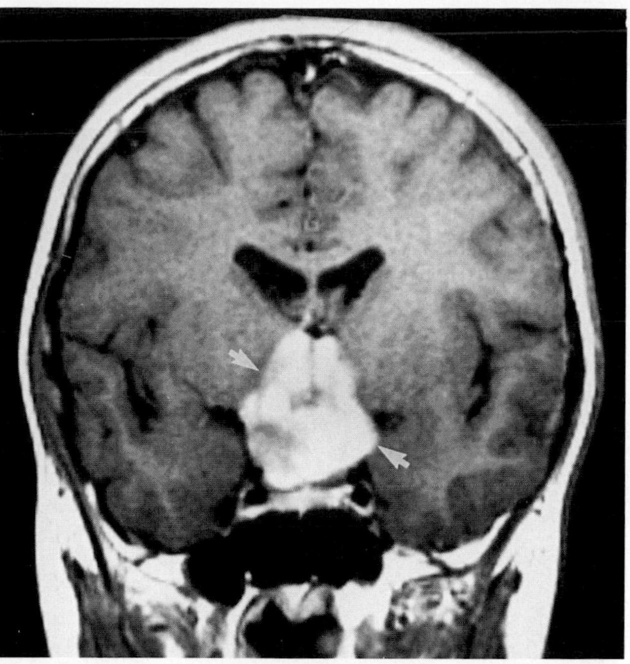

FIG. 8. Coronal postcontrast short TR/TE image defines enhancing chiasmatic-hypothalamic pilocytic astrocytoma (*arrows*) in patient with NF1.

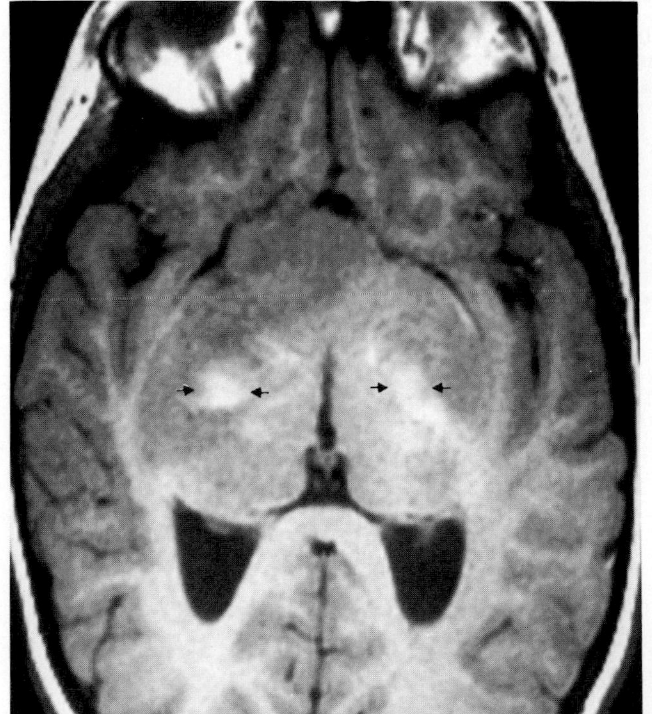

A

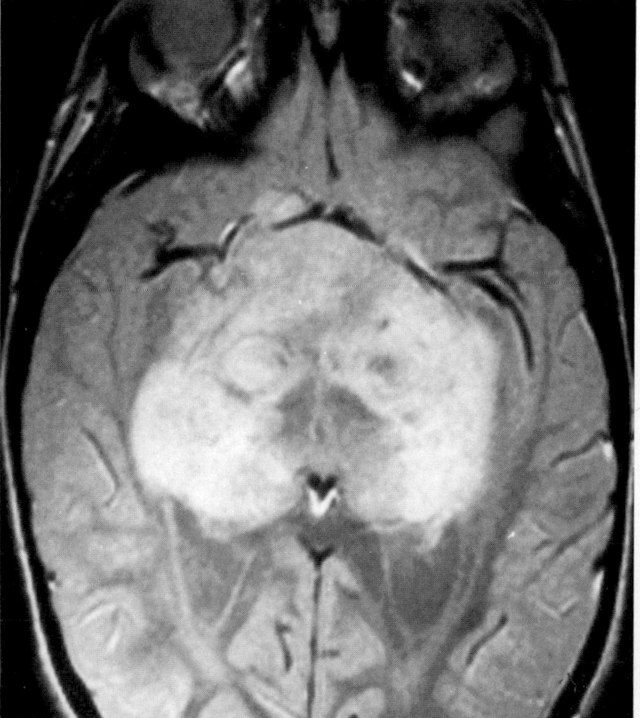

B

FIG. 9. Massive extension of bilateral optic gliomas into basal ganglia and medial temporal lobes, with focal regions of hyperintensity on short TR/TE image (*arrows*, **A**). The tumor extension is seen as diffuse high intensity on long TR/short TE image (**B**).

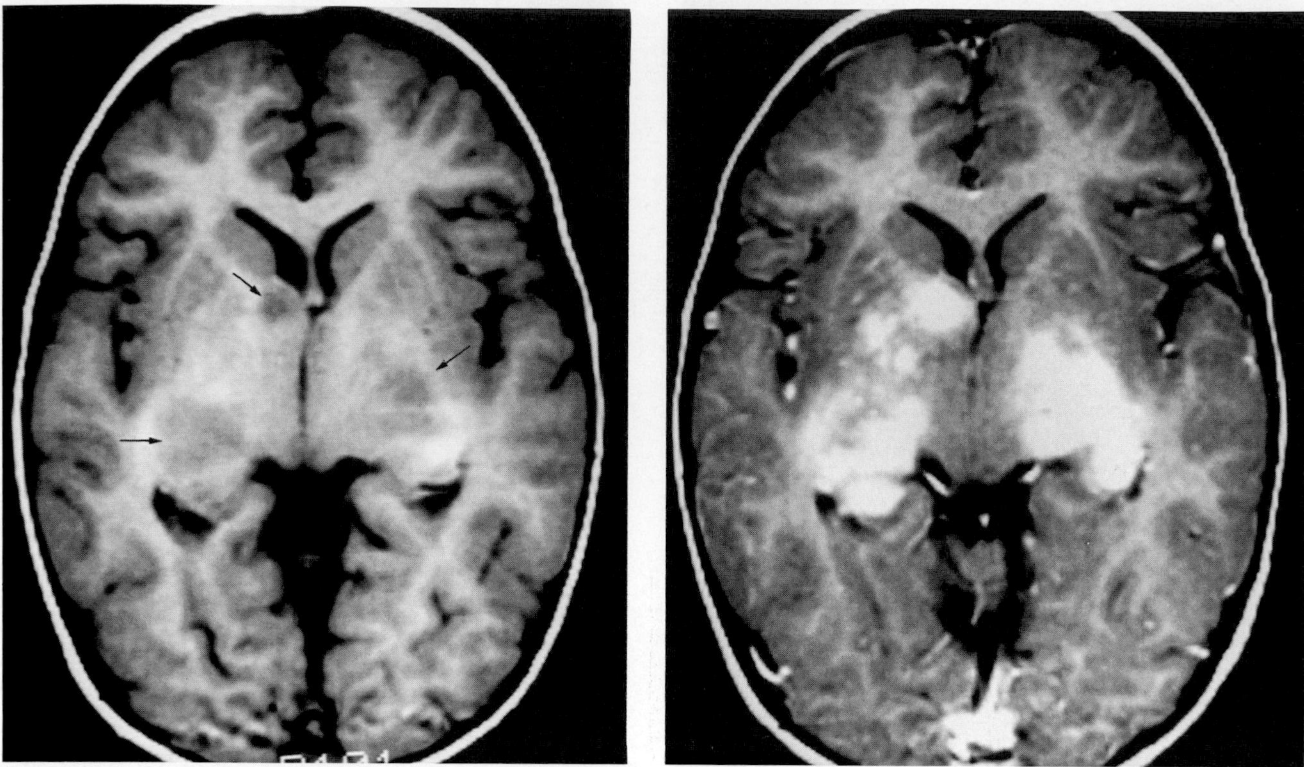

FIG. 10. Infiltrating cerebral gliomas in NF1 patient with bilateral ONG shown as hypointensity with mass effect (*arrows,* A) on precontrast short TR/TE image (A) and enhancement after contrast administration (B). The enhancement is highly suggestive of the neoplastic nature of masses.

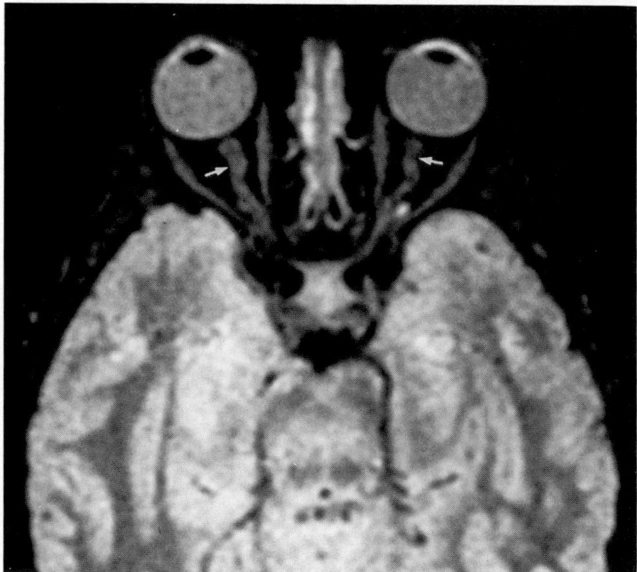

FIG. 11. Bilateral dural ectasia is seen on axial STIR MR image. Note normal size, but irregular, undulating outlines of nerve-sheath complexes (*arrows*).

In up to one third of patients with NF1, there will be neurofibromas affecting intraorbital and facial branches of the cranial nerves (CNN III–VI) and/or diffuse plexiform neurofibroma of the face and eyelids; and, in 5% to 10% of patients, there is proptosis of the globe because of dehiscence and dysplasia of the sphenoid bone (6,20,29,30) (Fig. 12). Sphenoid dysplasia is one of the "distinctive bone lesions" that can be used as a diagnostic feature for the diagnosis of NF1 using the NIH criteria (2) (Figs. 6 and 13).

Patients with von Recklinghausen neurofibromatosis develop several different lesions affecting the spinal column and cord. These include dysplastic neural foraminal enlargement, multiple nerve sheath tumors that are neurofibromas (rather than schwannomas, which are usually sporadic), and acquired meningoceles (Figs. 14 and 15). The lateral thoracic meningocele is strongly suggestive of NF1 (Fig. 16). These lesions represent a "pulsion diverticulum" of the spinal subarachnoid space. This occurs in the thorax because there are no paravertebral muscles overlying the neural foramina and because there is a larger pressure difference between the negative intrathoracic pressure and normal cerebrospinal fluid (CSF) pressure of the subarachnoid space (see Table 1).

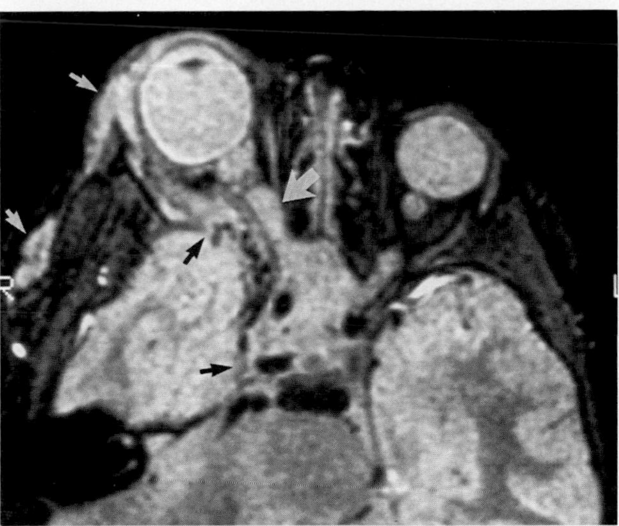

FIG. 13. STIR image of NF1 patient with enlargement of right orbit, buphthalmos of right globe, dysplasia and absence of right greater and lesser wings of sphenoid (*black arrows*), plexiform neurofibroma of skin and scalp in right temporal and periorbital regions (*small white arrows*), and right optic nerve glioma (*large white arrow*).

NEUROFIBROMATOSIS TYPE 2

Formerly called "bilateral acoustic neurofibromatosis," NF2 also has an autosomal dominant pattern of inheritance, and it has no known racial or sexual predilection (31,32). However, female patients may experience exacerbations during pregnancy (33). Multiple cranial nerve schwannomas are the hallmark of this type of "neurofibromatosis," and peripheral and cutaneous neurofibromas are uncommon, if they truly occur at all. The most common site for cranial nerve schwannomas, either sporadic or in NF2, is the eighth (vestibulocochlear) cranial nerve (CNN VIII). Schwannomas represent approximately 5% of all intracranial neoplasms; however, only 5% occur in patients with NF2. In sporadic eighth nerve schwannomas, the tumor may be entirely limited to the vestibular division of the nerve. This localization creates the potential for hearing preservation after surgery, in addition to sparing the facial nerve function. There has been an attempt to subdivide NF2 into two types: the early-onset rapid-course or Wishart type, and the late-onset, more benign or Gardner type. The NIH Consensus Committee has defined a set of diagnostic criteria for NF2, which are met if the patient has one of the following (modified from ref. 2):

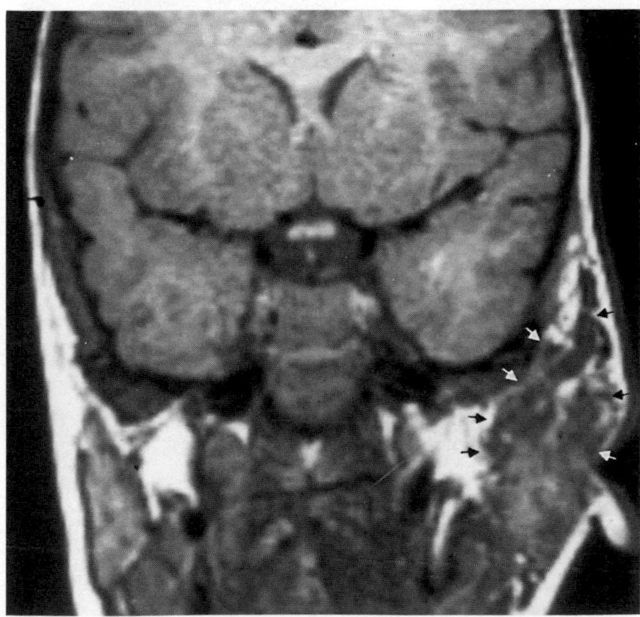

FIG. 12. Plexiform neurofibroma in left parotid is heterogeneous and somewhat ill-defined (*arrows*) on short TR/TE coronal image.

1. Bilateral masses of the eighth cranial nerve (biopsy not needed)
2. A first-degree relative with NF2 and either a single eighth nerve mass or any two of the following—schwannoma, neurofibroma, meningioma, glioma, or juvenile posterior subcapsular lens opacity.

With or without NF2, the cells in some of these associated neoplasms (meningiomas and schwannomas) exhibit deletions from chromosome 22, and it was suggested in 1986 and established in 1987, that a loss of genetic material on this chromosome was an inherited familial trait in "bilateral acoustic neurofibromatosis" (34,35). Analagous to the situation for NF1, individuals

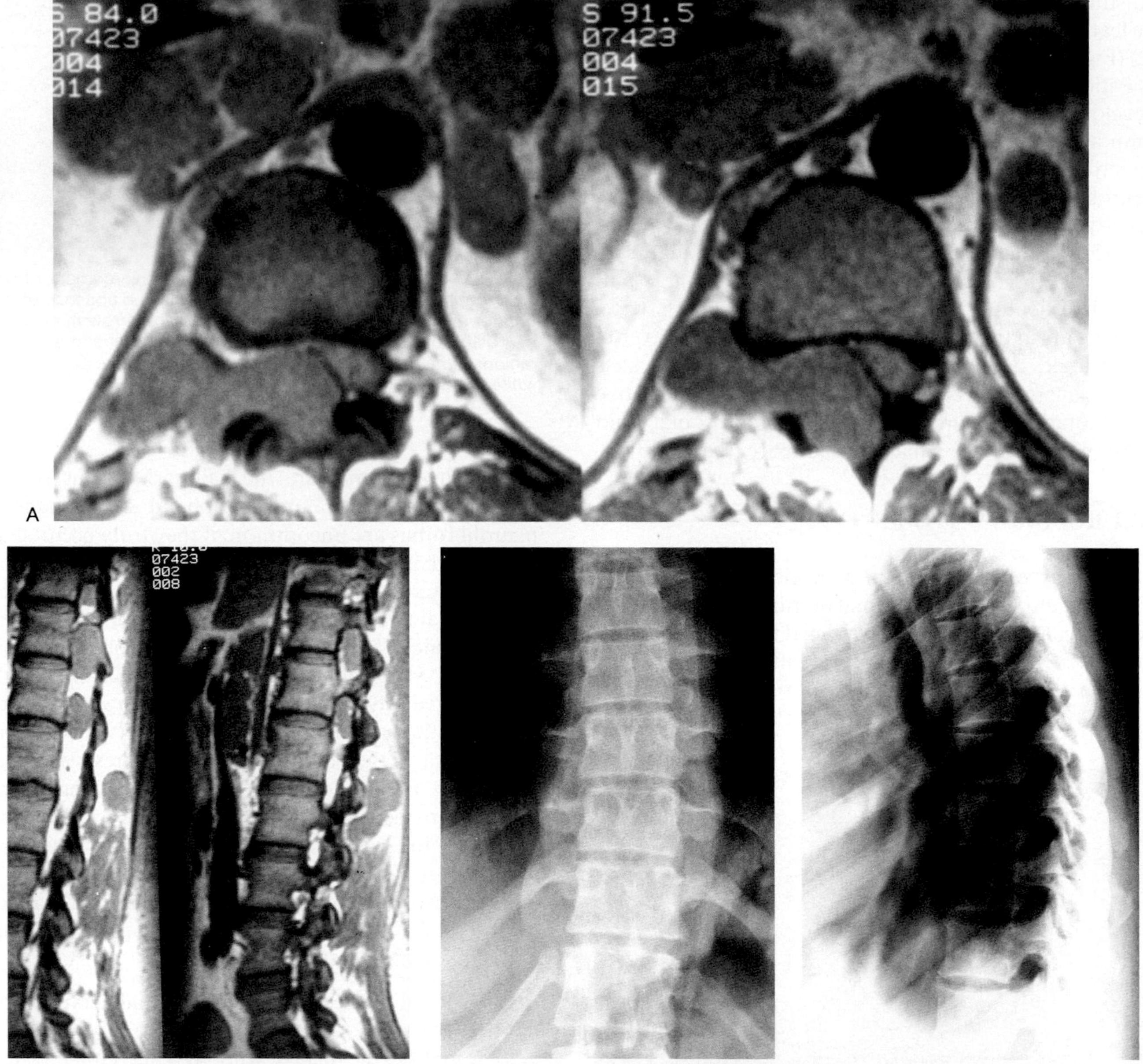

FIG. 14. Multiple spinal neurofibromas. **A:** NF1. The axial T1-weighted image demonstrates a dumbbell-shaped soft tissue mass passing through the right neural foramen. **B:** The sagittal T1-weighted image demonstrates multiple soft tissue masses occupying the neural foramina at multiple levels. The frontal (**C**)) and lateral (**D**) views of the thoracic spine demonstrate bilateral paravertebral soft tissue masses and enlargement of multiple neural foramina.

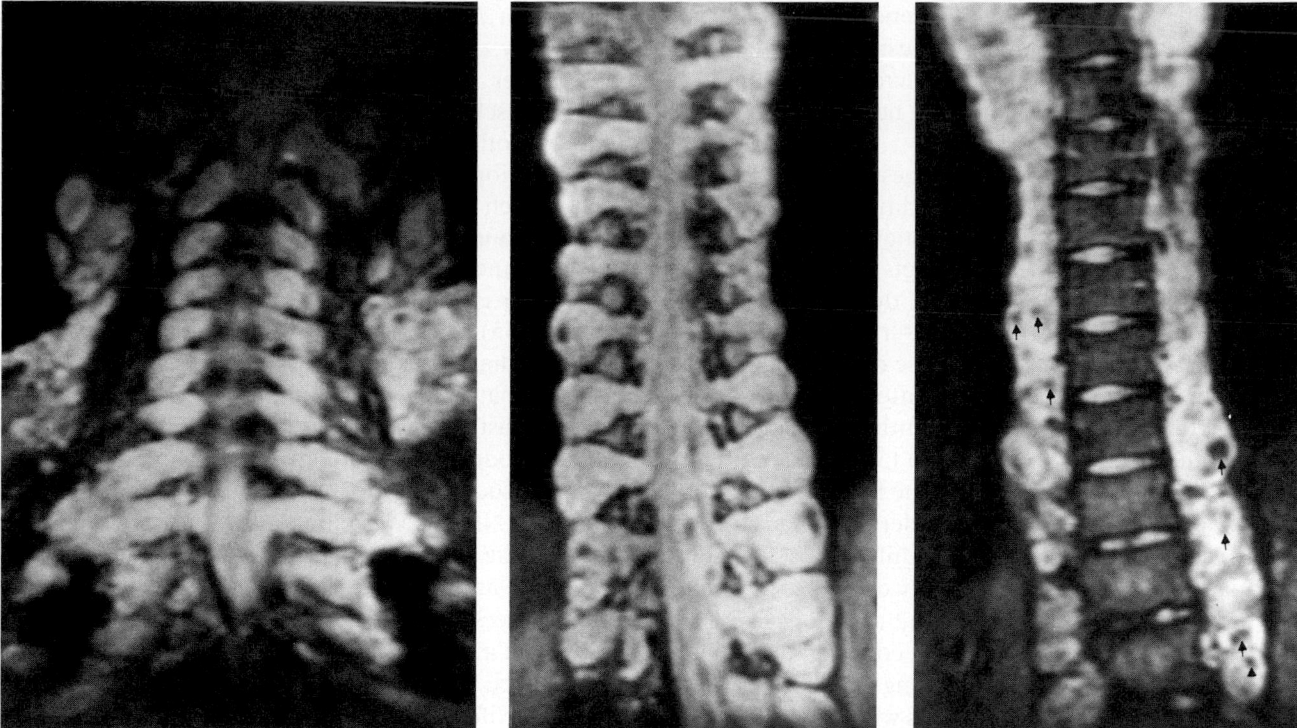

FIG. 15. Innumerable paraspinal neurofibromas comprise an entity known as "plexiform neurofibromatosis." Note that lesions are markedly hyperintense on coronal long TR/short TE images in cervical (**A**) and thoracic (**B**) regions. Characteristic central hypointensity (*arrows,* **C**) is seen on long TR/long TE image (*see text*).

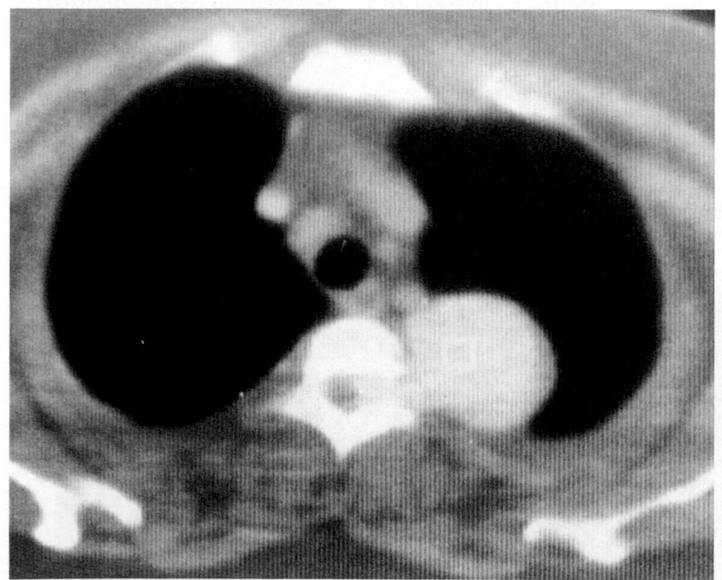

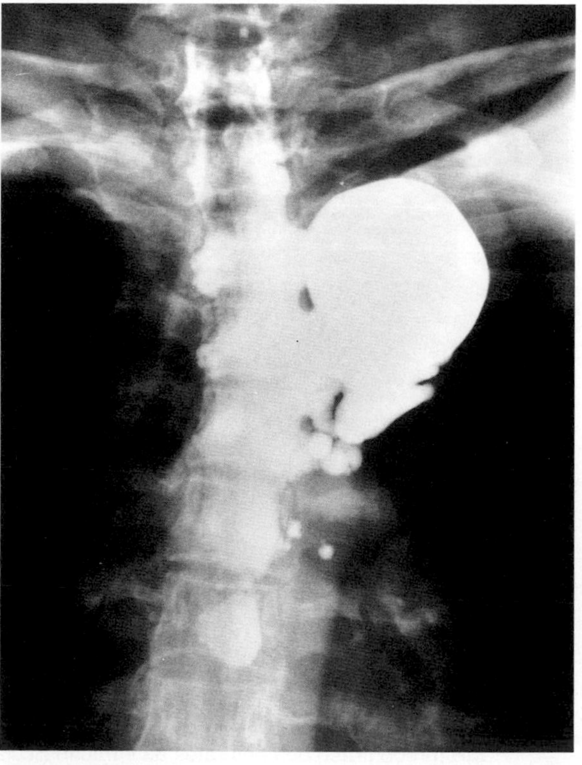

FIG. 16. NF1. Lateral thoracic meningocele. **A:** Axial CT after metrizamide myelogram demonstrates a contrast-opacified cystic mass in the left apex. This communicates with the intraspinal SAS through an enlarged neural foramen. **B:** Frontal view of the chest from a pantopaque myelogram demonstrates a large contrast-opacified left apical mass. In addition, many adjacent axillary root sleeves, at multiple levels, also show some degree of enlargement of the SAS.

who are heterozygous for the NF2 gene (at chromosome 22) are at risk for developing acoustic schwannomas, meningiomas, ependymomas, intracranial nontumoral calcification, and, less commonly, neurofibromas (32, 36,37).

Evans et al. have reported the largest series of patients (150 patients) with NF2 (38). In addition to the vestibular schwannomas, the affected patients have juvenile subcapsular lens opacities (cataracts) and a "specific type of cutaneous tumor" that is distinct from both schwannoma and neurofibroma—resembling "skin tags" (38). The diagnosed prevalence of NF2 is approximately 1 in 210,000; this translates into a calculated birth incidence for NF2 of almost one tenth that reported for NF1 (about 1 in 30,000 to 40,000) (38). Most patients (44%) present with hearing loss as the first manifestation of NF2, followed in descending order by balance problems (8%) and seizures (8%). (38). Unlike most sporadic vestibular schwannomas that merely compress the adjacent nerves, those occurring in NF2 are more likely to invade into, or even arise from, the cochlear and the facial nerves; thus, preserving hearing and facial nerve function is more difficult in patients with NF2 (39,40).

Acoustic schwannomas (ASs) are the hallmark of NF2. In the absence of this congenital syndrome, ASs present as solitary lesions in the fifth decade; with NF2 they present as bilateral masses in the second and third decades (41). Acoustic schwannomas almost invariably arise either within the internal auditory canal (IAC) or at its orifice, the porous acousticus (Fig. 17). Deformity and/or enlargement of the IAC is noted on routine CT in more than 70% of cases (42,43). Schwannomas are histologically composed of dense areas (Antoni A tissue) and looser areas (Antoni B tissue). As they enlarge and age, schwannomas tend to become heterogenous masses, both grossly and on imaging, because of "cystic degeneration" and hemorrhage (15,41,44). Schwannomas, which are the principle neoplasms of NF2, both centrally and peripherally, tend to show prominent contrast enhancement, which may be homogeneous when the tumor is small and heterogeneous when the tumor is large (45) (Figs. 18 and 19). Schwannomas are more vascular than neurofibromas, and both hemorrhage and "cystic change" are more common than in NF1. On noncontrast CT, there is a tendency for both neoplasms to be hypodense compared to skeletal muscle, and hypodense to isodense compared to brain (42,43,45). Schwannomas in NF2 also develop in the dorsal (sensory) nerve roots of the spinal cord (Fig. 20). Intramedullary spinal cord schwannomas also occur in NF2, either as a primary process or through secondary extension into the cord from a site of origin in the nerve root (31). The MR appearance of peripheral nerve sheath tumors (SCH, NFB, plexiform NFB, and MNS) are nonspecific; they tend to be smooth, well-demarcated masses that are mildly heterogeneous with increased signal intensity that progresses from intermediate, through moderate, to clearly bright, as the pulse sequence is changed from T1-weighted, through "proton density" (PD), to T2-weighting (46). Because they are relatively vascular neoplasms without a blood–brain barrier, the vast majority of acoustic schwannomas will enhance on both CT and

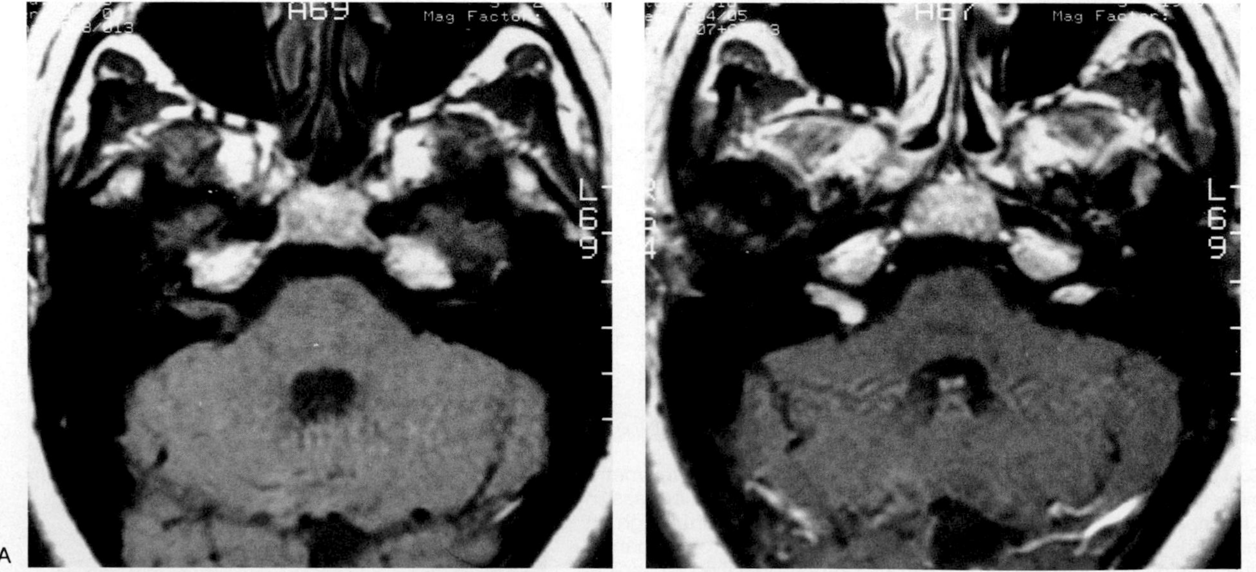

FIG. 17. NF2. Twenty-eight-year-old woman with NF2, bilateral vestibular schwannomas. **A:** The axial T1-weighted MR (precontrast) demonstrates an intracanalicular mass with focal enlargement of the right IAC. This tumor is contiguous with a rounded mass in the cerebellopontine angle cistern. The left IAC is of normal size. **B:** After gadolinium enhancement, the axial T1-weighted image demonstrates bilateral abnormal enhancement involving the IACs. The rounded mass in the right cerebellopontine angle cistern is also enhancing.

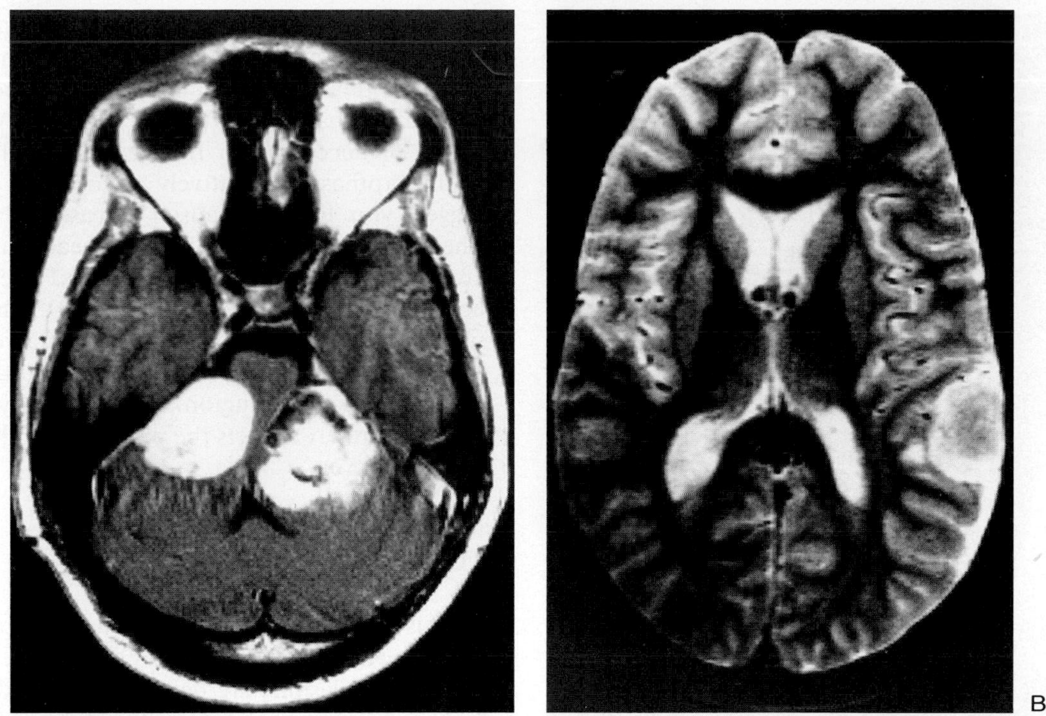

FIG. 18. NF2. Bilateral vestibular schwannomas and multiple meningiomas. **A:** Gadolinium-enhanced T1-weighted axial scan shows bilateral cerebellopontine angle masses, heterogeneous on the patient's left, and homogeneous on the right. Note that a "dural tail" can be seen on the posterior aspect of the left lesions, and on the anterior margin on the left. These were both schwannomas of the eighth cranial nerve. **B:** Axial T2-weighted image shows a dural-based hemispheric extraaxial mass, with a prominent posterior "dural tail." This was a meningioma.

MR scans performed after contrast infusion. Small intracanalicular acoustic schwannomas, which formerly required gas or positive-contrast CT-cisternography for identification, can now be confidently diagnosed or excluded using gadolinium-enhanced MR (47).

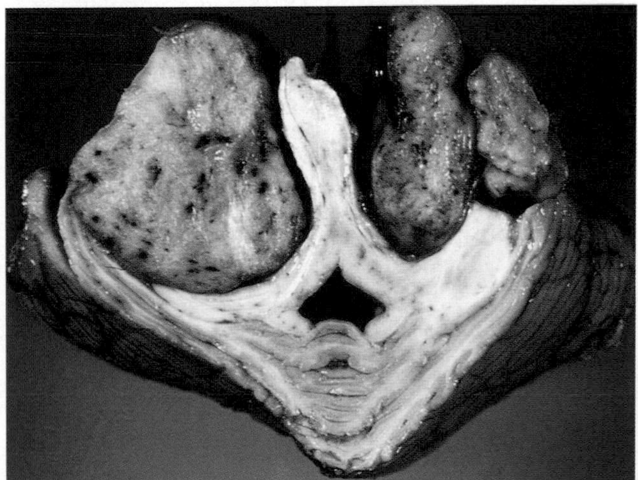

FIG. 19. NF2. Gross—bilateral vestibular schwannomas. This gross brain demonstrates bilateral cerebellopontine angle masses. There is significant pontine compression and molding around these masses that would not be possible if they were not slowly growing lesions. The mass on the right appears to be bilobate.

In addition to acoustic schwannomas, patients with NF2 will develop intracranial meningiomas and schwannomas involving other cranial nerves (10). Patients with NF2 may present with intracranial meningiomas that may be multiple and can present in the lateral ventricle more commonly than sporadic meningiomas (16% vs. 5% intraventricular location) (37). Any meningioma presenting in childhood should alert the physician to be particularly suspicious for NF2 (48). The meningiomas that develop in association with NF2 are similar to sporadic tumors in their histology and radiologic appearance, differing only by their multiplicity and perhaps by a younger age at presentation. Young patients may be examined because of symptoms related to other features of the disease, or as part of family screening. Meningiomas are usually slowly growing benign tumors that can be resected for cure. However, some have suggested that the meningiomas occurring in NF2 may have a worse prognosis. The multiple meningiomas may be few and large, or appear as a myriad of small masses, producing a nodular studding along the dural surfaces. It has also been suggested that true multiple meningiomas (without accompanying schwannomas) may be an entity separate from NF2, rather than being a forme fruste of that disease (49), whereas others have disagreed, suggesting that most cases of multiple meningioma merely represent one end of the spectrum of NF2 (50).

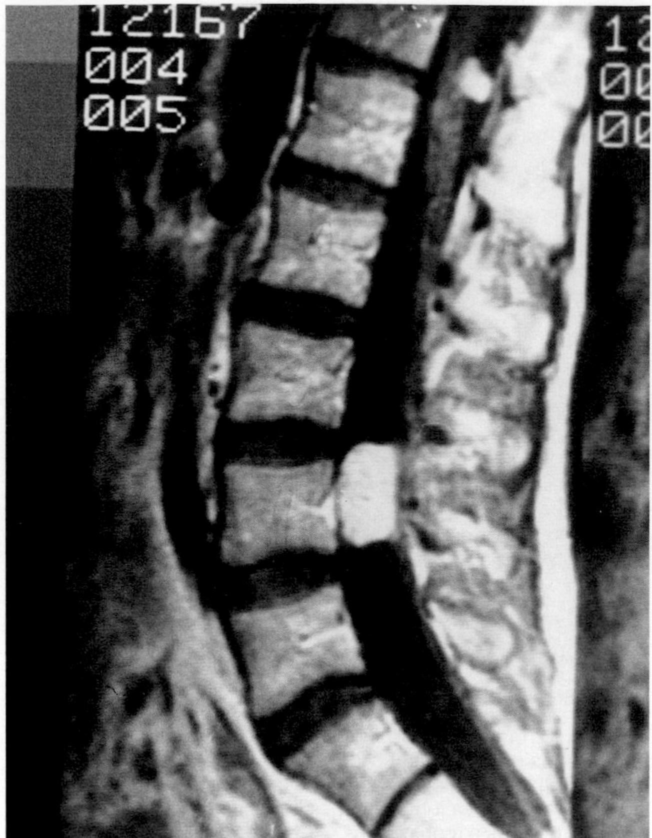

FIG. 20. Thirty-six-year-old man with NF2. This sagittal T1-weighted MR after gadolinium demonstrates two intradural-extramedullary rounded enhancing masses. Both of these were schwannomas. Solitary schwannomas are usually sporadic; however, multiple primary nerve sheath tumors indicate NF1 if they are neurofibromas and NF2 if they are schwannomas. The radiologic features of these two types of benign nerve sheath tumor are often indistinguishable.

The meningiomas are usually dural based, homogeneous, and hyperdense to brain before contrast, and enhancement is usually homogeneous after contrast infusion. On MR, meningiomas may appear relatively isointense compared to brain, but may nonetheless be identified because of secondary displacement of the adjacent brain or by associated calvarial changes of hyperostosis and, less commonly, erosion. Meningiomas enhance brightly after gadolinium infusion, but perhaps a little less intensely than schwannomas.

In comparing the two types of "neurofibromatosis," NF1 is characterized by pathology of the nervous system including the neurons (heterotopias) and astrocytes (ONGs), as well as multiple neurofibromas of the spinal and peripheral nerves. These patients also have prominent cutaneous lesions, most notably café-au-lait spots and neurofibromas of or under the skin. NF1 patients are also at significant risk for various visceral and skeletal problems (the "distinctive bone lesions"). In contrast, patients with NF2 are prone to develop neoplasia not of the astrocyte and neuron, but rather from other cells. NF2 patients develop multiple schwannomas (of the cranial and spinal nerves), meningiomas, and ependymomas (rather than astrocytomas) (1,37,51). When the histology of nerve sheath tumors is carefully evaluated, neurofibromas are relatively uncommon in NF2, and suggest von Recklinghausen disease (NF1) (1,32,36). The spinal and peripheral nerve sheath tumors in NF2 are usually schwannomas. Perhaps NF2 (central neurofibromatosis) should be rechristened "schwannomatosis," or better still a new and distinct acronym can be proposed, for example, M.I.S.M.E.—*m*ultiple *i*nherited *s*chwannomas, *m*eningiomas, and *e*pendymomas, that more accurately reflects the pathology of this congenital syndrome (52).

TUBEROUS SCLEROSIS

TS is an inherited systemic disease with prominent cutaneous, visceral, and CNS manifestations. The vast majority of the lesions are hamartomas—indolent, slowly growing masses composed of a disorganized arrangement of cells that are otherwise relatively normal and that are appropriate for the tissue or site of origin. Although von Recklinghausen was the first to describe this entity, the disease is often referred to as "Bourneville disease," after the French physician who described in several reports a series of such cases. Other eponyms for tuberous sclerosis include "cerebral sclerosis," "Pringle's disease," and "epiloia"—a contraction for the almost constant feature of epilepsy and the less frequently noted "anoia" (mindlessness). TS is autosomal dominant, without any racial or sexual preponderance. More than 50% of cases appear to arise from new spontaneous mutations (i.e., the disease is not clinically evident in the parents). The prevalence of TS in some populations is quite high, varying from 1 in 20,000 to 1 in 150,000, and the incidence has been reported to be as high as 1 in 10,000 (53,54). In some series a chromosome 9 deletion has been reported in association with TS; however, chromosome 11 may also play a role (55,56). Before the development of sophisticated imaging and clinical evaluation, only the more handicapped individuals were recognized, while many less severely affected patients were classified as bearing a forme fruste of the disease. The original diagnostic criteria for TS required all three elements of the classic Vogt triad: adenoma sebaceum, epilepsy, and mental handicap. However, the work of Gomez and others has revealed that TS has a variable expression of mental retardation. TS can now be diagnosed by the presence of even a single lesion from a list of several unique findings that are common in TS and that are only rarely (if ever) seen in the normal population. The classic Vogt triad has now been replaced by this modern and more inclusive set of diagnostic criteria (57) (Table 2).

Imaging features, without any physical findings or symptoms, can also be used to make the diagnosis of TS. These unique diagnostic findings include the presence (on CT, MR or US) of multiple subependymal nodules (especially when calcified) and multiple cortical "tubers" (especially if associated with subcortical white matter "edema") (Fig. 21). Somewhat less specific, but nonetheless highly suggestive of TS, are imaging features that include an intraventricular tumor consistent with subependymal giant cell astrocytoma (SGCA), focal cortical calcifications (especially wedge-shaped) in either the cerebrum or cerebellum, and multiple cortical or subcortical foci of "edema" (hypodense on CT, hyperintense on T2-weighted MR).

The retinal lesion of TS (van der Hoeve's "phakoma") occurs in roughly half the patients. It is a histologically benign proliferation of astrocytes on the surface of the retina. This lesion may present in children and can produce leukokoria—a yellow-white reflection of light from the back of the eye. Childhood leukokoria has many other causes, and the differential diagnosis includes malignant neoplasm (retinoblastoma), infection (toxocariasis), and other congenital lesions (Coates' disease, persistent hyperplastic primary vitreous). On ocular examination (fundoscopic, ultrasound, CT, and MR) the hamartomatous lesion of TS can often be differentiated by the experienced observer. These retinal "phakomata" may be either flat or slightly raised, semitransparent, and can be calcified (58–60). They may be similar to retinoblastoma in location (retina), age at presentation (childhood), frequent multiplicity and bilaterality, and the common presence of calcification. However, unlike retinoblastoma, they are not necrotic, do not hemorrhage, do not fungate and grow into either the vitreous nor invade through the retina into the surrounding choroid or sclera. They may diminish visual acuity, but usually without causing complete blindness.

TABLE 2. *Common findings in tuberous sclerosis*[a]

Brain
Cortical tubers
Subependymal nodules ("candle gutterings")
Ventriculomegaly ("idiopathic or obstructive")
Radial-glia abnormalities
Subependymal giant cell astrocytoma
Seizures
Infantile spasms (hypsarrhythmia)
Mental handicap
Eye
Retinal hamartoma (phakoma of van der Hoeve)
Skin
Angiofibroma (of face) ("angiofibroma")
Ungual fibroma (angiofibroma of nailbed)
Hypomelanotic macules (ash leaf macule)
Shagreen patch (subepidermal fibrosis)
Fibrous forehead plaque
Heart
Cardiac rhabdomyoma
Kidney
Multiple angiomyolipoma
Multiple cysts
Lung
Lymphangiomyomatosis
"Honeycomb lung"
Pneumothorax
Bone
Bone islands (sclerotic calvarial patches)
"Cystic" bone lucencies (small tubular bones—hands, etc.)

Modified from Gomez, ref. 57, with permission.

[a] Primary diagnostic criteria (only one necessary) are in italics. Many of those features not in italics are "secondary diagnostic criteria"—two or more of which, and/or a family history, can also be used to make a clinical diagnosis of the tuberous sclerosis complex.

There are several different, yet interrelated, processes that occur within the brain in TS: cortical hamartomas (CH) (these are the "tubers"); white-matter lesions; subependymal nodules (SEN); ventriculomegaly; and the intraventricular tumor—the subependymal giant cell astrocytomas (SGCA) (Figs. 21 and 22) (61–63). With the exception of the SGCA, which is a true neoplasm (low grade, WHO grade I) the other lesions have been variously described as benign hamartomas and/or migration anomalies. Bender and Yunis reported that the cellular components of the subependymal nodules are identical to those of the cortical tubers (63). The primary differences are the size and the location. The cortical tubers are large, potato or tuber-like, misshapen gyri, that are firm to the touch and prone to calcification. The affected cerebral gyri are composed of disorganized tissue without the normal laminar arrangement of the neurons into six layers. In the traditional definition of a "hamartoma," the cells are cytologically normal but the tissue organization is haphazard or otherwise abnormal. However, the cortical hamartomas of TS contain unusually large cells that may be either neurons or bizarre giant astrocytes. A similar cerebellar cortical disorganization is seen in the posterior fossa in about 20% of patients. The SEN are histologically similar to the CH, but are smaller and arise primarily in the striothalamate groove (between the caudate and thalamus) along the lateral margin of the lateral ventricles (61). The SEN do not appear to grow; however, they do calcify progressively during the first two decades, so that by age 20 virtually 100% are hyperdense. The calcifications in SEN and CH may be dense enough for a plain film diagnosis (64–66). This presence of calcification allows SEN to be distinguished from the otherwise similar-appearing subependymal gray-matter heterotopias. Heterotopic gray matter is isodense and isointense to normal gray matter, without contrast enhancement. The theory that the SEN and cor-

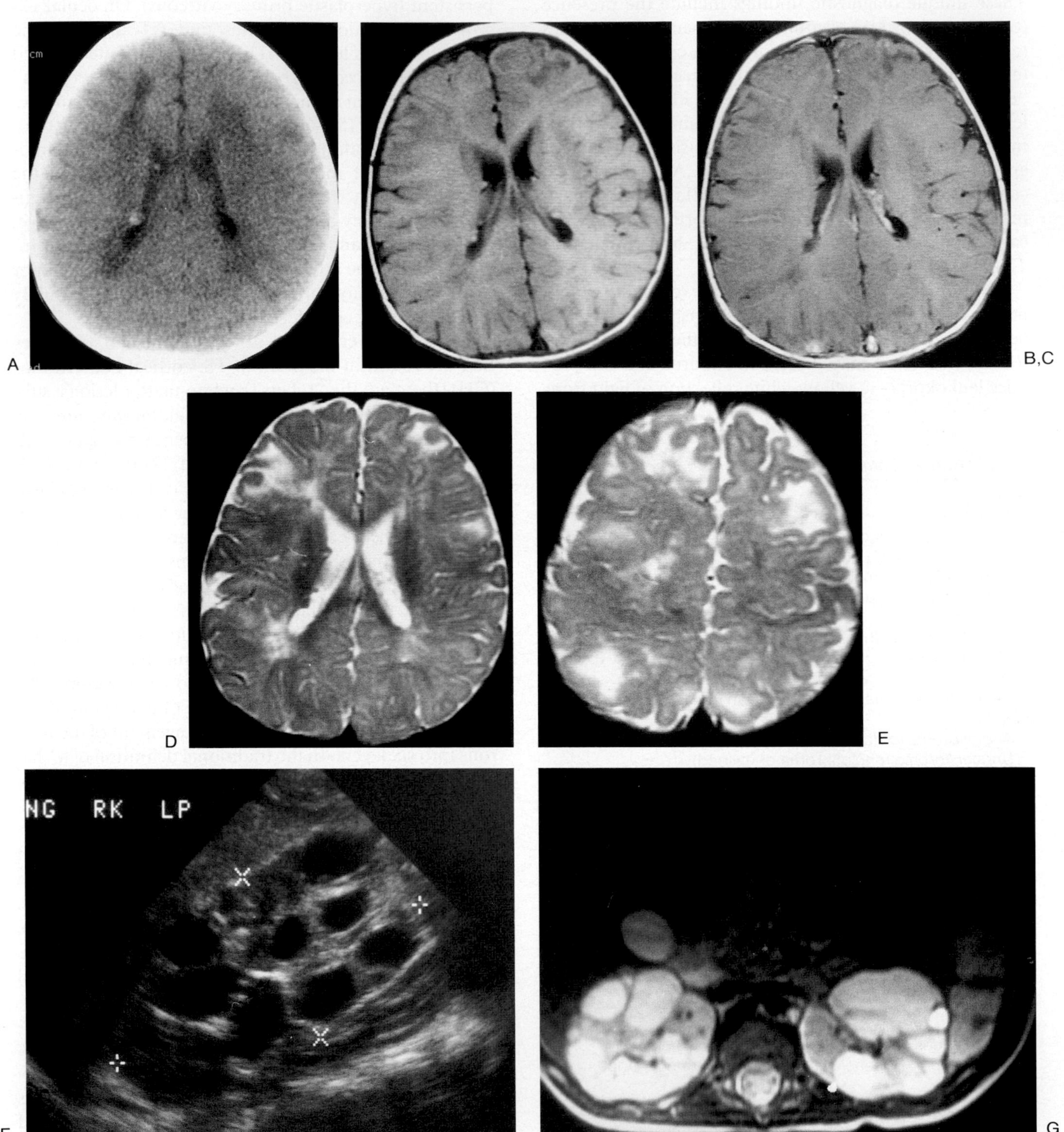
A
B,C
D
E
NG RK LP
F
G

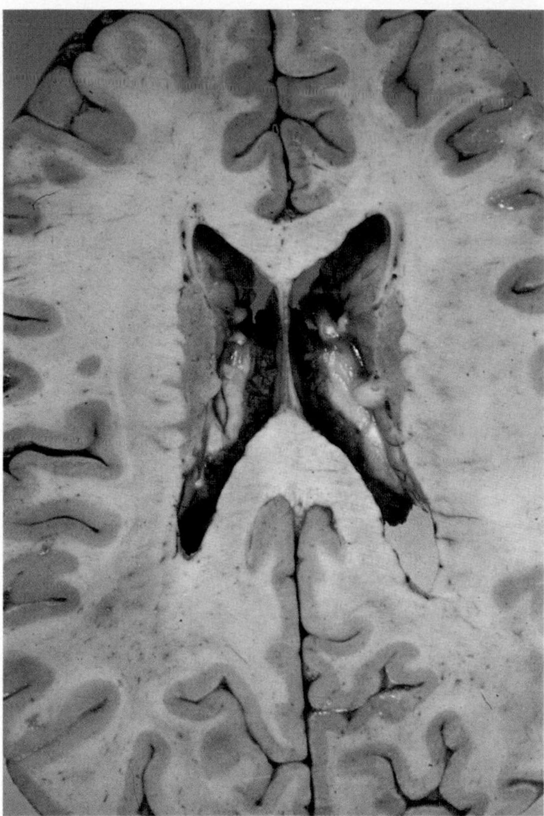

FIG. 22. Gross specimen TS. This axial gross brain section demonstrates multiple nodular masses protruding into both lateral ventricles along the groove between the caudate and the thalamus (striothalamate groove). There is an enlarged gyrus in the right frontal lobe that is a cortical tuber.

tical lesions arise from abnormal neuronal migration is bolstered not only by the absence of a layered cortex, but also by the occasional appearance of bands of curvilinear white matter signal abnormalities that appear to connect from the periventricular subependymal nodules to the superficial cortical tubers (67). This appearance suggests a track along the course of the radial glia, a persistent remnant from the abnormal migration of neuroblasts from the germinal matrix zone to the developing cerebral cortex.

Multiple cortical tubers are diagnostic of TS. However, similar-appearing solitary sporadic cortical hamartomas can occur without any other features of TS, and these can be histologically similar to the lesions of TS. The CH only rarely show contrast enhancement on MR with gadolinium. They are usually visualized as large misshapen gyri. Various patterns of signal abnormalities have been reported for the cortical tubers, including the "gyral core" appearance on T1-weighted MR and the "sulcal island" on T2-weighted scans described by Nixon et al. (67–69). The abnormal hamartomatous tissue of the cortical tubers usually has prolonged T1 and T2, so they are bright on T2-weighted images. The characteristic "gyral core" is an isointense expanded gyrus of gray matter surrounding a central hypointense white matter center, and, the "sulcal island" is both a geometric and signal intensity inversion of the "gyral core"—the subcortical white matter is abnormally bright, and surrounds a sulcus with its gray matter borders of normal intensity (68).

The subependymal nodules, although quite obvious on CT (contrast against CSF and/or because of calcifications) can be subtle on MR. The signal intensity patterns are variable, and can change over time. Some SEN may have a "target" appearance on T2-weighted MR, with a central hyperintensity—reminiscent of the "gyral core" seen in the cortical tubers. Occasionally the center of an SEN can be bright on the T1-weighted image. This appearance could be related to the paradoxical T1 shortening that occurs with dispersed microscopic calcifications (see Fig. 21). The SEN have been reported to have variable patterns of enhancement. On CT, the SEN enhancement has been viewed as diagnostic of the conversion of the hamartoma into a neoplasm, the subependymal giant cell astrocytoma. On MR, however, multiple SEN show gadolinium enhancement, often clustered about the foramen of Monro (70). Since multiple SGCAs are distinctly uncommon, it is unlikely that all the en-

FIG. 21. Tuberous sclerosis (TS). **A:** An enhanced CT scan demonstrates two subependymal nodules along the lateral border of the right lateral ventricle. They are partially calcified. There are multiple and bilateral regions of abnormally lucent white matter. Some are deep, affecting the periventricular white matter and some peripheral, within cortical tubers. **B:** Plain T1-weighted MR at approximately the same plane as the CT in A. Note that there is slight hyperintensity to the subependymal nodules, probably because of the presence of microcalcification. There are multiple cortical tubers, with a large and prominent lesion in the left frontal lobe. However, close inspection demonstrates multifocal areas of abnormal hypointensity involving both subcortical and deeper white matter. **C:** After gadolinium infusion, there is a small focus of abnormal cortical enhancement in the right occipital region. The subependymal nodules in this case are not enhancing, but continue to be slightly hyperintense. (This could easily be mistaken for enhancement, without benefit of a precontrast scan for comparison). **D:** T2-weighted MR. The subependymal nodules along the right lateral ventricle are now seen as relative hypointensities. However, there is a small central hyperintensity within one of these nodules, creating a "target" lesion. There is abnormal central signal hypointensity in multiple cortical tubers. In addition, there are periventricular areas of abnormal white matter hyperintensity. **E:** Axial section through the upper centrum semiovale. There are multiple enlarged gyri with abnormal central signal hyperintensity—the "gyral core" sign. **F:** Abdominal ultrasound in this patient demonstrates multiple renal cysts. **G:** The axial T2-weighted MR also demonstrates the bilateral multiple renal cysts. TS is one of a number of inherited diseases that produce multicystic kidneys in childhood.

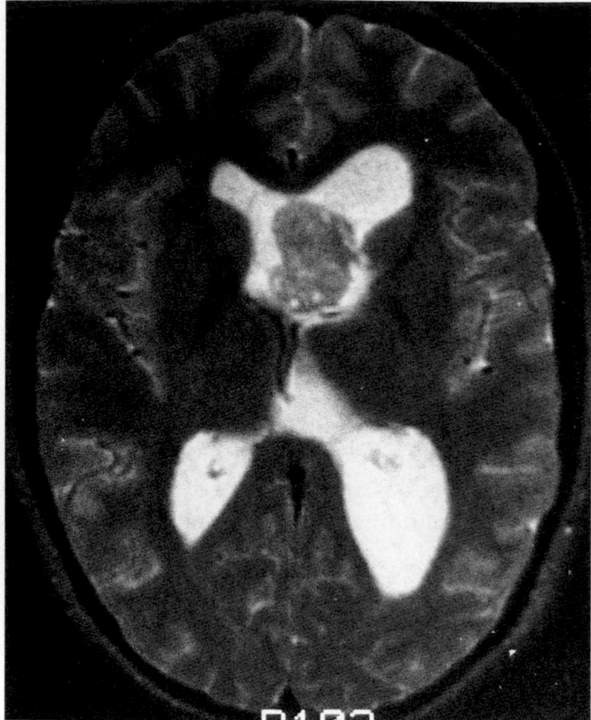
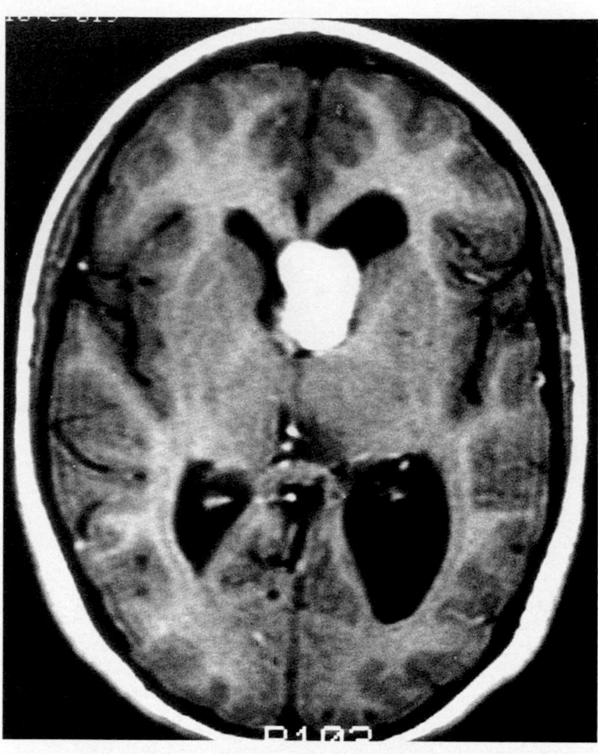

FIG. 23. TS. Subependymal giant cell astrocytoma. **A:** This T2-weighted axial image shows a lobulated intraventricular mass in the left lateral ventricle near the foramen of Monro. The lesion is slightly heterogeneous, but is basically isointense to gray matter and hypointense compared to CSF. **B:** This gadolinium-enhanced T1-weighted axial MR shows intense enhancement in the mass. It is attached to the left caudate head. The remainder of the brain, at this level, is grossly normal. However, the patient has TS, and the neoplasm is a subependymal giant cell astrocytoma.

hancing subependymal nodules are undergoing neoplastic transformation into SGCA, because these are usually solitary tumors. The SGCA is a benign and slowly growing tumor. The major morbidity is related to ventricular obstruction, which is common, considering this tumor has a predilection to arise attached to the caudate head, near the foramen of Monro. Although the SGCA is usually attached to the caudate, this tumor does not invade into the neural parenchyma, preferring to grow as a polypoid mass, free within the ventricular lumen (Fig. 23). The SGCA does not seed the CSF, and it is unlikely to recur after adequate resection. The spinal cord and peripheral nerves are not affected in TS.

The visceral changes of TS are summarized in Table 2. The findings with the greatest clinical significance are the rare, but often fatal, pulmonary changes of lymphangiomyomatosis. This benign smooth muscle proliferation along pulmonary arteries can produce pulmonary hypertension and even cor pulmonale. The secondary reorganization of the lung parenchyma is associated with a "honeycomb" appearance of interstitial thickening, surrounding abnormally large "cystic" air spaces. Although appearing fibrotic, the lung volume is expanded, rather than contracted, and these patients may suffer multiple episodes of spontaneous pneumothorax.

The kidney may harbor multiple simple cysts and/or angiomyolipomas (AMLs). TS is one of many inherited causes of polycystic kidney disease. If there is an unusually large number of cysts, the kidneys enlarge and renal function may be compromised. The AMLs are composed of blood vessels, smooth muscle, and mature adult fat. The composition varies among the three components but, when the fat predominates, a confident imaging diagnosis is possible. The bizarre vascularity of the AML is prone to spontaneous hemorrhage that can be clinically occult (without hematuria). The blood may accumulate in the subcapsular space of the kidney or in the retroperitoneum (see Table 2).

ENCEPHALOTRIGEMINAL ANGIOMATOSIS

Encephalotrigeminal angiomatosis is a descriptive term for a vascular malformation that affects the CNS (brain and eye) as well as the soft tissues of the face and head, in an approximation of the territory innervated by the trigeminal (Vth) cranial nerve. It is a congenital lesion of uncertain origin that has been reported with a variety of inheritance patterns (dominant, recessive, mixed). However, it may in fact be an isolated and sporadic vascular malformation. The Sturge-Weber Foundation is actively collecting blood specimens in an effort to identify possible genetic linkage features. Two of the common eponyms for encephalotrigeminal angiomatosis are "Sturge-

Weber syndrome" (SWS) and "Sturge-Weber-Dimitri disease." The nature of this phakomatosis appears to be rooted in an abnormal vascular development of the cephalic mesenchyme: the cerebral (telencephalic) circulation is impaired, a vascular plexus of immature vessels occupies the affected portions of the subarachnoid space, and a cutaneous plexus of dilated vessels creates a facial discoloration. The original clinical triad for the diagnosis of SWS included seizures, mental handicap, and a "port-wine" nevus of the face. The most constant features are the association of seizures with the intracranial findings of unilateral cerebral atrophy and cortical calcification. In some series most patients have normal mentation, and the facial lesion can be absent in cases that have otherwise typical intracranial features.

The classical clinical diagnosis was based on observing

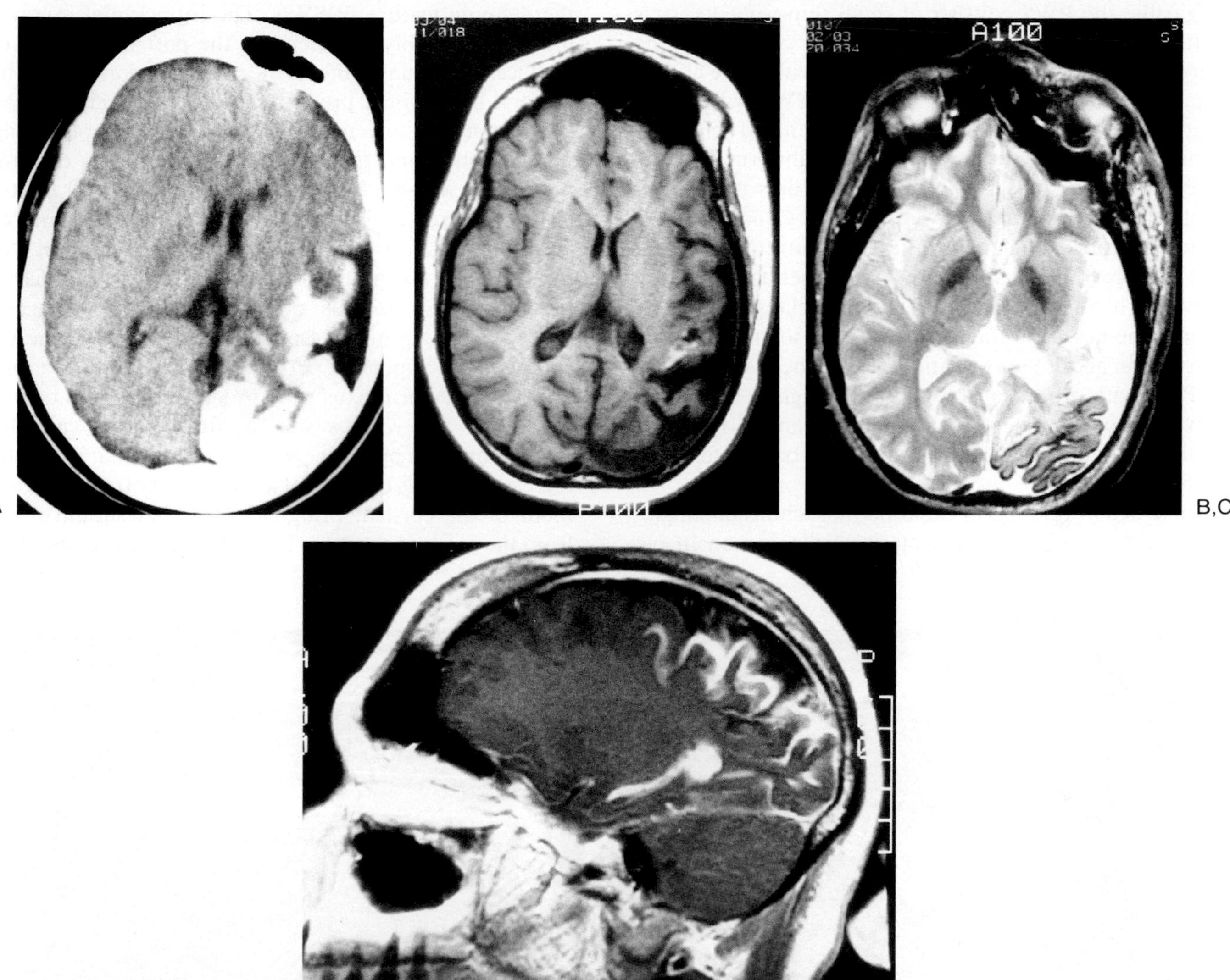

FIG. 24. Twenty-four-year-old woman with Sturge-Weber disease. **A:** Plain CT scan demonstrates left hemispheric atrophy. There is an asymmetric increase in the pneumatization of the left frontal sinus. Notice the unusually dense calcification affecting the atrophic portions of the occipital and temporal lobes. **B:** T1-weighted MR at approximately the same level as the CT also demonstrates asymmetric pneumatization of the left frontal sinus overlying an atrophic frontal lobe. The extensive atrophy of the left hemisphere is seen to better advantage. There is a small focus of hyperintensity in the posterior of the left temporal lobe, which may be related to T1 shortening from dispersed calcification within the cortex. **C:** The T2-weighted image demonstrates a curvilinear gyriform hypointensity outlining the surface of the atrophic left occipital lobe. It is surprising to see how remarkably narrow and linear the hypointensity bands are in comparison to the apparently massive tissue calcification noted on the previous CT in A. Notice that there is a "spongy" enlargement and hyperintensity of the left temporalis muscle. This may represent hemangiomatous telangiectasias within the muscle. **D:** Sagittal gadolinium-enhanced T1-weighted MR demonstrates superficial gyriform enhancement overlying the surface of the atrophic portions of the left hemisphere. Notice the round and mass-like enlargement of the left choroid plexus (in the trigone region). Anteriorly, there is widening of the diploic space in the frontal bone (anterior to the coronal suture). Although this has been described as another compensatory change (part of the Dyke-Davidoff-Masson syndrome) it may be a hemangiomatous telangiectasia, similar to the lesions in the muscle and skin of the face.

seizures and/or mental retardation in association with a "port-wine" stain of the face. The "port-wine" stain (PWS) or nevus flammeus can be pink to reddish brown, and roughly conforms to the topography of the trigeminal nerve dermatome. The PWS will be present at birth. The nevus flammeus follows the dermatome of the trigeminal nerve as a fortuitous geographic result of embryology, and not from a causal relationship between the Vth cranial nerve and vascular development. Pathologically, the PWS consists of small thin-walled vessels within the skin. The reddish-brown color comes from the largely deoxygenated blood contained within the abnormal vessels. The cutaneous "stain" in SWS will blanch with pressure, as the largely deoxygenated blood is squeezed from the small vessels. These abnormal vessels are immature, and have histologic features resembling both dilated capillaries as well as small veins. They are often described as telangiectasias. In addition to the skin, the linings of the nasal cavity and sinuses as well as the choroid of the eye may have similar telangiectasias. A port wine nevus on the face can be an isolated sporadic process in about 90% of patients (71). The association of a PWS with other features of SWS is highest if all three divisions of the trigeminal are affected, and virtually nil if the medial portion of the ophthalmic branch territory is not involved.

The ocular findings of buphthalmos, choroidal angiomas, and episcleral telangiectasias are common in patients with SWS. Buphthalmos (literally "Ox-eye") occurs in up to 15% of patients, and is caused by congenital glaucoma that causes the ocular globe to enlarge because of increased intraocular pressure. This increased pressure may be related to impaired reabsorption of ocular fluid due to abnormal vasculature of the choroid. In almost one third of cases either the sclera and/or the ocular choroid may show a dilated plexus of small vessels (72).

The brain is affected in 100% of cases because that is the defining feature of SWS. The intracranial involvement is invariably ipsilateral to the port-wine nevus of the face, and usually affects the posterior portions of the cerebral hemisphere predominantly. The occipital lobe is preferentially affected, followed by the temporal and parietal lobes, and frontal lobe involvement is uncommon (Figs. 24 and 25). The posterior fossa (infratentorial) structures are not affected in SWS, presumably because their embryologic development is different. Although there are many theories and possible explanations for SWS, the most appealing hypothesis suggests that the telangiectatic vasculature of the syndrome results from an abnormal persistence of the primitive/primordial vascular plexus. The process appears to be primarily on the venous side of the cerebral capillary circulation. The primitive vascular plexus that normally regresses, persists because of a failure of normal development of the cortical bridging veins that should drain from the cerebral capillary bed into the dural sinuses (es-

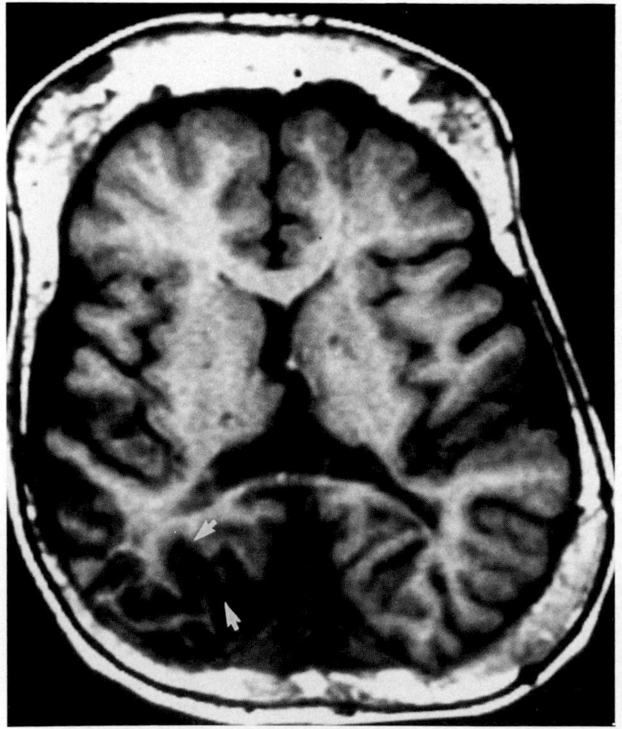

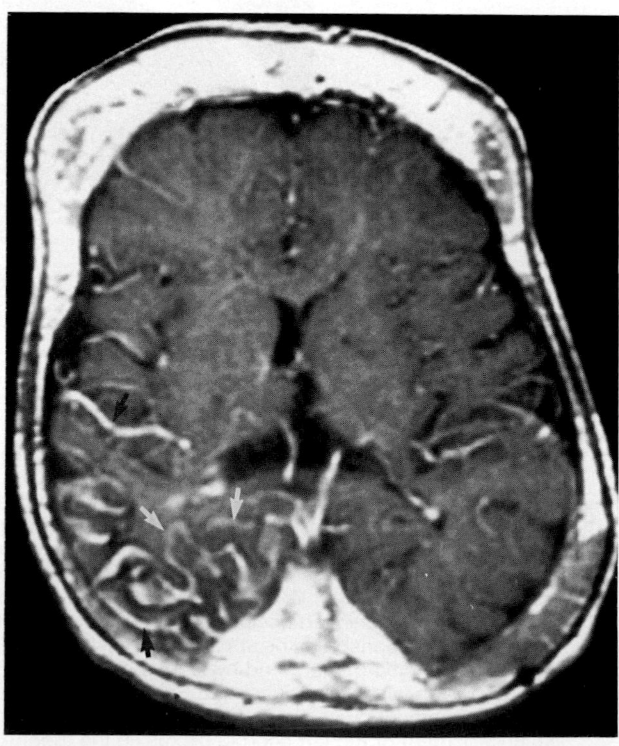

FIG. 25. Sturge-Weber syndrome with cortical atrophy (**A,B**), thickened calvarium, and areas of hypointense serpentine calcifications involving right occipital lobe (*white arrows*) and prominent cortical veins (*black arrows*, B) involving right temporo-occipital regions, seen on postgadolinium image (B).

pecially into the posterior half of the superior sagittal sinus). The cerebral capillary outflow is thus impaired and the cortical capillary bed drains into a plexus of small vessels in the subarachnoid space (SAS) instead of directly into the dural sinuses. In addition, there may be prominent medullary veins that drain the cortex in a centripetal (retrograde) fashion to the periventricular vein (Fig. 26). The abnormal cortical venous drainage—through the collaterals described—is well tolerated by the fetus until birth, allowing the brain itself to develop

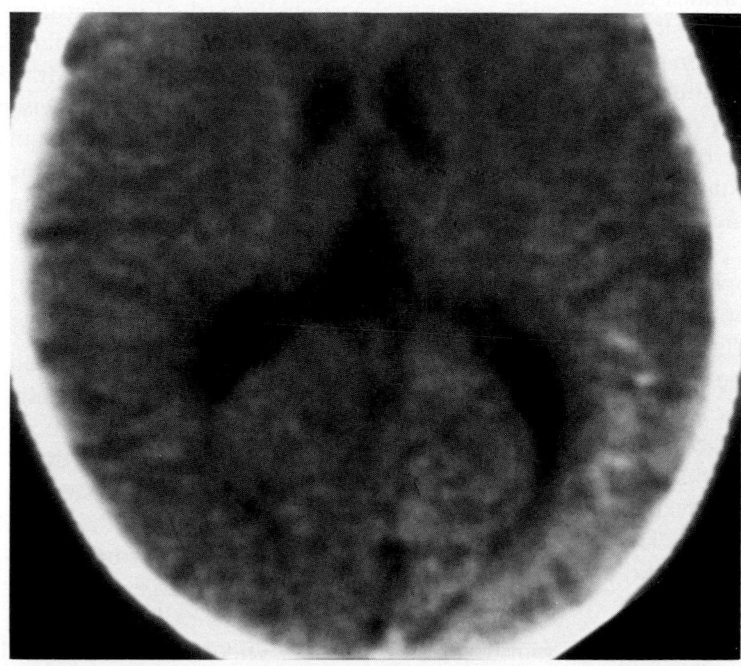

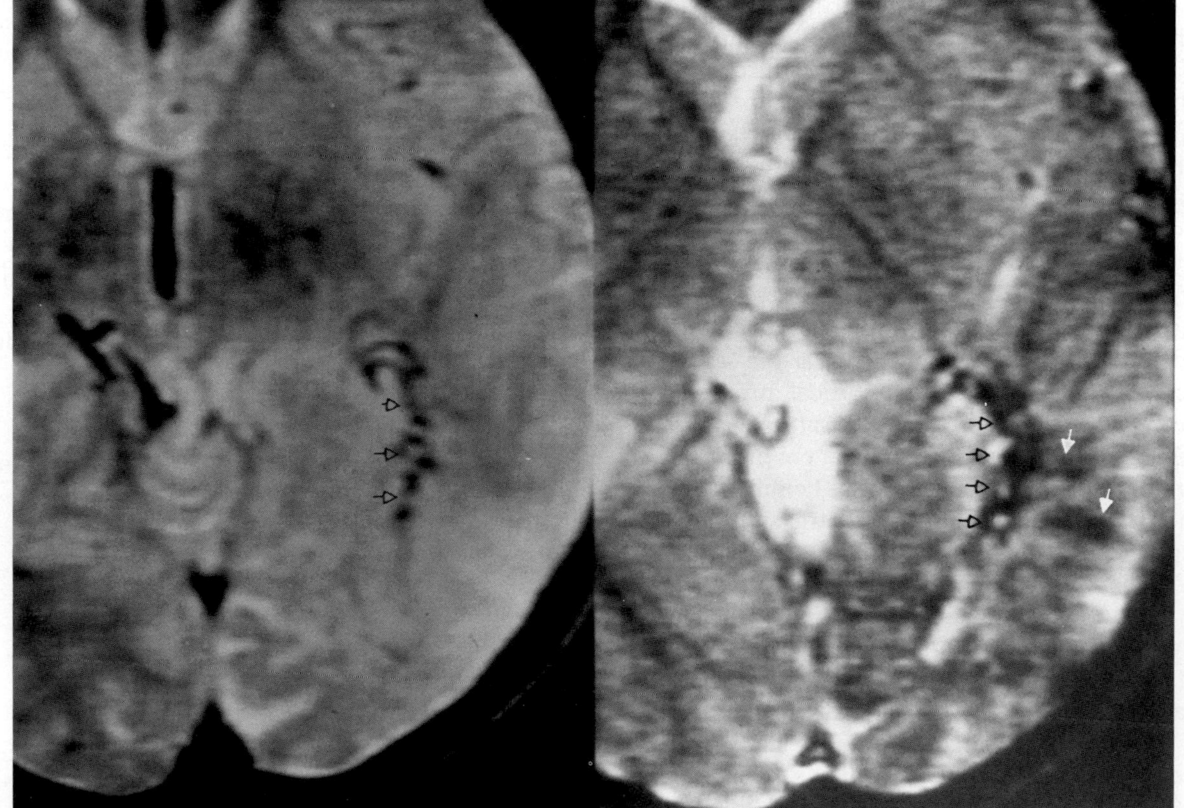

FIG. 26. Infant with Sturge-Weber syndrome. Note minimal calcification in left parieto-occipital lobe (**A**) on CT. Long TR/TE MRI (**B**) shows hyperintense, abnormal white matter and cortex, and absent sulci. Gradient-echo image shows hypointensity due to calcification (*closed arrows,* **C**). Also note vascular malformation (*open arrows,* B, C).

normally. At birth, however, when the oxygen demands and therefore the cerebral blood flow dramatically increase, the abnormalities in the venous drainage of the circulation become significant and lead to progressive pathologic changes. The central veins are overloaded and there may be secondary venous hypertension. The impaired cortical circulation and reduced oxygen tension lead to electrical instability of the cortex and ultimately to seizures. The seizure activity aggravates the process because of further increases in oxygen and blood flow demands. The chronically impaired circulation produces cerebral ischemia that in turn leads to a failure of the blood–brain barrier in the affected posterior regions of the hemisphere. Eventually, the imbalance between metabolic needs and blood supply causes cellular death and the subsequent deposition of dystrophic calcification into the atrophic cortex.

The layering of calcification within the atrophic brain produces the characteristic "tram-track" or railroad track appearance seen on plain films. The earliest calcifications may be within the middle layers of the cerebral cortex, or even in the subcortical white matter (73,74). As the child ages, further growth of the brain, complicated by seizure activity, leads to episodic exacerbations of the ischemia with atrophy and calcification affecting progressively larger areas of the cortex (see Fig. 24). The child may gain—and then lose—developmental milestones. The density and extent of calcification increases over time, and advances from posterior to anterior. However, controlling or eliminating the aggravating effects of the seizures may prevent further progression of both the atrophy and the calcification. For this reason, partial hemispherectomy for seizure control may be more beneficial than harmful, especially in patients under the age of 5 years. Removing the brain regions with the abnormal circulation may allow seizure control and reduce venous hypertension. The remaining brain is thus granted a better chance to develop normally.

MR is the most sensitive test for revealing the full extent of the lesions in SWS, as well as for direct visualization of the persistent embryologic plexus in the SAS (75). However, both CT and MR can reveal the secondary changes, which include cerebral cortical atrophy, gyriform cerebral calcification, compensatory ventricular enlargement, "angiomatous" enlargement of the ipsilateral choroid plexus, and calvarial hemihypertrophy (widened diploic spaces and asymmetric sinus enlargement ipsilateral to the cortical atrophy). Superficial "gyriform" enhancement is common in SWS (see Fig. 24D). There are two possible causes for this enhancement: slowly flowing blood within the persistent plexus of the SAS, and/or loss of the blood–brain barrier within the cerebral cortex itself, from the chronic ischemia. Overall, MR is much more sensitive than CT in identifying the affected areas. CT, MR, and even plain skull films often reveal a hemangiomatous thickening of the diploic space and facial soft tissues (e.g., the temporalis muscle) in patients with SWS.

VON HIPPEL-LINDAU DISEASE

Von Hippel-Lindau disease (VHL) was originally described as the association of multiple vascular "angiomas" of the retina (von Hippel disease) and hemangioblastomas of the cerebellum (the Lindau tumor). It was soon recognized that this association was familial, and that affected individuals also presented with multiple cysts and neoplasms of the solid abdominal viscera (kidney, liver, pancreas, adrenal gland) as well as in the epididymis in men and affecting the ovarian adnexa in women. There are no cutaneous findings in von Hippel-Lindau disease. VHL is an autosomal dominant disorder without any racial or sexual predilection. The chromosome responsible is on the short arm of chromosome 3p. The prevalence is approximately 1 in 40,000 to 1 in 50,000 people. Although the disease causes multiple lesions in multiple different organ systems, Neuman et al. reported that the dominant feature, and the most common cause of death, is the CNS lesion—the cerebellar hemangioblastoma (76). Hemangioblastoma was the cause of death in 82% of patients in that series. Pheochromocytoma is 10 times more common in VHL patients than in the population at large; however, this particular manifestation appears to breed true in certain families, yet is distinctly uncommon in others. The current diagnostic criteria are summarized in Table 3.

The ocular lesions of VHL, often called angiomas, is actually a hemangioblastoma—identical to those occurring in the cerebellum and elsewhere. Retinal hemangioblastomas may be asymptomatic or cause a blind spot. However, they may hemorrhage and can cause retinal detachment with secondary changes, including blindness. They are often diagnosed by ophthalmoscopy and/or fluorescein angiography rather than by CT or MR. Chronic ocular changes from complications of the hemangioblastomas (or their treatment) may lead to phthisis bulbi—indistinguishable from that produced by other causes, for example, trauma.

TABLE 3. *Diagnostic criteria for von Hippel-Lindau disease*[a]

1. CNS and retinal hemangioblastomas ("angiomas")
2. Hemangioblastoma and at least one:
   a. Renal, pancreatic, hepatic, epididymal cyst
   b. Pheochromocytoma
   c. Renal cancer
3. A family history (of VHL) and at least one:
   a. Hemangioblastoma
   b. Visceral cyst (see 2a above)
   c. Pheochromocytoma
   d. Renal cancer

[a] Only one criterion needed for diagnosis of von Hippel-Lindau disease.

The hallmark lesion of VHL is the hemangioblastoma (HBL) (Fig. 27) These are most common in the cerebellum, but occasionally present in the medulla oblongata, pons, spinal cord, and supratentorially in the optic nerves and cerebral hemispheres. Overall, with and without VHL, hemangioblastomas account for up to 3% of intracranial neoplasms, and 5% to 8% of posterior fossa masses in adults—about as common as cerebellar metastasis. Only approximately 20% or less of patients with a solitary cerebellar HBL will fulfill other diagnostic criteria for VHL. However, any patient with multiple HBLs should have a thorough evaluation (including abdominal imaging) because of the high likelihood of having von Hippel-Lindau disease.

Grossly, the HBL varies from completely solid to almost entirely cystic (Figs. 28, 29, and 30). The "classic" appearance is that of a fluid-filled cystic lesion, with a reddish hypervascular "mural nodule" embedded in the wall. The "cyst" is not lined by an epithelium; instead, the wall is usually formed by compressed (but otherwise normal) cerebellar tissue. In some cases there is a reactive gliosis in the rim, and in other cases the fluid accumulates as a cyst completely surrounded by the neoplastic tissue. A truly "cyst with nodule" appearance occurs in about one third of HBLs either with or without VHL. The remainder are divided almost equally between completely solid masses, and those with a complex morphology—a heterogeneous combination of solid and cystic components. The neoplastic tissue is extremely vascular, composed of multiple capillary and/or sinusoidal vessels. Three cells proliferate in this neoplasm: endothelial cells, pericytes, and the so-called stromal cells. These stromal cells have a lipid-filled cytoplasm, and are interposed between the myriad vascular channels (Fig. 31). The presence of these stromal cells distinguishes the HBL from both cavernous hemangiomas (all vessels) and arteriovenous malformations (gliotic brain between vessels). The hypervascular neoplastic nodule is usually identified in a superficial subpial location, allowing for confusion with meningioma.

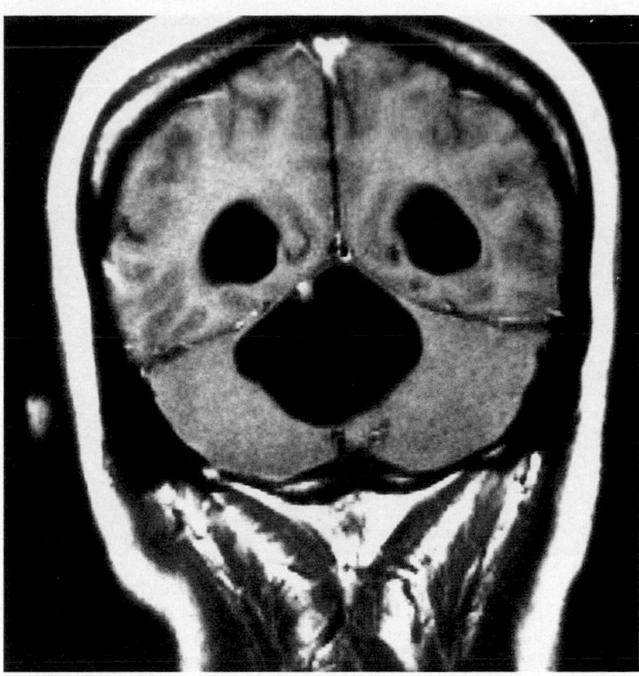

FIG. 28. HBL. This coronal T1-weighted gadolinium-enhanced image demonstrates an unusually large cyst with a very small enhancing mural nodule. Again, the characteristic feature that suggests the HBL is the absence of significant wall enhancement—the "cyst with nodule" appearance. In an adult, this is usually due to an HBL. The childhood juvenile pilocytic astrocytoma can have an identical appearance. However, this large cyst-to-nodule ratio is rare for pilocytic astrocytomas, and much more likely to be seen in an HBL.

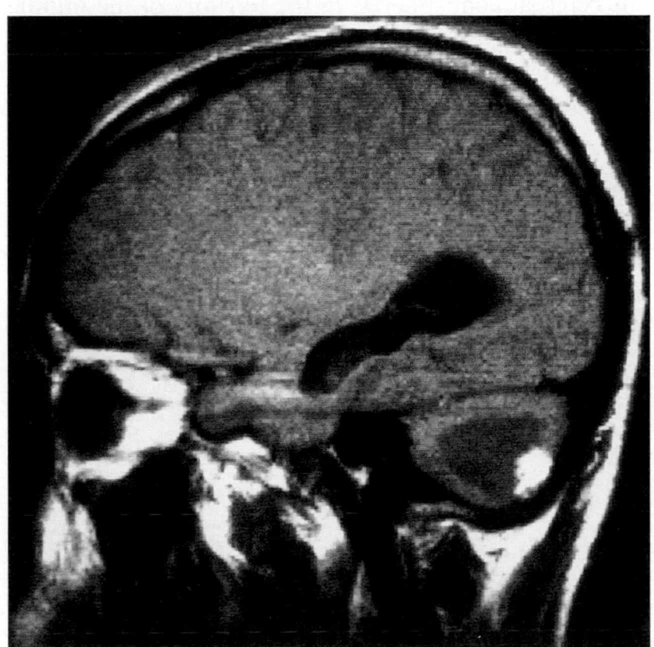

FIG. 27. Hemangioblastoma (HBL). This sagittal T1-weighted gadolinium-enhanced scan demonstrates a typical "cyst with nodule" morphology for a cerebellar HBL. Most of the cyst lining is non-neoplastic tissue that does not enhance. The mural nodule of the HBL is typically found in a subpial location, as in this case. The cyst fluid commonly has a signal intensity higher than that of CSF because of a protein content, and occasionally from bleeding into the fluid.

Angiographically, the solid portions of an HBL are hypervascular, and may mimic the appearance of a meningioma. The flow pattern includes a dense capillary tumor blush that may appear early after the injection. The contrast appears to "hang up" within the tumor, and there may be delayed and/or persistent venous opacification in draining vessels. These angiographic characteristics, combined with the typical superficial location, may mimic the appearance of a meningioma. On CT, the solid portions of the HBL can be isodense to hyperdense compared to the brain—they are usually not hypodense. The cyst fluid, when present, typically has an attenuation

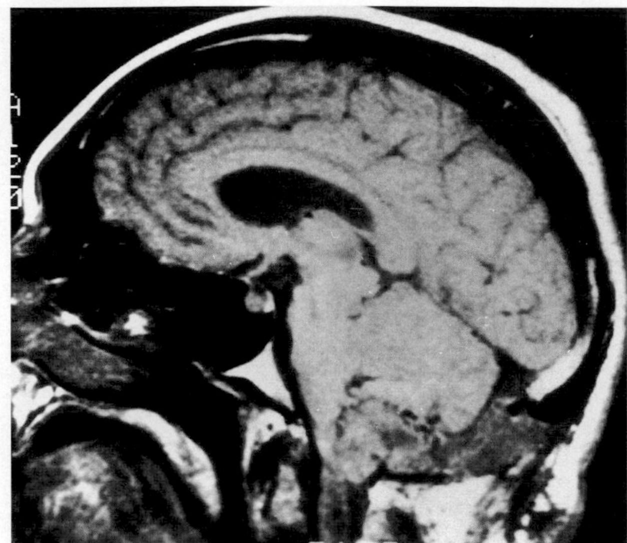

A

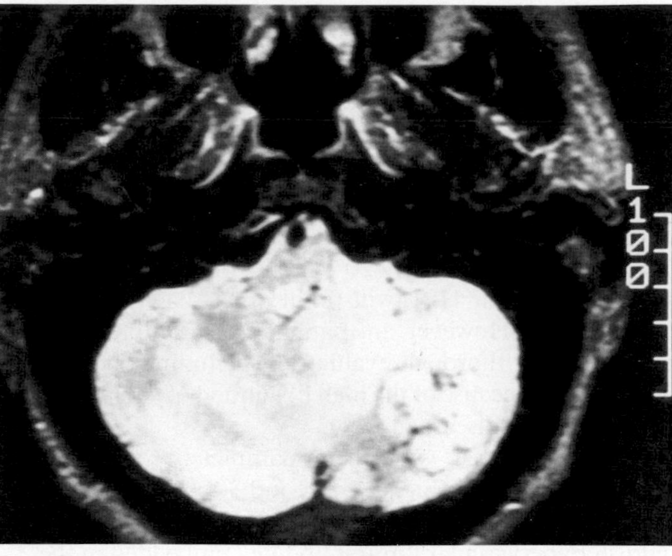

B

FIG. 29. HBL. **A:** This sagittal T1-weighted MR demonstrates a heterogeneous solid cerebellar mass. Note the peripheral curvilinear signal voids. These are most likely flow related and represent either large tumor sinusoids or vessels feeding or draining the neoplasm. An alternate possibility is that the peripheral hypointensities are related to hemosiderin deposition. **B:** An axial T2-weighted MR demonstrates a heterogeneous and lobulated mass. Again notice that there are multiple peripheral curvilinear hypointensities, consistent with flow voids. A solid HBL can mimic a cavernous hemangioma. However, when there is a significant cystic component (with large, >1 cm fluid collections) and associated vascular flow voids, HBL should be suspected.

greater than CSF. This is most often related to a high protein concentration—although some HBLs are complicated by small amounts of hemorrhage. The solid portions of the tumor show intense enhancement after contrast infusion. The portions of the cyst margin that are compressed or gliotic cerebellum do not enhance. Multiple-enhancing cerebellar masses, without accompanying supratentorial lesions, are suggestive of VHL with multiple HBLs. Most hematogenous metastases are distributed in rough approximation to blood flow, with most lesions presenting near the gray-white junction of the cerebral hemispheres, in the territory of the middle cerebral artery.

On MR, HBLs may be solid, cystic, or complex. The

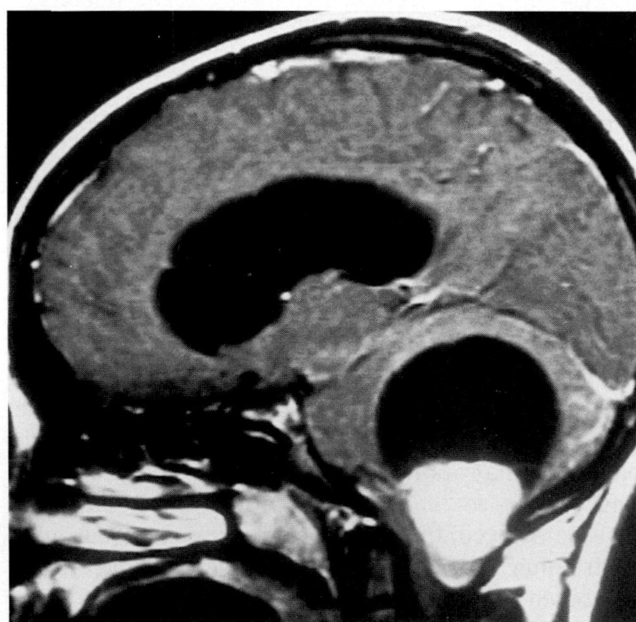

FIG. 30. Densely enhancing solid nodule with associated nonenhancing cyst of HBL herniates down through foramen magnum in patient with von Hippel-Lindau syndrome on sagittal short TR/TE postcontrast scan.

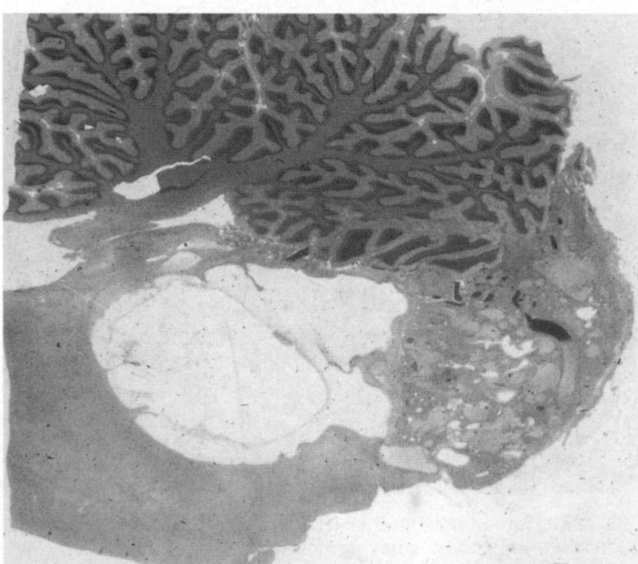

FIG. 31. Gross—HBL. This subgross H&E–stained HBL demonstrates the superficial (subpial) location of the mural nodule. Most of the fluid-filled "cyst" is lined by normal cerebellar tissue, and not by neoplasm. The "mural nodule" is extremely vascular, and several large sinusoids are visible.

hypervascular tumor nodule usually, but not always, presents with tubular flow voids that may be internal, but are more typically seen around the margin of the mass. In some cases the T1-weighted image may show focal hyperintensities within the tumor. These hyperintensities have been ascribed to the paramagnetic effect of methemoglobin from subacute hemorrhage. However, it is also possible that the high signal represents the lipid-laden stromal cells. On T2-weighted MR the cyst fluid is usually as bright as CSF. The solid tumor nodule, however, may be heterogeneous, with hypointensities that can be central and focal or peripheral and curvilinear. These hypointense areas may be caused by flow voids in large sinusoids, or feeding and draining vessels. However, as a chronic result of hemorrhage, hemosiderin can be deposited in a rim around the lesion. Therefore, solid HBLs may have a heterogeneous black-and-white speckled or salt-and-pepper appearance that mimics a cavernous hemangioma or hemorrhagic metastasis.

HBLs have also been reported to occur outside the CNS. HBLs in the liver and lung were first reported by McGrath et al. (77). HBLs, with and without VHL, are often associated with erythrocytosis. Production of erythropoietin by the tumor has been documented by Horton et al. (78).

Annual screening examinations of the abdomen, by ultrasound or CT, has been recommended for some patients with VHL. Almost 75% of adult patients will develop pancreatic cysts and more than half will have renal cysts or renal cell carcinoma (RCC). The RCCs that arise in the setting of VHL are usually multiple, often bilateral, and frequently are partially cystic carcinomas. Because of the low rate of recurrence, frequent bilaterality, and the rarity of hematogenous metastasis, the RCCs of VHL are often treated with conservative renal-sparing surgery. In one series of 28 patients, followed with serial abdominal studies, most of the renal cystic lesions (80%) were stable and either did not change (71%) or regressed (9%); however, 20% did increase in size (79). In that same series, 12 patients had purely solid, or mixed cystic and solid lesions, and the solid component always contained RCC.

The vast majority of patients with VHL will develop pancreatic masses. Most of these patients will harbor pancreatic cysts. Some patients will form benign pancreatic neoplasms called microcystic cystadenomas. These microcystic tumors produce serous secretions, and do not secrete mucin. Thus, they are quite distinct from the more common, and usually sporadic, macrocystic cystadenomas that are premalignant lesions. The microcystic tumors typically have a low attenuation on CT and may simulate a cyst or pseudocyst. However, in many cases they will have a characteristic central, often stellate, scar of more dense fibrous tissue. Occasionally the central scar may contain calcifications. On ultrasound the microcystic adenomas reveal themselves as echogenic solid masses, because the size of the "cystic" components is quite small (1–15 mm). In addition to the pancreatic cysts and serous microcystic adenomas just described, VHL patients may develop islet cell tumors. Binkovitz et al. reported six islet cell tumors among a group of 35 patients with VHL examined by CT (80). Pancreatic carcinoma has also been reported in association with VHL, but the true nature of this (causal vs. fortuitous) has not been definitively established.

ATAXIA-TELANGIECTASIA

Ataxia-telangiectasia (AT) is an autosomal recessive inherited disorder described by Louis-Bar in 1941 (81,82). It is a progressive disorder with involvement of the CNS, skin, respiratory, and immune systems. It is characterized by telangiectasias involving the skin (face) and eyes, with cerebellar ataxia, immunodeficiencies, and recurrent infections of the paranasal sinuses and lungs. It occurs in children and produces progressive ataxia. The telangiectasia commonly involves the pia mater and white matter of the brain and predominantly affects the cerebellum. The major MR findings consist of severe atrophy of the cerebellum, with enlarged cerebellar sulci, enlarged fourth ventricle, and enlarged CSF cisterns of the posterior fossa (Fig. 32) (81–83).

MISCELLANEOUS SYNDROMES

Miller-Dieker Syndrome

Miller-Dieker (MD) syndrome, or the lissencephalic syndrome, was first described by Miller in 1963 and later

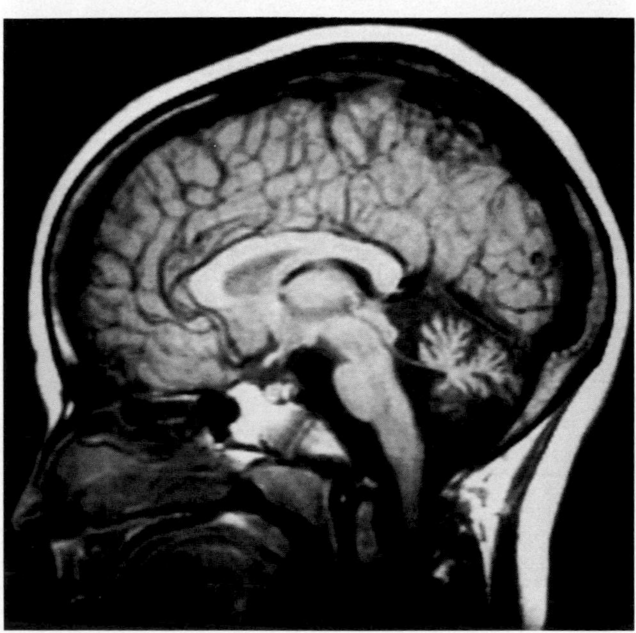

FIG. 32. Severe cerebellar vermian atrophy is identified in a patient with ataxia-telangiectasia on sagittal short TR/TE image.

by Dieker to include a disorder consisting of characteristic dysmorphic facies in a child with a lissencephalic brain. This disease can be inherited as an autosomal recessive disorder and is due to a deletion of part of chromosome 17 (84–87). MD syndrome presents at birth with microcephaly and classic facies, which consist of bitemporal grooving, vertical midline wrinkling of the forehead, anteverted nares, ear anomalies with low-set ears, and micrognathia. The symptomatology of these patients begins at birth with hypotonia, which may progress to hypertonia and intractable seizures. The prognosis is poor, and most infants die at birth or within 6 to 24 months. Patients die from associated cardiac and/or respiratory problems or from general failure to thrive. At autopsy, brains of these patients show characteristic features of lissencephaly (see Chapter 8).

MRI is clearly the best antemortem modality to evaluate this syndrome. The lissencephalic brain shows the following characteristics: (a) smooth cerebral surface with total agyria or mixed areas of agyria and pachygyria; (b) oval or hour-glass configuration of the brain with shallow sylvian grooves, due to lack of opercularization of the brain; and (c) normal gray-white matter distribution. The cortex is often thickened diffusely with loss of the normal gray-white matter interdigitation (Fig. 33) (87).

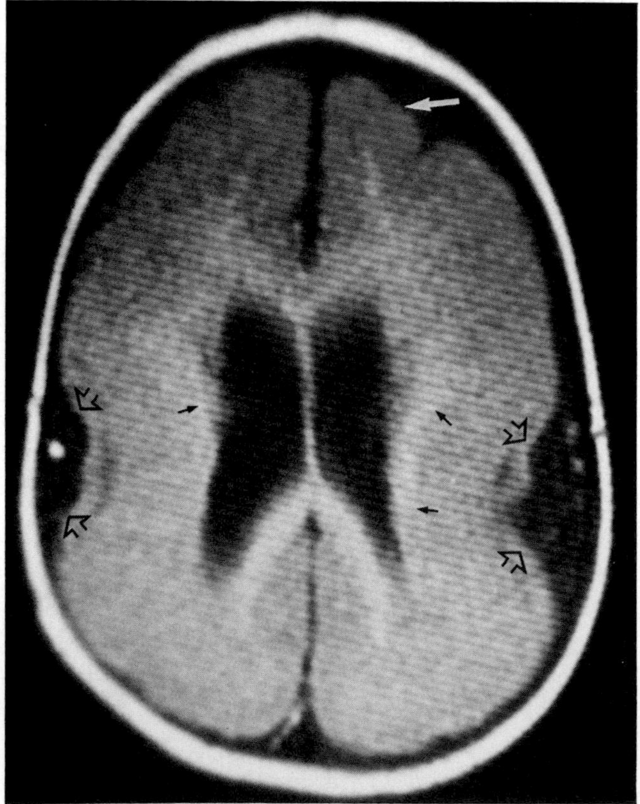

FIG. 33. Miller-Dieker syndrome patient demonstrates near total agyria, except for focal areas of pachygyria involving left frontal lobe (*large arrow*); increased gray matter involves almost all the brain with relative paucity of white matter (*small arrows*) and extremely shallow grooves (*open arrows*).

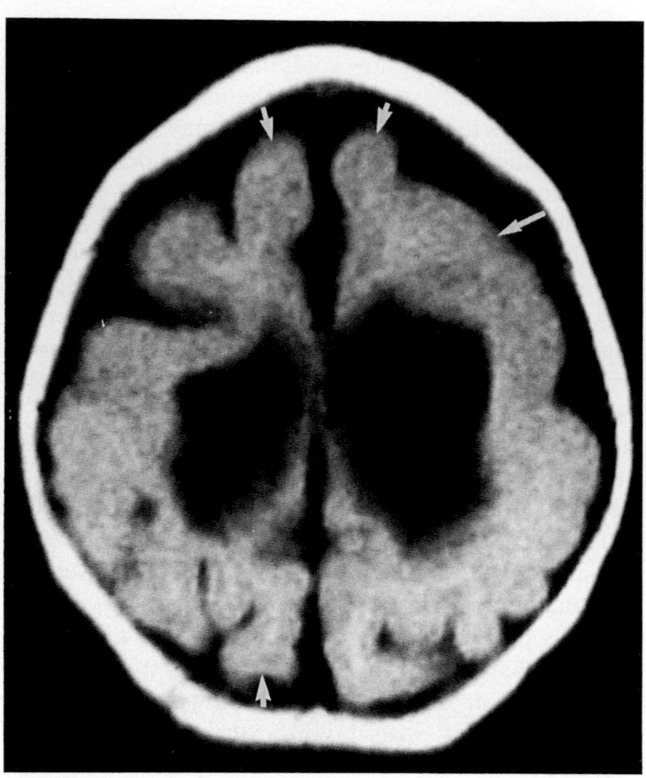

FIG. 34. Abnormal cortical sulci with large (*long arrow*) and small (*short arrows*) regions of pachygyria throughout the brain in a patient with Zellweger's syndrome.

Zellweger's Syndrome (Cerebrohepatorenal Syndrome)

Zellweger's syndrome (ZW) is an autosomal recessive disorder. ZW children present at birth with muscle hypotonia and weak or absent Moro's reaction, tendon, sucking, and swallowing reflexes. Typical facies consist of high bulging forehead, upslanting palpebral ridges, epicanthal folds, and hypotelorism, which gives these children a resemblance to those with Down syndrome. Additional findings consist of micrognathia, glaucoma, macrocephaly with split sutures and enlarged fontanelle, hepatomegaly, renal cysts, and abnormal bone and patellar calcification. The great majority of these patients (85%) die within the first year of life. On laboratory analysis, there is an increased level of long-chain fatty acids within serum plasma and urine (81,86).

On gross examination, the brain may be megaloencephalic. There is evidence of apparent pachygyria, but histologic analysis of these areas of pachygyria actually reveals polymicrogyria. There may also be evidence of increased gray matter involving cortical surfaces with microgyria, with a general decrease in cerebral white matter. Laboratory abnormalities consist of deficiencies in peroxisomal enzymes (86).

Characteristic MR findings include broad-based areas of thickened cortex looking like pachygyria, with focal increases in gray matter thickness, loss of normal cortical subjacent white matter interdigitation, and reduction in the relative quantity of white matter (Fig. 34) (81,86,88).

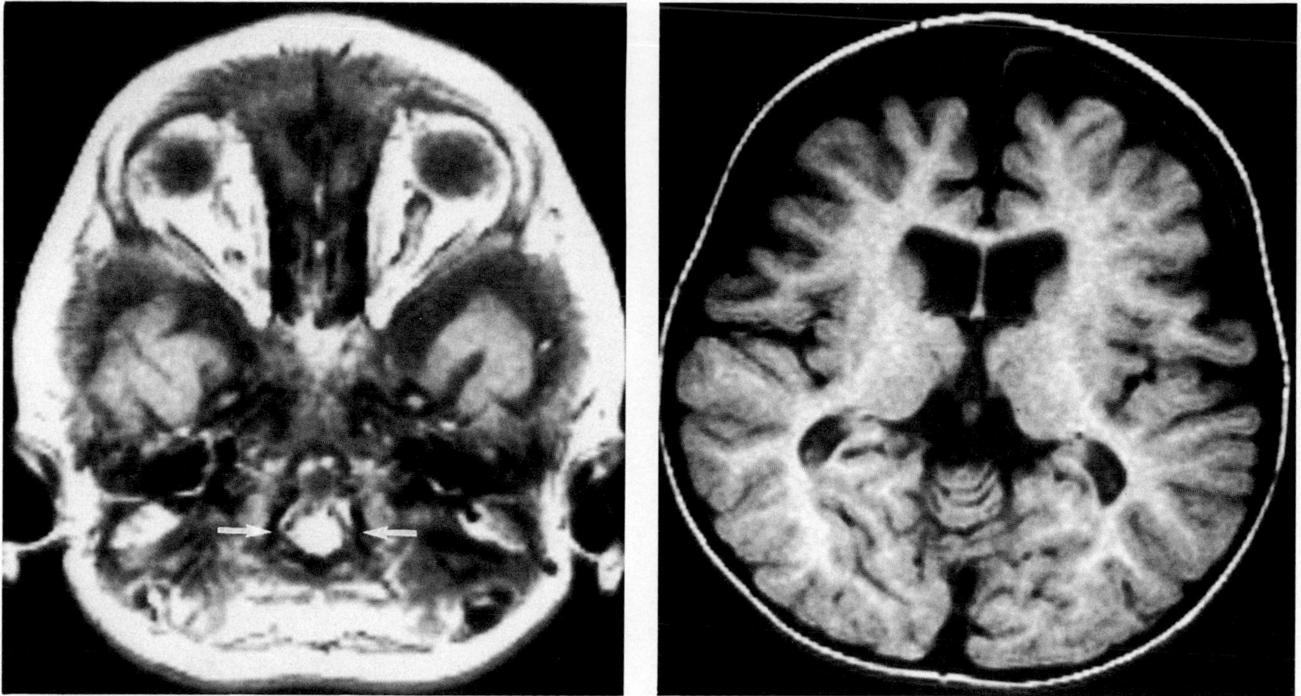

FIG. 35. Achondroplasia patient shows small foramen magnum (*arrows*, **A**) and communicating hydrocephalus (**B**) on short TR/TE images.

Achondroplasia

Achondroplasia is a relatively rare form of dwarfism. It is the most common form of chondrodysplasia and occurs in 1 in 26,000 births. It is an abnormality of endochondral bone formation and affects primarily the skull, spine, and long bones. Achondroplasia is inherited as an autosomal dominant trait, although more than 90% of cases are thought to represent sporadic mutations. The infant is born with characteristic craniofacial and skeletal abnormalities. Macrocephaly, which is due to true megalencephaly in most cases, can also be a reflection of communication hydrocephalus secondary to retardation of the cartilaginous growth of the skull base,

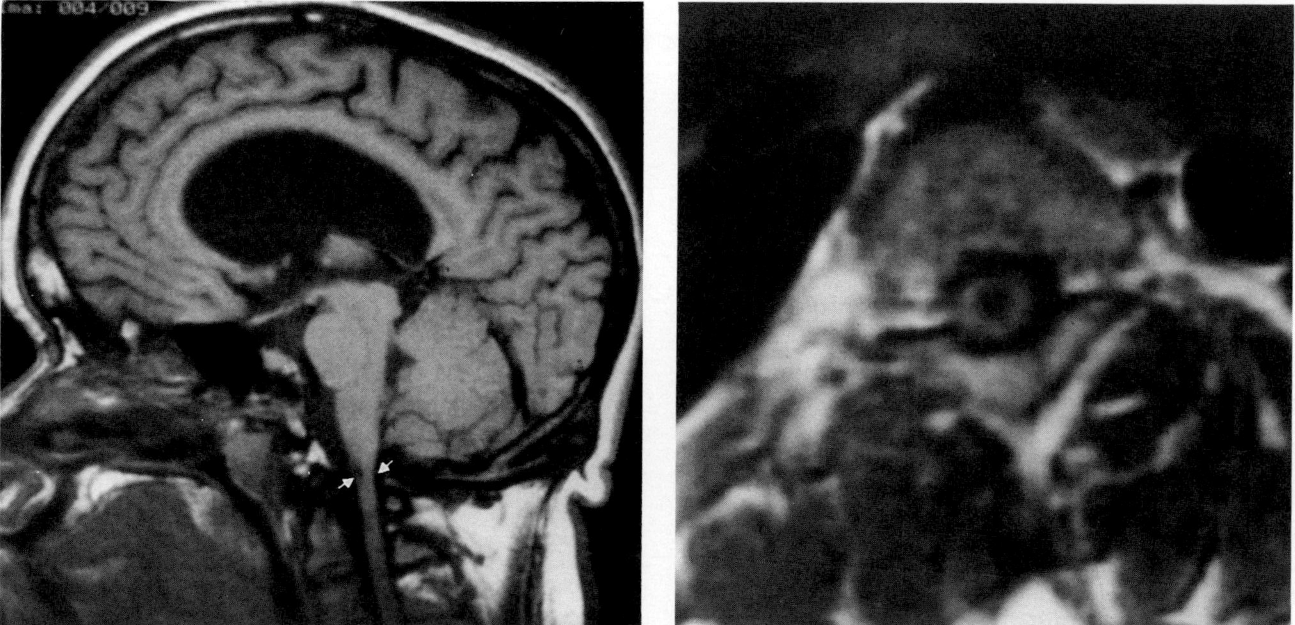

FIG. 36. Sagittal short TR/TE image (**A**) in achondroplasty reveals extremely tight foramen magnum (*arrows*, A) and hydrocephalus. Note hydromyelia on axial short TR/TE image through thoracic cord (**B**).

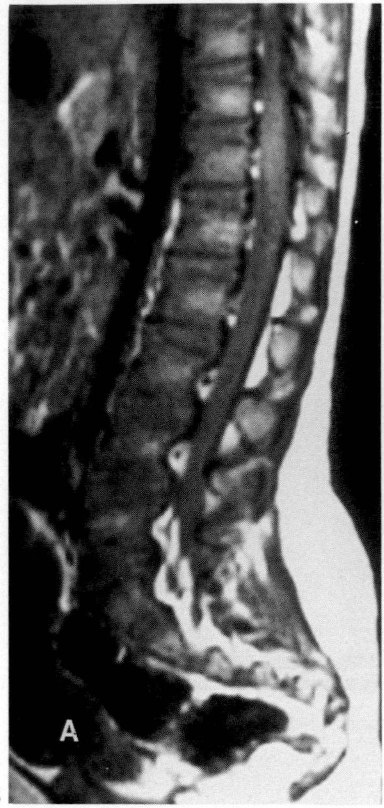

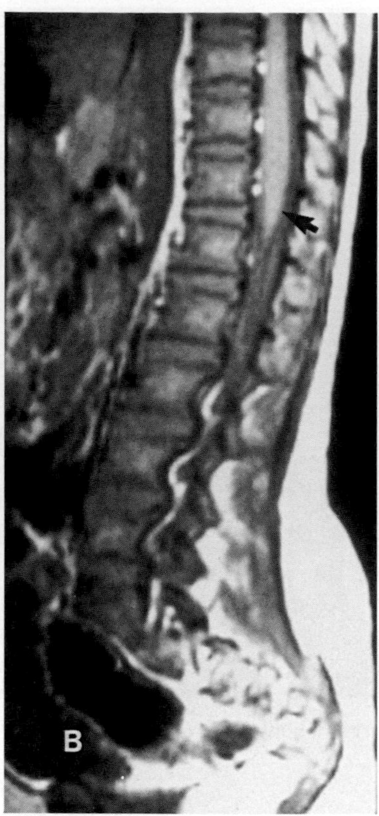

A,B

FIG. 37. Thoracolumbar spinal canal stenosis is seen in this achondroplasia patient on sagittal short TR/TE images (**A,B**). Note exaggerated lumbosacral lordosis.

resulting in a small foramen magnum and small jugular foramen. Spinal abnormalities consist of often severe spinal stenosis, with an increase in lordosis of the normal lordotic curvature in the lumbar region and at times kyphoscoliosis in the thoracic spine. Vertebral bodies may have a cuboid shape. Patients also show a low nasal bridge, short humeri and femurs, and trident hand deformities (89).

MRI clearly shows small foramen magnum and jugular foramen (Figs. 35 and 36). Communicating hydrocephalus can also be seen. Sagittal spine images demonstrate the notable spinal canal stenosis and vertebral body abnormalities (Fig. 37) (81,89,90).

CONCLUSIONS

The phakomatoses are a diverse group of disorders, because they do not obey the original dictum of "inherited neurocutaneous disorders." The most common phakomatoses (excluding Sturge-Weber syndrome) are autosomal dominant; therefore, a correct diagnosis has genetic implications that should prompt a screening evaluation of all first-degree relatives to see if they are also affected. After the affected individuals are identified and an initial survey is obtained, a routine follow-up surveillance program should be established. This typically includes annual CNS imaging studies and, where appropriate, abdominal ultrasound, CT, or MR.

ACKNOWLEDGMENTS. The authors would like to acknowledge Steve Kruger for photographic support and Phyllis Hickey for manuscript preparation.

DISCLAIMER. The views and opinions expressed herein are solely those of the authors and should not be construed as official or as reflecting those of the Departments of the VA Army or Defense.

REFERENCES

1. Mulvihill JJ, Parry DM, Sherman JL, Pikus A, Kaiser-Kupfer MIE. Neurofibromatosis 1 (Recklinghausen disease) and neurofibromatosis 2 (bilateral acoustic neurofibromatosis)—an update. *Ann Intern Med* 1990;113:39–52.
2. National Institutes of Health Consensus Development Conference. Neurofibromatosis, Conference Statement. *Arch Neurol* 1988;45:575–578.
3. Riccardi V. *Neurofibromatosis. Phenotype, Natural History, and Pathogenesis.* 2nd ed. Baltimore: The Johns Hopkins University Press; 1992.
4. Tibbles JA, Cohen MM Jr. The proteus syndrome: the elephant man diagnosed. *Br Med J* 1986;293:683–685.
5. Cohen MM. Further diagnostic thoughts about the elephant man. *Am J Med Genet* 1988;29(4):777–782.
6. Gardeur D, Palmieri A, Mashaly R. Cranial computed tomography in the phakomatoses. *Neuroradiology* 1983;25:293–304.
7. Barker D, Wright E, Nguyen K, Cannon P. Gene for von Recklinghausen neurofibromatosis is in the pericentromeric region of chromosome 17. *Science* 1987;236:1100–1102.
8. Seizinger BR, Rouleau GA, Ozelius LJ, Lane AH. Genetic linkage of von Recklinghausen neurofibromatosis to the nerve growth factor receptor gene. *Cell* 1987;49:589–594.
9. DiMario FJ, Ramsby G, Greenstein R, Langshur S, Dunham B.

Neurofibromatosis type 1: magnetic resonance imaging findings. *J Child Neurol* 1993;8:32–39.

10. Aoki S, Barkovich AJ, Nishimura K, Kjos B. Neurofibromatosis types 1 and 2: cranial MR findings. *Radiology* 1989;172:527–534.
11. Brown EW, Riccardi VM, Mawad M, Handel S, Goldman S, Bryan RN. MR imaging of optic pathways in patients with neurofibromatosis. *AJNR* 1987;8:1031–1036.
12. Hurst RW, Newman SA, Cail WS. Multifocal intracranial MR abnormalities in neurofibromatosis. *AJNR* 1988;9:293–296.
13. Bognanno JR, Edwards MK, Lee TA, Dunn DW, Roos KL, Klatte EC. Cranial MR imaging in neurofibromatosis. *AJNR* 1988;9: 461–468.
14. Pomeranz SJ, Shelton JJ, Tobias J, Soila K, Altman D, Viamonte M. MR of visual pathways in patients with neurofibromatosis. *AJNR* 1994;8:831–836.
15. Russell DS, Rubinstein LJ. Dysgenetic syndromes (phacomatoses) associated with tumors and hamartomas of the nervous system. In: *Pathology of Tumors of the Nervous System.* Baltimore: Williams & Wilkins; 1989:766–784.
16. Mirowitz SA, Sartor K, Gado M. High-intensity basal ganglia lesions on T1-weighted MR images in neurofibromatosis. *AJNR* 1989;10:1159–1163.
17. Ferner RE, Chaudhuri R, Bingham J, Cox T, Hughes RAC. MRI in neurofibromatosis 1. The nature and evolution of increased intensity T2 weighted lesions and their relationship to intellectual impairment. *J Neurol Neurosurg Psychiatry* 1993;56:492–495.
18. Lee Y, Van Tassel P, Bruner JM, Moser RP, Share JC. Juvenile pilocytic astrocytomas: CT and MR characteristics. *AJNR* 1989;10:363–370.
19. Listernick R, Charrow J, Greenwald M. Emergence of optic pathway gliomas in children with neurofibromatosis type 1 after normal imaging results. *J Pediatr* 1992;121:584–587.
20. Jacoby CG, Go RT, Beren RA. Cranial CT of neurofibromatosis. *AJNR* 1980;1:311–315.
21. Imes RK, Hoyt WF. Magnetic resonance imaging signs of optic nerve gliomas in neurofibromatosis 1. *Am J Ophthalmol* 1991;111: 729–734.
22. Brzowski AE, Bazan C 3d, Mumma JV, Ryan SG. Spontaneous regression of optic glioma in a patient with neurofibromatosis. *Neurology* 1992;42:679–681.
23. Hoyt WF, Baghdassarian SA. Optic glioma of childhood: natural history and rationale for conservative management. *Br J Opthalmol* 1969;53:793–798.
24. DeSousa AL, Kalsbeck JE, Mealey J, Ellis FD, Muller J. Optic chiasmatic glioma in children. *Am J Ophthalmol* 1979;87:376–381.
25. Tenny RT, Laws ER, Younge BR, Rush JA. The neurosurgical management of optic glioma. Results in 104 patients. *J Neurosurg* 1982;57:452–458.
26. Wright JE, McDonald WI, Call NB. Management of optic nerve gliomas. *Br J Ophthalmol* 1980;64:545–552.
27. Dosoretz DE, Blitzer PH, Wang CC, Linggood RM. Management of glioma of the optic nerve and/or chiasm. *Cancer* 1980;45:1467–1471.
28. Wong JYC, Uhl V, Wara WM, Sheline GE. Optic gliomas, a reanalysis of the University of California, San Francisco experience. *Cancer* 1987;60:1847–1855.
29. Reed D, Robertson WD, Rootman J, Douglas G. Plexiform neurofibromatosis [sic] of the orbit: CT evaluation. *AJNR* 1986;7: 259–263.
30. Harkens K, Dolan KD. Correlative imaging of sphenoid dysplasia accompanying neurofibromatosis. *Ann Otol Rhinol Laryngol* 1990;99:137–141.
31. Martuza RL, Eldridge R. Neurofibromatosis 2 (bilateral acoustic neurofibromatosis). *N Engl J Med* 1988;318:684–688.
32. Wertelecki W, Rouleau GA, Superneau DW, Forehand LW. Neurofibromatosis 2: clinical and dna linkage studies of a large kindred. *N Engl J Med* 1988;319:278–283.
33. Kanter WR, Eldridge R, Fabricant R, Allen JC, Koerber T. Central neurofibromatosis with bilateral acoustic neuroma: genetic, clinical and biochemical distinctions from peripheral neurofibromatosis. *Neurology* 1980;30:851–859.
34. Seizinger BR, Martuza RL, Gusella JF. Loss of genes on chromosome 22 in tumorigenesis of human acoustic neuroma. *Nature* 1986;322:644–647.
35. Rouleau GA, Wertelecki W, Hains JL, Hobbs WJ. Genetic linkage of bilateral acoustic neurofibromatosis to a dna marker on chromosome 22. *Nature* 1987;329:246–248.
36. Halliday AL, Sobel RA, Martuza RL. Benign spinal nerve sheath tumors: their occurrence sporadically and in neurofibromatosis types 1 and 2. *J Neurosurg* 1991;74:248–253.
37. Rodriguez HA, Berthrong M. Multiple primary intracranial tumors in von Recklinghausen's neurofibromatosis. *Arch Neurol* 1966;14:467–475.
38. Evans DGR, Huson SM, Donnai D, et al. A clinical study of type 2 neurofibromatosis. *Q J Med* 1992;84:603–618.
39. Baldwin D, King TT, Chevretton E, Morrison AW. Bilateral cerebellopontine angle tumors in neurofibromatosis type 2. *J Neurosurg* 1991;74:910–915.
40. Miyamato RT, Campbell RL, Fritsch M, Lochmueller G. Preservation of hearing in neurofibromatosis 2. *Otolaryngol Head Neck Surg* 1990;103:619–624.
41. Kasantikul V, Netsky MG, Glasscock ME, Hays JW. Acoustic neurilemmoma, clinicoanatomical study of 103 patients. *J Neurosurg* 1980;52:28–35.
42. Kendall B, Symon L. Investigation of patients presenting with cerebellopontine angle syndromes. *Neuroradiology* 1977;13:65–84.
43. Wu E, Tang Y, Zhang Y, Bai R. CT in diagnosis of acoustic neuromas. *AJNR* 1986;7:645–650.
44. Harkin JC, Reed RJ. *Tumors of the Peripheral Nervous System. Fascicle 3, Second Series, Atlas of Tumor Pathology.* Washington DC: AFIP; 1969:97.
45. Chui MC, Bird BL, Rogers J. Extracranial and extraspinal nerve sheath tumors: computed tomographic evaluation. *Neuroradiology* 1988;30:47–53.
46. Stull MA, Moser RP, Kransdorf MJ, Bogumill GP, Nelson MC. Magnetic resonance appearance of peripheral nerve sheath tumors. *Skeletal Radiol* 1991;20:9–14.
47. Price AC, Runge VM, Carollo BR, Braun IF. Contrast enhancement in the evaluation of the cerebellopontine angle (*Abst.*). *AJNR* 1989;10:879.
48. Merten D, Gooding C, Newton T, Malamud N. Meningiomas of childhood and adolescence. *J Pediatr* 1974;84:696–700.
49. Domenicucci M, Santoro A, D'Osvaldo DH, Delfini R, Cantore GP, Guidetti B. Multiple intracranial meningiomas. *J Neurosurg* 1989;70:41–44.
50. Eljamel MSM, Foy PM. Multiple meningiomas and their relation to neurofibromatosis. Review of the literature and report of seven cases. *Surg Neurol* 1989;32:131–136.
51. Ilgren EB, Kinnier-Wilson LM, Stiller CA. Gliomas in neurofibromatosis: a series of 89 cases with evidence for enhancement malignancy in associated cerebellar astrocytoma. *Pathol Ann* 1985;20: 331–358.
52. Smirniotopoulos J, Murphy F. The phakomatoses. *AJNR* 1992;13:725–746.
53. Shepherd CW, Beard CM, Gomez MR, Kurland LT, Whisnant JP. Tuberous sclerosis complex in Olmsted County, Minnesota. *Arch Neurol* 1991;48:400–401.
54. Sampson JR, Scahill SJ, Stephenson JBP, Mann L, Connor JM. Genetic aspects of tuberous sclerosis in the west of Scotland. *J Med Genet* 1989;26:28–31.
55. Winship IM, Connor JM, Beighton PH. Genetic heterogeneity in tuberous sclerosis: phenotypic correlations. *J Med Genet* 1990;27: 418–421.
56. Stefansson K. Tuberous sclerosis (*editorial*). *Mayo Clin Proc* 1991; 66:868–872.
57. Gomez MR. Diagnostic criteria. In: Gomez MR, ed. *Tuberous Sclerosis*, 2nd ed. New York: Raven Press; 1985:9–20.
58. van der Hoeve J. Eye symptoms in tuberose sclerosis of the brain. *Trans Ophthalmol Soc UK* 1923;40:329–334.
59. van der Hoeve T. Eye diseases in tuberose sclerosis of the brain and in Recklinghausen's disease. *Trans Ophthalmol Soc UK* 1923;43: 534–541.
60. Nyboer JH, Robertson DM, Gomez MR. Retinal lesions in tuberous sclerosis. *Arch Ophthalmol* 1976;94:1277–1280.
61. Boesel CP, Paulson GW, Kosnik EJ, Earle KM. Brain hamartomas and tumors associated with tuberous sclerosis. *Neurosurgery* 1979;4:410–417.

62. Reagan TJ. Neuropathology. In: Gomez MR, ed. *Tuberous Sclerosis,* 2nd ed. New York: Raven Press; 1985:63–74.
63. Bender BL, Yunis EJ. The pathology of tuberous sclerosis. *Pathol Annu* 1982; 17:339–382.
64. Fitz CR, Harwood-Nash DCF, Thompson JR. Neuroradiology of tuberous sclerosis in children. *Radiology* 1974; 110:635–642.
65. Schafer JA, Berg BO, Norman D. Cerebellar calcification in tuberous sclerosis. *Arch Neurol* 1975; 32:642–643.
66. Lee BCP, Gawler J. Tuberous sclerosis, comparison of computed tomography and conventional neuroradiology. *Radiology* 1978; 127:403–407.
67. Iwasaki S, Nakagawa H, Kichikawa K, Fukusumi A. MR and CT of tuberous sclerosis: linear abnormalities in the cerebral white matter. *AJNR* 1990; 11:1029–1034.
68. Nixon J, Houser O, Gomez M, Okazaki H. Cerebral tuberous sclerosis: MR imaging. *AJNR* 1994; 170:869–873.
69. Altman NR, Purser RK, Donovan Post MJ. Tuberous sclerosis: characteristics at CT and MR imaging. *Radiology* 1988; 167:527–532.
70. Martin N, Debussche C, DeBroucker T, Mompoint D, Marsault C, Nahum H. Gadolinium-DTPA enhanced MR imaging in tuberous sclerosis. *Neuroradiology* 1990; 31:492–497.
71. Enjolras O, Rich MC, Merlan JJ. Facial port-wine stains and Sturge-Weber syndrome. *Pediatrics* 1985; 76:48–51.
72. Peterman AF, Hayles AB, Dockerty MB, Love JG. Encephalotrigeminal angiomatosis (Sturge-Weber disease). *JAMA* 1958; 167: 2169–2176.
73. Wohlwill FJ, Yakovlev PI. Histopathology of meningo-facial angiomatosis (Sturge-Weber's disease). *J Neuropathol Exp Neurol* 1957; 16:341–364.
74. Welch K, Naheedy MH, Abroms IF, Strand RD. Computed Tomography of Sturge-Weber Syndrome in Infants. *J Comput Assist Tomogr* 1980;4:33–36.
75. Schmauser I, Bittner R. MR-imaging findings in children with Sturge-Weber syndrome. *Neuropediatrics* 1990; 21:146–152.
76. Neumann HPH, Eggert HR, Schumacher M, Mohadjer M, Wakhloo AK, Volk B, et al. Central nervous system lesions in von Hippel-Lindau syndrome. *J Neurol Neurosurg Psychiatry* 1992; 55:898–901.
77. McGrath FP, Givney RG, Owen DA, Erb SR. Case report: multiple hepatic and pulmonary hemangioblastomas—a new manifestation of von Hippel-Lindau disease. *Clin Radiol* 1992;45:37–39.
78. Horton JC, Harsh GR, Fisher JW, Hoyt WF. Von Hippel-Lindau disease and erythrocytosis: radioimmunoassay of erythropoietin in cyst fluid from a brainstem hemangioblastoma. *Neurology* 1991; 41:753–754.
79. Choyke PL, Glenn GM, Walther MM, et al. The natural history of renal lesions in von Hippel-Lindau disease: a serial CT study in 28 patients. *AJR* 1992; 159:1229–1234.
80. Binkovitz LA, Johnson CD, Stephens DH. Islet cell tumors in von Hippel-Lindau disease: increased prevalence and relationship to the multiple endocrine neoplasias. *AJR* 1990; 155:501–505.
81. Jones KL, Smith S. *Recognizable Patterns of Human Malformation,* 4th ed. Philadelphia: WB Saunders C; 1988.
82. McFarlin DW, Strober W, Waldmann TA. Ataxia-telangiectasia. *Medicine* 1972; 51:281–314.
83. Paller A. Ataxia-telangiectasia. *Neurol Clin* 1987; 5:447–449.
84. Dobyns WB, Stratton RF, Parke JT, Greenberg F, Nussbaum RL, Ledbetter DH. Miller-Dieker syndrome: lissencephaly and monosomy 17. *J Pediatr* 1983; 102:552–558.
85. Stratton RF, Dobyns WB, Airhart SE, Ledbetter DH. New chromosomal syndrome: Miller-Dieker syndrome and monosomy. *Hum Genet* 1984;67:143–200.
86. Barth PG. Disorders of neuronal migration. *Can J Neurol Sci* 1987; 14:1–16.
87. Byrd SE, Bohan TP, Osborn RE, Naidich TP. The CT and MR evaluation of lissencephaly. *AJNR* 1988;9: 923–927.
88. Optitz JM, Zurhein GM, Vitale L. The Zellweger syndrome. *Birth Defects* 1969; 2:144–158.
89. Cohen ME, Rosenthal AD, Matson DD. Neurological abnormalities in achondroplastic children. *J Pediatr* 1967; 73:367–376.
90. Silverman FN. *Caffey's Pediatric X-ray Diagnosis,* 8th ed. Chicago: Yearbook Medical Publishers; 1985.

Magnetic Resonance Imaging of the Brain and Spine, Second Edition, edited by Scott W. Atlas. Lippincott-Raven Publishers, Philadelphia © 1996.

18

The Aging Brain and Neurodegenerative Diseases

Frank J. Lexa, John Q. Trojanowski, Bruce H. Braffman, and Scott W. Atlas

F. J. Lexa, M.D.: Department of Radiology, University of Pennsylvania Medical Center, Philadelphia, PA 19104.

J. Q. Trojanowski, M.D., Ph.D.: Division of Anatomic Pathology, Department of Pathology and Laboratory Medicine, Hospital of the University of Pennsylvania, Philadelphia, PA 19104.

B. H. Braffman, M.D.: Department of Radiology, Memorial Hospital, Hollywood, FL 33021.

S. W. Atlas, M.D.: Neuroradiology Division, Department of Radiology, Oregon Health Sciences University, Portland, OR 97201.

Degenerative disorders represent a major challenge for the neuroradiologist. This chapter includes a wide spectrum of diseases—some that are now becoming well understood at the molecular level as well as many that are still poorly understood—remaining "idiopathic" entities. As research continues, the latter list will shrink as those disorders are reclassified into other categories. The neurodegenerative diseases also represent some of the most interesting pathologic entities encountered in the field of neuroscience. The past few years have seen very active and productive research into the mechanisms that lead both to the death of individual neurons as well as networks of interconnected neurons. Recently, there has also been enormous progress in developing the ability of magnetic resonance (MR) imaging to detect many of the events that underlie this common theme of cellular dysfunction and neuronal degeneration.

Normal aging constitutes the most common form of neuronal degeneration. Programmed cell death is part of both the normal early development of the brain as well as a normal component of senescence as humans live to old age. Life span refers to the average age in a species which would be achieved in the absence of accidental death from illness or injury. For humans this is thought to be between 85 to 120 years of age (1). Life expectancy (i.e., the number of years of life any individual may statistically expect from birth onward) has increased significantly in the past century due to a variety of factors including improvements in sanitation, nutrition, and health care. In industrialized countries with high standards of living, life expectancy is now approaching the life span (1). In those nations, the elderly now constitute a very rapidly growing proportion of the population. This demographic change will continue to grow in importance with a profound impact on the practice of medicine. In particular, it is important for the neuroradiologist to be aware of the wide range of "normal" in older patients, to understand what constitutes normal and abnormal aging, and to be aware of the findings in neurodegenerative disorders that present in late middle age and in elderly patients.

Normal aging of the brain and many neurodegenerative disorders are characterized by the death of subsets of specific classes of neurons (1). A wide variety of mechanisms have been invoked to explain the senescence and death of cells including loss of hormonal stimulation, accumulation of toxins, and/or genetic errors, and internal cellular clocks that program death.

In neurodegenerative disorders this occurs prematurely. Loss of neural tissue leads to the neuroimaging findings of focal and/or diffuse atrophy. As the brain shrinks, the cerebrospinal fluid (CSF) spaces appear capacious with prominence of the ventricles, cisterns, and sulci. In the brain, normal aging and the neurodegenerative disorders share other MR imaging changes including hyperintense foci in the white matter on long TR/TE images and loss of signal intensity in the deep gray matter nuclei. This chapter will discuss the MRI and neuropathologic findings in the brain due to aging and the neurodegenerative disorders.

THE AGING BRAIN

The normal appearance of the brain on MR imaging changes in several significant ways from young adulthood into old age. The following sections address these changes by category and where possible discuss the significance with regard to overlap with pathologic processes.

Global White Matter Changes with Age

At 1.5 Tesla, slight lengthening of T1 and T2 values for both white and gray matter appears to occur during normal aging (2). A report using low field strength showed a more complex relationship to age with a minimum T1 between 40 and 45 years and an increase with advancing age in both gray and white matter structures (3). Another study at low field strength examined aged individuals (75–85 years old) with above average health and intellectual function. This report showed a positive correlation between measured T1 and advanced age (4).

Focal Areas of Hyperintense Signal in White Matter

MR imaging is more sensitive than CT in the detection of focal abnormalities of cerebral white matter (5–8). Focal areas of high signal intensity on long TR images can be seen routinely in several normal locations, can be scattered within the deep white matter during normal aging, and are much more widespread and prominent in a variety of pathological disorders. The interpretation of these foci of high signal intensity requires analysis of size, shape, location, and overall number. Given the correlation of size and severity of these periventricular hyperintense lesions with age, the radiologist needs to cultivate an overall sense of how much is allowable before invoking superimposed pathology at a given age.

Even the normal white matter of the adult is not uniformly dark on long TR/TE images. Some high signal intensity foci are physiologic and found in younger patients (terminal areas of myelination) or in virtually all ages (ependymitis granularis and relative hyperintensity of the posterior aspect of the posterior limb of the internal capsule on long TR/TE images). Virchow-Robin perivascular spaces are also normal findings which can be found in patients of all ages. These Virchow-Robin spaces may show an age- or atrophy-related increase in prominence in the same fashion as other CSF spaces.

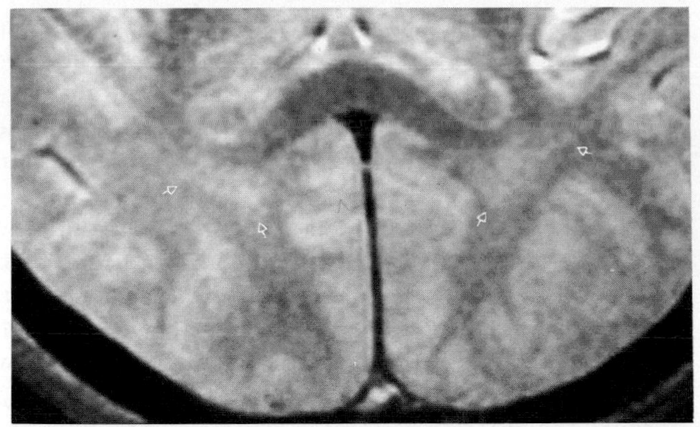
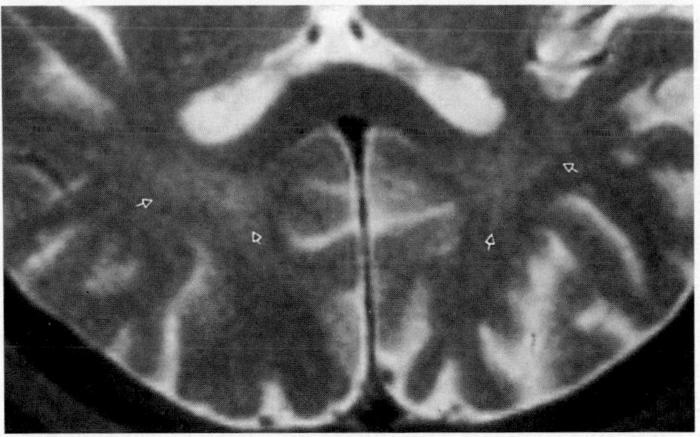

FIG. 1 Terminal areas of myelination. Axial plane, long TR, short (**A**) and long (**B**) TE. The mild hyperintense signal of the white matter (*arrows*) posterosuperior to the trigones is normal and is thought to represent the terminal areas of myelination.

NORMAL CNS FOCI OF HIGH SIGNAL INTENSITY ON LONG TR/TE IMAGES

The Trigone: Terminal Areas of Myelination

Triangular-shaped regions posterior and superior to the trigones that are variably hyperintense on long TR images are normal in patients in their first and second decades (Fig. 1) (9). They are thought to represent the known delayed myelination of the fiber tracts involving the association areas of the convexities of the posterior and inferior parietal and posterolateral temporal cortex, i.e., the "terminal areas" (9,10). Occasionally, some of these regions lack myelin staining until the fourth decade (10).

The Frontal Horns: Ependymitis Granularis

Hyperintense foci on long TR sequences exist in virtually all normal patients anterior and lateral to the frontal horns (Fig. 2) (11). These may be punctate or up to a centimeter in width (11). They are of uniform triangular shape, with the base resting on the tops of the frontal horns and with the apex pointing anteriorly into the adjacent white matter. The medial aspect of the triangle is defined by the genu of the corpus callosum, while the lateral border extends along the white matter, terminating posteriorly at the head of the caudate in the most prominent cases (11).

Several mechanisms may contribute to the hyperintense signal seen in this location (11). First, the myelin content is decreased. Second, this region displays ependymitis granularis, which refers to a focal breakdown of the ependymal lining with adjacent astrocytic gliosis. Third, periependymal and extracellular fluid is increased. Interstitial fluid in the brain preferentially drains to the subependymal region, especially to the dorsolateral angle of the lateral ventricle. This region serves as a natural funnel for extracellular fluid produced in the brain interstitium, an organ which lacks hemispheric lymphatics (11).

The Posterior Aspect of the Posterior Limb of the Internal Capsule

The posterior portion of the internal capsule shows focal areas of variable signal intensity compared to the remainder of the internal capsule. In one report, approximately one-half of normal patients demonstrated this

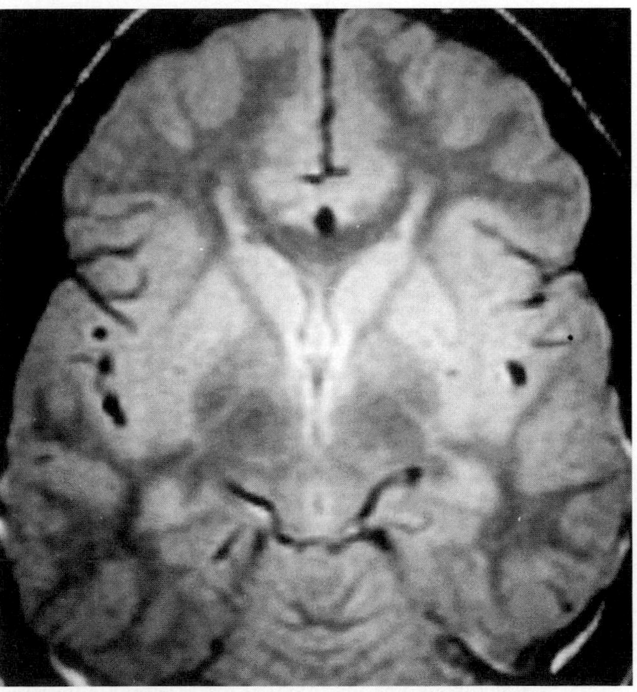

FIG. 2. A 12-year-old girl with normal ependymitis granularis. Image using TR/TE 2300/30 in the axial plane. Note the normal triangular-shaped hyperintense foci anterolateral to the frontal horns of the lateral ventricle.

finding. These foci were well circumscribed, round or oval, symmetrical, appeared comparable to cortical gray matter on T2, and iso- or hypointense on proton-density images (Fig. 3). Histopathologic correlation suggests that this corresponds to the parietopontine tracts with less intense myelin staining (12). The presence of the pars retrolenticularis of the optic tract (13) and absence of iron (14) are other postulated contributors.

On axial images at the level of the velum interpositum, they are consistently medial to the distal putamen near the junction of the posterior limb and retrolenticular portion of the internal capsule. They do not demonstrate intravenous contrast enhancement (12). These foci are not seen in patients under the age of 10 years; otherwise they show no definite relation to age (12). Pathologic lesions are more variable in size, shape, and location, are more inhomogeneous and ill-defined, uncommonly are bilaterally symmetric, and may enhance with Gd-DTPA (12).

Perivascular Spaces of Virchow and Robin

Pestalozzi (15) and later Virchow in 1851 (16) and Robin in 1859 (17), characterized the perivascular space of Virchow-Robin (VRS). This is an extension of the subarachnoid space that accompanies penetrating vessels into the brain to the level of the capillaries (15,18). The word lacunae carries with it many connotations and has created some semantic confusion. One classification system is shown in Table 1 (19,20). Type I lacunae are small infarcts, type II are small hemorrhages, and type III are dilated VRS. CT studies can demonstrate large dilated VRS (21) while MR imaging permits the routine visualization of normal VRS due to greater resolution and contrast (15,18,22).

On MR, VRS are small foci which remain isointense to CSF on all pulse sequences and conform to the path of penetrating arteries (15,18,22). They lack mass effect, and are round, oval, or curvilinear with well-defined, smooth margins. The VRS at the base of the brain follow the lenticulostriate arteries as they enter the basal ganglia through the anterior perforated substance. On axial images they are typically adjacent to the anterior or posterior surface of the lateral portion of the anterior commissure (Fig. 4) (22). In the coronal or sagittal plane they are adjacent to the superior surface of the commissure or just lateral to the putamen. Those in the high convexity (Fig. 5) follow the course of the penetrating cortical arteries and arterioles from the high-convexity gray matter into the centrum semiovale (15). High signal intensity foci in the midbrain can also be seen from enlarged perivascular spaces, in this case from branches of the collicular and accessary collicular arteries (23).

Small VRS (less than 2 mm) are found in all age groups and probably represent a normal anatomic finding (15). With advancing age, VRS are found with increasing frequency and larger apparent size (15). In one report, lenticulostriate VR spaces had a mild correlation

A 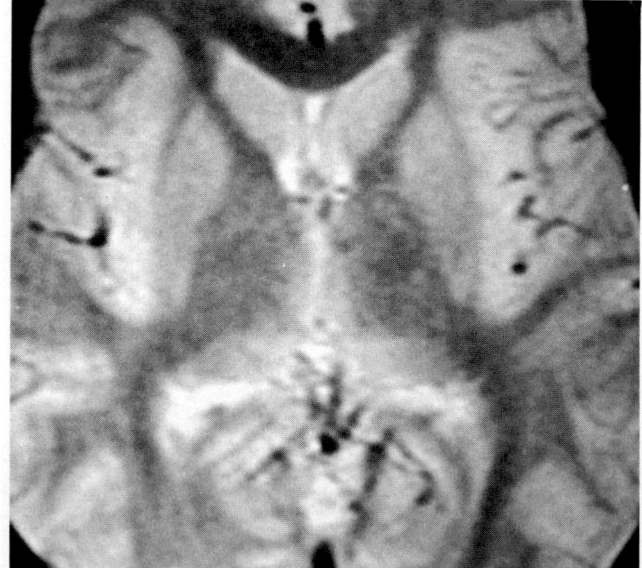

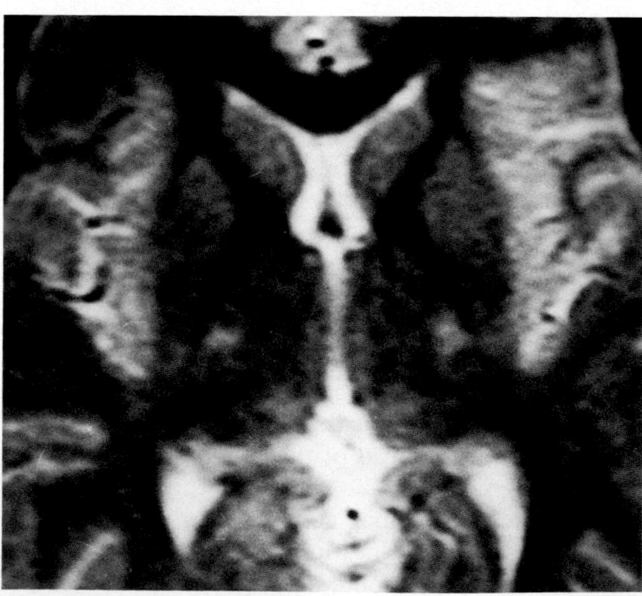 B

FIG. 3. A 33-year-old with normal hyperintensity in the posterior limb of the internal capsule imaged on an 0.5 T unit. Axial plane, long TR, short (**A**) and long (**B**) TE. On the second echo of the long TR sequence (B), bilateral symmetric hyperintense foci are noted in the posterior internal capsule medial to the distal putamen near the junction of the posterior limb or retrolenticular portion of the internal capsule. On the first echo of the long TR sequence (A), however, these normal foci are isointense (or hypointense) to the remainder of the internal capsule. Most pathologic processes cause hyperintense signal on both echoes of the long TR sequences. See Fig. 45 for comparison.

TABLE 1. *New pathologic classification of cerebral lacunae*[a]

Type	Pathologic criteria
1	Old small deep cerebral infarcts with irregular cavities containing macrophages and parenchymal fragments surrounded by gliosis
2	Old small hemorrhages with hemosiderin-laden macrophages and iron pigmentation of their walls
3	Dilated perivascular spaces; they are round, very regular cavities that always contain one or two sections of an artery with a patent lumen and usually normal walls; the cavity is lined by a single layer of epithelial cells that correspond to the leptomeningeal cells forming the normal lining of the perivascular spaces; according to their number and size, four varieties of type 3 exist.
3a	Numerous small round perivascular spaces (état criblet or status cribosus)
3b	Perivascular dilatation destroying the adjacent brain (lacunes de desintegration, vaginalité destructive)
3c	Solitary subputaminal cavities surrounding the lenticulostriate arteries at their entrance into the lentiform nucleus
3d	Expanding perivascular spaces that cause mass effect with possible reactive lesions such as gliosis, spongiosis, swollen oligodendroglia, and myelin loss with edema

From Poirier et al., ref. (19), and Benhaeim-Sigaux et al., ref. (20).

[a] Cerebral lacunae classically have been considered to be old, small deep infarcts due to occlusion of penetrating arteries. However, some also referred to old hemorrhages and dilated perivascular spaces as lacunae (i.e., cavities). To avoid the semantic confusion that is associated with the term cerebral lacunae, the above neuropathologic classification was proposed.

with age, while high-convexity VR spaces, though rarer, had a much stronger correlation with age (15). Age, hypertension, dementia, and incidental subcortical white matter lesions were significantly associated with large (>2 mm) VRS (15). More detailed analysis using logistic regression showed age to be the significant variable (15). Two mechanisms can account for this age-related increase in size. First, aging is associated with enlargement of ventricles and sulci. The VRS, an extension of the subarachnoid space, enlarges as the subarachnoid space does elsewhere in the brain with aging (15,20,24). Second, age-related vascular changes may play an important role. Atherosclerotic changes in the brain are common in elderly patients, occurring in over 50% of patients over 50 years of age (25). This can be found in normotensive patients, but is more diffuse and widespread in hypertensives (1). Even without atherosclerosis, vessels become larger and more tortuous with aging (1). The unfolding of these tortuous vessels may account for the vacuolated parenchyma around the vessels and ultimately lead to increased prominence of the perivascular space (20,24).

On MR it may be difficult to distinguish a lacunar infarct from a prominent VRS. In many cases, the following rules can be useful for correct identification. Lacunar infarcts occur in the upper two-thirds of the putamina (22), are not isointense to CSF on all pulse sequences unless they have undergone cystic change (18) (Fig. 4), and usually are larger (18) (5 mm or more) (22). VRS typically are smaller (18) [usually under 5 mm (22)], are bilateral and often symmetric (15), and are in the inferior one third of the putamen (22).

PERIVENTRICULAR HYPERINTENSE WHITE MATTER LESIONS

Periventricular hyperintense white matter lesions (PVH) are contiguous with the margins of the lateral ventricles (6). They range in extent from small focal lesions to cloaking of most of the lateral ventricular margins (Fig. 6) to irregular confluent high signal extending into the deep white matter (see Fig. 24) (6). PVH increases with increasing age and in patients with a variety of cerebral pathologies (6). They may be present in up to 10% to 30% of cognitively normal elderly patients (26). The larger lesions may represent true infarcts with associated gliosis increasing the apparent size of the lesion (27).

A physiologic process (6), corroborated in pathologic investigations (28,29), may help to explain these findings. Water escapes from the vascular system into the extracellular space in aging, and in pathological processes (6). The cerebral hemispheres lack a lymphatic system to drain this interstitial space. This extracellular water flows in a centripetal fashion from more peripheral sites within the white matter to the more confined periventricular region to drain into the lateral ventricles. The higher concentration of interstitial water at the ventricular lining likely contributes to the high signal on long TR sequences. With aging and in association with a variety of cerebral pathologic conditions, interstitial water is increased, contributing to the increase in PVH. In hydrocephalus, the distribution of PVH is similar to that in patients with increased interstitial water from parenchymal abnormalities but the direction of flow is the opposite (ventriculofugal) (6). In hydrocephalus, ependymal cells flatten and stretch, ultimately becoming denuded, which facilitates entry of CSF into brain (11).

Deep White Matter

Hyperintense white matter lesions can also be seen in the corona radiata, centrum semiovale, and subcortical regions—with distinct sparing of the subcortical arcuate

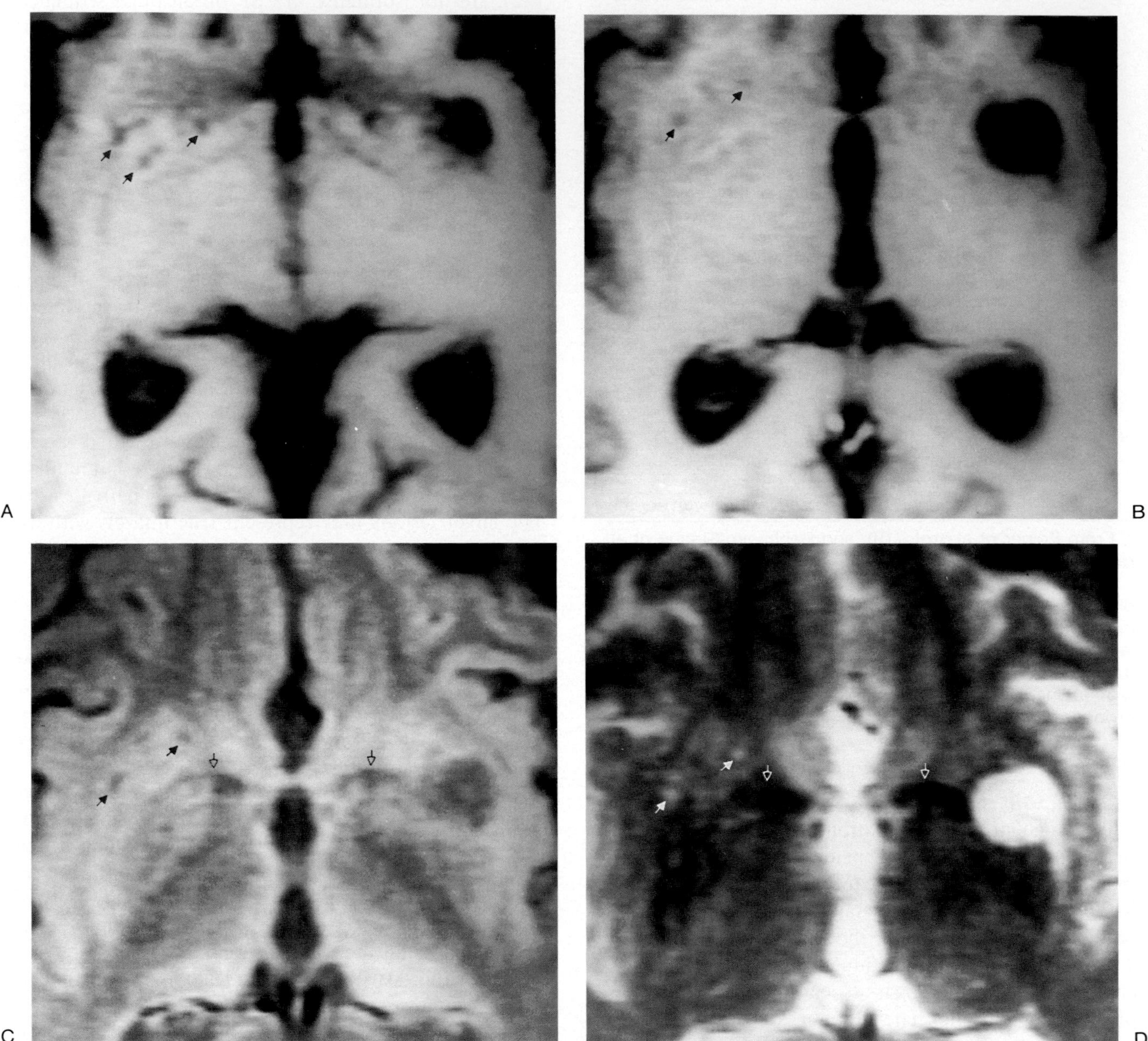

FIG. 4. Prominent VRS in right putamen, cystic lacunar infarct in left putamen. **A–D:** Axial MR images before death (A,B) 600/20, (C) 2500/30, and (D) 2500/80, (×2 magnification). VRS are very small, are round or linear, and are isointense to CSF. Note relationship of VRS to the anterior commissure (*open arrows*). The cystic infarct is also isointense to CSF.

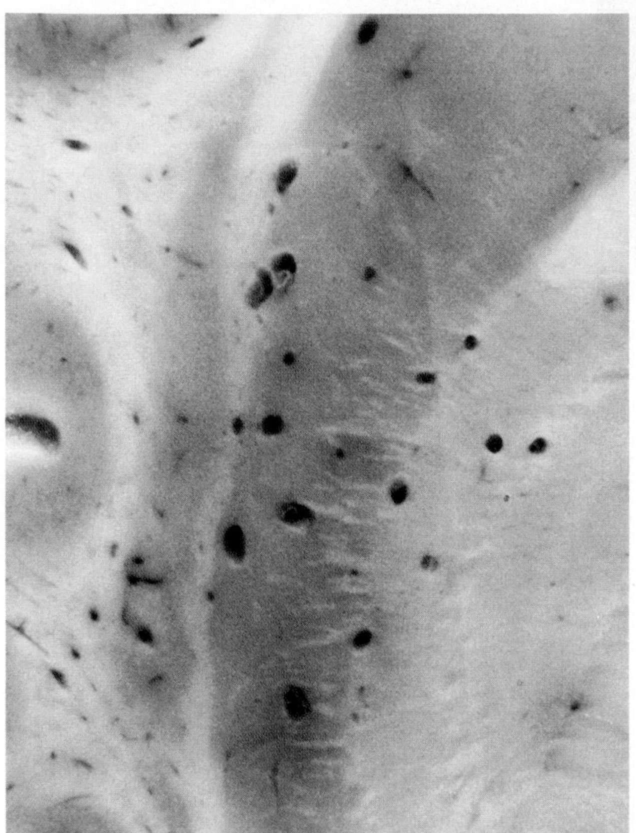
E

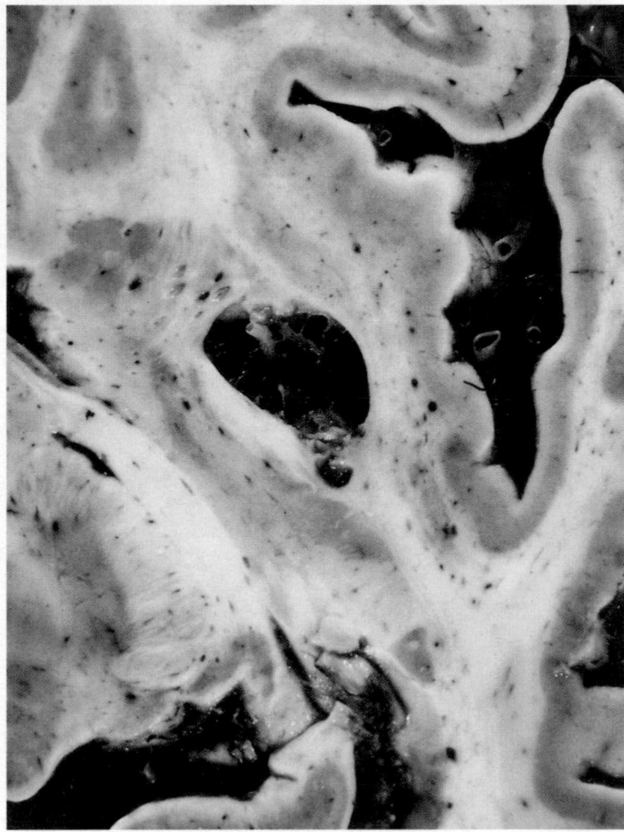
F

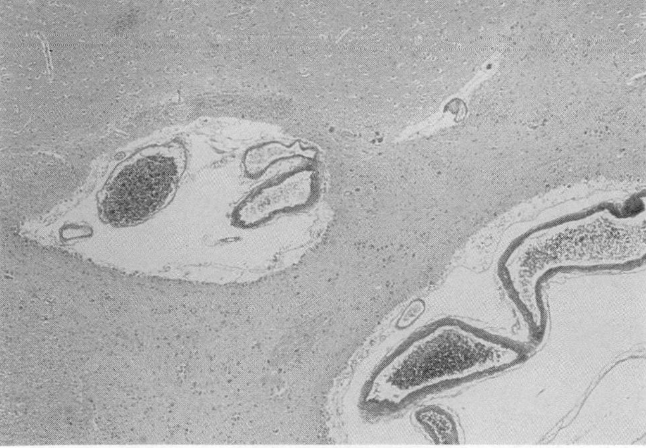
G

FIG. 4. (*Continued.*) **E,F:** Gross pathology. Dilated VRS in the putamen (E) and cavitated, round infarct (F). Histopathology (not shown) revealed reactive astrocytes in the wall of this old healed infarct. **G:** Stained section (H&E) of basal forebrain of a different elderly patient illustrates degree of perivascular spaces frequently occurring in these individuals. (From Braffman et al., ref. 18, with permission.)

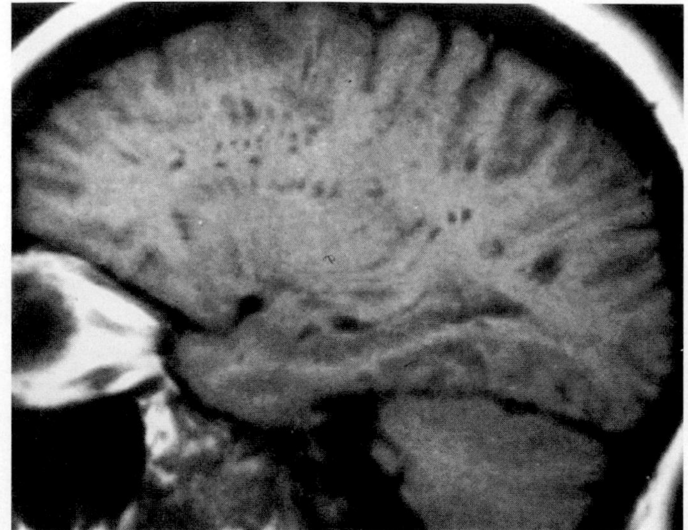

A

FIG. 5. High convexity VRS. **A:** Sagittal plane, TR/TE 600/20. Axial (**B,C**) and coronal (**D,E**) planes. TR/TE 2500/30 (B,D) and TR/TE 2500/80 (C,E). Dilated VRS are well-defined, small, foci isointense to CSF on all pulse sequences. In this patient they appear round (A), and curvilinear (B–E). On the first echo of the long TR sequence, in which CSF is nearly isointense to white matter, the VRS are virtually undetectable (B, D). Note subcortical lesion (SCL, *arrow,* D,E), in contrast, is hyperintense on both first and second echoes of the long TR sequence.

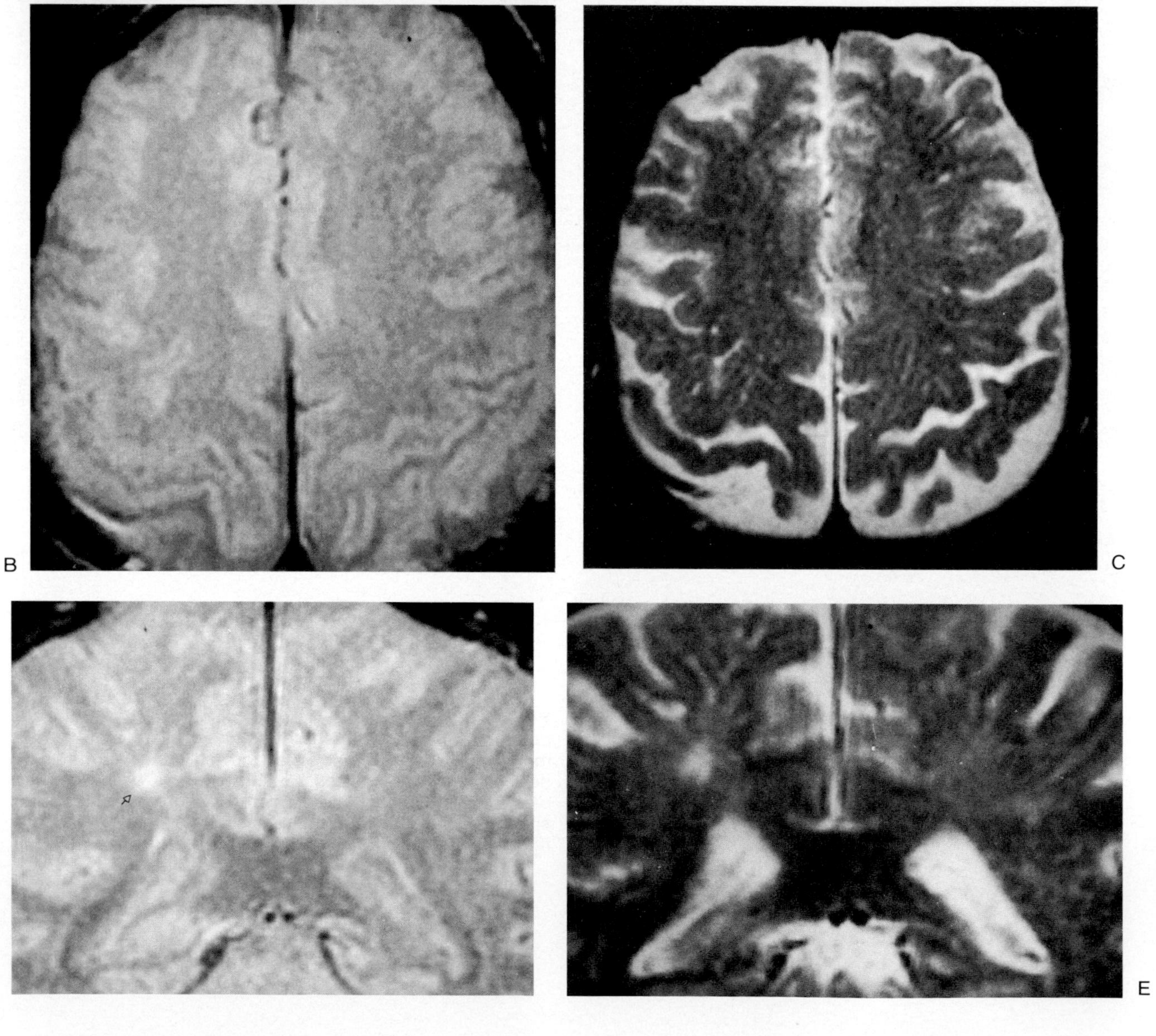

B

C

D

E

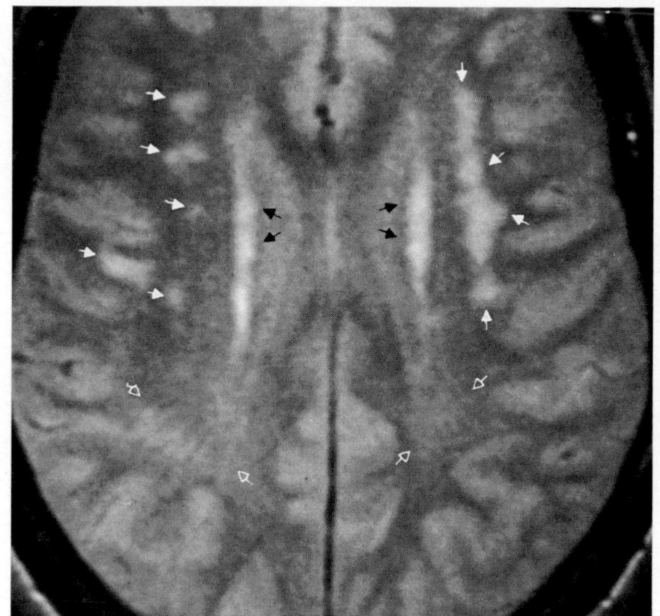

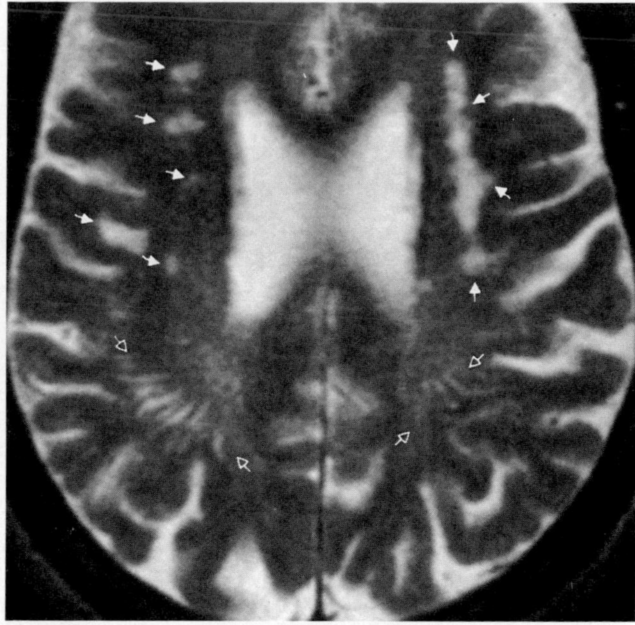

FIG. 6. Axial, long TR, short (**A**) and long (**B**) TE. Curvilinear foci in the white matter posterior to the lateral ventricles (*white open arrows*) have morphology, size, and configuration of dilated VRS, but are at least partly hyperintense to CSF on the first echo of the long TR sequence (A), particularly on the right. They do become brighter on the second echo (B). The hyperintense signal on both first and second echoes may correspond to gliosis and/or demyelination surrounding the dilated perivascular spaces. Alternatively, T1 and T2 shortening may be due to association of water in the confined perivascular spaces to proteins. Other types of hyperintense white matter foci are also present. Subcortical and deep white matter lesions (SCL) (*closed white arrows*) are hyperintense to brain on both echoes (A,B), range in size from punctate (several in right hemisphere) to larger patchy irregular foci (in left hemisphere) and invariably spare the subcortical U fibers (55). They are particularly prevalent at the upper portions of the lateral ventricles (30). Periventricular hyperintensity (PVH) (*black arrows,* A) are also hyperintense to brain on both echoes (A,B), but are difficult to differentiate from hyperintense CSF of the adjacent lateral ventricles on the long TR/TE sequence (B). They are contiguous with the margins of the lateral ventricles.

U fibers (Figs. 6 and 7) (30). Similar to the periventricular findings, these also increase in number and extent with increasing age (6,8,30–35). The lesions range from punctate (smaller than 0.5 cm) to larger, patchy, irregular lesions (greater than 1 cm in size) (30). They are hyperintense to brain parenchyma on both echoes of the long TR sequences and are not usually seen on the short TR sequence (36). In contrast to some other pathologic entities, these do not enhance with Gd-DTPA (37), and do not exert mass effect. Leukoaraiosis appears to have nonspecific neurologic sequelae according to some authors (38); however, some investigators have correlated lesion sites with certain abnormalities, for example frontal lesions and subtle motor deficits (26).

The exact histologic correlate of these deep white matter lesions remains controversial. However, the results of several pathologic investigations (27,39–44) suggest that these findings represent a variety of pathologies ranging from ischemic foci to infarctions. These have been variably described pathologically as perivascular atrophic demyelination (43), incomplete infarcts (40), "état criblé" (39) or lesions intermediate between white matter gliosis and small infarcts (44) (Fig. 7). The role of this histologic substrate is supported by analysis of the vascular anatomy in typical sites (see discussion below) (36,45,46) and by positive correlation of the presence of these lesions with cerebrovascular risk factors (i.e., hypertension, carotid artery stenosis, high Hachinski ischemic score, transient ischemic attack, or completed stroke), documented in multiple investigations (30–34,47–50). Measurement of local cerebral blood flow has shown diminished blood flow in areas of periventricular high signal and leukoaraiosis (8). A common clinical problem is the differentiation of age-related hyperintense white matter foci from ischemia, demyelinating disorders, and other multifocal neuropathologic processes. While this distinction on MR often may not be possible, differential features, based on published investigations, are summarized in Table 2. Idiopathic white matter lesions demonstrate longer T1, higher proton density, and longer T2 than normal white matter (60).

A study of asymptomatic volunteers suggested that both age and the use of antihypertensive medication were associated with the number of focal hyperintensities (61). However, interobserver variability in analyzing high-signal foci is high unless a preliminary consensus is

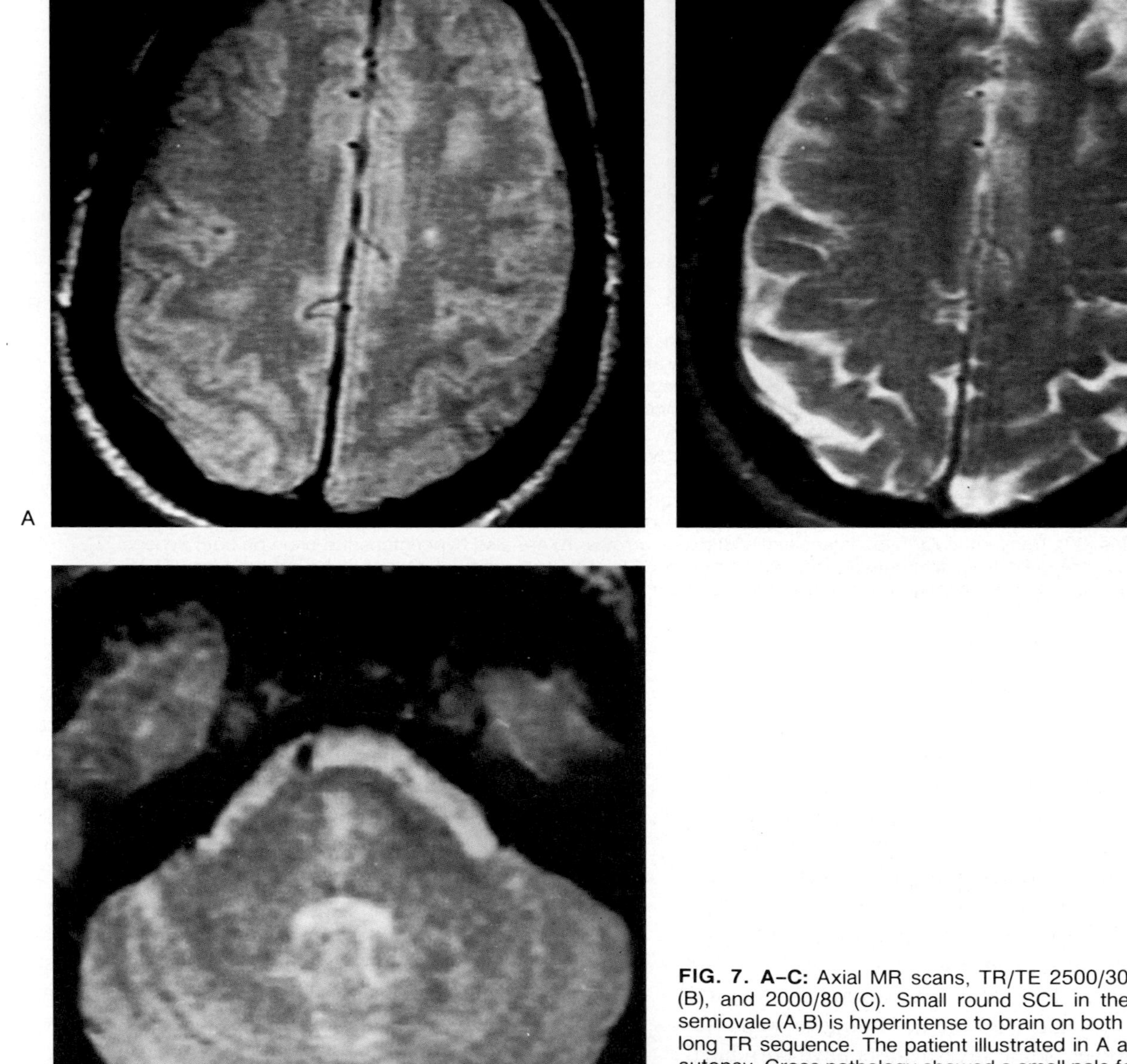

FIG. 7. A–C: Axial MR scans, TR/TE 2500/30 (A), 2500/80 (B), and 2000/80 (C). Small round SCL in the left centrum semiovale (A,B) is hyperintense to brain on both echoes of the long TR sequence. The patient illustrated in A and B came to autopsy. Gross pathology showed a small pale focus. Histopathology revealed a focus difficult to categorize and was described as either gliosis or infarction. In the brainstem (C), these hyperintense foci predominate in the central portion of the mid and upper pons (56), reflecting the vascular anatomy to this region (see text). (From Braffman et al., ref. 44, with permission.)

established in advance (62). A study at low field strength examined aged individuals (75–85 years old) with above average health and intellectual function. This group demonstrated less than 9% incidence of white matter lesions (4).

An autopsy study of six patients with incidental foci of high-signal intensity on MRI revealed that small, punctate foci of high-signal intensity showed areas of reduced myelination and neuropil atrophy. These were centered on hyalinized arteries. In addition, myelin rarefaction and demyelination was observed in a perivenous distribution (63).

Anatomic Predisposition to Ischemia

Detection of deep white matter lesions on MRI and pathologic changes of subacute arteriosclerotic encephalopathy (SAE—discussed below) typically occur in the centrum semiovale (particularly in the upper portions of the lateral ventricles) (30), basal ganglia, lateral one-quarter of the corpus callosum (51), and the central portions of the mid and upper pons (45,53) (Fig. 7). These lesions usually spare the cortex, subcortical U fibers, central corpus callosum (51), medulla, midbrain, cerebellar peduncles, and cerebellar hemispheres (53). The anatomy of the blood supply to these areas and their variable vulnerability to hypoperfusion may account for these differences (51,53).

Two anatomic patterns provide protection from hypoperfusion to selected cerebral areas (64). The first is collateral blood supply from cortical vessels, which supplies the subcortical U fibers and the external capsule, claustrum, and extreme capsule (64). This supplements the supply from deep penetrating vessels coming from the inferior surface of the brain. The second involves short arterioles (approximately 8 mm) that do not experience a significant pressure drop with hypoperfusion, and are not subject to aging and hypertensive changes such as spirals, loops, or kinks (64). This afferent supply exists in the corpus callosum (including the splenium), cortical gray matter (64), medulla, and midbrain (53). These protective vascular features do not exist in the basal ganglia, extreme lateral corpus callosum, thalamus, or centrum ovale. These latter regions are supplied by noninterdigitating long arteries and long arterioles (20 to 50 mm) (64). Hypoperfusion quickly overwhelms the ability of these vessels to autoregulate because arteries are more vulnerable than arterioles to vascular changes

TABLE 2. *MR differential features of multiple sclerosis and age-related subcortical and periventricular lesions*[a]

	Multiple sclerosis	SCL and PVH
Location		
Subcortical arcuate "U" fibers	Yes (6)	No (51)
Corpus callosum	Yes (51)	No (51)
Basal ganglia	Uncommon (52)	Common (52)
Brainstem	Any site (53)	Frequently central and midportion upper pons (53)
Cerebellar peduncles	Common (53)	Uncommon (53)
Cerebellar white matter	Common (53)	Uncommon (53)
Adjacent to aqueduct	Common (52)	Uncommon (52)
Adjacent to 4th ventricle	Common (52)	Uncommon (52)
Signal characteristics		
Short TR sequence	Often hypointense (52), but variable	Often not seen (53) on routine short TR/TE sequences
Short TR with Gd-DTPA	Active lesions enhance (54)	No enhancement (37)
Long TR sequence	Hyperintense	Hyperintense
Lesion orientation	Variable; occasionally seen as Dawson's fingers (55) [i.e., thin or plump elliptically shaped lesions in the periventricular white matter with their major axes pointed perpendicular to the anteroposterior axis of the head (56).]	Variable
Morphology	Variable	Variable, ranging from smooth (57) to irregular
Size	Often greater than or equal to 6 mm, but variable (58)	Typically less than 6 mm, but variable (58)
Clinical data		
Age	Younger adults (50,59)	Older adults (50,59)
Symptoms	Often symptomatic, but variable correlation between symptoms and lesions	Absence of widespread symptoms (50)

[a] These criteria sometimes permit differentiation of multiple sclerosis from age-related hyperintense white matter foci on MRI. In most cases, however, this distinction may not be possible on MRI, and clinical information, in fact, is essential to MR interpretation. SCL, subcortical lesions; PVH, periventricular hyperintense lesions.

from aging and hypertension, and a greater pressure drop occurs with a long penetrating arteriole or artery than with a short arteriole (64). As a result the regions supplied by these vessels are more susceptible to hypoperfusion. Common conditions that may cause a reduction in perfusion pressure are cardiac disease (arrhythmias, congestive heart failure, myocardial infarction), hypotensive shock, respiratory insufficiency, and vascular occlusive disease (i.e., distal to a high-grade arteriole stenosis (64).

HYPOINTENSITY OF EXTRAPYRAMIDAL NUCLEI DUE TO IRON DEPOSITION

The changing signal intensities of the deep gray matter nuclei with normal aging have been documented at 1.5 T (14,65) (Figs. 8–10). During the first 10 years of life the extrapyramidal nuclei studied are isointense to cortical gray matter (65) (Fig. 8). In most patients by age 25, the globus pallidus, followed by the red nucleus and pars reticulata of the substantia nigra, become hypointense relative to cortical gray matter and to white matter on the long TR/TE sequence (65) (Fig. 9). The dentate nucleus decreases in signal intensity more slowly and inconsistently; only $\frac{1}{3}$ of patients' dentate nuclei are hypointense relative to white matter by age 25 (65). With further aging, hypointensity in the caudate and putamen progresses and may equal that in the globus pallidus in individuals in their eighth decade (Fig. 10) (66).

A report using a carefully screened pool of normal adult volunteers showed that the volume of deep gray matter hypointensity on long TR/TE images in the red nucleus, substantia nigra, and dentate nucleus was relatively stable, showing no definite relationship to age. However, the globus pallidus showed increased volume of hypointensity in middle-aged and older patients, while the putamen showed measurable hypointensity only in elderly patients. None of the normals had hypointensity in the thalamus or caudate (67).

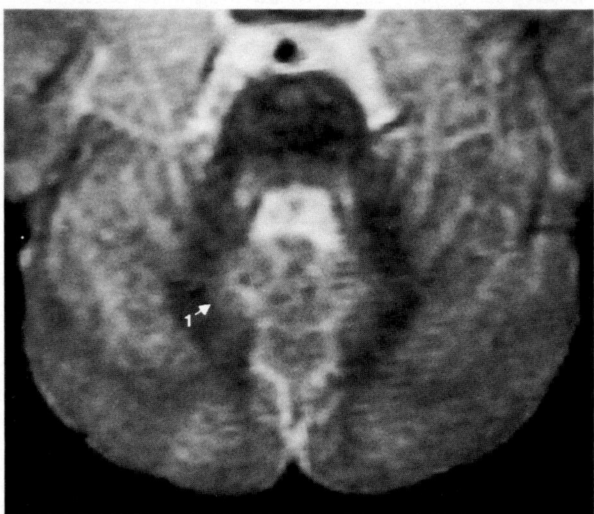

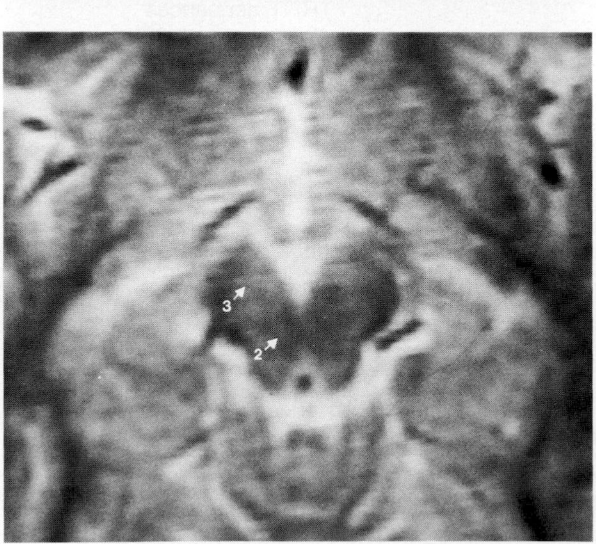

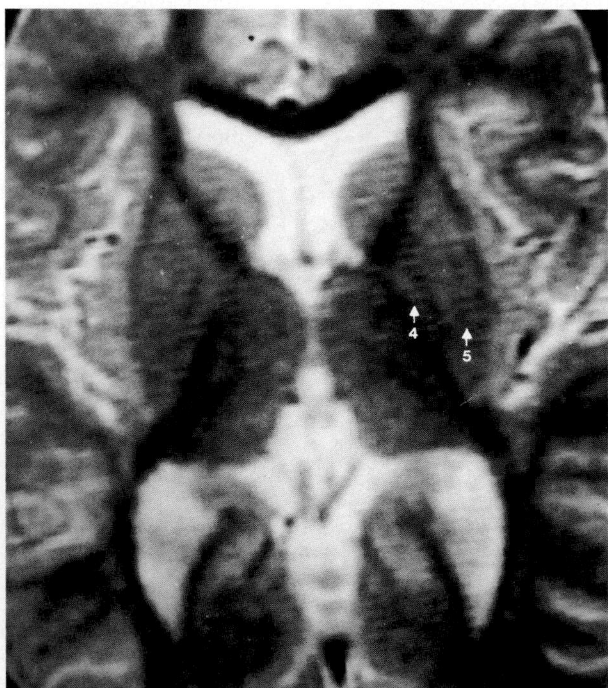

FIG. 8. Age-related signal intensity on long TR/TE at 1.5 T sequences of dentate nuclei (*1* in **A**), red nuclei, and pars reticulata of the substantia nigra (*2* and *3*, respectively, in **B**), and globus pallidus and putamen (*4* and *5*, respectively, in **C**). At 2 years old these gray matter nuclei are isointense to cortical gray matter and hyperintense to white matter.

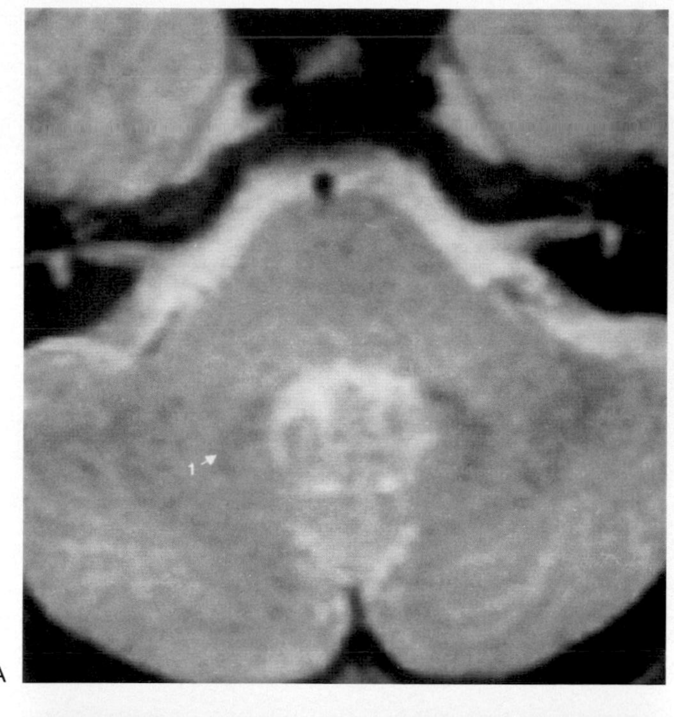

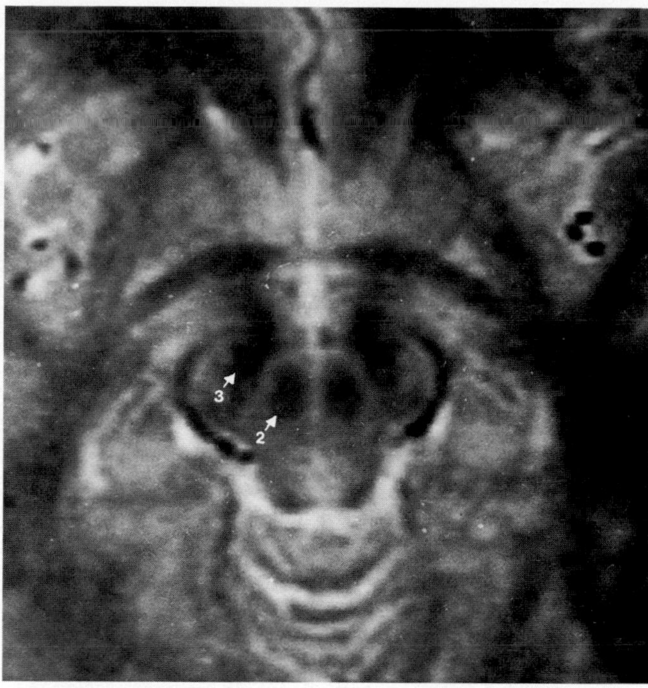

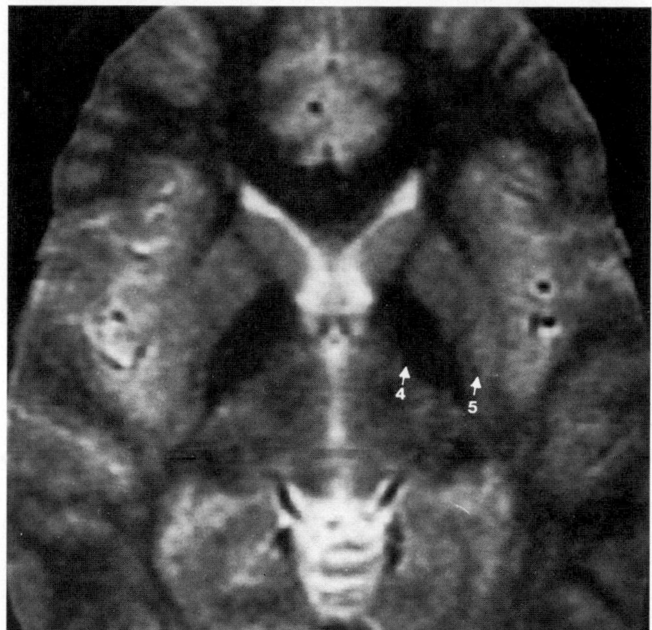

FIG. 9. At age 27 years, the globus pallidus, red nucleus, pars reticulata of the substantia nigra, and, to a lesser extent, the dentate nuclei are hypointense to cortical gray and to white matter. Note the greater degree of hypointensity of the globus pallidus in this 27-year-old imaged at 1.5 T to that of a 33-year-old patient at 0.5 T in Fig. 3. The hypointense signal of the anterior commissure in Fig. 9B is not due to iron but is secondary to heavy myelination and fiber density (433). Note the normal PVS anterior to anterior commissure.

While the cause of this age-related apparent T2 shortening has been controversial (68–73), iron deposition most likely accounts for these MR observations in aging (25,66,67,74,75) as well as in a wide variety of pathologic disorders (13,66,76–91; F. J. Lexa, S. W. Atlas, W. Milton et al., *unpublished data*).

The hypointense signal correlates with Perls' staining for ferric iron (13,14) and follows the same anatomic and age-related trend of iron deposition documented by other investigations of pathologic material (74). This signal loss probably arises from proton diffusion through local areas of magnetic homogeneity due to the iron-containing moieties (92,93).

The magnitude of this effect is dependent upon several technical factors. Factors that increase the conspicuousness of the hypointense signal include a greater concentration of compartmentalized paramagnetic substance, an increased signal-to-noise ratio [e.g., increasing the (TR) repetition time], a prolonged (TE) echo time, a longer interecho interval, use of gradient reversal for signal acquisition, and higher field strength (compare Figs. 3 and 9) (88,94,95). The dependence of T2 shortening

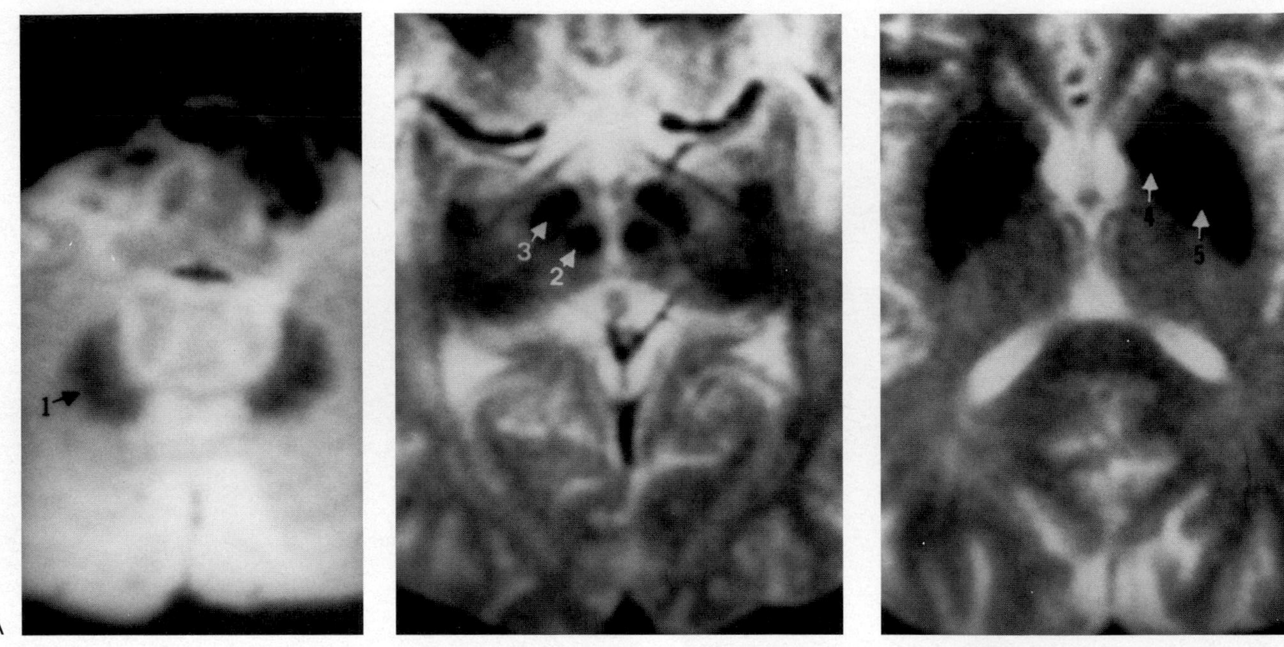

FIG. 10. This healthy 80-year-old displays hypointensity of the putamen almost as pronounced as in the globus pallidus. (From Cross et al., ref. 88, with permission.)

from inhomogeneity on field strength may in part resolve some of the conflicting reports regarding iron and apparent hypointensity. Brooks et al. showed that the T2 of the basal ganglia only decreased 50% with increases of Tesla from 2.35 to 8.5 (70). Another group examined Rhesus monkeys at field strengths from 0.5 to 4.7 Tesla and again found that there was less than the expected quadratic effect, with a "saturation" at higher strengths that they felt was due to more complicated super or antiferromagnetic effects in the core of the iron deposits (71). Mathematical modeling (96) and more recent in vitro and in vivo work support the role of iron as the cause of observed hypointensity on long TR/TE imaging in the basal ganglia (97,98).

Many processes lead to the final common pathway of marked hypointensity on long TR/TE images in the extrapyramidal nuclei, thalami, and deep white matter. These include demyelinating [multiple sclerosis (Fig. 11) (85)] and dysmyelinating processes (Pelizaeus-Merzbacher disease) (99), trauma (F. J. Lexa, S. W. Atlas, W. Milton, et al., *unpublished data*), and cerebral infarcts (Fig. 12) (86,88). The mechanism by which iron accumulates in these sites is not completely understood (86,88). Insights from research on the transport pathway for brain iron, however, provide an interesting hypothesis. Intracellular iron has an important role in the metabolism of neurotransmitters, and is normally found in the basal ganglia (100–104). Iron is taken up by capillary endothelial cells in the thalamus and extrapyramidal system after transferrin (the main iron-containing protein of the plasma) binds to a specific receptor on the cell surface (105,106). Iron is thought to be subsequently transported along neuronal axons to their sites of projection (86). It is possible that iron continues to accumulate at sites of uptake (i.e., in the extrapyramidal nuclei) despite interruptions of specific axonal projections by multiple causes (i.e., infarction, demyelination, and/or neurodegenerative disorders) (86,88). Since iron is still taken up but can no longer be transported, increased amounts would accumulate proximally (86).

Iron may also be deposited directly in hemorrhagic areas of the brain (88,107–109) or from a variety of other insults including multiple sclerosis (110). Following an anoxic injury, calcium ion homeostasis is lost, followed by a loss of control of the intracellular iron pool during reperfusion. Low molecular weight iron species, as a transition metal catalyst, can then initiate free radical-mediated lipid peroxidation reactions, resulting in additional brain tissue injury (88,107,109).

THE INJURED BRAIN: WALLERIAN DEGENERATION

Degenerative changes in the distal axonal segment occur after it is separated from the proximal axon or when the neuronal cell body is damaged or killed. This occurs as a series of events that was first described at the histologic level by Waller almost 150 years ago (111). Wallerian degeneration occurs in several discreet stages (112,113). The earliest event consists of interruption of axonal transport, collapse of the axon, and opening of Schmidt-Lantermann incisures in the overlying myelin (114). This leads to physical breakup and degradation of

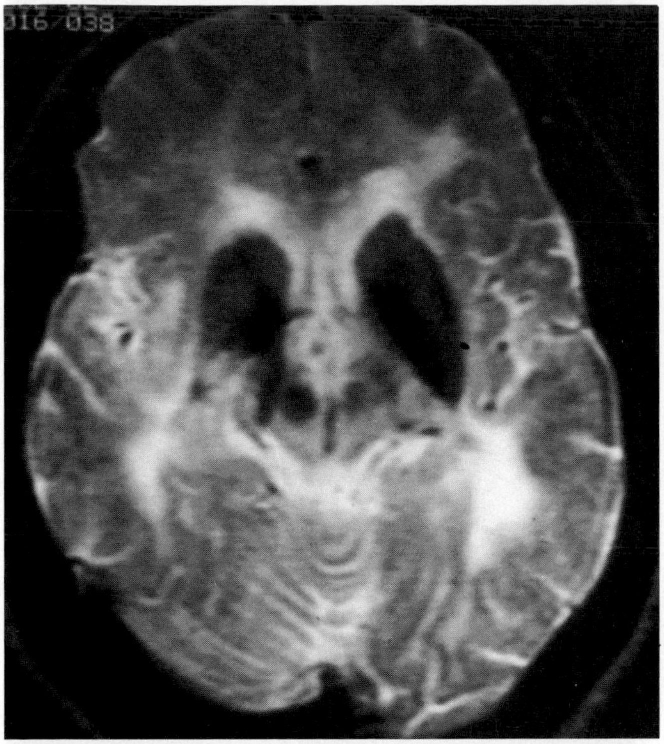

A

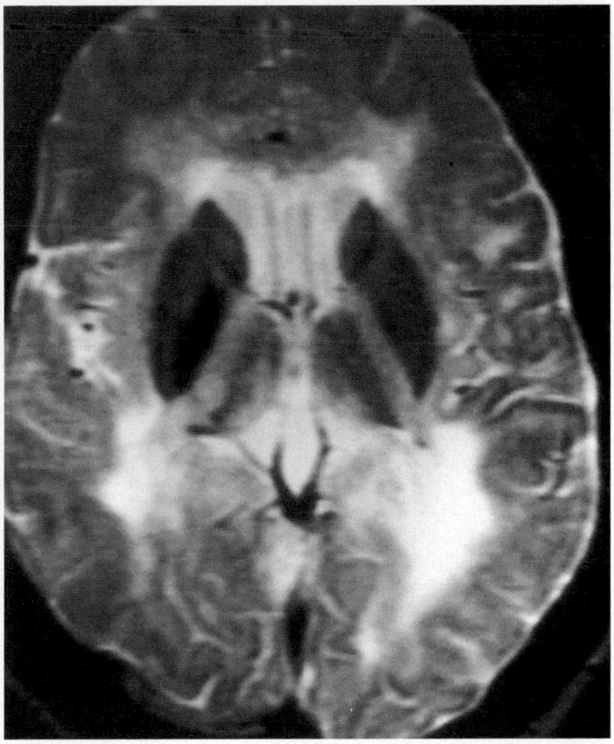

B

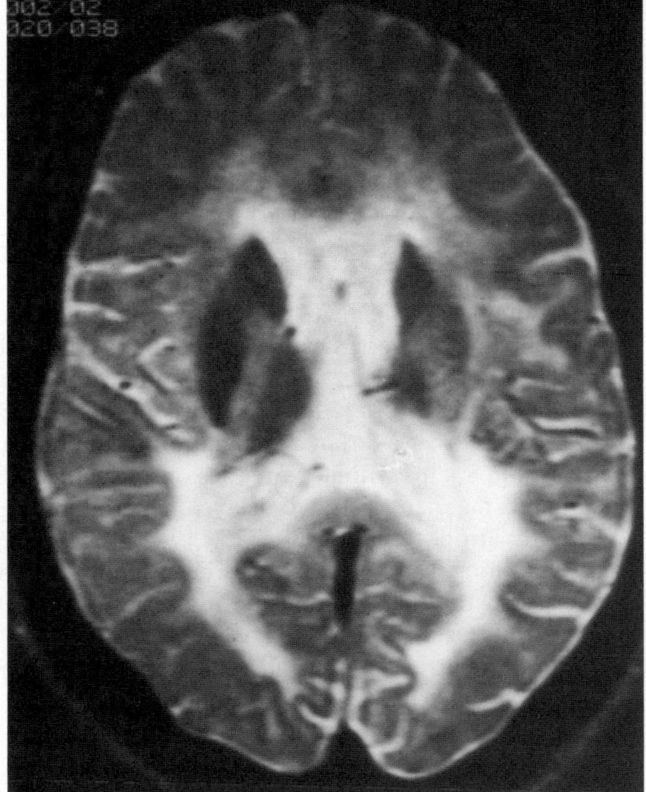

C

FIG. 11. In this patient with a clinical diagnosis of multiple sclerosis, white matter involvement (hyperintense on this long TR/TE sequence) is extensive. Note the marked hypointense signal of the red nuclei, pars reticulata of the substantia nigra, thalami, globus pallidi, caudate, and putamen (**A–C**).

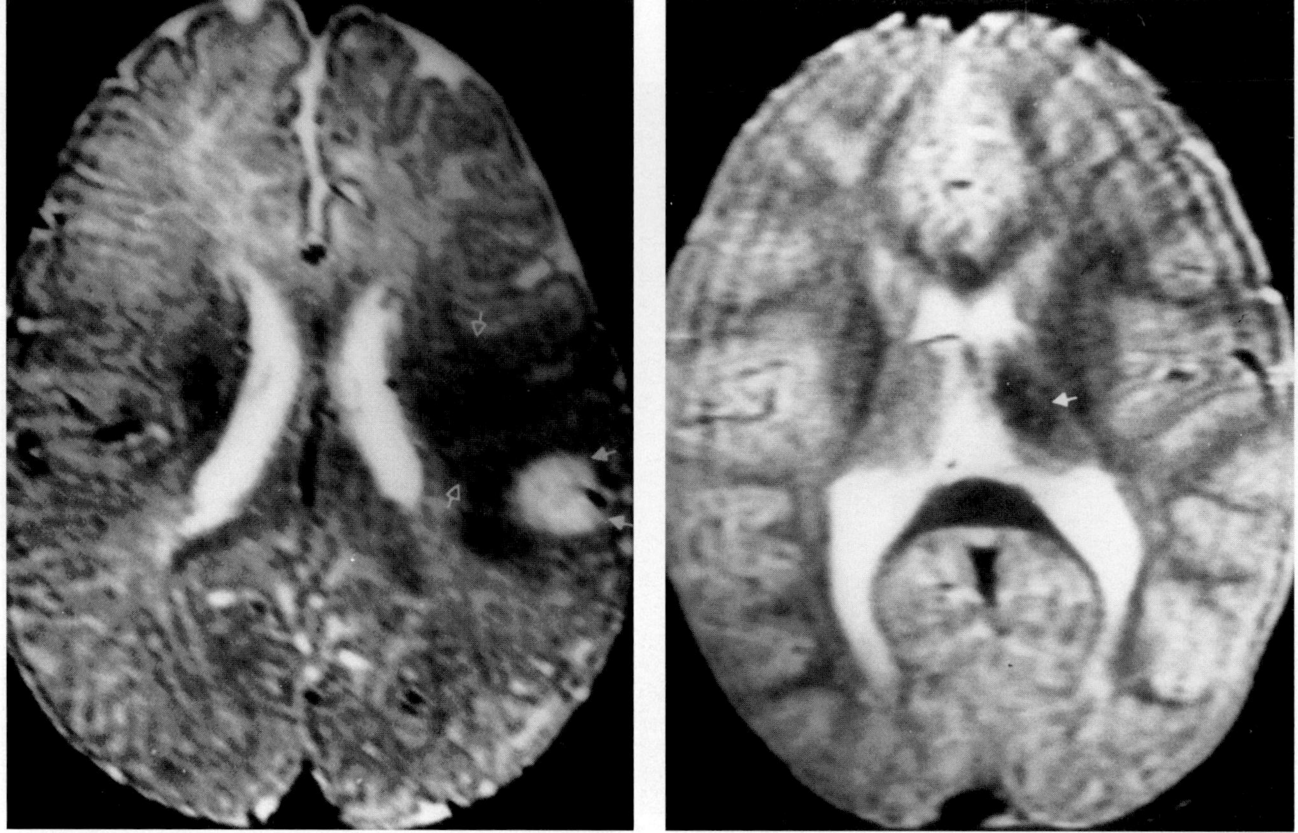

FIG. 12. Infarctions in two infants, aged 7 months (**A**), and $1\frac{1}{2}$ years (**B**), respectively, showing associated abnormal hypointensity on long TR/TE sequences at 1.5 T. TR/TE 2500/80 (A). Diffuse white matter hypointensity (*open arrows*), probably due to iron deposition, is adjacent to hyperintense left parietal lobe infarct (*closed arrows*). TR/TE 3000/90 (B). Hypointense signal in left thalamus (*arrow*) is present $1\frac{1}{2}$ months after clinical infarction. Abnormal hypointensity in both of these infants is present at an age in which virtually no physiologic cerebral iron was found in pathologic investigation (74) and no normal hypointensity on an MR investigation (65). (From Cross et al., ref. 88, with permission.)

the surrounding myelin sheath. Later, there is a cellular stage with cell proliferation and edema. At this point, the myelin is chemically broken down and removed. Finally, there is resultant volume loss with gliosis (Fig. 13).

Detection of axonal degeneration is important for many reasons in clinical neuroradiology. The ubiquitous nature of this process means that this represents an "injury signal" in the central nervous system. A better understanding of the signal characteristics of its components will lead to improved sensitivity and specificity in the detection of most of the diseases that attack the CNS. Moreover, the lack of significant regeneration of axonal tracts in the human CNS means that the presence of the final stage of degeneration would be expected to have important prognostic implications in certain critical pathways. In particular, it should be possible to discriminate between reversible and irreversible forms of neuronal injury. Work investigating this hypothesis with regard to motor recovery from middle cerebral artery infarction has shown that detectable degeneration in the corticospinal projection pathways is associated with significantly poorer prognosis (115,116).

Conventional MR scanning is far superior to CT for the detection and staging of wallerian degeneration. It is capable of detecting changes in the physical structure of the myelin tracts, whereas with few exceptions CT is only capable of detecting the volume loss and atrophy that occur late in the process. Initial reports of the MR appearance of CNS wallerian degeneration in the human came from patients with acquired lesions, usually cortical infarcts that demonstrated delayed hyperintense signal and/or atrophy on long TR/TE (117–120). Hyperintensity on long TR/TE images has been reported to be associated with T1 hypointensity in a series of infarcts that were at least 3 months old (121).

In a later study, Kuhn et al. (122) reported a more complex signal pattern with no abnormality before 4 weeks, decreased signal intensity on T2-weighted images at 4 weeks, and elevation of signal intensity at 10–14 weeks with a corresponding drop in signal intensity on T1 imaging. The drop in signal intensity on T2-weighted images was ascribed to a transitory increase in lipid-protein ratio. Uchino et al. (123) also reported a multiphase effect at 1.5 Tesla with loss of signal intensity seen as

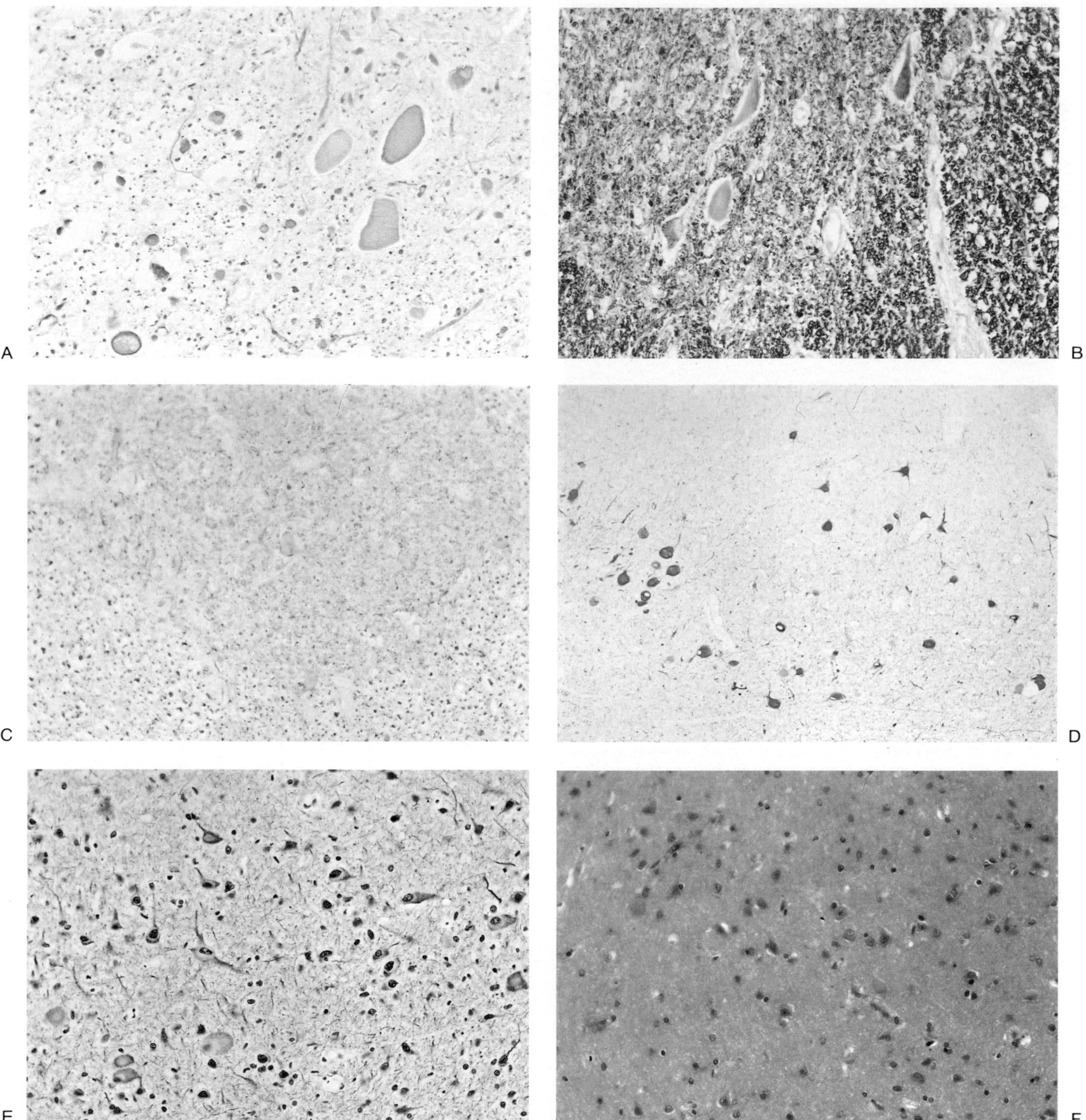

FIG. 13. Wallerian degeneration following injury. **A,B:** Consecutive sections of cervical spinal cord near the site of an epidural abscess that compressed and damaged the cord. The section in A was stained with antibodies to neurofilament (NF) proteins and shows swollen, chromatolytic neurons in gray matter (*to the right*), and axons undergoing wallerian degeneration in the white matter (*to the left*). These findings are less obvious in the adjacent section in B stained by Luxol fast blue—H&E. **C:** Uninjured spinal cord stained with the same anti-NF protein antibodies used in A. Note that neuronal perikarya are not NF positive or swollen (*upper portion*), while axons in the white matter are NF positive but show no evidence of swelling and fragmentation (*lower portion*). **D–F:** Chromatolytic cortical neurons following a white matter lesion that disrupted the axons of these cells. The section in D is stained with anti-NF antibodies that label normal axons but not normal neuronal perikarya, and all of the labeled neurons seen in D are swollen and undergoing chromatolysis. These neurons are not seen as well in sections stained with the Bodian method (E) or H&E (F).

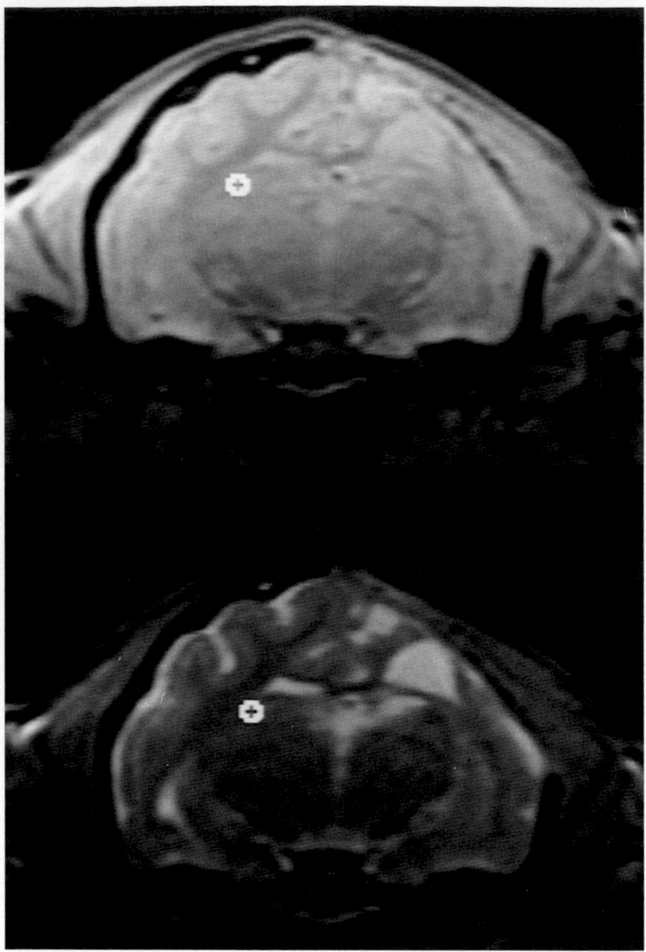

FIG. 14. Region of interest on the control side of the brain over white matter immediately superolateral to the lateral geniculate nucleus. (From Lexa et al., ref. 132, with permission.)

early as 25 days in the expected site of wallerian degeneration on proton-density images (2000/20/1) which later normalized at 70–80 days. Beyond 80 days increased signal intensity was seen on T2-weighted images, some with and some without corresponding signal loss on T1-weighted images. Pujol et al. (124) examined 24 patients at 1.5 Tesla in which 11 had definite and 6 possible evidence of T1 and T2 lengthening in the pyramidal tracts from infarcts of the internal capsule, all of whom were at least 3 months in age.

Similarly, Inoue et al. (125) noted T1 and T2 lengthening as the primary signal-intensity abnormality at 0.5 Tesla. In their study of 150 patients, 33 had this finding, which was observed as early as 5 weeks and was present in all 33 by 10 weeks, the prominence of which was said to be maximal at 3–6 months. Danek et al. (120) observed high signal intensity on T2-weighted images at 1.0 Tesla along the corticofugal pathways. In one patient, this was not seen at 17 days, appeared at 4–7 months, and normalized at 20 months. A second patient also demonstrated high signal at 4–7 months. In a report discussing the use of coronal imaging to examine the pyramidal tract, Orita et al. (127) examined 21 patients at 0.5 Tesla all at least 3.5 months status post a basal ganglia or cortical insult. All of these demonstrated high signal intensity on proton-density or T2-weighted images (2000/50/100). Resection of the dentate nucleus resulted in high signal intensity along the expected pathway of the dentato-rubro-thalamic tract with high signal intensity in the contralateral red nucleus, which was presumed to represent wallerian degeneration and anterograde transneuronal degeneration, respectively (128). Recent work suggests that FSE imaging shows early wallerian degeneration more conspicuously than conventional proton-density imaging (A. Kumar and F. J. Lexa, *unpublished data*).

Animal models have been used to address the controversies raised by the above studies. MR spectroscopy of peripheral nerve showed significant increases in T1- and T2-relaxation times 15 days after sectioning the sciatic nerve (129). Imaging of the tibial nerve confirmed that T2-signal intensity was elevated on long TR/TE images at day 15 in a crush injury model (20). Grossman et al. obtained histologic confirmation of wallerian degeneration in a feline model of radiation injury (130). These areas showed high signal intensity on long TR/TE images over 200 days after radiation injury. Using a cat ablation model another group reported hypointensity on

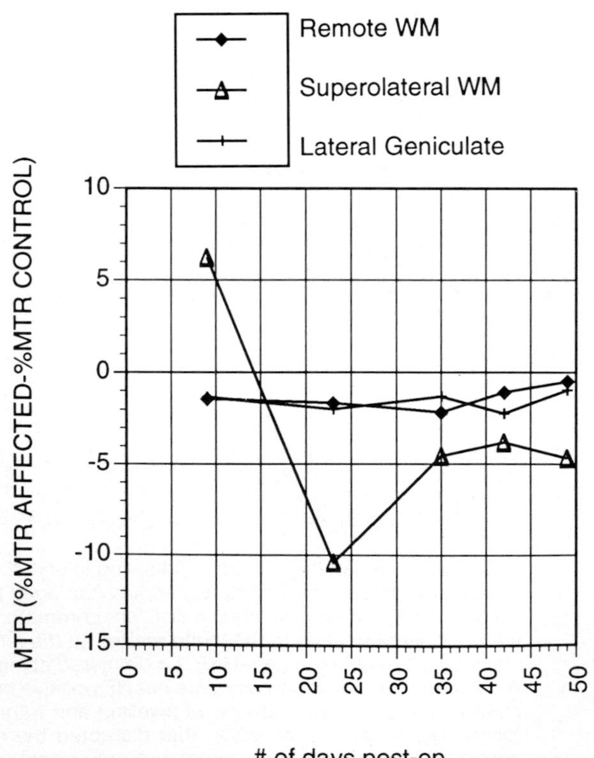

FIG. 15. Magnetization transfer ratio changes versus postoperative time. Complete data from animal 3. (From Lexa et al., ref. 132, with permission.)

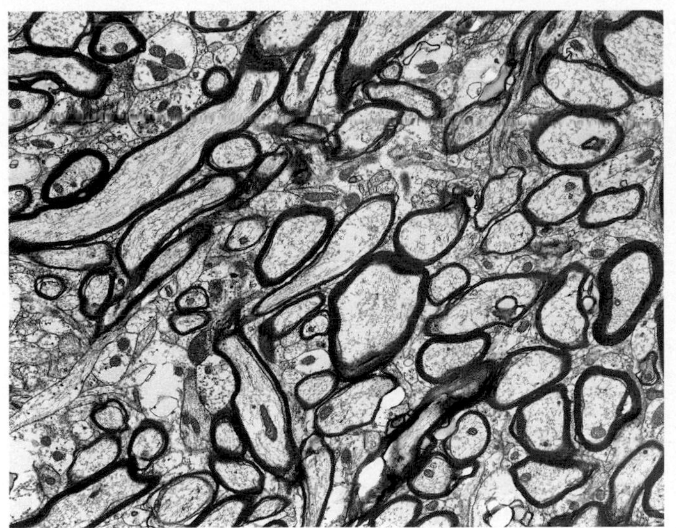

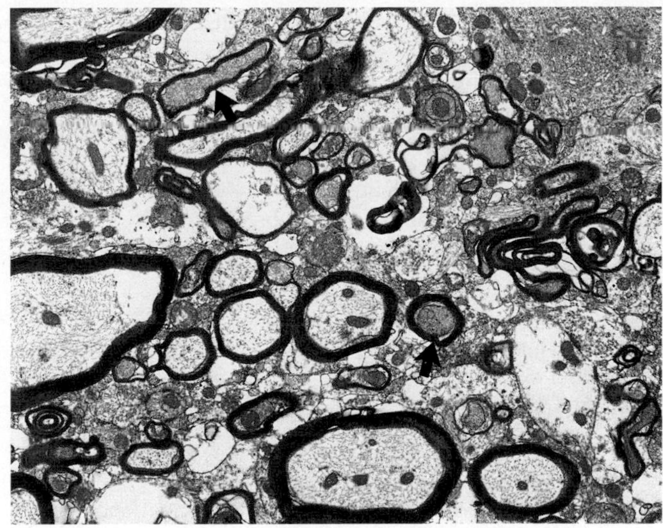

FIG. 16. A: Electron micrograph from white matter immediately superolateral to the lateral geniculate nucleus, contralateral to the ablated hemisphere. Normal findings at 8 days after surgery, no evidence of edema, inflammation, or degenerative changes. **B:** Electron micrograph from white matter immediately superolateral to the lateral geniculate, ipsilateral to ablation of the visual cortex, 8 days after surgery. Arrows demonstrate several examples of early changes of wallerian degeneration with increased axonal staining and irregularity and collapse of axons. (From Lexa et al., ref. 132, with permission.)

proton-density and T2-weighted images from 13 to 48 days in projection fiber pathways (131). Nothing was detectable for the first 12 days and these areas became undetectable in the period from 49 to 175 days. Histologic confirmation of the later stages of myelin loss and glial proliferation was obtained.

Newer techniques utilizing magnetization transfer techniques (discussed elsewhere) appear very promising for the early detection and separation of some of these changes. Using a cortical ablation model, Lexa et al. were able to demonstrate changes as early as the first week after injury (132). Magnetization transfer images detected degenerating tracts at a distance from the primary injury site before conventional spin-echo images or even routine light microscopy showed significant evidence of injury (Figs. 14 and 15). Electron microscopy confirmed that the first phase of wallerian degeneration was underway (Fig. 16). Myelin degeneration and cellular degeneration were not detectable by light microscopic techniques until significantly later. Moreover, the biphasic nature of the early changes in magnetization transfer suggest that it may be possible to separate some of the processes occurring early in axonal injury with these techniques.

NEURODEGENERATIVE DISEASES

Neurodegenerative diseases generally encompass disorders that currently have no known cause and are characterized by gradual progressive disintegration of part(s) of the nervous system. Some occur sporadically, while others depend on known genetic factors, and may be designated heredo-degenerative (1). By definition, neurodegenerative diseases begin insidiously, after a period of normal nervous system function. Their symptomatic expressions become possible only when the degree of neuronal loss reaches or exceeds the "safety factor" for a particular neuronal system (1).

For example, clinical manifestations of parkinsonism are thought to first become apparent following a loss of 80% of nigral dopaminergic neurons (133). With aging about half the nigral dopaminergic neurons are lost with a consequent reduction of basal ganglia dopamine levels to around 50% of that measured in young to middle-aged controls (133). This reduction during senescence is still far from reaching the critical value of 20% of function that would lead to a clinical state of parkinsonism. Neurodegenerative diseases pursue a gradually progressive course that may continue for many years (1). They are generally subdivided according to their pathologic anatomy and consequent clinical syndromes (1,134). Common related disorders with known causes that share significant clinical, pathologic, and radiologic features with primary neurodegenerative disorders are also presented (Table 3).

Gross pathology and neuroimaging in general are characterized by focal atrophy due to neuronal loss. MRI of most neurodegenerative disorders also shows abnormal hyperintensity or hypointensity in affected areas on long TR sequences (13,135). The former is due to prolongation of the T2-relaxation time secondary to an increased water content in the setting of neuronal loss, gliosis, demyelination, and wallerian degeneration. The

TABLE 3. *Neurodegenerative and related disorders*

I. Dementias
  A. Primary neurodegenerative disorders
    1. Alzheimer's disease
    2. Pick's disease
  B. Related disorders
    1. Multi-infarct dementia
    2. Normal pressure hydrocephalus
    3. Creutzfeldt-Jacob disease
II. Degeneration of extrapyramidal nuclei
  A. Primary neurodegenerative disorders
    1. Huntington's disease
    2. Hallervorden-Spatz disease
    3. Leigh's syndrome
  B. Related disorders
    1. Mitochondrial encephalomyelopathies
    2. Wilson's disease
    3. Acquired hepatocerebral syndromes
    4. Hypoxic-ischemic insults (e.g., carbon monoxide poisoning)
III. Degeneration of the substantia nigra and related systems: parkinsonisms
  A. Primary neurodegenerative disorders
    1. Parkinson's disease
    2. Striatonigral degeneration
    3. Shy-Drager syndrome
    4. Progressive supranuclear palsy
    5. Multiple system atrophy
  B. Secondary parkinsonisms
    1. Infarction
    2. Infection
    3. Trauma
    4. Drug or toxin-induced
IV. Degeneration of cerebellum, brainstem, and spinal cord
  A. Primary neurodegenerative disorders
    1. Olivopontocerebellar degeneration
    2. Cerebellar-olivary degeneration
    3. Infantile cerebellar ataxia
    4. Acetazolamide-responsive familial ataxia
    5. Friedreich's ataxia
  B. Acquired cerebellar degenerations
    1. Alcohol abuse
    2. Paraneoplastic disorders
    3. Drug toxicity (dilantin, diphenylhydantoin, high-dose cytosine arabinoside)
    4. Chronic poisoning with thallium or toluene (rare)
    5. Following influenza vaccination (rare)
V. Degeneration of motor system
  A. Primary neurodegenerative disorders
    1. Amyotrophic lateral sclerosis
    2. Progressive spinal muscular atrophy
    3. Progressive bulbar palsy
    4. Juvenile amyotrophy of distal upper extremity
  B. Related disorders
    1. Wallerian degeneration

Data from Adams and Victor, ref. (1), and Schoene, ref. (134).

[a] This table includes neurodegenerative disorders (which, by definition, have no known cause) and common, related disorders with known causes that share significant clinical, pathologic, and radiologic features. They are classified according to pathologic anatomy and consequent clinical syndrome(s). This table does not include rare neurodegenerative or related disorders.

latter is due to deposition of iron and/or other paramagnetic substances that induce preferential T2-proton relaxation shortening.

Additional histologic hallmarks of many neurodegenerative disorders (as well as normal aging) are extracellular deposits of β-amyloid peptides in neuritic or diffuse plaques and various abnormal neuronal inclusions (Table 4) (131,136–146). These include neurofibrillary tangles (NFTs) first described by Alzheimer in 1907 (147) and Lewy bodies (LBs) in Parkinson's disease, first reported by Lewy in 1913 (148). Recent immunocytochemical techniques utilizing monoclonal and polyclonal antibodies have established that these abnormalities are selective disorganized states of the neuronal cytoskeleton (i.e., tau in NFTs and neurofilament proteins in LBs) (136,140–146) (Fig. 17). These cytoskeletal lesions are thought to arise from abnormal proteolysis and phosphorylation (140–146).

Dementia

Intelligence or intelligent behavior is "the aggregate or global capacity of the individual to act purposefully, to think rationally, and to deal effectively with his environment" (1,149). In dementia, intellectual faculties and higher integrative faculties are impaired, such that it interferes with the activities of daily living (1,15). The precise prevalence of dementia in the elderly population is unknown but is estimated to be approximately 15% (34,66,150). Approximately 5% of the population over 65 years of age has severe dementia, with an additional 10% of individuals having mild to moderate dementia (66). The reported prevalence of severe dementia further increases with age to 15% at 85 years (66), but much higher percentages have been reported (151).

Routine neuroimaging of patients with dementia may not be necessary when the clinician is certain regarding the underlying etiology (152). Usually, however, there is enough uncertainty regarding the diagnosis that imaging is performed. This also ensures that additional or superimposed treatable conditions are not overlooked in a patient with deteriorating mental status. In particular, imaging should be performed in patients in whom a potentially treatable structural disorder is suspected (hemorrhage, neoplasm, and hydrocephalus) (66), when signs or symptoms suggest superimposed pathology (stroke, trauma, multi-infarct dementia), or when an abrupt onset of dementia or acute deterioration of mental status occurs (152,153).

A discussion of the primary degenerative dementias (Alzheimer's disease and Pick's disease), and some other

TABLE 4. *Cytoskeletal abnormalities*[a]

Abnormality	Conditions found	Composition
Neurofibrillary tangles	Alzheimer's disease Progressive supranuclear palsy Pick's disease Normal aging Parkinson's dementia of Guam Postencephalitic Parkinson's disease Dementia pugilistica Down's syndrome	Paired helical and straight filaments, comprised of tau proteins (low molecular weight microtubule associated protein)
Pick's bodies	Pick's disease	Round inclusions that contain straight fibrils comprised of tau and neurofilament proteins
Lewy bodies	Parkinson's disease Normal aging Diffuse Lewy body disease	Round inclusions with peripheral halo comprised of neurofilament triplet proteins
Spheroids	Amyotrophic lateral sclerosis Animal models of motor neuron disease Normal individuals of all ages Increases with aging	Neurofilament-rich inclusions
Hirano bodies	Alzheimer's disease Amyotrophic lateral sclerosis Pick's disease Kuru Normal	Rod-shaped inclusions that arise as a consequence of perturbations of the microfilament system
Granulovacuolar change	Alzheimer's disease Normal aging	Tau
Neuroaxonal dystrophy	Hallervorden-Spatz disease Infantile neuroaxonal dystrophy Juvenile neuroaxonal dystrophy Neuroaxonal leukodystrophy	Swellings of terminal portions of axons due to accumulation of cellular products, vesicular profiles, and neurofilaments

Modified from Goldman and Yen, ref. (136), Trojanowski et al., ref. (137), and Seitelberger, ref. (138).

[a] The abnormal intraneuronal inclusions (left column) are characteristic of aging, and of many neurodegenerative and related disorders (middle column). Only the major conditions are listed in the middle column. While these inclusions have been recognized since the fundamental histopathologic features of these disorders were described, only recent ultrastructural and immunocytochemical techniques have revealed their precise composition (summarized in the third column). These diverse abnormalities are all selective disorganized states of the neuronal cytoskeleton.

common causes of dementia (multi-infarct dementia, normal pressure hydrocephalus) follows.

Alzheimer's Disease

Epidemiology

Alzheimer's disease (AD) is the commonest degenerative disease of the brain and the commonest cause of dementia (1). The incidence rate for dementia in general is 187 new cases per 100,000 population per year, and for AD it is 123 new cases per 100,000 population per year (1). As a consequence of the increasing number of individuals living beyond the seventh decade, AD has become the fourth leading cause of death in the United States (140–146). Males and females are affected about equally (1).

Previously, patients with AD aged 65 years or older were classified as senile dementia or senile dementia of the Alzheimer type (SDAT), with the distinction being that those who developed symptoms earlier were said to have AD (154). Currently, the illness in both age groups is referred to as AD (154). The familial occurrence of early-onset AD may be due to an autosomal dominant mode of inheritance (1).

A number of mutations in the β-amyloid precursor protein (APP) gene and in β-amyloid itself have been identified in a few familial AD (FAD) cases (143–146) but these account for a small percentage of FAD cases that have been linked to chromosomes 14,19, and 21. Recently, homozygosity for the apolipoprotein E4 (Apo E4) allele has been shown to be a risk factor for FAD and sporadic AD but the reasons for this are unclear (143–146,155) (Fig. 18).

Clinical Presentation

The major symptom is the gradual onset and progression of forgetfulness (1). Other failures of cognitive function are language disturbances, conceptual loss, visuospatial disorientation, and ideational and ideomotor apraxia (1). The course of this tragic illness usually extends over a period of 5 or more years (1). Patients with a clinical diagnosis of AD on the basis of Hachinski isch-

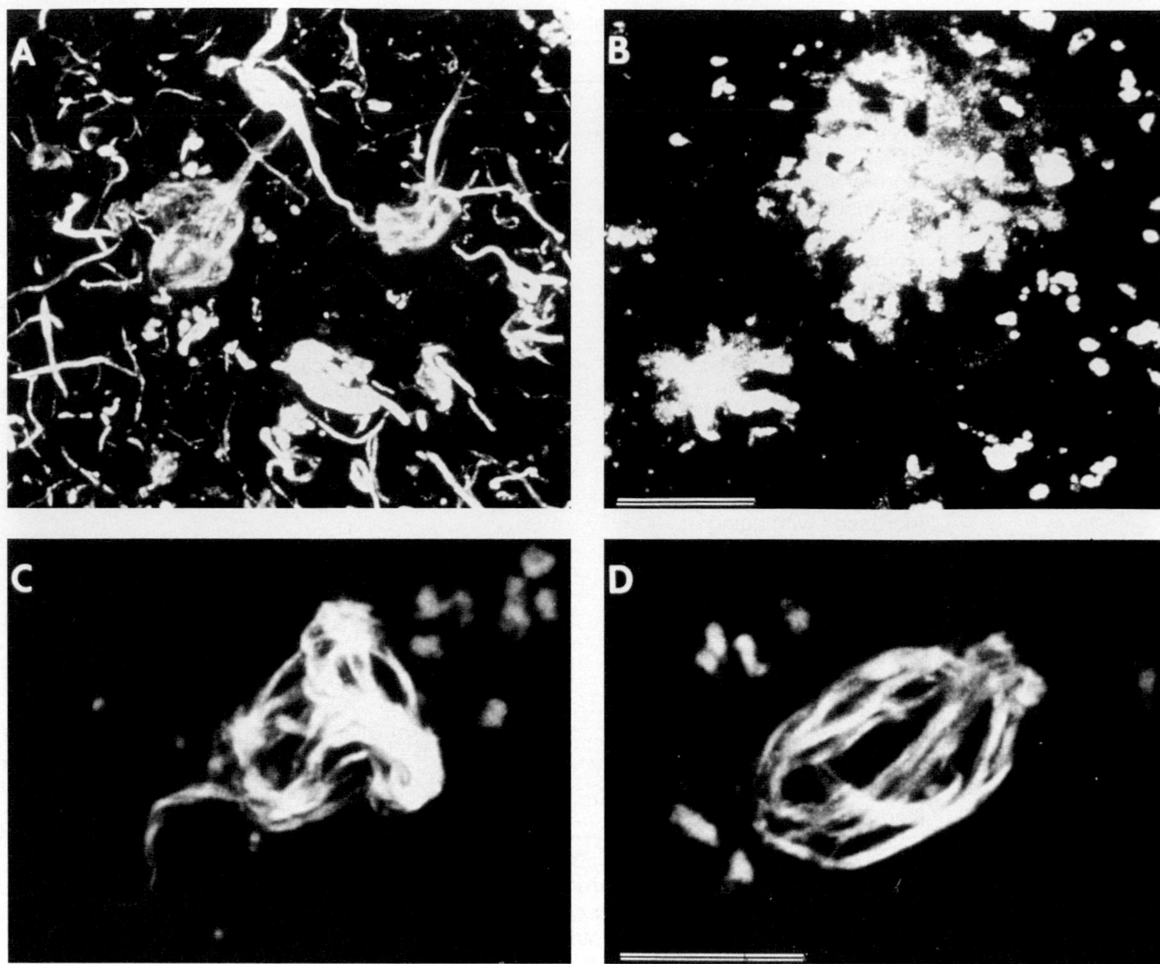

FIG. 17. Microscopy of AD neocortex (**A,C,D**) showing neurofibrillary tangles (NFTs) stained with antibodies to tau proteins, the subunit proteins of the paired helical filaments (PHFs) in AD NFTs. Amyloid plaques (**B**) stained with antibodies to Aβ in a section of AD neocortex. (From Trojanowski et al., ref. 140, with permission.)

emic scores of 4 or less truly have this diagnosis alone in 80% to 90% of cases, as documented in neuropathologic studies (156,157).

Neuroimaging and Pathology

Hypothetical mechanisms to account for the formation of plaques and tangles are illustrated in Fig. 18. Based on current insights into the pathogenesis of AD, plaques and tangles are thought to result from the altered metabolism of normal brain proteins (i.e., the Aβ peptide and the microtubule-associated protein tau, respectively) (Fig. 19).

Atrophy

Neuroimaging studies (154,158–165) and gross pathology (166) (Fig. 20A) have both demonstrated diffuse cerebral atrophy with enlarged lateral ventricles and widened sulci in patients with AD. The degree of atrophy generally increases in parallel with the progress of the clinical stage (160–162). These changes are attributed to neuronal loss histologically (1,162). Normal aging, beginning around the fifth to sixth decade, also shows enlargement of cerebrospinal fluid spaces (167) due to age-related neuronal loss (1,162,168). While this process in AD is greater (158,159,165,167) and evolves more rapidly (as documented on longitudinal neuroimaging studies) (158,159,161), overlap with normal aging exists, especially after 65 years (166). In neurodegenerative disorders and normal aging, portions of the brain vary in their susceptibility to degeneration. Specifically, the hippocampal formation is consistently and heavily involved in the pathology of AD (169), and considerably less affected in normal aging. Consequently, focal, symmetric or asymmetric (163) enlargement of the temporal horns (Fig. 20B and C) [particularly well seen on coronal MR (66)], choroidal/hippocampal fissure, suprasellar cisterns, and sylvian fissures may be more useful discriminators between AD patients and the normal elderly (154,163,164,170,171). The loss of hippocampal functions may be the cause of the memory deficits that are a hallmark of AD (139).

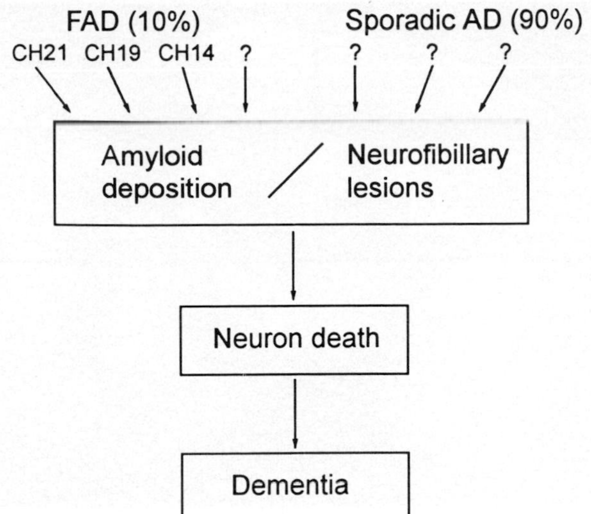

FIG. 18. Putative factors leading to the development of AD, and a hypothetical scenario for the convergence of different initiating events on the generation of AD brain lesions (i.e., amyloid deposits, neurofibrillary lesions, neuron death). Amyloid and neurofibrillary lesions are thought to result in the progressive death of neurons and dementia in AD. Although the sequence of events illustrated here is hypothetical, familial AD (FAD), which accounts for about 10% of all AD cases, has been linked to chromosome 21 (CH21), 19 (CH19), and 14 (CH14), and the apolipoprotein E4 allele (not illustrated) is a risk factor for FAD and sporadic AD. (From Trojanowski and Lee, ref. 142, with permission.)

Measurement of the interuncal distance on cross-sectional imaging of the brain has been proposed as an easy-to-use discriminating measure for the detection of hippocampal atrophy in AD (172). Age-related normative data is available for normal interuncal distance demonstrating increases with advancing age, with 30 mm appearing to be a useful demarcation for separating normals from affected. However, the specificity of these measurements for AD is still unknown (173) and the issue remains controversial, as a recent journal forum discussed (174).

Computer-driven volumetric methods for segmenting the brain (175) have been applied to the study of aging and AD. One group reported that affected patients had higher total CSF and lower brain volumes on MR than controls as well as a more accelerated change in these values with age than controls (176). Previous work with CT data comparing SDAT and controls showed too much overlap to predict presence or prognosis of SDAT (177). A study that compared CT and MRI in this setting showed that MR was superior for discriminating AD patients from age-matched controls (178). Volumetric examination of the brain has also shown significant reductions in the percentage of gray matter in patients with AD relative to controls. This is particularly significant

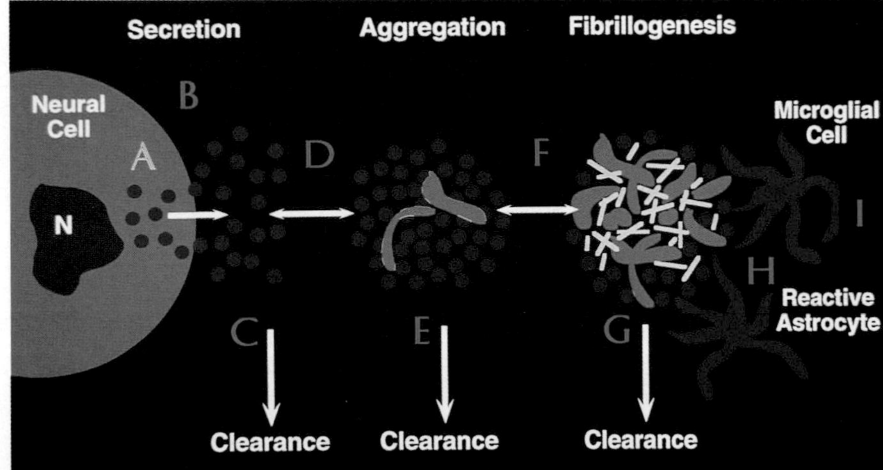

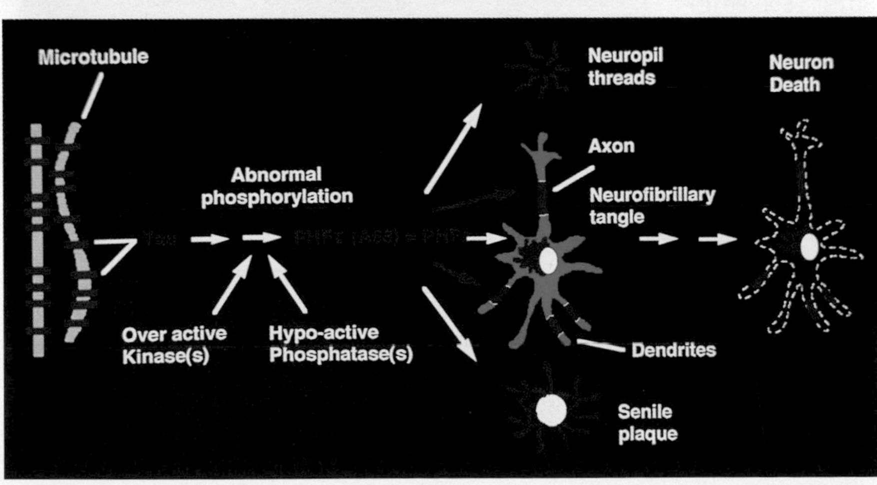

FIG. 19. A: Series of events leading to the formation of SPs in AD. Soluble Aβ (*filled circles*) is produced in one or more neural cells (e.g., neurons) in the brain (N, nucleus) and secreted into the extracellular space (b) from whence it is cleared in normal younger individuals (c). With age, soluble Aβ aggregates (d) into pre-amyloid plaques (*closely packed filled circles* to the right of d). Some aggregated Aβ also may form amyloid plaques and reactive changes (f–h). **B:** Hypothetical mechanism for the conversion of normal brain tau (*rectangles* overlying 2 microtubules on the left) into PHFtau. PHFtau is generated in neuronal perikarya and their processes as a consequence of the overactivity or inappropriate activation of kinase(s) and/or the hypoactivity or loss of phosphatase(s) that regulate the phosphorylation state of CNS tau. PHFtau accumulates in neuronal processes as neuropil threads (*top*), in neuronal perikaryal as NFTs (*middle*), and in plaque-associated dystrophic neurites (*bottom*). PHFtau loses the ability to bind microtubules, and this could lead to the depolymerization of microtubules, followed by the disruption of axonal transport, and the dysfunction and/or degeneration of neurons in AD. The accumulation of PHFs in neurons could exacerbate this process by sequestering normal tau and by physically blocking the transport of proteins and organelles in neuronal perikarya, axons, and dendrites. The death of the neuron (*on the right*) would be the ultimate outcome of all of these events. (From Trojanowski and Lee, ref. 142, with permission.)

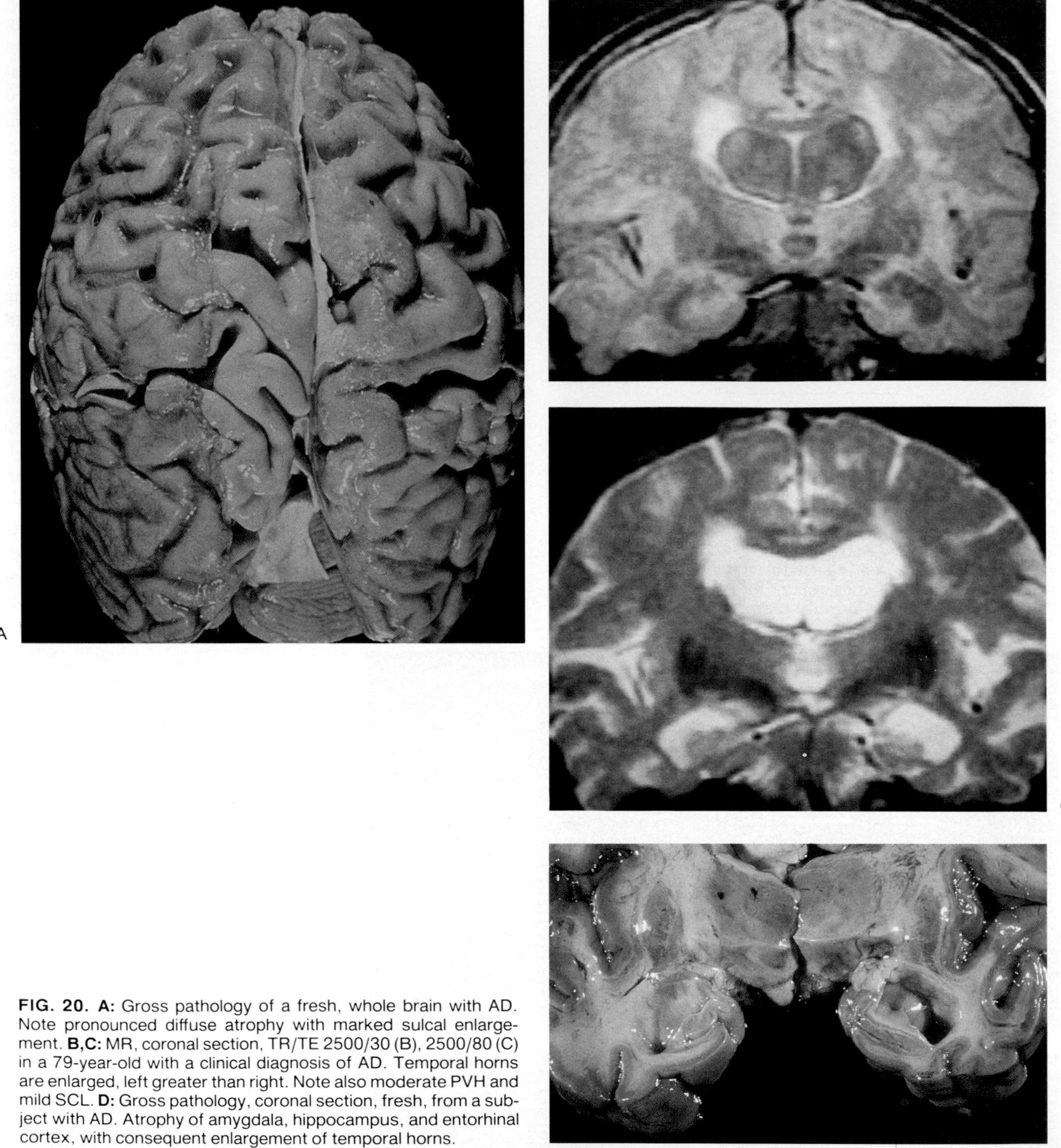

FIG. 20. A: Gross pathology of a fresh, whole brain with AD. Note pronounced diffuse atrophy with marked sulcal enlargement. **B,C:** MR, coronal section, TR/TE 2500/30 (B), 2500/80 (C) in a 79-year-old with a clinical diagnosis of AD. Temporal horns are enlarged, left greater than right. Note also moderate PVH and mild SCL. **D:** Gross pathology, coronal section, fresh, from a subject with AD. Atrophy of amygdala, hippocampus, and entorhinal cortex, with consequent enlargement of temporal horns.

in the temporal lobes and the central structures—basal ganglia, thalamus, and adjacent white matter, with lesser changes noted in the frontal and occipital gray matter. CSF volume was increased, and white matter volume was the same as controls (179). A study of eight patients using volumetric techniques showed that measurements of the hippocampus, temporal horn of the lateral ventricle, and temporal lobe distinguished affected and normals (180). This is supported by work with measurements of the anterior temporal lobe and hippocampal formation that were corrected for overall brain volume. Although these indices declined with age in both normals and affecteds, the hippocampal measurement was capable of distinguishing AD from normals in 85% (181). Recent work at low field strength has shown that volumetric measurements of CSF spaces were substantially larger in patients with SDAT versus controls in particular in the temporal horns. Lateral ventricular measurements also correlated with severity of dementia and memory impairment (182). Finally, a study of an 81-year-old monozygotic twin pair, one of whom had AD, showed marked differences in the magnitude of atrophy and parenchymal signal abnormalities on MR, with the unaffected twin considered to be in the normal range (183).

Parenchymal Signal Abnormality

Some AD patients (as well as multi-infarct dementia patients) show hyperintense sylvian and/or hippocampal-uncal cortex on long TR sequences (Fig. 21) (34). This signal may reflect in part the histopathology of AD (34). An increase in water content could be due to many of the known histologic substrates of AD, including neuronal loss, gliosis, neurofibrillary tangles, senile (neuritic) plaques, congophilic (amyloid) angiopathy, granulovacuolar degeneration of neurons, and Hirano bodies (1,166). Others have observed subtle gyral hypointense bands on long TR/long TE sequences, particularly in parietal regions in AD patients (184), possibly due to iron or other paramagnetic accumulation (66).

In addition to the relatively specific findings described in the last section, many (30,32,34,185–187), but not all (8,33,35) MR and CT investigations found that nonspecific white matter lesions are more common in AD patients than in normal elderly controls. An MR investigation found the severity of SCL and PVH in AD (Figs. 20 and 21) (30) to be intermediate between the findings in aged normals and patients with multi-infarct dementia. A pathologic study (40) found incomplete white matter infarctions more commonly in AD than in non-AD subjects. The pathogenetic mechanism underlying these lesions in AD is uncertain (30,40). As in nondemented elderly patients, SCL may be due to the vulnerability of medullary and other penetrating arteries to hypoperfusion. A study that noted increased white matter lesions in patients with AD, vascular dementia, and normal aging did show a correlation of both periventricular and subcortical lesions with dementia and memory disorders. Subcortical white matter lesions were more associated with vascular disease than with AD as a cause of cognitive dysfunction (30).

The increased incidence of SCL and PVH in AD compared to age-matched controls has led to the hypothesis that normal aging and AD, at least in part, represent a continuum, with AD reflecting accelerated brain aging (30). PVH in part reflects bulk centripetal flow of interstitial water into the ventricles (6). This presumably is increased due to cortical pathology of AD and/or white matter incomplete infarcts (34).

Several important caveats regarding white matter lesions in the normal and demented elderly exist. First, although AD probably is associated with an increased incidence of white matter pathology, several groups have reported that there is a lack of correlation between lesion burden and the severity of dementia (7,30,187). In a study that did report such a correlation this was stronger for vascular causes of white matter lesions than from AD (30). Second, extensive white matter changes may be found both on CT (188–190), MR (32,190–192), and on autopsy (193) in the absence of neurologic or cognitive deficits. Finally, a demented patient with prominent SCL and PVH (and basal ganglionic and cortical infarcts) is more likely to have a diagnosis of multi-infarct dementia (MID) or mixed MID and AD than of isolated AD (30,34,194).

The absence or mild extent of hyperintense white matter lesions on MR in a demented individual favors the diagnosis of AD over MID (7,30,34,191). A comparison of patients with presenile and senile onset of dementia also suggests that the senile onset form of the disease is associated with significantly more white matter lesions on MR versus age-matched controls. It is inferred that this may represent a "mixed" form of the disease, with a significant vascular component (195).

MR Spectroscopy in AD

Some investigations using phosphorous ^{31}NMR spectroscopy (196–198) have reported elevated levels of phosphomonoesters and phosphodiesters in AD brains, possibly reflecting hyperphosphorylation of neuronal cytoskeletal components. However, other reports using proton and phosphorous spectroscopy have stated that changes in phosphocreatine, ATP, inorganic phosphate, and phosphomonoesters and diesters could be explained on the basis of atrophy alone in patients with dementia (199). In support of this, a study of AD patients, patients with ischemic disease and age-matched normals showed no differences in phosphorous spectroscopy measurements between the normals and the AD affecteds, while the patients with ischemia had elevations in high-energy phosphate compounds (64). Another comparison of PET and MR spectroscopy in AD showed decreased glucose utilization, but no significant alteration in phosphorous metabolites (200).

Other work with proton spectroscopy suggests that myo-inositol is elevated and *N*-acetylaspartate is decreased in patients with mild to moderate dementia relative to healthy age-matched controls (201). The increase in myo-inositol suggests that the inositol polyphosphate messenger pathway is disrupted in AD, while the decrease in NAA, a marker of neuronal cell populations, suggests loss of neurons.

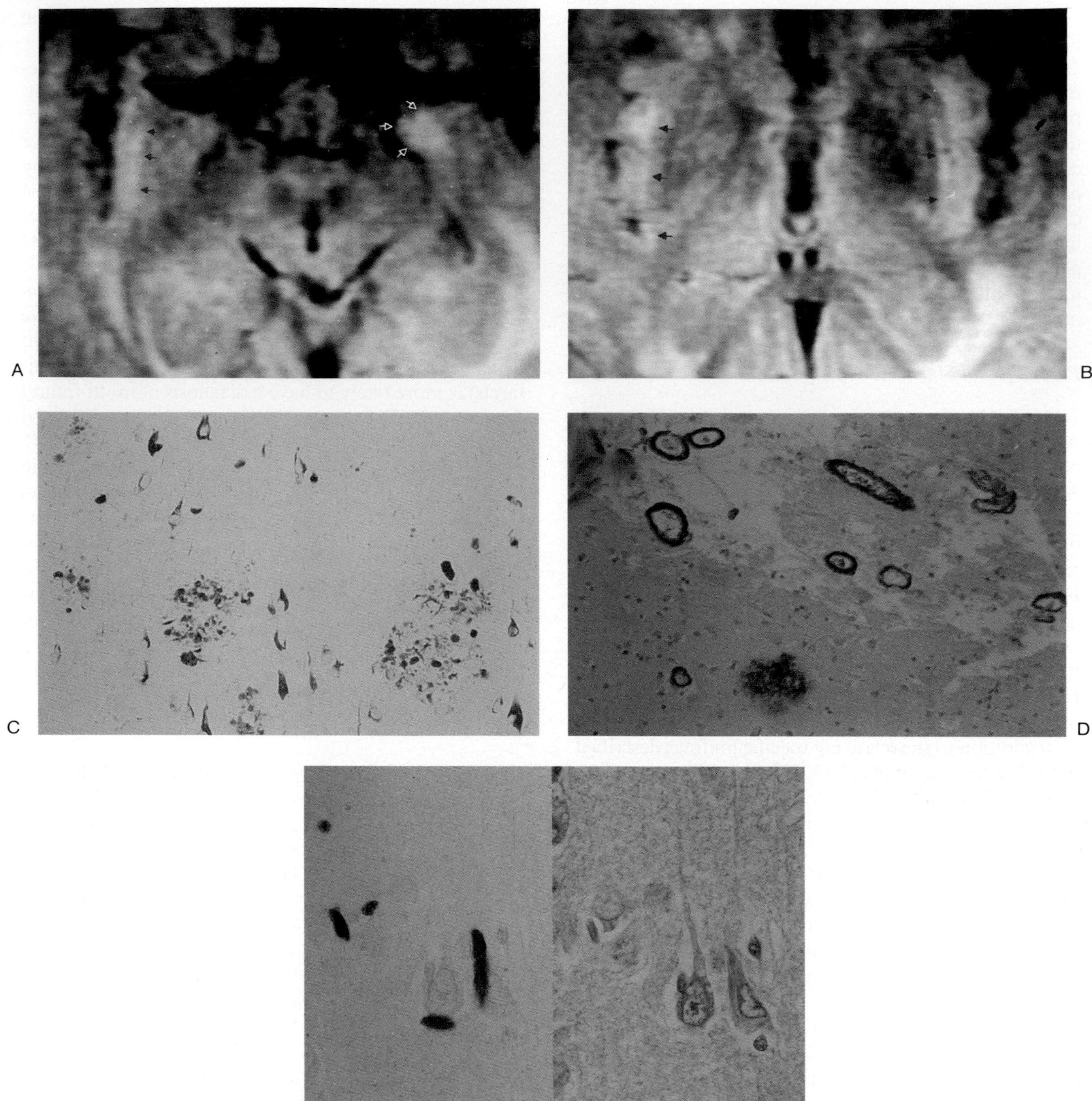

FIG. 21. MR signal changes and histopathology of AD. **A,B:** TR/TE 2500/35. Note the cortical hyperintensity in the left medial temporal lobe (*white arrows*) and insula cortex (*black arrows*) bilaterally. These signal abnormalities possibly reflect the cortical histopathology of AD. Note also moderate PVH and mild to moderate SCL. **C:** Neurofibrillary tangles (elongated brown staining structures) and senile plaques (irregular brown staining structures) in the subiculum (retrocommissural hippocampus) in AD subject, labeled with tau antibody. **D:** Low-power micrograph of a section of AD cortex was probed with antibodies to Aβ by immunohistochemistry. Numerous diffuse and neuritic amyloid plaques are labeled with the antibody throughout the cortex but not in the subjacent white matter. **E:** Hirano bodies in the hippocampus. The right half of the section is stained with a standard H&E preparation. The left half is the same section, which was immunostained following removal of H&E dyes. These intraneuronal rod-shaped inclusions are easily seen on the immunostained section (*left*) as brown, rod-like structures. The same section was stained by routine H&E technique; Hirano bodies are eosinophilic and more subtle. Hirano bodies arise as a consequence of perturbations of the microfilament system (i.e., actin, tropomyosin, vinculin, and alpha actinin).

Cerebral Amyloid Angiopathy (Congophilic Angiopathy)

Two forms of amyloid deposits are recognized in the central nervous system due to the accumulation of β-amyloid (Aβ) peptides (143–146). One is the amyloid deposition in senile plaques, which is discussed above in the section on AD. The second is a vascular deposition of amyloid called cerebral amyloid angiopathy (CAA). CAA has a predilection for the elderly and of note is more frequent in patients with AD (25,202). The reported incidence of CAA varies from 5% to 23% in patients over 60 and may be greater than 60% in individuals over age 80 (203–206). CAA shows no correlation with hypertension, atherosclerosis, or diabetes mellitus (202) (Fig. 22).

Familial and sporadic forms exist and a missense mutation in the APP gene has been implicated in the Dutch form of CAA (143–146). Patients with CAA occasionally present with slowly progressive dementia and/or with multiple small infarcts; more typically they present with an intracerebral hemorrhage (154,207–209). CAA is an important cause of atraumatic lobar hemorrhage in the normotensive elderly population (204). In fact, it may account for as many as 5% to 12% of sporadic intracerebral hemorrhages (208,209).

CAA is characterized by the presence of homogeneous eosinophilic deposits in cortical and meningeal vessels (210). Pathologically, amyloid infiltrates and replaces the adventitia and media and subsequently the elastic lamina and the entire vascular wall (208). The vessel may then undergo secondary degenerative changes of intimal fibrosis with luminal stenosis or occlusion and fibrinoid necrosis. The latter often leads to microaneurysm formation (207–209). The resultant fragile vessels may rupture in response to otherwise incidental factors, including a bump on the head, transient elevation of blood pressure, anticoagulant therapy, or surgical manipulation (208, 209). Very rarely, cerebral amyloid may be associated with a granulomatous angiitis (211).

The neuroradiologic and gross pathologic manifestations of CAA are superficial lobar hematomas (Fig. 22), commonly with subcortical white matter and/or subarachnoid extension (202,211). While some reports have shown predilection for certain locations, these hematomas may occur in any lobe of the cerebrum and often they are multiple (25,154,202,208,212). Superficial lobar hematomas are typical because CAA affects small and medium-sized cerebral cortical and leptomeningeal vessels, with sparing of subcortical and deep white matter, basal ganglionic, and cerebellar vessels (202,206,213). In addition to the well-known presentation of lobar hemorrhage, several groups have observed that CAA is associated with extensive patchy or confluent white matter disease with a particular predominance in the periventricular regions (214,215). It is hypothesized that this represents another manifestation of a generalized vasculopathy.

Pick's Disease

(Lobar Atrophy, Lobar Sclerosis, and Circumscribed Cerebral Atrophy)

Pick's disease is also a primary dementing illness, but it is far less common than AD. The cognitive deficits may be similar in AD and Pick's (1). In Pick's, however, abnormal behaviors, apathy, abulia, difficulty with language and Klüver-Bucy syndrome (oral tendencies, emotional blunting, altered dietary habits, hypermetamorphosis, hypersexuality, and agnosia) are more common than memory disturbances (1,154,216). The disease is probably transmitted as a dominant trait with polygenic modification (1). Women probably are more often affected than men (1). The course of the illness is usually 2 to 5 years, occasionally longer.

Neuroimaging and Pathology

Neuroimaging (216–218) and gross pathology (1,134) both show dramatic focal atrophy affecting one or more cerebral lobes, with severe reduction of affected gyri to a paper-thin edge referred to as "knife blade atrophy" (Fig. 23) (1,134). The atrophic lobe has also been likened to the kernel of a desiccated walnut. The circumscribed, lobar predilection, first described by Pick in 1892, most commonly involves the frontal and/or temporal lobes (1) or frontoparietal region (134), and affects the left hemisphere more frequently than the right. In striking contrast to these severely atrophic regions, the posterior two-thirds of the superior temporal gyrus, occipital lobes, pre- and postcentral gyri, and usually the parietal lobes are relatively unaffected (134,154). The vulnerable regions for atrophy seem to be phylogenetically newer parts of the brain (134). The atrophic process may also extend to the extrapyramidal nuclei (especially the caudate nucleus, which may be as atrophic as in Huntington's chorea), island of Reil, amygdaloid-hippocampal structures, corpus callosum, and anterior commissure (1,134,154).

MR also shows mild hyperintense signal on the long TR sequences of the cortex and adjacent white matter of the affected lobes (Fig. 23B). The histologic changes of swollen neurons with intracytoplasmic Pick bodies, loss of myelin in the subjacent white matter, and extensive gliosis of the cortex and subjacent white matter that accompany neuronal loss (1,134) likely account for this hyperintensity on MR. The MR findings of circumscribed lobar atrophy with these signal changes may support a diagnosis of Pick's disease in the appropriate clinical setting.

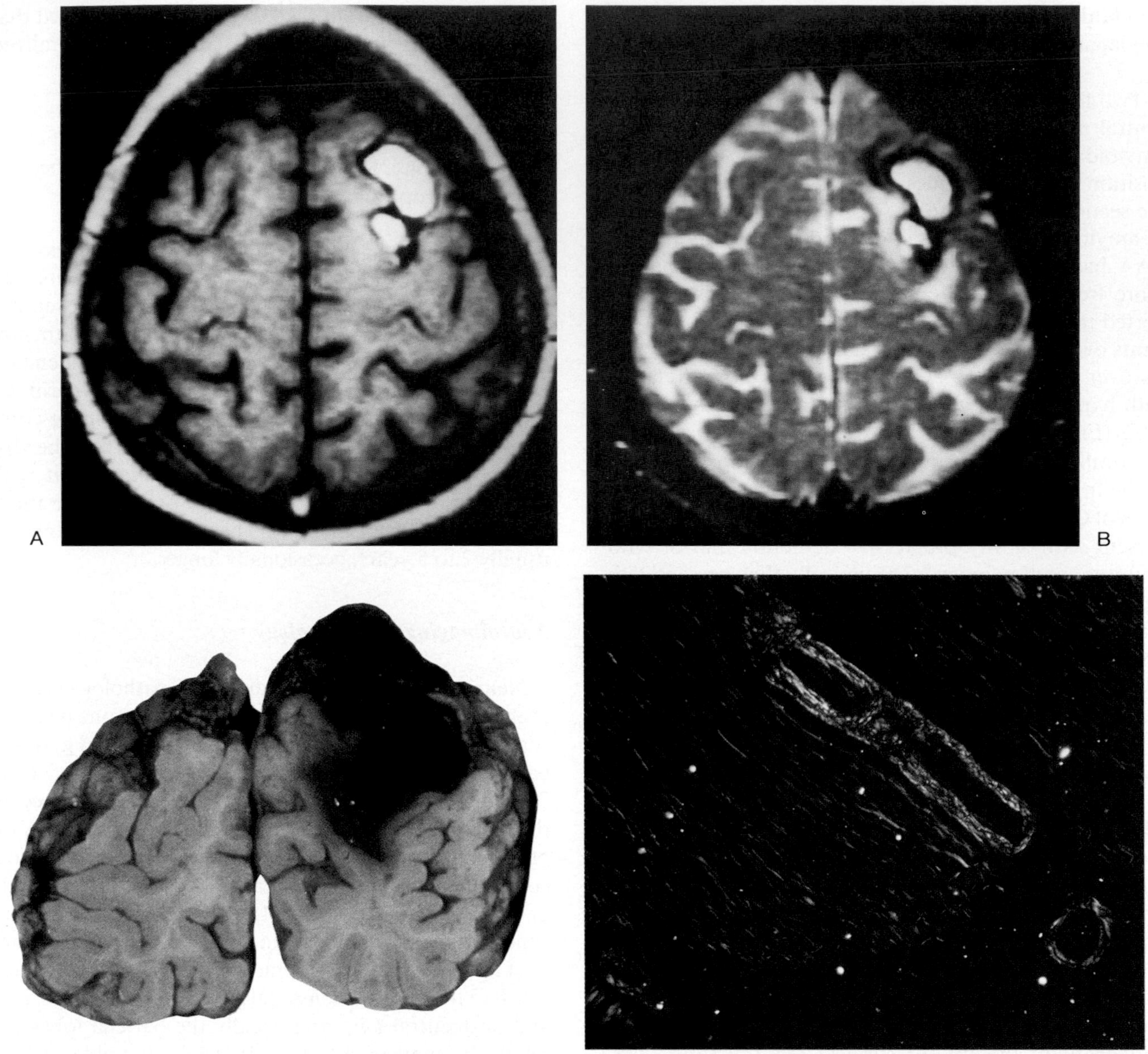

A

B

C

D

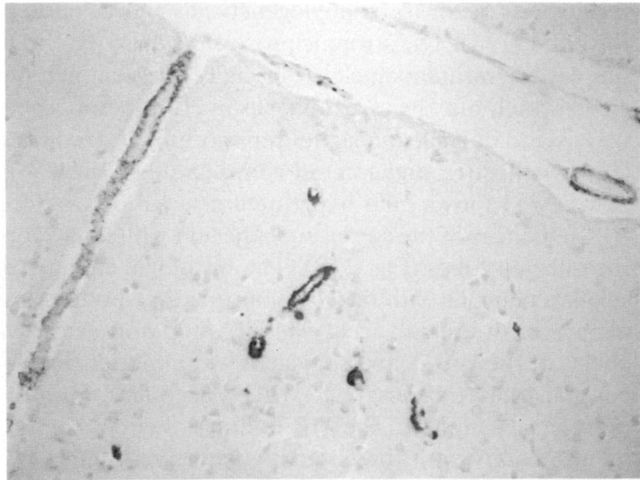

FIG. 22. Cerebral amyloid angiopathy. Axial plane, TR/TE 600/20 (**A**), 2500/90 (**B**). A 75-year-old patient with superficial left frontal lobar hematoma probably due to CAA. The lesion meets the criteria on MRI for a benign hematoma; i.e., presence of a complete rim of hypointense signal, most pronounced on the long TR/TE sequence due to hemosiderin, central hyperintensity on both short and long TR sequences representing extracellular methemoglobin, and resolving peripheral-most hyperintensity on long TR sequences due to resolving edema. **C:** Gross pathology of CAA with superficial lobar hematoma in the occipital lobe. These typical locations illustrated on MRI (A,B) and gross pathology (C) contrast with hypertensive hematomas, which much more commonly affect deep structures (e.g., basal ganglia, thalamus, pons, cerebellum). While hematomas due to CAA often rupture into the subarachnoid spaces of adjacent sulci, hypertensive hematomas may rupture into the ventricular system (147,200). **D:** Histology of CAA. Congo red stain of blood vessels shows characteristic apple-green birefringence under polarized light; hence the name congophilic angiopathy (195). **E:** Low-power photomicrograph of a section of cortex demonstrates congophilic angiopathy visualized with immunohistochemistry and antibodies to β amyloid (Aβ), which forms the amyloid fibrils in congophilic blood vessels. Several cortical vessels are stained with these antibodies.

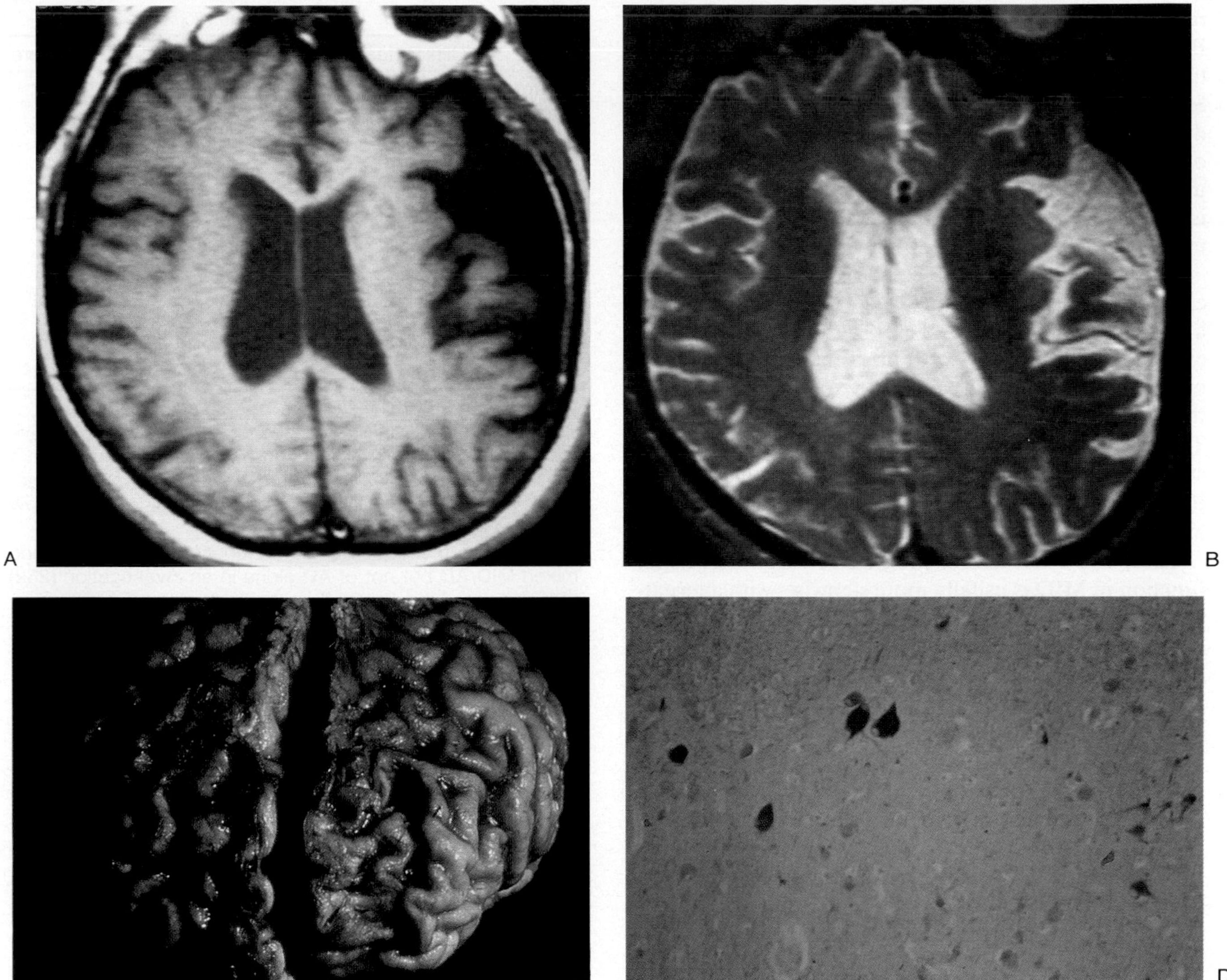

FIG. 23. Pick's disease. Axial MR TR/TE 600/20 (**A**) and 3000/80 (**B**) of a 74-year-old man. Note the pronounced circumscribed atrophy of the left frontal and parietal opercula and insula cortex (island of Reil) with consequent focal enlargement of the left sylvian fissure. On the long TR sequence (B) the mild hyperintense signal of the left insula cortex and adjacent white matter (compare to unaffected right side) is probably due to cortical and subcortical gliosis with myelin loss of Pick's disease and possibly due to swollen surviving neurons. **C:** Gross pathology, fixed brain, of a different subject with Pick's disease. Circumscribed atrophy of the left frontal pole is striking, and has been likened to the kernel of a desiccated walnut. The extreme gyral atrophy has also been called knife blade atrophy. **D:** Microscopic pathology of Pick's disease, neurofilament stain. Ballooned neurons contain Pick's bodies. Pick's bodies are round cytoplasmic inclusions that contain straight fibrils ultrastructurally (*1*) and stain (*brown*) with antiserum to neurofilaments (136).

Multi-Infarct Dementia

Cerebral vascular disease is the third leading cause of death in the U.S., after myocardial infarction and cancer (219). Dementia is a common sequelae of infarction in older people, and may be the single most common risk factor for age-associated dementias worldwide (220). Occlusive cerebrovascular damage presents most often as a stroke with sudden loss of cerebral function (219). Multiple small or large infarcts may result in dementia, depending on their number, size, and location (221). Among elderly patients with a history of stroke, 23% to 28% meet the criteria for vascular dementia (222). Hachinski popularized the term multi-infarct dementia (MID), referring to demented patients with cortical and subcortical infarcts and decreased cerebral blood flow (223). Two other forms of MID are état lacunaire, first described by Marie in 1901 (224), and subcortical arteriosclerotic encephalopathy (SAE), first described by Binswanger in 1894 (225). In a large autopsy investigation, 3.8% of elderly subjects had pathologic changes of SAE (193). However, most patients with this pathology do not have clinical dementia (188,189). Dementia secondary to multiple lacunae is thought to be extremely unusual (226). However, the role of more subtle forms of ischemic damage is controversial, and this may contribute to vascular dementia (220).

The pathogenesis of the cerebrovascular lesions that cause dementia is uncertain (221). In those patients with a mixed disorder of AD and MID a threshold effect may exist (221,227). Patients with functionally compensated or unrecognized AD may experience one or more strokes that may precipitate clinically overt dementia (221). Transcranial doppler ultrasound measurements demonstrated decreased blood flow velocity and pulsatility in patients with MID versus AD patients, and may provide an additional way of discriminating these entities (228).

Compared with AD, the progressive decline in mental function in MID is usually more stepwise, with alternating periods of clinical stability and progression; a history of focal neurologic deficits due to one or more strokes can usually be elicited (1,154). Additional features of SAE include pseudobulbar palsy and prominent motor signs (229). The classic description of état lacunaire includes pseudobulbar palsy, marché à petits pas, dementia, incontinence, episodic laughing and crying, dysarthria, and imbalance; this clinical picture is extremely unusual in patients with multiple lacunae (226).

All forms of MID are associated with hypertension (154,190). SAE may also occur in a setting of hypotension and other processes that cause hypoperfusion (229). MID can be prevented or arrested by measures that prevent recurrent infarction (i.e., control of hypertension, antiplatelet therapy) (150). Cognition may even improve following control of these factors (189), suggesting that at least a portion of dementia is caused by reversible physiologic changes and not infarction (230). Therefore, clinical and radiologic tests that aid in distinguishing MID from less treatable forms of dementia may be beneficial (189).

When MID is diagnosed on a Hachinski ischemic score of 7 or greater (Table 5), this pathologic diagnosis alone is confirmed in about 25% of cases; more commonly, a mixed disorder with neuropathologic changes of both AD and MID is found (30,156). Therefore the Hachinski ischemic score is useful but limited (221). A low score can rule out MID, since it is unlikely that an ischemic lesion can produce intellectual dysfunction yet be neurologically silent. A high ischemic score correlates with one or more cerebral infarcts; a high score, however, does not establish that the patient's dementia was caused by the cerebral infarctions (230).

TABLE 5. *Hachinski ischemic score*[a]

Clinical feature	Score
Abrupt onset[b]	2
Stepwise deterioration[b]	1
Fluctuating course	2
Nocturnal confusion	1
Relative preservation of personality	1
Depression	1
Somatic complaints[b]	1
Emotional incontinence[b]	1
History of hypertension[b]	1
History of strokes[b]	2
Evidence of associated atherosclerosis	1
Focal neurologic symptoms[b]	2
Focal neurologic signs[b]	2

Modified from Hachinski et al., ref. (231).

[a] The Hachinski ischemic score provides an objective means for clinically differentiating demented patients with a probable diagnosis of AD from those with a probable diagnosis of MID or mixed MID/AD. The former group has a low score, while the latter has a high score.

[b] Features found to be characteristic of both MID and mixed MID/AD but not of AD alone in an investigation (232) that correlated the above clinical criteria with histologic diagnosis.

Neuroimaging and Pathology

MR is also useful but limited in the diagnosis of MID. Extensive PVH, SCL, cortical infarcts, and basal ganglia lacunar infarcts in a patient with dementia favor a clinical diagnosis of MID or mixed MID/AD over AD. The absence or mild extent of these changes in a patient with dementia militates against a diagnosis of MID (30,34). However, among patients with significant cerebrovascular risk factors (i.e., stroke, transient ischemic attack, hypertension) (222), both those with and without dementia have extensive PVH and SCL on MR. Neither the presence nor extent of white matter lesions distinguishes demented and nondemented patients.

SAE is characterized by marked cerebral arteriosclerosis with arteriolar sclerotic changes in the white matter, loss of myelin and axons, and frank infarctions of the cerebral white matter (with a spectrum between these two processes), and basal ganglionic lacunar infarcts (40,189,193). Notably the subcortical arcuate U fibers and the cortex are spared (Fig. 24A,B). The vascular anatomy and circulatory disturbance that are thought to account for this selective involvement are discussed in the SCL section.

Lacunar infarcts (i.e., type 1 cerebral lacunae, see Table 1) may be found in all forms of MID. They are small infarcts lying in the deep portions of the cerebrum (basal ganglia, thalami, white matter) and the dentate nuclei of the cerebellum and brainstem (226,233). They are due to occlusion of penetrating arteries. The causes of the vas-

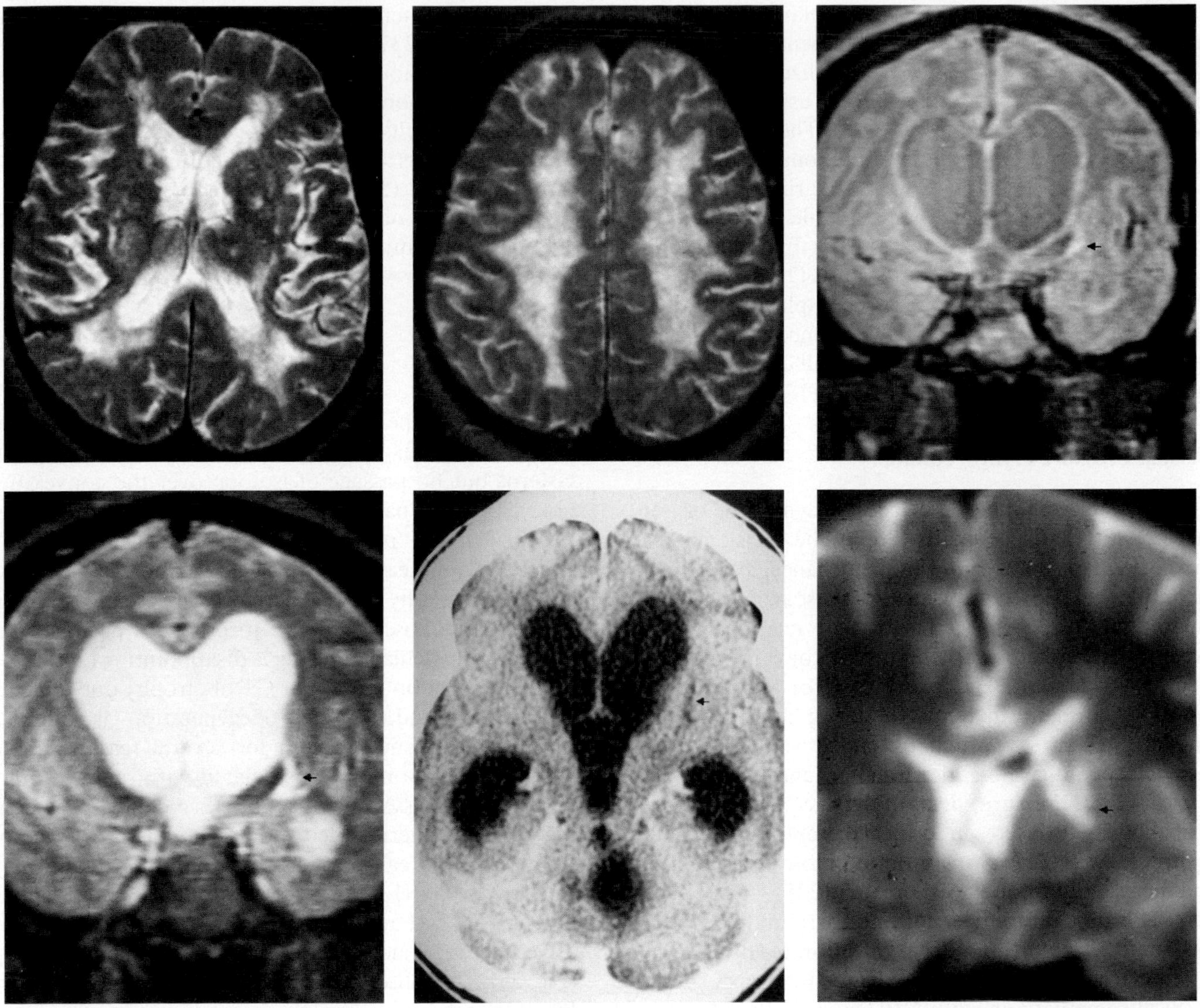

A B,C

D E,F

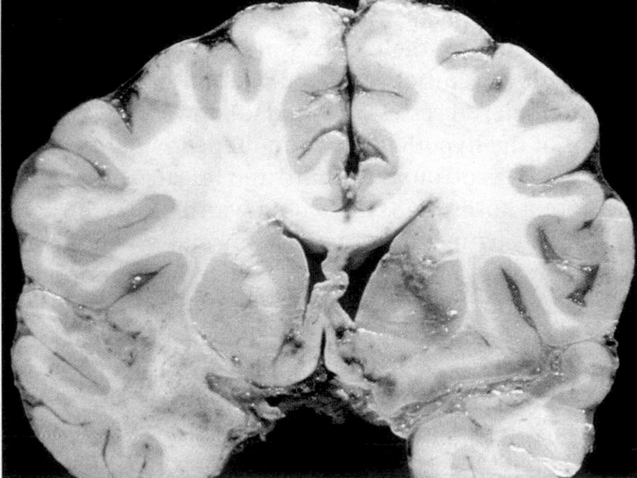

G

FIG. 24. A,B: Elderly demented patient with probable SAE, axial long TR/TE sequence. Note that extensive SCL and large, confluent PVH with irregular margins extends into the deep white matter with characteristic sparing of subcortical arcuate U fibers. **C–G:** Left basal ganglia lacunar infarct (*arrow*) in a patient who did not have MID. Coronal MR images, TR/TE 2500/30 (C) and 2500/80 (D), prior to death. Slit-like lacuna is hyperintense relative to brain parenchyma on both long TR sequences. Axial CT scan (E). Note slit-like hypodensity. Coronal MR image (F), TR/TE 2500/80 after death and subsequent formalin fixation of brain. Compared with MR studies before death, orientation of left lacuna has changed, likely because of decompression of ventricles. Gross pathology (G). Slit-like, irregular cavity in left basal ganglia transects head of caudate nucleus, anterior limb of internal capsule, and putamen. (C–G from Braffman et al., ref. 18, with permission.)

cular occlusion are atheromata, lipohyalinosis, fibrinoid necrosis, and embolization (226). Pathologically (226,233) and on MRI (18) lacunar infarcts most commonly are linear, ovoid, and less frequently round. Unlike SCL, which typically are not visualized on short TR sequences, lacunae, like most infarcts, usually are hypointense on short TR sequences (234). They are hyperintense to brain on both echoes of the long TR sequence (18,234) (Fig. 24C–G). With time, the rim remains hyperintense on long TR sequences while the center becomes isointense to cerebrospinal fluid; this is due to central cavitation with surrounding gliosis (234). In the late chronic stage lacunae may become completely cavitated, and are isointense to CSF on all sequences; at this stage pathologically verified gliosis in the wall of the cavitated infarct may not be detectable on MRI (18) (Fig. 4).

Normal Pressure Hydrocephalus

Adams, in 1965, first described the syndrome of normal pressure hydrocephalus (235). The classic clinical triad of NPH is dementia, gait disturbance, and urinary incontinence (236). One or more of these symptoms may predominate (237–239). The causal relationship between hydrocephalus and these symptoms is substantiated by documented improvement or resolution of symptoms in some patients following shunting (238). The mechanism by which distended ventricles cause their effects on gait, bladder function and mentation is unclear (238). Pressure effects of the distended ventricles probably are exerted on critical cerebral sites (238). Symptomatic NPH is uncommon before the age of 60 and increases in frequency thereafter (238).

NPH is thought to most commonly result from previous hemorrhage or meningeal infection resulting in interference with absorption of CSF (154). Autopsy studies (238) of some patients with NPH support this hypothesis. A second view postulates that periventricular white matter ischemic damage or edema fluid decreases the tensile strength of the ventricular walls and leads to ventricular dilatation (240). Other hydrocephalic states may also result in this reversible clinical syndrome. Hydrocephalus associated with spinal tumors is a well-known but uncommon phenomenon (241–243) and these patients may present with the clinical syndrome of NPH (244). Patients with compensated congenital hydrocephalus who function well throughout most of their lives may develop the syndrome of NPH as they age (245).

Since both dementia and the other symptoms may reverse with shunting, and since patients with NPH who are not shunted may progress symptomatically (246), distinction between responders and nonresponders is important. This distinction, however, by clinical, laboratory, and neuroimaging techniques can be difficult (240).

Lumbar puncture with removal of 20 to 30 cc of CSF may be a useful therapeutic test (237,246). If clinical signs improve following CSF removal, the diagnosis of NPH is strengthened and shunting usually is beneficial to the patient (237,246). Failure to respond to this test, however, does not exclude the diagnosis; some of these patients may, nonetheless, improve following shunting (237,246). Results of shunting are favorable when the disorder presents as gait disturbance or when this feature is predominant (246). Nonresponders tend to have a longer duration of symptoms prior to shunting than responders, presumably because of irreversible changes caused by longer-standing disease (247).

Neuroimaging

Positive isotope cisternography in NPH demonstrates ventricular influx and occasional flow into the sylvian cisterns but no passage of isotope over the convexities (243). Delayed passage of isotope over the convexities is considered a "mixed" pattern (243). However, some degenerative diseases also may show abnormal CSF flow on cisternography (154). Therefore, the use of cisternography to diagnose NPH and to predict a positive outcome to ventricular shunting is disappointing (240).

The distinction on MR or CT of atrophy due to aging versus NPH-induced neurodegeneration is often a difficult diagnostic problem for several reasons. First, CSF obstruction may be associated with brain atrophy (i.e., both processes coexist) (248). Second, while widening of hemispheric sulci and sylvian fissures is commoner in other causes of atrophy than in NPH (247), a minority of NPH patients have similar features. Third, patterns of PVH and SCL in NPH, aging, neurodegenerative disorders (such as AD), and SAE (190) may overlap (Fig. 25). The following features, however, may diagnose hydrocephalus with or without concomitant atrophy in the elderly. Lateral ventricular distention in patients with hydrocephalus causes uniform smooth thinning and elevation of the corpus callosum (248). Distention of the third ventricle causes dilatation of the optic and infundibular recesses (248), and downward displacement of the hypothalamus. Transependymal migration of CSF may surround the third and fourth ventricles and temporal horns (248). Increased width of the third ventricle and temporal horns with normal sylvian fissures are more common in responders than in nonresponders (247). Normal CSF flow void sign (CFVS) in the aqueduct may be augmented in NPH. This is believed to be secondary to decreased compliance (ventricular elasticity) in NPH (249). The ventricles have a more limited capacity to expand in response to systolic expansion of the choroid. As a result, relative outflow of CSF through the aqueduct and the intraventricular pressure pulsations increase (249). Resultant increased velocity and increased turbulence cause increased signal loss (249).

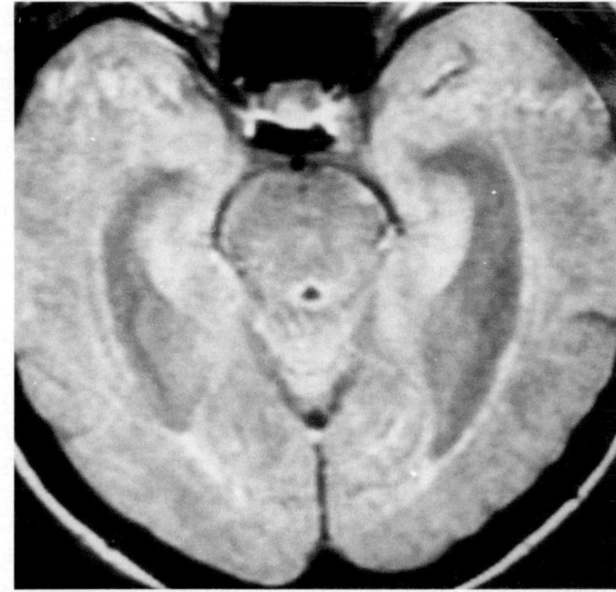

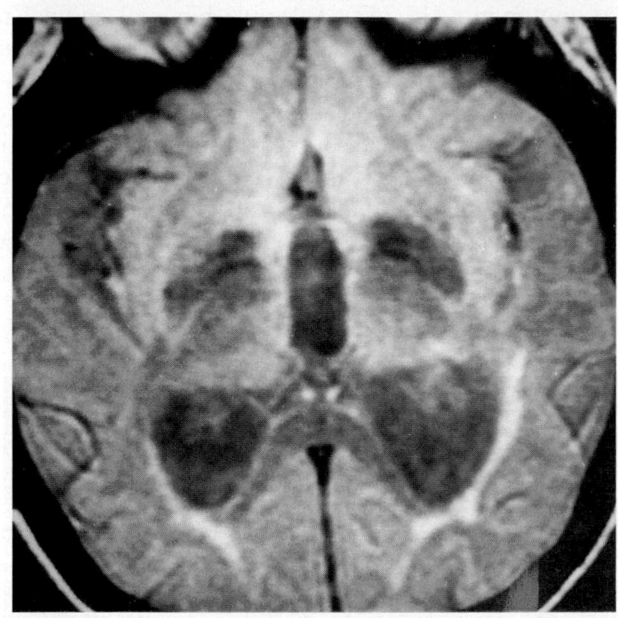

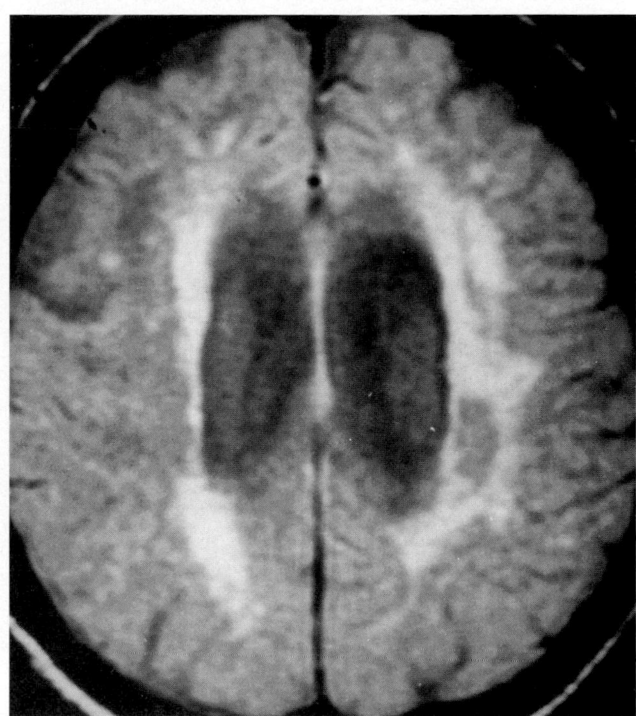

FIG. 25. Elderly patient with NPH with resolution of symptoms following shunting. **A–C:** Axial MR, TR/TE 2500/35. Note enlarged ventricles, including temporal horns (A) and third ventricle (B) with relatively small sulci. PVH is extensive at the levels of the bodies of the lateral ventricles (C). A thin rim of PVH extends to the temporal horns (A) and questionably surrounds the third ventricle. SCL are present (C), moderate in extent. Note CSF flow void (A) in the aqueduct. (Compare signal void within aqueduct to the signal of CSF in the lateral ventricles.)

While the presence of moderate or marked CFVS does not differentiate NPH from atrophic ventriculomegaly, the absence of either militates against a diagnosis of NPH (189). The magnitude of signal loss also depends on several operator-dependent factors, including TE, FOV, slice thickness, cardiac gating, field strength, and use of gradient echo for signal acquisition (189,250). These factors must be considered when using CFVS in diagnosis. Degrees of CFVS are broader on low field strength MR units; CFVS may not be a useful parameter at high field strength (189).

A further caveat is that a statistically significant association between NPH and deep white matter infarction has been reported. The degree of severity of the two diseases also appears to correlate (251). The authors have proposed that infarction leads to loss of tensile strength in the periventricular white matter and results in communicating hydrocephalus.

DEGENERATIVE DISEASES OF THE EXTRAPYRAMIDAL AND BRAINSTEM NUCLEI

The extrapyramidal nuclei are large subcortical gray matter masses that constitute, with their emerging fiber systems, a number of interrelated loops or circuits that in turn send output to affect other neuronal systems (252). Since modulation of the corticospinal tract is the most prominent of these control systems (134,252), lesions of the extrapyramidal nuclei typically result in motor dysfunction. The motor symptoms can be grouped into 4 categories: (i) impaired voluntary movements (akinesia, hastening phenomena such as festinating gait), (ii) abnormal muscle tone (rigidity, hypotonia, dystonia), (iii) involuntary movements (resting tremor, chorea, athetosis, ballismus), and (iv) abnormal postures and postural reflexes (253).

The striatum (i.e., the caudate and putamen) is the largest subcortical gray matter structure in the brain (252). These two nuclei are of telencephalic origin, and histologically similar containing a homogeneous structure with predominantly small neurons. The striatum is currently thought to have a role in the selection and activation of certain patterns of muscles required in any planned voluntary or automatic activity and the inhibition of others. This occurs through a prefrontal corticostriatal-pallidal-thalamic-motor cortical circuit prior to activation of the motor cortex and corticospinal system (254). Removal of striatal influence causes choreoathetosis, if the corticospinal system and substantia nigra are still intact (254). Athetosis is an involuntary movement of cranial, trunk, or limb muscles characterized by slow mobile spasms (254). Chorea refers to more rapid involuntary movements of the same type (254). Chorea may merge imperceptibly with athetosis in diseases such as Huntington's disease, hence the term choreoathetosis (254). Relatively restricted caudatal lesions tend to be more choreic without rigidity whereas putaminal lesions with involvement of pallidal and thalamic connections are more likely to cause both rigidity and athetosis (13,254). As rigidity becomes extreme the athetotic and choreic movements are suppressed and converted into fixed postures, with abnormal sustained muscle tone, also called dystonia (1,253). Dystonia commonly occurs with putaminal lesions in Leigh's disease and Wilson's disease (13,255). No clear line separates the fluctuant movements of athetosis from the fixed postures of dystonia (1).

The globus pallidus forms the smaller part of the lentiform nucleus, lying medial to the putamen (256). Both the lateral and medial segments of the globus pallidus, separated by medullary lamina, are of diencephalic origin (256). This nucleus is chiefly composed of large, widely spaced, fusiform cells (252). Pallidal lesions can result in akinesia (i.e., a poverty and slowness of initiation and execution of voluntary movements), rigidity, dystonia, and postural disorders, but sometimes they are asymptomatic (13,257). Selective bilateral pallidal necrosis is considered an organic hallmark of hypoxic-hypotensive insults of various origin (Fig. 26) (257).

The subthalamic nucleus is a lens-shaped nucleus on the dorsomedial surface of the peduncular part of the internal capsule (256). It is derived from the most caudal part of a lateral hypothalamic cell column (256). Lesions of this nucleus, usually due to infarction, typically result in contralateral hemiballistic movements. These consist

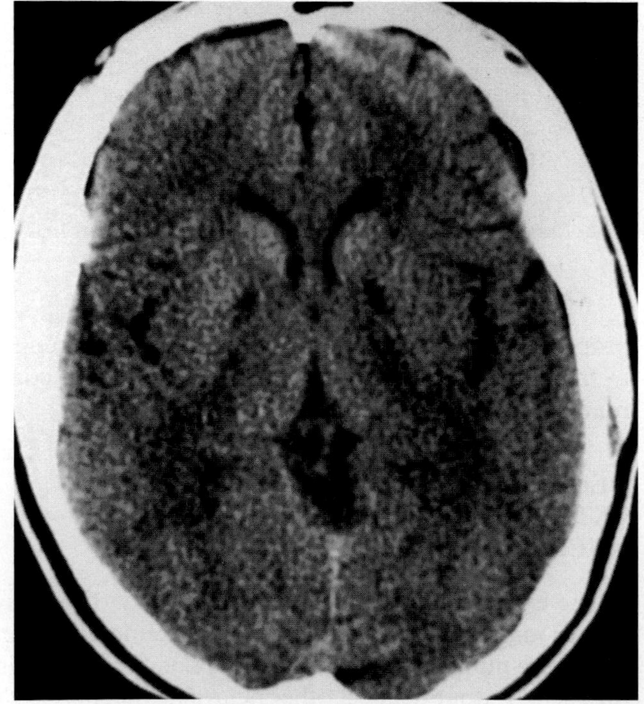
A

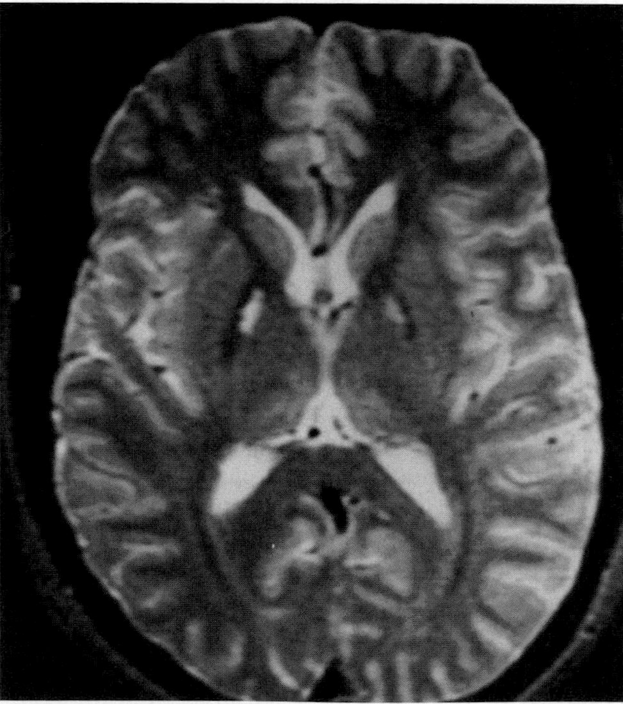
B

FIG. 26. Bilateral pallidal necrosis secondary to carbon monoxide poisoning. **A:** Axial noncontrast CT. **B:** Axial MR, TR/TE 2500/80. Note bilateral symmetric lesions of the globus pallidus, hypodense on CT, hyperintense on long TR MR. The pallidal lesions typically do not affect the entire nucleus, but predominate in the anterior two-thirds, with occasional extension into the contiguous internal capsule, striatum, and subthalamic nucleus, suggesting a preferential vulnerability of these sites to hypoxic-hypotensive insults.

of ceaseless and continuous violent and flinging involuntary movements of the limbs (253).

The substantia nigra is the largest nucleus in the mesencephalon (256). It can be divided into the pars compacta, a cell-rich region containing melanin pigment, and the pars reticulata, a cell-poor region (256). The former is implicated in Parkinsonian syndromes, while the latter is involved in Hallevorden-Spatz disease.

Huntington's Disease

While reports of the disease had appeared earlier, George Huntington in 1872 (1) gave the first accurate and complete description of the disease that bears his name. Huntington's disease (HD) occurs in approximately 4 to 5 persons per million (1). While some reports have shown a male predominance, others have found no sex predominance (1). The usual age of onset is in the fourth and fifth decades, although earlier and later ages of onset may occur (1). It is inherited in an autosomal dominant fashion with complete penetrance (1). A marker linked to the Huntington gene is localized to the short arm of chromosome 4 (258). This discovery has made the development of a test for the detection of carriers of the defective gene possible (1).

Clinical manifestations are a choreoathetosis (typically), rigidity (less commonly), dementia, and emotional disturbance (1,253). Once begun, the disease progresses relentlessly, and death occurs an average of 15 years after onset, although sometimes much earlier or later (1,253).

Neuroimaging and Pathology

Neuroimaging and pathology studies both show characteristic atrophy of the caudate and putamen (Fig. 27) (259). Both of these nuclei may be affected or one of them may be more selectively involved (134). Caudatal atrophy results in loss of the usual bulge of the inferolateral borders of the frontal horns of the lateral ventricles created by the head of the caudate nucleus (1). Striatal atrophy is imaged on MRI (260) with improved definition compared to CT (259). Diffuse cerebral atrophy may coexist with the more focal striatal process and may correlate with clinical dementia (134). A comparison of at-risk patients with and without the gene for HD showed progressive development of caudate atrophy as measured by the bicaudate ratio in affected patients (261).

MR also shows signal changes of the striatum, either hyperintensity or hypointensity (Fig. 27) on long TR/TE images (13,184). As in the case of other neurodegenerative processes, these signal changes reflect different histologic processes of the same disease. Neuronal loss of the striatum [particularly of the small neurons with lesser involvement of the large neurons (262)] is accompanied by loss of myelinated fibers and by gliosis (1). These changes likely result in the hyperintense signal on MR. Iron accumulation (13,184,263,264) in the striatum likely account for the hypointense signal.

Volumetric studies of patients with HD show marked reductions in the volume of striatal structures as well some reduction in the thalamus and mesial temporal lobes (171). In a study of mildly affected patients, the putamen showed the greatest magnitude of atrophic change (50.1%) versus a 27.7% reduction in caudate volume. The putaminal measurement when corrected for head volume allowed the investigators to distinguish affecteds and controls in 100% (265).

^{31}P NMR studies demonstrated significant elevations in the levels of phosphomonoesters and phosphodiesters in HD over controls, possibly representing molecular alterations with corresponding metabolic correlates and possibly reflecting a subcellular molecular neuropathology (266).

Hallervorden-Spatz Disease

Hallervorden-Spatz disease (HSD) is an unusual metabolic disorder characterized clinically by relentless progression of gait impairment, rigidity of all limbs, slowing of voluntary movements, dystonic posturing, choreoathetosis, dysarthria, dysphasia, optic nerve atrophy, and mental deterioration (138,267–269). Familial occurrence has been reported in approximately half of all cases (267) with autosomal recessive transmission (268). Onset of symptomatology generally occurs in late adolescence with occasional younger and older cases (138,268). The index patient reported by Hallervorden and Spatz in 1924 was 24 years old when she died from this progressive neurologic disease (270).

Neuroimaging and Pathology

At least two types of HSD exist (271). The pathology affects both the globus pallidus and the pars reticulata of the substantia nigra in group 1 but involves only the globus pallidus in group 2 (271). Long TR/TE MR images show signal changes in these extrapyramidal nuclei (Fig. 28), either hypointense (267,272), hyperintense, or mixed (13,268,273). Gross pathology shows bilaterally symmetric rust-brown discolorations due to deposition of iron pigment (138). The latter accounts for the hypointense signal on MR through preferential T2-proton relaxation enhancement. The pathology of HSD is also characterized by axonal spheroids (neuroaxonal dystrophy), which are swellings of the terminal portions of the axons due to accumulation of cellular constituents and products (Fig. 28) (138) The spheroid expands the myelin sheath and ultimately causes its disintegration (138). This demyelination is accompanied by reactive gliosis (138). These changes likely account for the hyperintense signal of involved nuclei on MR.

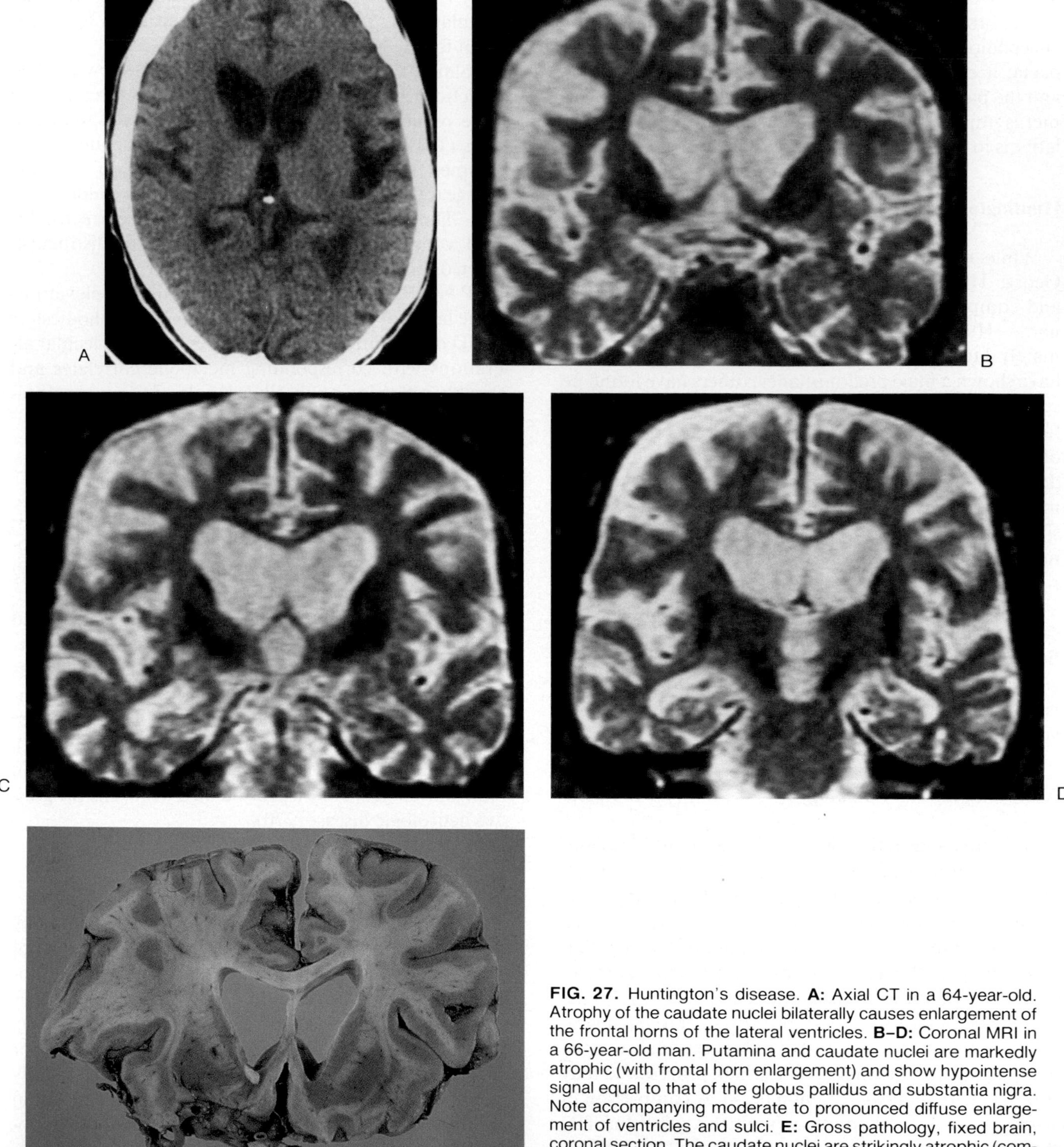

FIG. 27. Huntington's disease. **A:** Axial CT in a 64-year-old. Atrophy of the caudate nuclei bilaterally causes enlargement of the frontal horns of the lateral ventricles. **B–D:** Coronal MRI in a 66-year-old man. Putamina and caudate nuclei are markedly atrophic (with frontal horn enlargement) and show hypointense signal equal to that of the globus pallidus and substantia nigra. Note accompanying moderate to pronounced diffuse enlargement of ventricles and sulci. **E:** Gross pathology, fixed brain, coronal section. The caudate nuclei are strikingly atrophic (compare to Fig. 28) with resultant loss of the usual bulge of the inferolateral borders of the frontal horns. The putamina are relatively spared.

One MR investigation on a 0.5 T unit documented the evolution of these signal intensities (274). Initially, long TR/TE sequences disclosed bilateral and symmetric hyperintense pallidal signal (274) (Fig. 28G,H). Over a period of 3 years this evolved to a peripheral hypointense ring with a central hyperintensity, suggesting that iron is scanty or absent early in HSD and progressively increases during pathologic evolution (274). These obser-

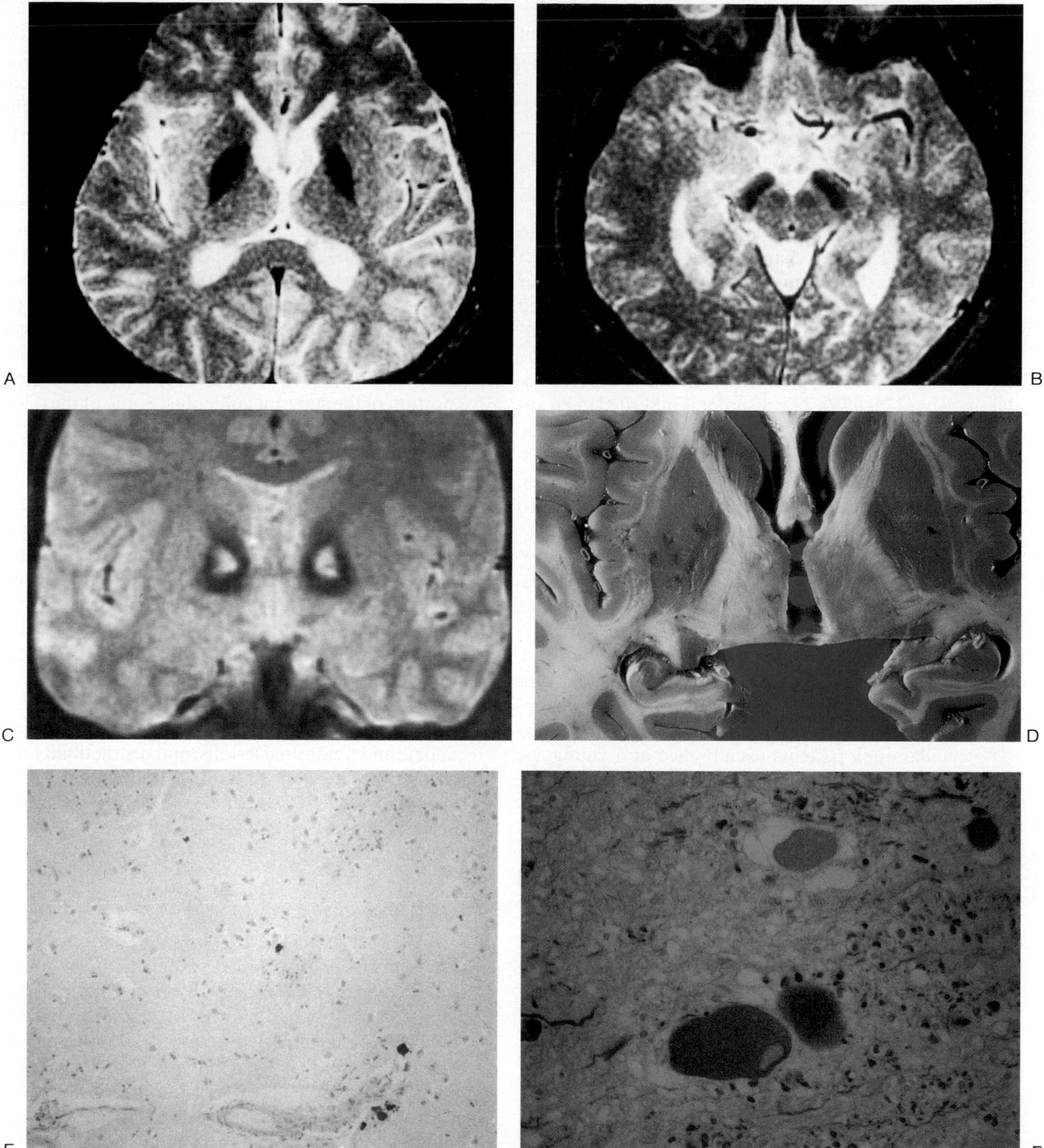

FIG. 28. Hallervorden-Spatz disease. **A,B:** Axial MR, TR/TE 2000/80. Note pronounced hypointensity of both the globus pallidus (A) and substantia nigra (B). **C:** Coronal MR, TR/TE 2000/50. Note the "eye of the tiger" sign (265) with pronounced bilateral pallidal hypointensity peripherally and hyperintensity centrally. **D:** Gross pathology, coronal section. The globus pallidi show bilaterally symmetric dark brown discoloration with diminished size. **E:** Histopathology, Perls' stain. Iron in the globus pallidus stain blue green. **F:** Histopathology, antiserum to neurofilament. In contrast to normal axons (small, punctate brown staining structures, right side of micrograph), the much larger brown oval structures are spheroids (i.e., swellings of the terminal portion of these axons). (A,B is from Mutoh et al., ref. 267; C from Sethi et al., ref. 273.)

vations support the view (138) that neuroaxonal degeneration is the basis of the pathology, and pallidonigral pigmentation follows (274).

Wilson's Disease
(Hepatolenticular Degeneration)

Wilson's disease (WD) or hepatolenticular degeneration is an uncommon genetic disorder that localizes to chromosome 13 (275) characterized by a deficiency of ceruloplasmin, the serum transport protein for copper (276,277). As a result, copper is abnormally deposited in various tissues with resultant toxicity to these organs (276,277). The most pronounced involvement is in the liver and brain, with typical involvement of the lenticular nucleus (276–279). The disorder is inherited in an autosomal recessive fashion (1,255). It results from genetic expression at a locus on chromosome 13 (275). The disease can present at any age from 5 to 50 years or older, but the peak age at presentation is between 8 and 16 years (279).

Although symptomatology may be variable, neurologic and psychiatric findings associated with liver disease predominate (255,280). Typical neurologic signs include tremor, rigidity, dystonia, gait difficulty, incoordination, difficulty with fine motor tasks, and dysarthria. Superimposed hepatic dysfunction may lead to additional neurologic dysfunction from hepatic encephalopathy. Before the discovery of effective chelation therapy (D-penicillamine), patients usually died at a young age (277,279). The Kayser-Fleischer ring, a granular deposit of copper in Descemet's membrane, is virtually diagnostic of WD (279). The definitive diagnosis is made biochemically, with low levels of serum ceruloplasmin, increased rate of urinary copper excretion, and elevated hepatic copper levels (255,277,280).

Neuroimaging and Pathology

Neuroimaging studies and gross pathology can show diffuse or focal atrophy (277,281). Typical sites of cerebral involvement are deep gray matter and central white matter (276,280,282–284). Gray matter nuclei involvement is more common, usually bilaterally symmetric in the putamen, caudate, thalamus, globus pallidus, dentate nucleus, pons, and mesencephalon (substantia nigra, periaqueductal gray matter, tectum, red nucleus). In contrast, white matter lesions usually are asymmetric, located in the subcortical regions or the centrum semiovale, and are commonest in the frontal lobes with a frontal-temporal-occipital-parietal gradient. Lesions are hypodense on CT, hypointense on short TR MR sequences (285,286), and variably hyperintense, hypointense, or both on long TR sequences (255,276,277, 280,283–287) (Fig. 29). Pathologically, gliosis, edema, and variable necrosis with cavitation occur (255,276). This may be due to the toxicity of copper and/or secondary to ischemia (255). These changes likely account for the hyperintense signal on long TR sequences, hypointensity on short TR images, and hypodensity on CT. Hypointensity on long TR sequences is either due to the paramagnetic effects of copper deposition itself, associated iron deposition, or some other agent resulting in preferential T2-proton-relaxation enhancement (277, 281,285). Mesencephalic involvement can be characteristic—the so-called face of the giant panda sign (284). This consists of high signal throughout the mesencephalon except for sparing of the red nucleus and the lateral portion of the pars reticulata of the substantia nigra and a portion of the superior colliculus. Some of these lesions appear to improve or reverse during treatment (283, 288–290).

Cerebral MR findings correlate well with neurologic findings. Most patients without neurologic symptoms have normal MR scans, while most patients with neurologic symptoms have abnormal studies (255,276,280, 286,291). In a comparison study, white matter lesions were seen in 60% of symptomatic patients and 19% of asymptomatic patients, with the basal ganglia the most frequent site. Atrophy was present in 68% of symptomatic patients and 6% of asymptomatics (291). Lesion location is also useful in that bradykinesia and dystonia correlate with putaminal lesions, dysarthria with both caudate and putaminal lesions, and distractibility of gaze fixation with frontal lobe involvement (280,291). Another report subdivided patients into three subgroups on the basis of neuropsychiatric symptoms and lesion location (292).

Wernicke-Korsakoff Syndrome

Wernicke's encephalopathy refers to an acute or subacute syndrome characterized by disorientation, gaze paralysis, ataxia, and nystagmus. Korsakoff psychosis manifests as impaired ability to acquire new information and retrograde amnesia. It is thought that Korsakoff syndrome is a later sequela of the acute encephalopathy. The syndrome of Wernicke-Korsakoff is almost always encountered in longstanding alcoholics, but the etiology is due to an associated thiamine deficiency, rather than a toxic effect of alcohol itself.

Neuroimaging and Pathology

Lesions on pathologic examination of the brain as well as MRI are typically found in the mamillary bodies, periventricular thalamus, periaqueductal gray, and hypo-

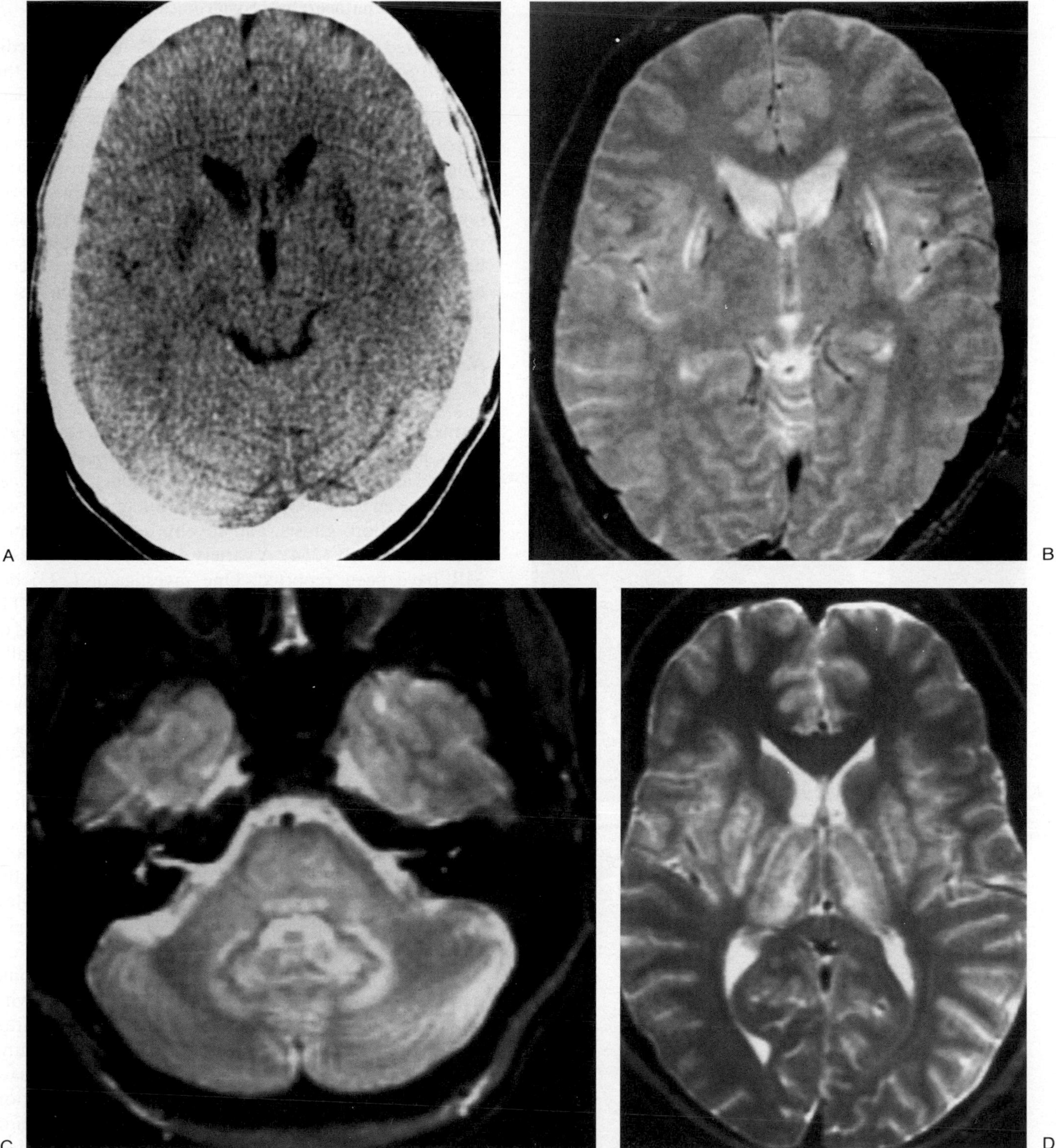

FIG. 29. Wilson's disease. **A,B:** A 28-year-old man with bilateral symmetric striatal involvement. Axial CT (A), Axial MR, TR/TE 3000/70 (B). Putaminal hypodensity on CT (A) and hyperintensity on long TR MR images (B) likely reflect pathologic changes on gliosis, edema, and/or necrosis. Hypointensity on MR in the medial putamen and caudate (B) is due to preferential T2 proton relaxation enhancement of copper itself or some other paramagnetic substance. Atrophy of the caudate results in enlargement of the frontal horns of the lateral ventricles. (A and B courtesy of Dr. David Yousem.) **C,D:** A 14-year-old boy with thalamic, putaminal, pallidal, dentate nuclei, and pontine lesions. Axial MR TR/TE 3000/80. In contrast to patient illustrated in A and B, all lesions are hyperintense on this long TR/TE sequence at 1.5 T. Note also the variable sites of involvement from patient to patient.

thalamus (134). In the acute stages of the disease, hemorrhage, necrosis, and edema are encountered, whereas in the later stages atrophy of these regions, particularly the mamillary bodies, may be the sole manifestation. Specific dorsal-median involvement of the thalami, with or without enhancement, is typical (Fig. 30A). The key to the diagnosis rests on the recognition of mamillary body abnormality (Fig. 30B), as well as the clinical history of alcoholism, since the syndrome can be easily misdiagnosed by the clinician.

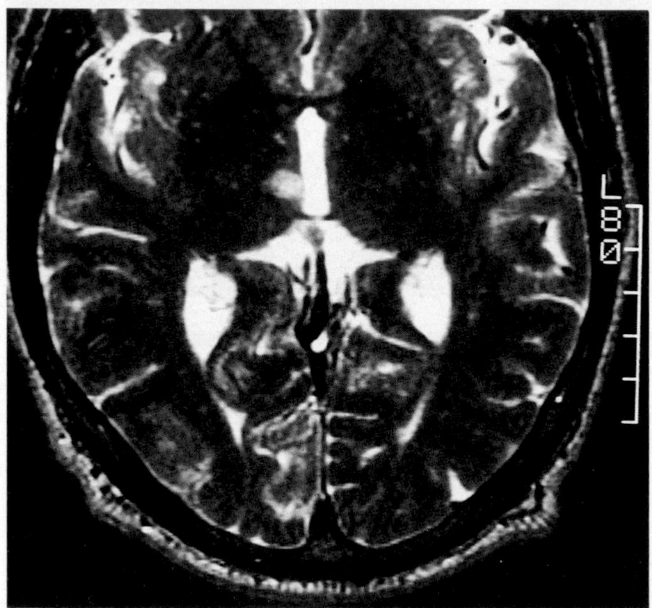
A

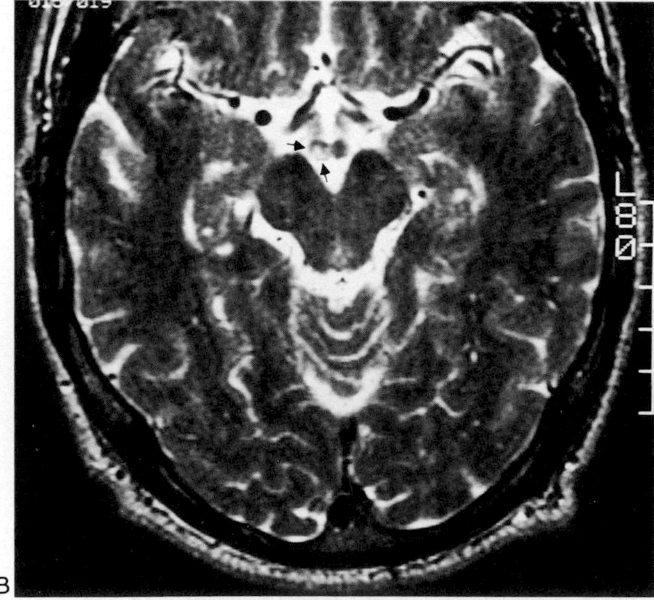
B

FIG. 30. A–C. Cerebral lesions associated with alcoholism. **A,B:** Wernicke-Korsakoff syndrome. Note right thalamic lesion (A) and necrosis of right mamillary body (B) in alcoholic patient with confusion, gaze paralysis, and ataxia.

Acquired Hepatocerebral Syndromes

Acquired hepatocerebral syndromes are nonhereditary disorders in which a primary derangement of the liver affects cerebral function (254). Most of the disorders of cerebral function develop rapidly, over a period of days, and result mainly in a disturbance of consciousness ranging from confusion through stupor to coma and death (254). Others may present with progressive movement disorders (characteristic of basal ganglia damage) or dysarthria, tremor, and ataxia (characteristic of cerebellar impairment). The patient's neurologic status correlates best with serum ammonium levels; progressive deterioration occurs after each insult (293).

Neuroimaging and Pathology

The most significant neuropathologic change in acute forms of acquired hepatocerebral syndromes is enlargement and hyperplasia of protoplasmic astrocytes in the cerebral and cerebellar cortex, basal ganglia, and diencephalic nuclei (254,293). Gray and white matter necrosis with cavitation, gliosis, and myelin degeneration may occur chronically (254). A variety of different findings on MR have been reported. One investigator (293) described bilateral hyperintense dentate nuclei on long TR images. Another study (294) found symmetric lesions of the white matter. A third investigator (295) found pallidal hypointensity on MR with calcification on CT. Other patients in this same series had hyperintensity on short TR sequences in the globus pallidus (Fig. 30C), putamen, subthalamic region, surrounding the red nucleus, quadrigeminal plate, and anterior pituitary.

In another study, 9 out of 16 patients with cirrhosis and portal-systemic encephalopathy had lesions that were high signal intensity on short TR/TE imaging and low on long TR imaging (296). These were seen in the basal ganglia, cerebral peduncles, and internal capsules. They appeared well marginated and did not exert mass effect.

A proton spectroscopic study of patients with chronic hepatic encephalopathy showed elevated glutamine with reductions in choline metabolites and myo-inositol (297). The authors hypothesized that this last finding may relate to the postulated role of myo-inositol as a glucuronic acid precursor. Glucuronic acid conjugation is an important detoxification pathway, and its depletion may occur with long-term exposure to hepatic toxins. Furthermore, this depletion may in part explain the sensitivity of the brain to other neurotoxins in hepatic disease.

DISEASES OF THE SUBSTANTIA NIGRA

Parkinsonism

Parkinsonism, or Parkinson's syndrome, is a clinical term that refers to the neurologic abnormalities, in part

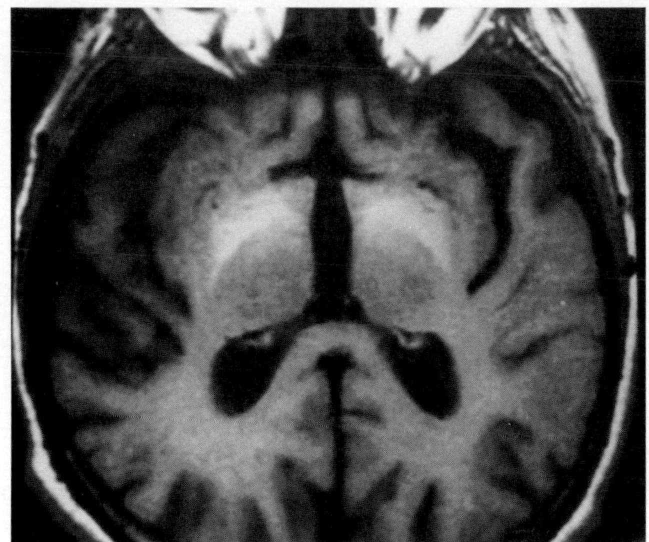

FIG. 30. (*Continued.*) **C:** Acquired hepatocerebral degeneration. Axial MR, TR/TE 600/20. Note bilateral hyperintense signal of globus pallidi.

or complete, elucidated by James Parkinson, i.e., an "involuntary tremulus motion, with lessened muscular power, in parts not in action and even when supported; with a propensity to bend the trunk forward, and to pass from a walking to a running pace. . ." (298–133). These neurologic signs are due to malfunction of the major efferent projection of the substantia nigra—the nigrostriatal tract (134). The cell bodies of this dopaminergic system are in the pars compacta of the substantia nigra, and its axons ascend to the striatum (252). Clinical manifestations of parkinsonism are thought to first become apparent following a loss of 80% of nigral dopaminergic neurons (133). Primary parkinsonian syndromes include Parkinson's disease (PD), progressive supranuclear palsy (PSP), and striatonigral degeneration (SND). [The latter may be associated with olivopontocerebellar degeneration (OPCD) and/or Shy-Drager syndrome (SDS) in multiple system atrophy (MSA).] Secondary parkinsonism can occur following infarction, infection, trauma, or be drug or toxin-induced (13). MR may show increased signal on long TR sequences in the midbrain or upper pons in patients with stroke-induced parkinsonism (13).

Idiopathic Parkinson's Disease

Idiopathic Parkinson's disease (PD) (also known as paralysis agitans) is relatively common (133). Each year about 1 in 4000 of the total population and about 1 in 1000 in the population 50 years and over are newly affected (133). Two to three percent of the population may be expected to develop parkinsonism at some time during life. The age of onset in most series ranges between 50 and 60 years of age (133).

The principal symptoms are tremor, rigidity, akinesia, and postural difficulties (133). Patients with PD generally respond well, at least initially, to medication. Neurologic improvement may occur in some PD patients following autografting of adrenal medullary tissue (299,300). The disorder is progressive, without remissions or exacerbations; however, the course and prognosis are often not uniform (133).

Neuroimaging and Pathology

The neuropathologic hallmark of the disease is loss of neuromelanin-containing neurons,with gliosis and Lewy body (LB) formation in the substantia nigra (primarily the pars compacta) (Figs. 31E–G and 32), the locus coeruleus, the dorsal nucleus of the vagus, the substantia innominata, and several other regions. A hypothetical mechanism to account for the formation of Lewy bodies is shown in Fig. 33).

On MR (Fig. 27A–C) the width of the pars compacta is diminished in PD patients compared to controls; overlap between both groups, however, does exist (301,302). This diminished width, also found in PSP and SND (135,303), either reflects selective neuronal loss of the pars compacta and/or iron or other paramagnetic deposition. Unusually, patients with PD have hyperintense foci on long TR sequences in the substantia nigra (Fig. 31D), possibly due to gliosis that accompanies cell loss (302). One investigator (13) found that the normal hypointense signal of the dorsal lateral substantia nigra was changed to a signal similar to that of brain parenchyma without iron. This is thought to be due to depletion of iron by increased cellular metabolic activity or by local cell death. In contrast to other Parkinsonian syndromes, most PD patients do not have putaminal hypointensity on long TR images greater than expected with normal aging (13,302).

Pathologic (133,304) and radiologic investigations (13,133,302,305) found that central and cortical atrophy is more common in patients with PD than in controls, although an overlap exists with that observed during normal aging (305). However, in younger PD patients atrophy is more evident than in controls. This is at a time when the normal, age-dependent atrophy is still of small magnitude.

An association of AD with PD exists. Clinical and neuropathologic changes of AD are commoner in patients with PD than in the brains of age-matched controls (1,306). Alternatively, 8% to 45% of patients with AD are reported to have the clinical and or neuropathologic manifestations of PD (133,152). Additionally, a form of dementia due to the accumulation of cortical LBs known as diffuse LB disease has been recognized (142,307). It is characterized clinically by dementia and pathologically by diffuse cerebral LBs in the absence of plaques, tangles, or other lesions (142,307,308). Recent recognition of this common disorder will likely prompt a re-evaluation of

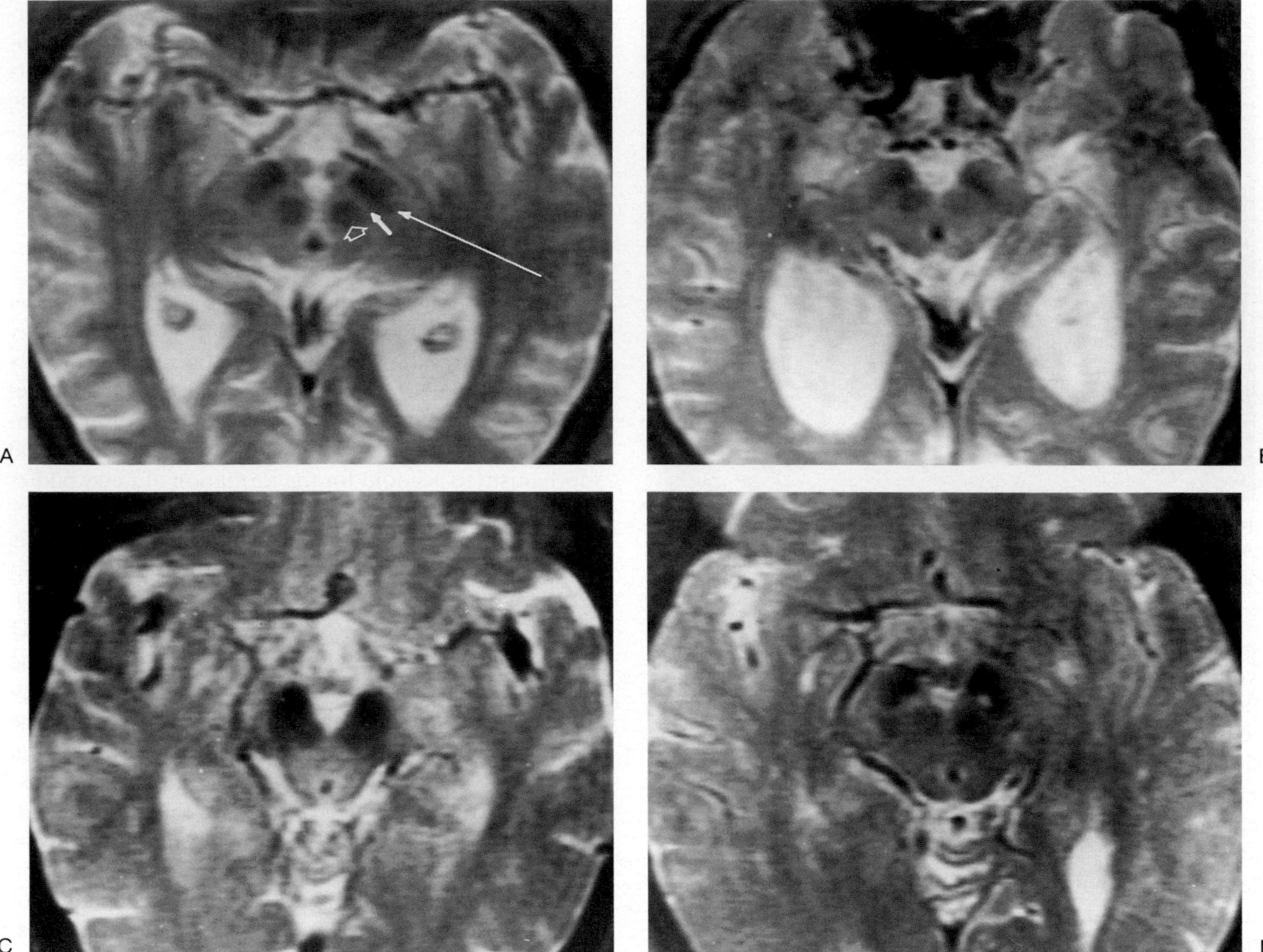

FIG. 31. Parkinson's disease (B–G), control subject (A). A–D: Axial MR, TR/TE 2500/80, 0 to 20° positive to inferior orbitomeatal line. **A:** Pars compacta (*short solid arrow*) of substantia nigra is the relatively hyperintense band between hypointense pars reticulata (*long solid arrow*) of substantia nigra and hypointense red nucleus (*open arrow*). **B:** Note narrowed hyperintense band (pars compacta of substantia nigra) between hypointense pars reticulata of substantia nigra and red nucleus. **C:** The hyperintense bands between the pars reticulata and the red nuclei are completely lost bilaterally. **D:** Punctate hyperintense foci are present in the substantia nigra bilaterally. **E:** Gross pathology, axial section of midbrain. Proceeding from top to bottom of figure, the cerebral peduncles, substantia nigra, red nuclei, cerebral aqueduct, and superior colliculi (partly cut off) are successively seen. The substantia nigra shows pronounced depigmentation (compare to normal specimen, Fig. 35). **F:** Histopathology of pars compacta of substantia nigra in PD. Brown pigments are neuromelanin in neurons of pars compacta. This section shows marked neuronal loss and loss of neuromelanin; normally brown pigments would encompass the entire field. **G:** Lewy body in pigmented neuron of the substantia nigra in PD, antiserum to neurofilament. Lewy body is the brown-stained, round intraneuronal inclusion with a peripheral halo toward the bottom of the figure. Neurofilament triplet proteins are the major cytoskeletal proteins found in Lewy body (131). The small brown punctate pigment is neuromelanin in neurons of the pars compacta. (A–D from Braffman et al., ref. 302, with permission.)

the overlap between PD and AD. MR investigations have compared PD patients with and without dementia. One found that the presence of dementia in patients with PD was not associated with any specific pattern of MR abnormalities (309). The other study found more profound white matter changes in PD patients with dementia (310).

Striatonigral Degeneration

Striatonigral degeneration (SND), coined by Adams, van Bogaert, and Vandereecken (311), is characterized clinically by parkinsonian symptoms with prominence of rigidity and with an absent or poor response to antiparkinsonian medication (1).

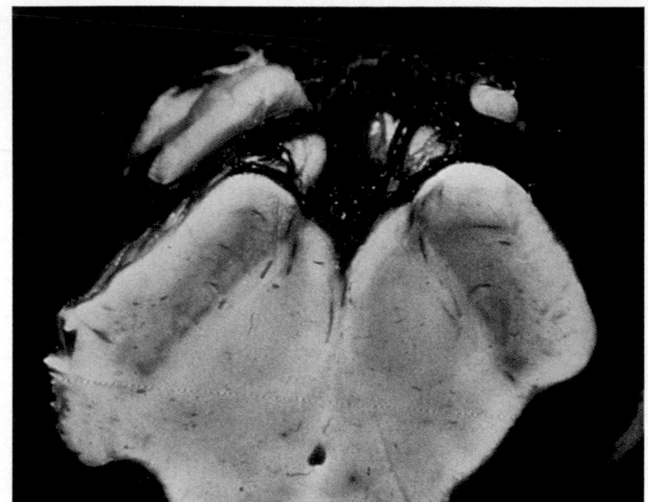

E

F

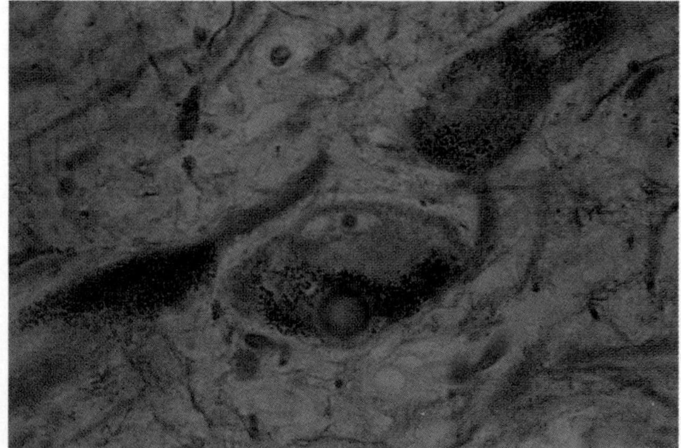

G

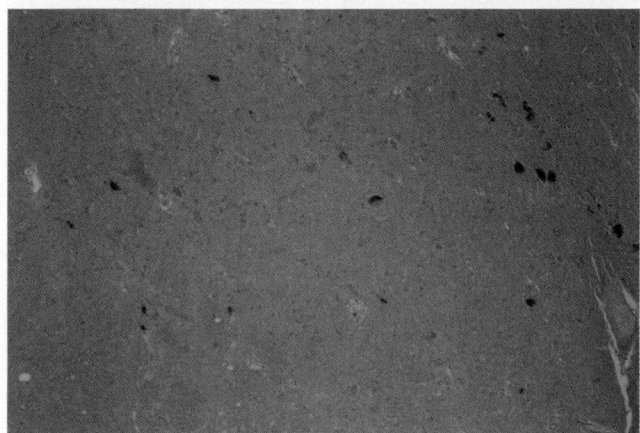

FIG. 31. *Continued.*

Neuroimaging and Pathology

Neuroimaging and gross pathology show atrophy of the striatum, due to neuronal loss particularly of small neurons, with the putamen more involved than the caudate (134,254). On MR, signal changes of the putamen vary with the magnetic field strength (135). At 1.5 T, the putaminal hypointensity, particularly along its posterolateral margin, is equal to or more evident than pallidal hypointensity on long TR/TE images (Fig. 34) (77,79, 135,303,312). The degree of hypointense signal correlates significantly with the severity of rigidity, suggesting a causative or associating role for putaminal degeneration with this clinical feature (313). This hypointensity at 1.5 T may be accompanied by a thin rim of hyperintense signal (135). With low or intermediate field strength, the putamina are hyperintense on these pulse sequences (254). Apparently, the magnetic susceptibility effect is not detected on the lower strength magnet. The hyperintense signal at 0.5 T likely reflects increased amounts of water due to gliosis and/or cell loss (135). At 1.5 T, magnetic susceptibility effects predominate. Pathologically, the shrunken putamina are gray or tan, and contain a variety of abnormal deposits, including hematin, neuromelanin, lipofuscin, cobalt, magnesium, silicon, sodium, strontium, tin, zirconium potassium, manganese, and/or copper (314).

Like other primary parkinsonian syndromes, the width of the pars compacta is diminished in SND patients on MR (135,303). A histologic difference between the nigral lesions of SND and PD exists—unlike PD, the remaining neurons do not contain Lewy bodies in SND (1,134). When SND is associated with OPCD (i.e., in MSA), characteristic MR changes of OPCD also occur.

Shy-Drager Syndrome

Shy-Drager syndrome (SDS) is characterized by autonomic nervous system failure (orthostatic hypotension, urinary incontinence, and inability to sweat) (135). While the pathologic changes are somewhat variable, neuronal loss in the substantia nigra and the intermediolateral cell column of the spinal cord (134), accompanied by gliosis, commonly occurs. SDS may occur alone or in association with the clinical, pathologic, and radiologic features of striatonigral degeneration and/or olivopontocerebellar degeneration (i.e., MSA) (313). On MR, patients with SDS associated with SND had typical findings of SND (i.e., putaminal atrophy and/or signal changes). MR exams in pure autonomic failure patients were normal (313). These observations may be useful in diagnosis (313). The clinical distinction between MSA and pure SDS may be impossible in early stages, since MSA patients may initially only present with autonomic findings. Since the prognosis of MSA is significantly different than that of isolated autonomic failure, the diagnosis is important (313).

Progressive Supranuclear Palsy

Although reported in previous communications, Richardson, Steele, and Olszewski, in 1963, were the first to

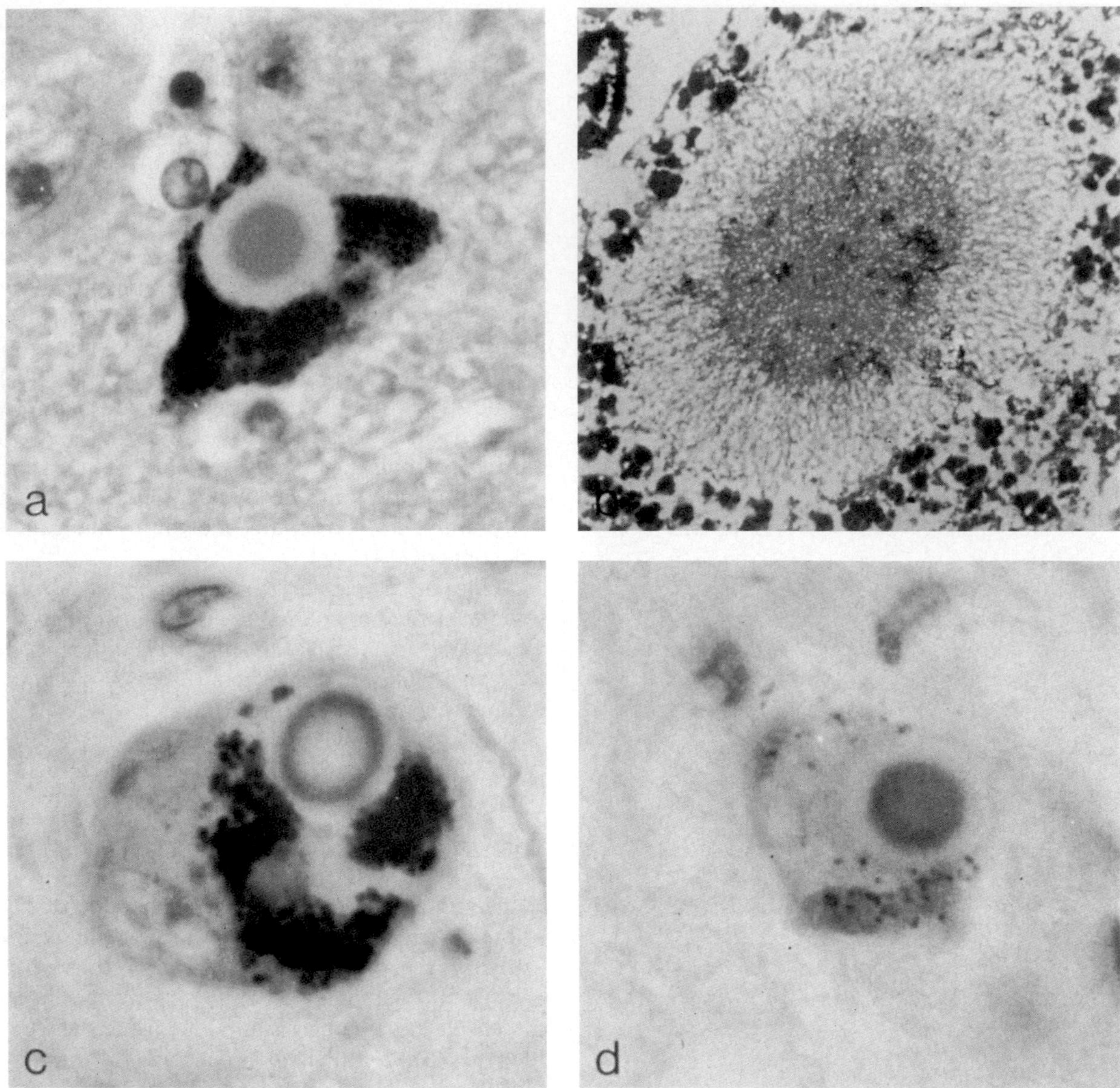

FIG. 32. Light (**a,c,d**) and electron (**b**) micrographs of substantia nigra Lewy bodies from a patient with Parkinson's disease (PD) stained with H&E (**a**) or antibodies to neurofilament protein (**c** and **d**). (From Trojanowski et al., ref. 137, with permission.)

clearly describe progressive supranuclear palsy (PSP) (315,316). The disease usually begins in the sixth decade, with a range from the mid-40s to the mid-70s (1). The diagnosis can be established by the symptoms of axial rigidity with neck extension, supranuclear ophthalmoplegia with particular impairment of vertical eye movements, pseudobulbar palsy, extrapyramidal symptoms, and occasional dementia (135). MR findings can sometimes support the clinical diagnosis (135).

Neuroimaging and Pathology

Pathologic and neuroimaging studies have documented atrophy of the mesencephalon in PSP (13,135, 317–324). More specifically, focal atrophy and/or signal changes of midbrain structures may occur on MR (13,135). The superior colliculi comprise the subcortical region of oculomotor control that is impaired in PSP (135). Some, but not all PSP patients on MR show corresponding superior collicular focal atrophy (Fig. 35) and/or hypointense signal on the second echo of the long TR sequence (135). The latter observation presumably reflects iron or other paramagnetic deposition. The periaqueductal region of the midbrain is also implicated in the pathology of PSP with histologic changes of gliosis and NFTs (134,135,318). The composition of these tangles is similar but not identical to the NFTs in AD (325). On MR, some patients show slight hyperintense signal on the long TR sequences of the periaqueductal gray matter (13,135). Severity of MR findings correlated well with severity and duration of disease.

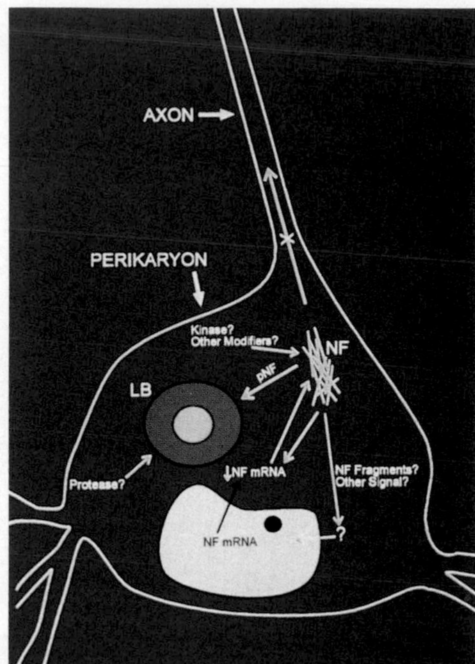

FIG. 33. Hypothetical series of events leading to the formation of LBs in cortical and subcortical neurons as well as potential deleterious consequences of LB formation in neurons. Neurofilaments (NFs) may aggregate into perikaryal LBs due to aberrant phosphorylation of NFs or NF subunits (pNF) in the perikaryon where proteases fail to degrade these inclusions completely. Proteolytic NF fragments in perikarya or other signals may downregulate NF mRNA levels leading to reduced NF subunit synthesis. This and the diversion of NFs into LBs may deplete the axon of NFs leading to the "dying back" of axons, the degeneration of affected neurons, and functional impairments in LB disorders. (From Trojanowski and Lee, ref. 142, with permission.)

MR also shows diminished width of the pars compacta of the substantia nigra in PSP patients (Fig. 35C). As in the other primary parkinsonian syndromes, this either reflects neuronal loss of the pars compacta (Fig. 35D) or iron deposition. The presence of abnormal signal changes of the putamen in PSP vary in MR investigations. Some found prominent hypointense signal of the putamen on the second echo of the long TR sequence on 1.5 T (77,303) (Fig. 35). Others observed this change only in a minority of patients with PSP (135). No definite pathologic changes of the putamen are described in this entity.

Leigh's Syndrome

(Subacute Necrotizing Encephalomyelopathy)

Subacute necrotizing encephalomyelopathy (SNE) or Leigh's syndrome presents early in life with psychomotor regression, abnormal muscle tone, weakness, dystonia, brainstem and cerebellar dysfunction (ataxia), visual loss, missed milestones of development, tachypnea, and seizures (326–329). Clinical findings, however, can be variable and nonspecific (269). SNE is usually inherited in an autosomal recessive fashion, and the underlying defect can be at any of a number of sites in the enzyme pathway for respiratory metabolism. Age of onset of symptoms is typically less than 2 years (infantile form), but others may present in childhood (juvenile form) and unusually in adulthood (330,331). Death usually occurs within a few years after onset of symptoms, typically from progressive respiratory failure (269). Laboratory

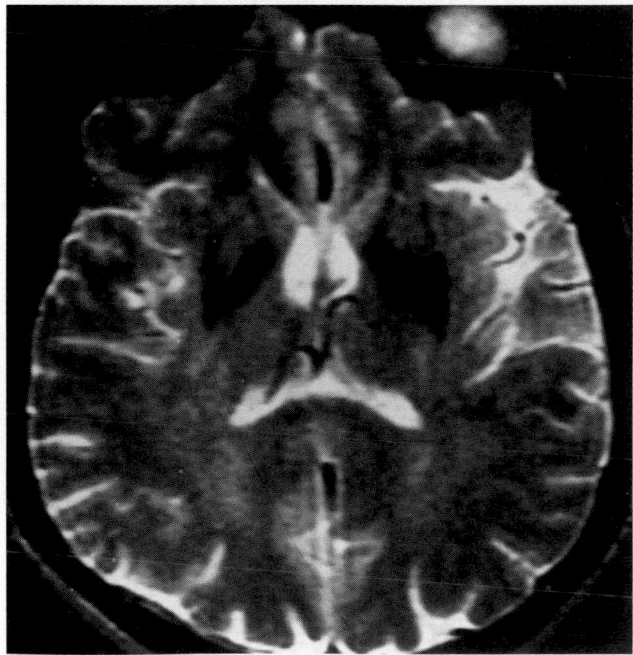

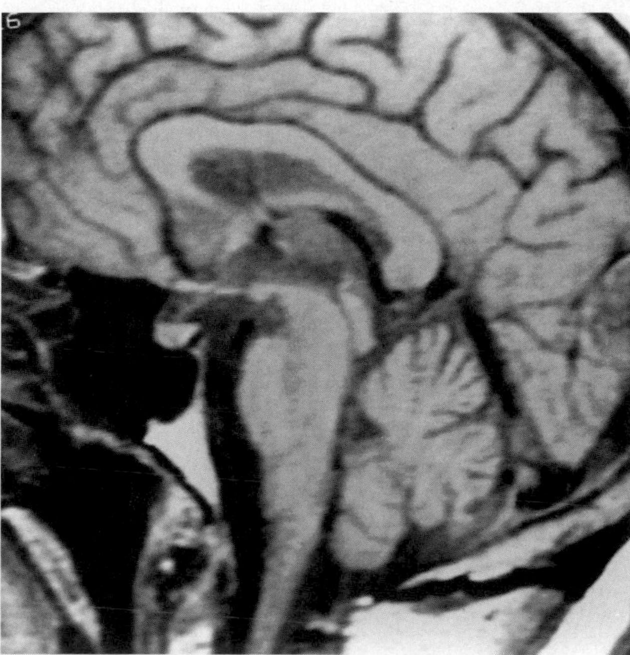

FIG. 34. Striatonigral degeneration. **A:** Axial MR, TR/TE 2500/80. In this 56-year-old woman, the signal of the lateral aspect of the putamen is as hypointense as the globus pallidus. **B:** Sagittal MR, TR/TE 600/20. Note absence of atrophy of the midbrain, pons, and cerebellum (compare with PSP, Fig. 35 and OPCD, Fig. 38, respectively).

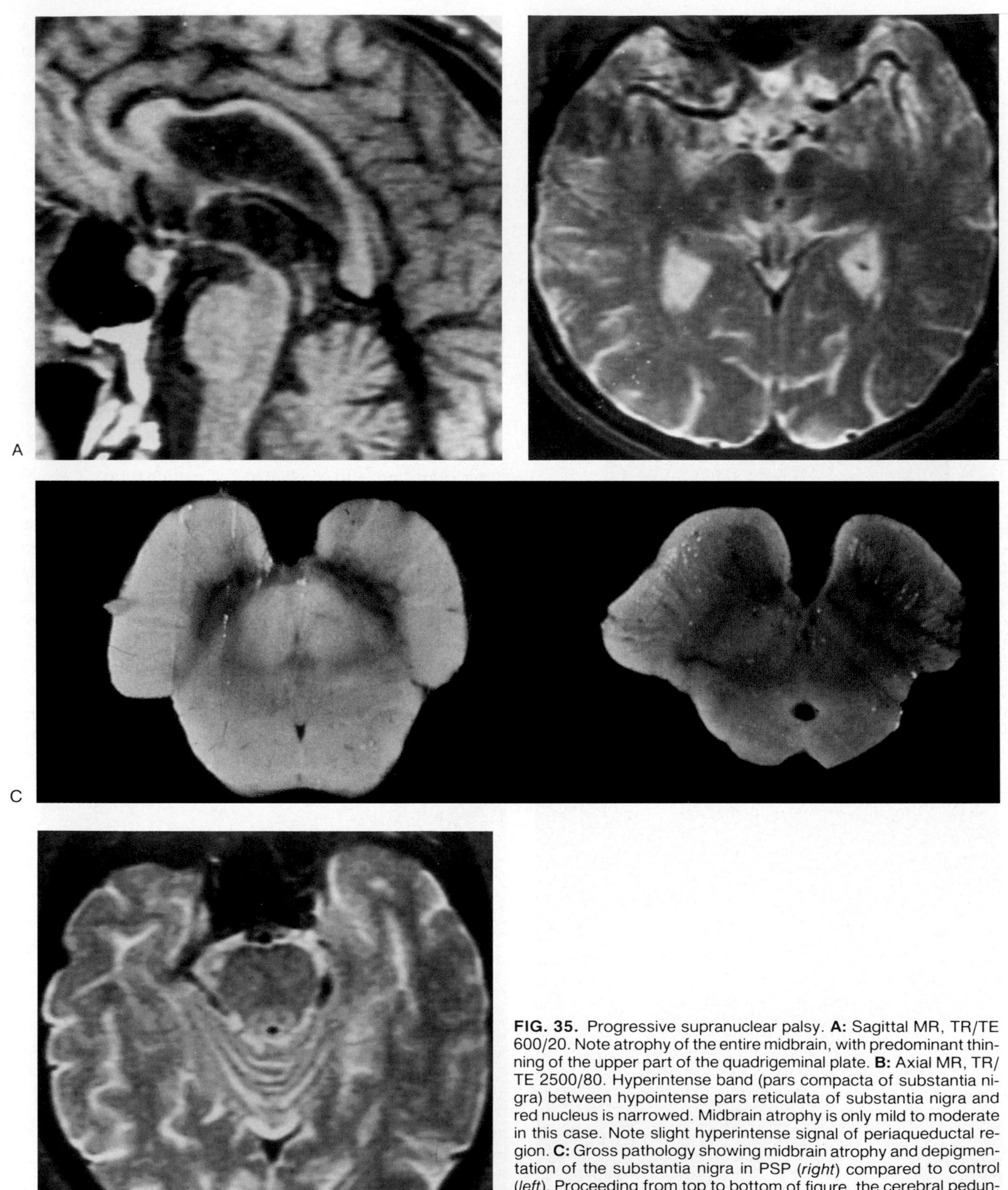

FIG. 35. Progressive supranuclear palsy. **A:** Sagittal MR, TR/TE 600/20. Note atrophy of the entire midbrain, with predominant thinning of the upper part of the quadrigeminal plate. **B:** Axial MR, TR/TE 2500/80. Hyperintense band (pars compacta of substantia nigra) between hypointense pars reticulata of substantia nigra and red nucleus is narrowed. Midbrain atrophy is only mild to moderate in this case. Note slight hyperintense signal of periaqueductal region. **C:** Gross pathology showing midbrain atrophy and depigmentation of the substantia nigra in PSP (*right*) compared to control (*left*). Proceeding from top to bottom of figure, the cerebral peduncles, substantia nigra, red nuclei, cerebral aqueduct, and superior colliculi are successively seen. Midbrain atrophy with enlargement of the cerebral aqueduct and depigmentation of the substantia nigra in PSP are striking when contrasted with the control specimen. **D:** Axial MR, TR/TE 2500/80.

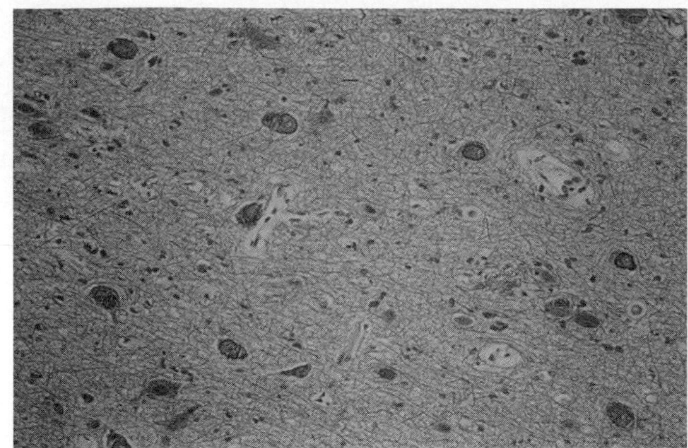
E

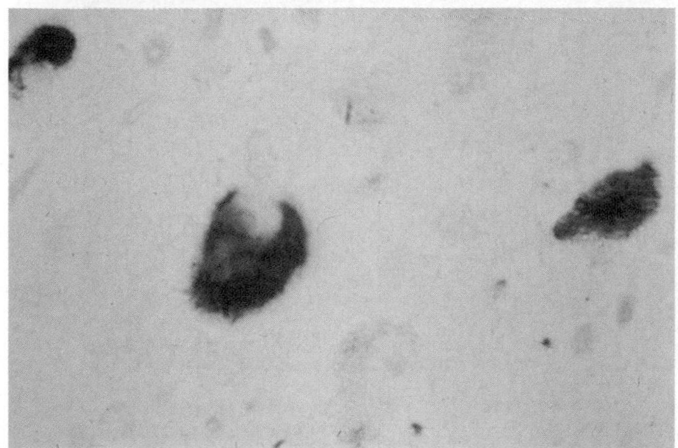
F

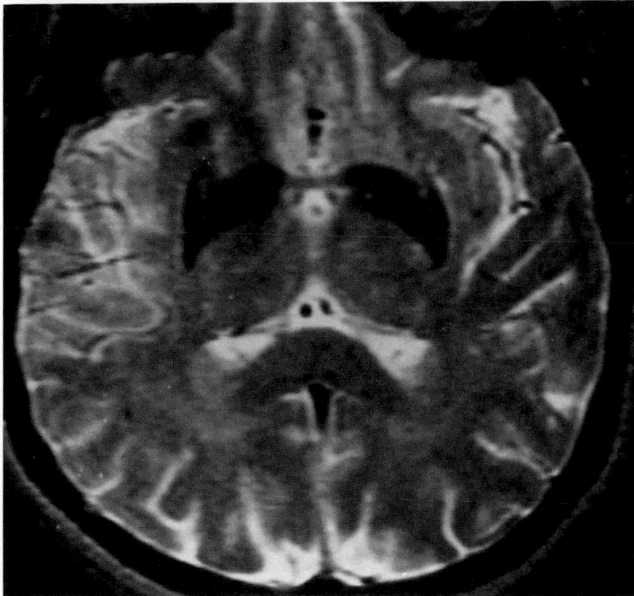
G

FIG. 35. (*Continued.*) The periaqueductal region shows moderate hyperintense signal. **E:** Neurofibrillary tangles in third nerve nucleus, Bodian stain. Violet stained round structures are neurofibrillary tangles. **F:** Neurofibrillary tangles in pons labeled with tau antibody. Neurofibrillary tangles in AD and PSP differ in location (hippocampal and brainstem in AD, brainstem in PSP) and in morphology [paired helical filaments in AD and straight filaments in PSP (317)]. Immunologic studies have documented similarities and dissimilarities between PSP and AD neurofibrillary tangles (317). **G:** Axial MR, TR/TE 2500/80. Signal intensity of lateral putamen is as hypointense as globus pallidus.

analysis shows metabolic acidosis with elevated blood, CSF lactate, and pyruvate concentrations (328,332). Associated mitochondrial enzyme deficiencies are pyruvate carboxylase, pyruvate dehydrogenase, cytochrome C oxidase, and Complex 1 (nicotinamide-adenine dinucleotide-coenzyme Q reductase) deficiencies (328,329,332); however, specific metabolic abnormalities are variable (327). It is possible to come to a diagnosis of probable SNE during life on the basis of clinical signs and symptoms, mode of inheritance, metabolic abnormalities, and neuroimaging findings (333,334).

Neuroimaging and Pathology

The pathology of SNE is characterized by capillary proliferation with bilaterally symmetric gray and white matter necrosis, spongiform degeneration or vacuolization, and demyelination (328,331,335). [Thus the descriptive term coined by Leigh—subacute necrotizing encephalomyelopathy (326).] These lesions result in nonenhancing hypodensities on CT (336–338). The sensitivity is significantly improved with MR imaging, with lesions appearing hypointense on short TR and hyperintense on long TR sequences (327,328,331,333,339,340) (Fig. 36). The pathologic findings overlap with Wernicke's encephalopathy; sparing of the mammillary bodies in SNE is an important differential feature (328,331).

MR imaging shows bilateral areas of abnormal high signal intensity on long TR/TE images in the basal ganglia, periventricular white matter, corpus callosum, and brainstem. Although lesions may occur variably in a wide range of locations (327,328,331,334,341), the commonest sites in a large pathologic series (335) were the brainstem tegmentum (98%), spinal cord (74%), basal ganglia (67%), and optic pathways (65%). In the basal ganglia, the putamen is particularly involved (Fig. 36). Hypointense signal on long TR/TE images of the thalami and lentiform nuclei in an infant with SNE has been observed, presumably due to deposition of iron or another paramagnetic substance. In one series, 100% of preschool-aged patients with proven SNE had putaminal involvement (328). In that report, a patient with congenital lactic acidosis of undetermined origin also had multiple abnormal areas of high signal intensity, but no evidence of putaminal lesions.

Some lesions on MR or CT are transient, and resolve with time; this may reflect detection of active lesions with vascular proliferation that pathologically resolve and do not progress to cavitation with necrosis (339). Another group reported a juvenile-onset patient studied serially through the acute phase of an attack. The lesions appear to have a dynamic component, with resolution of abnormalities observed acutely as well as the development of new lesions on a follow-up scan three months later. No putaminal involvement was seen in this patient (342). Proton spectroscopy has demonstrated elevated brain

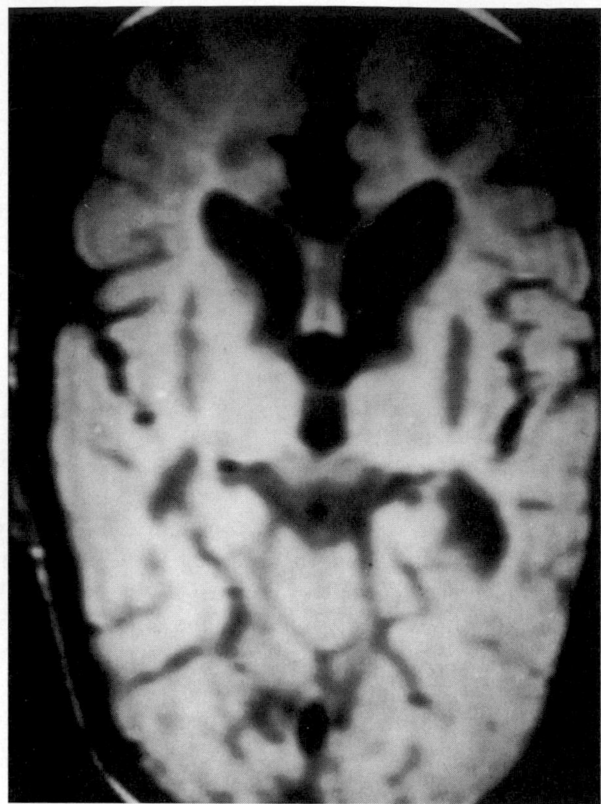

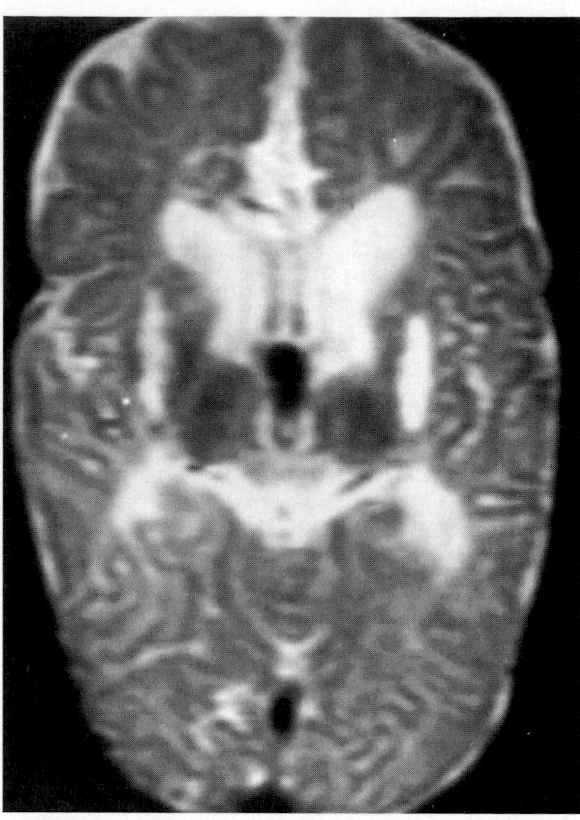

FIG. 36. Infantile form of SNE. Note bilateral putaminal lesions, hypointense on the short TR sequence (**A**), hyperintense on the long TR/TE image (**B**). Note also hypointense signal of the thalami and globus pallidi bilaterally and lateral aspect of the right putamen, probably due to iron or other paramagnetic deposition.

lactate levels in the basal ganglia, occipital cortex, and brainstem. This abnormality was greatest at sites of abnormal signal intensity on T2-weighted images (343).

Other Mitochondrial Encephalomyelopathies

The mitochondrial encephalomyelopathies comprise a group of disorders that have in common structural or functional mitochondrial abnormalities resulting in multisystem disorders of the central and peripheral nervous systems, skeletal muscles, heart, endocrine glands, gastrointestinal tract, hematopoietic system, and kidneys (269,344,345). Muscle biopsy may display characteristic "ragged red fibers" (344,345). In addition to Leigh's syndrome, these disorders include mitochondrial cytopathy, mitochondrial myopathy, Kearns-Sayre (K-S) syndrome, MERRLA (myoclonus, epilepsy, ragged red fibers, and lactic acidosis), MELAS (mitochondrial myopathy, lactic acidosis, and stroke), and Alpers' and Menke's diseases (269,346). They show heterogeneity and overlap with regard to their clinical, biochemical, pathologic, and radiologic features, making classification of the mitochondrial encephalomyeopathies somewhat difficult (347). In addition, newly discovered rarer diseases such as hereditary spastic dystonia are considered putative forms of mitochondrial encephalopathy on the basis of shared findings such as basal ganglia involvement (348). Biopsy of brain and muscle tissue has led to the suggestion that a mitochondrial angiopathy may underlie the ischemic episodes in this family of illnesses (349). This hypothesis is supported by work with SPECT and MRI showing dysfunction of the capillary endothelium at the sites that were abnormal on MR (350).

Clinical presentation of Leigh's syndrome, and Alpers', and Menkes' diseases occur in infants and early childhood, while MELAS, MERRF, and Kearns-Sayre (K-S) syndrome tend to present in older children and adults (269,346). Progression of disease is usually slow (269). Typical features are short stature, dementia, weakness, sensorineural hearing loss, and serum lactic acidosis (347). MELAS can be clinically differentiated from other mitochondrial disorders by the presence of cortical blindness and hemiparesis and absence of ophthalmoplegia, heart block, and myoclonus (347).

Neuroimaging and Pathology

MELAS syndrome shows bilateral symmetric and asymmetric infarct-like lesions that do not strictly correlate with vascular territories (347,351) (Fig. 37). MR is more sensitive than CT for their detection (352). Common sites of involvement are the basal ganglia, parietal, occipital, and temporal lobes, and cerebellar hemispheres. Involvement of optic radiations and occipital cortex account for cortical blindness in MELAS (347). The frontal lobes and brainstem are typically spared (347). With progression of disease, diffuse atrophy develops (347). When the white matter is involved, particularly in MELAS, MERRF, K-S syndrome, and Leigh's syndrome, there is a predilection for peripheral and retrotrigonal white matter (346,353).

The histology of the brain lesions in MELAS is referred to as spongy degeneration with neuronal loss, gliosis, spongy alteration of cortical layers, and microcystic liquefaction (347). Basal ganglionic lesions in MELAS (and in MERRF and K-S syndrome) not uncommonly calcify (347). In MELAS, it is possible to follow patients from presentation of an acute stroke through to either resolution (338,354) or more commonly later develop-

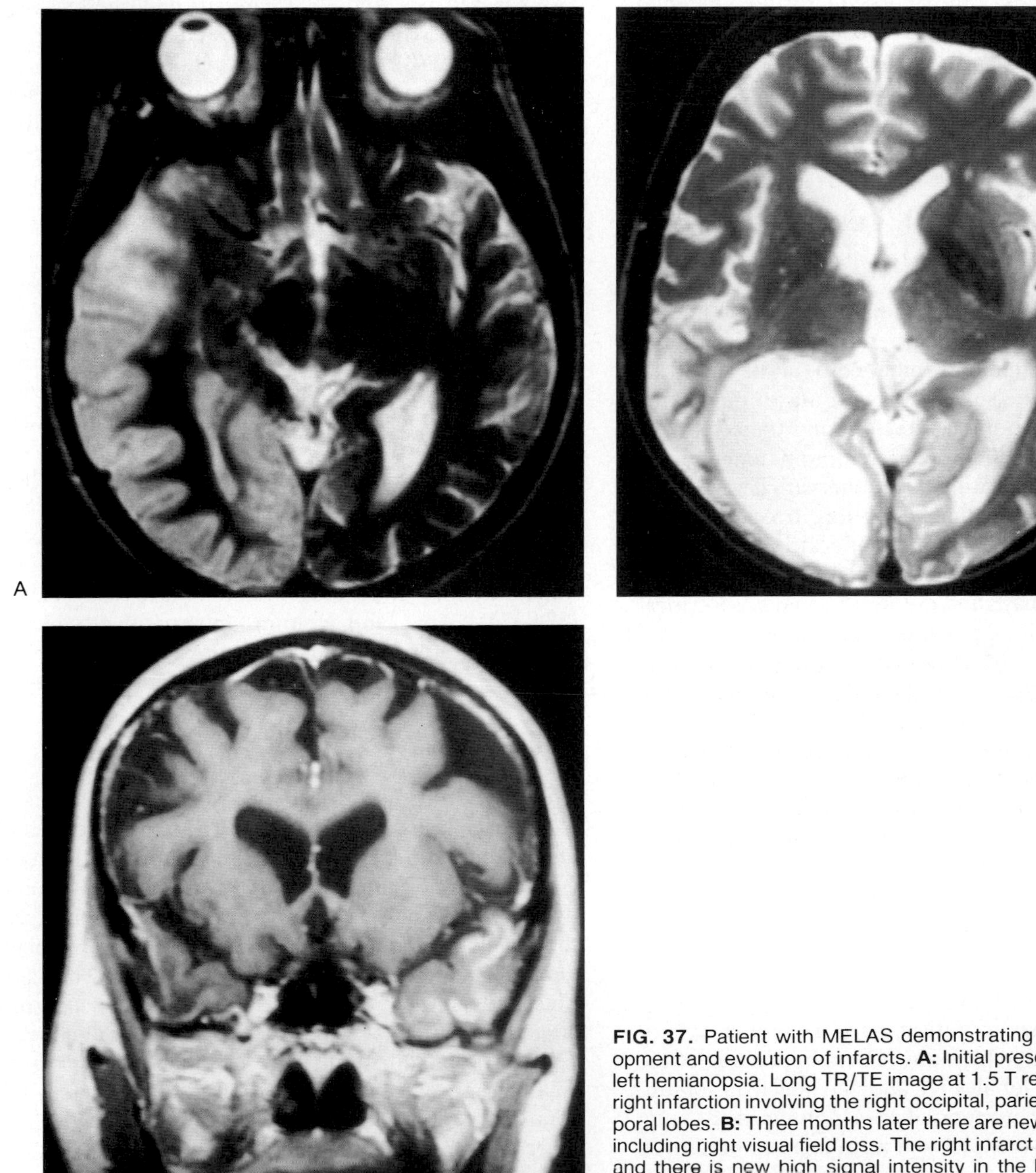

FIG. 37. Patient with MELAS demonstrating serial development and evolution of infarcts. **A:** Initial presentation with left hemianopsia. Long TR/TE image at 1.5 T reveals a large right infarction involving the right occipital, parietal, and temporal lobes. **B:** Three months later there are new symptoms, including right visual field loss. The right infarct has evolved, and there is new high signal intensity in the left calcarine cortex. **C:** Enhanced image from the same day as figure B shows enhancement in the left temporal lobe, confirming the presence of a recent infarct.

ment of focal atrophy at the site of infarction, as well as the development of progressive generalized atrophy (Fig. 37).

MERRF typically involves the basal ganglia, cerebellum, brainstem, and spinal cord (347). Lesions in the basal ganglia and in the cerebral and cerebellar white matter have been reported in K-S syndrome (355). Menke's kinky hair disease is an X-linked disorder of copper metabolism. Clinically, patients present with arrested motor development, seizures, and mental retardation. The hair has a characteristic kinking and friability. MR imaging and MRA reveal progressive cerebral atrophy in the first years of life, markedly tortuous cerebral vessels, ischemic changes, extra-axial hematomas, and hygromas—presumably from shearing of bridging veins (356–358). Other forms of copper deficiency (non-Menke's) may also demonstrate atrophy and periventricular ischemia (359).

DEGENERATION OF THE CEREBELLUM, BRAINSTEM, AND SPINAL CORD

Ataxia typically is a predominant neurologic finding in patients with cerebellar degenerative processes (1). Lesions of the brainstem and spinal cord (and even of the parietal lobe) may also present with ataxia due to the many links between the cerebellum and the cerebrum, brainstem, and spinal cord (1). Symptomatology, however, may differ. For example, patients with degenerative changes in the cerebellum have more frequent occurrence of ophthalmoplegia and optic atrophy than patients with spinal cord degenerative processes (1). The cerebellum in humans and in lower primates is a critical relay station for foveal pursuits and visual-vestibular interaction requiring foveal pursuit (360). Neuroimaging of degenerative processes of the cerebellum, brainstem, and/or spinal cord has dramatically improved with MR imaging compared to CT (361,362) because of absence of bone artifact, the possibility to evaluate in the three orthogonal planes, the ability to directly visualize the spinal cord, and an increased sensitivity of imaging atrophy as well as underlying degenerative parenchymal abnormalities (with consequent signal changes).

Autism

The MR findings in autism have generated controversy in the scientific literature. Focal hypoplasia of the superior vermian lobules VI and VII (declive, folium, and tuber) has been reported in a nonretarded young adult with autism (364) as well as in a group of autistic children, both retarded and nonretarded (365). In the cerebrum, volume loss of the parietal lobe cortex and white matter, as well as the posterior corpus callosum, has also been reported (365). Another group reported that the midbrain and medulla were significantly smaller in retarded autistic children and nonautistic mentally retarded children than in controls (366). Furthermore, in another report, the brainstem and cerebellar vermis (lobules VIII to X) were significantly smaller in autistics than in controls (367).

However, in a large study of 53 patients with autism no single pattern predicted the presence or severity of the disease. Specifically, the vermian pattern described above was not confirmed (368). This alternative conclusion is supported by a study that reported no significant anatomic abnormalities or differences from controls (369) as well as a study of 15 autistic children by visual inspection of MR images that showed no detectable abnormalities (370). A more recent report showed no significant anatomic findings in high-functioning autistics versus controls matched for several variables including IQ and socioeconomic status (371), while another study showed no differences when patients were matched for IQ (372).

Fragile X

Fragile X or Martin-Bell syndrome consists of mental retardation, hyperactivity, repetitive stereotyped movements, language dysfunction, self-destructive behavior, and autism in males. Female carriers are less likely to be mentally retarded; however, psychiatric symptoms can occur, and neuroanatomic findings can be intermediate between normals and affected males (373–375). MR studies have shown decreased size of the posterior cerebellar vermis (lobules VI/VII and to a lesser degree lobules VIII–X) and increased size of the fourth ventricle (374,376). Area and volume measurement showed vermian atrophy and enlargement of the fourth ventricle (377).

Rett's Syndrome

Rett syndrome is a disease of young females with loss of language skills, autistic behaviors, stereotypical hand movements, and loss of motor skills. Frontal atrophy is detectable on CT and MR (378). In another study, quantitative MR analysis relative to normal volunteers showed global brain hypoplasia. In addition, the cerebellum showed progressive atrophy with increasing age. This may represent the disease process itself or superimposed factors such as seizure activity, use of anticonvulsants, or poor nutrition (379). Another group used an area measuring technique and found reductions in the hemisphere and caudate nuclei sizes versus controls; other measurements including those for the cerebellum were not significantly different compared to controls (380). Another quantitative study showed reduced cerebral volume (gray greater than white matter) but, without evidence of ongoing degeneration (381).

Down Syndrome

Down syndrome is one of the major genetic causes of mental retardation. The vast majority of cases is due to nondisjunction of chromosome 21 with a few percent due to translocation or mosaicism.

Quantitative techniques utilizing MR show reductions in volume of the brain, cortex, white matter, and cerebellum (382). These findings continued to be significant after correction for cranial cavity volume.

Down syndrome is also a significant risk factor for developing AD since virtually all Down syndrome patients develop AD pathology by age 40 (383). This is particularly interesting in that the gene for amyloid-β protein is present on the 21st chromosome (384,385). A study of older patients with Down syndrome (29 to 64 years old) showed significant widening of the temporal horns in the majority over the age of 50 (386). Proton spectroscopy investigations in patients with Down syndrome have shown a rapid decline in the NAA:choline ratio after the age of 40. This preceded identifiable marked atrophic changes on CT and correlates with the timing of clinical decline (387,388). Rarely, Down syndrome may be associated with moyamoya phenomena (389).

Olivopontocerebellar Degeneration

Both an inherited form of olivopontocerebellar degeneration (OPCD), first described by Menzel (390), and a sporadic type, first described by Dejerine and Thomas (391) exist. The former is inherited in a dominant fashion (134), although transmission in a recessive mode has been reported (1). Onset of OPCD varies between early childhood and old age, with most cases evenly spread from the first through the fifth decades (134). The duration of illness is between 10 and 20 years (134). The main manifestation is ataxia, first in the legs, then the arms and hands, and finally the bulbar musculature. This symptomatology is common to all the cerebellar atrophies (1). Because the clinical symptoms and signs of OPCD may overlap with other cerebellar degenerative and nondegenerative diseases, and since a unifying biochemical marker is lacking, positive neuroimaging findings are essential in the in vivo diagnosis of OPCD (392).

Neuroimaging and Pathology

The primary degeneration in OPCD centers in pontine nuclei, with a subsequent progressive anterograde degeneration of pontocerebellar fibers and of the cerebellar cortex, hemispheric greater than vermian (134,392, 393) (Fig. 38E–G). Pontocerebellar fibers originate in the pontine nuclei, have a transverse course in the pons (thus they are called transverse pontine fibers), run to the cerebellum through the middle cerebellar peduncles (134,392,393), and terminate in all lobules of the cerebellar hemisphere and in the declive, folium, and tuber of the cerebellar vermis (252). The degeneration in OPCD is characterized by myelin sheath loss and gliosis of this pontocerebellar pathway and neuronal loss of the cerebellar cortex (134). The cortical lesions cause a retrograde degeneration of the inferior olives (392–393). [These fibers originate in the contralateral inferior olive and reach the cerebellum via the inferior cerebellar peduncle (252).] As a result, the inferior olive loses its normal bulge due to neuronal loss accompanied by gliosis (134). Clinically (1), pathologically (134), and radiologically (392), SND and/or SDS may coexist with OPCD in patients with multiple system atrophy (MSA).

On MR, atrophy and abnormal signal occur in these selectively involved structures (392) (Fig. 31A–D). The midline sagittal section shows selective pontine atrophy with flattening of its inferior part and loss of the normal pontine bulge (392). Atrophy of the middle cerebellar peduncles, the cerebellum (hemispheric greater than vermian), and the inferior olives is also well seen on MR (13,392,394). On long TR sequences a slight hyperintense signal, best appreciated on the first echo, involves the pontocerebellar pathway (Fig. 38B and D) (392) and the olives (Fig. 31C). Adjacent tracts not involved in the pontocerebellar pathway (i.e., the tegmentum, pyramidal tracts, and superior cerebellar peduncles) are spared pathologically (393) and on MRI (392) (Fig. 31B and D). Cerebellorubral degeneration is detectable after resection of the dentate nucleus (128). Loss of the contralateral dentate nucleus can also lead to a hypertrophic degeneration of the olivary nucleus with palatal myoclonus (395). This is manifested as enlargement and hyperintensity on MR of the hypertrophied olivary nucleus.

Cerebello-Olivary Degeneration
(Cerebellar Cortical Degeneration)

A familial form, first described by Holmes in 1907, and a sporadic form, initially reported by Marie, Foix, and Alajouine in 1922, exist. The onset of the familial form is usually around age 35, but onset can occur between infancy and old age (134). The onset of the sporadic form is 10–20 years later than that of the inherited form (134). Progression is extremely slow (survival 15 to 20 years) (1). The clinical picture is a progressive cerebellar ataxia (1) with ataxia of gait, instability of trunk, tremor of hands and head, and slightly slowed, hesitant speech.

Neuroimaging and Pathology

Neuroimaging and gross pathology of cerebello-olivary or cerebellar cortical degeneration (CCD) shows

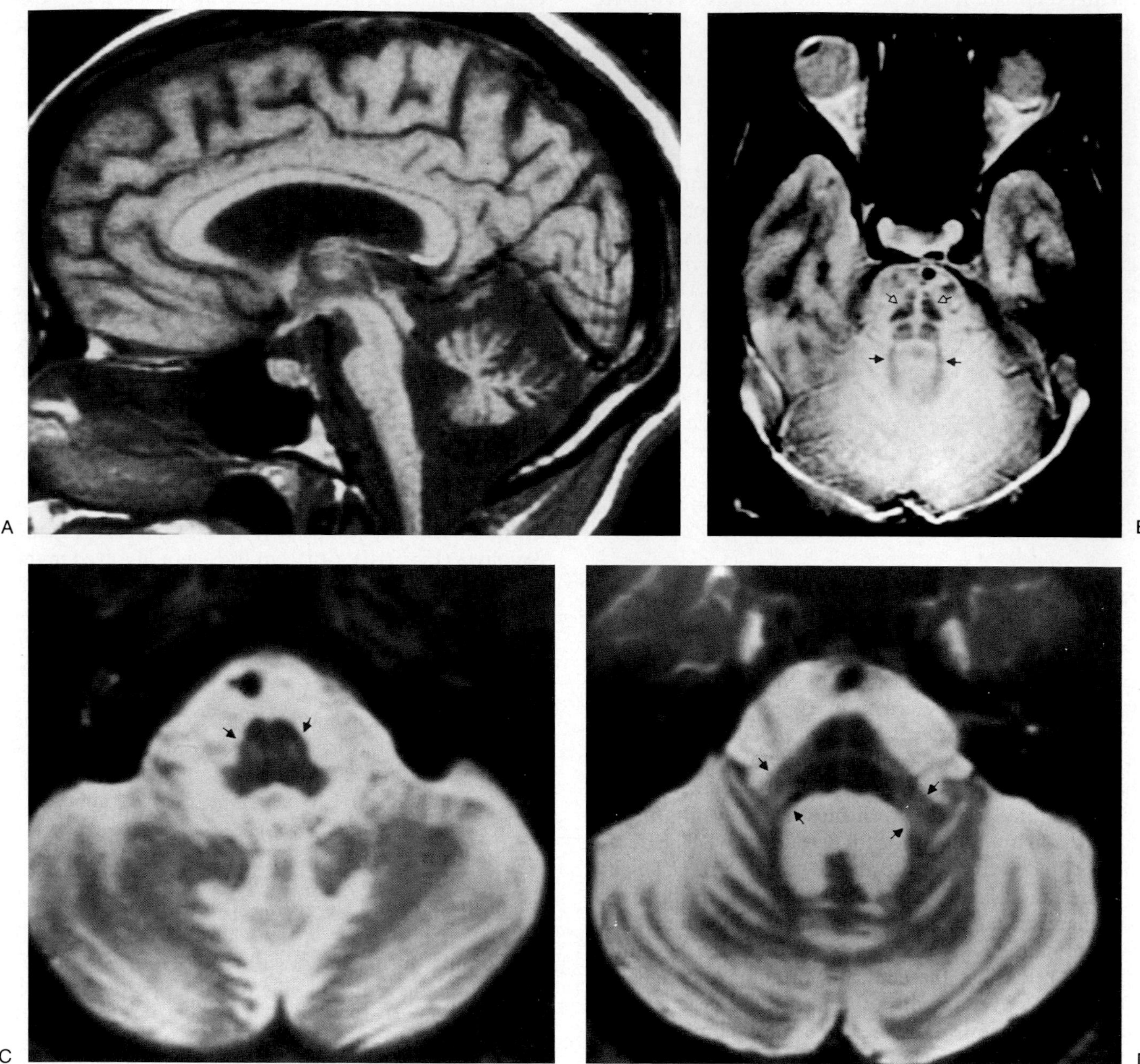

FIG. 38. Olivopontocerebellar degeneration. **A:** Sagittal MR, TR/TE 600/20. The normal bulge of the pons is reduced with flattening of its inferior part. Moderate atrophy is also seen in the cerebellum. **B–D:** Axial MR, TR/TE 2500/20 (B), 2500/80 (C,D). On first echo of long TR sequence through the pons (B) note abnormal hyperintense signal of transverse pontine fibers (between the tegmentum posteriorly and the base of the pons anteriorly), the raphe, the anterior and lateral portions of the pons merging with the middle cerebellar peduncles and extending to the cerebellum. In contrast, the superior cerebellar peduncles (*black arrows*), tegmentum of the pons, and pyramidal tracts (*open black arrows*) are spared and show normal signal. In the medulla (C), note loss of the normal olivary bulge with slight underlying hyperintense signal (*black arrow*). **D:** Abnormal hyperintense signal of transverse pontine fibers, the raphe, and on the anterior and lateral portions of the pons merging with the middle cerebellar peduncles (*arrows*) is more subtle in this case. Also note atrophy of middle cerebellar peduncle, cerebellum, and pons with marked enlargement of the prepontine cistern, fourth ventricle, and sulci of the cerebellar hemispheres.

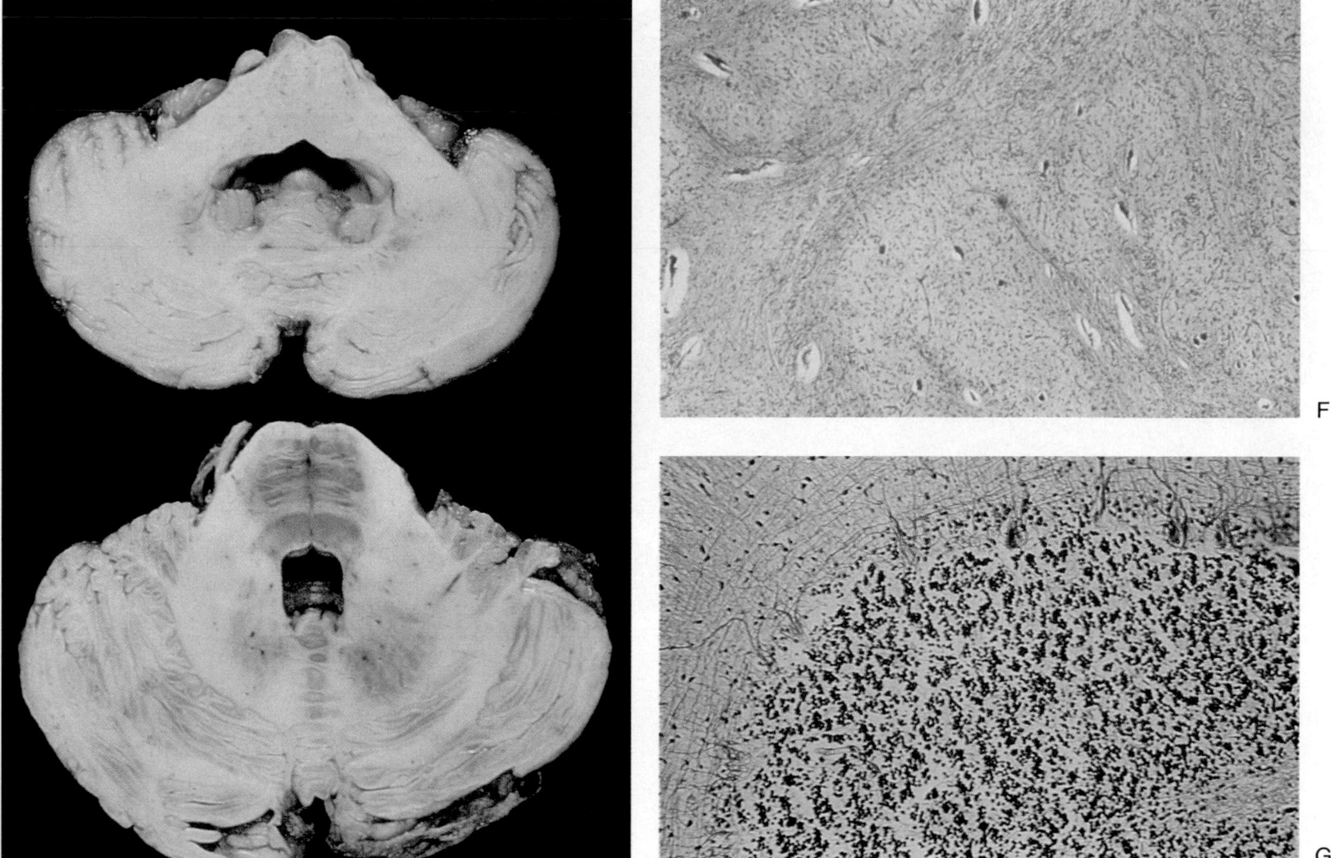

FIG. 38. (*Continued.*) **E:** Gross pathology olivopontocerebellar degeneration top, with normal specimen on bottom. Note marked loss of the normal rounded ventral bulge of the pons, moderate diminished width of the middle cerebellar peduncles, and significant atrophy of the cerebellum. **F:** Histopathology of inferior olives. Nissl and Luxol fast blue stain show neuronal loss and gliosis. The portions staining darker blue are white matter; the paler staining serpentine component is the inferior olivary nucleus. The larger cells in the inferior olive are neurons, and are greatly reduced in number. The smaller cells are glial cells, and are increased (i.e., gliosis). **G:** Histopathology of cerebellum at corticomedullary junction. Bodian stain, showing "empty" basket cells. Purkinje cells are large cells at the corticomedullary junction in the upper right portion and normally abut basket cells. In lower left, basket cells are "empty" due to Purkinje cell loss.

selective cerebellar atrophy due to loss of Purkinje cells, granule cells, and myelinated fibers (134). While these changes may occur throughout the cerebellum, they predominate in the vermis (Fig. 31), particularly the anterior vermis (360,396). As a result, the primary fissure (which separates the anterior and posterior parts of the cerebellar vermis) and the superior cerebellar cistern are enlarged. CCD is believed to represent a primary degeneration of the cerebellar cortex with secondary retrograde transsynaptic degeneration of the inferior olives (134,360). Olivary atrophy, due to neuronal loss and gliosis, consequently occurs (134).

Selective atrophy of the cerebellar vermis, particularly of its anterior part, also occurs with other primary cerebellar neurodegenerative disorders [acetazolamide-responsive familial paroxysmal ataxia (ARFPA) and infantile cerebellar ataxia] and with acquired cerebellar degenerations. ARFPA is a rare, dominantly inherited disorder, characterized clinically by lifelong recurrent attacks of cerebellar ataxia, dysarthria, and nystagmus (396). A unique feature of this disorder among the heredoatrophic degenerations of the brain is its relatively benign natural history, characterized by intermittency of clinical manifestations. The first documentation of the neuroanatomical abnormality in this condition (i.e., atrophy of the cerebellar vermis, particularly the anterior vermis) was achieved in an MR investigation (396). Infantile cerebellar atrophy is a unique type of dominantly

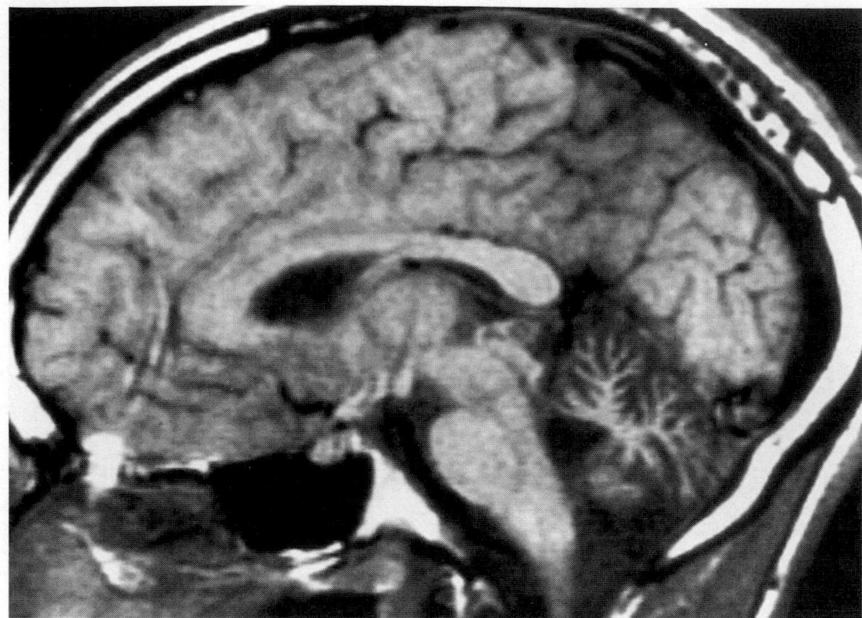

FIG. 39. Sagittal MRI, TR/TE 600/20. A 17-year-old with probable primary cerebellar cortical degeneration. Note pronounced vermian atrophy. Unlike OPCD (Fig. 38), the basis pontis is preserved.

inherited, early-onset, nonprogressive cerebellar degeneration (397).

Differential Diagnosis of Neurodegenerative Cerebellar Atrophy: Acquired Cerebellar Degeneration

Causes of acquired cerebellar degeneration include alcohol abuse (398) (Fig. 39), paraneoplastic disorders (399), toxic effects of drugs [dilantin, diphenylhydantoin (134) (Fig. 40), high-dose cytosine arabinoside (400)], and rarely with thallium or chronic toluene poisoning, or following influenza vaccination (401). The selective atrophy common to all these disorders suggests that the anterior cerebellar vermis is unusually susceptible to various degenerative processes that primarily affect the cerebellum (397). Sparing of pontocerebellar tracts and vermian atrophy predominating over hemispheric involvement are useful in differentiating cerebellar cortical

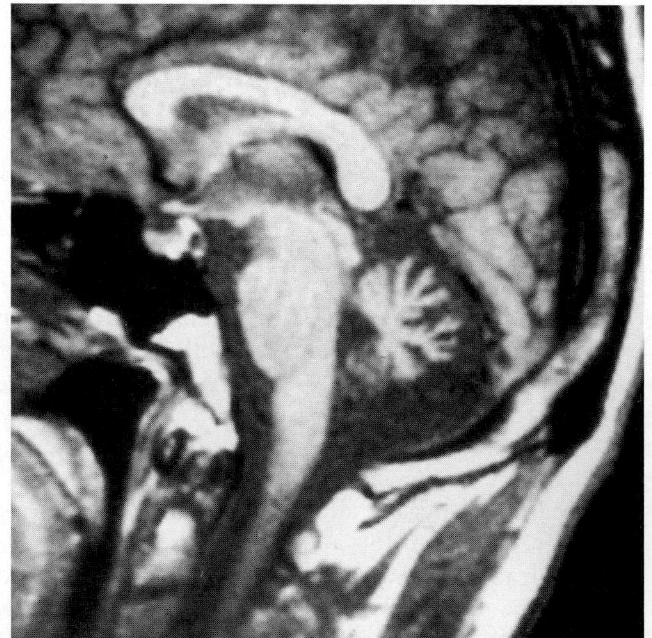

A

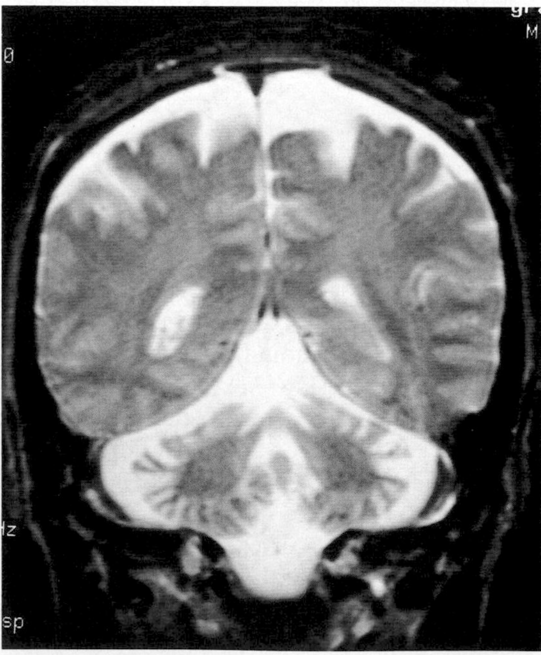

B

FIG. 40. A: Sagittal MR, TR/TE 600/20. In this patient on long-standing anti-seizure medication, note significant vermian atrophy. **B:** Chronic alcoholism: coronal long TR/TE images showing marked infratentorial atrophy.

TABLE 6. *Uncommon cerebellar degenerations*[a]

Disorder	Pathology and/or MRI
Gerstmann-Straussler-Sheinker disease	Atrophy of cerebellum, spinocerebellar, and corticospinal tracts and posterior columns of spinal cord, caudate, and cerebrum (1). MR also shows hypointensity on long TR sequences of basal ganglia (87)
Infantile X-linked ataxia and deafness	Cell loss and gliosis of cerebellar cortex, inferior olives, dentate nucleus, red nucleus, dorsal motor nucleus of vagus, and central auditory pathways (402)
Hereditary branchial myoclonus with spastic paraparesis and cerebellar ataxia	Severe atrophy of medulla and spinal cord with mild cerebellar and cerebral cortical atrophy (403)
Infantile neuroaxonal dystrophy	Cerebellar atrophy, demyelination, and intra-axonal spheroid. Cerebellum hyperintense on long TR MR (399)
Machado Joseph disease	Multisystem degeneration of neurons with gliosis: spinocerebellar tracts, anterior horn cells, Clarke's column of the spinal cord, cerebellum, brainstem, basal ganglia, and cerebrum (134,404)

[a] The predominant neuropathologic and/or MR findings of these less common cerebellar degenerations are described in the second column.

degenerations from OPCD (394). Other uncommon cerebellar degenerations are described in Table 6.

In addition to causing cerebral and cerebellar degeneration and atrophy (405–407), toluene exposure from chronic abuse by so-called spray heads can lead to particular atrophy of the corpus callosum with multifocal areas of hyperintense signal in the cerebral white matter (408–410) and symmetric hypointensity of the thalami (411) and other central gray matter structures suggestive of iron deposition has been reported on long TR/TE images (412).

Friedreich's Ataxia

Friedreich, in 1861, first described this progressive familial ataxia (1). Both autosomal recessive (more common) and dominant inheritance patterns occur. The gene mutation is assigned to chromosome 9 (1). The average age of onset is between 10 and 20 years (1). This syndrome is considered the prototypical progressive ataxia (1). Ataxia of gait (typically mixed sensory and cerebellar) with arm clumsiness and dysarthria are typical symptoms (1). Within 5 years of the onset walking is no longer possible. Pes cavus and kyphoscoliosis are characteristic features (1). Mean age of death ranges from 25 to 40 years. Kyphoscoliosis and restricted respiratory function may contribute to death (1). Kyphoscoliosis is probably due to spinal muscular imbalance (1). Tabetic aspects of the disease are explained by degeneration of posterior columns (i.e., fasciculi gracilis and cuneatus). Cerebellar ataxia is due to degeneration of the spinocerebellar tracts, the superior vermis, and the dentatorubral pathways; sensory impairment and loss of tendon reflexes are due to loss of large neurons in the sensory gan-

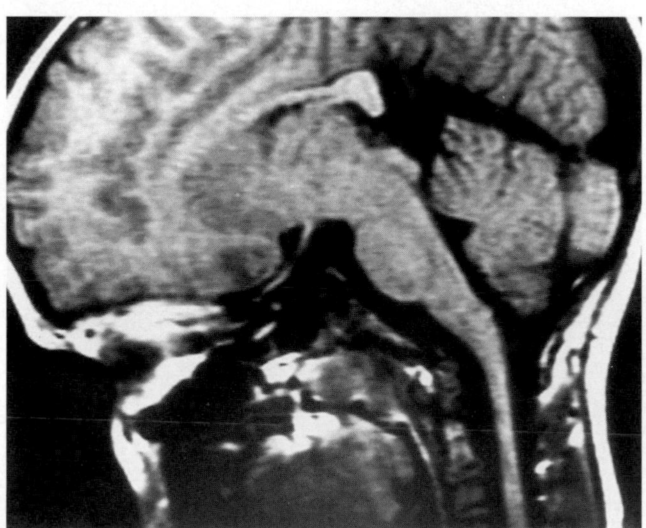
A

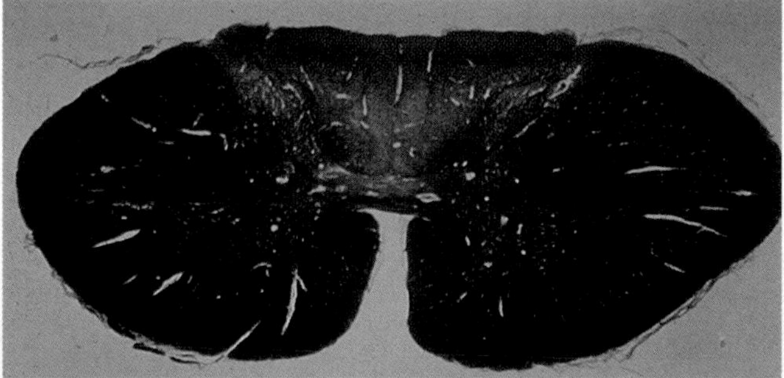
B

FIG. 41. A: Sagittal MR, TR/TE 600/20. Unclassified spinal form of hereditary ataxia. Note spinal cord atrophy with preservation of basis pontis and of cerebellum. **B:** Myelin-stained axial section of cervical spinal cord in Friedreich's ataxia. Note paler staining due to myelin loss of the posterior columns (i.e., fasciculus gracilis, fasciculus cuneatus). More mild pallor occurs at the extreme lateral margins (anterior spinocerebellar tracts) anteromedially (anterior corticospinal tract) and posterolaterally (lateral corticospinal tract).

TABLE 7. *Other spinal degenerations*

Disorder	Pathology
Hereditary spastic paraplegia (Strümpell-Lorrain disease)	Atrophic spinal cord with degeneration of posterior columns and corticospinal tract (134)
Hereditary posterior column ataxia (Biemond's disease)	Atrophic spinal cord with degenerated posterior columns (11)
Spinopontine degeneration	Pontine, cerebellar peduncles, spinocerebellar, and pontocerebellar tracts are atrophic and degenerated with sparing of cerebellum and inferior olives (11)

glia. Corticospinal lesions account for weakness and Babinski signs.

Neuroimaging and Pathology

Gross pathology and neuroimaging reveal a small spinal cord (134). These atrophic changes are due to degeneration with myelin loss and gliosis of the posterior columns and roots and spinocerebellar and corticospinal tracts (1,134) (Fig. 33). Some but not all patients exhibit cerebellar atrophy (361). These variable changes are due to slight to moderate neuronal loss of Purkinje cells in the superior vermis and of neurons in corresponding parts of the inferior olive (1). The absence or milder nature of the cerebellar atrophy in Friedreich's ataxia serves as a useful differential feature from primary cerebellar degenerative processes (compare Figs. 39–40 with 41) (361). Additional degenerative processes of the spinal cord are listed in Table 7.

DISEASES OF THE MOTOR SYSTEM

The corticospinal tract (pyramidal tract) is the crucial pathway for voluntary movement (252). This tract arises from the precentral and nearby gyri of the cerebral cortex; its fibers descend through the corona radiata, converge on the posterior limb of the internal capsule (252,413), course through the cerebral peduncles, the basis pontis (where the fibers are separated by the transverse pontine fascicles), and once again converge on the medullary pyramids (252,413). (Their course through the latter structure is the origin of the other name for this pathway, the pyramidal tract.) Most of the fibers cross at the pyramidal decussation in the lower medulla and descend in the contralateral corticospinal tract of the spinal cord (252,413); a small proportion of fibers do not decussate at this level but descend in ipsilateral anterior or lateral corticospinal tracts.

The primary neurodegenerative disorders of this group are motor neuron diseases. Wallerian degeneration of the corticospinal tract can be recognized pathologically and with neuroimaging because this tract is a discrete, compact collection of large numbers of axons. This is discussed in more detail in the section on wallerian degeneration.

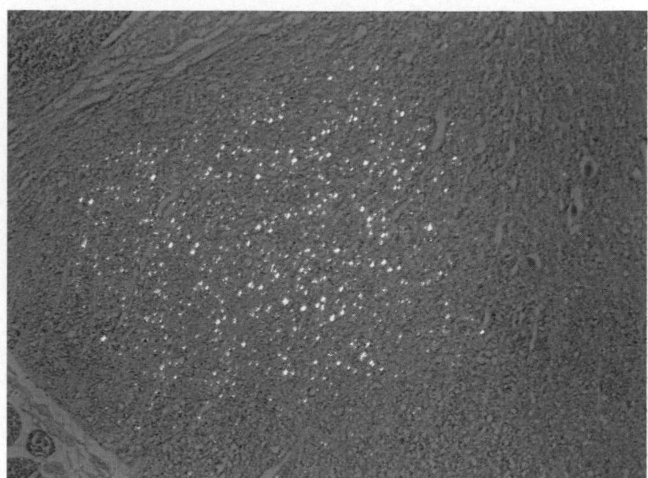

FIG. 42. Amyotrophic lateral sclerosis. Photomicrograph using a fat stain to demonstrate myelin and axonal breakdown products in the cervical cord. This section uses polarizing filters, and the breakdown products appear as white stipples against the blue background.

Amyotrophic Lateral Sclerosis

Motor neuron diseases are a heterogeneous group of syndromes in which the upper and/or lower motor neurons degenerate (414). Cortical motor neurons, including the pyramidal Betz cells, constitute the upper motor neuron in the circuit (134). The descending pathways include the corticospinal, and the indirect corticorubrospinal, corticoreticulospinal, corticovestibulospinal, and

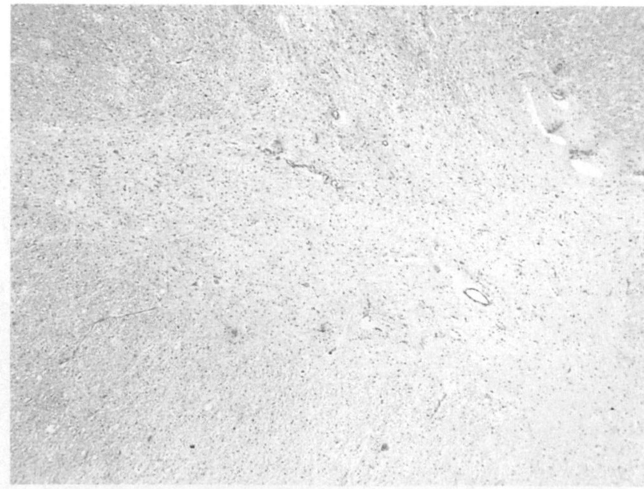

FIG. 43. Amyotrophic lateral sclerosis. Luxol fast blue—H&E stain in a case of ALS shows a complete loss of motor neurons in the anterior horn of the cervical spinal cord.

corticotectospinal tracts (1). The upper motor neurons synapse with cell bodies of the lower motor neurons in either motor nuclei of the brainstem or anterior horn cells (134). Axons of brainstem motor nuclei form the motor cranial nerves, and axons of anterior horn cells run out through the spinal ventral root and into the peripheral nerves to the end organ muscle (134).

Amyotrophic lateral sclerosis (ALS) is the most frequent type of degenerative motor neuron disease, with an annual incidence rate of 0.4 to 1.76 per 100,000 people (1). Most patients are 50 years and older at the onset of symptoms, and the incidence increases with aging. Most cases are sporadic; in about 5% of cases it is inherited in an autosomal dominant fashion (1). Its pathogenesis is unknown. However, a recent report that mutations in the superoxide dismutase (SOD) gene may account for some cases of familial ALS suggests a role for free-radical associated damage as a cause of this neurodegenerative disease (415).

Studies of transgenic mice suggest that altered neurotransmitter metabolism may be implicated in other cases (416,417). Recent success with a clinical trial utilizing the antiglutamate agent riluzole supports the role of the putative neurotransmitter glutamate in the disease pro-

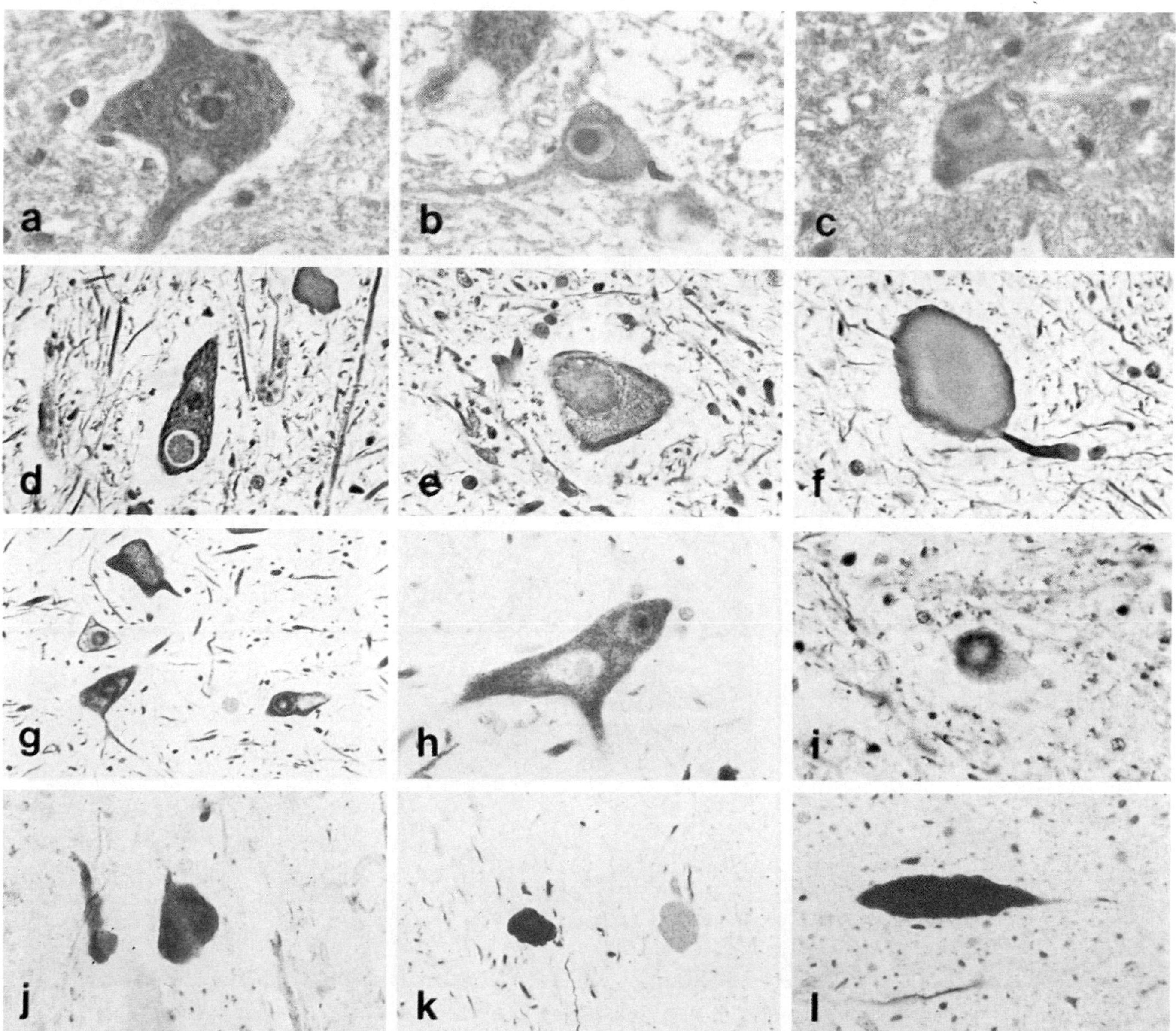

FIG. 44. Amyotrophic lateral sclerosis. Series of photomicrographs showing spheroids and inclusions in neurons and their processes in the cervical spinal cord of an ALS patient. **a–c:** Eosinophilic intra-neuronal inclusions (some of which resemble LBs) stained with hematoxylin and eosin. **d,e:** Similar inclusions stained with the Bodian method and the same stain reveals a spheroid in **f**. **g–i** show intra-neuronal inclusions (some of which resemble LBs), and **j–l** show spheroids. The sections in **g–i** were stained with antibodies to NF proteins. (From Schmidt et al., ref. 434, with permission.)

cess (418). The clinical triad of atrophic weakness of the hands and forearms, slight spasticity of the legs, and generalized hyper-reflexia is characteristic (1). Muscles are affected by amyotrophy, i.e., denervation atrophy. The disorder progresses relentlessly; about half of ALS patients are dead within 3 years and 90% within 6 years (1).

Neuroimaging and Pathology

Although many parts of the brain may be affected, ALS is characterized predominantly by degeneration of both the corticospinal tract as well as lower motor neurons. Microscopic examination shows motor neuron loss and accumulation of spheroids composed of neurofilaments in remaining motor neurons (Figs. 42–44). The extent of corticospinal tract degeneration varies along the neuraxis. At autopsy, it can usually be traced from the lower portion of the spinal cord up through the medulla. Occasionally, degeneration of motor fibers proceeds further cephalad sequentially through the pyramidal tracts of the brainstem and cerebral peduncles, the posterior part of the posterior limb of the internal capsule, corona radiata, to the motor cortex (134). On MR,

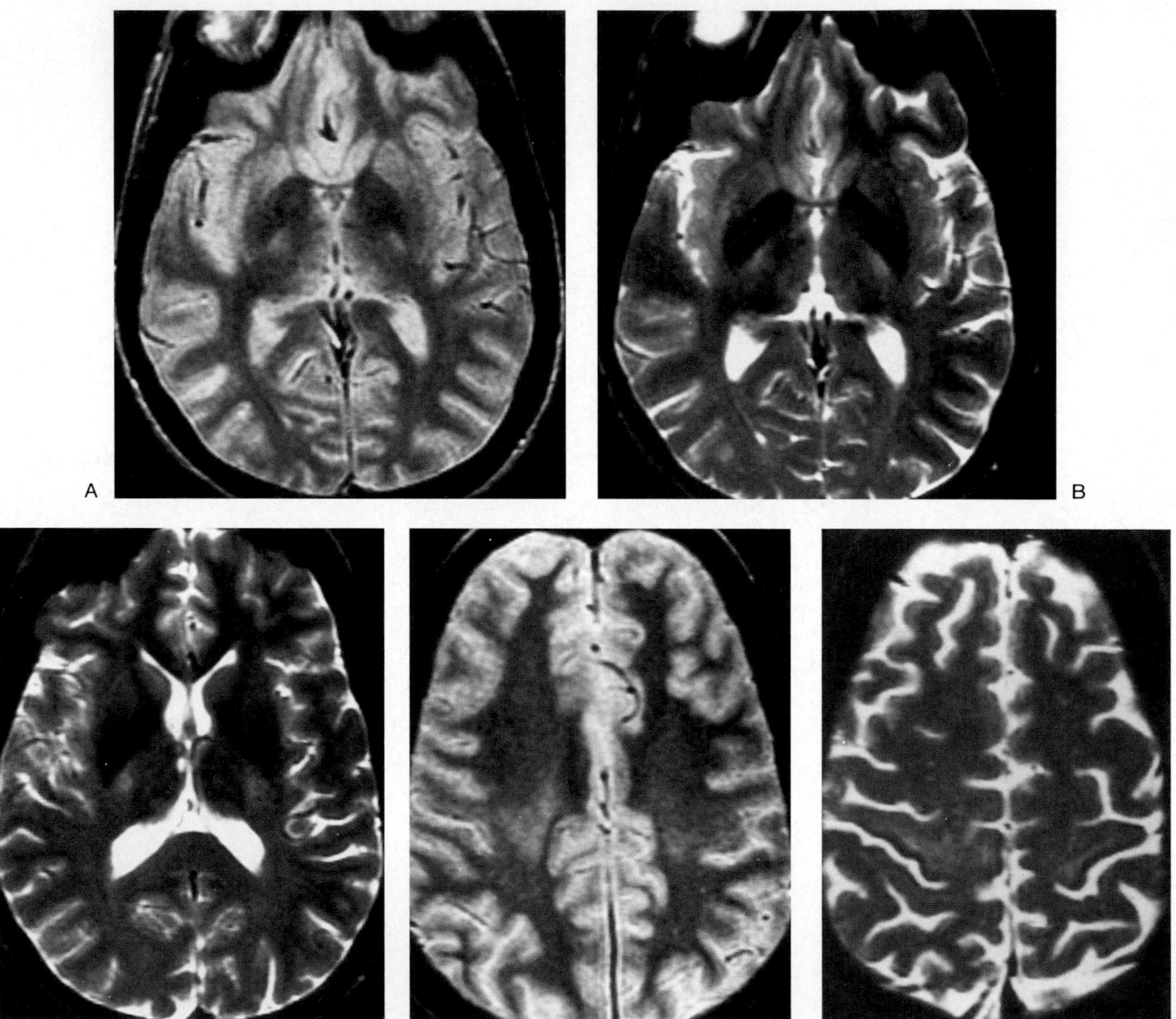

FIG. 45. Amyotrophic lateral sclerosis. **A–F:** A 38-year-old patient, long TR sequences, short (A,D) and long (B,C,E,F) TE. A–E: Axial plane. F: Coronal plane. Note bilateral symmetric hyperintense signal extending from the posterior portion of the posterior limb of the internal capsule (A,B,C,F), coronal radiata (F), and centrum semiovale (E,F) to the precentral gyrus (E). The lateral margins of the putamen show hypointense signal on the second echo of the long TR sequence, more pronounced than usual at age 38. Note that the abnormal signal in the corticospinal tract of the internal capsule is hyperintense on both the first (A) and second (B) echoes of the long TR sequence, in contrast to the normal hyperintense signal of the posterior internal capsule, which is only of high signal on the second echo (see Fig. 3).

corresponding hyperintense foci are seen on long TR sequences along the course of the corticospinal tract from the precentral gyrus to the level of the cord (Fig. 45) (384,419–424). This high signal likely reflects histologic changes of myelin loss and gliosis (134). Another report discussed the presence of nonspecific white matter changes in younger patients with more severe clinical involvement (425). Hypointense signal on the long TR/TE

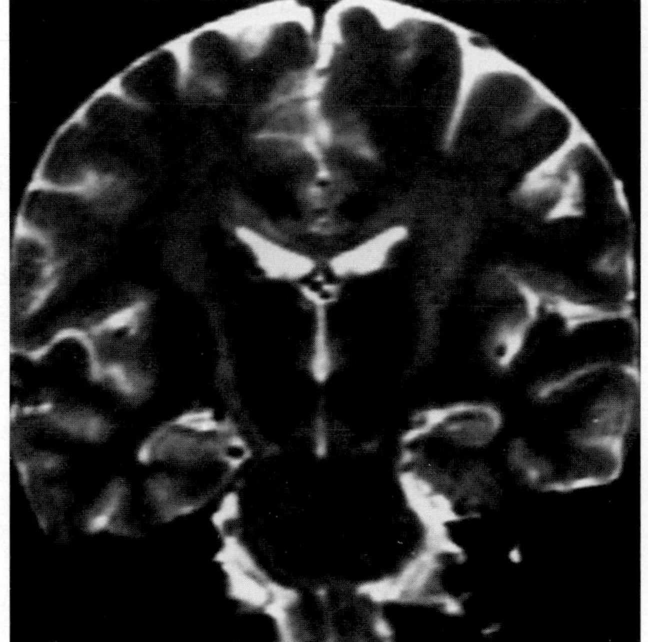
F

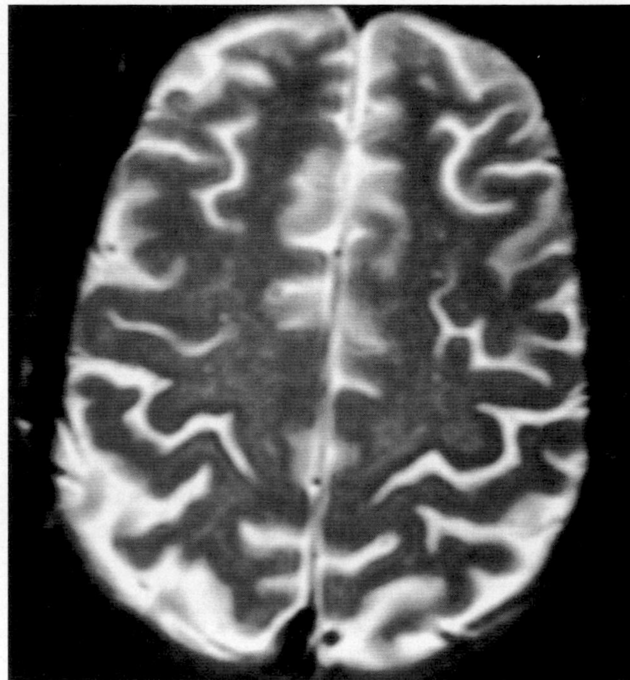
G

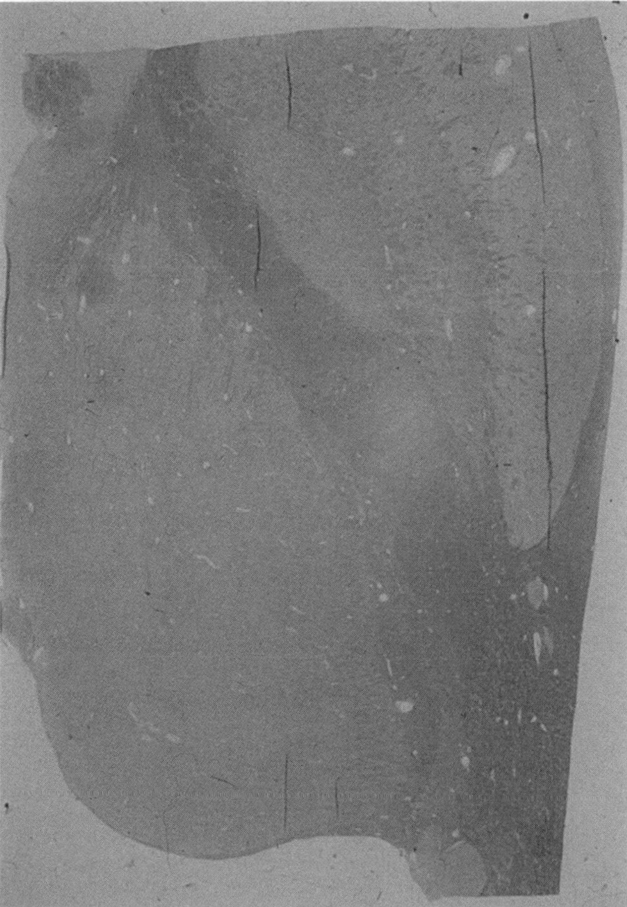
H

FIG. 45. (*Continued.*) **G:** In addition to the areas of hyperintense signal on the long TR/TE it is possible to discern a strip of low signal intensity underlying the motor strip. **H:** Luxol fast blue—H&E stain. Blue staining structure coursing obliquely is the posterior limb of the internal capsule. Predominantly pink structures are the lentiform nuclei and thalami anterolateral and posteromedial, respectively, to the internal capsule. Note the pale blue component of the posterior portion of the posterior limb of the internal capsule due to degeneration with myelin loss of the corticospinal tract. This corresponds to the site of hyperintense signal on long TR MR (A–C).

sequence may also be found in the motor cortex (425,426), possibly due to iron or other ion deposition (Fig. 45G). Gross pathology (134) and imaging (414) may also show focal atrophy along the course of the corticospinal tract. The anterior and lateral portions of the spinal cord may be atrophic and flattened due to cell loss of motor neurons in the anterior horns and corticospinal tracts. Variable loss of motor neurons is seen in brainstem nuclei, particularly of the hypoglossal motor neuron cells. The latter results in neurogenic atrophy of the tongue. Abnormalities of size, shape, position, and internal structure of the tongue are all well documented on MR (427).

Less Common Motor Diseases

There are also related but less common forms of motor neuron disease. The term primary lateral sclerosis has been given to isolated involvement of the corticospinal and corticobulbar tracts with sparing of the lower motor neurons (428). MR studies have reported high signal intensity along the course of the corticospinal tracts into the brainstem (429) and shrinkage of the precentral gyrus (430).

Progressive spinal muscular atrophy is isolated involvement of the lower motor neurons, characterized by weakness and atrophy *without* corticospinal tract dysfunction (1). In a case of progressive juvenile segmental spinal muscular atrophy, MR was capable of detecting atrophy in the cervical and thoracic cord (431). Progressive bulbar palsy shows denervation atrophy of muscles innervated by motor nuclei of the lower brainstem (1).

Juvenile amyotrophy of the distal upper extremity (monomelic amyotrophy, benign focal amyotrophy) is a separate entity among motor neuron diseases (414). It typically causes unilateral muscular atrophy in the hand and forearm due to selective involvement of the anterior horn cells in the lower cervical cord. It occurs most commonly in young males and stabilizes after an initial progressive course lasting 1 to 3 years. This latter benign feature contrasts with the relentlessly progressive course of ALS. MR shows focal atrophy of the lower cervical cord, often limited to the anterior horn region (414).

SENSORY DEGENERATION

Subacute combined degeneration of the spinal cord is caused by vitamin B_{12} deficiency. In the United States the most common cause of this deficiency is lack of absorption in the setting of pernicious anemia from antibodies to intrinsic factor and gastric parietal cells. This can lead to demyelination of the dorsal and lateral columns of the spinal cord with a resulting sensory ataxia. High signal on long TR/TE MR can be seen in the spinal cord, and these lesions may decrease in conspicuousness with treatment (432).

CONCLUSION

MR imaging has made enormous strides in the past decade in the detection and classification of neurodegenerative diseases of the central nervous system. Advances in MR technique now allow earlier and more accurate assessment of degenerative damage to brain tissue. This progress has occurred due to both advances in technology and in the human ability to interpret and use the information provided.

ACKNOWLEDGMENTS. We thank our colleagues in the Departments of Pathology and Laboratory Medicine, Neurology, Psychiatry, and the Penn Alzheimer Center for their many contributions to the work reviewed here, which was supported by grants from the DANA Foundation and the NRA. FJL's research has been supported by NIH EY-02654, NS 29029, ASNR Basic Science Fellowship Award, and RSNA Seed Grant Award.

REFERENCES

1. Adams RD, Victor M. *Principles of Neurology*, fourth ed. New York: McGraw-Hill Information Services Company, Health Professions Division; 1989:35–77,334–346,488–500,921–967.
2. Breger R, Yetkin F, Fischer M, et al. T1 and T2 in the cerebrum: correlation with age, gender, and demographic factors. *Radiology* 1991;181:545–547.
3. Agartz I, Saaf J, Wahlund L-O, et al. T1 and T2 relaxation time estimates in the normal human brain. *Radiology* 1991;181:537–543.
4. Wahlund L-O, Agartz I, Almqvist O, et al. The brain in healthy aged individuals: MR imaging. *Radiology* 1990;174:675–679.
5. George AE, de Leon MJ, Kalnin A, et al. Leukoencephalopathy in normal and pathologic aging. I. MR of brain lucencies. *AJNR* 1986;7:567–570.
6. Zimmerman RD, Fleming CA, Lee BCP. Periventricular hyperintensity as seen by magnetic resonance: prevalance and significance. *AJNR* 1986;7:13–20.
7. Erkinjuntti T, Ketonen L, Sulkava R, et al. Do white matter changes on MRI and CT differentiate vascular dementia from Alzheimer's disease? *J Neurol Neurosurg Psychiatry* 1987;50:37–42.
8. Kobari M, Meyer JS, Ichijo M, et al. Leukoaraiosis: correlation of MR and CT findings with blood flow, atrophy, and cognition. *AJNR* 1990;11:273–281.
9. Barkovich AJ, Kjos BO, Jackson DE. Normal maturation of the neonatal and infant brain: MR imaging at 1.5 T. *Radiology* 1988;166:173–180.
10. Yakovlev PI, Lecours AR. The myelogenetic cycles of regional maturation of the brain. In: Mankowski A, ed. *Regional Development in Early Life*. Philadelphia: Davis; 1967:3–69.
11. Sze G, DeArmond SJ, Brant-Zawadzki M, et al. Foci of MRI signal (pseudolesions) anterior to the frontal horns: histologic correlations of a normal finding. *AJNR* 1986;7:381–387.
12. Mirowitz S, Sartor K, Gado M, et al. Focal signal-intensity variations in the posterior internal capsule: normal MR findings and distinction from pathologic findings. *Radiology* 1989;172:535–539.
13. Rutledge JN, Hillal SK, Silver AJ, et al. Study of movement disorders and brain iron by MR. *AJNR* 1987;8:397–410.
14. Drayer BP, Burger P, Darwin R, et al. Magnetic resonance imaging of brain iron. *AJNR* 1986;7:373–380.
15. Heier LA, Bauer CJ, Schwartz EA. Large Virchow-Robin spaces: MR-clinical correlation. *AJNR* 1989;10: 929–936.
16. Virchow R. Uber die Erweiterung kleinerer geffase. *Virchows Arch A Pathol Anat Histopathol* 1851;3:427–462.

17. Robin C. Recherches sur quelques particularites de la structure des capillaries de l'encephale. *J Physiol Paris* 1859:536–548.
18. Braffman BH, Zimmerman RA, Trojanowski JQ, et al. Brain MR: pathologic correlation with gross and histopathology. I. Lacunar infarction and Virchow-Robin spaces. *AJNR* 1988;9:621–628.
19. Poirier J, Gray F, Gherardi R, et al. Cerebral lacunae. A new neuropathological classification. *J Neuropathol Exp Neurol* 1985;44: 312(abst).
20. Benhaiem-Sigaux N, Gherardi R, Roucayrol AM, et al. Expanding cerebellar lacunae due to dilatation of the perivascular space associated with Binswanger's subcortical arteriosclerotic encephalopathy. *Stroke* 1987;18:1087–1092.
21. Mirfakhraee M, Crofford MJ, Guinto SC Jr., et al. Virchow-Robin space: a path of spread of neurosarcoidosis. *Radiology* 1986;158:715-720.
22. Jungreis CA, Kanal E, Hirsch WL, et al. Normal perivascular spaces mimicking lacunar infarction: MR imaging. *Radiology* 1988;169:101–104.
23. Elster A, Richardson D. Focal high signal on MR scans of the midbrain caused by enlarged perivascular spaces: MR-pathologic correlation. *AJNR* 1990;11:1119–1122.
24. Challa VR. White matter lesions in MR imaging of elderly subjects [letter]. *Radiology* 1987;164:874.
25. Drayer BP. Imaging of the aging brain. Part I. Normal findings. *Radiology* 1988;166:785–796.
26. Kluger A, Gianutsos J, de Leon MJ, et al. Significance of age-related white matter lesions. *Stroke* 1988;19:1054–1055.
27. Marshall VG, Bradley WG Jr, Marshall CE, et al. Deep white matter infarction: correlation of MR imaging and histopathologic findings. *Radiology* 1988;167:517–522.
28. Gado M, Torack R, Morris J. Periventricular high signal (PVHS) and correlation with histologic examination: a post-mortem study. *Proceedings of the Twenty-Sixth Annual Meeting of the American Society of Neuroradiology,* Chicago. 1988.
29. Heier LA, Morgello S, Farrar JT, et al. Periventricular hyperintensities: MR pathologic correlations between subcortical and subependymal hyperintensities. *AJNR* 1988;9:1034(abst).
30. Bowen B, Barker W, Loewenstein D, et al. MR signal abnormalities in memory disorder and dementia. *AJNR* 1990;11:283–290.
31. Bradley WG, Waluch V, Brant-Zawadzki M, et al. Patchy periventricular white matter lesions in the elderly: common observation during NMR imaging. *Noninvasive Med Imaging* 1984;1:35–41.
32. Brant-Zawadzki M, Fein G, Dyke CV. MR imaging of the aging brain: patchy white-matter lesions and dementia. *AJNR* 1985;6: 675–682.
33. Awad IA, Spetzler RF, Hodak JA, et al. Incidental subcortical lesions identified on magnetic resonance imaging in the elderly. I. Correlation with age and cerebrovascular risk factors. *Stroke* 1986;17:1084–1089.
34. Fazekas F, Chawluk JB, Alavi A, et al. MR signal abnormalities at 1.5T in Alzheimer's dementia and normal aging. *AJNR* 1987;8:421–426.
35. Hendrie HC, Farlow MR, Austrom MG, et al. Foci of increased T2 signal intensity on brain MR scans of healthy elderly subjects. *AJNR* 1989;10:703–707.
36. Salomon A, Teates AE, Burger PC, et al. Brain MR: pathologic correlation with gross and histopathology. 2. Hyperinense white-matter foci in the elderly. *AJNR* 1988;165:625–629.
37. Hesselink JR, Press GA. MR contrast enhancement of intracranial lesions with Gd-DTPA. *Radiol Clin North Am* 1988;26:873–887.
38. Prencipe M, Marini C. Leuko-araiosis: definition and clinical correlates—an overview. *Eur Neurol* 1989;29(Suppl):27–29.
39. Awad IA, Johnson PC, Spetzler RF, et al. Incidental subcortical lesions identified on magnetic resonance imaging in the elderly. II. Postmortem pathologic correlations. *Stroke* 1986;17:1090–1097.
40. Brun A, Englund E. A white matter disorder in dementia of the Alzheimer type: a pathoanatomical study. *Ann Neurol* 1986;19: 253–262.
41. Brun A, Gustafson L, Englund E. Subcortical pathology of Alzheimer's disease. *Adv Neurol* 1990;51:73–77.
42. Englund E, Brun A, Persson B. Correlations between histopathologic white matter changes and proton MR relaxation times in dementia. *Alzheimer Dis Assoc Disord* 1987;1:156–170.
43. Kirkpatrick JB, Hayman LA. White-matter lesions of clinically healthy brains of elderly subjects: possible pathologic basis. *Radiology* 1987;162:509–511.
44. Braffman BH, Zimmerman RA, Trojanowski JQ, et al. Brain MR: pathologic correlation with gross and histopathology. 2. Hyperintense white-matter foci in the elderly. *AJNR* 1988;9:629–636.
45. Burger PC, Burch JG, Kunze U. Subcortical arteriosclerotic encephalopathy (Binswanger's disease). A vascular etiology of dementia. *Stroke* 1976;7:626–631.
46. Moody DM. Morphological features of the cerebral vascular supply. Categorical Course on Cerebrovascular Disease. *Proceedings of the Twenty-Seventh Annual Meeting of the American Society of Neuroradiology,* Orlando, March 18–19. 1989.
47. Gerard G, Weisberg LA. MR periventricular lesions in adults. *Neurology* 1986;36: 998-1001.
48. Fazekas F, Niederkorn K, Schmidt R, et al. White matter signal abnormalities in normal individuals: correlation with carotid ultrasonography, cerebral blood flow measurements, and cerebrovascular risk factors. *Stroke* 1988;19:1285–1288.
49. Heier LA, Barbut DR, Deck MDF. MR clinical correlation of transient ischemic attacks. *AJNR* 1989;10:872.
50. Lechner H, Schmidt R, Bertha G, et al. Nuclear magnetic resonance imaging white matter lesions and risk factors for stroke in normal individuals. *Stroke* 1988;19:263–265.
51. Moody DM, Bell MA, Challa VR. The corpus callosum, a unique white-matter tract: anatomic features that may explain sparing in Binswanger disease and resistance to flow of fluid masses. *AJNR* 1988;9:1051–1059.
52. Uhlenbrock D, Sehlen S. The value of T1-weighted images in the differentiation between MS, white matter lesions, and subcortical arteriosclerotic encephalopathy (SAE). *Neuroradiology* 1989;31: 203-212.
53. Salomon A, Teates AF, Burger PC, et al. Subcortical arteriosclerotic encephalopathy: brain stem findings with MR imaging. *Radiology* 1987;165:625–629.
54. Grossman RI, Gonzalez-Scarano F, Atlas SW, Galetta S, Silberberg DH. Multiple sclerosis: gadolinium enhancement in MR imaging. *Radiology* 1986;161:721–725.
55. Dawson JW. The histology of disseminated sclerosis. *Trans R Soc Edinb* 1916;50:517–740.
56. Horowitz AL, Kaplan RD, Grewe G, et al. The ovoid lesion: a new MR observation in patients with multiple sclerosis. *AJNR* 1989;10:303–305.
57. Ormerod IEC, Miller DH, McDonald WI, et al. The role of NMR imaging in the assessment of multiple sclerosis and isolated neurological lesions. A quantitative study. *Brain* 1987;110:1579–1616.
58. Fazekas F, Offenbacher H, Fuchs S, et al. Criteria for an increased specificity of MRI interpretation in elderly subjects with suspected multiple sclerosis. *Neurology* 1988;38:1822–1825.
59. Awad IA, Spetzler RF, Hodak JA, Awad CA, Williams F Jr, Carey R. Incidental lesions noted on magnetic resonance imaging of the brain: prevalence and clinical significance in various age groups. *Neurosurgery* 1987;20:222–227.
60. Geis J, Hendrick R, Lee S, et al. White matter lesions: role of spin density in MR imaging. *Radiology* 1989;170:863–868.
61. Yetkin F, Fischer M, Papke R, et al. Focal hyperintensities in cerebral white matter on MR images of asymptomatic volunteers: correlation with social and medical histories. *AJR* 1993;161:855–858.
62. Yetkin F, Haughton V, Fischer M, et al. High-signal foci on MR images of the brain: observer variability in their quantification. *AJR* 1992;159:185–188.
63. Fazekas F, Kleinert R, Offenbacher H, et al. The morphologic correlate of incidental punctate white matter hyperintensities on MR images. *AJNR* 1991;12:915–921.
64. Brown GG, Garcia JH, Gdowski JW. Altered brain energy metabolism in demented patients with multiple subcortical ischemic lesions. Working hypothesis. *Arch Neurol* 1993;50:384–388.
65. Aoki S, Okada Y, Nishimura K, et al. Normal deposition of brain

iron in childhood and adolescence: MR imaging at 1.5 T. *Radiology* 1989;172:381–385.
66. Drayer B. Imaging of the aging brain. Part II. Pathologic conditions. *Radiology* 1988;166:797–806.
67. Milton W, Atlas S, Lexa F, et al. Deep gray matter hypointensity patterns with aging in healthy adults: MR imaging at 1.5 T. *Radiology* 1991;181:715–719.
68. Chen J, Hardy P, Cluberg M, et al. T2 values in the human brain: comparison with quantitative assays of iron and ferritin. *Radiology* 1989;173:521–526.
69. Drayer BP. Basal ganglia: significance of signal hypointensity on T2-weighted MR images. *Radiology* 1989;173:311–312.
70. Brooks D, Luthert P, Gadian D, et al. Does signal-attenuation on high-field T2-weighted MRI of the brain reflect regional cerebral iron deposition? Observations on the relationship between regional cerebral water proton T2 values and iron levels. *J Neurol Neurosurg Psychiatry* 1989;52:108–111.
71. Bizzi A, Brooks R, Brunetti A, et al. Role of iron and ferritin in MR imaging of the brain: a study in primates at different field strengths. *Radiology* 1990;177:59–65.
72. Chen J, Hardy P, Kucharczyk W, et al. MR of human postmortem brain tissue: correlative study between T2 and assays of iron and ferritin in Parkinson and Huntington disease. *AJNR* 1993;14:275–281.
73. Gomori J, Grossman R. The relation between regional brain iron and T2 shortening. *AJNR* 1993;14:1049–1050.
74. Hallgren B, Sourander P. The effect of age on the non-haemin iron in the human brain. *J Neurochem* 1958;3:41–51.
75. Thomas L, Boyko O, Anthony D, et al. MR detection of brain iron. *AJNR* 1993;14:1043–1048.
76. Drayer BP. Magnetic resonance imaging and extrapyramidal movement disorders. *Eur Neurol* 1989;29:9–12.
77. Drayer BP, Olanow W, Burger P, et al. Parkinson plus syndrome: diagnosis using high field MR imaging of brain iron. *Radiology* 1986;159:493–498.
78. Bartzokis G, Garber H, Marder S, et al. MRI in tardive dyskinesia: shortened left caudate T2. *Biol Psychiatry* 1990;28:1027–1036.
79. De Volder AG, Francart J, Lateere C, et al. Decreased glucose utilization in the striatum and frontal lobe in probably striatonigral degeneration. *Ann Neurol* 1989;26:239–247.
80. Hall S, Rutledge JN, Schallert T. MRI, brain iron and experimental Parkinson's disease. *J Neurol Sci* 1992;113:198–208.
81. O'Brien C, Sung J, McGeachie R, et al. Striatonigral degeneration: clinical MRI and pathologic correlation. *Neurology* 1990;40:710–711.
82. Arena JF, Schwartz C, Stevenson R, et al. Spastic paraplegia with iron deposits in the basal ganglia: a new X-linked mental retardation syndrome. *Am J Med Genet* 1992;43:479–490.
83. Olanow CW. Magnetic resonance imaging in parkinsonism. *Neurol Clin* 1992;10:405–420.
84. Antonini A, Leenders KL, Meier D, et al. T2 relaxation time in patients with Parkinson's disease. *Neurology* 1993;43:697–700.
85. Drayer B, Burger P, Hurwitz B, et al. Reduced signal intensity on MR images of thalamus and putamen in multiple sclerosis: increased iron content? *AJR* 1987;149:357–363.
86. Dietrich R, Bradley W Jr. Iron accumulation in the basal ganglia following severe ischemic-anoxic insults in children. *Radiology* 1988;168:203–206.
87. Farlow M, Yee R, Dlouhy S, et al. Gerstmann-Sträussler-Scheinker disease. I. Extending the clinical spectrum. *Neurology* 1989;39:1446–1452.
88. Cross P, Atlas S, Grossman R. MR evaluation of brain iron in children with cerebral infarction. *AJNR* 1990;11:341–348.
89. Osbourne A, Harnsberger H, Smoker W, et al. Multiple sclerosis in adolescents: CT and MR findings. *AJNR* 1990;11:489–494.
90. Silverstein A, Hirsh D, Trobe J, et al. MR imaging of the brain in five members of a family with Pelizaeus-Merzbacher disease. *AJNR* 1990;11:495–499.
91. Chang KH, Han MH, Kim HS, et al. Delayed encephalopathy after acute carbon monoxide intoxication: MR imaging features and distribution of cerebral white matter lesions. *Radiology* 1992;184:117–122.
92. Hardy P, Kucharczyk W, Henkelman R. Cause of signal loss in MR images of old hemorrhagic lesions. *Radiology* 1990;174:549–555.
93. Thulborn K, Sorensen A, Kowall N, et al. The role of ferritin and hemosiderin in the MR appearance of cerebral hemorrhage: a histopathologic biochemical study in rats. *AJR* 1990;154:1053–1059.
94. Gomori JM, Grossman RI, Yu-Ip C, et al. NMR relaxation times of blood: dependence on field strength, oxidation state, and cell integrity. *J Comput Assist Tomogr* 1987;11:684–690.
95. Norfray JF, Couch JR, Elble RJ, et al. Visualization of brain iron by mid-field MR. *AJNR* 1988;9:77–82.
96. Schenker C, Meier D, Wichmann W, et al. Age distribution and iron dependency of the T2 relaxation time in the globus pallidus and putamen. *Neuroradiology* 1993;35:119–124.
97. Vymazal J, Brooks RA, Zak O, et al. T1 and T2 of ferritin at different field strengths: effect on MRI. *Magn Reson Med* 1992;27:368–374.
98. Bartzokis G, Aravagiri M, Oldendorf WH, et al. Field dependent transverse relaxation rate increase may be a specific measure of tissue iron stores. *Magn Reson Med* 1993;29:459–464.
99. Penner NW, Li KC, Gebarski SS, et al. MR imaging of Pelizaeus-Merzbacher disease. *J Comput Assist Tomogr* 1987;11:591–593.
100. Hill J, Sitzer R. The regional distribution and cellular localization of iron in the rat brain. *Neuroscience* 1984;11:595–603.
101. Harrison W, Netsky M, Brown M. Trace elements in human brain: copper, zinc, iron, and magnesium. *Clin Chim Acta* 1968;21:55–60.
102. Cumings J. The copper and iron content of brain and liver in the normal and in hepato-lenticular degeneration. *Brain* 1948;71:410–414.
103. Gans A. Iron in the brain. *Brain* 1923;46:128–136.
104. Francois C, Nguyen-Legros J, Percheron G. Topographical and cytological localization of iron in rat and monkey brains. *Brain Res* 1981;215:317–322.
105. Jeffries W, Brandon M, Hunt S, et al. Transferrin receptor density on endothelium of brain capillaries. *Nature* 1984;312:162–163.
106. Hill J, Ruff M, Weber R, et al. Transferrin receptors in rat brain: neuropeptide-like pattern and relationship to iron distribution. *Proc Natl Acad Sci USA* 1985;82:4553–4557.
107. White B, Aust S, Afors K, et al. Brain injury by ischemic anoxia: hypothesis extension—a tale of two ions? *Ann Emerg Med* 1984;13:862–867.
108. Babbs C. Role of iron ions in the genesis of reperfusion injury following successful cardiopulmonary resuscitation: preliminary data and a biochemical hypothesis. *Ann Emerg Med* 1985;14:777–783.
109. Komara J, Nayini N, Bialick H, et al. Brain iron delocalization and lipid peroxidation following cardiac arrest. *Ann Emerg Med* 1986;15:384–389.
110. Craelius W, Migdal M, Luessenhop C, et al. Iron deposits surrounding multiple sclerosis plaques. *Arch Pathol Lab Med* 1982;106:397–399.
111. Waller AV. Experiments on the section of the glossopharyngeal and hypoglossal nerves of the frog, and observations of the alterations produced thereby in the structure of the primitive fibres. *Philos Trans R Soc Lond* 1850;140:423–429.
112. Rossiter RJ. The chemistry of wallerian degeneration. In: Folch-Pi J, ed. *Chemical Pathology of the Nervous System.* New York: Pergamon Press; 1961:207–227.
113. Daniel PM, Strich SJ. Histological observations on wallerian degeneration in the spinal cord of the baboon, *Papio papio. Acta Neuropathol (Berl)* 1969;12:314–328.
114. Webster H, De F. The relationship between Schmidt-Lanterman incisures and myelin segmentation during wallerian degeneration. *Ann N Y Acad Sci* 1964;122:29–41.
115. Sonoda S, Tsubahara A, Saito M, et al. Extent of pyramidal tract wallerian degeneration in the brain stem on MRI and degree of motor impairment after supratentorial stroke. *Disabil Rehabil* 1992;14:89–92.
116. Inagaki M, Koeda T, Takeshita K. Prognosis and MRI after ischemic stroke of the basal ganglia. *Pediatr Neurol* 1992;8:104–108.
117. DeWitt LD, Kistler JP, Miller DC, et al. NMR-neuropathologic correlation in stroke. *Stroke* 1987;18:342–351.
118. Cobb SR, Mehringer CM. Wallerian degeneration in a patient

with Schilder disease: MR imaging demonstration. *Radiology* 1987;162:521–522.
119. Kuhn MJ, Johnson KA, Davis KR. Wallerian degeneration: evaluation with MR imaging. *Radiology* 1988;168:199–202.
120. Bouchareb M, Moulin T, Cattin F, et al. Wallerian degeneration of the descending tracts. *J Neuroradiol* 1988;15:238–252.
121. Uchino A, Onomura K, Ohno M. Wallerian degeneration of the corticospinal tract in the brain stem: MR imaging. *Radiat Med* 1989;7:74–78.
122. Kuhn MJ, Mikulis DJ, Ayoub DM, et al. Wallerian degeneration after cerebral infarction: evaluation with sequential MR imaging. *Radiology* 1989;172:179–182.
123. Uchino A, Imada H, Ohno M. MR imaging of wallerian degeneration in the human brain stem after ictus. *Neuroradiology* 1990;32:191–195.
124. Pujol JE, Mari-Vilata JL, Junque C, et al. Wallerian degeneration of the pyramidal tract in capsular infarction studied by magnetic resonance imaging. *Stroke* 1990;21:404–409.
125. Inoue Y, Matsumura Y, Fukuda T, et al. MR imaging of wallerian degeneration in the brainstem: temporal relationships. *AJNR* 1990;11:897–902.
126. Danek A, Bauer M, Fries W. Tracing of neuronal connections in the human brain by magnetic resonance imaging in vivo. *Eur J Neurosci* 1990;2:112–115.
127. Orita T, Tsurutani T, Izumihara A, et al. Coronal MR imaging for visualization of wallerian degeneration of the pyramidal tract. *J Comput Assist Tomogr* 1991;15:802–804.
128. Bontozoglou NP, Chakeres DW, Martin GF, et al. Cerebellorubral degeneration after resection of cerebellar dentate nucleus neoplasms: evaluation with MR imaging. *Radiology* 1991;180:223–228.
129. Jolesz FA, Polak JF, Ruenzel PW, et al. Wallerian degeneration demonstrated by magnetic resonance spectroscopy. *Radiology* 1984;152:85–87.
130. Grossman RI, Hecht-Leavitt CM, Evans SM, et al. Experimental radiation injury: combined MR imaging and spectroscopy. *Radiology* 1988;169:305–309.
131. Rafto SE, Wallace SE, Grossman RI, et al. Magnetic resonance imaging: an animal model of CNS wallerian degeneration. *AJNR* 1988;9:1025–1026(abst).
132. Lexa FJ, Grossman RI, Rosenquist AC. MR of wallerian degeneration in the feline visual system: characterization by magnetization transfer rate with histopathologic correlation. *AJNR* 1994;15:201–212.
133. Barbeau A. Parkinson's disease: clinical features and etiopathology. In: Vinken PJ, Bruyn GW, Klawans HL, eds. *Handbook of Clinical Neurology*, vol 49. Amsterdam: Elsevier Science; 1986;87–152.
134. Schoene WC. Degenerative diseases of the central nervous system. In: Davis RL, Robertson DM, eds. *Textbook of Neuropathology*. Baltimore: Williams & Wilkins; 1985:788–823.
135. Savoiardo M, Strada L, Girotti F, et al. MR imaging in progressive supranuclear palsy and Shy-Drager syndrome. *J Comput Assist Tomogr* 1989;13:555–560.
136. Goldman JE, Yen S-H. Cytoskeletal protein abnormalities in neurodegenerative diseases. *Ann Neurol* 1986;19:209–223.
137. Trojanowski JQ, Schmidt ML, Otvos L, et al. Vulnerability of the neuronal cytoskeleton in aging and Alzheimer's disease: widespread involvement of all three major filament systems. *Annu Rev Gerontol Geriatr* 1990;10:167–182.
138. Seitelberger F. Neuroaxonal dystrophy: its relation to aging and neurological diseases. In: Vinken PJ, Bruyn GW, Klawans HL, eds. *Handbook of Clinical Neurology, vol. 49.* Amsterdam: Elsevier Science; 1986:391–415.
139. Schmidt ML, Lee VM-Y, Trojanowski JQ, et al. Analysis of epitopes shared by Hirano bodies and neurofilament proteins in normal and Alzheimer's disease hippocampus. *Lab Invest* 1989;60:513–522.
140. Trojanowski JQ, Schmidt ML, Shin RW, et al. PHF, (A68): From pathological marker to potential mediator of neuronal dysfunction and degeneration in Alzheimer's disease. *Clin Neurosci* 1994;1:184–191.
141. Trojanowski JQ, Lee VMY. Paired helical filament in Alzheimer's disease: the kinase connection. *Am J Pathol* 1994;144:449–453.
142. Trojanowski JQ, Lee VMY. Phosphorylation of neuronal cytoskeletal proteins in Alzheimer's disease and Lewy body dementias. *Ann N Y Acad Sci* 1994;747:92–109.
143. Hardy J. Genetic mistakes point the way for Alzheimer's disease. *J NIH Res* 1993;5:46–49.
144. Mullan M, Crawford F. Genetic and molecular advances in Alzheimer's disease. *Trends Neurosci* 1993;16:398–403.
145. Price DL, Borchelt DR, Sisodia SS. Alzheimer's disease and the prion disorders amyloid-β-protein and prion protein amyloidoses. *Proc Natl Acad Sci USA* 1993;90:6381–6384.
146. Selkow DJ. Physiological production of the β-amyloid protein and the mechanisms of Alzheimer's disease. *Trends Neurosci* 1993;16:403–409.
147. Alzheimer A. Ueber eine eigenartige Erkrankung der Hirnrinde. *Allg Z Psychiatry* 1907;64:146–148.
148. Lewy FH. Zur pathologischen Anatomie der Paralysis agitans. *Dtsch Z Nervenheilkd* 1913;50:50–55.
149. Wechsler D. *The Measurement of Adult Intelligence*, 3rd ed. Baltimore: Williams & Wilkins; 1944.
150. Glatt SL, Lantos G, Danziger A, et al. Efficacy of CT in the diagnosis of vascular dementia. *AJNR* 1983;4:703–705.
151. Evans DA, Funkenstein H, Albert MS, et al. Prevalence of Alzheimer's disease in a community population of older persons: higher than previously reported. *JAMA* 1989;262:2551–2556.
152. Larson EB, Reifler BV, Sumi SM, et al. Diagnostic tests in the evaluation of dementia. A prospective study of 200 elderly outpatients. *Arch Intern Med* 1986;146:1917–1922.
153. Hollister LE, Boutros N. Clinical use of CT and MR scans in psychiatric patients. *J Psychiatry Neurosci* 1991;16:194–198.
154. Le May M. CT changes in dementing diseases: a review. *AJNR* 1986;7:841–853.
155. Saunders AM, Strittmatter WJ, Schmechel D, et al. Association of apolipoprotein E allele epsilon 4 with late-onset familial and sporadic Alzheimer's disease. *Neurology* 1993;43:1467–1472.
156. Wade JPH, Mirsen TR, Hachinski VC, et al. The clinical diagnosis of Alzheimer's disease. *Arch Neurol* 1987;44:24–29.
157. Molsa PK, Paljarvi L, Rinne JO, Rinne UK, Sako E. Validity of clinical diagnosis in dementia: a prospective clinicopathological study. *J Neurol Neurosurg Psychiatry* 1985;48:1085–1090.
158. Gado M, Patel J, Hughes CP, et al. Brain atrophy in dementia judged by CT scan ranking. *AJNR* 1983;4:499–500.
159. Gado M, Hughes CP, Danziger W, et al. Aging, dementia, and brain atrophy: a longitudinal computed tomographic study. *AJNR* 1983;4:699–702.
160. Ichimiya Y, Kobayashi K, Arai H, et al. A computed tomography study of Alzheimer's disease. *J Neurol* 1983;229:69–77.
161. de Leon MJ, George AE, Reisberg B, et al. Alzheimer's disease: Longitudinal CT studies of ventricular change. *AJNR* 1989;10:371–376.
162. Creasey H, Schwartz M, Fredrickson H, et al. Quantitative computed tomography in dementia of the Azheimer type. *Neurology* 1986;36:1563–1568.
163. Kido DK, Caine ED, LeMay M, et al. Temporal lobe atrophy in patients with Alzheimer's disease: a CT study. *AJNR* 1989;19:551–555.
164. Sandor T, Albert M, Stafford J, et al. Use of computerized CT analysis to discriminate between Alzheimer patients and normal control subjects. *AJNR* 1988;9:1181–1187.
165. Johnson KA, Davis KR, Buonannon FS, et al. Comparison of magnetic resonance and roentgen ray computed tomography in dementia. *Arch Neurol* 1987;44:1075–1080.
166. Terry RD. Alzheimer's disease. In: Davis RL, Robertson DM, eds. *Textbook of Neuropathology*. Baltimore: Williams & Wilkins; 1985:824–841.
167. Tomlinson BE, Blessed G, Roth M. Observations on the brains of nondemented old people. *J Neurol Sci* 1968;7:331–356.
168. Schwartz M, Creasey H, Grady CL, et al. Computed tomographic analysis of brain morphometrics in 30 healthy men aged 21–81 years. *Ann Neurol* 1985;17:146–157.
169. Hyman BT, Van Hoesen GW, Damasio AR, et al. Alzheimer's disease: cell-specific pathology isolates the hippocampal formation. *Science* 1984;225:1168–1170.

170. George AE, deLeon MJ, Stylopoulos L, et al. CT diagnostic features of Alzheimer's disease: importance of the choroidal/hippocampal fissure complex. *AJNR* 1990;11:101–107.
171. Jernigan TL, Salmon DP, Butters N, et al. Cerebral structure on MRI. Part II. Specific changes in Alzheimer's and Huntington's diseases. *Biol Psychiatry* 1991;29:68–81.
172. Dahlbeck JW, McCluney KW, Yeakley JW, et al. The interuncal distance: a new MR measurement for the hippocampal atrophy of Alzheimer's disease. *AJNR* 1991;12:931–932.
173. Doraiswamy P, McDonald W, Patterson L, et al. Interuncal distance as a measure of hippocampal atrophy: normative data on axial MR imaging. *AJNR* 1993;14:141–143.
174. Ishii K, Howieson J, de Leon MJ, et al. Value of interuncal distance measure in diagnosis of Alzheimer's disease questioned. *AJNR* 1994;15:1286–1290.
175. Kohn M, Tanna N, Herman G, et al. Analysis of brain and cerebrospinal fluid volumes with MR imaging. Part 1. Methods, reliability and validation. *Radiology* 1991;178:115–122.
176. Tanna N, Kohn M, Horwich D, et al. Analysis of brain and cerebrospinal fluid volumes with MR imaging. Part II. Aging and Alzheimer dementia. *Radiology* 1991;178:123–130.
177. Wippold F II, Gado M, Morris J, et al. Senile dementia and healthy aging: a longitudinal CT study. *Radiology* 1991;179:215–219.
178. Sandor T, Jolesz F, Tieman J, et al. Comparative analysis of computed tomographic and magnetic resonance imaging scans in Alzheimer patients and controls. *Arch Neurol* 1992;49:381–384.
179. Rusinek H, de Leon MJ, George AE, et al. Alzheimer's disease: measuring loss of cerebral gray matter with MR imaging. *Radiology* 1991;178:109–114.
180. Killiany RJ, Moss MB, Albert MS, et al. Temporal lobe regions on magnetic resonance imaging identify patients with early Alzheimer's disease. *Arch Neurol* 1993;50:949–954.
181. Jack CR, Petersen RC, O'Brien PC, et al. MR-based hippocampal volumetry in the diagnosis of Alzheimer's disease. *Neurology* 1992;42:183–188.
182. Wahlund LO, Anderson-Lundman G, Basun H, et al. Cognitive functions and brain structures: a quantitative study of CSF volumes on Alzheimer patients and healthy control subjects. *Magn Reson Imaging* 1993;11:169–174.
183. Small GW, Leuchter AF, Mandelkem MA, et al. Clinical, neuroimaging, and environmental risk differences in monozygotic female twins appearing discordant for dementia of the Alzheimer type. *Arch Neurol* 1993;50:209–219.
184. Drayer BP. Magnetic resonance imaging and brain iron: implications in the diagnosis and pathochemistry of movement disorders and dementia. *BNI Q* 1987;3:15–30.
185. De Leon MJ, George AE, Ferris SH. CT and PET study of leukoencephalopathy in Alzheimer's disease. *AJNR* 1985;6:468(abst).
186. Rezek DL, Morris JC, Fulling KH, et al. Periventricular white matter lucencies in senile dementia of the Alzheimer type and in normal aging. *Neurology* 1987;37:1365–1368.
187. George AE, de Leon MJ, Gentes CI, et al. Leukoencephalopathy in normal and pathologic aging: 1. CT of brain lucencies. *AJNR* 1986;7:561–566.
188. Lotz PR, Ballinger WE, Quisling RG. Subcortical arteriosclerotic encephalopathy: CT spectrum and pathologic correlation. *AJNR* 1986;7:817–822.
189. Jack CR, Mokri B, Laws ER, et al. MR findings in normal pressure hydrocephalus: significance and comparison with other forms of dementia. *J Comput Assist Tomogr* 1987;11:923–931.
190. Kinkel WR, Jacobs L, Polachini I. Subcortical arteriosclerotic encephalopathy (Binswanger's disease): computed tomographic, nuclear magnetic resonance, and clinical correlations. *Arch Neurol* 1985;42: 951–959.
191. Drayer BP. Microangiopathic leukoencephalopathy: MR imaging. Categorical Course on Cerebrovascular Disease. *Proceedings of the Twenty-Seventh Annual Meeting of the American Society of Neuroradiology*, Orlando, March 18–19. 1989.
192. Rao SM, Mittenberg W, Bernardin L, et al. Neuropsychological test findings in subjects with leukoaraiosis. *Arch Neurol* 1989;46:40–44.
193. Tomonaga M, Yamanouchi H, Toghi H, et al. Clinicopathologic study of progressive vascular encephalopathy (Binswanger type) in the elderly. *J Am Geriatr Soc* 1982;30:524–529.
194. Erkinjuntti T, Sipponen JT, Livanainen M, et al. Cerebral NMR and CT imaging in dementia. *J Comput Assist Tomogr* 1984;8:614–618.
195. Scheltens P, Barkhof F, Valk J, et al. White matter lesions on magnetic resonance imaging in clinically diagnosed Alzheimer's disease. *Brain* 1992;115:735–748.
196. Pettegrew JW, Withers G, Panchalingam K, et al. 31P nuclear magnetic resonance (NMR) spectroscopy of brain in aging and Alzheimer's disease. *J Neural Transm Suppl* 1987;24:261–268.
197. Pettegrew JW, Panchalingam K, Moosy J, et al. Correlation of phosphorous-31 magnetic resonance spectroscopy and morphologic findings in Alzheimer's disease. *Arch Neurol* 1988;45:1093–1096.
198. Brown GG, Levine SR, Gorell JM, et al. In vivo 31P NMR profiles of Alzheimer's disease and multiple subcortical infarct dementia. *Neurology* 1989;39:1423–1427.
199. Bottomley PA, Cousins JP, Pendrey DL, et al. Alzheimer dementia: quantification of energy metabolism and mobile phosphoesters with P-31 NMR spectroscopy. *Radiology* 1992;183:695–699.
200. Murphy GMD, Bottomley PA, Salerno JA, et al. An in vivo study of phosphorus and glucose metabolism in Alzheimer's disease using magnetic resonance spectroscopy and PET. *Arch Gen Psychiatry* 1993;50:341–349.
201. Miller B, Moats R, Shonk T, et al. Alzheimer's disease: depiction of increased cerebral myo-inositol with proton MR spectroscopy. *Radiology* 1993;187:433–437.
202. Patel DV, Hier DB, Thomas CM, et al. Intracerebral hemorrhage secondary to cerebral amyloid angiopathy. *Radiology* 1984;151:397–400.
203. Glenner CG. Amyloid deposits and amyloidosis: the beta-fibriloses. *N Engl J Med* 1980;302:1333-1343.
204. Wagle WA, Smith TW, Weiner M. Intracerebral hemorrhage caused by cerebral amyloid angiopathy: radiographic-pathologic correlation. *AJNR* 1984;5:171–176.
205. Wright JR, Calkins E. Relationship of amyloid deposits in the human aorta to aortic artherosclerosis: a postmortem study of 100 individuals over 60 years of age. *Lab Invest* 1974;30:767–773.
206. Vinters HV, Gilbert JJ. Cerebral amyloid angiopathy: incidence and complications in the aging brain. II. The distribution of amyloid vascular changes. *Stroke* 1983;14: 924–928.
207. Okazaki H, Reagan TJ, Campbell RJ. Clinicopathologic studies of primary cerebral amyloid angiopathy. *Mayo Clin Proc* 1979;54:22–31.
208. Case records of the Massachusetts General Hospital. Case 49-1982. *N Engl J Med* 1982;307:1507–1514.
209. Ishii N, Nishihara Y, Horie A. Amyloid angiopathy and lobar cerebral hemorrhage. *J Neurol Neurosurg Psychiatry* 1984;47(11):1203–1210.
210. Vanley C, Aguilar M, Kleinhenz R, et al. Cerebral amyloid angiopathy. *Hum Pathol* 1981;12:609–616.
211. Mandybur TI, Bates RD. Fatal massive intracerebral hemorrhage complicating cerebral amyloid angiopathy. *Arch Neurol* 1978;35:246–248.
212. Cosgrove G, Leblanc R, Meagher-Villemure K, et al. Cerebral amyloid angiopathy. *Neurology* 1985;35:625–631.
213. Esiri MM, Wilcock GK. Cerebral amyloid angiopathy in dementia and old age. *J Neurol Neurosurg Psychiatry* 1986;49:1221–1226.
214. Gray F, Dubas F, Roullet E, et al. Leukoencephalopathy in diffuse hemorrhagic cerebral amyloid angiopathy. *Ann Neurol* 1985;18:54–59.
215. Loes D, Biller J, Yuh W, et al. Leukoencephalopathy in cerebral amyloid angiopathy: MR imaging in four cases. *AJNR* 1990;11:485–488.
216. Cummings JL, Duchen LW. Klüver-Bucy syndrome in Pick disease: clinical and pathologic correlations. *Neurology* 1981;31:1415–1422.
217. Weschler AF, Verity MA, Rosenschein S, et al. Pick's disease. A clinical, computed tomographic, and histologic study with Golgi impregnation observations. *Arch Neurol* 1982;39:287–290.
218. Groen JJ, Hekster REM. Computed tomography in Pick's disease: findings in affected in three consecutive generations. *J Comput Assist Tomogr* 1982;6:907–911.
219. Kricheff I. Arteriosclerotic ischemic cerebrovascular disease. *Radiology* 1987;162:101–109.

220. Roman GC, Tatemichi TK, Erkinjuntti T, et al. Vascular dementia: diagnostic criteria for research studies. *Neurology* 1993;43:250–260.
221. Liston EH, La Rue A. Clinical differentiation of primary degenerative and multi-infarct dementia: a critical review of the evidence. Part II: pathologic studies. *Biol Psychiatry* 1983;18:1467–1484.
222. Hershey LA, Modic MT, Greenough G, et al. Magnetic resonance imaging in vascular dementia. *Neurology* 1987;37:29–36.
223. Hachinski VC, Lassen NA, Marshall J. Multi-infarct dementia. A cause of mental deterioration in the elderly. *Lancet* 1974;2:207–210.
224. Marie P. Des foyers lacunaires de desintegration et de differents autres etats cavitaire du cerveau. *Rev Med* 1901;21:281–298.
225. Binswanger O. Die Abgrenzung der algemeinen progressiven Paralyse (Referat, Erstattet auf der Jahresversammlung des Vereins deutscher irrenartzte zu Dresden am 20 Sept 1894). *Ber Klin Wochenschr* 1894;31:1103–1105, 1137–1139, 1180–1186.
226. Fisher CM. Lacunar strokes and infarcts: a review. *Neurology* 1982;32:871–876.
227. Rothschild D. Neuropathologic changes in arteriosclerotic psychoses and their psychiatric significance. *Arch Neurol Psychiatry* 1942;48:417–436.
228. Ries F, Horn R, Hillekamp J, et al. Differentiation of multi-infarct and Alzheimer dementia by intracranial hemodynamic parameters. *Stroke* 1993;24:228–235.
229. McQuinn BA, O'Leary DH. White matter lucencies on computed tomography, subacute arteriosclerotic encephalopathy (Binswanger's disease), and blood pressure. *Stroke* 1987;18: 900–905.
230. Scheinberg P. Dementia due to vascular disease: a multifactorial disorder. *Stroke* 1988;19:1290–1299.
231. Hachinski VC, Iliff LD, Zilkha E. Cerebral blood flow in dementia. *Arch Neurol* 1975;32:632–637.
232. Rosen WG, Terry RD, Fuld PA, Katzman R, Peck A. Pathologic verification of the ischemic score in the differentiation of dementias. *Ann Neurol* 1980;7:486–488.
233. Fisher CM. Lacunae: small deep cerebral infarcts. *Neurology (NY)* 1965;15:76–80.
234. Brown JJ, Hesselink JR, Rothrock JF. MR and CT of lacunar infarcts. *AJNR* 1988;9:477–482.
235. Adams RD, Fisher CM, Hakim S, et al. Symptomatic occult hydrocephalus with "normal" cerebrospinal fluid pressure (a treatable syndrome). *N Engl J Med* 1965;273:117–126.
236. Sypert GW, Leffman H, Ojemann GA. Occult normal pressure hydrocephalus manifested by parkinsonism-dementia complex. *Neurology* 1973;23:234–238.
237. Fisher CM. Communicating hydrocephalus. *Lancet* 1978;1:1–37.
238. Fisher CM. Hydrocephalus as a cause of disturbances of gait in the elderly. *Neurology* 1982;32:1358–1363.
239. Ojemann RG, Fisher CM, Adams RD, et al. Further experiences with the syndrome of "normal" pressure hydrocephalus. *J Neurosurg* 1969;31:279–294.
240. Huckman MS. Normal pressure hydrocephalus: evaluation of diagnostic and prognostic tests. *AJNR* 1981;2:385–395.
241. Messer HD, Brinker RA. Hydrocephalus and dementia complicating spinal tumor. *J Neurosurg* 1980;53:544–547.
242. Mittal MM, Gupta NC, Sharman ML. Spinal epidural meningioma associated with increased intracranial pressure. *Neurology* 1970;20:818–820.
243. Bamford CR, Labadie EL. Reversal of dementia in normotensive hydrocephalus after removal of a cauda equina tumor. *J Neurosurg* 1976;45:104–107.
244. Feldmann E, Bromfield E, Navia B, et al. Hydrocephalic dementia and spinal cord tumor. *Arch Neurol* 1986;43:714–718.
245. Graff-Radford NR, Godersky JC. Symptomatic congenital hydrocephalus in the elderly simulating normal pressure hydrocephalus. *Neurology* 1989;39:1596–1600.
246. Rasker JJ, Jansen ENH, Haan J, et al. Normal pressure hydrocephalus in rheumatic patients. *N Engl J Med* 1985;312:1239–1241.
247. Wikkelso C, Andersson H, Blomstrand C, et al. Computed tomography of the brain in the diagnosis and prognosis in normal pressure hydrocephalus. *Eur Arch Psychiatry Clin Neurosci* 1989;31:160–165.
248. El Gammal T, Allen MB, Brooks BS, et al. MR evaluation of hydrocephalus. *AJNR* 1987;8:591–597.
249. Bradley WG Jr, Kortman KE, Burgoyne B. Flowing cerebrospinal fluid in normal and hydrocephalic states: appearance on MR images. *Radiology* 1986;159:611–616.
250. Malko JA, Hoffman JC Jr, McClees EC, et al. A phantom study of intracranial CSF signal loss due to pulsatile motion. *AJNR* 1988;9:83–89.
251. Bradley WG Jr, Whittemore A, Watanabe A, et al. Association of deep white matter infarction with chronic communicating hydrocephalus: implications regarding the possible origin of normal-pressure hydrocephalus. *AJNR* 1991;12:31–39.
252. Nieuwenhuys R, Voogd J, van Huijzen C. *The Human Central Nervous System. A Synopsis and Atlas.* New York: Springer-Verlag; 1981.
253. Kanazawa I. Clinical pathophysiology of basal ganglia disease. In: Vinken PJ, Bruyn GW, Klawans HL, eds. *Handbook of Clinical Neurology*, vol. 49. Amsterdam: Elsevier Science; 1986:65–86.
254. Adams RD, Salam-Adams M. Striatonigral degeneration. In: Vinken PJ, Bruyn GW, Klawans HL, eds. *Handbook of Clinical Neurology*, vol. 49. Amsterdam: Elsevier Science; 1986:205–212.
255. Starosta-Rubinstein S, Young AB, Kluin K, et al. Clinical assessment of 31 patients with Wilson's disease. Correlations with structural changes on magnetic resonance imaging. *Arch Neurol* 1987;44:365–370.
256. Carpenter MB. Anatomy of the basal ganglia. In: Vinken PJ, Bruyn GW, Klawans HL, eds. *Handbook of Clinical Neurology*, vol. 49. Amsterdam: Elsevier Science; 1986;1–18.
257. Jellinger K. Exogeneous lesions of the pallidum. In: Vinken PJ, Bruyn GW, Klawans HL, eds. *Handbook of Clinical Neurology*, vol. 49. Amsterdam: Elsevier Science; 1986;465–492.
258. Gusella JF, Wexler NS, Conneally PM. A polymorphic DNA marker genetically linked to Huntington's disease. *Nature* 1983; 306:234–238.
259. Simmons JT, Pastakia B, Chase TN, et al. Magnetic resonance imaging in Huntington disease. *AJNR* 1986;7:25–28.
260. Sax DS, Bird ED, Gusella JF, et al. Phenotypic variation in two Huntington's disease families with linkage to chromosome 4. *Neurology* 1989;39:1332–1336.
261. Grafton ST, Mazziotta JC, Pahl JJ, et al. Serial changes of cerebral glucose metabolism and caudate size in persons at risk for Huntington's disease. *Arch Neurol* 1992;49:1161–1167.
262. Roos RAC. Neuropathology of Huntington's chorea. In: Vinken PJ, Bruyn GW, Klawans HL, eds. *Handbook of Clinical Neurology*, vol. 49, Amsterdam: Elsevier Science; 1986:315–326.
263. Klintworth GK. Huntington's chorea: morphologic contributions of a century. In: Barbeau A, Chase TN, Paulson GW, eds. *Advances in Neurology*, vol 1. New York: Raven Press; 1973:353–368.
264. Hallervorden J. *Handbuch der speziellen pathologischen Anatomie und Histologie*, Berlin: Springer-Verlag; 1957:793.
265. Harris GJ, Pearlson GD, Peyser CE, et al. Putamen volume reduction on magnetic resonance imaging exceeds caudate changes in mild Huntington's disease. *Ann Neurol* 1992;31:69–75.
266. Pettegrew JW, Koop SJ, Minshew NJ, et al. 31P nuclear magnetic resonance studies of phosphoglyceride metabolism in developing and degenerating brain: preliminary observations. *J Neuropathol Exp Neurol* 1987;46:419–430.
267. Mutoh K, Okuno T, Ito M., et al. MR imaging of a group I case of Hallervorden-Spatz disease. *J Comput Assist Tomogr* 1988;12:851–853.
268. Gallucci M, Bozzao A, Splendiani A, et al. Wernicke encephalopathy: MR findings in five patients. *AJNR* 1990;11:887–892.
269. Barkovich AJ. Toxic and metabolic brain disorders. In: *Pediatric Neuroimaging*. New York: Raven Press; 1995:55–106.
270. Hallervorden J, Spatz H. Eigenartige Erkrankung im extrapyramidalen System mit besonderer Beteiligung des Globus Pallidus und der Substantia Nigra. *Z Neurol Psychiatr* 1922;79:254–302.
271. Dooling EC, Schoene WC, Richardson EP. Hallervorden-Spatz syndrome. *Arch Neurol* 1974;30:70–83.
272. Littrup PJ, Gerbarski SS. Imaging of Hallervorden-Spatz disease. *J Comput Assist Tomogr* 1985;9:491–493.
273. Sethi KD, Adams RJ, Loring DW, et al. Hallervorden-Spatz syndrome: clinical and magnetic resonance imaging correlations. *Ann Neurol* 1988;24:692–694.
274. Gallucci M, Cardona F, Arachi M, et al. Follow-up MR studies in

Hallervorden-Spatz disease. *J Comput Assist Tomogr* 1990;14: 118–120.
275. Frydman M, Bonne-Tamir B, Farer I, et al. Assignment of the gene for Wilson's disease to chromosome 13: linkage to the esterase D locus. *Proc Natl Acad Sci USA* 1984;82:1819–1821.
276. Aisen AM, Martel W, Gabrielsen TO, et al. Wilson disease of the brain: MR imaging. *Radiology* 1985;157:137-141.
277. Yuh WT, Flickinger FW. Unusual MR findings in CNS Wilson disease (letter). *AJR* 1988;151:834.
278. Wilson SAK. Progressive lenticular degeneration: a familial nervous disease associated with cirrhosis of the liver. *Brain* 1912;34: 295-309.
279. Walshe JM. Wilson's disease. In: Vinken PJ, Bruyn GW, Klawans HL, eds. *Handbook of Clinical Neurology,* vol. 49. Amsterdam: Elsevier Science Publishers; 1986:223–238.
280. Lennox G, Jones R. Gaze distractibility in Wilson's disease. *Ann Neurol* 1989;25:415–417.
281. Hitoshi S, Iwata M, Yoshikawa K. Mid-brain pathology of Wilson's disease: MRI analysis of three cases. *J Neurol Neurosurg Psychiatry* 1991;54:624–626.
282. Starosta-Rubinstein S, Young AB, Kluin K, et al. Clinical assessment of 31 patients with Wilson's disease. Correlations with structural changes on magnetic resonance imaging. *Arch Neurol* 1984;44:365–370.
283. Prayer L, Wimberger D, Kramer J, et al. Cranial MRI in Wilson's disease. *Neuroradiology* 1990;32:211–214.
284. Bang-sen S, Yan-bing C, Jin S, et al. Magnetic resonance imaging in hepatolenticular degeneration. *Chin Med J (Engl)* 1992;105: 73–76.
285. De Haan J, Grossman RI, Civitello L, et al. High-field magnetic resonance imaging of Wilson's disease. *J Comput Assist Tomogr* 1987;11:132–135.
286. Lawler GA, Pennock JM, Steiner RE, et al. Nuclear magnetic resonance (NMR) imaging in Wilson disease. *J Comput Assist Tomogr* 1983;7:1–8.
287. Singcharoen T, Chakkaphak K, Udompanich O. Unusual magnetic resonance findings in Wilson's disease. *Br J Radiol* 1991;64: 752–754.
288. Linne T, Agartz I, Saaf J, et al. Cerebral abnormalities in Wilson's disease as evaluated by ultra-low-field magnetic resonance imaging and computerized image processing. *Magn Reson Imaging* 1990;8:819–824.
289. Thuomas KA, Aquilonius SM, Bergstrom K, et al. Magnetic resonance imaging of the brain in Wilson's disease. *Neuroradiology* 1993;35:134–141.
290. Nazer H, Brismar J, Al-Kawi MZ, et al. Magnetic resonance imaging of the brain in Wilson's disease. *Neuroradiology* 1993;35: 130–133.
291. Grimm G, Prayer L, Oder W, et al. Comparison of functional and structural brain disturbances in Wilson's disease. *Neurology* 1991;41:272–276.
292. Oder W, Prayer L, Grimm G, et al. Wilson's disease: evidence of subgroups derived from clinical findings and brain lesions. *Neurology* 1993;43:120–124.
293. Hanner JS, Li KCP, Davis GL. Acquired hepatocerebral degeneration: MR similarity with Wilson disease. *J Comput Assist Tomogr* 1988;12:1076–1077.
294. Gilbert GJ. Acute ammonia intoxication 37 years after ureterosigmoidostomy. *South Med J* 1988;81:1443–1445.
295. Brunberg JA, Kanal E, Hirsch W, et al. Chronic acquired hepatic failure: MR imaging of the brain. *AJNR* 1988;9:1034–1035.
296. Inoue E, Hori S, Narumi Y, et al. Portal-systemic encephalopathy: presence of basal ganglia lesions with high signal intensity on MR images. *Radiology* 1991;179:551–555.
297. Kreis R, Ross BD, Oxon DP, et al. Metabolic disorders of the brain in chronic hepatic encephalopathy detected with H-1 MR spectroscopy. *Radiology* 1992;182:19–27.
298. Parkinson J. *An essay on the shaking palsy.* London: Sherwood Neely and Jones; 1817.
299. Madrazo I, Drucker-Colin R, Diaz V, et al. Open microsurgical graft of adrenal medulla to the right caudate nucleus in two patients with intractable Parkinson's disease. *N Engl J Med* 1987; 317:831–834.
300. Hurtig H, Joyce J, Sladek JR, et al. Postmortem analysis of adrenal-medulla-to-caudate autograft in a patient with Parkinson's disease. *Ann Neurol* 1989;25:607–614.
301. Duguid JR, De La Paz R, DeGroot J. Magnetic resonance imaging of the midbrain in Parkinson's disease. *Ann Neurol* 1986;20:744–747.
302. Braffman BH, Grossman RI, Goldberg HI, et al. MR imaging of Parkinson disease with spin-echo and gradient-echo sequences. *AJNR* 1988;9:1093–1099.
303. Stern MB, Braffman BH, Skolnick BE, et al. Magnetic resonance imaging in Parkinson's disease and parkinsonian syndromes. *Neurology* 1989;39:1524–1526.
304. Alvord EC. The pathology of parkinsonism. In: Minckler J, ed. *Pathology of the Nervous System, vol 1.* New York: McGraw Hill; 1968;1152–1161.
305. Steiner I, Gomori JM, Melamed E. Features of brain atrophy in Parkinson's disease. *Neuroradiology* 1985;27:158–160.
306. Hakim AM, Mathieson G. Dementia in Parkinson disease: a neuropathologic study. *Neurology* 1979;29:1209–1214.
307. Pollanen MS, Dickson DW, Bergeron C. Pathology and biology of the Lewy Body. *J Neuropathol Exp Neurol* 1993;52:183–191.
308. Dickson DW, Crystal H, Mattiace LA, et al. Diffuse Lewy body disease: light and electron microscopic immunocytochemistry of senile plaques. *Acta Neuropathol* 1989;78:572–584.
309. Huber SJ, Shuttleworth EC, Christy JA, et al. Magnetic resonance imaging in dementia of Parkinson's disease. *J Neurol Neurosurg Psychiatry* 1989;52:1221–1227.
310. Besson JA, Mutch WJ, Smith FW, et al. The relationship between Parkinson's disease and dementia. A study using proton NMR imaging parameters. *Br J Psychiatry* 1985;147:380–382.
311. Adams RD, Van Bogaert L, Vandereecken H. Degenerescence nigro-striee et cerebello-nigro-striee. *Psychiatr Neurol* 1961;142: 219-259.
312. Pastakia B, Polinsky RJ, DiChiro G, et al. Multiple system atrophy (Shy-Drager syndrome): MR imaging. *Radiology* 1986;159: 499–505.
313. Brown R, Polinsky RJ, Di Chiro G, et al. MRI in autonomic failure. *J Neurol Neurosurg Psychiatry* 1987;50: 913–914.
314. Borit A, Rubinstein LJ, Urich H. The striatonigral degenerations: putaminal pigments and nosology. *Brain* 1975;98:101–112.
315. Steele JC, Richardson JC, Olszewski J. Progressive supranuclear palsy. *Arch Neurol* 1964;10:333–359.
316. Steele JC. Progressive supranuclear palsy. *Brain* 1972;95:693–704.
317. Polsby M, Patronas NJ, Dweyer A. Progressive supranuclear palsy and magnetic resonance imaging. *Neurology* 1985;35:136.
318. Kristensen MO. Progressive supranuclear palsy—20 years later. *Acta Neurol Scand* 1985;71:177–189.
319. Ambrosetto P, Kim M. Progressive supranuclear palsy [Letter]. *Arch Neurol* 1981;38:672.
320. Ambrosetto P, Michelucci R, Forti A. CT findings in progressive supranuclear palsy. *J Comput Assist Tomogr* 1984;8:406–409.
321. Ambrosetto P. CT in progressive supranuclear palsy. *AJNR* 1987;8:849–851.
322. Masucci EF, Borts FT, Smirniotopoulos J, et al. Thin-section CT of midbrain abnormalities in progressive supranuclear palsy. *AJNR* 1985;6:767–772.
323. Schonfeld SM, Safer JN, Sage JI, et al. Computed tomography findings in progressive supranuclear palsy. *AJNR* 1985;6: 462(abst).
324. Duvoisin RC, Golbe LI, Lepore FE. Progressive supranuclear palsy. *Can J Neurol Sci* 1987;14 (3 Suppl):547–554.
325. Schmidt ML, Lee VM, Hurtig H, Trojanowski JQ. Properties of antigenic determinants that distinguish neurofibrillary tangles in progressive supranuclear palsy and Alzheimer's disease. *Lab Invest* 1988;59:460–466.
326. Leigh D. Subacute necrotizing encephalomyelopathy in an infant. *J Neurol Neurosurg Psychiatry* 1951;14:216.
327. Davis PC, Hoffman JC Jr., Braun IF, et al. MR of Leigh's disease (subacute necrotizing encephalomyelopathy). *AJNR* 1987;8:71–75.
328. Medina L, Chi T, DeVivo D, et al. MR findings in patients with subacute necrotizing encephalomyelopathy (Leigh syndrome): correlation with biochemical defect. *AJNR* 1990;11:379–384.
329. Macaya A, Munell F, Burke RE, et al. Disorders of movement in Leigh syndrome. *Neuropediatrics* 1993;24:60–67.
330. Fulham M, Lawrence C, Harper C. Diagnostic clues in an adult case of Leigh's disease. *Med J Aust* 1988;149:320–322.
331. Geyer CA, Sartor KJ, Prensky AJ, et al. Leigh disease (subacute

necrotizing encephalomyelopathy): CT and MR in five cases. *J Comput Assist Tomogr* 1988;12:40–44.

332. Fujii T, Ito M, Okuno T, et al. Complex I (reduced nicotin-amide-adenine dinucleotide-coenzyme Q reductase) deficiency in two patients with probable Leigh syndrome. *J Pediatr* 1990;116:84–87.
333. van Erven PM, Cillessen JP, Eekhoff EM, et al. Leigh syndrome, a mitochondrial encephalo (myo)pathy. A review of the literature. *Clin Neurol Neurosurg* 1987;89:217–230.
334. Kissel JT, Kolkin S, Chakeres D, et al. Magnetic resonance imaging in a case of autopsy-proved adult subacute necrotizing encephalomyelopathy (Leigh's disease). *Arch Neurol* 1987;44:563–566.
335. Montpetit VJA, Anderman F, Carpenter S, et al. Subacute necrotizing encephalomyelopathy. *Brain* 1971;94:1–30.
336. Hall K, Gardner-Medwin D. CT scan appearances in Leigh's disease (subacute necrotizing encephalomyelopathy). *Neuroradiology* 1978;16:48–50.
337. Palteil HJ, O'Gorman AM, Meagher-Villemure K, et al. Subacute necrotizing encephalomyelopathy (Leigh disease): CT study. *Radiology* 1987;162:115–118.
338. Abe K, Inui T, et al. Fluctuating MR images with mitochondrial encephalopathy, lactic acidosis, stroke-like syndrome (MELAS). *Neuroradiology* 1990;32:77.
339. Koch TK, Yee MHC, Hutchinson HT, et al. Magnetic resonance imaging in subacute necrotizing encephalomyelopathy (Leigh's disease). *Ann Neurol* 1986;19:605–607.
340. Martin JJ, Van de Vyver FL, Scholte HR, et al. Defect in succinate oxidation by isolated muscle mitochondria in a patient with symmetrical lesions in the basal ganglia. *J Neurol Sci* 1988;84:189–200.
341. Onuma A, Miyabayashi S, Iinuma K, et al. Comparative appraisal of CT scan and MRI in the diagnosis of Leigh encephalomyelopathy in two siblings. *J Child Neurol* 1987;2:324–326.
342. Heckmann J, Eastman R, Handler L, et al. Leigh disease (subacute necrotizing encephlomyelopathy): MR documentation of the evolution of an acute attack. *AJNR* 1993;14:1157–1159.
343. Detre J, Wang Z, Bogdan A, et al. Regional variation in brain lactate in Leigh syndrome by localized ^{1}H magnetic resonance spectroscopy. *Ann Neurol* 1991;29:218–221.
344. Egger J, Lake BD, Wilson J. Mitochondrial cytopathy. A multisystem disorder with ragged red fibers on muscle biopsy. *Arch Dis Child* 1981;56:741–752.
345. Egger J, Kendall BE. CT in mitochondrial cytopathy. *Neuroradiology* 1981;22:73–78.
346. Barkovich AJ, Good WV, Koch TK, et al. Mitochondrial disorders: analysis of their clinical and imaging characteristics. *AJNR* 1993;14:1119–1137.
347. Allard JC, Tilak S, Carter AP. CT and MR of MELAS syndrome. *AJNR* 1988;9:1234–1238.
348. Bruyn GW, Vielvoye GJ, Went LN. Hereditary spastic dystonia: a new mitochondrial encephalopathy. *J Neurol Sci* 1991;103:195–202.
349. Forster C, Hubner G, Miller-Hocker J, et al. Mitochondrial angiopathy in a family with MELAS. *Neuropediatrics* 1993;23:165–168.
350. Suzuki T, Koizumi J, Shiraishi H, et al. Mitochondrial encephalomyopathy (MELAS) with mental disorder CT, MRI and SPECT findings. *Neuroradiology* 1990;32:74–76.
351. Hausegger KA, Millner MM, Ebner F, et al. Mitochondrial encephalomyopathy—two years follow-up by MRI. *Pediatr Radiol* 1991;21:231–233.
352. Rosen L, Phillips S, Enzmann D. Magnetic resonance imaging in MELAS syndrome. *Neuroradiology* 1990;32:168–171.
353. Matthews PM, Phil D, Tampieri D, et al. Magnetic resonance imaging shows specific abnormalities in the MELAS syndrome. *Neurology* 1991;41:1043–1046.
354. Chen R-S, Huang C-C, Lee C-C, et al. Overlapping syndrome of MERRF and MELAS: molecular and neuroradiological studies. *Acta Neurol Scand* 1993;87:494–498.
355. Elsas T, Rinck PA, Isaksen C, et al. Cerebral nuclear magnetic resonance (MRI) in Kearns syndrome. *Acta Ophthalmol (Copenh)* 1988;66:469–473.
356. Johnsen DE, Coleman J, Poe L. MR of progressive neurodegenerative change in treated Menkes' kinky hair disease. *Neuroradiology* 1991;33:181–182.
357. Jacobs DS, Smith AS, Finelli DA, et al. Menkes kinky hair disease: characteristic MR angiographic findings. *AJNR* 1993;14:1160–1163.
358. Takahashi S, Ishii K, Matsumoto K, et al. Cranial MRI and MR angiography in Menkes' syndrome. *Neuoradiology* 1993;35:556–558.
359. Fujii T, Okuno T, Ito M. Non-Menkes-type copper deficiency with regression, lactic acidosis, and granulocytopenia. *Neurology* 1991;41:1263–1266.
360. Baloh RW, Yee RD, Honrubia V. Late cortical cerebellar atrophy. Clinical and oculographic features. *Brain* 1986;109:159–180.
361. Ramos A, Quintana F, Diez C, et al. CT findings in spinocerebellar degeneration. *AJNR* 1987;8:635–640.
362. Bradac GB, Riva A, Mortora P, et al. Primary progressive cerebellar ataxia. *Neuroradiology* 1989;31:16–18.
363. Courchesne E, Hesselink JR, Jernigan TL, et al. Abnormal neuroanatomy in a nonretarded person with autism. *Arch Neurol* 1987;44:335–341.
364. Courchesne E, Yeung-Courchesne R, Press G, et al. Hypoplasia of cerebellar vermal lobules VI and VII in autism. *N Engl J Med* 1988;318:1349–1354.
365. Courchesne E, Press G, Yeung-Courchesne R. Parietal lobe abnormalities detected with MR in patients with infantile autism. *AJR* 1993;160:387–393.
366. Hashimoto T, Murakawa K, Miyazaki M, et al. Magnetic resonance imaging of the brain structures in the posterior fossa in retarded autistic children. *Acta Pediatr* 1992;81:1030–1040.
367. Hashimoto T, Tayama M, Miyazaki M, et al. Brainstem and cerebellar vermis involvement in autistic children. *J Child Neurol* 1992;7:149–153.
368. Nowell MA, Hackney DB, Muraki AS, et al. Varied MR appearance of autism: fifty-three pediatric patients having the full autistic syndrome. *Magn Reson Imaging* 1990;8:811–816.
369. Garber HJ, Ritvo ER. Magnetic resonance imaging of the posterior fossa in autistic adults. *Am J Psychiatry* 1992;149:245–247.
370. Ekman G, Chateau P, Marions O, et al. Low field magnetic resonance imaging of the central nervous system in 15 children with autistic disorder. *Acta Paediatr Scand* 1991;80:243–247.
371. Holttum JR, Minshew NJ, Sanders RS, et al. Magnetic resonance imaging of the posterior fossa in autism. *Biol Psychiatry* 1992;32:1091–1101.
372. Piven J, Nehme E, Simon J, et al. Magnetic resonance imaging in autism: measurement of the cerebellum, pons, and fourth ventricle. *Biol Psychiatry* 1992;31:491–504.
373. Reiss AL, Freund S. Fragile X syndrome. *Biol Psychiatry* 1990;27:223–240.
374. Reiss AL, Aylward EH, Freund LS, et al. Neuroanatomy of fragile X syndrome: the posterior fossa. *Ann Neurol* 1991;29:26–32.
375. Reiss AL, Freund S, Tseng JE, et al. Neuroanatomy in fragile X females: The posterior fossa. *J Hum Genet* 1991;49:279–288.
376. Reiss AL, Patel S, Kumar A, et al. Preliminary communication. Neuroanatomical variations of the posterior fossa in adult males with the fragile X (Martin-Bell) syndrome. *Am J Med Genet* 1988;31:407–414.
377. Aylward EH, Reiss AL. Area and volume measurement of posterior fossa structures in MRI. *J Psychiatr Res* 1991;25:159–168.
378. Nihei K, Naitoh H. Cranial computed tomographic and magnetic resonance imaging studies on the Rett syndrome. *Brain Dev* 1990;12:101–105.
379. Murakami J, Courchesne E, Haas R, et al. Cerebellar and cerebal abnormalities in Rett syndrome: a quantitative MR analysis. *AJR* 1992;159:177–183.
380. Casanova MF, Naidu S, Goldberg TE. Quantitative magnetic resonance imaging in Rett syndrome. *J Neuropsychiatry Clin Neurosci* 1991;3:66–72.
381. Reiss AL, Faruque F, Naidu S, et al. Neuroanatomy of Rett syndrome: a volumetric imaging study. *Ann Neurol* 1993;34:227–234.
382. Weiss S, Weber G, Neuhold A, et al. Down syndrome: MR quantification of brain structures and comparison with normal control subjects. *AJNR* 1991;12:1207–1211.
383. Lai F. Clinicopathologic features of Alzheimer's disease in Down syndrome. *Prog Clin Biol Res* 1992;379:15–34.
384. Abe K, Yorifuji S, Nishikawa Y. Reduced isotope uptake re-

stricted to the motor area in patients with amyotrophic lateral sclerosis. *Neuroradiology* 1993;35:410–411.

385. Tanzi RE, St George-Hyslop PH, Haines JL, et al. The genetic defect in familial Alzheimer's disease is not tightly linked to the amyloid beta-protein gene. *Nature* 1987;329:156–157.
386. LeMay M, Alvarez N. The relationship between enlargement of the temporal horns of the lateral ventricles and dementia in aging patients with Down's syndrome. *Neuroradiology* 1990;32:104–107.
387. Koshino Y, Murata T, Omori M, et al. In vivo proton magnetic resonance spectroscopy in adult Down's syndrome. *Biol Psychiatry* 1992;32:625–627.
388. Murata T, Koshino Y, Omori M, et al. In vivo proton magnetic resonance spectroscopy study on premature aging in adult Down's syndrome. *Biol Psychiatry* 1993;34:290–297.
389. Storm UD. Magnetic resonance imaging of moyamoya disease in a child with Down's syndrome. *J Mental Deficiency Res* 1988;33:507–510.
390. Menzel P. Beitrag zur kenntnis der hereditaren ataxie und kleinhirnatrophie. *Arch Psychiatr Nervenker* 1891;22:160.
391. Dejerine J, Thomas A. L'atrophie olivo-ponto-cerebelleuse. *Nouv Iconogr Salpet* 1900;13:330.
392. Savoiardo M, Strada L, Girotti F, et al. Olivopontocerebellar atrophy: MR diagnosis and relationship to multisystem atrophy. *Radiology* 1990;174:693–696.
393. Oppenheimer DR. Diseases of the basal ganglia, cerebellum and motor neurons. In: Hume AJ, et al., eds. *Greenfield's Neuropathology*, 4th ed. New York: Wiley; 1984:699–747.
394. Nabatame H, Fukuyama H, Akiguchi I, et al. Spinocerebellar degeneration: qualitative and quantitative MR analysis of atrophy. *J Comput Assist Tomogr* 1988;12:298–303.
395. Revel M, Mann M, Brugieres P, et al. MR appearance of hypertrophic olivary degeneration after contralateral cerebellar hemorrhage. *AJNR* 1991;12:71–72.
396. Vighetto A, Froment JC, Trillet M, et al. Magnetic resonance imaging in familial paroxysmal ataxia. *Arch Neurol* 1988;45:547–549.
397. Furman JM, Baloh RW, Chugani H, et al. Infantile cerebellar atrophy. *Ann Neurol* 1985;17:399–402.
398. Torvik A, Lindboe CF, Rogde S. Brain lesions in alcoholics. *J Neurol Sci* 1982;56:233–248.
399. Barlow JK, Sims KB, Kolodny EH. Early cerebellar degeneration in twins with infantile neuroaxonal dystrophy. *Ann Neurol* 1989;25:413–415.
400. Miller L, Link MP, Bologna S, et al. Cerebellar atrophy caused by high-dose cytosine arabinoside: CT and MR findings. *AJR* 1989;152:343–344.
401. Saito H, Yanagisawa T. Acute cerebellar ataxia after influenza vaccination with recurrence and marked cerebellar atrophy. *Tohoku J Exp Med* 1989;158: 95–103.
402. Schmidley JW, Levinsohn MW, Manetto V. Infantile X-linked ataxia and deafness: a new clinicopathologic entity? *Neurology* 1987;37:1344–1349.
403. de Yebenes JG, Vazquez A, Rabano J, et al. Hereditary bronchial myoclonus with spastic paraparesis and cerebellar ataxia: a new autosomal dominant disorder. *Neurology* 1988;38:569–572.
404. Kitamura J, Kubuki Y, Tsuruta K, et al. A new family with Joseph disease in Japan. Homovanillic acid, magnetic resonance, and sleep apnea studies. *Arch Neurol* 1989,46:425–428.
405. Lazar RB, Ho SU, Melen O, et al. Multifocal central nervous system damage caused by toluene abuse. *Neurology* 1983;33:1337–1340.
406. Formazzari L, Wilkinson DA, Kapur BM, et al. Cerebellar cortical and functional impairment in toluene abusers. *Acta Neurol Scand* 1983;67:319–329.
407. Metrick SA, Brenner RP. Abnormal brainstem auditory evoked potentials in chronic paint sniffers. *Ann Neurol* 1982;12:553–556.
408. Rosenberg NL, Kleinschmidt-Demasters BK, Davis KS, et al. Toluene abuse causes diffuse central nervous system white matter changes. *Ann Neurol* 1988;23:611–614.
409. Filley CM, Heaton RK, Rosenberg NL. White matter dementia in chronic toluene abuse. *Neurology* 1990;40:532–534.
410. Ikeda M, Tsukagoshi H. Encephalopathy due to toluene sniffing; report of a case by MRI. *Eur Neurol* 1990;30:347–349.
411. Xiong L, Matthes JD, Li J, et al. MR imaging of "spray heads": toluene abuse via aerosol paint inhalation. *AJNR* 1993;14:1195–1199.
412. Caldemeyer KS, Pascuzzi RM, Moran CC, et al. Toluene abuse causing reduced MR signal intensity in the brain. *AJR* 1993;161:1259–1261.
413. Carpenter MB, Sutin J. *Human Neuroanatomy*, 8th ed. Baltimore: Williams & Wilkins; 1982:282–288.
414. Biondi A, Dormont D, Weitzner I Jr, et al. MR imaging of the cervical cord in juvenile amyotrophy of distal upper extremity. *AJNR* 1989;10:263–268.
415. Rosen DR, Siddique T, Patterson D, et al. Mutations in Cu/Zn superoxide dismutase gene are associated with familial amyotrophic lateral sclerosis. *Nature* 1993;362:59–62.
416. Cote F, Collard JF, Julien JP. Progressive neuronopathy in transgenic mice expressing the human neurofilament heavy gene: a mouse model of amyotrophic lateral sclerosis. *Cell* 1993;73:35–46.
417. Xu Z, Cork LC, Griffin JW, et al. Increased expression of neurofilament subunit NF-L produces morphological alterations that resemble the pathology of human motor neuron disease. *Cell* 1993;73:23–33.
418. Bensimon G, Lacomblez L, Meininger V. A controlled trial of riluzole in amyotrophic lateral sclerosis. ALS/Riluzole Study Group. *N Engl J Med* 1994;330:585–591.
419. Goodin DS, Rowley HA, Onley RK. Magnetic resonance imaging in amyotrophic lateral sclerosis. *Ann Neurol* 1988;23:418–420.
420. Bernstein EF. Proposed method for analyzing carotid endarterectomy results. *Stroke* 1988;19:1054–1055.
421. Sales Luis ML, Hormigo A, Mauricio C, et al. Magnetic resonance imaging in motor neuron disease. *J Neurol* 1990;237:471–474.
422. Udaka F, Sawada H, Seriu N, et al. MRI and SPECT findings in amyotrophic lateral sclerosis. *Neuroradiology* 1992; 34:389–393.
423. Friedman DP, Tartaglino LM. Amyotrophic lateral sclerosis: hyperintensity of the corticospinal tracts on MR images of the spinal cord. *AJR* 1993;160:604–606.
424. Kato S, Hayashi H, Yagishita A. Involvement of the frontotemporal lobe and limbic system in amyotrophic lateral sclerosis: as assessed by serial computed tomography and magnetic resonance imaging. *J Neurol Sci* 1993;116:52–58.
425. Iwasaki Y, Kinoshita M, Shiojima T. MRI in primary lateral sclerosis. *Neurology* 1991;41:951(abst).
426. Ishikawa K, Nagura H, Yokota T, et al. Signal loss in the motor cortex on magnetic resonance images in amyotrophic lateral sclerosis. *Ann Neurol* 1993;33:218–222.
427. Cha CH, Patten BM. Amyotrophic lateral sclerosis: abnormalities of the tongue on magnetic resonance imaging. *Ann Neurol* 1989;25:468–472.
428. Hudson AJ, Kierman JA, Munoz DG, et al. Clinicopathological features of primary lateral sclerosis are different from amyotrophic lateral sclerosis. *Brain Res Bull* 1993;30:359–364.
429. Marti-Fabregas J, Pujol J. Selective involvement of the pyramidal tract on magnetic resonance imaging in primary lateral sclerosis. *Neurology* 1990;40:1799–1800.
430. Pringle CE, Hudson AJ, Munoz DG, et al. Primary lateral sclerosis. *Brain* 1992;115:495–520.
431. Liu GT, Specht LA. Progressive juvenile segmental spinal muscular atrophy. *Pediatr Neurol* 1993;9:54–56.
432. Timms SR, Cure JK, Kurent JE. Subacute combined degeneration of the spinal cord: MR findings. *AJNR* 1993; 14:1224–1227.
433. Curnes JT, Burger PC, Djang WT, et al. MR imaging of compact white matter pathways. *AJNR* 1988;9:1061–1068.
434. Schmidt ML, Carden MJ, Lee VM-Y, Trojanowski JQ. Phosphate dependent and independent neurofilament epitopes in the axonal swellings of patients with motor neuron disease and controls. *Lab Invest* 1987;56:282–294.

Magnetic Resonance Imaging of the Brain and Spine, Second Edition, edited by Scott W. Atlas. Lippincott-Raven Publishers, Philadelphia © 1996.

19

The Sella Turcica and Parasellar Region

Walter Kucharczyk, Walter J. Montanera, and Laurence E. Becker

NORMAL ANATOMY

The sella turcica is a spherical depression in the superior surface of the sphenoid bone. The sphenoid sinus is inferior and anterior to the sella turcica, the paired cavernous sinuses are lateral, the suprasellar cistern and its contents are superior, and the basilar artery and brainstem are posterior (Fig. 1). The pituitary gland, which weighs about 0.5 g in the adult, is the only structure of significance within the sella turcica (1). The dimensions of the pituitary gland are extremely variable, particularly its height. On average it is 12 mm in width, 8 mm in anteroposterior diameter, and 3 to 8 mm in height. It achieves its greatest size in adolescent and pregnant women because of normal physiologic hypertrophy (2). At puberty, particularly in girls, the gland enlarges tremendously and may reach 10 mm in height. In boys the increase is more modest, with a height limit of about 8 mm (3–5). Even more marked changes occur in pregnancy. The gland increases progressively in size with ges-

W. Kucharczyk, M.D., F.R.C.P.(C): Department of Medical Imaging, University of Toronto, Toronto, Ontario, Canada M5S 1A8.
W. J. Montanera, M.D., F.R.C.P.(C): Department of Radiology, Toronto Hospital, Toronto, Ontario, Canada, M5T 2S8.
L. E. Becker, M.D., F.R.C.P.(C): Department of Pathology, The Hospital for Sick Children, Toronto, Ontario, Canada, M5G 1X8.

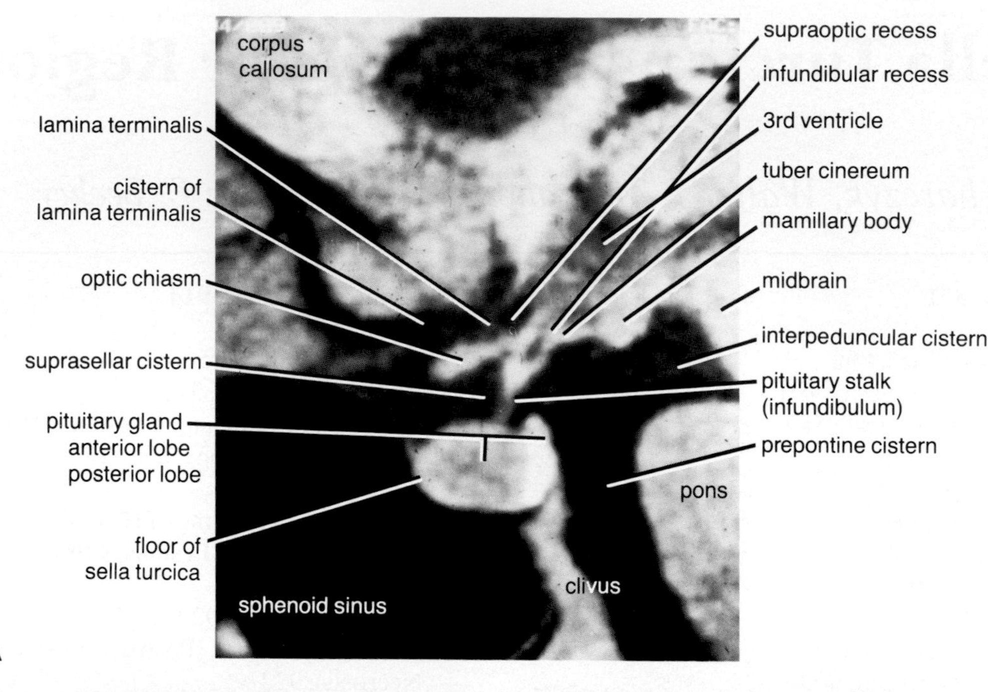

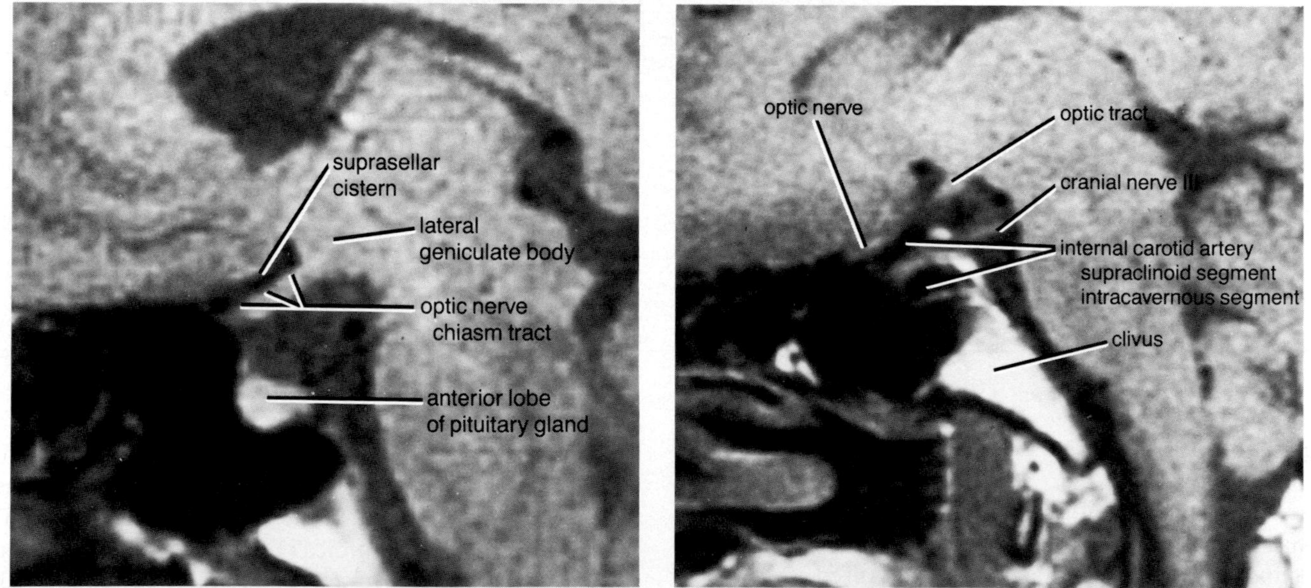

FIG. 1. Normal anatomy. The anatomy of the sella turcica and parasellar region is illustrated in sagittal (**A–C**), coronal (**D–G**), and axial (**H–K**) planes using T1-weighted images. The most important structures are labeled.

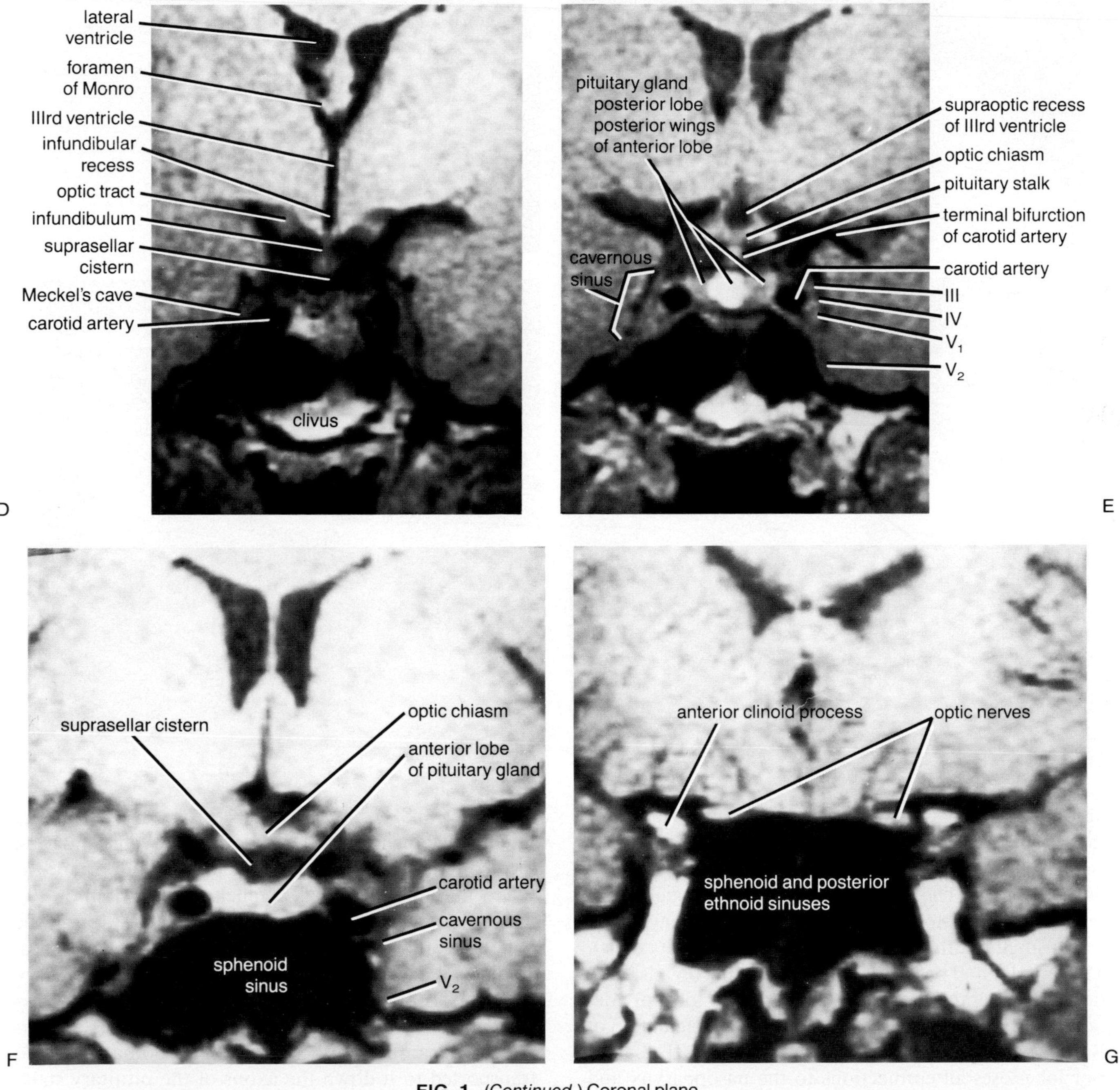

FIG. 1. (*Continued.*) Coronal plane.

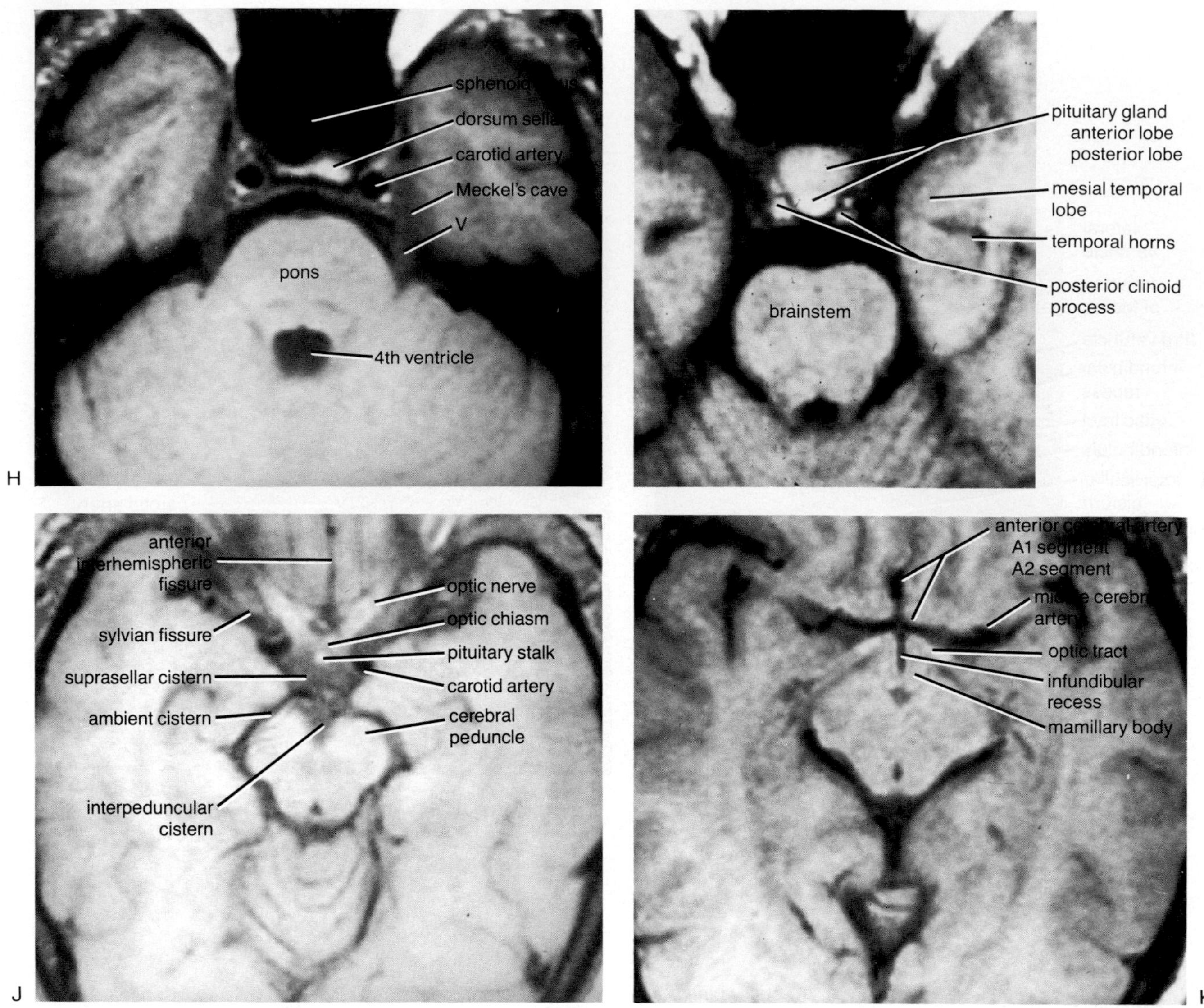

tation, reaching its maximum immediately postpartum (6–8). The maximum height may be as much as 12 mm.

The pituitary gland has anterior, intermediate, and posterior lobes. The intermediate lobe is vestigial in humans and serves no physiologic purpose but may be the site of small nonfunctional cysts (pars intermedia cysts). The anterior and posterior lobes are distinct organs functionally and embryologically. The anterior lobe, or adenohypophysis, originates from a superior invagination of Rathke's pouch from the fetal nasopharynx. The anterior lobe loses all connections to the nasopharynx and develops into a true endocrine organ. The anterior lobe synthesizes many hormones under the influence of hypothalamic stimulatory and inhibitory controls. Adenohypophyseal cells have a definite topographical representation within the gland (9). Prolactin and growth hormone-secreting cells predominate laterally; adrenocorticotropic hormone (ACTH), thyroid-stimulating hormone (TSH), and follicle-stimulating hormone/luteinizing hormone (FSH/LH)-secreting cells tend to be located centrally. This is a finding of some importance as the location of adenomas parallels this distribution (9). The posterior lobe, or neurohypophysis, arises from the hypothalamus as a down-growth into the sella turcica. The posterior lobe retains its connections to the hypothalamus throughout life via the pituitary stalk (the hypothalamohypophyseal tract) and functions as a reservoir for hormones synthesized in the hypothalamus and transported to it down the axons of the pituitary stalk. The posterior lobe itself does not synthesize any hormones.

Although functionally distinct, the anterior and posterior lobes are anatomically closely related, apposed to one another within the confines of the sella turcica. The latter is the much smaller of the two lobes and occupies only 10% to 20% of the volume of the sella turcica, almost always in the midline and directly applied to the dorsum sella. The anterior lobe fills the anterior and central portions of the sella turcica, and has two lateral wings that extend posteriorly, often to the dorsum sella. On rare occasions the lateral wings of the anterior lobe completely envelop the posterior lobe, so that the posterior lobe assumes a central location within the gland.

The pituitary gland receives its blood supply principally from the hypophyseal portal venous system (10). Small branches of the internal carotid artery, the inferior and superior hypophyseal arteries, do provide some direct arterial supply: the inferior hypophyseal artery to the posterior lobe and the lateral surfaces of the anterior lobe; the superior hypophyseal artery to the pituitary stalk and the superior surface of the gland. This combination of arterial and portal venous blood supply explains the differential rates of enhancement of the pituitary gland on dynamic scans after bolus administration of intravenous (i.v.) contrast agents (Fig. 2) (11,12). Within the gland, the vascular pattern is one of a loosely organized network of capillaries. The capillaries are lined by fenestrated endothelium, a characteristic feature of endocrine organs and one that is clearly visible in the pituitary gland (13). On the venous side, the gland is drained by the cavernous sinuses, and afterward the petrosal sinuses. There is preferential venous drainage of the gland to the ipsilateral cavernous sinus, but because there are extensive intercavernous venous connections, anterior, posterior, and inferior to the gland without any valves to restrict directionality of flow, contralateral mixing of venous blood is possible.

The anterior and posterior lobes of the pituitary gland are easily distinguished from one another on magnetic resonance imaging (MRI). Except in the neonate and in pregnancy, the anterior lobe is similar in signal intensity to cerebral white matter on all pulse sequences, whereas the posterior lobe is distinctly hyperintense on T1-weighted images (14–16) (see Figs. 1 and 2). Upon administration of i.v. contrast, the anterior lobe, the posterior lobe, and the pituitary stalk all enhance intensely.

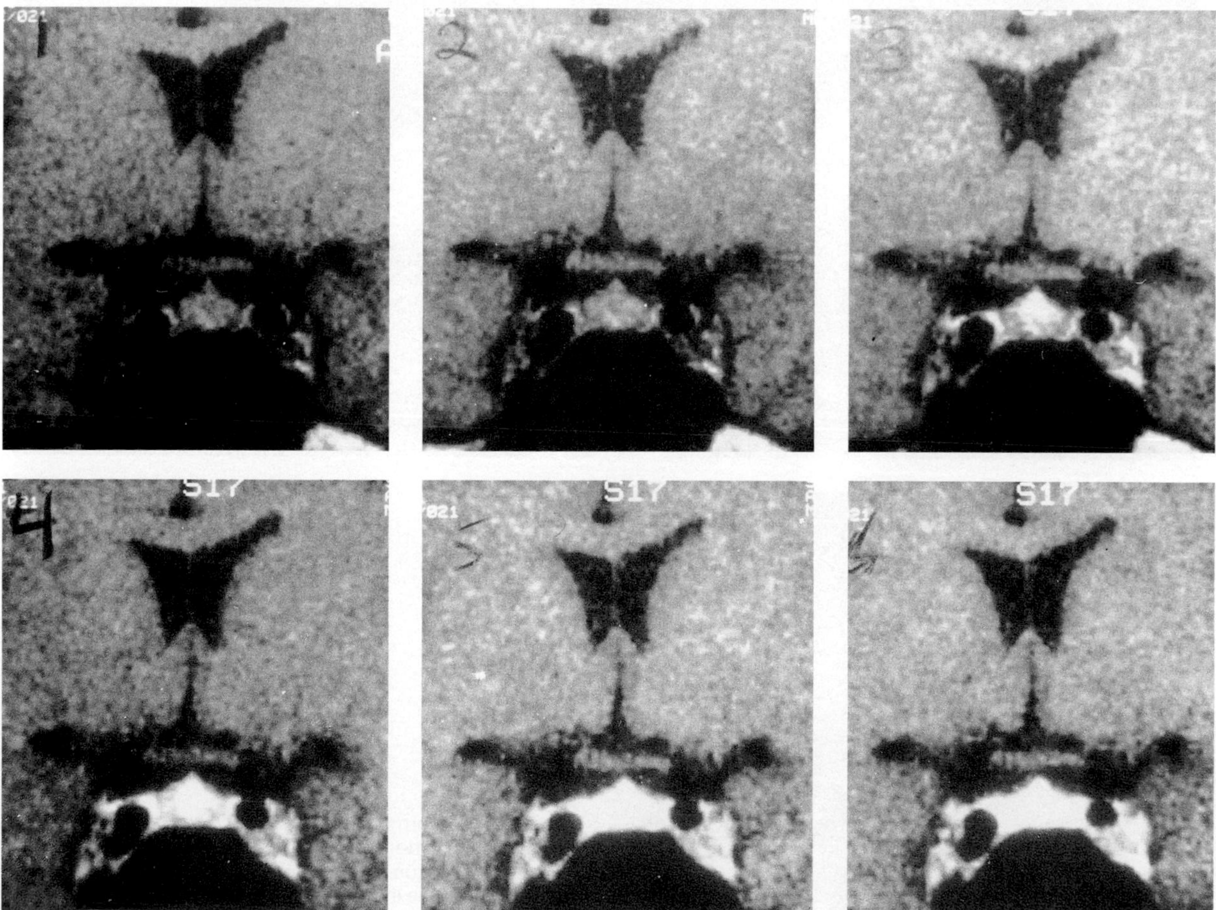

FIG. 2. Normal pituitary gland. Dynamic contrast-enhanced fast spin-echo T1-weighted images. Following a bolus injection of i.v. Gd-DTPA, six consecutive sets of three images were obtained in the coronal plane every 10 sec. The middle image of each of these six three-image sets is shown. The order of the images proceeds from top left to bottom right. Note that enhancement occurs first in the pituitary stalk, then in the pituitary tuft (the junction point of the stalk and gland), and finally there is centrifugal opacification of the entire anterior lobe. By 60 sec the entire gland is enhanced.

In neonates the anterior lobe is brighter than in the adult (Fig. 3). At about 2 months of age the intensity begins to diminish. By about 4 to 6 months of age it resembles that of the adult (Fig. 3). In both pregnancy and in the neonate, lactotroph hypertrophy and increased protein synthesis in the pituitary gland have been invoked to explain the high signal (17–20).

The material within the posterior lobe responsible for the high signal intensity has not been conclusively identified and remains the subject of debate (14,15,21–29). Various constituents of the neurohypophysis have been examined as possible sources of this signal, including vasopressin, phospholipid, neurophysin, and various combinations of the above. To date no one material has been shown to be able to reproduce the appropriate MR signal and be uniquely related to the neurohypophysis. For example, vasopressin is an obvious consideration because of its presence in the posterior lobe. Furthermore, in cases of vasopressin depletion, as in diabetes insipidus, the hyperintensity is not visible. Yet, experiments with concentrated solutions of vasopressin have failed to demonstrate any effect of vasopressin on the relaxation of water (27). Studies with phospholipid vesicles similar in size to those found in the posterior lobe have shown significant T1 shortening without chemical shift. Therefore, phospholipid has the physical properties that could account for the appearance of the posterior lobe (27) yet phospholipid is found in all tissues, not just the posterior lobe. The other constituent of the posterior lobe that merits consideration is the vasopressin-associated carrier protein, "neurophysin". Neurophysin is a 10,000-dalton molecular weight glycoprotein that complexes with vasopressin to form insoluble crystal aggregates. Tien et al. have recently identified neurophysin in the anterior lobe

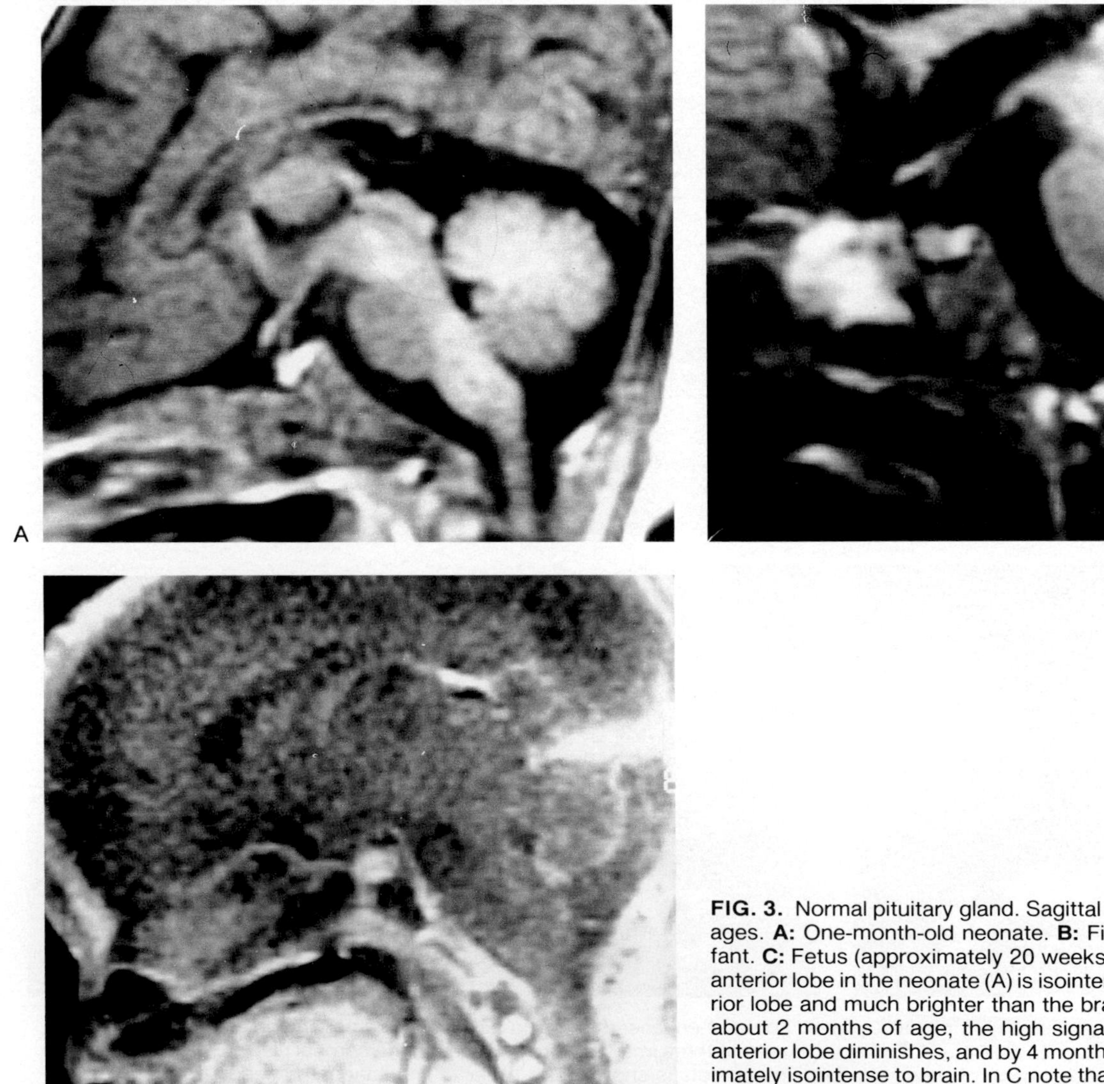

FIG. 3. Normal pituitary gland. Sagittal T1-weighted images. **A:** One-month-old neonate. **B:** Five-month-old infant. **C:** Fetus (approximately 20 weeks' gestation). The anterior lobe in the neonate (A) is isointense to the posterior lobe and much brighter than the brain. Beginning at about 2 months of age, the high signal intensity of the anterior lobe diminishes, and by 4 months (B) it is approximately isointense to brain. In C note that in the fetus the anterior lobe is also very hyperintense. This is expected as the metabolic activity of the fetal gland is similar to that of the neonate.

of the fetus. This is of interest because the fetal anterior lobe, like the posterior lobe at all ages, is also hyperintense on T1-weighted MRI, thus leading to speculation that neurophysin is the agent responsible for the high signal intensity in both the posterior lobe and the fetal anterior lobe (30). No studies to date have investigated the MR characteristics of neurophysin; therefore, its role remains uncertain. Finally, the hyperintensity may not correspond precisely to the entire extent of the posterior lobe. Early postcontrast images in the sagittal plane show enhancement of an area in the posterior sella turcica larger than the posterior lobe hyperintensity visible on noncontrast images. This has led to the suggestion that the hyperintensity on non-contrast MRI may only be located in the posterior portion of the posterior lobe, which contains more neurosecretory granules than the anterior part of the neurohypophysis (31).

The sella turcica and the pituitary gland contained therein are completely covered by the fibrous diaphragma sellae except for a small opening, the diaphragmatic hiatus, which allows passage of the pituitary stalk. Above the diaphragma sellae lies the suprasellar cistern. In axial cross-section the cistern resembles a six-pointed star: the interhemispheric fissure is anterior, the interpeduncular cistern is posterior, the paired sylvian fissures are anterolateral, and the ambient cisterns are posterolateral (see Fig 1). The suprasellar cistern contains all the vascular anastomoses of the circle of Willis, the optic chiasm and nerves, the inferior hypothalamus, and the pituitary infundibulum with its investing venous plexus.

The pituitary stalk is a central landmark in the suprasellar cistern. It is approximately 2 mm thick, wider superiorly and tapering inferiorly. It slopes forward as it descends from the inferior hypothalamus, through the diaphragma sellae, to insert onto the superior surface of the pituitary gland at the junction of the anterior and posterior lobes (see Fig. 1). The optic chiasm is horizontally oriented and is immediately anterior to the pituitary stalk. When viewed from below, the chiasm resembles the letter "X." Anteriorly the chiasm divides into the optic nerves; these are closely applied to the inferior surface of the frontal lobes. Posteriorly the chiasm divides into the optic tracts. The paired optic tracts pass on either side of the midline stalk and paired mamillary bodies to enter the inferolateral aspect of the thalamus at the lateral geniculate bodies. The signal intensity of the optic chiasm, nerves, and tracts is similar to other compact white matter tracts on MR images (see Fig. 1).

The internal carotid artery enters the suprasellar cistern upon emerging from the cavernous sinus just medial to the anterior clinoid process. The carotid artery then gives off three medium-sized branches: ophthalmic, posterior communicating, and anterior choroidal arteries. Finally, the carotid artery terminally bifurcates into the anterior and middle cerebral arteries. The middle cerebral artery (MCA) turns immediately laterally into the sylvian fissure while the anterior cerebral artery (ACA) turns medially and traverses the suprasellar cistern along the superior surface of the optic chiasm and nerves, crosses those structures from lateral to medial, then anastomoses with its contralateral companion via the anterior communicating artery. The internal carotid artery, MCA, and ACA are obvious on MRI because of their relatively large caliber and the absence of signal from the rapidly flowing blood in the vascular lumen ("flow void") (see Fig. 1). The smaller ophthalmic, anterior choroidal, and posterior communicating arteries are also often visible, particularly with newer high resolution techniques and with MR angiography.

The paired cavernous sinuses are located immediately lateral to the sella turcica. These are venous structures that are functionally part of the dural venous system but anatomically are much more complex than any other dural sinus. They extend from the orbital fissures anteriorly to Meckel's cave posteriorly and consist of an intricate network of small endothelial-lined spaces. They may communicate with one another via a network of intercavernous connections, anterior, inferior, and posterior to the pituitary gland, through the sella turcica (the "circular sinus"). Laterally the cavernous sinuses are delimited by a well-defined dural reflection separating the sinus from the middle cranial fossa. Medially, the dural reflection is much more tenuous and it may be difficult to distinguish the exact boundary between cavernous sinus and the pituitary gland. The lateral wall of the cavernous sinus contains (from superior to inferior) cranial nerves III, IV, V1, and V2. These cranial nerves are occasionally recognizable on MRI as nodular prominences in the lateral cavernous sinus wall (32,33) (see Fig. 1). Within the sinus the internal carotid artery is easily recognized as the largest structure contained therein (see Fig. 1). Cranial nerve VI is also within the sinus, directly beneath the internal carotid artery. It is usually not visible on MRI. The appearance of the venous spaces themselves are heterogeneous. Much of the sinus is gray whereas some parts display a more typical flow void (32–34). Presumably the latter is from larger channels with higher rates of blood flow, the former from smaller channels with sluggish flow. The entire cavernous sinus, except for the internal carotid artery, enhances intensely with i.v. contrast administration.

Meckel's cave is anatomically distinct but its position is closely related to the cavernous sinus. It is a dural invagination that arises from the vertical surface of the anterior wall of the posterior cranial fossa. The orifice through which it communicates with the basal cisterns is inferior to the petroclinoid ligament. It is immediately lateral to the posterior third of the cavernous sinus and houses the trigeminal ganglion. Cranial nerve V_3 is identified passing inferolaterally from Meckel's cave through the foramen ovale directly beneath and slightly lateral to Meckel's cave (see Fig. 1).

TECHNIQUE

Suspected abnormalities of the pituitary gland and sella turcica are one of the most frequent indications for MRI. An effective imaging strategy that is cognizant of image contrast and spatial resolution requirements yet does not place an undue burden on imaging time is necessary. The objective is to obtain the most spatially detailed images, in the appropriate plane, with the best possible signal to noise ratio, and the highest image contrast, and accomplish this in the shortest period of time.

It is generally accepted that the single best imaging plane is the coronal. The coronal plane allows visualization of the pituitary gland free of partial averaging effects from the carotid arteries, sphenoid sinus, and suprasellar cistern. Coronal images are commonly supplemented by an imaging series in the sagittal plane, primarily for display of midline structures.

Exact specifications of technique are not provided because the constantly improving capabilities of modern scanners require that technique be continually revised. However, high spatial detail is important in this area and should be achieved through the use of thin slices, a fine matrix size, and a relatively small field of view. Requirements for spatial detail need to be balanced against signal to noise and imaging time. We prefer to limit individual sequences to 5 to 6 minutes, and certainly to no longer than 10 minutes.

The pulse sequence for best tissue contrast is still somewhat controversial. Spin-echo (SE) methods were the first to gain widespread popularity and continue to be the most widely used. Several groups have shown that short TR, short TE SE images (i.e., T1-weighted) generate very good contrast for visualizing pituitary pathology (16,35–38). Long TR, long TE SE (i.e., T2-weighted) images have been less successful in demonstrating pituitary lesions, in particular small adenomas (35,39). However, there are an increasing number of cases in which only the T2-weighted image has been positive (Fig. 4). Because fast spin-echo (FSE) methods are now readily available, and do not incur the time penalty of conventional T2-weighted SE sequences, we are resorting to T2-weighted FSE with increasing frequency as a supplementary sequence for pituitary adenomas.

A variety of other pulse sequences have met with varying degrees of success, including inversion recovery and gradient-echo methods. Multislice inversion recovery sequences have not been widely available and have been infrequently used. Two-dimensional (2D) FT GE images have been unsuccessful primarily because of the marked susceptibility artifacts generated from the interface between the skull base and air-containing sphenoid sinus. On the other hand, three-dimensional (3D) FT GE images have achieved greater success; these have been found to provide results comparable to T1-weighted SE methods (40,41). They have the advantage of thinner slices compared to conventional 2DFT SE methods, yielding better spatial resolution. Also, the voxels are more nearly isotropic and truly contiguous slices are possible. However, they are prone to motion and truncation artifacts in the two dimensions that are phase-encoded.

Paramagnetic contrast-enhanced images are widely used and are very useful. Although most adenomas are visible without the injection of i.v. contrast, several stud-

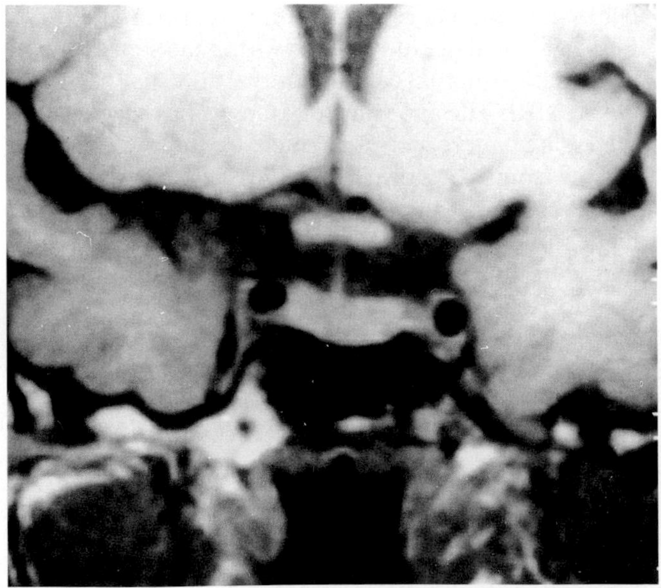

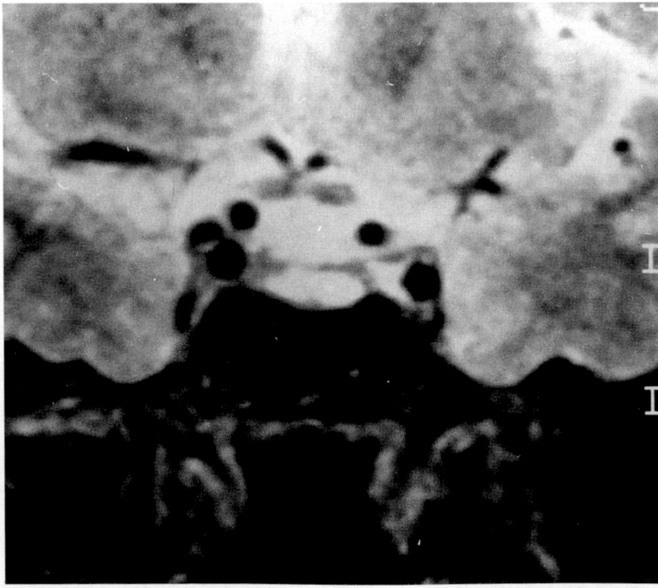

FIG. 4. Pituitary microadenoma. T1- (**A**) and T2-weighted (**B**) images. In this case only the T2-weighted image was positive. Although it is unusual to detect microadenomas on T2-weighted images that are occult on T1-weighted images, these situations do occur. The widespread availability of T2-weighted FSE images may make T2-weighted images a routine part of pituitary examinations to cover cases such as these.

ies have shown that small adenomas may become visible only after contrast injection (42–47). Many radiologists, including ourselves, have reduced the amount of contrast used for the investigation of pituitary adenomas to half the usual dose (to 0.05 mmol/Kg). It has been demonstrated that half-dose studies have comparable results to full-dose studies in terms of pituitary gland opacification and microadenoma detection (48,49).

Because of the differential rates of contrast enhancement between adenomas and normal pituitary gland, the degree of image contrast can be accentuated by scanning immediately after administration of the contrast agent.

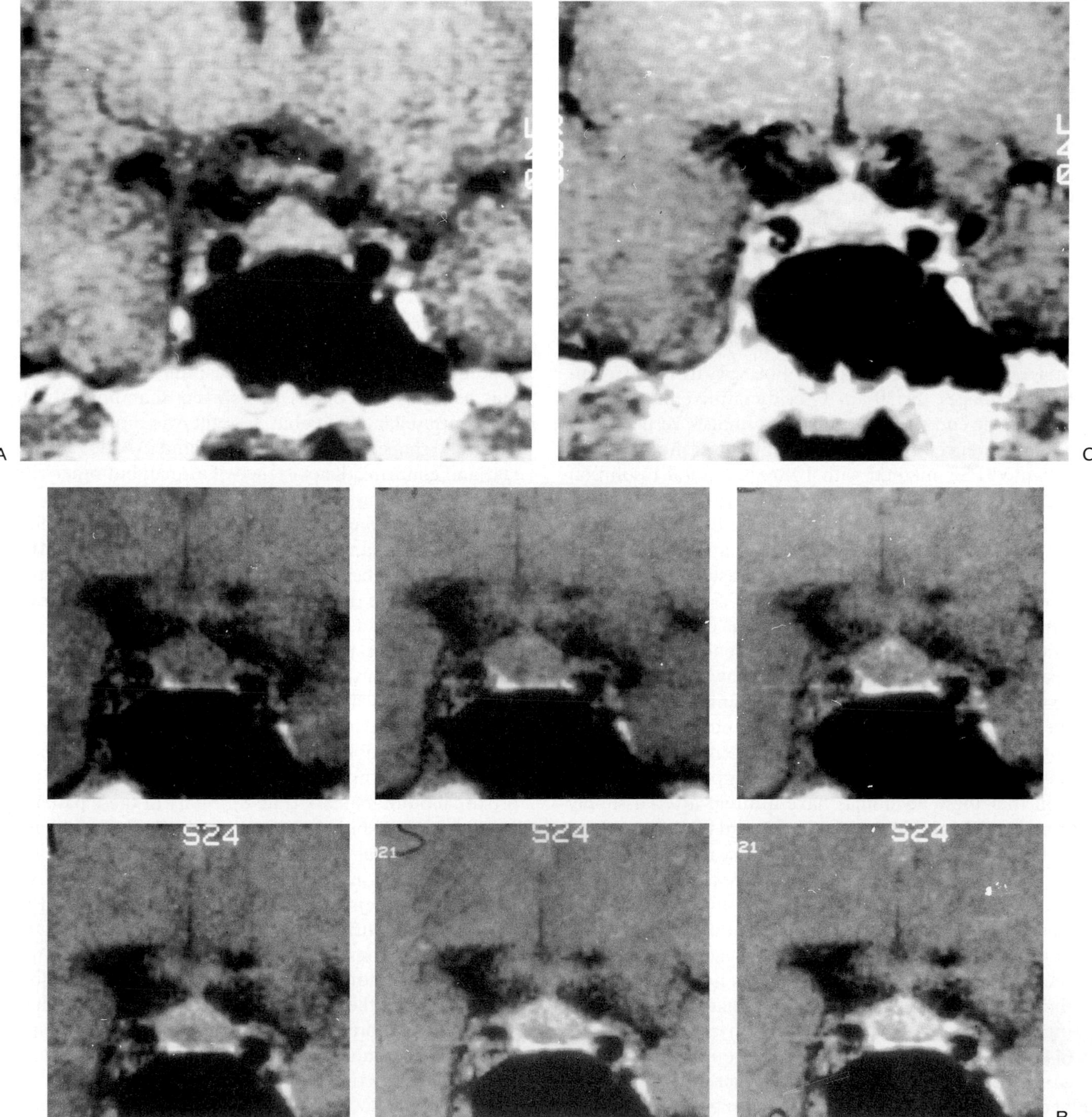

FIG. 5. ACTH microadenoma. **A:** Unenhanced, (**B**) dynamic-enhanced set, and (**C**) conventional enhanced images. Both the unenhanced and conventional contrast-enhanced sequences were negative, whereas the dynamic images obtained 30 to 50 sec after contrast injection clearly show a 4-mm right paracentral microadenoma. By the time of the last image, the adenoma is becoming less conspicuous as it slowly becomes more hyperintense.

Immediately after contrast injection most adenomas will appear as relatively nonenhancing (dark) lesions within an intensely enhancing pituitary gland. However, soon afterward this image contrast begins to dissipate and the adenoma may no longer be detectable. The development of faster and faster imaging sequences has popularized "dynamic imaging" of the pituitary gland. Dynamic imaging sequences may have temporal resolution as fast as 1 to 2 sec per set of images, although protocols range from images every second to images every minute (12,50–53). Our own experience with dynamic scanning has shown that the contrast enhancement behavior of microadenomas is not constant from case to case. Some microadenomas display the most lesion-to-gland contrast on unenhanced scans. With these, the image contrast begins to diminish the moment the contrast-enhancing agent arrives in the pituitary gland. In about 20% of cases the maximum image contrast between normal pituitary tissue and microadenomas is attained about 30 to 50 sec after the bolus injection of i.v. contrast, whereas others have the best image contrast 1 to 2 min after contrast agent injection (52). Thus, the best images for microadenoma detection vary from the unenhanced images, the 30- to 50-sec dynamic-enhanced images, to the conventional enhanced images, respectively. Our preference for dynamic scanning is a modified T1-weighted FSE method with 10-sec temporal resolution (52). We have found an incremental yield in microadenoma detection of about 10% above and beyond that detected on a combination of plain and conventional contrast-enhanced MRI (Fig. 5). Faster dynamic sequences with temporal resolution of 5 to 10 sec have demonstrated an early component of enhancement in microadenomas not visible on sequences with slower resolution. These fast images have shown that some microadenomas have subtle enhancement early, at about the same time as the posterior lobe, and long before the anterior lobe. This confirms earlier computed tomography (CT) work of Bonneville and supports the conclusion that these adenomas have a direct arterial supply from branches of the carotid artery, and therefore, would not be subject to the normal regulatory influences of the hypothalamus via the portal venous system (53).

Delayed scans (i.e., longer than 30 minutes after contrast injection) occasionally may demonstrate a reversal of this image contrast. As the contrast agent diffuses into the adenoma, the adenoma becomes hyperintense and the intensity of the normal pituitary gland fades, allowing the adenoma to stand out as a hyperintense focus (44). Unfortunately, delayed scans are not practical because they require that the patient either wait in the scanner or return for re-examination 30 to 60 minutes later. Thus, they are infrequently used.

Our current practice is to perform unenhanced T1-weighted SE sagittal and coronal sequences. If these are positive for an intrapituitary lesion the examination stops. If negative or equivocal, a bolus of i.v. contrast is given synchronously with the beginning of a dynamic T1-weighted FSE sequence. At the completion of the dynamic study we immediately proceed to a conventional T1-weighted SE sequence. If these are negative, equivocal, or discordant with one another, or if there is evidence of a suprasellar or hypothalamic lesion, T2-weighted images are obtained; otherwise, the examination ends.

CONGENITAL ABNORMALITIES

Pituitary Gland Hypoplasia

Congenital abnormalities of the pituitary gland and hypothalamus are often associated with anomalies of other midline cranial, orbital, and facial structures such as the optic nerves, septum pellucidum, osseous skull base, and palate (54). In many cases there is a small, shallow sella turcica (Fig. 6). Pituitary and hypothalamic dysfunction is most often recognized clinically by growth failure, which occurs with variable frequencies in these conditions (55). The hypoplastic pituitary gland itself may be recognized on CT as a smaller than normal soft tissue intrasellar density but it is otherwise normal in position and shape. MRI displays the gland to better advantage and confirms the existence of a small but otherwise normal-appearing gland and pituitary stalk (Fig. 7).

A group of congenital pituitary deficiency disorders has become apparent with the widespread use of MRI (56,57). A number of patients with short stature and growth hormone deficiency (GHD) have highly characteristic features on MRI. Many of these patients have additional anterior pituitary hormone deficiencies. The MR findings consist of one or more of the following: small sella turcica, small anterior pituitary gland, absence of the usual high signal intensity from the posterior pituitary gland, absence or hypoplasia of the distal pituitary stalk, and an anomalous high signal area in the proximal pituitary stalk (Fig. 8). Many of these patients have a history of breech presentation at birth, some have other intracranial midline anomalies, and some have both midline anomalies and history of breech presentation. Those patients with all the above findings tend to have multiple pituitary hormone deficiencies (MPHD).

Two theories have emerged to explain the MR findings and the associations with breech deliveries and midline anomalies. One theory presumes that the head "trauma" associated with breech delivery causes rupture of the pituitary infundibulum with its investing vascular plexus as the stalk is stretched between the pituitary gland (which is fixed to the skull base) and the more mobile brain. This theory does not adequately explain the associated midline anomalies because these develop long before birth. The alternate theory invokes early fetal maldevelopment of midline structures including the fetal

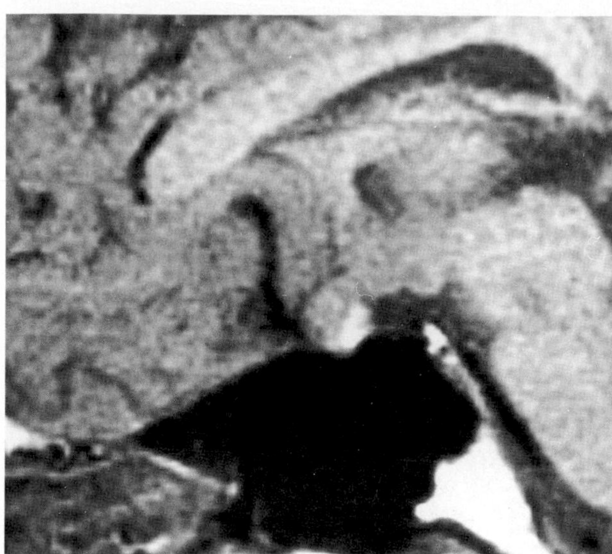

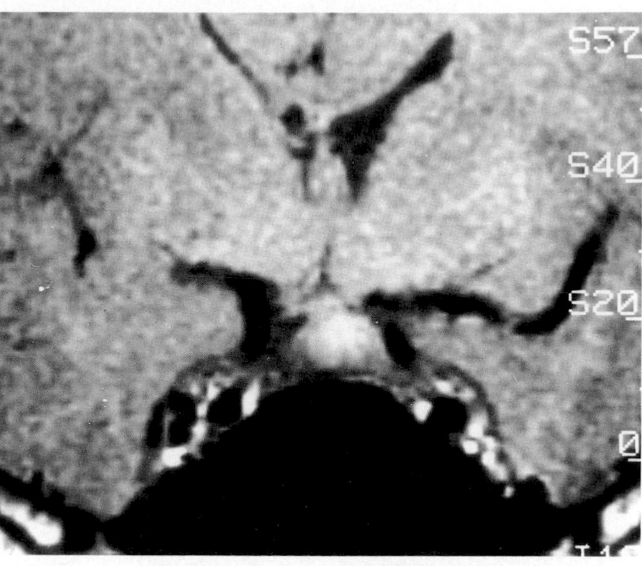

FIG. 6. Undeveloped sella turcica. **A:** Sagittal T1-weighted and (**B**) coronal T1-weighted image. A suprasellar enhancing mass was incidentally "discovered" on a CT scan of this teenaged boy (CT not shown). A presumptive diagnosis of craniopharyngioma was made and the boy was referred to MRI before biopsy. The MRI shows that the sella turcica is extremely shallow. The pituitary gland is situated in the suprasellar cistern but otherwise appears normal in morphology and is easily recognized on the sagittal images because of the characteristic high signal intensity in the posterior lobe. A diagnosis of a "normal suprasellar pituitary gland" was made and the biopsy was canceled.

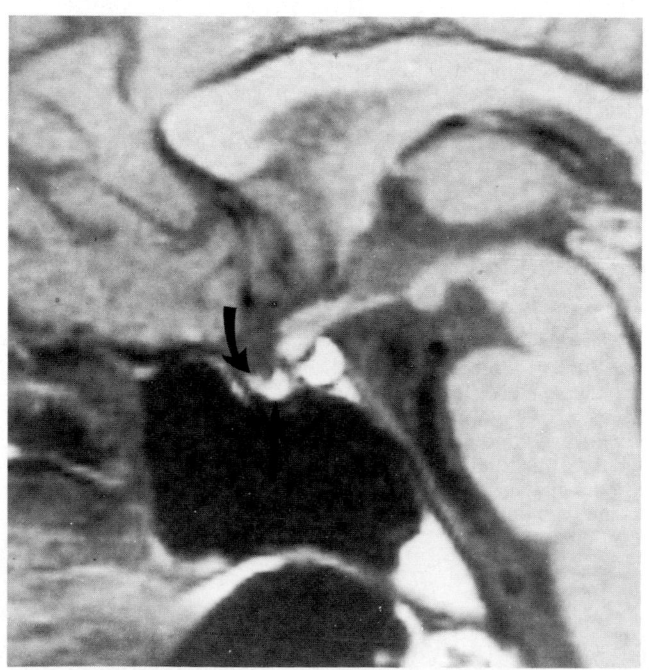

FIG. 7. Pituitary hypoplasia. Midline sagittal T1-weighted image. This young adult had a history of hypopituitarism dating from infancy. The sella turcica is shallow and reduced in anteroposterior diameter. The high signal intensity of the posterior lobe is easily identified in the posterior half of the sella turcica (*arrow*). The anterior lobe is a vestige of its normal size and it is visible as a tiny remnant of tissue in the anteroinferior portion of the sella turcica (*curved arrow*). The semilunar high intensity structure dorsal to the pituitary gland is the dorsum sella. The small sella turcica distinguishes pituitary hypoplasia from an "empty sella" wherein the sella is normal or large in size.

hypothalamic-pituitary axis with failure of the neurohypophysis and its investing vascular plexus to descend completely into the sella turcica and come into contact with the adenohypophysis (58–60). Anterior lobe dysfunction results because the anterior lobe is deprived of part of its blood supply (via the portal veins) and also is deprived of hypothalamic stimulating hormones (also normally transmitted via the portal veins). Proponents of this latter theory suggest that fetal position and the normal progress of labor require a normally functioning fetal pituitary gland. If the fetal gland is dysfunctional, breech presentation and delivery may result. Thus, this theory can explain the associations with both breech presentations and midline anomalies.

Regardless of which etiology is correct, the resultant functional and morphologic derangement can be understood on the basis of the failure of hypothalamic axons and surrounding venous plexus to connect in the normal fashion with the adenohypophysis. With failure of this connection to develop, the anterior lobe is deprived of hypothalamic stimulating factors and some of its blood supply. The deficiency of anterior lobe hormones is thus not surprising. On the other hand, posterior lobe function is preserved in this condition. The most plausible explanation is that the neurosecretory vesicles normally transported to the posterior lobe from their synthetic site in the hypothalamus are simply dammed up above the level of the stalk discontinuity, usually in the proximal portion of the stalk. This "ec-

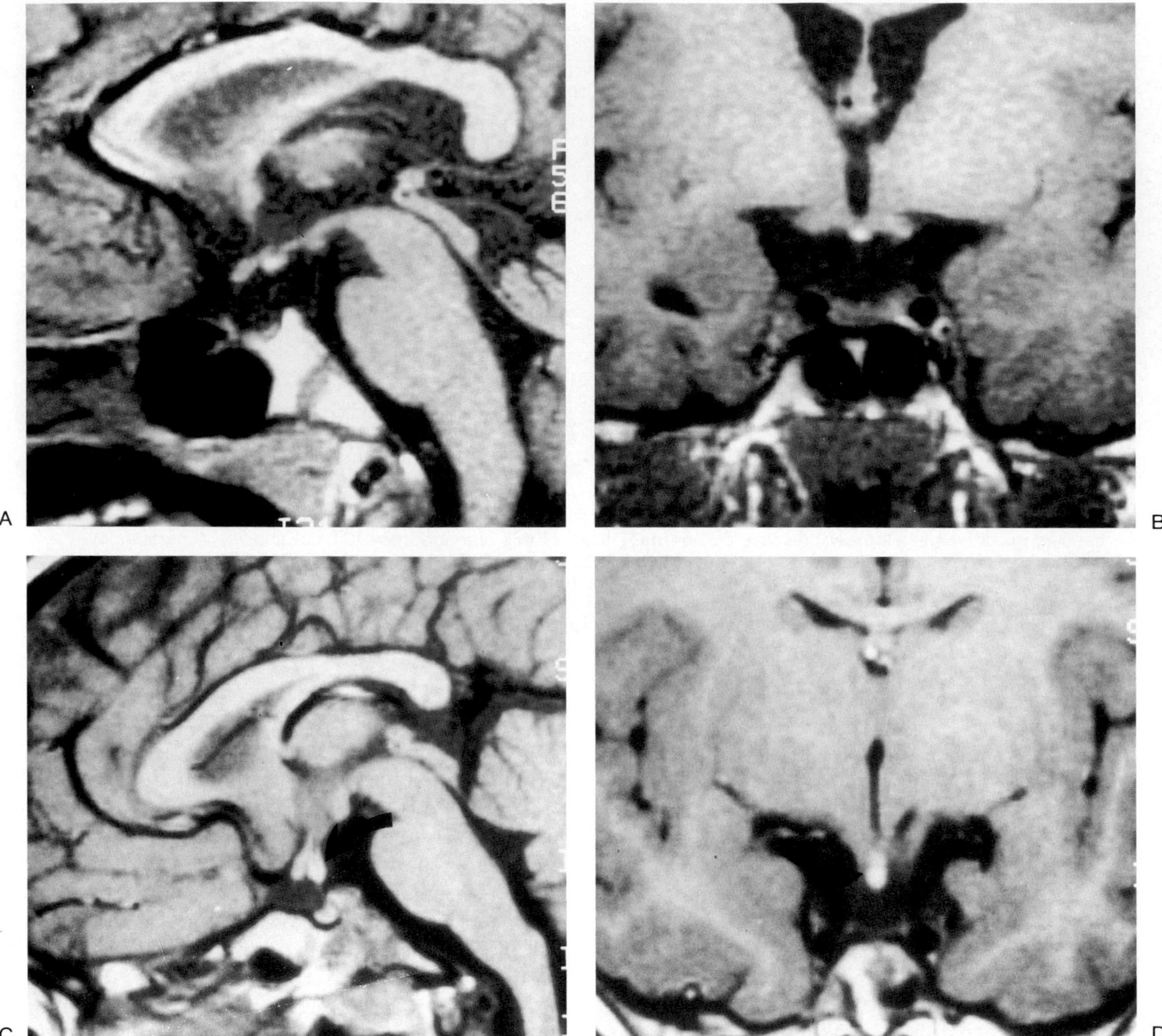

FIG. 8. Growth hormone–deficient dwarfism (two cases). **A:** Sagittal T1-weighted image. The sella turcica is extremely small and contains virtually no pituitary tissue. The entire pituitary stalk is absent. There is a focal area of high intensity at the proximal infundibulum demarcating the ectopic location of the posterior pituitary lobe. This combination of findings is specific for this diagnostic entity. **B:** Coronal T1-weighted image. The high intensity nodule is visualized at the level of the infundibular recess directly between the optic tracts. The distal stalk is absent and the sella turcica is poorly formed. **C,D:** This is a second example of the same disorder. In this case the sella turcica and pituitary gland are larger than in the first case but the imaging findings are otherwise the same.

topic" location functions as the posterior lobe and is represented on MRI as the high signal area. This "regeneration" of an ectopic posterior lobe is known to occur in animal experiments after distal stalk transection, and a similar high signal nodule often becomes apparent after pituitary surgery (61). If an anatomically normal posterior lobe develops at all (i.e., within the sella turcica), it is depleted of neurosecretory vesicles and does not have its normal high signal. Diagnostically these findings are specific for this disorder. The high signal intensity in the suprasellar cistern should not be misinterpreted as a craniopharyngioma or other suprasellar or hypothalamic mass. The only pathologic confirmation of the nature of the tissue in the bright nodule is described in a report by Kaufman et al. (62). In this case a patient with anterior pituitary deficiencies was discovered to have a retrochiasmatic mass and no tissue in the sella. Biopsy of the mass revealed normal pituitary stalk tissue. The authors recommend that the term "posterior pituitary ectopia" not be used to describe the suprasellar tissue as the tissue more closely resembles the pituitary stalk than the posterior lobe.

A classification scheme has been proposed that divides GHD patients into three groups based on morphology as defined on MRI (59). The first group in this scheme has the most severe morphologic derangement, consisting of posterior lobe "ectopia", aplasia of the stalk, and hypoplasia of the anterior lobe. These patients are most likely to have or develop MPHD. It is proposed that the underlying cause is developmental, probably early in fetal life. The second group demonstrates only anterior lobe hypoplasia. The cause may be a perinatal event or birth trauma, or a less severe developmental defect. The third group has normal morphology on MRI and the mildest clinical and biochemical deficit; derangement of neuroendocrine mechanisms controlling GH secretion is the proposed mechanism. MRI may also have a role in determining the prognosis of patients with GHD by establishing which patients are at risk for developing MPHD versus those who are likely to have only isolated GHD (60).

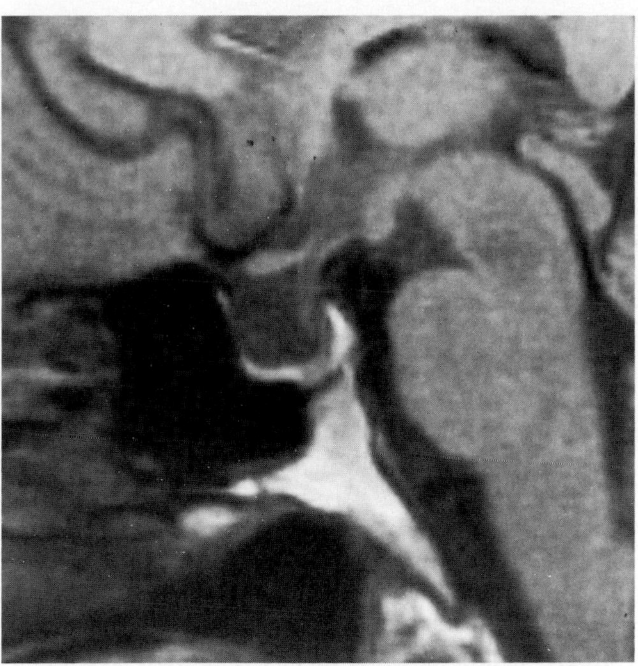

FIG. 10. Empty sella turcica. Sagittal T1-weighted image. The sella turcica is enlarged and filled with CSF from the suprasellar cistern. The pituitary gland is flattened into a thin rim of tissue along the floor of the sella turcica. Of importance is that the pituitary stalk can be visualized in its entire course from the hypothalamus to the pituitary gland, thereby excluding the presence of an intrasellar cyst.

The "Empty Sella Turcica"

The empty sella turcica refers to an anatomic finding of a severely flattened pituitary gland (Fig. 9). The term "empty sella" arises because the superior portion of the sella turcica appears empty [it is actually filled with cerebrospinal fluid (CSF)]. The diaphragma sella is thin and the diaphragmatic hiatus enlarged. In many cases the volume of the sella turcica is expanded. It is the deficiency of the diaphragma that is the primary defect. This allows the suprasellar cistern to herniate into the sella, exposing it to CSF pulsation and eventually resulting in enlargement of the sella turcica.

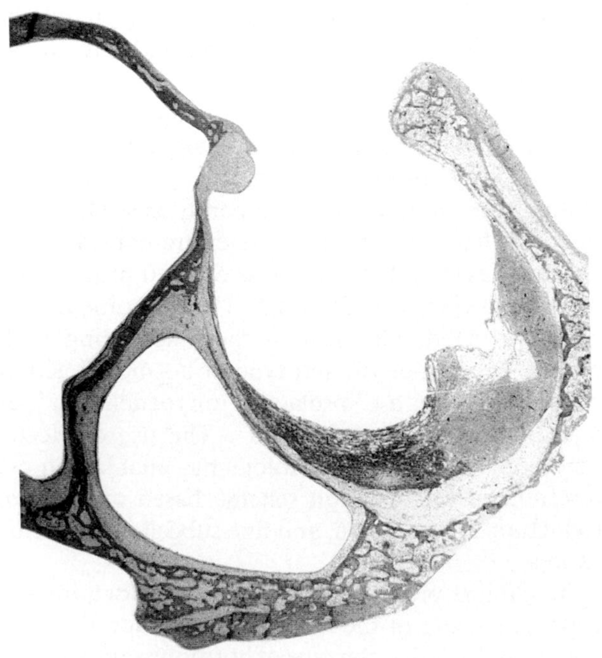

FIG. 9. "Empty sella turcica." This is a midline sagittal section through the sella turcica. The pituitary gland is compressed into a semilunar-shaped layer of tissue along the floor of the sella turcica.

Patients with an empty sella may have symptoms referable to the area of the sella turcica such as endocrine dysfunction (63), CSF rhinorrhea (64,65), or visual field loss (66). However, these clinical findings are all rare compared to nonspecific complaints such as headache, memory loss, and dizziness. Most frequently the empty sella is an incidental finding of little or no clinical significance.

The finding of an empty sella turcica is particularly common on MRI, in no small part because of the frequent use of T1-weighted sagittal images and the ease of visualization of the pituitary gland, stalk, and sella turcica. The pituitary gland is variably flattened; frequently it is only a thin rim of tissue along the sella floor (Fig. 10). The only differential diagnosis is that of a cyst occupying the superior portion of the sella turcica. To that end, it is important to determine the position of the pituitary stalk. In the empty sella the stalk is normal in position, whereas space-occupying cysts cause it to be obliterated or displaced.

Cephaloceles

Cephaloceles are herniations of the meninges ("meningocele") or of the meninges and brain ("meningoencephalocele" or simply "encephalocele") through a developmental defect in the cranium. Cephaloceles in the sellar region, or "transsphenoidal encephaloceles," are very rare; their estimated incidence is 1 per 700,000 live births (67). Most of these are associated with other midline anomalies, particularly agenesis of the corpus callosum. Children with transsphenoidal encephaloceles present with craniofacial deformities, CSF rhinorrhea, or meningitis; patients reaching adulthood experience hypothalamic—pituitary dysfunction or chiasmatic syndromes because of herniation of the pituitary gland, and/or optic chiasm into the hernial sac (67–70).

MRI clearly demonstrates the aberrant anatomy, much more so than is possible on CT, particularly because of the ability to distinguish solid and fluid components within the hernial sac, and identify the specific structures within the sac (Fig. 11). With MRI it is important to assess accurately the position of the optic chiasm, pituitary gland, and aberrant vessels in patients that develop CSF leaks or progressive visual loss—these patients require surgical repair of their skull base defects and it is extremely helpful to have knowledge of the position of these vital structures preoperatively. T1-weighted sagittal and coronal images generally suffice for diagnosis.

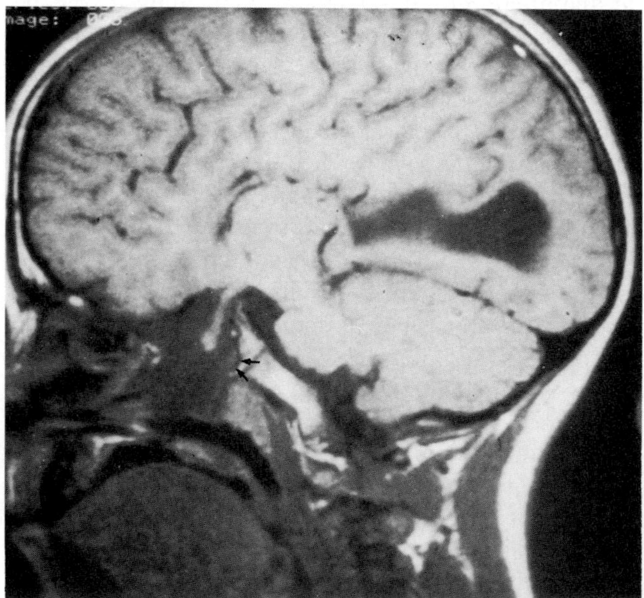

FIG. 11. Transsphenoidal encephalocele. Sagittal T1-weighted image. There is herniation of intrasellar and suprasellar tissue into the nasopharynx through a bony defect in the skull base. The anterior wall of the sella turcica is completely deformed by the encephalocele and only a remnant of pituitary tissue can be identified (*small arrows*). There is also agenesis of the corpus callosum. These midline anomalies are frequently associated with one another.

TUMORS

Pituitary Adenoma

Pituitary adenomas are slow-growing, benign neoplasms of epithelial origin that arise from the adenohypophysis. They are the most common tumors of the sella turcica. In clinical series they represent 10% to 15% of all intracranial neoplasms (71). Their estimated incidence in nonselected autopsy series has varied between 2.7% and 27% (72). In a recent report of 1,000 nonselected autopsy specimens, incidental pituitary adenomas were found in 3.1% of glands (73). Pituitary adenomas are predominantly tumors of adulthood; in distinction from Rathke cleft cysts, incidental adenomas were found exclusively in subjects older than 40 years of age in Teramoto's autopsy study (73). Virtually all pituitary tumors are benign adenomas but on rare occasions adenohypophyseal cells give rise to carcinoma. The histologic criteria of malignancy are not well established, and the morphologic diagnosis is often difficult. Cellular pleomorphism and mitotic figures indicate a rapid growth rate but can be apparent also in benign tumors. Invasion of adjacent tissue is not regarded as unequivocal proof of malignancy. Conventionally, the diagnosis of carcinoma is used only when distant metastases occur (71).

Pituitary adenomas are usually well demarcated lesions that are separated from the normal pituitary gland by a pseudocapsule of compressed tissue containing condensed reticulin; there is no true fibrous capsule (Fig. 12). In some instances the margins of the adenoma are poorly defined, the pseudocapsule is not well formed, and nests of adenoma cells extend the into "normal" gland adjacent to the lesion (71). Of incidentally discovered pituitary adenomas larger than 2 mm at autopsy, 85% were situated in the lateral wings of the gland (Fig. 13) (73). Furthermore, of all laterally situated masses in that study, 74% were pituitary adenomas.

Pituitary adenomas are conveniently classified by size; those less than 10 mm in diameter are considered *micro*adenomas (Fig. 12), and those over 10 mm are *macro*adenomas (Fig. 14). Clinically it has become the convention to subdivide each of these according to the presence or absence of, and type of hormonal activity, with terms such as "prolactin microadenoma" and "nonfunctional macroadenoma". The use of electron microscopy and immunocytology has enabled an even more refined classification scheme based on hormone production, cell of origin, and fine subcellular structural features.

The clinical presentation of pituitary adenomas depends on the size of the lesion, the presence or absence of hormonal activity, the type of hormone produced, and the degree of extrasellar extension. Approximately 25% of patients with pituitary adenomas have "nonfunctioning tumors"; the remaining 75% display clinical signs or

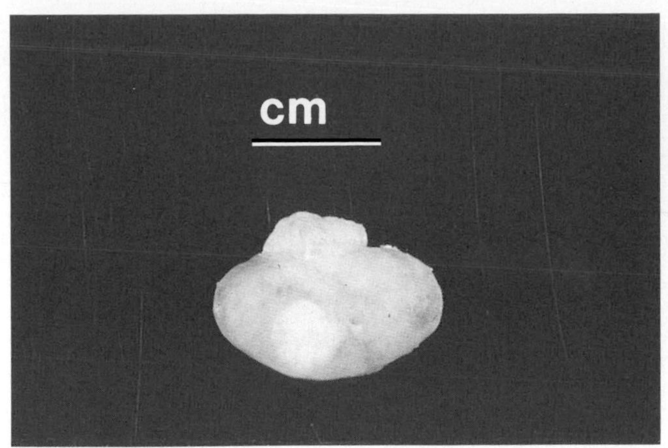

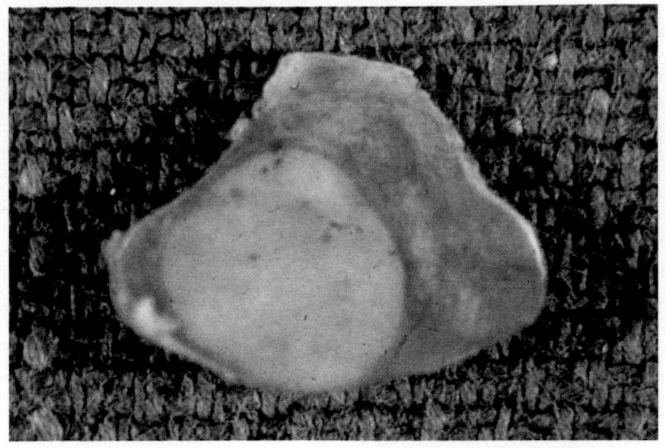

FIG. 12. Pituitary microadenomas. **A:** This 3-mm to 4-mm microadenoma is located just to the right of the midline. Its coloration is different from normal anterior lobe tissue, thereby clearly demarcating it from the normal anterior lobe. However, the external contours of the gland are not deformed in any way; therefore, the detection of this size of adenoma usually requires an imaging method that provides good image contrast between normal and abnormal tissue. (Courtesy of Dr. Sylvia Asa, Mount Sinai Hospital, Toronto.) **B:** This is a larger adenoma, approximately 9 mm in diameter, and occupying about 60% of the volume of the pituitary gland. Although the lesion does not have a true capsule around it, compression of pituitary tissue by the tumor creates an apparent pseudocapsule. Lesions this size almost always distort the external contours of the gland, as is apparent in this case.

symptoms of hormone excess (71). In general, hormonally active adenomas usually present earlier in the course of their evolution with signs and symptoms of endocrine hyperfunction. The most common of these is the prolactinoma, a tumor that originates from prolactin-secreting cells (lactotrophs) of the adenohypophysis and accounts for approximately 50% of hormonally active adenomas. Prolactin hypersecretion may result in amenorrhea, galactorrhea, infertility, loss of libido, or impotence. In men and postmenopausal women, the effects of elevated prolactin levels are less conspicuous. The tumors often present only when they are large and cause dysfunction of the normal pituitary gland or optic tract through compression.

Elevated prolactin levels are not always due to increased production by a hormonally active adenoma.

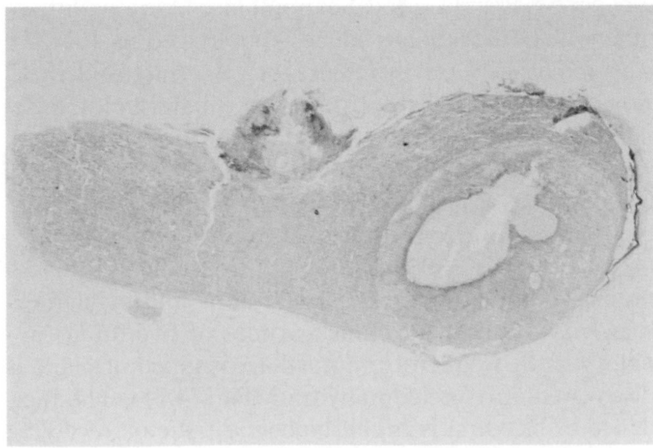

FIG. 13. Incidental pituitary microadenoma with cystic degeneration is seen within lateral wing of gland. (From Teramoto, et al., ref. 73, with permission.)

Any process that interferes with the production, release, or pituitary portal venous transport of prolactin-inhibiting factors from the hypothalamus will result in hyperprolactinemia because of disinhibition of normal prolactin cells. This is most commonly due to suprasellar tumors that compress the hypothalamus or pituitary stalk ("stalk section effect"), certain drugs (particularly phenothiazines), and primary hypothyroidism. Nevertheless, the degree of hyperprolactinemia caused by these latter processes is at most moderate; serum prolactin levels above 150 ng/ml are almost always due to an underlying autonomously secreting adenoma (normal serum prolactin <20 ng/ml). However, the converse is not true because many patients with prolactinomas have serum prolactin levels between 20 and 150 ng/ml.

The next most prevalent hormonally active adenomas are those that produce growth hormone and ACTH. They are of approximately equal incidence (71). Tumors arising from growth hormone–secreting cells (somatotrophs) cause acromegaly in the adult and gigantism in children; those arising from ACTH-producing cells (corticotrophs) produce Cushing's disease, the most serious of the endocrinopathies. Cushing's disease is more common in women (75%) and the high morbidity is usually due to the complications of prolonged hypercortisolism. Nelson's syndrome is also caused by ACTH hypersecretion; it results from continued growth of an ACTH-producing pituitary adenoma in an adrenalectomized patient. Continued secretion of ACTH results in stimulation of cutaneous melanocytes with resultant hyperpigmentation. Adenomas causing Nelson's syndrome are often large and extend outside the sella when discovered (Fig. 15). Rarely adenomas arise from thyrotrophs (TSH-secreting) or gonadotrophs (FSH and/or LH-

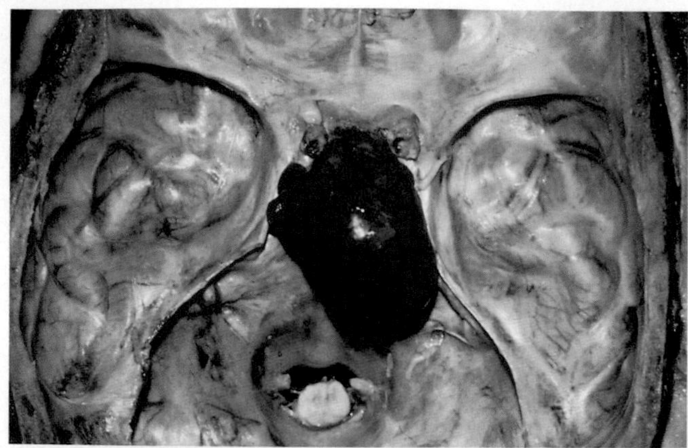

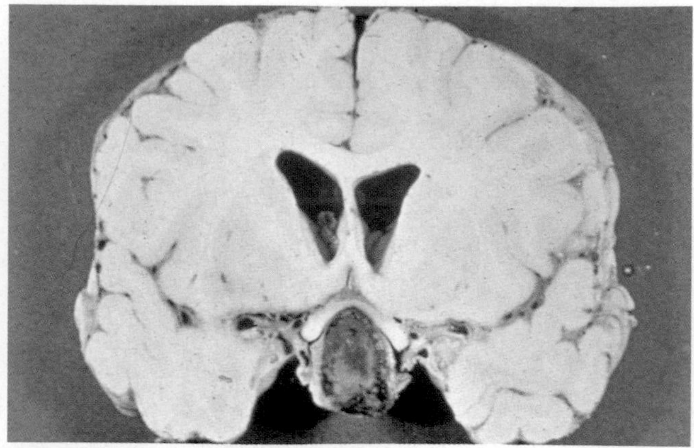

A B

FIG. 14. Pituitary macroadenomas. **A:** This is a view of the intracranial surface of the skull base with the brain removed. A large adenoma is spilling out of the sella turcica with compression of adjacent structures. **B:** Coronal section (different case). This large adenoma is compressing the optic chiasm.

secreting). In addition, approximately 10% are plurihormonal adenomas that secrete more than one type of pituitary hormone (71,72). The prolactin-growth hormone adenoma is the most common of the plurihormonal adenomas.

In contrast to the signs and symptoms of specific hormone excess in the case of hormonally active tumors, nonfunctional pituitary adenomas present because of compression or invasion of structures adjacent to the adenoma. These adenomas are usually large and have grown superiorly into the suprasellar cistern, laterally into the cavernous sinus, or inferiorly into the sphenoid sinus by the time of clinical presentation. Compression of the optic nerve, chiasm, or optic tract produces visual disturbances. Further growth superiorly compresses or distorts the third ventricle. Obstruction at the foramen of Munro results in hydrocephalus. Lateral extension with invasion or compression of the cavernous sinus can result in cranial nerve palsies with diplopia, and facial sensory disturbances, but this is infrequent. Compression of normal pituitary tissue causes anterior pituitary gland failure. Interference with neurohypophyseal function can cause diabetes insipidus, but this is a very rare and late finding in pituitary adenomas (H. S. Smyth, *personal communication*). Rarely, a pituitary adenoma may present acutely with pituitary apoplexy because of intratumoral hemorrhage (see the section entitled, "Pituitary Apoplexy").

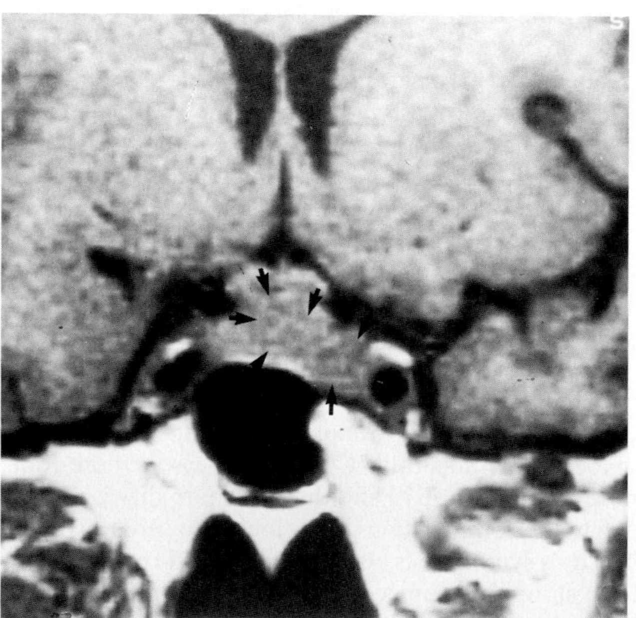

FIG. 15. Nelson's syndrome. Coronal T1-weighted image. This patient had both adrenal glands resected several years before this scan for uncontrolled hypercorticalism. Several months after surgery increasing skin pigmentation was documented. This image demonstrates the presence of a left-sided adenoma extending superiorly into the suprasellar cistern, laterally toward the cavernous sinus and inferiorly remodeling the floor of the sella turcica (*arrows*).

The MR image of the pituitary adenoma is characterized by evidence of lengthening of both T1 and T2 relaxation when compared to normal pituitary tissue. In 80% to 95% of cases, T1-weighted images of pituitary microadenomas show a focal hypointense lesion within an otherwise homogeneous adenohypophysis (Fig. 16) (35). The remainder are isointense or hyperintense. Small isointense adenomas constitute the majority of false-negative MRI examinations. Many of these can be detected on contrast-enhanced MR studies. Hyperintensity in adenomas is accounted for by the presence of old blood in the tumor (Fig. 17). Intratumoral hemorrhage occurs in 20% to 30% of adenomas, usually macroadenomas. Although pituitary infarction and/or hemorrhage may result in the clinical syndrome of pituitary apoplexy, more frequently hemorrhage is subclinical and is discovered only incidentally on MRI (74,75). The incidence of bleeding is much higher in patients receiving bromocriptine. Yousem et al. reported a 45% incidence of hemorrhage in patients treated with bromocriptine, compared to 13% in those who did not receive the drug

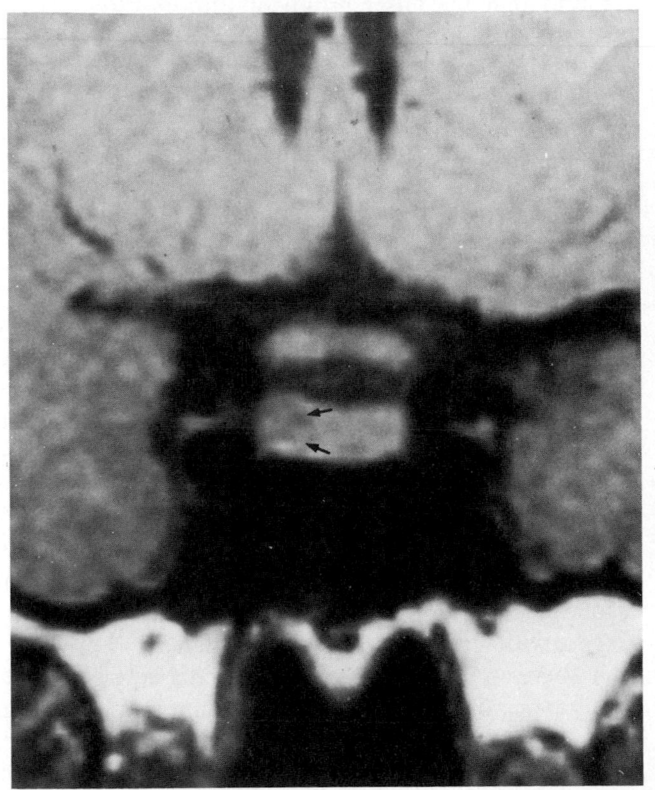

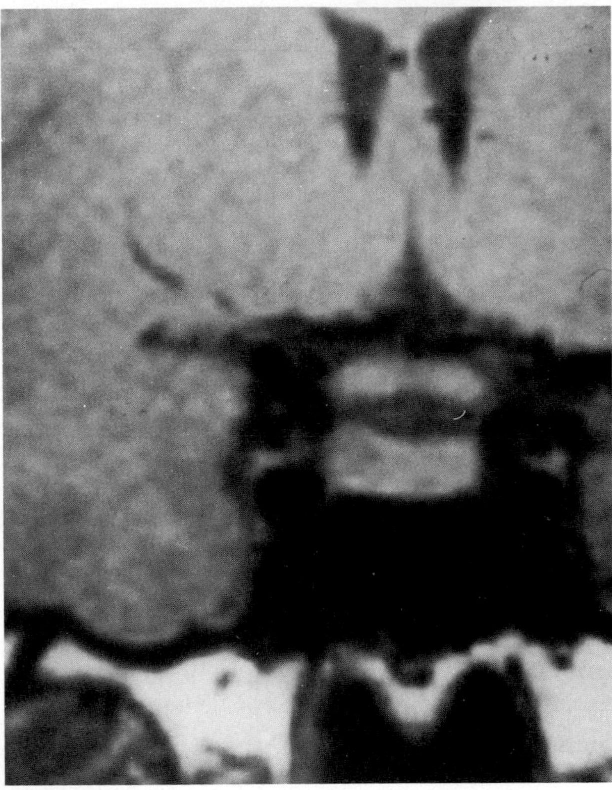

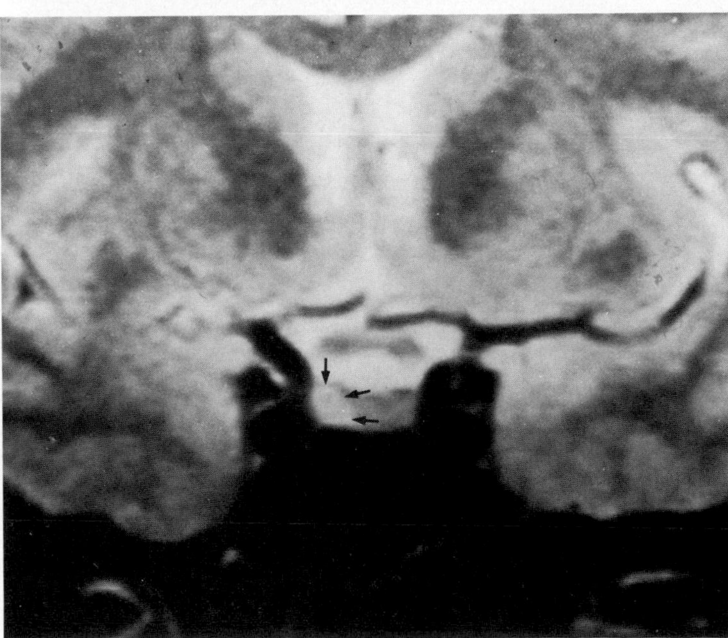

FIG. 16. Pituitary microadenoma. **A,B:** Coronal T1-weighted images. There is a distinct 4-mm hypointense lesion in the right side of the pituitary gland (*small arrows*). There is no distortion of the gland contour. This is the typical appearance of a pituitary microadenoma. Most adenomas are not high contrast lesions and relatively narrow windows must be used to demonstrate the margins of the adenoma. **C:** Coronal T2-weighted image. The same adenoma is again clearly visible but with the T2-weighted technique the image contrast is reversed, the adenoma now being hyperintense compared to the normal pituitary gland (*small arrows*). In most cases, the T1-weighted image is more reliable than the T2-weighted image.

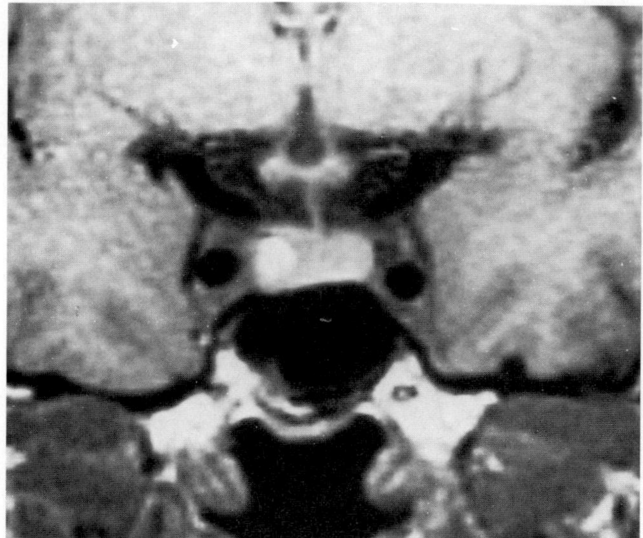

FIG. 17. Cystic microadenoma with hemorrhage. Coronal T1-weighted image. This patient presented with the syndrome of amenorrhea—galactorrhea accompanied by hyperprolactinemia. There was no clinical episode suggestive of a hemorrhagic event. The MRI clearly demonstrates a hyperintense focus about 4 mm in diameter on the right side of the gland. At surgery an adenoma was discovered in this location that was predominantly cystic and filled with dark brown fluid.

(76). About one-third to one half of microadenomas are hyperintense with T2 weighting; most of the remainder are isointense (Fig. 16) (35). Macroadenomas are more often hyperintense on T2-weighted images than are microadenomas. Hyperintensity on the T2-weighted images may be useful in predicting that a macroadenoma is soft or partially necrotic, and thus easily removed by suction and curettage. Snow et al. found 32 of 35 "soft" macroadenomas to be hyperintense, whereas 7 of 7 "firm" macroadenomas were isointense (77). They found that the latter group of tumors often required sharp dissection, the use of laser, and in five of seven cases the tumor could not be removed in a single transsphenoidal procedure. Our own experience with assessing tumor consistency by signal intensity has not yielded such a strong correlation with T2-weighted images, but we have found that tumors that are hyperintense on T1-weighted images are always cystic, with the cyst containing old blood.

The T1-weighted sequence is the more reliable for microadenoma detection than the T2-weighted sequence. On both T1- and T2-weighted images the differential signal intensity between normal and abnormal tissue is often subtle. It is therefore important to scrutinize the gland at narrow display windows so as to not overlook the abnormality (Fig. 18). As a general rule, the contrast between adenoma and normal tissue is equal to that between gray and white matter; on T1-weighted images the adenomatous tissue is isointense to adjacent temporal lobe gray matter whereas normal pituitary tissue is isointense with temporal lobe white matter.

There are no imaging features to distinguish the various types of adenomas from one another except that ACTH-secreting microadenomas are on average the smallest of all adenomas (mean size = 3 mm) (Fig. 19)

A

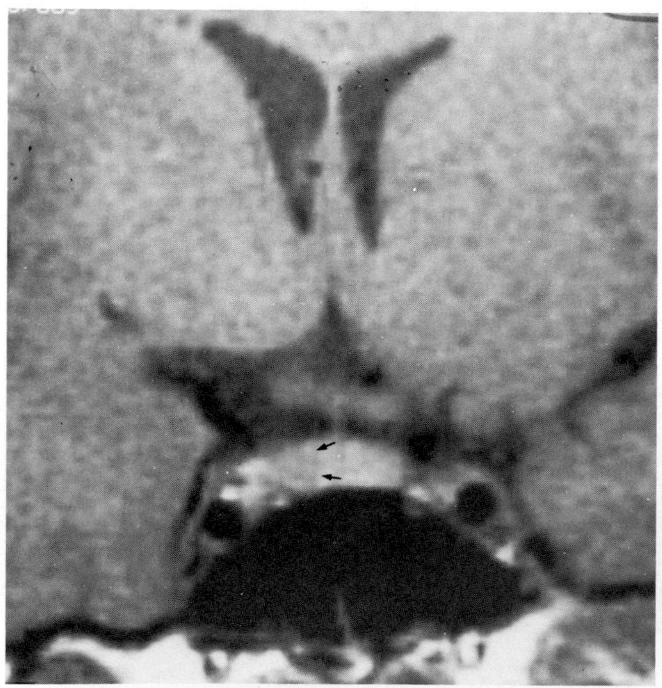

B

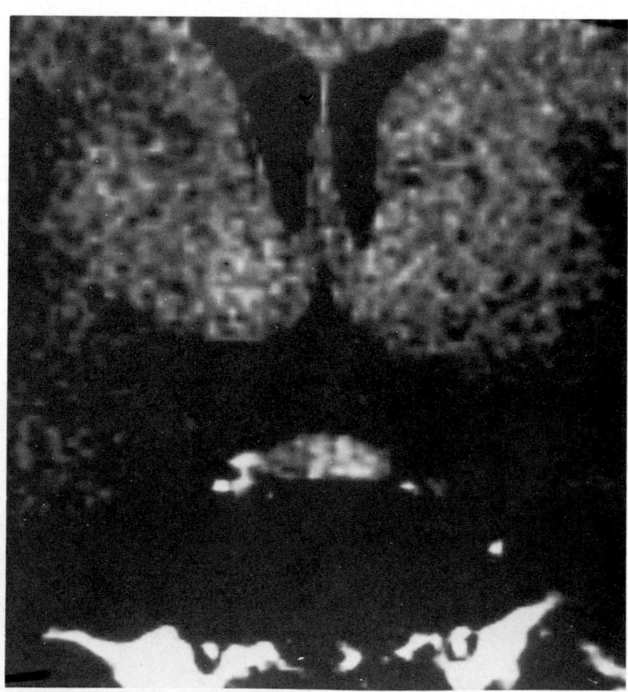

FIG. 18. Prolactin microadenoma. Photography at regular and narrow windows. **A:** Coronal T1-weighted image. The right-sided adenoma is barely visible when photographed at regular window widths (*small arrows*). **B:** Extremely narrow window displays are at times required to demonstrate adenoma convincingly. Although this image is extremely noisy, the adenoma is distinctly visible on the right side of the gland.

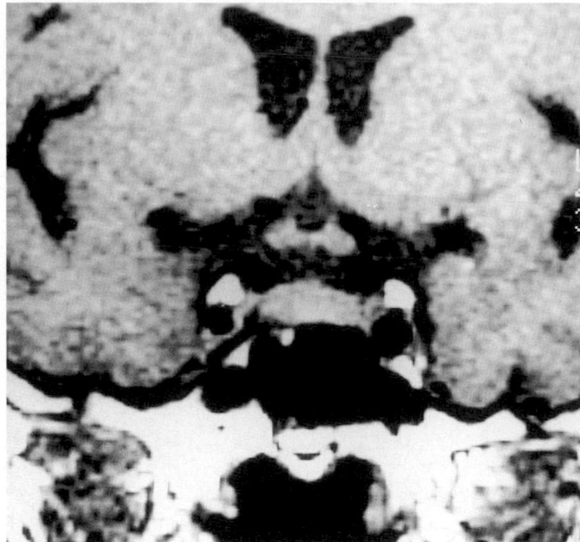

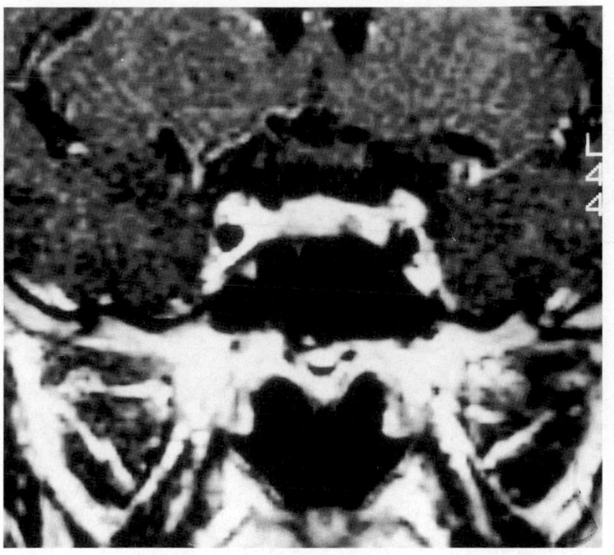

A B

FIG. 19. Cushing's disease. **A:** Coronal T1-weighted image, noncontrast study. The pituitary gland appears normal. **B:** Coronal T1-weighted image following i.v. contrast enhancement (*narrow windows*). This image was obtained immediately following the i.v. injection of 0.1 mmol/Kg of gadolinium-DTPA. A distinct 4-mm hypointense abnormality is seen on the left side of the gland (*small arrows*). Surgically this was proven to be an ACTH-secreting microadenoma.

and all hormonally active adenomas have a certain topographic bias within the gland that parallels the distribution of the normal secretory cells. Therefore, prolactin and growth hormone microadenomas have a predilection to a lateral position within the gland, whereas ACTH, TSH, and LH/FSH microadenomas tend to be centrally located (Figs. 20 and 21). Laterally placed lesions are often accompanied by unilateral contour deformities of the gland such as an eccentric bulge of the superior or inferior surface of the gland on the side of the adenoma and contralateral deviation of the pituitary stalk (Fig. 22). However, these latter two signs are less reliable than internal changes in signal intensity. On occasion, the stalk may actually deviate toward the side of the adenoma (Fig. 23). Almost half of all patients undergoing MRI have tilt of the pituitary stalk, even those without any symptoms referable to the pituitary gland (78). Tilt is therefore a poor lateralizing sign of intrapitu-

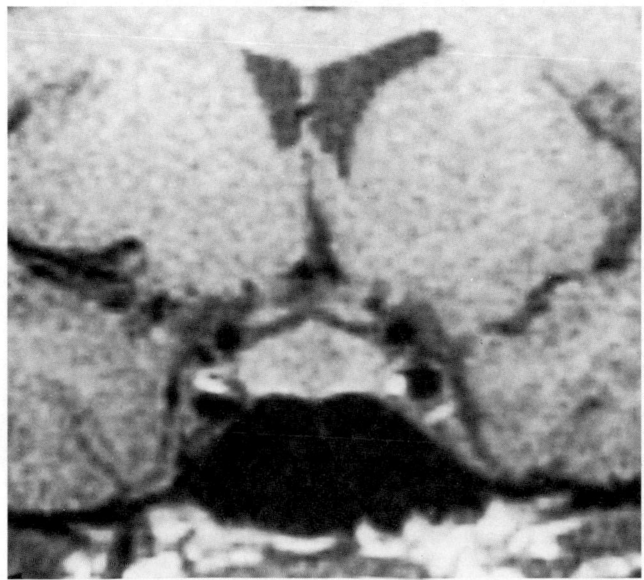

FIG. 20. Cushing's disease. Coronal T1-weighted image. There is a 10-mm microadenoma centrally located in the gland causing a prominent bulge of the gland into the suprasellar cistern. A central location is typical for ACTH-secreting microadenomas. The size is atypical in that most are considerably smaller with a mean size of 3 mm to 4 mm.

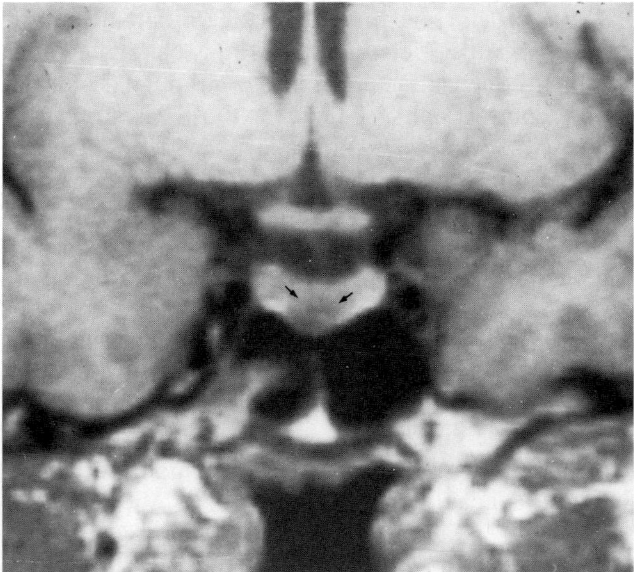

FIG. 21. TSH adenoma. Coronal T1-weighted image. There is a 5-mm centrally positioned adenoma associated with a focal deformity in the sella floor (*small arrows*). TSH adenomas are one of the rarest types. Their appearance is identical to other microadenomas except that their position is more frequently central than lateral.

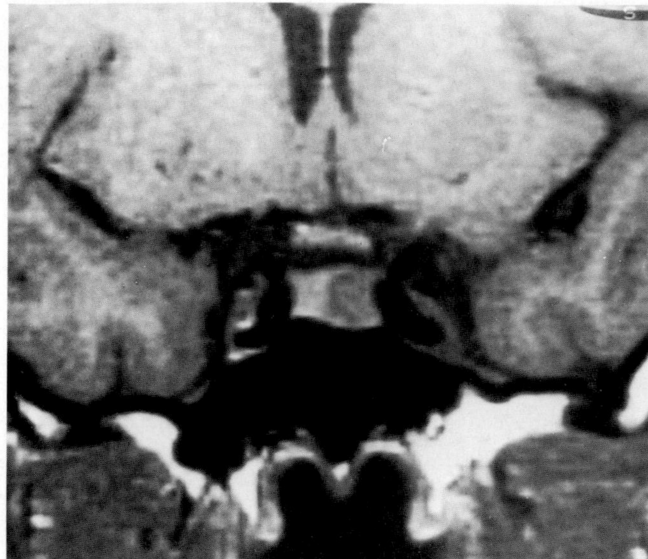

FIG. 22. Pituitary microadenoma. Coronal T1-weighted image. Typical of most microadenomas, this left-sided microadenoma is hypointense in comparison to the normal pituitary gland. The degree of signal difference is greater than found in most microadenomas and in this way this lesion almost mimics the appearance of a cyst. Also, this lesion is associated with contour deformities in both the superior and inferior surfaces of the gland. These signs of a "mass" aid in the confirmation of an intrapituitary tumor.

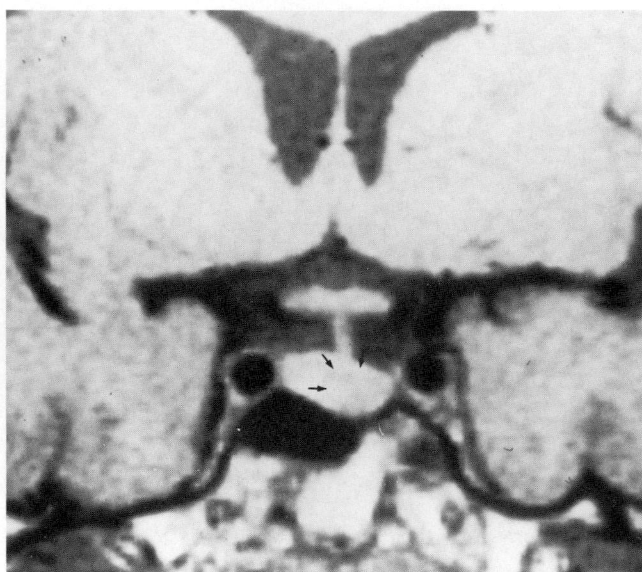

FIG. 23. Adenoma with ipsilateral stalk movement. Coronal T1-weighted image. There is a microadenoma present on the left side of the gland extending inferiorly and laterally (*small arrows*). This case is unusual in that the stalk is displaced toward the side of the adenoma, illustrating that the position of the stalk is not as reliable a finding as focal abnormalities in signal intensity within the gland.

itary pathology. The tilt of the stalk is usually due to developmental lateral eccentricity of the pituitary gland in relationship to the midline of the brain. A minority of cases of tilt is due to eccentric insertion of the infundibulum off the midline of the gland.

The excellent sensitivity of plain (unenhanced) T1-weighted SE MRI for microadenomas has made it the first-line sequence for imaging the pituitary gland. We reserve contrast enhancement for those cases in which there is good clinical and biochemical evidence of a pituitary adenoma with a negative or equivocal plain MRI. In these circumstances gadolinium–diethylenetriamine pentaacetic acid (Gd-DTPA) enhancement has been documented to detect adenomas that would otherwise have remained occult (43–47). This is especially important in Cushing's disease because ACTH-secreting adenomas are the smallest and the most difficult to detect, yet accurate documentation of the presence and the position of these tumors is essential as surgical removal is the only effective means of therapy. Enhanced MRI is the best available means of detecting these tumors (37,43–45,47). In most cases the best imaging routine is to perform a plain scan and then repeat a T1-weighted coronal sequence immediately after i.v. injection of contrast. Because of the differential rates of enhancement between normal pituitary tissue and adenomas, the adenoma will stand out as a hypointense focus within the enhancing gland (see Fig. 19). Dynamic scanning of the

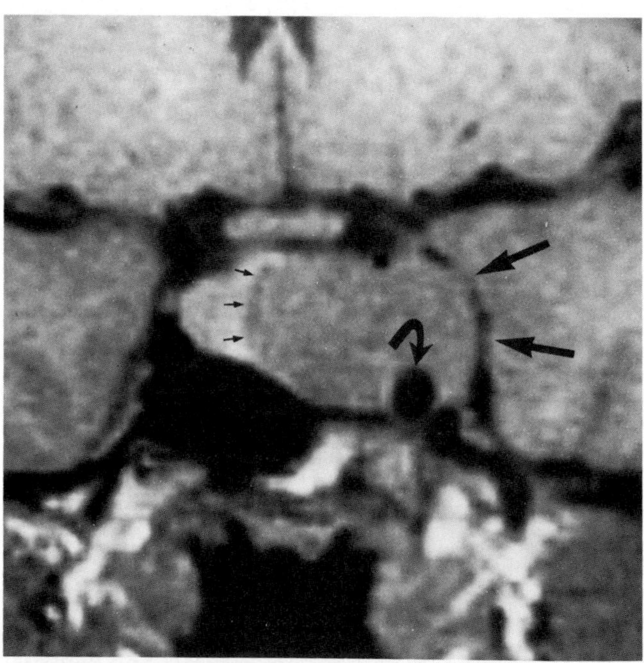

FIG. 24. Pituitary macroadenoma. Coronal T1-weighted image. There is an adenoma originating on the left side of the pituitary gland, extending superiorly into the suprasellar cistern and laterally through the medial cavernous sinus wall into the cavernous sinus and encircling the carotid artery (*curved arrow*). The lateral wall of the left cavernous sinus is displaced and has a distinct lateral convexity (*large arrows*). Note the clear visualization of the lateral cavernous sinus dura on the right and the left. The lateral walls are relatively thick dural structures that are clearly visualized on MRI examinations, forming a useful landmark. The medial cavernous sinus wall, on the other hand, is too thin to be reliably visualized, making subtle degrees of cavernous sinus invasion difficult to assess. Note also the clear distinction between normal and abnormal pituitary tissue (*small arrows*).

pituitary gland may be temporally interposed between a bolus injection of i.v. contrast and the regular postcontrast scan. In a small number of cases the dynamic study will demonstrate an adenoma that is otherwise occult (see Fig. 5). If these images are all negative or equivocal, delayed images (30–60 min after injection) can in some instances demonstrate reversal of this image contrast because of the accumulation of Gd-DTPA in the adenoma and washout from the normal gland (44).

The accuracy of MRI for the diagnosis of pituitary microadenomas is difficult to establish, particularly because of the high incidence of incidental lesions found in pituitary glands (73). Our own experience correlating MRI with surgical findings has been excellent. In an early report of histologically proven cases, more than 90% of microadenomas were detected and accurately localized with MRI (35). This early report continues to reflect accurately our experience to this day. Less favorable statistics have also been published (36,38) but generally results have improved as the use of high field strength scanners has become more prevalent, finer spatial resolution has been achieved, and experience with technique and interpretation has increased. Most published studies (including our own) suffer from small numbers of patients and the inability to ascertain the true number of false negatives. Similar variability in accuracy is evident in the CT literature (36,79–82). There still has not been a large prospective blinded study of MRI of pituitary adenomas, nor any large series comparing MRI and CT in the same group of patients (83). It seems apparent, however, that MRI has for the most part replaced CT as the preferred method of investigation and in our opinion it is the superior technique. The major limitations are in the detection of very small adenomas (3–4 mm), particularly in Cushing's disease.

The discussion of the modern radiologic investigation of pituitary microadenomas would not be complete without considering petrosal venous sampling. Petrosal venous sampling is a useful adjunct in localizing the source of ACTH secretion in the preoperative work-up of patients with Cushing's disease, particularly when imaging tests have failed to reveal a pituitary adenoma (84–87). Petrosal sinus sampling is an extremely reliable test for distinguishing Cushing's disease from ectopic ACTH syndrome and autonomous adrenal disease, with accuracy close to 100% (88). The same accuracy is not achieved in lateralizing an adenoma within the pituitary gland. In 128 patients, the higher level of ACTH was on the side of the tumor in only 70%, whereas it was opposite the tumor in 23%, and nonlateralizing in 6%. However, the contralateral gradients occurred most commonly with larger microadenomas (>6 mm), probably because the low pressure valveless intercavernous sinuses are compressed by tumors of this size. On the other hand, lateralization is most reliable for the smallest lesions (<4 mm), the very cases in which MRI is likely to be negative, and lateralization is otherwise most difficult (88).

Before proceeding to macroadenomas there are two practical issues that warrant comment: "pituitary incidentalomas" and the appropriate interval for follow-up of microadenomas. With respect to the first matter, it is well known that focal abnormalities may be seen incidentally in the pituitary gland. At autopsy, incidental pituitary lesions greater than 2 mm were found in 5.8% to 8.3% of all subjects over the age of 30 years (73). This is increasingly true on MRI as ever better resolution is achieved. The discovery of these focal abnormalities may be due to several factors—the presence of asymptomatic coincidental cysts or microadenomas, or artifactual hypointensities caused by magnetic susceptibility–induced signal distortions in the gland that mimic pathology (89,90). Most of these incidental "lesions" are small, usually less than 3 mm in size. It should be noted that incidental pituitary lesions greater than 2 mm are nearly always either pituitary adenomas or Rathke cleft cysts from autopsy studies (73). Focal susceptibility artifacts are particularly common near the junction of the sphenoid sinus septum and the sellar floor (90). Thus, the interpretation of pituitary MRI must be related to knowledge of typical imaging artifacts in the sella turcica and be closely tied to the clinical and biochemical findings.

The other practical clinical issue is the question of the appropriate interval between MR scans for microadenomas. We are often asked to repeat MR imaging of microadenomas at annual intervals. It has been our experience that there is rarely any significant change in tumor size over such intervals. The literature supports our observations, particularly with microprolactinomas. One study of 38 untreated patients who were followed with prolactin radioimmunoassay and high resolution CT over an average period of 32 months showed no evidence of tumor growth in any patient, not even in two patients with exuberant rises in prolactin (91). The authors concede that gradual tumor growth over decades may be possible. Although a similar study has not been performed using MRI, the implication is that the imaging follow-up interval for microprolactinomas should probably not be any more often than every several years.

Macroadenomas share some of the MRI characteristics as their smaller counterparts. MRI typically demonstrates a mass arising from the pituitary fossa, hypointense on T1-weighted images and compressing the higher intensity normal pituitary tissue (Fig. 24). In many instances the adenoma completely fills the sella; the normal tissue is so compressed that it is virtually obliterated and cannot be identified (Fig. 25).

The multiplanar capabilities, lack of bone and surgical clip artifact, and ability to demonstrate large arterial structures make MRI a powerful tool in the pre- and postoperative assessment of pituitary macroadenomas (Fig. 26). Furthermore, direct visualization of the cav-

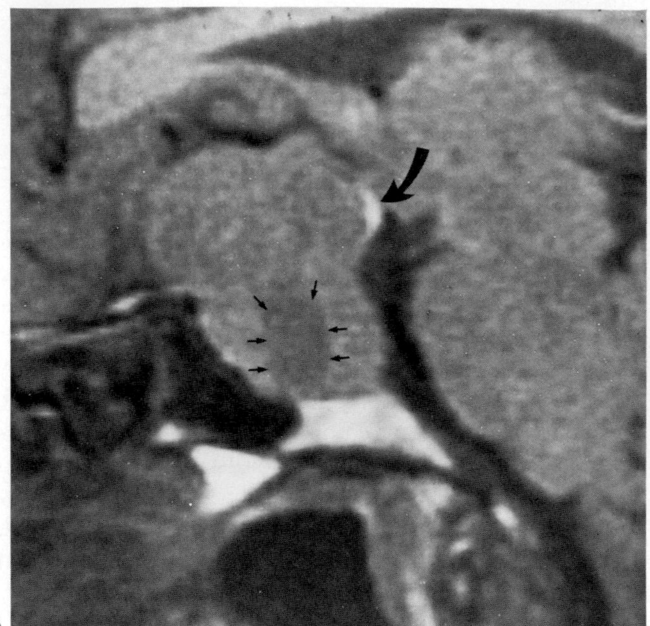

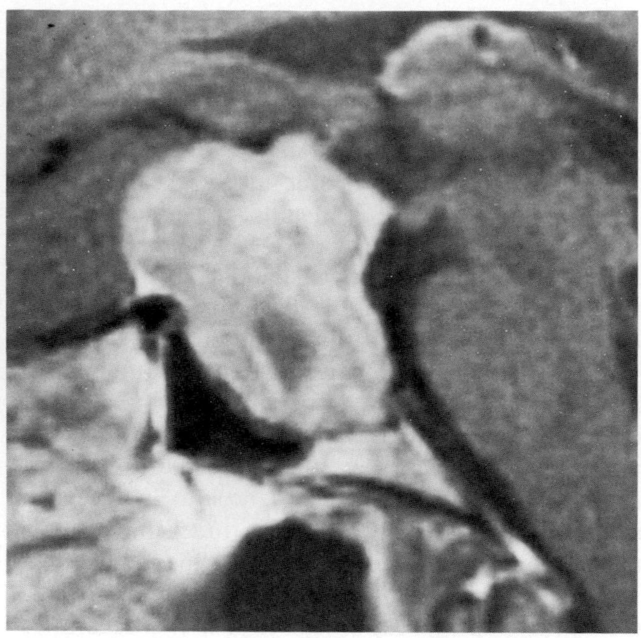

FIG. 25. Pituitary macroadenoma. **A:** Sagittal T1-weighted image. There is a large, soft tissue mass (*small arrows*) in the sella turcica and suprasellar cistern. The sella turcica itself is expanded—a good sign that the tumor originated from within the sella rather than above it. The optic chiasm and third ventricle are elevated. Note the high intensity band along the posterior margin of the superior aspect of the tumor (*curved arrow*). This is thought to represent the material normally present in the posterior lobe; however, because of the large size of the tumor, this material cannot descend all the way through the stalk to the normal intrasellar position and remains at the site of "stalk obstruction". Within the tumor there is a focal necrotic area of low intensity. **B:** Following contrast enhancement, the entire tumor enhances rather intensely but not completely homogeneously. In particular, the area of necrosis shows no enhancement.

ernous portion of the internal carotid arteries as well as the middle and anterior cerebral arteries makes routine preoperative angiography for delineation of these vessels unnecessary. Superior extension into the suprasellar cistern is particularly well delineated because of the superb image contrast between the adenoma against the markedly hypointense CSF. The optic nerves, chiasm, and tracts are directly visualized as they are draped over the tumor. Lateral extension of the adenoma into the cavernous sinus is a common phenomenon, but in contrast to suprasellar extension is less well delineated with MRI (92,93). The principal reason is that the medial wall of the cavernous sinus is very thin and in most cases not directly visualized. In many instances coronal MRI demonstrates that a pituitary adenoma extends above or below the sagittal plane of the cavernous segment of the carotid artery yet it is impossible to determine if the cavernous sinus is invaded or only compressed by the adenoma (Figs. 27 and 28). On the other hand, the lateral dural wall of the cavernous sinus is a reliable landmark; it is relatively thick and directly visible. Lateral extension and interposition of abnormal tissue between the lateral wall of the cavernous sinus and the artery is the most reliable indicator of cavernous sinus invasion (see Fig. 24). Significant asymmetry between cavernous sinuses also correlates well with invasion, as does very high serum prolactin levels (93). Levels over 1,000 ng/ml almost always indicate cavernous sinus involvement. It is important to note that although lateral extension and invasion of the cavernous sinus by adenomas is not uncommon, constriction or occlusion of the cavernous portion of the internal carotid artery is very rare. This is of some differential diagnostic significance in distinguishing adenomas from meningiomas (see "meningiomas").

Extension inferiorly is easily documented by the visualization of the moderate signal intensity of the adenoma protruding into the air-containing sphenoid sinus. Similarly, extension into the marrow space of the clivus is visible as replacement of the normal high signal intensity of marrow on T1-weighted images by tumor. On the other hand, subtle abnormalities in the cortical bone are difficult to evaluate by MRI. Because of the insensitivity to fine bony detail, osseous invasion cannot be distinguished from remodeling and expansion of the sella. This is one disadvantage of MRI relative to CT but it is of little surgical importance. With regard to the sphenoid sinus, narrow display windows can define the septal anatomy (because of the mucoperiosteum lining these septa) (Fig. 29). These septa can be used as landmarks to aid in planning transsphenoidal surgery.

Larger pituitary adenomas may be accompanied by cystic degeneration or hemorrhage. Cystic degeneration in an adenoma is evident as sharply defined regions of very low signal intensity on T1-weighted images that are

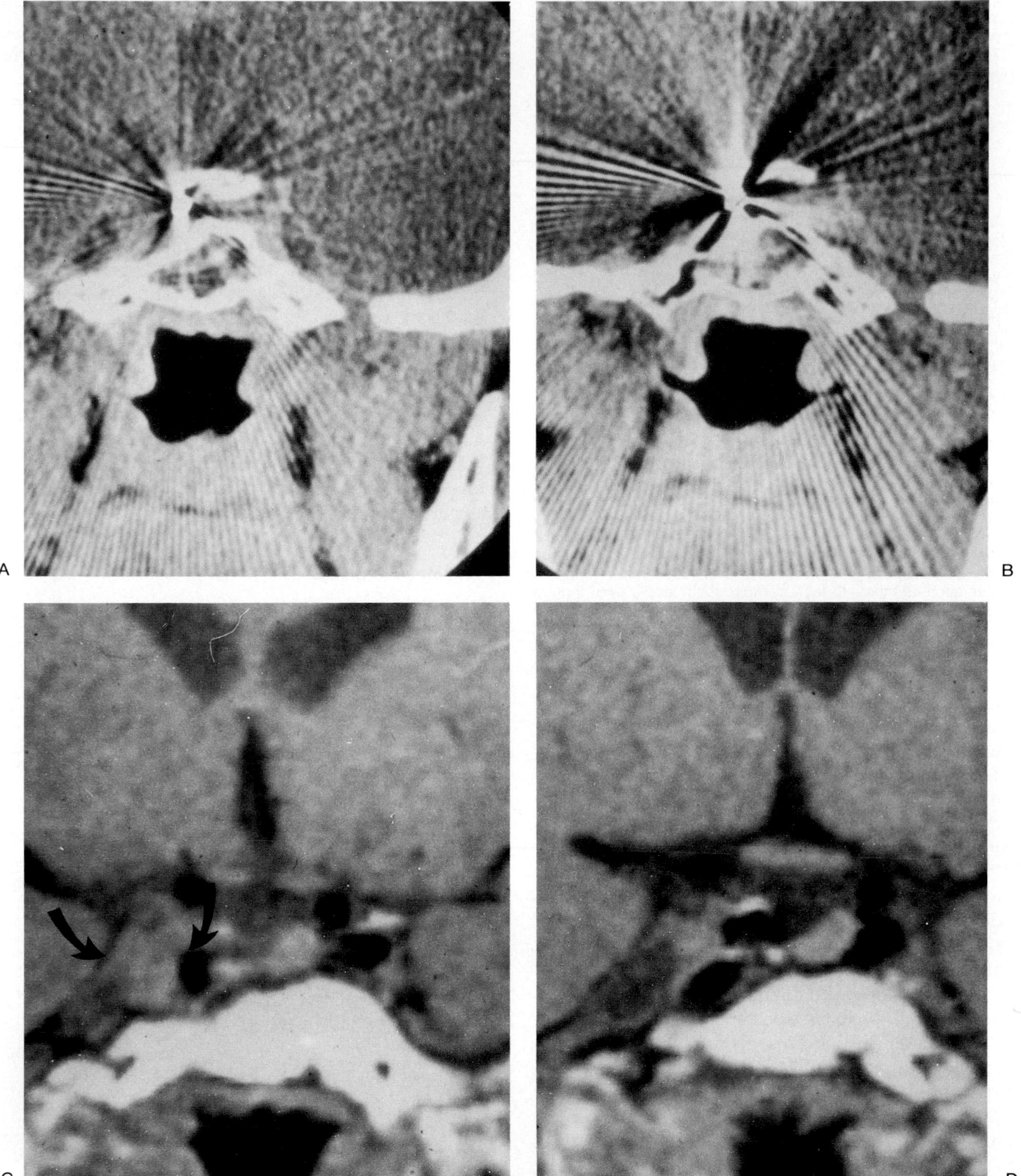

FIG. 26. Surgical clip artifact and tumor recurrence. **A,B:** CT scans. This patient had a prolactinoma resected 10 years before this CT scan. At the time of surgery a clip was placed in the operative site. Recently the patient's symptoms returned and she was found to have markedly elevated prolactin levels. The CT scan was nondiagnostic because of the artifact from the clip in the sella turcica. **C,D:** Coronal T1-weighted MRI. These nonferromagnetic surgical clips cause virtually no artifact on the MR scan. This makes this type of patient an ideal candidate for MRI assessment. The tumor recurrence is clearly visible in the right cavernous sinus, as evidenced by the abnormal amount of soft tissue interposed between the lateral wall of the cavernous sinus and the internal carotid artery (*curved arrows*).

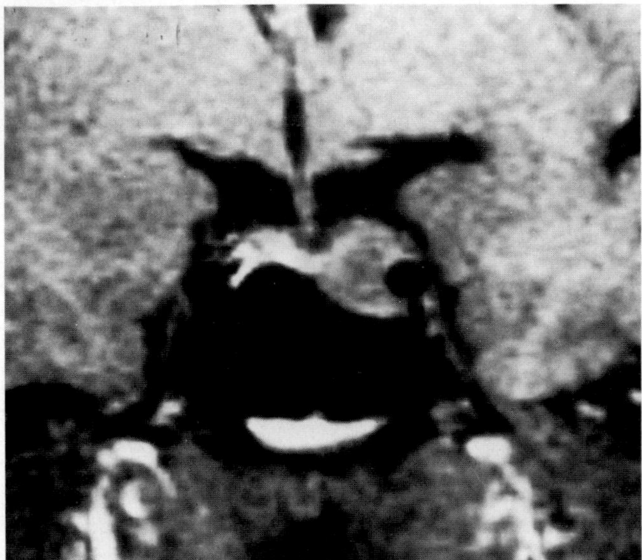

FIG. 27. Lateral extension of pituitary adenoma. Coronal T1-weighted image. There is a 1-cm pituitary adenoma on the left. It extends laterally above and below the left internal carotid artery. It appears that the tumor has extended into the cavernous sinus but at surgery the medial wall of the cavernous sinus was merely displaced laterally and was not breached. The failure to visualize consistently the medial cavernous sinus wall on MR images makes it difficult to predict reliably cavernous sinus invasion in cases such as these. In fact, in most such cases, even though the tumor extends to the sagittal plane of the cavernous portion of the carotid artery, the cavernous sinus is usually not invaded.

markedly hyperintense on the T2-weighted sequence. A fluid-fluid level is a more specific sign of cystic degeneration but is infrequently present. Occasionally noncystic adenomas possess similar signal characteristics and mimic a cyst (see Fig. 22). Hemorrhage into macroadenomas is not uncommon and the MRI features are characteristic. A focal area of hyperintensity on both T1- and T2-weighted images is demonstrated in the otherwise homogeneous, intermediate signal intensity of the adenoma. Only a small fraction of these patients have clinical findings of pituitary apoplexy (see the section entitled, "Pituitary Apoplexy") (94).

An area of continued difficulty in pituitary and parasellar imaging is that of the postoperative examination in search of residual or recurrent pituitary adenoma. In these cases, it may be difficult to distinguish postoperative scarring, or graft material, from the normal gland or adenomatous tissue. This is especially true in the first 6 months after surgery. In these cases, progressive growth of a soft tissue mass on sequential postoperative MR scans is the best imaging sign of recurrent tumor. This must also be interpreted in conjunction with endocrinologic markers.

The use of positron emission tomography (PET) for the study of pituitary adenomas has been limited to a few institutions. Despite this limited use, proponents of PET have demonstrated that C^{11}-methionine PET can give valuable complementary information in the diagnosis of adenomas because of PET's ability to distinguish viable tumor from fibrosis, cysts, and necrosis, and it also gives valuable information about treatment effects. Also PET with dopamine D2 receptor ligands can characterize the degree of receptor binding and thus give some prognostic information about the likelihood that bromocriptine (a dopamine agonist) therapy will be successful (95). The spatial resolution of PET is not nearly as good as CT or MRI, yet PET with fluorodeoxyglucose (FDG) tracers has been used for microadenoma detection with some success (96). The ability to detect small adenomas arises because the low metabolic activity of the normal pituitary gland renders it invisible on PET. Thus, on a background of no activity, even a tiny focus of hyperactivity in a microadenoma is very conspicuous. In one study, 12 of 20 surgically verified microadenomas were visible with PET, compared with 13 on MRI. Although MRI had a higher sensitivity overall, five of the lesions visible on PET were negative or equivocal on MRI. Thus, PET may be useful when there is strong clinical evidence of an adenoma and MRI is negative or equivocal.

Craniopharyngioma

Craniopharyngiomas are epithelially derived neoplasms that occur exclusively in the region of the sella

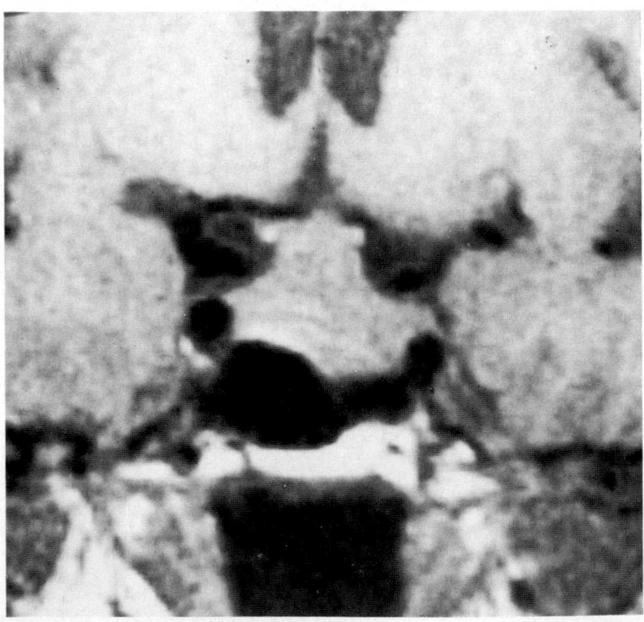

FIG. 28. Lateral extension of pituitary adenoma. Coronal T1-weighted image. In this case the tumor extends even farther laterally than the previous case. Clinically the patient had an acute left cranial nerve III palsy. On these clinical grounds the lateral wall of the cavernous sinus was thought to be involved. Yet, without therapy the cranial nerve III palsy resolved and the adenoma was resected transsphenoidally. At operation, there was no evidence of cavernous sinus involvement. This once again illustrates the difficulty in predicting cavernous sinus invasion.

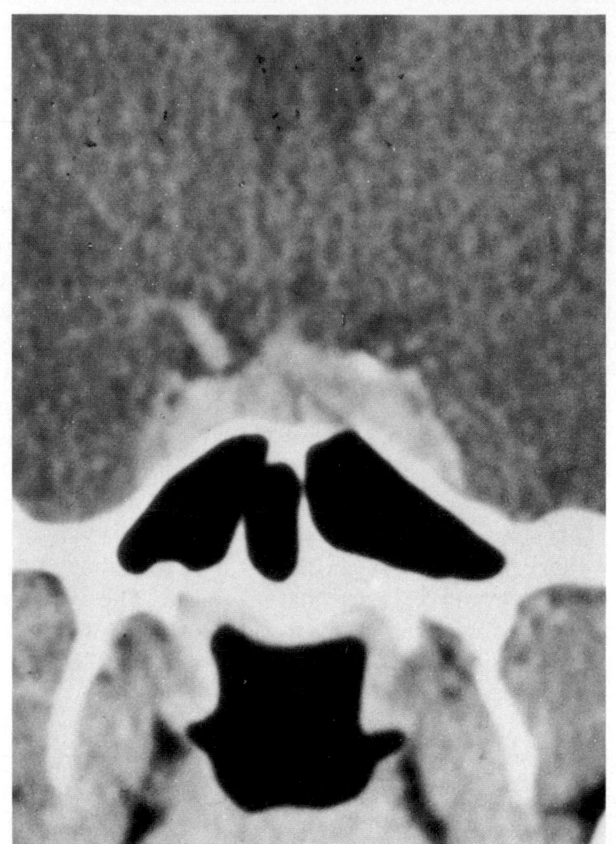

A

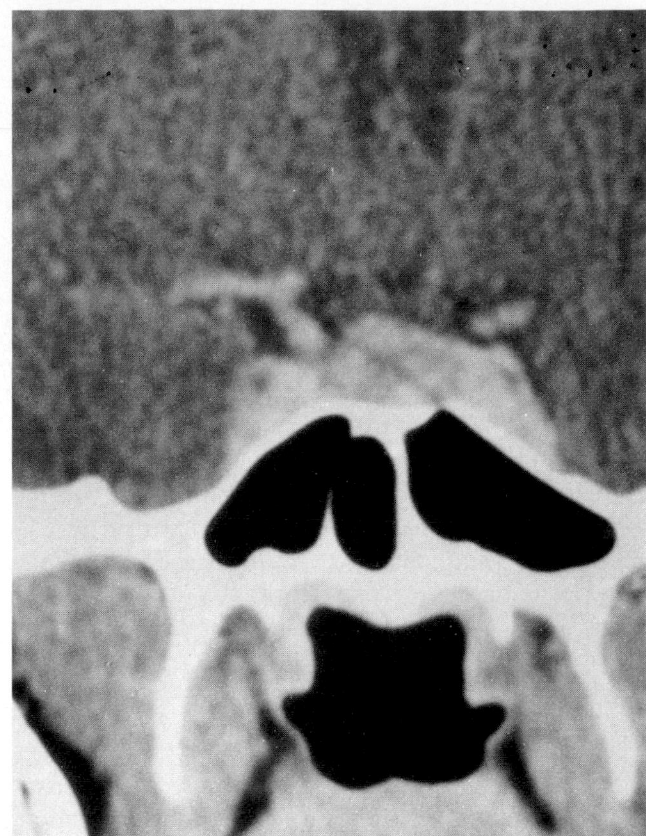

B

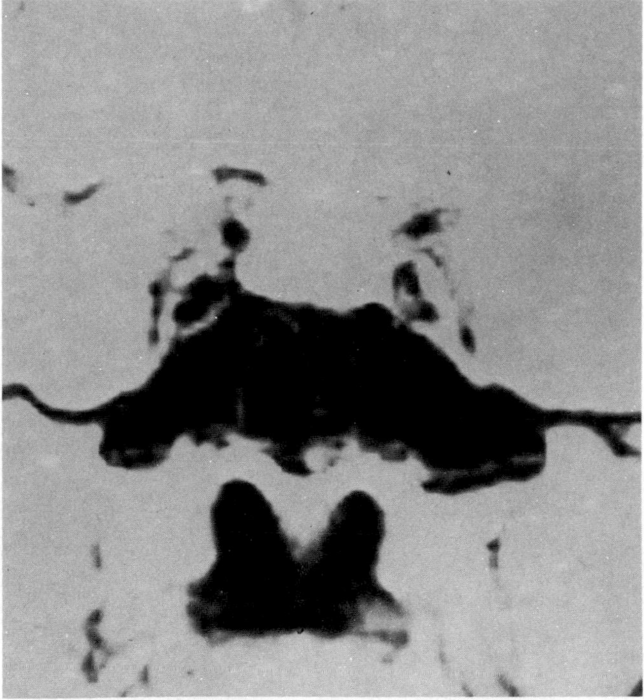

C

FIG. 29. Sphenoid sinus septa. MRI bone windows. **A,B:** Coronal CT scans. Coronal CT is clearly superior in demonstrating the anatomy of the sella turcica floor and the bony anatomy of the sphenoid sinus. Two distinct vertical septations are noted within the sphenoid sinus, useful anatomic landmarks for the surgeon approaching the sella turcica transsphenoidally. In most cases these septations are not visible on MRI. **C:** Photography at extremely narrow display windows can demonstrate these septations because of the mucoperiosteum on the septa. Clearly the visualization is not as good as with CT, yet MRI suffices and removes the necessity for obtaining preoperative CT.

turcica and suprasellar cistern or in the third ventricle. Craniopharyngiomas account for approximately 3% of all intracranial tumors and show no sex predominance. Craniopharyngiomas are hormonally inactive lesions. They have a bimodal age distribution; more than half occur in childhood or adolescence, with a peak incidence between 5 and 10 years of age; there is a second smaller peak in the sixth decade (97). The tumors vary greatly in size, from a few millimeters to several centimeters in diameter. The epicenter of most is in the suprasellar cistern (Fig. 30). Infrequently, the lesions are entirely within the sella or in the third ventricle (98).

Most discussions of craniopharyngiomas in the literature are confined to the most frequent form, the classic *adamantinomatous* type, but a distinct squamous or *papillary* type is becoming recognized with increasing frequency. The two forms of craniopharyngioma are distinct in terms of clinical presentation, imaging features, histopathology, and treatment outcome (99), so they must be considered separately. Regardless of which form of the entity is being considered, the histogenesis of these lesions remains a subject of investigation.

Adamantinomatous Craniopharyngioma

The classic form of craniopharyngioma is the adamantinomatous type, which is the most frequently encountered form of the lesion. Typically, cases are identified as suprasellar masses during the first two decades of life. These children most often present with symptoms and signs of increased intracranial pressure: headache, nausea, vomiting, and papilledema. Visual disturbances due to compression of the optic apparatus are also frequent but difficult to detect in young children. Others present with pituitary hypofunction because of compression of the pituitary gland, pituitary stalk, or hypothalamus. Occasionally, lesions rupture into the subarachnoid space and evoke a chemical meningitis. Rarely, adamantinomatous craniopharyngiomas are found outside the suprasellar cistern, including the posterior fossa, pineal region, within the third ventricle, and in the nasal cavity.

Adamantinomatous tumors are almost always grossly cystic and usually have both solid and cystic components. Cyst contents vary in color and viscosity, but the typical content of the cyst is a dark brown "machine-oil" that contains characteristic suspended cholesterol crystals. Calcification is seen in the vast majority of these tumors. The diagnostic histopathological finding is the clumps of "wet keratin" often with dystrophic calcification. They contain cords of columnar or squamous epithelium with keratin formation. Extensive fibrosis and signs of inflammation are often found with these lesions, particularly when they are recurrent, so that they adhere to adjacent structures, including the vasculature at the base of the brain. Moreover, adamantinomatous craniopharyngiomas are often invasive into adjacent brain, which evokes a dense gliosis that may be difficult to distinguish from a primary glial neoplasm. The inflammatory and fibrotic nature of the lesions makes recurrence a not uncommon event, typically occurring within the first 5 years after surgery.

The most characteristic MRI finding is a suprasellar mass that is itself heterogeneous but contains a cystic component that is well defined, internally uniform, and hyperintense on both T1- and T2-weighted images (Fig. 31) (100,101). The lesions often encase nearby cerebral vasculature. The solid portion, which is frequently partially calcified, is represented as the heterogeneous region. On rare occasions the cyst is absent and the solid component is completely calcified (Fig. 32). These calcified types of tumors can be entirely overlooked on MRI unless close scrutiny is paid to subtle distortion of the normal suprasellar anatomy. Contrast enhancement will cause a moderate degree of enhancement of the solid

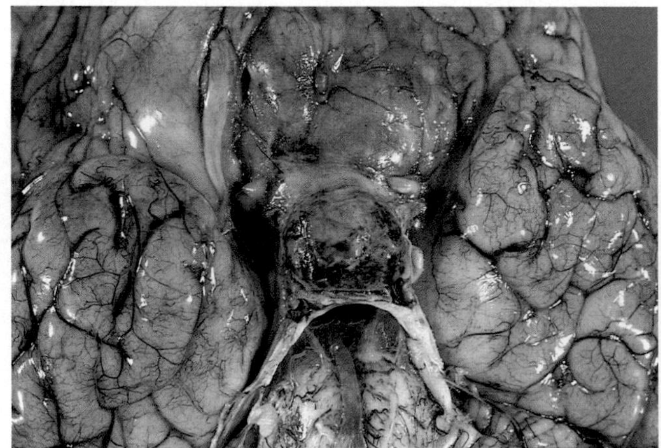
A

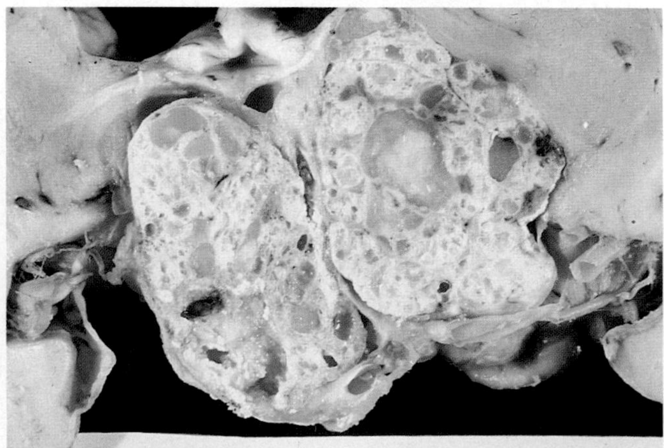
B

FIG. 30. Craniopharyngioma (adamantinomatous type). **A:** View of excised brain from below. **B:** Coronal section through the tumor. There is compression of hypothalamic structures and striking solid and cystic components.

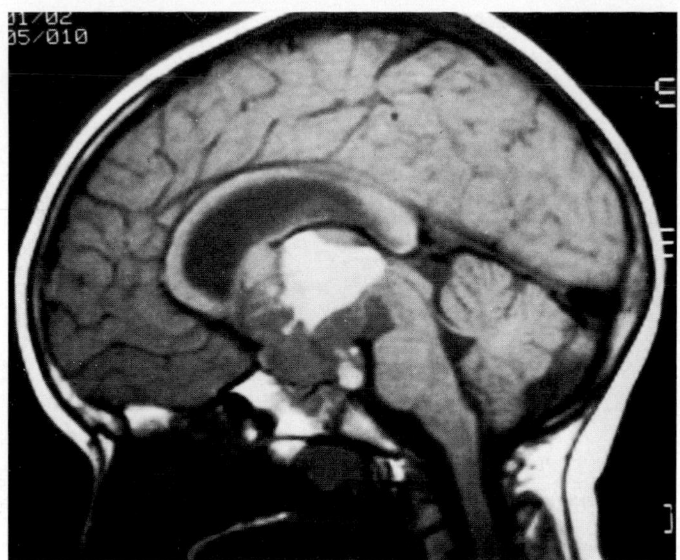
A

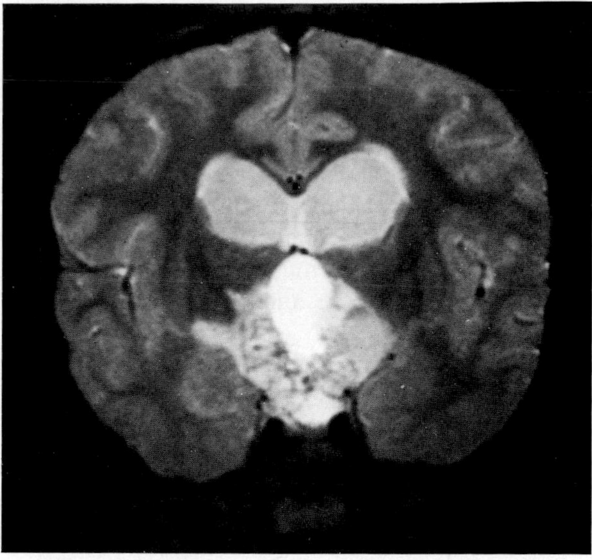
B

FIG. 31. Craniopharyngioma. **A:** Sagittal T1-weighted image. There is a large, complicated suprasellar mass causing obstructive hydrocephalus. This appearance is virtually pathognomonic of craniopharyngioma. The signal intensity is mixed; the lower half is low signal whereas the upper half is markedly hyperintense. The high signal intensity corresponds to the "machine-oil" cyst so often found in these tumors. **B:** Coronal T2-weighted image. The cystic component of the tumor remains hyperintense; the solid portion is irregular and slightly hyperintense as well. The ventricles are dilated and capped by regions of periventricular edema secondary to transependymal absorption of CSF.

portion of the tumor, which otherwise may be difficult to see.

Papillary Craniopharyngioma

Papillary craniopharyngiomas are typically found in the adult patient. These lesions are solid, without calcification, and often found within the third ventricle. Although surgery remains the definitive mode of therapy for all craniopharyngiomas, papillary variants are encapsulated and are readily separable from nearby structures and adjacent brain, so they are generally thought to recur much less frequently than the adamantinomatous type.

On pathologic examination, papillary lesions do not show the features characteristic of the adamantinomatous variant; that is, the cholesterol crystals in a cystic component, wet keratin nodules, fibroinflammatory tissue, keratin, calcification, and nuclear pali-

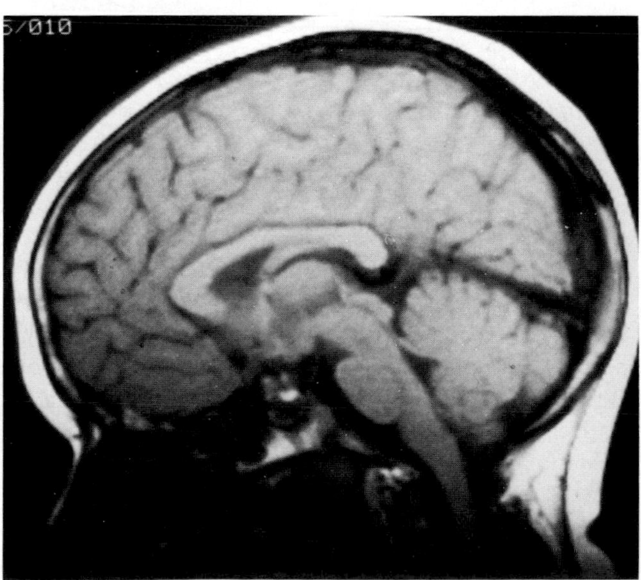
A

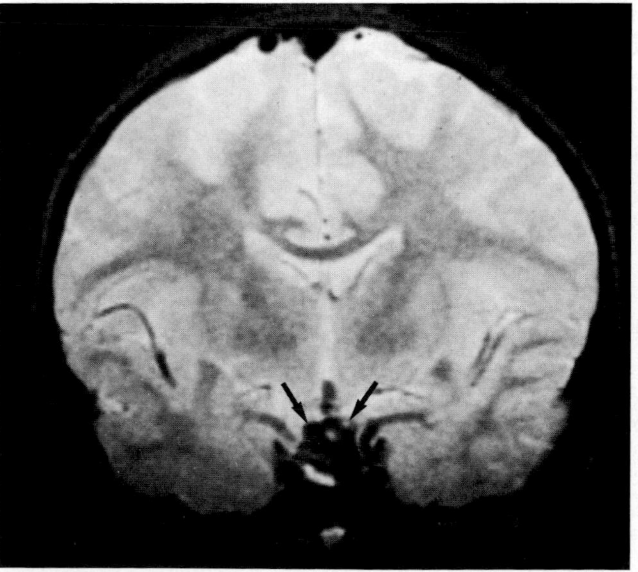
B

FIG. 32. Calcified craniopharyngioma. **A:** Sagittal T1-weighted image. On T1-weighted image the calcified tumor can easily be overlooked because of the lack of image contrast between it and the suprasellar CSF. **B:** Coronal T2-weighted image. The marked hypointensity of the tumor is more clearly evident with T2-weighting because the area of dark signal stands out in relief against the white CSF (*arrows*).

sades. In papillary lesions, there is extensive squamous differentiation.

In distinction from their adamantinomatous counterpart, MRI shows papillary craniopharyngiomas as solid lesions. As noted above, they are often situated within the third ventricle. These lesions demonstrate a nonspecific signal intensity pattern, without the characteristic hyperintensity on T1-weighted images of the cystic component of adamantinomatous tumors. Like all craniopharyngiomas, papillary lesions typically enhance.

Rathke Cleft Cyst

Symptomatic cysts of Rathke's cleft are much less frequent than craniopharyngiomas, although they are a common incidental finding at autopsy. In a recent evaluation of 1,000 nonselected autopsy specimens, 113 (11.3%) of pituitary glands harbored incidental Rathke cleft cysts (73). These cysts are predominantly intrasellar in location. Of incidental Rathke cysts larger than 2 mm in a large autopsy series, 89% were localized to the center of the gland (Fig. 33), whereas the remaining 11% extended to show predominant lateral lesions (Fig. 34). In that series, of all incidental pituitary lesions localized to the central part of the gland, 87% were Rathke cysts (73). Others may be centered in the suprasellar cistern, usually midline and anterior to the stalk. Rathke cysts are found in all age groups. They share a common origin with some craniopharyngiomas in that they are thought to originate from remnants of squamous epithelium from Rathke's cleft. The cyst wall is composed of a single cell layer of columnar, cuboidal, or squamous epithelium on a basement membrane. The epithelium is often ciliated and may contain goblet cells. The cyst contents are typically mucoid, less commonly filled with serous fluid, or desquamated cellular debris (102,103). Calcification in the cyst wall is rare.

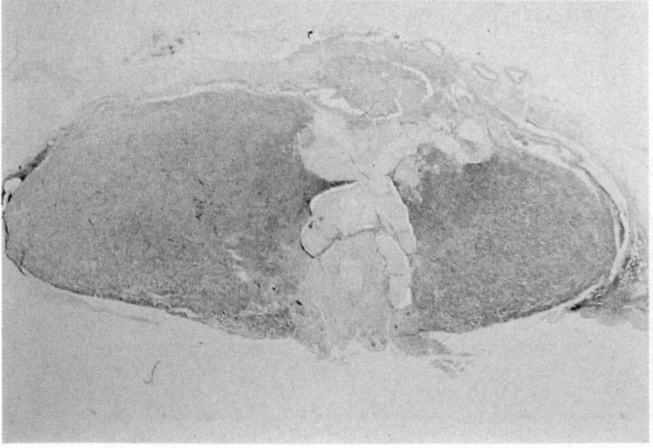

FIG. 33. Typical Rathke cleft cyst is localized within the central portion of the gland. (From Teramoto, et al., ref. 73, with permission.)

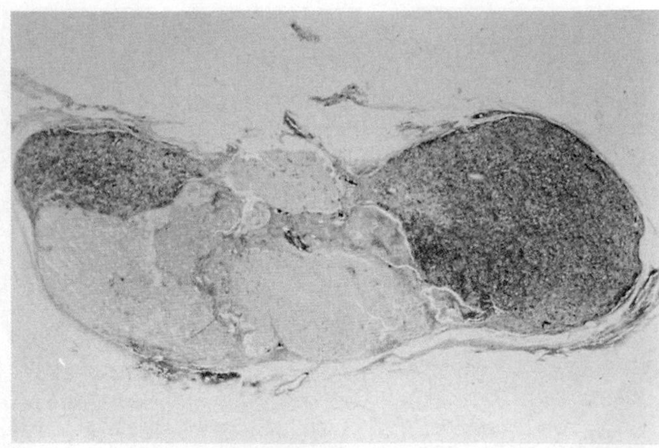

FIG. 34. The Rathke cleft cyst is seen extending into the lateral aspect of the gland. (From Teramoto, et al., ref. 73, with permission.)

Most Rathke's cleft cysts are small, asymptomatic, and discovered only at autopsy. Symptoms occur if the cyst enlarges sufficiently to compress the pituitary gland or optic chiasm. The cysts with mucoid fluid are indistinguishable from cystic craniopharyngiomas on MRI: both are hyperintense on both T1- and T2-weighted images (Fig. 35). The serous cysts match the signal intensity of CSF and are the only subtype that have the typical imaging features of benign cysts (Fig. 36). Those containing cellular debris pose the greatest difficulty in differential diagnosis for they resemble solid nodules. However, Rathke cleft cysts do not enhance except for occasional, thin, marginal enhancement of the cyst wall. This feature can be used to advantage to separate these cysts from craniopharyngiomas in difficult cases.

Meningioma

Approximately 10% of meningiomas occur in the parasellar region (72,104). These tumors arise from a variety of locations around the sella including the tuberculum sellae, clinoid processes, medial sphenoid wing, and cavernous sinus (Fig. 37). Meningiomas can also extend into the juxtasellar region from more distant sources. For example, optic sheath meningiomas often extend intracranially and involve the cavernous sinus, and meningiomas of the planum sphenoidale or olfactory grooves extend posteriorly into the suprasellar cistern, or downward into the sella turcica.

Meningiomas are usually slow-growing lesions that present because of compression of vital structures. Patients may suffer visual loss because of compression of the optic nerves, chiasm, or optic tracts; ophthalmoplegia due to cranial nerve involvement; or proptosis due to venous congestion at the orbital apex. Accurate differentiation between meningioma and pituitary adenoma is important because meningioma requires crani-

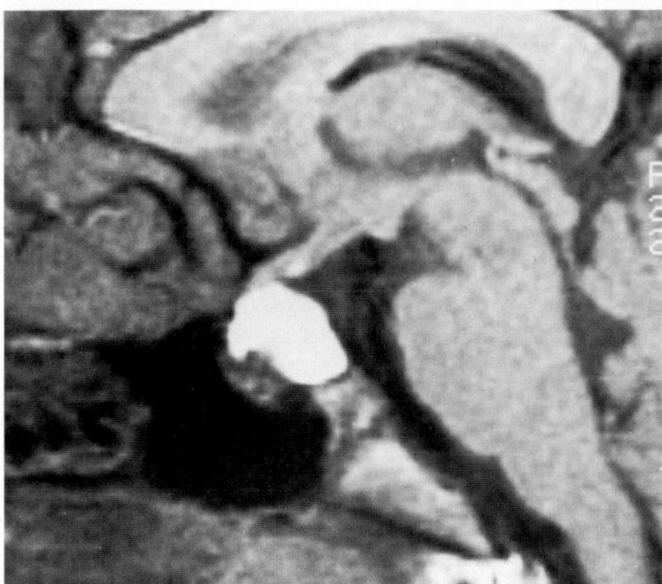

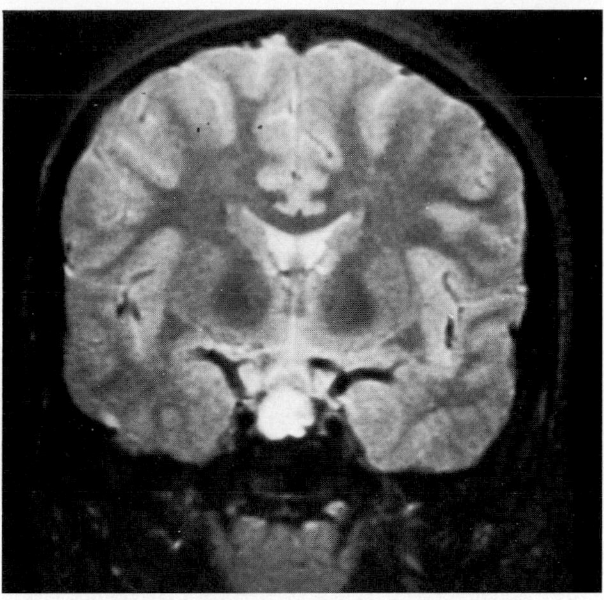

A B

FIG. 35. Rathke cleft cyst. **A:** Sagittal T1-weighted image. A 15-mm hyperintense lesion is present in the superior half of the sella turcica, extending into the suprasellar cistern. It is uniform in signal intensity and has a well-defined border. **B:** Coronal T2-weighted image. The cyst is also hyperintense on the T2-weighted image. This signal intensity pattern is the most common type in Rathke's cyst, although the cyst contents can also be hypointense or isointense on either T1- or T2-weighted images. The main differential diagnoses are craniopharyngioma and hemorrhagic pituitary adenoma.

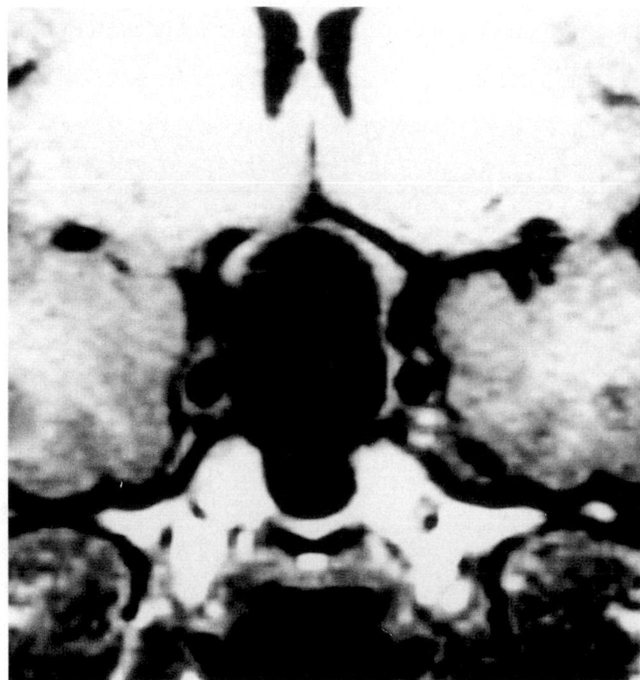

FIG. 36. Rathke's cleft cyst. Coronal T1-weighted images. The cyst in this case exactly matches the signal characteristics of CSF, typical of about 50% of Rathke's cleft cysts. A diagnosis of a benign cyst can be confidently established when the MRI has this appearance, with the differential diagnosis being an arachnoid cyst.

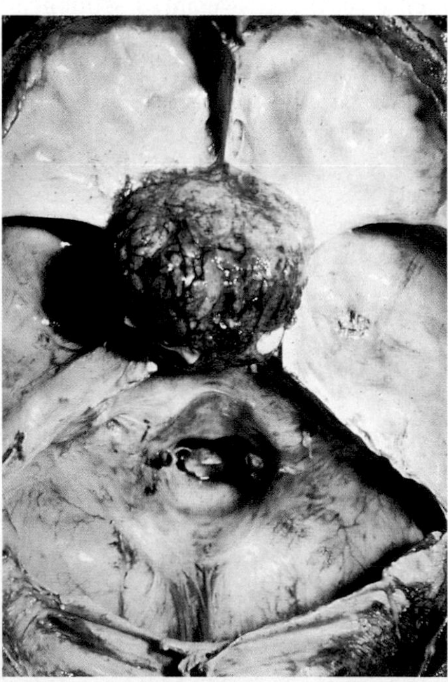

FIG. 37. Large suprasellar meningioma. This is a view of the intracranial surface of the skull base with the brain removed. The tumor is well encapsulated and its surface is covered by a network of vessels. The potential for compression of the optic chiasm and hypothalamus is obvious.

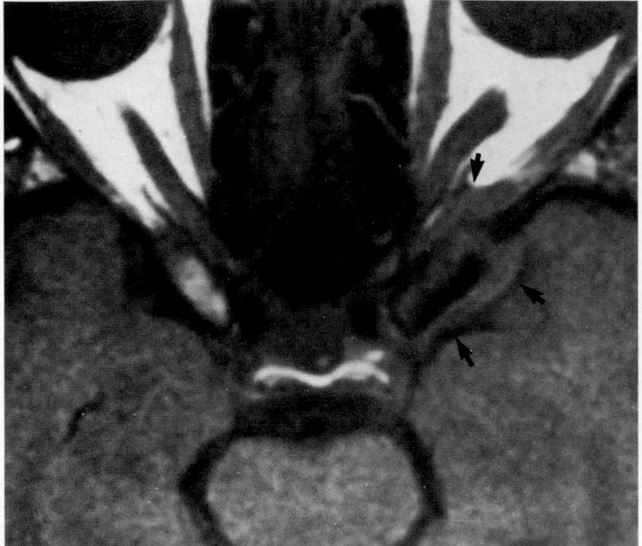

FIG. 38. Sphenoid wing meningioma. Axial T1-weighted image. There is a subtle mass on the medial one third of the left sphenoid wing. It has a wide dural base on the intracranial and intraorbital surfaces of the sphenoid bone (*arrows*) and it enlarges the left cavernous sinus. The signal intensity is equal to that of adjacent gray matter, typical of meningioma.

otomy, whereas a transsphenoidal route is preferred for removing most pituitary macroadenomas (105).

Meningiomas are most frequently isointense relative to gray matter on unenhanced T1-weighted sequences, and less commonly hypointense. Approximately 50% remain isointense on the T2-weighted sequence, whereas 40% are hyperintense (106–111). Because there is little image contrast to distinguish meningiomas from brain parenchyma, indirect signs such as a mass effect, thickening of the dura, buckling of adjacent white matter, white matter edema, and hyperostosis are important diagnostic features (Fig. 38). Other diagnostic signs include visualization of a cleft of CSF separating the tumor from the brain (thus denoting that the tumor has an extra-axial location), and a clear separation of the tumor from the pituitary gland (Fig. 39), thus indicating that the tumor is not of pituitary gland origin. The latter sign is particularly well assessed on sagittal views of planum sphenoidale meningiomas. A peripheral black rim has been described on the edges of these meningiomas. This is thought to be related to surrounding veins (109). Hyperostosis and calcification are features that may be apparent on MRI but are better assessed with CT scan. Vascular encasement is not uncommon, particularly with meningiomas in the cavernous sinus. The pattern of encasement is of diagnostic value. Meningiomas commonly constrict the lumen of the encased vessel. This is rare with other tumors (Fig. 40). As on CT, the administration of i.v. contrast markedly improves the visualization of basal meningiomas. They enhance intensely and homogeneously with gadolinium (Fig. 41), often with a trailing edge of thick surrounding dura (the "dural tail sign"). This feature, together with the characteristic wide dural base, are the most distinctive imaging features of parasellar meningiomas. If MRI cannot distinguish a meningioma from a pituitary adenoma, phosphorus MR spectroscopy may be of help because pituitary adenomas have a much higher phosphate monoester peak than meningiomas (112).

A

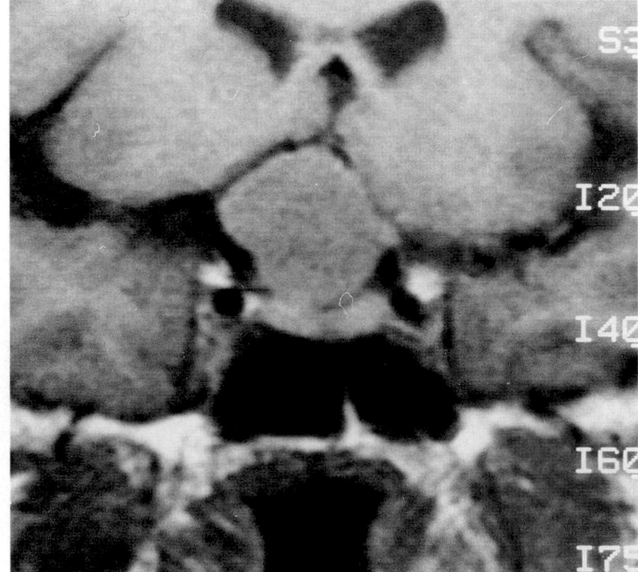

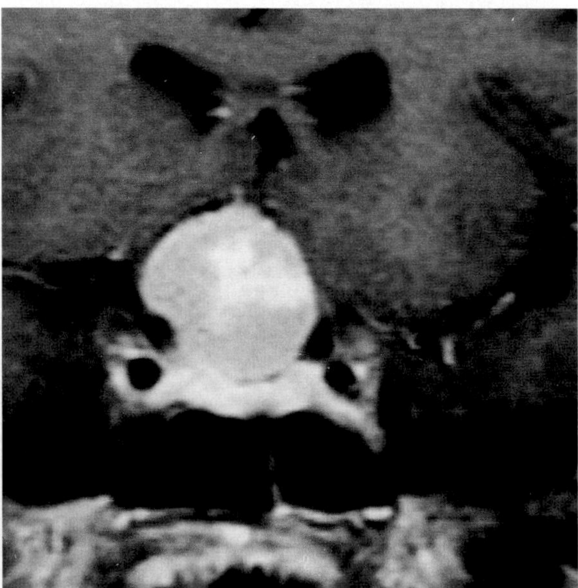

B

FIG. 39. Suprasellar meningioma. **A:** Unenhanced and, (**B**), contrast-enhanced T1-weighted coronal images. The MRI was performed to assist in the differential diagnosis of a mass discovered on CT: meningioma, versus pituitary macroadenoma, versus aneurysm. Aneurysm can be excluded on the basis of signal intensity and morphology; macroadenoma can be excluded because the mass is clearly separate from the pituitary gland. The normal pituitary gland is clearly visualized inferior to and separate from the mass.

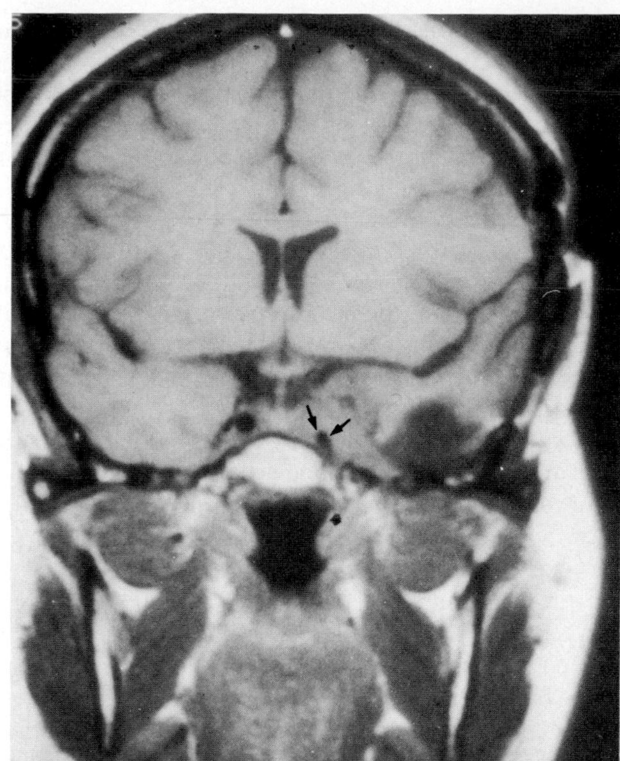

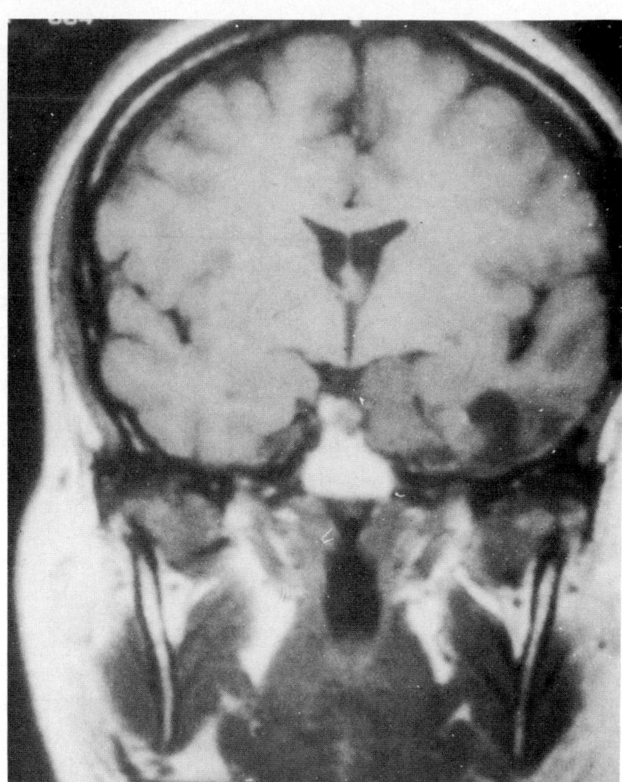

FIG. 40. Cavernous sinus meningioma. **A,B:** Coronal T1-weighted images. There has been partial resection of the tumor with evidence of left temporal lobe encephalomalacia. There is residual tumor in the left cavernous sinus and suprasellar cistern. Note the encasement and constriction of the left internal carotid artery (*small arrows*), a feature that is very infrequent in tumors other than meningiomas.

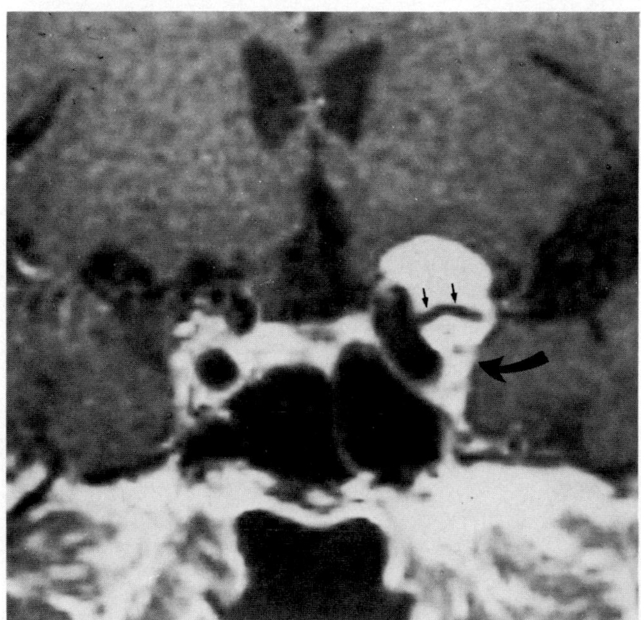

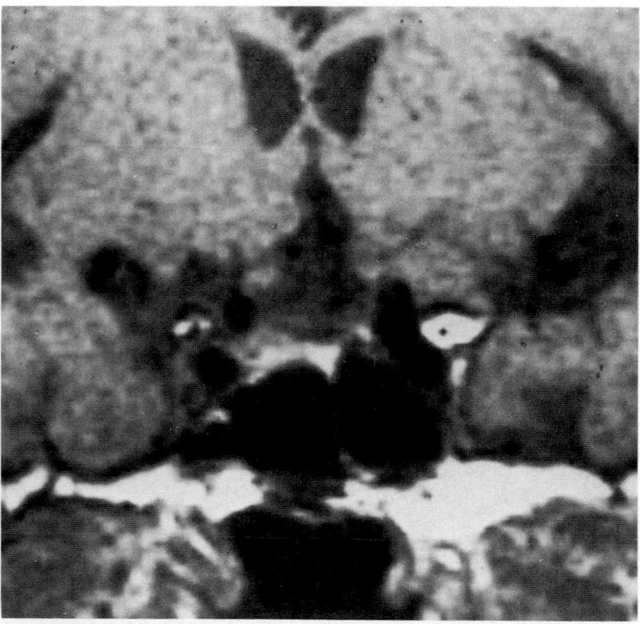

FIG. 41. Meningioma. **A:** Contrast-enhanced coronal T1-weighted image. The tumor enhances intensely, typical of meningiomas. This makes it difficult to separate the tumor from the marrow fat of the anterior clinoid process and the venous enhancement of the cavernous sinus. On this image it appears that the tumor envelops a branch of the carotid artery (*arrows*) and extends inferiorly into the cavernous sinus (*curved arrow*). **B:** Unenhanced coronal T1-weighted image. The meningioma is much less conspicuous on the unenhanced study but its true extent is more obvious. The horizontal band of low signal is, in fact, shown to be the cortical surface of the clinoid process (not an arterial branch) and the tumor does not extend inferiorly; marrow fat is mimicking tumor extension.

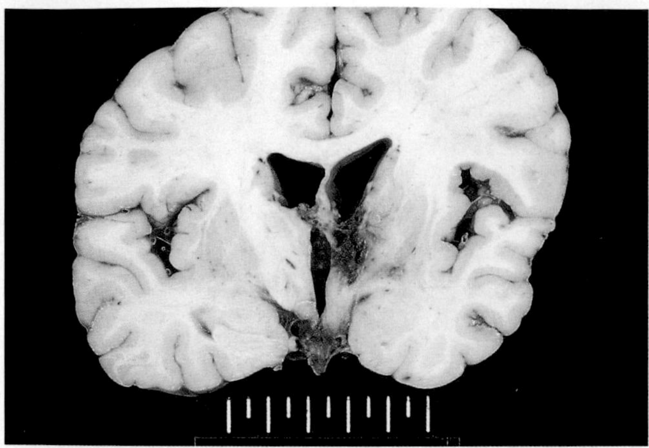

FIG. 42. Germinoma. The tumor is adherent to the hypothalamus. It has spread via the CSF to involve the periventricular region, a well known method of dissemination of the tumor.

Germinoma and Teratoma

Germinomas are tumors of germ cell origin that account for approximately 0.5% to 2% of primary intracranial tumors. Roughly 20% of these occur in the suprasellar cistern or pituitary fossa (113). Other common locations include the pineal region (the most frequent site) and posterior third ventricle. Suprasellar germinomas occur either as a metastatic deposit from a pineal region tumor or arise primarily in the suprasellar cistern (114). Metachronous occurrence in the pineal gland and suprasellar cistern is possible. Germinomas are tumors of children or young adults. Most patients present between 5 and 25 years of age. Pineal germinomas affect males predominantly. No sex predominance is seen in the suprasellar variety.

Most patients present with diabetes insipidus as the earliest symptom. This indicates that the tumor has involved the floor and walls of the third ventricle. Visual field defects and optic atrophy are almost as common. Hydrocephalus, pituitary insufficiency, and diplopia are other frequent manifestations of tumor extension into the parasellar region.

Germinomas are composed of large polygonal germ cells and clusters of lymphocytes in a dense connective tissue stroma. Their histology is similar to ovarian dysgerminoma and testicular seminoma. Other tumors of germ cell origin also occur in this region, including yolk sac tumors, choriocarcinoma, embryonal carcinomas, and teratomas. Suprasellar germinomas are not encapsulated, very infiltrative, adherent to the ventral surface of the brain, and often closely related to the optic nerves. They have a propensity to spread through the subarachnoid space with metastatic deposits to the walls of the ventricles and the basal cisterns (Fig 42).

Most suprasellar germinomas are readily evident on MRI because their size is considerable by the time of clinical presentation. They are typically midline, centered at or just behind the pituitary infundibulum. In

A

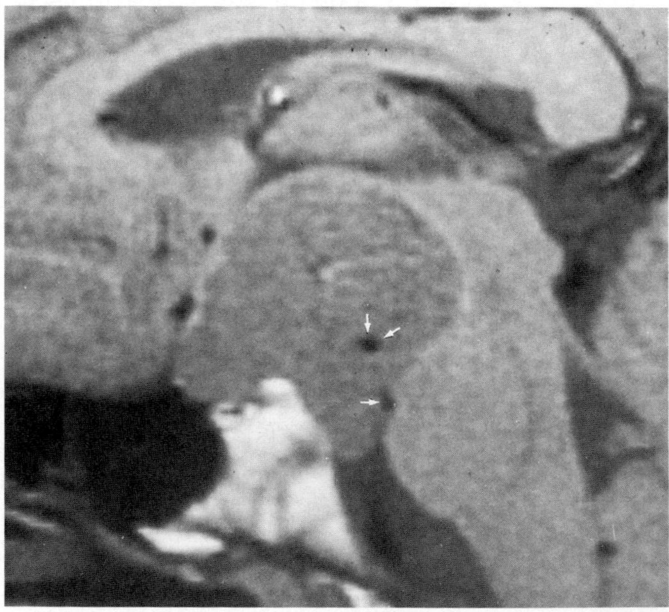

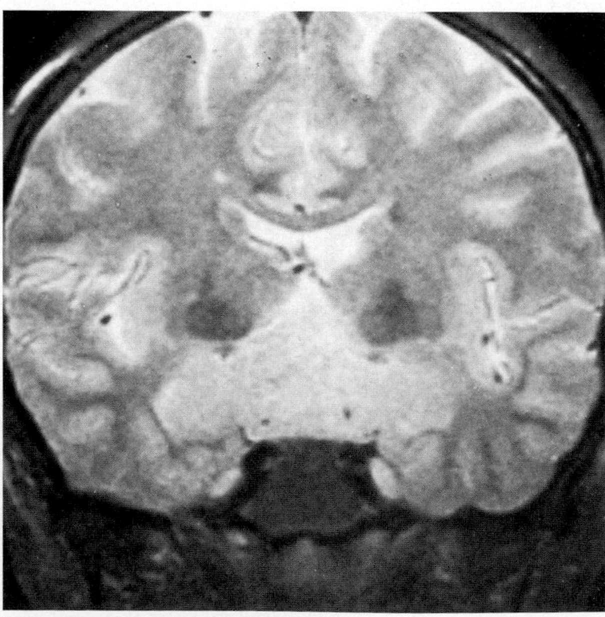

B

FIG. 43. Germinoma. **A:** Sagittal T1-weighted image. This teenaged boy presented with diabetes insipidus. The MRI demonstrates a large suprasellar mass elevating the optic chiasm and floor of the third ventricle. Tongue-like projections of the tumor extend into the sella turcica and prepontine cistern, and encase the basilar artery (*arrows*). The signal intensity is slightly lower than brain and is quite homogeneous. **B:** Coronal T2-weighted image. The tumor is slightly hyperintense compared to cortex. Given the age and clinical presentation of the patient, the suprasellar location of the tumor, and the relative signal uniformity, germinoma is the prime consideration in the differential diagnosis.

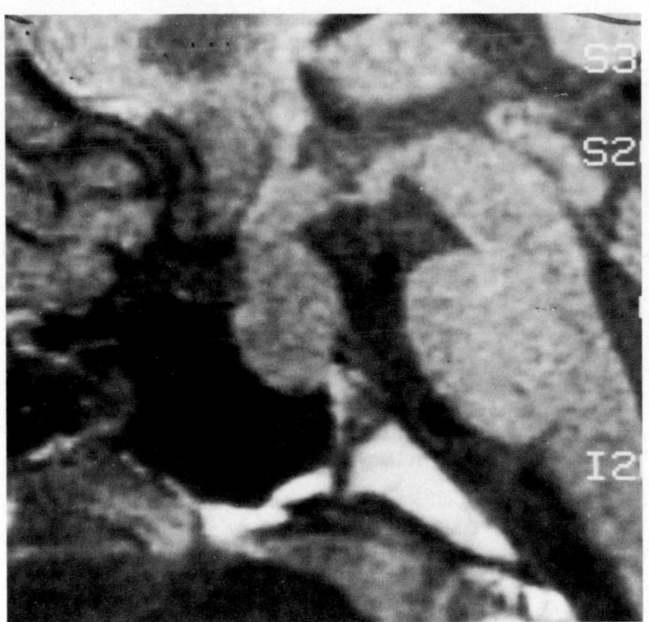

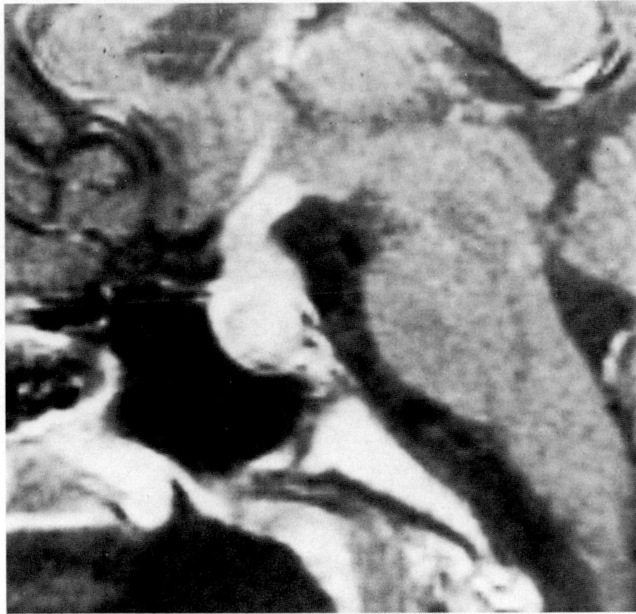

A B

FIG. 44. Germinoma. **A:** Sagittal T1-weighted image. In this case the germinoma completely fills the sella turcica as well as infiltrating the pituitary stalk (note the marked stalk thickening). The signal intensity is identical to the previous case. **B:** Contrast-enhanced T1-weighted image. There is marked uniform enhancement of the tumor.

contrast to craniopharyngiomas, germinomas are homogeneous and only rarely have cystic components. The signal is slightly different from brain: mildly hypointense on T1-weighted images and hyperintense on T2-weighted images (Fig. 43). Marked contrast enhancement is the rule (Fig. 44). If a pineal lesion is discovered in conjunction with a suprasellar lesion in a young person, the diagnosis of germinoma is virtually assured (Fig 45). Teratomas have mixed, heterogeneous signal and most have evidence of fat or calcification.

Epidermoid and Dermoid

Epidermoids and dermoids are benign, slow-growing "inclusion tumors" that can occur intracranially or intraspinally. Epidermoids account for approximately 0.5% to 1.5% of all intracranial neoplasms. Dermoids are approximately one fifth as common. Both of these tumors are thought to result from inclusions of epithelium during the time of neural tube closure during the third to fifth week of embryogenesis (115).

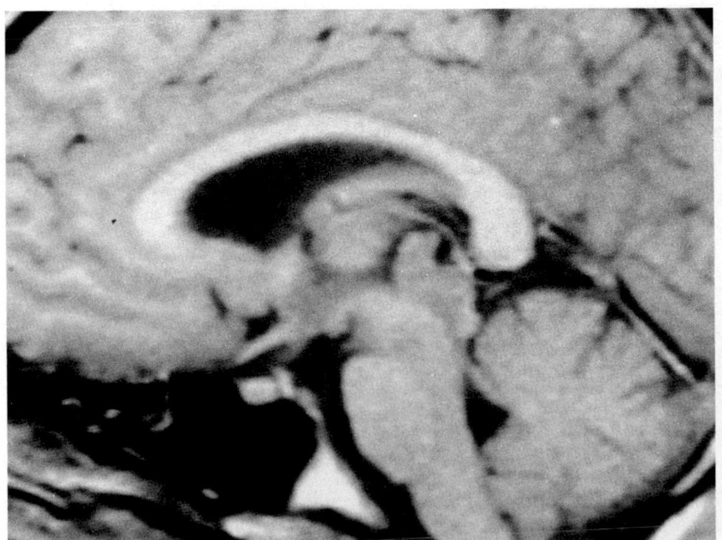

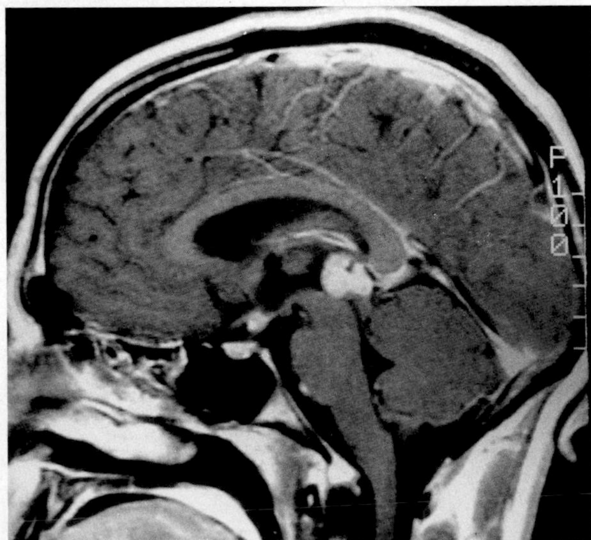

A B

FIG. 45. Germinoma, suprasellar, and pineal. **A:** Unenhanced and, (**B**), enhanced T1-weighted MRI. There are lesions in both the suprasellar cistern and the pineal gland. In this case, the suprasellar component can be diagnosed confidently only on the enhanced study.

Epidermoids are lesions of adulthood, most commonly in the second to fourth decade (115). They are predominantly located in the basal cisterns and are lateral in position. The cerebellopontine angle is the most frequent site of occurrence followed by the parasellar region. The walls of these cysts are composed of simple stratified squamous epithelium resting on an outer layer of connective tissue (59). The interior of the cyst is composed of a waxy material composed of the desquamative keratin products of the cyst wall.

Dermoids are more likely to be discovered in the pediatric age group and are more commonly located in the midline, most frequently in the IVth ventricle or vermis. Less frequently they are in the subfrontal or juxtasellar region. The cyst wall contains various dermal appendages such as hair follicles and sebaceous and sweat glands, in addition to stratified squamous epithelium.

Slow, expansile growth is characteristic of these tumors and they tend to insinuate within and around adjacent neural structures, conforming to the space within which they are situated. They become symptomatic because of compression of neural or vascular structures. Suprasellar tumors most often present with visual disturbances. Less common signs are hypopituitarism, diabe-

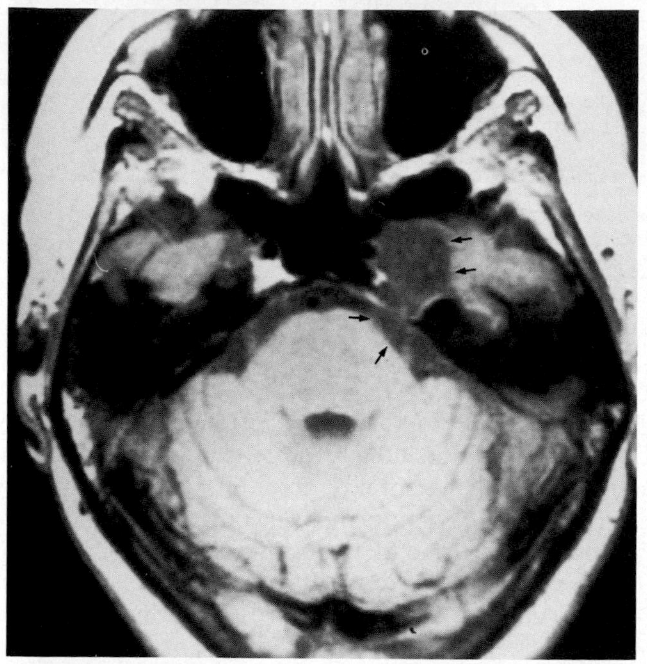
A

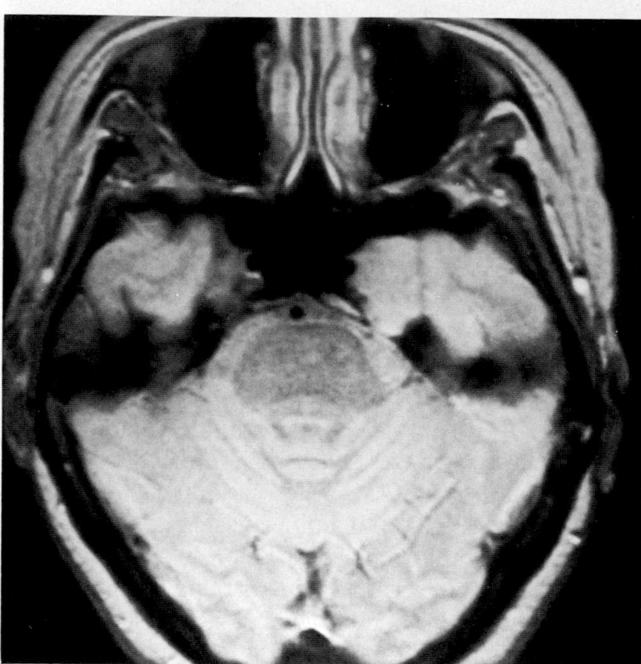
B

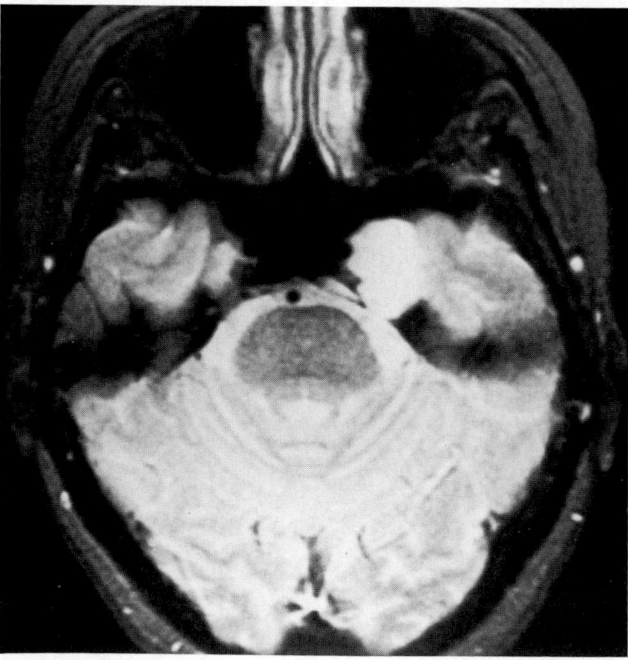
C

FIG. 46. Left paracavernous epidermoid cyst. **A:** Axial T1-weighted image. This 50-year-old woman had a slowly progressive, 20-year history of left facial pain. A cystic lesion is obvious in the medial portion of the left middle cranial fossa, with a small component extending into the left cerebellopontine angle cistern adjacent to the cisternal portion of cranial nerve V (*arrows*). The lesion is well defined and almost identical to CSF in intensity, although close inspection reveals it is not as dark as the CSF. **B,C:** Axial proton density-weighted image and T2-weighted image. The lesion is again only minimally hyperintense compared to CSF on these two sequences. At surgery a typical epidermoid cyst filled with "cheesy, keratinous material" was found and excised. This is the usual signal intensity pattern on MR in epidermoids (i.e., minimally different from CSF) but in most cases the differential signal intensity between epidermoid and CSF is more obvious. In this case a simple arachnoid cyst was the main differential diagnosis.

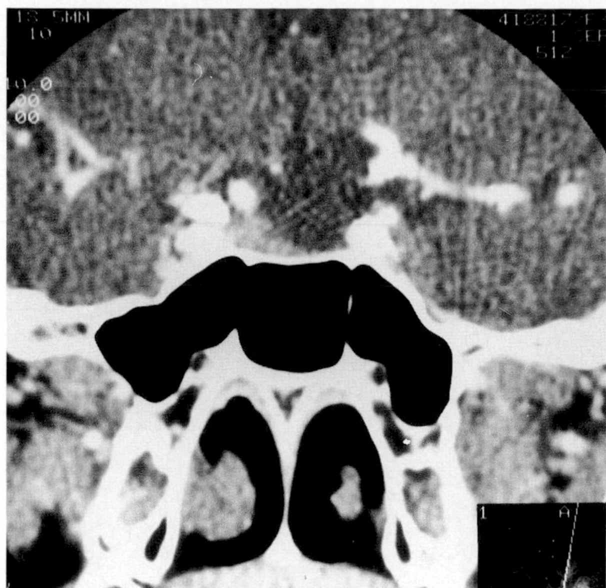

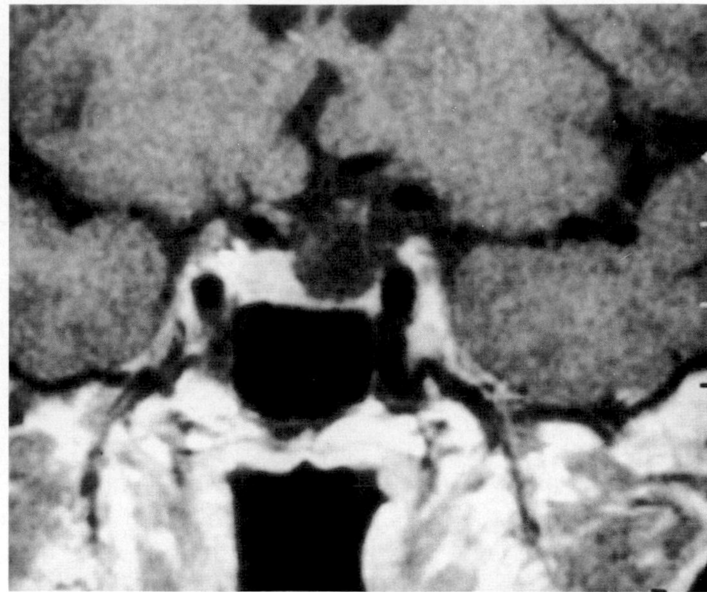

FIG. 47. Epidermoid. **A:** Coronal contrast-enhanced CT and, (**B**), T1-weighted coronal MRI. This patient presented with a visual field defect. There is a 1- to 2-cm mass elevating the optic chiasm on the left and involving the left side of the pituitary gland. The mass is very hypointense but, unlike arachnoid cysts, it has internal strands and reticulations. This internal structure is not apparent on the CT.

tes insipidus, and cranial nerve deficits. Extension laterally into the sylvian fissure or temporal lobe may cause seizures. Rarely, the cyst ruptures and produces a chemical granulomatous meningitis.

Epidermoids are typically slightly hyperintense to CSF on T1- and T2-weighted images but the proton-density image is the most valuable for differential diagnostic purposes. Epidermoids are characteristically hyperintense to brain and CSF on this sequence in distinction to arachnoid cysts, which remain isointense to CSF (116–123). Unfortunately, this is not an infallible criterion—we have encountered cases in which epidermoids are identical to CSF on all sequences (Fig. 46). Other features include a slightly inhomogeneous internal architecture and scalloped margins (Fig. 47). Calcification is very rare. Enhancement occurs only along the periphery.

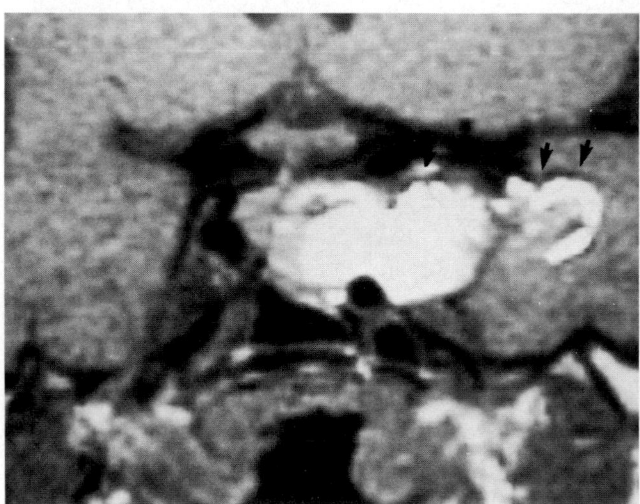

FIG. 48. Intrasellar/parasellar dermoid. Coronal T1-weighted image. A hyperintense mass is located in the sella turcica, superior portion of the left cavernous sinus, and mesial left temporal lobe. Note the chemical shift artifact along the superior aspect of the lesion (the frequency-encoding direction is in the superior-inferior direction) (*arrows*). This artifact identifies fat (rather than hemorrhage) as the source of the high intensity signal. The patient had only minimal symptoms (partial cranial nerve III palsy).

Dermoids are more heterogeneous (117). Most have evidence of a fatty component (hyperintense on T1-weighted images) and small areas of dense calcification (Figs. 48 and 49), but on those occasions when fat or calcium are not in the tumor, dermoids may mimic the appearance of epidermoids, or even arachnoid cysts.

Chiasmatic and Hypothalamic Glioma

The distinction between chiasmatic and hypothalamic gliomas often depends on the predominant position of the lesion. In many cases the origin of larger gliomas cannot be definitively determined as the hypothalamus and chiasm are inseparable; therefore, hypothalamic and chiasmatic gliomas are discussed as a single entity. These tumors are for the most part tumors of childhood; 75% occur in the first decade of life. There is an equal male to female distribution. There is a definite association of optic nerve and chiasmatic gliomas with neurofibromatosis, more so for tumors that arise from the optic nerve rather than from the chiasm or hypothalamus. Tumors of chiasmal origin are also more aggressive than those originating from the optic nerves and tend to in-

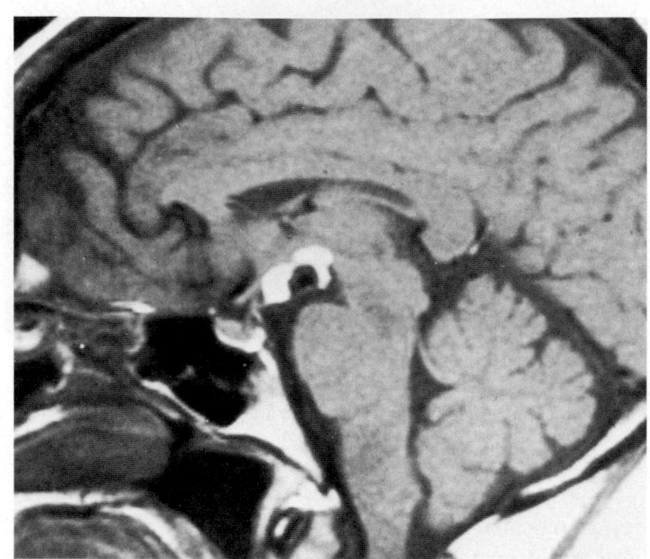

A

FIG. 49. Suprasellar dermoid. **A:** Sagittal T1-weighted image. The lesion has two components. The largest is predominantly fatty (high signal) with a smaller central area of marked hypointensity corresponding to a dense calcific nodule. **B,C:** Axial T1-weighted image and T2-weighted image. Typical of fat-containing lesions, the signal decays to a very low level on the long TE study (T2-weighted). Compare the signal intensity of the lesion to that of subcutaneous fat.

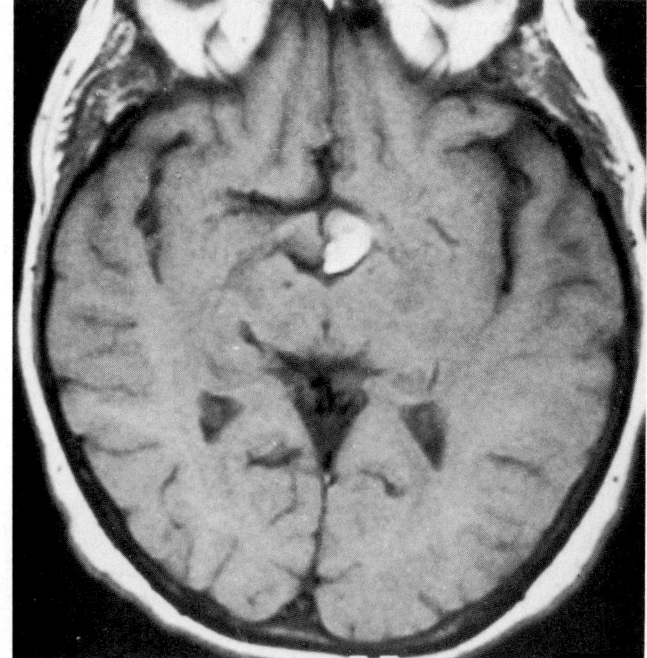

B

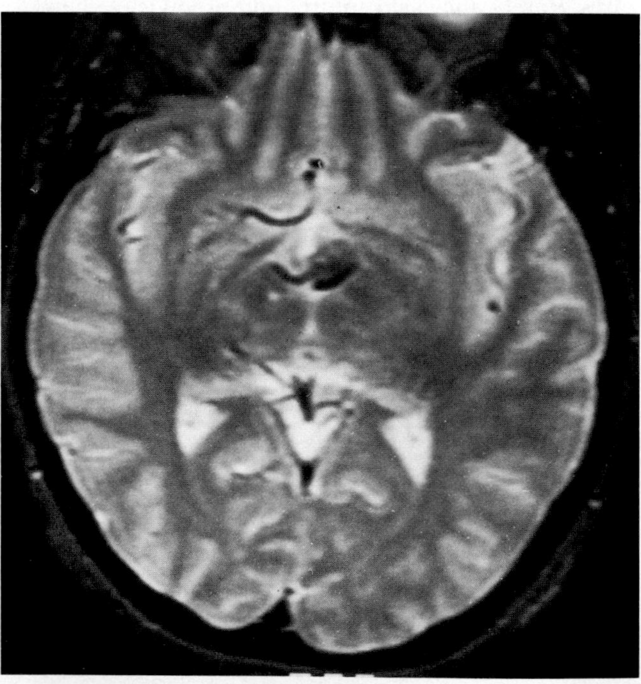

C

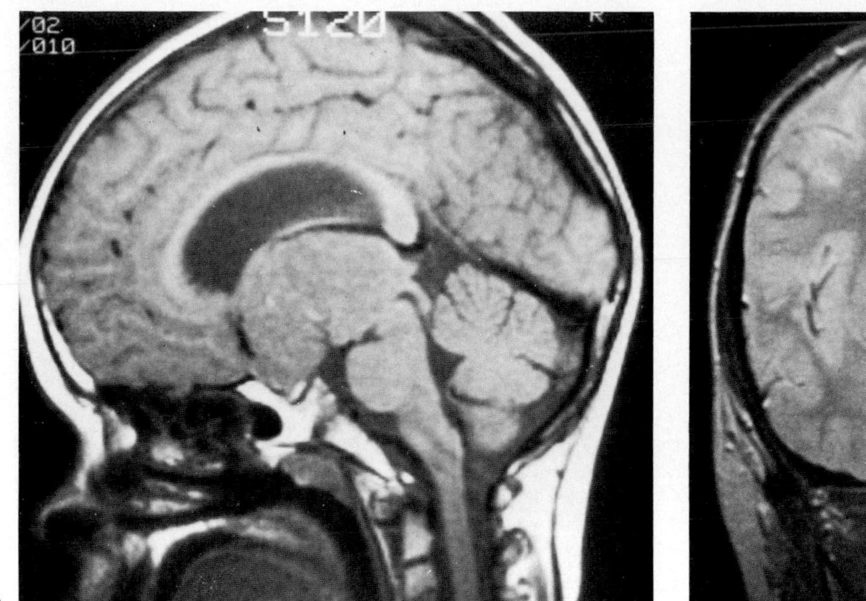

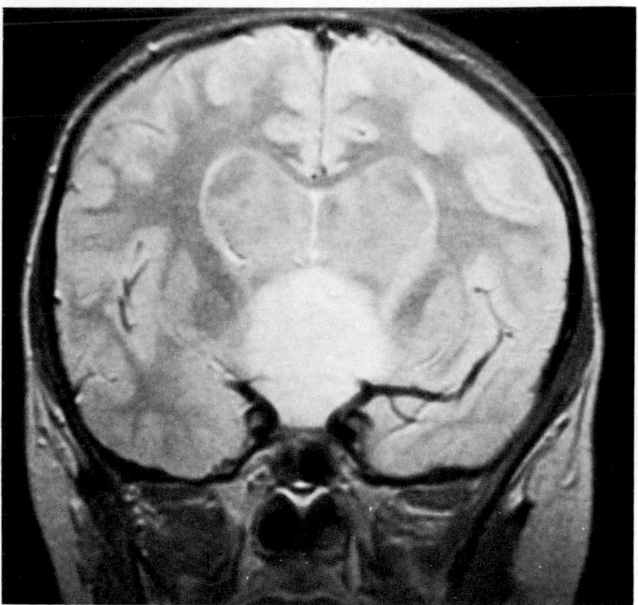

FIG. 50. Hypothalamic glioma. A,B: Sagittal T1-weighted image and coronal T2-weighted image. A huge mass involves both hypothalami and the optic chiasm, and fills the suprasellar cistern. There is also obstructive hydrocephalus. The tumor is hypointense on the T1- and hyperintense on the T2-weighted image, a signal pattern common to most intra-axial tumors. With large tumors such as these, it is impossible to determine whether the hypothalamus or the optic chiasm is the primary site of origin.

vade the hypothalamus and floor of the third ventricle and cause hydrocephalus. Patients suffer from monocular or binocular visual disturbances, hydrocephalus, or hypothalamic dysfunction (124).

The appearance of the tumor depends on its position and direction of growth. It can be confined to either the chiasm or the hypothalamus; however, because of their slow growth the tumor has usually attained a considerable size by the time of presentation and the site of origin is frequently conjectural (Fig. 50). Smaller nerve and chi-

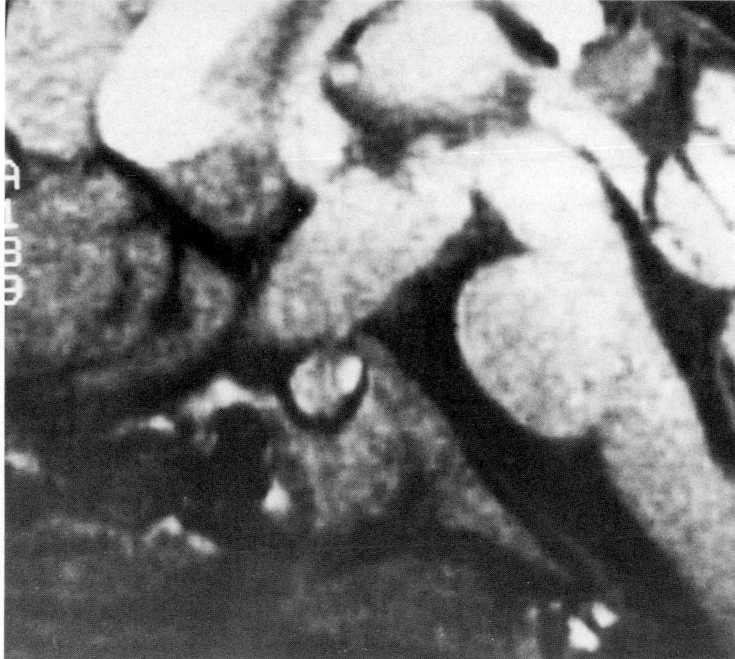

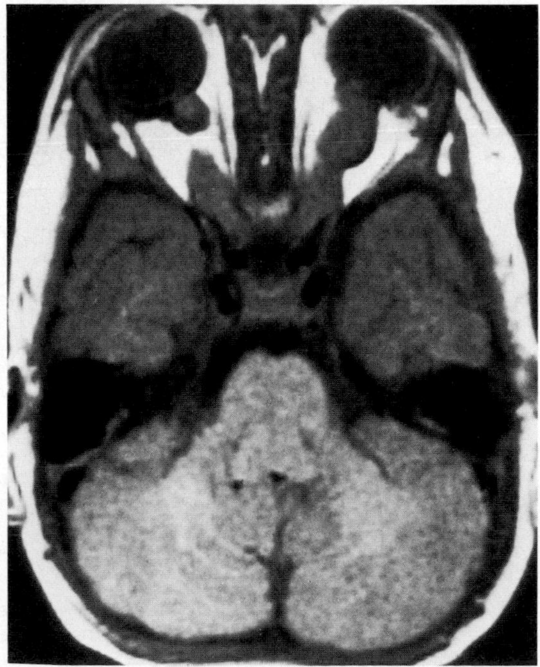

FIG. 51. Optic glioma. A: Sagittal T1-weighted image. The chiasm and floor of the third ventricle are thickened by tumor. B: Axial T1-weighted image. The tumor extends along both optic nerves all the way to the globes. The nerves are thick and tortuous. Optic nerve extension generally does not occur with tumors of hypothalamic origin and is a good indicator that the neoplasm is primarily from the chiasm or nerves.

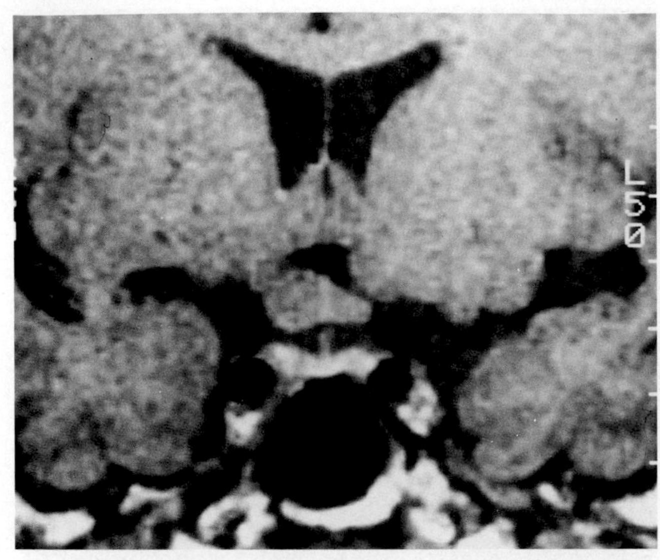

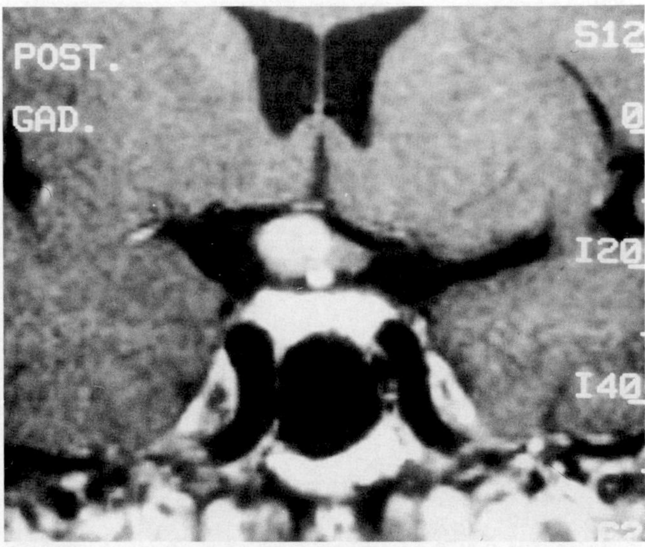

FIG. 52. Optic chiasm glioma. **A:** Coronal T1-weighted and, (**B**), coronal enhanced MRI. There is marked enlargement and enhancement of the right side of the optic chiasm with a clear plane of separation between the chiasm and the hypothalamus.

asmal tumors are visually distinct from the hypothalamus and their site of origin is more clear-cut (Figs. 51 and 52). From the point of view of differential diagnosis, these smaller tumors can be difficult to distinguish from optic neuritis, which can also cause optic nerve enlargement. The clinical history is important in these cases (neuritis is painful, tumor is not) and, if necessary, interval follow-up of neuritis will demonstrate resolution of optic nerve swelling (Fig. 53). T1-weighted images are most often isointense with moderate hyperintensity on T2 weighting. Calcification and hemorrhage are not features of these gliomas but cysts are seen, particularly in

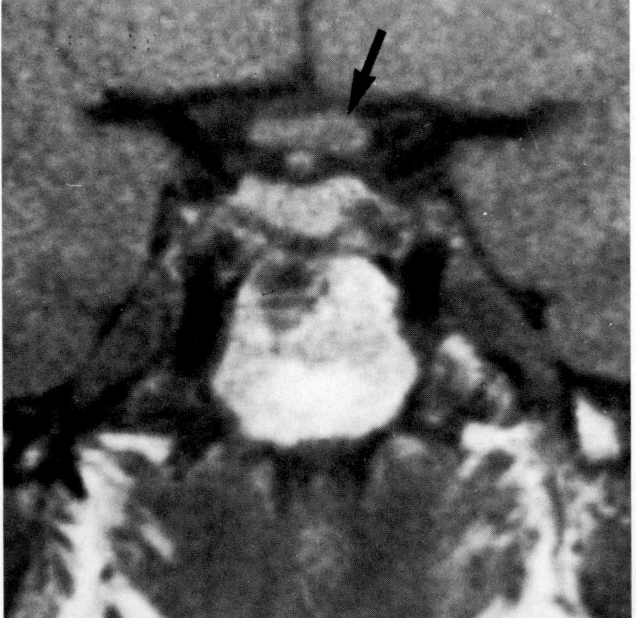

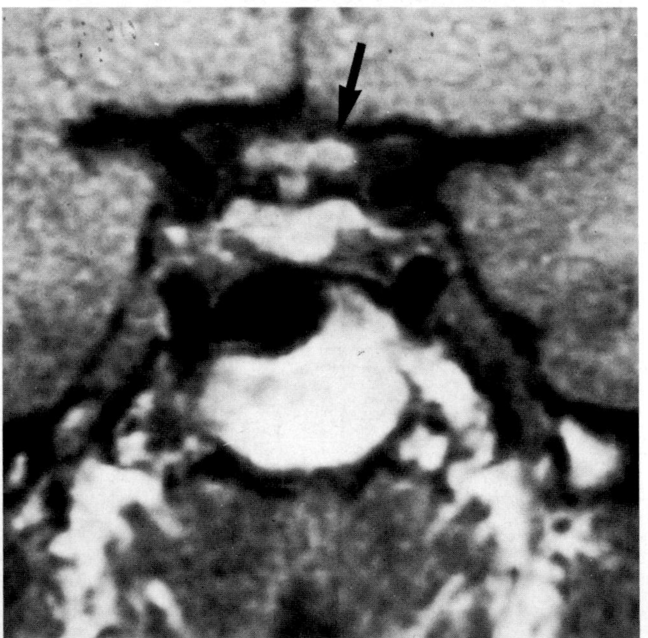

FIG. 53. Optic neuritis. **A:** Coronal T1-weighted image. This young adult gentleman suffered from a 2-month history of painless progressive visual loss in the left eye. Ophthalmoscopic examination was normal. The MRI shows definite enlargement of the left optic nerve with reduction in signal intensity (*arrow*). This same area was hyperintense on the T2-weighted image (not shown). The differential diagnosis was between an atypical neuritis (atypical because there was progressive visual loss and no pain) and an early optic nerve glioma. **B:** Four-month follow-up study. After several months the patient's symptoms resolved and a repeat MRI demonstrates that the left optic nerve has returned to normal size (*arrow*). This is the expected temporal evolution in the appearance of neuritis and differentiates neuritis from a glioma. Glioma would show no change in size or progressive enlargement with time.

the larger hypothalamic tumors. Contrast enhancement occurs in about half of all cases. Because of their known propensity to invade the brain along the optic radiations, T2-weighted images of the entire brain are necessary. This pattern of tumor extension is readily evident as hyperintensity on the T2-weighted image; however, patients with neurofibromatosis (NF) present a problem in differential diagnosis (Fig. 54). This is because there is a high incidence of benign cerebral hamartomas and/or atypical glial cell rests in NF that can exactly mimic glioma. These gliomas can be confused with these benign lesions that also occur in the optic radiations (125,126). Lack of interval growth and possibly the presence or absence of contrast enhancement are the best means of differentiating the two entities.

Chordoma

Cranial chordomas are rare intracranial neoplasms derived from remnants of the primitive notochord. They account for about 0.2% of intracranial tumors and are more common in males. The mean age of presentation is 38 years, but these tumors can present at any age. Almost all cranial chordomas are found in relation to the clivus, although rare lesions may be found exclusively in the pituitary fossa or laterally in the petrous bone.

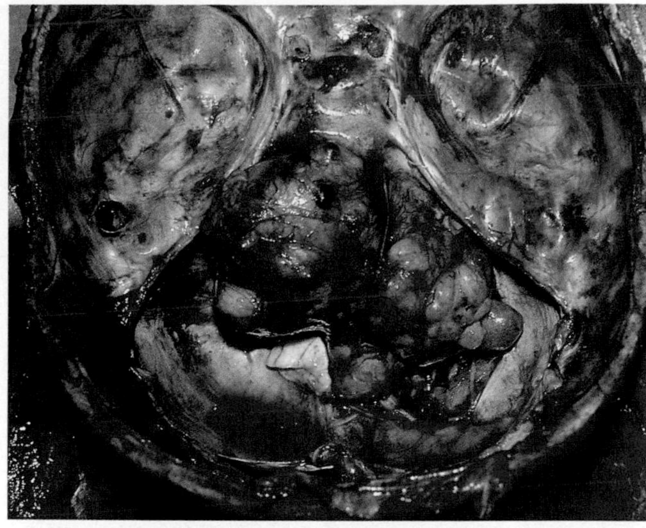

FIG. 55. Chordoma. The brain has been removed and the tumor is viewed from above. The tumor arises from the clivus but has grown exophytically out of the bone into the retroclival portion of the posterior fossa. Note the multiple lobulations.

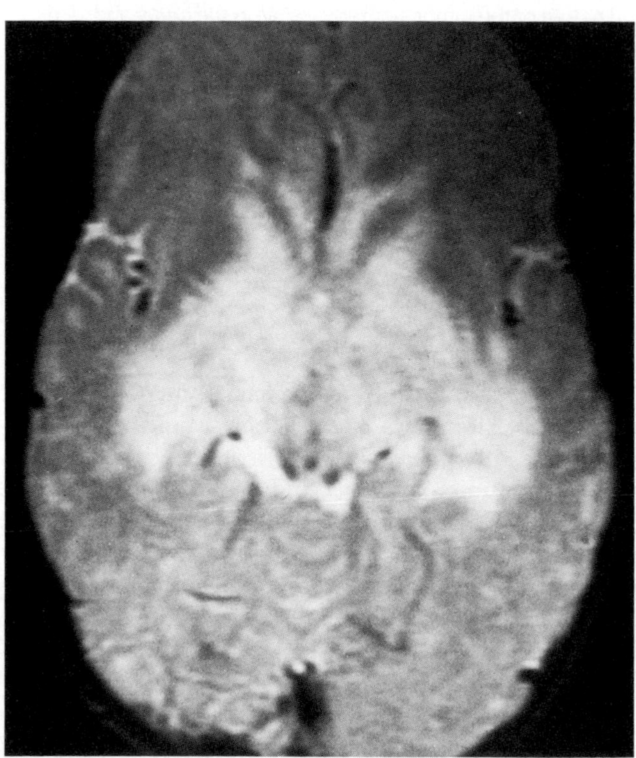

FIG. 54. Neurofibromatosis. Axial proton density–weighted image. This child with neurofibromatosis had bilateral optic nerve gliomas. MRI demonstrated multiple lesions in the cerebrum, diencephalon, brainstem, and cerebellum. A representative section through the optic radiations is shown here. Large bilateral lesions are obvious. This appearance should not be automatically accepted as evidence of tumor infiltration into the optic radiations. That is a significant possibility, but the alternative diagnosis of hamartomas, dysplasia, or atypical glial cell rests should be considered in the differential diagnosis. Interval follow-up is probably the best means of refining the differential diagnosis to the point of confirming or excluding the presence of tumor. The significance of contrast enhancement in this type of abnormality is still uncertain.

These tumors form soft, lobulated, gray masses that are histologically benign but locally invasive and destructive (103). They are composed of clear cells with large intracytoplasmic vacuoles. Thick strands of fibrous connective tissue can give the mass a "lobular" appearance.

Chordomas of the sella or parasellar region present with visual disturbances, pituitary insufficiency, or cavernous sinus syndrome. Lesions of the body of clivus can extend ventrally and present as a parapharyngeal mass, or extend dorsally and cause cranial nerve palsies, brainstem compression, or hydrocephalus (Fig. 55). Lateral clival chordomas may present as a mass in the cerebellopontine angle.

Chordomas are characteristically isointense (75%) or hypointense (25%) on T1-weighted MRI sequences (127). Extension into the marrow space of the clivus with replacement of the normal high signal of marrow fat is clearly shown. There is moderate to extreme hyperintensity on the T2-weighted sequence. Septations composed of fibrous connective tissue form low intensity strands separating lobulated areas of high intensity of T2-weighted images (Fig. 56). MRI is superior to CT in delineating the full extent of the tumor, the relationship to the adjacent neurovascular structures, and extension along the epidural space. However, residual ossified fragments, tumor calcification, and the status of the cortical bone of the clivus is less adequately shown.

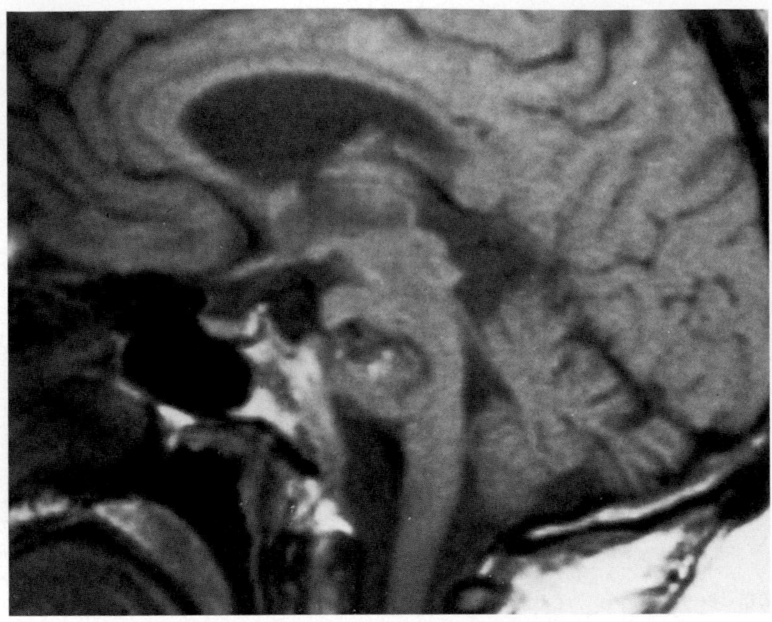

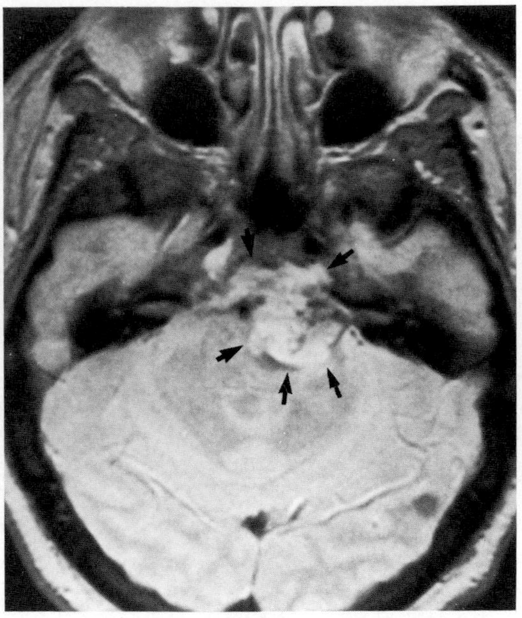

FIG. 56. Chordoma. **A:** Sagittal T1-weighted image. The normally high signal intensity clivus is permeated by the chordoma, which extends in an exophytic manner into the prepontine cistern and displaces the brainstem dorsally. **B:** Axial proton density–weighted image. The irregular, lobulated nature of the tumor is clearly visible in the clivus and in the posterior fossa (*arrows*).

Ecchordosis

Ecchordosis refers to a nodule of benign cells of notochordal origin, usually the size of a pea, that occurs in or attached to the clivus (Fig. 57). Although related to chordoma embryologically, ecchordosis differs from chordoma in that it is not a neoplasm and has no potential for growth or dissemination. We have scanned one proven case (not the case illustrated above). The patient was a woman who presented with CSF rhinorrhea. MRI demonstrated a 1-cm nodule in the midline of a congenitally thin clivus. The nodule bridged the prepontine cistern and sphenoid sinus. It was dark on T1 weighting and bright on T2 weighting, without the whorls or heterogeneity visible in many chordomas. We are unaware of any MRI literature describing this entity.

FIG. 57. Ecchordosis. This view of the inferior aspect of the brain demonstrates a pea-sized nubbin of notochordal tissue.

Choristoma

Choristoma (also referred to as 'granular cell tumor' and 'myoblastoma') is a rare neoplasm of the neurohypophysis. Although small 'choristoma nests' are relatively common autopsy findings, neoplasms large enough to cause symptoms are rare. They are composed of large polygonal cells with small nuclei and granular cytoplasm. Presenting symptoms include decreased vision and pituitary endocrine hypofunction. Since these lesions can be extremely vascular, the preoperative diagnosis is important to surgical planning. The transsphenoidal approach can be hazardous with choristomas because of their propensity to bleed extensively. MRI features are nonspecific, demonstrating a well defined mass within the sella, often extending into the suprasellar cistern. The specific anatomic site of the mass is the most telling feature; in fact, the diagnosis should be suspected when the pituitary mass is situated posteriorly within the gland and the normal posterior lobe hyperintensity cannot be identified. Of course, the most common posteriorly situated pituitary tumor is still the adenoma. No "typical" signal intensity pattern of choristoma can be described because of the rarity of these lesions. There is a single case report; the tumor was isointense to brain on

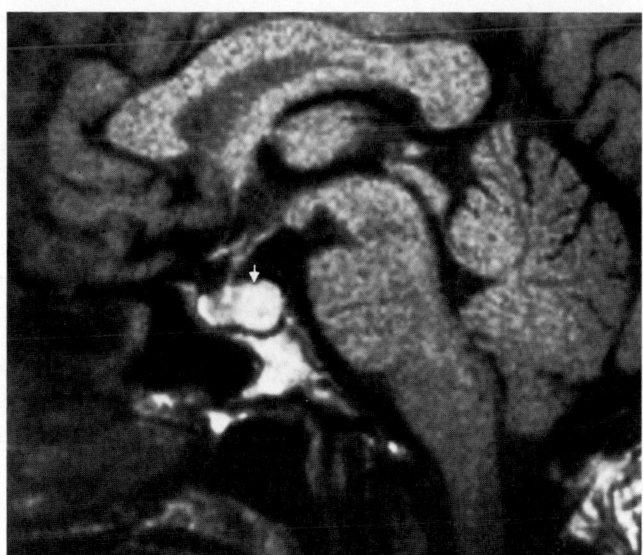

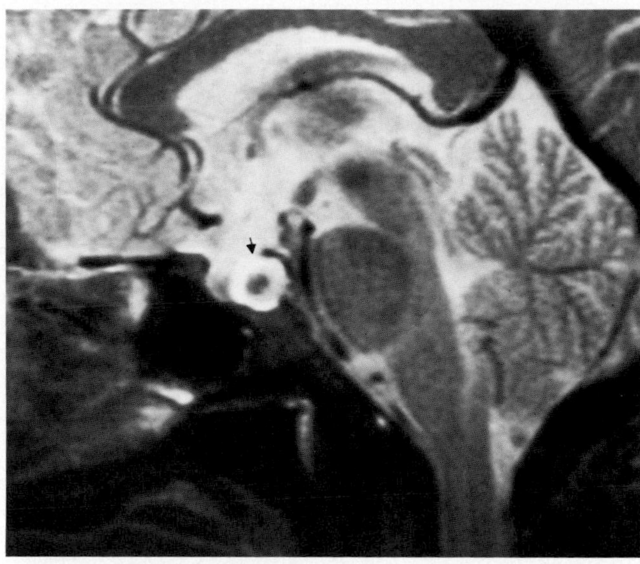

FIG. 58. Choristoma. Sagittal T1-weighted image. **A** shows a posterior pituitary mass (*arrow*), which is hyperintense. Note absence of the normal thin hyperintensity, which corresponds to posterior lobe in normal glands. The tumor is heterogeneous on T2-weighted image (**B**).

both T1- and T2-weighted sequences (128). The case illustrated here (Fig. 58) shows hyperintensity throughout the tumor on T1-weighted images and heterogeneity on T2-weighted images.

Schwannoma

Intracranial schwannomas occasionally occur in the region of the pituitary fossa and present as a parasellar mass. In general, these benign tumors originate from the sensory nerves. The most common site is from the vestibular division of the eighth cranial nerve in the internal auditory canal. The fifth cranial nerve is the second most common site of intracranial "neuroma" and the most frequent cranial nerve tumor to cause a parasellar mass (129,130).

The most common clinical finding is a sensory disturbance in the distribution of the affected cranial nerve. Weakness of the muscles of mastication, or facial pain, are less common. Diplopia may result from compression of adjacent cranial nerves in the cavernous sinus. Unsteadiness, dizziness, vertigo, and multiple palsies of the lower cranial nerves can be caused by compression of posterior fossa structures.

The most characteristic feature of neuromas is that they follow the course of the nerve from which they arise (Fig. 59). By and large they are isointense to brain on T1-weighted images and hyperintense on T2-weighted images. Small tumors are homogeneous; large tumors frequently have heterogeneous internal signal. Like meningiomas, they enhance intensely.

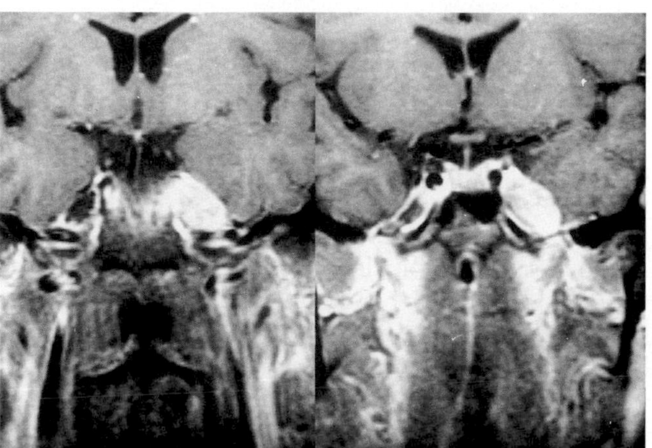

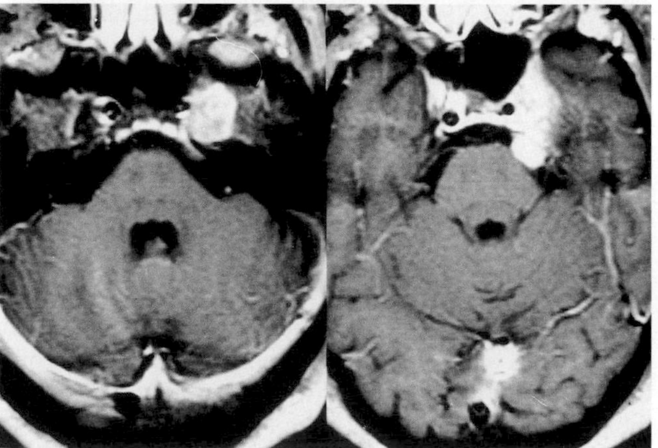

FIG. 59. Left fifth nerve schwannoma. Axial and coronal contrast-enhanced images. The tumor is situated in the cistern and Meckel's cave. Contrast enhancement greatly facilitates determining the full extent of the tumor.

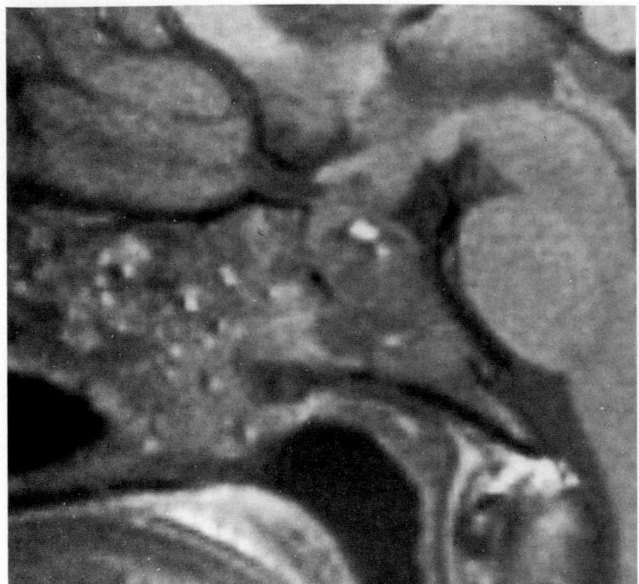

FIG. 60. Metastatic breast carcinoma. Sagittal T1-weighted image. A heterogeneous destructive tumor mass fills the sphenoid sinus and posterior ethmoid sinuses, and infiltrates the clivus and pituitary gland and stalk (note the stalk thickening). The loss of tissue planes is an indication of an aggressive lesion.

Metastases

One to five percent of cancer patients have symptomatic metastases to the pituitary gland. These are primarily patients with advanced, disseminated malignancy, particularly breast and bronchogenic carcinoma. The vast majority die of their underlying disease before becoming symptomatic of pituitary disease. Autopsy series have demonstrated a much higher incidence, but these by and large are small and asymptomatic lesions.

Intrasellar and juxtasellar metastases arise via hematogenous seeding to the brain (in the hypothalamus or medial temporal lobes), or to the dura around the sphenoid bone, by CSF seeding, and by direct extension from head and neck neoplasia. There are no distinctive MRI characteristics of metastases, although bone destruction is a prominent feature (Fig. 60).

TUMOR-LIKE CONDITIONS

Arachnoid Cyst

Arachnoid cysts are frequent incidental findings on cranial MRI and are most common in the anterior one third of the temporal fossa. Approximately 15% are in the juxtasellar region (122). Suprasellar arachnoid cysts are thought to be developmental in origin and arise from an imperforate membrane of Liliequist in the suprasellar cistern. This causes a relative obstruction of CSF flow. The membrane develops into a diverticulum and further expansion may cause it to lose its communication with the subarachnoid space, thus forming a cyst (131).

Most patients with symptomatic cysts present in infancy with signs of hydrocephalus. Smaller cysts that do not obstruct the CSF pathways present later with seizures, hypopituitarism, or compression of adjacent neural structures.

The MRI examination demonstrates a homogeneous, well-marginated lesion that is isointense to CSF on all imaging sequences (122,123). There is no abnormal signal intensity in the nearby neural structures. Presence of a long-standing suprasellar arachnoid cyst can also result in remodeling of the skull base. They show no calcification in the cyst wall and there is no enhancement. Isointensity on all sequences differentiates this lesion from other suprasellar cystic masses such as epidermoid and craniopharyngioma. Similar MRI appearances may occur with parasitic or ependymal cysts.

Tuber Cinereum Hamartoma

Tuber cinereum hamartomas are sessile or pedunculated masses attached to the posterior hypothalamus between the pituitary stalk and mammillary bodies (Fig. 61). They are composed of disorganized neural tissue often resembling cerebral cortex with little histologic similarity to normal hypothalamus. They are not neoplasms. Although they do not invade surrounding tissues, they do have the potential for slow growth and may be quite large. The most frequent presenting complaint is that of precocious puberty.

Hamartomas have been consistently reported as isointense to gray matter on T1-weighted MRI, but isointensity and hyperintensity have both been reported as features on T2-weighted images (132–134). One large series

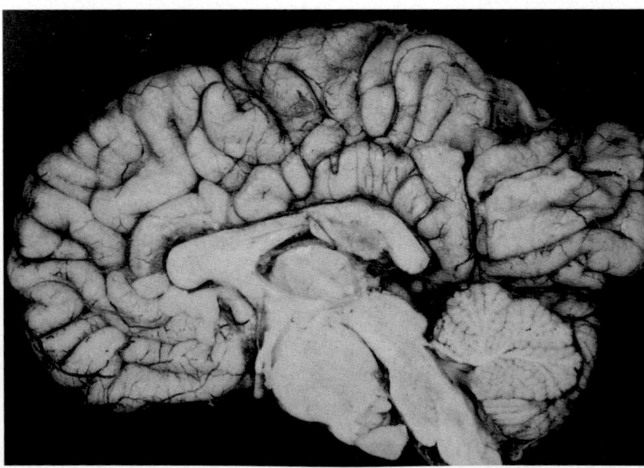

FIG. 61. Large hypothalamic hamartoma. On sagittal section, the attachment site of the tumor to the floor of third ventricle immediately posterior to the pituitary stalk is clearly seen. The optic chiasm is elevated and compressed.

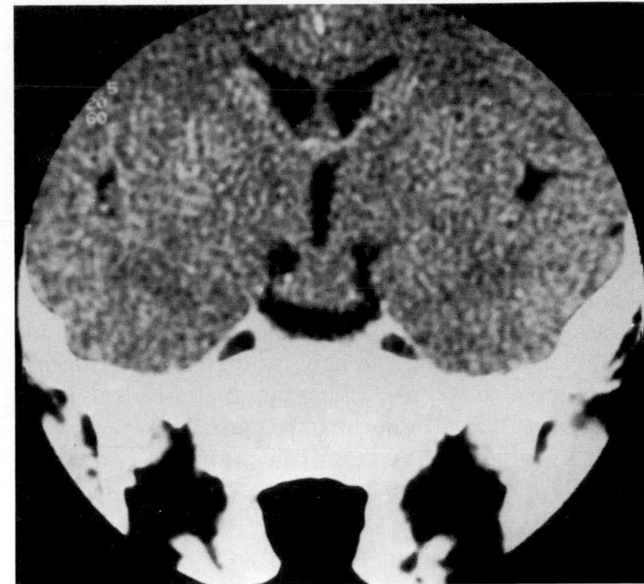

FIG. 62. Hypothalamic hamartoma. **A–D:** Coronal contrast-enhanced CT, sagittal T1-weighted image, coronal T2-weighted image, and sagittal contrast-enhanced MRI. The features of a hypothalamic hamartoma are well illustrated here: well defined margins, origin from the tuber cinereum (posterior to the stalk), lack of contrast enhancement, and signal that is isointense to brain on both T1- and T2-weighted images. **E:** Autopsy specimen, coronal section. This pathology specimen is a different case than the MRI shown in A–D, but it has a strikingly similar morphology, displaying the typical appearance of a small pedunculated hamartoma. Note that the brain parenchyma and the hamartoma have a similar coloration and gross appearance.

A

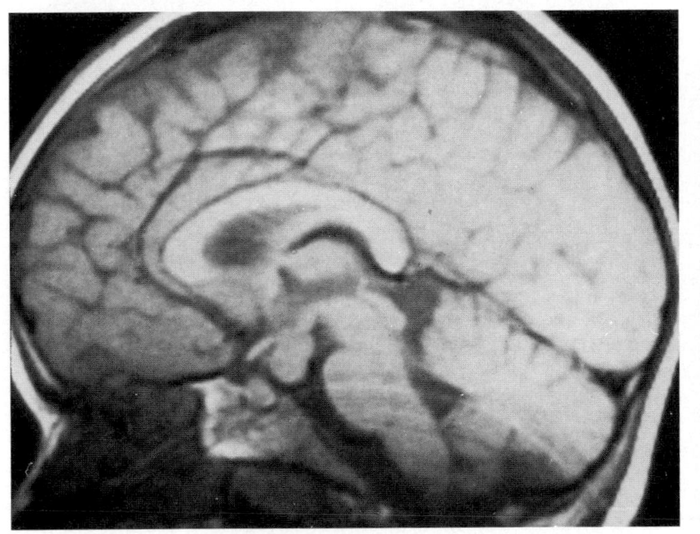

B

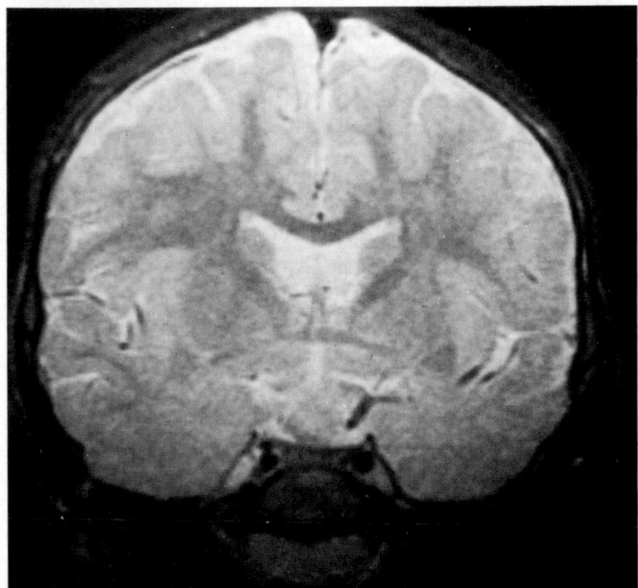

C

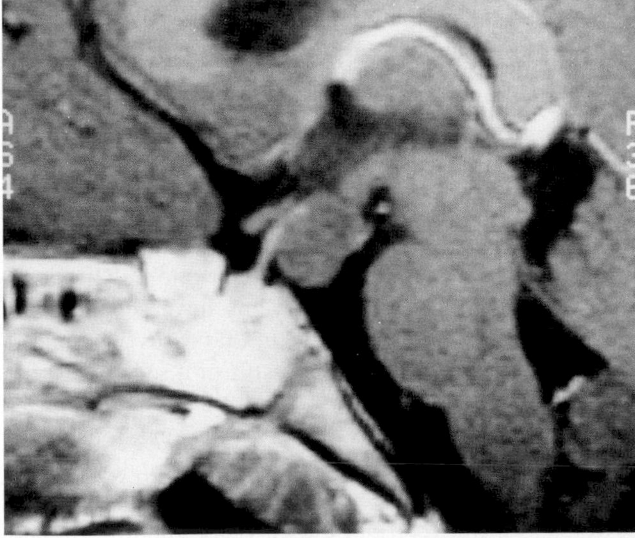

D

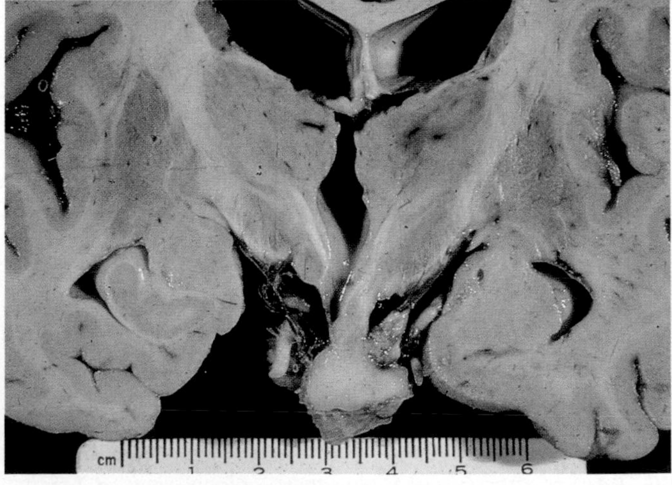

E

of cases noted that 80% of lesions were hyperintense to grey matter (135). No lesions changed in size during a mean follow-up of 5.4 years. Our own experience with three cases has been that hamartomas are isointense to gray matter on all sequences (Fig. 62). Contrast enhancement should not occur as hamartomas should possess an intact blood–brain barrier, equivalent to that of normal brain tissue. There is some controversy as to whether this is an inviolable rule, and it could even be argued that because the blood–brain barrier in the normal tuber cinereum is permeable, tuber cinereum hamartomas should enhance. However, hamartomas are not histologically similar to the tuber cinereum; therefore, this argument seems weak. In our own practice, we would view contrast enhancement in any hypothalamic mass as atypical for hamartoma, and would watch it closely.

Eosinophilic Granulomatosis (Histiocytosis X)

This is a group of diseases characterized by proliferation of histiocytes (macrophages). The term in popular usage, "histiocytosis X," has been supplanted. The preferred terms now are "eosinophilic granulomatosis" or "Langerhans' cell granulomatosis", the Langerhans' cell being the common cell in all these disorders (136–138). There are unifocal and multifocal forms of this disease. Unifocal eosinophilic granulomatosis is a benign disease characterized by a solitary lytic bone lesion. Although the skull may be the site of involvement, the hypothalamic pituitary axis is spared. Multifocal eosinophilic granulomatosis is a more aggressive disorder, usually occurring in childhood. Twenty-five percent of cases develop the classical clinical triad of diabetes insipidus, exophthalmos, and lytic bone lesions (the Hand-Schüller-Christian syndrome). In these cases granulomas may be found in the hypothalamus or pituitary stalk (Fig. 63). CT demonstrates thickening and enhancement of the involved structures. MRI findings include thickening of the pituitary stalk and hyperintensity on T2-weighted images (Fig. 64) (137,139). Involved areas display intense contrast enhancement (140). Diagnosis is by biopsy of one of the bone lesions.

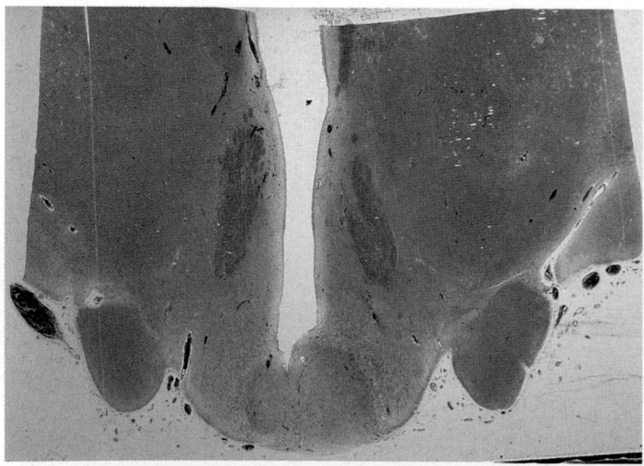

FIG. 63. Langerhans' cell histiocytosis (coronal view, H & E stain). There is thickening and infiltration of the hypothalamus, in the region of the floor of the third ventricle (*arrows*).

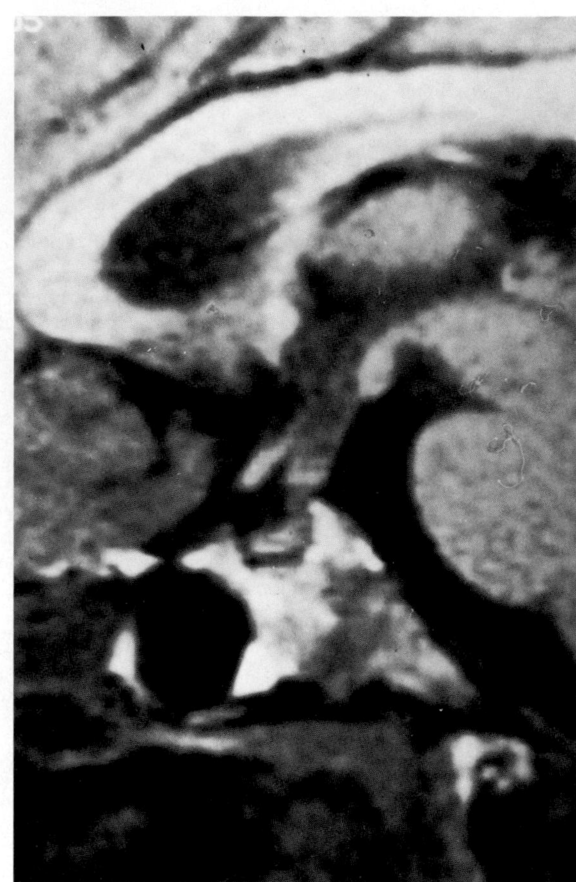

FIG. 64. Eosinophilic granuloma. Sagittal T1-weighted image. This 12-year-old boy presented with diabetes insipidus. The pituitary stalk is abnormally thick and the normal signal intensity of the posterior pituitary is absent. Diagnosis was made by biopsy of a bone lesion. (Courtesy of Dr. Donald Lee, University of Western Ontario.)

INFLAMMATORY LESIONS

Infections

Infections of the pituitary gland, regardless of etiologic agent, are distinctly uncommon. For example, direct viral infection of the hypophysis has never been established. There has been speculation that cases of acquired diabetes insipidus may be the result of a select viral infection of the hypothalamic supraoptic and paraventricular nuclei. Tuberculosis and syphilis, previously encountered in this region because of the higher general prevalence of these diseases in the population, are now rare (141). Even bacterial infections are uncommon and usually only become clinically manifest once an abscess has formed.

Pituitary Abscess

Gram-positive cocci are the most frequently identified organisms in pituitary abscesses, although the entity itself is rare. The infection may be blood borne or spread into the sella turcica contiguously from an infected sphenoid or cavernous sinus. Pituitary abscesses usually occur in the presence of other sellar masses such as pituitary adenomas, Rathke's cleft cysts, and craniopharyngiomas, indicating that these mass lesions function as predisposing factors to infection (142,143). Surprisingly, transsphenoidal surgery is rarely complicated by infection, presumably because of the effectiveness of perioperative prophylactic antibiotics.

Clinically, abscesses have similar presentations to large nonfunctioning adenomas, headache and visual loss being the most common symptoms. Systemic signs of sepsis are uncommon. There are few reports on CT of pituitary abscesses. These indicate that the lesion is similar in appearance to an adenoma. Because of the frequent coincidental occurrence of abscesses with adenomas, and because of their common clinical presentations, the correct preoperative diagnosis of abscess is difficult and rarely made. Noncontrast MRI demonstrates a sellar mass indistinguishable from an adenoma. With i.v. contrast there is rim enhancement of the mass with persistence of low intensity in the center (Fig. 65). Hopefully, contrast-enhanced MRI will prove beneficial if, as with abscesses in other sites, the rim enhancement is a common and distinctive feature.

Parasellar Infections

Infection in the suprasellar cistern and cavernous sinuses is usually part of a disseminated process, or occurs by means of intracranial extension of an extracranial infection. The basal meninges in and around the suprasellar cistern are susceptible to tuberculous and other forms of granulomatous meningitis (Fig. 66). The cistern may also be the site of parasitic cysts, in particular cysticercosis (Fig. 67) (144,145). Infection of the cavernous sinus, albeit rare, is usually secondary to venous spread of a septic embolus from a periorbital or perinasal source such as a furuncle with resultant cavernous sinus thrombophlebitis.

NONINFECTIOUS INFLAMMATORY LESIONS

Lymphocytic Hypophysitis

Lymphocytic hypophysitis is a rare, noninfectious inflammatory disorder of the pituitary gland. It occurs almost exclusively in women and particularly during late pregnancy or in the postpartum period. It is probably an autoimmune disorder; many cases are associated with other autoimmune endocrine disorders such as Hashimoto's thyroiditis. Circulating antibodies to prolactin have been demonstrated in some cases (146–149). Pathologically it is characterized by diffuse infiltration of the adenohypophysis by lymphocytes and occasional

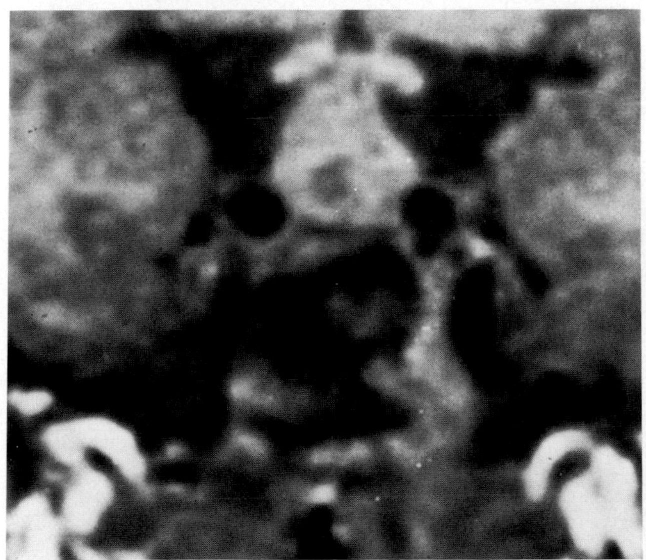

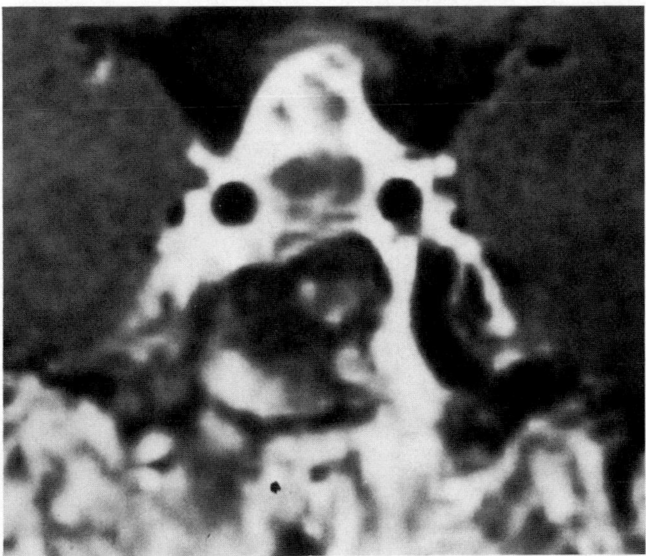

FIG. 65. Pituitary abscess. **A:** Coronal T1-weighted image. This patient developed fever, headache, and diabetes insipidus following transsphenoidal resection of an adenoma. An abnormal amount of soft tissue is identified in and around the sella turcica. There is a low intensity component centrally. **B:** Contrast-enhanced T1-weighted image. Following administration of Gd-DTPA there is rim enhancement of the intrasellar component and irregular enhancement of the suprasellar portion. At surgery purulent material was drained from the sella. Although the "low intensity center, rim enhancement" appearance is what one would expect from an abscess, it can also be seen with pituitary adenomas because areas of necrosis are common in adenomas. (Courtesy of Dr. Robert Tien, UCSD Medical Center.)

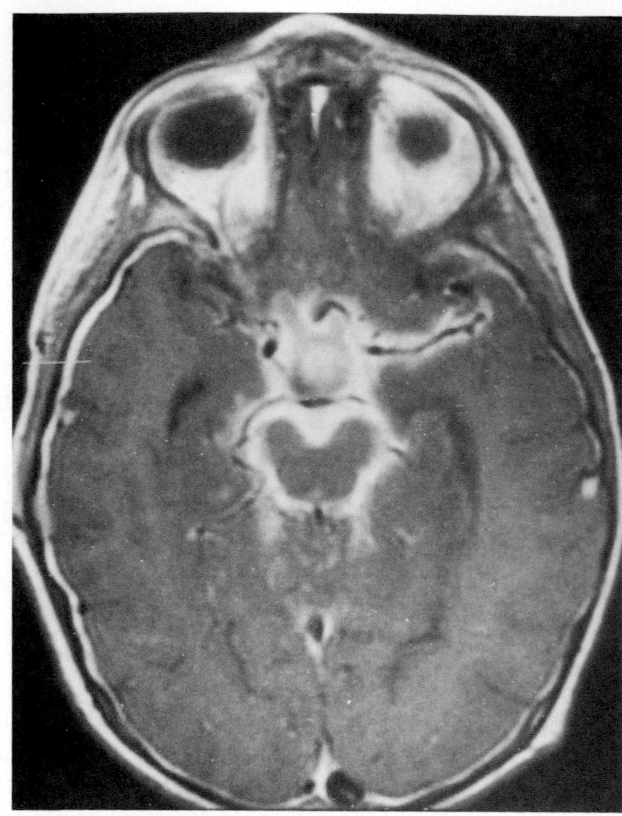

FIG. 66. Tuberculous basal meningitis. Contrast-enhanced axial T1-weighted image. The basal cisterns in and around the optic chiasm and midbrain enhance intensely. There is also enhancement over the convexities and in the sylvian fissures. The diagnosis was established by CSF aspiration. (Courtesy of Dr. William Kelly, UCSF Medical Center.)

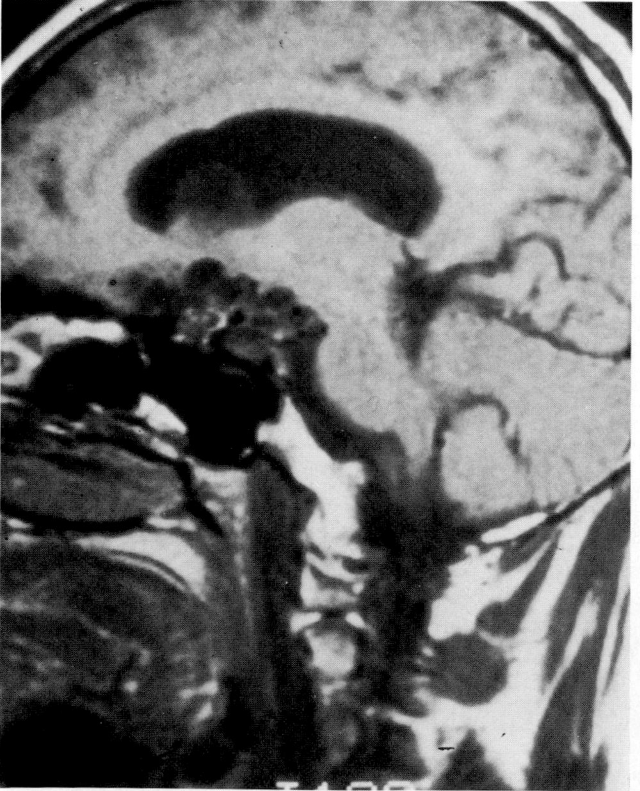

A

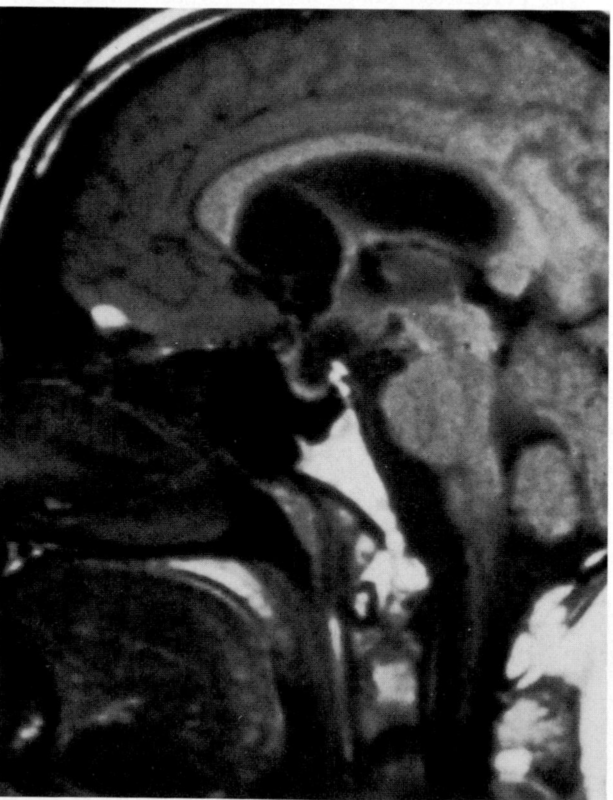

B

FIG. 67. Cysticercosis. Sagittal T1-weighted image. **A,B:** There is a large, multilobulated cyst in the suprasellar cistern, and an intraventricular cyst at the foramen of Monro. The signal intensity of cysticercal cysts such as this one resembles that of CSF. This characteristic feature, together with the difficulty in visualizing their thin walls, causes problems in identifying small cisternal lesions because there is little contrast between the cyst and the surrounding CSF. Large cysts, such as in this case, are readily apparent by the displacement of the brain.

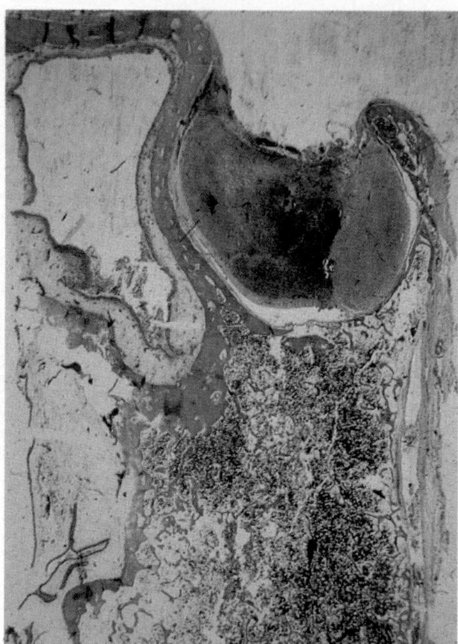

FIG. 68. Lymphocytic hypophysitis. This midline sagittal section demonstrates diffuse infiltration of the anterior lobe with lymphocytes, particularly apparent in the posteroinferior aspect of the lobe (dark blue staining cells).

plasma cells (Fig 68). The diagnosis should be considered in a female patient who is in the peripartum period with a pituitary mass, particularly when the degree of hypopituitarism is greater than that expected with the size of the mass. It is believed that, if untreated, the disease results in panhypopituitarism.

Clinically the patient complains of headache, visual loss, failure to resume menses, inability to lactate, or some combination thereof. Pituitary hormone levels are depressed. CT and MRI demonstrate diffuse enlargement of the anterior lobe without evidence of any focal abnormality or change in internal characteristics of the gland (Fig. 69) (146–150). The distinction between simple pituitary hyperplasia and lymphocytic hypophysitis may be difficult on MRI alone, so clinical correlation is required in this setting.

Sarcoidosis

Sarcoidosis is a chronic, multisystem, inflammatory disease of unproven etiology pathologically characterized by noncaseating granulomas. Evidence suggests that sarcoidosis results from an aberrant immune response to a variety of antigens. The lung and hilar lymph nodes are the organs most often involved, with involvement of the skin and eye next most frequent. It is a relatively common disorder affecting both sexes, females outnumbering males slightly. In the United States blacks outnumber whites by more than 10 to 1 (151).

Any part of the central nervous system (CNS) can be involved. There are neurologic findings in approximately 5% of patients with sarcoidosis, most frequently a cranial nerve dysfunction, especially a facial nerve palsy. Affliction of the hypothalamic-pituitary axis usually manifests itself clinically as diabetes insipidus, or occasionally as a deficiency of one or more anterior lobe hormones. The clinical presentation of neurologic disease is completely dependent on the site affected. Onset is usually indolent with a progressive course. The disease process is usually extremely steroid responsive.

Protean MRI manifestations are possible: multiple small lesions, large solitary masses, or thickening or distortion of the cranial nerves or meningeal surfaces (Figs. 70 and 71) (152–156). The imaging characteristics of the individual CNS lesions are insufficiently distinct to allow any precision in differential diagnosis, unless of course there is evidence of systemic sarcoidosis. The presence of multiple, scattered intraparenchymal lesions should raise the possibility of the diagnosis, as should diffuse or multifocal lesions of the basal meninges. The latter are best defined on coronal contrast-enhanced T1-weighted images.

Tolosa-Hunt Syndrome (THS)

The Tolosa-Hunt syndrome (THS) refers to a painful ophthalmoplegia caused by an inflammatory lesion of

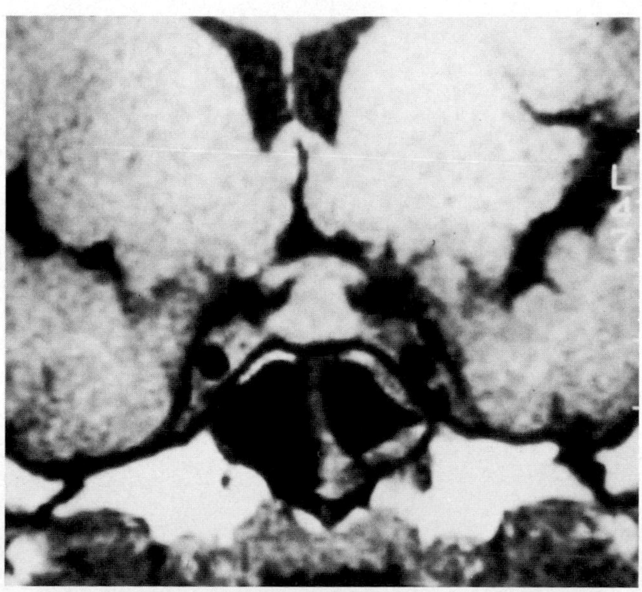

FIG. 69. Lymphocytic hypophysitis. Coronal T1-weighted image. This postpartum patient complained of a visual field defect and inability to lactate. The pituitary gland is diffusely enlarged and bulges through the suprasellar cistern to compress the optic chiasm. The signal intensity is identical to normal glandular tissue and no focal lesion is identified within the gland. Lymphocytic hypophysitis is probably an autoimmune disorder that is histologically characterized by diffuse lymphocytic infiltration of the pituitary gland.

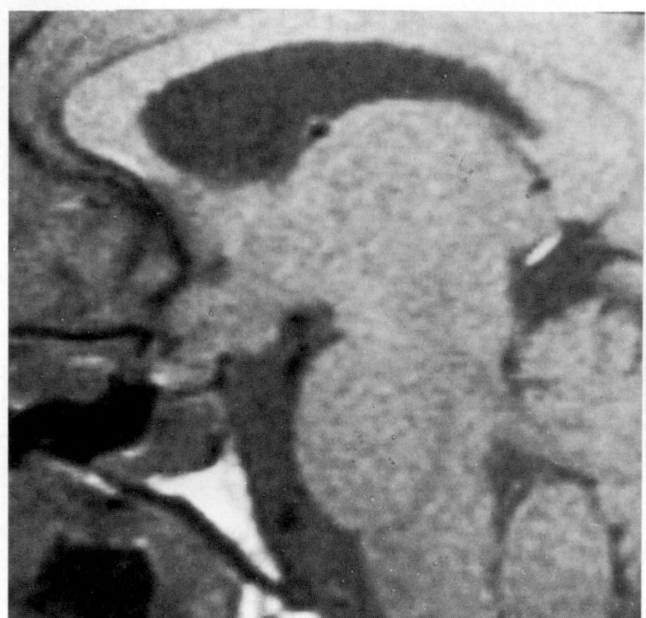

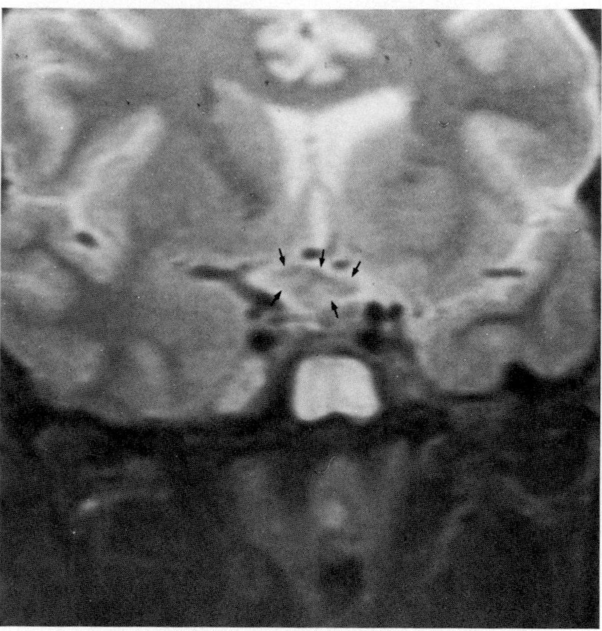

FIG. 70 Sarcoid. **A:** Sagittal T1-weighted image. This young woman presented with diabetes insipidus and visual loss. The MRI was obtained following transsphenoidal biopsy. It shows marked lobulated thickening of the optic chiasm and pituitary stalk, and absence of the normal posterior lobe signal, as well as postoperative changes in the sphenoid sinus. **B:** Coronal T2-weighted image. The lesion is slightly hypointense to cortex, a feature most commonly seen in lymphoma, sarcoid, and other forms of granulomatous inflammation (*arrows*).

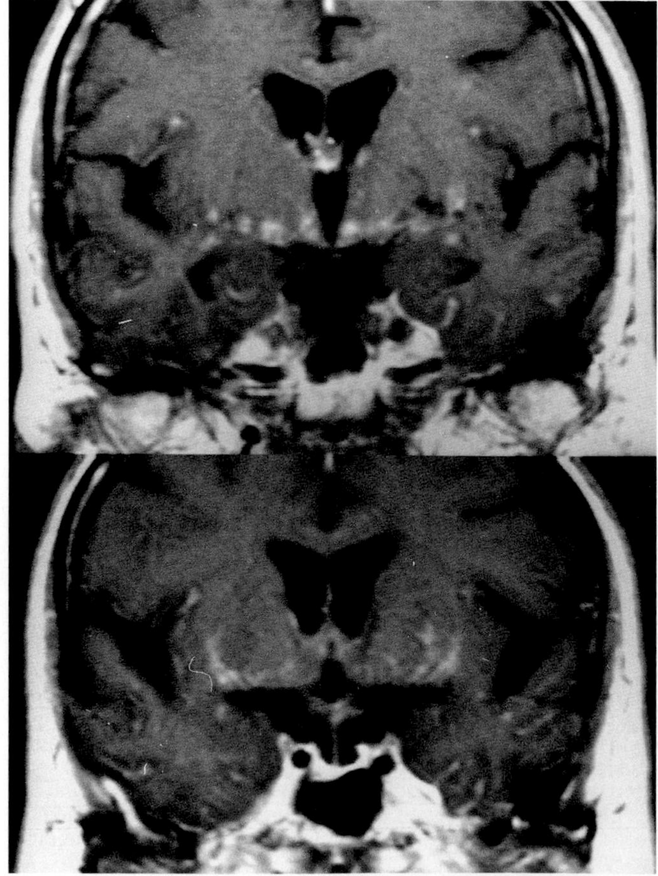

FIG. 71. Sarcoidosis. Enhanced T1-weighted coronal images. There are multiple, small, enhancing lesions in the brain parenchyma. Many of these lesions are in the hypothalamus; others are in the optic chiasm and the brain parenchyma immediately adjacent to the perivascular spaces that accompany the perforating lenticulostriate arteries.

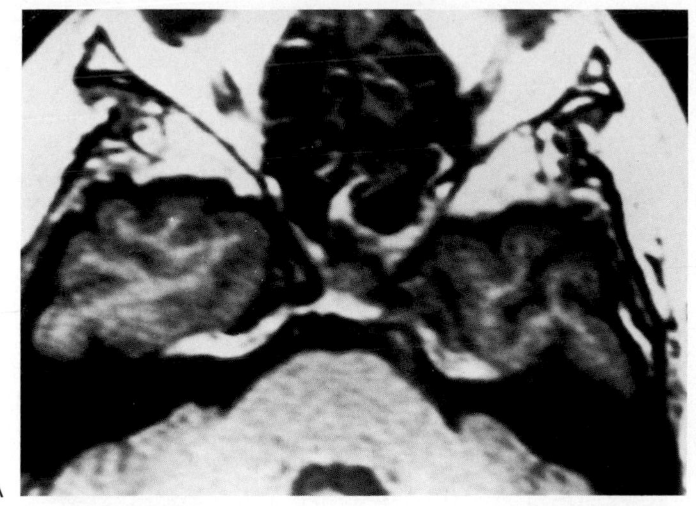

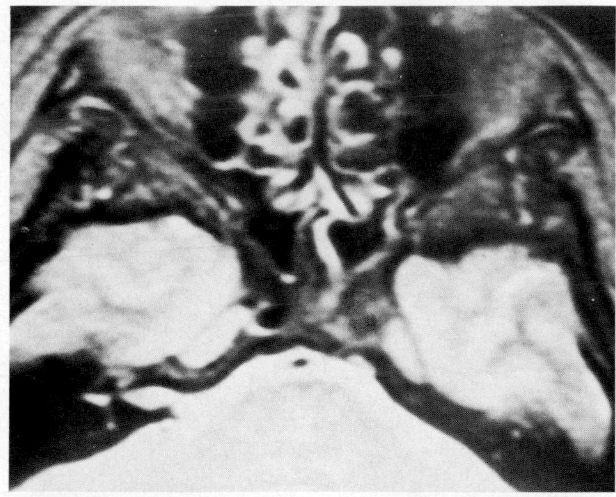

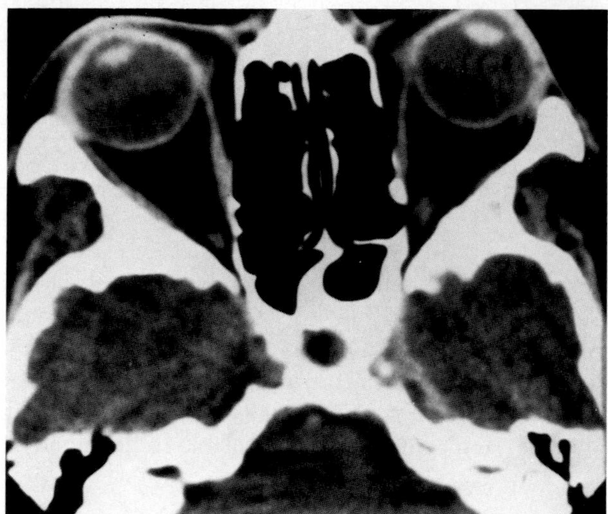

FIG. 72. Tolosa-Hunt syndrome. **A,B:** Axial T1- and T2-weighted image. The inflammatory process fills the left cavernous sinus. It is characterized by enlargement of the sinus contents and hypointensity on both T1- and T2-weighted image. **C:** Contrast-enhanced CT. The CT scan shows only enlargement of the cavernous sinus. (Courtesy of Dr. Scott W. Atlas, Oregon Heath Sciences University.)

the cavernous sinus that is steroid responsive. Pathologically the process is similar to orbital pseudotumor.

CT investigations in this disorder are often normal (157) or show subtle findings such as asymmetric enlargement of the cavernous sinus, enhancement of the prepontine cistern, or abnormal soft tissue density in the orbital apex (158). Yousem et al., in a report of 11 cases of THS, demonstrated positive MRI findings in nine patients (159). They found the affected side to have an enlarged cavernous sinus containing abnormal soft tissue, isointense to muscle on T1-weighted images, and isointense to fat on T2-weighted images (hypointense to muscle on T2-weighted images) (Fig. 72). In 8 of 11 cases the lesion extended to the orbital apex, reinforcing the belief that THS and orbital pseudotumor may be manifestations of the same disease. The lesion resolves promptly with steroid therapy (157). The hypointensity on T2-weighted images is an uncommon feature in all but a few diseases. These include meningioma, lymphoma, and sarcoidosis. Clinical history allows further precision in differential diagnosis. Meningioma does not respond to steroids and the latter two entities have evidence of their primary disease elsewhere in almost all cases.

VASCULAR AND ISCHEMIC LESIONS

Aneurysms

Saccular aneurysms in the sella turcica and parasellar area arise from either the cavernous sinus portion of the carotid artery or its supraclinoid segment; occasionally anterior communicating, posterior communicating, and basilar artery tip aneurysms project into the suprasellar cistern. These are extremely important lesions to identify correctly. Confusion with a solid tumor can lead to surgical catastrophes. Fortunately, their MRI appearance is distinctive and easily appreciated (Fig. 73) (160,161). Aneurysms are well defined and lack any internal signal on SE images, the so-called signal void created by rapidly flowing blood. This blood flow may also cause substantial artifact on the image, usually manifest as multiple

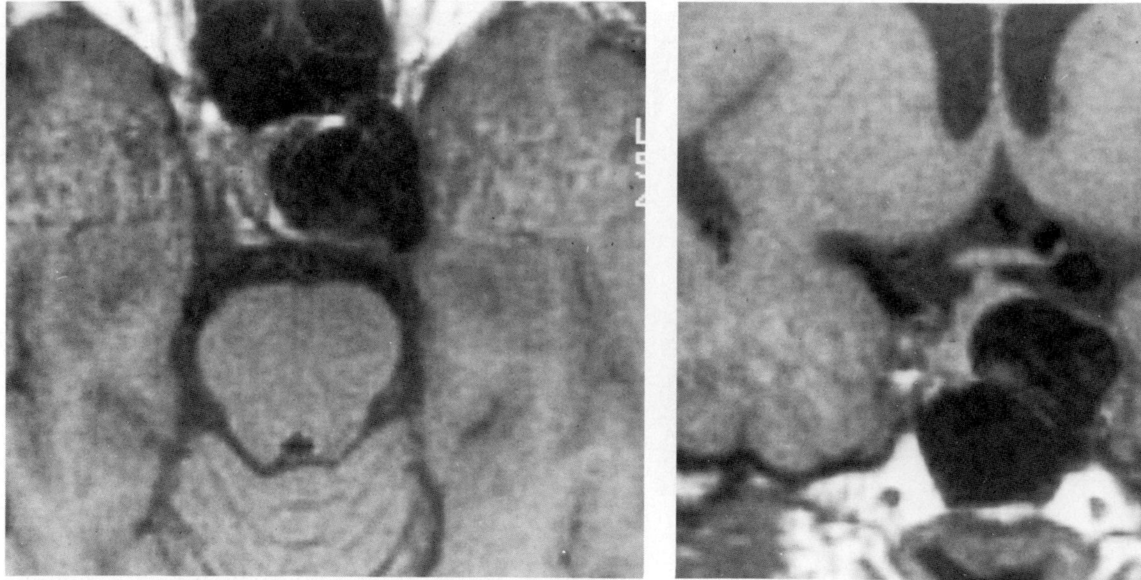

FIG. 73. Aneurysm. **A,B:** Axial and coronal T1-weighted image. There is a large, slightly lobulated low signal intensity lesion centered in the left cavernous sinus with intrasellar extension. It is virtually devoid of signal and is associated with a band of artifactual signal ghosting running from side to side across the image. The latter a is phase-encoding artifact induced by flow through the aneurysm. It is seen only in lesions that have flow through them and is confirmation of the presence of blood flow through the left cavernous sinus lesion.

ghosts in the phase-encoding direction and in itself is a useful diagnostic sign (Fig. 73). Thrombus in the aneurysm lumen fundamentally alters these characteristics, the clot usually appearing as multilamellated high signal on T1-weighted SE images, partially or completely filling the lumen. Hemosiderin may be visible in the adjacent brain, evident as a rim of low signal intensity on T2-weighted SE images, or on GE images. If confusion exists as to the vascular nature of these lesions, GE images may be used as a simple supplement to demonstrate in-flow enhancement of the aneurysm lumen. MR angiography is a more elegant means of confirming the diagnosis, de-

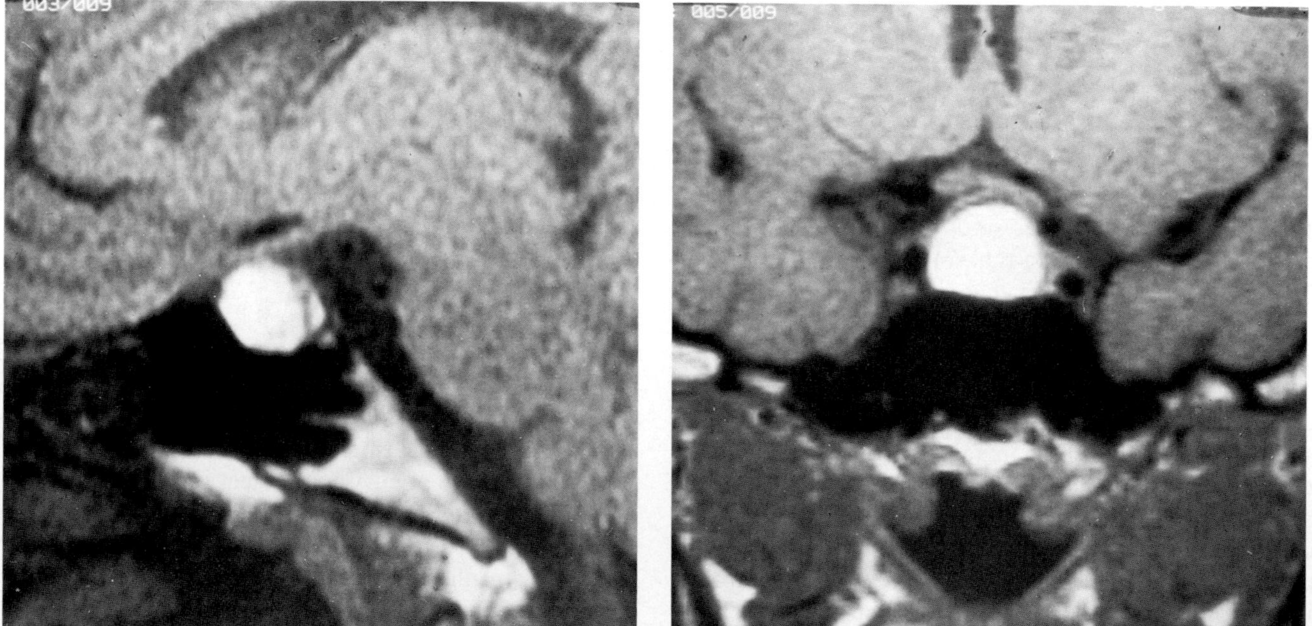

FIG. 74. Subacute pituitary hemorrhage (asymptomatic). **A,B:** Sagittal and coronal T1-weighted image. This middle-aged man complained of decreased libido but was otherwise asymptomatic. The MRI shows an enlarged sella containing a uniformly hyperintense lesion. Surgery revealed a cystic adenoma containing chocolate brown fluid from an old hemorrhage. Even in retrospect, no history of a hemorrhagic event could be elicited from the patient.

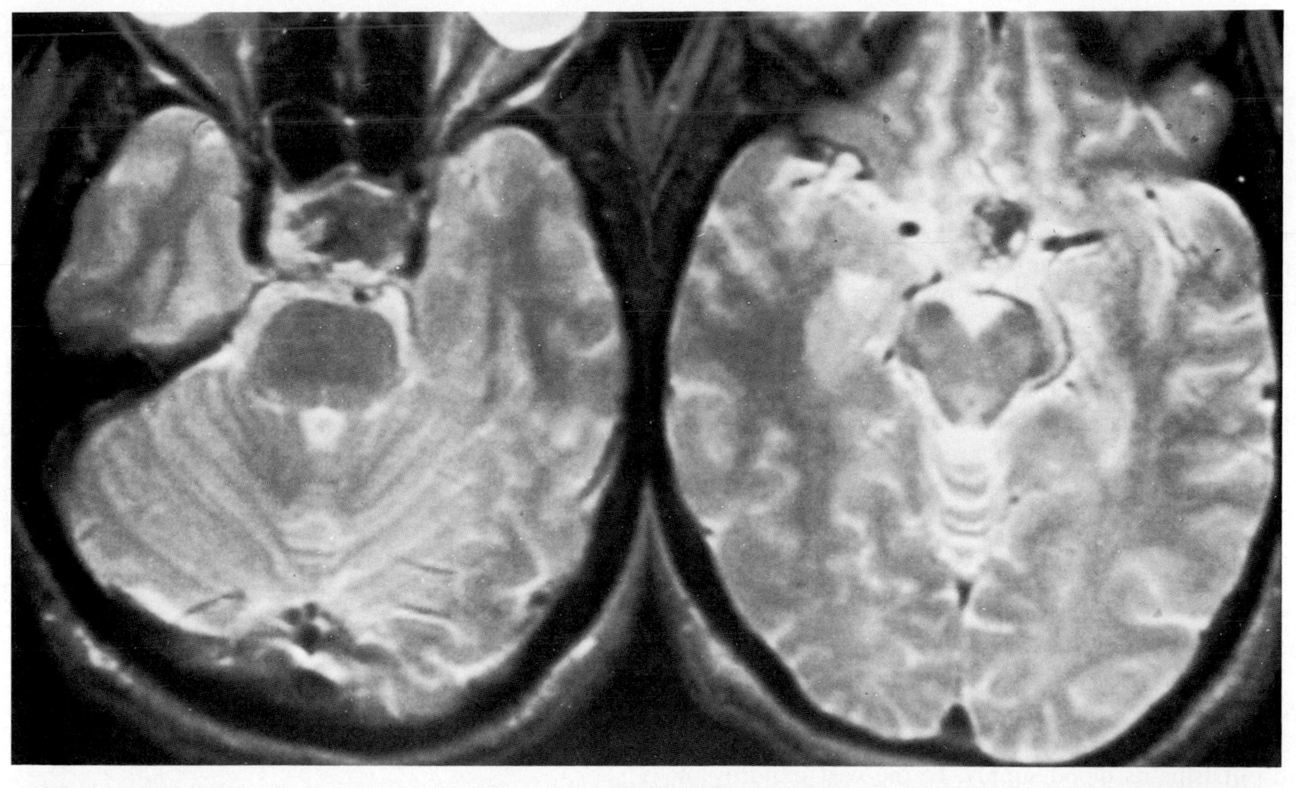

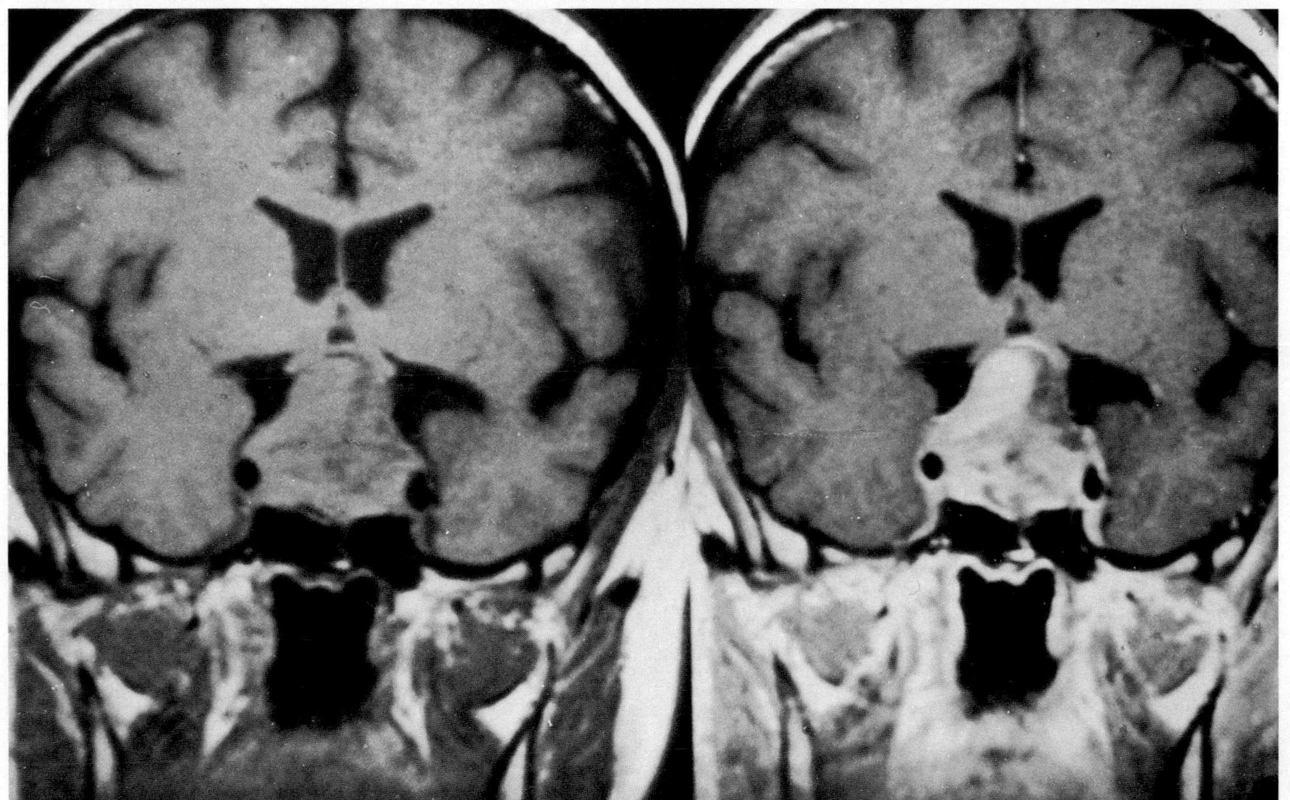

FIG. 75. Acute pituitary hemorrhage. **A,B:** Axial T2-weighted images. One day before this scan the patient developed severe headache and sudden visual loss. There is an enlarged sella turcica with a markedly hypointense lesion indicative of an acute hematoma in a pituitary adenoma. **C:** Coronal T1-weighted image. The gland is tremendously enlarged, compressing the chiasm. The left side of the gland (containing the hematoma) is low in intensity. **D:** Contrast-enhanced coronal T1-weighted image. The solid portion of the tumor enhances, the hematoma does not. (Courtesy of Dr. William Kelly, UCSF Medical Center.)

fining the neck of the aneurysm and establishing the relationship of the aneurysm to the major vessels.

Pituitary Apoplexy

Acute degeneration in a pituitary adenoma is termed "pituitary apoplexy" (162). While pituitary necrosis and hemorrhage may be accompanied by an apoplectiform clinical event (severe headache, hypotension, sudden visual loss), in many cases the patient is asymptomatic. Despite there being radiologic or pathologic evidence of hemorrhage or infarction, the patient cannot recall any clinical event, even in retrospect, to match the pathologic findings (Fig. 74). Indeed, in our own series of macroadenomas, almost 20% have evidence of cystic changes, necrosis, or hemorrhage, yet a history of sudden clinical deterioration is present in less than 1% (unpublished data). Ostrov et al. have reported that only 3 of 12 patients with MR evidence of intratumoral hemorrhage had clinical apoplexy (94).

The pathogenesis of this entity is due to sudden expansion of the tumor mass because of infarction or hemorrhage within the tumor. This occurs as the tumor grows and outstrips its blood supply. In the vast majority of cases the hemorrhage is contained within the pituitary gland. Rupture into the subarachnoid space is rare.

MRI demonstrates an enlarged sella turcica containing a macroadenoma. In most cases there is considerable suprasellar extension of the tumor with the optic chiasm draped over the dome of the tumor. There is always some heterogeneity in the tumor because of the hemorrhage within. If only a short interval has elapsed between the hemorrhage and MRI, the hematoma will be most notable as an area of low signal intensity on T2-weighted images (Fig. 75). If imaging is delayed (more than 3 days), the same hematoma is most evident as an area of high signal intensity on the T1-weighted images (see Fig. 74).

Sheehan's Syndrome (Postpartum Pituitary Necrosis)

Pregnancy induces substantial changes in the structure and function of the adenohypophysis. During pregnancy, the pituitary increases in size because of prolactin cell hyperplasia. The hyperplastic pituitary gland of pregnancy seems especially vulnerable to circulatory disturbances. Postpartum ischemic necrosis after complicated deliveries associated with hemorrhage and shock is well recognized (163). The MRI appearance is similar to that described for pituitary apoplexy except that the sella is of normal size and there is no evidence of an adenoma (Fig. 76).

Carotid Cavernous Fistulas and Cavernous Sinus Dural Arteriovenous Malformations

Carotid cavernous fistulas are abnormal communications between the carotid artery and cavernous sinus. Most cases are due to trauma; less frequently they are "spontaneous". These "spontaneous" cases are due to a variety of abnormalities, including atherosclerotic degeneration of the arterial wall, congenital defects in the media, or rupture of an internal carotid aneurysm within the cavernous sinus (164). Dural arteriovenous malfor-

A 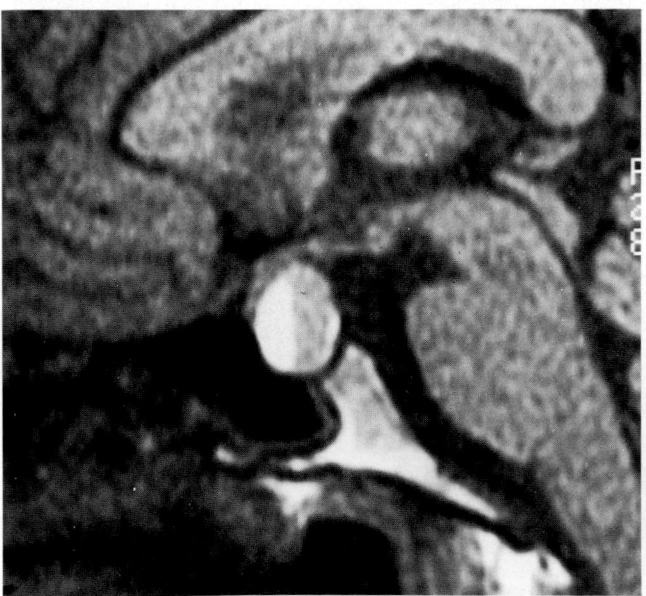

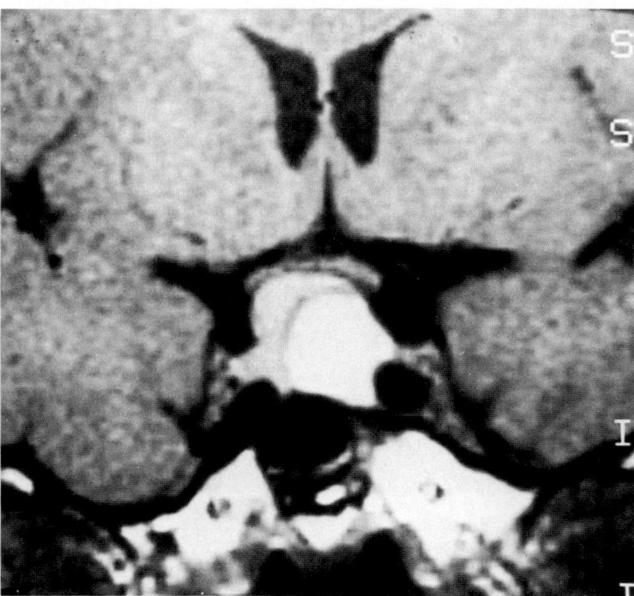 B

FIG. 76. Sheehan's syndrome. **A,B:** Sagittal and coronal T1-weighted image. This woman developed headache, hypopituitarism, and visual loss following delivery of her child. A frank hematoma is evident in the gland with a fluid/fluid level. The normal gland is displaced upward and to the right.

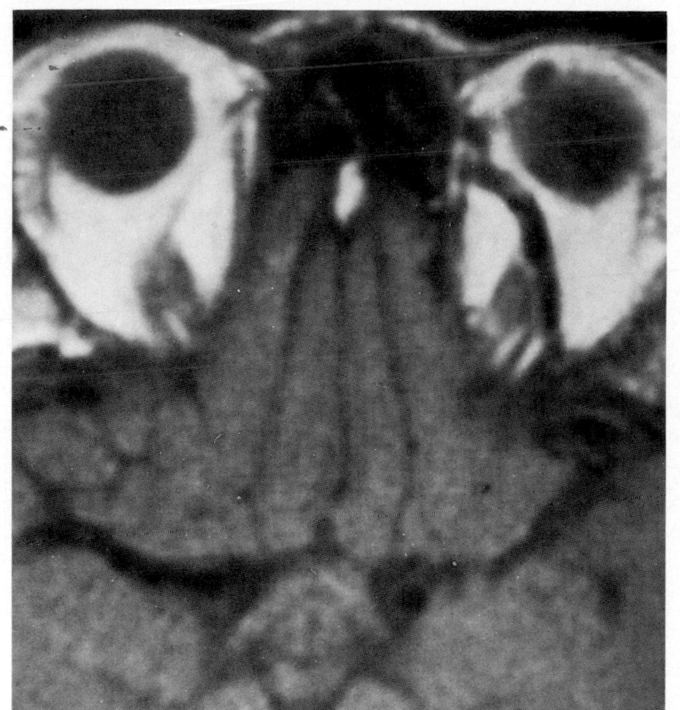

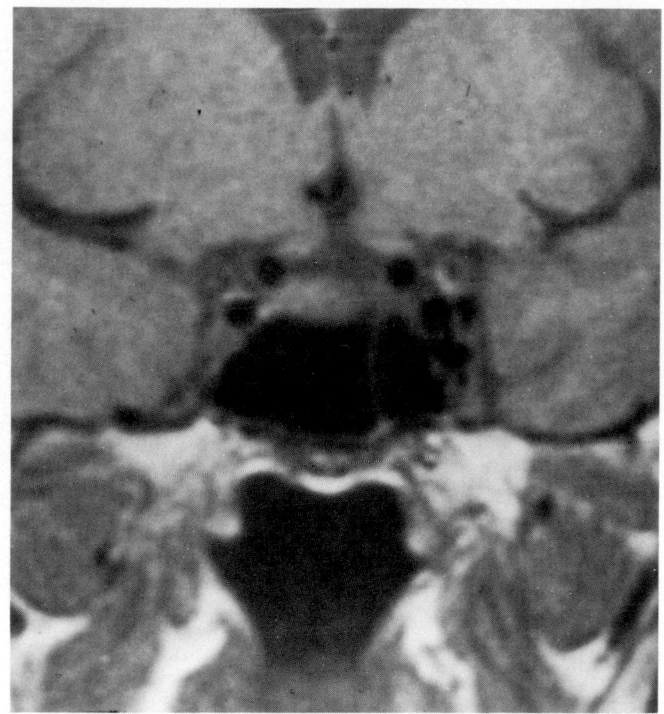

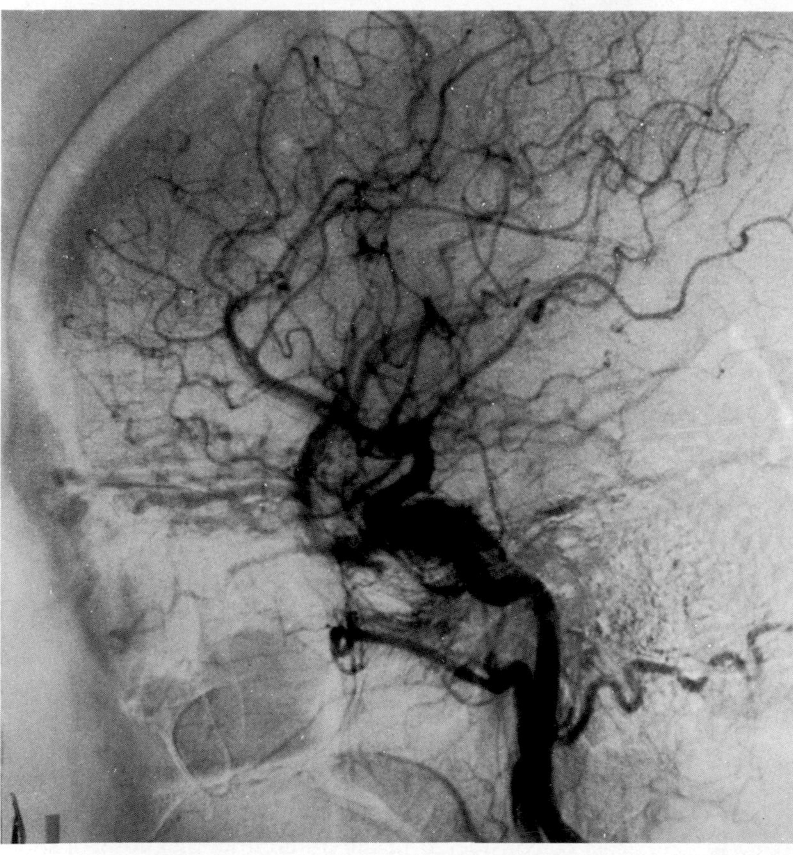

FIG. 77. Left carotid cavernous fistula. **A:** Axial T1-weighted image. The left superior ophthalmic vein is markedly enlarged. **B:** Coronal T1-weighted image. Multiple vascular channels are evident in the left cavernous sinus (compare this to the normal right side). **C:** Left carotid angiogram. The angiogram demonstrates a fistulous communication with arteriovenous shunting between the carotid artery and the cavernous sinus. (Courtesy of Dr. William Kelly, UCSF Medical Center.)

mations (AVMs) of the cavernous sinus are another form of abnormal arteriovenous (A-V) communication in this region. Clinically patients complain of redness, swelling, proptosis, and bruits. Physical examination most frequently reveals chemosis, and occasionally visual loss. Angiography readily demonstrates the fistulous connection between the artery and the cavernous sinus. The ipsilateral cavernous sinus, orbital veins, and petrosal sinus fill prematurely because of A-V shunting and are dilated (Fig. 77). If flow is of sufficiently high volume, the contralateral venous structures also enlarge because of multiple communicating channels between the two sides (intercavernous venous connections and petrosal venous plexus) (Fig. 78). Rarely venous drainage is exclusively to the contralateral side. On MRI the dilatation of the venous structures, in particular the ophthalmic vein and cavernous sinus, is usually clearly visible. The intercavernous venous channels dilate in carotid cavernous fistulas and may also be seen on MR images (165). Furthermore, the internal character of the cavernous sinus is altered; definite flow channels become evident secondary to the arterial rates of flow within the sinus. The fistulous communication itself is most often occult on MRI.

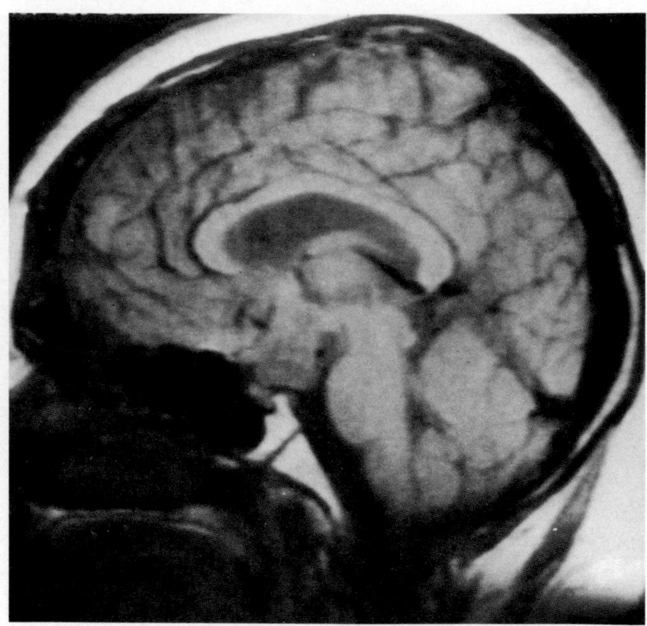

FIG. 79. Cavernous hemangioma. Sagittal T1-weighted image. There are no distinct features to this extra-axial hemangioma. In fact, it lacks the characteristic features normally seen in its intra-axial counterparts. This makes prospective diagnosis very difficult.

Cavernous Malformations

It is rare for any type of cavernous malformation to occur in or around the sella turcica except for carotid cavernous fistulas. As previously discussed, these are acquired lesions and not true malformations. However, there have been a few reports of extra-axial cavernous hemangiomas occurring in the suprasellar cistern (166–168). Of importance is that one of these hemangiomas did not have the features usually associated with, and so highly characteristic of, cavernous hemangiomas in the brain (166). It lacked the dark peripheral hemosiderin ring on the T2-weighted image and the internal "mulberry-like" mixed high signal/slow signal intensity on T1-weighted images. In our own practice we have had one similar case, identical in appearance (Fig. 79).

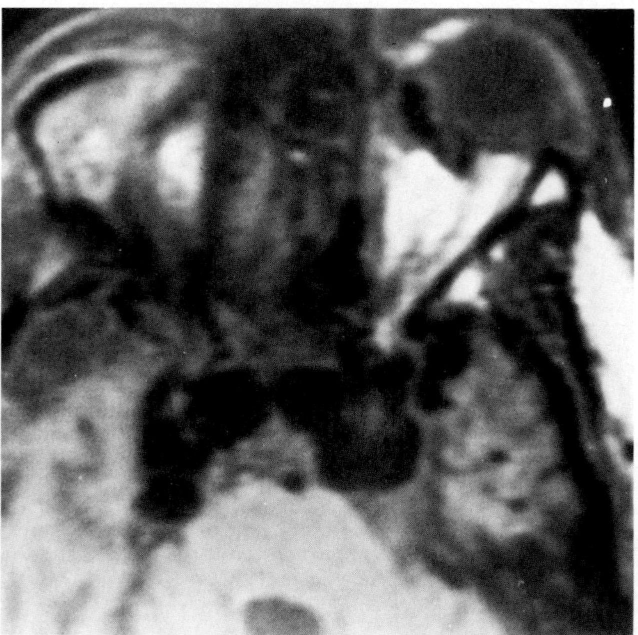

FIG. 78. Left carotid cavernous fistula. Axial T1-weighted image. There is tremendous enlargement of not only the left cavernous sinus and superior ophthalmic vein, but also the right cavernous sinus. Dilatation of both cavernous sinuses is not uncommon with carotid cavernous fistulae as there are transellar venous communications between the two sides. (Courtesy of Dr. Scott W. Atlas, Oregon Health Sciences University.)

Presumably extra-axial hemangiomas can lack these features because hemoglobin breakdown products are cleared more effectively from the subarachnoid space than from the brain parenchyma. Hence, hemoglobin breakdown products do not accumulate and are not evident around the lesion. The atypical appearance of extra-axial cavernous hemangiomas indicates that some caution must be exercised in the differential diagnosis of parasellar masses, because even though cavernous hemangiomas in this location are rare, failure of the surgeon to appreciate their vascular nature can lead to unanticipated hemorrhage. Cavernous hemangiomas should at least be considered in the differential diagnosis of solid, suprasellar masses that do not have the classic features of more common lesions, in particular craniopharyngiomas or meningiomas. Furthermore, T2-weighted images should be a routine part of the MRI protocol for suprasellar masses because visualization of a peripheral dark rim may be the only sign of the nature of the lesion.

METABOLIC DISORDERS

Diabetes Insipidus

Pituitary diabetes insipidus results from a lack of sufficient vasopressin (antidiuretic hormone; ADH) to effect water conservation. It is characterized by the persistence of an inappropriately dilute urine even in the presence of strong stimuli to ADH secretion, the absence of renal concentrating effects, and by a rise in urine osmolality upon vasopressin administration (169). The nephrogenic form is due to end-organ unresponsiveness (the renal collecting tubule) to vasopressin.

The inability to release vasopressin in response to normal stimuli is due to either primary failure to synthesize the hormone in the paraventricular nuclei of the hypothalamus, destruction of these nuclei or proximal transport pathways in the hypothalamus and proximal pituitary stalk, or dysfunction of hypothalamic osmoreceptors such that despite adequate vasopressin reserves, the hormone is not released appropriately. Eighty percent or more of the vasopressin-secreting cells must be affected before clinical diabetes insipidus develops.

Approximately one-third of cases of diabetes insipidus are idiopathic. Suprasellar and intrasellar neoplasms (craniopharyngiomas, germinomas, hypothalamic gliomas, metastases), head trauma, cranial and transsphenoidal surgery each account for 10% to 20% (169,170). There is also a rare hereditary form that is transmitted as an autosomal dominant trait (170). Once a clinical and biochemical diagnosis of diabetes insipidus is made, diagnostic efforts are directed toward establishing an etiology. Since the cause of diabetes insipidus in cases of head trauma and pituitary surgery are self-evident, imaging is usually pursued only in nontraumatic cases and is directed at excluding a neoplastic or infiltrative lesion of the suprasellar cistern or hypothalamus. Both CT and MRI demonstrate such pathology satisfactorily, but it is important to be aware of the fact that diabetes insipidus may be the first symptom of hypothalamic or suprasellar disease. Hypothalamic lesions have appeared as long as 10 years after the onset of "idiopathic" diabetes insipidus. Relative to CT, MRI has the added advantages of showing the pituitary stalk more clearly and documenting the status of the posterior pituitary gland, the storage site for the neurosecretory vesicles containing vasopressin. It is a unique imaging feature of this gland that it is hyperintense on T1-weighted images and that the signal disappears in diabetes insipidus, whatever the cause (Fig. 80) (14,15,22,23,171–173).

The diagnostic significance of visualization and nonvisualization of high signal intensity in the posterior lobe remains an interesting point of discussion. A high percentage of MRIs will demonstrate high signal intensity in the posterior lobe of normal individuals on routine sagittal T1-weighted views. This percentage has been reported as high as 98% to 100% (15,174), and as low as 60% (175). Arguments have been made, therefore, particularly by the "high percentage" reporters, that nonvisualization of the posterior lobe high signal should be interpreted as a sign of neurohypophyseal dysfunction. We subscribe partially to this viewpoint but with a qualification. Because the posterior lobe is small and occasionally eccentrically positioned, it may not be visualized on relatively thick, midline cuts simply because of geometry and partial volume averaging effects. Unless thin, contiguous cuts are obtained, preferably in all three orthogonal planes, confirm the finding, we tend to ignore the finding. If the signal is still not visible under the more stringent conditions, we view the absence as abnormal.

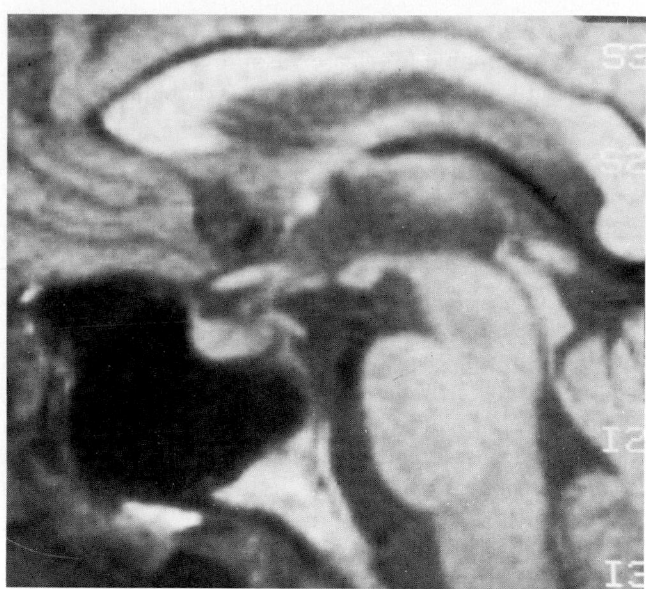

FIG. 80. Diabetes insipidus. Sagittal T1-weighted image. The high signal intensity normally seen in the posterior lobe is conspicuously absent. No other abnormality is present. In all cases of diabetes insipidus reported to date the posterior lobe high signal intensity has been absent.

Nonvisualization has been reported in nephrogenic diabetes insipidus (174), a disorder in which the neurohypophysis is functionally intact. This seems a paradox in that there should be abundance of neurosecretory activity to compensate for the insensitivity of the end organ, but Moses et al. (174) have proposed that in nephrogenic diabetes insipidus there is continuous stimulation and release of hormones, thus depleting the posterior lobe of neurosecretory vesicles, and hence the lack of signal. This is an entirely plausible explanation and would be akin to the depletion demonstrated by Fujisawa et al. in chronically stimulated rabbits (25). Maghnie et al. have found that not all cases of neurogenic diabetes insipidus are accompanied by absent posterior lobe signal (176). They describe a small subset of patients with neurogenic diabetes insipidus who have reserves of neurosecretory vesicles in the posterior lobe, but have an abnormal response to stimulation (osmoreceptor dysfunction), and thereby are unable to release vasopressin appropriately, which in turn is clinically manifest as diabetes insipidus.

Primary Hypothyroidism

Primary hypothyroidism is known to be associated with pituitary gland enlargement and hyperprolactinemia (177,178). The low serum levels of thyroxine lead to high levels of thyroid-releasing hormone (TRH). TRH not only stimulates pituitary thyrotrophs, but also causes lactotroph hyperplasia because of its prolactin-releasing factor effect. Treatment of the primary condition with thyroid hormone replacement therapy has been shown to result in a prompt reduction in the size of the pituitary gland (177).

Hemochromatosis

Hemochromatosis is a metabolic disorder characterized by iron overload. It is subdivided into a primary form, in which there is inappropriate intestinal absorption of iron relative to body needs, and secondary forms, particularly chronic disorders of erythropoiesis such as thalassemia. The excess iron is deposited throughout the body, but particularly in the liver, heart, and pancreas. The pituitary gland is frequently involved. For some unknown reason, there is a relatively preferential deposition of iron in FSH- and LH-secreting cells (gonadotrophs), leading to depressed secretion of these hormones. Dysfunction is most commonly manifest as loss of libido and hypogonadism.

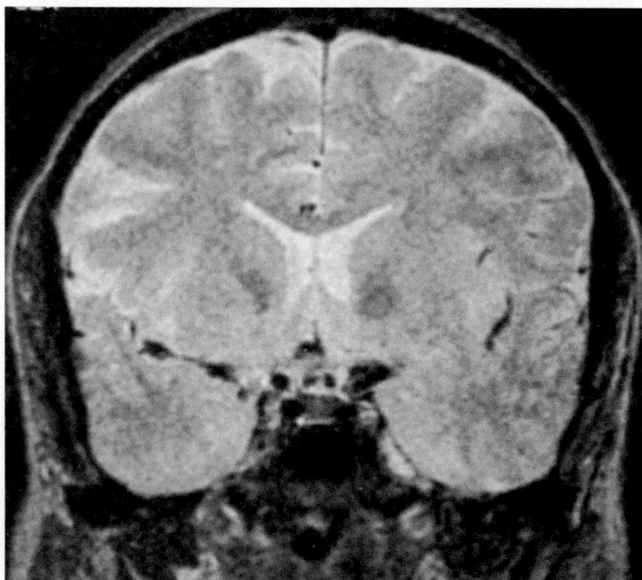

FIG. 81. Hemochromatosis. Coronal T2-weighted image. The pituitary gland is very hypointense because of iron deposition in the parenchyma of the gland. Iron deposition reduces signal intensity on all imaging sequences but particularly on T2-weighted images.

MRI is the only imaging modality that has demonstrated abnormalities of the pituitary gland in this disorder. The gland is abnormally dark on MRI, particularly on T2-weighted images (Fig. 81) (179). This is because of the high levels of iron deposited in the gland that, as expected, reduces signal intensity especially on late echoes. The hypointensity can be qualitatively assessed by comparing it to a nearby reference tissue. Temporal lobe white matter is the most convenient reference tissue to use as its signal intensity is unaffected by hemosiderosis and it is the field of view of coronal MR images of the sella. The most severely affected pituitary glands are darker than white matter on all imaging sequences, including short echo T1-weighted images, whereas the mildly overloaded glands are hypointense only on those sequences most sensitive to the presence of iron, namely T2-weighted sequences with late echoes. We have used the above gradation scheme to assess the severity of disease in patients with transfusional siderosis and we have obtained a good correlation between gonadotroph dysfunction as measured by gonadotrophin stimulation tests and the degree of MRI hypointensity (180).

REFERENCES

1. Williams PL, Warwick R, Dyson M, Bannister LH. The hypophysis cerebri. In: *Gray's Anatomy,* 37th ed. New York: Churchill Livingstone; 1989:1451–1456.
2. Elster AD, Chen MYM, Williams DW, Key LL. Pituitary gland: MR imaging of physiologic hypertrophy in adolescence. *Radiology* 1990;174:681–685.
3. Konishi Y, Kuriyama M, Sudo M, et al. Growth patterns of the normal pituitary gland and in pituitary adenoma. *Dev Med Child Neurol* 1990;32:69–73.
4. Elster AD, Chen MYM, Williams DW III, Key LL. Pituitary gland: MR imaging of physiologic hypertrophy in adolescence. *Radiology* 1990;174:681–685.
5. Doraiswamy PM, Potts JM, Figiel GS, et al. MR imaging of physiologic pituitary gland hypertrophy in adolescence. *Radiology* 1991;178(1):284–285.
6. Goluboff LG, Ezrin C. Effect of pregnancy on the somatotroph and the prolactin cells of the human adenohypophysis. *J Clin Endocrinol Metal* 1969;29:1533–1543.
7. Elster AD, Sanders TG, Vines FS, Chen MYM. Size and shape of the pituitary gland during pregnancy and post partum: measurement with MR imaging. *Radiology* 1991;181:531–535.
8. Elster AD, Sanders TG, Vines FS, Chen MYM. Size and shape of the pituitary gland during pregnancy and post partum: measurement with MR imaging. *Radiology* 1991;181:531–535.
9. Hardy J. *Transsphenoidal Operations on the Pituitary.* Randolph, Mass: Codman and Shurtleff; 1975.
10. Renn WH, Rhoton AL, Jr. Microsurgical anatomy of the sellar region. *J Neurosurg* 1975;43:288–298.
11. Tien R. Sequence of enhancement of various portions of the pituitary gland on Gd-enhanced MR images: correlation with regional blood supply. *AJR* 1992;158(3):651–654.
12. Sakamoto Y, Takahashi M, Korogi Y, et al. Normal and abnormal pituitary glands: gadopentetate dimeglumine–enhanced MR imaging. *Radiology* 1991;178(2):441–445.

13. Okado N, Yokota N. An electron microscopic study on the structural development of the neural lobe in the human fetus. *Am J Anat* 1980;159:261–273.
14. Colombo N, Berry I, Kucharczyk J, et al. Posterior pituitary gland: appearance in MRI in normal and pathologic states. *Radiology* 1987;165:481–485.
15. Fujisawa I, Asato R, Nishimura K, et al. Anterior and posterior lobes of the pituitary gland: assessment by 1.5 T MR imaging. *J Comput Assist Tomogr* 1987;11:214–220.
16. Chakeres DW, Curtin A, Ford G. Magnetic resonance imaging of pituitary and parasellar abnormalities. *Radiol Clin North Am* 1989;27:265–281.
17. Wolpert SM, Osborne M, Anderson M, Runge VM. The bright pituitary gland: a normal MR appearance in infancy. *AJNR* 1988;9:1–3.
18. Cox TD, Elster AD. Normal pituitary gland: changes in shape, size, and signal intensity during the 1st year of life at MR imaging. *Radiology* 1991;179:721–724.
19. Miki Y, Asato R, Okumura R, et al. Anterior pituitary gland in pregnancy: hyperintensity at MR. *Radiology* 1993;187:229–231.
20. Hayakawa K, Konishi Y, Matsuda T, et al. Development and aging of brain midline structures: assessment with MR imaging. *Radiology* 1989;172:171–177.
21. Colombo N, Berry I, Kucharczyk J, Kucharczyk W. MR imaging findings in the posterior pituitary gland: reply. *Radiology* 1988;168:282.
22. Fujisawa I, Nishimura K, Asato R, et al. Posterior lobe of the pituitary in diabetes insipidus.: MR findings. *J Comput Assist Tomogr* 1987;11:221–225.
23. Fujisawa I, Asato R. MR imaging findings in the posterior pituitary gland [*Letter*]. *Radiology* 1988;168:282.
24. Fujisawa I, Asato R, Kawata M. Hyperintense signals of the posterior lobe of the pituitary gland on MR images [*Letter*]. *AJNR* 1989;10:1280–1281.
25. Fujisawa I, Asato R, Kawata M, et al. Hyperintense signal of the posterior pituitary on T1-weighted MRI: an experimental study. *J Comput Assist Tomogr* 1989;13:371–377.
26. Kucharczyk J, Kucharczyk W, Berry I, et al. Histochemical characterization and functional significance of the hyperintense signal on MR images of the posterior pituitary. *AJNR* 1988;9:1079–1083.
27. Kucharczyk W, Lenkinski RE, Kucharczyk J, Henkelman RM. The effect of phospholipid vesicles on the NMR relaxation of water: an explanation for the appearance of the neurohypophysis? *AJNR* 1990;11:693–700.
28. Norman D, Kucharczyk J, Kucharczyk W, Newton TH. Hyperintense signals of the posterior lobe of the pituitary gland on MR images [*Reply*]. *AJNR* 1989;10:1281–2.
29. Kim BJ, Kido DK, Simon JH, et al. Chemical shift MR imaging of posterior lobe of pituitary gland (a). *AJNR* 1989;10:892.
30. Tien R. Neurophysins in the neonatal adenohypophysis. ASNR Annual Meeting, May 1993, Vancouver.
31. Miki Y, Asato R, Okumura R, et al. Contrast enhanced area of posterior pituitary gland in early dynamic MRI exceeds hyperintense area on T1-weighted images. *J Comput Assist Tomogr* 1992;16(6):845–848.
32. Daniels DL, Pech P, Mark L, et al. Magnetic resonance imaging of cavernous sinus. *AJNR* 1985;6:187.
33. Daniels EL, Czervonike LF, Bonneville JF, et al. MRI of the cavernous sinus value of spin-echo and gradient recalled echo images. *AJR* 1988;151:1009–1014.
34. Komiyama M, Yasui T, Baba M, et al. MR imaging of blood flow in the cavernous sinus. *Radiation Med* 1988;6:124–129.
35. Kucharczyk W, Davis DO, Kelly WM, et al. Pituitary adenoma: high-resolution MRI at 1.5 T. *Radiology* 1986;161:761–765.
36. Davis PC, Hoffman JC Jr, Spencer T, et al. MR imaging of pituitary adenoma: CT, clinical, and surgical correlation. *AJNR* 1987;8:107.
37. Peck WW, Dillon WP, Norman D, et al. High-resolution MR imaging of pituitary microadenomas at 1.5T: experience with cushing disease. *AJNR* 1988;9:1085.
38. Pojunas KW, Daniels DL, Williams AL, Haughton VM. MR imaging of prolactin-secreting microadenomas. *AJNR* 1986;7:209.
39. Kulkarni MV, Lee KF, McArdle CB, et al. 1.5–T MR imaging of pituitary microadenomas: technical considerations and CT correlation. *AJNR* 1988;9:5.
40. Rao VM, Vinitski S, Barbaria A, et al. Enhanced resolution of pituitary fossa with 3D fat suppressed gradient echo MRI: pre- and post gadolinium enhancement (a). *AJNR* 1989;10:892.
41. Stadnik T, Stevenaert A, Beckers A, et al. Pituitary microadenomas: diagnosis with two- and three-dimensional MR imaging at 1.5T before and after injection of gadolinium. *Radiology* 1990;176:419–428.
42. Davis PC, Hoffman JC Jr, Malko JA, et al. Gadolinium-DTPA and MR imaging of pituitary adenoma: a preliminary report. *AJNR* 1987;8:817.
43. Doppman JL, Frank JA, Dwyer AJ, et al. Gadolinium DTPA enhanced MR imaging of ACTH-secreting microadenomas of the pituitary gland. *J Comput Assist Tomogr* 1988;12:728.
44. Dwyer AJ, Frank JA, Doppman JL, et al. Pituitary adenomas in patients with Cushing Disease: initial experience with GD-DTPA-enhanced MR imaging. *Radiology* 1987;163:421.
45. Nakamura T, Schorner W, Bittner RC, et al. Value of paramagnetic contrast agent gadolinium-DTPA in the diagnosis of pituitary adenomas. *Neuroradiology* 1988;30:481–486.
46. Newton DR, Dillon WP, Norman D, et al. GD-DTPA-enhanced MR imaging of pituitary adenomas. *AJNR* 1989;10:(5)949–954.
47. Steiner E, Imhof H, Knosp E. Gd-DTPA enhanced high resolution MR imaging of pituitary adenomas. *Radiographics* 1989;9:587.
48. Davis PC, Gokhale KA, Joseph GJ, et al. Pituitary adenoma: correlation of half-dose gadolinium-enhanced MR imaging with surgical findings in 26 patients. *Radiology* 1991;180(3):779–784.
49. Giacometti AR, Joseph GJ, Peterson JE, Davis PC. Comparison of full- and half-dose gadolinium-DTPA: MR imaging of the normal sella. *AJNR* 1993;14(1):123–127.
50. Finelli DA, Kaufman B. Ultrafast, contrast-enhanced, dynamic scanning of the pituitary: the first thirty seconds. SMRM Annual Meeting 1992, San Francisco.
51. Miki Y, Matsuo M, Nishizawa S, et al. Pituitary adenomas and normal pituitary tissue: Enhancement patterns on gadopentetate-enhanced MR imaging. *Radiology* 1990;177(1):35–38.
52. Kucharczyk W, Bishop JE, Plewes DB, et al. Dynamic MR imaging of pituitary microadenomas with FSE T1-weighted shared view MRI. SMRM Annual Meeting 1993, New York.
53. Yuh WTC, Tali ET, Nguyen H, et al. Sequential MR enhancement pattern in normal pituitary gland and pituitary adenoma. SMRM Annual Meeting 1993, New York.
54. Naidich TP, McLane DG, Bauer BS, et al. Midline craniofacial dysraphism: midline cleft upper lip, basal encephalocele, callosal agenosis, and optic nerve dysplasia. *Concept Pediatr Neurosurg* 1983;4:186–207.
55. Hoyt WF, Kaplan S, Grumbach MM, et al. Septo-optic dysplasia and pituitary dwarfism. *Lancet* 1970;1:893–894.
56. Kelly WM, Kucharczyk W, Kucharczyk J, et al. Posterior pituitary ectopia: an MR feature of pituitary dwarfism. *AJNR* 1988;9:453–460.
57. Fujisawa I, Kikuchi K, Nishimura K, et al. Transection of the pituitary stalk: development of an ectopic posterior lobe assessed with MR imaging. *Radiology* 1987;165:487.
58. Triulzi F, Scotti G, di Natale B, et al. Evidence of a congenital midline brain anomaly in pituitary dwarfs: an MRI study in 101 patients. *Pediatrics* 1994;93:409–416.
59. Maghnie M, Triulzi F, Larizza D, et al. Hypothalamic-pituitary dwarfism: comparison between MR imaging and CT findings. *Pediatr Radiol* 1990;20:229–235.
60. Maghnie M, Triulzi F, Larizza D, et al. Hypothalamic-pituitary dysfunction in growth hormone-deficient patients with pituitary abnormalities. *J Clin Endocrinol Metab* 1991;73(1):79–83.
61. Gammal TE, Brooks BS, Hoffman WH. MR imaging of the ectopic bright signal of posterior pituitary regeneration. *AJNR* 1989;10:323–328.
62. Kaufman BA, Kaufman B, Mapstone TB. Pituitary stalk agenesis: Magnetic resonance imaging of 'ectopic posterior lobe' with surgical correlation. *Pediatr Neurosci* 1988;14:140–144.
63. Carmel PW. The empty sella syndrome: In: Wilkins RH, Regan-

chary SS, eds. *Neurosurgery*, New York: McGraw-Hill; 1985: 884–888.

64. Ommaya AK, DiChiro G, Baldwin M, Pennybacher JB. Nontraumatic cerebrospinal fluid rhinorrhea. *J Neurol Neurosurg Psychiatry* 1968;31:214–225.
65. Weisberg LA, Zimmerman EA, Fratnz AG. Diagnosis and evaluation of patients with an enlarged sella turcica. *Am J Med* 1976;61:590–596.
66. Kaufman B, Tumsak RL, Kaufman BA, et al. Herniation of suprasellar visual system and and third ventricle into empty sellae: morphologic and clinical considerations. *AJNR* 1989;10:65–69.
67. Smith DE, Murphy MJ, Hitchon PW, et al. transsphenoidal encephaloceles. *Surg Neurol* 1983;20:471–480.
68. Rice JF, Eggers DM. Basal transsphenoidal encephalocele: MR findings. *AJNR* 1989;10:S79–S80.
69. Diebler C, Dulac. Cephaloceles: clinical and neuroradiologic appearance. *Neuroradiology* 1983;25:199–216.
70. Boulanger T, Mathurin P, Doans, G et al. Sphenopharyngeal meningoencephalocele; unusual clinical and radiologic features. *AJNR* 1989;10:S81–S82.
71. Kovacs K, Horvath E, Asa SL. Classification and pathology of pituitary tumors. In: Wilkins RH, Rengachary SS, eds. In: *Neurosurgery*. New York: McGraw-Hill; 1985:834–842.
72. Russell DS, Rubinstein LJ. *Pathology of Tumours of the Nervous System*, 5th ed. Baltimore: Williams & Wlikins; 1989.
73. Teramoto A, Hirakawa K, Sanno N, Osamura Y. Incidental pituitary lesions in 1000 unselected atutopsy specimens. *Radiology* 1994;193:161–164.
74. Ostrov SG, Quencer RM, Hoffman JC, et al. Hemorrhage within pituitary adenomas: how often associated with pituitary apoplexy syndrome? *AJNR* 1989;10:503–510.
75. Kyle CA, Laster RA, Burton EM, Sanford RA. Subacute pituitary apoplexy: MR and CT appearance. *J Comput Assist Tomogr* 1990;14:40–44.
76. Yousem DM, Arrington JA, Zinreich SJ, et al. Pituitary adenomas: possible role of bromocriptine in intratumoral hemorrhage. *Radiology* 1989;170:239–243.
77. Snow RB, Johnson CE, Morgello S, et al. Is magnetic resonance imaging useful in guiding the operative approach to large pituitary tumors? *Neurosurgery* 1990;26:801–803.
78. Ahmadi H, Larsson EM, Jinkins JR. Normal pituitary gland: coronal MR imaging of infundibular tilt. *Radiology* 1990;177:389–392.
79. Marcovitz S, Wee R, Chan J, et al. Diagnostic accuracy of preoperative CT scanning in the evaluation of pituitary ACTH-secreting adenomas. *AJNR* 1987;8:641.
80. Marcovitz S, Wee R, Chan J, et al. Diagnostic accuracy of preoperative CT scanning of pituitary prolactinomas. *AJNR* 1988;9: 13.
81. Marcovitz S, Wee R, Chan, J, et al. Diagnostic accuracy of preoperative CT scanning of pituitary somatotroph adenomas. *AJNR* 1988;9:19.
82. Syvertsen A, Haughton VM, Williams AL, Cusick JF. The computed tomography appearance of the normal pituitary gland and pituitary microadenomas. *Radiology* 1979;133:385–391.
83. Johnson MR, Hoare RD, Cox T, et al. The evaluation of patients with a suspected pituitary microadenoma: computer tomography compared to magnetic resonance imaging. *Clin Endocrinol* 1992;36:335–338.
84. Doppman JL, Oldfield EH, Krudy AG, et al. Petrosal sinus sampling for Cushing syndrome: anatomical and technical considerations. *Radiology* 1984;150:99–103.
85. Miller DL, Doppman JL. Petrosal sinus sampling: technique and rationale. *Radiology* 1991;178:37–47
86. Miller DL, Doppman JL, Nieman LK, et al. Petrosal sinus sampling: discordant lateralization of ACTH-secreting pituitary microadenomas before and after stimulation with corticotropin-releasing hormone. *Radiology* 1990;176:429–431.
87. Miller DL, Doppman JL, Peterman SB, et al. Neurologic complications of petrosal sinus sampling. *Radiology* 1992;185:143–147.
88. Doppman JL. Inferior petrosal sinuses sampling: origins, history and personal experience with over 500 cases. *Rivista Neuroradiol* 1994;7:17–26.
89. Chong BW, Kucharczyk W, Singer W, George S. Distinguishing focal signal hypointensities in the pituitary glands of normal volunteers from microprolactinomas. In: *Book of Abstracts, 30th Annual Meeting*. Oak Brook, III: ASNR 1992:34–35.
90. Elster AD. Sellar susceptibility artifacts: theory and implications. *AJNR* 1993;14:129–136.
91. Sisam DA, Sheeham JP, Sheeler LR. The natural history of untreated microprolactinomas. *Fertil Steril* 1987;48(1):67–71.
92. Ahmadi J, North CM, Segall HD, et al. Cavernous sinus invasion by pituitary adenomas. *AJNR* 1985;6:893.
93. Scotti G, Yu CY, Dillon WP, et al. MRI of cavernous sinus invasion by pituitary adenomas. *AJR* 1988;151:799–806.
94. Ostrov SG, Quencer RM, Hoffman JC, et al. Hemorrhage within pituitary adenomas: how often associated with pituitary apoplexy syndrome? *AJNR* 1989;10:503–510.
95. Bergstrom M, Muhr C, Lundberg PO, Langstrom B. PET as a tool in the clinical evaluation of pituitary adenomas. *J Nucl Med* 1991;32(4):610–615.
96. De Souza B, Brunetti A, Fulham MJ, et al. Pituitary microadenomas: a pet study. *Radiology* 1990;177:39–44.
97. Carmel PW, Antunes JL, Chang CH. Craniopharyngiomas in children. *Neurosurgery* 1982;11:382–389.
98. Matthews FD. Intraventricular craniopharyngioma. *AJNR* 1983;4:984.
99. Crotty T, Sheithauer BW, Young WF, et al. Papillary craniopharyngiomas: a morphology and clinical study of 46 cases. *Endocrin Pathol* 1992;3(suppl 1):S6.
100. Pusey E, Kortman KE, Flannigan BD, et al. MR of craniopharyngiomas: tumor delineation and characterization. *AJNR* 1987;8:439–444.
101. Price AC, Runge V, Allen JH, et al. Craniopharyngioma: correlation of high resolution CT and MRI (a). *AJNR* 1985;6:465.
102. Kucharczyk W, Peck WW, Kelly WM, et al. Rathke cleft cysts: CT, MR imaging, and pathologic features. *Radiology* 1987;165: 491.
103. Maggio WW, Cail WS, Brookeman JR, Persing JA, Jane JA. Rathke's cleft cyst: computed tomographic and magnetic resonance imaging appearances. *Neurosurgery* 1987;21:60–62.
104. Rubinstein LJ. *Atlas of Tumor Pathology; Second Series, Fascicle 6: Tumors of the Central Nervous System*. Washington, D.C.: Armed Forces Institute of Pathology; 1972.
105. Taylor SL, Barakos JA, Harsh GR 4th, Wilson CB. Magnetic resonance imaging of tuberculum sellae meningiomas: preventing preoperative misdiagnosis as pituitary macroadenoma. *Neurosurgery* 1992;31(4):621–627.
106. Bradac GB, Riva A, Schoiner W, Stura G. Cavernous sinus meningiomas: an MRI study. *Neuroradiology* 1987;29:578–581.
107. Castillo M, Davis PC, Ross WK, Hoffman JC Jr. Meningioma of the chiasm and optic nerves: CT and MR findings. *J Comput Assist Tomogr* 1989;13:679–681.
108. Yeakley JW, Kulkarni MV, McArdle CB, et al. High-resolution MR imaging of juxtasellar meningomas with CT and angiographic correlation. *AJNR* 1988;9:279.
109. Zimmerman RD, Fleming CA, Saint-Louis LA, Lee BCP, Manning JJ, Deck MDF. Magnetic resonance imaging of meningiomas. *AJNR* 1985;6:149–157.
110. Bydder GM, Kingsley DPE, Brown J, Niendorf HP, Young IR. MR imaging of meningiomas including studies with and without gadolinium-DTPA. *J Comput Assist Tomogr* 1985;9:690–697.
111. Mawhinney RR, Buckley JH, Holloand IM, Worthington BS. The value of magnetic resonance imaging in the diagnosis of intracranial meningiomas. *Clin Radiol* 1986;37:429–439.
112. Arnold DL, Emrich JF, Shoubridge EA, et al. Characterization of astrocytomas, meningiomas, and pituitary adenomas by phosphorus magnetic resonance spectroscopy. *J Neurosurg* 1991; 74(3):447–453.
113. Jellinger K. Primary intrasellar germ cell tumors. *Acta Neuropathol* 1973;25:291–306.
114. Takeuchi J, Handa H, Nagata I. Suprasellar germinoma. *J Neurosurg* 1978;49:41–48.
115. Conley FK. Epidermoid and dermoid tumors: clinical features and surgical management. In: Wilkins RH, Rengachary SS, eds. *Neurosurgery*. New York: McGraw-Hill; 1985:668–670.

116. Latack JT, Kartush JM, Kemink JL, et al. Epidermoidoma of the cerebello-pontine angle and temporal bone: CT and MR aspects. *Radiology* 1985;157:361–366.
117. Newton DR, Larson TC III, Dillon WP, Newton TH. Magnetic resonance characteristics of cranial epidermoid and teratomatous tumors (a). *AJNR* 1987;8:945.
118. Tampieri D, Melanson D, Ethier R. MR imaging of epidermoid cysts. *AJNR* 1989:351.
119. Vion-Dury J, Vincentelli F, Jiddane M, et al. MR imaging of epidermoid cysts. *Neuroradiology* 1987;29:333–338.
120. Houston LW, Hinke ML. Neuroradiology case of the day: suprasellar epidermoid. *AJR* 1986;146:1094–1095.
121. Rooney MS, Poon PY, Wortzman G. Magnetic resonance imaging of intracranial epidermoids: report of two cases. *J Can Assoc Radiol* 1987;38:283–287.
122. Wiener SN, Pearlstein AE, Eiber A. MR imaging of intracranial arachnoid cysts. *J Comput Assist Tomogr* 1987;11:236–241.
123. Kjos B, Brant-Zawadzki M, Kucharczyk W, et al. Cystic intracranial lesions: magnetic resonance imaging. *Radiology* 1985;155: 363.
124. Houspian EM, Marquardt MD, Behrens M. Optic gliomas. In: Wilkins RH, Rengachary SS, eds. *Neurosurgery*. New York: McGraw-Hill; 1985:916–920.
125. Bognanno JR, Edwards MK, Lee TA, et al. Cranial MR imaging in neurofibromatosis. *AJNR* 1888;9:461.
126. Hurst RW, Newman SA, Cail WS. Multifocal intracranial abnormalities in neurofibromatosis. *AJNR* 1988;9:293.
127. Sze G, Uichanco LS, Brant-Zawadzki MN, et al. Chordomas: MR imaging. *Radiology* 1988;166:187–191.
128. Cone L, Srinivasan M, Romanul FCA. Granular cell tumor (choristoma) of the neurohypophysis: two cases and a review of the literature. *AJNR* 1990;11(2):403–406.
129. Bordi L, Compton J, Symon L. Trigeminal neuroma: a report of eleven cases. *Surg Neurol* 1989;31:272–276.
130. Yuh WTC, Wright DC, Barloon TJ, et al. MR imaging of primary tumors of trigeminal nerve and meckel's cave. *AJNR* 1988;9:665.
131. Fox JL, Al-Mefty O. Suprasellar arachnoid cysts: an extension of the membrane of Liliequist. *Neurosurgery* 1980;7:615–618.
132. Burton EM, Ball WS Jr, Crane K, Dolan LM. Hamartomas of tuber cinereum: comparison of MR and CT findings in 4 cases. *AJNR* 1989;10:497.
133. Hahn FJ, Leibrock LG, Huseman CA, Makos MM. The MR appearance of hypothalamic hamartoma. *Neuroradiology* 1988;30: 65–68.
134. Hubbard AM, Egelhoff JC. MR Imaging of large hypothalamic hamartomas in two infants. *AJNR* 1989;10:1277.
135. Rothman M, Akhtar N, Bush C, et al. MR imaging of hamartomas of the tuber cinereum. ASNR 1995 Annual Meeting, paper #37, Chicago, IL.
136. Haynes EF. Enlargement of lymph nodes and spleen: In: Braunwald E, Isselbacher KJ, Petersdorf RG, et al., eds. *Harrison's Principles of Internal Medicine*, 11th ed. New York: McGraw-Hill; 1987:272–278.
137. Moore JB, Kulkarn R, Crutcher DC, Bhimani S. MRI in multifocal eosinophilic granulomatosis: staging disease and monitoring response to therapy. *Am J Pediatr Hematol Oncol* 1989;11:174–177.
138. Daughaday WH. The anterior pituitary. In: Wilson JD, Foster DW, eds. *William's Textbook of Endocrinology*, 7th ed. Philadelphia: WB Saunders; 1985:568–612.
139. Tien RD, Newton TH, McDermott MW, et al. Thickened pituitary stalk on MR images in patients with diabetes insipidus and Langerhans' cell histiocytosis. *AJNR* 1990;11:703–708.
140. Rosenfield NS, Abrahams J, Komp D. Brain MR in patients with Langerhans' cell histiocytosis: findings and enhancement with Gd-DTPA. *Pediatr Radiol* 1990;20(6):433–436.
141. Gupta RK, Jena A, Sharma A. Cranial, sellar abscess associated with tuberculous osteomyelitis of skull: MR findings. *AJNR* 1989;10:448.
142. Daningue JN, Wilson CB. Pituitary abscesses: report of 7 cases and review of the literature. *J Neurosurg* 1977;46:601–608.
143. Selosse P, Mahler, Klaes RL. Pituitary abscess: case report. *J Neurosurg* 1980;53:851–852.
144. Martinez HR, Rangel-Guerra R, Elizondo G, et al. MR imaging in neurocysticercosis: study of 56 cases. *AJNR* 1989;10:1011.
145. Suss RA, Maravilla KR, Thompson J. MR imaging of intracranial cysticercosis: comparison with CT and anatomopathologic features. *AJNR* 1986;7:235.
146. Asa SL, Bilbao JM, Kovacs K, et al. Lymphocytic hypophysitis of pregnancy resulting in hypopituitarism: a distinct clinicopathologic entity. *Ann Intern Med* 1981;95:166.
147. Goudie RB, Pinkerton PH. Anterior hypophysitis and Hashimoto's disease in a young woman. *J Pathol Bacteriol* 1962;83: 584–585.
148. Hungerford GD, Biggs PJ, Levine JH, et al. Lymphoid adenohypophysitis with radiologic and clinical findings resembling a pituitary tumor. *AJNR* 1982;3:444.
149. Quencer RM. Lymphocytic adenohypophysitis: autoimmune disorder of the pituitary gland. *AJNR* 1980;1:343.
150. Levine SN, Benzel EC, Fowler MR, et al. Lymphocytic hypophysitis: clinical, radiological, and magnetic resonance imaging characterization. *Neurosurgery* 1988;22(5):937–941.
151. Crystal RG. Sarcoidosis: In: Braunwald E, Isselbacher KJ, Petersdorf RG, et al., eds. *Harrison's Principles of Internal Medicine,* 11th ed. New York: McGraw-Hill; 1987:1445–1450.
152. Cooper SD, Brady MB, Williams JP, et al. Neurosarcoidosis: evaluation using CT and MRI. *J Comput Assist Tomogr* 1988;12:96–99.
153. Hayes WS, Sherman JL, Stern BJ, et al. MR and CT evaluation of intracranial sarcoidosis. *AJR* 1987;149:1043–1049.
154. Lewis R, Wilson J, Smith FW. Diabetes insipidus secondary to intracranial sarcoidosis confirmed by low-field MRI. *Magn Res Med* 1987;5:466–470.
155. Miller DH, Kendall BE, Barter S, et al. MRI in central nervous system sarcoidosis. *Neurology* 1988;38:378–383.
156. Smith AS, Meisler DM, Weinstein MA, et al. High signal periventricular lesions in patients with sarcoidosis: neurosarcoidosis or multiple sclerosis? *AJR* 1988;153:147–152.
157. Aron-Rosa D, Doyon D, Salamon G, Michotey P. Tolosa-Hunt syndrome. *Ann Ophthalmol* 1978;10:1161–1168.
158. Kwan ESK, Wolpert SM, Hedges TR III, Lancella M. Tolosa-Hunt syndrome revisited: not necessarily a diagnosis of exclusion. *AJNR* 1987;8:1067–1072.
159. Yousem DM, Atlas SW, Grossman RI, et al. MR imaging of Tolosa-Hunt syndrome. *AJNR* 1989;10:1181–1184.
160. Atlas SW, Mark AS, Fram EK, Grossman R. Vascular intracranial lesions: applications of gradient-echo MR imaging. *Radiology* 1988;169:455–461.
161. Biondi A, Scialfa G, Scotti G. Intracranial aneurysms: MR imaging. *Neuroradiology* 1988;30:214–218.
162. Brougham M, Heusner AP, Adams RD. Acute degenerative changes in adenomas of the pituitary body—with special reference to pituitary apoplexy. *J Neurosurg* 1950;7:421–439.
163. Sheehan HL, Stanford JP. The pathogenesis of post-partum pituitary necrosis of the anterior lobe of the pituitary gland. *Acta Endocrinol* 1961;37:479–510.
164. Newton TH and Trost BT. Arteriovenous malformations and fistulas. In: Newton TH and Potts DG, eds. *Radiology of the Skull and Brain*. St. Louis: Mosby; 1974:2490–2565.
165. Elster AD, Chen MYM, Richardson DN, Yeatts PR. Dilated intercavernous sinuses: an MR sign of carotid-cavernous and carotid-dural fistulas. *AJNR* 1991;12:641–645.
166. Kaard HP, Khangure MS, Waring P. Extraaxial parasellar cavernous hemangioma. *AJNR* 1990;11:1259–1261.
167. Zentner J, Grodd W, Hassler W. Cavernous angioma of the optic tract. *J Neurol* 1989;236:117–119.
168. Tien R, Dillon WP. MR imaging of cavernous hemangioma of the optic chiasm. *J Comput Assist Tomogr* 1989;13(6):1087–1100.
169. Streeten DHP, Moses AM, Miller M. Disorders of the neurohypophysis: In: Braunwald E, Isselbacher KJ, Petersdorf RG, et al., eds. *Harrison's Principles of Internal Medicine*, 11th ed. New York: McGraw-Hill; 1987:1722–1732.
170. Martin MR. Familial diabetes insipidus. *Q J Med* 1959;28:573–582.
171. Halimi P, Sigal R, Doyon D, et al. Post-traumatic diabetes insip-

idus: MR demonstration of pituitary stalk rupture. *J Comput Assist Tomogr* 1988;12:135.
172. Massol J, Humert P, Cattin F, et al. Post-traumatic diabetes insipidus and amenorrhea galactorrhea syndrome after pituitary stalk rupture. *Neuroradiol* 1987;29:299.
173. Gudinchet F, Brunelle F, Barth MO, et al. MR imaging of the posterior hypophysis in children. *AJNR* 1989;10:511.
174. Moses AM, Clayton B, Hochhauser L. Use of T1-weighted MR imaging to differentiate between primary polydipsia and central diabetes insipidus. *AJNR* 1992;13:1273–1277.
175. Brooks BS, Gammal TE, Allison JD, Hoffman WH. Frequency and variation of the posterior pituitary bright signal on MR images. *AJNR* 1989;10:943–948.
176. Maghnie M, Villa A, Arico M, et al. Correlation between magnetic resonance imaging of posterior pituitary and neurohypophyseal function in children with diabetes insipidus. *J Clin Endocrinol Metab* 1992;74(4):795–800.
177. Hutchins WW, Crues JV III, Miya P, Pojunas KW. MR demonstration of pituitary hyperplasia and regression after therapy for hypothyroidism. *AJNR* 1990;11:410.
178. Kuroiwa T, Okabe Y, Hasuo K, et al. MR imaging of pituitary hypertrophy due to juvenile primary hypothyroidism: a case report. *Clin Imag* 1991;15:202–205.
179. Fujisawa I, Morikawa M, Nakano Y, Kanishi J. Hemochromatosis of the pituitary gland: MR imaging. *Radiology* 1988;168:213–214.
180. Kucharczyk W, Olivieri NF, Liu P, Henkelman RM. MRI of the anterior pituitary gland in thalassemia major: correlation of T2 relaxation with clinical and hormonal status. ASNR 28th Annual Meeting, Washington, D.C., 1991.

Magnetic Resonance Imaging of the Brain and Spine, Second Edition, edited by Scott W. Atlas.
Lippincott-Raven Publishers, Philadelphia © 1996.

20

The Skull Base

Hugh D. Curtin and Joseph J. Wehner

Magnetic resonance imaging (MRI) has become an essential part of the evaluation of skull base lesions. There are two primary issues that must be addressed by the radiologist. First, the identity of the tumor is important. The radiologist uses both anatomic location (Fig. 1) and imaging characteristics to arrive at a best approximation of the diagnosis preoperatively. Second, with the advent of the newer surgical techniques, the precise definition of the extent of a lesion has assumed far greater importance and has provided a further challenge to the radiologist. The first section of the chapter discusses general concepts about differentiating tumor from the normal structures of the skull base. In particular, we will focus on the detection of a tumor margin as the tumor spreads either by direct encroachment or by perineural (transforaminal) extension. The next section is devoted to identifying specific tumor types, using their position and various imaging characteristics as a guide. Finally, brief mention is made of miscellaneous non-neoplastic pathologies.

H. D. Curtin, M.D.: Department of Radiology and Otolaryngology, University of Pittsburgh School of Medicine, and Department of Radiology, Pittsburgh, PA 15213.

J. J. Wehner, M.D.: Neuroradiology Division, Department of Radiology, University of Pittsburgh School of Medicine, Pittsburgh, PA 15213.

EVALUATION OF MASS LESIONS

General Concepts: Normal versus Abnormal

The radiologist tries to differentiate a lesion from the myriad of normal structures making up the skull base. The interface of the tumor with bone, muscle, and fat must be defined in the same way as it is in other regions of the body. Problems specific to the skull base include showing the margin of the tumor relative to the cavernous sinus and differentiating tumor from an obstructed paranasal sinus. The relationship of the tumor to the carotid artery is of extreme importance, often determining the feasibility of resection and the necessity of further radiologic investigation.

Bone

The cortical bone of the skull base is represented as a signal void. The bone may or may not have a medullary cavity. For example, the clivus has a significant marrow cavity whereas the roofs of the orbit and the ethmoid do not. If the medullary cavity is filled with fatty yellow marrow, then tumor can usually be differentiated from either cortex or marrow based on signal difference. On nonenhanced T1-weighted images, the tumor is usually

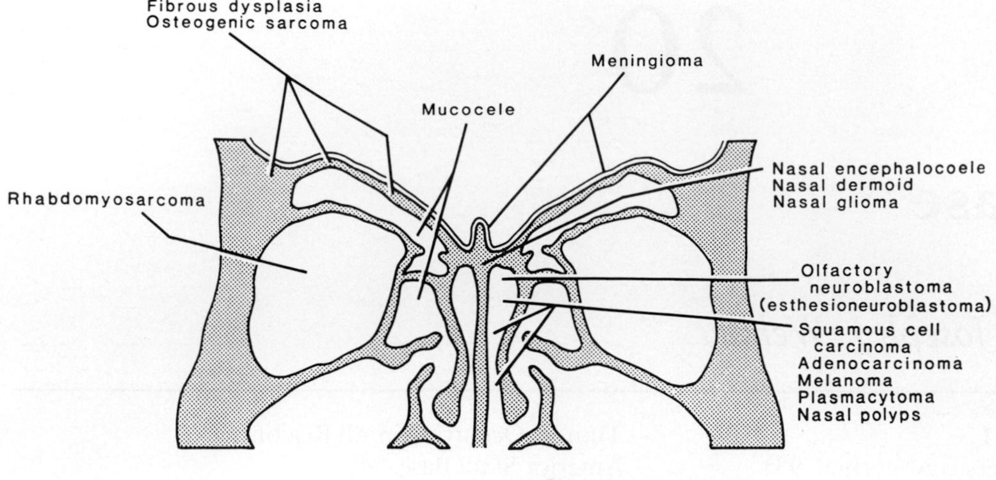

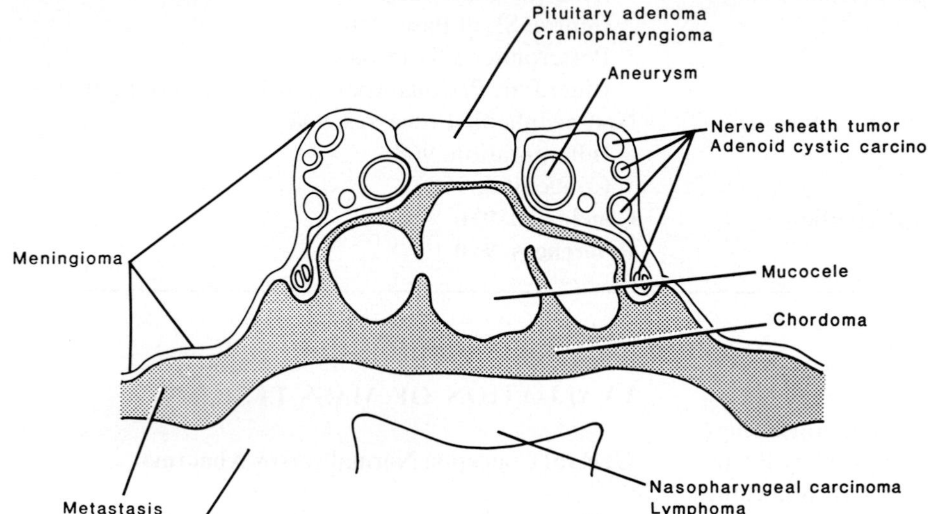

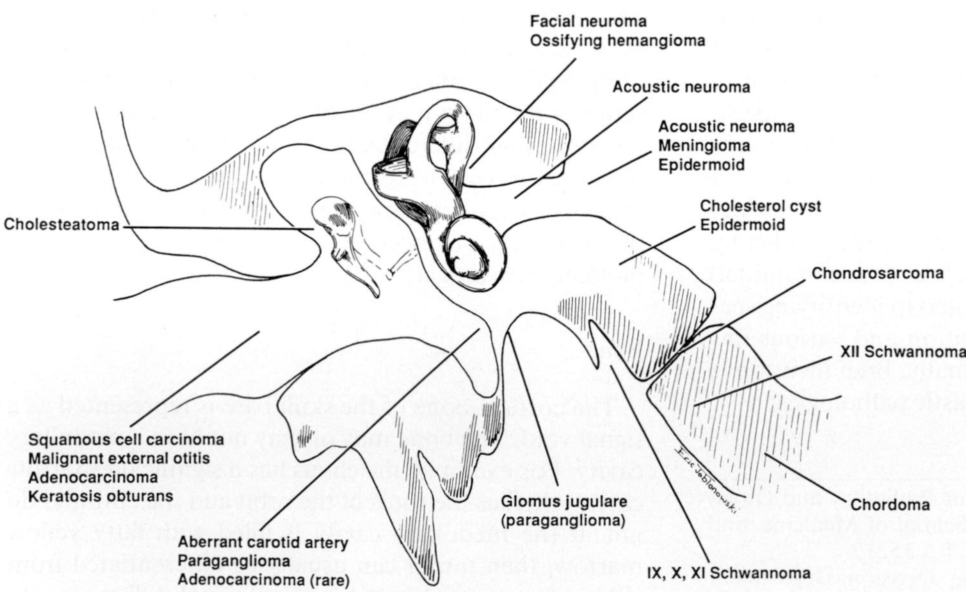

FIG. 1. Anatomic sites of skull base masses. **A:** Coronal schematic section through orbits. **B:** Coronal section through cavernous sinuses. **C:** Coronal schematic section through right temporal bone.

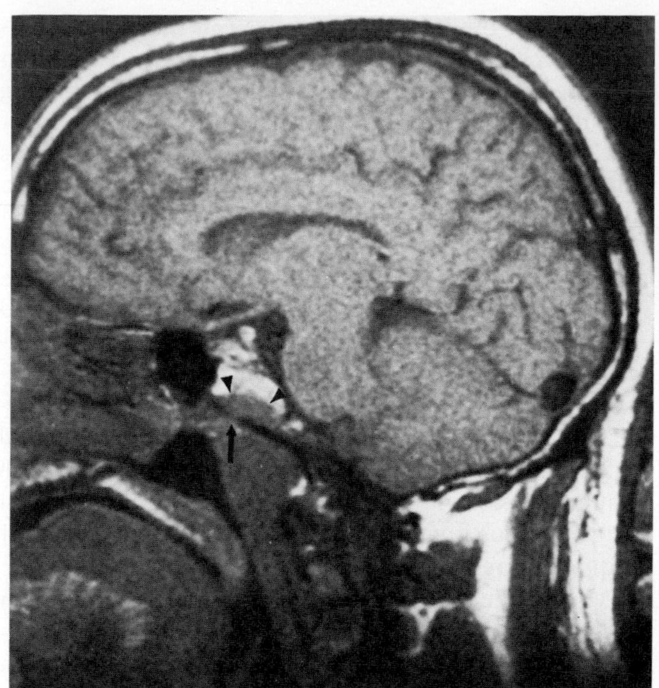

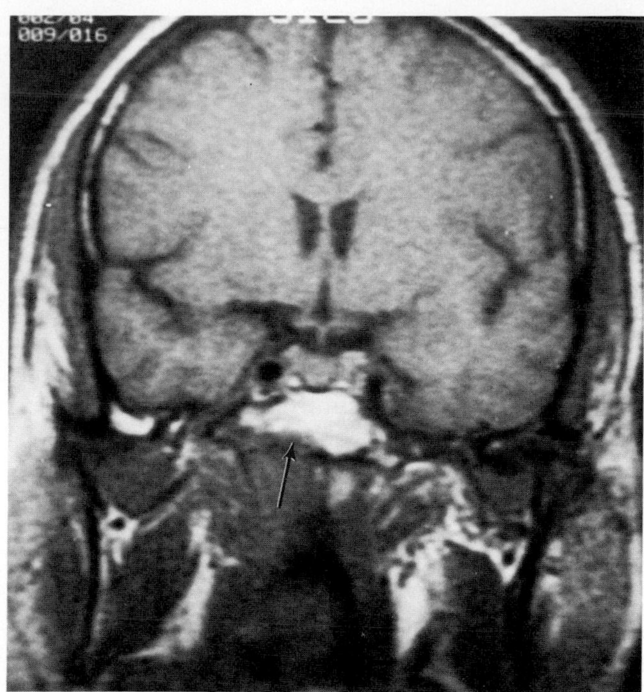

FIG. 2. Nasopharyngeal lesion. **A:** Sagittal SE (400/20) MRI shows a mass passing through the signal void of the nasopharyngeal cortex of the clivus (*arrow*). The high signal of the marrow is replaced by the intermediate-signal tumor (*arrowheads*). **B:** Coronal view shows the minimal erosion of the cortex and extension into the marrow (*arrow*).

intermediate in signal intensity. The tumor can be seen passing through the signal void of the cortex or can replace the high signal of the fatty marrow (Fig. 2) (1).

There can be several problems in making this determination. First, if the marrow has not yet been replaced with fat, as in a young child, differentiation can be more difficult (Fig. 3). The tumor may have a very similar appearance to this hematopoietic marrow on the various sequences (1,2).

Second, if a thin bony cortex does not completely fill a voxel, then normal soft tissue immediately adjacent to the thin bone will give enough signal so that the signal void is not present. This is especially true when a thin bone is oblique to the plane of imaging.

Third, the contiguous area may have no signal or low enough signal that the cortical bone cannot be confidently distinguished. This is a particular problem in the roof of the ethmoid. Air in the sinus below is a signal void and the cerebrospinal fluid (CSF) above is also low enough in signal that the ethmoid roof disappears. Definition of fine cortical bony structures, such as the ethmoid septations, roof of the ethmoid, or the wall of the carotid canal still requires high resolution computed tomography (CT).

Other sequences can be helpful in determining bone

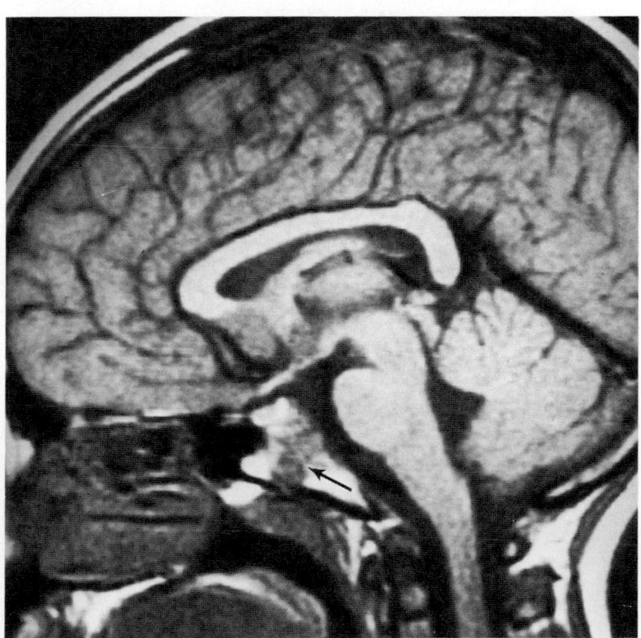

FIG. 3. Normal clivus in a young child. Sagittal SE (500/20) MR scan shows fatty replacement of basiocciput but residual hematopoietic marrow in the basisphenoid (*arrow*). The red marrow could be confused with neoplastic involvement of the basisphenoid. Fatty replacement of the clivus generally occurs by age 6 years.

invasion. Tumor frequently will enhance after administration of gadolinium. If the tissue on the opposite side of the bone (such as the dura) enhances more than usual then one can tell that the bone is involved even though the cortex is not actually visualized. If fat suppression is used after gadolinium, the enhancing tumor may be visualized within the marrow as well. The tumor enhances whereas the fat within the marrow is suppressed.

Care must be taken when using fat suppression in skull base imaging. Susceptibility effects caused by an air/tissue interface may cause artifacts obscuring important structures. The susceptibility effect shifts the resonant frequency of nonfat tissues into the suppression range. This can be seen in the area of the cavernous sinus where "blooming" of the sphenoid sinus obscures the normal structures (Fig. 4).

On T2-weighted sequences, tumor may be relatively brighter than normal tissues. With conventional spin-echo sequences fat is dark on T2 and so tumor in the medullary cavity of bone may also be seen. The fat may remain bright if fast spin-echo (FSE) sequences are used. Using a fat suppression pulse with the FSE can eliminate this problem.

Soft Tissues

The soft tissues beneath the skull base are similar to soft tissues anywhere in the body. Tumor, although variable in appearance, can usually be separated from muscle and fat using the combination of T1, T2, and proton spin-density images (Fig. 5). Usually, the tumor has about the same signal on the short TR sequence as does muscle, but the long TR sequence can make the differentiation. Often, both early and late echoes are useful in this regard. Gadolinium can be very helpful in finding the interface of tumor and normal soft tissue.

Considerable fat surrounds the various muscle groups in the infratemporal fossa, orbit, and elsewhere beneath the skull base. As tumor invades this fat, the normal high signal on the short TR sequence is obliterated by the more intermediate signal of tumor. Indeed, the interface between tumor and fat is so crucial that, in head and neck tumor imaging, gadolinium enhancement can actually interfere with tumor visualization. Fat and enhancing tumor can have the same signal, making the lesion less obvious. Gadolinium enhancement is helpful in evaluating some features such as tumor margins with brain and cavernous sinus. Therefore, we use contrast as part of our imaging protocol but a nonenhanced T1 sequence is included as well.

More recently, fat suppression techniques have been used with gadolinium enhancement to define better tumor extent in the region below the skull base. Often, with this technique, the tumor can be made more conspicuous and imaging time can be saved by allowing the examination to be done with fewer sequences. With fat suppression, the tumor, which usually enhances, has a different signal than either fat or muscle and both important interfaces can be assessed at the same time.

As previously discussed, there can be problems with fat suppression. Regions surrounding the sphenoid sinus, or other air-containing structures, are prone to obscuration by artifact on fat suppression sequences because of susceptibility effects at the air/tissue interface (see Fig. 4).

A 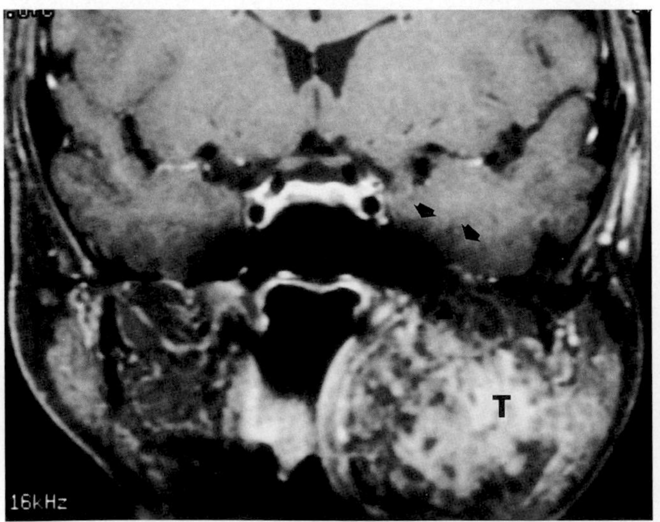

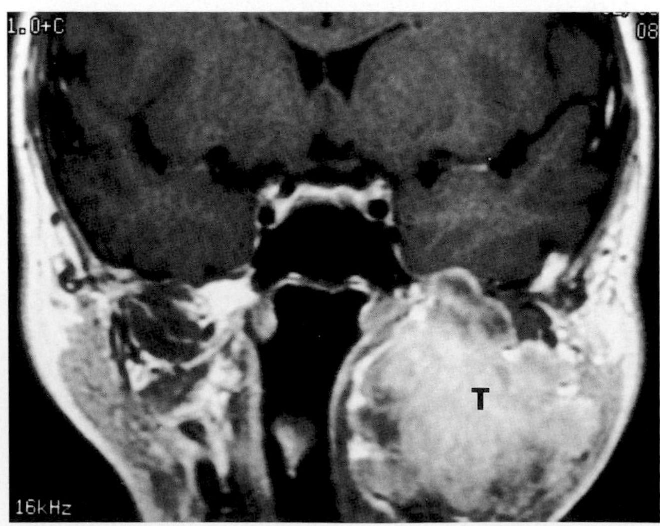 B

FIG. 4. A: Parotid tumor (*T*) extending into skull base. Postgadolinium coronal T1-weighted images with fat saturation pulse shows artifactual water signal suppression of the area of interest because of susceptibility effect related to air in sphenoid sinus (*arrows*). **B:** Similar sequence without fat saturation shows extension of tumor into left middle cranial fossa in region of foramen ovale.

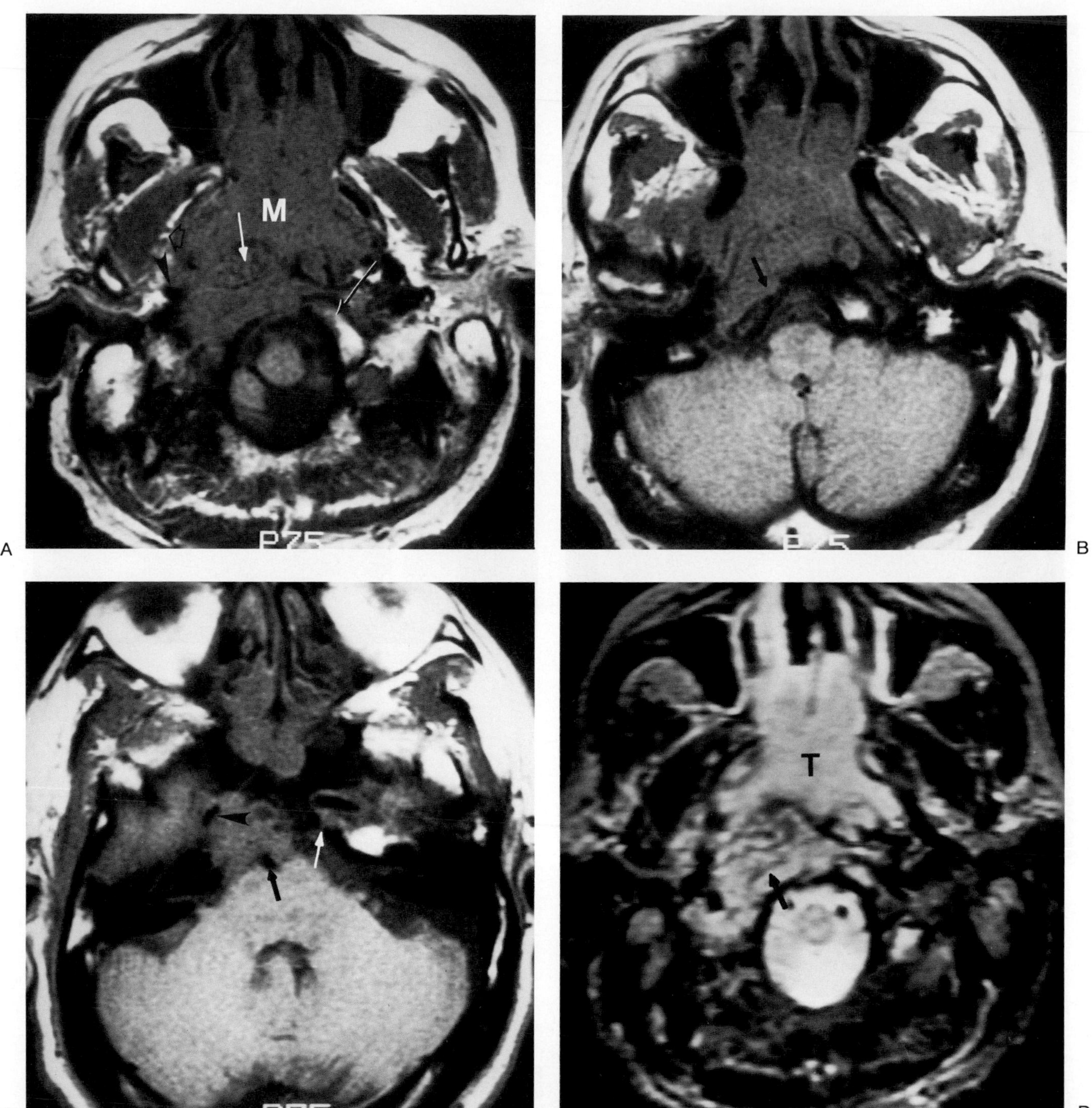

FIG. 5. A–G. Nasopharyngeal carcinoma with skull base involvement. **A:** Axial (short TR/TE) MRI. Large tumor mass fills the nasopharynx. There is extension into the prevertebral muscles (*white arrow*). There is invasion of the occipital condyles on the right (compare with the intact cortex and medullary cavity at the same level on the left) (*black arrow*). The parapharyngeal fat (*open arrow*) is displaced but not invaded. The tumor abuts the carotid artery (*arrowhead*). **B:** Slightly higher slice, same sequence. There is involvement of the basiocciput (*arrow*). **C:** Higher slice, same sequence. There is extension through the petro-occipital suture. The tumor abuts the basilar artery (*black arrow*) as well as the carotid (*arrowhead*). Note the petro-occipital suture (*white arrow*) on the opposite side. **D:** Long TR/long TE MRI shows brightening of the primary tumor (*T*) as well as the involved area of the skull base (*arrow*).

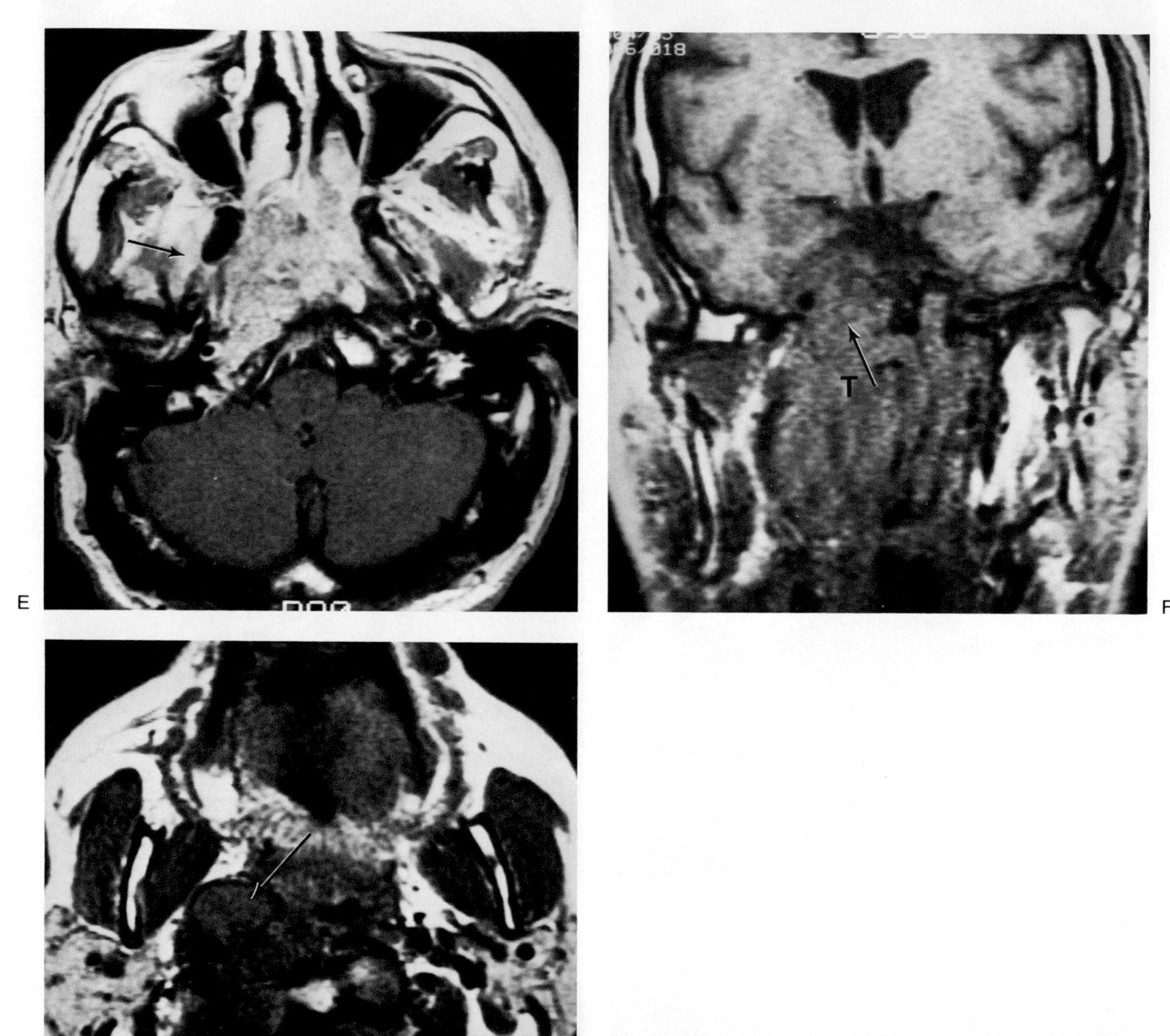

FIG. 5. (*Continued.*) **E:** Postgadolinium short TR/short TE MRI (same level as B). The tumor enhances. It is now more difficult to identify the tumor (*arrow*) in the infratemporal fossa. **F:** Coronal image shows the tumor mass (*T*) extending through the region of the petro-occipital suture and foramen lacerum (*arrow*). Note the involvement of the cavernous sinus with the outward bulging of the lateral wall. **G:** Inferior slice short TR/ short TE shows a lateral retropharyngeal node (*arrow*) (node of Rouvière).

Paranasal Sinuses

As a tumor grows within a sinus, the signal void of air is replaced by signal representing tumor. However, inflammation or obstruction also give signal in the sinus. If the tumor margin is to be clearly identified, the radiologist must separate inflammatory/obstructive from neoplastic changes. Since the tumor may actually cause the obstruction of the sinus, both tumor and nontumor changes can be found within the same sinus cavity.

One can be relatively sure that a sinus is obstructed rather than involved by tumor if the signal is very bright on the late echo of a long TR sequence (T2) (Fig. 6). Some tumors are also relatively bright, but very seldom are they as intense as an obstructed sinus (3). One can be even more confident if the high signal area conforms exactly to the expected configuration of the sinus in question.

However, as more experience is gained with MRI, the variations in the appearance of benign sinus disease have grown significantly. A simple obstruction often has low or intermediate signal on T1 and a high signal on T2 weighting (see Fig. 6). A sinus obstructed for a longer time may have a very different appearance. As the protein content of the secretions increases, the sinus may become fairly bright on both T1-weighted and T2-weighted images (Fig. 7). Further increases can cause gradually decreasing signal until, finally, as the protein content reaches approximately 35%, there is a relative signal void (Fig. 8). This can mimic air even though the sinus is completely obstructed. At our institution, this phenomenon has been seen most often with aspergillosis, but other observers have described similar findings in long-standing obstruction without the fungus (4–6). Hemorrhage into the sinus, at any time during the course of the disease, may further complicate the appearance of the non-neoplastic sinus (7).

Intravenous contrast can help. In an obstructed sinus, the mucosal lining around the circumference of the sinus enhances but the central mucus-filled cavity will not (see Fig. 8B). Tumors, by comparison, almost always enhance to some degree. Caution must be exercised as the mucosa may be quite thick or the tumor may not enhance uniformly. Even though both tumor and benign changes can have a wider spectrum of appearance than was initially hoped, MRI can, in most cases, make a reliable determination of the margin of a tumor relative to the obstructed sinus. As each case is analyzed using multiple pulse sequences, the signal characteristics of the tumor differ enough from the sinus in question so that an accurate determination can be made (see Fig. 7). Tumor extension through the wall of the sinus interrupts the signal void of the cortical bony wall and tumor will be seen on the opposite side of that wall. In most cases, the outer surface of the sinus wall abuts fat, CSF, or air in another sinus. In these situations, tumor can easily be differen-

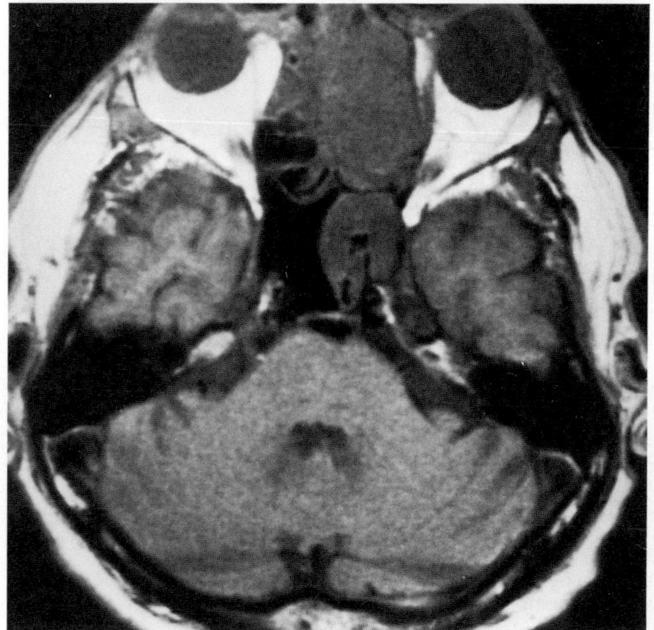

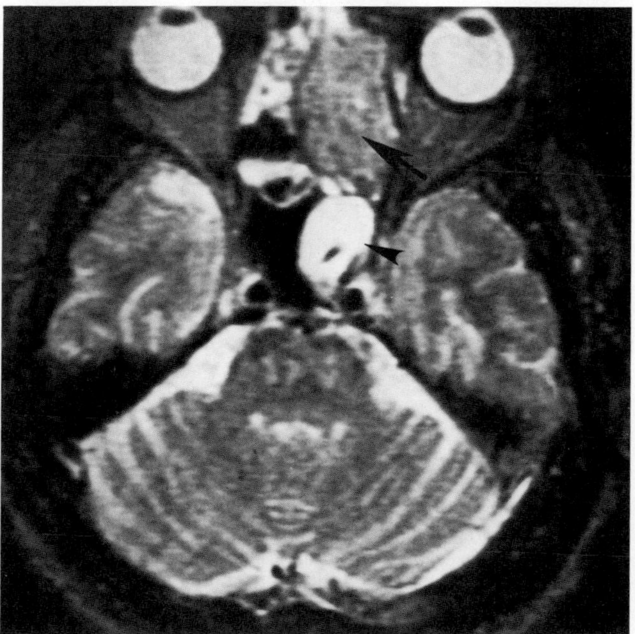

FIG. 6. Carcinoma of the ethmoid. **A:** Axial SE (500/20) short TR/short TE MRI shows abnormal tissue in the ethmoid and sphenoid air cells. It is difficult to differentiate the tumor from the adjacent obstructed air cells. **B:** Axial SE (2500/100) MRI. On this T2-weighted image the neoplasm (*large arrow*) is low signal. The adjacent obstructed air cell in the right sphenoid sinus is high signal (*arrowhead*). The high signal abnormality conforms to the expected configuration of the air cells.

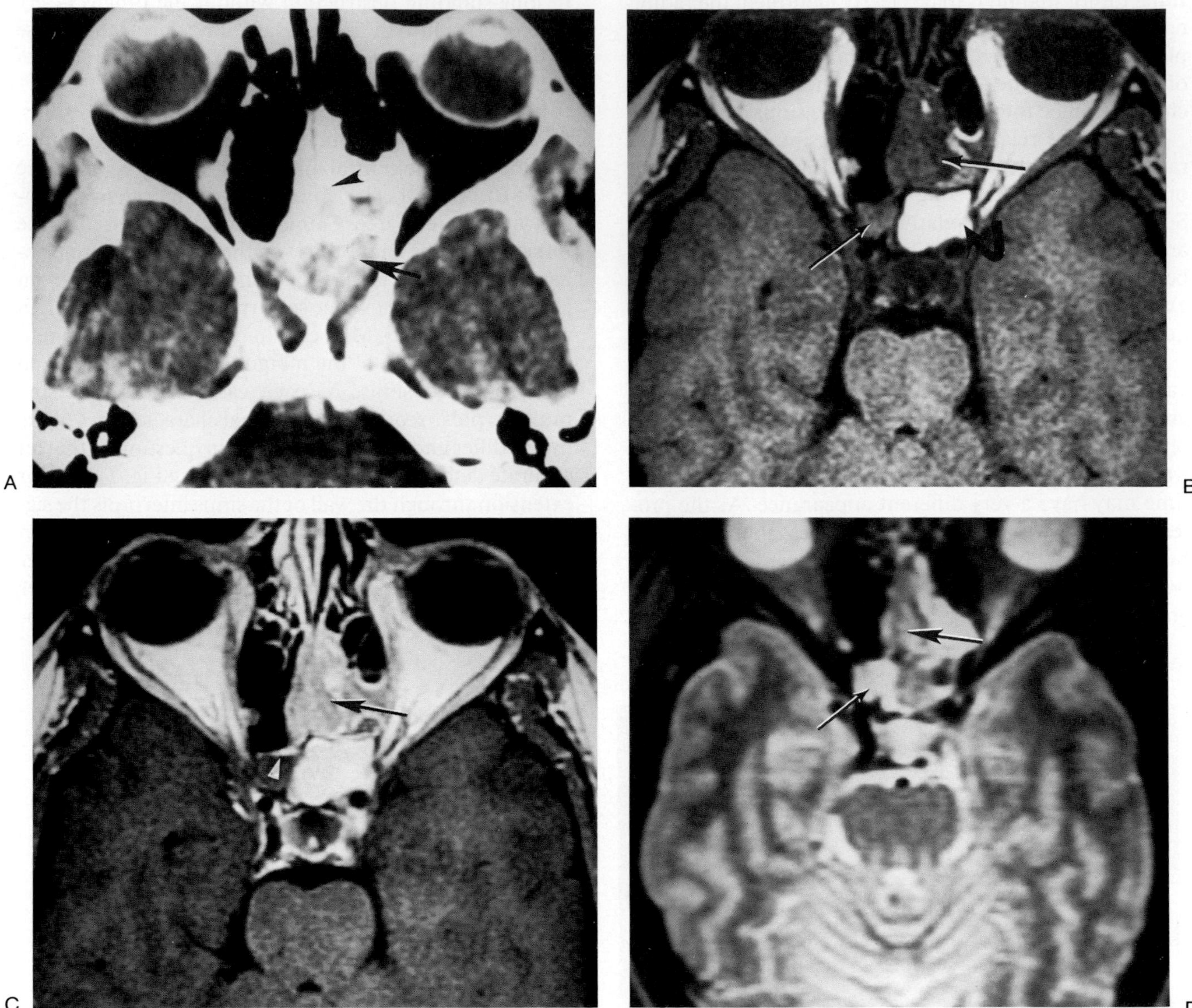

FIG. 7. Esthesioneuroblastoma. **A:** Axial enhanced CT scan shows opacification of the upper nasal cavity and sphenoid air cells. Beam-hardening artifact (*arrow*) gives the impression that the enhancing mass protrudes into the sphenoid air cells. Actual tumor (*arrowhead*) **B:** Unenhanced SE (500/20) MRI. There is a mass in the nasal cavity (*large arrow*) of intermediate-signal intensity. The right sphenoid air cell (*small arrow*) is obstructed, but on this T1-weighted image its contents cannot be differentiated from tumor. The left sphenoid air cell (*curved arrow*) is also obstructed but has high signal contents, easily differentiated from tumor. **C:** After gadolinium the esthesioneuroblastoma enhances (*large arrow*). There is peripheral enhancement of the obstructed right sphenoid air cell (*arrowhead*). **D:** Axial SE (2200/90) MRI. The neoplasm (*large arrow*) is isointense with brain. Some of the obstructed air cells have high signal (*small arrow*), whereas the left sphenoid air cell has a signal intensity similar to the tumor. With MRI tumor can be differentiated from obstructed sinus in most cases by comparing the various pulsing sequences.

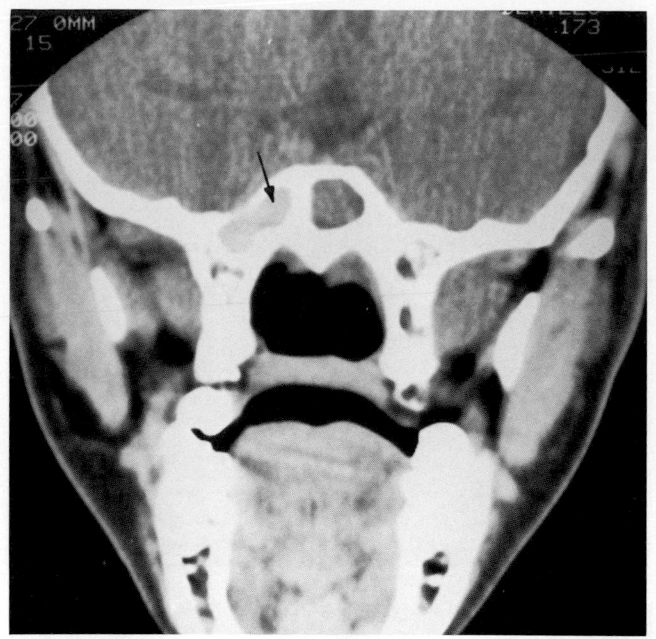

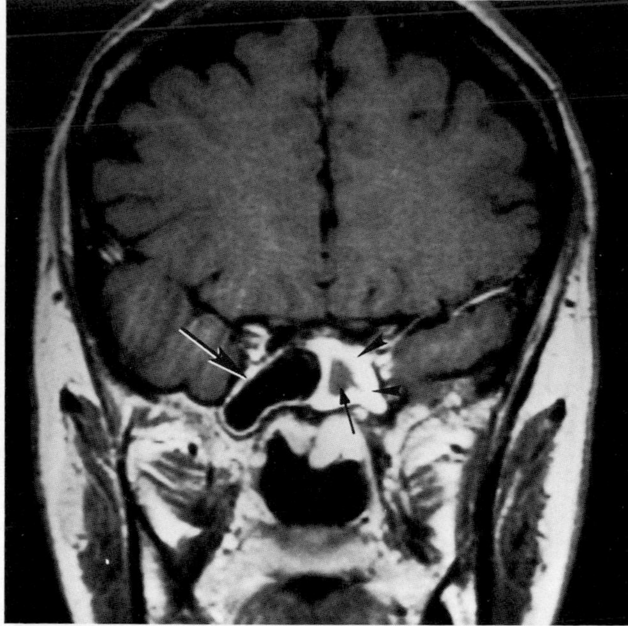

A B

FIG. 8. Fungal sinusitis. **A:** Coronal nonenhanced CT. The sphenoid sinus is opaque, but the air cell on the right (*arrow*) is denser than the one on the left. **B:** Postcontrast SE (500/20) MRI. The right-sided air cell has a thin enhancing mucosa surrounding a signal void (*large arrow*). Even though it is completely obstructed, this sinus appears to be aerated, having similar signal characteristics to the air in the nasopharynx. At surgery this sinus contained an aspergillus mycetoma. The left sphenoid air cell has a more typical appearance of an obstructed sinus with a thick enhancing mucosal lining (*arrowheads*) surrounding nonenhancing secretions (*small arrow*). On long TR/long TE there was no signal in the right sinus.

tiated from the normal tissues. Tumor breaking out of the sphenoid sinus may involve the cavernous sinus. As we discuss below, differentiation of tumor from the cavernous sinus is often difficult.

Cavernous Sinus (Including Perineural Extension)

The cavernous sinus is a plexus of small veins and venous sinusoids adjacent to the sella. In common usage, the term "cavernous sinus" encompasses the entire parasellar region including the investing dura, Meckel's cave, and the parasellar segments of the cranial nerves III through VI. Tumor can reach the region either by direct extension or by following the many nerves that traverse the sinus and Meckel's cave. If the tumor first reaches the cave, the signal of the CSF usually found there is replaced, and thus the tumor is identified (8) (Fig. 9). Demonstration of the interface of a tumor with the rest of the cavernous sinus is more difficult. The cavernous sinus may have the same signal characteristics as tumor. By comparing the multiple sequences, however, the edge of the tumor can usually be defined (Fig. 9). Frequently, gadolinium enhancement is helpful because a tumor enhances differently than the normal cavernous sinus, thus allowing definition of the tumor edge.

A change in the shape of the cavernous sinus is a strong indication of tumor involvement (see Fig. 11C). Increased bowing of the lateral wall is seen best on the coronal image but can be appreciated on the axial image as well. Tumor contiguous to Meckel's cave can compress the normal oval or triangular CSF space even if it does not extend into the cave itself (9).

Complete evaluation of the cavernous sinus requires careful inspection of the pathways by which tumor can reach the cavernous sinus/Meckel's cave region. Other than by direct encroachment, the most frequent pathway is along the branches of the trigeminal nerve. This so-called perineural spread may be from tumors arising in the paranasal sinuses, face, orbit, palate, oral cavity, or any area that receives branches of the trigeminal nerve. Each of the branches traverses at least a small amount of fat immediately after exiting the skull base. As tumor replaces this fat, the characteristic high signal on the T1-

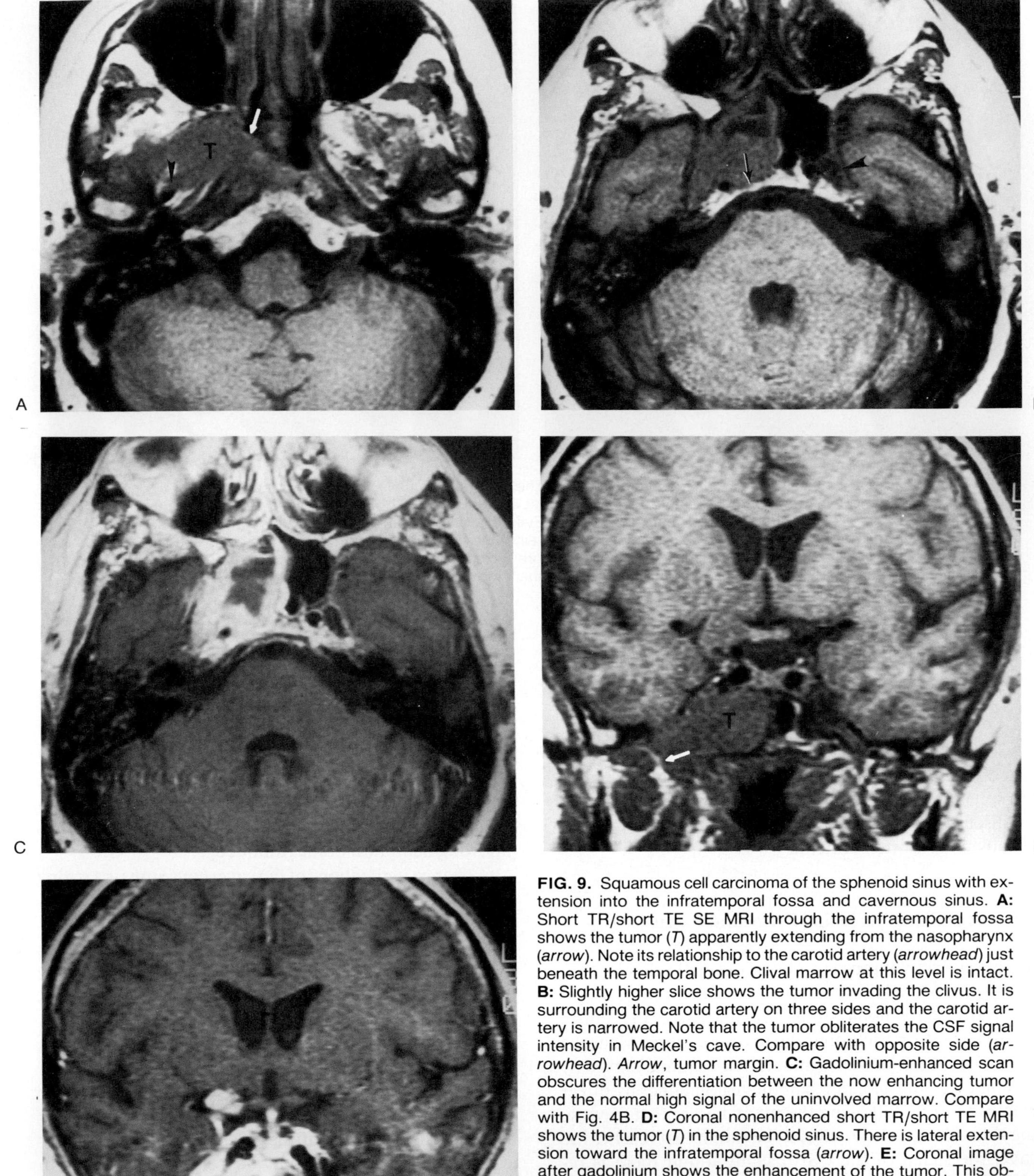

FIG. 9. Squamous cell carcinoma of the sphenoid sinus with extension into the infratemporal fossa and cavernous sinus. **A:** Short TR/short TE SE MRI through the infratemporal fossa shows the tumor (*T*) apparently extending from the nasopharynx (*arrow*). Note its relationship to the carotid artery (*arrowhead*) just beneath the temporal bone. Clival marrow at this level is intact. **B:** Slightly higher slice shows the tumor invading the clivus. It is surrounding the carotid artery on three sides and the carotid artery is narrowed. Note that the tumor obliterates the CSF signal intensity in Meckel's cave. Compare with opposite side (*arrowhead*). *Arrow*, tumor margin. **C:** Gadolinium-enhanced scan obscures the differentiation between the now enhancing tumor and the normal high signal of the uninvolved marrow. Compare with Fig. 4B. **D:** Coronal nonenhanced short TR/short TE MRI shows the tumor (*T*) in the sphenoid sinus. There is lateral extension toward the infratemporal fossa (*arrow*). **E:** Coronal image after gadolinium shows the enhancement of the tumor. This obscures the margin between enhancing tumor and infratemporal fossa fat. Note again the normal low signal intensity representing the CSF in Meckel's cave on the normal side (*arrowhead*). Meckel's cave is obliterated on the involved side, and there is outward bowing of the lateral wall of the cavernous sinus. The mucosa in the nasopharynx also enhances (*arrow*), but the lesion does not appear to be arising from this tissue.

weighted image is obliterated (Fig. 10). If the fat is normal just outside a particular neural foramen, then it is highly unlikely that tumor has reached or more importantly traversed the foramen.

Perhaps the most important of these small fat-containing structures is the pterygopalatine fossa (Fig. 10A). Tumors can travel along the second branch of the trigeminal nerve through the pterygopalatine fossa to reach the foramen rotundum and thus the cavernous sinus and Meckel's cave (10). Assessment of this area is an important part of the evaluation of any tumor of the face, paranasal sinuses, or palate.

Fat in the superior orbital fissure protrudes into the anterior aspect of the cavernous sinus. A tumor growing along the nerves that pass through the fissure obliterates this fat and is therefore detectable. Although less obvious than in the superior orbital fissure or the pterygopalatine fossa, there is a small amount of fat just below the foramen ovale and below the stylomastoid foramen (11). Thus, perineural extension entering the skull base via the mandibular branch of the trigeminal nerve or via the facial nerve can be detected as well.

Tumor actually in the foramen can be detected in several ways. The tumor usually enlarges the foramen. Enhancement of the tissue within the foramen is presumed to represent tumor even if the foramen is not enlarged (Fig. 11). Of course, tumor visualized at the endocranial opening of the foramen also indicates that the foramen is involved.

Carotid Artery

Preoperative imaging has proven to be very valuable in demonstrating the relationship of skull base tumors to the carotid artery. The radiologist must decide whether the artery will be at risk by the planned surgical procedure. Will a study such as a balloon test occlusion with blood-flow mapping be necessary to determine the feasibility of carotid sacrifice (12)?

At our institution, we begin with the MRI. Usually the boundaries of a lesion can be defined by using the three planes available with MRI. The carotid is well seen as a signal void passing through the skull base. With MRI areas of contact between the tumor and the carotid artery can be defined. If the tumor surrounds the artery, then the vessel is clearly involved. The artery may even be narrowed as the tumor surrounds and compresses it. Luminal narrowing may also indicate invasion of the arterial wall itself. At surgery, tumor may have to be picked piecemeal off the involved segment. This technique is accompanied by the risk of carotid tear and possible tumor recurrence. Alternatives include carotid sacrifice and resection of the involved segments or a bypass graft. With tumors close to the intrapetrous carotid, CT with bone algorithms has an advantage over MR because CT can assess the very fine cortical bony wall of the carotid canal (see Fig. 34). Similarly, CT may be required to determine whether or not there is bony separation between a tumor in the sphenoid sinus and the cavernous carotid artery.

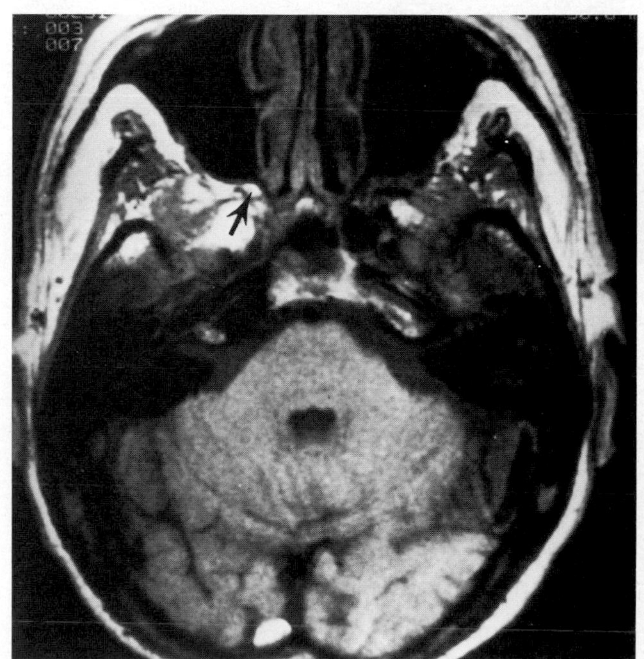

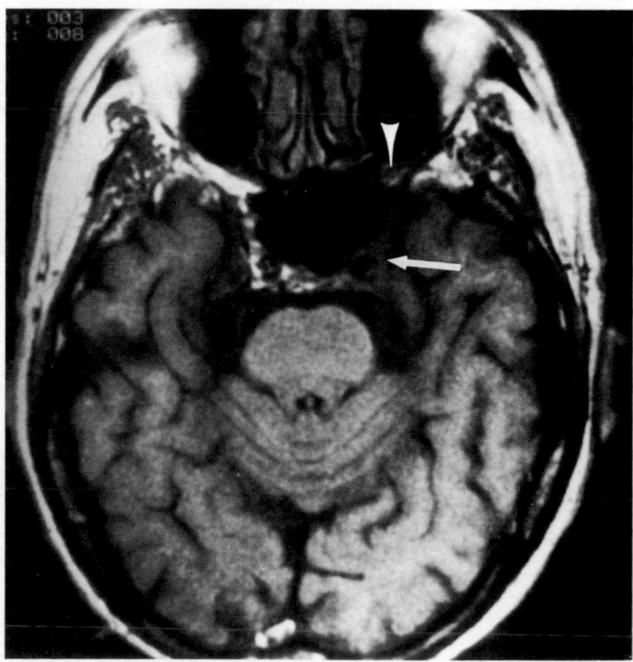

FIG. 10. Adenoid cystic carcinoma with perineural spread. **A:** Axial SE (500/20) MRI. The right pterygopalatine fossa contains normal fat signal (*arrow*). On the left the fat is replaced by neoplasm. **B:** Slightly higher cut shows involvement of the left cavernous sinus (*arrow*) and obliteration of the fat in the upper pterygopalatine fossa (*arrowhead*).

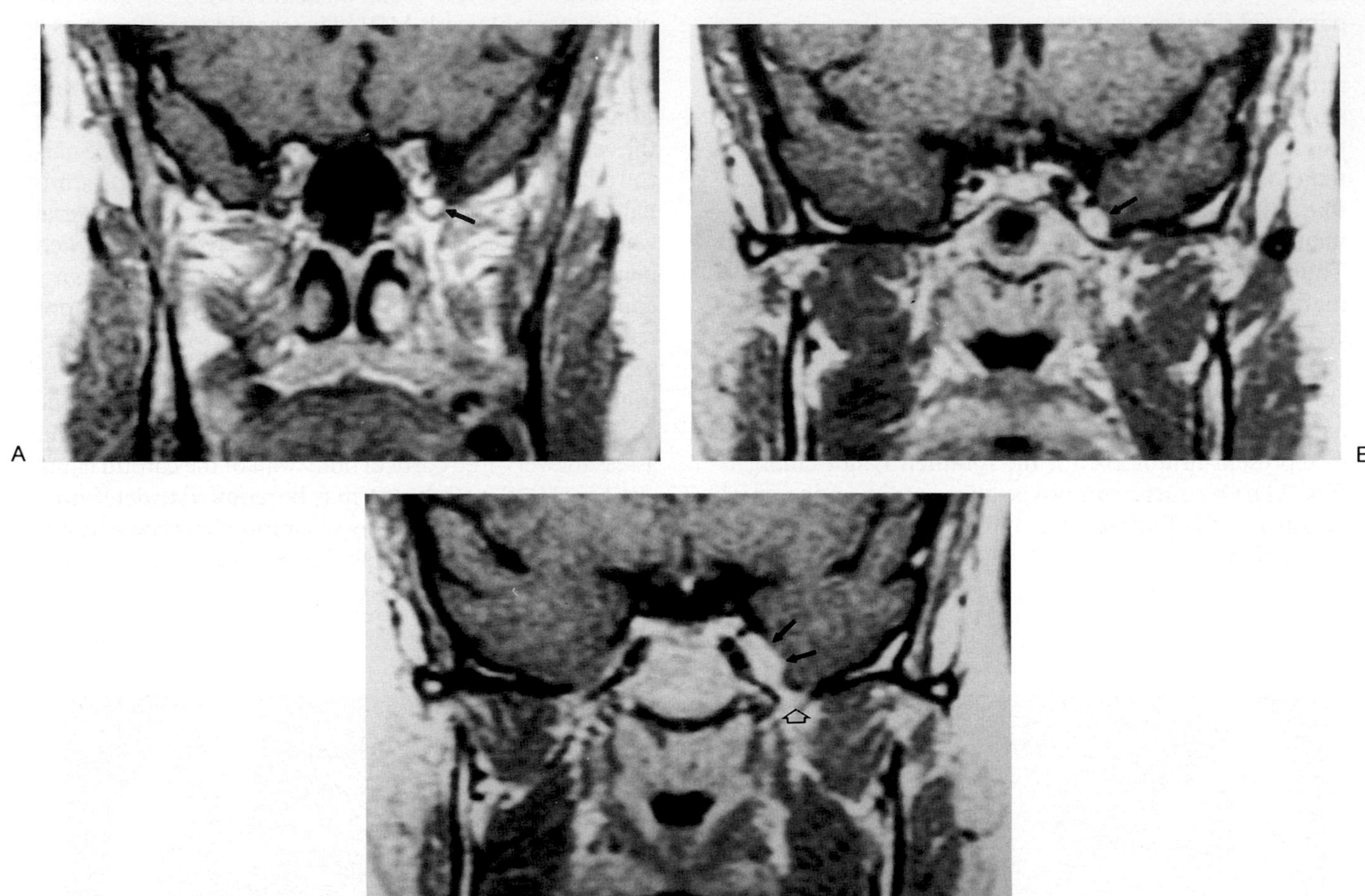

FIG. 11. Coronal T1-weighted gadolinium enhanced images. Adenoid cystic carcinoma of the hard palate including left ptergopalative fossa (not shown). **A:** *Arrow* shows enhancement within foramen rotundum without expansion of the foramen, indicating perineural spread along V_2. **B:** *Arrow* shows enlargement and enhancement of cranial aspect of foramen rotundum. **C:** *Arrows* show asymmetry of the cavernous sinus indicating intracavernous tumor extension. *Hollow arrowhead*, foramen ovale.

TUMOR IDENTIFICATION AND EVALUATION IN SPECIFIC REGIONS

Although the final determination of the identity of a tumor almost always requires biopsy, the radiologist is usually called on to predict the tumor type preoperatively. Using the apparent site of origin and the MRI appearance, the radiologist can often be quite accurate in making such a determination, or in at least limiting the possibilities. One of the most important predictors of tumor identity is the apparent site of origin. Some tumors have a strong tendency to arise at particular locations in the skull base but almost never occur in other regions. Other tumors, such as meningiomas and metastatic disease, can occur almost anywhere. For the purposes of this discussion, the skull base can be divided into three regions. The anterior region includes the floor of the anterior cranial fossa or the orbital roofs and the cribriform region. The central region includes the clivus, sella, planum sphenoidale, cavernous sinus, and, more laterally, the greater wing of the sphenoid. The posterolateral region is the temporal bone. This classification is based on commonality of tumor type and, to some extent, surgical approach.

Tumors Occurring in All Regions

Although the site of origin certainly narrows the list of likely diagnoses, some lesions may involve any part of the skull base.

Meningiomas arise from the dura covering the intracranial surface of the skull base or from the dural sleeves following some of the cranial nerves. Although signal characteristics vary, meningiomas are often isointense with brain on both T1-weighted and T2-weighted images (Fig. 12). On T2-weighted images, about 10% are low signal, 50% are intermediate, and 40% are hyperintense relative to brain (Fig. 13) (13).

After gadolinium administration meningiomas enhance, often intensely. The enhancement may taper out or appear to extend along the dura beyond the edge of the main tumor mass (Fig. 13). There are various opinions about the significance of this enhancement. Tumor cells spreading along the dural sheet may be responsible for local recurrence.

Although more readily apparent on CT, hyperostosis can often be appreciated on MR as a thickening of the cortical surface of the skull (Figs. 13A,B). Calcification may be present in meningiomas and, if large enough,

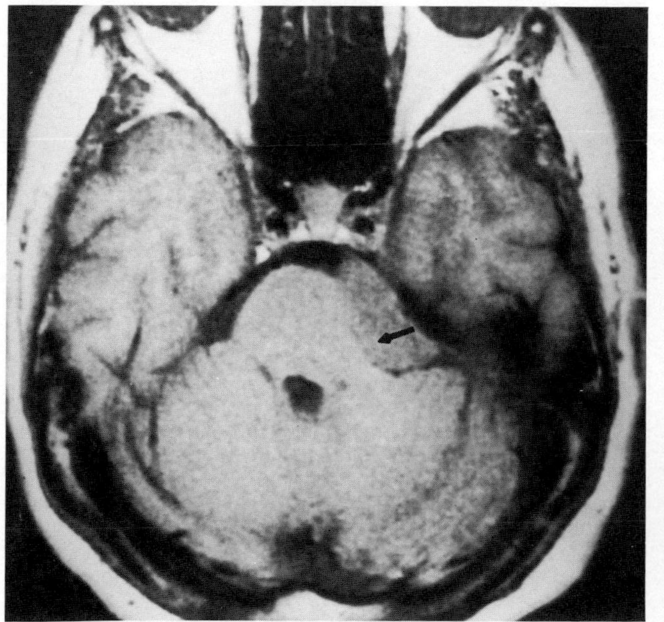

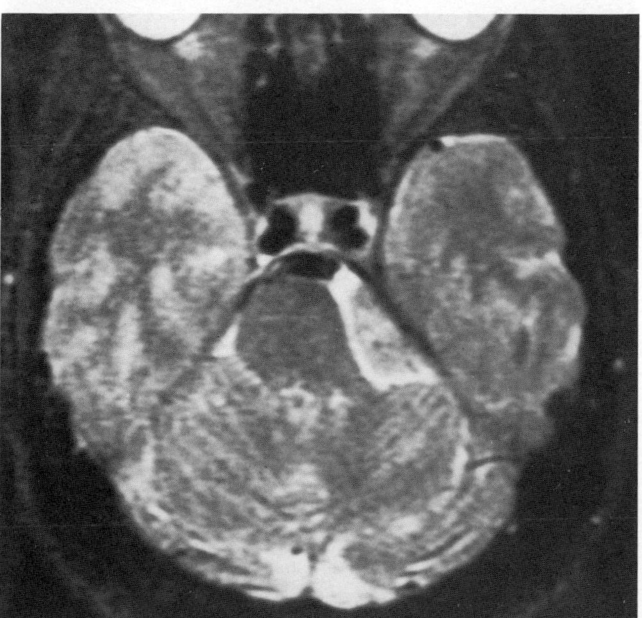

FIG. 12. Typical meningioma. **A:** Axial SE (550/20) MRI. Meningioma protruding into the cerebellopontine angle cistern and compressing the pons (*arrow*). The mass is similar in intensity to gray matter. **B:** T2-weighted (2500/100) MRI shows the mass again to be isointense with brain.

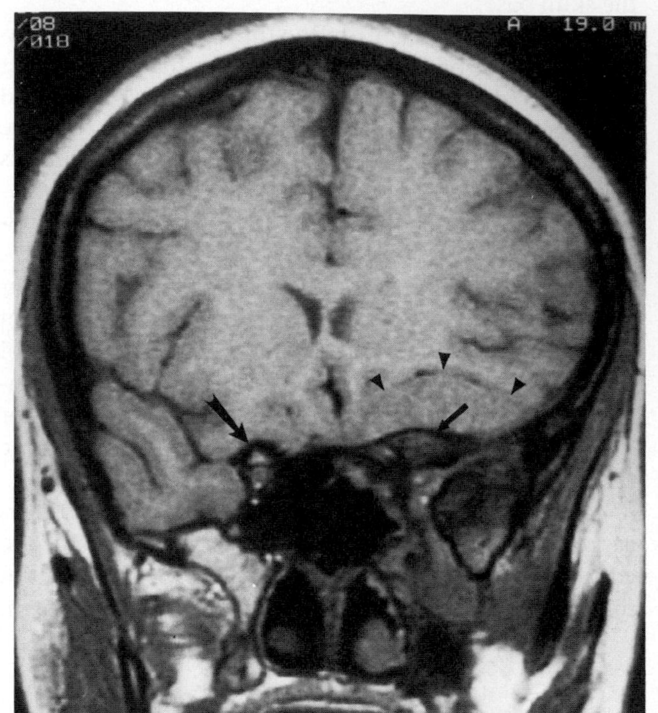

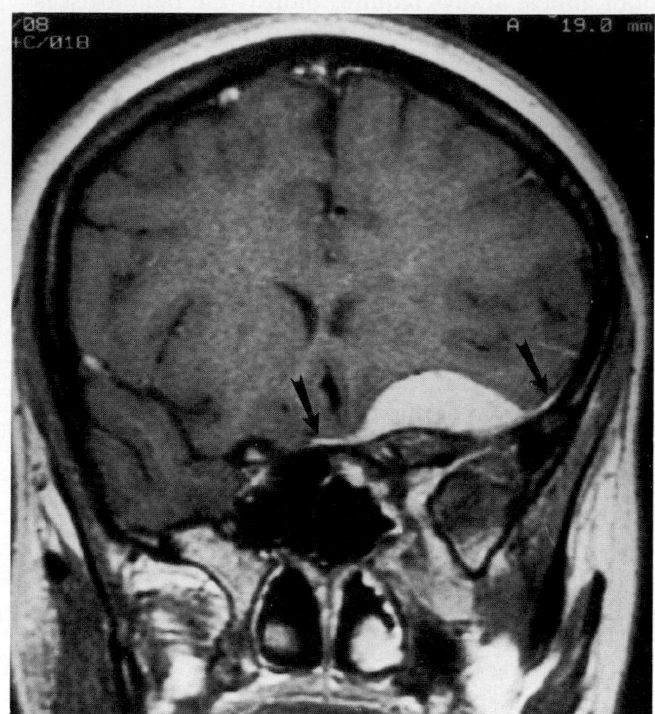

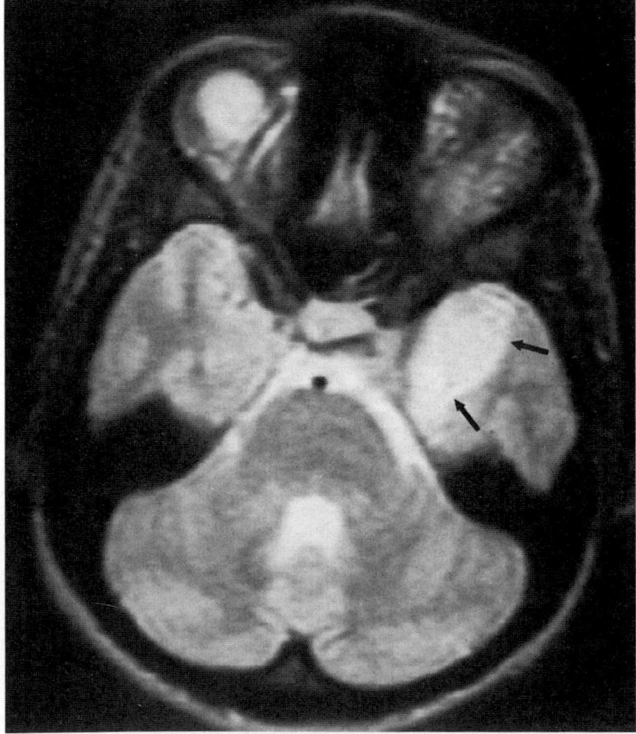

FIG. 13. Meningioma. **A:** Coronal SE (500/20) MRI. The left anterior clinoid (*small arrow*) is enlarged due to hyperostosis [compare with the normal right anterior clinoid (*large arrow*)]. The soft tissue component of the meningioma Is difficult to see because it is isointense with adjacent brain. The arrowheads indicate the margin of the tumor. **B:** Coronal enhanced MRI at the same level as A. The intracranial component of the lesion is much more conspicuous following contrast. Note that there is a "halo" of abnormally enhancing but only minimally thickened meninges surrounding the main tumor bulk (*large arrows*). This may represent infiltration of the meninges surrounding the lesion by tumor. **C:** Axial T2-weighted SE (2000/500/90) MRI. The meningioma spreads posteriorly along the lateral wall of the cavernous sinus. This meningioma has high signal (*arrows*).

may be detectable as absence of signal. Small calcifications are often undetectable. Even a small amount of soft tissue within the same voxel as the small calcification will negate the signal void effect. Extracranial extension is seen most often when meningiomas involve the greater wing of the sphenoid or the floor of the anterior cranial fossa. Bone lesions can be benign or malignant and include sarcomas (Fig. 14), benign fibro-osseous tumors, fibrous dysplasia, and other bony dysplasias (Figs. 15–17). Depending on the degree of calcification, bone tumors may be either relatively dark or may have enough signal to be easily confused with various soft tissue neoplasms. Various soft tissue sarcomas arise inferior to the skull base and involve the skull by direct encroachment. Sarcomas may arise in the orbit, nasopharynx, infratemporal fossa, or indeed almost anywhere. Any part of

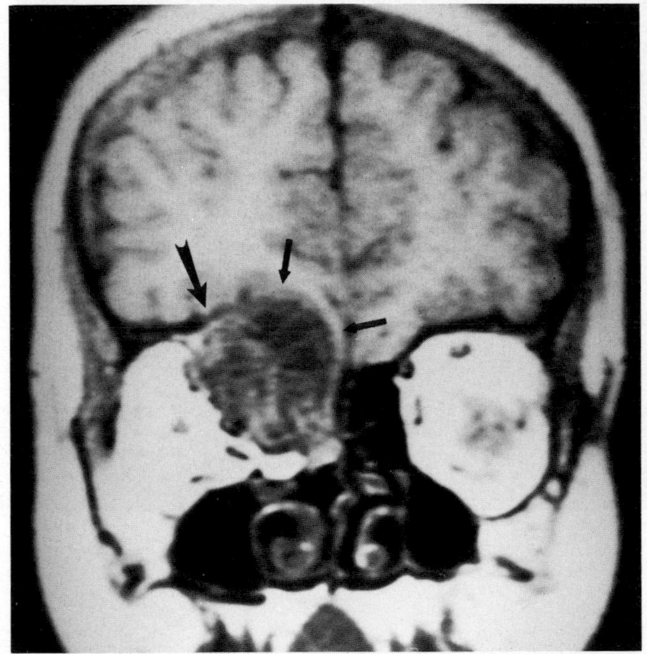
A

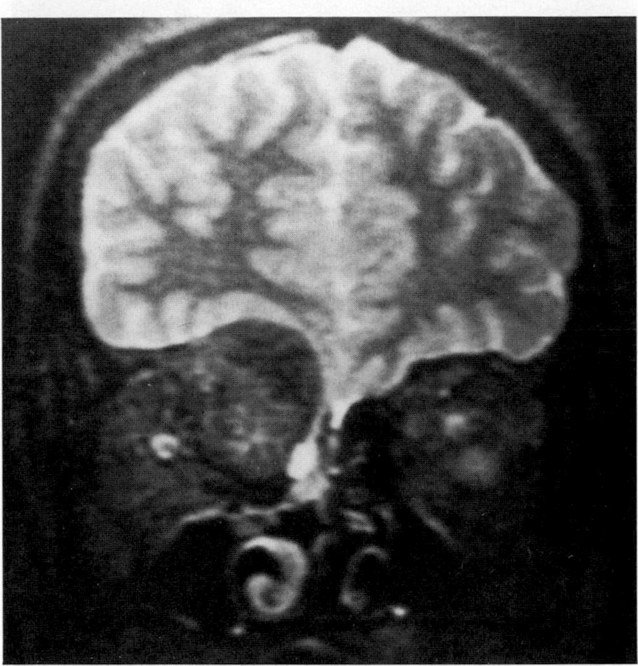
B

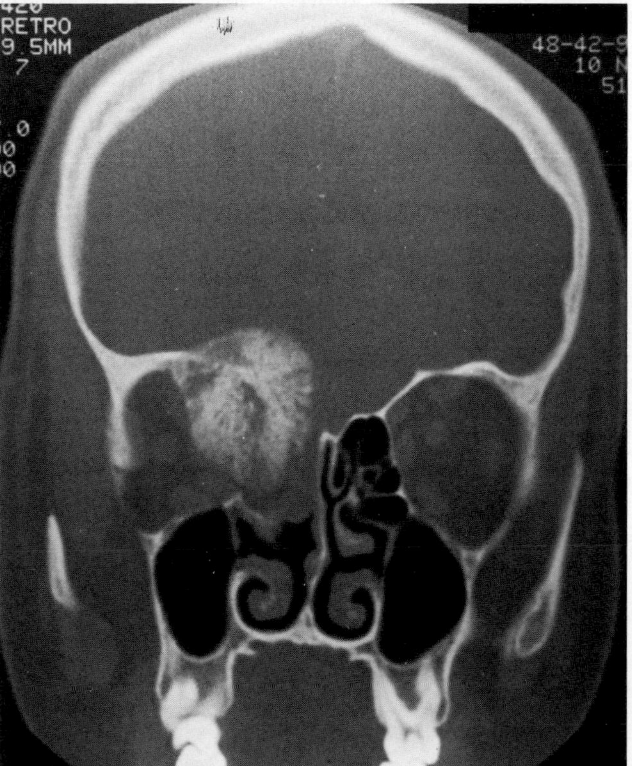

C

FIG. 14. Osteogenic sarcoma. **A:** Coronal SE (600/25) MRI shows a heterogeneous mass involving the roof of the right orbit (*small arrows*). Note that the low signal of the cortical bone is interrupted by this process (*large arrow*). **B:** Coronal T2-weighted image (2400/90) shows the mass to have areas of low and intermediate-signal intensity. **C:** Coronal CT (bone algorithm) shows that the mass consists largely of an ossified matrix. This is very characteristic of osteogenic sarcoma. The bony nature of the mass was difficult to discern with MRI alone, but such a diagnosis can be suspected, however, when a skull base mass is primarily low signal.

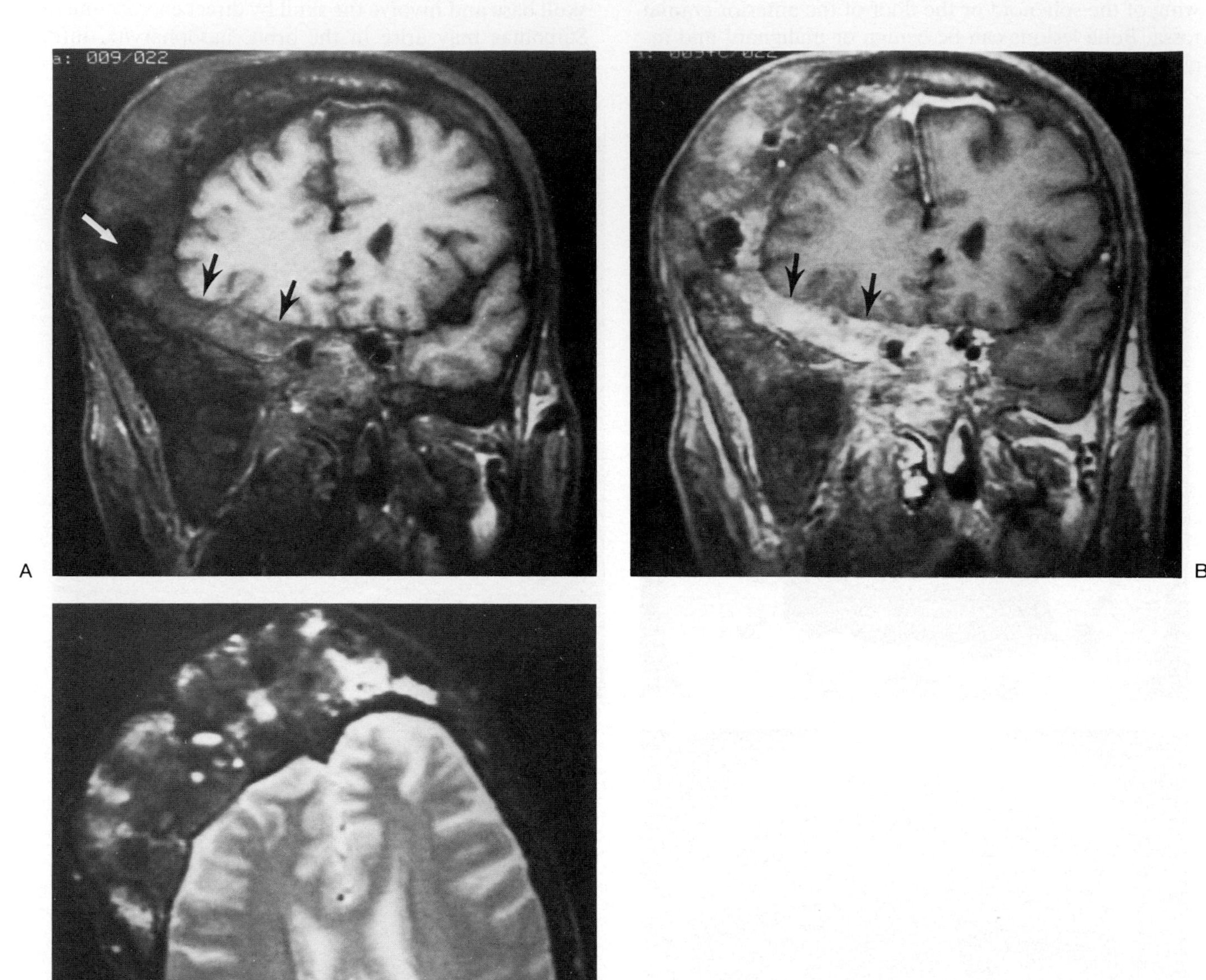

FIG. 15. Fibrous dysplasia. **A:** Coronal SE (500/20) MRI shows enlargement of the greater and lesser wings of the sphenoid (*black arrows*) and of the right calvaria. The enlarged bone has variable signal characteristics with some areas of very low signal (*white arrow*). **B:** Contrasted exam at the same level shows marked enhancement in most of the involved bone (*arrows*). **C:** Axial T2-weighted SE (2500/100) MRI. There is great variability in the signal characteristic of the dysplastic bone with some areas of very high signal and other areas of intermediate or near absent signal.

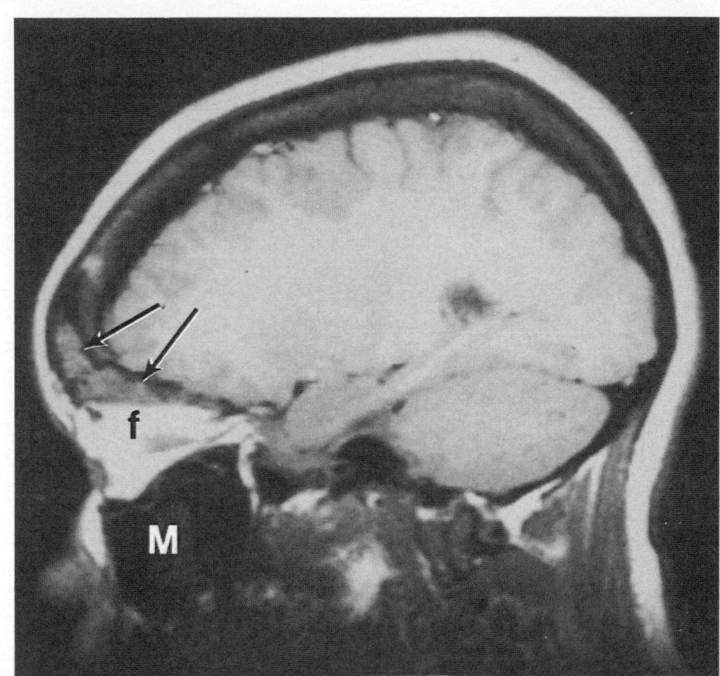

FIG. 16. Fibrous dysplasia. **A:** Sagittal SE (400/20) MRI shows variable signal intensity involving the roof of the right orbit (*arrows*). M, maxillary sinus; *f*, orbital fat. **B:** Coronal SE (600/20) MRI. There is abnormal thickening of the roof of the right orbit (*arrows*). **C:** Coronal CT scan (bone algorithm) demonstrates diffuse thickening and amorphous increased density (ground glass appearance) of the right orbital roof.

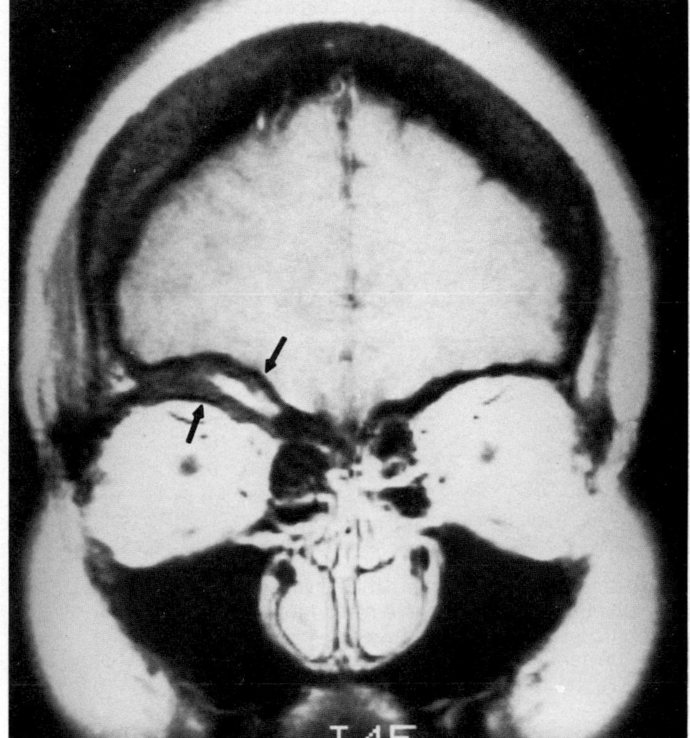

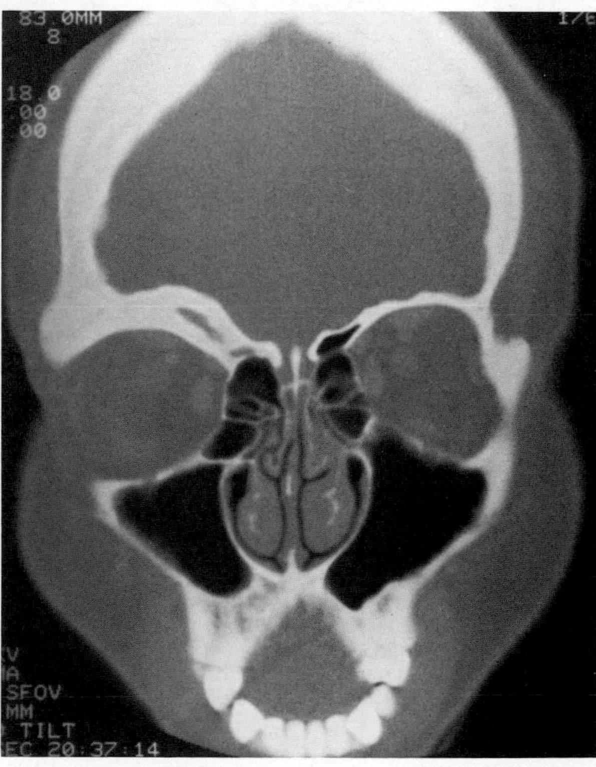

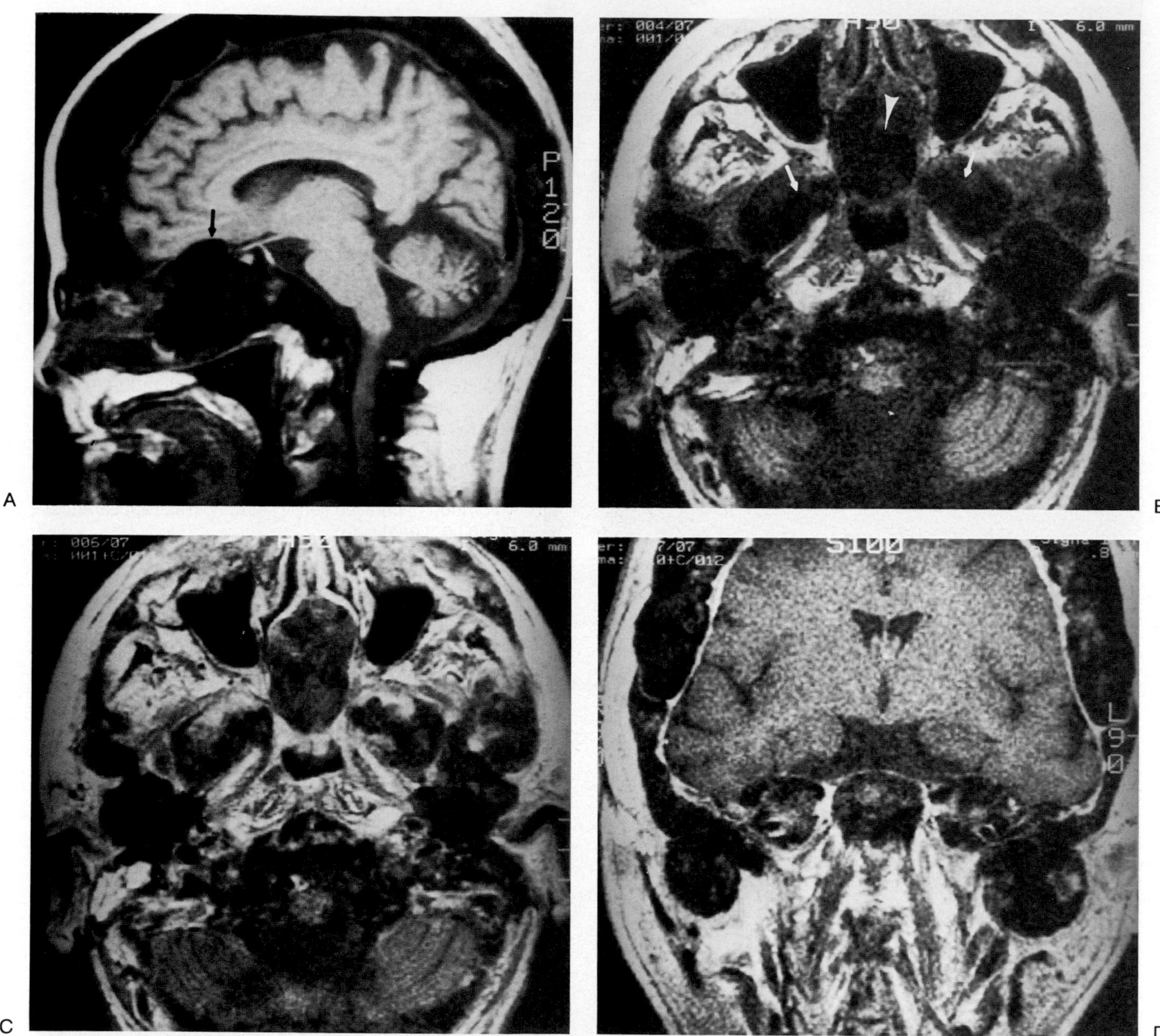

FIG. 17. Engelmann's disease. **A:** Sagittal SE (500/20) MRI scan shows marked thickening of the clivus and calverium. There is a thick bony mass in the posterior ethmoid (*arrow*). The sphenoid sinus has not developed. **B:** Axial SE (500/20) MRI shows enlargement of the pterygoid processes (*arrows*) and a large low signal mass in the region of the nasal septum (*arrowhead*). **C:** Enhanced MRI at the same level as B. There is mottled enhancement of the hypertrophic bone. **D:** Gadolinium-enhanced coronal short TR/short TE MR image. (Courtesy of Laura Applegate, M.D.)

the skull can be eroded (Fig. 18). Fissures and foramina represent potential lines of least resistance and so may be the site of initial tumor spread. More aggressive sarcomas can result in destructive patterns with erosion of large segments of bone.

Anterior Skull Base

Tumors involving the anterior skull base arise from the meninges, the olfactory nerves and mucosa, the upper nasal cavity and paranasal sinuses, the orbit, or the bone itself. Thus, the tumors that occur may be meningiomas, olfactory neuroblastomas (esthesioneuroblastomas), and various sinus, orbit, and bone tumors. Primary tumors of the nasal cavity include squamous cell carcinoma, adenocarcinoma, and a variety of rare lesions such as melanoma and plasmacytoma. Although squamous cell carcinoma is still the most common lesion, adenocarcinoma is more common in the upper nasal cavity than it is in the lower. Rhabdomyosarcoma, usually seen in children, can extend through the skull base, usually from the orbit (14).

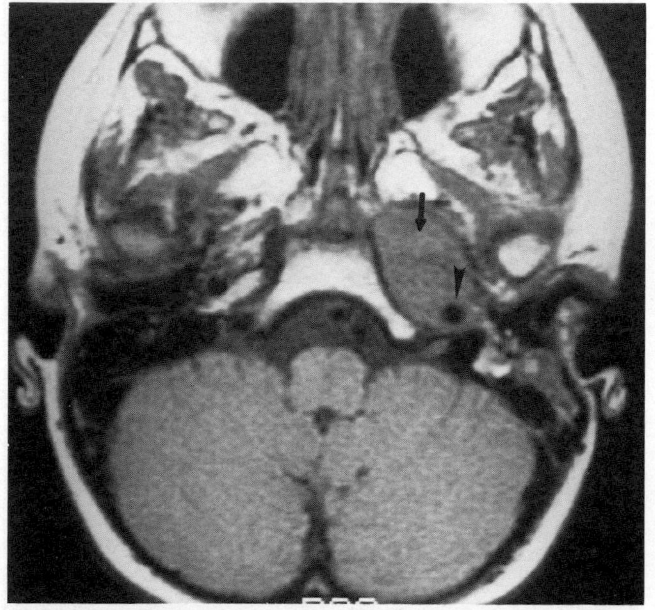

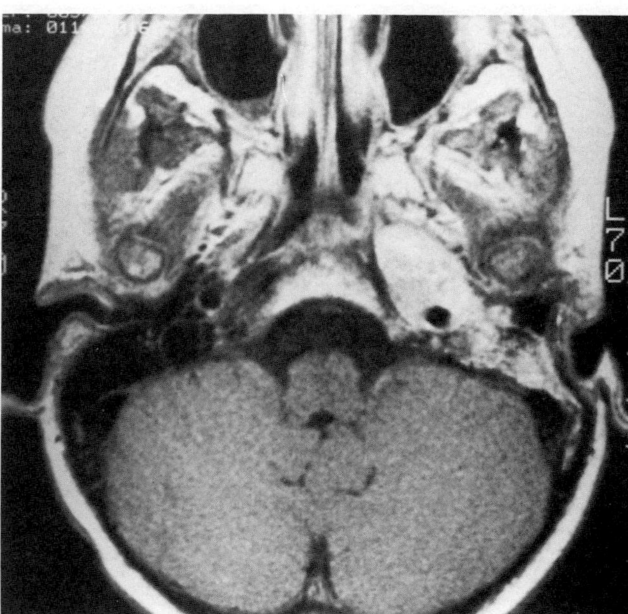

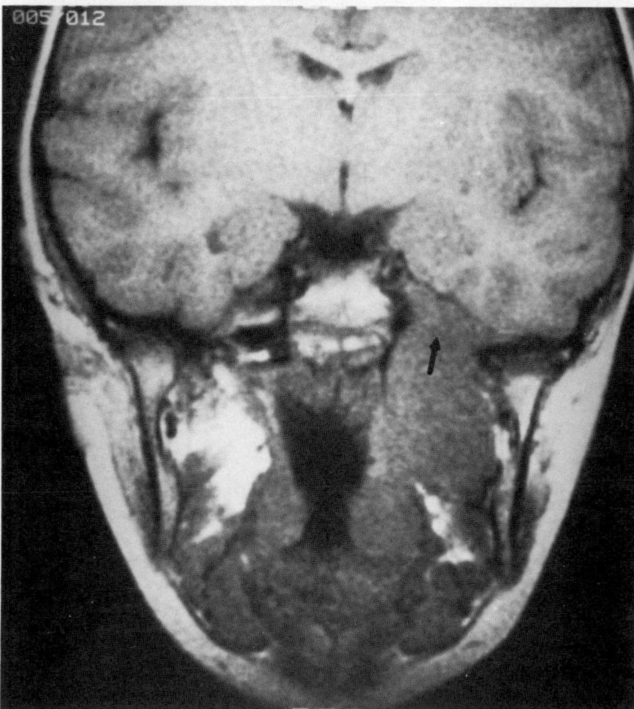

FIG. 18. Rhabdomyosarcoma. **A:** Axial short TR/short TE shows the tumor mass (*arrow*) extending into the petrous apex and surrounding the carotid artery (*arrowhead*). **B:** After gadolinium enhancement the same level shows enhancement of the tumor around the carotid. **C:** Coronal view shows the tumor from the infratemporal fossa extending through the skull base (*arrow*).

Currently, we cannot make a definite differentiation among these tumor types using signal characteristics alone. In some melanomas, the diagnosis may be suggested by bright signal on the T1-weighted image and low signal on the T2-weighted image (15) (Fig. 19).

Again, imaging evaluation of these types of lesions requires definition of the extent rather than absolute identification of the cell type. Does the tumor arising in the nasal cavity or sinuses extend through the skull base into the anterior cranial fossa (Figs. 20–22)? Does the tumor involve the brain? Because of the shape of the floor and anterior wall of the anterior fossa, multiple sequences in multiple planes are required. An alternative strategy is to use a three-dimensional 3D volume acquisition that achieves high resolution images in several planes using one sequence. Axial, coronal, and sagittal views are generated from one data set. Oblique planes may be chosen to optimally demonstrate the tumor margin.

The roof of the orbit and the cribriform plate is well evaluated by coronal imaging. More anteriorly, the transition from the floor to the anterior wall of the anterior cranial fossa represents a smooth curve. Along this

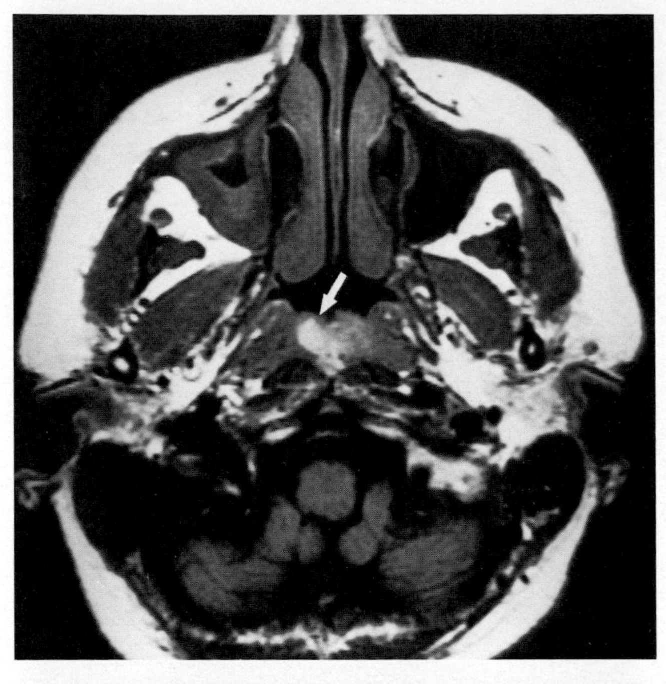

A

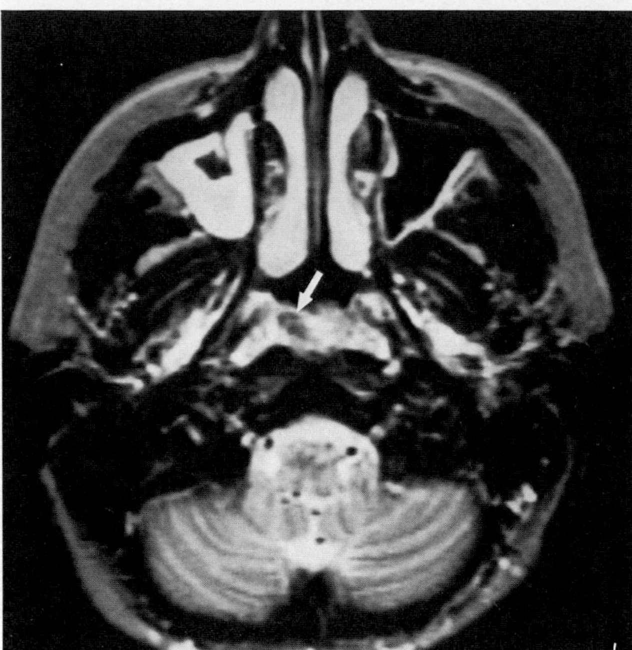

B

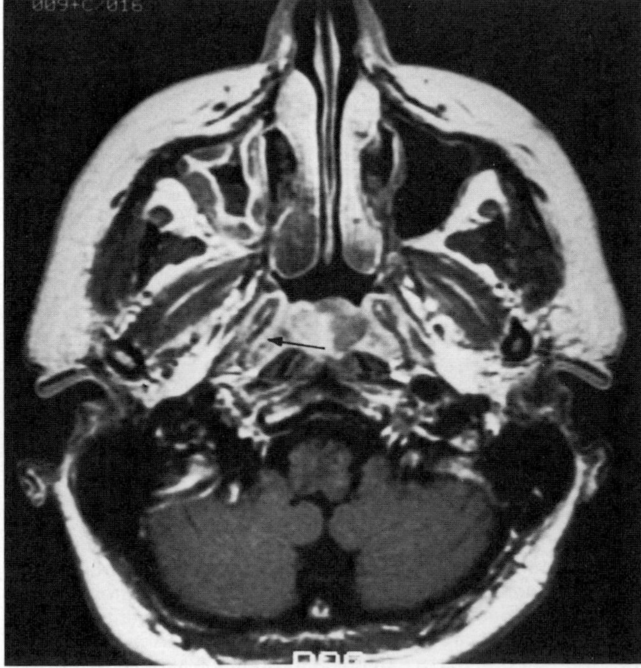

C

FIG. 19. Melanoma of the nasopharynx. **A:** Unenhanced axial SE (550/20) MRI at the level of the torus tubarius. There is a high signal lesion in the nasopharynx (*arrow*). Incidentally, there is mucosal thickening in the right maxillary sinus. **B:** T2-weighted SE (2300/90) MRI at the same level. The lesion (*arrow*) has low signal. This signal pattern is characteristic of melanoma. Hemorrhagic lesions can also have this appearance. **C:** Gadolinium-enhanced short TR/short TE MRI. The lesion has approximately the same signal as the enhancing mucosa (*thin arrow*) passing into the fossa of Rosenmüller.

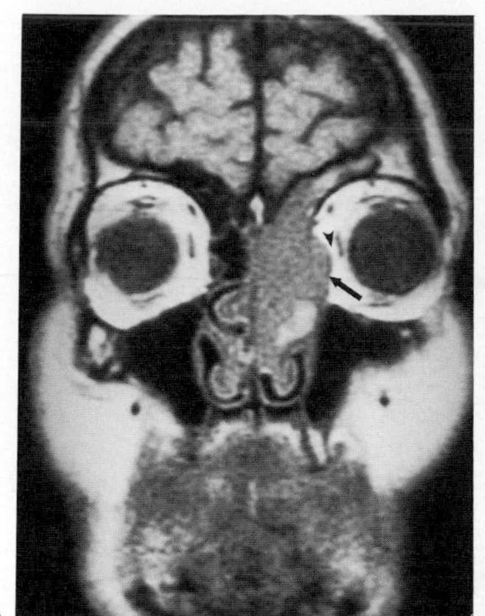

A

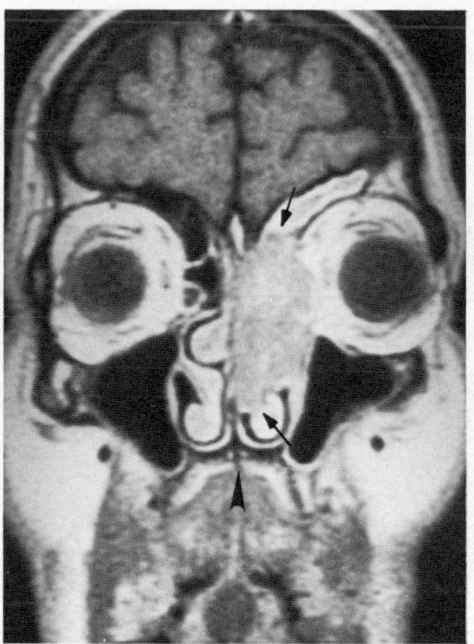

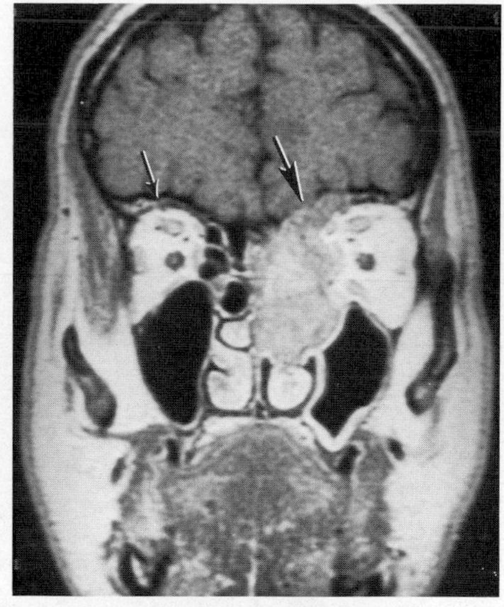

B,C

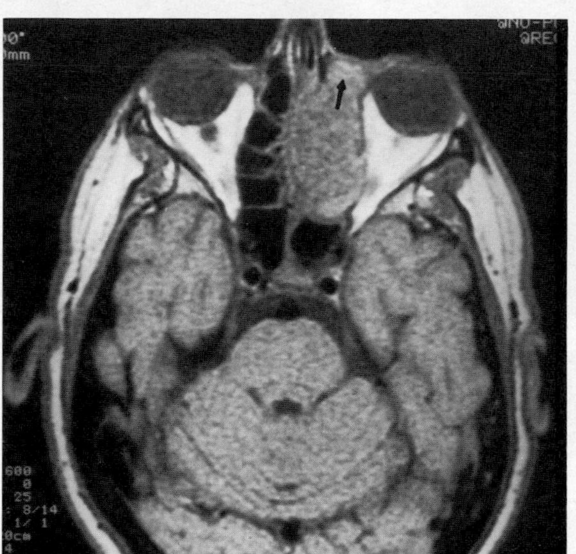

D

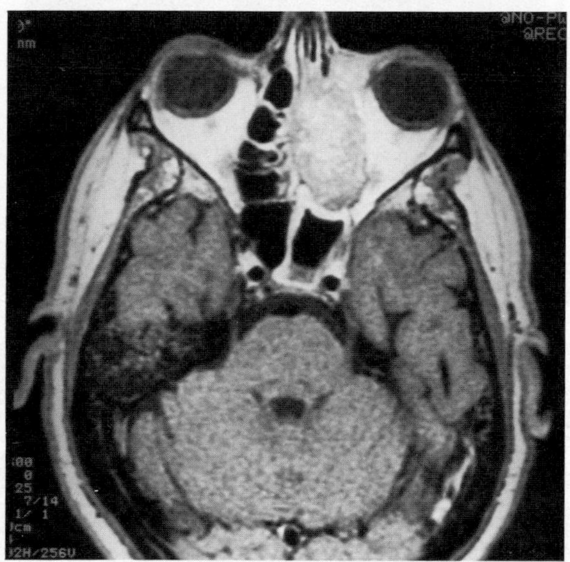

E

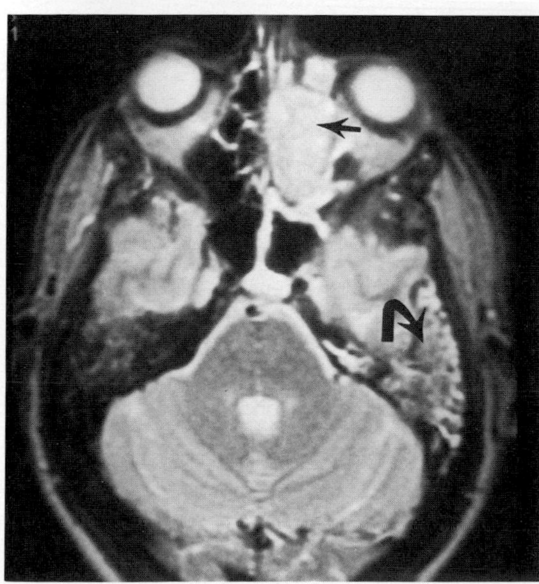

F

FIG. 20. Undifferentiated malignancy (rhabdomyosarcoma). **A:** Coronal short TR/short TE MRI shows the tumor extending into the orbit. The periorbita is deviated (*arrow*) but limits the tumor extension into the orbital fat. There is still a small amount of fat (*arrowhead*) between the lesion and the medial rectus muscle. At this level there is no evidence of intracranial extension. **B:** Gadolinium-enhanced scan same level. The tumor enhances slightly. The mucosa enhances more than the tumor. Thus the tumor margin (*arrows*) can be separated from normal inferior turbinate below and the obstructed supraorbital air cell above. Note that the hard palate (*arrowhead*) is not invaded. **C:** Slightly more posterior cut. There is invasion of the roof of the orbit (*large arrow*). The brain immediately above is slightly displaced. Compare with the intact supraorbital roof on the opposite side (*small arrow*). **D:** Axial short TR/short TE unenhanced MRI. The tumor is seen extending anteriorly (*arrow*) toward the skin. In this region it is difficult to differentiate tumor from an obstructed nasolacrimal duct and lacrimal sac. The fact that the tissue here has exactly the same signal as the tumor suggested tumor involvement. **E:** Enhanced axial short TR/short TE MRI. The abnormality in the region of the lacrimal sac behaves the same as does the tumor. **F:** Long TR/long TE MRI. Tumor (*large arrow*) again has the same signal as the abnormality in the lacrimal sac region. Increased signal (*curved arrow*) in the region of the mastoid indicates obstruction of the eustachian tube.

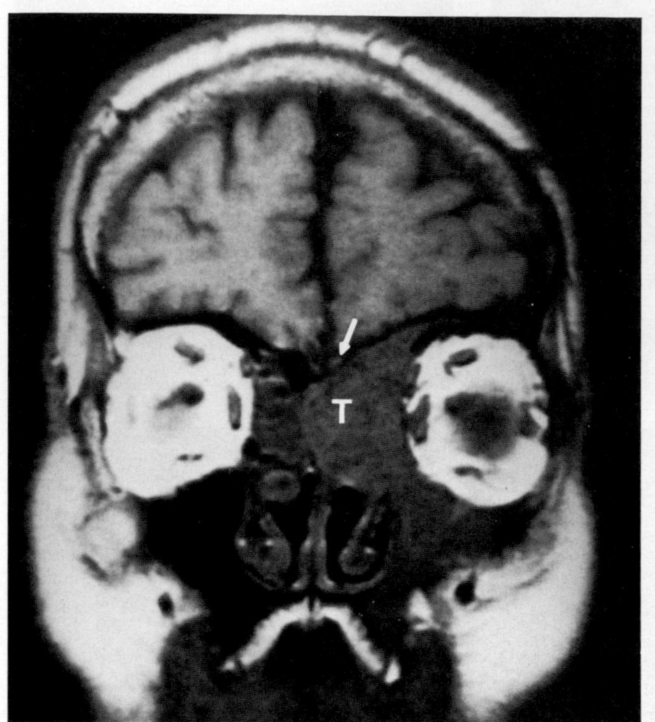

A

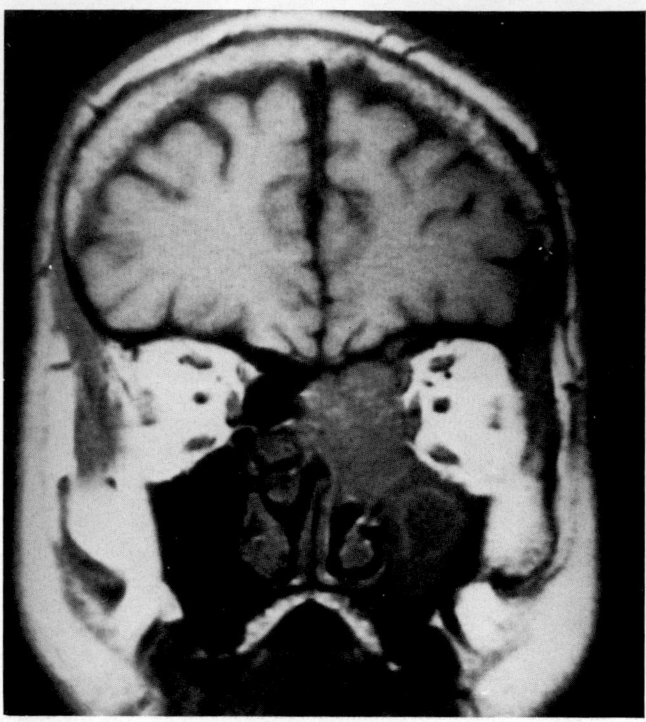

B

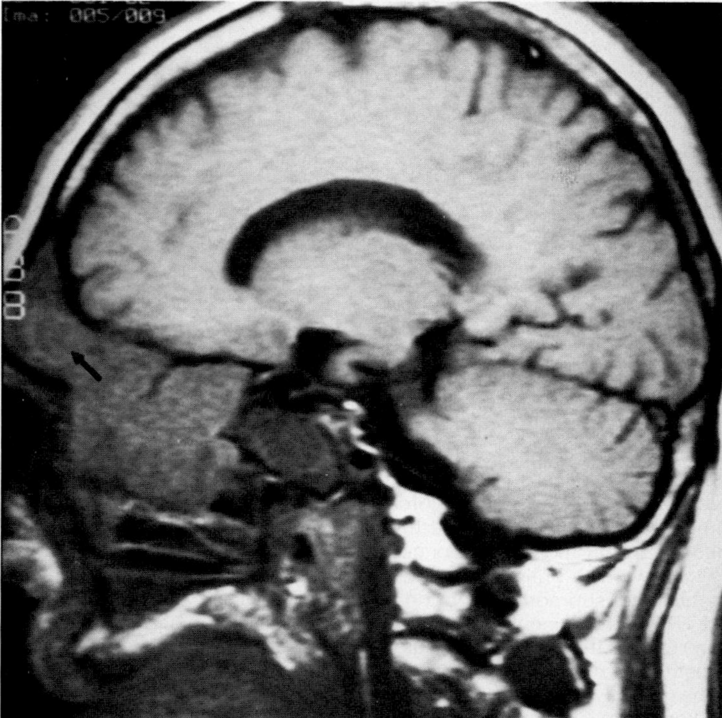

C

FIG. 21. Carcinoma of the nasal cavity and ethmoids with minimal intracranial extension. **A:** The tumor (*T*) extends through the cribriform plate and roof of the orbit. There is a clear separation between the tumor and the brain. The olfactory bulb (*arrow*) is displaced upward. **B:** Slightly more posteriorly the olfactory bulb can be seen in the normal position. Note that the lamina papyracea cannot be identified as a cortical line. **C:** Sagittal image shows a tumor extending up into the frontal sinus (*arrow*).

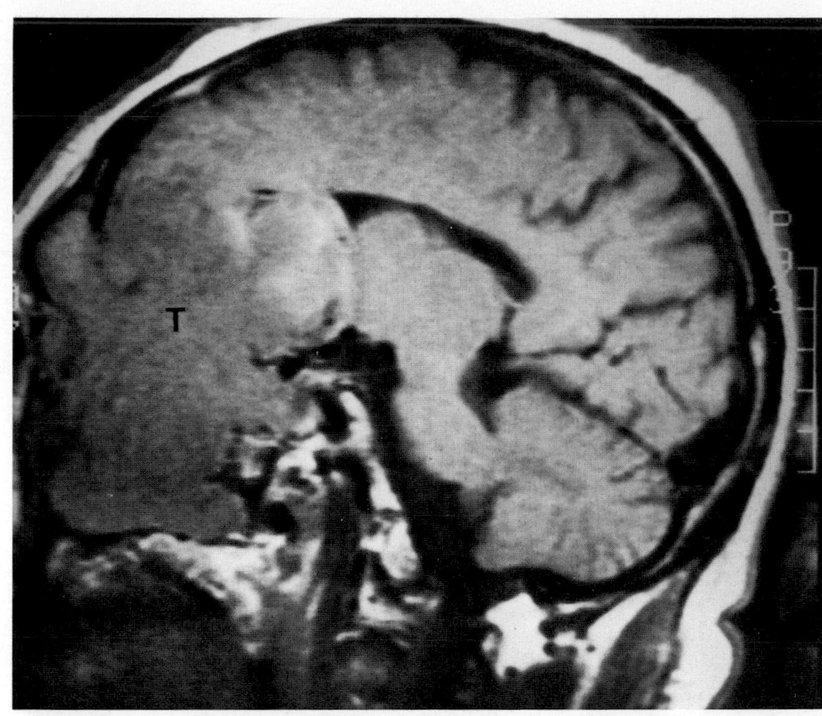

FIG. 22. Sagittal short TR/short TE MR image of a large carcinoma of the nasoethmoid region with extensive intracranial spread and involvement of the frontal bones. *T*, tumor.

curve, neither axial nor coronal images represent a perpendicular slice and, so, the cortical line may not be obvious. Sagittal images may be helpful in this region (Fig. 23).

Does the lesion extend into the orbit? Often the tumor may extend through the bony lamina papyracea and elevate the periorbita without extending through this fibrous layer into the orbital fat (see Fig. 20). Demonstration of the proximity of a tumor to the optic nerve or the optic canal is always of considerable importance.

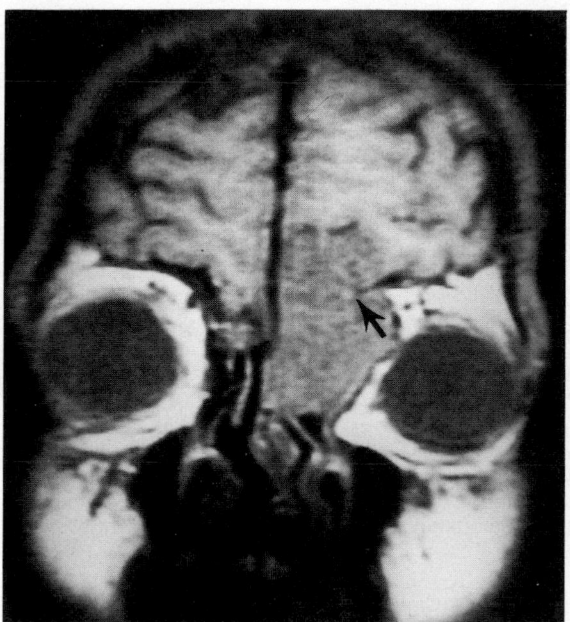

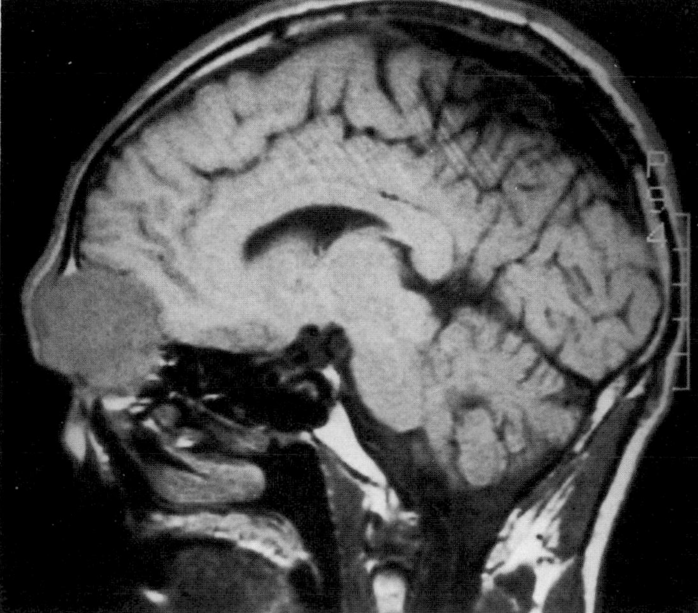

FIG. 23. Lymphoma of the frontoethmoid region. **A:** Coronal short TR/short TE MRI. The lesion interrupts the signal void of the orbital roof (*arrow*) and extends intracranially. We cannot tell if there is invasion of the brain. **B:** Sagittal image shows that the brain is displaced by the tumor.

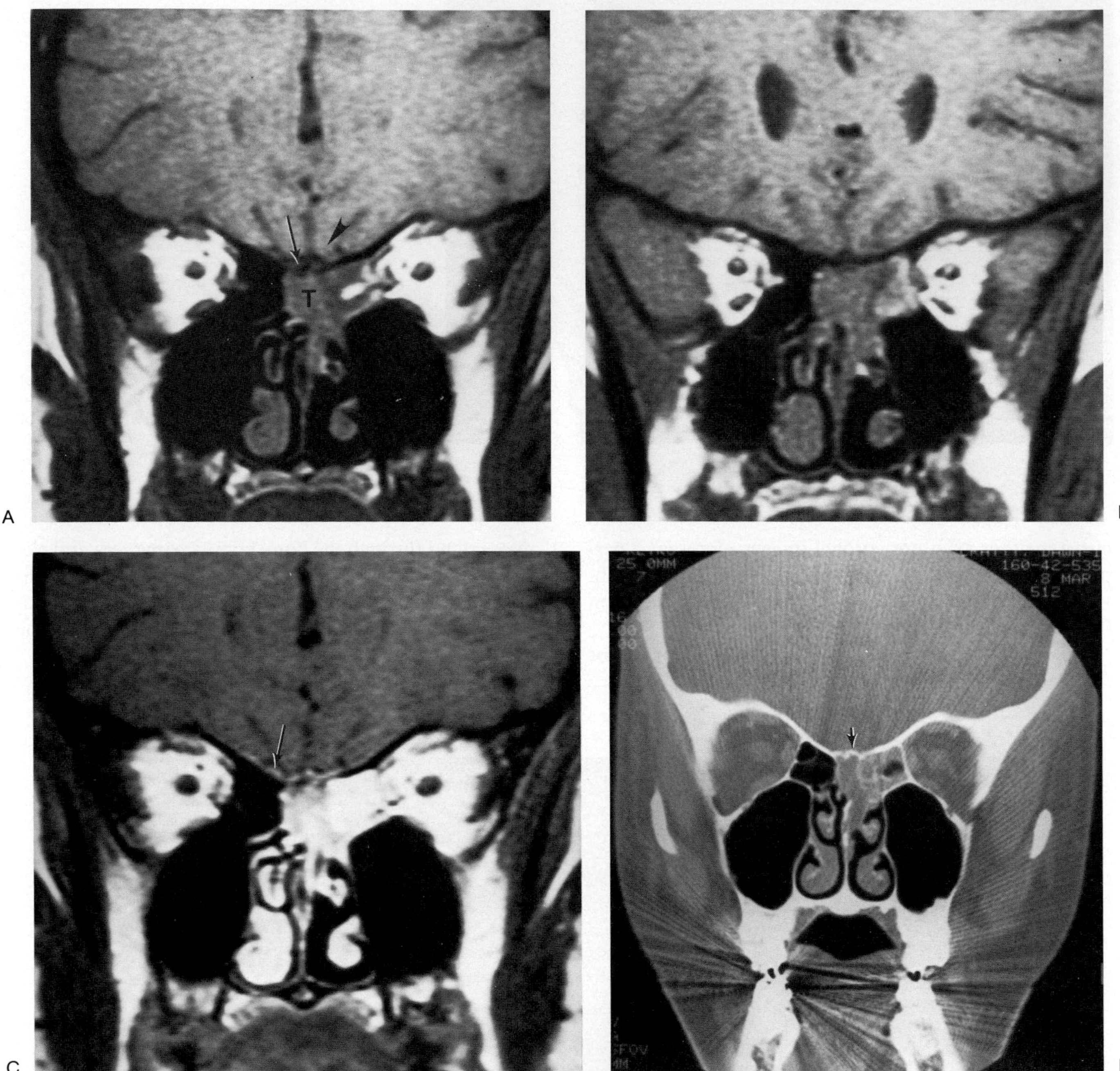

FIG. 24. Esthesioneuroblastoma. **A:** The tumor of the upper nasal cavity (*T*) involves the nasal septum. It is difficult to appreciate intracranial extension. The olfactory nerves/bulbs (*arrow*) are visualized. The gyrus rectus (*arrowhead*) is definitely uninvolved. **B:** The signal void of the floor of the anterior cranial fossa appears to be intact. **C:** There is slight enhancement of the dura (*arrow*), indicating intracranial involvement. **D:** Coronal CT image shows that the bone at the junction of the planum sphenoidale and cribriform plate (*arrow*) is remodeled superiorly. This fine bony change is more easily appreciated on the CT

Special note should be made of olfactory neuroblastomas (esthesioneuroblastomas) (Figs. 24–26). These lesions arise either just above or just below the cribriform plate from the olfactory nerves or the olfactory mucosa. Even if the lesion cannot be radiographically demonstrated above the cribriform plate, involvement of both sides of the plate is presumed, and surgical approaches include removal of this area. The completeness of initial tumor resection appears to correlate with long-term survival (16,17). The MRI appearance may be similar to other neoplasms of the upper nasal cavity. These lesions may be bright on T2-weighted images (Fig. 25); hyperostosis may occur but is rare (Fig. 26) (16). Again, the position of the lesion in the upper nasal cavity adjacent to the cribriform plate suggests this possibility.

Benign lesions of the sinonasal tract can affect the skull base. Mucoceles can expand the sinus and extend intracranially (Fig. 27). Nasal polyps have been reported to protrude through the floor of the anterior cranial fossa (18).

Meningiomas and bone tumors have been discussed in the previous section.

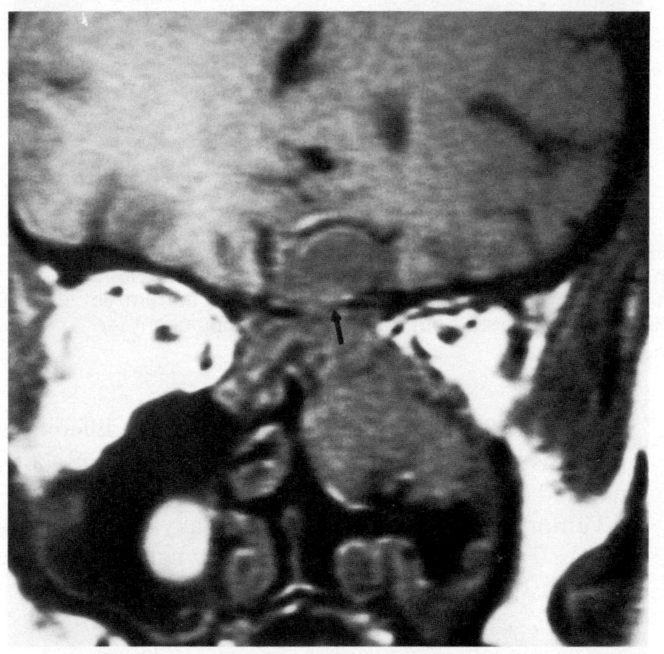
A

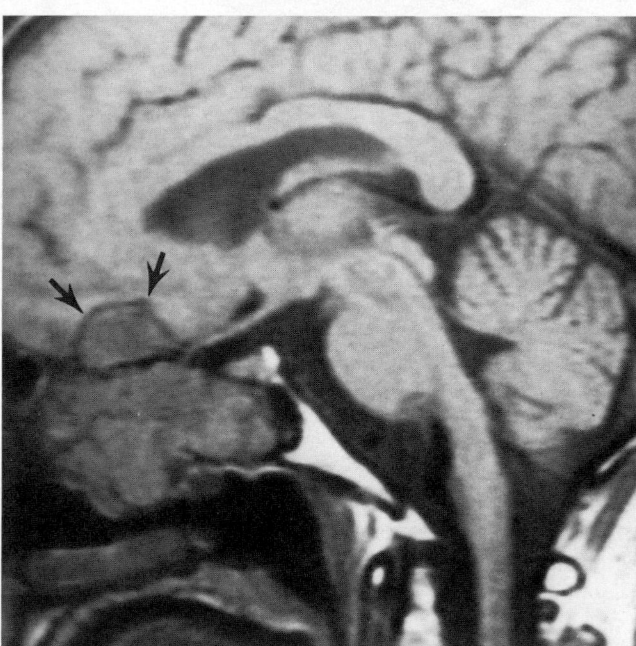
B

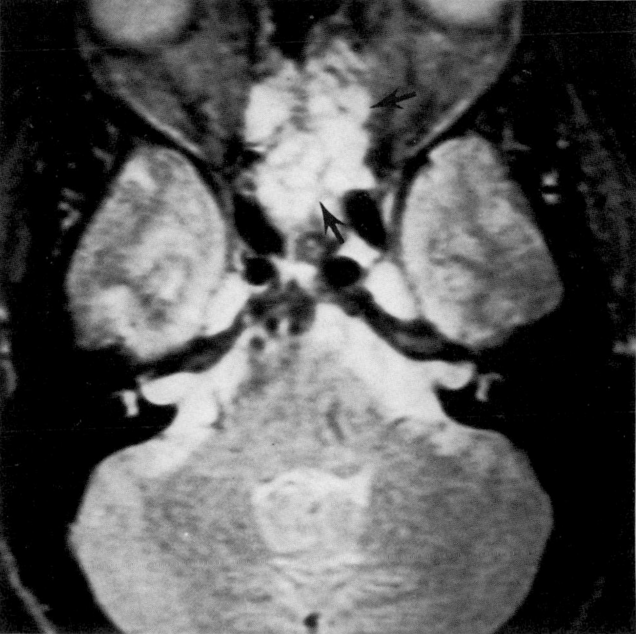
C

FIG. 25. Esthesioneuroblastoma. **A:** Coronal SE (500/20) MRI shows a mass involving the upper nasal cavity, which erodes the cribriform plate (*small arrow*) and protrudes into the anterior cranial fossa. **B:** Sagittal SE (500/20) MRI showing intracranial extension (*arrows*). **C:** Axial SE (2500/100) MRI. The nasal component of the mass is quite lobulated and has high signal (*arrows*). At surgery the tumor along with the cribriform plate and medial walls of both orbits was removed en bloc.

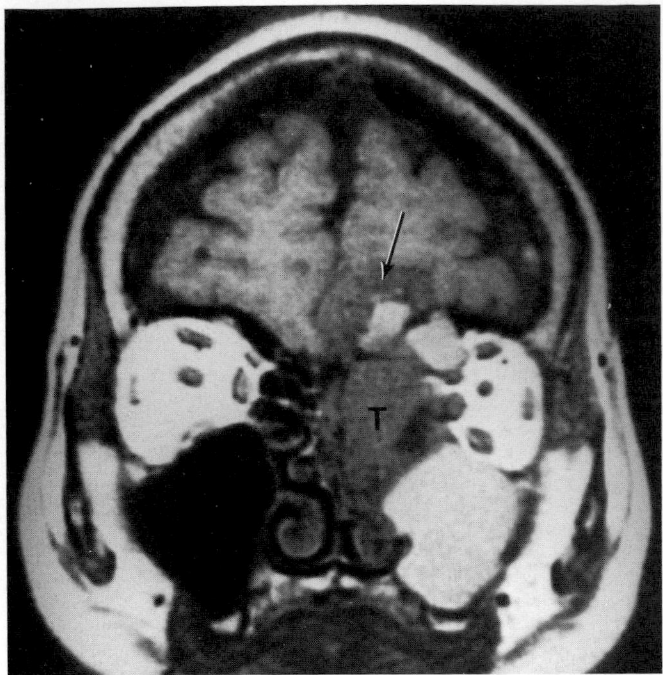

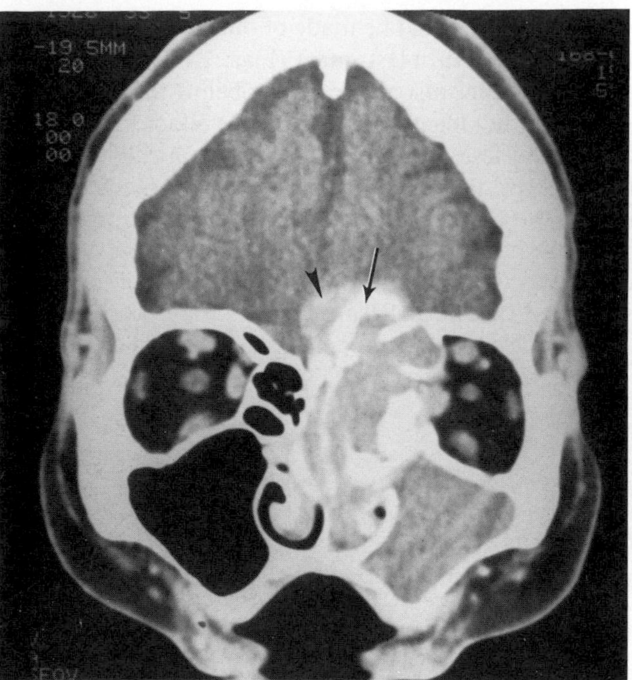

A B

FIG. 26. Esthesioneuroblastoma. **A:** Short TR/short TE MRI. Tumor (*T*) of the nasoethmoid region with intracranial extension. Note the hyperostosis (*arrow*) and compare with B. Some of the "hyperostosis" may be an inflammatory reaction related to obstructed neighboring air cells. Note the high signal of the secretions in the maxillary antrum. **B:** Coronal CT scan shows the hyperostosis (*arrow*) more clearly differentiated from the soft tissue component (*arrowhead*) of the intracranial extension.

Central Skull Base

The central skull base consists mainly of the sphenoid bone. Meningioma, one of the more common neoplasms occurring in the area, is one of the most likely possibilities when a lesion involves almost any part of the sphenoid bone. However, other possibilities in the differential diagnosis depend on the part of the sphenoid bone involved.

Tumors involving the sella are usually pituitary adenomas. Twenty percent of craniopharyngiomas involve the sella and may erode bone. The clivus is the point of

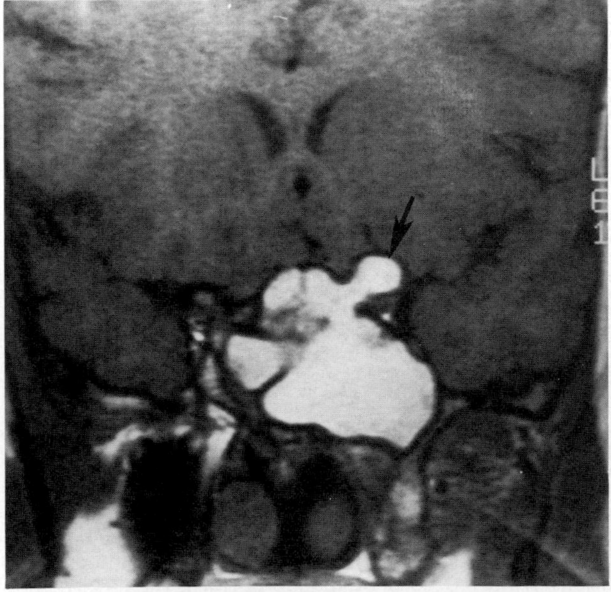

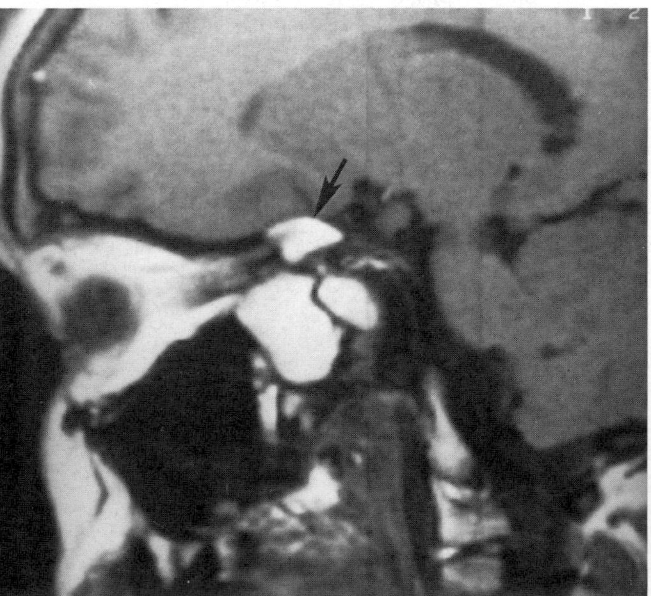

A B

FIG. 27. Mucocele. **A:** Coronal SE (600/20) MRI. The sphenoid sinus is enlarged and its contents are of high signal. Mucocele also involves the left anterior clinoid (*arrow*), which is markedly expanded and filled with the same high signal contents as the rest of the sinus. **B:** Sagittal SE (500/20) MRI again shows marked enlargement of the left anterior clinoid (*large arrow*).

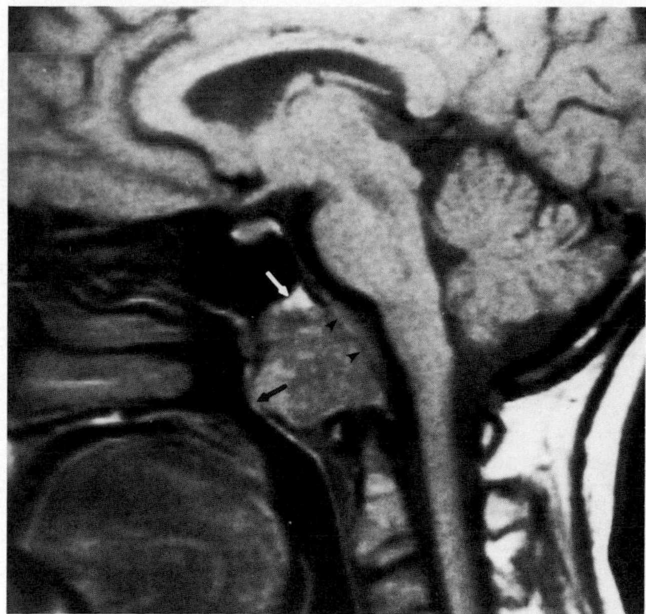

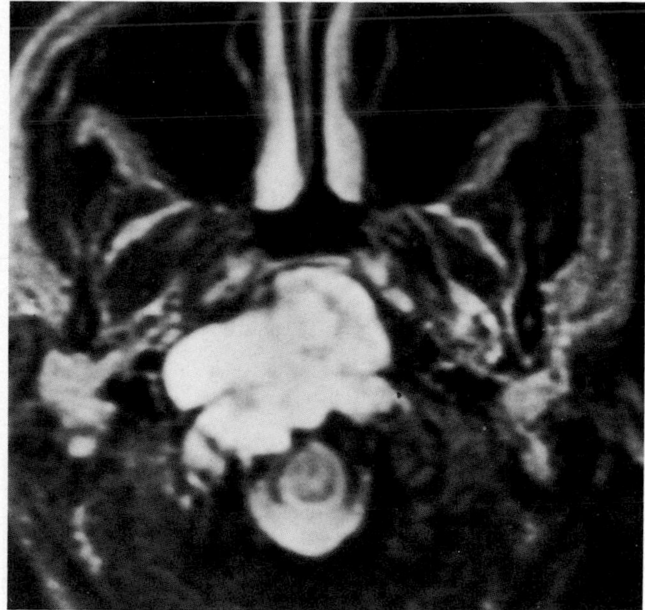

A B

FIG. 28. Chordoma. **A:** Sagittal SE (600/20) MRI shows a large mass involving the clivus. Only a small amount of normal clival marrow persists (*white arrow*). The intracranial surface of the clivus (*arrowheads*) has been violated and there is tumor protruding into the CSF cistern. The tumor also displaces the nasopharyngeal mucosa (*black arrow*). **B:** T2-weighted SE (2500/90) axial MRI. The tumor is primarily high signal.

origin of the chordoma. Chondrosarcomas arise in the same area but tend to be more lateral in position, involving the petroclival suture.

The sella and parasellar region is covered in a separate chapter, as are pituitary adenomas and craniopharyngiomas. Some statements are made here about chordoma and chondrosarcoma.

Chordomas arise from remnants of the notochord, usually in the clivus. Chordomas completely within the nasopharynx have been reported on rare occasions. The appearance of chordomas can be somewhat variable; some are fairly homogeneous in signal (Fig. 28) but there are often cyst-like components that have high signal on T1-weighted images (Fig. 29). Signal void within the le-

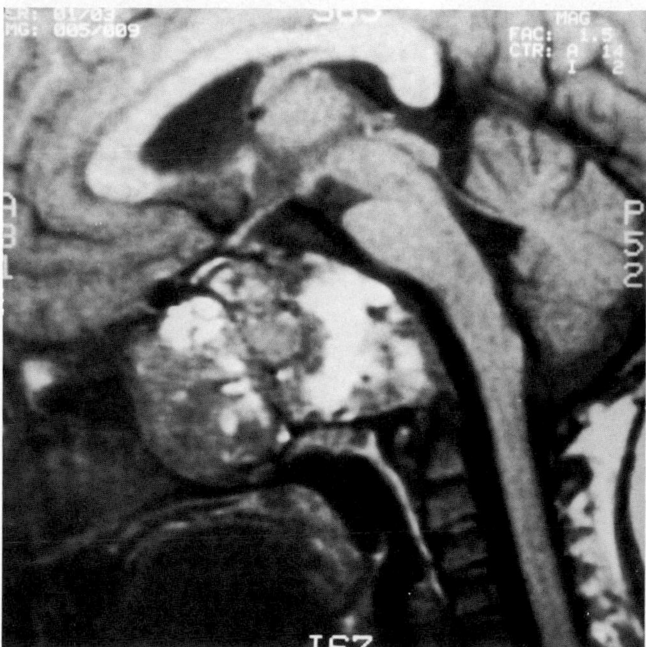

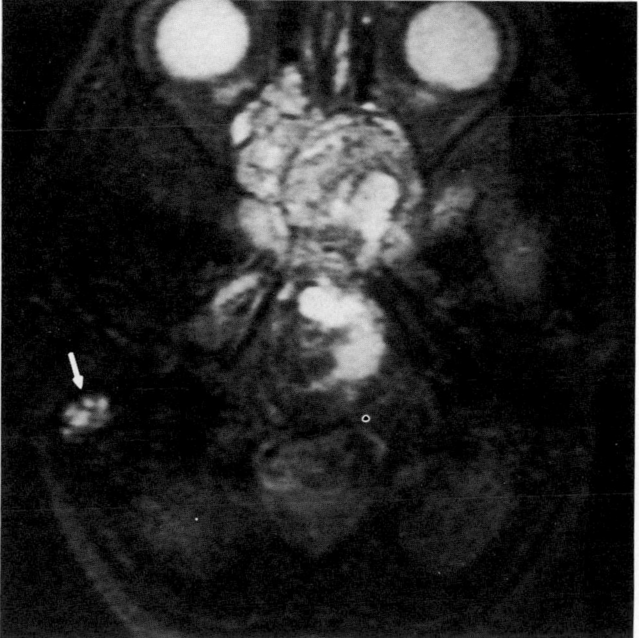

A B

FIG. 29. Chordoma. **A:** Sagittal SE (600/20) MRI shows a large irregular mass replacing the marrow of the clivus and protruding into the nasopharynx as well as the prepontine cistern. Certain components have high signal and others have intermediate signal. **B:** Axial T2-weighted SE (2500/90) MRI shows mixed intermediate and high signal within the mass. There is obstruction of the right eustachian tube with resultant opacification of the right mastoid air cells (*arrow*).

sion may represent sequestrations of cortical bone rather than new bone formation (19).

Chondrosarcomas may have an appearance very similar to chordoma. They can occur in the midline but are usually more lateral, arising in the petrooccipital (petroclival) suture (Fig. 30). These tumors often contain tumoral calcification (19), but this may not be obvious on the MRI. Chondromatous lesions usually have a bright signal on T2-weighted images.

Chondrosarcomas can arise in different locations often associated with sutures. For instance, chondrosarcomas may arise in the posterior nasal septum where sutures separate the vomer, ethmoid, and sphenoid (20).

Lesions of the nasopharynx erode into the central skull base (21). In our experience, the malignancy erodes directly into the bone involving the nasopharyngeal surface of the sphenoid (see Fig. 5). The sutures extending from the foramen lacerum are the most common lines of least resistance. Tumor can extend through the petroclival suture and foramen lacerum into the posterior fossa and into inferior aspect of the cavernous sinuses.

Most malignancies invading the central skull base

A

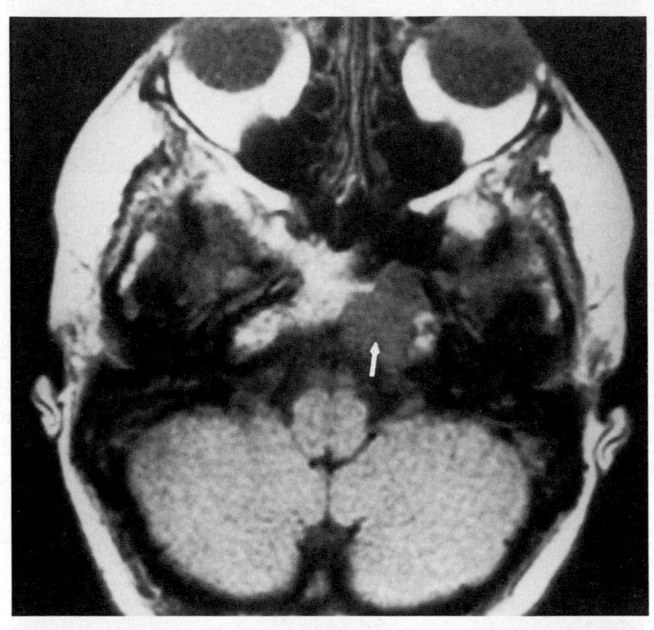

B

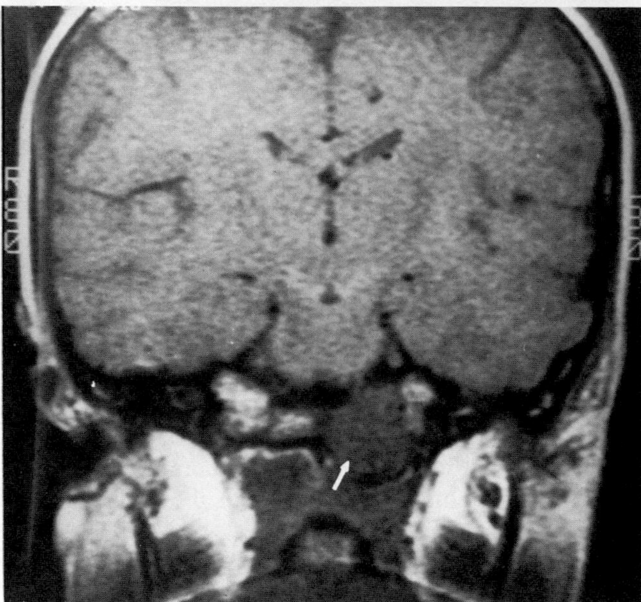

C

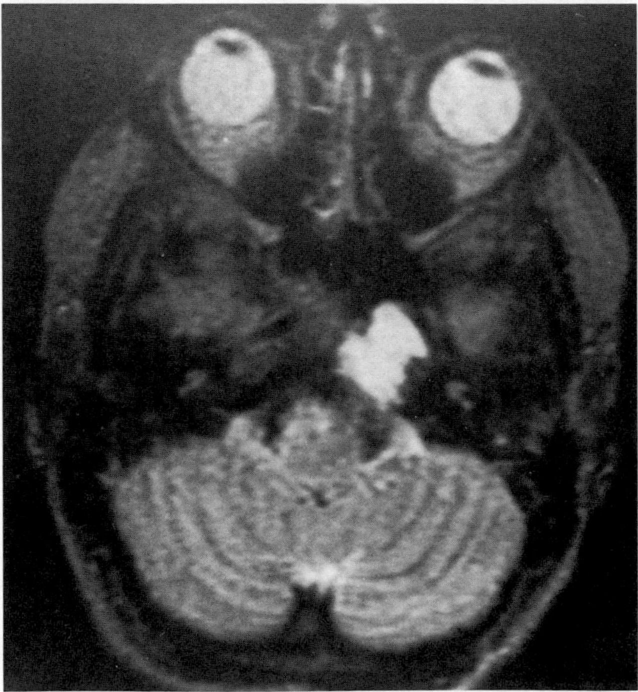

FIG. 30. Typical chondrosarcoma. **A:** Axial SE (550/20) MRI. An intermediate signal mass (*arrow*) replaces the high signal of the marrow fat of the clivus and left petrous apex. **B:** Coronal SE (800/20) MRI again demonstrates the mass (*arrow*). This location, in the region of the petro-occipital synchondrosis, is characteristic of chondrosarcomas. **C:** T2-weighted (2500/90) axial MRI shows that the mass is high signal.

from below are nasopharyngeal carcinomas. Lymphoma and a variety of rare tumors must also be considered. Diagnosis is made by direct biopsy.

The cavernous sinus and Meckel's cave region is the site of tumors arising from the cranial nerves that traverse this area. Meckel's cave contains the trigeminal ganglion and its divisions that communicate via numerous foramina and fissures with the regions immediately beneath the skull base. These extracranial regions include the pterygopalatine fossa and infratemporal fossa (specifically the masticator space) (22). Thus, as was described more completely in the previous section on the

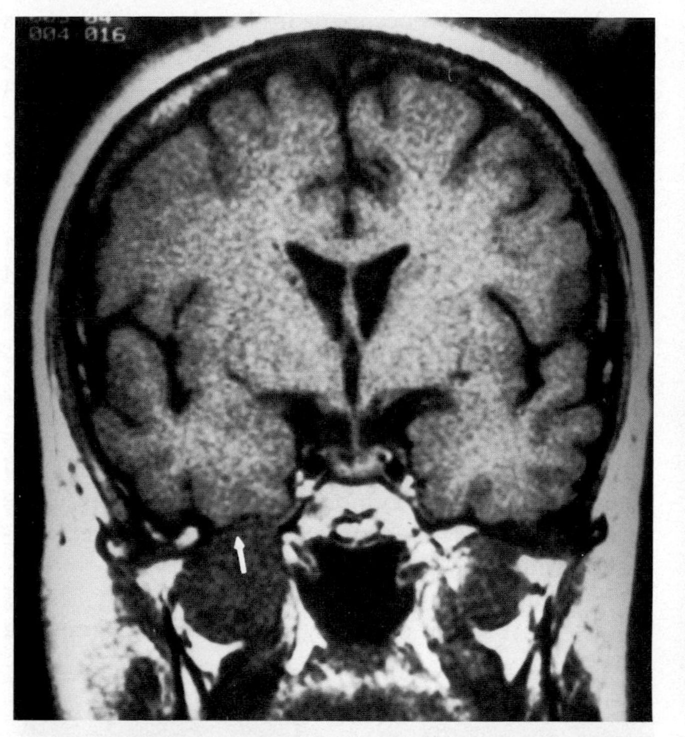
A

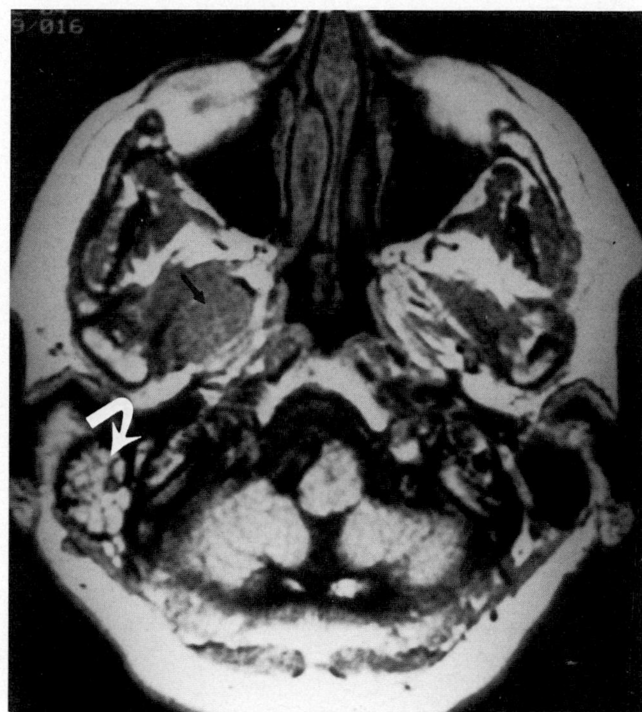
B

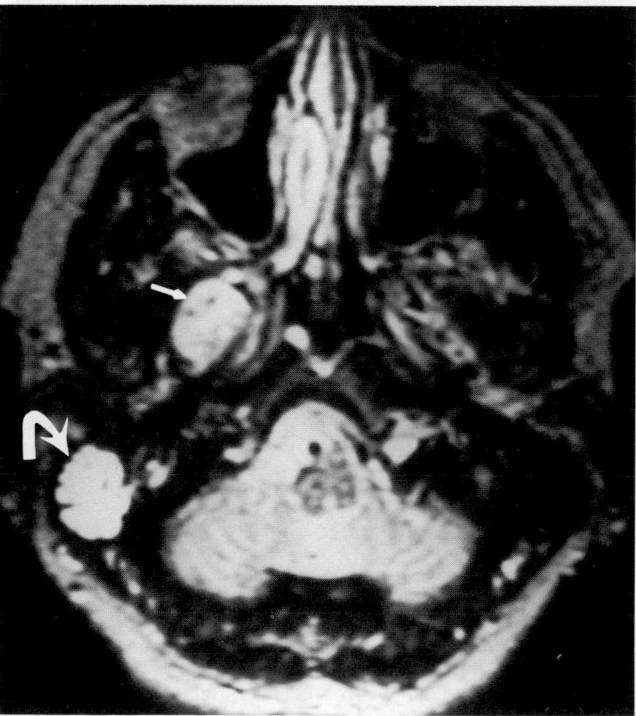
C

FIG. 31. Nerve sheath tumor. **A:** Coronal SE (800/20) MRI shows a smoothly marginated mass of the superior masticator space that remodels the floor of the middle cranial fossa (*arrow*). It is less intense than brain but of similar intensity to the muscle of mastication. **B:** Axial SE (550/20) MRI. The mass (*small arrow*) disrupts the normal fat planes of the superior masticator space (compare with normal left side). The mass compresses the eustachian tube orifice and there is resultant build-up of secretions in the right mastoid air cells (*curved arrow*). **C:** Axial T2-weighted image (2500/90) at the same level as B. The mass (*arrow*) has high signal intensity. Again note the obstructed right mastoid (*curved arrow*).

cavernous sinus, Meckel's cave becomes the target site for tumors spreading along the branches of the trigeminal nerve.

The tumor most commonly implicated in perineural extension is adenoid cystic carcinoma (see Fig. 10). This phenomenon has been described in squamous cell carcinoma and lymphomas as well (10). The signs of transforaminal spread include obliteration of the fat just outside the neural foramina and enlargement of the actual bony canal. Occasionally, slight enhancement of the tumor can be seen within the canal itself (Fig. 11A).

Nerve sheath tumors may also exhibit transforaminal spread. These tumors may be either homogeneous or inhomogeneous. They are low or intermediate on T1-weighted images and may be bright on a T2-weighted image (Fig. 31). They tend to be fairly smoothly marginated and enhance intensely after gadolinium (23). The carotid artery passes through the cavernous sinus so aneurysms must be included in the differential diagnosis for lesions found in the parasellar area (Fig. 32). Meningioma must be included in the differential diagnosis of a tumor arising in any part of the sphenoid bone. This includes the clivus, cavernous sinus, tuberculum sella, planum sphenoidale, and greater wing of the sphenoid. Meningiomas involving the greater wing of the sphenoid often have an extracranial component.

Most of the greater wing of the sphenoid is lateral to the foramen ovale. In our experience, tumors actually appearing to arise from the bone in this region are either meningiomas or metastatic lesions. Metastatic tumors can reach this area by direct extension from tumors arising below the skull base or by hematogenous spread from more remote sites. Often a subtle soft tissue component is seen at all margins of the bone. The dura enhances in the middle cranial fossa and soft tissue tumor impinges on the fat planes of the temporalis space laterally and infratemporal fossa inferiorly. Blastic metastases may have the same appearance as en plaque meningiomas.

Juvenile angiofibroma can also extend into the central skull base and anterior part of the cavernous sinus. Diagnosis of this tumor, occurring in the adolescent male, is seldom in question. Its appearance on MRI is fairly characteristic. The lesion almost always obliterates the fat in the pterygopalatine fossa (Fig. 33). Signal voids representing large vascular structures are seen throughout the tumor (24). The lesion can extend through the root of the pterygoid (junction of the pterygoid process with the body of the sphenoid). The lesion involves the bone in the region of the foramen rotundum and Vidian's canal and can extend into the anterior portion of the cavernous sinus.

Posterolateral Skull Base

The posterolateral region consists almost entirely of the temporal bone. Tumors within the temporal bone can be further subdivided, depending on their precise location within the bone.

Laterally, in the region of the external auditory canal, a destructive lesion is usually squamous cell carcinoma

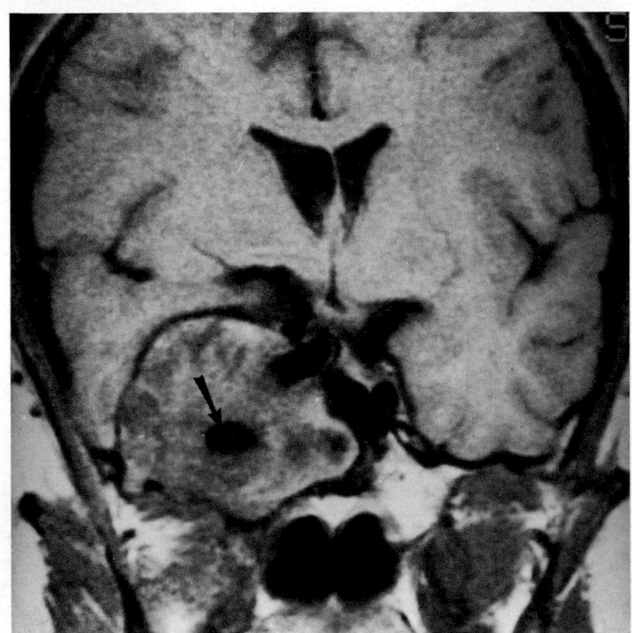

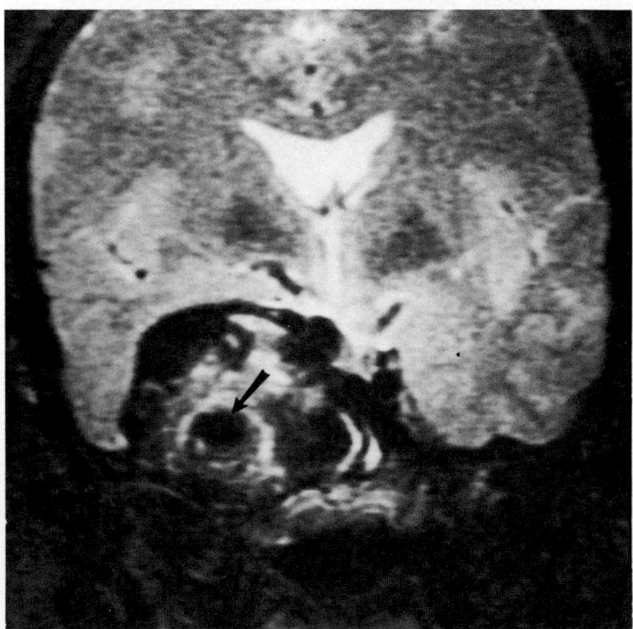

FIG. 32. Cavernous carotid aneurysm. **A:** Coronal SE (700/20) MRI. There is a large mass enlarging the right cavernous sinus and remodeling the middle cranial fossa floor. The residual lumen within the aneurysm is a signal void (*large arrow*). **B:** T2-weighted SE MR image (2500/100) at the same level as A shows mixed high and low signal within the thrombus of the aneurysm. The patient lumen still appears as a signal void (*large arrow*). The variable signal of the thrombus and evidence of hemorrhage in the wall help distinguish aneurysms from other parasellar masses.

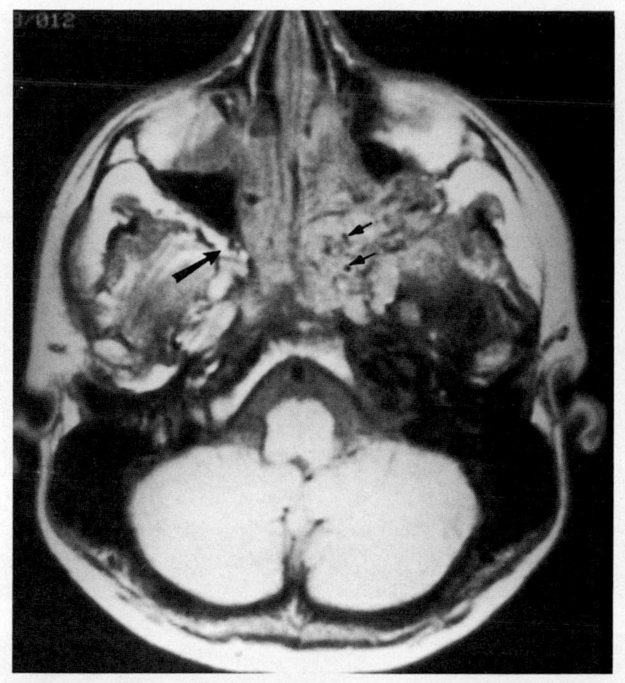

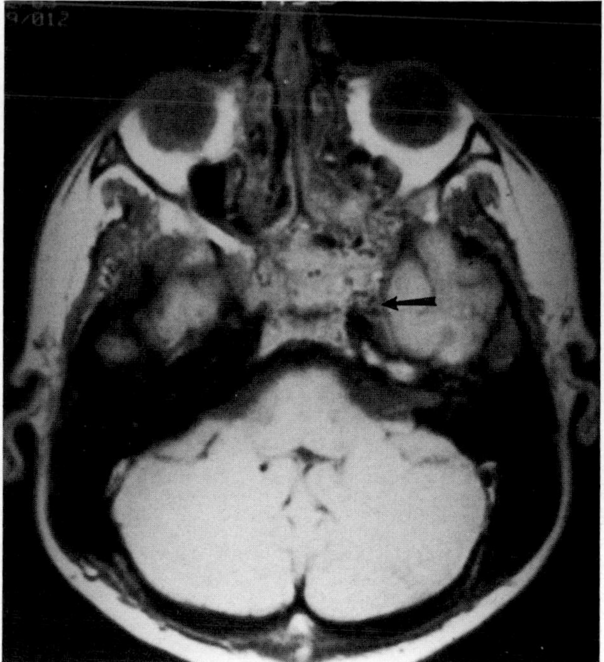

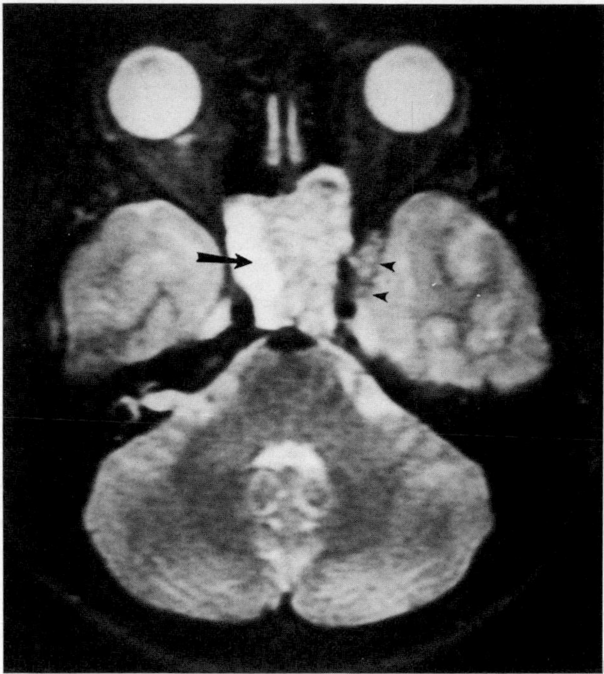

FIG. 33. Juvenile angiofibroma. **A:** Axial SE (600/20) MRI shows an irregular mass expanding the pterygopalatine fossa. The normal fat located here is replaced by the mass [compare with the normal right pterygopalatine fossa (*large arrow*)]. There are small flow voids (*small arrows*) in the mass. **B:** Axial SE (600/20) MRI, slightly higher slice, shows tumor in the pterygopalatine fossa extending through the bone and reaching (*arrow*) Meckel's cave. **C:** Axial T2-weighted SE (2500/100) MRI. The mass is slightly more intense than brain. Note the differentiation from obstructed sphenoid on the right (*large arrow*). There is extension into the left cavernous sinus (*arrowheads*).

(Fig. 34) or malignant external otitis. Other possibilities, such as adenocarcinoma (ceruminoma), are very rare. Tumors can erode into the external auditory canal from contiguous areas such as the parotid.

In most cases, the diagnosis is made by biopsy because the external auditory canal is superficial and accessible to direct visualization. The diagnosis of malignant external otitis can, however, be quite difficult. This lesion is a *Pseudomonas* infection and occurs almost exclusively in elderly diabetics. Many of these patients have already been treated with antibiotics, so isolation of the *Pseudomonas* bacteria can be difficult. The typical histologic pattern of carcinoma, however, is not found at biopsy.

Imaging is used to define the extent of the lesion rather than to make the diagnosis. Extension of either tumor or malignant external otitis (MEO) into the mastoid is seen as a defect through the cortical external canal. Separation of abnormality from fluid-filled mastoid air cells can be difficult, but the distinction can often be made based on signal differences. Anterior extension brings the proces-

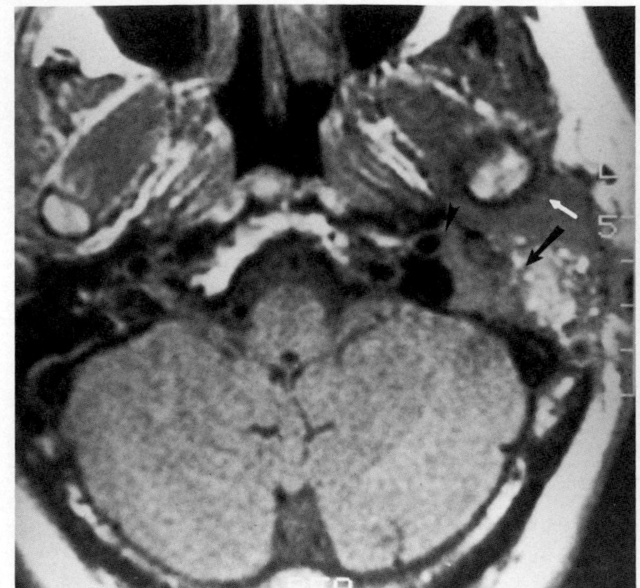

A

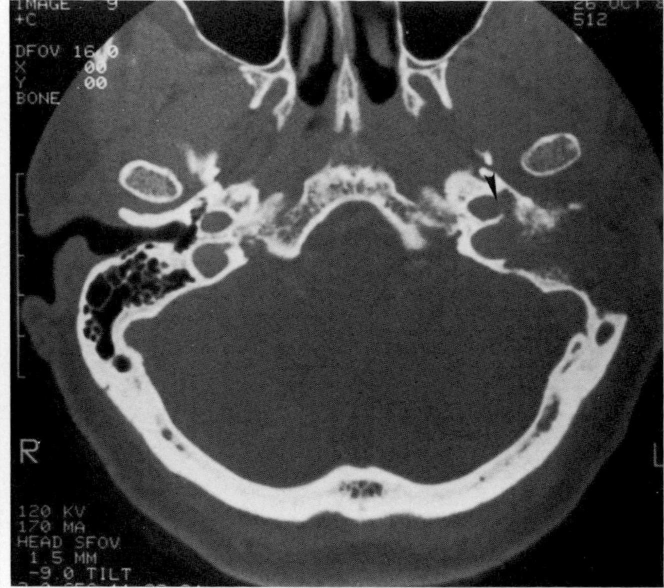

B

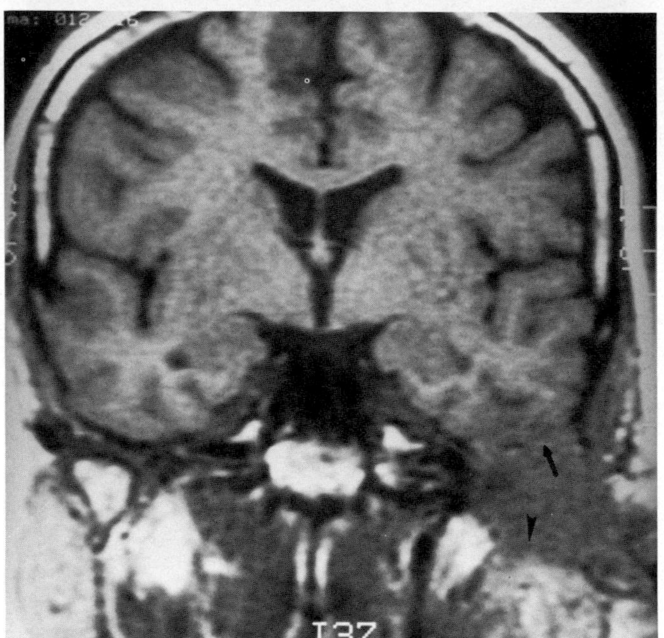

C

FIG. 34. Squamous cell carcinoma of the external auditory canal and middle ear. **A:** Axial short TR/short TE MRI shows tumor of the external ear (*black arrow*) extending into the region of the temporomandibular joint (TMJ) (*white arrow*). The tumor reaches the carotid canal. It is difficult to tell if there is erosion of the canal itself (*arrowhead*). **B:** Bone algorithm CT shows erosion of the carotid canal (*arrowhead*) as well as the jugular bulb immediately posteriorly. **C:** Coronal image shows extension into the middle cranial fossa (*arrow*) and inferior extension to the tissues below the temporal bone (*arrowhead*).

sor into the region of the temporomandibular joint (Figs. 34A,B). Superior extension brings the lesion into the middle cranial fossa (Fig. 34C). If the abnormality extends inferiorly, the fat planes just beneath the temporal bone are obliterated either by tumor or by MEO. MEO can preferentially extend along the undersurface of the skull base after escaping the external auditory canal. The lesion can first involve cranial VII and then cranial nerves IX, X, XI, and XII as the disease process extends medially.

Keratosis obturans and cholesteatoma of the external auditory canal are often considered to be the same disease. Some authors indicate subtle differences. The external canal is obstructed and expansion is more sharply defined than in squamous cell carcinoma or MEO.

In the middle ear, only a few tumors need to be considered. The most common diagnoses are cholesteatoma and paraganglioma (glomus tumor). The differentiation can certainly be made radiographically, but this is not useful as the two entities are not confused clinically. As with tumors involving the external ear, the role of the radiologist is often to define the extent of the lesion rather than to make the initial diagnosis. In the case of cholesteatoma, the clinician may or may not know that there is a cholesteatoma but certainly knows that there is chronic middle ear disease. The radiologist looks for subtle bone erosions of the scutum or ossicles or for expansion of the attic to indicate that indeed a cholesteatoma is present. Erosion of the lateral bony margin of the horizontal semicircular canal is particularly important. If the surgeon tries to remove the wall of the cholesteatoma that has eroded into the semicircular canal, the patient may lose all hearing in the ear. Erosion may be suspected on MRI, when the lesion intersects the lumen of labyrinth. More subtle erosions are more confidently identified using bone algorithm CT.

In the case of a paraganglioma, the clinician has already seen a reddish mass behind the tympanic membrane. The radiologist looks for subtle bony changes that will indicate that this is a glomus jugulotympanicum with extension into the middle ear from the jugular bulb (Fig. 35), rather than a glomus tympanicum, which is confined to the middle ear. Clinically, it is difficult to differentiate glomus tumor from an aberrant carotid artery. In the latter, the bony carotid canal is more lateral than usual. The lateral wall of the canal may be incomplete and the artery bulges into the middle ear. These subtle bony changes are difficult to appreciate on MRI.

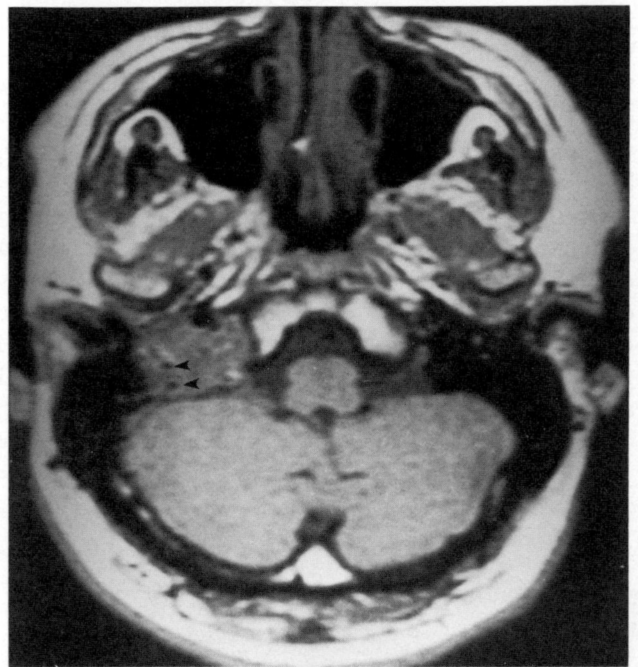
A

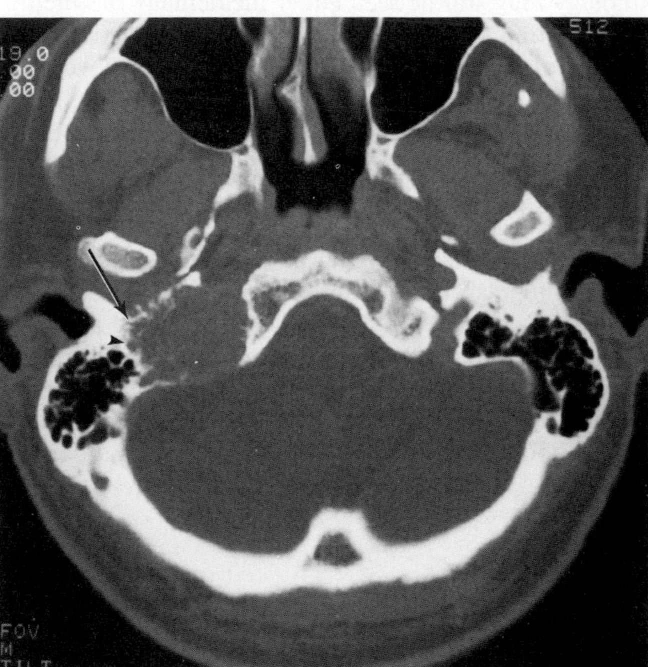

B

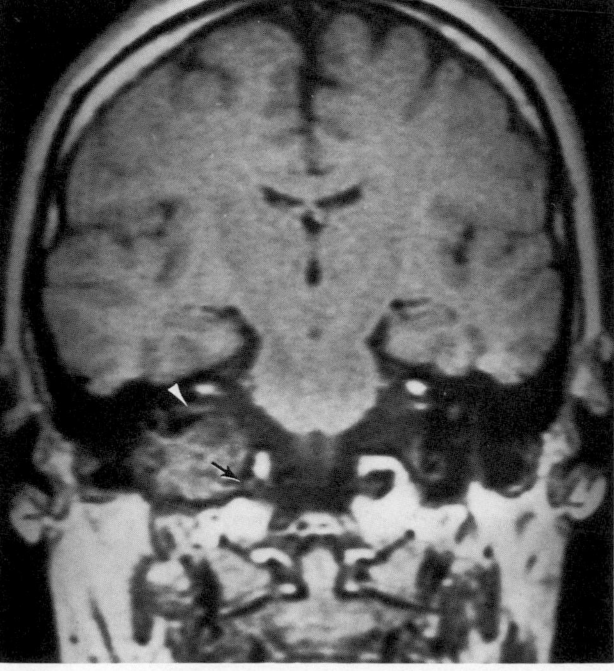
C

FIG. 35. Glomus jugulotympanicum. **A:** Axial SE (700/20) MRI shows a mass in the right jugular bulb. The mass involves both the lateral and medial aspects of the jugular fossa. There are several small flow voids (*arrowheads*) within the mass. **B:** CT with bone algorithm at the same level. There is extensive erosion of the jugular bulb. Note the "smudgy erosion" of bone (*arrow*). There is involvement of the mastoid segment of the facial nerve canal (*arrowhead*). **C:** Coronal SE (700/20) MRI. The mass replaces the right jugular bulb. On any one pulsing sequence this signal within the bulb could be due to a flow defect, but visualization of the mass in multiple planes and on multiple pulse sequences confirms its presence. This glomus tumor has eroded the right hypoglossal canal (*arrow*). The mass does not involve the internal auditory canal (*arrowhead*).

Other tumors that present in the middle ear are nerve sheath tumors related to the facial nerve canal (Fig. 36) or the rare adenomatous tumor of the middle ear. Although usually benign, the adenomatous tumor can be locally destructive.

Because the evaluation of the middle ear requires such attention to fine bony detail, CT is usually the first choice in imaging this area (see Fig. 34). With MRI, the signal void of the fine cortical bony structures cannot be differentiated from the signal void of air in the middle ear or mastoid air cells. Even though MRI is not used as the first imaging modality in suspected middle ear disease, pathology may still be seen either incidentally or when the presenting symptoms suggest more central pathology. In most cases, the pathology is seen as signal where there should be none. That is, the pathology replaces the signal void of the air or the cortical bone (Fig. 36).

Inner Ear, Petrous Apex, and Jugular Foramen

The more central temporal bone contains the bony labyrinth, jugular, carotid, internal auditory, and facial nerve canals as well as the medullary cavity and a variable number of air cells in the petrous apex. The differential diagnosis depends on the precise position of the pathology. For example, an acoustic neuroma (nerve sheath tumor) is not likely to be confused with a paraganglioma (25,26). Their different sites of origin, although separated by only a few millimeters, are clearly evident on imaging (see Fig. 35). Glomus jugulare tumors (paraganglioma) arise in the lateral portion of the jugular foramen. Growth can be in any direction. There can be significant inferior extension beneath the temporal bone or there can be intracranial growth. In our experience, all the glomus jugulare tumors have had significant extension laterally into the middle ear region (Fig. 37). We have not seen a paraganglioma that involved only the medial portion of the jugular foramen (without affecting the lateral boundary of the jugular canal) unless this medial involvement represented superior extension from a glomus vagale (Fig. 38) arising below the skull base. Paragangliomas are often intermediate signal intensity on T1-weighted images and are relatively bright on T2-weighted images (Figs. 35 and 38) (25). Small signal voids, scattered throughout, are very characteristic, but may not be present in small tumors (<2 cm) (25).

On the other hand, nerve sheath tumors arising from cranial nerves IX, X, or XI do arise in the medial part of the jugular foramen, the so-called pars nervosa. They expand superiorly and inferiorly and usually spare the lateral wall of the jugular foramen. The enlargement of the medial segment of the foramen is smooth. The MRI signal characteristics are variable (23,26).

Lesions of the petrous apex that seem to arise in the

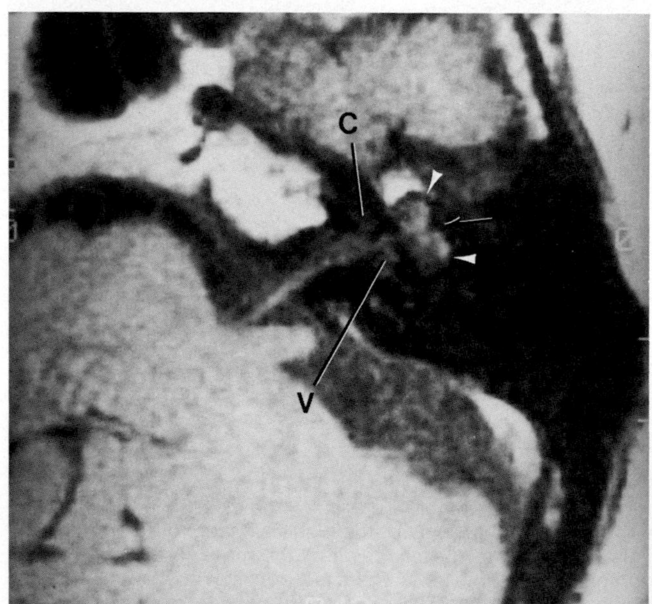

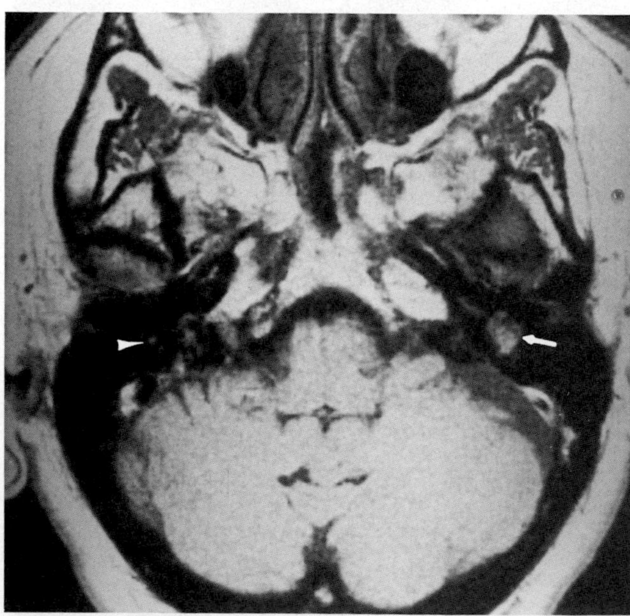

FIG. 36. Facial nerve sheath tumor. **A:** Short TR/short TE MRI. Axial image through the bony labyrinth shows a lobulated abnormal signal (*arrowheads*) representing an enlarged tympanic segment of the facial nerve canal. Some signal is usually present in the labyrinth representing fluid in the cochlea (*C*) and vestibule (*V*). The indentation on the tumor (*arrow*) represents a signal void of the ossicular chain. Note that the ossicular chain cannot be clearly separated from residual air in the mastoid. **B:** More inferior section shows the enlarged vertical segment of the facial nerve canal (*arrow*) compared with the normal canal on the opposite side (*arrowhead*).

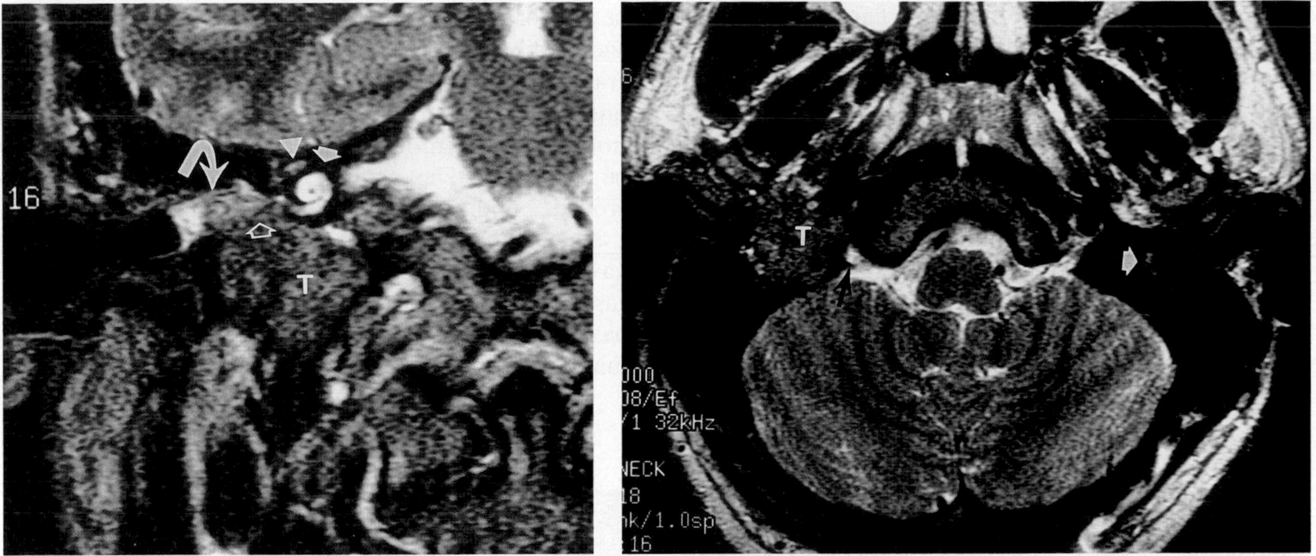

FIG. 37. **A:** Coronal T2-weighted image shows extension of tumor mass (glomus jugulare) into middle ear and external auditory canals. *White arrowhead*, facial nerve; *white arrow*, cochlea; *T,* tumor; *curved white arrow*, tumor extension into external auditory canal; *hollow arrow*, tumor extension into middle ear. **B:** Axial T2-weighted image shows gross extension of glomus juglare beyond lateral jugular foramen into temporal bone. *T,* tumor; *black arrow*, pars nervosa; *white arrow*, normal left facial nerve. *Note:* Signal from right facial nerve is not seen because of invasion by tumor.

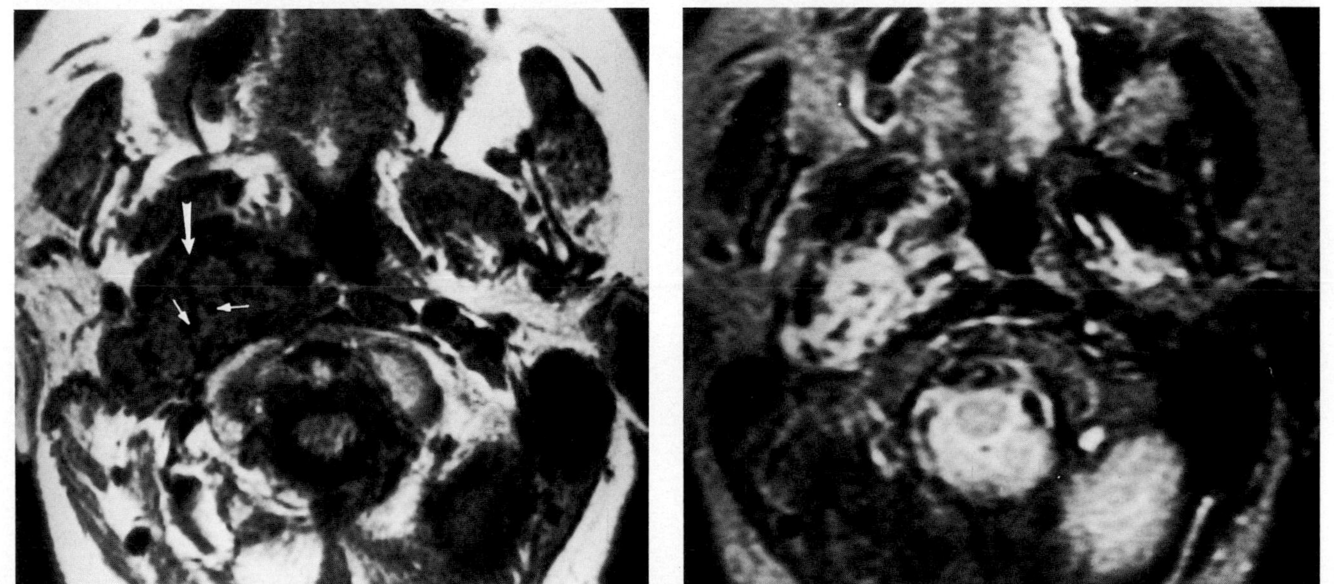

FIG. 38. Glomus vagale. **A:** Axial SE (800/20) MRI shows an irregular mass involving the right poststyloid parapharyngeal space (*large arrow*). Several flow voids are present within the mass (*small arrows*). **B:** T2-weighted SE (2500/100) MRI at the same level shows the mass as high signal with internal flow voids.

bone but not in the various traversing canals tend to be cholesterol cysts (cholesterol granulomas) (Fig. 39) (27). In the past, these were considered to be epidermoids, but most of these are actually air cells that have been partially obstructed and are now filled with liquid and cellular debris and recurrent hemorrhage. The wall of cholesterol cyst is lined by fibrous tissue. True epidermoids certainly do occur in the apex, but they are much less common than was previously thought. Their walls consist of stratified squamous epithelium, which surrounds more solid keratin debris. They may have a connection to the middle ear. Epidermoids (cholesteatomas) tend to be dark or intermediate in signal on the T1-weighted images and bright on T2-weighted images. The cholesterol granuloma is bright on both sequences (Fig. 39) but will often have dark areas within, representing hemosiderin from current hemorrhage (28). The carotid artery may be displaced. The wall of the carotid canal may be eroded, a finding more easily appreciated on CT.

Aneurysms of the petrous carotid artery are rare, but have a similar appearance to a cholesterol cyst. In the case of an aneurysm, the carotid may be demonstrated passing through the abnormality rather than along the margin, as in the case of a cholesterol cyst.

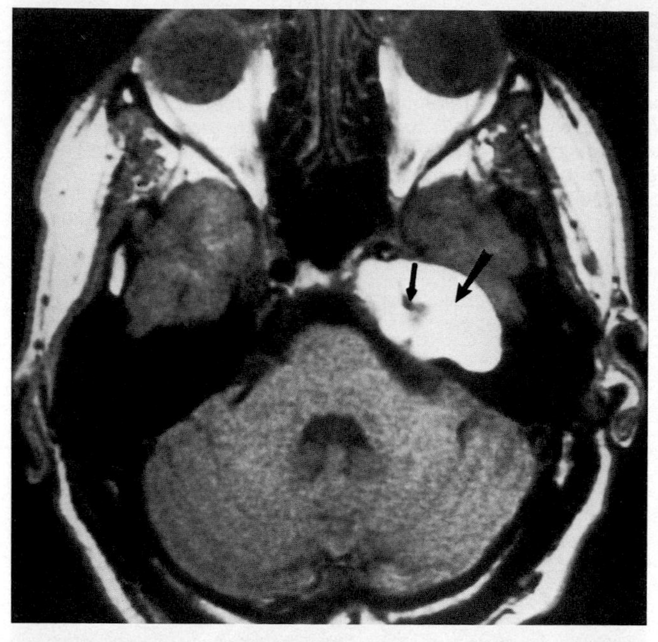

A

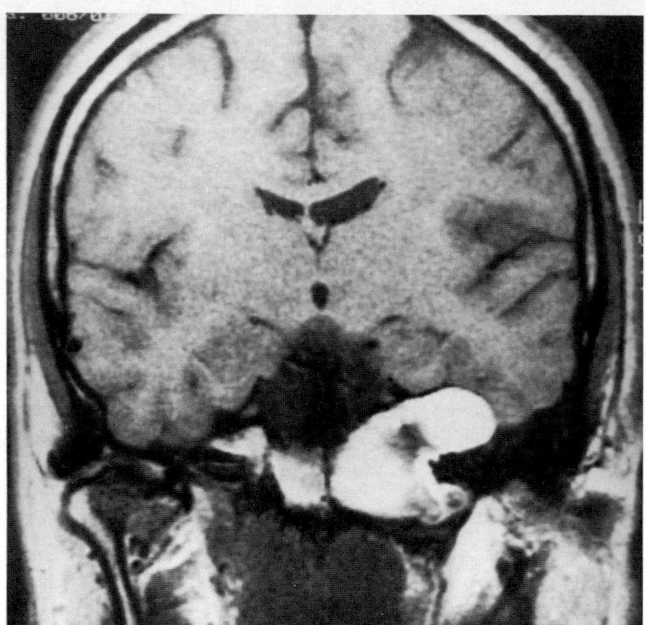

B

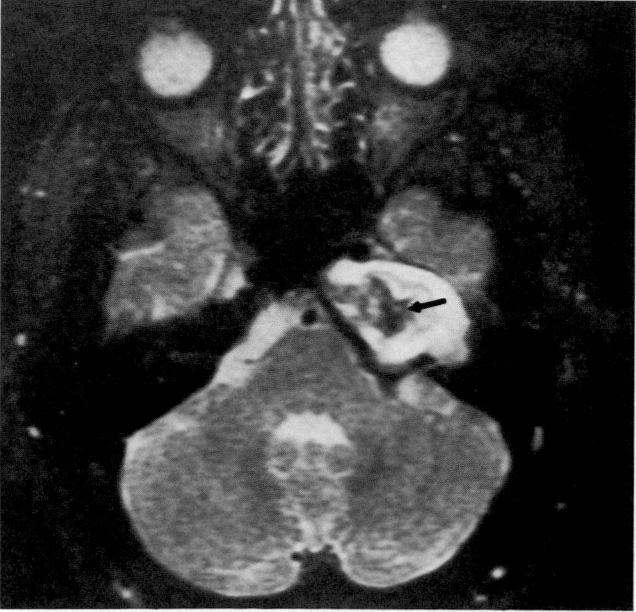

C

FIG. 39. Cholesterol cyst. **A:** Axial SE (700/20) MR [shows a high signal lesion expanding the left petrous apex (*large arrow*). There is some low signal within the center of the mass (*small arrow*). **B:** Coronal T1-weighted SE (600/20) MRI shows superior extension of the mass with remodeling of the petrous apex. **C:** T2-weighted SE image (2500/100) shows that the mass is largely high signal but has a central area of lower signal (*arrow*). The high signal on both T1-weighted and T2-weighted images is characteristic of cholesterol cysts and is seldom seen in other pathologies of the petrous bone. It may be due to the products of hemorrhage within this chronically obstructed petrous apex. The signal void may represent hemosiderin.

The arachnoid villi may invaginate into the petrous apex. Eventually the CSF pulsations may form a small CSF collection in the apex. The cavity has the signal characteristics of CSF and a communication with the subarachnoid space is identified.

The internal auditory canal is the site of origin of the eighth nerve sheath tumor (acoustic neuroma, vestibular schwannoma). Seventh nerve tumors, meningiomas, epidermoids, and lipomas also occur here but are much less common. Tumors of this area as well as extra-axial posterior fossa tumors are covered in another chapter (*this volume*).

The seventh nerve canal (Fallopian canal) winds its way through the temporal bone, passing around the labyrinth and through the middle ear and mastoid before exiting at the stylomastoid foramen. Most often lesions involving this canal are nerve sheath tumors (Fig. 40; see Fig. 36) or hemangiomas (29). Meningiomas also occur in the region of the canal but are less common. The subtle differences between these lesions are best appreciated on CT.

Tumors that follow the entire length of the canal are most frequently nerve sheath tumors (see Fig. 31). Perineural extension of tumor may also do this. Adenoid cys-

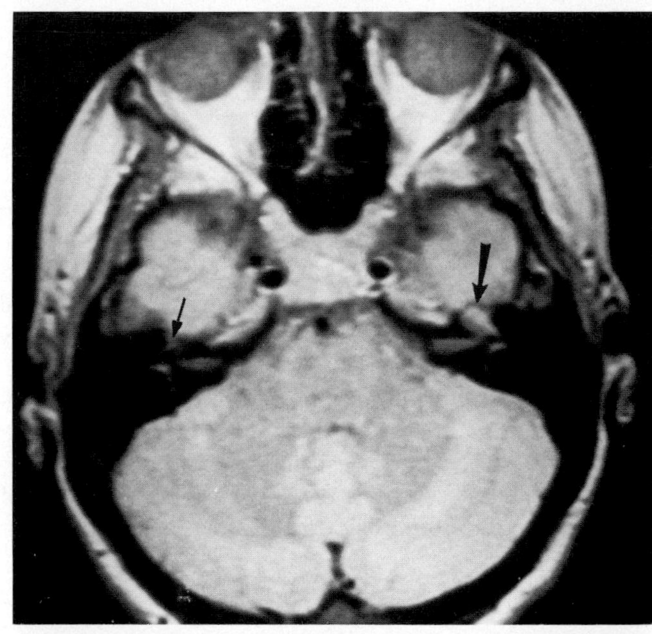

A

FIG. 40. Facial neuroma. **A:** Axial long TR/short TE (2500/20) MRI. There is a mass expanding the facial canal in the region of the geniculate ganglion (*large arrow*). Note the normal facial nerve on the contralateral side (*small arrow*). **B:** Postcontrast coronal SE scan (600/20). The lesion enhances following contrast (*arrow*). **C:** Enhancement not only can be seen in the region of the geniculate ganglion (*arrowhead*), but also there is abnormal enhancement in the internal auditory canal (IAC) (*arrow*). The enhanced scan is very helpful in showing the involvement of IAC.

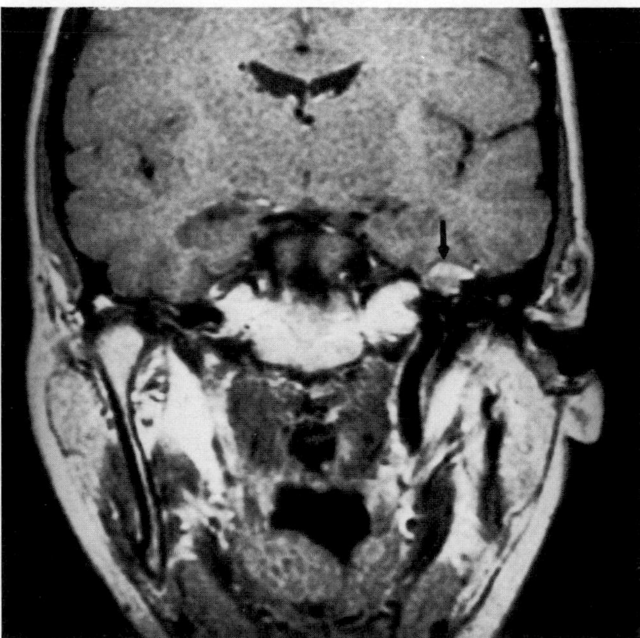

B

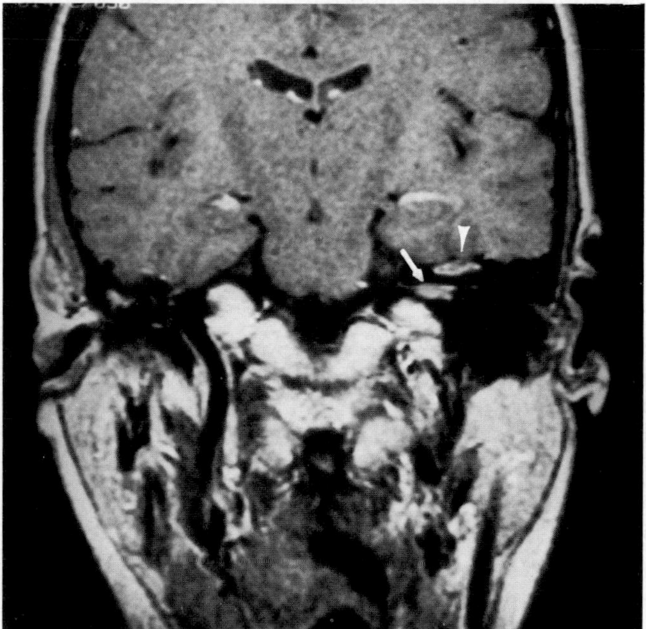

C

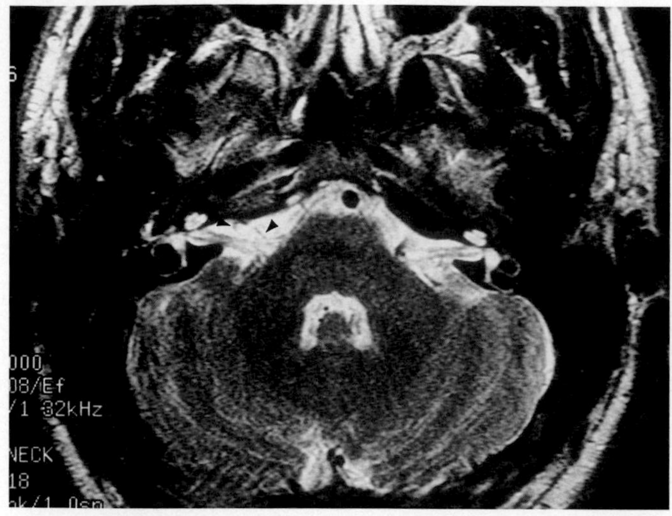

FIG. 41. Axial FSE T2-weighted image shows the normal neural structures within the internal auditory canals. *Arrowheads*, anterior inferior cerebellar artery.

tic carcinoma of the parotid gland can follow the facial nerve all the way to the internal auditory canal.

Finally, at the extreme medial margin of the petrous apex is the petro-occipital (petroclival) suture. Chondromatous tumors have a predilection for this area (see Fig. 30). As the lesion grows, differentiation from the tumors of the clivus becomes more difficult.

In the temporal bone, CT is almost always used because of the importance of fine bony detail. The internal auditory canal is an exception. Here, MRI with gadolinium is the modality of choice for excluding acoustic neuromas. T2-weighted high resolution FSE sequences are also routinely used at our institution for evaluation of the internal auditory canals. This provides highly detailed imaging of the internal auditory canal contents and actual visualization of the eighth cranial nerve within the cerebellopontine angle and within the canal (Fig. 41).

NON-NEOPLASTIC PROCESSES

Inflammation

Obstruction of a sinus can lead to mucocele formation. A mucocele represents an expanded sinus. This expansion can impinge on neural structures and actually displace the brain. Signal characteristics are variable (see Fig. 27). Secondary inflammatory change within an obstructed sinus can also result in osteomyelitis of the skull base. An intracranial abscess may develop. These abscesses are usually epidural at least initially. Usually we image these pathologic processes with CT scans, as the bony detail can be quite important. However, gadolinium-enhanced MRI is considered to be more sensitive in detecting an epidural abscess.

Various fungi such as actinomycoses and invasive aspergillosis can cause considerable destruction of the skull base and extend intracranially. These infections may mimic a neoplastic process.

The various granulomatous pathologies such as Wegener's granulomatosis lead to nonspecific mucosal thickening, but there can be destruction of bony walls, especially the nasal septum. We have not seen a case of Wegener's granulomatosis on MRI.

Congenital

Congenital lesions anterior to the cribriform plate include encephalocele, nasal dermoid, and the so-called nasal glioma. They are related to aberrant closure of the neuropore. They present as a mass at the bridge of the nose. In most cases, the surgeon will need to determine whether there is an intracranial connection. A bony canal, if present, connects the intracranial and extracranial components (Fig. 42). The anterior margin of the crista galli is bifid. These lesions represent a broad spectrum. They may be dumbbell-shaped and have a large intra- and extracranial component. At other times, there is only an extracranial mass and the bony canal is occupied by a small, blind-ending fibrous tract. CT is superior to MRI in showing the actual bone changes, but MRI has the advantage of multiplanar imaging and superior soft tissue discrimination. For example, the CSF in an encephalocele can be differentiated from the more solid material in a nasal glioma. The relationship to the inferior surface of the frontal lobe is well seen on MRI.

Defects in the anterior portion of the sphenoid bone

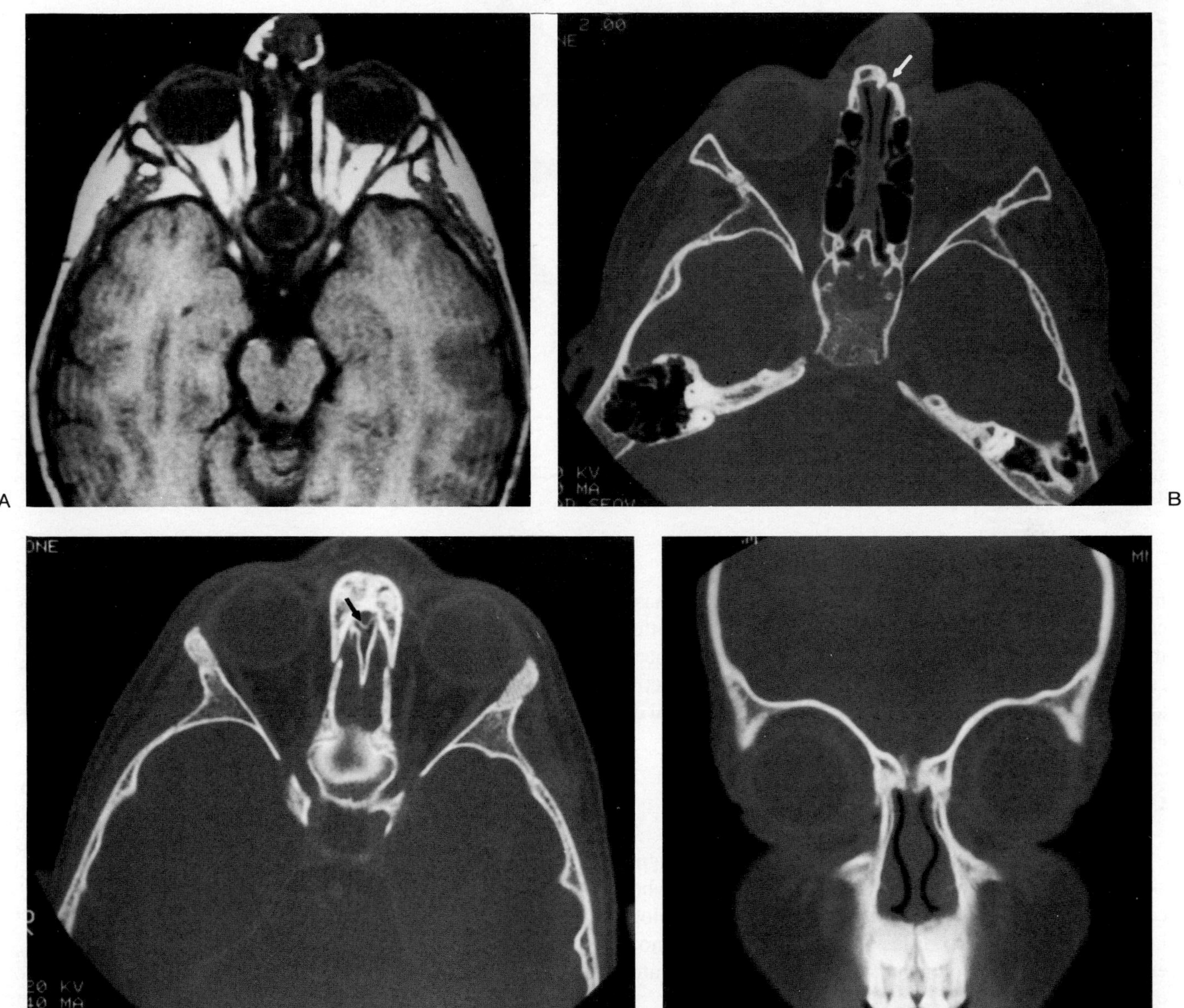

FIG. 42. Nasal dermoid. **A:** Axial SE (600/25) MRI shows a mass of intermediate-signal intensity at the bridge of the nose. The bony canal is difficult to detect with MRI. **B:** Bone algorithm of an axial CT scan shows a small bony canal connecting the dermoid with the nasal septum (*arrow*). **C:** Axial slice at a slightly higher level shows the bifid crista galli (*arrow*). **D:** Coronal CT (bone algorithm) shows a bony defect in the midline. However, neither MRI nor CT showed an intracranial component. This lesion was removed with an extracranial procedure.

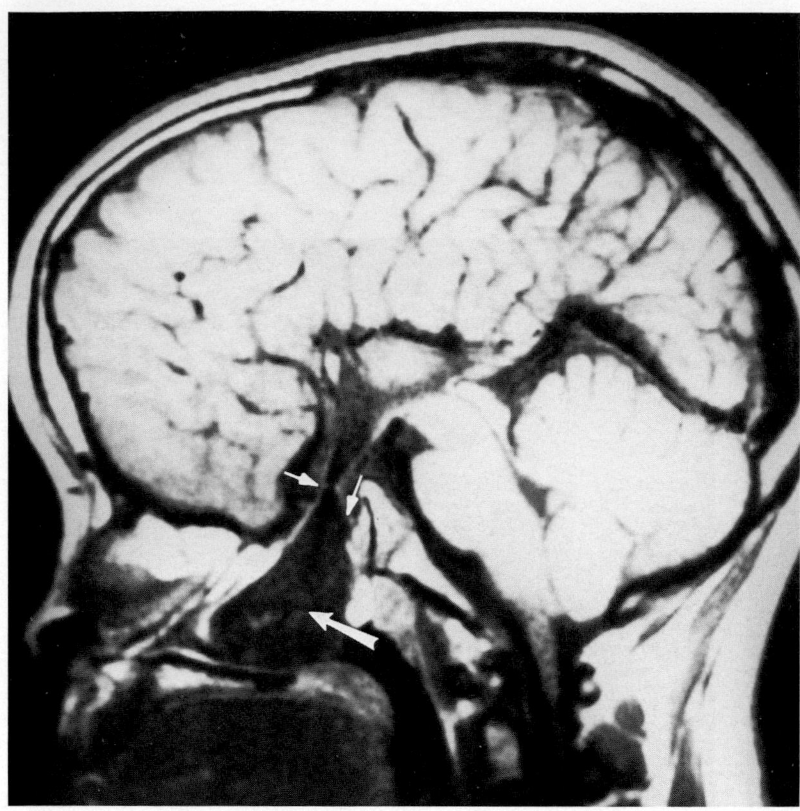

FIG. 43. Sphenoid encephalocele. Sagittal SE (600/25) MRI. There is a midline defect in the sphenoid bone in the region of the sella (*small arrows*). A sac protrudes through this defect into the nasal cavity (*large arrow*). The sac abuts the soft palate.

may present as encephaloceles protruding into the nasal cavity or nasopharynx (Fig. 43). These can mimic other masses, such as nasal polyps. Biopsy of an encephalocele can result in CSF leak and meningitis; therefore, encephalocele should always be considered in the differential diagnosis of nasopharyngeal masses.

CONCLUSION

MRI has become the preferred modality for imaging skull base lesions. The rapid advances of imaging when coupled with similar advances in surgical technology have allowed resection of lesions once considered inoperable. Further technological advances and accumulated experience should improve our diagnostic abilities.

REFERENCES

1. Okada Y, Aoki S, Barkovich AJ, et al. Cranial bone marrow in children: assessment of normal development with MR imaging. *Radiology* 1989;171:161–164.
2. Shigeki A, Dillon WP, Barkovich AJ, Norman D. Marrow conversion before pneumatization of the sphenoid sinus: assessment with MR imaging. *Radiology* 1989;172:373–375.
3. Som PM, Shapiro MD, Biller HF, Sasaki C, Lawson W. Sinonasal tumors and inflammatory tissues: differentiation with MR imaging. *Radiology* 1988;167:803–808.
4. Dillon WP, Som PM, Fullerton GD. Hypointense MR signal in chronically inspissated sinonasal secretions. *Radiology* 1990;174:73–78.
5. Som PM, Dillon WP, Fullerton GD, Zimmerman RA, Rajagopalan B, Marom Z. Chronically obstructed sinonasal secretions: observations on TI and T2 shortening. *Radiology* 1989;172:515–520.
6. Zinreich SJ, Kennedy DW, Malat J, et al. Fungal sinusitis: diagnosis with CT and MR Imaging. *Radiology* 1988;169:439–444.
7. Som PM, Shugar JM, Troy K, et al. The use of magnetic resonance and computed tomography in the management of a patient with intrasinus hemorrhage. *Arch Otolaryngol Head Neck Surg* 1988;114:200–202.
8. Laine FJ, Braun IF, Jensen ME, Nadel L, Som PD. Perineural tumor extension through the foramen ovale: evaluation with MR imaging. *Radiology* 1990;174:65–71.
9. Hirsch WL, Hryshko FG, Sekhar LN, et al. Comparison of MR imaging, CT, and angiography in the evaluation of the enlarged cavernous sinus. *AJNR* 1988;9:907–915.
10. Curtin HD, Williams R, Johnson J. CT of the perineural tumor extension: pterygopalatine fossa. *AJR* 1985;144:163–169.
11. Curtin HD, Wolfe P, Snyderman N. Facial nerve between the stylomastoid foramen and the parotid: computed tomographic imaging. *Radiology* 1983;149:165–169.
12. Erba SM, Horton JA, Latchaw RE, et al. Balloon test occlusion of the internal carotid artery with stable xenon/CT cerebral blood flow imaging. *AJNR* 1988;9:533–538.
13. Elster AD, Challa VR, Gilbert TH, Richardson DN, Contento JC. Meningiomas: MR and histopathologic features. *Radiology* 1989;170:857–862.
14. Latack JT, Hutchinson RJ, Heyn RM. Imaging of rhabdomyosarcomas of the head and neck. *AJNR* 1987;8:353–359.
15. Atlas SW, Grossman RI, Gomori JM, et al. MR imaging of intracranial metastatic melanoma. *J Comput Assist Tomogr* 1987;11:577–582.
16. Regenbogen VS, Zinreich J, Kim KS, et al. Hyperostotic esthesioneuroblastoma: CT and MR findings. *J Comput Assist Tomogr* 1988;12:52–56.
17. Mills SE, Frierson HF. Olfactory neuroblastoma: a clinicopathologic study of 21 cases. *Am J Surg Pathol* 1985;9:317–327.
18. Som PM, Dillion WP, Sze G, Lidov M, Biller HF, Lawson W. Be-

nign and malignant sinonasal lesions with intracranial extension: differentiation with MR imaging. *Radiology* 1989;172:763–766.

19. Oot RF, Melville GE, New PFJ, et al. The role of MR and CT in evaluating clival chondroma and chondrosarcomas. *AJNR* 1988;9:715–723.
20. Lee Y, Tassel PV. Craniofacial chondrosarcomas: imaging findings in 15 untreated cases. *AJNR* 1989;10:165–170.
21. Teresi LM, Lufkin RB, Vinuela F. MR imaging of the nasopharynx and floor of the middle cranial fossa, part II. Malignant tumors. *Radiology* 1987;164:817–821.
22. Curtin HD. Separation of the masticator space from the para pharyngeal space. *Radiology* 1987;163:195–204.
23. Watabe T, Azuma T. T1 and T2 measurements of meningiomas and neuromas before and after GD-DTPA. *AJNR* 1989;10:463–470.
24. Lloyd GAS, Phelps PD. Juvenile angiofibroma: imaging by magnetic resonance, CT and conventional techniques. *Clin Otolaryngol* 1986;11:247–259.
25. Olsen WL, Dillon WP, Kelly WM, Norman D, Brant-Zawadzki M, Newton TH. MR imaging of paragangliomas. *AJNR* 1986;7: 1039–1042.
26. Press GA, Hesselink J. MR imaging of cerebellopontine angle and internal auditory canal lesions at 1.5 T. *AJR* 1988;150:1371–1381.
27. Lo WW, Solti-Bohman LG, Brackmann DE, Gruskin P. Cholesterol granuloma of the petrous apex: CT diagnosis. *Radiology* 1984;153:705–711.
28. Martin N, Sterkers 0, Mompoint D, Julien N, Nahum H. Cholesterol granulomas of the middle ear cavities: MR imaging. *Radiology* 1989;172:521–525.
29. Curtin HD, Jensen JE, Barnes LJ, May M. Ossifying hemangiomas of the temporal bone: evaluation with CT. *Radiology* 1987;164: 831–835.

Magnetic Resonance Imaging of the Brain and Spine, Second Edition, edited by Scott W. Atlas. Lippincott-Raven Publishers, Philadelphia © 1996.

21

Anatomy and Diseases of the Temporal Bone

Alexander S. Mark

Until recently, the only appropriate imaging modality for diseases affecting the temporal bone was high-resolution computed tomography (HRCT). Although this technique is obviously still important and in fact relied on by most centers for imaging many temporal bone diseases, the advent of magnetic resonance (MR) contrast agents has clearly expanded the role of MR imaging (MRI) in this region. Recent technical innovations in fast imaging and high resolution techniques have finally made MRI appropriate for many of these conditions, and in some cases uniquely so. This chapter discusses the pertinent anatomy and the role of MRI in the evaluation of the labyrinth and the internal auditory canal (IAC), cranial nerve VII, and a variety of miscellaneous conditions of the temporal bone itself. The reader is also referred to Chapter 20, "Base of the Skull."

THE LABYRINTH

Anatomy of the Inner Ear

The Bony Labyrinth

The bony labyrinth develops from the primitive otic capsule and consists of the vestibule, semicircular canals, and cochlea. The vestibule leads anteriorly into the cochlea and posteriorly into the semicircular canals. The wall of the vestibule is marked by the elliptical recess for the utricle and the spherical recess for the saccule. Between these recesses lies the vestibular crest, which divides posteriorly into two limbs that locate the cochlear recess for the vestibular cecum of the cochlear duct. The cribrose areas of the vestibule consist of groups of small foramina through which the vestibular nerve bundles enter the vestibule. Other openings in the vestibule are the vestibular aqueduct and the oval window.

Each of the three bony semicircular canals makes two thirds of a circle; each lies at right angles to the other two, and each measures about 1 mm in diameter. An enlargement at one end forms the bony ampulla. The nonampullated ends of the superior and posterior semicircular canals join to form the common crus. The bony cochlea contains a base lying at the anterolateral aspect of the IAC and an apex directed anterolaterally and inferiorly. It is a spiral canal with two and one half turns around a bony core, the modiolus, and ends at the apex in the hook-like hamulus. The osseous lamina spirals about the modiolus and incompletely subdivides the spiral canal into the scala vestibuli and scala tympani, which join at the helicotrema (1). The normal anatomy and abnormalities of the bony labyrinth are best imaged with HRCT.

The Membranous Labyrinth

The membranous labyrinth (Fig. 1) is enclosed within the bony labyrinth. The outer layer is generally separated

A. S. Mark, M.D.: Neuroradiology Section, Department of Radiology, George Washington University Medical Center, and Department of Radiology, Washington Hospital Center, Washington, D.C. 20010.

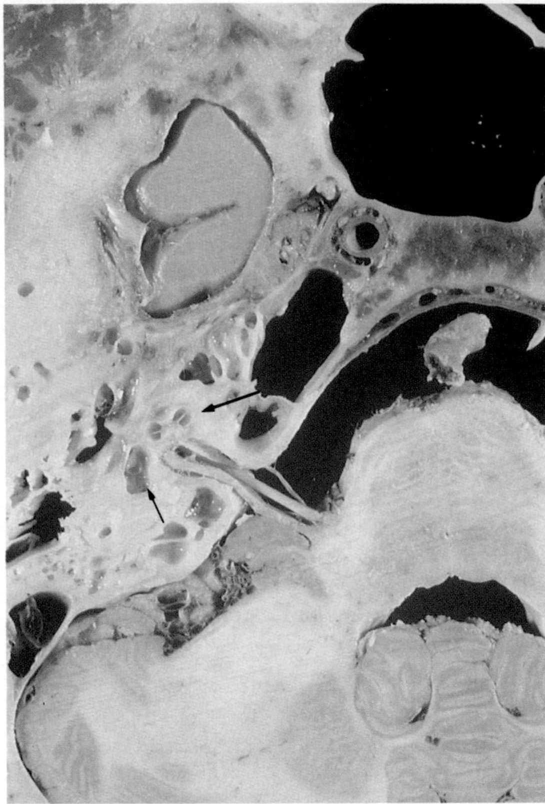

FIG. 1. Normal anatomy. Axial histologic section through the labyrinth, internal auditory canal, and cerebellopontine angle. *Long arrow*, cochlea; *short arrow*, vestibule. (Courtesy of Dr. J. De Groot, San Francisco, CA.)

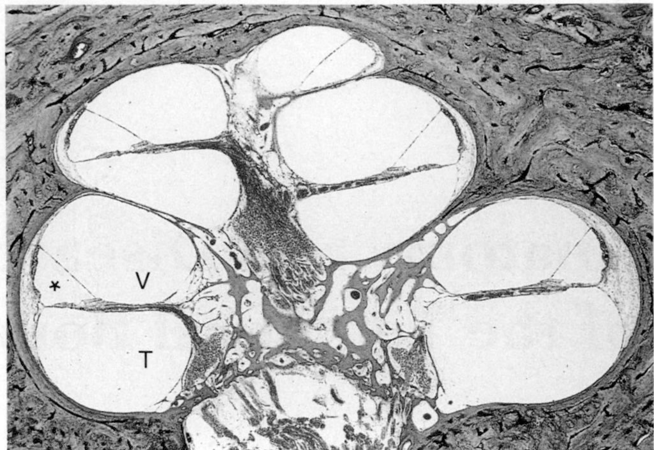

FIG. 2. Normal anatomy. Axial histologic section through the cochlea demonstrating the cochlear duct (or scala media) containing endolymph (*asterisk*), the scala vestibuli (*V*), and the scala tympani (*T*) containing perilymph. The cochlear duct (endolymph) is considerably smaller than the scala vestibuli and scala tympani.

from the periosteum of the bony labyrinth by a space containing perilymphatic fluid.

The Cochlear Duct

The cochlear duct is a spiral membranous canal located between the osseous spiral lamina and external bony wall of the cochlea. With the osseous spiral lamina, it completes the subdivision of the bony spiral canal into the scala vestibuli and scala tympani. Reissner's membrane is a thin membrane extending obliquely from the vestibular crest of the spiral ligament to the spiral limbus (Fig. 2) (1). The spiral ligament is located in a sulcus on the external wall of the bony cochlear duct and is lined on its internal surface by the stria vascularis, spiral prominence, and external sulcus cells. It provides for the external attachments of the basilar membrane and Reissner's membrane. The basilar membrane extends from the tympanic lip of the osseous spiral lamina to the basilar crest of the spiral ligament and supports the organ of Corti on the scala media side.

The Vestibular Sense Organs

The saccule is a flattened, irregularly shaped sac that lies on the medial wall of the vestibule. Its membranous wall projects superiorly in the wall of the utricle, where it has a broad attachment without any communication. The lateral part of the saccular wall, adjacent to the vestibular wall, has a well defined thickening termed the "macula" (Fig. 3). The utricle is an irregular oval-shaped tube superior to the saccule in the elliptical recess of the wall of the vestibule. The three semicircular ducts communicate with the utricle via five openings, one of which is formed by the union of the nonampullated ends of the superior and posterior canals and is termed the "common crus" (1).

The Endolymphatic Duct and Sac

The endolymphatic sac (Fig. 4) lies partly within a bony niche on the posterior surface of the petrous bone

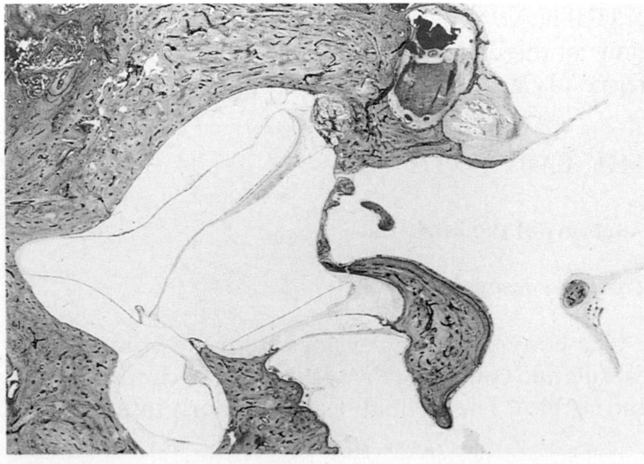

FIG. 3. Normal anatomy. Vertical section through the vestibule showing the relationship between the round window and the oval window. Notice also the location of the facial nerve. (From Schuknecht, ref. 1, with permission.)

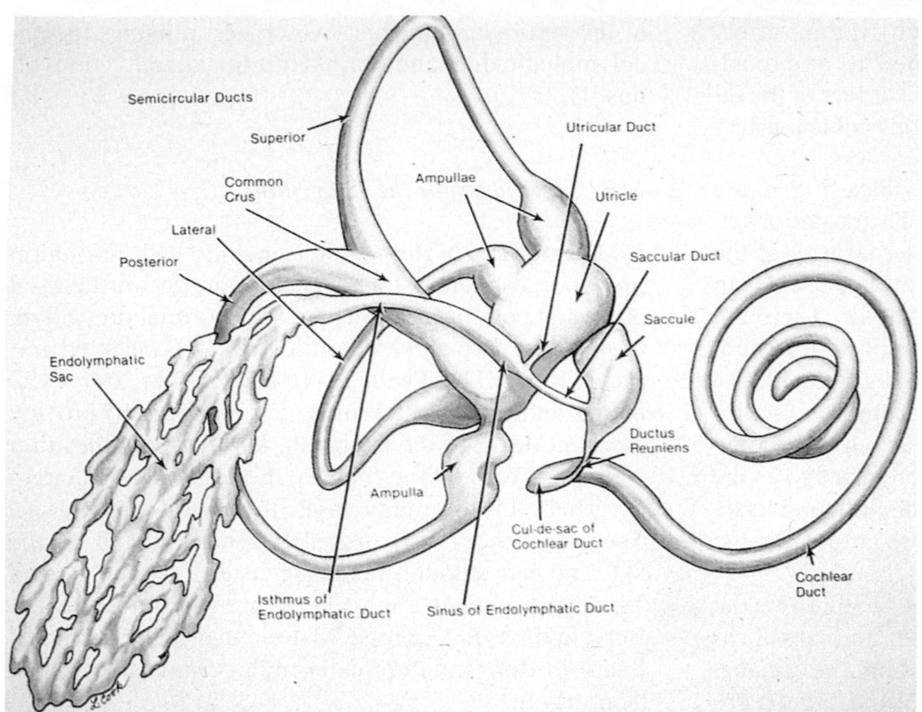

FIG. 4. Normal anatomy. The endolymphatic sac and its relationship to the rest of the membranous labyrinth. (From Schuknecht, ref. 1, with permission.)

and partly within the layers of the dura mater of the posterior cranial fossa. It is connected to the endolymphatic system by the endolymphatic duct, which lies in a bony canal known as the vestibular aqueduct. The duct is lined mainly by squamous and cuboidal cells and its lumen at the isthmus (narrowest region) measures 0.1 to 0.2 mm in diameter. The presence of lateral intercellular spaces in the sac epithelium is strong evidence of a fluid transport function for the sac.

The Vascular System

An arterial loop supplying the labyrinth (Fig. 5) is consistently found in the region of the IAC. This loop is found inside the IAC in 40%, at the meatus in 27%, and in the cerebellopontine angle in 33% of cases. The anterior inferior cerebellar artery gives rise to the labyrinthine artery (also termed internal auditory artery) and also frequently the subarcuate artery before taking a re-

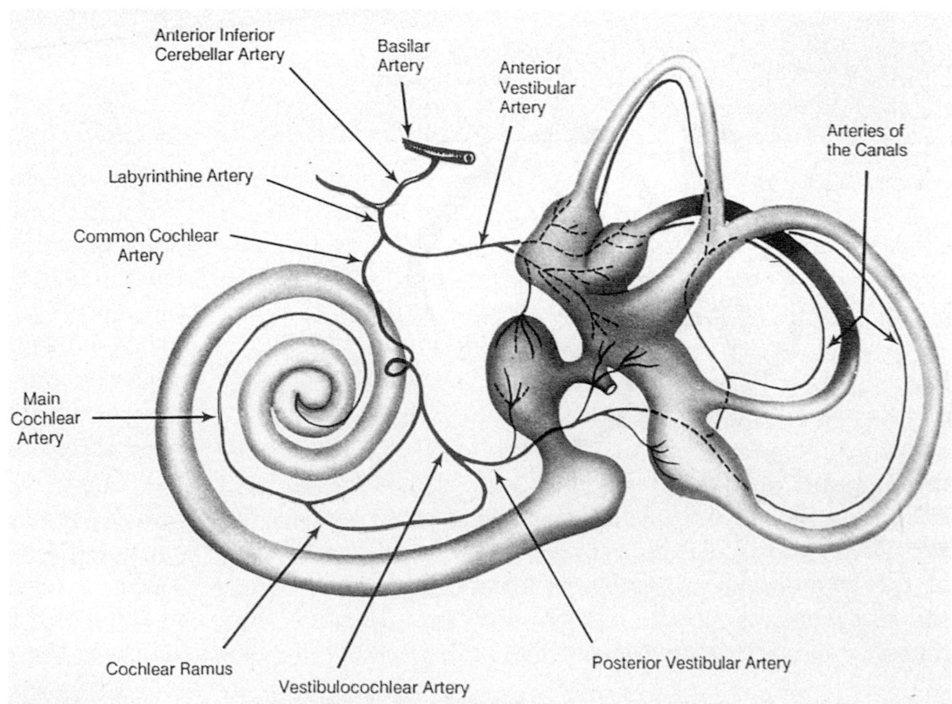

FIG. 5. Normal anatomy. Principal arteries of the inner ear. (From Schuknecht, ref. 1, with permission.)

current course to the cerebellum. The labyrinthine artery distributes to the dura and nerves in the IAC and to adjacent bone around the IAC and medial aspect of the inner ear before dividing into the common cochlear artery and the anterior vestibular artery

The main venous channels of the cochlea (Fig. 6) are the posterior and anterior spiral veins. The posterior spiral vein drains the spiral ganglion, external wall of the scala media, and scala tympani. The anterior spiral vein drains the spiral lamina and scala vestibuli. There are several shunts from the anterior to the posterior spiral vein before they join near the basal end of the cochlea to form the common modiolar vein. The common modiolar vein is joined by the vestibulocochlear vein to become the vein at the cochlear aqueduct, also referred to as the inferior cochlear vein. This main channel then enters a bony canal near the cochlear aqueduct to empty into the inferior petrosal sinus.

The anterior vestibular vein carries blood from the utricle and the ampullae of the superior and lateral canals. The posterior vestibular vein drains the saccule, ampulla of the posterior canal, and basal end of the cochlea. The confluence of these two vessels is joined by the vein of the round window to become the vestibulocochlear vein. The semicircular canals are drained by vessels that pass toward their utricular ends to form the vein of the vestibular aqueduct, which accompanies the endolymphatic duct and drains into the lateral venous sinus (1).

MRI Techniques for the Labyrinth

MRI of the labyrinth should include high resolution pre- and post-contrast T1-weighted images in the axial plane and postcontrast images in the coronal projection. Conventional spin-echo 3-mm thick T1-weighted images (TR 600/TE 13 with 14–16 field of view, 256 × 192 matrix and four excitations on a 1.5-T imager) provide excellent detail of the labyrinth, allowing identification of different turns of the cochlea, the vestibule, semicircular canals, and, in many cases, the endolymphatic sac. These sequences also provide exquisite detail of the IAC and cerebellopontine angle cistern. Fat-suppressed T1-weighted images may be a useful adjunct to exclude lipoma. Precontrast T1-weighted images are necessary to differentiate enhancement from labyrinthine hemorrhage.

Several authors recently described the use of high resolution three-dimensional (3D) volume T2-weighted images that permit submillimeter-thick sections through the temporal bone (2–4). Three-dimensional reconstruc-

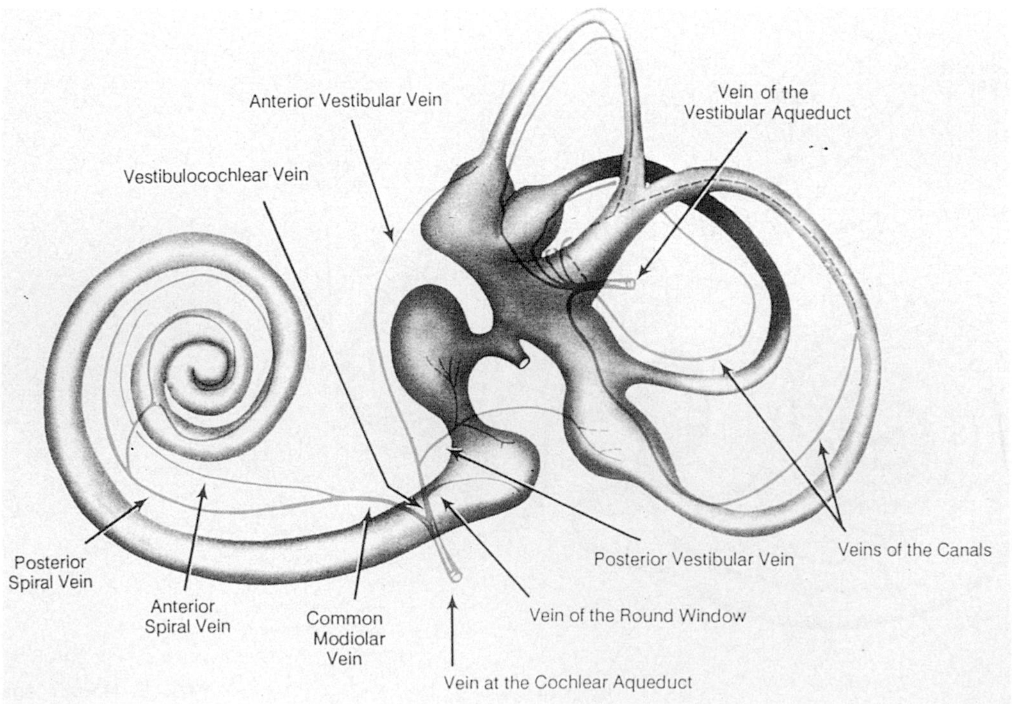

FIG. 6. Normal anatomy. Principal veins of the inner ear. (From Schuknecht, ref. 1, with permission.)

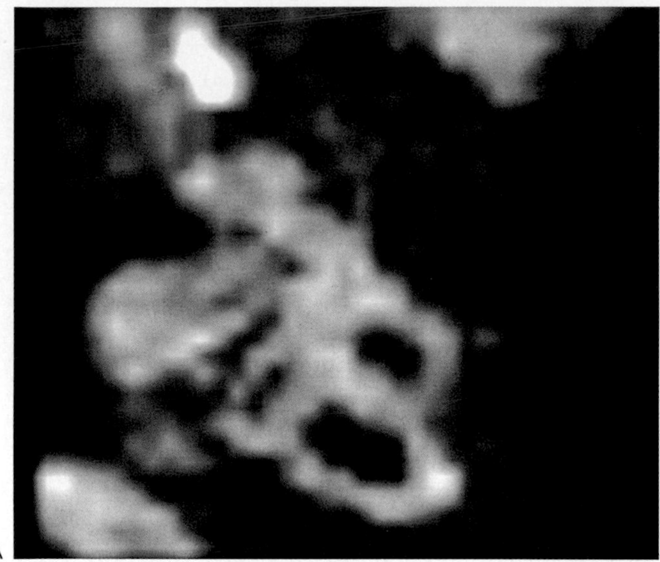

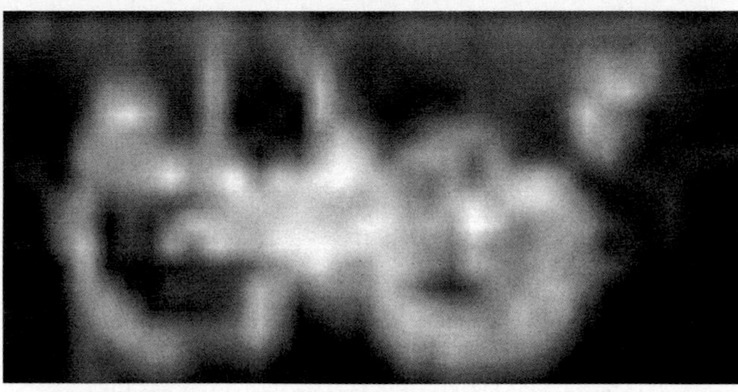

FIG. 7. Normal anatomy. **A:** Craniocaudal and, **B,** anteroposterior 3D volume reconstruction from 0. 7-mm thick T2-weighted high resolution axial gradient-echo images (3). (Courtesy of Dr. J. Casselman, Bruges, Belgium.)

tions of the fluid-containing membranous labyrinth may also be obtained (Fig. 7). These images exhibit exquisite anatomic detail and are mostly used to demonstrate the appearance of the fluid-filled endolymphatic and perilymphatic spaces. T1-weighted 3D volume gradient-echo images may also be obtained with 1-mm thick sections through the labyrinth in conjunction with intravenous contrast administration to look for inflammatory or neoplastic lesions. Axial T2-weighted images are also obtained to exclude an intra-axial lesion (Fig. 8) (5–9).

Labyrinthine Lesions

Until recently, the labyrinth was almost exclusively imaged with high resolution CT. CT remains the clear imaging modality of choice for the evaluation of congenital sensorineural hearing loss. Recently, because of a number of technical advances coupled with the availability of intravenous contrast agents, a number of inflammatory and neoplastic lesions of the labyrinth diagnosed previously only at autopsy or at surgery could be imaged. This section describes some of the labyrinthine diseases that can be diagnosed by imaging modalities and emphasizes the respective strengths of high resolution CT and MRI.

Labyrinthine Hemorrhage

Labyrinthine hemorrhage can occur in patients with coagulopathies, leukemia (Fig. 9) (10), after fistulization of an adjacent tumor (e.g., hemangioma, cholesterol granuloma, or carcinoma of the endolymphatic sac) (Figs. 10 and 11) or secondary to trauma with or without an associated fracture. Viral labyrinthitis may also be hemorrhagic (Fig. 12) (11). Labyrinthine hemorrhage

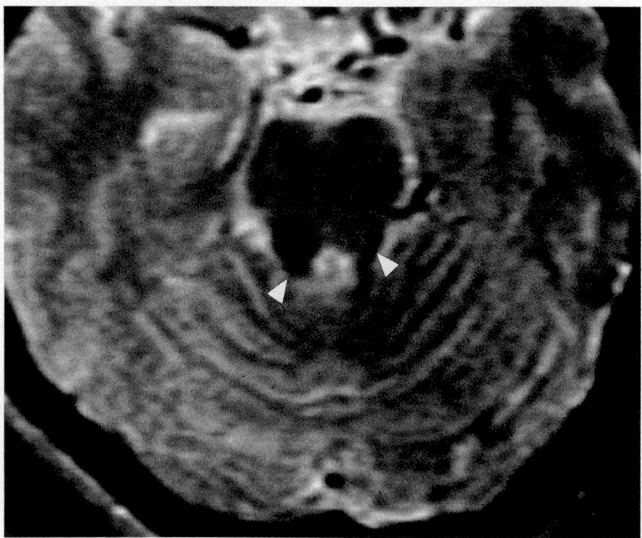

FIG. 8. Tectal contusion causing bilateral sensorineural hearing loss following trauma. Axial T2-weighted MRI demonstrates bilateral hemorrhagic contusions of the superior cerebellar peduncles (*arrowheads*).

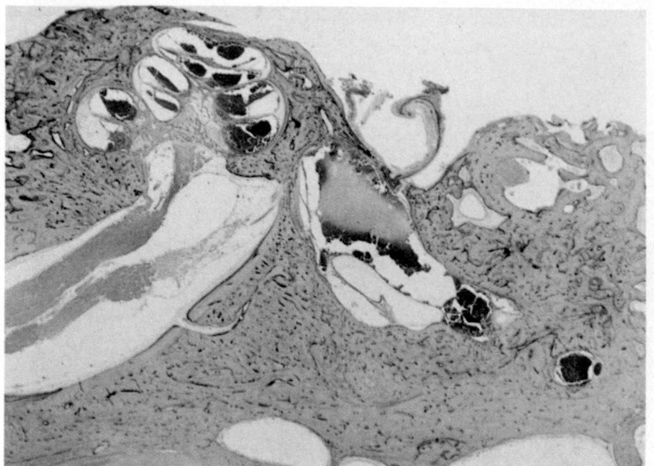

FIG. 9. Labyrinthine hemorrhage. Eleven-year-old girl with leukemia and sudden total right-sided sensorineural hearing loss. Fine horizontal nystagmus to the left on left lateral gaze. Temporal bone specimen demonstrates hemorrhage in the cochlea and vestibule. (From Schuknecht, ref. 1, with permission.)

cannot be demonstrated by CT. However, it can be suspected when a fracture of the temporal bone (12) is identified passing through the labyrinth (13). MR is uniquely suited to the demonstration of labyrinthine hemorrhage. Precontrast studies demonstrate high signal intensity in the labyrinth consistent with subacute hemorrhage (14). Theoretically, acute hemorrhage should be diagnosed on T2-weighted images as a very low signal intensity signal, but we have not encountered such cases in our experience. Realistically, most patients will be studied at the subacute stage.

Labyrinthitis

The term *labyrinthitis* describes any inflammatory process of the membranous labyrinth. It is most often due to viruses (Fig. 13) (15–17) such as rubella (18),

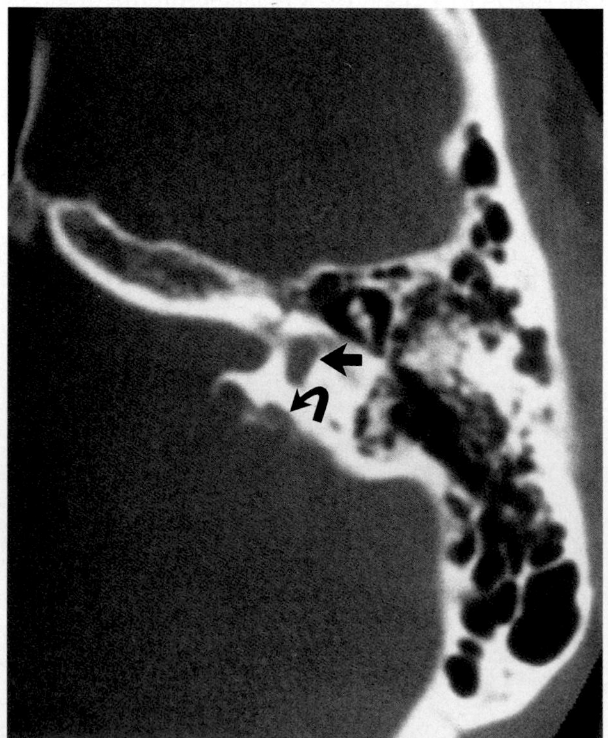

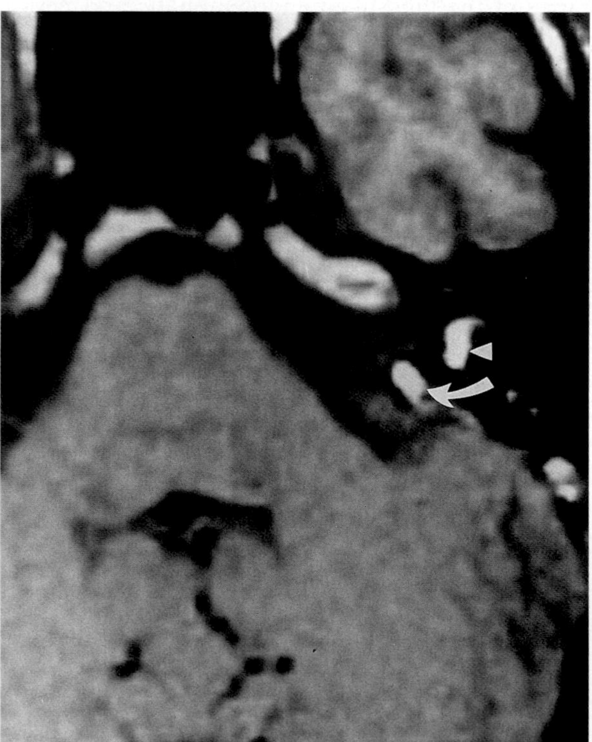

FIG. 10. Hemorrhagic low grade adenocarcinoma of the endolymphatic sac within the medial temporal bone fistulizes to the membranous labyrinth with subacute blood in vestibule. **A:** Axial CT image of the left temporal bone at the level of the vestibule (*arrow*) shows the adenomatous tumor (*curved arrow*) as an area of scalloping along the medial surface of the temporal bone. **B:** T1 axial MRI at the same level as A reveals the high signal tumor (*curved arrow*) with high signal within the vestibular membranous labyrinth (*arrowhead*), presumed to represent methemoglobin. (From Mark et al., ref. 30a, with permission.)

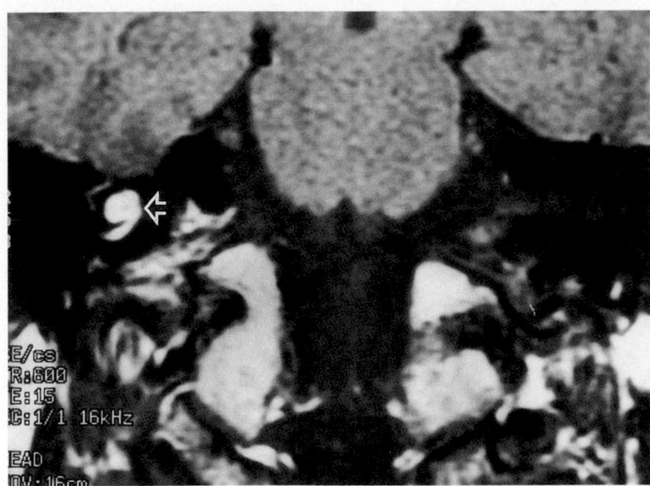

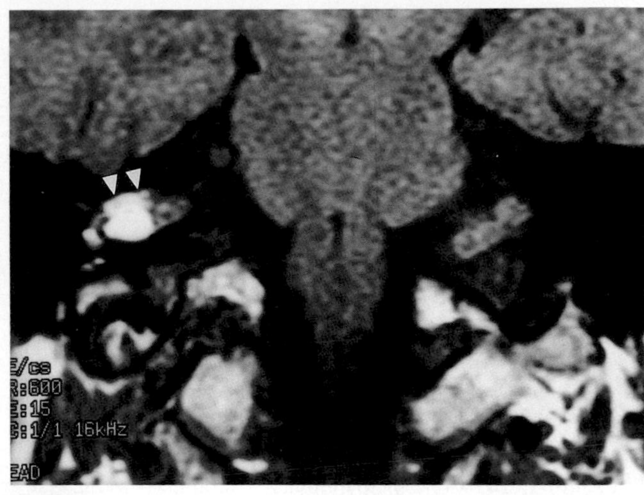

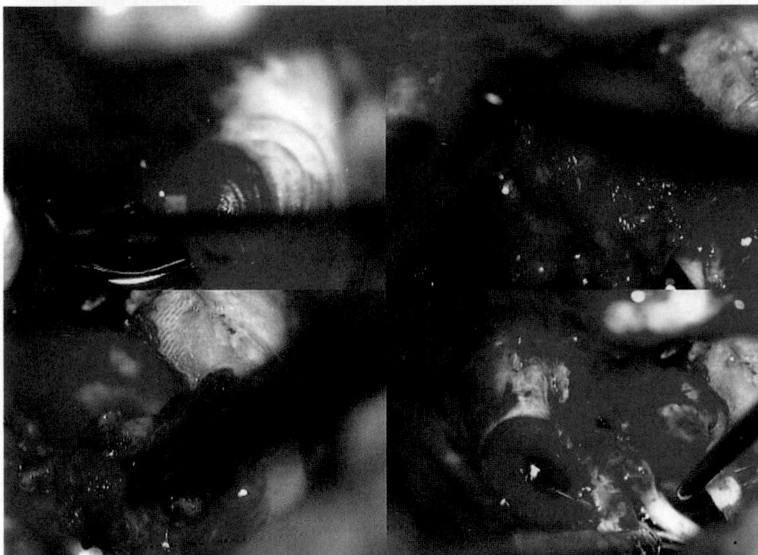

FIG. 11. Cochlear hemorrhage secondary to an surgically proven intracanalicular AVM. **A:** Coronal nonenhanced T1 MRI shows high signal (*open arrow*) presumed to represent methemoglobin in the cochlea. **B:** Coronal T1 MRI through the IAC shows high signal within it (*arrowheads*). **C:** Intraoperative photograph confirms the hemorrhage. (Courtesy of Dr. D. Fitzgerald, Washington, D.C.)

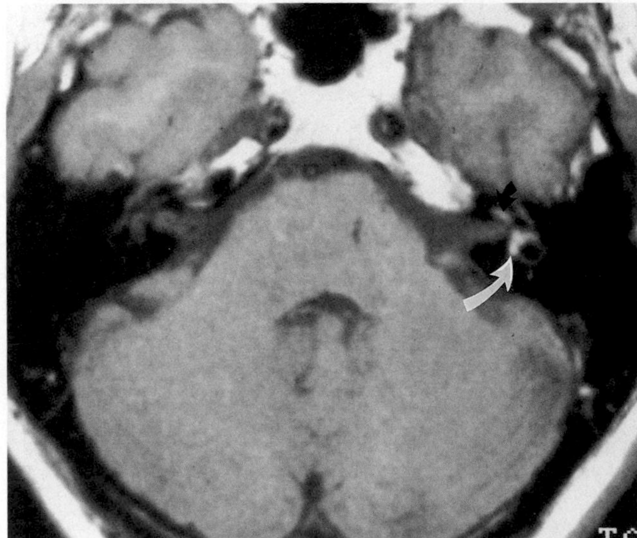

FIG. 12. Acute hemorrhagic viral labyrinthitis. Thirty-year-old woman with acute sensorineural hearing loss on the left and vertigo during the course of a viral illness. Axial unenhanced T1-weighted image reveal high signal intensity in the left cochlea (*black arrow*) and vestibule (*curved white arrow*) consistent with subacute hemorrhage. (Courtesy of Dr. D. Schellinger, Washington, D.C.)

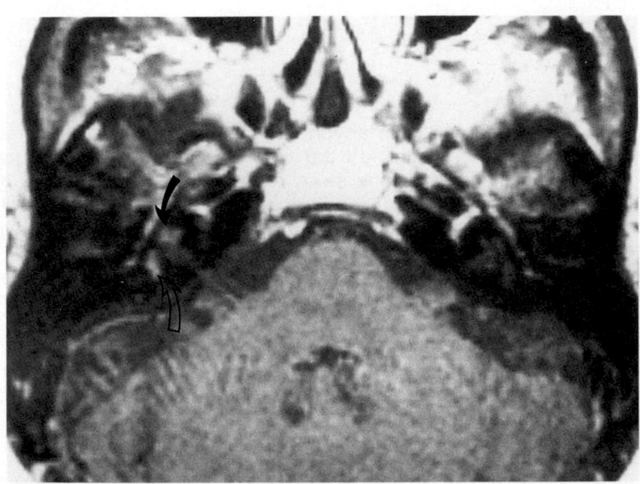

FIG. 13. A 73-year-old woman with right-sided hearing loss and vertigo following a viral illness. T1-weighted, gadolinium-enhanced image shows enhancement of the right cochlea (*solid arrow*) and vestibule (*open arrow*). No enhancement is seen on the opposite side.

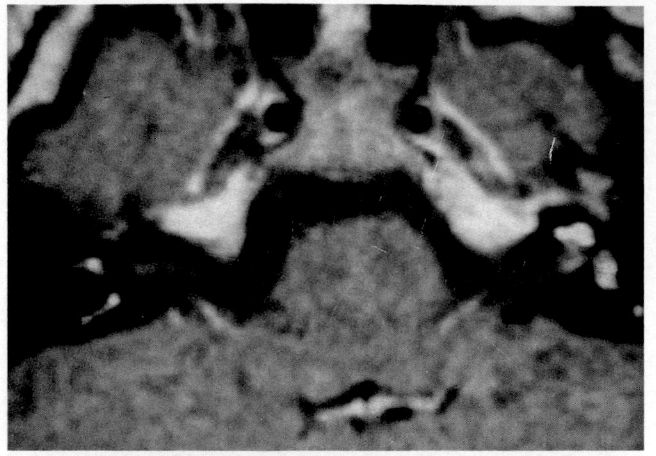
A

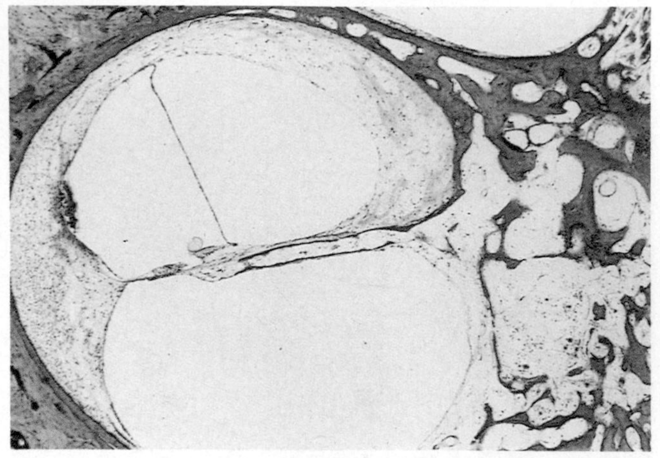
B

FIG. 14. Mumps labyrinthitis. Young child with bilateral sensorineural hearing loss and vertigo 3 weeks following mumps orchitis. **A:** Axial T1-weighted image postcontrast demonstrates intense enhancement of the cochlea and membranous labyrinth. **B:** Late sequelae of measles labyrinthitis from another patient who had severe sensorineural hearing loss since age 4 years following measles infection. The study shows severe atrophy of the organ of Corti and endolymphatic hydrops. (From Schuknecht, ref. 1, with permission.)

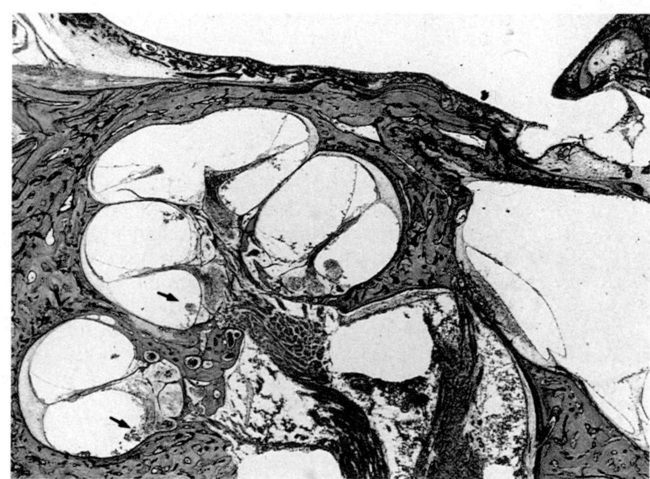
A

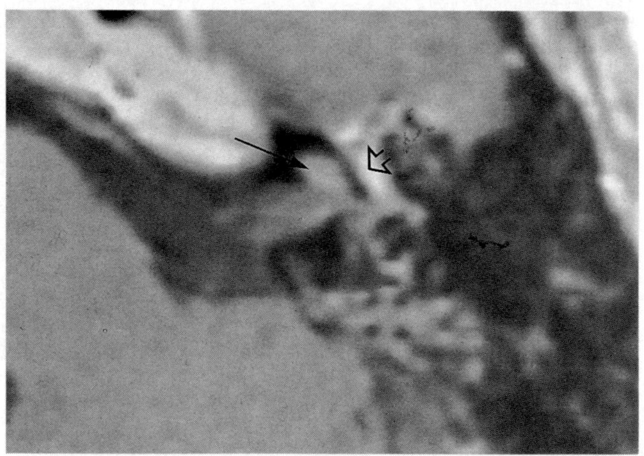
B

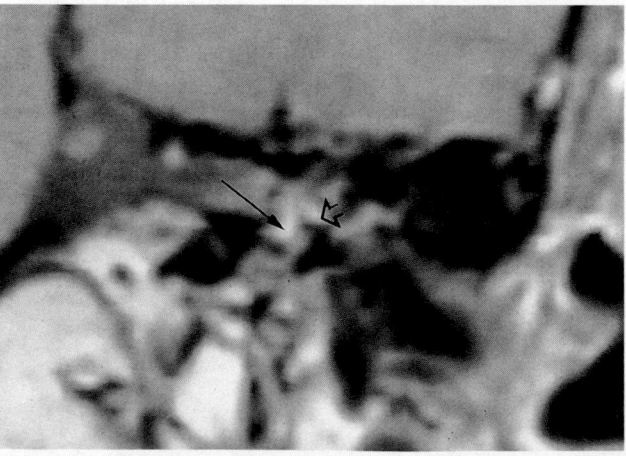
C

FIG. 15. Pneumococcic labyrinthitis. **A:** Fifty-three-year-old man with severe pain in the left ear who developed pneumococcal meningitis. Temporal bone study reveals large collections of inflammatory cells, in particular in the scala tympani (*arrows*) with partial necrosis of the membranous labyrinth and a precipitate in the perilymphatic and endolymphatic spaces. (Courtesy of Dr. H. Schuknecht, Boston, MA.) **B:** Bacterial labyrinthitis. Middle-aged man with left middle ear infection, acute hearing loss, and facial nerve paralysis. Gadolinium-enhanced axial T1-weighted image demonstrates enhancement of the left cochlea (*arrow*) and tympanic segment of the facial nerve (*open arrow*). Adjacent mastoiditis is seen as enhancement in the mastoid air cells. **C:** Coronal images confirm these findings.

mumps (Fig. 14) (19), herpes zoster (20), measles (21), or Lassa fever (22), but it may be secondary to pyogenic bacterial infections (Fig. 15) (23) or syphilis (Fig. 16) (24,25). The hallmark of labyrinthitis on MRI is demonstration of enhancement of the cochlea or vestibule on the postcontrast study (26,27). The final diagnosis of the etiology of labyrinthitis is established by clinical and laboratory findings.

Bacterial labyrinthitis can result either from extension to the labyrinth of a middle ear infection (otogenic suppurative labyrinthitis), in which case the infection usually penetrates the labyrinth through the oval window, or after meningitis, in which case it is usually bilateral (meningococcal bacterial labyrinthitis). Otogenic suppurative labyrinthitis is characterized pathologically in the acute phase by a polymorphonuclear infiltrate in the perilymphatic space followed by a fine fibrillar precipitate and endolymphatic hydrops. Necrosis of the membranous labyrinth and, if the patient survives. healing with new bone formation (labyrinthitis ossificans) develop in the later stages (28).

In the preantibiotic era, *syphilis* was a major cause of sensorineural hearing loss. The disease could be acquired perinatally, resulting in congenital hearing loss, or in adult life. The pathology includes a meningoneurolabyrinthitis in the early stages of congenital syphilis and in the acute meningitides of the secondary and tertiary stage, and temporal bone osteitis in the late congenital forms and in tertiary syphilis. The chronic lesions are identical regardless of the acquisition mode and are characterized by endolymphatic hydrops and degeneration of the sensory and neural structures (29).

Immune-mediated inner ear disease may be isolated or seen in the context of a systemic autoimmune disease. Primary autoimmune labyrinthitis is a relatively new cause of sensorineural hearing loss (24,30). The diagnosis is based on a positive lymphocyte transformation test to inner ear preparation and a positive response to steroid treatment.

Systemic autoimmune disorders that may affect the inner ear include Cogan's syndrome, polyarteritis nodosa, Wegner's granulomatosis, and relapsing polychondritis. Cogan's syndrome is an autoimmune disease characterized by interstitial keratitis and hearing loss in

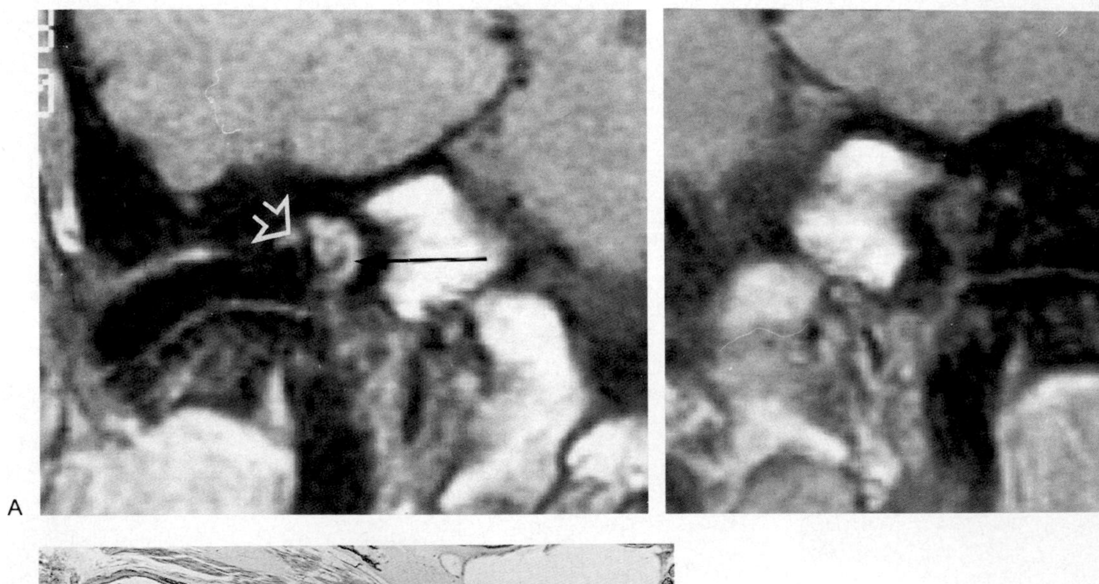

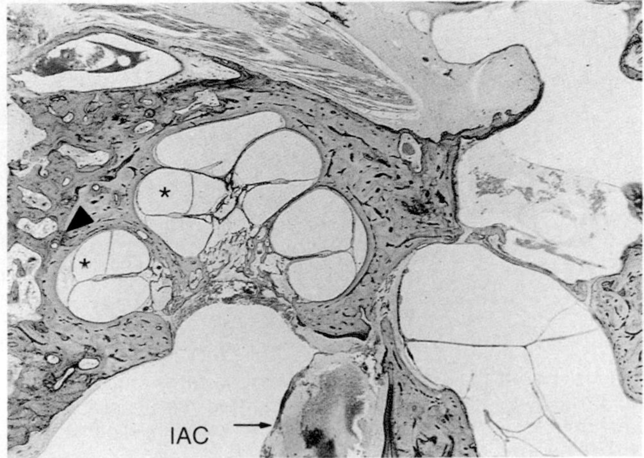

FIG. 16. Syphilitic labyrinthitis. A 30-year-old man with decreased hearing and facial palsy on the right. **A:** Coronal T1-weighted, Gd-DTPA–enhanced images. Enhancement of the right cochlea (*solid arrow*) and of the right facial nerve (*open arrow*). The left cochlea and facial nerve are normal. **B:** Congenital syphilis. Progressive bilateral hearing loss since age 18 years, progressing over 10 years. Extensive microgummata are noted in the pericochlear bone (*arrowhead*). A large gumma is noted in the internal auditory canal (*IAC*) in the place vacated by degenerated vestibular and cochlear nerves (*arrow*). There is marked endolymphatic hydrops (*asterisks*) and advanced atrophy of all structures in the IAC. (From Schuknecht, ref. 1, with permission.)

Venereal Disease Research Laboratory (VDRL)-negative patients. The disease responds to steroids. Enhancement of the cochlea and vestibule as well as obliteration of the membranous labyrinth have recently been reported in autoimmune labyrinthitis and in patients with Cogan's syndrome (Fig. 17) (31). Relapsing polychondritis is an autoimmune disease characterized by multiple episodes of cartilage inflammation, in particular the earlobe. The condition may be associated with hearing loss and vertigo. We have recently demonstrated labyrinthine enhancement in this entity (Fig. 18).

Contrast Enhancement of the Labyrinth

Study of the functional correlation between labyrinthine enhancement and objective and subjective cochlear and vestibular symptoms reveals that the enhancement is a highly specific finding of labyrinthine pathology (26). Indeed, *all* patients with enhancement of the cochlea and/or vestibule have cochlear and/or vestibular findings, both subjectively and objectively. Furthermore, these symptoms and signs are severe when the standard dose of contrast (0.1 mmol/Kg) was used. We have recently used triple-dose contrast in the setting of only moderate sensorineural hearing loss. This study demonstrated marked enhancement of the cochlea and vestibule. Our anecdotal observation suggests that the use of higher doses may increase the sensitivity for such abnormalities. Thus, similar to enhancement in the meninges, there is a threshold effect (Fig. 19), with only the most severe inflammatory processes producing labyrinthine enhancement. The resolution of the enhancement may parallel resolution of the patient's symptoms (Fig.

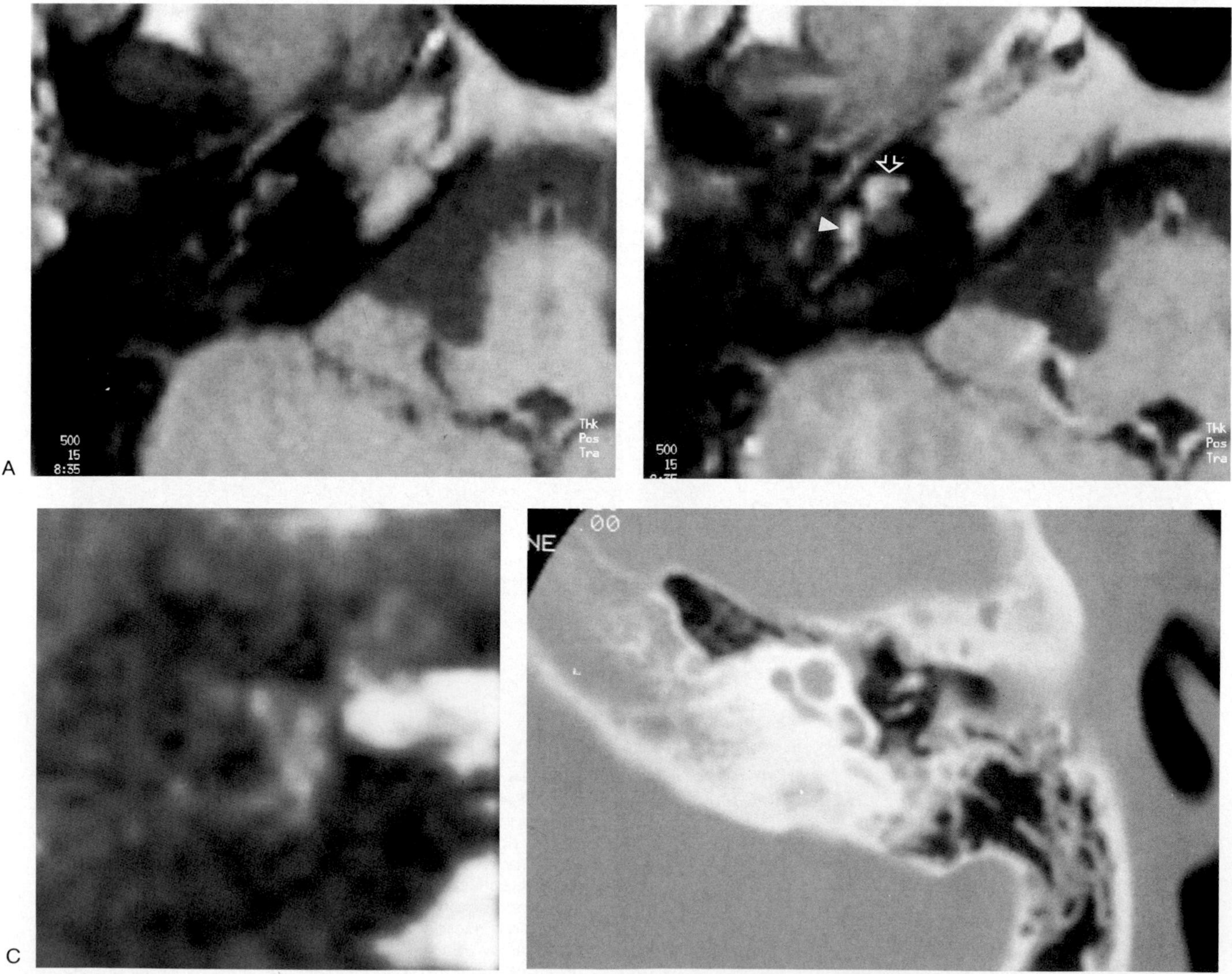

FIG. 17. Cogan's syndrome. **A:** Precontrast and, **B,** postcontrast axial T1-weighted image demonstrates enhancement of the right cochlea (*arrow*) and vestibule (*arrowhead*). **C:** 0. 7-mm high resolution T2-weighted image demonstrates obliteration of the normal fluid in the cochlea and vestibule. **D:** High resolution CT demonstrates ossification in the basal turn of the cochlea. (From Casselman, ref. 30a, with permission.)

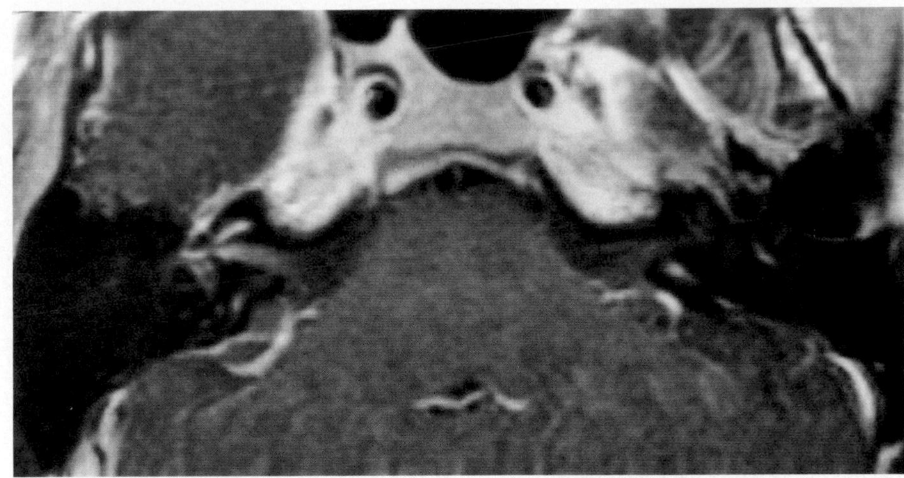

FIG. 18. Relapsing polychondritis. Thirty-year-old man with sudden sensorineural hearing loss and a history of recurrent pain and inflammation in the ear lobe. Axial postcontrast T1-weighted image demonstrates marked enhancement of the cochlea and vestibule and faint enhancement of the IAC.

20) (24,26) or, if the inflammatory process has resulted in permanent damage to the labyrinthine membrane, the enhancement may resolve but the patient's symptoms persist indefinitely. Enhancement may also recur if the inflammatory process is reactivated, even in patients who have been deaf for years (Fig. 21).

In a subset of patients with sensorineural hearing loss, we have demonstrated *segmental enhancement* of different turns of the cochlea (33) . In certain patients the level of enhancement correlates with the range of frequency of the hearing loss, that is, enhancement of the basal turn of the cochlea results in high frequency hearing loss (Figs. 22 and 23) (33) and enhancement of the apical turn results in low frequency hearing loss (Fig. 24). This correlation is not always present because certain patients with isolated enhancement of the basal turn will have complete hearing loss over all frequencies. The remarkable degree of correlation between high resolution–enhanced MRI and clinical examination in many cases should prompt further investigations using MRI in this highly specialized anatomic region.

Perilymphatic Fistula

Perilymphatic fistula is a controversial entity defined as an abnormal communication between perilymph of the inner ear and the middle ear typically involving injury to the membranes of the oval window, round window, or both (24,34,35). This condition is one of the many causes of sudden hearing loss and vertigo. It is a difficult condition to diagnose even at surgery because the leakage of perilymph may be intermittent and such small amounts of fluid are involved that its direct observation may be difficult. The condition is associated with either direct trauma to the ear or barotrauma. Experimental studies in guinea pigs have shown that barotrauma can induce ruptures of the round window and oval window membranes and intralabyrinthine hemorrhage, which predominates in the basal turn of the cochlea (36), where the round window opens. We have seen three patients with perilymphatic fistulae suspected clinically and/or surgically proven in whom labyrinthine enhancement was present (33). As suggested in the experi-

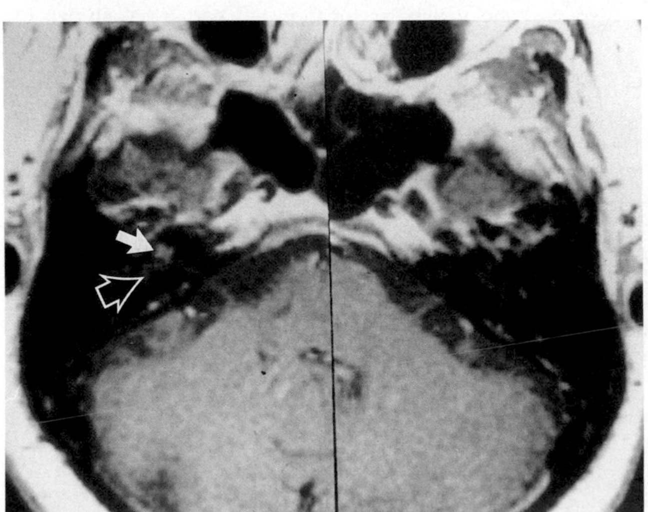

FIG. 19. Selective enhancement of the cochlea. Viral labyrinthitis, 70-year-old woman with severe right-sided hearing loss and vertigo but only minimally abnormal ENG. T1-weighted, Gd-DTPA-enhanced image. Enhancement of the cochlea (*solid arrow*) but not the vestibule (*open arrow*) on the right side. No enhancement of the asymptomatic side. The enhancement and her symptoms resolved 6 months later. (From Seltzer and Mark, ref. 27, with permission.)

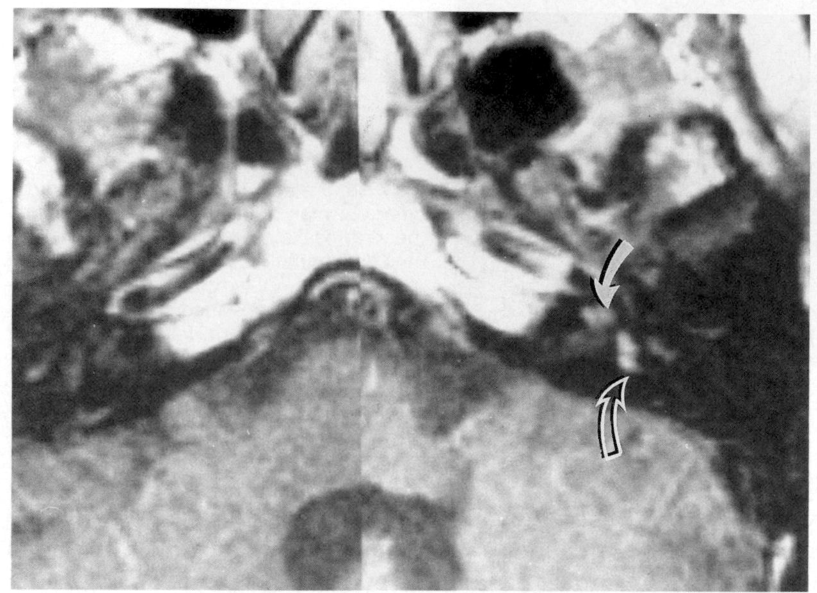

A

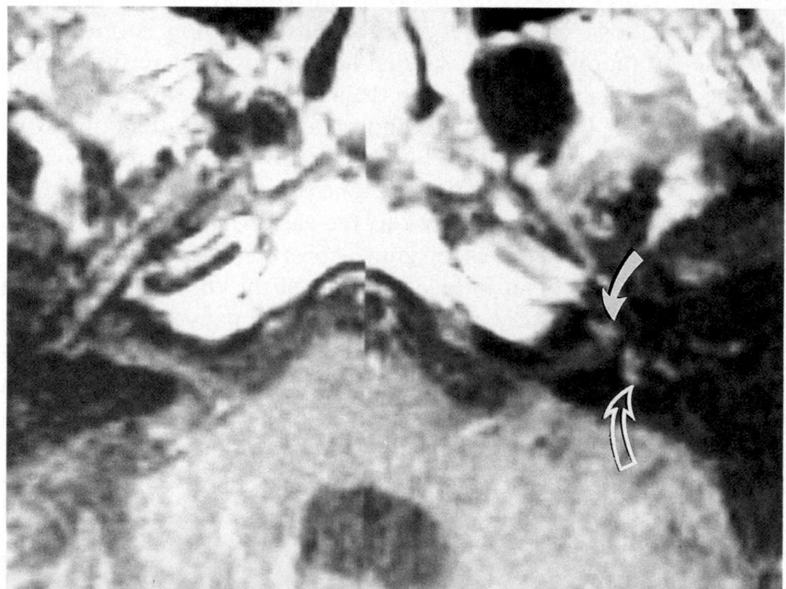

B

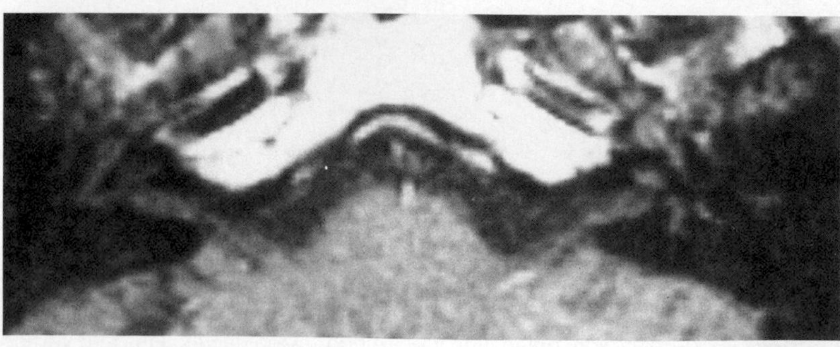

C

FIG. 20. Viral labyrinthitis. **A:** Abnormal cochlear and vestibular function left ear; initial study. T1-weighted, Gd-DTPA-enhanced image. Enhancement of the left cochlea (*solid arrow*) and vestibule (*open arrow*). No enhancement is seen on the contralateral side. **B:** One month after initial study, at which time the patient had some improvement in hearing and slight improvement on ENG testing. T1-weighted, Gd-DTPA-enhanced image. There is persistent labyrinthine enhancement. **C:** Five months after initial study, at which time the patient had marked improvement in hearing and resolution of vestibular symptoms. Axial T1-weighted, Gd-DTPA-enhanced image. The previously noted enhancement of the left cochlea and vestibule is no longer present. (From Seltzer and Mark, ref. 27, with permission.)

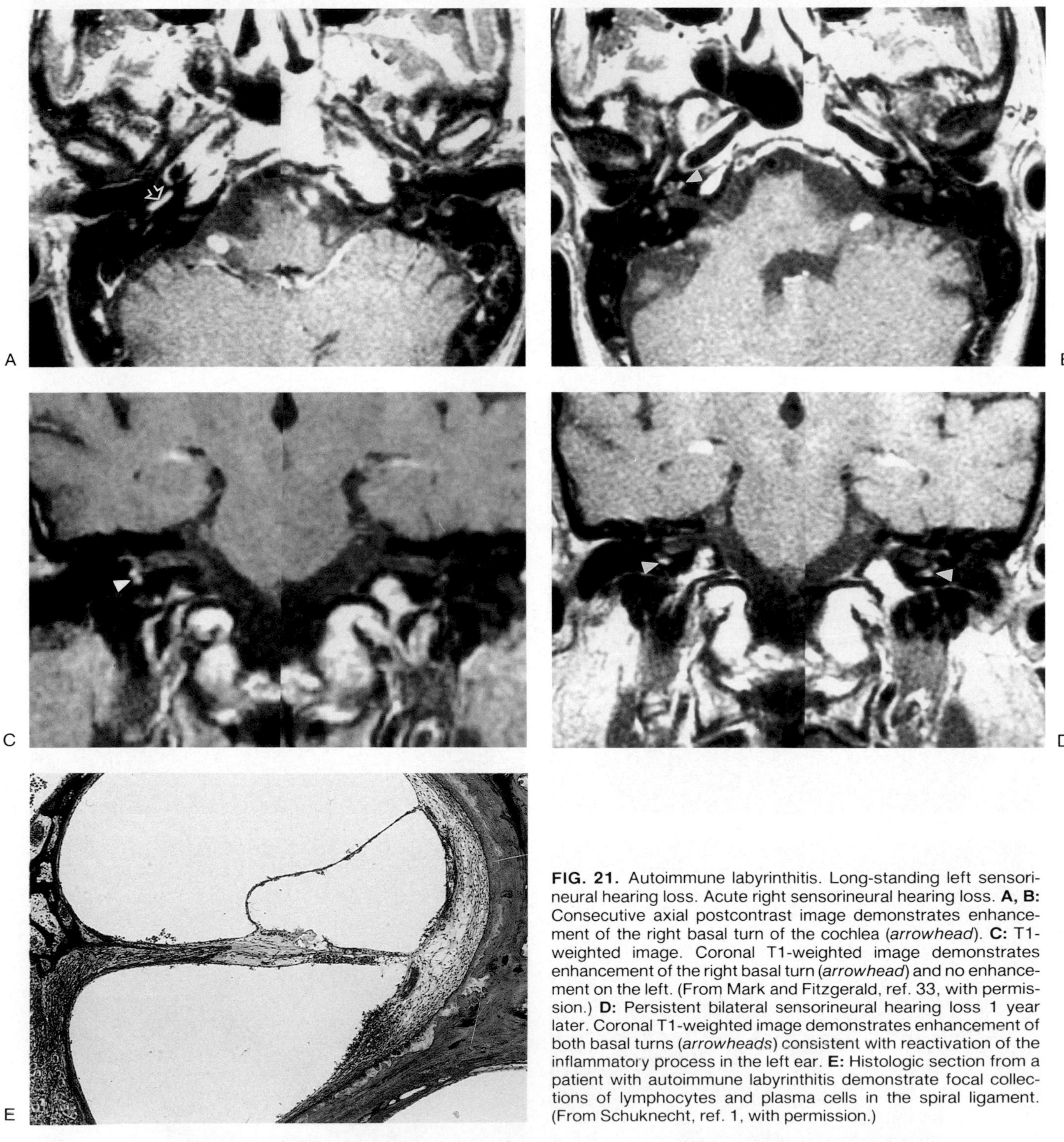

FIG. 21. Autoimmune labyrinthitis. Long-standing left sensorineural hearing loss. Acute right sensorineural hearing loss. **A, B:** Consecutive axial postcontrast image demonstrates enhancement of the right basal turn of the cochlea (*arrowhead*). **C:** T1-weighted image. Coronal T1-weighted image demonstrates enhancement of the right basal turn (*arrowhead*) and no enhancement on the left. (From Mark and Fitzgerald, ref. 33, with permission.) **D:** Persistent bilateral sensorineural hearing loss 1 year later. Coronal T1-weighted image demonstrates enhancement of both basal turns (*arrowheads*) consistent with reactivation of the inflammatory process in the left ear. **E:** Histologic section from a patient with autoimmune labyrinthitis demonstrate focal collections of lymphocytes and plasma cells in the spiral ligament. (From Schuknecht, ref. 1, with permission.)

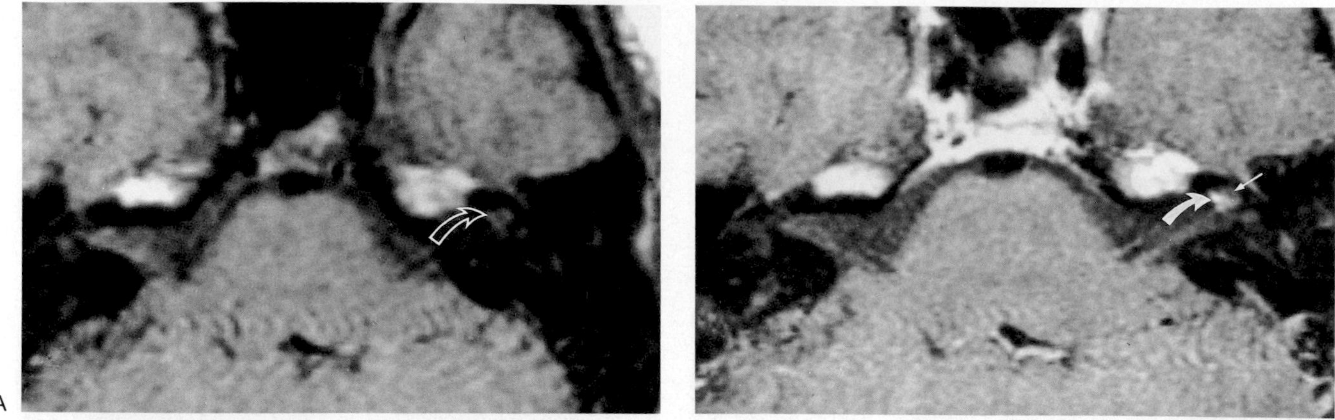

FIG. 22. Selective enhancement of the basal turn of the cochlea. Forty-year-old woman with high frequency sensorineural hearing loss. **A:** Precontrast axial T1-weighted image demonstrates no cochlear anomaly (*curved arrow*). **B:** Postcontrast T1-weighted image demonstrates selective enhancement of the basal turn of the cochlea (*curved arrow*). Notice the lack of enhancement in the apical turn (*straight arrow*). (From Mark et al., ref. 26, with permission.)

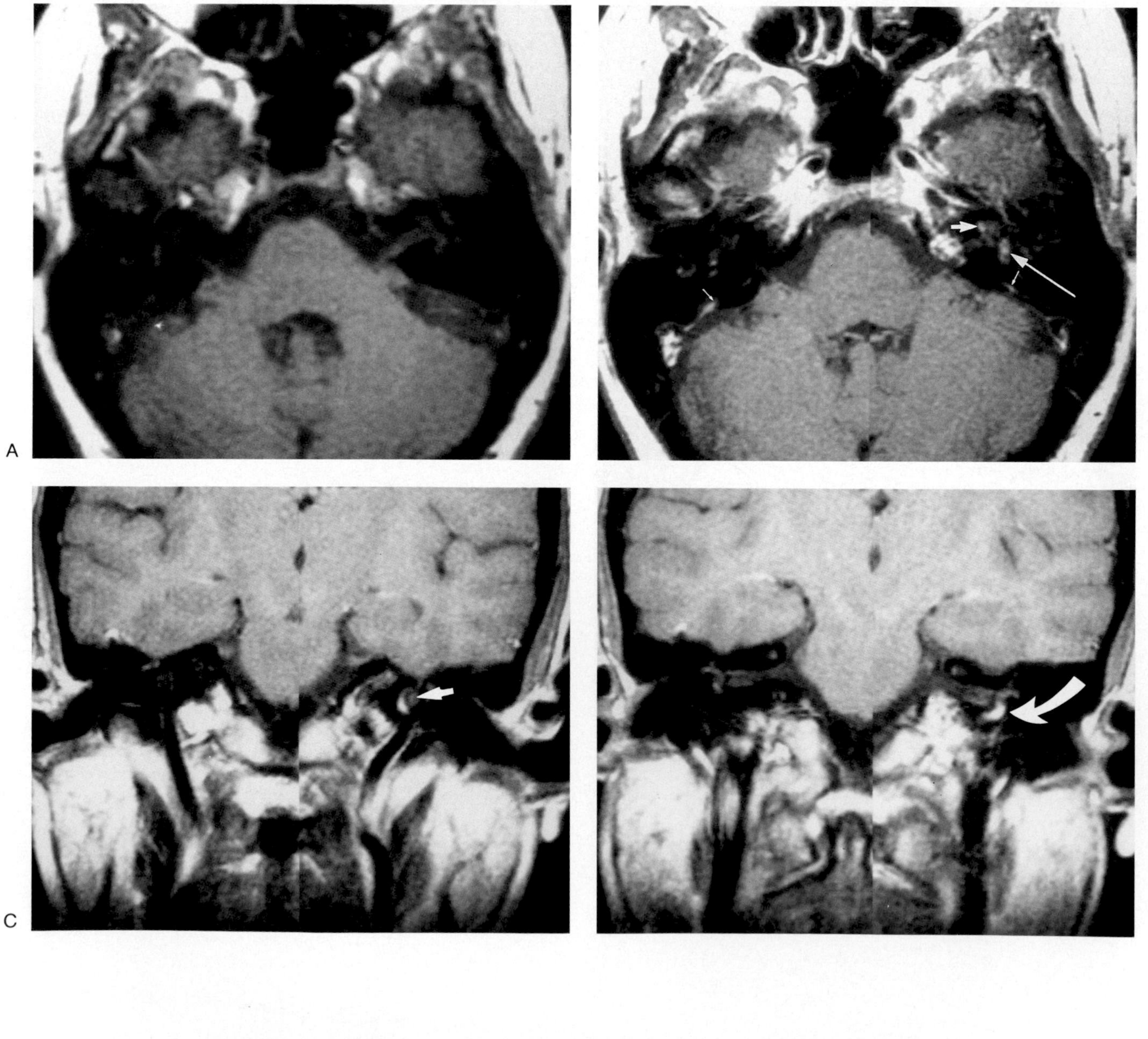

A

B

C

D

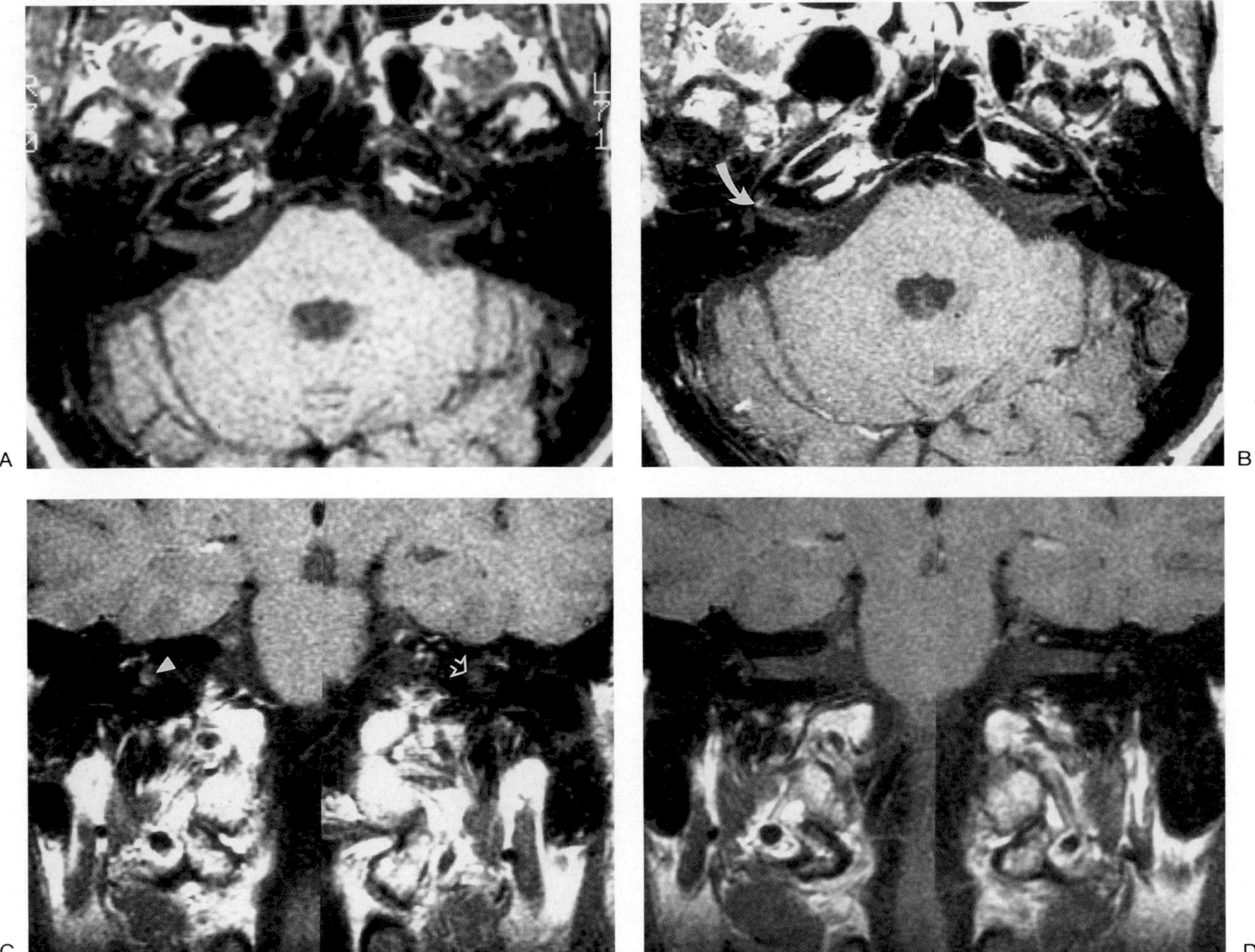

FIG. 24. Forty-year old man with low frequency sensorineural hearing loss. **A:** Axial precontrast T1-weighted image is normal. **B:** Postcontrast axial T1-weighted image demonstrates a small focus of enhancement in the apical turn of the cochlea (*arrow*). **C:** Coronal T1-weighted image postcontrast through the anterior aspect of the cochlea demonstrates enhancement of the right apical turn of the cochlea (*arrowhead*) and normal apical turn of the left cochlea (*open arrow*). **D:** Coronal T1-weighted image postcontrast through the basal aspect of the cochlea is normal. (From Mark and Fitzgerald, ref. 33, with permission.)

FIG. 23. Selective enhancement of the basal turn of the cochlea. A 35-year-old woman with left-sided high frequency hearing loss. Pre- (**A**) and postgadolinium (**B**) axial T1-weighted images demonstrate enhancement of the basal turn (*medium arrow*) of the cochlea and vestibule (*long arrow*). Notice also the enhancement of the endolymphatic sac bilaterally (*small arrows*). **C, D:** Postgadolinium consecutive coronal T1-weighted images. Notice enhancement of the basal turn (*curved arrow*) but not of the apical turn (*straight arrow*) of the left cochlea, correlating with the patient's high frequency hearing loss. (From Mark and Fitzgerald, ref. 33, with permission.)

mental studies, the enhancement predominated in the basal turn of the cochlea but was also seen in the vestibule in some patients (Figs. 25 and 26). Some of these patients had improved following surgical patching of the oval window.

Labyrinthine Neoplasms

Labyrinthine Schwannomas. Labyrinthine schwannomas are the most common benign neoplasms of the labyrinth (37,38). They are histologically identical to their counterparts in the IAC. In our experience and reviewing the literature, they are more common in the vestibule, which is not surprising because the schwannomas in the IAC originate most commonly from the vestibular nerve. Labyrinthine schwannomas can present with sensorineural hearing loss and/or vertigo and clinically be indistinguishable from Meniere's disease. In fact, in the past these lesions were mostly diagnosed during destructive labyrinthectomy for intractable "Meniere's disease" (37). In the past, the diagnosis on CT could be made only in the later stages when there was bony expansion of the cochlea or vestibule. Now these lesions can be easily diagnosed using contrast-enhanced MRI, which demon-

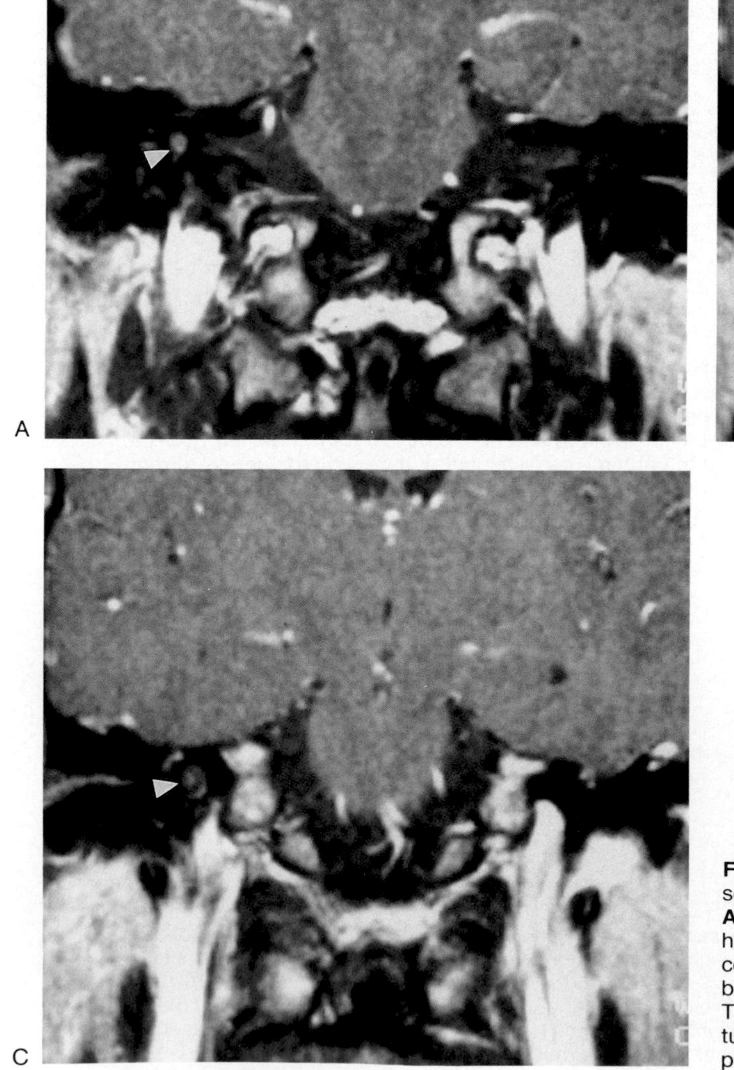
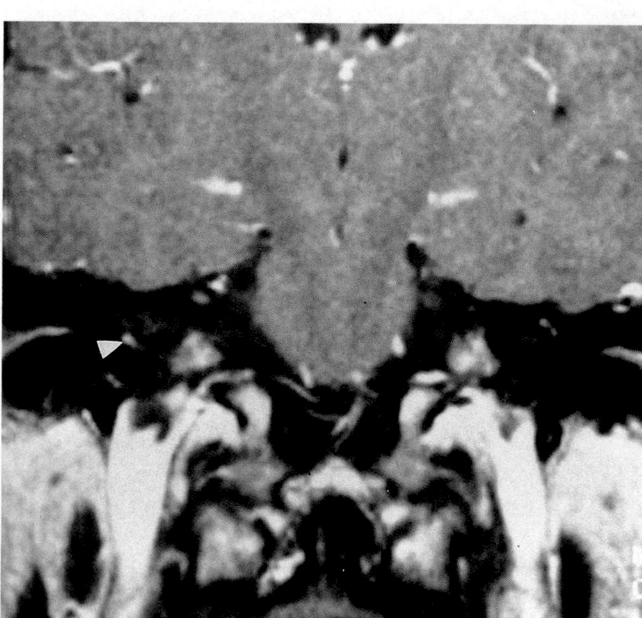

FIG. 25. Perilymphatic fistula. Thirty-year-old man with sudden sensorineural hearing loss after lifting heavy weights at the gym. **A:** Coronal postcontrast T1-weighted image demonstrates enhancement of the right vestibule (*arrowhead*). **B:** Coronal postcontrast T1-weighted image demonstrates enhancement of the basal turn of the cochlea (*arrowhead*). **C:** Coronal postcontrast T1-weighted image demonstrates enhancement of the apical turn of the cochlea (*arrowhead*). The patient's symptoms improved following surgical patching of the oval window.

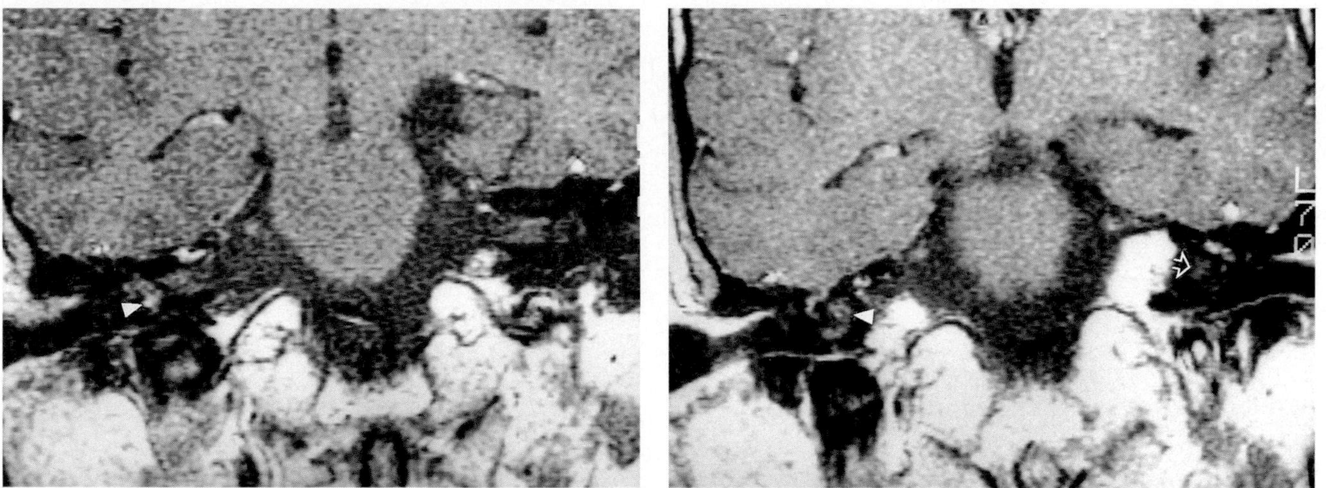

FIG. 26. Labyrinthine concussion. Young man with sensorineural hearing loss following a motorcycle accident 1 month before the MRI. High resolution temporal bone CT was normal. **A:** Coronal-enhanced T1 MRI demonstrates enhancement of the vestibule (*arrowhead*) **B:** Coronal-enhanced T1 MRI demonstrates enhancement of the cochlea (*arrowhead*). The left cochlea (*open arrow*) is normal. A fistula was suspected but the patient did not improve after patching of the oval window.

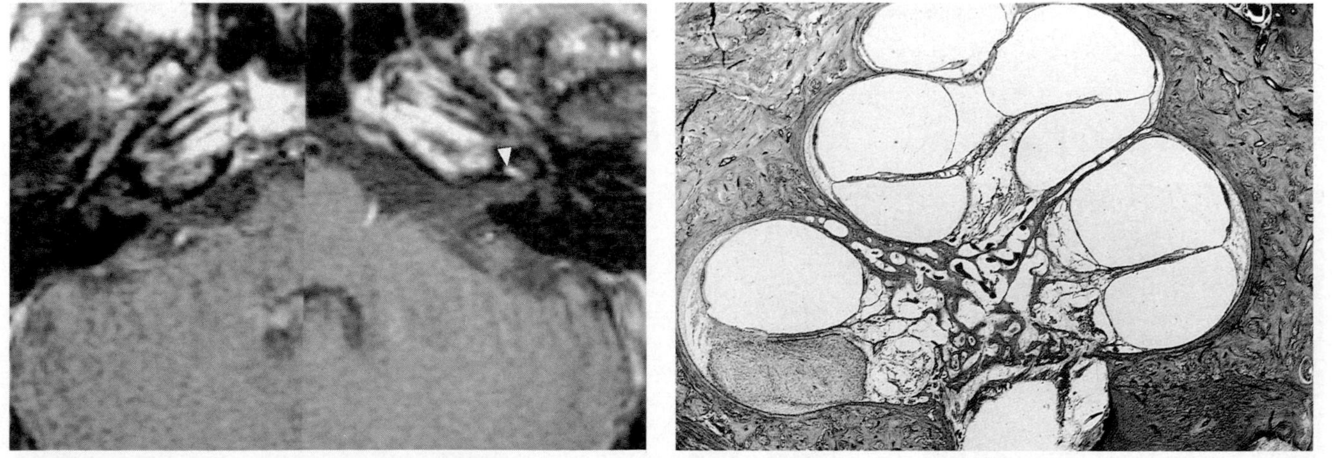

FIG. 27. Presumed left cochlear schwannoma. Fifty-year-old man with slowly progressive high frequency sensorineural hearing loss. **A:** Axial T1-weighted image demonstrates a 1-mm enhancing mass in the middle turn of the cochlea (*arrowhead*). The lesion remained unchanged over 3 years while the patient's symptoms slowly progressed. **B:** Pathologic specimen from another patient demonstrates a 1-mm intracochlear schwannoma. (Courtesy of Dr. H. Schuknecht, Boston, MA.)

strates a markedly enhancing mass in the cochlea (Fig. 27) or vestibule (Fig. 28) (2,39).

The major differential diagnosis of labyrinthine schwannoma is labyrinthitis. Schwannomas usually enhance much more intensely, the enhancement persists over many months, and the lesions may expand, contrary to labyrinthitis, where the enhancement resolves over several months with or without resolution of the patient's symptoms. In patients with labyrinthine schwannomas, a soft tissue mass is always present in the labyrinth on very thin (<1 mm) T2-weighted images (3), whereas normal labyrinthine fluid isointense to cerebrospinal fluid (CSF) is seen on these sequences in patients with labyrinthitis (J.W. Casselman, *personal communication*, 1994). Patients with vestibular schwannomas have stable or progressively worsening symptoms. Vestibular schwannomas may be associated with intracanalicular and cerebellopontine angle schwannomas (Fig. 29) in patients with neurofibromatosis (11). Recently, a synchronous intracochlear and intracanalicular schwannoma was reported (D. Brown, *personal communication*, 1994) (Fig. 30).

Malignant Neoplasms

Malignant neoplasms of the cochlea are exceptional. Squamous cell carcinoma in the adult or rhabdomyosarcoma (Fig. 31) of the temporal bone in the child may extend into the labyrinth. Metastasis may extend peri-

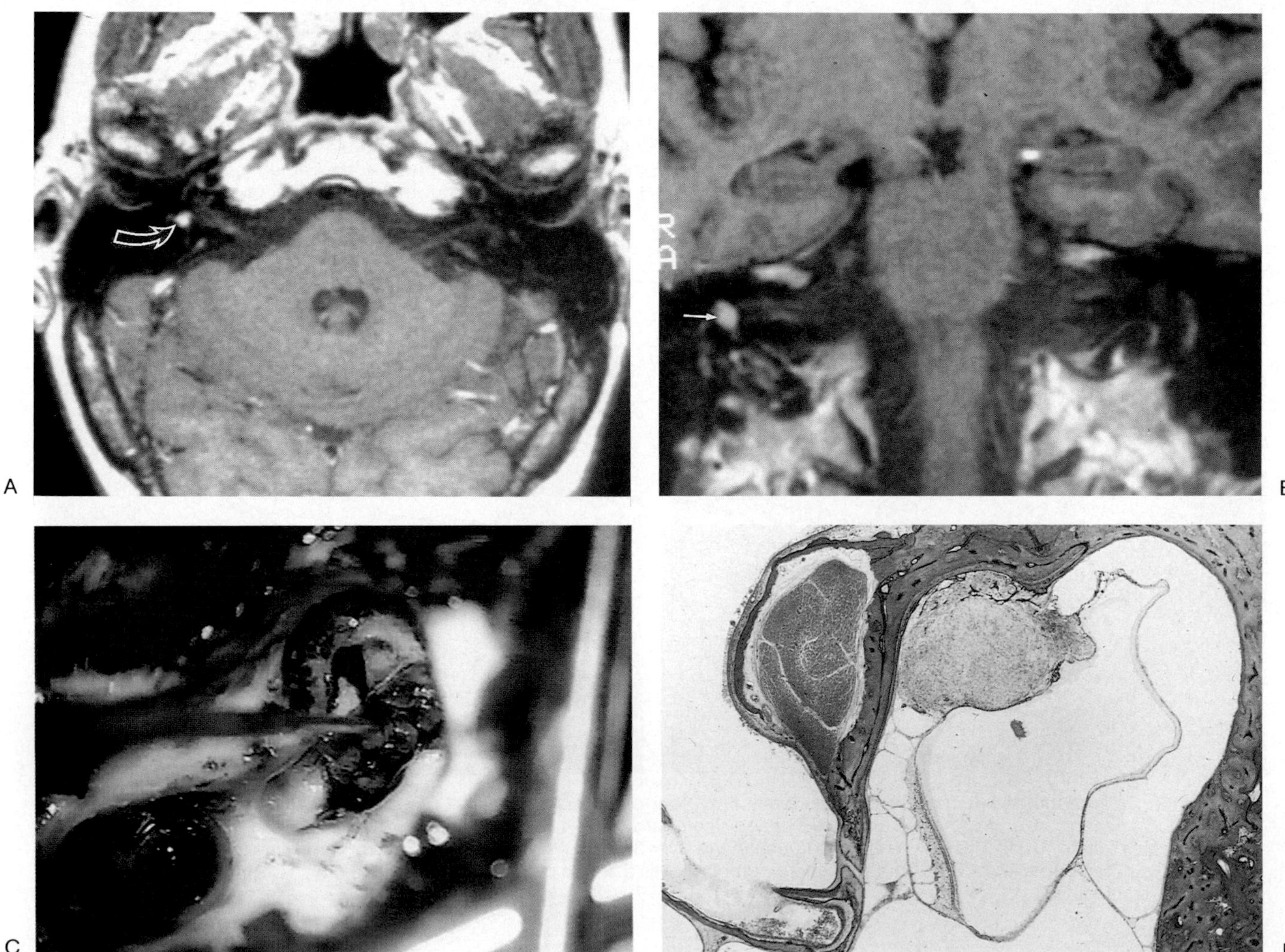

FIG. 28. Right vestibular schwannoma in a patient with a 1-year history of vertigo and hearing loss. **A:** Axial and, **B**, coronal T1-weighted images show globular enhancement of the right vestibule (*arrow*). The long-standing history and the focal enhancement suggest schwannoma rather than labyrinthitis. **C:** Intraoperative photograph from another patient with an intravestibular schwannoma. (Courtesy of Dr. D. Fitzgerald, Washington, D.C.) **D:** Histologic section through the vestibule reveals a small intravestibular schwannoma that had been asymptomatic. (From Schuknecht, ref. 1, with permission.)

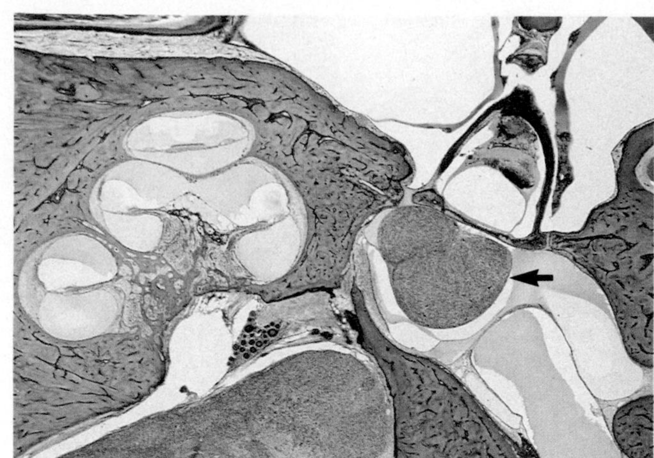

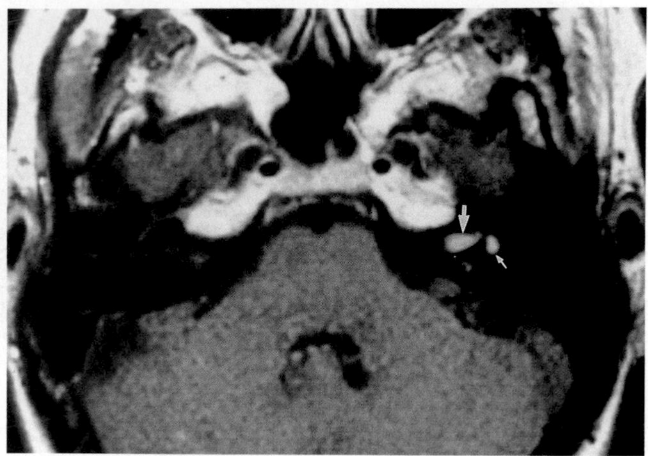

FIG. 29. Twenty-three-year-old man with neurofibromatosis type II. **A:** Temporal bone specimen. Simultaneous schwannoma in the right IAC and a 2 × 2.5-mm vestibular schwannoma (*arrow*) is present between the footplate of the stapes and the lateral wall of the saccule. (From Schuknecht, ref. 1, with permission.) **B:** Presumed left vestibular schwannoma (*small arrow*) and intracanalicular schwannoma (*large arrow*) in another patient with left-sided sensorineural hearing loss and vertigo and no history of neurofibromatosis Type II. (Courtesy of Dr. D. Brown, Washington, D.C.)

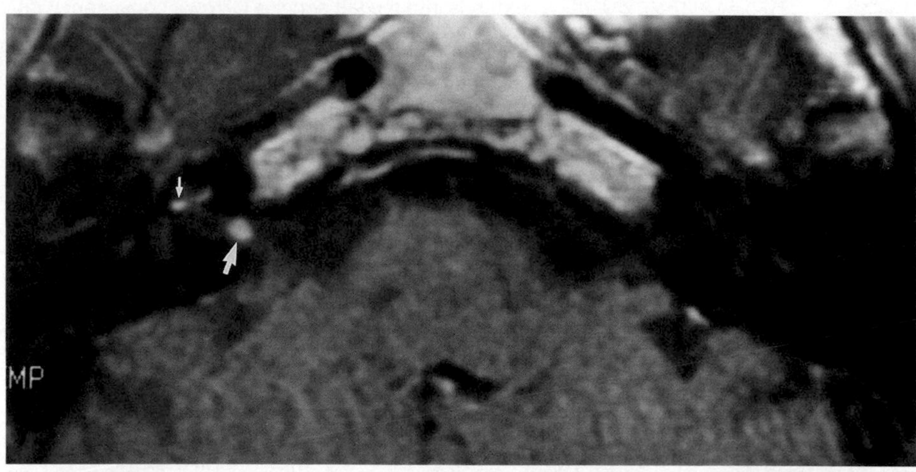

FIG. 30. Presumed right intracochlear schwannoma and intracanalicular schwannoma of the cochlear nerve. Axial T1-weighted MRI reveals enhancing masses in the basal turn of the cochlea (*small arrow*) and in the anterior aspect of the IAC (*large arrow*). (Courtesy of Dr. D. Brown, Washington, D.C.)

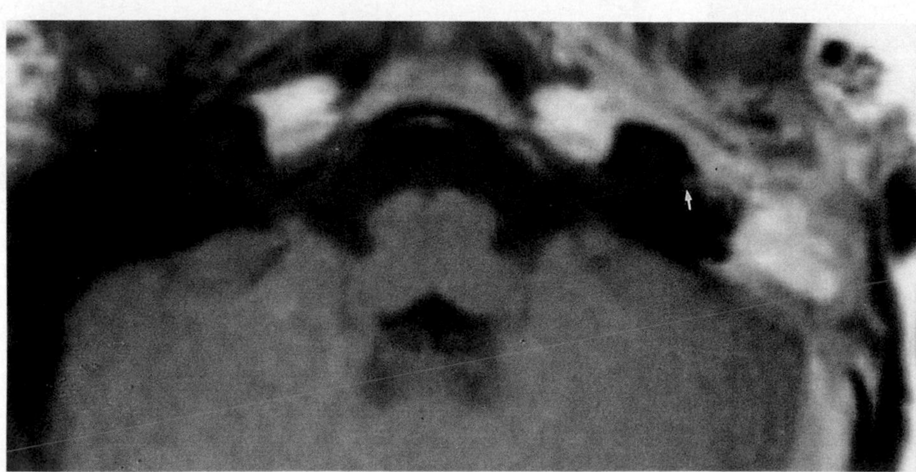

FIG. 31. Rhabdomyosarcoma invading the vestibule in a 6-year-old girl. Axial T1 MRI demonstrates an enhancing mass in the left mastoid and middle ear invading the left vestibule (*arrow*) and horizontal semicircular canal.

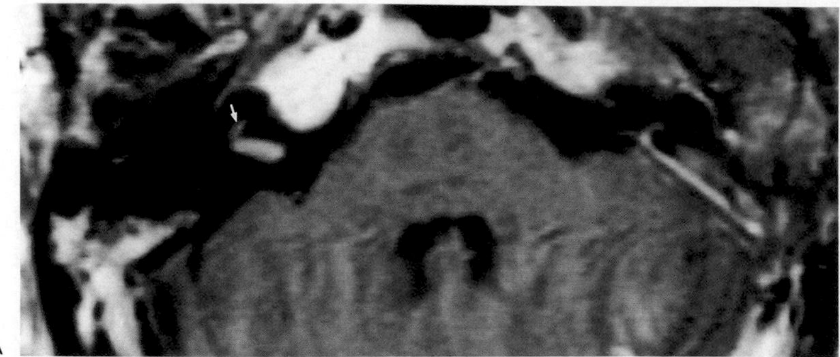
A

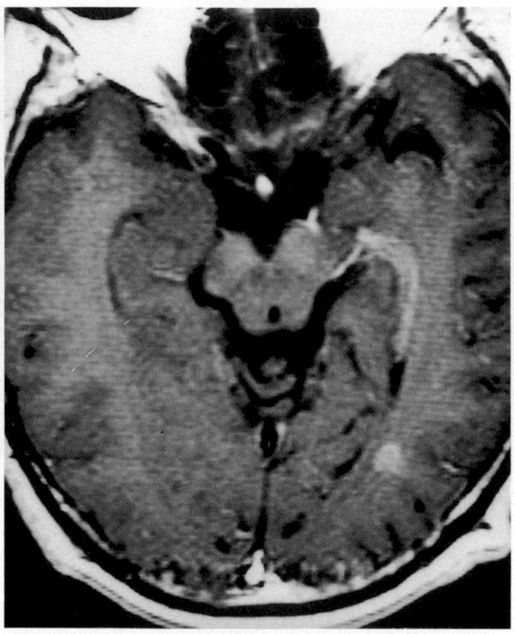
B

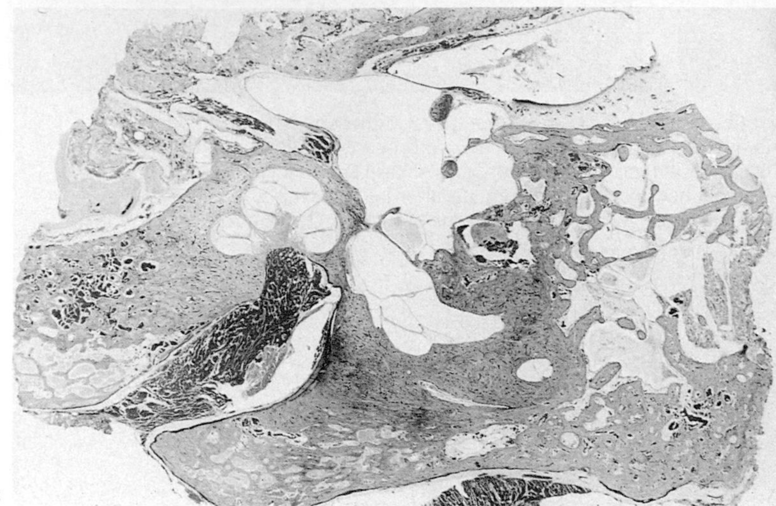
C

FIG. 32. Metastatic lung carcinoma to the left IAC and left cochlea. **A:** Axial T1-weighted image demonstrates an enhancing mass fills the left IAC and extends into the left cochlea (*arrow*), consistent with leptomeningeal tumor spread extending into the patient's cochlea. **B:** Higher level image shows the associated parenchymal metastasis. (Courtesy of Dr. C. Truwit, Minneapolis, MN). **C:** Metastatic adenocarcinoma of the breast in a 75-year-old patient who presented with acute hearing loss and facial palsy. (From Schuknecht, ref. 1, with permission.)

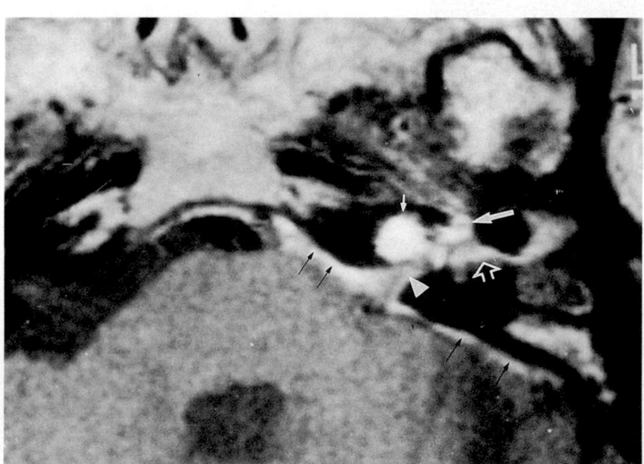

FIG. 33. Cholesteatoma invasion of bony labyrinth in a 60-year-old retarded man with long-standing hearing loss. Axial enhanced T1 MRI reveals enhancement within the destroyed cochlea (*large white arrow*) and vestibule (*open white arrow*), the IAC (*arrowhead*), the adjacent meninges (*small black arrows*), and anterior temporal bone (*small white arrow*). (From Mark et al., ref. 32, with permission.)

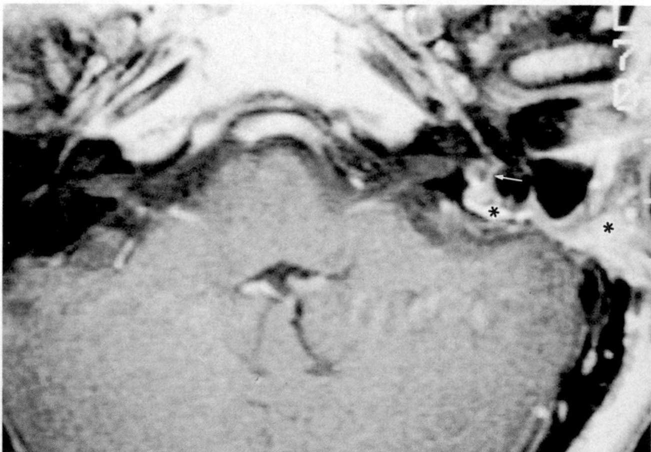

FIG. 34. Postoperative labyrinthine enhancement following destructive labyrinthectomy for intractable vertigo in Meniere's disease. Postoperative axial enhanced T1 MRI demonstrates enhancement of the right vestibule (*arrow*) and enhancing soft tissue in the left mastoid (*asterisks*). Without proper clinical history, this finding was thought to represent a cholesteatoma invading the vestibule.

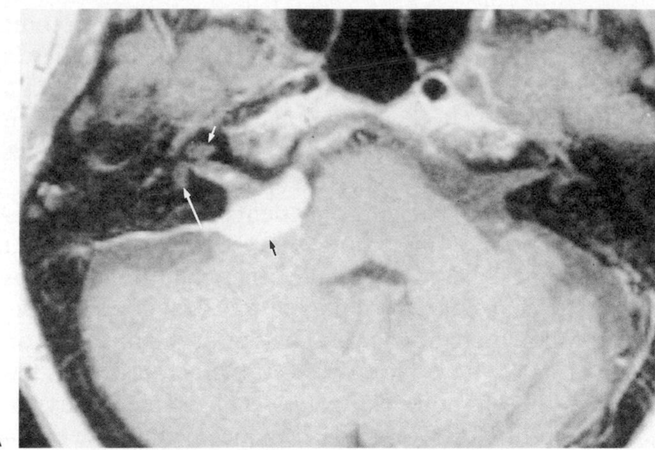

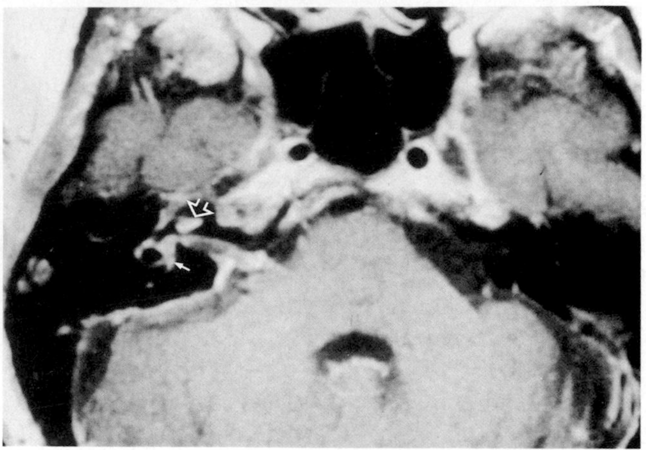

FIG. 35. Postoperative labyrinthine enhancement following CPA surgery. **A:** Axial enhanced T1 MRI before surgery demonstrates a right CPA meningioma (*small black arrow*) and normal cochlea (*small white arrow*) and labyrinth (*long white arrow*). **B:** Postoperative axial enhanced T1 MRI demonstrates enhancement of the cochlea (*open arrow*) and labyrinth (*small arrow*).

neurally along the cochlear nerve and penetrate the cochlea (Fig. 32) (11). Middle ear cholesteatomas in the later stages may also invade the inner ear, but the patient's history and the CT findings are usually obvious (Fig. 33).

Postoperative Changes

Enhancement of the vestibule may be seen in patients who have undergone destructive vestibulectomies for incurable Meniere's disease (Fig. 34). In this case, an enhancing "mass" may be seen in the vestibule communicating with the mastoid. Clinical correlation is necessary not to confuse this finding with extension of middle ear infection into the vestibule. Postoperative enhancement of the labyrinth may also be seen in patients who have undergone surgery in the IAC or cerebellopontine angle cistern for acoustic schwannomas or meningiomas (Fig. 35). The enhancement is usually not clinically relevant because these patients have lost their hearing from their original tumor and/or the surgery. However, this finding may be significant in a patient with a small intracanalicular tumor in whom a hearing-sparing procedure was attempted, that is, "chemical labyrinthitis" from perioperative extension of hemorrhage from the IAC into the cochlea or vestibule. This finding, rather than direct injury to the cochlear nerve at the time of surgery, may explain some of the surgical failures in these cases.

Endolymphatic Hydrops

Endolymphatic hydrops is defined pathologically as dilatation of the endolymphatic spaces. Extensive experimental evidence suggests that endolymphatic hydrops is the result of a functional failure of the endolymphatic sac to resorb the endolymph (40–45), resulting in dilatation of the endolymphatic spaces with or without rupture of Reissner's membrane and communication of the endolymph and the perilymph (42).

Schuknecht and Gulya (42) classified endolymphatic hydrops in congenital, acquired, and idiopathic forms. Any congenital malformation can result ultimately in endolymphatic hydrops. Among the best known is the *large vestibular aqueduct syndrome* (Fig. 36), in which a markedly dilated endolymphatic sac and vestibular aqueduct are associated with other inner ear malformations and congenital sensorineural hearing loss and vertigo. Any of the inflammatory or traumatic lesions mentioned earlier may have, as the end result, labyrinthine hydrops.

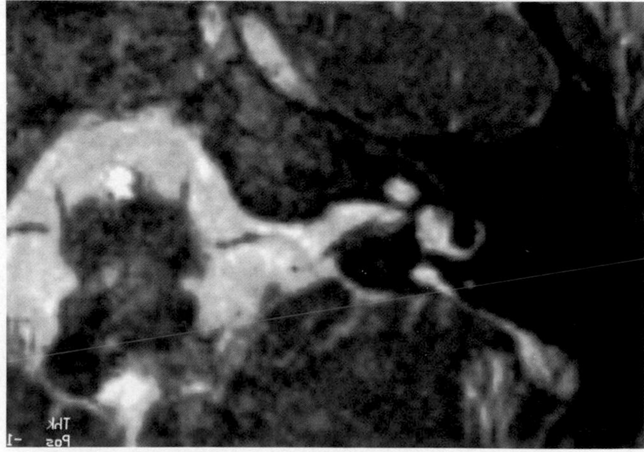

FIG. 36. Probable congenital hydrops. Large vestibular aqueduct syndrome. 0.7-mm high resolution T2-weighted image (3) demonstrates a large left vestibular aqueduct. (Courtesy of Dr. J. W. Casselman, Bruges, Belgium.)

Among the idiopathic forms of labyrinthine hydrops, *Meniere's disease* is the best known. This condition is clinically characterized by fluctuating sensorineural hearing loss with or without vertigo and tinnitus. It is most often unilateral and, when bilateral, it is usually asynchronous. There is ample laboratory evidence that Meniere's disease is caused by a functional failure of the endolymphatic sac to resorb the endolymph. Electromicroscopy study of biopsies of the endolymphatic sac (40) in patients with Meniere's have revealed a wide spectrum of findings from a near normal sac to an inflammatory reaction to fibrosis and complete atrophy and obliteration of the endolymphatic sac. This spectrum of histologic findings explains the great heterogeneity of the clinical findings in these patients from mild forms with occasional episodes of vertigo to severe vertigo and hearing loss and intractable vertiginous symptoms requiring hospitalization. The clinicopathologic correlation is complicated further by the discovery of labyrinthine hydrops at autopsy in patients with no reported symptoms of vertigo during their lifetime. The concept of Meniere's disease being the consequence of a viral infection with a predilection for the endolymphatic sac is appealing in the sense that it may explain both the histologic findings and the patient's clinical symptoms.

Until recently, imaging of patients with Meniere's disease has been disappointing and CT (46–48) and MRI were primarily used to exclude other conditions such as acoustic neuroma, which may mimic Meniere's disease. The endolymphatic sac can be seen on high resolution MRI (2). We have recently encountered a series of patients with symptoms compatible with Meniere's disease in whom MRI demonstrated enhancement of the endolymphatic sac (Fig. 37) (49). Similar to enhancement of the cochlea and vestibule, enhancement of the endolymphatic sac is consistent with an inflammatory process in this location, such as a viral infection, and may correlate with the acute stage of the disease. It is possible that in

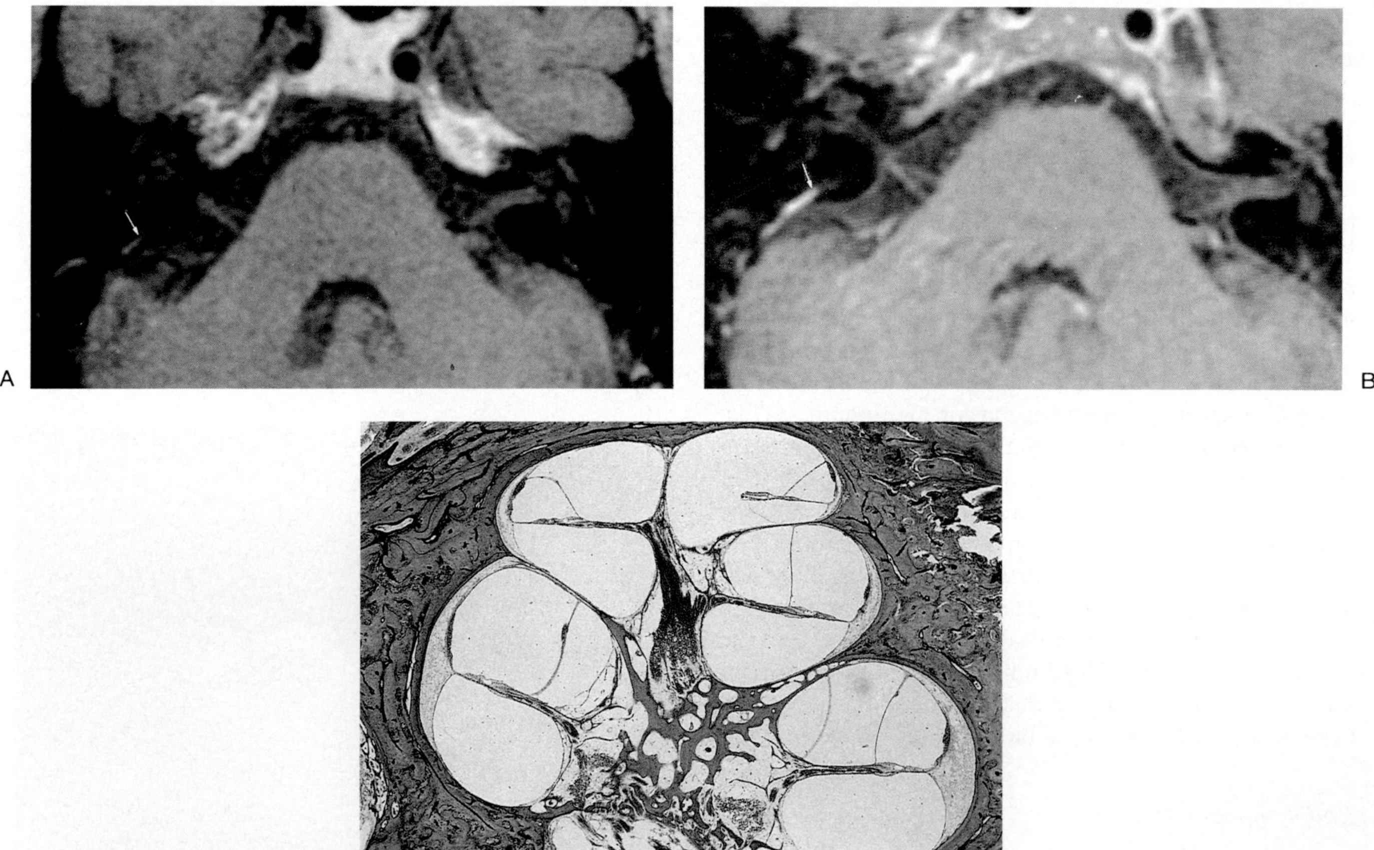

FIG. 37. Probable Meniere's disease. Fifty-year-old woman with sudden onset sensorineural hearing loss and vertigo. Hearing improved after 4 days. The patient had a similar episode 5 years earlier. **A:** Axial T1 MRI is normal. **B:** Axial enhanced fat-saturated T1 MRI reveals enhancement of the right endolymphatic sac (*arrow*). **C:** Pathologic specimen from another patient showing endolymphatic hydrops. (Courtesy of Dr. H. Schuknecht, Boston, MA.)

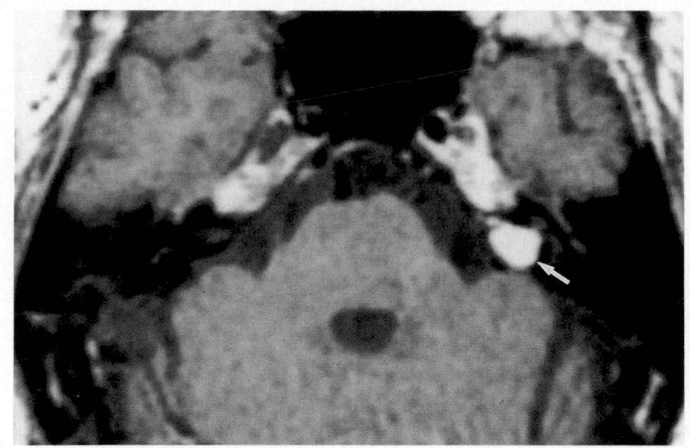

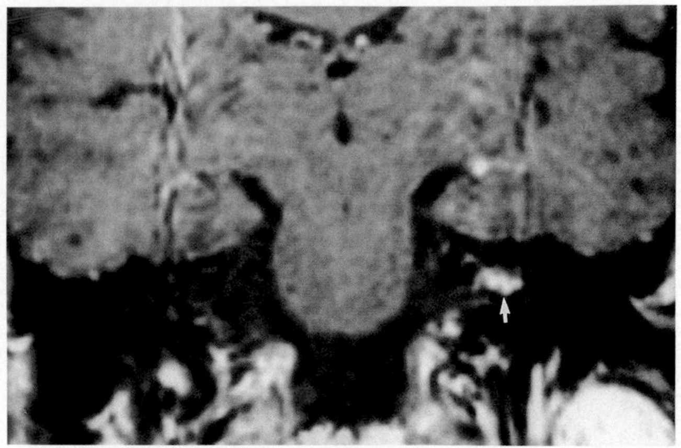

FIG. 38. Osseous hemangioma in the IAC in a patient with sensorineural hearing loss. **A:** Axial enhanced T1 MRI reveals an enhancing mass in the right IAC (*arrow*) . **B:** Coronal postcontrast T1-weighted image shows the serpiginous nature of the mass (*arrow*).

later stages the enhancement resolves and the fibrotic sac may not be seen at all on MRI in the later stages of the disease.

INTERNAL AUDITORY CANAL AND CEREBELLOPONTINE ANGLE LESIONS

Lesions of the internal auditory canal/cerebellopontine angle (IAC/CPA) lesions have been extensively described. Contrast-enhanced MRI has made a major impact on the detection and diagnosis of acoustic schwannoma (50), meningioma (51–53), and epidermoid (54) of the IAC/CPA area (55–57).

The most common lesion in the IAC is the schwannoma of cranial nerve VIII (also known as acoustic neuroma). These lesions develop from the Schwann sheath cells of sensory nerves. The vast majority of schwannomas arise from the vestibular division of the VIIIth cranial nerve, most commonly in the region of Scarpa's ganglion at the glial-Schwann junction. They account for 8% to 10% of all intracranial tumors and 80% to 90% of all CPA tumors. Grossly, these tumors are encapsulated and firm. Sudden sensorineural hearing loss is the presenting symptom in 10% of patients (58). On MRI, larger lesions may be diagnosed without contrast. Small intracanalicular lesions markedly enhance following gadolinium administration.

Although most enhancing lesions in the IAC are acoustic schwannomas, care must be taken not to misdiagnose other causes of enhancement in the IAC as "early acoustic schwannoma." The converse is also true, that is, lesions that appear as more linear "neuritis" may transform to more globular acoustic neuroma over time (31). Osseous hemangiomas (Fig. 38) (59) and arteriovenous malformation (Fig. 39) are two lesions that may

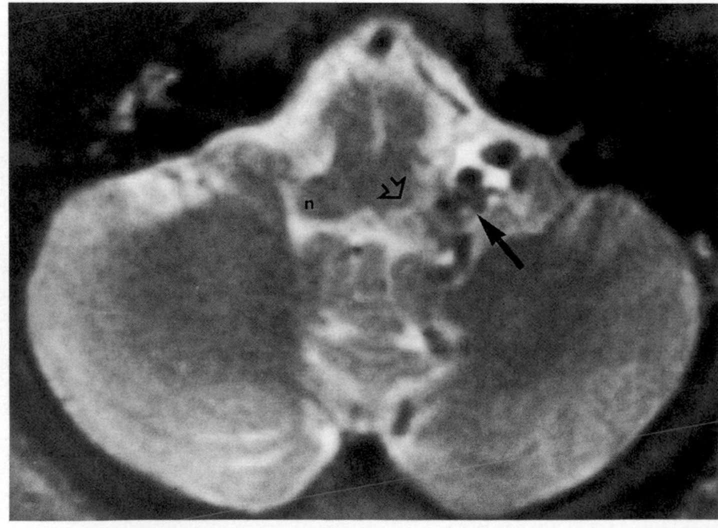

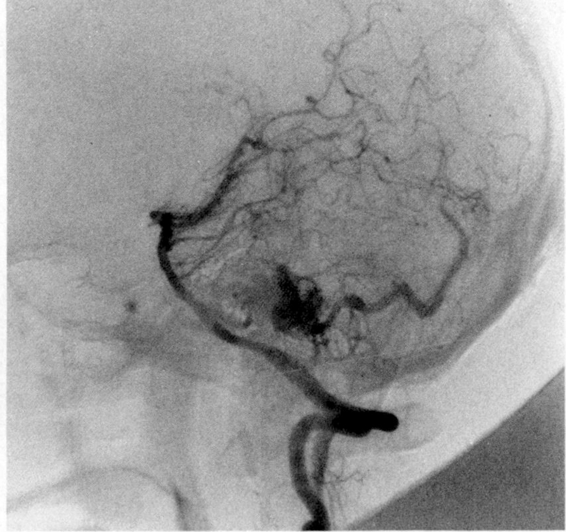

FIG. 39. Arteriovenous malformation of the CPA cistern. **A:** Axial T2 MRI of the CPA cistern reveals the malformation nidus (*arrow*) within the cistern; inferior cerebellar peduncle containing the cochlear nuclei (*n*). Notice the edema in the left inferior cerebellar peduncle (*open arrow*). **B:** Left vertebral angiogram confirms the arteriovenous malformation.

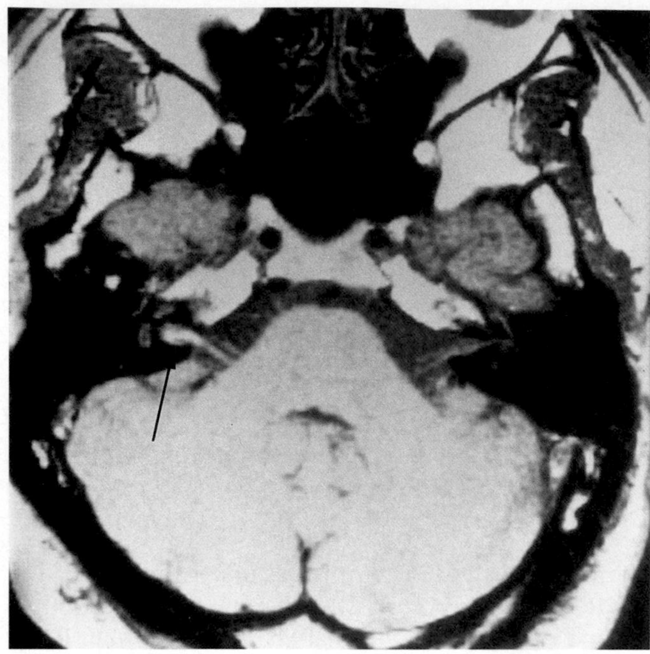

FIG. 40. Forty-year-old man with sudden right-sided sensorineural hearing loss. Axial T1-weighted images demonstrate subacute hemorrhage in the right IAC (*arrow*), probably from a hemangioma. (From Mark et al., ref. 32, with permission.)

enhance in the IAC, thereby mimicking acoustic schwannoma. Furthermore, as they can present with hemorrhage, precontrast T1 images become important in study interpretation to differentiate enhancement from subacute hemorrhage (Fig. 40). Lipomas of the IAC (60,61) can also mimic enhancing lesions and will be readily diagnosed on the precontrast T1 images (Fig. 41) or on the fat-suppression images.

The meninges of the IAC may be involved in a variety of inflammatory [sarcoid (Fig. 42), toxoplasmosis (62), neuroborelliosis (63), cryptococcosis (64), Sjögren's syndrome (Fig. 43) (65) post–shunt meningeal fibrosis, idio-

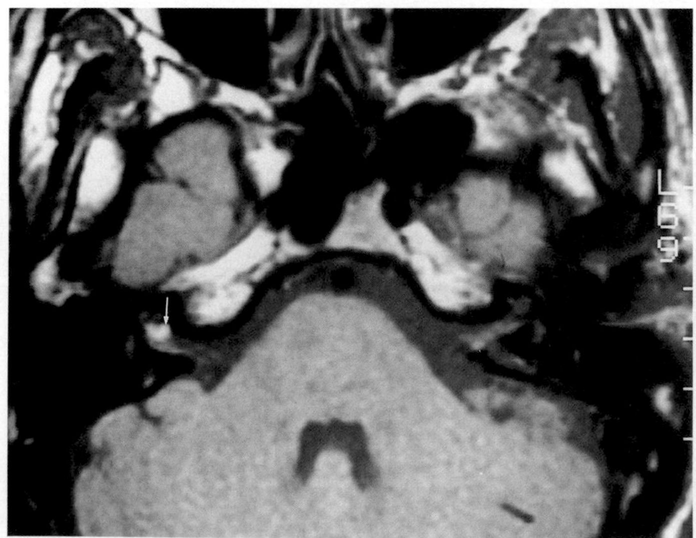

A

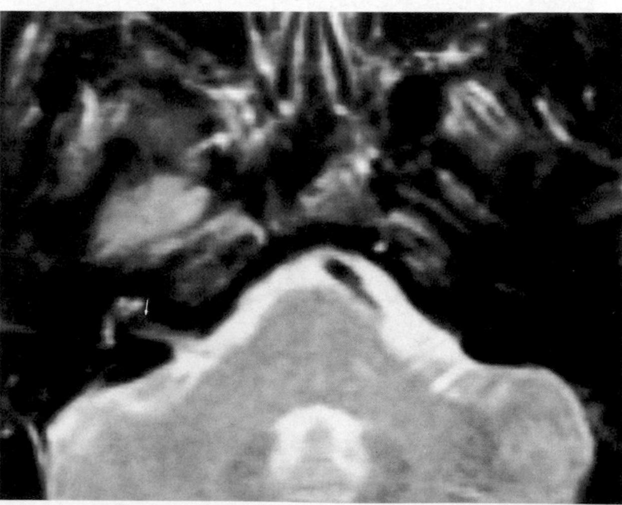

B

FIG. 41. Intracanalicular lipoma. Thirty-four-year-old man with very mild right-sided sensorineural hearing loss. **A:** Precontrast axial T1-weighted image reveals a small high signal intensity mass in the fundus of the IAC (*arrow*) along the cochlear nerve consistent with a lipoma. **B:** The lesion (*arrow*) is isointense with fat on T2-weighted images.

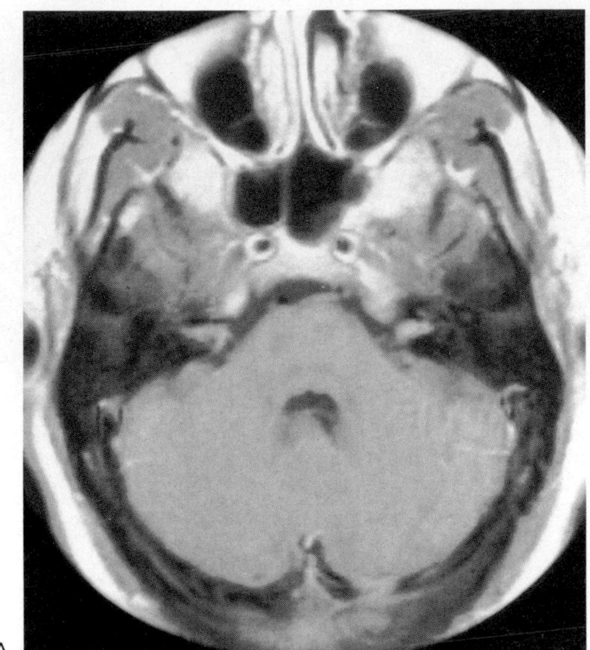
A

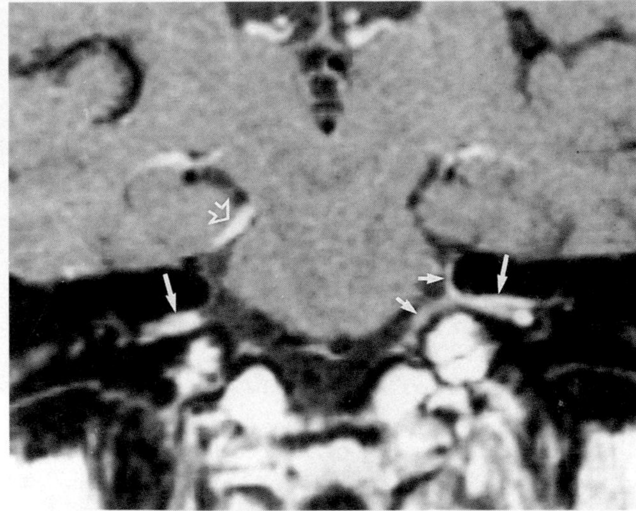
B

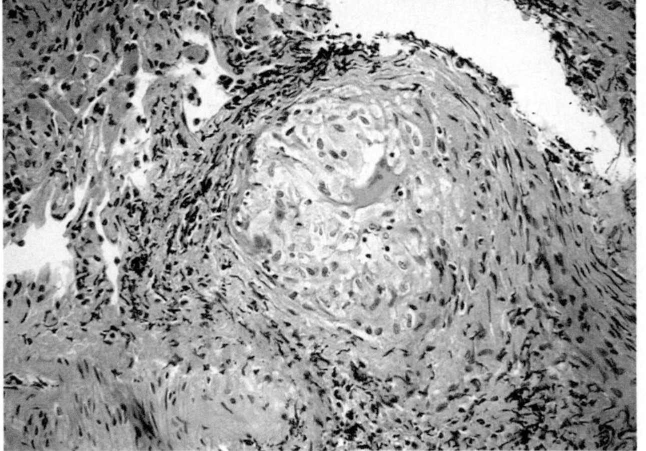
C

FIG. 42. Sarcoidosis of the IACs. **A:** Young woman with bilateral hearing loss demonstrates enhancement within both IACs on axial T1-weighted contrast-enhanced images. (Courtesy of Dr. J. Schwartz, Philadelphia, PA.) **B:** Coronal T1-weighted image in another patient with sarcoidosis reveals enhancement of the IACs (*long arrows*) as well as the meninges of the left CP angle (*short arrows*) and the tentorium (*open arrow*). **C:** Histologic section from another patient showing the typical features of a noncaseating granuloma.

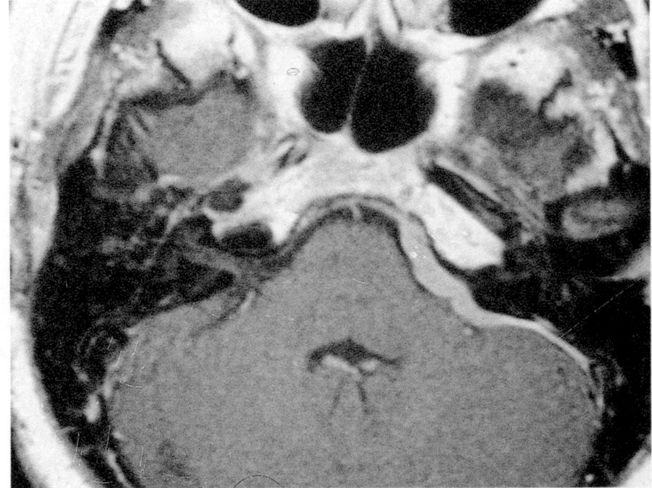

FIG. 43. Sjögren's syndrome. Fifty-six-year-old woman with left sensorineural hearing loss and Sjögren's syndrome. Axial postcontrast T1-weighted image demonstrates an enhancing lesion in the left CP cistern. Surgery demonstrated a nonmalignant lymphocytic infiltrate (pseudolymphoma).

pathic arachnoiditis (66)] and neoplastic [lymphoma (Fig. 44), metastasis (see Fig. 32)] conditions and the meningeal enhancement may mimic an acoustic schwannoma (67).

Symptomatic central nervous system (CNS) sarcoidosis (68,69) has been reported in 5% of patients with sarcoidosis and meningeal involvement was seen in 8 of 12 patients in a recent article (70). The disease may present as sudden sensorineural hearing loss (71). The enhancement may involve only the IAC or extend into the IAC from the adjacent CPA cistern. The thickened, enhanced meninges may touch each other in the midline, mimicking an acoustic schwannoma. It is important to scrutinize the remainder of the meninges in the posterior fossa and supratentorial level to find other evidence of meningeal enhancement that would point to the correct diagnosis. Repeat MR examination after steroids can demonstrate marked reduction in the enhancement and convert the homogeneously enhancing lesion filling the IAC into two thin layers of enhancement along the meninges of the IAC and/or CPA.

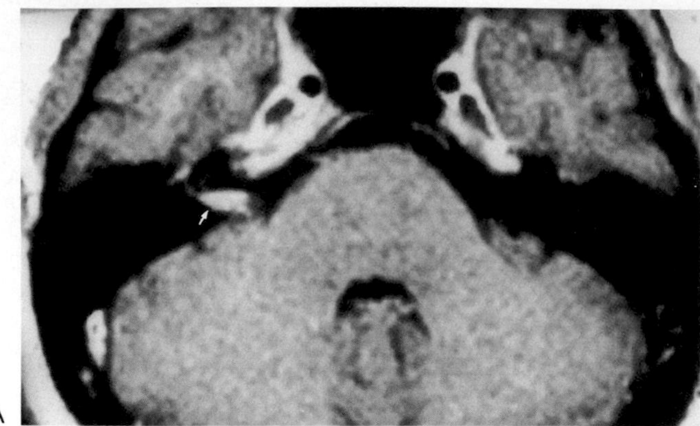

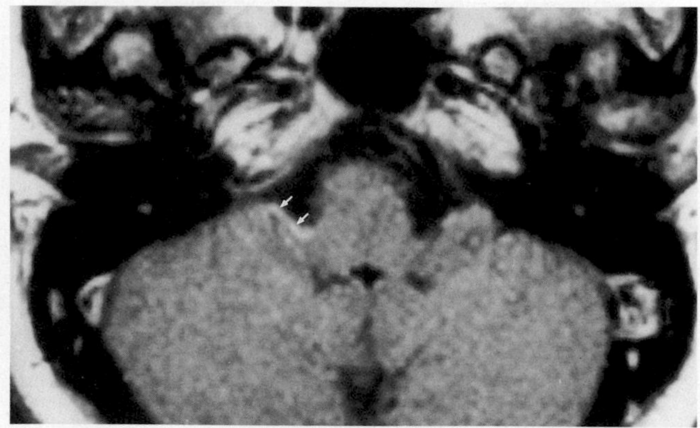

FIG. 44. Lymphoma involving the left IAC. Forty-year-old woman with 1 year history of back pain and right sensorineural hearing loss. CSF cytology confirmed the diagnosis of lymphoma. **A:** Axial postcontrast T1-weighted image demonstrates an enhancing lesion in the right IAC (*arrow*). **B:** Axial postcontrast T1-weighted image 6 mm lower demonstrates subtle pial enhancement (*arrows*).

THE FACIAL NERVE

Anatomy

The fibers of the facial nerve serve several functions. Efferent fibers enervate the striated musculature of the face and neck, the stylohyoid muscle, the posterior belly of the digastric muscle, and the stapedius muscle. Efferent preganglionic fibers of secretory function serve the lacrimal glands and seromucinous glands of the nasal cavity via the greater superficial petrosal nerve and the submandibular and sublingual glands via the chorda tympani nerve. Afferent fibers convey taste impulses from the anterior two thirds of the tongue via the chorda tympani nerve and from the palate and tonsillar fossae via the greater superficial petrosal nerve. Afferent fibers carry proprioceptive sensation from the facial muscles and cutaneous sensation from the external auditory canal and adjacent conchal region.

In its course in the IAC and labyrinthine segment, the nerve is usually separated into bundles by the endoneurial sheaths; however, more distally in the tympanic and mastoid segments, the endoneurium is less distinct or missing. The upper part of the motor nucleus receives bilateral enervation from the motor cortex and supplies the frontal and orbicularis oculi muscles. The inferior part of the motor nucleus receives unilateral uncrossed cortical enervation. The facial nerve fibers closely loop around abducens nucleus to form the internal genu. The superior salivary nucleus is located dorsal to the motor nucleus and conveys parasympathetic secretory impulses to the lacrimal glands, seromucinous glands of the nasal cavity, and submandibular and sublingual glands. The nucleus of the solitary tract lies in the medulla oblongata and receives taste, proprioceptive, and cutaneous sensory fibers from the facial nerve.

The facial nerve fibers exit the brain at the inferior border of the pons. As the nerve trunk proceeds toward the IAC, it lies in a groove on the superior surface of the cochlear nerve. This *intracranial segment* is 23 to 24 mm in length. The proximal segment is located in the IAC and is 7 to 8 mm in length and lies in a superior relationship to the cochlear nerve, passing above the transverse crest to enter the area nervi facialis. The *labyrinthine segment*, which is 3 to 4 mm in length, begins at the area nervi facialis and passes forward and laterally at nearly right angles to the petrous pyramid, just superior to the cochlea and vestibule, to reach the geniculate ganglion. At the geniculate ganglion the nerve makes a sharp posterior angulation known as the *external genu*, which marks the beginning of the *tympanic segment*, which is 12 to 13 mm in length and passes posteriorly and laterally, parallel to the longitudinal axis of the petrous bone, on the medial wall of the tympanic cavity superior to the oval window and inferior to the lateral semicircular canal. At the pyramidal eminence the nerve turns inferiorly. This bend in the nerve trunk, known as the pyramidal turn, marks the beginning of the *mastoid segment*, which is 15 to 20 mm in length and passes vertically downward in the posterior wall of the tympanic cavity and anterior wall of the mastoid to reach the stylomastoid foramen, where it exits from the skull.

The greater superficial petrosal nerve arises from the geniculate ganglion and ends in the sphenopalatine ganglion in the pterygopalatine fossa. The nerve to the stapedius muscle leaves the mastoid segment in the region of the pyramidal eminence to supply this muscle. The chorda tympani nerve normally leaves the facial nerve about 5 mm above the stylomastoid foramen and ends in the lingual nerve.

Topographic diagnosis of lesions in patients with facial palsy may be attempted by studying the special functions

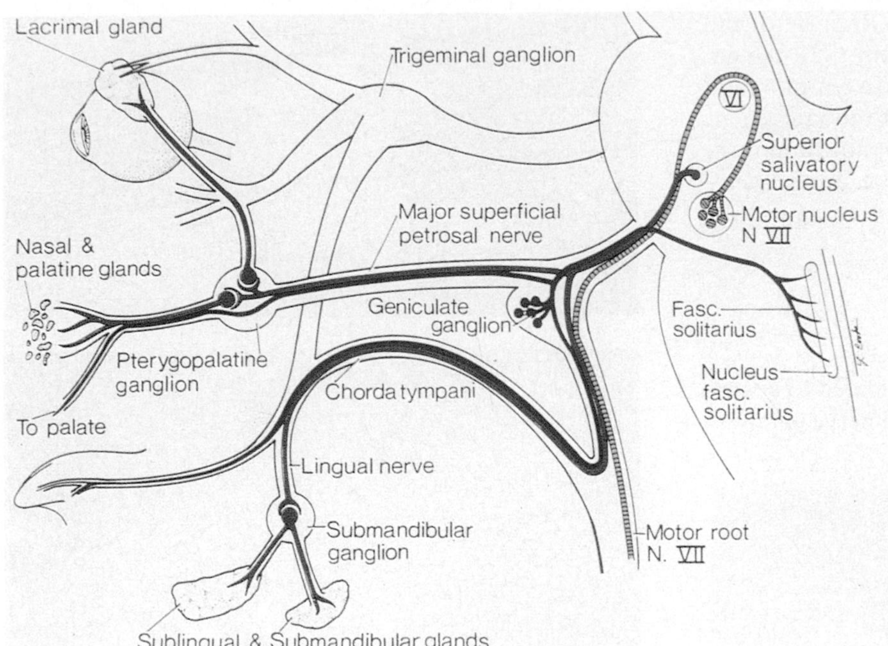

FIG. 45. Schematic representation of the facial nerve and its branches. (From Schuknecht, ref. 1, with permission.)

of the nerve (Fig. 45): infrachordal lesions are located inferior to the chorda tympani branch and do not alter taste, lacrimation, or the stapedial reflex; infrastapedial lesions are located between the chorda tympani branch and the nerve to the stapedius muscle and affect taste but have no effect on lacrimation or the stapedial reflex; suprastapedial lesions are located between the nerve to the stapedius muscle and the geniculate ganglion and affect taste and the stapedial reflex but have no effect on lacrimation; and suprageniculate lesions are located between the geniculate ganglion and motor nucleus and affect taste, lacrimation, and the stapedial reflex. This topographic approach is useful for lesions that completely transect all the components of the nerve trunk at the site of involvement. However, some disorders of the facial nerve affect the several functional components differentially, in which case topographic diagnosis is invalid (72).

The intratemporal course of the facial nerve can be

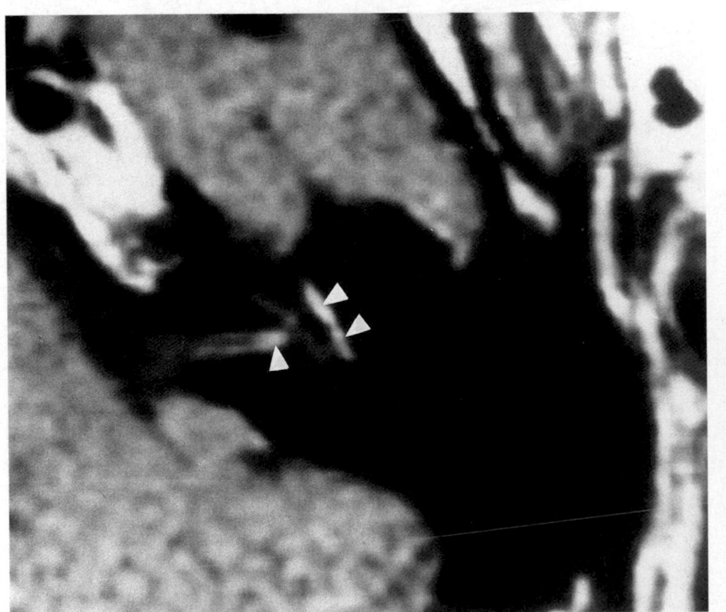

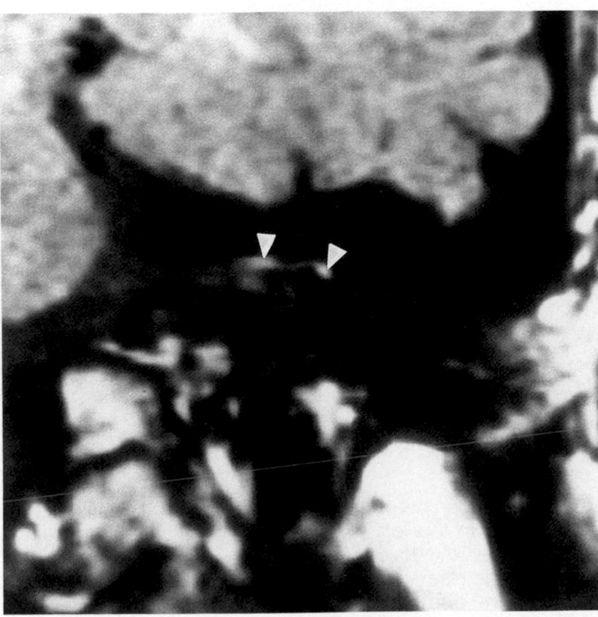

FIG. 46. Left Bell's palsy. Thirty-year-old man with acute peripheral left VIIth nerve palsy. **A:** Postcontrast T1-weighted image demonstrates enhancement of the horizontal segment of the facial nerve and of the distal intracanalicular segment (*arrows*). **B:** Coronal postcontrast T1-weighted image confirms these findings (*arrows*). (From Mark, ref. 76, with permission.)

easily defined by high resolution MRI. Because of the abundant and highly vascular epineurium (72), the geniculate ganglion enhances commonly in asymptomatic patients after contrast administration. The enhancement is usually mild and symmetric. The tympanic and mastoid segments may also enhance, but the intracanalicular segment of the facial nerve does not enhance normally (82).

Facial Nerve Pathology

Peripheral facial nerve palsy may be related to a variety of conditions. Eighty percent of facial nerve paralysis

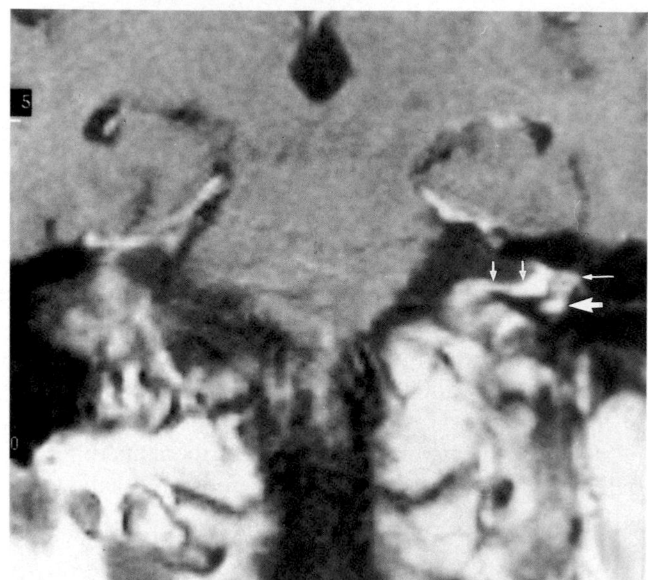

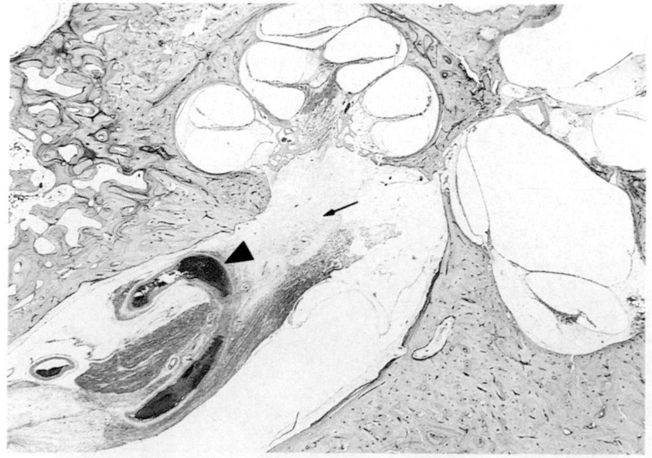

FIG. 47. Sudden hearing loss and left facial nerve palsy. Patient had vesicles in the left external auditory canal consistent with herpes zoster oticus. **A:** Coronal T1-weighted image postcontrast demonstrates enhancement of the meninges in the IAC (*small arrows*) and of the left cochlea (*large arrow*) and vestibule (*long thin arrow*). (Courtesy of Dr. C. Citrin, Washington, D.C.) (From Mark, ref. 76, with permission.) **B:** Pathologic specimen from another patient with herpes zoster oticus demonstrates degeneration of the cochlear nerve, which is replaced by fibrous tissue and a round cell infiltrate (*arrow*). Notice the loop of the AICA (*arrowhead*) (From Schuknecht, ref. 1, with permission.)

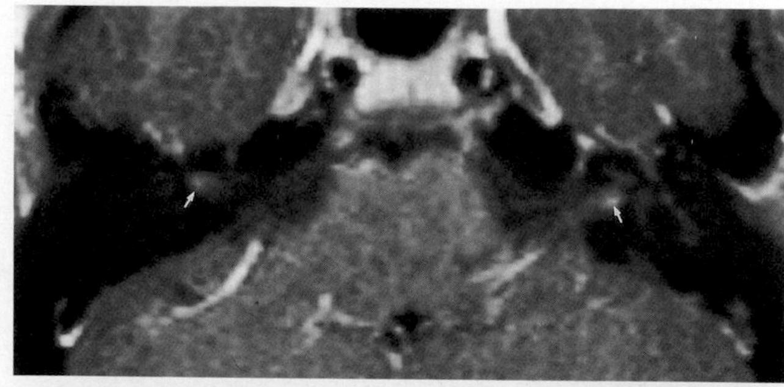

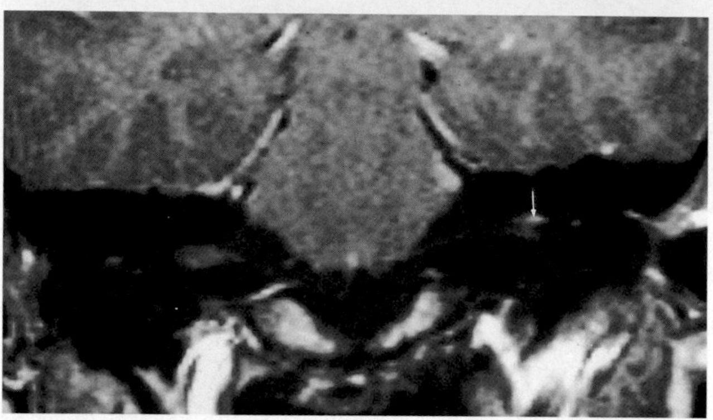

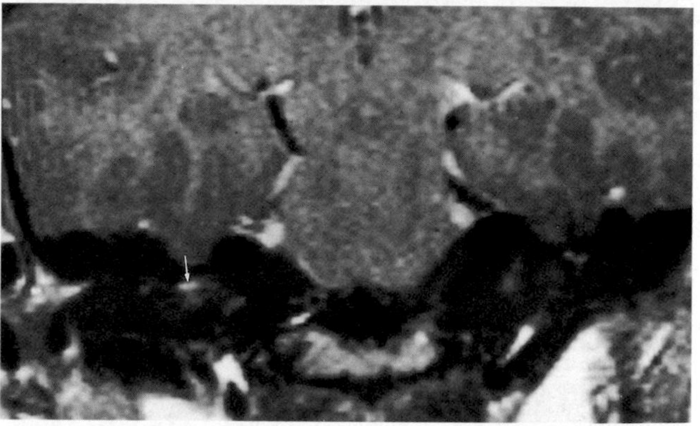

FIG. 48. Lyme disease and bilateral facial palsy. **A:** Axial postgadolinium T1-weighted image demonstrates bilateral enhancement in the IACs (*arrows*). **B,C:** Consecutive coronal T1-weighted image through the IACs confirm the enhancement of the facial nerves (*arrows*). Notice also the bilateral enhancement of the trigeminal nerves. (Courtesy of Dr. S. Seltzer, Boston, MA.)

is idiopathic, that is, caused by Bell's Palsy. This is a presumed viral illness resolving spontaneously within 8 weeks. If the palsy lasts longer, it is termed "atypical Bell's palsy" and these patients should definitely be imaged with contrast-enhanced MR. Patients with idiopathic Bell's palsy may demonstrate enhancement of various segments of the facial nerve in the temporal bone (Fig. 46) (73). Usually the nerve is not enlarged. Clinically, the symptoms develop acutely and usually resolve in 8 to 10 weeks.

Many inflammatory conditions and a host of other etiologies account for the remainder of peripheral facial palsies. Herpes zoster involvement of the VIIth and VIIIth nerves (17,83) may produce sudden hearing loss and facial palsy (Ramsay-Hunt syndrome) (Fig. 47). Lyme disease (Fig. 48) and syphilis (see Fig. 16) may also in-

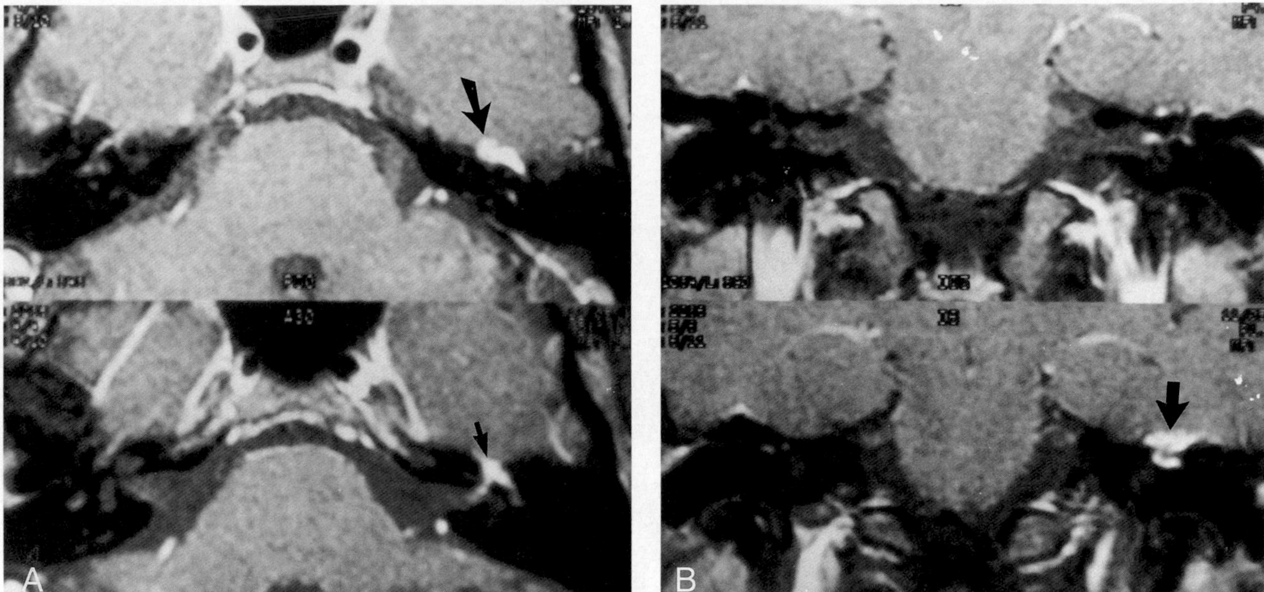

FIG. 49. Facial nerve schwannoma. Twenty-nine-year-old woman with progressive dryness of the left eye. The patient then developed progressive left facial nerve palsy. **A:** Two consecutive 3-mm thick sections postcontrast axial T1-weighted images demonstrate an enhancing mass (*arrows*) in the left geniculate ganglion, consistent with a facial nerve schwannoma. **B:** Coronal postcontrast T1-weighted images confirm these findings (*arrow*). Notice the subtle "normal" enhancement of the right VIIth nerve. (From Mark, ref. 76, with permission.)

volve the facial nerve and enhancement of the facial nerve may be observed on contrast-enhanced images. Enhancement of the facial nerve may also be seen secondary to trauma (73). Neoplasms of the facial nerve result in a progressive facial palsy. The most common primary neoplasm of the facial nerve is a schwannoma (Fig. 49) (74). It can occur along any segment of the nerve but it has a predilection for the geniculate ganglion. These lesions markedly enhance after contrast administration. Other lesions that can produce facial nerve palsy in the temporal bone include cavernous hemangiomas, sclerosing hemangioma, epidermoid (Fig. 50), hemartoma, meningioma, and chemodectoma. Cavernous hemangiomas also have a predilection for the geniculate ganglion. Patients often present with hemifacial spasm; meningiomas of the facial nerve are unusual lesions that also enhance after contrast administration. Metastasis to the facial nerve, especially perineural tumor spread from parotid adenoid cystic carcinoma, should be a prime consideration in elderly patients with progressive facial nerve palsy. The imaging studies should always include the parotid gland in order not to miss such a lesion.

MISCELLANEOUS ENHANCING LESIONS OF THE TEMPORAL BONE

Both inflammatory (75) and neoplastic (55) lesions of the temporal bone may enhance after contrast administration. Although CT remains the imaging modality of choice for inflammatory diseases of the middle ear because of its superior ability to detect bone erosions, contrast-enhanced MRI may be very helpful in assessing the adjacent intracranial extension of the infection, in particular, an epidural abscess. Lateral sinus thrombophlebitis may also be detected by MRI with or without intravenous contrast. MR angiography may be an easy, noninvasive way to diagnose this condition. Extension of middle ear infection to the petrous apex (76,77) is rare now in the antibiotic era, but was a common condition in the past. The infection results in a paralysis of the VIth nerve and deep pain along the trigeminal nerve (Gradenigo syndrome). In the appropriate clinical context, an enhancing lesion of the petrous apex is strongly suggestive of this condition (Fig. 51). MRI may demonstrate focal enhancement of the meninges over the petrous apex and extension of the infection into Meckel's cave.

Otosclerosis is a condition of unknown origin in which the normal endochondral bone is replaced by foci of spongy, vascular, irregular new bone that is less dense (78). These spongy decalcified foci in the later stages become less vascular and more solid. The condition is bilateral in most patients and often symmetric. There is a 2 to 1 female predominance. The disease usually appears in the second or third decade of life. There are two major clinical categories. The fenestral type of otosclerosis involves the lateral wall of the labyrinth, including the promontory, facial nerve canal, and both the oval and round window niche. The involvement of the oval window results in fixation of the footplate of the stapes and conductive hearing loss. Retrofenestral otosclerosis occurs when the process of demineralization involves the

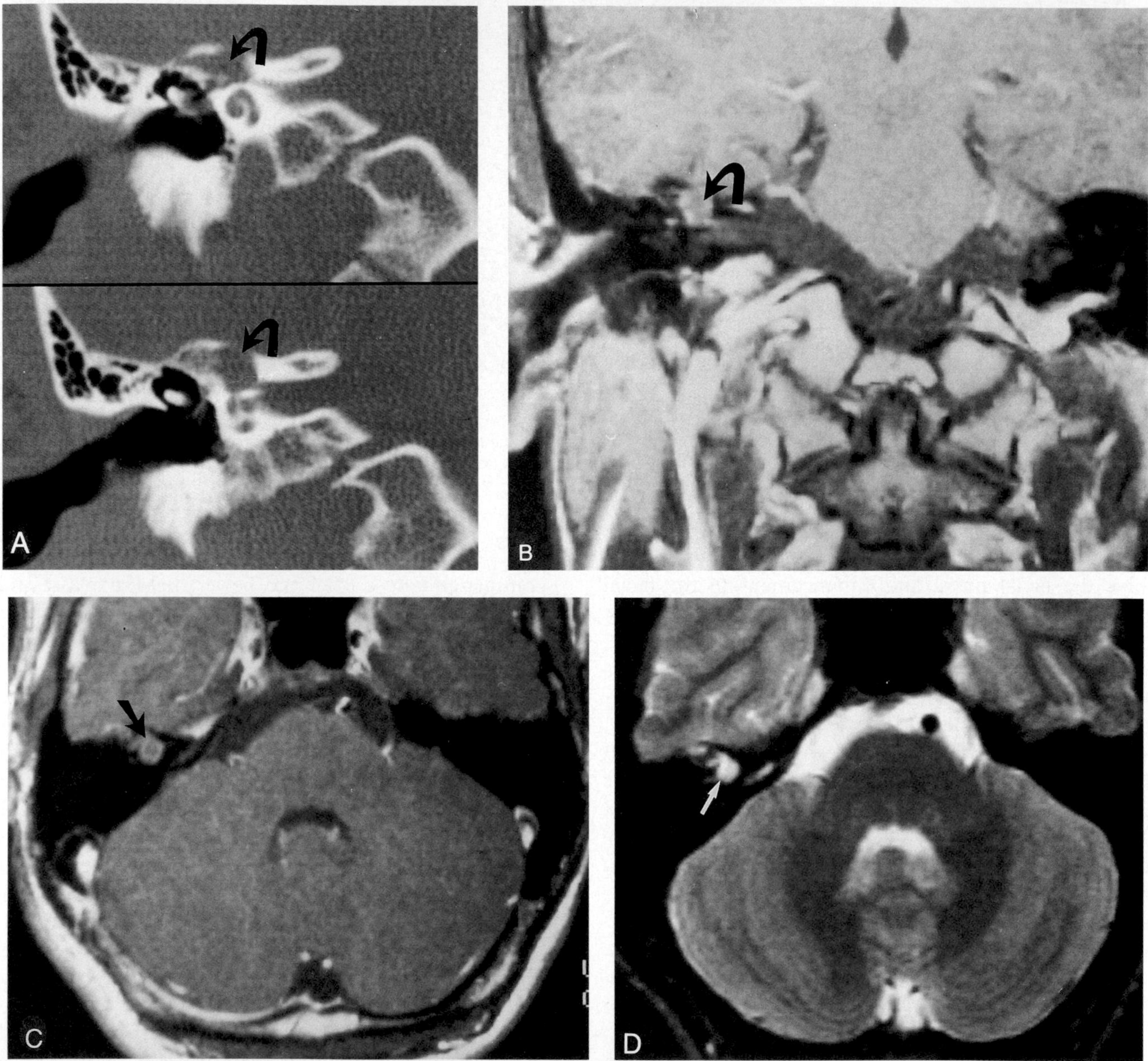

FIG. 50. Sixteen-year-old boy with right peripheral facial nerve palsy. **A:** High resolution coronal CT through the IAC. Two consecutive sections 1 mm apart. A destructive mass (*arrow*) is noted in the superior aspect of the temporal bone affecting the labyrinthine segment of the facial nerve. Differential diagnosis includes a VIIth nerve schwannoma, a hemangioma, or an epidermoid. **B:** Coronal postcontrast T1-weighted image through the right IAC demonstrates an 8-mm mass (*arrow*) above the superior aspect of the canal compressing the labyrinthine segment of the right facial nerve. Axial T1- (**C**) and T2- (**D**) weighted image 3 mm above the IAC confirms this mass (*arrow*), does not enhance, and has a signal intensity consistent with an epidermoid. (Courtesy of Dr. G. Vezina, Washington, D.C.) (From Mark, ref. 76, with permission.)

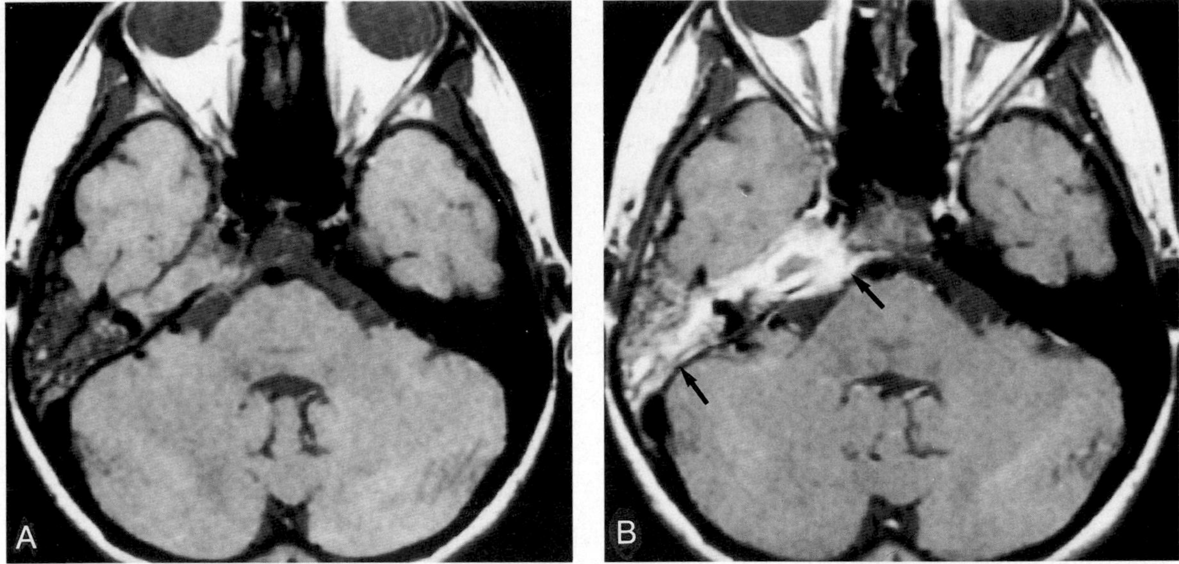

FIG. 51. Gradenigo syndrome. Ten-year-old girl with right VIth nerve palsy, sensorineural hearing loss, and severe right facial pain. **A:** Precontrast axial T1-weighted image through the temporal bone demonstrates an isointense mass in the right petrous apex and fluid or mass in the mastoid air cells. **B:** Postcontrast axial T1-weighted image demonstrates marked enhancement of the right petrous apex (*arrows*), of the dura over the right petrous apex including Dorello's canal, and of the right mastoid. (Courtesy of Dr. H. R. Harnsberger, Salt Lake City, UT.) (From Mark, ref. 76, with permission.)

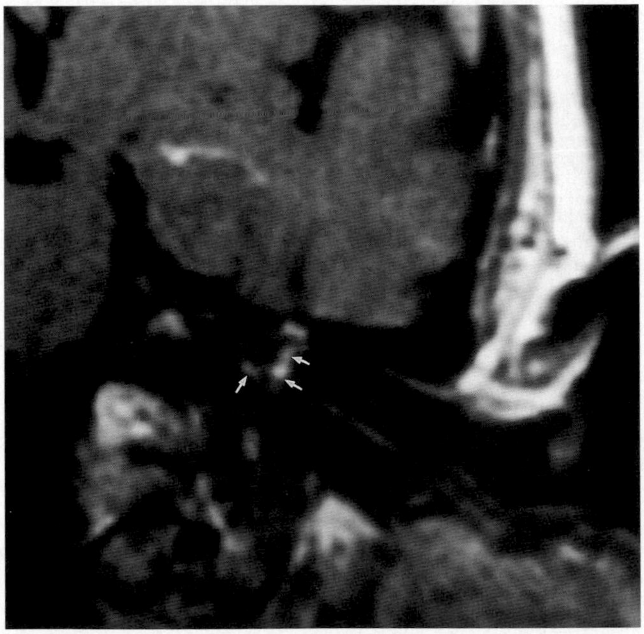

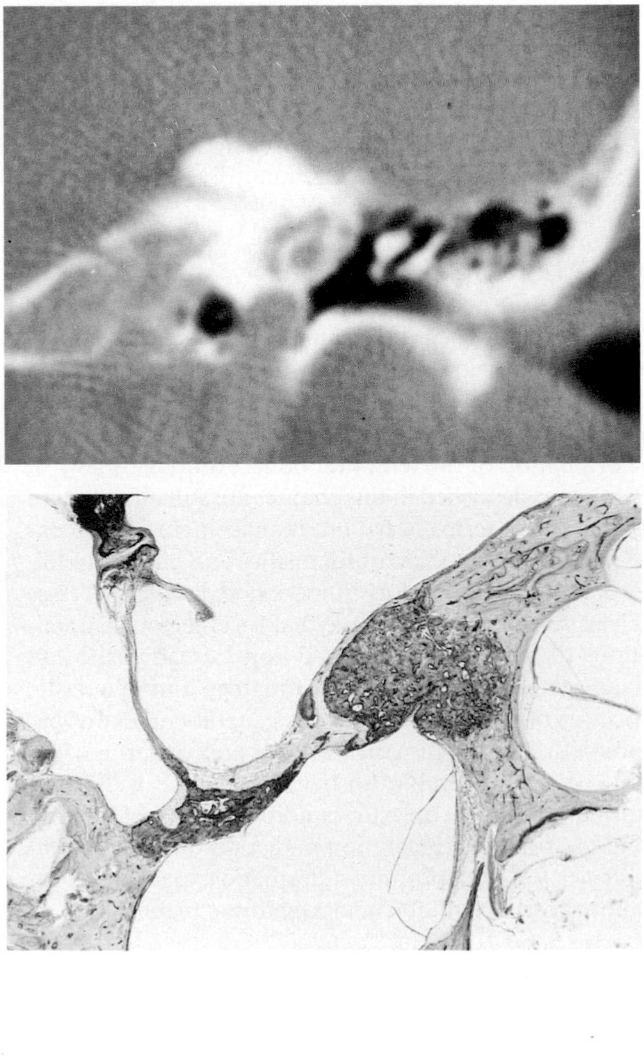

B

A

C

FIG. 52. Cochlear otosclerosis. **A:** Enhanced coronal T1-weighted image of the right temporal bone in a patient with the clinical and CT diagnosis of cochlear otosclerosis shows foci of enhancement within the bony labyrinth (*arrows*) surrounding the cochlea. **B:** CT shows the typical findings of otosclerosis. (From Mark, Seltzer, and Harnsberger, ref. 31, with permission.) **C:** Pathologic specimen shows a focus of otosclerosis anterior to the oval window. (From Schuknecht, ref. 1, with permission.)

otic capsule itself. These changes in the bone may affect the spiral ligament at the surface of the membranous labyrinth and result in sensorineural hearing loss; thus, a patient with otosclerosis may have a combined conductive and sensorineural hearing loss depending on the relative distribution and severity of the disease. CT is the imaging modality of choice for diagnosing otosclerosis (79,80). Depending on the location of the foci of demineralization along the cochlea, specific frequency ranges may be affected more than others (80). Recently, we have described a case of typical cochlear otosclerosis on CT with pericochlear and perivestibular areas of enhancement on MRI (Fig. 52) (31). This finding probably reflects the leakage of gadolinium in the highly vascular spongiotic bone during the early stages of the disease. In the later stages of the disease, when the spongiotic bone is replaced by dense bone, the enhancement disappears.

Both benign and malignant neoplasms may affect the temporal bone (81). Paragangliomas may affect the middle ear (glomus tympanicum) or the jugular foramen (glomus jugulare). These lesions markedly enhance after contrast administration. When large enough, they exhibit a characteristic flow void pattern on precontrast MRI. Metastatic diseases from any source may affect the temporal bone. The appearance of metastatic disease to the temporal bone is that of a nonspecific enhancing mass that needs to be differentiated from an inflammatory process. Other masses affect the temporal bone such as chondrosarcoma and lymphoma, and a carcinoma and rhabdomyosarcoma in children may also enhance. CT may be very useful in demonstrating the characteristic "popcorn" calcifications of chondrosarcoma.

CONCLUSION

The availability of intravenous contrast agents sensitive to the disruption of the blood–brain and blood–labyrinth barrier coupled with high resolution imaging have significantly expanded the potential role of MRI in the evaluation of the temporal bone. Although many of the findings described in this chapter are still of uncertain significance in terms of patient management, the potential for insight into the natural history and pathophysiology of many of these poorly understood disease processes is clear. At present, we believe that several clinical applications of MRI in the temporal bone already exist and include the evaluation of inflammatory and neoplastic processes of the labyrinth (in the general context of patients with sensorineural hearing loss and/or vertigo), patients with peripheral VIIth nerve palsies, as well as inflammatory and neoplastic conditions of the temporal bone itself. Higher resolution and faster imaging methodologies for MRI promise a dramatic expansion of capabilities for this unique neuroanatomic region.

ACKNOWLEDGMENT. The author thanks Nancy Carnes for her editorial assistance.

REFERENCES

1. Schuknecht HF. Anatomy of the inner ear. In: Schuknecht HF, ed. *Pathology of the Ear*, 2nd ed. Philadelphia: Lea and Febiger; 1993: 45–66.
2. Brogan M, Chakeres DW, Schmalbrock P. High-resolution 3DFT MR imaging of the endolymphatic duct and soft tissues of the otic capsule. *AJNR* 1991;12:1–11.
3. Casselman JW, Kuhweide R, Deimling M, Ampe W, Dehaene L, Meeus L. Constructive interference in steady state (CISS)-3DFT MR imaging of the inner ear and cerebellopontine angle. *AJNR* 1993;14:47–57.
4. Casselman JW, Kuhweide R, Ampe W, Meeus L, Steyaert L. Pathology of the membranous labyrinth: comparison of T1- and T2-weighted and gadolinium-enhanced spin-echo and 3DFT-CISS imaging. *AJNR* 1993;14:59–69.
5. Armington WG, Harnsberger HR, Smoker WRK, Osborn AG. Normal and diseased acoustic pathway: evaluation with MR imaging. *Radiology* 1986;167:509–515.
6. Cure JK, Cromwell LD, Case JL, Johnson GD, Musiek FE. Auditory dysfunction caused by multiple sclerosis: detection with MR imaging. *AJNR* 1990;11:817–820.
7. Fox AJ, Bogousslavsky J, Carey LS, et al. Magnetic resonance imaging of small medullary infarctions. *AJNR* 1986;7:229–233.
8. Jani NN, Laureno R, Mark AS, Brewer CC. Deafness after bilateral midbrain contusion: a correlation of magnetic resonance imaging with auditory brain stem evoked responses. *Neurosurgery* 1991;29: 106–109.
9. Kumar A, Maudelonde C, Mafee M. Unilateral sensorineural hearing loss: analysis of 200 consecutive cases. *Laryngoscope* 1986;96:14–18.
10. Sando I, Egami T. Inner ear hemorrhage and endolymphatic hydrops in a leukemic patient with sudden hearing loss. *Ann Otol Rhinol Laryngol* 1977;86:518–524.
11. Mark AS. Vestibulocochlear system. *Neuroimag Clin North Am* 1993;3:153–170.
12. Swartz JD, Swartz NG, Korsvik H, et al. Computerized tomographic evaluation of the middle ear and mastoid for post traumatic hearing loss. *Ann Otol Rhinol Laryngol* 1985;94:263–266.
13. Zimmerman RA, Bilaniuk LT, Hackney DB, Golberg HI, Grossman RI. Magnetic resonance imaging in temporal bone fracture. *Neuroradiology* 1987;29:246–251.
14. Weissman JL, Curtin HD, Hirsch BE, Hirsch WL Jr. High signal from the otic labyrinth on unenhanced magnetic resonance imaging. *AJNR* 1992;13:1183–1187.
15. Massab HF. The role of viruses in sudden deafness. *Adv Otorhinolaryngol* 1970;20:229–235.
16. Nomura Y, Hiraide F. Sudden deafness: a histopathological study. *J Laryngol Otol* 1976;90:1121–1142.
17. Schuknecht HF. Viral infections. In: Schuknecht HF, ed. *Pathology of the Ear*, 2nd ed. Philadelphia: Lea and Febiger; 1993:235–244.
18. Hemenway WG, Sando I, Mochesnay D. Temporal bone pathology following maternal rubella. *Arch Klin Exp Ohren-Nosen-Kehlkopfheiekol* 1969;193:287–300.
19. Westmore GA, Pickard BH, Stern H. Isolation of mumps virus from the inner ear after sudden deafness. *Br Med J* 1977;1:14–15.
20. Blackley B, Friedmann I, Wright I. Herpes zoster auris associated with facial nerve paralysis and auditory nerve symptoms. *Acta Otolaryngol* (Stockh) 1967;63:533–550.
21. Lindsay JR, Hemenway W. Inner ear pathology due to measels. *Ann Otol Rhinol Laryngol* 1954;63:754–771.
22. Liao BS, Byl FM, Adour KK. Audiometric comparison of lassa fever hearing loss and idiopathic sudden hearing loss: evidence for viral cause. *Otolaryngol Head Neck Surg* 1992;106:226–229.
23. Schacher PA, et al. Bacterial labyrinthitis, meningitis, and sensorineural damage. *Arch Otolaryngol Head Neck Surg* 1992;118:53–57.

24. Cole RR, Jahrsdoerfer RA. Sudden hearing loss: an update. *Am J Otol* 1988;9(3):211–215.
25. Hendershot E. Luetic deafness. *Otolaryngol Clin North Am* 1978;11:43–47.
26. Mark AS, Seltzer S, Nelson-Drake J, et al. Labyrinthine enhancement on GD-MRI inpatients with sudden hearing loss and vertigo: correlation with audiologic and electronystagmographic studies. *Ann Otol Rhinol Laryngol* 1992;101:459–464.
27. Seltzer S, Mark AS. Contrast enhancement of the labyrinth on MR scans in patients with sudden hearing loss and vertigo: evidence of labyrinthine disease. *AJNR* 1991;12:13–16.
28. Schuknecht HF. Infections of the inner ear. In: Schuknecht HF, ed. *Pathology of the Ear*, 2nd ed. Philadelphia: Lea and Febiger; 1993:212–218.
29. Schuknecht HF. Infections of the inner ear. In: Schuknecht HF, ed. *Pathology of the Ear*, 2nd ed. Philadelphia: Lea and Febiger; 1993:248–253.
30. McCabe BF. Autoimmune sensorineural hearing loss. *Ann Otol* 1979;88:585–589.
31. Casselman JW, Mojoor MHJM, Albers FW. MR of the inner ear in patients with Cogan syndrome. *AJNR* 1994;15:131–136.
32. Mark AS, Seltzer S, Harnsberger HR. MRI of sensory neural hearing loss: more than meets the eye? *AJNR* 1993;14:37–45.
33. Mark AS, Fitzgerald D. Segmental enhancement of different turns of the cochlea on Gd-enhanced MRI: correlation with the frequency of hearing loss and a possible sign of perilymphatic fistula. *AJNR* 1993;14:991–996.
34. Althaus SR. Perilymph fistulas. *Laryngoscope* 1981;91:538–562.
35. Gussen R. Sudden deafness associated with bilateral Reisner's membrane ruptures. *Am J Otolaryngol* 1983;9:27–32.
36. Nakoshima T, Itoh M, Sato M, Natanabe Y, Yanogita N. Auditory and vestibular disorders due to barotrauma. *Ann Otol Rhinol Laryngol* 1988;97:146–152.
37. Babin RW, Harker LA. Intralabyrinthine acoustic neurinomas. *Otolaryngol Head Neck Surg* 1980;88:455–461.
38. DeLozier HL, Gacek RR, Dana ST. Intralabyrinthine schwannoma. *Ann Otol* 1979;88:187–191.
39. Mafee MF, Lachenauer CS, Kumar A, Arnold PM, Buckingham RA, Valvassori GE. CT and MR imaging of intralabryinthine schwannoma: report of two cases and review of the literature. *Radiology* 1990;174:395–400.
40. Arenberg IK, Marovitz WF, Shambaugh Jr GE. The role of the endolymphatic sac in the pathogenesis of endolymphatic hydrops in man. *Acta Oto-Laryngologica* 1970;275(Suppl):1–49.
41. Lundquist PG. Aspects on endolymphatic sac morphology and function. *Arch Oto-Rhino-Laryngol* 1976;212:231–240.
42. Schuknecht HF, Gulya AJ. Endolymphatic hydrops—an overview and classification. *Ann Otol Rhinol Laryngol* 1983;(Suppl)106: 1–20.
43. Schuknecht HF. Pathophysiology of endolymphatic hydrops. *Arch Oto-Rhino-Laryngol* 1976;212:253–262.
44. Shea TT. Surgery of the endolymphatic sac. *Otolaryngol Clin North Am* 1968;1:613–621.
45. Tomiyama S, Harris JP. The endolymphatic sac: its importance in inner ear immune responses. *Laryngoscope* 1986;96:685–691.
46. Clemis JD, Valvassori GE. Recent radiographic and clinical observations on the vestibular aqueduct. *Otolaryngol Clin North Am* 1968;1:339–346.
47. Hall SF, O'Connor AF, Thakkar CH, Wylie IG, Morrison AW. Significance of tomography in Meniere's disease: visualization and morphology of the vestibular aqueduct. *Laryngoscope* 1983;93: 1546–1550.
48. Valvassori GE, Dobben GD. Multidirectional and computerized tomography of the vestibular aqueduct in Meniere's disease. *Ann Otol Rhinol Laryngol* 1984;93:547–550.
49. Mark AS, Seltzer S, Fitzgerald D. MRI of endolymphatic hydrops. Presented at the RSNA meeting November, 1992, Chicago, Ill.
50. Curati WL, Graif M, Kingsley DPE, Niendorf HP, Young IR. Acoustic neuromas: GD-DTPA enhancement in MR imaging. *Radiology* 1986;158:447–451.
51. Demaerel P, Wilms G, Lammens M, Marchal G, Plets C, Goffin J, et al. Intracranial meningiomas: correlation between MR imaging and histology in fifty patients. *J Comput Assist Tomogr* 1991;15(1):45–51.
52. Tien RD, Yang PJ, Chu PK. "Dural tail sign": a specific MR sign for meningioma? *J Comput Assist Tomogr* 1991;15(1):64–66.
53. Bydder GM, Kingsley DPE, Brown J, Niendorf HP, Young IR. MR imaging of meningiomas including studies with and without gadolinium DTPA. *J Comput Assist Tomogr* 1985;9(4):690–697.
54. Steffey DJ, De Filipp GJ, Spera T, Gabrielsen TO. MR imaging of primary epidermoid tumors. *J Comput Assist Tomogr* 1988;12(3): 438–440.
55. Lo WWM. Tumors of the temporal bone and the cerebellopontine angle. In: Som PM, Bergeron RT, eds. *Head and Neck Imaging*, 2nd ed. St. Louis: Mosby Year-Book; 1991.
56. Mikhael MA, Ciric IS, Wolff AP. Differentiation of cerebellopontine angle neuromas and meningiomas with MR imaging. *J Comput Assist Tomogr* 1985;9(5):852–856.
57. Press GA, Hesselink JR. MR imaging of cerebellopontine angle and internal auditory canal lesions at 1.5T. *AJNR* 1988;9:241–251.
58. Satloff RT, Davies B, Myers DL. Acoustic neuromas presenting as sudden deafness. *Am J Otol* 1985;95:67–69.
59. Glasscock ME, Smith PG, Schwoher MK, Nissen AJ. Clinical aspects of osseous hemangiomas of the skull base. *Laryngoscope* 1984;94:869–873.
60. Wong ML, Larson TI, Brockman DE, Lo WWM. Lipoma of internal auditory canal. *Otolaryngol Head Neck Surg* 1992;107:374–376.
61. Cohen TI, Powers SK, Williams DW III. MR appearance of intracanalicular eighth nerve lipoma. *AJNR* 1992;13:1188–1190.
62. Katholm M, Johnsen NJ, Siim C, Willumsen L. Bilateral sudden deafness and acute acquired toxoplasmosis. *J Laryngol Otol* 1991;105:115–118.
63. Hanner P, Rosenhall U, Edstrom S, Kaijser B. Hearing impairment in patients with antibody production against *Borrelia Burgdorferi* antigen. *Lancet* 1989;101:13–15.
64. Kwartler JA, Linthicum FH, Jahn AF, Hawke M. Sudden hearing loss due to AIDS-related cryptococcal meningitis—a temporal bone study. *Otolaryngol Head Neck Surg* 1991;104:265–269.
65. Tzioufas AG, et al. Lymphoid malignancy and monoclonal proteins. In: Taial N, et al., eds. *Sjogren's Syndrome*. Berlin: Springer-Verlag; 1987;129–136.
66. Reid E. Enhancing lesions in the internal auditory canal mimicking acoustic neuroma. Presented at the Fourth International Meniere Society Meeting Snowmass, CO, July 18–23th.
67. Han MH, Jabour BA, Andrews JC, et al. Non-neoplastic enhancing lesions mimicking intracanalicular acoustic neuroma on gadolinium-enhanced MR images. *Radiology* 1991;179:795–796.
68. Hayes WS, Sherman JL, Stern BJ, Citrin CM, Pulaski PD. MR and CT evaluation of intracranial sarcoidosis. *AJNR* 1987;8:841–847.
69. Sherman JL, Stern BJ. Sarcoidosis of the CNS: comparison of unenhanced and enhanced MR images. *AJNR* 1990;11:915–923.
70. Seltzer S, Mark AS, Atlas SW. CNS sarcoidosis: evaluation with GD-DTPA enhanced MRI. *AJNR* 1991;12:1227–1233; *AJR* 1992;158.
71. Kava CR, Varrs DM, Bell AF. Sudden hearing loss as the sole manifestation of neurosarcoidosis. *Otolaryngol Head Neck Surg* 1991;105:376–381.
72. Schuknecht HF. The facial nerve. In: Schuknecht HF, ed. *Pathology of the Ear*, 2nd ed. Philadelphia: Lea and Febiger; 1993:42–45.
73. Daniels OL, Czervionke LP, et al. Facial nerve enhancement in MR imaging. *AJNR* 1987;8:605–607.
74. Conley J, Janecka I. Schwann cell tumors of the facial nerve. *Laryngoscope* 1983;84:958–962.
75. Zizmor J, Noyek AM. Inflammatory diseases of the temporal bone. *Radiol Clin North Am* 1974;12:491–504.
76. Mark AS. Contrast-enhanced magnetic resonance imaging of the temporal bone. *Neuroimaging Clin North Am* 1994;4:117–131.
77. Jackler RK, Parker DA. Radiographic differential diagnosis of petrous apex lesions. *Am J Otol* 1992;13:561–574.
78. Wiet RJ, Rasian W, Shambugh GE. Otosclerosis 1981 to 1985, our four year review and current perspective. *Am J Otol* 1986;7:221–228.

79. Blakley BW, Hilger PA, Taylor S, Hilger J. Computed tomography in the diagnosis of cochlear otosclerosis. *Otolaryngol Head Neck Surg* 1986;94:434–438.
80. Swartz JD, Mandell DW, Berman SE, Wolfson RJ, Marlowe FL, Popky GL. Cochlear otosclerosis (otospongiosis): CT analysis with audiometric correlation. *Radiology* 1985;155:147–150.
81. Mafee MF, Valvassori GE, Kumar A, et al. Tumors and tumor-like conditions of the middle ear and mastoid: role of CT and MRI. An analysis of 100 cases. *Otolaryngol Clin North Am* 1988;21:349–375.
82. Gebaiski SS, Telian SA, Niparko JK. Enhancement along the normal facial nerve in the facial canal: MR imaging and anatomic correlation. *Radiology* 1992;183:391–394.
83. Sartoretti-Schefer S, Wichmann W, Valavanis A. Idiopathic, herpetic ann HIV-associated facial nerve palsies: abnormal MR enhancement patterns. *AJNR* 1994;15:479–485.

Magnetic Resonance Imaging of the Brain and Spine, Second Edition, edited by Scott W. Atlas.
Lippincott-Raven Publishers, Philadelphia © 1996.

22

The Orbit and Visual System

Scott W. Atlas and Steven L. Galetta

The visual system represents an intricately organized and important region of the central nervous system (CNS). It has critical sensory and motor functional components that are commonly affected by a wide variety of neurologic diseases, so it is frequently the specified region of interest on magnetic resonance imaging (MRI) examinations. It is therefore essential for the neuroradiologist to have a working knowledge of this system's anatomy, physiology, and pathology. This chapter covers three general areas of the visual system that can be involved with pathologic processes that are often manifested on MRI: lesions of the globe and orbit, gaze disorders, and abnormalities affecting the visual fields.

THE ORBIT

The eye and orbit comprise a unique and complex region of the nervous system, which presents a challenge to the neuroradiologist because of its highly specialized anatomy, pathology, and physiology. It is obvious from the radiologic and ophthalmologic literature that MR can demonstrate virtually the entire spectrum of orbital and ocular diseases (1–22). Although orbital MRI was initially regarded with a great deal of skepticism, the advent and subsequent improvement of small diameter surface coils (Fig. 1) (23–25) represented a major step in the maturation of MR. It is generally held that the development and refinement of surface coil technology has proved critical for the success of MR in the orbit. MRI has certainly progressed technically since the first edition of this chapter, and many of these technical innovations are directly applicable to evaluation of the visual system. These technical advances have brought attention to situations where MR provides information that is not available on computed tomography (CT) alone. Despite recent improvements in such areas as rapid imaging and high resolution techniques, our endorsement of MR for the orbit must remain a qualified one, because CT undeniably shows excellent contrast between normal retrobulbar fat and disease, and because MR is so sensitive to globe and lid motion. These two facts are not likely to change, regardless of any refinements in MR technology. Despite these uncertainties

S. W. Atlas, M.D.: Neuroradiology Division, Department of Radiology, Oregon Health Sciences University, Portland, Oregon 97201.
S. L. Galetta, M.D.: Departments of Neurology and Ophthalmology, Hospital of the University of Pennsylvania, Philadelphia, PA 19104.

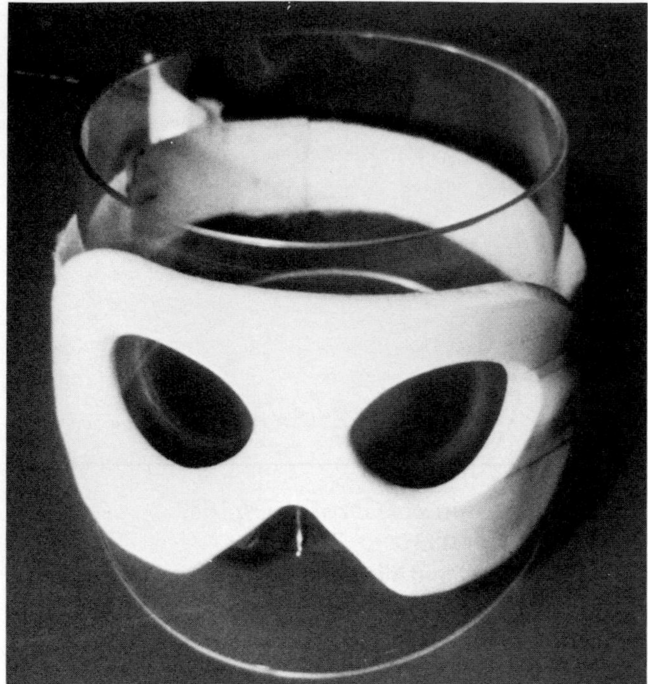

FIG. 1. Flexible binocular surface coil. Wrap-around soft mask configuration coil allows imaging of both orbits with minimal patient discomfort and reduces problems from asymmetric coil placement. (From Atlas, ref. 34, with permission.)

and concerns regarding limitations, contraindications (26,27), and artifacts (Figs. 2–4) (1,28,29), it is clear that MR is a powerful tool in state-of-the-art imaging of the orbit and can provide important information that is unavailable on CT scanning.

In this section, the normal anatomy of the eye and orbit are briefly reviewed, with particular attention to features that are of relevance to MR imaging. The diagnosis of ocular and orbital pathology, as depicted by high resolution MR, is discussed and related to pathologic and clinical findings. Overall advantages and limitations of MR as compared to other imaging modalities, as well as its current indications and contraindications, are discussed and illustrated. Clinical applications of adjunctive pulse sequences also are noted.

Basic Orbital MRI Techniques

We believe that optimal MR evaluation of most orbital lesions necessitates the use of small diameter surface coils. Surface coils should be employed for evaluating superficial periorbital and lid lesions, the globe, and all retrobulbar structures as far posterior as the orbital apex. The advantage of surface coil imaging lies in its resultant increase in the signal-to-noise ratio (SNR) (23–25). This is accomplished in two ways. First, the signal is stronger because the receive-coil (the surface coil) is closer to the area of interest. Second, unwanted patient-generated noise from areas outside the region of interest is reduced. The marked increase in SNR has permitted thinner sections and higher spatial resolution without the penalty of prolonged imaging time that often results in motion artifacts that particularly degrade orbit images (1).

Orbital surface coils vary greatly in shape and size. Both monocular and binocular coils have been successfully used and each type of coil has its own particular strengths and weaknesses. Our orbital surface coils range in diameter from 7 cm to 9 × 14 cm, and are oval, round, mask, or figure-of-eight in configuration. The shape and size of the coil are both clinically important, so the particular coil should be chosen with consideration of the clinical setting. First, it may be useful to compare the

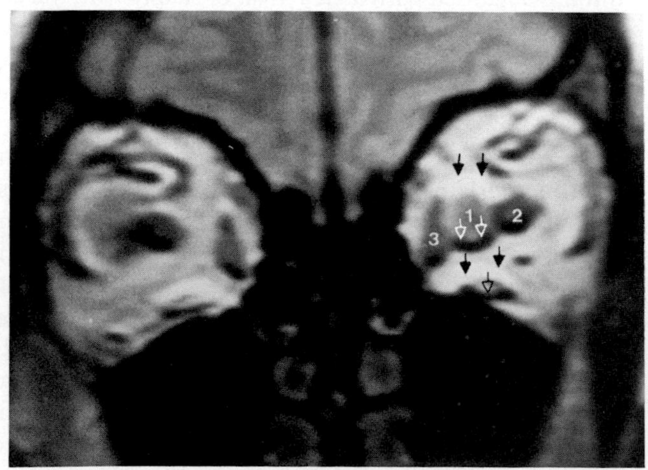

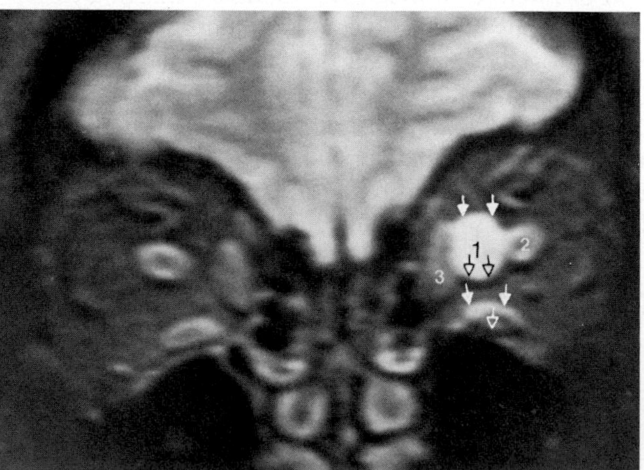

FIG. 2. Chemical shift misregistration artifact. **A:** Coronal long TR/short TE MRI. **B:** Coronal long TR/TE MRI. Note hyperintense bands (*closed arrows*) at fat–water interfaces and hypointense bands at water-fat interfaces (*open arrows*) along the frequency-encoding axis (superior-inferior), more evident on long TR/short TE image (A). Patient has intraconal mass (*1*) between left optic nerve (*2*) and left medial rectus muscle (*3*). (From Atlas, ref. 34, with permission.)

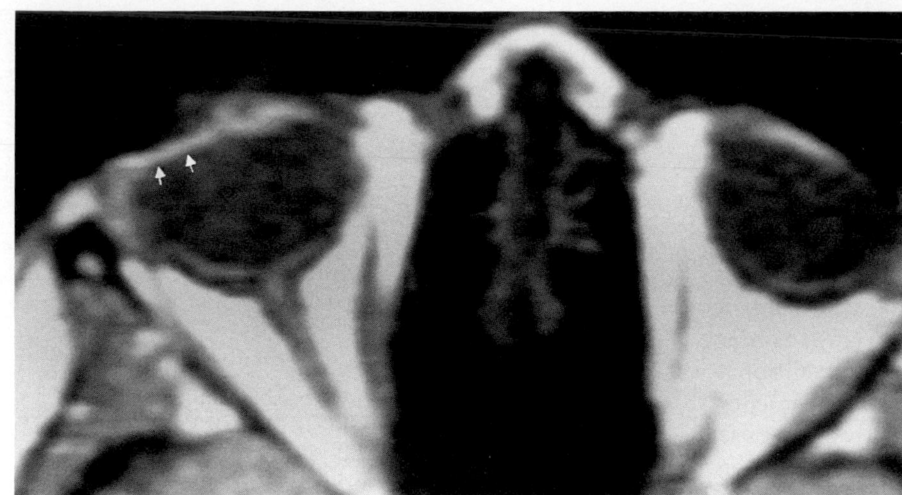

FIG. 3. Ferromagnetic artifact from mascara (600/20). Hyperintense linear region (*arrows*) posterior to adjacent region of signal void obscures part of right globe and lens, due to metallic particles in lid mascara. (From Atlas, ref. 34, with permission.)

contents of both orbits, so, in these cases, the coil ideally must be large enough to encompass the region of both orbits (see Fig. 1). In practice, many patients have unilateral symptoms or have already had CT scans. Those patients who have CT-documented unilateral lesions usually can be evaluated with a monocular coil, whereas bilateral abnormalities should be imaged with a coil that can be placed over the area of both orbits simultaneously. Second, the depth from which useful signal is received is highly dependent on the diameter of the signal receiver (i.e., the surface coil) (23–25). The radiologist must be cognizant of the fact that the signal drop-off also depends strongly on the distance of the region of interest from the surface coil (23–25). The farther from the coil that the lesion is situated, and the smaller the coil diameter, the greater the signal drop-off. Therefore, the area of interest should be ascertained, if possible, at the start of the examination so that the appropriate coil can be selected. Orbital apex pathology requires either a larger surface coil, a standard head coil, or both (1) for optimal imaging. It should be noted that the optic chiasm is not optimally imaged with a surface coil, because this structure is nearly in the center of the intracranial space. In fact, the ideal coil for imaging the sella and parasellar region is the standard head coil. In all orbit cases, the radiologist should take an active role in the selection of the coil, because the quality of the MR examination can be drastically changed by the coil selection alone (see Fig 4).

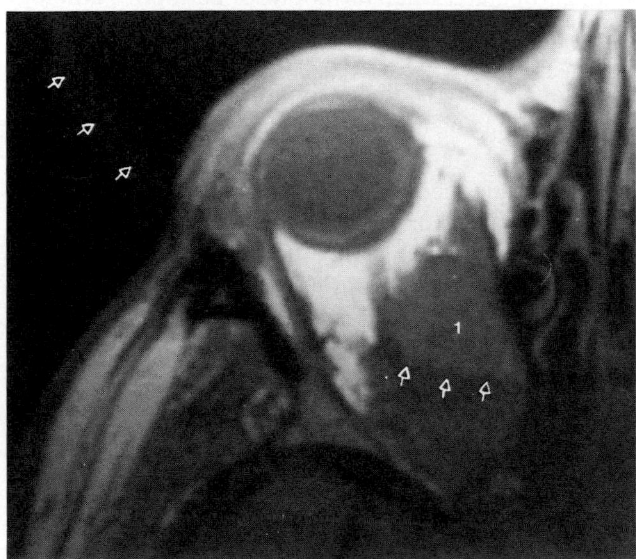

FIG. 4. Aliasing causing artifactual intralesional signal heterogeneity (600/20). Apparent high intensity in anterior part of retrobulbar mass (*1*) is due to aliasing of signal from the back of the patient's head (*arrows*). This was caused by unwanted coupling of the surface coil to the body coil. (From Atlas, ref. 34, with permission.)

In our experience, the nemesis of surface coil orbital MR and the major cause of a suboptimal examination is still artifact from globe and lid motion. There are two principal methods of minimizing artifacts from this nonperiodic orbital motion: (a) attempt to reduce the motion itself, and (b) keep the imaging time short. We instruct each patient to fix their gaze with their eyes open in one direction during the entire scan time when we are scanning with a surface coil. Perhaps most importantly, however, the scan time must be kept to a minimum (while maintaining the quality of the image). The scanning time depends on three factors: (a) repetition time (TR), (b) number of excitations (NEX), and (c) number of phase-encoding steps. Because of the high SNR when using a small diameter surface coil, high quality, thin, short TR/TE (T1-weighted) spin-echo (SE) scans can be obtained in approximately 3 minutes (especially at high field strength) (at the time of this writing, we use 1 NEX, with TR of 500 and 512 × 256 matrix). Cooperative patients can usually fix their gaze for up to 3 to 4 minutes. Although increased SNR would result from increasing the number of excitations or prolonging TR, we have found that the vast majority of surface coil studies of the orbits are suboptimal when all these parameters are "maximized" for that purpose. Just as in all MR protocols, all parameter changes have potential drawbacks, and the added imaging time required for increasing SNR in the orbit is invariably accompanied by motion artifacts (1). We usually opt for interslice gaps of 20% to 50% of the slice thickness when using SE imaging (i.e., for a 3-mm thick scan, slices are separated by 0.6–1.5 mm), since interslice gaps minimize cross-talk. The field of view should be small (approximately 12–16 cm), in order to maximize spatial resolution. Since conventional 3DFT volume acquisitions are typically too time consuming for routine use in the orbit, we nearly always use 2DFT techniques. Newer fast spin echo (FSE) imaging has permitted 3DFT high resolution in short acquisition times; it remains to be seen whether there is significant clinical advantage to 3DFT methods for orbital disease.

All SE MR examinations should include both short TR and long TR sequences for full lesion characterization, as one of the unique strengths of MR over other imaging modalities is the ability to provide information beyond anatomic localization (i.e., signal intensity patterns for tissue characterization). Since conventional long TR SE imaging sequences result in a significant increase in imaging time (approximately 8–12 minutes), marked image degradation from globe motion has usually resulted, in our experience, in poor scans when these sequences were used with surface coils (1,3). We now routinely employ FSE for T2-weighted imaging of the eye and orbit (Fig. 5). This technique can generate high resolution (512 × 256) thin sections in less than 2 minutes, thereby allowing T2-weighted imaging in virtually all patients. Since fat is hyperintense on FSE scans, we recommend combining fat suppression with all T2-weighted imaging in the orbit when FSE sequences are used.

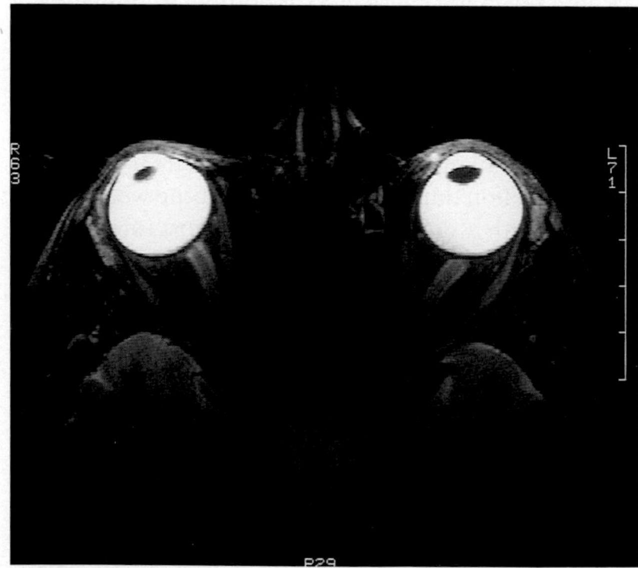

FIG. 5. T2-weighted FSE of orbit. Note anatomic detail in an essentially motion-free image even though T2-weighted technique was used.

TABLE 1. *Indications for i.v. contrast enhancement in orbital MRI*

Ocular lesions	Retrobulbar disease
R/O intraocular tumor	Perioptic vs. optic nerve mass
Tumor vs. non-neoplastic detachment	R/O meningioma
R/O episcleral extension	R/O optic neuritis
R/O endophthalmitis	R/O orbital inflammation
R/O multiple lesions	Mass lesion characterization

i.v., intravenous; R/O, rule out.

Plane of section should be chosen to optimally visualize the specific structure or area in question, as in all other regions of the body. This is especially important in orbital MR because the initial series of images is often the least affected by motion. We feel that, ideally, all orbital MR examinations should include T1-weighted images in at least two planes. Our standard protocol always includes axial and coronal scans. The optimal plane for lesion visualization (as depicted by the T1-weighted sequences) should then be selected for imaging with a long TR multi-echo FSE sequence.

It has become apparent that intravenous (i.v.) contrast plays a significant role in imaging orbital and ocular disease, particularly since fat suppression techniques are now routinely implemented. We do not believe that all orbit cases necessarily require i.v. contrast. In many settings, particularly when intraoptic or perioptic pathology is suspected, however, i.v. contrast is important (Table 1).

Although there is obviously no single "correct" technique for imaging any part of the body in MRI, we believe that the standard MR examination of the orbit should include the following: T1-weighted and FSE T2-weighted images using small diameter surface coils, with (a) thin (3 mm or less) slice thickness, (b) at least two scan planes, (c) short scanning times (preferably under 3 minutes), (d) small field of view (12–16 cm) and (e) a high resolution matrix (at least 256 × 256). We also routinely use fat suppression in all cases where i.v. contrast is administered. Finally, we believe that the vast majority of cases should also undergo long TR/multi-echo images of the brain.

Normal Anatomy

The anatomy of the orbit and its contents have been thoroughly reviewed by many authors (30–32) and have been described as depicted by high resolution CT (33). The ease of imaging in multiple planes, coupled with the high inherent contrast of intraorbital structures as visualized by SE MR imaging, makes the anatomy of the orbit ideal for evaluation by this modality.

The characteristic intensity of retrobulbar fat (high intensity using T1-weighted sequences, and low intensity using T2-weighted sequences with fat suppression when FSE is used) and the absence of signal from cortical bone and (in most cases) flowing blood provides an excellent background for depiction of intraorbital anatomy and pathology using SE pulse sequences. Newer, ultrahigh resolution MR techniques combined with high gradient strength systems offers the potential to depict anatomic detail approaching that of low-power microscopic examination. Since MR allows recognition of some previously nonvisualized structures on conventional imaging modalities (4,34,35), a thorough knowledge of normal orbital and ocular anatomy (Figs. 6–8) is essential to the understanding and recognition of disease entities involving this region.

Orbital Walls and Canals

The orbits are pyramid-shaped bony compartments that contain the globes and their associated muscles, nerves, and blood vessels, as well as retrobulbar fat and the lacrimal glands (30,31). The orbital apex is directed posteriorly, and its base projects anteriorly. The four walls of the orbit separate intraorbital contents from the surrounding brain and facial structures, and are seen as signal void on all MR images, because they are essentially dense cortical bone.

The roof of the orbit is triangular in shape and is formed by the orbital plate of the frontal bone and by the lesser wing of the sphenoid, separating the orbit from the anterior cranial fossa. The lacrimal gland resides in the lacrimal fossa in the superolateral aspect of the orbit anteriorly. At the superomedial aspect of the orbit anteriorly is a small fossa (the trochlear pit) at the site of attachment of the cartilaginous pulley (trochlea) of the superior oblique muscle tendon (see Fig. 6). In the posterior portion of the roof of the orbit lies the optic canal, situated between the roots of the lesser wing of the sphenoid (the optic struts) and lying lateral to the body of the sphenoid bone. This canal transmits the optic nerve and its meninges, as well as the ophthalmic artery and sympathetic nerves, from the middle cranial fossa. The optic strut separates the optic canal from the superior orbital fissure. The signal void from these bony structures on MR serves to highlight the intracanalicular optic nerve and other structures coursing through the fissures and canals. Importantly, these areas are often suboptimally visualized on CT because of beam-hardening artifacts.

The floor of the orbit is comprised of the maxilla, but also has contributions from the zygomatic and palatine bones. The infraorbital nerve (from the second division of the Vth cranial nerve) and its accompanying artery course along the floor of the orbit in the infraorbital groove, as they pass from the inferior orbital fissure to the infraorbital foramen. This nerve is clearly delineated as a soft tissue structure on coronal MR and should be sought in cases of maxillary sinus processes or trauma because it is commonly affected clinically. From the anteromedial angle of the floor of the orbit, lateral to the nasolacrimal canal, arises the inferior oblique muscle. Anteriorly, the orbital rim is in continuity with the anterior wall of the maxillary sinus below.

The lateral wall of the orbit, the thickest and strongest orbital wall, separates the orbital contents from the temporal fossa, which contains the temporalis muscle. This wall is formed by the zygomatic bone and the greater wing of the sphenoid. Two major fissures are present in the later wall of the orbit. The superior orbital fissure lies between the greater and lesser sphenoid wings and is separated medially from the optic canal by the optic strut. The wider, more medial portion of the superior orbital fissure transmits the superior ophthalmic vein, cranial nerves III, IV, VI, and the ophthalmic division of V, and sympathetic nerve fibers between the orbit and the middle cranial fossa. The inferior orbital fissure connects the orbit with the infratemporal and the pterygopalatine fossae. It is between the maxilla and the palatine bone below and the greater sphenoid wing above. The inferior orbital fissure transmits the infraorbital artery, nerve, and the venous connection between the inferior ophthalmic vein and the pterygoid venous plexus.

The medial wall, the thinnest wall of the orbit, separates the ethmoid and sphenoid sinus air cells from the orbit. The largest component of the medial wall is formed by the ethmoidal orbital plate and is termed the "lamina papyracea."

The orbital septum is a thin fibrous sheath continuous with periosteum that is attached to the anterior orbital margin (see Figs. 6–8). It extends to the levator superioris of the upper eyelid and the tarsal plate of the lower eyelid. This low intensity structure divides the orbit into pre- and postseptal compartments and is important in limiting spread of infection. The extensive orbit fat is delimited anteriorly by the orbital septum.

Muscles of the Globe

Six skeletal extraocular muscles insert on the sclera and control motion of the eyeball (see Figs. 6–8). The four rectus muscles (superior, inferior, lateral, and medial) arise from a common tendinous ring, the annulus of Zinn, and form a muscle cone that runs forward and inserts onto the front of the sclera. The superior rectus is the longest muscle, being approximately 40 mm in length, and the medial rectus has the largest diameter in the normal orbit. The medial and lateral recti lie in the

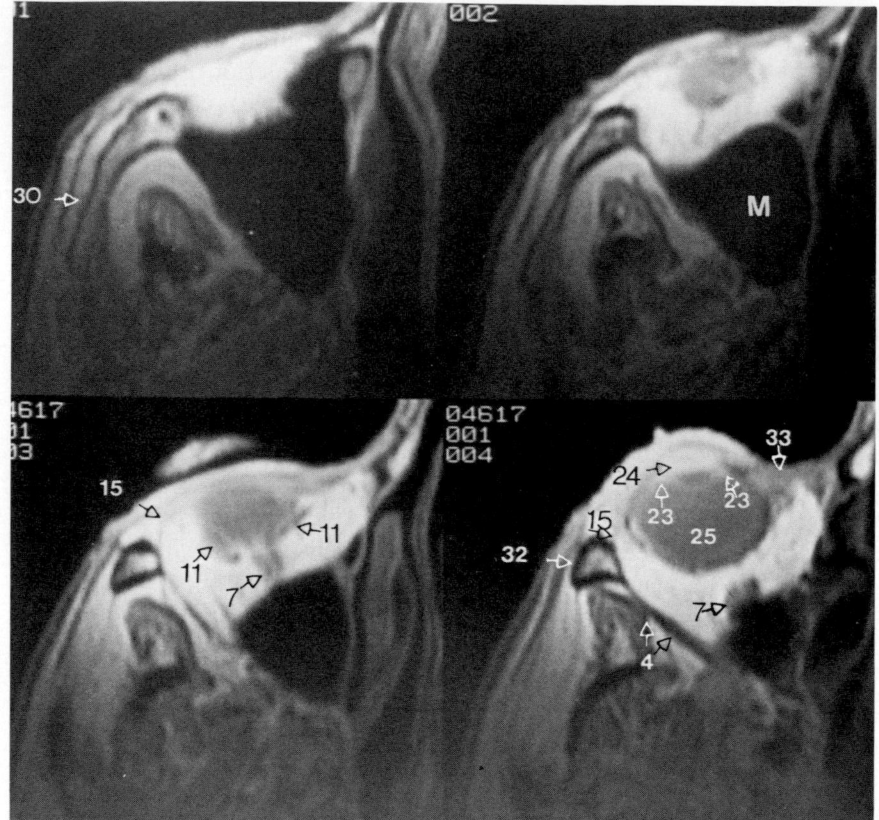

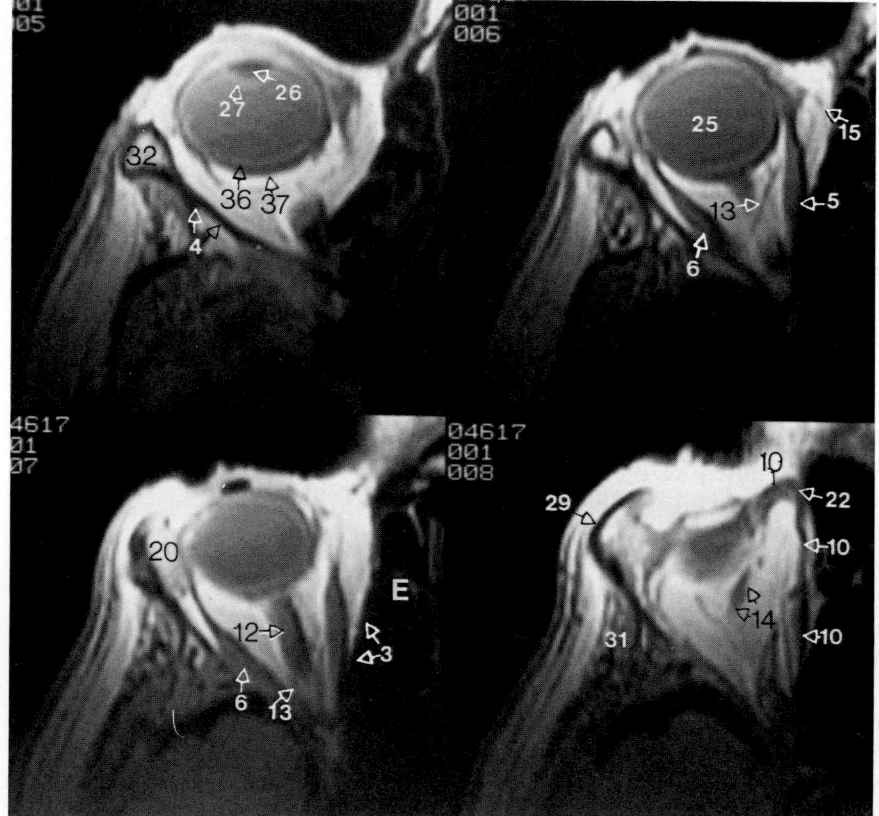

FIG. 6. Normal axial MR anatomy (600/20, inferior to superior). *1,* floor of orbit; *2,* roof of orbit; *3,* medial wall; *4,* lateral wall; *5,* medial rectus; *6,* lateral rectus; *7,* inferior rectus; *8,* superior rectus; *9,* levator palpebrae superioris; *10,* superior oblique; *11,* inferior oblique; *12,* optic nerve; *13,* ophthalmic artery; *14,* superior ophthalmic vein; *15,* orbital septum; *16,* frontal nerve; *17,* supraorbital nerve and artery; *18,* infraorbital nerve; *19,* lacrimal nerve and artery; *20,* lacrimal gland; *21,* (probable) oculomotor nerve branches; *22,* trochlea of superior oblique; *23,* ciliary body and iris; *24,* anterior chamber; *25,* vitreous; *26,* lens (nucleus); *27,* lens (cortex); *28,* frontozygomatic suture; *29,* frontal bone; *30,* zygoma; *31,* temporalis muscle, *32,* malar eminence; *33,* medial palpebral ligament; *34,* upper eyelid; *35,* lower eyelid; *36,* choroid/retina; *37,* sclera; *F,* frontal sinus; *E,* ethmoid sinus; *M,* maxillary sinus. (From Atlas, ref. 34, with permission.)

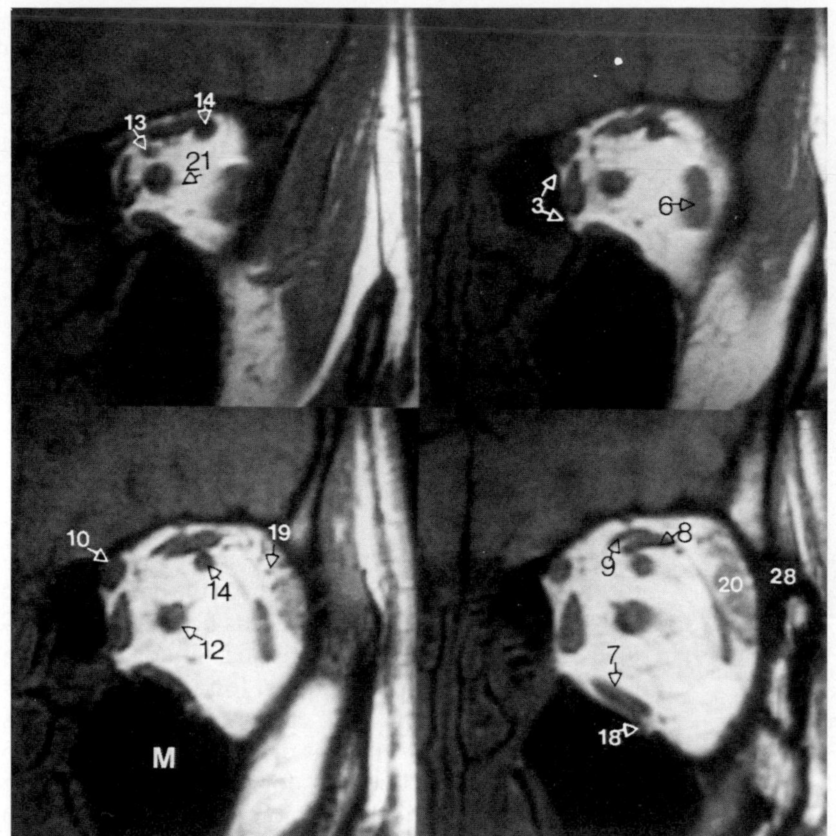

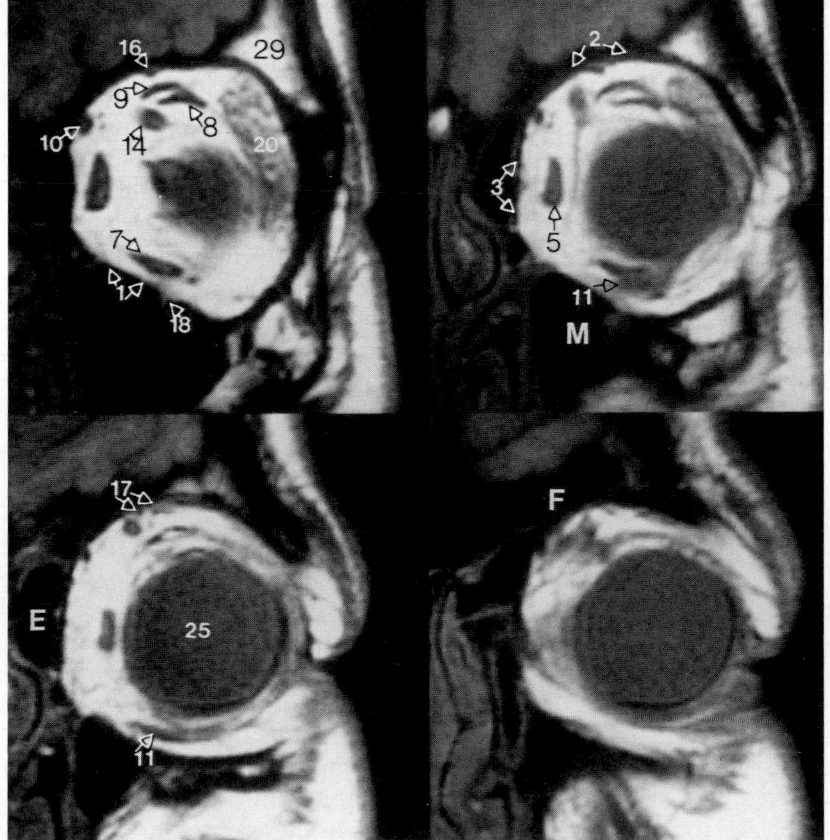

FIG. 7. Normal coronal MR anatomy (short TR/TE, posterior to anterior). (See legend to Fig. 6.) (From Atlas, ref. 34, with permission.)

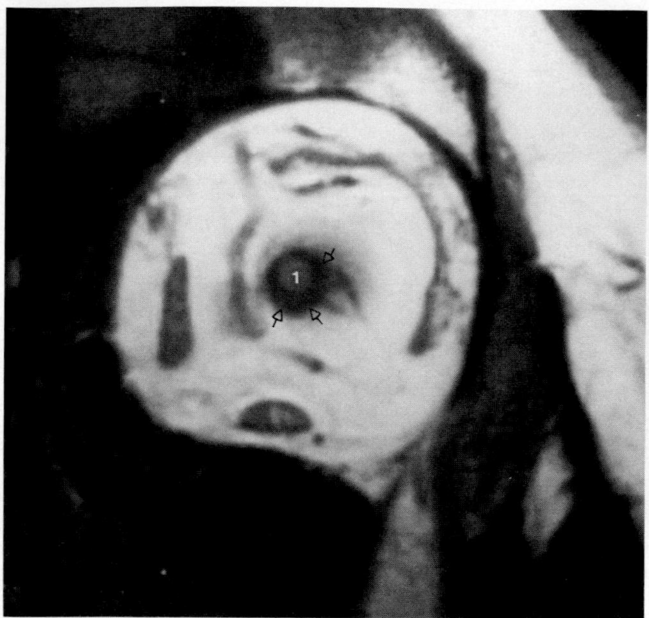

FIG. 8. Normal optic nerve and perioptic subarachnoid space, coronal MRI (short TR/TE). Coronal short TR/TE surface-coil image clearly depicts perioptic CSF (*arrows*) surrounding optic nerve (*1*) in normal patient. (From Atlas, ref. 34, with permission.)

same axial plane, and the superior and inferior recti lie in the same vertical plane (31). The oblique muscles insert into the posterior portion of the sclera. The superior oblique is the thinnest extraocular muscle and lies in the superomedial aspect of the orbit, coursing forward above the medial rectus muscle. Its tendon passes through the cartilaginous trochlea, turns laterally, posteriorly, and downward and inserts into the posterolateral aspect of the sclera. The course of this muscle is well delineated by MR (see Fig. 6). The inferior oblique muscle, the only muscle to arise from the front of the orbit (31), originates from a depression in the upper surface of the maxilla, lateral to the nasolacrimal canal. This muscle passes backward and laterally, inferior to the inferior rectus, to insert onto the posterolateral sclera. Its course is best seen on coronal images. The superior oblique muscle is supplied by the trochlear nerve and the lateral rectus is supplied by the abducens nerve, whereas all other extraocular muscles are supplied by the oculomotor nerve (see Fig. 7).

The levator palpebrae superioris muscle can usually be distinguished from the superior rectus muscle with high resolution coronal MR. It is also supplied by the oculomotor nerve, and lies just under the roof of the orbit, above the superior rectus muscle. This muscle controls the upper eyelid. Below the superior rectus lies the superior ophthalmic vein and below it lies the optic nerve, all clearly seen on coronal images.

The normal extraocular muscle has intermediate intensity on short TR/TE images and stands out as hypointense against the background high intensity orbital fat. On long TR/TE images, normal muscle is isointense or minimally hyperintense to fat (Fig. 9). If one uses FSE sequences for T2-weighted imaging of the orbit, retrobulbar fat is hyperintense and therefore would obscure most lesions. We routinely use fat suppression in this sequence. It should be noted that normal muscles enhance significantly after i.v. contrast; this enhancement is dramatic on fat-suppressed images (Fig. 10).

Nerves of the Orbit

The optic nerve (the second cranial nerve) interconnects the retina with the brain and extends approximately 3.5 to 5 cm in length between the posterior globe and the optic chiasm.

Approximately 90% of its fibers are afferent (36) arising in the retinal ganglion cell layer. In the orbit, the optic nerve lies intraconally and proceeds backward and medially from the globe in an oblique, sinuous course to gain entry into the middle cranial fossa via the optic canal, and ending in the optic chiasm. The optic nerve is fully myelinated by 7 months of age, but it continues to increase in size and thickness for the first 8 years of life (37). The intracanalicular portion of the nerve (Fig. 11) measures 4 to 9 mm and enters the optic canal superior to the ophthalmic artery. The intraorbital optic nerve is surrounded by continuations of the three layers of meninges and is surrounded by a subarachnoid space filled with cerebrospinal fluid (CSF). The outermost dura fuses with orbital periosteum and with the annulus of Zinn, perhaps explaining the finding of pain associated with eye movement in optic neuritis (37). Perioptic arachnoid is adherent to pia and dura within the optic canal except along its inferior side, which is the only site of free communication between periotic and intracranial subarachnoid spaces (37). Although opacification of the perioptic subarachnoid space has been recognized on CT following intrathecal contrast administration (38), high resolution MR has essentially obviated this procedure. The normal intraorbital optic nerve is usually clearly separable from surrounding CSF on SE images (see Fig. 8).

The ophthalmic nerve (the first division of the Vth cranial nerve) is a sensory nerve that receives input from the globe and its conjunctivae, the lacrimal gland, the nose and nasal mucosa, the upper lid, frontal sinus, scalp, and forehead (30,31). Arising from the trigeminal ganglion, it traverses the dura in the lateral aspect of the cavernous sinus to divide near the superior orbital fissure into its three branches: lacrimal, frontal, and nasociliary. These small branches subsequently pass through the superior orbital fissure into the orbit, and can often be seen on short TR/TE MR images as they course through the orbital fat. The lacrimal nerve enters the orbit superior to the annulus of Zinn (a tendinous ring from which the

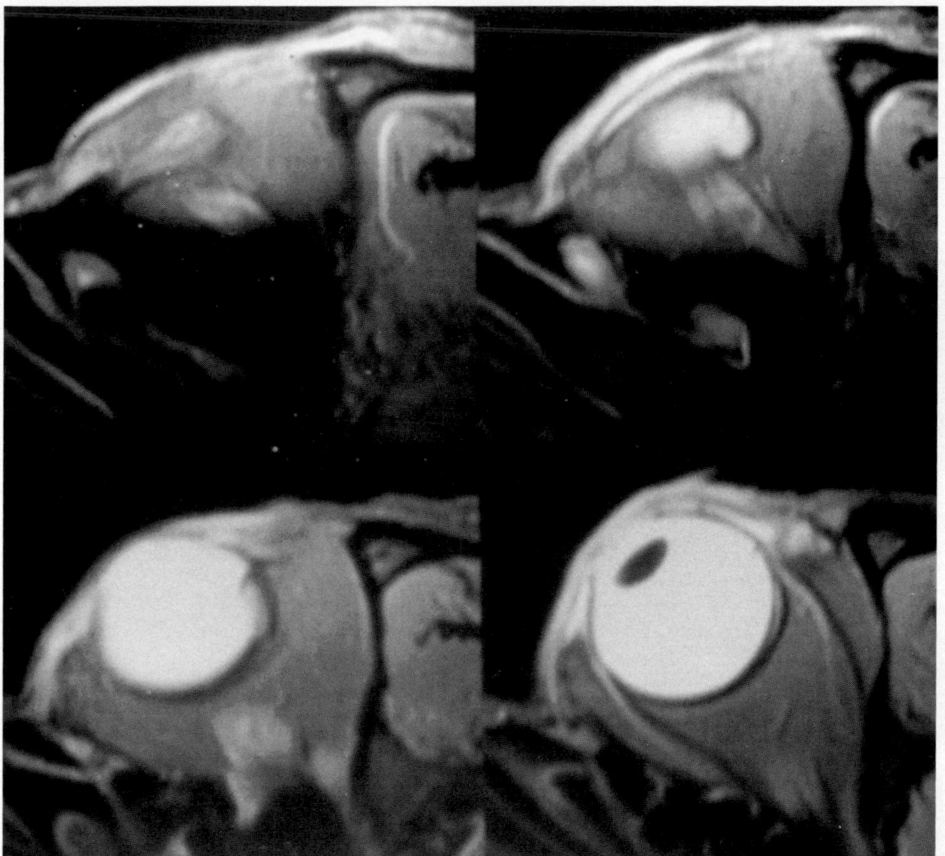

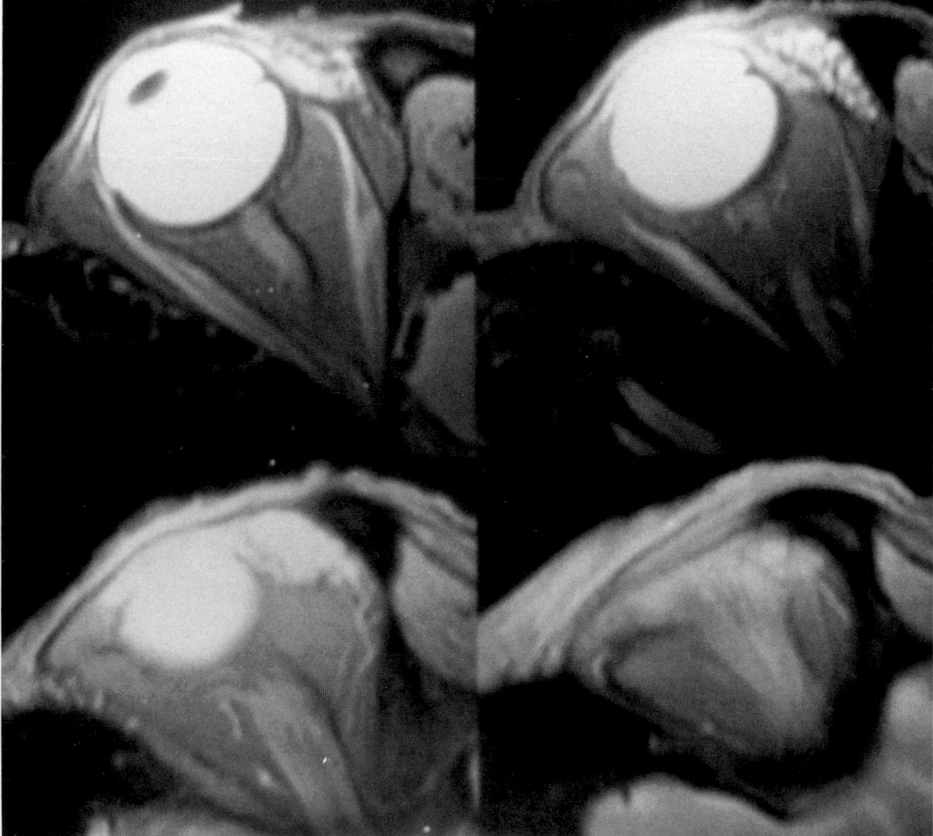

FIG. 9. Normal orbital structures, long TR/TE MR images, inferior to superior. **A,B:** Normal muscles are only minimally hyperintense to retrobulbar fat on long TR/TE images. Superolaterally situated lacrimal gland is heterogeneous but also hyperintense, mainly due to proximity to coil.

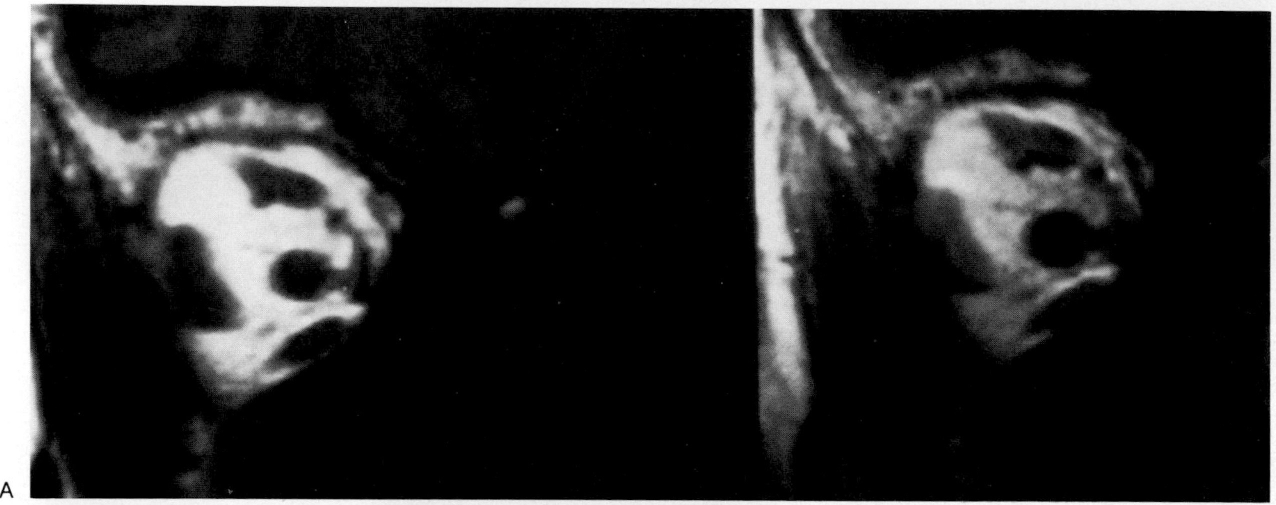

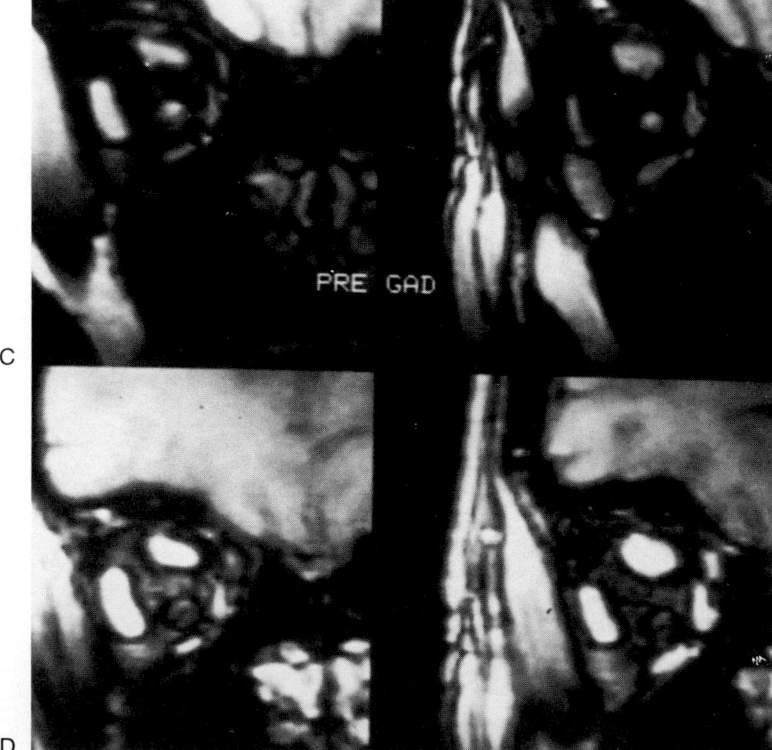

FIG. 10. Normal retrobulbar enhancement after i.v. contrast. **A:** Coronal MRI (short TR/TE). **B:** Coronal MRI (short TR/TE), after i.v. contrast administration. **C:** Coronal fat-suppressed MRI (600/23). **D:** Coronal fat-suppressed MRI (600/23), after i.v. contrast administration. Enhancement of extraocular muscles is subtle on conventional SE images (compare B with A). Fat-suppressed images show definite increase in intensity after contrast in muscles, but not in nonenhancing nerve.

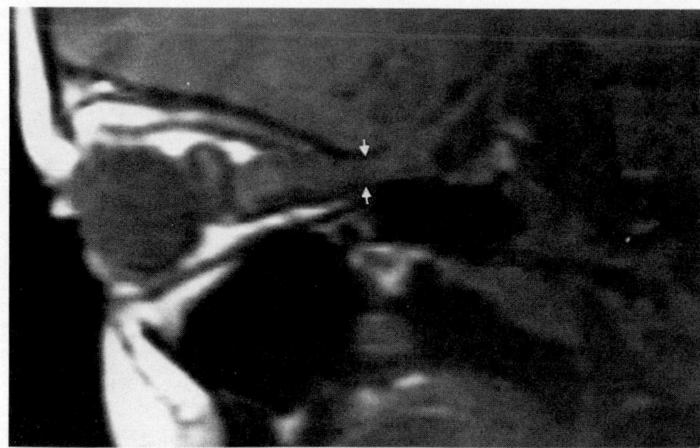

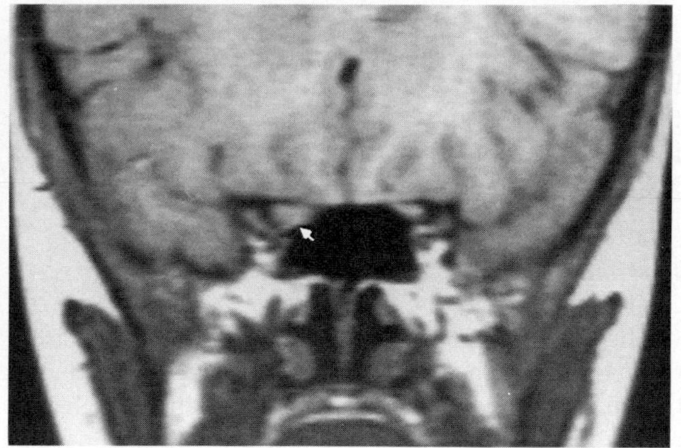

FIG. 11. Intracanalicular optic nerve glioma. **A:** Sagittal oblique MRI (short TR/TE). **B:** Coronal MRI (short TR/TE). Enlarged optic nerve is seen extending into the optic canal (*arrows*) on oblique sagittal image (A). Note the asymmetry in size of the intracanalicular nerves depicted on the coronal view (B). (From Atlas, ref. 34, with permission.)

rectus muscles arise) and proceeds along the lateral aspect of the extraconal space (with the lacrimal artery), above the superior border of the lateral rectus muscle, to give branches to the lacrimal gland, upper eyelid, and conjunctiva. The frontal nerve is also extraconal in location and courses anteriorly on the levator palpebrae superioris muscle (superior to the superior rectus muscle). The nasociliary nerve, the sensory nerve for the globe, enters the orbit via the superior orbital fissure to its intraconal location, between the two divisions of the oculomotor nerve. It runs anteriorly under the superior rectus muscle and courses medially to lie between the superior oblique and the medial rectus muscles. The nasociliary nerve forms part of the afferent limb of the corneal reflex (31).

The IIIrd cranial nerve, or oculomotor nerve, is the major motor supply for eye movements, supplying extraocular muscles except the superior oblique and lateral rectus muscles. After emerging from the midbrain just medial to the cerebral peduncle, it runs just lateral to the posterior communicating artery and then traverses the cavernous sinus. The nerve divides into a superior and inferior division, which enter the superior orbital fissure to lie within the muscle cone of the orbit, flanking the nasociliary nerve. The trochlear nerve (IVth cranial nerve), the only motor nerve that arises from the dorsal aspect of the CNS, decussates and emerges from the back of the brainstem below the inferior colliculus. Because of its peculiar site of origin, it is commonly contused after severe closed head trauma. It passes from the brainstem through the lateral cavernous sinus to traverse the superior orbital fissure, entering the orbit extraconally to supply the superior oblique muscle. The abducens nerve is the VIth cranial nerve and supplies only the lateral rectus muscle. Originating at the pontomedullary junction, it also traverses the cavernous sinus and enters the orbit intraconally via the superior orbital fissure, entering the medial aspect of the lateral rectus muscle.

Vessels of the Orbit

Vascular structures containing flowing blood emit variable signal intensities on SE MR, dependent on the pulse sequence parameters, the velocity of the flow, and physical properties of the state of flow (i.e., laminar, turbulent, etc.). In the orbital vessels detected by MRI, relevant normal flow phenomena (39–41) include (a) signal void, identified on most SE pulse sequences when flow is rapid or sufficiently complex (e.g., turbulent), (b) flow-related enhancement, seen as high intensity in patent, but relatively slow flow states, at entry level slices (i.e., at one end of a stack of acquired slices) or on gradient-echo images (42), and (c) second-echo rephasing (39), identified as high signal intensity within patent, but again relatively slowly flowing systems; whereby early echo images demonstrate low (or absent) signal and delayed, second-echo images show a marked increase in signal.

The ophthalmic artery is the chief artery of the orbit arising medial to the anterior clinoid process from the supraclinoid internal carotid artery. It passes anterolaterally through the optic canal, below the optic nerve. Intraorbitally, its course and relation to the optic nerve is variable until it divides into the supratrochlear and dorsal nasal arteries near the front of the orbit. It is usually visible on thin-section MR images as a very thin, serpentine structure with internal signal void.

The superior and inferior ophthalmic veins drain the orbital structures. The superior ophthalmic vein, the largest and most consistently visualized intraorbital vessel on MR images, forms at the root of the nose from the union of the supraorbital and angular veins and enters the intraconal space of the orbit to lie adjacent to the inferior aspect of the superior rectus muscle, above the optic nerve. It then turns medially and enters the superior orbital fissure at the orbital apex to drain into the cavernous sinus. The diameter of the superior ophthalmic vein varies from 2 to 3.5 mm and can change somewhat with head position or Valsalva maneuver. Asymmetry may be present in a normal patient (33). The inferior ophthalmic vein originates as a plexus on the floor of the orbit and drains either directly or indirectly into the cavernous sinus (30,31). It is not easily seen on MR unless pathologically enlarged.

Lacrimal Gland

The lacrimal gland lies in the lacrimal fossa, a postseptal, extraconal space in the superolateral aspect of the orbit anteriorly (see Figs. 5–9). The gland abuts the lateral rectus and levator superioris muscles. Although usually not a palpable structure unless involved with pathology, it is often located more anteriorly and therefore palpable in African-Americans, which is ascribed to a slightly shallower configuration of the orbit (37). The gland may normally be somewhat lobulated and heterogeneous on MR, but it is generally isointense to muscle on short and long TR/TE images. Therefore, normal lacrimal tissue can be minimally hyperintense to fat on long TR/TE scans. Note that if one uses a surface coil, the lacrimal gland, because of its proximity to the coil, may be hyperintense without true pathologic involvement (see Fig. 9), particularly when fat suppression is also used. Tears drain medially into superior and inferior canaliculi, which empty into the lacrimal sac in a small fossa at the inferomedial margin of the orbit, usually visualized only if pathologically enlarged (i.e., obstructed). The nasolacrimal duct measures 2 cm in length and empties into the inferior nasal meatus (31).

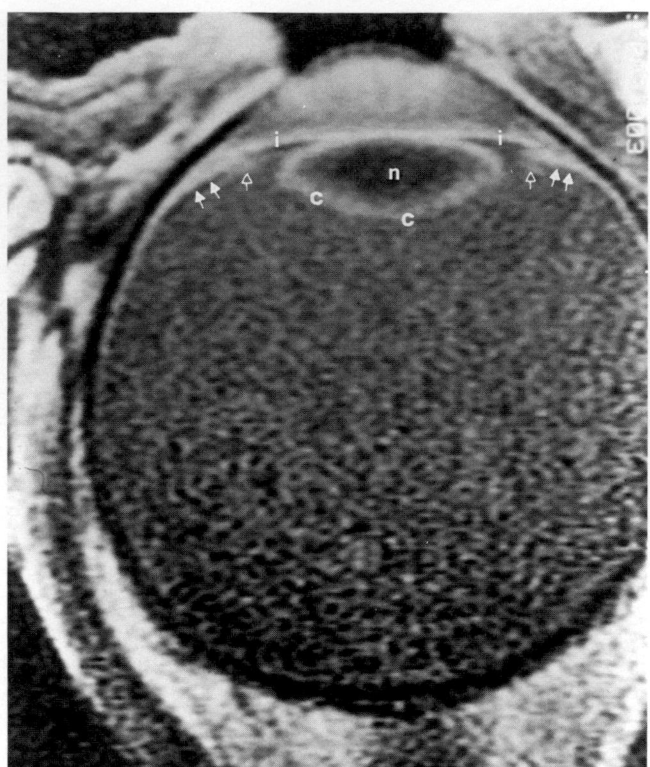

FIG. 12. Ultrahigh-resolution MR anatomy of globe (field-of-view 4 cm, 600/20, 3 mm thick). Extremely small field-of-view surface-coil image of globe shows high intensity of lens cortex (c) with low-intensity nucleus (*n*); hyperintense iris (*i*), pars plana (*closed arrows*), and pars plicata (*open arrows*) of ciliary body. The hyperintensity of aqueous in the anterior chamber probably is artifactual due to proximity to coil.

The Globe

Fine anatomic detail can be delineated by conventional surface-coil NM imaging of the globe (35) (see Figs. 6, 7, 9). Ultrahigh resolution techniques have shown promise in investigations of the "microanatomy" of the eye (Fig. 12) using either extremely small (e.g., 4 cm) fields of view (43) or very thin (1 mm) contiguous sections with a 3DFT acquisition (S.W. Atlas, *unpublished data*). As already noted, high gradient strength systems becoming commercially available offer further high resolution capabilities.

The eye occupies approximately one third (or less) of the volume of the orbit (31). The wall of the globe consists of three layers. The most outer layer is a fibrous protective layer that constitutes the sclera and, anteriorly, the transparent cornea. The cornea forms the anterior one sixth of the outer circumference of the globe. Its average diameter in the adult measures 10.5 mm vertically and 11.5 mm in the horizontal dimension (37). Centrally, the cornea is only 0.5 mm thick, where the anterior and posterior surfaces are in parallel. Whereas the cornea is composed of five distinct layers, the stroma (or substantia propria) forms 90% of its thickness. This layer is mainly interlacing, parallel bundles of avascular collagen fibrils, surrounded by mucopolysaccharide ground substance (37). The functions of the cornea are twofold: to protect the anterior segment of the eye, and to be a component of the eye's refractive system. The curvature of the cornea is stable throughout adult life in the absence of pathology, but it is significantly greater in newborns and young infants. The cornea on MR is mainly a low intensity structure because it is fibrocollagenous and very low in mobile water proton density. The cornea is highlighted by a thin rim of slight hyperintensity on short TR/TE images, which may represent the thin coat of adherent tear film, rather than corneal tissue itself (see Fig. 12). The rigid sclera comprises the remaining outer protective coat of the globe. It merges with the cornea at the limbus anteriorly. The sclera is also mainly composed of collagen bundles. Its thickness varies from 0.3 mm to 1.0 mm. It functions to protect the globe, maintain intraocular pressure, and serve as sites of attachment for extraocular muscles (37). The outer layer of sclera is continuous posteriorly with the optic nerve dura. The sclera changes shape and thickness throughout life. During early childhood, it thickens and becomes opaque, enlarging with the growth of the eye. With a sustained increase in intraocular pressure during this time, the sclera may stretch and result in an enlarged globe. In contrast, the adult sclera is less likely to stretch diffusely, but focal thinning with ectasia can result in staphylomas, or focal protrusions in areas of thinned sclera (37). In elderly patients, the sclera becomes even more rigid, owing to a decrease in hydration; scleral calcification can occur, commonly at sites of rectus muscle insertion (37). On MR, the sclera is similar to the cornea and other fibrocollagenous structures, and is seen as a thin, low intensity region at the periphery of the globe (see Fig. 12).

The uveal tract consists of the choroid, ciliary body, and iris, a set of structures having vascular and nutritive function. It contains, in addition to blood vessels, numerous nerves, connective tissue, and pigmented melanocytes. The vascular supply of the uveal tract is important to the neuroradiologist, because "blood–ocular barriers", analogous to the blood–brain barrier, are present at several points, including the retinal pigment epithelium (for the choroid), the retinal blood vessel endothelium (for the retina), vessel endothelium of the iris, and the pial and retinal vessels at the optic nerve head (37). The iris is a pigmented diaphragm that separates the region between the peripheral aspects of the lens and the superficial cornea into an anterior and posterior chamber. Both these chambers contain aqueous humor, and are depicted as fluid-containing spaces on MR. The peripheral part of the iris attaches to the ciliary body. Two major parts of the ciliary body are the pars plicata, which forms the most anterior 2 mm, and the pars plana, comprising the more posterior, flat portion (Fig. 13). The main source of aqueous is the pars plicata (37). The ciliary body extends from the iris to merge with the choroid at the ora serrata, which also marks the point of tight fusion between sensory retina and retina pigment epithelium. The ciliary body connects to the lens via the zonule, a suspensory ligament. These structures are involved in lens accommodation. The choroid extends from the ora serrata to the optic nerve head and is the major vascular and pigmented tissue of the "middle coat" of the globe (37). It ranges in thickness from 0.1 to

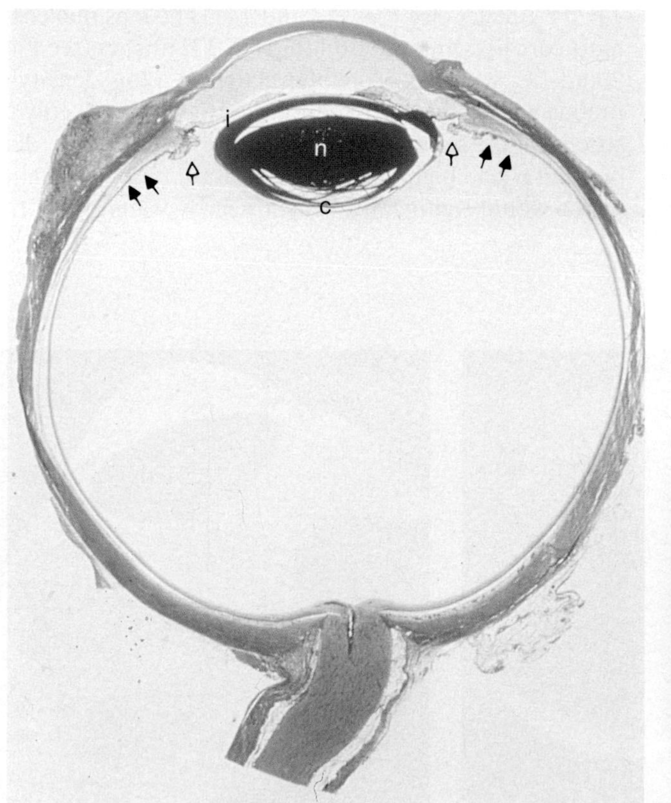

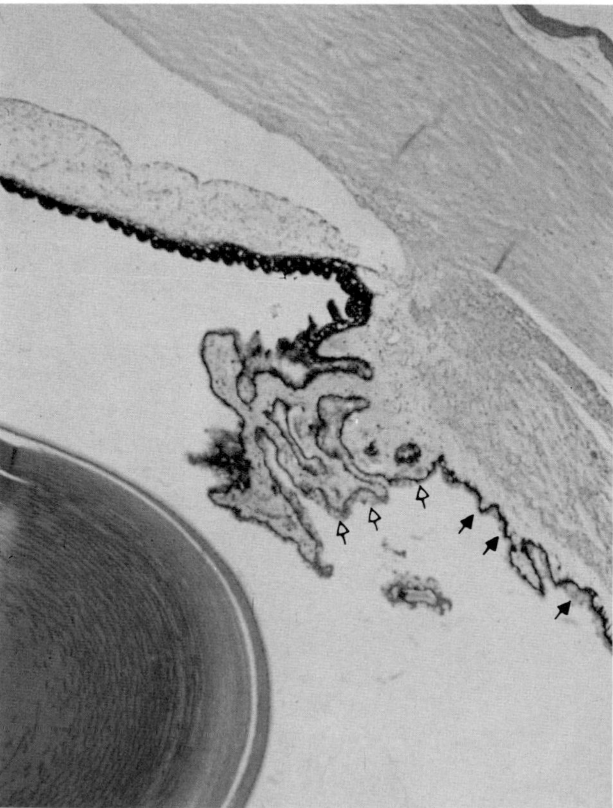

FIG. 13. Anatomic sections of globe. **A:** Low-power microscopic section of globe. **B:** High-power microscopic section of anterior chamber structures. Note that hyperintense structures of choroid have pigmented epithelium, perhaps accounting for shortened relaxation (refer to Fig. 11 legend for abbreviations). (Courtesy of Dr. A. Laties, Philadelphia, PA.)

0.22 mm. The entire uveal tract is hyperintense on short TR/TE MR images (Figs. 12 and 14). These structures stand out on long TR/TE images as low intensity against the hyperintense vitreous and aqueous (see Figs. 9 and 14). The retina consists of a thin, outer retinal pigment epithelium layer and an innermost sensory retina, which contains neural elements for visual perception. These two retinal layers are bound tightly only at the ora serrata and at the optic disc; otherwise, they are maintained in close apposition by the intraocular pressure and weak contact points. In young patients, the vitreous is rather firmly held to the inner sensory retina, but this bonding becomes tenuous with aging. MR can routinely separate the sclera from the choroid and retina because the fibrous sclera is low intensity on short TR images, in contrast to the hyperintense choroid/retina (see Fig. 12). High resolution conventional MR can often delineate the iris and ciliary body in cooperative patients. Ultrahigh resolution imaging (43) can separate the pars plana from the pars plicata of the ciliary apparatus (see Fig. 12). It has been hypothesized by the author that the high intensity of portions of the choroid, iris, and ciliary apparatus on short TR/TE images is related to their pigmented (i.e., melanin-containing) epithelium (see Fig. 13). Furthermore, it has been shown by electron microscopy that retinal pigment epithelium may contain other naturally occurring metallic (paramagnetic) ions, including iron and copper (44).

The lens is a normally transparent, biconvex crystalline structure approximately 1 cm in greatest diameter that transmits light and separates the aqueous from the vitreous. It forms part of the posterior boundary of the anterior chamber. Zonular fibers of the suspensory ligaments hold the lens in place by attaching it to the ciliary body. During fetal development, the lens is nearly spherical in shape, but eventually it assumes an elliptical configuration because of selective growth in the equatorial diameter into adult life. The infantile lens is usually seen as a globular and spherical shape. The adult lens, measuring approximately 4 μm in thickness, consists of multiple layers of cells arranged in a concentric pattern (30). These zones are acquired in a circumferential pattern with age, and their formation may depend on periods of slow growth (34). Cells forming the adult lens nucleus grow during childhood, whereas the lens cortex surrounding the nucleus continues to develop throughout life (37). The lens cortex is surrounded by a 2- to 20-μm thick lens capsule, essentially an acellular insoluble protein-polysaccharide material. The lens itself contains approximately two thirds water and one third structural protein. These proteins are synthesized in the cortex and precipitate in the nuclear region (45,46). Although the great majority of lens protein is soluble, the amount of insoluble protein increases in concentric layers toward the central part of the lens (37). The development of lens opacification (i.e., cataract), although of several diverse etiologies, seems to be related more to conformational changes in protein structure rather than to an increase in amount of insoluble protein (37). MR appears to be able to distinguish the low intensity lens nucleus from the external cortex, a more hyperintense structure on short TR/TE images (see Figs. 12 and 14). The lens nucleus is markedly hypointense on long TR/TE images (see Figs. 9 and 14), which is probably related to a low density of mobile water protons, in combination with markedly restricted motion of water by macromolecules (i.e., lens proteins). The highly structured nature of lens proteins, which would significantly affect nearby water, is a strik-

A,B
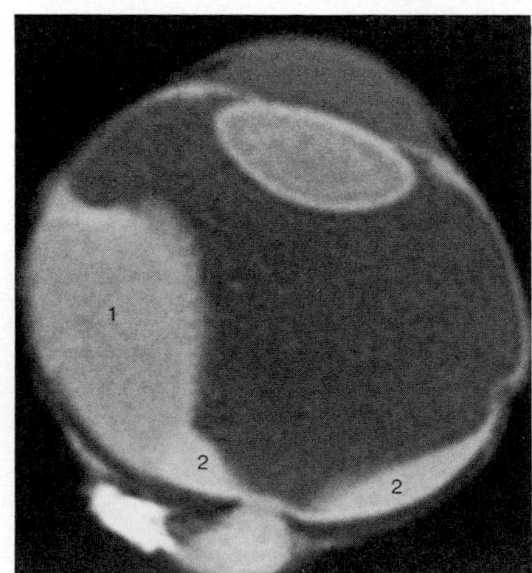

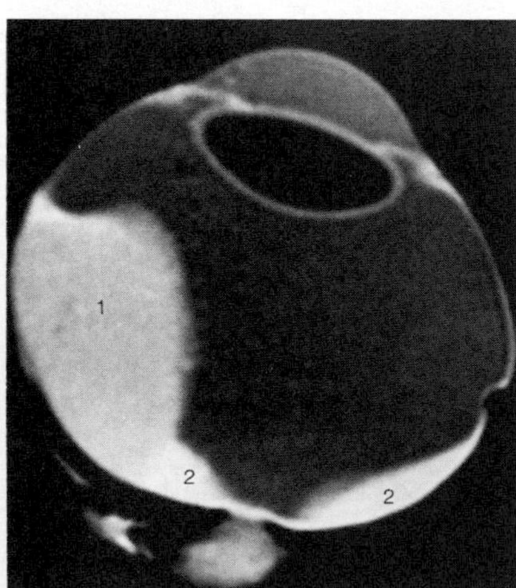

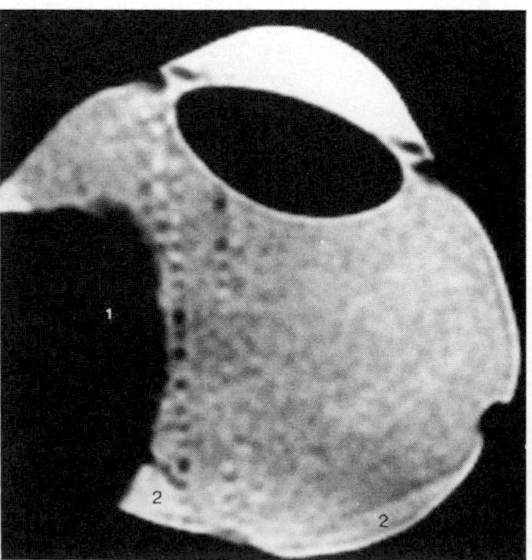

C

FIG. 14. Choroidal melanoma with detachment (ex vivo). **A:** Short TR/TE MRI (400/15). **B:** Long TR/short TE MRI (2000/15). **C:** Long TR/TE MRI (2000/75). Large choroidal melanoma (*1*) is hyperintense on short TR/TE (A) and hypointense on long TR/TE (C) due to presence of melanin. Note associated hemorrhagic detachment (2). (From Gomori et al., ref. 57, with permission.)

ing example of the importance of water motion, rather than merely water content, to the signal intensity on MR images (47).

Ocular Lesions

Ocular Melanoma

Malignant melanoma of the uveal tract (iris, choroid, ciliary body) is the most common intraocular malignancy in adults (48). Nearly always unilateral, melanomas usually occur in older patients and are uncommon in the pediatric age group. The clinical presentation varies from decreased visual acuity to pain or inflammation. After funduscopic diagnosis, the mainstay of imaging evaluation of ocular melanoma has been CT scanning. These lesions usually appear as focal masses of slightly increased attenuation, often showing slight enhancement with i.v. contrast (49,50). Associated retinal detachment is common but often indistinguishable from the neoplasm without i.v. contrast on CT scanning. Even ophthalmoscopy may fail to distinguish detachment or other benign entities from melanoma. The role of MRI in intraocular melanoma is based on its ability to aid differential diagnosis, as many benign and malignant lesions can simulate melanoma both funduscopically and on CT scanning (Tables 2 and 3). In addition, the detection of episcleral extent, which reportedly occurs in 13% of cases (51), or tumor recurrence is extremely important in these patients. Local recurrence of melanoma following orbital exenteration is extremely high if extraocular extension has already occurred.

The typical appearance of ocular melanoma on MR consists of a focal mass extending into the vitreous. These intraocular lesions have no characteristic morphology: they may be polypoid, flat, or crescentic (Figs. 14 and 15). Since they may arise from regions with pigmented epithelium, the entire uveal tract must be inspected for focal masses on MR. They enhance after i.v. contrast, as do most globe neoplasms, since the tumors are usually associated with an abnormal (or absent) "blood–ocular barrier" (52). In a study of 55 uveal melanomas, Peyster et al. (53) reported that 93% were markedly hyperintense to normal vitreous on short TR/TE images, whereas all four choroidal metastases were isointense or minimally hyperintense. On long TR/TE images, melanotic melanomas are typically (mildly) hypointense, whereas choroidal hemangioma has been reported as hyperintense on all SE sequences (53). It is well known, however, that melanoma varies significantly in its degree of pigmentation, and lesions may be virtually amelanotic, so amelanotic melanoma is indistinguishable from other amelanotic lesions on MR. Furthermore, mucinous ocular lesions (metastases) can appear similar to melanotic melanoma.

TABLE 2. *Differential diagnosis of choroidal melanoma in adult*

Malignant neoplasm	Malignant melanoma (melanotic or amelanotic)
	Choroidal metastasis (esp. breast or lung)
Benign neoplasm	Benign melanocytoma
	Choroidal hemangioma
	Astrocytic hamartoma
Inflammation	Sarcoidosis
	Granuloma
	Endophthalmitis
Other	Choroidal detachment
	Choroidal hematoma
	Retinal cyst
	Arterial macroaneurysm

Modified from Atlas et al., ref. 33, with permission.

TABLE 3. *Signal intensity patterns of melanoma versus hemorrhage*

	Signal intensity (relative to gray matter)	
	Short TR/TE	Long TR/TE
Amelanotic tumor	↓	= or sl.↑
Melanotic tumor	↑↑	= or sl.↓
Early subacute blood (intracellular methemoglobin)	↑↑	↓↓
Late subacute blood (extracellular methemoglobin)	↑↑	↑↑

sl., slightly.
Modified from Atlas et al., ref. 55, with permission.

Although ocular melanomas can display nearly pathognomic signal intensity patterns on MR, they can be confusing lesions because they exhibit paramagnetic behavior when they are melanotic or hemorrhagic (54–57), and are often associated with hemorrhagic detachments. Melanotic melanoma has a shorter T1 and T2 than the vast majority of other malignant tumors (54,55,57). The paramagnetic relaxation enhancement in melanin-containing tumors behaves as a dipole-dipole interaction, increasing 1/T1 and 1/T2 equally (55,57). Selective T2 shortening has not been observed at field strengths of up to 1.9T (56,57). Therefore, melanotic melanoma is high signal intensity on T1-weighted images (see Figs. 14 and 15) and usually only mildly hypointense on T2-weighted images (55,57). The degree of relaxation enhancement seems to be related to the degree of pigmentation of these neoplasms (55–57), although the etiology of the paramagnetic effect of melanin has never been completely elucidated. It has been documented that melanin contains relatively stable free radicals (58) which, by definition, have unpaired electrons. Enochs and others (59) have proposed that the relaxation enhancement in melanin-containing lesions may be related to the pres-

FIG. 15. Choroidal melanoma. **A:** Short TR/TE MRI (500/20). (From Atlas, ref. 127, with permission.) **B:** Resected specimen, amelanotic choroidal melanoma. **C:** Resected specimen, densely melanotic choroidal melanoma. Crescentic area of hyperintensity (*arrows,* A) in temporal aspect of right globe is compatible with known ocular melanotic melanoma. Note that melanomas can range from virtually amelanotic (*arrows,* B) to densely melanotic (*arrows,* C).

A

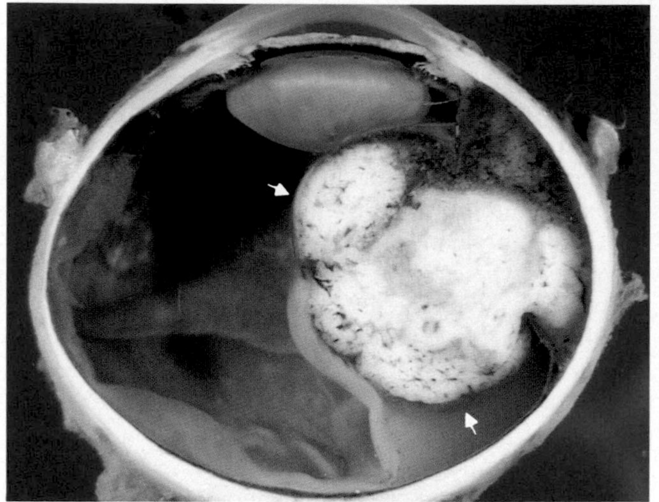

B

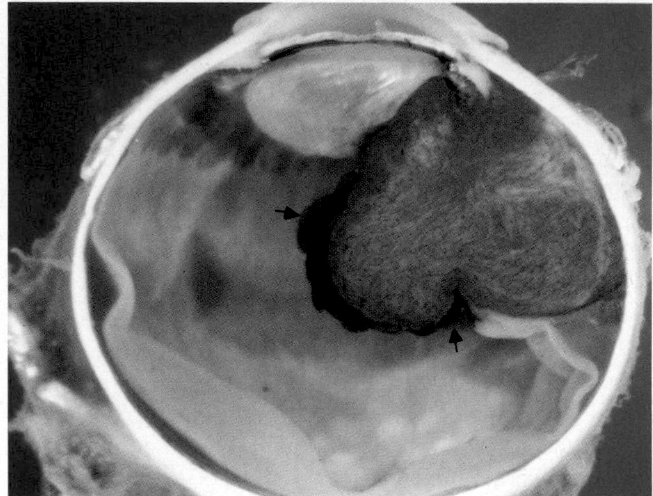

C

ence of associated paramagnetic metal cations rather than free radicals. On the other hand, in a study of human melanomas implanted in nude mice, Atlas and colleagues did not detect any paramagnetic substance with electron paramagnetic resonance in melanotic lesions, other than melanin, to account for the observed relaxation enhancement (56).

In general, especially at high field strengths, SE MR images can usually distinguish melanotic melanoma from their associated hemorrhagic (or nonhemorrhagic) subretinal fluid collections and from amelanotic neoplasms on the basis of signal intensity patterns (5,53,55–57) (Table 3). The distinction between melanotic melanoma from subretinal fluid collections by MR (53) can often be made without i.v. contrast, as opposed to the experience on CT (Figs. 14 and 16).

However, it is clearly advantageous to study the eye with i.v. contrast in the search for this lesion because the vast majority of ocular neoplasms will enhance but isolated detachments with fluid collections typically do not. It should be recognized that the appearance of choroidal hematomas and effusions may resemble melanoma if the MR examination is limited to a noncontrast short TR/TE series (7), since high intensity on short TR/TE images can be related to many factors (Table 4). Methemoglobin in subacute-chronic hemorrhage is high signal intensity on short TR/TE images, as is melanotic melanoma (55). Long TR/TE sequences can often distinguish these entities at high field strengths (55), as intracellular (early) methemoglobin is markedly hypointense (60), extracellular (chronic) methemoglobin is markedly hyperintense (60,61), and melanin is only minimally hypointense (55,57) on this pulse sequence. To fully characterize and differentiate these tumors and their associated fluid collections, both short and long TR/TE sequences must be performed, preferably with at least two echo delays.

Ocular Metastases

In the adult patient harboring a malignancy, the globe is the most frequent site of metastases to the orbit; in fact,

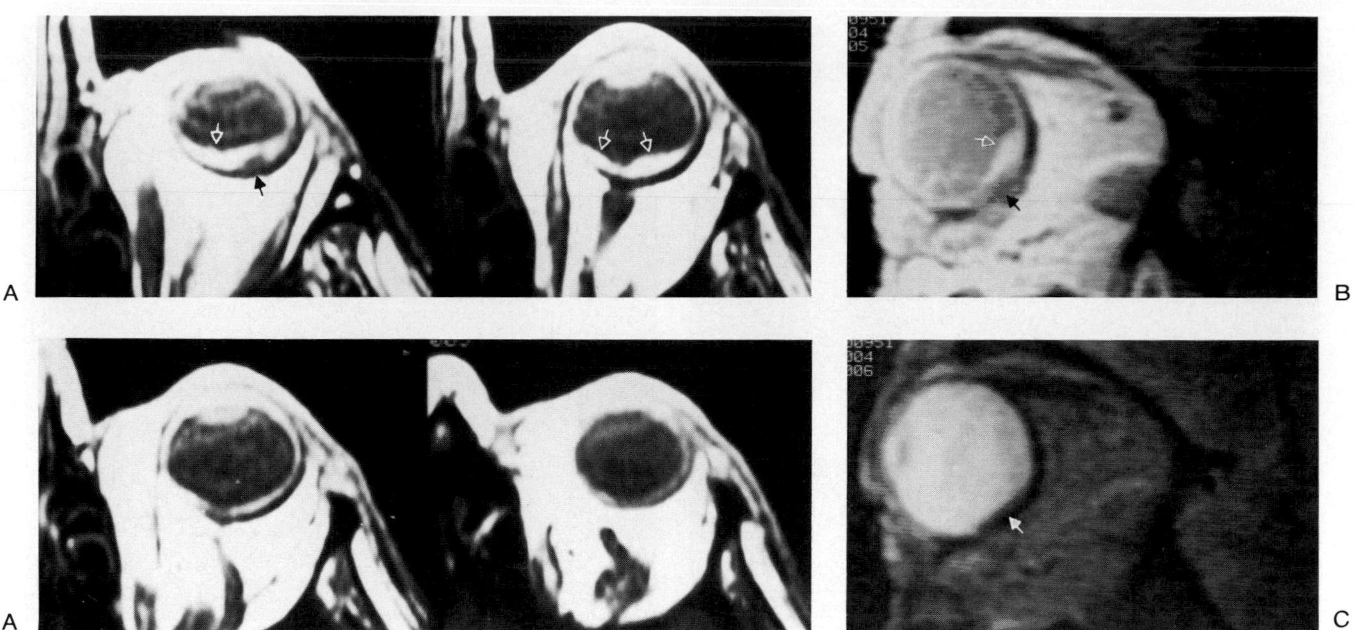

FIG. 16. Choroidal metastasis from lung carcinoma with detachment. **A:** Serial axial short TR/TE MRI, inferior to superior. **B:** Sagittal short TR/TE MRI. **C:** Sagittal long TR/TE MRI. Note low-intensity inferotemporal choroidal mass in left globe (*closed arrows,* A–C) with associated high-intensity hemorrhagic detachment (*open arrows,* A,B). Small metastasis is low intensity on long TR/TE image (C). (Courtesy of Dr. R. Peyster, Philadelphia, PA.)

up to 90% of orbital metastases are intraocular in this age group (62). Hematogenously disseminated metastases to the globe are usually located within the uveal tract, in concordance with its highly vascular nature. The most common sites of primary carcinoma are breast and lung (Figs. 16 and 17), but a variety of neoplasms can spread to this region. It is quite common for choroidal metastases to be accompanied by nonhematogenous detachment (see Figs. 16 and 17). In all patients suspected of harboring intraocular metastases, i.v. contrast should be given to distinguish mass from detachment on imaging studies.

TABLE 4. *High-intensity ocular lesions on short TR/TE MR images*

Type of pathology	Specific lesion	Etiology of hyperintensity
Neoplasm	Melanotic melanoma	Melanin Hemorrhage Necrosis
	Retinoblastoma	Hemorrhage Ions associated with calcification Necrosis
	Choroidal metastasis	Hemorrhage Mucinous content Necrosis
	Capillary hemangioma	Hemorrhage
Detachment	Coats' disease	Lipoproteinaceous material
	PHPV	Associated hemorrhage
	Traumatic	Hemorrhage
	Associated with neoplasms	Hemorrhage
	Rhegmatogenous	Markedly high protein content or hemorrhage
Infection	Endophthalmitis	Hemorrhage
Degenerative	Phthisis bulbi	Ions associated with calcification Old hemorrhagic detachment
Iatrogenic	Intravitreal silicone oil (treatment for detachment)	Lipid

PHPV, persistent hyperplastic primary vitreous.

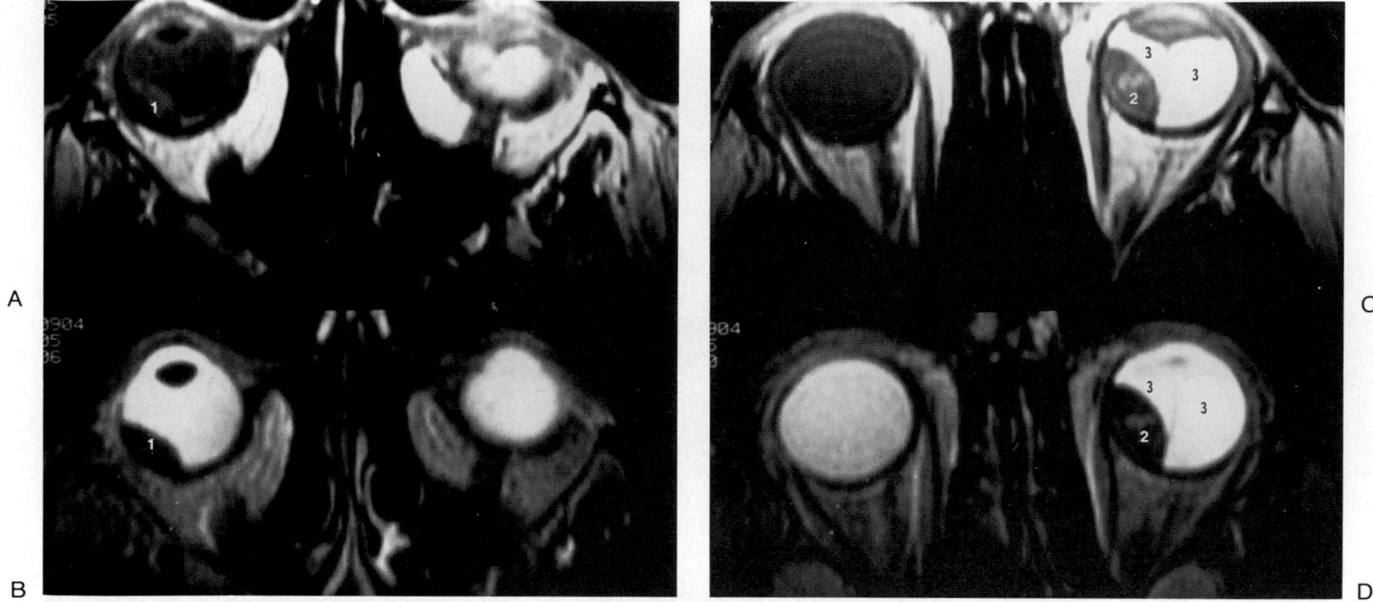

FIG. 17. Choroidal metastasis from small bowel carcinoid tumor with detachment. **A:** Short TR/TE MRI through right globe mass. **B:** Long TR/TE MRI through right globe mass. **C:** Short TR/TE MRI through left globe mass. **D:** Long TR/TE MRI through left globe mass. Note slightly hyperintense temporal choroidal mass in right globe (*1*, A) with marked hypointensity on long TR/TE image (*1*, B). Left eye metastasis (*2*, C,D) is mainly hypointense on short TR/TE (C) with marked hypointensity on long TR/TE image (D), and is associated with extensive hemorrhagic detachment (*3*) nearly filling vitreous. (Courtesy of Dr. R. Peyster, Philadelphia, PA.)

Although no specific signal intensity on MR has been described in uveal metastases, the major differential diagnosis is malignant melanoma [although there is a long list of diagnostic possibilities to be considered (Tables 2 and 4)]. Both metastatic disease and melanoma will enhance with i.v. contrast because the normal blood–ocular barrier is deficient in the region of the neoplasm (52). These focal masses can be distinguished from melanotic melanoma by its intensity on short TR/TE images: metastases are usually isointense to vitreous (see Fig. 16), whereas melanotic melanoma is markedly hyperintense (5,6,53). Melanoma has a higher incidence of intratumoral hemorrhage than metastases overall, so a hemorrhagic uveal mass is also more likely to represent melanoma. Mucinous adenocarcinoma metastases can simulate melanotic melanoma and show high intensity on short TR/TE images (see Fig. 17) (53).

Retinoblastoma

Retinoblastoma is the most common intraocular malignancy of childhood. Although this tumor is thought to be congenital, it is not necessarily recognized at birth. The average age at diagnosis is 18 months (63). The typical clinical presentation of leukokoria, strabismus, glaucoma, or vision loss occurs in 90% of cases, and the remaining 10% manifest as systemic illness (64). There are several important roles for imaging in retinoblastoma, despite the classical clinical presentation. First, there is an extensive clinical differential diagnosis of leukokoria, and imaging can limit the diagnostic possibilities significantly. Second, retinoblastoma spreads in a variety of ways, most of which are readily detectable by imaging with i.v. contrast. These include (a) intraocular dissemination, (b) along perineural and perivascular spaces to the retrobulbar orbit, (c) via the perioptic CSF space to seed the CNS, and (d) rarely, through the hematogenous route (64). Bilaterality is extraordinarily common in retinoblastoma (Fig. 18), occurring in up to one third of patients, especially those who are familial. In addition, intracerebral metastases (Fig. 19) (65) and the rare "trilateral" retinoblastoma (bilateral retinoblastoma with associated pineal tumor) (66) could also be detected by MR. Furthermore, there has been an appreciation that survivors of bilateral retinoblastoma have a predisposition to the development of radiation-induced neoplasms (67), occurring in about one fifth of survivors who have been irradiated. These tumors are most commonly manifested within 10 years of radiation therapy and are most commonly sarcomas or carcinomas. In addition, second malignancies in nonirradiated patients apparently occur more frequently than in the general population (68).

Retinoblastoma has been reported to have variable signal intensities on SE MR (22,69). Since retinoblastoma shares many histopathologic features with other primitive neuroectodermal tumors of the CNS (e.g., medulloblastoma, pinealoblastoma) (70), its signal intensity

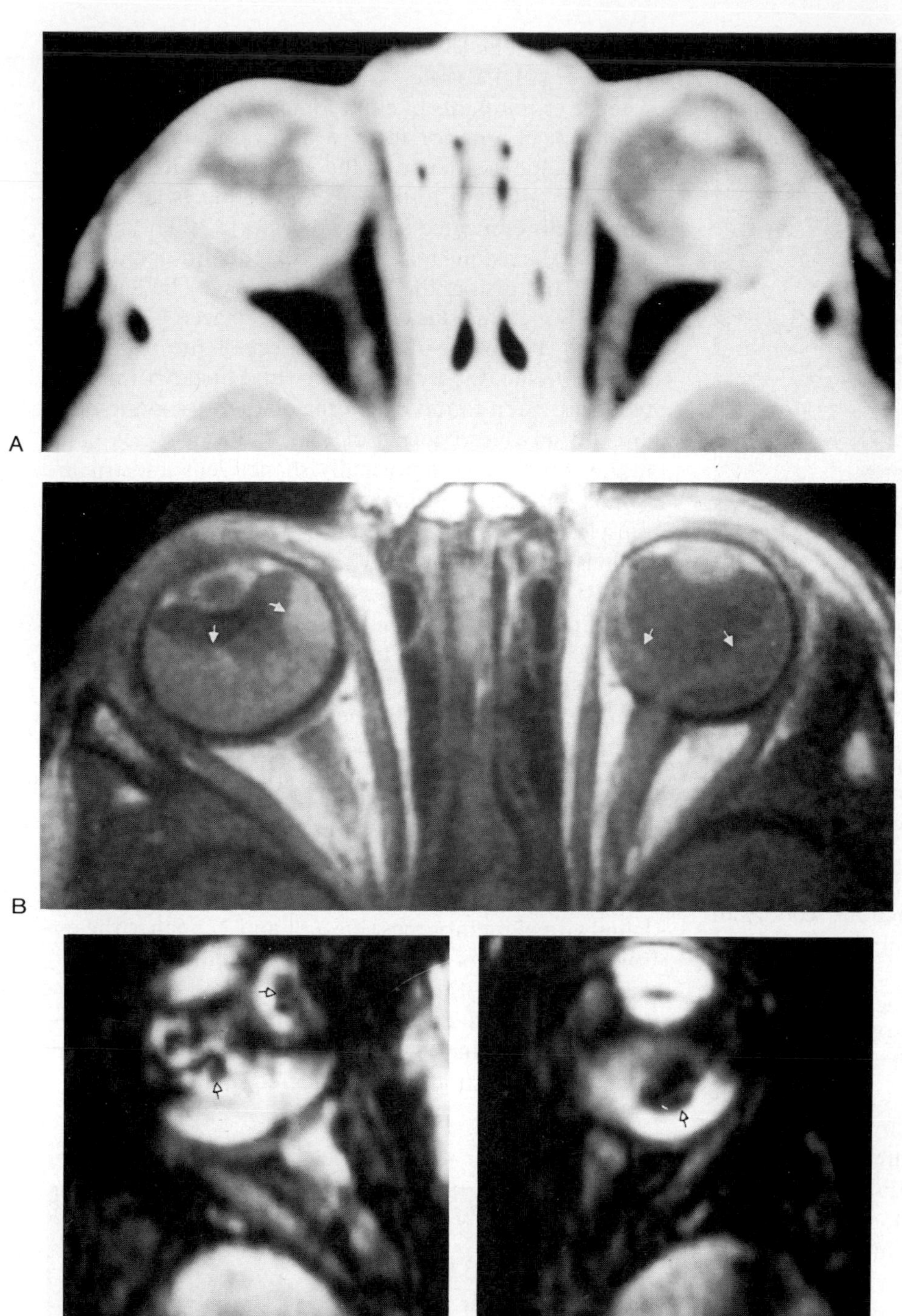

FIG. 18. Bilateral calcified retinoblastoma. **A:** Axial CT. **B:** Axial MRI (SE short TR/TE). **C:** Axial MRI (gradient-echo 200/50/100). Nodular calcification in bilateral retinoblastoma on CT (A) is not identified on SE MRI (B), although bilateral retinal detachments (*closed arrows*) with nodularity in right globe are demonstrated. Gradient-echo MRI (C) clearly depicts focal regions of marked hypointensity (*open arrows*) in areas of CT-documented calcification. (From Atlas, ref. 34, with permission.)

may be similar to them on MR. These pediatric lesions may also appear similar to adult melanomas on short and long TR/TE MR images (21): high intensity on short TR/TE and low intensity on long TR/TE. The hyperintensity on short TR/TE images may be related to the fact that retinoblastoma commonly demonstrates necrosis and hemorrhage pathologically, or that paramagnetic substances are associated with calcium deposition in this entity (71). Hypointensity on T2-weighted images is also multifactorial because it may be at least partially due to any of several factors: hemorrhage, necrosis with liberation of cellular iron, low free water as a concomitant of hypercellularity and scant cytoplasm content, etc. Importantly, however, the classic CT sign of retinoblastoma in a young patient is retinal calcification. Since CT is extremely sensitive for calcification, and SE MR is well known to be insensitive for demonstrating calcification (72,73), CT remains the initial diagnostic imaging modality of choice for this entity. Furthermore, in one fourth to one third of patients there is bilateral disease,

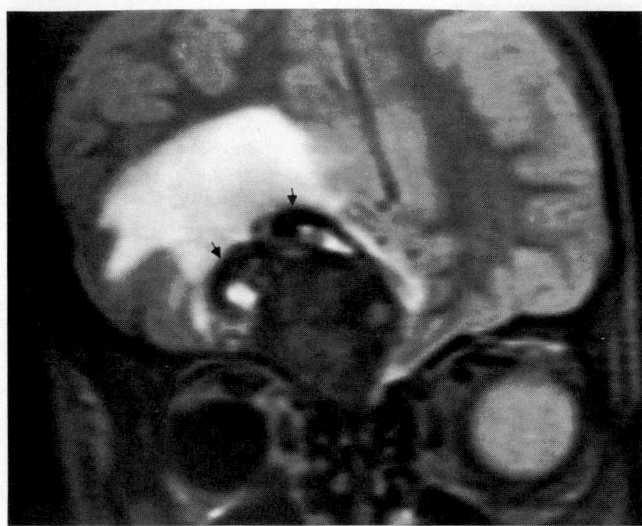

FIG. 19. Hemorrhagic intracranial retinoblastoma metastasis, long TR/TE coronal MRI (2500/80). Large hemorrhagic intracranial metastasis from right ocular retinoblastoma (now enucleated) demonstrates marked intralesional heterogeneity, incomplete iron rim (*arrows*), and extensive peritumoral edema.

which may be seen only as a tiny focus of calcification, so the role of MR in evaluating this entity may be very limited. Gradient-echo techniques can demonstrate calcification as marked hypointensity due to magnetic susceptibility effects (71) (see Fig. 18). The efficacy of 3DFT techniques with ultrathin, contiguous sections in this entity remains to be evaluated. Again, i.v. paramagnetic contrast enhancement may be useful, as the vast majority of retinoblastomas with noncalcified portions enhance. Episcleral extension of retinoblastoma is critical to exclude, and fat-suppressed MR with the use of i.v. contrast is presumed to be sensitive to document this ominous sign of spread. Retinal detachment should be readily differentiated from retinoblastoma with i.v. contrast, but benign masses (e.g., choroidal hemangioma, astrocytic hamartoma, inflammation), most of which are extremely rare, may be virtually indistinguishable (Fig. 20).

Other Causes of Leukokoria

Persistent Hyperplastic Primary Vitreous

Virtually all developmental anomalies of the vitreous are related to a persistence of the vascular components of the "primary vitreous." The primary vitreous forms from the third to ninth gestational weeks and essentially regresses completely during the latter stages of fetal life (37). In the normal globe after birth, the only residual structure of the primary vitreous may be the 1- to 2-mm wide canal of Cloquet. It extends from the optic nerve head to a point just inferior and nasal to the posterior pole of the lens (37). "Persistent hyperplastic primary vitreous" (PHPV) refers to an abnormal congenital persistence of remnants of embryonic hyaloid vessels. In its most typical anterior form, a fibrovascular connective tissue plaque is situated in the vitreous immediately behind and adherent to the lens and connects laterally to abnormally elongated ciliary processes (37). The anterior aspect of the plaque may actually extend through the lens capsule and distort the lens morphology. The lens may also show cataractous change or be replaced by fatty tissue (37). From the posterior aspect of the retrolental mass of tissue, the hyaloid artery and linear connective tissue are often found extending all the way to the optic disc. In advanced forms of PHPV, the globe is commonly small. The abnormally shaped lens and iris are shifted anteriorly to narrow the anterior chamber. Fat, muscle, and cartilage have all been found in the retrolental mass (37).

MRI can reflect all these described pathologic changes and can be highly specific in this entity. The specific diagnosis hinges on the demonstration of the low intensity fibrocollagenous retrolental plaque in intimate association with an abnormally configured lens within a small globe (Fig. 21). The classically described hyaloid vasculature remnants are seen on MR as linear, low intensity structures extending directly from the posterior part of the lens/plaque complex all the way to the optic nerve head (see Figs. 20 and 21). The vitreous is often high intensity, because of associated hemorrhage within retrolental vitreal membranes (Figs. 21 and 22). Since the retrolental plaque is highly vascular, it would presumably demonstrate contrast enhancement. Note that the lens configuration should be abnormal in this entity; if a normal lens is seen in the presence of a retrolental mass, another diagnosis should be considered (Fig. 23).

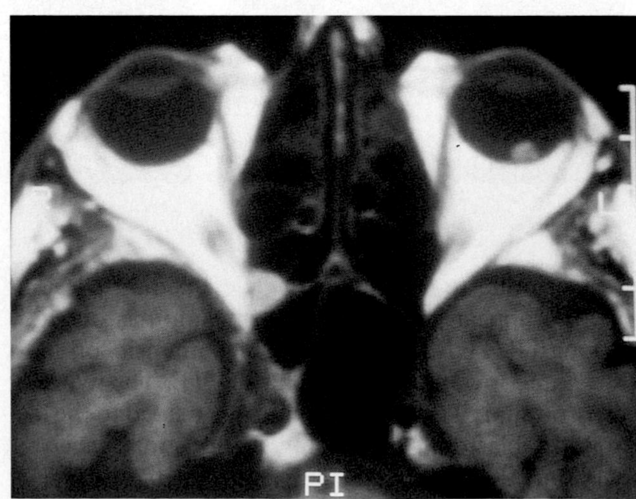

FIG. 20. Intraocular cysticercosis. (Courtesy of Dr. M. Castillo, Chapel Hill, NC.). Hyperintense mass in left globe on T1-weighted image represents ocular cysticercosis.

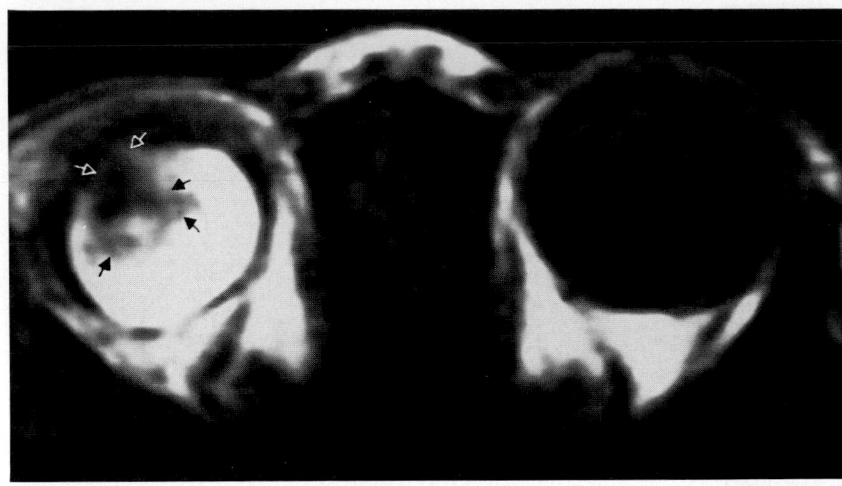

FIG. 21. Persistent hyperplastic primary vitreous, unilateral. Short TR/TE image shows malformed right lens (*open arrows*) with retrolental fibrovascular mass (*closed arrows*) in otherwise diffusely hyperintense vitreous. (Courtesy of Dr. E. Fram, Phoenix, AZ.)

Coats' Disease

This idiopathic, benign entity consists of unilateral retinal telangiectasia with an associated massive subretinal exudative (nonhematogenous) fluid accumulation causing retinal detachment. Boys (80%) aged 6 to 8 years are typically affected (63). It has been put forth that there is a breakdown in the normal blood–retina barrier at the endothelial level, allowing diffuse leakage of plasma into a subsequently disorganized vessel wall. It is thought that aneurysmal dilatations and telangiectasia formation are consequences of the abnormal permeability of the retinal vessels (37). In Coats' disease, a lipoproteinaceous effusion accumulates, which has been reported as hyperintense on short and long TR/TE sequences (69). The entire globe is abnormal in signal intensity, because the retinal detachment is complete. High intensity, massive effusions can distend the subretinal space to the extent that the detached leaves of the retina are in contact in the midline, at the level of the optic disc. The low intensity leaves of the retina apposed in the midline could simulate the linear low intensity hyaloid vasculature remnants seen in PHPV, a congenital globe lesion. The normal morphology of the lens, the failure to identify the retrolental mass, and the normal shape and size of the globe distinguish this entity radiologically from PHPV.

Choroidal and Retinal Hemangioma

Cavernous hemangiomas of the choroid are very uncommon, nonprogressive, benign lesions, usually seen in patients 10 to 20 years of age. As these lesions are histologically cavernous hemangiomas, they demonstrate benign behavior similar to their retrobulbar counterpart (37) (Fig. 24). Occasionally, cavernous hemangiomas exert traction on vitreous and cause rhegmatogenous detachments. Capillary hemangiomas of the retina are distinct lesions, histologically similar to the cerebellar hemangioblastoma (37). Approximately 25% to 50% of these patients have von Hippel-Lindau syndrome (63). Retinal angiomas are bilateral in up to one half of cases

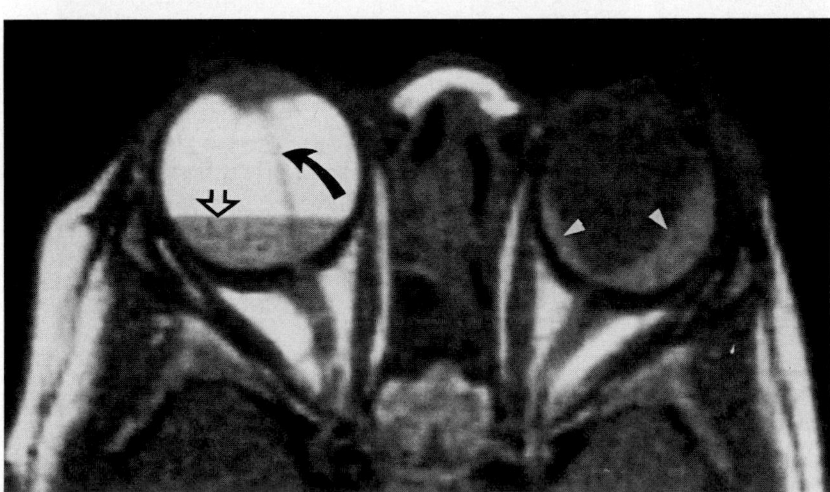

FIG. 22. Warburg syndrome with subretinal fluid, short TR/TE MR (600/25). Dependent portion of right globe (*open arrow*) may represent intracellular blood products in serosanguinous collection. Thin, linear hypointensity coursing through vitreous (*curved arrow*) suggests Cloquet's canal, which is seen in persistent hyperplastic primary vitreous. Also note hyperintense subretinal fluid in left globe (*arrowheads*). (Courtesy of Dr. M. Mafee, Chicago, IL.) (From Atlas, ref. 34, with permission.)

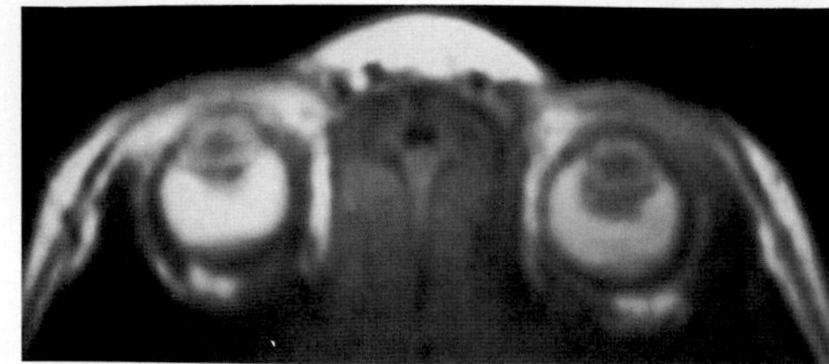

A

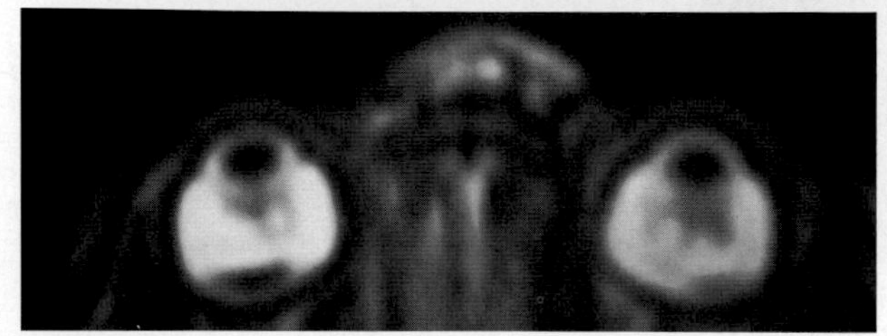

B

FIG. 23. Bilateral retrolental masses, retinoblastoma. T1-weighted (**A**) and T2-weighted (**B**) images show massive intraocular hemorrhage bilaterally, masses behind lenses, and hemorrhagic detachments. Normal shape of lenses confirms diagnosis of retinoblastoma rather than PHPV.

and multiple in the affected eye in one third (37). Although considered hamartomatous in nature, these lesions can enlarge. Furthermore, their propensities to bleed and cause exudative retinal detachments often results in abrupt symptomatology. These lesions can be minimally hyperintense on T1-weighted images, occasionally appearing similar to melanotic melanoma. They also seem to become high signal intensity on long TR/TE images (53) and therefore are distinguishable from melanoma on this basis. Since some of these lesions can spontaneously hemorrhage and are often associated with subretinal collections, MRI can demonstrate a variety of signal intensity patterns. All choroidal and retinal hemangiomas demonstrate intense contrast enhancement (Fig. 25), and small lesions can be inapparent on noncontrast scans.

Retinal and Choroidal Detachment

The retina is comprised mainly of sensory and pigment epithelium layers. These two components are only firmly attached at two points: the optic disc posteriorly and the ora serrata anteriorly (37). The entire course of the delicate sensory retina is otherwise only weakly and tentatively apposed to the retinal pigment epithelium by intraocular pressure, microscopic villi, and mucopolysaccharide substance (37). In the strict sense, the term "retinal detachment" implies separation of retinal pigment epithelium from Bruch's membrane of choroid. It is generally stated, however, that when the pigmented epithelial layer of the retina is separated from the sensory retina by fluid accumulation, a retinal detachment results. Choroidal detachment implies separation of sclera from subjacent choroid (or ciliary body, hence the term "ciliochoroidal detachment"). Retinal detachments are due to fluid in the subretinal space; ciliochoroidal detachments show collections in the suprachoroidal space.

Retinal detachments are classified as rhegmatogenous or nonhematogenous, depending on whether a rhegma (hole) exists in the sensory retina (37). Most detachments are rhegmatogenous, and are secondary to either accu-

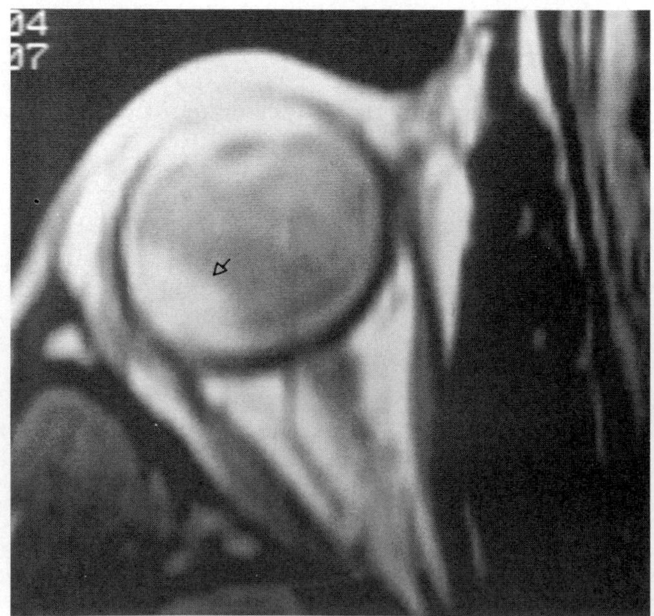

A

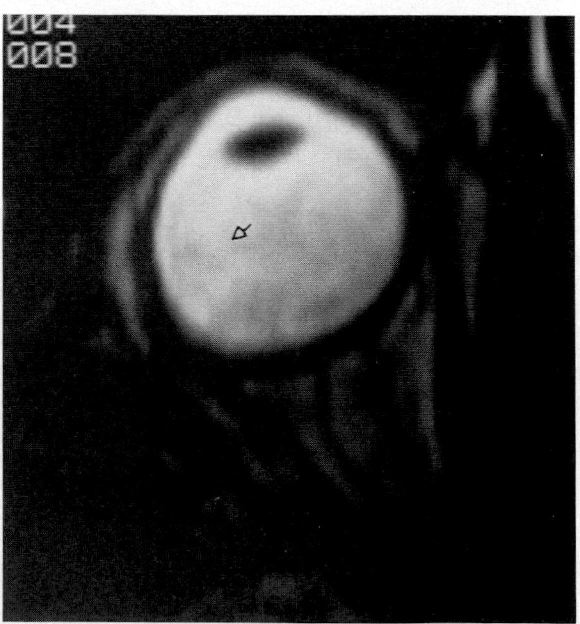

B

FIG. 24. Choroidal hemangioma. **A:** Long TR/short TE MR. **B:** Long TR/TE MR. Focal choroidal hemangioma (*arrow*) in 14-year-old boy is hyperintense on long TR images (A,B). (Courtesy of Dr. R. Peyster, Philadelphia, PA.)

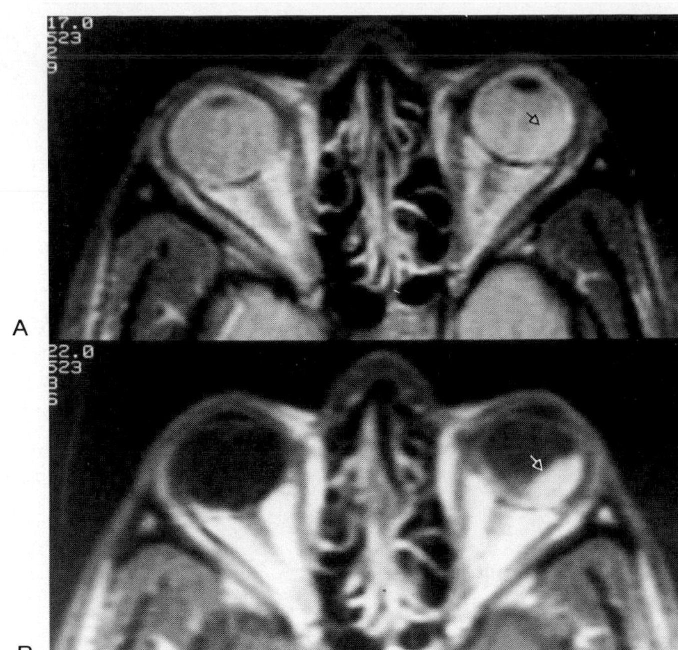

FIG. 25. Choroidal hemangioma, contrast-enhancing. **A:** Long TR/short TE MR, before contrast administration. **B:** Short TR/TE MR, after contrast administration. The lesion (*arrow*) is only minimally hyperintense to vitreous on long TR/short TE (A), but enhances densely with i.v. contrast (B). (Courtesy of Dr. M. Mafee, Chicago, IL.)

mulation of subretinal fluid via a retinal tear, or vitreal degeneration and retraction of the retina from condensation and fibrosis of the underlying vitreous. Nonhematogenous retinal detachments are caused by subretinal fluid accumulation leaking from abnormal small vessels, frequently secondary to neoplastic disease (melanoma, metastases, hemangioma, or retinoblastoma). In addition, nonhematogenous detachments may occur in Coat's disease and inflammation. Although the role of tears in the retina in the pathogenesis of retinal detachment is widely accepted, the significance of finding the tear alone is not clear (37). The cause of the retinal hole is most commonly degenerative change secondary to vitreoretinal adhesions and vitreous degeneration. Spontaneous detachments are said to occur in less than 10 per 100,000 per year (74). Patients are predisposed to retinal detachment if they have severe axial myopia, surgical aphakia (lens absence), or a history of contralateral retinal detachment. Gradual vision loss is a common clinical presentation. The treatment of retinal detachment resides in either scleral buckling procedures or pars plana vitrectomy. Temporary tamponade may also be obtained with intraocular silicone oil (75).

Ciliochoroidal detachments can be due to either serous effusions or hemorrhagic collections. Hemorrhagic choroidal detachment, or choroidal hematoma, is usually related to trauma or surgical intervention. Ciliochoroidal serous effusions are commonly secondary to trauma, especially vitreous surgery, and inflammation (37). In the great majority of ciliochoroidal effusions, ocular hypotony is present and, in fact, is thought to represent a significant contributing factor to the development of the effusion itself (37).

The MR appearance of retinal and ciliochoroidal detachments (see Figs. 14, 16–19, 21, and 22) depends on the ability of MR to distinguish fluid collections from hemorrhagic collections (60), as well as on the variable protein content of subretinal or suprachoroidal fluid. It appears that MR usually cannot distinguish suprachoroidal from subretinal collections (7), although ciliochoroidal detachments frequently extend anteriorly into the ciliary body, while retinal detachments characteristically are limited anteriorly at the ora serrata (7). Nonhemorrhagic retinal detachments should appear as subretinal fluid, but marked elevation of protein content may shorten relaxation time somewhat (76,77). In fact, MR has been reported to be able to distinguish subretinal collections of varying protein content because of this differential relaxation time shortening (76). Serous ciliochoroidal effusions in the suprachoroidal space have also been reported as being hyperintense to vitreous on long TR/short TE MR images (7). [It should be noted that many clinically diagnosed ciliochoroidal effusions are more accurately only choroidal edema (37); these lesions are seen as only slight thickening of the entire hyperintense choroid on MR images.] Therefore, even nonhemorrhagic collections may occasionally be more intense than normal vitreous on certain SE pulse sequences. Okabe et al. (76) correlated the appearance on SE MR of rhegmatogenous and nonrhegmatogenous collections to their protein content. Short T1 and T2 were noted in chronic rhegmatogenous and nonrhegmatogenous effusions, being present in those lesions with markedly elevated protein concentrations, in contrast to recently acquired rhegmatogenous detachments that contained low protein. As described earlier, the appearance of hemorrhage varies with its evolutionary stage and environment. Practically speaking, funduscopic examination can detect retinal detachments, so the essential role of MR is to exclude unsuspected neoplasm, such as choroidal melanoma (see earlier section), and i.v. contrast should be administered in all such cases. MR may play a role in delineating the etiology of retinal detachments (i.e., rhegmatogenous vs. nonrhegmatogenous).

Globe Shape Abnormalities

Axial myopia is characterized by elongation of the globe in the anteroposterior dimension. It can be distinguished from staphyloma (an acquired defect in the globe wall, resulting in focal protrusion of a thinned cornea or sclera, usually posterotemporal to the disc) by the absence of focal bulge in the elongated globe (Fig. 26).

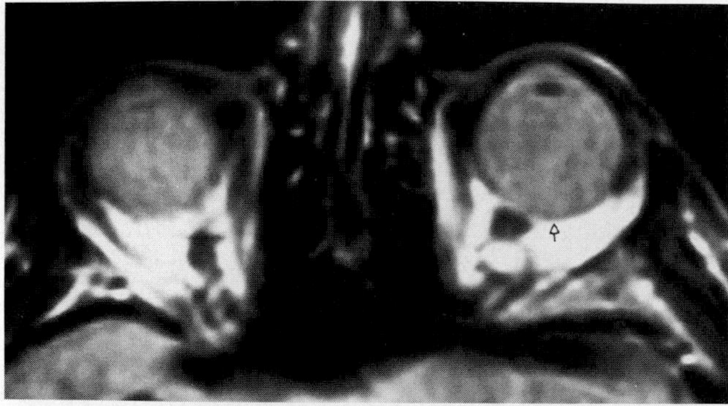

FIG. 26. Axial myopia with staphyloma, long TR/short TE MRI. Left globe has elongated shape in anteroposterior dimension. Note focal thinning of sclera indicating staphyloma on temporal side of disc (*open arrow*).

Staphylomas are lined with iris or choroidal tissue. Retinal detachment and/or staphyloma commonly accompany a severely myopic globe (Fig. 27). Colobomas are congenital defects in the retina, choroid, iris, lens, and/or optic nerve situated inferonasally and are often seen as excavations into the optic nerve head that result from failure of closure of the fetal optic fissure (37). These lesions are bilateral in up to 60% of cases. Colobomas are transmitted as an autosomal dominant trait with variable penetrance. The utility of MR imaging in the work-up of these lesions lies in its ability to reveal any additional associated CNS anomalies that are frequently seen with colobomatous lesions, such as encephalocele or callosal agenesis and its spectrum of concurrent malformations (78,79). Microphthalmia is a condition that can be classified as either simple or complex, depending on whether the small eye is anatomically intact or if it is malformed (80). Microphthalmos and retinal cysts may occur in conjunction with coloboma (colobomatous cyst) and are clearly detected with MR (see Fig. 27) (81). If a colobomatous cyst is present, the cyst lies inferior to the site of exit of the nerve from the globe, and is often the cause of superior displacement and proptosis of a microphthalmic eye (37). The major differential diagnoses in that case are meningocele or congenitally cystic globe. Coloboma may also occur in association with a choristoma, a malformation composed of heterotopic mesodermal elements usually within or adjacent to the coloboma (37). Microphthalmia may also occur secondary to intrauterine infection or as an isolated anomaly, where it is often bilateral. Buphthalmos, or congenital glaucoma, is a result of maldevelopment of the outflow channels in the anterior chamber angle. Glaucoma in a young child results in an enlarged globe, due to the distensibility of the sclera. Macrophthalmos may be unrelated to intraocular pressure, however, and may be seen as an isolated entity, secondary to massive intraocular tumor, or in association with neurofibromatosis (Fig. 28). Phthisis bulbi represents an end-stage, atrophic globe that has undergone extensive degenerative changes. This condition can result from any of a variety of insults, including prior inflammation and trauma. In phthisic eyes, the sclera becomes markedly thickened, irregular, and calcified. These globes are easily recognized on MRI by their characteristic morphology, as well as by their signal intensity patterns: peripheral hyperintensity on short TR/TE and marked hypointensity on long TR/TE images (Fig. 29), reflecting iron and other paramagnetic ion deposition along with the dystrophic calcification. Finally, a characteristic distortion of globe shape is seen in patients who have had prior scleral banding procedures as treatment for retinal detachment, often in patients with high myopia.

Orbital Inflammatory Disease

Idiopathic Inflammatory Pseudotumor

In the adult population, the most common cause of an intraorbital mass lesion is idiopathic orbital pseudotumor (82). These lesions, by definition, have no definable local cause and are unassociated with a systemic illness. Orbital pseudotumor is usually a clinical diagnosis with a symptom triad of pain, ophthalmoparesis, and proptosis. Although pseudotumor is one of the most common

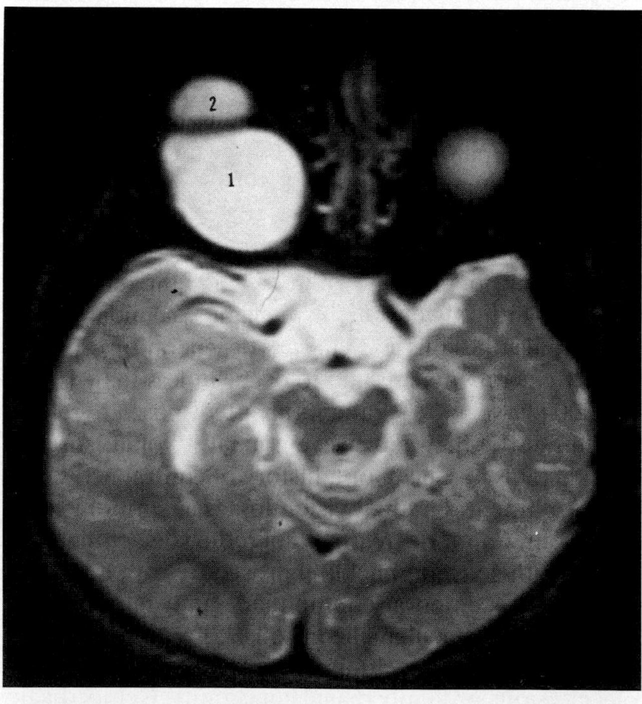

FIG. 27. Coloboma with retinal cyst and microphthalmos. On this long TR/TE MR image, note large cyst (*1*) displacing microphthalmic globe (*2*) in patient with coloboma and Aicardi syndrome.

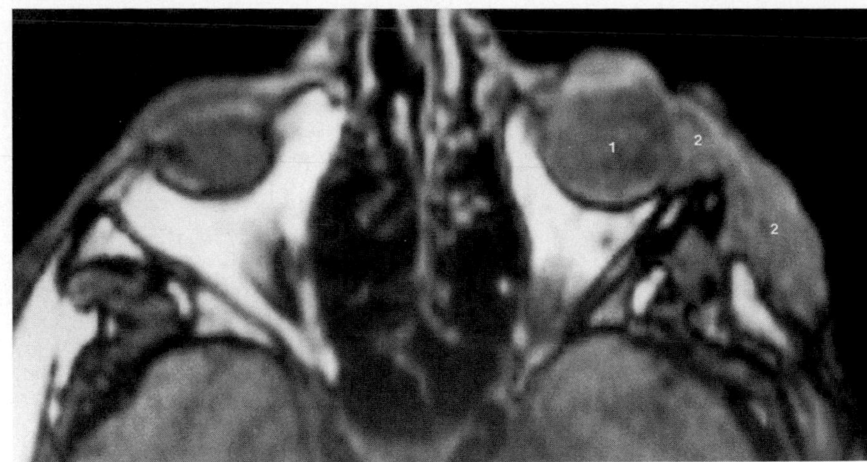

FIG. 28. Macrophthalmos and plexiform neurofibroma in neurofibromatosis (Dixon method MRI, 600/25). Note enlarged left globe (*1*) in patient with neurofibromatosis but without glaucoma, and left plexiform neurofibroma (*2*). (From Atlas, ref. 34, with permission.)

causes of unilateral proptosis (probably second after Graves' disease), bilateral disease is not uncommon (3,83,84), but when identified should raise suspicions about an underlying systemic disorder (i.e., Wegner's disease, Trichinella, collagen-vascular disorder). Unusual clinical presentations of pseudotumor often require radiographic evaluation and occasionally biopsy, especially if steroid response is lacking and radiation therapy is contemplated (85,86). Pathologic findings are diverse and depend on the tissue sampled or on the site of inflammation (37). In the very early stages of the disease, edema and inflammatory infiltrate are evident; as the disease evolves, fibrosis and collagen fibrils are laid down. The degree of fibrosis can be extensive and helps distinguish pseudotumor from lymphoid tumors (37).

CT is typically nonspecific (83) (Table 5) and is extremely variable in depicting the spectrum of abnormalities seen in this entity, as the disease process may present in many forms: uveal-scleral thickening (periscleritis) (Fig. 30), obliteration of retrobulbar fat planes, rectus muscle enlargement (myositis) (Fig. 31), isolated lacrimal mass (dacryoadenitis), or even as a discrete retrobulbar mass lesion (Fig. 32) (33). Pseudotumor may involve any part of one or multiple muscles; if the insertion of the muscle is involved, pseudotumor is more likely than thyroid orbitopathy, but a normal muscle insertion with enlargement of the muscle belly has no differential utility (84). Uveal-scleral thickening may be seen in connection with other causes of intraorbital inflammation (i.e., trauma, surgery, bacterial infection, sarcoidosis), as well as infiltrating neoplasms (i.e., lymphoma or metastatic disease) (33). Orbital pseudotumor usually shows dramatic resolution with steroid therapy; in fact, the final diagnosis is often based on response to steroids.

A

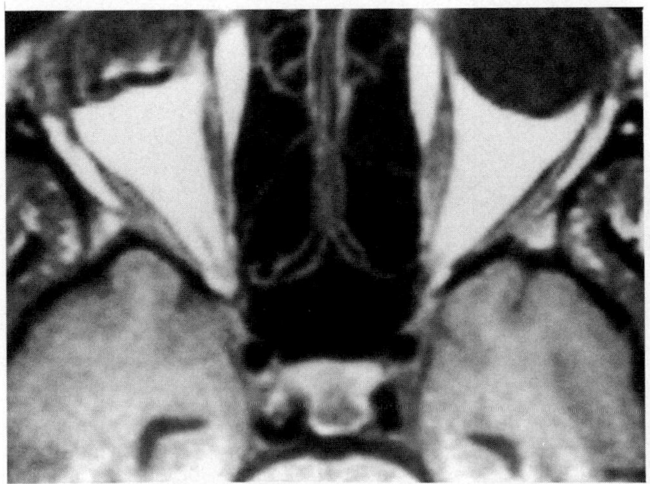

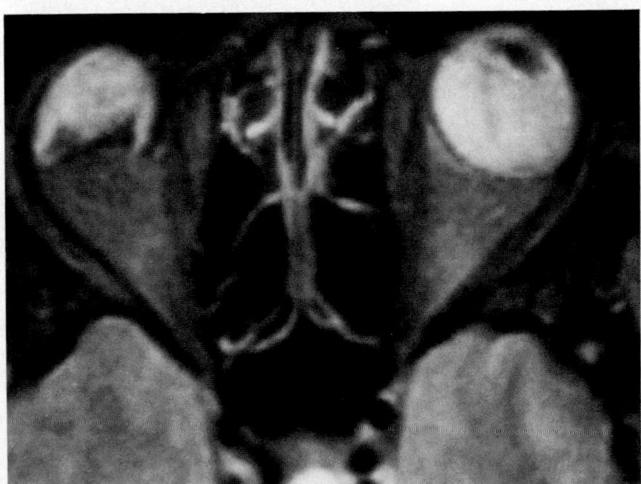

B

FIG. 29. Phthisis bulbi. **A:** Short TR/TE MRI. **B:** Long TR/TE MR. Note heterogeneous hyperintensity of small and irregularly shaped right globe, probably reflecting paramagnetic ions, which are deposited with calcification in this end-stage degenerative globe.

TABLE 5. *Causes of extraocular muscle enlargement*

Thyroid eye disease	
Myositis	Idiopathic inflammatory pseudotumor
	Bacterial (from sinus extension)
	Other (e.g., Lyme disease)
Vascular congestion	Traumatic carotid–cavernous fistula
	Dural arteriovenous malformation
	Superior ophthalmic vein (or cavernous sinus) thrombosis
	Orbital apex mass
Malignant neoplasm	Metastases (esp. breast carcinoma)
	Infiltrating adenoid cystic carcinoma
	Lymphoma
	Leukemia
	Rhabdomyosarcoma
Lymphangioma	
Trauma	Edema
	Hemorrhage
Acromegaly	

From Atlas et al., ref. 33, with permission.

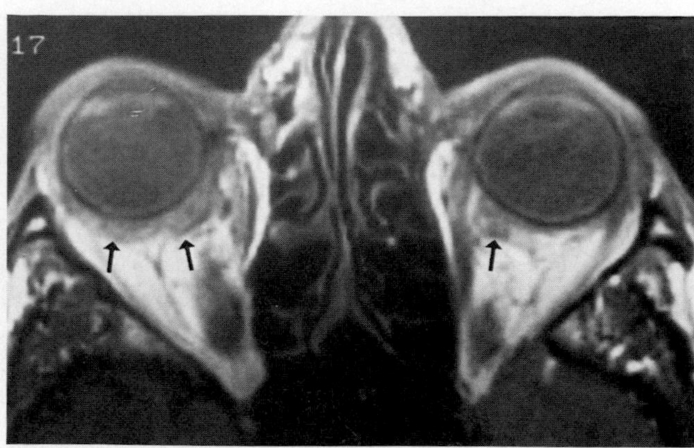

FIG. 30. Orbital pseudotumor with uveal-scleral thickening. Short TR/TE MRI. Uveal-scleral thickening (*arrows*) is clearly depicted by MRI. (From Atlas et al., ref. 3, with permission.)

The MR appearance of idiopathic orbital pseudotumor has been evaluated prospectively in a series of patients who presented with clinical symptoms and signs consistent with orbital pseudotumor (3). These lesions were isointense to normal muscle on T1-weighted images and isointense or only minimally hyperintense to orbital fat on T2-weighted images in 10 of 11 patients with proven orbital pseudotumor (see Figs. 31 and 32). In that study, patients who were proven to have retrobulbar metastatic disease had lesions that were markedly hyperintense to fat on T2-weighted images (Fig. 33). Therefore, in this group of patients who had identical clinical presentations, MR added specificity to the imaging appearance of these lesions (Table 6). On the other hand, from larger retrospective series (1), some malignant orbital lesions (such as lymphoma and myeloma) may have identical signal intensity patterns to pseudotumor, i.e., relatively low intensity on T2-weighted images. The relatively low intensity of pseudotumor on long TR/TE images is probably related to the common pathologic finding of fibrocollagenous deposition in this lesion. The similar appearance of some neoplasms (e.g., myeloma, lymphoma, neuroblastoma metastases) may be due to histopathologic features shared by these tumors, including marked hypercellularity, coupled with a notably scant amount of cytoplasm on a cellular level, thereby

A

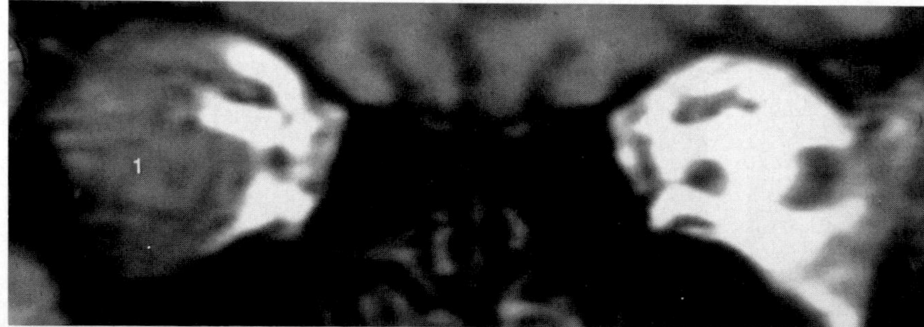

B

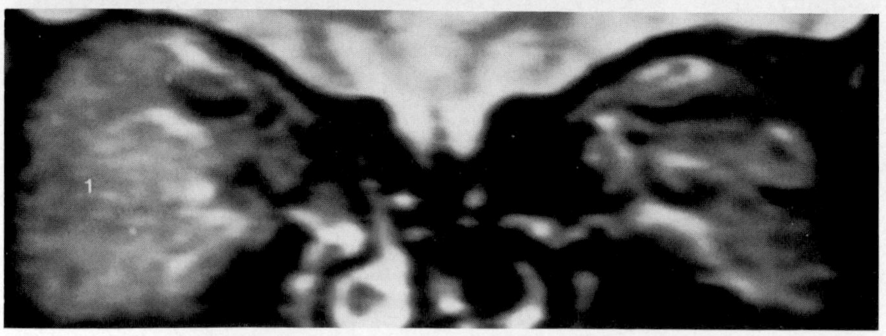

FIG. 31. Orbital pseudotumor with lateral rectus mass. **A:** Short TR/TE MRI (600/20). **B:** Long TR/TE MRI (2500/80). Large lateral mass (*1*) is isointense to muscle on short TR/TE (A) and remains low intensity (i.e., isointense to fat) on long TR/TE image (B), different from the hyperintensity seen in metastases. (From Atlas et al., ref. 3.)

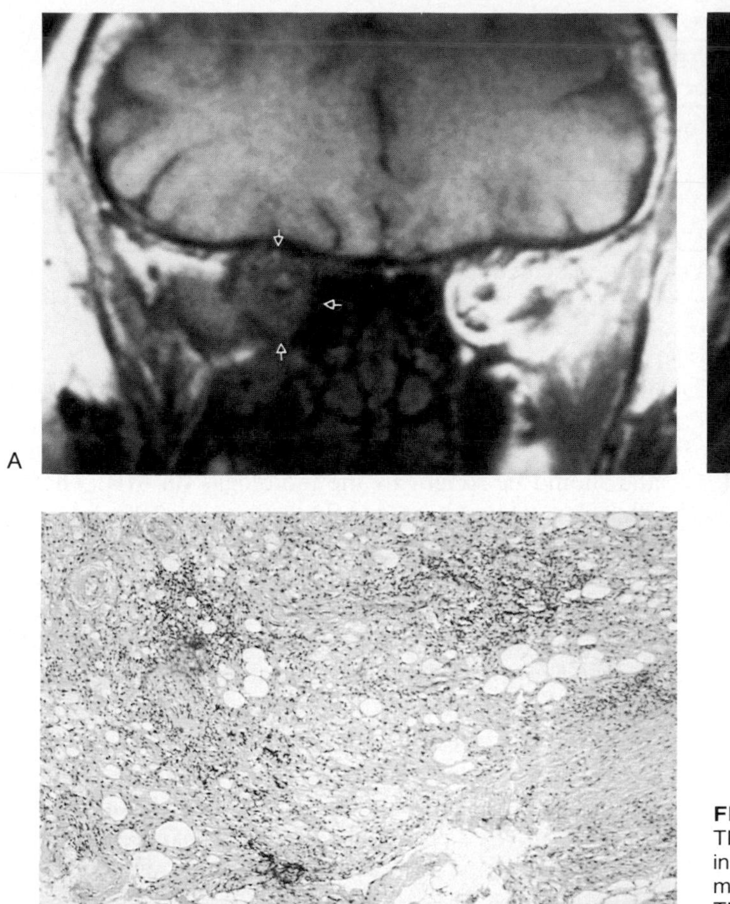

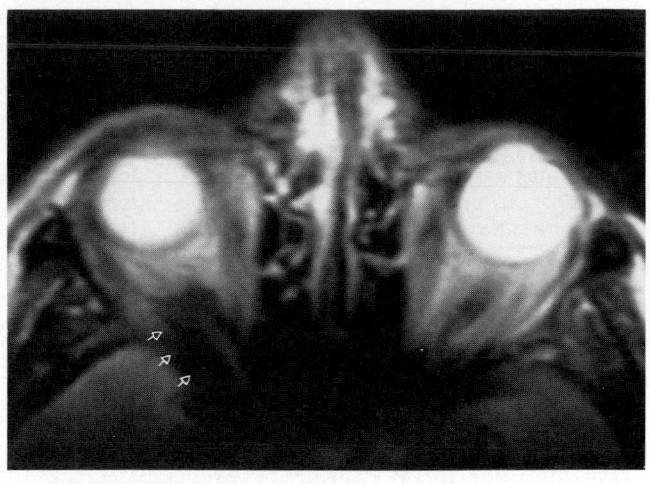

FIG. 32. Inflammatory orbital pseudotumor. **A:** Coronal short TR/TE MRI. **B:** Axial long TR/TE MRI. **C:** Pathologic specimen in another patient with inflammatory pseudotumor (H&E). Note marked hypointensity of apex mass (*arrows,* A,B) on long TR/TE image (B). This hypointensity probably relates to the intense desmoplastic fibrosis often present on histopathology (C).

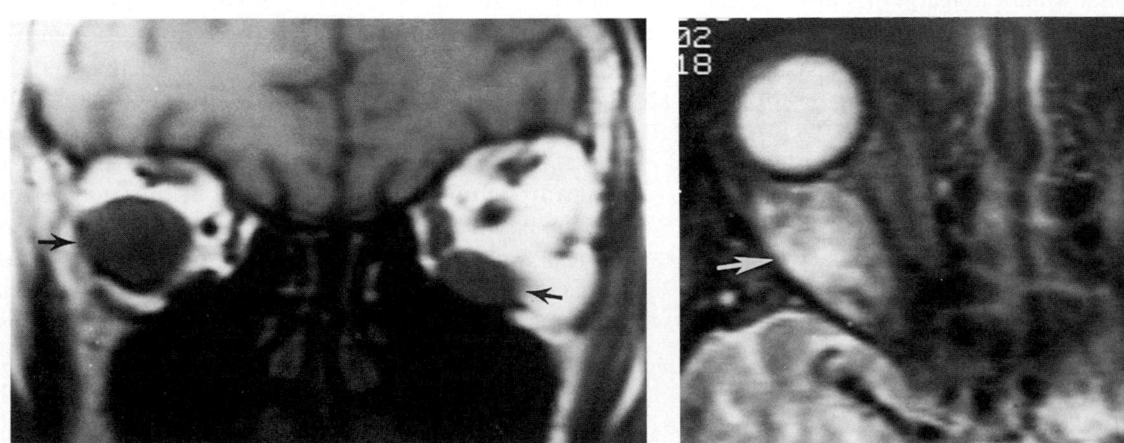

FIG. 33. Breast carcinoma metastases to rectus muscles. **A:** Coronal short TR/TE MR (600/20). **B:** Axial long TR/TE MRI (2500/80). Bilateral rectus muscle masses (*arrows*) are isointense to muscle on short TR/TE (A), but are markedly hyperintense on long TR/TE image (B), distinguishing these metastases from pseudotumor. (From Atlas et al., ref. 3, with permission.)

TABLE 6. *Signal intensity patterns in extraocular muscle enlargement*

Lesion	Short TR/TE (relative to normal muscle)	Long TR/TE (relative to normal muscle)
Thyroid eye disease	Isointense or hyperintense	Isointense to minimally hyperintense
Idiopathic inflammatory pseudotumor	Isointense	Hypointense to minimally hyperintense
Metastases (carcinoma)	Isointense	Hyperintense
Vascular congestion	Isointense	Isointense to minimally hyperintense
Intramuscular hematoma	Hyperintense[a]	Hyperintense[a]

[a] Signal intensity of intramuscular hematoma depends on stage of hemorrhage.

resulting in a shorter T2 than most neoplasms (Fig. 34). Other inflammatory entities (e.g., sarcoidosis) can also have the identical appearance (Fig. 35). In the clinical setting, low intensity on T2-weighted images can be used as supportive evidence for pseudotumor in the appropriate clinical setting, but a differential diagnosis for lesions with low intensity on T2-weighted images should be given (Table 7).

Cellulitis and Abscess

Bacterial infections of the orbit are usually secondary to adjacent sinus infection, skin infection, bacteremia, or perforating injury and retained foreign body (87). The orbital septum (see Figs. 6 and 7), the periosteum reflected from the anterior bony margin of the orbit, is a strong barrier preventing preseptal cellulitis from entering the postseptal orbital compartment. Since the veins draining the face, orbit, and sinuses have no valves, elevated pressure and infection can be readily transmitted between the skin or sinus and orbit. Infections may therefore extend into the orbit via these venous pathways or through the orbital wall. Extension of sinus infection through osseous dehiscences (congenital or secondary to osteomyelitis) often leads to subperiosteal abscess formation. Intraorbital infections can be classified as intraconal, extraconal, or subperiosteal. Most cases of postseptal cellulitis are extraconal, whereas most discrete abscesses are subperiosteal. Orbital myositis as a solitary lesion is usually considered to be an idiopathic inflammation (as in inflammatory pseudotumor), but it has been reported in association with Lyme disease (88).

MR can clearly demonstrate orbital infection as focal or diffuse regions of abnormal signal intensity, due to an increase in water (edema) in the involved regions. Areas of inflammation should enhance with i.v. contrast and are easily seen on fat-suppressed T1-weighted images. Ill-defined orbital cellulitis can appear as a subtle decrease in the normal high signal intensity of orbital fat on short TR/TE images (2). This appearance can be accentuated by using any of a variety of fat-suppression methods (2) (Fig. 36). This appearance of diffuse decrease in signal intensity of the orbital fat on T1-weighted images has also been described in idiopathic pseudotumor (3), and can be seen in any infiltrative process.

Complications of orbital infection are not uncommon and should be sought by the radiologist on MR. These often devastating events include secondary thrombosis of the superior ophthalmic vein (2) (see Fig. 36) and cavernous sinus thrombosis (89). In addition, bone destruction, seen as interruption of the expected linear signal void seen where intact cortical bone is present (1), should be searched for and would indicate intracranial extension. Enhancement of intracranial meninges in regions bordering the orbit (or sinus) can also be an indicator of intracranial extension through bone, but this finding can also be seen by virtue of transvenous extension of inflammation. We believe that in all cases of orbital infection, therefore, i.v. contrast should be administered.

Thyroid Orbitopathy

The major clinical signs of thyroid disease of the orbit can be categorized as either congestive or toxic (74). The primary manifestation of thyrotoxicosis is upper lid retraction, resulting in a characteristic stare that may resolve after treatment of hyperthyroidism. Congestive signs include exophthalmus, periorbital edema, and decreased range of globe motion, often accompanied by diplopia. Motility problems often predominate over proptosis. Pain is not a common feature of this entity. The clinically significant visual sequelae of thyroid eye disease are based on the potential loss of vision, either from corneal exposure due to lid retraction and exophthalmus, or from compressive optic neuropathy (Fig. 37) due to increased extraocular muscle size and often massive increases in orbital fat. Optic neuropathy that fails to respond to medical therapy can be treated surgically by orbital decompression (i.e., bony wall removal near the orbital apex) or by radiotherapy (90).

The histopathologic features of muscles in Graves' disease are often similar to those found in orbital pseudotumor (64). Inflammatory infiltration of muscles and other orbital connective tissues are seen, with interstitial edema and lymphocytic infiltration accounting for muscle enlargement. Fatty infiltration of atrophic muscles,

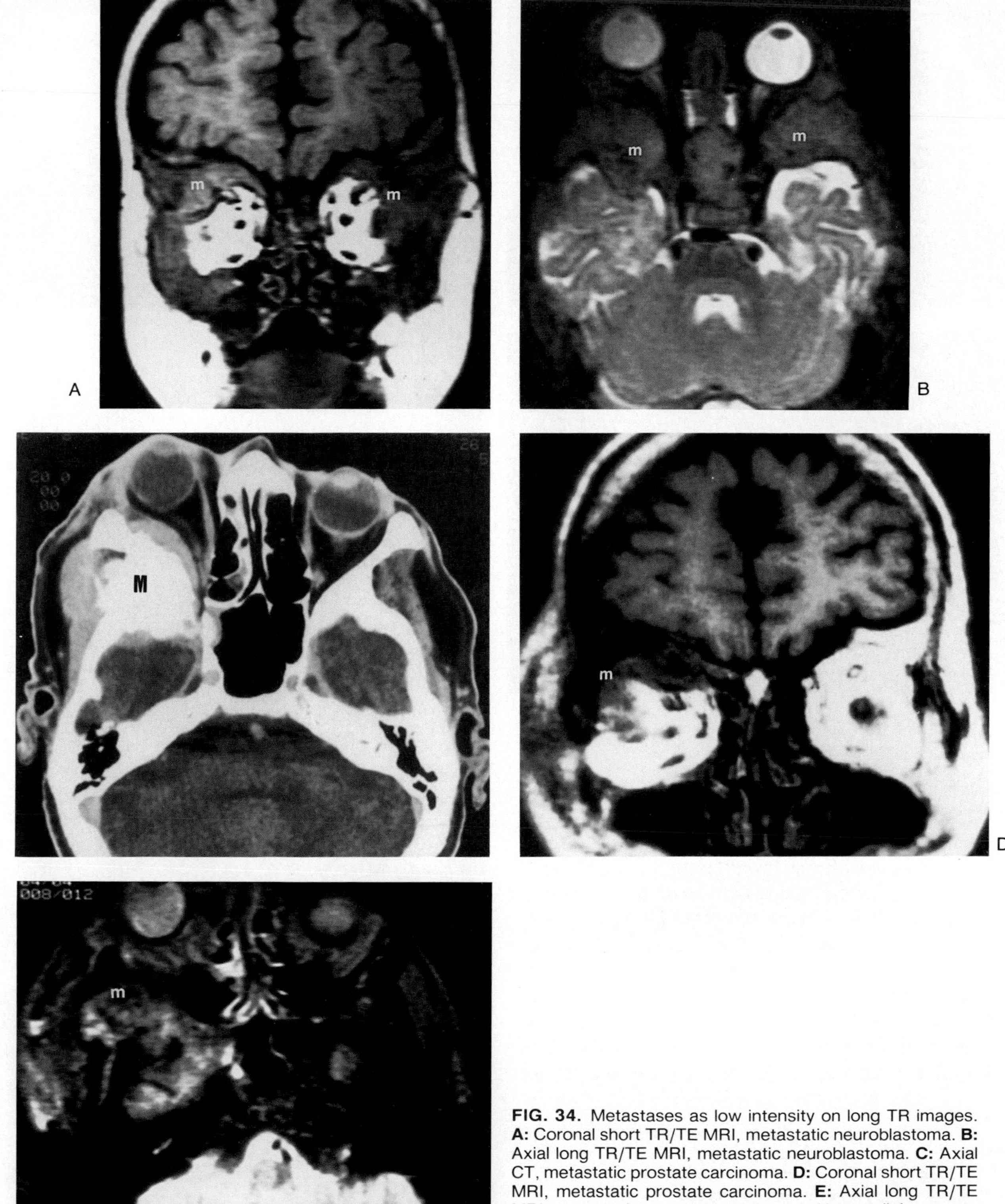

FIG. 34. Metastases as low intensity on long TR images. **A:** Coronal short TR/TE MRI, metastatic neuroblastoma. **B:** Axial long TR/TE MRI, metastatic neuroblastoma. **C:** Axial CT, metastatic prostate carcinoma. **D:** Coronal short TR/TE MRI, metastatic prostate carcinoma. **E:** Axial long TR/TE MRI, metastatic prostate carcinoma. Hypercellular neuroblastoma (*m*) is low intensity on both short TR/TE (A) and long TR/TE (B) MR images. Similarly, blastic metastasis from prostate carcinoma (*m,* C–E) has large regions of hypointensity on both short TR/TE (D) and long TR/TE (E) images.

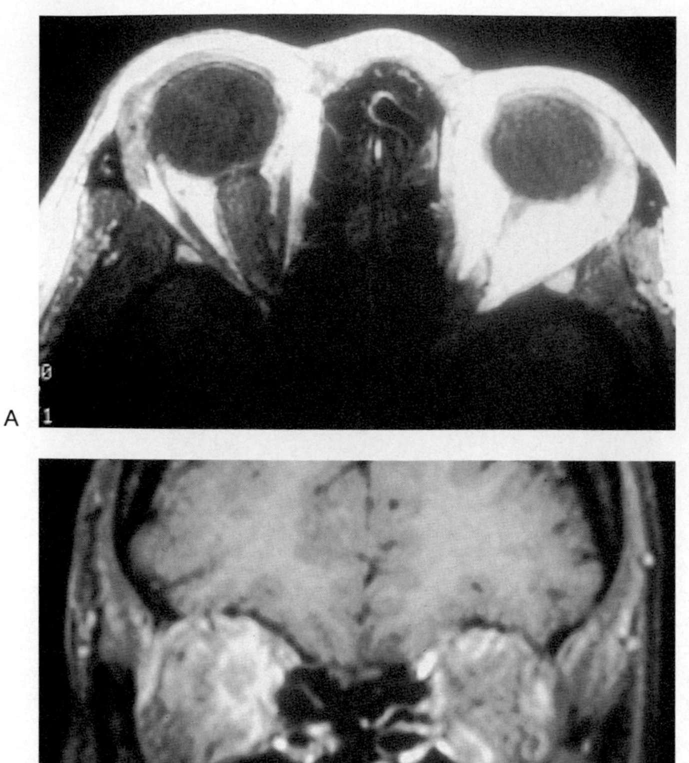

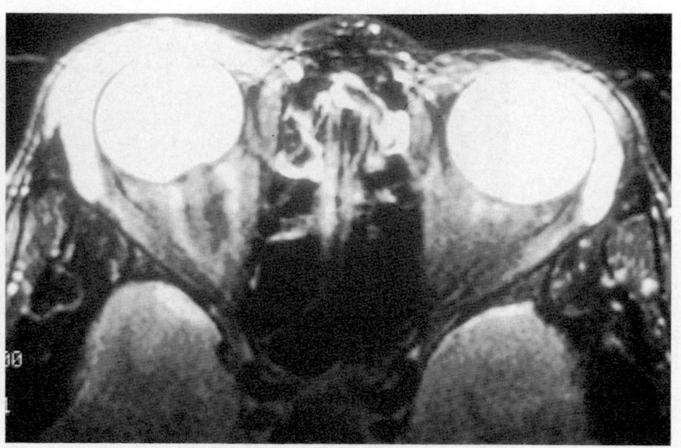

FIG. 35. Sarcoidosis as low intensity on T2-weighted images. Optic/perioptic mass is inseparable from optic nerve on T1-weighted image (**A**). Bulk of lesion is low intensity on T2-weighted image (**B**). After i.v. contrast (**C**), most of enhancement is perioptic. Pathology showed intraoptic and perioptic sarcoidosis.

as well as fibrosis, can occur in late stages of the disease (91). The exact incidence of thyroid exophthalmus is not known, but it may occur in both hyperthyroid and euthyroid individuals. It has been reported to be bilateral in up to 90% of cases (83), and females predominate. Imaging, either by CT or more recently MR, can demonstrate the extent of muscle involvement and its bilaterality (Fig. 37), and it is useful in patients with ophthalmopathy without clinical or laboratory evidence of thyroid disease (92). It is often difficult to separate the muscle enlargement of thyroid disease from other causes of muscle enlargement (83); although the majority of

TABLE 7. *Hypointense retrobulbar masses on T2-weighted images*

Inflammatory pseudotumor
Lymphoma
Sarcoidosis
Metastases from small cell or mucinous tumors
Fungal infection (abscess or cellulitis)
Retrobulbar hematoma (acute)
Meningioma

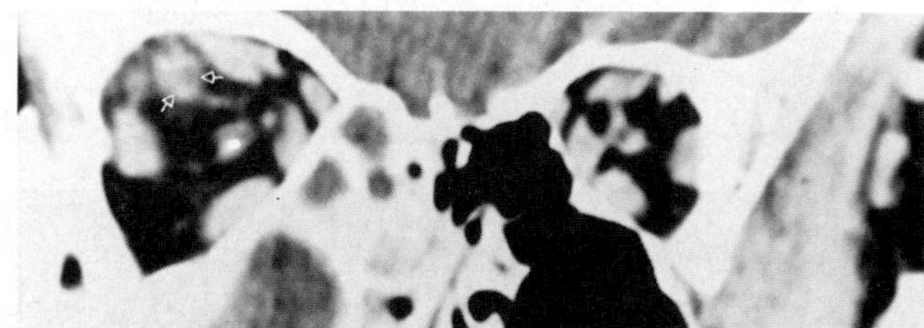

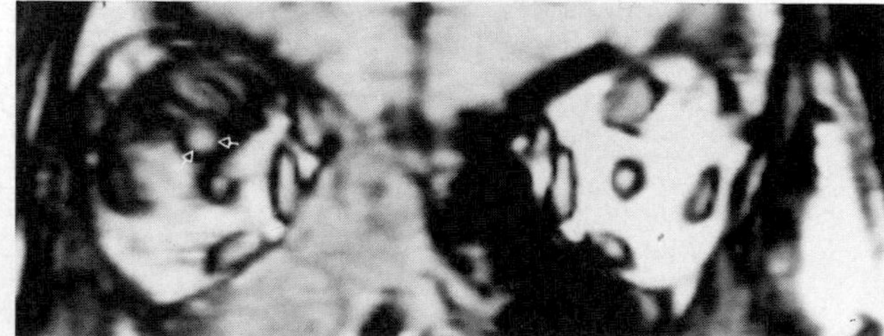

FIG. 36. Superior ophthalmic vein thrombosis and orbital cellulitis. **A:** Coronal CT. **B:** Coronal short TR/TE MRI (Dixon method opposed image 600/25). Enlarged right superior ophthalmic vein (*arrows*) on CT (A) is clearly seen on opposed MR image (B) as high-intensity clot, outlined by peripheral rim of signal void due to edge effect of Dixon method. Also note generalized decrease in intensity in superior aspect of right orbit from increased water content of inflamed orbital fat. (From Atlas et al., ref. 2, with permission.)

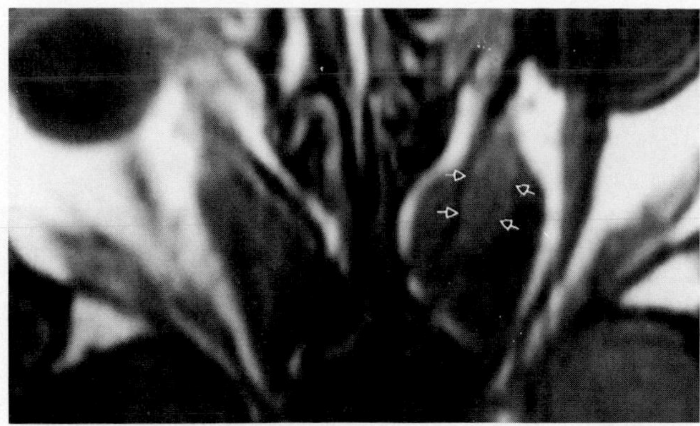

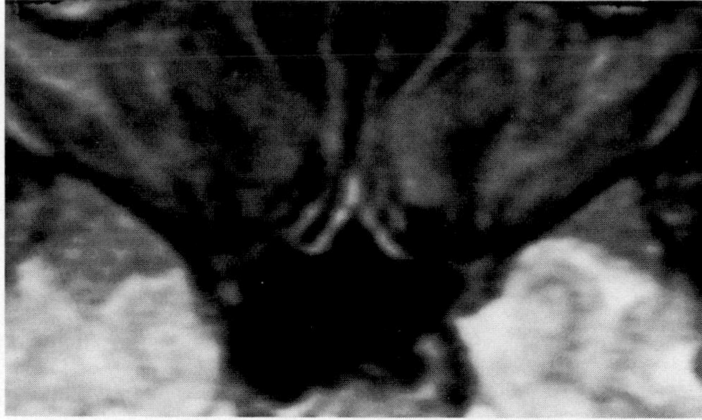

A B

FIG. 37. Thyroid orbitopathy. **A:** Axial short TR/TE MRI (600/25). **B:** Axial long TR/TE MRI (2500/80). Bilateral enlarged medial rectus muscles are low intensity on long TR/TE MR image (B). Note focal areas of hyperintensity on short TR/TE image (*arrows,* A), due to fatty infiltration of involved muscles. (From Atlas, ref. 34, with permission.)

cases of thyroid orbitopathy are bilateral, any or all extraocular muscles may be involved in nearly any combination. Typically, the inferior and medial recti are the earliest and most severely involved. It is said that muscle belly involvement usually predominates and tendinous insertion points are characteristically spared (see Fig. 37). If isolated lateral rectus muscle enlargement is present, another etiology should be considered (33). In most cases of thyroid disease of the orbit, the referring clinician is aware of the diagnosis, so the simple documentation of the orbital involvement is not of particular importance to the clinician.

MR identifies similar morphologic alterations to extraocular muscles that have been well documented on CT. The MR signal intensity pattern of muscle enlargement from thyroid disease has varied somewhat in the literature. Involved muscles can appear identical in signal intensity to other benign inflammatory entities (e.g., pseudotumor) (1) on SE MR (see Table 6): isointense to normal muscle on short TR/TE and low intensity or mildly hyperintense on long TR/TE images. One study has noted an increase in calculated T2 in the muscles of 50% of patients with Graves' disease (93). In that study, 9 of 23 patients had visible hyperintensity in involved muscles on long TR/TE images. These authors (93) postulate that the MR finding of prolonged T2 (or high intensity on long TR/TE images) in involved muscles may be predictive for response to anti-inflammatory therapy, since edematous muscles would presumably respond with a higher rate than nonedematous fibrotic muscles. In addition, 2 of 23 patients had high intensity within involved muscles on short TR/TE images (see Fig. 37), consistent with fatty infiltration, a finding previously reported on pathology in chronic cases. The MR finding of focal or irregular fatty infiltration in extraocular muscles may be a previously neglected clue to the underlying diagnosis of thyroid eye disease, and may be the only differentiating feature between thyroid disease and pseudotumor for the radiologist (Fig. 38). Perhaps the most important reason for imaging the orbit in cases of thyroid orbital disease is to identify optic nerve compression in the orbital apex by the enlarged muscles. The assessment of optic nerve compression is also readily made from MRI (see Fig. 37) and is clearly seen in the area of the orbital apex, thereby providing useful information to the ophthalmologist considering orbital decompressive procedures.

Optic Neuritis and Optic Neuropathy

Inflammation of the optic nerve itself is one of the many causes of unilateral (or bilateral) visual impairment. Its etiologies are numerous (Fig. 39), but by far the most common is demyelinating disease. A large percentage of cases are idiopathic. The optic nerve is a favored site for demyelination, but of patients who experience a solitary, isolated attack of optic neuritis, only 40% to 50% develop multiple sclerosis (MS) (94). In optic neuri-

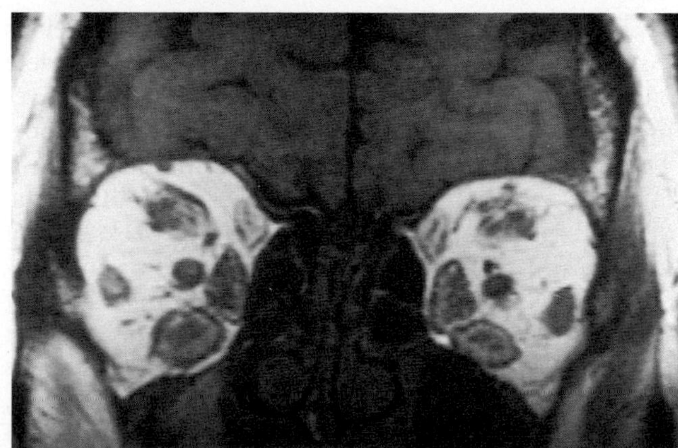

FIG. 38. Thyroid disease with muscle enlargement and fatty infiltration. Note multiple enlarged extraocular muscles with hyperintense fatty infiltration bilaterally, highly suggestive for thyroid disease.

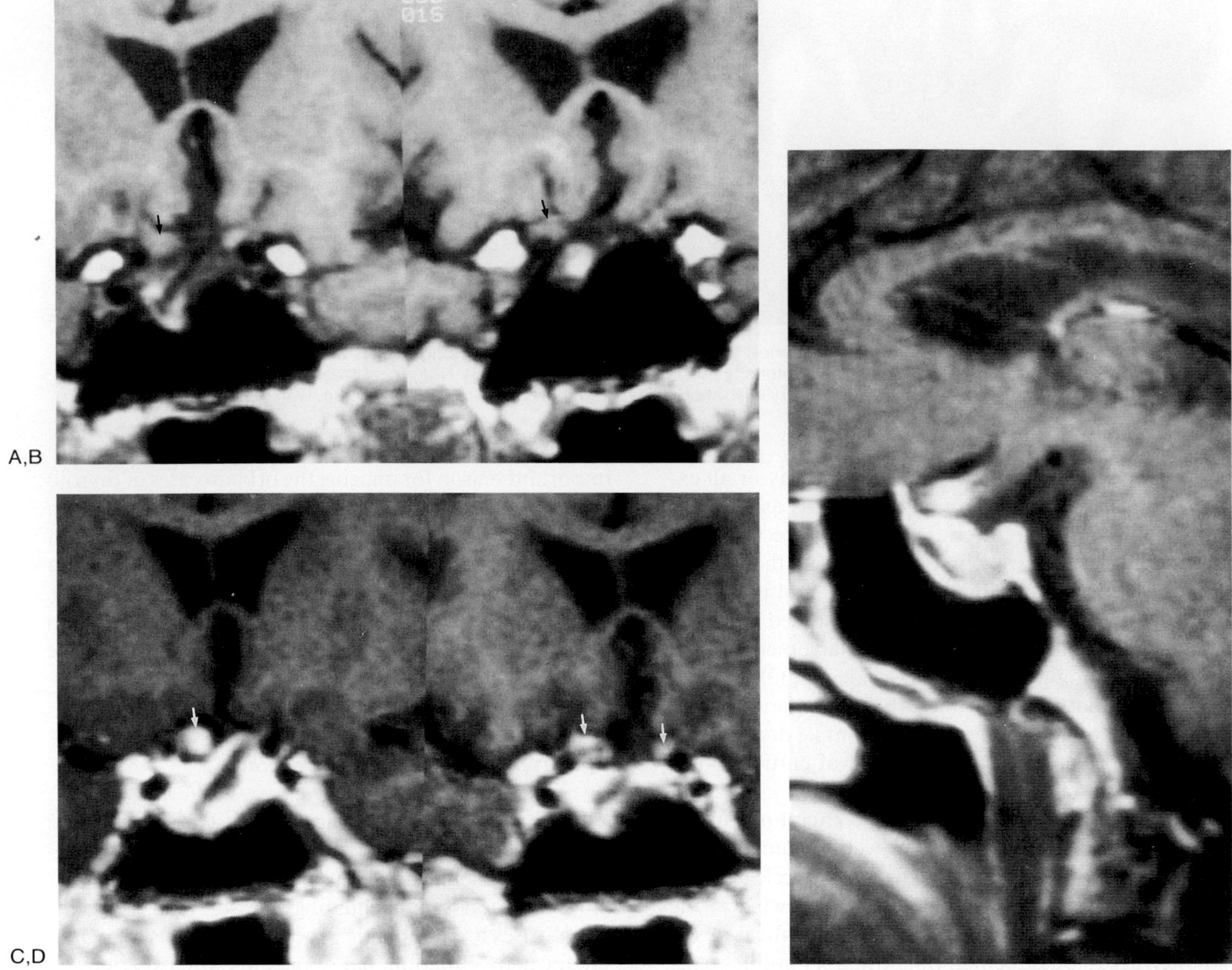

FIG. 39. Optic neuritis due to radiation therapy. Coronal T1-weighted images (**A,B**) show enlargement of intracranial prechiasmatic right optic nerve (*arrow*). After i.v. contrast (**C,D**), both optic nerves enhance (*arrows*). Sagittal image (**E**) shows right prechiasmatic enhancement.

tis, a decrease in visual acuity or field defect develops over hours to days, sometimes progressing to complete blindness. Other symptoms include pain on eye movement and tenderness on pressure applied to the globe. The presence or absence of optic disc findings on funduscopic examination depend on the proximity of the disease process to the nerve head. Within weeks, vision improves in most patients. Recovery occurs spontaneously but is hastened slightly by i.v. administration of steroids. However, the ultimate visual prognosis is not affected by the administration of steroids. In most cases of suspected demyelinating disease of the optic nerve, conventional SE MR is normal, but occasionally focal high intensity lesions are demonstrated on long TR images, particularly when T2-weighted FSE images in conjunction with fat suppression are obtained (Fig. 40). Some investigators have noted a higher sensitivity for detecting optic neuritis on MR by using inversion recovery sequences with short inversion times (STIR) (Fig. 41) (95). Acute lesions can enhance with i.v. contrast (Figs. 40, 42, and 43). Contrast enhancement of the involved optic nerve is seen more easily when fat suppression is employed (Fig. 44). The enhancement can be within the nerve substance or at its periphery, simulating the "tram track" sign more commonly associated with perioptic meningioma and other lesions (Table 8).

It may not be the detection of the optic neuritis itself that is important for the neuroradiologist in cases of clinically diagnosed optic neuritis; rather, data suggest that MRI of the brain may be more relevant to patient management and outcome (see Fig. 40). In the optic neuritis treatment trial, 46.9% of patients with monosymptomatic optic neuritis had abnormal brain MRI scans and 26.7% had two or more white matter lesions (96). The

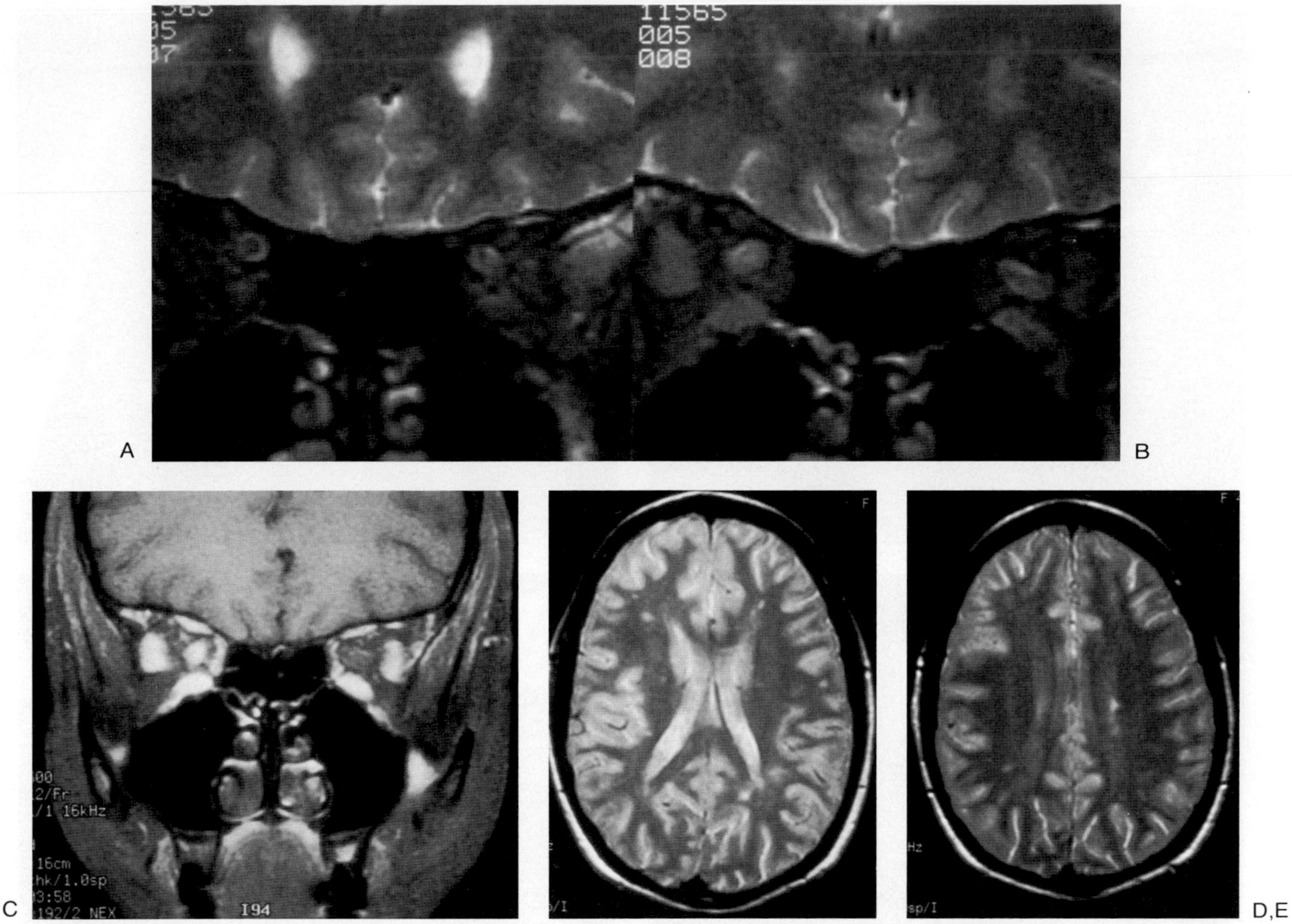

A B

C D,E

FIG. 40. Optic neuritis, hyperintense on T2-weighted FSE in MS. Coronal fat-suppressed T2-weighted FSE images (**A,B**) show subtle hyperintensity within right optic nerve. Note obvious enhancement after gadolinium (**C**). Brain images (**D,E**) demonstrate multiple focal hyperintensities compatible with the clinical diagnosis of MS.

presence of an abnormal MRI was associated with more severe visual loss and a higher occurrence of retrobulbar neuritis as opposed to papillitis. In the large cohort of more than 400 patients, MRI was helpful in correcting the misdiagnosis of only one patient (96). However, a follow-up analysis found high signal abnormalities on initial brain MRI to predict a higher rate of developing MS in a 2-year follow-up (97). MS subsequently developed in 4.9% of patients with normal brain MRI scans compared to 30.3% with three or more periventricular or ovoid white matter lesions. The administration of i.v. methylprednisolone also appeared to convey short-term benefit, reducing the risk of MS when compared to placebo and oral prednisone therapy (97). This was particularly true of those patients with intracranial white matter lesions on their initial MRI. Further work is warranted in a study specifically designed to evaluate the prophylactic benefits of i.v. steroids and beta-interferon therapy in those with isolated optic neuritis. The authors of the optic neuritis treatment trial conclude that brain MRI may not be helpful in the diagnosis of optic neuritis, but it appears valuable in defining the 2-year risk of developing multiple sclerosis (97).

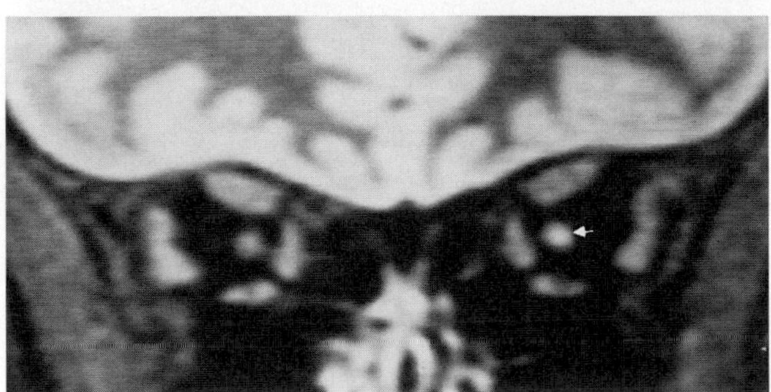

FIG. 41. Optic neuritis on STIR, coronal MRI (2500/150/60). Note marked hyperintensity in left optic nerve (*arrow*), as compared with normal contralateral nerve, in patient with left optic neuritis. (From Atlas, ref. 34, with permission.)

One important consideration in evaluating optic neuritis is distinguishing it from optic neuropathy of other causes, especially compression from a mass lesion. In el-

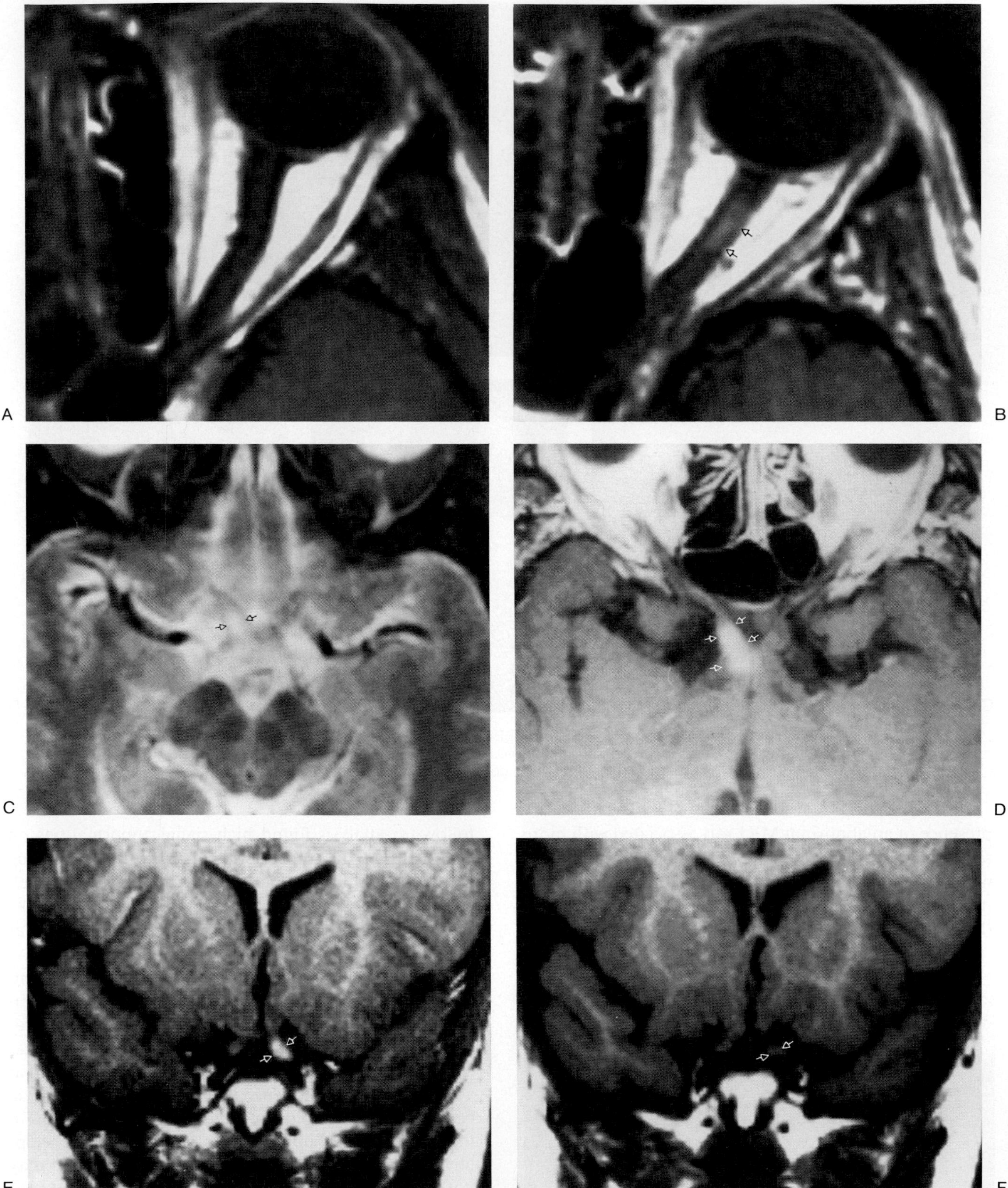

FIG. 42. Acute optic neuritis in demyelinating disease, with contrast enhancement. **A,B:** In a patient with probable MS. **C,D:** In a patient with definite MS. **E,F:** Acute disseminated encephalomyelitis. In patient with probable MS (A,B), enhancement is noted in the optic nerve (*arrows,* B), despite normal appearance on precontrast image (A). Similarly, in different patient with MS (C,D), note high intensity on long TR/TE image in prechiasmatic right optic nerve (*arrows,* C) with focal enhancement in right intracranial optic nerve and chiasm (*arrows,* D). Different patient with acute disseminated encephalomyelitis (ADEM) demonstrates focal enhancement in left intracranial portion of optic nerve (*arrows,* E), which is of normal size precontrast (*arrows,* F). (A,B, courtesy of Dr. A. S. Mark, Washington, DC.)

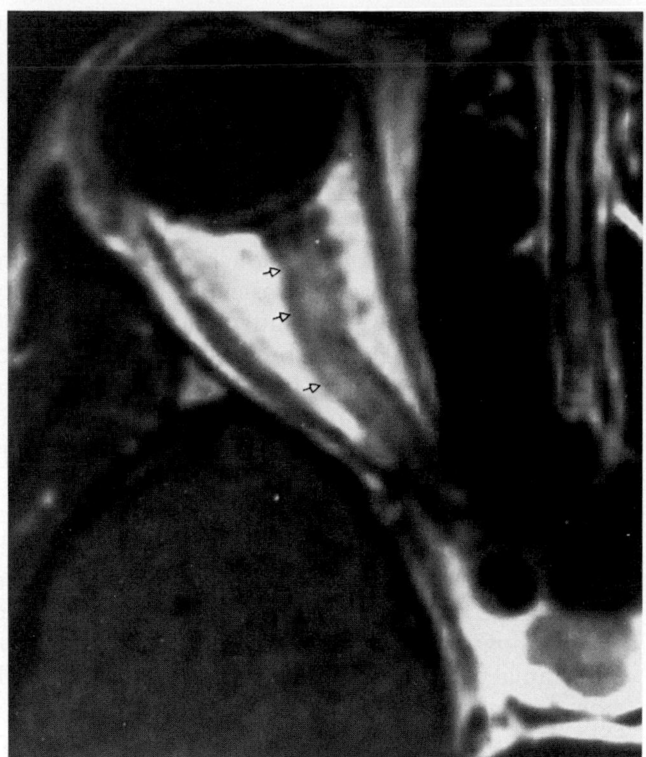

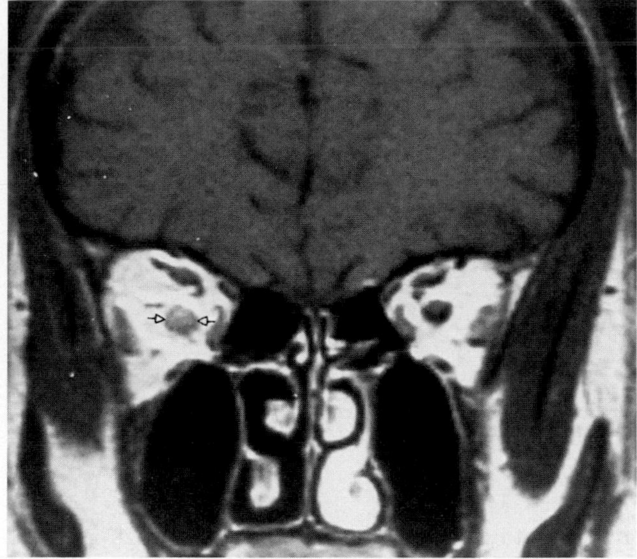

FIG. 43. Acute optic neuritis, with contrast enhancement in AIDS patient with syphilis, note enhancing lesion involving entire right optic nerve (*arrows,* **A,B**). (Courtesy of Dr. A. S. Mark, Washington, DC.)

derly and hypertensive patients who present with rapid onset of unilateral vision loss, optic nerve ischemia has been purported to be the underlying mechanism of injury. Interestingly, one small series of patients with this diagnosis (nonarteritic ischemic optic neuropathy) was evaluated with MR, and no significant increase in cerebral deep white matter lesions was seen as compared to

FIG. 44. Optic neuritis as tram-track enhancement. Coronal fat-suppressed postgadolinium T1-weighted image shows clear but thin peripheral enhancement around right optic nerve in patient with acute optic neuritis.

controls (98). The visual loss in these patients has been considered untreatable and is usually permanent. MRI is mainly used in this setting to exclude a mass lesion.

Tumors of the Orbit

It is of paramount importance to consider the clinical history when formulating a differential diagnosis of orbital mass lesions. The clinician usually has a good idea of the presence or absence of a focal mass; the role of the radiologist is to provide some diagnostic specificity and lesion localization. It is not rare, however, for benign orbital masses, particularly cavernous hemangiomas, to be diagnosed as incidental lesions on brain MRI.

Generally, lesions with abrupt onset of symptomatology are either malignant or inflammatory, whereas those with long periods of constant symptoms are usually be-

TABLE 8. *Etiologies of the "tram-track" sign of enhancement*

Perioptic nerve meningioma
Optic neuritis
Idiopathic inflammatory pseudotumor
Sarcoidosis
Leukemia
Lymphoma
Perioptic hemorrhage
Metastases
Normal variant

Modified from Atlas et al., ref. 33, with permission.

TABLE 9. *Causes of enlarged optic nerve/sheath complex*

Neoplasm	Optic nerve glioma
	Optic nerve hemangioblastoma
	Perioptic meningioma
	Plexiform neurofibroma
	Leukemia
	Lymphoma
	Metastases
Inflammation	Idiopathic inflammatory pseudotumor
	Thyroid eye disease
	Sarcoidosis
	Tuberculosis
	Optic neuritis
	Toxoplasmosis
Trauma	Perioptic hematoma

Modified from Atlas et al., ref. 33, with permission.

nign. Exceptions to this general rule are benign lesions that are prone to bleed, such as lymphangioma. Orbital structures are well demonstrated by both CT and MR, so their enlargement, displacement, and precise anatomic relationship to mass lesions can usually be readily appreciated. The ease of direct multiplanar imaging and high inherent contrast between retrobulbar fat and other structures (and lesions) with MR affords optimal anatomic information with little or no patient manipulation or discomfort in the great majority of cases. MR allows easier distinction between optic nerve masses and perioptic lesions (Table 9). MR may also have some specificity for certain lesions based on signal intensity patterns, especially in those that contain hemorrhage (1), fat, or melanin, and might help differentiate benign inflammatory lesions from malignant lesions in certain patients (3). In general, however, it seems that signal intensity patterns are usually not specific for differentiating most benign orbital masses from one another, or in distinguishing benign from malignant lesions in most cases (1,21). Fat suppression techniques in combination with i.v. contrast administration is clearly more sensitive than conventional imaging to subtle tumor extension (99).

Meningioma

Orbital meningiomas most commonly arise from the optic nerve sheath (Fig. 45), although extraconal meningiomas from orbital wall periosteum or randomly located arachnoidal nests are infrequently seen as well. Secondary extension into the orbit from intracranial meningiomas may also occur. These tumors comprise approximately 5% of primary orbital tumors (33); perioptic meningiomas account for one third of primary tumors of the optic nerve or sheath (63). Bilateral perioptic meningiomas may be associated with neurofibromatosis. These lesions are most common in females (80%) in their third to fifth decades and usually present with loss of vision followed by proptosis (100). Perioptic meningiomas have been reported to occur at an earlier age than their intracranial counterpart and, when encountered in children, are found commonly to be associated with neurofibromatosis (37). Papilledema or optic atrophy may accompany perioptic meningiomas, and visual field defects may occur.

The method of choice for evaluating orbital and perioptic meningiomas has traditionally been high resolution CT. These lesions are frequently calcified and usually enhance markedly on CT. However, at times it may still be difficult to distinguish perioptic masses from intrinsic optic nerve tumors on CT (although to a large extent, optic nerve gliomas occur in children, whereas perioptic meningiomas are most common in adults). Furthermore, a distended subarachnoid space may mimic optic nerve or sheath mass lesions on CT. One of the major advantages of MR in evaluating these lesions

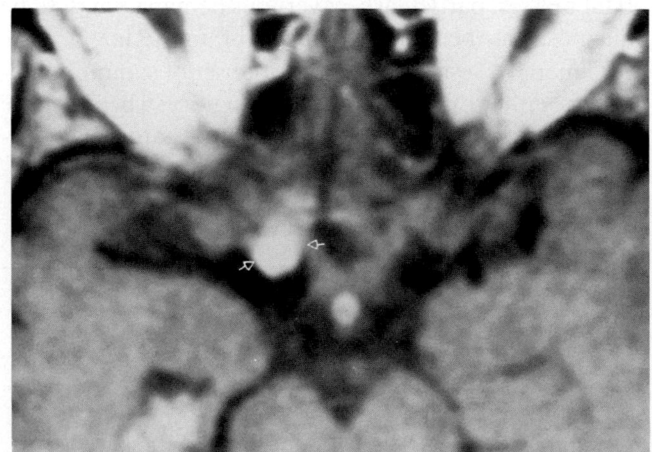

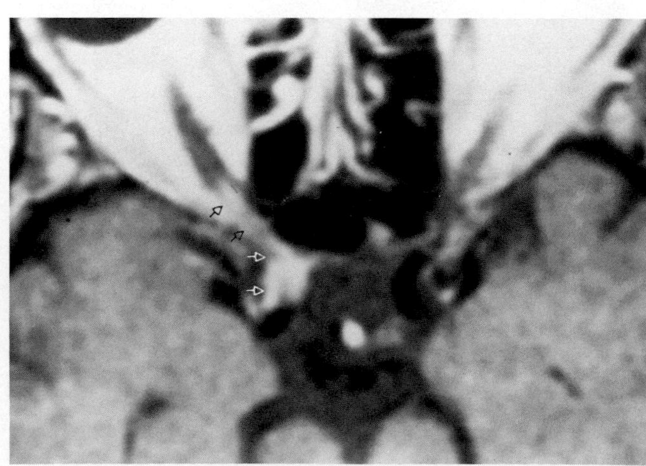

FIG. 45. Perioptic meningioma extending into intracranial compartment. Short TR/TE images (**A,B**) show enhancing perioptic meningioma (*arrows*) extending along and separate from intracranial nerve, well seen on these contrast-enhanced images.

lies in its ability to directly visualize the optic nerve and separate it from surrounding subarachnoid CSF space (1,8,101) (see Fig. 8), thereby easily distinguishing optic nerve lesions from sheath lesions. MR is also clearly superior to CT for visualizing the intracanalicular portion of the optic nerve (see Fig. 11) (1), an important area to evaluate for defining the posterior extent of perioptic and optic nerve lesions as they enter the superior orbital fissure and/or optic canal (Fig. 46). MR images do not suffer from artifacts arising from apical bony structures, which frequently interfere with the interpretation of CT scans in this region. In addition, direct oblique parasagittal imaging can provide exquisite anatomic delineation of the course of the optic nerve through the orbital apex (see Fig. 11), although we do not believe this is necessary in the vast majority of cases. Note that the head coil is usually needed for delineating the intracanalicular optic nerve and its entrance into the intracranial space.

Signal intensity patterns on MR have been described for orbital meningiomas (1,9,22) and are somewhat variable, depending on the site of the lesion. In one series (1), perioptic meningiomas appeared isointense to muscle on short TR/TE images and isointense to fat (i.e., relatively low signal intensity) on long TR/TE images. In contrast, extraconal intraorbital meningiomas were hyperintense to fat (i.e., high intensity) on long TR/TE images. The use of fat-suppression techniques has been quite helpful in defining the full anterior and posterior extent of perioptic meningiomas (2). Despite the fact that MR is not sensitive to the calcification often found in these lesions, the vast majority of perioptic meningiomas enhance with i.v. contrast. In conjunction with fat suppression, gadolinium-enhanced MR is clearly the most sensitive imaging technique for the detection of intraorbital meningioma, regardless of whether perioptic or not. In addition, fat-suppressed T2-weighted FSE imaging has been successful in delineating intraoptic signal abnormalities that can be found in the presence of perioptic nerve meningiomas (Fig. 47). We believe this hyperintensity represents the sequela of vascular compromise of the nerve itself and may correlate to vision loss in these patients.

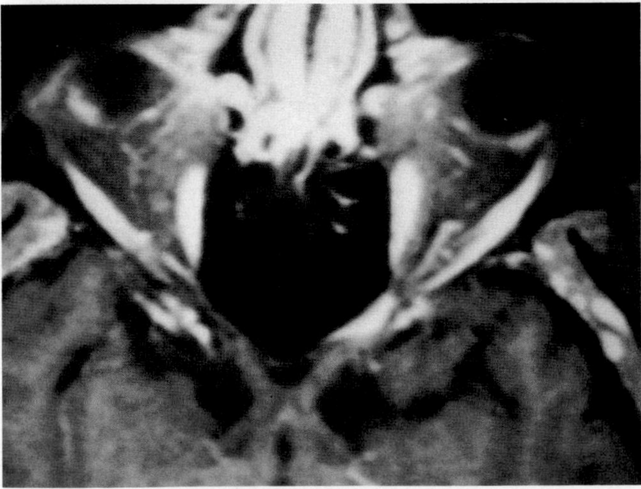

FIG. 46. Intracanalicular meningioma, on fat-suppressed T1-weighted image. Broad-based enhancing mass within left optic canal compresses optic nerve.

Secondary bone changes from orbital meningiomas (i.e., canal widening, bone disruption, and hyperostosis) can also be seen with MR (1,102) (Fig. 48). The high signal intensity on short TR/TE images of fat in the marrow of the boundaries of the superior orbital fissure and optic canal easily highlight their widened margins. Hyperostosis, representing either actual tumor infiltration or blastic response to adjacent tumor (70), is often seen in orbital wall meningiomas, and can be identified as intermediate or high signal intensity within an area of expected signal void (i.e., in an area of cortical bone). This has been reported in both orbital meningiomas and extraorbital, intracranial meningiomas. En plaque meningiomas involving orbital walls are most definitively evaluated with fat-suppression and contrast-enhanced studies (see Fig. 48).

There are still important limitations when using MR to evaluate meningiomas in the orbit. Since SE MR cannot easily detect calcification (72,73), the classic CT finding of calcification in a perioptic meningioma would not be confidently identified using SE MR. Furthermore, small, entirely calcified lesions might be missed entirely by MR (1). Gradient-echo imaging has been able to detect calcification in brain lesions, due to susceptibility-induced signal loss (71), so this technique may have a role in perioptic lesions. In addition, chemical shift misregistration artifact (29,101), seen in the orbit primarily as a black line that occurs at one interface between orbital fat and optic nerve in the frequency-encoding direction and a bright line at the water-fat interface (see Fig. 2), could obscure small perineural lesions. Although most perioptic meningiomas seem to have a noncalcified component that can be detected by MR (1), i.v. contrast should be administered to any patient suspected of harboring a perioptic meningioma. The classically described "tram-track" sign of perineural enhancement is nonspecific and cannot be used in isolation as diagnostic for meningioma (see Table 8).

Optic Nerve Glioma

Optic gliomas are usually low grade pilocystic astrocytomas (70) that, in 12% to 38% of cases, are associated with neurofibromatosis, especially when they are bilateral. These lesions are usually found in patients between 2 and 6 years of age, with three quarters presenting by age 10, and 90% by age 20. Initial symptoms include progressive, nonpulsatile exophthalmus with decreased eye movement and optic atrophy. Proptosis usually precedes the recognition of visual loss and the onset of strabismus,

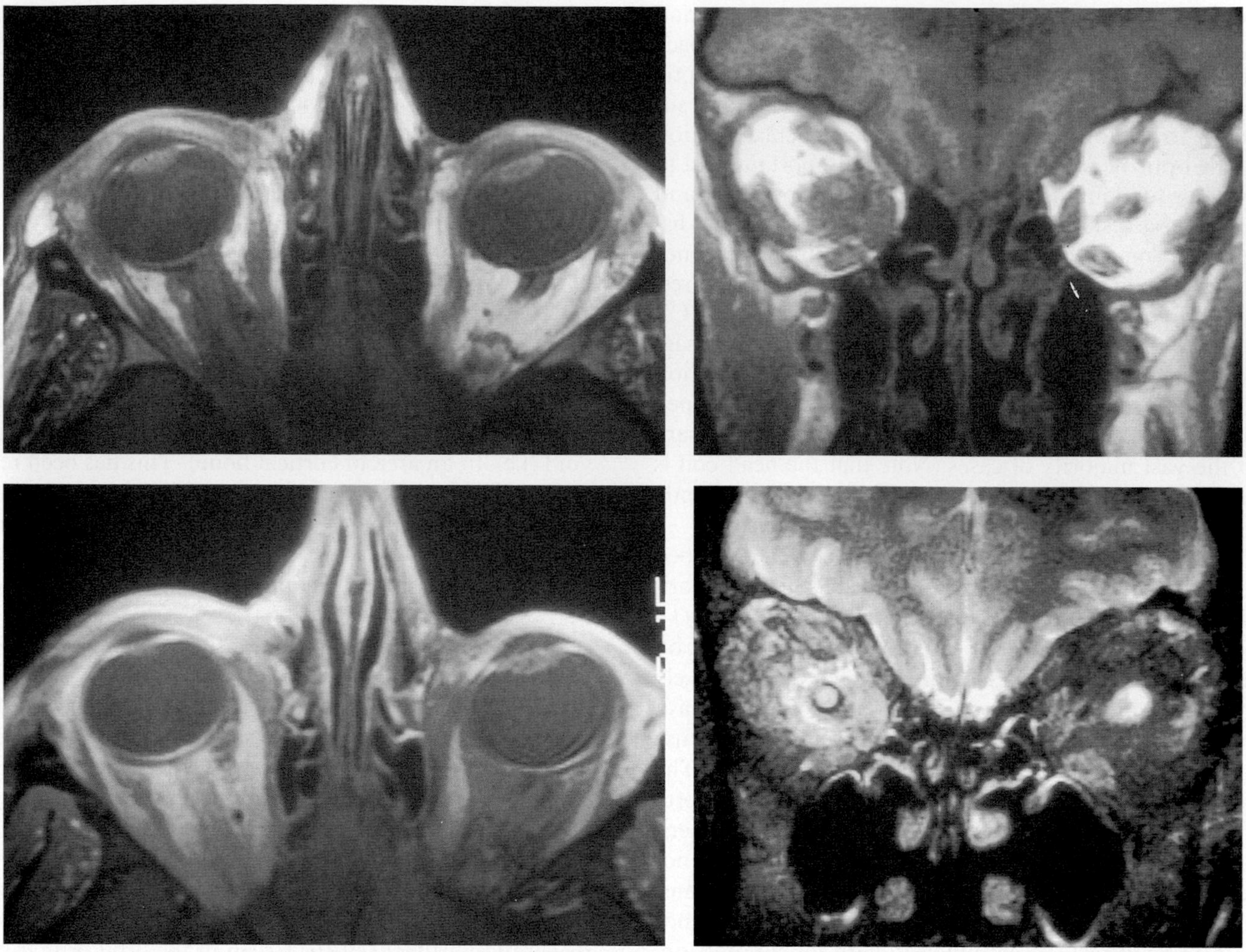

FIG. 47. Perioptic meningioma with ischemic change within optic nerve. Axial (**A**) and coronal (**B**) T1-weighted images show right perioptic mass. Note tram-track enhancement after i.v. contrast (**C**). Coronal T2-weighted image (**D**) shows hyperintensity of tumor and reveals high signal abnormality within compressed optic nerve in patient with significant vision loss, presumably due to ischemia.

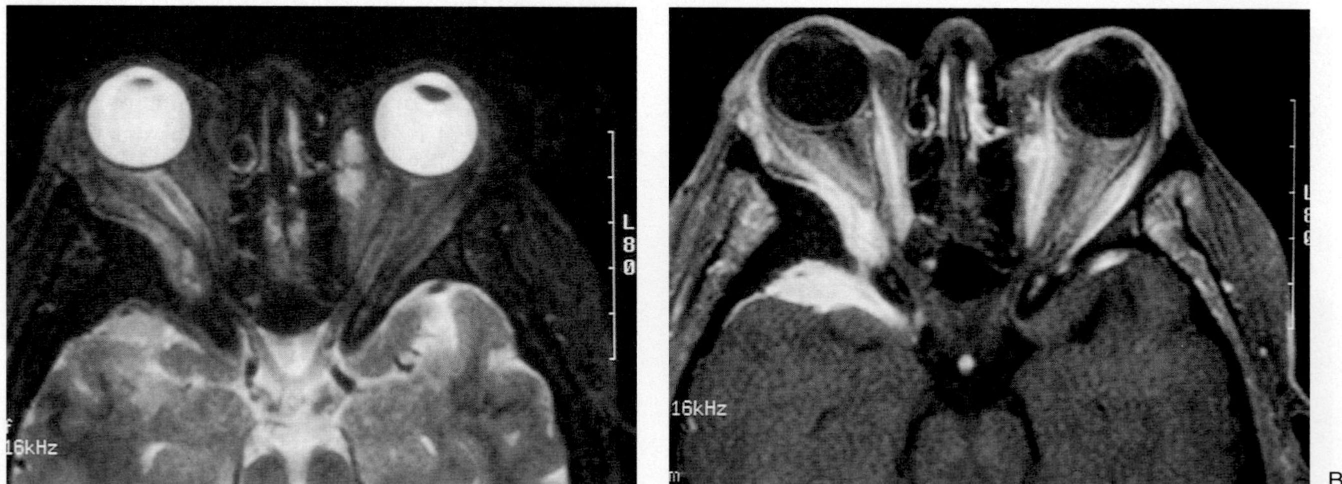

FIG. 48. En plaque meningioma. T2-weighted image (**A**) shows marked hyperostosis in right sphenoid wing with small amount of abnormal tissue within right posterolateral orbit. After i.v. contrast (**B**), fat-suppressed image shows intracranial and intraorbital meningioma. Absence of enhancement within hyperostotic bone implies reactive bony change, rather than actual tumor within bone.

but visual loss is common on detailed physical examination. Visual field deficits are notably variable, regardless of the site of the lesion (103). Although the differential diagnosis of this lesion is lengthy (see Table 9), the main diagnostic challenge to the clinician and the radiologist is the perioptic meningioma. Traditional teaching has described a very benign course for patients with these lesions, but more recent studies note a much poorer long-term prognosis than originally thought (104).

On pathologic examination, gliomas of the optic nerve are usually fusiform, intradural masses that stretch, rather than disrupt, the overlying meninges. At the tapering margins of the mass, it may be impossible to separate tumor from normal nerve by gross inspection. Furthermore, many optic gliomas contain areas where tumor merges with normal nerve on microscopy, in which neoplastic glial cells are virtually impossible to distinguish from reactive gliosis (37). This concept is perhaps the pathologic finding of most significance to the radiologist who interprets MRIs of these patients. Intratumoral hemorrhage and necrosis are said to be distinctly unusual (37). Some optic gliomas are accompanied by extensive thickening of the perioptic meninges, comprised of meningothelial cells, fibroblasts, and neoplastic astrocytes (Fig. 49). This peritumoral reactive change has been called arachnoidal hyperplasia or arachnoidal gliomatosis. It has been reported that a thick perineural cuff of reactive meningeal change is characteristic of patients with neurofibromatosis (105), although it remains controversial whether this represents a diagnostic sign of the syndrome.

MR is especially suited to evaluate optic pathway gliomas because MR clearly shows the intracanalicular and prechiasmatic intracranial nerve without artifact from nearby bony structures and is ideal for demonstrating the extension of the posterior portion through the optic canal and into the chiasm (see Fig. 11). This is another instance where the question of intracranial extension of the tumor often necessitates the use of supplementary head coil short TR/TE images. Enlargement of the optic nerve can readily be distinguished from prominent perioptic CSF spaces, as well as from perineural mass lesions. In most cases, optic nerve gliomas are isointense to normal white matter on short TR/TE and long TR/TE SE images (1,106), whereas prominent CSF spaces are high intensity on long TR/TE images. It is apparent that CSF clearly outlines optic gliomas, especially on long TR/TE sequences. The enhancement of optic gliomas with i.v. contrast is variable, but pilocystic astrocytic astrocytomas as a rule enhance frequently despite their relatively

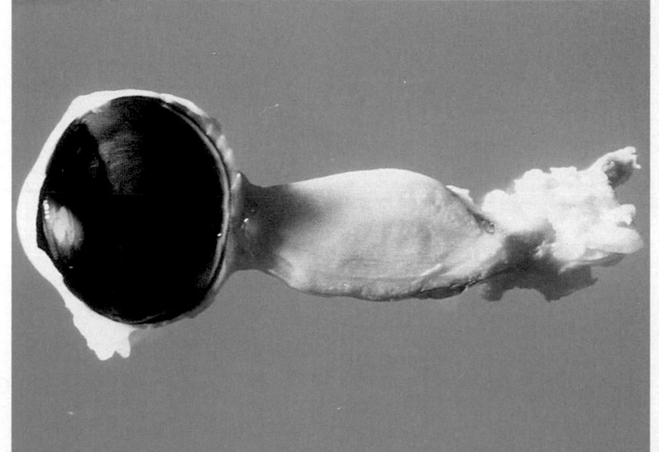
A

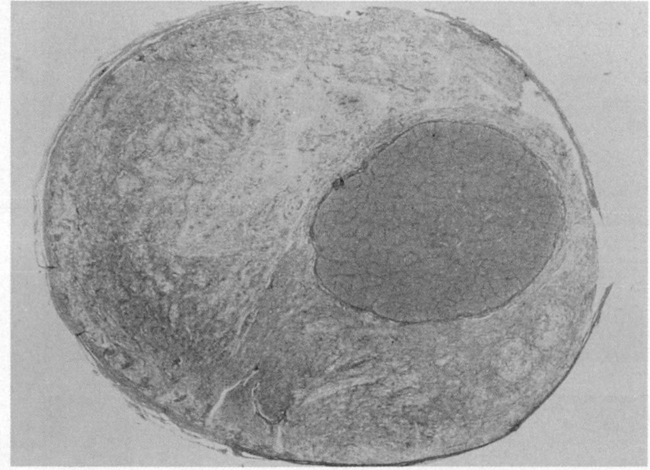
B

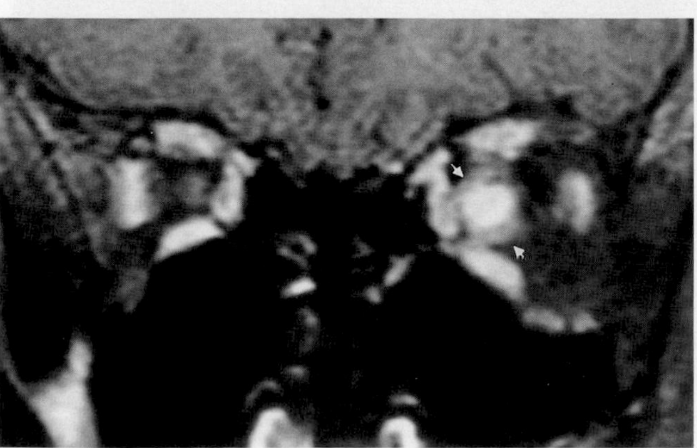
C

FIG. 49. Pathologic specimen, optic glioma in neurofibromatosis. **A:** Gross specimen. **B:** Transverse microscopic section, H&E. Note fusiform enlargement of involved nerve (A). Although the tumor is within the optic nerve itself, prominent thickening of perioptic arachnoid (arachnoidal hyperplasia) is forming most of the mass. (From Okazaki and Scheithauer, ref. 175, with permission.) **C:** Coronal postcontrast fat-suppressed T1-weighted image in similar case shows enhancement of optic nerve tumor centrally with thick peripheral region of enhancement (*arrows*) correlating to arachnoidal reactive change. (Courtesy of Dr. V. Mathews, Winston-Salem, NC.)

low grade (Fig. 50). Those optic nerve gliomas that are histologically of the diffuse (infiltrative) type are those that show more variable enhancement.

In evaluating a patient suspected of having an optic pathway glioma, the entire visual pathway must be evaluated, because a considerable proportion of these tumors involve the chiasm and retrochiasmal pathways, and frequently extend to the level of the lateral geniculate bodies (106,107). While CT literature states that visual pathway gliomas involved the optic tracts and lateral geniculate bodies in approximately one fourth of cases, MR has detected more frequent posterior extension of these lesions (106,107). In fact, a significant proportion of visual pathway gliomas are primarily isolated to the chiasm and retrochiasmal tracts, sparing intraorbital optic nerves. Retrochiasmal abnormal high signal intensity on long TR SE MR has been reported to be demonstrated without evidence of posterior extension on contrast-enhanced CT.

The signal intensity of these lesions varies with the site of involvement in the visual pathway (108) (Fig. 51). Optic nerve masses are isointense to white matter (i.e., relatively low intensity) on long TR/TE images, particularly in patients with neurofibromatosis. The relative hypointensity of the orbital portion of optic gliomas in these patients may correlate with the pathologic finding of peritumoral arachnoidal hyperplasia and relate to fibrocollagenous reactive change in association with neoplastic tissue. When the lesion invades the chiasm, there is an abrupt change in signal (108) to hyperintensity. Retrochiasmatic involvement is also characteristically high intensity on long TR/TE images. In our experience, we have only occasionally seen abnormal signal intensity extending beyond the geniculate bodies (i.e., into the optic radiations) on MR imaging (108). Pathologic correlation of the true etiology of abnormal signal intensity in the posterior retrochiasmal pathways in patients with optic pathway gliomas is not clearly defined because pathology is difficult to obtain from these relatively stable patients. Hamartomatous change, demyelination, gliosis, Wallerian degeneration, and neoplasm have all been proposed as responsible for these areas of abnormal signal intensity.

Neurofibroma and Schwannoma

There are numerous nerve branches other than the optic nerve within the orbit, including cranial nerves III,

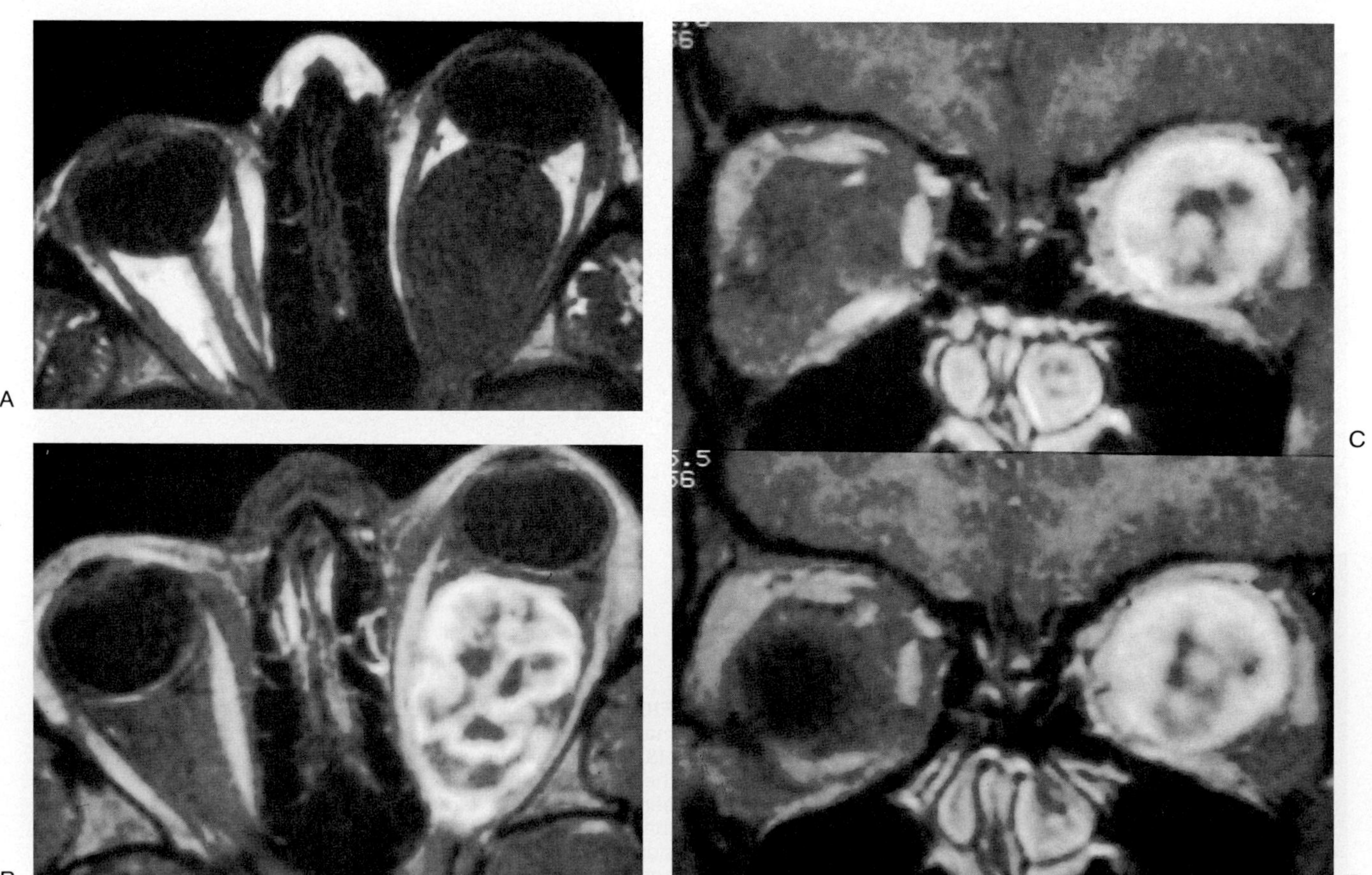

FIG. 50. Optic glioma with peripheral enhancement. Large intraconal mass inseparable from optic nerve (**A**) enhances in periphery (**B–D**).

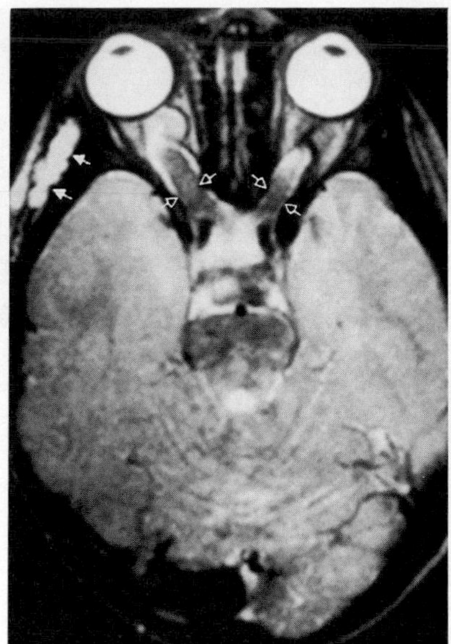

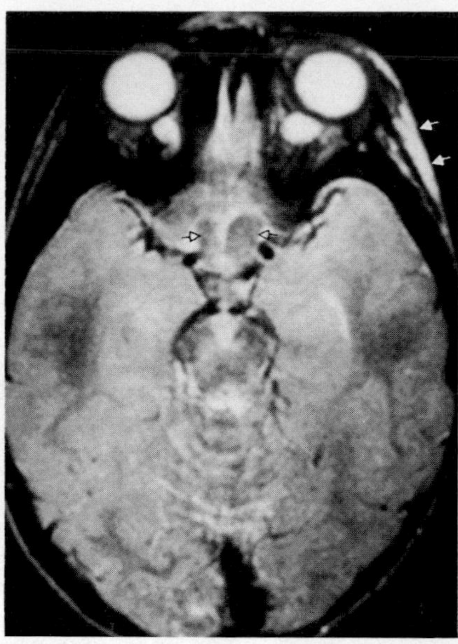

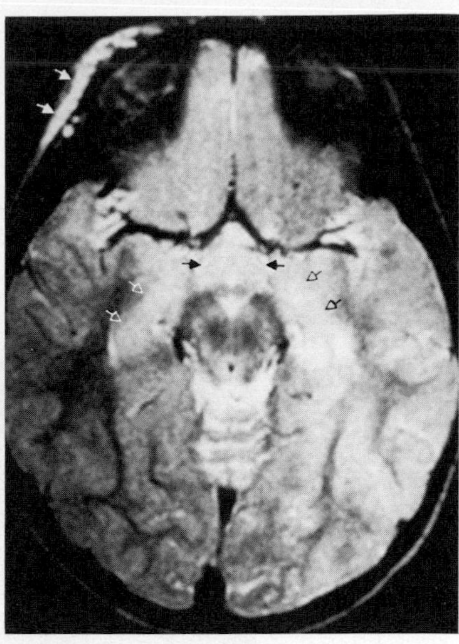

A B,C

FIG. 51. Visual pathway glioma signal intensity patterns. **A:** Long TR/TE MRI (2500/80). **B:** Long TR/TE MRI (2500/80). **C:** Long TR/TE MRI (2500/80). Enlarged intraorbital (*open arrows,* A) and intracranial (*open arrows,* B) optic nerves are isointense to normal white matter on long TR/TE images. In contrast, chiasm mass (*closed black arrows,* C) and retrochiasmatic extension (*open arrows,* C) demonstrate hyperintensity. Also note right frontal-temporal plexiform neurofibroma (*closed white arrows,* A–C). (From Atlas, ref. 34, with permission.)

IV, V, and VI, as well as sympathetic and parasympathetic fibers. Peripheral nerve sheath tumors comprise about 4% of orbital tumors and most often arise from sensory branches, especially those of the trigeminal nerve (37). The vast majority are benign and can be classified as either plexiform neurofibromas, schwannomas, or circumscribed neurofibromas. The plexiform neurofibroma is thought to be virtually pathognomonic of neurofibromatosis. It is an ill-defined, infiltrative lesion presenting in childhood that can involve all the orbital soft tissues, including the lacrimal gland. It is commonly associated with overgrowth of the lid and adjacent cutaneous tissues, and sphenoid wing dysplasia. The lesion is difficult to resect because it is highly vascular and so poorly circumscribed; therefore, there is a high rate of recurrence. On MR, plexiform neurofibromas are characteristic in their poor demarcation and infiltrative appearance. The diagnosis is certain when one notes enlargement of the ipsilateral orbital wall or lid and sphenoid wing defect (see Fig. 28). The lesions are somewhat heterogeneous on long TR/TE images, and could appear somewhat similar to lymphangiomas or even capillary hemangiomas if one failed to note the associated anomalies. Circumscribed neurofibromas are also benign masses, most commonly affecting the branches of the Vth cranial nerve. These appear as well-delineated and frequently multiple mass lesions that are discovered in the third to fifth decades. Generally, circumscribed neurofibromas are not associated with neurofibromatosis (109). They appear as many other sharply demarcated, benign masses on MR images: isointense to muscle on short TR/TE and markedly hyperintense on long TR/TE images. They may be indistinguishable on imaging studies from schwannoma, which also arises from sensory nerve branches in the orbit. Slowly progressive symptomatology and imaging studies cannot distinguish these lesions from isolated neurofibromas in the vast majority of cases. Schwannomas are somewhat less likely to undergo malignant degeneration and are less likely to be multiple (37). Histologically, schwannomas are unique in that they are truly encapsulated; they may also be partially cystic and occasionally demonstrate intratumoral hemorrhage (37). In occasional cases, MR can identify focal heterogeneities consistent with intratumoral hemorrhage or cystic change and lead one to favor schwannoma (Fig. 52) over neurofibroma. All these tumors enhance with some heterogeneity with i.v. contrast.

Retrobulbar Orbital Metastases

Metastases to the orbit are relatively uncommon in clinical imaging practices (110), and sites of involvement, as well as the origin of the primary neoplasm, differ between children and adults. In the child, metastases to the orbit are much more common than those that involve the globe, with neuroblastoma, leukemia, and Ewing's sarcoma being the most common primary neoplasms involved. In the adult, up to 90% of metastases are ocular and only 10% are retrobulbar in location (37). In only 50% of these patients is the origin of the primary

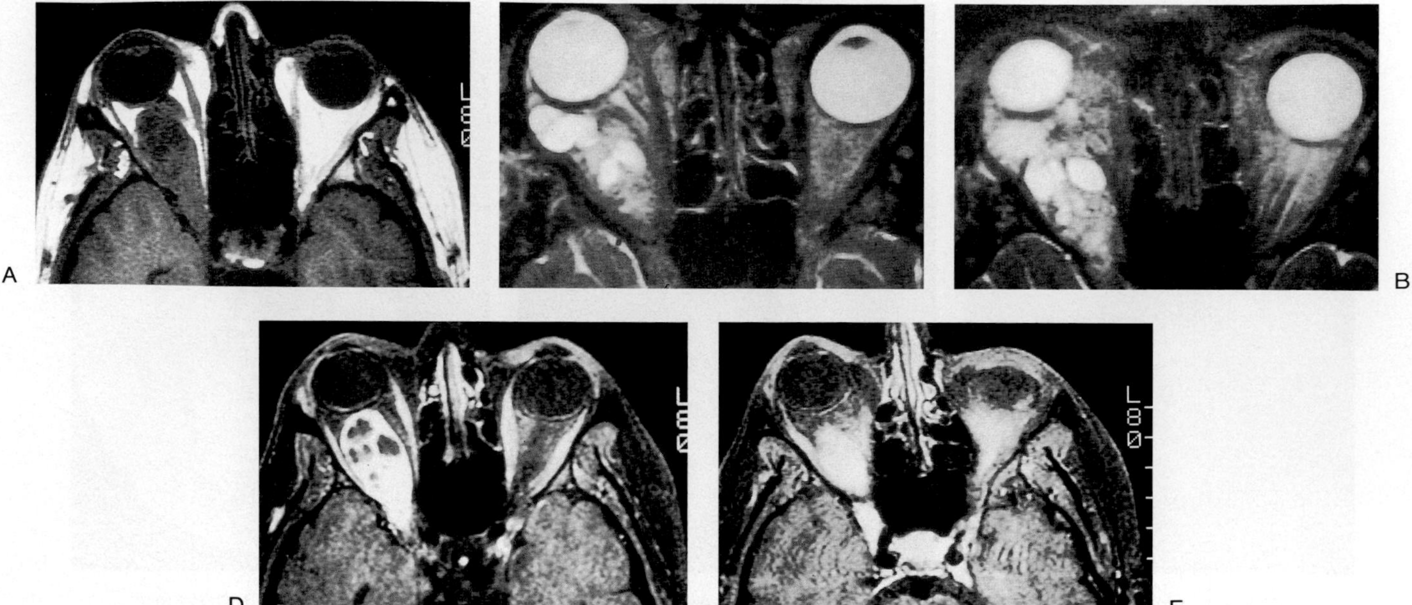

FIG. 52. Schwannoma. Large intraconal mass separate from optic nerve (A–C) is markedly heterogeneous and partially enhances (D) reflecting cystic changes. Note extension into cavernous sinus (E), revealing its origin from cranial nerve III, IV, V, or VI.

tumor known, and these are usually carcinomas of the breast or lung (110). In children, orbital metastases usually involve orbital wall destruction and often extend into a subperiosteal location. Although metastatic disease is usually bilateral, unilateral metastases are common. Of particular note is metastatic disease from scirrhous carcinoma of the breast, where extensive fibrous response can result in enophthalmos, often a clue to the diagnosis.

Symptoms of orbital metastatic disease include sudden onset of proptosis, ophthalmoplegia, and pain, often mimicking the clinical presentation of inflammatory pseudotumor. Unfortunately, the CT appearance of metastatic disease to the retrobulbar region is well known to be indistinguishable from that of pseudotumor, in the absence of gross bone destruction. In one series of patients with clinical presentations compatible with orbital pseudotumor, the investigators (3) were able to distinguish malignant metastases from benign inflammatory conditions on the basis of signal intensity patterns on T2-weighted images. Metastases demonstrated markedly high signal intensity compared to that of orbit fat on long TR/TE sequences (see Fig. 33) (see Table 6), whereas benign inflammatory lesions were isointense or minimally hyperintense in all but one case (Fig. 53).

Some malignant retrobulbar lesions are certainly not distinguishable from pseudotumor on the basis of signal intensity alone (1). Myeloma involving the orbit can appear as low signal intensity (isointense to fat) on long TR/TE images, as can lymphoma and neuroblastoma (see Fig. 34). The explanation for the low intensity of some neoplasms on long TR/TE sequences may reside in the fact that these neoplasms histopathologically show a very hypercellular, monotonous infiltration of tumor cells with very scant cytoplasm and, consequently, little free water content, thereby resulting in a relatively shorter T2 than other lesions.

Another common neoplasm to metastasize to the orbit is prostate carcinoma. A favorite site of prostate carcinoma metastasis is the greater wing of the sphenoid, often producing large intraorbital mass lesions and secondary sclerotic bone reaction. Although MR is generally regarded as being inferior to CT for detecting bony abnormalities, some authors have noted that MR can clearly document orbital bone destruction and hyperostotic change (1) as either clear interruption of an expected rim of cortical bone signal void, suggesting overt destruction, or the presence of signal contained within an expected region of signal void, as seen in hyperostosis from meningiomas (1). Blastic metastatic disease is usually hypointense on MR images (see Fig. 34). It should be noted that hypointensity from chemical shift misregistration at fat–water interfaces can occasionally be confused with cortical bone.

Orbital Hemangioma and Lymphangioma

Vascular tumors and malformations are among the most common causes of proptosis. The three most common vascular tumors in the orbit are the adult-type cav-

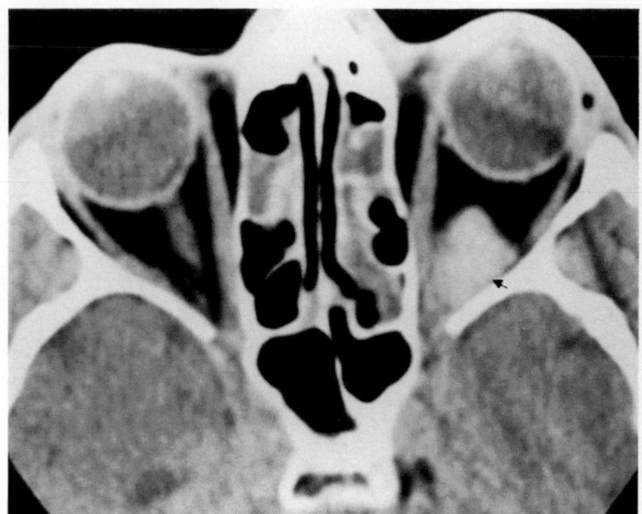

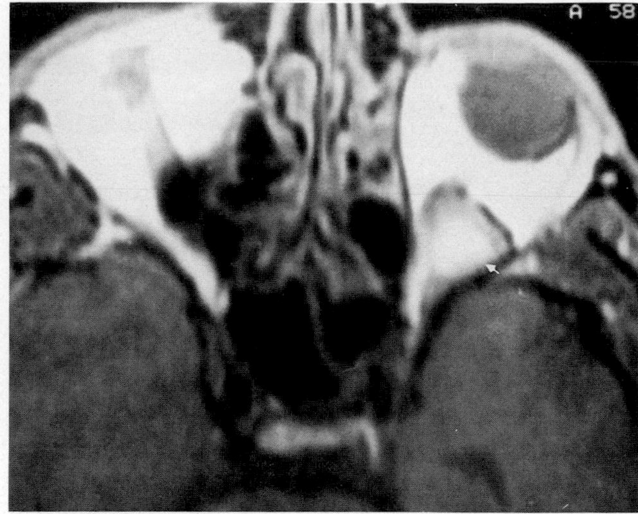

FIG. 53. Inferior rectus muscle hematoma. **A:** CT. **B:** Short TR/TE MRI (600/20). High attenuation orbital apex mass (*arrows*) on CT (A) is hyperintense on short TR/TE MR (B), due to methemoglobin in traumatic intramuscular hematoma. (From Atlas et al., ref. 3, with permission.)

ernous hemangioma, the pediatric-type capillary hemangioma, and lymphangioma (37). These lesions all differ in their imaging appearance, but the most useful clue to the differential diagnosis is the age of the patient (Table 10).

The most common retrobulbar mass lesion in the adult, excluding inflammatory pseudotumor, is the cavernous hemangioma. It most frequently occurs in young to middle-aged females and is characterized by very slowly progressive, painless proptosis. These lesions are usually intraconal (Fig. 54), but extraconal hemangiomas are not uncommon. Cavernous hemangiomas are composed of large endothelium-lined dilated vascular channels with variable amounts of fibrous tissue and a fibrous capsule. Since the blood "flow" in the vascular spaces is essentially stagnant, thrombosis is common; spontaneous bleeding does not occur. Since these lesions are soft [described as "spongy" on gross examination (37)], they often do not deform the globe, even when abutting its surface; however, expansion of adjacent orbital walls can occur with long-standing lesions. Cavernous hemangiomas are the most common orbital mass in the adult who is asymptomatic and should be very high on the list of possibilities in all cases of incidentally discovered lesions.

The MR appearance of cavernous hemangiomas are smooth or slightly lobulated, well circumscribed masses of low intensity (Fig. 55) on short TR/TE images (i.e., isointense to muscle). Occasionally, these lesions contain regions of high signal intensity on short TR/TE images, raising the possibility of areas of thrombosed vascular spaces (see Fig. 54). Cavernous hemangiomas are usually markedly hyperintense on long TR/TE images (Fig. 56). If evidence of intralesional flow is seen, another diagnosis should be suggested (such as vascular hemangiopericytoma, varix, or arteriovenous malformation). High resolution imaging may occasionally demonstrate the calcified phlebolith (Fig. 56), a nearly pathognomonic sign of cavernous hemangioma. Cavernous hemangiomas always enhance with i.v. contrast. The major role of MR in the evaluation of cavernous hemangiomas is to provide the precise anatomic delineation of the mass and its relationships to the optic nerve and other orbital structures, since these lesions are surgically curable (i.e., they are encapsulated and do not recur).

In the pediatric patient, orbital hemangiomas are usually classified as capillary rather than cavernous on histopathology. These lesions are also known as benign hemangioendothelioma or infantile hemangioblastic hemangioma (37). They usually concomitantly involve the periocular tissues and lid and are diagnosed within the first weeks of life. Although these lesions may undergo fairly rapid enlargement early and occasionally simulate rhabdomyosarcoma, they plateau in size within

TABLE 10. *Vascular masses in the retrobulbar region*

Lesion	Age of patient	Location	Morphology
Capillary hemangioma	Infant (birth–2 yrs)	Often preseptal	Infiltrative
Lymphangioma	Child (1–15 yrs)	Mixed; involves muscle cone	Infiltrative
Cavernous hemangioma	Adult (young–middle-aged)	Intraconal or extraconal	Well circumscribed

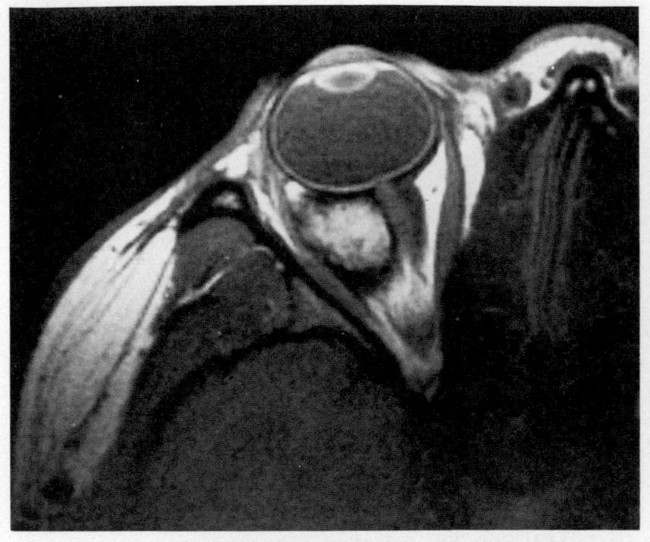

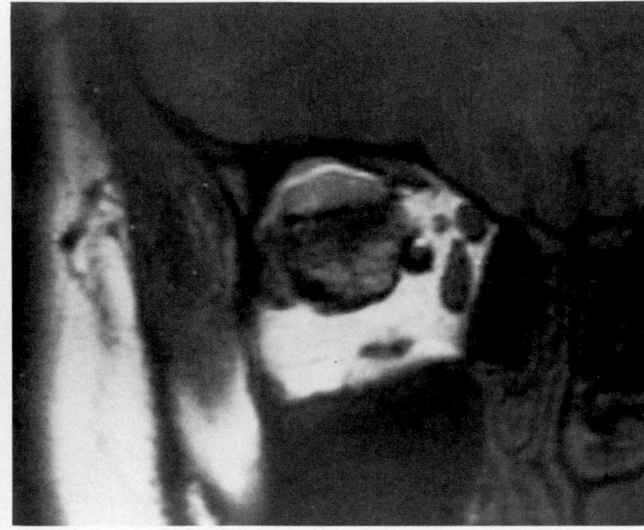

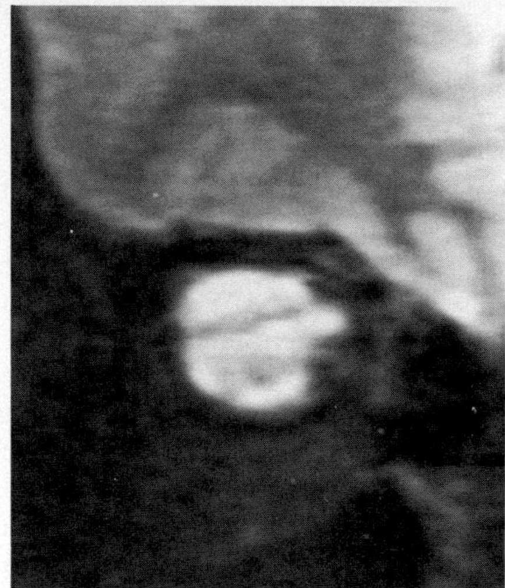

FIG. 54. Partially thrombosed cavernous hemangioma. **A:** Axial short TR/TE MRI (600/20). **B:** Coronal short TR/TE MRI (600/20). **C:** Coronal long TR/TE MRI (2500/80). Large intraconal mass is markedly hyperintense at its periphery on short TR/TE images (A,B), probably due to intralesional thrombosis of cavernous spaces. Entire lesion is hyperintense on long TR/TE image (C).

the first year or two and often go on to involute significantly. These are infiltrative lesions with highly vascular channels throughout, presenting a distinctly different appearance from the adult cavernous hemangioma in many respects. In view of the virtually exclusive appearance of capillary hemangiomas during infancy, the diagnosis should be suspect if made in an adult (in whom a more likely diagnosis is arteriovenous malformation or hemangiopericytoma) (37). The MR appearance of capillary hemangiomas mirrors their gross pathologic features. These lesions are poorly demarcated and often extend into the anterior periocular tissues. The key finding is the identification of numerous vascular channels, seen as linear or focal regions of signal void on SE images (Fig. 57). MR angiography depicts these areas as markedly hypervascular and clinch the diagnosis (Fig. 57) (111).

It is important to differentiate lymphangioma from cavernous hemangioma because lymphangiomas are not removed easily because of the lack of a well-defined capsule and therefore often recur. Lymphangiomas are much less common than hemangiomas and are usually extraconal or involve the muscle cone itself. They generally occur in younger patients. In fact, because of the wide separation of ages at diagnosis for capillary and cavernous hemangiomas, lymphangiomas represent the most likely diagnosis if a vascular tumor appears in the orbit between the ages of 1 and 15 years (37). These lesions can be classified according to their location (i.e., deep vs. superficial); superficial lesions are not diagnostic or therapeutic dilemmas, but deep lesions are both difficult to remove and often cause marked symptomatology (112). These lesions commonly involve lid and conjunctivae. Although lymphangiomas can present with slow and progressive proptosis, they have a propensity to intermittently hemorrhage (Fig. 58), sometimes producing acute symptoms such as pain and rapidly progressive proptosis. They tend to infiltrate adjacent soft tissues. MR identifies lymphangiomas by their charac-

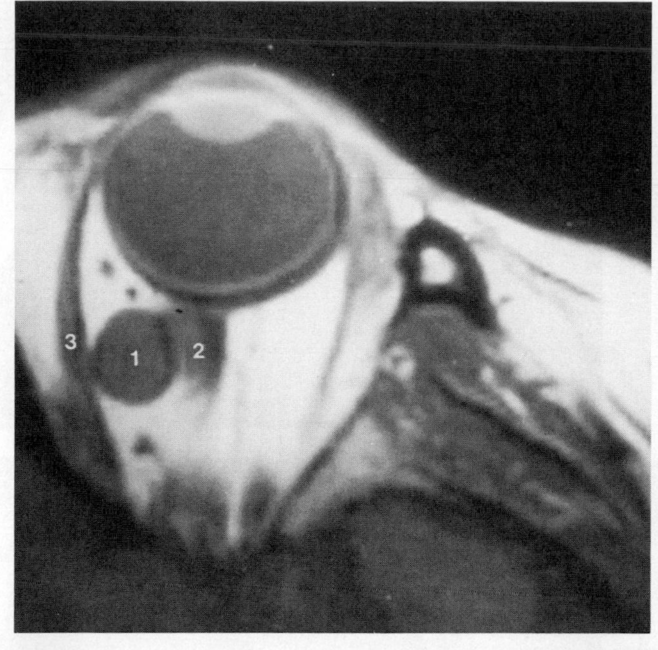

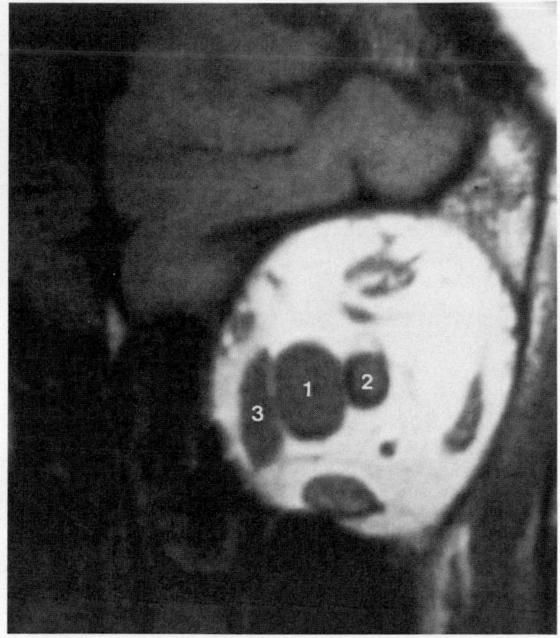

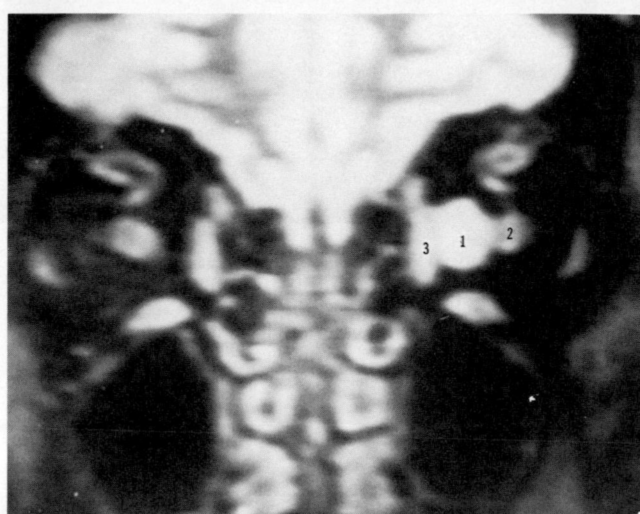

FIG. 55. Intraconal cavernous hemangioma, SE vs. STIR. **A:** Axial short TR/TE MRI (600/20). **B:** Coronal short TR/TE MRI (600/20). **C:** Coronal MRI (STIR, 2500/150/30). Mass (*1*) between optic nerve (*2*) and medial rectus (*3*) is clearly seen on both short TR/TE (A,B) and STIR (C) images. Note all retrobulbar structures are markedly hyperintense on STIR (C) obtained at null point for fat. (From Atlas et al., ref. 176, with permission.)

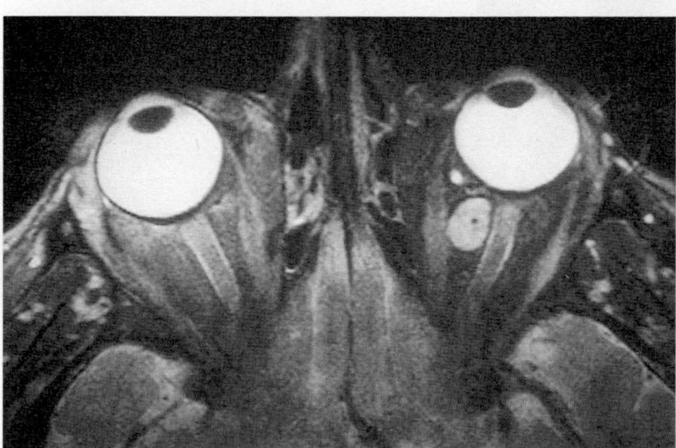

FIG. 56. Cavernous hemangioma with calcified phlebolith. Tiny focal hypointensity on high resolution FSE T2-weighted image represents calcified phlebolith in cavernous hemangioma.

teristic heterogeneity (1) with hemorrhagic foci of varying ages, cystic regions, and conal-extraconal location (see Fig. 50).

Dermoid and Epidermoid Cysts

Dermoid cysts are the most common congenital lesion of the orbit. They are usually found in the first decade of life, especially when superficial (113), and present with proptosis or progressive upper lid swelling. Although most commonly in the region of the lacrimal fossa, they can be located anywhere in the orbit. They arise as a result of intrasutural sequestration during orbital development, so are frequently found in intimate association with eroded bone. These lesions can extend through the bone into the extradural space of the anterior or middle

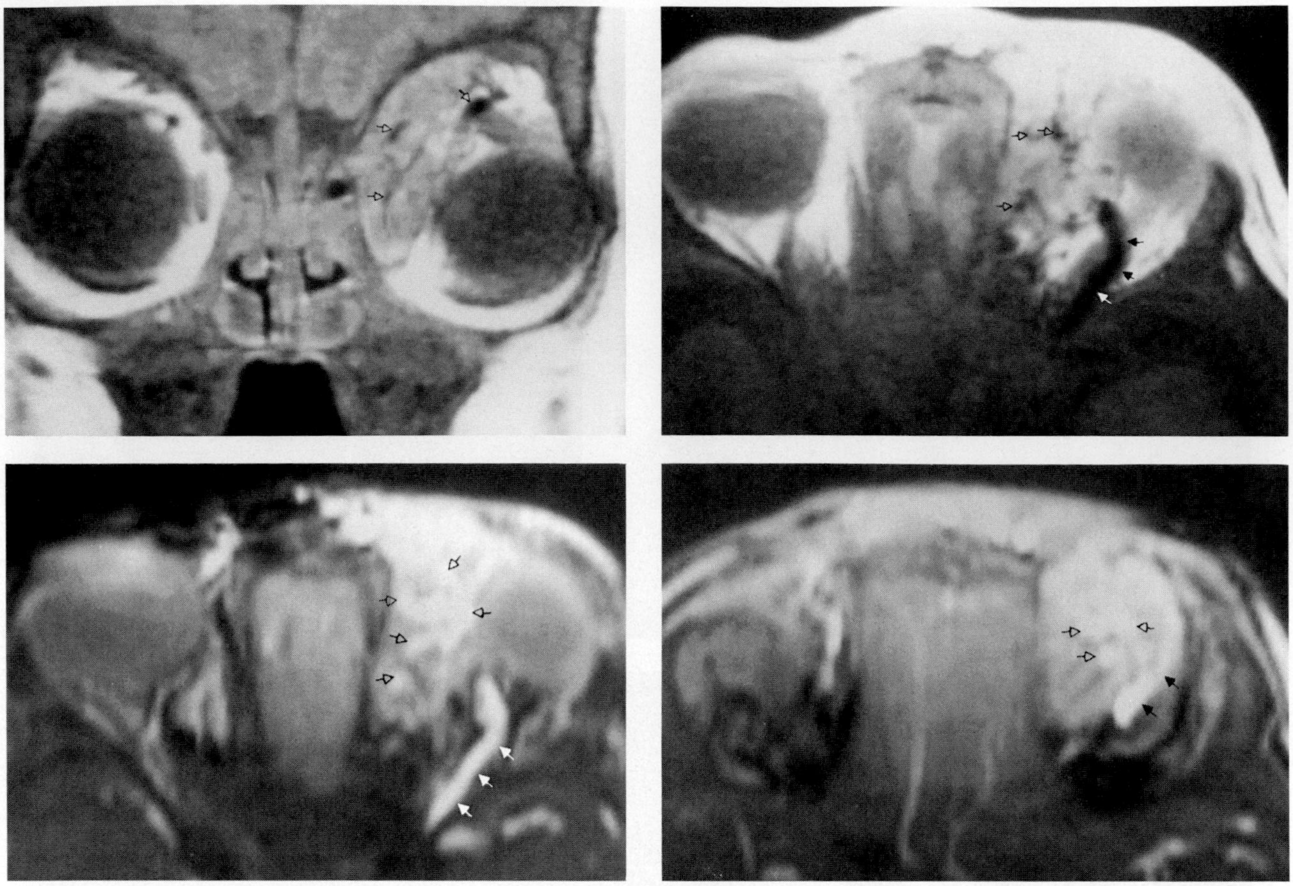

FIG. 57. Vascular capillary hemangioma, SE vs. GRASS. **A:** Coronal short TR/TE MRI (600/20). **B:** Axial short TR/TE MRI (600/20). **C:** Axial MRI (gradient echo 150/15/500). **D:** Axial MRI (gradient echo 150/15/500). Left extraconal mass has focal areas of low signal (*open arrows*) and is associated with enlarged superior ophthalmic vein (*closed arrows*). Gradient-echo images (C,D) depict these areas as high intensity due to flow and confirm vascular nature of this capillary hemangioma. (From Atlas, ref. 34, with permission.)

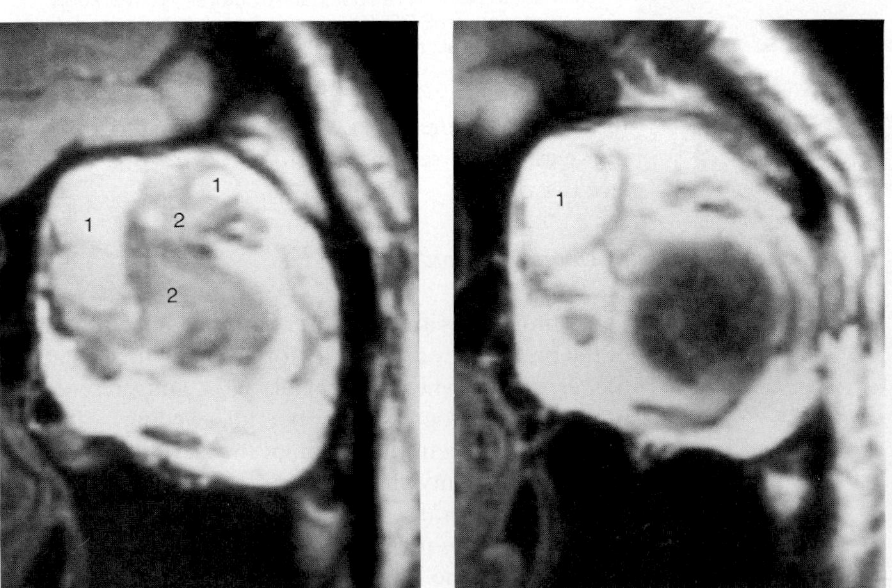

FIG. 58. Extraconal/intraconal lymphangioma with hemorrhage. **A:** Short TR/TE MRI (600/20). **B:** Short TR/TE MRI (600/20). Superonasal extraconal/intraconal mass has ill-defined margins and foci of high intensity hemorrhage (*1*) and lower intensity soft tissue components (*2*). (From Atlas, ref. 34, with permission.)

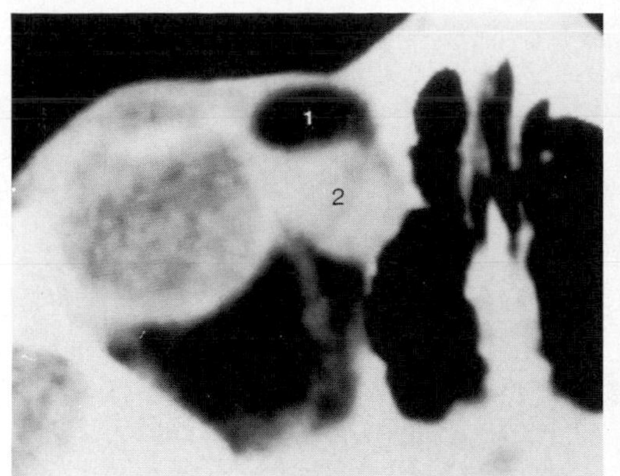

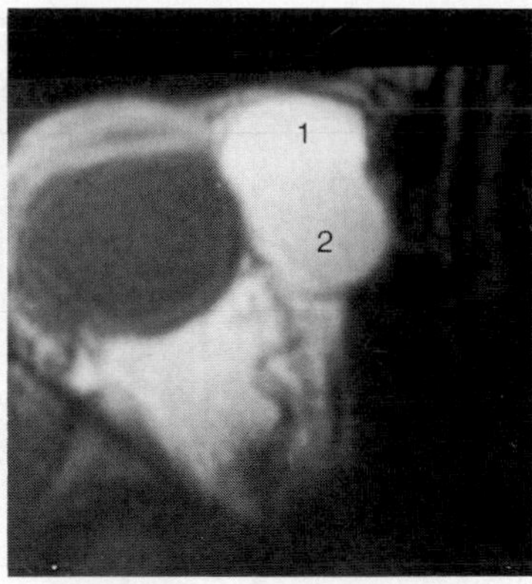

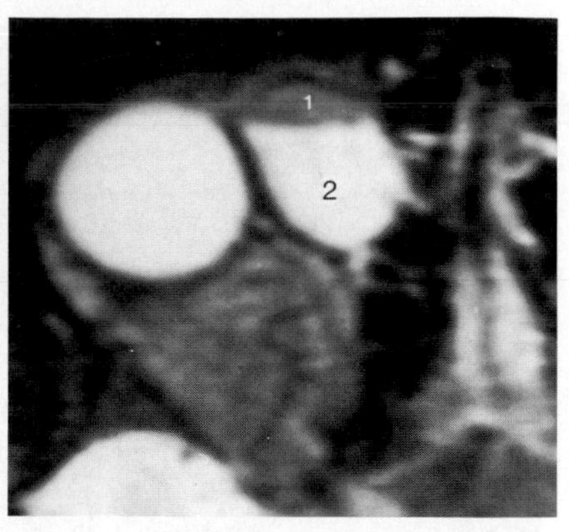

FIG. 59. Fat-fluid level in dermoid. **A:** CT. **B:** Short TR/TE MRI (600/20). **C:** Long TR/TE MRI (2500/80). Pathognomonic appearance of fat (*1*)-fluid (*2*) level on CT (A) and MRI (B,C). (From Atlas, ref. 34, with permission.)

cranial fossa. Dermoid cysts may become acutely symptomatic following rupture, which can elicit a significant inflammatory reaction and mimic more ominous entities. If no adnexal structures, such as hair or sweat glands, are found in the wall of pathologic specimens, the lesion is called an epidermoid cyst (37). Orbital dermoids can show pathognomonic fat-fluid levels on MR (Fig. 59). Focal areas of fat are easily identified when compared to adjacent orbital fat on both short and long TR/TE sequences. Ruptured orbital dermoid would demonstrate the associated inflammatory reactive changes and may not be distinguishable from cellulitis. Dense enhancement is not typical. When enhancement is present it may relate to secondary perilesional inflammation (113) and therefore be peripheral rather than central within the lesion (Fig. 60). One of the roles of MR in evaluating these congenital lesions is to exclude other lesions that also produce proptosis and have associated bony change, such as orbital meningocele or encephalocele. Epidermoid cysts in the orbit are also well-demarcated, round lesions with fluid content, but they do not contain fat (Fig. 61). These masses are typically somewhat hyperintense on short TR/TE images because of minor intralesional hemorrhage or proteinaceous debris.

Lacrimal Gland Masses

The lacrimal fossa is extraconal but postseptal in location, in the superolateral aspect of the orbit and just behind the superotemporal rim (see Figs. 6 and 7). Although normally the gland resides completely within its fossa, lacrimal gland tissue may occasionally appear anteriorly displaced, a normal variant commonly found in African-Americans that falsely implies pathologic enlargement and is ascribed to an anatomically shallower orbit (37). Since the gland is histologically considered analogous to a minor salivary gland, pathologic processes are similar to those found in other minor salivary glands of the head and neck. Approximately one half of

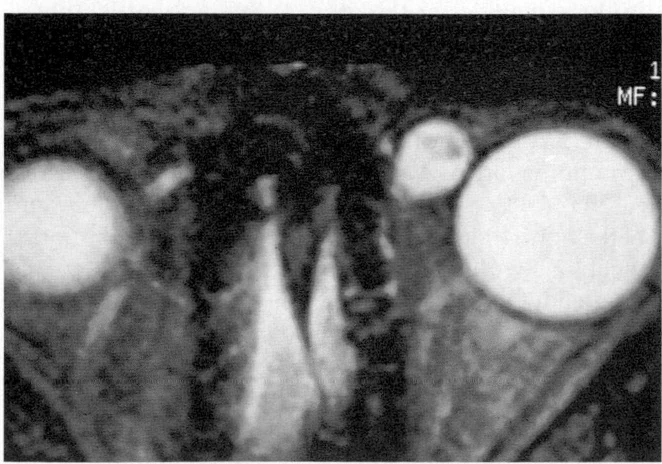

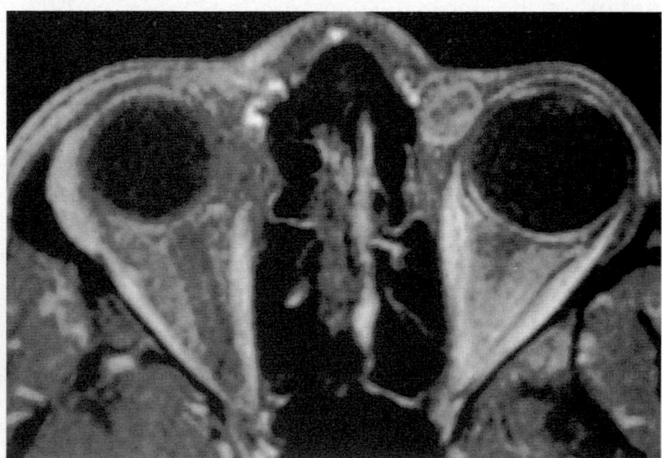

FIG. 60. Dermoid with peripheral enhancement. Heterogeneous mass in nasal aspect of left orbit (**A**) shows peripheral enhancement on fat suppressed T1-weighted image (**B**).

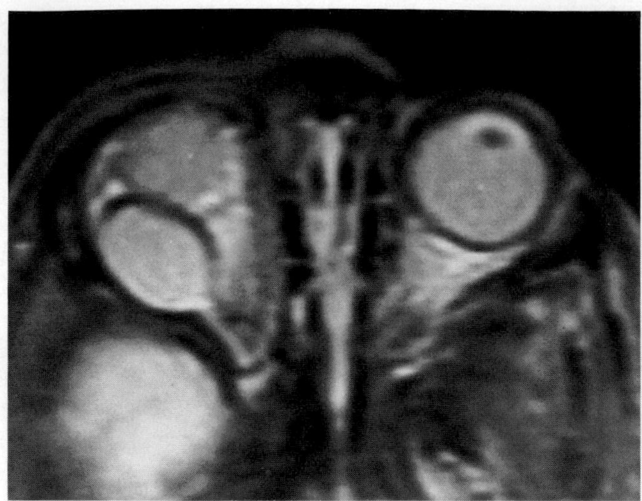

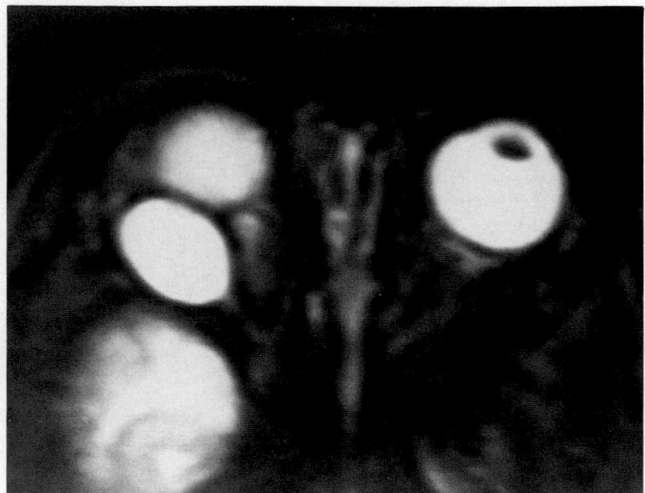

FIG. 61. Orbital epidermoid. **A:** Long TR/short TE MRI. **B:** Long TR/TE MRI. Laterally situated right extraconal mass has remolded lateral margin of orbit and is nearly isointense to vitreous.

neoplasms that primarily arise within the lacrimal gland are epithelial cell tumors, with half of these being benign mixed tumors and half being carcinomas. The remaining one half of primary masses of the lacrimal gland are lymphomatous or inflammatory. It has been estimated, however, that in routine (nonreferral) clinical practices, inflammatory and lymphomatoid masses are at least five times as common as epithelial tumors (37).

Epithelial Neoplasms

Benign mixed lacrimal tumors (pleomorphic adenomas) are usually clinically noted as slowly progressive upper lid swelling without pain in patients usually ranging in age from the fourth to the seventh decades (114). Grossly, these tumors appear encapsulated and often produce smooth remodeling of the lacrimal fossa because of their long-standing growth. Almost all epithelial tumors of the lacrimal gland arise in the deep portion of the gland, so it is unusual for these lesions to project significantly beyond the margin of the orbital rim (37). They often are collagenous in areas of hypercellularity. Patient survival rates are essentially 100% at 15 years, even in cases of recurrence (37).

Lacrimal gland carcinomas usually have a rapidly worsening course that lasts less than 9 months. Adenoid cystic carcinoma is the most common malignant epithelial cell tumor of the lacrimal gland (115), comprising 25% to 30% of all epithelial tumors in this area. Patients average 40 years of age at diagnosis, but these lesions can present within the first two decades of life (37). They are somewhat more common in females. These lesions are highly malignant and often show perineural infiltration with extensive soft tissue invasion. Only one half of patients survive more than $2\frac{1}{2}$ years after diagnosis, although this varies somewhat with the precise histology. Adenoid cystic carcinomas are unilateral and infiltrative, rather than having the encapsulated appearance of benign mixed tumors.

Lymphomatoid Tumors and Inflammatory Lesions

Lymphomatoid neoplasms of the lacrimal gland as a group constitute a controversial and often difficult diagnosis for the clinician, radiologist, and pathologist. Reasons for this include the tendency for many physicians to group lymphoid tumors together with inflammatory disorders, the difficulty in predicting whether the orbital tumor will become part of a more ominous systemic disorder, and overlapping histopathologic features shared by many of the neoplastic and inflammatory entities. Histologically, lymphocytes are present normally only in the conjunctivae and the lacrimal gland, and are absent in the remainder of the orbit. It follows that lymphoid tumors found in conjunctivae, for example, have a distinctly different significance than those found in retrobulbar soft tissues: more than 90% of conjunctival lymphomas are localized, but more than 50% of orbital lymphomas are part of systemic lymphoproliferative disease (116,117). In the orbit, nearly all lymphomas are of the non-Hodgkin's type (37). Lymphomatoid tumors, including lymphoma and reactive lymphoid hyperplasia or pseudolymphoma, are usually detected because of painless swelling, rather than overt signs of inflammation. Patients are usually in their fifth or sixth decades. Proptosis or dysmotility is present for relatively short periods of time, generally less than 6 months. The lacrimal fossa is the most common site of all lymphomatoid tumors in the orbit. There is no clinical sign of malignancy rather than benignity in lymphoid tumors, aside from

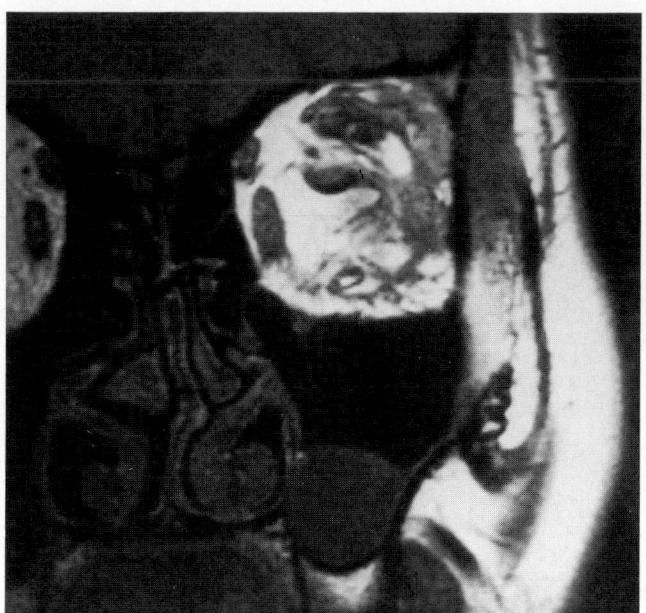

FIG. 62. Infiltrating adenoid cystic carcinoma, coronal short TR/TE MRI (600/20). Left lacrimal mass infiltrates muscle cone medially and is both extraconal and intraconal.

metastases, but recurrence and bilateral disease suggest malignancy (117). Lymphomatoid tumors are usually soft, solitary masses that mold to the contour of the globe and orbital wall, rather than cause overt destruction or focal distortion. Pathologically, these neoplasms are friable and have a conspicuous absence of fibrocollagenous stroma (37), a distinguishing feature from inflammatory pseudotumor.

Dacryoadenitis refers to inflammation of the lacrimal gland. This may be acute, subacute, or chronic, and is seen as a nonspecific inflammatory enlargement of the gland on imaging studies. It may occur in isolation or in association with autoimmune inflammatory syndromes, notably Sjögren's syndrome. Sarcoidosis is another etiology of nonacute inflammatory masses of the lacrimal glands. Up to 80% of patients with sarcoidosis have involvement of the lacrimal glands, but many are asymptomatic (37). Interestingly, both sarcoidosis and lymphoma characteristically involve both lacrimal glands in patients with systemic disease elsewhere in the body. The lacrimal gland is also the most frequent site of orbital lymphoma and orbital sarcoidosis. Both these entities usually present with painless swelling in a palpable, relatively firm mass. The lacrimal gland is commonly involved by idiopathic orbital pseudotumor and is occasionally the only site of the disease. Inflammatory pseudotumor most commonly is manifested by pain and tenderness, but subacute and chronic cases can occur in the absence of significant pain. This lesion is difficult at times to distinguish from other lymphomatoid lacrimal masses, even by histopathology.

Imaging Features of Lacrimal Masses

The clear significance of bone changes to the determination of whether a lacrimal lesion is malignant or not suggests that CT scanning plays an important role in the evaluation of these tumors because it is more sensitive than MR to subtle bone destruction. In the diagnostic evaluation of lacrimal gland disease, in fact, there are essentially only two important factors to consider for differential diagnosis: symptoms (both type and duration) and the presence or absence of bony change adjacent to the mass (37). If symptoms are of short duration, then the diagnosis is usually either inflammatory, lymphomatoid tumor, or malignant epithelial neoplasm. If pain is a prominent feature of the symptomatology, then inflammatory lesion or epithelial malignancy is likely. If the disease duration is short and there are bony changes identified, the most likely diagnosis is malignant epithelial tumor. Bone erosion (as opposed to destruction) suggests either benign epithelial tumor or lymphomatoid neoplasm.

In general, although both CT and MR can show the precise location and extent of lacrimal masses (Figs. 62 and 63), specific etiologies cannot be discerned in the vast majority of cases (1,118), even with i.v. contrast enhancement (119). Infiltrative, destructive masses are certainly more likely to represent adenoid cystic carcinoma (Figs. 62 and 64), but focal and well-demarcated lacrimal masses can represent any etiology, including inflammatory, benign, and malignant neoplasm. Bilaterality suggests either lymphoma or sarcoidosis as the most likely diagnosis. Overall, morphology is not a helpful criterion in the differential diagnosis in most cases.

The MR signal intensities of various lacrimal gland masses have been described in only a small number of cases, but these preliminary data suggest that there is

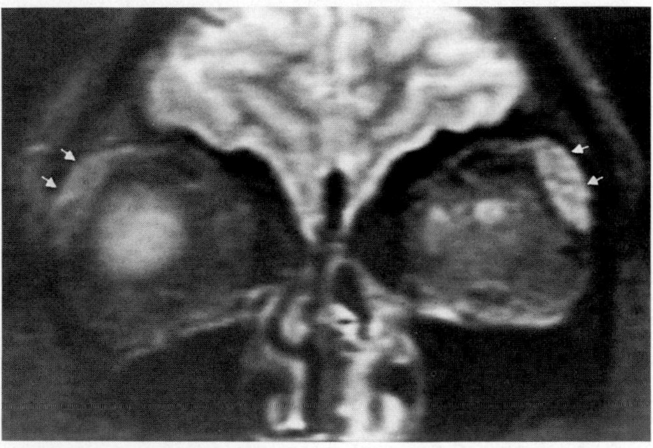

FIG. 63. Sarcoidosis with lacrimal masses, coronal long TR/TE MRI (2500/80). Bilateral lacrimal involvement with sarcoidosis depicted as hyperintense lacrimal glands (*arrows*) on long TR/TE image.

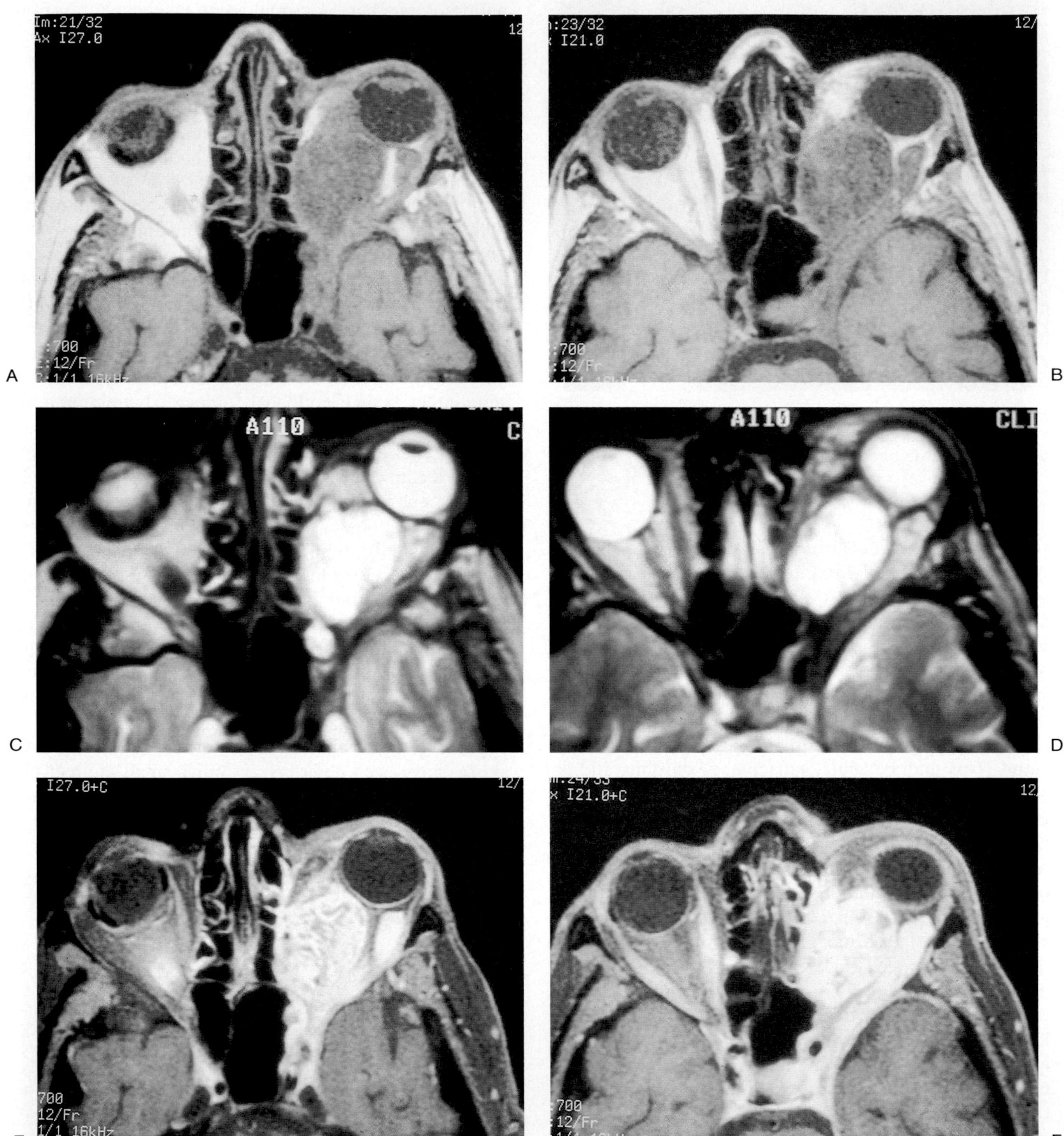

FIG. 64. Adenoid cystic carcinoma extending into orbit. Large retrobulbar mass completely replaces retrobulbar fat (**A,B**) and extends into left cavernous sinus. Lesion is markedly hyperintense and heterogeneous on T2-weighted images (**C,D**) and enhances diffusely (**E,F**).

marked variation in intensity patterns. The signal on long TR/TE images probably reflects differences in edematous inflammation with high water content (giving high intensity) versus high fibrocollagenous stromal content (giving low intensity). For example, inflammatory pseudotumor, which can present as an isolated lacrimal mass, is usually low intensity on long TR/TE images. This lesion has, as a dominant part of its histopathologic picture, extensive fibrotic tissue (37). MR of other lacrimal inflammations are usually more reflective of acute inflammation, showing hyperintensity on long TR/TE images. Unfortunately, sarcoidosis of the lacrimal gland can be either low intensity or high intensity on long TR/TE images (see Fig. 63). Lymphoma has been demonstrated as low intensity, as well as high intensity on long TR/TE images (1). Epithelial neoplasms are generally high intensity on long TR/TE images. It appears that MR may not be able to accurately discern specific lacrimal mass lesion histologies and may not add specificity to the notoriously nonspecific CT in evaluating lacrimal lesions.

Vascular Anomalies

The most apparent and largest vascular structure within the orbit is the superior ophthalmic vein.

Its enlargement is relatively common and nonspecific; in fact, mild asymmetry can be present in a normal individual, and placing the head in a dependent position (as in the coronal position for CT scanning) can enlarge these veins without indicating true pathology. A long list of entities can be associated with enlargement of the superior ophthalmic vein (33) (Table 11). Intravascular flow abnormalities in the orbit can often be diagnosed with SE MR and do not require i.v. contrast (1,2). In confusing cases, gradient-echo imaging with sequential slice acquisition (111,120) can be used to clarify ambiguous SE signal patterns.

Carotid Cavernous Fistula

When a direct communication between the internal carotid artery (or branches of the external carotid artery) and the venous cavernous sinus develops, a fistula occurs. Subsequent transmission of arterial pressure into the superior ophthalmic vein leads to symptoms and signs of carotid-cavernous fistula, which include proptosis, motility disturbances, pulsatile exophthalmos (often accompanied by a bruit), and suffusion of the globe, sclera, and conjunctiva. Fistulae can be traumatic in etiology (Fig. 65), but often occur spontaneously, either secondary to atherosclerotic disease or from communication between dural branches of the external carotid artery and the basilar venous plexus (i.e., dural arteriovenous malformation). Exophthalmos and other symptoms, including a disturbing noise audible only to the patient, are usually ipsilateral to the fistula, but can be bilateral (because of the presence of intercavernous sinus connections) and are predominantly contralateral in 10% of cases.

While carotid arteriography remains the definitive method for demonstrating the precise site of the fistula and its drainage, noninvasive imaging is contributory in the initial diagnosis of cases that are not clinically obvious. Findings on MR include enlargement of the superior ophthalmic vein, engorgement of muscles, proptosis, and distended cavernous sinuses. Signal void in dilated superior ophthalmic veins and cavernous sinuses due to rapidly flowing blood in a traumatic carotid cavernous fistula can be clearly seen on MR (Fig. 66). Furthermore, clarification of secondary parasellar "masses" (as seen on CT) in such a patient can be made on MR because of the characteristic signal void of rapidly flowing blood.

A more interesting and elegant diagnosis that can be made by MRI is the documentation of thrombosis of the dural arteriovenous malformation, as implied by the visualization of clot in the superior ophthalmic vein (Fig. 67) and/or cavernous sinus (89). In these patients, although the bothersome noise heard by the patient often disappears, there is seemingly paradoxical worsening of the proptosis and motility disturbance due to thrombosis. Angiography can be avoided by MR demonstration of thrombosis in these patients. Although traumatic carotid cavernous fistula usually requires surgical or neurointerventional treatment, dural fistulas often thrombose spontaneously, sometimes after diagnostic arteriography.

TABLE 11. *Etiologies of enlargement of superior ophthalmic vein*

Carotid–cavernous fistula
Traumatic
Dural arteriovenous malformation
Superior ophthalmic vein (or cavernous sinus) thrombosis
Varix
Orbital apex mass
Thyroid eye disease
Idiopathic inflammatory pseudotumor
Normal variant

Modified from Atlas et al., ref. 33, with permission.

Superior Ophthalmic Vein Thrombosis

Thrombosis in the superior ophthalmic vein can be readily identified by SE MRI (1,2,89). The key to the diagnosis is the recognition of the absence of expected signal void in this normal structure (Figs. 67 and 68). In addition, secondary signs of thrombosis, such as enlargement of the superior ophthalmic vein, diffuse extraocular muscle prominence, and proptosis, can be present.

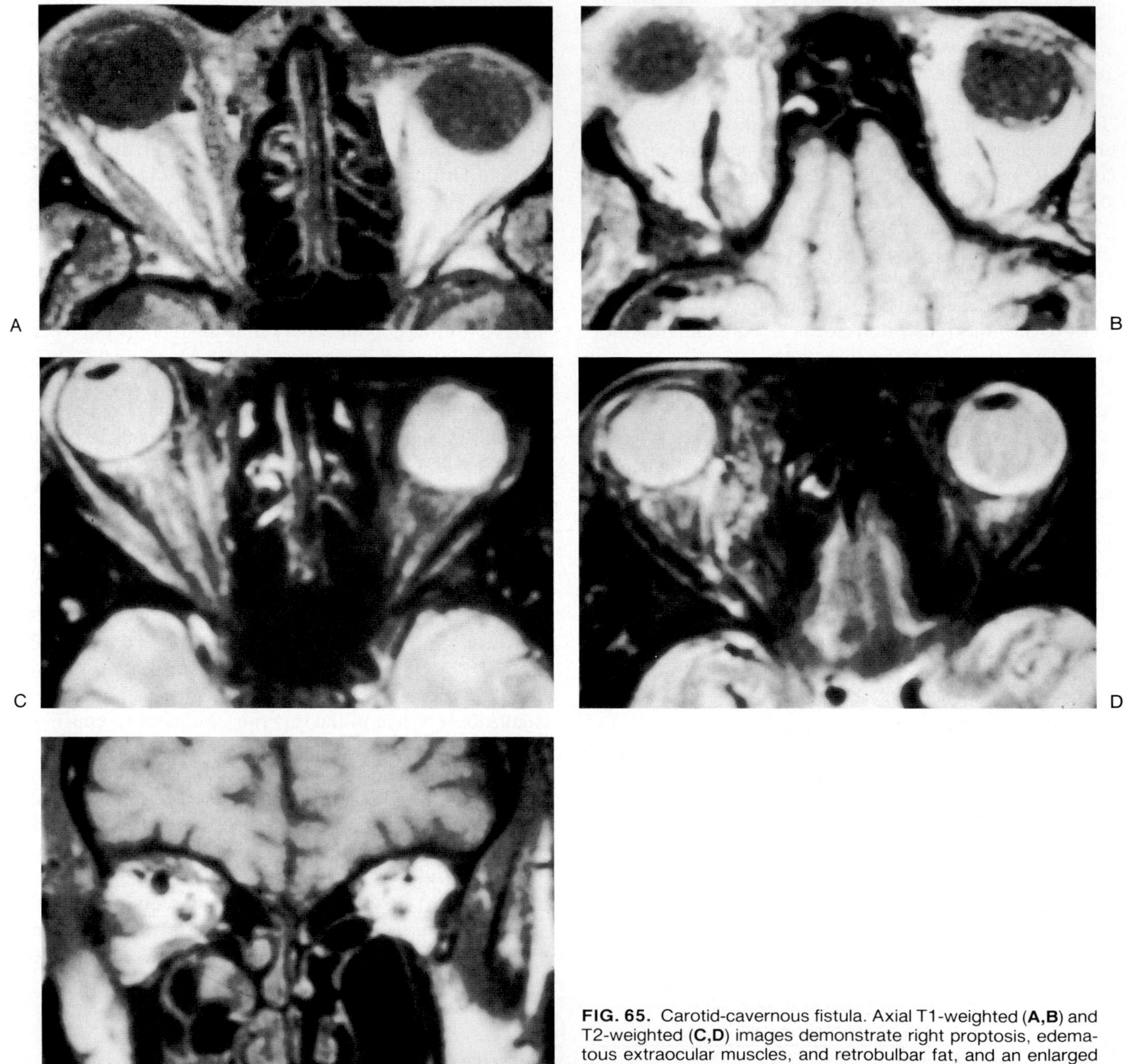

FIG. 65. Carotid-cavernous fistula. Axial T1-weighted (**A,B**) and T2-weighted (**C,D**) images demonstrate right proptosis, edematous extraocular muscles, and retrobulbar fat, and an enlarged superior ophthalmic vein, particularly well seen on coronal image (**E**).

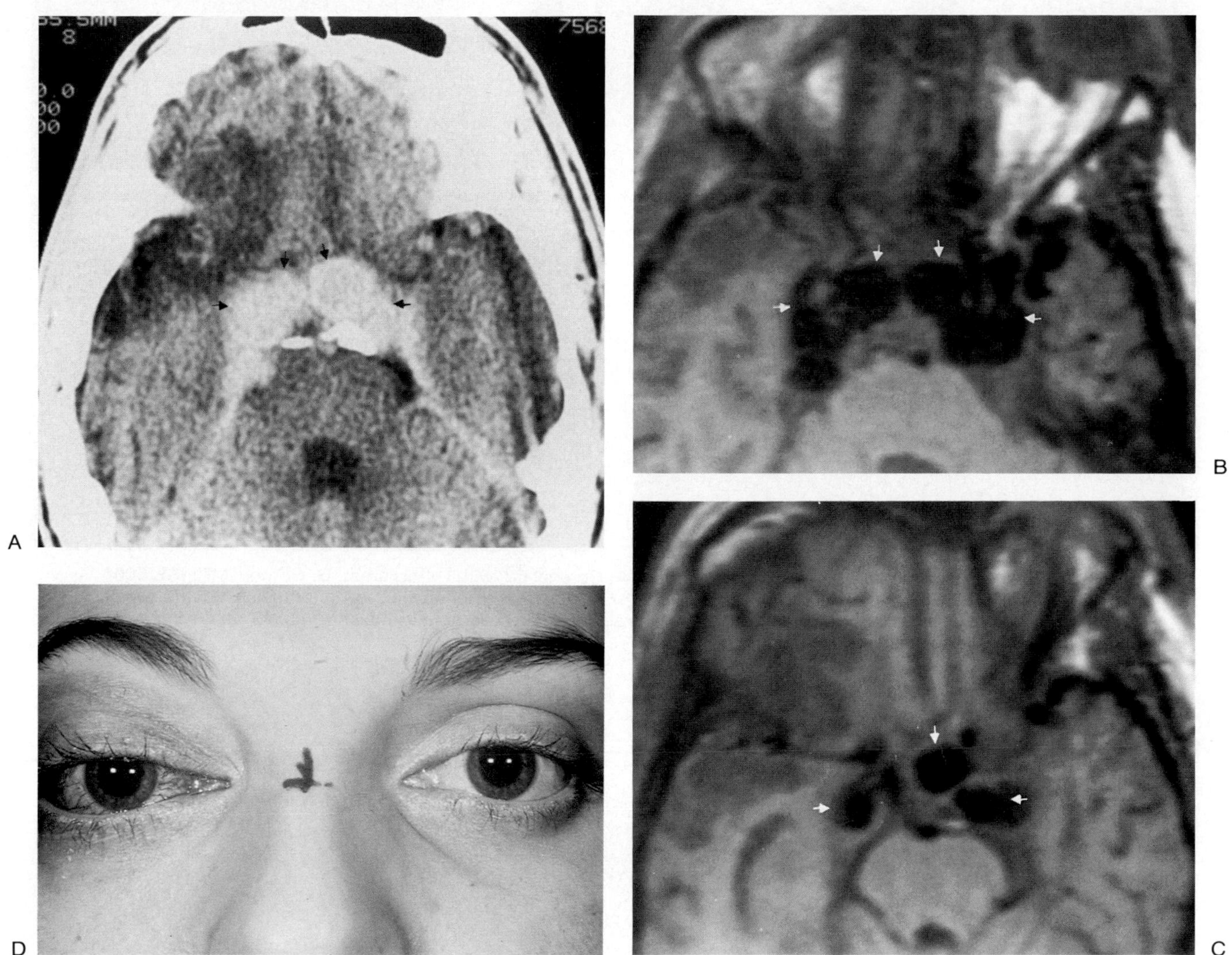

FIG. 66. Traumatic carotid-cavernous fistula. **A:** CT with i.v. contrast. **B:** Short TR/TE MRI (600/20). **C:** Short TR/TE MRI (600/20). **D:** Patient with traumatic CCF. Enhancing sellar/suprasellar masses (*arrows*) on CT (A) show signal void, indicating vascular nature, on MRI (B,C). This diagnosis is not a dilemma for the clinician and typically presents with chemosis, proptosis, and arterialization of the involved conjunctival vessels, as seen in right eye (D). (From Atlas, ref. 34, with permission.)

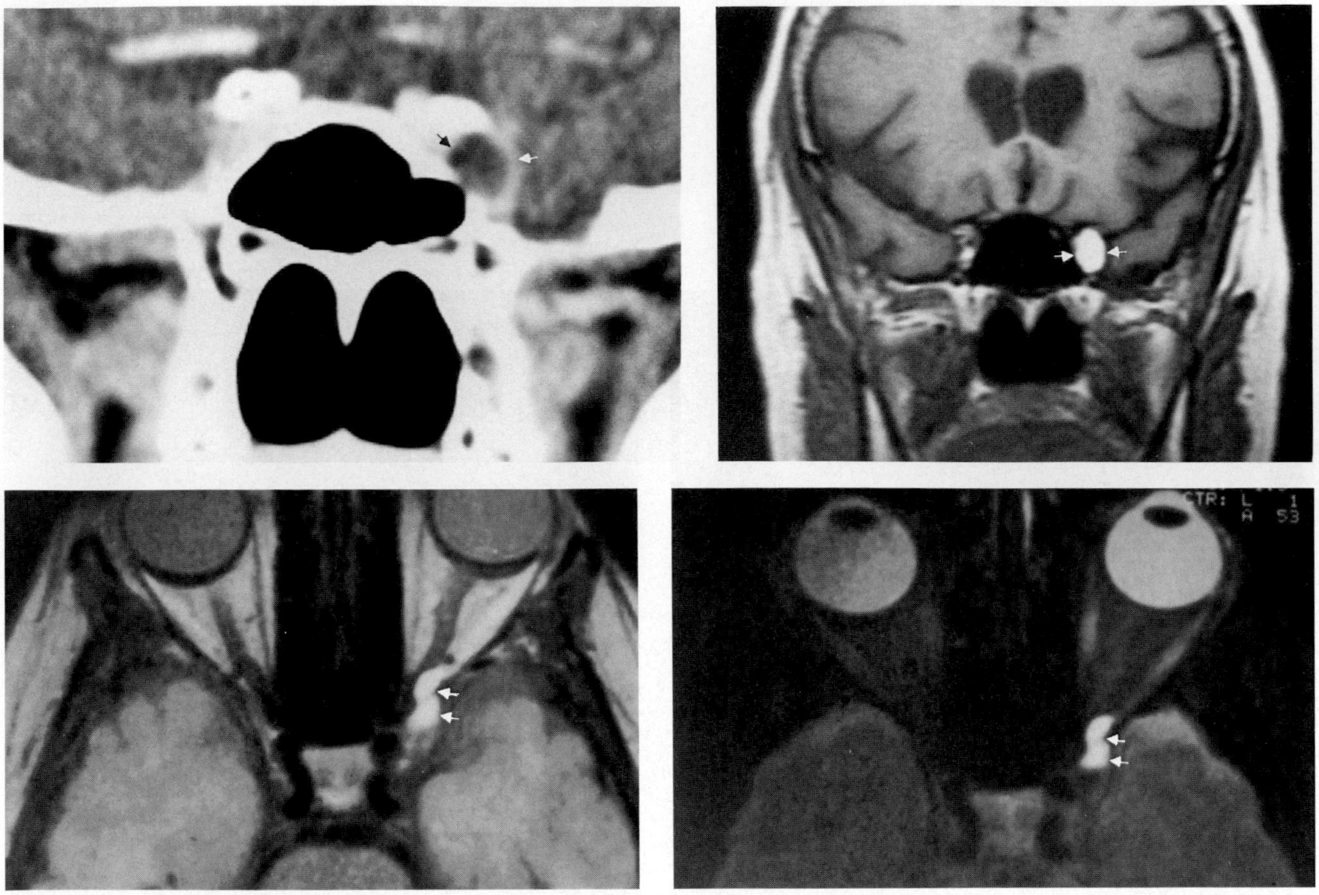

FIG. 67. Cavernous sinus dural AVM with thrombosis. **A:** Coronal CT with i.v. contrast. **B:** Coronal MRI (SE 600/25). **C:** Axial MRI (SE 2500/40). **D:** Axial MR (SE 2500/80). CT (A) shows a nonspecific low attenuation mass (*arrows*) in the left cavernous sinus. MRI (B–D) demonstrates high signal clot in cavernous sinus and superior ophthalmic vein (*arrows*). (From Savino et al., ref. 89, with permission.)

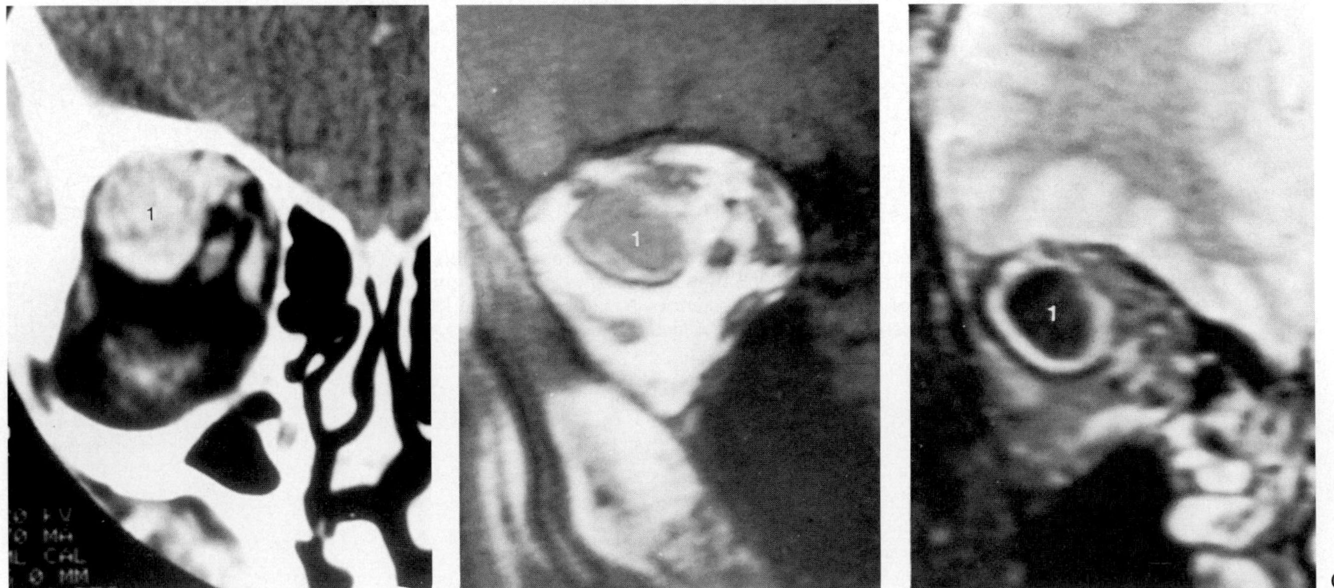

FIG. 68. Thrombosed superior ophthalmic vein varix. **A:** Coronal CT. **B:** Coronal MRI (600/20). **C:** Coronal MRI (2500/80). Massively enlarged varix with relatively acute thrombosis (*1*). (From Atlas, ref. 34, with permission.)

The diagnosis of thrombosis of the superior ophthalmic vein can still be elusive, however, because of confusion from chemical shift misregistration artifact (1). Since chemical shift misregistration places a dark line at a fat–water interface, signal void from this artifact could be misinterpreted as signal void within the superior ophthalmic vein and falsely imply patency of the vein (Fig. 69). This confusion can be clarified with the use of adjunctive sequences and other technical maneuvers. Gradient-echo imaging can clearly depict flow as high intensity (111,120). To distinguish high intensity on SE images due to slow flow from true clot, perhaps the most efficient approach is to employ saturation pulses to eliminate signal from incoming spins, thereby causing any flow-related enhancement to appear as signal void.

There are many causes of superior ophthalmic vein thrombosis. These include dural arteriovenous malformation, cavernous sinus thrombosis (secondary to tumor, inflammation, or trauma), and adjacent orbital infection. In addition, a markedly dilated superior ophthalmic vein varix could spontaneously clot because of venous flow stagnation.

Orbital Varix

Vascular malformations involving the venous system are uncommon in the orbit and include varix, varicocele, and venous angioma. These lesions are manifested usually by intermittent exophthalmos, often associated with activities that produce marked increases in venous pressure, such as coughing or the Valsalva maneuver. The absence of valves in the internal jugular vein allows free transmission of back pressure into the orbit venous system, which distends when part of a vascular malformation. Venous variceal malformations associated with arteriovenous fistula (i.e., carotid cavernous or dural fistula) are often pulsatile and do not regress intermittently.

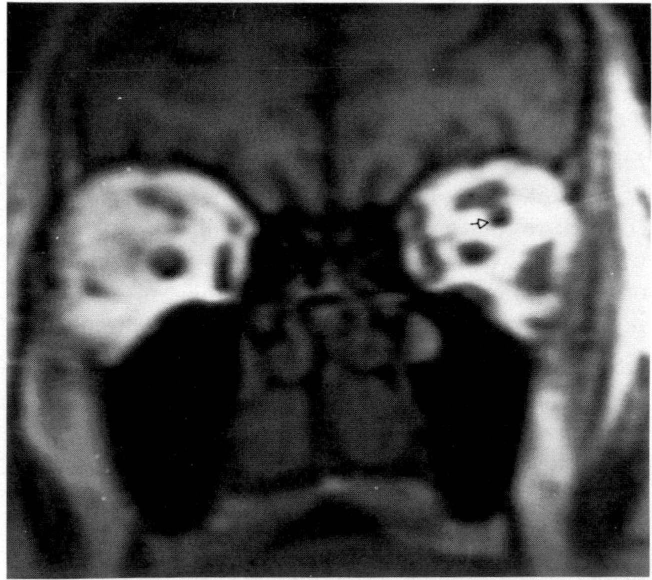

FIG. 69. Chemical shift artifact masquerading as patent vein, coronal MRI (600/20). Signal void (*arrow*) due to chemical shift misregistration was misinterpreted as void from rapid flow in patient with angiographically proven venous thrombosis. (From Atlas et al., ref. 2, with permission.)

Although rarely containing calcified phleboliths, venous varices are often only demonstrated by maneuvers that increase the orbital venous pressure so that imaging in the absence of such maneuvers may not delineate the lesion. Imaging must therefore be performed both at rest and during Valsalva (Fig. 70) or, alternatively, with the head in such a position as to increase significantly venous pressure. These lesions can be clearly demonstrated by their intermittent appearance on MR, but the true vascular nature of the evanescent mass can also be documented by its flow characteristics (i.e., flow-related signal void if rapid, or flow-related enhancement or second-echo rephasing if slow flow) (39). Large venous varices may contain essentially stagnant blood during maneuvers that cause variceal distention, so intralesional flow may not be seen even on flow-sensitive MR techniques. Distended varices with stagnant, nonclotted blood can appear as soft tissue masses with no evidence of paramagnetic constituents (since oxygenated blood is diamagnetic) (see Fig. 70). Orbital varices can also spontaneously thrombose (1) and appear as constant mass lesions whose signal characteristics indicate clot (see Fig. 68).

Foreign Bodies and Trauma

Overlying, superficial soft tissue swelling and hemorrhage often preclude thorough physical examination of the orbit and globe in patients suffering sequelae of trauma to the face and orbit. CT is the initial modality of choice in orbital trauma because it can clearly delineate fractures and document the presence of small or retained opaque foreign bodies. In fact, the possibility of intraorbital metallic foreign body is an absolute contraindication to MR (Fig. 71) because of the possibility of ocular injury from movement of a ferromagnetic substance (27). Both CT and MR show wooden foreign bodies as air (i.e., signal void on MR) (121). Prognostic information may be obtained by demonstrating penetrating injuries of the globe (122,123), since double penetration of the globe and optic nerve injury are important to surgical planning and prognosis.

Bone fragments, although potentially visible on MR as signal void, are certainly more confidently detected by CT. MR can demonstrate bony fractures as interruptions of cortical bone signal void with linear high intensity hemorrhage or fluid (124), and implicate fractures by delineating prolapsed orbital fat into adjacent sinuses (Figs.

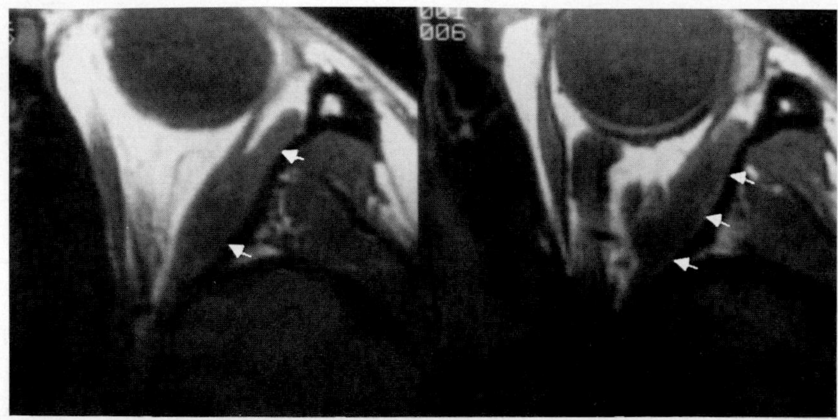

A,B

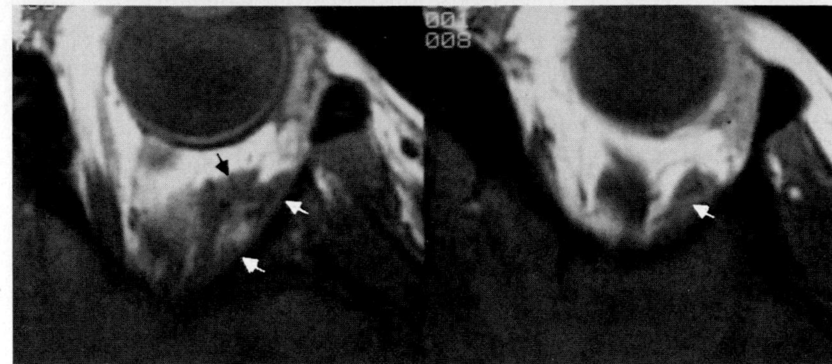

C,D

FIG. 70. Orbital varix with stagnation during Valsalva maneuver, axial MRI (600/20). **A–D:** Inferior to superior. Mainly extraconal mass (*arrows*) is isointense to muscle and represents stagnant flow in distended venous varix, only visible during Valsava maneuver. (From Atlas, ref. 34, with permission.)

72 and 73) (125). More importantly, muscle and nerve entrapment secondary to blow-out fractures can be clearly documented by MR (Figs. 72 and 73). Intraocular (Fig. 73) and retrobulbar hemorrhage can be readily demonstrated by MR, and in fact MR is often more specific for its appearance (2,126) than CT (see Fig. 74). Perioptic hemorrhage and optic nerve contusion are more evident on MR (Fig. 72) (127). Small retinal hemorrhages have not been detected by either CT or MR to date, although detachments with subretinal fluid accumulation can be well visualized by both modalities (5,7,76). Severe sequelae of blunt trauma, such as ruptured globe and lens disruption, are identifiable by both

FIG. 71. Ocular metallic foreign body. Ferromagnetic artifact emanating from left ocular metallic foreign body in patient who had forgotten prior incident.

CT and MR as gross morphologic distortion of the globe. Since these patients might be less able to fully cooperate for MRI, however, CT remains the more practical initial imaging modality in acute globe trauma in most patients.

EYE MOVEMENT AND DISORDERS OF GAZE

The final neural pathway for the control of eye movements occurs through cranial nerves III, IV, and VI (Figs. 75 and 76). The continuing improvements in spatial and contrast resolution in MRI has permitted for the first time clear visualization of these cranial nerves from their origin in brainstem nuclei through their intracisternal portions, into the cavernous sinus, and occasionally into the orbital apex. Clinical localization of a given oculomotor nerve palsy is established by the accompanying neurologic signs, and recognizing these associated signs and symptoms aids significantly in the search for causative intracranial pathology. For instance, the presence of a contralateral hemiparesis would indicate a brainstem lesion. Involvement of multiple cranial nerves, particularly when bilateral, would suggest a process in the subarachnoid space. Ipsilateral IIIrd, IVth, and VIth nerve palsies indicate a cavernous sinus process, whereas concomitant involvement of the optic nerve and proptosis implicate the orbital apex. Knowledge of the anatomy

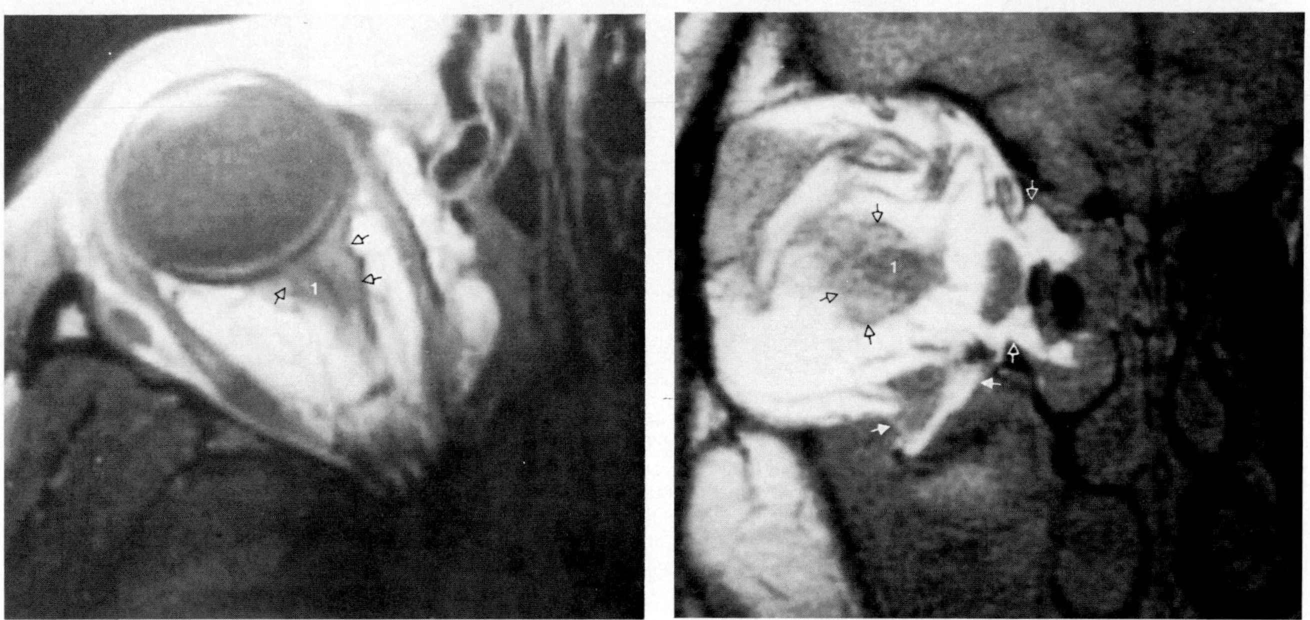

FIG. 72. Optic sheath hematoma. **A:** Axial short TR/TE MRI (600/20). **B:** Coronal short TR/TE MRI (600/20). Surrounding optic nerve (*1*) is slightly hyperintense perioptic hematoma (*open black arrows*). Note herniation of fat and infraorbital nerve through inferior wall blow-out (*closed white arrows*) and medial wall blow-out (*open white arrows*) fractures. (From Atlas, ref. 34, with permission.)

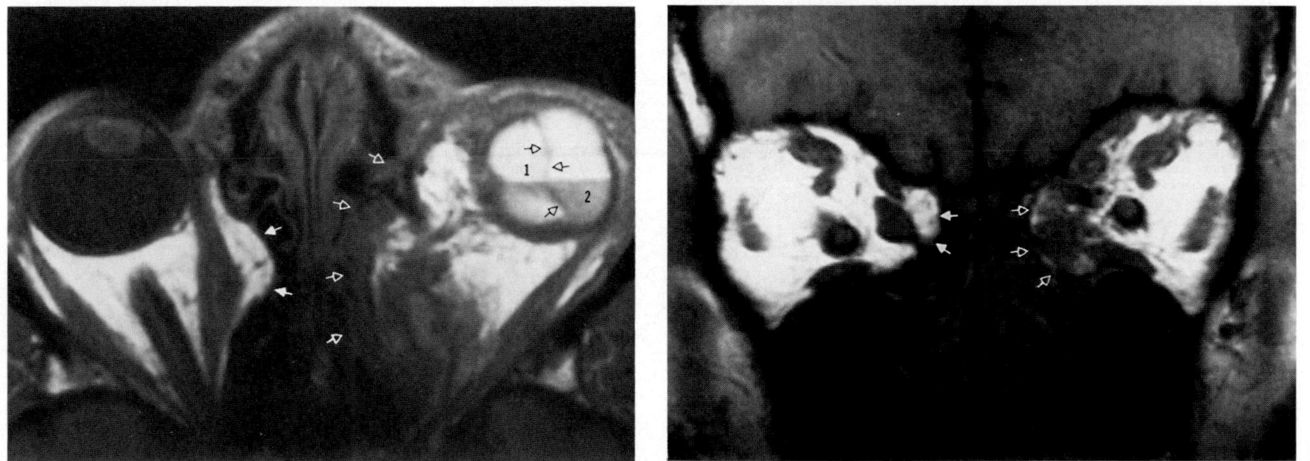

FIG. 73. Hemorrhagic total retinal detachment from blunt trauma. **A:** Axial short TR/TE MRI (500/20). **B:** Coronal short TR/TE MRI (500/20). Complete retinal detachment in left globe is seen on axial image (A), with high-intensity hemorrhage (methemoglobin) (*1*) filling the anterior half of the globe, including the anterior and posterior chambers. Detached retinal leaves (*open black arrows*) are identifiable within hemorrhage. Lens is not seen. Dependent level of lower intensity blood (*2*) was markedly hypointense on long TR/TE image (not shown), indicating acute blood. Also note disrupted left medial rectus muscle herniating into left ethmoid sinus from medial wall blow-out fracture (*open white arrows*). Previous right medial wall blow-out fracture with herniation of fat and medial rectus is also seen (*solid white arrows*). (From Atlas, ref. 127, with permission.)

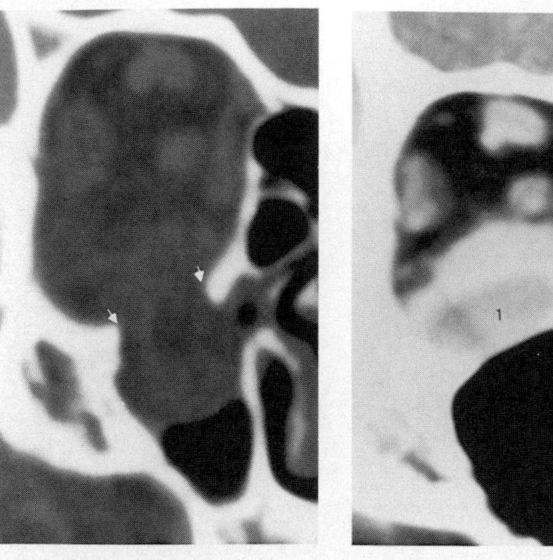

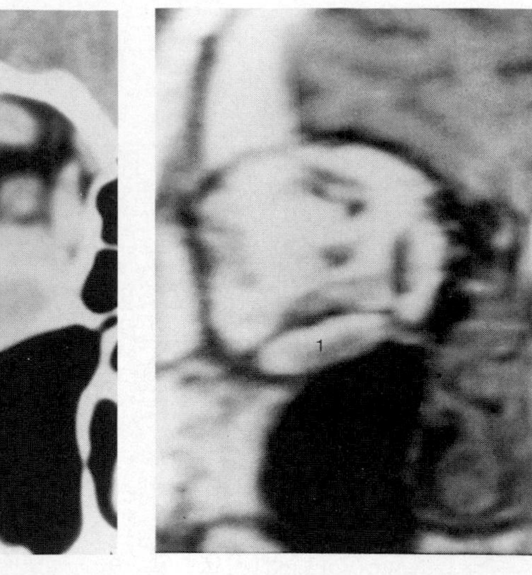

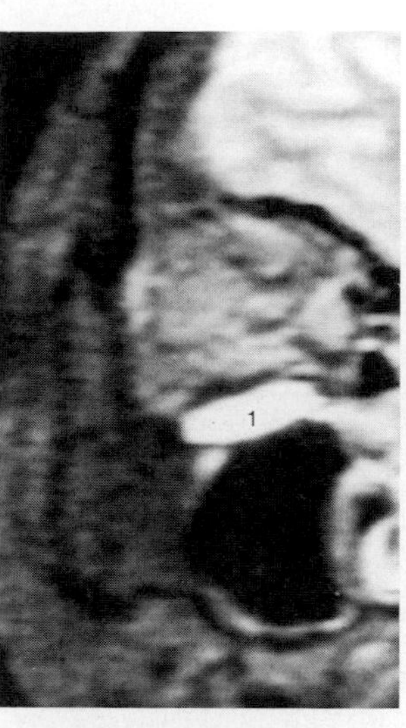

FIG. 74. Post-traumatic hemorrhagic subperiosteal cyst. **A:** Coronal CT immediately after trauma. **B:** Coronal CT 5 months after trauma. **C:** Coronal short TR/TE MRI (600/20). **D:** Coronal long TR/TE MRI (2500/80). Floor of right orbit blow-out fracture (*arrows*) with inferior herniation of orbital contents into right maxillary sinus (A). Five months later, inferior orbital mass (*1*) with peripheral enhancement on CT (B) is high intensity on short TR/TE (C) and long TR/TE (D) MRI representing chronic subperiosteal hematoma. (From Atlas, ref. 34, with permission.)

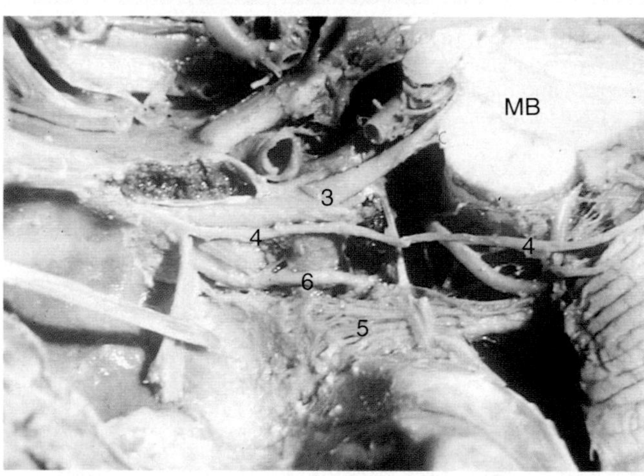

FIG. 75. Anatomic dissection of cranial nerves controlling gaze. Oblique view from the anterolateral aspect of the midbrain (MB) allows visualization of cranial nerves III (*3*), IV (*4*), and VI (*6*) (*5* denotes gasserian ganglion) as these nerves course from the brainstem toward the cavernous sinus. Note the extremely long course of the cranial nerve IV from the dorsal midbrain. (Courtesy of Dr. W. Hoyt, San Francisco, CA.)

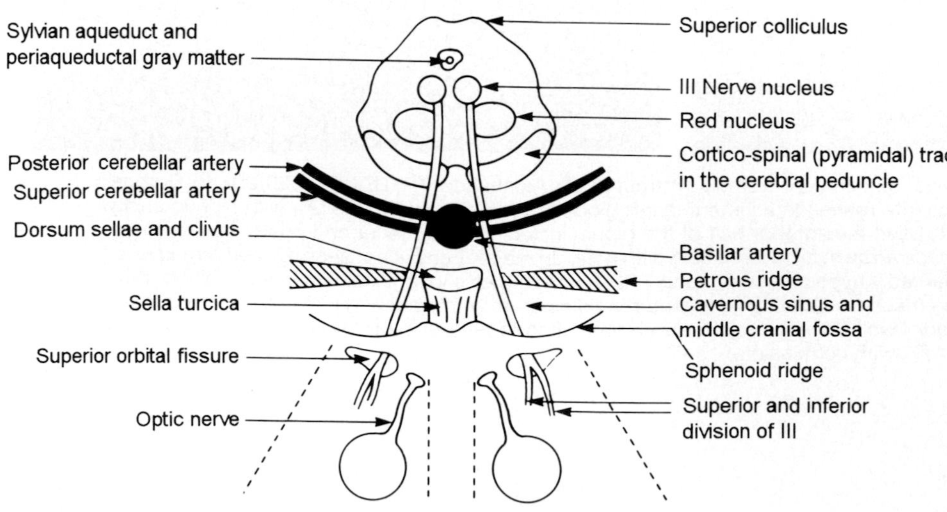

FIG. 76. Course of the third nerve from brainstem to superior orbital fissure. (From Bajandas and Kline, ref. 177, with permission.)

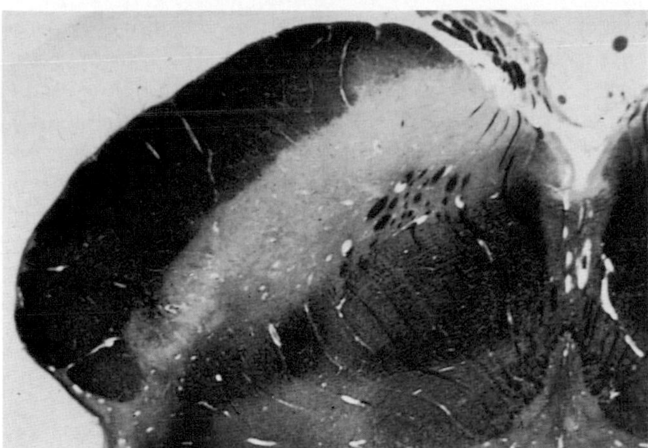

FIG. 77. Anatomic specimen through fascicle of the third nerve in midbrain. Fascicle of the right third nerve (*dark fibers*) crosses the red nucleus and peduncle before exiting the brainstem to become a cisternal segment of the third nerve.

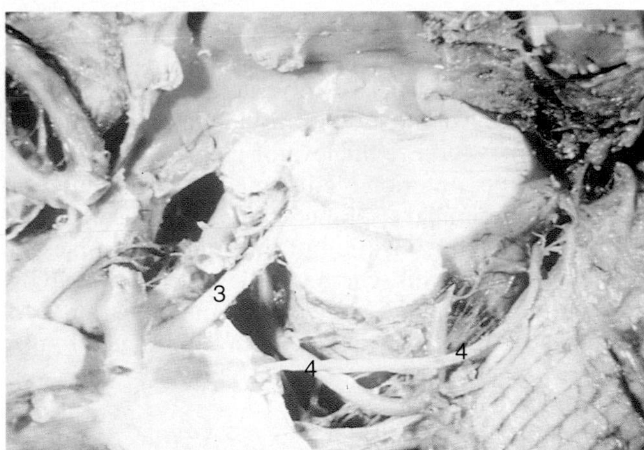

FIG. 78. Anatomic specimen showing exiting of the third nerve from the brainstem. Note cranial nerves III (*3*) and IV (*4*) as they course toward the cavernous sinus. (Courtesy of Dr. W. Hoyt, San Francisco, CA.)

of the Vth nerve is also useful in localization. Since the mandibular division exits the skull base via the foramen ovale, involvement of this branch indicates a lesion posterior to the cavernous sinus (see Chapter 19). Moving anteriorly, the maxillary division leaves the base of the skull within the cavernous sinus via the foramen rotundum and the ophthalmic division travels through the superior orbital fissure along with cranial nerves III, IV, and VI. In every motility disorder, one has to consider other disorders that mimic lesions of the oculomotor nerves, such as thyroid eye disease and myasthenia gravis. Furthermore, conditions such as drug intoxication, hysteria, and refractive error may be associated with diplopia without impairment of extraocular motility. A full discussion of these entities is beyond the scope of this chapter.

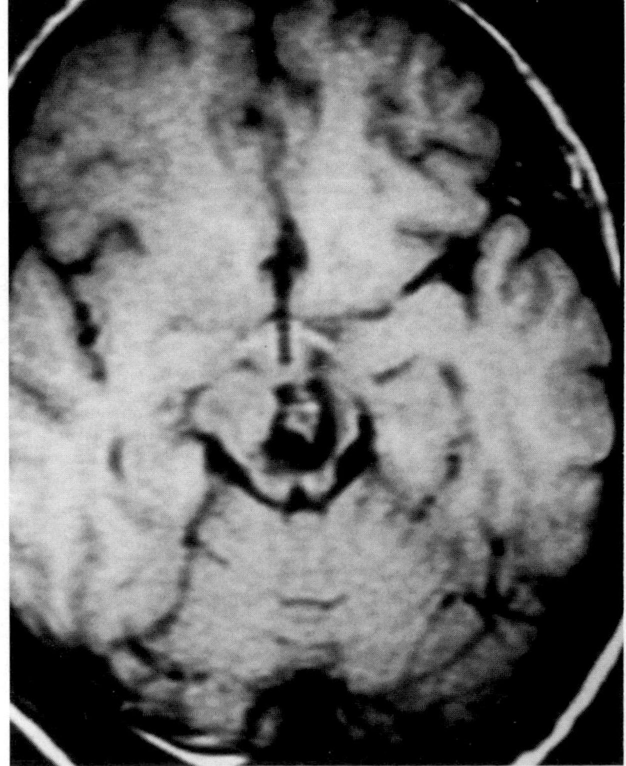

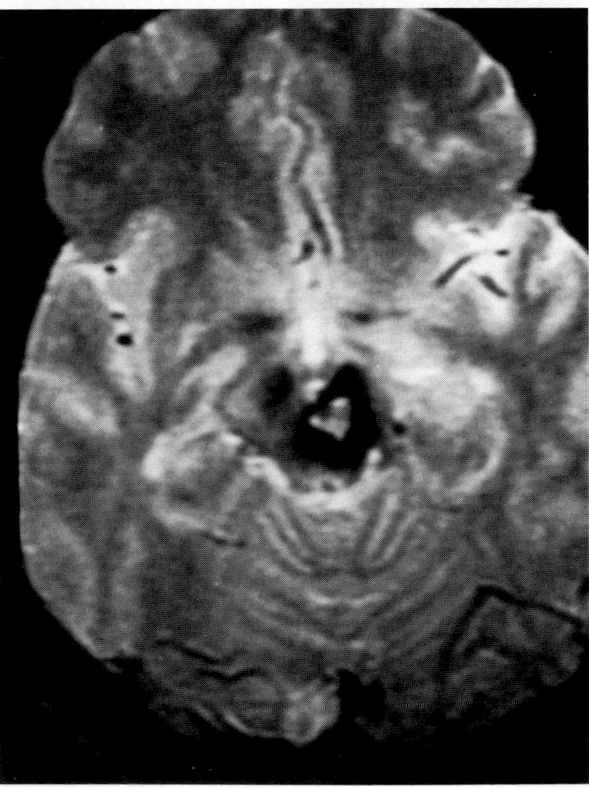

FIG. 79. Weber's syndrome. **A:** Short TR/TE MRI. **B:** Long TR/TE MRI. Cavernous hemangioma in left midbrain involved fascicle of left third nerve and resulted in third nerve palsy with contralateral hemiparesis.

Third Nerve Palsy

The third nerve nuclear complex is located in the midbrain at the level of the superior colliculus and ultimately supplies innervation to the levator palpebrae superioris, superior rectus, inferior rectus, medial rectus, inferior oblique, and pupillary sphincter muscles. Warwick has determined the organization of this nuclear complex in primates (128). In this scheme, the levator is supplied by a single midline caudal nucleus and the innervation to the superior rectus muscle is by a contralateral subnucleus. Thus, nuclear lesions are suggested by the presence of bilateral ptosis and a contralateral superior rectus palsy. Leaving this nuclear complex, the fibers of the third nerve coalesce ventrally into a fascicle (Fig. 77), which crosses the red nucleus and then the cerebral peduncle before exiting the brainstem (Fig. 78). A lesion in the region of the red nucleus results in an ipsilateral third nerve palsy and contralateral rubral tremor (Benedikt's syndrome), whereas a more ventral lesion is associated with a contralateral hemiparesis (Weber's syndrome) (Fig. 79). Common lesions of the brainstem parenchyma

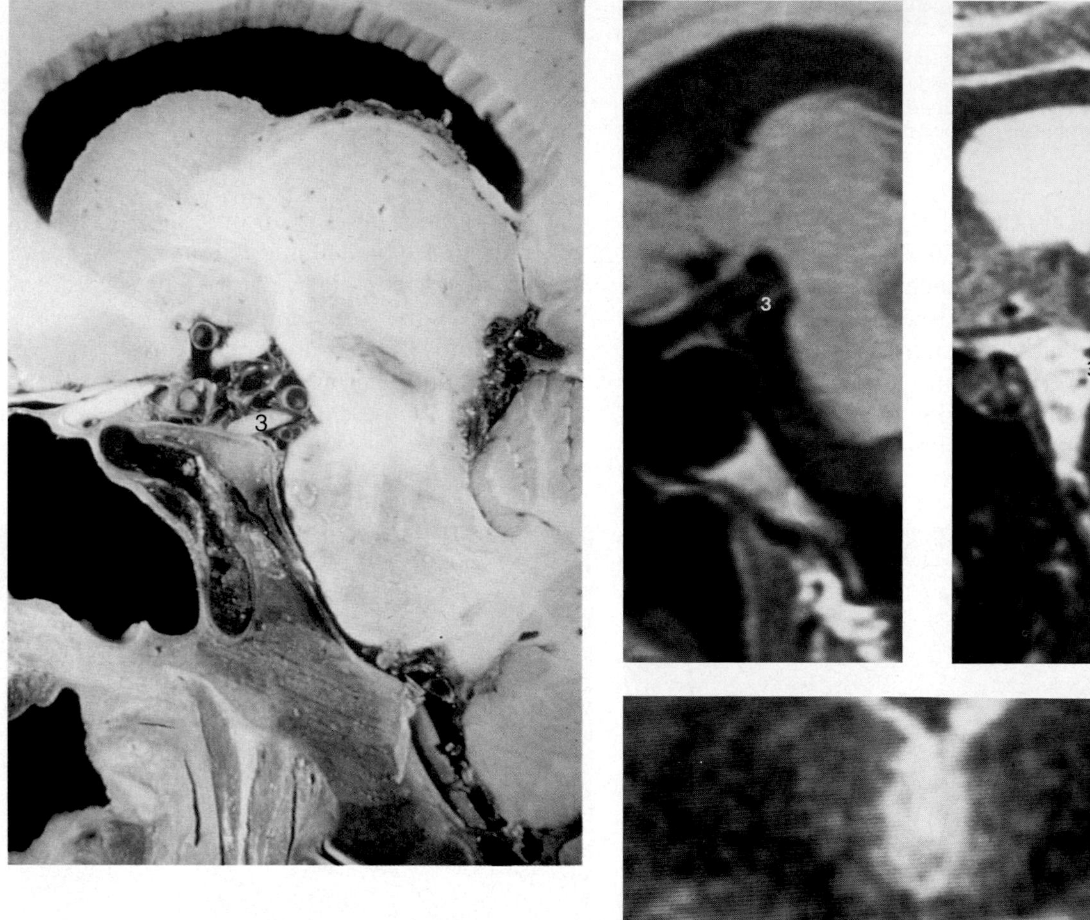

FIG. 80. Cisternal portion of third nerve is seen on sagittal anatomic section (**A**) and short TR/TE (**B**) and long TR/TE. **C**: MRI as it courses between posterior cerebral artery and superior cerebellar artery. Coronal long TR/TE MR (**D**) also shows relationship of third nerve (*3*) to arteries.

include infarction, hemorrhage, and demyelination. Recently, brainstem ocular motility defects have been documented in the acquired immunodeficiency syndrome (129).

The third nerve exits the brainstem between the posterior cerebral and superior cerebellar arteries (Fig. 80). At this level the third nerve may be compromised by a posterior communicating artery aneurysm or a meningeal process. Traveling from the interpeduncular fossa, the third nerve enters the superior portion of the cavernous sinus (Fig. 81). The superficial location of the pupillary fibers within the third nerve substance has been suggested as a cause of early pupillary involvement in compressive lesions, such as a posterior communicating aneurysm or transtentorial herniation (130). However, third nerve lesions in the cavernous sinus may completely spare pupillary function. These observations suggest that pupillary involvement may be related to the temporal profile of a given lesion as well as to the location of the pupillary fibers in the third nerve (131). Thus, in a rapidly expanding lesion such as an aneurysm or a transtentorial herniation, pupillary involvement is anticipated, whereas slowly expanding tumors of the cavernous sinus may spare pupillary function. The third nerve anatomically separates into a superior division (controlling the levator and superior rectus muscles) and inferior division (controlling pupillary fibers medial rectus, inferior rectus, and inferior oblique muscles) in the anterior cavernous sinus. Despite this anatomic separation within the cavernous sinus, a divisional palsy may be observed from a lesion affecting the third nerve at any point posterior to this location, including the brainstem parenchyma (132).

The most common cause of an isolated pupil-involving third nerve palsy is an aneurysm at the junction of the internal carotid artery and posterior commu-

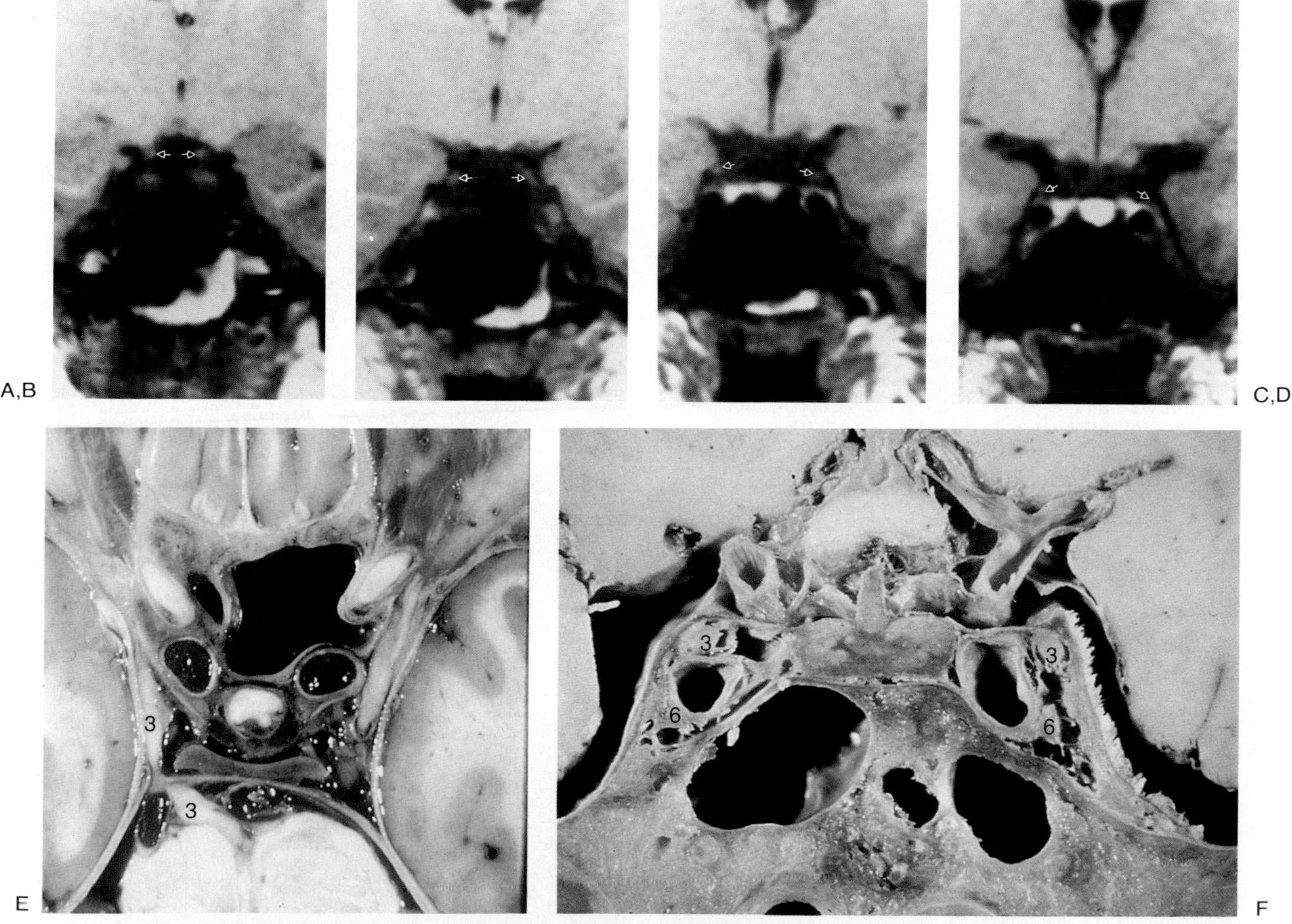

FIG. 81. Serial coronal MR images (**A–D**) demonstrate the course of the third nerve as it traverses the interpeduncular cisterns (*arrows*). Axial (**E**) and coronal (**F**) anatomic sections document the third nerve position as it enters the cavernous sinus. (E and F, Courtesy of Dr. W. Hoyt, San Francisco, CA.)

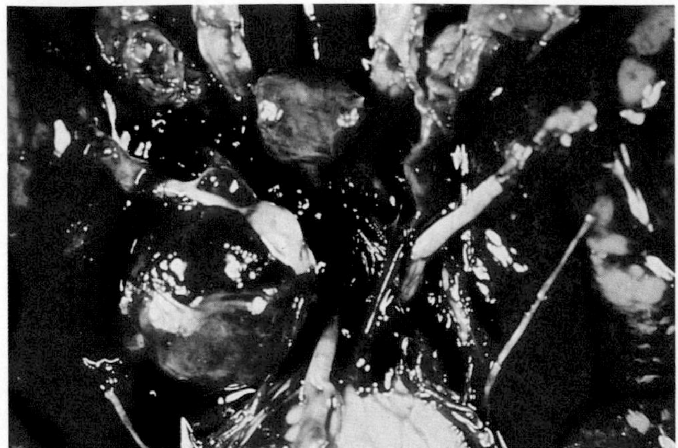

FIG. 82. Aneurysmal compression of third cranial nerve, autopsy specimen. Note large posterior communicating artery aneurysm compressing precavernous segment of right third nerve. (Courtesy of J. Lawton Smith, Miami, FL.)

nicating artery (Figs. 82 and 83) (133,134). In contrast, microvascular occlusion is the most common cause of a pupil-sparing third nerve palsy (133,134). Other causes of an oculomotor palsy include trauma, neoplasm (Figs. 84 and 85), and infection (Fig. 86) (Table 12). In children, congenital origin and trauma (Fig. 87) are the leading causes of isolated third nerve palsy. Aberrant regeneration of the third nerve usually occurs following an acute oculomotor palsy either from an aneurysm or trauma. A variety of anomalous innervation patterns may ensue and include elevation of the lid on downgaze, globe retraction in attempted vertical gaze, and light near dissociation of pupils. Rarely, these misdirected phenomena are observed with meningiomas of the cavernous sinus (135).

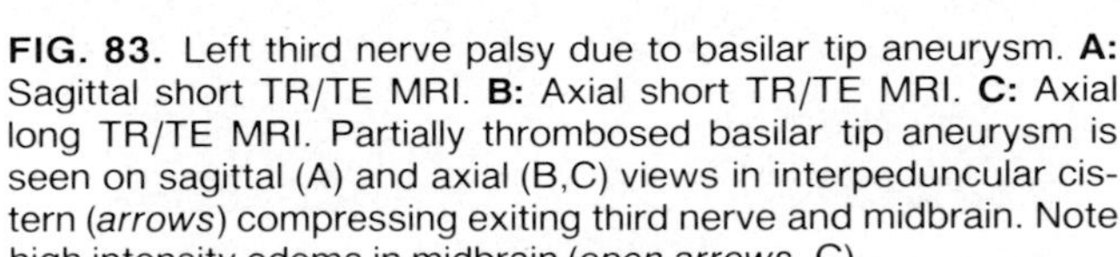

FIG. 83. Left third nerve palsy due to basilar tip aneurysm. **A:** Sagittal short TR/TE MRI. **B:** Axial short TR/TE MRI. **C:** Axial long TR/TE MRI. Partially thrombosed basilar tip aneurysm is seen on sagittal (A) and axial (B,C) views in interpeduncular cistern (*arrows*) compressing exiting third nerve and midbrain. Note high intensity edema in midbrain (*open arrows,* C).

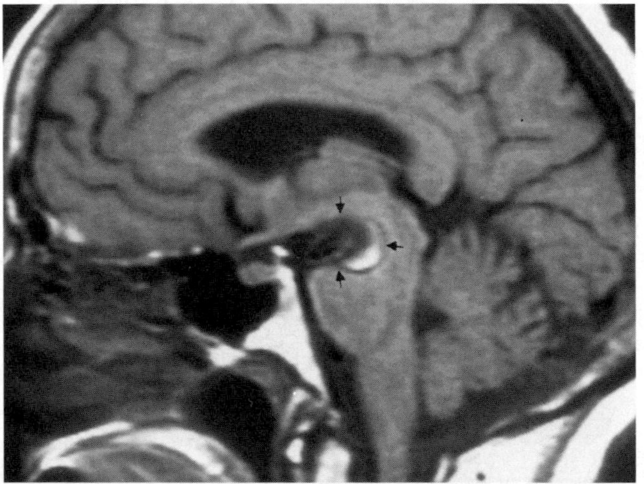

A

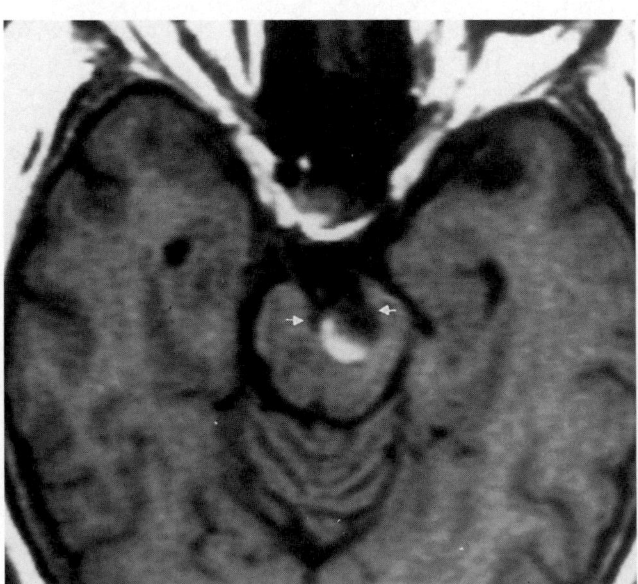

B

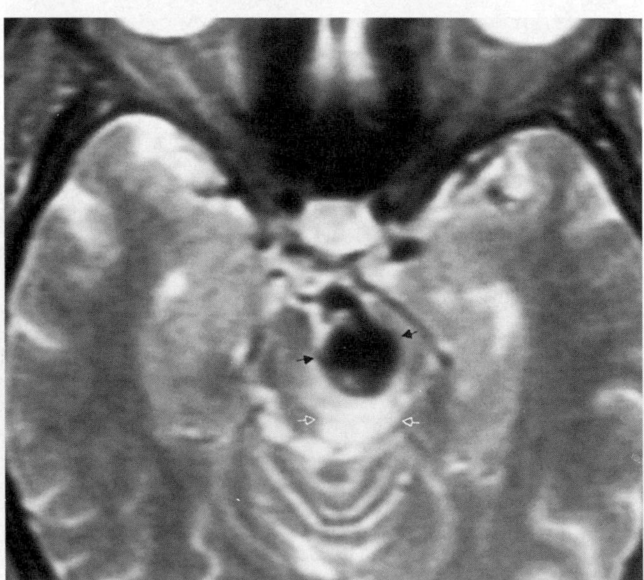

C

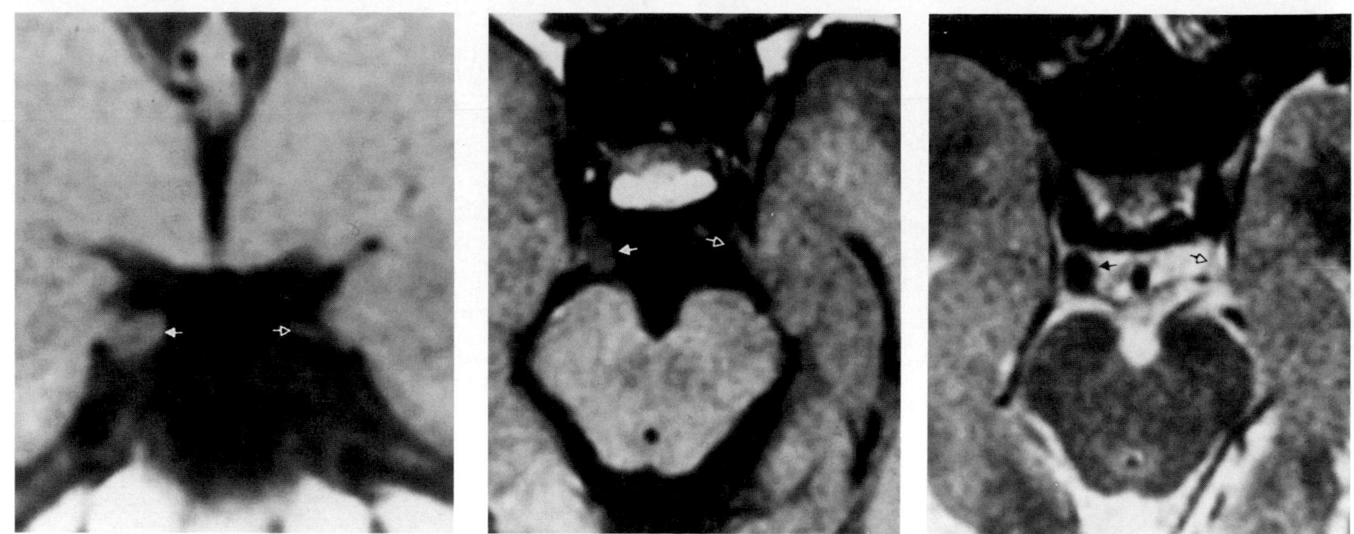

FIG. 84. Intrinsic right third nerve mass in patient with chronic palsy. **A:** Coronal short TR/TE MRI. **B:** Axial short TR/TE MRI. **C:** Axial long TR/TE MRI. Mass lesion involving right third nerve (*closed arrow*) may represent hemorrhagic cavernous hemangioma of third nerve. Normal third nerve on left is seen (*open arrow*).

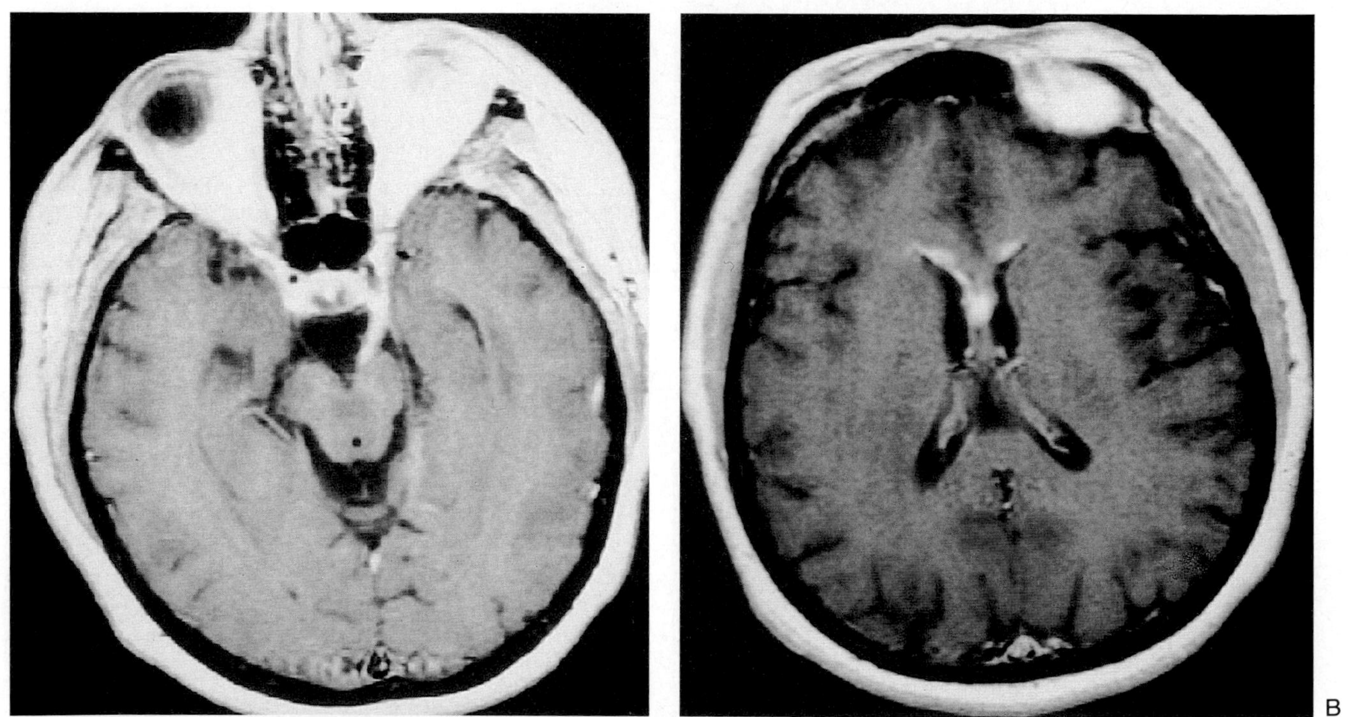

FIG. 85. Left third nerve palsy in lymphoma. Note densely enhancing left third nerve (**A**) extending from interpeduncular cistern to cavernous sinus in patient with supependymal and subarachnoid spread of lymphoma (**B**).

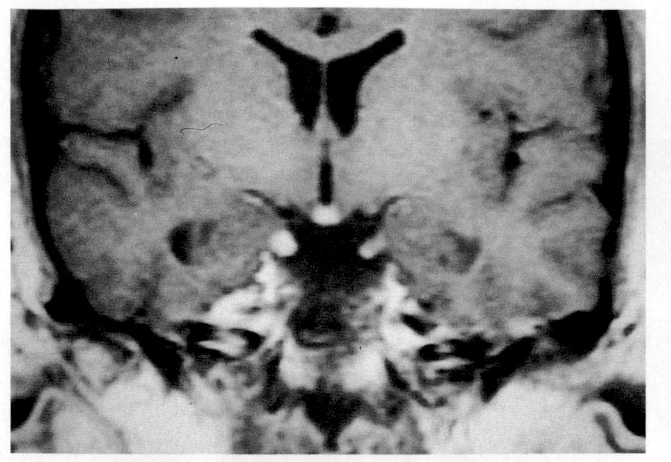
A

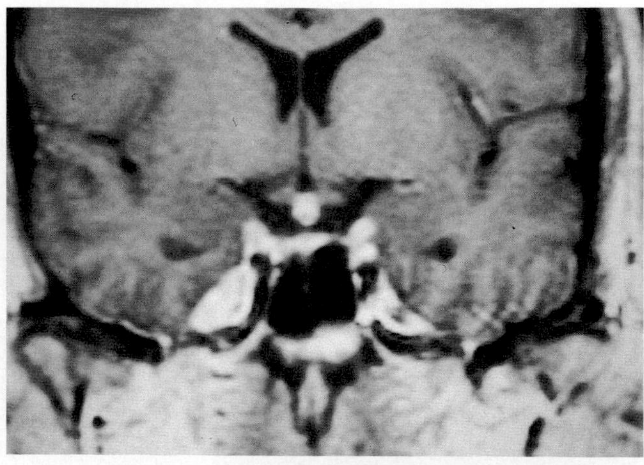
B

FIG. 86. Bilateral third and fourth nerve palsies in TB meningitis. Coronal postgadolinium images (**A,B**) show enlarged, enhancing third and fourth nerves bilaterally. Also note similar abnormality in pituitary infundibulum.

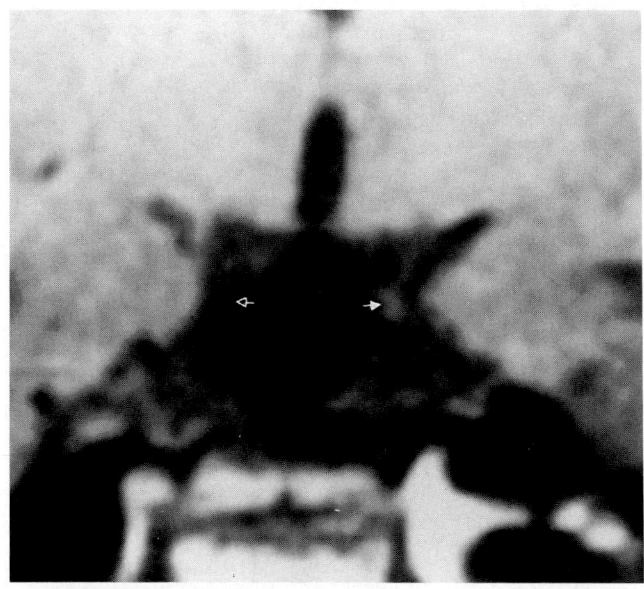
A

FIG. 87. Severe head trauma causing right third nerve avulsion. **A:** Coronal short TR/TE MRI. **B:** Sagittal short TR/TE MRI. **C:** Midline sagittal short TR/TE MRI. Years after this child was hit by moving train, note absence of right third nerve (*open arrows* show expected location, A,B). Left third nerve is well seen (*closed arrow,* A). Also note hypothalamic tear (*arrows,* C) and corpus callosum lesion.

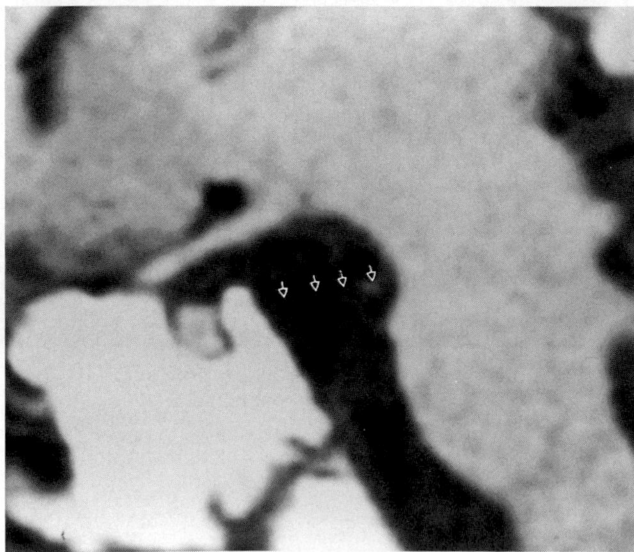
B

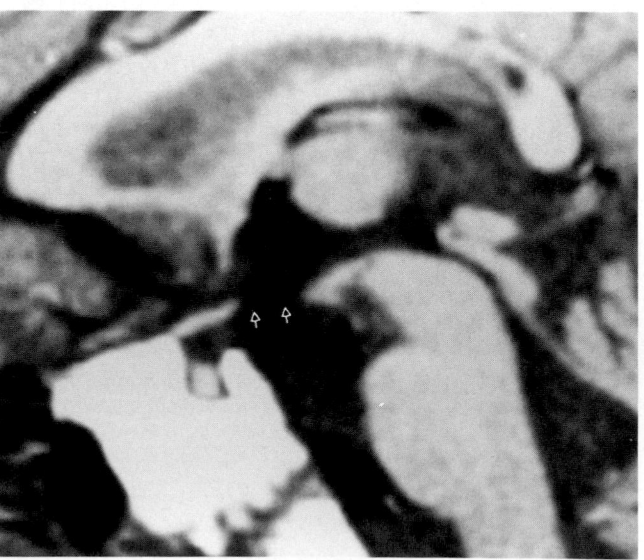
C

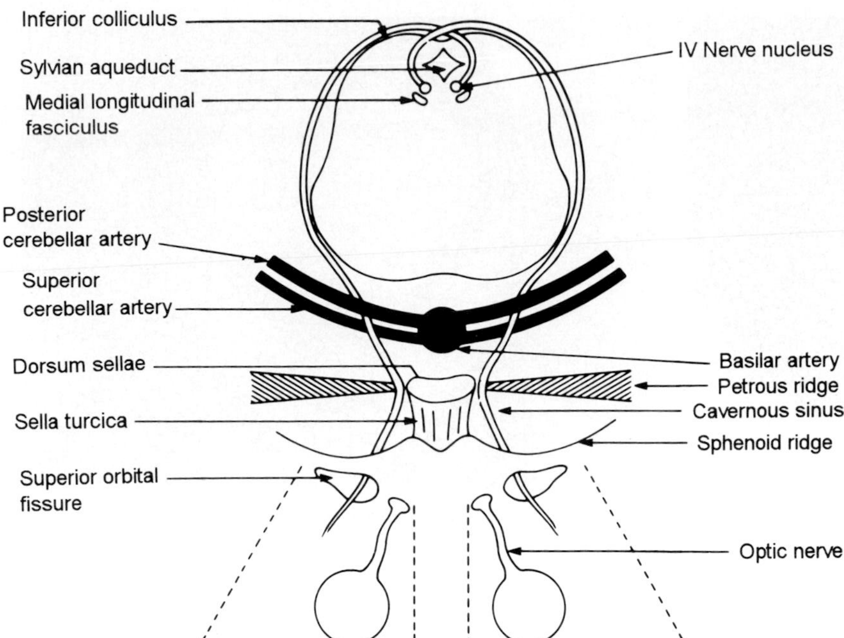

FIG. 88. Course of the fourth cranial nerve from brainstem to cavernous sinus. (From Bajandas and Kline, ref. 177, with permission.)

Fourth Nerve Palsy

This is the least common of the oculomotor palsies. The fourth nerve nucleus is located in midbrain at the level of the inferior colliculus (Figs. 88 and 89). The fascicles from this nucleus cross in the anterior medullary velum to supply the contralateral superior oblique muscle (Fig. 90). This is the only cranial nerve to exit the brainstem dorsally (Fig. 91), and it is susceptible to damage in head trauma. In trauma to the forehead, the dorsal midbrain may be contused against the rigid tentorium (Fig. 92) resulting in a unilateral or bilateral fourth nerve palsy. Other common causes of an isolated fourth nerve palsy are microvascular occlusion and congenital (Table 13) (136–138). A superior oblique palsy combined with a contralateral Homer's syndrome signifies a lesion in the dorsal mesencephalon on the side of the sympathetic interruption (139). In hydrocephalus, a trochlear nerve paresis may result from dilatation of the aqueduct or compression of the dorsal midbrain by an expanded suprapineal recess (140). Rarely, an isolated fourth nerve palsy may result from a ruptured midbrain vascular malformation (141) (Fig. 93).

TABLE 12. *Differential diagnosis of an acquired third nerve palsy*

Etiology	"Isolated" III (130 patients) (%)	Combined nonisolated and isolated III (290 patients) (%)
Aneurysm	30	14
Vasculopathy	19	21
Tumor	4	12
Trauma	11	16
Undetermined	23	23
Other	13	14

Data from Green, ref. 133, and Rush and Younge, ref. 136, with permission.

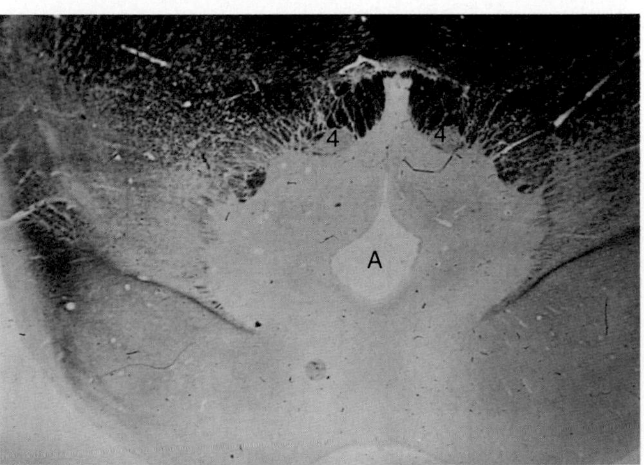

FIG. 89. Microscopic section through nuclei of fourth cranial nerves (*4*) in midbrain. Note the dark-staining medial longitudinal fasciculus just ventral to the nuclei of fourth nerves, both of which lie ventral to the aqueduct (*A*).

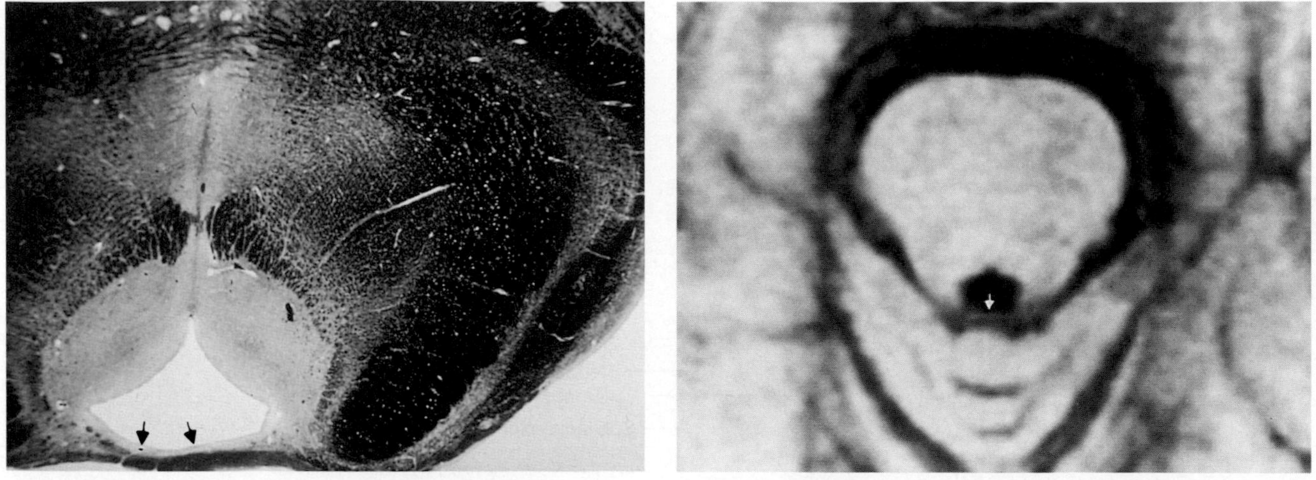

FIG. 90. Decussation of fourth nerves. Microscopic section (**A**) and axial short TR/TE MRI (**B**) both clearly demonstrate the anterior medullary velum (*arrows*), the site of the decussation of the fourth nerve fibers.

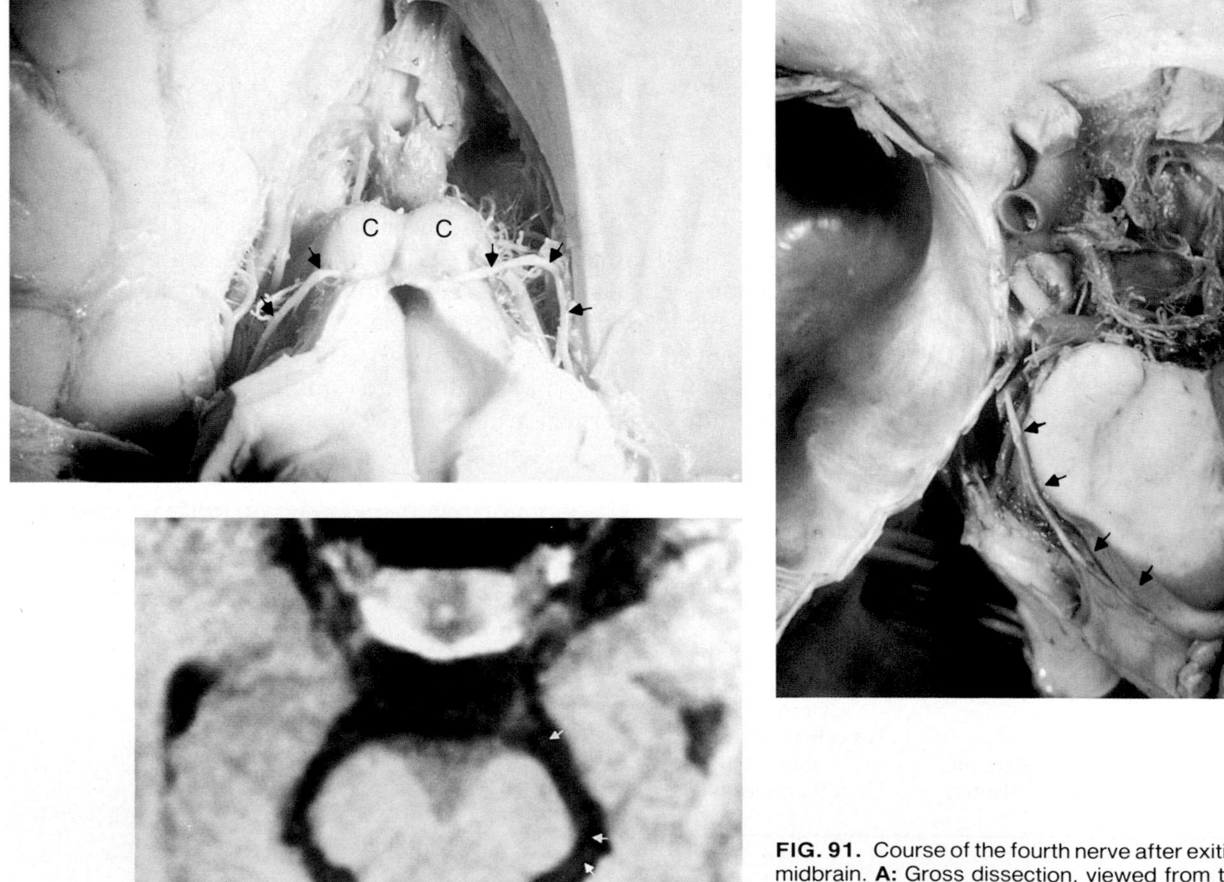

FIG. 91. Course of the fourth nerve after exiting dorsal midbrain. **A:** Gross dissection, viewed from the dorsal and superior aspect of the brain. **B:** Gross dissection, viewed from above. **C:** Axial short TR/TE MRI through the midbrain. Note that thin fourth nerves (*arrows*) exit just under colliculi (*C* in A) and traverse around dorsolateral midbrain (B and C). Occasionally, the entire course of the fourth nerve is visible on MR (*arrows,* C). (A,B, courtesy of Dr. W. Hoyt, San Francisco, CA.)

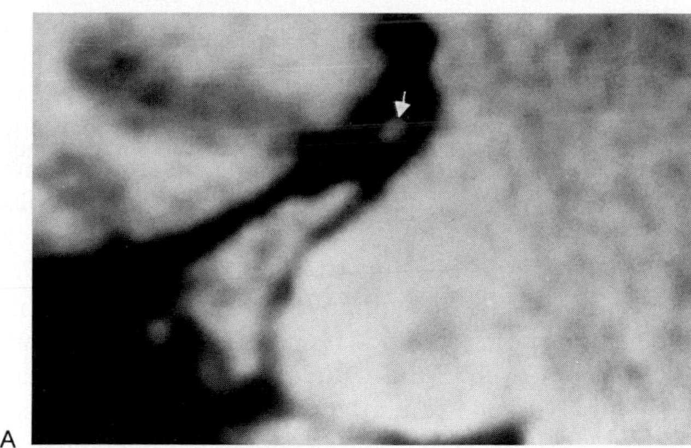

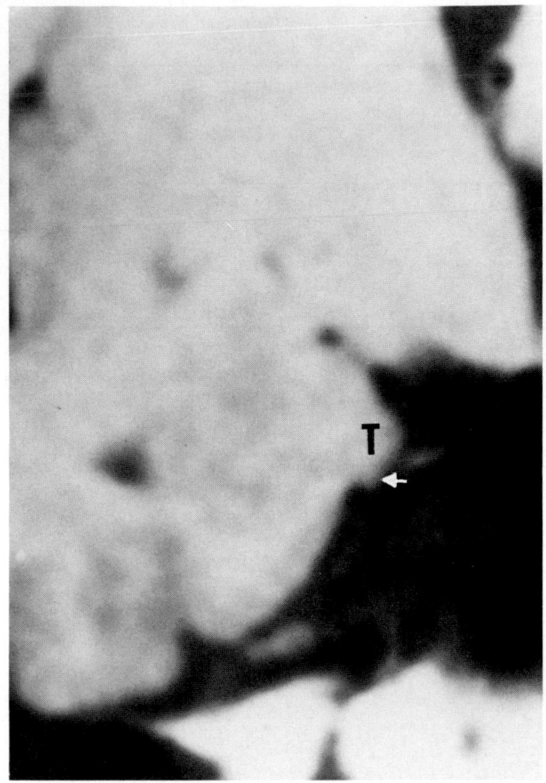

FIG. 92. Proximity of fourth nerve to tentorial edge. Note on serial coronal short TR/TE MR images (**A,B**) that small fourth nerve (*arrows*) comes from behind brainstem, lies immediately adjacent to tentorial edge, and is next to medial temporal lobe (*T*).

Sixth Nerve Palsy

The abducens nuclei lie in the dorsomedial part of the pons near the paramedian pontine reticular formation (horizontal gaze center). Along the floor of the fourth ventricle, the seventh nerve fascicles wind around the sixth nerve nucleus to form the facial colliculus (Figs. 94 and 95). Since the sixth nerve nucleus also contains interneurons to form the medial longitudinal fasciculus, a lesion in this region results in an ipsilateral facial palsy and horizontal gaze palsy. The fascicles of the sixth nerve then proceed ventrally from their nucleus to cross the

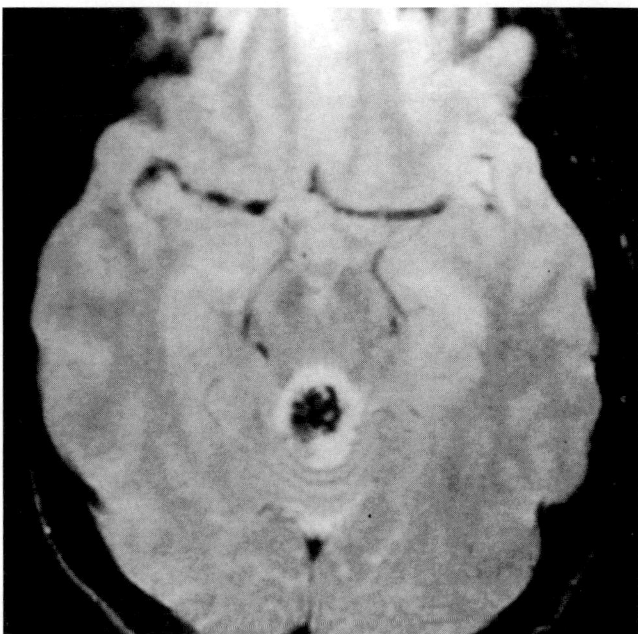

FIG. 93. Isolated right fourth nerve palsy in young patient with cavernous hemangioma in tectum (long TR/TE MRI).

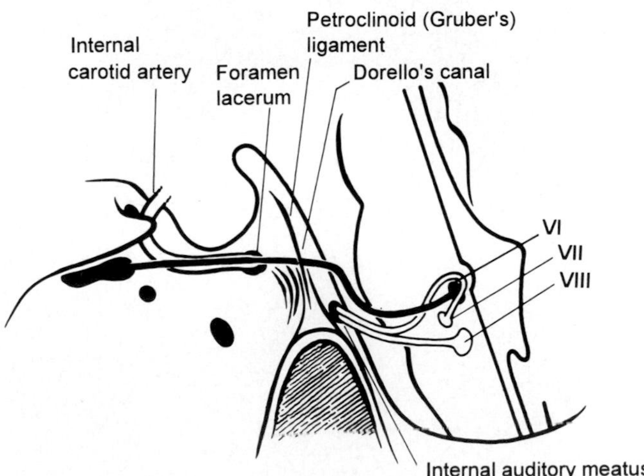

FIG. 94. Course of the sixth cranial nerve from brainstem to cavernous sinus. (From Bajandas and Kline, ref. 177, with permission.)

TABLE 13. *Differential diagnosis of an acquired fourth nerve palsy*

Etiology	Combined isolated and nonisolated IV (172 patients) (%)	Isolated IV (100 patients) (%)
Vasculopathy	19	39
Tumor	4	—
Trauma	32	24
Undetermined	36	23
Other	8	14[a]

[a] Includes two patients classified as compressive.

Data from Rush and Younge, ref. 136, and Kziazek et al., ref. 137, with permission.

fibers of the corticospinal tracts as they exit the brainstem. A lesion in this region causes an ipsilateral sixth nerve palsy and a contralateral hemiparesis.

In the subarachnoid space, the sixth nerve may be involved in a variety of neoplastic or infectious meningeal processes such as tuberculosis, syphilis, Lyme disease, and lymphomas. Disorders that involve multiple bilateral cranial nerves imply a process in the subarachnoid space until proven otherwise. Leaving the area of the subarachnoid space (Fig. 96), the sixth nerve ascends the clivus, traveling beneath the petroclinoid ligament (within Dorello's canal) to enter the confines of the cavernous sinus. Here the sixth nerve lies freely just lateral

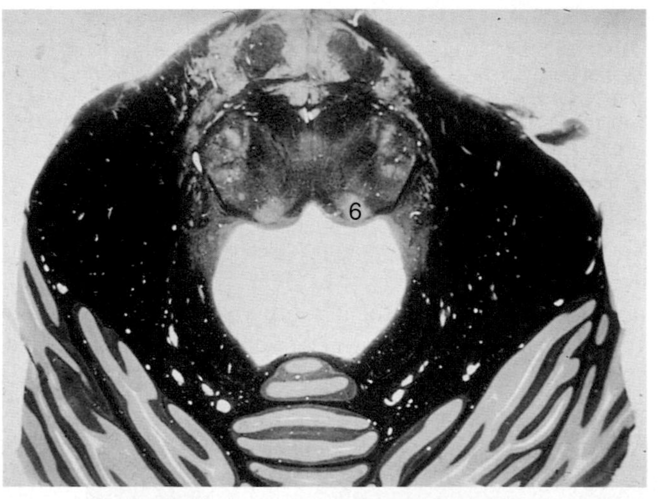

A

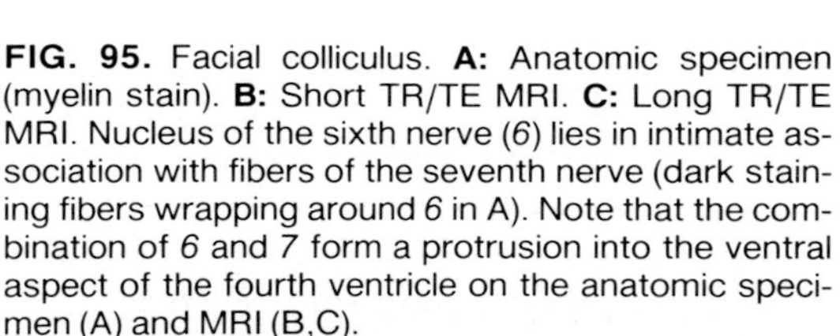

FIG. 95. Facial colliculus. **A:** Anatomic specimen (myelin stain). **B:** Short TR/TE MRI. **C:** Long TR/TE MRI. Nucleus of the sixth nerve (*6*) lies in intimate association with fibers of the seventh nerve (dark staining fibers wrapping around *6* in A). Note that the combination of *6* and *7* form a protrusion into the ventral aspect of the fourth ventricle on the anatomic specimen (A) and MRI (B,C).

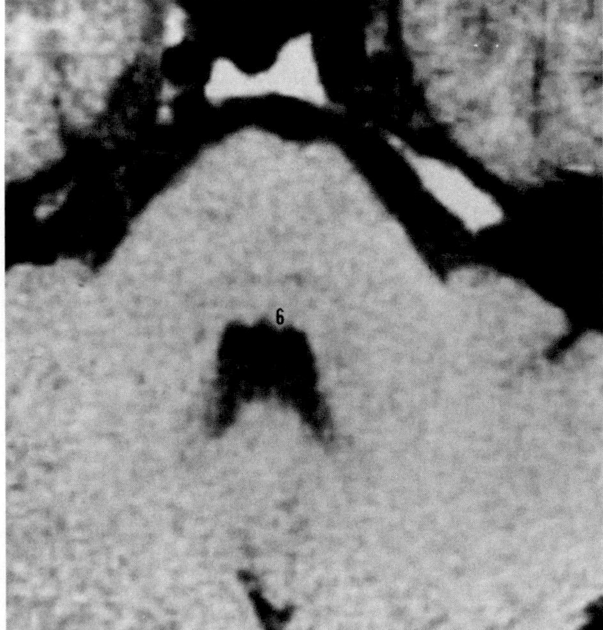

B

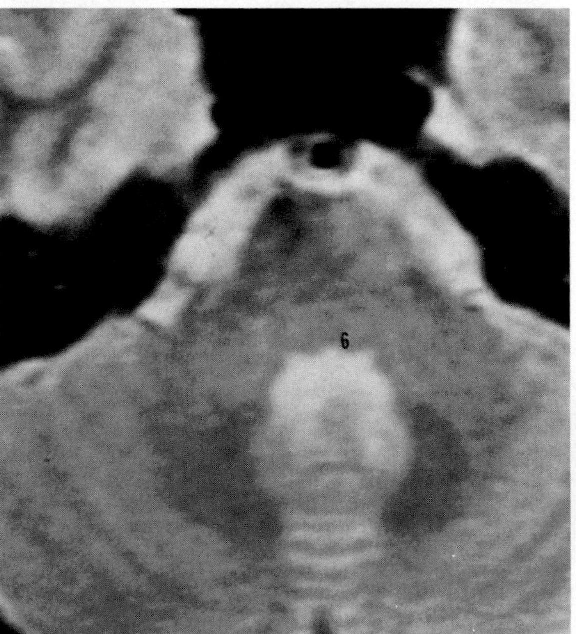

C

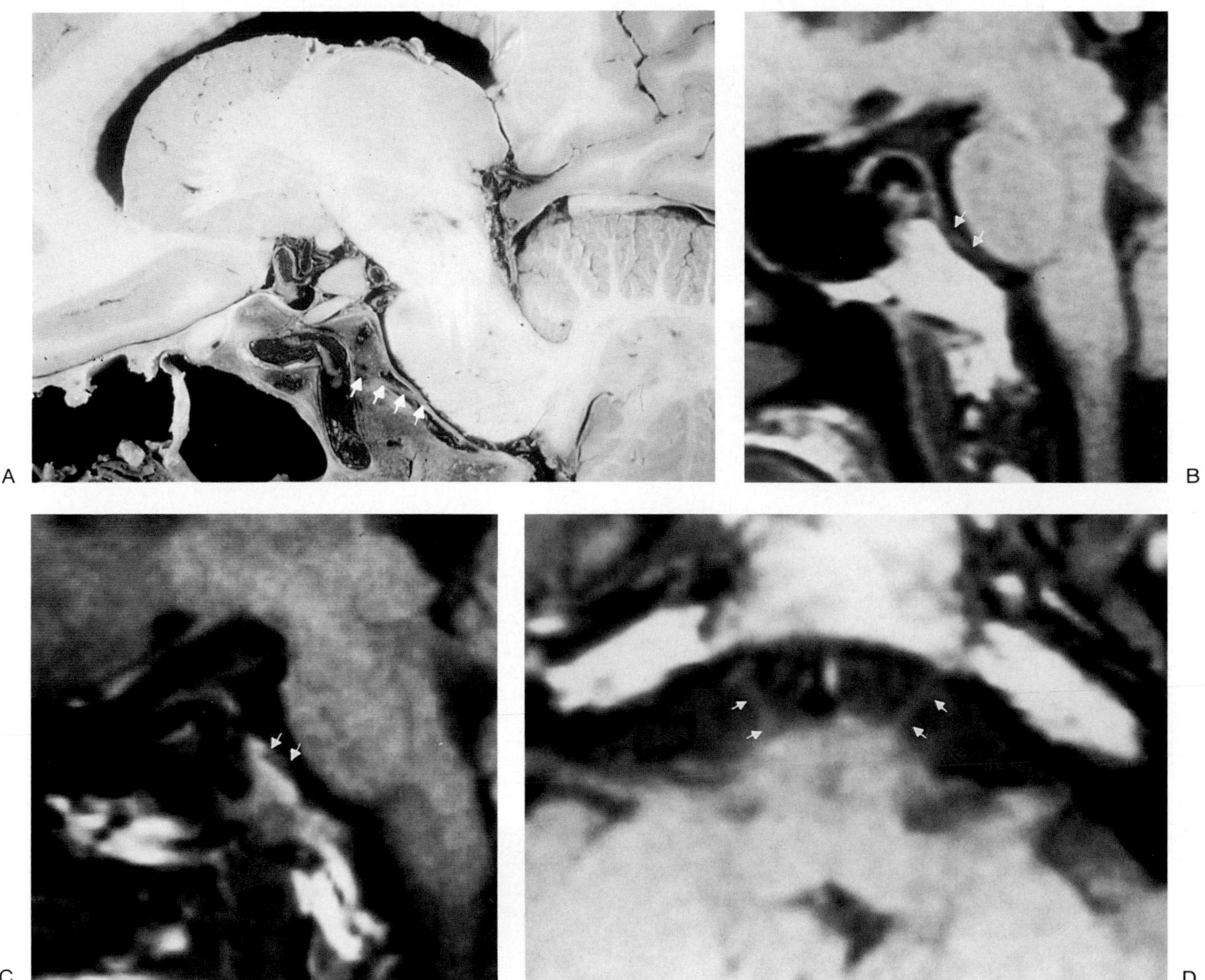

FIG. 96. Intracisternal course of sixth nerve into Dorello's canal. **A:** Sagittal anatomic specimen. **B:** Sagittal short TR/TE MRI. **C:** Sagittal short TR/TE MRI. **D:** Axial short TR/TE MRI. Sixth nerve ascends subarachnoid space and traverses Dorello's canal (*arrows,* A–C) under petroclinoid ligament on its way to cavernous sinus. Rarely, sixth nerve can be seen in prepontine cistern on MRI (D).

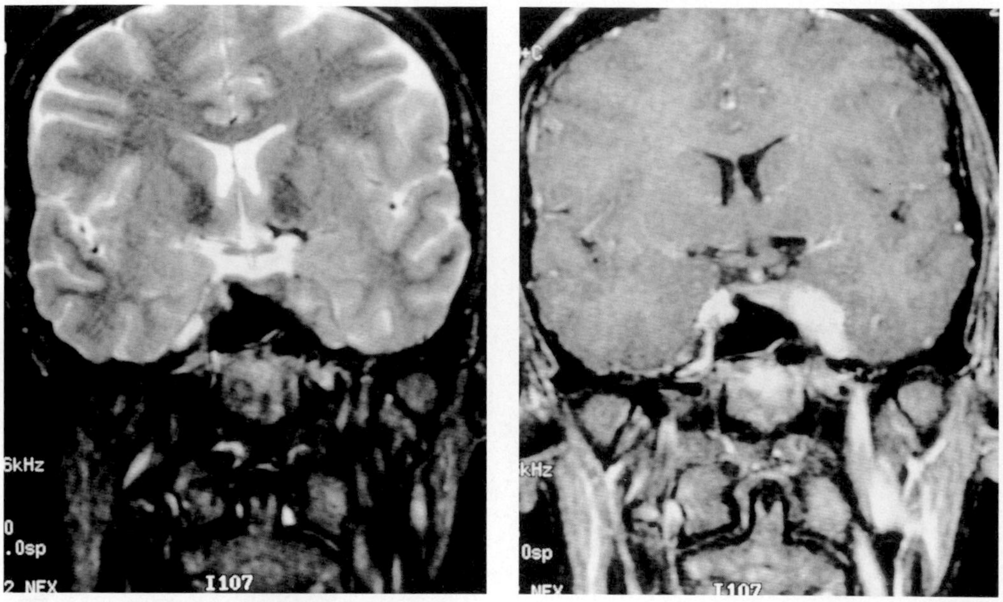

FIG. 97. Cavernous sinus involvement of Hodgkin's lymphoma. Isointense mass in left cavernous sinus (**A**) enhances homogeneous after i.v. contrast (**B**) and extends slightly along tentorial margin (**C**). Note absence of carotid narrowing (C), distinguishing this lesion from cavernous meningioma.

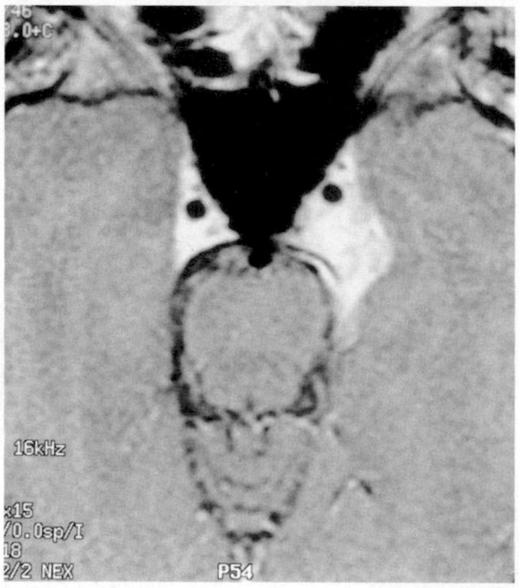

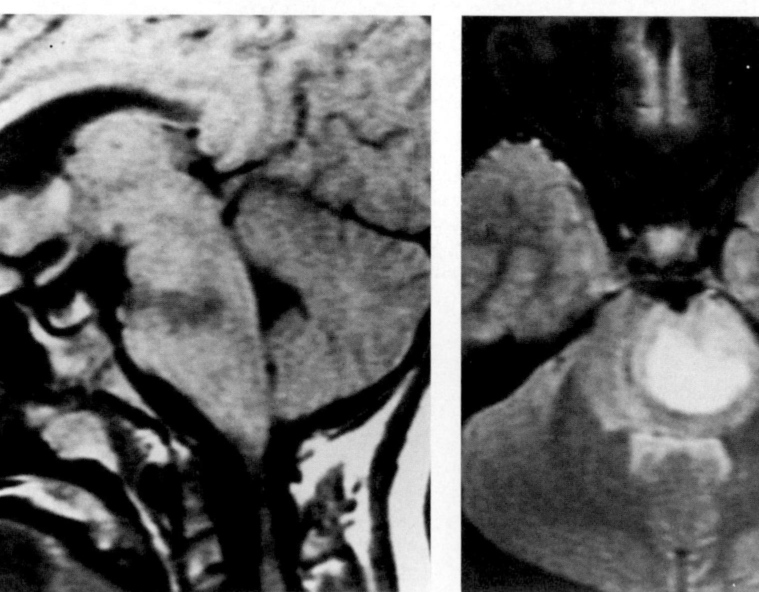

FIG. 98. Left sixth nerve palsy in child. Note intra-axial mass on sagittal short TR/TE MRI (**A**) and axial long TR/TE MRI (**B**), denoting presence of brainstem glioma.

TABLE 14. *Differential diagnosis of an acquired abducens palsy*

Etiology	"Isolated" VI (104 patients) %	Combined nonisolated and isolated VI (419 patients) %	Isolated VI in young adults (49 patients) %
Vasculopathy	36	18	29
Undetermined	24	30	22
Tumor	7	15	16
Aneurysm	—	3	—
Trauma	3	17	6
Multiple sclerosis	13	4	12
Other	18	18	15

Data from Schrader and Schlezinger, ref. 144; Rush and Younge, ref. 136; and Moster et al., ref. 143, with permission.

to the carotid artery. The sympathetic fibers traveling along the carotid plexus will briefly join the abducens nerve in this region. Thus, the presence of an ipsilateral Horner's syndrome in conjunction with abducens palsy implicates a lesion in the cavernous sinus (142). Lesions of both the cavernous sinus and superior orbital fissure are characterized by variable, but ipsilateral, involvement of cranial nerves I, IV, V, and VI (Fig. 97). When the sixth nerve is damaged within the orbit, optic nerve dysfunction and proptosis are usually found.

The etiology of abducens palsies is often age-dependent. In children, a sixth nerve palsy may occur following a viral infection or in the presence of an intracranial (e.g., brainstem) tumor (Fig. 98). In young adults, common causes include microvascular occlusion, demyelinating lesions, tumors, and idiopathic sixth nerve palsy (143). In patients over 40 years of age, microvascular occlusion predominates (Table 14) (144).

Chronic isolated sixth nerve palsies pose a special diagnostic problem and careful attention must be paid to the base of the skull and cavernous sinus region (145). Chordomas, cavernous sinus meningiomas (Fig. 99) and aneurysms, nasopharyngeal tumors, and trigeminal neuromas may be responsible for a persistent abducens palsy (Figs. 100, 101, and 102). Finally, it should be remembered that thyroid eye disease, myasthenia gravis, congenital Duane retraction syndrome, spasm of the near reflex, and orbital trauma may cause a lateral rectus or pseudoabducens palsy (Fig. 103).

Internuclear Ophthalmoplegia

The medial longitudinal fasciculus (MLF) connects the nuclei of the third, fourth, and sixth cranial nerves (Fig. 104). The MLF is a paired structure located dorsally and near the midline throughout the brainstem (Fig. 105). A lesion in the MLF typically results in an internuclear ophthalmoplegia (Fig. 105). This eye move-

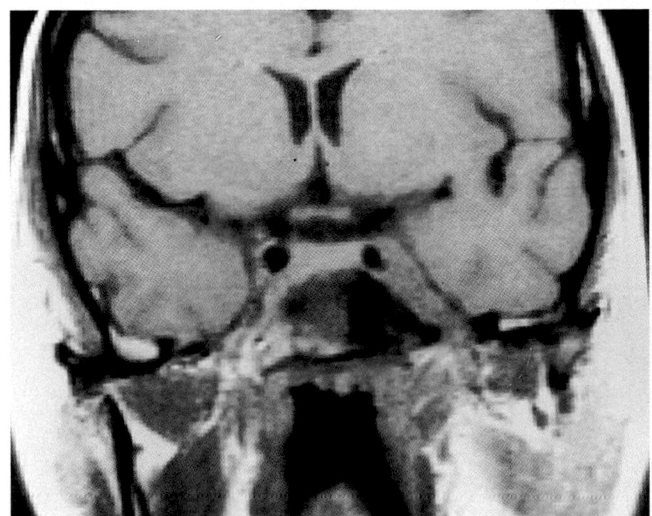

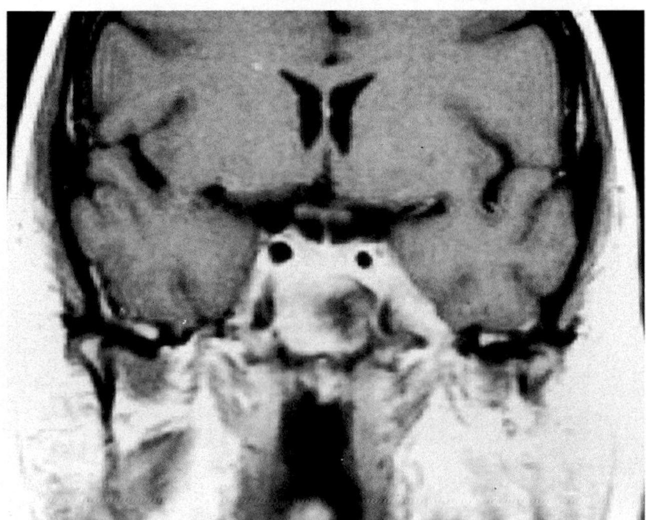

FIG. 99. Isolated left sixth nerve palsy in cavernous sinus meningioma. Coronal pre- (**A**) and post- (**B**) gadolinium enhanced T1-weighted images show left cavernous soft tissue mass that enhances homogeneously. As is typical in meningioma, not mild but definite cavernous carotid narrowing (small focus of low intensity superolateral to left carotid in B is left third nerve).

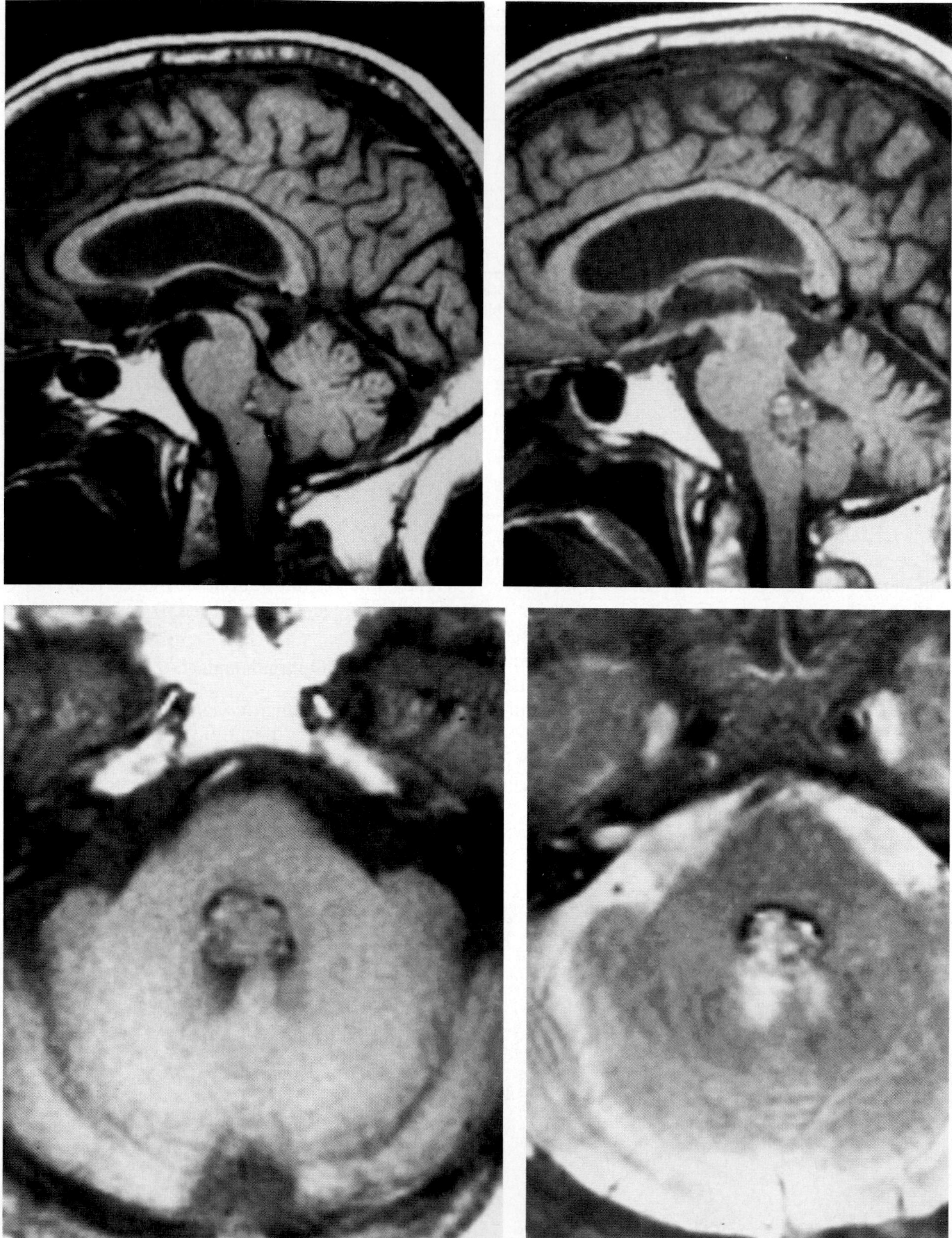

FIG. 100. Sixth and seventh nerve palsies in adult. Heterogeneous subpial exophytic mass protruding into fourth ventricle represents cavernous hemangioma, arising in facial colliculus.

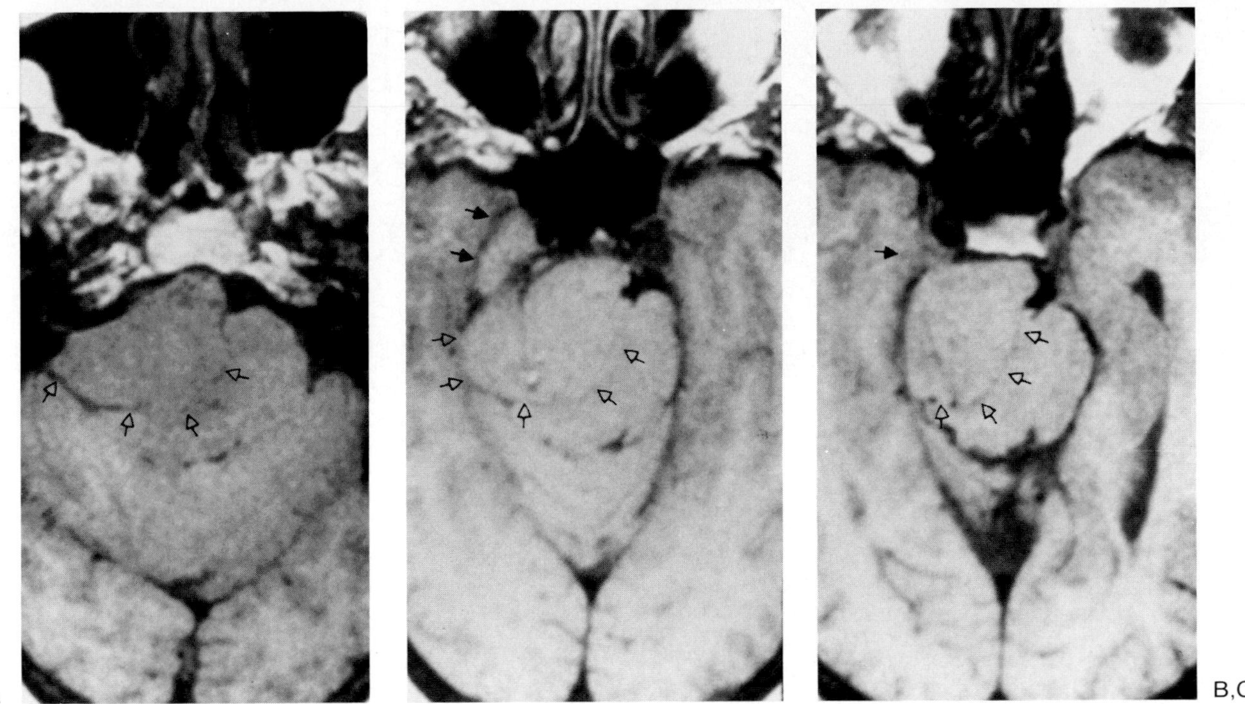

FIG. 101. Isolated right sixth nerve palsy in adult. Note large cerebellopontine angle meningioma (*open arrows,* **A–C**) extending into cavernous sinus (*closed arrows*) and compressing brainstem on serial short TR/TE MR images.

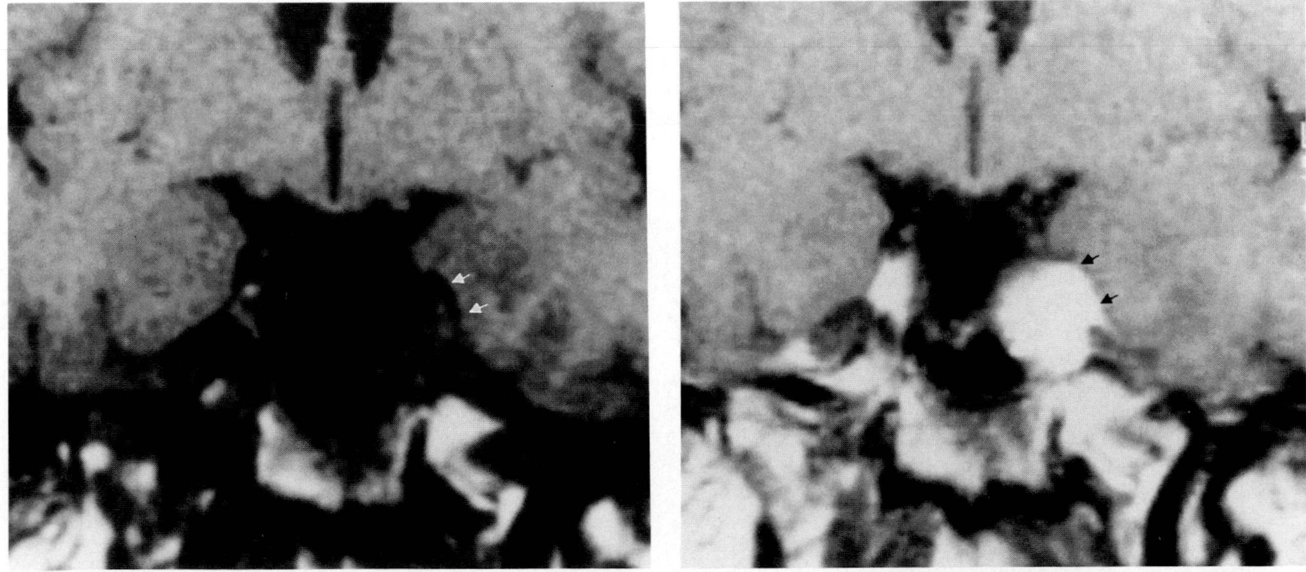

FIG. 102. Left sixth nerve palsy in adult. Precontrast short TR/TE image (**A**) depicts low intensity mass displacing left medial temporal lobe (*arrows*). Note dense enhancement after contrast (*arrows,* **B**) in this proven chordoma. (Courtesy of Dr. W. Hoyt, San Francisco, CA.)

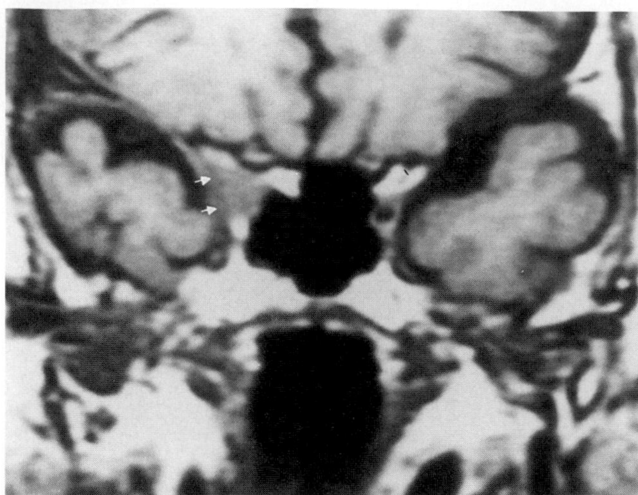

FIG. 103. Right sixth nerve palsy in patient with metastatic breast carcinoma. Coronal short TR/TE image through orbital apex shows mass (*arrows*) causing lateral gaze palsy, due to metastatic carcinoma.

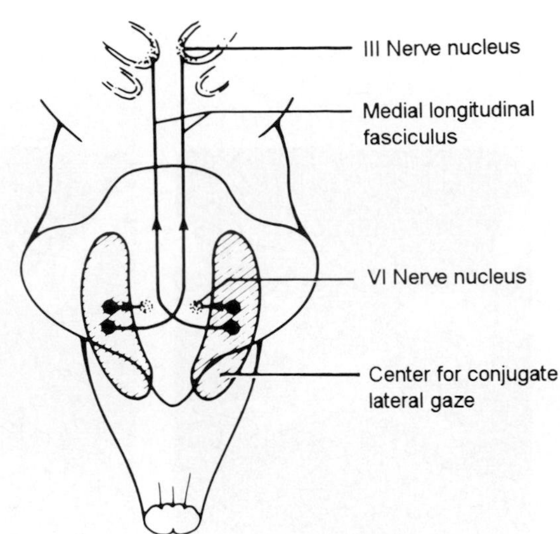

FIG. 104. Medial longitudinal fasciculus. Note that MLF runs from level of sixth nerve nucleus, crosses, and ascends to third nerve nucleus. (From Atlas et al., ref. 146, with permission.)

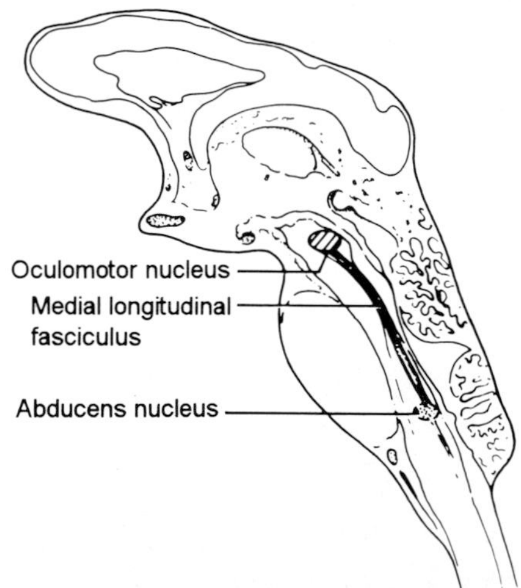

FIG. 105. Sagittal view, MLF. **A:** Artist's conception. **B:** Myelin-stained anatomic specimen. **C:** Sagittal long TR/short TE MRI in patient with intranuclear ophthalmoplegia (INO) and medial longitudinal fasciculus (MLF) lesion. MLF is situated in dorsal aspect of brainstem (*arrows,* B). Patient with MS (MS) and INO shows focal lesion in region of MLF (*arrow,* C). (A,B, from Atlas et al., ref. 146, with permission.)

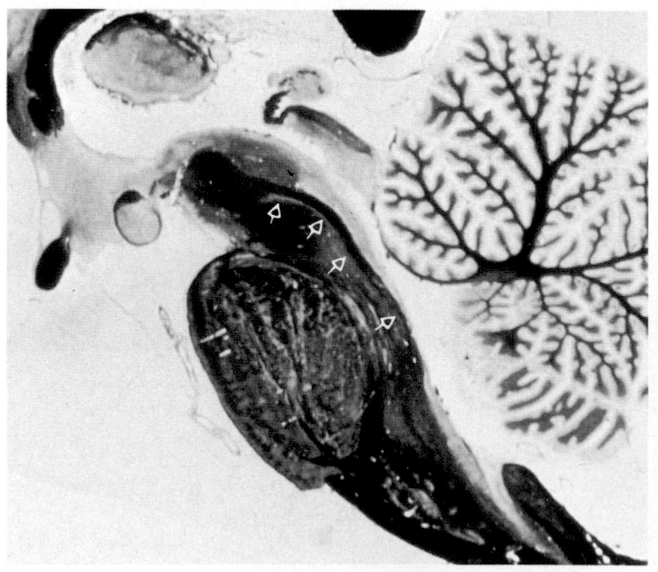

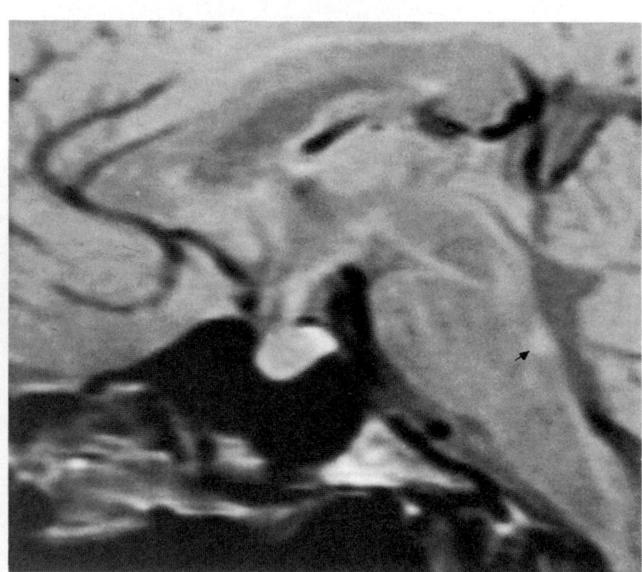

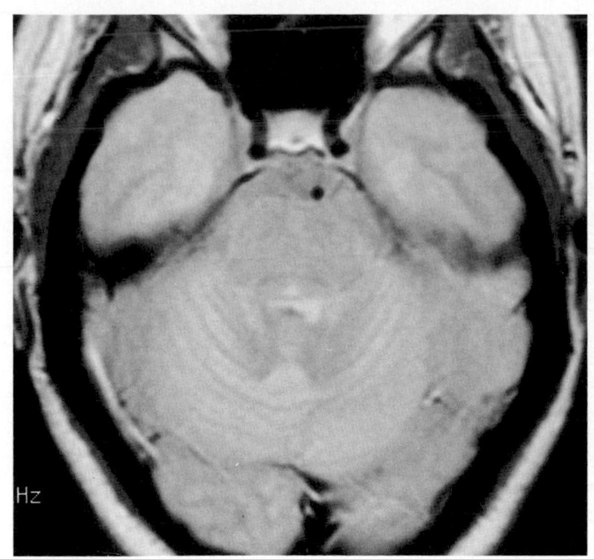

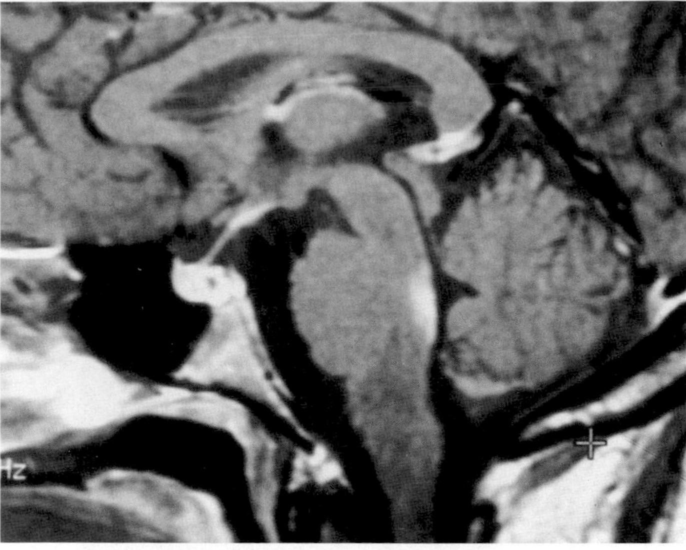

FIG. 106. Internuclear ophthalmoplegia in MS. Axial long TR/short TE image (**A**) shows left-sided hyperintensity in floor of fourth ventricle in patient with recent onset of unilateral INO. Sagittal image after i.v. contrast (**B**) shows clear enhancement in region of MLF in dorsal pons.

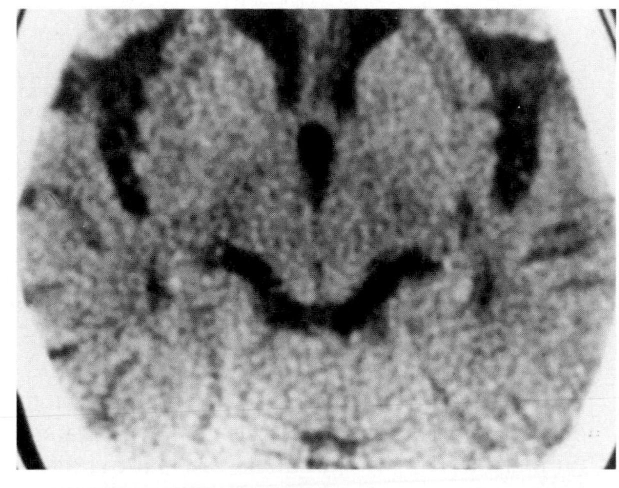

FIG. 107. Infarction and unilateral INO, CT vs. MRI. **A:** CT. **B:** Sagittal long TR/short TE MRI. **C:** Sagittal long TR/TE MRI. CT is normal (A). MRI (B,C) shows focal area of hyperintensity (*arrow*) consistent with infarction in the cephalad aspect of MLF in this elderly patient. (From Atlas et al., ref. 146, with permission.)

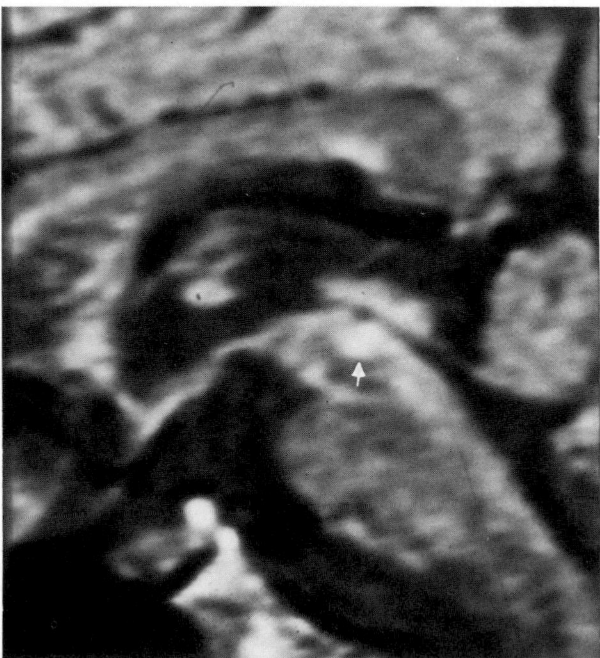

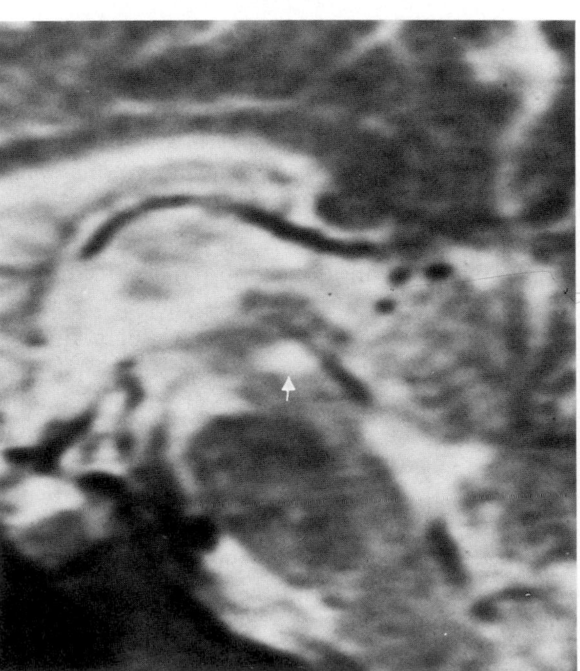

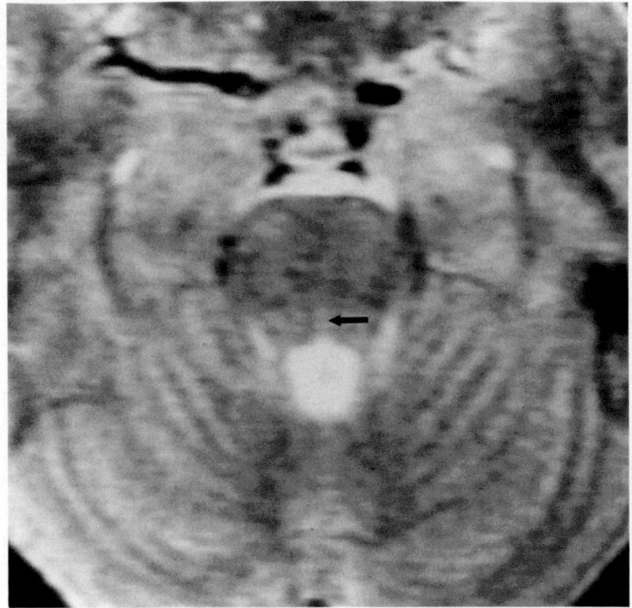

FIG. 108. "Pseudo-MLF lesion" in normal patient. Long TR/TE MRI shows thin, strictly midline region of slight hyperintensity, a normal finding that is probably related to signal from the nuclei of the median raphe. (From Atlas et al., ref. 146, with permission.)

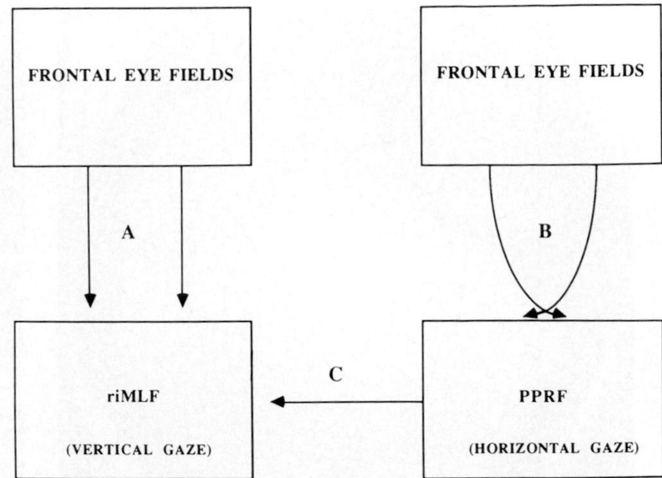

FIG. 109. Supranuclear pathways for control of vertical and horizontal gaze. **A:** Both frontal eye fields project to the rostral interstitial nucleus of the medial longitudinal fasciculus (riMLF) for control of vertical gaze. **B:** Frontal eye fields project to contralateral paramedian pontine reticular formation (PPRF) for control of horizontal saccades. **C:** PPRF may influence vertical saccades by projecting to riMLF.

ment disorder is characterized by an ipsilateral decrease in adduction and contralateral abducting nystagmus. In a young person with a bilateral internuclear ophthalmoplegia, a demyelinative disorder should be considered likely (Fig. 106). In contrast, an elderly individual with a unilateral internuclear ophthalmoplegia often has a brainstem infarction (Fig. 107). Note that MRIs commonly show a thin band of slight hyperintensity precisely in the midline in normal patients (Fig. 108); this probably relates to the nuclei of the median raphe and should not be confused with a paramedian MLF lesion (146).

Clinical Features of Gaze Palsies

The supranuclear fibers for horizontal gaze originate in the frontal eye fields and travel caudally to decussate at the pontine-mesencephalic junction before proceeding to the paramedian pontine reticular formation (PRRF). Thus, a horizontal gaze palsy in one direction may result from a lesion of the contralateral frontomesencephalic pathway or a disturbance of the ipsilateral pontine tegmentum involving the PPRF or abducens nucleus (147) (Fig. 109). In a frontomesencephalic lesion, the gaze palsy can be overcome by oculocephalic maneuvers. When the supranuclear tracts are disturbed, the eyes will typically deviate in the direction opposite the hemiparesis. In pontine lesions, the eyes usually deviate toward the side of the hemiparesis.

The presence of a vertical gaze palsy implies a lesion in the midbrain. The midbrain structure known as the rostral interstitial nucleus of the medial longitudinal fasciculus (riMLF) is considered to be the vertical gaze center (Fig. 109). Bilateral disruption of riMLF may result in a downgaze palsy or a complete vertical gaze palsy (148,149). An isolated upgaze palsy typically results from a lesion of the posterior commissure, but may rarely follow a unilateral thalamus or midbrain disturbance (150). When a vertical gaze palsy is combined with light near dissociation of the pupils, lid retraction, and convergence retraction nystagmus, a lesion in the dorsal midbrain is suggested. Common causes of the dorsal midbrain syndrome include pineal tumors and aqueductal stenosis. Other etiologies include intramedullary tumors, brainstem infarctions, vascular malformations,

TABLE 15. *Localizing nystagmus*

Type	Location
Brun's nystagmus[a]	Cerebellopontine angle
Convergence retraction	Dorsal mesencephalon
Dissociated	Medial longitudinal fasciculus
Downbeat	Craniocervical junction
Gaze-evoked	Vestibular, cerebellum
Oculopalatal myoclonus	Dento-rubro-olivary connections (central tegmental tract)
Periodic alternating	Craniocervical junction
Rebound	Cerebellum
Seesaw	Parasellar, mesencephalon
Spasmus nutans	Exclude chiasmal glioma
Torsional	Central vestibular or cerebellum
Upbeat	Pontomesencephalic, pontomedullary, cerebellar

[a] Refers to ipsilateral gaze paretic and contralateral high-frequency, low-amplitude nystagmus.

demyelinating disorders, and infection. Although a monocular elevation palsy is most commonly caused by an orbital process such as thyroid eye disease, a rare supranuclear paresis may result from a midbrain lesion. The lesion is usually contralateral to the elevation palsy (151).

Nystagmus

Nystagmus refers to an abnormal to-and-fro movement of the eyes. When the oscillations are smooth and sinusoidal, the nystagmus is referred to as pendular, and when a slow phase alternates with a quick phase, it is known as jerk nystagmus. Many forms of nystagmus have exquisite localizing value (Table 15). Other eye oscillations such as ocular dysmetria, macrosquare-wave jerks, ocular flutter, and opsoclonus are often associated with cerebellar disorders. Ocular bobbing is typically seen with extensive pontine lesions causing a horizontal gaze palsy, but may be observed with diffuse processes affecting the CNS (152). Familiarity with the localization of specific nystagmus types increases the diagnostic acumen of the neuroradiologist because high resolution studies can then be tailored to regions of expected pathology.

VISUAL PATHWAY AND VISUAL FIELD DEFECTS

Knowledge of the anatomy and blood supply of the visual pathway is essential for both the clinician and the neuroradiologist (Fig. 110, Table 16).

Optic Nerve

In the anterior portion of the visual pathway, the optic nerve head is formed from approximately 1 million axons derived from retinal ganglion cells. The optic nerve can be divided into intraocular, intraorbital, intracanicular, and intracranial segments measuring approximately 1 mm, 30 mm, 6 mm, and 10 mm, respectively. Optic nerve dysfunction is manifested by unilateral visual loss and may result from ischemia, inflammation, extrinsic compression, and hereditary conditions (Leber's optic neuropathy). The five clinical features of an optic neuropathy are decreased color vision, an afferent pupillary defect, a visual field defect, optic disc change, and decreased visual acuity. The optic nerve head may appear normal in early retrobulbar processes. The etiology of an optic neuropathy is best determined by documenting the temporal profile of visual loss. For example,

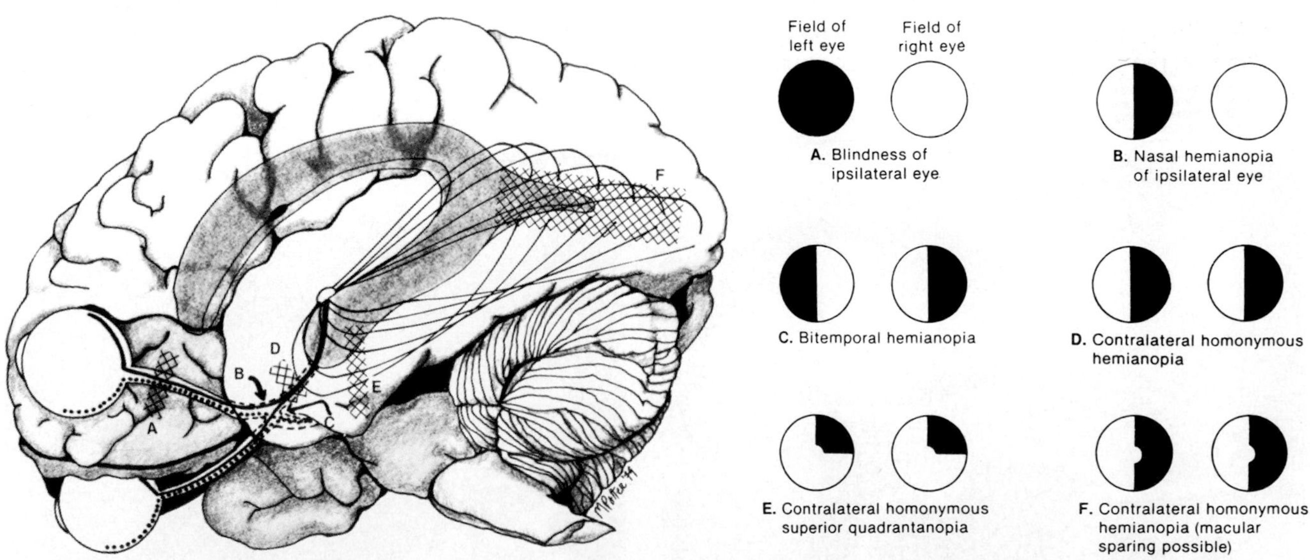

FIG. 110. Visual field deficits caused by lesions at various points along the visual pathway. **A:** Destruction of one optic nerve causes blindness of the eye in which that nerve arises. **B:** Damage to one side of the optic chiasm destroys the noncrossing fibers from the ipsilateral eye; these fibers arise in the temporal retina, so a nasal hemianopia of the ipsilateral eye results. **C:** Pressure on the middle of the optic chiasm, typically from a pituitary tumor, destroys the crossing fibers from both eyes, causing a bitemporal hemianopia (one type of heteronymous hemianopia). **D:** Destruction of one optic tract causes contralateral homonymous hemianopia. **E:** Damage to one temporal lobe could destroy part of the optic radiation, specifically the fibers representing the contralateral superior quadrant of each visual field; since the optic radiation is rather spread out at this point, some fibers are likely to be spared (e.g., in this case the macular fibers remain intact). **F:** Massive damage to one occipital lobe (such as might be caused by occlusion of one posterior cerebral artery) causes contralateral homonymous hemianopia; the macular representation is quite large, and some of it is likely to survive, resulting in macular sparing. (From Nolte, ref. 178, with permission.)

TABLE 16. *Localization of visual field defects*

Field defect	Localization
One eye only	Retina or optic nerve
Bitemporal hemianopia	Chiasm
Junctional scotoma (central defect one eye, temporal defect other eye)	Junction of optic nerve and chiasm
Incongruous hemianopia	Optic tract or lateral geniculate
Horizontal sectoranopia	Usually lateral geniculate
Congruous hemianopia	Occipital lobe
Complete homonymous hemianopia	Anywhere in retrochiasmal pathway
Superior quadrantanopsia	Temporal or occipital lobe (V1 or V2/V3)
Inferior quadrantanopsia	Parietal or occipital lobe (V1 or V2/V3)
Macular-sparing hemianopia	Occipital lobe
Temporal crescent	Anterior visual cortex
Achromatopsia or prosopagnosia	Bilateral occipitotemporal lesions
Alexia without agraphia	Left occipital cortex and splenium of corpus callosum

patients with optic neuritis typically lose vision over hours to days with eventual spontaneous recovery in a large majority of patients over months. Tumors involving the optic nerve such as meningiomas or gliomas result in progressive visual decline. Ischemic lesions occur abruptly and are not usually associated with visual recovery.

A wide variety of visual deficits are seen in optic neuropathies and include generalized constriction, arcuate, altitudinal, central, centrocecal, temporal, and nasal scotomas. These field defects are usually nondiagnostic with regard to etiology, but altitudinal field loss suggests a vascular process, central scotomas support an inflammatory or infiltrative lesion, and hemianopic defects imply a compressive process (153). The cause of compressive optic neuropathies is diverse and includes the entire gamut of mass lesions in the vicinity of the optic nerve, such as meningiomas, hemangiomas, lymphoma, metastatic disease, aneurysm, mucoceles, thyroid eye disease, and disorders of the bone such as fibrous dysplasia and osteopetrosis (154).

Optic Chiasm

The two optic nerves meet at the optic chiasm, where the axons from the nasal retina (temporal field) of each eye join. The position of the optic chiasm is usually directly above the sella turcica in 80% of patients, but may lie over the tuberculum in 9% of cases or over the dorsum sellae in 11% (155). The superior portion of the chiasm

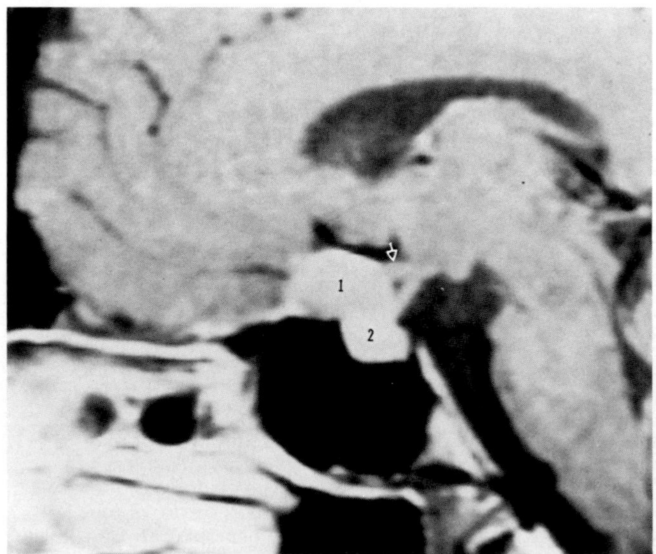

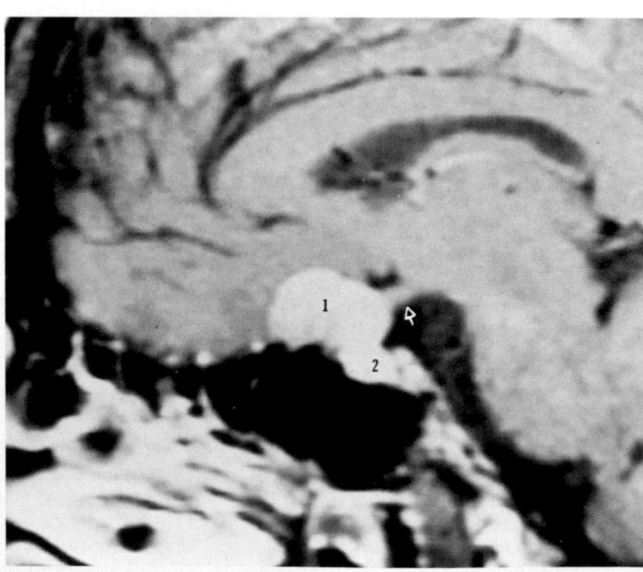

FIG. 111. Meningioma compressing prechiasmatic intracranial nerve resulting in temporal hemianopic scotoma of left eye. Sagittal postgadolinium short TR/TE images (**A,B**) show densely enhancing mass (*1*) arising separate from pituitary (*2*), which is impinging on medial aspect of prechiasmatic left optic nerve (chiasm indicated by *open arrow*). There was no superior field defect in the right eye, since crossing fibers of the anterior chiasm (anterior knee of Wilbrand) were spared.

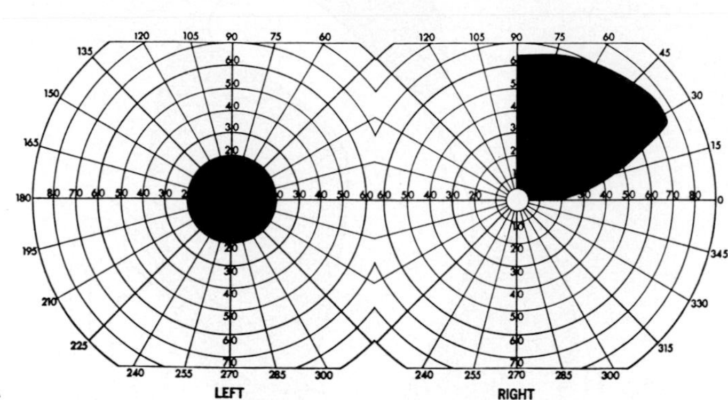

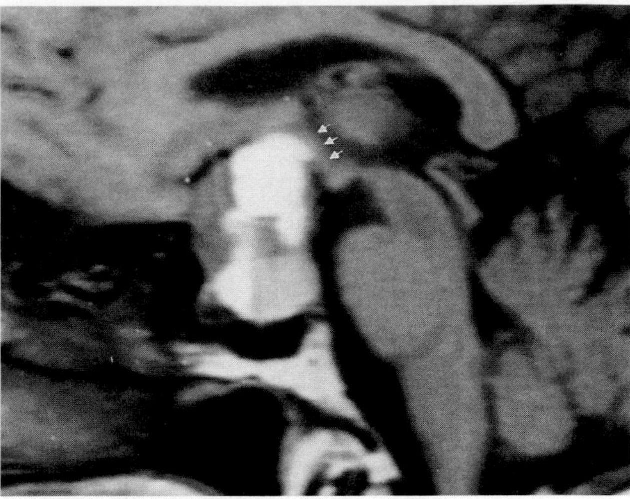

FIG. 112. Anterior chiasmal compression with field defect. **A:** Central scotoma in left eye with superior temporal defect in right eye consistent with left anterior chiasmal syndrome. **B:** Sagittal short TR/TE MRI shows massive hemorrhagic pituitary adenoma elevating chiasm (*arrows*) from anteroinferior aspect.

derives its blood supply from the anterior communicating and anterior cerebral arteries while the undersurface is supplied by branches of the internal carotid and posterior communicating arteries (156). A bitemporal hemianopsia is the classic field defect associated with a chiasmal lesion, but important variations exist. The anterior or junctional chiasmal syndrome is characterized by an ipsilateral central scotoma with contralateral superior temporal field loss (Figs. 111 and 112). This highly localizing visual defect usually results from a pituitary adenoma arising from the sella. Since the optic chiasm is angled upward at a 45° angle from the horizontal plane (posterior and superior to the tuberculum), lesions arising from the sella have tended to encroach on the anterior bar of the chiasm (154) (Fig. 113). Since these fibers are derived from the inferior nasal retinae of both eyes, the corresponding field is a bitemporal superior quadrantanopia. In contrast, lesions arising from above or behind the chiasm (e.g., craniopharyngioma) typically produce a bitemporal inferior quadrantanopia. Bitemporal paracentral scotomas may also indicate a lesion in the posterior portion of the chiasm (Fig. 114). Although a binasal hemianopia usually does not indicate an intracranial process, this field defect may rarely result from lateral compression of the optic chiasm by a carotid aneurysm.

Causes of chiasmal lesions include pituitary adenomas, aneurysms, craniopharyngiomas, metastatic disease, ectopic pinealomas (suprasellar germinoma), sarcoidosis, gliomas, trauma, demyelinating disease, and ischemia of the chiasm. In addition, there are several disorders that may give rise to a pseudobitemporal hemianopsia, which include tilted optic nerves, upper lid ptosis, sector retinitis pigmentosa, enlargement of the physiologic blind spot, and centrocecal scotomas with

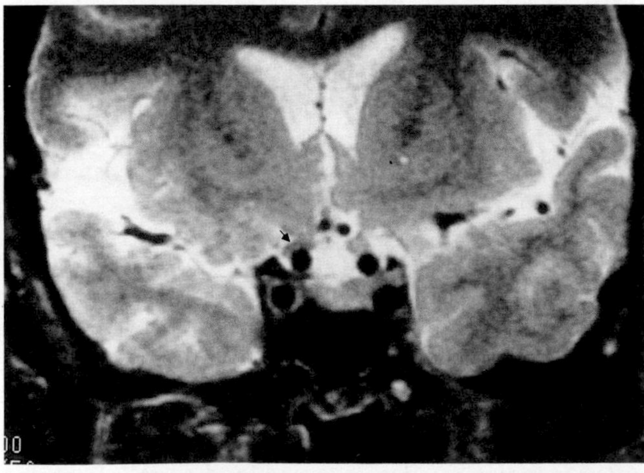

FIG. 113. Compression of prechiasmatic optic nerve by ectatic supraclinoid carotid artery. High resolution coronal MRI shows clear compression and deformity of prechiasmatic right optic nerve (*arrow*).

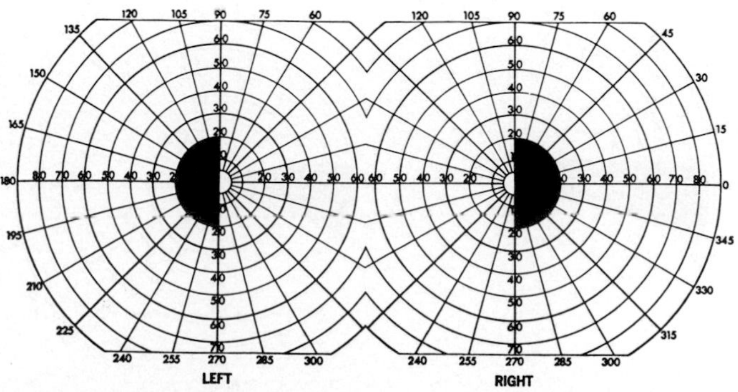

FIG. 114. Bilateral paracentral scotomas respecting vertical meridian consistent with posterior chiasmal lesion.

eccentric fixation (154). Normal neuroimaging studies would be anticipated in such cases.

Optic Tract

Fibers of the optic tract are derived from the optic chiasm and synapse in the lateral geniculate body. The major blood supply of the optic tract is from the branches of the internal carotid, in particular from the anterior choroidal artery. The anterior portion of the optic tract also derives some of its supply from the posterior communicating artery. Field defects resulting from optic tract lesions are generally incongruous homonymous hemianopias. There may be an afferent pupillary defect on the side of the greater visual field loss and optic atrophy may occur in long-standing lesions. In some optic tract lesions, a complete homonymous hemianopia ensues and congruity can no longer be assessed. It should be emphasized that a complete homonymous hemianopia may occur anywhere in the retrochiasmal visual pathways and is nonlocalizing. The most common cause of an optic tract lesion is craniopharyngioma, but other etiologies include aneurysm, infarction, trauma, pituitary tumor, and demyelinating disease (157,158). An infarction of the optic tract may occasionally follow temporal lobectomy for refractory seizures, perhaps resulting from irritative vasospasm of the anterior choroidal artery induced by surgical manipulation (159).

Lateral Geniculate Nucleus

Fibers from the optic tract synapse in several locations including the lateral geniculate body (primary visual pathway), pretectum (pupillomotor pathway), superior colliculus (subcortical visual pathway), accessory optic tract, and suprachiasmatic nucleus. Lesions of the lateral geniculate nucleus (LGN) may produce incongruous or congruous field cuts, depending on their underlying etiology. For instance, occlusion of the lateral choroidal artery may produce a congruous horizontal sectoranopia

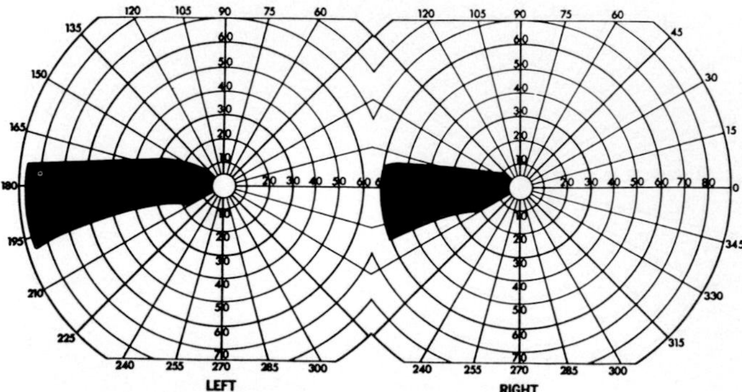

FIG. 115. Left homonymous horizontal sector defect in a right lateral geniculate lesion.

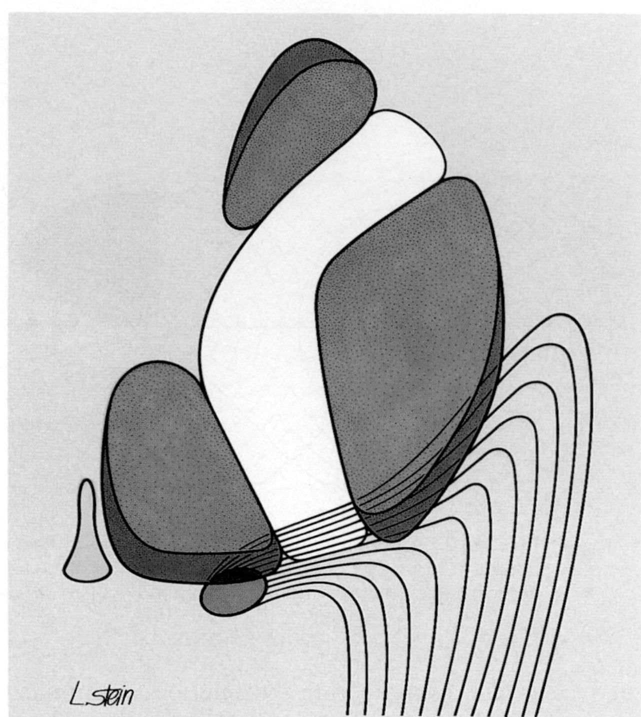

FIG. 116. Optic radiations exiting lateral geniculate nucleus and their relationship to the posterior limb of the internal capsule and basal ganglia.

(160) (Fig. 115). This unique field cut was thought to be specific for a disturbance in the lateral geniculate body, but recent reports provide evidence that a strategically placed lesion in the retrogeniculate pathways may also produce this field deficit (161,162). Rarely, gliomas and arteriovenous malformations may involve the lateral geniculate body, and they typically produce incongruous homonymous hemianopias. Disruption of the anterior choroidal artery supply to LGN may produce another specific field defect known as an upper and lower quadrant sectoranopia (163). In this field defect, the horizontal sector is spared. Patients with lateral geniculate lesions may have hemianesthesia if the ventral-posterior nuclei of the thalamus is involved. Tandem lesions of the lateral geniculate body and occipital cortex are also possible with proximal posterior cerebral artery occlusion. In this situation, it may be difficult to determine which site is responsible for the field defect.

Optic Radiations

After departing the lateral geniculate body, the anterior optic radiations course laterally behind the posterior limb of the internal capsule and basal ganglia. This region has been referred to as the carrefour (Fig. 116). The anterior radiations derive their blood supply from the anterior choroidal and thalamogeniculate arteries. Fortunately, the radiations of the carrefour are usually spared from lacunar infarction. However, occlusion of the anterior choroidal artery may produce a homonymous hemianopia in combination with hemianesthesia and hemiparesis.

The fibers of the anterior optic radiations that subserve the contralateral superior quadrant of field bend forward around the lateral ventricle to form Meyer's loop of the temporal lobe. Lesions of the temporal lobe usually cause a superior quadrantanopia and patients typically have associated language, motor, or sensory dysfunction (Fig. 117). Field defects from temporal lobe dysfunction may also be minimally incongruous or complete homonymous hemianopias. Tumors and cerebral infarctions are the most common lesions of the temporal lobe to produce such superior field defects.

Parietal Lobe

Geniculocalarine fibers subserving the contralateral inferior field travel through the parietal lobe. Blood supply to the parietal radiations is from branches of the middle cerebral artery whereas the most posterior radiations derive their supply from the posterior cerebral artery. Field defects of parietal lobe origin are often associated with body neglect or constructional apraxia when right-sided. Patients with left hemisphere lesions may have features of Gerstmann's syndrome (right-left confusion, finger agnosia, acalculia, and agraphia). Pursuit and optokinetic responses are often depressed toward the side of the parietal lesion. Patients may also show spasticity of conjugate gaze, in which the eyes will deviate away from the side of the lesion with Bell's phenomenon. Surprisingly, ischemic and demyelinating periventricular lesions easily seen on MRI only rarely produce a clinically evident field defect (164). Presumably, the fibers of the optic radiations are so spread apart that it requires a large lesion to produce a field defect.

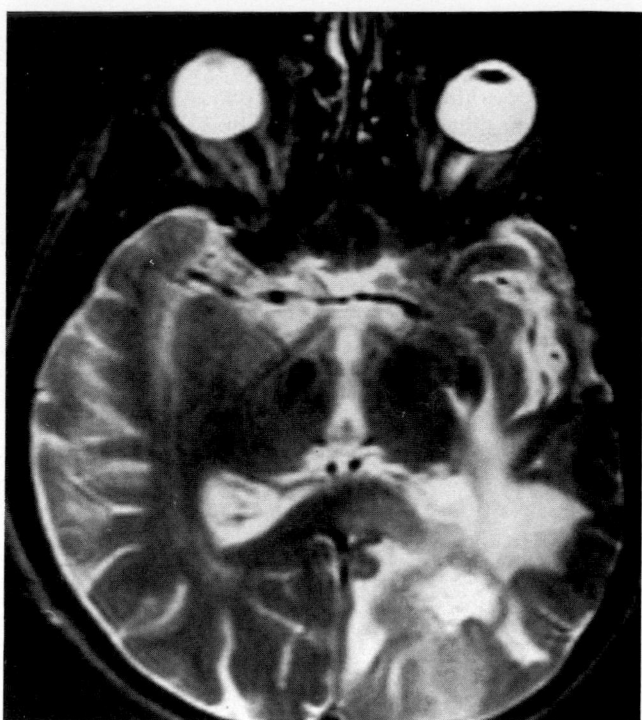

FIG. 118. Complete homonymous hemianopia in patient with left occipital glioblastoma. Note extensive infiltration of entire occipital lobe by left-sided glioblastoma in this patient with complete homonymous field defect.

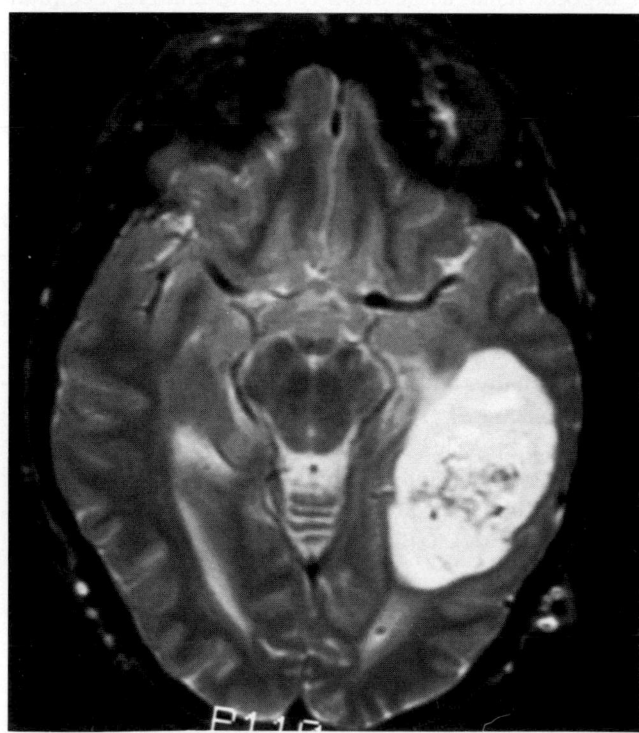

FIG. 117. Astrocytoma affecting temporal lobe radiations. Note large mass lesion in left posterior temporal-occipital lobe on long TR/TE image, producing a right homonymous hemianopia from optic radiation involvement.

Occipital Lobe

Fibers from the optic radiations terminate in the primary visual cortex of the occipital lobe. In the occipital cortex, the most peripheral visual field is represented in the anterior mesial aspect of the occipital lobe while the macular representation lies at the occipital pole. The map of the primary visual cortex has been recently revised by careful correlation of field defects and circumscribed MRI lesions (165). Accordingly, the visual cortex devoted to the macular region has been expanded. Human and animal data suggest that the central 100 of the visual field occupies approximately 55% to 60% of the striate cortex surface area (165). Field defects of the occipital cortex are characterized by their congruity (Fig. 118). Distinct field defects from occipital lobe lesions include homonymous hemianopias with macular sparing and preservation of the temporal crescent. Macular sparing probably results from the dual blood supply of the posterior occipital pole, since this region is nourished by both the middle and posterior cerebral arteries. Thus, in posterior cerebral artery occlusions, the middle cerebral artery may provide adequate blood supply to the macular representation of the occipital cortex to allow for preservation of function. Bilateral cortical representation of the macula is an alternative explanation. Since the temporal field of an eye is larger than the nasal field, preservation of the temporal crescent occurs in lesions that spare the anterior visual cortex, which is monocularly represented (Fig. 119). Isolated quadrant defects may be the consequence of injury to the primary visual cortex, but lesions of the optic radiations and area V2-V3 may also produce quadrant defects, especially when there is a sharp horizontal border in the field cut (166,167). Area V2-V3 comprises the cortical tissue lying just above or below the primary visual cortex (V-1).

Smith has studied 100 patients with homonymous hemianopia, regardless of their other neurologic findings, and found occipital lobe lesions in 39%, parietal lesions in 33%, temporal lobe lesions in 24%, optic tract lesions in 3%, and a single lateral geniculate nucleus lesion (168). Other studies have shown when a homonymous field defect is an isolated neurologic finding, it is likely to be of occipital lobe origin (169). Patients who suffer cortical blindness from a variety of causes may show a denial of blindness. This has been referred to as Anton's syndrome and patients may become quite elaborate in confabulating a visual scene.

Most occipital cortical lesions are the result of thromboembolic disease, watershed infarctions, or trauma. Severe traumatic injury may also produce a secondary occipital infarction as brain herniation leads to compromise of the posterior circulation. Reversible occipital lobe dysfunction may be seen in trauma, migraine, postangiography, hypertensive encephalopathy, eclamptic encephalopathy, and toxic-metabolic processes such as uremia and cyclosporin toxicity (170–172). Rare causes of occipital lobe dysfunction include primary and secondary tumors and degenerative processes such as Alzheimer's and Creutzfeldt-Jakob disease. When injury is diffuse to the visual cortex and visual association areas, conventional MRI may be normal. Disorders such as Alzheimer's disease, Creutzfeldt-Jakob disease, cerebral anoxia, carbon monoxide poisoning, and trauma may produce field defects or visual agnosia without focal findings on MRI (173). In this situation functional studies such as SPECT or PET may prove helpful diagnostically (173,174). Functional MRI (see Chapter 30) also holds great promise to enhance our diagnostic sensitivity for these conditions.

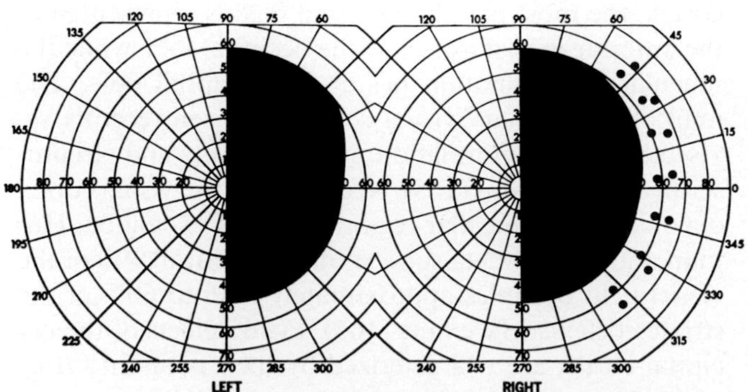

FIG. 119. Right homonymous hemianopia with sparing of temporal crescent (indicated by *dots*).

Higher Visual Cortical Dysfunction

In alexia without agraphia, the patient is unable to read but has intact language function, including the ability to write. This disorder results when the visual cortex is disconnected from the language area (angular gyrus). The lesion usually occurs with damage to the left occipital cortex in conjunction with damage to the splenium of the corpus callosum. Thus, visual information from the intact right occipital cortex cannot reach the language areas.

Color anomia is another feature of this disorder. Both prosopagnosia (inability to recognize familiar faces) and cerebral dyschromatopsia (inability to recognize colors) may result from bilateral lesions affecting the occipital temporal visual association cortex. Unilateral occipital-temporal lesions may produce a hemidyschromatopsia. In contrast, lesions affecting both parieto-occipital visual association areas result in Balint's syndrome, which is characterized by simultagnosia and visual misreaching phenomena. Palinopsia is an unusual disorder that may occur in either occipital or parietal lobe lesions. This visual illusion frequently occurs in a defective hemifield and lesions tend to be right-sided. Patients with palinopsia experience a recurrence of a visual scene after they have looked away from it. This may be considered a form of visual perseveration (154).

Visual hallucinations may occur in patients with decreased vision of any cause, dementia psychiatric disorders, focal brain lesions, seizures, migraine, and as a side effect from a variety of medications. Unformed visual hallucinations suggest an occipital lobe localization whereas formed hallucinations tend to be of temporal lobe origin.

CONCLUSIONS

Complete evaluation of the visual system can now be performed with a previously unavailable degree of sensitivity for a variety of pathologic processes. Exquisite neuroanatomic localization of the entire spectrum of disease entities involving the eye and orbit, or indeed any structure that influences the visual pathways and control of eye movement, can be directly demonstrated with MRI. New techniques in functional MRI promise to provide insight into the natural history of diseases and, more fundamentally, may answer questions about the basic cortical and subcortical workings of the brain in vision. Therefore, it is incumbent on the neuroradiologist and anyone else who is involved with discussing the results of intracranial MR examinations to be familiar with the neuropathology, neuroanatomy, and now neurophysiology of this highly specialized and complex system.

REFERENCES

1. Atlas, SW Bilaniuk, LT Zimmerman, RA Hackney, DB Goldberg, HI Grossman, RI. Orbit: Initial experience with surface coil spin-echo MR imaging at 1.5T. *Radiology* 1987;164:501–509.
2. Atlas SW, Grossman RI, Axel L, et al. Orbital lesions: proton spectroscopic phase-dependent contrast MR imaging. *Radiology* 1987;164:510–514.
3. Atlas SW, Grossman RI, Savino PJ, et al. Surface-coil MR of orbital pseudotumor. *AJR* 1987;148:803–808.
4. Atlas SW, Bilaniuk LT, Zimmerman RA. MR imaging of the orbit. In: Stark D, Bradley WG, eds. *Magnetic Resonance Imaging.* St Louis: CV Mosby; 1988.
5. Mafee MF, Peyman GA, Grisolano JE, et al. Malignant uveal melanomas and simulating lesions: MR imaging evaluation. *Radiology* 1986;160:773–780.
6. Mafee MF, Peyman GA, Peace JH, et al. Magnetic resonance imaging in the evaluation and differentiation of uveal melanoma. *Ophthalmology* 1987;94:341–348.
7. Mafee MF, Linder B, Peyman GA, et al. Choroidal hematoma and effusion: evaluation with MR imaging. *Radiology* 1988;168: 781–786.
8. Daniels DL, Herfkens R, Gager WE, et al. Magnetic resonance imaging of the optic nerves and chiasm. *Radiology* 1984;152:79–83.
9. Bilaniuk LT, Schenck JF, Zimmerman RA, et al. Ocular and orbital lesions: surface coil MR imaging. *Radiology* 1985;156:669–674.
10. Braffman BH, Bilaniuk LT, Eagle RC, et al. MR imaging of a carcinoid tumor metastatic to the orbit. *J Comput Assist Tomogr* 1987;11:891–894.
11. Daniels DL, Yu S, Pech P, et al. Computed tomography and magnetic resonance imaging of the orbital apex. *Radiol Clin North Am* 1987;25:803–817.
12. Fries PD, Char DH, Norman D. MR imaging of orbital cavernous hemangioma. *J Comput Assist Tomogr* 1987;11:418–421.
13. Han JS, Benson JE, Bonstelle CT, et al. Magnetic resonance imaging of the orbit: a preliminary experience. *Radiology* 1984;150: 755–759.
14. Hawkes RC, Holland GN, Moore WS, et al. NMR imaging in the evaluation of orbital tumors. *Am J Neuroradiol* 1983;4:254–256.
15. Mafee MF, Putterman A, Valvassori GE, et al. Orbital space-occupying lesions: role of computed tomography and magnetic resonance imaging. Analysis of 145 cases. *Radiol Clin North Am* 1987;25:529–559.
16. Linder B, Campos M, Schafer M. CT and MRI of orbital abnormalities in neurofibromatosis and selected craniofacial anomalies. *Radiol Clin North Am* 1987;25:787–802.
17. Peyster RG, Shapiro MD, Haik BG. Orbital matastasis: role of magnetic resonance imaging and computed tomography. *Radiol Clin North Am* 1987;25:647–662.
18. Rootman J, Damji KF, Dimmick JE. Malignant rhabdoid tumor of the orbit. *Ophthalmology* 1989;96:1650–1654.
19. Sobel DF, Mills C, Char D, et al. NMR of the normal and pathologic eye and orbit. *Am J Neuroradiol* 1984;5:345–350.
20. Sobel DF, Kelly W, Kjos BO, et al. MR imaging of orbital and ocular disease. *Am J Neuroradiol* 1985;6:259–264.
21. Sullivan JA, Harms SE. Surface-coil MR imaging of orbital neoplasms. *Am J Neuroradiol* 1986;7:29–34.
22. Sullivan JA, Harms SE. Characterization of orbital lesions by surface coil MR imaging. *Radiographics* 1987;7:9–28.
23. Schenck JF, Hart HR, Foster TH, et al. High resolution magnetic resonance imaging using surface coils. In: Kressel HY, ed. *Magnetic Resonance Annual 1986.* New York: Raven Press; 1986: 123–160.
24. Schenck JF, Hart HR Foster TH, et al. Improved imaging of the orbit at 1.5T with surface coils. *AJNR* 1985;6:193–196.
25. Axel L. Surface coil magnetic resonance imaging. *J Comput Assist Tomogr* 1984;8:381–384.
26. New PFJ, Rosen BR, Brady TJ, et al. Potential hazards and artifacts of ferromagnetic and nonferromagnetic surgical and dental materials and devices in nuclear magnetic resonance imaging. *Radiology* 1983;147:139–148.
27. Kelly WM, Paglen PG, Pearson JA, et al. Ferromagnetism of intraocular foreign body causes unilateral blindness after MR study. *AJNR* 1986;7:243–245.
28. Pusey E, Lufkin RB, Brown RLJ, et al. Magnetic resonance imaging artifacts: mechanism and clinical significance. *RadioGraphics* 1986;6:891–911.
29. Brateman L. Chemical shift imaging: a review. *AJR* 1986;146: 971–980.
30. Duke-Elder S, Wybar KC. The anatomy of the visual system. In: Duke-Elder S, ed. *System of Ophthalmology.* London: Kimpton; 1961.
31. Gardner, E, Gray, DJ, O'Rahilly, R. *Anatomy,* 4th ed. Philadelphia: WB Saunders; 1975.
32. Whitnall, SE. *The Anatomy of the Human Orbit and Accessory Organs of Vision,* 2nd ed. London: Oxford University Press; 1932.
33. Atlas SW, Zimmerman RA, Bilaniuk LT. The orbit. In: Lee SH, Rao KCVG, eds. *Cranial Computed Tomography and MRI.* New York: McGraw-Hill Book Co; 1987.
34. Atlas SW. MR imaging of the orbit: current status. *Magn Reson Q* 1989;5:39–96.
35. Gomori JM, Grossman RI, Shields JA, et al. Ocular MR imaging and spectroscopy: an ex vivo study. *Radiology* 1986;160:201–205.
36. Wolter JR, Knoblich RR. Pathway of centrifugal fibres in the human optic nerve, chiasm and tract. *Br J Ophthalmol* 1965;49: 246–250.
37. Spencer WH. *Ophthalmic Pathology. An Atlas and Textbook.* Philadelphia: WB Saunders; 1985.
38. Fox AJ, Debrun G, Vinuela F, et al. Intrathecal metrizamide enhancement of the optic nerve sheath. *J Comput Assist Tomogr* 1979;3:653–656.
39. Axel L. Blood flow effects in magnetic resonance imaging. *AJR* 1984;143:1157–1166.
40. Bradley WG. MR appearance of flowing blood and CSF. In: Brant-Zawadzki M, Norman D, eds. *Magnetic Resonance Imaging in the Central Nervous System.* New York: Raven Press; 1987:83–96.
41. von Schulthess GK, Higgins CB. Blood flow imaging with MR: Spin-phase phenomena. *Radiology* 1985;157:687–695.
42. Fram EK, Dimick R, Hedlund LW, et al. Parameters determining the signal of flowing fluid in gradient refocused MR imaging: flow velocity, TR and flip angle. *Book of Abstracts,* SMRM Annual Meeting 1986. Montreal, 1986:84–85.
43. Yousem D, Atlas SW, Dougherty L, Listerud J. Ultrahigh resolution MR imaging of the anterior ocular structures. *Annual Meeting of the RSNA.* Chicago: 1988.
44. Ulshafer RJ, Allen CB, Rubin ML. Distributions of elements in the human retinal pigment epithelium. *Arch Ophthalmol* 1990;108:113–117.
45. Young RW, Fulhorst HW. Regional differences in protein synthesis within the lens of the rat. *Ophthalmol Vis Sci* 1966;5:288–297.
46. Dische Z, Borenfreund E, Zelmenis G. Changes in lens proteins of rats during aging. *Arch Ophthalmol* 1956;55:471–483.
47. Koenig SH, Brown RD. The raw and the cooked, or the importance of the motion of water for MRI revisited. *Invest Radiol* 1988;23:495–497.

48. Shields JA. Current approaches to the diagnosis and management of choroidal melanomas. *Surv Ophthalmol* 1977;21:443–463.
49. Mafee MF, Peyman GA, McKusick MA. Malignant uveal melanoma and similar lesions studied by computed tomography. *Radiology* 1985;156:403–408.
50. Peyster RG, Augsburger JJ, Shields JA, et al. Choroidal melanoma: comparison of CT, fundoscopy and US. *Radiology* 1985;156:675–680.
51. Starr H, Zimmerman L. Extrascleral extension and orbital recurrence of malignant melanomas of the choroid and ciliary body. *Int Ophthalmol Clin* 1962;2:369.
52. Frank JA, Girton M, Dwyer AJ, et al. Ocular and cerebral metastases in the VX2 rabbit tumor model: contrast-enhanced MR imaging. *Radiology* 1987;164:527–530.
53. Peyster RG, Augsburger JJ, Shields JA, Hershey BL, Eagle R Jr, Haskin ME. Intraocular tumors: evaluation with MR imaging. *Radiology* 1988;168:773–779.
54. Damadian R, Zaner K, Hor D. Human tumors by NMR. *Physiol Chem Phys* 1973;5:381–402.
55. Atlas SW, Grossman RI, Gomori JM, et al. MR imaging of intracranial metastatic melanoma. *J Comput Assist Tomogr* 1987;11: 577–582.
56. Atlas SW, Braffman BH, LoBrutto R, Elder D, Herlyn D. Human malignant melanomas with varying melanin content in nude mice: correlations of MR with histopathology and electron paramagnetic resonance. *J Comput Assist Tomogr* 1990;14:547–554.
57. Gomori JM, Grossman RI, Shields JA, Augsburger JJ, Joseph PJ, DeSimone D. Choroidal melanomas: correlation of NMR spectroscopy and MR imaging. *Radiology* 1986;158:443–445.
58. Jimbow K, Miyake Y, Homma K, et al. Characterization of melanogenesis and morphogenesis of melanosomes by physicochemical properties of melanin and melanosomes in malignant melanoma. *Cancer Res* 1984;44:1128–1134.
59. Enochs WS, Hyslop WB, Bennett HF, Brown RD, Koenig SH, Swartz HM. Sources of the increased longitudinal relaxation rates observed in melanotic melanoma: an in vitro study of synthetic melanins. *Invest Radiol* 1989;24:794–804.
60. Gomori JM, Grossman RI, Goldberg HI, Zimmerman RA, Bilaniuk LT. Intracranial hematomas: imaging by high-field MR. *Radiology* 1985;157:87–93.
61. Bradley WGJ, Schmidt PG. Effect of methemoglobin formation on the MR appearance of subarachnoid hemorrhage. *Radiology* 1985;156:99–103.
62. Spencer G, Lufkin R, Simons K, Straatsma B, Foos R, Hanafee W. MR of a melanoma-simulating ocular neoplasm. *AJNR* 1987;8:991–992.
63. Reese AB. *Tumors of the Eye.* New York: Harper and Row; 1976.
64. Jones JS, Jakobiec FA. *Diseases of the Orbit.* Hagerstown, MD: Harper and Row; 1979.
65. Atlas SW, Kemp SS, Grossman RI, et al. Hemorrhagic intracerebral retinoblastoma metastases: MR-pathology correlation. *J Comput Assist Tomogr* 1988;12:286–289.
66. Johnson DL, Chandra R, Fisher WS, et al. Trilateral retinoblastoma: ocular and pineal retinoblastomas. *J Neurosurg* 1985;63: 367–370.
67. Solloway HB. Radiation-induced neoplasms following curative therapy for retinoblastoma. *Cancer* 1966;12:1984–1988.
68. Abramson DH, Ellsworth R, Kitchin S. Second non-ocular tumors in retinoblastoma survivors. *Ophthalmology* 1984;91: 1351–1355.
69. Mafee MF, Goldberg MF, Greenwold MJ, et al. Retinoblastoma and simulating lesions: role of CT and MR imaging. *Radiol Clin North Am* 1987;25:667–682.
70. Russell DS, Rubinstein LJ. *Pathology of Tumors of the Nervous System,* 5th ed. Baltimore: Williams and Wilkins; 1989.
71. Atlas SW, Grossman RI, Hackney DB, et al. Calcified intracranial lesions: Detection with gradient-echo acquisition rapid MR imaging. *AJNR* 1988;9:253–259.
72. Holland BA, Kucharcyzk W, Brant-Zawadzki M, Norman D, Haas DK, Harper PS. MR imaging of calcified intracranial lesions. *Radiology* 1985;157:353–356.
73. Oot RF, New PFJ, Pile-Spellman J, et al. The detection of intracranial calcifications by MR. *AJNR* 1986;7:801–809.
74. Gittinger JW. *Ophthalmology: A Clinical Introduction.* Boston: Little, Brown, and Co; 1984.
75. Gonvers M. Temporary silicone oil tamponade in the management of retinal detachment with proliferative vitreoretinopathy. *Am J Ophthalmol* 1985;100:239–245.
76. Okabe H, Kizosawa M, Yamada S. Nuclear magnetic resonance imaging of subretinal fluid. *Am J Ophthalmol* 1986;102:640–646.
77. Hackney DB, Grossman RI, Zimmerman RA, et al. Low sensitivity of clinical MR imaging to small changes in the concentration of nonparamagnetic protein. *AJNR* 1987;8:1003–1008.
78. Atlas SW, Zimmerman RA, Bilaniuk LT, et al. Corpus callosum and limbic system: neuroanatomic-MR evaluation of developmental anomalies. *Radiology* 1986;160:355–362.
79. Corbett J, Savino PJ, Schatz NJ, Orr LS. Cavitary developmental defects of the optic disc. *Arch Neurol* 1980;37:210–213.
80. Weiss AH, Kousseff BG, Ross EA, Longbottom J. Complex microphthalmos. *Arch Ophthalmol* 1989;107:1619–1624.
81. Wright DC, Yuh WTC, Thompson HS, et al. Bilateral microphthalmos with orbital cysts: MR findings. *J Comput Assist Tomogr* 1987;11:727–729.
82. Bernardino ME, Dunn RD, Citrin CM, Davis DO. Scleral thickening: a sign of orbital pseudotumor. *AJR* 1977;129:703–706.
83. Rothfus WE, Curtin HD. Extraocular muscle enlargement: a CT review. *Radiology* 1984;151:677–681.
84. Dresner SC, Rothfus WE, Slamovitz TL, et al. Computed tomography of orbital myositis. *AJR* 1984;143:671–674.
85. Leone CR, Lloyd WC. Treatment protocol for orbital inflammatory disease. *Ophthalmology* 1985;92:1325–1331.
86. Sergott RC, Glaser JS, Charyulu K. Radiotherapy for idiopathic inflammatory pseudotumor: indications and results. *Arch Ophthalmol* 1981;99:853–856.
87. Krohel GB, Krauss HR, Winnick J. Orbital abscess: presentation, diagnosis, therapy, and sequelae. *Ophthalmology* 1982;89:492–498.
88. Seidenberg KB, Leib ML. Orbital myositis with Lyme disease. *Am J Ophthalmol* 1990;109:13–16.
89. Savino PJ, Grossman RI, Schatz NJ, et al. High-field magnetic resonance imaging in the diagnosis of cavernous sinus thrombosis. *Arch Neurol* 1986;43:1081–1082.
90. McCord CD. Current trends in orbital decompression. *Ophthalmology* 1985;92:21–33.
91. Riley FC. Orbital pathology in Graves disease. *Mayo Clin Proc* 1972;47:975–979.
92. Enzmann DR, Donaldson SS, Dris JP. Appearance of Graves' disease on orbital computed tomography. *J Comput Assist Tomogr* 1979;3:815–819.
93. Hosten N, Sander B, Cordes M, et al. Graves ophthalmopathy: MR imaging of the orbits. *Radiology* 1989;172:759–762.
94. Sandberg-Wollheim M, Bynke H, Cronqvist S, Holtas S, Platz P, Ryder LP. A long term prospective study of optic neuritis: evaluation of risk factors. *Ann Neurol* 1990;27:386–393.
95. Johnson G, Miller DM, MacManus D, et al. STIR sequences in NMR imaging of the optic nerve. *Neuroradiology* 1987;29:238–245.
96. Beck R, Arrington J, Murtagh F. Brain magnetic resonance imaging in optic neuritis: experience of the optic neuritis study group. *Arch Neurol* 1993;50:841–846.
97. Beck RW, Cleary PA, Trobe JD, et al. The effect of corticosteroids for acute optic neuritison the subsequent development of multiple sclerosis. *N Engl J Med* 1993;329:1764–1769.
98. Jay WM, Williamson MR. Incidence of subcortical lesions not increased in nonarteritic ischemic optic neuropathy on magnetic resonance imaging. *Am J Ophthalmol* 1987;104:398–400.
99. Simon JH, Szumowski J. Chemical shift imaging with paramagnetic contrast material enhancement for improved lesion depiction. *Radiology* 1989;171:539–543.
100. Wright JE. Primary optic nerve meningiomas: clinical presentation and management. *Trans Am Acad Ophthalmol Otolaryngol* 1977;83:617–624.
101. Daniels DL, Kneeland JB, Shimakawa A. MR imaging of the optic nerve and sheath: correcting the chemical shift misregistration effect. *AJNR* 1986;7:249–253.
102. Spagnoli MV, Goldberg HI, Grossman RI, et al. Intracranial meningiomas: high-field MR imaging. *Radiology* 1986;161:369–375.
103. Glaser JS, Hoyt WF, Corbett J. Visual morbidity with chiasmal glioma. *Arch Ophthalmol* 1971;85:3–12.

104. Alvord EC, Lofton S. Gliomas of the optic nerve or chiasm. *J Neurosurg* 1988;68:85–98.
105. Stem J, Jakobiec FA, Housepien EM. The architecture of optic nerve gliomas with and without neurofibromatosis. *Arch Ophthalmol* 1980;98:505–511.
106. Brown EW, Riccardi VM, Mawad M, et al. MR imaging of optic pathways in patients with neurofibromatosis. *AJNR* 1987;8:1031–1036.
107. Pomeranz SJ, Shelton JJ, Tobias J, et al. MR of visual pathways in patients with neurofibromatosis. *AJNR* 1987;8:831–836.
108. Dowd CP, Atlas SW, Hoyt WF. Chiasm gliomas in neurofibromatosis patients: MR characteristics. *Annual Meeting of the ASNR*. Boston: 1988.
109. Shields JA, Shields CL, Lieb WE, Eagle RC. Multiple orbital neurofibromas unassociated with von Recklinghausen's disease. *Arch Ophthalmol* 1990;108:80–83.
110. Appelboom T, Durso F. Tumor metastases to the eye. 1. Incidence in 213 adult patients with generalized malignancy. *Am J Ophthalmol* 1967;63:723–726.
111. Atlas SW, Fram EK, Mark AS, Grossman RI. Vascular intracranial lesions: applications of fast scanning. *Radiology* 1988;169:455–461.
112. Rootman J, Hay E, Graeb D, Miller R. Orbital adnexal lymphangiomas. *Ophthalmology* 1986;93:1558–1570.
113. Nugent RA, Lapointe JS, Rootman J, Robertson WD, Graeb DA. Orbital dermoids: features on CT. *Radiology* 1987;165:475–478.
114. Wright JE, Stewart WB, Krohel GB. Clinical presentation and management of lacrimal gland tumors. *Br J Ophthalmol* 1979;63:600–606.
115. Lee DW, Campbell RJ, Waller RR, Ilstrup OM. A clinicopathologic study of primary adenoid cystic carcinoma of the lacrimal gland. *Ophthalmology* 1985;92:128–134.
116. Knowles DMI, Jakobiec FA. Orbital lymphoid neoplasms: a clinicopathologic study of 60 cases. *Cancer* 1980;46:576–589.
117. Jakobiec FA, McLean I, Font R. Clinicopathologic characteristics of orbital lymphoid hyperplasia. *Ophthalmology* 1979;86:948–966.
118. Balchunas WR, Quencer RM, Byrne SF. Lacrimal gland and fossa masses: evaluation by computed tomography and A-mode echography. *Radiology* 1983;149:751–78.
119. Forbes GS, Sheedy PF, Waller RR. Orbital tumors evaluated by computed tomography. *Radiology* 1980;136:101–111.
120. Wehrli FW. *Introduction to Fast-Scan Magnetic Resonance*. Milwaukee: General Electric Co; 1986.
121. Bodne D, Quinn SF, Cochran CF. Imaging foreign glass and wooden bodies of the extremities with CT and MR. *J Comput Assist Tomogr* 1988;12:608–611.
122. Brown GC, Tasman WS, Benson WE. BB-gun injuries to the eye. *Ophthalmic Surg* 1985;16:505–508.
123. Stemberg P, DeJuan E, Michels RG, Auer C. Multivariate analysis of prognostic factors in penetrating ocular injuries. *Am J Ophthalmol* 1984;98:467–472.
124. Zimmerman RA, Bilaniuk LT, Hackney DB, et al. Paranasal sinus hemorrhage: evaluation with MR imaging. *Radiology* 1987;162:199–203.
125. Tonarni H, Nakagawa T, Ohguchi M, et al. Surface coil MR imaging of orbital blow-out fractures: a comparison with reformatted CT. *AJNR* 1987;8:445–449.
126. Chen JC, Kucharczyk W. Nontraumatic orbital subperiosteal hematoma in a scuba diver: CT and MR findings. *J Comput Assist Tomogr* 1988;12:504–506.
127. Atlas SW. MR of the orbit: current imaging applications. *Semin US CT MR* 1988;9:381–400.
128. Warwick R. Representation of the extraocular muscles in the oculomotor nuclei of the monkey. *J Comp Neurol* 1953;98:449–495.
129. Hamed LM, Schatz NJ, Galetta SL. Brainstem ocular motility defects and AIDS. *Am J Ophthalmol* 1988;106:437–442.
130. Kerr FW, Hollowell OW. Location of pupillomotor and accommodation fibers in the oculomotor nerve: experimental observations on paralytic mydriases. *J Neurol Neurosurg Psychiatry* 1964;27:473–481.
131. Glaser JS. *Neuro-Ophthalmology*. Philadelphia: JB Lippincott; 1990:364.
132. Kziazek SM, Repka MY, Maguire A, et al. Divisional oculomotor nerve paresis caused by intrinsic brainstem disease. *Ann Neurol* 1989;26:714–718.
133. Green WR, Hackett ET, Schlezinger NE. Neuro-ophthalmologic evaluation of oculomotor nerve paralysis. *Arch Ophthalmol* 1964;72:154–167.
134. Trobe JD. Third nerve palsy and the pupil. *Arch Ophthalmol* 1988;106:601–602.
135. Schatz NJ, Savino PJ, Corbett JJ. Primary aberrant oculomotor regeneration: a sign of intracavemous meningioma. *Arch Neurol* 1977;34:29–32.
136. Rush JA, Younge BR. Paralysis of cranial nerves III, IV and VI. *Arch Ophthalmol* 1981;99:76–79.
137. Kziazek S, Behar P, Savino P, et al. Isolated acquired fourth nerve palsies. *Neurology* 1988;38(Suppl):246.
138. Von Noorden GK, Murray E, Wong SY. Superior oblique paralysis: A review of 270 cases. *Arch Ophthalmol* 1986;104:1771–1776.
139. Guy J, Day AL, Mickle JP. Contralateral trochlear nerve paresis and ipsilateral Homer's syndrome. *Am J Ophthalmol* 1989;107:73–76.
140. Guy JR, Friedman WF, Mickle JP. Bilateral trochlear nerve paresis in hydrocephalus. *J Clin Neuroophthalmol* 1989;9:105–111.
141. Gonyea EF. Superior oblique palsy due to a midbrain vascular malformation. *Neurology* 1990;40:554–555.
142. Striph GG, Burde RM. Abducens nerve and Homer's syndrome revisited. *J Clin Neuroophthalmol* 1988;8:13–17.
143. Moster NL, Savino PJ, Sergott RD, Bosley TM, Schatz NJ. Isolated sixth nerve palsies in younger adults. *Arch Ophthalmol* 1984;102:1328–1330.
144. Schrader EC, Schlezinger NE. Neuro-ophthalmologic evaluation of abducens nerve paralysis. *Arch Ophthalmol* 1960;63:108–115.
145. Galetta SL, Smith JL. Chronic isolated sixth nerve palsies. *Arch Neurol* 1989;46:79–82.
146. Atlas SW, Grossman RI, Savino PJ, et al. Internuclear ophthalmoplegia: neuroanatomic—MR correlation. *AJNR* 1987;8:243–247.
147. Daroff RB, Troost BT, Leigh RJ. Supranuclear disorders of eye movements. In: Glaser JS, ed. *Neuro-Ophthalmology*. Philadelphia: JB Lippincott; 1990:299–323.
148. Buttner-Ennever JA, Buttner U, Cohen B. Vertical gaze paralysis and the rostral interstitial nucleus of the medial longitudinal fasciculus. *Brain* 1982;105:125–149.
149. Pierrot-Deseilligny CH, Chain F, Gray F, et al. Parinaud's syndrome. *Brain* 1982;105:667–696.
150. Bogousslavsky J, Milossy J, Deruaz JP, et al. Unilateral left paramedian infarction of thalamus and midbrain: a clinicopathological study. *J Neurol Neurosurg Psychiatry* 1986;49:686–694.
151. Lessell S. Supranuclear paralysis of monocular elevation. *Neurology* 1975;25:1134–1136.
152. Susac JO, Hoyt WF, Lawrence W. Clinical spectrum of ocular bobbing. *J Neurol Neurosurg Psychiatry* 1970;23:771–775.
153. Trobe JD, Glaser JS. Quantitative perimetry in compressive optic neuropathy and optic neuritis. *Arch Ophthalmol* 1978;96:1210–1216.
154. Glaser JS. *Neuro-Ophthalmology*. Philadelpha: J.B. Lippincott; 1990:83–238.
155. Bergland RM, Ray BS, Torack RM. Anatomical variations in the pituitary gland and adjacent structures in 225 human autopsy cases. *J Neurosurg* 1968;28:93–99.
156. Harrington D, Drake M. *The Visual Fields: Text and Atlas of Clinical Perimetry*, 6th ed. St. Louis: CV Mosby; 1990.
157. Savino PJ, Paris M, Schatz NJ, et al. Optic tract syndrome: a review of 21 cases. *Arch Ophthalmol* 1978;96:656–663.
158. Newman SA, Miller N. Optic tract syndrome: neuro-ophthalmologic considerations. *Arch Ophthalmol* 1983;101:1241–1250.
159. Anderson DR, Trobe JD, Hood TW, et al. Optic tract injury after temporal lobectomy. *Ophthalmology* 1989;96:1065–1070.
160. Shacklett DE, O'Connor PS, Dorwart RH, et al. Congruous and incongruous sectoral visual field defects with lesions of the lateral geniculate nucleus. *Am J Ophthalmol* 1984;98:283–290.
161. Carter JE, O'Connor P, Shacklett D, et al. Lesions of the optic radiations mimicking lateral geniculate nucleus visual field defects. *J Neurol Neurosurg Psychiatry* 1985;48:982–988.
162. Grossman M, Galetta SL, Nichols CW, et al. Horizontal homon-

ymous sectoral field defect after ischemic infarction of the occipital cortex. *Am J Ophthalmol* 1990; 109:234–236.

163. Helgason C, Caplan L, Goodwin J, et al. Anterior choroidal artery-territory infarction: report of cases and review. *Arch Neurol* 1986;43:681–686.
164. Plant G, Kermode A, Turano G, et al. Symptomatic retrochiasmal lesions in multiple sclerosis: clinical features, visual evoked potentials, and magnetic resonance imaging. *Neurology* 1992;42: 68–76.
165. Horton J, Hoyt W. The representation of the visual field in human striate cortex: a revision of the classic Holmes map. *Arch Ophthalmol* 1991; 109:816–824.
166. Borruat F, Siatkowski R, Schatz N, et al. Congrous quadrantanopsia and optic radiation lesion. *Neurology* 1993;43:1430–1432.
167. Horton J, Hoyt W. Quadrantic visual field defects: a hallmark of lesions in extrastriate (V2/V3) cortex. *Brain* 1991; 114:1703–1718.
168. Smith JL. Homonymous hemianopia: a review of one hundred cases. *Am J Ophthalmol* 1960; 54:616–622.
169. Trobe JD, Lorber ML, Schlezinger NS. Isolated homonymous hemianopia: a review of 104 cases. *Arch Ophthalmol* 1973;89: 377–381.
170. Wilson SE, de Groen P, Aksamit A, et al. Cyclosporin A–induced reversible cortical blindness. *J Clin Neuroophthalmol* 1988;8: 215–220.
171. Lantos G. Cortical blindness due to osmotic disruption of the blood–brain barrier by angiographic contrast material: CT and MRI studies. *Neurology* 1989;39:567–571.
172. Raps E, Galetta S, Broderick M, Atlas S. Delayed peripartum vasculopathy: cerebral eclampsia revisited. *Ann Neurol* 1993;33: 222–225.
173. Silverman I, Galetta S, Gray L, et al. SPECT in patients with cortical visual loss. *J Nucl Med* 1993;34:1447–1451.
174. Zeki S, Watson JDG, Lueck CJ, Friston KJ, Kennard C, Frackowiak RSJ. A direct demonstration of functional specialization in human visual cortex. *J Neurosci* 1991; 11:641–649.
175. Okazaki H, Scheithauer B. *Atlas of Neuropathology.* New York: Gower Medical Publishing, 1987.
176. Atlas SW, Grossman RI, Hackney DB, et al. STIR MR imaging of the orbit. *AJNR* 1988;9:969.
177. Bajandas FJ, Kline LB. *Neuro-ophthalmology Review Manual.* Thorofare: Slack Publishers, 1987.
178. Nolte J. *The Human Brain.* St Louis: C.V. Mosby, 1988.

Magnetic Resonance Imaging of the Brain and Spine, Second Edition, edited by Scott W. Atlas.
Lippincott-Raven Publishers, Philadelphia © 1996.

23

Degenerative Disease of the Spine

Leo F. Czervionke and Victor M. Haughton

Magnetic resonance imaging (MRI) has become the optimal imaging modality for evaluation of degenerative disorders of the cervical, lumbar, and thoracic spine. The intervertebral disc, vertebrae, ligaments, spinal canal, and neural foramen may all be evaluated using current MRI techniques. Paramagnetic contrast agents are valuable for differentiating scar and recurrent disc herniation in the postoperative setting and have limited use preoperatively for detecting annular tears and enhancing nerve roots.

This chapter deals with the spectrum of degenerative disease of the spine including disc herniation, disc degeneration, spinal stenosis, spondylosis deformans, and osteoarthritis, as well as other degenerative disorders affecting the spinal column. MR techniques used to evaluate the spine are discussed.

MR PULSE SEQUENCE CONSIDERATIONS

It is important to be aware of the array of basic MR pulse sequences available when designing protocols for examining the spine because the optimal MR technique will vary considerably, depending on the region of interest, as well as on the pathologic process being studied.

Spin echo (SE) remains the standard pulse sequence to which all others are compared (1). SE images (Fig. 1) have high signal-to-noise and high contrast-to-noise ratios when the appropriate parameters are used, but require relatively long acquisition times compared to gradient-echo (GE) or fast spin echo (FSE) techniques. Because SE and FSE sequences have a 180° refocusing pulse, they are not sensitive to magnetic field inhomogeneities and are therefore less prone to magnetic susceptibility artifacts than are GE sequences.

GE sequences lack a 180° pulse, and the signal is generated instead by reversing the polarity of the frequency-encoding (read-out) gradient (2). GE sequences are generally acquired in shorter times than are SE sequences. The shorter acquisition time is related to the fact that very short repetition times (TR) can be used. The signal-to-noise ratio (SNR) is maintained at a reasonably high level by utilization of small flip angles (usually less than 90°). Contrast between bony spine, spinal cord, cerebrospinal fluid (CSF), and disc is strongly influenced by the choice of flip angle. GE scans are more sensitive to chemical shift artifacts (3) and to all perturbations in the mag-

L. F. Czervionke, M.D.: Department of Diagnostic Radiology, Mayo Clinic Jacksonville, Jacksonville, FL 32224.
V. M. Haughton, M.D.: Department of Radiology, Medical College of Wisconsin, Milwaukee, WI 53226.

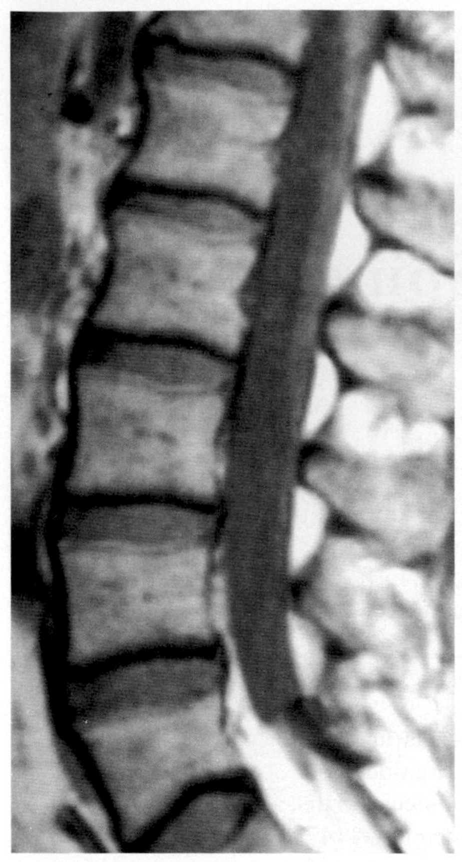

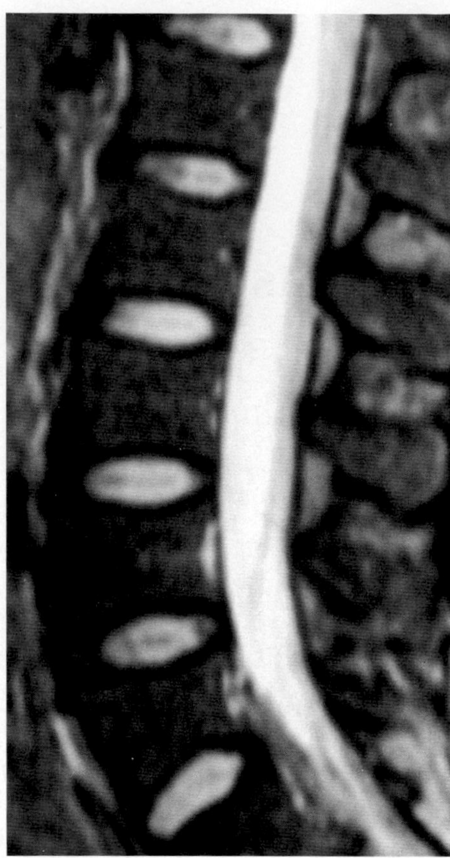

A,B

FIG. 1. Normal (**A**) sagittal T1-weighted SE image and sagittal conventional (**B**) T2-weighted SE image. Intervertebral disc is slightly hypointense with respect to the vertebral body marrow in A. The inner annulus and nucleus have high signal intensity on B, whereas the outer annulus has low signal intensity relative to the vertebral body and nucleus. Note epidural fat ventral to the thecal sac from L4-S1.

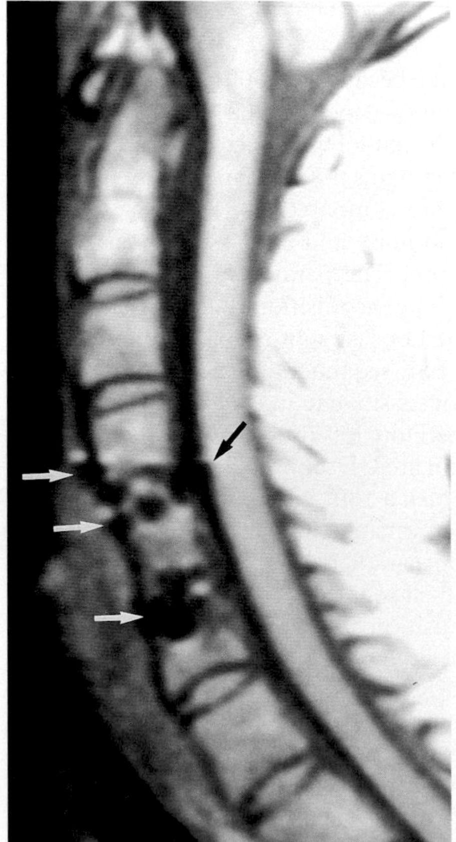

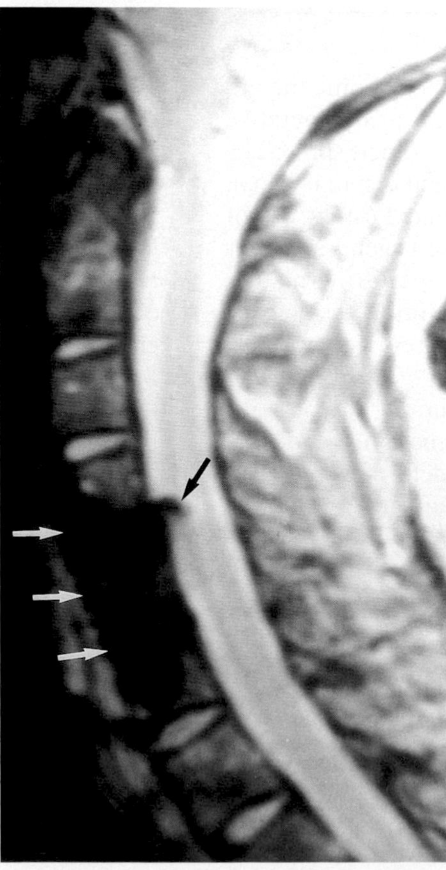

A,B

FIG. 2. Sagittal T1-weighted SE (**A**) and sagittal 2D GE (**B**) obtained with 30° flip angle demonstrates ferromagnetic artifact (*arrows*) having low signal intensity with curvilinear bright signal intensity adjacent to the artifact representing misregistration along the frequency and coding axis. The signal intensity loss is much greater on the GE, and the artifact (*black arrow*) encroaches on the spinal canal.

netic field (4) than are SE scans, whether due to main B_0 inhomogeneities, or due to intrinsic susceptibility gradients in the imaged volume. This enhanced sensitivity to magnetic susceptibility limits the use of GE techniques in evaluating postoperative spines because surgical drilling and fixation devices leave ferromagnetic particles, which significantly degrade GE images (Fig. 2).

In the lumbar spine, the SE technique remains the best sequence to diagnose degenerative disc disease. The major reason for the success of SE imaging in this region is that epidural fat is abundant and stands out as high intensity on T1-weighted SE images compared to the relatively lower intensity of the adjacent thecal sac, herniated disc, or other tissue. On most GE and FSE images, the intensity of the epidural fat is similar to or less than that of CSF and does not provide adequate contrast between the other tissues in the spinal canal (Fig. 3).

Compared to the lumbar spine, the epidural space in the cervical and thoracic spine have little epidural fat. In the cervical spine, contrast is provided by the presence of prominent epidural veins and from CSF in the thecal sac. Therefore, GE imaging is an important tool in the cervical spine for defining extramedullary disease. Furthermore, on conventional SE and FSE images, it is difficult to differentiate osteophytes from disc material. On GE images these can usually be differentiated because bone is markedly hypointense and disc is hyperintense, regardless of flip angle (Figs. 4 and 5) (5).

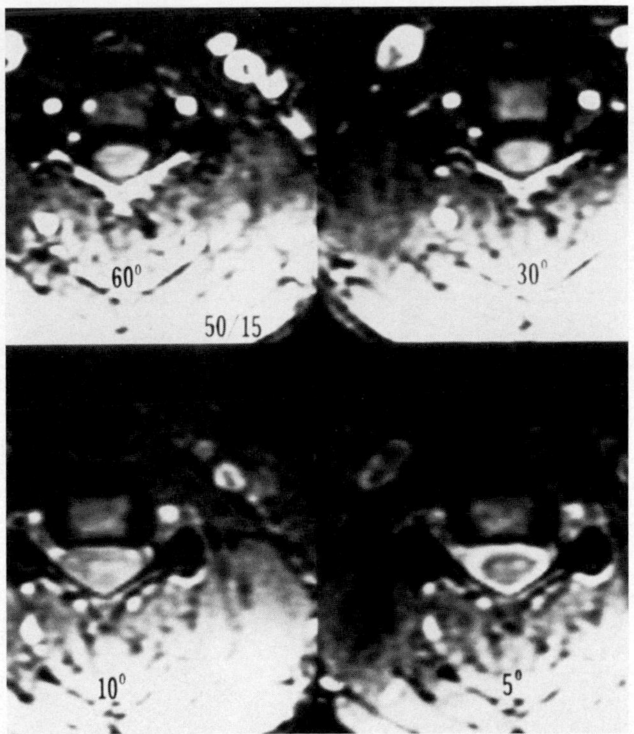

FIG. 4. Axial images through the cervical spine (3DFT GE MRI; 50/15/60°, 30°, 10°, and 5°) show that at a high flip angle, the cord is hyperintense and CSF is of low intensity. At 10°, the cord and surrounding CSF are isointense, and at 5° the CSF is hyperintense to low intensity cord. Note that neural foramina are clearly depicted on 5° flip angle image. Also note that bone is always of low intensity, whereas disc material is always of high intensity regardless of flip angle.

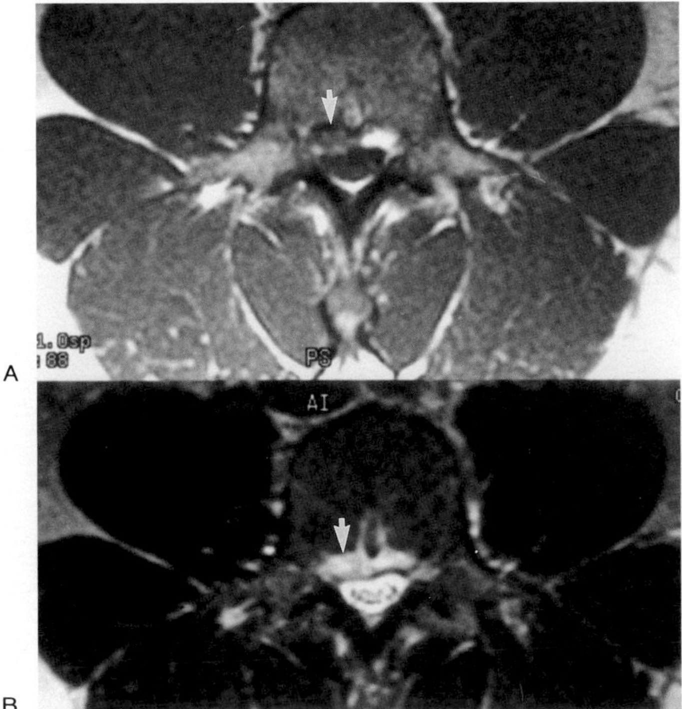

FIG. 3. Axial SE image (**A**) and T2-weighted FSE image (**B**) demonstrating a herniated disc (*arrow*) at the L5 level on the right obscuring the normally bright signal of the epidural fat. In B, the herniated disc is difficult to differentiate from the epidural fat because they both have similar signal intensity.

FSE T2-weighted images are routinely obtained in the sagittal axial plane to evaluate the lumbar spine. These can be obtained in one third to one half the acquisition time required for conventional T2-weighted SE sequences. FSE images are typically obtained using a single echo pulse sequence with an effective TE of approximately 100 msec. The TR interval (determined by the patient's heart rate) is generally in the range of 3500 to 4500 seconds. Axial FSE images are useful in the lumbar region to evaluate spinal canal size and particularly to evaluate the nerve roots of the cauda equina within the thecal sac as well as the facet joints (see Fig. 3). A major disadvantage of axial FSE imaging is the difficulty in differentiating disc from bone (Fig. 6). For this reason, GE axial images are preferable to axial FSE images in the cervical spine. However, sagittal FSE sequences can

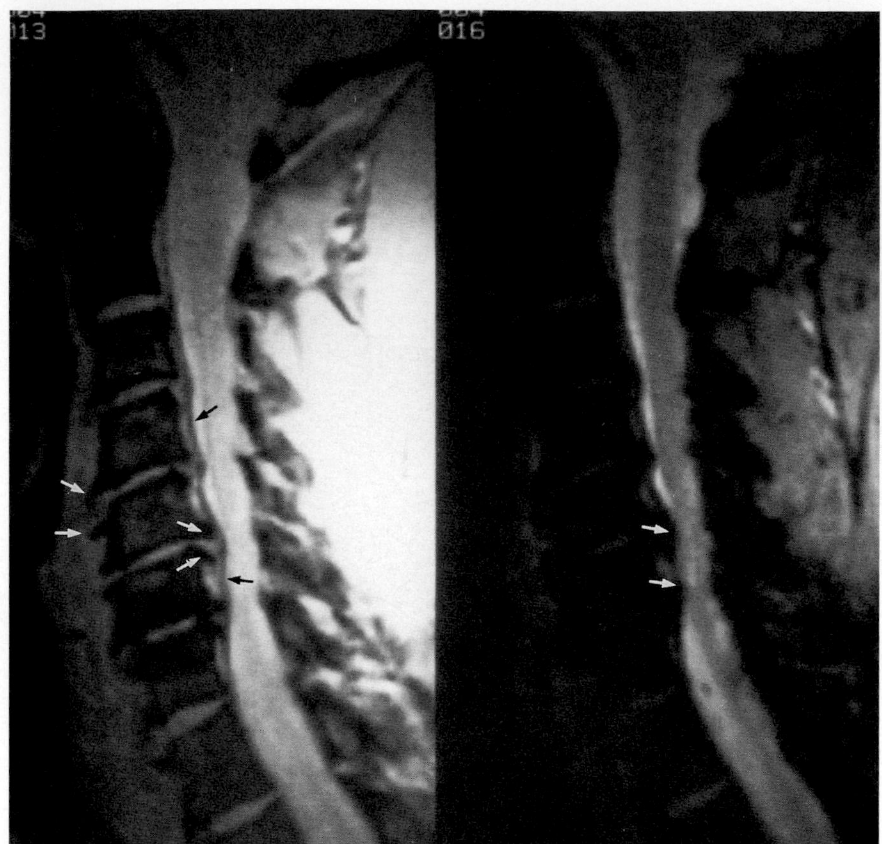

A,B

FIG. 5. A,B: Cervical spondylosis with osteophytes and bulging discs noted at multiple levels in GE images (A, TE = 9 ms) (B, TE = 27 ms). Note that the osteophyte (*white arrows*) appears larger in B because of accentuation of their size by magnetic susceptibility artifact. This makes the spinal canal appear narrower in B than in A. *Black arrows* in A, posterior longitudinal ligament.

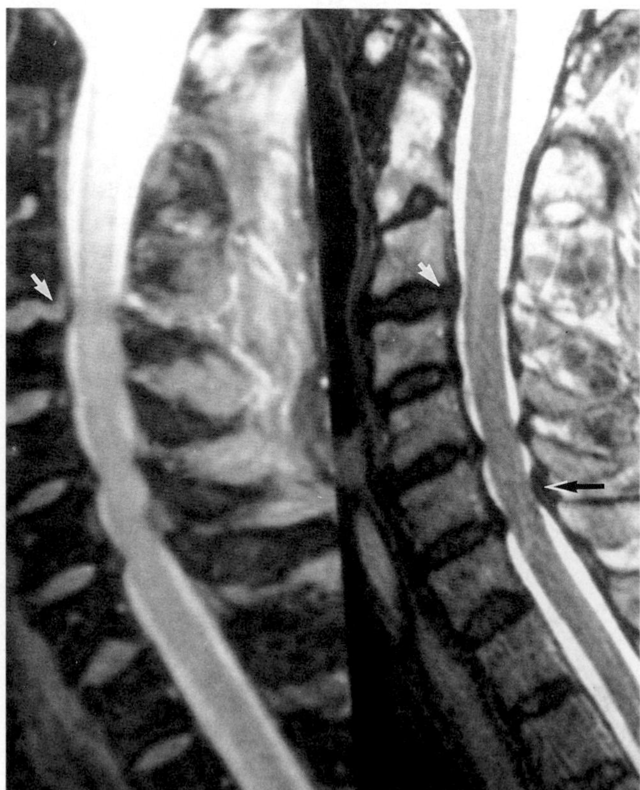

A,B

FIG. 6. Cervical disc bulging shown on sagittal GE (**A**) obtained with 30° flip angle and on corresponding sagittal T2-weighted FSE (**B**). Because the intervertebral disc (*white arrow*) has high signal intensity in A compared to B, it is easier to differentiate the vertebral body from the disc material in A on the GE. The spinal cord is visualized better in B, as is the thickened ligamentum flavum (*black arrow*).

produce images with exquisite spinal cord detail (Fig. 7) and are not nearly as sensitive to magnetic susceptibility artifacts as are GE sequences.

We also use a linear phased array spine coil and 512 × 256 matrix to produce images of the spine with excellent signal-to-noise and spatial resolution, and larger portions of the spine may be evaluated with this coil compared to conventional surface coils.

Anatomic considerations also impact highly on the choice of MR pulse sequence. First, there is less of a need for ultrathin section, very high resolution scans in the lumbar spine because disc spaces are relatively thick and foramina are large. Therefore, a 5-mm slice thickness is adequate for evaluation of the lumbar spine. In the cervical and thoracic spine, disc spaces are thinner and the neural foramina are smaller, so thinner slice thicknesses are necessary. Cervical spine imaging requires the use of contiguous slices, a factor that also favors GE sequences, because contiguously acquired conventional SE scans are degraded by cross-excitation artifacts ("cross-talk") or necessitate very long scan times.

The sagittal plane is adequate for demonstrating lumbar spine neural foramina because of the anatomic orientation of these canals, whereas the cervical foramina are obliquely oriented and require either oblique sectioning or three-dimensional (3D) reformatted images for optimal visualization.

Two-Dimensional Fourier Transform Versus Three-Dimensional Fourier Transform Imaging

Although most degenerative disorders of the spine may be evaluated adequately with two-dimensional Fourier Transform (2DFT) MR sequences, there are certain disadvantages of 2D techniques especially in the evaluation of the cervical neural foramina. Most notable is the inability to generate extremely thin slices with standard 2D sequences. Thinner sections are preferable because spatial resolution is improved and partial volume averaging artifacts are thereby reduced to allow better visualization of small structures. Furthermore, thin slices are advantageous when using GE sequences, because magnetic susceptibility artifacts that might falsely exaggerate foraminal stenosis or central canal stenosis are minimized with thinner slices.

Although computed tomography (CT) scanning using thin sections (1 mm or less) and 3D reformatting remains the gold standard for evaluation of the cervical neural foramen, 3DFT GE MRI of the cervical neural foramen has become an acceptable alternative (Fig. 8). The 3D images are acquired using either T2*-weighted GE or T1-weighted GE (spoiled grass) sequences. The 3D spoiled grass (SPGR, GE Medical Systems, Milwaukee, WI) sequence with intravenous (i.v.) gadolinium is especially valuable for evaluating the foramen because the epidural veins, prevalent in the cervical foramen, enhance with paramagnetic contrast agents whereas nerve roots do not enhance. However, the dorsal root ganglia do enhance with contrast, because they lack a "blood–nerve barrier." The size of the cervical neural foramina can be accurately measured, and any impinging osteophytes may be detected using the 3D SPGR technique (Fig. 9).

3DFT GE scans are obtained using an anisotropic 3D technique in which the slab volume is acquired optimally in coronal plane. (Coronal plane acquisition is optimal

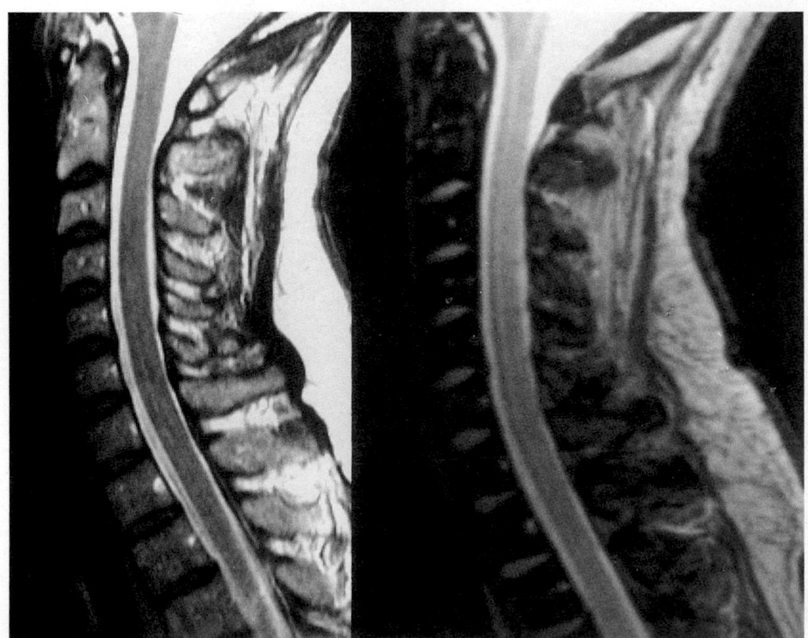
A,B

FIG. 7. Comparison of sagittal T2-weighted FSE image (**A**) and GE image (**B**). The intervertebral discs have higher signal intensity relative to bone on the GE image. However, the spinal cord and ligaments are better visualized in A.

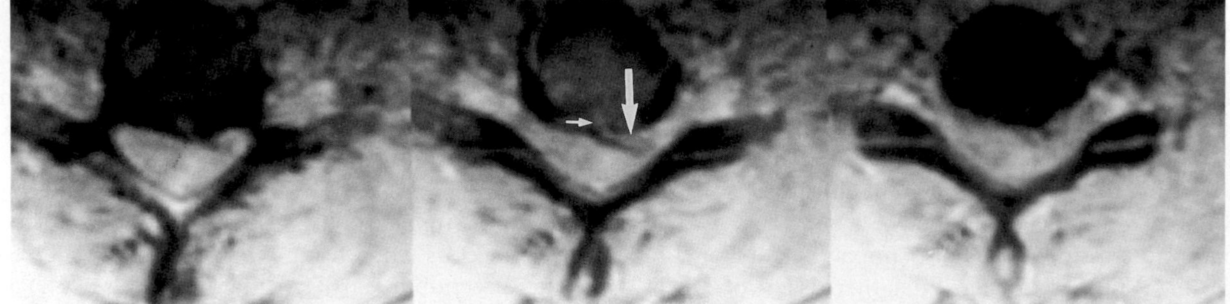

FIG. 8. 3DFT images showing a herniated disc (*large arrow*) at the C5-C6 level to the left of midline. Note that the cervical neural foramen are well shown on two image slices. The site of annular tear (*small arrow*) is also well shown. However, there is poor differentiation between the cervical spinal cord and the CSF despite the 5° flip angle used.

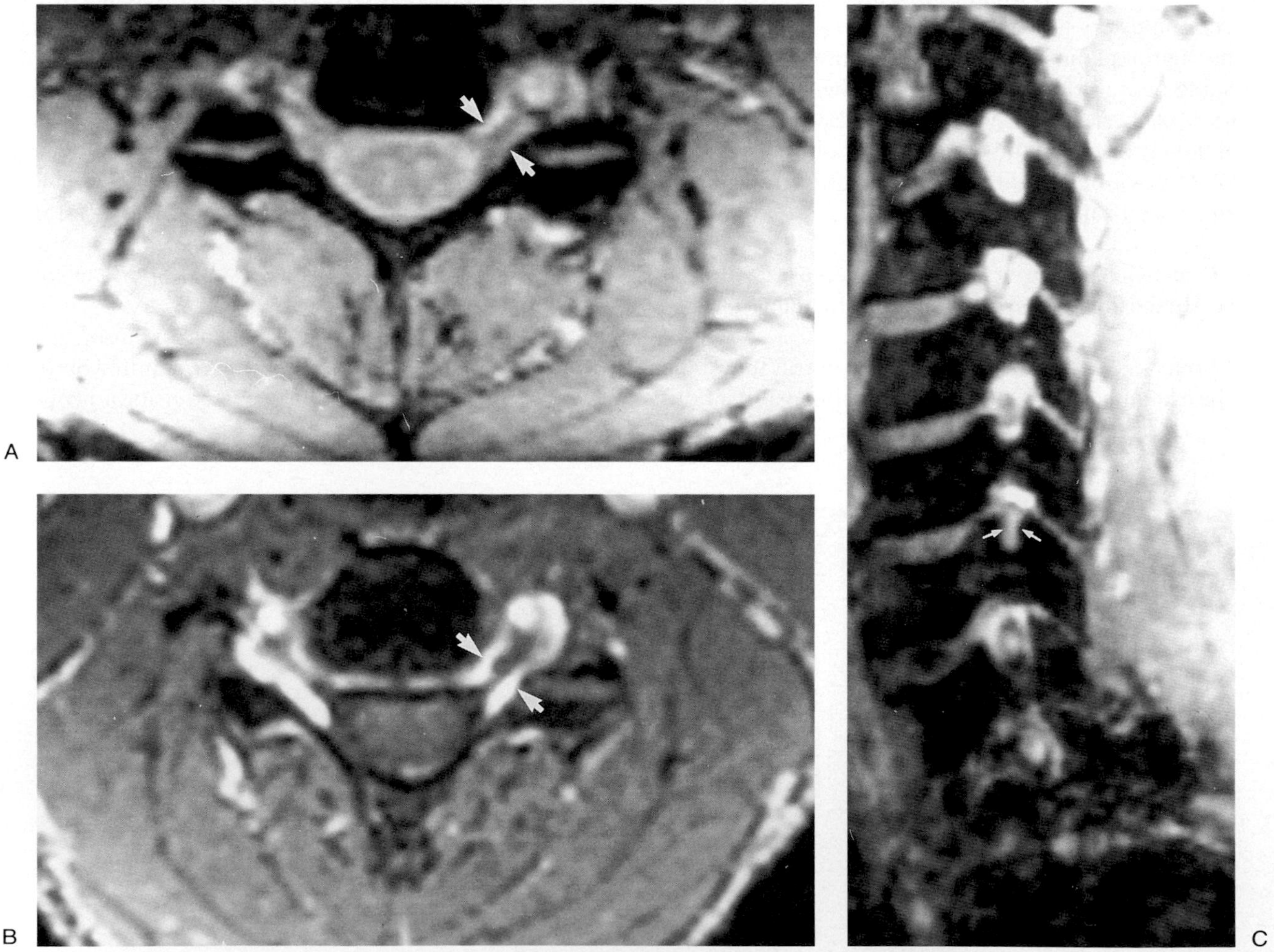

FIG. 9. Evaluation of cervical neural foramen using 3DFT imaging in axial 3D GE image (**A**) with a 1-mm slice thickness and 5° flip angle. The neural foramen (between *arrows*) is well demonstrated, and there is adequate contrast between the CSF and the spinal cord. In axial 3D spoiled grass (**B**) following administration of i.v. gadolinium DTPA, the epidural venous network and other connective tissues enhance surrounding the nerve root and nerve root sheath in the neural foramen (*arrows*). **C:** Reformatted 45° oblique coronal image with gadolinium enhancement demonstrates the size of the neural foramen and indicates the presence of mild neural foraminal narrowing (*arrows*) at the C5-C6 level on the left due to uncinate and facet hypertrophy.

because sagittal plane acquisition results in too many CSF motion artifacts, and axial plane acquisition is insufficient to cover the entire cervical spine unless multiple axial slabs are obtained.) 3DFT techniques result in images that are contiguous, but not degraded from "cross-talk" artifact seen in conventional 2DFT techniques. Additionally, thinner slices are possible (less than 1 mm) in 3DFT imaging, because the thickness of each slice is limited only by signal-to-noise, whereas in 2DFT imaging, the slice thickness (usually no less than 3 mm) is limited by gradient strength. Volume 3DFT images have very high signal-to-noise because the entire volume is excited and the signal-to-noise is proportional to yet another factor not inherent in 2DFT imaging: the square root of the number of slices. Therefore, in 3DFT sequences, choosing more slices results in images with higher signal-to-noise. On the down side, choosing more slices means longer acquisition time, so there are tradeoffs with this technique.

One important benefit of 3D MRI is the ability to generate high-quality reformatted images with any obliquity in any plane from the original acquired volume with very good anatomic resolution, provided that the slice thickness, matrix size, and field of view are chosen so that the voxels are approximately cubic. Although 3DFT volume scanning may be performed with conventional SE sequences, imaging times are prohibitively long unless very short TR intervals are chosen. However, in the near future 3D FSE sequences may be available that would theoretically provide high-detail images with negligible magnetic susceptibility artifact.

Although 3DFT techniques have many theoretical advantages, these techniques have not gained universal acceptance in routine screening of the spine with MRI because important disadvantages also exist in current 3DFT spine imaging: (a) smaller flip angles (5–10°) are required in 3DFT imaging to achieve high-intensity CSF (so-called myelogram effect). This is because 2D techniques benefit more from inflow of unsaturated spins, because each 2D slice is generally thinner than the 3D slab chosen. Hence, the intensity enhancement effect of fresh unsaturated spins is greater using 2D techniques (Fig. 10); (b) the lower flip angle needed to generate high-intensity CSF on 3DFT sacrifices some signal-to-noise; (c) aliasing, or "wrap-around" artifacts, superimpose one end of the excited slab of tissue on the other and produce image degradation on several slices on each end of the slab, so the useful number of slices, in practice, is less than the number being generated in 3D volume acquisitions. Despite these shortcomings, 3DFT imaging can reliably delineate cervical disc and foraminal disease and is an important adjunct to standard 2DFT imaging of the spine.

Motion Suppression Methods

Several techniques are available to reduce motion artifacts caused by CSF and vascular pulsations. These include gradient moment nulling, peripheral pulse gating, and presaturation pulses (6). In general, all conventional T2-weighted SE sequences should use either a gradient

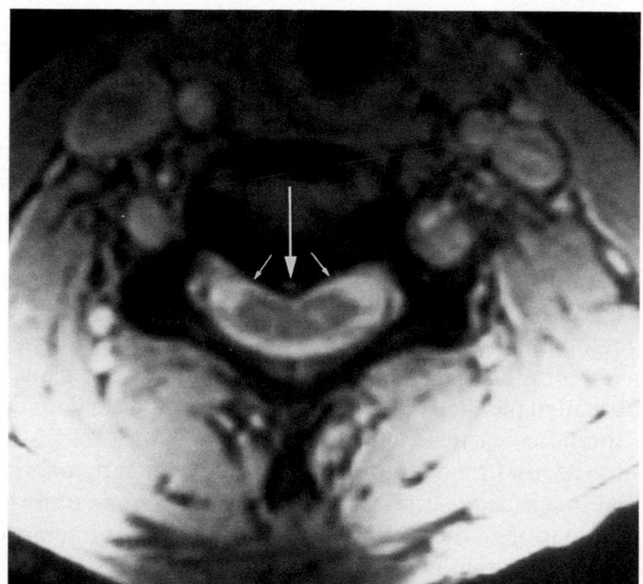
A

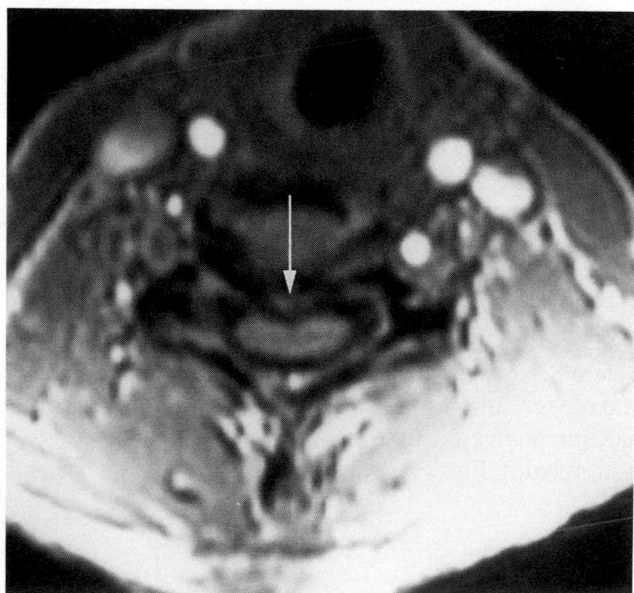
B

FIG. 10. 2D vs. 3D GE images. Comparison of herniated disc and osteophyte. **A:** 2D axial GE image obtained with 30° flip angle and 3-mm slice thickness demonstrates a prominent bilaterally symmetric osteophytic ridge (*small arrows*) and a small midline herniated disc showing higher signal intensity (*long arrow*) causing cord compression. **B:** In 3D axial image obtained with a 20° flip angle, it is difficult to distinguish the herniated disc in the midline from the adjacent bone because of improper choice of flip angle. Note the CSF is dark in B and bright in A.

moment nulling technique, peripheral pulse gating, or both. Gradient moment nulling cannot be implemented with current FSE sequences. Peripheral pulse gating can be performed with FSE sequences but is often not necessary. We do not routinely use pulse gating with T2 FSE sequences for spine imaging.

Gradient moment nulling modifies the gradient waveform to compensate for the phase change that a moving spin accumulates in the presence of a bipolar gradient (such as the slice-select gradient). The phase change depends on the type of motion the spin in question is experiencing; that is, constant velocity motion causes a different phase shift than acceleration. In general, more complex (higher order) movement, such as acceleration, requires more complex alterations of the flow-compensating gradients (7). The trade-off for implementing flow-compensating gradients is that these gradients take some time to play out. The end result is that gradient moment nulling necessitates a higher minimum TE and cannot be used with some sequences such as FSE, which does allow enough time to play out the compensating gradients.

More complex gradient moment nulling techniques such as MAST (Picker International) will compensate for motion artifact from accelerating spins but require even more time within the pulse sequence to apply the compensating gradients. The use of higher-order gradient moment nulling techniques results in only minimal improvement in image quality over first-order (velocity correction) gradient moment nulling.

Saturation techniques use a selective pulse that is applied to tissue either inside or outside the field of view. Their purpose is to excite (saturate) moving spins that lie outside the imaging plane, so that these spins will not contribute signal when they eventually enter the plane of interest and are subjected to the 90° rf pulse. Saturation techniques are extremely useful to eliminate motion-induced artifacts arising from motion outside of the spine. In the cervical spine, saturation pulses should be applied to the soft tissues of the oropharynx and larynx to reduce motion artifacts from swallowing and breathing. Saturation pulses are also routinely used to minimize respiratory and cardiac artifacts, which are a problem in thoracic and lumbar spine imaging. It is preferable to place two smaller saturation bands in the field of view anterior to the spine because two bands produce more effective tissue saturation than one larger saturation band (Fig. 11).

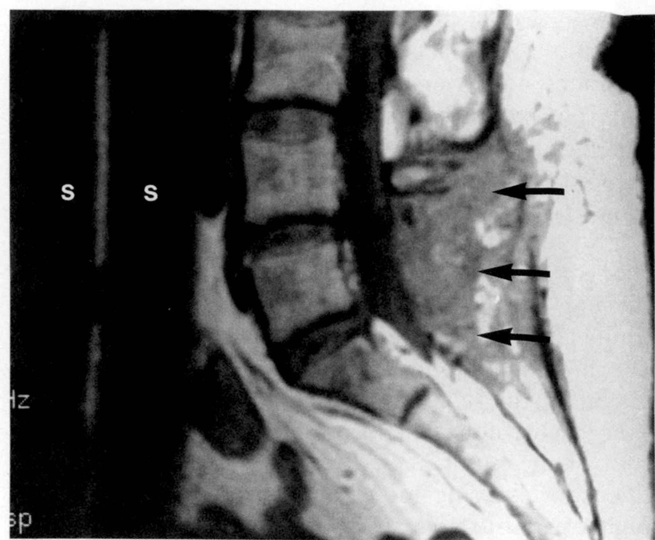

FIG. 11. Two saturation bands (*S*) have been placed anterior to the lumbar spine. Incidentally noted is a laminectomy defect (*arrows*) extending from L4-S1 containing scar tissue.

Imaging Strategies

When imaging degenerative disease of the lumbar spine with MR, there are several generalizations that can be made to ensure adequate imaging protocols. In the lumbar region, it is clear that SE and FSE sequences are the most useful to depict the relevant anatomy. All patients evaluated for spinal disease should first be scanned with a T1-weighted SE sequence. In MRI, one should capitalize on the unique ability to image the spine in multiple planes, which allows us to see the nerve roots in the foramina, the cephalocaudad extent of herniated disc material, and changes in the disc architecture itself. In the lumbar spine a 5-mm slice thickness is sufficient, although a 3-mm slice thickness is preferable for adequate resolution of the disc and neural foramen in the sagittal and axial planes. In the cervical and thoracic spine, a 3-mm slice thickness is the minimum requirement necessary for routine sagittal and axial imaging. 3DFT reformatted images are necessary to optimally evaluate the cervical neural foramen, although axial 2D images are satisfactory for screening purposes.

Coverage on the sagittal images should include foramen to foramen, and the conus must also be imaged, because it is not rare for a conus mass to present as radiculopathy or low back pain. In the axial plane, the intervertebral disc is best shown when the imaging plane is oriented parallel to each respective disc, and axial images should cover pedicle-to-pedicle through at least L3-L4, L4-L5, and L5-S1. However, nonangled, contiguous axial image acquisition is preferable to angled sections for evaluation of the vertebrae. For example, pars interarticularis defects may not be detected if contiguous axial sections are not obtained.

FSE sequences are excellent for evaluating the spinal cord and cauda equina as well as for measuring the spinal canal. However, FSE sequences are less effective for evaluating marrow-infiltrating disease unless the FSE tech-

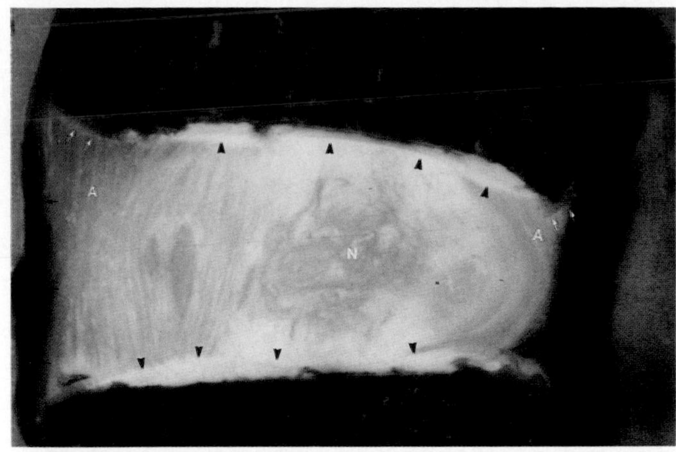

FIG. 12. Sagittal anatomic section through a normal lumbar intervertebral disc illustrating the cartilaginous endplate (*arrowheads*), the annulus fibrosus (*A*), nucleus pulposus (*N*), ring apophysis (*white arrows*), anterior longitudinal ligament (*black arrows*), and adjacent vertebral bodies.

A
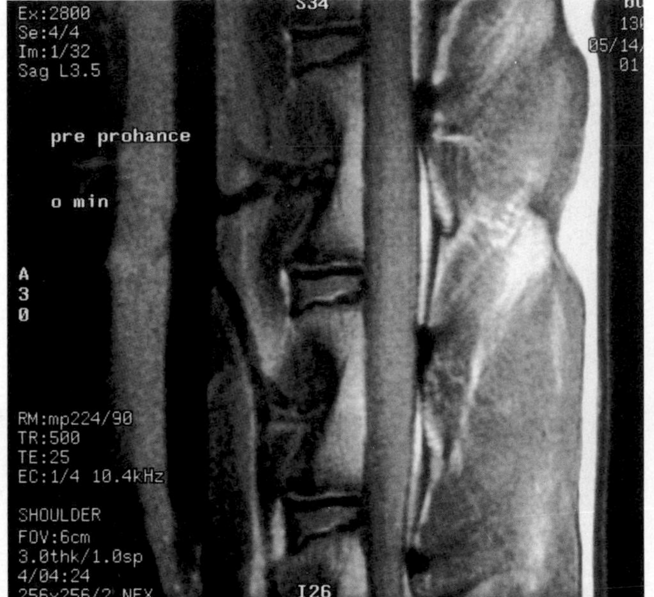

B
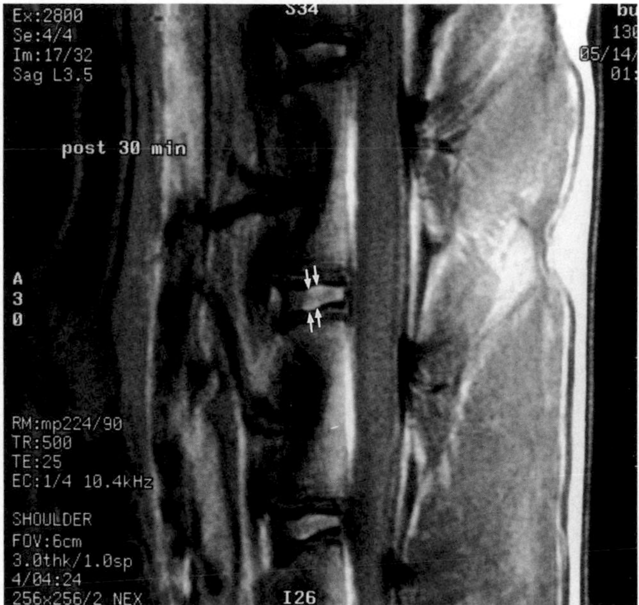

C
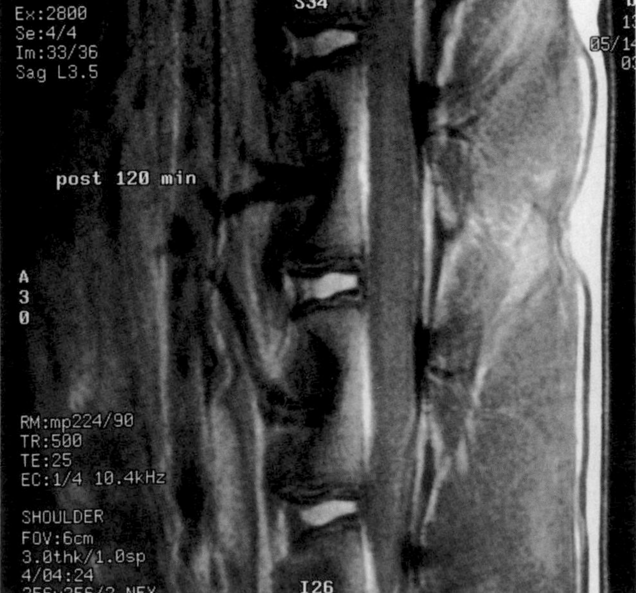

FIG. 13. Sagittal MR images of a rabbit spine obtained before (**A**) and at 30 (**B**) and 120 (**C**) minutes after i.v. administration of gadoteridol 0.3 mmol/Kg. Note that contrast enhancement is evident first at the endplate (*arrows,* B) and then throughout the intervertebral disc (C).

nique is acquired with a fat-suppression technique. In the cervical spine, GE images are more useful than FSE images in evaluating disc disease, particularly in the axial plane.

In cervical and thoracic spine imaging, the initial sequence should include a thin-section (3 mm), sagittal T1-weighted SE scan with minimal or no interslice interval. Sagittal T2-weighted FSE and GE images with short flip angle (to generate high-intensity CSF) are routinely obtained. Axial images should be performed using either 2D or 3D GE techniques, especially in the cervical spine, where a low flip angle is selected to generate high-intensity CSF (5° flip angle for 3DFT and 30° flip angle for 2DFT techniques). Slice thickness should be as thin as possible without sacrificing too much signal-to-noise.

Thoracic imaging often is accomplished by the use of sagittal, thin-section SE images, and is optimized with the concomitant use of saturation pulses and gradient moment nulling, as already discussed. In imaging for thoracic disc and spinal cord disease, T1-weighted SE and T2-weighted FSE sequences are obtained routinely. Axial images are optionally obtained if the sagittal scans show an abnormality.

ANATOMY OF THE INTERVERTEBRAL DISC

The intervertebral disc is a complex structure consisting of several highly specialized connective tissues (8). A combination of hyaline cartilage, fibrocartilage, mucopolysaccharide, and dense collagenous fibrous tissue give the discs the properties that confer flexibility and stability to the spine (9). The disc structure is usually described in terms of three components: the cartilaginous endplate, nucleus pulposus, and annulus fibrosus.

The cartilaginous endplate is a layer of hyaline cartilage that covers most of the vertebral endplate (Fig. 12). Surrounding the cartilaginous endplate is a ring of dense bone, the ring apophysis, which fuses to the vertebra in the second decade of life. The cartilaginous endplate attaches firmly to the osseous endplate by means of numerous collagenous fibers, and strengthens the osseous endplate, which contains multiple perforations. Because of the perforations, Schmorl suggested that it should be classified with cancellous bone. Within the pores of the vertebral endplate are numerous vascular channels, which are the major source for the nutrients and, during imaging studies, the contrast medium, which diffuses into the disc (10,11) (Fig. 13). With degeneration of the disc, the perforations become less well defined and less conspicuous. One of the theories of disc degeneration is that endplate changes that impair diffusion into and out of the disc hinder the function of chondrocytes and fibroblasts in the disc.

The annulus fibrosus is a complex fibrous and fibrocartilaginous structure that consists of 12 to 15 layers, each with well developed dense parallel fibrous bands (12) (see Fig. 12). For descriptive purposes, it can be divided into outer and inner rings. The outer ring contains the densest fibrous lamellae. The fibers in this portion of the annulus originate and insert in the compact cortical bone in the ring apophysis (Fig. 14). These fibers, because of their osseous attachments, may be described as Sharpey's fibers after the English anatomist who described the collagenous structure of bone. The lamellae consist almost exclusively of dense Type I collagen with little ground substance, unlike other portions of the disc. This portion of the disc on T2- or T1-weighted images has a low signal intensity (Fig. 15). The approximately 8000 cells in each cubic millimeter of tissue within the outer ring of the annulus are almost exclusively fibroblasts. The outer annulus is thicker anteriorly than posteriorly.

The inner ring of the annulus fibrosus contains fibrocartilage. Unlike the outer ring of the annulus, the inner ring contains predominantly chondrocytes, and has plentiful ground substance. The collagen in the inner ring is less plentiful than in the outer ring. Because of the ground substance, the inner ring has a high signal intensity like the nucleus pulposus in T2-weighted images (Fig. 15) (13). The lamellae are less well defined and less fibrous than in the peripheral ring. The lamellae be-

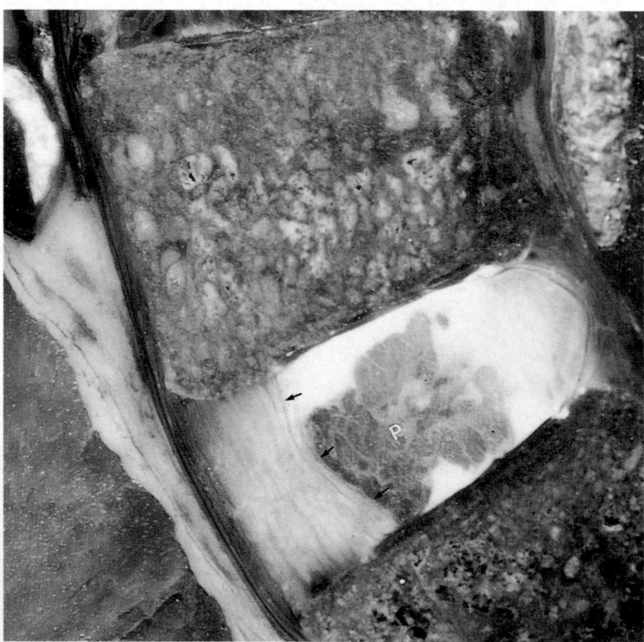

FIG. 14. Sagittal anatomic section of the L5-S1 intervertebral disc illustrating dense collagenous lamellar structure in the peripheral annulus fibrosus (*arrows*). These dense fibers originate and insert in the ring apophysis. Medial to this dense collagenous structure is the central portion of the annulus fibrosus with a less well defined lamellar structure and fibrocartilage. The nucleus pulposus occupies a small portion of the intervertebral disc. The dark pigment (*P*) stains part of the nucleus and the inner annulus.

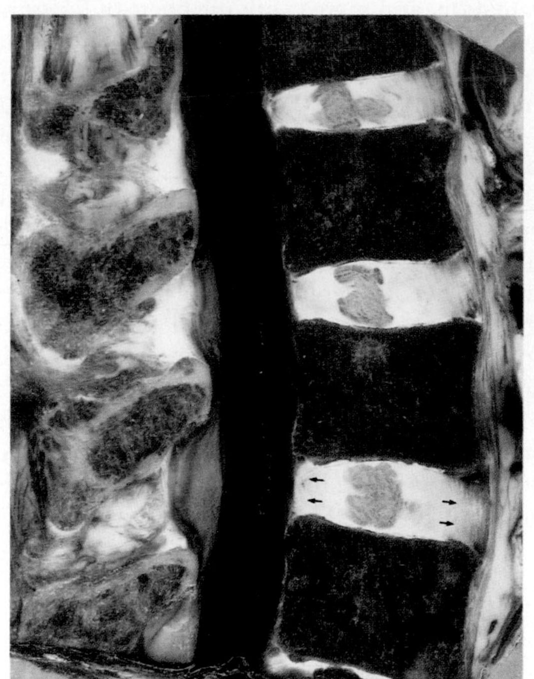

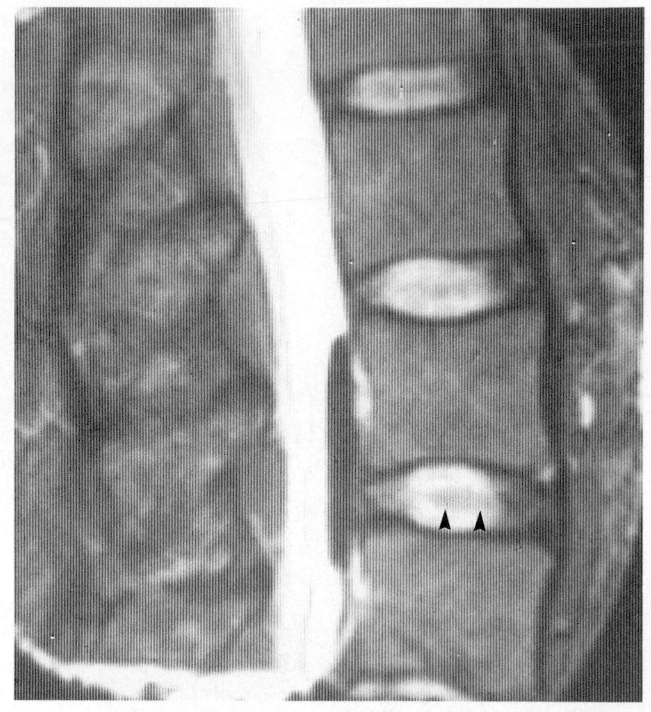

FIG. 15. Comparison of a sagittal anatomic section with the exact corresponding MR image (TR 2000, TE 80 SE). Note that the peripheral annulus has a low signal intensity (*arrows*) whereas the inner annulus and the nucleus pulposus, which have a mucopolysaccharide matrix, have a higher signal intensity. The lower signal intensity in the equator of the nucleus and annulus (*arrowheads*) is due to a higher concentration of collagen.

come less and less well defined toward the center of the disc. As the lamellar structure changes, the annulus becomes gradually less and less distinguishable from the nucleus pulposus (Fig. 16). The fibers in each layer of the inner or outer annulus run radially at an angle of about 30° with respect to the endplates. Fibers in adjacent lamellae are nearly perpendicular to each other.

The nucleus pulposus is also composed of fibrocartilage. It has approximately the same amount of ground substance as the inner annulus, and approximately the same signal intensity as the inner annulus in T2-weighted images (Fig. 15). The collagen present in the nucleus is Type II, which is stronger in compression and less strong in tension compared to Type I. The collagen in the nucleus is less well structured than in the annulus, giving it an amorphous appearance rather than a lamellar structure. The equator of the disc contains a higher collagen concentration than the remainder of the disc. The region of greater collagen concentration has a lower signal intensity than the remainder of the disc on T2-weighted images (13) (Fig. 14). The ground substance in the nucleus pulposus consists of hyaluronic acid and glycosaminoglycans, which contain the polysaccharides keratin and chondroitin sulfate. These substances have a high concentration of fixed negative charges that cause the disc to absorb water even in the presence of a high-pressure gradient (14). The mucopolysaccharide gel in the nucleus pulposus gives the disc its high intrinsic pressure, which allows it to resist compressive forces. When the nucleus is removed from the disc, it readily absorbs water and expands. Water in the disc is normally determined by the intradiscal pressure and the capacity of the disc to absorb water. When the load on the disc increases, water leaves the disc, and when the intradiscal pressure diminishes, water returns (15). These changes in water content result in a diurnal variation in height. The glycosaminoglycans are synthesized by the chondrocytes present in the nucleus pulposus. Diffusion through the vertebral endplates provides the nutrients necessary for the metabolism and function of these cells (11).

The composition of the fibrocartilage in the intervertebral disc explains the observed phenomenon of contrast enhancement. Normally, with doses of contrast medium in the range of 0.1 mmol/Kg and images obtained promptly after i.v. injection of contrast medium, enhancement is not observed in the intervertebral disc. With larger doses of contrast medium and with longer elapsed times before imaging, enhancement may be observed because of the slow accumulation of contrast medium by diffusion (10). The enhancement is observed first near the periphery of the disc, and subsequently near the center (see Fig. 13). Enhancement is greater when nonionic contrast media such as gadoteridol or gadodiamide are used, because diffusion of the ionic medium is

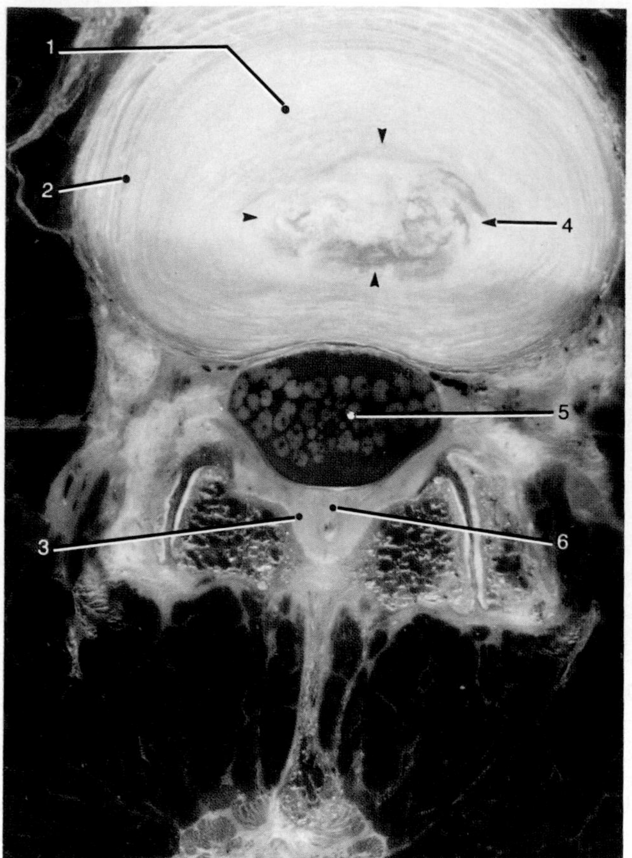

FIG. 16. Axial cryomicrotome section through L3-L4 intervertebral disc. No clear distinction exists between the inner annulus and nucleus pulposus. Concentric fiber bundles make up the outer annulus. The posterior disc margin is concave and does not deform the thecal sac. *1*, inner annulus; *2*, outer annulus; *3*, ligamentum flavum; *4*, nucleus pulposus; *5*, thecal sac containing cauda equina nerve rootlets; *6*, epidural fat.

hindered by the fixed negative charges in the intervertebral disc (16) (Fig. 17).

The anterior and posterior longitudinal ligaments (PLL), although not normally considered part of the disc, are not easily distinguished from the disc (Fig. 16). The anterior longitudinal ligament, consisting of fibroblasts and collagen, forms a thin layer over the anterior and lateral surfaces of the disc (see Fig. 12). Its fibers are in contact with the outermost layer of the annulus fibrosus. It contains some fibers that originate and insert in the compact cortical bone in the vertical portion of the vertebrae. The low signal intensity of the PLL is difficult to distinguish from the low signal intensity of the peripheral annulus fibrosus in either T1- or T2-weighted MRI. The PLL has a similar composition and signal intensity. The thin band of collagenous fibers in the PLL is difficult to distinguish from the annulus fibrosus along the posterior aspect of the disc (see Fig. 12). At the intervertebral disc level the fibers of the PLL diverge, have a horizontal orientation, and merge with the fibers of the annulus fibrosus. Between disc spaces, the PLL has mostly longitudinally oriented fibers. It forms a band approximately 1 mm thick and 3 mm wide between intervertebral discs, posterior to the retrovertebral plexus and ventral to the dural sac.

The disc normally lacks innervation and vascularity. Nerves, which may be nociceptors, have been identified in the anterior and PLLs, in the facet joints, in the vertebral endplates, and arguably in the peripheral layer of the annulus fibrosus (9). Therefore, the disc is not normally a source of pain, although degeneration in the disc may lead to pain by means of stretching of nociceptor as well as nerve compression of the production of inflammation. Blood vessels are not normally found in cartilage. The nutrition of the intervertebral disc, as in other cartilaginous structures, is provided by diffusion.

AGE-RELATED CHANGES IN THE INTERVERTEBRAL DISC

The intervertebral disc undergoes marked changes with aging, which must be distinguished from the changes due to degeneration of the intervertebral disc (15,17–20). When age-related and degenerative changes are not distinguished, the incidence of degeneration is grossly exaggerated. The incidence of intervertebral disc degeneration increases with age, but most intervertebral discs in normal individuals do not show the changes in height, signal intensity, and morphology that characterize degenerating intervertebral discs. Despite increasing numbers of small tears and amount of pigment and col-

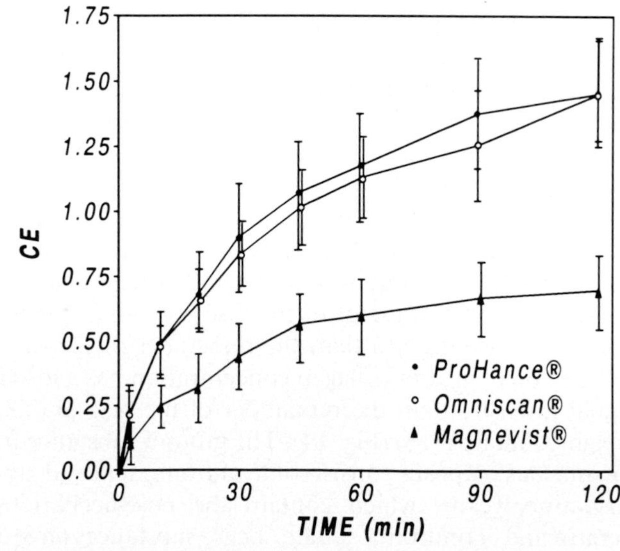

FIG. 17. Contrast enhancement of normal rabbit intervertebral discs after the administration of a non-ionic or ionic Gd-containing chelate (0.3 mmol/Kg). Contrast enhancement is greater from non-ionic ProHance or Omniscan than ionic Magnevist.

lagen and decreasing amounts of glycosaminoglycans in the nucleus pulposus, most discs retain normal biomechanical function into the seventh and eighth decades of life (12,19). The magnitude of the age-related changes in the intervertebral disc can be illustrated by comparing the appearance of the neonatal, transitional and young adult, and older adult intervertebral discs.

In the neonate, with an incompletely ossified vertebral body, the space between vertebrae appears large. A portion of that space consists of unossified cartilaginous vertebral body. The disc itself contains a thin peripheral rim with a distinct lamellar structure, which corresponds to the peripheral annulus fibrosus (Fig. 18). This rim and the ossification centers in the vertebrae have low signal intensity on T1- and T2-weighted images. The remainder of the disc has moderately high signal intensity (21). Medial to the peripheral annulus is a thin layer of tissue with little lamellar structure that grossly has the same appearance as vertebral cartilage. It represents the inner portion of the annulus fibrosus. The remainder of the disc consists of a translucent substance, the nucleus pulposus. In the equator of the disc are thin streaks of tissue with syncytial cells that are remnants of the primitive notochord (19). The nucleus and annulus are sharply demarcated in the newborn. On gross inspection, vessels are evident in the vertebral cartilage near the future ring apophysis and in the ossifying center of the vertebra (see Fig. 18). Otherwise the disc appears avascular as in the adult.

During the first two decades of life, the disc develops the fibrous structure that characterizes the adult disc (22). During the second decade of life, the intervertebral disc can be characterized as transitional between the newborn and the adult disc. The transitional disc has lamellae of fibrocartilage with a distinct fibrous structure. The nucleus pulposus, which has an ill-defined border within the annulus, has become opaque rather than translucent because of the development of collagen fibers within it. The collagen content of the inner annulus and the equator of the disc has increased to the degree that

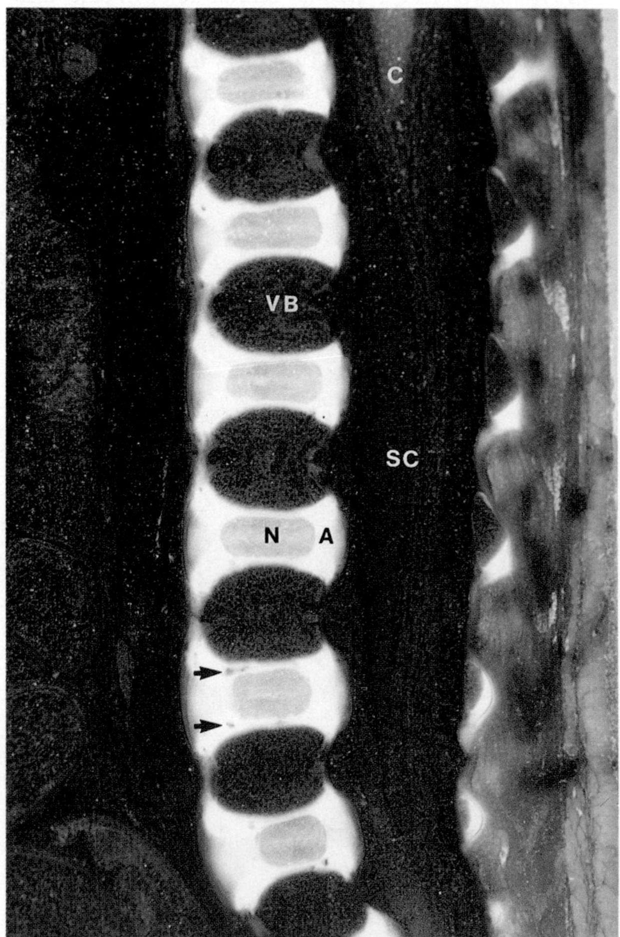

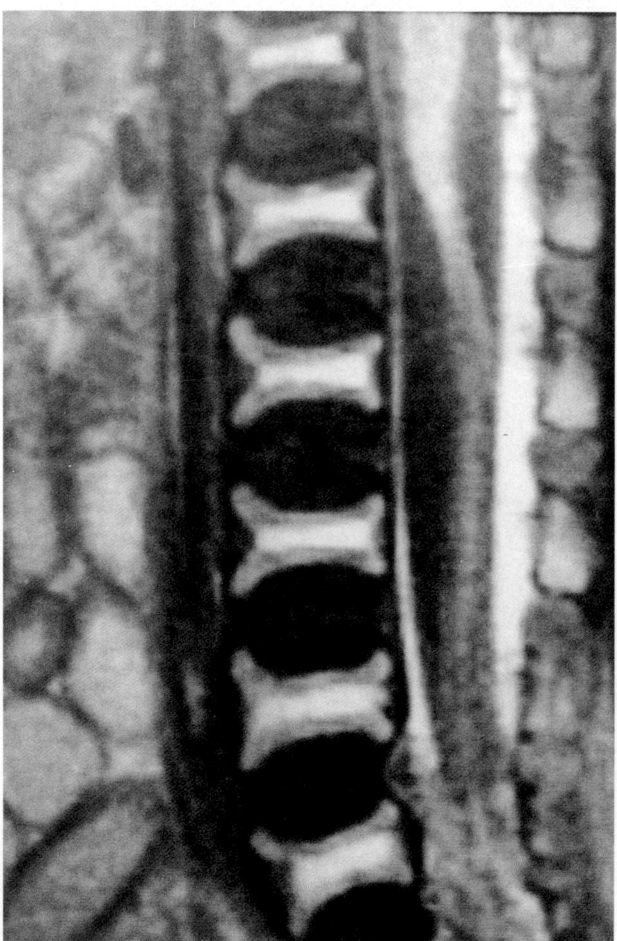

FIG. 18. In the cryomicrotome (**A**) and MRI (**B**) of the neonatal intervertebral disc, the unossified portion, small vascular channels can be identified (*arrows*). The annulus and nucleus are sharply demarcated. In the peripheral annulus, a lamellar structure is evident.

these regions are less translucent and lower in signal intensity in T2-weighted MRI (Fig. 19). The vertebral body and the ring apophysis have not yet ossified completely. In MRI, the marked difference in signal intensity between the fibrous and fibrocartilaginous portions of the disc are evident.

Once the adult intervertebral disc has appeared, it continues to change with age. With aging, small concentric and transverse tears develop in the annulus (20,22) (Fig. 20). The former is characterized as delamination of the lamellae in the annulus fibrosus with the development of a mucoid substance or fluid in the space. These tears may be visualized on MRI as a narrow band of higher intensity signal, indicating the location of the mucoid substance or fluid. The latter are short disruptions in the annulus near the insertion of Sharpey's fibers into the ring apophysis. These may be visualized on MR or CT as small collections of fluid. Rarely, gas may be identified in these tears. Both types of tears are common in adult discs with or without other signs of degeneration. These are therefore aging changes rather than degenerative changes.

With aging, the composition of the intervertebral disc changes (14,23). Collagen increases and glycosaminoglycans decrease in the disc. These changes result in a lower affinity of the disc for water and therefore a decrease in the water content of the disc. The water content of the disc may diminish by 10% or 15% over five decades. Therefore with aging, the signal intensity of the disc diminishes by a few percent. Loss of the normal high signal intensity in T2-weighted images or loss of the normal intervertebral disc height are, however, not explained by aging.

DEGENERATION OF THE INTERVERTEBRAL DISC

The pathogenesis of intervertebral disc degeneration is not well understood. Trauma is not likely the major factor in degeneration. Epidemiologic studies show that a history of trauma is obtained in a small minority of patients with herniated intervertebral discs. Biomechanical studies show that the disc is less likely than the vertebral body to fail as the result of trauma (24). Repetitive cyclical loading of the disc may result in failure of annular fibers (25). Decreasing permeability of the vertebral endplates has been suggested as a cause for disc degeneration.

Despite the lack of consensus on the cause of disc degeneration, one morphologic feature characterizes discs with herniations, bulging, loss of height, and loss of signal intensity (26,27). The radial tear of the annulus, which is found consistently with the other degenerative changes in the intervertebral disc, is characterized in the biomechanical engineering studies of the disc as a primary failure of the annulus (28,29). The radial tear in-

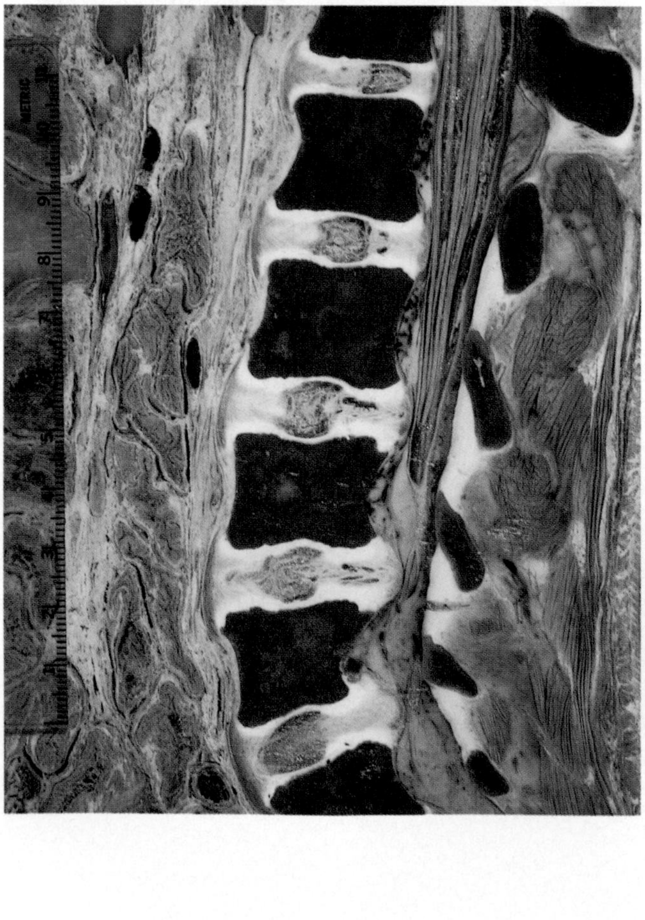

FIG. 19. Sagittal anatomic image of the spine of a 13-year-old child. Note the decreased translucency of the nucleus pulposus.

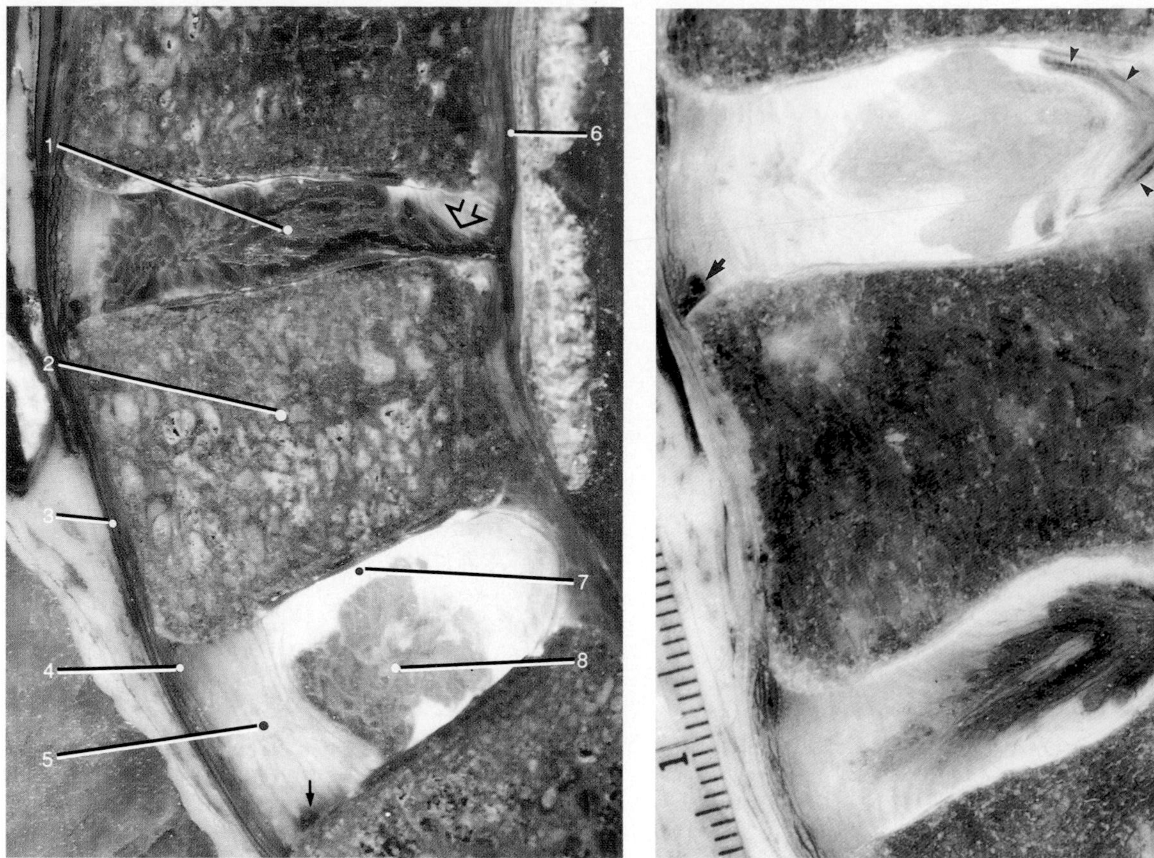

FIG. 20. Sagittal anatomic and MR images. **A:** Sagittal cryomicrotome section of lower lumbar spine in an adult. With advancing age, the disc loses water and becomes fibrotic (*1*). A more normal disc is seen at the L5-S1 level. There are early degenerative changes seen in the nucleus pulposus at this level. The normal annulus fibrosus has 12–15 concentric lamellae (5). *1*, degenerated L4-L5 disc; *2*, L% vertebral body; *3*, anterior longitudinal ligament; *4*, Sharpey's fibers; *5*, anterior annulus; *6*, posterior longitudinal ligament; *7*, cartilaginous endplate; *8*, nucleus pulposus. **B**: Sagittal anatomic sections illustrating transverse (*arrow*) and concentric tears (*arrowheads*) that develop in many older intervertebral discs. For comparison, a radial tear is illustrated (*open arrows*) at levels where disc degeneration is present.

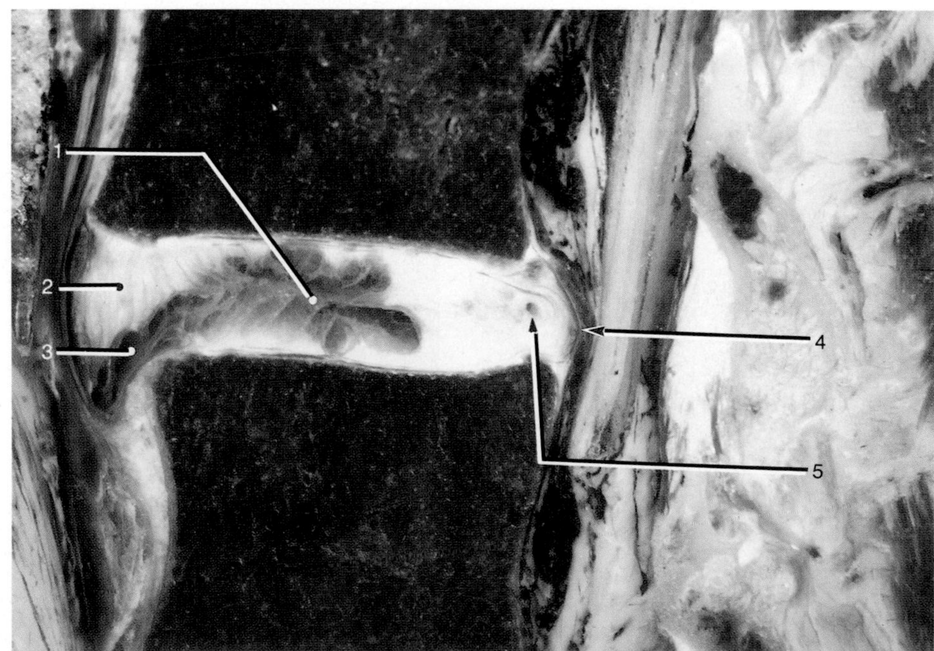

FIG. 21. Sagittal cryomicrotome section through the lumbar intervertebral disc. The nucleus (*1*) is desiccated and there is a type 2 tear (*3*) in the outer annulus (*2*). The posterior disc margin (*4*) bulges into the spinal canal. A tiny type 1 tear (*5*) is seen in the posterior annulus.

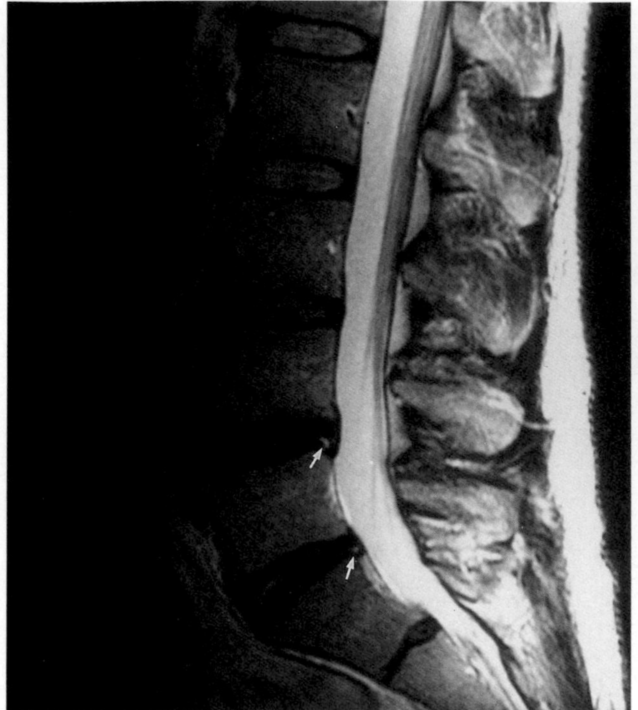

FIG. 22. Sagittal T2-weighted FSE image (TR 2000 msec, TE 80 msec) shows annular tears with high signal intensity (*arrows*) in the posterior annulus of L4-L5 and L5-S1. The interventional portions of the disc diminished signal intensity because of disc degeneration.

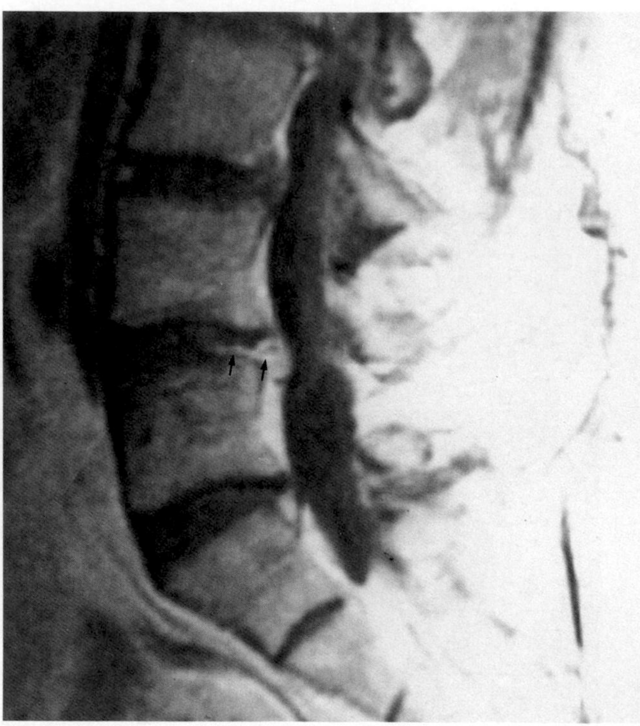

FIG. 23. Sagittal T1-weighted SE image after i.v. administration of gadolinium demonstrates enhancement in a radial tear (*arrows*) of the posterior annulus fibrosus at the L4-L5 level.

volves all layers of the annulus fibrosus in its anterior, posterior, or possibly lateral portion (Figs. 20 and 21). The radial tear can be seen effectively with precise anatomic sectioning techniques such as cryomicrotomy. It may be detected by MRI as a band of high-signal-intensity tissue in the region of the disc normally characterized by low signal intensity (Fig. 22). It may also be visualized on contrast-enhanced MRI as a strip of enhancement in the normally nonenhancing disc (Figs. 23 and 24). The radial tear may therefore be a marker of

A

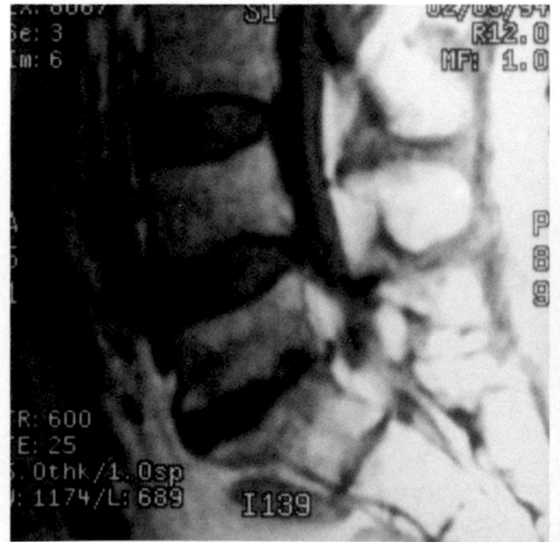

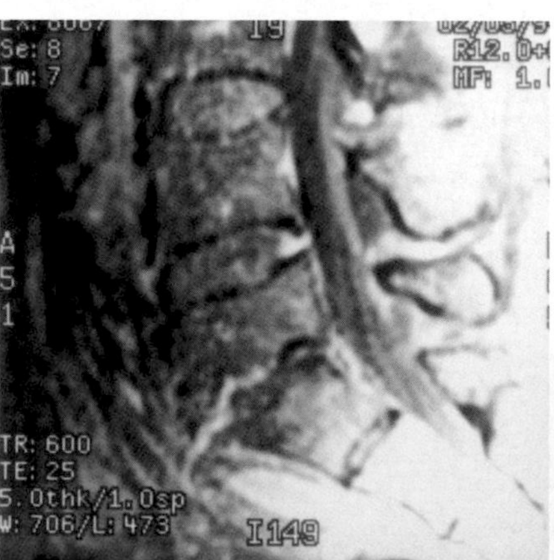

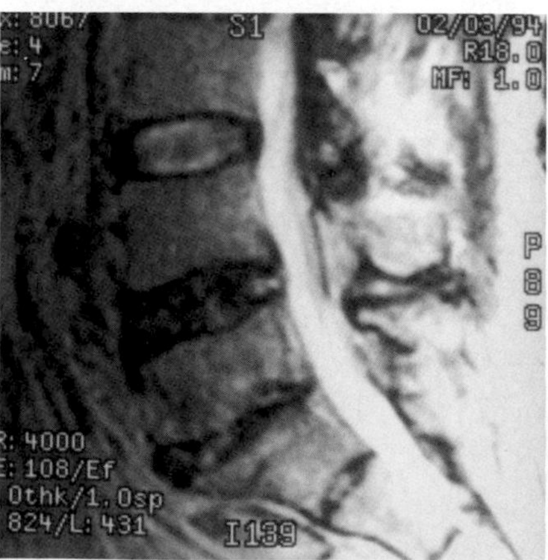

B,C

FIG. 24. A composite of a T1-weighted SE image (**A**), a contrast-enhanced and fat-suppressed T1-weighted image (**B**), and a T2-weighted image (**C**) illustrating a radial tear of the posterior annulus at L4-L5 characterized by contrast enhancement and high signal intensity in T2-weighted images.

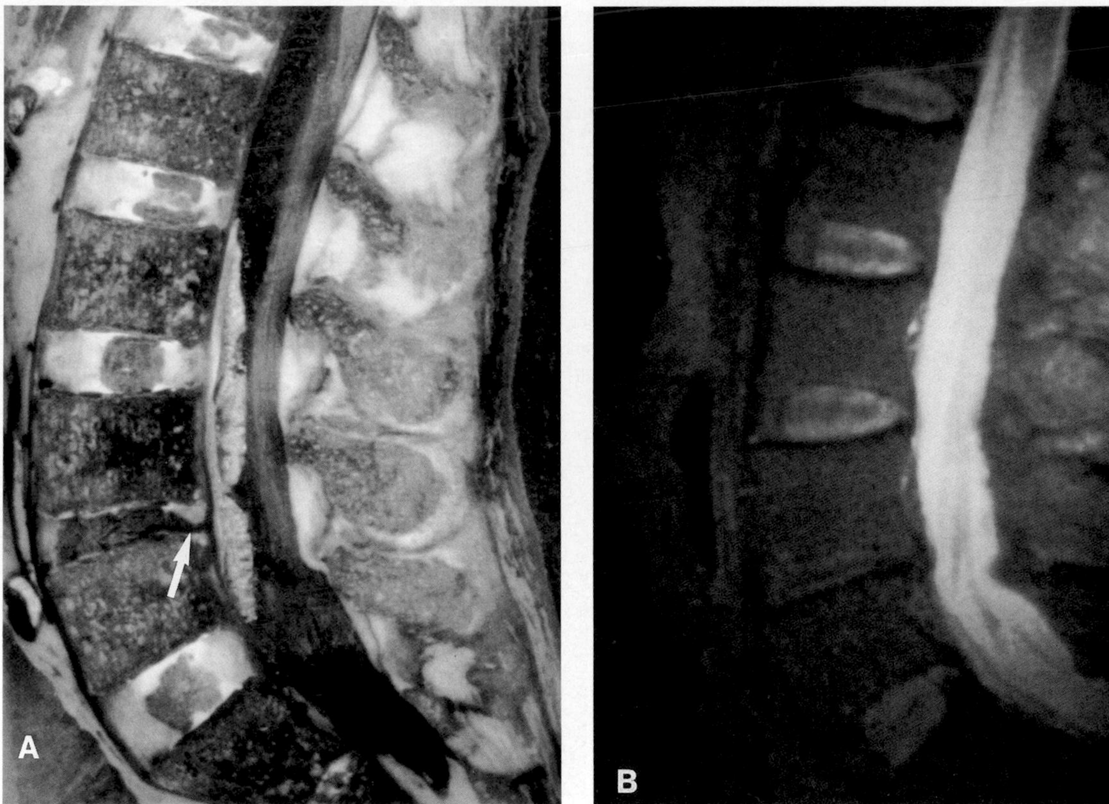

FIG. 25. Anatomic (**A**) and exactly correlating MRI (**B**) illustrating degenerative changes associated with a radial tear of the annulus fibrosus in a cadaver. At L4-L5, the intervertebral disc has diminished height, diminished signal intensity, and slight bulging of the posterior annulus. The radial tear (*arrow*) is evident on the anatomic sections as a dark band extending through the annulus.

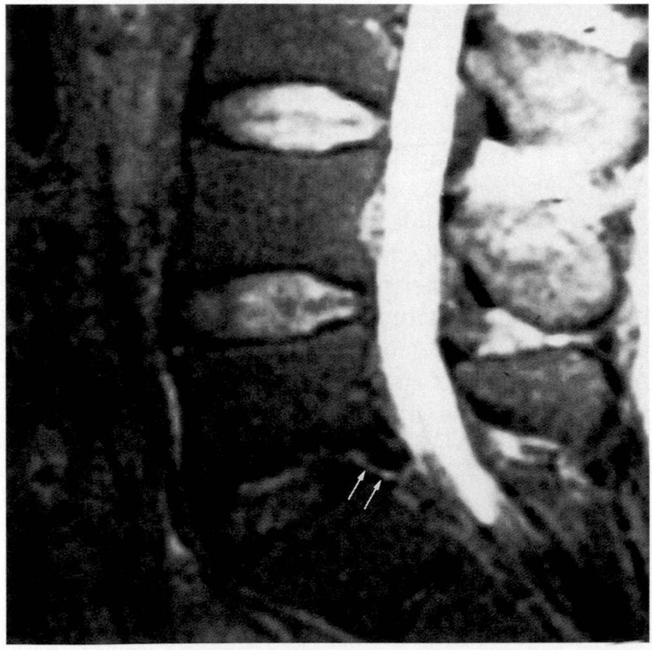

FIG. 26. Sagittal T2-weighted SE image showing early degenerative disc disease at L4-L5 and marked signal intensity loss in the intervertebral disc at L5-S1 indicating advanced disc degeneration at this level. A posterior radial tear (*arrows*) has high signal intensity relative to adjacent bone and degenerating disc.

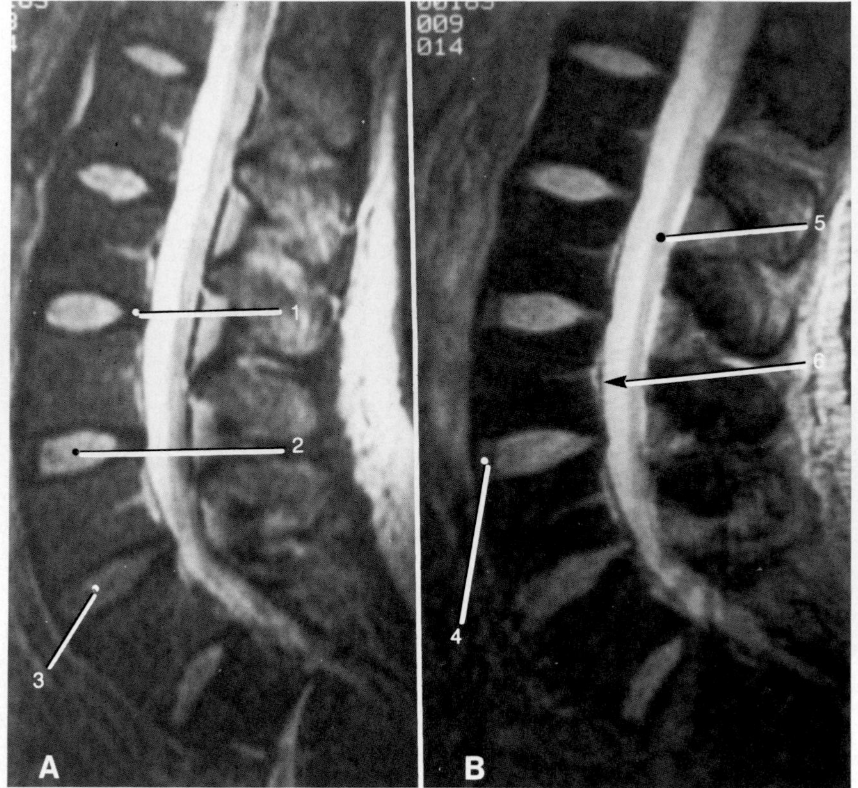

FIG. 27. Comparison of T2-weighted sagittal SE image (**A**) and GE image (**B**) (30° flip angle). The signal intensity of the degenerating disc is relatively lower than the normal disc on the conventional SE image (A) compared to the GE image (B), where the degenerating disc (*3*) is only slightly less intense than the normal disc. *1*, the outer annulus; *2*, the inner annulus and nucleus; *4*, anterior annulus; *5*, cauda equina; *6*, posterior longitudinal ligament.

disc degeneration. MR is less sensitive than cryomicrotomy or discography in detecting radial tears.

MRI of Degenerative Disc Disease

As a disc degenerates it loses water, fissures develop in the annulus, and the structural integrity of the annulus becomes compromised (Fig. 25). On MRI, these changes are manifested as a decrease in disc space vertical height and decreased signal intensity on T2-weighted image (Fig. 26). Diffuse disc bulging may or may not be present. The loss of signal intensity is more apparent on T2-weighted SE images than in T2*-weighted images, because GE images are more sensitive to the presence of water (Fig. 27). In severe disc degeneration, the disc is collapsed, and often contains gas (believed to be nitrogen), which is difficult to see with MR. Gas may be better seen on T2*-weighted GE images because of signal intensity loss related to magnetic susceptibility effects. However, CT remains the procedure of choice to detect gas in a degenerating facet or disc (Fig. 28).

Another characteristic of disc degeneration (also known as intervertebral osteochondrosis) is alterations of the adjacent vertebral body architecture (Fig. 29). Affected vertebrae show increased density ("discogenic sclerosis") on radiographs and CT. The MR appearance of degenerative discogenic vertebral changes has been classified (20). Type I endplate changes represent vascularized marrow and are seen as low signal intensity on T1-weighted images and high signal intensity on T2-weighted images (Fig. 28). Type II changes represent more chronic discogenic disease with proliferation of fatty marrow in the vertebral body adjacent to the degenerating disc and are characterized by high signal intensity

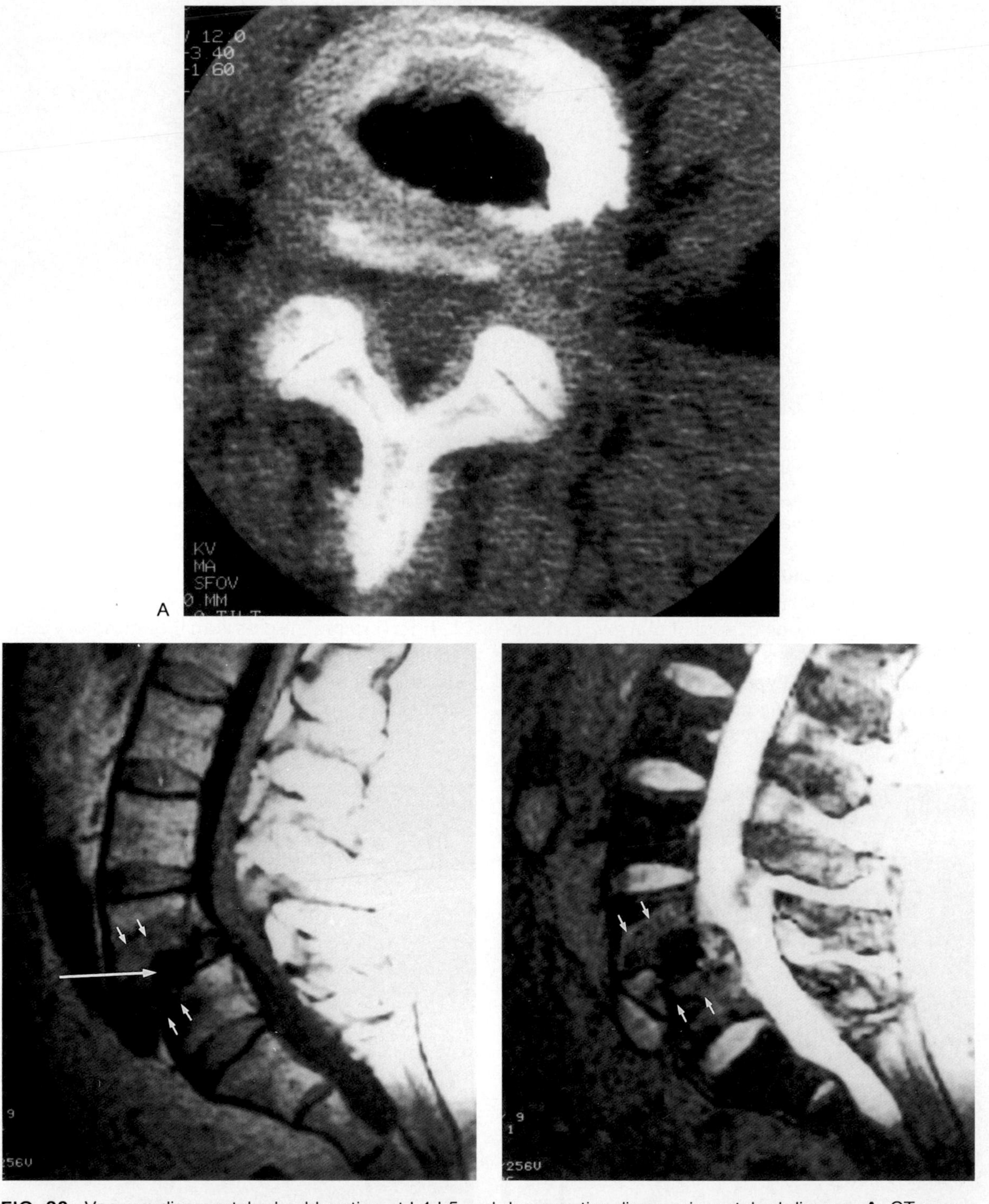

FIG. 28. Vacuum disc, vertebral subluxation at L4-L5 and degenerative discogenic vertebral disease. **A:** CT scan demonstrates gas in the L4-L5 intervertebral disc. Sagittal T1-weighted SE image (**B**) and GE image (**C**) demonstrate gas (*long arrow*) in the L4-L5 disc, and has low signal intensity. Type I degenerative vertebral disease (*small arrows*) are seen in the adjacent vertebrae. Note anterior subluxation of L4 on L5.

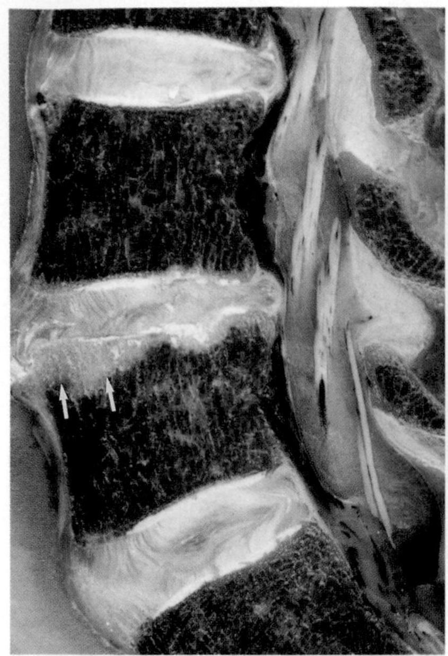

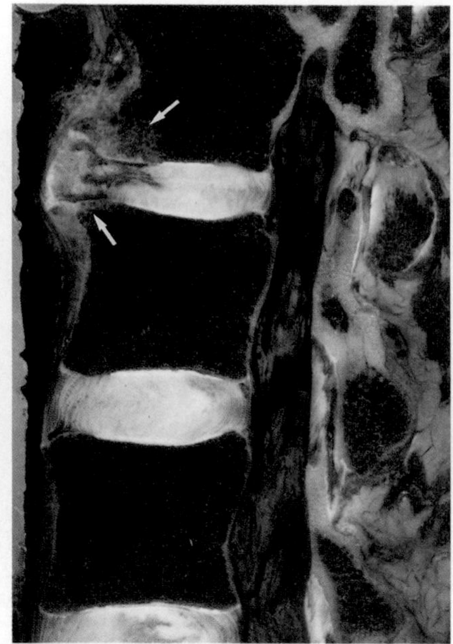

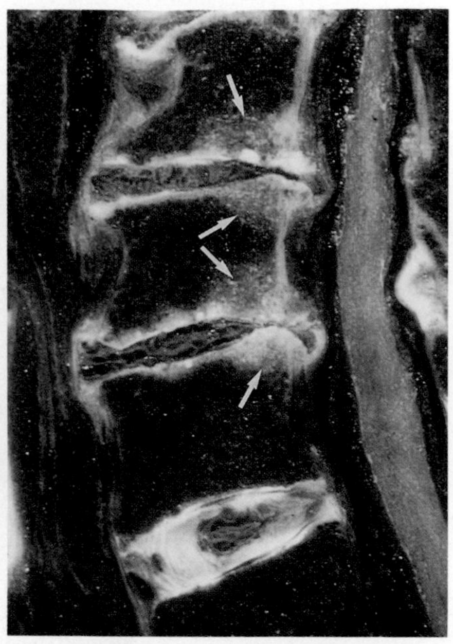

A B,C

FIG. 29. Vertebral marrow and endplate changes associated with degenerative disc disease. In the vertebrae adjacent to a degenerating L4-L5 disc (**A**), fatty degeneration (*arrows*) is noted in the marrow. A different type of reaction characterized by fibrosis and hyperemia of the marrow (*arrows*) is noted adjacent to another degenerating intervertebral disc with a radial tear (**B**). Sclerosis of the adjacent vertebral endplates (*arrows*) is illustrated by this anatomic section through the cervical spine (**C**).

on T1-weighted images and isointense or slightly hyperintense on T2-weighted images (Fig. 30). Type III changes represent dense bone devoid of marrow, and are dark on T1-weighted images and T2-weighted images. The vertebral endplates in Type I or II may enhance with Gd-DTPA and must not be confused with the endplate enhancement that is commonly seen with disc infection.

Intervertebral Disc Infection

Intervertebral discitis is an inflammatory condition resulting in disc and vertebral endplate destruction and usually osteomyelitis in the adjacent vertebral bodies. In adults, the process is caused by infection that initially involves the cancellous bone adjacent to the vertebral end-

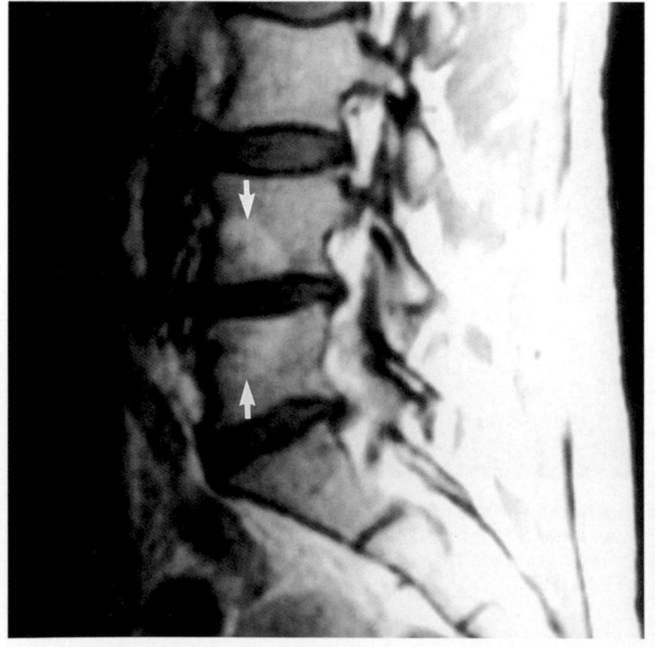

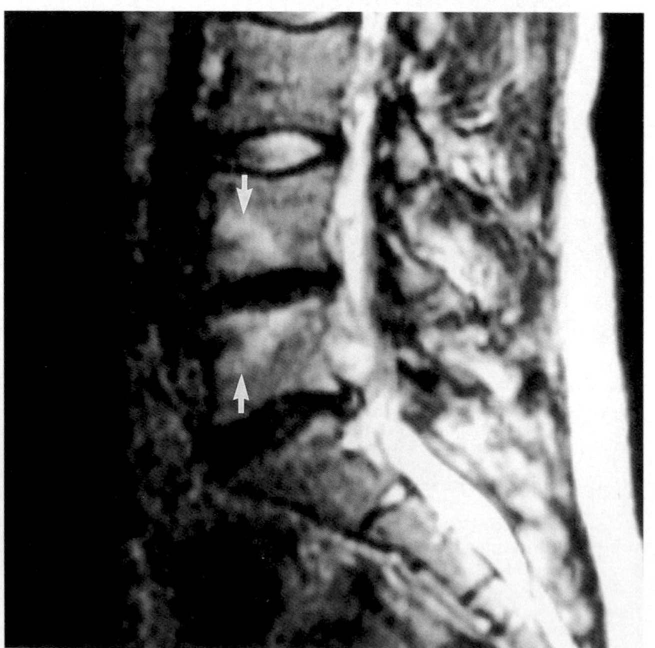

A B

FIG. 30. Type II discogenic vertebral disease. The distorted vertebral architecture (*arrows*) has high intensity on T1-weighted (**A**) and T2-weighted (**B**) SE images. Loss of signal intensity in the intervertebral disc at L4-L5 and L5-S1 indicates disc degeneration.

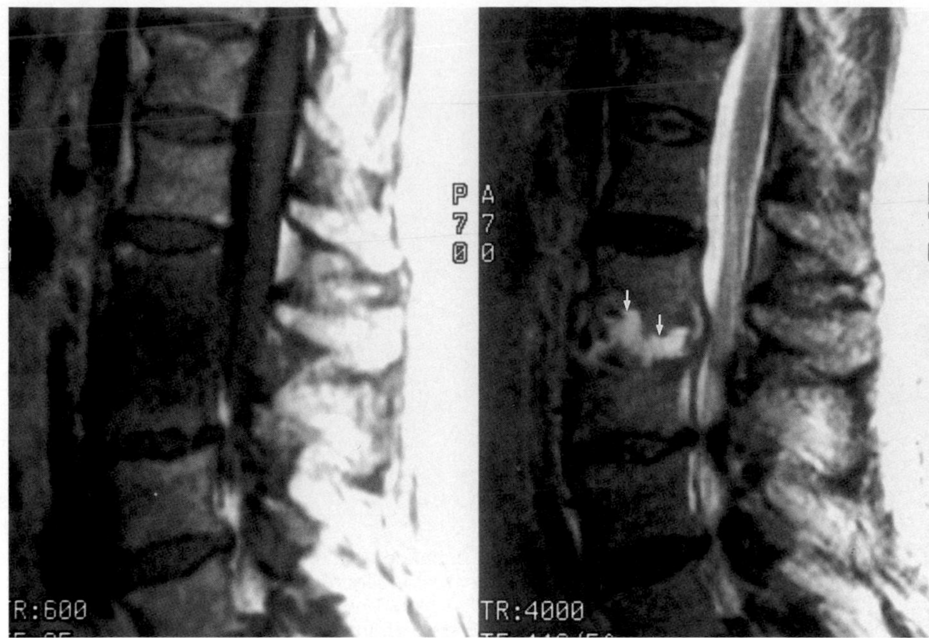

A,B

FIG. 31. L2-L3 disc space infection and osteomyelitis. The vertebral endplates are destroyed and the adjacent vertebral bodies have abnormal signal intensity secondary to osteomyelitis on T1-weighted sagittal SE image (**A**) and T2-weighted FSE image (**B**). The infected disc space (*small arrows*) has higher intensity than normal intervertebral disc.

plate; as the endplate is destroyed the disc is destroyed and fluid accumulates in the disc space. A paraspinal mass is often present at the affected level, but 25% have other disc levels involved also.

On T1-weighted images, the vertebral body endplates in discitis are hypointense and sometimes slightly hyperintense and the endplate cortex is destroyed (Fig. 31). The signal intensity within the disc is decreased on T1-weighted images, but is almost always increased on T2-weighted images (Fig. 31). This is an important differential diagnostic point, because in uncomplicated degenerative discogenic disease, the intervertebral disc has low signal intensity (30). Vertebral osteomyelitis, seen as high signal intensity on T2-weighted images, often enhances intensely with Gd-DTPA (Fig. 32). Endplate enhancement due to degenerative disease tends to be more subtle unless a fat-suppression technique is used. The intervertebral disc itself typically enhances intensely in discitis unless the disc space contains fluid sequestered from the contrast agent (Figs. 33 and 34). An inflammatory paraspinal and peridiscal mass usually accompanies discitis, and the paraspinal mass enhances with Gd-DTPA. In chronic osteomyelitis and discitis, the disc space can be totally obliterated.

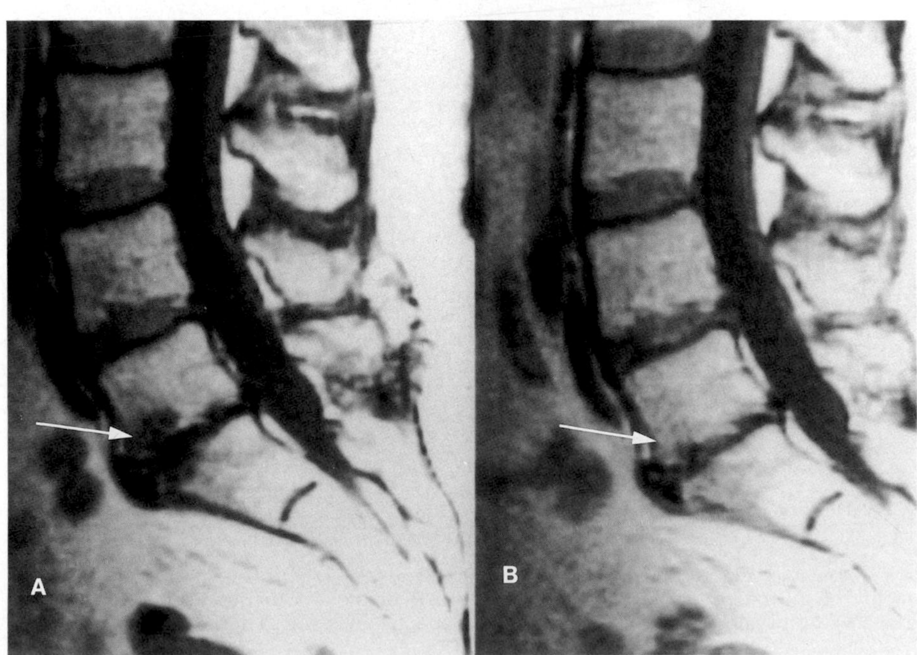

FIG. 32. Enhancing degenerative endplate disease. Unenhanced image (**A**) shows low signal intensity (*arrow*) in the vertebral bodies adjacent to the degenerating L5-S1 disc. Gadolinium-enhanced image (**B**) shows subtle enhancement in the adjacent endplates and vertebral body, but no appreciable enhancement of the intervertebral disc itself.

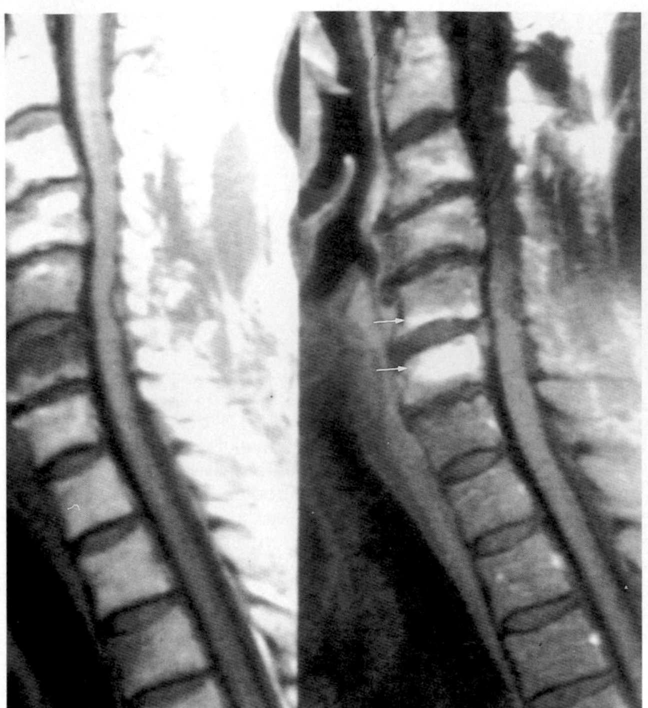

A,B

FIG. 33. Intense enhancement of vertebral endplates and vertebral bodies adjacent to degenerating disc at C5-C6. Unenhanced image (**A**) shows low signal intensity in the vertebral bodies adjacent to the C5-C6 disc. **B:** Intense enhancement (*arrows*) in C5 and C6 vertebral bodies adjacent to the disc is accentuated by fat-suppression technique. The intervertebral disc endplates appear intact.

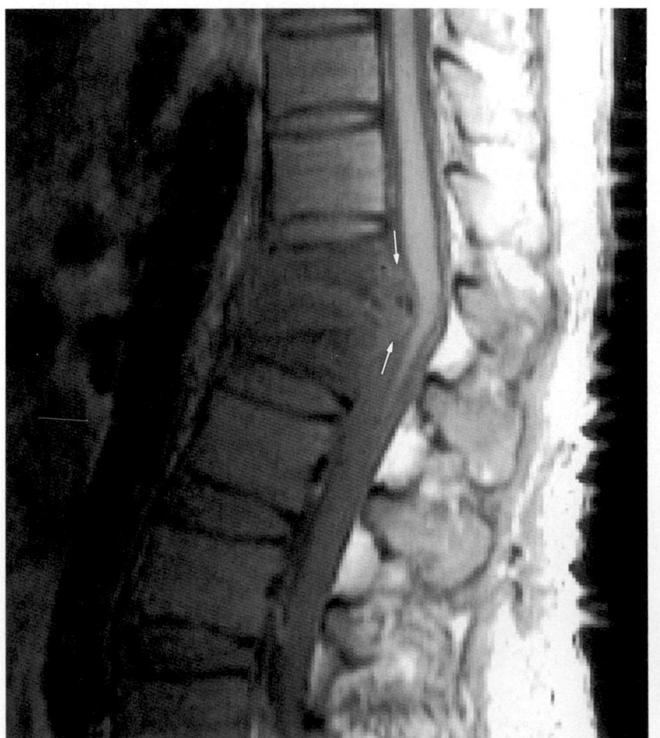

A

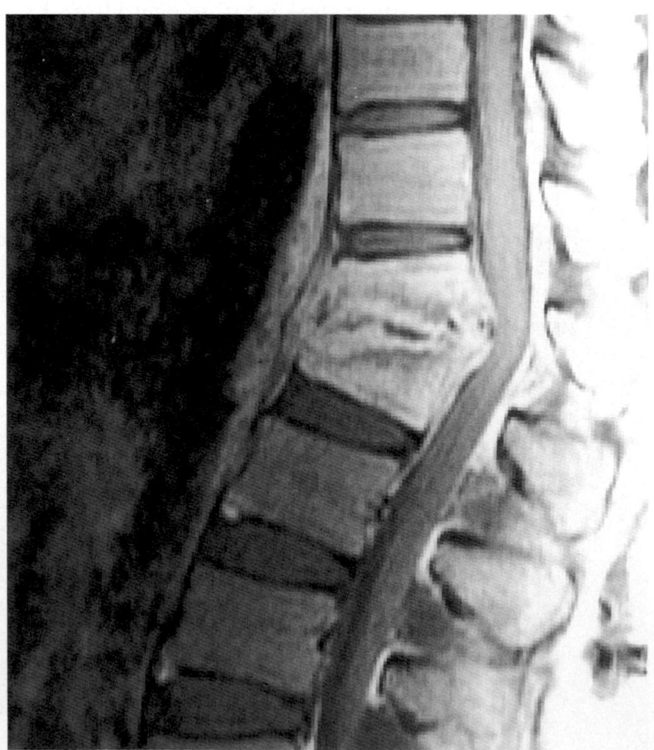

B

FIG. 34. Disc space infection, osteomyelitis, and epidural abscess (*arrows*, **A**) at T12-L1 level compresses the conus medullaris. Note intense enhancement in **B** of the vertebral bodies and vertebral endplates. A thin dark band of nonenhancement at the disc space level in B probably represents fluid in the disc space that is sequestered from the blood supply.

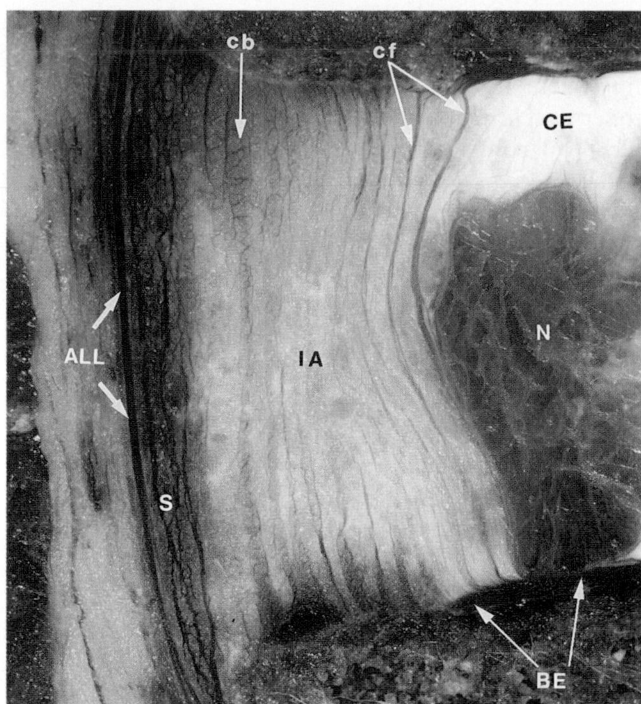

FIG. 35. Sagittal cryomicrotome image through anterior portion of the L4-L5 intervertebral disc demonstrating nucleus pulposus (*N*), inner annulus (*IA*), and cartilaginous endplate (*CE*); vertically oriented annular fibers are called concentric fibers. These are joined by oblique and transverse collagen bridges (*cb*). Densely compacted outer collagen fibers (*cf*) are called Sharpey's fibers (*S*). ALL, anterior longitudinal ligament. *BE*, vertebral body endplate.

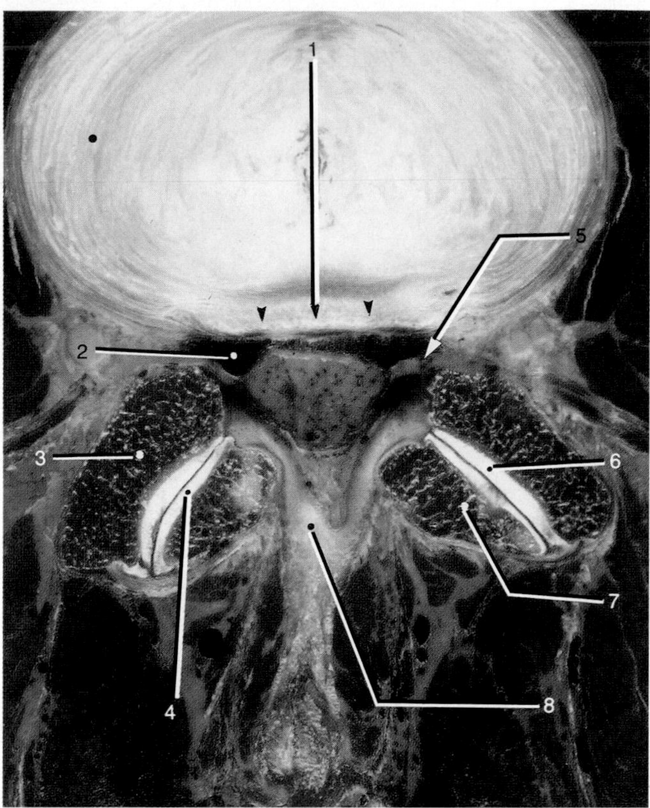

FIG. 36. Axial cryomicrotome section through L3-L4 disc. The disc bulges diffusely in all directions and has a flattened or slightly convex posterior margin (*1*). *2*, anterior epidural venous space; *3*, superior articular process of L4; *4*, inferior articular cartilage of L3; *5*, nerve root; *6*, superior articular cartilage L4; *7*, inferior articular process; *8*, ligamentum flavum.

CLASSIFICATION OF DISC HERNIATION

The terms used to describe bulging and herniated discs are somewhat confusing and are widely misused. It is important to understand a morphologic definition of the various stages of disc herniation and then to adopt a practical working definition for reporting purposes. A widely accepted structural classification (31,32) is as follows:

1. *Bulging disc.* A bulging disc represents a disc that extends diffusely beyond the adjacent vertebral body margins in all directions. This is probably due to tears that have occurred in the oblique collagen bridges between the concentric annular fibers (Fig. 35), producing diffuse laxity of the annulus. The concentric annular fibers remain intact (Fig. 36). The MR appearance of disc bulging is symmetric extension of the outer disc margin circumferentially (Fig. 37).

2. *Protruding disc.* The term "protruding disc" has been used to mean anything from a bulging disc, which one could say "protrudes" diffusely to a herniated disc, which "protrudes" focally. A better term for this category would be "intra-annular protrusion" (32). I consider two subcategories: (a) *Inner annular disruption*

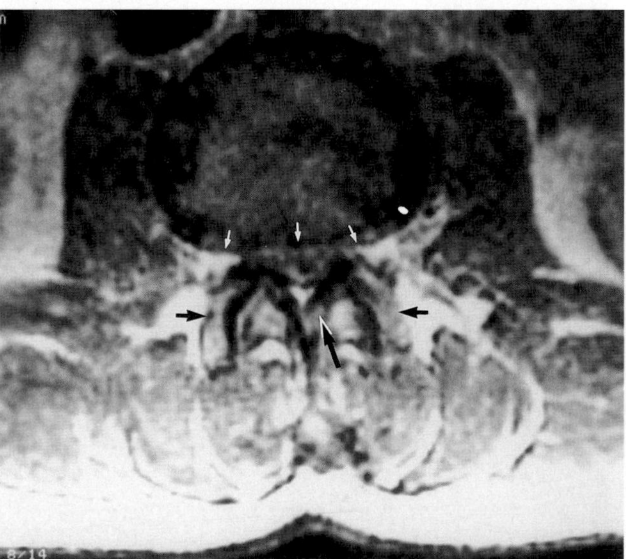

FIG. 37. Diffusely bulging disc and central spinal canal stenosis. The disc margin (*small white arrows*) bulges in all directions symmetrically. Bilateral facet hypertrophy (*small black arrows*) and thickening of the ligamentum flavum (*larger black arrow*) all contribute to produce moderate central canal stenosis.

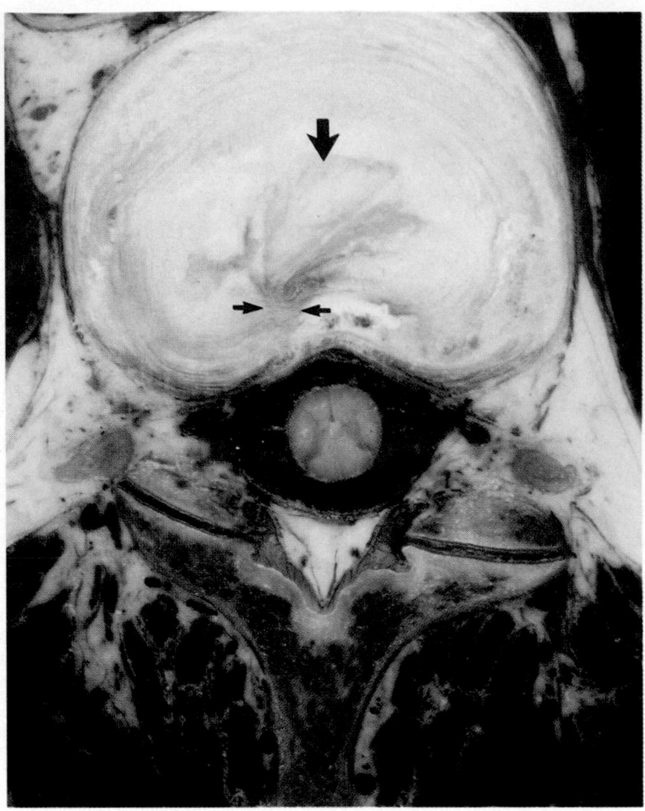

FIG. 38. Anatomic section, disc protrusion. The nuclear material (*large arrow*) protrudes through a defect in the inner annulus (*small arrows*) but does not extend through the outer annular fibers.

(Fig. 38). This is similar to the term "intradiscal mass displacement," which represents a shift in the location of nuclear material within the disc due to ruptures in the innermost fibers of the annulus. This causes no appreciable focal contour abnormality of the disc margin on MRI; (b) *Subtotal annular disruption.* In this situation there is displacement of nuclear and inner annular material through a defect (radial tear) involving the inner annular fibers and some outer annular fibers. However, a few overlying outer annular fibers remain intact. On MRI, this causes a tiny focal abnormality of the disc margin and may be associated with localized or referred pain. Based on MRI alone, it is difficult or impossible to differentiate a small herniated disc that has extended through the inner annulus from a small herniated disc that has penetrated all layers of the annulus, because either may produce a small focal contour abnormality along the posterior disc margin (Fig. 39). It is likely that many so-called midline bulging discs represent annular disc protrusions. The term "prolapsed disc" is often used synonymously with protruding disc or herniated disc, and therefore its use should probably be avoided.

3. *Extruded disc.* This is a true herniated disc that has extended through all layers of the annulus and appears as a focal epidural mass obscuring the epidural fat. The term "herniated nucleus pulposus" is widely used but is actually a misnomer because the herniated disc material often contains not only the nuclear material but also portions of the annulus and even the cartilaginous endplate.

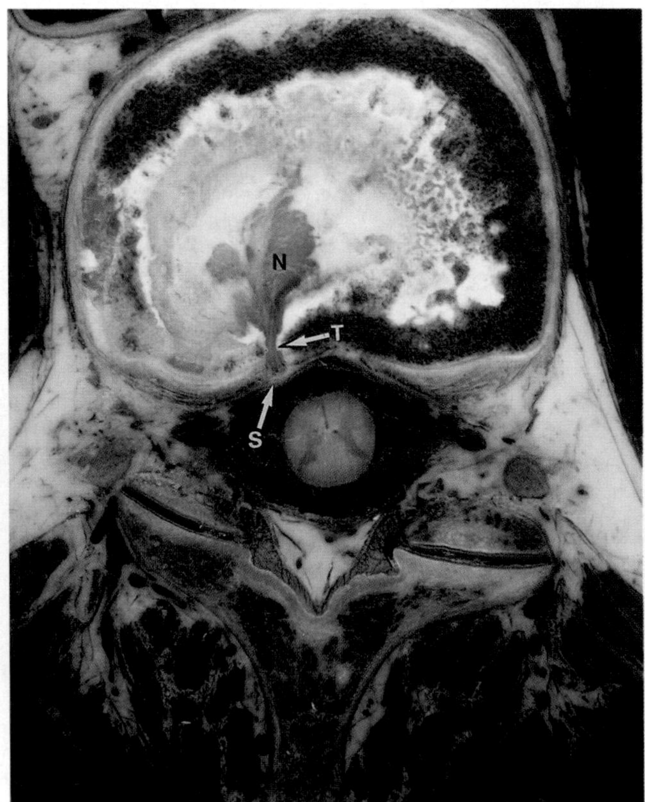

A

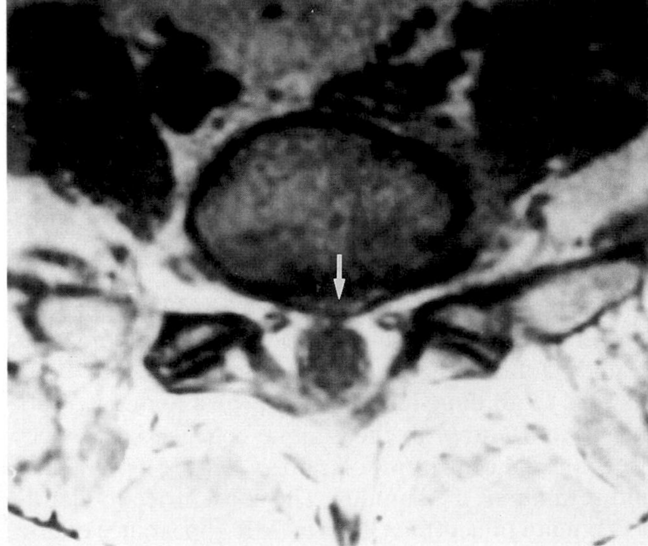

B

FIG. 39. Anatomic section showing partial annular disruption. Nuclear material (*N*) extends through a radial tear (*T*) in the posterior annulus on the right. **A:** Some overlying Sharpe's fibers (*S*) remain intact in axial cryomicrotome. **B:** An axial T1-weighted SE image. There is a small focal protrusion of disc material centered slightly to the left of midline at the L5-S1 level in a patient. It is difficult to say whether this represents a "protruding disc" with some outer annular fibers intact or a true "extruded disc," which has extended through all layers of the annulus.

True extruded discs may lie either anterior or posterior to the PLL or both. Extruded discs that lie anterior to the posterior longitudinal ligament are often termed "subligamentous" herniations. The term "extruded disc" is sometimes erroneously used to indicate a free disc fragment.

4. *Free disc fragment (sequestered disc).* A free disc fragment is one that is no longer in continuity with the parent disc material. The free fragment may lie at the disc level either anterior or posterior to the PLL or can migrate inferiorly or less commonly superiorly to the parent disc level. Rarely, free disc fragments may extend into the thecal sac and then represent true intradural disc herniations.

Because it is not always possible to apply the above anatomic classification to image interpretation, it is reasonable to adopt a simplified classification for reporting. A *bulging disc* refers only to generalized or diffuse disc bulging and can be modified by the terms mild, moder-

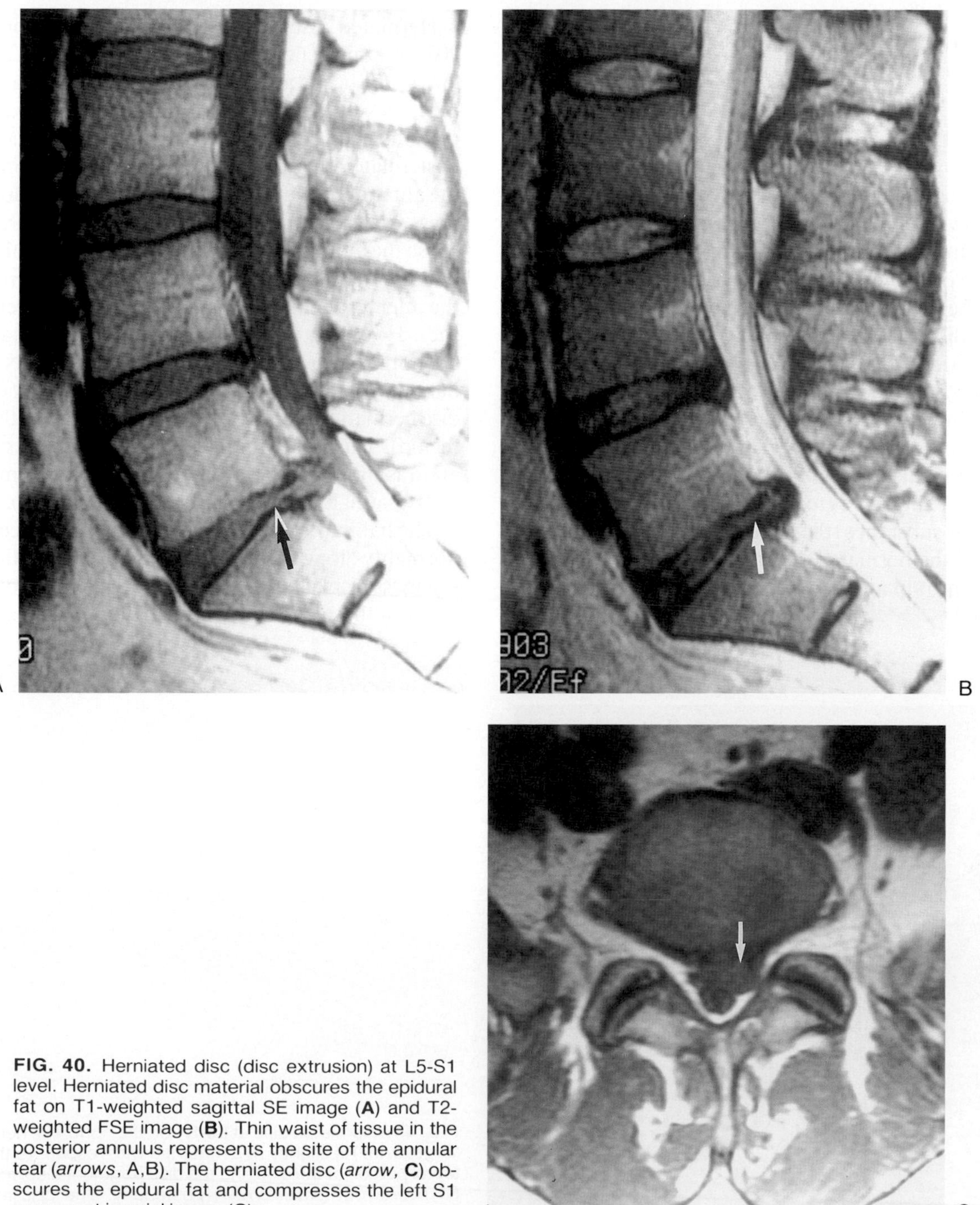

FIG. 40. Herniated disc (disc extrusion) at L5-S1 level. Herniated disc material obscures the epidural fat on T1-weighted sagittal SE image (**A**) and T2-weighted FSE image (**B**). Thin waist of tissue in the posterior annulus represents the site of the annular tear (*arrows*, A,B). The herniated disc (*arrow*, **C**) obscures the epidural fat and compresses the left S1 nerve root in axial image (C).

ate, or severe, depending on the degree of disc bulging. A *herniated disc* by convention causes a focal contour abnormality along the disc margin. The disc fragment size should be further characterized into small, medium, or large. The relationship of the disc fragment to surrounding structures should also be mentioned in describing a herniated disc. It is also important to describe the precise location of the disc fragment in relation to the PLL and whether or not the disc fragment has migrated superior or inferior to the disc space level. The term "herniated nucleus pulposus" is thoroughly entrenched in the literature, and is somewhat of a misnomer because the herniated disc fragment typically contains components of nuclear and annular material and sometimes even portions of the cartilaginous endplate.

LUMBAR DISC HERNIATION

The etiology of disc herniation in the lumbar spine is still unknown, but certainly degenerative disc disease, repeated trauma, and genetic factors have been implicated. Even more obscure is the etiology of the pain associated with disc herniation. While mechanical pressure of the herniated disc on the nerves is certainly an important factor, this does not explain all symptoms in every case (33). Lindahl has shown that pressure on normal nerves is insufficient to cause pain unless the nerves are already hypersensitive to pain (34). Inflammation caused by release of chemicals or metabolites when the disc herniates may sensitize the nerves to pain (35,36). Since the disc is an avascular substance (the largest in the body), the body may regard the herniated disc material as a foreign substance and mount an autoimmune response to it in some cases (37).

Nerve endings are known to exist in the periphery of the annulus, and when cracks develop in the annulus these nerve endings may be irritated, causing low back pain (38) . Stretching of the PLL by bulging or herniated discs has been implicated as a cause of low back pain and referred pain. Instability of the spine with movement at the facet joints eventually develops because of degenerative disc disease, and undoubtedly plays a major role in causing low back pain and sciatica.

MRI of Herniated Lumbar Discs

Herniated discs are rare in children. Approximately 90% of lumbar herniated discs occur at L4-L5 or L5-S1 levels; 7% occur at the L3-L4 level and 3% at L1-L2 or L2-L3 levels (39). The vast majority of lumbar disc herniations extend through defects in the posterior annulus posterolaterally or in the midline. Herniations through the anterior annulus also occur, but usually do not compress vital structures and are less common, probably because the annulus is thicker anteriorly. Virtually all lumbar disc herniations are associated with degeneration of the intervertebral portion of the disc on T1-weighted images. However, the vast majority of degenerating discs are not associated with disc herniation (40). Normal signal intensity on T2-weighted images virtually excludes a disc herniation (this is not necessarily true in the cervical region). This signal intensity loss reflecting disc degeneration is more apparent on T2-weighted SE images than on T2*-weighted GE images (41) (see Fig. 27).

The hallmark of a herniated disc is a focal contour abnormality along the posterior disc margin with a soft tissue mass displacing the epidural fat, nerve root, epidural veins, or thecal sac. The herniated disc material is usually

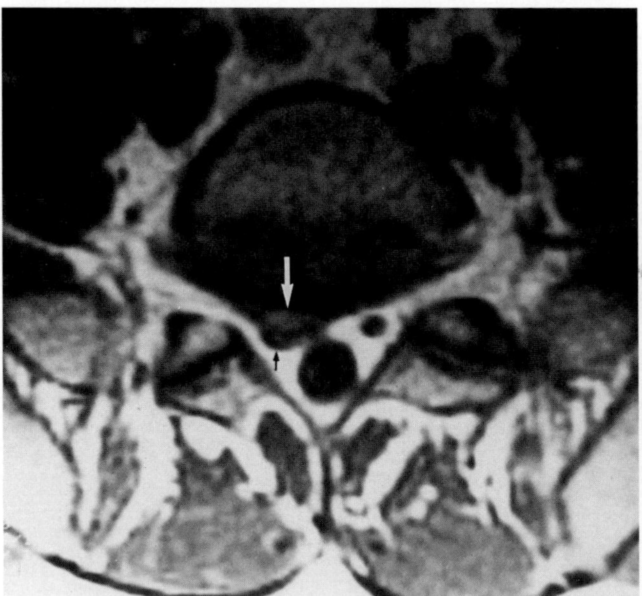

FIG. 41. Herniated disc at L5-S1 on the right. The herniated disc (*large arrow*) is slightly hyperintense with respect to the intervertebral portion of the disc and the disc fragment displaces the right S1 nerve root (*small arrow*) posteriorly. The disc material obscures the epidural fat normally seen anterior to the nerve root.

contiguous with the intervertebral portion of the disc by a narrow waist, which is the site of a radial tear in the annulus (Fig. 40). Midline, posterolateral, and lateral disc herniations are well seen on T1-weighted images because of displacement of high signal intensity fat in the epidural space or foramen. Fat displacement is an especially important sign in the evaluation of small disc herniations (Fig. 41).

MR not only provides morphologic information, but also improves visualization of disc herniations because of better soft tissue contrast of MR relative to CT. On T1-weighted images, the herniation appears isointense or slightly hyperintense relative to the intervertebral portion of the disc (see Fig. 37). On T2-weighted images, the herniated portion is typically more intense than the degenerating intervertebral disc (Fig. 42). This may be due to increased water content or granulation tissue infiltrating the disc. On GE images, it is difficult to visualize the herniated disc in the epidural space because the signal intensity of fat and disc material is similar. How-

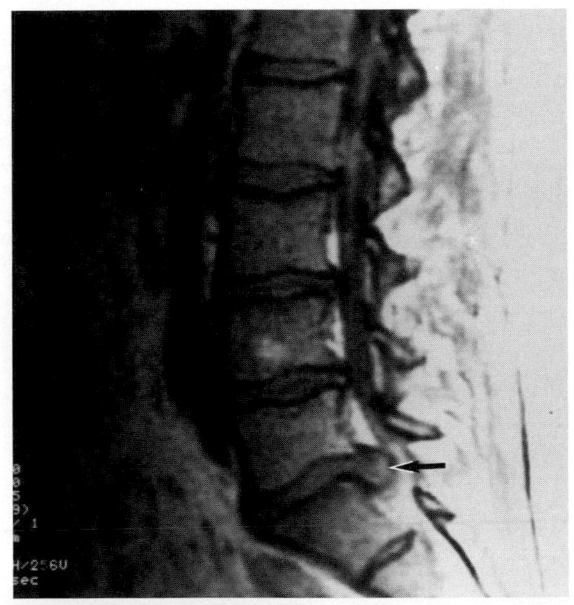
A

FIG. 42. Herniated disc at L5-S1. **A:** There is a large herniated disc (*black arrows*) that displaces the epidural fat in sagittal T1-weighted image. **B:** On GE, the herniated disc (*black arrow*) has high intensity relative to the degenerating intervertebral portion of the disc (*small white arrow*). Degenerating discs (*long arrows*) are also noted at L4-L5 and L5-S1. In axial image (**C**), the herniated disc (*arrows*) has a broad base, and causes significant compression of the thecal sac.

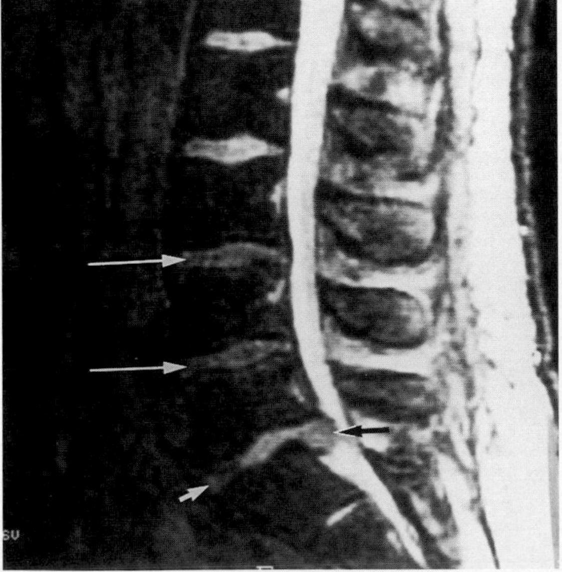
B

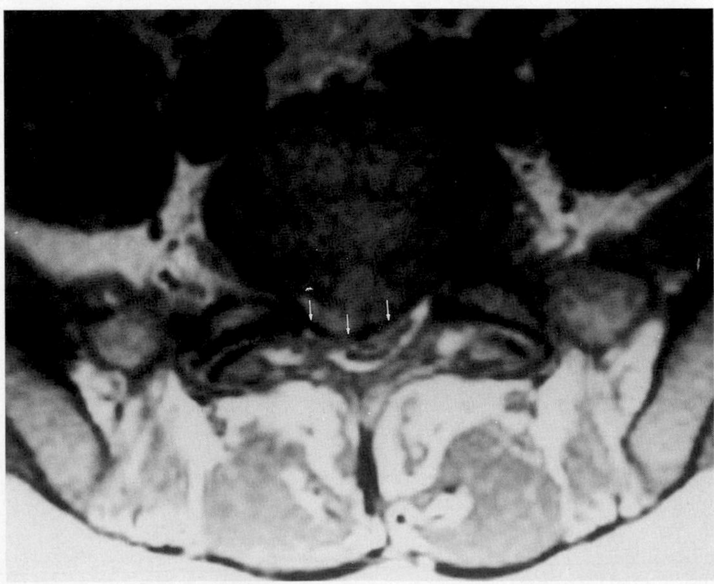
C

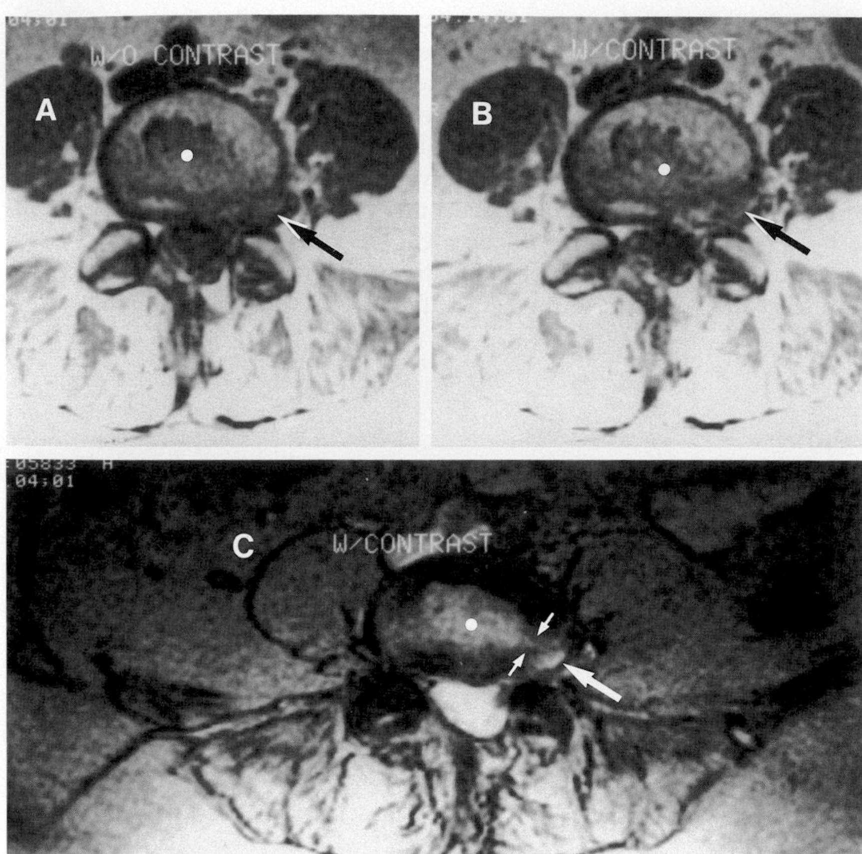

FIG. 43. Lateral disc herniation, axial plane at L3-L4. **A:** In unenhanced axial image the herniated disc (*arrow*) is seen as a soft tissue mass in the neural foramen on the left, which does not enhance with gadolinium (**B,** *arrow*). **C:** T2-weighted GE image at same level demonstrates defect (*small arrows*) in annulus and disc fragment (*large arrow*), which has high signal intensity similar to the intervertebral portion of the disc (*dot*).

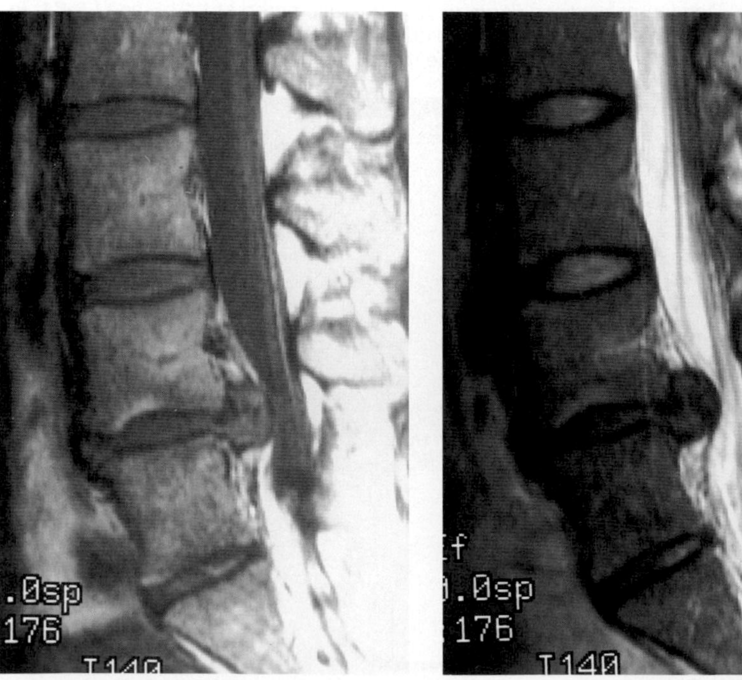
A,B

FIG. 44. Large herniated disc at L4-L5 causing cauda equina syndrome. **A:** Large midline herniated disc fragment compresses the thecal sac at the L4-L5 level obscuring the epidural fat in T1-weighted SE image. **B:** Herniated disc fragment has very low signal intensity on FSE image (TR 4000, effective TE = 102).

ever, annular tears may be better seen with GE sequences (Fig. 43). GE images show bone abnormalities better than do conventional SE images, because normal bone is very dark relative to disc material on T2*-weighted GE images.

FSE sequences are routinely used to evaluate lumbar disc disease. Herniated discs typically have very low signal intensity on sagittal and axial T2-weighted FSE images (Figs. 44 and 45). In some cases, small herniated discs are easier to detect on T1-weighted SE images (Fig. 46).

Nerve root and thecal sac compression are well shown on T1-weighted SE images particularly in the axial plane, which is necessary to show the side of the disc displacement (Fig. 47). Occasionally the nerve root sleeve will have slightly higher signal intensity than normal, possibly indicating an inflammatory response to the disc material (Fig. 48). The nerve root adjacent to the herniated disc may enhance with gadolinium (see below).

MR is very sensitive in detecting *sequestered disc* fragments (40). Sequestered fragments (free fragments) at the disc level in the spinal canal often have the appearance of two distinct fragments (Fig. 49). Herniated discs that

A

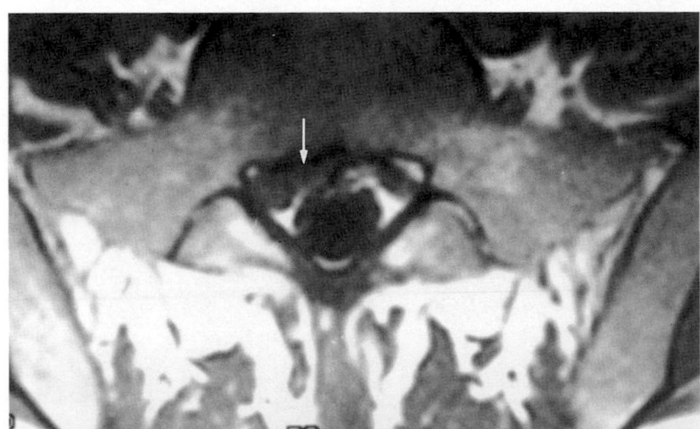

B

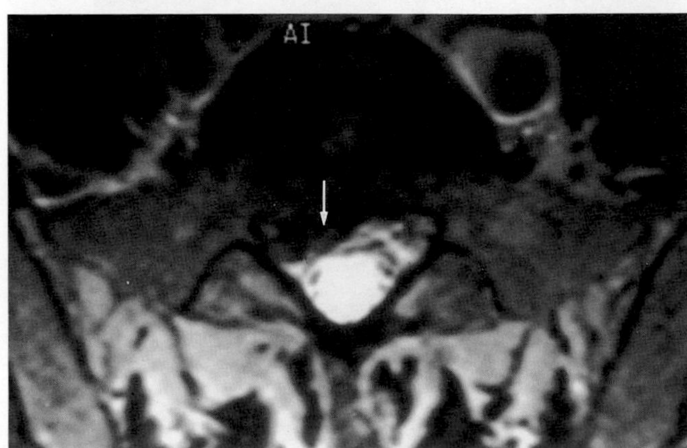

FIG. 45. Herniated disc below L5-S1 disc level on the right. **A:** The herniated disc fragment (*arrow*) obscures the epidural fat medial to the right S1 nerve root. **B:** The herniated disc fragment has very low signal intensity (*arrow*) on FSE image.

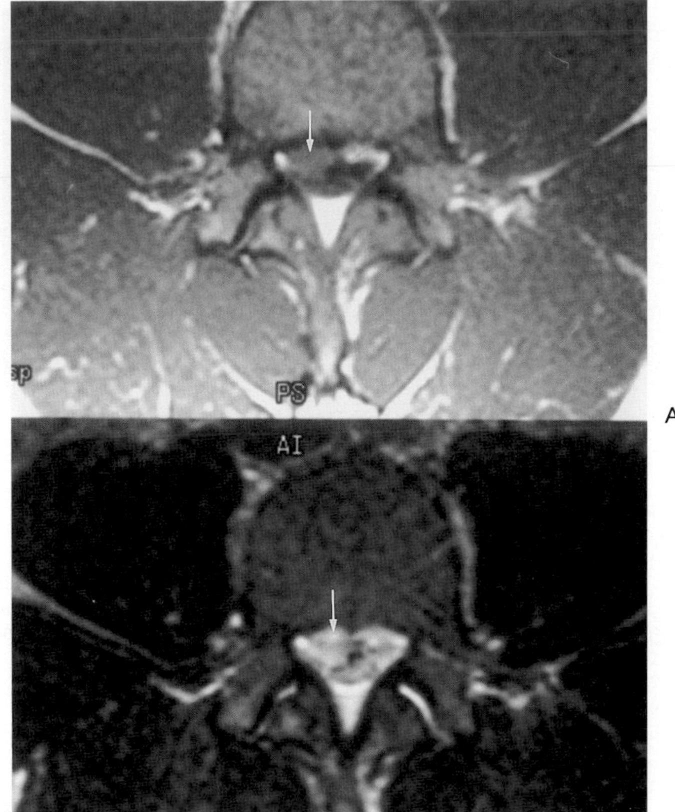

A

B

FIG. 46. Herniated disc (*arrow*) in lateral recess on the right at L4 level is easier to visualize on T1-weighted axial SE image (**A**) compared to FSE image (**B**).

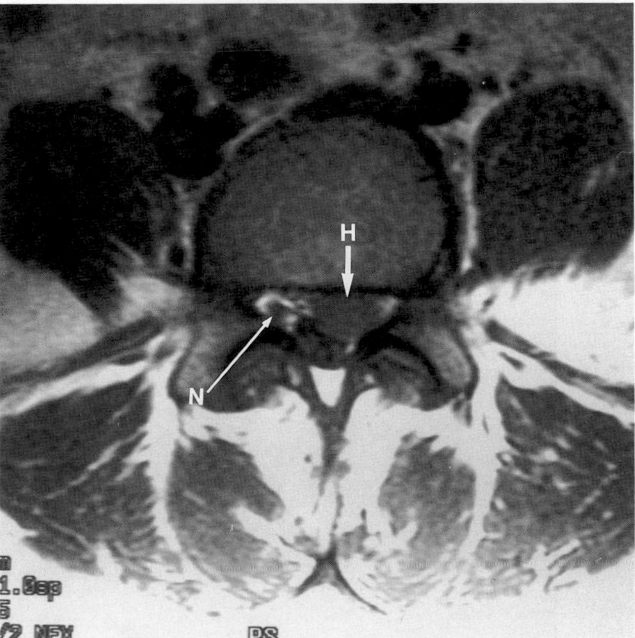

FIG. 47. Herniated disc (*H*) obscures the epidural fat and nerve root on the left above the L4-L5 level. The thecal sac is also deformed ventrally on the left. *N*, normal right L4 nerve root and sheath.

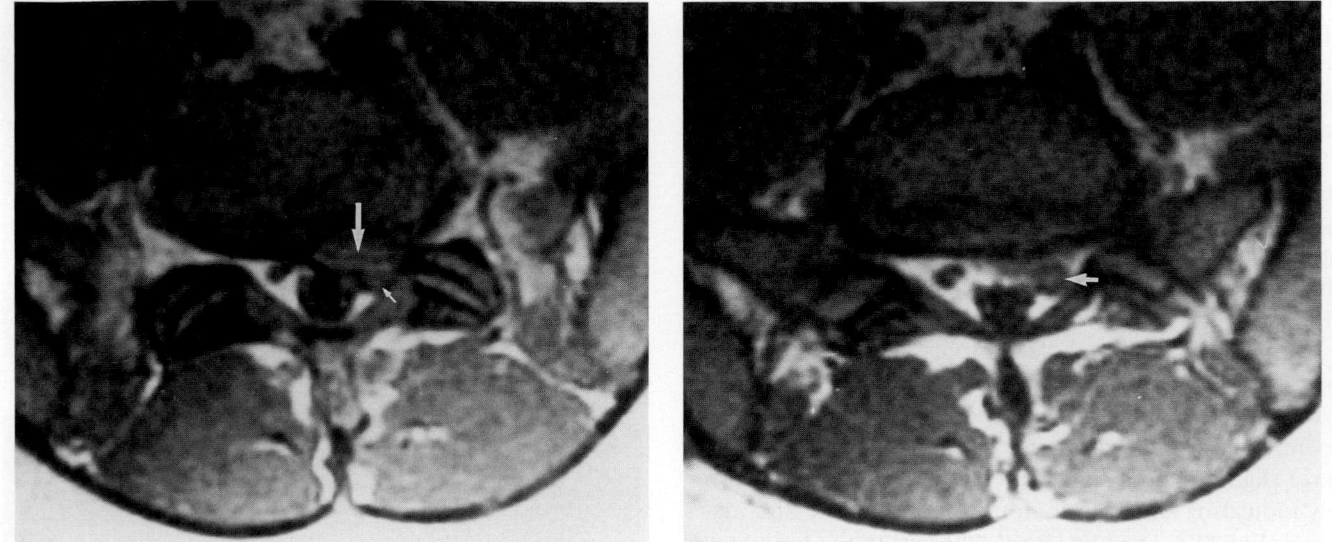

FIG. 48. A: Herniated disc at L4-L5 on the left has higher signal intensity (*long arrow*) than the intervertebral portion of the disc. The disc fragment displaces the left L5 nerve root (*small arrow*) posteriorly. **B:** Below the disc level, the L5 nerve root (*arrow*) is enlarged and slightly hyperintense relative to the right nerve root and sheath.

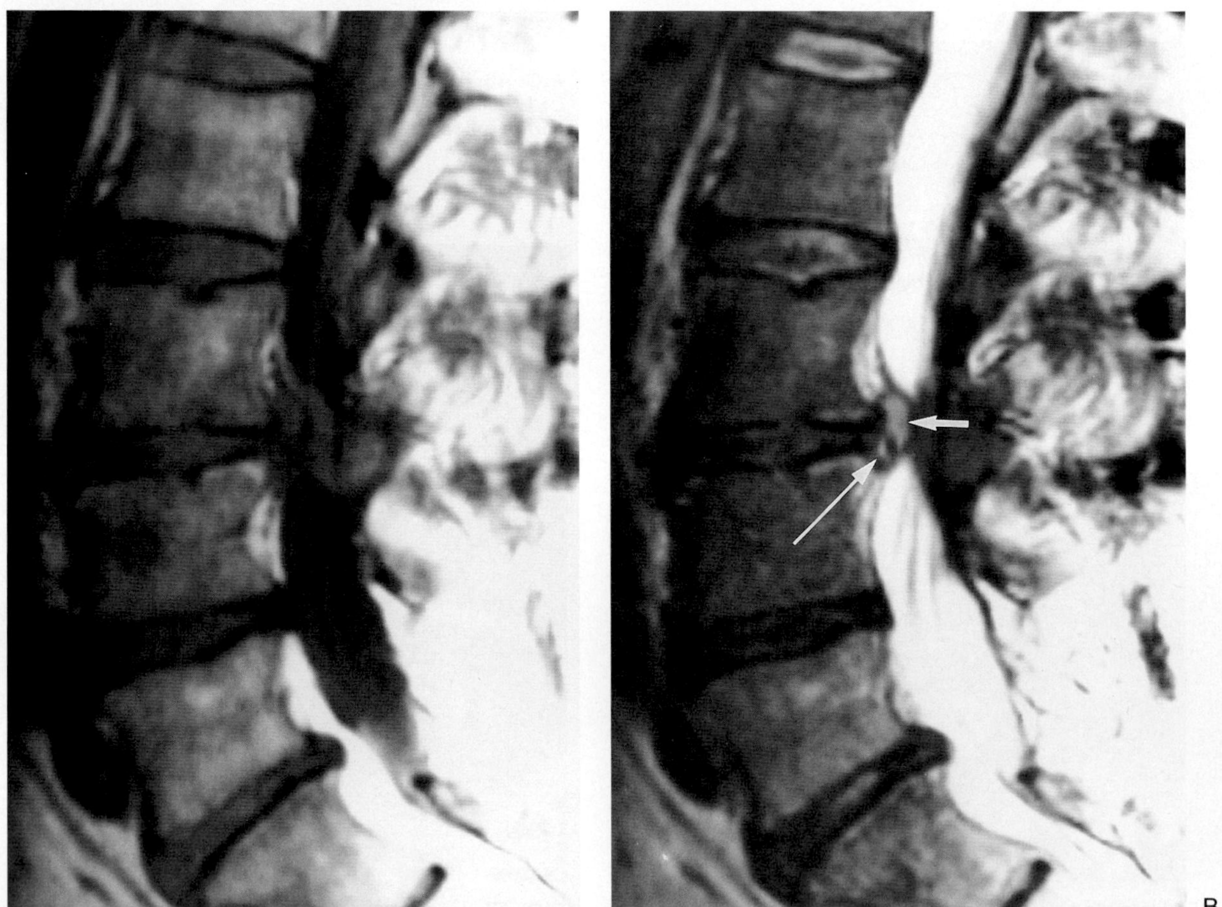

FIG. 49. Sequestered disc fragment at L3-L4 level. **A:** Vague soft tissue mass is seen on the T1-weighted sagittal image. **B:** In T2-weighted image, two discrete fragments (*arrows*) are seen posterior to the disc in the spinal canal. This "double fragment" appearance is a sign of a sequestered disc.

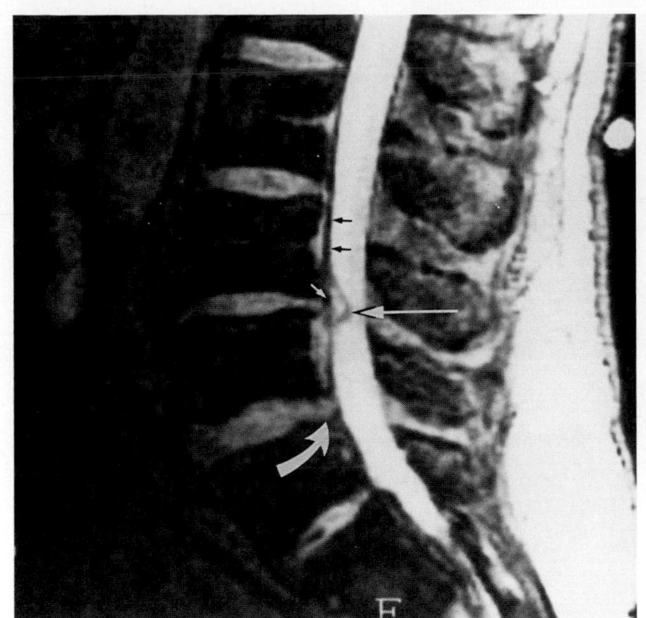

FIG. 50. Free disc fragment in the spinal canal at the L3-L4 level shown in sagittal GE image. The posterior longitudinal ligament (PLL) (*small black arrows*) is displaced posteriorly by the herniated disc. A thin dark line (*small white arrow*) separates the protruding disc fragment from the free fragment more posteriorly (*long white arrow*). A small subligamentous herniation (*curved arrow*) is seen at the L4-L5 level.

penetrate the PLL often represent sequestered fragments (free fragments) and can be diagnosed by a thin dark line between the free fragment and the parent disc, which implies a breech in the PLL (Fig. 50). Not all free disc fragments represent nuclear material; a fragment of the annulus may also be separated from the disc by herniating nuclear material (Fig. 51). Free fragments more commonly migrate inferiorly than superiorly, can be found anterior or posterior to the PLL, and are best seen on sagittal MRI (Fig. 52).

The intradural herniated disc represents a rare type of free fragment that penetrates the dura to reside in the subarachnoid space and is seen as a vague region of increased signal intensity in the spinal canal or in the thecal sac on T1-weighted images (42) (Fig. 53).

Acute traumatic disc herniations can occur anywhere

A,B

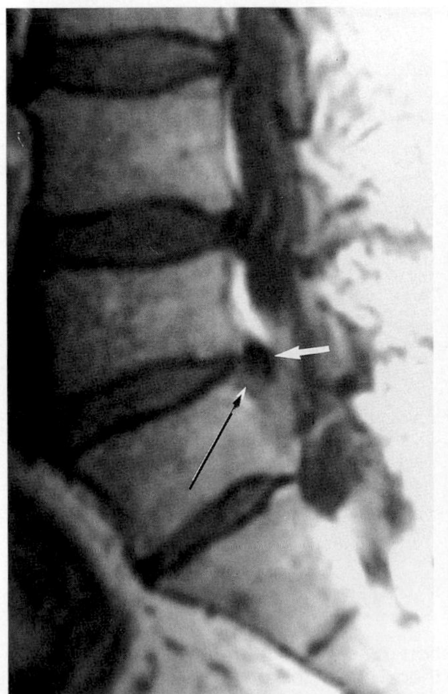

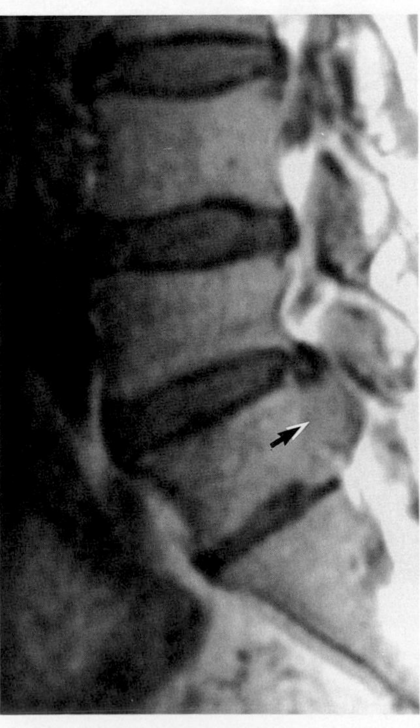

FIG. 51. Parasagittal SE images of herniated disc at the L4-L5 level with an inferiorly migrated fragment (*arrow*, **B**). The fragment has extended to a radial tear (*long arrow*, **A**). A small annular fragment (*white arrow*, **A**) is positioned superior to the annular tear.

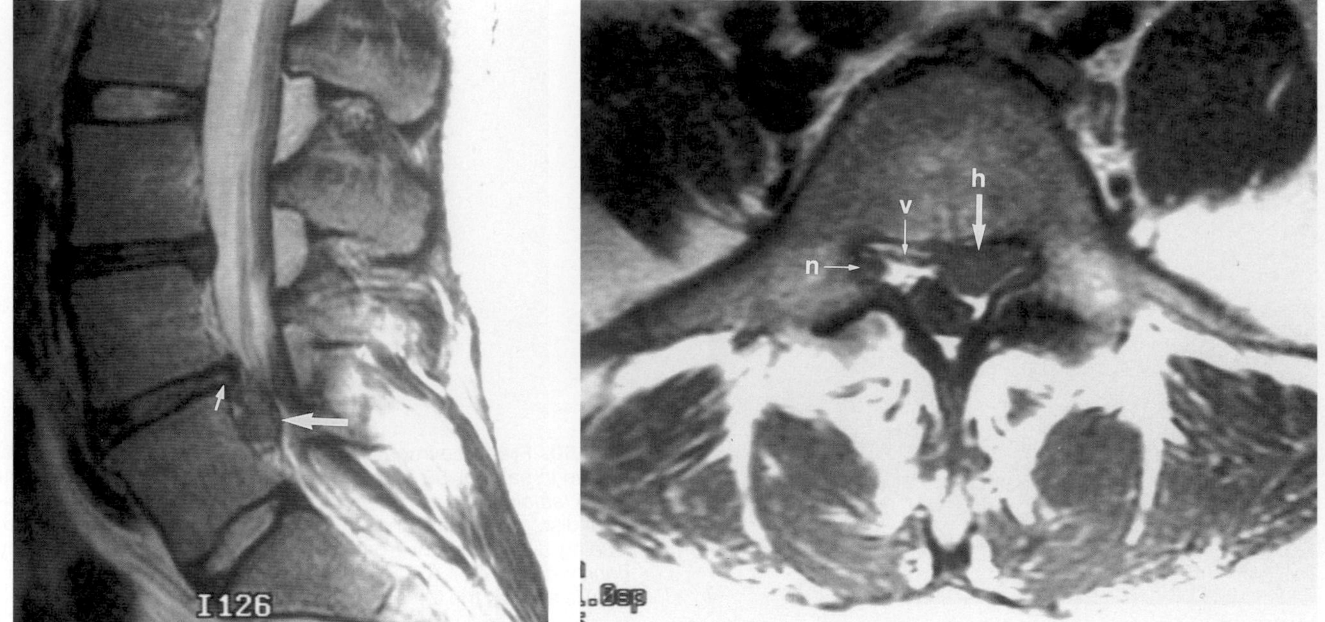

FIG. 52. Herniated disc with inferior migration of disc fragment behind L5 vertebral body. **A:** On sagittal T2-weighted FSE image, a small tear (*small arrow*) is seen in the posterior annulus of the L4-L5 disc. The disc fragment (*large arrow*) is seen behind the L5 vertebral body within the spinal canal. **B:** In axial image, the herniated disc (*h*) is located on the left, and deforms the left ventral aspect of the thecal sac. *v*, epidural veins; *n*, right L5 nerve root/nerve root pouch.

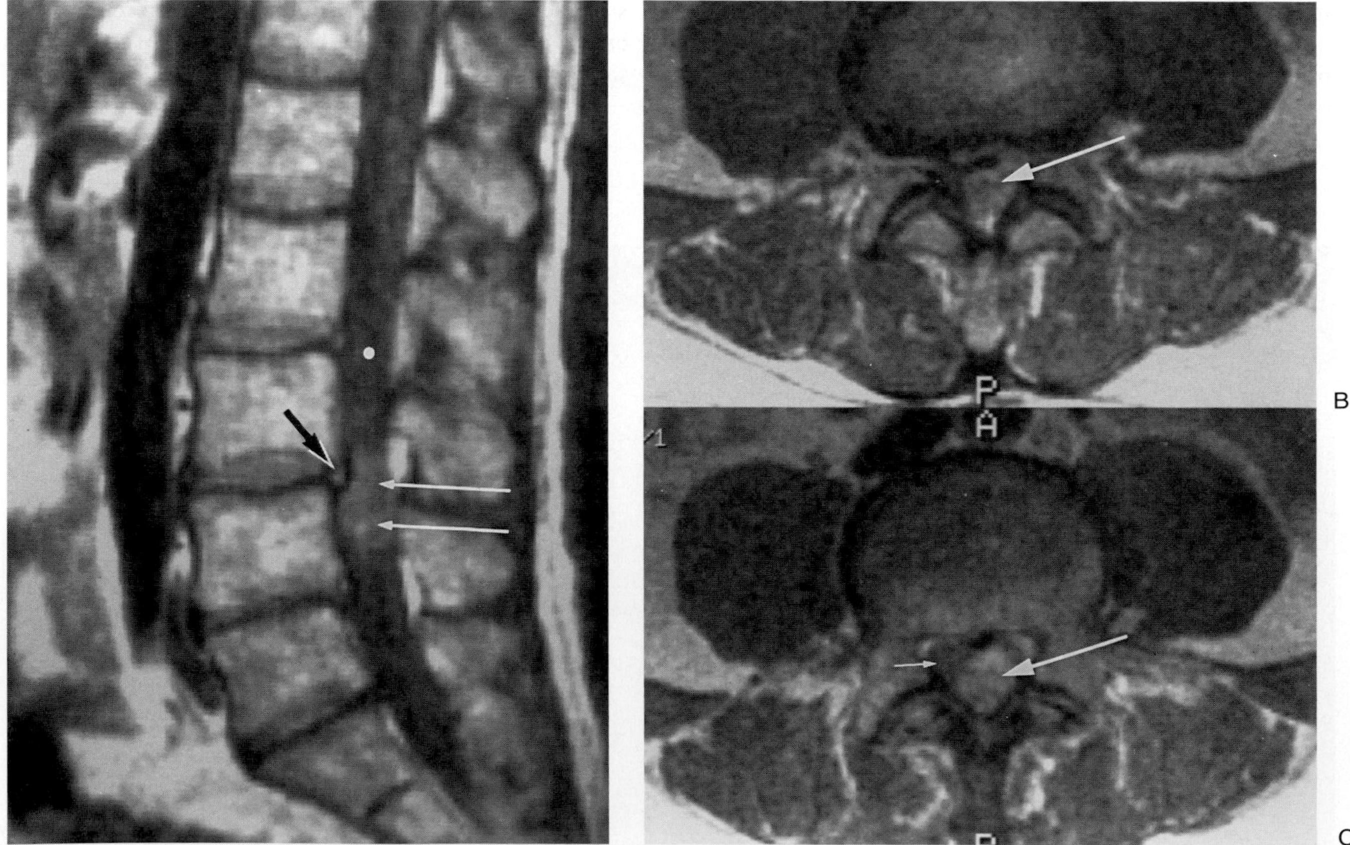

FIG. 53. Intradural disc herniation at L3-L4 level. **A:** A small disc bulge or herniation (*black arrow*) in sagittal T1-weighted image extends from the intervertebral disc. A vague soft tissue mass in the thecal sac at this level represents an intradural disc herniation (*white arrows*). **B,C:** The intradural fragment (*long arrows*) has higher intensity than the CSF (*dot*), and occupies the majority of the spinal canal, displacing the thecal sac (*small arrow,* C) into the right lateral recess. (Case contributed by Brian S. Puglisi, Phoenix, AZ.)

along the spine, and are often associated with spine fracture or subluxation. A migrated disc fragment is typically seen posterior to the subluxed vertebrae (Fig. 54). The limbus vertebra probably represents the sequela of a traumatic herniated disc that extended beneath the ring apophysis early in life.

Lateral disc herniations in the neural foramen often go undetected by myelography, causing minimal or no root pouch deformity; they require CT or MR for detection. Lateral disc fragments compress the exiting nerve roots as they course below the pedicle at a given lumbar disc level. For example, a far lateral disc herniation at the L4-L5 level will produce L4 radiculopathy, whereas a posterolateral disc herniation compressing the thecal sac at the same level causes L5 radiculopathy. MR has advantages over CT for detection of lateral disc herniation (Figs. 43 and 55). In addition to the axial T1-weighted images, which show excellent contrast between

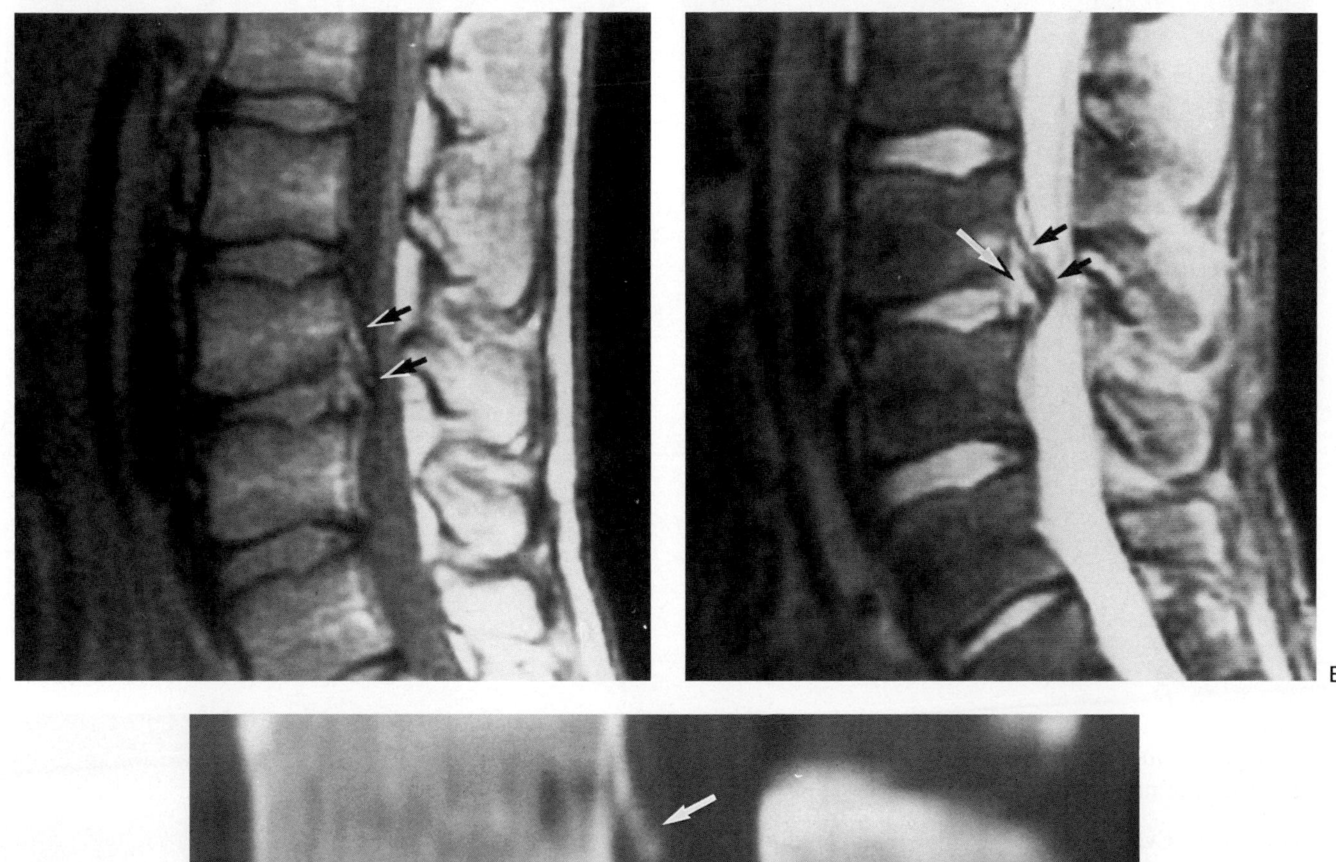

C

FIG. 54. Traumatic disc herniation, vertebral fracture. The ruptured disc and L3 vertebral body fracture (*arrows*) are difficult to differentiate on T1-weighted SE image (**A**). In GE image (**B**) obtained with 30° flip angle, the bone fragment has low signal intensity compared to the CSF and herniated disc fragment (*long arrow*). CT scan (**C**) confirms the displaced fragment of bone (*white arrows*) and correlates well with B. *Black arrows* denote site of bone avulsion from the right apophysis.

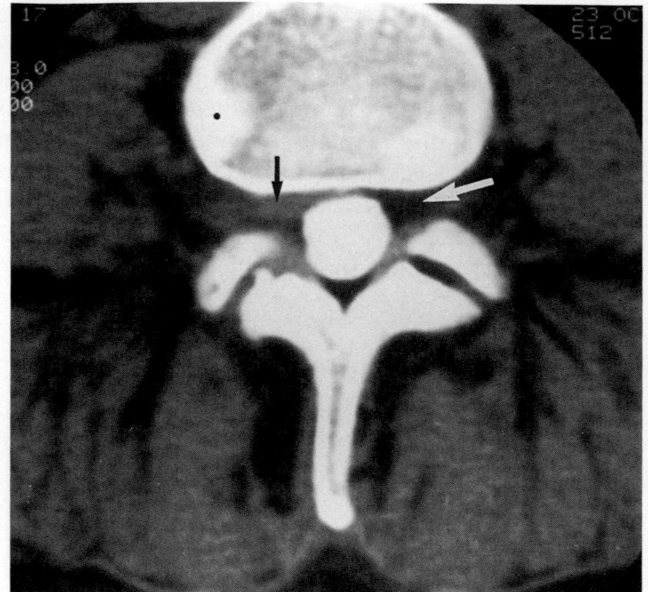

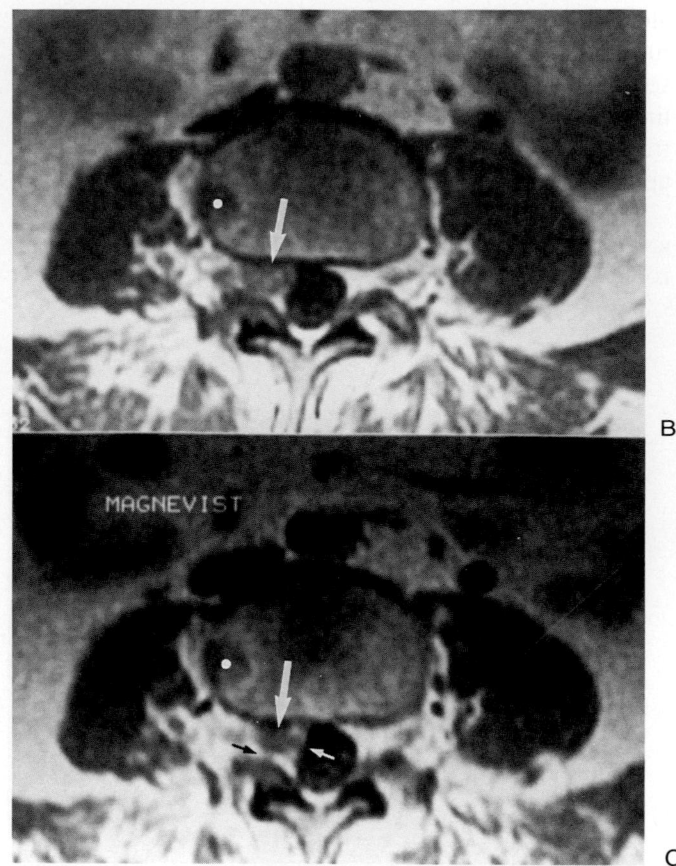

FIG. 55. Herniated disc into medial neural foramen. **A:** Axial CT scan at L3-L4 demonstrates herniated disc material (*black arrow*) obscuring the epidural fat in the medial portion of the neural foramen compared to the normal epidural fat (*white arrow*) on the left. **B:** Unenhanced axial T1-weighted image shows herniated disc (*arrow*) obscuring epidural fat. **C:** The disc fragment (*large white arrow*) does not enhance but there is enhancing tissue (*small black arrow*) posterior to the disc fragment. The thecal sac is compressed (*small white arrow*). A Schmorl's node (*dot*) is sclerotic on the CT scan and has low intensity on the MRI.

the disc material and the fat, sagittal MR T1-weighted SE images through the foramen are valuable for defining the amount of nerve root compression.

Preoperative Evaluation of the Spine with Gadolinium

It is difficult to justify the routine use of paramagnetic contrast agents in the diagnosis of intervertebral disc disease preoperatively. However, there are situations in which gadolinium-enhanced images are valuable: (a) contrast-enhanced scans are clearly indicated for differentiating a lateral disc herniation from a nerve sheath tumor (e.g., schwannoma) in the neural foramen, because both can occupy the lateral recess (Figs. 56 and 57). Lateral disc herniations may cause minimal or no root pouch deformity on myelography and are often difficult to distinguish from a nerve sheath schwannoma by CT. Lateral disc fragments compress the exiting nerve roots in the lateral recess or beneath the pedicle. The neural foramen in the lumbar region is optimally evaluated on sagittal and axial T1-weighted MR scans before and after administration of i.v. gadolinium-DTPA (Fig. 58). The

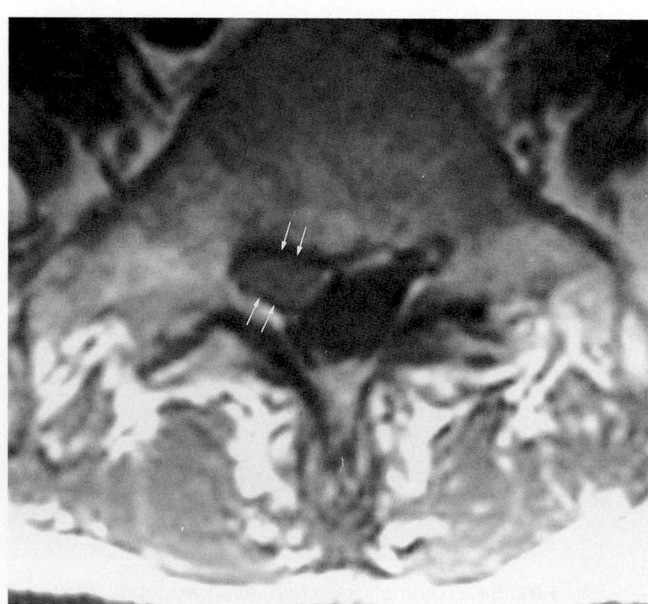

FIG. 56. Herniated disc material causing widening of the right lateral recess (*arrows*) of L5. This appearance may be mistaken for a nerve sheath tumor.

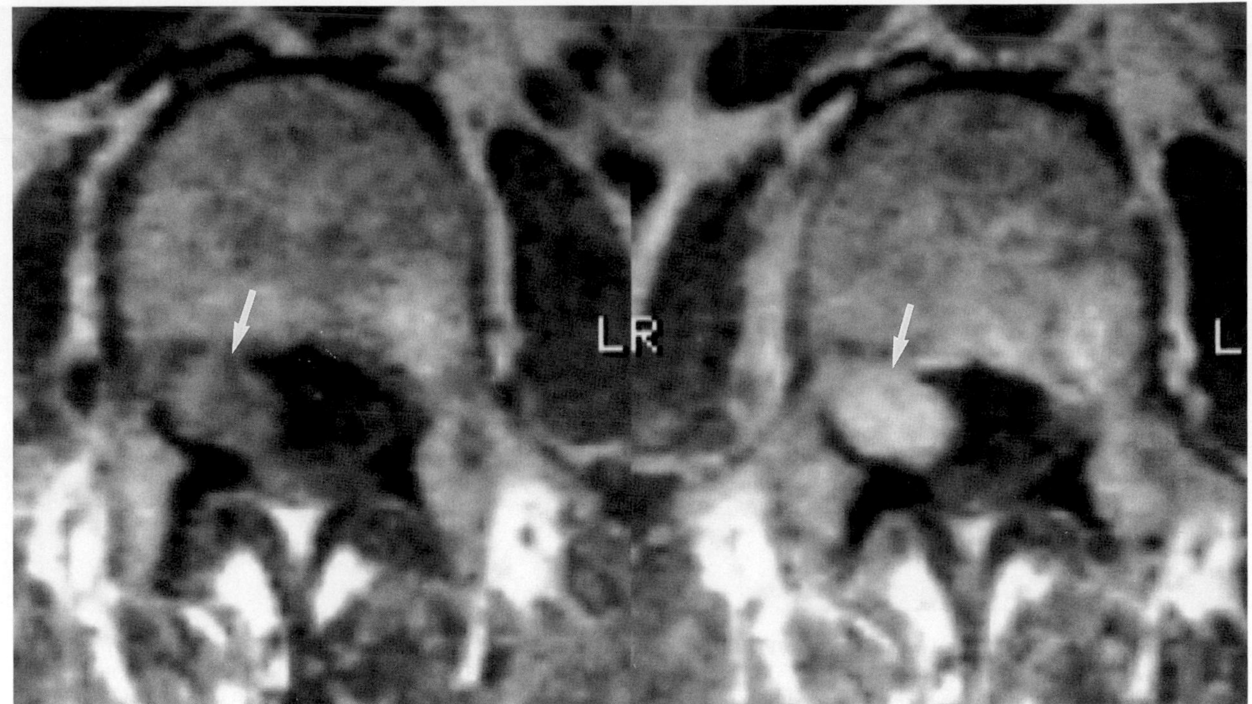

FIG. 57. Schwannoma in the lateral recess of L3 on the right. Unenhanced image (**A**) and enhanced image (**B**) demonstrate a homogeneously enhancing mass (*arrow*) in the lateral recess of L3 on the right causing widening of the lateral recess and neural foramen.

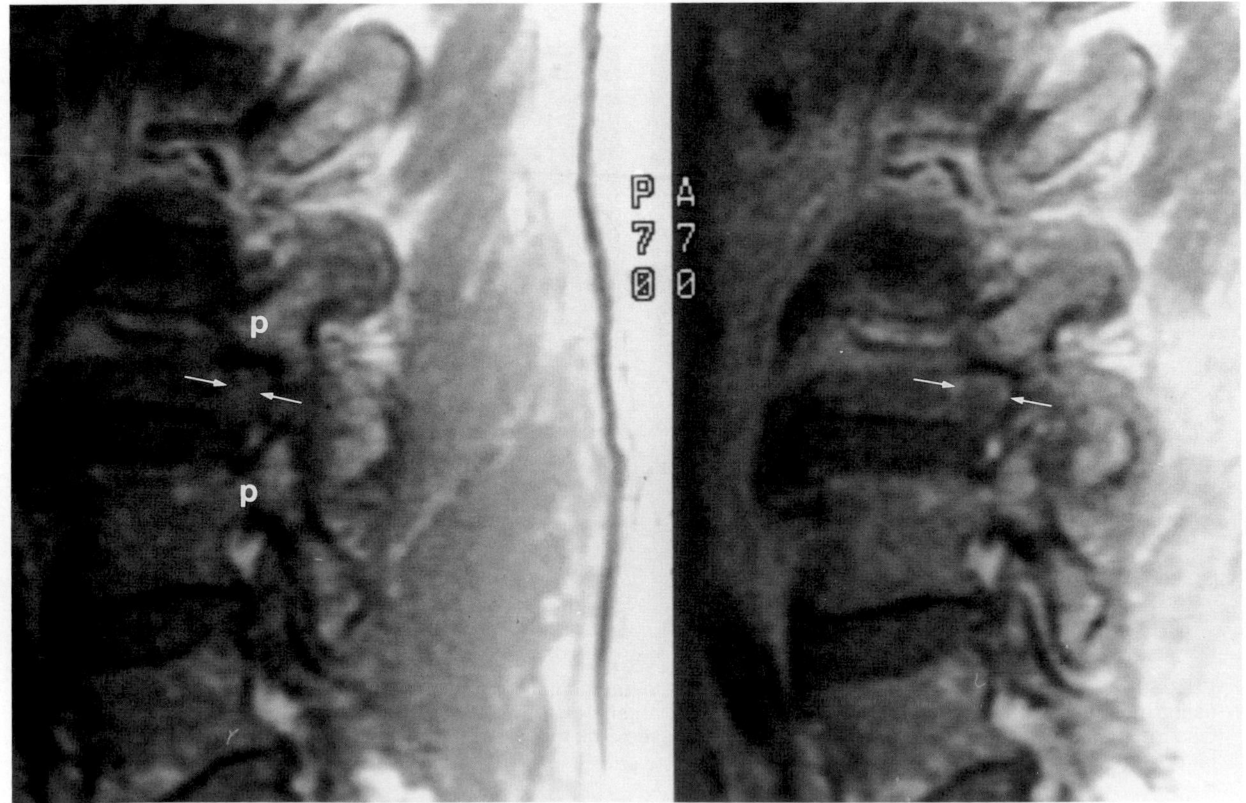

FIG. 58. Herniated disc in the neural foramen at L3-L4 level. Right parasagittal unenhanced image (**A**) and enhanced image (**B**) demonstrate a nonenhancing soft tissue mass (*arrows*) in the neural foramen. *p*, pedicle of L3 and L4, respectively.

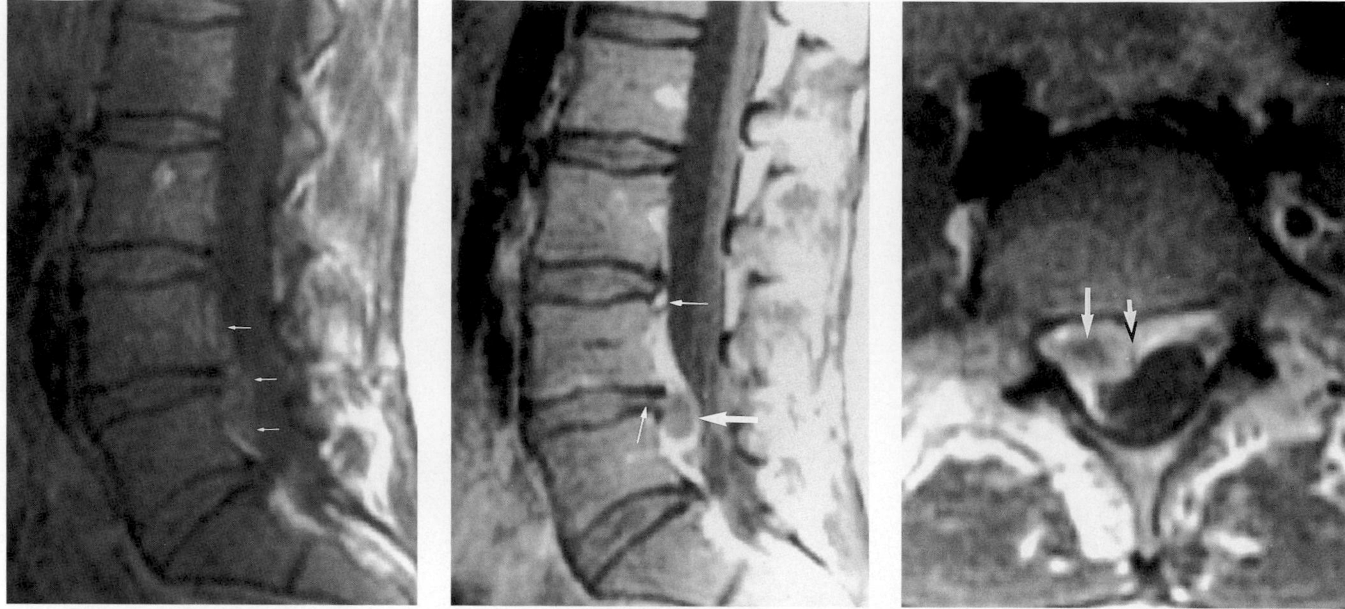

FIG. 59. Herniated disc at L4-L5 level with prominent inflammatory component. **A:** Unenhanced sagittal image shows a vague soft tissue mass (*arrows*) ventral to the thecal sac at L4 and L5. Most of this tissue is seen to enhance with contrast material (**B**) except for the disc fragment (*large arrow*). Small arrows indicate the site of radial tears in the posterior annulus at L3-4 and L4-5. In axial image (**C**), the herniated disc fragment (*larger arrow*) is surrounded by a rim of enhancing tissue. The *small arrow* indicates a thin dark linear structure representing a midline septum that limits the migration of the disc fragment across midline.

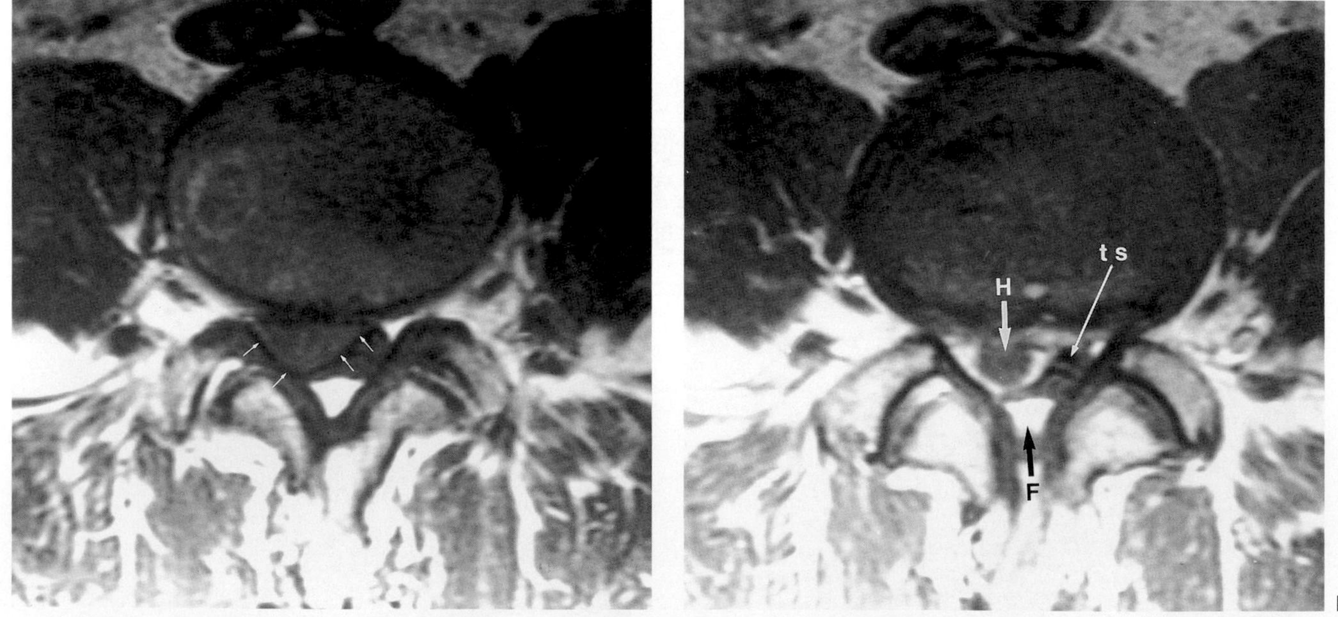

FIG. 60. Preoperative rim enhancement of herniated disc fragment. Unenhanced image (**A**) shows a prominent soft tissue mass (*arrows*) obscuring the epidural fat in the spinal canal on the right. In the enhanced image (**B**), the herniated disc fragment (*H*) is surrounded by a rim of enhancing tissue. The thecal sac (*ts*) is markedly compressed. *F*, epidural fat posterior to thecal sac.

herniated disc fragment generally does not enhance, although there often is subtle enhancement at the periphery of the disc fragment (see Fig. 55); (b) a herniated disc may incite an intense inflammatory response that may mimic an epidural abscess or tumor ventral to the thecal sac but centered at the intervertebral disc level (Fig. 59); (c) contrast-enhanced MR scans are useful to differentiate a herniated disc from a disc space infection or tumor. If one performs contrast-enhanced scans routinely on patients with herniated discs, peripheral enhancement around the nonenhancing disc fragment is usually seen (Fig. 60). A herniated disc fragment may rarely enhance centrally if granulation tissue infiltrates the fragment; (d) nerve roots in the thecal sac near a herniated disc may enhance either because of compression or from an inflammatory response caused by the disc herniation (43) (Fig. 61). Occasionally, a patient will have symptoms on the opposite side of a large herniated disc. Gadolinium-

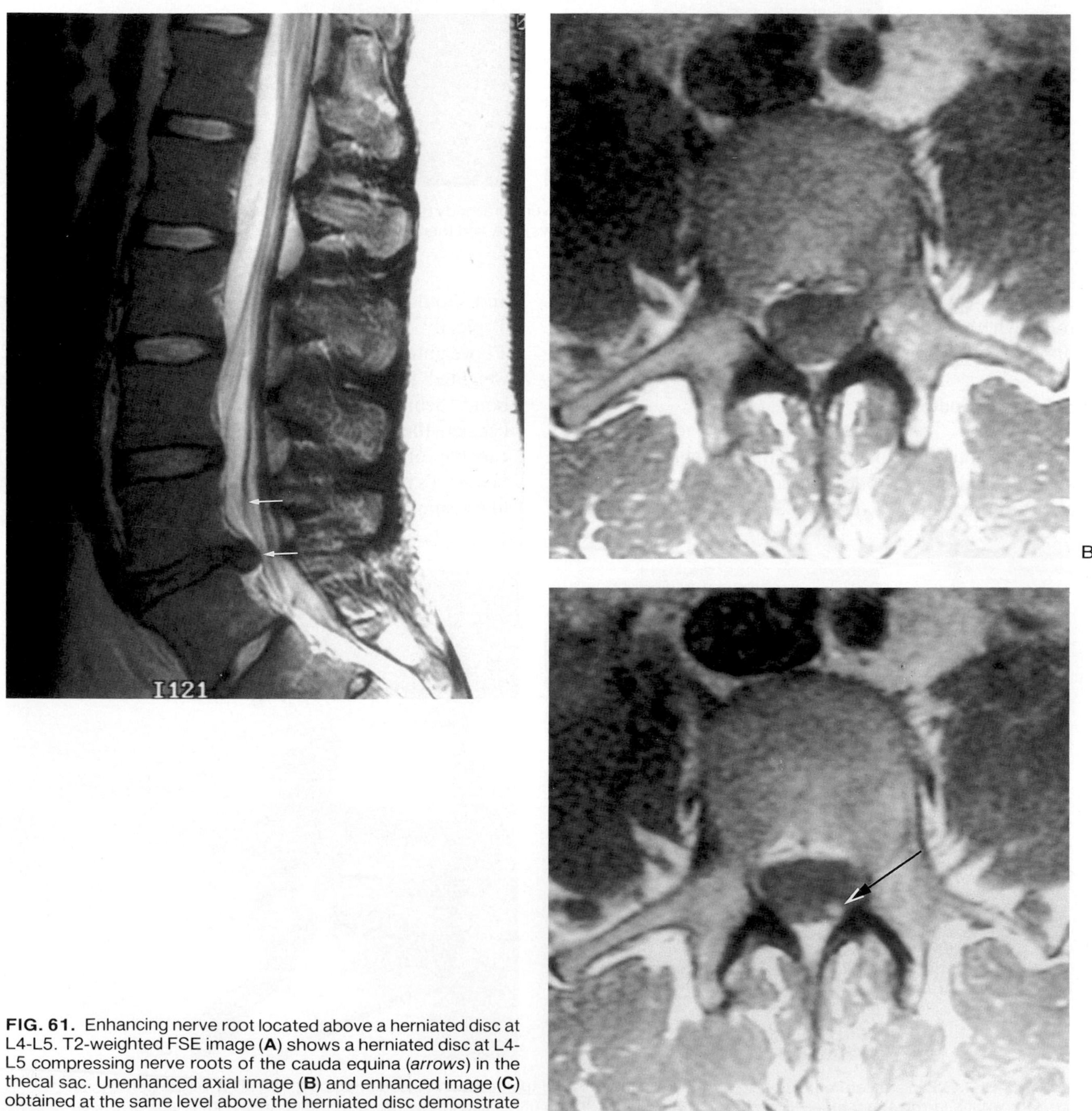

FIG. 61. Enhancing nerve root located above a herniated disc at L4-L5. T2-weighted FSE image (**A**) shows a herniated disc at L4-L5 compressing nerve roots of the cauda equina (*arrows*) in the thecal sac. Unenhanced axial image (**B**) and enhanced image (**C**) obtained at the same level above the herniated disc demonstrate an enhancing nerve root (*arrow*) on the left within the thecal sac.

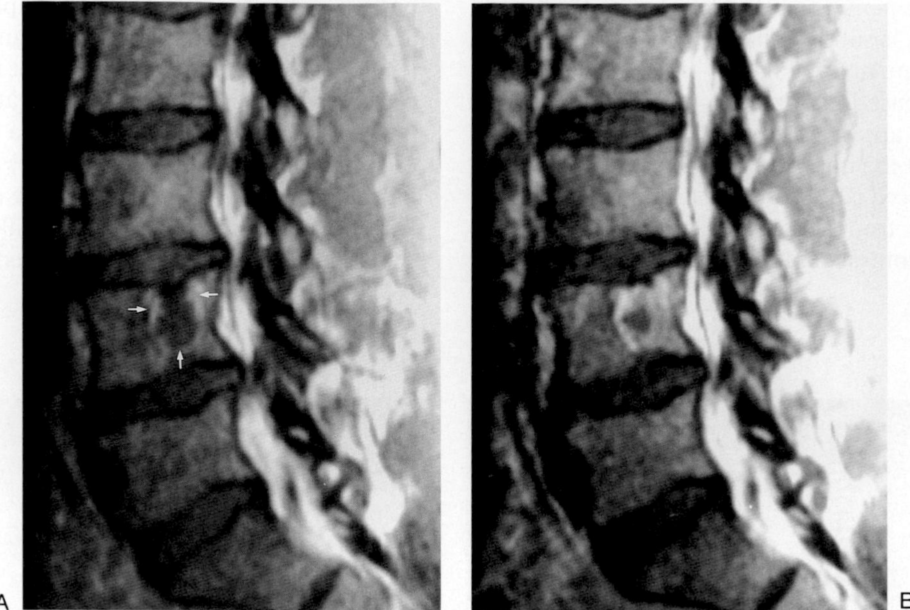

FIG. 62. A Schmorl's node is seen extending into the L4 vertebral body on unenhanced (**A**) and enhanced (**B**) images. The Schmorl's node has a slightly hyperintense rim (*arrows*) in A and there is ring enhancement shown in B.

enhanced scans may be useful in this situation to determine whether there is an enhancing nerve root on the opposite side of the herniated disc (44).

Schmorl's Node

Herniations that extend into the vertebral endplates are called Schmorl's nodes. These are usually asymptomatic, but are well seen on MRI adjacent to the endplate and should not be confused with vertebral metastases. Typically, Schmorl's nodes have low signal intensity on T1-weighted images and high signal intensity on T2-weighted images with respect to cancellous vertebral bone. Schmorl's nodes can enhance with Gd-DTPA because there is a rich vascular supply in the endplates capable of infiltrating the herniated disc (Fig. 62). Schmorl's nodes may enhance homogeneously, in a ring-like fashion or not at all (see Fig. 55).

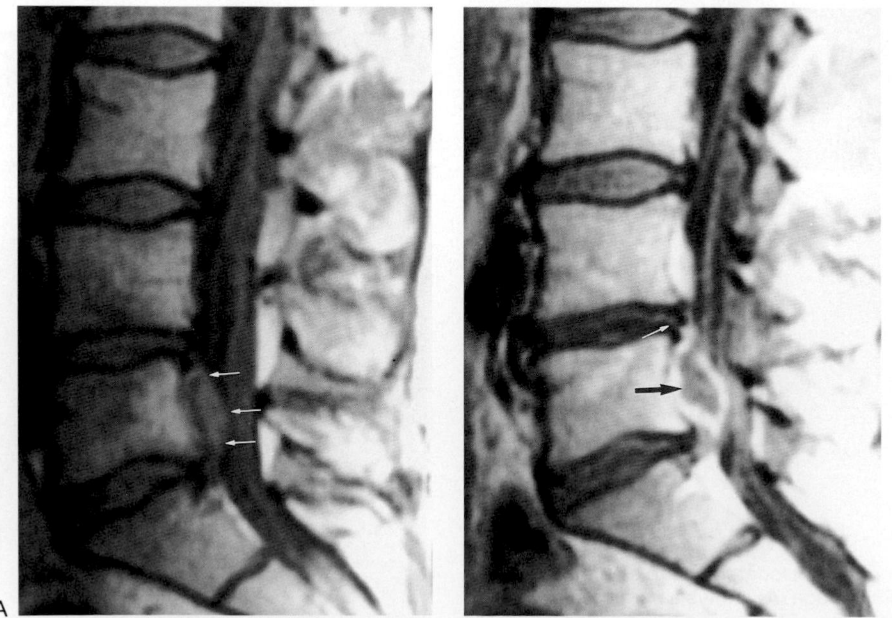

FIG. 63. Sequestered disc fragment mimicking epidural tumor. Unenhanced image (**A**) reveals a vague soft tissue mass (*arrows*) posterior to the L5 vertebral body. In the enhanced image (**B**), a free disc fragment (*black arrow*) is seen posterior to the vertebral body. A rim of enhancement surrounds the disc fragment. A tear (*small white arrow*) is seen in the posterior annulus of the L4-L5 disc.

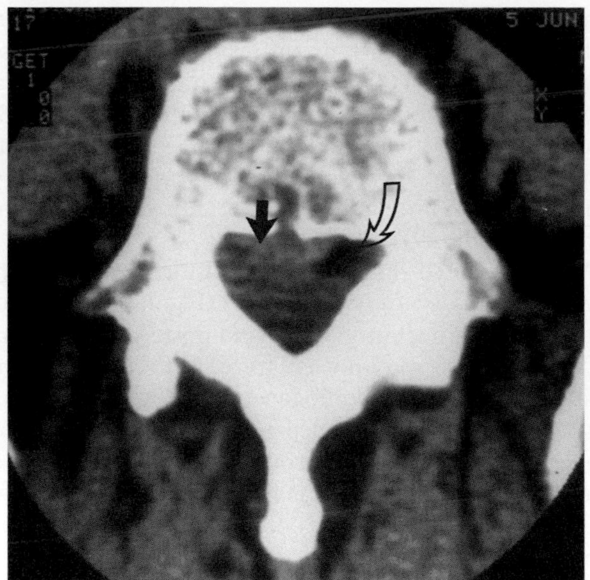

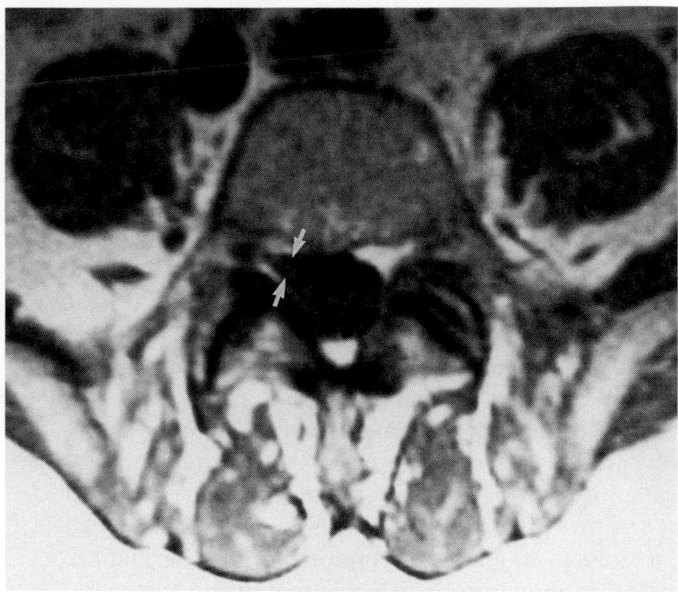

FIG. 64. Conjoined root mimics herniated disc on CT scan. Axial CT scan (**A**) reveals soft tissue density obscuring epidural fat on the right (*black arrow*). The epidural fat on the left (*open arrow*) is seen as a region of low density. In the axial T1-weighted image (**B**) the conjoined root pouch (*arrows*) has the same signal intensity as the thecal sac and is clearly delineated by adjacent high intensity fat.

Conditions that Mimic Lumbar Disc Herniation

It is usually not difficult with present MR techniques to differentiate lumbar disc herniation from other conditions. Epidural metastasis will occasionally resemble a herniated disc on axial images, but the distinction is easily made on sagittal scan. The epicenter of the epidural tumor in the spinal canal tends to be located away from the disc level, whereas herniated discs generally are located at the disc level unless the fragment has migrated. A free disc fragment that has migrated away from the disc level may mimic epidural neoplasm. Contrast-enhanced scans are needed to differentiate a tumor from a sequestered disc in this situation (Fig. 63).

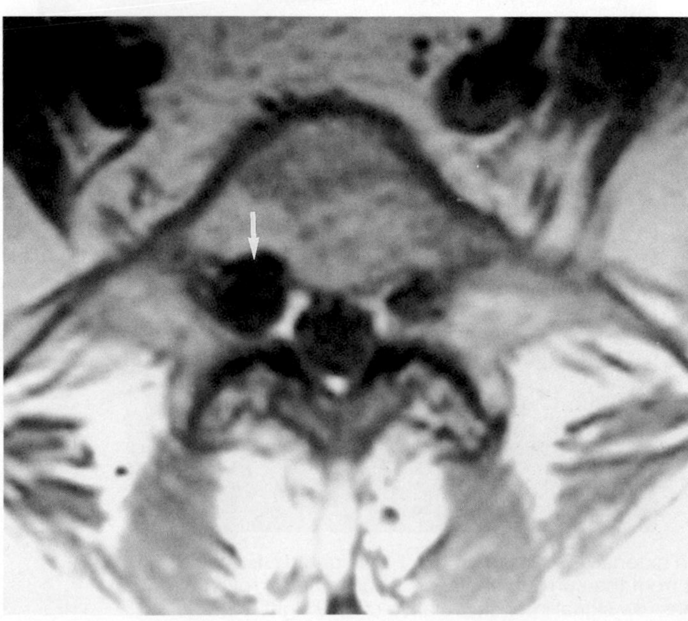

FIG. 65. A Tarlov cyst has low signal intensity (*arrow*) similar to that of the CSF in the thecal sac on this T1-weighted SE image.

Conjoined roots, sometimes difficult to distinguish from disc herniation by plain CT, are easily seen on MR because they have the same signal intensity as the thecal sac on T1-weighted images (Fig. 64). Synovial cysts, enlarged root pouches, and Tarlov cysts also have similar signal intensity as CSF (Fig. 65). It is rarely if ever a problem to distinguish epidural hematoma or abscess from herniated disc because of typical signal intensity characteristics and patterns of enhancement seen in these conditions.

The Postoperative Lumbar Spine and Gd-DTPA

Some herniated disc fragments will involute spontaneously, and this can occur in the cervical lumbar and thoracic spine. The incidence of spontaneous regression of a disc fragment is unknown. However, many patients go on to surgery to alleviate symptoms of disc herniation, and MR is an extremely valuable tool in the postoperative setting provided that there is no metallic hardware adjacent to the spine. The use of gadolinium-based paramagnetic contrast agents for MRI has dramatically improved the evaluation of the postoperative spine for recurrent disc herniation. Contrast-enhanced MR scanning is the most valuable imaging method for differentiating scar and recurrent or residual herniated disc. Contrast-enhanced CT scanning has not been proven as effective as MRI for differentiating scar and disc (45–48). On unenhanced images, epidural scar is isointense with respect to disc on T1-weighted images and relatively hypointense on T2-weighted images, but the distinction can be difficult (49) (Fig. 66).

Most herniated discs detected postoperatively at the site of surgery do not enhance (50) (Fig. 67). Scar tissue within the laminectomy defect and posterior paraspinal soft tisse may or may not enhance, but scar in the epidural space enhances homogeneously (Fig. 68). Normal tissues in the epidural space or foramen that also enhance include epidural fat, connective tissue, dura, root sleeves, and the dorsal root ganglia. The nerve roots and spinal cord do not enhance because a blood–neural barrier exists for these tissues.

It is important to obtain sagittal and axial images before and after paramagnetic contrast is given. Scanning should be performed immediately after the contrast material is administered. If scanning is delayed postinjection, the disc fragment may enhance, making it very difficult to differentiate scar from disc material. It is ex-

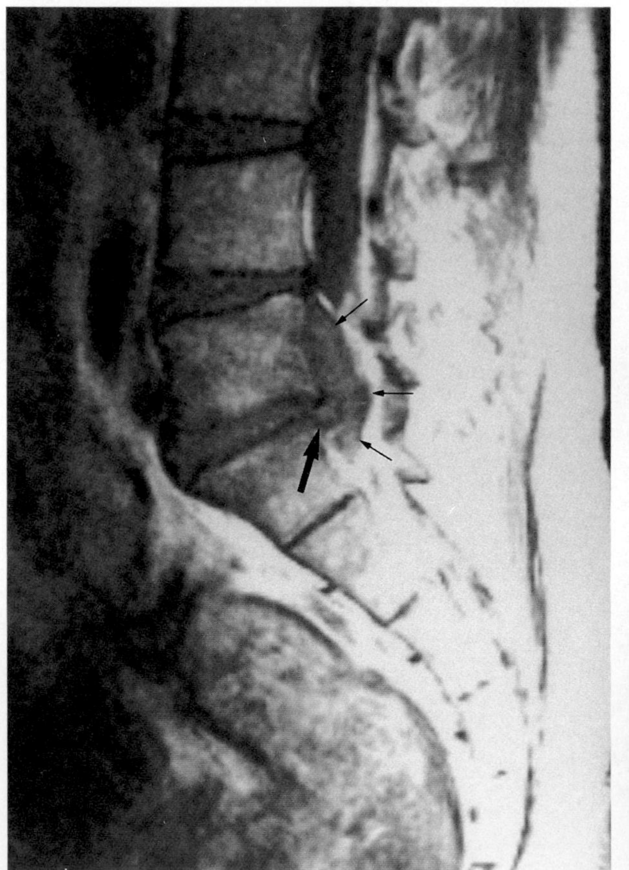

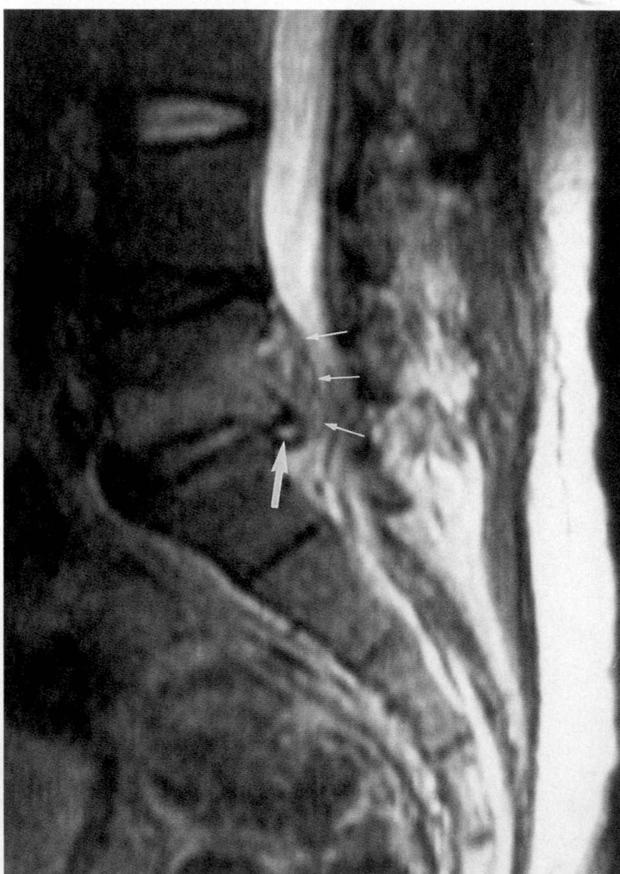

FIG. 66. Postoperative herniated disc at L5-S1 level with extensive scarring. In the T1-weighted SE image (**A**), the herniated disc (*large straight arrow*) can be distinguished from the surrounding scar tissue (*small arrows*) by a dark rim of annular fibers. **B:** The scar tissue has inhomogeneous low signal intensity relative to the bright CSF.

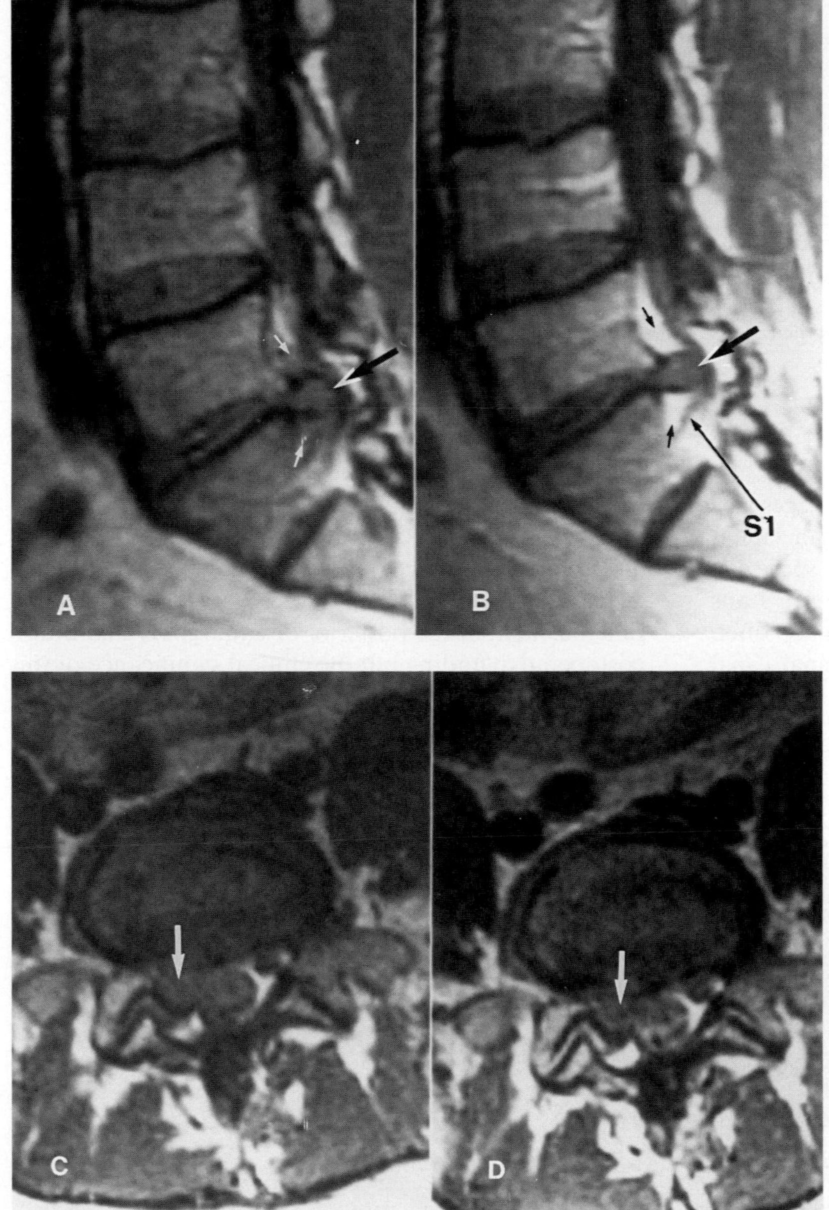

FIG. 67. Large herniated disc and enhancing scar at L5-S1. **A:** Unenhanced image shows a herniated disc (*black arrow*) poorly distinguished from adjacent scar (*small white arrows*). **B:** In the enhanced image, the herniated disc (*black arrow*) is clearly demarcated by enhancing scar above and below (*tiny black arrows*). The S1 root (*S1*) is posteriorly displaced. **C:** The unenhanced image reveals the herniated disc (*arrow*) lateral to the thecal sac. **D:** In the enhanced image, the disc fragment (*arrow*) does not enhance, which is typical of most recurrent disc herniations.

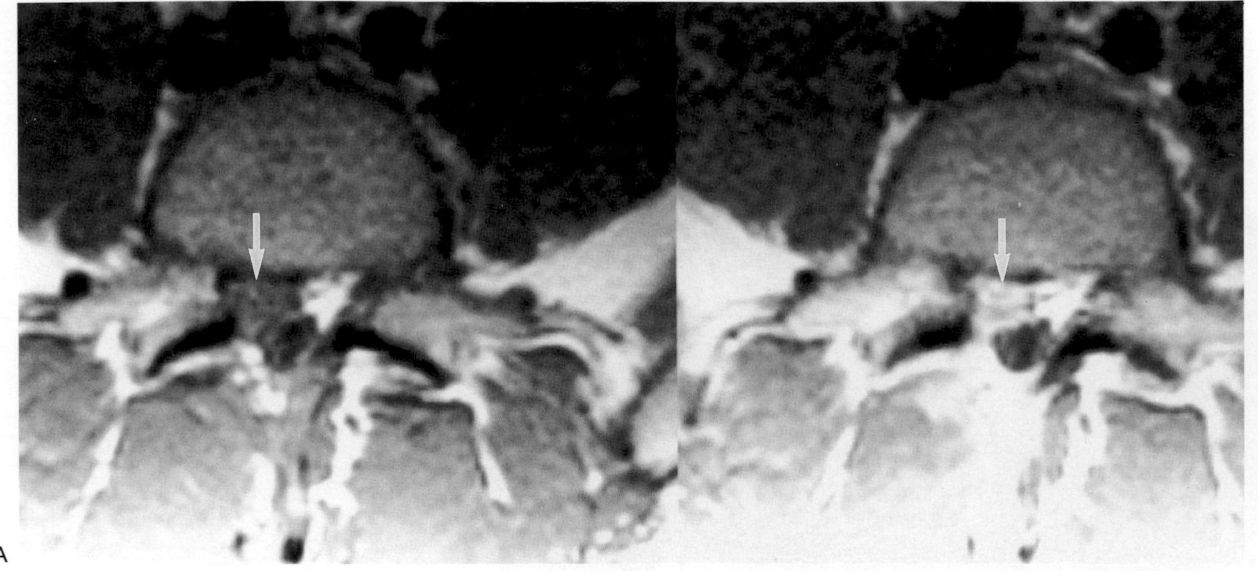

FIG. 68. A: Scar tissue (*arrow*) mimics a herniated disc in the axial image. **B:** This tissue enhances almost homogeneously in the gadolinium-enhanced image.

tremely useful to film pre- and postcontrast images side by side to detect subtle differences in the enhancement pattern (Fig. 69). Focal scarring in the epidural space can mimic disc herniation on precontrast MR or CT scans (Fig. 68). Diffuse scarring in the epidural space often masks all normal anatomic detail in the spinal canal (Fig. 70).

The most common pattern we observe in patients with low back pain or radiculopathy following surgery for disc disease is the presence of both scar and recurrent herniated disc material in the epidural space (Figs. 67 and 71). Enhancement of the posterior disc margin is a common postoperative finding but the clinical significance of this is unknown. This probably represents scar or granula-

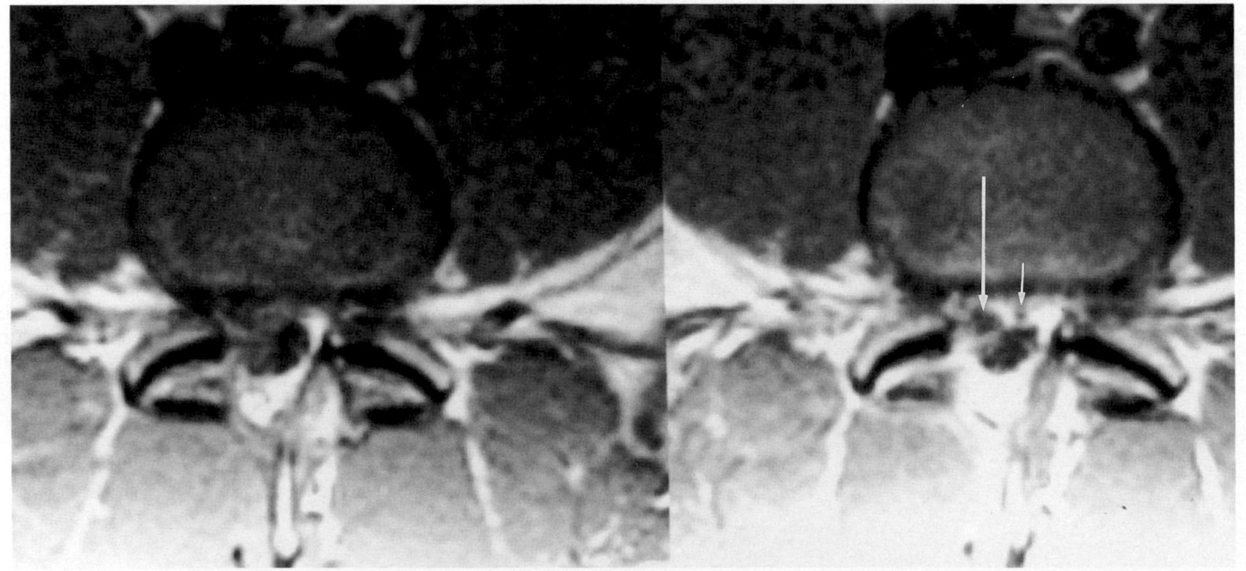

FIG. 69. Herniated disc and scar at L3-L4 on the right. **A:** Unenhanced axial image demonstrates soft tissue obscuring the epidural fat and thecal sac on the right. **B:** In the enhanced image, enhancing scar tissue surrounds the recurrent disc fragment (*long arrow*). *Small arrow* indicates the presence of a midline septum extending between the thecal sac and the posterior vertebral body margin.

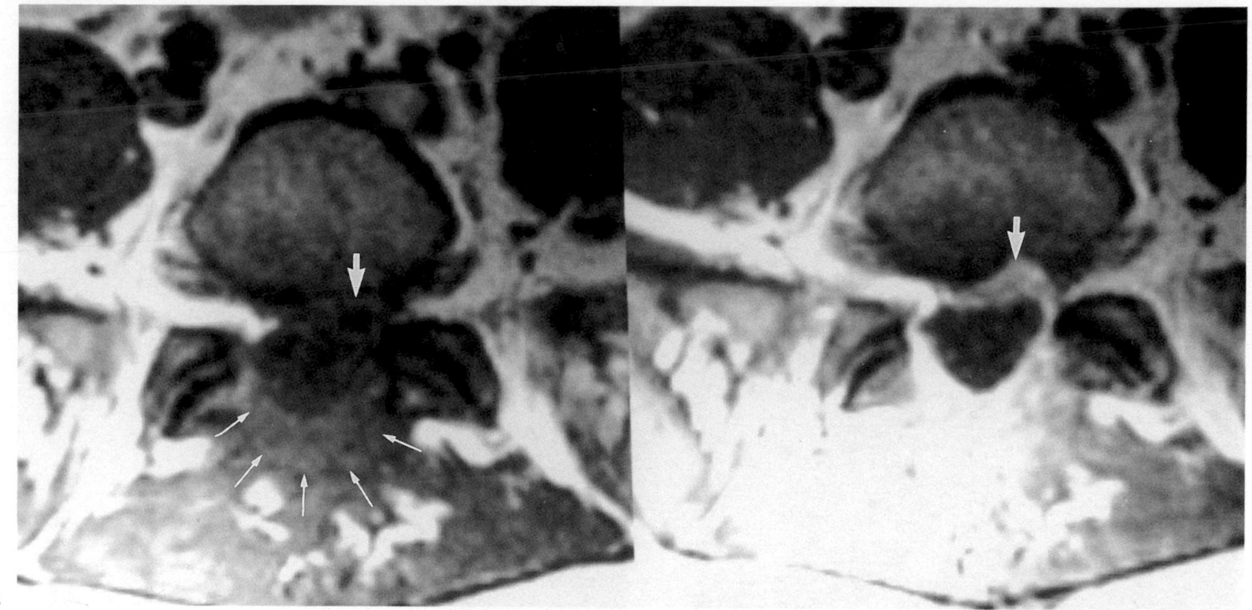

FIG. 70. Scar tissue encases the thecal sac. Unenhanced axial image (**A**) and enhanced image (**B**) at the L4-L5 level demonstrate extensive scar tissue surrounding the thecal sac, which enhances in B. *Small arrows* in A represent scar tissue in the laminectomy defect. Focal-enhancing scar tissue (*arrow,* B) might be mistaken for a recurrent disc herniation in unenhanced image A.

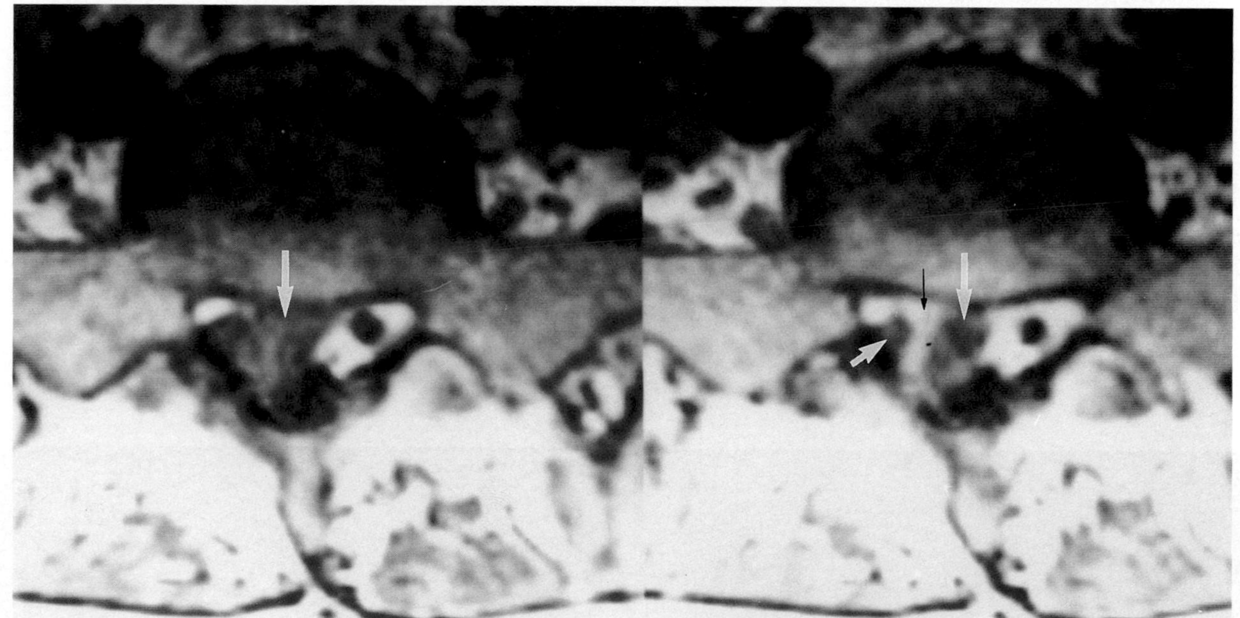

FIG. 71. Postoperative recurrent disc herniation and scar tissue at L5-S1. In the axial unenhanced image (**A**), the soft tissue mass obscures the epidural fat between the thecal sac and nerve root. The gadolinium-enhanced image (**B**) reveals enhancing scar tissue (*small black arrow*) between the disc fragment (*longer white arrow*) and the S1 root (*smaller white arrow*).

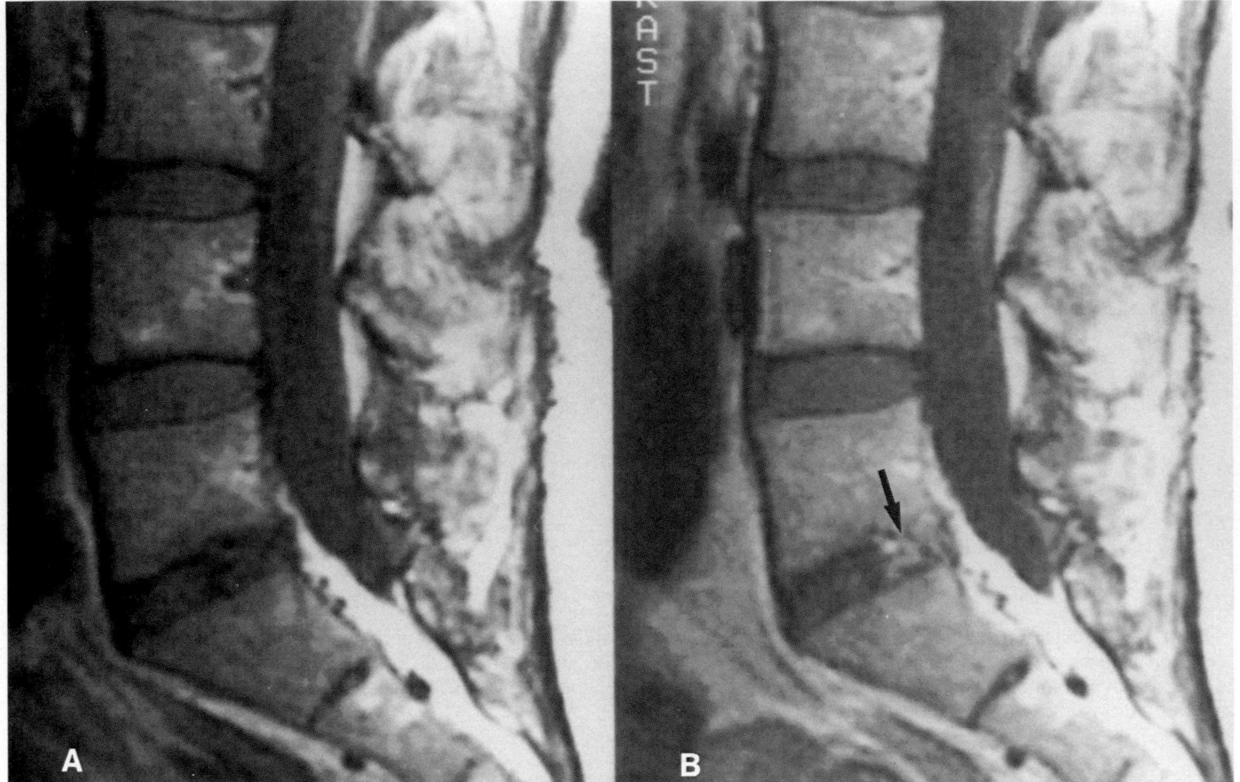

FIG. 72. Enhancing L5-S1 intervertebral disc postoperatively. Unenhanced sagittal T1-weighted image (**A**) shows no evidence of thecal sac deformity in the midline at L5-S1. Enhanced image (**B**) reveals inhomogeneous enhancement in the posterior one third of the L5-S1 disc, presumably due to infiltration of the disc by granulation tissue and scarring, but no evidence of recurrent disc herniation. Enhancement of a small portion of the intervertebral disc postoperatively is common.

tion tissue infiltrating the disc through a defect in the posterior annulus (47) (Fig. 72). Herniated discs can enhance with Gd-DTPA, but this enhancement is generally along the margins of the disc (Fig. 73), although rarely the entire disc fragment will enhance (Fig. 74). In these cases it is usually possible to make the diagnosis because of nerve root or thecal sac displacement, which is usually not seen to any significant degree in scarring alone. Pre-

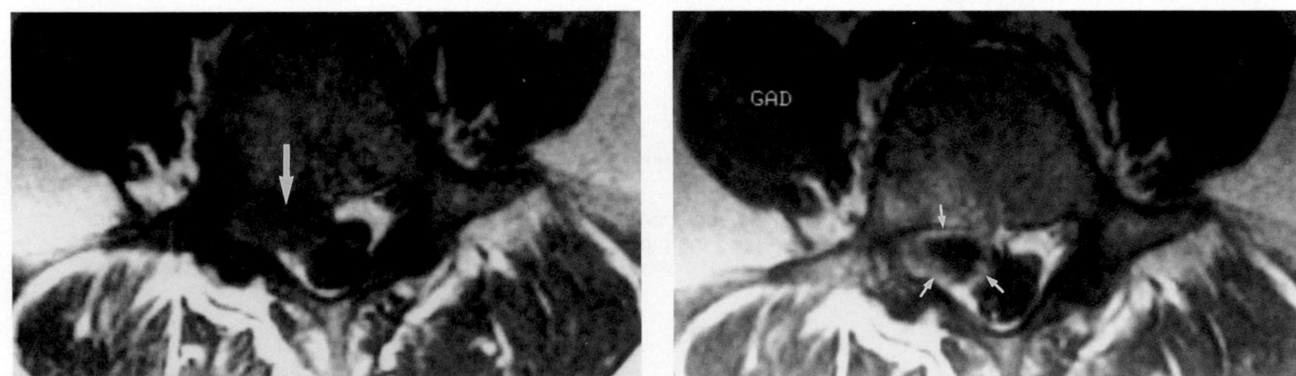

FIG. 73. Postoperative herniated disc with surrounding scar tissue in the lateral recess of L5. **A:** In the unenhanced image, soft tissue (*arrow*) obscures the epidural fat on the right. **B:** In the enhanced image, there is enhancing scar tissue (*arrows*) surrounding a nonenhancing recurrent disc fragment.

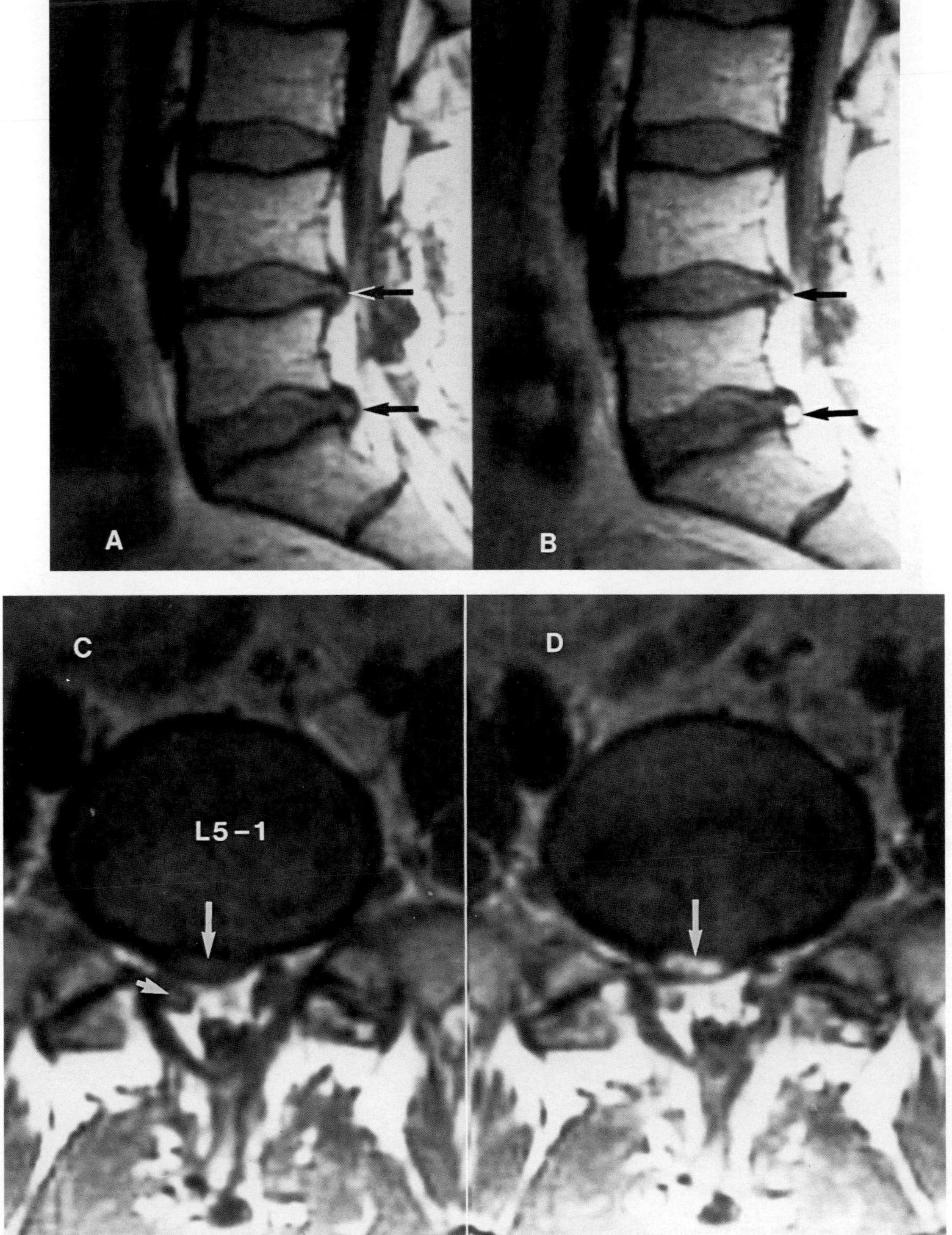

FIG. 74. Postoperative enhancing disc herniations at L4-L5 and L5-S1. Compared to the unenhanced sagittal T1-weighted image (**A**) and the enhanced image (**B**), the herniated disc (*arrows*) at L4-L5 and L5-S1 enhances (*black arrows*). **C:** The axial unenhanced image reveals a focal herniated disc (*large arrow*) and posterior S1 root displacement (*small arrow*). **D:** The herniated disc at L5-S1 (*arrow*) enhances.

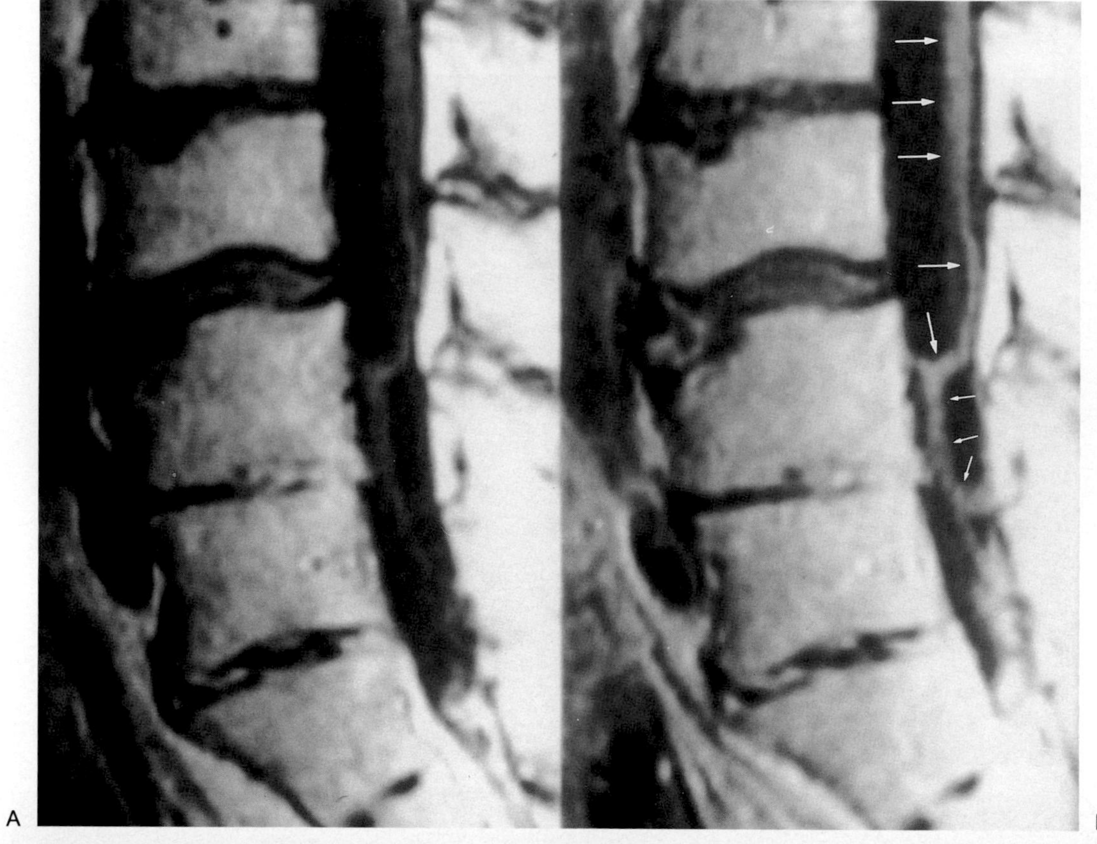

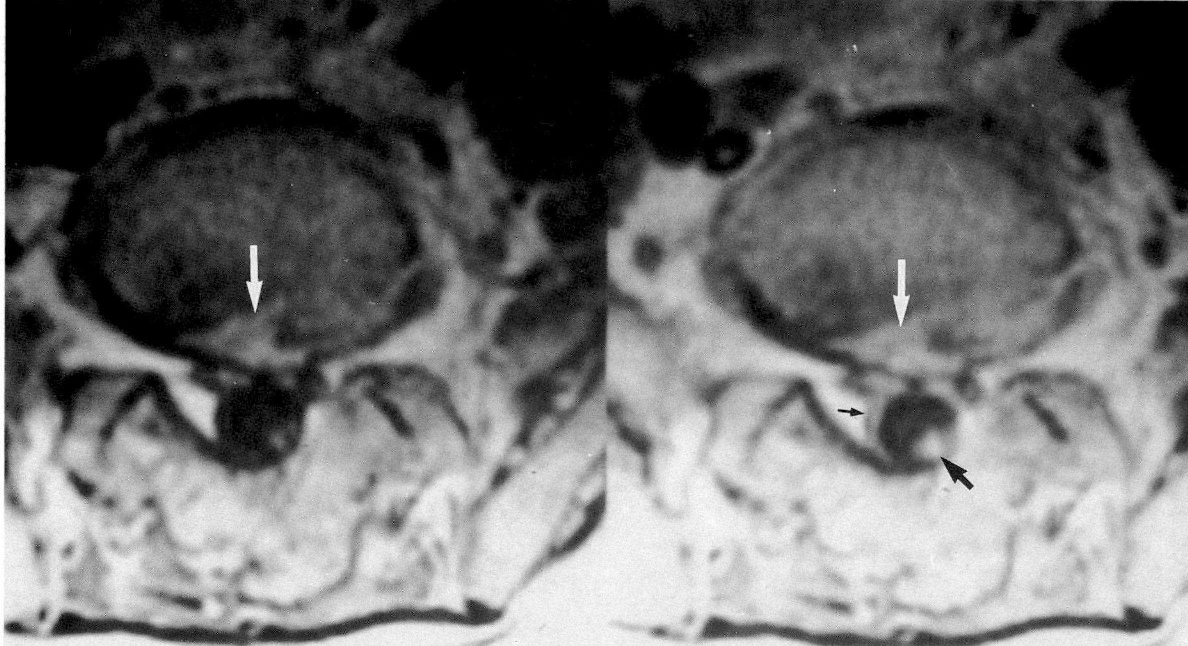

FIG. 75. Postoperative arachnoiditis. The thickened and clumped nerve roots of the cauda equina in the unenhanced image (**A**) shows subtle enhancement (*arrows*) in **B.** In both the axial unenhanced image (**C**) and the enhanced image (**D**), there is a region of hyperintensity (*white arrow*) in the posterior portion of the disc. This probably represents granulation tissue infiltrating the disc. There is enhancement of a thickened cluster of nerve roots in the thecal sac on the left (*large black arrow*) and there is a crescentic band of enhancing tissue along the right lateral margin of the thecal sac, which probably represents thickened dura with adherent nerve roots (*small black arrow*, D).

or postoperative enhancement of the vertebral body endplates is occasionally seen and can be confused with discitis, as already mentioned.

The role of Gd-DTPA in the evaluation of postoperative arachnoiditis is controversial. The pathogenesis of arachnoiditis is still poorly understood and the clinical diagnosis can be difficult, usually presenting with vague, nonspecific back pain with radiation into the lower extremities. Arachnoiditis is an inflammatory process that causes the nerve rootlets of the cauda equina to adhere to the thecal sac and to each other. The most common finding is clumping of nerve rootlets in the thecal sac; this finding is seen on myelography, postmyelogram CT scans, or with MR, particularly T2-weighted FSE images. The pattern of enhancement in arachnoiditis is variable from no enhancement to minimal or even pronounced enhancement of the nerve rootlets. The nerve roots may be clumped centrally or peripherally (51) (Fig. 75).

A common cause of postoperative low back pain is abnormal mobility of the vertebra due to incomplete fusion following laminectomy. MR is useful to exclude a disc herniation, but plain radiographs and CT are best to show any associated bone abnormalities.

THORACIC DISC HERNIATION

Degenerative disc disease of the thoracic spine is extremely common in older age groups manifested by multilevel osteophytosis (spondylosis deformans) and degenerating discs seen as narrowed discs having low signal intensity on T2-weighted images. Herniated discs in the thoracic region are not uncommon and are being increasingly recognized because of the ease of screening the thoracic spine with MR (52).

A thoracic herniated disc usually presents with myelopathy or referred back pain rather than a radiculopathy. Because of the normal dorsal kyphotic curvature, the thoracic cord is positioned in the subarachnoid space anteriorly, close to the vertebral bodies. Therefore, a small disc herniation in the thoracic region can produce significant myelopathy. Even minimal deformity of the cord anteriorly suggests significant cord compression (Fig. 76). Large herniations also occur in the thoracic re-

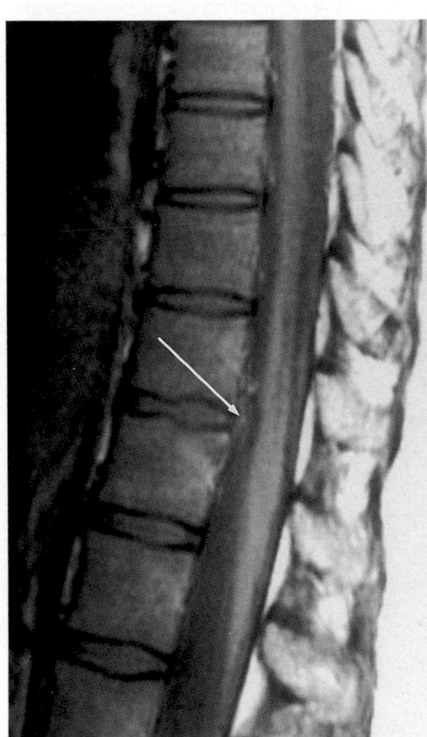
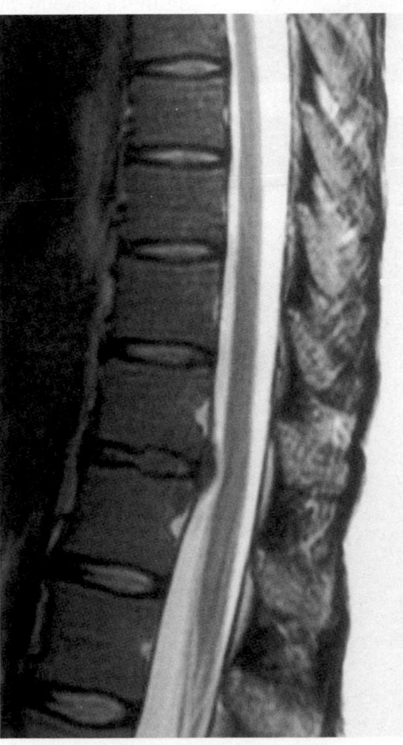
A,B

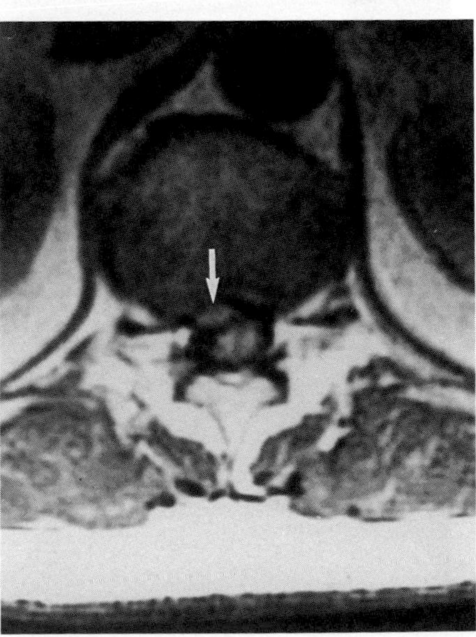
C

FIG. 76. Herniated disc at T10-T11 level. **A:** The herniated disc (*arrow*) extends into the ventral aspect of the spinal canal in the T1-weighted sagittal SE image. **B:** In the T2-weighted FSE image, the herniated disc fragment has low signal intensity relative to the CSF. **C:** In the axial image, the herniated disc fragment is positioned to the right of midline and the spinal cord is deformed slightly on the right.

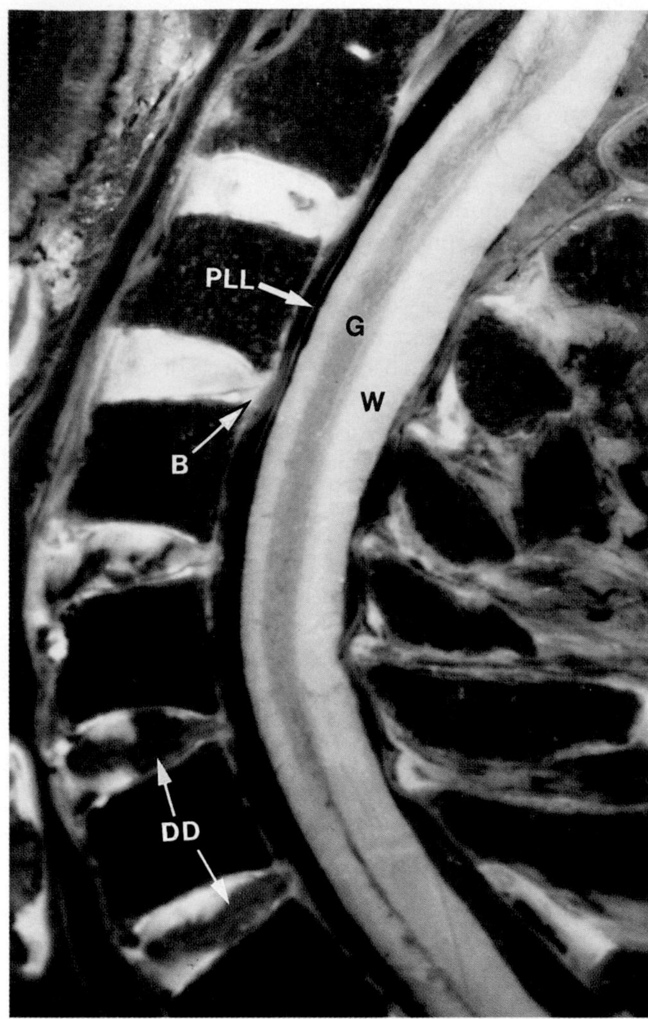

FIG. 77. Sagittal anatomic section of the cervical spine demonstrates a bulging disc (*B*) at C3-C4 contacting the posterior longitudinal ligament (*PLL*). The spinal cord containing gray (*G*) and white (*W*) matter does not appear deformed. Degenerating discs (*DD*) are present at lower cervical levels.

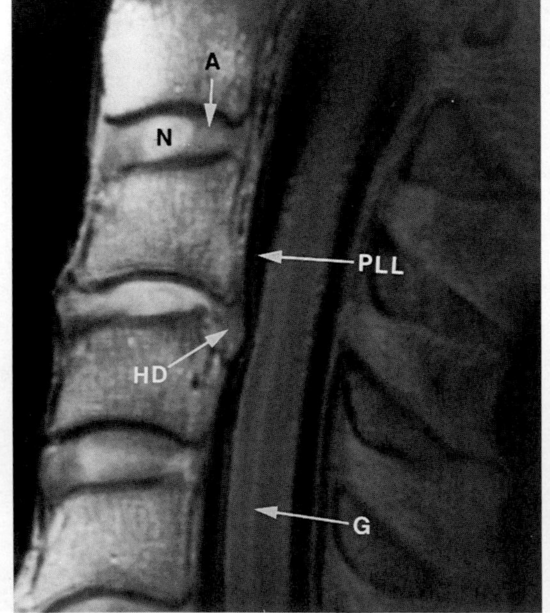

A

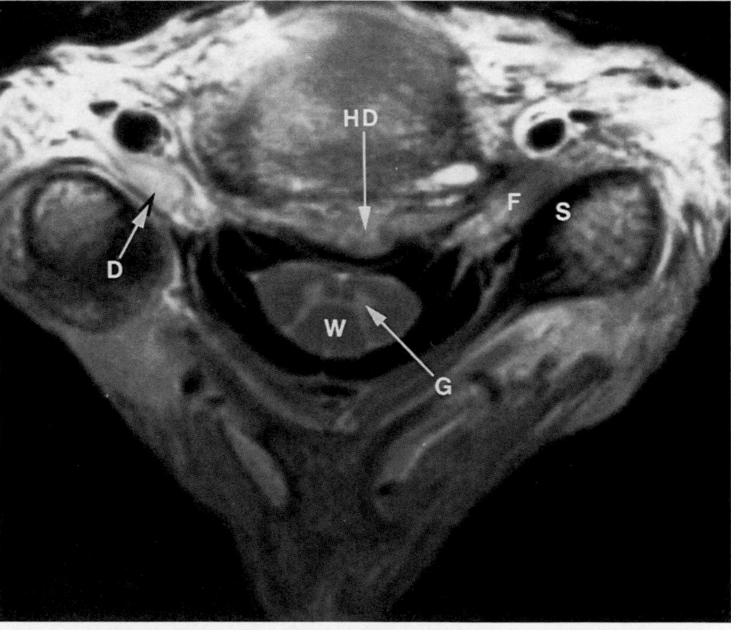

B

FIG. 78. MR scan of herniated disc in cadaver on sagittal (**A**) and axial (**B**) SE images. Herniated disc (*HD*) displaces the posterior longitudinal ligament (*PLL*) posteriorly. *A*, normal annulus; *N*, normal nucleus at level above; *G*, cord gray matter stripe; *D*, dorsal root ganglion; *F*, neural foramen; *S*, superior articular process; *W*, white matter of posterior columns.

gion but are rare. A thoracic disc herniation may calcify and mimic a calcified tumor in the spinal canal on CT (53).

CERVICAL DISC HERNIATION

The morphologic characteristics of cervical disc herniations are similar to those seen in the lumbar spine (Fig. 77). A focal displacement of the disc margin represents a disc herniation (Fig. 78), whereas diffuse bulging of the disc is seen as a broad, convex posterior disc margin extending between uncinate processes. It may not be possible to differentiate a bulging cervical disc from a small herniated disc based on the sagittal images alone, and therefore axial images are essential (4). In addition, large bulging cervical discs can produce significant myelopathy and even cord edema. MRI is very sensitive to cervical degenerative disc disease and spondylosis deformans (54,55).

Small herniated discs may be difficult to detect on standard T1-weighted SE images. They are easier to detect in 2D or 3D GE images (see Fig. 8) than on T1-weighted SE images because there is a paucity of epidural fat and foraminal fat in the cervical region and instead a rich venous plexus surrounds the thecal sac and nerve root sheaths. Because GE images display fluid-containing structures with very high signal intensity, and bone has very low signal intensity relative to the disc, disc herniations are very obvious on GE sequences in the cervical region and can be differentiated from osteophytes (Fig. 79). Herniated cervical disc fragments have very low signal intensity on FSE images (Fig. 80).

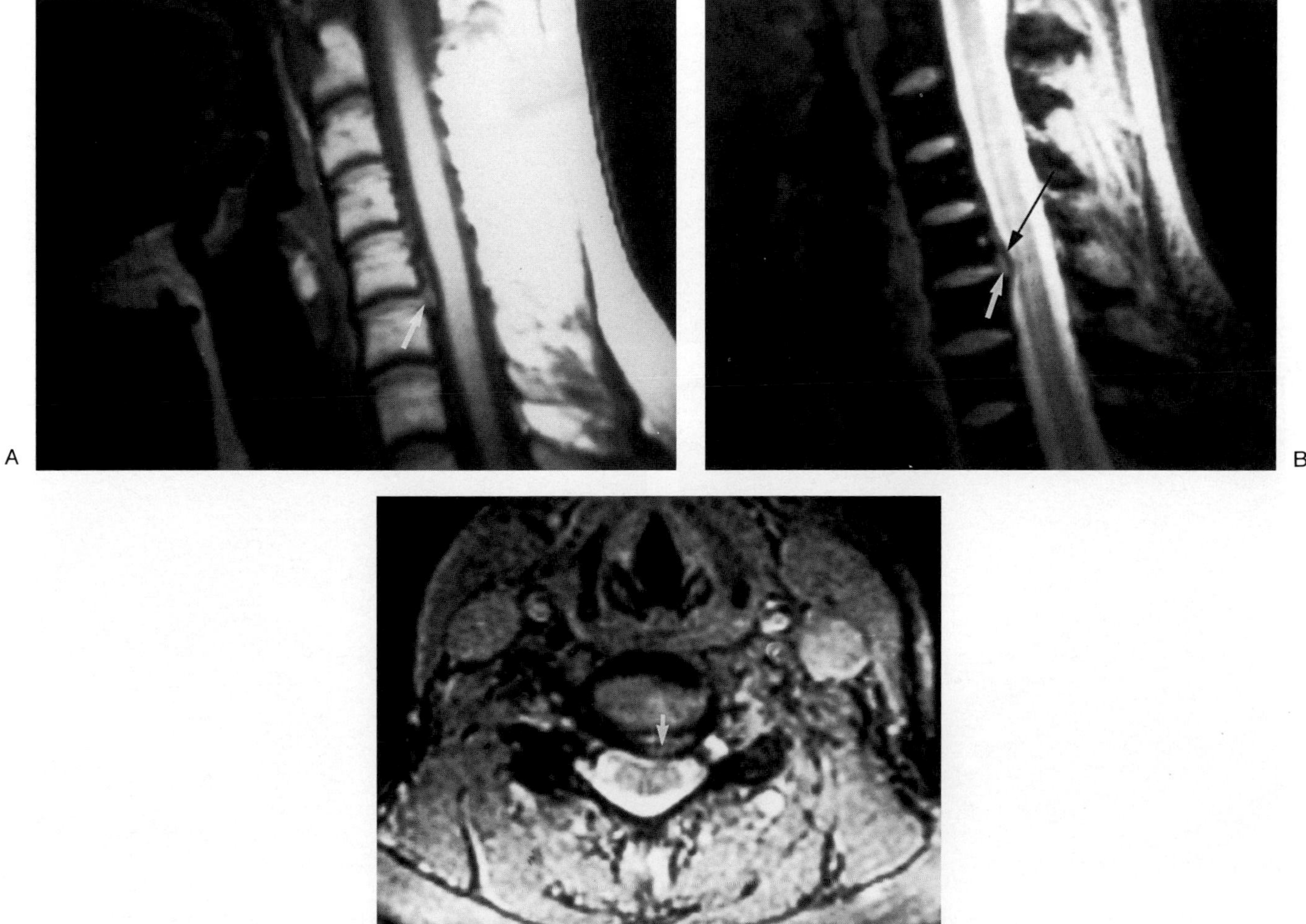

FIG. 79. C5-C6 disc herniation. Sagittal T1-weighted SE (**A**) and GE image (**B**) demonstrate disc herniation (*white arrow*) displacing posterior longitudinal ligament (*black arrow*) and indenting the thecal sac. Disc herniation (*arrow*) is located to the left of the midline in the axial GE image (**C**).

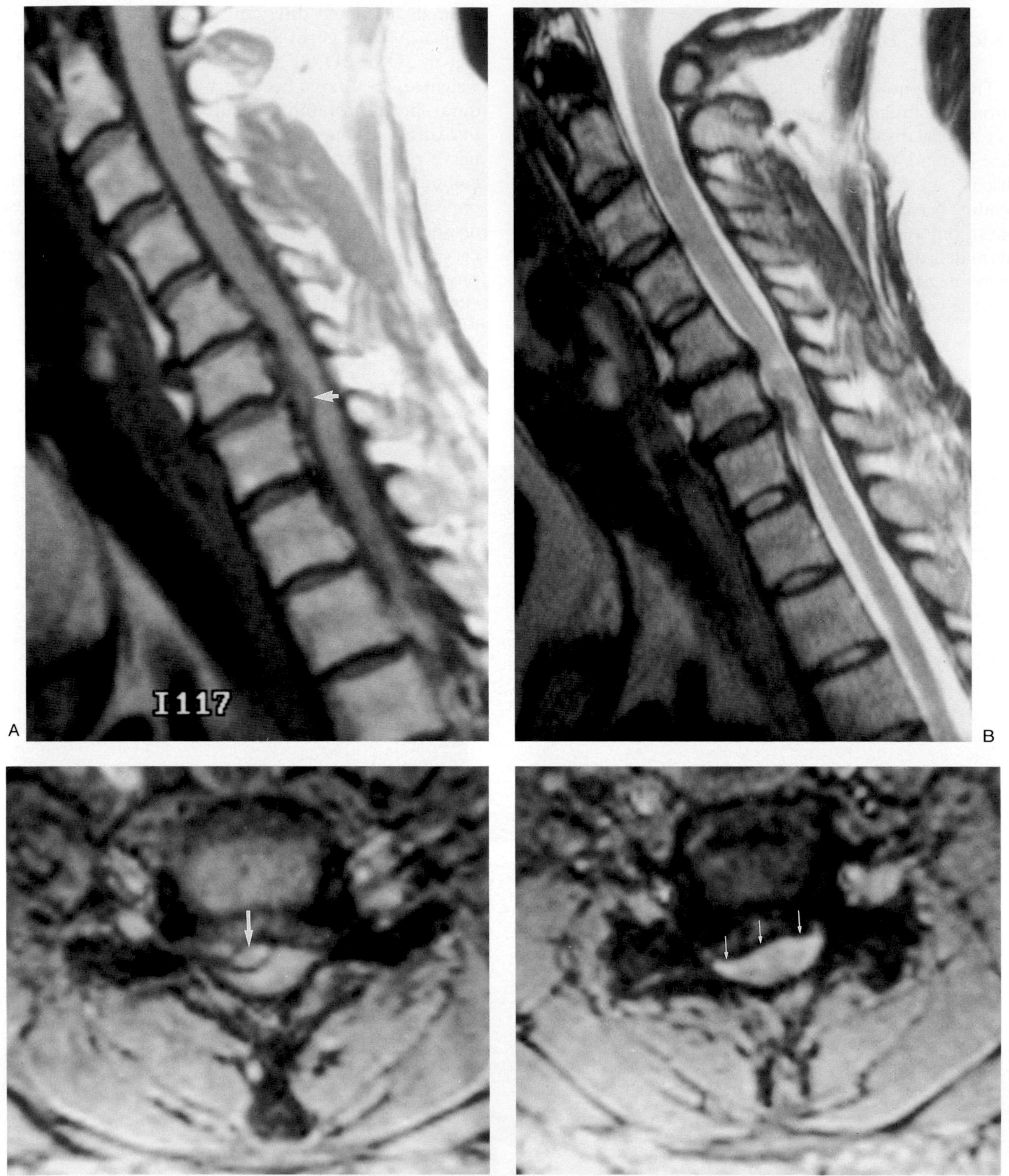

FIG. 80. Cervical spondylosis, herniated disc, and cord compression. Generalized disc bulging, disc degeneration, and osteophyte formation is seen on sagittal T1-weighted SE image (**A**) and T2-weighted FSE image (**B**). A herniated disc (*arrow*) in A has low intensity in image B. Focal areas of high signal in the cord at C5-C6 and C6-C7 represent either edema or myelomalacia from chronic cord compression. In the axial GE image (**C**), the herniated disc (*arrow*) has higher intensity than the bone. **D:** This image, obtained adjacent to the herniated disc, shows an osteophytic ridge (*arrows*) encroaching on the spinal canal more on the right.

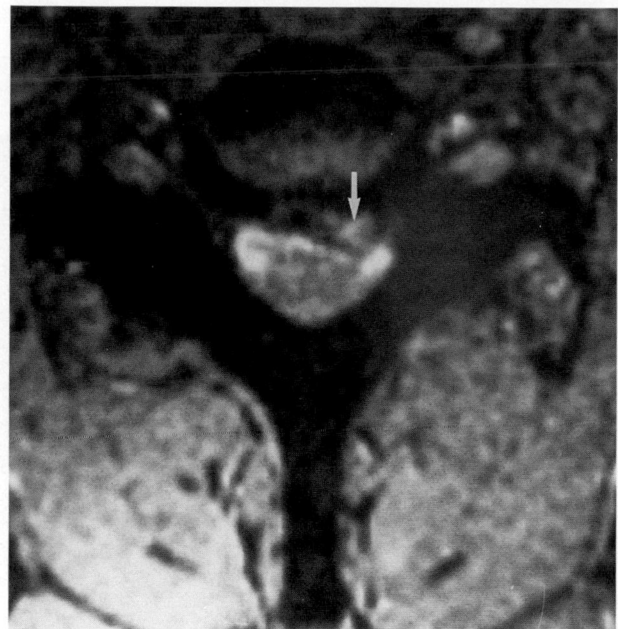

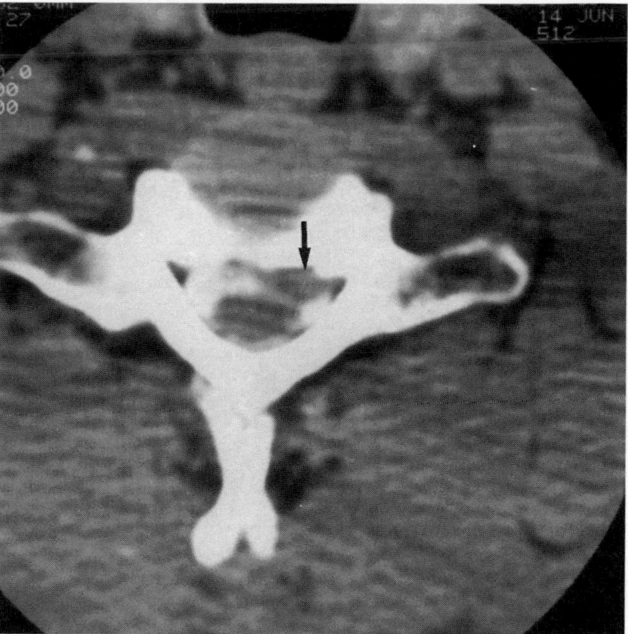

FIG. 81. Herniated disc at C6-C7 level on the left. Axial CT scan (**A**) shows the disc fragment as a soft tissue mass (*arrow*) compressing the contrast-filled thecal sac on the left. **B:** The herniated disc (*arrow*) has high signal intensity, a GE image obtained with a 30° flip angle, and the bone is relatively dark compared to the disc fragment.

Asymptomatic cervical disc herniations are common (63), and therefore the significance of a disc herniation seen on MR must be judged based on associated clinical findings. The most common symptoms found with cervical disc herniation are neck pain, radiculopathy, and myelopathy if the cord is compressed. Cervical herniations most commonly (90%) occur at C5-C6 or C6-C7 levels. Midline cervical disc herniations are more common than in the lumbar region, but posterolateral herniations are also common (Fig. 81). Far lateral herniated discs are rare, probably because of buttressing by the uncinate processes (Fig. 82).

Herniated disc fragments may migrate inferiorly or superiorly, and are best seen on T2*-weighted images (Fig.

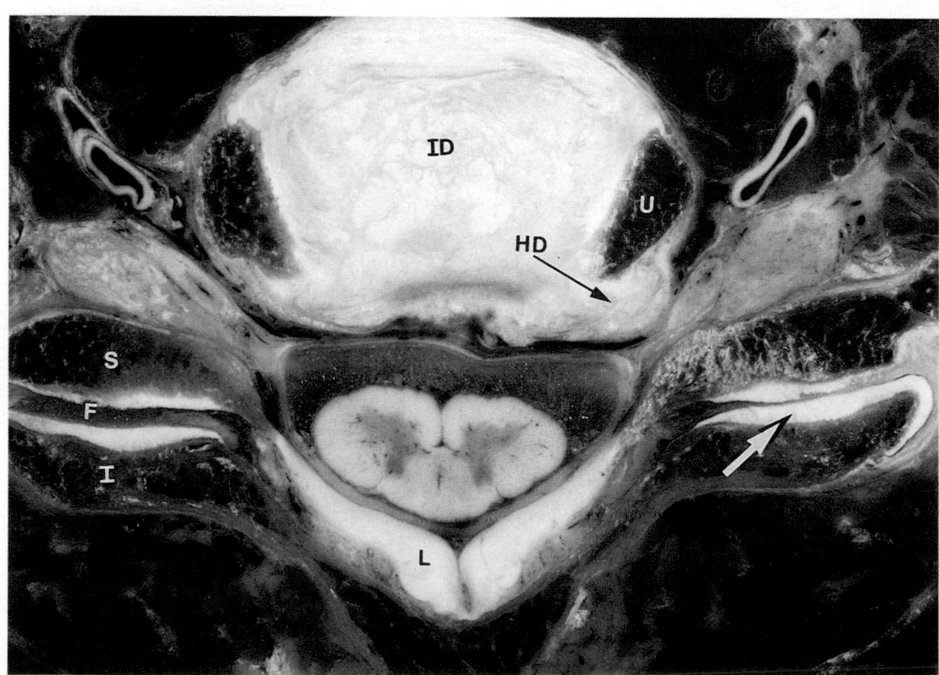

FIG. 82. Axial cryomicrotome section in cadaver. A lateral herniated disc (*HD*) extends into the medial aspect of the left neural foramen posterior to the uncinate process (*U*) and compresses the ventral root (*V*). *ID*, intervertebral disc; *HD*, dorsal root ganglion; *S*, superior articular process; *F*, facet joint; *I*, inferior articular process; *L*, ligamentum flavum. *White arrow* indicates articular cartilage of inferior facet of C5 on left.

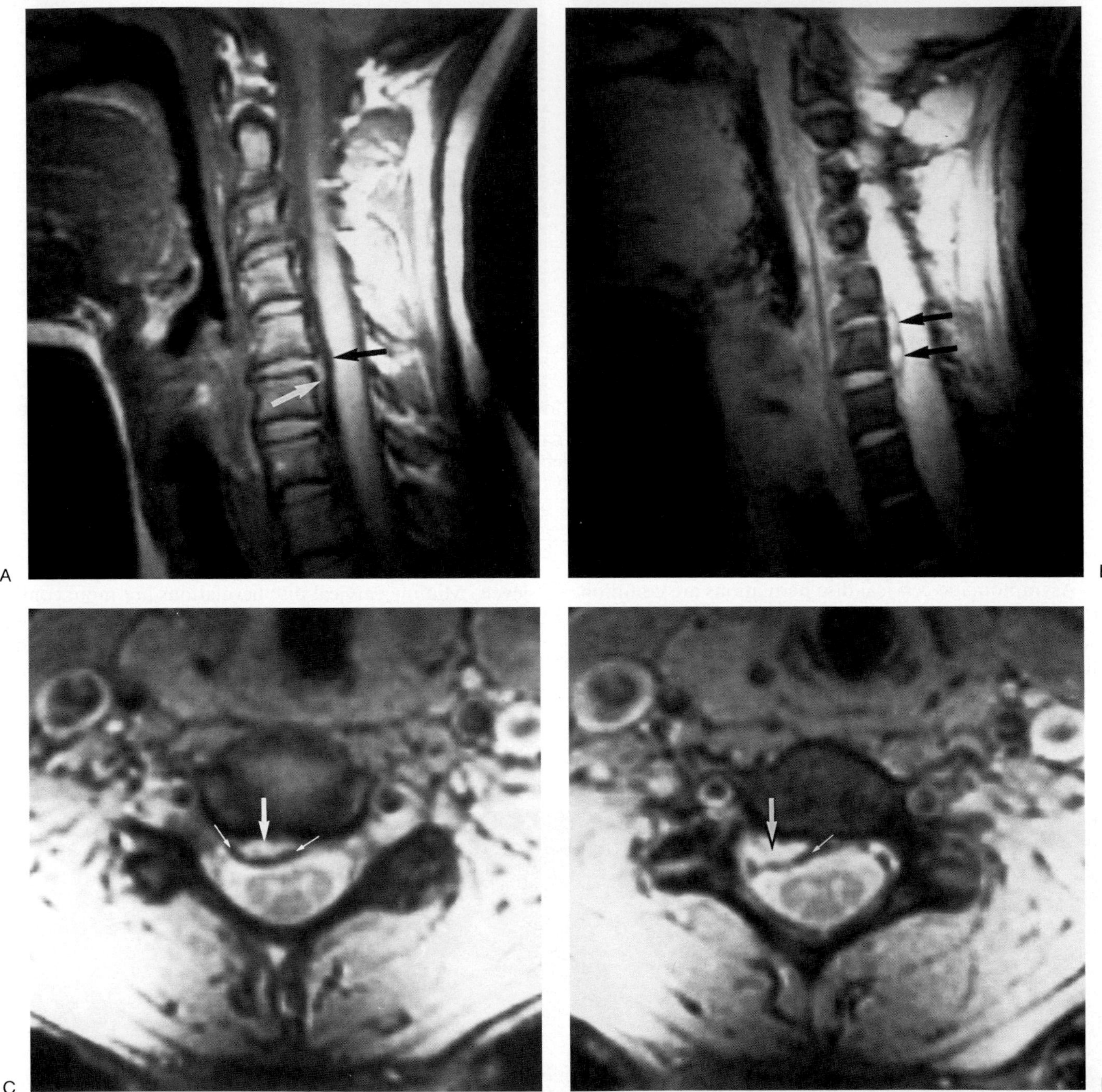

FIG. 83. Herniated disc C5-C6 level with inferior migration. Sagittal T1-weighted SE image (**A**) reveals disc material extending from the intervertebral disc level inferiorly (*white arrow*) and causing mild deformity of the cervical cord anteriorly (*black arrow*). The disc fragment is best seen on parasagittal GE image (**B**) where the fragment (*black arrows*) extends inferiorly from the C5-C6 level to the C6-C7 level. **C:** Axial GE image obtained with 30° flip angle at the C5-C6 level demonstrates the disc herniation (*large white arrow*) to have higher intensity than adjacent bone. Dark band (*tiny white arrows*) between the disc fragment and the cord represents posteriorly displaced posterior longitudinal ligament and dura.

83). If the disc fragment penetrates the PLL, a thin dark band is sometimes seen between the parent disc and the free fragment similar to that seen in the lumbar region (Fig. 84). If the PLL appears to be thin and diminished in intensity on the sagittal T2*-weighted images, this is a sign of disc herniation, and is more commonly seen in the acute stage after disc herniation. In chronic cervical disc disease, the PLL may be thickened or heavily calcified, which can contribute to spinal cord compression. A compressed spinal cord may show areas of increased signal intensity, representing edema in the acute stage and myelomalacia or gliosis in the case of chronic cord compression (see Fig. 80).

Herniated disc fragments may calcify (so-called hard

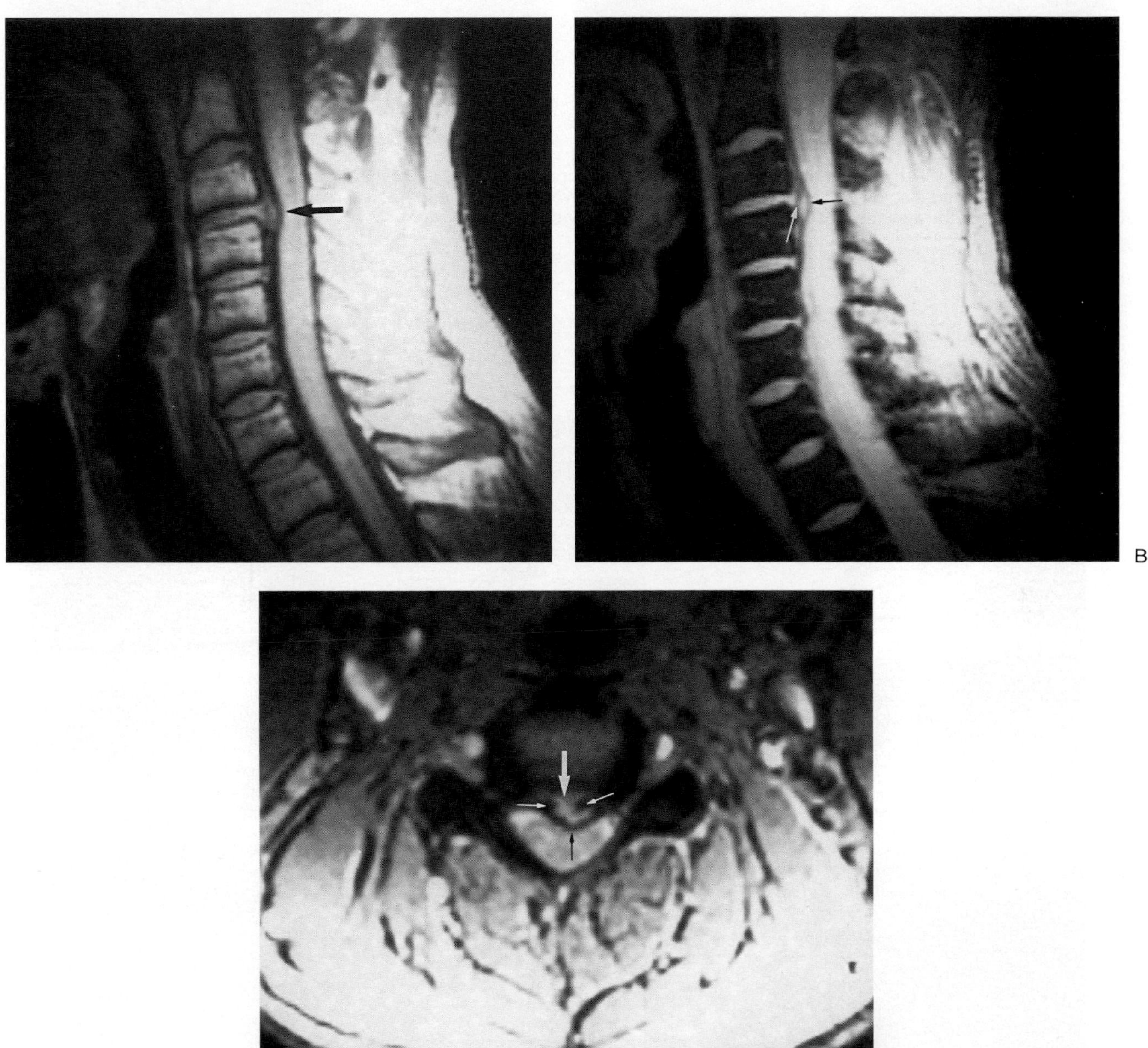

FIG. 84. A: Large herniated disc C3-C4 level, "double fragment sign." A large herniated disc compresses the spinal cord ventrally. **B:** Sagittal GE image demonstrates a thin dark line (*white arrow*) separating two apparent disc fragments at the C3-C4 level. A dark line is also located behind the second aberrant disc fragment (*black arrow*). In axial GE image (**C**), the herniated disc (*large white arrow*) has high signal intensity relative to bone. *Tiny white arrows* point to defect in annulus and posterior longitudinal ligament. *Black arrow* points to dark line between disc fragment and spinal cord, representing thickened posterior longitudinal ligament fragment and dura.

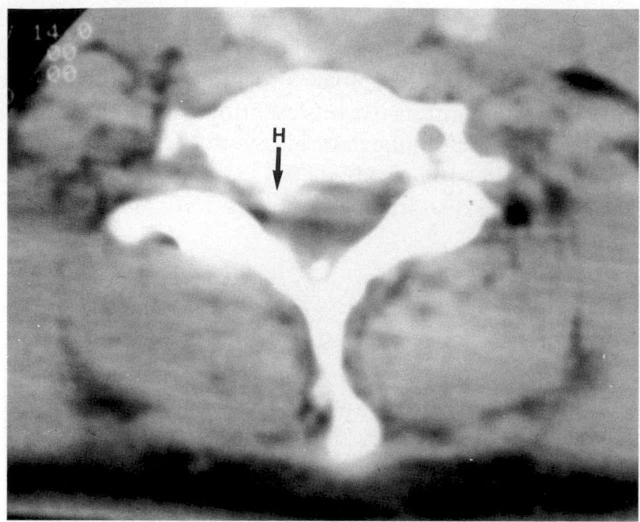

A

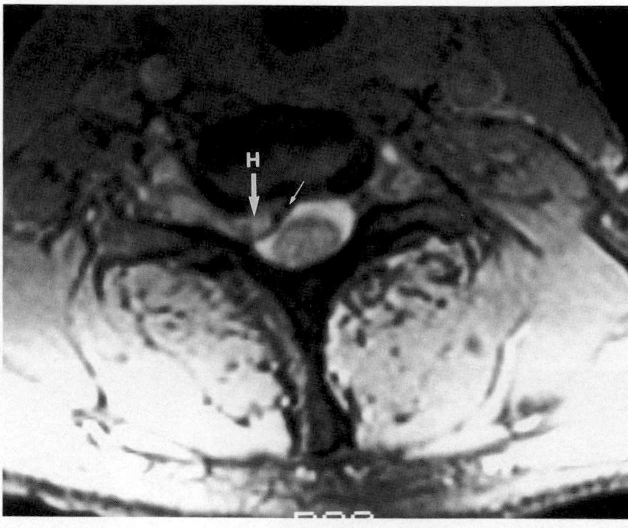

B

FIG. 85. Calcified herniated disc (*H*) resembles an osteophyte on axial CT scan (**A**) but has the typical appearance of a herniated disc on 2-D GE image (**B**). *Small white arrow* indicates dark medial margin of disc fragment due to remnant of the annulus, posterior longitudinal ligament, or dural thickening.

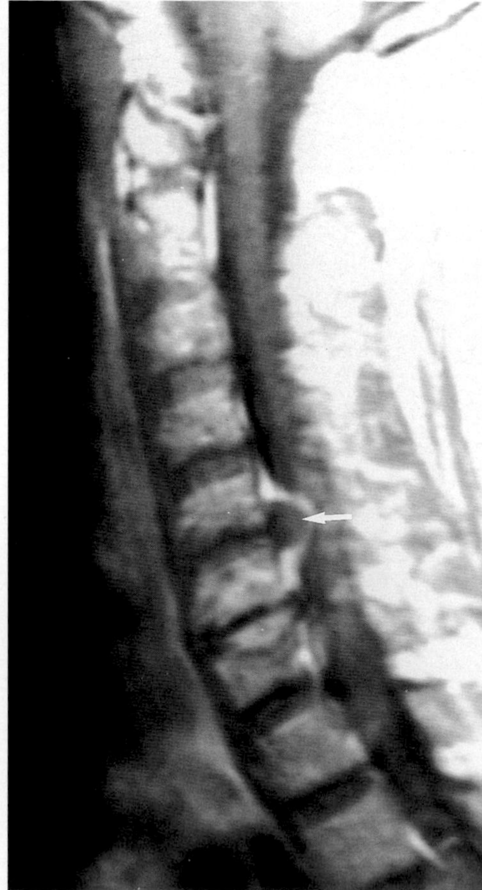

A

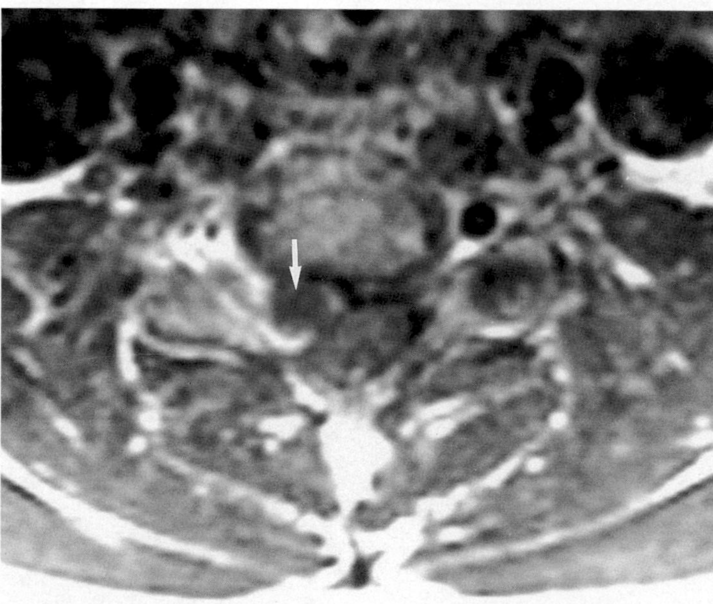

B

FIG. 86. Postoperative enhancement of the tissue surrounding a herniated disc fragment at the C5-C6 level. Herniated disc (*arrow*) does not enhance with gadolinium, similar to that seen in unoperated lumbar disc herniations.

disc) and these may occur anywhere in the spine. CT scans may be misleading because calcified herniated discs resemble osteophytes (Fig. 85). Calcified herniated discs on MRI have the typical appearance of a herniated disc. The role of gadolinium-enhanced MRI in the cervical region is still unclear. Normal structures that enhance include the dural sac, epidural veins, fat, connective tissue, and dorsal root ganglia (56). Because the epidural venous network is so extensive, contrast enhancement by CT and MR has been advocated in the diagnosis of herniated discs (Fig. 86). Although this technique is a useful adjunct in the diagnosis of cervical disc herniation, contrast-enhanced scans are usually not required to make the diagnosis; in fact, midline and paramidline cervical herniated discs are often seen better on T2*-weighted gradient images (Fig. 87).

SPINAL STENOSIS, OSTEOARTHRITIS, AND SPONDYLOSIS

The changes seen in spinal stenosis are best evaluated with a combination of T1-weighted SE, FSE, and 3D reformatted images. The most common degenerative process of the spine is spondylosis deformans. Osteophytes probably arise secondary to degenerative disc disease. When Sharpey's fibers are torn from their attachments along the vertebral body margins, stress is placed on the bone as the disc moves and osteophytes form in reaction to this stress (57). Osteoarthritis refers to a degenerative arthritis involving synovial joints, so the affected joints in the spine are the apophyseal (facet) joints (58) (Fig. 88). Spondylosis and osteoarthritis are terms often used synonymously because they often coexist and have similar predisposing factors. Both conditions result in bone proliferation and enlargement, which narrow either the spinal canal or neural foramen producing spinal stenosis.

LUMBAR SPINAL STENOSIS

Lumbar spinal stenosis includes central spinal canal stenosis, lateral recess stenosis, and foraminal stenosis. These conditions may coexist or occur independently in any given patient. Central canal stenosis is most common at the L2-L3, L3-L4, and L4-L5 levels (59) and patients present with symptoms of radiculopathy or myelopathy, often with bilateral lower extremity claudication on exertion. The degenerative complex in acquired spinal stenosis includes diffuse disc bulging, facet

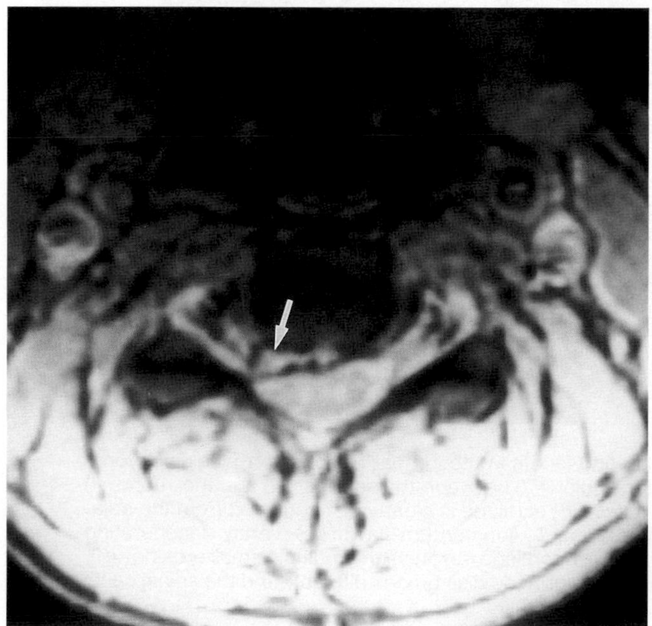

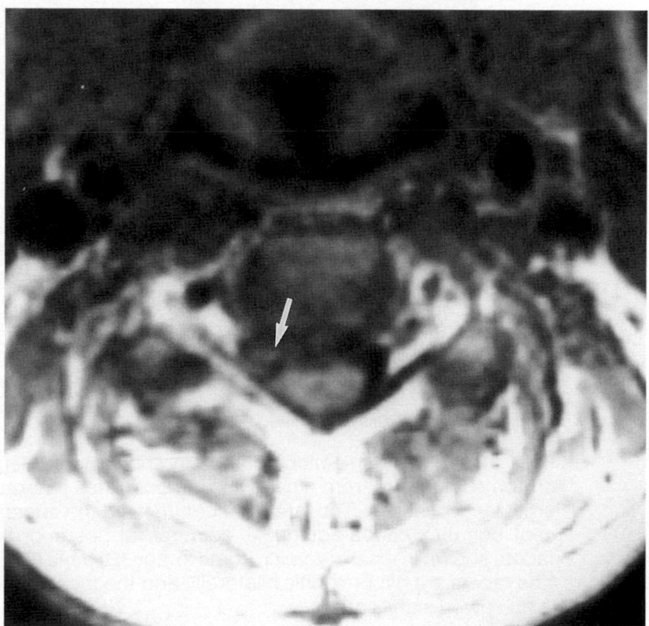

FIG. 87. Herniated cervical disc GE vs. gadolinium-enhanced SE comparison. A herniated disc (*arrow*) has high signal intensity on axial GE image (**A**) obtained with 30° flip angle. Enhancement of foraminal structures including foraminal veins is seen in axial T1-weighted SE image (**B**) but the herniated disc does not enhance, and is more difficult to visualize in B compared to A.

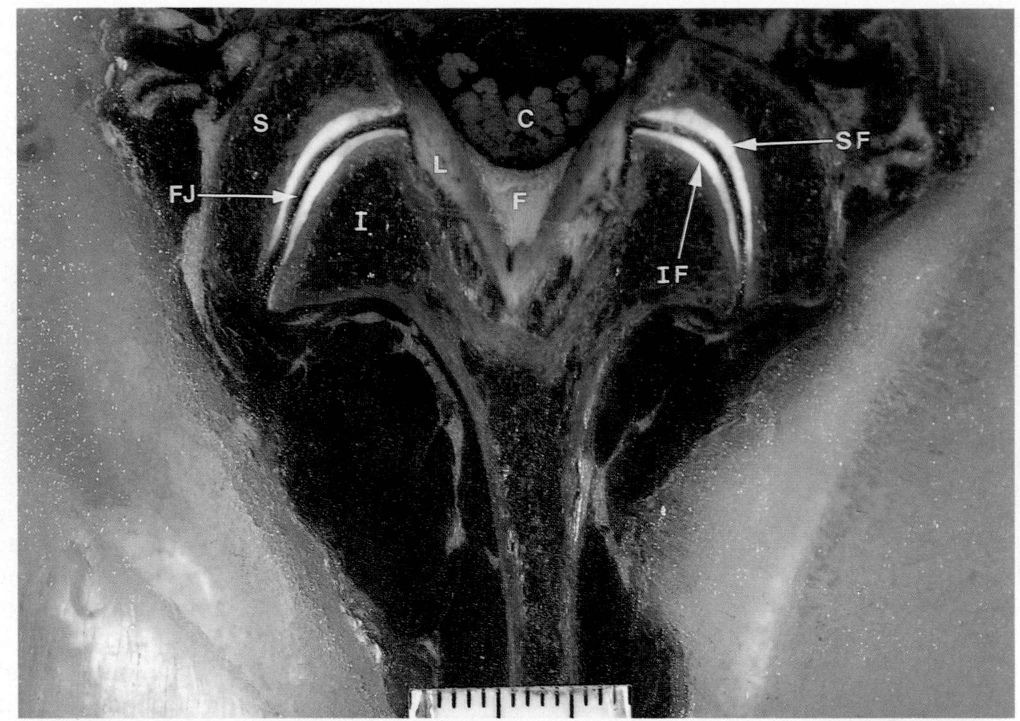

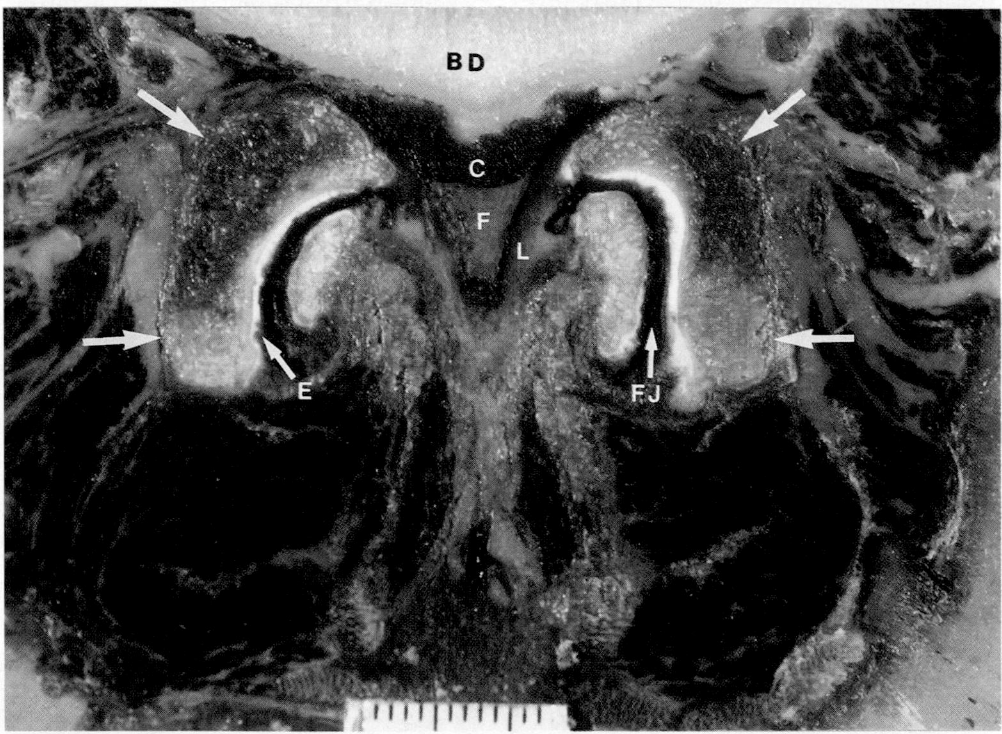

FIG. 88. Anatomic sections comparing normal and degenerating facets in the lumbar region. Normal axial cryomicrotome image (**A**) from a cadaver demonstrates a normal facet joint (*FJ*) between the superior (*S*) and the inferior (*I*) articular processes. The inferior facet (*IF*) and the superior facet (*SF*) cartilage is clearly distinguished from the adjacent bone. *C*, cauda equina; *F*, epidural fat posterior to thecal sac; *L*, ligamentum flavum. Severely degenerating facets shown in axial cryomicrotome image (**B**) have loss of articular cartilage (*arrows*) and multiple small erosions (*E*). The facets are hypertrophic bilaterally and the facet joints are widened. The disc bulges diffusely and the spinal canal is narrowed significantly.

hypertrophy and ligamentous thickening, and redundancy (60). In patients who have "short pedicles" on a developmental basis, minimal degenerative disease will result in symptoms of spinal stenosis at an earlier age than in those patients with purely acquired spinal stenosis.

Lumbar central stenosis is characterized by circumferential ("napkin-ring") narrowing of the central canal to an area less than 1.5 cm^2 or an anteroposterior diameter of less than 11.5 mm (61). The thecal sac narrowing is well seen on myelography, CT, or MR in the sagittal and axial planes (Fig. 89). The nerve rootlets of the cauda equina are compressed by this process, resulting in neurogenic claudication. The affected nerve roots and engorged veins may enhance with paramagnetic contrast (44).

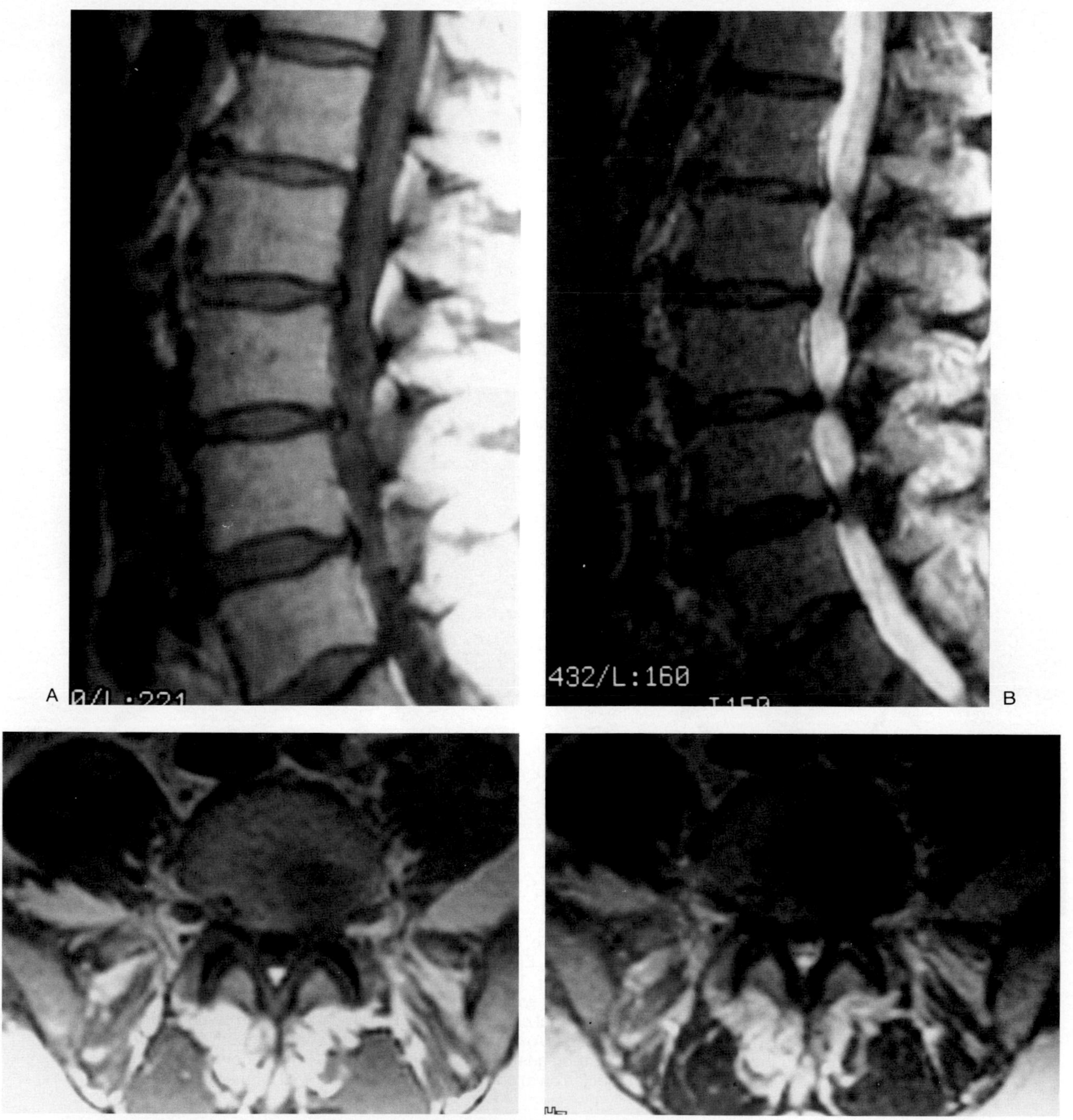

FIG. 89. Severe multilevel spinal stenosis in the lumbar region. Sagittal T1-weighted image (**A**) and T2-weighted FSE image (**B**) reveal multiple bulging and degenerating discs along with thickening of the ligamentum flavum, causing circumferential narrowing of the thecal sac, more pronounced at L3-L4 and L4-L5. Central canal stenosis is more apparent on the T2-weighted axial FSE image (**D**) than on the T1-weighted SE image (**C**).

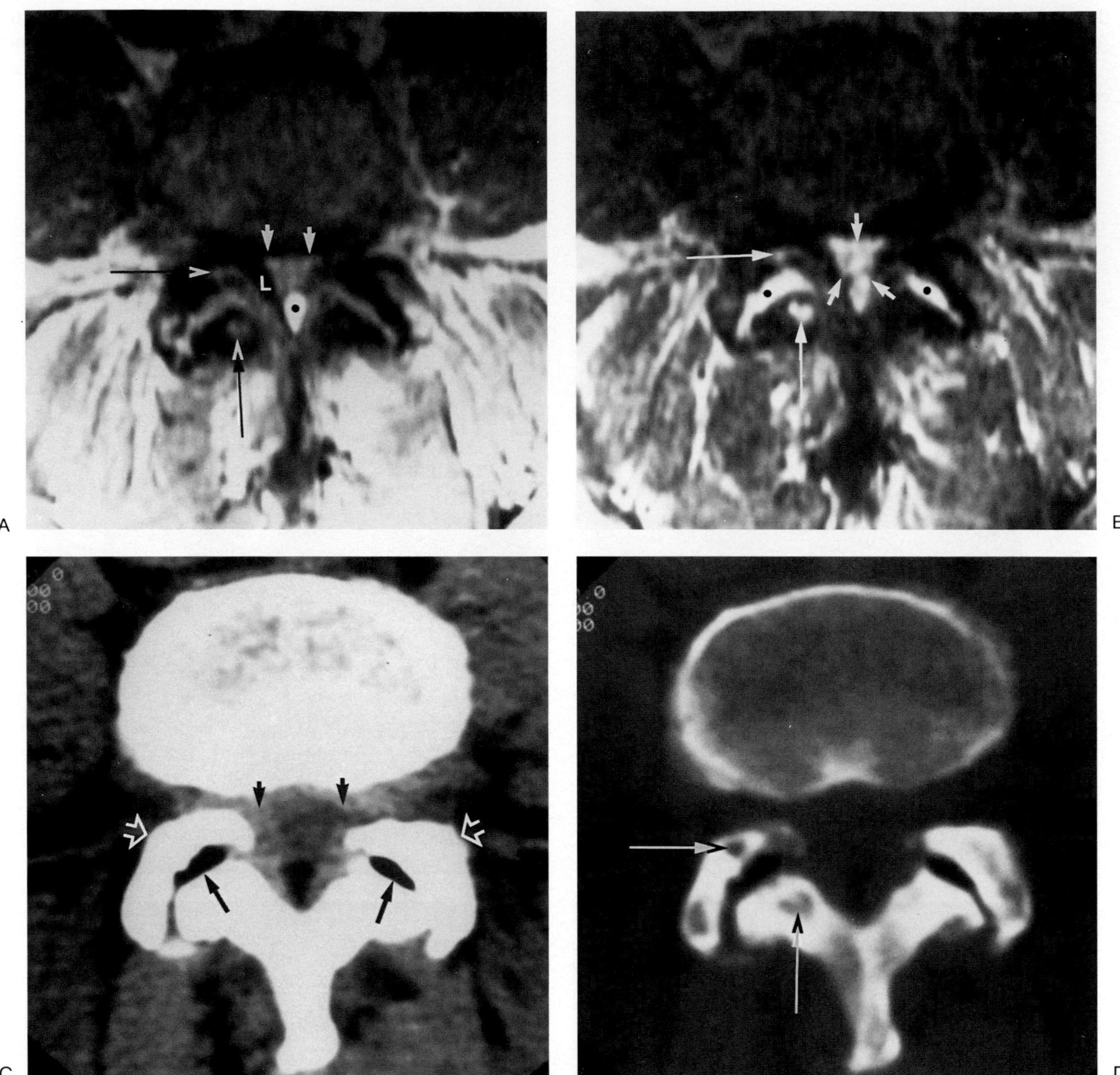

FIG. 90. Severe lumbar spinal stenosis and facet disease, MR vs. CT. A diffusely bulging disc (*small arrows*) narrows the spinal canal anteriorly on T1-weighted SE image (**A**). Epidural fat (*dot*) is located posterior to the thecal sac. The facets are bilaterally enlarged and the facet joints irregular. The long arrows in A indicate facet erosions. *L*, ligamentum flavum. In T2-weighted SE image (**B**), the erosions (*long arrows*) have high signal intensity probably containing fluid. Facet joint effusions are seen bilaterally (*dots*). The spinal canal (*small arrows*) is markedly narrowed and triangular in shape. CT scans obtained 1 year later with soft tissue (A) and bone (B) windows reveal vacuum facet (*long arrows*, **C**). At the site of previous joint effusions, the disc bulges diffusely (*small arrows*). The facets are enlarged (*open arrows*). Erosions in the superior and inferior facet (*arrows*) on CT scan (**D**) correlate well with erosion seen on MRI 1 year earlier (B).

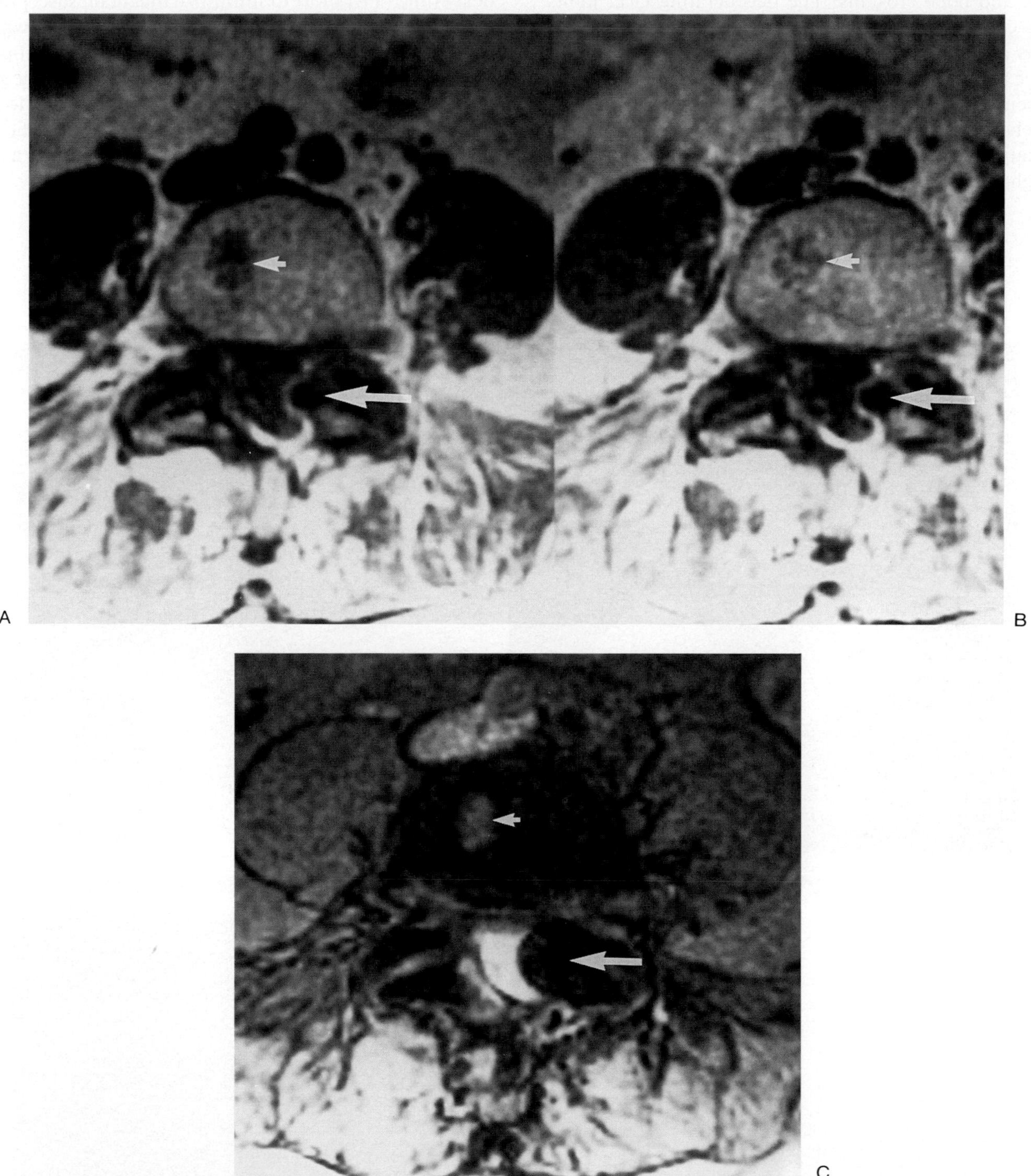

FIG. 91. Artifact mimicking facet hypertrophy and stenosis, incidental Schmorl's node. **A:** Unenhanced T1-weighted axial image at L3-L4 demonstrates a metallic object (*large arrow*) that might be confused for facet hypertrophy. This does not enhance in gadolinium-enhanced image (**B**). There is enhancement of the Schmorl's node (*small arrow* in A and B). In GE image (**C**), the apparent increased size of the metallic clip is due to magnetic susceptibility artifact, which might be confused with severe facet hypertrophy causing central stenosis. The Schmorl's node (*small arrow*) has high intensity in C.

Osteoarthritic disease of the facets is a contributing factor producing facet hypertrophy, cartilage destruction, and bone erosions. The degenerating facet joints may contain effusions or gas (vacuum facets), and erosions are present in advanced disease. The facet joint space is widened when acute inflammatory effusions are present, but is often narrowed in chronic facet disease. The bone abnormalities and vacuum discs are easiest to visualize with CT (62), but can be detected with T2*-weighted sequences, which depict bone as low signal intensity, and fluid, erosions, and bone defects as high signal intensity (Fig. 90). It is important to keep the echo delay time (TE) short to minimize magnetic susceptibility artifacts from bone or ferromagnetic material, which can simulate spinal stenosis or make the facets appear larger than they are (Fig. 91). The obliteration of the epidural fat that accompanies spinal stenosis is easier to see on T1-weighted SE images. However, bone detail is poorly seen on T1-weighted SE images, and this is a disadvantage in visualizing calcified discs or ligaments.

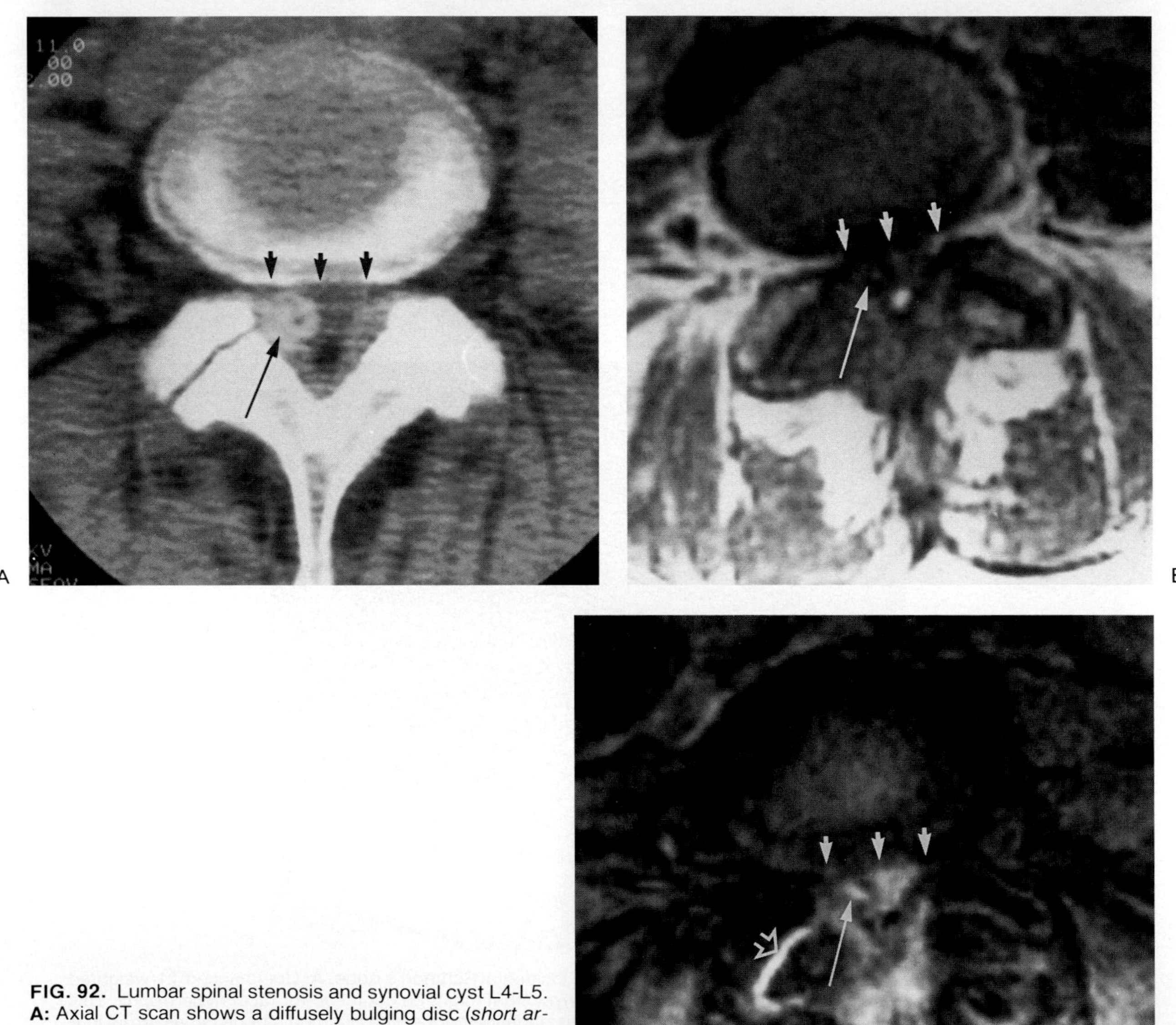

FIG. 92. Lumbar spinal stenosis and synovial cyst L4-L5. **A:** Axial CT scan shows a diffusely bulging disc (*short arrows*) and a calcified synovial cyst (*long arrow*) on the right encroaching on the spinal canal. **B:** In T1-weighted SE image, the synovial cyst (*long arrow*) is difficult to distinguish from adjacent bone. **C:** The synovial cyst has high signal intensity as a fluid (*long arrow*) in GE image. A facet joint effusion (*open arrow*) is present on the right. The bulging disc has low intensity along its margins (*small arrows* in B and C).

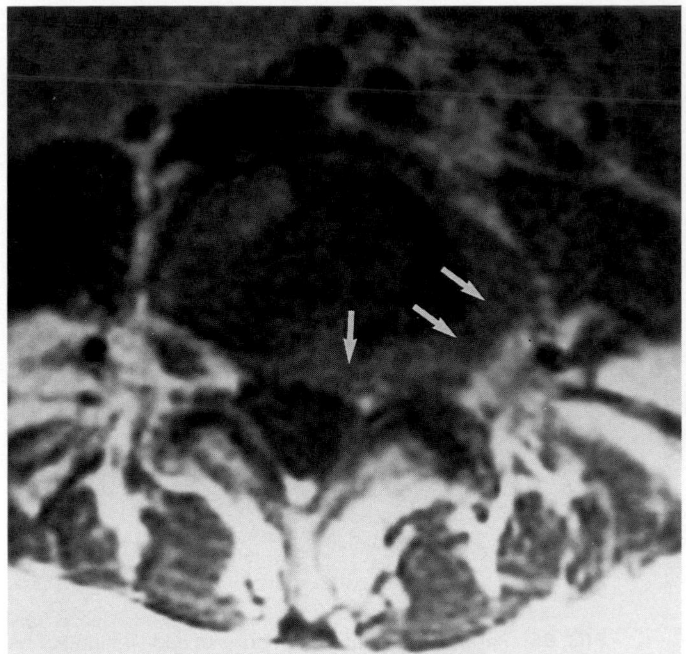

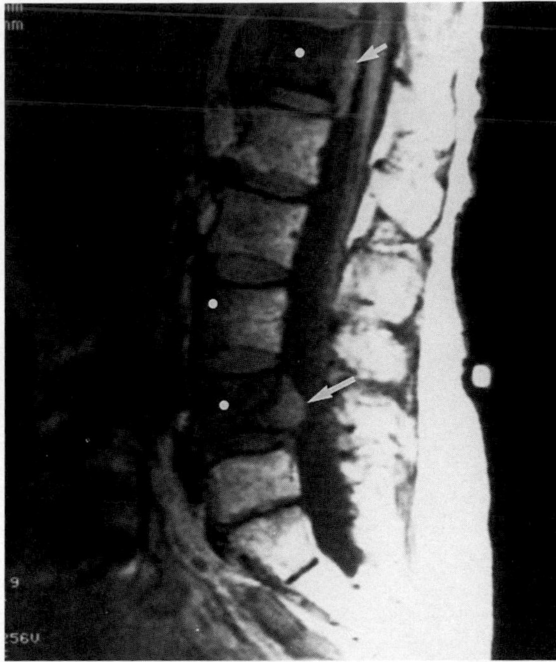

FIG. 93. Epidural tumor simulating a herniated disc in an axial plane. **A:** In T1-weighted SE MR image, abnormal soft tissue (*arrows*) compresses the thecal sac ventrally, obliterates the epidural fat on the left, and extends into the left neural foramen. This may be confused with a large extruded disc. **B:** In sagittal T2-weighted scan, the epidural mass (*long arrow*) is centered above the disc space level, typical of epidural metastasis. The tumor is seen in multiple vertebral bodies (*dots*) as low signal–intensity material replacing the normally high intensity fatty marrow. The epidural tumor is also present in the spinal canal at the T12 level (*short arrow*).

Synovial cysts arise at the L4-L5 or L5-S1 level more commonly on the right, and are probably related to facet degeneration of trauma. Synovial cysts are easier to visualize on CT because they are often calcified (Fig. 92). On MR the cysts are isointense or slightly hyperintense with respect to CSF on T1-weighted SE images and hyperintense on T2-weighted images (63,64). Sometimes, synovial cysts can bleed, and are seen as low intensity on T2-weighted images (Fig. 93). Synovial cysts can be difficult to see with MR on any pulse sequence, but are important because they can produce thecal sac compression and contribute to central canal stenosis.

Lateral recess stenosis (LRS) is present when the distance between the superior facet anteromedially and the posterior vertebral body margin is less than 4 mm. Lateral recess stenosis is caused by the hypertrophic superior facet encroaching on the lateral recess, and produces symptoms by compressing the nerve root before it exits the neural foramen. Hypertrophic inferior facets narrow the lateral recess by reducing the interlaminar angle (65) (Fig. 94).

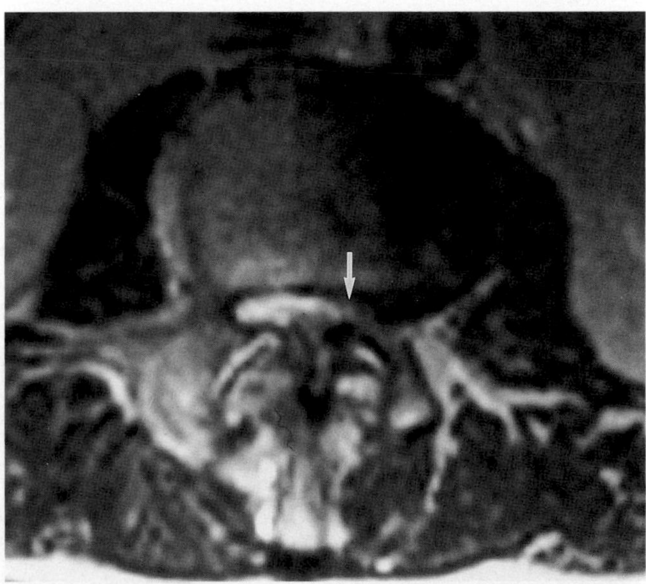

FIG. 94. Lateral recessed stenosis on the left at L4 obscures the epidural fat (*arrow*) at the L4 level on the left on this T2-weighted axial FSE image. Central canal stenosis is also present due to facet hypertrophy bilaterally.

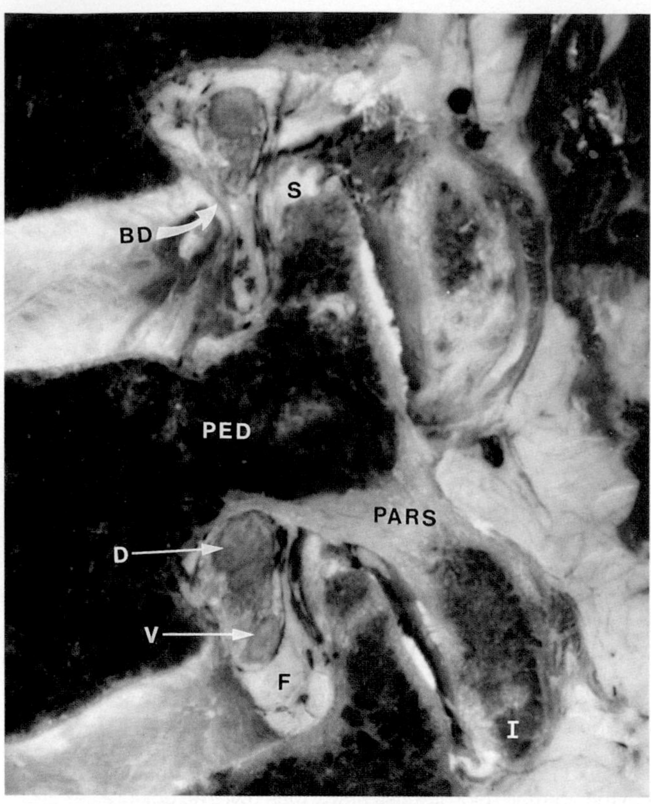

FIG. 95. Parasagittal anatomic images of cadaver lumbar neural foramen showing bulging disc (*BD*) encroaching on the inferior aspect of the upper foramen. The normal disc annulus at the lower level does not encroach on the epidural fat (*F*) of the lower foramen. *D*, dorsal root ganglion; *V*, ventral root; *S*, superior articular process; *I*, inferior articular process; *PARS*, pars interarticularis; *PED*, pedicle.

Foraminal stenosis occurs when a bulging disc, hypertrophic facet, or vertebral body osteophyte encroaches on the neural foramen (Figs. 95 and 96). Foraminal size is best assessed on sagittal-unenhanced or gadolinium-enhanced T1-weighted SE images because fat outlines the nerve root and dorsal root ganglia in the foramen. A bulging or herniated disc first encroaches on the lower portion of the neural foramen, largely composed of fat and veins. The lumbar nerve roots are located in the superior portion of the foramen (Fig. 97).

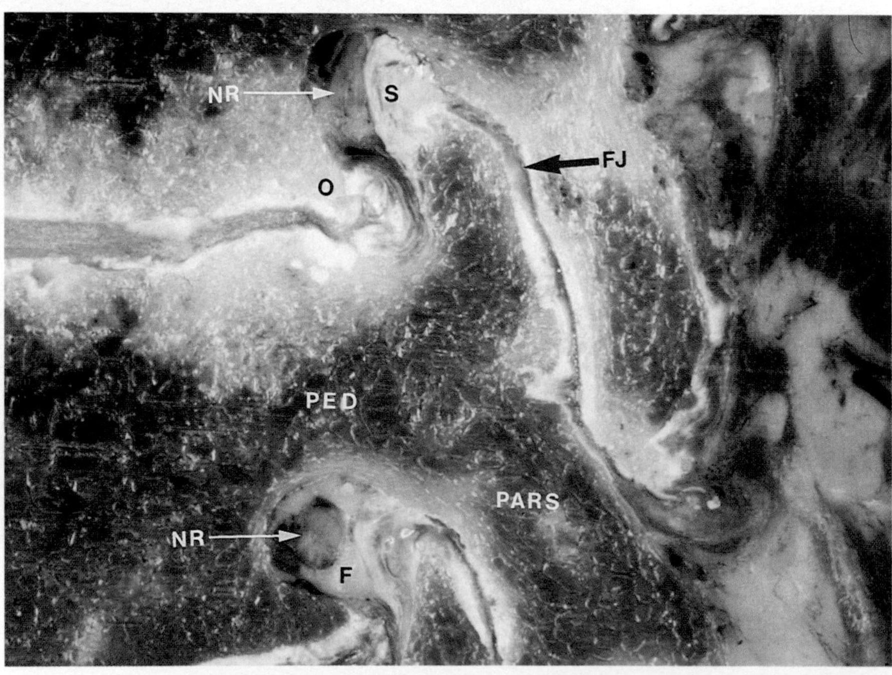

FIG. 96. Severe foraminal stenosis in anatomic parasagittal section through lumbar neural foramina obtained with cryomicrotome. A vertebral body osteophyte (*O*) and bulging disc encroach on the inferior portion of the upper neural foramen. A hypertrophied superior articular process (*S*) compresses the nerve roots in the foramen. *F*, foraminal fat; *FJ*, facet joint; *PARS*, pars interarticularis; *PED*, pedicle.

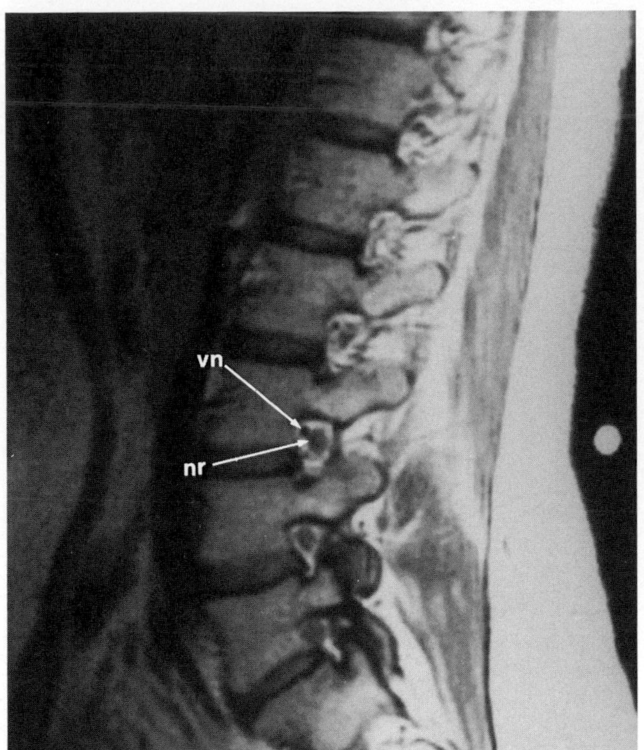

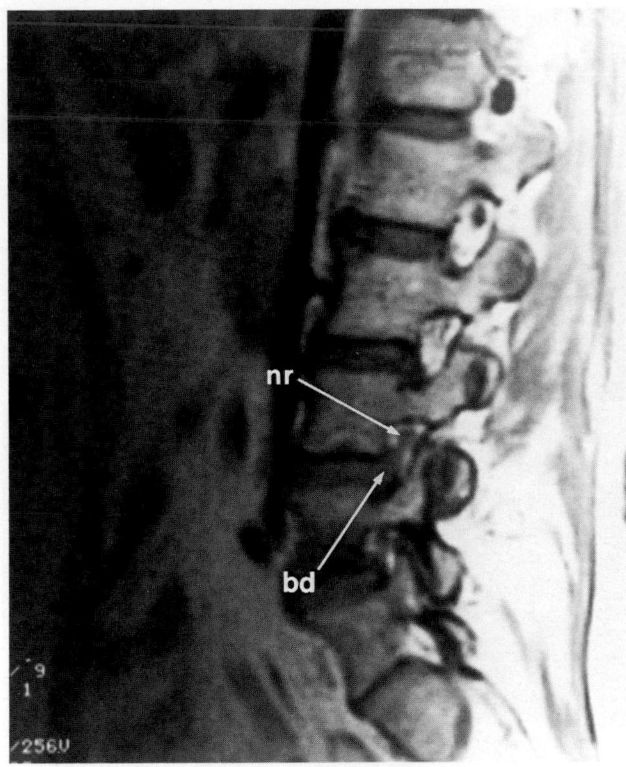

FIG. 97. Disc bulging into foramen shown in parasagittal T1-weighted lumbar SE images. **A:** A slightly bulging disc encroaches on the L4-L5 foramen inferiorly (*nr*, nerve root in foramen; *vn*, foraminal. **B:** In a different patient, a bulging disc (*bd*) abuts the nerve root (*nr*) in the L4-L5 foramen.

CERVICAL SPINAL STENOSIS

Central canal stenosis in the cervical spine is most often secondary to spondylosis deformans (osteophytosis) and ligamentous thickening (Figs. 98 and 99). Foraminal stenosis is usually caused by uncinate process hypertrophy and enlargement of the superior articular facet. MRI is well suited for screening the cervical spine for cervical stenosis. Patients generally experience symptoms of myelopathy or radiculopathy if the anteroposterior diameter of the cervical canal is less than 11 mm.

Assuming magnetic susceptibility artifact can be minimized, T2*-weighted GE images are well suited for evaluating cervical spondylosis because osteophytes are clearly distinguished from discs. However, the most accurate assessment of spinal canal size can be obtained from T2-weighted sagittal FSE images. Osteophytes have low signal intensity relative to higher signal intensity disc material on GE images. The constellation of findings in spinal stenosis includes bulging discs, osteophytic ridging (spondylosis deformans), and thickening or redundancy of the ligaments (posterior longitudinal ligament and ligamentum flavum) (Fig. 100). If the spinal cord is compressed over a long period, irrevocable change in the spinal cord architecture occurs manifested by gliosis and myelomalacia. These changes are seen as focal areas of increased signal intensity in the cord on T2-weighted im-

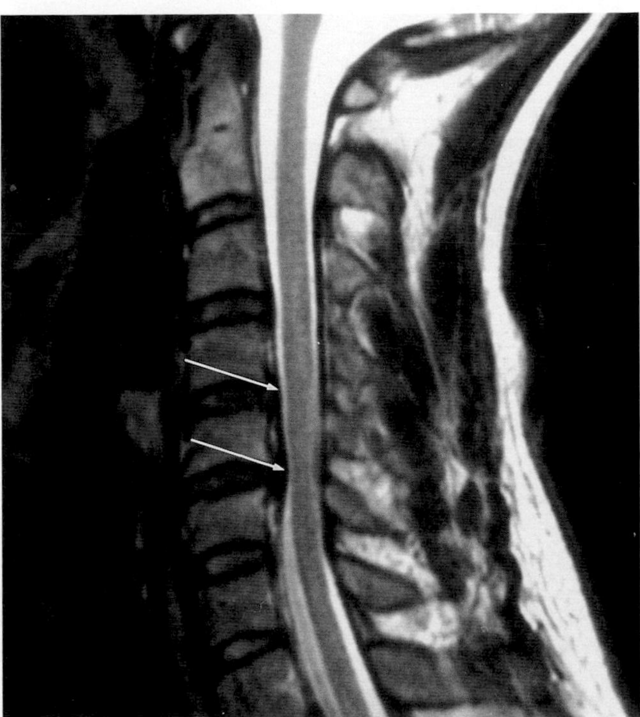

FIG. 98. Spinal stenosis at the C4-C5 and C5-C6 levels demonstrated on sagittal T2-weighted FSE image. In addition to disc bulging at these levels, there is thickening of the posterior longitudinal ligament (*arrows*), which contributes to the spinal stenosis.

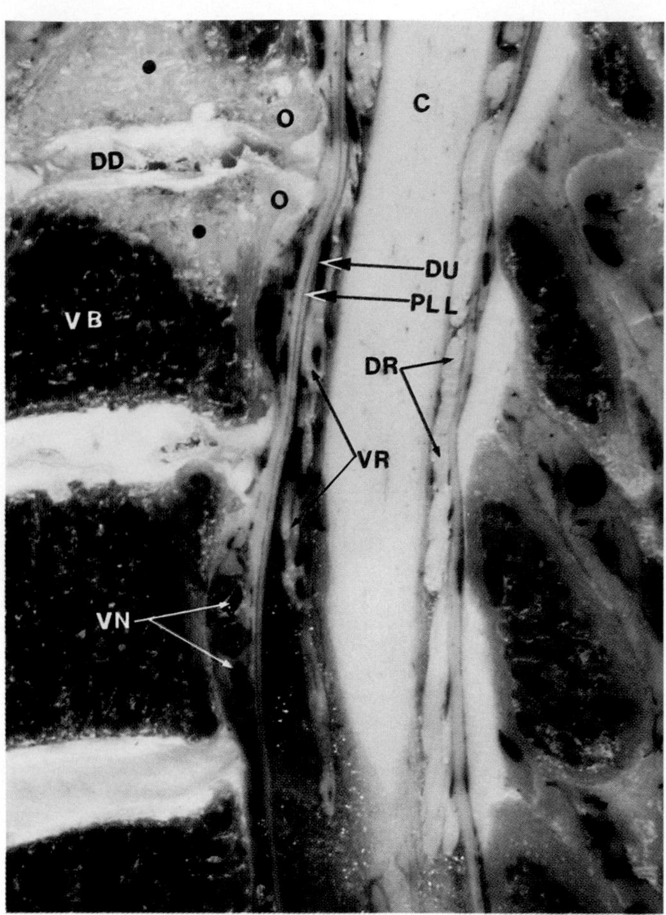

FIG. 99. Sagittal cryomicrotome section of a cadaver. Cervical spine with osteophytes (*O*) displacing dura (*DU*) and posterior longitudinal ligament (*PLL*) posteriorly. *DD*, degenerating disc; *VB*, vertebral body; *VN*, anterior epidural veins; *black dots*, sclerotic vertebral endplates; *DR*, dorsal rootlets; *VR*, ventral rootlets; *C*, spinal cord.

A,B

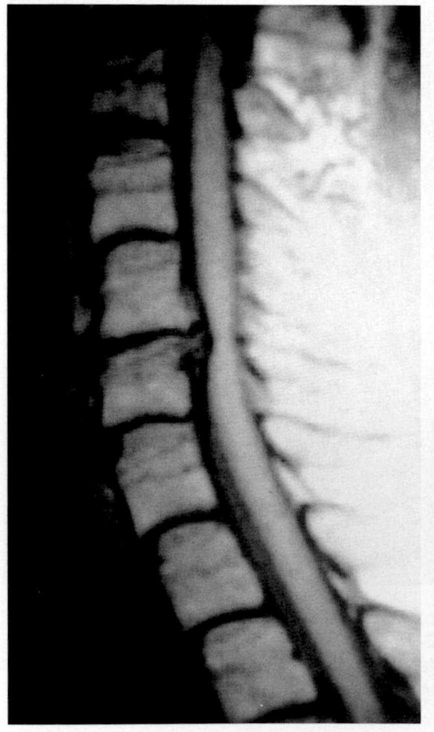

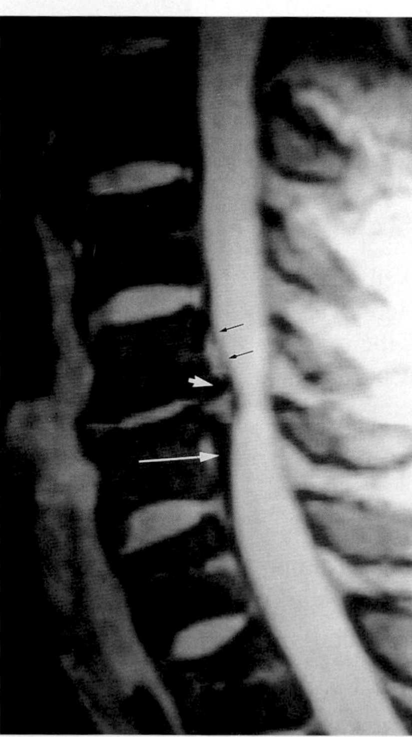

FIG. 100. Herniated disc, osteophyte, and ligamentous thickening, causing cord compression at the C5-C6 level. **A:** The herniated disc is seen to cause cord compression on the T1-weighted sagittal SE image. **B:** In GE image obtained with a 30° flip angle, the bulging disc has high signal intensity relative to the adjacent osteophyte (*small white arrow*). Below the herniated disc, there is thickening of the posterior longitudinal ligament (*long arrow*). The normal posterior longitudinal ligament (*small black arrows*) is seen above the disc level.

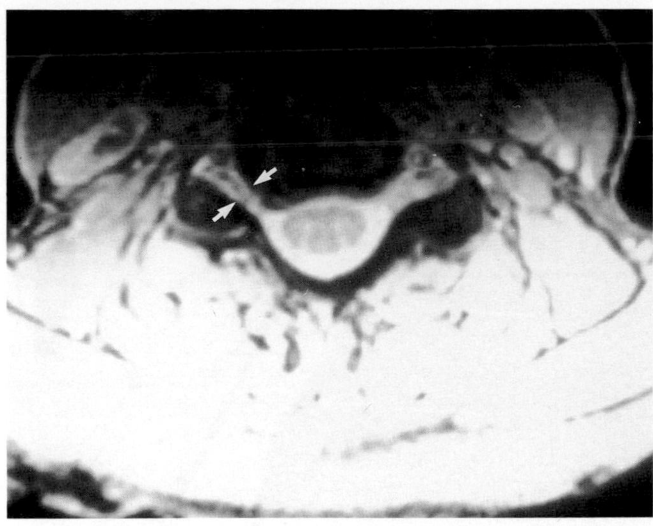

FIG. 101. Foraminal stenosis (*arrows*) is shown at the C5-C6 level on the right because of uncinate hypertrophy and facet hypertrophy on this axial 2D GE image with 30° flip angle and 3-mm slice thickness.

ages and they are indicative of a poor prognosis (see Fig. 80) (66).

Degenerative involvement of the adjacent vertebral bodies has a similar MR appearance in the cervical spine to that already described in the lumbar spine, and often accompanies advanced cervical spondylosis deformans. Degenerative disease of the vertebral endplates should not be confused with cervical discitis, in which the infected disc space has high signal intensity and vertebral endplate destruction is present (see Fig. 96).

CT scanning has been considered the procedure of choice for diagnosing foraminal stenosis because the margins of the normal foramen, spinal canal, and osteophytes are so well demonstrated. Assuming motion and magnetic susceptibility artifacts can be controlled, GE sequences represent a viable alternative to CT in the evaluation of cervical radiculopathy. Using volume 3D GE techniques, thin sections (1 mm or less) can be obtained, which is ideal for evaluating the cervical neural foramen (67). Contrast-enhanced MR scanning with gadolinium enhancement using 3D or 2D pulse sequences represents an important adjunct to CT in evalu-

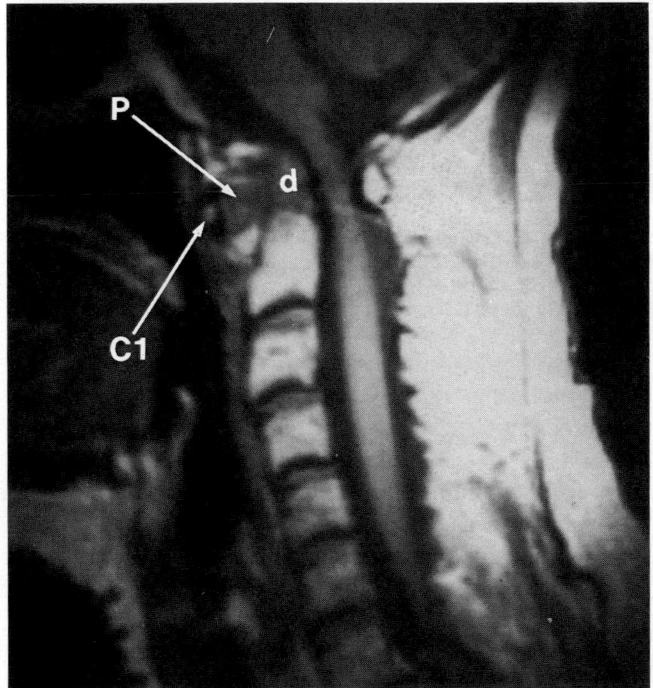

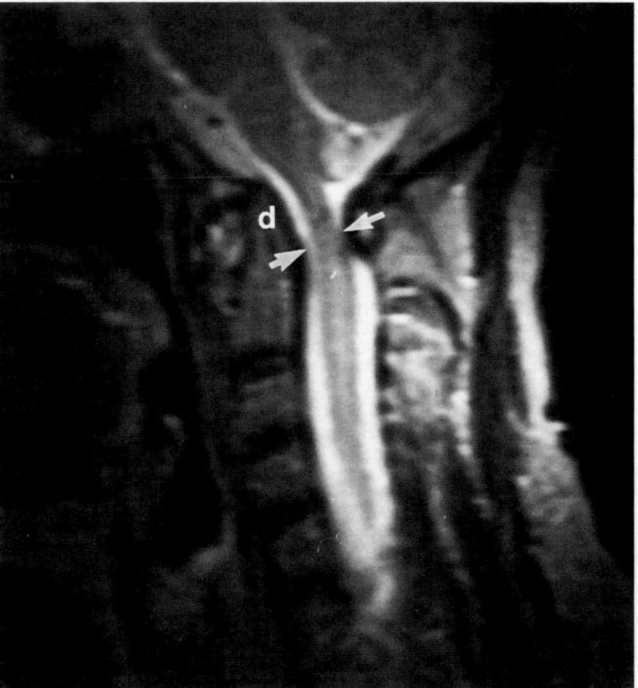

FIG. 102. Rheumatoid arthritis. Sagittal T1- (**A**) and T2-weighted (**B**) SE images show separation of the dens (*d*) and anterior arch of C1 by pannus (*P*). The spinal canal (*arrows*, B) is narrowed because of dens displacement, resulting in spinal cord compromise.

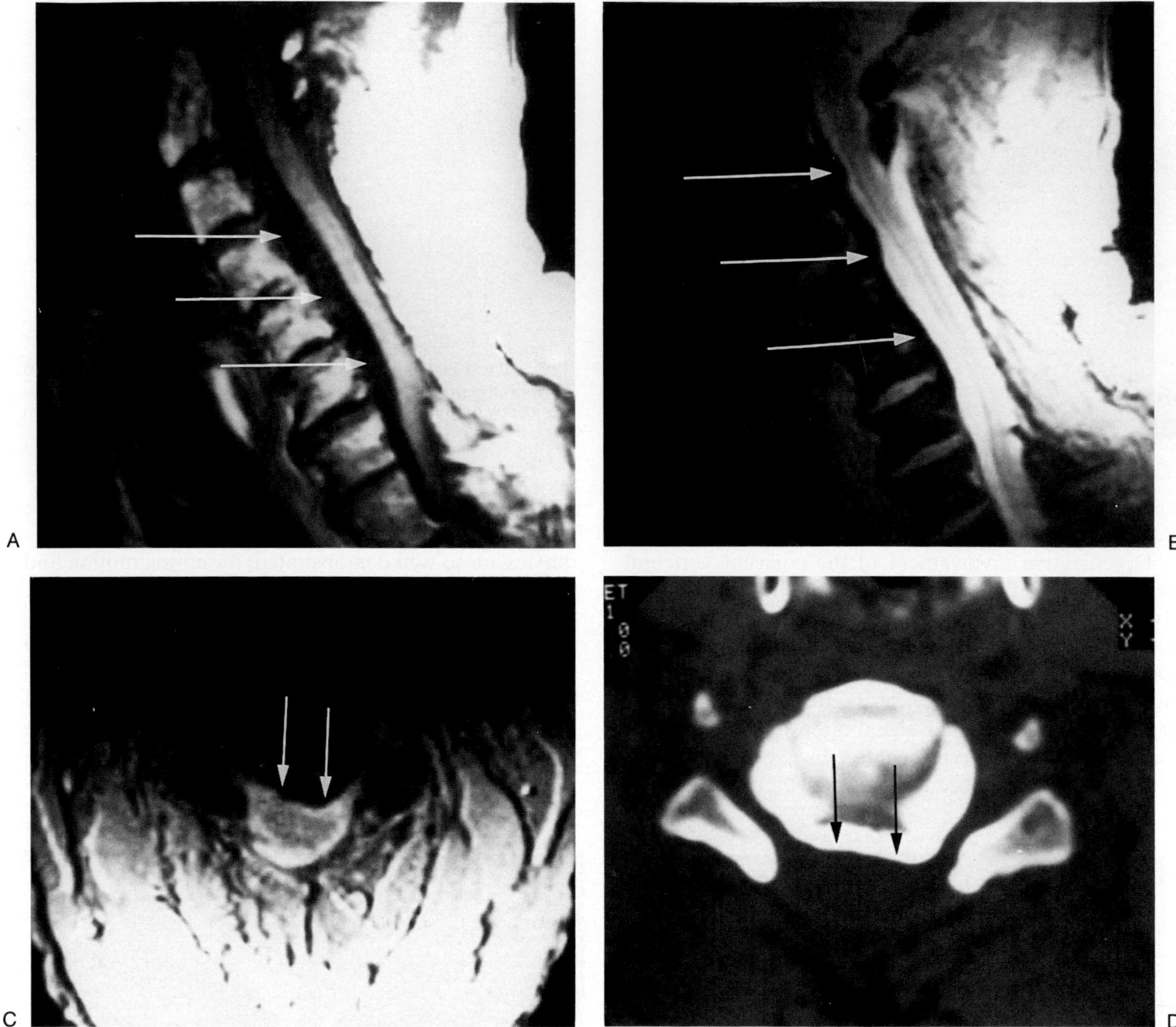

FIG. 103. Ossified posterior longitudinal ligament. Patient had wide laminectomy for cervical myelopathy. The ossified ligaments (*arrows*) in **A** and **B** are difficult to visualize in the SE image (A), but are seen as a thickened band of low intensity, representing an ossified posterior longitudinal ligament, in the GE image (B). Axial GE scan (**C**) demonstrates the calcified ligament (*arrows*) encroaching on the spinal canal anteriorly. Axial CT scan (**D**) included for comparison.

ating foraminal disease of all types, including cervical radiculopathy (Fig. 101). Although CT scanning is the preferred method, MR can be used to screen for neural foraminal narrowing on axial GE or contrast-enhanced MRI. 3D volume imaging with oblique reformatting is reserved for difficult cases to minimize examination time (see Fig. 9).

Rheumatoid arthritis and other arthritides can also be associated with spondylosis and canal narrowing (Fig. 102) (68,69). In rheumatoid arthritis, pannus formation, odontoid erosion, and cord compression, if present, are well shown with MR (Fig. 103). Since plain radiographs are fine for assessing the degree of atlantoaxial subluxation, MR is most valuable for assessing the degree of cord compression. Atlantoaxial subluxation can be diagnosed on T1-weighted images obtained in neck flexion and extension.

Ossification of the posterior longitudinal ligament (OPLL) can produce significant myelopathy because of severe spinal canal stenosis (70). In this condition, segmental or diffuse ossification of the posterior longitudinal ligament is responsible for the cord compression. The ossified ligaments have high or low signal intensity depending on whether or not they contain bone marrow elements (71,72). Diffuse idiopathic skeletal hyperostosis (DISH) is manifested by exuberant calcification of the anterior longitudinal ligament in the absence of apophyseal joint ankylosis, and relatively minimal degenerative disc disease is present (73). DISH and OPLL often coexist.

REFERENCES

1. Edelman RR, Shoukimas GM, Stark DD, et al. High-resolution surface-coil imaging of lumbar disk disease. *AJR* 1985;144:1123–1129.
2. Frahm J, Haase A, Matthaei D. Rapid NMR imaging of dynamic processes using the FLASH technique. *Magn Reson Med* 1986;3:321–327.
3. Wehrli FW. Fast-scan magnetic resonance imaging: principles and contrast phenomenology. In: Higgons C, Hricak H, eds. *Magnetic Resonance Imaging of the Body*. New York: Raven Press; 1987.
4. Czervionke LF, Daniels DL. Cervical spine anatomy and pathologic processes. *Radiol Clin North Am* 1988;26:921–947.
5. Yousem D, Atlas SW, Goldberg HI, Grossman RI. Degenerative narrowing of the cervical spine neural foramina: evaluation with high resolution 3DFT gradient-echo MR imaging. *AJNR* 1991;12:229–236
6. Felmlee J, Ehman R. Spatial presaturation; a method for suppressing flow artifacts and improving depiction of vascular anatomy in MR imaging. *Radiology* 1987;164:559–564.
7. Pattany P, Phillips J, Chiu L, et al. Motion artifact suppression technique (MAST) for MR imaging. *J Comp Assist Tomogr* 1987;11:369–377.
8. Peacock A. Observations on the postnatal structure of the intervertebral disc in man. *J Anat* 1952;86:162–179.
9. Rabischong P, Louis R, Vignaud J, et al. The intervertebral disc. *Anat Clin* 1978;1:55–64.
10. Ibrahim MA, Jesmanowicz A, Hyde JS, Estkowski L, Haughton VM. Contrast enhancement in normal intervertebral discs: time and dose dependence. *AJNR* 1994;15:419–423.
11. Urban JPG, McMullen JF. Fifth international congress on biorheology symposium: some biorheological aspects of joint diseases. *Biorheology* 1985;22:145–157.
12. VanDenHooff A. Histological age changes in the annulus fibrosus of the human intervertebral disk with a discussion of the problem of disk herniation. *Gerontologia* 1964;9:136–149.
13. Pech P, Haughton VM. Lumbar intervertebral disc: correlative MR and anatomic study. *Radiology* 1985;156:679–702.
14. Adams P, Eyre D, Rand Muir H. Biochemical aspects of development and aging of human lumbar intervertebral discs. *Rheumatol Rehab* 1977;16:22–29.
15. Pritzker KPH. Aging and degeneration in the lumbar intervertebral disc. *Orthop Clin North Am* 1977;8:65–77.
16. Ibrahim MA, Haughton VM, Hyde JS. Enhancement of normal intervertebral discs with gadolinium complexes: comparison of an ionic and a non-ionic medium. *AJNR* [*in press*].
17. Peacock A. Observations on the pre-natal development of the intervertebral disc in man. *J Anat* 1951;85:260–278.
18. Taylor JR. Growth of human intervertebral discs and vertebral bodies. *J Anat* 1975;120:49–68.
19. Twomey LT, Taylor JR. Age changes in lumbar vertebrae and intervertebral discs. *Clin Orthop Rel Res* 1987;224:97–104.
20. Modic MT, Steinberg, PM, et al. Degenerative disc disease assessment of changes in vertebral marrow with imaging. *Radiology* 1988; 166:193–199.
21. Ho PSP, Yu S, Sether LA, Wagner M, Ho KC, Haughton VM. Progressive and regressive changes in the nucleus pulposus. Part I: The neonate. *Radiology* 1988;169:87–91.
22. Yu S, Haughton VM, Sether LA, Wagner M. Comparison of MR and diskography in detecting radial tears of the annulus: a postmortem study. *AJNR* 1989;10:1077–1081.
23. Gower WE, Pedrini V. Age-related variations in protein polysaccharides from human nucleus pulposus, annulus fibrosus, and costal cartilage. *J Bone Joint Surg* 1969;51A:1154–1162.
24. Taylor TKF, Akeson WH. Intervertebral disc prolapse: a review of morphologic and biochemic knowledge concerning the nature of prolapse. *Clin Orthop* 1971;76:54–79.
25. Adams MA, Hutton WC. Gradual disc prolapse. *Spine* 1985;10:524–531.
26. Hirsch C, Schajowicz F. Studies on structural changes in the lumbar annulus fibrosus. *Acta Orthop Scand* 1952;22:184–231.
27. Yu S, Haughton VM, Sether LA, et al. Criteria for classifying normal and degenerated lumbar intervertebral discs. *Radiology* 1989;170:523–526.
28. Virgin WJ. Experimental investigations into the physical properties of the intervertebral disc. *J Bone Joint Surg* 1951;33:607–611.
29. Nachemson A. Some mechanical properties of the lumbar intervertebral discs. *Bull Hosp Joint Dis* 1962;23:130–143.
30. Modic MT, Feiglin DH, Pirainao DW, et al. Vertebral osteomyelitis; assessment using MR. *Radiology* 1985;157:157–166.
31. Modic MT. Degenerative disorders of the spine. In: Modic M, Masaryk T, Ross J, eds. *Magnetic Resonance Imaging of the Spine*. Chicago: Year Book Medical Publishers; 1989.
32. Kramer J. *Intervertebral Disk Disease*, 2nd ed, New York: Thieme Medical Publishers; 1992.
33. Harris RI, Macnab I. Structural changes in the lumbar intervertebral discs: their relationship to low back pain and sciatica. *J Bone Joint Surg* 1954;36:304–323.
34. Lindahl O. Hyeralgesia of the lumbar nerve roots in sciatica. *Acta Orthop Scand* 1966;37:367–374.
35. Nachemson AL. Intradiscal measurements of ph in patients with lumbar rhizopathies. *Acta Orthop Scand* 1969;40:23–42.
36. Crock HV. Internal disc disruption: a challenge to disc prolapse fifty years on. *Spine* 1986;11:650–655.
37. Bobechko WP, Hirsch C, Auto-immune response to nucleus pulposus in the rabbit. *J Bone Joint Surg* 1965;47:574–580.
38. Jinkins JR, Whittemore AR, Bradley WG. The anatomic basis of vertebrogenic pain and the autonomic syndrome associated with lumbar disc extrusion. *AJR* 1989;152:1277–1289.
39. Shapiro, R. *Myelography*. Chicago: Year Book Medical Publishers; 1975.
40. Sylven B. 1951. On the biology of the nucleus pulposus. *Acta Orthop* 1975;20:275–279.
41. Murayama S, Numaguchi Y, Robinson AE. The diagnosis of herniated intervertebral disks with MR imaging: a comparison of gradient-refocused-echo and spin-echo pulse sequences. *AJR* 1990;11:17–22.
42. Holtas S, Nordström CH, Larsson EM, Pettersson H. MR imaging of intradural disk herniation. *J Comput Assist Tomgr* 1987;11:353–356.
43. Jinkins JR. MR of enhancing nerve roots in the unoperated lumbosacral spine. *AJNR* 1993;14:193–202.
44. Jinkins JR. Magnetic resonance imaging of benign nerve root enhancement in the unoperated and postoperative lumbosacral spine. *Neuroimag Clin North Am* 1993;3(3):525–541.
45. Teplick JG, Haskin ME. Intravenous contrast-enhanced CT of the postoperative lumbar spine: improved identification of recurrent disk herniation, scar, arachnoiditis, and diskitis. *AJNR* 1984;5:373–383.
46. Braun IF, Hoffman JC, Davis PC, Landman JA, Tindall GT. Contrast enhancement in CT differentiation between recurrent disk herniation and postoperative scar: prospective study. *AJR* 1985;6:607–612.
47. Yang PJ, Seeger JF, Dzioba RB, et al. High-dose i.v. contrast in CT scanning of the postoperative lumbar spine. *AJNR* 1986;7:703–707.
48. Bundschuh CV. Imaging of the postoperative lumbosacral spine. *Neuroimag Clin North Am* 1993;3(3):499–516.
49. Bundschuh CV, Modic MT, Ross JS, Masaryk TJ, Bohlman H. Epidural fibrosis and recurrent disk herniation in the lumbar spine: MR imaging assessment. *AJNR* 1988;9:169–178.

50. Hueftle MG, Modic MT, Ross JS, et al. Lumbar spine: postoperative MR imaging with Gd-DTPA . *Radiology* 1988; 167:817–824.
51. Bangert BA, Ross JS. Arachnoiditis affecting the lumbosacral spine. *Neuroimag Clin North Am* 1993;3(3):517–524.
52. Ross JS, Perez-Reyes N, Masaryk TJ, Bohlman H, Modic MT. Thoracic disc herniation: MR imaging. *Radiology* 1987; 165:511–515.
53. Roosen N, Uwe D, Nicola N, Irlich G, Gahlen D, Stork W. MR imaging of calcified herniated thoracic disk. *J Comput Assist Tomogr* 1987; 11:733–735.
54. Teresi LM, Lufkin RB, Reicher MA, et al. Asymptomatic degenerative disk disease and spondylosis of the cervical spine: MR imaging. *Radiology* 1987; 164:83–88.
55. Hedberg MC, Drayer BP, Flom RA, Hodak JA, Bird CR. Gradient echo (grass) MR imaging in cervical radiculopathy. *AJNR* 1988; 150:683–689.
56. Czervionke LF, Daniels DL, Ho PSP, et al. The cervical neural foramina: a correlative anatomic and MR study. *Radiology* 1988; 1:753–759.
57. McRae, DL. Asymptomatic intervertebral disc protrusions. *Acta Radiol* 1956; 46:9–27.
58. Resnick D, Niwayama G. Degenerative diseases of the spine. In: Resnick D, ed. *Bone and Joint Imaging.* Philadelphia: WB Saunders; 1989:413–439.
59. Newton TH, Potts DG. *Computed Tomography of the Spine and Spinal Cord.* San Anselmo, CA: Clavadel Press; 1983.
60. Major NM, Helms CA. Central and foraminal stenosis of the lumbar spine. *Neuroimag Clin North Am* 1993;3(3):557–566.
61. Ullrich CG, Binet EF, Sanecki MG, Kieffer SA. Quantitative assessment of the lumbar spinal canal by computed tomography. *Radiology* 1980; 134:137–143.
62. Grenier N, Grossman RI, Schiebler ML, Yeager BA, Goldberg HI, Kressel HY. Degenerative lumbar disk disease: pitfalls and usefulness of MR imaging in detection of vacuum phenomenon. *Radiology* 1987; 164:861–865.
63. Jackson DE, Atlas SW, Mani JR, Norman D. Intraspinal synovial cysts: MR imaging. *Radiology* 1989; 170:527–530.
64. Liu SS, Williams KD, Drayer BP, Spetzler RF, Sonntag VK. Synovial cyst of the lumbosacral spine: diagnosis by MR imaging. *AJNR* 1989; 10:163–166.
65. Mikhael MA, Ciric I, Tarkington JA, Vick NA. Neuroradiological evaluation of lateral recess syndrome. *Radiology* 1981; 140:97–107.
66. Takahashi M, Yasuyuki Y, Yuji S, Ryutaro K. Chronic cervical cord compression: clincal significance of increased signal intensity on MR images. *Radiology* 1989; 173:219–224.
67. Tsuruda JS, Norman D, Dillon W, Newton TH, Mills DG. Three-dimensional gradient-recalled MR imaging as a screening tool for the diagnosis of cervical radiculopathy. *AJNR* 1989; 10:1263–1271.
68. Pettersson H, Larsson EM, Holtas S, et al. MR imaging of the cervical spine in rheumatoid arthritis. *AJNR* 1988;9:573–577.
69. Bundschuh CV, Modic MT, Kearney F, et al. Rheumatoid arthritis of the cervical spine: surface-coil MR imaging. *AJNR* 1988;9:565–571.
70. Resnick D. Calcification and ossification of the posterior spinal ligaments and tissues. In: Resnick D, ed. *Bone and Joint Imaging.* Philadelphia: WB Saunders; 1989:452–457.
71. Luetkehans TJ, Coughlin BF, Weinstein MA. Ossification of the posterior longitudinal ligament diagnosed by MR. *AJNR* 1987;8: 924–925.
72. Widder DJ. MR imaging of ossification of the posterior longitudinal ligament. *AJR* 1989; 153:194–195.
73. Resnick D, Niwayama G. Diffuse idiopathic skeletal hyperostosis (DISH). In: Resnick D, ed. *Bone and Joint Imaging.* Philadelphia: WB Saunders; 1989:440–451.

Magnetic Resonance Imaging of the Brain and Spine, Second Edition, edited by Scott W. Atlas. Lippincott-Raven Publishers, Philadelphia © 1996.

24

Spinal Trauma

Adam E. Flanders and Sidney E. Croul

Magnetic resonance imaging (MRI) has changed the diagnostic evaluation of spinal injuries. While many of the established therapies for spinal cord injuries (SCI) are based on radiologic classifications of osseous injury to the spinal column, the extent of associated soft tissue injury to the intervertebral discs, ligaments, and spinal cord has been determined primarily by inference from known biomechanical principles rather than by direct imaging of the affected tissues (1,2). Moreover, whereas most therapeutic interventions for SCI are directed primarily by radiographic findings such as re-establishment of normal anatomic alignment of the spinal canal and removal of bone fragments, conventional therapies often do not directly address correction of the associated soft tissue and spinal cord damage (3–6).

The greatest impact that MRI has made in the evaluation of SCI has been in assessment of the intracanalicular and paraspinal soft tissues (3–5,7–15). The integrity of the intervertebral discs and ligamentous complexes can be routinely evaluated following trauma. In addition, MRI permits direct visualization of the morphology of the injured cord parenchyma and the relationship of the surrounding structures to the spinal cord (2,16). No other imaging modality has been able to faithfully reproduce the internal architecture of the spinal cord and it is this particular feature of MRI that promises to have the greatest impact on the management of the SCI patient in the future.

Despite its imaging potential, MRI has not supplanted conventional radiologic imaging in the initial evaluation of SCI (16). The conventional diagnostic algorithm of plain radiography supplemented by computed tomography (CT) is the most appropriate and cost effective method to evaluate most cases of spinal trauma (7,10,16–18). An MRI examination in the acute period is warranted in any patient who has a persistent neurologic deficit after spinal trauma (10,11,17). MRI is advocated as a supplemental method of evaluation because it depicts associated soft tissue injury with particular clarity. Acute traumatic disc herniations and epidural hematomas are often difficult, if not impossible, to resolve on conventional radiographs and CT. MRI has replaced

A. E. Flanders, M.D.: Department of Radiology, Division of Neuroradiology, Thomas Jefferson University Hospital, Philadelphia, PA 19107.

S. E. Croul, M.D.: Department of Pathology and Laboratory Medicine, Medical College of Pennsylvania and Hahnemann University Hospital, Philadelphia, PA 19102.

myelography and CT myelography (CTM) as the primary imaging option available to assess for residual soft tissue compression of the spinal cord (10,12,14,19). Identification of residual compression of the spinal cord has significant implications in regard to timing of subsequent surgery and the type of surgical approach that is required (8,12). MRI is well suited to confirming the diagnosis by depicting these soft tissue injuries. MRI is also an essential diagnostic modality in cases of SCI without radiographic abnormality (SCIWORA) (11,17,20–23).

The focus of this chapter is the application of MRI in the evaluation of injuries of the spinal axis and spinal cord. For a comprehensive reference of the radiology of spine trauma, the reader is encouraged to pursue several excellent reviews (24–26).

SCI is a significant cause of disability in the United States. Although the number of individuals who sustain paralysis yearly is substantially less than the number of people who sustain moderate to severe traumatic brain injury (TBI), (10,000 to 20,000 SCI per year versus 70,000 to 90,000 TBI per year), the financial costs to society for SCI are significant. Since most patients survive the acute SCI, there are approximately 180,000 to 225,000 SCI patients with partial or complete paralysis currently being cared for in the United States. The total lifetime costs for medical treatment and rehabilitation range from $200,000 to $800,000 per individual. These costs may exceed $1 million, depending on the severity of the initial injury (27). Nearly 60% of all SCI occur in young adults between the ages of 16 to 30 years. Most SCI victims are white males (82.3%). The etiology of SCI are vehicular (44.8%), falls (21.7%), acts of violence (16%), and sports injuries (13%) (National Spinal Cord Injury Statistical Center, 1990). Since SCI primarily affects employed (63%) young adults, there is a tremendous financial loss to society in terms of overall lifetime productivity. The total lifetime costs of all new cases of SCI in 1989 was estimated at $6 billion (27).

Tetraplegia (quadriplegia) is defined as an injury to one of the eight cervical segments of the spinal cord with paralysis of all four limbs. Paraplegia usually results from injury to the thoracic, lumbar, or sacral segments of the spinal cord with dysfunction of both legs. A neurologically complete lesion is one in which there is no motor or sensory function three segments below the neurologic level of injury.

Injuries to the spinal axis can be subdivided into *spinal injuries* (damage to the spinal axis without neurologic injury) and *SCI* (damage to the spinal cord with or without spinal axis abnormality). An accurate estimate of the total number of SCI is difficult to define because patients who expire in the field from a fatal SCI (i.e., high cervical cord) or from related injuries (e.g., cerebral trauma) are not included in the national statistics. Of those spinal cord–injured persons who survive to reach a medical facility, the most frequent neurologic deficit is incomplete tetraplegia (30.6%), followed by complete paraplegia (25.8%), complete tetraplegia (22.1%), and incomplete paraplegia (19.3%). Less than 1% of SCI patients recover completely during the initial hospitalization.

MRI TECHNIQUES

Imaging Considerations

The spinal cord–injured patient requires special consideration before MR imaging with regard to patient transfer, life support, monitoring of vital signs, fixation devices, choices of surface coils, and pulse sequences. All potential risks for imaging the medically unstable patient must be carefully weighed against the need for the diagnostic information provided by MRI. Most SCI patients can be accommodated with minimal risk to the patient as long as appropriate precautions are adhered to. As with all critical care patients, a myriad of life-sustaining devices accompany the SCI patient to the MRI suite. Many of these devices are incompatible with the MRI environment. Conventional ventilatory equipment is safe to use only in the fringe field of ultralow field strength units. For mid- and high-field strength MRI units, several manufacturers offer MRI-compatible ventilators. The unit itself is operated remotely and the ventilator controls remain inside the control room. Similarly, MRI-compatible monitors are now available that can relay heart rate, respiration, blood pressure, and oxygenation information directly into the MRI control area. Indwelling central venous catheters with thermocouples and conventional intravenous medication pumps are prohibited in the MRI environment.

External spinal fixation devices warrant special attention because, if used improperly in the MRI suite, they can pose a significant safety hazard to both the patient and personnel (28). Moreover, fixation devices that are composed of ferromagnetic alloys may destroy the static magnetic field close to the region of interest, resulting in image degradation.

Most patients will arrive for an MRI examination following closed reduction of the spinal injury and fixation with the appropriate external spinal stabilization device. Occasionally, traction will be applied using cranial tongs and a system of pulleys and weights. Although it is possible to maintain traction on the scanning table, it is not advisable to do so for several reasons: (a) it is cumbersome to attach the weights and pulleys to the scanning table, (b) the traction device may interfere with table motion, and (c) conventional traction weights ("sandbags") contain metallic pellets that pose a significant projectile hazard to patient and personnel (28). Only MRI-compatible weights are permitted inside the scanning area (29).

Patients with cervical spine injuries are usually stabilized with a fiberglass cervical collar or, in more severe injuries, a halo and halo vest are used (30). For thoracic and lumbar injuries the patient may arrive on a rigid spine board, a body cast, or in traction. MRI-compatible halo vests are composed of a graphite composite, aluminum, and plastic, and are devoid of stainless steel components (31,32). If the fixation pins used for femoral traction are ferrous, they usually do not interfere to any noticeable degree with the images of the spine, although tissue heating can occur.

Transfer of a patient with spine instability to and from the scanning table should be performed only by properly trained personnel. Patient motion should be minimized as there is potential risk for further neurologic deterioration from moving of an unstable spine.

Patient motion (voluntary or involuntary) can also be detrimental to the quality of any MRI study. Even a patient with acute tetraplegia can seriously degrade a cervical MRI examination either by movement of the head and neck or from irregular ventilation. Sedation may be necessary to complete an examination.

Choice of surface coil is determined by the location(s) of injury, access to the area of interest, and the types of coils available. The proximity of the surface coil to the area of interest is a key factor in determining image quality. Temporary removal of a cervical collar, for example, will permit the use of specially designed quadrature or anterior/posterior neck coils. When the neck is fixed in a halo frame, a 5-inch circular surface coil closely applied to the back of the neck can be used effectively. For thoracic and lumbar evaluation, the patient should be placed over a sliding surface coil tray, which permits repositioning of the coil without moving the patient. The conventional 5″ × 11″ "license plate" surface coil provides adequate coverage for sagittal fields of view up to 32 cm. When available, a quadrature lumbar coil and phased array transmit/receive coil system can produce exceptional results.

MRI evaluation of the spine following penetrating trauma requires special consideration for two reasons: (a) retained metallic fragments within the spinal canal may be regarded as a safety hazard to the patient, and (b) these fragments can produce significant local image degradation. Most firearm projectiles are nonferrous and therefore will not move in the static magnetic field (33). A ferrous fragment in the spinal canal could theoretically migrate, producing further neurologic injury. Although we are not aware of any reports of ascending paralysis from retained bullet fragments in the spinal canal, any MRI examination following penetrating trauma to the spine should be performed at the discretion of the radiologist after review of radiographs and/or CT of the area of interest. If there are sufficient safety concerns, then myelography or CTM should be used instead.

Imaging Methods

At a minimum, evaluation of the injured spine should be performed both in the axial and sagittal planes using a combination of pulse sequences. Both T1- and T2-weighted information are necessary to completely assess the spinal axis and the spinal cord. Additional sequences are performed as needed, depending on the portion of the spine that is injured, the degree of injury, and patient tolerance. Conventional spin-echo and gradient-echo pulse sequences are used most often. The development of rapid spin-echo pulse sequences [e.g., rapid acquisition with relaxation enhancement (RARE), fast spin-echo (FSE)] has effectively replaced conventional spin-echo methods for obtaining T2-weighted information in many clinical applications (34,35). In the evaluation of SCI, T2-weighted FSE images demonstrate as much (or more) diagnostic information, fewer artifacts, and improved resolution in less time than conventional spin-echo (CSE) methods (36).

An inherent property of the rapid spin-echo pulse sequences (RSE) is that the images exhibit less magnetic susceptibility artifact as compared to conventional spin-echo and gradient-echo images. Although this property may seem theoretically disadvantageous when searching for small areas of acute spinal cord hemorrhage, RSE images have been shown to be comparably sensitive to conventional spin-echo images for detecting intramedullary hemorrhage (37). The decrease in magnetic susceptibility with RARE or FSE may be advantageous when imaging postoperative spines that otherwise would be obscured by artifacts (Fig. 1) (34).

Imaging of the cervical, thoracic, or lumbar regions begins with a low resolution gradient-echo localizer in the coronal plane. This image(s) can be obtained in less than 1 minute and can be used subsequently to prescribe the sagittal sequences. A maximum of 9 to 12 images are needed and the outermost sagittal images should include both facet joints. Sagittal images should be no more than 3 to 4 mm thick with a 0- to 1-mm slice gap. The field of view of the area of interest is adequate at 22 to 24 cm. In the thoracic spine, a large low resolution sagittal localizer is needed (48 cm) for accurate labeling of the involved levels.

The prescribed spatial resolution depends on the type of sequence used and acquisition time limitations. For conventional T2-weighted spin-echo imaging, 128 phase-encoding steps (y_{res}) and two excitations are recommended. The phase-encoding axis is oriented parallel to the spine so that phase ghosting is not propagated across the spinal canal. A form of gradient moment nulling (GMN) should also be employed in the cervical and thoracic regions to compensate for cerebrospinal fluid (CSF) flow artifacts. Cardiac gating is another option for correcting cerebrospinal flow artifacts on T2-weighted sequences. Appropriately placed saturation pulses are

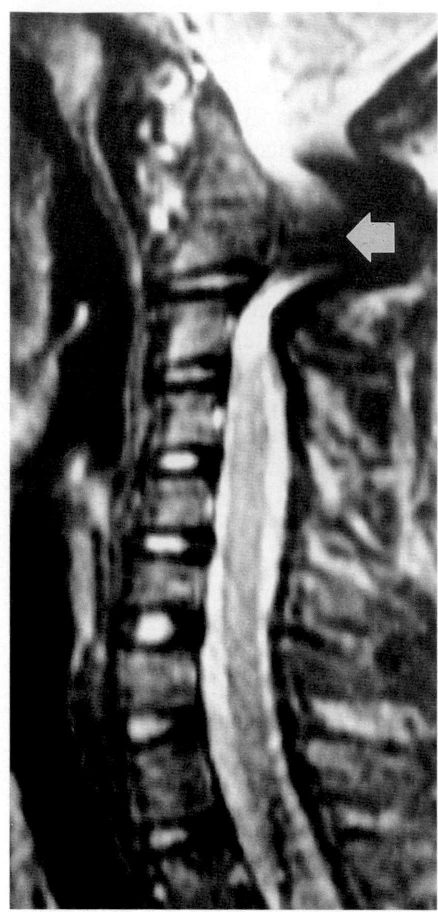

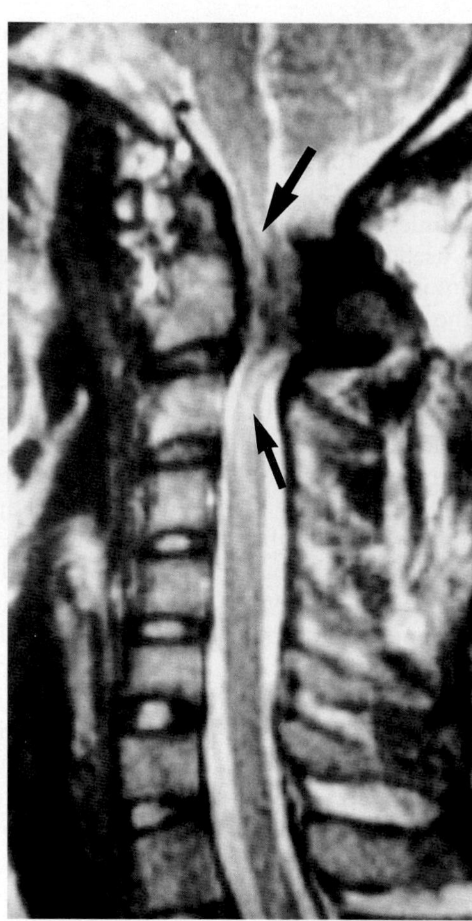

A,B

FIG. 1. Comparison of SE and FSE to reduce artifacts from fixation hardware. **A:** Sagittal SE T2-weighted image (2000/80/2 NEX) shows marked field inhomogeneity artifact from stainless steel wires that transfix the posterior elements of C2 and C3. The spinal canal is completely obscured by the field distortion (*arrow*). **B:** Sagittal FSE T2-weighted image (2500/85Ef/4 NEX/ETL8) shows a decrease in the artifact. Although there is still artifact present, it has diminished substantially when compared to the SE image. Note the residual spinal cord edema (*arrows*). (Courtesy of Lisa M. Tartaglino, M.D.)

helpful in reducing artifacts produced by swallowing, breathing, and cardiac motion. Respiratory compensation may be of benefit when imaging the thoracic and lumbar regions. Resolution can be maintained with reduced imaging times by implementing options that vary the number of phasing encoding steps and field of view.

When a RSE sequence is available, it is the preferred acquisition method for T2-weighted images. T2-weighted information is obtained using two separate RSE sequences. For the short TE_{eff} image an echo train of 4 with two excitations is suggested, whereas for the long TE_{eff} image an echo train of 8 with four excitations is recommended. For each sequence, 256 steps are prescribed in both the frequency (x_{res}) and phase (y_{res}) axes. Fat suppression may be employed on the long TR sequences to improve visualization of edema in the posterior ligamentous complexes.

Cross-sectional information is desirable, especially when evaluating for spinal cord pathology in the cervical and thoracic regions. The choice of axial pulse sequence varies, depending on the part of the spine being evaluated, extent of injury, type of tissue contrast required, and time constraints. Usually, axial images are obtained using gradient-echo (GE) or spin-echo (SE) pulse sequences. In the cervical spine, a myelographic-like image is produced using an axial three-dimensional (3-D) FT GE pulse sequence to obtain 28 or 64 contiguous images, at 1.5-mm thickness. Technical parameters include 5° flip angle, minimum TR/TE, 256 × 128 matrix and two excitations. The TE should be less than 15 msec in order to minimize unwanted susceptibility effects that might exaggerate bony stenoses (37). To maximize detection of acute intramedullary hemorrhage, at least one GE sequence should be performed when RSE sequences are used to obtain T2-weighted images. High-resolution cross-sectional imaging of the spinal cord can be performed using RSE techniques in the study of the cervical and thoracic spine. An alternative method is to prescribe short TR axial images angled parallel through the level of injury.

As a supplement to the cervical examination, a survey of the extracranial vasculature is useful to detect post-traumatic occlusion or dissection of the carotid and vertebral arteries. This may be achieved with T1-weighted sequences, two-dimensional (2D) time-of-flight (TOF) magnetic resonance angiography (MRA), 3D TOF MRA, or a combination of these techniques.

Although there are reported cases in which gadolinium was useful in the evaluation of acute SCI, the justi-

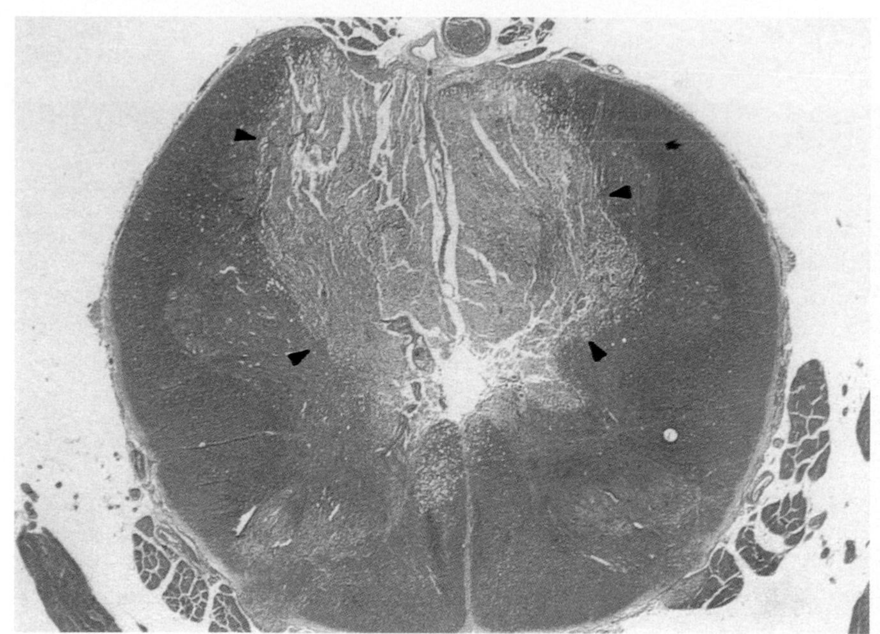

FIG. 2. Anterior cord syndrome. The ventral aspect of the spinal cord shows infarction with necrosis (*arrowheads*). In this case, the most medial portions of the anterior horns bear the brunt of the injury with relative preservation of the remainder of the anterior circulation. Quite often, the area of damage spreads more laterally to involve the entire anterior horn and the white matter comprising spinothalamic and corticospinal tracts. (Luxol fast blue–periodic acid Schiff. Material courtesy of A. Hirano, M.D., Division of Neuropathology Montefiore Medical Center, Bronx, N.Y. and Igaku-Shoin Publishers.)

fication for routine use is unsubstantiated (38,39). In our experience, contrast agents are not useful in the MRI evaluation of acute spinal trauma.

Clinical Measures of Spinal Cord Injury

The American Spinal Injury Association (ASIA) has devised standards for both neurologic and functional classification of spinal injuries (40). A standardized set of examination procedures allows the determination of sensory/motor deficits and a spinal level for the lesion. From these, a clinical spinal cord syndrome and an impairment scale are derived, including a measure of functional independence.

Lesions of the spinal cord have been classically divided into five neuroanatomic syndromes: anterior cord, central cord, Brown-Séquard, conus medullaris, and cauda equina.

Anterior cord syndromes most commonly result from occlusion of the anterior spinal artery (Fig. 2) (41–44). Lesions that collapse a vertebral body with resultant canal compromise and compression of the cord may also result in this syndrome, probably on the basis of vascular insufficiency. Patients experience profound loss of motor function and pain and temperature sensation below the level of lesion. There is relative preservation of vibration and position sense. Since the anterior two thirds of the spinal cord is supplied by the anterior spinal artery, this syndrome has been correlated anatomically with damage to the corticospinal and lateral spinothalamic tracts with relative sparing of the posterior columns.

The *central cord syndrome* (45–47) usually follows an acute cervical injury and is characterized by greater weakness in the arms than the legs, with almost constant sacral sensory sparing. Patients with cervical spondylosis/stenosis are predisposed to central cord injuries (Fig. 3) (23). The proposed mechanism of injury suggests

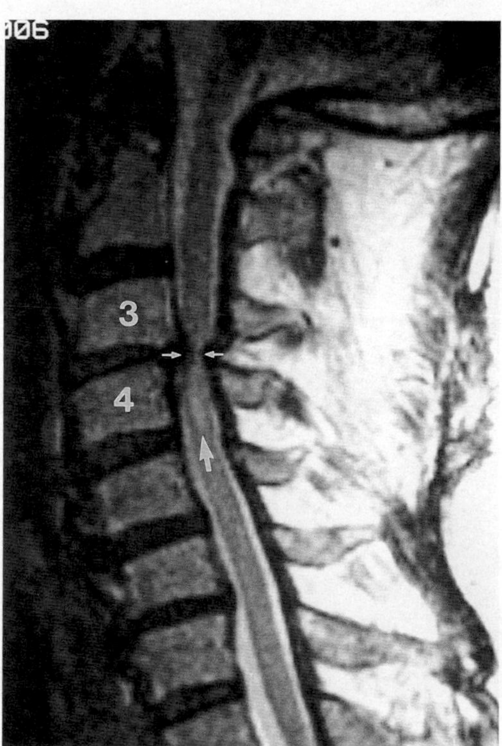

FIG. 3. Central cord injury. Sagittal FSE T2-weighted image (2500/85Ef/2 NEX/ETL8) shows compression of the cervical spinal cord between a retropulsed disc fragment and a buckled ligamentum flavum at the C3-C4 interspace (*small arrows*). There is a small area of spinal cord edema noted at the C4 level (*arrow*). Of incidental note are generalized changes of cervical spondylosis with large anterior endplate spurs.

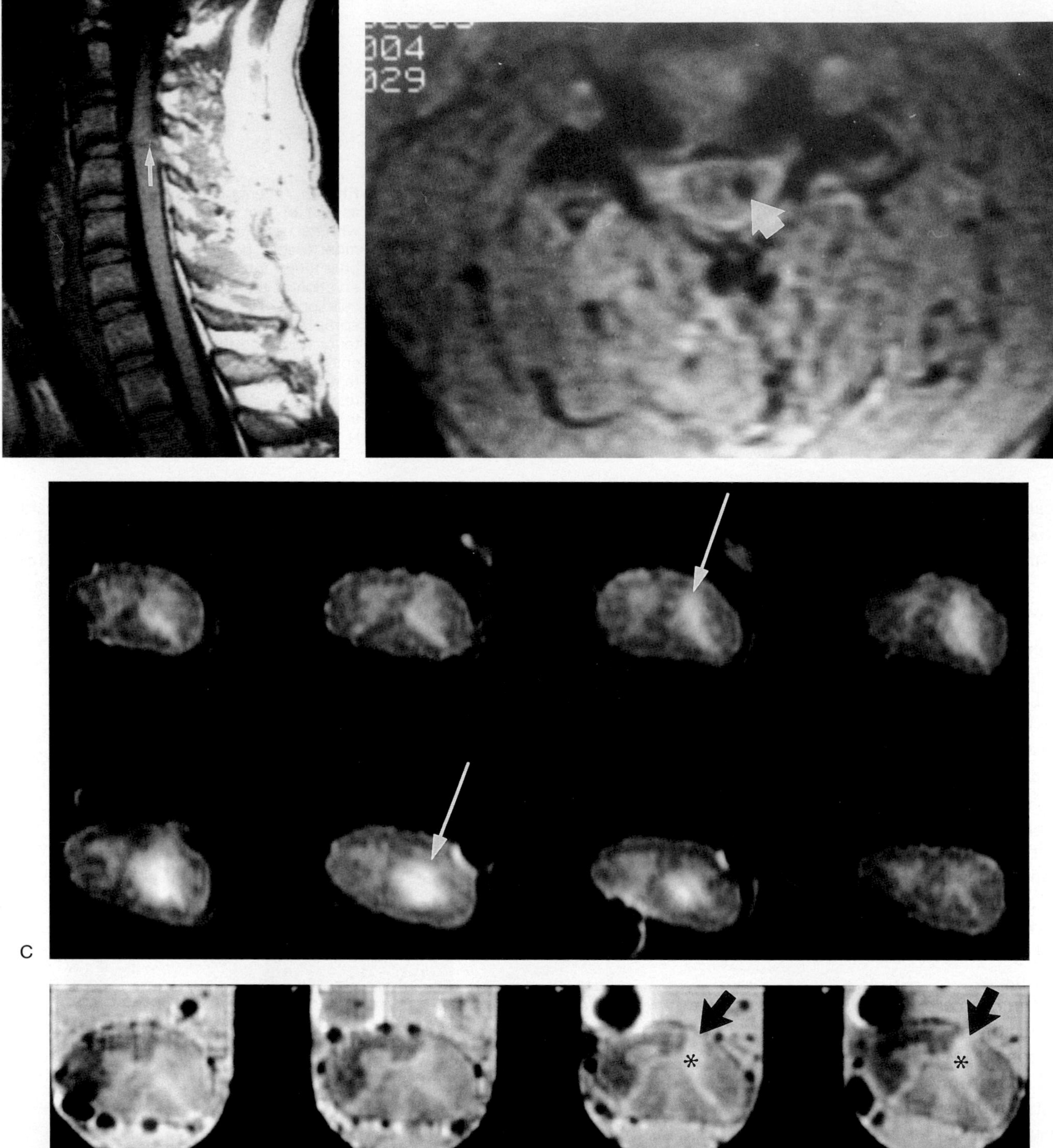

FIG. 4. Brown-Séquard syndrome. **A:** Sagittal T1-weighted image (500/20/4 NEX) shows an obliquely oriented hypointense band that traverses the width of the spinal cord between C3 and C4 (*arrow*), which represents the path of a knife blade. There is a mild degree of cord swelling at this level. **B:** Axial GE 3DFT (35/15/5°) in another patient shows a discrete hypointense focus in the central gray matter of the spinal cord on the left side (*arrow*) representing deoxyhemoglobin. **C:** Serial axial T1-weighted images (700/14/3 NEX) of a human spinal cord specimen with a Brown-Séquard lesion. A focal area of hyperintensity is noted within the central gray matter on the left side secondary to hemorrhage (methemoglobin). **D:** Serial axial intermediate-weighted FSE images (1800/24Ef/2 NEX, ETL 4) shows abnormal morphology of the central gray matter on the left (*asterisks*). Tissue damage extends into the ventral white matter approximating the spinothalamic tracts (*arrow*). (Multiple magnetic susceptibility artifacts are present surrounding the specimen presumably from metal in solution during preparation).

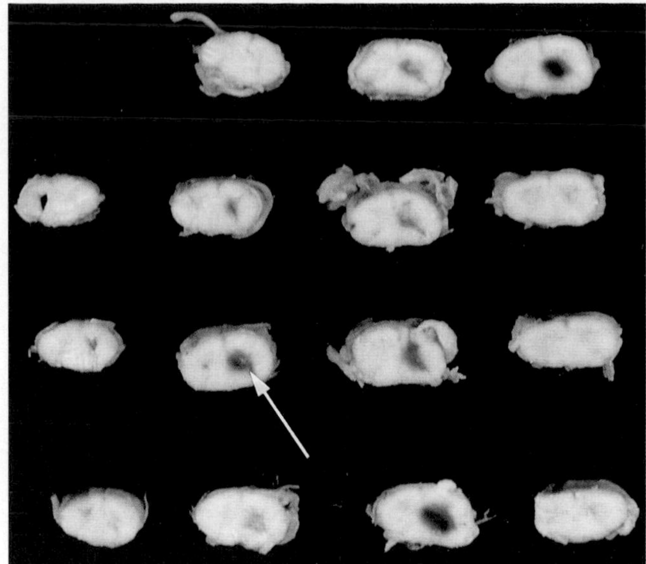

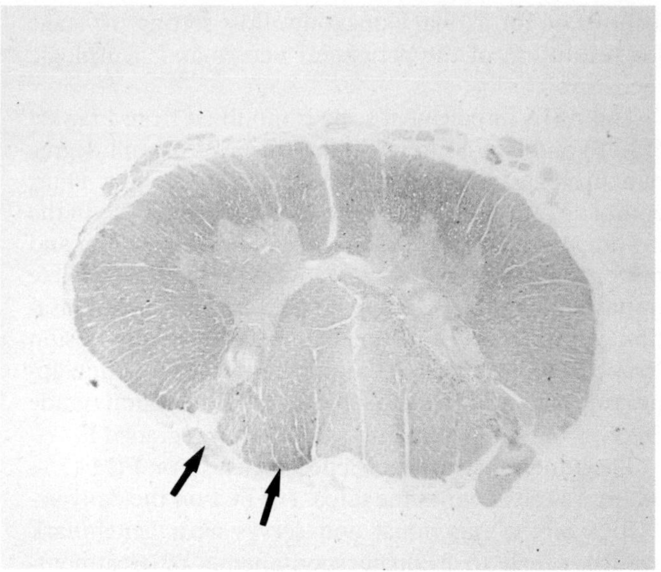

FIG. 4. (*Continued.*) **E:** Gross specimen of C and D. Note the asymmetrical hemorrhagic lesion involving the gray matter (*arrow*). **F:** Photomicrograph of a stained section taken from the case illustrated in E. Note the area of tissue destruction in the left dorsal horn and dorsal columns (*arrows*). Although the lesion was hemorrhagic, the blood pigments fail to show with this method. (Luxol fast blue.)

that the spinal cord is pinched between a dorsally displaced vertebral body and a buckled ligamentum flavum during hyperextension (48). Classically, the underlying pathology has been felt to consist of contusion, hemorrhage, and/or necrosis of the central cervical gray matter. Since both the corticospinal and spinothalamic tracts in primates and probably in man are laminated such that the most rostral projections are most medial, the central damage in the cervical cord would injure the cervical laminations most severely and spare the sacral laminations, resulting in the characteristic pattern of deficit. Recent work questions this traditional view. One study described 11 cases of acute central cord syndrome, 9 of which had MRI correlation and 3 of which had pathologic examination (49). In none of these cases was blood or blood products found by imaging or pathology. In all cases, the most severe changes occurred in the white matter and included demyelination with or without axonal loss. No necrotic lesions were reported in the central gray matter. Since these findings are at variance with what has been previously accepted, they challenge other investigators to attempt independent confirmation.

The *Brown-Séquard syndrome* is due to a purely unilateral transverse lesion above midlumbar spinal cord levels. Probably the most common trauma associated with this syndrome is a fall on the back from a considerable height (50), although stab wounds may also be responsible (Fig. 4) (51). The resultant loss of proprioception and motor control ipsilateral to the lesion reflects damage to the corticospinal tract and posterior columns on the side of the lesion, whereas contralateral loss of sensitivity to pin and temperature is due to damage to the crossing spinothalamic tracts.

Traumatic lesions of the lower spinal canal rarely affect the sacral spinal cord or conus medullaris exclusively, but they may also damage the surrounding cauda equina (52,53). Damage to the sacral spinal segments alone produces a pure *conus medullaris syndrome* resulting in an areflexic bladder, fecal incontinence, and saddle anesthesia. Additional cauda equina injury may result in a variable degree of flaccid paralysis in the legs with accompanying multimodal sensory loss. Lesions that occur higher in the sacral cord may effectively isolate the distal-most cord and thus these injuries exhibit preservation of bowel, bladder, and genital reflexes.

Injuries below the level of the sacral segments cause a pure *cauda equina syndrome*. Damage to lumbosacral nerve roots results in flaccid paralysis of the bowel, bladder, and legs. All forms of sensory input are also affected. The cauda equina is said to be more resistant to trauma than the spinal cord and certainly shows a greater propensity for recovery. The fact that it is composed of peripheral nerve roots rather than central nervous system tissue may account for its resistance to injury. Nerve roots are ensheathed by a substrate that includes fibrous tissue; this covering renders them more resistant to trauma than the spinal cord. The fact that peripheral axons are myelinated by Schwann cells rather than the oligodendrocytes found in the spinal white matter is a major factor that accounts for the unique ability of peripheral nerves to regenerate following trauma. Following injury to the cauda equina, Schwann cells provide a substrate for axonal elongation, thus setting the stage for restitution of the peripheral nerves and neurologic recovery.

The ASIA impairment scale is modified from Frankel (54,55) and is used to grade the patient's overall degree of neurologic impairment due to the spinal lesion. Thus, complete (grade A) impairment connotes paralysis in the lower extremities and the absence of both sensation and motor function in the sacral segments S4-S5. Incomplete impairment (grades B,C,D) ranges from preserved sensation without motor function below the level of the lesion (grade B) to preserved sensation with motor function approximating normal below the level of the lesion (grade D). Normal sensory and motor function is graded E.

The functional independence measure or FIM (56–58) more fully defines the impact of SCI on the daily activities of the individual and serves as a benchmark against which to evaluate spontaneous or treatment-associated changes in overall function. By focusing on 18 items in six areas of function (self-care, sphincter control, mobility, locomotion, communication, and social cognition) a 7-point scale is constructed ranging from complete independence [7] to total assistance [1] for each item. The total score summed across all items gives a more complete estimate of total disability.

CHARACTERIZATION OF SPINAL INJURY USING MRI

Although the biomechanics and types of injuries to the spine vary by location, the observed soft tissue and osseous changes to the spinal axis and spinal cord on MRI are relatively similar. Any interpretation of an MRI examination performed for spinal injury should include a discussion of the integrity of the intervertebral discs, vertebral bodies, vertebral alignment, ligaments, and neural elements. Specifically, the types of changes that are observed with MRI in SCI can be grouped into osseous injuries, ligamentous and joint disruption, intervertebral disc injury, fluid collections, vascular injury, and SCI. The force of injury is often dissipated primarily at one level in the spine; therefore, injury to all the tissues (e.g., bone, ligament, disc, and spinal cord) is usually anticipated at one to two isolated levels. Identification of injury to one tissue type should prompt the observer to scrutinize the same level for injuries to other tissues.

Most of the diagnostic information is derived from the sagittal images. Axial images serve as a supplement (2). Sagittal T1-weighted images offer an excellent anatomic overview. Disc herniations, epidural fluid collections, subluxations, vertebral body fractures, cord swelling, and cord compression are also visualized (18). Sagittal T2-weighted images depict most of the soft tissue abnormalities including spinal cord edema and hemorrhage, ligamentous injury, disc herniation, and epidural fluid collections (13). Axial and sagittal GE images aid in the identification of acute spinal cord hemorrhage, disc herniations, and fractures. MRI has not been successful in demonstrating traumatic nerve root avulsions. CT with intrathecal contrast remains the diagnostic method of choice for demonstrating the characteristic empty nerve root sheath and the periradicular cavities (59,60).

Osseous Injury

Currently, MRI does not offer any advantage over plain radiography and/or high-resolution CT in the evaluation of associated osseous injuries following spinal trauma (8,16,18,23). Moreover, even when MRI is available, it should only be performed *after* appropriate radiographic evaluation of the osseous injury.

The traumatic osseous changes to the spinal axis on MRI are divided into subluxations, fracture deformities, and compressive injuries. Relative loss of alignment at a specific level of the spinal axis is readily depicted on a mid-sagittal MRI image. The sensitivity of MRI in detecting anterior subluxation is probably better than conventional radiography or CT because the morphology of the thecal sac is also demonstrated (16).

Nondisplaced fracture lines through the vertebral bodies and posterior elements are poorly demonstrated on MRI. The fracture line is sometimes visible on GE im-

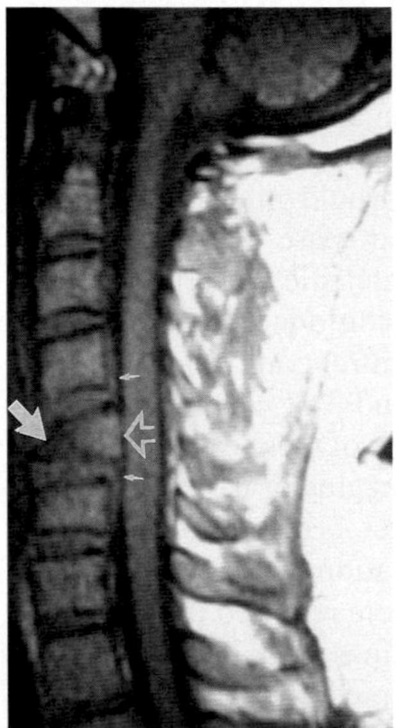

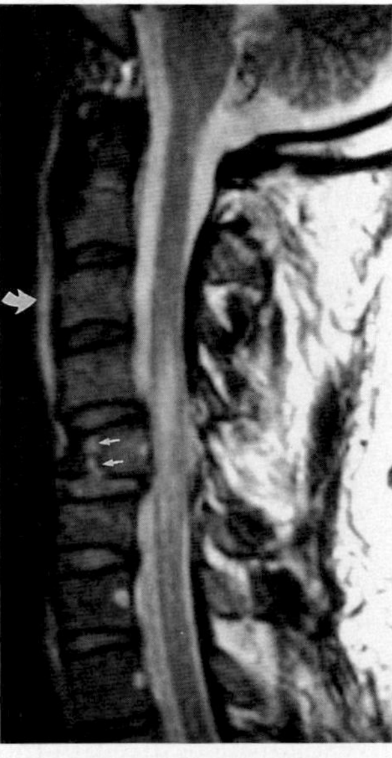

A,B

FIG. 5. Flexion teardrop fracture of C5. **A:** Sagittal T1-weighted image (416/11/2 NEX) shows loss of height of the C5 vertebral body anteriorly (*large arrow*). The marrow signal of the compressed segment is hypointense. The posterior aspect of the vertebral body is retropulsed into the spinal canal (*open arrow*). There is associated elevation of the PLL (*small arrows*) and there is mild swelling of the spinal cord. **B:** Sagittal FSE T2-weighted image (2000/85Ef, 4 NEX/ETL8) depicts the hyperintense vertically oriented fracture line that interrupts the inferior endplate (*small arrows*). A small amount of prevertebral edema is also present (*curved arrow*). There is edema in the spinal cord without a discrete focus of hemorrhage. (Hypointense focus in brainstem is artifactual.)

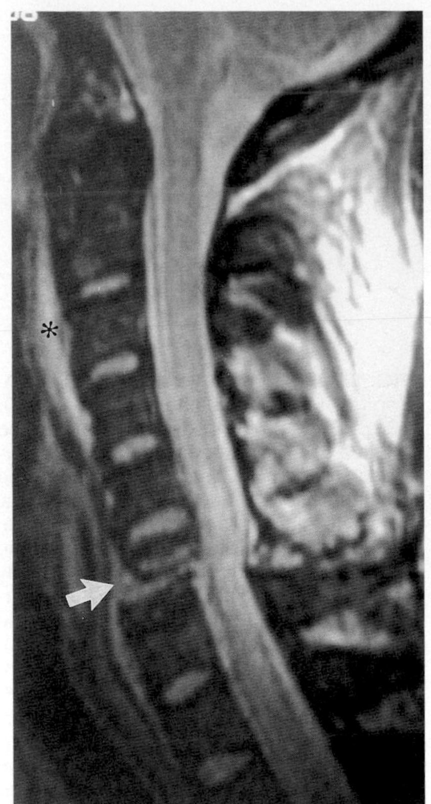

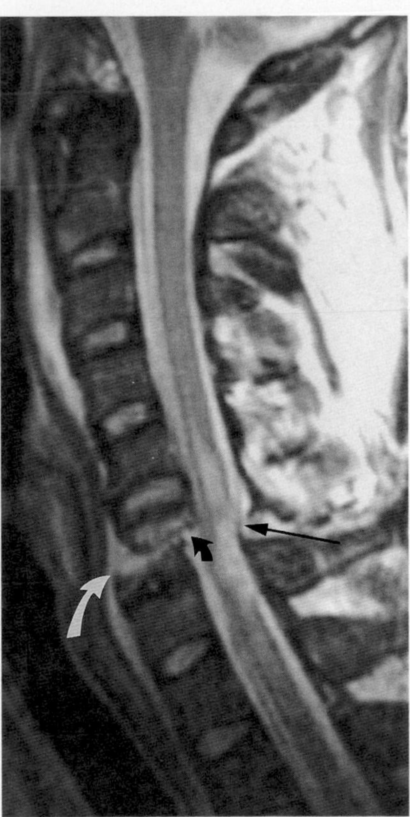

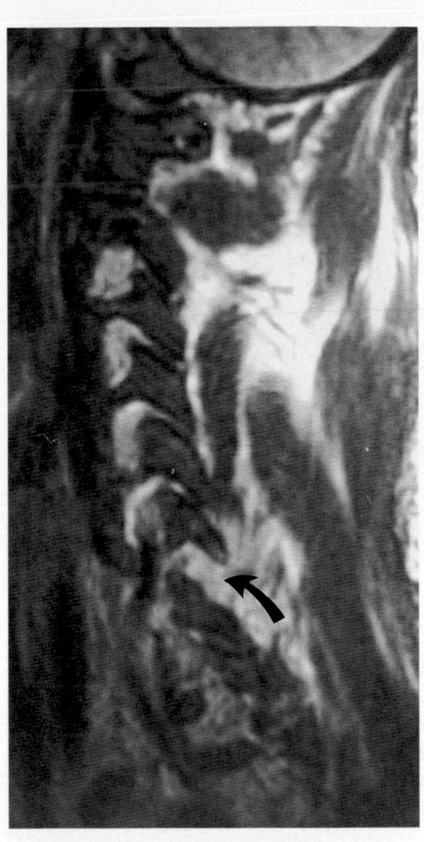

FIG. 15. Fracture dislocation at C6 in a 29-year-old man. **A:** Sagittal T2-weighted image (2000/80/2 NEX, 256×128) reveals a horizontal fracture line that extends through the C6 vertebral body (*arrow*). There is offset of the upper segment relative to the lower segment. Spinal cord edema is present, extending the length of three vertebral segments. There is a mound of prevertebral soft tissue swelling/hemorrhage (*asterisk*). **B:** Sagittal FSE T2-weighted image (2500/85Ef/4, ETL 8, 256×256) shows the details of the injury with better clarity than the SE image. There is disruption of the ALL (*curved white arrow*), the PLL (*curved black arrow*), and the LF (*straight black arrow*). Note that the borders defining the spinal cord edema are better defined than in A. **C:** Parasagittal FSE T2-weighted image shows distraction of the C6 and C7 facet joints on the right (*curved arrow*).

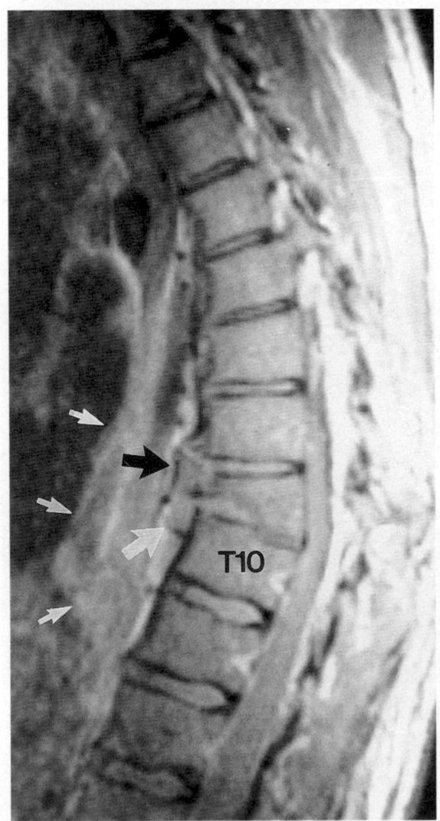

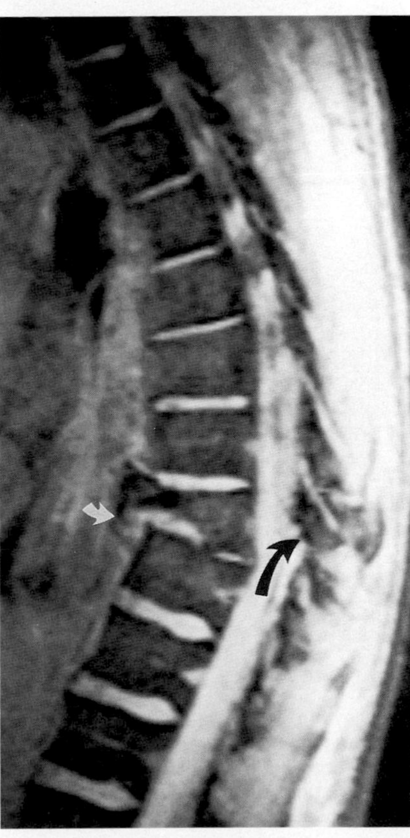

FIG. 16. Fracture dislocation T9-10. **A:** Sagittal FSE intermediate weighted image (2200/16Ef/2 NEX/ETL4). There is severe loss of height of the T9 vertebral body secondary to a fracture-dislocation of T9-T10. A large fracture fragment originating from T9 is displaced anteriorly (*black arrow*). An anterior disc herniation that has migrated in front of the T10 body is also demonstrated (*white arrow*). A paraspinal hematoma is also present (*small white arrows*). **B:** Sagittal GE image (400/15/15°). The hypointense cortical margins are sharply delineated against the hyperintense disc material and CSF. The ALL is stretched over the fracture fragment but appears intact (*curved white arrow*). The posterior elements are misaligned after reduction because of fractures (*curved black arrow*).

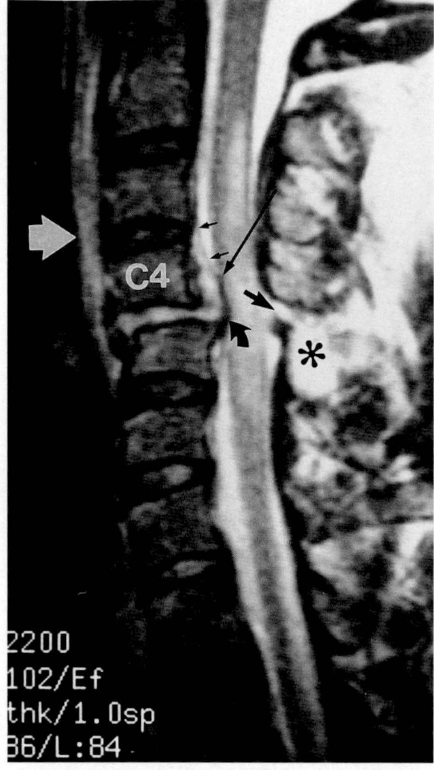

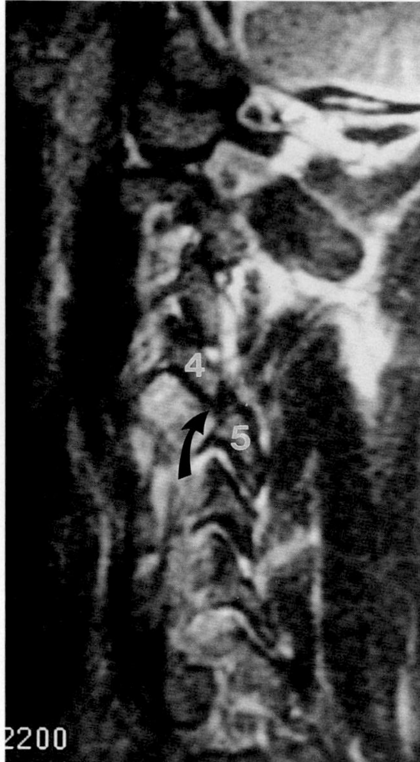

A,B

FIG. 17. Flexion-rotation injury at C4-5. **A:** Sagittal FSE T2-weighted image (2200/102Ef/3 NEX). The body of C4 is subluxed relative to C5. A moderate-sized disc herniation (*curved black arrow*) has impacted on the swollen and edematous spinal cord. No blood products are identified in the spinal cord. Note the separation of the PLL from the midportion of the C4 body (*long black arrow*). The ventral dura margin is represented by a thin hypointense line (*small black arrows*). There is associated disruption of the ligamentum flavum (*black arrow*) and the interspinous ligaments (*asterisk*). Prevertebral edema is also present (*white arrow*). **B:** Right parasagittal image (same sequence as A). The right C4 inferior facet is jumped and locked in front of the C5 superior facet (*arrow*).

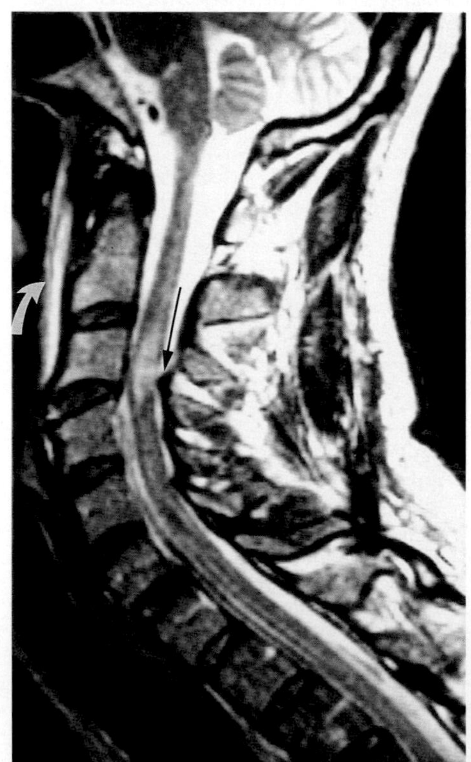

A

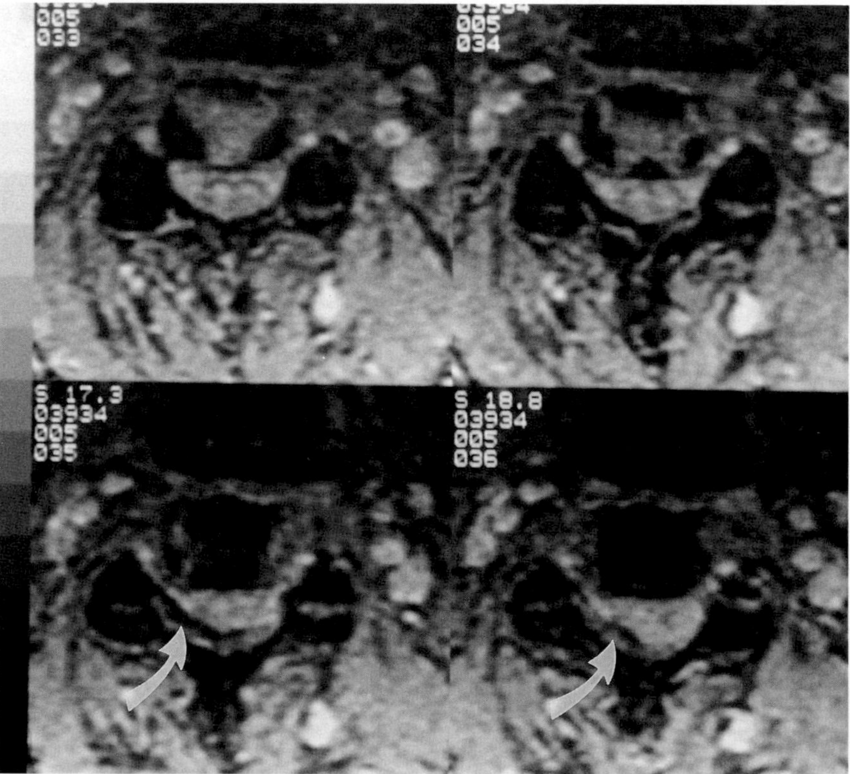

B

FIG. 18. Hyperextension strain injury at C3/4. **A:** Sagittal FSE T2-weighted image (3000/85Ef/4 NEX, ETL 8) shows anterior widening of the C3/4 disc space and an associated prevertebral hematoma (*curved arrow*). There is buckling of the LF (*arrow*). A discrete area of spinal cord edema is also present. **B:** Axial GE axial images, 3DFT (35/15/5°), show deformity of the right posterolateral aspect of the thecal sac by the buckled LF. The spinal cord was compressed between the vertebral body anteriorly and the LF posteriorly.

that lies ventral to the anterior cortical surface of the vertebral bodies (65,66). Normally, the ALL may be indiscernible from the cortex or the outer annulus of the intervertebral disc; however, when elevated by fluid, disc, or bone, it may be more apparent. Portions of the ligament merge with Sharpey's fibers at the vertebral endplate and with the outer annular fibers. The ALL may rupture as the result of hyperextension injury (17,23, 65,67,68). This is seen on all pulse sequences as a focal discontinuity of the hypointense band that is adherent to the ventral aspect of the vertebral bodies (Figs. 14–16). This finding may be associated with an avulsion of the vertebral endplate or hemorrhage in the prevertebral musculature (17,65,67,68). The accumulation of hemorrhage and fluid in the prevertebral space is seen on T2-weighted or GE sequences as a crescent-shaped mass of high signal intensity centered over the segment of injured ligament (Figs. 5, 14–16) (14,23,65).

Unlike the ALL, the PLL is much more variable in width. The PLL is widest at the level of the intervertebral disc and thinner as it passes behind the vertebral bodies (66). Therefore, the PLL may normally appear discontinuous on sagittal MRI images (14). The PLL is represented on MRI as a thin, hypointense band that is interposed between the ventral dural sac and the posterior margin of the vertebral bodies and intervertebral discs. It is best visualized on T2-weighted and intermediate-weighted sagittal images, however, the PLL is often impossible to resolve as a separate structure from the ventral dura or annulus on mid-sagittal images. When elevated away from the posterior cortex by a herniated disc or post-traumatic fluid collection, the PLL is better delineated (Figs. 7, 15, and 17). As with the ALL, rupture of the PLL is identified as a focal region of discontinuity. Rupture of the PLL can occur in association with hyperflexion and hyperextension injuries.

The LF forms a continuous strip of fibroelastic tissue that bridges adjacent lamina. Along with the ISP, they act as check ligaments to oppose hyperflexion and distraction of the posterior elements and maintain alignment. Normally, the LF are small structures (especially in the cervical and thoracic regions), which are oriented parallel to the adjacent lamina. The LF may enlarge either on a degenerative basis or physiologically by bulging into the spinal canal in hyperextension. LF rupture is often associated with fractures of the posterior elements. The injured LF can be easier to visualize when the damaged segment projects into the spinal canal and distorts the posterolateral aspect of the thecal sac. This finding is best seen on parasagittal and axial images (Figs. 7, 14, 17, and 18). Disruption of the ISP is best appreciated on the mid-sagittal views. High signal intensity is demonstrated in the ligaments that are interposed between the widened spinous processes (Figs. 11, 17) (16).

The facet joint complexes are easily identified on sagittal and axial images, particularly in the cervical and lumbar region where the structures are somewhat larger in size and the joint plane is oriented in the sagittal direction. In the thoracic spine, the facet joints are small in size and the joint is oriented in the coronal plane.

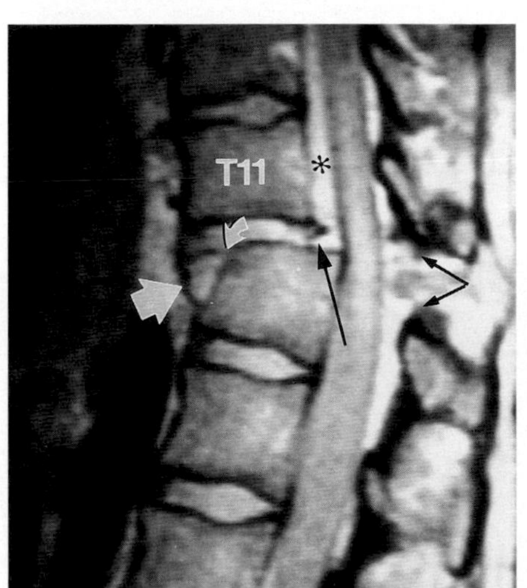

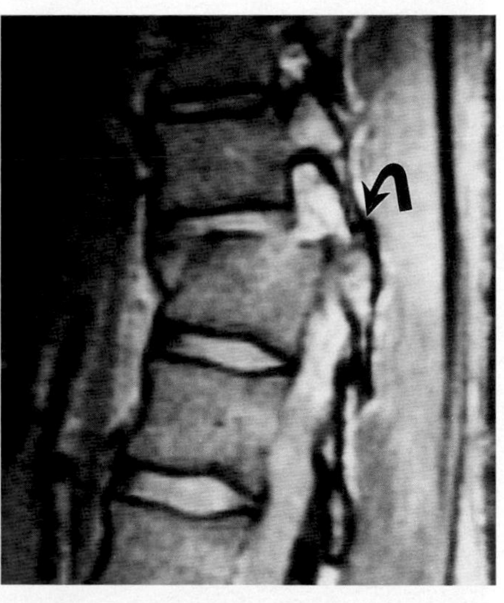

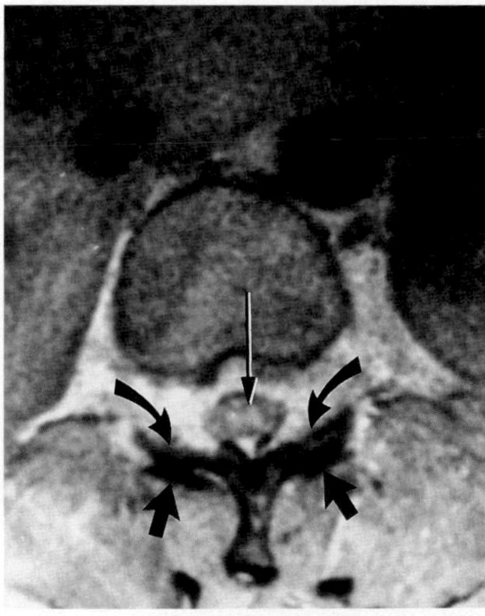

FIG. 19. Fracture dislocation at T11-12 with locked facets. **A:** Sagittal intermediate weighted FSE image (2250/24Ef/2 NEX/ETL4) shows subluxation and angulation at T11-12. There is a fracture deformity of the T12 vertebral body. The disc at T11/12 is damaged with interruption of the annulus anteriorly (*curved white arrow*) and posteriorly (*long black arrow*). There is an anterior disc herniation that appears contained by the ALL (*large white arrow*). The LF is ruptured (*black arrows*). A hematoma is present in the ventral epidural space (*asterisk*) that extends cephalad from the disc injury. **B:** Parasagittal intermediate-weighted FSE image shows the right inferior facet of T11 dislocated anterior to the superior facet of T12 (*curved arrow*). The same finding was present on the left side. **C:** Axial intermediate-weighted FSE image (3300/18Ef/2 NEX/ETL8) of T11 demonstrates the abnormal relationship of the facet joints. The inferior facet surfaces (*curved arrows*) are displaced anterior to the superior facet surfaces (*arrows*). Note the edema in the central gray matter of the spinal cord (*long arrow*).

The facet joint complex is a dynamic structure that permits limited compression and distraction of the posterior elements during extension and flexion while resisting rotation and translation. Although fractures that involve the facet surfaces are better detected with plain radiographs, tomography, and CT, subtle damage to the synovial capsule and cartilaginous surface of the joint is best appreciated with MRI. The facets are demonstrated on the far left and right parasagittal images of any well centered sagittal sequence. Normally, the articular surface of the superior facet maintains close apposition to the inferior facet surface. Widening of this space is suggestive of a distraction injury (Figs. 13, 15, 17, and 19). Loss of facet alignment or subluxation is usually an obvious finding. Increased fluid within the joint space is suggested by a well demarcated hyperintense focus interposed between the articular surfaces on T2-weighted and GE images (Fig. 15). The increased fluid is contained within the joint space and joint capsule.

Disc Injury

The identification and classification of a traumatic disc injury are important factors in determining the timing of and type of surgical decompression and stabilization (69). Although post-traumatic disc herniation does not correlate with the degree of associated injuries or neurologic deficit, unrecognized disc herniation is a cause of neurologic deterioration after stabilization (8,69,70). Myelography, plain CT, and post-CTM formerly played an important role in determining whether disc material extruded into the epidural space and compressed the thecal sac. Plain CT is relatively insensitive to disc herniation compared to MRI (8,10,62). As a result, the incidence of post-traumatic disc herniation was probably underestimated in the pre-MRI era.

Although degenerative disc herniations are probably more common in the lumbar spine, post-traumatic disc herniations are encountered more frequently in the cervical and thoracic regions (17,65,69). In the cervical region, disc herniations most commonly occur at the C4-C7 levels (8,71). Disc herniations from thoracic trauma are more common than previously estimated, and they may occur in up to one half of these injuries (69). When only CT and CTM were available for the evaluation of spine trauma, cervical disc herniations were estimated to occur in 3% to 9% of all cervical spine injuries. In addition, a large number of false-positive disc herniations were reported using CT and myelography (69). With the routine use of MRI in this application, the reported incidence ranges from 5% to 54% (8,70,71). In one MRI series, cervical disc herniations were found in association

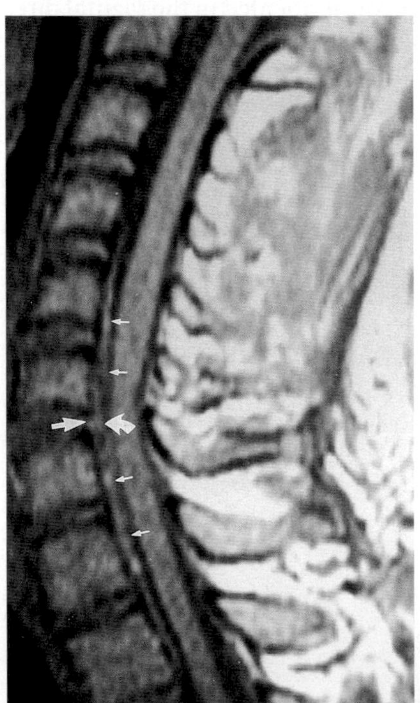

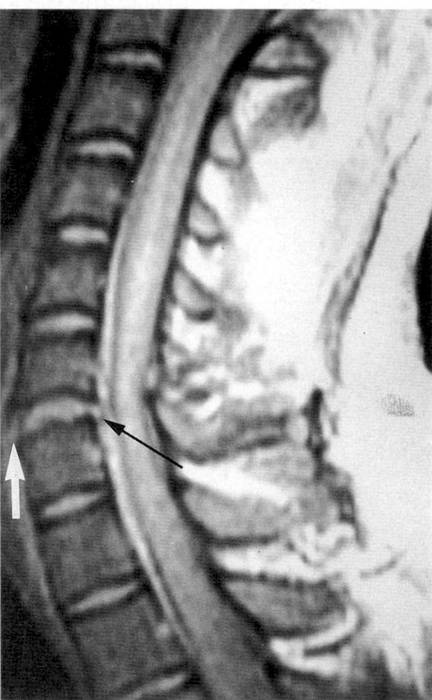

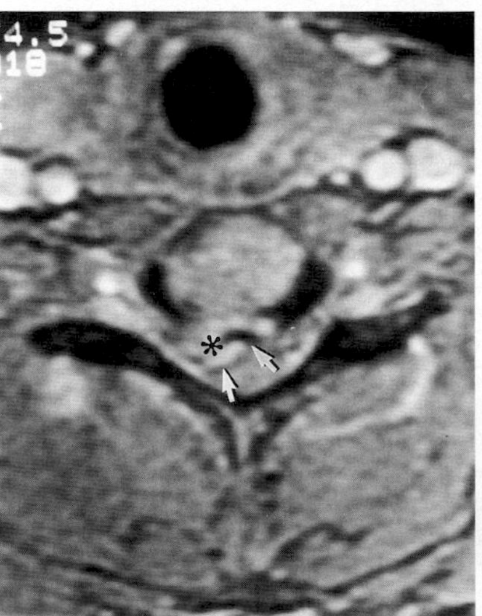

A,B C

FIG. 20. Traumatic disc herniation with epidural hematoma. **A:** Sagittal SE T1-weighted image (500/11/4 NEX) shows interruption of the posterior annulus at the C6/7 level (*white arrow*). A mound of tissue projects behind and above the disc space (*curved arrow*) representing herniated material bounded by the elevated PLL. The associated epidural hematoma (*small arrows*) is minimally hyperintense. Also note the marked swelling of the spinal cord. **B:** Sagittal SE (2000/30/2 NEX) image shows that the epidural fluid collection is hyperintense. The margins around the herniated disc are better demonstrated (*black arrow*). Note the associated interruption of the ALL (*white arrow*). **C:** Axial 3DFT GE image (35/15/5°) in another patient shows a large extruded disc fragment (*asterisk*) that is compressing the right anterior margin of the thecal sac (*arrows*).

with 80% of bilateral facet dislocations, 60% of hyperextension injuries, 47% of central cord injuries, and all cases of anterior cord syndromes. In this same report, 22% of neurologically normal patients demonstrated disc herniations on MRI (71). Cervical disc herniation is reported to occur more frequently in flexion-distraction and flexion-compression type injuries (72). The presence of herniated disc material compressing the thecal sac is a significant factor in determining whether a discectomy should be performed at the time of stabilization (72). In addition, residual cord compression from a disc herniation is associated with more severe neurologic injuries than disc herniation without cord compression (8,73).

Post-traumatic disc changes on MRI can be classified as either disc injury or disc herniation. Normally, the well hydrated intervertebral disc is hypointense relative to bone marrow on T1-weighted images and hyperintense on T2-weighted images. The nondegenerated disc is uniform and symmetric in height and the peripheral fibers of the annulus fibrosus merge imperceptibly with the longitudinal ligaments. *Disc injury* is implied whenever there is asymmetric narrowing or widening of an isolated disc space on sagittal images and focal hyperintensity of the disc material on T2-weighted images. The injured disc is often higher in signal intensity than the adjacent discs on T2-weighted images and the level of injury is usually contiguous with other damaged tissues (Fig. 17). The observed signal changes in the disc may be the result of tearing of the disc substance during hyperflexion, hyperextension, or subluxation (8,14,65). In adults, the intervertebral disc is an avascular structure; the observed MR signal changes of a damaged disc may be, in part, due to damage to the adjacent endplates. The signal changes of the injured disc may be easier to identify in patients with hypointense discs from pre-existing degenerative disc disease.

An acute, post-traumatic disc herniation has a similar MRI appearance to nontraumatic disc herniation. The nucleus pulposus is forced under pressure to extrude into the peripheral annulus fibrosus and, in some instances, extend beyond the outer annulus into the anterior epidural space. The herniation may be broad-based or eccentric and may or may not be associated with a vertebral body fracture. On sagittal MRI images, the disc herniation is isointense and contiguous with the disc of origin (2,8,10,12,14,18). A small herniated disc fragment often appears as a focal area of expansion of the annulus beyond the border of the posterior cortical margin (Figs. 17, 19, 20). Occasionally, a small rent in the annulus may appear that allows passage of nuclear material into the epidural space. On axial images, the herniated disc produces focal distortion of the ventral theca (Fig. 20). Depending on the size and location of the disc herniation, the fragment may be demonstrated on multiple sagittal and axial images.

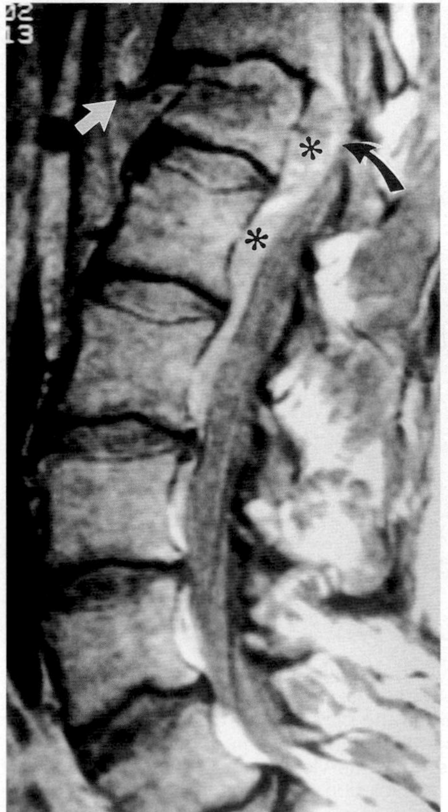

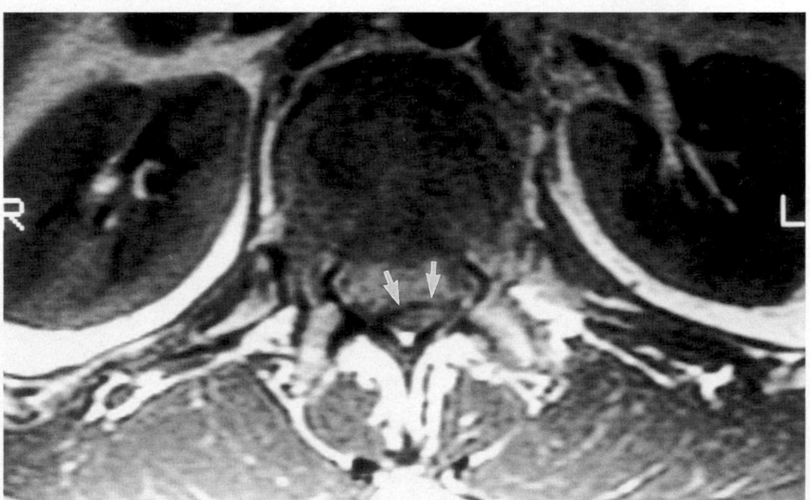

FIG. 21. Large epidural hematoma. **A:** Sagittal FSE intermediate weighted image (2000,17Ef/2 NEX/ETL4). There is a fracture of the T12 vertebral body with resultant kyphous deformity of the spine. The ALL is ruptured at the T12 level (*white arrow*). A large hyperintense fluid collection is present in the ventral epidural space that extends caudally to approximately the L3 level (*asterisks*). There is marked compression of the thecal sac (*curved arrow*). **B:** Axial T1-weighted image (600/14/4 NEX). The epidural hemorrhage is forcing the thecal sac dorsally and causing severe compression of the conus medullaris (*arrows*).

The degree of compressive injury to the neural elements depends on the size of the herniated fragment, the width of the spinal canal at the level of injury, and the diameter of the spinal cord. For example, a small disc herniation in the thoracic region may cause more neural impingement than an identical fragment would cause in the lumbar or cervical regions (74).

Identification of an acute disc herniation can be difficult in the setting of superimposed degenerative spondylotic changes (17). In such instances, multiple chronic spondylotic disc herniations associated with osteophytes may complicate the identification of an acute traumatic disc (23). Imaging factors that may aid in the identification of an acute disc herniation with superimposed spondylosis include signal changes suggestive of disc injury, asymmetric width of the intervertebral disc space, subluxation, and associated injuries at the same level. In some circumstances, definitive identification may be impossible.

Epidural Hematoma

MRI reveals more post-traumatic epidural hematomas in the spine than were previously recognized clinically (16). They have been reported to occur in up to 41% of spine injuries (16). Spinal epidural hematomas occur as the result of tearing of a portion of the epidural venous plexus with focal extravasation of blood into the anterior epidural space. Most epidural hematomas from closed trauma are found in association with other injuries, are relatively small in size, and are probably not clinically significant (14). Since the spinal dura is not firmly adherent to the vertebral canal, relatively large epidural hematomas may remain clinically silent because they extend

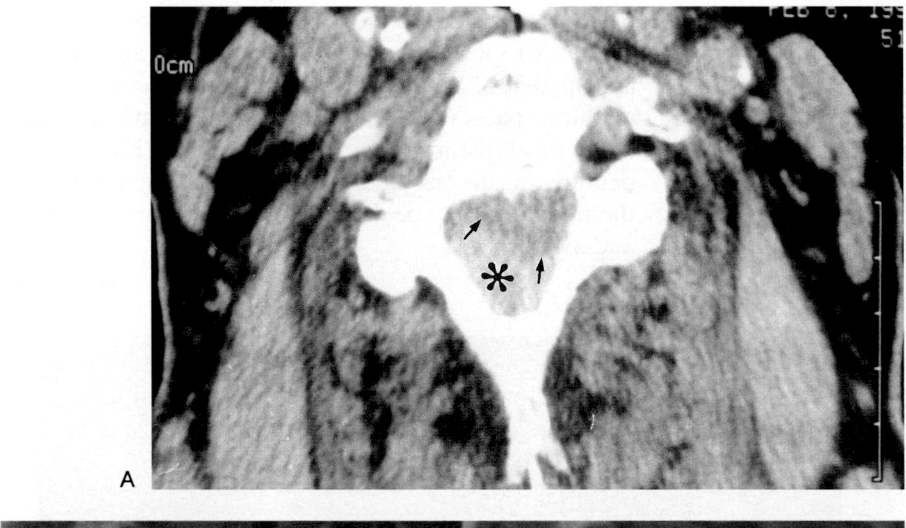

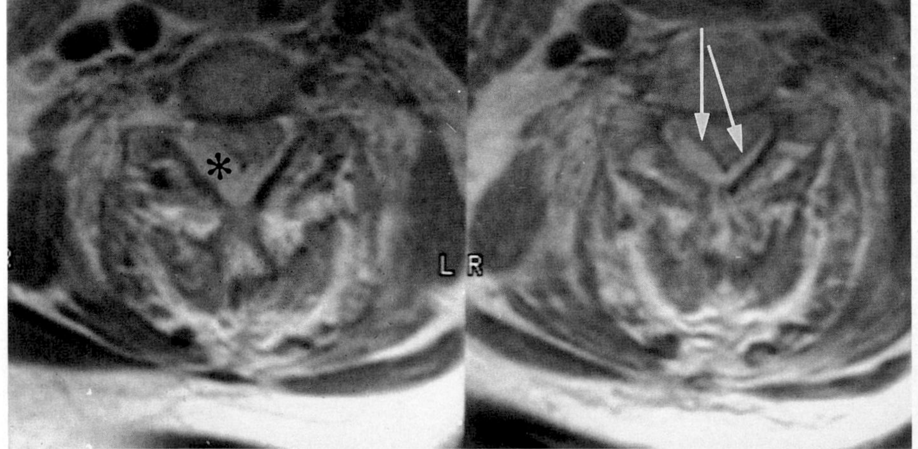

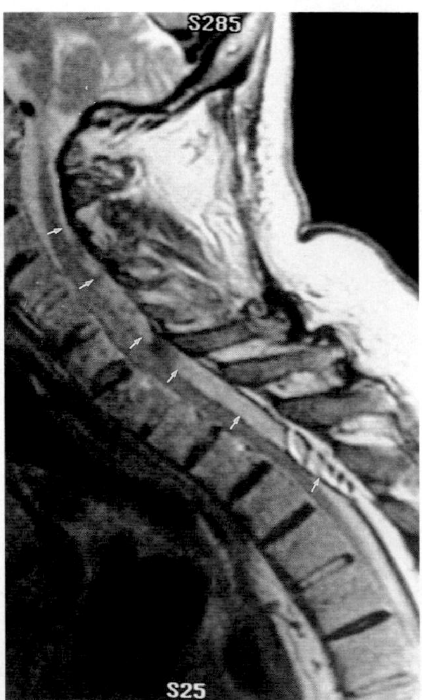

FIG. 22. Dorsal epidural hematoma in patient with ankylosing spondylitis. **A:** Oblique axial CT image through lower cervical spine shows a large biconvex hyperdense collection (*asterisk*) dorsal to the thecal sac. The theca is displaced anteriorly (*arrows*). **B:** Axial FSE MRI images (2200/102Ef/2 NEX/ETL8) confirms the presence of the epidural hematoma (*asterisk*) and the compression of the posterior dura (*arrows*). **C:** Sagittal FSE T2-weighted image (2200/102Ef/4 NEX/ETL8) shows the broad extent of the hemorrhage through the entire cervical region (*arrows*). The heterogeneous signal characteristics are secondary to heme in various stages of evolution. The accentuated configuration of the cervical spine is secondary to ankylosing spondylitis.

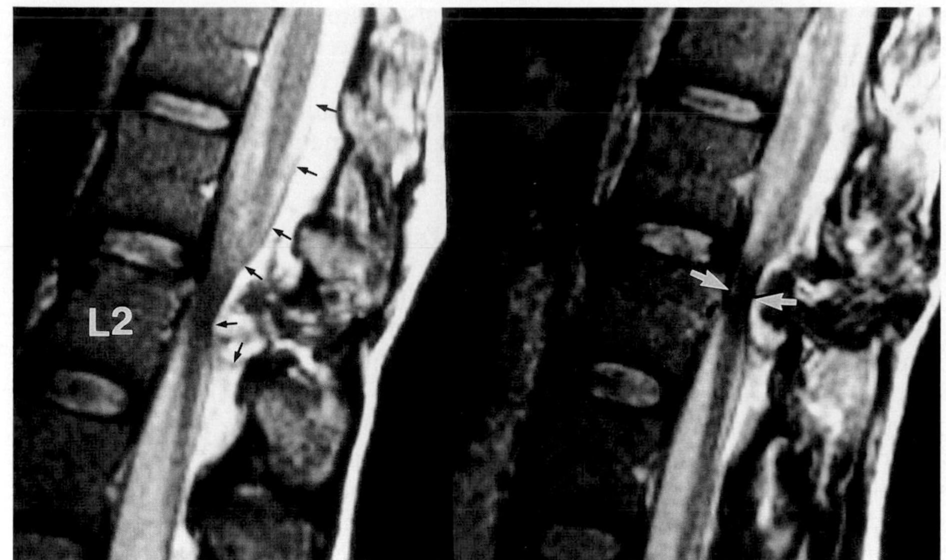

FIG. 23. Chance fracture with epidural hematoma. Sagittal FSE T2-weighted images (2200/102EF/4NEX/ETL8). A large dorsal epidural hematoma is displacing the posterior margin of the dura (*small black arrows*). The hematoma is heterogeneous with both hypointense and hyperintense components. The roots of the cauda equina are compressed against the vertebral body by the hematoma (*white arrows*).

over multiple levels and therefore do not significantly compromise the thecal sac and contents. The imaging characteristics of epidural hematomas are variable, they depend on the oxidative state of the hemorrhage and the separation of hematocrit from plasma (Figs. 6, 11, and 18–24) (63,75,76). In the acute phase, the epidural hematoma is isointense with spinal cord parenchyma on T1-weighted images and isointense with CSF on intermediate- and T2-weighted sequences (2). The epidural collection may be difficult to distinguish from the adjacent CSF in the subarachnoid space. This distinction can often be made by the hypointense dura, which separates the two compartments (Figs. 11, 20, 22).

Vascular Injury

The true incidence of associated post-traumatic dissection or thrombosis of the extracranial carotid and ver-

A

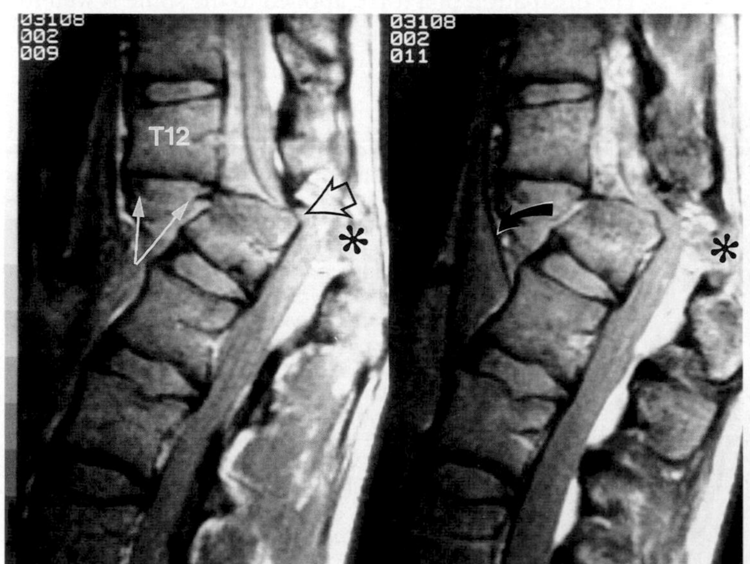

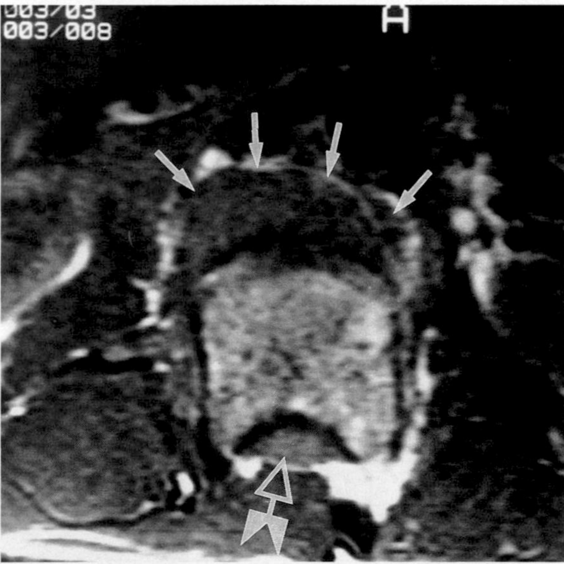

B

FIG. 24. Complete dislocation at T12-L1. **A:** Sagittal intermediate-weighted FSE image (2000/17Ef/2 NEX/ETL8). The body of T12 is dislocated relative to L1. The T12/L1 disc is avulsed and free edges of the annular fibers are demonstrated (*white arrows*). The posterior ligamentous complex is disrupted (*asterisk*). The spinal cord is markedly distorted and compressed at the level of the dislocation (*open arrow*). Hematoma is present in the anterior epidural space (*curved black arrow*). The ALL is stretched over the dislocated segments but appears intact (*curved white arrow*). **B:** Axial T1-weighted image (500/14/4 NEX) shows the avulsed disc (*arrows*) displaced anteriorly to the L1 vertebral body. The spinal cord (*open arrow*) is draped over the vertebral body. Note the absence of the posterior elements.

tebral arteries following cervical spine injury is unknown because the vascular injury often remains clinically occult. Prior investigations have suggested that damage to the vertebral arteries can be demonstrated angiographically in up to 40% of patients following cervical subluxation/dislocation (77). Dissection of the vertebral artery is more frequent than carotid artery dissection following fracture/subluxation because a portion of the cervical vertebral artery is contained within the foramen transversarium. A fracture that extends through the foramen transversarium may compress the ipsilateral vertebral artery. Because the artery is rigidly contained within the foramen, it may also be subject to severe stretching and torsional forces from cervical subluxation (Figs. 25 and 26) (78). In our case material, vertebral artery injury was identified in nine patients in a review of 37 neck MRAs from SCI patients over a 6-month period. One patient expired secondary to embolic infarction of the right cerebellar hemisphere (78a).

Conventional angiography cannot be justified to evaluate all patients with cervical trauma for occult vascular injury, in view of the small percentage of clinically symptomatic patients. However, MRA is an appropriate screening test to identify patients who may require subsequent catheter angiography. For example, a 2D TOF sequence is effective in screening the extracranial vasculature. No special surface coil is required. A walking superior saturation pulse is used to suppress venous inflow. This technique is adequate to evaluate vascular occlusion or significant narrowing, however, resolution limits the effectiveness of detecting subtle intimal injuries associated with dissection (Fig. 26). In cases of vertebral artery occlusion, axial GE images reveal replacement of normal flow-related enhancement in the foramen transversarium by a hypointense clot (deoxyhemoglobin) (Figs. 25 and 26). The indications for prophylactic anticoagulation for asymptomatic vertebral injury are controversial.

Biomechanics and Distribution of Injuries

Most SCI reported in any given year result in tetraparesis due to damage to the cervical spinal cord. Most victims of thoracic and lumbar spine trauma suffer no neurologic sequelae (74,79). The type of injuries that occur in the cervical, thoracic, and lumbar regions differ because of regional structural differences, biomechanical variations, and mechanisms of injury. Factors that may predispose to SCI include developmental or acquired spinal stenosis, degenerative spondylosis, and ankylosing spondylitis (65,68,80).

The pathophysiology of spinal injury can be better understood in a biomechanical framework (81). The spine is made up of relatively rigid components (vertebral bodies and posterior elements) and flexible components (intervertebral discs and ligaments). All the spinal segments work in concert with the adjacent segments to allow for reasonable amounts of flexion, extension, and rotation. The response of any substance to stretching or compression by an external force is defined by its *elastic modulus*. The application of too great a force over a short period of time results in tissue stress and eventual failure. Bone and ligament have different failure characteristics (1). The dissipation of a force applied to the spine is well tol-

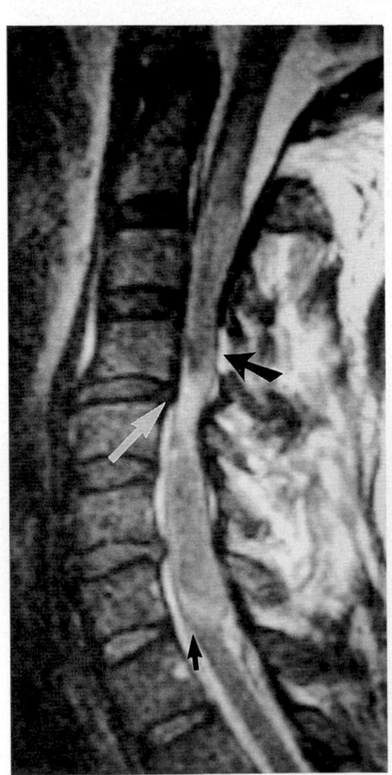

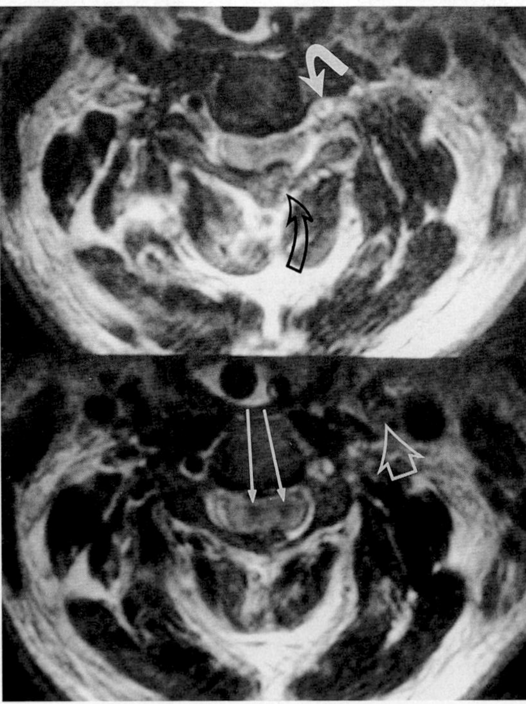

A,B

FIG. 25. A–J. Crush injury from fork lift in a 49-year-old man. **A:** Sagittal FSE T2-weighted image (3000/85Ef/2NEX, ETL 8) shows a massive hemorrhagic injury of the cervical spinal cord. The edema extends up to the level of the foramen magnum. A disc herniation is present at C4-C5 (*white arrow*) and there is offset of the cervical segments at that level. The ligamentum flavum is disrupted at the C4 level (*black arrow*). Note the sharp change in caliber of the spinal cord caudally (*small black arrow*). **B:** Axial FSE T2-weighted images (4400/90Ef/2NEX, ETL 8) at the C3-C4 level shows buckling of the lamina with encroachment on the posterior epidural space (*open black arrow*). The spinal cord is enlarged, deformed, and devoid of all normal internal anatomic features. Portions of the central gray matter are hypointense secondary to hemorrhage (*long white arrows*). Note the absence of normal flow void in the left vertebral artery (*curved white arrow*) and left internal carotid artery (*open white arrow*) suggestive of slow flow or occlusion (compare with normal right side).

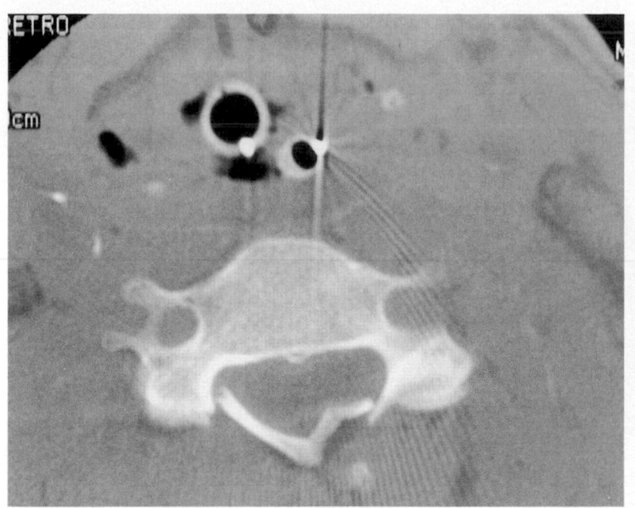

C

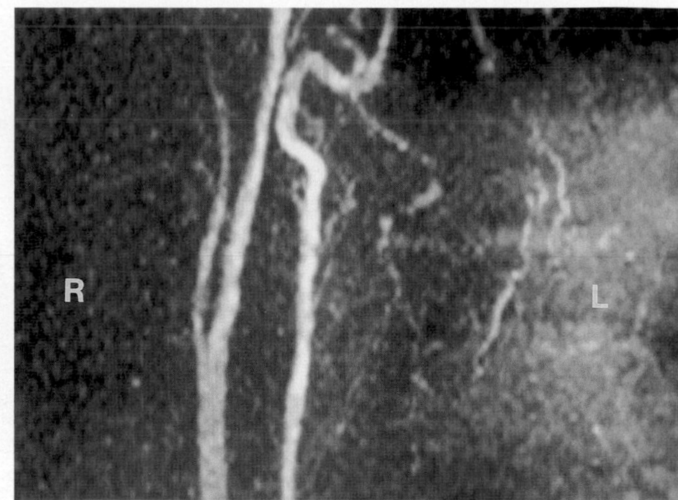

D

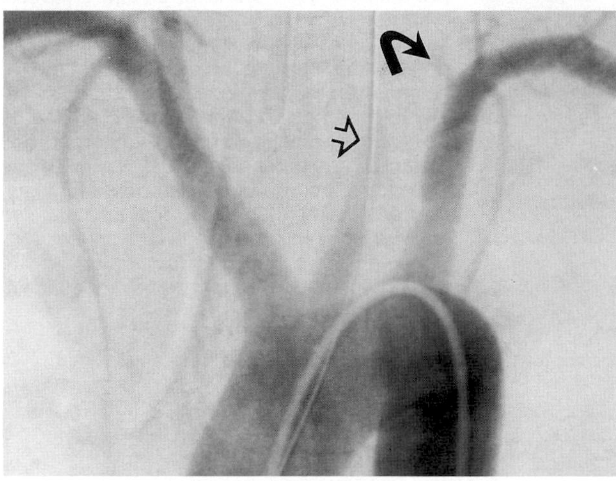

E

FIG. 25. (*Continued.*) **C:** Axial CT image at the C4 level shows comminuted fractures of the lamina bilaterally with resultant narrowing of the spinal canal. **D:** MIP image from axial 2D TOF acquisition (45/8.7/1 NEX, 60° flip) reveals normal flow-related enhancement of the right carotid artery and right vertebral artery with absence of the left carotid and vertebral arteries. **E:** RPO view from arch arteriography confirms the traumatic occlusion of the left common carotid artery (*open arrow*) and left vertebral artery (*curved arrow*).

erated under the following circumstances: (a) the force is applied gradually over a prolonged period, and (b) the resultant motion of the spine by the force does not exceed the design specifications in terms of length of travel. If either of these rules is violated, then the elastic modulus of the tissues may be exceeded and tissue failure results. This phenomenon is well illustrated in the cervical region: the cervical spine supports a large free weight (the head) that allows for a full range of motion (flexion, extension, and rotation). During periods of rapid acceleration/deceleration, the head develops to large amounts of kinetic energy that must be completely dissipated by the cervical spine. In this setting, a lower segment of the cervical spine may behave as a fulcrum against the fixed thoracic spine, resulting in tissue failure. Tissue failure allows for focal dissipation of this kinetic energy; therefore, the osseous, ligamentous, and spinal cord damage tend to be in anatomic proximity (8,65,68).

Classification systems have been developed to help simplify the description of spinal injuries as an aid in diagnosis, prognosis, and treatment (82,83). These systems are used to infer the amount of "invisible" soft tissue damage based on radiographic appearance. Some of these schemata are based on mechanisms of injury, i.e., hyperflexion, hyperextension, rotation, flexion-rotation, extension-rotation, axial loading, or lateral translation (81). A major limitation of this method of analysis is that few injuries can be explained by "pure" mechanisms. Moreover, the biomechanics of the spine differ drastically by location and therefore the types of injuries produced by the same force vectors differ by location. A classification based on mechanism alone does not directly relate either to treatment or prognosis.

Other schemes are based solely on the presence of stability or instability of an injury. Potential instability is an important determining factor in the type of surgical stabilization. Instability is defined as the loss of ability of the spine to maintain normal anatomic alignment under normal physiologic loads (74,84). The properties of spinal instability are based on the three-column model of spine trauma suggested by Holdsworth and revised by Denis, and applied to the thoracic and lumbar spine (82,83). This model was devised so that inferences could be made about the status of soft tissue injury based solely

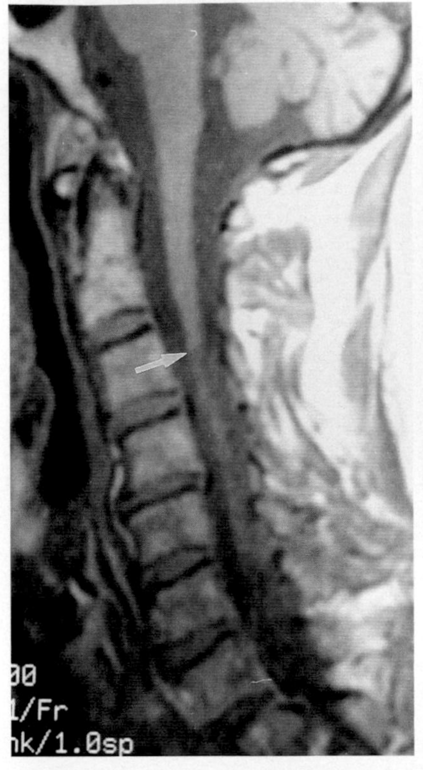

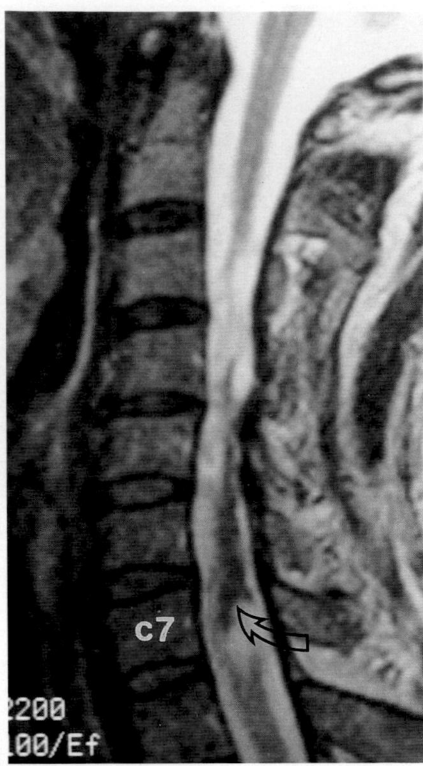

F,G

FIG. 25. (*Continued.*) **F:** Sagittal T1-weighted image (600/11/2 NEX) obtained approximately 10 months after injury reveals marked atrophy of the damaged segment of cervical cord with a sharp transition in morphology beginning at the midportion of the C3 vertebral body (*arrow*). **G:** Sagittal FSE T2-weighted image (2200/102Ef/4 NEX, ETL 8), 10 months postinjury, shows the atrophic and malacic cord parenchyma between C3 and T1 levels. The hypointense portion of the spinal cord is secondary to hemosiderin staining (*curved arrow*).

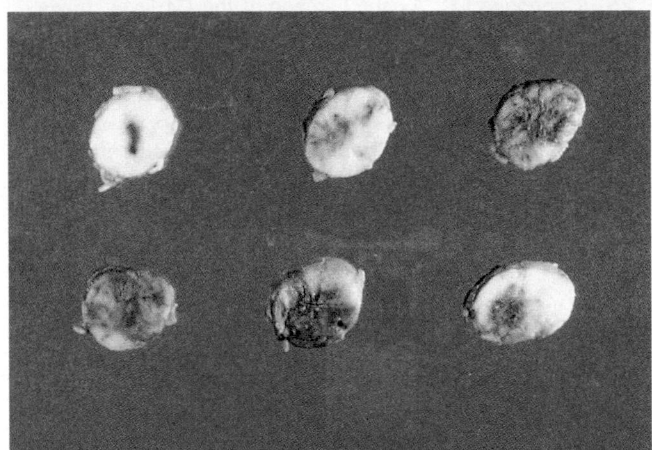

H

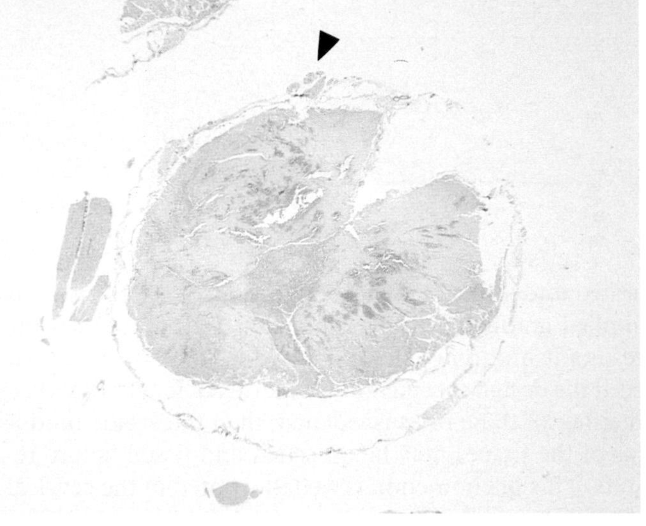

I

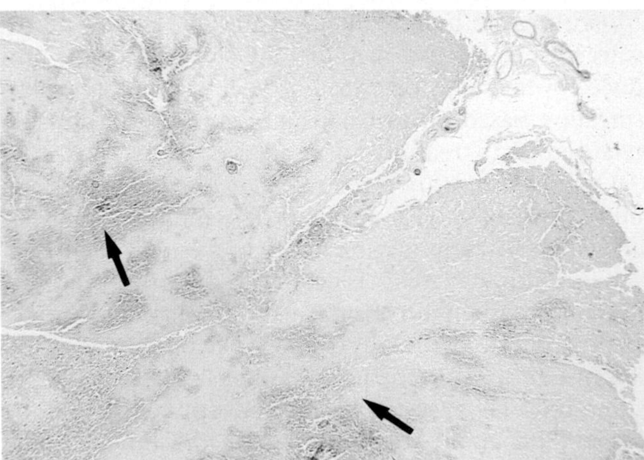

J

FIG. 25. (*Continued.*) **H:** Sections of cervical spinal cord taken from a patient who died 6 days following a neurologically complete C6-C7 anterior dislocation that did not come to medical attention immediately. Note that the hemorrhage occupies the complete extent of gray and white matter over several centimeters of spinal cord. **I:** Micrograph of spinal cord from case illustrated in H. Even in this histologic preparation, the hemorrhage has distorted the spinal anatomy almost beyond recognition. For orientation, note preserved anterior spinal artery (*arrowhead*) (H & E). **J:** Impregnation for axons (Bodian stain). Case previously illustrated in H and I. The axonal profiles (*arrows*) have been destroyed by the mechanical force of the cervical dislocation. Axonal profiles which would normally stain as black dots in white matter are not seen. Hemorrhage stains green in this preparation (*arrows*).

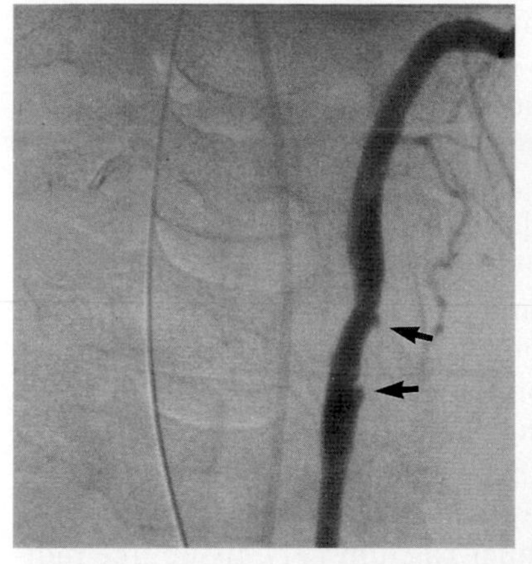

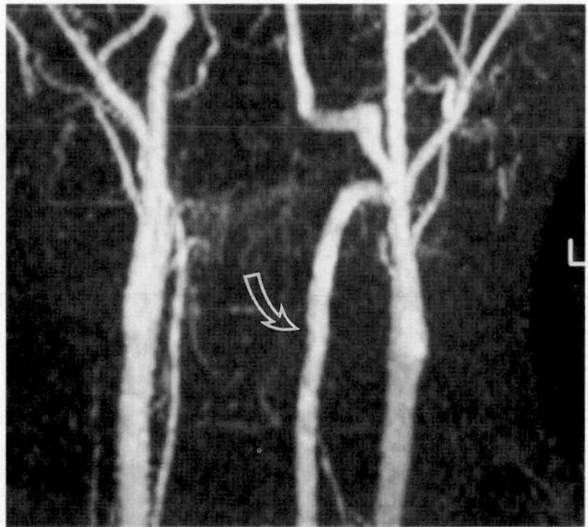

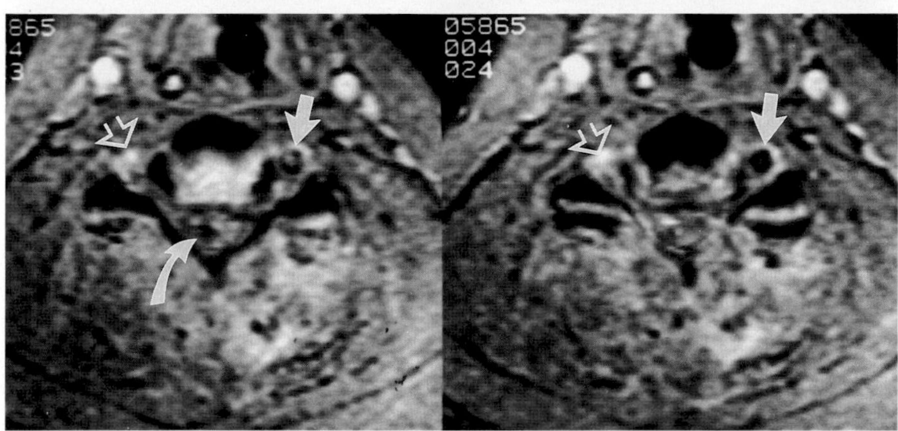

FIG. 26. Traumatic intimal injury of vertebral artery. **A:** AP radiograph from a left vertebral arteriogram shows irregularity of the lateral wall (*arrows*) of the contrast column secondary to distractive injury at C3-C4. (No associated fracture at this level.) **B:** Single projection from a 2D TOF MRA (45/8.7/60°) shows normal flow-related enhancement in all vessels. There is minimal irregularity of the left vertebral artery (*arrow*) but the intimal damage is not apparent. **C:** Axial 3DFT GE images (35/15/5°) in another patient with traumatic occlusion of the left vertebral artery. Hypointense acute clot is demonstrated within the lumen of the left vertebral artery (*arrows*). Compare with normal flow-related enhancement in the right vertebral artery (*open arrows*). Also note the massive hemorrhage in the spinal cord (*curved arrow*).

on radiologic changes. In this model, the spine is represented by three columns: the *anterior column*, which is made up of the anterior one half of the vertebral body, the anterior annulus fibrosus, and the ALL; the *middle column*, composed of the posterior half of the vertebral body and the PLL; and the *posterior column*, which contains the posterior bony arch, ligamentum flavum, facets, and interspinous ligaments. Isolated disruption of the posterior column does not constitute instability; the structures of the middle column must also be involved to invoke instability in the thoracic and lumbar spine (83).

Although this type of classification offers information that aids in the diagnosis and treatment of specific injuries, it is an oversimplification that is probably not valid biomechanically (74). Tears of the posterior longitudinal ligament, LF, interspinous and supraspinous ligaments, and facet joint disruption are potentially unstable (85). Some fractures that would be classified as stable can still harbor components that would render the injury unstable if not adequately treated (86). Furthermore, MRI may supersede this type of assessment since it directly depicts all soft tissue components of an injury.

Degenerative spondylosis alters the biomechanical properties of the spine by decreasing elasticity, thereby diminishing the ability of the tissues to safely tolerate applied force (68). The loss of spinal elasticity in ankylosing spondylitis is so severe that even minor trauma can result in a fracture-dislocation.

Because of biomechanical differences, the pathophysiology of upper cervical spine injuries (C1-C2) differs from lower cervical spine injuries (C3-C7) (20,79). Therefore, it is more appropriate to discuss upper and lower cervical spine injuries separately. Upper cervical spinal cord injuries are more common in children than adults because the head size for children is proportionally larger than for adults (20). Furthermore, in adults, the probability of developing a permanent neurologic deficit is much higher in the lower cervical spine injuries.

The classification system devised by Allen et al. (1) is the most widely used classification scheme for lower cervical injuries. Injuries are classified by major and minor injury force vectors and then are subclassified into degree of severity. The common classification groups are compressive flexion, vertical compression, distractive flexion, compressive extension, distractive extension, and lateral flexion (1). Most injuries to the cervical spine are the result of hyperflexion mechanisms (79%) (75).

Although fractures of the thoracic spine are not unusual, they comprise only a small proportion of all fractures of the spinal column (16%) (74,87). The biomechanics of the upper thoracic spine (T1-T10) differ from the cervical spine as well as from the lower thoracic spine

(T10-T12). Most thoracic fractures occur at the thoracolumbar junction and remain neurologically intact (79). The thoracic cage offers a protective effect to the upper thoracic spine by adding stiffness and providing additional energy-absorbing capacity. The rib cage alters the moment of inertia of the spine and therefore imparts resistance to rotational forces. In addition, the facet joints have a coronal orientation in the upper thoracic spine that resist anterior translational forces. Considerable force is therefore necessary to fracture or dislocate the thoracic spine. It is estimated that these anatomic features increase the compression tolerance of the thoracic spine by a factor of four (74). These factors contribute to the lower overall incidence of fracture-dislocations in the upper thoracic spine compared to other areas (74).

Since the thoracic spinal canal is relatively narrow in dimension, there is a high association of complete SCI (63%) with fractures of the upper thoracic spine (87). Most of these injuries occur via hyperflexion mechanisms (74,87). When there are associated bilateral fractures of the posterior elements with resultant autodecompression of the spinal canal, the spinal cord sometimes escapes injury (74).

In adults, SCI without radiographic abnormality (SCIWORA) is a well recognized syndrome of the cervical spine that is thought to occur secondary to hyperextension dislocations or hyperextension sprain associated with cervical spondylosis (47,65,67,68). This type of mechanism is reproduced in rear-end motor-vehicle collisions and direct anterior craniofacial trauma (65). In one report, 96% of patients over the age of 40 years with SCIWORA had severe cervical spondylosis (68). Common to this type of injury is momentary compression of the thecal sac between the edge of the dorsally displaced vertebral body or disc and the buckled LF (23,65,67,68). Minimal changes that may be appreciated on radiographs include prevertebral swelling, focal widening of the disc space anteriorly, or avulsion of a small portion of the vertebral endplate. MRI is of particular diagnostic value in this type of injury because it depicts abnormalities that are invisible on conventional radiographs, including separation of the intervertebral disc, rupture of the ALL and annulus, prevertebral hemorrhage, and parenchymal SCI (23,65).

SPINAL CORD INJURY

Pathology of SCI

The extent of damage to the spinal cord depends to a great degree on the mechanism and severity of the individual injury. The changes that occur in the acute phase after injury are divided into direct effects and secondary or reactive effects (76). Direct effects are related to sudden impaction or compression of the spinal cord by retropulsed bone, disc, or translational forces from ligamentous rupture. In instances where no radiologic abnormality is demonstrated in association with SCI (SCIWORA), it is postulated that spinal cord stretching may be the responsible mechanism (9).

Following contusion or compression of the spinal cord, there is mechanical disruption of tissue that can lead directly to neurologic dysfunction through damage to axons, dendrites, or neuronal cell bodies. Other tissue components, including blood vessels and glial cells, may be damaged as well. Secondary effects that may add to the degree of tissue destruction include ischemia (88,89), edema (90), extracellular calcium (91), tissue free radicals (92), products of arachidonic acid metabolism (93–96), and the release of excitatory amino acids (4,97).

Experimental SCI can be created by a variety of methods, including spinal column distraction, graded contusion, crush, and surgical sectioning. Except for surgical sectioning, most other models produce an anatomically incomplete lesion that features a central zone of damage over a length of several spinal segments. Contusive injuries have been the focus of much work because the amount of kinetic energy involved in the lesion can be graded. The most mild of these injuries will cause only a transitory paralysis, reminiscent of clinical spinal cord concussion, and may give us a clue to pathologic changes underlying SCIWORA. The tissues from these experimental animals show no gross lesions. When greater amounts of kinetic energy are employed, the area of tissue destruction may vary from a small region just dorsal to the central canal to a large lesion involving all the central gray and a variable amount of the surrounding white matter tracts (98). Regardless of the size of the zone of greatest injury, the damage rostral and caudal to this zone tapers off so that the entire lesion resembles a spindle aligned along the long axis of the spinal cord (3,39,76).

Although tissue changes are not grossly evident in those animals with minimal concussive lesions, electron microscopic studies have shown definite abnormalities. Sludging in the gray matter microcirculation is evident within 5 minutes of the injury, gray matter microhemorrhages by 1 hour postcontusion, and capillary and venule abnormalities throughout the cord by 4 hours after the injury (99). The myelin sheaths in approximately one fourth of the axons of the spinal white matter also showed some degree of damage by 4 hours after the injury (100).

Following greater concussive lesions, early changes are again seen in the microcirculation. Gray matter blood flow falls off rapidly during the first hour following injury (101,102). Flow to the lateral columns is variable during that period but falls to about one half of control values by 3 hours after injury (88). In keeping with the blood flow data, the earliest lesions seen are gross and microscopic gray matter hemorrhages (99,103), which may appear within minutes of the injury. Edema also occurs within the acute period, in some cases as soon as 1 hour after trauma (104), and spreads from the site of tissue injury to adjacent segments. Acute inflammatory changes, neuronal swelling, and neuronal necrosis are also noted within hours of injury. The chronic stage of histologic progression lasts from several weeks to months as macrophages ingest and remove tissue debris, new vessels are formed, and the glial scar is deposited.

Paralleling the time course of histologic change, animals reach their nadir of neurologic function between 1 and 2 days following injury (105), although in more severe injuries the loss of function may be almost immediate (106). Abnormal recovery of neurologic function in these experimental models occurs between 1 and 4 weeks (105) and seems to occur earlier for milder lesions (107). Particularly in cases of severe injuries, the survival of spinal white matter around the area of tissue destruction may be the determining factor for the preservation of function in the period immediately following injury and for the ultimate recovery of function. Thus, in studies correlating morphology with locomotor behavior, both the cross-sectional area of tissue lost and the number of myelinated axons surviving the injury positively correlate with the behavioral outcome (108,109). In addition, demyelinated and thinly myelinated axons are present in the surviving white matter around the injury (105). These may represent remyelinating axons and form a crucial substrate for those animals whose eventual recovery of locomotor function is most substantial (88,110).

In human SCI, the acute changes following injury are similar to those seen in animal models as manifested by disruption of axons, effects on neuronal cell bodies, hemorrhage, necrosis, edema, and cellular reaction (Figs. 25H,I). In post-mortem preparations, the axonal damage can be clearly seen with silver impregnation stains and appears as swelling or beading of the stained processes. In severely damaged spinal cords, the normal axonal staining in the white matter may be reduced to a fine dust (Fig. 25J). Stains for myelin will often show corresponding degeneration, ranging from a subtle bubbly appearance to complete and obvious fragmentation. Surviving neuronal cell bodies with damaged axons may show classic microscopic evidence of active reaction to the axonal injury (chromatolysis).

The true incidence of tissue necrosis and/or hemorrhage is much more difficult to estimate in human than in experimental spinal cord injury. In the case of spinal cord concussion, tissue is not available for examination because all patients completely recover function. In the acute stage of SCI, it has been generally accepted that both hemorrhage and necrosis are seen (111,112). However, a recent study (49) challenges this notion in regard to central cord injuries.

Classically, the term hematomyelia has been reserved for injuries that involve only hemorrhage into the substance of the cord without evidence of tissue necrosis. The interest in distinguishing this injury from hemorrhagic necrosis stems from the belief that it may represent the most appropriate circumstance for surgical drainage of the cord, since the presence of blood without tissue necrosis may imply a better prognosis compared with other hemorrhagic spinal injuries for eventual return of locomotor function. Some sources (111) assert that true hematomyelia following cord trauma is extremely infrequent, on the order of 1% or less. In other injuries in which hemorrhage is not grossly evident, petechial perivascular hemorrhage may be seen microscopically. The frequency of tissue necrosis and hemorrhage following spinal injury was previously estimated almost solely from autopsy specimens.

Whether hemorrhage or necrosis is part of the lesion, edema and cellular reaction in human patients are almost certainly present as they are in animal models. The most minimal edema may be perivascular in distribution. More commonly, it affects the entire cross-sectional area of the cord and results in a spindle with its long axis in the rostrocaudal sagittal plane (similar to the pattern in experimental models) (3,39,76). This deformation results in obliteration of the spinal subarachnoid and subdural spaces in the area of injury. Compression of draining veins may cause venous stasis, which is grossly manifested as a purplish discoloration of the cord. The inflammatory infiltrate at this early stage consists of polymorphonuclear leukocytes and lymphocytes.

The acute pathologic changes subside after several weeks and give way to a phase of tissue healing which, at the gross and microscopic levels, may last up to 2 or 3 years (Fig. 27). The acutely necrotic tissue is resorbed. First, fresh hemorrhage is converted to hemosiderin and then resorbed. Polymorphonuclear leukocytes and lymphocytes are replaced by large numbers of macrophages, many of which contain lipid breakdown products or hemosiderin. Damaged neurons are no longer easily recognized. The areas of tissue loss become cystic and are surrounded by areas of gliosis. In regions of the cord that have been most severely damaged, a true fibroblastic response can also be seen.

In the spinal cords that have been examined after long-term survival, the damaged areas are completely replaced by a mixed glial and fibrocytic scar. Evidence of continued cellular reaction is manifested by only a few residual macrophages. The subarachnoid and subdural spaces may be completely obliterated by scar tissue. The area of tissue loss often is manifested by a cavity with a thick glial and fibroblastic capsule (Fig. 28D). This cavity can be clinically significant as the nidus for a pro-

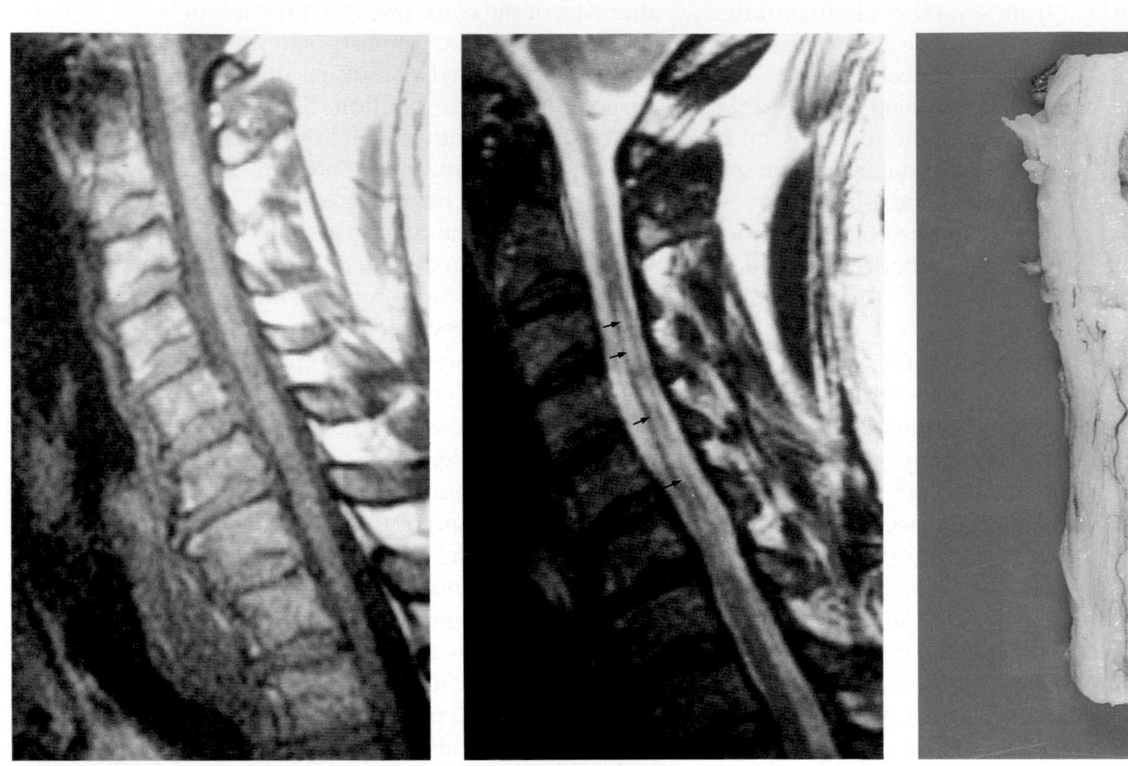

A,B C

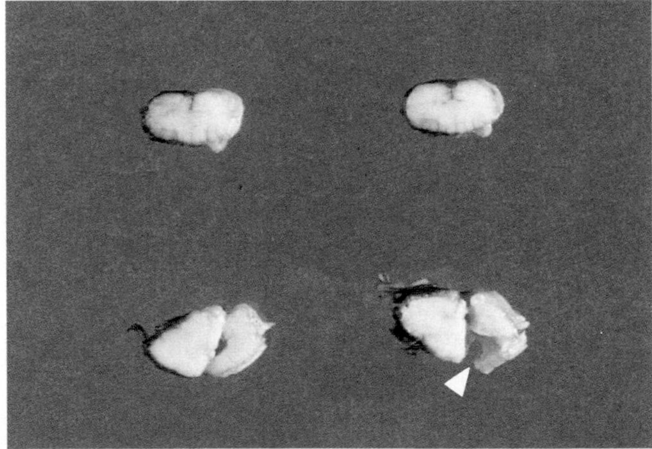

D

FIG. 27. Myelomalacia/atrophy from prior injury. **A:** Sagittal T1-weighted image (500/14) shows an atrophic spinal cord without parenchymal changes. **B:** Sagittal FSE T2-weighted image (2000/102Ef/4 NEX/ETL8) demonstrates a markedly atrophic spinal cord. There is a patchy band of high signal intensity that occupies most the cervical spinal cord (*arrows*). Note that there is no evidence of cord expansion or residual compression. **C:** Cervical spinal cord specimen from another patient who suffered a C3-C4 lesion after a fall 5 months before death. The cord is viewed dorsally, which reveals a cavity (without a cyst) (*arrow*). **D:** Cross-sections of the cord, shown in C, show a softened area of tissue.

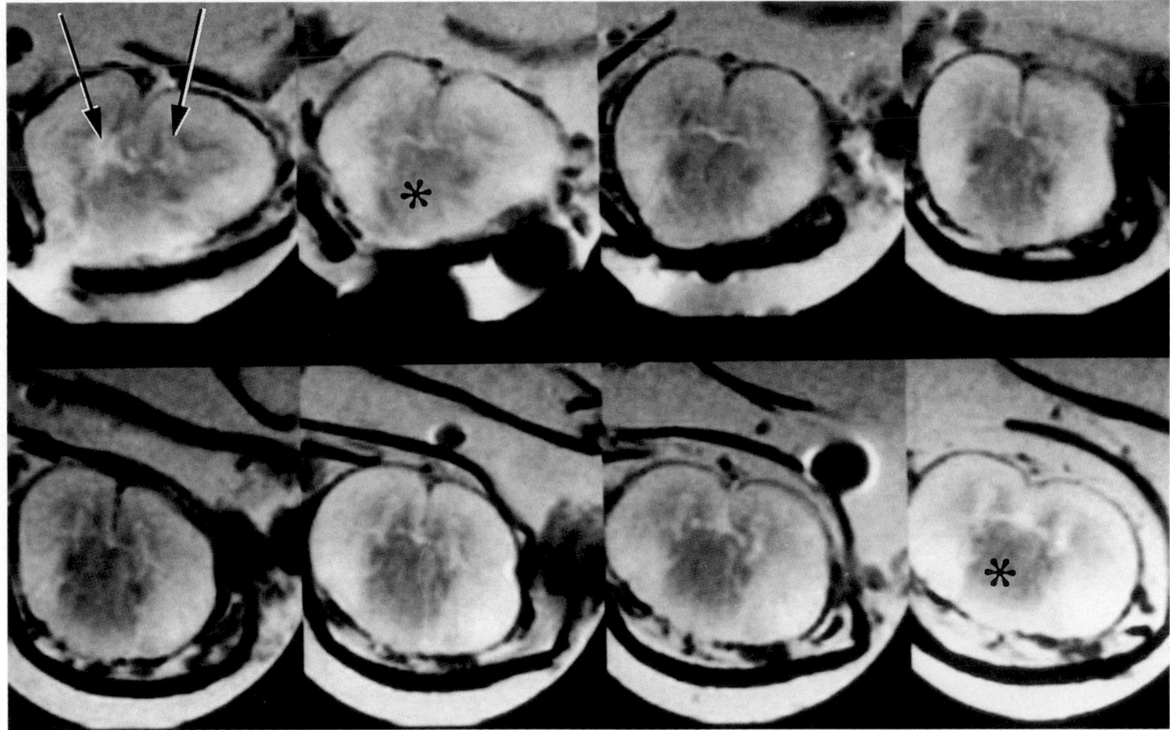

FIG. 27. (*Continued.*) **E:** Serial axial T2-weighted image SE images (2000/100/2 NEX) of the specimen in C and D shows distortion of the ventral horns of the central gray matter (*arrows*). There is a well defined focus of hypointensity that involves the middle third of the posterior cord, which corresponds pathologically to the area of parenchymal softening (*asterisk*).

gressive syringomyelia. There are multiple reports of progressive neurologic deficit from expansion of such cavities (113–117).

Following injury, tract degeneration occurs in the portions of spinal cord both rostral and caudal to the lesion. Degeneration stains show such events quite clearly more than a year after injury (Fig. 29) (118). Although correlations have been made between white matter survival and locomotion in animals (see above), the correlation between tract degeneration, white matter survival, and eventual functional status following human spinal injury has not been made.

MRI Findings of SCI

MRI has had a greater impact on our understanding of SCI than any other diagnostic modality developed in the past decade. The clarity with which MRI is able to depict the internal architecture of the spinal cord is unmatched by any other imaging modality. Moreover, the depiction of parenchymal SCI on MRI not only correlates well with the degree of neurologic deficit, but it also bears significant implications in regard to prognosis and potential for neurologic recovery (4,8,9,39,70,73, 119–122).

Although the spinal cord can be reliably visualized with conventional MRI, it does not always allow one to distinguish between spinal gray and white matter. The image obtained is homogeneous in signal intensity on all sagittal pulse sequences. In routine clinical use, the gray-white matter interface is sometimes demonstrated on long TR SE and GE axial images. Despite these limitations, there are basic MRI features of SCI that correlate with the pathology and severity of the initial injury.

In animal models, correlation of MRI with histopathology has shown that MRI provides excellent definition of intramedullary hemorrhage and edema (3,38,76). Imaging of the excised vertebral column and spinal cord of the rat has allowed resolution to approach 75 μm per pixel edge (123). Magnetic resonance spectroscopy has also been used to monitor metabolic events following experimental spinal trauma and has been able to demonstrate lactic acid accumulation, intracellular acidosis, and loss of high energy phosphates (124). Post-mortem studies of human pathology have correlated MR scans of cords following autopsy removal and tissue fixation (49,125,126). In this setting, commercially available scanners will reliably show the definition of spinal gray from white matter. These series also show a high correlation of MRI evidence of hemorrhage, edema, necrosis, and cystic change with histopathology (125,126).

The foundation for understanding MRI patterns of SCI were developed initially with animal models (3,4,39,76,127). It has been shown in a rat model of SCI that the areas of low and high signal intensity in the cord

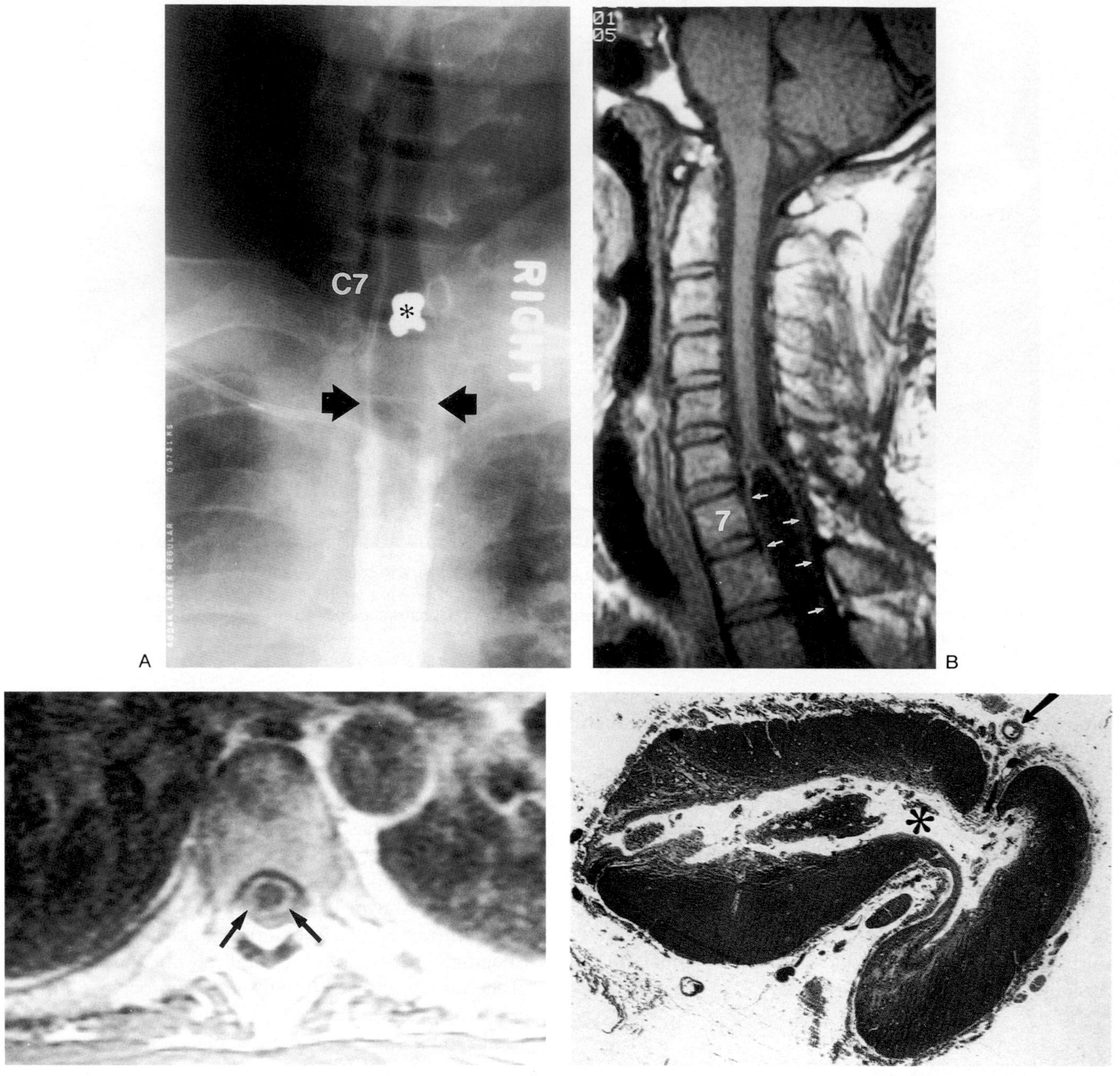

FIG. 28. Syringomyelia secondary to gun-shot wound 10 years prior. **A:** AP radiograph from a myelogram shows a bullet fragment lodged in the spinal canal at C7-T1 (*asterisk*). There is a complete intradural block noted at the T1-T2 level with enlargement of the spinal cord (*arrows*). **B:** Sagittal T1-weighted image (550/11/2 NEX) obtained 4 years later following removal of bullet fragment shows marked enlargement of the spinal cord extending from the C6-C7 level with extension into the thoracic region. The internal signal characteristics are isointense with CSF. There is a thin peripheral rim of tissue around the cyst (*arrows*). **C:** Axial T1-weighted image (400/12/4 NEX) obtained in the upper thoracic region shows the central cystic cavity in the expanded spinal cord. The residual tissue is compressed peripherally (*arrows*). **D:** This cross-section of cervical spinal cord from a different patient shows a syrinx cavity lined by astrocytes (*asterisk*). The necrotic material has been removed. Although most of the gray matter is gone, some of the surrounding white matter is preserved. The anterior spinal artery is visible at the upper right (*arrow*) (H & E). (Courtesy of A. Hirano, M.D., Division of Neuropathology, Montefiore Medical Center, Bronx, N.Y., and Igaku-Shoin Publishers.)

A

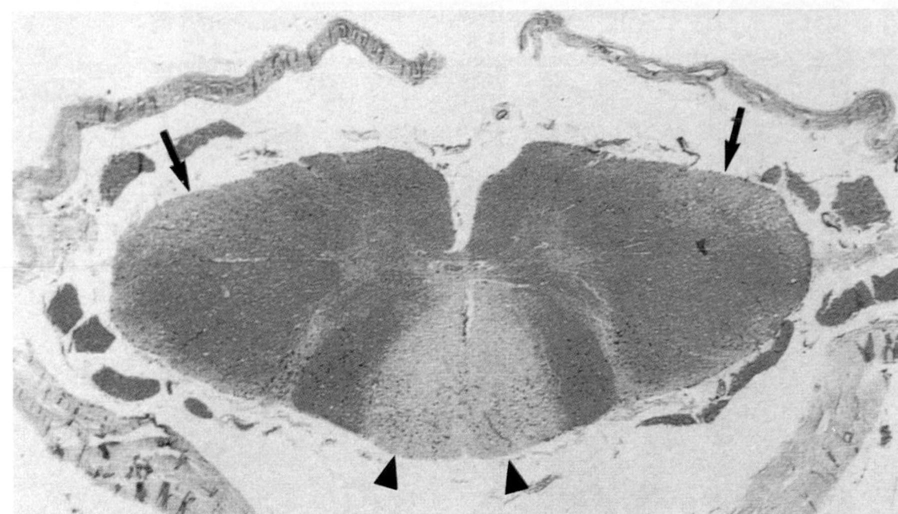

B

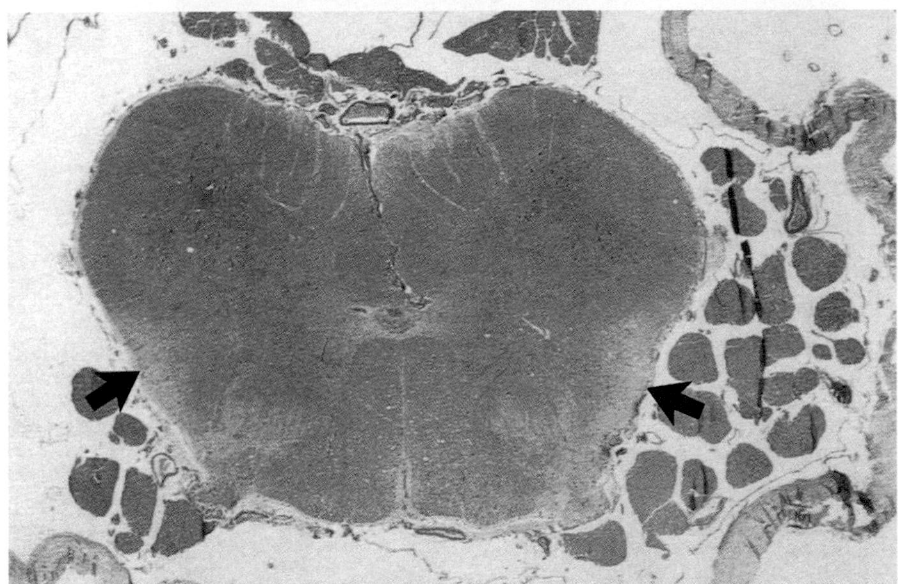

FIG. 29. Ascending and descending tract degeneration. **A:** This section from the upper thoracic spinal cord is taken from a patient who suffered a transection of the lower thoracic spinal cord. There is pallor of the more medial dorsal columns (*arrowheads*) and the spinothalamic tracts (*arrows*) due to degeneration. (Luxol fast blue–periodic acid Schiff.) **B:** Descending tract degeneration. From the same case as A. The lumbar spinal cord shows wallerian degeneration of the corticospinal tracts (*arrows*) (Luxol fast blue–periodic acid Schiff). (Material courtesy of A. Hirano, M.D., Division of Neuropathology, Montefiore Medical Center, Bronx, N.Y., and Igaku-Shoin Publishers.)

on T2-weighted images were confirmed histologically as foci of intramedullary hemorrhage and edema, respectively (3,76). These findings were corroborated in dogs using a weight-drop technique (4,39). The more severe lesions had greater longitudinal and cross-sectional involvement of the spinal cord and evidence of central hemorrhage (39). One study (125) also demonstrated the sensitivity of MRI to post-traumatic tract degeneration.

In the clinical setting, several MRI injury classification schemes have been proposed by prior investigators (4,5,9). Kulkarni et al. first described three basic patterns of acute SCI on MR (9). Schaeffer et al. described a four-tiered classification system (7,70). Common to these schemes are three imaging observations: spinal cord hemorrhage, spinal cord edema, and spinal cord swelling (4,5,8–10,18,70). Using these schemes, any injury can be accurately defined by the length of spinal cord involved and anatomic location of each of these three characteristics. Thus, a typical complete SCI is composed of an epicenter of hemorrhage surrounded by a halo of edema; the latter has a greater rostrocaudal extent than the central hemorrhage. Spinal cord swelling usually involves a slightly larger length of spinal cord than edema or hemorrhage alone. The degree of neurologic deficit is directly correlated with these MRI findings. Since spinal cord transection from closed trauma is unusual, it is not included in this system (18).

Spinal Cord Hemorrhage

Post-traumatic spinal cord hemorrhage (i.e., hemorrhagic contusion) is defined as the presence of a discrete focus of hemorrhage within the substance of the spinal cord after an injury. The most common location is within the central gray matter of the spinal cord, and centered at the point of mechanical impact (Figs. 4, 25, 30,

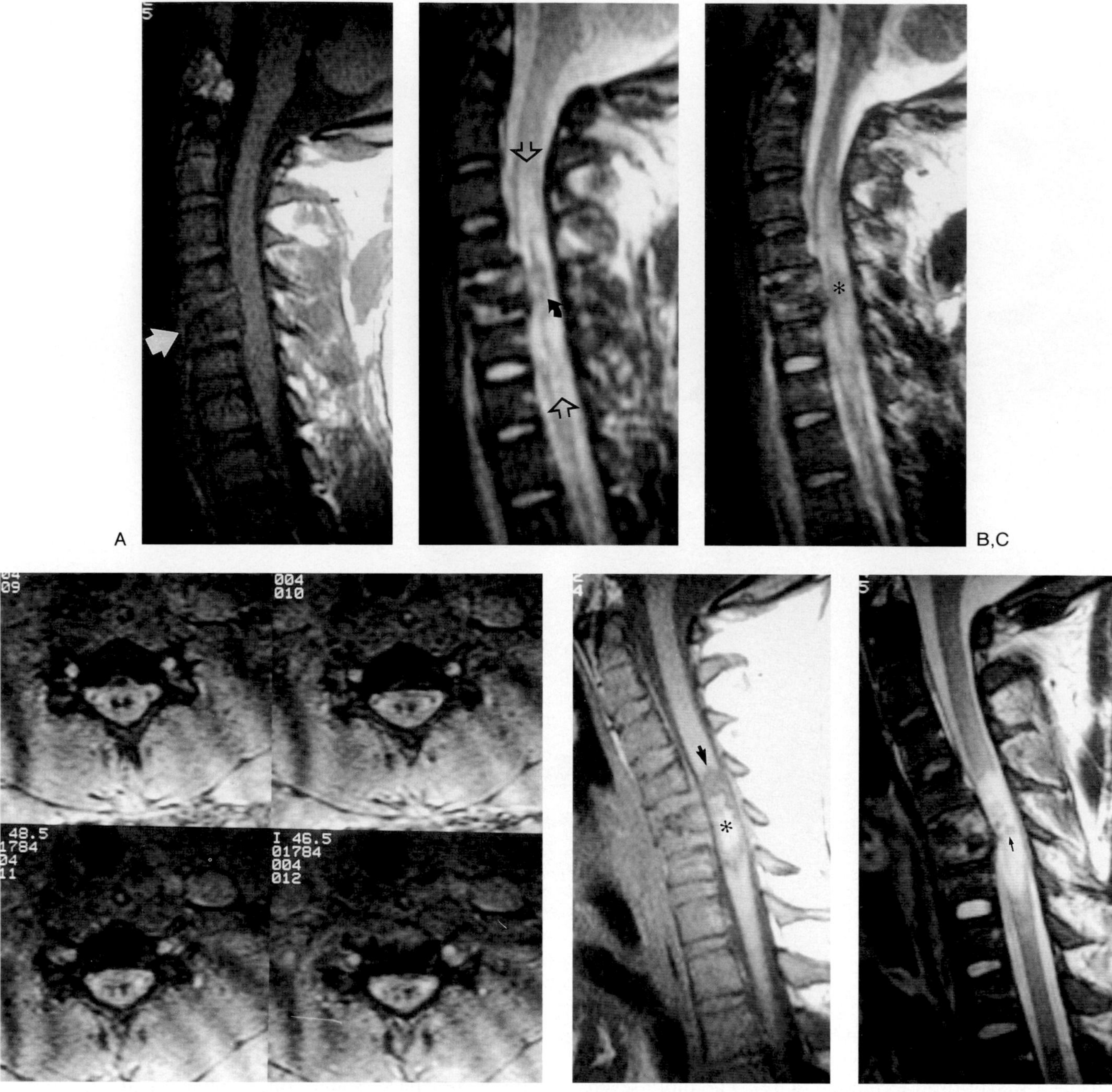

FIG. 30. Evolution of intramedullary hemorrhage (18-year-old man). **A:** Sagittal T1-weighted image (500/11/2 NEX) shows fracture deformity of C5 (*arrow*) with loss of height anteriorly. Extensive spinal cord swelling is present with effacement of the subarachnoid space. Note the lack of cord signal abnormality. **B:** Sagittal T2-weighted image (2000/80/2 NEX) shows a long segment of signal abnormality in the spinal cord. The hyperintensity that extends from C2 to T1 represents spinal cord edema (*open arrows*). The central focus of hypointensity centered at the C5 level is intramedullary hemorrhage (deoxyhemoglobin) (*curved arrow*). **C:** Sagittal FSE T2-weighted image (2500/102Ef/4 NEX, ETL 8) also depicts the spinal cord signal abnormalities. Note that the intramedullary hemorrhage (*asterisk*) is not as hypointense as it is in B. Acquisition time was half that of B. **D:** Four 1.5-mm thick continuous axial images from a 3DFT GE sequence (35/15/2 NEX) through the epicenter of the injury show discrete hypointense foci of hemorrhage within the central gray matter of the spinal cord. **E:** Sagittal T1-weighted image (500/11/2 NEX) obtained 2 months after injury shows a well defined area of cavitation within the still swollen spinal cord. The central portion of the cavity is now hyperintense (*asterisk*) from retained hemorrhagic breakdown products. The cavity is surrounded by a rind of myelomalacia/gliosis (*arrow*). **F:** Sagittal FSE T2-weighted image (2500/102Ef/4 NEX, ETL 8) shows the persistent swelling of the spinal cord. The necrotic cavity and malacic tissue are all hyperintense. Several discrete foci of low signal intensity are noted within the cavity (*arrow*) from hemorrhagic residue.

and 31) (3,7–9,128). Drawing from experimental and autopsy pathologic studies, the underlying lesion most often will be hemorrhagic necrosis of the spinal cord. True hematomyelia will rarely be found (39).

In the acute phase following injury, deoxyhemoglobin is the most common species generated (3,7,8,10,39,76). Thus, the hemorrhagic component of the SCI on high field strength scanners is depicted as a discrete area of hypointensity on the T2-weighted and GE images (Figs. 4, 25, 30, 31) (4,5,7–9,12,17,70,128). This represents the imaging manifestations of hemorrhagic necrosis of the spinal cord (8,9,18,129). The oxidative process in which deoxyhemoglobin evolves to methemoglobin is prolonged in the injured spinal cord. Methemoglobin is pre-

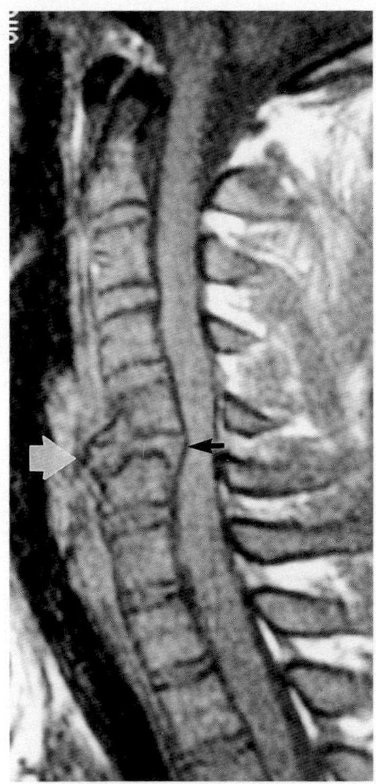
A

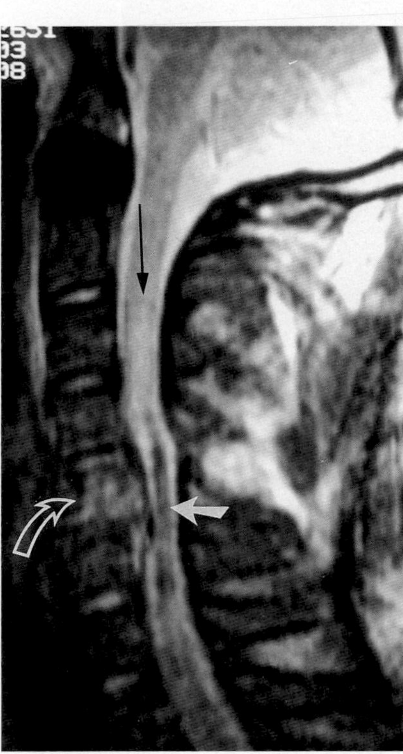

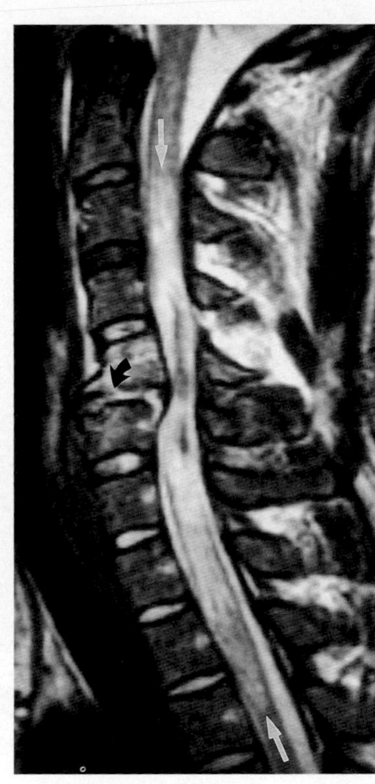
B,C

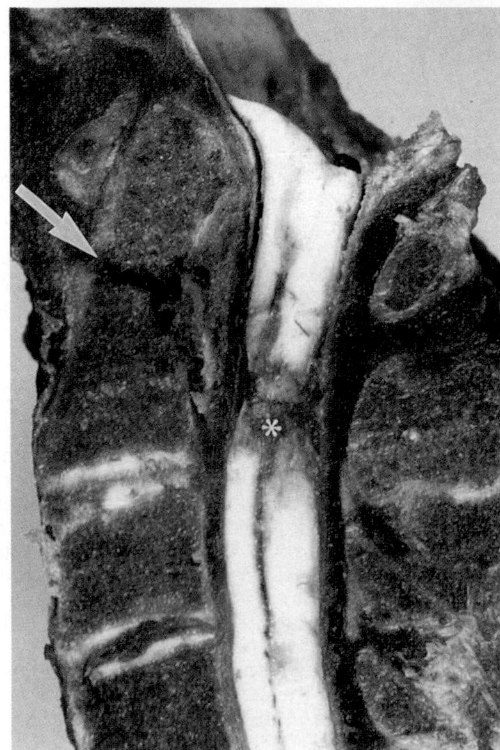
D

FIG. 31. Hyperflexion injury in a 20-year-old man; comparison of SE and FSE techniques. **A:** Sagittal SE T1-weighted image (400/11/2 NEX) shows a flexion deformity centered at the C5-C6 interspace (*white arrow*). There are fractures that extend through the inferior endplate of C5 and superior endplate of C6. Disc material is retropulsed into the anterior epidural space (*black arrow*). **B:** Sagittal SE T2-weighted image (2000/80/2 NEX,256×128) shows that the compressed marrow space of C5 reverts to hyperintensity (*open arrow*). A large hypointense focus of spinal cord hemorrhage (deoxyhemoglobin) is present extending from C4 to T1 (*white arrow*). The upper margin of spinal cord edema is indistinct (*black arrow*). **C:** Sagittal FSE T2-weighted image (2000/85Ef/4NEX, ETL 8, 256×256) shows the injury with improved clarity due to increased matrix size and improved signal. This image shows interruption of the inferior endplate at C5 (*black arrow*). The upper and lower boundaries of the spinal cord edema are very distinct (*white arrows*). Note that the spinal cord hemorrhage is not as hypointense as it is in the SE image because of decreased magnetic susceptibility effects. **D:** This sagittal section of the cervical spine and cord was taken from a patient who died 3 hours after trauma. The odontoid process is fractured and displaced posteriorly (*arrow*). The cord is transected just caudal to the fracture with obvious tissue distortion and fresh hemorrhage (*asterisks*). Additional blood can be seen tracking centrally for several centimeters rostral and caudal to the transection. (Material courtesy of R.O. Weller M.D., University of Southampton, UK, and Harvey Miller Publishers.)

dicted to appear 3 to 5 days after an initial hemorrhage in the brain; however, appearance of the intramedullary high signal intensity of methemoglobin on T1-weighted images may be delayed for 8 days or more in the spinal cord following injury (Fig. 32) because degradation of deoxyhemoglobin is delayed due to local hypoxia (7–9,76). Early investigations in animal and human SCI suggested that identification of acute hemorrhage was

A,B

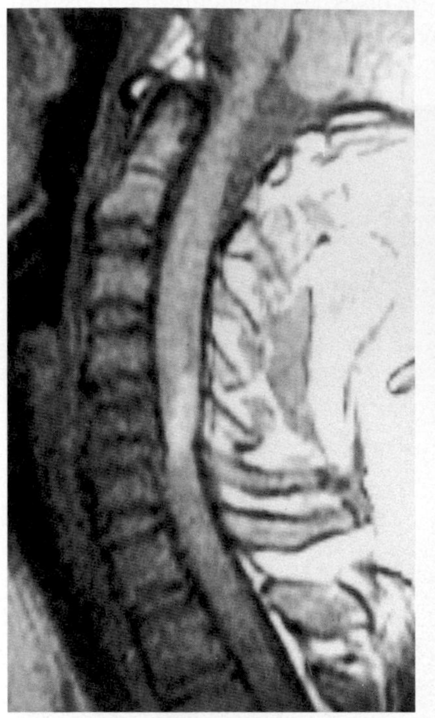

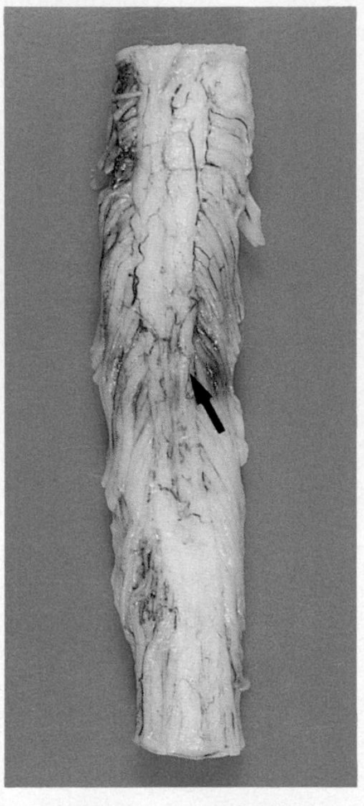

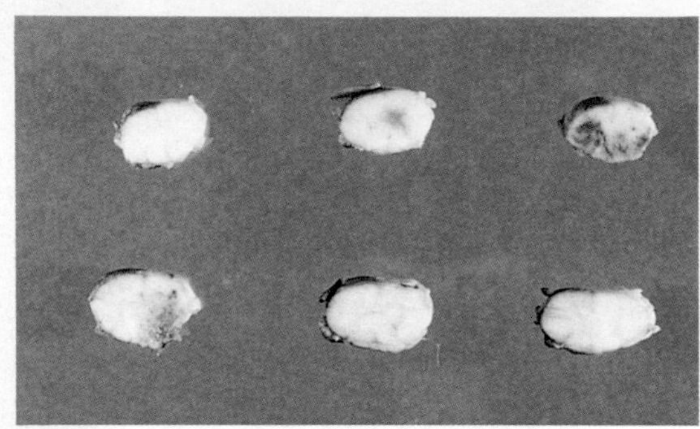

C

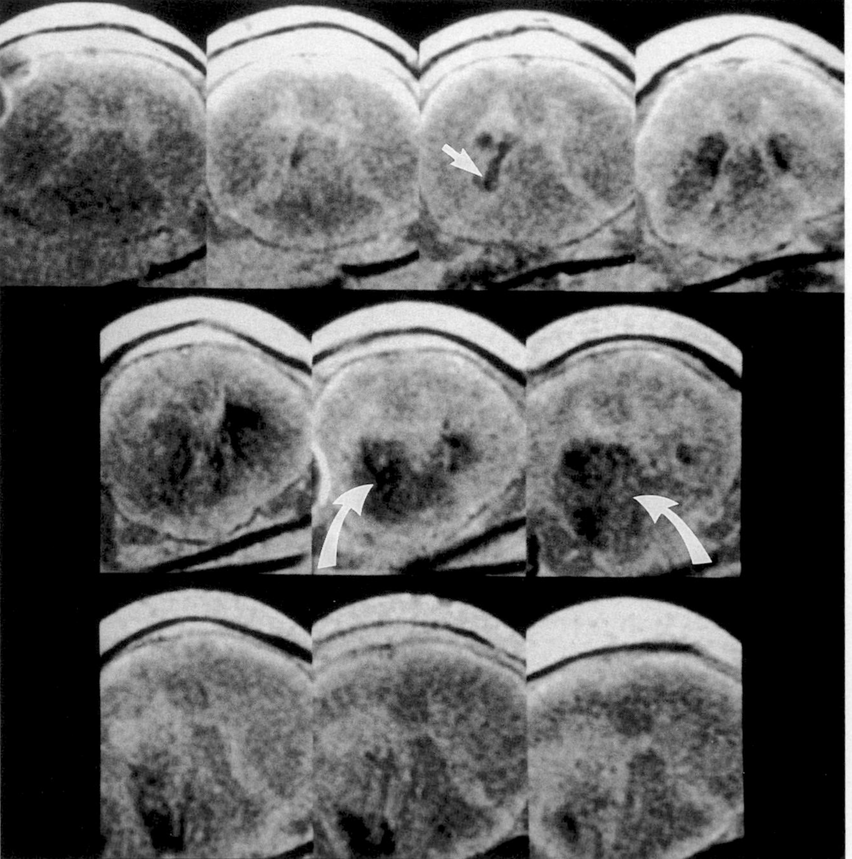

D

FIG. 32. Methemoglobin in a 9-day-old spinal cord injury. **A:** Sagittal SE T1-weighted image (500/20/4 NEX) demonstrates a markedly swollen spinal cord that effaces the surrounding subarachnoid space. There is associated herniation of disc material at C5-C6. The large hyperintense focus within the spinal cord at the level of injury is extracellular methemoglobin. **B:** Cervical spinal cord from another patient who sustained a C6 lesion 1 week before demise. Dorsal view of the cord reveals a hematoma (*arrow*). **C:** Cross-sections of the cord shown in B demonstrate extension of the contusion into the dorsal spinal white and gray. **D:** Serial axial T2-weighted SE images (3000/100/2 NEX) of specimen in B and C show well demarcated areas of hypointense hemorrhage involving the central gray matter (*arrow*) as well as the surrounding white matter (*curved arrows*).

unusual and that methemoglobin was the most prevalent species (7–9,39). The low overall incidence of detecting deoxyhemoglobin in these early reports was a technical limitation rather than a direct contradiction of known pathologic evidence. These variations most likely are due to the use of low static field strength magnets in prior studies (4,7,8,12,39).

The MRI identification of hemorrhage in the spinal cord following trauma has significant clinical implications. It was originally thought that detection of intramedullary hemorrhage was predictive of a complete injury. However, the increased sensitivity and spatial resolution of current MRI techniques has shown that small amounts of hemorrhage can be identified in incomplete lesions. Therefore, the basic construct has been altered such that the detection of a sizable focus of blood (>10 mm in length on sagittal images) in the cord usually is indicative of a complete neurologic injury at the anatomic location of the hemorrhage and it often implies that there is poor potential for neurologic recovery (7–9,73,119,128).

Spinal Cord Edema

Spinal cord edema is defined on MRI as a focus of abnormal high signal intensity on T2-weighted images within the substance of the cord (17). This signal abnormality presumably reflects a focal accumulation of intracellular and interstitial fluid in response to injury (3–5,7–10,12,17,39,70,76). Definition of this abnormality is usually optimal on the mid-sagittal long TR image (Figs. 5–7, 14, 15, 17–19, 25, 33). Axial T2-weighted images offer supplemental information in regard to involvement of structures in cross-section. Edema involves a variable length of spinal cord above and below the level of injury, with discrete boundaries adjacent to uninvolved parenchyma. Spinal cord edema on MRI is invariably associated with some degree of spinal cord swelling; however, it can occur without MRI evidence of intramedullary hemorrhage. Simple edema within the spinal cord in the setting of trauma has been referred to as a contusion by some investigators or as a hemorrhagic contusion when blood products are identified on MRI

A,B
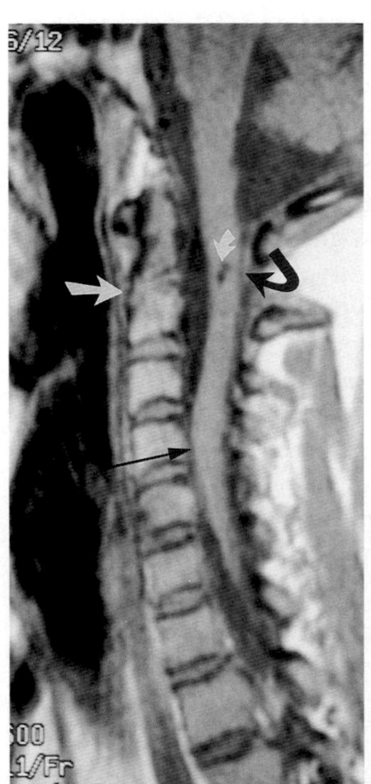
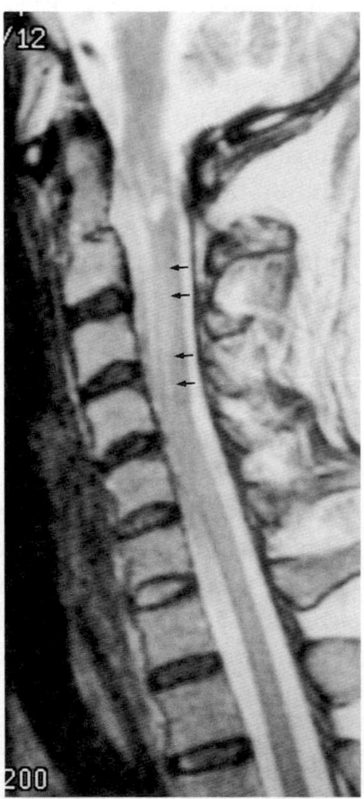
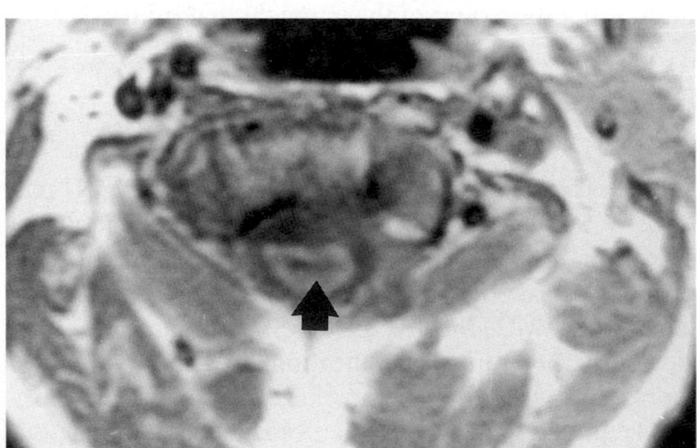
C

FIG. 33. Spinal cord tethering with adhesions and intramedullary cyst. **A:** Sagittal T1-weighted image (600/11/2 NEX) shows deformity of the C2 vertebral body at the base of the dens (*white arrow*) from prior fracture. A small intramedullary cyst is present at the C2 level (*curved white arrow*). The spinal cord is dorsally displaced at the C2 level and appears adherent to the posterior aspect of the spinal canal (*curved black arrow*). The spinal cord is displaced ventrally at the C4 level and is adherent to the ventral aspect of the spinal canal (*long black arrow*). **B:** Sagittal FSE T2-weighted image (2200/102Ef/2 NEX, 8 ETL) demonstrates that the intramedullary cyst appears larger in size compared to the T1-weighted image because of peripheral gliosis around the cyst. There is a vague area of increased signal intensity noted along the anterior aspect of the cord (*arrows*) secondary to changes of myelomalacia. **C:** Axial T1-weighted image (500/13/2 NEX) at the C2 level shows the hypointense central intramedullary cyst (*arrow*).

(18,70,76,128). The length of spinal cord affected by edema is directly proportional to the degree of initial neurologic deficit (8,70). Cord edema alone signifies a more favorable prognosis than cord hemorrhage (9,75, 119,128).

Spinal Cord Swelling

Spinal cord swelling is the most nondescriptive imaging finding associated with SCI. It is defined as a focal increase in caliber of the spinal cord centered at the level of an injury. By itself, swelling does not specifically describe any signal changes in the spinal cord. Spinal cord swelling is best demonstrated on the T1-weighted sagittal images (8,9,18,70); the parenchyma may be normal to slightly hypointense (8,70). Unfortunately, the T1-weighted images do not usually show the other elements of SCI.

The spinal cord is normally relatively uniform in caliber, although it increases slightly in diameter at the lower cervical and lower thoracic areas. This normal enlargement may be difficult to discern on MR images. The change in caliber of the injured spinal cord is usually maximal at the level of trauma and tapers gradually cranially and caudally from the epicenter of the injury (Figs. 5, 20, 25, 30, 31). In some instances, the swelling abruptly begins at the level of impact and progresses cranially only. Spinal cord swelling may be difficult to appreciate at a level of acute compression or when superimposed spinal canal stenosis is present. In this instance, the surrounding subarachnoid space is completely effaced, obscuring the upper and lower borders of the swelling. Although identification of spinal cord swelling alone is an indicator of spinal cord dysfunction, it does not predict the extent of the parenchymal injury (8,73).

MRI Correlates of SCI

Several investigators have reported that the MRI patterns of SCI correlate with the neurologic deficit at presentation (7–9,70,73,75,128). Kulkarni et al. initially proposed three MRI injury patterns for SCI and correlated these with the five-part ASIA impairment scale [formerly the Frankel classification (54)] and total motor scores. Intramedullary hemorrhage (Type I pattern of injury) equated with a severe neurologic deficit and a poor prognosis. Cord edema alone (Type II pattern of injury) was found in patients with mild to moderate initial neurologic deficits who subsequently improved (7,9,75,128).

Schaefer et al. refined the MRI patterns of SCI by including the size of the injured segment (70). Cord edema that extended for more than the span of one vertebral segment was associated with a more severe initial deficit than smaller areas of edema. Cord hemorrhage was associated with the most severe neurologic abnormalities (70).

Flanders et al. (8) demonstrated that spinal cord hemorrhage in the cervical region was a strong predictive finding for a complete neurologic injury. The location of the hemorrhage corresponded anatomically to the level of neurologic injury. Although the location of spinal cord edema related imprecisely to the neurologic level, the proportion of spinal cord affected by edema was directly related to the severity of initial neurologic injury. The presence of vertebral body fractures, disc herniation, and ligamentous injury was not predictive of the neurologic deficit; however, the presence of residual spinal cord compression by bone, disc, or fluid was predictive of a hemorrhagic spinal cord lesion located at the level of the compression. This last finding supports the controversial concept of early decompressive surgery for SCI patients (8,12,72).

The imaging changes observed in the spinal cord parenchyma with MRI show a close correlation with the initial neurologic deficit. Furthermore, substantial evidence suggests that these changes also portend prognostic factors in terms of potential for neurologic recovery (7,9,46,73,75,119,122,128,130,131). Yamashita et al. (130,131) showed that poor recovery from SCI was associated with severe cord compression, cord swelling, and abnormal signal on T1-weighted and T2-weighted images. Moreover, patients with persistent signal changes in the spinal cord on follow-up MRI examinations demonstrated little or no clinical improvement whereas prognosis was improved for patients who demonstrated resolution of signal abnormalities (130,131). Signal patterns that correlate with the best prognosis include normal spinal cord signal or hyperintensity on T2-weighted images (intramedullary edema). Hypo- or hyperintensity on T1-weighted images with hyperintense parenchyma on T2-weighted images is a poor prognostic indicator (73,130,131).

Silberstein et al. found that the presence of associated spinal fractures, subluxation, ligamentous injury, prevertebral swelling, and epidural hematoma was associated with a more severe clinical deficit at presentation and a poorer prognosis. All these associated imaging features suggested that residual spinal cord compression may be an important factor in determining poor neurologic recovery (73).

Schaefer et al. correlated the MRI appearance of the spinal cord on admission to the change in total motor index score (MIS) in 57 patients. Patients with hemorrhagic spinal cord lesions showed no statistical improvement in motor index score at follow-up. The group of patients with small areas of edema (less than one vertebral segment in length) demonstrated the largest improvement in MIS (72% recovery), whereas larger areas of edema showed intermediate recovery of MIS (42%) (121).

In a similar study, Marciello et al. compared the presence or absence of intramedullary hemorrhage to change in individual motor scores for the upper and lower extremities in 24 subjects. For patients with spinal cord hemorrhage, only 16% of muscles in the upper extremities and 3% of muscles in the lower extremities improved to a useful grade ($>\frac{3}{5}$) at follow-up and only 7% improved one or more motor levels. For patients without MRI evidence of spinal cord hemorrhage, 73% of upper extremity and 74% of lower extremity muscles improved to useful grade and 78% of subjects improved one or more motor levels (119).

Chronic Changes of SCI

Many clinical factors have to be considered in making a determination regarding neurologic recovery following SCI. The most significant of these are the degree of initial deficit (motor complete or incomplete) and the neurologic level. The most severe injuries usually demonstrate the least clinical improvement. The age of the patient is also an important determining factor, since most elderly tetraplegic patients are dead within 1 year after injury. Unfortunately, a segment of patients who improve after their initial injury will succumb to progression of neurologic symptoms many years after injury (122).

Post-traumatic progressive myelopathy (PTPM) describes a clinical syndrome in which spontaneous deterioration of the neurologic status of an SCI patient occurs after a long period of clinical stability (132). The most frequent clinical findings are increasing myelopathy and ascending neurologic level (122). This deterioration can be physically catastrophic for the patient with marginally useful function. The common imaging correlates described in association with PTPM include spinal cord atrophy, syringomyelia, residual/recurrent spinal cord compression, myelomalacia, and tethering/subarachnoid adhesions of the spinal cord (16,122,131–134). All of these entities encompass a continuum of repair processes of the spinal cord that may continue for several years after injury. The most severe SCI (tetraplegia) have twice the risk of developing syringomyelia as compared to motor-incomplete injuries (135). It is important to recognize these potential sequelae because they are not infrequent after SCI and because at least one condition (syringomyelia) is potentially treatable.

Myelomalacia/cord atrophy is an endstage of cord trauma that features loss of neurons, microcyst formation, and gliosis at the level of injury. It is the result of the concussive effects of trauma, ischemia, and the release of vasoactive substances and cellular enzymes (132). There is sufficient pathologic evidence that spinal cord myelomalacia progresses for several years after injury, in parallel with a progressive loss of neurons. Myelomalacia has been reported to produce symptoms as early as 2 months and as late as 25 years after injury (135). Cystic myelomalacia may be a precursor of syringomyelia (135).

On MRI, myelomalacia can be distinguished from a syrinx. Although both entities produce hyperintensity in the cord parenchyma on T2-weighted images, a syrinx cavity is isointense to cerebrospinal fluid on T1-weighted images, well-defined, and associated with cord enlargement (136,137). In contradistinction, myelomalacia is poorly demonstrated on T1-weighted images, is poorly marginated, and is associated with spinal cord atrophy (Figs. 25, 27, 33, 34) (49,136,137). Myelomalacia and syringomyelia are not unrelated. The microcysts that develop in myelomalacia may ultimately coalesce into a true spinal cord cyst (132). There is a strong causal relationship between persistent/recurrent spinal cord compression and cystic myelomalacia (122,138). The mechanism by which spinal cord compression produces myelomalacia and cyst formation is poorly understood, but the histologic changes of long tract demyelination, gliosis, cyst formation, and necrosis may be explained by secondary vascular insufficiency initiated by ongoing compression and edema (138).

The incidence of syringomyelia following SCI was previously estimated to be 0.9% to 2% (132). More recent studies that incorporate MRI into the diagnostic evaluation suggest that the incidence is much higher (47–59%) in patients presenting with new symptoms (122,135, 139). The most frequent symptoms reported at the time of diagnosis are pain, numbness, increased motor deficit, increased spasticity, hyperhidrosis, and autonomic dysreflexia (15,79,114). The most common signs found on clinical examination include ascent of the previous sensory level, depressed tendon reflexes, and increased motor deficits (79).

The pathogenesis of syringomyelia is not completely understood, although many investigators feel that the process begins shortly after the initial injury (73). Microcysts develop within the spinal cord parenchyma during the period of hemorrhagic necrosis. These cysts eventually coalesce into a common cavity. Cysts that are 5 mm in size or less are termed intramedullary cysts, while cysts larger than 5 mm are regarded as a true syrinxes (122). Progressive enlargement of the cavity may occur if there is direct transmission of CSF pulsation into the cavity via the central canal (16,135). Alternatively, subarachnoid adhesions may alter the CSF dynamics such that CSF is preferentially shunted into Virchow-Robin spaces, which provide a pathway for syrinx formation (16).

Before the advent of MRI, delayed contrast CT was the diagnostic method of choice for syringohydromyelia (132,136,137). Syrinx cavities are easy to identify on MRI. They are well marginated lesions within the cord parenchyma that are isointense to CSF on all pulse sequences (Figs. 11 and 28). Diminished pulsatility within the cyst cavity and the presence of protein may produce mild alterations in signal characteristics such that the

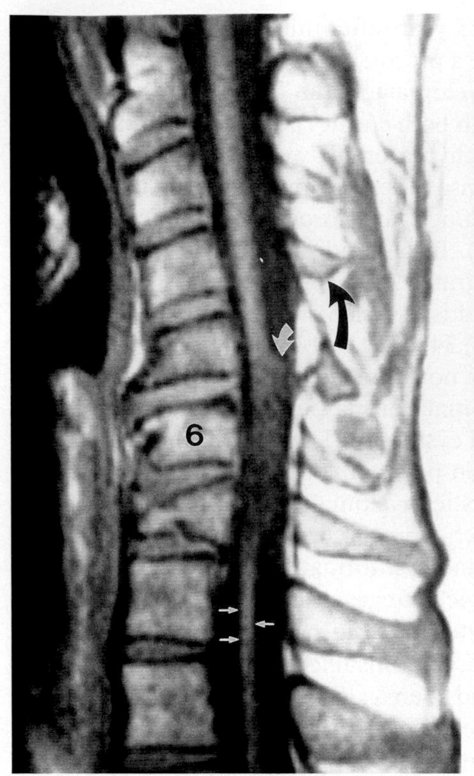

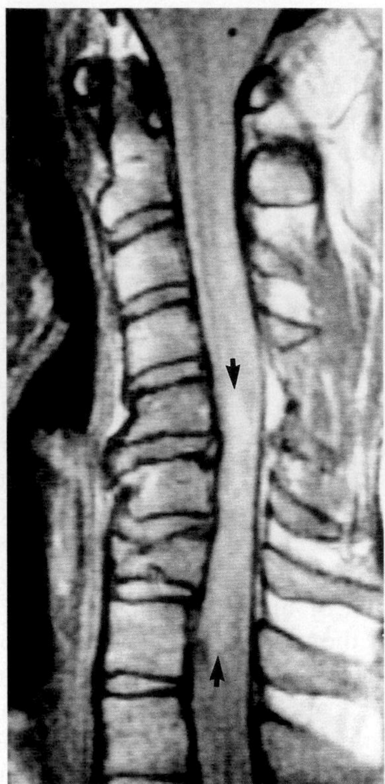

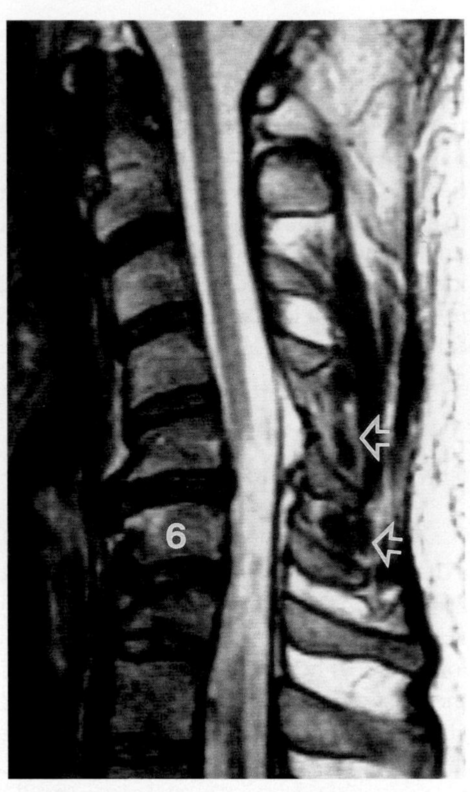

A,B C

FIG. 34. Progressive instability with cystic myelomalacia and atrophy 3 years postinjury. **A:** Sagittal T1-weighted image (500/11/2 NEX) shows an old fracture of the C7 vertebral body with loss of height anteriorly. There is loss of the normal cervical lordosis with flexion deformity centered at the C5-C6 interspace. There is splaying of the spinous processes between C4 and C5 secondary to disruption of the interspinous ligament complex (*curved black arrow*) and LF. There is partial dissolution of the cord parenchyma between the C5-6 interspace and C7 without evidence of a discrete cavity or rim of spared peripheral tissue. The distal spinal cord is markedly atrophic (*small white arrows*). The dorsal aspect of the injured cord segment appears adherent to the posterior theca (*curved white arrow*). **B:** Sagittal FSE intermediate-weighted image (2000/17Ef/2 NEX/ELT4) shows that the damaged segment (*arrows*) is hyperintense relative to CSF. **C:** Sagittal FSE T2-weighted image (2500/78Ef/4 NEX/ELT8). The damaged segment of spinal cord is isointense to CSF. There is no evidence of a peripheral rim of spared tissue as seen with syringomyelia. Note the hypointense areas within the interspinous ligament complexes between C4-C5 and C5-C6 secondary to scar tissue (*open arrows*).

syrinx is mildly hyperintense to CSF on all pulse sequences. Syrinx cavities vary considerably in size, ranging from less than 1 cm to the entire length of the spinal cord. When the cavity is large there is marked expansion of the cord with thinning of the residual parenchyma. Internal septations are often demonstrated. Syrinx cavities can enlarge progressively until they manifest clinically. The size threshold for syringomyelia to produce symptoms is variable. Large cavities may progress for years with few symptoms while small cavities may manifest profound neurologic changes (140). The average latency interval between injury and new neurologic symptoms is extremely variable, ranging from 3 months to 30 years (15,79,122,131,136). While the incidence of syringomyelia increases with severity of injury, there is a lack of relationship with the site of injury (135). At least one half of syringes extend nine or more vertebral segments in length (135).

Relief or reduction of symptoms is accomplished by surgical drainage and shunting of symptomatic cysts that are larger than 1 cm (79,139). There is evidence that MRI demonstration of a flow void or turbulence within a cyst cavity increases the likelihood that shunting may improve a patient's symptoms (140).

Several investigators have attempted to identify the initial MRI patterns of injury that predict chronic changes in the spinal cord parenchyma that ultimately lead to PTPM (122,131,138). Of the five imaging patterns described by Yamashita, lesions that were low in signal intensity on T1-weighted images and hyperintense on T2-weighted images predicted the worst prognosis (Fig. 35) whereas normal cords or simple cord edema showed the most improvement (131,138). Moreover, the severe SCI have a greater propensity to subsequently develop a syrinx (122,131,135,138).

Pediatric Injuries

The incidence and distribution of SCI in children differ from adults (20,21,141). Upper cervical spine in-

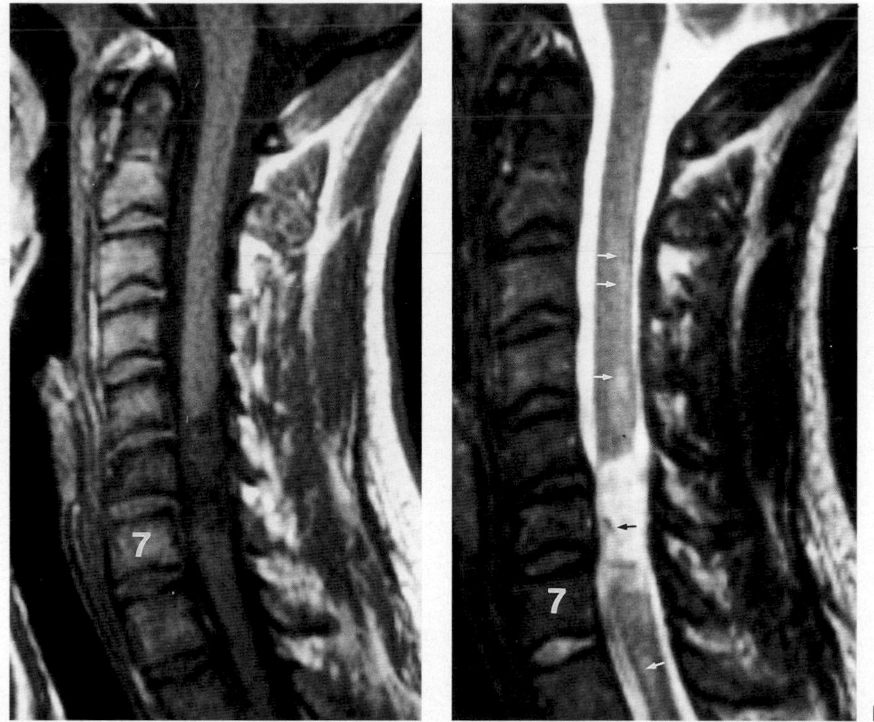

FIG. 35. Evolution of spinal cord injury 2 months after trauma. **A:** Sagittal T1-weighted image (500/11/2 NEX) shows a discrete focus of hypointense parenchyma, extending from C5-C6 to C7. Note the absence of subacute blood products. **B:** Sagittal FSE T2-weighted image (3000/102Ef/4 NEX, ETL 16) shows that most of the cord lesion reverts to hyperintensity; however, there is a small area ventrally that represents resolving hemorrhage (*black arrow*). This defines the area of necrosis. Foci of edema persist in the parenchyma above and below the injury (*white arrows*). Note that the borders around the lesion are extremely well defined at this stage as the cord undergoes repair. This injury pattern has been shown to correlate with a poor prognosis.

jury is more common in children because of anatomic differences, which include hypermobility due to ligamentous laxity, open ossification centers, horizontal orientation of the facets, underdeveloped neck musculature, and an increased cranial-thoracic ratio (20). These biomechanical differences help to explain the occurrence of SCIWORA in children (20,21,22,141,142). Although no abnormality is detectable on plain radiographs, SCI in these children is well demonstrated on MRI (20,22,141). SCIWORA accounts for 4% to 67% of all pediatric SCI (141). The pathophysiologic mechanism of SCIWORA in children may be related to cord stretching rather than cord compression. Biomechanical studies on neonatal spines have shown that the spinal column can be stretched up to 5 cm without loss of structural integrity, whereas the spinal cord can only tolerate approximately 6.25 mm of elongation before rupture (142). In addition, a rare but well described complication following breech or difficult cephalic deliveries is spinal cord transection (143,144) (Figs. 36 and 37). Other conditions that may predispose a child to SCI include Chiari malformation, achondroplasia, congenital cervical stenosis, Down or Klippel-Feil syndrome, basilar invagination, spondyloepiphyseal dysplasia, Morquio syndrome, and Conradi syndrome (20).

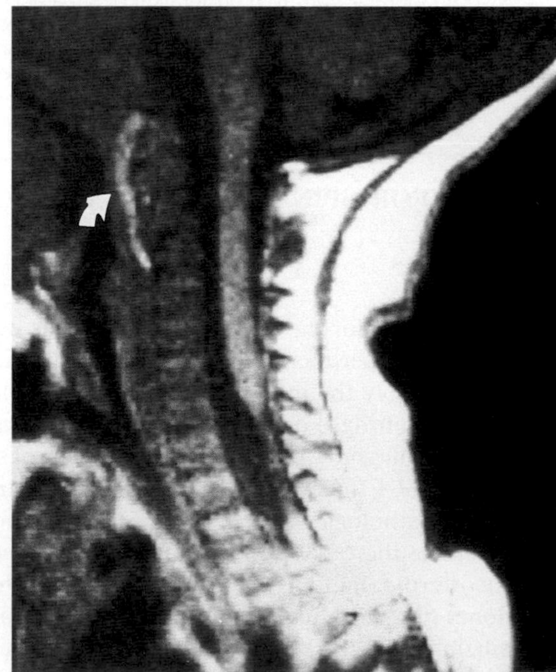

FIG. 36. Cervicothoracic spinal cord "near transection" injury following breech delivery. Sagittal T1-weighted image. Note marked focal thinning of spinal cord at cervicothoracic junction and posterior tethering of cord (*arrow*).

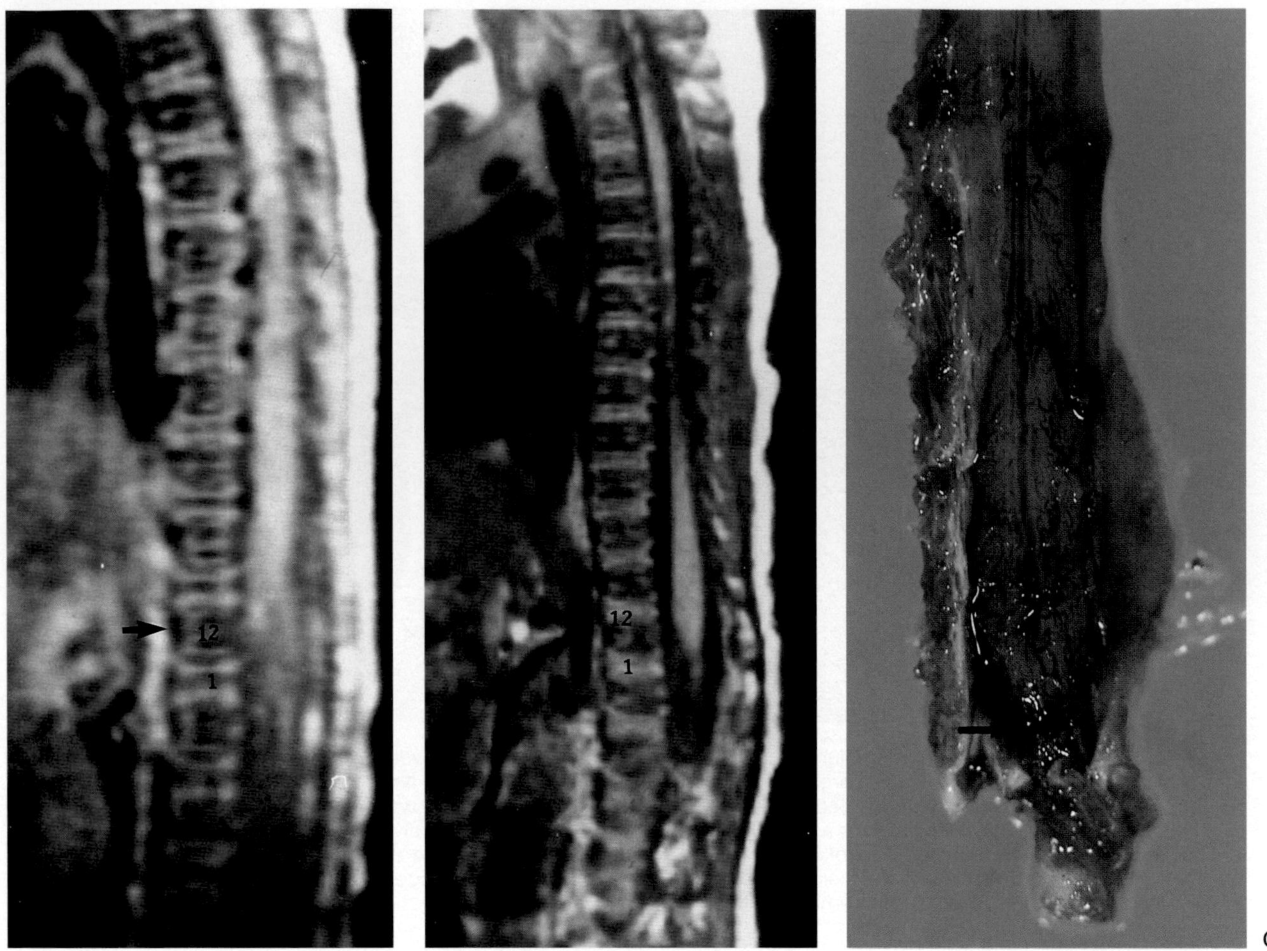

FIG. 37. Conus and cauda equina avulsion 1 month after breech delivery. **A:** Sagittal T1-weighted MRI scan shows swollen thoracic cord with obliteration of subarachnoid space and indistinct, irregular termination at T12 (*arrow*), as compared to expected normal appearance (B). **B:** Normal sagittal T1-weighted MRI in 1-month-old baby for comparison. **C:** Pathologic specimen from another child shows avulsion of tip of conus (*arrow*) and cauda equina. (Courtesy of Juan Sanches, M.D., University of Geneva, Switzerland.)

THERAPIES FOR SPINAL TRAUMA AND SCI

Medical Therapies

Pharmacotherapy for the acute stage of SCI has been investigated both experimentally and clinically. Corticosteroids are probably the most extensively studied class of drugs in this setting. For more than 20 years, many experimental studies have reported salutary effects of steroid therapy in SCI that include improved ambulation and decreased pathologic damage (98,145). In the more recent literature, there has been enthusiasm for megadose corticosteroid therapy (30–60 mg/kg of methylprednisolone) (91). Although doses in this range clearly have stabilizing effects on spinal blood flow, extracellular calcium, and lipid peroxidation, questions still remain as to whether the side effects from these high doses will outweigh potential clinical benefits. Other classes of drugs that have received experimental attention include opiate antagonists [most notably naloxone (146)], thyrotropin-releasing hormone (147), calcium channel blockers, antioxidants, and free radical scavengers. Following these experimental leads, the most convincing study to date remains the Second National Acute Spinal Cord Injury Study (NASCIS 2) (148–150). In this multicenter study, high doses of methylprednisolone (30 mg/kg bolus followed by 5.4 mg/kg per hr × 23 hr) were compared with naloxone and placebo in the acute phase following SCI. The most beneficial effects occurred in patients in whom methylprednisolone therapy was initiated within 8 hours of the trauma. A surprising result of that study was that the possibility for improved function extended to patients with both complete and incomplete lesions at the time of initiation of therapy.

Surgical Therapies

Surgical intervention has been aimed at both stabilization of the vertebral column and decompression of the spinal canal. MRI clearly plays an important role in surgical management by corroborating the status of alignment as shown on plain radiographs and in detecting any soft tissue causes of cord compression (6,69).

Surgical stabilization is directed toward restoration of structural integrity of the spine because osseous and ligamentous elements have been disrupted. One third of injuries treated with closed reduction alone will spontaneously misalign (86). Stabilization is accomplished primarily by fusion of the posterior elements using a combination of autologous bone and metallic devices. In the cervical spine, stainless steel wire is wrapped over the posterior elements above and below the injured segment. Titanium alloy wire has also been used successfully in this application, with the added benefit of diminished magnetic susceptibility artifacts on MRI imaging (33,151,152). In thoracic and lumbar stabilization, paired stainless steel rods are affixed to the posterior elements with wires over multiple levels. Paired metallic plates that lay over the posterior elements can be affixed with transpedicular screws.

A second procedure may need to be performed in conjunction with posterior fusion to stabilize the anterior elements (vertebral bodies). This may be necessary when there is severe loss of height of the anterior column or a disc herniation in the cervical or thoracic region (69). The stabilization procedure is often performed electively during the initial hospitalization.

The need for, and the timing of, decompressive surgery is more controversial (72,153–158). In the acute period following trauma, osseous fragments, disc fragments, foreign bodies, or blood may complicate the therapeutic picture by presenting as extra- or intradural compressive masses. Moreover, the literature suggests that residual compression of the injured spinal cord is a significant factor in predicting neurologic outcome. Therefore, early restitution of the integrity of the vertebral column both in terms of reducing any distraction and assuring stability are of key importance (6,8,15,72,73,139,154). Blood in the form of hematomyelia may be present within the cord. Although there are sporadic reports of improvement following myelotomy to drain cord hemorrhage, surgical attempts to relieve this mass effect in the acute period may prove counterproductive (139,156,159).

Although a patient may derive the most clinical benefit from early decompressive surgery, this is also the period in which the spinal cord may be most sensitive to further damage from surgical manipulation (160,161). Regardless, some centers advocate early decompressive surgery without myelotomy for acute SCI as a measure to preserve function or prevent deterioration, especially when there is residual compression of the spinal cord (156,159,162). Other centers pursue a more conservative approach and perform decompression several weeks after injury (163,164). At the Regional Spinal Cord Injury Center of the Delaware Valley, immediate decompression is felt to be most warranted in an incomplete injury that begins to deteriorate neurologically. Otherwise, early elective stabilization is performed. Stabilization procedures provide statistically better motor recoveries than conservative therapies (162–164).

Different surgical alternatives are available in the lumbar region because of the increased tolerance of the cauda equina to compressive injury compared to the spinal cord (16). Empirical evidence suggests that clinical benefit is derived from decompression of the lumbar spinal canal from bone fragments when there is more than a one-third reduction in diameter. Clinical trials that are currently in progress may provide a more definitive answer in this area.

Novel Therapies

While most drug therapies that have received experimental and clinical attention are directed toward limiting damage during the acute phase of SCI, a slightly different approach has been taken with pharmacotherapy in the more chronic phase. Several drugs have been in clinical use for some time that reduce spasticity, which interferes with rehabilitation of the patient. More recently, clinical and experimental investigations have drawn attention to groups of neurotransmitters and transmitter receptors (most notably of adrenergic and serotonergic subtypes) that are felt to play central roles in locomotor behavior. Drugs directed at these subtypes (such as clonidine, L-DOPA, yohimbine, quipizine, and cyproheptadine) can markedly alter the expression of locomotor behavior in experimental animals. Preliminary data in SCI patients suggest that clonidine and cyproheptadine are effective in decreasing spasticity and even improving locomotor function (165).

A more radical and novel therapy for SCI is embryonic spinal cord transplantation. In animal models, embryonic spinal transplants have been shown to survive and integrate with the host (Fig. 38) (166). These transplant models have allowed transected newborn rats and cats to develop impressive degrees of locomotor function (167–169). MRI studies of transplanted cats have been able to visualize the transplants. In vivo SE images reveal homogeneous, slightly hyperintense signal at the graft site in most cases and isointense or hypointense signal in a minority of cases. When compared with histopathology, hyperintense and isointense signals correlate with graft survival, whereas hypointense signal implies rejection (170). The degree to which transplant technology will succeed in restoring locomotor function to adult animals following SCI is an area of active research. Therapeutic trials in humans are not in progress at this time and probably await evaluation of more animal data. Nonetheless, it would appear that MRI will play a role in both the experimental and clinical settings for the evaluation of transplant anatomy and viability.

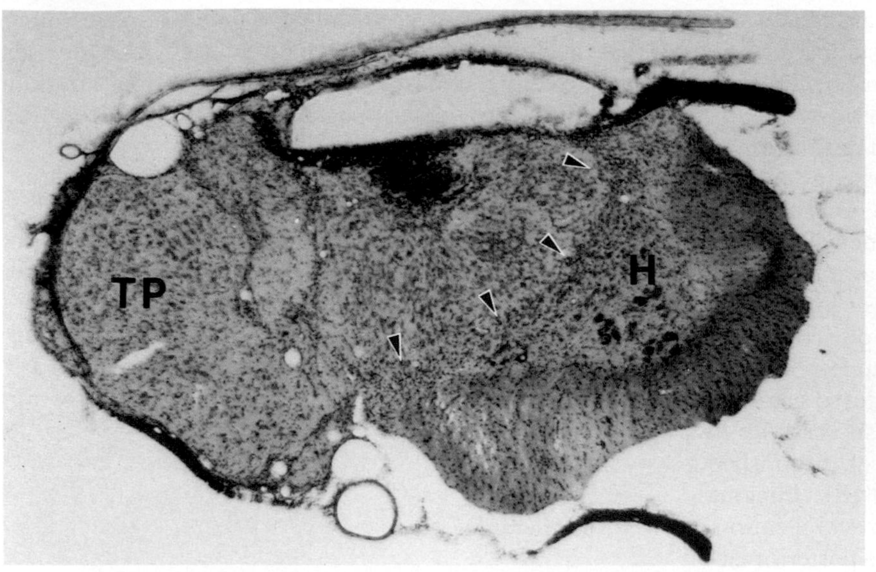

FIG. 38. Embryonic spinal cord transplant. In this cross-section of rat thoracic spinal cord, a surgical cavity on the left had been filled with a transplant of embryonic rat spinal cord. The specimen is taken several weeks following surgery. The transplanted tissue (marked *TP* and delineated by *arrowheads*) has clearly survived in the adult spinal cord environment. The remaining host spinal cord (marked *H*) shows survival of both gray and white matter (Cyanin R/Hematoxylin). (Material courtesy of A. Tessler, M.D., Medical College of Pennsylvania.)

Prognosis of SCI

Survival of SCI patients has dramatically changed in the last 50 years. During World War I, SCI was associated with an 80% mortality, whereas today, 94% of patients survive the initial hospitalization. When there is a sudden worsening of the neurologic deficit in the acute period, the most common etiology is vascular insufficiency to the spinal cord (161). This occurs in approximately 3% of patients (161). Approximately 95% of patients with SCI are able to return to the community and nearly one half of those patients who were employed before their injury are able to return to work (171). Although the average life expectancy for individuals with a SCI is less than the general population, it is gradually increasing. The 10-year survival rates are highest for those who were less than 30 years of age when injured. The survival rates decline substantially after age 30; less than 20% of those above the age of 70 years are alive 10 years after injury (171).

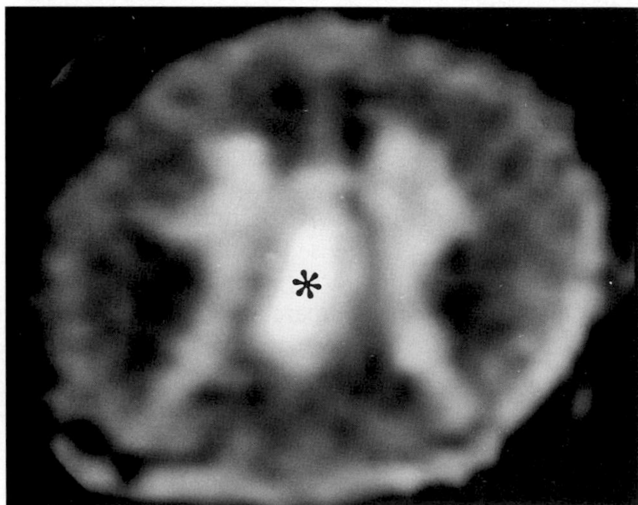

FIG. 39. Cervical spinal cord specimen with hemorrhage in the posterior columns. Axial T1-weighted image (500/20/4 NEX) shows a large focus of hemorrhage (*asterisk*) that involves the posterior columns bilaterally, with greater involvement on the right.

The cumulative survival during the first 12 years after SCI is more than 88% of that expected in absence of injury. Causes of death include septicemia, pulmonary embolism, and pneumonia (171).

The clinical impact of MRI in the evaluation of SCI is just being realized. Faster imaging times and higher spatial resolution may ultimately allow for routine evaluation of individual tracts of the spinal cord (Fig. 39). This may provide additional insight into spinal cord function and response to injury. As newer techniques are refined and become widely available, functional imaging and spinal cord spectroscopy (124) may become part of the routine diagnostic evaluation. As experimental therapies for SCI reach the stage of clinical trials, MRI may play a pivotal role in helping to select for a particular therapy as well as to monitor the therapeutic response.

ACKNOWLEDGMENTS. This work was supported by NIH/NINDS grants 5KO8 NS01564 and Ns24707 (SC) and (AF). We thank John F. Ditunno, Michelle Cohen, Gerald J. Herbison, David P. Friedman, Robert J. Rapoport, Marion Murray, and Alan Tessler for their continuing support and critical input and the Regional Spinal Cord Injury Center of the Delaware Valley for clinical support.

REFERENCES

1. Allen BL, Ferguson RL, Lehmann TR, O'Brien RP. A mechanistic classification of closed, indirect fractures and dislocations of the lower cervical spine. *Spine* 1982;7(1):1–27.
2. McArdle CB, Crofford MJ, Mirfakhraee M, Amparo EG, Cal-

houn JS. Surface coil MRI of spinal trauma: preliminary experience. *Am J Neuroradiol* 1986;7(5):885–893.

3. Weirich SD, Cotler HB, Narayana PA, et al. Histopathologic correlation of magnetic resonance imaging signal patterns in a spinal cord injury model. *Spine* 1990;15(7):630–638.
4. Wittenberg RH, Boetel U, Beyer HK. Magnetic resonance imaging and computed tomography of acute spinal cord trauma. *Clin Orthop* 1990;260:176–185.
5. Chakeres DW, Flickinger F, Bresnahan JC, et al. MRI imaging of acute spinal cord trauma. *Am J Neuroradiol* 1987;8(1):5–10.
6. Robertson PA, Ryan MD. Neurological deterioration after reduction of cervical subluxation; mechanical compression by disc tissue. *J Bone Joint Surg* [*Br*] 1992;74-B:224–227.
7. Bondurant FJ, Cotler HB, Kulkarni MV, McArdle CB, Harris JH. Acute spinal cord injury. A study using physical examination and magnetic resonance imaging. *Spine* 1990;15(3):161–168.
8. Flanders AE, Schaefer DM, Doan HT, Mishkin MM, Gonzalez CF, Northrup BE. Acute cervical spine trauma: correlation of MRI imaging findings with degree of neurologic deficit. *Radiology* 1990;177(1):25–33.
9. Kulkarni MV, McArdle CB, Kopanicky D, et al. Acute spinal cord injury: MRI imaging at 1.5T. *Radiology* 1987;164(3):837–843.
10. Mirvis SE, Geisler FH, Jelinek JJ, Joslyn JN, Gellad F. Acute cervical spine trauma: evaluation with 1.5-T MRI imaging. *Radiology* 1988;166(3):807–816.
11. Tracy PT, Wright RM, Hanigan WC. Magnetic resonance imaging of spinal injury. *Spine* 1989;14(3):292–301.
12. Beers GJ, Raque GH, Wagner GG, et al. MRI imaging in acute cervical spine trauma. *J Comput Assist Tomogr* 1988;12(5):755–761.
13. Goldberg AL, Daffner RH, Schapiro RL. Imaging of acute spinal trauma: an evolving multi-modality approach. *Clin Imag* 1990;14(1):11–16.
14. Flanders AE, Tartaglino LM, Friedman DP, Aquilone L. Magnetic resonance imaging in acute spinal injury. *Semin Roentgenol* 1992;27(4):271–298.
15. Sett P, Crockard HA. The value of magnetic resonance imaging (MRI) in the follow-up management of spinal injury. *Paraplegia* 1991;29(6):396–410.
16. Kerslake RW, Jaspan T, Worthington BS. Magnetic resonance imaging of spinal trauma. *Br J Radiol* 1991;64:386–402.
17. Goldberg AL, Rothfus WE, Deeb ZL, et al. The impact of magnetic resonance on the diagnostic evaluation of acute cervicothoracic spinal trauma. *Skeletal Radiol* 1988;17(2):89–95.
18. Kalfas I, Wilberger J, Goldberg A, Prostko ER. Magnetic resonance imaging in acute spinal cord trauma. *Neurosurgery* 1988;23(3):295–299.
19. Larsson EM, Holtas S, Cronqvist S. Emergency magnetic resonance examination of patients with spinal cord symptoms. *Acta Radiol* 1988;29(1):69–75.
20. Riviello JJ, Marks HG, Faerber EN, Steg NL. Delayed cervical central cord syndrome after trivial trauma. *Pediatr Emerg Care* 1990;6(2):113–117.
21. Pang D, Wilberger JE. Spinal cord injury without radiographic abnormalities in children. *J Neurosurg* 1982;57:114–129.
22. Mendelsohn DB, Zollars L, Weatherall PT, Girson M. MRI of cord transection. *J Comput Assist Tomogr* 1990;14(6):909–911.
23. Goldberg AL, Rothfus WE, Deeb ZL, Frankel DG, Wilberger JE, Daffner RH. Hyperextension injuries of the cervical spine. Magnetic resonance findings. *Skeletal Radiol* 1989;18(4):283–288.
24. Harris JH, Edeiken-Monroe B. *The Radiology of Acute Cervical Spine Trauma*. 2nd ed. Baltimore: Williams & Wilkins; 1987.
25. Rogers LF ed. *Radiology of Skeletal Trauma*. 2nd ed. New York: Churchill Livingstone; 1992.
26. Mirvis SE, Young JW, eds. *Imaging in Trauma and Critical Care*. Baltimore: Williams & Wilkins; 1992.
27. Pope AM, Tarlov AR. *Disability in America: Toward a National Agenda for Prevention*. Washington, DC: National Academy Press; 1991.
28. Mani RL. Potential hazard of metal-filled sandbags in MRI imaging. *Radiology* 1992;182:286–287.
29. Brunberg JA, Papadopoulos SM. Technical note. Device to facilitate MRI imaging of patients in skeletal traction. *Am J Neuroradiol* 1991;12(4):746–747.
30. Ballock RT, Hajed PC, Byrne TP, et al. The quality of magnetic resonance imaging, as affected by the composition of the halo orthosis. *J Bone Joint Surg* [*Am*] 1989;71:431–434.
31. Shellock FG, Slimp G. Halo vest for cervical spine fixation during MRI imaging. *Am J Radiol* 1990;154:631–632.
32. Shellock FG, Morisoli S, Kanal E. MRI procedures and biomedical implants, materials, and devices: 1993 update. *Radiology* 1993;189:587–599.
33. Teitelbaum GP, Yee CA, Van Horn DD, et al. Metallic ballistic fragments: MRI imaging safety and artifacts. *Radiology* 1990;175:855–859.
34. Tartaglino LM, Flanders AE, Vinitski S, Friedman DP. Metallic artifacts on MRI images of the postoperative spine: reduction with fast spin-echo techniques. *Radiology* 1994;190:565–569.
35. Jones KM, Mulkern RV, Schwartz RB, Oshio K, Barnes PD, Jolesz FA. Fast spin-echo MRI imaging of the brain and spine: current concepts. *Am J Radiol* 1992;158:1313–1320.
36. Flanders AE, Tartaglino LM, Friedman DP, Vinitski S. Application of fast spin-echo MRI imaging in acute cervical spine injury. *Radiology* 1992;185(P):220.
37. Yousem DM, Atlas SW, Goldberg HI, Grossman RI. Degenerative narrowing of the cervical spine neural foramina: evaluation with high-resolution 3DFT gradient-echo MRI imaging. *Am J Neuroradiol* 1991;12(2):229–236.
38. Perovitch M, Perl S, Wang H. Current advances in magnetic resonance imaging (MRI) in spinal cord trauma: review article. *Paraplegia* 1992;30:305–316.
39. Schouman-Claeys E, Frija G, Cuenod CA, Begon D, Paraire F, Martin V. MRI imaging of acute spinal cord injury: results of an experimental study in dogs. *Am J Neuroradiol* 1990;11(5):959–965.
40. DiTunno J, ed. *Standards for Neurological and Functional Classification of Spinal Cord Injury*. 4th ed. Chicago: American Spinal Injury Association; 1992.
41. Spiller, WG. Thrombosis of the cervical anterior median spinal artery: syphilitic acute anterior poliomyelitis. *J Nerv Ment Dis* 1909;36:601–613.
42. Austin G, Rouhe S, Horn N. Vascular diseases of the spinal cord. In: Austin G, ed. *The Spinal Cord*. Springfield, IL: Charles C Thomas; 1972:455–469.
43. Hughes J, Brownell B. Cervical spondylosis complicated by anterior spinal artery thrombosis. *Neurology* 1964;14:1073.
44. Hughes J, Brownell B. Spinal cord ischemia due to arteriosclerosis. *Arch Neurol* 1966;15:189–202.
45. Schneider RC, Cherry GL, Pantek HE. The syndrome of acute central cervical spinal cord injury. *J Neurosurg* 1954;11:546–577.
46. Schneider, RC, Thompson JM, Bebin J. The syndrome of the acute central cervical spinal cord injury. *J Neurol Neurosurg Psychiatry* 1958;21:216–227.
47. Rand RW, Crandall P. Central cord syndrome in hyperextension injuries of the cervical cord. *J Bone Joint Surg* 1962;44:1415–1422.
48. Taylor AR. The mechanism of injury to the spinal cord in the neck without damage to the vertebral column. *J Bone Joint Surg* [*Br*] 1951;33:543–547.
49. Quencer RM, Bunge RP, Egnor M, et al. Acute central cord syndrome: MRI-pathological correlations. *Neuroradiology* 1992;34:85–94.
50. Austin, G. *The Spinal Cord: Basic Aspects and Surgical Considerations*. Springfield, IL: Charles C Thomas; 1961.
51. St. John JR, Rand CW. Stab wounds of the spinal cord. *Bull Los Angeles Neurol Soc* 1953;18:1–24.
52. Haymaker W. *Bing's Local Diagnosis in Neurological Diseases*. 15th ed. St. Louis: CV Mosby; 1969.
53. Hartwell JB. An analysis of 133 fractures of the spine treated at the Massachusetts General Hospital. *Boston Med Surg J* 1917;177:31–41.
54. Frankel HL, Hancock DO, Hyslop G. The value of postural reduction in the initial management of closed injuries of the spine with paraplegia and tetraplegia. *Paraplegia* 1969;7:179–192.
55. Tator CH, Rowed DW, Schwartz ML, eds. *Sunnybrook Cord Injury Scales for Assessing Neurological Injury and Neurological Recovery in Early Management of Acute Spinal Cord Injury*. New York: Raven Press; 1982.
56. Ditunno JF. Functional assessment measures in CNS trauma. *J Neurotrauma* 1992;9:S301–S305.

57. Hamilton BB, Fuhre MJ, eds. *Rehabilitation Outcomes: Analysis and Measurement*. Baltimore: Brooks; 1987:137–147.
58. Hamilton BB, Laughlin JA, Fiedler RC, Granger CV. Interrater reliability of the seven level functional independence measure (FIM). *Scand J Rehab Med* 1994;26:115–119.
59. Nussbaum ES, Sebring LA, Wolf AL, Mirvis SE, Gottlieb R. Myelographic and enhanced computed tomographic appearance of acute traumatic spinal cord avulsion. *Neurosurgery* 1992;30:43–48.
60. Volle E, Assheuer J, Hedde JP, Gustorf-Aeckerle R. Radicular avulsion resulting from spinal injury: assessment of diagnostic modalities. *Neuroradiology* 1992;34:235–240.
61. Wagner A, Albeck MJ, Madsen FF. Diagnostic imaging in fracture of lumbar vertebral ring apophyses. *Acta Radiol* 1992;33:72–75.
62. Levitt MA, Flanders AE. Diagnostic capabilities of magnetic resonance imaging and computed tomography in acute cervical spinal column injury. *Am J Emerg Med* 1991;9(2):131–135.
63. Tarr RW, Drolshagen LF, Kerner TC, Allen JH, Partain CL, James AE. MRI imaging of recent spinal trauma. *J Comput Assist Tomogr* 1987;11(3):412–417.
64. Baker LL, Goodman SB, Perkash I, Lane B, Enzmann DR. Benign versus pathologic compression fractures of vertebral bodies: assessment with conventional spin-echo, chemical shift, and STIR MRI imaging. *Radiology* 1990;174:495–502.
65. Davis SJ, Teresi LM, Bradley WG, Ziemba MA, Bloze AE. Cervical spine hyperextension injuries: MRI findings. *Radiology* 1991;180(1):245–251.
66. Gardner E, Gray DJ. The back. In: Gardner E, Gray DJ, O'Rahilly Ronan, eds. *Anatomy*. 4th ed. Philadelphia: WB Saunders; 1975;508–540.
67. Edeiken-Monroe B, Wagner LK, Harris JH. Hyperextension dislocation of the cervical spine. *Am J Radiol* 1986;146:803–808.
68. Regenbogen VS, Rogers LF, Atlas SW, Kim KS. Cervical spinal cord injuries in patients with cervical spondylosis. *Am J Radiol* 1986;146:277–284.
69. Pratt ES, Green DA, Spengler DM. Herniated intervertebral discs associated with unstable spinal injuries. *Spine* 1990;15(7):662–666.
70. Schaefer DM, Flanders A, Northrup BE, Doan HT, Osterholm JL. Magnetic resonance imaging of acute cervical spine trauma: correlation with severity of neurologic injury. *Spine* 1989;14(10): 1090–1095.
71. Rizzolo SJ, Piazza MRI, Cotler JM, Balderston RA, Schaefer DM, Flanders AE. Intervertebral disc injury complicating cervical spine trauma. *Spine* 1991;16(6):187–189.
72. Harrington JF, Likavec MJ, Smith AS. Disc herniation in cervical fracture subluxation. *Neurosurgery* 1991;29:374–379.
73. Silberstein M, Tress BM, Hennessy O. Prediction of neurologic outcome in acute spinal cord injury: the role of CT and MRI. *Am J Neuroradiol* 1992;13:1597–1608.
74. El-Khoury GY, Whitten CG. Trauma to the upper thoracic spine: anatomy, biomechanics, and unique imaging features. *Am J Radiol* 1993;160:95–102.
75. Kulkarni MV, Bondurant FJ, Rose SL, Narayana PA. 1.5 tesla magnetic resonance imaging of acute spinal trauma. *Radiographics* 1988;8(6):1059–1082.
76. Hackney DB, Asato LR, Joseph P, et al. Hemorrhage and edema in acute spinal cord compression: demonstration by MRI imaging. *Radiology* 1986;161:387–390.
77. Greiner FG, Orrison WW, King JN, et al. Vertebral artery injury association with cervical spine fractures. *Proceedings of the 29th Annual Meeting of the American Society of Neuroradiology*. Washington, DC; 1991:171.
78. Friedman DP, Flanders AE. Unusual dissection of the proximal vertebral artery: description of three cases. *Am J Neuroradiol* 1992;13:283–286.
78a. Friedman DP, Flanders AE, Thomas C, Millar W. Vertebral artery injury after acute cervical spine trauma: rate of occurrence as detected by MR angiography and assessment of clinical consequences. *AJR* 1995;164:443–447.
79. Greenberg MS. *Handbook of Neurosurgery*. 3rd ed. Lakeland, Fl: Greenberg Graphics; 1994.
80. Matsura P, Waters RL, Adkins RH, Rothman S, Gurbani N, Sie I. Comparison of computerized tomography parameters of the cervical spine in normal control subjects and spinal cord-injured patients. *J Bone Joint Surg* 1989;71(2):183–188.
81. Atlas SW, Regenbogen V, Rogers LF, Kwang SK. The radiographic characterization of burst fractures of the spine. *Am J Radiol* 1986;147:572–582.
82. Holdsworth F. Fractures, dislocations and fracture-dislocations of the spine. *J Bone Joint Surg [Am]* 1970;52A:1534–1551.
83. Denis F. The three column spine and its significance in the classification of acute thoracolumbar spinal injuries. *Spine* 1983;8: 817–831.
84. White AA III, Panjabi MM. *Clinical Biomechanics of the Spine*. Philadelphia: JB Lippincott; 1978.
85. McAfee PC, Yuan HA, Fredrickson BE, Lubicky JP. The value of computed tomography in thoracolumbar fractures. *J Bone Joint Surg [Am]* 1983;65:461–473.
86. Dorr L, Harvey J, Nickel V. Clinical review of the early stability of spine injuries. *Spine* 1982;7(6):545–550.
87. Meyer PR. Fractures of the thoracic spine: T1 to T10. In: Meyer PR, ed. *Surgery of Spine Trauma*. New York: Churchill Livingstone; 1989:525–571.
88. Senter HJ, Venes JL. Altered blood flow and secondary injury in experimental spinal cord trauma. *J Neurosurg* 1978;49:569–578.
89. Tator CH, Fehlindgs MJ. Review of the secondary injury theory of acute spinal cord trauma with emphasis on vascular mechanisms. *J Neurosurg* 1991;75:15–26.
90. Kwo S, Young W, DeCrescito V. Spinal cord sodium, potassium, calcium and water concentration changes in rats after graded contusion injury. *J Neurotrauma* 1989;6:13–24.
91. Young W, Flamm ES. Effect of high dose corticosteroid therapy on blood flow, evoked potentials and extracellular calcium in experimental spinal cord injury. *J Neurosurg* 1982;57:667–673.
92. Hall ED, Yonkers PA, Horan KL, Braughler JM. Correlation between attenuation of posttraumatic spinal cord ischemia and preservation of tissue vitamin E by the 21-aminosteroid U74006F. *J Neurotrauma* 1989;6:169–176.
93. Pietronigro DD, Housepian M, Demopoulos HB, Flamm ES. Loss of ascorbic acid from injured feline spinal cord. *J Neurochem* 1983;41:1072–1076.
94. Saunders RD, Dugan LL, Demediuk P, Means ED, Horrocks LA, Anderson DK. Effects of methylprednisolone and the combination of alpha tocopherol and selenium on arachidonic acid metabolism and lipid peroxidation in traumatized spinal cord tissue. *J Neurochem* 1987;49:24–31.
95. Hsu CY, Halushka PV, Spicer KM, Hogan EL, Martin HF. Temporal profile of thromboxane-prostacyclin imbalance in experimental spinal cord injury. *J Neurol Sci* 1988;83:55–62.
96. Hall ED, Braughler JM. Central nervous system trauma and stroke. II. Physiological and pharmacological evidence for involvement of oxygen radicals and lipid peroxidation. *Free Radical Biol Med* 1989;6:303–313.
97. Meldrum B. Possible therapeutic applications of antagonists of excitatory amino acid neurotransmitters. *Clin Sci* 1985;68:113–122.
98. Ducker TB, Hamit HF. Experimental treatments of acute spinal cord injury. *J Neurosurg* 1966;30:693–700.
99. Dohrmann GJ, Wagner FC, Bucy PC. The microvasculature in transitory traumatic paraplegia. *J Neurosurg* 1971;35:263–271.
100. Dohrmann GJ, Wagner FC, Bucy PC. Transitory traumatic paraplegia: electron microscopy of early alterations in myelinated nerve fibers. *J Neurosurg* 1972;36:407–415.
101. Dohrmann GJ, Wick KM, Bucy PC. Spinal cord blood flow patterns in experimental traumatic paraplegia. *J Neurosurg* 1973;38: 52–58.
102. Rivlin AS, Tator CH. Regional spinal cord blood flow in rats after severe cord trauma. *J Neurosurg* 1978;49:844–853.
103. Assenmacher DR, Ducker TB. Experimental traumatic paraplegia: the vascular and pathological changes seen in reversible and irreversible spinal cord lesions. *J Bone Joint Surg* 1971;53:671–680.
104. Yashon D, Bingham WG, Faddoul EM. Edema of the spinal cord following experimental impact trauma. *J Neurosurg* 1973;38: 693–697.
105. Blight AR. Remyelination, revascularization and recovery of

function in experimental spinal cord injury. *Adv Neurol* 1993;59: 91–104.

106. Young W. Blood flow, metabolic and neurophysiological mechanisms in spinal cord injury. In: Beckerand D, Poulishock J, eds. *NIH Central Nervous System Status Report*. Bethesda: NINDS-NIH; 1985:463–473.
107. Noble L, Wrathall J. Spinal cord contusion in the rat: morphometric analysis of alterations in the spinal cord. *Exp Neurol* 1985;88:135–149.
108. Blight AR, De Crescito V. Morphometric analysis of experimental spinal cord injury in the cat: the relation of injury intensity to survival of myelinated axons. *Neuroscience* 1986;19:321–341.
109. Blight AR. Morphometric analysis of a model of spinal cord injury in guinea pigs, with behavioral evidence of delayed secondary pathology. *J Neurol Sci* 1991;103:156–171.
110. Koles ZJ, Rasminsky M. A computer simulation of conduction in demyelinated nerve fibers. *J Physiol* 1972;227:351–364.
111. Kakulas BA. Pathology of spinal injuries. *CNS Trauma* 1984;1: 117–129.
112. Hughes JT. *Pathology of the Spinal Cord*. Philadelphia: WB Saunders; 1978.
113. Barnett HJM, Botterell EH, Jousse AT, Wynn-Jones M. Progressive myelopathy as a sequel to traumatic paraplegia. *Brain* 1966;89:159–173.
114. Rossier AB, Foo D, Shillito J, et al. Progressive late post-traumatic syringomyelia. *Paraplegia* 1981;19:96–97.
115. Watson N. Ascending cystic degeneration of the cord after spinal cord injury. *Paraplegia* 1981;19:89–95.
116. Williams B, Terry AF, Francis Jones HW, McSweeny T. Syringomyelia as a sequel to traumatic paraplegia. *Paraplegia* 1981;19: 67–80.
117. Vernon JD, Silver JR, Ohry A. Post-traumatic syringomyelia. *Paraplegia* 1982;20:339–364.
118. Nathan PW, Smith MC, Deacon P. The corticospinal tracts in man: course and location of fibres at different segmental levels. *Brain* 1990;113:303–324.
119. Marciello M, Flanders AE, Herbison GJ, Schaefer DM, Friedman DP, Lane JI. Magnetic resonance imaging related to neurologic outcome in cervical spinal cord injury. *Arch Phys Med Rehabil* 1993;74:940–946.
120. Flanders AE, Schaefer DM, Friedman DP, Lane JI, Herbison GR. Predictive value of MRI imaging in the determination neurologic recovery in acute cervical spinal cord injury. *Radiology* 1991;181(P):172.
121. Schaefer DM, Flanders AE, Osterholm JL, Northrup BE. Prognostic significance of magnetic resonance imaging in the acute phase of cervical spine injury. *J Neurosurg* 1992;76(2):218–223.
122. Silberstein M, Tress BM, Hennessy O. Delayed neurologic deterioration in the patient with spinal trauma: role of MRI imaging. *Am J Neuroradiol* 1992;13:1373–1381.
123. Duncan EG, Lemaire C, Armstrong RL, Tator CH, Potts DG, Linden RD. High-resolution magnetic resonance imaging of experimental spinal cord injury in the rat. *Neurosurgery* 1992;31: 510–519.
124. Vink R, Noble LJ, Knoblach SM, Bendall MRI, Faden AI. Metabolic changes in rabbit spinal cord after trauma:magnetic resonance spectroscopy studies. *Ann Neurol* 1989;25(1):26–31.
125. Ohshiop I, Hatayama A, Kaneda K, Takahara M, Nagashima K. Correlations between histopathologic features and magnetic resonance images of spinal cord lesions. *Spine* 1993;18:1140–1149.
126. Bunge RP, Puckett WR, Becerra JL, Marcillo A, Quencer RM. Observations on the pathology of human spinal cord injury: a review and classification of 22 new cases with details from a case of chronic cord compression with extensive focal demyelination. *Adv Neurol* 1993;59:75–89.
127. Ford JC, Hackney DB, Joseph PM. A method for in vivo high resolution MRI of rat spinal cord injury. *Magn Reson Med* 1994;31:218–223.
128. Cotler HB, Kulkarni MV, Bondurant FJ. Magnetic resonance imaging of acute spinal cord trauma: preliminary report. *J Orthop Trauma* 1988;2(1):1–4.
129. Blackwood W. Vascular disease of the central nervous system. In: Blackwood W, McMenemey WH, Meyer A, Norman RM, Russell DS, eds. *Greenfield's Neuropathology*. Baltimore: Williams & Wilkins; 1963:71–115.
130. Yamashita Y, Takahashi M, Matsuno Y, et al. Chronic injuries of the spinal cord: assessment with MRI imaging. *Radiology* 1990;175(3):849–854.
131. Yamashita Y, Takahashi M, Matsuno Y, et al. Acute spinal cord injury: magnetic resonance imaging correlated with myelopathy. *Br J Radiol* 1991;64(759):201–209.
132. Gebarski SS, Maynard FW, Gabrielsen TO, et al. Posttraumatic progressive myelopathy: clinical and radiologic correlation employing MRI imaging, delayed CT metrizamide myelography, and intraoperative sonography. *Radiology* 1985;157:379–385.
133. Falcone S, Quencer R, Green BA, Patchen S, Post MJ. Progressive posttraumatic myelomalacic myelopathy. *AJNR* 1994;15: 747–754.
134. Waters RL, Adkins RH, Yakura JS. Definition of complete spinal cord injury. *Paraplegia* 1991;9:573–581.
135. Curati WL, Kingsley DPE, Kendall BE, Moseley IF. MRI in chronic spinal cord trauma. *Neuroradiology* 1992;35:30–35.
136. Quencer RM, Sheldon JJ, Post MJD, et al. MRI of the chronically injured cervical spinal cord. *AJR* 1986;147:125–132.
137. Quencer RM. The injured spinal cord. Evaluation with magnetic resonance and intra-operative ultrasonography. *Radiol Clin North Am* 1988;26:1025–1045.
138. Silberstein M, Hennessy O. Implications of focal spinal cord lesions following trauma: evaluation with magnetic resonance imaging. *Paraplegia* 1993;31:160–167.
139. Nidecker A, Kocher M, Maeder M, et al. MRI-imaging of chronic spinal cord injury. Association with neurologic function. *Neurosurg Rev* 1991;14:169–175.
140. Silberstein M, Hennessy O. Cystic cord lesions and neurological deterioration in spinal cord injury: operative considerations based on magnetic resonance imaging. *Paraplegia* 1992;30:661–668.
141. Matsumura A, Meguro K, Tsurushima H, Kikuchi Y, Mitsuyoshi W, Nakata Y. Magnetic resonance imaging of spinal cord injury without radiologic abnormality. *Surg Neurol* 1990;33:281–283.
142. Leventhal HR. Birth injuries of the spinal cord. *J Pediatr* 1960;56:447–453.
143. MacKinnon JA, Perlman M, Kirpalani H, et al. Spinal cord injury at birth: diagnostic and prognostic data in twenty-two patients. *J Pediatr* 1993;122:431–437.
144. Shulman ST, Madden JD, Esterly JR, Shanklin DR. Transection of spinal cord: a rare obstetrical complication of cephalic delivery. *Arch Dis Child* 1971;46:291–294.
145. Means ED, Anderson DK, Waters TR. Effect of methylprednisolone in compression trauma to the feline spinal cord. *J Neurosurg* 1981;55:200–208.
146. Faden AI, Jacobs TP, Mougey E, Holaday JW. Endorphins in experimental spinal injury: therapeutic effect of naloxone. *Ann Neurol* 1981;10:326–332.
147. Faden AI, Jacobs TP, Holaday JW. Thyrotropin-releasing hormone improves neurologic recovery after spinal trauma in cats. *N Engl J Med* 1981;305:1063–1067.
148. Bracken MB, Shepard MJ, Collins WF, et al. A randomized controlled trial of methylprednisolone or naloxone in the treatment of acute spinal cord injury: results of the Second National Acute Spinal Cord Injury Study. *N Engl J Med* 1990;322:1405–1411.
149. Bracken MB, Shepard MJ, Collins WF, et al. Methylprednisolone or naloxone in the treatment of acute spinal cord injury: one year follow up results of the Second National Acute Spinal Cord Injury Study. *J Neurosurg* 1992;76:23–31.
150. Young W, Bracken MB. The Second National Acute Spinal Cord Injury Study. In: Jane J, Torner J, Anderson D, Young W, eds. *NIH Central Nervous System Status Report*. New York: Mary Ann Liebert; 1991:5429–5451.
151. Mirvis SE, Geisler F, Joslyn JN, Zrebeet H. Use of titanium wire in cervical spine fixation as a means to reduce MRI artifacts. *Am J Neuroradiol* 1988;9(6):1229–1231.
152. Geisler FH, Mirvis SE, Zrebeet H, Joslyn JN. Titanium wire internal fixation for stabilization of injury of the cervical spine: clinical results and postoperative magnetic resonance imaging of the spinal cord. *Neurosurgery* 1989;25(3):356–362.
153. Donovan WH, Kopaniky D, Stolzmann E, Carter RE. The neu-

rological and skeletal outcome in patients with closed cervical spinal cord injury. *J Neurosurg* 1987;66:690–694.
154. Harris P, Karmi MZ, McClemont E, Mathoko D, Paul KS. The prognosis of patients sustaining severe cervical spine injury (C2-C7 inclusive). *Paraplegia* 1980;18:324–330.
155. Wagner FC, Chehrazi B. Early decompression and neurological outcome in acute cervical spinal cord injuries. *J Neurosurg* 1982;56:699–705.
156. Fox JL, Wener L, Drennan DC, Manz HJ, Won DJ, Al-Mefty O. Central spinal cord injury: magnetic resonance imaging confirmation and operative considerations. *Neurosurgery* 1988;22(2): 340–347.
157. Dall D. Injuries of the cervical spine. I. Does the type of bony injury affect spinal cord recovery? *SA Med J* 1972;46:1048–1056.
158. Dall D. Injuries of the cervical spine. II. Does anatomical reduction of the bony injuries improve the prognosis for spinal cord recovery? *SA Med J* 1972;46:1083–1090.
159. Koyanagi I, Iwasaki Y, Isu T, Akino M, Abe H. Significance of spinal cord swelling in the prognosis of acute cervical spinal cord injury. *Paraplegia* 1989;27:190–197.
160. Levi L, Wolf A, Rigamonti D, Ragheb J, Mirvis S, Robinson W. Anterior decompression in cervical spine trauma: does the timing of surgery affect the outcome? *Neurosurgery* 1991;29(2):216–222.
161. Ducker T, Bellegarrigue R, Saloman M, Walleck C. Timing of operative care in cervical spinal cord injury. *Spine* 1984;9(5): 525–531.
162. Anderson PA, Bohlman HH. Anterior decompression and arthrodesis of the cervical spine: long-term motor improvement. Part II—improvement in complete traumatic quadriplegia. *J Bone Joint Surg* 1992;74(5):683–692.
163. Bohlman HH, Anderson PA. Anterior decompression and arthrodesis of the cervical spine: long-term motor improvement. Part I—improvement in incomplete traumatic quadriparesis. *J Bone Joint Surg* 1992;74(5):671–682.
164. Bose B, Northrup BE, Osterholm JL, Cotler JM, Ditunno JF. Reanalysis of central cervical cord injury management. *Neurosurgery* 1984;15(3):367–372.
165. Rossignol S, Barbeau H. Pharmacology of locomotion: an account of studies in spinal cats and spinal cord injured subjects. *J Am Paraplegia Soc* 1993;16:190–196.
166. Tessler A, Himes BT, Houle J, Reirer PJ. Regeneration of adult dorsal root axons into transplants of embyonic spinal cord. *J Comp Neurol* 1988;270:537–548.
167. Bregman BS, Kunkel-Bagden E, Reier PJ, Dai HN, McAtee M, Gao D. Recovery of function after spinal cord injury: mechanisms of underlying transplant-mediated recovery of function differ after spinal cord injury in newborn and adult rats. *Exp Neurol* 1993;123:3–16.
168. Howland DR, Bregman BS, Tessler A, Goldberger ME. Anatomical and behavioral effects of transplants in kittens. *Soc Neurosci* 1991;17:236.
169. Iwasshita Y, Kawaguchi S, Murata M. Restoration of function by replacement of spinal cord segments in the rat. *Nature* 1994;367: 167–170.
170. Wirth ED, Theele DP, Mareci TH, Anderson DK, Brown SA, Reirer, PJ. In vivo magnetic resonance imaging of fetal cat neural tissue transplants in the adult cat spinal cord. *J Neurosurg* 1992;76:261–274.
171. DiTunno JF, Formal CS. Chronic spinal cord injury. *N Engl J Med* 1994;330(8):550–556.

Magnetic Resonance Imaging of the Brain and Spine, Second Edition, edited by Scott W. Atlas.
Lippincott-Raven Publishers, Philadelphia © 1996.

25

Infectious and Inflammatory Diseases of the Spine

Alexander S. Mark

There is no doubt that imaging of spinal infections and other spinal inflammatory diseases, regardless of the compartment of involvement, must be performed by magnetic resonance imaging (MRI). Vertebral body and disc space changes are clearly evident on MRI, even when only subtle or no abnormalities are detected by computed tomography (CT). Associated paraspinal and epidural masses are routinely depicted by MRI and findings pointing to their precise etiologies (e.g., infectious vs. neoplastic) are usually rather obvious. Beyond spinal column disease, MRI is the first imaging modality able to directly visualize the spinal cord. Its wide clinical use has enabled radiologists to demonstrate a number of intramedullary inflammatory and infectious conditions that previously required the injection of intrathecal contrast for even indirect evidence of disease. In spinal cord inflammation, notwithstanding its unsurpassed sensitivity, MRI has very limited specificity and cannot usually differentiate between the wide array of possible causes of intramedullary lesions. Despite its recognized lack of specificity, MRI has nearly completely supplanted all other imaging modalities in these patients.

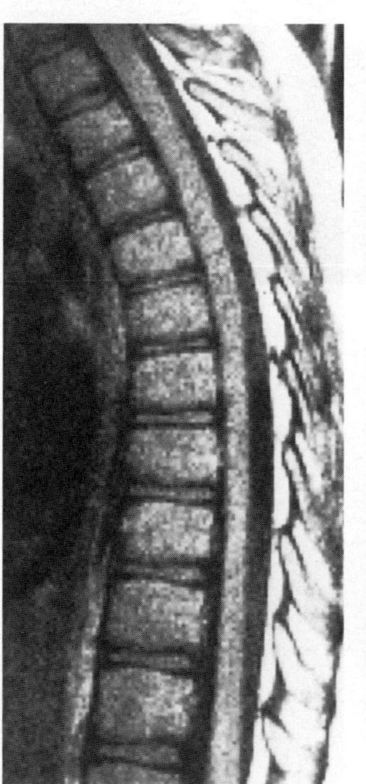
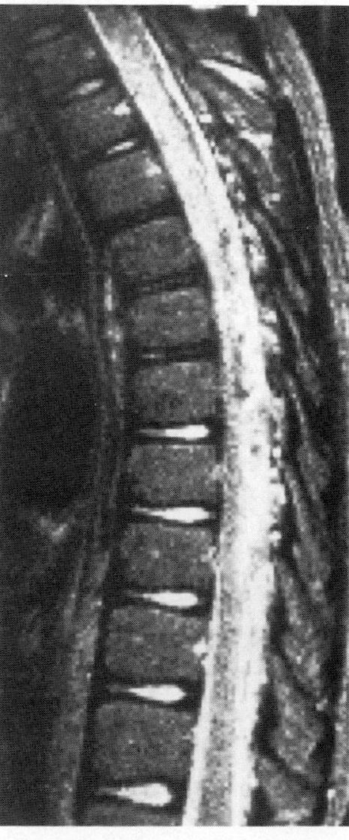

A,B

FIG. 1. Transverse myelitis in a 9-year-old boy with rapid onset of back pain and paraplegia. He had had a viral illness 3 weeks before. **A:** Sagittal T1-weighted image reveals questionable enlargement of the cord. **B:** T2-weighted image demonstrates diffuse increase in the signal intensity of the cord consistent with edema. (From Barakos et al., ref. 2, with permission.)

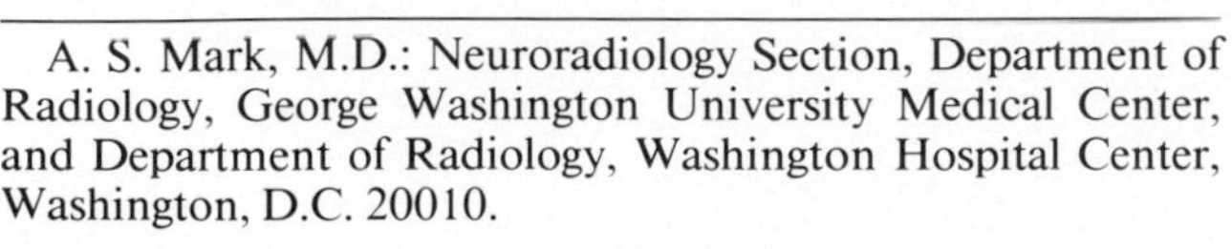
A. S. Mark, M.D.: Neuroradiology Section, Department of Radiology, George Washington University Medical Center, and Department of Radiology, Washington Hospital Center, Washington, D.C. 20010.

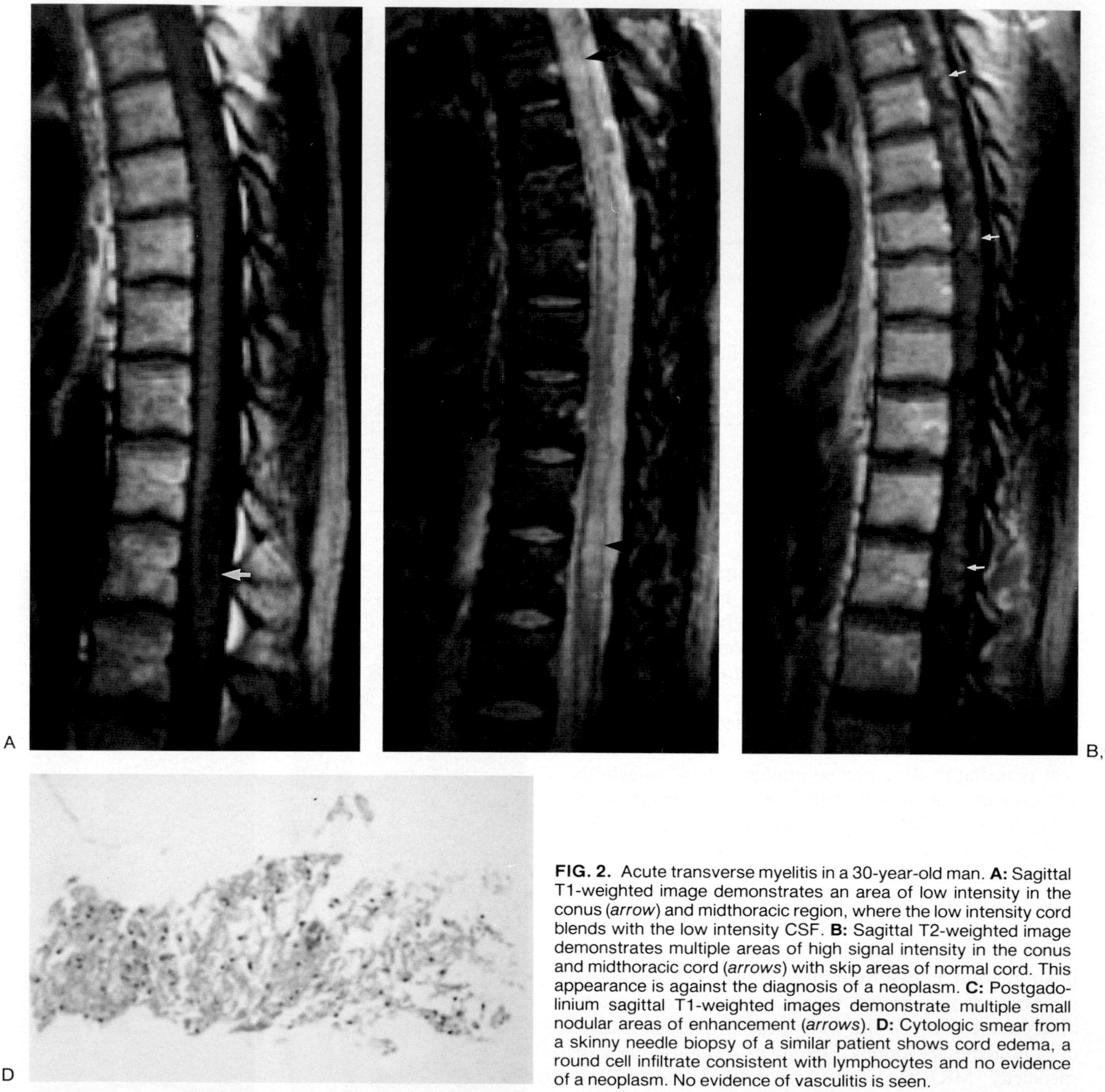

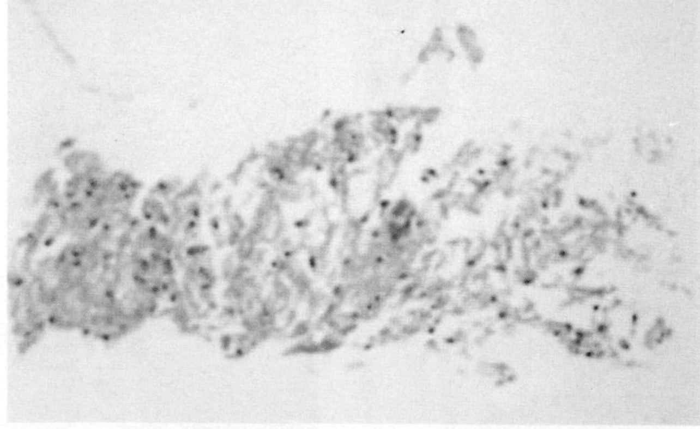

FIG. 2. Acute transverse myelitis in a 30-year-old man. **A:** Sagittal T1-weighted image demonstrates an area of low intensity in the conus (*arrow*) and midthoracic region, where the low intensity cord blends with the low intensity CSF. **B:** Sagittal T2-weighted image demonstrates multiple areas of high signal intensity in the conus and midthoracic cord (*arrows*) with skip areas of normal cord. This appearance is against the diagnosis of a neoplasm. **C:** Postgadolinium sagittal T1-weighted images demonstrate multiple small nodular areas of enhancement (*arrows*). **D:** Cytologic smear from a skinny needle biopsy of a similar patient shows cord edema, a round cell infiltrate consistent with lymphocytes and no evidence of a neoplasm. No evidence of vasculitis is seen.

Infection of the spinal column is most often part of the discitis/osteomyelitis spectrum of disease. This entity is common only in bacteria-induced discitis in a limited spectrum of patients. However, numerous other organisms can involve the spine. Spinal cord inflammation is only rarely due to infectious agents; most spinal cord inflammation is in the setting of demyelinating disease. This chapter covers a spectrum of inflammatory and infectious lesions of the spine, the spinal cord, and the various compartments delimited by spinal meninges. The reader is also referred to Chapter 15, White Matter Diseases, and Chapter 16, Intracranial Infection.

INFLAMMATORY AND DEMYELINATING DISEASES

Transverse Myelitis

Inflammatory and demyelinating lesions of the spinal cord are often grouped into the clinical syndrome of acute transverse myelitis. The term usually does not refer to a unique pathologic entity; rather, it is a clinical syndrome that has many etiologies. In idiopathic cases, acute transverse myelitis is characterized by an acutely developing ascending or static spinal cord lesion affecting both halves of the cord in the absence of any known neurologic disease or cord compression. In the past, acute transverse myelitis was a diagnosis of exclusion after spinal cord compression was ruled out. Today, MRI may directly demonstrate abnormal intramedullary signal, that is, low intensity on T1-weighted images and high intensity on T2-weighted images (1–4) (Fig. 1). The spinal cord may be of normal caliber or slightly expanded, which in the latter case may suggest a neoplasm. The disease may affect the cervical, thoracic (Fig. 2), or both segments (Fig. 3) of the cord. The abnormal signal may extend above the level of clinical deficit. After gadolinium administration, the abnormal areas may show enhancement (Figs. 2–4).

Transverse myelitis may be associated with infections (5), vaccination (6,7) (Fig. 5), disorders of the immune system such as systemic lupus (8–10) (Figs. 6 and 7), and multiple sclerosis (MS) or paraneoplastic syndromes. The prognosis of transverse myelitis is variable, but recovery may occur over several weeks or months. Follow-up MRI in these patients may demonstrate resolution of the abnormal signal and return of the cord to a normal caliber or cord atrophy. The association of transverse myelitis and optic neuritis is called Devic's syndrome, or neuromyelitis optica (11). Although MS is the most common cause of this condition, Devic's syndrome may be associated with viral infections (12–14), tuberculosis (15), and lupus (16) (Fig. 8).

All the inflammatory and demyelinating diseases we will discuss in this section can produce a clinical picture

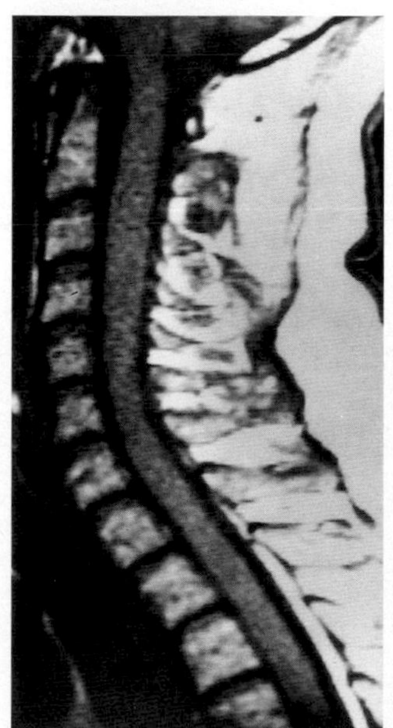

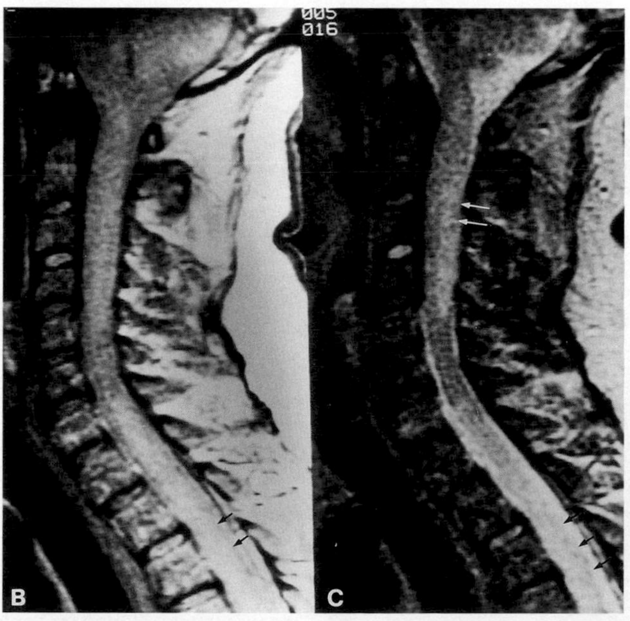

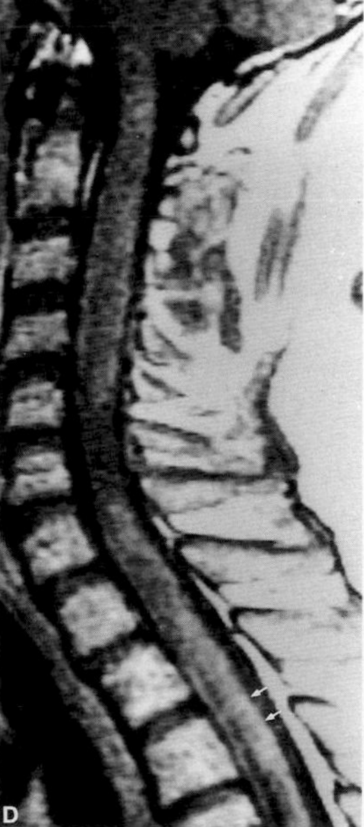

FIG. 3. Inflammatory myelitis in a 28-year-old woman with acutely progressive arm and truncal numbness, inability to walk, and urinary and fecal incontinence. **A:** Sagittal T1-weighted image demonstrates expansion of the cervical and upper thoracic cord. Sagittal proton (**B**) and T2-weighted (**C**) images demonstrate areas of high signal intensity in the cervical and upper thoracic cord (*arrows*) separated by an area of normal signal at the C5 and C6 level. **D:** Postgadolinium sagittal T1-weighted images demonstrate enhancement of the cervical and thoracic cord separated (*arrows*) by a nonenhancing area at the C6 level. Open biopsy demonstrated inflammatory myelitis without a syrinx. (From Gero et al., ref. 38, with permission.)

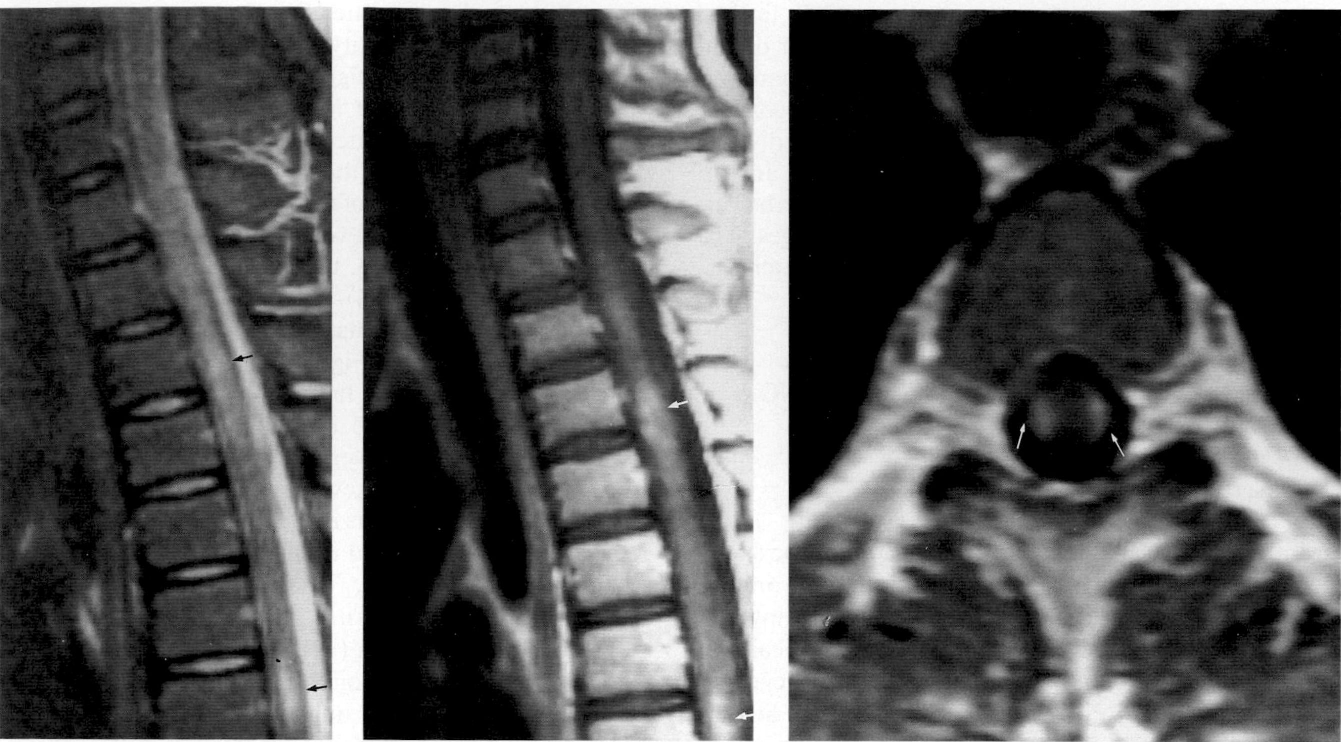

FIG. 4. Acute transverse myelitis in an 11-year-old child. **A:** Sagittal T2-weighted image demonstrates several foci of high signal intensity in the upper thoracic cord (*arrows*). The cord is of normal caliber. **B:** Postgadolinium sagittal T1-weighted image demonstrates several areas of enhancement (*arrows*) separated by a nonenhancing area. **C:** Axial T1-weighted image postcontrast demonstrates patchy enhancement of both sides of the cord (*arrows*).

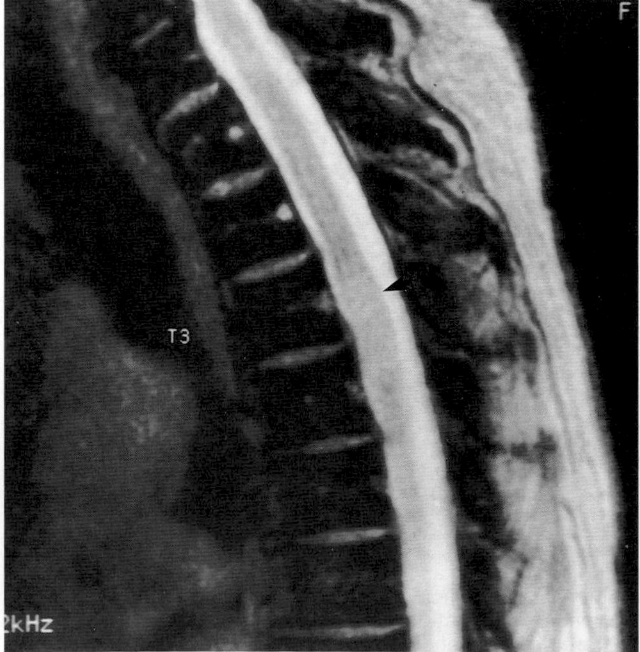

FIG. 5. Transverse myelitis following flu vaccination. A 40-year-old woman developed an acute thoracic myelopathy 3 weeks following a flu vaccination. Sagittal T2*-weighted image demonstrates mild cord swelling and an area of increased signal in the midthoracic cord (*arrow*).(Courtesy of Dr. W. Aulin, Washington, D.C.)

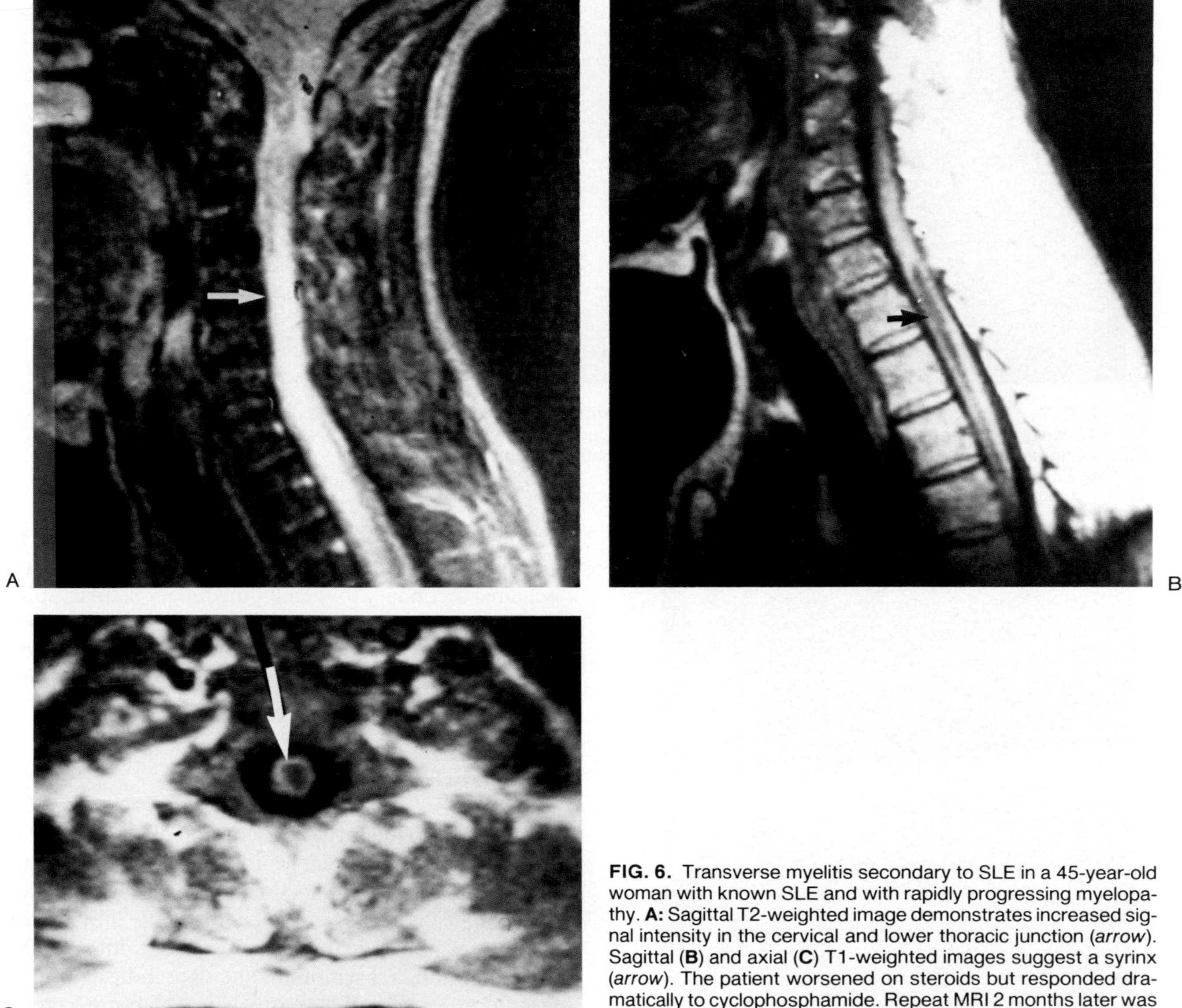

FIG. 6. Transverse myelitis secondary to SLE in a 45-year-old woman with known SLE and with rapidly progressing myelopathy. **A:** Sagittal T2-weighted image demonstrates increased signal intensity in the cervical and lower thoracic junction (*arrow*). Sagittal (**B**) and axial (**C**) T1-weighted images suggest a syrinx (*arrow*). The patient worsened on steroids but responded dramatically to cyclophosphamide. Repeat MRI 2 months later was normal.

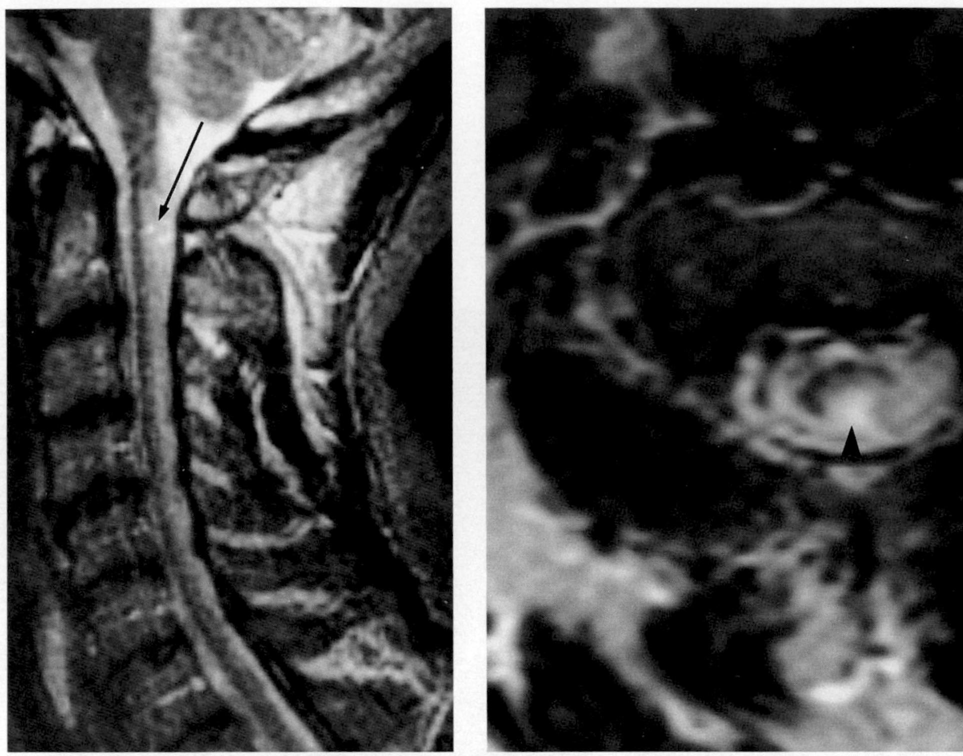

FIG. 7. SLE myelopathy. A 45-year-old woman with a known history of SLE and loss of proprioception. **A:** Sagittal T2-weighted image demonstrates an area of increased signal intensity in the posterior aspect of the cord correlating with a lesion in the posterior columns. **B:** Axial T2-weighted image in the same patient confirms the high intensity lesion in the posterior aspect of the cord.

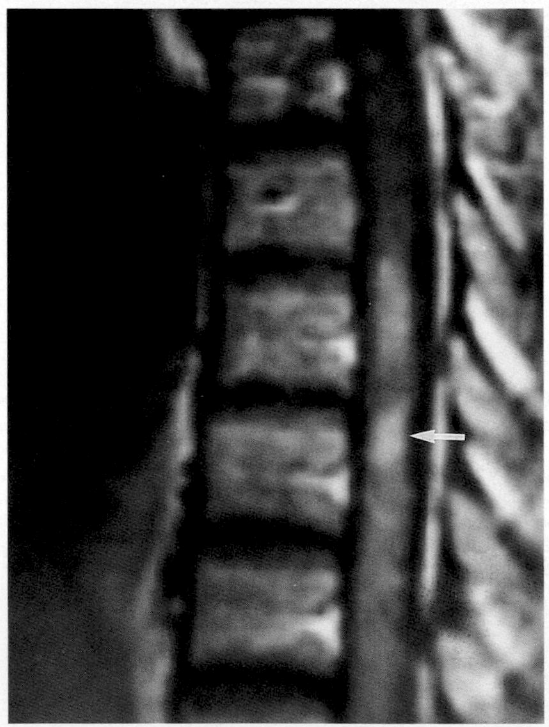

FIG. 8. Devic syndrome secondary to SLE. A 30-year-old woman with prior history of optic neuritis in the left eye and new onset optic neuritis in the right eye. Sagittal T1-weighted image postcontrast demonstrates enhancement of the midthoracic cord (*arrow*) consistent with the clinical impression of transverse myelitis.

of transverse myelitis; however, they are by no means the exclusive causes of this syndrome; in particular, venous ischemia secondary to radiculomedullary fistulae, spinal cord infarction due to occlusion of the anterior spinal artery, and the infectious myelitides should be excluded before the diagnosis of idiopathic transverse myelitis is made.

Multiple Sclerosis

Even though the earliest description of MS in 1849 involved lesions of the spinal cord, most of the initial literature about MRI in MS focused on the intracranial findings. Clinically, it is estimated that one third of MS patients exhibit spinal symptoms only, although it is most common that symptoms and signs indicate a mixed form of the disease, that is, involving cerebrum, cerebellum, optic nerves, brainstem, and spinal cord (17).

On gross pathologic examination of the spinal cord in MS patients, the great majority show evidence of disease regardless of the clinical history and, indeed, the extent of involvement usually far exceeds that which would be suspected by the patient's history. The lesions in the cord demonstrate no particular functional correlation with topographic localization, except that it is generally recognized that the cervical spinal cord is twice as likely to be involved than the lower levels (18). Lesions within the

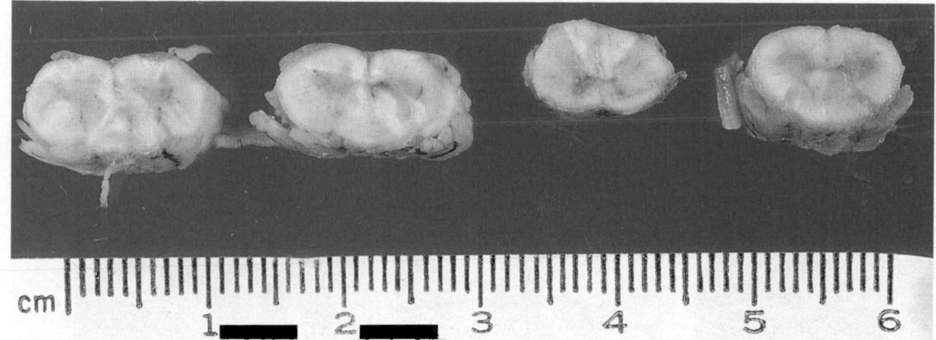

FIG. 9. MS. Gross pathology. Notice the multiple patchy areas of yellowish white discoloration corresponding to areas of demyelination.

cord are usually firm and brittle in texture and there is often gross atrophy with disseminated superficial patches of disease along the entire length (Fig. 9). Histologically, the early lesions are characterized by fragmentation of myelin, axonal preservation, and microglial proliferation. In the following weeks, the loss of myelin and oligodendrocytes becomes total, neutral fat can be demonstrated free and within macrophages, and there is marked proliferation of astrocytes with perivascular inflammation. If the plaques involve the gray matter, there is a striking preservation of the neuronal cell bodies. Several months later, fibrillary gliosis is established. In the very old plaques, there is evidence of wallerian degeneration, especially in the long tracts of the spinal cord. Iron deposition has been demonstrated at the edge of the plaques (18). The significance of this histologic finding is uncertain in regard to its correlate on MRI, but it may explain some foci of low intensity on T2-weighted images (Fig. 10).

The correlation between the clinical symptoms and the MS plaques is not fully understood. Experimental studies suggest that slowing of the nerve conduction following demyelination is probably the major factor in the symptomatology of MS. Occasionally, MS is clinically silent and is discovered unexpectedly at necropsy (18).

MS lesions in the cord appear as areas of increased signal intensity on T2-weighted images (18), with (see Fig. 14) or without corresponding areas of low intensity on

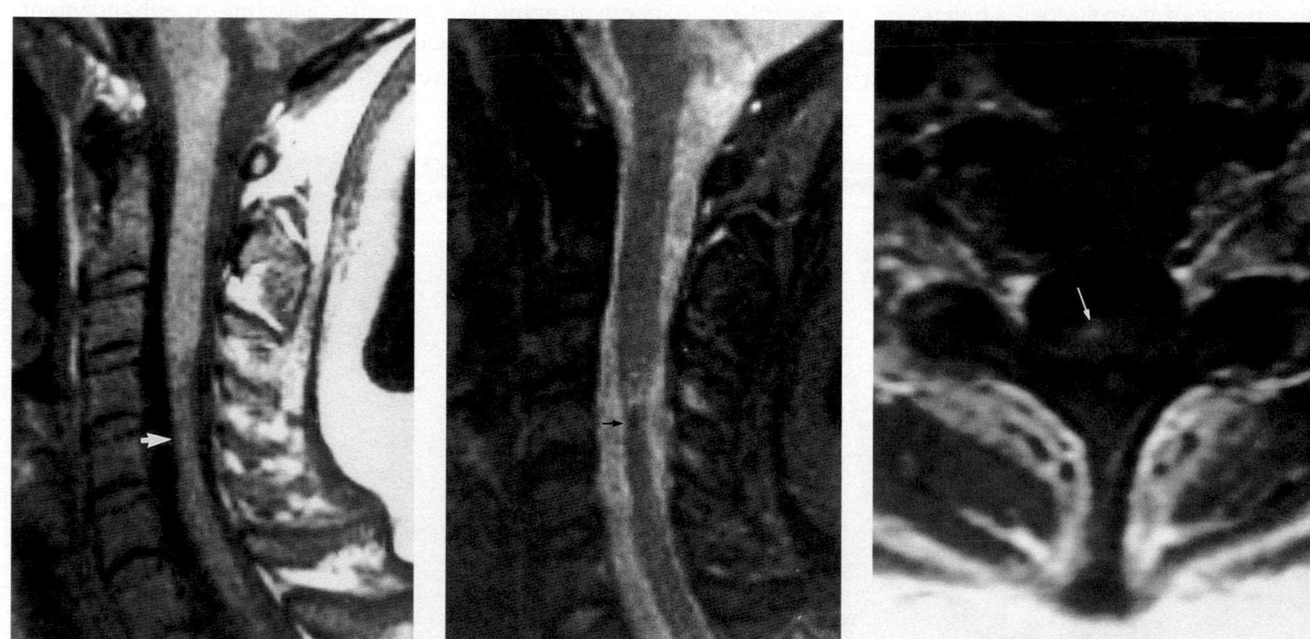

FIG. 10. Sequelae of transverse myelitis, possibly MS in a patient who presented with acute myelopathy 2 months before this study. He did not respond to steroids. **A:** Sagittal T1-weighted image demonstrates severe atrophy (*arrow*) of the cervical cord at the C3 and C4 level with relatively normal cord above and below. **B:** Sagittal T2-weighted image demonstrates the cord atrophy (*arrow*). There is a questionable focal area of low signal intensity (*arrow*) at the C3-C4 level. **C:** Axial T1-weighted image postcontrast at the C3 level demonstrates the severe cord atrophy. A small focus of enhancement is noted in the anterior aspect of the cord (*arrow*).

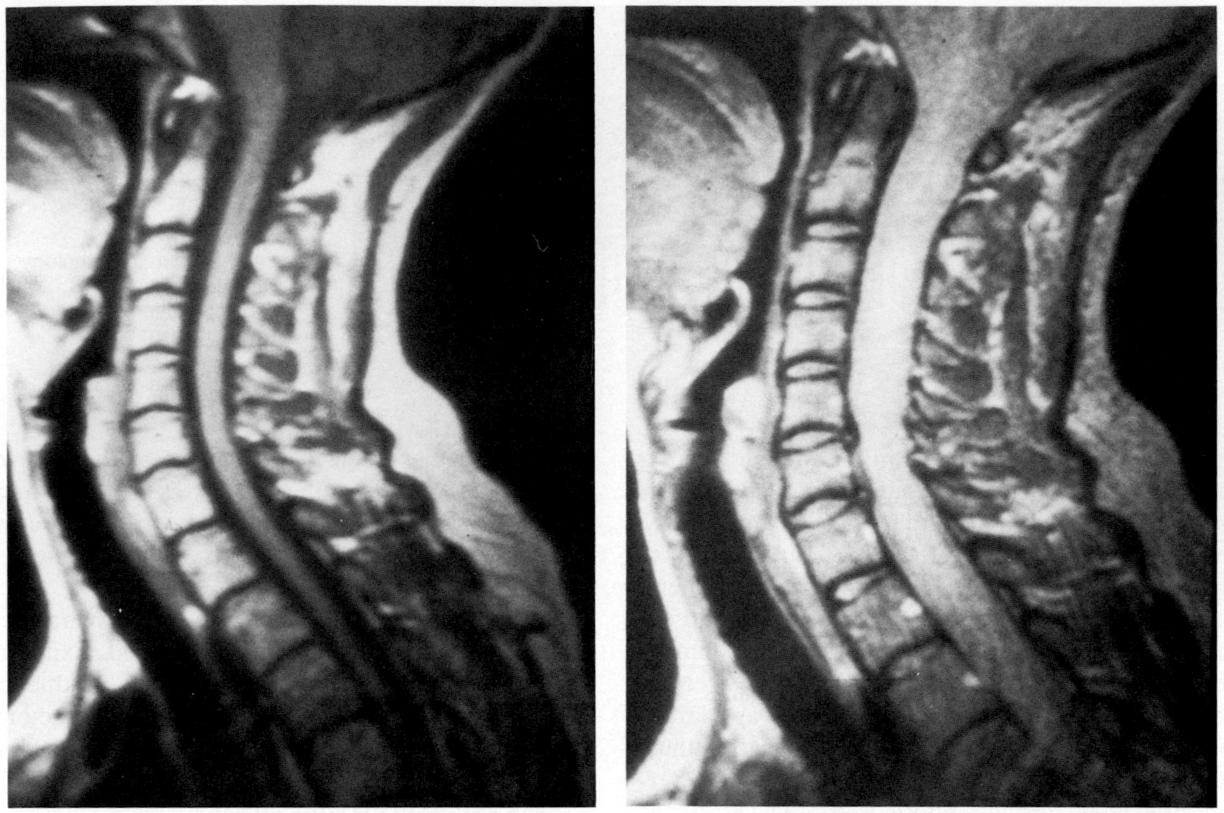

FIG. 11. MS. **A:** Sagittal T1-weighted images are normal. **B:** Sagittal proton-density image. Note diffuse increase in the signal intensity of the cord.

T1-weighted images (Fig. 11). These lesions may be seen in the absence of morphologic changes on T1-weighted image (Fig. 11) or be associated at the acute phase with swelling of the cord, which can mimic an intramedullary neoplasm (Fig. 12). In the late stages the cord may become atrophic (see Fig. 10). Gadolinium enhancement seems to correlate with active disease (19). One third of patients with MS presenting clinically with myelopathy

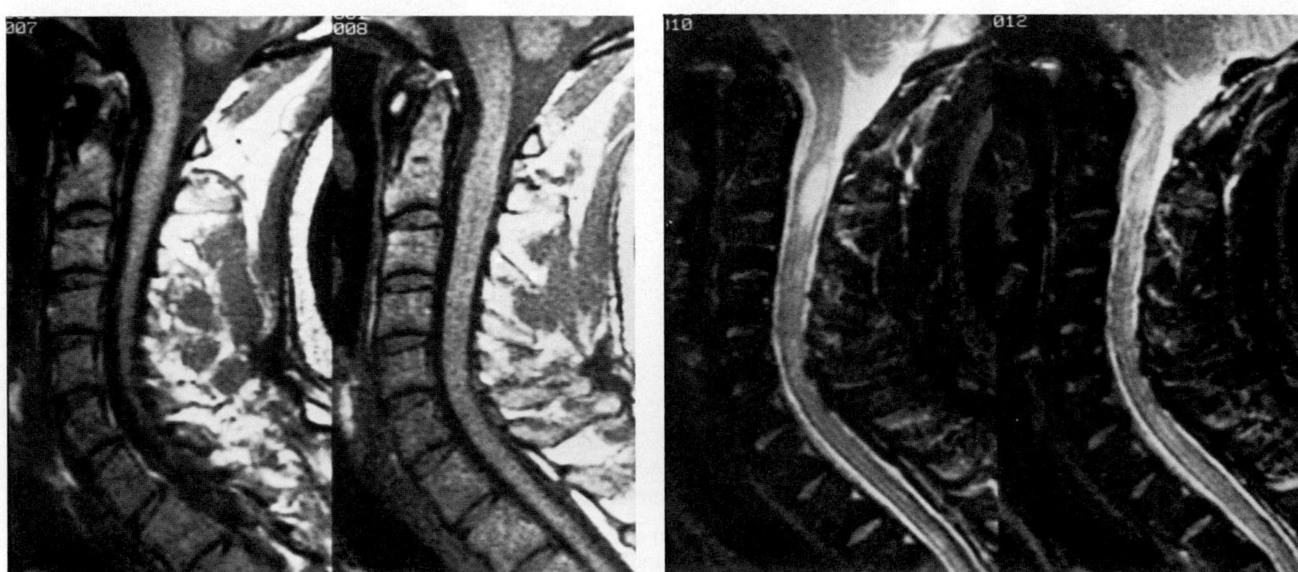

FIG. 12. MS presenting as transverse myelitis. **A:** Sagittal T1-weighted image. Focal enlargement of the cord at the C2 level. **B:** T2-weighted image. The area of swelling is of high signal intensity. (From Barakos et al., ref. 2, with permission.)

will have no associated periventricular lesions on brain MRI. Furthermore, a normal brain or spinal cord MRI does not exclude the diagnosis of MS, which is made clinically according to specific criteria (19) requiring neurologic symptoms involving multiple areas of the nervous system and/or neurologic episodes at different separations in time.

Acute Disseminated Encephalomyelitis

The term "acute disseminated encephalomyelitis" (ADEM) can be used to refer collectively to a group of inflammatory demyelinating diseases that share pathologic features and clinical course. These entities show multiple foci of inflammation that involve perivenous regions of white matter and are accompanied by perivenous and subpial demyelination (18). Clinically, these diseases are severe and sometimes fatal, and usually relate to prior viral illness or vaccination. The basis of the inflammatory response and subsequent demyelination is thought to be an autoimmune phenomenon. When severe hemorrhagic necrosis is identified as a major component, the disease is referred to as "acute hemorrhagic leukoencephalopathy" and a rapid progression to a fatal outcome is usual. The disease is clinically differentiated from MS by its clinical monophasic course, contrary to MS, which classically has periods of exacerbation and remission. If the patients recover, there is usually no further neurologic deficit; however, the outcome may be fatal.

Although spinal ADEM is uncommon, the MRI findings in cases of spinal involvement are nonspecific and indistinguishable from acute MS or other myelitides (Fig. 13). Hemorrhage may occur in the more severe forms, although it is not specific. In fact, the presence of a mass lesion in the spinal cord with hemorrhage in the absence of trauma would most likely represent an intramedullary neoplasm unless the classic history of a viral illness occurring 10 days to 2 weeks previously can be elicited.

Radiation Myelopathy

Radiation myelopathy is an uncommon complication of radiation therapy to lesions of the spine or adjacent tissues when the treatment plan does not allow for protection of the spinal cord, such as radiation for nasopharyngeal carcinoma. The incidence of radiation myelopathy correlates positively with a total radiation dose, dose per fraction, and length of the spinal cord irradiated. The incidence of radiation myelopathy after radiotherapy for nasopharyngeal carcinoma is estimated to be between 1% and 10%. A 50% incidence of radiation myelopathy may be expected when the cord receives between 68 and 73 GY and only 5% when the cord receives between 57 and 61 GY (20). The latent period of radiation myelopathy has two distinctive peaks, one at 12 to 14 months and the other 24 to 28 months, and the latent periods decrease with an increasing dose (21). The histopathology of radiation myelopathy can be classified as primarily

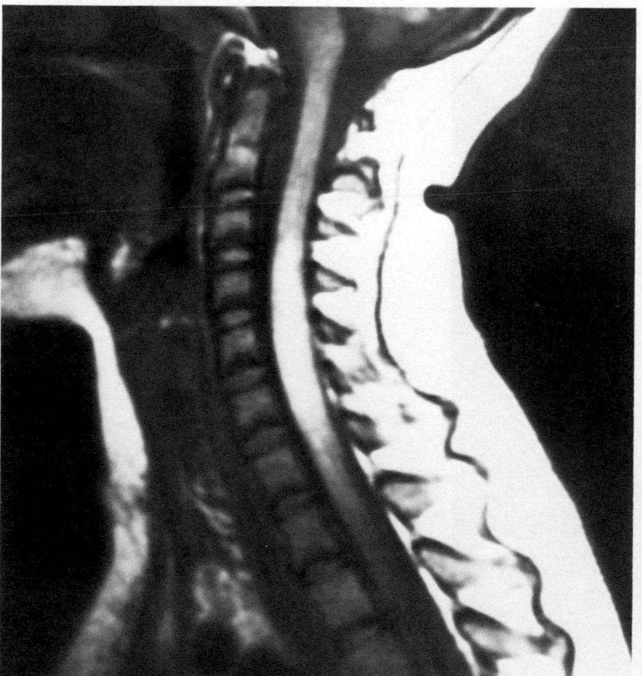

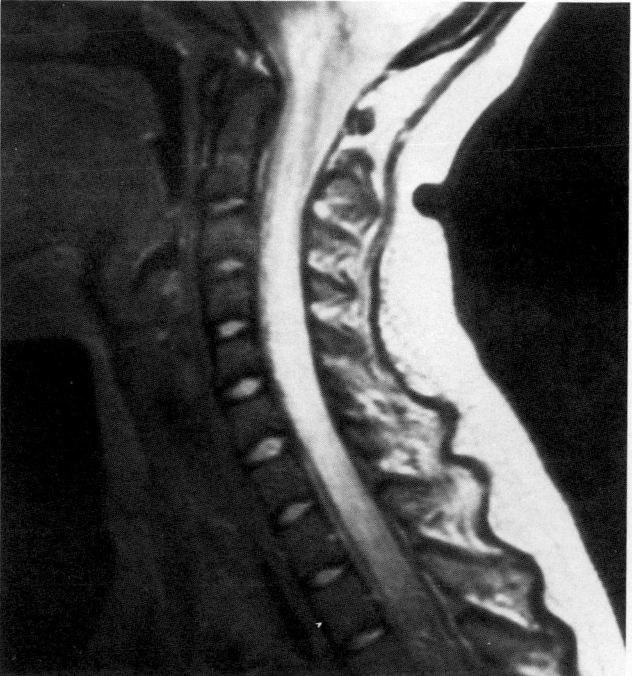

FIG. 13. Presumed acute disseminated encephalomyelitis with hemorrhage. Sagittal T1-weighted image (**A**) shows enlarged high intensity cervical cord, consistent with hemorrhagic lesion. Note extensive high intensity on long TR/short TE image (**B**) extending throughout entire cervical cord and up into brainstem. (Courtesy of Dr. Clark Carrol, Houston, TX.)

white matter parenchymal lesions, primary vascular lesions, or a combination of vascular and white matter lesions. The white matter lesions and the combination of vascular and white matter lesions have the shorter latent period corresponding to the earliest peak at 12 to 14 months, whereas the vascular lesions are associated with a longer latent period corresponding to the second peak, 24 to 28 months. Pathologic studies in experimental rabbit models reveal demyelination, focal astrocytosis, erythrodiapedesis, and perineuronal edema. In autopsy studies the typical histopathologic finding associated with radiation myelopathy is leukomalacia. The gray matter is rarely involved and never is it involved to the exclusion of the white matter. Treatment for radiation myelopathy has been disappointing. Steroids have been helpful in some patients.

A spectrum of MR findings has been described in patients with radiation myelopathy (22). There is no correlation between the MR findings and the latency of radiation myelopathy; however, there appears to be correlation between the time of MR imaging after the onset of symptoms and the MR findings. Within less than 8 months after the onset of symptoms, MR demonstrated low intensity on T1- and high intensity on T2-weighted images in a long segment of the cervical cord. Swelling of the cord and/or focal enhancement after contrast administration (Fig. 14) may also be seen. Imaging longer than 3 years after the onset of symptoms usually reveals atrophy of the cord. The diagnosis of radiation myelopathy remains a diagnosis of exclusion. MR is extremely helpful in excluding tumor recurrence or carcinomatous meningitis. Chemotherapy-induced myelitis should also be considered in the appropriate clinical context. Occasionally, it may not be possible to describe a single cause to a treatment-related myelopathy in cancer patients.

Sarcoidosis

Sarcoidosis is a multisystem disease of unknown etiology characterized by noncaseating granulomas. Young adults are most frequently affected, usually presenting with pulmonary symptoms. Bone involvement is seen in 1% to 13% of cases in various series, is usually late, and is commonly associated with cutaneous lesions. The tubular bones of the hand and feet are most often involved. Sarcoidosis of the vertebral bodies is rare, with only 20 cases reported in a recent review. The thoracolumbar spine region is affected most commonly. Typically, plain radiographs reveal lytic lesions with variable regions of surrounding sclerosis involving single multiple bones. An associated paraspinal mass may be present and disc space involvement is rare. These findings usually suggest tuberculosis or a neoplasm. When the disc is involved (23), pyogenic discitis is the most common diagnosis. Biopsy is necessary for a definitive diagnosis.

Clinical involvement of the central nervous system occurs in 5% of patients with sarcoid. Primary involvement of the spinal cord is very rare, with only 72 cases reported in the literature in a recent review article (24). In two thirds of the cases, the diagnosis was not known before the onset of symptoms. Approximately 35% of cases

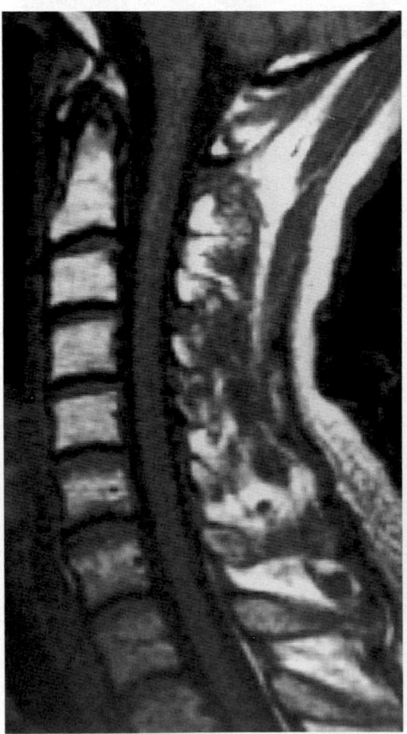

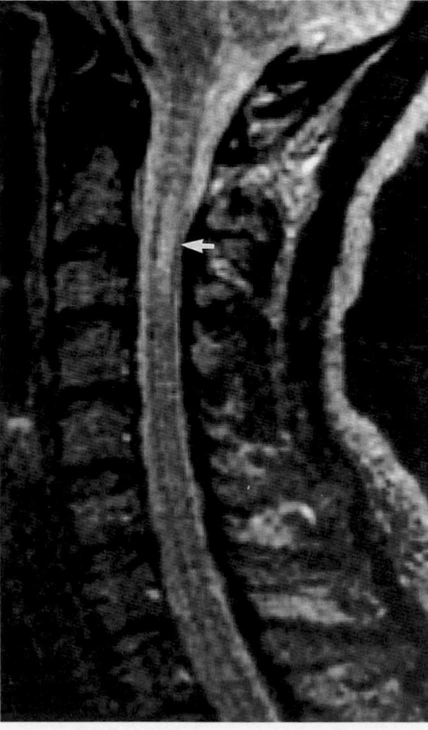

A,B

FIG. 14. Radiation myelopathy. A 60-year-old man 2 years S/P radiation therapy for laryngeal cancer presented with cervical myelopathy. **A:** Sagittal T1-weighted image demonstrates increased signal intensity in the upper cervical vertebral bodies consistent with postradiation changes. No definite abnormalities are noted in the cord. **B:** Sagittal T2-weighted image demonstrates a focus of high signal intensity in the upper cervical cord at the C2-C3 level (*arrow*).

showed intramedullary (Figs. 15 and 16) and 35% extramedullary disease; involvement of both was present in 23%. Gadolinium MRI is extremely helpful, and may actually suggest the diagnosis in the appropriate clinical setting if, in addition to areas of intramedullary enhancement, pial enhancement (Fig. 17) is demonstrated. The MRI findings, however, are not specific and may be seen in tuberculous, toxoplasmic, or human immunodeficiency virus (HIV)-related meningitis (25), leptomeningeal metastasis (26), and post-shunting meningeal fibrosis.

Behçet Syndrome

Behçet syndrome is characterized by recurrent ulcerations of the mouth and genitalia accompanied by uveitis or iridocyclitis, but 20% to 30% of the patients may have a disseminated central nervous system (CNS) disease affecting the brain and spinal cord. Because of the diversity of the lesions, the condition may simulate MS. The neuropathology is that of multifocal necrotizing lesions with marked inflammatory cell reactions. In addition, necrosis may affect the gray and white matter, probably secondary to vasculitis (18,27).

Necrotizing Myelopathy

Necrotizing myelopathy is a pathologic condition characterized by coagulative necrosis and thickening and hyalinization of the vascular walls (28). The most common cause is venous hypertension (29) in the medullary veins secondary to a dural arteriovenous fistula. Factors predisposed to its development include hypercoagulability, migratory thrombophlebitis, and polycythemia. The condition corresponds to the description by Foix and Alajouanine (30) (Foix-Alajouanine syndrome) and was given a variety of names, including subacute necrotic myelitis.

While most commonly secondary to a dural fistula, necrotizing myelopathy is also associated with inflammatory and demyelinating conditions such as MS, acute disseminated encephalomyelitis, varicella-zoster (6), mumps, rubeola, infectious mononucleosis, systemic lupus erythematosus (SLE) (10), pulmonary tuberculosis (31), and clioquinol intoxication (32).

For instance, in 15% to 20% of patients with SLE, the myelopathy is the presenting feature. Typically, the course of the illness is rapidly progressive and is characterized by remissions and relapses. The most common

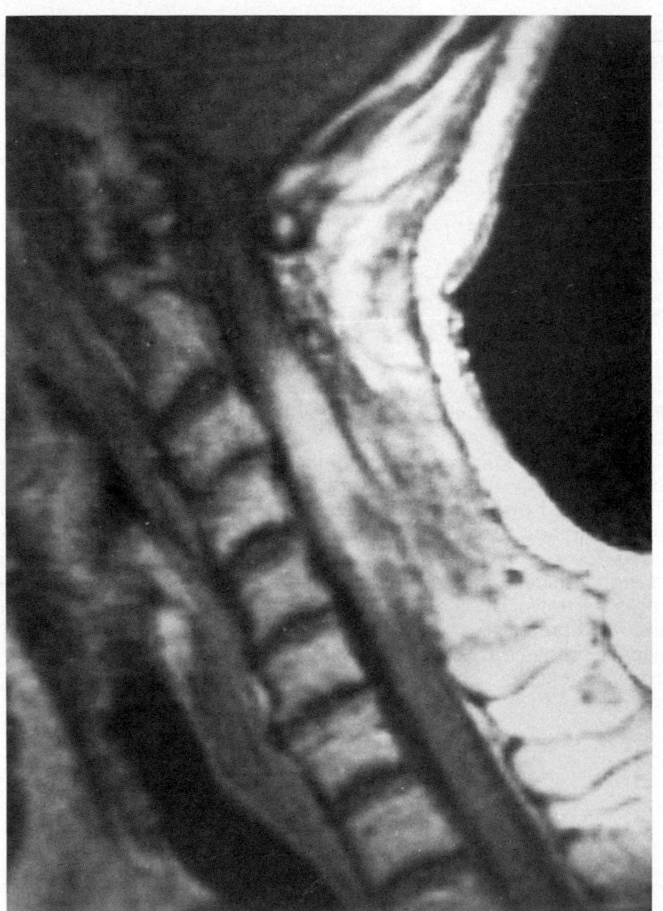

A

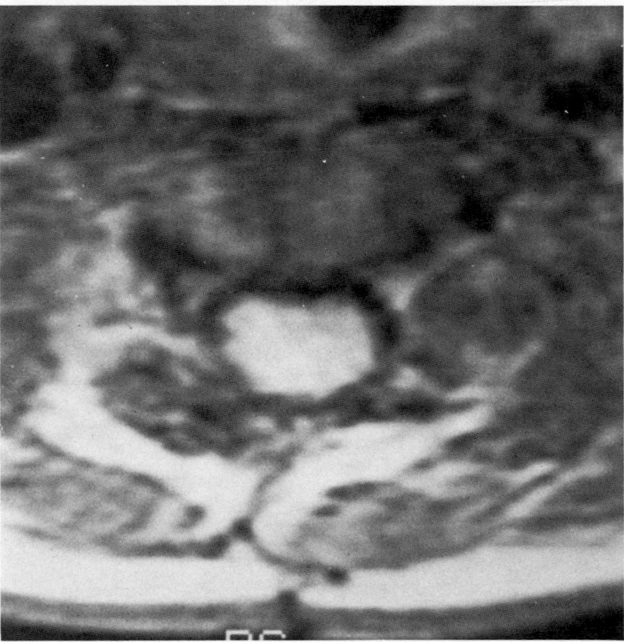

B

FIG. 15. Intramedullary sarcoidosis in a 54-year-old woman with progressive myelopathy. Sagittal (**A**) and axial (**B**) T1-weighted image following GD-DTPA. Enhancing intramedullary mass is indistinguishable from a glioma.

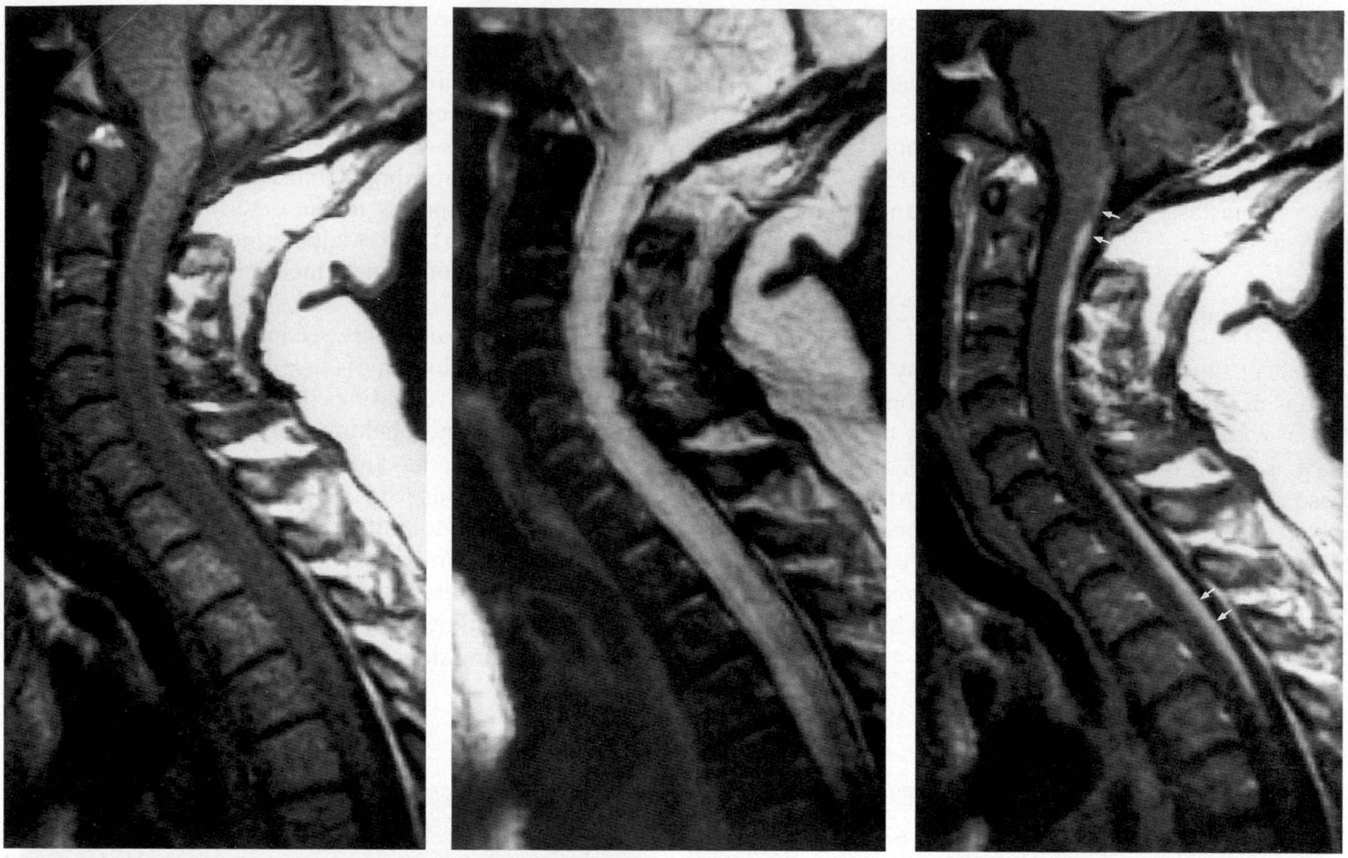

A

B,C

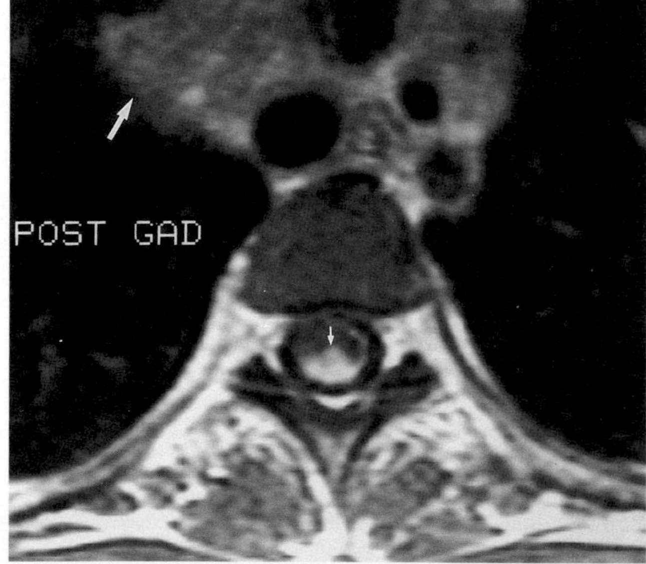

D

FIG. 16. Intramedullary sarcoidosis. A 40-year-old woman with acute paraplegia and sensory loss below C3. **A:** Sagittal T1-weighted image pregadolinium demonstrates marked enlargement of the cord in the entire cervical and upper thoracic region. **B:** Sagittal T2-weighted image demonstrates increased intramedullary signal in the entire cervical and upper thoracic region. **C:** Sagittal T1-weighted image postgadolinium demonstrates marked enhancement in the posterior aspect of the cord in the entire cervical and upper thoracic region (*arrows*). **D:** Axial T1-weighted image postgadolinium through the midthoracic spine demonstrates enhancement in the posterior aspect of the cord (*small arrow*). Note the mediastinal adenopathy consistent with sarcoidosis (*large arrow*).

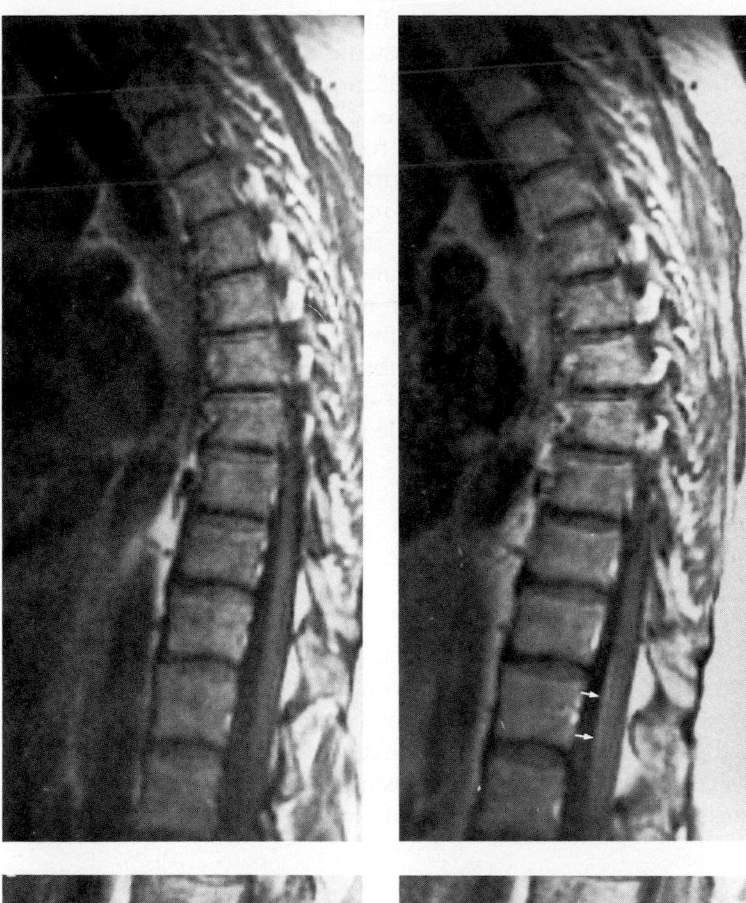

A,C

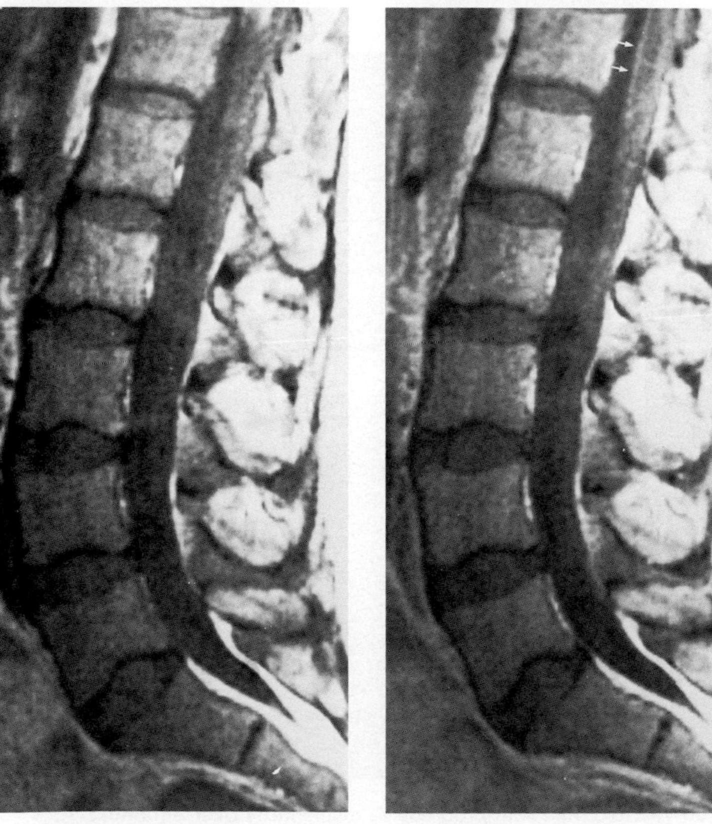

B,D

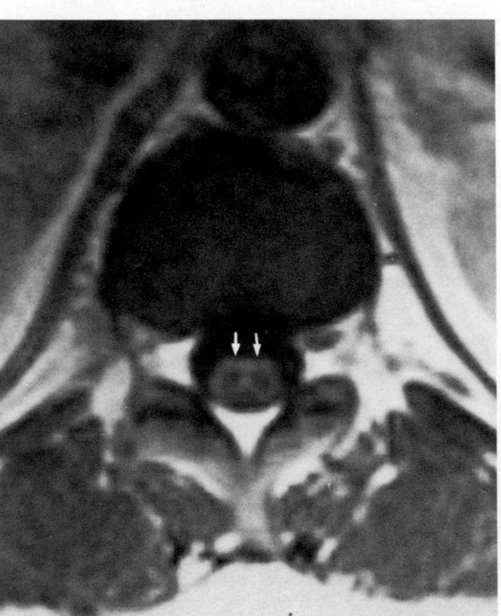

E

FIG. 17. Pial sarcoidosis in a 42-year-old woman with known sarcoid and bilateral lower extremity numbness. Sagittal thoracic (**A**) and lumbar (**B**) T1-weighted images precontrast are normal. Thoracic (**C**) and lumbar (**D**) sagittal and axial **(E)** T1-weighted images postcontrast enhancement demonstrate pial enhancement *(arrows)* along the conus. The numbness resolved on steroid therapy.

segment of the spinal cord to be affected is the thoracic level, but in one quarter of the patients the cervical spine is involved. Pathologically, the lesions consist of one or more foci of subtle coagulative or liquefactive necrosis, although on occasion circumferentially distributed pallor of the white matter with ballooning degeneration of myelin sheath and destruction of the axons has been described. The pathogenesis is not fully understood, but the presence of antiphospholipid antibodies has been implicated (33).

A paraneoplastic necrotizing myelopathy not associated with radiation therapy, cord compression, or tumor infiltration has also been described (34). The condition is associated with a variety of neoplasms, most commonly bronchopulmonary carcinoma and lymphoma (35). It is characterized pathologically by massive or patchy multifocal areas of coagulative necrosis in both the gray and the white matter, with a paucity of inflammatory cells. The pathogenesis is unknown, but recently two such cases have been associated with the presence of herpes virus type II (36). Finally, in a number of cases, no specific cause for the necrotic myelopathy can be determined.

The MRI findings in patients with necrotic myelopathy are nonspecific, with diffuse areas of increased signal intensity on T2-weighted images (Fig. 18) and decreased signal intensity on T1-weighted images with variable enhancement on postcontrast studies (37). The similar MRI appearance of most of the inflammatory and demyelinating diseases of the spine probably reflects the limited number of responses to a variety of insults that the spinal cord can mount. Most of these responses macroscopically result in increased water concentration responsible for the increased signal intensity on T2-weighted images and occasionally disruption of the cord–blood barrier responsible for enhancement. The confusion caused by the noninflammatory necrotizing myelopathy is attributable to our lack of knowledge of the pathogenesis of most of the disorders and the difficulty of access to adequate amounts of tissue for diagnostic purposes.

Summary

From a practical point of view, when enlargement of the spinal cord and increase in the signal intensity on T2-weighted images with or without enhancement is demonstrated on MR in a patient with an acute or subacute myelopathy, it is incumbent upon the neuroradiologist to consider foremost the treatable causes for such a condition. It is imperative to exclude a dural vascular mal-

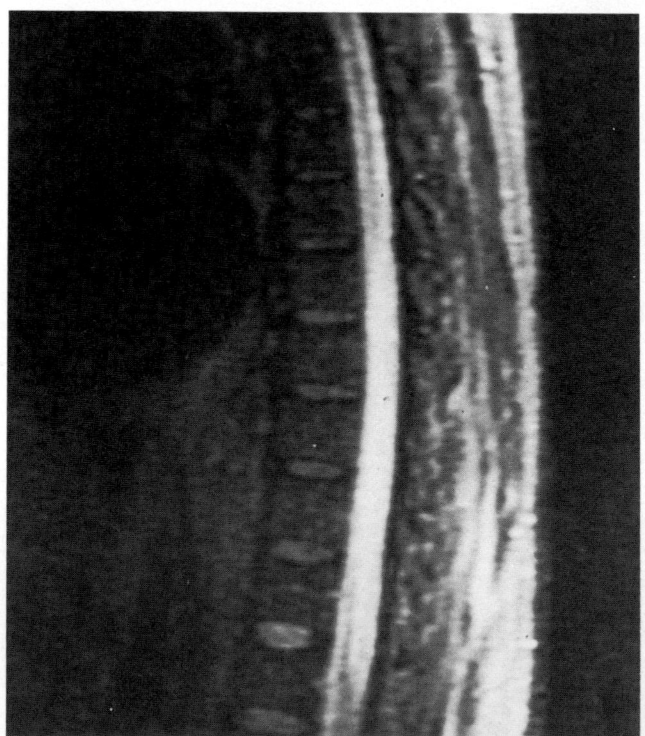
A

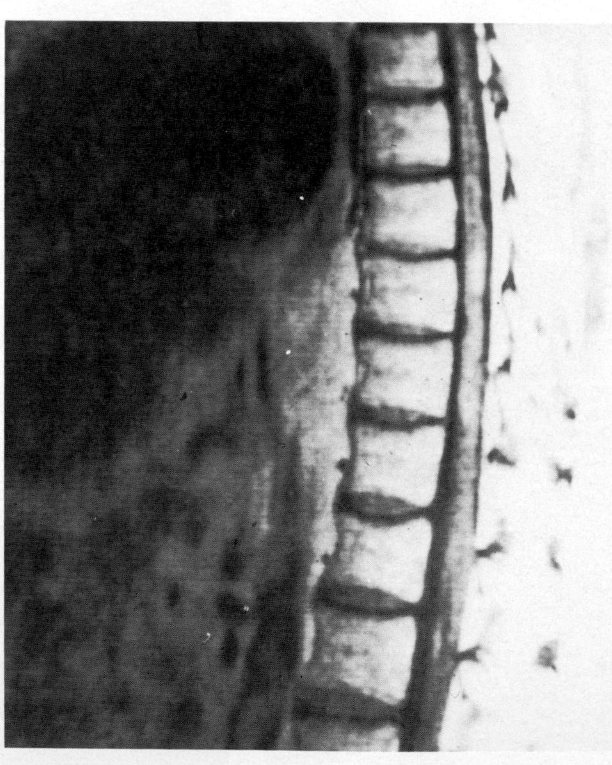
B

FIG. 18. Probable thrombosed dural fistula in a 60-year-old man with progressive myelopathy over 9 months. **A:** Sagittal T2-weighted image demonstrates high signal in the mid- and lower thoracic cord. **B:** Postcontrast sagittal T1-weighted image shows intramedullary enhancement. Myelography with the patient in the supine position was normal. At surgery, a thrombosed dorsal vein was found. There was no intramedullary neoplasm. Sagittal long TR/short TE image.

formation by scrutinizing the posterior subarachnoid space for dilated vessels (see Chapter 28). In difficult cases, myelography with the patient supine may be helpful in planning the site for spinal angiography. Treatable infectious myelitides such as bacterial, that is, pyogenic, syphilitic, or Lyme disease, should be excluded by direct examination of the cerebrospinal fluid (CSF) via spinal tap. Finally, noninfectious inflammatory conditions such as MS and SLE, which may respond to steroid treatment, should be considered. In a recent article (38), it has been suggested that the pattern of enhancement may be somewhat helpful in the differential diagnosis of various spinal cord lesions. Focal nodular areas of enhancement have been associated with granulomatous conditions such as tuberculosis, toxoplasmosis, or other fungal infections. Diffuse areas of abnormal signal intensity and/or enhancement were associated with viral infections or inflammatory and/or demyelinating processes.

INFECTIONS

Infections of the spine can be separated into infections of the vertebral bodies and discs, epidural space, intradural space, and infections of the spinal cord itself.

Pathophysiology of Spinal Infections

Hematogenous spread of infection to the vertebral body can occur via arterial or venous routes. The initial suggestion that Batson's plexus served as the principal route of infection has been refuted. It has been shown through selective retrograde injection in both human and rabbit cadavers that the bony vertebral tributaries of Batson's plexus were too small and the injection could be achieved only with considerable pressure. Injection into the arterial nutrient vessels was much easier and demonstrated a rich vascular network. The lack of associated meningitis and extradural thrombophlebitis in patients with osteomyelitis suggests that the venous route of infection is unlikely and hematogenous spread via the arterial route is the primary mechanism of osteomyelitis (39).

In children, because of the richly vascularized endplate, the infection starts in the endplate and disc, resulting in "discitis" (40). In adults, the blood supply to the intervertebral disc involutes and the primary site of infection becomes the vertebral body, particularly the metaphyseal area close to the anterior longitudinal ligament (41). From there the infection can spread in a subligamentous fashion or extend to the disc and involve the adjacent vertebral body. Most disc space infections are limited to one interspace and adjacent vertebral body. Approximately 25% involve more than one level. A primary source of infection can be found in approximately 50% of patients, with the most common sources being in the skin, upper respiratory tract, and genitourinary tract.

Contiguous spread of vertebral and disc infection can result from soft tissue infection such as psoas abscess, decubitus ulcer, or paravertebral abscess. Tuberculous and fungal infections most frequently extend from the spine to the adjacent soft tissues and from there may extend in a subligamentous fashion to other vertebral bodies.

Direct inoculation can result during surgical procedures or diagnostic invasive procedures such as discograms or lumbar punctures. Postdisc surgery infections can also occur.

Pyogenic Infections

Vertebral Osteomyelitis and Discitis

Pyogenic infections of the spine involve primarily the disc space in children and the vertebral bodies in adults. Adults in the sixth and seventh decade are more frequently affected and men are affected twice as often as women. The lumbar spine is most frequently involved. Most cases of juvenile discitis occur in children younger than 2 years old, are more common in girls than boys, and are usually self-limited (42).

Staphylococcus aureus accounts for 60% of adult infection. *Escherichia coli, Pseudomonas aeruginosa,* and *Klebsiella* account for another 30%. *Salmonella* osteomyelitis is seen with increasing frequency in patients with sickle cell. The patient's symptoms often precede the radiographic findings by several weeks. Paraplegia develops in less than 1% of patients with osteomyelitis. Cultures of the disc material obtained by needle biopsy are negative in 50% to 70% of patients.

The MRI findings of discitis and osteomyelitis closely match the pathologic findings (43). The signal alterations reflect the early inflammatory response characterized by infiltration of polymorphonuclear leukocytes and fibrin deposition in the adjacent endplates. Bony destruction secondary to lytic enzymes and the associated increased water content are reflected by the increased signal intensity on T2-weighted images and decreased signal intensity on T1-weighted images (Figs. 19 and 20). The signal alterations often precede the destructive changes (44–47).

The aim of any imaging modality is to make the diagnosis as early as possible (48). Clearly, MRI is the most sensitive technique. However, the MR findings may lag behind the clinical symptoms of severe back pain. When the diagnosis is uncertain, a follow-up MRI in 1 week may be helpful to show the evolution of the early changes.

In the same way the MRI findings lag behind the early signs of disc space infection, the MRI findings also lag in the healing phase of vertebral osteomyelitis. Once ade-

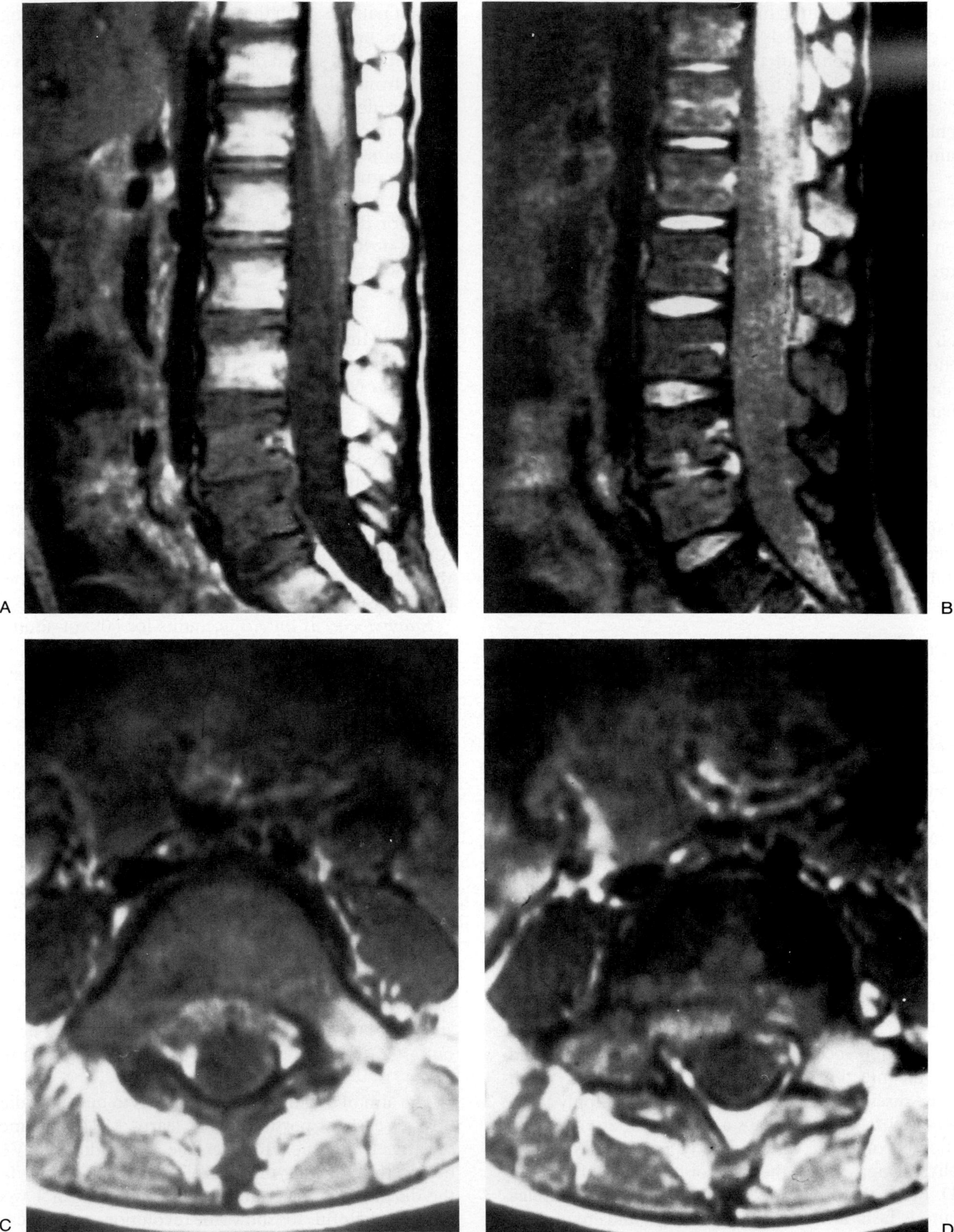

FIG. 19. Discitis and epidural abscess. **A:** Sagittal T1-weighted image demonstrates loss of height of the L4-L5 disc and decreased intensity of the adjacent vertebral body marrow. **B:** Sagittal T2-weighted image demonstrates increased signal intensity in the disc and adjacent vertebral bodies. **C,D:** Axial T1-weighted images at the L5 level visualize an epidural mass consistent with an abscess and granulation tissue.

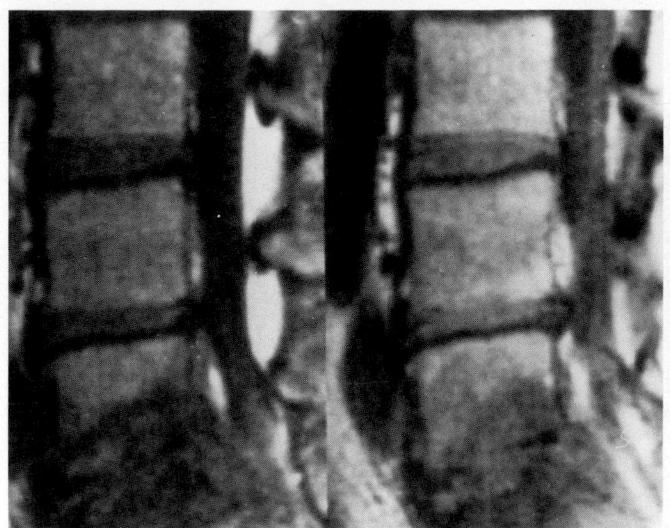

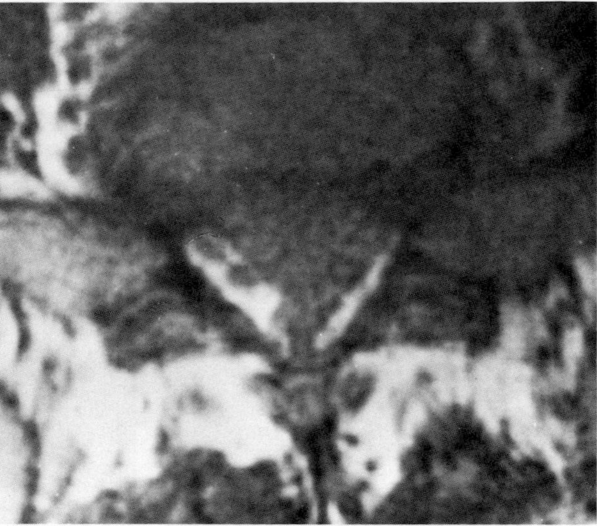

FIG. 20. Discitis and epidural abscess at the L5-S1 level. **A:** Sagittal T1-weighted image demonstrates loss of height of the disc and decreased intensity of the adjacent vertebral body marrow. **B:** Axial T1-weighted image at the L5 level visualizes an epidural mass consistent with an abscess or granulation tissue.

quate antibiotic treatment has been instituted, the clinical symptoms improve dramatically, whereas the MRI findings evolve much more slowly (Fig. 21). The findings of healing osteomyelitis include persistent disc space narrowing, decreased signal intensity of the disc on T2-weighted images consistent with disc degeneration, fusion of the adjacent vertebral bodies, and resolution of the high signal intensity in the adjacent endplates corresponding to resolution of the edema. If an epidural abscess was present (see below), the epidural space also returns to normal. Thus, in the early stages of treatment, laboratory findings such as sedimentation rate and white count are more helpful in monitoring the response to treatment than the MRI findings.

A number of conditions other than discitis can produce similar changes and should be considered in the differential diagnosis. Modic et al. (49) have described three types of simple *degenerative changes in the vertebral endplates* secondary to degenerative changes. Type I changes are characterized by low signal intensity on T1-weighted images and high signal intensity on T2-weighted images, which can mimic infection. The histologic correlation demonstrates fissures of the vertebral endplates with the presence of fibrous granulation tissue richly vascularized, as confirmed by the increase in the signal intensity after gadolinium injection. A degenerated disc can also enhance even in its central portion or in the periphery adjacent to the vertebral endplates. However, the disc is usually of low signal intensity on T2-weighted images. A follow-up study in several weeks should demonstrate no change in contrast to the changes of discitis that will progress. The type II and type III changes have signal characteristics that can easily be differentiated from discitis and osteomyelitis.

Patients with *osteomalacia secondary to renal osteodystrophy* can present with noninfectious disc space erosions and partial collapse of the adjacent vertebral bodies, mimicking an aggressive osteomyelitis. This condition is particularly worrisome because patients with renal osteodystrophy are at an increased risk for infection. In this setting, disc space aspiration and/or vertebral biopsy is often necessary to exclude infection.

Patients with *ankylosing spondylitis* may develop pseudoarthrosis, which can mimic an infectious discitis by MRI (50). Again, follow-up MRI may help differentiate these two conditions.

Postoperative discitis occurs in 0.75% to 2.8% of postdiscectomy patients in various series (51,52). The cause is assumed to be direct inoculation of the avascular disc space. *S. aureus* is the most frequently recovered pathogen but in many cases no organism is recovered, suggesting an alternative inflammatory disc process in some cases. Boden et al. (53) compared the postoperative findings in asymptomatic patients undergoing discectomy with those in patients who developed postoperative discitis. Although there was some overlap in the disc space abnormalities and adjacent bone marrow abnormalities between the normal and abnormal group, the most reliable MR finding of postoperative discitis was the decrease in the signal intensity of adjacent vertebral bone marrow on T1-weighted images (Fig. 22), followed by enhancement of the same areas on postcontrast images (Fig. 23). The marrow enhancement appeared as a homogeneous horizontal band on either side of the disc space. Unenhanced T2-weighted sequences were less reliable because they were not present in the bone marrow of some patients with discitis. Enhancement of the annulus fibrosus was an unreliable finding. High sig-

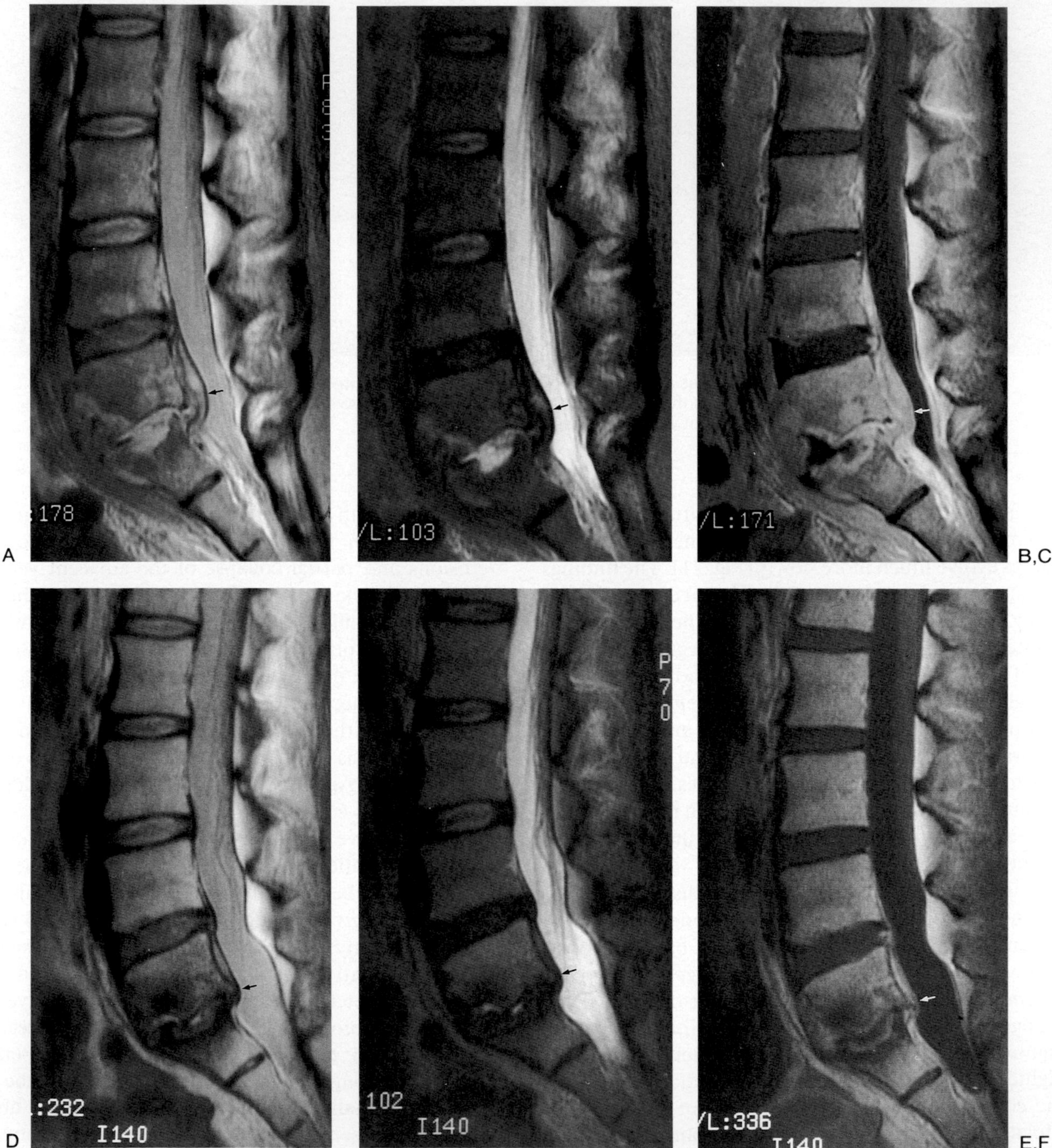

FIG. 21. Discitis: evolution following therapy. A 55-year-old woman with no infectious risk factors presenting with severe low back pain. **A,B:** Sagittal proton-density and T2-weighted images demonstrate typical findings of L5-S1 discitis and a large epidural mass suggesting epidural abscess (*arrow*). **C:** Postgadolinium T1-weighted images demonstrate no area of low intensity in the epidural mass to suggest pus. This appearance is more suggestive of granulation tissue. **D,E:** Sagittal proton-density and T2-weighted images. **F:** Sagittal postcontrast T1-weighted image images following antibiotic treatment demonstrates almost complete resolution of the disc infection and epidural granulation (*arrow*). Note the complete loss of disc height with fusion of the L4-L5 vertebral body. The patient was asymptomatic.

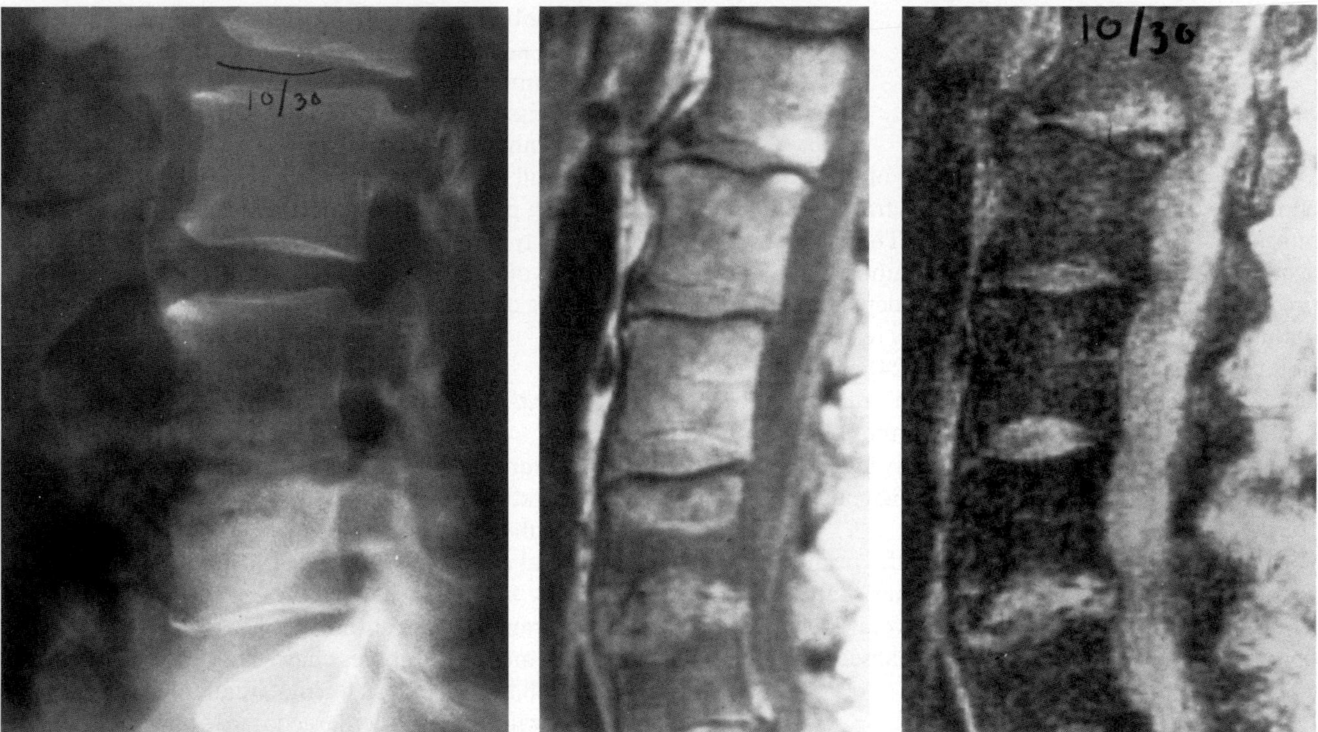

A B,C

FIG. 22. Postoperative discitis. **A:** Plain films show erosion of the vertebral endplates at L4-L5. **B:** Sagittal T1-weighted image demonstrates loss of height of the disc and decreased intensity of the adjacent vertebral body marrow. **C:** Sagittal T2-weighted image demonstrates increased signal intensity in the adjacent vertebral endplates.

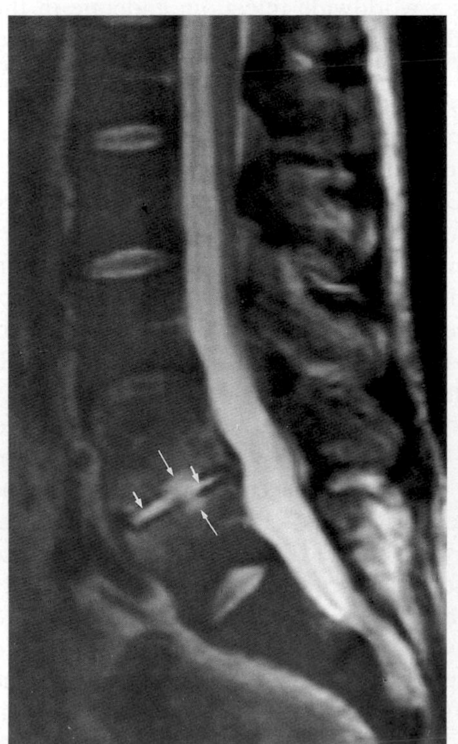

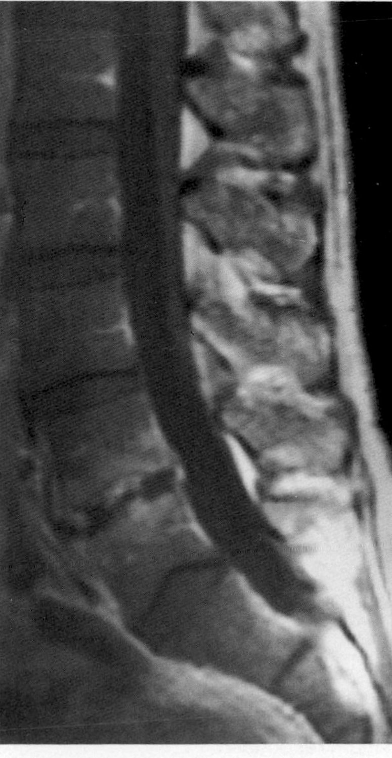

A,B

FIG. 23. Fifty-year-old man with back pain. **A:** Sagittal T2-weighted images demonstrate narrowing of the L4-L5 intervertebral disc (*arrows*), irregularity, and slight increase in the signal intensity of the adjacent endplates (*long-stem arrows*) consistent with signs of early infection. There is no evidence of an epidural abscess. **B:** Postcontrast T1-weighted images demonstrate patchy areas of enhancement within the disc and enhancement of the adjacent endplates. Note the lack of an epidural abscess.

nal intensity on T2-weighted images developing in a previously dehydrated disc was also a useful finding suggesting discitis.

Epidural Abscess

Acute epidural abscess is the result of direct hematogenous seeding of the epidural space from a cutaneous, pulmonary, or urinary tract source. The most common agent is *S. aureus*. Diabetes and immunosuppression are predisposing factors. The symptoms depend on the level of the infection. Epidural abscess may result in compression of the cord in the cervical (Fig. 24) and thoracic region and thecal sac compression with cauda equina syndrome in the lumbar spine. Thrombophlebitis of the epidural veins or adjacent arteries may lead to infarction of the cord (Fig. 25). At surgery, frank pus is often encountered (43).

Chronic epidural abscess is often the result of discitis and contains granulation tissue rather than frank pus. The infection often extends over several levels. MRI is helpful in the diagnosis of epidural abscess by demonstrating an extradural mass (54) (Fig. 26). The complete extent of involvement and the degree of cord compression are both clearly delineated by MRI. Gadolinium is usually not necessary for the diagnosis, but may be helpful in subtle cases (55–57) to distinguish epidural granulation tissue from a frank abscess. Epidural granulation tissue enhances homogeneously, whereas an epidural abscess will enhance in the periphery and contain nonenhancing pus in its center (58) (Fig. 27). This differentiation may be useful in surgical planning (59). Areas of signal void within the epidural collection suggest a gas-forming organism (60).

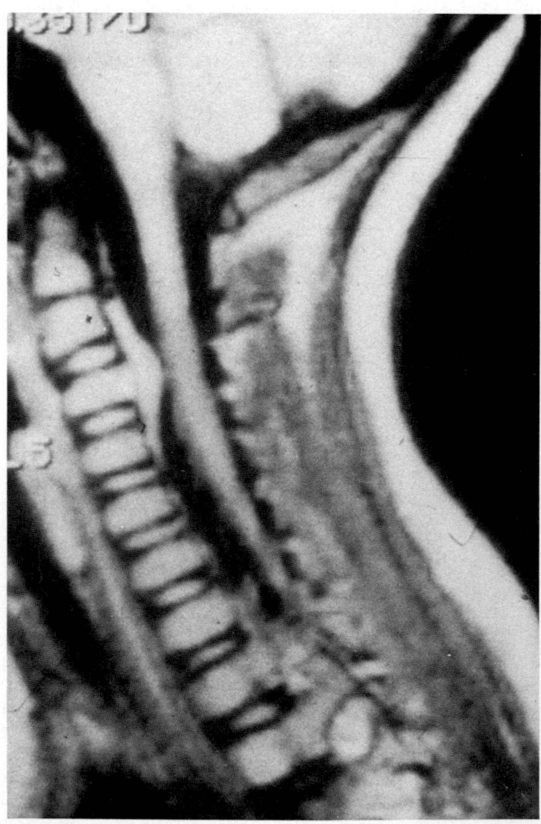

FIG. 24. Acute cervical epidural abscess in a 4-year-old boy with neck pain and fever. Sagittal T1-weighted image demonstrates an anterior epidural mass centered at C4. The patient responded to antibiotics. (From Colombo et al., ref. 45, with permission.)

Subdural and Intramedullary Abscesses

Subdural and intramedullary abscesses are extremely rare conditions secondary to hematogenous spread of the organism to these structures. The clinical presentation of subdural abscesses (Fig. 28) is similar to that of epidural abscess. Intramedullary abscesses can cause back pain and a transverse myelitis-type picture.

Intramedullary abscess has been reported on gadolinium-enhanced MRI as a ring-enhancing intramedullary lesion with a slightly enlarged cord. Infected syrinx can also appear as an intramedullary abscess (Fig. 29).

Brucellosis

Brucellosis is a worldwide infection, endemic in the Midwest United States. The infection in humans follows the ingestion of unpasteurized milk. The organism penetrates the lymphatics from the gastrointestinal tract and spreads to the reticuloendothelial system. The bone involvement is rare and involves the lumbar spine (61).

Even though both tuberculosis and brucellosis induce a granulomatous inflammatory reaction in the spine, certain distinguishing features often allow differentiation of the two conditions by MRI. Brucellosis has a predilection for the lower lumbar spine (Fig. 30), whereas tuberculosis tends to favor the lower thoracic spine. In brucellosis the height of the vertebral bodies is usually preserved even though signal abnormalities are noted consistent with osteomyelitis. In tuberculosis the vertebral bodies are severely damaged, with marked gibbus deformity. Brucellosis tends to spare the posterior elements that may be affected by tuberculosis. The disc tends to be preserved in brucellosis whereas it is severely destroyed by tuberculosis. Brucellosis rarely extends into the epidural space whereas tuberculosis often extends to form epidural abscesses and involve the meninges. The paraspinous soft tissues are rarely affected by brucellosis and commonly affected by tuberculosis, which causes cold abscesses. Spinal deformities are rare with brucello-

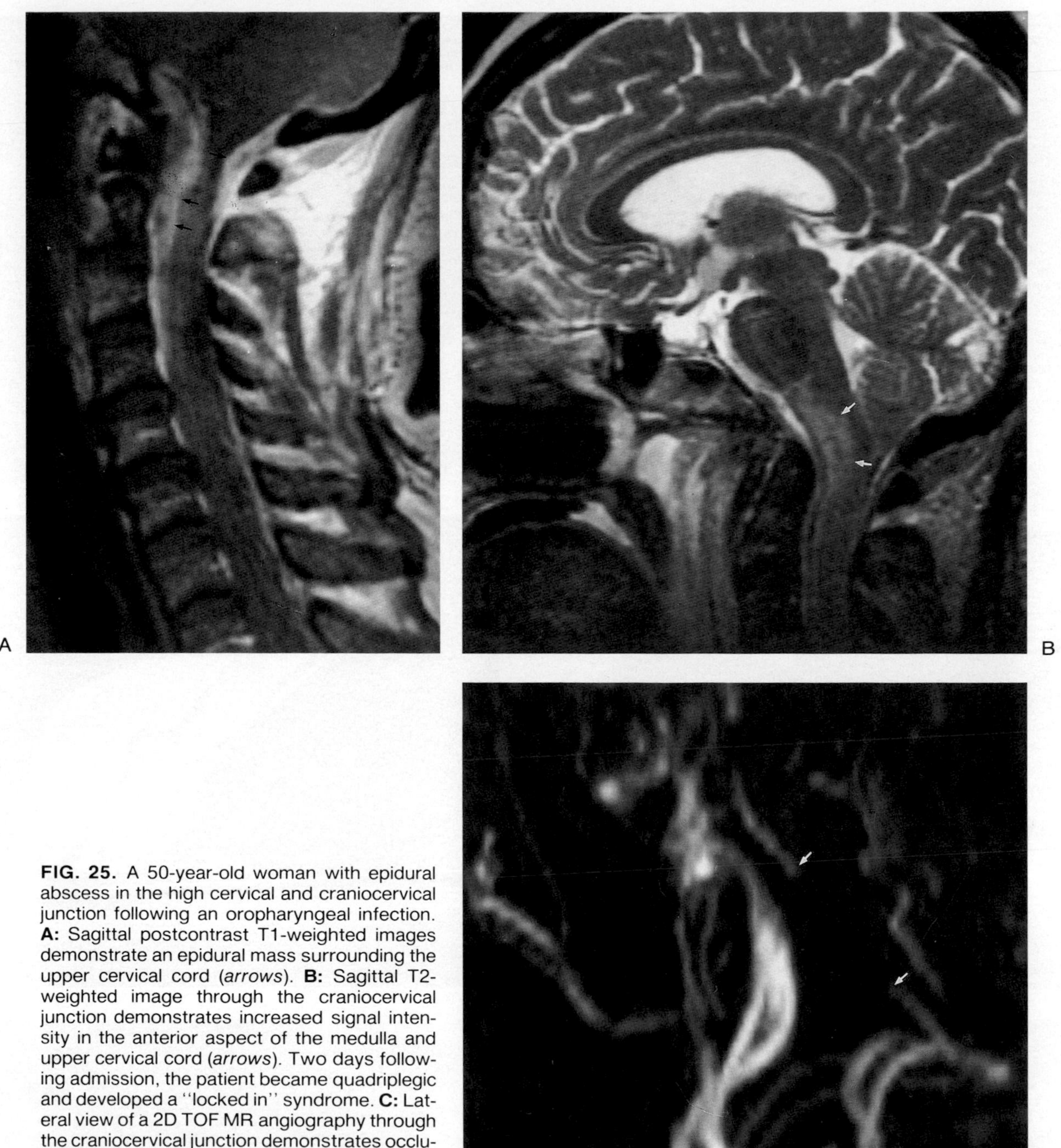

FIG. 25. A 50-year-old woman with epidural abscess in the high cervical and craniocervical junction following an oropharyngeal infection. **A:** Sagittal postcontrast T1-weighted images demonstrate an epidural mass surrounding the upper cervical cord (*arrows*). **B:** Sagittal T2-weighted image through the craniocervical junction demonstrates increased signal intensity in the anterior aspect of the medulla and upper cervical cord (*arrows*). Two days following admission, the patient became quadriplegic and developed a "locked in" syndrome. **C:** Lateral view of a 2D TOF MR angiography through the craniocervical junction demonstrates occlusion of the lower aspect of the basilar artery (*arrows*).

sis and common in tuberculosis. These radiographic findings enabled correct prediction of the type of infection in 94% of cases (62). The imaging findings are important because the percutaneous biopsy of the affected spinal region is of little use because the organisms are difficult to culture and the pathology shows a nonspecific granulomatous reaction. The diagnosis is confirmed by positive serologic results and/or positive blood cultures.

Actinomycosis

Actinomycosis is caused by an anaerobic organism found normally in the mouth flora. It usually disseminates from the oral cavity in debilitated individuals. Osseous involvement results from contiguous extension from adjacent tissues with the mandible and spine more commonly affected. The posterior elements of the spine

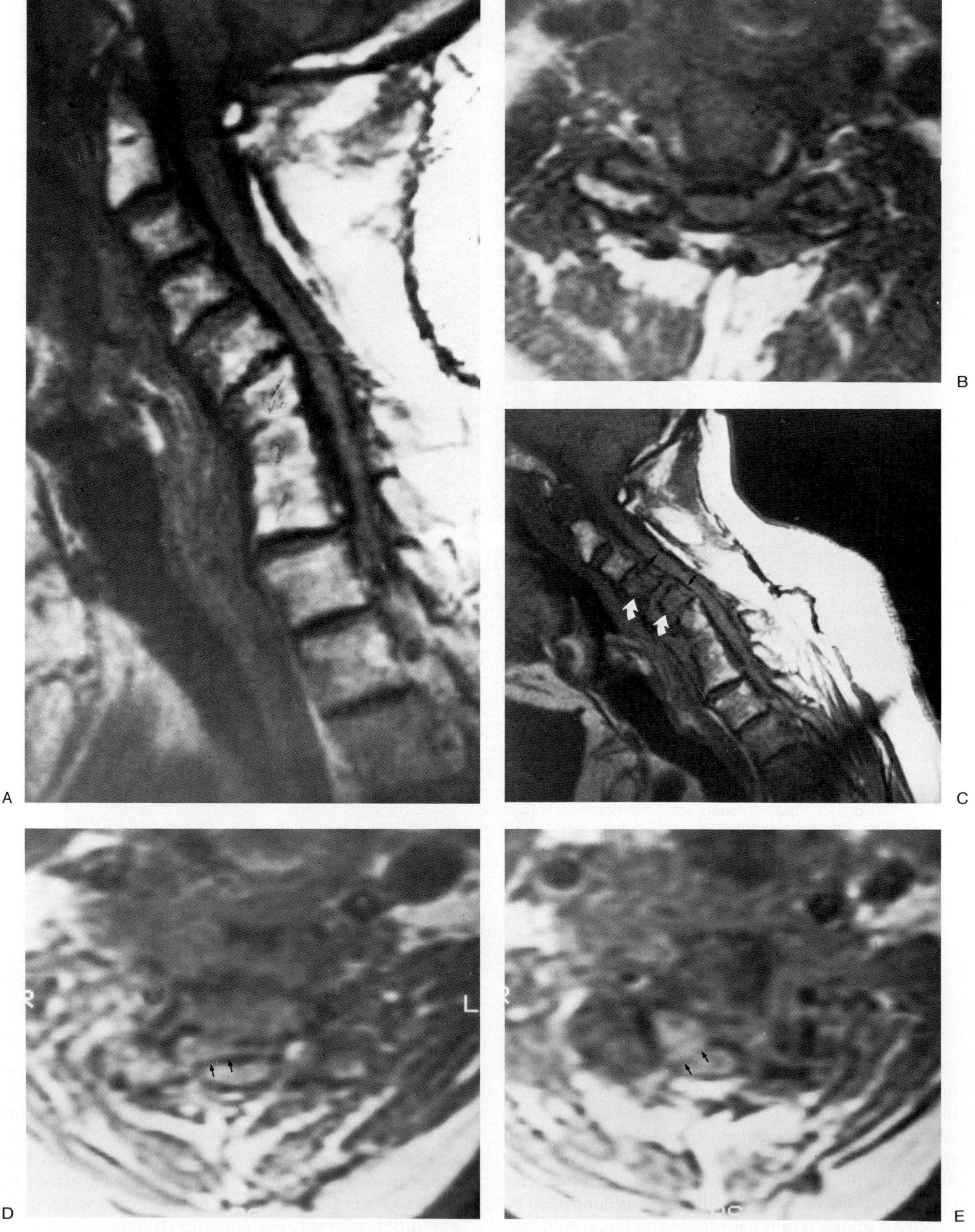
A
B
C
D
E
R
L
R

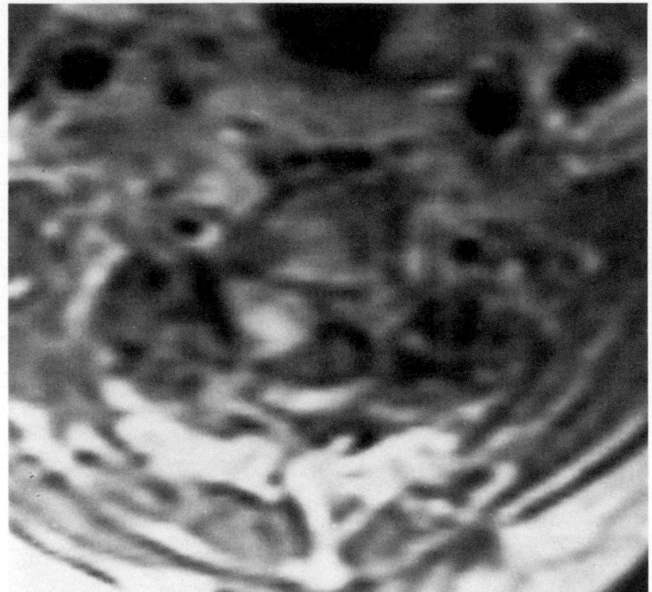
F

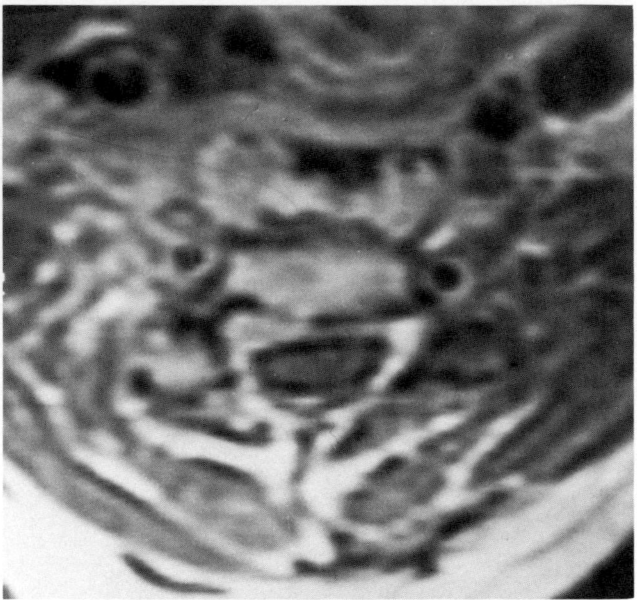
G

FIG. 26. Chronic epidural abscess in a 70-year-old diabetic patient. Sagittal (**A**) and axial (**B**) T1-weighted images demonstrate previous laminectomy and C6 to T1 fusion. Sagittal (**C**) and axial (**D, E**) T1-weighted images 6 weeks later; the patient had persistent pain and right shoulder weakness. Interval decrease in the intensity of C4 and C5 vertebral bodies (*white arrows*) and new anterior epidural mass (*black arrows*) compressing the cord and the C5 root. **F,G:** Axial T1-weighted images. The periphery of the epidural abscess enhances after gadolinium administration.

and ribs can be affected and the association of such findings with sinus tracts should suggest the diagnosis (41).

Syphilis

Syphilis caused by *Treponema pallidum* infection rarely affects the spine. Syphilitic transverse myelitis and polyradiculitis are rare manifestations of secondary syphilis. The disease is characterized pathologically by a plasmocytic infiltrate surrounding the vessels and affects primarily the meninges and the pia. The clinical manifestations are indistinguishable from transverse myelitis from any other cause.

MRI in patients with syphilitic myelitis has been reported (39,62). The precontrast images demonstrated a nonspecific increase in the signal intensity of the cord on T2-weighted images. After contrast there was enhancement of the pia and of the spinal cord nerve roots (Fig. 31). The lesions in one case resolved on follow-up imaging following adequate therapy with penicillin. The high intensity area in the cord on T2-weighted images may reflect ischemic changes secondary to the severe vasculitis, which may lead to cord infarction.

Neuroborreliosis (Lyme Disease)

Lyme disease is a tick-transmitted, spirochetal, infectious disease with multisystem inflammatory manifestations. It was first identified as a distinct entity in the United States in 1975 (63), and is the most commonly reported vector-transmitted disease in the United States. The causative organism, *Borrelia burgdorferi,* is transmitted by the nymph stage of infected ticks (*Ixodes dammini, Ixodes pacificus,* or *Ixodes ricinus*). These ticks are three-host organisms; in successive life stages, a tick may parasitize and infect a number of different animals, including mice, raccoons, and several other small mammals, in addition to the deer, which is the preferred host and breeding ground for the adult ticks.

In most patients, the first evidence of Lyme disease is the appearance of a skin lesion, erythema chronicum migrans (ECM), at the site of a tick bite. Other signs and symptoms commonly associated with the early stage of Lyme disease include fever, chills, myalgias, arthralgias, headache, stiff neck, and exhaustion. Several weeks to a few months after the onset, most untreated patients have signs and symptoms of disseminated Lyme disease. In general, the sequence of organ involvement is predictable, but it can vary. Many patients do not seek treatment until late in the disease; therefore, initial clinical presentation with carditis, meningoencephalitis, or Lyme arthritis is not uncommon.

The neurologic manifestations of Lyme disease are variable (64) and may occur anytime from a few days after the onset of the disease to years later. In the United States, neurologic signs develop within the first few months of illness in 10% to 15% of persons not treated during the early stage of the disease. These include, in various combinations, meningitis, encephalitis, sensory

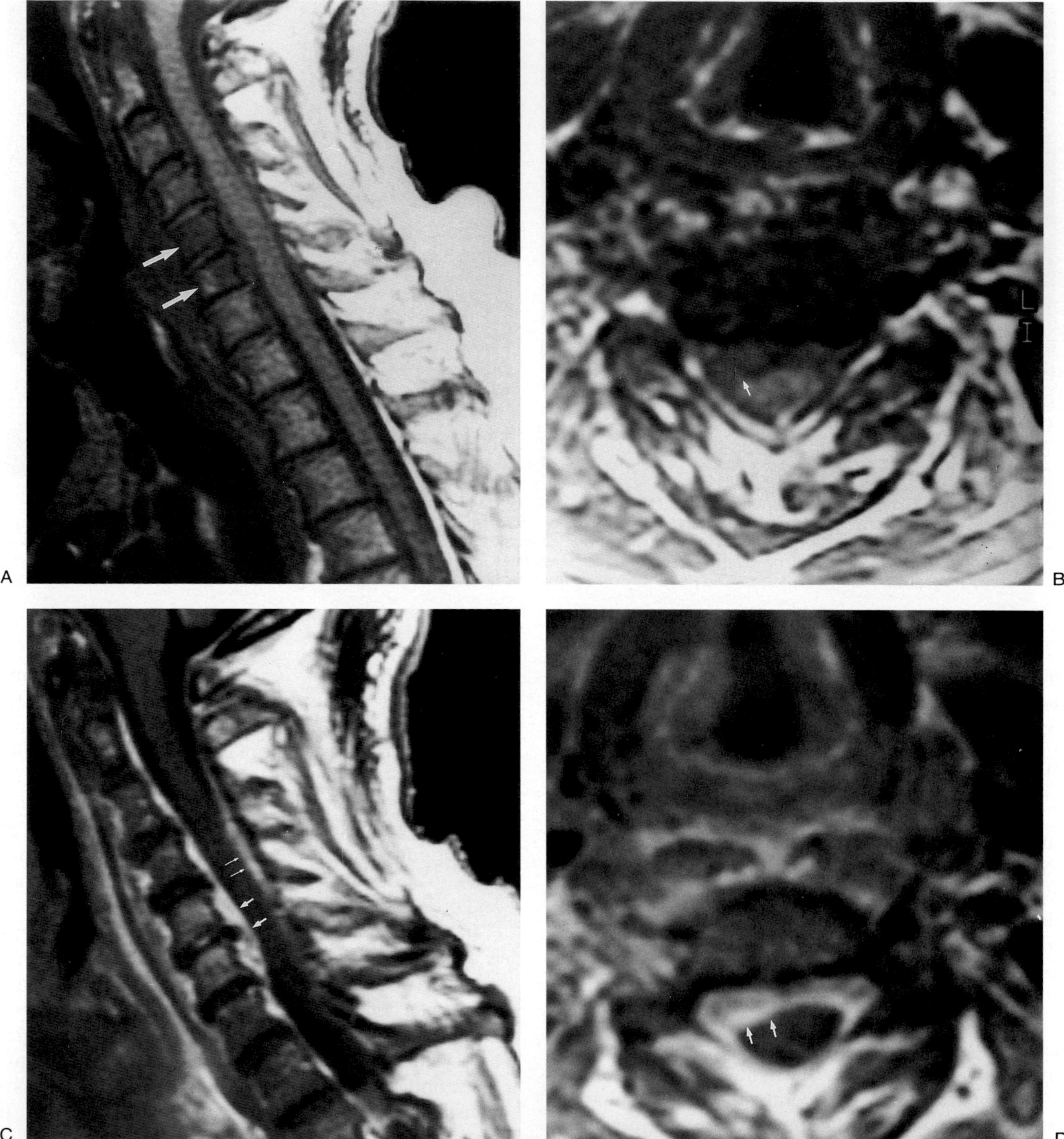

FIG. 27. Cervical epidural abscess following discography. A 50-year-old woman with severe neck pain 10 days following discography. **A:** Sagittal T1-weighted image demonstrates a decrease in the signal intensity of C5 and C6 vertebral bodies (*arrows*) and a questionable anterior epidural soft tissue at the C5-6 level. **B:** Axial T1-weighted image precontrast demonstrates definite anterior epidural lesion (*arrow*) with slight cord compression. **C:** Postcontrast sagittal T1-weighted image demonstrates an enhancing anterior epidural mass (*arrows*) and slight enhancement of the C5 and C6 vertebral bodies consistent with an epidural abscess and osteomyelitis. Note also slight enhancement of the posterior epidural space at the C4 level (*small arrows*). **D:** Axial T1-weighted images confirm the enhancing lesion. Note the slight low density of the anterior epidural lesion (*arrows*) suggesting pus rather than granulation tissue.

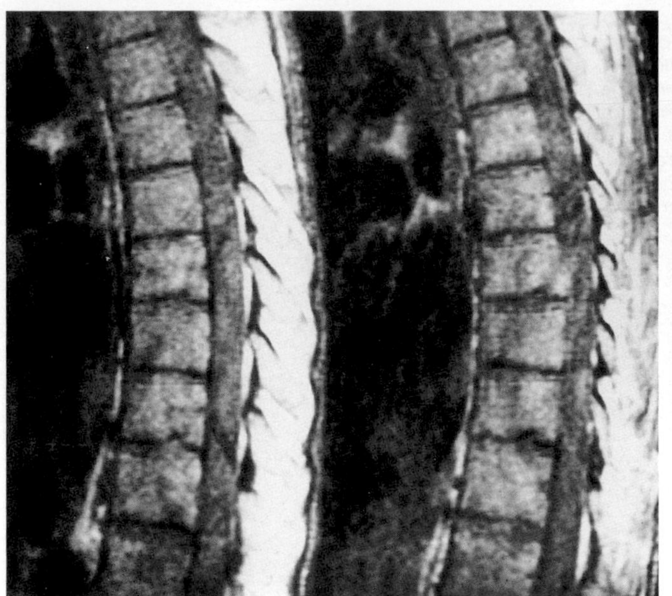

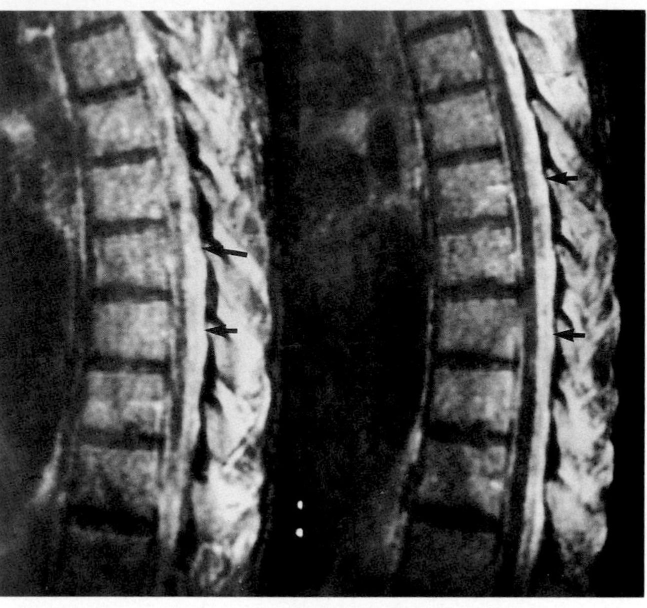

FIG. 28. Enterococcal meningitis. A 26-year-old man with fever who subsequently developed sepsis and tetraparesis. Gram-positive cocci in CSF smear and enterococci grown from blood confirmed enterococcal meningitis. **A,B:** Two adjacent sagittal pre- (A) and post- (B) contrast T1-weighted images of thoracic spine. Precontrast image (A) shows loss of normal spinal cord–CSF interface and poor characterization of the type or location of the abnormality. On postcontrast image (B), diffuse, thick, intradural enhancement (*arrows*) outlining the spinal cord locates the disease in the intradural extramedullary compartment. (From Gero et al., ref. 38, with permission.)

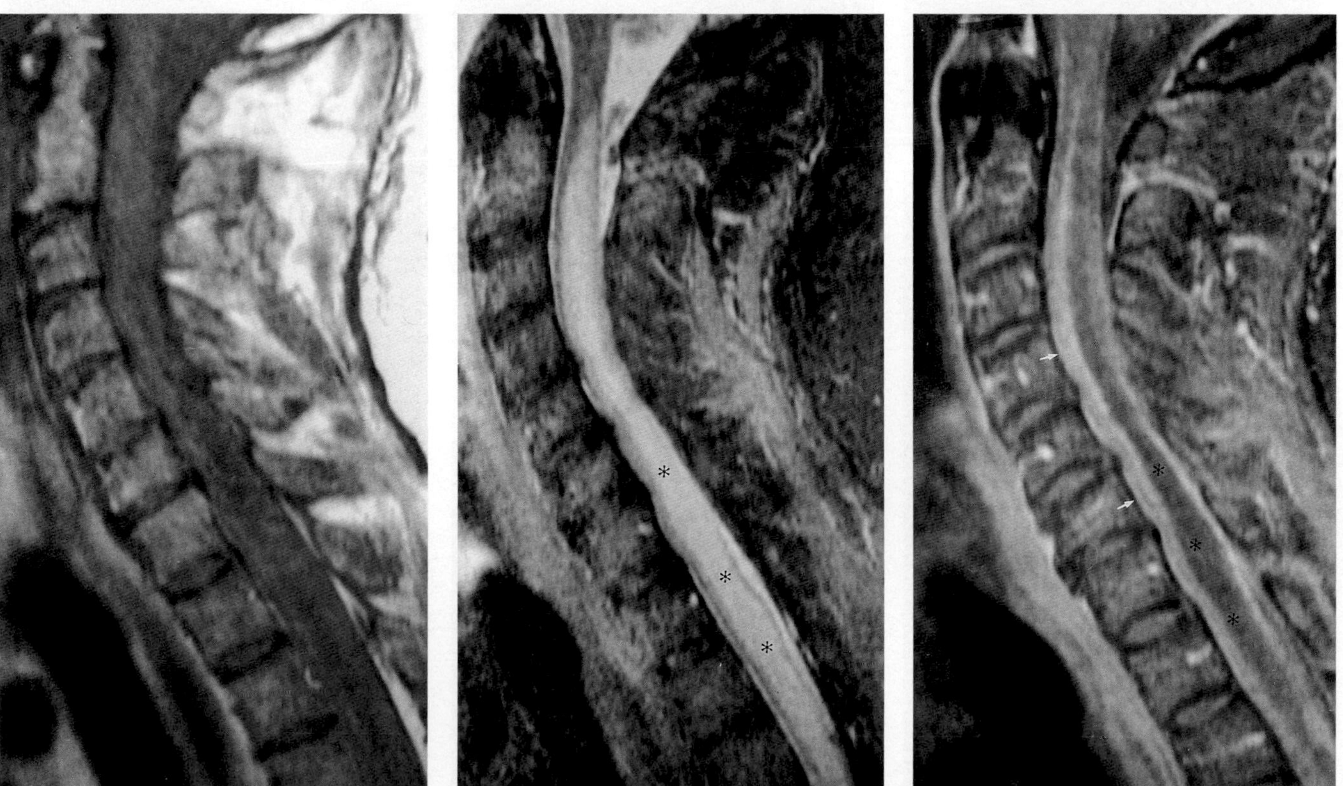

FIG. 29. Intramedullary abscess in a 60-year-old man with long-standing paraplegia who became quadriplegic over 6 hours. **A:** Sagittal T1-weighted image demonstrates marked expansion of the cord. **B:** Sagittal T2-weighted image demonstrates diffuse hyperintensity of the cervical cord (*asterisks*). **C:** Postcontrast sagittal T1-weighted image demonstrates diffuse enhancement of the periphery of the cord (*arrows*) and a low intensity center (*asterisks*). At surgery, the posterior columns were split open and pus was coming out from the central cavity.

FIG. 30. Brucellosis in a 30-year-old man. **A:** Coronal STIR image demonstrates a focus of high intensity in the L4 vertebral body (*small arrow*) and a paraspinous high intensity lesion consistent with granulation (*large arrow*). Pre- (**B**) and post- (**C**) contrast axial T1-weighted images, and axial (**D**) T2-weighted image confirm the paraspinous granulation (*arrow*). Follow-up MRI 8 weeks later demonstrates considerable extension of the disease. **E:** Coronal STIR image demonstrate enlargement of the paraspinous granulation area and increased signal in the L3, L4, and L5 vertebral bodies consistent with osteomyelitis (*asterisks*). Sagittal T2-weighted image (**F**) and postcontrast T1-weighted image (**G**) show the associated epidural granulation (*arrows*) and the disc space enhancement as well as the disc herniation at L3-L4.

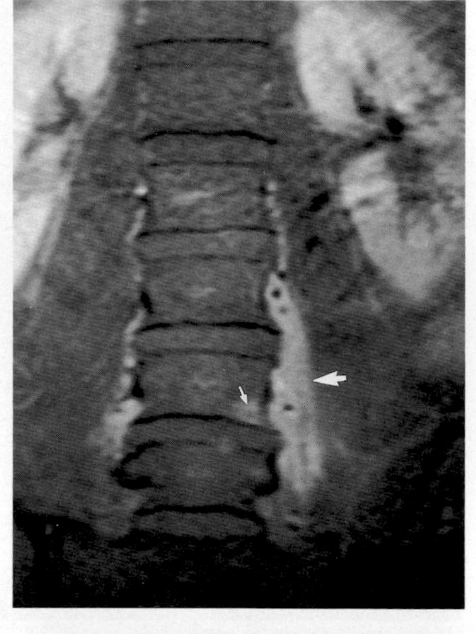

A

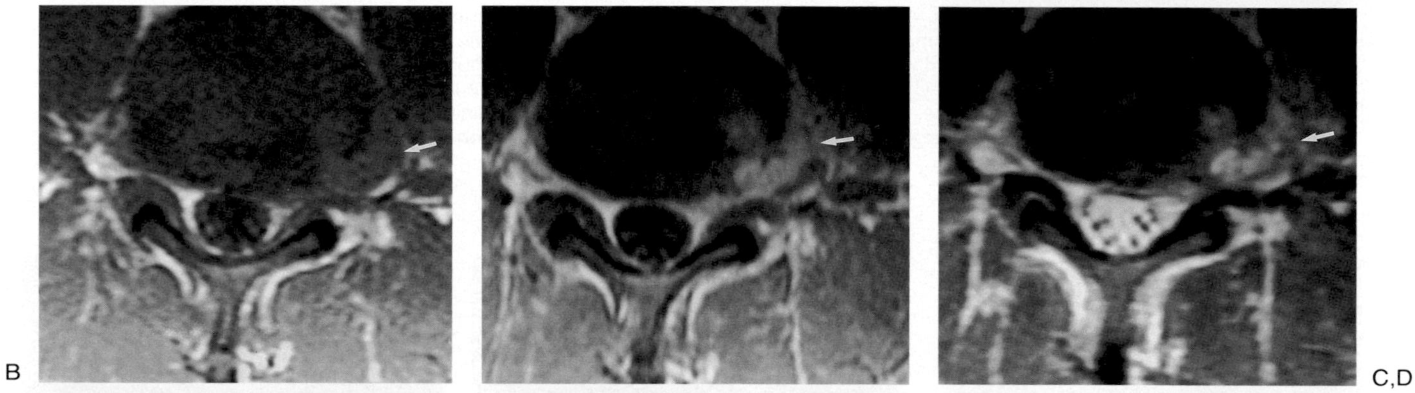

B

C,D

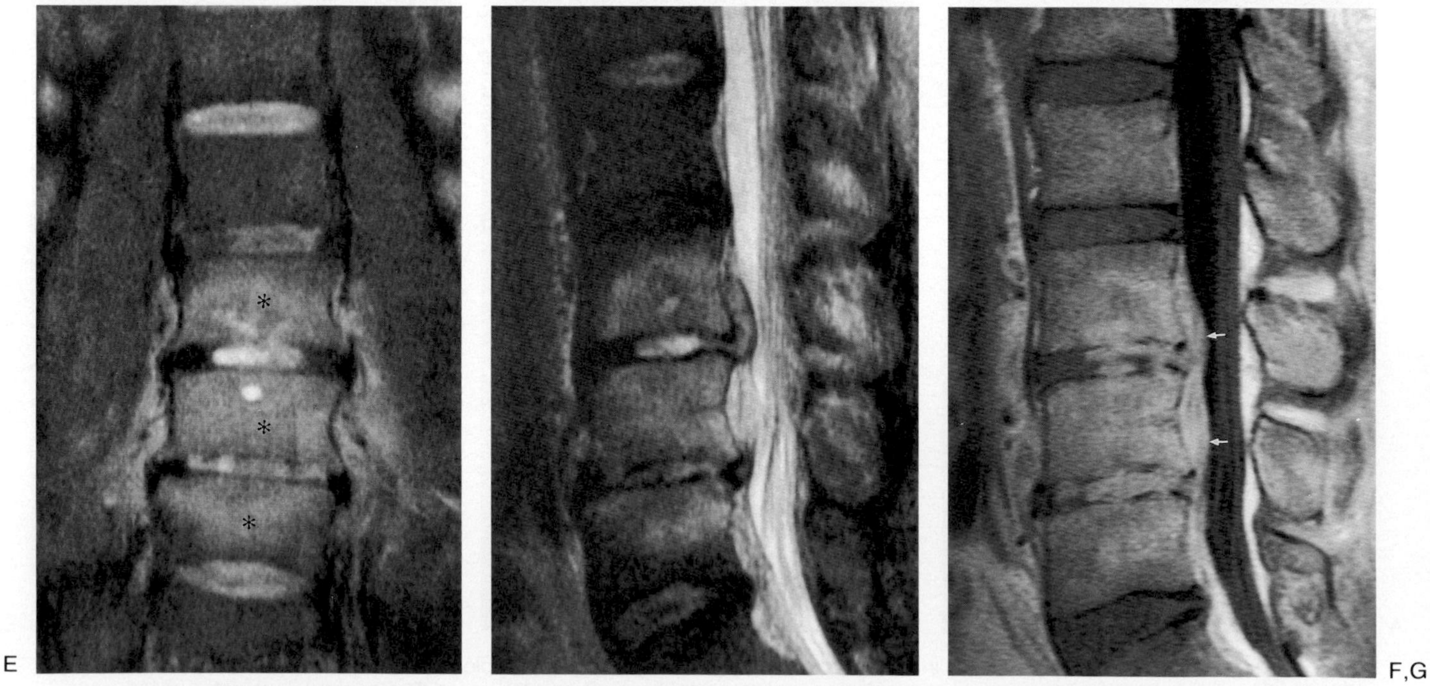

E

F,G

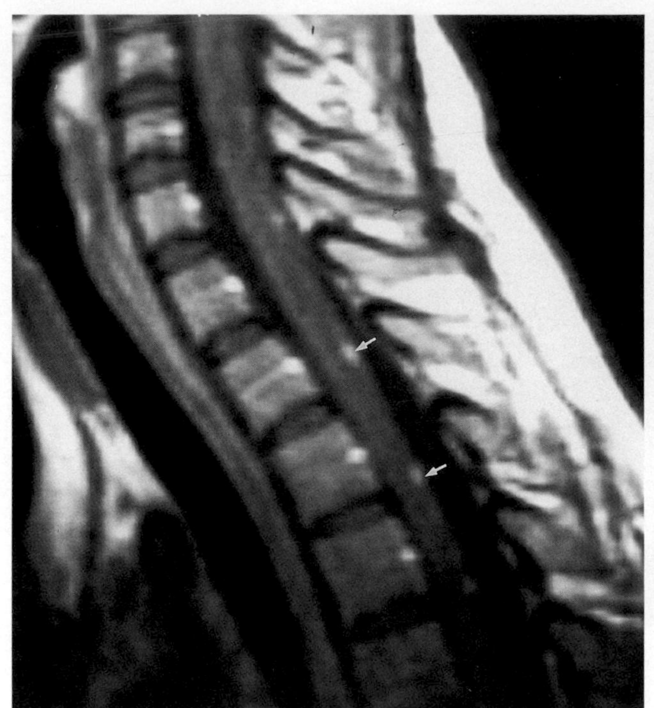
A

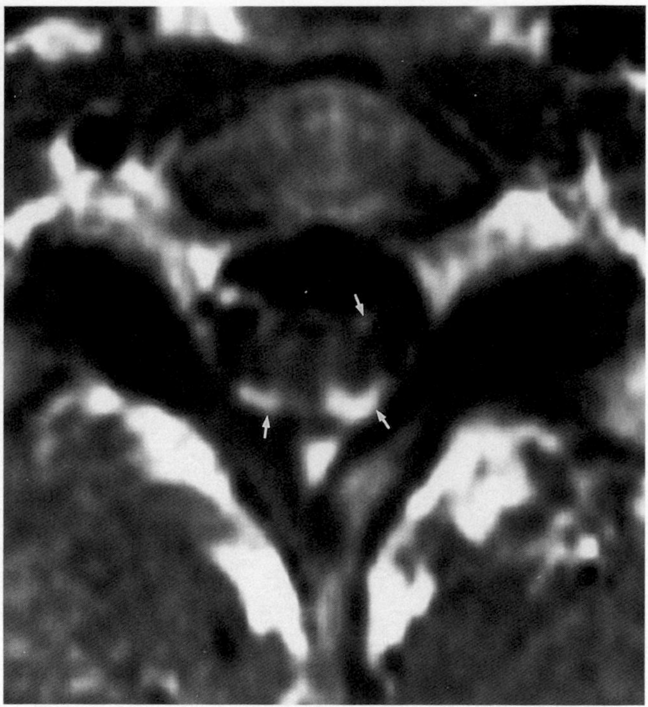
B

FIG. 31. Syphilitic polyradiculopathy. A 23-year-old HIV-positive Ethiopian woman with sudden onset of profound bilateral polyradiculopathy. **A:** Sagittal T1-weighted image postcontrast demonstrates multiple foci of pial enhancement on the dorsal aspect of the lower cervical and upper thoracic cord (*arrows*). **B:** Axial T1-weighted image postcontrast demonstrates enhancement of the cervical roots (*arrows*). CSF studies confirmed the diagnosis of syphilis. A follow-up study after antibiotic therapy demonstrated resolution of the enhancement and the patient's condition improved. (Courtesy of Dr. P. Blake, Washington, D.C.)

and motor radiculoneuritis, and cranial neuritis. MRI may show enhancement of the leptomeninges and nerve roots as they exit the cord (Fig. 32). Lyme meningitis and encephalitis seem to be caused by direct borrelial infection of the CNS, and generally appropriate antibiotic therapy is rapidly effective.

Listeriosis

Listeria monocytogenes commonly causes meningitis in the immunocompromised core host and less frequently brain or spinal cord abscesses. The disease may occur in individuals with occupational exposure to farm animals and occasionally in patients with no predisposing factors. The diagnosis is often difficult and the organism is rarely identified from CSF cultures but, more commonly, from blood cultures. In a recent case report (65), an intramedullary listeria abscess was demonstrated on MR as an area of increased signal intensity on T2-weighted images and an elongated ring-enhancing lesion on postcontrast T1-weighted images.

Tuberculosis

Over the world, tuberculosis is the most common cause of vertebral body infection, particularly in Third World countries. The current acquired immunodeficiency syndrome (AIDS) epidemic is responsible for a recrudescence of tuberculosis cases in the United States and, in particular, of spinal tuberculosis. Seventy-five percent of cases of tuberculous spondylitis occur before the age of 20 years. The involvement of the vertebral body occurs through hematogenous spread of mycobacterium tuberculosis from a pulmonary source that may go unrecognized. Cord compression (Fig. 33) and neurologic deficit due to epidural extension occurs in 10% to 20% of patients. These neurologic symptoms may be reversed more easily than in pyogenic infections. Infection usually starts anteriorly in the vertebral body and in 50% of the cases spreads through the disc space to the adjacent vertebral body. Extension to distant vertebra can occur secondary to subligamentous spread. The posterior elements are less frequently involved than in pyogenic or fungal infection. Massive bone destruction and severe gibbus deformity (Fig. 33) is characteristic of this infection. Paraspinous masses that may calcify are also strongly suggestive of tuberculous abscess (Fig. 34). Typical features on MRI include destruction of the anterior aspect of one or two vertebral bodies (66). In the early stages, differentiation from pyogenic infection or a small neoplasm may be difficult.

Tuberculous radiculomyelitis is most commonly a secondary tuberculous lesion, although it may rarely oc-

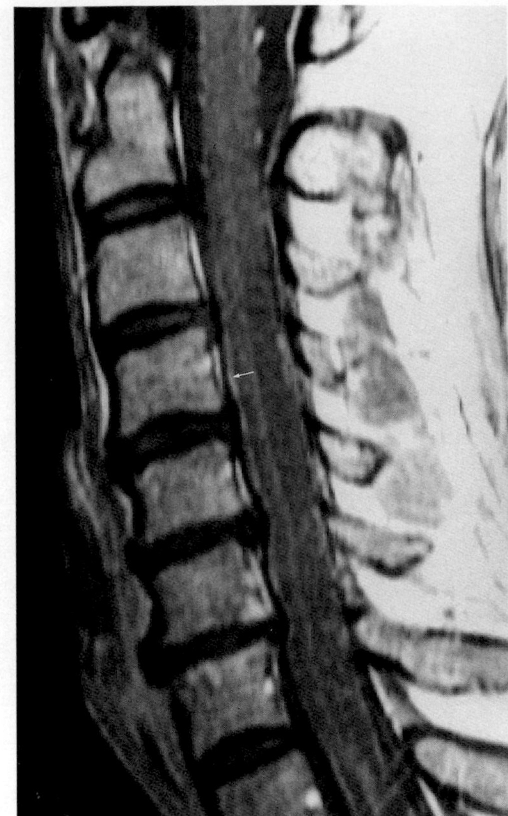
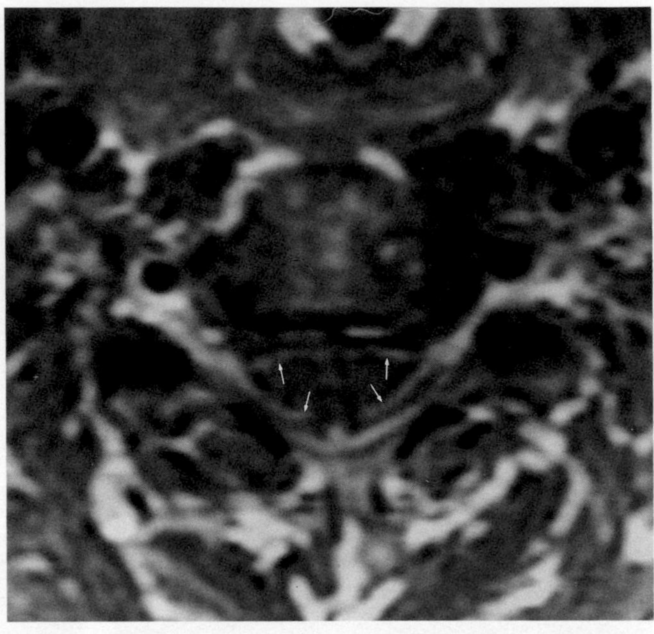

A B

FIG. 32. Lyme meningitis. **A:**. Sagittal T1-weighted image post-contrast demonstrates pial enhancement (*arrow*). **B:** Axial post-contrast T1-weighted image demonstrates enhancement of the roots (*arrows*). (Courtesy of Dr. Monteserrante, Washington, D.C.)

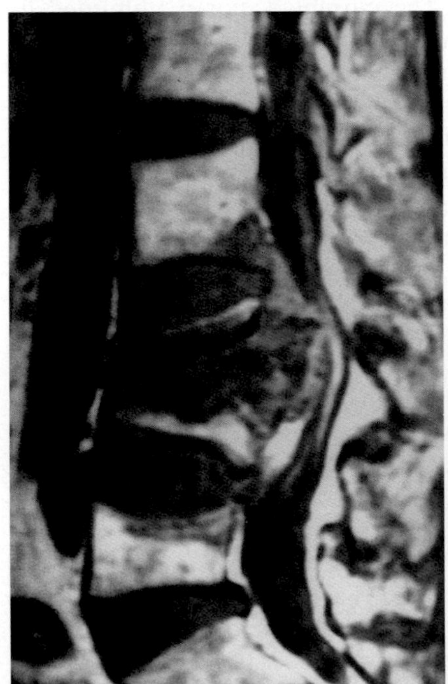
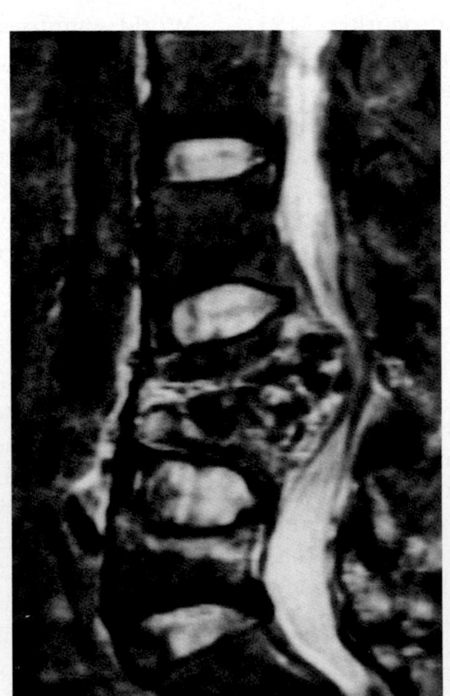
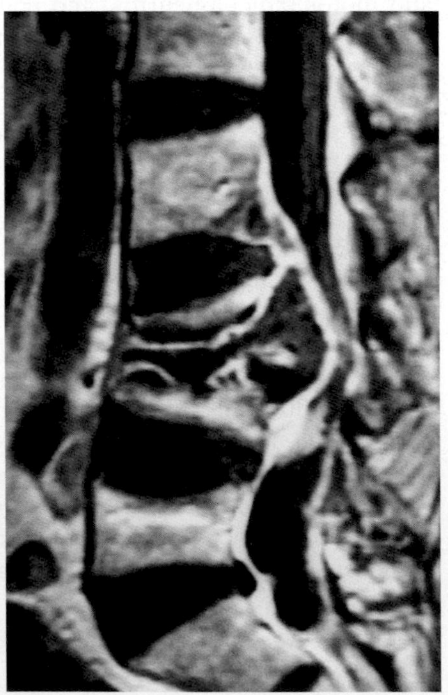

A B,C

FIG. 33. Pott's disease **A:** Sagittal T1-weighted image demonstrates destruction of the L3-L4 disc and adjacent vertebral bodies, with the large epidural abscess compressing the sac. **B:** Sagittal T2-weighted image. The high signal in the vertebral body is consistent with tuberculous osteomyelitis. **C:** Postcontrast sagittal T1-weighted image. (Courtesy of Dr. Sung Lee, Seoul, Korea.)

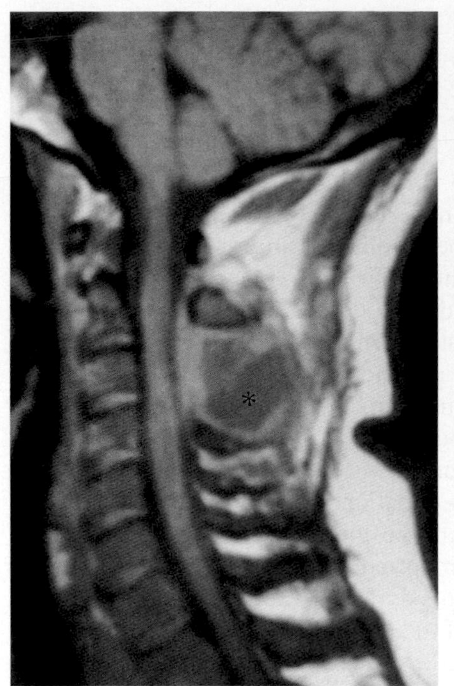

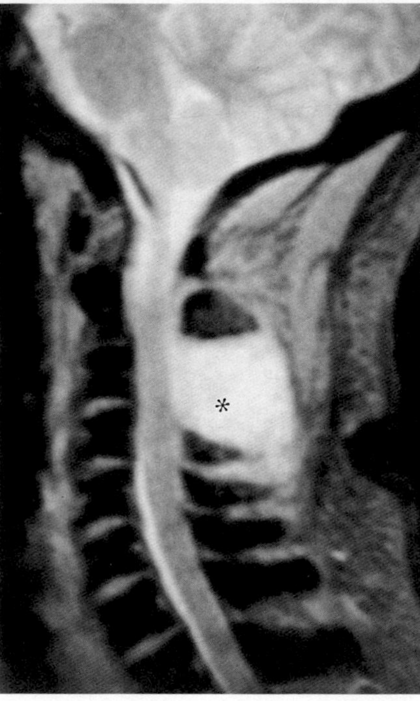

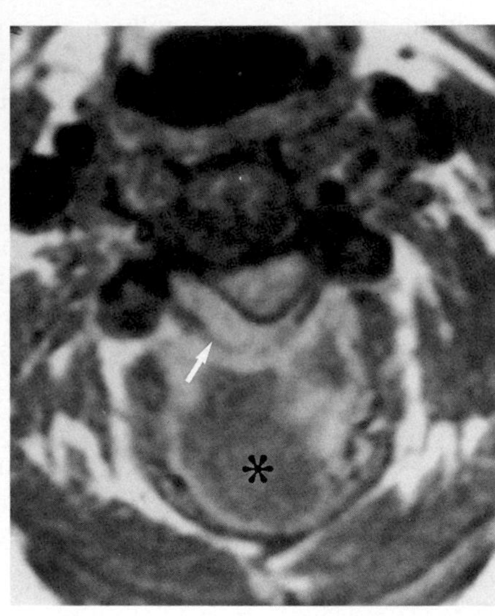

A,B C

FIG. 34. Cervical tuberculous abscess in a migrant farmer with neck pain. **A,B:** Sagittal T1- and T2*-weighted images demonstrate a posterior collection replacing the C3 spinous process (*asterisk*) and compressing the posterior epidural space (*arrow*). **C:** Axial T1-weighted image in the same patient confirms these findings. (Courtesy of Drs. M. Koby and C.S. Zee, Los Angeles, CA.)

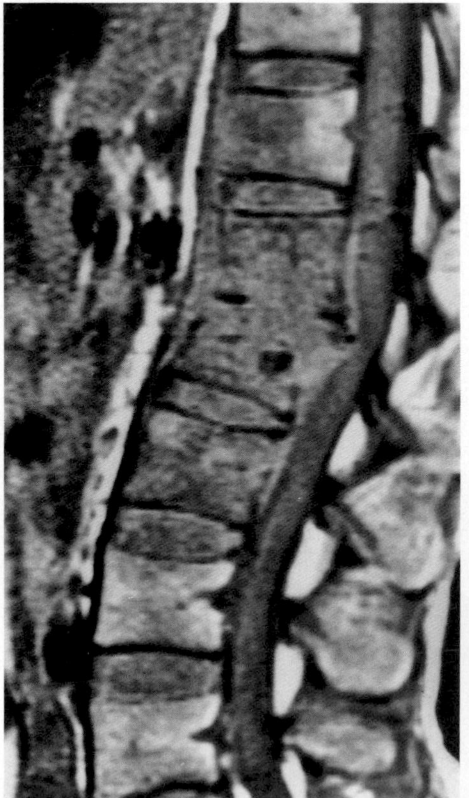

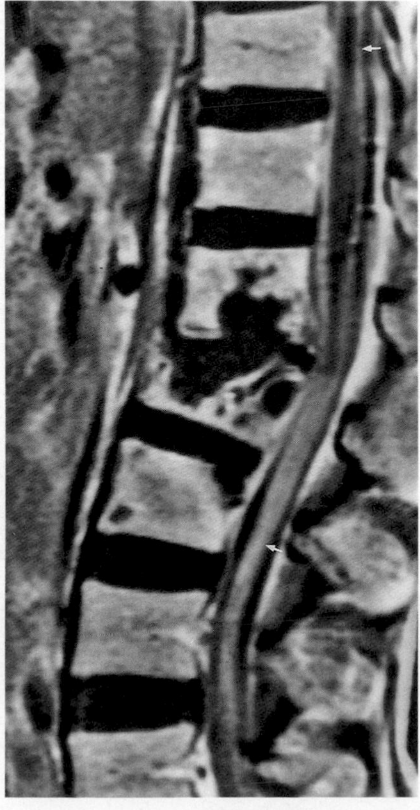

A,B

FIG. 35. Tuberculous discitis and polyradiculopathy. **A,B:** Sagittal pre- (A) and post- (B) contrast T1-weighted images of lumbar spine. Precontrast image (A) shows destruction of the disc and adjacent endplates with mild gibbus deformity. Postcontrast image (B) demonstrates marked enhancement of the nerve roots of the cauda equina and of the pia along the lower thoracic spine (*arrows*). (Courtesy of Dr. Sung Lee, Seoul, Korea.)

cur primarily. The disease may appear during the acute state of primary tuberculosis or in variable periods after the onset of the disease. Most patients with spinal radiculomyelitis secondary to tuberculosis are less than 30 years old, in contrast to the typical form of spinal arachnoiditis, which is seen usually in older patients. The clinical features of this condition include paraplegia and quadriplegia, pain, and other radicular symptoms depending on the site involved.

The meninges of the cord show variable degrees of congestion and inflammatory exudates throughout their course. The spinal root and nerve roots are surrounded by gelatinous exudates and may be edematous. The tuberculoma may be located anywhere within the thecal sac. It is usually closely adherent to the inner aspect of the dura and may dig a crater in the cord, making it difficult to determine whether an intradural tuberculoma is extramedullary or intramedullary (67). In the chronic stages, fibrin-covered roots stick to each other and to the thecal sac, forming dense collagen adhesions by proliferating fibrocytes.

Contrast-enhanced MR demonstrates enhancement of the dura-arachnoid complex (Fig. 35), indicating the presence of active meningeal inflammation (Fig. 36) and may demonstrate the intramedullary tuberculoma (Fig. 37) as nodular areas of enhancement (38,68). Expansion of the cord with diffuse increase in intensity on T2-weighted images may reflect cord edema without an intramedullary tuberculoma or infarction secondary to vasculitis or myelitis. During the chronic stages the roots and the thickened dura do not enhance; these changes are difficult to distinguish from postsurgical or postpyogenic infection arachnoiditis.

Mycobacterium avium-intracellulare complex (MAC) was previously considered a rare condition, but it has recently been recognized with increased frequency among immunosuppressed patients, in particular patients infected with human immunodeficiency virus (HIV). The disease has been reported in up to 30% of living patients and 50% of patients dying of AIDS. In addition to massive infiltration of the lymph nodes, the marrow may be diffusely infiltrated (69) with MAC, resulting in diffuse

A,B

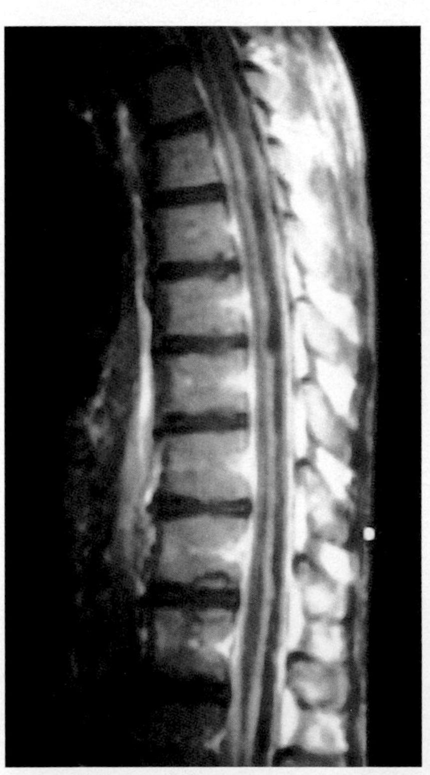

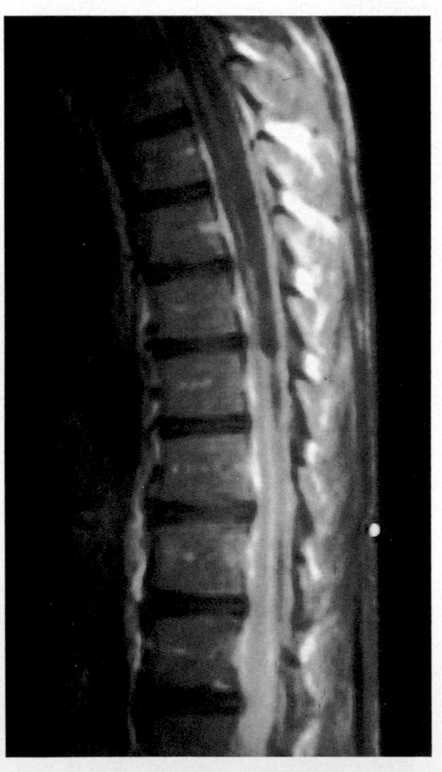

C

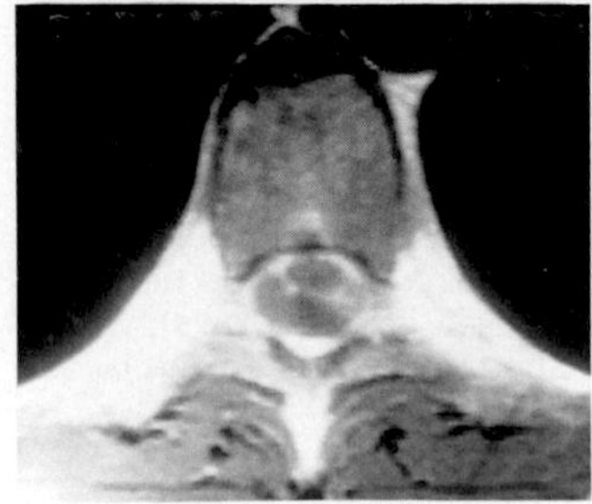

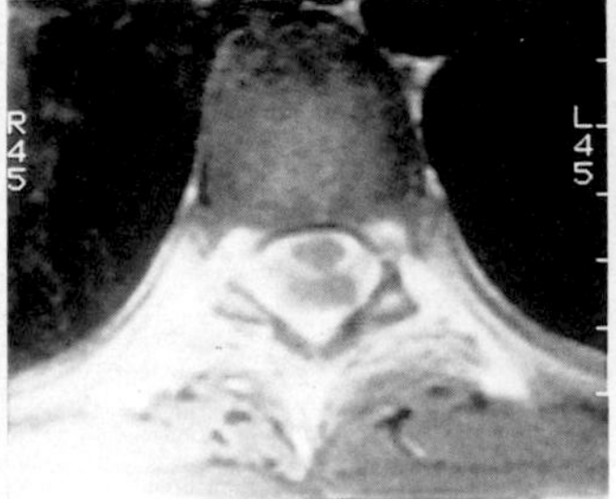

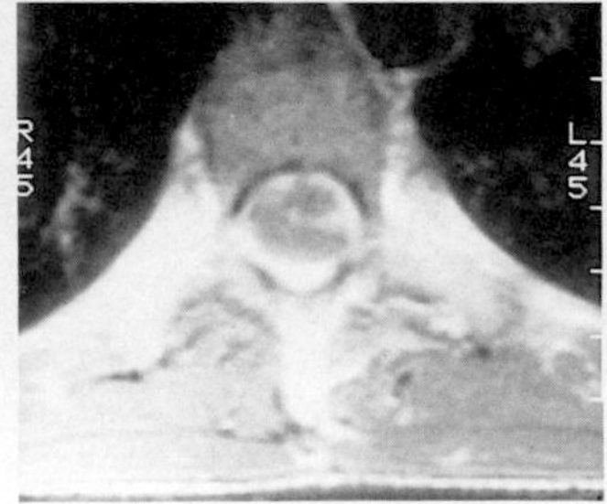

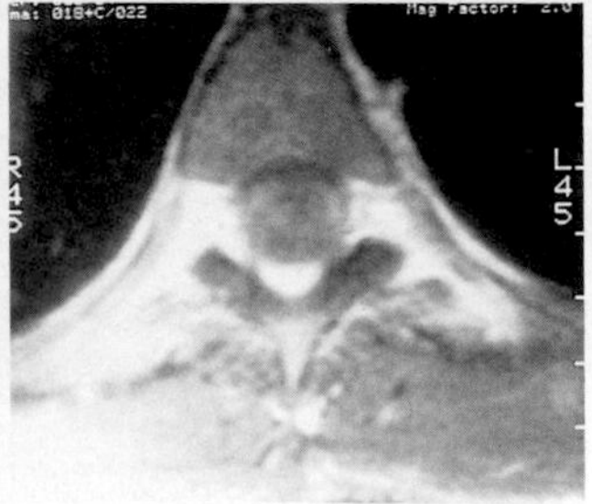

FIG. 36. TB meningitis in a 16-year-old with progressive lower extremity weakness and paresthesias. **A–C:** MRI after gadolinium shows extensive diffuse enhancement along surfaces of spinal cord. Note loculations on axial images (C). (Courtesy of Dr. Renato Mendonça, São Paulo, Brazil.)

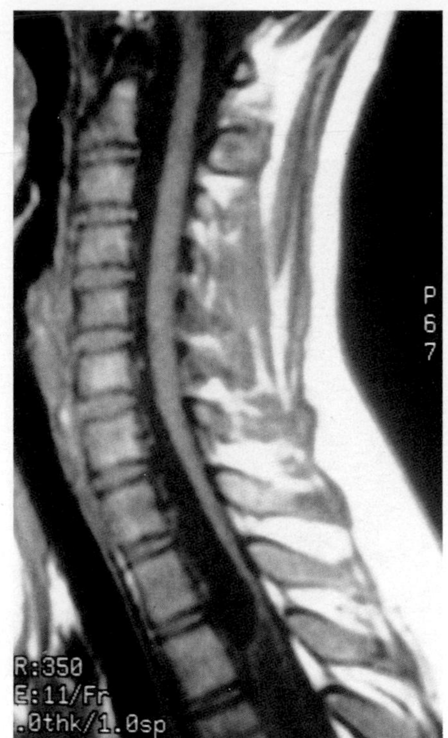

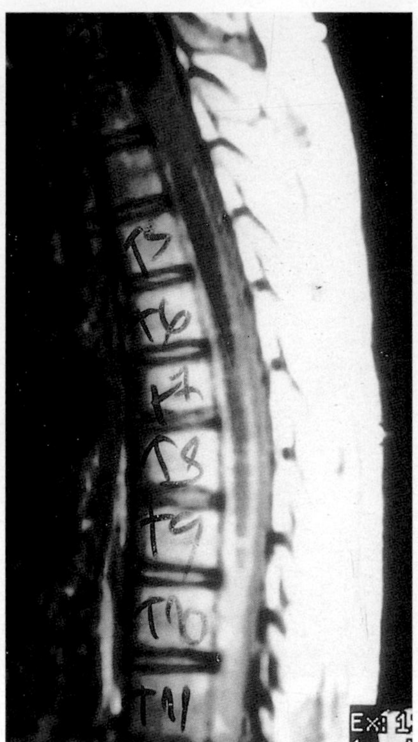

A,B

FIG. 37. Intradural extramedullary TB with syrinx in a 15-year-old complaining of progressive lower extremity paresthesias and weakness. (Courtesy of Dr. Renato Mendonça, São Paulo, Brazil.) Extramedullary intradural lesion in upper thoracic region is associated with large syrinx in mid- to lower thoracic spinal cord and extensive intradural enhancement (**A,B**).

decreased intensity on T1-weighted image. This appearance, however, is nonspecific because it may be seen with any diffuse inflammatory or neoplastic process involving the marrow. Epidural extension of the MAI infection indistinguishable from other infections may be seen (Fig. 38).

Fungal Infections

Fungal infections of the spine can be divided into two principal categories: those induced by pathogens, and those produced by saprophytes in patients who are immunocompromised by conditions such as diabetes, leukemia, lymphoma, prolonged use of antibiotics, steroids, or HIV infection (70). These infections are called opportunistic and include meningitis, formation of abscesses and granulomas, and, because of the invasion of the walls of the vessels, thrombosis leading to cord infarction.

Blastomycosis

North American blastomycosis is caused by *Blastomyces dermatitides.* The disease is found in southern Africa, South America, and in the south, central, and mid-Atlantic states in the United States (71). Disease is acquired by inhalation of spores with bone involvement in about 50% of patients with systemic disease. The disease may be both a primary infection and occur as an opportunistic infection. In the nervous system, the disease can present as meningitis or as single or multiple abscesses. The meninges may be involved in the form of an extradural lesion that causes pachymeningitis leading to compression of the underlying cord. The fibropurulent exudates may result in obstruction of the CSF flow of the foramen magnum and hydrocephalus. The prognosis is exceedingly poor (71). The center of the abscess contains caseous necrotic material, neutrophiles, and lymphocytes, and is surrounded by epithelioid and multinucleated giant cells of the Langhans type. The fungus is identifiable in sections stained with hematoxylin and eosin.

The radiologic features are nonspecific and similar to tuberculosis (71). The adjacent ribs are frequently involved (Fig. 39).

Coccidioidomycosis

Coccidioidomycosis is caused by *Coccidioides immitis* and is endemic in the southwestern United States (70). The primary focus is the lung. The disease is not an opportunistic infection. It usually causes a mild upper respiratory illness. Osseous manifestation occurs in 10% to 50% of patients with disseminated disease (72). The disease does not result in gibbus deformity. This organism seems to occur frequently at bony protuberances. Aside from this observation, the MR findings are nonspecific (Fig. 40) and diagnosis is made by biopsy in a patient from an endemic area. In addition to the bone

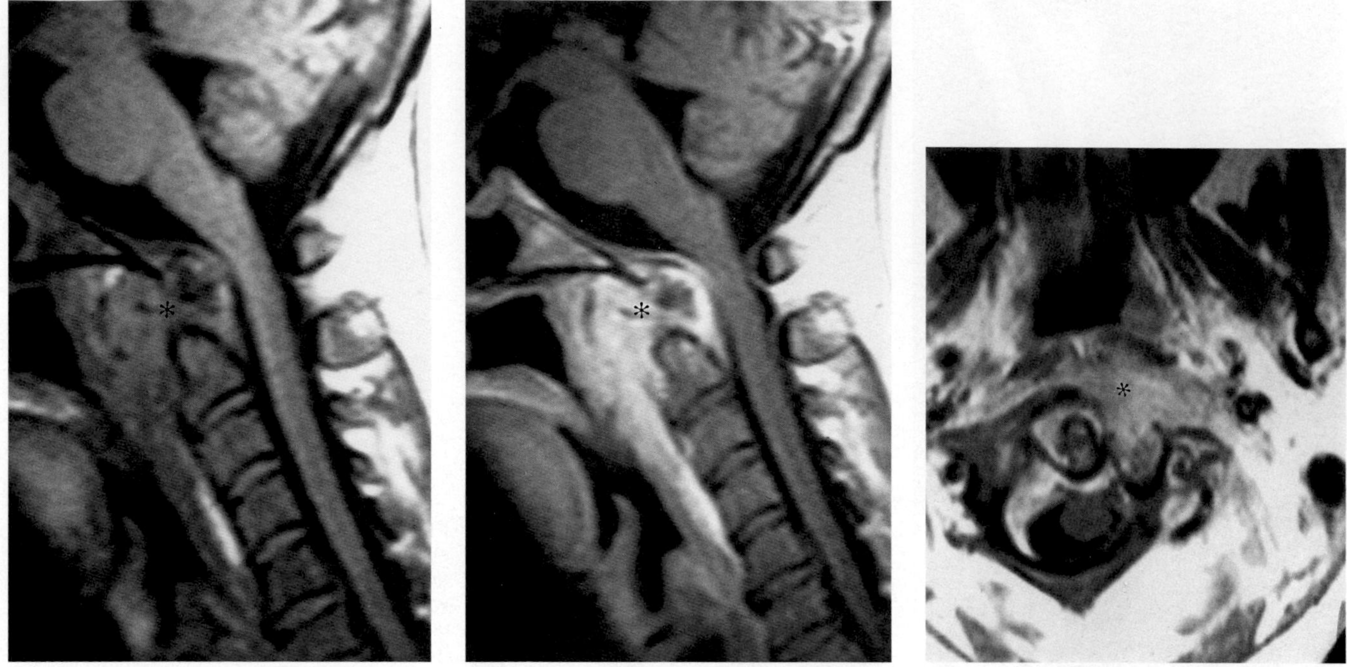

FIG. 38. Mycobacterium avium intracellulare (MAI) epidural abscess in an immunosuppressed patient. **A:** Sagittal T1-weighted image demonstrates abnormal signal intensity and destruction in the C2(*asterisk*) vertebral body and an anterior epidural abscess. **B:** Postcontrast sagittal and, **C,** axial T1-weighted image demonstrate the abscess to better advantage. (Courtesy of Drs. N. Petronas and M. Koby, Bethesda, MD.)

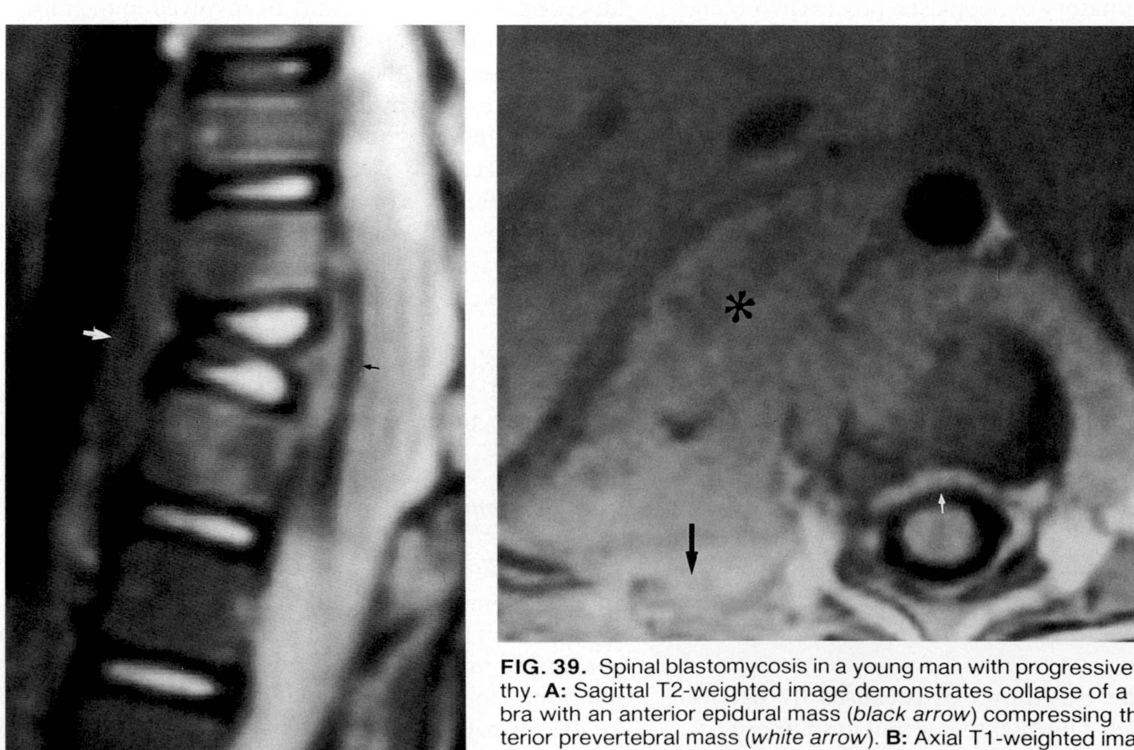

FIG. 39. Spinal blastomycosis in a young man with progressive thoracic myelopathy. **A:** Sagittal T2-weighted image demonstrates collapse of a midthoracic vertebra with an anterior epidural mass (*black arrow*) compressing the cord and an anterior prevertebral mass (*white arrow*). **B:** Axial T1-weighted image confirms these findings. Note also the anterior prevertebral mass (*asterisk*) and the rib destruction (*black arrow*). (Courtesy of Dr. Azmi Hamzaoglu, Istanbul, Turkey.)

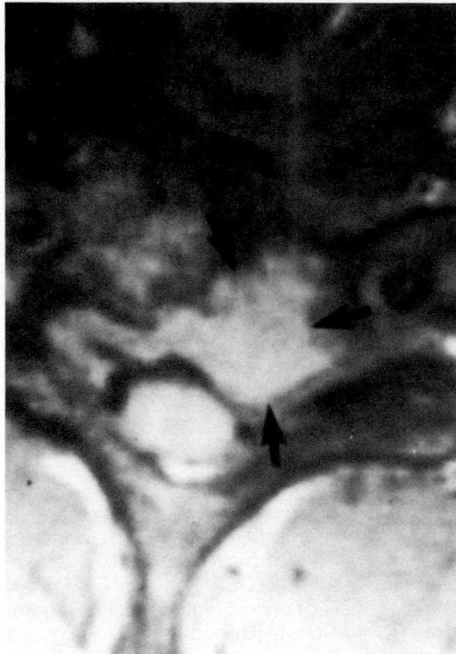
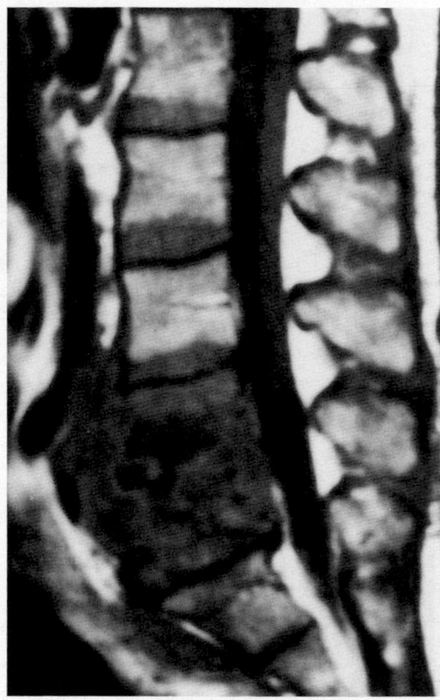
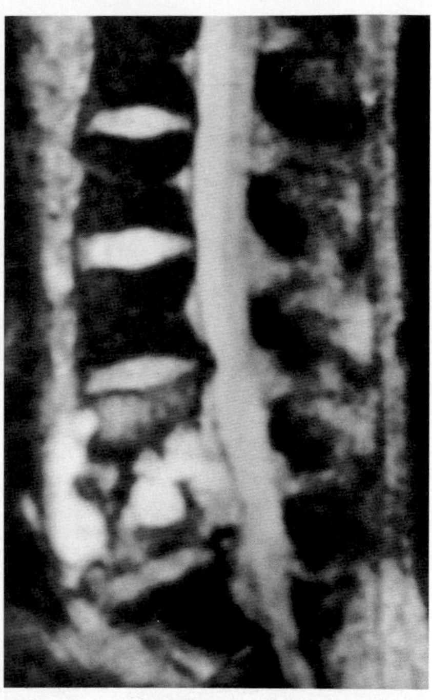

A B,C

FIG. 40. Coccidioidomycosis. **A:** A 22-year-old man with a 3-month history of neck pain, fever, and left C8 radiculopathy. Axial T2-weighted image demonstrates a left anterior epidural mass originating in the vertebral body. **B,C:** Coccidioidomycosis of the lumbar spine in another patient. Sagittal (B) T1-weighted image and (C) T2-weighted image demonstrate severe destruction of the L4 and L5 vertebral bodies and intervertebral disc and a prevertebral and anterior epidural mass. The radiographic appearance is not specific. (Courtesy of Dr. M. Koby, Bethesda, MD.)

involvement, the CNS manifestation includes meningitis primarily of the skull base, and granulomatous lesions may involve the spinal cord and the roots of the cauda (Fig. 41).

Nocardiosis

Nocardia asteroides is the causative agent of this infection. It is an opportunistic parasite associated with patients who are immunosuppressed. The CNS is invaded from a primary pulmonary lesion. The disease results in an abscess and/or meningitis and the spinal cord has been occasionally involved (73).

Aspergillosis

Aspergillosis is ubiquitous, with more than 350 species known, although the most common pathogen is *Aspergillus fumigatus,* consisting of branching septate hyphae with a diameter of 3 to 10 μm. It is estimated that 60% to 70% of patients with disseminated aspergillosis have neurologic lesions (70). The disease may produce a granulomatous reaction, but commonly results in abscess formation. The gross appearance is either that of a pale, soft area sometimes with petechiae or necrotic and hemorrhagic lesions with central cavitation. Histologically, the most striking feature is the intensity of the vascular invasion with thrombosis. Aspergillus spinal cord abscess has been reported on MRI in an immunosuppressed patient (74). The lesion appeared as a nonspecific ring-enhancing medullary mass. An epidural abscess with cord compression secondary to aspergillosis has also been reported (75).

Candidiasis

Candida albicans is a worldwide cause of opportunistic fungal infection. The CNS is only occasionally involved by hematogenous dissemination, with primary focus in the respiratory gastrointestinal tract. The disease can occasionally occur in previously healthy individuals. The fungus usually produces a chain of elongated cylindrical cells and oval buds. The early brain lesions described resemble hemorrhagic infarcts with abscesses and granulomas without central foci of necrosis occurring later. The disease has been reported in the spinal cord (76), and may involve the disc space (Fig. 42).

Histoplasmosis

Histoplasmosis is caused by *Histoplasma capsulatum* and can be isolated from soil from domestic and wild animals. Epidemics have occurred as a result of exposure to chicken, pigeon, and starling manure and bat guano. The disease is endemic in some regions of the United States such as the Ohio Valley and central Mississippi

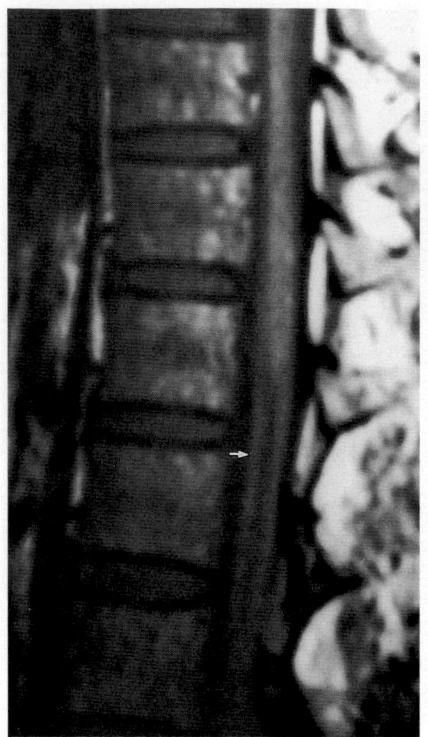

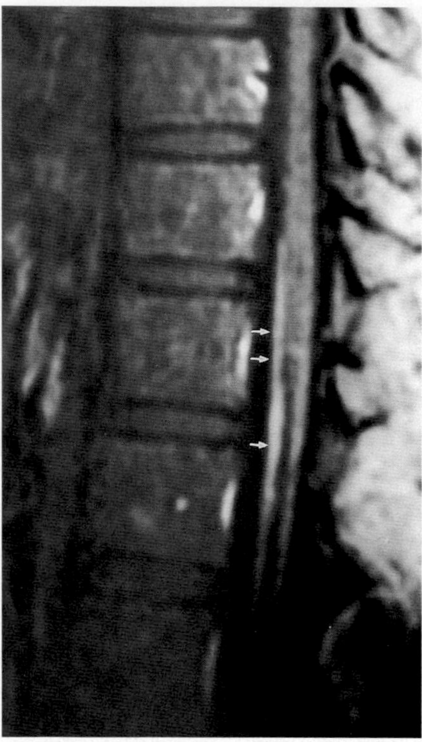

A,B

FIG. 41. Coccidioidomycosis polyradiculopathy. A 30-year-old HIV-positive man with a 3-month history of back pain and lower extremity weakness. CSF analysis confirmed the diagnosis of coccidioidomycosis. Sagittal pre- (**A**) and post- (**B**) contrast T1-weighted images demonstrate enhancement of the pia over the conus and of the roots of the cauda equina (*arrows*). (Courtesy of Dr. C. Lindan, San Francisco, CA.)

Valley. The disease may occur as an isolated benign infection or disseminated infection, which is usually due to reinfection involving the lungs. Involvement of the CNS is uncommon. A case of intramedullary histoplasma granuloma has been reported (77).

Parasitic Infections

Parasitic infections of the spine are uncommon, but should be considered in endemic areas in patients with signs and symptoms of spine or spinal cord disease.

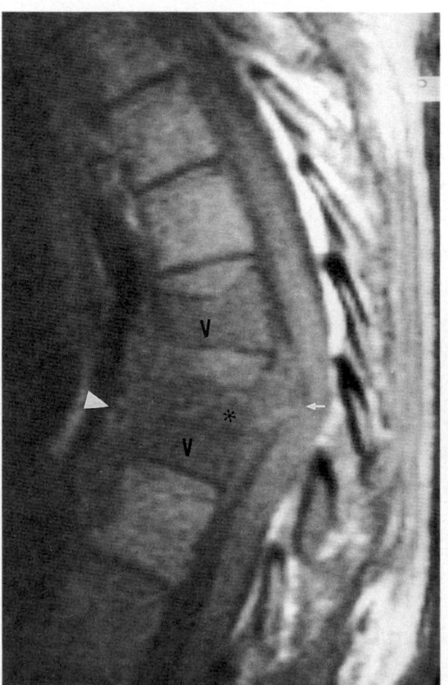

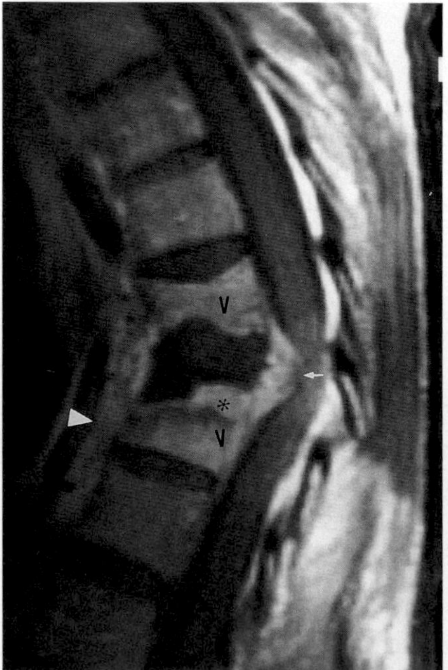

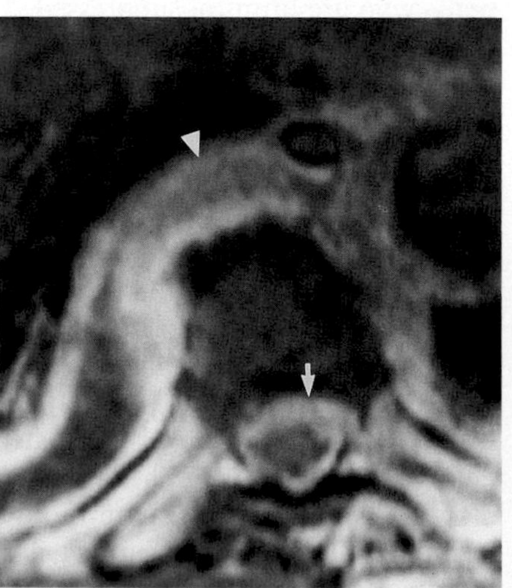

A,B C

FIG. 42. Candida discitis. A 70-year-old diabetic man with back pain and paraplegia. **A:** Sagittal T1-weighted image demonstrates destruction of the disc, vertebral body (*asterisk*), and adjacent end plates (*V*), and a prevertebral (*arrowhead*) and an epidural mass compressing the cord (*arrow*). Postcontrast (**B**) sagittal and (**C**) axial T1-weighted image demonstrate the epidural mass to better advantage. (Courtesy of Dr. P. Baum, Sacramento, CA.)

Cysticercosis

Cysticercosis is a world-wide disease particularly prevalent in South America and India. With increases in the number of immigrants from these countries, the disease has increased in frequency in the United States. The organism responsible for the disease is *Taenia solium,* a tape worm. In the duodenum, the shells of the ova are dissolved and the embryos penetrate the wall of the intestine and are carried by the circulation to all organs, including occasionally the spine. In the CNS the cysts can take several forms. In most cases, they remain small, sequestered, and eventually die. Less frequently, thin-walled racemose cysts develop in the subarachnoid space and basal cistern, causing hydrocephalus in the brain or cord compression (Figs. 43 and 44) in the spine (78,79).

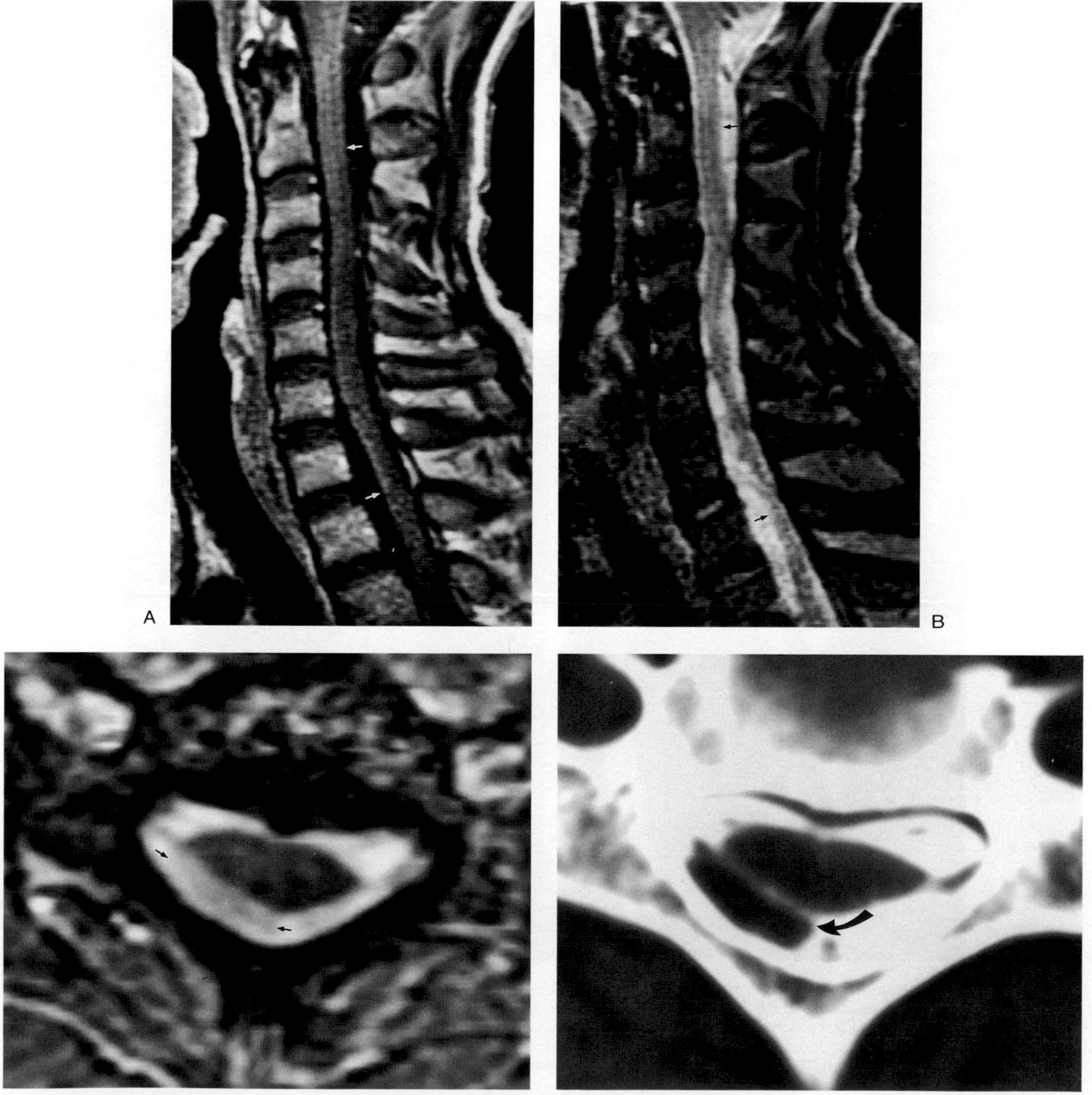

FIG. 43. Extramedullary cervical spinal cysticercosis. Sagittal T1-weighted image (**A**) and T2-weighted image (**B**) demonstrate multiple subarachnoid lesions with signal intensity close to that of CSF displacing the cord (*arrows*). Axial T2-weighted image (**C**) demonstrates a subarachnoid mass (*arrows*). Postmyelogram CT (**D**) shows the subarachnoid cysts to better advantage (*curved arrow*). (Courtesy of Dr. Sung Lee, Seoul, Korea.)

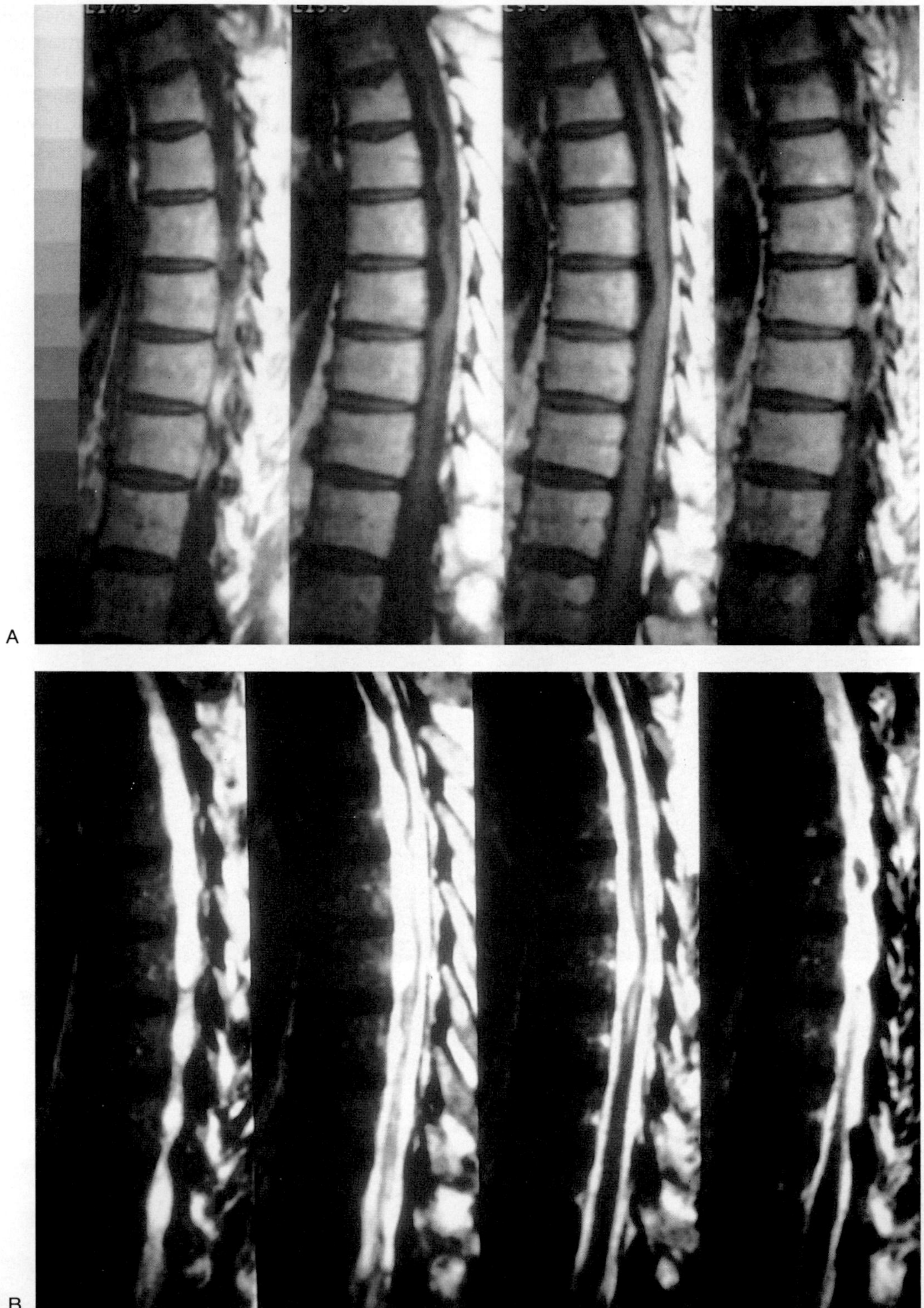

FIG. 44. Intradural extramedullary cysticercosis in a 51-year-old man with radiating low back pain and symptoms referable to the conus. Sagittal T1-weighted (**A**) and T2-weighted (**B**) images of the thoracic spine show irregular intradural extramedullary loculations with associated hyperintensity in parenchyma (A). Axial T2-weighted images (**C**) demonstrate loculated intradural collections in the lower thoracic region that mimic epidural disease in their configuration. After gadolinium (**D**), extra-axial enhancement is seen. Surgery confirmed racemos cysticercosis. (Courtesy of Dr. Renato Mendonça, São Paulo, Brazil.)

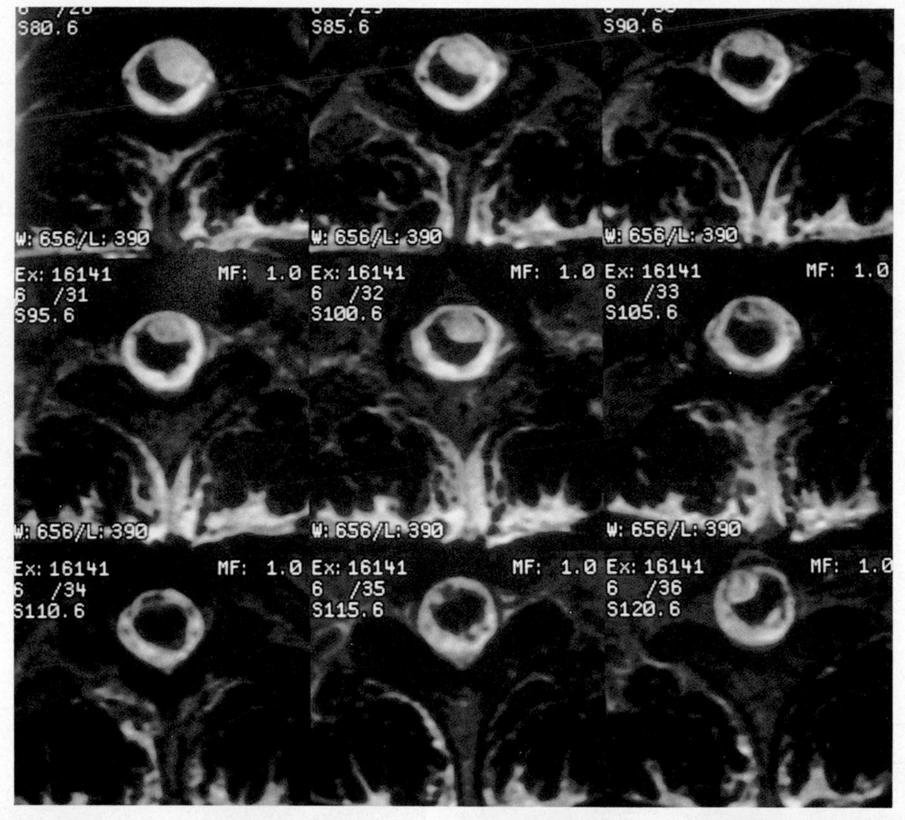

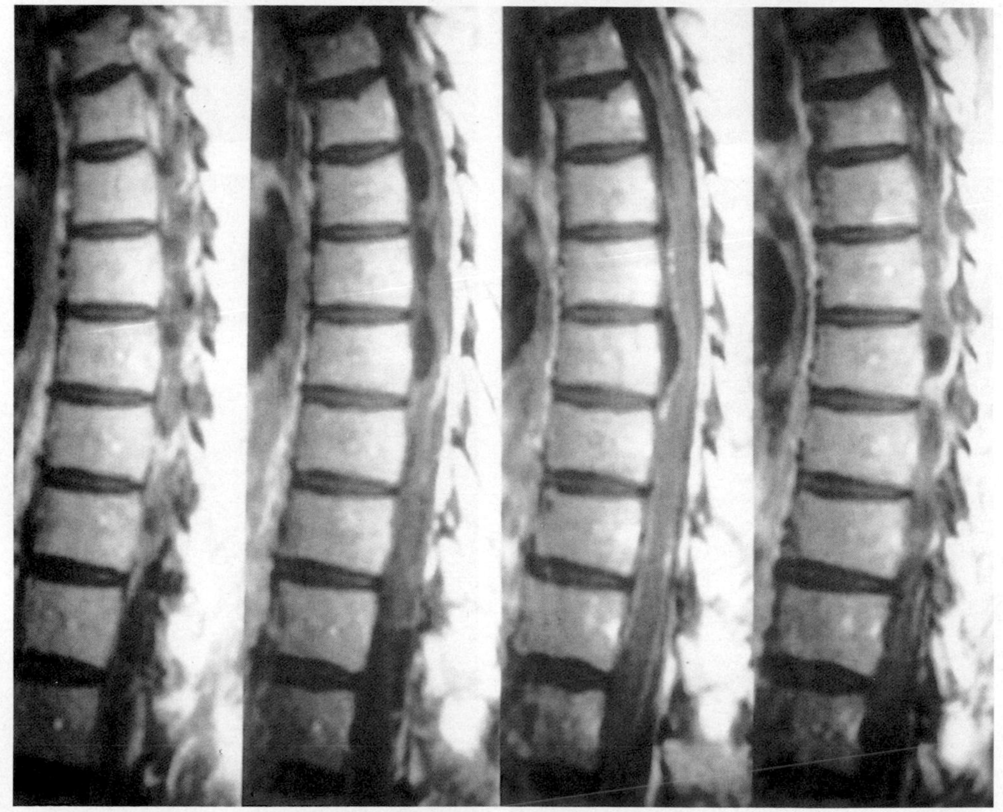

FIG. 44. *Continued.*

In the meninges the cysts appear as small, colorless structures adherent to the pia or floating freely in the subarachnoid space. Most subarachnoid racemose cysts are sterile. Intracerebral or intramedullary cysts (80,81) (Fig. 45) are surrounded by a collagenous capsule produced by the host and elicit a slight inflammatory reaction that becomes more evident after the death of the parasite.

Cryptococcosis

Cryptococcosis is caused by *Cryptococcus neoformans,* also known as *Torula histolytica,* which is harbored in fruit, milk, soil, and manure of some birds. The disease has a world-wide distribution but is most commonly reported in southern parts of the United States and Aus-

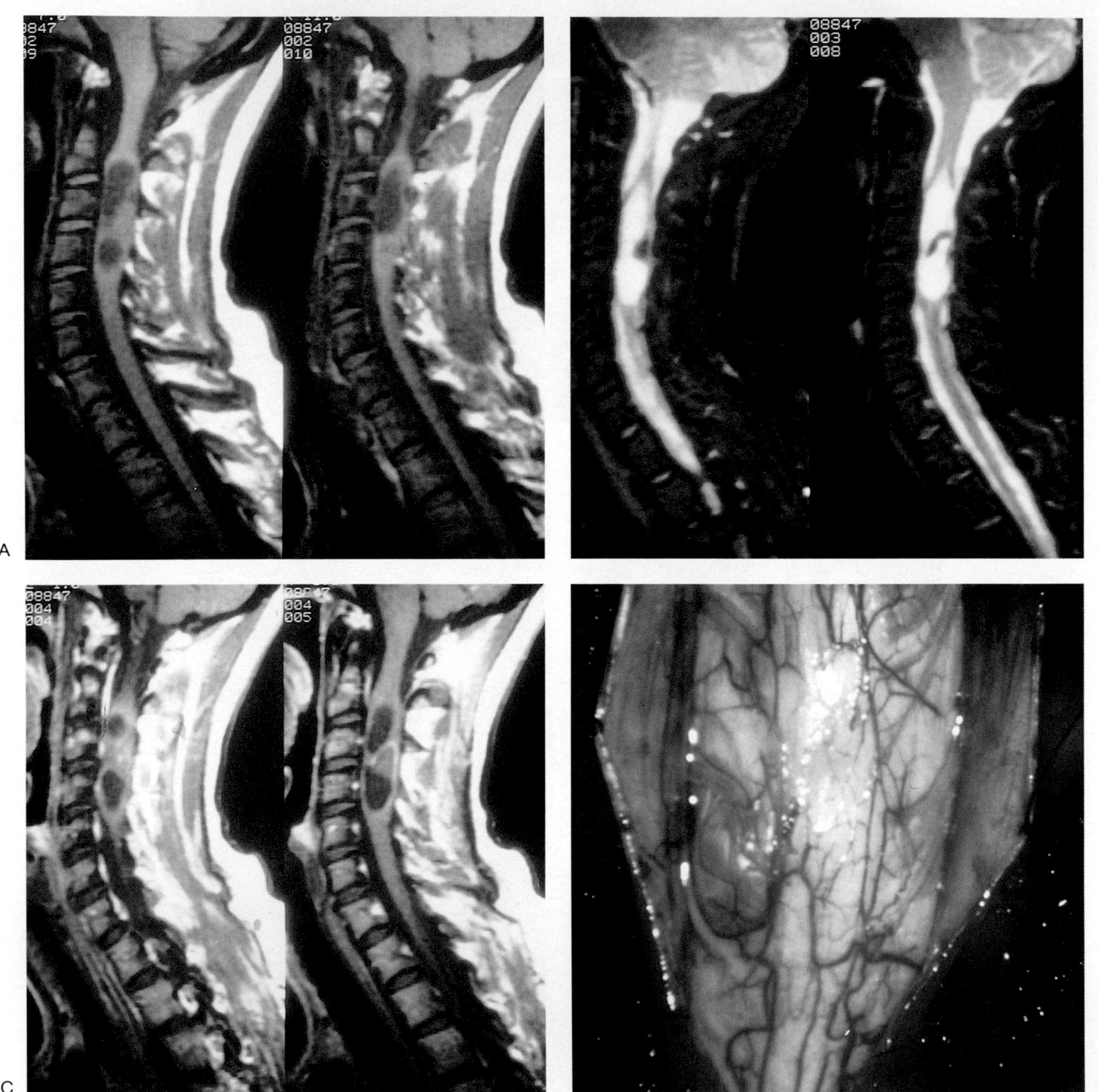

FIG. 45. Intramedullary cysticercosis in a 46-year-old woman with 9 months of lower extremity weakness and paresthesias. Sagittal T1-weighted (**A**) and T2-weighted (**B**) images of the cervical spine show a heterogeneous, loculated, multicystic intramedullary lesion with marked expansion of the cervical spinal cord. After gadolinium (**C**), intramedullary disease with heterogeneous enhancement is noted. Intraoperative photographs (**D**) show the multicystic, loculated nature of the lesion, proven to be cysticercosis. (Courtesy of Dr. Renato Mendonça, São Paulo, Brazil.)

tralia. The disease may develop in previously healthy individuals, but in 85% of patients it is an opportunistic infection. Although cryptococcal meningitis is extremely common in HIV-positive patients, cryptococcal spondylitis is a rare condition usually seen in immunosuppressed patients, and occasionally reported in immunocompetent patients (82). In a recent review of the literature, 11 documented cases were found up to 1989. A current report described the MR features of a case of cryptococcal spondylitis (83). The findings were indistinguishable from tuberculous spondylitis, with involvement of the vertebral body and extensive involvement of the posterior elements and paraspinous and perivertebral soft tissues with relative preservation of the disc (Fig. 46).

The CNS lesions consist primarily of meningitis involving the skull base and occasionally the spinal cord. In the acute cases, there is often very little inflammatory reaction, with no meningeal enhancement (70).

Schistosomiasis

Schistosoma mansoni and *Schistosoma haematobium* may rarely involve the spine. Four separate syndromes have been distinguished: medullary compression, acute transverse myelitis, granulomatous root involvement, and anterior spinal artery occlusion. In a recent article (84), 53 histologically proved cases of spinal cord involvement by *S. mansoni* and 15 cases of *S. haematobium* have been reported.

The disease involves the spine by extension from the inferior mesenteric venules or the perivesical venules. Host granulomatous reaction to the ova is the major factor in the pathogenesis of schistosomiasis. The importance of an early diagnosis is undermined by the relatively good response to praziquantel and steroids, which may reverse some of the symptoms early in the disease.

MR reports (84,85) of schistosomal myelitis secondary to *S. mansoni* revealed nonspecific enlargement of the lower thoracic spine and conus and increased signal intensity on the T2-weighted images (Figs. 47 and 48). Following gadolinium administration, there was enhancement of the lower thoracic cord (Fig. 49). Follow-up examination after treatment with praziquantel demonstrated resolution of these findings.

Granulomatous root involvement and medullary compression should also be easily demonstrated by MRI. Occlusion of the anterior spinal artery may also result in enlargement of the spinal cord and increased signal intensity on long TR sequences.

Echinococcosis

Hydatid disease in man is caused by the larvae of *Echinococcus granulosus*. Humans may contract infection by direct contact with dogs or ingestion of food or drink containing the ova. After ingestion, the larvae have to penetrate through the liver barrier and then through the pulmonary capillaries to reach the systemic blood circulation, from where they can disseminate. Hydatid disease of the bone is, therefore, uncommon, being encountered between 0.5% and 4% of patients. The vertebrae are most commonly involved (44%), the long bones of the limbs

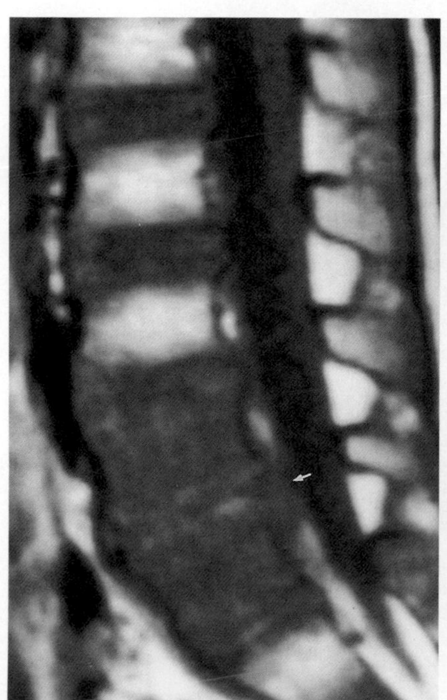

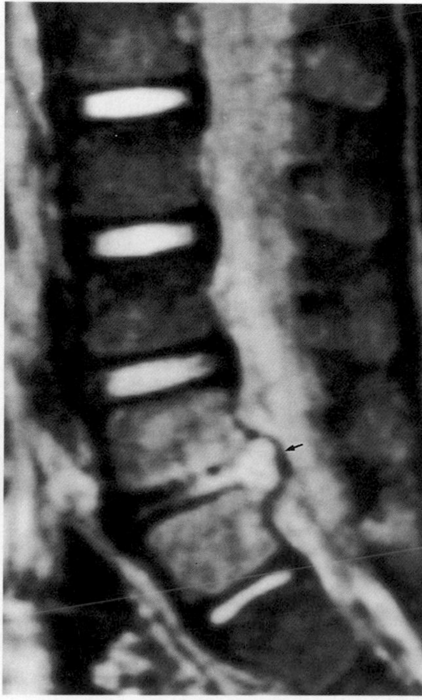

A,B

FIG. 46. Cryptococcosis of the spine. Three-year-old HIV-positive child with back pain. Sagittal T1-weighted (**A**) and T2-weighted (**B**) images demonstrate abnormal signal in the L4 and L5 vertebral bodies and loss of disc height, and a small epidural mass at the disc level (*arrow*), a nonspecific finding consistent with diskitis of any cause. Biopsy revealed cryptococcus. (Courtesy of Dr. J. Ahmadi and M. Koby, Los Angeles, CA.)

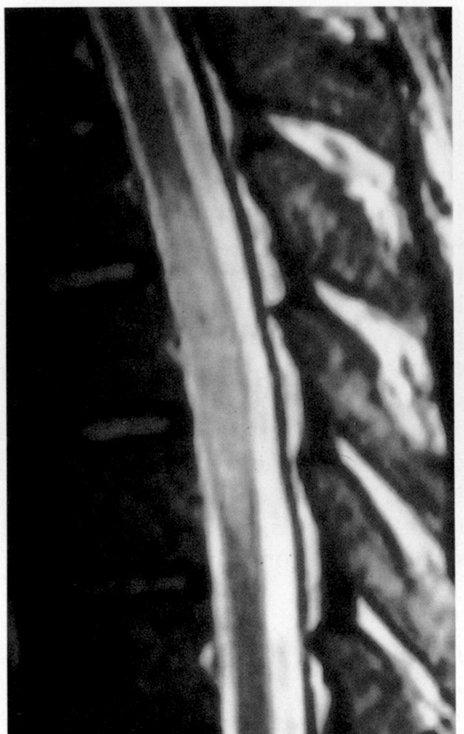

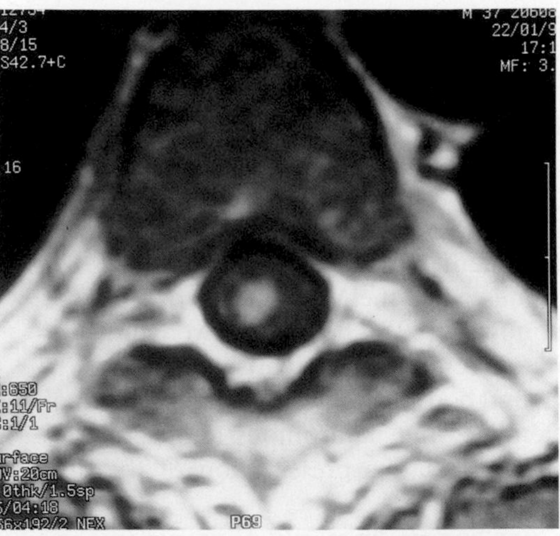

FIG. 47. Intramedullary *S. mansoni* in a 37-year-old man with bilateral lower extremity pain and paresthesias. Hyperintense intramedullary lesion (**A**) shows focal nodular enhancement (**B**). Schistosomiasis was confirmed by surgery. (Courtesy of Dr. Renato Mendonça, São Paulo, Brazil.)

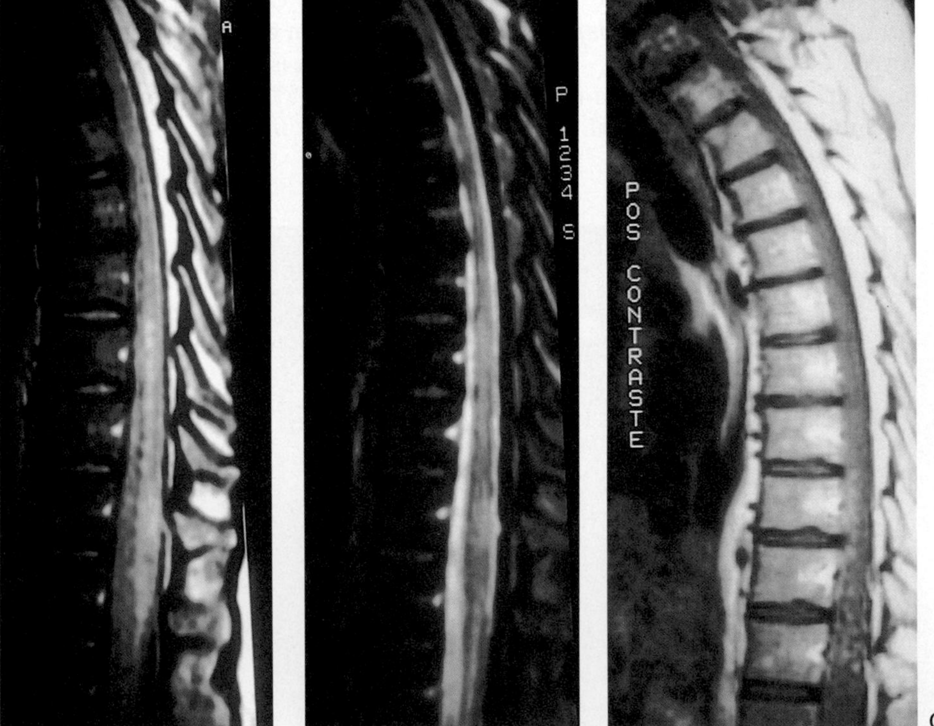

FIG. 48. *S. mansoni* in a 49-year-old man with progressive lower extremity weakness, paresthesias, and bowel and bladder dysfunction. Proton density–weighted (**A**) and T2-weighted (**B**) images show extensive hyperintensity throughout lower thoracic spinal cord and conus. After gadolinium (**C**), multiple nodules of enhancement are seen within conus and proximal cauda equina. Schistosomiasis confirmed by serology and rectal biopsy; there was a complete recovery with therapy. (Courtesy of Dr. Renato Mendonça, São Paulo, Brazil.)

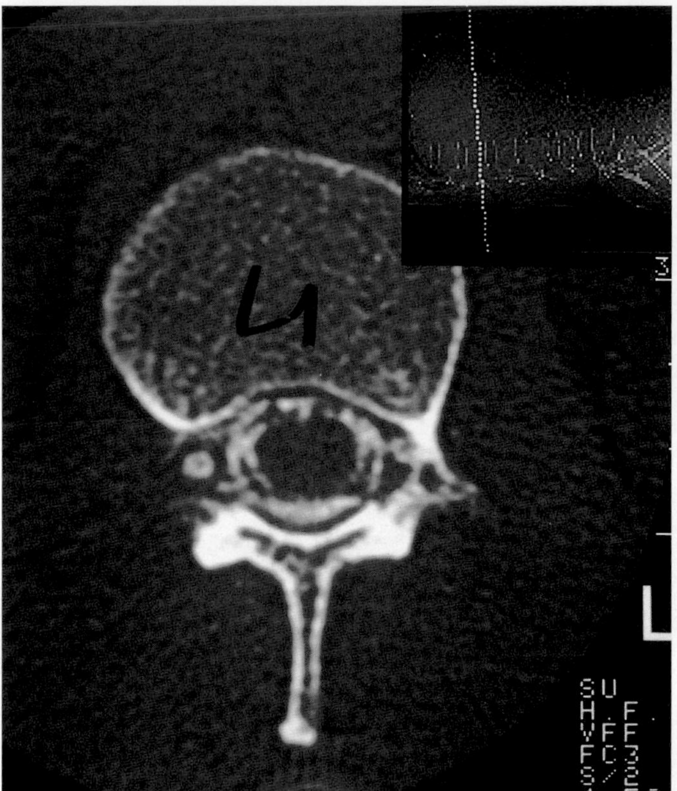

A

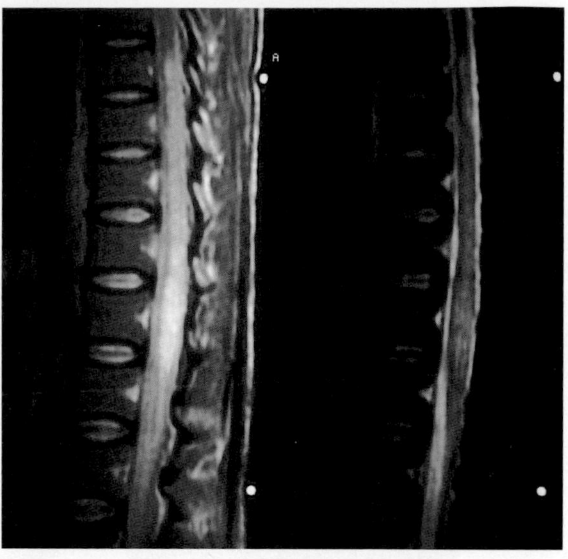

B,C

FIG. 49. *S. mansoni* in a 42-year-old man with radiating low back pain, sensory disturbance, and impotence. **A:** CT myelogram shows expansion of conus. **B,C:** MRI shows intramedullary hyperintensity on long TR images. Schistosomiasis confirmed by serology, rectal biopsy, and response to therapy. (Courtesy of Dr. Renato Mendonça, São Paulo, Brazil.)

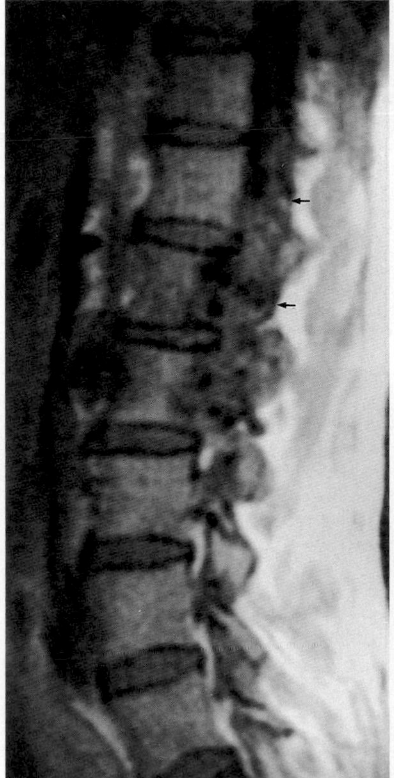

A

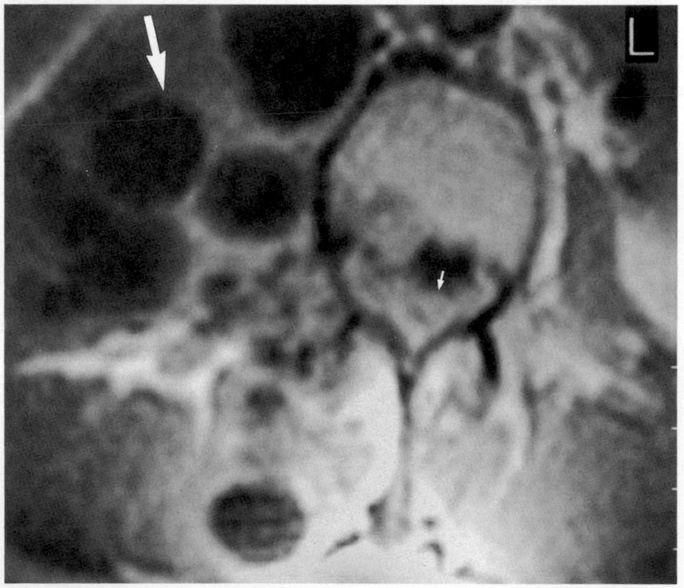

B

FIG. 50. Hydatid cyst. **A:** Sagittal T1-weighted image demonstrates an intradural mass completely obliterating the conus (*arrows*). **B:** Axial T1-weighted image demonstrates a multiloculated cyst (*large arrow*) in the right paraspinous region extending into the spinal canal surrounding the conus (*small arrow*). (Courtesy of Dr. Izzet Rosanes, Istanbul, Turkey.)

in 28% the pelvis, and hip joints 16%, the ribs and scapula in 8%, and the calvarium and phalanges in 4%. Contrary to cysts in other parts of the body, hydatid disease is always multilocular. Within cancellous bone the parasite develops as multiple small cysts that grow along the path of least resistance and, with time, may destroy the cortex and extend into the adjacent soft tissues. The differential diagnosis includes spinal tuberculosis, which may be difficult to distinguish preoperatively.

The plain radiographs show nonspecific bony destruction. MRI and CT may demonstrate the massive bone destruction. The cysts on MR demonstrate inhomogeneous low signal intensity on T1-weighted images and high intensity on T2-weighted images. The T2 measurements are not helpful in differentiating quiescent from active cysts. MRI may demonstrate the intradural extension to better advantage than CT (Figs. 50 and 51) without the need for subarachnoid contrast (86). CT is superior to MRI in demonstrating calcified lesions (Fig. 52).

Sparganosis

Sparganosis is a rare infection caused by the migrating larvae of a tapeworm of the genus *Spirometra*. Most infections involve the subcutaneous soft tissues and the or-

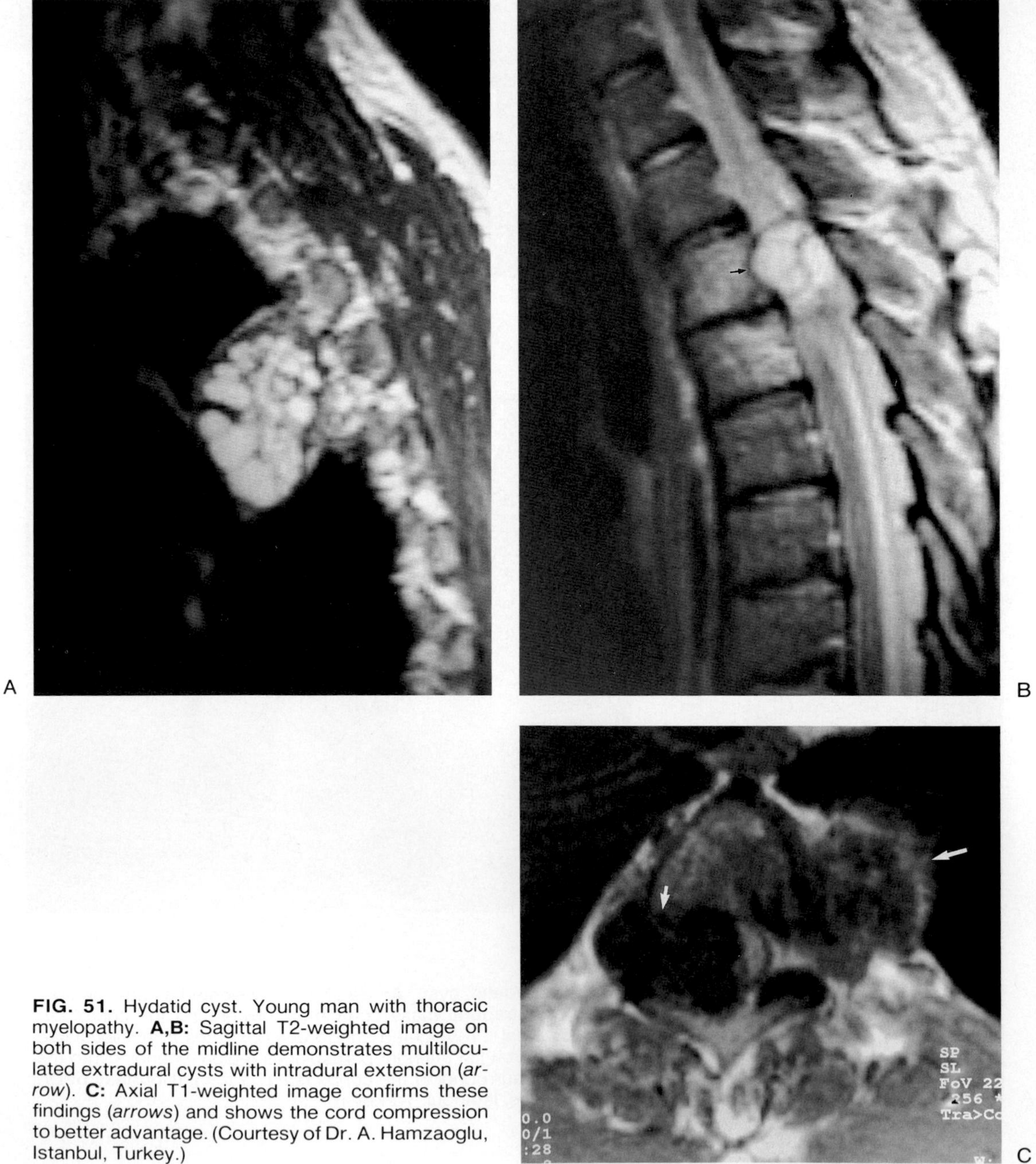

FIG. 51. Hydatid cyst. Young man with thoracic myelopathy. **A,B:** Sagittal T2-weighted image on both sides of the midline demonstrates multiloculated extradural cysts with intradural extension (*arrow*). **C:** Axial T1-weighted image confirms these findings (*arrows*) and shows the cord compression to better advantage. (Courtesy of Dr. A. Hamzaoglu, Istanbul, Turkey.)

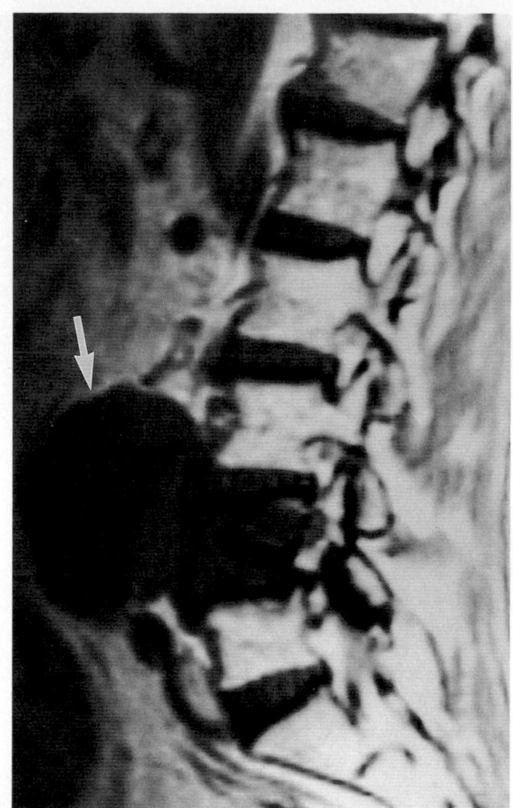

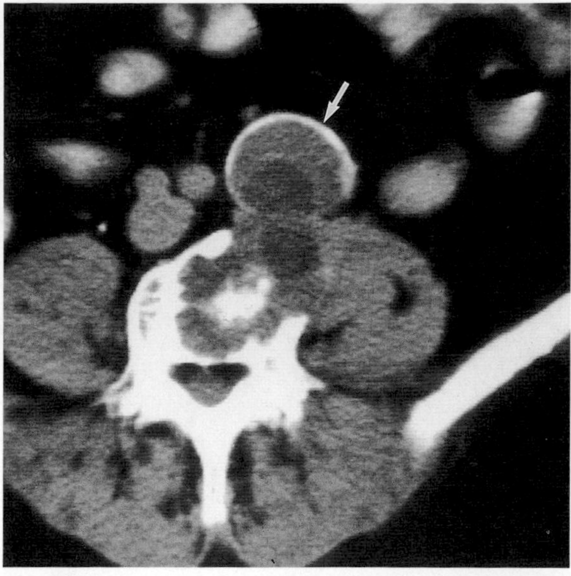

FIG. 52. Hydatid cyst. **A:** Sagittal T1-weighted image demonstrates a destructive lesion of L4 with a large anterior prevertebral mass (*arrow*). **B:** Axial CT demonstrates the calcification in the periphery of the mass (*arrow*) not seen on MRI. (Courtesy of M. Koby, Bethesda, MD.)

ganisms rarely invade the CNS. The involvement of the spine has been reported exceptionally. Approximately 65 cases have been reported in the United States, and the disease is endemic in China, Korea, Europe, and South America. Most human infections are caused by larvae of *Spirometra mansonoides.* The definitive hosts are domestic (and wild) cats and dogs. The orbit, pleura, brain, and spinal canal may also be infected. Pathologic findings include focal necrosis along the tortuous tract of migration. In the rare cases where the infection involves the subarachnoid space, the worm induces a granulomatous reaction that may be indistinguishable from other granulomas, including tuberculosis, which is often endemic in the same geographic area.

In a case report (87), the authors demonstrated effacement of the subarachnoid space on precontrast T1-weighted images and multiple subarachnoid-enhancing nodules following the administration of contrast. The diagnosis is made by a highly sensitive and specific enzyme-linked immunoadsorbent assay (ELISA) test.

Toxoplasmosis

Toxoplasmosis is due to the infection with *Toxoplasma gondii* and is the most common focal infection of the brain in AIDS patients. Toxoplasmosis of the spinal cord is rare (88), but it has been reported on MRI (89,90). The lesions present as focally enhancing masses in the cord (Figs. 53 and 54) mimicking an intramedullary tumor. Pathologically, an eosinophilic and granulomatous reaction has been noted on biopsy. The diagnosis may be considered in HIV-positive patients when the coexistence of an intramedullary mass and high serum toxoplasma titers are noted. A therapeutic trial of antitoxoplasma medication may be warranted before biopsy.

Viral Diseases

Viruses may affect the spinal cord or the nerve roots. Some viral effects on the spinal cord were discussed in the section on transverse myelitis and necrotic myelopathy. This section discusses some of the common viruses affecting the spine such as the Herpes family of viruses and HIV.

Herpes Virus

The family of herpes viruses consists of a large group of double-stranded DNA viruses, which includes herpes simplex virus type 1 (HSV-1), herpes simplex virus type 2 (HSV-2), cytomegalovirus (CMV), Epstein-Barr virus (EBV), varicella-zoster virus (VZV), B virus, herpesvirus 6, and herpesvirus 7. In addition to producing infection

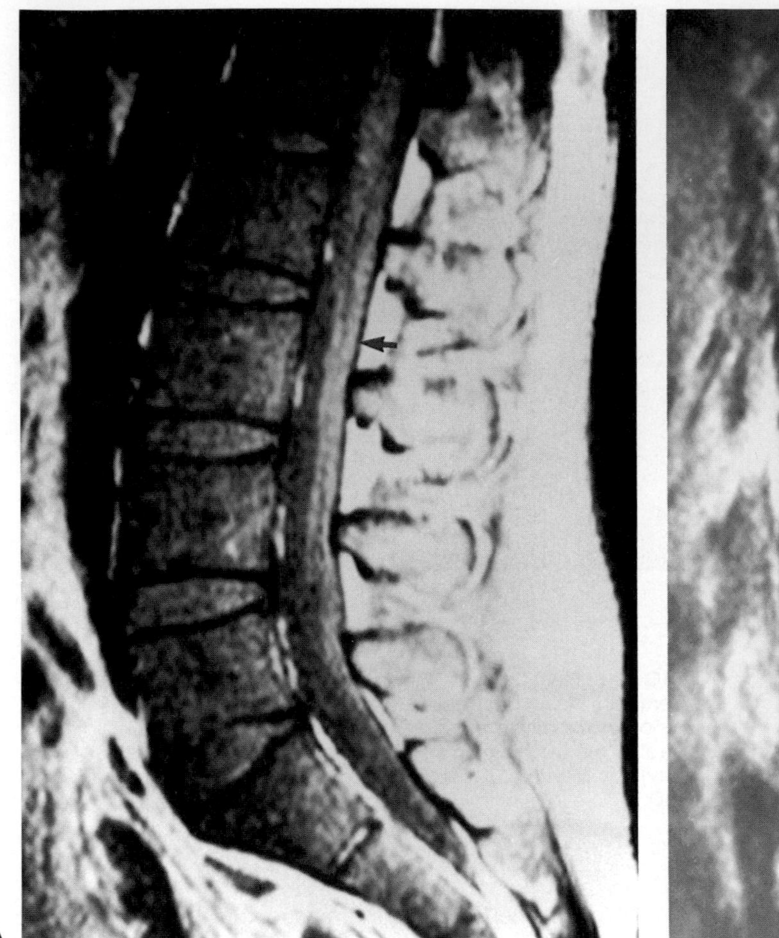

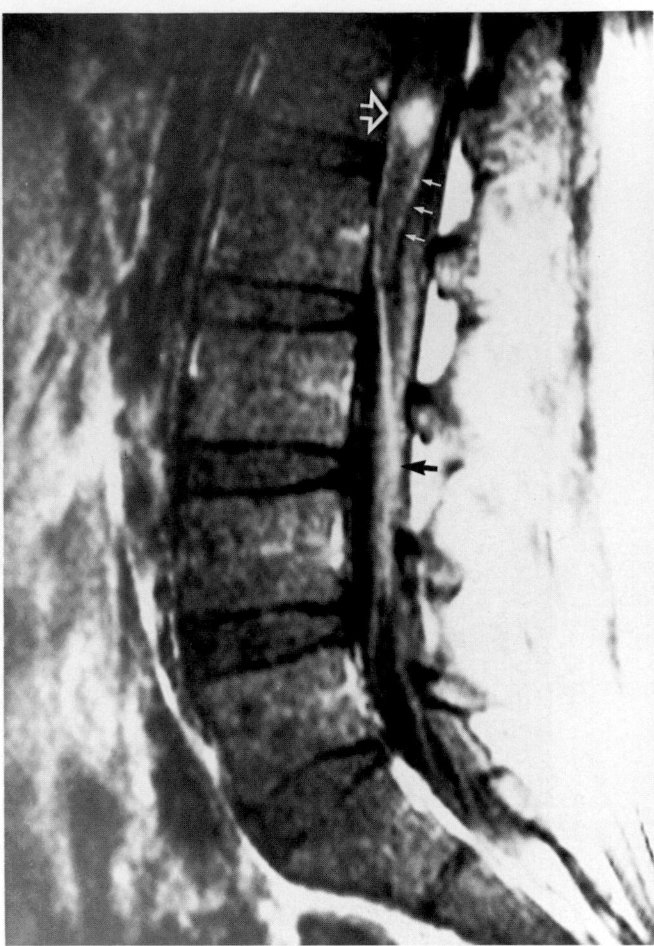

A B

FIG. 53. Intramedullary toxoplasmosis in a hemophiliac patient with AIDS. **A:** Sagittal T1-weighted image suggests thickened nerve roots (*arrow*). **B:** Postgadolinium sagittal T1-weighted image demonstrates intramedullary enhancement (*open arrow*) proved to represent toxoplasmosis at biopsy. Notice also the enhancement of the nerve roots (*black arrow*) and of the pia along the conus (*small white arrows*). (Courtesy of Mary K. Edwards, Indianapolis, IN.)

when the host initially acquires the virus, an important property shared by these viruses is the ability to produce latent infection and to be reactivated.

Although encephalitis is the most common manifestation some herpes viruses may produce myelitis, and polyradiculitis. Myelitis associated with herpes zoster is an unusual complication (91). The pathogenesis may involve a direct viral invasion of the spinal cord (92) (Fig. 55), a vasculitic process with ischemic necrosis or an immunologic, parainfectious mechanism. The onset of the myelitis can occur weeks to months after an episode of herpes zoster.

Epstein-Barr Virus

EBV is the cause of a common disease, infectious mononucleosis. EBV has been associated with Guillain-Barré syndrome and transverse myelitis (93).

Cytomegalovirus

CMV can cause HIV-related spinal polyradiculopathy (subacute progressive weakness, hyporeflexia, and mild sensory symptoms), which can be diagnosed with contrast-enhanced MR. Enhancement of nerves and leptomeninges of the conus region can be identified (94) (Figs. 56 and 57). Finally, CMV infection has been incriminated as the cause of Guillain-Barré syndrome.

Herpes B Virus (**Herpesvirus Simiae***)*

The B virus (*Herpesvirus simiae*) is an alpha herpes virus that is endemic among monkeys of the Macaca species and usually causes stomatitis or conjunctivitis in these primates. Most reported human cases have resulted from bites by rhesus monkeys. Among other manifestations, transverse myelitis may occur (95).

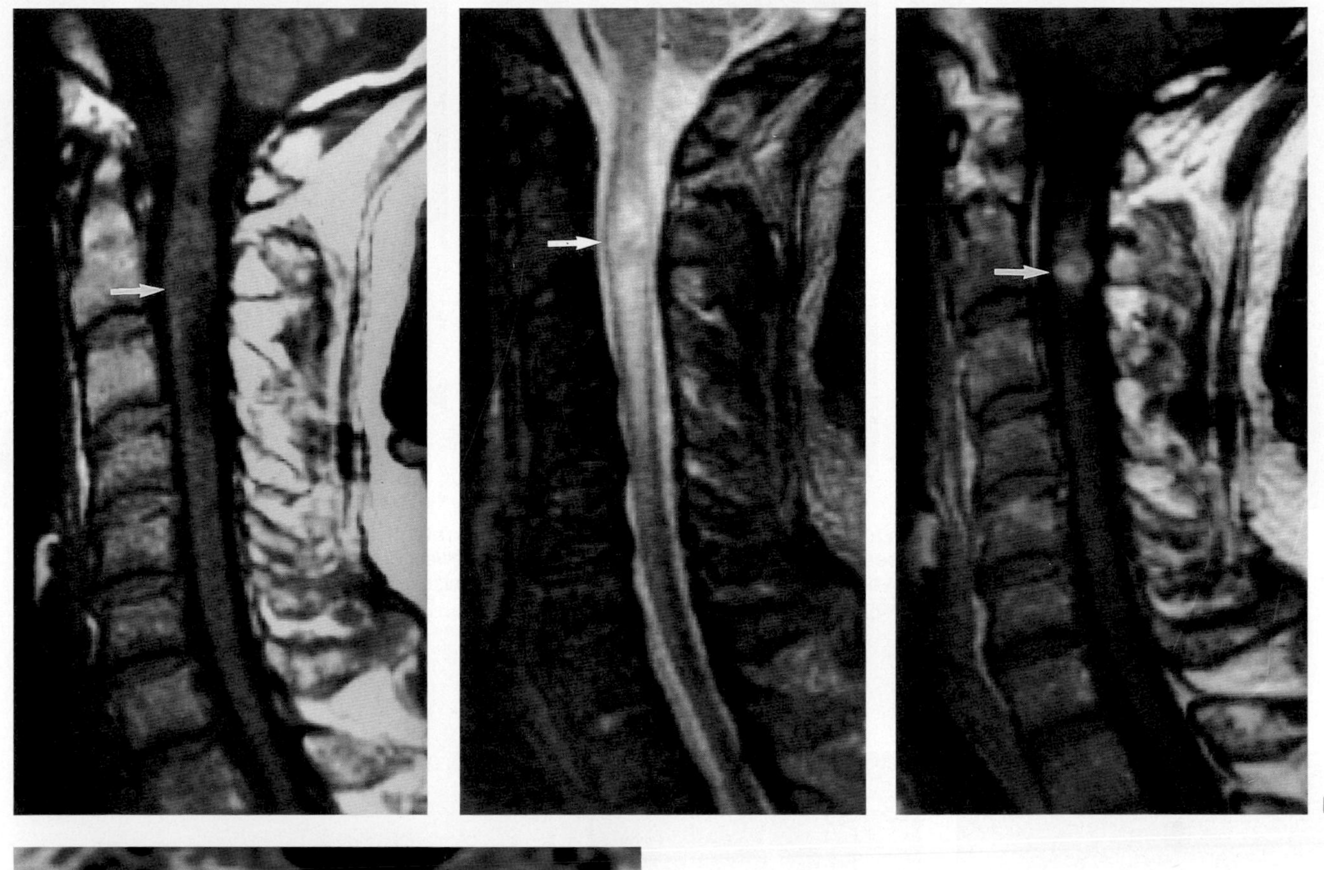

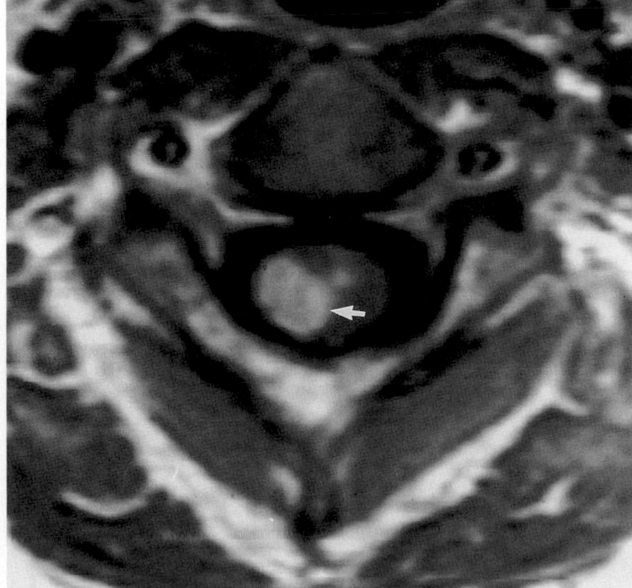

FIG. 54. Intramedullary toxoplasmosis in an HIV-positive 40-year-old man with acute quadriparesis and high toxoplasmosis titers. **A:** Sagittal T1-weighted image demonstrates expansion of the cord at the C2 level. **B:** Sagittal T2-weighted image demonstrates expansion of the cord and increased signal intensity in the cord between C2 and C4 and a central hypointense center. **C:** Postcontrast sagittal T1-weighted image demonstrates a nodular enhancing lesion in the cord at the C2 level. **D:** Axial image demonstrate a well-defined lesion in the right aspect of the cord at the C2 level. This nodular enhancement has been associated with granulomatous infections or neoplasms rather than idiopathic or viral-induced transverse myelitis.

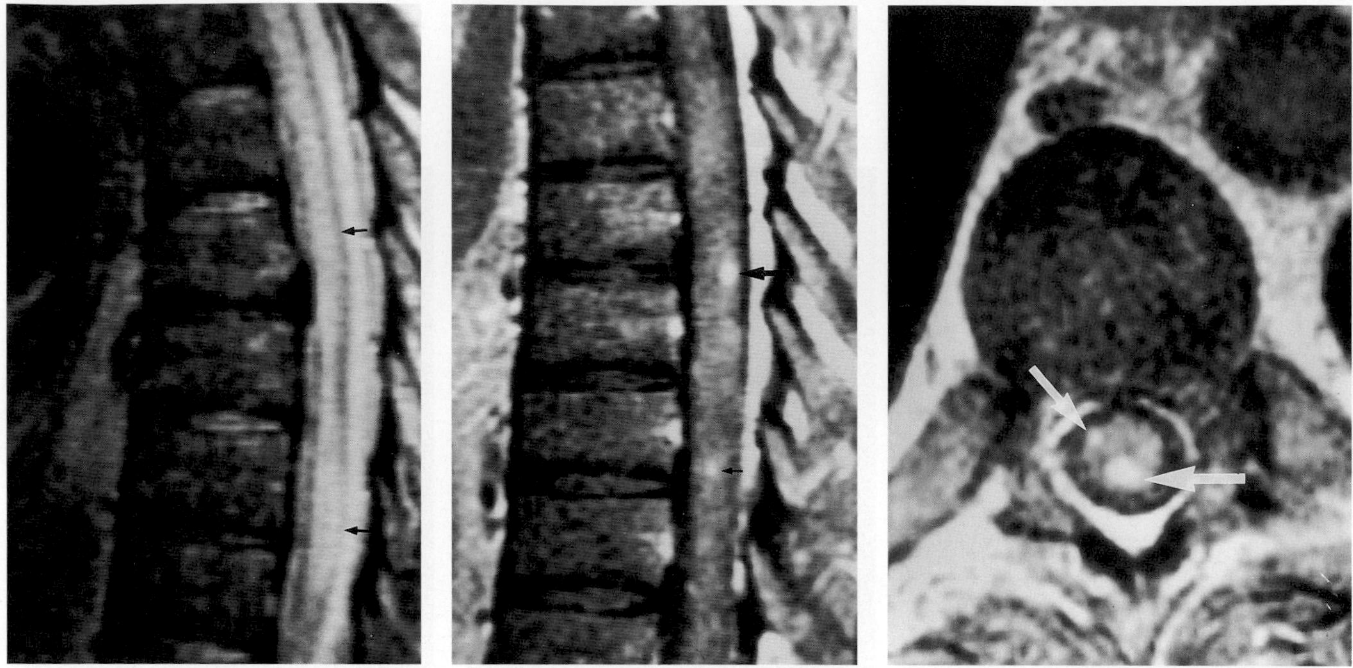

FIG. 55. Herpes zoster myelitis in a 41-year-old man with progressive urinary retention and bilateral leg weakness. The patient had concomitant herpes zoster skin papules in some of the involved dermatomes. Acyclovir therapy resulted in moderate clinical improvement. (From Gero et al., ref. 38, with permission.) Note extensive lesion on T2-weighted image (**A**, *arrows*) with irregular foci of enhancement (**B,C**).

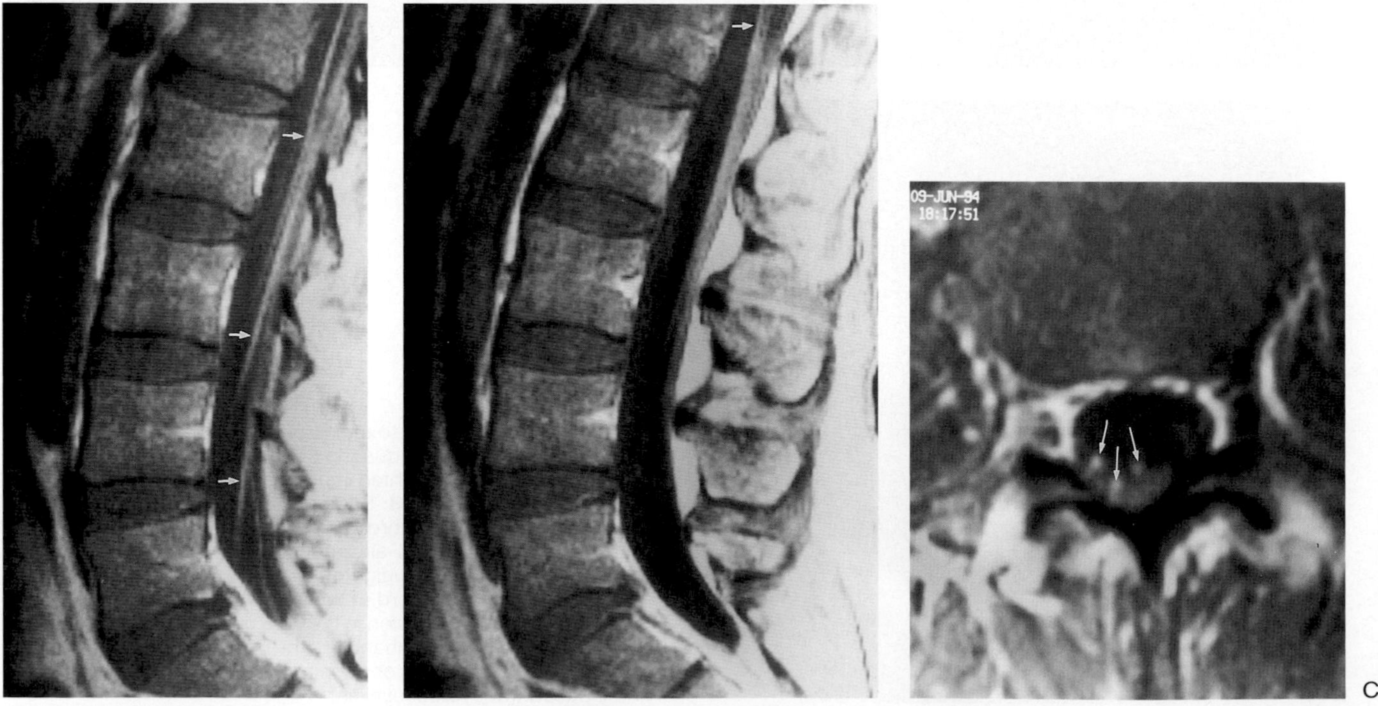

FIG. 56. CMV polyradiculopathy in an HIV-infected patient. Sagittal precontrast T1-weighted image were normal (not shown). Parasagittal (**A,B**) and axial postcontrast T1-weighted images (**C**) demonstrate marked enhancement of the roots in the cauda equina (*arrows*). (Courtesy of Dr. Charles Lanzieri, Cleveland, OH.)

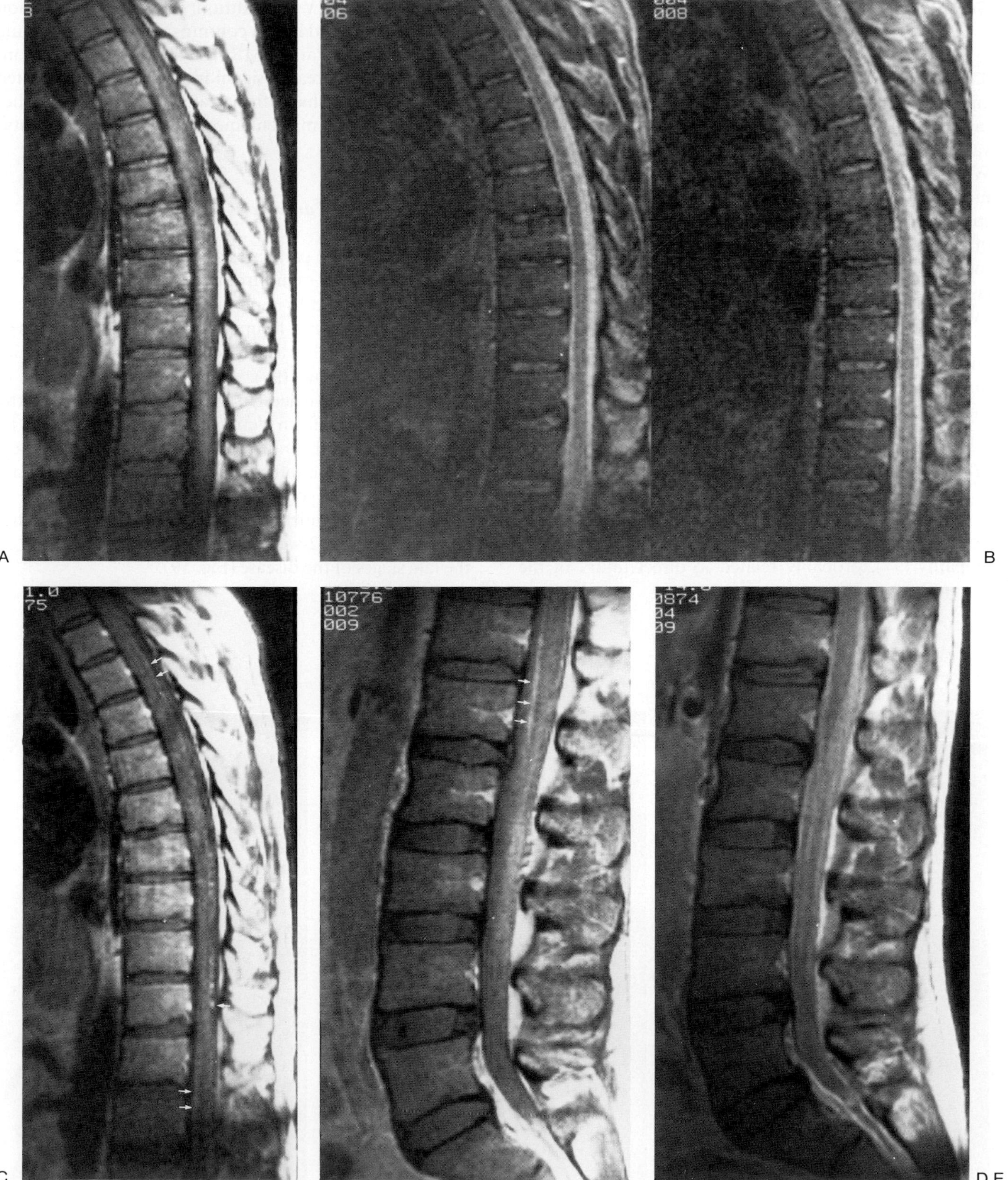

FIG. 57. AIDS radiculitis and meningitis, probably secondary to CMV. A 40-year-old HIV-positive man with new onset bowel and bladder incontinence. Sagittal (**A**) T1-weighted image and (**B**) T2-weighted image are normal. No intramedullary lesion is seen. **C:** Postgadolinium sagittal T1-weighted image demonstrates subtle enhancement of the pia (*arrows*). **D:** Postgadolinium sagittal T1-weighted image of the lumbar spine confirms the pial enhancement of the conus (*arrows*) and distal roots. **E:** Postgadolinium sagittal T1-weighted image 1 week later demonstrates marked enhancement of the entire subarachnoid space and nerve roots. The lumbar puncture revealed severe lymphocytosis (4000/mm^3). Routine bacterial and tuberculosis cultures were negative. Cytology was negative for lymphoma. The intracranial meninges did not enhance.

Guillain-Barré Syndrome

Guillain-Barré syndrome, also known as acute inflammatory demyelinating polyradiculoneuropathy, is an acquired demyelinating neuropathy characterized by rapid onset weakness, hyporeflexia or areflexia, and elevated levels of protein in the CSF without pleocytosis. Weakness may progress for up to 4 weeks, is usually symmetrical and involves the lower extremities before spreading to the upper extremities and face. Involvement of cranial nerves and autonomic dysfunction are common. Although the cause of Guillain-Barré syndrome is unclear, most evidence now supports an immune-mediated phenomenon.

MRI in Guillain-Barré syndrome can show marked enhancement of thickened nerve roots of the conus medullaris and cauda equina (96). However, MRI is usually unremarkable in this entity.

HIV Infection

In addition to the many cerebral neurologic complications, patients with AIDS may develop a vacuolar myelopathy (97), probably related to direct injury of the neurons by the HIV. In addition, there is demyelination of the posterior and lateral columns resembling subacute combined degeneration. MRI may be normal or demonstrate areas of increased signal intensity on T2-weighted image indistinguishable from transverse myelitis of other causes. The lesion may enhance after gadolinium administration (Fig. 58).

Tropical Spastic Paraparesis

Tropical spastic paraparesis (TSP) is a neurologic disorder endemic in many tropical and subtropical countries, characterized by a progressive myelopathy associated with a retrovirus, human T-lymphotropic virus type 1 (HTLV1), which was found in 68% of patients with TSP in Martinique (98). Neuropathologic studies in these patients revealed an inflammatory myelopathy with focal spongiform demyelinating and necrotic lesions, perivascular and meningeal infiltrates, and focal gray matter destruction with a predilection for the posterior columns and corticospinal tracts. The spectrum of MRI findings includes nonspecific cord swelling and hyperintensity on T2-weighted image to cord atrophy in the late stages of the disease (Fig. 59).

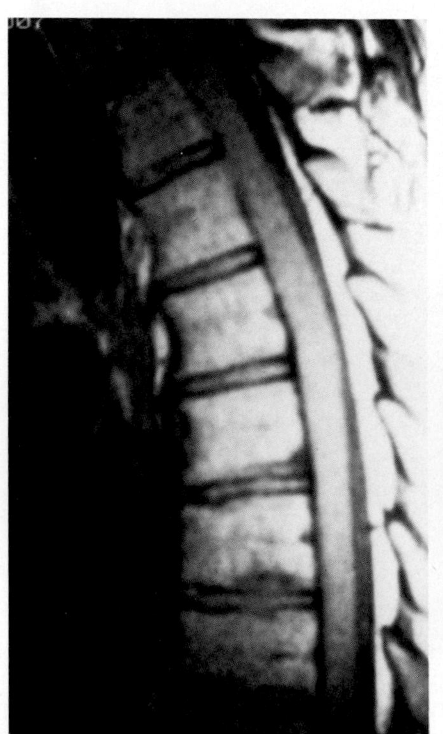

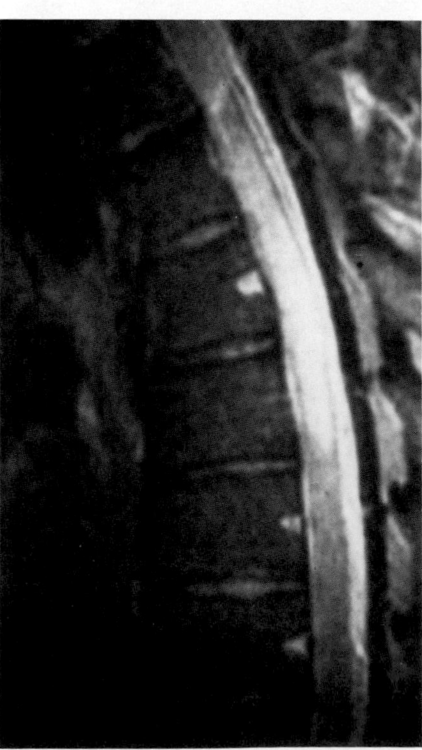

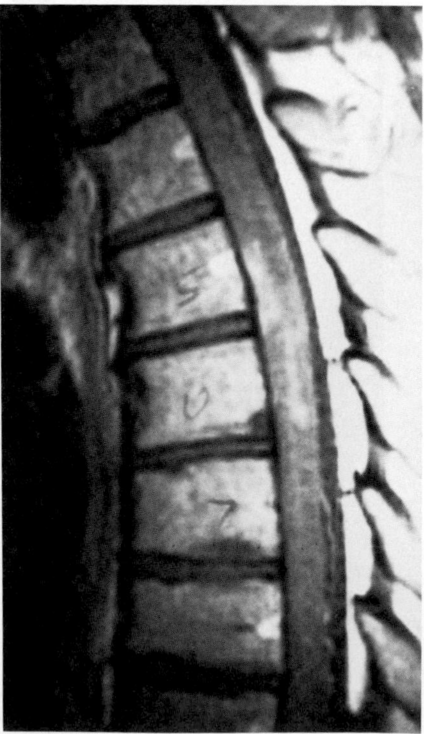

A,B C

FIG. 58. AIDS myelopathy. **A:** Sagittal T1-weighted image. The thoracic cord is slightly swollen. **B:** Sagittal T2-weighted image. High intramedullary signal in the same area. **C:** Postgadolinium sagittal T1-weighted image shows patchy areas of intramedullary enhancement at the same level.

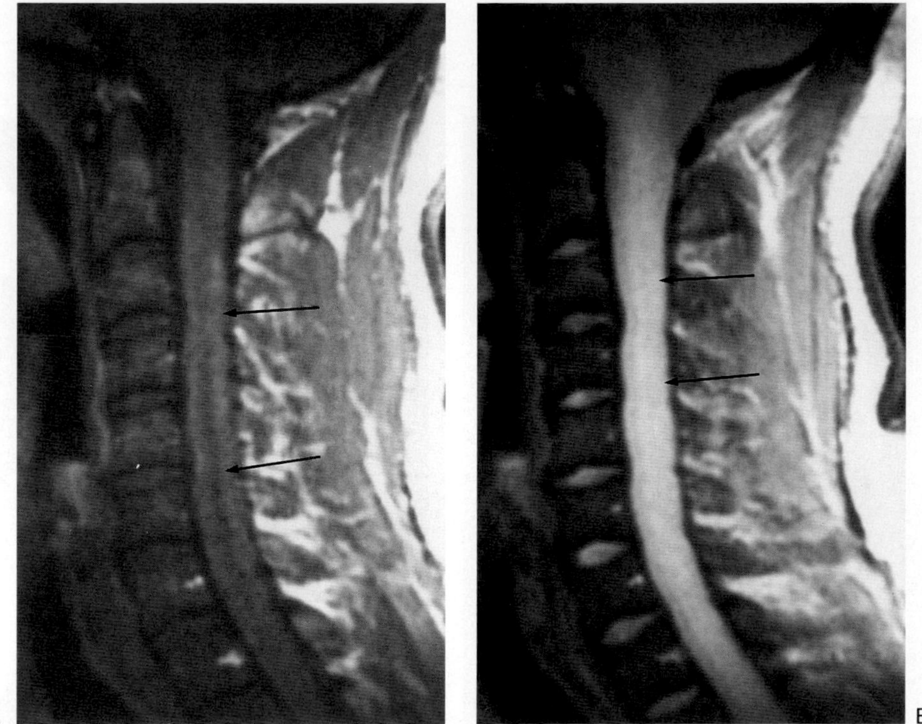

FIG. 59. Tropical spastic paraparesis (HTLV-1 myelopathy) in a 34-year-old man from Barbados who presented with progressive quadriparesis HTLV-1 infection was proved by CSF titers. **A:** Sagittal precontrast T1-weighted image shows diffuse swelling of cervical spinal cord (*arrows*). **B:** Sagittal T2-weighted image shows high intensity in the cord (*arrows*). (From Gero, ref. 38, with permission.)

ARACHNOIDITIS

Arachnoiditis (arachnoid adhesions) may develop secondary to infections such as syphilis (pachymeningitis cervicalis hypertrophica), tuberculosis (Fig. 60) (both Pott's disease and healed tuberculous meningitis), pyogenic meningitis (Fig. 61), trauma, surgery, nontraumatic subarachnoid hemorrhage, spinal anesthetic agents, reaction to radiopaque material such as Pantopaque (Fig. 62), or reactions to detergents in syringes used to introduce anesthetic or radiopaque substances; in a large group of patients no cause can be found (99–101). Surgery is probably the largest current cause because of the large number of operations for herniated disc and the decrease in the number of postinfectious arachnoiditis. Arachnoiditis may cause persistent symptoms following surgery in 6% to 16% of patients. The pathogenesis of postoperative arachnoiditis includes predominantly a fibrinous exudate with little cellular exudate. The fibrin-covered roots adhere to each other and to the thecal sac. Dense collagen adhesions are formed during the repair stage (101).

The appearance of arachnoiditis is well known on myelography and postmyelogram CT (102,103). Two groups of patients have been described based on the myelographic findings: group 1, caused by adhesions of the roots inside the meninges producing thickened "sleeveless" roots, and group 2 presenting with filling defects and narrowing of the thecal sac and myelographic block. On postmyelogram CT, the clumping of the roots can be directly visualized. The adherence of the roots to the thecal sac produces an empty sac appearance. The findings of postoperative arachnoiditis have also been described by MRI (104). MRI is able to demonstrate the individual roots of the cauda equina in 78% of cases (105) and detect moderate to severe arachnoiditis, correlating well with the myelographic and postmyelogram CT findings. The axial T1-weighted images have been the most helpful. However, more recent fast spin-echo techniques delineate the morphology of intrathecal nerve roots extremely well. Therefore, T2-weighted imaging using fast spin-echo acquisitions should be performed in all suspected cases.

The findings can be separated into three types: (a) type 1 shows conglomerates of adherent roots in the center of the sac, (b) type 2 demonstrates the roots adherent to the thecal sac peripherally (empty sac appearance), and (c) type 3 demonstrates soft tissue masses obliterating

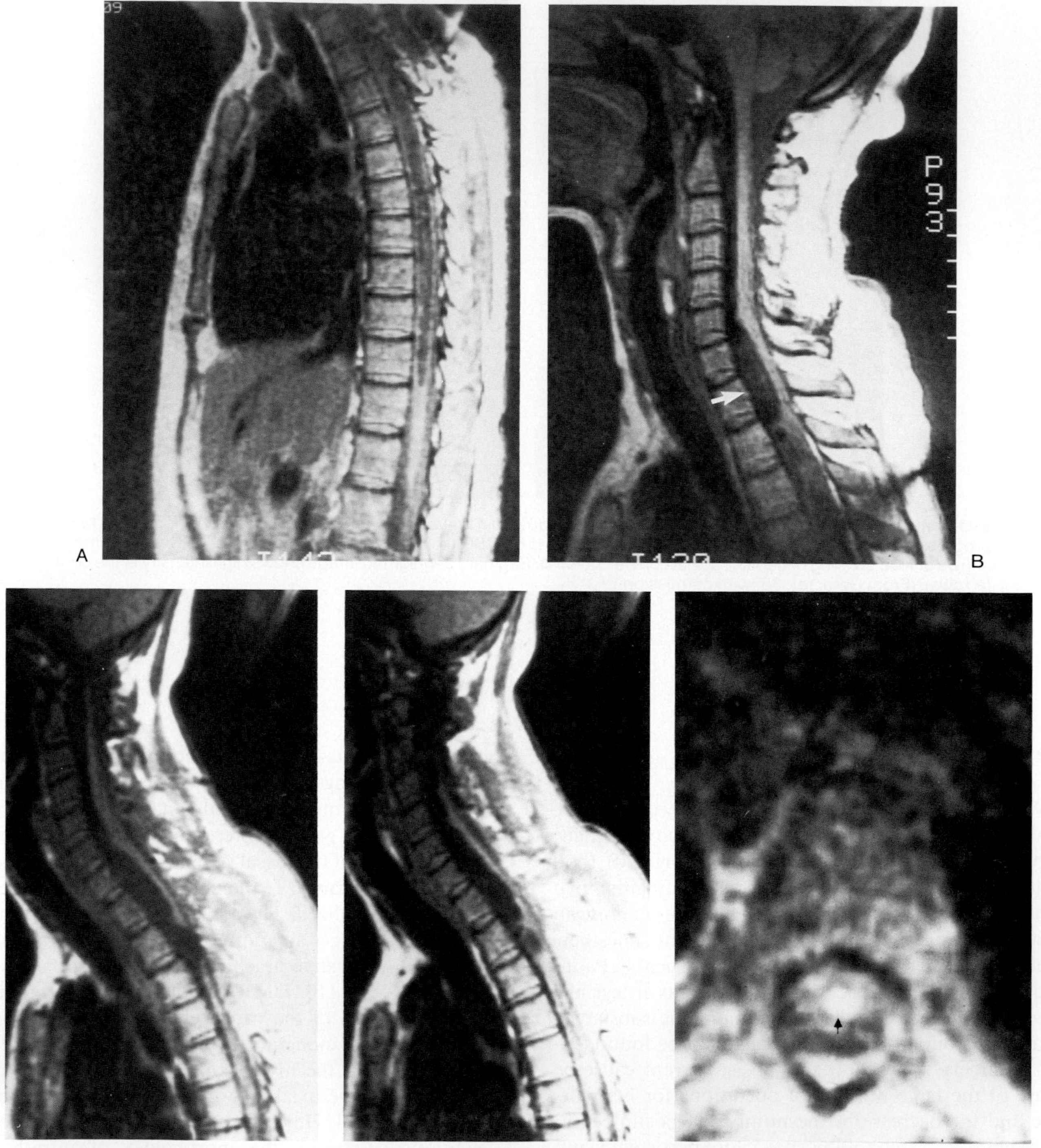

FIG. 60. Syringomyelia secondary to arachnoid adhesions in a middle-aged woman with a history of tuberculous meningitis 20 years earlier and progressive myelopathy over the past months. **A:** Sagittal T1-weighted image visualizes the thoracic syrinx. **B:** Sagittal T1-weighted image in the cervical spine demonstrates a large anterior arachnoid cyst (*arrow*) compressing the cord. Postoperative sagittal (**C**) and axial (**D**) T1-weighted images demonstrate the collapse of the syrinx, residual cord deformity at the level of the cyst, and a small area of hemorrhage in the midthoracic cord (*arrow,* **E**).

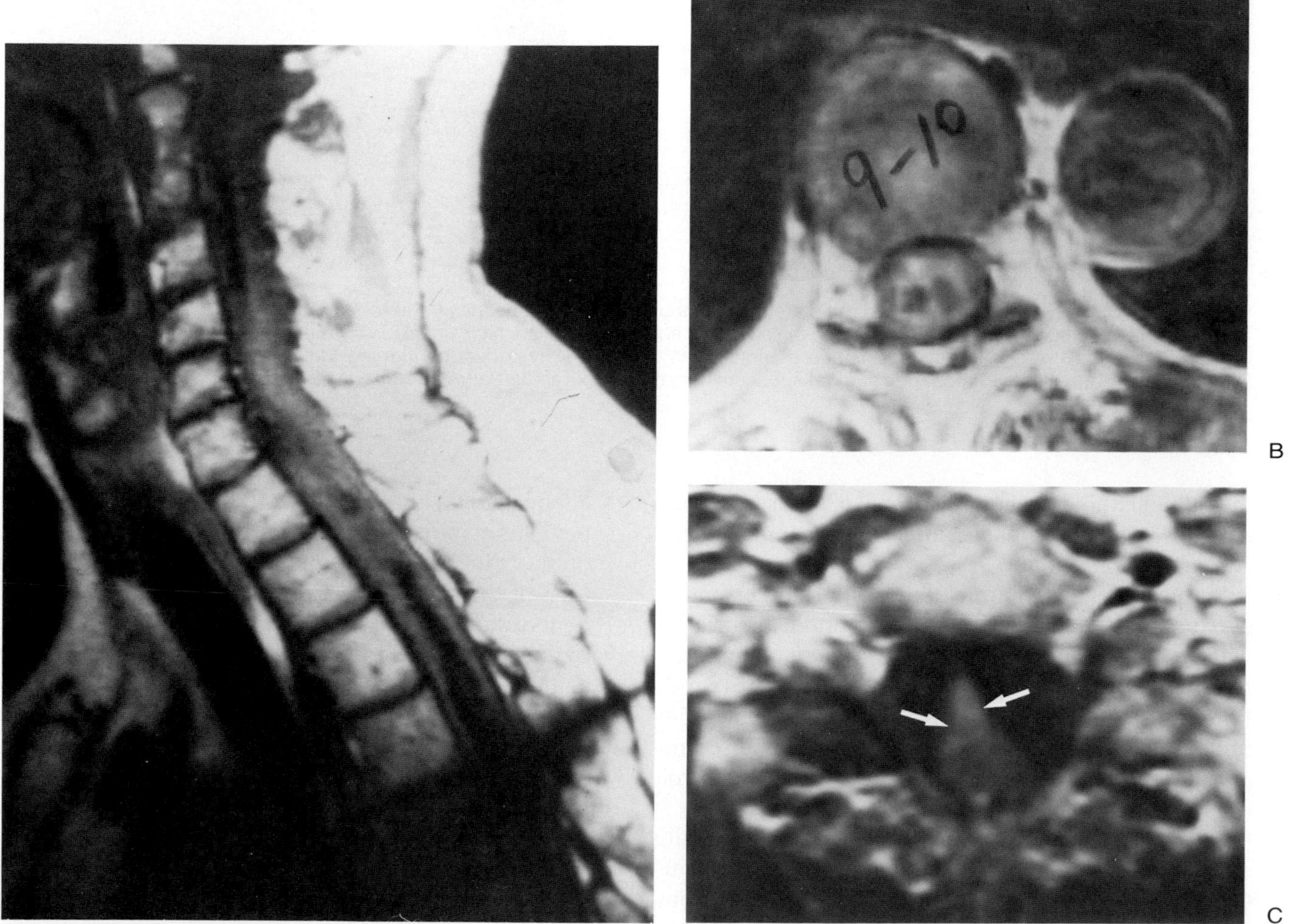

FIG. 61. Syringomyelia secondary to arachnoid adhesions in a middle-aged woman with a history of bacterial meningitis. **A:** Sagittal T1-weighted image. Large syrinx with ill-defined cord–CSF interface. **B:** Axial T1-weighted image in the thoracic spine. Notice the septated aspect of the syrinx most likely representing two parallel areas of cavitation. **C:** Axial T1-weighted image in the cervical region. The cord has a triangular shape because of compression by arachnoid loculations (*arrows*).

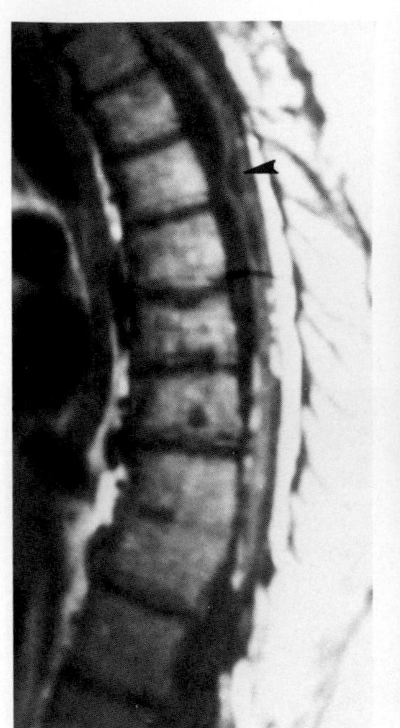

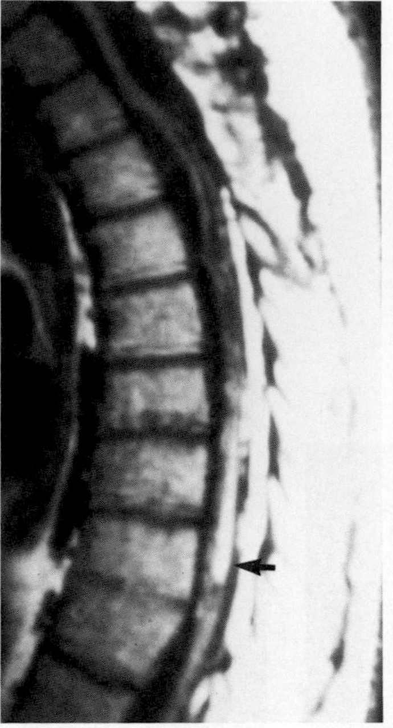

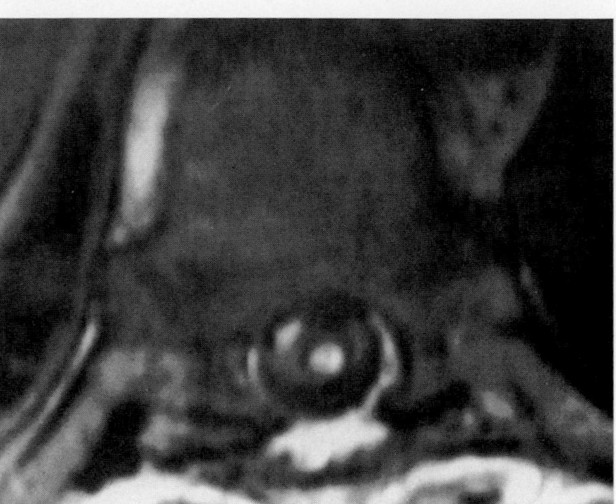

A B

FIG. 62. Syringomyelia secondary to arachnoid adhesions and intramedullary Pantopaque. **A:** Sagittal T1-weighted image demonstrates a thoracic syrinx (*arrowhead*), and intramedullary high signal (*arrow*) consistent with fat or hemorrhage. **B:** Axial T1-weighted image demonstrates chemical shift artifact confirming that the intramedullary high signal represents Pantopaque and not subacute hematoma. Extramedullary Pantopaque is also present ventrally and to the right.

the subarachnoid space (104) (Fig. 63). Arachnoiditis may or may not enhance after intravenous contrast administration.

Syringomyelia, cavitation of the spinal cord extending over several vertebral levels, can be found in association with arachnoiditis [syringomyelia secondary to arachnoid adhesions (SSAA)]. The pathogenesis of this condition is still incompletely understood, but the obliteration of the subarachnoid space by the adhesions and secondary alteration in CSF flow is thought to play a major role (106–108).

This condition was first reported as chronic meningitis or hypertrophic cervical pachymeningitis and the cavitation was attributed to venous stasis and arterial thrombosis in the late 19th century (108).

Compared with the earlier literature, in our experience (109) the proportion of the cases secondary to infection was much smaller, reflecting the marked decrease in the incidence of both syphilis and tuberculosis. Most of the patients had arachnoid lesions secondary to trauma or previous spinal surgery. Regardless of the origin of the adhesions, the clinical presentation is similar (110). Symptoms develop months to years after the initial episode and the condition that caused the adhesions may have been forgotten.

Most of these syrinxes are located in the thoracic cord. Thoracic predilection for arachnoiditis had been described before in patients with arachnoiditis without cavitation. Sixty-eight percent of 41 cases in one series were confined to the thoracic area (108). The MR characteristics of this type of syrinx differ from the usual appearance of the syringomyelia secondary to Chiari malformation. Loss of the sharp cord CSF interface seen in these patients results from obliteration of the subarachnoid space by arachnoid adhesions. The metameric haustrations encountered within the syrinx on sagittal T1-weighted images in patients with Chiari malformation are not present in patients with SSAA. The syrinx in patients with Chiari malformation is usually central and smooth, most likely representing at least initially hydromyelia, rather than syringomyelia. In patients with SSAA, the syrinx may be septated on axial T1-weighted images, probably representing parallel areas of cavitation rather than septa within the same cavity.

The most striking finding in SSAA is the high incidence of associated extramedullary arachnoid cysts (arachnoid loculations) (109). Arachnoid adhesions containing cystic loculations were first described by Schwartz in 1897 and the condition was termed "meningitis serous spinalis" by Mendel and Adler in 1908 (108). These cysts have been encountered in 44% of patients operated for arachnoiditis. In a recent review of 14 cases of syringomyelia secondary to arachnoiditis, 5 of the 14 patients had associated cysts (109). The high incidence of arachnoid cysts recently noted on MRI probably reflects their better detection. Most of the cysts are located at the upper aspect of the syrinx, suggesting that they may play a role in the development of cord cavita-

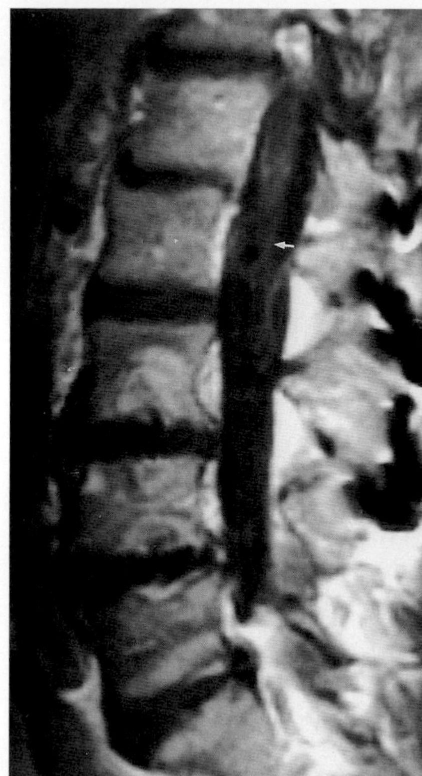
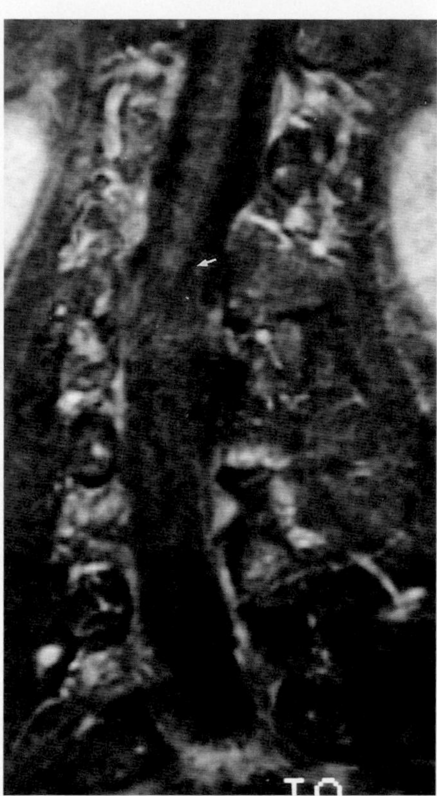

A,B

FIG. 63. Lumbar arachnoiditis. A 60-year-old man with progressive lower extremity weakness and pain. Sagittal T1-weighted images postcontrast (**A**) and coronal (**B**) demonstrate hazy strand densities in the thecal sac, in particular, the L2 level without any compression (*arrow*). On myelography there was a complete block at the L2 level.

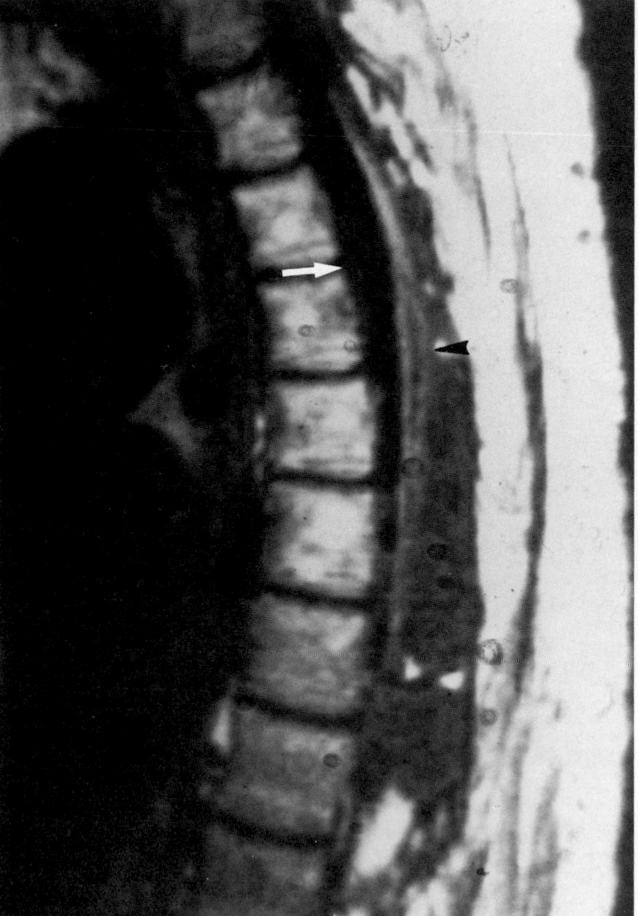

A

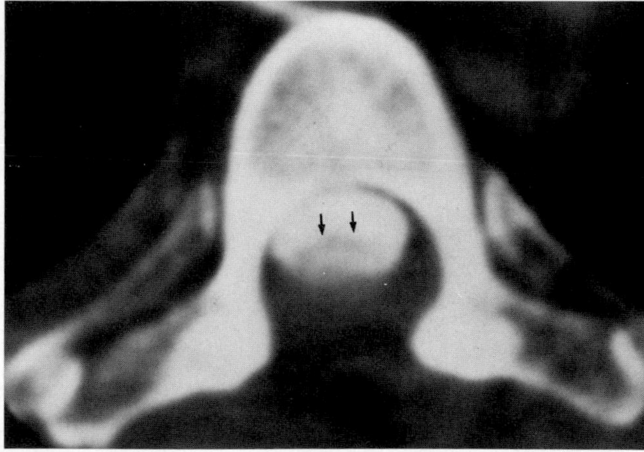

B

FIG. 64. Syringomyelia secondary to arachnoid adhesions in a 30-year-old man with a history of trauma and previous midthoracic laminectomy. **A:** Sagittal T1-weighted image demonstrates an atrophic cord with a small syrinx (*arrowhead*). The anterior subarachnoid space is large, possibly suggesting an arachnoid loculation (*arrows*). **B:** Axial delayed postmyelogram CT. The anterior surface of the cord (*arrows*) is convex anteriorly, consistent with a posteriorly tethered cord and not an arachnoid cyst. (From Andrews et al., ref. 111., with permission.)

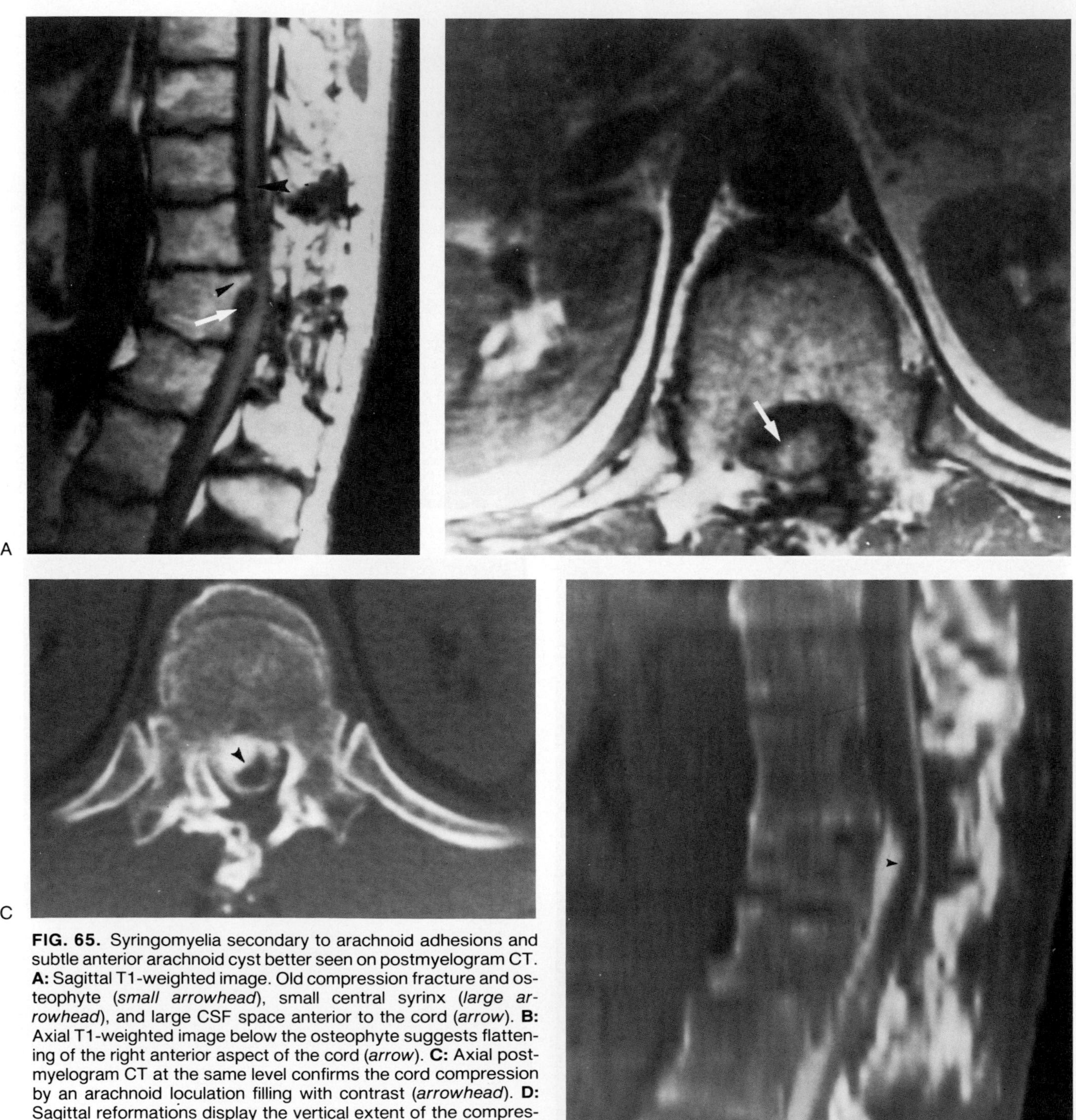

FIG. 65. Syringomyelia secondary to arachnoid adhesions and subtle anterior arachnoid cyst better seen on postmyelogram CT. **A:** Sagittal T1-weighted image. Old compression fracture and osteophyte (*small arrowhead*), small central syrinx (*large arrowhead*), and large CSF space anterior to the cord (*arrow*). **B:** Axial T1-weighted image below the osteophyte suggests flattening of the right anterior aspect of the cord (*arrow*). **C:** Axial postmyelogram CT at the same level confirms the cord compression by an arachnoid loculation filling with contrast (*arrowhead*). **D:** Sagittal reformations display the vertical extent of the compression to better advantage. The superiority of CT in this case is due to the thinner sections. (From Andrews et al., ref. 111, with permission.)

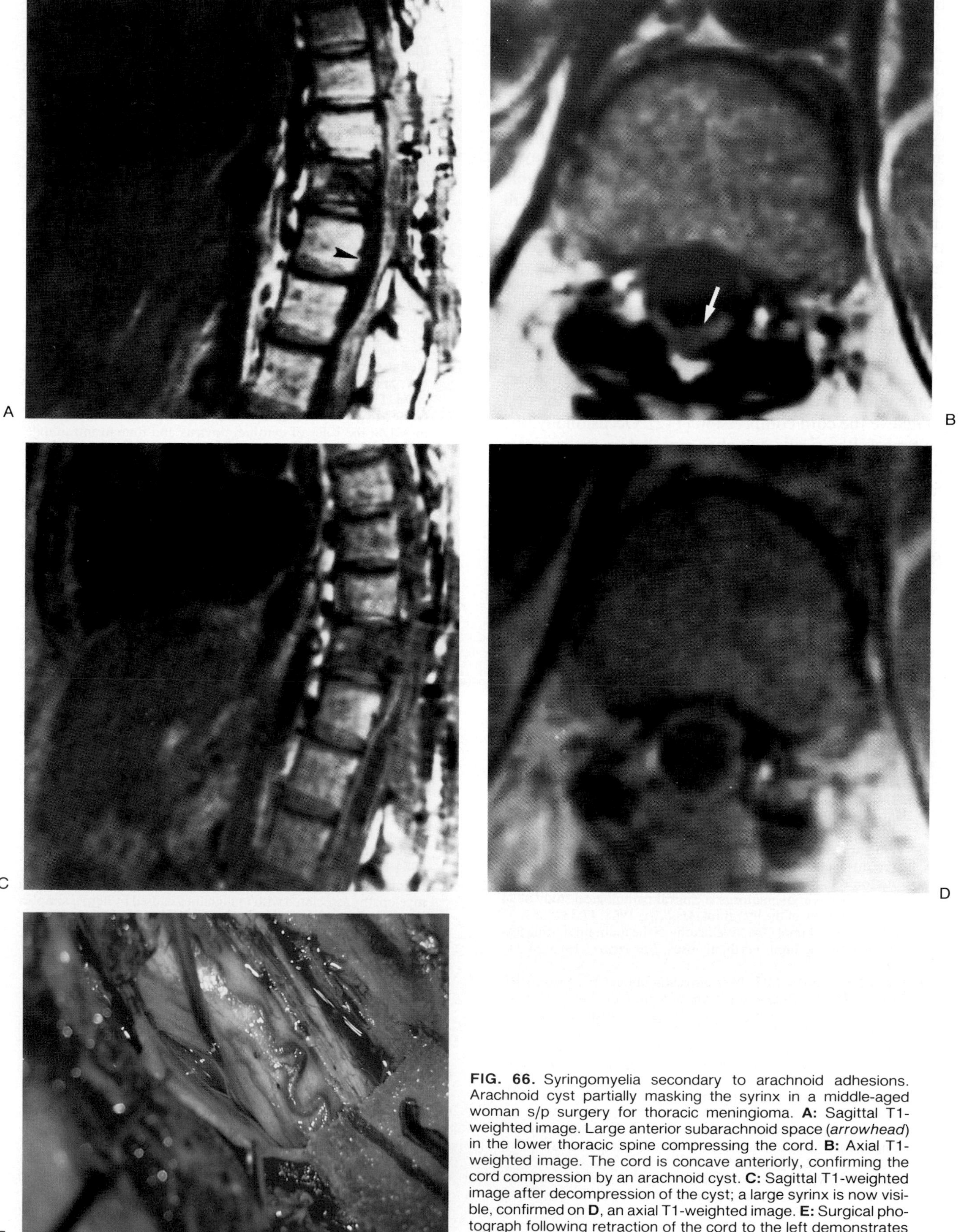

FIG. 66. Syringomyelia secondary to arachnoid adhesions. Arachnoid cyst partially masking the syrinx in a middle-aged woman s/p surgery for thoracic meningioma. **A:** Sagittal T1-weighted image. Large anterior subarachnoid space (*arrowhead*) in the lower thoracic spine compressing the cord. **B:** Axial T1-weighted image. The cord is concave anteriorly, confirming the cord compression by an arachnoid cyst. **C:** Sagittal T1-weighted image after decompression of the cyst; a large syrinx is now visible, confirmed on **D**, an axial T1-weighted image. **E:** Surgical photograph following retraction of the cord to the left demonstrates the anterior arachnoid cyst compressing the cord.

tion. The diagnosis of an arachnoid cyst is made by demonstrating compression of the cord by a mass with CSF signal characteristics. The anterior subarachnoid space may also appear enlarged when the cord is tethered posteriorly by adhesion, thus mimicking an arachnoid cyst. However, in this case, the anterior aspect of the cord is convex anteriorly and not concave, as in the case of an arachnoid loculation (Fig. 64). In difficult cases, delayed CT following subarachnoid injection of water-soluble contrast agents may be helpful (Fig. 65) (111). When all these signs are present in a patient with a history of a previous event that might have resulted in arachnoid adhesions, the MR is virtually pathognomonic. However, the initial trauma might have been minor and overlooked; and if an arachnoid cyst is not present, SSAA may be difficult to differentiate from a tumor-related syrinx. A gadolinium-enhanced study is then indicated to exclude a neoplasm. The surgical treatment includes both shunting of the syrinx and fenestration of the cyst to relieve the cord compression (112). Occasionally, the cyst masks the syrinx, which is revealed once the cyst is decompressed (Fig. 66). Post-traumatic arachnoid cysts may also occur in the absence of syringomyelia (113,114).

REFERENCES

1. Pardatscher K, Fiore DL, Lavano A. MR imaging of transverse myelitis using GD-DTPA. *J Neuroradiol* 1992;19:63–67.
2. Barakos JA, Mark AS, Dillon WP, Norman D. MR imaging of acute transverse myelitis and AIDS myelopathy. *J Comput Assist Tomogr* 1990;14:45–50.
3. Shen WC, Lee SK, Ho YJ, et al. MRI of sequela of transverse myelitis. *Pediatr Radiol* 1992;22:382–383.
4. Holtas S, Basibuyuk N, Fredriksson K. MRI in acute transverse myelopathy. *Neuroradiol* 1993;35:221—226.
5. Friedman DP. Herpes zoster myelitis: MR appearance. *AJNR* 1992;13:1404–1406.
6. Owen NL. Myelitis following type A2 influenza. *JAMA* 1971;215:1986–1987.
7. Harrington RB, Olin R. Incomplete transverse myelitis following rabies duck embryo vaccination. *JAMA* 1971;216:2137–2138.
8. Yamamoto M. Recurrent transverse myelitis associated with collagen disease. *J Neurol* 1986;233(3):185–187.
9. Johnson RT, Richardson EP. The neurological manifestations of systemic lupus erythematosus: a clinical-pathological study of 24 cases and review of the literature. *Medicine* 1968;47:337–369.
10. Al-Husaini A, Jamal GA. Myelopathy as the main presenting feature of systemic lupus erythematosus. *Eur Neurol* 1985;24:94–106.
11. Cloys DE, Netsky MG. Neuromyelitis optica. In: Vinken PJ, Bruyn GW, eds. *Handbook of Clinical Neurology, Vol. 9. Multiple Sclerosis and Other Demyelinating Diseases.* Amsterdam: North-Holland; 1970:426–436.
12. Chusid MJ, Williamson SJ, Murphy JV, Ramey LS. Neuromyelitis optica (Devic disease) following varicella infection. *J Pediatr* 1979;95:737–738.
13. Williamson PM. Neuromyelitis optica following infectious mononucleosis. *Proc Aust Assoc Neurol* 1975;12:153–155.
14. McAlpine D, Kuroiwa Y, Toyokura Y, Araki S. Acute demyelinating disease complicating herpes zoster. *J Neurol Neurosurg Psychiatry* 1959;22:120–123.
15. Silber MH, Wilcox PA, Bowen RM, Unger A. Neuromyelitis optica (Devic's syndrome) and pulmonary tuberculosis. *Neurology* 1990;40:934–938.
16. April RS, Vansonnenberg E. A case of neuromyelitis optica (Devic's syndrome) in systemic lupus erythematosus: clinicopathologic report and review of the literature. *Neurology* 1976;26:1066–1070.
17. Allen IV. Demyelinating diseases. In: Hume Adams J, Corsellis JAN, Duchen LW. *Greenfield's Neuropathology*, 4th ed. New York: John Wiley and Sons; 1984:337–339.
18. Larsson E-M, Holtas S, Nilsson 0. GD-DTPA-enhancement of suspected spinal multiple sclerosis. *AJNR* 1989;10:1071–1076.
19. Poser CM, Paty DW, Scheinberg L, et al. New diagnostic criteria for multiple sclerosis: guidelines for research protocols. *Ann Neurol* 1983:13:227–231.
20. Marcus RB Jr, Million RR. Incidence of myelitis after irradiation of the cervical spinal cord. *Int J Radiat Oncol Biol Phys* 1990;19:3–8.
21. Wang P-Y, Shen W-C, Jan J-S. MR imaging in radiation myelopathy. *AJNR* 1992;13:1049–1055.
22. Sze G, Russell E, Lee D. MR imaging of chronic radiation myelopathy. Presented at the 75th Annual meeting and scientific assembly of the RSNA, Chicago, Ill, 1989.
23. Kenney CM III, Goldstein SJ. MRI of sarcoid spondylodiskitis. *J Comput Assist Tomogr* 1992;16:660–662.
24. Nesbit GM, Miller GM, Baker HL, Eberson MJ, Scheithauer BW. Spinal cord sarcoidosis: a new finding at MR imaging with GD-DTPA enhancement. *Radiology* 1989;173:839–843.
25. Grafe MR, Wiley CA. Spinal cord and peripheral nerve pathology in AIDS: the roles of cytomegalovirus and human immunodeficiency virus. *Ann Neurol* 1989;25:561–566.
26. Lim V, Sobel DF, Zyroff J. Spinal cord pial metastasis: MR imaging with gadopentetate dimeglumine. *AJNR* 1990;11:975–982.
27. Morrissey SP, Miller DH, Hermeszewski R, et al. MRI of the CNS in Behçet's disease. *Eur Neurol* 1993;33(4):287–293.
28. Kim RC. Necrotizing myelopathy. *AJNR* 1991;12:1084–1086.
29. Henderson FC, Crockard HA, Stevens JM, et al. Spinal cord oedema due to venous stasis. *Neuroradiology* 1993;35:312–315.
30. Foix C, Alajouanine T. La myelite necrotique subaigue. *Rev Neurol* 1926;33:1–42.
31. Hughes RAC, Mair WGP. Acute necrotic myelopathy with pulmonary tuberculosis. *Brain* 1977;100:223–238.
32. Tateishi J, Kuroda S, Saito A, Otsuki S. Experimental myelo-optico neuropathy induced by clioquinol. *Acta Neuropathol* 1973;24:304–320.
33. Lavalle C, Pizarro S, Drenkard C, Sanchez-Guerrero J, Alarcon Segovia D. Transverse myelitis: a manifestation of systemic lupus erythematosus strongly associated with antiphospholipid antibodies. *J Rheumatol* 1990;17:34–37.
34. Norris FH Jr. Remote effects of cancer on the spinal cord. In: Vinken PJ, Bruyn GW, Klawans HL, eds. *Handbook of Clinical Neurology, Vol. 38. Neurological Manifestations of Systemic Diseases, Part 1.* Amsterdam: North-Holland; 1979:669–677.
35. Ojeda VJ. Necrotizing myelopathy associated with malignancy: a clinicopathologic study of two cases and literature review. *Cancer* 1984;53:1115–1123.
36. Iwamasa T, Utsumi Y, Sakuda H, et al. Two cases of necrotizing myelopathy associated with malignancy caused by herpes simplex virus type 2. *Acta Neuropathol* 1989;78:252–257.
37. Mirich DR, Kucharczyk W, Keller MA, et al. Subacute necrotizing myelopathy: MR imaging in four pathologically proved cases. *AJNR* 1991;12:1077–1083.
38. Gero B, Sze G, Sharif H. MR imaging of intradural inflammatory diseases of the spine. *AJNR* 1991;12:1009.
39. Wiley AM, Trueta J. The vascular anatomy of the spine and its relationship to pyogenic vertebral osteomyelitis. *J Bone Joint Surg* 1959;41(8):796–809.
40. Hossler 0. The human intervertebral disc. *Acta Ortho Scand* 1969;40:765–772.
41. Resnick D, Niwayama G. Osteomyelitis, septic arthritis, and soft tissue infections: the axial skeleton. In: Resnick D, Niwayama G, eds. *Diagnosis of Bone and Joint Disorders.* Philadelphia: WB Saunders; 1981:2130–2153.
42. Hensey OJ, Coad N, Carty HM, Sills JM. Juvenile discitis. *Arch Dis Child* 1983;58:983–987.
43. Angelo CM, Whisler WW. Bacterial infections of the spinal cord

and its coverings. In: Vinken PJ, Bruyn GW, eds. *Handbook of Clinical Neurology*. Amsterdam: North-Holland; 1978.
44. Modic MT, Feiglin DH, Piraino DW, et al. Vertebral osteomyelitis: assessment using MR. *Radiology* 1985;157:157–166.
45. Colombo N, Berry I, Norman D. Infections of the spine. In: Manelfe C, ed. *Imaging of the Spine and Spinal Cord*. New York: Raven Press; 1992:489–512.
46. Thrush A, Enzmann D. MR imaging of infectious spondylitis. *AJNR* 1990;11:1171–1180.
47. Smith AS, Blaser SI. Infectious and inflammatory processes of the spine. *Radiol Clin North Am* 1991;29:809–827.
48. Sharif HS. Role of MR imaging in the management of spinal infections. *AJR* 1992;158:1333–1345.
49. Modic MT, Steinberg PM, Ross JS, Masaryk TJ, Carter JR. Degenerative disc disease: assessment of changes in vertebral body marrow with MR imaging. *Radiology* 1988;166:193–199.
50. Eschelman DJ, Beers GJ, Naimark A, et al. Pseudoarthrosis in ankylosing spondylitis mimicking infectious diskitis: MR appearance. *AJNR* 1991;12:1113–1114.
51. Lindholm TS, Pylkkanen P. Diskitis following removal of intervertebral disk. *Spine* 1982;7:618–622.
52. Fernand R, Lee CK. Post-laminectomy disk space infection: a review of the literature and a report of three cases. *Clin Orthop* 1986;209:215–218.
53. Boden SD, Davis DO, Dina TS, Sunner JL, Wiesel SW. Postoperative diskitis: distinguishing early MR imaging findings from normal postoperative disk space changes. *Radiology* 1992;184: 765–771.
54. Angtuaco EJC, McConnell JR, Chadduck WM, Flanigan S. MR imaging of spinal epidural sepsis. *AJNR* 1987;8:879–883.
55. Sandhu FS, Dillon WP. Spinal epidural abscess: evaluation with contrast-enhanced MR imaging. *AJNR* 1991;12:1087–1093.
56. Martijn A, van der Vliet AM, van Waarde WM, et al. Gadolinium-DTPA-enhanced MRI in neonatal osteomyelitis of the cervical spine. *Br J Radiol* 1992;65:720–722.
57. Shen WC, Lee SK, Ho YJ, et al. Acute spinal epidural abscess in the whole spine: case report of a 2 year old boy. *Eur Radiol* 1992;26:589.
58. Numaguchi Y, Rigamonti D, Rothman MI, Sato S, Mihara F, Sadato N. Spinal epidural abscess: evaluation with gadolinium-enhanced MR imaging. *RadioGraphics* 1993;13:545–559.
59. Quencer RM. Spinal epidural abscess: evaluation with gadolinium-enhanced MR imaging: invited commentary. *RadioGaphics* 1993;13:559.
60. Kokes F, Iplikcioglu AC, Camurdanoglu M, et al. Epidural spinal abscess containing gas: MRI demonstration. *Neuroradiology* 1993;35:497–498.
61. Sharif HS, Clark DC, Aabed MY, et al. Granulomatous spinal infections: MR imaging. *Radiology* 1990;177:101–107.
62. Nabatame H, Nakamura K, Matuda M, et al. MRI of syphilitic myelitis. *Neuroradiology* 1992;34:105–106.
63. Steere AC, Malawista SE, Snydman DR. et al. Lyme arthritis: an epidemic of oligo-articular arthritis in children and adults in three Connecticut communities. *Arthritis Rheum* 1977:20:7–17.
64. Coyle PK, Neurologic Lyme disease. *Semin Neurol* 1992;12(3): 200–208.
65. King SJ, Jeffree MA. MRI of an abscess of the cervical spinal cord in a case of Listeria meningoencephalomyelitis. *Neuroradiology* 1993;35:495–496.
66. Smith AS, Weinstein MA, Mizushima A, et al. MR imaging characteristics of tuberculous spondylitis vs vertebral osteomyelitis. *AJNR* 1989;10:619–625.
67. Golkap HZ, Ozkal E. Intradural tuberculoma of the spinal cord. Report of two cases. *J Neurosurg* 1981;55:289–292.
68. Chang KH, Han MH, Choi YW, Kim 10, Han MC, Kim CW. Tuberculous arachnoiditis of the spine: findings on myelography, CT, and MR imaging. *AJNR* 1989;10:1255–1266.
69. Gorbach SL, Bartlett JG, Blacklow NR. *Infectious Diseases*. Philadelphia: WB Saunders; 1992:1254–1255.
70. Scaravilli F. Parasitic and fungal infections of the nervous system. In: Hume Adams J, Corsellis JAN, Duchen LW, eds. *Greenfield's Neuropathology*, 4th ed. New York: John Wiley and Sons; 1984: 305–333.
71. Gehweiler JA, Capp MP, Chick EW. Observation on the roentgen pattern in blastomycosis of bone. A review of cases from the blastomycosis cooperative study of the Veteran's Administration and Duke University Medical Center. *AJR* 1970;108:497–510.
72. McGahan JP, Graves DS, Palmer PES. Coccidioidal spondylosis; usual and unusual radiographic manifestations. *Radiology* 1980;136:5–9.
73. Welsh JD, Rhodes ER, Jacques W. Disiminated nocardiosis involving the spinal cord. Case report. *Arch Intern Med* 1961;108: 73–79.
74. Parker SL, Laszewski MJ, Trigg ME, et al. Spinal cord aspergillosis in immunosuppressed patients. *Pediatr Radiol* 1990;20:351.
75. Reich JM. Aspergillus epidural abscess and cord compression in a patient with aspergilloma and empeyema [*Letter*]. *Am Rev Respir Dis* 1993;147(5):1322–1323.
76. Ho KC, Williams A, Gronseth G, Aldrich M. Spinal cord swelling and candidiasis. A case report. *Neuroradiology* 1982;2:117–118.
77. Voelker JL, Muller J, Worth RM. Intramedullary spinal histoplasma granuloma. Case report. *J Neurosurg* 1989;70:959–961.
78. Firemark HM. Spinal cysticercosis. *Arch Neurol* 1978;35:250–251.
79. Palasis S, Drevelengas A. Extramedullary spinal cysticercosis. *Eur J Radiol* 1991;12:216.
80. Akiguchi I, Fujiwara T, Matsuyama H, Muranaka H, Kameyama M. Intramedullary spinal cysticercosis. *Neurology* 1979;29:1531–1534.
81. Castillo M, Quencer RM, Post MJD. MR of intramedullary spinal cysticercosis. *AJNR* 1988;9:393–395.
82. Lie KW, Yu YL, Cheng IKP, Woo E, Wong WT. Cryptococcal infection of the lumbar spine. *J Roy Soc Med* 1989;83:172–173.
83. Cure JK, Mirich DR. MR imaging in cryptococcal spondylisis. *AJNR* 1991;12:1111.
84. Dupuis MJM, Atrouni S, Dooms GC, et al. MR imaging of schistosomal myelitis. *AJNR* 1990;11:782.
85. Silbergleit R, Silbergleit R. Schistosomal granuloma of the spinal cord: evaluation with MR imaging and intraoperative sonography. *AJR* 1992;158:1351–1353.
86. Ogut AG, Kanberoglu K, Altug A, et al. CT and MRI in hydatid disease of cervical vertebrae. *Neuroradiology* 1992;34:430.
87. Cho YD, Huh JD, Hwang YS, et al. Sparganosis in the spinal canal with partial block: an uncommon infection. *Neuroradiology* 1992;34:241.
88. Nag S, Jackson AC. Myelopathy: an unusual presentation of toxoplasmosis. *Can J Neurol Sci* 1989;16:422–425.
89. Poon TP, Tchertkoff V, Pares GF, et al. Spinal cord toxoplasma lesion in AIDS: MR findings. *J Comput Assist Tomogr* 1992;16: 817.
90. Mehren M, Burns PJ, Mamani F, Levy CS, Laureno R. Toxoplasmic myelitis mimicking intramedullary spinal cord tumor. *Neurology* 1988;38:1648–1650.
91. Reichman RC. Neurological complications of varicella-zoster infections. *Ann Intern Med* 1978;89:375–388.
92. Hogan EL, Krigman MR. Herpes zoster myelitis: evidence for viral invasion of spinal cord. *Arch Neurol* 1973;29:309–313.
93. Silverstein A, Steinberg G, Nathanson M. Nervous system involvement in infectious mononucleosis: the heralding and/or major manifestation. *Arch Neurol* 1972;26:353–358.
94. Talpos D, Tien RD, Hesselink JR. Magnetic resonance imaging of AIDS related polyradiculopathy. *Neurology* 1991;41:1996–1997.
95. Holmes GP, Hilliard JK, Klontz KC, et al. B virus infection in humans: epidemiologic investigation of a cluster. *Ann Intern Med* 1990;112:833–839.
96. Baran GB, Sowell MK, Sharp GB Glasier CM. MR findings in a child with Guillain-Barré syndrome. *AJR* 1993;161:161–163.
97. Petito CK, Navia BA, Cho E-S, Jordan BD, George DC, Price RW. Vacuolar myelopathy pathologically resembling subacute combined degeneration in patients with acquired immunodeficiency syndrome. *N Engl J Med* 1985;312(14):874–879.
98. Victor M, Adams RD. Tropical spastic paraparesis and HTLVI infection. In: Victor M, Adams RD. *Principles of Neurology*, 5th ed. New York: McGraw-Hill; 1993;665:1109.
99. Wolman L. The neuropathological effects resulting from the intrathecal injection of chemical substances. *Paraplegia* 1966;4: 97–115.

100. Hoffman GS, Ellsworth CA, Wells EE, Franck WA, Mackie RW. Spinal arachnoiditis: what is the clinical spectrum? II. Arachnoiditis induced by pantopaque/autologous blood in dogs, a possible model for human disease. *Spine* 1983;8(5):541–551.
101. Shaw DM, Russell JA, Grossart KW. The changing pattern of spinal arachnoiditis. *J Neurol Neurosurg Psychiatry* 1978;41:97–107.
102. Jorgensen J, Hansen PH, Steenskov V, Ovesen NA. Clinical and radiological study of lower spinal arachnoiditis. *Neuroradiology* 1975;9:139–144.
103. Simmons JD, Newton TH. Arachnoiditis. In: Newton TH, Potts DG, eds. *Computed Tomography of the Spine and Spinal Cord.* San Anselmo, CA: Clavadel; 1983:223–229.
104. Ross JS, Masaryk TJ, Modic MT. MR imaging of lumbar arachnoiditis. *AJR* 1987;8:885–892.
105. Monajati A, Wayne WS, Rauschning W, Ekholm SE. MR of the cauda equina. *AJNR* 1987;8:893–900.
106. Barnett JHM, Foster JB, Hudgson P. *Syringomyelia.* Philadelphia: WB Saunders; 1973:179–225.
107. Barnett HJM. Syringomyelia associated with spinal arachnoiditis. In: *Non-Communicating Syringomyelia.* 220–243.
108. Barnett HJM. The pathogeneous of syringomyelic cavitation associated with arachnoiditis localized to the spinal canal. In: *Non-Communicating Syringomyelia.* 245–259.
109. Mark AS, Andrews BT, Sanchez J, Manelfe C, Peck W, Norman D. MRI of syringomyelia secondary to arachnoid adhesions (arachnoiditis) with emphasis on associated arachnoid cysts. VIth Annual Meeting of the Society of Magnetic Resonance in Medicine, New York, Aug. 1987, p. 251.
110. Savoiardo M. Syringomyelia associated with postmeningetic spinal arachnoiditis. *Neurology* 1975;26:551–554.
111. Andrews BT, Weinstein PR, Rosenblum ML, Barbaro NM. Intradural arachnoid cysts of the spinal canal associated with intramedullary cysts. *J Neurosurg* 1988;688(4):544–549.
112. Barbaro NM, Wilson CB, Gutin PH, Edwards MSB. Surgical treatment of syringomyelia: favorable results with syringoperitoneal shunting. *J Neurosurg* 1984;61:53–538.
113. Cilluffo JM, Miller RH. Posttraumatic arachnoidal diverticula. *Acta Neurochirurg* 1980;54:77–87.
114. Palmer JJ. Spinal arachnoid cysts: report of six cases. *J Neurosurg* 1974;41:728–735.

Magnetic Resonance Imaging of the Brain and Spine, Second Edition, edited by Scott W. Atlas. Lippincott-Raven Publishers, Philadelphia © 1996.

26

Congenital Anomalies of the Spine and Spinal Cord

Embryology and Malformations

Thomas P. Naidich, Robert A. Zimmerman, David G. McLone, Charles A. Raybaud, Nolan R. Altman, and Bruce H. Braffman

In the spine, the most common congenital lesions presenting to medical attention are (a) the diverse forms of spinal dysraphism and (b) the diverse forms of caudal spinal anomalies (1). Most commonly, these conditions are discovered at birth or in early childhood. Less commonly, they first present to medical attention in adulthood (2–4). Widespread use of magnetic resonance imaging has reduced the incidence of delayed diagnosis of these conditions and disclosed surprising numbers of adult dysraphics.

Congenital malformations of the spine are grouped into three broad categories (1,5,6):

1. Spina Bifida Aperta. Those lesions in which the neural tissue is exposed to view in the midline of the back are designated spina bifida aperta. The most common forms of spina bifida aperta are the myelocele and myelomeningocele; simple meningoceles without skin cover are less common.

2. Occult Spinal Dysraphism. Those lesions in which the neural tissue lies deep to an intact skin cover are designated occult spinal dysraphism (1,7). This is a heterogeneous group of lesions which includes dorsal dermal sinus, spinal lipoma, tight filum terminale syndrome, neurenteric cyst, and diastematomyelia. These lesions

T. P. Naidich, M.D.: Department of Radiology, Baptist Hospital of Miami, Miami, FL 33176.
R. A. Zimmerman, M.D.: Department of Radiology, Children's Hospital of Philadelphia, Philadelphia, PA 19104.
D. G. McLone, M.D., Ph.D.: Department of Neurosurgery, Children's Memorial Hospital, Chicago, IL 60614.
C. A. Raybaud, M.D.: Department of Radiology, Groupe Hospitalier de la Timon, Marseille, France.
N. R. Altman, M.D.: Department of Radiology, Miami Children's Hospital, Miami, FL 33136.
B. H. Braffman, M.D.: Department of Radiology, Memorial Hospital, Hollywood, FL 33021.

share the common features that the spinal cord is cleft and/or is tethered in an abnormally low position by a fibrous band, a bone spur or a caudal mass (8). The specific cause of the tethering is often unknown (9). Midline cutaneous stigmata such as skin dimples, skin tags, hemangiomatous naevi, and patches of hypertrichosis frequently overlie the zone of abnormal nervous tissue and signal the presence of "hidden" pathology.

3. Caudal Spinal Anomalies. Those lesions in which malformations of the distal end of the spine, spinal cord, and meninges are associated with disorders of the hindgut, kidneys, urinary bladder, and genitalia are designated caudal spinal anomalies. These include sacral agenesis, terminal myelocystocele, and anterior sacral meningocele, among others.

This chapter addresses the most common forms of dysraphism and the most common caudal spinal anomalies (10,11). It provides an overview of embryology for orientation and then groups the anomalies in terms of the specific derangements of embryology that are believed to give rise to the anomalies (12,13). It is hoped that this approach will provide greater understanding of these lesions and better long-term retention of information about them. A conceptual framework of embryology and pathogenesis may eliminate the need for rote memorization; certainly it is a more satisfying approach intellectually (1,14–29).

OVERVIEW OF NORMAL EMBRYOGENESIS

By the end of the second week of gestation, the embryo has taken the form of a two-layered cell disc (Fig. 1). The ectodermal layer faces the amniotic cavity. The subjacent entodermal layer faces the yolk sac (also called vitelline sac or future gut). At one end of the ectodermal layer, a slight thickening known as the prochordal plate indicates the future cephalic region, the cranio-caudal axis of the embryo and the left-right axis of the embryo (10–13, 30).

By day 14 or 15, a linear midline primitive streak forms at the caudal end of the amniotic side of the ectodermal disc (Fig. 1). Ectodermal cells migrate toward the primitive streak, pass through it to the interface of ectoderm and entoderm, and then migrate laterally along the interface to form an intermediate "mesodermal" germ layer (Fig. 2A). This migration converts the bilaminar disc to a trilaminar disc. The mesodermal cells migrate along defined routes to each side of the midline. No mesodermal cells migrate along the midline between the primitive streak and the prochordal plate.

As the mesoderm migrates laterally, the cephalic end of the primitive streak shows a marked thickening known variously as Hensen's node, the primitive node or the primitive knot. This contains a small primitive pit. Ectodermal cells pass inward at the primitive pit and migrate cephalically in the midline to reach the prochordal plate (Fig. 2B). By a series of steps detailed later, these midline cells establish the notochord directly between the entoderm and the ectoderm. The notochord induces the overlying ectoderm to differentiate into specialized neural ectoderm (Fig. 2C). The notochord will also direct the organization of the future vertebral centra and discs (31,32). From these simple beginnings, subsequent steps will form the cephalic portion of the spinal cord and then the caudal (or distal) cord (10–13).

A

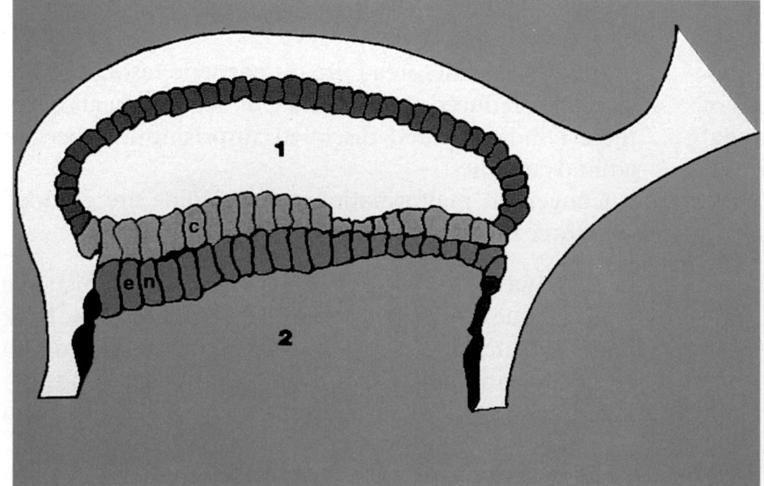

B

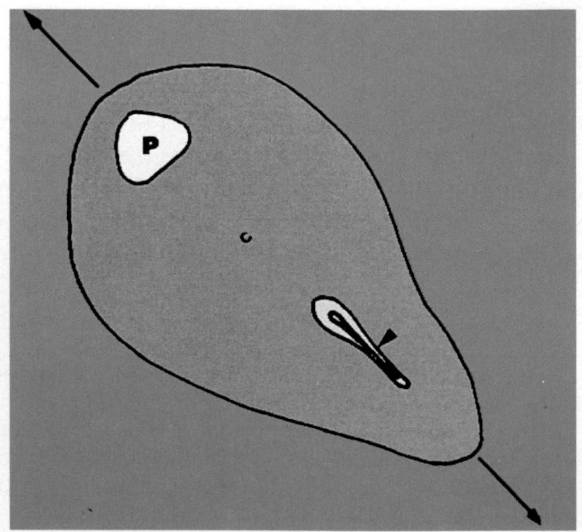

FIG. 1. Bilaminar disc. Prochordal plate. **A:** Longitudinal section. **B:** View of the ectodermal surface that faces the amnion. By the end of the second week of gestation, the two-layered embryo consists of an ectodermal layer (*c*) that faces the amnionic cavity (*1*) and an entodermal layer (*en*) that faces the yolk (vitelline) sac (*2*). The prochordal plate (*P*) establishes the cephalic end of the bilaminar disc and the first craniocaudal, left-right axes of the embryo. The primitive streak (*arrowhead*) forms in the midline toward the caudal end of the embryo. The thickening at the cephalic end of the streak, designated Hensen's node, contains a small primitive pit. (From Raybaud et al., ref. 13, with permission.)

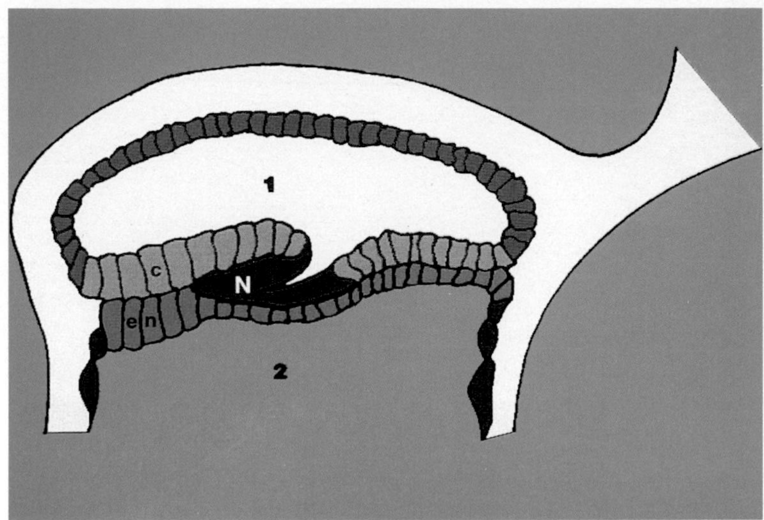

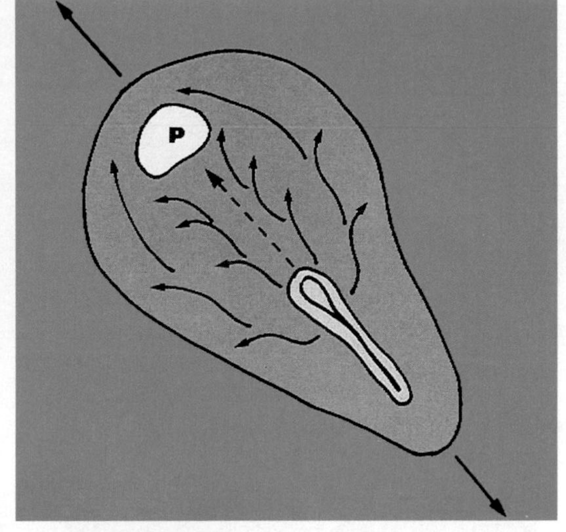

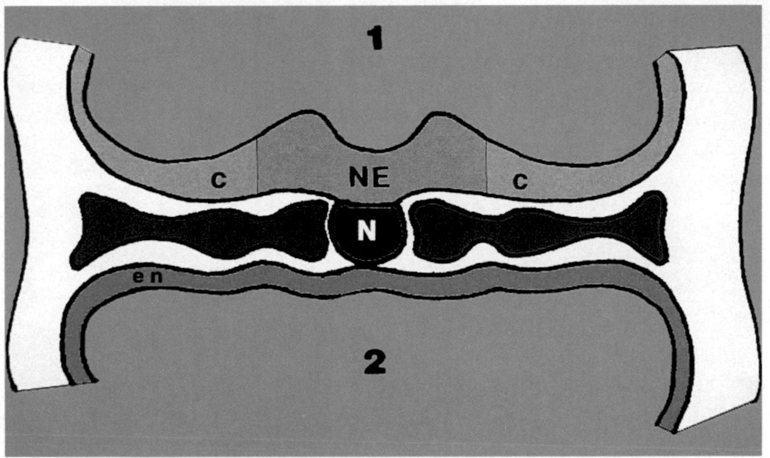

FIG. 2. Trilaminar disc. Migrations. **A:** Longitudinal section. **B:** View of the ectodermal surface that faces the amnion. **C:** Transverse section through the notochord at a slightly later time when the notochord has begun to induce formation of neural ectoderm (*NE*). Ectodermal cells pass medially to enter the primitive streak, descend to the interlaminar level, and then migrate cephalically and laterally between the ectoderm (*c*) and the entoderm (*en*). This migration converts the bilaminar disc to the trilaminar disc. Those cells that migrate in the true midline between Hensen's node and the prochordal plate (*P*) will form the notochordal process (*N*). The primitive pit will deepen and invaginate into this process to form the notochordal canal. Cells that migrate in the paramedian location will form the paraxial mesoderm (*M*), which becomes somites. Cells that migrate in the intermediate and the lateral locations will form the intermediate and lateral mesenchyme. (From Raybaud et al., ref. 13, with permission.)

The cephalic portion of the spinal cord forms by the mechanism of neurulation: an orderly sequence of steps in which the neural ectoderm forms a neural plate that then folds up into a neural tube. This mechanism establishes the cervical and thoracic segments of spinal cord and the upper portion of the lumbar cord to the midlumbar enlargement. The smaller, more distal portion of the lumbar cord, the conus medullaris and the filum terminale form by a far-less well-organized sequence of agglomeration of cells, vacuolation, and involution that is designated canalization and retrogressive differentiation.

Because the cephalic and caudal portions of the spinal cord are formed by distinctly different mechanisms, they are heir to distinctly different types of malformation.

NEURULATION AND DERANGEMENTS OF NEURULATION

Normal Neurulation

By the end of the third week, the notochord induces formation of a slipper-shaped plate of ectodermal cells in the midline just cephalic to Hensen's node (Fig. 2C). This neural plate is directly contiguous laterally with the superficial ectoderm from which it differentiated (Figs. 3A and 4A). During the next few days, active contraction of actin filaments flexes the lateral portions of the plate, elevating the neural folds. The midline portion remains depressed as the ventral neural groove (Figs. 3B and 4B). Progressive flexion and folding cause the left and right

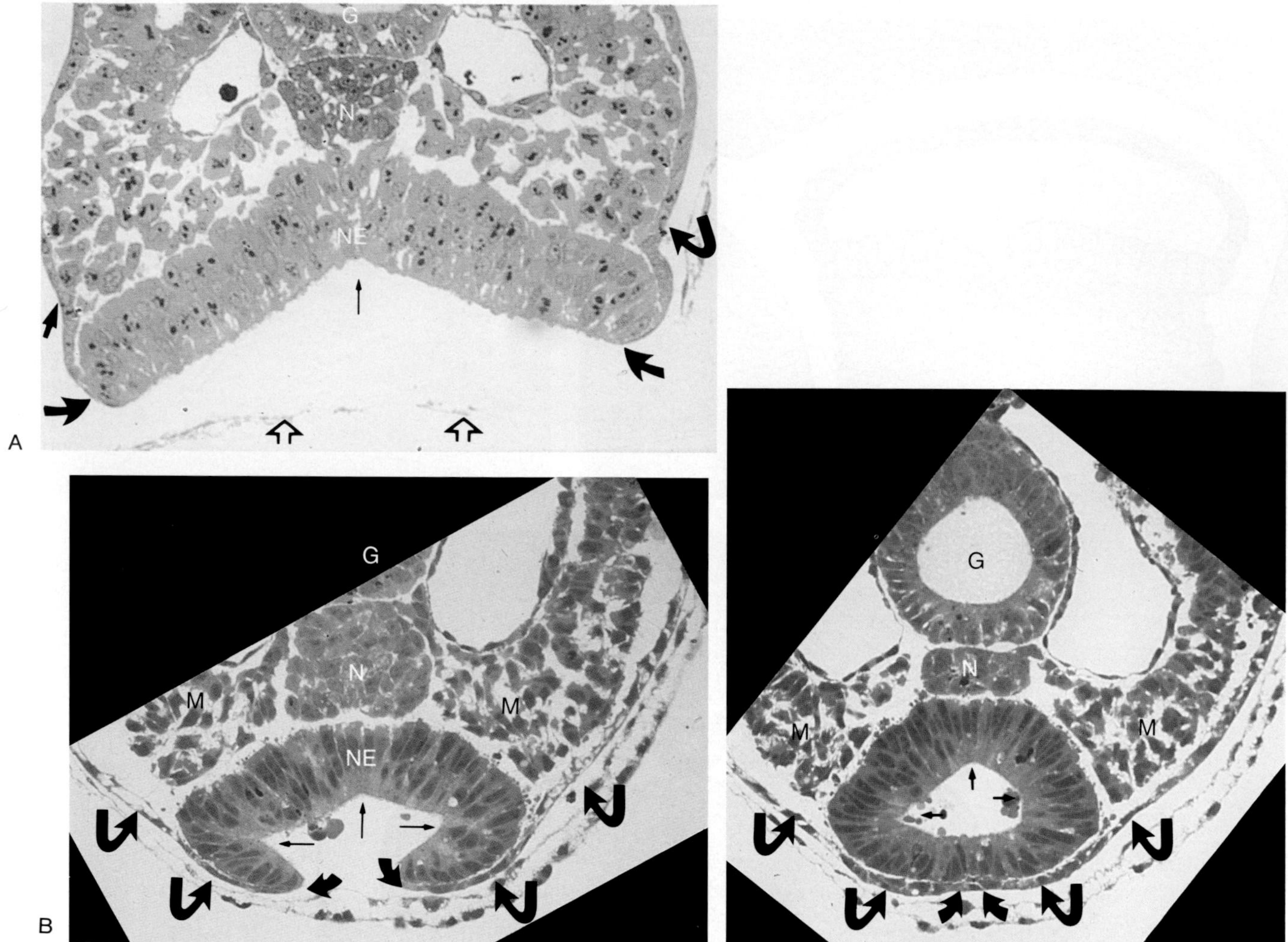

FIG. 3. Three stages of neurulation. Axial sections of mammalian embryos oriented like axial MRI with ventral toward the top. **A:** Neural plate. The primitive CNS originates as a "flat" plate of neural ectoderm (*NE*) composed of a single layer of cells with two distinct surfaces. The *ventral* surface of the neural plate faces the interior of the embryo. With folding, the ventral surface will form the entire external surface of the spinal cord. This ventral surface is contiguous with the notochord (*N*) in the midline and with the loose mesenchyme (*M*) to each side. The *dorsal* surface of the neural plate faces the exterior of the embryo and the amniotic cavity (*open arrows* indicate the amnion). With folding, the dorsal surface will form the inner surface of the spinal cord around the central canal of the cord. This dorsal surface exhibits a midline sulcus (*black arrow*) that is called the ventral neural groove, because it will become the ventral groove of the central canal of the cord. The cutaneous ectoderm (*large curved arrows*) forms a thin layer of cells that encloses the embryo ventrally and laterally. This cutaneous ectoderm is tightly adherent (*small curved arrows*) to the neural ectoderm at the lateral edges of the neural plate, precisely at the junction of the ventral and dorsal surfaces of the neural plate. At this stage the mesenchyme is restricted to two paramedian zones ventral to the neural plate: mesenchyme is excluded from the midline by the contiguity between the primitive gut (*G*), the notochord (*N*), and the ventral surface of the neural epithelium. Mesenchyme is prevented from passing posterolaterally by the tight adherence of the cutaneous ectoderm with the neural ectoderm at the margins of the neural plate. No mesenchyme can pass around to the dorsal aspect of the neural epithelium. **B:** Neural folds. With further development, active contraction of actin filaments concentrated near the dorsal surface of the neural plate begins to flex the plate dorsally, creating the neural folds. The ventral surface of the neural epithelium is beginning to assume the appearance of the external surface of the future spinal cord. The future central canal appears between the folds as a dorsal channel with a ventral neural groove (*vertical black arrow*) and two lateral sulci called the sulci limitans (*horizontal black arrows*). The cutaneous ectoderm (*large curved arrows*) remains tightly adherent to the neural ectoderm (*NE*) precisely at the neural ridge (*small curved arrows*) and passes dorsally with the ridge as the neural plate folds. This tight adherence of cutaneous with neural ectoderm prevents mesenchyme from migrating to the dorsal surface of the neural epithelium. The primitive gut remains contiguous with the notochord and the notochord with the ventral surface of the neural plate, excluding mesenchyme from the midline. The mesenchyme remains restricted to the two paramedian zones ventral to the developing neural tissue. The superficial membranes external to cutaneous and neural ectoderm are the amnion. **C:** Neural tube. Further flexion of the neural folds brings the two neural ridges into apposition. Molecules of glycosaminoglycans on the surface of the neural epithelium contact each other, recognize, and fuse together, closing the neural tube. The old dorsal surface of the neural plate has now become the wall of the primitive central canal. The old ventral surface of the neural plate has now become the entire exterior of the neural tube. The cutaneous ectoderm now lies in the dorsal midline but is still attached to the neural ectoderm. In a very carefully orchestrated series of events, first the neural folds fuse, closing the neural tube. Then, and only then, can the cutaneous ectoderm of each side separate from the neural ectoderm in a process called disjunction. Following disjunction, the left and right layers of cutaneous ectoderm also fuse in the midline dorsal (*superficial*) to the neural tube, enclosing the future CNS beneath the future skin.

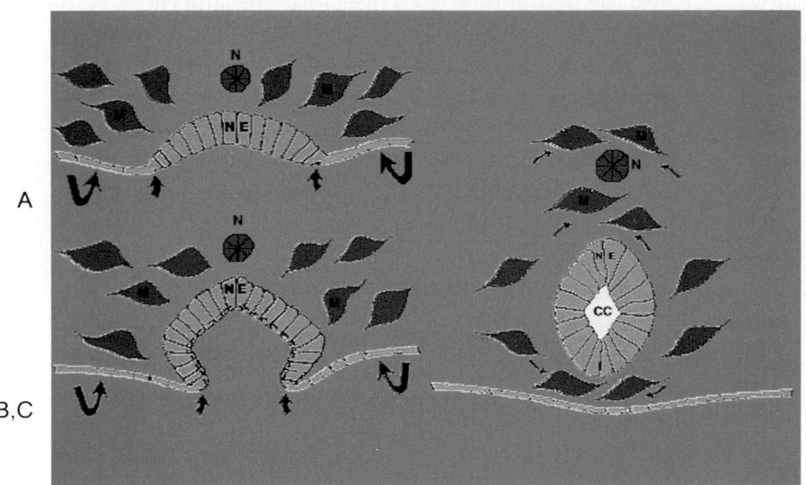

FIG. 4. Diagrammatic representation of neurulation. **A,B:** Summary of events illustrated in Fig. 3A and B. *curved arrows*, cutaneous ectoderm. The horizontal lines at the dorsal surfaces of the individual neuroectodermal cells indicate the actin filaments that act on the cytoskeleton to flex the neural plate. **C:** Following closure of the neural tube and successful disjunction of cutaneous from neural ectoderm, the cutaneous ectoderm fuses in the dorsal midline superficial to the neural tube. Then (*1*) the notochord (*N*) and the primitive gut migrate ventrally. They separate from each other and from the neural tube, permitting mesenchyme (*M*) to migrate around the notochord. This perichordal mesenchyme will be induced by the notochord to form the vertebral centra and intervertebral discs. (*2*) The cutaneous ectoderm separates more widely from the neural ectoderm, permitting the mesenchyme (*M*) to migrate dorsal to the neural tissue. This mesenchyme will be induced by the neural tube to make the neural arches and lateral elements. Mesenchyme condensing ventrolateral and dorsolateral to the developing vertebrae will become the paraspinal musculature. CC, central canal. (From Naidich et al., ref. 22, with permission.)

neural folds to approximate each other and fuse together in the midline. This process forms a neural tube (future spinal cord) with a central channel (future central canal of the cord) (Figs. 3C and 4C).

Traditionally the folds are thought to meet first and fuse in the future occipital region at about postovulatory day 22. Thereafter the entire process of flexion and fusion is believed to proceed cranially and caudally as a "wave," such that the level of fusion corresponds to the level of the most recently formed somite. At approximately 24 and 26–27 postovulatory days, respectively, the cephalic and caudal ends of the neural tube close at the anterior and posterior neuropores (13,33).

More recently, experimental data in mice and study of human malformations have led to a postulate that the neural tube closes independently at multiple sites, perhaps 4–5 sites (34). These closures would include the traditional first closure between somites 2–4 to form the cervical-thoracic cord down to a posterior neuropore at L2 and an additional closure distal to L2 (and distal to the posterior neuropore) to form a caudal segment of neurulated spinal cord between L2 and S2. Below S2 the cord would not be formed by neurulation. These postulates require further substantiation.

Immediately following fusion of the neural folds into the neural tube, the superficial ectoderm of each side separates from the neural ectoderm in a process designated disjunction. The two portions of superficial ectoderm then fuse together in the midline dorsal to the neural tube to establish the integrity of the superficial ectoderm (future skin) (Fig. 4C). As mesenchyme migrates dorsally between the neural tube and the skin, the entire cord becomes buried beneath a thick layer that ultimately forms the meninges, neural arches and paraspinal muscles.

Deranged Neurulation

Spina Bifida Aperta: Myelocele and Myelomeningocele

The term spina bifida aperta designates those forms of spinal dysraphism in which the neural tissue and/or meninges are exposed to the environment, because the skin, fascia, muscle, and bone are deficient in the midline of the back. Myelocele and myelomeningocele are the two commonest forms of spina bifida aperta.

Myelocele and myelomeningocele occur in 1–2 patients per 1,000 live births, up to 8 per 1,000 live births in specific populations (35). Such high incidence may be reduced sharply by providing supplements of dietary folic acid to the mother prior to and during pregnancy (36).

Myelomeningocele afflicts females slightly more commonly than males (35,37) and is evident at birth in all cases. The lesion involves the lower back predominantly: thoracic 2%, thoracolumbar 32%, lumbar 22%, and lumbosacral 44% (35). Since studies of embryos indicate that cervical and holocord myeloceles and myelomeningoceles actually occur more commonly than lumbosacral lesions, the predominance of caudal lesions evident at birth reflects their lesser severity and greater survival to term (38).

Patients with myelomeningocele manifest a number of neurological signs including sensorimotor deficits of the lower extremities, incontinence of bladder and bowel, hindbrain dysfunction, intellectual-perceptual impairments, and hydrocephalus (39–43). A component of the motor deficit appears to result from birth trauma and spinal shock. Infants delivered by Cesarian section prior to onset of labor manifest less severe deficits than those delivered vaginally or those delivered by C-section after some period of labor (44). Motor strength typically improves 1–2 levels after the initial repair of the myelomeningocele and then stabilizes at a set motor level. Deterioration thereafter is regarded as evidence of a secondary complication.

Myelocele and myelomeningocele appear to result from deranged neurulation. If the neural folds fail to flex and to fuse into a tube, they persist instead as a flat plate of neural tissue (Fig. 5) (45,46). This flat plate of unneurulated neural tissue is designated the neural placode. Because the neural tube does not close, the superficial ectoderm cannot disjoin from the neural ectoderm and remains in lateral position. Therefore the skin that develops from the ectoderm also lies lateral in position, leaving a midline defect. Mesenchyme then cannot migrate behind the neural tube, so the bony, cartilaginous, muscular, and ligamentous elements are also deficient in the midline. Instead, the bones, cartilage, muscle, and ligament develop in an abnormal position ventral-lateral to the neural tissue, and appear bifid and "everted." The

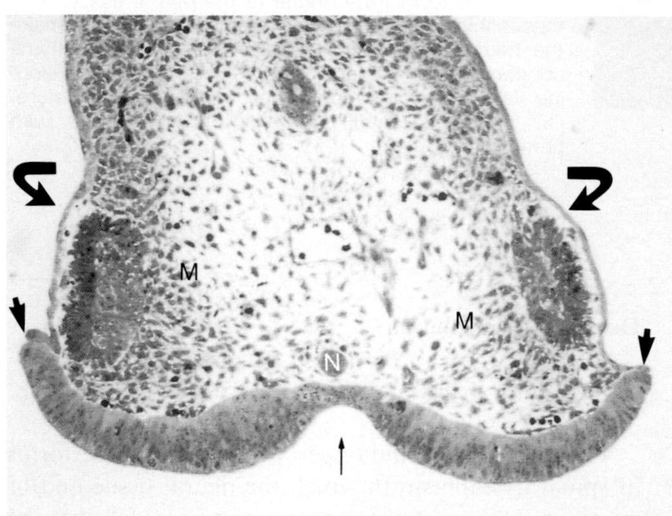

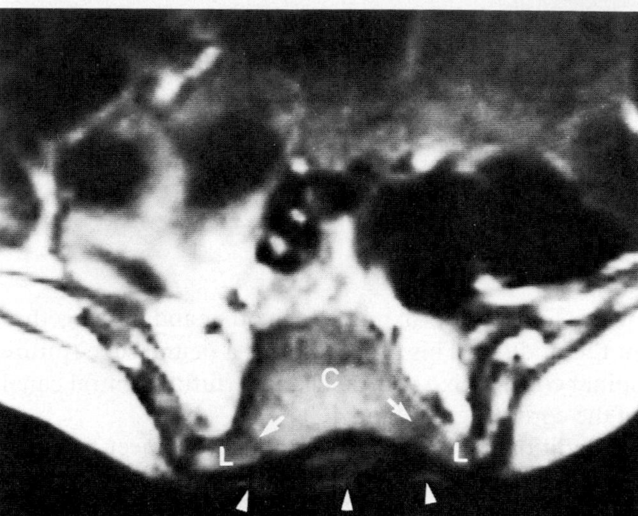

C

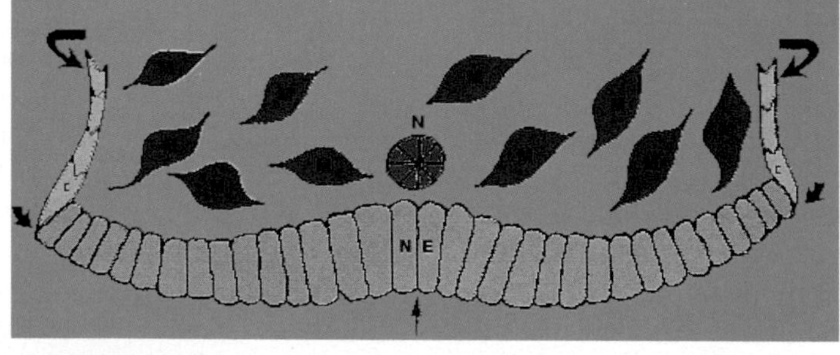

B

FIG. 5. Unneurulated neural placode. Proposed embryogenesis for spina bifida aperta by failure to neurulate the neural plate with consequent nondisjunction of cutaneous from neural ectoderm. Mammalian embryo (**A**); diagrammatic representation (**B**). Images oriented like axial MRI with ventral toward the top. **C:** Resulting spina bifida with widely everted laminae. Axial T1 MRI in a 4-year-old girl. If the neural folds fail to close, the neural plate appears to open widely and to evert with the lateral margins ventral to the rest of the plate. The neural placode thus remains in a nearly coronal plane. The cutaneous ectoderm (*c*) (*large curved arrows*) cannot disjoin from the neural ectoderm (*NE*). Instead, it remains attached to the neural ectoderm far laterally and does not pass dorsal to the neural tissue. With future development, the skin that arises from the cutaneous ectoderm will also lie far laterally, leaving a midline defect in the skin cover. Adherence of the cutaneous ectoderm to the neural ectoderm prevents migration of mesenchyme behind the neural plate (*placode*). Therefore, no bone, muscle, or fascia can develop in the midline dorsal to the neural tissue; all skin, fascia, muscle, and bone must lie lateral or ventral to the neural tissue. Thus the dorsal surface of the unneurulated neural placode will remain visible in the midline. Despite absence of neurulation, the notochord on the ventral aspect will still migrate ventrally to become separated from the neural plate. Perichordal mesenchyme will develop into vertebral centra and discs ventral to the neural tissue. The mesenchyme that should have migrated dorsal to the neural tube must, instead, condense in abnormal position, ventral-lateral to the neural tissue, forming widely everted (bifid) laminae (*L, L*). *C*, vertebral centrum. Compare the contours of the bifid laminae with the mesenchyme ventral-lateral to the recurved neural placode. Because the laminae (*L*) are widely everted, the sagittal dimension of the spinal canal is markedly reduced, crowding the neural structures. Acutely angled kyphosis, often associated with wide spina bifida, stretches the skin and subcutaneous tissue and prevents the surgeon from mobilizing enough tissue to cover the spina bifida. There is consequently little tissue and no high-signal subcutaneous fat overlying the spina bifida (*arrowheads*). The neurocentral synchondroses (*white arrows*) have nearly fused. (B from Naidich et al., ref. 22; C from Naidich and McLone, ref. 66; with permission.)

unfused neural plate is thus exposed to view in the midline of the back at the site of the midline deficiency of skin, bone, cartilage, muscle and ligament.

The neural tissue appears as a raw, reddish, vascular oval plate (Fig. 6A). The raw surface represents the interior of what should have been the spinal cord. A midline groove runs down the center of this plate. This groove is the residuum of the ventral neural groove and is directly continuous with the central canal of the normally formed cord above.

The pia-arachnoid membrane that covers the ventral surface of the neural plate and encloses the CSF may present at the surface of the back as a thin ring encircling the neural tissue. The size of this membranous ring varies. When the subarachnoid space is small, the membranous ring is narrow and the neural plate lies flush with the back. This situation is designated myelocele (Figs. 6A and 7A). When the subarachnoid space is very large, the membranous ring is wide and the neural plate is elevated far above the skin surface. This condition is designated myelomeningocele (Fig. 6B and 7B). Together, myelocele and myelomeningocele are the commonest forms of spinal dysraphism. When used colloquially, spina bifida usually means myelocele or myelomeningocele.

In both myelocele and myelomeningocele, the membranous ring itself is encircled by normal skin peripheral to the midline defect. Epithelial cells may grow inward from the skin margins to cover the membranes and even the neural tissue that lie within the defect (Fig. 6B). If infection does not cause early death, the entire site may become epithelialized secondarily by a thin dysplastic skin layer (Fig. 8A).

Deep to the visible surface, the ventral face of the neural plate represents the neural tissue that should have formed the entire outer circumference of the spinal cord. The two ventral motor nerve roots arise from the ventral surface of the neural plate just to each side of the midline ventral sulcus. The paired dorsal sensory roots also arise from the ventral surface of the neural plate, lateral to the corresponding ventral roots. They arise in this position because the neural plate has failed to fold dorsally. The ventral and dorsal nerve roots traverse the subarachnoid space and exit via the neural foramina in the usual manner.

The pia-arachnoid membrane covers the ventral surface of the neural plate and continues around the entire subarachnoid space as one continuous sheet (Fig. 7) (45). This membrane is given the name pia mater where it is contiguous with neural tissue and the name arachnoid mater where it is separated from the neural tissue. The relationship of pia to arachnoid mater is analogous to the relationship of visceral to parietal pleura. The dura mater lies peripheral to the arachnoid. The dura forms a distinct layer ventrally but becomes lost in the margins of the defect dorsally. Because the neural plate and meninges are anchored to the skin surface, the spinal cord is tethered and relatively immobile.

Rarely, one is able to study the untreated myelomeningocele (Fig. 8B). Nearly always, however, patients with myelocele and myelomeningocele do not require detailed radiological evaluation in the newborn period, because the pathology is so clearly visible. The back is simply repaired surgically (i) to protect against infection and (ii) to free the spinal cord so later growth of the child

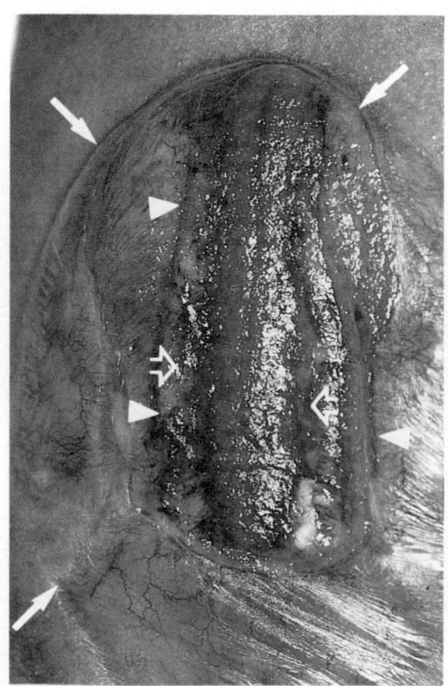

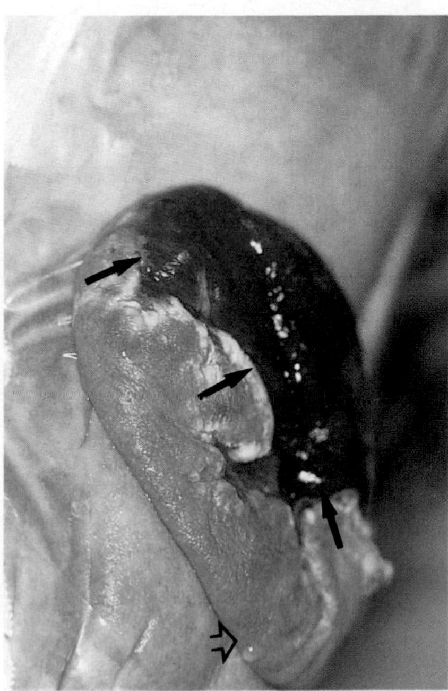

A,B

FIG. 6. Myelocele and myelomeningocele. Photographs of the backs of two newborn patients. **A:** In myelocele, the neural placode lies nearly flush with the surrounding skin surface. The edges of the skin (*white arrows*) are separated from the edges of the neural plate (*white arrowheads*) by variably epithelized membranes. Note the midline groove, and the two paramedian grooves (*open white arrows*). These would have formed the ventral neural groove and the sulci limitans of the ventral canal of a closed, well-neurulated spinal cord. **B:** In myelomeningocele, expansion of the subjacent subarachnoid space is associated with elevation of the neural plate well above the surrounding back. In this patient, skin partially encloses the meningocele, so the edge (*black arrows*) of the skin lies along the lateral margins of the neural plate with little intervening nonepithelialized membrane. Note the drop of CSF (*open arrow*) that has passed from the central canal over the external surface of the neural placode and run down the slope of the myelomeningocele.

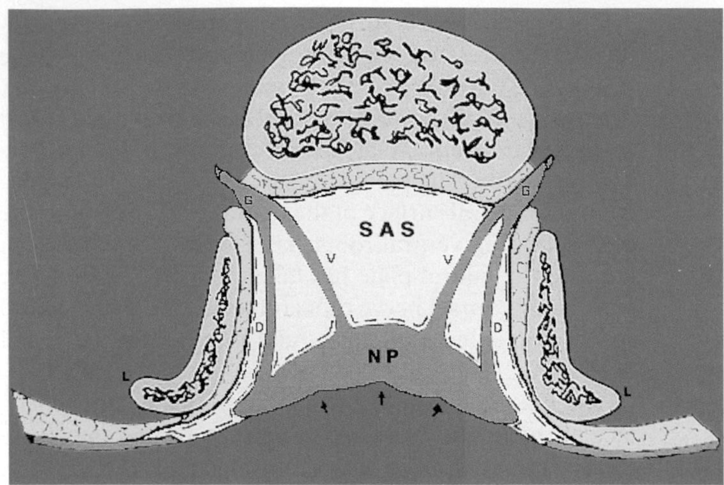

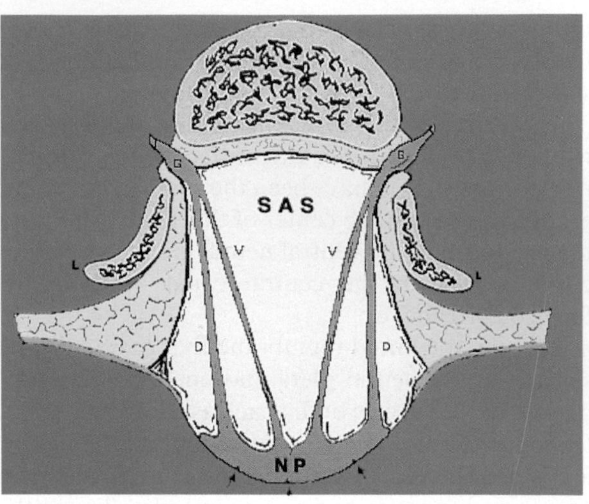

FIG. 7. Diagrammatic representation of myelocele (**A**) and myelomeningocele (**B**). The myelocele (A) is nearly flush with the surface of the back. The neural tissue has the flat configuration of the unneurulated neural placode. The dorsal surface, exposed to the exterior, exhibits midline and paramedian sulci (*arrows*) corresponding to the ventral neural groove and sulci limitans (unless secondary trauma or infection distort the tissue further). The ventral surface is lined by pia that becomes continuous with arachnoid at the lateral edge of the neural plate. This pia-arachnoid (*dashed line*) is one continuous sheet of membrane that encloses the subarachnoid space (*SAS*). The dorsal roots (*D*) arise from the ventral surface of the neural plate lateral to the ventral roots (*V*), not dorsal to them, because the plate has not flexed into a tube. *G*, the dorsal root ganglion. The pia-arachnoid continues along the ventral and dorsal roots, but is not shown there in order to simplify the diagram. The dura (*dark line* superficial to the pia arachnoid) encloses the CSF ventrally and laterally, and then becomes lost in the tissue lateral to the neural placode. No dura forms dorsal to the neural placode. The laminae (*L*) are widely everted (wide posterior spina bifida). The myelomeningocele (B) exhibits the same basic anatomy, but expansion of the subarachnoid space (*SAS*) displaces the neural placode posteriorly, everts it, and elevates it well above the surface of the surrounding back. (From Naidich et al., refs. 22 and 65, with permission.)

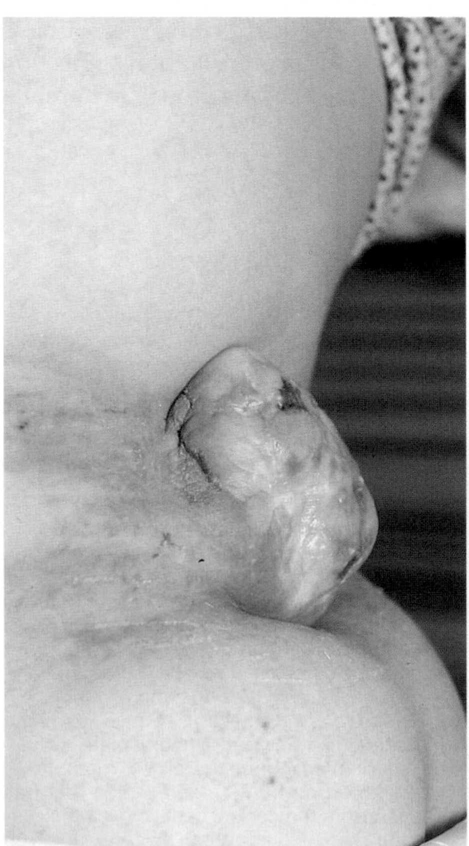

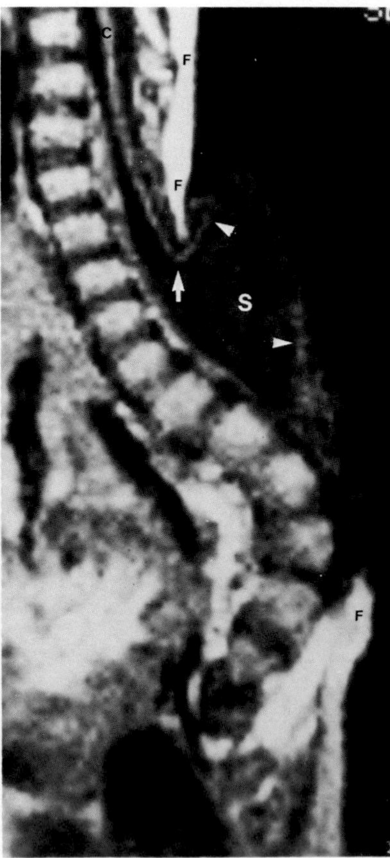

FIG. 8. Untreated myelomeningocele. **A:** Patient photograph. The surface of the myelomeningocele has become covered by skin through secondary epithelialization from the margins of the defect. **B:** Sagittal T1-weighted MRI demonstrates features characteristic of untreated myelomeningocele: dehiscence of high signal subcutaneous fat (*F*), fascia, muscle, and bone in the zone of spina bifida, low position of the spinal cord (*C*), acute angulation (*arrow*) of the cord under the last intact lamina at the upper margin of the spina bifida, and posterior herniation of the neural tissue (*white arrowheads*) forming the dorsal wall of the CSF space (*S*) that protrudes through the spina bifida. This patient also exhibits thoracolumbar kyphos. (B from Naidich et al., ref. 92, with permission.)

does not cause neurological dysfunction by cord stretching. As a result of this primary repair, the child's neurological function is stabilized or is improved to some "best" level for the child. Thereafter, the child should maintain that level of function (39).

Any subsequent deterioration in neurological function represents a complication that must be evaluated for potential surgical correction. The usual role of radiology is to elucidate the cause for late deterioration in patients who have already undergone primary repair of the myelomeningocele. Such complications include retethering of the cord to the wall of the spinal canal by abnormal spinal curvature, inclusion epidermoid, inclusion lipoma, hydromyelia, and arachnoid cyst.

Devascularization of the Placode

In patients with myelomeningocele, the placode is supplied by radicular branches and by many large vessels which pass directly to the neural tissue via the lateral dural reflections. Surgery may injure these lateral dural vessels, especially superiorly at the junction between the neurulated cord and placode, leading to focal cord infarction and atrophy (1,28,40).

Local Wound Site

Brau et al. have reported a 20% incidence of complications at the local wound, including skin necrosis, CSF leak, and wound infection (35). Herman et al. report CSF leak at the repair site in 6%, CSF pseudocyst in 2%, and local wound infection in 3% (47).

Latex Anaphylaxis

Eighteen percent to 40 percent of patients with myelomeningocele (and up to 6% of medical personnel) are now showing latex sensitivity, occasionally leading to life-threatening anaphylaxis during surgery (48). The powder on surgical gloves may be a vehicle for transmitting protein allergens from the latex gloves to the patients. Careful washing of gloves and careful histories of prior reactions need to be obtained to avoid these problems.

Retethering by Scar

When the spinal cord is freed from the back at the time of primary repair, it is replaced into the spinal canal. The dura and skin are closed over it. Because dura and skin are deficient in the midline, it may be technically difficult to mobilize sufficient tissue to provide a relaxed cover over the spinal canal, subarachnoid space, and cord. The raw surfaces of the neural tissue may adhere to the surgical closure and scar densely to it (Figs. 9 and 10).

In approximately 27% of patients with repaired myelomeningocele, retethering of the cord by scar causes new symptoms which necessitate a second procedure to release the cord at an average age of 6 years (49). These symptoms include new or progressive weakness of the lower extremities (55%), change of gait requiring added mechanical support (54%), new or progressive scoliosis (51%), pain localized to the back and legs (32%), progressive orthopedic deformities of the foot or hip (11%), and/or new urinary incontinence (6%) (47).

In such cases, radiological studies show that the posterior surface of the spinal cord becomes lost at the level of closure (Fig. 11) (50). The spinal cord remains attached to the dorsal wall of the spinal canal despite placing the patient prone and flexing the back. The subarachnoid space is obliterated dorsal to the cord and is unusually wide ventral to the cord.

The entire thecal sac lies unusually far posteriorly and protrudes partially through the posterior spina bifida. The ventral epidural fat space is consequently enlarged (Figs. 11 and 12). The cord itself appears thin and pursues a very straight, stretched, "bow-string tight" course down the length of the spinal canal. Because the cord extends so far caudal, there is no cauda equina. Instead, the nerve roots that arise from the cord at the level of the spina bifida pass horizontally or even cephalically to their root sleeves. These roots tend toward a plexiform arrangement (Fig. 10).

Reoperation for tethering after primary myelomeningocele repair may be complicated by coexisting pathology. In 123 patients, Reigel et al. (51) found concurrent lipoma (50%), fibrolipoma (9%), dermoid (12%), epidermoid (16%), arachnoid cyst (11%), and diastematomyelia (11%). Approximately 10% of these patients had 2 concurrent lesions (51).

Surgical release of the adherent cord is effective, leading to improved motor function in 79% (including unexpected improvement in many patients who had been considered "stable" prior to untethering). Reoperated patients show: improved gait and stance in 72% of cases, improvement of orthopedic deformities in 54%, improved scoliosis in 51%, and improved urinary and social continence in 33% (47). However, 16% of patients initially untethered will later require surgical procedures to again untether a rescarred cord (51).

Spinal Curvature

The incidence of spinal curvature in patients with myelomeningocele depends on the level of the myelomeningocele, patient age, and the type of curvature assessed (Fig. 12) (Table 1) (52–56).

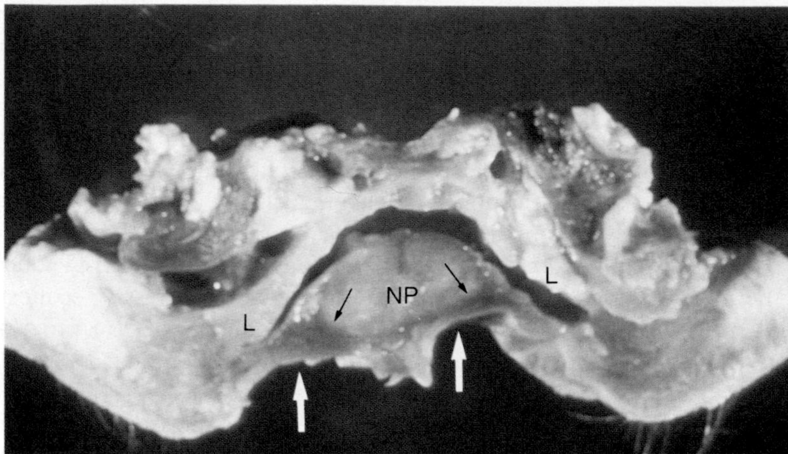

FIG. 9. Repaired myelocele. Retethering by scar. Axial anatomic specimen oriented like MRI. The site of repair exhibits thinner, atrophic skin with a thin subcutaneous layer (*white arrows*). The neural tissue (*NP*) is tethered to the surgical repair site by thick collagenous scar (*black arrows*). *L*, *L*, everted, widely bifid laminae. Specimen courtesy of Harry M. Zimmerman, M.D., New York, NY. (From Naidich et al., ref. 22, with permission.)

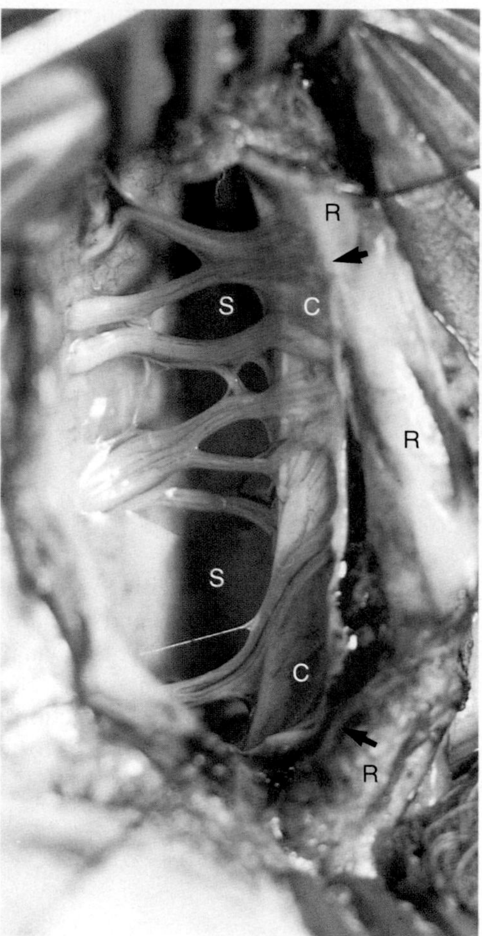

FIG. 10. Repaired myelocele. Retethering by scar, 2-year-old girl. Sagittal surgical exposure demonstrates the low-lying distal spinal cord (*C*), horizontal segmental origin and course of the lumbosacral roots through the subarachnoid space (*S*) with no cauda equina, somewhat plexiform arrangement of these roots, dorsal surface of the spinal canal along the zone of repair (*R*), adherence (*black arrows*) of the distal neural tissue to the repair zone at two sites, and clear CSF-filled space behind the neural tissue between the two sites of adherence.

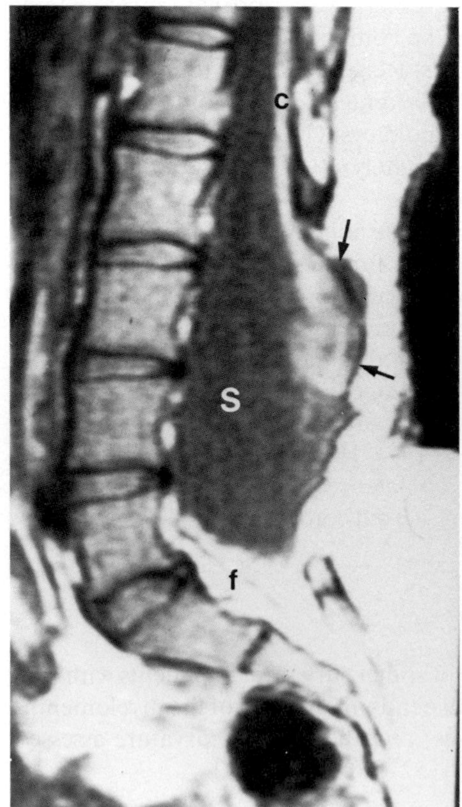

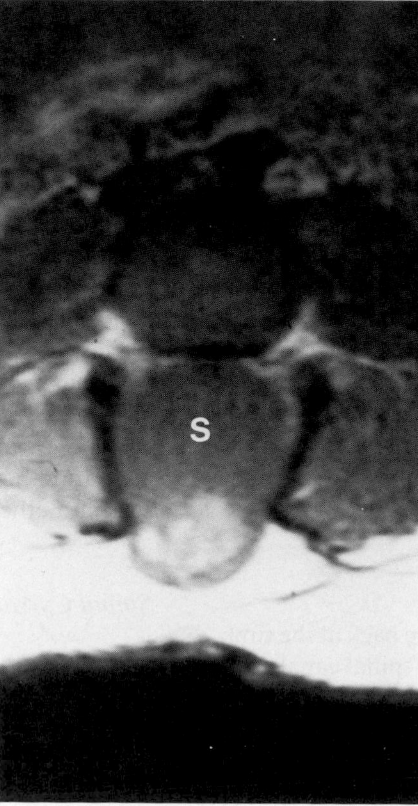

A,B

FIG. 11. Repaired myelomeningocele retethered by scar, 18-year-old girl. Sagittal T1-weighted MRI (**A**) and axial T1-weighted MRI (**B**) reveal increased lumbar lordosis with enlarged ventral epidural fat (*f*), expanded lumbosacral spinal canal and subarachnoid space (*S*), posterior spina bifida with dehiscent posterior wall of the spinal canal, bulging of the thecal sac into the spina bifida, low-lying tethered spinal cord (*c*) closely applied (and presumably adherent) to the low-signal, heavily collagenized scar (*arrows*), and a rather generous subcutaneous fat layer suggesting good skin–subcutaneous cover at the repair site. (From Zimmerman et al., ref. 8, with permission.)

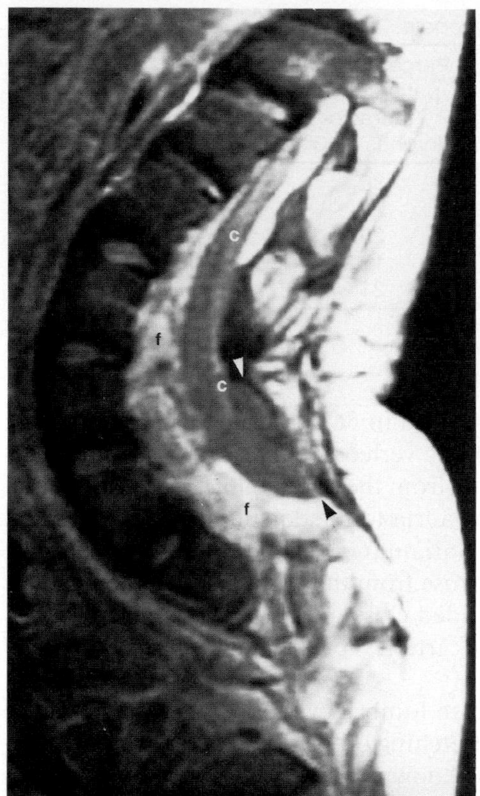

FIG. 12. Repaired myelomeningocele. Kyphoscoliosis. Sagittal proton-density-weighted MRI, 15-year-old girl. In this patient, there is severe kyphoscoliosis with exaggerated lumbar lordosis and remarkable increase in ventral epidural fat (*f*). The tethered spinal cord (*c*) is visualized in only part of its course. Absence of posterior elements between the *white* and *black arrowheads* indicates posterior spina bifida.

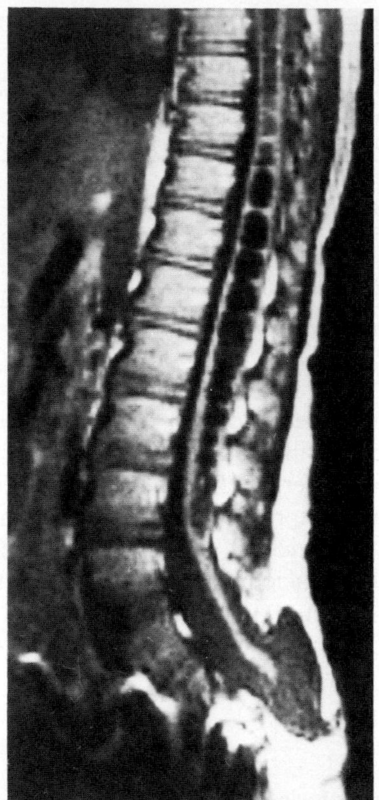

FIG. 13. Holocord hydromyelia complicating repaired myelomeningocele, 3-year-old boy. Sagittal T1-weighted MRI reveals protrusion of the subarachnoid space outside the lumbosacral spinal canal via the posterior spina bifida, surgical repair with good skin and subcutaneous fat cover for the meningocele, low-lying spinal cord extending into the sacral canal at the ostium of the meningocele (in this slice), and expansion of the length of the cord with a "bamboo" or "haustral" appearance that indicates hydromyelia. Note that the anterior wall of the hydromyelic cord is visualized more easily than the posterior wall. (From Naidich et al., ref. 66, with permission.)

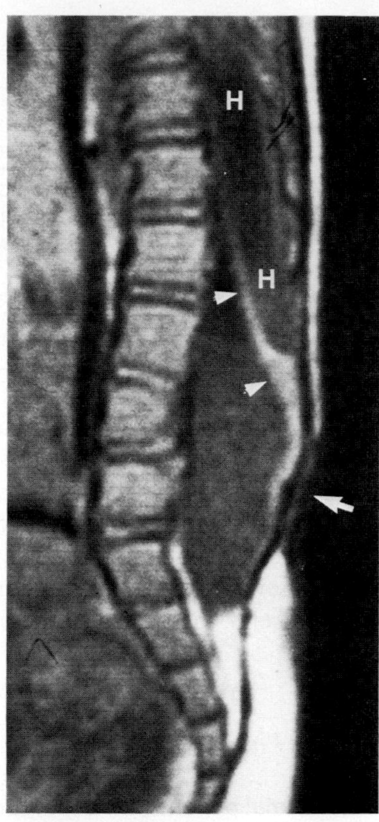

FIG. 14. Repaired thoracolumbar myelomeningocele with marked hydromyelia. Sagittal T1-weighted MRI, 3-week-old girl. In patients with repaired myelomeningocele, detection of a thin "cord" (*arrowheads*) situated anteriorly, abrupt arcing of the cord posteriorly to the upper end of the spina bifida, and a large CSF intensity space posterior to the "cord" suggests that the supposed "thin" cord is only the anterior wall of a cord expanded by hydromyelia (*H*). Note poor skin and subcutaneous fat coverage of the spina bifida (*white arrow*). (From Naidich et al., ref. 92, with permission.)

Scoliosis

Twenty-three percent of the scolioses are congenital structural scolioses which result from vertebral anomalies such as hemivertebrae, solid bony bars and unilateral unsegmented bars. In such cases the arc of curvature is very sharp and the apex of the curve lies at the site of the bony anomaly (1,57). Sixty-five percent of scolioses are developmental scolioses which result from muscle imbalance and distal pelvic and extremity malformations in the absence of congenital spinal anomalies (Fig. 12) (57). In these patients the arc of curvature is usually less sharp and lies in the dorsolumbar region.

By functional spinal level the incidence of scoliosis associated with myelomeningocele is 85% for thoracic levels, 100% for L1–L2 levels, 50% for L3–L4 levels, and 6% for sacral levels (58). Overall, 80% of patients with myelomeningocele have scoliosis by age 10 years (49). Progression of scoliosis occurs in the first decade and dramatically increases during the second decade for patients with functional levels at the thoracic or upper lumbar (L1–L3) spine (51). After 10 years of age, 43% of myelomeningocele patients have scoliosis of 20° or greater (48).

Although spinal curvatures are widely thought to be most rapidly progressive at the time of growth spurts, careful study of spinal curvatures in 23 patients receiving growth hormone showed no significant change in the scoliotic curve and no evidence of neurologic change over 3 years, despite patient growth at a rate of 7–8 cm/year (51).

TABLE 1. *Spinal curvatures and myelomeningocele*

Functional level of myelomeningocele	Percent of 216 patients with scoliosis >30° (COBB angle)	Percent of 169 patients with lumbar lordosis >55°	Percent of 188 patients with thoracic kyphus >40°
Thoracic	77	60	36
Lumbar 1–3	40	53	20
Lumbar 4–5	13	40	29
Sacral	3	27	10
Total percent	25	43	21

Data tabulated from Reigel et al., ref. 51.

In patients with myelomeningocele retethering of the spinal cord should always be considered the likely cause of scoliosis. In these patients, surgical untethering of the cord stabilizes most cases and actually improves the curve in 21% of patients (49). The greatest incidence and greatest severity of scoliosis occur with thoracic myelomeningoceles; these are also the most refractory to therapy (51).

Lumbar Lordosis

In normal patients, the usual lumbar lordosis develops rapidly during infancy and again at puberty, reaching a plateau of about 50° at maturity. Significant lordosis, defined as >55°, develops by age 20 in 43% of patients with repaired myelomeningocele and tethered cord. As with scoliosis, more cephalic lesions show a greater incidence of lordosis and a more rapid progression. After release of the tether, the improvement of lordosis is greatest for the those patients with severe thoracic myelomeningocele.

Thoracic Kyphosis

In myelomeningocele patients a thoracic kyphosis develops slowly and "normally" reaches 40° by 20 years. Thoracic kyphosis >40° is seen in 21% of patients with tethered cord following myelomeningocele repair, and exhibits the same cranio-caudal gradient of incidence and severity as do scoliosis and lumbar lordosis. However, release of the cord does not seem to affect the progression and incidence of thoracic kyphosis.

Lumbar Kyphosis

Congenital lumbar kyphos is a major deformity in 8% of patients with myelomeningocele and is frequently associated with compensatory thoracic lordosis (53,59). It is usually located in the upper lumbar region, measures 80° or more at birth, and progresses thereafter. The vertebra at the apex of the curve is typically hypoplastic and anteriorly wedged (Fig. 8B) (1). The aorta lies well away from the kyphos and in 56% is strung like a bow-string across the kyphotic vertebral curve (60). The lumbar arteries originating from the aorta follow a long horizontal course from the aorta to the dorsum of the kyphos and are commonly variant (60,61); in one case for example, a single trunk arose from the aorta distal to the renal arteries and ascended close to the vertebrae giving rise to two intercostal arteries per segment over 5 lumbar segments.

In patients with lumbar kyphosis the sharp curvature leads to tight stretching of the skin over the closure, skin ulceration, breakdown, and infection. These patients suffer progressive respiratory difficulty, because of incompetence of inspiratory muscles, crowding of abdominal content, and upward pressure on the diaphragm (59). Excision of the proximal lordosis stabilizes their curvature and facilitates ambulation. Children born with a thoracolumbar kyphos who function at or below L4 should have kyphectomy before their second birthday (49).

Inclusions

(Epi)dermal inclusion cysts are found in both the unoperated newborn and the previously repaired back (41,62,63). Prior to closure of the myelomeningocele, the placode and central canal are open to the environment and exposed to desquamated skin, laguno, and hair in the amniotic fluid. Storrs. (62) found epidermoid cysts in 29% and dermoid cysts in 6% of newborns during the initial closure of their myelomeningocele. Free-floating-epidermoid "pearls" may even be found in the spinal subarachnoid space.

During the repair of a myelomeningocele, the surgeon must trim all the skin away from the cord, lest some skin elements be included within the closure. This is hard, probably impossible, to do perfectly. In some cases, therefore, these included (epi)dermal elements may grow into epidermoid (12% to 13%) and dermoid cysts (2% to 5%) (51,62). Scott et al. has suggested that (epi)dermoids found within the scar, dorsal to the placode, may be inclusion epidermoids resulting from surgery, whereas those found ventral to the neural tissue and those containing unusual features such as respiratory epithelium might well be congenital (64).

Lipomas are found in 6% of newborn untreated myelomeningoceles and 7% of operations performed to release tethered cords. It may be difficult to distinguish inclusion lipomas from inclusion dermoids by imaging procedures alone (1,65–67).

Hydromyelia

Before the back is repaired, the central canal of the spinal cord is directly continuous with the midline groove on the dorsal surface of the neural plate. As a result, CSF passes freely down the central canal to discharge over the dorsal (external) surface of the neural plate (Fig. 6B). Following repair of the back, this egress for CSF is blocked. Perhaps as a result, dilation of the central canal of the spinal cord (i.e., hydromyelia) is observed at necropsy in 30% to 50% of patients with myelomeningocele (68–72). The precise incidence varies from series to series (70,72). The hydromyelia is holocord, or nearly holocord in 11%, cervical in 2%, cervicothoracic in 7%, thoracic in 7%, thoracolumbar in 11%, and lumbar in 9%. Seven percent of patients show hydromyelia at two different levels (72).

When severe, hydromyelia may cause neurological dysfunction and rapidly progressive scoliosis (73). In any patient with myelomeningocele and rapidly progressive scoliosis, cranial imaging studies should be performed to rule out hydrocephalus or occult shunt malfunction. Spinal imaging should be performed to detect any hydromyelia present.

On MRI, hydromyelia usually appears as a CSF-intensity space within the center of a dilated cord. The sides of the cavity may be indented periodically by bands that resemble the haustra of the colon (Fig. 13). Hydromyelia may also present as an ovoid, sagittally flattened atrophic cord (collapsed hydromyelia). In some cases, the central canal is so wide and the cord so thin, that only one wall of the cord is visible, usually the anterior wall. In these cases the thin anterior wall may be mistaken for the entirety of a very atrophic cord (Fig. 14). In other cases it may be very difficult to distinguish hydromyelia with scoliosis from intraspinal arachnoid cyst. Such arachnoid cysts are found in 2% of patients with myelomeningocele (Fig. 15) (24,74).

Diastematomyelia and Hemimyelocele

Diastematomyelia is seen in 31% to 46% of patients with myelomeningocele (69,70). It affects the cord cephalic to the plaque in 31%, the plaque itself in 22%, and the cord caudal to the plaque in 25% (70). Hemimyelocele is a special form of myelomeningocele with diastematomyelia reported in 9% of patients with Chiari II malformations (75). In 1%, paired hemicords each exhibit a myelomeningocele at different levels. In the other 8%, one posteriorly situated hemicord exhibits a myelomeningocele while the other hemicord is normal. The normal hemicord is usually smaller, usually lies ventrally, and may be isolated within a separate ventrolateral hemicanal by an oblique bone spur. In such cases, the visible hemimyelocele may be mistaken for a complete myelomeningocele, so that the diastematomyelia and other hemicord are not recognized until the child presents with tethering sometime after the initial repair. However, strikingly asymmetric motor strength in the lower extremities, with one normal or nearly normal leg, should suggest the diagnosis of hemimyelocele in the newborn period.

Chiari II Malformation

Myelocele and myelomeningocele are nearly always associated with a specific deformity of the brainstem, cerebellum, and upper cervical spinal cord designated the Chiari II malformation (Fig. 16) (24,74,76–78). This malformation presents clinically with hindbrain dysfunction which is severe in 4% to 13% of all patients with myelomeningocele (79), (7% of infants and 2% of older patients) (42,79). Clinical signs include swallowing difficulty (71%), strider (59%), apneic spells (29%), aspiration (12%), weak cry (18%), and arm weakness (53%) (80). The apnea may result from bilateral abductor vocal cord paralysis (obstructive apnea), from central neural dysfunction (centrally mediated expiratory apnea with cyanosis) (81), or both together.

Hindbrain dysfunction is the major cause of mortality in the myelomeningocele patient, and accounts for 11% of the total of 15% of deaths observed in the first 2 years of life (42). Overall infant and childhood mortality are high in the immediate perinatal period, stabilize at 15% by 2 years of age, but then increase to 18% to 19% by 15 years (37,49,82), predominantly because of deaths related to surgical procedures (3%) (81).

Multiple diverse theories have been offered to explain the diffuse manifestations of the Chiari II malformation and myelomeningocele (24,82). To date, no single theory has proven satisfying, so none has been accepted widely.

Recently, McLone and Knepper (82) presented experimental data that suggest the Chiari II malformation could be the result of diversion of ventricular CSF to the amnion with consequent "collapse" of the developing ventricular system. This theory is based on the following facts.

1. The fluid-filled space of the developing brain and spinal cord is called the neurocele.
2. The medial walls of the neural tube normally appose

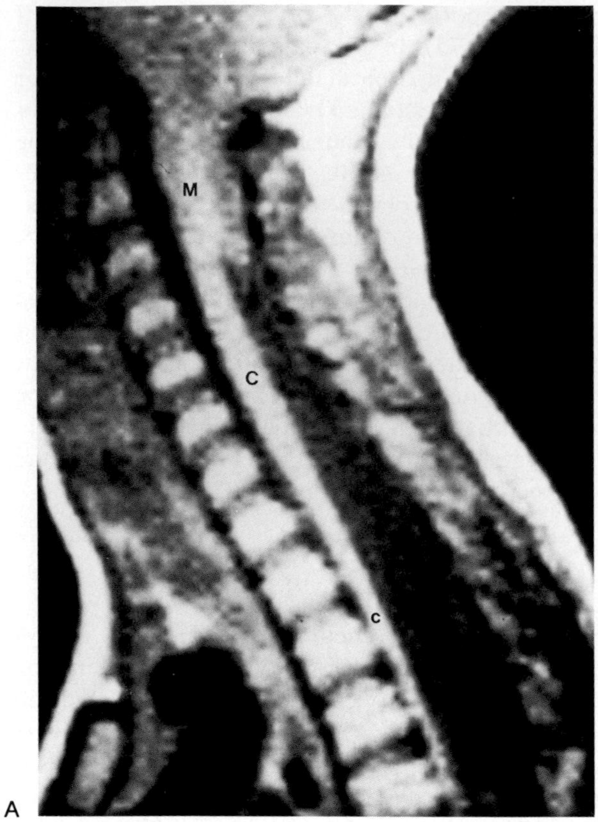

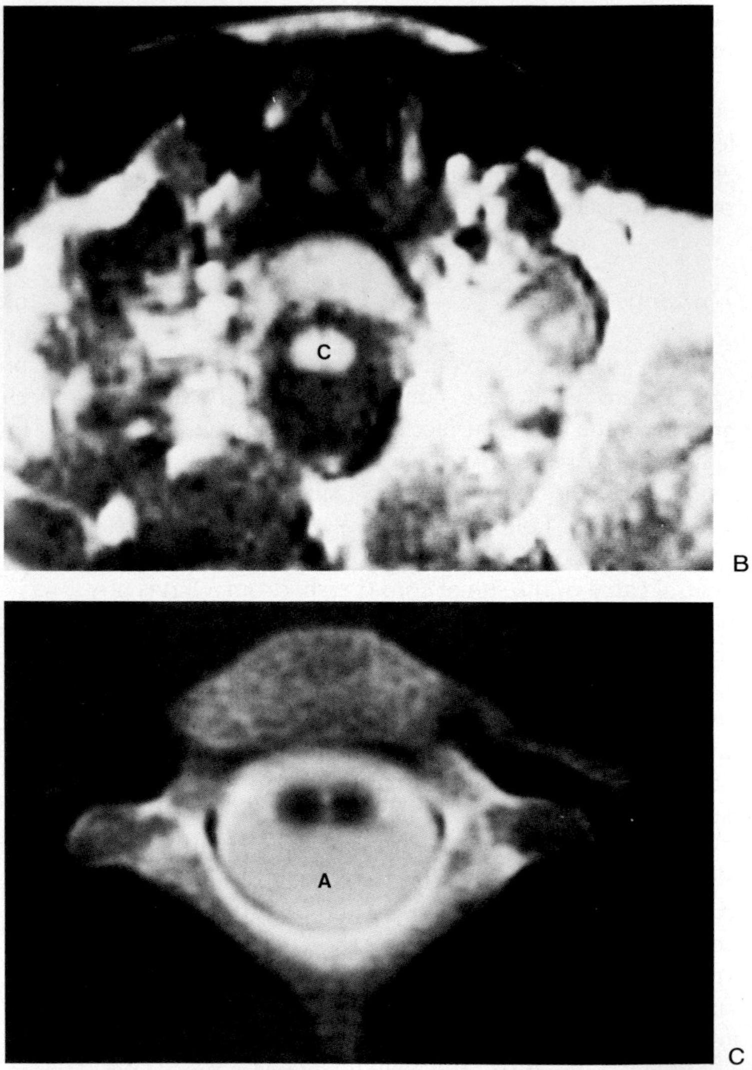

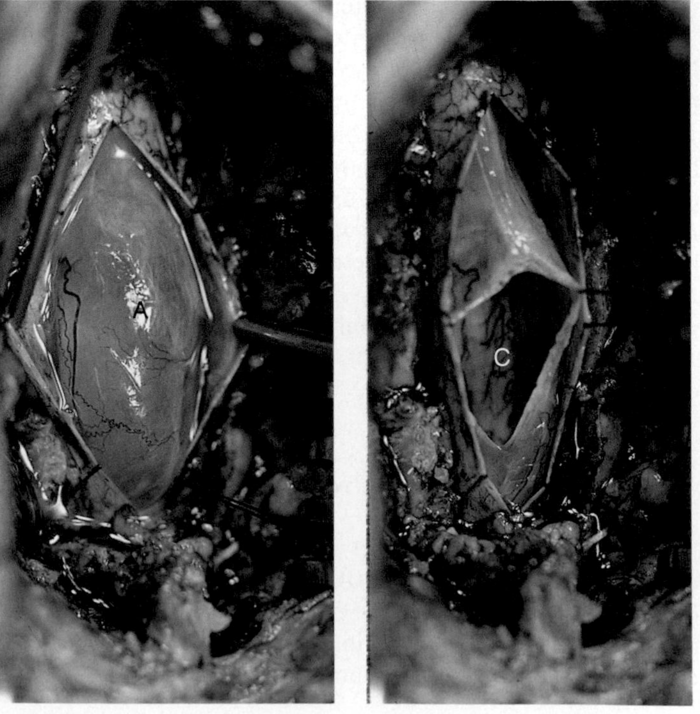

FIG. 15. Chiari II malformation with cervicothoracic arachnoid cyst. **A:** Sagittal T1-weighted MRI reveals the Chiari II malformation with kink and spur where medulla (*M*) buckles behind the cord (*C*) (cf. Figs. 16–19). The tapering of the cord inferiorly could indicate scoliosis alone, hydromyelia with thin, undetectable posterior wall, and/or dorsal arachnoid cyst. **B:** Axial T1-weighted MRI demonstrates a large low-signal space posterior to the cord (*C*) and suggests that the space does not represent hydromyelia at that level. Cord contour is slightly "dumbbell." **C:** CT myelography reveals a less well-communicating compartment dorsal to the cord representing a subdural arachnoid cyst (*A*). The cord exhibits a mild form of diastematomyelia. **D:** Operative exposure in another patient with Chiari II malformation and myelomeningocele, 3-year-old boy. The dura is tented laterally by stay sutures. The thin-walled, transparent sausage-shaped arachnoid cyst lies within the subdural space and displaces the spinal cord anteriorly. It contained clear fluid resembling cerebrospinal fluid. **E:** Opening the cyst reveals the spinal cord (*C*) situated ventral to the cyst. The dorsal surface of the spinal cord was deeply indented by the cyst. (D and E from Naidich et al., ref. 24, with permission.)

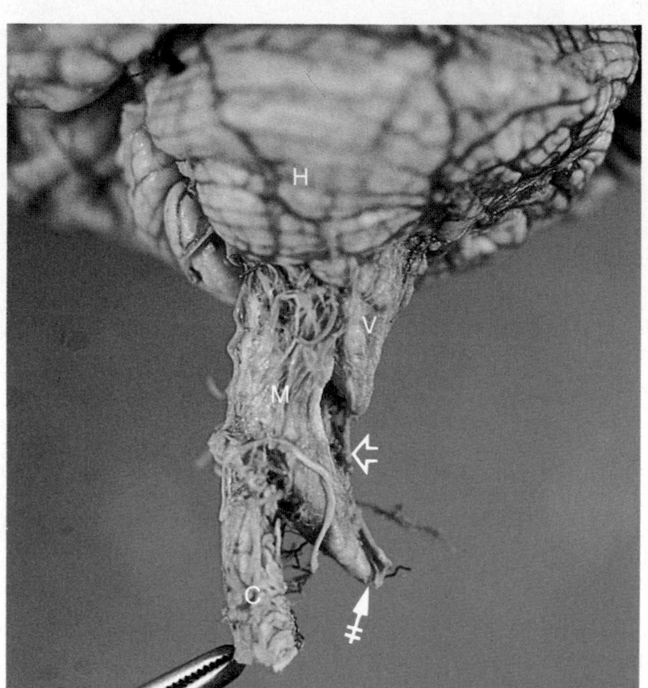

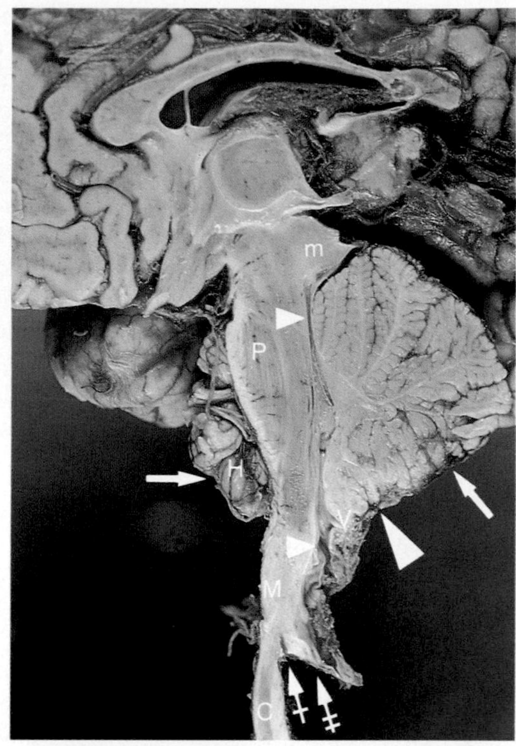

FIG. 16. Chiari II malformation. Medullary protrusion and the cervicomedullary kink, 11-month-old boy. **A:** Left lateral view of the uncut hindbrain. **B:** Midsagittal section of the same brain (larger field of view includes corpus callosum). Anterior is to the reader's left. *White arrows* indicate the position of foramen magnum. *White arrowhead* indicates the site of the posterior arch of C1. The Chiari II medulla (*M*) protrudes below foramen magnum and C1 into the cervical spinal canal. The medulla buckles dorsal to the cervical spinal cord, and forms a kink (*crossed white arrow*) where it forces the upper cervical cord to recurve on itself and forms a spur (*double crossed white arrow*) at the true cervicomedullary junction. The medullary hernia overlaps the cervical cord. The fourth ventricle (*white arrowheads*) is greatly elongated, extends into the cervical canal, and widens there. Choroid plexus (*open white arrowheads*) lies along the dorsal aspect of the intraspinal fourth ventricle. The vermis protrudes downward through the large foramen magnum, rests upon the posterior arch of C1 (*white arrowhead*), and extends a tongue or peg of tissue (*V*) through the C1 ring dorsal to the medulla and fourth ventricle. Note the sharp notch (*white arrowhead*) where the posterior lip of the C1 ring indents the vermian peg. The cerebellar hemispheres (*H*) pass anteriorly to lie in front of and encompass the brainstem. Also demonstrated are the beaked midbrain (*m*), and the pons (*P*). (From Naidich et al., ref. 24, with permission.)

and occlude the neurocele transiently during brain development in humans, mice, and chicks.

3. Experimental animals with distal myelomeningocele fail to occlude the neurocele, even at sites remote from the myelomeningocele.
4. This failure to appose the walls appears to result from the same biosynthetic defect in cell surface glycosaminoglycans that prevents the neural tube from closing. That is, the mechanism that causes failure of neurulation also causes failure of apposition of the medial walls of the neurocele. Based on these findings, the theory proceeds as follows:
5. Because the neurocele is not occluded, CSF passes freely down the central canal and out the myelomeningocele to the amnionic cavity.
6. This abnormal shunt collapses the developing primitive ventricular system.
7. Therefore, the volume of the ventricular system and surrounding neural tissue is less than normal.
8. The mesenchyme condenses in relation to an abnormally small volume of developing CNS. This establishes a smaller-than-normal posterior fossa with low tentorium.
9. The developing CNS must then grow within an envelope of membrane, cartilage, and bone that is too small for it.
10. This leads to failure to form the pontine flexure, downward growth of the cervicomedullary junction, medulla, and cerebellum through the foramen magnum, and upward growth of the cerebellum through the incisura.
11. Reduced size of the third ventricle means closer approximation of the thalami with larger massa intermedia.
12. Collapse of the cerebral ventricles leads to disorganization of the developing hemispheres with gray matter heterotopias, disorganization of cerebral gyri, and dysgenesis of the corpus callosum.

13. The collapse of the ventricular system leads to disordered development of the membranous bone of the vault (82). Normally, the skull develops from centers in each cranial plate. As the brain expands, the collagen bundles are drawn out from those centers in an orderly radial fashion, much like the uniform expansion of the surface of an inflating balloon. As radial expansion proceeds, the collagen bundles become calcifiable and membranous bone forms. Lack of distension of the brain mass by increasing volumes of CSF produces disordered arrays of collagen bundles. Thus, instead of radial lines of collagen, whorls and coils of collagen form with varying density between them. Ossification of this disorganized collagen mat then leads to lükenshädel.

In the Chiari II malformation the upper cervical cord is displaced caudally, so that the cervical nerve roots ascend retrograde to their exit foramina. The brainstem is also displaced caudally so that the medulla and even the low pons lie within the cervical spinal canal.

The medulla may descend purely vertically, so it remains in line above the spinal cord (30%). More commonly the medulla buckles backward and downward as it descends, forcing the dorsal surface of the uppermost cervical cord to kink back on itself (the "kink") and forming a spur of tissue at the cervicomedullary junction (the "spur") (70%) (Figs. 15 and 16). The cuneate and gracile tubercles at the upper ends of the dorsal columns form the apex of the spur and point caudally, not cephalically.

Emery and McKenzie (74) demonstrated that the deformities at the cervicomedullary junction form a spectrum of pathology that falls into 5 major groups. In order of increasing severity (Fig. 17), these may be categorized as:

Group a. In 4% of Chiari II patients the medulla and fourth ventricle do not descend below foramen magnum. The sole evidence of hindbrain deformity is mild inferior displacement of the spinal cord with ascending course of the cervical nerve roots.

Group b. In 26% of cases, the medulla and fourth ventricle descend vertically, in line with and above the displaced cervical cord. In these cases the fourth ventricle leads directly inferiorly into the central canal of the cord.

Group c. In another 26% of cases the medulla shows mild buckling behind the cervical cord, so there is less than 5 mm of overlap of medulla on cord. Because of the buckling, the fourth ventricle lies partly behind the cord and the central canal arises from the anterior surface of the cord (Fig. 18).

Group d. In 23% of cases the medulla shows greater buckling with greater than 5 mm overlap of medulla behind the cord (Figs. 15A and 19).

Group e. In a further 21% of cases, severe buckling of medulla is associated with a sac-like process or diverticulum of the dorsal surface of the fourth ventricle. This protrudes behind the cord caudal to the kink.

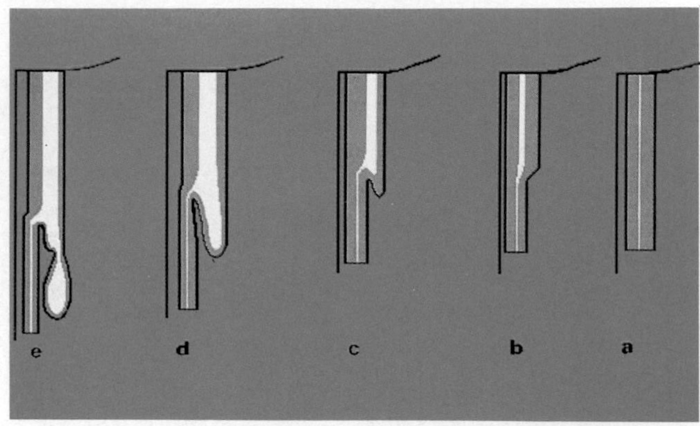

FIG. 17. Diagrammatic representation of the spectrum of cervicomedullary deformities in the Chiari II malformation. Lateral views oriented with anterior to the reader's left. Diagrams **a-e** represent a graded series of increasingly more severe deformities discussed fully in the text. Curved lines at the top indicate the foramen magnum. *Black shading* indicates the fourth ventricle and central canal of the spinal cord. (From Emery and MacKenzie, ref. 74, with permission.)

The fourth ventricle descends with the brainstem and forms a cranio-caudally elongated, tubular structure that lies partially within the posterior fossa and partially within the spinal canal. The cerebellum usually protrudes caudally into the spinal canal behind the medulla. The major portion of the cerebellum that protrudes below the foramen magnum cannot fit into the C1 ring and appears to rest or "sit" upon the posterior arch of C1. A smaller, thinner portion of cerebellum designated the cerebellar "peg" or "tongue" or "tail" does extend further caudally within the C1 ring. Typically the peg is formed by the nodulus (most inferiorly), the uvula (more superiorly), and the pyramis (often situated within the foramen magnum). The length of the peg is variable and does not correlate with the length of the medullary spur. In 75% of cases, the cerebellar tail terminates cephalic to the kink (Figs. 15 and 19). In 25%, the tail extends below the kink, behind the lower cervical cord. The overlapping herniations of cerebellum on medulla and of medulla on cord form a "cascade" of hernias each of which displaces anteriorly and compresses all structures ventral to it. All of the herniations are compressed in turn by impaction in foramen magnum and the small C1 ring. The tectum of midbrain is typically molded into a conical "beak." Numerous other anatomic distortions, also present, are delineated in the references (24,77,78).

Patients symptomatic from Chiari II malformation are potential candidates for surgical decompression of the hindbrain (73). However, in the neonate and young infant, surgical decompression of the cervicomedullary junction for hindbrain dysfunction remains controversial. The infants are clearly at risk from their brainstem problems, but the surgical procedure itself is associated

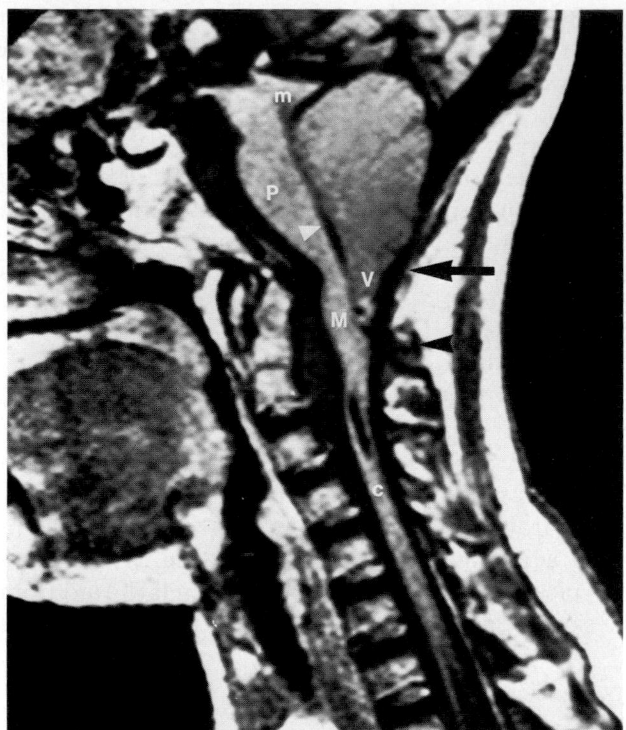

A

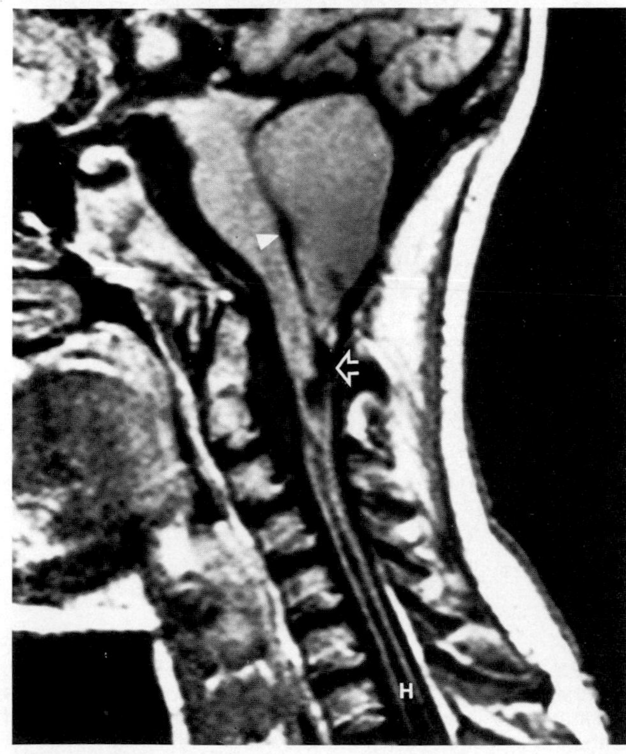

B

FIG. 18. A,B: Chiari II malformation with hydromyelia. Sagittal T1-weighted MRI, 15-year-old girl. The vermian peg does not protrude far caudally. The kink and spur are mild, and there is severe hydromyelia (*H*). The peculiar concavity in the posterior aspect of the C2–C3 vertebral bodies is commonly observed in Chiari II malformations and cannot be interpreted as evidence for arachnoid cyst or other mass. *c*, cord; *m*, midbrain; *M*, medulla; *P*, pons; *V*, vermis.

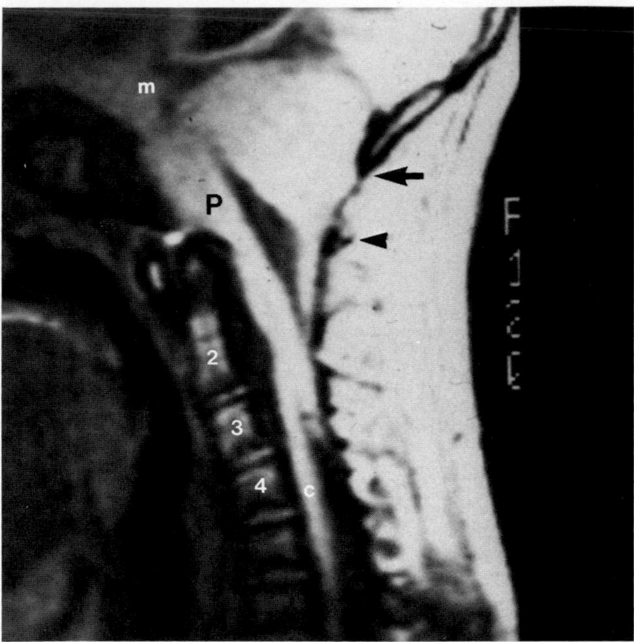

FIG. 19. Chiari II malformation, 11-year-old girl. Sagittal T1-weighted MRI reveals beaking of the midbrain, low position of the brainstem, compression of the pons (*P*) by the dens, marked buckling of the medulla behind the cord (*white c*) with kink at the level of mid C3 and spur at the level of C3–C4, protrusion of cerebellum caudally through the large foramen magnum (*black arrow*), further caudal extension of the vermian peg through the C1 ring (*arrowhead*) to the level of lower C2, enlarged fourth ventricle, and prominent posterior concavity of the C2–C3 vertebral bodies with wide ventral subarachnoid space. In Chiari II malformation, the greatest sagittal dimension of the fourth ventricle frequently lies below the foramen magnum. Enlargement of the intracervical portion of the fourth ventricle is seen in about 5% of Chiari II malformations. It suggests possible associated hydromyelia. (From Zimmerman et al., ref. 8, with permission.)

with a high operative mortality and may not provide definitive, long-term relief. Vandertop et al. report complete recovery from hindbrain dysfunction in 88% of treated infants, with only 2 deaths; one 8 months after surgery from respiratory arrest and a second from shunt infection with peritonitis 7 years after decompression (80). In Bell's series of 14 patients decompressed surgically for symptomatic hindbrain dysfunction before age 6 months, however, only 29% became asymptomatic (79), 50% died, and 21% improved partially.

In older patients, there is no controversy about surgical decompression of the hindbrain. The incidence of hindbrain dysfunction is smaller, the patients withstand the procedure more easily and decompression of the cervicomedullary junction is nearly always successful in alleviating the symptoms. The reduced incidence of symptoms may result from the disproportionately greater growth of the sagittal dimension of the C1 ring than the lower cervical segments (83) or from other factors relating to the changing proportion of the size of the foramen magnum to the length of the cerebellar hernia (84).

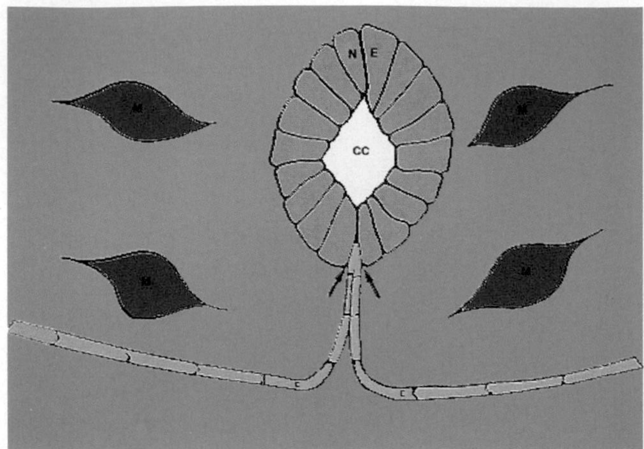

FIG. 20. Proposed embryogenesis of dorsal dermal sinus by incomplete disjunction. Diagrammatic representation. Focal failure of cutaneous ectoderm (*c*) to disjoin from neural ectoderm (*NE*) results in a persistent segmental adhesion (*arrows*). As the mesenchyme migrates dorsally to thicken the retroneural tissue and as the cord ascends, this adhesion is drawn out into a long epithelial-lined tube. *M*, mesenchyme; *CC*, central canal. (From Naidich et al., ref. 22, with permission.)

The Dorsal Dermal Sinus

If the superficial ectoderm fails to separate from the neural ectoderm at one point, then a focal segmental adhesion is created. As the spinal cord becomes buried beneath the surface by the developing spinal column and as different rates of growth between neural and spinal tissue lead to "ascent" of the cord, the local adhesion or "spot-weld" is drawn out into an elongated epithelial-lined tube that still connects the spinal cord with the skin of the dorsal surface of the child (Fig. 20) (1,5,85). Such an elongated segmental epithelial tract is designated a dorsal dermal sinus. The points of attachment of skin and cord remain segmental or metameric, so the dermatome of involvement predicts the site of neural abnormality. In Wright's collected series of 127 dermal sinuses: 57% were lumbosacral, 24% were occipital (86). The rest occur at uncommon sites.

Clinically the sinus most frequently appears as a pinpoint hole or a small atrophic zone in the skin. The sinus ostium is typically midline, but may be paramedian in unusual cases. A tuft of short sparse wiry hairs may emerge from the ostium (85). Small hemangiomas commonly adjoin or surround the ostium (Fig. 21).

Typically the dermal sinus tract extends inward from the skin surface for a variable depth (Fig. 22). It passes

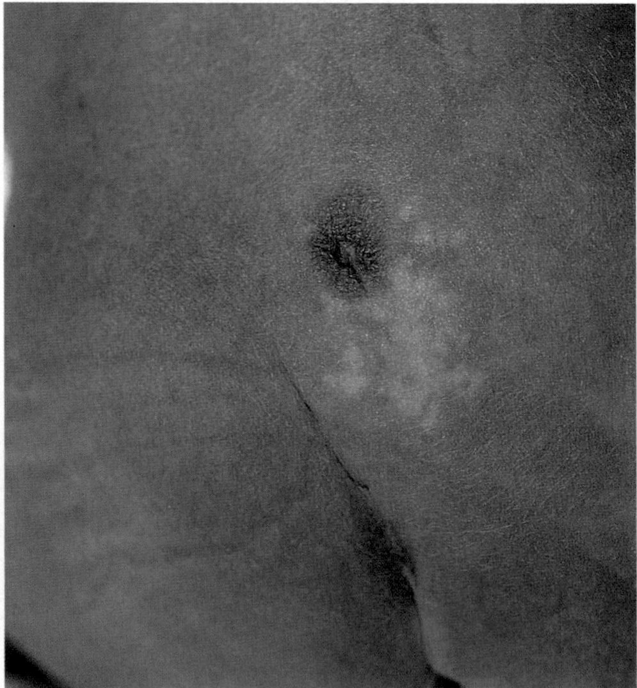

FIG. 21. Dorsal dermal sinus, 1-month-old boy. Posterior view of the patient reveals the typical midline lumbosacral hemangioma. The hemangioma surrounds a small atrophic dimple that was the external end of the dermal sinus in this patient. These stigmata lie well above the anus and coccyx.

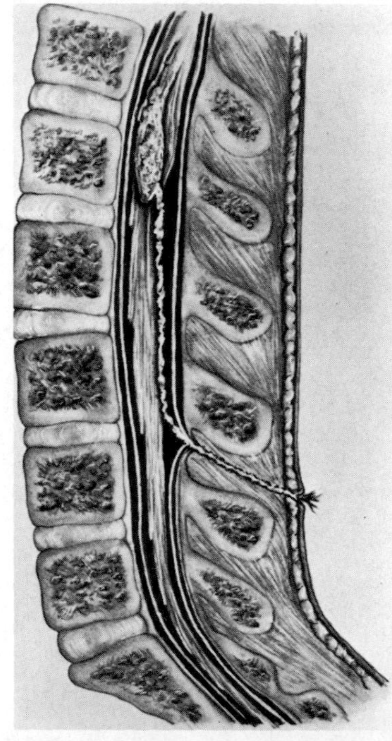

FIG. 22. Dorsal dermal sinus. Diagrammatic representation. Note the cutaneous ostium, variable uncommon presence of a small tuft of wiry hairs protruding from the ostium, the course of the tract to the lumbodorsal fascia through the median raphe (or between bifid spinous processes), and passage of the tract through the dura and arachnoid leaving a small triangular dorsal outpouching of the meninges akin to a root sleeve. The tract may then ascend within the spinal canal, incorporate one or several (epi)dermoid lesions, and end (variably) in an (epi)dermoid at the conus. The ascent of the *extraspinal* component of the sinus tract shown here is unusual in imaging studies. It may represent, in part, Matson's experience with placing the patient in a prone, flexed position for surgery. In our experience, imaging studies routinely show that the extraspinal component of the tract passes inferiorly and ventrally to the lumbodorsal fascia, before the deeper portion turns upward to ascend within the spinal canal (cf. Fig. 24). (From Matson, ref. 85, with permission.)

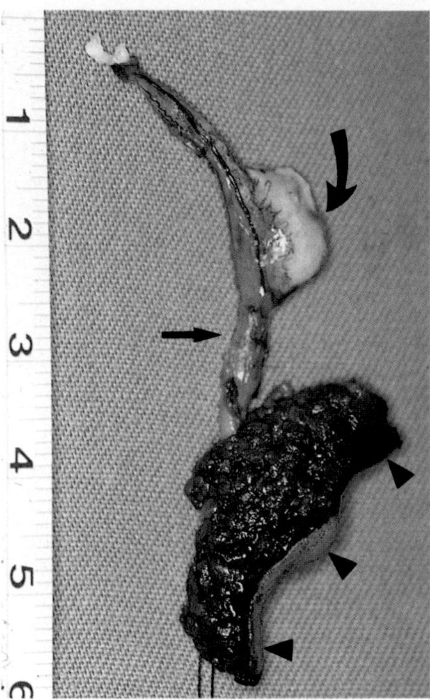

FIG. 23. Dorsal dermal sinus, 22-month-old boy. Pathological specimen resected in toto. From the skin surface (*arrowheads*), the tract passed ventrally through the subcutaneous fat to the lumbodorsal fascia, traversed the spina bifida, pierced the dura (*arrow*), ascended within the thecal sac, expanded into a dermoid (*curved arrow*) within the distal thecal sac, and then continued as a tract toward the conus, where it was ligated and resected.

deeply through the subcutaneous layer and through the median raphe (or between bifid laminae) toward the dura. It may end superficial to the dura, at dura or deep to dura. In one-half to two-thirds of cases, the tract extends into the spinal canal (1,86,87). A small midline sleeve of dura and arachnoid, directed dorsally, marks the point at which the tract attaches to or penetrates the dura (Fig. 22). Rarely the tract ends in the subarachnoid space as an open tube through which CSF discharges and through which infection may ascend retrograde to the spinal canal (87). Such infection may lead to arachnoiditis, epidural/subdural abscess, and intramedullary spinal cord abscess (88,89). The dermal sinus may also end in a fibrous nodule among the roots of cauda equina. In up to 60% of cases, the tract incorporates or ends in one or multiple dermoid or epidermoid tumor(s) (Fig. 23). Approximately 25% of all spinal (epi)dermoids are associated with dermal sinuses (14). The (epi)dermoids may act as masses. Cyst rupture may cause sterile chemical meningitis and obliterative arachnoiditis.

Lumbosacral dermal sinuses are usually associated with tethering of the spinal cord and low position of the conus (80%) (14,22). Thoracic and cervical dermal sinuses do not appear to influence conal position. Some 15% to 20% of patients with dermal sinus have concurrent lipoma, and vice versa, presumably because both lesions result from deranged disjunction of cutaneous from neural ectoderm. An error in disjunction could then lead to failed disjunction (dermal sinus), premature disjunction (spinal lipoma), or both at slightly different sites.

Imaging studies typically demonstrate the small depression in the skin at the ostium. The extraspinal portion of the dermal sinus tract may appear as a single line or as double parallel (railroad) lines that traverse the midline and correspond to the lumen and walls of the tract. Infrequently, the tract is filled by the included (epi)dermoid. Lumbosacral sinuses typically course inferiorly as well as ventrally as they pass from the skin surface to the lumbodorsal fascia, and then reverse direction to course superiorly as they pass further ventrally into the spinal canal (Figs. 24 and 25). Less commonly the superficial portion of the tract appears horizontal or even ascends from the skin toward the spine. The precise course may depend on the degree of lumbar lordosis and the position of each sinus with respect to that curvature.

The intraspinal portion of the tract is hard to identify. It may be indistinguishable from the filum or from the roots of cauda equina unless it is expanded by (epi)dermoids or contains fat (14).

True dermal sinus tracks must be distinguished from the sacral dimple or pilonidal sinus (Figs. 26 and 27). These are nearly identical to the dermal sinus but always

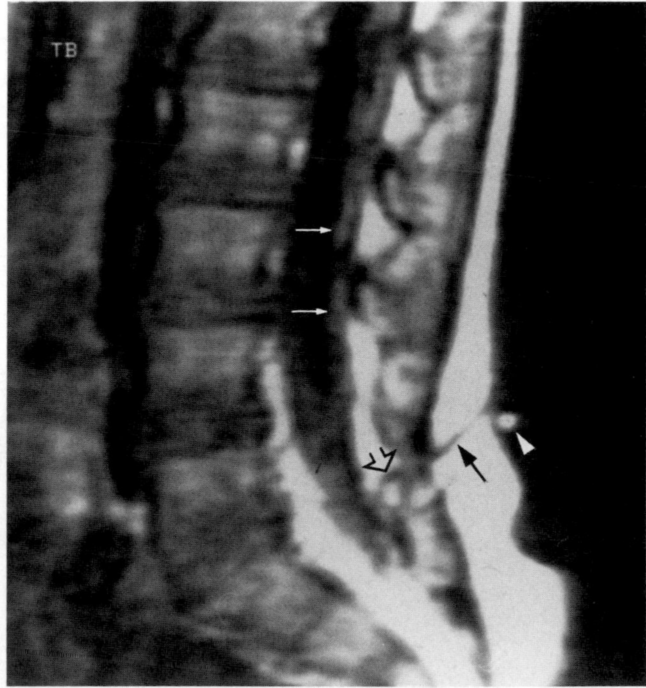

FIG. 24. Dorsal dermal sinus, 6-month-old infant. Sagittal T1-weighted MRI reveals the oblique course (*black arrow*) of the superficial portion of the dermal sinus. It descends as it passes anteriorly from the skin surface to the lumbodorsal fascia. A skin tag (*white arrowhead*) is detected at the inferior margin of the ostium. A hypodense epidermoid (*open black arrow*) is detected within the epidural space. Nodular tissue (*white arrows*) within the dorsal subarachnoid space proved to be a series of epidermoid tumors. (From Zimmerman et al., ref. 8, with permission.)

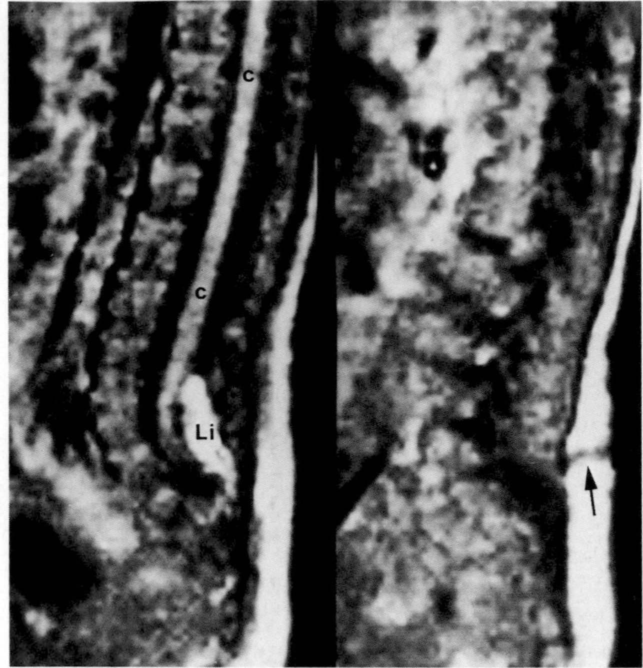

FIG. 25. A,B: Dorsal dermal sinus and lipoma, 22-month-old boy. Same patient as in Fig. 21. Sagittal T1-weighted MRI reveals a low-signal sinus tract (*arrow*) that traverses the subcutaneous tissue to the lumbodorsal fascia (where it is lost to view) and a high-signal lipoma (*Li*) related to the dorsal aspect of the low-lying spinal cord (*C*).

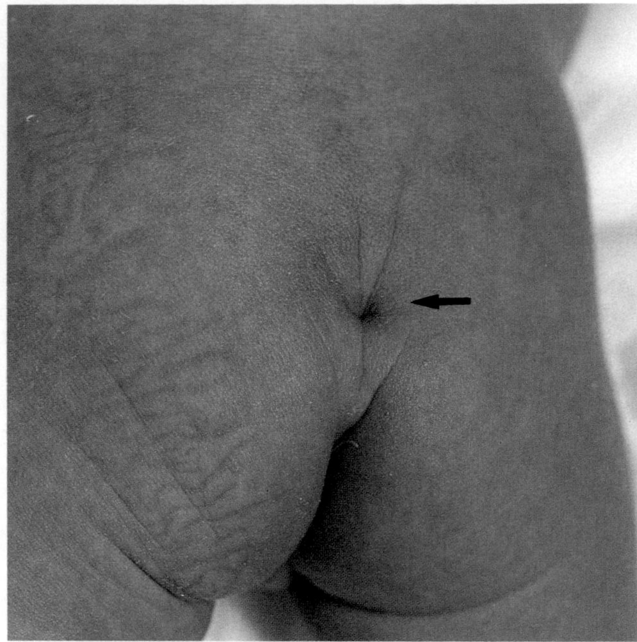

FIG. 26. Sacral dimple, 1-month-old girl. An ostium situated near to the anus may be a "sacral" dimple or a dorsal dermal sinus.

lie in low location, near to anus, and extend inferiorly or horizontally toward or to the dorsal surface of the coccyx (90–92). Pilonidal sinuses are nearly always incidental and asymptomatic; they do not enter the spinal canal. However, sacral dimples may occur together with spinal dysraphism and do appear to be more frequent in patients with diverse forms of dysraphism. A few sacral dimples become infected or develop painful cysts that require excision of the tract (Fig. 28).

Dermoid and Epidermoid Tumors

Epidermoid cysts are masses lined by a membrane composed only of superficial (epidermal) elements of the skin. Dermoid cysts are unilocular or multilocular cystic masses lined by a simple or stratified squamous epithelium which contains skin appendages such as hair follicles, sweat glands, and sebaceous glands. These (epi)dermoid tumors may arise as congenital rests in the absence of dermal sinuses (Fig. 29), or as the result of iatrogenic implantation of viable skin elements during back surgery or during spinal taps performed with needles that lack a

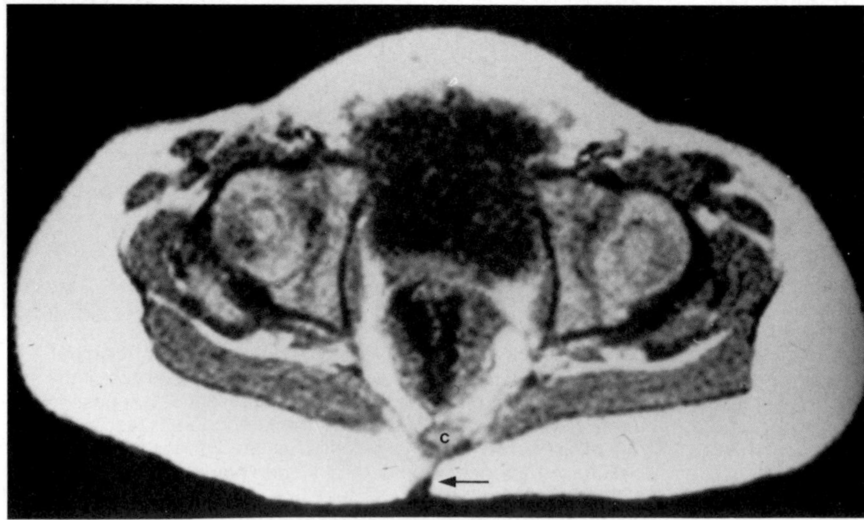

FIG. 27. Sacral dimple. Axial T1-weighted MRI, 2-month-old girl. MR demonstration that the dimple and tract (*arrow*) run directly to the coccyx (*c*) indicates that the lesion is a sacral dimple, not a dermal sinus tract.

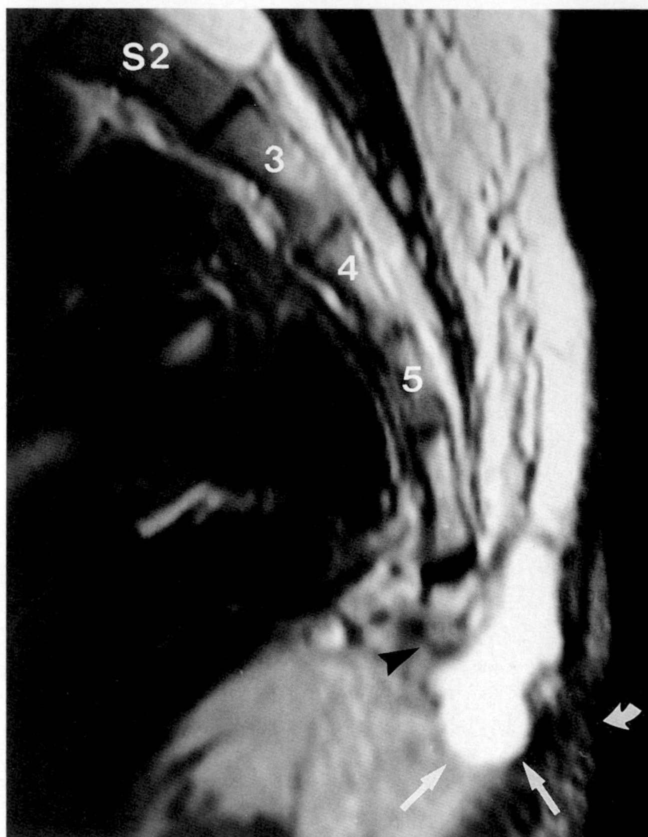

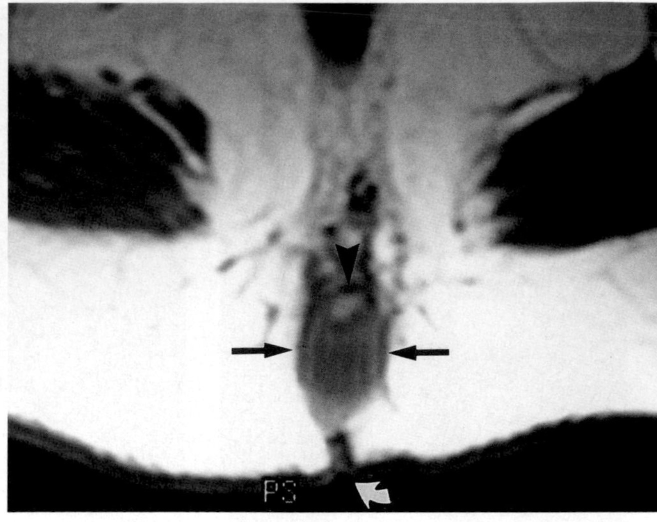

FIG. 28. Pilonidal cyst, 16-year-old girl. New infection of a pilonidal sinus present since birth. **A:** Sagittal MRI, T2-weighted fast spin-echo image. **B:** Axial MRI, T1-weighted image. The sharply marginated, thick-walled cyst (*arrows*) expands the midline and extends inward from the superficial portion of the sinus (*curved white arrows*) to lie immediately posteroinferior to the distal coccyx (*arrowheads*). *S2*, second sacral body; *3, 4, 5*, third, fourth, and fifth sacral bodies.

trocar (1). Approximately 25% of (epi)dermoid tumors form in association with dermal sinuses (1,88).

Spinal dermoid and epidermoid tumors constitute about 15% of all CNS (epi)dermoids, a cranial to spinal ratio of 6:1 (93). They account for 1% to 2% of spinal cord tumors below age 15 years (93). Dermoid and epidermoid tumors occur equally frequently (93). Approximately 40% are single epidermoids, 35% single dermoids, and 5% multiple dermoid or epidermoid tumors. In Lunardi's series, epidermoids were most frequently lumbar in location; dermoids were most frequently dorsal (25%) or dorsolumbar (75%) (93). Thirty-eight percent were intramedullary and 63% intradural extramedullary (93). Of (epi)dermoids associated with dermal sinus, approximately 60% have both intramedullary and intradural extramedullary components (14).

Epidermoid tumors are usually isointense with CSF or just slightly hyperintense to CSF, so they may be difficult to discern within the spinal canal. Intramedullary components do stand out in relation to the expanded cord (14,94), but extramedullary components may be invisible or may be detectable only by secondary displacements of the roots of cauda equina (14). Epidermoids that fill nearly the entire spinal canal may prove indetectable by routine spin-echo series (14). Fat-containing portions of dermoids will manifest as lesions with high signal on T1 series and reduced signal on T2 series (95). Infected (epi)dermoids exhibit intense contrast enhancement within the tumor and at other sites to which the inflammation may spread (88,96,97).

Spinal Lipoma

By definition, spinal lipomas are distinct collections of fat and connective tissue that are at least partially encapsulated and have a definite connection with the spinal cord (1,25,98,99). Spinal lipomas are the most common type of occult spinal dysraphism and account for some 35% of skin-covered lumbosacral masses (Fig. 30). Typically the mass lies in the midline just cephalic to the intergluteal crease (Fig. 30), and extends caudally, asymmetrically, into one buttock.

Spinal lipomas are more common in females, with a sex ratio of about 1.5:1 to 2:1 in some series (46,100). The chief complaints are usually a mass on the back (59%), urinary incontinence (23%), or weak/deformed lower extremity, perhaps with trophic ulceration (11%) (100). Those patients with prominent subcutaneous lipomas and cutaneous stigmata (Table 2) usually present at a younger age. Patients who are "missed" early present at older ages with neurological deterioration (100,101).

McLone has suggested that spinal lipomas result from focal premature disjunction of cutaneous ectoderm from

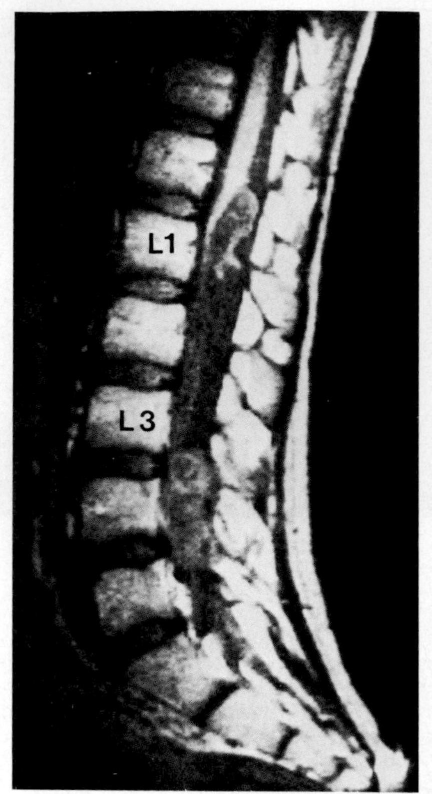

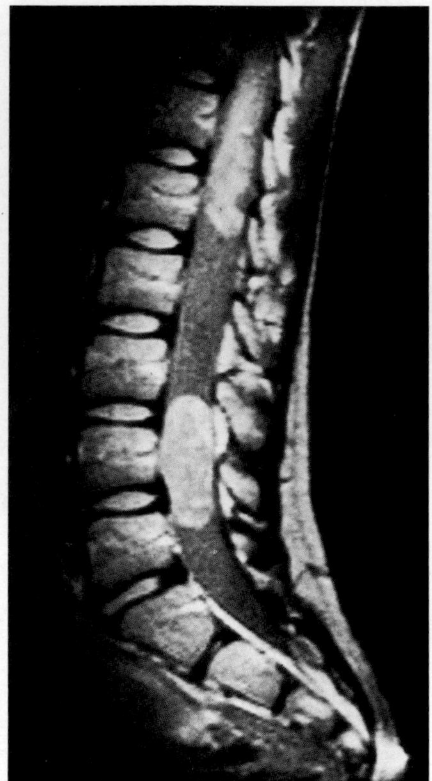

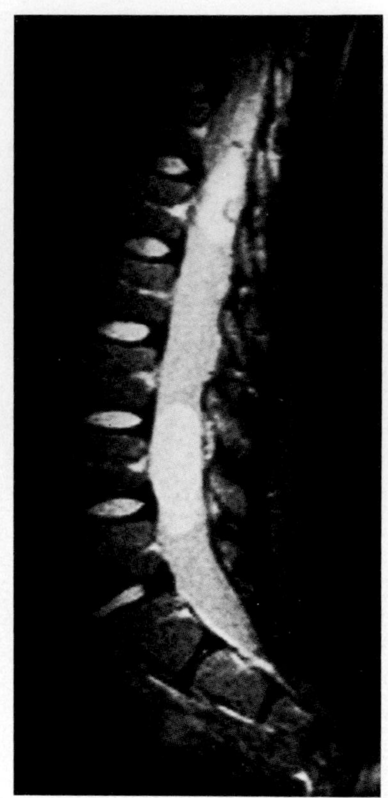

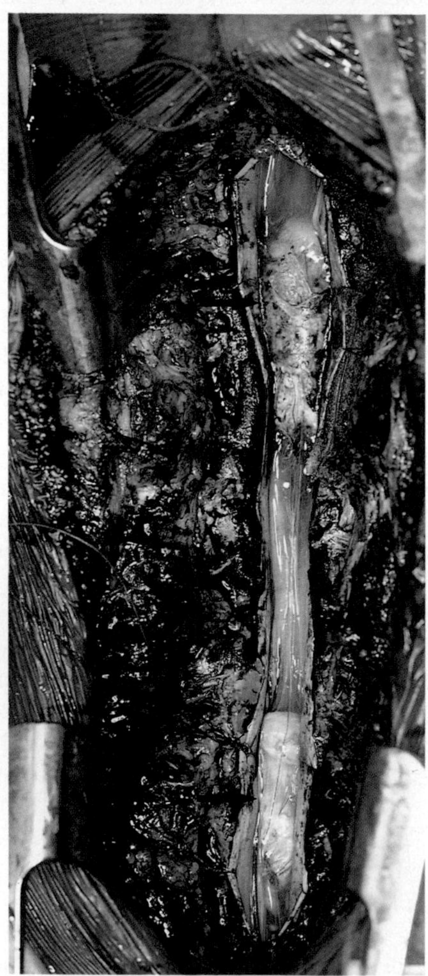

FIG. 29. Intraspinal epidermoids, 12-year-old boy. **A-C:** Sagittal MRI. T1-weighted image (A), proton-density-weighted image (B), and T2-weighted image (C). Well-defined ovoid masses are related to the dorsal aspect of the conus medullaris at T12–L1 and to the cauda equina at L3–L4. No dermal sinus was identified on imaging studies or at surgery. **D:** Operative exposure after opening the dura in the midline reveals the two, separate (epidermoids (*black arrows*). (From Naidich et al., ref. 22, with permission.)

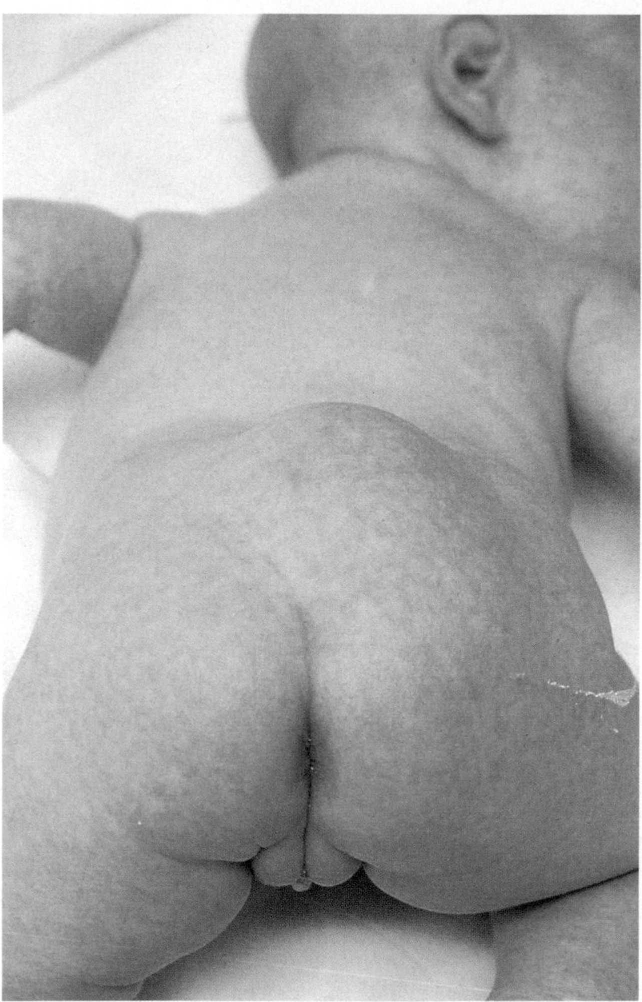

FIG. 30. Spinal lipoma, 1-month-old girl. Photograph of the patient's back reveals a skin-covered lumbosacral mass situated cephalic to the intergluteal cleft in the midline and extending asymmetrically to the reader's right. (From Naidich et al., ref. 25, with permission.)

TABLE 2. *Cutaneous stigmata in spinal lipoma*

	Hoffman et al.[a]	Pierre-Kahn et al.
	$N = 97$	$N = 73$
Subcutaneous mass[b]	100%	75%
Skin dimple	27%	30%
Hemangioma	25%	23%
Tail-like appendage	5%	8%
Hairs or hairy-nevus	1%	8%
Denuded skin patch	1%	7%
Scar-like patch	3%	3%
No cutaneous stigma	—[a]	5.5%

Combined data from two large series, refs. 100 and 101.

[a] Hoffman et al. excluded lipomas associated only with "tethered spinal cord" and fatty filum.

[b] The mass is lumbar in 20%, lumbosacral in 34%, and sacral in 46% of Hoffman's series.

neural ectoderm as follows (1): If the superficial ectoderm separates from the neural ectoderm prematurely, before the neural tube has closed completely, then mesenchyme may gain access to the interior of the closing neural tube (Fig. 31). Such mesenchyme could prevent closure of the neural tube focally, leading to dorsal myeloschisis. The dorsal and ventral surfaces of the closing neural plate are fundamentally different, and are postulated to induce mesenchyme to differentiate in two distinct ways (Fig. 32). The mesenchyme adjacent to the dorsal surface of the closing plate, i.e., the future interior of the cord, is induced by the dorsal surface to form fat. This fat would "insert" into the entire dorsal surface of the neural plate. It would fill the complete dorsal cleft. Its lateral extent would necessarily be limited by the lateral edge of the dorsal surface, because only the dorsal surface would induce differentiation of the mesenchyme into fat.

The mesenchyme surrounding the ventral surface of the closing plate, i.e., the future exterior of the neural tube, is induced by the ventral surface to form meninges. The dorsal-medial extent of the meninges would be limited by the lateral margin of the ventral surface at the neural ridge, since only the ventral surface would induce differentiation of the mesenchyme to meninges. Therefore, the meninges would attach to the neural tissue laterally, exactly at the neural ridge. No meninges would form in the midline dorsally since there is no ventral surface to induce them there, unless successful neurulation closes the folds into a tube. This would leave a midline dorsal defect in the meninges. Similarly, improper neurulation would prevent proper development of the neural arches, fascia, and muscle, creating a posterior spina bifida.

The fat induced by the dorsal surface of the neural plate could then extend directly posteriorly, through the gap in the meninges and through the spina bifida into

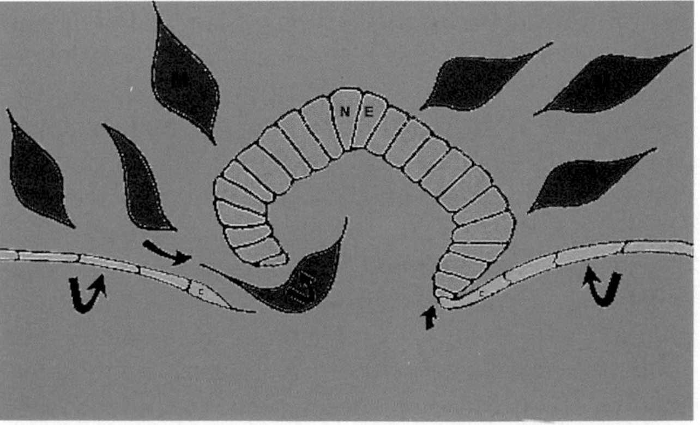

FIG. 31. Spinal lipoma. Proposed embryogenesis by focal premature disjunction of cutaneous from neural ectoderm. The mechanism proposed is detailed in the text. Labels as in Figs. 3 and 4, except that *curved arrows* are also used to indicate the course of mesenchyme migrating through the focal disjunction to the dorsal surface of the closing neural folds. (From Naidich et al., ref. 24, with permission.)

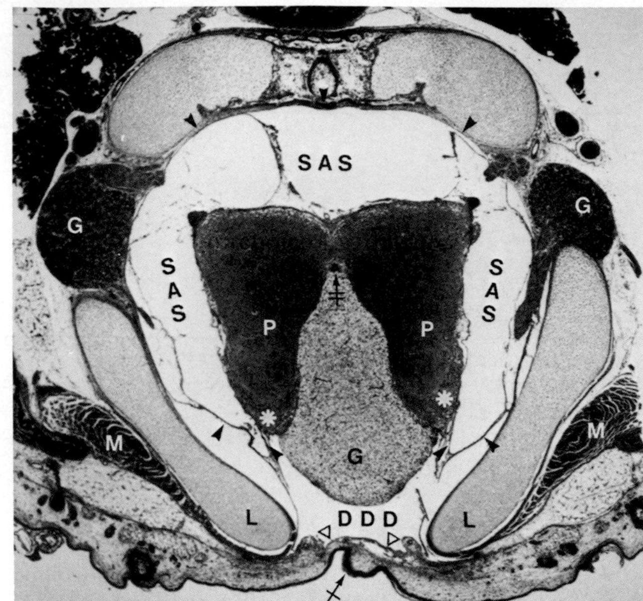

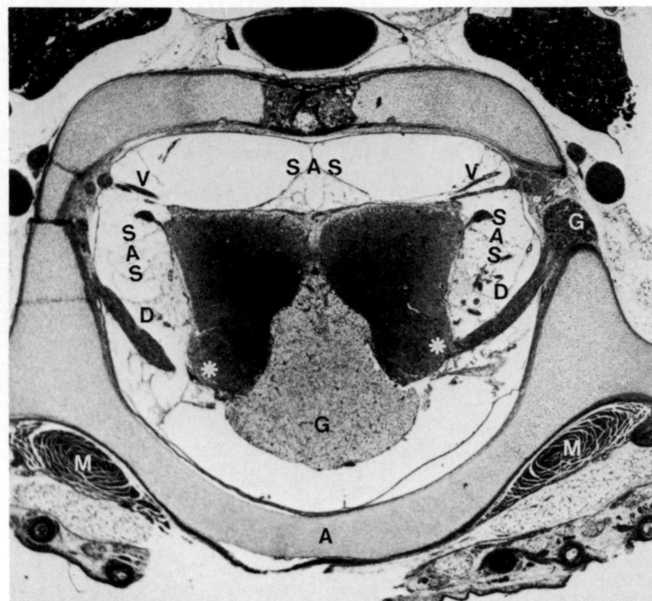

FIG. 32. Animal model for spinal lipoma. Axial anatomic sections of 21-day-old myeloschistic chicken embryo with dorsal glycogen body. Myelin stain. Ventral lies toward the top. The relations of the normal avian lumbosacral glycogen body and dura depicted here are believed to be a paradigm for human lipomyeloschisis. **A:** Intact skin (*single crossed arrow*) covers the spina bifida. Bifid laminae (*L*) are joined by a fibrovascular band (*open arrowheads*). Dura (*black arrowheads*) underlies the entire inner surface of the vertebral canal except directly beneath the spina bifida. Instead of crossing under the spina bifida, dura is reflected onto the posterolateral aspect of the neural placode (*P*) at the ipsilateral neural ridge, just behind the ipsilateral dorsal nerve root entry zone (*asterisks*). This leaves a median dorsal dural deficiency (*DDD*). The left and right halves of the neural tissue are joined only ventral to the remnant of the central canal (*double crossed arrow*) of the spinal cord. The pia-arachnoid lines the deep surface of the dura and is reflected from the lateral wall of the canal (where it is called arachnoid mater) onto the ventral surface of the neural plate (where it is called pia mater) as one continuous sheet. This is exactly analogous to the arrangement of pia-arachnoid in myelocele and myelomeningocele. The subarachnoid space (*SAS*) has the shape of a horseshoe, open end directed posteriorly. The subarachnoid space is crossed by multiple arachnoid trabeculae. The normal avian glycogen body (*black G*) occupies the midline between the dorsal halves of the neural placode and projects posterior to the neural tissue within the dorsal deficiency of leptomeninges and dura. Note that the lateral extent of the glycogen body lies exactly at the neural ridge. *White Gs* and *Ms* indicate the dorsal root ganglia and the paraspinal musculature, respectively. **B:** The neural arch (*A*) is intact 5-mm cephalad. Paired ventral (*V*) and dorsal (*D*) nerve roots arise from the pial surface of the neural tissue. The glycogen body has ascended within the dorsal myeloschisis and within a pocket-like extension of the meningeal defect to underlie the intact laminae of the more cephalic vertebra. While the glycogen body appears to be intradural at this level, it remains anatomically extradural. (From Naidich et al., ref. 25, with permission.)

the subcutaneous tissue of the back. The fat would be anatomically extradural. The junction of fat and meninges would necessarily lie at the neural ridge that divides the dorsal and ventral surfaces of the neural folds. Depending on the degree of spina bifida, size of the spinal canal and the subarachnoid space, and volume of the lipoma, the spinal cord and placode could remain in the canal, herniate partially, or herniate completely. The lipo-neural junction could be intracanalicular or extracanalicular. Depending on whether the premature disjunction was unilateral or bilateral, the spinal lipoma could be asymmetric to either side or nearly midline. Depending on "packing" considerations, the lipoma could remain truly posterior to the placode or the lipoma could bulge laterally, bilaterally, to compress the posterolateral borders of the placode. The dorsal surface of the placode could rotate to either side or become folded.

The mechanism of premature disjunction, and the subsequent mechanical effects considered above, appear to account for all the features observed in spinal lipomas which involve the portion of the cord formed by neurulation (1,25,102). Since the process of neurulation creates all the spinal cord except the distalmost conus medullaris and filum terminale, premature disjunction could account for all spinal lipomas affecting the mid conus or higher. Lipomas that involve the distal conus and filum must be explained differently, as a disorder of canalization and retrogressive differentiation (vide infra).

Spinal lipomas are usually considered in 3 groups: lipomas with intact dura, deficient dura, and filar lipomas.

Spinal Lipomas with Intact Dura

The intradural lipomas are a small group of intramedullary tumors that appear to arise in the dorsal midline of a cleft spinal cord and then bulge outward to form subpial masses of fat (Figs. 33A and 34). They constitute

A

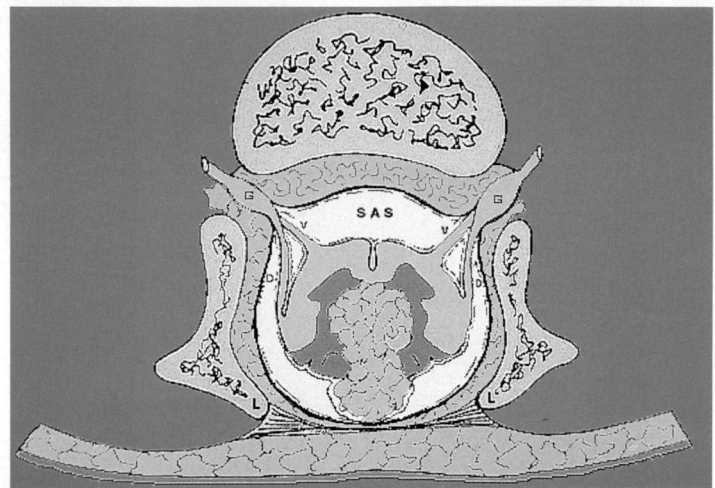

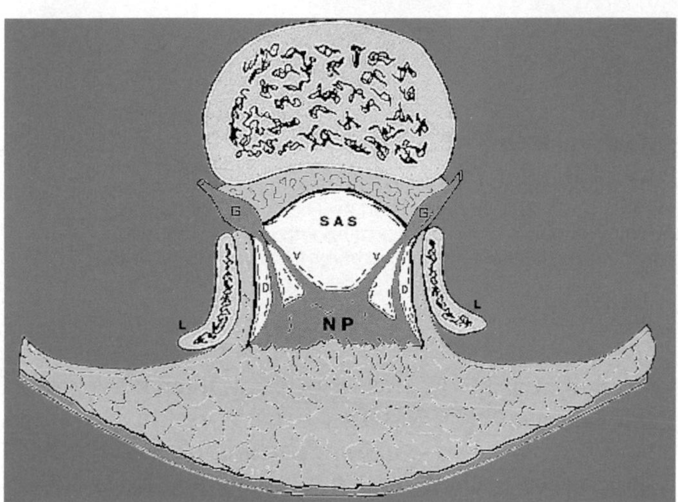

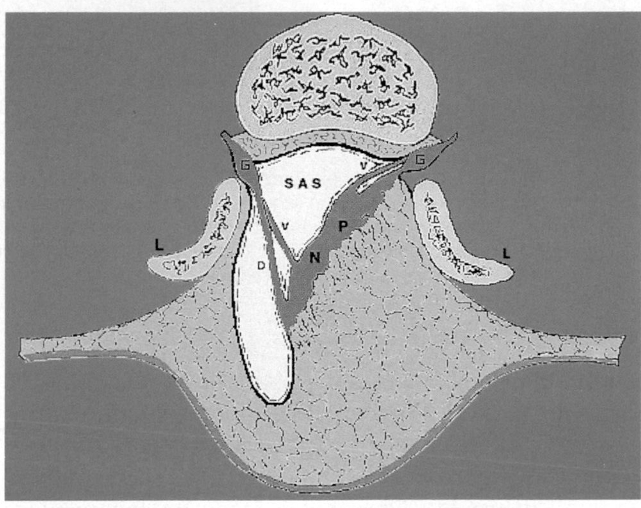

FIG. 33. Diagrammatic representations of spinal lipomas. **A:** Intradural lipoma. The laminae (*L*) are bifid. The dura (*dark line*) is intact. The pia-arachnoid (*dashed line*) encloses the spinal cord and the lipoma. The lipoma lies predominantly within a midline cleft in the dorsal spinal cord but fungates *beneath* the pia to bulge into the dorsal subarachnoid space (*SAS*). *D*, dorsal root; *V*, ventral root; *G*, dorsal root ganglion. **B:** Lipomyelocele. There is posterior spina bifida with everted laminae. The spinal cord is cleft dorsally and oriented like the original unneurulated neural placode (*NP*) in a nearly coronal plane. The dura (*heavy line*) inserts into the lateral aspect of the cord just lateral to the edge of the cleft and just dorsal to the entry zones of the dorsal roots (*D*). The pia and arachnoid (*light dashed line*) are one continuous membrane that lines the inside of the dura and the ventral surface of the spinal cord, enclosing the subarachnoid space (*SAS*). This pia-arachnoid membrane also encloses the nerve roots but is not drawn there to simplify the diagram. The nerve roots arise directly from the cord and traverse the subarachnoid space to their root sleeves. They do not cross through fat. The skin is intact. The lipoma passes ventrally from the subcutaneous space through the spina bifida toward the spinal cord. As it nears the cord, the lipoma becomes increasingly fibrous and inserts along the dorsal face of the cleft, reaching the midline groove that should have become the central canal of the spinal cord. As shown, the lipoma lies entirely outside the dura and the arachnoid. From this site it may ascend into the central canal of the "normal" cord above and/or into the extradural space of the spinal canal. No fat lies within the subarachnoid space. A pseudocapsule usually delineates portions of the superficial surface of the lipoma. **C:** Lipomyelomeningocele. The basic anatomic relationships remain. Gross expansion of the subarachnoid space (*SAS*) causes the cord and pia-arachnoid to herniate out of the spinal canal, either symmetrically or asymmetrically. When the lipoma lies partially off midline, it tethers the spinal cord to one side, so that the cord rotates as it herniates posteriorly. The meningocele bulges to the contralateral side. As a consequence the nerve roots on the side of the meningocele are unusually long and easy to mobilize at surgery. The nerve roots on the side of the lipoma may be very short and may pass out of the spinal canal into the neural foramina nearly immediately. Such short roots may be very hard to mobilize at surgery and may themselves limit cord mobility after complete "untethering" of the cord from the lipoma. (From Naidich et al., refs. 22 and 65, with permission.)

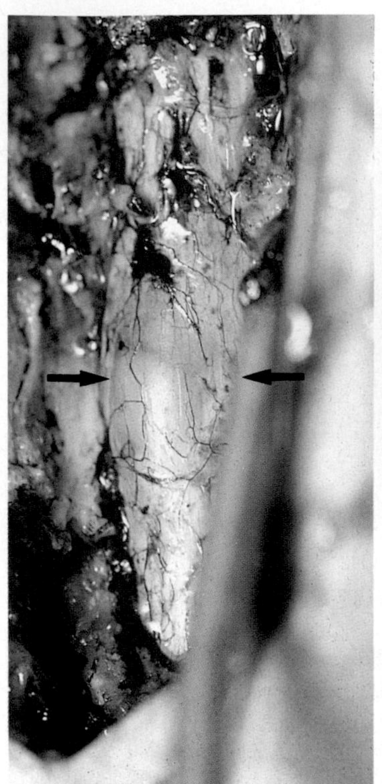

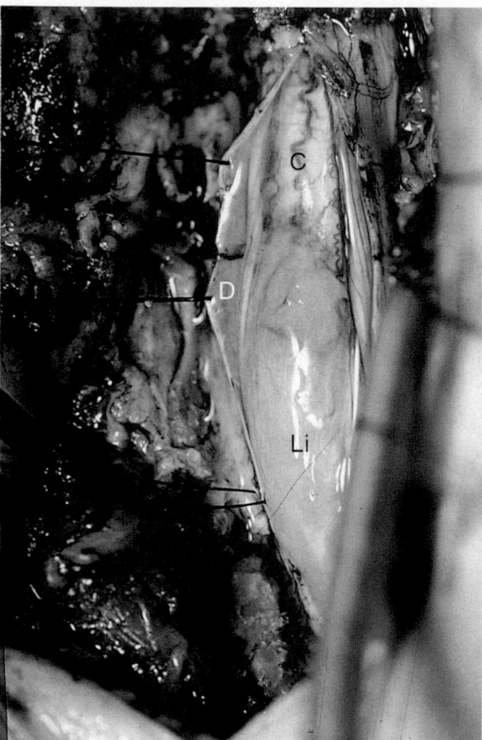

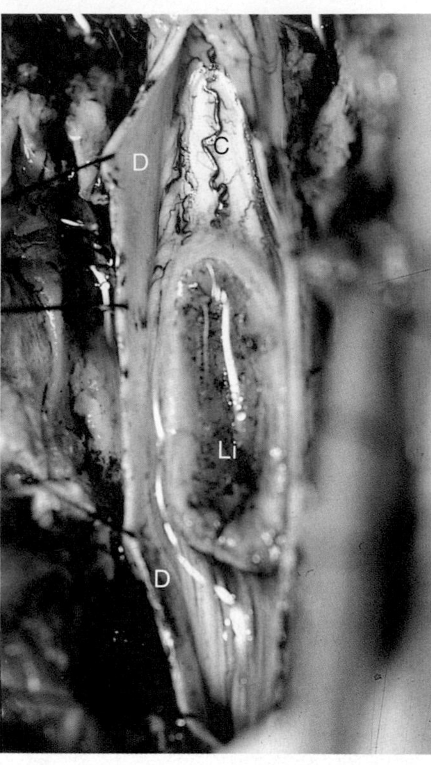

A B,C

FIG. 34. Operative exposure of intradural lipoma, 2-year, 11-month-old girl. **A:** Dissection of midline structures uncovers the intact dura (*arrows*). The dura is thin and translucent. **B:** Midline dural incision and retraction of dura (*D*) with tenting sutures reveals the glistening pia-arachnoid that covers the spinal cord (*C*) and lipoma (*Li*). **C:** Following dissection of pia-arachnoid and partial laser vaporization of the lipoma, one sees the insertion of the lipoma (*Li*) into the midline cleft in the dorsal aspect of the distal cord (*C*).

approximately 4% of the lipomas in our series and affect the cervical and thoracic spinal cords predominantly (1,66,103). In this group the spinal canal is usually nearly normal with narrow spina bifida or focal segmentation anomalies (Fig. 35). The canal itself may be expanded by the mass. The dura is thinned, perhaps translucent, but remains intact and is displaced peripherally by the combined mass of cord and lipoma (Fig. 34). The lipoma typically lies dorsal or dorsolateral to the cord, frequently causes cord rotation and frequently causes high-grade stenosis or block. Often it is the upper or lower pole of the lipoma that protrudes from the surface of the cord as an intradural extramedullary mass. These lesions can be regarded as formes fruste of the more common lipoma.

Spinal Lipomas with Deficient Dura

The most common forms of spinal lipoma (84%) are associated with definite defects in the dura through which the lipoma may extend from the spinal cord to the subcutaneous tissue (Figs. 33B and 36) (25,104). In these cases, the subcutaneous component of the mass typically forms a lump in the low back. The subjacent spinal canal usually shows a wide spina bifida. Segmentation anomalies and anomalies of the sacrum and sacro-iliac joint are present in nearly 50% of cases. The spinal cord beneath the lipoma is cleft dorsally (partial dorsal myeloschisis) and very closely resembles the neural plate of a myelomeningocele. The dura that normally forms a complete tube around the cord is deficient in the dorsal midline, deep to the lipoma. The medial edges of the dura attach along the edges of the neural plate just dorsal to the entry zones of the dorsal roots. Thus the raw, cleft surface of the neural plate lies medial to and outside of the dural sac in an anatomically extradural location. The arrangement of arachnoid and of nerve roots in such lipomas is identical with that seen in myeloceles and myelomeningoceles. Lipomyelocele (Figs. 33B, 37, and 39) and lipomyelomeningocele (Figs. 33C, 38, and 40) are exactly analogous to the myelocele (Fig. 7A) and the myelomeningocele (Fig. 7B), with the addition of fat inserting into the dorsal surface of the neural plate and closure of the skin over the fat. The lipoma inserts into the exposed, dorsal, "extradural" face of the neural plate and extends from there to the subcutaneous space. Since the exposed surface of the neural plate is directly continuous with the central canal of the normal cord above, lipoma may also extend in continuity from the dorsal surface of the neural plate into the central canal of the cord. While the portion of lipoma within the central canal is certainly intramedullary, it is also extradural in the sense that it is not sur-

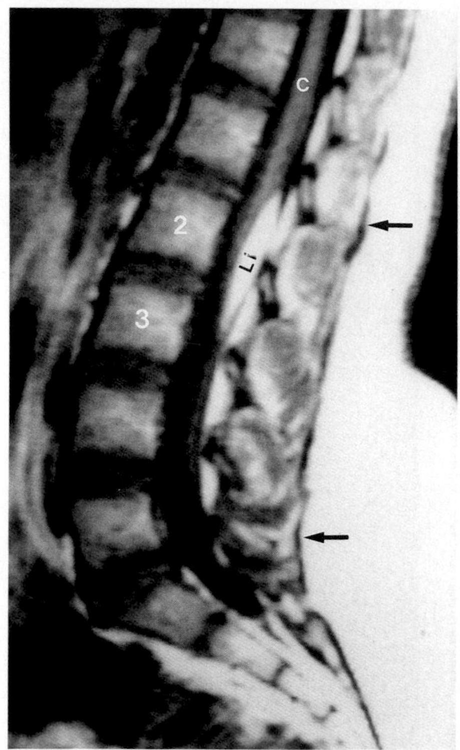

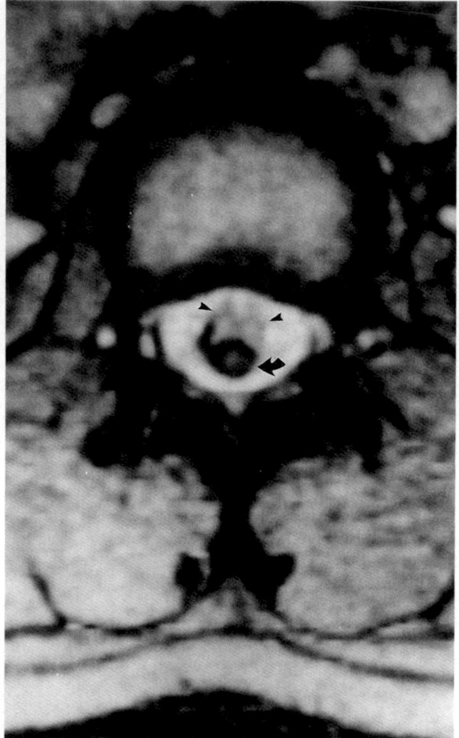

FIG. 35. Intradural lipoma. **A:** Sagittal T1-weighted MRI. **B:** Axial T2-weighted MRI. A: The dorsal subcutaneous fat, lumbodorsal fascia (*black arrows*) and posterior spinal elements are intact. The normal dorsal epidural fat appears as discontinuous patches of high signal. The lipoma (*Li*) lies deep to and is separate from the epidural fat, has a longer continuous extent, and is adherent to the dorsal surface of the distal cord (*c*) at the conus. *2,3*, L2 and L3 bodies. B: The lipoma (*curved arrow*) is identified by its markedly reduced signal intensity on T2-weighted images and its location within a partial cleft in the dorsal midline of the cord (*arrowheads*). The high-signal spinal fluid, dura, and spine are intact posterior to the lipoma. T2-weighted images often show the anatomic relationships of neural tissue, lipoma, spinal fluid, and spinal canal most clearly.

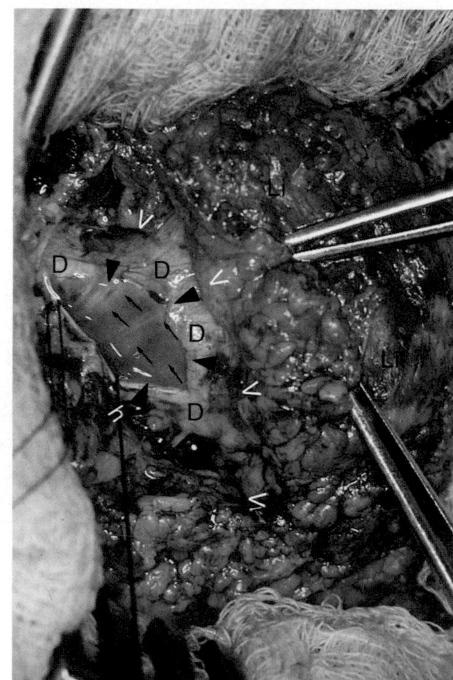

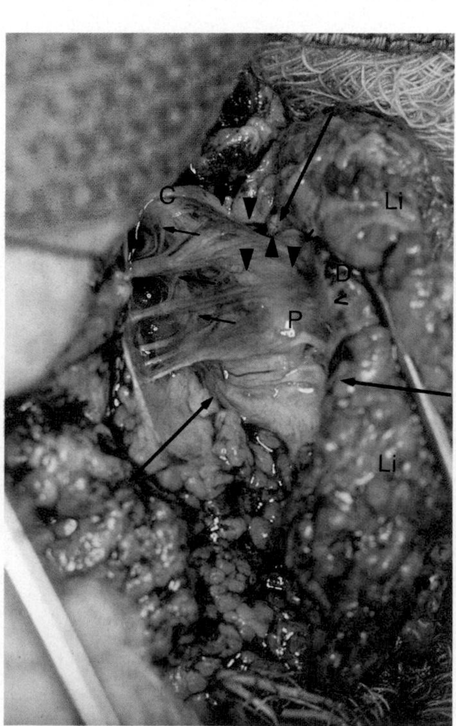

FIG. 36. Spinal lipoma (lipomyelomeningocele), 1-month-old girl. (Same patient as in Fig. 30.) **A:** Operative field viewed from the patient's left side and posterior. The skin has been incised and retracted, and the bone resected, to expose the lipoma (*Li*) that passes into the spinal canal medial (and external to) the dura (*D*) through the dorsal dural deficiency. The dura is incised (*black arrowheads*) well ventral and away from the dorsal root entry zone (*open white arrowheads*) that lies beneath the lipodural junction. This incision exposes the glistening arachnoid and the dorsal and ventral nerve roots (*small black arrows*) that run in the subjacent subarachnoid space. **B:** Circumferential incision of dura and arachnoid exposes the distal well-neurulated spinal cord (*C*), the expanded (dorsally cleft) placode (*P*, *long arrows*), the dorsal nerve roots (*small black arrowheads*), the ventral nerve roots (*small black arrows*), and their passage through the subarachnoid space to their exit foramina. The flap of dura (*D*) has been lifted up and reflected medially to expose the dorsal nerve root entry zone (*open black arrowheads*). Note that the lipoma (*Li*) passes into the cord extradurally, medial and external to the insertion of the dura into the edge of the cleft in the cord. The lipoma (*Li*) lies entirely outside the subarachnoid space. Because the cord is tethered and low-lying, there is no cauda equina. Note also that the lipodural junction lies immediately dorsal to the dorsal root entry zone and serves as a landmark for that zone. (From Naidich et al., ref. 25, with permission.)

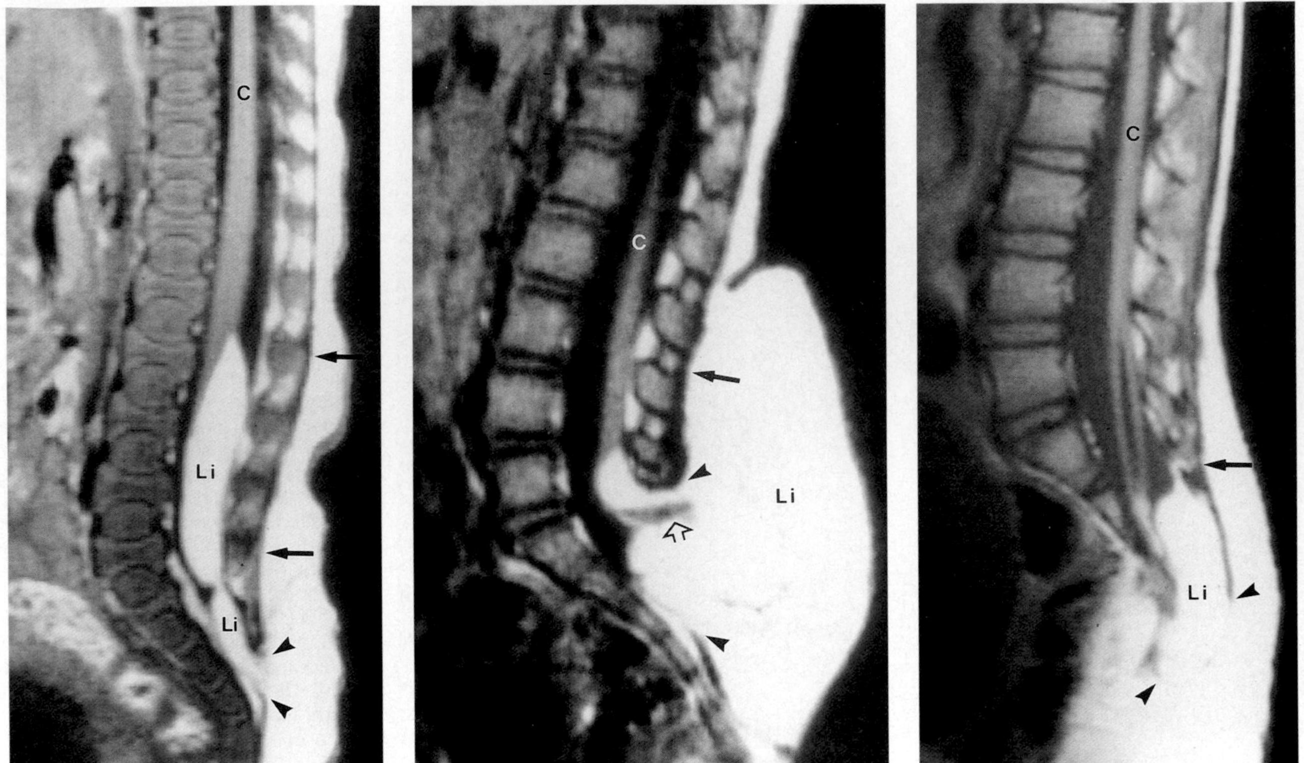

FIG. 37. Lipomyoceles. Midline sagittal T1-weighted MRI of three patients. In each the high-signal lipoma (*Li*) extends inward from the subcutaneous plane, through a defect (*arrowheads*) in the lumbodorsal fascia (*arrows*) into the spinal canal, where it inserts into the dorsal surface of a low-lying, tethered spinal cord (*c*). In A, the posterior defect is narrow. The lipoma has an elongated bilobed cylindrical configuration. The cord remains entirely within the canal. In B, the posterior spinal bifida is larger. The cord (*c*) extends (*open arrow*) out of the canal into the defect, but there is no meningocele. In C, there is concurrent hydromyelia of the distal cord.

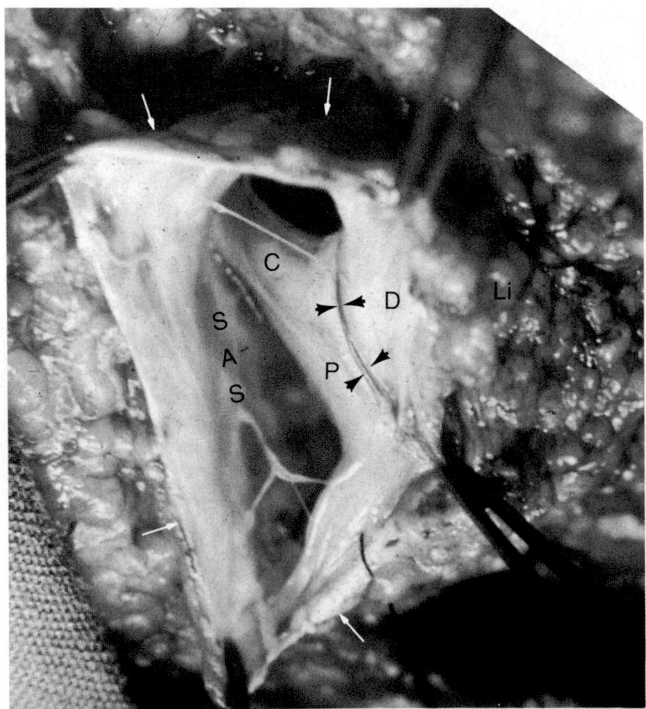

FIG. 38. Large lipomyelomeningocele. Operative exposure. Broad opening into the meningocele (*white arrows*) reveals the subarachnoid space (*SAS*), the distal cord (*C*) that widens into the placode, the typical shape of the placode resembling the bowl of a porcelain Chinese soup spoon, the insertion of dura (*D*) into the edge (*black arrowheads*) of the placode (*P*), and the entry of the lipoma (*Li*) into the placode extradurally, medial and external to the dura via the dorsal dural deficiency. Case courtesy of Francisco Gutierrez, M.D., Chicago, IL. (From Naidich et al., ref. 25, with permission.)

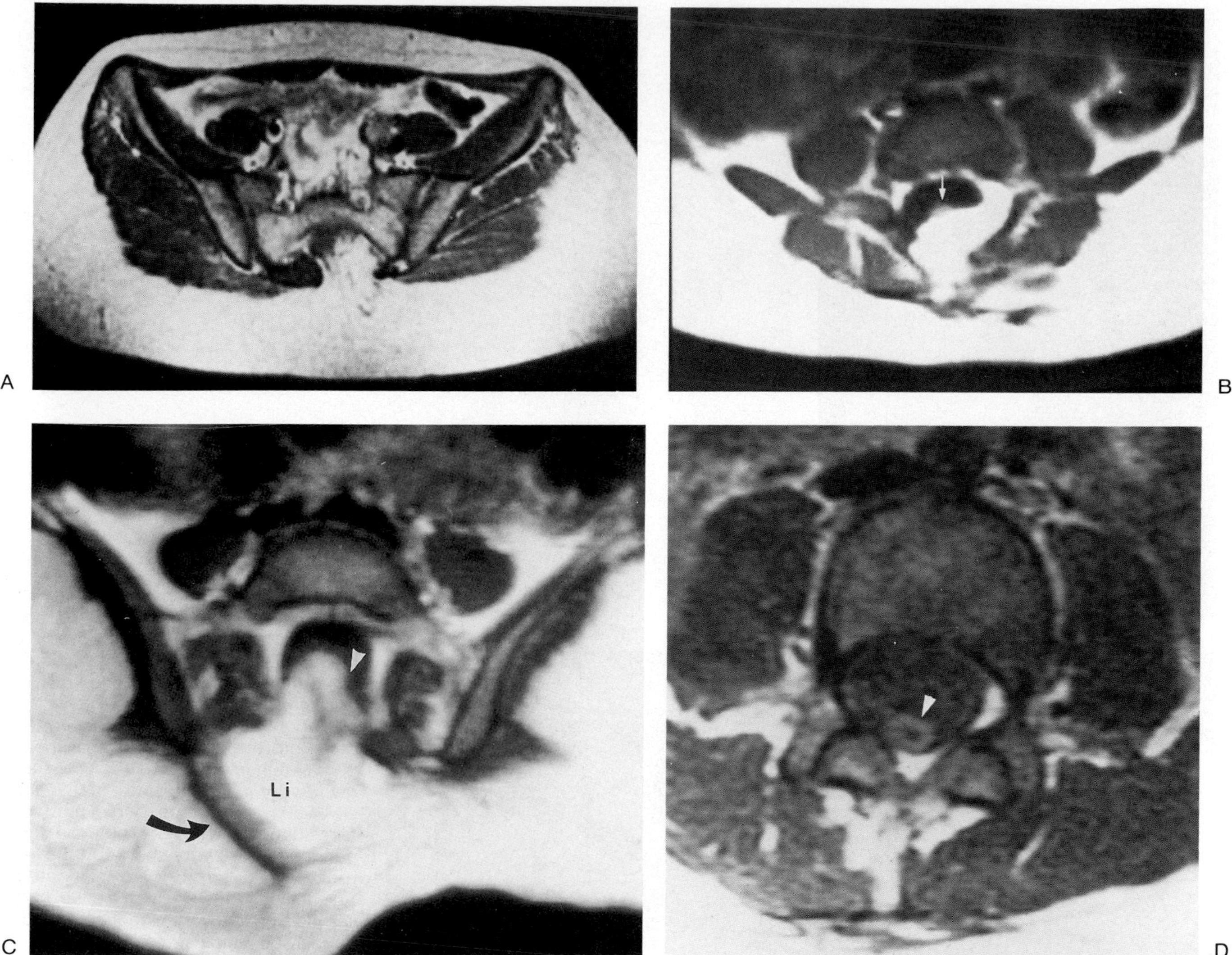

FIG. 39. Lumbosacral lipomyeloceles. Axial T1 -weighted MRI, in three patients, an 11-year-old girl (A), a 16-month-old girl (B), and a 9-year-old girl (D). The shape of the liponeural interface varies widely. **A:** When the lipoma is prominent and the distal cord is thin the neural tissue may be difficult to discern. One still detects entry of high-signal lipoma into the spinal canal via the midline spinal dysraphism. **B:** When the lipoma remains as a single dorsal mass, it displaces the cord (*white arrow*) anteriorly and thins it sagittally. **C:** When the lipoma bulges toward each side, deformation of the distal cord (*white arrowhead*) causes it to resemble an arrowhead with the tip pointing posteriorly. There is a keel-shaped iliac bone (*black arrow*) articulating with the right sacroiliac joint. **D:** This patient also exhibits hydromyelia with expansion of the central canal of the cord (*white arrowhead*) just superior to the liponeural junction (D). (A from Naidich et al., ref. 24; B from Naidich and McLone, ref. 66; D from Zimmerman et al., ref. 8; with permission.)

rounded on all sides by dura; it is directly continuous caudally with the extradural portion of the lipoma.

The lipo-neural junction may be relatively smooth or stellate. A variably thick band of low signal is often observed at the lipo-neural junction and appears to represent (i) collagenous tissue that separates the fat and nervous tissue elements, and (ii) phase-shift artifacts related to the fat-soft tissue interface.

Filar Lipomas (*see also page 1299*)

Dermal sinuses may concur in up to 20% of cases of spinal lipoma, and vice versa, probably because both lesions result from deranged disjunction of cutaneous from neural ectoderm. Thus insults may lead to premature disjunction (spinal lipoma), incomplete disjunction (dermal sinus), or both at the same or adjacent sites (Figs. 25 and 41). Dermoids and teratomas are seen in 3% to 7% of patients with spinal lipoma, diastematomyelia in 1% to 6% and hydromyelia in 2.5% to 24% of patients with spinal lipoma, often as a terminal dilatation of the cord (Figs. 39D) (25,100,101,105). Chiari I malformation has been seen in 1% to 3% of cases in some series (25,101) but not in others (1,17,22,65–67,100). Extraspinal genito-urinary lesions (4%) and genito-anal lesions (4%) are also seen with spinal lipomas (101).

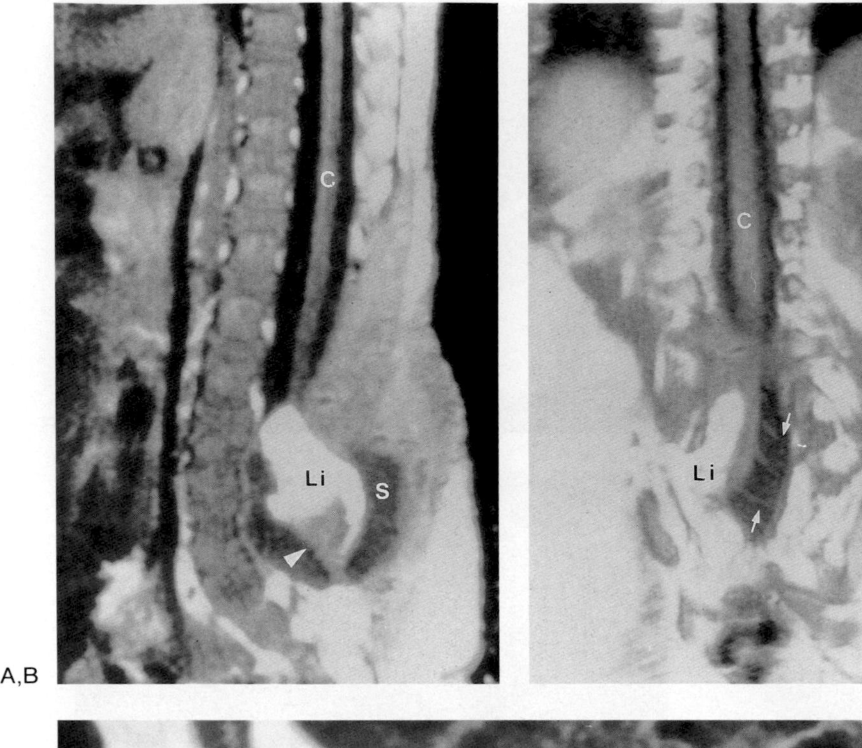

A,B

C

FIG. 40. Lipomyelomeningocele. T1-weighted sagittal (**A**), coronal (**B**), and axial (**C**) MRI demonstrate an asymmetric right-sided high-signal lipoma (*Li*) with a substantial left-sided meningocele (*S*) that extends into the midline posterior to the cord (*C*). The lipoma inserts into the dorsal surface of the lipoma, tethers the cord (*C*, *white arrowheads*) inferiorly, and rotates the cord 90° so that its dorsal surface faces rightward (see C). Thus, the right nerve roots are very short and the left roots (*white arrows*) are elongated. See also Fig. 33C. In such a case, midline incision to the meningocele may be dangerous since it comes down directly onto the dorsal roots of the rotated cord. The short deep roots may prevent complete "untethering" and mobilization of the cord despite successful resection of the lipoma.

Patients with lipomyelomeningoceles are typically neurologically intact at birth, but develop neurological deficits with increasing age. In Hoffman's series of 97 patients, none remained neurologically intact by age 4 years and many had significant deficits (100). For that reason, corrective surgery is recommended early in life—perhaps at 2–3 months of age—even in asymptomatic patients. The risk of surgery is small. Review of nearly 400 surgical procedures showed only 1 death (from meningitis) and 3 instances of immediate postoperative deterioration (0.8%) (101).

Symptoms appear to result from the mass effect of the adipose tissue and from cord ischemia secondary to repetitive stretching of the tethered cord. The cells of the lipoma appear biochemically identical to normal subcutaneous lipoma cells in their ability to store, synthesize, and mobilize fat (101). Therefore, the lipoma may increase in bulk (101), occasionally rapidly (106), and low caloric diets may aid in limiting lipoma mass. Tethering of the cord subjects it to repetitive mild stretching with normal daily activities and unusually severe stretching with trauma or sports. Stretching of the cord constricts cord vascularity, reduces blood flow, and leads to mitochondrial anoxia (107) with decreased oxidative phosphorylation. Release of tethering stabilizes or improves this situation. The two goals of surgery are to debulk the lipoma and to free the tethered cord.

Otherwise-successful surgical release of a tethered cord may be frustrated by two circumstances: (i) second tethering lesions and (ii) anomalously short lumbosacral nerve roots which themselves anchor the cord in a low, stretched position (25,108). Hoffman et al. (100) have

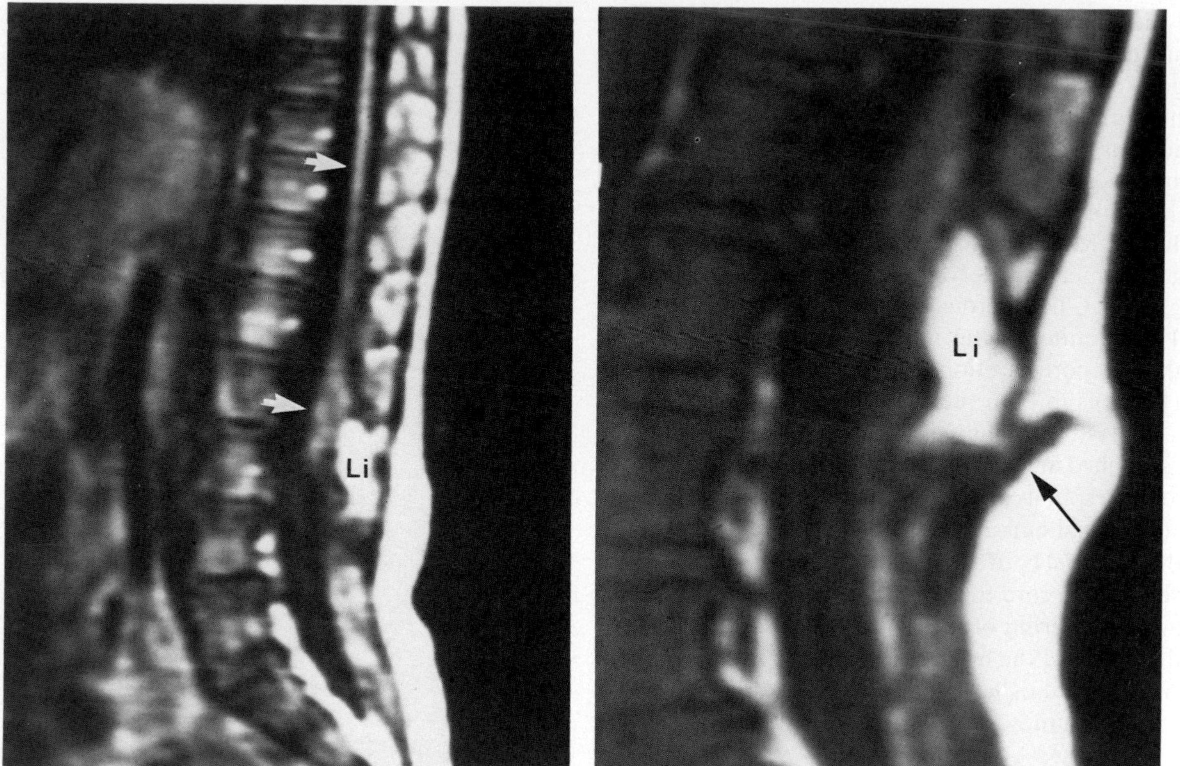

FIG. 41. A,B: Concurrent spinal lipoma and dermal sinus. Sagittal T1-weighted MRIs reveal high-signal fat inserting into the dorsal surface of a low-lying, tethered spinal cord (*white arrows*) and a low-signal tract (*black arrow*) that traverses the lipoma to merge with the zone of spina bifida. (From Zimmerman et al., ref. 8, with permission.)

reported that 8% of patients with spinal lipoma have a concurrent short thick filum that is a secondary cause of cord tethering. These thickened fila were seen most frequently in patients with rostrally situated lipomas of the thoracolumbar, lumbar, or upper lumbosacral region. In such circumstances, the thick fila must also be sectioned to effect complete cord release.

In patients with distal lumbosacral anomalies and with lipomyelomeningoceles that rotate the cord, it is not uncommon to find that the nerve roots which have rotated anteriorly, closer to their exit foramina, are far shorter than those that have rotated posteriorly, away from their exit foramina. These short anterior roots may pass nearly directly from the cord into the extradural space, so that their mobile intra-arachnoid course is negligible. In such circumstance the roots themselves anchor the cord inferiorly and, unless sectioned, cannot be addressed surgically (25,109). In our experience, the group of patients with sacral lipomas, sacral scoliosis, wide sacroiliac joints, and other sacral anomalies more commonly suffer this circumstance and may have less successful surgical repair.

Up to 10% of patients with spinal lipoma show retethering of the cord months to years after the primary repair (47,109). This is seen most often in the lumbosacral region and results from dense adhesions between the distal cord and the posterolateral walls of the spinal canal at the site of the previous repair (47). The adhesions are often asymmetrical and are predominant on the side of greater symptomatology (101).

The major clinical signs of retethering may appear at the time of growth spurts and include pain localized to the back and legs (57%), new or progressive weakness of the lower extremities (47%), change in gait (44%), progressive foot deformities or hip dislocation (32%), new urinary incontinence (21%), and new or progressive scoliosis (11%) (47).

Greater than 90% of patients reoperated for retethering have stabilization of their deficits or improvement (47). Reoperation improves motor strength by at least one spinal segment in 52%, improves gait and stance in 59%, reduces scoliosis in 33%, and permits urinary continence and social continence in 36%. In 8% of cases the retethered cord may not be completely released due to extensive adhesions and entrapment of nerve roots (47).

Since the low-lying cord nearly always retethers to the posterior or posterolateral wall of the canal near to the upper margin of the old surgical defect, new surgical techniques may employ fine stay sutures between the ventral pia and the ventral dura in order to keep the distal cord centered in the subarachnoid space, away from the posterior wall of the canal. In addition, the dorsal wall of the canal is reconstructed and dorsal tenting sutures are used to hold the dorsal dura and any fascial patch graft posteriorly, away from the distal cord itself.

In the untreated case, MRI displays the position and extensions of the lipoma, any tethered cord, the relation of lipoma to cord, and any concurrent lesion such as terminal hydromyelia and diastematomyelia. Increasingly sophisticated MRI may display the precise relation of the lipoma to emerging nerve roots, but thus far post-myelographic CT still provides finer anatomic detail.

MRI has limited value in assessing retethering, because the low cord position and residual lipoma are expected findings in both successful surgery and retethering. A "bow-string tight" spinal cord suggests that the cord is stretched and thus tethered. Such cords appear to cut across the spinal canal along the shortest line between sequential spinal curvatures. Absence of CSF posterior to the distal spinal cord also suggests tethering of the dorsal surface of the cord to the canal wall. In patients with suspected retethering of the cord, MR detection of increased volume of the lipoma, progressive hydromyelia, concurrent dermoid, diastematomyelia, or other complicating condition may also assist in patient management.

NORMAL AND DERANGED CANALIZATION AND RETROGRESSIVE DIFFERENTIATION

The distal spinal cord (Fig. 42) forms by the processes of canalization and retrogressive differentiation (10–13).

Normal Canalization

After neurulation is complete on Day 26–27 the distal spinal cord has yet to be formed. The caudal end of the neural tube and the caudal end of the notochord blend into a large aggregate of undifferentiated cells designated the caudal cell mass (Fig. 43). The caudal cell mass extends into the tail fold, adjacent to the distal end of the developing hindgut and the mesonephros. This juxtaposition of developing genitourinary, notochordal, and neural structures within the tail fold appears to account for the common concurrence of distal vertebral, neural, anorectal, renal, and genital anomalies.

Within the caudal cell mass, small vacuoles form, coalesce, and eventually connect with the central canal of the spinal cord above, "canalizing" the caudal cell mass (Fig. 44A,B). A focal widening of this canal at the distal conus or proximal filum is designated the terminal ventricle (Fig. 44C) (111). Since vacuoles form at many sites and link up variably, accessory central canals, lateral or dorsolateral to the true lumen, are commonly observed in the distal cord of embryos. Normal adults show major forking of the canal in the conus medullaris in 10% of cases and minor forking in 35% of cases. Within the filum terminale, major forking of the canal is seen in 35% of individuals (112).

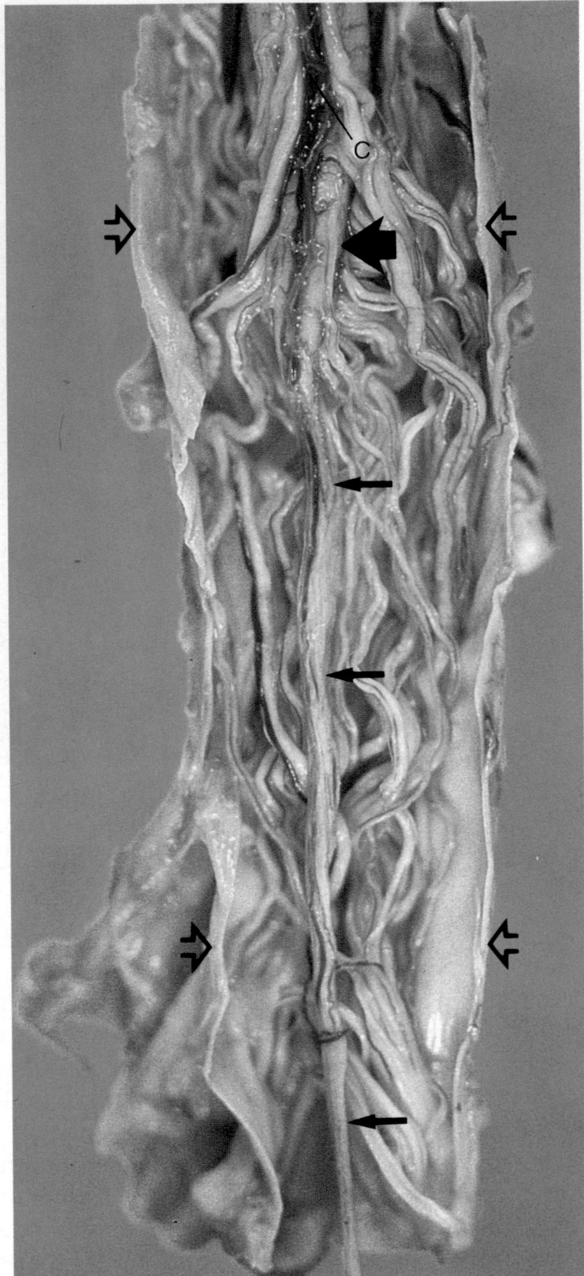

FIG. 42. Normal anatomic specimen of distal neural structures. Opening the dorsal dura and arachnoid (between *open black arrows)* exposes the dorsal aspect of the distal spinal cord (*C*), the tapering conus medullaris (*large black arrow*), and the filum terminale (*multiple small black arrows*). The roots of cauda equina are normally oriented nearly vertical, but appear here artifactually tortuous and redundant. The normal filum is as thick as two to three nerve roots combined.

As the vacuoles form, groups of cells orient themselves around the vacuoles and differentiate toward neural cells. By this method the distal cord and the central canal of the cord elongate far into the tail fold. The most cephalic portion of this distal cord forms the lower half of

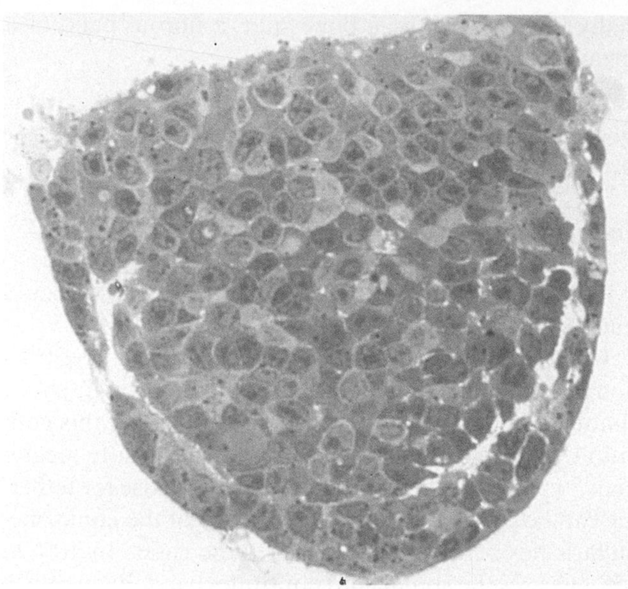

FIG. 43. Caudal cell mass. Mammalian embryo. At the start of canalization, the caudal end of the neural tube and the caudal end of the notochord lie within a large aggregate of undifferentiated cells—the caudal cell mass—that extends into the tail fold.

conus medullaris. In a process designated retrogressive differentiation, however, the major portion of this distal cord undergoes involution to a glio-ependymal strand called the filum terminale (Fig. 44B and C) (113–115).

The newly formed cord begins to involute before canalization is even complete. The embryonic tail disappears first. The lumen distal to future somite 32 (S3/4) becomes progressively narrower than the lumen above. This difference becomes exaggerated over time (13). The cells surrounding the narrowing distal lumen differentiate less completely than do those above. The thin caudal segment has only a single, ependymal zone about the lumen, while the thicker segment above differentiates into three distinct concentric zones: the deep ependymal zone, the intermediate mantel layer, and the superficial marginal zone. The primitive filum first appears as a bundle of nerve fibers on the ventral side of the distal cord. This extends caudally from the apex of the primitive conus to the 29th–30th vertebra. After involution of the distal cord to the filum terminale, the newly formed conus medullaris lies opposite the lower coccygeal segments. Thereafter, the spinal cord and filum do not shorten further. Rather, they elongate and thicken by interstitial growth.

The caudal spinal column also forms by a less well-organized process than that responsible for the more cephalic portions of the spine. The caudal cell mass formed by notochord, mesoderm, and neural tissue simply segments into somites to form the sacral, coccygeal, and tail vertebrae. Retrogressive differentiation then leads to reduction of most of these segments with loss of the tail. Thereafter the vertebral column elongates with growth and grows faster than the cord. All further "ascent" of the cord results from disproportionately greater longitudinal growth of the vertebrae, not involution; the bones simply grow faster and descend away from the cord.

The position of the tip of the conus medullaris is of significance in the diagnosis of the caudal spinal anomalies and the occult dysraphisms. Barson (116) studied the position of the tip of the conus medullaris with respect to the vertebral elements at different gestational ages (Fig. 45). Accepting a wide range of normal variation, he found that the tip "ascended" rapidly with respect to the vertebral elements from 12 to 16 weeks and rose more slowly thereafter. In his study, the tip of the conus lay at coccygeal 5 at 12 weeks, at L4–L5 by 18 weeks, at L2–L3 by term, and at adult levels of L1–L2 by about 3 months postpartum. Hawass et al. analyzed the position of the cord in situ in 146 "normal" fetuses (117), and found that the tip of the conus lay at the level of S5 at gestational age 7 weeks, ascended thereafter, and showed great variability in position between gestational ages 12–25 weeks. Between 35–38 weeks, the conus lay at or above the level of L3 (117). In collected series totaling 801 patients, James and Lassman (5) found that, by term, the tip of the spinal cord typically lay at or above the L2–L3

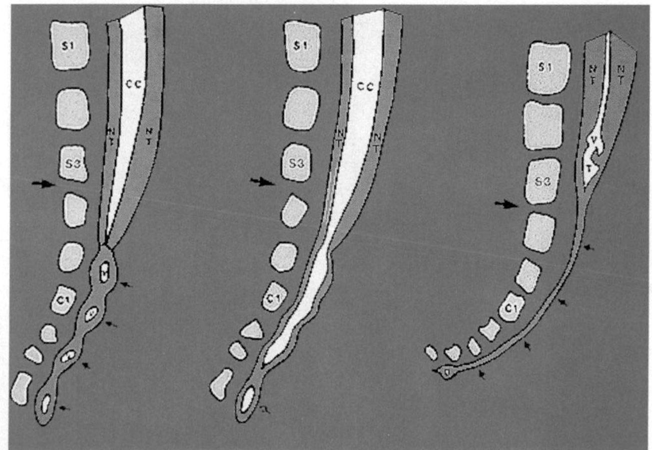

FIG. 44. Canalization and retrogressive differentiation. Diagrammatic representation of proposed embryogenesis. **A:** As small vacuoles (*v*) form in the caudal cell mass (*multiple small black arrows*), cells situated near to the vacuoles begin to orient themselves around the vacuoles and assume the configuration of ependymal cells. As more vacuoles form and coalesce, two to three layers of cells surrounding the vacuoles begin to resemble neural cells. **B,C:** The coalescing vacuoles merge with each other and with the central canal (*cc*) of the neurulated spinal cord (*NT*) above, canalizing the caudal cell mass. Accessory lumina may also form. The lumen of the spinal cord distal to the 32nd somite (*large black arrows*) (future S3/4) becomes narrower (*multiple small black arrows*) than the lumen cephalic to the 32nd somite. At about the 32nd somite (*large black arrow*), focal expansion of the hollow canal creates the terminal ventricle (*V.T.*). This may lie within the distal conus or the proximal filum terminale. The distalmost portion of the involuting tube remains hollow for long periods as the coccygeal medullary vestige (*small open arrow*). (From Naidich et al., ref. 22, with permission.)

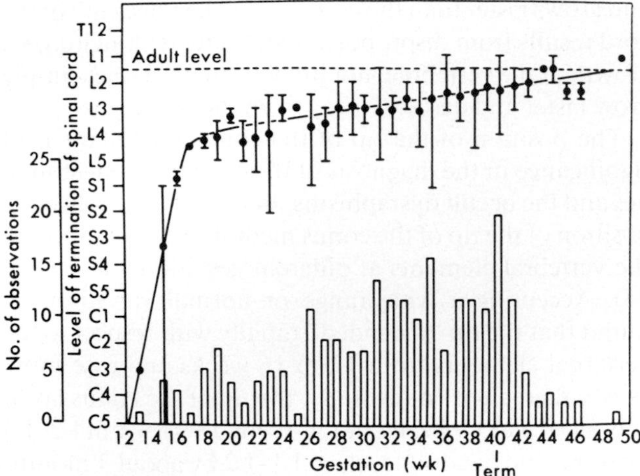

FIG. 45. Position of the tip of the conus medullaris (*dark circles* with error bars) with respect to the vertebral level and gestational age. (From Barson, ref. 52, with permission.)

interspace in 98% and overlay the L3 vertebra in 1.8% of cases (Fig. 46). Therefore a spinal cord that lies at or below L3 is best regarded as abnormal until study demonstrates that it is not anchored or "tethered" in abnormally low position by a bone spur, a fibrous band or a terminal mass such as lipoma.

Deranged Canalization and Retrogressive Differentiation

Tight Filum Terminale Syndrome

Failure of complete involution of the distal cord could lead to the tight filum terminale syndrome.

The term *tight filum terminale syndrome* signifies traction on the spinal cord as a result of an abnormally short, abnormally thick filum terminale (Fig. 47). In this condition, by definition (i) the filum must measure greater than 2 mm in diameter and (ii) no other cause for tethering can be present (1,110,118). The tip of the conus medullaris lies below L2 in 86% of these cases. In 10% to 15% of cases the spinal cord continues caudally to attach to the distal thecal sac without distinct termination. Filar fibrolipomas are present in 29% of cases. Kyphoscoliosis is present in 15% to 25% of these cases and improves following section of the filum in one-third of cases (110,119). In a large series, 100% of cases had midline defects in the arches of the lumbosacral spine, usually at

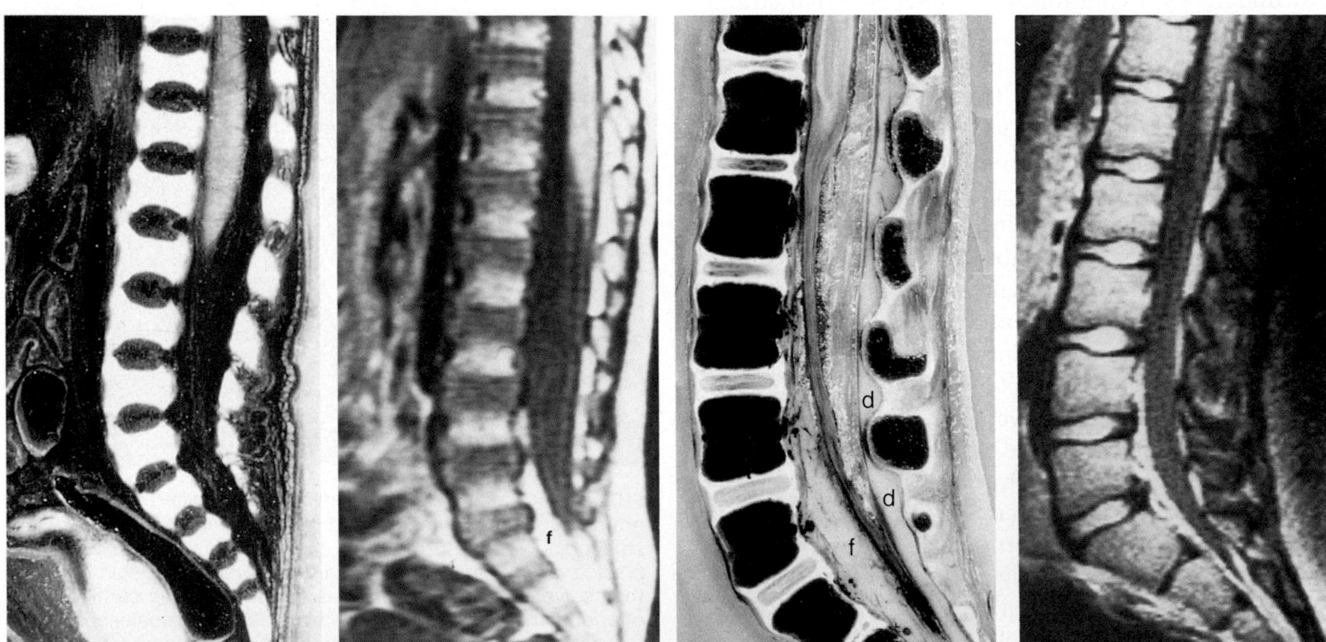

FIG. 46. Normal spinal canal and cord. Sagittal anatomic section, newborn (A), sagittal T1-weighted spin-echo MRI (B), sagittal anatomic specimen (C), and sagittal T1-weighted spin-echo MRI, 12-year-old boy (D). **A:** In the newborn, the marrow-containing central ossification centers (*V*) are relatively small compared with the cartilaginous end plates and the discs. The tip of the conus medullaris lies at L2–L3. The posterior elements are intact. The filum is not visualized. **B:** The tip of the conus lies at L1–L2. The ossification centers are thicker and more nearly rectangular. Note the normal pointed termination of the thecal sac and the ventral epidural fat (*f*) at the lumbosacral junction. **C:** The vertebral bodies are now more nearly adult in shape and are far larger than the intervertebral discs. The tip of the conus lies at L1. Ventral epidural fat (*f*) and dorsal epidural fat (*d*) are more prominent, partially because the section is off midline. The thecal sac tapers to a point. **D:** Sagittal image depicts the normal relationship among the vertebral bodies, discs, epidural fat, CSF, and cord. (A and C, courtesy of Victor Haughton, M.D., Milwaukee, WI; D from Naidich and McLone, ref. 66; with permission.)

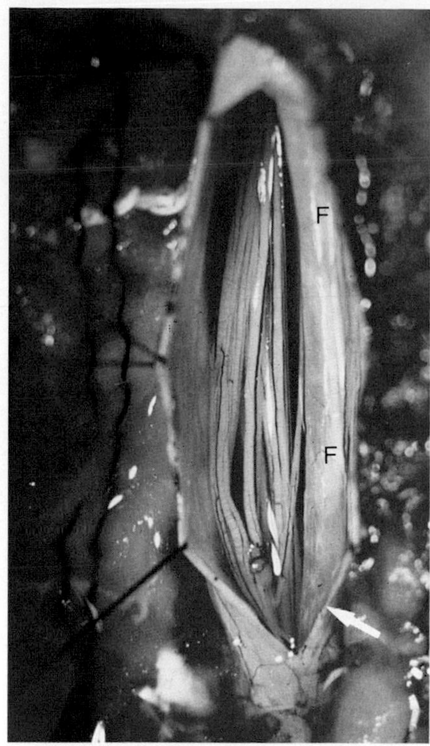

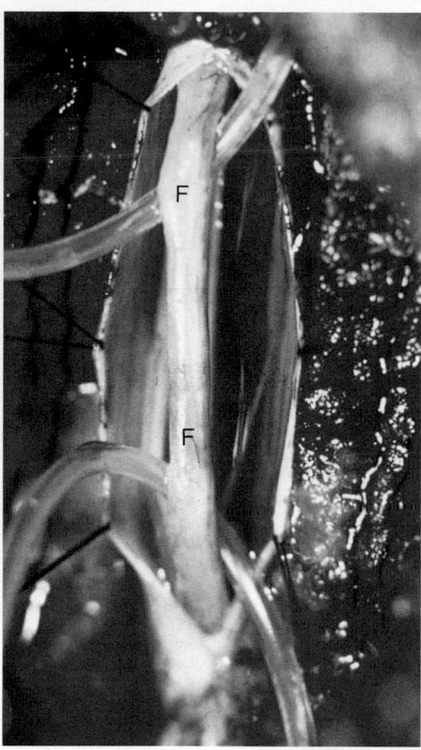

A,B

FIG. 47. A. Tight filum terminale syndrome. Intradural filar lipoma, 11-year-old girl with scoliosis. **A:** Midline entry into the thecal sac. The dura has been tented laterally by stay sutures. The filum terminale (*F*) is abnormally thick (cf. Fig. 40). The distal filum exhibits altered coloration (*white arrow*) representing fat. **B:** The thick filum has now been elevated and isolated in preparation for focal coagulation and section. Prior to section, it is essential to tease away from the filum lower sacral nerve roots that run with it and have filamentous adhesions to it.

L4, L5, and/or S1, leading Hendrick et al. (110) to suggest that normal spine radiographs almost exclude this diagnosis.

Lipoma of the Filum Terminale

Persistence of caudal cells that differentiate toward fat could produce filar lipomas. Indeed, such lipomas are observed incidentally in 4% to 6% of normal adults and may be considered a normal variation if they are not associated with cord tethering or neurological dysfunction.

Filar lipomas may involve the intradural portion of the filum, the extradural portion, or both. Intradural lipomas tend to be fusiform in shape and taper down toward a point where the filum pierces dura (Fig. 48). They exhibit increased signal intensity on T1-weighted images, progressively lower signal intensity with greater T2-weighting, and are easily observed on good sagittal and axial sections. Lipomas of the extradural portion of the filum (Fig. 49) are far more diffuse, tend to be larger and tend to merge with adjacent extradural fat. They commonly elevate and distort the distal thecal sac.

Filar lipomas may be associated with lipomas of the distal half of the conus medullaris—the portion of conus that is also formed by canalization and retrogressive differentiation (120). In some instances accessory fila are present and may also exhibit lipomas.

Sacrococcygeal Teratomas

Sacrococcygeal teratoma is a congenital tumor of the caudal pole of the body and, by definition, contains tissues derived from all three germ layers (121). It is the most common newborn tumor, the most common tumor of the sacrococcygeal region in childhood, and the most common sacrococcygeal germ cell tumor (Fig. 50) (122).

Sacrococcygeal teratomas most probably arise from totipotential cells derived from Hensen's node (11). The location of the majority of these at the distal coccyx raises suspicion that they may be related to the coccygeal medullary vestige (22). Because of the relation to the coccyx, coccygectomy is mandatory at the time of initial tumor resection (Feldman). Failure to excise the coccyx with the tumor is associated with increased incidence of tumor recurrence (as high as 37%) (123).

Sacrococcygeal teratomas occur in 1 per 35,000–40,000 births. Females predominate (80%) (91,92,99, 122,124–131). Hereditary forms have been reported (125,132,133). The incidence of twinning is increased to 10% to 53% in families with sacrococcygeal teratomas (123,132).

Patients may present clinically in utero with large-for-dates uterus, polyhydramnios, elevated amnionic alpha-fetoprotein (AFP), or visualization of the lesion by prenatal sonography (121). Such patients are best de-

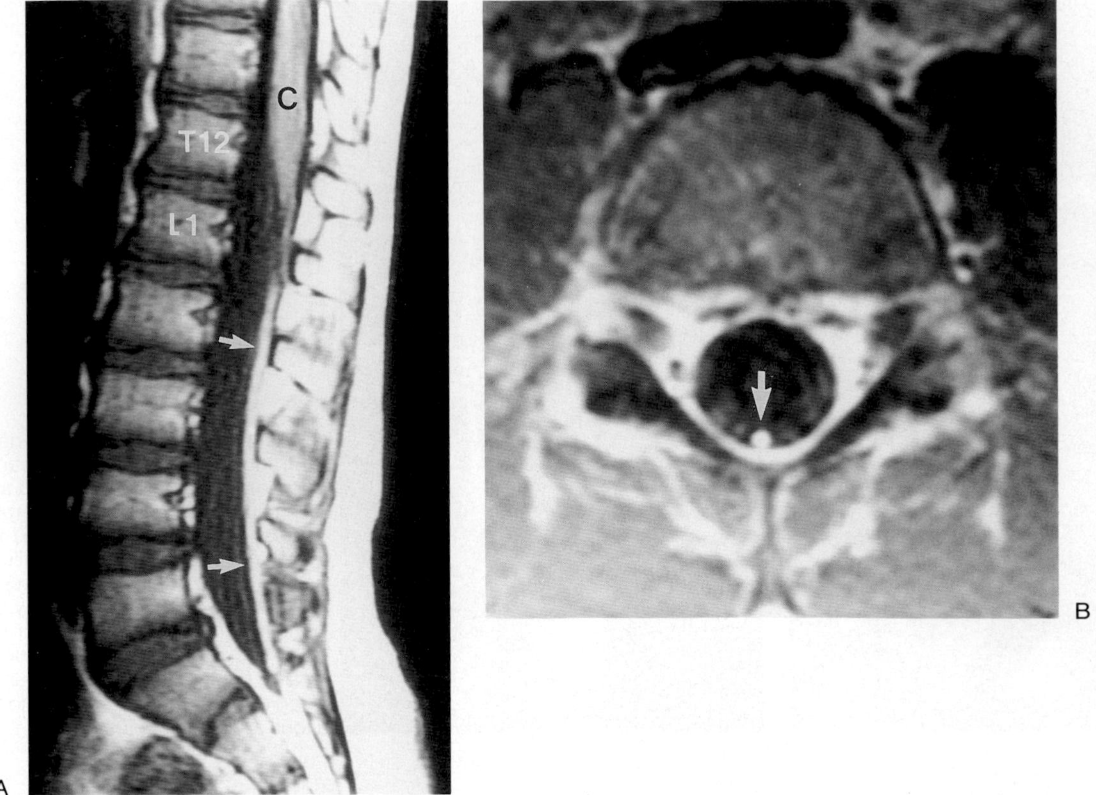

FIG. 48. Intradural filar lipoma. Sagittal (**A**) and axial (**B**) T1-weighted MRIs. The filum terminale (*white arrows*) is thickened by high-signal fat. It is closely applied to the dorsal surface of the canal but may be distinguished from normal dorsal epidural fat by its continuous extension over multiple segments, its slight line of separation from the segmented dorsal epidural fat and its classic round midline appearance in axial MRI (B). The conus (**C**) ends in normal portion at T12–L1, with no evidence of tethering. The subcutaneous fat, lumbodorsal fascia, and posterior spinal elements are normal.

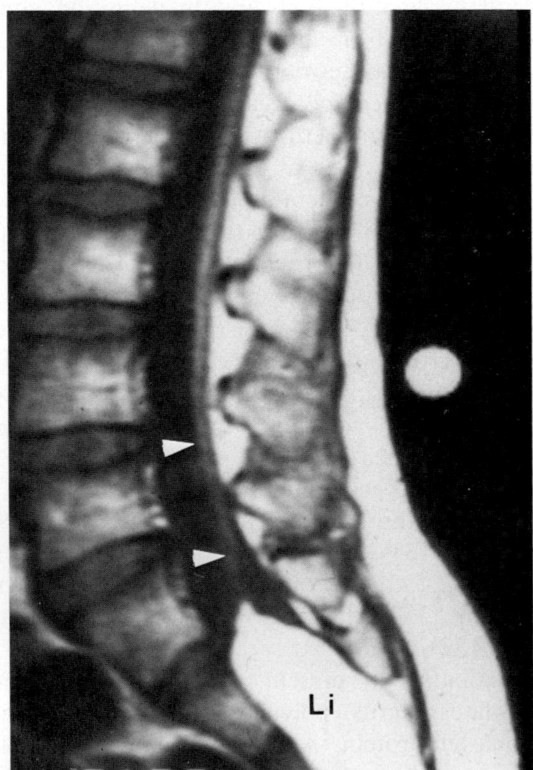

FIG. 49. Predominantly extradural filar lipoma with tethered cord. Sagittal T1-weighted MRI. The lipoma (*Li*) appears to arise within the distal filum (*white arrowheads*), enlarge progressively inferiorly, and expand the sacral canal.

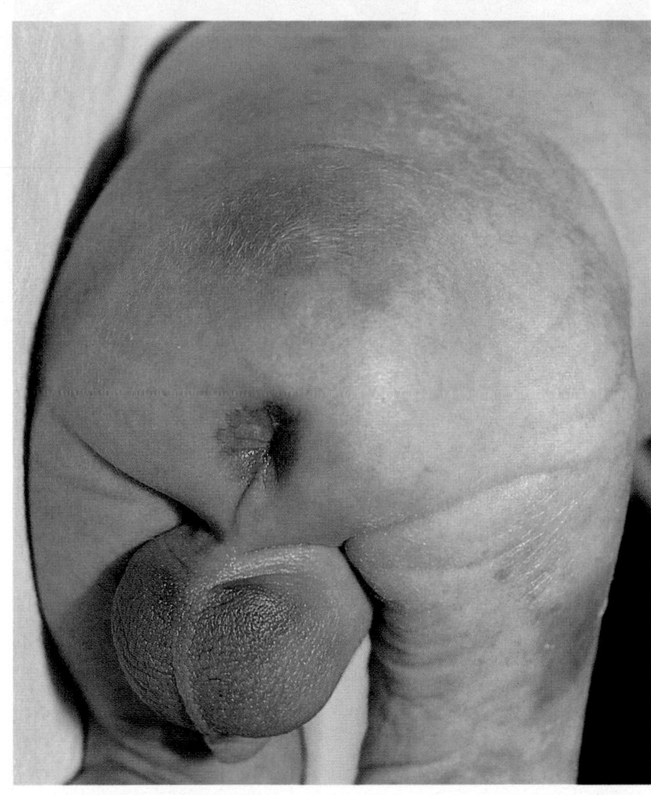

FIG. 50. Sacrococcygeal teratoma, 7-day-old boy. Posterior view. The intergluteal crease is obliterated and discolored by the dorsal component of a predominantly presacral teratoma. The mass obstructed the ureters leading to urine ascites, which communicated with the scrotum distending the scrotal sac.

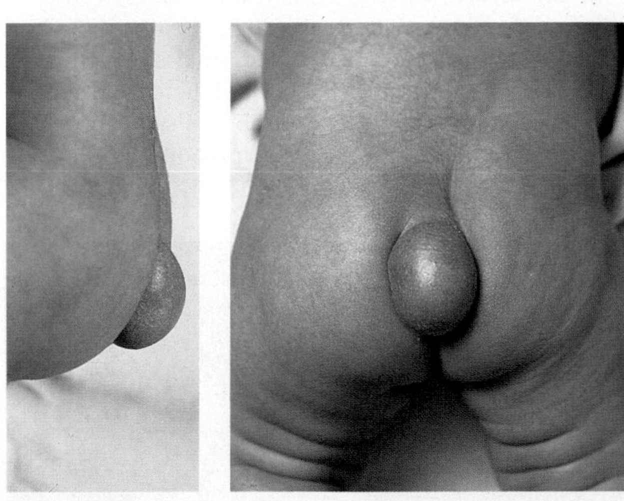

A,B

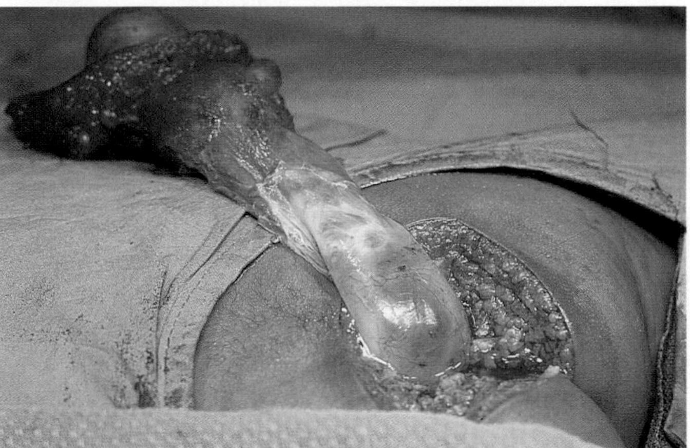

C

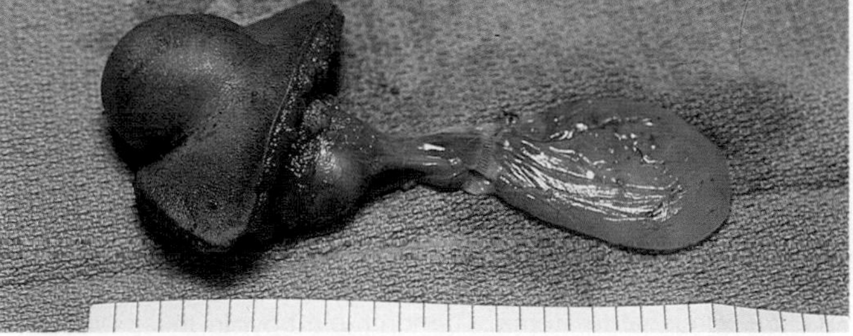

D

FIG. 51. Sacrococcygeal teratoma, 6-month-old boy. **A,B:** Lateral (A) and posterior (B) view of the patient shows a moderate-sized skin-covered mass within the midline intergluteal cleft suggesting teratoma, not lipoma. **C,D:** Specimen (C) and intraoperative photograph (D) shows the large cystic deep portion of the mass that had to be shaved away from the rectum to deliver it from the presacral space. The total mass was 14 cm in length, classified as Altman, type III.

livered by Cesarian section to avoid dystocia, tumor rupture, or bleeding into the tumor (134). In these patients, prenatal placentomegaly and hydrops at less than 30 weeks gestation is highly associated with fetal demise (134).

Postnatally, patients may present asymptomatically because of an external mass or they may manifest hydrops, high output cardiac failure, respiratory failure, and renal insufficiency related to the bulk and vascularity of the mass (134–136).

Most sacrococcygeal teratomas are visible externally (80% to 90%) (124). They may be small or huge (2.6 kg) representing 50% of total body weight (121). Sacrococcygeal teratomas account for 25% of skin-covered lumbosacral masses (11) and typically lie within or below the intergluteal cleft (Figs. 51 and 52). Conversely, spinal lipomas nearly always lie cephalic to the upper end of the intergluteal cleft.

Grossly, sacrococcygeal teratomas are classified by their relationship to the skin surface and the pelvis (124). Altman type I tumors (47%) lie predominantly external to the normal body and have minimal presacral component. Altman type II tumors (35%) are evident externally but have significant intrapelvic extension. Altman Type III tumors (9%) can be detected externally but lie predominantly within the pelvis and abdomen. Altman type IV tumors (10%) are entirely presacral. Only 2% of sacrococcygeal tumors grow into the spinal canal. Rare lesions connect to the distal filum terminale (137).

Most sacrococcygeal tumors are mixed solid and cystic lesions that form a large mass caudal to the coccyx (Fig. 53). Five percent are predominantly cystic. Calcification is found in about 50% of benign teratomas.

Histologically, sacrococcygeal teratomas may be mature (containing recognizable adult tissues only) (50% to 66%), immature (having embryonic tissues) (16% to 20%), or frankly malignant (30%) (138), including embryonal cell carcinomas, endodermal sinus tumors, and anaplastic carcinoma (Fig. 54). Malignant carcinoid has now been found within a number of sacrococcygeal teratomas (139). Tumors that are predominantly solid

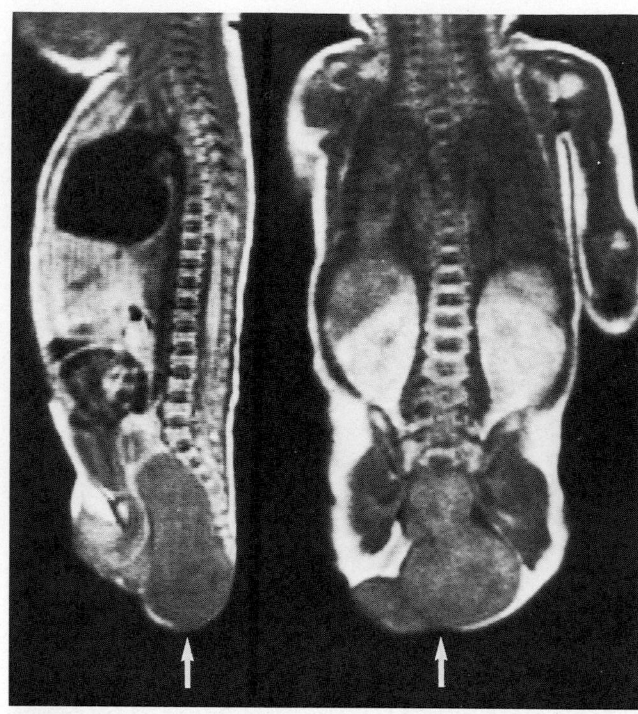

A,B

FIG. 53. Presacral teratoma, 6-day-old girl. Sagittal (**A**) and coronal (**B**) T1-weighted MRIs reveal a large, multicystic presacral mass bulging caudally below the coccyx. The spine is normal. (From Naidich et al., ref. 22, with permission.)

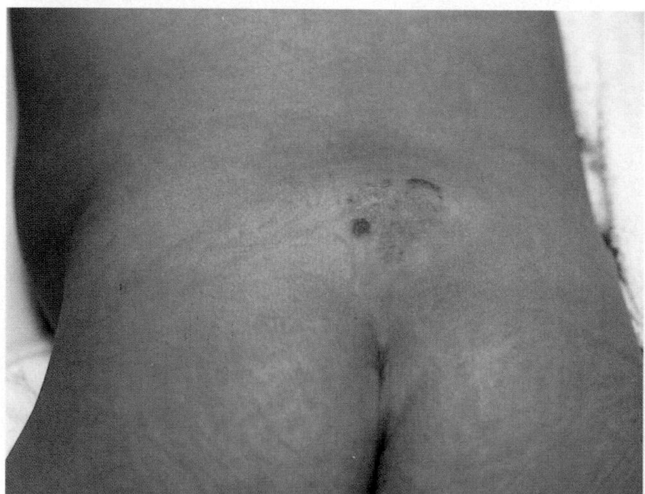

FIG. 52. Unusual teratoma, 10-month-old boy. In this patient, the skin-covered lumbosacral mass and hemangiomatous naevus signified a teratoma despite their location cephalic to the intergluteal cleft. There is an incidental concurrent sacral dimple.

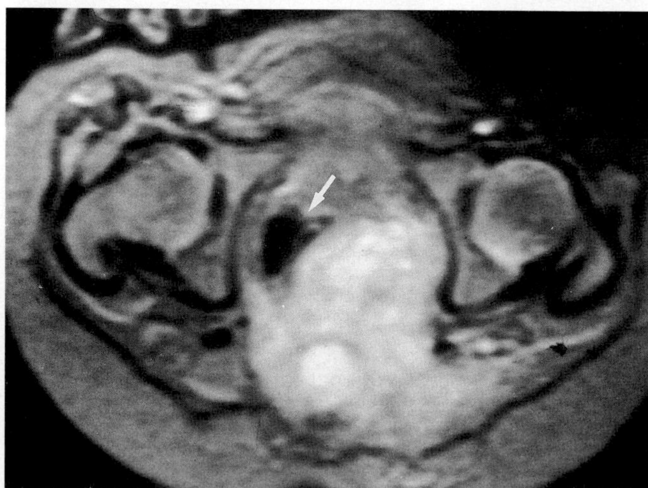

FIG. 54. Malignant teratoma, 11-month-old male. The large pelvic lesion shows heterogeneous signal consistent with calcification (*arrow*) and mixed solid tissue. It invades into the gluteal musculature on the left.

are more likely to be embryonal cell or anaplastic carcinoma than teratoma.

The incidence of malignancy is higher in males and increases with age in both sexes (122,124,126,127). At birth 90% to 94% of these tumors are benign (121,122). Malignant transformation appears to occur between 4 months and 5 years of age (121).

Long-term follow-up indicates that initially "benign" teratomas may recur locally or distally in 4% to 21% of cases. The "recurrences" may show either benign or malignant histology (122,131,140). Initial tumor size and Altman classification of extension do not predict recurrence rate (131). In Bilik's series, most recurrences were seen with mixed solid/cystic lesions. One totally solid tumor recurred. No purely cystic mass recurred (131).

The average survival of patients with malignant sacrococcygeal teratoma has been 9 months (range 1–28 months) (122). With modern chemotherapy initially malignant teratomas may have a 43% survival at a mean follow-up of 4–5 years (122). Serum alpha-fetoprotein levels and immunochemical markers do not predict malignancy during the first month of life (122,131). After the initial total tumor resection, elevation of serum alpha-fetoprotein is a (usually) reliable indicator of recurrent malignancy (131). However, teratoma may recur without elevation of alpha-fetoprotein (122).

Patients with completely successful resection of a benign sacrococcygeal teratoma may still suffer sciatic palsy with lower extremity weakness (7%), fecal and urinary incontinence (up 50%), and urinary tract infections (128,129,140). In one series, these complications have been found more often with larger tumors that extended into the pelvis and abdomen (128), but in other series tumor size and extension do not correlate with late dysfunction (129,140). It is unknown whether the dysfunction observed reflects some effect of the tumor or results from the surgical procedure itself.

In patients with sacrococcygeal teratoma, the spine may be normal, may show bone destruction, or, rarely, may show widening of the canal by intraspinal extension. Concurrent sacrococcygeal malformation suggests an autosomal dominant form of sacrococcygeal teratoma in which anorectal stenosis, retrorectal abscess, vesicoureteral reflux, and cutaneous stigmata concur (see also OEIS complex, Currarino Triad, VATER association, page 1332).

Terminal Ventricle and Terminal Syringohydromyelia

The terminal ventricle is the normal slight expansion of the central canal of the cord within the distal conus and/or proximal filum. It appears to represent the point of union between the portion of the central canal made by neurulation and the portion made by canalization of the caudal cell mass. MR studies often demonstrate a tiny drop of CSF at the site of the terminal ventricle. Slight expansion of this in patients without other pathology is presently regarded as normal (141,142).

Progressive expansion and cephalic extension of such a cavity may explain terminal hydrosyringomyelia, a variably large cystic expansion of the distal one-third of the cord found alone or in association with diverse forms of occult spinal dysraphism (Figs. 55 and 56) (143). Terminal hydrosyringomyelia may be seen by MRI in up to 30% of patients with occult spinal dysraphism. This terminal cavity is large in 19% and small in 11% (143) of patients. It is found most frequently in patients with concurrent anorectal anomalies (67%), meningocele manqué (54%), and diastematomyelia (38%), but is also seen with tight filum terminale syndrome (33%), lipomyelomeningocele (19%), and dermal sinus tract (17%) (143,144).

Caudal Spinal Anomalies with Anorectal and Urogenital Malformations

During normal embryogenesis, union of the hindgut, allantois, and wolffian duct forms a common cloaca just ventral to the notochord and near to the caudal cell mass (Fig. 57) (145–147). Appearance of a urorectal septum then divides the cloaca into a dorsal hindgut and a ventral urogenital sinus. At 7 weeks' gestation the cloacal membrane is bisected to form the anal membrane and the urogenital membranes (145–147). High and low imperforate anus, rectovaginal fistula and bladder, cloacal exstrophy, persistent cloaca, and genital anomalies all result from maldevelopment of the cloaca, urorectal septum, anal membrane, and urogenital membrane.

Perhaps 10% to 15% of patients with anorectal anomalies have concurrent spinal cord anomalies (145,147). Patients with more severe midline ventral caudal anomalies such as persistent cloaca, cloacal exstrophy, and imperforate anus have a markedly increased incidence of midline dorsal spinal malformations, including tethered cord (92%), myelocystocele (27%), lipomyelomeningocele (27%), blunt conus with terminal syrinx (40%), dorsal lipoma with short roots (4%), and fatty filum terminale (35%) (145,147). As a group those with cloacal exstrophy have more complex spinal cord anomalies. Those with high imperforate anus have more complex spinal lesions than those with low imperforate anus (145).

Terminal Myelocystocele (Syringocele)

Terminal myelocystocele is a complex malformation of the distal spine, meninges, and cord (Figs. 58 and 59). Terminal myelocystoceles constitute 1% to 5% of skin-covered lumbosacral masses (99,148). They are typically associated with the OEIS constellation (*O*mphalocele,

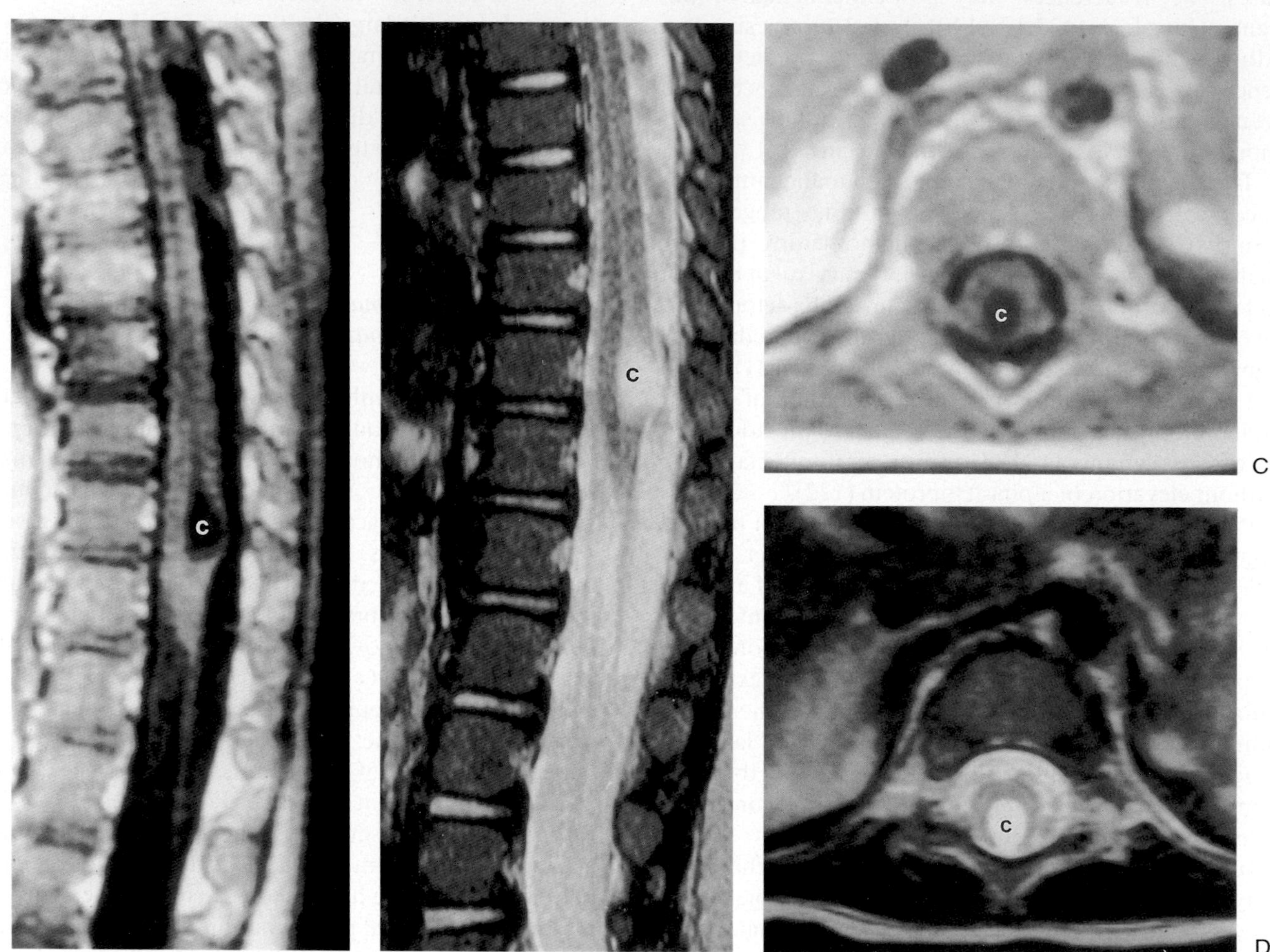

FIG. 55. Dilated terminal ventricle, asymptomatic 10-month-old boy with sacral dimple. **A,B:** Sagittal MRIs. T1-weighted image (A). Fast spin-echo T2-weighted image (B). **C,D:** Axial MRIs at conus. T1-weighted image (C). Fast spin-echo T2-weighted image (D). The minimally dilated central canal of the cord (*c*) expands into a symmetrical, dorsally directed terminal ventricle of CSF signal intensity. There is no tethering, no abnormal signal to suggest gliosis and no abnormal contrast enhancement (not shown). Over the next 12 months, the cyst and the central canal expanded slightly.

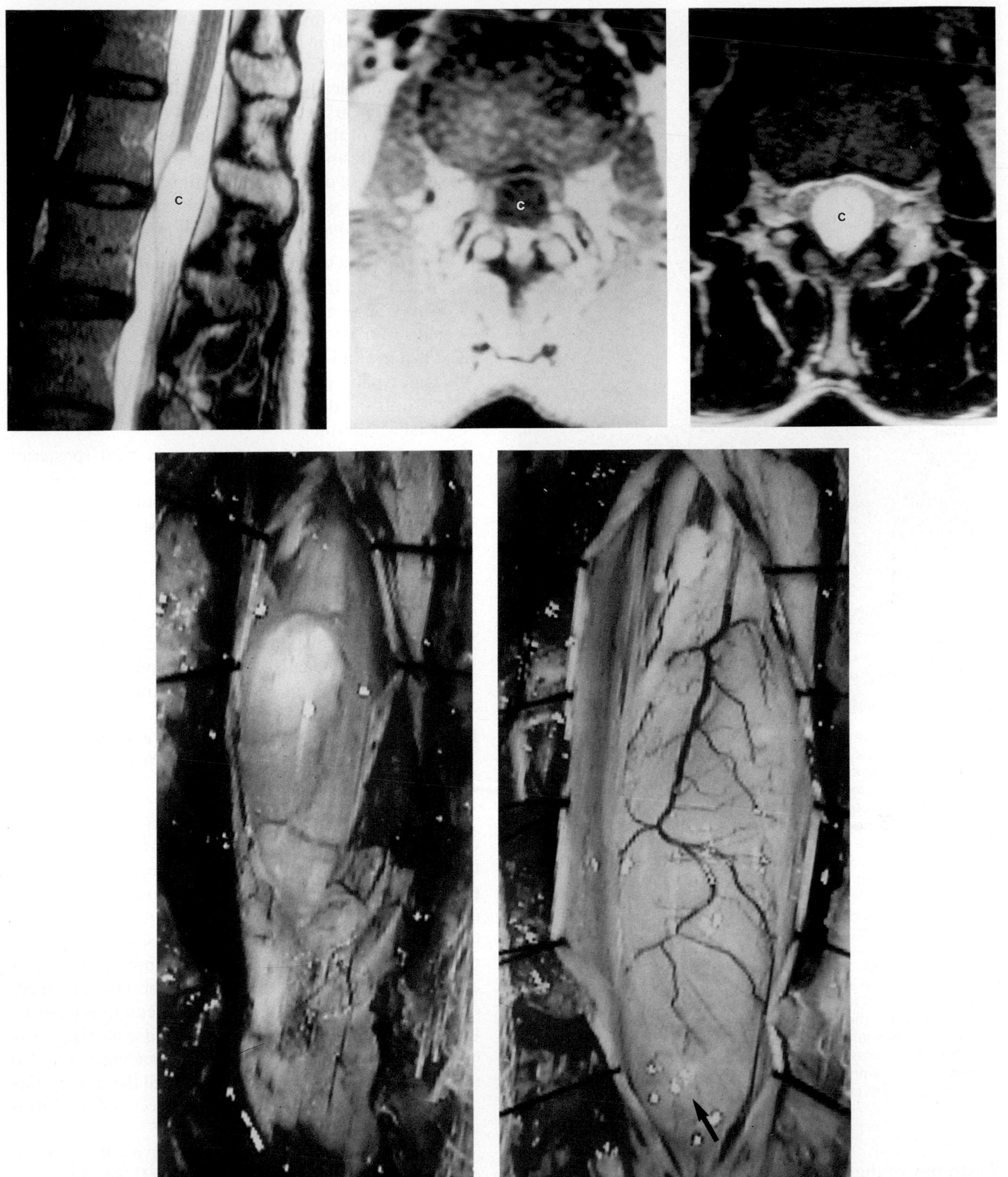

FIG. 56. Benign conal cyst, 42-year-old woman with perineal numbness and paraparesis. **A:** Sagittal T2-weighted fast spin-echo image. **B,C:** Axial T1-weighted (B) and T2-weighted fast spin-echo (C) images. The conus is tensely expanded by a CSF-intensity cyst not associated with tethering, gliosis, or abnormal enhancement (not shown). **D,E:** Intraoperative photographs (Courtesy of Dr. Sergio Gonzalez-Arias, Miami, FL). Opening and retraction of the dura with stay sutures exposes the glistening arachnoid and the expanded conus beneath (D). Opening the arachnoid exposes the conus and the translucent midline dorsal cyst wall (*arrow*) at the lower edge of the field (E). There was no discoloration and no sign of infection, inflammation, or tumor. Histology revealed an ependymal-lined cyst.

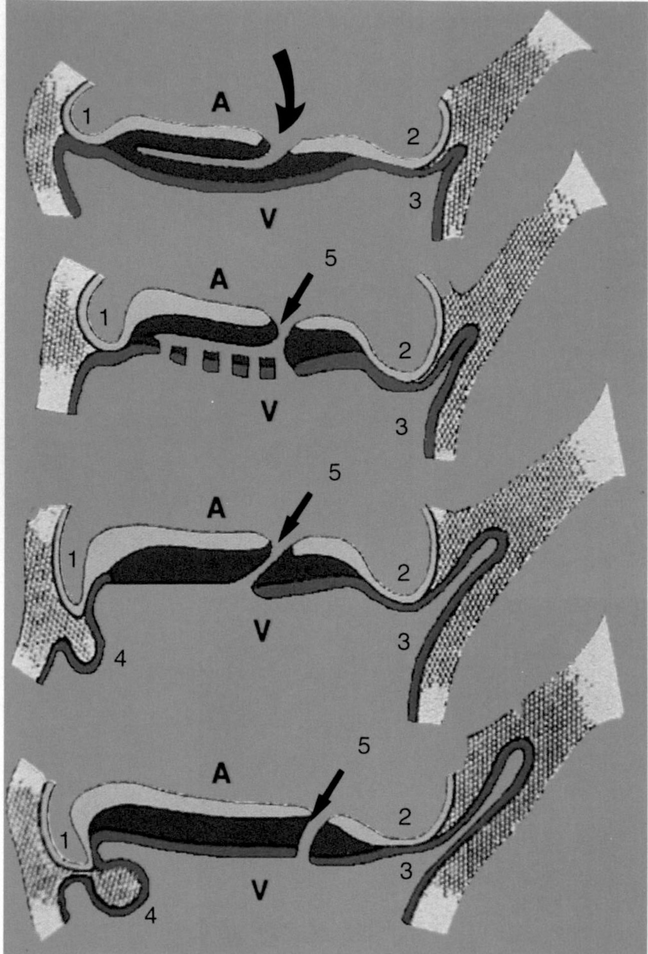

FIG. 57. Development of the notochord, notochordal canal, and canal of Kovalevsky, days 16–20. Diagrammatic representation of midsagittal sections. Cephalic is toward the reader's left; dorsal is toward the top. **A:** The cells that entered the primitive pit formed a midline cord of cells between the ectoderm and the endoderm. This is the notochordal process. The primitive pit deepens and invaginates into this process forming the notochordal canal (*curved arrow*). **B,C:** The ventral wall of the notochordal canal breaks down at one or multiple points affording communication between the notochordal canal and the primitive yolk sac (secondary vitelline sac). This communication between the amnion (dorsally) and the secondary vitelline sac (ventrally) is the canal of Kovalevsky (*5*). One canal or multiple accessory canals may be present. **D:** The endoderm then reforms a cell layer along the ventral surface of the notochord, obliterating much of the notochordal canal. This reestablishes a solid core of notochord, now designated the true notochord. The canal of Kovalevsky may persist for a time. *1*, buccopharyngeal membrane; *2*, cloacal membrane; *3*, allantois; *4*, cardiac evagination; and *5*, canal of Kovalevsky. *A*, amnionic cavity; *V*, vitelline sac. (From Raybaud et al., ref. 13, with permission.)

*E*xstrophy of the bladder, *I*mperforate anus, and *S*pinal anomalies in the same patient), with cloacal exstrophy, with caudal regression syndrome, and with other severe anomalies of the hindgut and genitourinary systems (Fig. 58) (14,148–150). Chromosomal studies are normal.

Terminal myelocystoceles may also be related to the teratogen retinoic acid (151). Experimentally, retinoic acid can produce myelocystoceles in golden hamster fetuses when the drug is given to the pregnant mother before or after the fetus closes the posterior neuropore (152). Pathologically, the changes induced by the retinoic acid appear to represent necrotizing damage to a limited zone of the spinal cord and adjacent mesoderm. The precise site and extent of involvement depend on the dose and time of drug administration.

Whatever the specific etiology, the pathogenesis of the lesion may be conceptualized as follows:

1. For unknown reasons, CSF is unable to exit from the early neural tube.
2. This CSF vents into the terminal ventricle after canalization occurs.
3. The terminal ventricle dilates.
4. The expanding terminal ventricle bulges into and disrupts the dorsal mesenchyme, but not the superficial ectoderm.
5. Consequently, the dorsal spine is bifid (posterior spina bifida) but the skin is intact.
6. As the terminal ventricle balloons into a cyst, it distends the arachnoidal lining of the distal cord, forming a meningocele.
7. The bulk of the cyst prevents ascent of the cord, producing tethered cord.
8. After formation of the arachnoid, progressive distention of the distalmost cord causes it to bulge caudally, below the end of the meningocele.
9. This portion then lies extra-arachnoid and is covered by fat.
10. The cyst also bulges cephalically to expand the distal cord, producing a trumpet-like flaring of the cord within the meningocele (148).

The anatomic components of this lesion are depicted diagrammatically in Fig. 59 and illustrated in Fig. 60. At the caudal end of the meningocele (compartment 1), the pia-arachnoid membrane is reflected from the "parietal" (arachnoid) wall of the meningocele onto the "visceral" (pial) wall of the spinal cord. The cord itself bulges caudal to this reflection into the extra-arachnoid space. This caudal portion of the cord contains the very enlarged, ependyma-lined cyst within a sac of edematous dysplastic glial tissue. The extra-arachnoid cord is partially covered by fat that merges with the subcutaneous tissue. No spinal nerves traverse the cyst. Rather all the spinal roots arise from the dorsal and ventral aspects of the intra-arachnoid segment of the cord.

In the cervical or cervicothoracic area, a different form of myelocystocele has been observed. In these cases, only the thinned, stretched dorsal wall of a hydromyelic cord may protrude into the meningocele to occupy the major portion of that sac (14,33,153). This type of myelocystocele is not associated with OEIS, cloacal exstrophy, or caudal regression syndrome. Instead, it is associated with Chiari II malformation (37), hydrocephalus, ectopic cer-

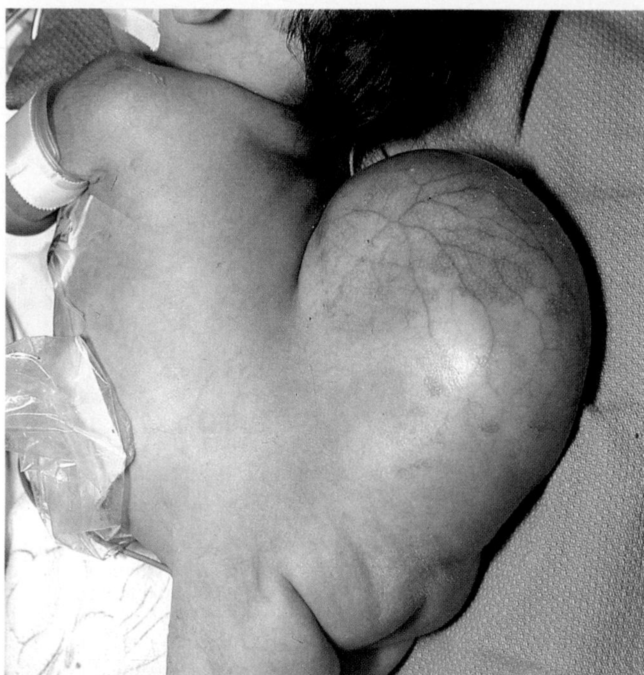

FIG. 58. Terminal myelocystocele. Left lateral view of patient reveals a tensely distended skin-covered lumbosacral mass. Patient is status post-partial repair of cloacal exstrophy. (From McLone and Naidich, ref. 148, with permission.)

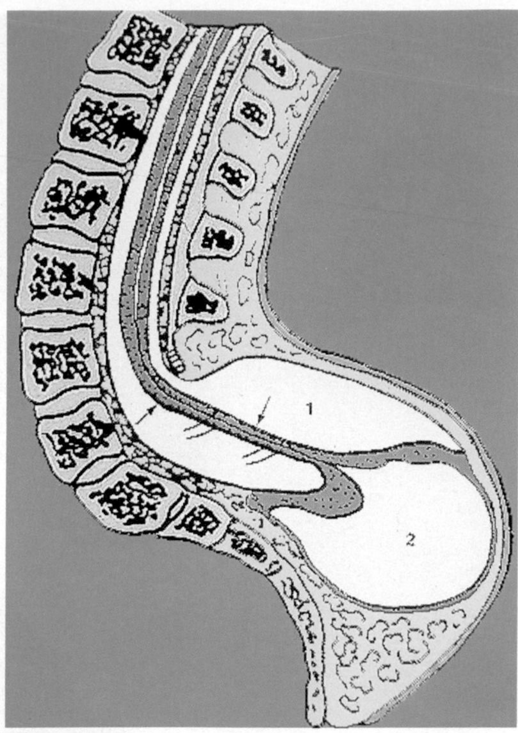

FIG. 59. Terminal myelocystocele. Left lateral view, diagrammatic representation. The lesion consists of posterior spina bifida, tethered spinal cord (*arrows*) with hydromyelia; protrusion of the spinal cord, meninges, and subarachnoid space (*1*) into the dorsal subcutaneous plane; compression of the cord and meningocele by a fibrous band (*hatch marks*) at the upper margin of the spina bifida; ballooning of the distal central canal into an ependyma-lined terminal cyst (*2*); bulging of the terminal cyst caudal to the arachnoid where it becomes covered by fat; origin of the nerve roots from the intra-arachnoid portion of the cord; absence of nerve roots in the terminal cyst; free communication of the cyst (*2*) with the central canal; free communication of the meningocele (*1*) with the spinal subarachnoid space; and no direct communication between the cyst (*2*) and the meningocele (*1*). (From McLone and Naidich, ref. 75, with permission.)

ebellar tissue, heterotopic nephrogenic tissue, and diastematomyelia (148). The cervical myelocystocele must be distinguished from the cervical meningocele.

Syndrome of Caudal Regression

The syndrome of caudal regression designates a constellation of anomalies of the hind end of the trunk, including partial agenesis of the thoracolumbosacral spine, imperforate anus, malformed genitalia, bilateral renal dysplasia or aplasia, pulmonary hypoplasia, and, in the most severe deformities, extreme external rotation and fusion of the lower extremities (sirenomelia) (1,154–161). Some recent communications question whether sirenomelia should be included in the caudal regression syndrome (162).

Sacral agenesis occurs in approximately 1 per 7,500 births (157). Males and females are affected equally. Nearly all cases are sporadic. It may be seen in one of otherwise identical monozygotic twins (163). Siblings are affected rarely (164).

There is a definite but incomplete association with diabetes mellitus including maternal prediabetes and latent diabetic states: One percent of offspring of diabetic mothers will have a form of this syndrome; 16% of patients with this syndrome have diabetic mothers (occasionally diabetic fathers) (165). The lesion may be related to hyperglycemia early in gestation in genetically predisposed fetuses (166,167), or to a teratogen or other insult acting on the caudal eminence (tail bud), after closure of the posterior neuropore (167). In animals, deficiencies of the caudal vertebrae have been created by subjecting the embryo to elevated temperatures, microtrauma, lithium salts, X-irradiation, and administration of insulin in the presence of 2-deoxy-D-glucose (168). These insults could cause failure of canalization and retrogressive differentiation, or excessive retrogression, leading to partial sacral agenesis, to distal thoracolumbosacral agenesis, and/or to concurrent anorectal and urogenital anomalies.

Clinically, most patients with sacral agenesis exhibit poorly developed "rumps" with short shallow intergluteal clefts and poor gluteal musculature (Fig. 61). They show narrow hips, distal leg atrophy, and talipes deformities (167). Approximately 20% have subcutaneous lesions such as skin-covered lipomeningoceles (6%), terminal myelocystoceles (9%), or limited dorsal myeloschises (3%) (167).

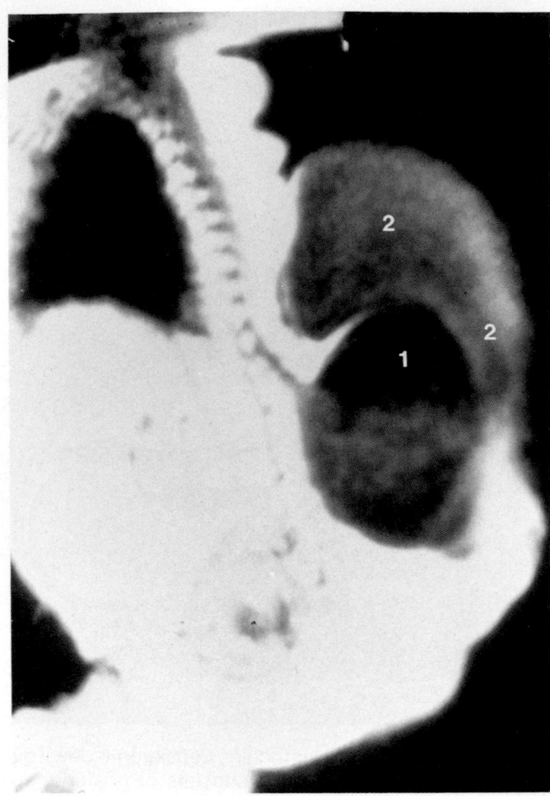

FIG. 60. Terminal myelocystocele. Same patient as in Fig. 58. **A:** Sagittal T1-weighted MRI reveals two separate fluid compartments (*1, 2*) within the large lumbosacral mass. In this case the embryologically more caudal, ependyma-lined sac (*2*) appears to have recurved cephalically to lie superior to the meningocele (*1*). **B,C:** Operative exposure (B). Opening the meningocele (*compartment 1*) (*white arrows*) exposes the distal cord (*C*) that traverses the sac to terminate in a grossly expanded sac. This sac is situated deep to the distal meningocele wall (behind the *white dot*). **C:** Reflecting that wall (*dot*) forward afforded entry into the large terminal cyst (*compartment 2*) (*white arrows*) revealing the smooth ependymal lining, the point of continuity (*white arrowhead*) with the hydromyelic central canal of the cord, and an almost colonic appearance of the lumen. Note the buttocks at the lower edge of the image, for orientation to the patient photograph. (A, courtesy of Eric Russell, M.D., Chicago, IL.)

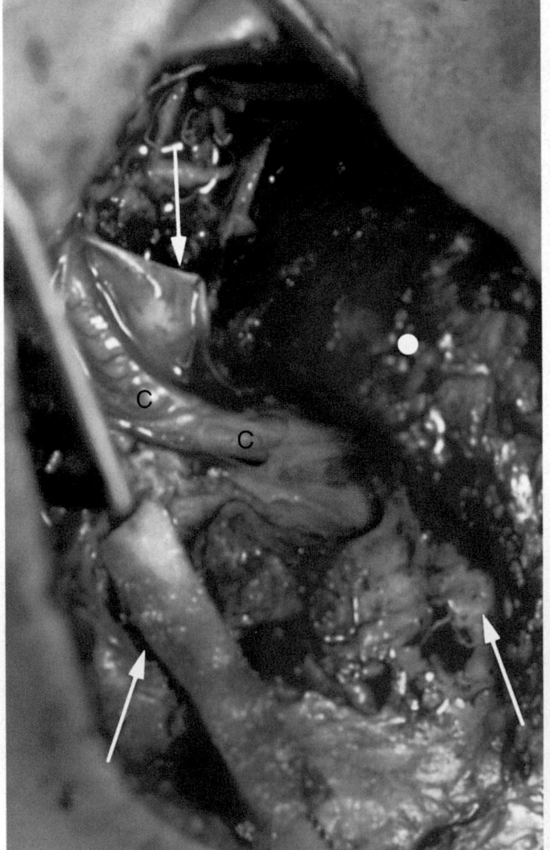

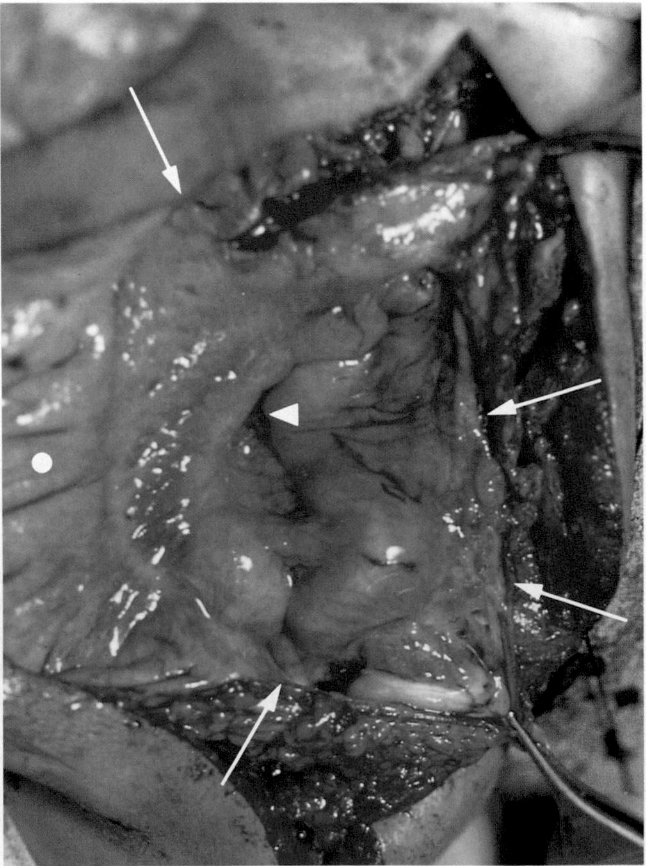

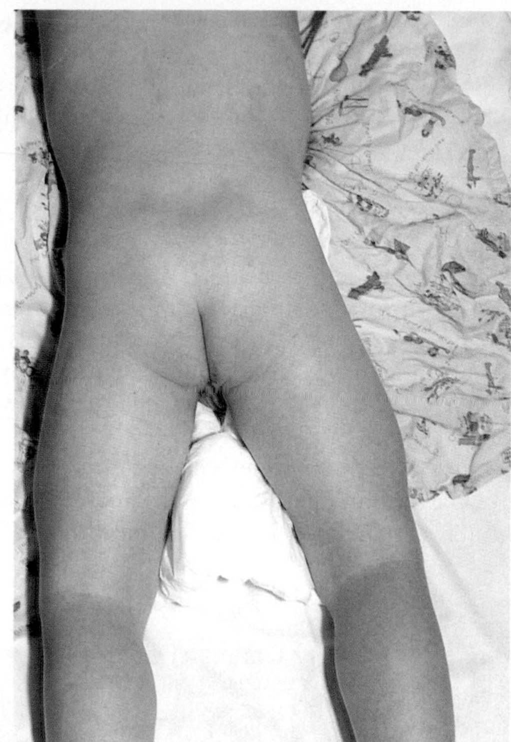

FIG. 61. Sacral agenesis, 4-year-old boy. Posterior view of the patient reveals the short, shallow intergluteal cleft and poorly developed gluteal musculature.

Sensation is better preserved than motor function in the lumbosacral region. (169) Total sacral agenesis may be associated with complete motor paralysis below the quadriceps, but relatively intact sensation in the perianal region (167). Function of the quadriceps and the hip girdle is typically preserved, unless there is concurrent lumbosacral dysraphism (167). Urinary and bladder dysfunction are constant (167).

Associated problems include: (i) multiple congenital malformations such as OEIS complex, VATER syndrome, and congenital heart defects (24%); (ii) genitourinary complaints with hydronephrosis, unilateral renal agenesis, pelvic and horseshoe kidneys, epispadias, and hypospadias (24%); (iii) orthopedic deformities such as hip dislocation, flexion contractures, genu recurvatum, posterior compartment atrophy, talipes deformities, and scoliosis (12%); and (iv) progressive neurological deficits and/or back and leg pain (38%) (167). Females show bicornate uterus, didelphic uterus, vaginal duplication, partial vaginal atresia, and rectovaginal rectovesicular fistulae.

The position of the conus defines two distinct groups of patients with sacral agenesis (167). In group 1 (41%) the conus ends cephalic to the lower border of L1 (Fig. 62) (167). The conus is typically deformed (92%) and terminates abruptly at T11 or T12, as if the normal distal "tip" were absent (14,167). It is nearly always club-shaped (64%) or wedge-shaped (extending lower dorsally) (28%), infrequently normal (8%). The median fissures are absent inferiorly (170–172). The normal subdivisions of gray and white matter become unrecognizable and there may be a terminal glial nubbin. The distal central canal may be slightly dilated and appear as a terminal ventricle, or substantially dilated as a terminal hydromyelia (173). In this group with high conus, the sacral deficit is typically large, and the sacrum usually ends at or above S1.

In group 2 (59%) the conus ends lower, below L1, and is elongated, stretched caudally, and tethered by thick filum (65%), terminal myelocystocele (15%), transitional lipoma (10%), or elongated cord with terminal hydromyelia (10%). In these patients the sacrum tends to be relatively well preserved, with identifiable portions of S2 or lower vertebral segments. The clinical courses of the two groups differ: Neurological deterioration is frequent in patients with low tethered cords, but not in those with short high blunt conuses (167). In this chapter, group 2 patients have been classified by their concurrent neural pathology rather than by the sacral defect alone.

In patients with sacral agenesis, the distal bony canal usually shows smooth tapering which does not constrict the thecal sac (35%). In 6% of cases hyperostosis indents the distal thecal sac. In 18% the distal sacral canal is enlarged and bifid dorsally (167,174). The lowest vertebra present is T11 or T12 in one-third of patients, L1 to L4

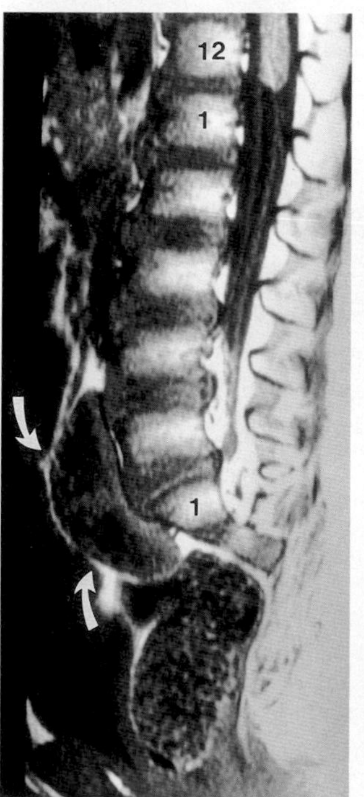

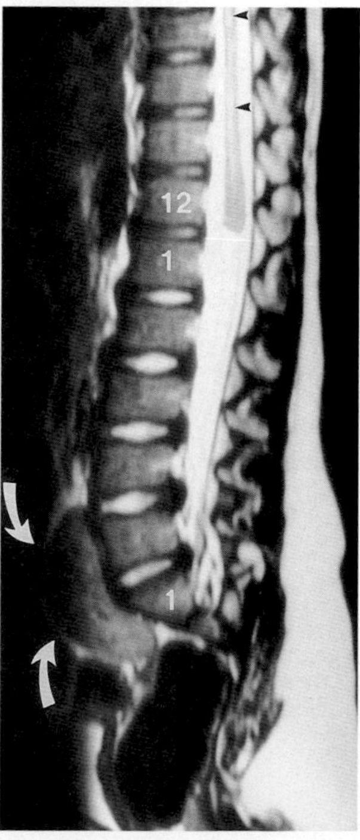

A,B

FIG. 62. Sacral agenesis, Group 1, 3-year-old boy. **A,B:** Midsagittal MRIs, T1-weighted (A) and T2-weighted (B) images. Only S1 (*1*) and a portion of S2 are present. The conus lies at T12–L1 (*12,1*) and shows bulbous, angulated termination. The distal central canal is slightly dilated (*small arrowheads* in B). The distal bony canal and thecal sac are narrow. Note the pelvic kidney (*curved white arrows*) anterior to L5 and S1.

in 40% of patients, and L5 or below in 27% of patients. The distal agenesis may be bilaterally symmetrical or unilateral.

The orthopedic deformity depends on the extent of the vertebral agenesis, the symmetry of involvement, and whether the ilia articulate with the sides of the last intact vertebra (relatively wide pelvis) or with each other inferior to the last vertebra (narrow pelvis) (Fig. 63) (167). Unilateral sacral agenesis leads to marked pelvic tilt and scoliosis. Isolated agenesis of the coccyx is an incidental finding in some patients. The diverse forms of sacral agenesis have recently been classified by Pang (Table 3) (167).

In most cases the dural sac shows nonstenotic tapering and shortening (47%). The tapering is greater and the sac ends higher with higher levels of spinal agenesis (167). In 9% of cases, severe dural stenosis constricts the caudal dural tube to pencil size and is associated with crowding of roots and neurogenic claudication (167,174).

Surgery may be required to decompress bony or dural stenosis for relief of pain and for preservation of neurological function.

Anterior Sacral Meningoceles

Anterior sacral meningoceles are diverticulae of the thecal sac that protrude anteriorly into the extraperitoneal presacral space. They usually have thin walls composed of an outer layer of dura and an inner layer of arachnoid, and typically communicate via a narrow stalk with the intraspinal thecal sac.

Most anterior sacral meningoceles occur sporadically. They may be seen in conditions with dural ectasia such as neurofibromatosis and Marfan's syndrome (175), or

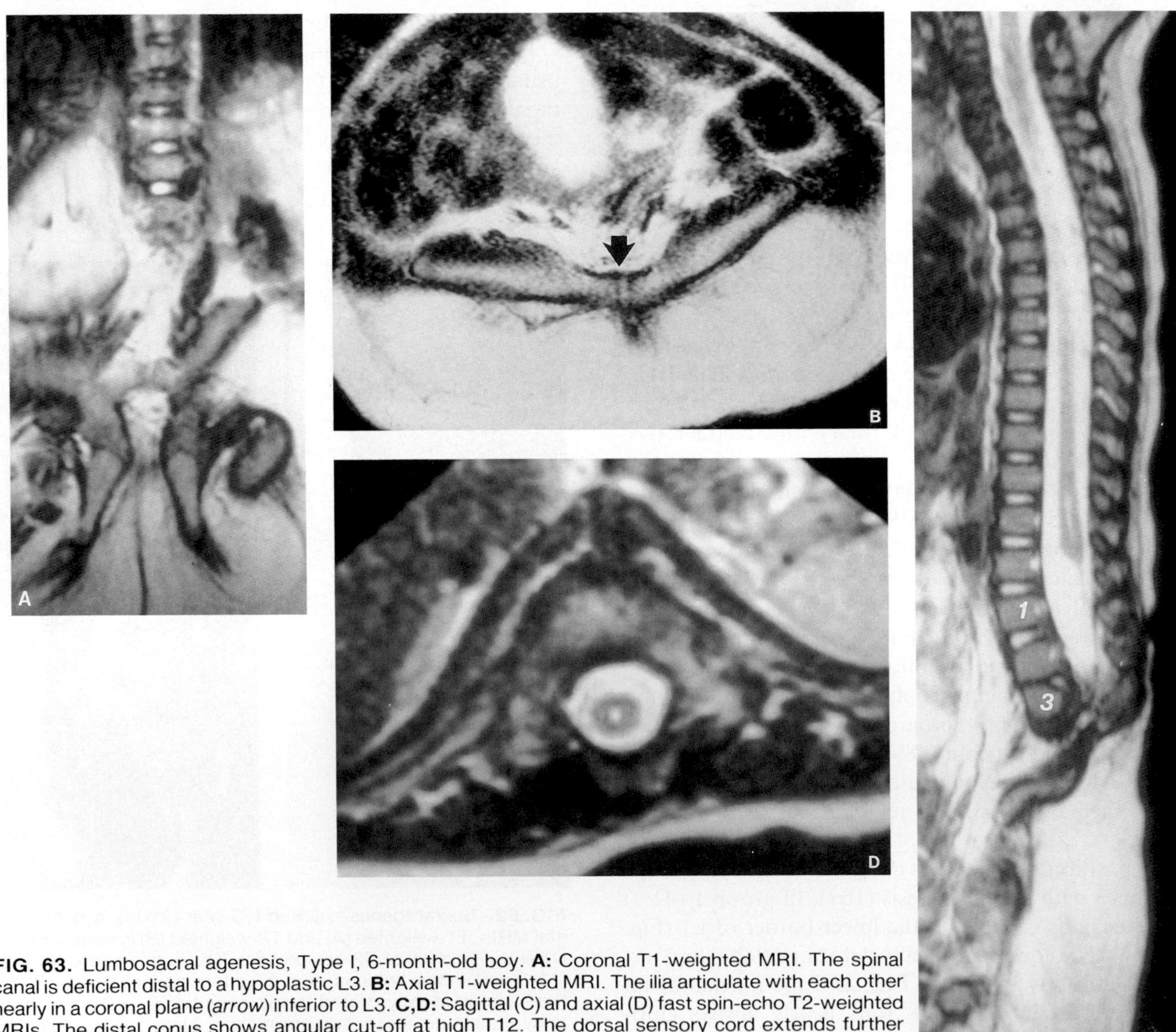

FIG. 63. Lumbosacral agenesis, Type I, 6-month-old boy. **A:** Coronal T1-weighted MRI. The spinal canal is deficient distal to a hypoplastic L3. **B:** Axial T1-weighted MRI. The ilia articulate with each other nearly in a coronal plane (*arrow*) inferior to L3. **C,D:** Sagittal (C) and axial (D) fast spin-echo T2-weighted MRIs. The distal conus shows angular cut-off at high T12. The dorsal sensory cord extends further caudally. The distal central canal is dilated.

TABLE 3. *Classification of lumbosacral agenesis*

Type	Subtype	Description
I		Total SA; some lumbar vertebrae also missing
	I_{W_a}	Ilia articulate with sides of the lowest vertebra, maintaining relatively normal transverse pelvic diameter
	I_{N_a}	Ilia articulate or fused with each other below last vertebra, severely shortening transverse pelvic diameter[a]
II		Total SA; lumbar vertebrae not involved
	I_{W_a}	Ilia articulate with sides of L5 vertebra maintaining relatively normal transverse pelvic diameter
	I_{N_a}	Ilia articulate or fuse with each other below L5 vertebra, severely shortening transverse pelvic diameter[a]
III		Subtotal SA; at least S1 is present, sacrum lacks four, three, two, or one of its caudal segments, ilia articulate with sides of rudimentary sacrum, maintaining normal transverse pelvic diameter
IV		Hemisacrum
	IV_A	Total hemisacrum; all sacral segments present on one side, but entire opposite side is missing
	IV_B	Subtotal hemisacrum, unilateral; all sacral segments present on one side, only part of opposite side is missing[b]
	IV_C	Subtotal hemisacrum, bilateral; part of each side is missing but to different extent
V		Coccygeal agenesis
	V_A	Total
	V_B	Subtotal

From Pang, ref. 167.

W, wide; N, narrow; both referring to the transverse pelvic diameter.

[a] Severe spinopelvic instability.

[b] Severe scoliosis.

may be associated with the Currarino triad of anorectal malformations, sacral defects, and presacral masses (176). A familial form with concurrent anterior sacral meningocele, tethered cord, lipomas, teratomas, and dermoids may be inherited in families as an autosomal dominant trait with incomplete penetrance (Fig. 64) (176–178).

Clinically, anterior sacral meningoceles account for 3.7% of retrorectal tumors (179). They may be detected at any age. In adults, females appear to be affected more commonly (approximately 10:6) (178). However, the lesion is equally frequent in boys and girls below age 15, suggesting that increased detection of anterior sacral meningoceles during pregnancy accounts for the female predominance in adult patients.

Local pressure on pelvic organs causes unremitting constipation, urinary frequency and incontinence, dysmenorrhea, dyspareunia, and back pain. Pressure on the nerve roots causes sciatica, diminished rectal and detrusor tone, numbness and paresthesias in the lower sacral dermatomes, reflex asymmetry, and occasional motor impairment (180–182). Severe headaches may result from fluid shifts related to changes in body position or to Valsalva maneuvers such as straining at stool. Women of childbearing age may present with a pelvic mass on prenatal examination or with dystocia at labor and delivery. Bicornate uterus, double vagina and uterus, bifid renal pelvis, imperforate anus, anal atresia and stenosis, and perianal fistulae are common (178). Meningitis may occur spontaneously, but is most often iatrogenic, secondary to manipulation of the sac.

In anterior sacral meningocele the spinal canal is usually widened with smoothly scalloped margins. The defect in the sacrum is typically asymmetrical (Fig. 64). The defect may be pinpoint, may be limited to one wide neural foramen, or may involve a large portion of the sacrum and affect multiple adjacent neural foramina. Serial studies over time show that the typical smooth curvilinear defect designated the "scimitar sacrum" often starts as a partial unilateral sacral agenesis that becomes remodeled around the hernia ostium with time (65). In approximately 20% the sacral defect is midline (183).

The sacral dural sac is often widened and patulous. The stalk is typically narrow. The meningocele sac may be unilocular or multilocular. Large meningoceles nearly fill the pelvis and may contain 1,500 cc of CSF (Fig. 65) (184). Small anterior sacral meningoceles just protrude beyond the sacral defect (Fig. 66). In 20% of cases nerve roots and the filum terminale may be contained within the meningocele sac, or nerve fibers and spinal ganglia may be present in the sac wall (178,182,184,185).

Surgery for anterior sacral meningoceles is now usually performed via a posterior trans-sacral approach, through the sacral thecal sac, with careful inspection of the stalk and the ostium of the sac to detect any contained neural structures and any thickened filum, tethered cord or concurrent lipoma and (epi)dermoid. If no nerve roots traverse the stalk the sac is aspirated and the stalk is closed in a watertight fashion to prevent recurrence. If nerve roots are present it may not be possible to obliterate the stalk of the meningocele.

Some anterior sacral meningoceles are treated via an anterior transabdominal approach with oversewing of the meningocele neck. This approach may be favored in cases associated with masses (176) or cases where adhesions between the sac and pelvic organs prevent sac collapse despite drainage of the contained CSF (184). Operative mortality, previously high, is now near zero (176).

Lateral Lumbar and Thoracic Meningoceles

These lesions are characterized by CSF-filled protrusions of dura and arachnoid through one or several en-

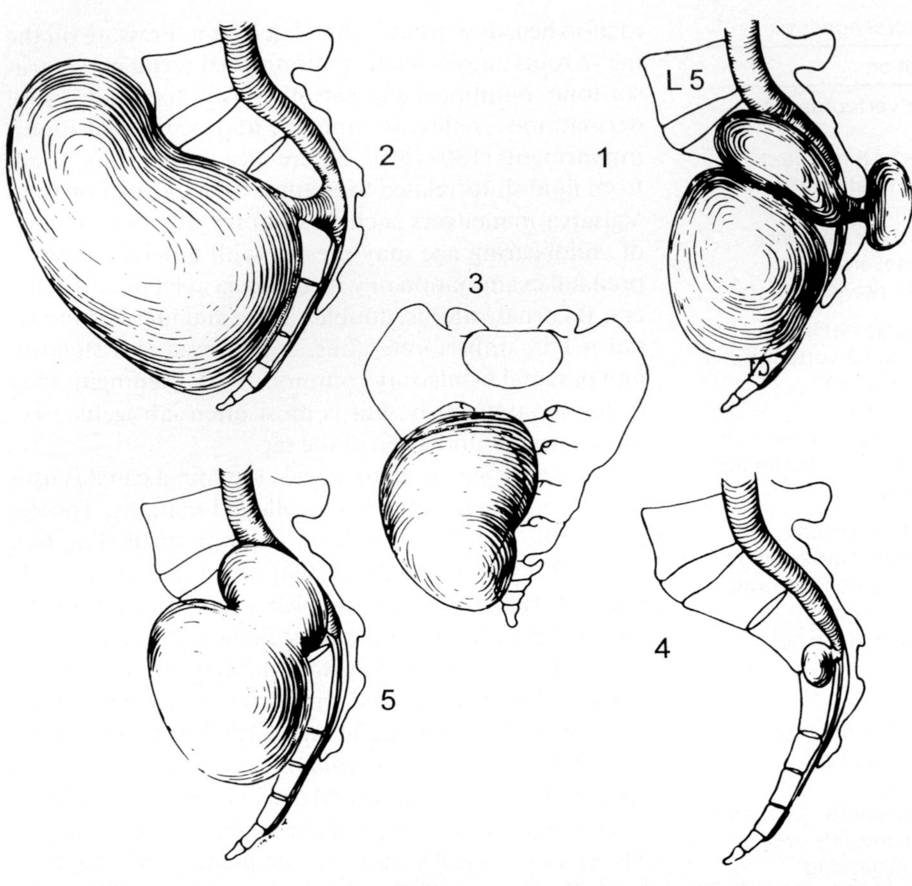

FIG. 64. Diagrammatic representation of five different anterior sacral meningoceles, some associated with intrasacral meningoceles as well. *1:* Cyst fills sacrum, extends anteriorly through the left third sacral foramen and posteriorly via prior laminectomy defect. *2:* Large intrapelvic anterior sacral meningocele with broad neck. *3:* Anterior sacral meningocele with crescentic sacral defect. *4:* Small anterior sacral meningocele found incidentally at myelography. *5:* Large intrasacral cyst and large presacral cyst communicating via broad neck extending through the right second sacral neural foramen. (From Amacher et al., ref. 180, and Naidich et al., ref. 182, with permission.)

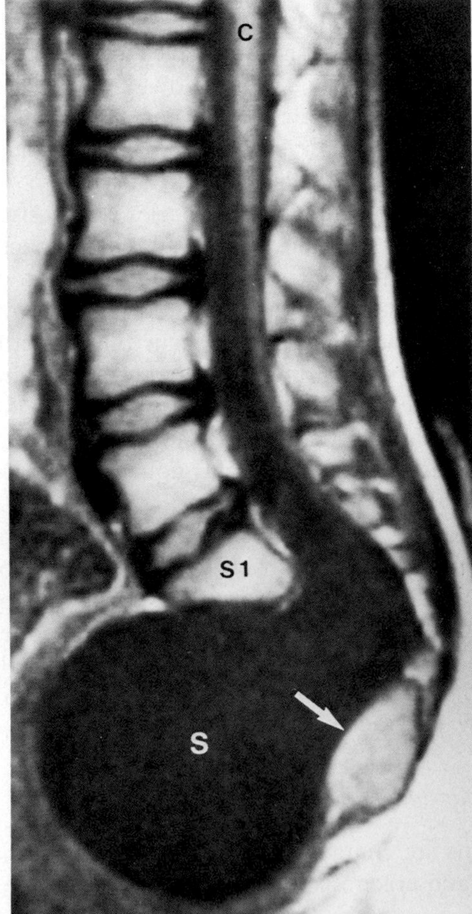

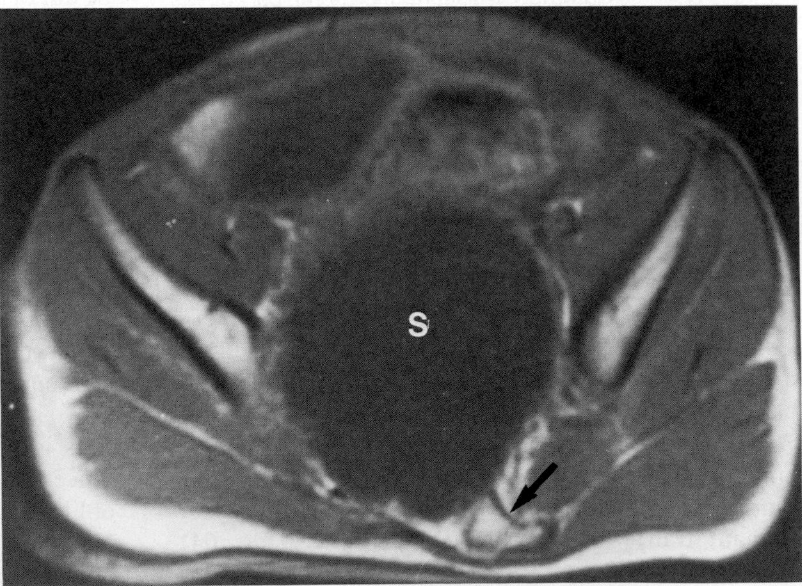

FIG. 65. Anterior sacral meningocele, 1-year-old girl. **A:** Sagittal T1-weighted MRI reveals partial hemisacral agenesis with anterior spina bifida, continuity of low-signal CSF into a bulbous anterior sacral meningocele (*S*), low-lying tethered spinal cord (*C*) that tapers progressively inferiorly, and mural cysts (*arrow*) that probably represent (epi)dermoids. **B:** Axial T1-weighted MRI reveals the lower portion of the scimitar hemisacrum (*arrow*) on the left and the large meningocele (*S*) that passes into the pelvis through the defect in the contralateral right half of sacrum. (From Naidich et al., ref. 22, and Naidich and McLone, ref. 66, with permission.)

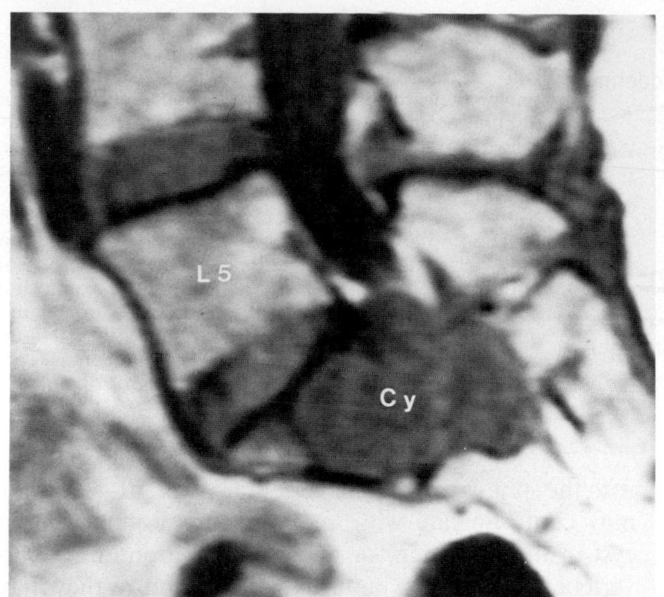

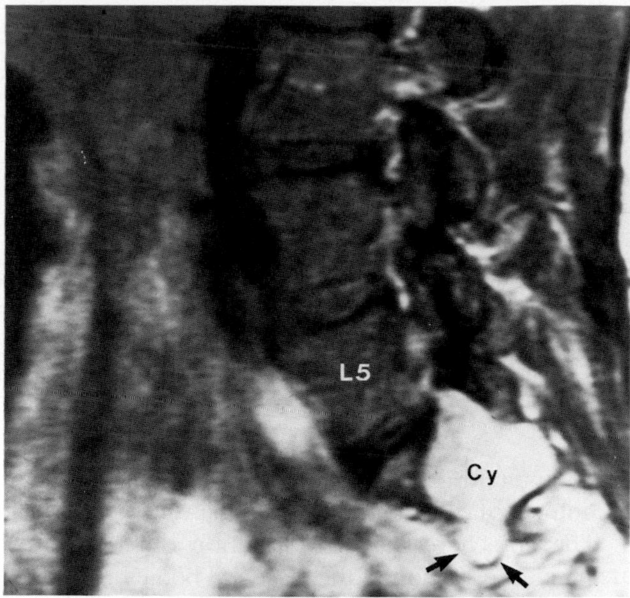

FIG. 66. Intrasacral meningocele bulging through a widened neural foramen, 62-year-old woman. Sagittal MRIs. T1-weighted image (**A**) and T2-weighted image (**B**) reveal erosion of S1 and expansion of the sacral canal by a lobulated CSF intensity cyst (*Cy*) that extends anteriorly (*arrows*) into the pelvis. (From Zimmerman et al., ref. 8, with permission.)

larged neural foramina into the paraspinal extrapleural and retroperitoneal tissue (1,186,187). They may be unilateral or bilateral, and are commonly associated with scoliosis (Fig. 67). Lateral meningoceles are most common in patients with mesenchymal disorders such as neurofibromatosis, Marfan's and Ehler-Danlos syndromes. Indeed, neurofibromatosis is present in 85% of lateral thoracic meningocele. (186). Depending on the level of the lesion and the degree of scoliosis, the spinal cord and cauda equina may lie away from the meningocele along the opposite side of the spinal canal, or may be pulled toward the meningocele by traction from the herniating meninges.

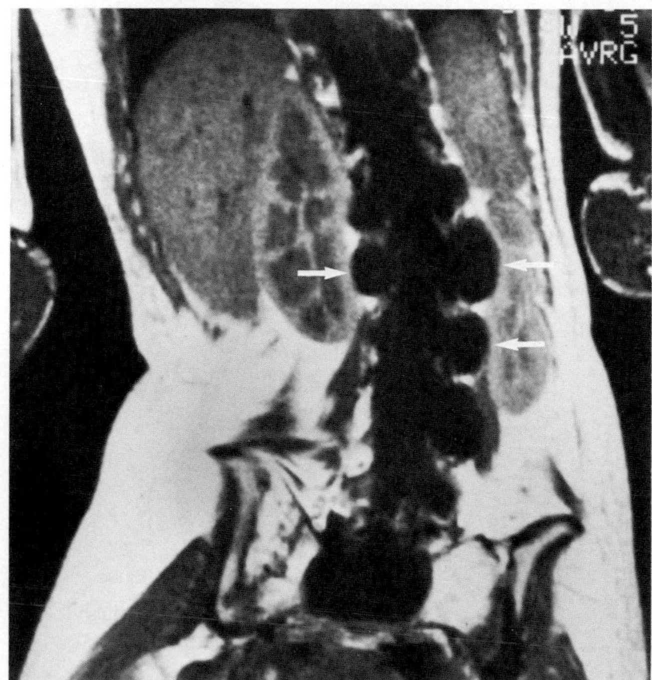

FIG. 67. Multiple lateral lumbar and thoracic meningoceles, 14-year-old girl. Coronal T1-weighted MRI demonstrates scoliosis and multiple bilateral low-signal diverticula (*arrows*) of the leptomeninges. These balloon through and enlarge the neural foramina and expand the sacral spinal canal. (From Naidich et al., ref. 22, and Naidich and McLone, ref. 66, with permission.)

NORMAL AND DERANGED EMBRYOGENESIS OF THE NOTOCHORD AND VERTEBRAE

Normal Embryogenesis of the Notochord

By Day 17 ectodermal cells that entered the primitive pit have advanced cephalically in the midline to the prochordal plate to create a notochordal process that extends along the midline from Hensen's node to the prochordal plate (Fig. 2) (10–13). The primitive pit then deepens and invaginates into the previously solid notochordal process, lengthening it into a hollow notochordal canal (Fig. 57). This quickly fuses with the entoderm. At the point(s) of fusion, breakdown of cells opens the notochordal canal to the yolk sac. As a result, there is a transient communication from the amnion through the notochordal canal to the yolk sac. This is the canal of Kovalevsky. Accessory canals may arise at other levels. Soon thereafter, the notochordal canal undergoes complex changes that close the communication with the yolk sac, re-establish complete layers of entoderm and of ec-

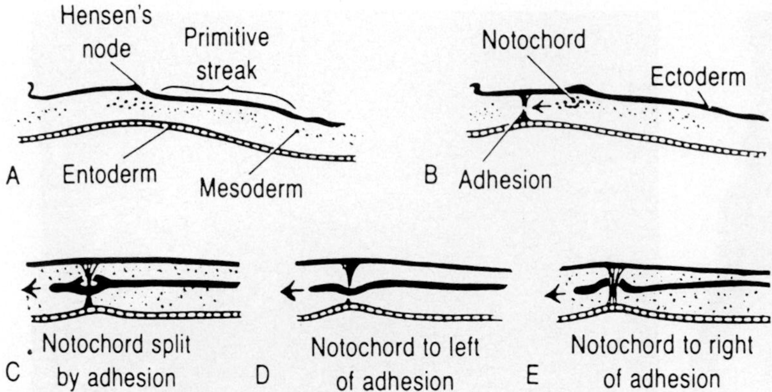

FIG. 68. Embryogenesis of split notochord syndrome. Diagrammatic representation of midsagittal section with cephalic toward the reader's left. **A:** Sagittal section displays the entoderm, which lines the primitive gut (archenteron), the ectoderm, which forms the outer surface of the embryo and which gives rise to the primitive streak, and the intervening mesoderm. Proliferating cells in Hensen's node, at the cephalic end of the primitive streak, form a cylindrical cell mass, the notochord. **B:** The primary event in the split notochord syndrome may be formation of an adhesion between ectoderm and endoderm. **C–E:** If such an adhesion exists, the notochord must split as it extends forward around the adhesion to form a focally ring-like notochord or it must deviate around the adhesion to one side. (From Beardmore and Wigglesworth, ref. 188, with permission.)

toderm, and reform a solid core of tissue designated the true notochord. The entoderm then ultimately forms gut. The notochord induces formation of the neural plate, guides formation of the vertebral bodies and contributes to the nuclei pulposi (31,32). The ectoderm forms spinal cord and skin.

Derangements in the Notochord (Split Notochord Syndrome)

Persistence of a midline adhesion between ectoderm and entoderm could cause derangement in the migration of notochordal cells with consequent deflection or splitting of the notochord (Fig. 68) (188,189). This appears to be the genesis of dorsal enteric fistula, neurenteric cyst, and diastematomyelia.

Dorsal Enteric Fistula and Neurenteric Cyst

Persistence of a patent notochordal canal (canal of Kovalevsky) would create a patent fistula from the mesenteric surface of gut through the mesentery and prevertebral tissue, through the vertebral bodies, spinal canal, and spinal cord, and through bifid laminae to an ostium in the midline skin of the back (Fig. 69). Such a complete communication is designated the dorsal enteric fistula. It is exceedingly rare. However, with variable site of the canal (or accessory canal) and with variable degrees of repair of the defect in the embryo, portions of the entire fistula might persist as (i) diverticula or patent duplications arising from the mesenteric border of gut and extending into mesentery or through diaphragm to mediastinum; (ii) as persistent cords between gut and vertebrae, (iii) enteric-lined cysts in the mesentery, mediastinum, spinal canal, and midline back; (iv) anterior and/or posterior spina bifida; (v) diastematomyelia; (vi) neurenteric cysts; or (vii) various combinations of these. Such a mechanism could also explain some of the dorsal dermal sinuses (presented earlier as a failure to disjoin cutaneous from neural ectoderm).

Neurenteric cysts are enteric-lined cysts that present within the spinal canal and exhibit a definite connection with the spinal cord and/or vertebrae (Figs. 70–72). They may communicate with an extraspinal component of cyst in the mesentery or mediastinum around a hemivertebra or through a butterfly vertebra and/or they may attach by a fibrous stalk to the vertebra, mesentery, or gut.

The vertebral column usually exhibits a wide spinal canal with widened interpediculate distance. Spina bifida and segmentation anomalies of the bodies are common, but not invariable. In older patients, the vertebrae

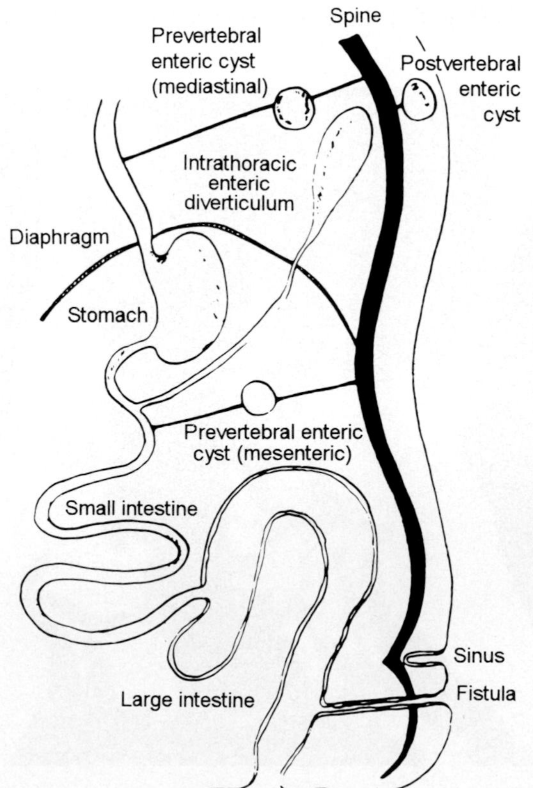

FIG. 69. Split notochord syndrome. Diagrammatic representation of developmental posterior enteric remnants. Varying segments of the prototypical dorsal enteric fistulae leave diverse posterior enteric remnants. Each of these types may happen at any segmental level. (From Bentley and Smith, ref. 190, with permission.)

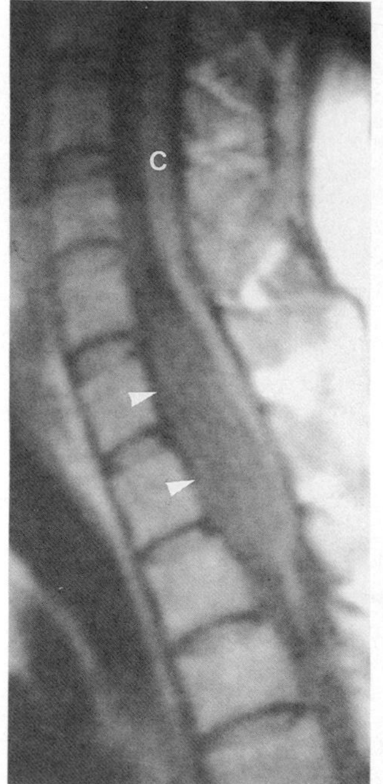

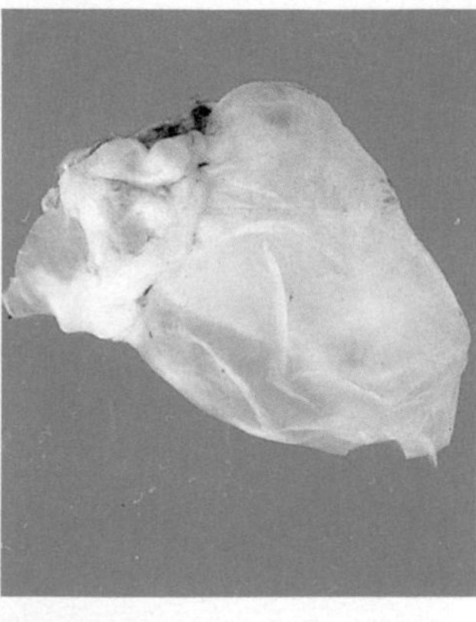

A,B

FIG. 70. Neurenteric cyst, 34-year-old man. **A:** Midsagittal T1-weighted MRI shows enlargement of the cervicothoracic spinal canal, posterior displacement of the cord (*C*), and marked cord compression by a sharply defined ventral cyst (*white arrowheads*). At surgery, the posterior wall of the cyst was attached to the ventral pia of the cord. **B:** Pathological specimen shows the thin-walled cyst. Histologically, the wall was composed of pseudostratified ciliated columnar epithelium resembling the lining of the respiratory tract. Courtesy of Glenn Geremia, Eric Russell, and Raymond Clase, Chicago, IL. (From Geremia et al., ref. 245, with permission.)

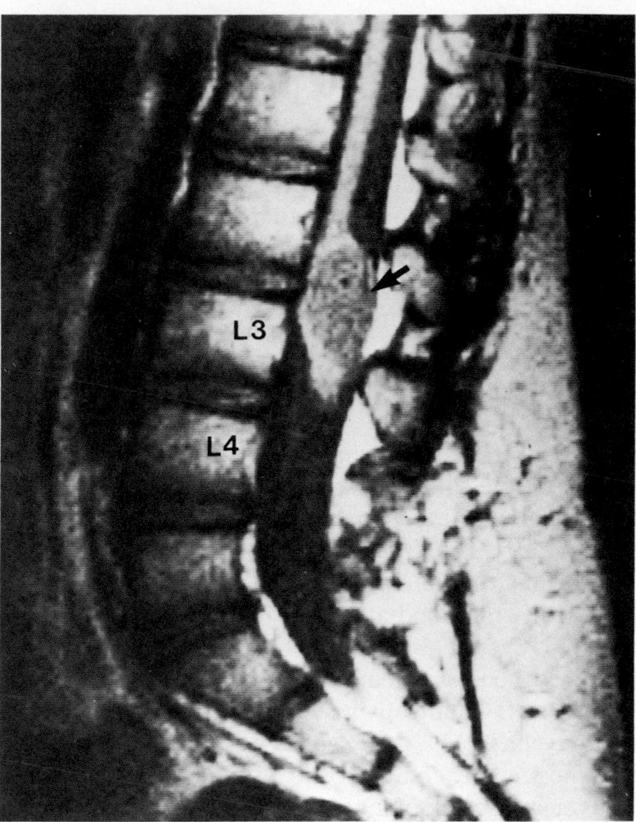

FIG. 71. Recurrent enteric cyst of the conus medullaris, 5-year-old boy. Sagittal T1-weighted MRI reveals prior extensive laminectomy, low position of distal cord (L3–L4), and the expansive cyst (*arrow*) within the dorsal portion of the conus medullaris.

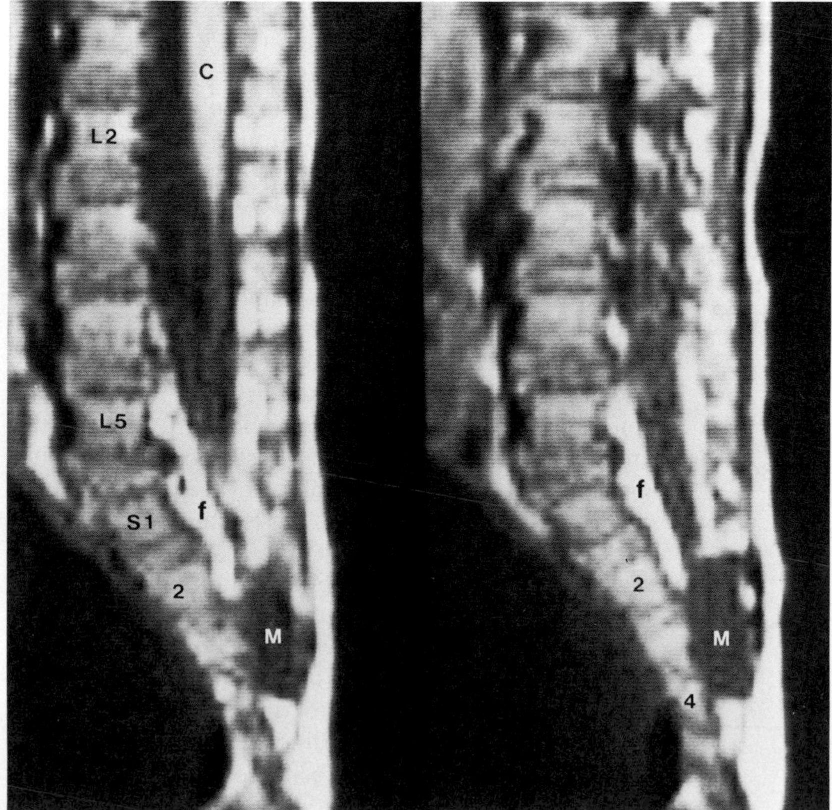

A,B

FIG. 72. A,B: Neurenteric cyst, 1-year-old girl. An ovoid mass (*M*) of low-signal intensity expands the midsacral canal in association with posterior spina bifida. The distal cord (*C*) lies slightly low. The lesion appears to communicate with the sacral subarachnoid space, but proved to be a separate enterogenous cyst with ciliated columnar epithelium. *f*, ventral epidural fat.

may be normal, aside from pressure erosion. Most cysts lie at the cervicothoracic junction or in relationship to the conus medullaris (1,190–192). The cyst usually lies ventral or ventrolateral to the cord and is usually either deeply invaginated into cord with firm attachment to the pia or is situated within the cleft between two hemicords. There is variable attachment to dura. MR displays the cyst and displaced cord plus any bone abnormalities. Flow studies reveal a high-grade stenosis or complete block to flow of CSF.

Diastematomyelia

By definition, diastematomyelia signifies a sagittal clefting of the spinal cord, conus medullaris, and/or filum terminale into two, not necessarily symmetrical, hemicords (1,23,193,194).

Clinically, patients with diastematomyelia usually present in childhood at one of 3 age ranges: 0–2 years (20%), 4–8 years (40%), and 12–13 years (17%) (195). Most cases occur in females: 80% overall, up to 94% in some series. Cutaneous naevi overlie the site of diastematomyelia in 45% to 85% of cases (Table 4) (196–199). The most nearly characteristic of these is the naevus pilosus, a large patch of long silky hairs (Fig. 73).

In children, the common presenting complaints are (i) musculoskeletal deformities (98%) including asymmetric lower extremities and pes cavus, (ii) neurologic deficits (84%) including weakness, reflex asymmetry, reduced sensation and incontinence of bladder and bowel, and (iii) scoliosis (79%) (196). In adults, sensorimotor changes (69%) and pain (58%) are the most frequent complaints (197).

Rilliet et al. studied the embryogenesis of diastematomyelia by microsurgical manipulation of chicken embryos (200). Simple incision of the distal neural plate and notochord in the midline to create a communication between the amnion and the yolk sac did not lead to diastematomyelia. The embryos healed, or showed an open posterior spina bifida. Similar incision plus placement into the cleft of a resorbable agar screen resulted in open anterior spina bifida, cleft notochord, and protrusion of a tongue-like process of the spinal cord into the anterior defect. This anterior process could coalesce with the primitive gut. The central canal of the cord could be dilated, but the central canal was not doubled. Therefore, this condition was judged not to represent diastematomyelia, despite intriguing similarities. Indeed, to the present authors, the condition has some similarities to the less severe cervicothoracic myelocystocele (syringocele).

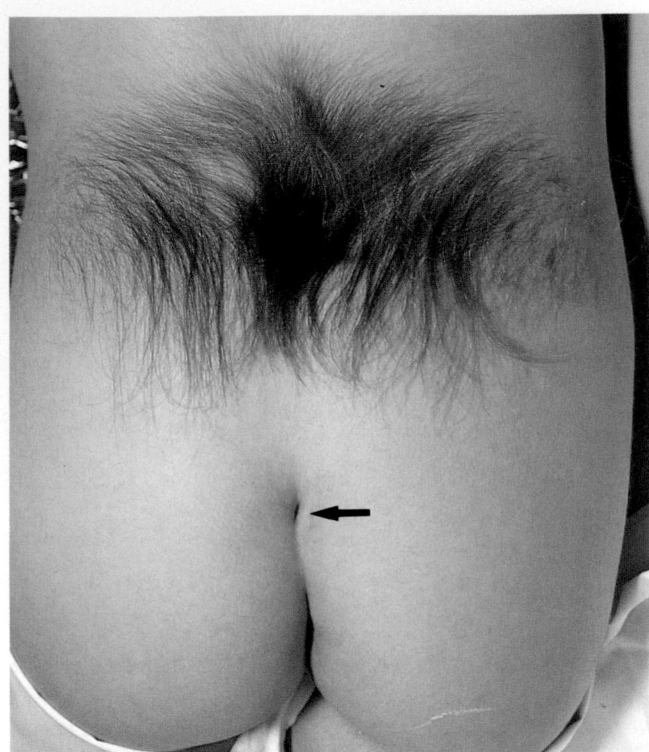

FIG. 73. Diastematomyelia, 4-year-old girl. Posterior view of patient reveals the large patch of long silky hairs overlying stematomyelia and a small sacral dimple (*arrow*). (From Schlesinger et al., ref. 205, with permission.)

TABLE 4. *Cutaneous stigmata in diastematomyelia*[a]

	Russell et al. (197)	Miller et al. (196)	Gower et al. (198)
	N = 45[b]	*N* = 43	*N* = 30
Hair patch	33%	40%	30%
Dimple/hemangioma	18%	28%	40%
(Myelo)meningocele	2%		23%
Subcutaneous mass	2%	5%	3%
Teratoma		2%	3%
Café-au-lait spots	9%		
No cutaneous stigmata	56%	44%	13%

[a] Combined data from 3 series.
[b] Several patients had multiple lesions.

When Rilliet et al. incised the embryo and placed into the gap a nonresorbable wedge-shaped piece of membranous shell, diastematomyelia resulted: there were two hemicords, each with its own central canal. Some canals had hydromyelia (200). Some embryos showed anterior spina bifida with protrusion of spinal cord through the anterior defect. Some had small cysts along the midline incision, and others had partial sacral agenesis.

The authors concluded that diastematomyelia cannot be a simple failure of neurulation. Instead, diastematomyelia requires in part, "the non-involution of a firm midline structure (probably the neurenteric canal, rapidly surrounded by mesodermal cells originating from the notochord) . . ." (200).

If the canal of Kovalevsky (or an accessory canal) persists (or there is another midline adhesion between the ectoderm and entoderm), then the notochordal cells would encounter an obstruction as they migrate cephalically (Fig. 68) (190,201). The notochordal cells might migrate leftward or rightward around the adhesion, or to both sides of the adhesion. As a result the notocord could develop with a focal left-sided or right-sided notch, or a central "donut hole." Since the notocord guides formation of the vertebrae, these alterations in the notochord would create, respectively, a local unilateral vertebral agenesis (i.e., contralateral hemivertebrae) or a ring vertebrae (i.e., butterfly vertebrae) with posterior spina bifida. Since the notochord also induces formation of the neural plate, a cleft notochord could induce formation of paired hemiplates leading to paired hemicords. This would lead to diastematomyelia.

Diastematomyelia affects the lumbar or lumbosacral spine in 45%, the thoracic spine in 31%, and the thoracolumbar spine in 12%. The cervical spine is affected in 7% and the sacrum in 1% (Table 5) (196–198). Lengthy diastematomyelias may extend widely over multiple segments in continuity (196–198). "Double" diastematomyelia at two separate sites is found in less than 1% of cases (196–198). A rare diastematomyelia has been seen to extend from the cervical spine into the spondylocranium, which is formed from the occipital somites (202,203).

In diastematomyelia, the conus medullaris is usually low in position. The two hemicords are each narrower than normal (Fig. 74). The two hemicords nearly always (91%) reunite distally into a reformed cord below the cleft (204). In 30% of cases the hemicords are grossly asymmetrical in size. When the hemicords are asymmetrical, the cord above and below the cleft is usually asymmetrically smaller on the side of the smaller hemicord and the smaller hemicord often lies ventral to the larger hemicord. The filum terminale is usually, perhaps always, thickened and may itself tether the reunited cord. Hydromyelia is present in up to 50% of cases of diastematomyelia. It may affect the cord above the cleft and extend into one or both hemicords (200,205).

The origins of the nerve roots from the hemicords varies. Each hemicord may give rise to the ipsilateral dorsal and ventral nerve roots. Alternatively, when the hemicords are asymmetrical, one "hemicord" may give rise to three of the four roots and the other only one. Accessory nerve roots may also be present.

The meninges that surround the cord may also be cleft, or not. The exact relationship of the arachnoid and dura to the hemicords is highly significant and defines two distinct forms of diastematomyelia that require two different approaches to treatment (Fig. 75) (23).

Single Dural-Arachnoid Tube

In the slight majority of all cases of diastematomyelia (50% to 60%), the two hemicords are enveloped together in a single arachnoid/dural sheath (Fig. 75B and 75C). In these cases, there is no bone spur. Surgical intervention may still be required to release a thick filum terminale or adhesions which tether the cord.

Dual Dural-Arachnoid Tubes

In the other 40% to 50% of cases, the meninges are also cleft, focally, so that each hemicord is contained in its own arachnoid/dural sheath (Fig. 75D). The single cord above the cleft is contained in a single meningeal sheath that divides to surround each hemicord and that then reunites to a single meningeal sheath when the hemicords reunite to one cord below the cleft. Typically, the spinal cord divides first into two hemicords within one coaxial arachnoid-dural tube. Further inferiorly, the arachnoid and dura also divide into paired, coaxial arachnoid-dural tubes, one coaxial meningeal tube surrounding each hemicord. Therefore, in this group with cleft meninges, the cleft in the cord is always longer than the cleft in the meninges; often it is far longer. In these cases the medial walls of the two dural tubes form a double layer of dura between the two hemicords, inside the

TABLE 5. *Diastematomyelia: sites of involvement*[a]

Site of involvement	Gower (198) $N = 30$	Russell (197) $N = 45$	Miller (196) $N = 43$	Total 118	Percentage
Cervical		8		8	6.7
Cervicothoracic	1	1		2	1.7
Thoracic	13	8	16	37	31
Thoracolumbar	13	1		14	12
Lumbar		24	27	51	43
Lumbosacral	3			3	2.5
Sacrum		1		1	0.8
Other[b]		2[b]		2	1.7

[a] Combined series, $N = 118$.
[b] In one case, the diastematomyelia extended from T7 to the sacrum, in the other case, two separate sites were involved: T2 and L3.

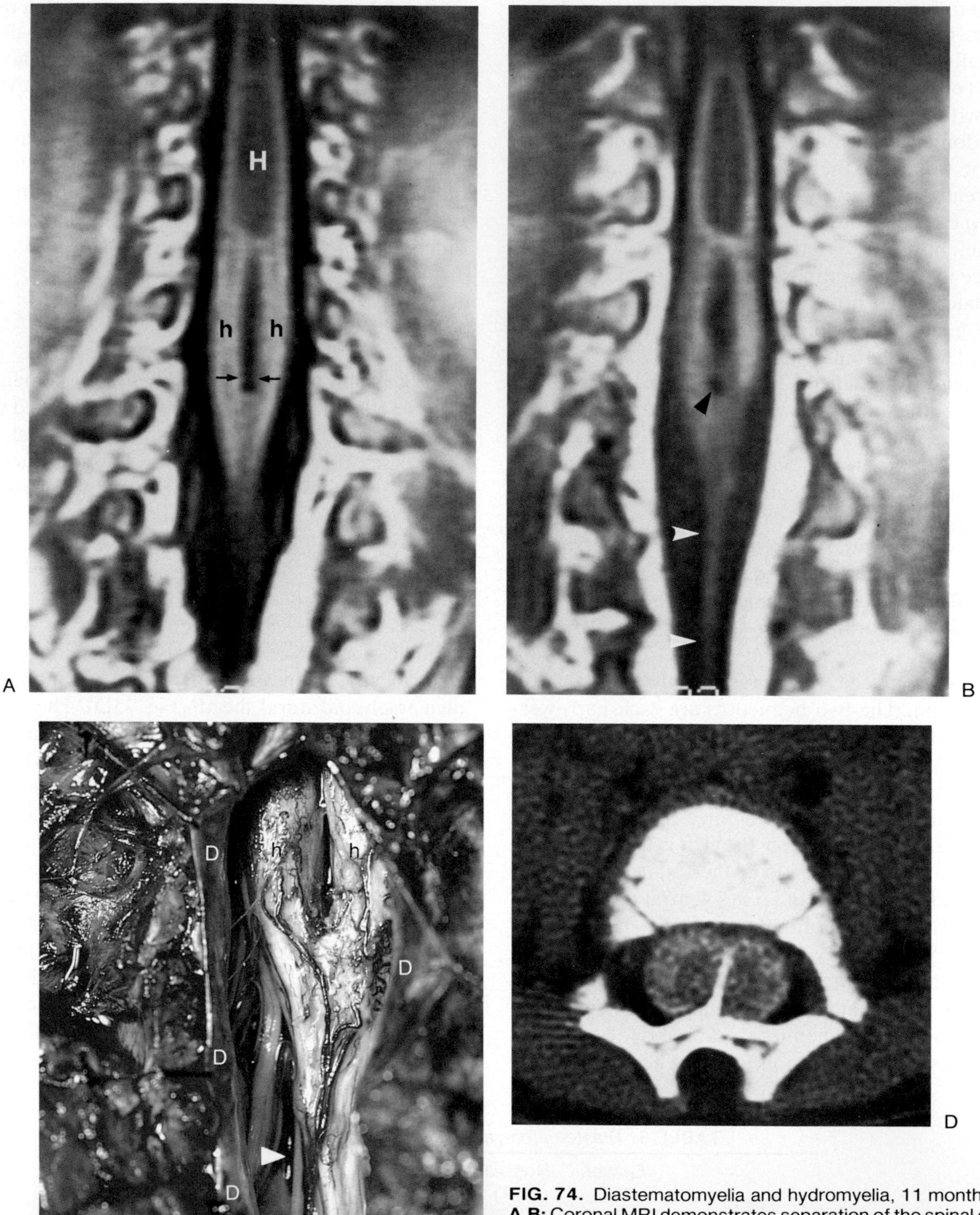

FIG. 74. Diastematomyelia and hydromyelia, 11 month-old girl. **A,B:** Coronal MRI demonstrates separation of the spinal cord into two hemicords (*h*) that reunite inferiorly and continue into a thick filum terminale (*white arrowheads*). The cord above the cleft exhibits hydromyelia (*H*). The bone spur (*black arrowhead*) appears as a small, round, low-signal structure at the lower end of the interdural cleft (between *small black arrows*). **C:** Surgical exposure of the dorsal aspect of the diastematomyelia (after resection of the bone spur). The dura (*D*) has been opened and retracted. The medial walls of the two dural tubes have been resected. The two hemicords (*h*) reunite below the cleft. A prominent blood vessel typically courses along the dorsal aspect of the thickened filum terminale (*white arrowheads*) partially obscuring it. **D:** Axial CT following myelography demonstrates the thin bone spur arising from the laminae and traversing the spinal canal between the two hemicords. (From Naidich et al., ref. 22, with permission.)

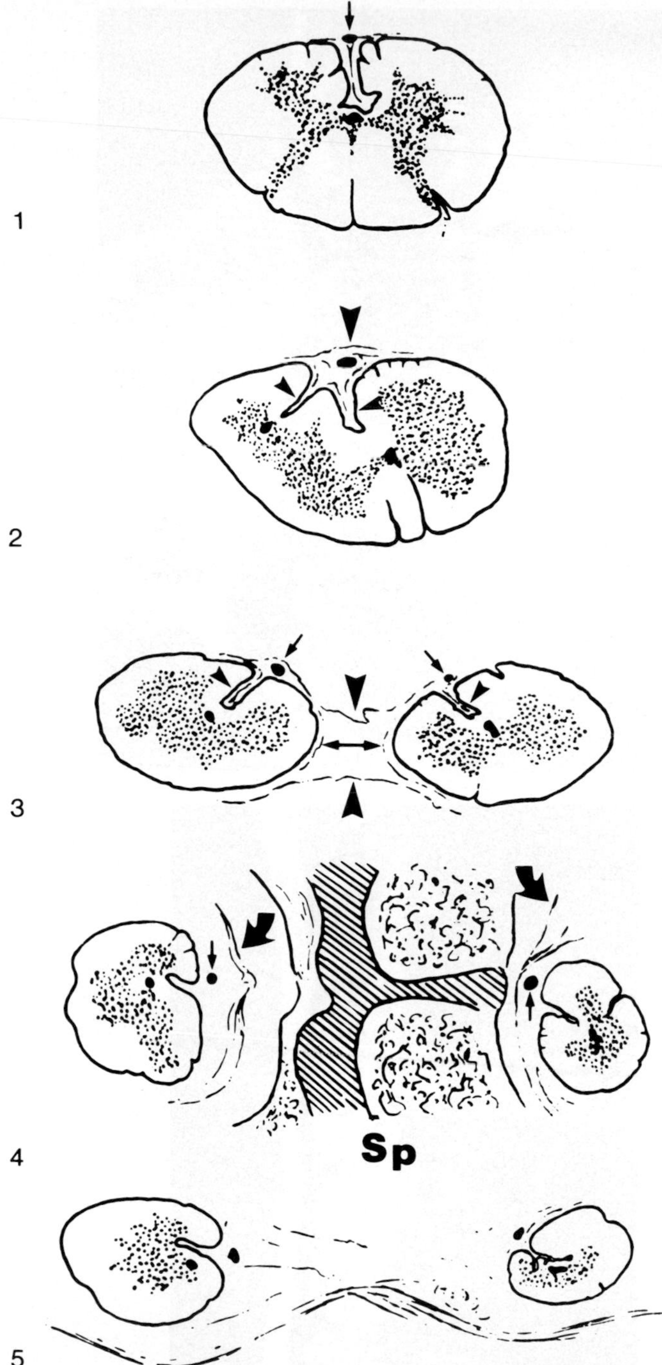

FIG. 75. Anatomic relationships in diastematomyelia. Sequential changes in the cord, meninges, and vessels as one passes from above the diastematomyelia into the region of abnormality. Ventral is toward the top. **Section 1:** The normal cervical cord above the lesion shows a single central canal (*black dot* in cord), single anterior and posterior horn on each side (*stippling*), a deep ventral median sulcus, and a single anterior spinal artery (*arrow*). The cord has normal pial investment. **Section 2:** Lower cervical cord. Partial ventral diastematomyelia at the zone of transition. The ventral median sulcus (*arrowheads*) shows dorsolateral invagination and beginning bifurcation. There is partial duplication of the anterior spinal artery representing persistence of the paired ventral longitudinal trunks of the embryo (*arrows*), formation of two well-separated central canals (*two black dots* in cord), and beginning separation of gray matter (*stippling*) into two not necessarily symmetrical parts. Each part may contain one ventral and one dorsal horn or they may separate asymmetrically. Pial investment follows the deepening ventral sulcus. The arachnoid (*large arrowhead*) lies more superficial. **Section 3:** Complete diastematomyelia with one arachnoid (and one coaxial dural) tube. Progressive dorsolateral invagination of the ventral sulcus (*small arrowheads*) causes complete sagittal diastematomyelia with formation of two adjacent, nearly symmetric thoracic hemicords, each containing one central canal (*black dot* in each hemicord). The anterior spinal artery (*arrows*) is duplicated. Each hemicord has its own pial investment (*double-headed horizontal arrow*). At this level, both hemicords are contained together in single arachnoid tube (*large arrowheads*) and single coaxial dural tube (not shown). In patients with diastematomyelia and single arachnoid and single dural tubes, the hemicords and meninges remain in this form for the length of the medullary cleft. **Section 4:** Complete diastematomyelia with double arachnoid and double dural tubes. In these patients, the two hemicords and anterior spinal arteries (*uncrossed arrows*) usually separate more widely. Arachnoid and dura (*curved arrows*) also become duplicated, forming separate arachnoid and dural tubes about each hemicord. The two medial walls of the two dural tubes form a double layer of dura between the two hemicords. This is the fibrous partition that separates the two hemicords. The region between the medial walls of the two dural tubes (i.e., between the *curved arrows*) is designated the interdural cleft. This is usually occupied by an osteocartilaginous bone spur (*Sp*). Depending on age, this spur may be purely cartilage, may be cartilage (*hatch lines*) with one or several ossification centers (as shown here), may be a nearly complete bone spur separated from the vertebral body by a thin layer of cartilage (the synchondrosis), or may be a completely united bone lamina. **Section 5:** Below the spur, the two hemicords may remain separate in separate dural and arachnoid tubes, may remain separate in a reformed single dural–single arachnoid tube, or may reunite to form a nearly normal distal spinal cord within nearly normal meninges. (From Cohen and Sledge, ref. 193, with permission.)

cleft in the cord. This dural partition is the so-called fibrous partition. The space between the two layers of dura may be called the interdural cleft.

In nearly all cases with cleft meninges, a bone spur forms in the interdural cleft between the two dural tubes—medial and external to the two dural tubes. The spur forms in cartilage from one or several ossification centers that mature with age (1,22,66,67). Depending on age, then, one may see no bone, several small fragments of bone separated by cartilage; a nearly complete bone spur still separated from the vertebra or laminae by cartilage, or a solid septum of bone completely crossing the spinal canal. The presence of cartilage along the spur signifies the site at which the bone spur will fracture away at surgery. In patients with several ossification centers, fracture between ossification centers could lead to regrowth of the spur, perhaps explaining the rare reports of regrowth of bone spurs after surgery.

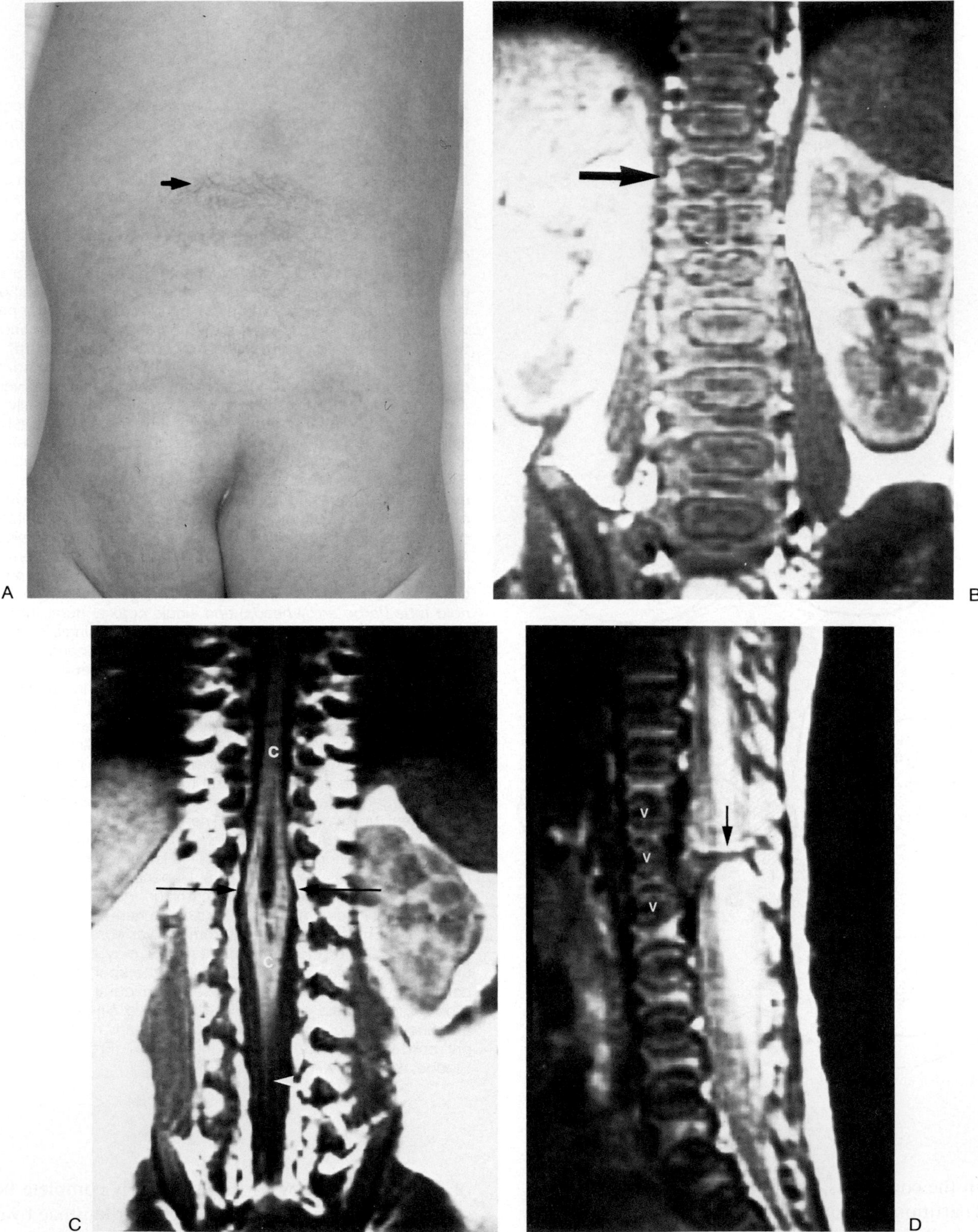

FIG. 76. Diastematomyelia, 2-month-old boy. **A:** Photograph of back showing early hairy patch (*arrow*). **B,C:** Coronal T1-weighted MRIs through the vertebrae (B) and cord (C) display slight scoliosis, butterfly ossification centers (*large arrow*), low position of the spinal cord (*C*), diastematomyelia with lateral separation of the hemicords (between the *arrows*), reunion of the two hemicords, thickened filum terminale (*white arrowhead*), and very low-signal "dot" in the lower end of the interdural cleft at the site of the bone spur. **D:** Sagittal proton-density-weighted MRI demonstrates three short, squat vertebral centra (*V*) with hypoplastic intervertebral discs and the bone spur (*arrow*) traversing the spinal canal between the two hemicords.

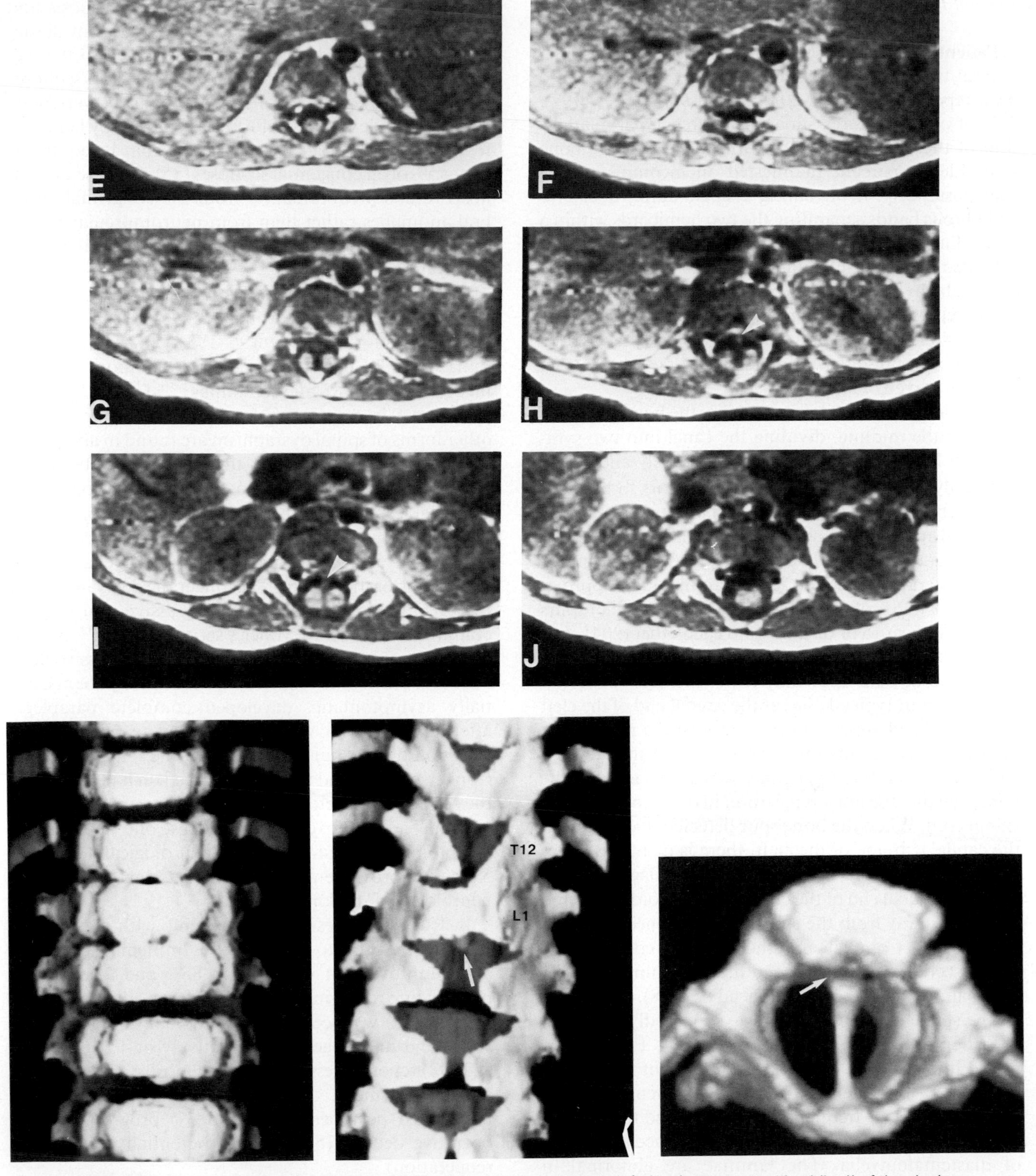

FIG. 76. (*Continued.*) **E–J:** Serial axial MRI displayed from superior to inferior demonstrate "budding" of the single cord (E) into two hemicords (F) that migrate laterally (G), passage of the bone spur (faintly seen at the *white arrowheads* in H and I) between the hemicords, and reunion of the hemicords below the bone spur (J). **K–M:** Three-dimensional CT in anterior (K), posterior (L), and axial (M) views displays the characteristic short squat vertebral bodies and hypoplastic discs, the intersegmental fusion of laminae (T12–L1), and the origin of the bone spur from the laminae with residual synchondrosis (*arrow*) anteriorly between the spur and the centrum. In L, note the relationship of the spur (*white arrow*) to the fused laminae.

Variant Forms

Patients with variant relationships of hemicords, meningeal tubes, fibrous bands, and bone spurs have also been reported (197,206–208). In Russell's series (197), 39% of operated cases showed the archetypal relationship of the two dural tubes with an intervening bone spur. Eleven percent manifested an incomplete bone spur posteriorly, invaginating a single dural tube; 11% had fibrous bands separating the two hemicords within a single dural tube; and 7% had a fibrous connection which extended from the subcutaneous tissue through a single dural tube to insert into the cleft in the cords. This cord could represent a meningocele manqué or obliterated dermal sinus (197). In one case (4%) a bone spur is stated to have been present within a single dural tube, but no details are given (197).

In patients with diastematomyelia, the bone spur may lie along the midline, dividing the canal into two symmetrical hemicanals or it may lie obliquely and asymmetrically. Nearly always, the spur appears to be more intimately associated with the laminae than the vertebral body and appears to arise from the laminae. It fuses with the vertebral body only later. In 6% of cases the spur projects posteriorly between bifid laminae. In approximately 5% to 6% of cases, double (rarely multiple) spurs are present near to or distant from each other (204).

In those patients with cleft meninges, the fibrous partition, and/or bone spur may tether the cord inferiorly. The bone spur typically lies at the caudal end of the cleft in the cord and appears to press against the medial surfaces of the two hemicords and the top of the reunited cord. In these cases, surgery may be required to resect the bone spur and the fibrous partition in order to release the spinal cord. When the bone spur detected does not lie at the caudal extreme of the cleft, there is increased likelihood that either (i) a second perhaps cartilaginous spur lies at the caudal end of the cleft or (ii) the cord is tethered inferiorly, away from the spur, by a thickened filum terminale (198). Complete untethering of the cord often requires section of the thickened filum terminale as well, by separate surgical incision if need be (198).

The spinal canal is nearly always markedly abnormal in patients with diastematomyelia (204). Focally narrowed intervertebral disc spaces are present in approximately 85% of patients. The sagittal dimension of the vertebral bodies is frequently decreased and the interpediculate distance is characteristically widened at the level of diastematomyelia. The laminae are abnormal in nearly all patients, and exhibit spina bifida, thickening of the laminae and fusion between laminae of adjacent segments. The combination of spina bifida and intersegmental fusion of laminae is present in 60% of patients and is highly suggestive of the diagnosis (Fig. 76).

Eight-five percent of patients with diastematomyelia show segmentation anomalies such as hemivertebrae, butterfly vertebrae, and block vertebrae. Scoliosis and kyphosis are present in 50% to 60% of cases of diastematomyelia and are usually directly related to the segmentation anomalies. In Miller's series, 41% of scolioses were caused by a unilateral bar, 31% by block vertebrae, 21% by complex spinal deformities, and 7% by hemivertebrae (196). Overall, diastematomyelia accounts for about 5% of all congenital scolioses (55). Because the scoliosis results predominantly from the congenital vertebral anomalies rather than from neuromuscular imbalance, untethering the cord does not affect the progress of the scoliosis (196).

Concurrent lesions seen with diastematomyelia include Klippel-Feil syndrome (2% to 7%) (196,198), Sprengel's deformity (7%) (196–198), Chiari I malformation (3%) (198), dermal sinus (3%) (198), lipomyelomeningocele (3%) (198), and teratomas (3%) (198). Spinal lipomas may be seen in relation to the bone spur. Diverse other forms of spinal dysraphism are found in about 35% of patients (196). However, the presence or absence of concurrent dysraphism is not related to the particular vertebral level affected by the diastematomyelia. Horseshoe kidneys are found in about 10% of patients (198).

Patients with untreated diastematomyelia usually show deterioration (196). The longer the delay in surgery the greater the likelihood of progressive neurological compromise (196). In Miller's series (196), 30% of children managed nonoperatively, showed progressive deterioration during the follow-up period. Two patients, initially asymptomatic, developed complete paraplegia after minor trauma, with nearly complete recovery after resection of the spur and release of the tethering (196). Conversely, no child that was operated on had damage to the cord or acute deterioration following surgery. Thirty-percent had improvement of at least one neurological symptom, 55% had no change in neurological status, and 3% had improvement in some but deterioration in other neurological functions.

In Russell's series of adult patients with diastematomyelia, 62% came to surgery (197). Immediate postoperative improvement was seen in 88% and delayed improvement (following initial deterioration or requiring reoperation) was seen in 13%. The clinical course was stable and unchanged postoperatively in 4%. Gower et al. (198) reported less encouraging results: 14% immediate improvement, 14% delayed improvement, 57% unchanged postoperatively, and 5% progressive postoperative decline (but refusing potentially remediable reoperation).

Normal Embryogenesis of the Vertebrae

The vertebrae form by a series of steps arbitrarily categorized as (1) membrane development, (2) chondrification, and (3) ossification. Each vertebra goes through

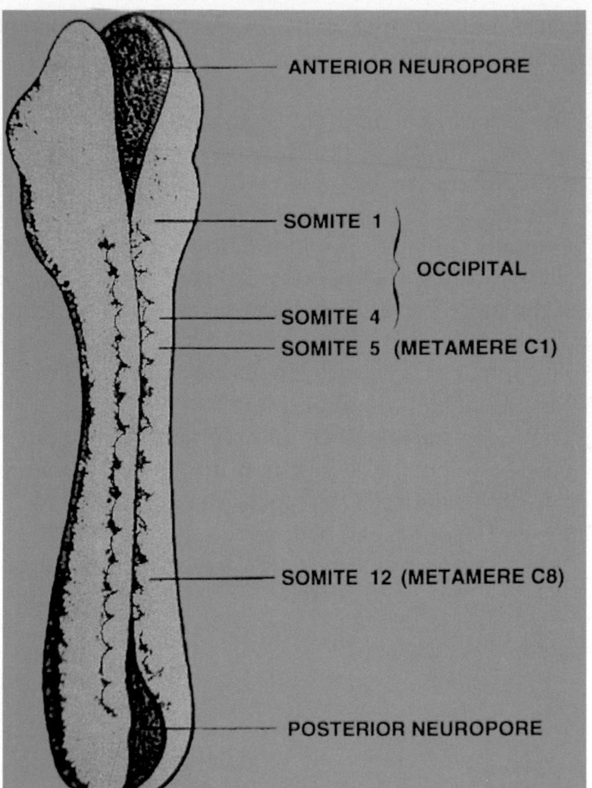

FIG. 77. Diagrammatic representation of an embryo of 23–24 days. Paired blocks of somites have formed to each side of the closing neural tube. Embryologists time events by the numbers of pairs of somites visible. After seven pairs of somites have formed (7-somite stage), the neural tube begins to close at the site of the third and fourth somite pairs (future occipital region). This closure sweeps cephalically to close the anterior neuropore at the lamina terminalis by Day 23 and posteriorly to close the posterior neuropore (at unknown site) at 25 days. (From Raybaud et al., ref. 13, with permission.)

these steps sequentially (10–13). The process starts in the future occipital region and sweeps along the length of the spine, so different parts of the spine exhibit different stages at any one moment in time.

Membrane Development

By Day 17, mesodermal cells at the cephalic end of the embryo form a thick mass of paraxial mesenchyme situated lateral to the notochord and ventrolateral to the neural plate. This paraxial mesoderm forms bilaterally symmetrical longitudinal columns of solid mesoderm that begin to segment into paired blocks called somites by Day 20 (Figs. 77 and 78). Somites first form in the future occipital region. They then continue to form as the embryo lengthens until, ultimately, 42–44 pairs are formed: 4 occipital, 8 cervical, 12 thoracic, 5 lumbar, 5 sacral, and 8–10 coccygeal. The first occipital and the last 5–7 coccygeal pairs later disappear.

The dorsolateral portion of each somite differentiates into the dermatomyotome. This will form the skeletal muscle and dermis. The ventromedial portion of each somite differentiates into the sclerotome that will form the cartilage, bone, and ligament of the vertebral column. This occurs as follows: During the fourth week of development the notochord separates from the ectoderm and the entoderm. Cells from the sclerotomes then migrate medially and surround the notochord to form a dense longitudinal column of perichordal mesenchyme (Fig. 4C). After the neural tube closes and separates from the superficial ectoderm, cells from the sclerotomes also migrate dorsal to the neural tube, between future cord

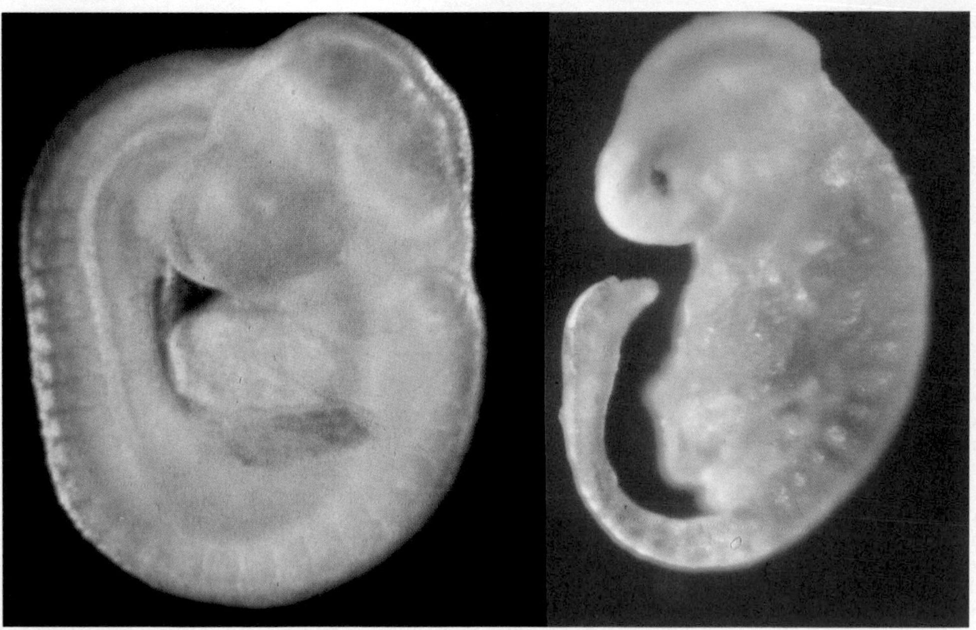

FIG. 78. Mouse embryo. The paired somites appear as segmented blocks of paramedian mesenchyme which curve along the dorsal surface of the embryo into the tail fold.

and future skin, to establish the precursors of the neural arches of the vertebrae. Migration of sclerotomic cells ventrolaterally forms the costal processes and ribs. Thus, at the end of the membranous stage, cell migration from the sclerotome forms the membranous anlagen of the vertebrae. These elements then undergo a complex resegmentation, chondrify and ossify as discussed below, creating the spinal column.

Starting at about Day 24, a major resegmentation occurs in the membranous vertebral bodies (Fig. 79). The caudal and cephalic halves of each segment differentiate from each other. Fissures form in the midportion of each segment, between the two halves, and the two halves cleave from each other. These halves then unite with adjacent half segments, such that the lower half of one old segment joins with the upper-half of the old segment below, forming a new structure designated the precartilaginous primitive vertebra. This entire process proceeds bilaterally and symmetrically. As a result of this new division and fusion:

1. The arteries situated between the two old segments become trapped within the middle of the new primitive vertebrae.
2. The less dense upper half-segments contribute substantially, possibly predominantly, to the formation of the future vertebral body. The precise contribution of the more dense caudal half-segment is still debated (209).
3. The spinal nerves and ganglia develop in relation to the cranial half-segment (209).
4. The lower halves of the old segments now abut the gaps between the adjacent primitive vertebrae and contribute the cells that form the annuli fibrosi and the cartilaginous end plates.
5. The dermatomyotomes that lay directly lateral to

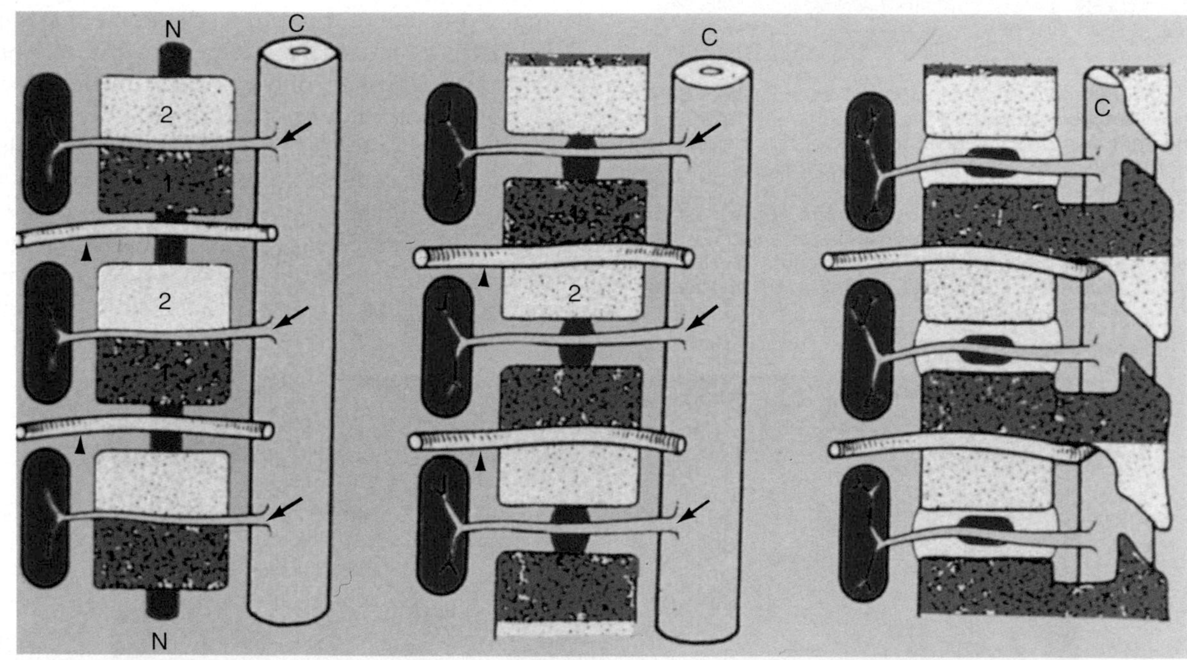

FIG. 79. Resegmentation of the sclerotomes into vertebrae. **A:** At the onset of resegmentation, each block of sclerotome consists of a denser, more cellular caudal half sclerotome (*1*) and a less dense, less cellular cranial half sclerotome (2). The cylindrical notochord (*N*) passes vertically through these and is of relatively uniform diameter. The nerve roots (*arrows*) arise from the spinal cord (*C*) and pass out in relation to the midportion of each sclerotome to innervate the muscle. The muscles are arranged segmentally opposite each sclerotomic block. The vessels (*arrowheads*) pass between the sclerotomic blocks. **B:** Then the sclerotomic blocks divide and reunite (resegment), so each dense caudal half sclerotome (*1*) unites with the next lower, less dense cranial half sclerotome (*2*) to make a new primitive precartilaginous vertebra. The old caudal half sclerotome thus becomes the top half of the new primitive vertebra. The notochord cylinder constricts within the vertebrae and expands at the levels of the newly formed gaps between the primitive vertebrae. The nerve roots (*arrows*) still arise from the cord (*C*) and pass to the muscles, but the nerves now course in relation to the new gaps and the muscles now bridge those gaps. The arteries (*arrowheads*) that ran between sclerotomes now course through the centers of the new primitive vertebrae. **C:** The portions of the notochord within the vertebrae degenerate to the mucoid streaks. The portions of the notochord within the gaps expand and undergo mucoid degeneration to help form the nuclei pulposi. Cells from the dense caudal half sclerotome (*1*) (new top half of the primitive vertebra) migrate into the adjacent gap to form the annulus fibrosus. The neural arches grow to encompass the cord. (From Raybaud et al., ref. 13, with permission.)

each old segment, now lie lateral to the new discs and are able to attach to adjacent vertebrae across the disc. This provides mechanical advantage.

The relationships between the somites, the vertebrae, and the nerves are given in Fig. 80.

Chondrification

The newly formed precartilaginous primitive vertebrae then chondrify (Fig. 81). Paired foci of chondrification appear just to each side of the midline within each precartilaginous centrum. Separate centers of chondrification also appear in each half of the neural arch, and at the junction of each neural arch with the centrum. Chondrification of the centra is associated with disappearance of the notochord at that level. However, a thin remnant of notochord persists in the centra as the mucoid streak.

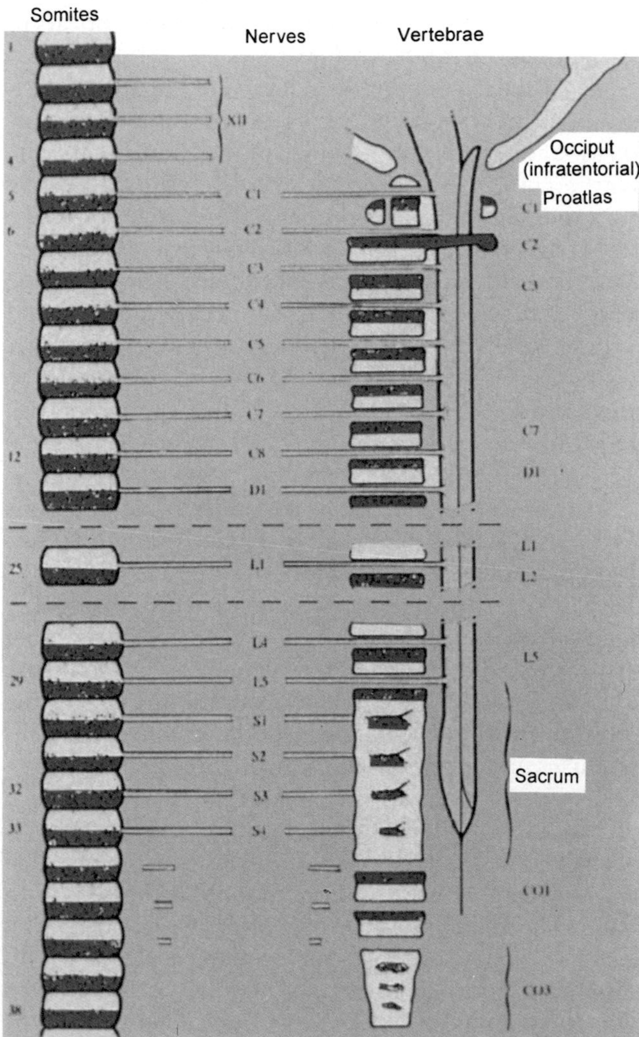

FIG. 80. Relation of somites to cranial-spinal nerves and to spinal cord. In humans, 42–44 pair of somites form. The most caudal five to seven pairs disappear during canalization and retrogressive differentiation. At term, the coccygeal vertebrae persist as vestiges without corresponding nerve roots. The conus medullaris probably represents somites 32–33, corresponding to the S3-S4 nerve level. The first pair of somites disappears in humans. The next three pairs form the portion of the skull designated the spondylocranium, i.e., the basiocciput and the exoccipital bones. Portions of the 5th, 6th, and 7th somites constitute C1 and C2. (Modified from Raybaud et al., ref. 13, with permission.)

Ossification

Each centrum initially has two ossification centers; one anterior to and the other posterior to the mucoid streak (Figs. 81C–D). These usually coalesce rapidly into a single ossification center for each centrum. These central ossification centers for the centra first appear, simultaneously, at about 9 weeks' gestation, in four sequential thoracolumbar vertebrae: T11, T12, and L1, plus either T10 or L2 (210). Additional ossification centers then arise within adjacent centra and extend, sequentially, in orderly fashion, cranially toward C2 (rapidly) and caudally toward S3 or S4 (more slowly) (210–214). The C1, S4, and S5 centers ossify later. All fetuses show ossification in the centrum of C2 by 15 weeks' gestation, and in C1 by 18 weeks' gestation (210). Caudally, all fetuses show ossification in the centrum of S2 by 11–12 weeks' gestation, S3 by 13–14 weeks' gestation, S4 by 17 weeks' gestation, and S5 after 19 weeks' gestation (210).

Within each vertebra enlargement of the ossification centers leaves residual plates of cartilage superior and inferior to the centrum. These plates become the cartilaginous end plates that face the intervertebral discs (Fig. 46). At approximately age 16 years, secondary centers of ossification form within the superior and inferior end plates of the vertebral bodies, and at the tips of the spinous processes and transverse processes. These secondary ossification centers generally fuse with the adjacent bone by age 25 years.

The vertebral arches ossify from distinct paired "neural" ossification centers, one within each hemiarch of each vertebra (215). Ossification of the neural arches is independent of ossification of the centra and, indeed shows no regular order of appearance or specific sequence pattern (210,214). In general, the first cluster of neural arch ossifications appears at about 9 weeks' gestation in a group of lower cervical–upper thoracic vertebrae. These ossifications tend to coincide with ossification in the superior nuchal line and squamous occipital bone and may reflect more active use of the attached musculature for head flexion and motion of the shoulder girdle (210). Shortly thereafter, a second cluster of neural ossifications appears in the upper cervical region. The remaining cervical arches may then "fill in" and the ossifications may extend inferiorly toward the midthoracic region (210). A third cluster of neural ossifications may then appear in the lower thoracic–upper lumbar verte-

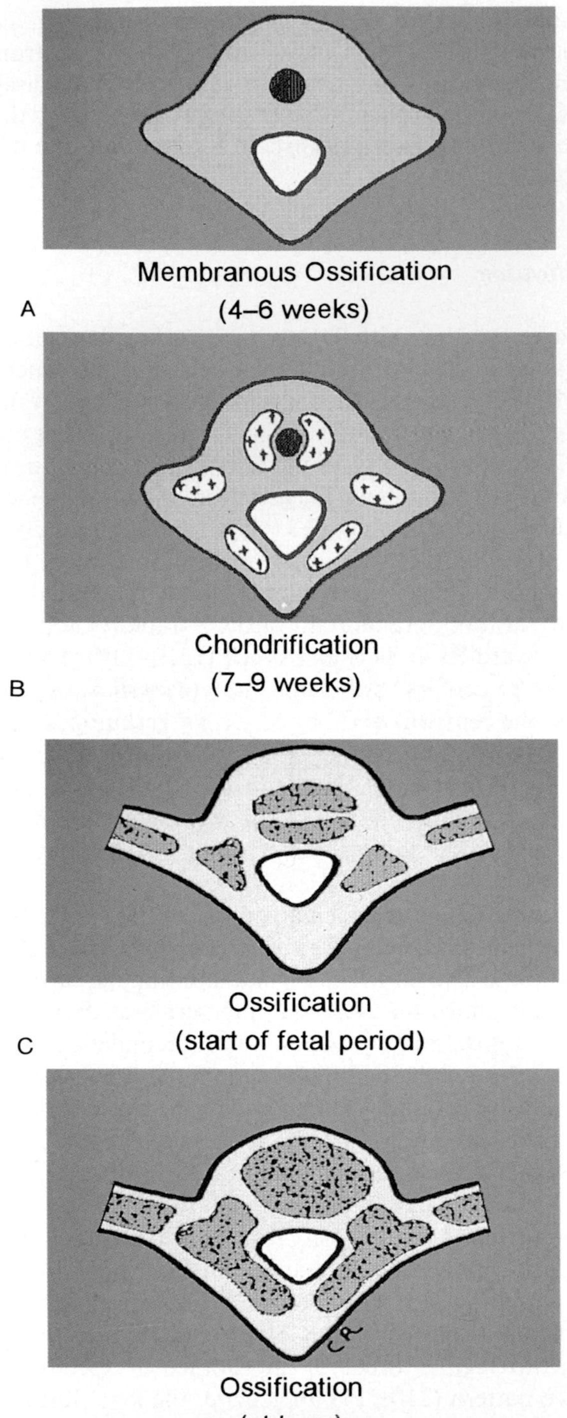

FIG. 81. Stages of formation of the vertebra. Diagrammatic representation oriented like axial MRI. **A:** Membranous stage (4th–6th weeks). The precartilaginous primitive vertebra (*pink*) contains a compressed, degenerate remnant of the notochord designated the mucoid streak (*purple*). **B:** Chondrification to the cartilaginous vertebra (7th–9th weeks). Paired centers of chondrification (*yellow with cross-marks*) usually appear lateral to the mucoid streak (*purple*) in the centrum, in each half of the neural arch and at the junctions of centrum with the neural arches. The centers for the centrum then merge together around the mucoid streak. The centers in the neural arch unite to form the cartilaginous neural arch and spinous process. The third pair extends laterally into the transverse processes. **C:** Ossification (*speckled gray*) of the centrum begins as two centers, one anterior to and the second posterior to the mucoid streak. These coalesce to form one center that enlarges from the 20th to the 24th week. Two additional pairs of ossification centers (*speckled gray*) arise in the neural arches, as shown. **D:** By term, these ossification centers (*speckled gray*) have enlarged to occupy a substantial portion of the cartilaginous vertebra (*hatch lines*). (Redrawn from Raybaud et al., ref. 13, with permission.)

brae and extend upward to meet those descending from the second cluster. In general, ossifications are seen histologically in all the neural arches C2–T2 by 9–10 weeks' gestation, T3–L2 by 10–11 weeks' gestation, and L3–S1 by 12 weeks' gestation (210,214).

Ossification of the lower sacral arches does proceed sequentially, caudally from S2 (at 15–16 weeks' gestation) toward S5 (19 weeks' gestation) (214). By using ultrasound in vivo Budorick et al. (216) actually displayed the sequential appearance of ossification within one new lumbosacral neural arch every 2–3 weeks of gestation: Substantial ossification of the neural arch was evident by ultrasound in all fetuses at L5 at 16 weeks' gestation, S1 at 19 weeks' gestation, S2 at 22 weeks' gestation, S3 at 24 weeks' gestation, S4 at 25 weeks' gestation, and S5 at 27 weeks' gestation (216). The rate of ossification appears to be slightly more rapid in females.

The cartilage between the neural and the central ossification centers on each side is designated the neurocentral synchondrosis. With growth of the centrum and the bony arches, the neurocentral synchondroses narrow and eventually fuse with the centra, well anterior to the sites of the pedicles (Figs. 82–84). Thus the "ossified vertebral bodies" include bone contributed from both the centra and the neural arches. The terms centrum and body are not interchangeable. The laminae in the lumbar region fuse after birth, followed by the remainder of the spine. It should be noted that the laminae at the L5 level may normally remain unfused until age five or six years (12,13,217–229).

The cervical spine exhibits several normal variations (Fig. 85). The atlas (C1) usually develops from one ossification center in the vertebral body and two centers in the neural arches. The center for the body is normally not ossified at birth but becomes visible during the first year of life. The neurocentral synchondroses usually fuse at about 7 years of age. If the ossification center in the body fails to develop, the ossification centers in the neural arches may grow forward to form the anterior portion of C1. If these do not fuse, a cleft may be visible in the anterior aspect of the vertebra.

The axis (C2) usually develops from four primary ossification centers: one for the dens, one for the body, and two for the neural arches. These primary centers fuse by age 3–6 years. A secondary ossification center for the tip of the dens normally appears at age 3–6 years and fuses with the dens by age 12 years. Occasionally the dens

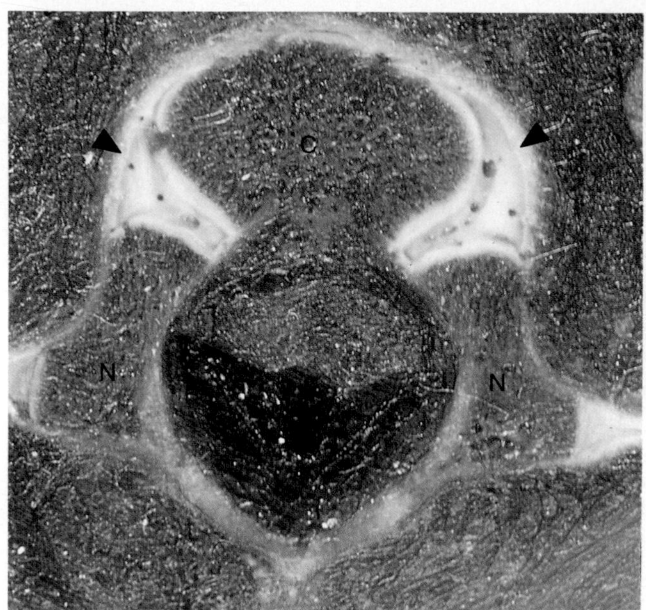

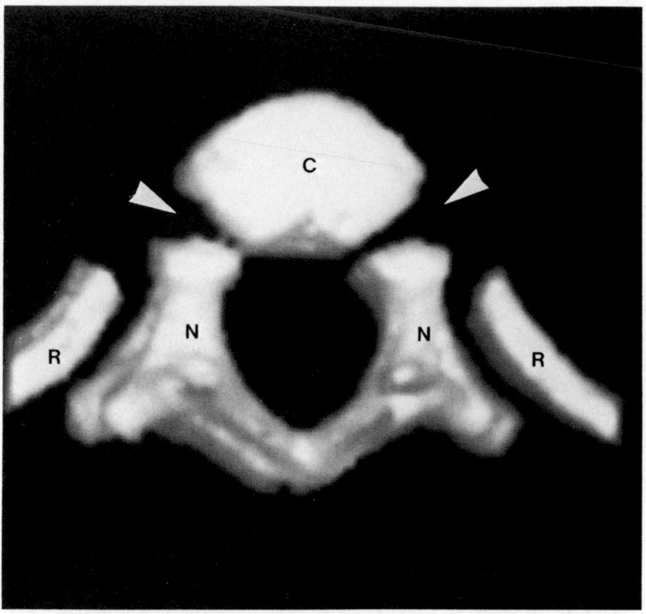

FIG. 82. Centers of ossification. **A:** Lumbar vertebra of newborn. Axial anatomic section. The darker, marrow-containing central (*C*) and neural (*N*) ossification centers develop within the cartilaginous vertebra. *Arrowheads* indicate the zones designated neurocentral synchondroses. The neural ossifications and posterior cartilage arch medially to close the dorsal spinal canal. **B:** Thoracic vertebra of a 2-month-old boy. Three-dimensional CT of bone shows the neural (*N*) and central (*C*) ossification centers, neurocentral synchondroses (*white arrowheads*), and costal ossification centers for the ribs (*R*).

arises instead from two ossification centers that may fail to fuse in the midline leaving a "bifid" dens.

The typical cervical vertebrae C3–C6 develop one ossification center for the body, and one for each half of the neural arch. The posterior synchondrosis between the two halves of the neural arches usually ossifies by age 2–3 years. The neurocentral synchondroses unite by age 3–6 years. The anterior portion of the transverse process may develop from a secondary center that arises in utero (6th month) and unites with the neural arch by age 6 years. At C7 a similar ossification center may persist separately and elongate to form a cervical rib. Secondary ossification centers for the bifid spinous process and the superior and inferior epiphyseal rings appear at puberty and fuse to the vertebra by age 25 years.

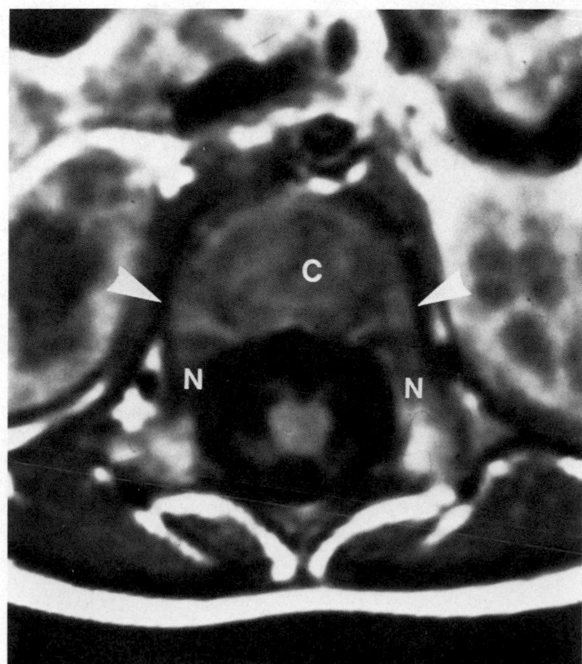

FIG. 83. Lumbar vertebra. Axial MRI demonstrates the neural (*N*) ossification centers, the centrum (*C*), and the residual neurocentral synchondroses (*white arrowheads*). Note the paired ventral and dorsal nerve roots arising from the cord.

Deranged Embryogenesis of the Spinal Column

With variable cell migration, segmentation, and ossification, it is possible to anticipate the presence of numerous spinal variants in the population. Patients with myelomeningocele and unneurulated spinal cords will condense mesenchyme in abnormal position making widely bifid posterior elements (Fig. 5C). Malsegmentation of the vertebrae and deranged formation of costal apophyses can lead to indeterminate vertebrae (219, 230,231). Thus the T12 vertebra may lack ribs in 2% of patients and the first lumbar vertebra may carry ribs, unilaterally or bilaterally, in 6% to 11% of cases. The last lumbar vertebra is sacralized in 6% of patients, while S1 is lumbarized in 2% of cases. Defective ossification of the laminae of the low lumbar and sacral vertebrae is common (although reported incidences vary from 0.2% to 34% of cases) (232–234). Most such defects are midline;

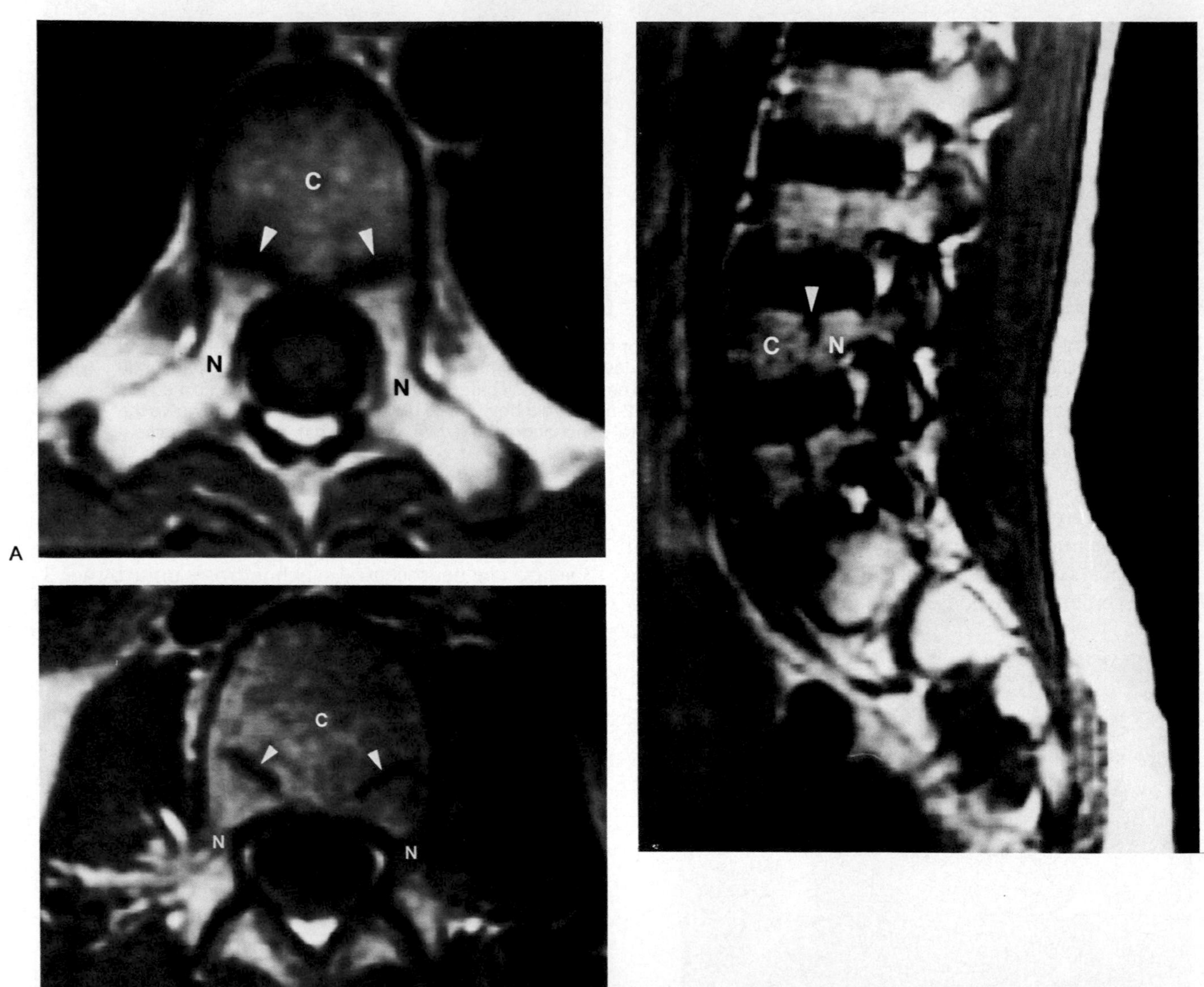

FIG. 84. Normal vertebra, 11-year-old boy. **A,B:** Axial T1-weighted MRI. **C:** Sagittal T1-weighted MRI. Nearly complete closure of central (*C*) and neural (*N*) ossification centers leaves the characteristic oblique low-signal fusion line (*arrowheads*) at the remnant neurocentral synchondroses. The vertebral body forms from both central and neural ossification centers.

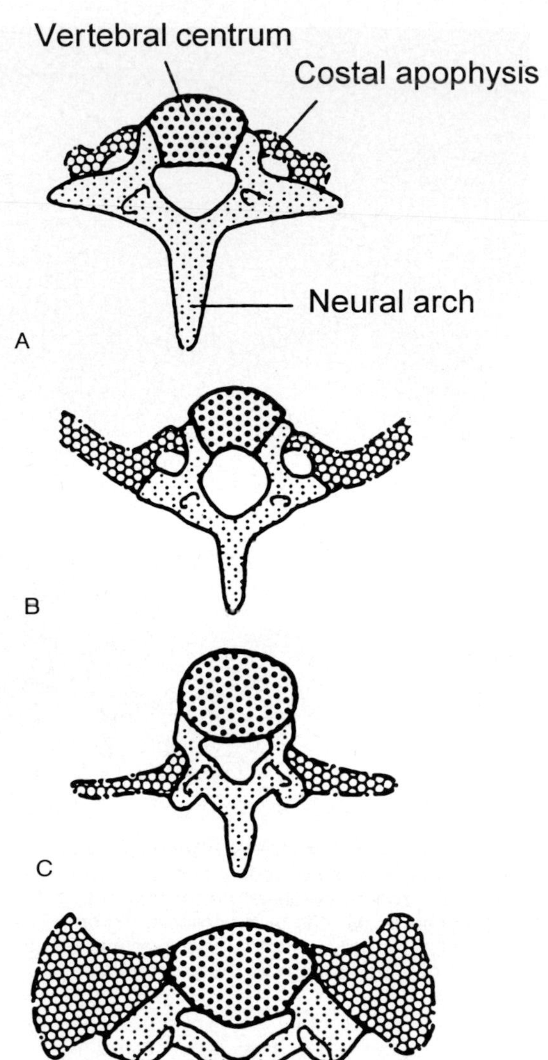

FIG. 85. Formation of the vertebra. Regional differentiation. Diagrammatic representations oriented like axial MRI. The centrum (*polka-dot*), the neural ossification centers (*light stipple*), and the costal apophyses (*circles*) give rise to characteristic and homologous portions of each of the cervical (**A**), thoracic (**B**), lumbar (**C**), and sacral vertebrae (**D**). In A the uncinate processes derive from the neural arch, not the costal apophyses. The size and proportion of each component vary from level to level, but the costal apophysis varies most widely. (From Raybaud et al., ref. 13, with permission.)

a few are paramedian at one or both sides of a well-formed spinous process.

Persistence of separate ventral and dorsal ossification centers for each centrum produces coronal cleft vertebrae. Such vertebrae occur more frequently in the thoracolumbar region of males. They may be a normal variant that disappears within a few months after birth. However, coronal cleft vertebrae appear in increased frequency in patients with imperforate anus, myelodysplasia, and chondrodystrophia calcificans.

Sagittal-cleft vertebral bodies appear to develop when separate ossification centers form in each of the paired paramedian chondrification centers. These also may disappear within 6 months after birth, or may persist as "butterfly" vertebra (Figs. 86–89). Hemivertebrae appear when the paramedian centers of chondrification fail to unite in the midline and the ossification center fails to develop on one side. These may lead to congenital mechanical scoliosis (Fig. 89).

Failure of bony union of the two neural arches posteriorly leads to spina bifida occulta. This is observed in the lumbar region in 9% of women and 1% of men. In descending order of frequency, the commonest sites of unfused spinous processes are L5 and S1, C1, C7, T1, and the lower thoracic region.

Formation of a complete or incomplete cleft in the vertebral arch may lead to unilateral absence or hypoplasia of a pedicle (235,236). In such patients, affected vertebrae may exhibit posterior position of the lateral mass and absence of the posterior transverse process. The contralateral pedicle is usually thicker than normal.

Block vertebrae may be single or multiple. They occur most commonly in the lumbar spine, then the cervical spine, and rarely in the thoracic spine. In larger series,

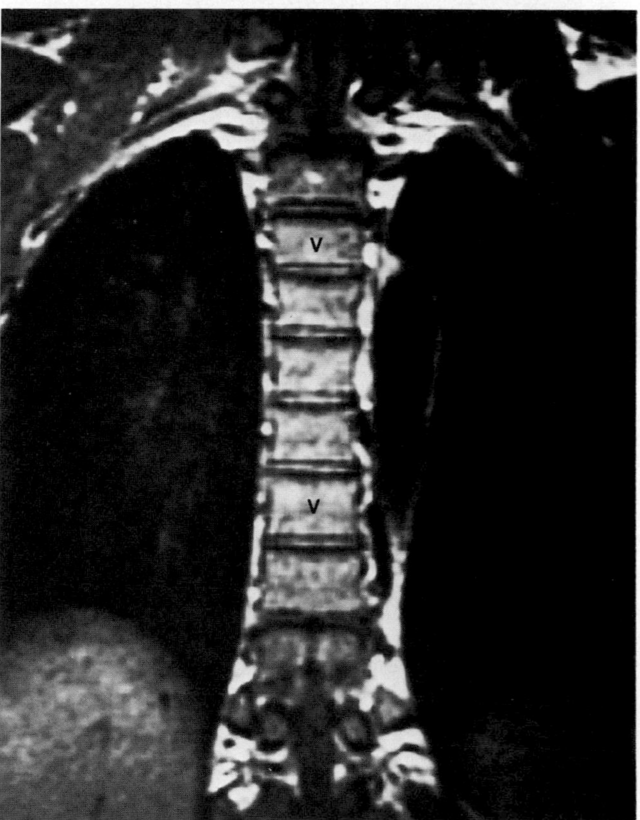

FIG. 86. Normal coronal MRI, 22-year-old woman. The vertebral bodies (*V*) exhibit normal, smoothly varying contour because the coronal section through the curved thoracic kyphosis intersects each vertebra at a slightly different portion of its sagittal dimension. This section through the greatest size of the upper and lower thoracic vertebrae includes only a smaller more anterior component of the midthoracic vertebrae.

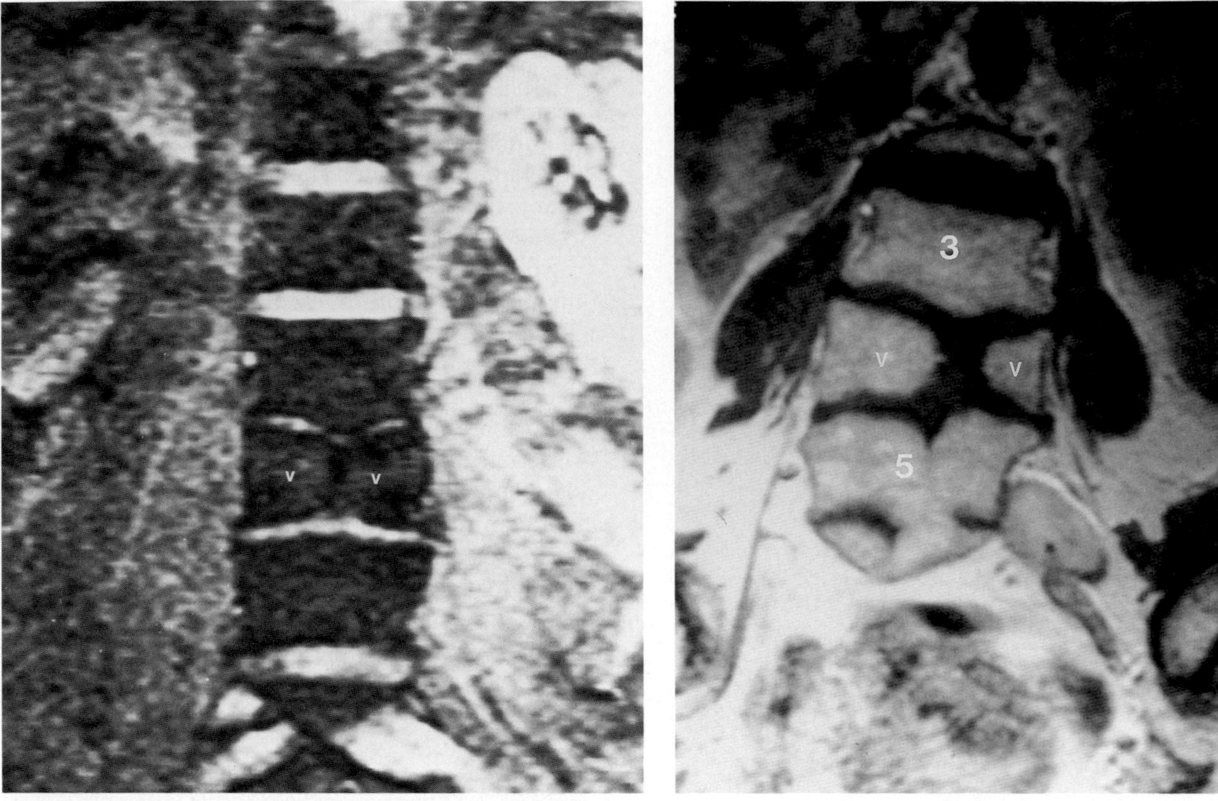

FIG. 87. Butterfly vertebra with consequent molding of the adjacent end plates. **A:** Mild malsegmentation, 55-year-old man. Coronal MRI of the lumbar spine shows paired hemivertebrae (*v*) with consequent constriction of the height of the midsagittal position of the vertebra. The adjacent vertebrae grow to compensate for that defect. Intervening discs are hypoplastic. **B:** More severe malsegmentation, 60-year-old woman with scoliosis. Coronal T1-weighted MRI demonstrates asymmetric separated hemivertebrae (*v*) at L4, partially united butterfly vertebra at L5, fusion between portions of L5 and S1, and molding of the inferior surface of L3 to conform to these changes.

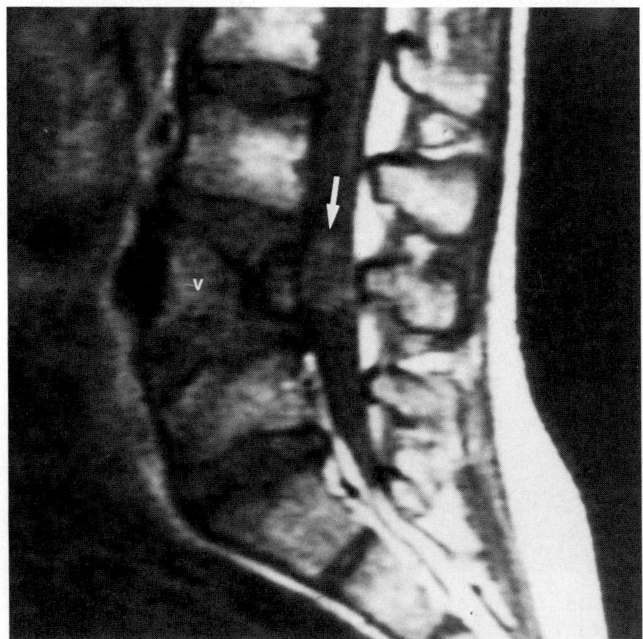

FIG. 88. Sagittal T1-weighted MRI, 15-year-old girl, reveals an anterior hemivertebra with dermoid (*arrow*). The apposing vertebrae exhibit no compensatory contour molding. (From Zimmerman et al., ref. 8, with permission.)

the incidence of congenital fusion of the cervical spine is 0.71% (217).

In block vertebrae, the intervertebral disc is absent or rudimentary. The combined vertebrae may be normal in height or tall. Deficient growth at the fusion site leads to narrow sagittal diameter and concave configuration of the block. Scalloping of the posterior surface may result from associated dural ectasia or (rarely) congenital mass. Disordered embryogenesis at adjacent levels may lead to hemivertebra or absent vertebra above or below the level of the block. Asymmetrical malsegmentation may lead to hemivertebrae and/or tripediculate vertebrae, often as a series of jumbled, mismatched half segments that extend along a substantial length of the spinal column.

The posterior elements are also malsegmented in many patients with block vertebrae. These posterior fusions may lead to severe, progressive kyphosis and scoliosis in unusual cases. Respiratory failure may result from thoracic lordosis created by the fused posterior elements.

The craniovertebral region requires special discussion because the embryology of this region is complex. The base of the skull around the foramen magnum is designated the spondylocranium, because it forms from the

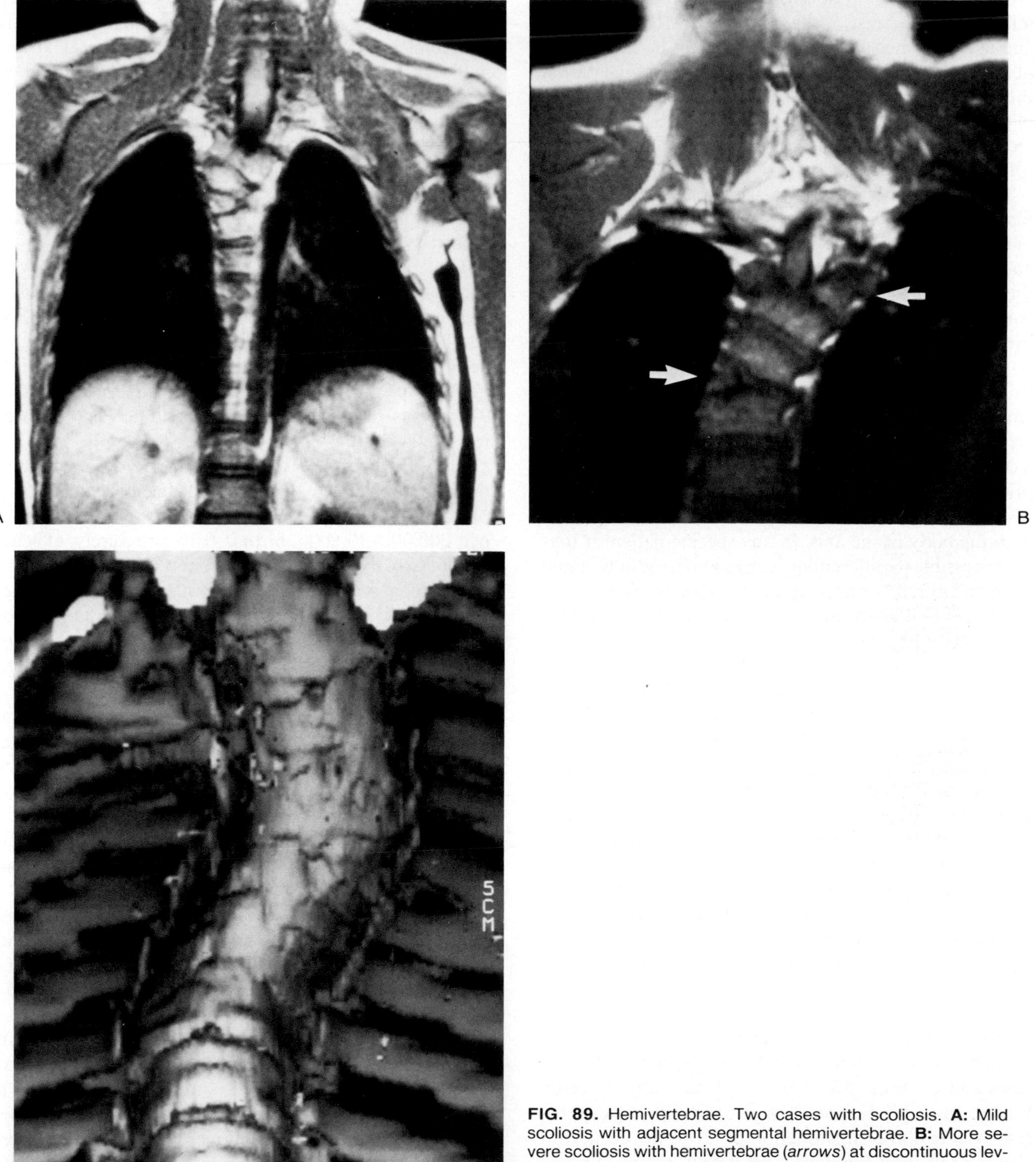

FIG. 89. Hemivertebrae. Two cases with scoliosis. **A:** Mild scoliosis with adjacent segmental hemivertebrae. **B:** More severe scoliosis with hemivertebrae (*arrows*) at discontinuous levels. **C:** Three-dimensional reformation of the scoliotic curve of patient B. Sagittal (A) and coronal (B) MRI. Multiple hemivertebra (*arrows*) cause congenital scoliosis on a mechanical basis. Three-dimensional image (C) depicts the full contour of the thoracic scoliosis.

union of "vertebral" elements derived from the occipital somites. The occipital condyles, superior facets of the atlas, and odontoid tip develop from the fourth occipital sclerotome. The rest of the dens and the lateral masses and neural arches of the atlas arise from the caudal part of the fourth occipital sclerotome plus the cranial part of the first cervical sclerotome. The body and neural arch of the axis derive from the caudal portion of the first cervical sclerotome plus the cranial portion of the second cervical sclerotome.

Faulty segmentation may cause unilateral or bilateral fusions of the occipital condyles with the lateral masses of the atlas or fusions between the neural arch of the atlas and the occiput. An occipital vertebra may form between the atlas and the occipital bone and present as a third condyle at the tip of the clivus or as multiple bone fragments in this region.

Absence of the dens is rare. Ossiculum terminale results from failure to fuse the apical portion of the dens with the body of the dens. Since the apical ossification center normally fuses with the base of the dens by age 12, a diagnosis of ossiculum terminale should not be made prior to this time. Os odontoideum results from failure to fuse the apical and basal portions of the odontoid process with the body of the axis. In any specific patient it may be impossible to differentiate congenital os odontoideum from "acquired" or post-traumatic os odontoideum.

Klippel-Feil syndrome is a congenital malformation characterized by failure in the segmentation of two or more cervical vertebrae (43,237). The condition occurs in between 1 in 233 births to 1 in 42,000 births, tends to run in families, and affects both sexes equally. Three types are described. Type 1 shows massive fusion of most of the cervical and upper thoracic spine. Severe neurological impairment and associated anomalies are most frequent in this group. Type 2 shows fusions of one or two interspaces, most often at C2–C3, next most often at C5–C6. Fusions at C2–C3 are inherited as an autosomal dominant trait with variable penetrance. Fusions at C5–C6 are inherited as an autosomal recessive trait. In 75% of cases fusions occur from C3 cephalad. Type 3 fusions involve cervical vertebrae and lower thoracic or lumbar vertebrae.

In Ulmer's series (43), 33% of patients exhibited the classic triad of short neck, low posterior hairline, and limited cervical motion. C2/3 was affected in 50% of cases and C5/6 in 33%. Hemivertebrae, butterfly vertebrae or spina bifida were seen in one-third of cases, basilar impression or assimilation of C1 to the occiput in one quarter, and Sprengel's deformity in 15%. Diastematomyelia with partial or complete cord clefting was found in 20% and Chiari I malformation in 8%. Up to 65% of patients have genitourinary tract abnormalities, most frequently unilateral renal agenesis (43).

Other classifications of vertebral anomalies are proposed and overlap with Klippel-Feil and with each other. These include the VATER association, the OEIS complex and the Currarino triad.

The VATER association is a nonrandom occurrence of multisystem congenital malformations, specifically Vertebral anomalies, Anal atresia, Esophageal atresia with Tracheoesophageal fistula, and Radial anomalies. Renal anomalies, a single umbilical artery, and cardiac malformations are commonly associated (238). Occult spinal dysraphism, especially filar-conal lipomas and lipomyelomeningoceles are also associated (238). Uncommonly, occipital cephalocele (239), callosal dysgenesis, olfactory bulb hypoplasia, and aqueductal stenosis are reported (239).

The VATER association overlaps in its features with hemifacial microsomia (HFM) and sirenomelia (240). Thirteen percent of patients with otherwise typical HFM also have three or more features of VATER and may be designated HFM-VATER phenotype (240). The HFM-VATER phenotype shows vertebral malformations in 97% versus 78% in VATER alone and versus 66% in sirenomelia (240).

The OEIS complex comprises a nonrandom combination of Omphalocele, Exstrophy of the cloaca, Imperforate anus, and Spinal defects. It occurs sporadically in 1 per 200,000–400,000 births. Ribs are rarely affected (241). Karyotypes are normal. The OEIS complex may be the most severe end of the exstrophy–epispadias sequence which includes epispadias, pubic diastasis, bladder exstrophy, cloacal exstrophy, and OEIS—in order of increasing severity and complexity (241). Posterior meningoceles may be associated (241).

The Currarino triad is an association of (partial) sacral agenesis and anorectal stenosis or other low anorectal malformation with presacral masses including meningocele, teratoma, enteric cyst, or a combination of these (133). The full Currarino triad may be one extreme of a spectrum of pathology inherited as an autosomal dominant trait with incomplete penetrance (242). The triad appears familial in more than 50% of cases (242). Of 40 reports of the complete triad (to 1984), 21 (53%) had meningocele alone, 17 (43%) had benign teratoma, and 2 (5%) had enteric cysts; 3 (7.5%) had a combination of anterior sacral meningocele and presacral teratoma (242).

Vertebral segmentation anomalies are also observed in a large number of other conditions including Goldenhar complex (243). In Goldenhar complex, 19% have cervical anomalies such as vertebral fusion, hemivertebrae, spina bifida occulta, and craniovertebral base anomalies. Less than 1% have vertebral anomalies below the cervical spine, or rib anomalies (243).

ACKNOWLEDGMENTS. The authors thank Antonio Chirinos and Mabel Rodriguez, Medical Photography in Media Services at Baptist Hospital of Miami, for their invaluable work overseeing the production of the images used in this contribution, as well as Susan DeBusk for manuscript and reference production.

REFERENCES

1. Naidich TP, McLone DG, Harwood-Nash DC. Spinal dysraphism. In: Newton TH, Potts EG, eds. *Modern Neuroradiology, vol 1, Computed Tomography of the Spine and Spinal Cord.* San Anselmo, CA: Clavadel Press; 1983:Ch. 17.
2. Kaplan JO, Quencer RM. The occult tethered conus syndrome in the adult. *Radiology* 1980;137:387–391.
3. Pang D, Wildberger JE. Tethered cord syndrome in adults. *J Neurosurg* 1982;57:32–47.
4. Simon RH, Donaldson JO. Ramsby GR. Tethered spinal cord in adult siblings. *Neurosurgery* 1981;8:241–244.
5. James CCM, Lassman LP. *Spinal Dysraphism, Spina Bifida Occulta.* New York: Appleton-Century-Crofts; 1972.
6. Friede RL. *Developmental Neuropathology*, 2nd ed. New York: Springer-Verlag; 1989:253–254.
7. Schut L, Pizzi FJ, Bruce DA. Occult spinal dysraphism. In: McLaurin Rl, ed. *Myelomeningocele.* New York: Grune & Stratton; 1977:349–368.
8. Zimmerman R A, Bilaniuk LT, Bury EA. Magnetic resonance of the pediatric spine. *Magn Reson Q* 1989;5:169–204.
9. Sarwar M, Virapongse C, Bhimani S. Primary tethered cord syndrome: a new hypothesis of its origin. *AJNR* 1984;5:235–242.
10. Langman J. Medical embryology. *Human Development—Normal and Abnormal.* Baltimore: Williams & Wilkins; 1963.
11. Lemire RJ, Leoser JD, Leech RW, et al. *Normal and Abnormal Development of the Human Nervous System.* Hagerstown, MD: Harper & Row; 1975.
12. Naidich TP, McLone DG. Growth and development. In: Kricun ME, ed. *Imaging Modalities in Spinal Disorders.* Philadelphia: WB Saunders; 1988:Ch. 1.
13. Raybaud CA, Naidich TP, McLone DG. Développement de la moelle et du rachis. In: Manelfe C, ed. *Imagerie du Rachis et de la Moelle.* Paris: Editions Vigot; 1989:chapter 1.
14. Barkovich AJ, Naidich TP. Congenital anomalies of the spine. In: Barkovich AJ, ed. *Contemporary Neuroimaging.* New York: Raven Press; 1990:Ch. 8:227–271.
15. Barnes PD, Lewster PD, Yamanashi WS, Prince JR. Magnetic resonance imaging in infants and children with spinal dysraphism. *AJNR* 1986;7:465–472.
16. Brunberg JA, Latchaw RE, Kanal E, Burk DL Jr, Albright L. Magnetic resonance imaging of spinal dysraphism. *Radiol Clin North Am* 1988;26:181–205.
17. Davis PC, Hoffman JC Jr, Ball TI, Wyly JB, Braun IR, Fry SM, Drvaric DM. Spinal abnormalities in pediatric patients: MR imaging findings compared with clinical myelographic, and surgical findings. *Radiology* 1988;166:679–685.
18. Harwood-Nash DC, Fitz CR. *Neuroradiology in Infants and Children.* St. Louis: CV Mosby; 1976.
19. Kuharik MA, Edwards MK, Grossman CB. Magnetic resonance evaluation of pediatric spinal dysraphism. *Pediatr Neurosci* 1985–86;12:213–218.
20. McLone DG. Embryonic deformation and caudal suppression. *Concepts in Pediatric Neurosurgery*, vol. 7. American Society for Pediatric Neurosurgeons. Basel: S. Karger; 1987:169–171.
21. Merx JL, Bakker-Niezen SH, Thijssen HOM, Walder HAD. The tethered spinal cord syndrome: a correlation of radiological features and preoperative findings in 30 patients. *Neuroradiology* 1989;31:63–70.
22. Naidich TP, Gorey MT, Raybaud C, McLone DG, Byrd S. Malformations congénitales de la moelle. In: Manelfe C, ed. *Imagerie du Rachis et de la Moelle.* Paris: Editions Vigot; 1989:Ch.18.
23. Naidich TP, Harwood-Nash DC. Diastematomyelia. Part I. Hemicords and meningeal sheaths. Single and double arachnoid and dural tubes. *AJNR* 1983;4:633–636.
24. Naidich TP, McLone DG, Fulling H. The Chiari II malformation. Part IV. The hindbrain deformity. *Neuroradiology* 1983;25: 179–197.
25. Naidich TP, McLone DG, Mutleur S. A new understanding of dorsal dysraphism with lipoma lipomyeloschisis: radiological evaluation and surgical correction. *AJNR* 1983;4:103–116.
26. Raghaven N, Barkovich AJ, Edwards M, Norman D. MR imaging in the tethered spinal cord syndrome. *AJNR* 1989;10:27–36.
27. Sarwar M, Kier EL, Virapongse C. Development of the spine and spinal cord. In: Newton TH, Potts, eds. *Modern Neuroradiology, Vol 1, Computed Tomography of the Spine and Spinal Cord.* San Anselmo, CA: Clavadel Press; 1983:Ch. 2.
28. Scatliff JH, Kendall BE, Kingsley DPE, Britton J, Grant DN, Hayward RD. Closed spinal dysraphism: analysis of clinical, radiological and surgical findings in 104 consecutive patients. *AJNR* 1989;10:269–277.
29. Sensenig EC. The early development of the human vertebral column. *Contrib Embryology, Carnegie Institute*, no. 214. 1949;33: 21–41.
30. England MA. Color atlas of life before birth. *Normal Fetal Development.* Chicago: Year Book Medical; 1983.
31. Ho PSP, Yu S, Sether LA, Wagner M, Ho K-C, Haughton VM. Progressive and regressive changes in the nucleus pulposis. Part I. The neonate. *Radiology* 1988;169:87–91.
32. Yu S, Haughton VM, Ho PSP, Sether LA, Wagner M, Ho K-C. Progressive and regressive changes in the nucleus pulposus. Part II. The adult. *Radiology* 1988;169:93–97.
33. Barkovich AJ. Congenital anomalies of the spine. In: Barkovich AJ, ed. *Pediatric Neuroimaging*, 2nd ed. New York: Raven Press; 1995:Ch. 9:477–540.
34. Van Allen ML, Kalousek DK, Chernoff GF, Juriloff D, Harris M, McGillivray BC, Yong S-L, Langlois S, MacLeod PM, Chitayat, D, Friedman JM, Wilson RD, McFadden D, Pantzer J, Ritchie S, Hall JG. Evidence for multi-site closure of the neural tube in humans. *Am J Med Genet* 1993;47:723–743.
35. Brau RH, Rafael R, Ramirez MV, Gonzalez R, Martinez V. Experience in the management of myelomeningocele in Puerto Rico. *J Neurosurg* 1990;72:726–731.
36. Smithells RW, Sheppard S, Schorah CJ, Seller MJ, Nevin NC, Harris R, Read AP, Fielding DW. Possible prevention of neural tube defects by periconceptional vitamin supplementation. *Lancet* 1980;1:339–340.
37. Steinbok P, Irvine B, Cochrane DD, Irwin BJ. Long-term outcome and complications of children born with meningomyelocele. *Child's Nervous System* 1992;8:92–96.
38. Osaka K, Matsumoto S, Tanimura T. Myeloschisis in early human embryos. *Child's Brain* 1978;4:347–359.
39. McLone DG. Results of treatment of children born with a myelomeningocele. *Clin Neurosurg* 1983;30:407–412.
40. McLone DG, Dias MS. Complications of myelomenigocele closure. *Pediatr Neurosurg* 1991–92;17:267–273.
41. McLone DG, Naidich TP. Myelomeningocele: outcome and late complications. In: McLaurin RL, Venes JL, Schut L, Epstein F, eds. *Pediatric Neurosurgery*, 2nd ed. Philadelphia: WB Saunders; 1989.
42. McLone DG, Naidich TP. Myelomeningocele. In: Hoffman HJ, Epstein F, eds. *Disorders of the Developing Nervous System: Diagnosis and Treatment.* Boston: Blackwell Scientific; 1986:Ch. 6.
43. Ulmer JL, Elser AE, Ginsberg LE, Williams DW III. Klippel-Feil syndrome: CT and MR of acquired and congenital abnormalities of cervical spine and cord. *J Comput Assist Tomogr* 1993;17: 215–224.
44. Luthy DA, Wardinsky TW, Shurtleff DB, Hollenbach KA, Hickok DE, Nyberg DA, Benedetti TJ. Cesarean section before the onset of labor and subsequent motor function in infants with meningomyelocele diagnosed antenatally. *N Engl J Med* 1991;324:662–666.
45. McLone DG. Technique for closure of myelomeningocele. *Childs Brain* 1980;6:65–73.
46. McLone DG, Suwa J, Collins JA, Poznanski S, Knepper PA. Neurulation: biochemical and morphological studies on primary and secondary neural tube defects. In: *Concepts in Pediatric Neurosurgery*, vol 4. Basel: S. Karger; 1983:15–29.
47. Herman JM, McLone DG, Storrs BB, Dauser RC. Analysis of

153 patients with myelomeningocele or spinal lipoma reoperated upon for a tethered cord. *Pediatr Neurosurg* 1993; 19:243–249.
48. Banta JV, Bonanni C, Prebluda JL. Latex anaphylaxis during spinal surgery in children with myelomeningocele. *Develop Med Child Neurol* 1993; 35:543–548.
49. McLone DG. Continuing concepts in the management of spina bifida. *Pediatr Neurosurg* 1992; 18:254–256.
50. Just M, Schwarz M, Ludwig B, Emert J, Thelen M. Cerebral and spinal MR findings in patients with post-repair myelomeningocele. *Pediatr Radiol* 1990; 20:262–266.
51. Reigel DH, Tchernoukha K, Bdazmi B, Kortyna R, Rotenstein D. Change in spinal curvature following release of tethered spinal cord associated with spina bifida. *Pediatr Neurosurg* 1994; 20:30–42.
52. Barson AJ. Radiological studies of spina bifida cystica: the phenomenon of congenital lumbar kyphosis. *Br J Radiol* 1965; 38: 294–300.
53. Hoppenfeld S. Congenital kyphosis in myelomeningocele. *J Bone Joint Surg [Br]* 1967; 49B:276–280.
54. Piggott H. The natural history of scoliosis in myelodysplasia. *J Bone Joint Surg [Br]* 1980; 62B:54–58.
55. Winter RB, Moe JH, Wang JF. Congenital kyphosis: its natural history and treatment as observed in a study of one hundred and thirty patients. *J Bone Joint Surg [Am]* 1973; 55A:223–256.
56. Winter RB, Moe JH, Bradford DS. Congenital thoracic lordosis. *J Bone Joint Surg [Am]* 1978; 60A:806–810.
57. Robin GC. Scoliosis of spina bifida and infantile paraplegia. *Isr J Med Sci* 1972; 8:1823–1829.
58. Banta JV, Becker GJ. The natural history of scoliosis in myelomeningocele. *Scoliosis Research Society Orthopaedic Transactions* 1986; 10:18.
59. Lindseth RE, Stelzer L Jr. Vertebral excision for kyphosis in children with myelomeningocele. *J Bone Joint Surg [Am]* 1979; 61A: 699–704.
60. Loder RT, Shapiro P, Towbin R, Aronson DD. Aortic anatomy in children with myelomeningocele and congenital lumbar kyphosis. *J Pediatr Ortho* 1991; 11:31–35.
61. Fromm B, Carstens C, Niethard, FU, Lang R. Aortography in children with myelomeningocele and lumbar kyphosis. *J Bone Joint Surg [Br]* 1992; 74B:691–694.
62. Storrs BB. Are dermoid and epidermoid tumors preventable complications of myelomeningocele repair? *Pediatr Neurosurg* 1994; 20:160–162.
63. Chadduck, WM, Roloson GJ. Dermoid in the filum terminale of a newborn with myelomeningocele. *Pediatr Neurosurg* 1993; 19: 81–83.
64. Scott RM, Wolpert SM, Bartoshesky LE, Zimbler S, Klauber GT. Dermoid tumors occurring at the site of previous myelomeningocele repair. *J Neurosurg* 1986; 65:779–783.
65. Naidich TP, Gorey MT, McLone D. Congenital anomalies of the spine and spinal cord. In: Putman CE, Ravin CE, eds. *Textbook of Diagnostic Imaging.* Philadelphia: WB Saunders; 1987:Ch. 27.
66. Naidich TP, McLone DG. Congenital pathology of the spine and spinal cord. In: Taveras JM, Ferucci JT, eds. *Radiology—Diagnosis/Imaging/Intervention.* Philadelphia: JB Lipincott; 1986: Ch. 103.
67. Naidich TP. McLone DG. Congenital pathology of the spine and spinal cord. In: Taveras JM, Ferucci JT, eds. *Radiology—Diagnosis/Imaging/Intervention.* Philadelphia, J. B. Lipincott; revised 1989:chap 103.
68. Batnitzky S, Hall PV, Lindseth RE, Wellman HN. Meningomyelocele and syringohydromyelia: some radiological aspects. *Radiology* 1976; 120:351–357.
69. Cameron AH. The Arnold Chiari and other neuroanatomical malformations associated with spina bifida. *J Pathol Bacteriol* 1957; 73:195–211.
70. Emery JL, Lendon RG. The local cord lesion in neurospinal dysraphism meningomyelocele. *J Pathol* 1973; 110:83–96.
71. Hall PV, Campbell RL, Kalsbeck JE. Meningomyelocele and progressive hydromyelia: progressive paresis in myelodysplasia. *J Neurosurg* 1975; 43:457–463.
72. Breningstall GN, Marker SM, Tubman DE. Hydrosyringomyelia and diastematomyelia detected by MRI in myelomeningocele. *Pediatr Neurol* 1992; 8:267–271.
73. Park TS, Hoffman HJ, Hendrick EB, Humphreys RP. Experience with surgical decompression of the Arnold-Chiari malformation in young infants with myelomeningocele. *Neurosurgery* 1983; 13: 147–152.
74. Emery JL, MacKenzie N. Medullo-cervical dislocation deformity Chiari II deformity related to neurospinal dysraphism meningomyelocele. *Brain* 1973; 96:155–62.
75. Duckworth T, Sharrard WJ, Lister J, Seymour N. Hemimyelocele. *Develop Med Child Neurol* 1968;(Suppl 10); 16:69–75.
76. El Gammel T, Mark EK, Brooks BS. MR imaging of Chiari II malformation. *AJNR* 1987; 8:1037–1044.
77. Wolpert SM, Anderson M, Scott RM, Kwan ES, Runge VM. Chiari II malformation: MR imaging evaluation. *AJNR* 1987; 8:783–792.
78. Wolpert SM, Scott RM, Platenberg C. Runge VM. The clinical significance of hindbrain herniation and deformity as shown on MR images of patients with Chiari II malformation. *AJNR* 1988; 9:1075–1078.
79. Bell WO, Charney EB, Bruce DA, Sutton LN, Schut L. Symptomatic Arnold-Chiari malformation: review of experience with 22 cases. *J Neurosurg* 1987; 66:812–816.
80. Vandertop WP, Asai A, Hoffman HJ, Drake JM, Humphreys RP, Rutka JT, Becker LE. Surgical decompression for symptomatic Chiari II malformation in neonates with myelomeningocele. *J Neurosurg* 1992; 77:541–544.
81. Cochrane DD, Adderley R, White CP, Normal M, Steinbok P. Apnea in patients with myelomeningocele. *Pediatr Neurosurg* 1990–91; 16:232–239.
82. McLone DG, Knepper PA. The cause of Chiari II malformation: a unified theory. *Pediatr Neurosci* 1989; 15:1–12.
83. Yousefzadeh DK, El-Khoury GY, Smith W L. Normal sagittal diameter and variation in the pediatric cervical spine. *Radiology* 1982; 144:319–325.
84. Ruge JR, Masciopinto J, Storrs BB, McLone DG. Anatomical progression of the Chiari II malformation. *Child's Nervous System* 1992; 8:86–91.
85. Matson DD. *Neurosurgery of Infancy and Childhood*, 2nd ed. Springfield, IL: Charles C Thomas; 1969.
86. Wright RL. Congenital dermal sinuses. *Prog Neurol Surg* 1971; 4: 175–191.
87. Scotti G, Harwood-Nash DC. Congenital thoracic dermal sinus: diagnosis by computer assisted metrizamide myelography. *J Comput Assist Tomogr* 1980; 4:675–677.
88. Benzil DL, Epstein MH, Knuckey NW. Intramedullary epidermoid associated with an intramedullary spinal abscess secondary to a dermal sinus. *Neurosurgery* 1992; 30:118–121.
89. Menezes AH, Graf CJ, Perret GE. Spinal cord abscesses: a review. *Surg Neurol* 1977; 8:461–470.
90. Haworth JC, Zachary RB. Congenital dermal sinuses in children: their relation to pilonidal sinuses. *Lancet* 1955; 2:10.
91. Naidich TP, McLone DG, Shkolnik A, Fernbach SK. Sonographic evaluation of caudal spine anomalies in children. *AJNR* 198; 4:661–664.
92. Naidich TP, Radkowski MA. Britton J. Real-time sonographic display of caudal spinal anomalies. *Neuroradiology* 1986; 28:512–527.
93. Lunardi P, Missori P, Gagliardi FM, Fortuna A. Long term results of the surgical treatment of spinal dermoid and epidermoid tumors. *Neurosurgery* 1989; 25:860–864.
94. Penisson-Besnier I, Guy G, Gandon Y. Intramedullary epidermoid cyst evaluated by computed tomographic scan and magnetic resonance imaging: case report. *Neurosurgery* 1989; 25:955–959.
95. Graham DV, Tampieri D, Villemure J-G. Intramedullary dermoid tumor diagnosed with the assistance of magnetic resonance imaging. *Neurosurgery* 1988; 23:765–767.
96. Algra PR, Hageman LM, Gadopentetate dimeglumine-enhanced MR imaging of spinal dermal sinus tract [Letter]. *AJNR* 1991; 12: 1025–1026.
97. Barkovich AJ. Gadopentetate dimeglumine-enhanced MR imaging of spinal dermal sinus tract [Letter]. *AJNR* 1991; 12:1026.
98. Gorey M, Naidich TP, McLone DG. Case report—double discontinuous lipomyelomeningocele: CT findings. *J Comput Assist Tomog* 1985; 9:584–591.

99. Lemire RJ, Graham CB, Beckwith JB. Skin-covered sacrococcygeal masses in infants and children. *J Pediatr* 1971;79:948–954.
100. Hoffman HJ, Taecholarn C, Hendrick EB, Humphreys RP. Management of lipomyelomeningoceles. Experience at the Hospital for Sick Children, Toronto. *J Neurosurg* 1985;62:1–8.
101. Pierre-Kahn A, Lacombe J, Pichon J, Giudicelli Y, Renier D, Sainte-Rose C, Perrigot M, Hirsch J-F. Intraspinal lipomas with spina bifida. Prognosis and treatment in 73 cases. *J Neurosurg* 1986; 65:756–761.
102. McLone DG, Mutluer S, Naidich TP. Lipomeningoceles of the conus medullaris. In: *Concepts in Pediatric Neurosurgery*, vol 3. American Society for Pediatric Neurosurgeons. Basel: S. Karger; 1982:170–177.
103. Guiffre R. Intradural spinal lipomas: review of the literature. 99 cases and report of an additional case. *Acta Neurochir* 1966;114: 69.
104. McLone DG, Naidich TP. Laser resection of fifty spinal lipomas. *Neurosurgery* 1986;118:611–615.
105. Brophy JD, Sutton LN, Zimmerman RA, Bury E, Schut L. *Neurosurgery* 1989;25:336–340.
106. Aoki N. Rapid growth of intraspinal lipoma demonstrated by magnetic resonance imaging. *Surg Neurol* 1990;34:107–110.
107. Yamada S, Zinke DE, Sanders D. Pathophysiology of "tethered cord syndrome." *J Neurosurg* 1981;54:491–503.
108. Barolat G, Schaefer D, Zeme S. Recurrent spinal cord tethering by sacral nerve root following lipomyelomeningocele surgery. Case report. *J Neurosurg* 1991;75:143–145.
109. Sakamoto H, Hakuba A, Fujitani K, Nishimura S. Surgical treatment of the retethered spinal cord after repair of lipomyelomeningocele. *J Neurosurg* 1991;74:709–714.
110. Hendrick EB, Hoffman HJ, Humphreys RP. The tethered spinal cord. *Clin Neurosurg* 1983;30:457–463.
111. Kernohan JW. The ventriculus terminalis: its growth and development. *J Comparative Neurol* 1924;38:107–125.
112. Lendon RG, Emery JL. Forking of the central canal in the equinal cord of children. *J Anat* 1970;106:499–505.
113. Kunitomo K. The development and reduction of the tail and of the caudal end of the spinal cord. *Contrib Embryol* 1918;8:161–198.
114. Streeter G. Factors involved in the formation of the filum terminale. *Am J Anat* 1919;25:1–11.
115. Tarlov IM. Structure of the filum terminale. *Arch Neurol Psychiatry* 1938;40:1–17.
116. Barson AJ. The vertebral level of termination of the spinal cord during normal and abnormal development. *J Anat* 1970;106: 489–497.
117. Hawass ND, El-Badawi MG, Fatani JA, Meshari AA, Abbas FS, Edrees YB, Jabbar FA, Banna M. Myelographic study of the spinal cord ascent during fetal development. *AJNR* 1987;8:691–695.
118. Fitz CR, Harwood-Nash DC. The tethered conus. *Am J Roentgenol Radium Ther Nucl Med* 1975;125:515–523.
119. Love JG, Daly DD, Harris LE. Tight filum terminale: report of condition in three siblings. *JAMA* 1961;176:31.
120. Emery JL, Lendon RG. Lipomas of the cauda equina and other fatty tumors related to neurospinal dysraphism. *Dev Med Child Neurol* 1969;(Suppl 11):20:62–70.
121. Feldman M, Byrne P, Johnson MA, Fischer J, Lees G. Neonatal sacrococcygeal teratoma: multi-imaging modality assessment. *J Pediatr Surg* 1990:25:675–678.
122. Schropp KP, Lobe TE, Rao B, Mutabagani K, Kay GA, Gilchrist BF, Philippe PG, Boles ET Jr. Sacrococcygeal teratoma: the experience of four decades. *J Pediatr Surg* 1992;27:1075–1079.
123. Gross RE, Clatworthy HW, Meeker IA. Sacrococcygeal teratomas in infants and children. *Surg Gynecol Obstet* 1951;92:341–354
124. Altman RP, Randolph JG, Lily JR. Sacrococcygeal teratoma: American Academy of Pediatrics Surgical Section Survey—1973. *J Pediatr Surg* 1974;9:389–398.
125. Hunt PT, Davidson KC, Ashcraft KW, Holder TM. Radiography of hereditary presacral teratoma. *Radiology* 1977;122:187–191.
126. Noseworthy J, Lack EE, Kozakewich HPW, et al. Sacrococcygeal germ cell tumors in childhood: an updated experience with 118 patients. *J Pediatr Surg* 1981;16:358–364.
127. Schey WL, Shkolnik A, White H. Clinical and radiographic considerations of sacrococcygeal teratomas: an analysis of 26 new cases and review of the literature. *Radiology* 1977;125:189–195.
128. Malone PS, Spitz L, Kiely EM, Brereton RJ, Duffy PG, Ransley PG. The functional sequelae of sacrococcygeal teratoma. *J Pediatr Surg* 1990;25:679–680.
129. Havránek P, Hedlund H, Rubenson A, Güth D, Husberg M, Frykberg T, Larsson LT. Sacrococcygeal teratoma in Sweden between 1978 and 1989: long-term functional results. *J Pediatr Surg* 1992;27:916–918.
130. Rintala R, Lahdenne P, Lindahl H, Siimes LM, Heikinheimo M. Anorectal function in adults operated for a benign sacrococcygeal teratoma. *J Pediatr Surg* 1993;28:1165–1167.
131. Bilik R, Shandling B, Pope M, Thorner P, Weitzman S, Ein SH. Malignant benign neonatal sacrococcygeal teratoma. *J Pediatr Surg* 1993;28:1158–1160.
132. Fiandaca MS, Ross WK, Pearl GS, Bakay RAE. Carcinoid tumor in a presacral teratoma associated with an anterior sacral meningocele: case report and review of the literature. *Neurosurgery* 1988;22:581–588.
133. Currarino G, Coln D, Votteler T. Triad of anorectal, sacral, and presacral anomalies. *AJR* 1981;137:395–398.
134. Teitelbaum D, Teich S, Cassidy S, Karp M, Cooney D, Gesner G. Highly vascularized sacrococcygeal teratoma: description of this atypical variant and its operative management. *J Pediatr Surg* 1994;29:98–101.
135. Nakayama DK, Killian A, Hill LM, Miller JP, Hannakan C, Lloyd DA, Rowe MI. The newborn with hydrops and sacrococcygeal teratoma. *J Pediatr Surg* 1991;26:1435–1438.
136. Calenda E, Bachy B, Guyard MD. Sacrococcygeal teratoma and venous shunting through a tumor: biological evidence [Letter]. *Anesth Anal* 1992;74:165–166.
137. Stringer DA, Sprigg A, Kerrigan D, Liu P, Daneman A, Sonley M. Malignant carcinoid within a recurrent sacrococcygeal teratoma in childhood. *Can Assoc Radiol* J 1990;41:105–107.
138. Powell RW, Weber ED, Manci EA. Intradural extension of a sacrococcygeal teratoma. *J Pediatr Surg* 1993;28:770–772.
139. Mahour GH. Sacrococcygeal teratoma: the experience of four decades. Discussion. *J Pediatr Surg* 1992;27:107–1079.
140. Lahdenne P, Heikinheimo M, Nikkanen V, Klemi P, Siimes MA, Rapola J. Neonatal benign sacrococcygeal teratoma may recur in adulthood and give rise to malignancy. *Cancer* 1993;72:3727–3731.
141. Sigal R, Denys A, Halimi P, Shapeero L, Doyon D, Boudghène F. Ventriculus terminalis of the conus madullaris: MR imaging in four patients with congenital dilatation. *AJNR* 1991;12:733–737.
142. Coleman LT, Zimmerman RA, Rorke LB. The fifth ventricle: ventriculus terminalis of the conus medullaris: MR findings in children. *AJNR* 1995;[*in press*].
143. Iskander BJ, Oakes WJ, McLaughlin C, Osumi ALK, Tien RD. Terminal syringohydromyelia and occult spinal dysraphism. *J Neurosurg* 1994;81:513–519.
144. Kaffenberger DA, Heinz ER, Oakes JW, Boyko O. Meningocele manqué: radiologic findings with clinical correlation. *AJNR* 1992;13:1083–1088.
145. Warf BC, Scott RM, Barnes PD, Hendren WH III. Tethered spinal cord with anorectal urogenital malformations. *Pediatr Neurosurg* 1993;19:25–30.
146. Davidoff AM, Thompson CV, Grimm JM, Shorter NA, Filston HC, Oakes WJ. Occult spinal dysraphism in patients with anal agenesis. *J Pediatr Surg* 1991;26:1001–1005.
147. Karrer FM, Flannery AM, Nelson MD Jr, Raffensperger JG. Anorectal malformations: evaluation of associated spinal dysraphic syndromes. *J Pediatr Surg* 1988;23:45–48
148. McLone DG. Naidich TP. Terminal myelocystocele. *Neurosurgery* 1985;16:36–43.
149. Vade A, Kennard D. Lipomeningomyelocystocele. *AJNR* 1987;8:375–377.
150. Carey JC, Greenbaum B, Hall BD. The OEIS complex omphalocele, exstrophy, imperforate anus, spinal defects. *Birth Defects* 1978;14:253–263.
151. Peacock WJ, Murovic JA. Magnetic resonance imaging in myelocystoceles: report of 2 cases. *Neurosurgery* 1989;70:804–807.

152. Tibbles L, Wiley MJ. A comparative study of the effects of retinoic acid given during the critical period for inducing spina bifida in mice and hamsters. *Teratology* 1988;37:113–125.
153. Bhargava R, Hammond DI, Benzie RJ, Carlos E, Ventureyra G,Higgins, MJ, Martin DJ. Prenatal demonstration of a cervical myelocystocele. *Prenatal Diagnosis* 1992;12:653–659.
154. Berdon WE, Hochberg B, Baker DH, Grossman H. Santulli TV. The association of lumbosacral spine and genitourinary anomalies with imperforate anus. *Am J Roentgenol* 1966;98:181–191.
155. Carlo WA, Kliegman RM, Dixon MS Jr, Fletcher, BD, Fanaroff AA. Vertebral agenesis: comprehensive care and outcome. *Am J Dis Child* 1982;136:533–537.
156. Duhamel B. From the mermaid to anal imperforation: the syndrome of caudal regression. *Arch Dis Child* 1961;36:152.
157. Kallen B, Winberg J. Caudal mesoderm pattern of anomalies: from renal agenesis to sirenomelia. *Teratology* 1974;9:99–111.
158. Renshaw TS. Sacral agenesis: a classification and review of twenty-three cases. *J Bone Joint Surg [Am]* 1978;60A:373–283.
159. Rubenstein MA, Bucy JG. Caudal regression syndrome: the urologic implications. *J Urol* 1975;114:934–937.
160. Sarnat HB, Case ME, Graviss R. Sacral agensis: neurologic and neuropathologic features. *Neurology* 1976;26:1124–1129.
161. Cohen AR. The mermaid malformation: cloacal exstrophy and occult spinal dysraphism. *Neurosurgery* 1991;28:834–843.
162. Twickler D, Budorick N, Pretorius D, Grafe M, Currarino G. Caudal regression versus sirenomelia. *J Ultrasound Med* 1993;12: 323–330.
163. Crawfurd M d'A, Cheshire J, Wilson TM, Woodhouse CRJ. The demonstration of monozygosity in twins discordant for sacral agenesis. *J Med Genet* 1992;29:437–438.
164. Muthukumar N, Gurunathan J, Sampathkumar M, Gajendran R, Sacral agenesis occurring in siblings: case report. *Neurosurgery* 1992;30:946–948.
165. Passarge E. Lenz W. Syndrome of caudal regression in infants of diabetic mothers: observations of further cases. *Pediatrics* 1966;37:672–675.
166. Pappas CTE, Seaver L, Carrion C, Rekate H. Anatomical evaluation of the caudal regression syndrome lumbosacral agenesis with magnetic resonance imaging. *Neurosurgery* 1989;25:462–465.
167. Pang D. Sacral agenesis and caudal spinal cord malformations. *Neurosurgery* 1993;32:755–779.
168. Meizner I, Press F, Jaffe A, Carmi R. Prenatal ultrasound diagnosis of complete absence of the lumbar spine and sacrum. *J Clin Ultrasound* 1992;20:77–80.
169. Hudson LP, Ramsay DA. Malformation of the lumbosacral spinal cord in a case of sacral agenesis. *Pediatr Pathol* 1993;13:421–429.
170. Price DL, Dooling EC, Richardson EP Jr. Caudal dysplasia caudal regression syndrome. *Arch Neurol* 1970;23:212–220.
171. Rusnak SL, Driscoll SG. Congenital spinal anomalies in infants of diabetic mothers. *Pediatrics* 1965;35:989–995.
172. Towfighi J, Housman C. Spinal cord abnormalities in caudal regression syndrome. *Acta Neuropathol* 1991;81:458–466.
173. O'Neill OR, Roman-Goldstein S, Piatt JH Jr. Sacral agenesis associated with spinal cord syrinx. *Pediatr Neurosurg* 1994;20;217–220.
174. Pang D, Hoffman HJ. Sacral agenesis with progressive neurological deficit. *Neurosurgery* 1980;7:118–126.
175. Schneider MB, Dittmar S, Boxer RA. Anterior sacral meningocele presenting as a pelvic/abdominal mass in a patient with Marfan syndrome. *J Adolesc Health* 1993;14:325–328.
176. Lee KS, Gower DJ, McWhorter JM, Albertson DA. The role of MR imaging in the diagnosis and treatment of anterior sacral meningocele. Report of 2 cases. *J Neurosurg* 1988;69:628–631.
177. Hafeez M, Tihansky DP. Intraspinal tumor with lumbosacral agenesis. *AJNR* 1984;5:481–482.
178. Thomas M, Halaby FA, Hirschauer JS. Hereditary occurrence of anterior sacral meningocele: report of ten cases. *Spine* 1987;12: 351–354.
179. Jackman RJ, Clark PLeM III, Smith ND. Retrorectal tumors. *JAMA* 1951;145:956–962.
180. Amacher AL, Drake CG, McLachin AD. Anterior sacral meningocele. *Surg Gynecol Obstet* 1968;126:986–994.
181. Smith HP, Davis CH Jr. Anterior sacral meningocele: two case reports and discussion of surgical approach. *Neurosurgery* 1980;7:61–67.
182. Naidich TP, McLone DG, Harwood-Nash DC. Arachnoid cysts, paravertebral meningoceles, and perineurial cysts. In: Newton TH, Potts EG, eds. *Modern Neuroradiology, vol 1, Computed Tomography of the Spine and Spinal Cord.* San Anselmo, CA: Clavadel Press; 1983:Ch. 20.
183. North RB, Kidd DH, Wang H. Occult, bilateral anterior sacral and intrasacral meningeal and perineurial cysts: case report and review of the literature. *Neurosurgery* 1990;27:981–986.
184. Chamaa MT, Berney JA. Anterior-sacral meningocele; value of magnetic resonance imaging and abdominal sonography. *Acta Neurochir (Wien)* 1991;109:154–157.
185. Dyck P, Wilson CB. Anterior sacral meningocele: case report. *J Neurosurg* 1980;53:548–552.
186. Erkulvrawatr S, El Gammal T, Hawkins J, Green JB, Srinivasan G. Intrathoracic meningoceles and neurofibromatosis. *Arch Neurol* 1979;36:557–559.
187. Fahrenkrug A, Hojgaard K. Multiple paravertebral lumbar meningocele. *Br J Radiol* 1963;36:574.
188. Beardmore HE, Wiglesworth FW. Vertebral anomalies and alimentary duplications: clinical and embryological aspects. *Pediatr Clin North Am* 1958;5:457–473.
189. Burrows FGO, Sutcliffe J. The split notochord syndrome. *Br J Radiol* 1968;41:844–847.
190. Bentley JFR, Smith JR. Developmental posterior enteric remnants and spinal malformations: the split notochord syndrome. *Arch Dis Child* 1960;35:76–86.
191. Brooks BS, Duvall ER, El Gammal T, Garcia JH, Gupta KL, Kapila A. Neuroimaging features of neurenteric cysts: analysis of nine cases and review of the literature. *AJNR* 1993;14:735–746.
192. Hoffman CH, Dietrich RB, Pais MJ, Demos DS, Pribram HFW. The split notochord syndrome with dorsal enteric fistula. *AJNR* 1993;14:622–627.
193. Cohen J. Sledge CB. Diastematomyelia: an embryological interpretation with report of a case. *Am J Dis Child* 1960;100:257–263.
194. Han JS, Benson JE, Kaufman B, Rekate HL, Alfidi RJ, Bohlman HH, Kaufman B. Demonstration of diastematomyelia and associated abnormalities with MR imaging. *AJNR* 1985;6:215–219.
195. Harwood-Nash DC, McHugh K. Diastematomyelia in 172 children: the impact of modern neuroradiology. *Pediatr Neurosurg* 1990–91;16:247–251.
196. Miller AW, Guille JT, Bowen JR. Evaluation and treatment of diastematomyelia. *J Bone Joint Surg [Am]* 1993;75A,1308–1317.
197. Russell NA, Benoit BG, Joaquin AJ. Diastematomyelia in adults. A review. *Pediatr Neurosurg* 1990–91;16:252–257.
198. Gower DJ, Curlin, OD, Kelly DL Jr, Alexander E Jr. Diastematomyelia—a 40-year experience. *Pediatr Neurosci* 1988;14:90–96.
199. Pang D. Split cord malformation. Part II: clinical syndrome. *Neurosurgery* 1992;31:481–500.
200. Rilliet B, Berney J, Schowing J, Berney J. Pathogenesis of diastematomyelia: can a surgical model in the chick embryo give some clues about the human malformation? *Child's Nervous System* 1992;8:310–316.
201. Pang D, Dias MS, Ahab-Barmada M. Split cord malformation. Part I: a unified theory of embryogenesis for double spinal cord malformations. *Neurosurgery* 1992;31:451–480.
202. Herman TE, Siegel MJ. Cervical and basicranial diastematomyelia. *AJR* 1990;154:806–808.
203. Pfeifer JD. Basicranial diastematomyelia: a case report. *Clin Neuropathol* 1991;10:232–236.
204. Hilal SK, Marton D, Pollack E. Diastematomyelia in children: radiographic study of 34 cases. *Radiology* 1974;112:609–621.
205. Schlesinger AE, Naidich TP, Quencer RM. Concurrent hydromyelia and diastematomyelia. *AJNR* 1986;7:473–477.
206. Beyerl BD, Ojemann RG, Davis KR, Hedley-Whyte ET, Mayberg MR. Cervical diastematomyelia presenting in adulthood: case report. *J Neurosurg* 1985;62:449–453.
207. Rawanduzy A, Murali R. Cervical spine diastematomyelia in adulthood. *Neurosurgery* 1991;28:459–461.
208. Azimullah PC, Smit LME, Rietveld-Kol E, Valk J. Malformations of the spinal cord in 53 patients with spina bifida studied by

magnetic resonance imaging. *Child's Nervous System* 1991;7:63–66.
209. O'Rahilly R, Meyer DB. The timing and sequence of events in the development of the human vertebral column during the embryonic period proper. *Anat Embryol* 1979:157:167–176.
210. Bagnall KM, Harris PF, Jones PRM. A radiographic study of the human fetal spine. 2. The sequence of development of ossification centres in the vertebral column. *J Anat* 1977;124:791–802.
211. O'Rahilly R, Müller F, Meyer DB. The human vertebral column at the end of the embryonic period proper. 3. The thoracicolumbar region. *J Anat* 1990;168:81–93.
212. Kjaer I, Kjaer TW, Graem N. Ossification sequence of occipital bone and vertebrae in human fetuses. *J Craniofac Genet Dev Biol* 1993;13:83–88.
213. Bareggi R, Grill, V, Sandrucci MA, Galdini G, De Pol A, Forabosco A, Narducci P. Developmental pathways of vertebral centra and neural arches in human embryos and fetuses. *Anat Embryol* 1993;187:139–144.
214. Noback CR, Robertson GG. Sequences of appearance of ossification centers in the human skeleton during the first five prenatal months. *Am J Anat* 1951;89:1–28.
215. Ford DM, McFadden,KD, Bagnall KM. Sequence of ossificiation in human vertebral neural arch centers. *Anat Rec* 1982;203:175–178.
216. Budorick NE, Pretorius DH, Grafe MR, Lou KV. Ossification of the fetal spine. *Radiology* 1991;181:561–565.
217. Bailey DK. The normal cervical spine in infants and children. *Radiology* 1982;59:712–719.
218. Brown MW, Templeton AW, Hodges FJ. The incidence of acquired and congenital fusions in the cervical spine. *Am J Roentgenol Radium Ther Nucl Med* 1964;92:1255–1259.
219. Cone RO, Flournoy J, MacPherson RI. The craniocervical junction. *Radiographics* 1981;1:1–37.
220. Epstein BS. *The Spine: A Radiological Text and Atlas,* 3rd ed. Philadelphia: Lea & Febiger; 1969.
221. Fielding JW. Disappearance of the central portion of the odontoid process: a case report. *J Bone Joint Surg* [*Am*] 1965;47A:1228–1230.
222. Gray SW, Romaine CB, Skandalakis JE. Congenital fusion of the cervical vertebrae. *Surg Gynecol Obstet* 1964;118:373–385.
223. Gunderson CH, Greenspan RH, Glaser GH, Lubo HA. The Klippel- Feil syndrome: genetic and clinical reevaluation of cervical fusion. *Medicine* 1967;46:491–512.
224. Gwinn JL, Smith JL. Acquired and congenital absence of the odontoid process. *Am J Roentgenol Radium Ther Nucl Med* 1962;88:424–431.
225. Juberg RC, Gershanik JJ. Cervical vertebral fusion Klippel-Feil syndrome with consanguineous parents. *J Med Genetics* 1976;13:246–249.
226. Klippel M, Feil A. Un cas d'absence des vertebres cervicales. *Nov Iconogr Salpet* 1912;25:223–250.
227. List CF. Developmental anomalies of the craniovertebral border. In: Khan EA, Crosby EC, Schneider RC, Turen JA, eds. *Correlative Neurosurgery*, 2nd ed. Springfield, IL: Charles C Thomas; 1969:432–443.
228. Sherk HH, Shut L, Chung S. Iniencephalic deformity of the cervical spine with Klippel-Feil and congenital elevation of the scapula. *J Bone Joint Surg* [*Am*] 1974; 56A:1254–1259.
229. Spillane JD, Pallis C, Jones AM. Developmental abnormalities in the region of the foramen magnum. *Brain* 1957;80:11–48.
230. Truex RC, Johnson CH. Congenital anomalies of the upper cervical spine. *Orthop Clin North Am* 1978;9:891–900.
231. Shands AR Jr, Bundens WD. Congenital deformities of the spine. An analysis of the roentgenograms of 700 children. *Bull Hosp Joint Dis* 1956;17:110.
232. Southworth JD, Bersack SR. Anomalies of the lumbosacral vertebrae in five hundred and fifty individuals without symptoms referable to the low back. *Am J Roentgenol* 1950;64:624–634.
233. Friedman MM, Fischer FJ, VanDemark RE. Lumbosacral roentgenograms of one hundred soldiers: a control study. *Am J Roentgenol* 1946;55:292–298.
234. Hadley HG. Frequency of spina bifida. *VA Med Monthly* 1941;68:43–46.
235. Sutow WW, Pryde AW. Incidence of spina bifida occulta in relation to age. *AMA J Dis Child* 1956;91:211–217.
236. Bardsley JL, Hanelin LG. The unilateral hypoplastic lumbar pedicle. *Radiology* 1971;101:315–317.
237. Yousefzadeh D, El-Khoury GY, Lupetin AR. Congenital aplastic-hypoplastic lumbar pedicle in infants and young children. *Skeletal Radiol* 1982;7:259–265.
238. Michie I, Clark M. Neurological syndromes associated with cervical and craniocervical anomalies. *Arch Neurol* 1968;18:241–247.
239. Chestnut R, James JE, Jones KL. The VATER association and spinal dysraphia. *Pediatr Neurosurg* 1992;18:144–148.
240. Duncan PA, Shapiro LR. Interrelationships of the hemifacial microsomia-VATER, VATER, and sirenomelia phenotypes. *Am J Med Genet* 1993;47:75–84.
241. Raffel C, Litofsky S, McComb JG. Central nervous system malformations and the VATER association. *Pediatr Neurosurg* 1990–91;16:170–173
242. Smith NM, Chambers HM, Furness ME, Haan EA. The OEIS complex omphalocele-exstrophy-imperforate anus-spinal defects: recurrence in sibs. *J Med Genet* 1992;29:730–732.
243. O'Riordain DS, O'Connell PR, Kirwan WO. Hereditary sacral agenesis with presacral mass and anorectal stenosis: the Currarino triad. *Br J Surg* 1991;78:536–538.
244. Rodriguez JI, Palacios J, Lapunzina P. Severe axial anomalies in the oculo-auriculo-vertebral Goldenhar complex. *Am J Med Genet* 1993;47:69–74.
245. Geremia GK, Russell EJ, Clasen RA. MR imaging characteristics of a neurenteric cyst. *AJNR* 1988;9:978–980.

Magnetic Resonance Imaging of the Brain and Spine, Second Edition, edited by Scott W. Atlas. Lippincott-Raven Publishers, Philadelphia © 1996.

27

Neoplastic Disease of the Spine and Spinal Cord

Gordon Sze

Of all areas of spinal pathology, it may be in the field of spinal tumors that magnetic resonance imaging (MRI) has had the most impact. Almost immediately after its inception, even with the poor quality of early scans, the potential of MRI in the evaluation of suspected neoplasms of the cord was recognized (1,2). With the advent of surface coils and improved imaging techniques, the superiority of MRI over myelography and postmyelography computed tomography (CT) in the assessment of intramedullary tumors was established. MRI also proved to be as efficacious as the traditional modalities in the evaluation of suspected extradural tumor impingement on the thecal sac, and is less invasive (3–5). MRI was found to be more sensitive than nuclear medicine in the detection of lesions within the vertebral bodies (6). Finally, with the advent of contrast agents, MRI proved to be at least as effective as myelography and postmyelography CT in the evaluation of suspected intradural extramedullary tumors (7).

Spinal tumors are often categorized as extradural, intradural extramedullary, or intramedullary in location. This classification represents somewhat of an overgeneralization for two reasons. First, a given lesion may reside in two compartments simultaneously. For example, a neurofibroma in one case may be dumbbell-shaped and extend into both the extradural and the intradural extramedullary spaces. Second, in different cases, two lesions with identical pathology may occur in different compartments. For example, neurofibromas may occur in any of the three compartments, including the intramedullary

G. Sze, M.D.: Department of Diagnostic Radiology, Yale University School of Medicine, New Haven, CT 06510.

space. Nevertheless, this classification scheme is useful, because it is traditional and helps to characterize spinal tumors.

In the extradural space, numerous primary bone tumors can occur. However, with few exceptions, such as hemangioma, most of the primary bone tumors are comparatively unusual. Secondary tumors, or metastases, are far more common in the extradural space.

In the intradural extramedullary space, primary tumors, such as neurofibroma and meningioma, are relatively common. Secondary tumors or leptomeningeal metastases were formerly considered quite rare. However, this entity is now seen with increasing frequency (8). The increase is probably due to several factors. First, clinicians have a higher awareness of leptomeningeal tumor and greater suspicion of it under the appropriate clinical circumstances. Second, laboratory tests are more precise in identifying tumor cells in the cerebrospinal fluid (CSF). Third, as patients live longer with their tumors, they have more opportunity to develop ancillary complications of their disease, such as leptomeningeal tumor. Therefore, the increase currently seen in leptomeningeal tumor is one of both better diagnosis and an actual increase in its incidence.

Finally, in the intramedullary space, primary tumors are far more common than secondary tumors or metastases. Metastases to the cord itself are comparatively unusual.

EXTRADURAL TUMORS

Technique

Two objectives exist in the MR evaluation of spinal tumors in the epidural space: a) the detection of vertebral body lesions, even if there is no suspicion of epidural impingement; and b) the delineation of possible thecal sac impingement.

Unenhanced MR scans are generally superb at delineating extradural tumors, whether they are primary or secondary (1–5,9–11). Vertebral body lesions are usually well defined as low intensity lesions surrounded by the higher intensity of normal fat-containing marrow on short TR images. Before the development of MRI, bone

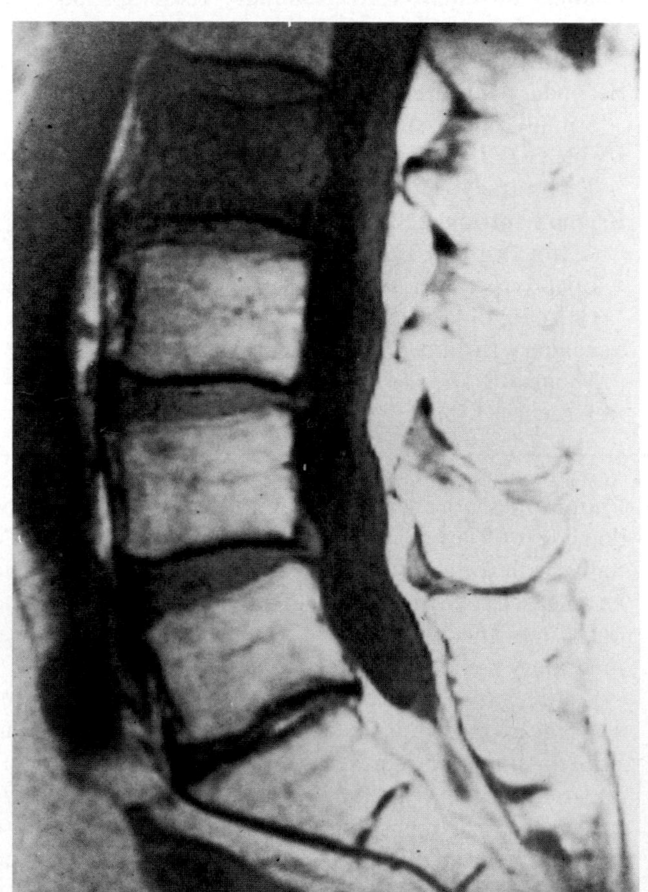

A

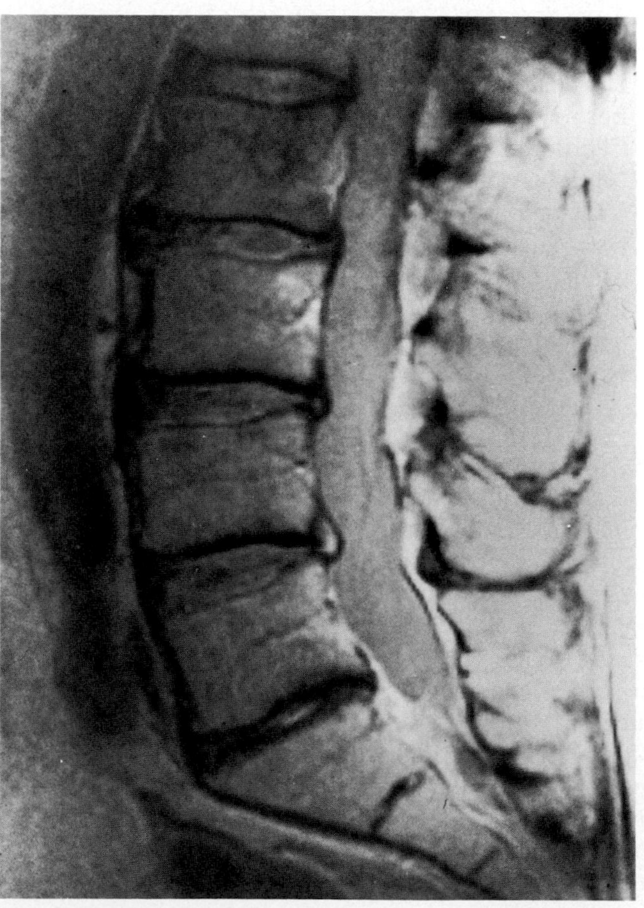

B

FIG. 1. Lung carcinoma metastasis. **A:** Short TR (600/20) sagittal MR scan shows low intensity in the L2 vertebral body, consistent with metastasis. **B:** Intermediate TR (1400/70) sagittal MR scan demonstrates increasing signal intensity of the L2 lesion. This lesion has now become virtually isointense with normal marrow. (From Sze, ref. 266, with permission.)

scans were considered the most sensitive means of detection of suspected tumors of the vertebral body. MRI, however, has been found to be more sensitive to marrow abnormalities (5,6,11). For example, very active lesions that might not be visible on a bone scan are generally detectable on MRI (5).

The standard MR parameters for the detection of vertebral body lesions generally consist of short TR/TE (T1-weighted) spin-echo (SE) sequences (3,5,9,11). These acquisitions are very sensitive to the high intensity of normal fat-containing marrow and show morphology in great detail. Intermediate TR scans are not generally useful because neoplasm and normal marrow can then appear isointense to each other (Fig. 1). Tumors usually are of low signal intensity on short TR sequences and of high signal intensity on long TR/TE (T2-weighted) sequences. Normal marrow, in contrast, generally is of high signal intensity on short TR scans and of less signal intensity on long TR scans. At intermediate repetition times, intensities of the lesion and of normal marrow may approach each other, dramatically decreasing the conspicuity of the tumor.

In occasional cases, uninvolved marrow appears of low signal, especially in young patients in whom the vertebral body marrow does not contain much fat or in patients with the anemia of chronic disease who are hypothesized to have altered metabolism of iron (11,12). In these cases, the low intensity lesions are not highlighted by the surrounding high intensity marrow, and it may be difficult to detect tumor (Fig. 2). Long TR SE sequences, short T1 inversion recovery sequences, or gradient-echo (GE) sequences may help for further evaluation (13,14). Fast spin-echo (FSE) sequences must be used with caution because the persistent high signal of surrounding fat on long TR images may decrease visualization of tumor.

Impingement on the thecal sac can occur by extension of vertebral body tumor or by neoplastic growth in the epidural space itself. Previously, myelography and post-myelography CT were standard in the evaluation of suspected epidural disease. However, current evidence suggests the MRI is competitive in accuracy and much less invasive (2–4). Good quality MR scans of the spine are generally very precise in showing impingement on the thecal sac. Short TR SE sequences are ideal, particularly when lesions are visualized in two orthogonal planes. However, in some cases, particularly when disease is extensive, long TR or GE acquisitions can also be of help. By producing a myelographic effect with the CSF of high signal, they can better delineate regions of impingement (Fig. 3).

MRI can also be useful in patients with compression fractures of the vertebral bodies in order to differentiate

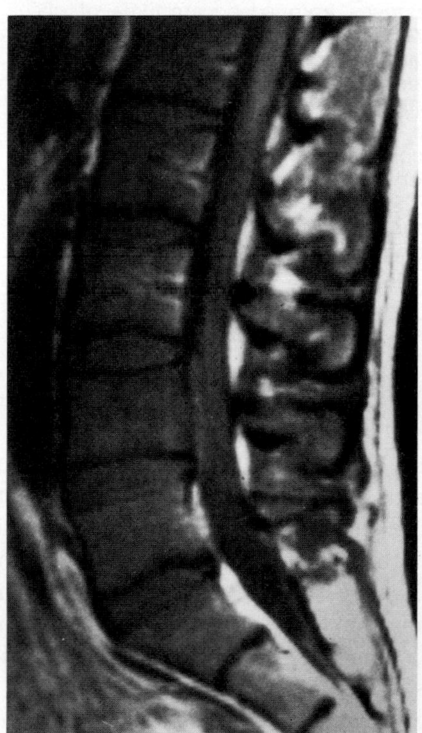
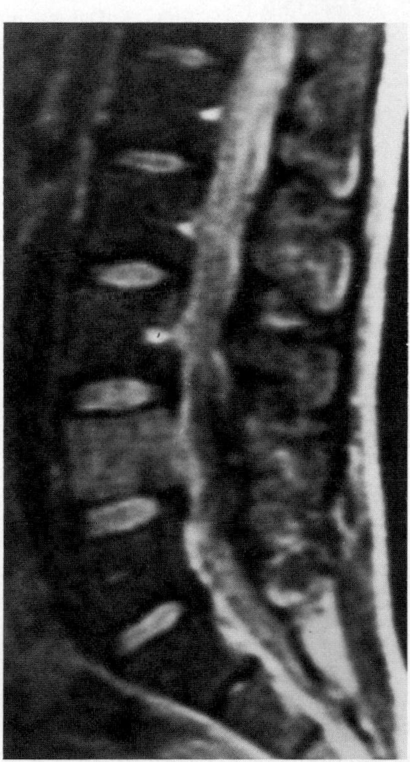
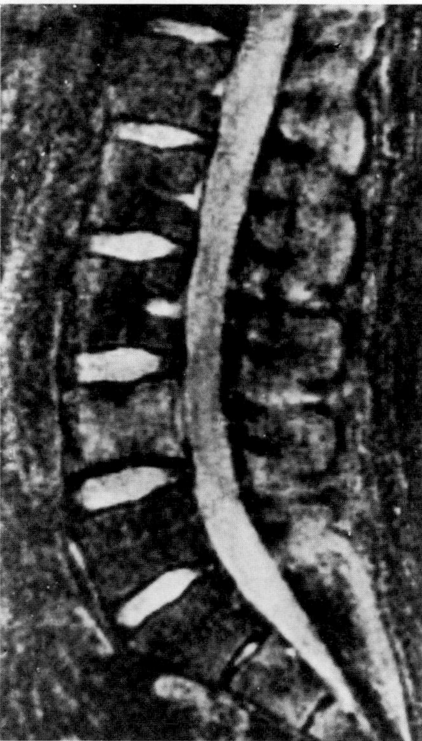

A B,C

FIG. 2. Seminoma metastases in a young man. **A:** Short TR (600/20) sagittal MR image discloses that all the vertebral bodies are nearly equal in signal intensity. In this young patient, even normal marrow appears somewhat low in signal intensity because of the paucity of fat in the red marrow. **B,C:** Long TR (2000/70) and short T1 inversion recovery (2000/40/140) sagittal MR scans disclose the lesion, which has now become of high signal intensity compared with the low signal intensity of normal marrow. (From Sze, ref. 266, with permission.)

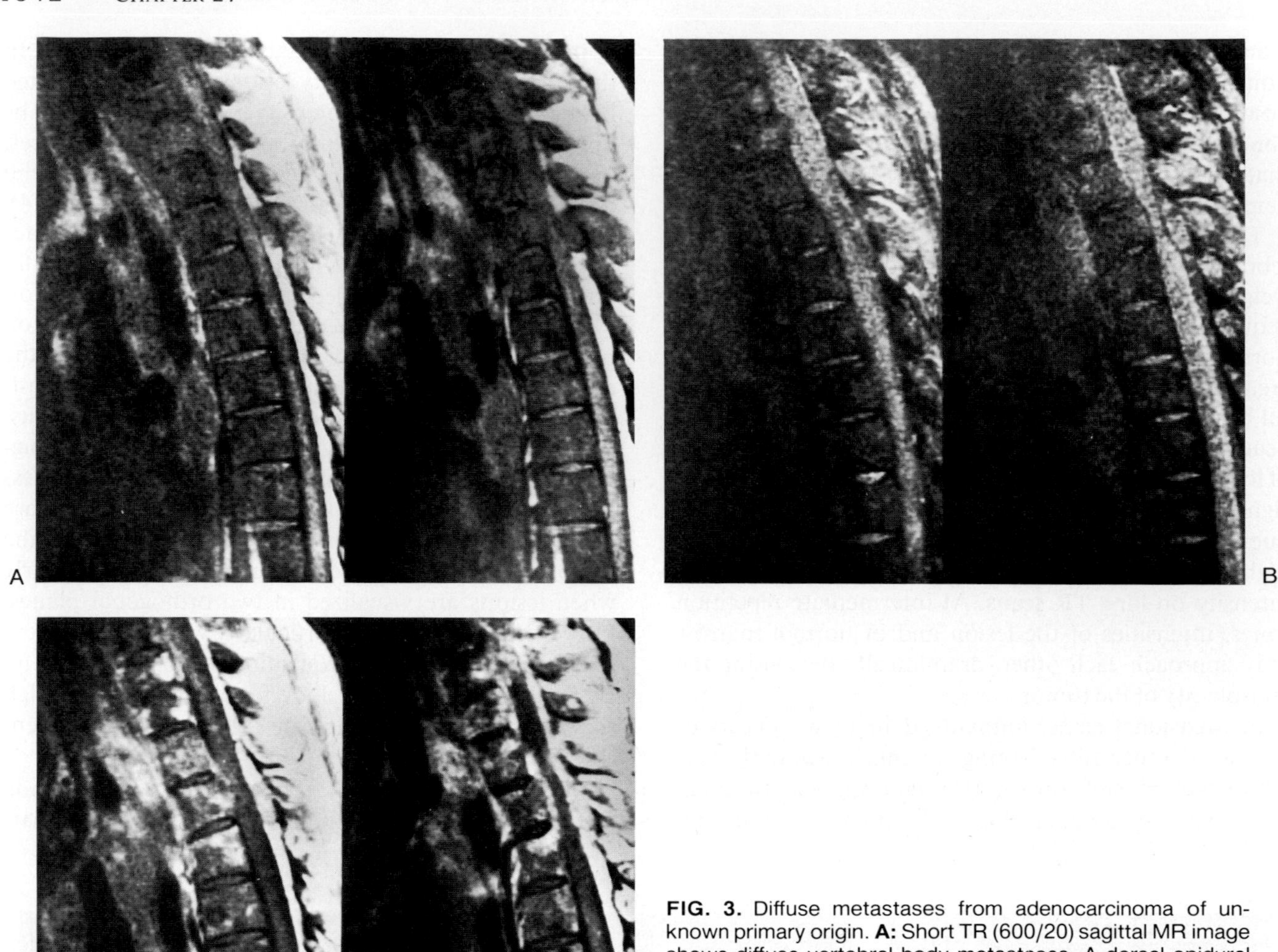

FIG. 3. Diffuse metastases from adenocarcinoma of unknown primary origin. **A:** Short TR (600/20) sagittal MR image shows diffuse vertebral body metastases. A dorsal epidural mass is also seen. Precise definition of the extent of spinal cord compromise is difficult to assess. **B:** Long TR (1333/70) MR image reveals the narrow spinal canal and spinal cord compression. **C:** Postcontrast short TR (600/20) MR images enhance tumor and better delineate its epidural extent than do precontrast short TR images. Nonenhanced spinal cord surrounded by enhanced tumor is easily identified. However, note that tumor displacing the dorsal epidural fat is less visible now. (From Sze et al., ref. 10, with permission.)

between benign osteoporotic collapse and neoplastic replacement as the cause (15). In the chronic situation, non-neoplastic involvement is typified by preservation of normal bone marrow, whereas tumor is characterized by replacement of marrow. The former appears of similar signal intensity to other normal vertebrae, whereas the latter appears of lower signal intensity on short TR images. Unfortunately, in more acute cases, the distinction between the two causes is more difficult because both may display low signal, because of marrow edema in non-neoplastic causes and because of tumor itself in neoplasms. In some cases of acute benign osteoporotic collapse, incomplete signal loss is seen. An even band of normal high signal marrow with smooth margins may remain adjacent to a band of lower signal in the same vertebral body. This appearance is suggestive of a non-neoplastic deformity.

When gadolinium compounds are given for spinal lesions, enhancement is extremely variable (10). Some tumors enhance mildly and remain hypointense to normal marrow; others enhance markedly and become hyperintense; still others enhance moderately and become isointense to normal marrow (Fig. 4). This variability of enhancement often occurs even in different metastatic lesions within the same patient.

Because low intensity lesions tend to enhance after the administration of gadolinium, they often become isointense with surrounding marrow and are less easily detectable (10,16). In fact, gadolinium can even obscure some lesions. For this reason, if the detection of vertebral body

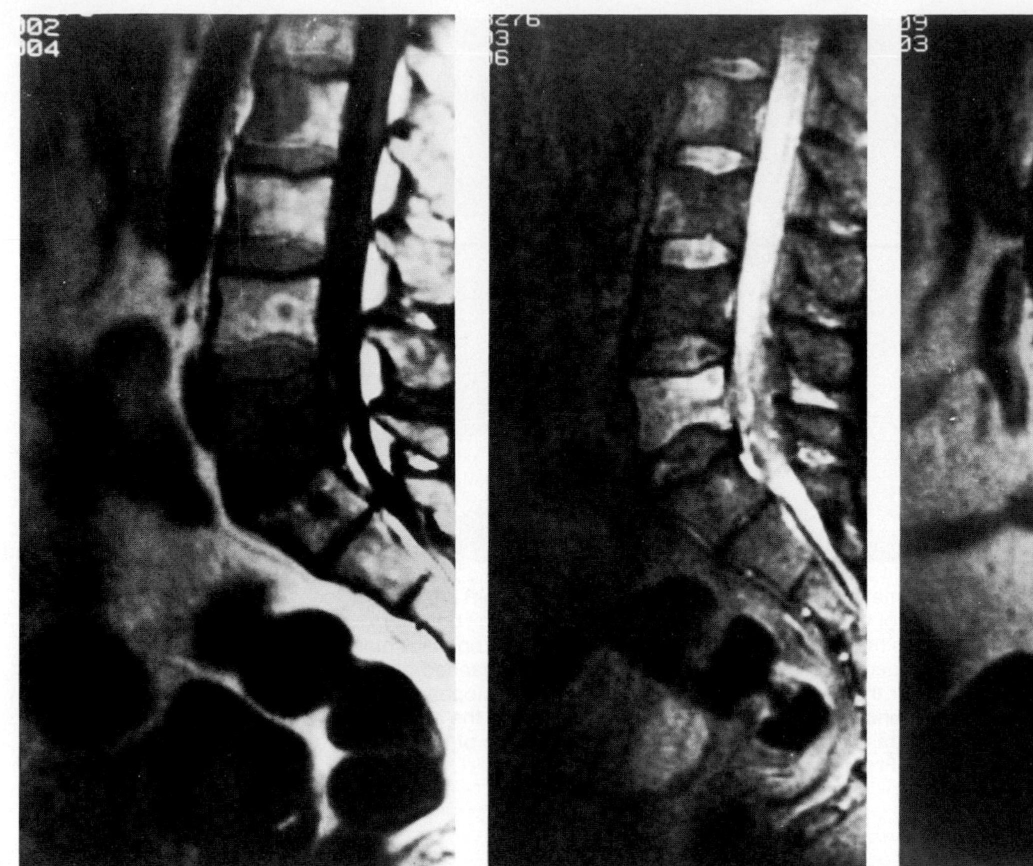

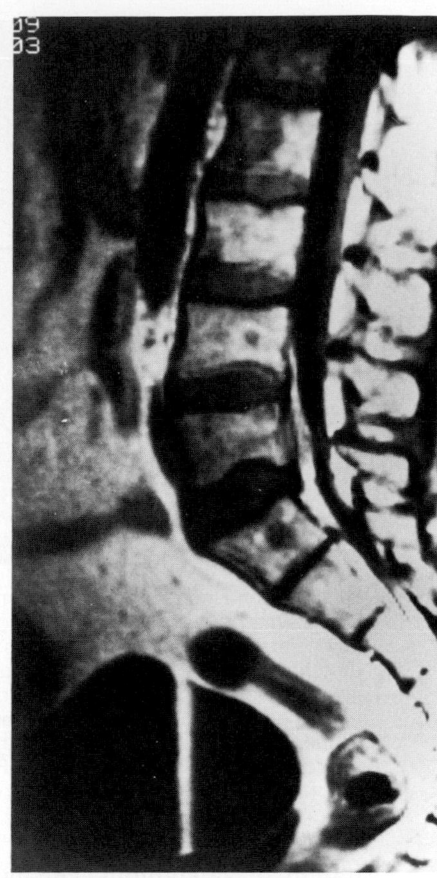

FIG. 4. Colon carcinoma metastases. **A:** Short TR (600/20) sagittal MR image reveals multiple foci of hypointensity within the vertebral bodies, consistent with known metastatic disease. Extension of tumor at L5 to the epidural space is also appreciated. **B:** Long TR (SE 1667/70) sagittal MR image demonstrates hyperintensity of the vertebral body metastases. **C:** Gadolinium-enhanced, short TR (600/20) sagittal MR image displays varying degrees of enhancement of lesions. Portions of L5 have now become nearly isointense with adjacent normal vertebra. Lesions in other vertebral bodies show mild enhancement but still appear hypointense compared with surrounding marrow. The epidural tumor is also enhanced to a similar extent as the adjacent tumor-infiltrated body of L5. The enhancing thin line continuing in the anterior epidural space from L5 superiorly to L4 may represent displaced enhancing epidural veins or extension of tumor. Note the layering of gadolinium in the bladder. (From Sze et al., ref. 10, with permission.)

lesions is a consideration, scans should either be performed without contrast or with sequences to suppress the signal of fat.

Although not helpful in the detection of vertebral lesions, gadolinium can be useful as an adjunct when epidural tumors are considered (10,16). Contrast may be helpful in a) more specifically characterizing possible epidural tumor, b) indicating regions of more active tumor for biopsy, and c) outlining areas of cord compression, when necessary. In specific cases it may also be helpful in a) differentiating diffuse marrow involvement with tumor from marrow that is hypointense for other reasons, and b) suggesting response to therapy.

Contrast can help to characterize further suspected epidural tumors (10,16). For example, although disc herniation is usually easily differentiated from epidural tumors on noncontrast MR scans, occasionally an epidural mass is seen adjacent to a narrowed disc. In these cases, the etiology of the mass may be in question. Gadolinium enhancement may prove helpful in this specific clinical situation (Fig. 5). Although discs and disc fragments generally do not enhance on immediately postcontrast scans (13), tumor does. Therefore, these cases may benefit from the administration of gadolinium, because enhancing tumor can be differentiated from nonenhancing disc material.

Enhancement with gadolinium can help to highlight areas of cord compression (10,15). Occasionally, especially in patients who have diffuse metastatic disease and congenitally narrow spinal canals, exact localization of areas of cord compression may be difficult on unenhanced short TR MR scans. This is particularly true in the cervical and thoracic regions, where a paucity of fat in the spinal canal prevents outlining of epidural lesions. Because of the extent of the vertebral body involvement, placement of the axial scans is also difficult. After the

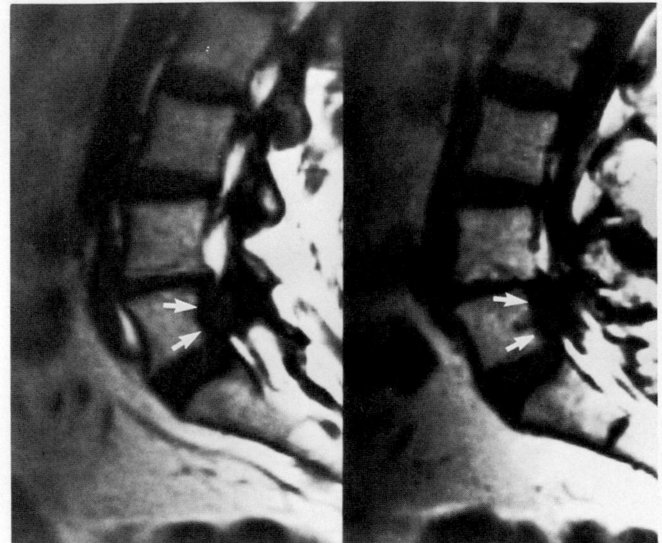
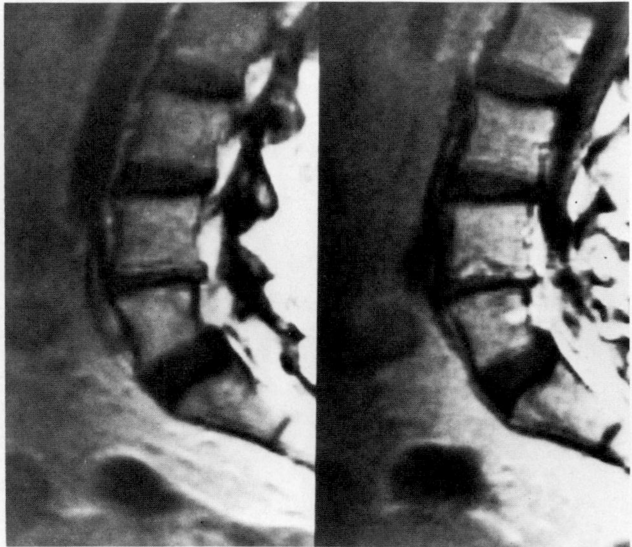

A B

FIG. 5. Non-Hodgkin's lymphoma metastasis. **A:** Short TR (600/20) sagittal MR images disclose a well defined mass with a signal intensity similar to that of the discs just posterior to the L5 vertebral body (*arrows*). The L4-L5 disc space immediately superior to the mass is markedly narrowed. Continuation of the epidural mass with the remaining disc material at L4-L5 cannot be excluded on these images. **B:** Gadolinium-enhanced short TR (600/20) sagittal MR images show a marked increase in the signal of the mass while the discs appear unchanged. If only a contrast-enhanced MR image had been obtained, it might have been difficult to detect the abnormality, but the enhancement of the mass on immediate postcontrast images confirms the neoplastic origin of the mass and makes the diagnosis of prolapsed disc material unlikely. (From Sze et al., ref. 10, with permission.)

administration of gadolinium, enhancing tumor surrounding nonenhancement cord is better delineated (see Fig. 3). Alternatively, high quality long TR scans or GE acquisitions can provide similar information.

PRIMARY EXTRADURAL TUMORS

Vertebral Hemangioma

Vertebral hemangiomas are benign vascular tumors in the spinal column, present in approximately 11% of all patients (17). In autopsies of 3,829 spines, Schmorl found hemangiomas in 409. Vertebral hemangiomas tend to increase in incidence with age (18). These lesions are solitary in 66% and multiple in 34% of cases (17). Sixty percent occur in the thoracic region, 29% in the lumbar region, 6% in the cervical region, and 5% in the sacrum. They are slightly more common in women.

The vast majority of vertebral hemangiomas are discovered incidentally (18–22). Rarely, they may be symptomatic. Symptomatic lesions tend to occur in the thoracic region (22). In one study, 13 of 14 cases (93%) of symptomatic vertebral hemangiomas were located in the thoracic region, specifically between T3 and T9 (23).

Initially, symptoms include localized pain and tenderness, often associated with muscle spasm. Radiculopathy may result from impingement on a nerve root (21). Myelopathic symptoms, such as motor and/or sensory abnormalities, can be seen with cord compression. Cord compression may occur secondary to a) mechanical compression of the spinal cord by the expansion of the tumor within the vertebral body and/or posterior elements, b) extension of tumor into the epidural space, c) epidural hematoma secondary to the hemangioma, and d) rarely, compression fracture of the involved vertebral body (18,21,22). Compression fractures in hemangiomas are unusual because the involved vertebrae usually have thickened vertical trabeculae, which tend to mitigate against axial collapse.

Pathology

Grossly, these lesions are characterized by their dark red color (17). Histologically, they consist of vascular structures within bony sinuses lined by endothelium and filled with blood. This angiomatoid tumor can destroy some bony trabeculae, resulting in compensatory thickening of the remaining vertical trabeculae.

Imaging

The thickened vertical trabeculae of hemangiomas cause parallel linear densities or a "jail bar" appearance in the vertebral body on plain films (18). Extension into the posterior elements can occur. On axial CT, the remaining thickened trabeculae give a typical spotted appearance to the vertebral bodies.

MRI is extremely sensitive in the detection of hemangiomas. On both short TR and long TR images, these lesions tend to have increased signal intensity (19). This high signal reflects the adipose tissue in these lesions, not a hemorrhagic component. Occasional hemangiomas within the bony confines can have a somewhat lower amount of adipose tissue and appear less intense. These lesions may be more aggressive and can enhance markedly with contrast (20).

MRI is able to show paravertebral and epidural extension of tumor (Fig. 6). Extraosseous components tend to lack adipose tissue and to appear isointense on short TR images. MRI readily defines spinal cord and/or thecal sac compression or displacement.

Treatment

Asymptomatic lesions are left untreated. Symptomatic lesions can be treated with surgical decompressive laminectomy. Preoperative angiography can be useful to identify and occlude feeding arteries (18). Radiation therapy may also be used, either preoperatively or by itself (18,21,22,24).

Osteochondroma

Although osteochondromas are the most common benign bone tumor (35.8%), only 3% of solitary and 7% of multiple osteochondromas occur within the spine (25–27). Nevertheless, because osteochondromas are much more common than many other bone tumors, they are actually encountered in the spine with regularity (28). Osteochondromas of the vertebral column are nearly always confined to the posterior elements, with a predilection for the spinous processes (25,28). Involvement of the vertebral body is unusual but has been reported (25,26). Most cases occur in the thoracic or lumbar region; the cervical spine is only rarely the primary site (26,29–31).

Three fourths of osteochondromas occur in patients younger than 20 years. There is a slight male predilection (25,32). Any bone preformed in cartilage can give rise to this lesion. These lesions occur in two different patterns. Solitary lesions have no known genetic component, whereas multiple lesions are seen in multiple hereditary exostosis.

Signs and symptoms are nonspecific. Frequently, pain is present. There may or may not be associated swelling or a palpable soft tissue mass (25). The lesions are usually large by the time they are symptomatic and come to medical attention (33).

Neurologic symptoms are rare, occurring in less than 0.1% of all patients. There is, however, a greater incidence of spinal cord symptoms in the teenage years, implying that growth spurts of the osteochondroma could compromise a marginally narrowed canal (27). Thoracolumbar lesions can present with bowel or bladder dysfunction and lower extremity weakness, but cervical lesions have a varied presentation (26,31). In addition to myelopathy, the presence of a mass may be noted. Dysphagia and even sudden death due to partial transection of the cervical cord from an osteochondroma of the dens have been reported (34,35). If lesions bridge multiple vertebrae, fusion and restricted motion can result, most evident in the cervical region (30).

Pathology

Osteochondromas are composed of cancellous bone surrounded by cortical bone (26,31). They have a pedicle that attaches to the adjacent bone, usually at the site of ligamentous insertions (25,33). Marrow is present within them. A thin layer of hyaline cartilage covers the tumor.

Imaging

Plain films show a pedunculated or sessile lesion with its cortex in direct contiguity with the cortex of the adjacent bone (25,36). These lesions generally originate from the posterior elements.

CT accurately delineates the exact site of attachment of the lesion to the adjacent bone, the presence of the cartilaginous cap, and any compromise of the spinal canal (25,33). In addition, CT can be helpful in distinguishing between benign osteochondromas and malignant degeneration into an osteosarcoma or chondrosarcoma (36). The incidence of malignant degeneration is 1% in cases of solitary osteochondroma and 5% to 25% in cases of multiple hereditary exostosis; rapid growth of the tumor should prompt suspicion of malignancy (25).

These tumors have a heterogeneous appearance on MRI. The cartilaginous portions of this lesion are of increased signal intensity on the long TR images, whereas the osteoid or calcified portions are of low signal intensity. Since a large portion of the tumor is bony, the extent of thecal sac impingement may be easier to delineate on long TR or GE sequences, rather than short TR sequences, in which the low intensity regions may blend into CSF. As with other imaging modalities, the rapid growth of the lesion is an ominous sign. Factors favoring benignity include cortical margins that are contiguous with the adjacent bone, well defined lobular surfaces, lack of adjacent bone involvement, and a thin cartilaginous cap (usually less than 1 cm) (36).

Treatment

Since these lesions are benign, no treatment is required unless they are large and compress adjacent structures (32). In this instance surgery can be performed and is

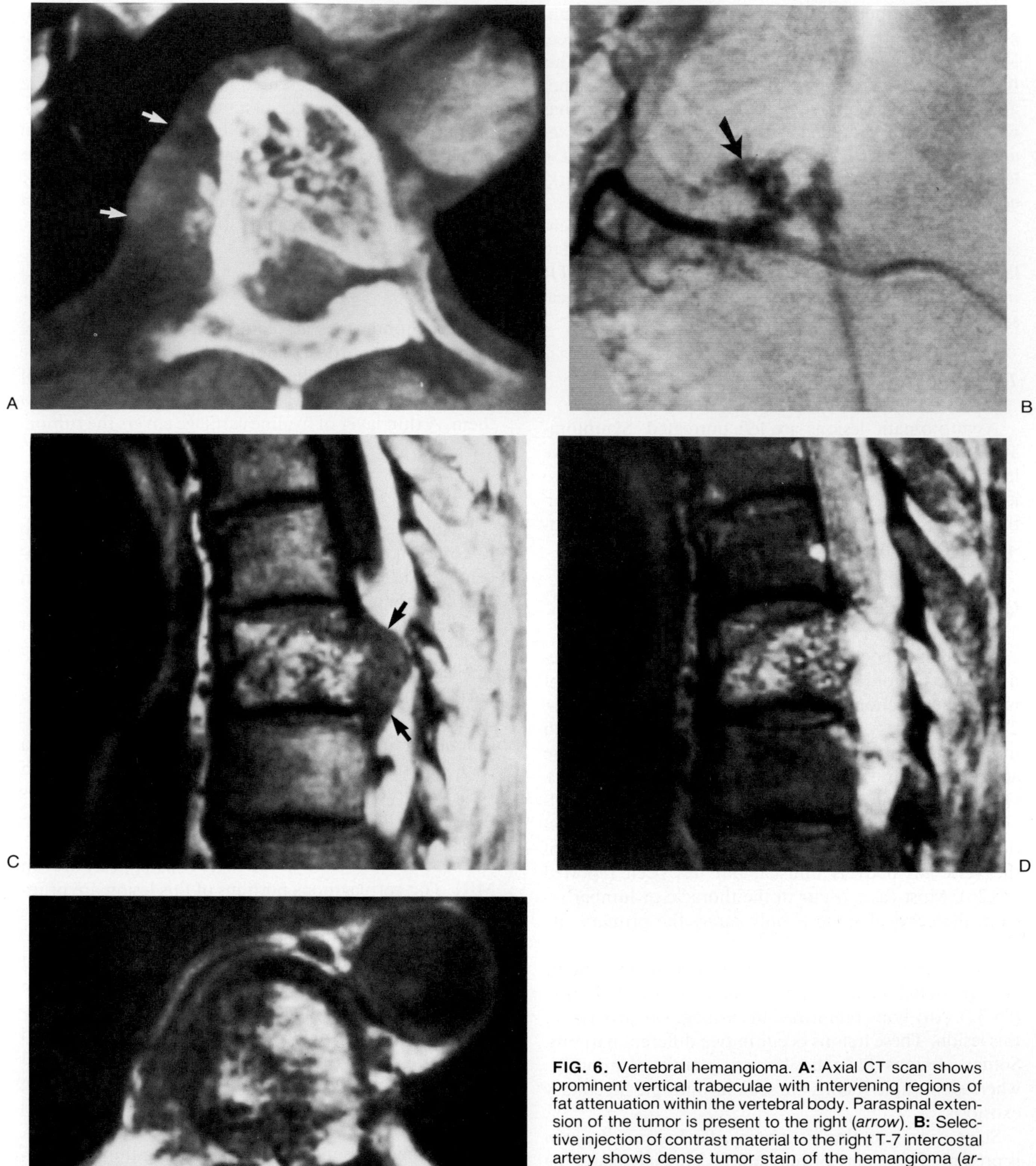

FIG. 6. Vertebral hemangioma. **A:** Axial CT scan shows prominent vertical trabeculae with intervening regions of fat attenuation within the vertebral body. Paraspinal extension of the tumor is present to the right (*arrow*). **B:** Selective injection of contrast material to the right T-7 intercostal artery shows dense tumor stain of the hemangioma (*arrow*). **C:** On sagittal short TR (400/17) MR images, osseous component of the hemangioma is of mottled high intensity signal, with the extraosseous extension demonstrating lower intensity signal (*arrows*). **D:** On sagittal long TR (1400/60) MR image, the osseous portion and extraosseous component are of high signal intensity. **E:** Axial short TR (400/17) image shows a mottled pattern in the vertebral body. (From Ross et al., ref. 19, with permission.)

usually curative, with only a 5% recurrence rate (36). Obviously, tumors with malignant degeneration require additional therapy.

Osteoid Osteoma

Osteoid osteoma comprises 11% to 12% of all benign bone tumors (37–39). It has been reported in virtually every bone, with a 0 to 25% incidence in the spine (average, approximately 10%) (38,40–44). The most common locations in the spine are the lumbar region (59%), followed by the cervical (27%), thoracic (12%), and sacral (2%) regions (41). Osteoid osteomas involve the posterior elements in 75% of cases. Thirty-three percent of cases involve the laminae, 19% affect the articular facets, and 15% the pedicles (41,42). The vertebral body is affected in only 7% (41,45,46).

Osteoid osteomas are more common in males than females, by a 2:1 to 4:1 ratio (40,44,47). This tumor is rare after age 30 years; 87% of the cases occur before this age (40). In MacLellan's review of the literature in 1967, of 36 documented cases of spinal osteoid osteoma, the average age was 16.7 years and 72% of the patients were between 10 and 25 years old (44).

The lesions almost always present with pain localized to the site of the lesion; rarely, they are symptom-free (1.6%) (31). Classically, the pain is worse at night and relieved by aspirin (42,44). Although it may be intermittent at first, it soon becomes constant and severe. Radicular pain can occur if the lesion encroaches on the neural foramina and is seen in 50% of patients (42–45).

There can be a significant delay in evaluation and diagnosis until the symptoms increase in severity (42,46). The average delay from initial symptoms to diagnosis in Jackson's series was 11.3 months (40). Back pain without a history of trauma is very unusual in a child and should prompt evaluation (48).

Focal tenderness is the most common sign of osteoid osteoma and is seen in 69% of patients (44,49). Also frequently seen are scoliosis due to muscle spasm and resultant pelvic tilt (42–46,48,49). Scoliosis was seen in 29 of 36 cases in one literature review (44).

Pathology

Grossly, this tumor has a central, vascular nidus that is reddish gray. Histologically, the tumor contains multinucleated giant cells (49). The nidus consists of very vascular fibrous connective tissue with surrounding osteoid matrix and can be calcified in an irregular fashion (39,48–50). The size of the nidus is less than 1.5 cm (if greater than 1.5 cm, the lesion would be classified as an osteoblastoma), with an average size of 0.9 cm (47). The nidus is surrounded by sclerotic bony reaction (48,51). The extent of sclerosis is extremely variable, but tends to be less in spinal lesions (44,48).

Imaging

The appearance of osteoid osteoma in the spine resembles its appearance elsewhere in the skeleton (40). Plain films, which demonstrate the classic findings in 66% to 75% of the cases, show a lucent nidus (47,48,52). Frequently, a small amount of calcium can be present in the nidus (42). Surrounding bony sclerosis can be seen but is variable in its extent. If there is extensive bony sclerosis, the exact location of the nidus can be difficult to discern on plain films, and further imaging is required to localize the nidus (42,53).

If the initial plain films are negative and clinical suspicion is still high for an osteoid osteoma, nuclear medicine bony scans are generally recommended. Osteoid osteomas are focally "hot" on bone scan (42,52,53). Once the level of the lesion is localized with the bone scan, then further cross-sectional imaging with either CT or MRI to confirm the precise location of the nidus preoperatively can be performed (42,52).

Frequently, the nidus can be seen only on cross-sectional imaging (42,53,54). CT shows a small rounded area of low attenuation, with or without calcification (42,54). Surrounding sclerosis is evident and can be extensive (42,53).

On MRI, osteoid osteomas demonstrate a heterogeneous appearance. The calcification within the nidus and the surrounding bony sclerosis are of low signal intensity on short TR and long TR images (39). The noncalcified portions of the nidus itself are of increased signal intensity on the long TR images (Fig. 7). The administration of gadolinium, like iodinated contrast material, causes intense enhancement within the very vascular nidus. This enhancement may help not only to localize the nidus but also to differentiate it from a nonenhancing lytic lesion such as Brodie's abscess (42,43). MR may also show an associated reactive soft tissue mass. This swelling is usually of inhomogeneous signal on short TR images, increasing on long TR images. Adjacent bone marrow may also demonstrate these signal changes (43). Both the soft tissue and the reactive marrow enhance with contrast. Because of the sensitivity of CT to bone detail, it is unlikely that MRI will supplant CT in the evaluation of suspected osteoid osteomas. However, in one case report, MRI was able to localize the nidus of a lesion that could not be defined on any other modality (53).

Osteoblastoma

Osteoblastomas are uncommon benign bone tumors accounting for 1% of all primary bone neoplasms (55–58). Although they have been described in almost every bone, there is a particular predilection for the spine, which accounts for 25% to 50% of cases (55,56,58–63). In the Mayo Clinic series, 39 of the 123 tumors were lo-

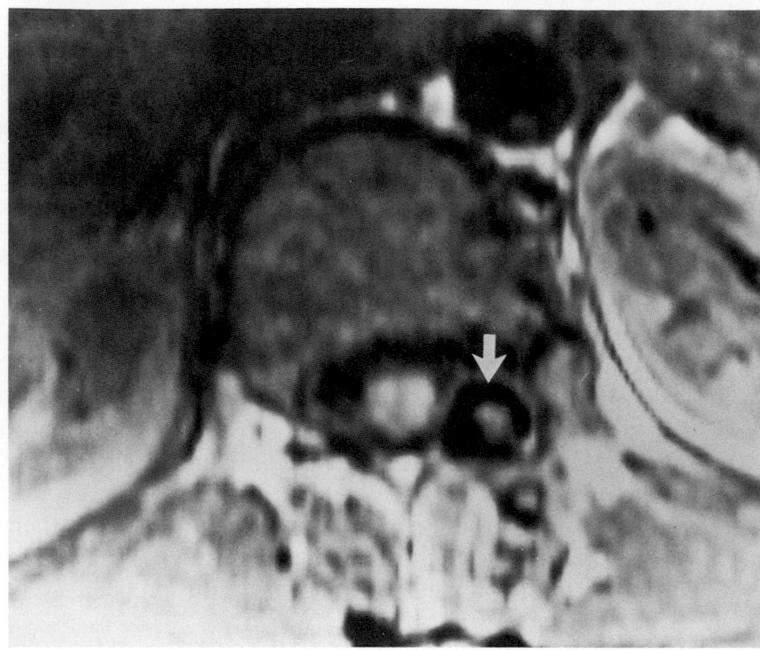

FIG. 7. Osteoid osteoma. Axial spin-density MR image shows leftward thoracic pedicular mass (*arrow*) with a hypointense cortical rim and central signal nidus. (From Pomeranz, ref. 67, with permission.)

cated in the spine (58). The lumbar spine is most often involved, followed by the thoracic and cervical spine (56,58,62).

Osteoblastomas occur most often in the posterior elements. In 1988, Myles reported 10 cases of spinal osteoblastoma in children and found that 9 were located in the posterior elements (56). In 14% of cases, the lesions were located in the vertebral body (56,58). In 24% of cases, both the vertebral body and posterior elements were involved (58). Epidural extension of tumor could be seen (56).

Osteoblastomas are more common in men (40,56, 62,63). In the Mayo Clinic series 87 of 123 cases were found in men (58). Ninety percent of the cases occur before age 30 years (40,58). This lesion usually presents in patients within the second or third decades of life (56,58,59,62,64).

Osteoblastomas most often present with pain and local tenderness (40,55–57). Scoliosis or torticollis may result. The symptoms may occur before the lesion becomes evident on plain films. Frequently there is a delay in diagnosis (average 9.3–12.3 months) (40,56,63,65).

Pathology

Grossly, these masses are soft, hemorrhagic, and very vascular and friable (40,59). Because of mineralized osteoid, they often have a granular texture (59). They also contain fibrovascular stroma (55,56,58,62,63).

Histologically, osteoblastomas appear similar to both osteoid osteoma and osteosarcoma (40,62). Osteoid osteoma and osteosarcoma are differentiated by their size. Osteoblastomas are larger than 1.5 cm. The average size of the nidus in one study was 2.4 cm (40). In another study, they ranged up to 10 cm (58). In addition, osteoblastomas may lack the identifiable central nidus and have less surrounding sclerosis than osteoid osteoma (55).

Imaging

On plain films and CT, these lesions tend to be expansile, with surrounding thinned cortex. In the spine, the lesions usually involve the posterior elements (56,57,63). The tumor may have a lucent or an ossified center (58,63). The margins are often, but not always, well defined. There can be dense sclerotic reaction associated with these lesions (58,63). CT also shows associated soft tissue masses and epidural extension (56,57,66).

MRI readily shows the lesion and any associated soft tissue mass. Impingement on the thecal sac can be detected. These lesions are inhomogeneous if areas of hemorrhage or calcification are present. A thin rim of signal void due to the bony shell may be visible (67). On long TR images, osteoblastomas are of high signal intensity, possibly corresponding to regions of vascularized stroma (Fig. 8). Irregular linear areas of signal void may be seen, corresponding to osseous trabeculae (67). On short TR images after the administration of contrast, osteoblastomas demonstrate enhancement.

Treatment

The treatment is aimed at total excision of the lesion (55,56,58). If the lesion is completely removed there is usually complete disappearance of symptoms with rela-

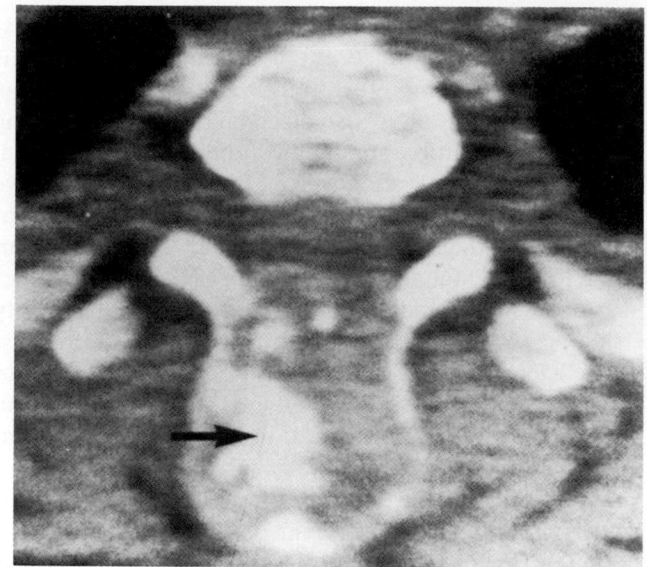

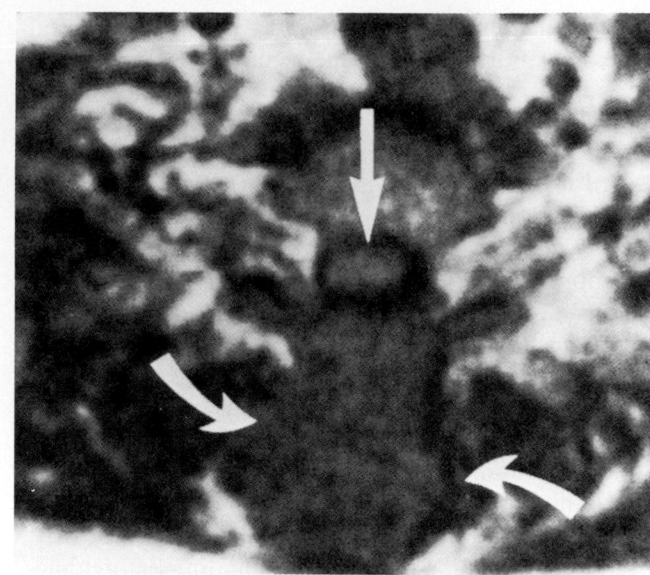

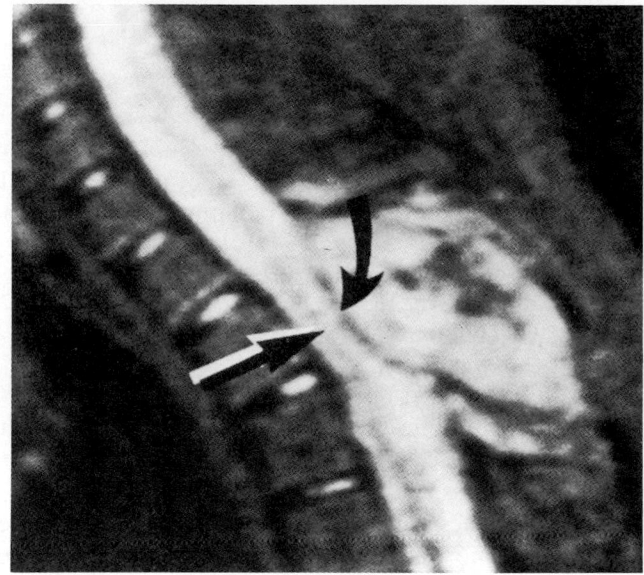

FIG. 8. Osteoblastoma of the spinous process of T2. **A:** Axial CT scan shows an expanded spinous process of T2 with internal amorphous calcifications (*arrow*). The anterior extent of the tumor and its relationship with the cord cannot be established. Axial short TR (600/25) (**B**) and sagittal long TR (2500/80) (**C**) MR images show the cord (*straight arrows*) and its relationship with the tumor (*curved arrows* in B). Note partial obliteration of the posterior subarachnoid space (*curved arrow*, C) on the sagittal MR image. (From Beltram et al., ref. 5, with permission.)

tively little chance for recurrence, although recurrence is more common in lesions involving the spine (55,56,63). Because recurrences may occur as long as 9 years after surgery, long-term follow-up is essential (68). Radiation therapy may be given for incompletely removed recurrent lesions (56). Rarely, malignant degeneration has been reported (40,69).

Aneurysmal Bone Cyst

Aneurysmal bone cysts (ABCs) are benign disorders of bone with an unknown etiology (70). These tumors represent 1.4% to 2.3% of primary bone neoplasms (37). Generally, these lesions arise de novo; however, they can be associated with other lesions (32%), such as giant cell tumor, chondroblastoma, chondromyxoid fibroma, fibrous dysplasia, and nonossifying fibroma (71–73). There is either a slight female predilection or no sexual predilection (71–75). The patients are usually in their first two decades, with 66% to 78% of the cases occurring in patients less than 20 years of age (37). In a study reviewing 81 cases of ABC in the spine, the average age was 16.6 years, and most occurred between 10 and 25 years of age (73,74,76,77). Giant cell tumors, which may appear similar, are usually seen in patients older than 30 years of age (72,73,75,78).

Although these lesions have been found in almost every bone, the spine is frequently involved. In the Mayo Clinic series of 134 cases of ABC, 27 were located in the spine, including 5 in the sacrum. In various other studies, between 3% and 20% of cases involve the spine (38,72,74,76). The neural arch is the most frequently affected site. Sixty percent of these lesions involve the posterior elements (40,70,74); 40% arise in the vertebral bodies (64). Forty-four percent occur in the lumbosacral region, 34% in the thoracic spine, and 22% in the cervical spine. They can cross the intervertebral disc space and involve an adjacent vertebral body (40,72,74,76). About 22% of lesions have extension into the paraspinal soft tissues. There may or may not be an associated soft tissue mass.

Symptomatology varies tremendously based on the size and degree of differentiation of the lesion. A small lesion can be entirely asymptomatic. When symptoms are present, they usually consist of localized pain and/or swelling (72–74,79). Large lesions can impinge on the spinal cord with resultant long tract symptoms and signs (74). In one study of 15 patients, compression fractures contributed to symptoms in four cases (76). In addition, neural foraminal narrowing can result in radiculopathy. Often the symptoms may be long-standing before diagnosis. The average duration of symptoms in one series was 8 months (74).

Pathology

Grossly, aneurysmal bone cysts are clearly delineated by the eggshell-thin cyst of subperiosteal new bone. The interior of the lesion can be solid and vascular or cystic and hemorrhagic. Aneurysmal bone cysts are composed of large anastomosing cavernous spaces filled with unclotted blood (76,78,80,81). The linings of these spaces lack normal features of blood vessels and do not contain endothelium, muscle fibers, or elastic laminae (73, 75,77,80,82–84). This benign lesion also has solid portions, which frequently are composed of osteoid material, sometimes intermixed with fibrous tissue (72,77). Histologically, these lesions can be mistaken for other entities, such as telangiectatic osteosarcoma. Giant cells are present within the trabeculae of this lesion and can lead to confusion with giant cell tumor (77).

Imaging

Plain films of aneurysmal bone cysts of the spine show an expansile lytic lesion usually involving the posterior elements (74,82). An eggshell-thin cortical margin is often seen (74). Severe lesions can destroy the vertebral body and result in collapse and vertebra plana (74,77). CT confirms the expansile appearance of the lesion and better defines any soft tissue extension (78,82). The absence of permeative bone destruction helps to lessen the possibility of more aggressive processes. In addition, multiple small fluid levels can sometimes be seen on CT (81). Frequently, to visualize these fluid levels best the patient must remain motionless for 10 minutes before scanning to allow the different components of blood to settle out within the cavernous spaces of the tumor (81,82).

MRI exhibits similar findings as those seen on CT. Expansile lesions are noted, often with internal septations and lobulations (Fig. 9). A thin, well-defined rim of low signal intensity is often visualized on both short and long TR images. Multiple small fluid/fluid levels and internal septations may be present (70,81,82). The fluid can have varying signal intensities based on the presence of intracystic hemorrhage of different ages (82). These vary from high to low signal on short and long TR images. In other cases, the lesions may appear of uniformly high intensity on long TR images. Paravertebral extension of the mass is well demonstrated on MRI. Any epidural extension or spinal cord compression is better depicted on MRI than on CT. After the administration of contrast, the septations within the lesion generally enhance (85).

In conclusion, the MR appearance of an ABC is characterized by involvement of the posterior elements of the spine, a rim of low signal intensity, and multiple fluid levels.

Treatment

Curettage is the initial treatment employed. Recurrence develops in from 10% to 20% of patients (37). If the lesion recurs several times, radiation therapy may be used.

Giant Cell Tumor

Giant cell tumors constitute approximately 4% to 5% of all primary bone tumors and 21% of the benign tumors (37). These lesions are most common in adults (86,87). There is no sex predilection (86).

Although these tumors occur most often at the knee, giant cell tumors are not infrequently seen in the spine. In the Mayo Clinic series of 2,276 bone tumors, they were the most common benign spinal column tumors, excluding hemangiomas (37). This lesion is the most frequent benign tumor to involve the sacrum (11 of 209 cases) (88,89). Giant cell tumors less often involve the rest of the spine (2 of 135 cases, 2 of 25 cases, and 3 of 209 cases) (86,88).

Pain is the most common symptom and is seen in up to 97% of patients (86,88–90). In giant cell tumors of the spine, radiculopathy may result from irritation of adjacent nerve roots. Initially the pain is intermittent and relieved by rest; however, eventually it becomes persistent (88). An associated soft tissue mass is often present (35 of 135 patients) (91).

Pathology

Although giant cell tumor is characterized by multinucleated giant cells, the presence of giant cells is not

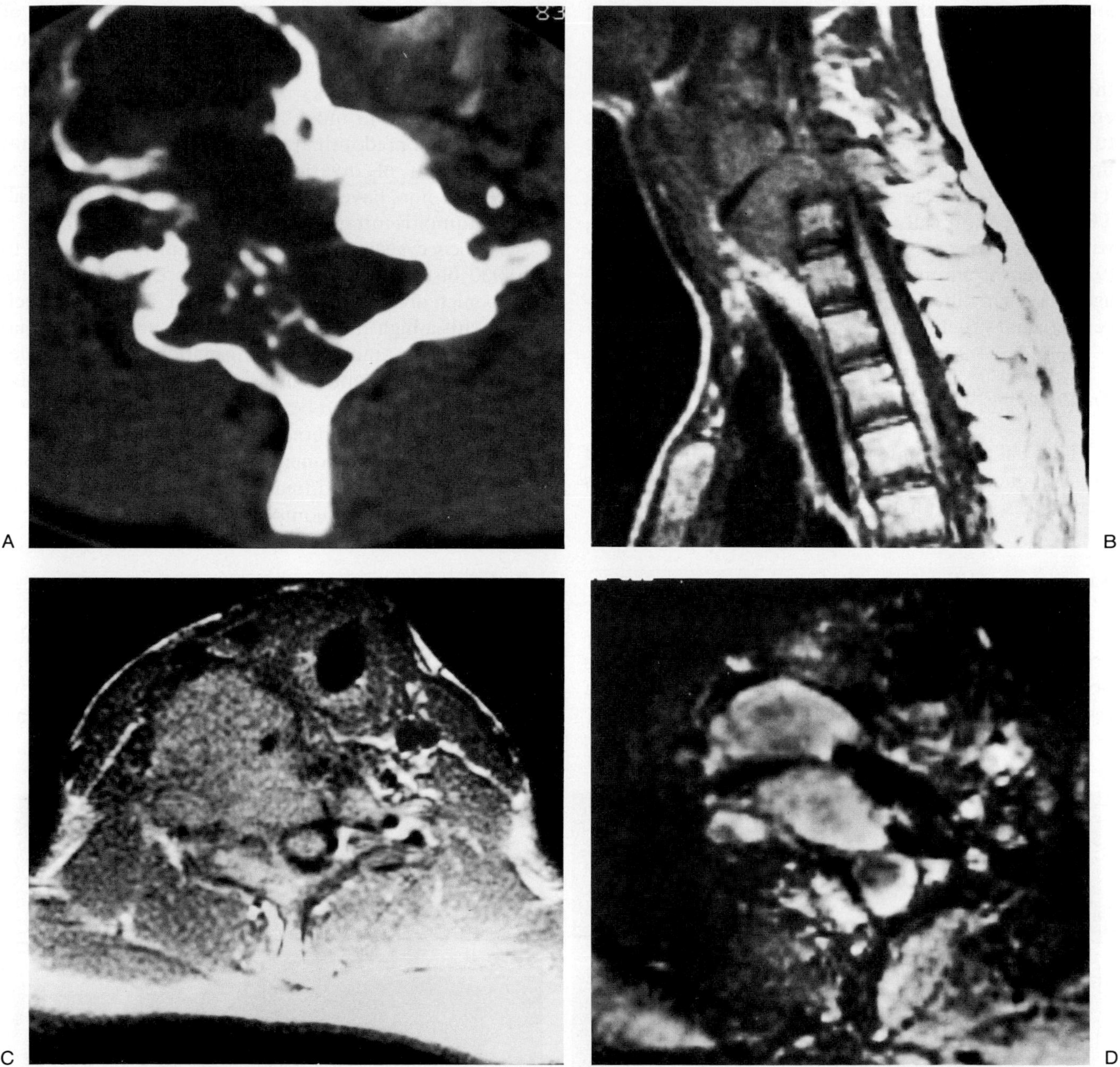

FIG. 9. Aneurysmal bone cyst. **A:** Axial CT scan demonstrates an expansile lesion with an intact cortical rim. Multiple loculations are present. **B,C:** Sagittal and axial short TR (600/20) MR images demonstrate a lobulated lesion of soft tissue intensity destroying portions of the vertebral body and extending anteriorly and laterally. **D:** Axial long TR (2400/70) MR image discloses a multiloculated lesion with high central intensity, surrounded by heterogeneous and low peripheral intensity. The central high intensity probably corresponds to cystic portions, whereas the peripheral low intensity most likely represents cortical rim and solid portions composed of osteoid material, intermixed with fibrous tissue. (Courtesy of Kenneth Maravilla, M.D.)

specific but may be seen in numerous other lesions, including chondroblastoma, chondromyxoid fibroma, aneurysmal bone cyst, and osteosarcoma (86,88). Most of the tumor is composed of mononuclear round or spindle-shaped fibroblastic mesenchymal cells (88). Jaffe states that the aggressiveness of this lesion is determined by the stromal cells (92). Many histologists divide giant cell tumors into three grades according to the degree of malignant features, but the presence of metastatic disease does not always correlate with the grade (86).

Imaging

Plain films show a lytic lesion with an expansile appearance (86). Rarely, the border of this lesion is sclerotic (86). In the spine, no definite characteristic radiographic appearance is seen (86). CT can show an associated soft tissue mass (91).

MRI is noninvasive and is able to demonstrate better the bony and soft tissue components of the lesion. Unenhanced short TR images can show the extent of the tumor within the bone because the lesion displaces the normal higher signal of fat-containing marrow (Fig. 10). The extent of the lesion is also readily assessed. On long TR images, giant cell tumors may be inhomogeneous, with areas of decreased and increased signal intensity (93). After the administration of contrast, short TR images may help differentiate enhancing tumor from adjacent normal structures (90).

Treatment

The usual treatment for this tumor is curettage (89). If surgery is not optimal because of location or numerous recurrences, then radiation therapy can be employed.

Sacrococcygeal Teratoma

Sacrococcygeal teratomas are rare tumors of childhood. They arise from multipotential cells of Hensen's node that migrate to lie within the coccyx (94,95). As a result, the soft tissue mass may be accompanied by bony abnormalities of the coccyx. The American Academy of Pediatrics has devised the following grading system (96). Type 1 tumors are almost always completely external and distort the buttocks. Type 2 tumors have an intrapelvic portion, but most of the tumor is external. Type 3 tumors are predominantly intrapelvic with significant displacement of invasion of surrounding structures. Type 4 tumors have no external portion and almost all of the tumor is intrapelvic.

Sacrococcygeal teratomas occur in 1 in 35,000 to 40,000 births (96–98). Most sacrococcygeal teratomas are benign and identified at birth (50). They are associated with a high frequency of other congenital anomalies, especially anorectal malformations (97). Females predominate over males in a ratio of 4:1 (94,96,97). Malignant lesions tend to be more common in males (96). Malignancy is also more frequent in lesions with a greater internal component (types 3 and 4), with a long delay in diagnosis and treatment and finally with more solid and fewer cystic components (50,96,97).

Pathology

Grossly, these tumors can be cystic, solid, or a combination of the two. Histologically, tissues arising from all three germ layers can be found. These tumors often contain squamous or intestinal epithelium, appendages, car-

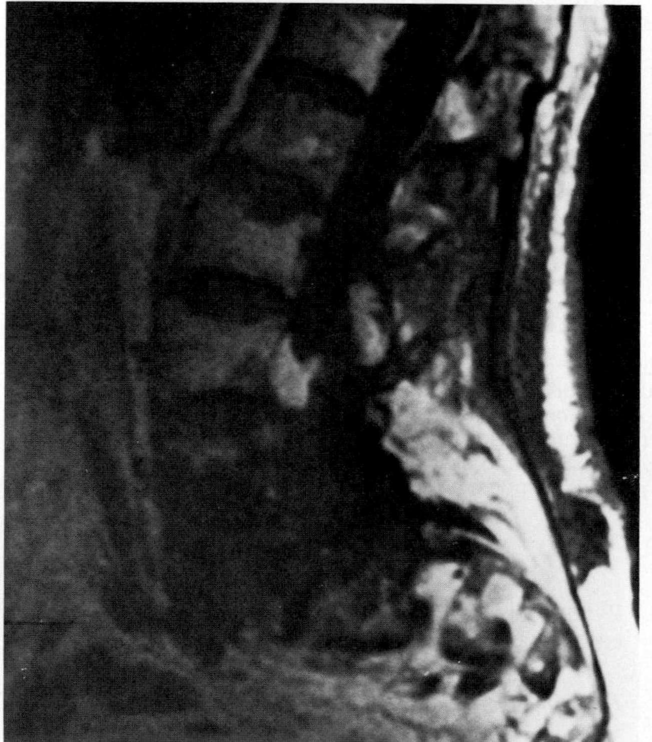
A

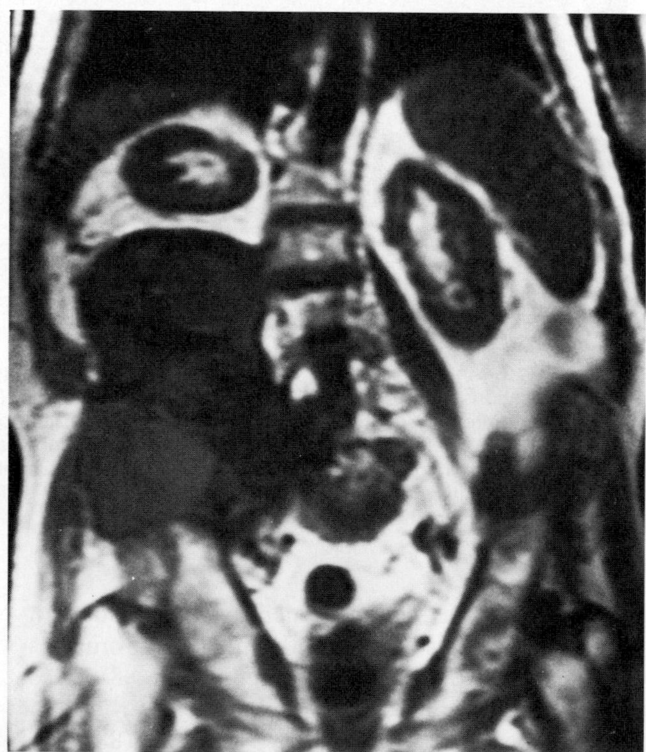
B

FIG. 10. Giant cell tumor. **A:** Short TR sagittal MR scan demonstrates a lesion invading and destroying much of the L5 vertebral body. **B:** Short TR coronal MR image demonstrates the marked extent of this lesion. Note the low-intensity structure extending from L5, the sacrum, and the iliac bone superiorly, elevating the kidney.

tilage, bone, or neuroglial fibers. They are often very vascular.

Imaging

Plain films may show a pelvic soft tissue mass. Coccygeal erosion may or may not be present. The mass can lie in a presacral location and displace the urinary bladder or bowel loops (96). The solid portions of this tumor are calcified in 60% of all cases (97,98).

MRI shows a mass adjacent to the coccyx (Fig. 11). Any intrapelvic or external components can be assessed. The lesion may be entirely solid or it may have cystic components. Although cysts generally appear of decreased intensity on short TR images or increased intensity on long TR images, some cysts may have different intensities if they contain hemorrhage. After the administration of gadolinium, solid portions of the tumor enhance.

Treatment

The treatment for both benign and malignant sacrococcygeal teratomas involves immediate surgical excision. These tumors have increased malignant potential with age; therefore, early surgery is advocated (96). The prognosis for benign lesions is excellent, although there may be morbidity secondary to surgical damage of the sacral plexus (99) or to severe blood loss at the time of surgery because of the vascular nature of these tumors

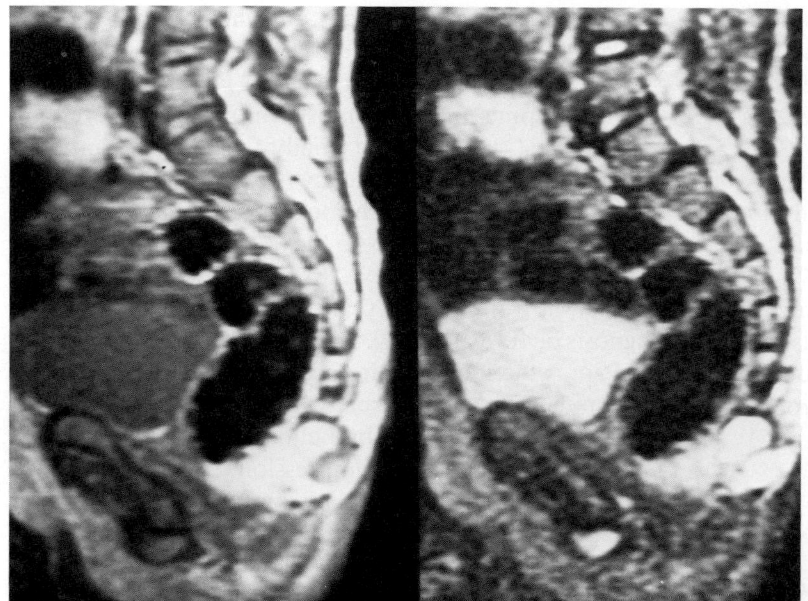
A

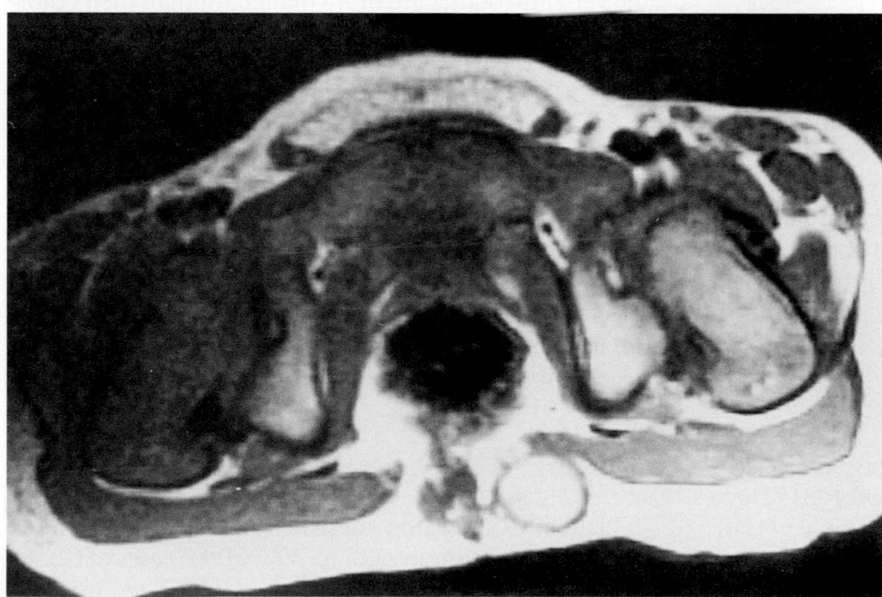
B

FIG. 11. Sacrococcygeal teratoma. **A:** Sagittal long TR (2000/80) MR images show small, well-defined high-signal lesions inferior to the sacrum. These lesions have signal intensity higher than fluid. **B:** Axial short TR (600/20) MR image shows a well-defined rounded mass posterior to the rectum. (From Twohig and Sze, ref. 268, with permission.)

(98). If metastases occur, these tumors have an extremely poor prognosis because there is limited response to chemotherapy or radiation therapy (96).

Eosinophilic Granuloma

Eosinophilic granuloma is a non-neoplastic condition with an unknown etiology (100). The disease is most common in children. In one series of 28 patients, the disorder was most frequently seen in the 6- to 10-year-old age group (101). In another series of 46 patients, 38% were less than 10 years of age, and an additional 26% were between 10 and 19 years old (98). Overall, there is a male predilection with 36 cases found in males and 7 cases in females in one review (100–103).

Symptoms are extremely variable, ranging from nonexistent to severe (100,101,103). The most common symptom is localized pain with or without an associated soft tissue mass (100–104). Systemic symptoms and signs, such as fever and weight loss, may also be present (100,101). The duration of the symptoms can be days to months (100).

These lesions can be single or multiple. In a study of 46 patients, 36 had solitary lesions and 10 had multiple lesions (100). Overall, the skull, pelvis, vertebrae, ribs, and long bones can be involved (100,101,103). When the lesions are multiple, the ribs and vertebrae are more commonly involved, frequently at numerous levels (100). With spinal lesions, collapse of the vertebral body can result in spinal cord compression, nerve root impingement, and deformity of the spine (100,103,105).

Pathology

Initially, these lesions are cystic and hemorrhagic (100,104). The cysts vary from 1 cm to 4 cm in size and have a yellow to reddish-brown appearance (100,106). As these lesions evolve, they develop increased amounts of lipid and appear friable and yellow. They heal into gray fibrous lesions, with bone formation in the later stages (100).

Histologically, these lesions are initially infiltrated by many eosinophils, accompanied by variable numbers of lymphocytes (100,107). Finally, in the healing stages, connective tissue is present, which in turn is transformed into bone.

Imaging

Plain films show round or oval, sharply marginated lytic lesions with well defined borders (100,103). There may or may not be an associated soft tissue mass (100). CT shows findings similar to the plain films and demonstrates better any associated soft tissue mass.

On MRI, lesions appear to have decreased signal intensity on short TR images and increased signal intensity on long TR images, unless hemorrhage is present (Fig. 12). Spinal cord compression is well delineated. When the vertebral body is involved, it is usually affected in its entirety. The weakened vertebral body can collapse, resulting in vertebra plana. A secondary kyphosis may develop. Associated epidural hematoma can also cause spinal cord compression. The lesions may be difficult to differentiate from metastatic disease.

Chordoma

Chordomas constitute 3% to 4% of all primary bony tumors (108,109). They arise from remnants of the notochord (110). Because the notochord, which forms the early fetal skeleton, extends from the clivus to the sacrum, chordomas can occur anywhere along the skull base and spine: 50% arise in the sacrum, 35% in the clivus, and 15% in the vertebrae (108,111).

In the spine, the areas most commonly involved are the cervical, lumbar, and finally the thoracic spine, in descending order of frequency (112). There is a definite male predominance, with roughly a 2:1 male-to-female ratio. Of 155 cases from the Mayo Clinic, 103 were male and 52 were female (112). In this same study, the age range was from 8 to 83 years, with an average age at diagnosis of 48 years (109).

Pain is the most common symptom in chordomas of the spine. The pain is usually localized to the site of origin. As they grow, vertebral chordomas can show signs and symptoms of cord compression. In one series of 46 cases, the average duration of symptoms to the time of diagnosis was almost 1 year (111).

Although chordomas invade adjacent structures, they metastasize less often. However, chordomas arising in the vertebral bodies are more malignant than their counterparts in the sacrum or the clivus. Although metastases have been reported in 10% to 15% of all cases, metastases occur in 80% of the vertebral body cases (111).

Pathology

Grossly, chordomas may be soft or firm. They often appear lobulated. Histologically, these lesions are composed of large vacuolated physaliferous cells. The cells are usually arranged in cords and contain abundant glycogen. Fibrous septae subdivide the tumors into lobules.

Imaging

Plain films show bony destruction with areas of amorphous calcification in 50% to 70% of the cases (112). In one study of 16 cases, seven patients exhibited involve-

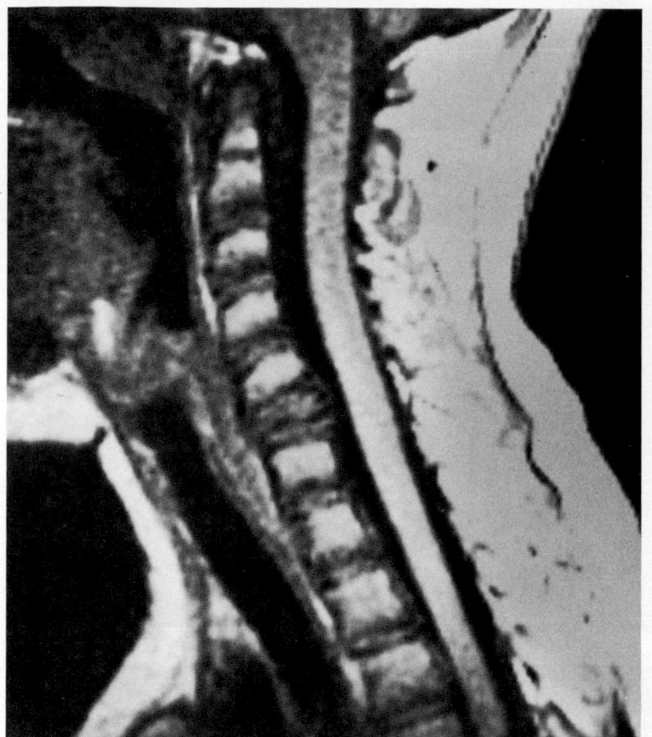
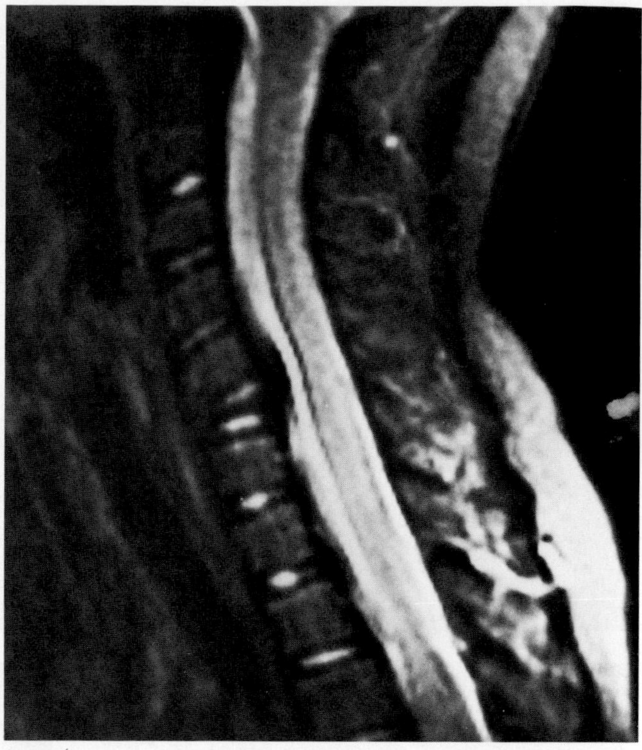

FIG. 12. Eosinophilic granuloma. **A:** Short TR (600/20) sagittal MR image demonstrates collapse of the C6 vertebral body. The remaining vertebral bodies appear normal in shape, although they are of increased intensity because of previous radiation therapy. **B:** Long TR (1922/70) sagittal MR image confirms the collapse of the C6 vertebral body and indicates mild epidural impingement. A mild kyphosis may be present.

ment of two or more adjacent vertebral bodies and the intervening disc, a finding generally associated with infectious etiologies and unusual in neoplasms (112). In addition, paravertebral masses can be seen.

CT can better show the calcification and paravertebral soft tissue masses. CT after intravenous contrast or after myelography can show an associated epidural component.

MRI is inferior to CT in showing bony destruction or calcification (113). MRI, however, is better able to show epidural disease and the true extent of disease involving the bone (Fig. 13). Seventy-five percent of chordomas are isointense to cord on short TR images and 25% are hypointense. The lesions are high signal on long TR images (113). Seventy percent of cases show internal septations and a surrounding capsule of low signal intensity. Areas of hemorrhage and cystic change are readily demonstrated if present. After the administration of contrast, prominent enhancement is usually seen (114).

Treatment

Treatment consists of surgical resection with radiation therapy (109). The prognosis is poor, with a 5-year survival rate of 10%. In one study, an average survival of 3 years after the time of diagnosis was seen (111). Although metastases are not common, local recurrence is the major problem, usually within 2 to 4 years after initial surgery and radiation therapy.

Neuroblastoma, Ganglioneuroma, and Ganglioneuroblastoma

Neuroblastoma is a tumor that originates from primitive cells called neuroblasts, which are of neural crest origin (115). These neural crest cells embryologically form the adrenal medulla and the paravertebral sympathetic chain. Therefore, neuroblastomas can originate in the adrenal medulla (36–40%) or in the paravertebral sympathetic chain (116). The adrenal medulla and upper abdominal parasympathetic chain are the primary sites of 65% of neuroblastomas (115–117).

Ganglioneuroma and ganglioneuroblastoma arise from the same cells as neuroblastoma. Ganglioneuroma is the most differentiated lesion and is composed almost entirely of mature ganglia cells.

Neuroblastoma is a disease of infancy and childhood that occurs once in every 10,000 births. Children less than 5 years of age are most often affected (115,116). Excluding central nervous system (CNS) tumors, neuroblastoma is the most common solid tumor of children (115,118,119). There is a slight male predilection in

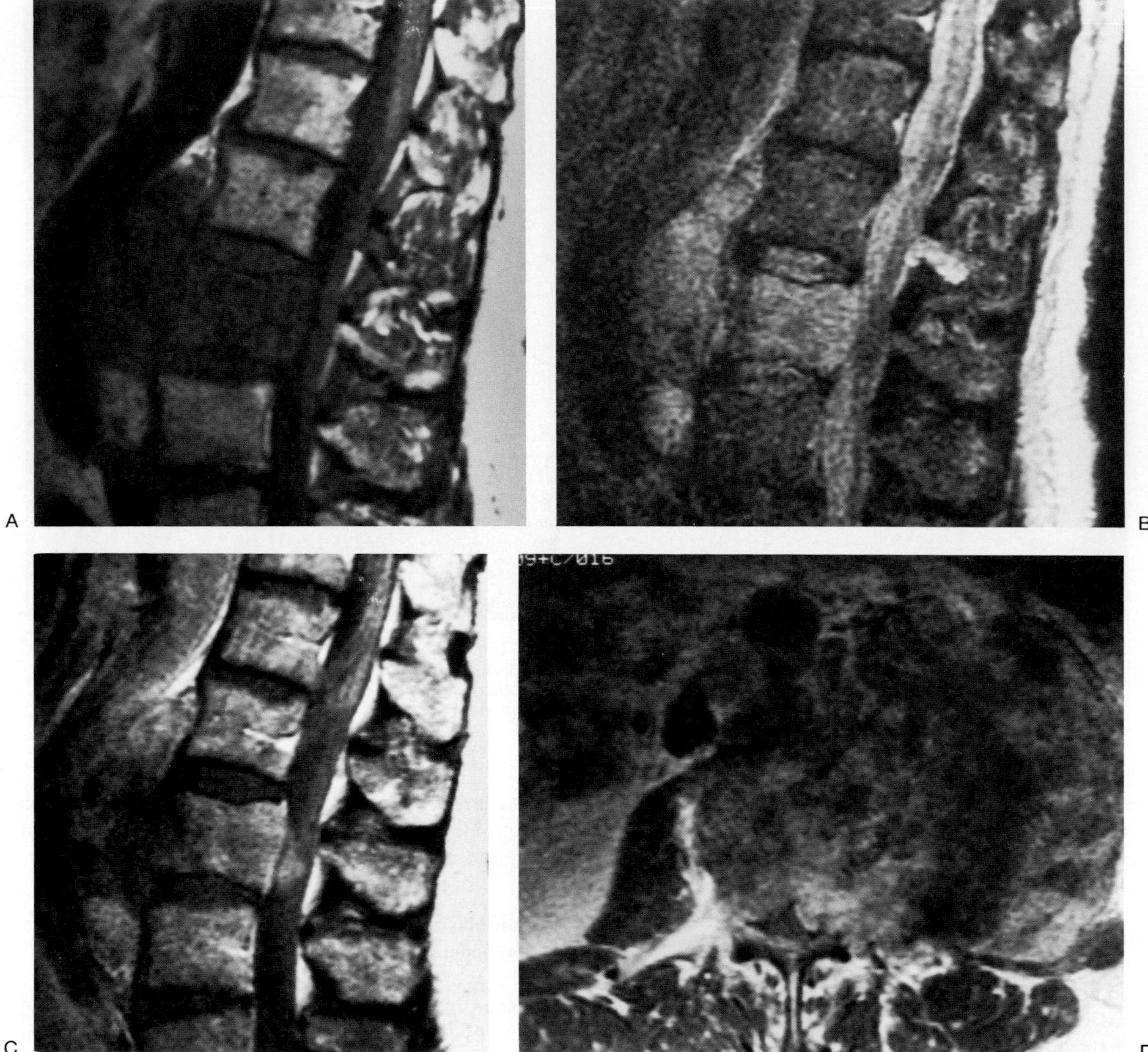

FIG. 13. Chordoma. **A:** Short TR (600/20) sagittal MR scan demonstrates a lesion extending from the L3 vertebral body into the surrounding paravertebral and anterior vertebral space. **B:** Long TR (2000/70) sagittal MR scans show that the lesion is increased in signal intensity and now approaches that of normal vertebral bodies. **C,D:** After the administration of gadolinium, short TR (600/20) sagittal and axial MR images disclose enhancement of the entire lesion.

some studies (51,115,117,120). Both ganglioneuroma and ganglioneuroblastoma tend to present later than neuroblastomas and are most often seen in the 5- to 8-year-old age group (121).

Because the tumors often originate in a paraspinal location, they can extend through the neural foramina to impinge on the thecal sac (116). Epidural extension occurred in 17 of 129 cases of neuroblastoma in a study from the Hospital for Sick Children (118). One to four percent of patients present with spinal cord compression. Punt reviewed the records of 21 children with neuroblastoma who presented with spinal cord compression (122). Four children had spinal cord compression at birth (122).

Involvement of the spine occurs most frequently in the thoracic and lumbar regions and is rare in the cervical area (121). In Punt's series of 21 cases with cord compression, 9 occurred in the thoracic region, 5 in the thoracolumbar, 6 in the lumbosacral, and only 1 in the cervical (122).

Symptomatology can vary tremendously according to the location and extent of disease (51). With intraspinal involvement, the most common presenting symptoms include local pain and spinal cord dysfunction (115,117). The patient may notice a paraspinal mass or may have signs of spinal cord compression (123). In one series of 11 cases, impaired motor and sphincter function were seen in 8, weakness of the lower extremities in 6, and weakness of the arms in 2 (51). Cord compression is also common in terminal stages of the disease because of the frequent occurrence of osseous metastases. Actual brain and spinal cord parenchymal metastases from neuroblastoma are rare, although leptomeningeal tumor spread is not unusual.

Pathology

Histologically, neuroblastomas are composed of small round cells with hyperchromatic dense nuclei, which can be confused with Ewing's sarcoma, rhabdomyosarcoma, lymphoma, and Wilms' tumor (115–117). Neuroblastoma is composed primarily of primitive cells and lacks elements characteristic of further maturation, such as increased size of nuclei, increased amount of cytoplasm, and production of fibrillar elements (115,117). The tumor is frequently hemorrhagic. Calcifications are seen in 10% of cases.

Ganglioneuroblastoma is a mixture of immature neuroblastoma and more mature elements, whereas ganglioneuroma is composed primarily of mature cells. The nuclei are large, and there is more cytoplasm present within the cells than in neuroblastoma. As the axonal processes develop, more mature fibrillary structures are seen (116,117). Calcifications are seen in 20% of cases (115,117). Neuroblastomas can differentiate into ganglioneuroma. In fact, neuroblastoma metastases can have ganglioneuroma elements within them.

Imaging

As tumor extends through the neural foramina, plain films disclose erosion of the pedicle, widening of the foramina, scalloping of the vertebral body, thinning of the ribs, or widening of the spinal canal (50,51,122). The intraspinal component of the tumor can spread through the epidural space over several levels, resulting in cord block remote from the site of the paravertebral mass (121). Rarely, these lesions can directly invade the intradural space (121).

MRI accurately demonstrates the intraspinal extension of tumor (Fig. 14). Tumor extending through the intervertebral foramina can be shown to displace the thecal sac and spinal cord (118). Areas of nonhemorrhagic necrosis have low signal intensity on short TR images and increased signal intensity on long TR images. Focal areas of hemorrhage can have a varied appearance. Acute hemorrhage is characterized by decreased signal intensity on both short TR and long TR images. Subacute hemorrhage initially tends to show increased signal on short TR images and decreased signal on long TR images, but it slowly progresses to display increased signal on all pulse sequences. Large areas of calcification may be visualized as areas of signal void. Finally, with contrast administration these tumors tend to enhance. Contrast frequently helps separate the epidural component from the normal thecal sac and spinal cord on short TR images.

Treatment

In the initial diagnosis, accurate assessment of intraspinal extension is crucial because symptoms referable to spinal cord compression can be permanent if not treated (118,122). In addition, when debulking the tumor, it is helpful to remove any epidural component because significant blood loss can occur if an unsuspected portion of the tumor remains within the spinal canal (118,122).

Prognostic factors in neuroblastoma depend on the age at diagnosis, the extent of the disease, the site of the primary tumor, and the degree of maturation of the cells. Factors consistent with a favorable outcome include younger age at diagnosis, extra-adrenal location, more differentiated histology, and more localized disease (51,115). There also appears to be a better prognosis for children presenting with spinal cord compression (51,122). Of 21 children with this presentation, 13 survived, 11 with long-term survival at the time of the report (122).

Osteosarcoma

Of all primary malignant bone tumors, osteosarcomas are one of the two most common. In the Mayo Clinic series of 2,276 primary bone tumors, there were 490 osteosarcomas (37). Osteosarcomas, however, are very unusual when they occur as primary tumors in the spine. Only 2 of 552 cases in the study from Memorial Sloan-Kettering Cancer Center and 10 of 600 cases from the Mayo Clinic series (1967) arose in the spine (124,125). In the latter series, an additional four cases involved the sacrum. Metastatic disease to the spine from osteogenic sarcoma arising elsewhere is very common, however.

Osteosarcomas occur most often in the 10- to 20-year-old age group (126). They are the most common primary malignant bone tumor in the pediatric population (124). In the Mayo Clinic series (1967) of 600 cases, 285 cases occurred in the 10- to 19-year-old age group (124).

There is a male predilection for this tumor (125–127). In the Mayo Clinic series (1967), 373 cases (62.2%) were seen in males and 227 (37.8%) were seen in females (124).

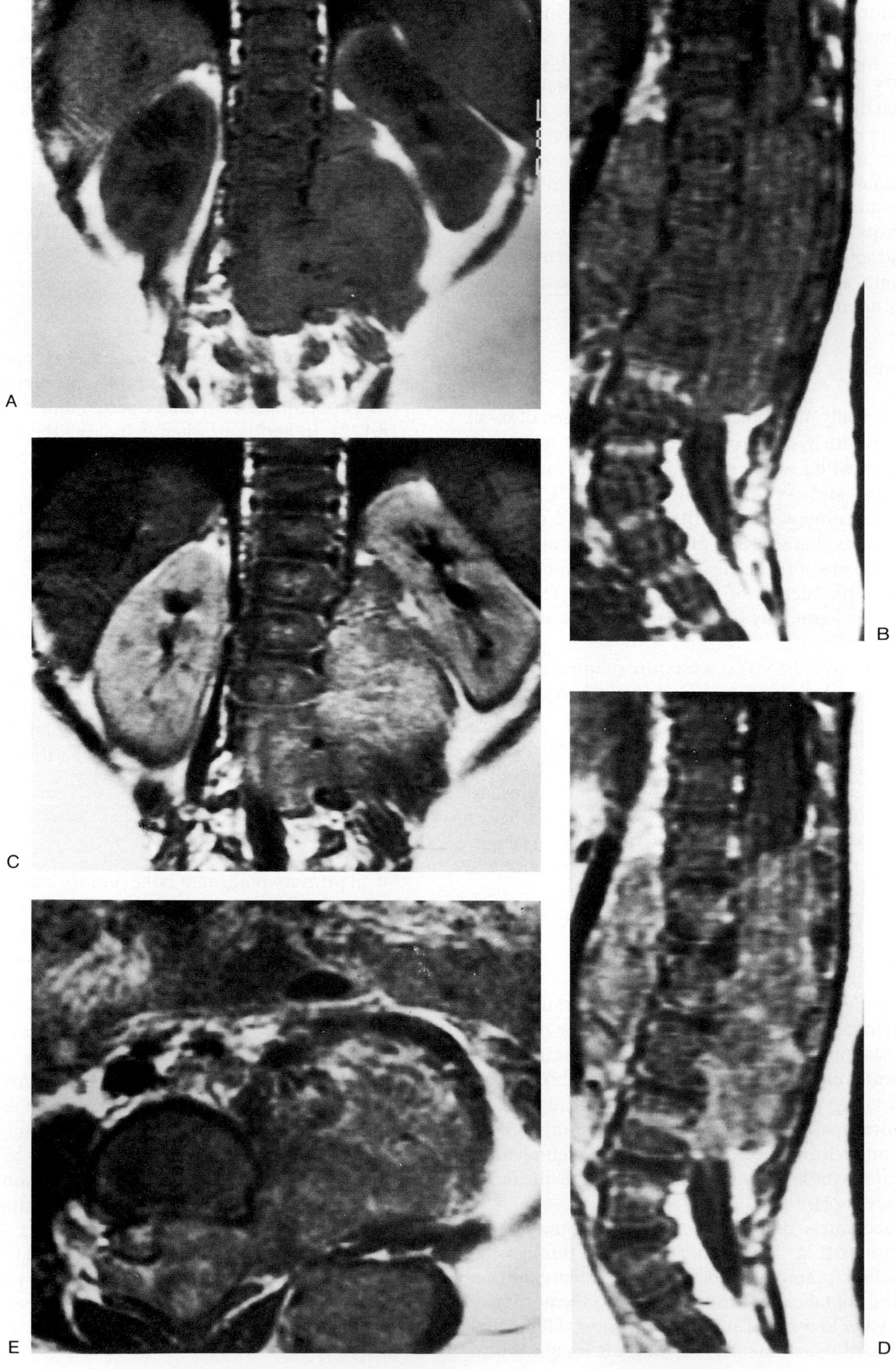
A
B
C
D
E

Osteosarcomas generally occur de novo. However, they may arise within bone that has been previously irradiated [16 of 600 cases in the Mayo Clinic series (1967)] (124,128). There is usually a 5- to 25-year latent period after the radiation before the development of the osteosarcoma (124). Osteosarcomas can arise in osteochondromas, as in 2 of the 600 cases reported in the Mayo Clinic series (124). Osteochondromas that become painful and show swelling should be regarded with suspicion (125). Finally, osteosarcomas can arise within pagetic bone in older patients over 60 years of age (124,128).

Pathology

Grossly, these lesions are calcified and firm. They are composed primarily of sarcomatous connective tissue that forms osteoid or bone (129). The amount of osteoid or bone may be extremely variable (125). These tumors can be further subcategorized based on their dominant histologic differentiation (129). In the Mayo Clinic series, 55% were osteoblastic, 23% fibroblastic, and 22% chondroblastic (124).

Imaging

Plain films of osteosarcoma arising in the vertebral bodies are nonspecific. CT can show osteoblastic or osteolytic bony changes. An associated soft tissue mass, either within the epidural space or paraspinal region, may be present (130).

On MRI, the degree of osteoid, bone, cartilage, or fibrotic tissue affects the appearance of osteosarcomas. On short TR sequences, tumor appears of low signal compared with the high signal in the marrow cavity (126). As with other invasive bone tumors, MRI is superior to CT in demonstrating the extent of osteosarcoma within the marrow space (131–133). On long TR sequences, intraosseous tumor can display low intensity, high intensity, or a combination of signal intensities. When the normal signal void of cortical bone is infiltrated by tumor, a mottled appearance will result (132). Short TR images after gadolinium are not as useful as unenhanced short TR images for showing bony extent of the tumor because the signal intensity of enhancing lesions can approach the signal intensity of fatty marrow unless fat suppression sequences are employed (134). Areas of periosteal reaction or areas of cortical thinning or cortical expansion can be shown with MRI as areas of low signal (126,131).

MRI is also extremely sensitive for delineating tumor extension into the paraspinal soft tissue masses (129). Although the tumor can be hypointense or isointense with muscle on short TR images, obliteration of normal fat planes can indicate extension of the neoplasm out of the vertebral bodies (126,133). On long TR images, extraosseous tumor is usually of high signal, permitting demarcation from uninvolved muscle (133). In addition, after the administration of gadolinium, these tumors often show immediate enhancement, again allowing separation from muscle, which only minimally enhances (129,134). Enhancing areas may reflect the more vascular and probably the more "aggressive" viable areas of the tumor (134). Biopsy is usually directed at these areas to characterize the mass best. Associated necrotic or sclerotic areas will either slowly enhance or fail to enhance (134). MRI is not as good as CT in showing associated calcification within the tumor or in defining the bony margins of the tumor (131).

Treatment

Although therapy for osteosarcoma in an extremity initially involves surgery, when the spine is involved, generally only chemotherapy and/or radiation therapy are given. Because curative amputation is not possible, the prognosis is poor. None of the nine cases in which follow-up was possible in the Mayo Clinic series survived 7 years (124).

Chondrosarcoma

Chondrosarcomas are malignant tumors arising from cartilage. They account for 7% to 20% of all primary malignant bone tumors (37,135,136).

Approximately two thirds of the patients are males. The peak incidence in Henderson and Dahlin's series of 288 cases was between 30 and 60 years of age (137). Chondrosarcomas can arise de novo as primary tumors or as secondary tumors from a pre-existing cartilaginous lesion, especially osteochondromas or enchondromas (138,139).

Chondrosarcomas rarely arise in the spine (135,140–143). Hovos found that only 3.8% of cases of children and 2.6% of cases in adults involved the spine (135). Torma studied 250 malignant tumors of the spine and extradural space and reported only 11 chondrosarcomas (144). All areas of the spinal column may be involved. Carmins found a fairly equal distribution of cases

FIG. 14. Neuroblastoma. **A:** Short TR (600/20) coronal MR image shows a large, low-intensity lesion in the left paravertebral space, with probable extension into the spinal canal. **B:** Short TR (600/20) sagittal MR scan demonstrates tumor extending in the epidural space within the spinal canal. **C–E:** Enhanced short TR (600/20) coronal, sagittal, and axial MR scans disclose enhancement of all the tumor, including the component within the spinal canal.

throughout the spine (143). Of 19 cases, 6 were located in the cervical region, 2 in the cervicothoracic junction, 3 in the thoracic region, 3 in the lumbar region, and 5 in the sacrum (143).

The signs and symptoms of chondrosarcomas are nonspecific. Pain is the most frequent symptom (140). The pain frequently is mild, leading to a delay in evaluation (140,143). Also, a palpable mass can be present (140,143). When the lesion involves the spine, there can be signs of spinal cord compression (141,143).

Pathology

The differentiation of chondrosarcoma from osteosarcoma has been controversial. However, chondrosarcomas are considered to arise from cartilage. Calcification or ossification of the cartilage may occur, but chondrosarcomas, unlike osteosarcomas, do not show neoplastic osteoid tissue or bone evolving from a sarcomatous matrix. Histologically, chondroblasts with varying nuclear pleomorphism and mitotic activity are surrounded by a myxoid matrix. In addition to conventional chondrosarcomas, variants include myxoid, mesenchymal, and dedifferentiated subtypes. Survival in chondrosarcoma is closely correlated with the grade of malignancy. Low-grade tumors are indolent and predisposed toward long-term survival. However, high-grade tumors are aggressive, and only 25% of patients with chondrosarcomas of this grade in any location survive 15 years.

Imaging

On plain films, chondrosarcomas cause lytic destruction. They often have a calcified matrix (140,143); the amount of calcification varies according to the differentiation of the tumor (138,143). Frequently, there is an associated soft tissue mass.

On MRI, the signal intensity of chondrosarcomas is heterogeneous because of the mixture of soft tissue, cartilage, calcification, and other components (144). Focal areas of decreased signal intensity on long TR images can be seen when the calcifications are very prominent (144). Areas of hemorrhage also contribute to the overall heterogeneity of this lesion. Again, MRI is excellent at defining associated soft tissue masses (133). Chondrosarcomas have also been reported in the extradural space, without bone involvement (146).

MRI may help in differentiating a malignant chondrosarcoma from a benign osteochondroma. This distinction is critical, especially in multiple hereditary exostosis. Malignant lesions tend to have large soft tissue masses, irregular disorganized calcifications, destruction of bone, and growth into adjacent soft tissues (143). The cortical margins may appear irregular and discontinuous with the parent bone. The thin cartilaginous cap typical of benign osteochondromas is usually not seen.

Treatment

Because of the location of chondrosarcomas of the spine, cure is difficult. However, radical surgery to remove the tumor is advocated if possible. Because total extirpation is difficult, recurrence, and ultimately metastasis, is common. In Camins's series, the 5-year survival rate for chondrosarcomas of the spine was 21%.

Ewing's Sarcoma

Ewing's sarcoma is a primary malignancy of bone affecting children and young adults, most commonly in patients 15 to 25 years of age (38,64,147–150). Ewing's sarcoma is rarely seen in patients less than 5 years of age (64,147–149).

Although Ewing's sarcoma is the second most common primary malignant bone tumor after osteosarcoma in younger individuals and represents 7% to 15% of all primary bone malignancies (38), it does not often originate in the spine (4%) or in the sacrum (1–2%) (147,149). Metastases, however, often involve the skeleton (92 of 229 cases), and when they occur, they frequently affect the spine (150).

Clinically, these lesions usually present with pain (147,148,150). Focal tenderness with swelling and a palpable mass can also be seen (150).

Pathology

Grossly, these tumors are soft, gray-white masses (150). There can be areas of hemorrhage, necrosis, and cyst formation within them. Histologically, they are composed of small, round cells, which may arise from mesenchymal connective tissue of bone (150).

Imaging

Plain films show mottled lytic changes (88 of 107 cases) and an associated soft tissue mass (52 of 107 cases) (52,148,150,151). The "onion peel" periosteal reaction is classic (148).

CT shows the soft tissue mass associated with the bony lesion; however, it is limited in its evaluation of the disease within the marrow cavity (152). MRI successfully demonstrates marrow invasion, which appears of decreased signal intensity on short TR images and increased signal intensity on long TR images. The tumor can be inhomogeneous secondary to hemorrhage, calcification, or necrosis. Its MR appearance is nonspecific.

Soft tissue paravertebral masses are readily assessed with MRI.

Treatment

Since amputation is not possible, the primary treatment for Ewing's sarcoma of the spine is radiation therapy. The tumor is extremely radiosensitive. Radiation therapy can also decrease symptoms such as pain and any associated soft tissue mass (148).

Leukemia

Leukemia is the most common malignancy in children, with an incidence of 42 cases per million in the United States (153,154). It is also the ninth most common malignancy in adults. One third of childhood neoplastic deaths are caused by leukemia (155). Acute lymphoblastic leukemia (ALL) represents 80% of all childhood leukemia; acute myelogenous leukemia accounts for another 10% (153,156,157). The remaining 10% is composed of less common histologic forms. ALL is most common in the 2- to 5-year-old age group, with a peak incidence at 3 years of age (157). There is a slight male predilection in ALL (156–158).

Children with leukemia are systemically ill (153). Because of the abnormally low production of all cellular components, as leukemic cells replace normal marrow cells patients display an increased susceptibility to infection, thrombocytopenia, and anemia (154,156,159). Spinal involvement can cause local pain and swelling (153,155,158). The pain can be migratory in nature, thus mimicking juvenile rheumatoid arthritis (158).

Imaging

Plain films disclose osteoporosis in 60% of cases due to infiltration of the marrow by leukemic cells (153, 155,159). Secondary compression fractures can result (155). Other findings in the spine include lucent bands and multiple focal defects (153,155). Osteosclerotic areas are rarely noted (155,158).

On MRI, patients with leukemia demonstrate homogeneous decreased signal on short TR images secondary to the replacement of the high signal fatty marrow by leukemic cells (160,161) (Fig. 15). Compression deformities of the vertebral bodies can also be seen. Foci of leukemic infiltration display increased signal intensity on long TR images (161). Although sclerotic foci are rare, they can be seen as low signal-intensity regions on both short and long TR images. Young children, especially less than 7 years of age, may have a paucity of fat in their marrow. In these cases, leukemic infiltration may be more difficult to detect. Enhancement with gadolinium may be useful because diffuse tumor infiltration enhances whereas normal marrow does not.

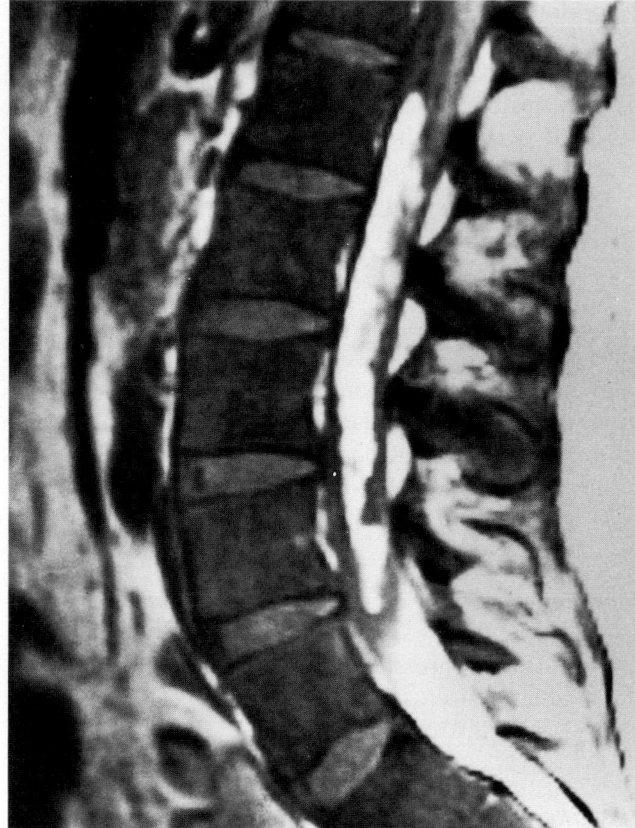

FIG. 15. Leukemia. Short TR (600/20) sagittal MR image discloses marked hypointensity in the marrow of this patient in relapse. Incidentally noted is high signal in the thecal sac due to bleeding after a lumbar puncture as a result of the patient's coagulopathy.

Moore et al. examined T1 relaxation times in 17 children with ALL in different stages: newly diagnosed, in relapse, or in remission (161). A significant increase in T1 relaxation times occurred in the marrow of patients with newly diagnosed ALL or ALL in relapse, when compared with those of healthy children or patients with ALL in remission. They suggest that MR relaxation times may be helpful in following progression of disease and in differentiating inactive disease from active disease, thus eliminating the necessity of serial bone biopsies. Long TR sequences were not helpful in distinguishing the different stages of the disease (161).

In patients with myelogenous leukemia, chloromas can occur. These collections of leukemia cells, often with a grossly green color, are unusual but, when they occur, they are often located in the spine. They appear as expanding masses, isointense on short TR images. To date, no reports have appeared regarding their appearance on long TR MR sequences in the spine, although they have been noted to be somewhat hypointense in the brain.

Non-Hodgkin's Lymphoma

Non-Hodgkin's lymphoma can involve the spine as an isolated primary lesion or as part of a systemic disease (153). It occurs with an incidence of approximately 7 cases per million population (162).

Primary non-Hodgkin's lymphoma, previously referred to as reticulum cell sarcoma of bone, is most frequently seen in adults. Ninety-five percent of cases occur after 20 years of age (153,163,164). Men are affected twice as often as women (165). Although primary non-Hodgkin's lymphoma usually occurs in long bones, review of several series demonstrated that 13 of 94 cases arose in the spine. Non-Hodgkin's lymphoma affects the spine much more often as metastatic disease. Patients frequently present with localized pain but characteristically lack constitutional symptoms (153,155,165,166).

Pathology

The tumor is grossly gray-pink in color and has frequent areas of necrosis (166). It is highly cellular and has a very vascular stroma (166).

Imaging

Plain films show a wide spectrum of radiographic manifestations of osseous non-Hodgkin's lymphoma, ranging from a permeative moth-eaten appearance to a more lytic geographic area of bony destruction to rare osteosclerotic lesions (153,155,164,167,168). On MRI, infiltration of the normal high signal–intensity fatty marrow of the vertebral bodies results in focal or diffuse areas of decreased signal intensity on short TR images (169). As the fatty marrow is replaced by cellular elements, the signal intensity decreases (170,171). On long TR images focal areas of tumor infiltrate have increased signal intensity. The appearance is nonspecific.

SECONDARY EXTRADURAL TUMORS

Metastatic Disease to the Spine and Extradural Space

The spine is the second most common location for metastatic disease to the CNS in patients with malignancies, after the brain (172). Thecal sac impingement as a result of tumor occurs in 5% of all patients with systemic cancer (173). Nearly every malignancy can involve the spine or the soft tissues in the epidural space, but myeloma, breast carcinoma, prostate carcinoma, lung carcinoma, and lymphoma are particularly often seen, both because of the frequency of these tumors and because of their propensity to metastasize to vertebral bodies (172). In autopsy series, the tumors that frequently affect the vertebrae, regardless of their overall frequency, are myeloma (77%), breast (61%), prostate (50%), stomach (44%), lymphoma (40%), melanoma (38%), uterus/cervix (36%), bladder (33%), pancreas (33%), and oropharynx (33%) (174).

The average age of patients with metastatic epidural disease ranges from 53 to 58 years of age (172,175). Metastatic involvement of the spine, however, can, of course, occur at any age. The site of epidural tumor is thoracic in approximately 68%, lumbar or sacral in 16%, and cervical in 15% (172). Different primary tumors appear to have a propensity to metastasize to different sites. For example, colon carcinoma metastasizes more frequently to the lumbosacral spine, whereas breast and lung tumors metastasize more often to the thoracic spine (172).

The most frequent symptoms of spinal cord compression are pain, weakness, autonomic dysfunction, and sensory loss (172). Back pain is the initial symptom in 80% to 96% of patients (172,166) and may be the *only* symptom present in patients with documented cord compression. The pain may be local or radicular. Weakness is a very common symptom at the time of diagnosis and is seen in 76% of patients (172). Bladder and bowel dysfunction occurs in 57% of patients and is an unfavorable prognostic sign (172). Sensory loss is noted in 35% to 51% of patients (172,175).

Imaging

Plain films can show a diversity of appearances. Although metastatic lesions are most often destructive and lytic, they can be sclerotic, especially in prostate carcinoma. On CT, destructive lesions of varying size, often with cortical breakthrough and extension into the paravertebral space, are seen.

MRI is extremely sensitive to the detection of metastasis in the vertebral bodies or extradural space (2–4,10). The multiplicity of lesions is strong evidence for a metastatic origin. However, in the case of single lesions, differentiation of a metastatic lesion from a primary tumor or from a lesion of another etiology is difficult. This evaluation is particularly important in patients who have had known malignancies but who have not had documented metastatic involvement. In these cases, biopsy is generally necessary.

On the basis of signal intensity alone, metastatic lesions appear identical to most primary bone tumors. They are generally of low intensity on short TR images. Rarely, metastatic lesions are hemorrhagic and appear of high signal intensity on short TR images. On long TR images, they may have a varied appearance and may be hypointense, isointense, or hyperintense. The presence of marked sclerosis predisposes to lesions that are hypointense on both short TR and long TR sequences.

Metastatic lesions may involve any portion of the vertebra. Because they usually spread hematologically, the large marrow space of the vertebral body is most often affected. However, metastases may also arise in the posterior elements. As with primary tumors, impingement on the thecal sac is well delineated on MRI.

Treatment

Patients with spinal metastases confined to the vertebral bodies without extradural or paravertebral extension are usually not treated or are treated with chemotherapy. Once thecal sac impingement occurs, however, patients are generally handled aggressively. Radiation therapy accompanied by the administration of steroids is the treatment of choice for most patients with extradural spinal cord compression (172). Decompressive laminectomy may be useful in patients who do not respond to radiation and in patients who relapse and cannot be treated with further radiation (172,175).

INTRADURAL EXTRAMEDULLARY TUMORS

Technique

Neoplastic disease in the intradural extramedullary space is best separated into primary and secondary disease. Primary tumors, such as meningiomas and neurofibromas, are generally well seen on noncontrast MR images (15,176). These tumors tend to be compact and to stand out against the lower intensity surrounding CSF on short TR sequences. On long TR sequences, contrast is reversed and the tumors often appear of lower signal intensity against the high intensity of CSF. Occasionally, small neuromas and meningiomas may be difficult to visualize without contrast. In addition, better delineation of tumor from cord may be possible with gadolinium (see Fig. 19).

Unlike the situation with primary tumors, noncontrast MRI frequently fails to evaluate adequately, and in some cases, even to detect, secondary tumors or leptomeningeal disease in the intradural extramedullary space (7,15,177–179). Myelography has been shown to be much more sensitive than noncontrast MRI (179). Of 15 positive myelograms for subarachnoid tumor, only 4 had positive findings on noncontrast MRI (178). A large number of the noncontrast MR images were equivocal or falsely negative (31% and 44%, respectively) because leptomeningeal tumor tends to blend with the adjacent CSF (178).

The reasons that leptomeningeal tumor is difficult to visualize on noncontrast MR images appear to be multiple (7). First, intradural extramedullary disease is characterized by marked elevations of protein levels in the CSF. In addition, leptomeningeal tumor spread is often delicate and friable, with a high water content. Both these factors combine to decrease the difference in the relaxation characteristics of the lesions from those of the surrounding CSF. Because of the marked protein elevation, the T1 and T2 relaxation times of the CSF decrease relative to pure CSF. Similarly, the high water content of the tumor acts to increase the relaxation times of the leptomeningeal tumor relative to more compact tumor. Therefore, even extensive tumor spread can often be poorly delineated on noncontrast MRI. Second, visualization of edema does not help in increasing sensitivity to detection. Although lesions in both the brain and the spinal cord are often highlighted by the presence of edema, no such mechanism can operate in the detection of intradural extramedullary disease. Third, technical difficulties often mar interpretation of MR spine images. Movement artifact particularly is a problem. CSF pulsation tends to blur lesion conspicuity (180). In addition, small nodules hanging off nerve roots can also move when the patient is positioned differently or with CSF pulsation. This movement degrades the delineation of lesions, although the use of the more recent cardiac gating and/or gradient moment nulling techniques can ameliorate the artifacts because of CSF flow.

Although noncontrast MRI can be equivocal in the detection and delineation of leptomeningeal tumor, contrast MRI is usually superb in this evaluation. The enhancement of intradural extramedullary lesions with gadolinium is often dramatic (7,15) (see Fig. 19). Even small nodules generally enhance brightly and are easily seen on short TR sequences. Mild enhancement stands out against the background of dark CSF and is readily detected. Leptomeningeal spread of tumor along nerve roots can also be demonstrated.

The ease and efficacy of administration of contrast are equally as important as its sensitivity (15). Most likely, if evidence of intradural extramedullary disease is sought, short TR sagittal sequences before and after the administration of gadolinium will be sufficient. Long TR scans may not be necessary. The enhancement of intradural extramedullary disease is generally most prominent on the immediate postcontrast scans, helping to shorten examination times (181).

PRIMARY INTRADURAL EXTRAMEDULLARY TUMORS

Nerve Sheath Tumor

Neurinoma, neurofibroma, neurilemoma, and schwannoma are various names for tumors that arise from Schwann cells of nerve sheaths. Schwannoma, neurinoma, and neurilemoma are synonyms. Schwannomas and neurofibromas are different entities, however (182). Schwannomas do not envelop the adjacent nerve root, which is usually the dorsal sensory root, generally are solitary, and clinically are not typical of neurofibromatosis (12,183,184). In contrast, neurofibromas envelop the dorsal sensory root, frequently are multiple, and are usually associated with neurofibromatosis, even when single (182,183,185). All these tumors may be referred to together as nerve sheath tumors.

In the general population, nerve sheath tumors are the most common intraspinal lesion, representing 16% to 30% of all intraspinal masses. These lesions most commonly present in the fourth decade of life (184,186,187). In the pediatric population, they probably constitute less than 10% of all intraspinal lesions, although some authors report an incidence as high as 29% (50,121). The youngest case was reported in a 13-month-old girl.

Nerve sheath tumors are most commonly intradural extramedullary in location (58%) (187). The remainder are purely extradural (27%), dumbbell-shaped with both an extradural and an intradural component (15%), and rarely, intramedullary (less than 1%) (121,187). Harwood-Nash reported 13 cases in children and found the most common location to be the cervical region, followed by the lumbar and thoracic regions (121).

The most frequent symptoms of nerve sheath tumors are pain and radiculopathy (185). These symptoms are present for an average of 26 months before diagnosis (187).

Neurofibromatosis is a phacomatosis that occurs spontaneously in 50% of cases and as an autosomal dominant in 50% of cases. Skin manifestations consist of café-au-lait spots that are greater than 15 mm in size. The presence of six or more spots is considered diagnostic. Patients with neurofibromatosis have a predisposition to other neoplasms in addition to neurofibromas, including intramedullary lesions, such as astrocytomas, ependymomas, and hamartomas.

Malignant degeneration is uncommon in nerve sheath tumors and is seen in 1% to 12% of cases (184,189,190). Malignant neoplasms arise either from pre-existing nerve sheath tumors or de novo from nerve sheaths. When they arise from pre-existing neoplasms, they probably have a latency period of 10 to 20 years (189,191). These tumors have a variety of names, including malignant schwannoma, malignant neuroma, nerve sheath fibrocarcinomas, and neurofibrosarcoma. The existence of numerous terms reflects controversy to their origin; however, they may all be grouped as malignant nerve sheath tumors. These malignant neural tumors are seen most often in the 15- to 39-year-old age group (189). The 5-year survival rate is poor and is between 15% and 30% (189,191,192). Those cases associated with neurofibromatosis tend to occur at a young age and to have a worse prognosis.

Pathology

Schwannomas appear as masses that project from one side of the nerve (Fig. 16) (182). Because they arise from a single focus, they displace normal nerve fibers to appear as lobulated, rather than fusiform, tumors. Cyst formation is common, although gross hemorrhage is not. Histologically, schwannomas are composed of Schwann cells that develop into neoplastic compact interlacing groups associated with fibrous strands. Fatty degeneration may occur.

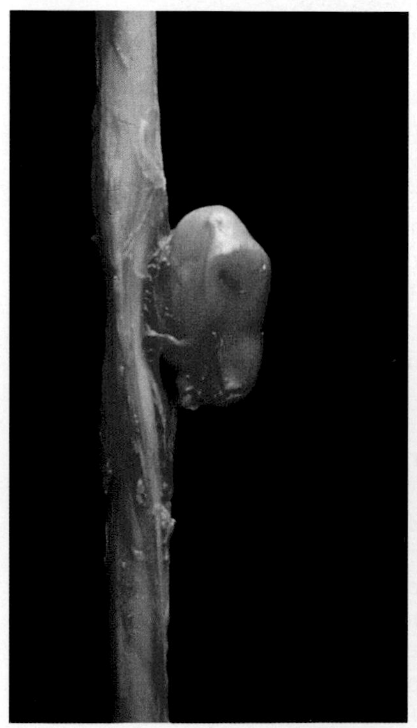

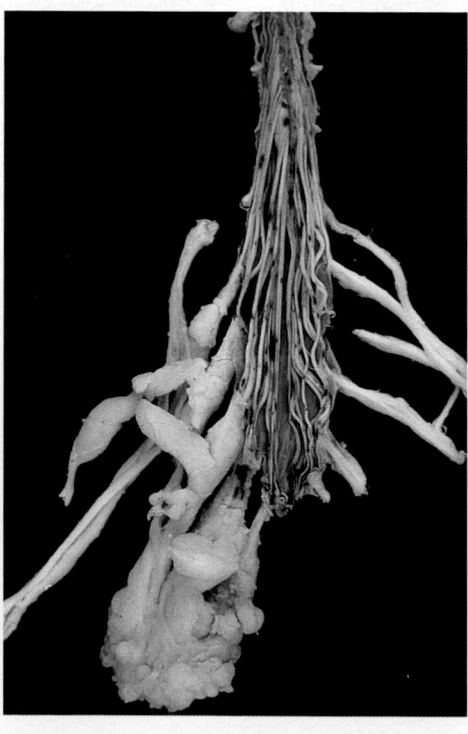

A,B

FIG. 16 Nerve sheath tumors. **A:** Intradural schwannoma involving a left upper thoracic posterior spinal root compresses spinal cord. **B:** Extensive plexiform neurofibromas involving the right lumbar and sacral plexuses in a child. (From Okazaki and Scheithauer, ref. 193, with permission.)

Neurofibromas consist of mixtures of fibroblasts and proliferated Schwann cells between dispersed nerve fibers. The matrix of a neurofibroma contains acid mucopolysaccharides and large amounts of tissue fluids with numerous fibrous strands. The matrix spreads apart the axons to produce the fusiform shape of the neurofibroma.

Imaging

Plain film findings of nerve sheath tumors include posterior scalloping of the vertebral bodies and widening of the neural foramina (182,194). On CT, they are of decreased attenuation and present as paraspinal or intraspinal masses. Differentiation of the intraspinal portion of the neurofibromas from the adjacent spinal cord and thecal sac can be difficult without instillation of intrathecal contrast material.

Nerve sheath tumors on MRI tend to have increased signal intensity compared with muscle on noncontrast short TR images (11 of 12 patients). The increased signal intensity on short TR images may be secondary to shortening of the T1 relaxation time by mucopolysaccharide molecules interacting with tissue water. On long TR images, these lesions can have markedly increased signal intensity secondary to the high water content of these lesions (177,195). Also frequently seen on long TR images are central areas of decreased signal intensity (7 of 12 patients), which may represent denser areas of collagen and Schwann cells, as shown pathologically. De-

A

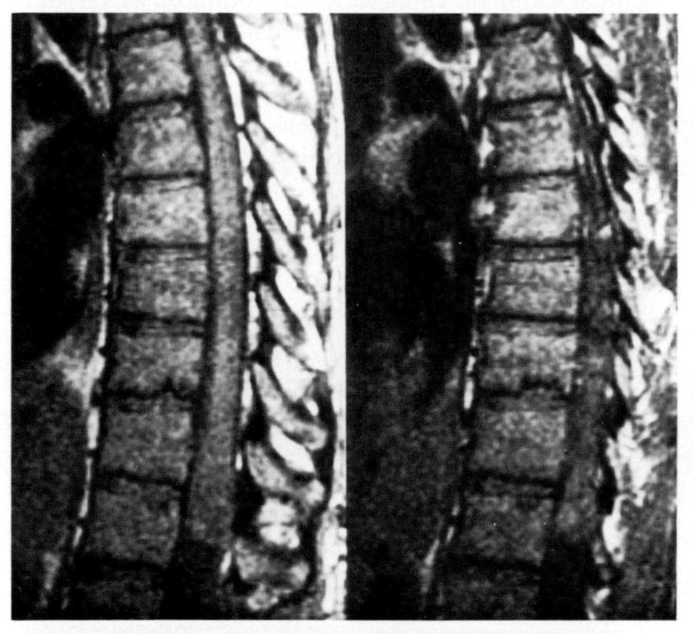

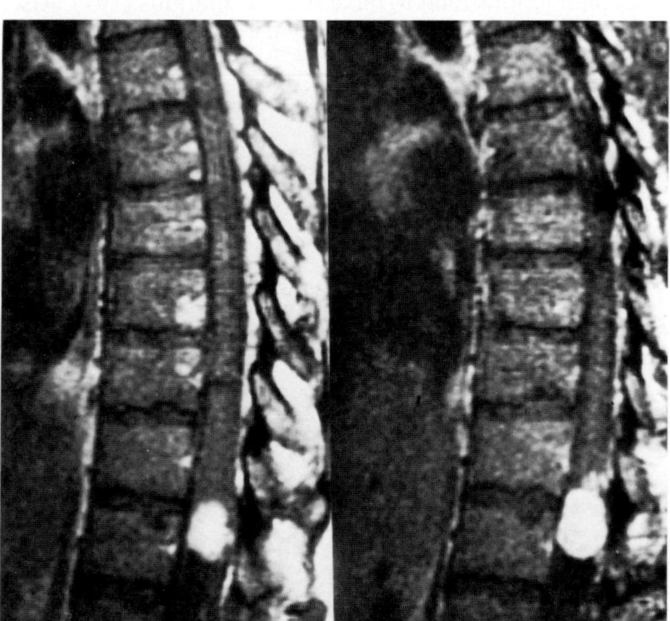

C

B

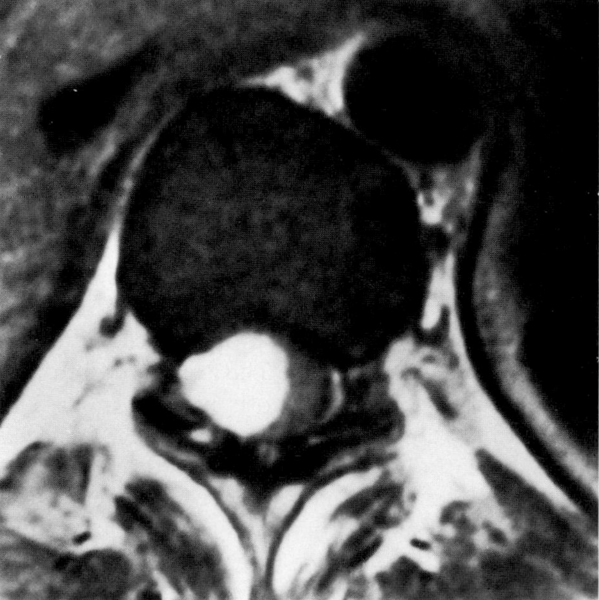

FIG. 17. Neurofibroma. **A:** Short TR (500/20) sagittal MR image depicts apparent widening of the distal cord and conus. **B:** Postcontrast short TR (500/20) sagittal MR image demonstrates a well defined enhancing mass, consistent with a neurofibroma. **C:** Postcontrast short TR (500/20) axial MR image confirms the intradural extramedullary location of the lesion, displacing cord to the left. (From Bronen and Sze, ref. 269, with permission.)

creased signal may result from the fact that fewer mobile protons are available within the fibrous matrix in the central portions of these lesions. These lesions usually enhance intensely and fairly homogeneously, although occasional schwannomas may initially enhance peripherally, sparing the central portion. They are frequently multiple. MRI is able to demonstrate with superb detail the intraspinal portions of these tumors, especially on short TR images after gadolinium, and to show any displacement or compression of the spinal cord (195) (Figs. 17 and 18).

Imaging modalities can help differentiate plexiform neurofibromas from malignant nerve sheath tumors. On CT and MRI both benign and malignant lesions show inhomogeneity. However, malignant schwannomas more often have irregular, infiltrative margins, whereas benign lesions tend to have smooth margins (191). Also, malignant nerve sheath tumors tend to lack the decreased central area of low signal intensity on long TR images that is frequently noted in benign schwannomas (191). Finally, malignant nerve sheath tumors tend to be larger than benign lesions.

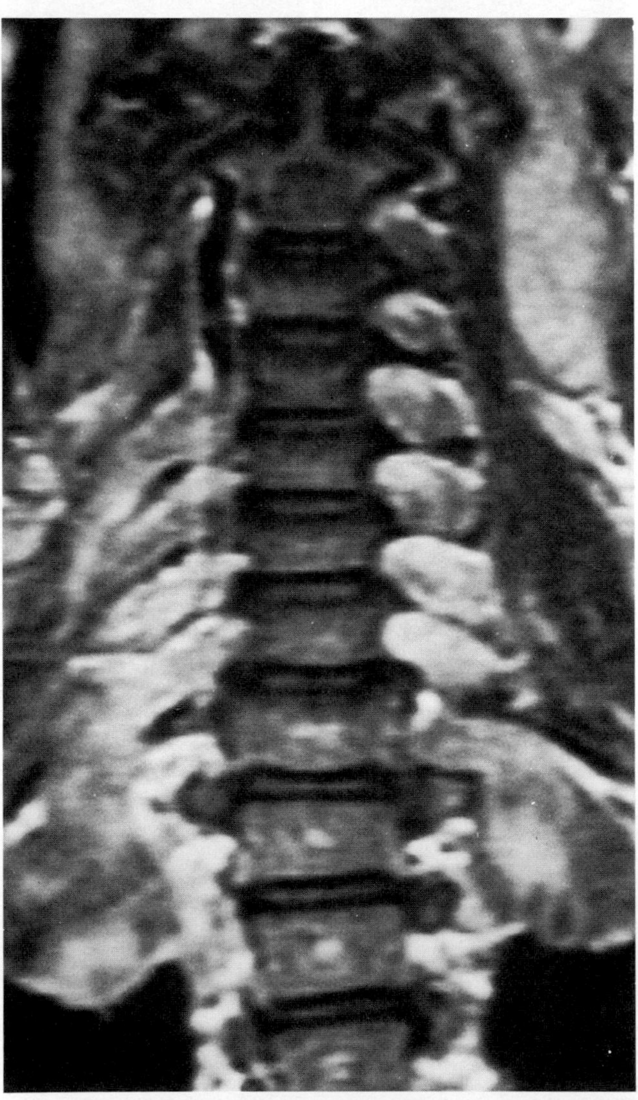

FIG. 18. Neurofibromatosis. Short TR (600/20) gadolinium-enhanced coronal MR image of the cervical and upper thoracic spine demonstrates enhancing neurofibromas at virtually every neural foramen.

Meningioma

Meningiomas of the spinal canal are generally lesions of adults (197–200). The average age of presentation is in the fifth and sixth decades, with 60% to 80% seen in females (197,198). Roughly 3% to 6% of all spinal meningiomas occur in children.

Meningiomas in the spine tend to be encapsulated and are attached to the dura. They do not invade the spinal cord but displace it (185). The location of spinal meningiomas within the canal varies depending on which study is cited. In general, these lesions are usually posterolateral in location except in the cervical region, where they are more likely to be anterior. They are primarily intradural extramedullary (76 of 84 cases) but can be both intradural and extradural (5 of 84 cases) or, less likely, purely extradural (3 of 84 cases) (198). When meningiomas are purely extradural, they tend to be malignant (198). Rarely, spinal meningiomas can be multiple (197).

In females, 83% of spinal meningiomas are in a thoracic location, with a 7:1 ratio of thoracic to cervical meningiomas. In males, approximately 47% of meningiomas are found in a thoracic location and another 41% at the cervical level (200). Considering the population as a whole, approximately 80% of meningiomas are found in the thoracic region, 16% are cervical, and 3% are lumbar (201). Within the cervical spine, excluding the foramen magnum, the segments most often affected are C3 and C4 (202).

The most common symptom is pain, either local or radicular (197). Other findings include paresthesias, numbness, weakness, and bowel or bladder abnormalities (197). Symptoms of cord compression are more frequent than those of root compression. In one study, only 21% of patients had distinctly radicular pain. When symptoms are unilateral, the tumor has been found to be on the ipsilateral side of the symptoms in 95% of cases. More rarely, symptoms can include headaches, dizziness, nausea, and vomiting. The intracranial symptoms are felt to result from elevated intracranial pressure due to an absorption block from high protein, recurrent hemorrhage, or venous obstruction. The average duration of symptoms before correct diagnosis is 28 months. The acute onset of symptoms may be indicative of a bleed into an angioblastic-type meningioma (200).

On physical examination, the nature of the neurologic deficit is reported as approximately 50% sensory and 50% motor (203). In one study only 17% of patients had intact motor function. Seventy-nine percent had abnormal reflexes, the most common being lower extremity hyperflexia. The high incidence of laterally positioned tumors is the explanation for the frequency of a Brown-Séquard syndrome with ipsilateral paralysis, decreased tactile and deep sensation, and a contralateral deficit in pain and temperature sensation (204,205).

Pathology

The tissue of origin of meningiomas other than the angiomatous type appears to be the covering cell of the arachnoid layer, known as the "cap cell" layer. Meningiomas arise from persistent arachnoid cell remnants in the spinal coverings, usually from arachnoid. Meningiomas usually adhere to, but do not arise from, dura. Because they arise from arachnoid, dural attachment is fortuitous and due to infiltration. Meningiomas may also become attached to dentate ligaments, nerve roots, or even cord itself (204,206,208–210).

Histologically, the meningothelial, fibroblastic, psammomatous, and angiomatous types are seen (206). Calcifications are present in up to 72% of the cases (201). The angiomatous (angioblastic) form differs from the other types of meningiomas in lacking arachnoid cap cells (210). The angioblastic form is subdivided into hemangioblastic and hemangiopericytic categories. The hemangioblastic form arises from capillary walls and is similar histologically to the cerebellar hemangioblastoma. The hemangiopericytic form arises from pericytes, tends toward recurrence at a younger age, has a higher rate of recurrence, and lacks psammoma bodies. Some have stated that it is more prone to metastasize than other forms (212,213), whereas others state that no valid correlation can be drawn between the histologic type and the tendency toward recurrence or metastasis (214).

Imaging

Plain films can show bony abnormalities associated with spinal meningiomas such as pedicle erosion and widening of the neural foramina, although these changes are more commonly seen with neurofibromas (206). On CT, an isodense or slightly hyperdense mass can be visualized. Prominent enhancement occurs after the administration of contrast.

On MRI, short TR images disclose lesions that are hypointense to isointense to the spinal cord (215) (Fig. 19). Meningiomas in the spine tend to be well circumscribed,

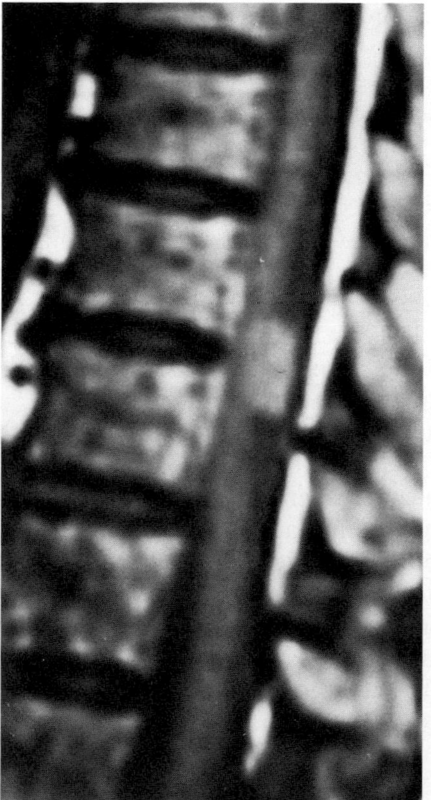
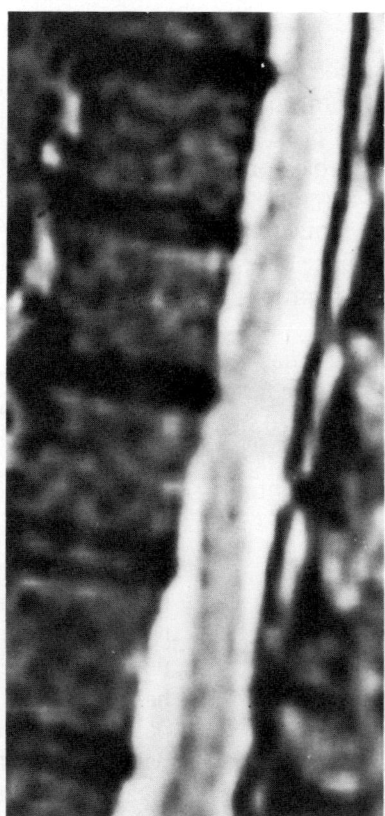
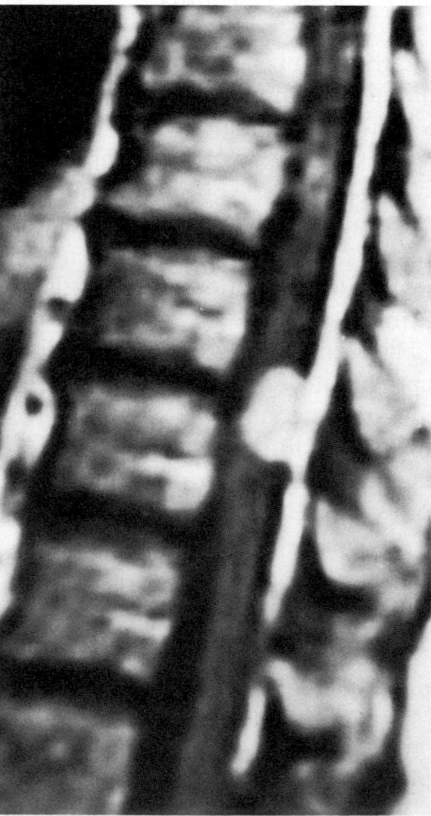

A B,C

FIG. 19. Spinal meningioma. **A:** Short TR (600/20) sagittal MR image, precontrast, shows intradural extramedullary lesion compressing the cord from its posterior location. **B:** Long TR (2000/70) sagittal MR image shows the lesion displacing the CSF column (high signal intensity) posterior to the cord. **C:** Short TR (600/20) sagittal MR image, postcontrast, shows the brightly enhancing lesion with excellent cord/lesion differentiation. (From Augenstein et al., ref. 196, with permission.)

frequently located anterolateral or posterolateral to the spinal cord, and tend to displace it (198). Long TR images show meningiomas to be slightly hyperintense to the spinal cord. In the intradural extramedullary location they are silhouetted against the high signal intensity of the CSF on the long TR images. These vascular tumors usually enhance immediately, intensely, and homogeneously after gadolinium administration (215,216). Finally, there may be areas of signal void, representing calcifications, especially in the psammomatous type (198).

The most common spinal lesion in the differential diagnosis with a meningioma is a nerve sheath tumor. Several criteria help to differentiate these two lesions. Neural tumors tend to be more anteriorly located within the spinal canal, whereas spinal meningiomas have a posterolateral location except when they are located in the cervical region where they are more likely to be anterior (197). Frequently, neurofibromas are multiple, whereas meningiomas tend to be solitary. Nerve sheath tumors are not attached to the dura and therefore have more mobility than meningiomas (185). Finally, neural tumors can have a central area of decreased signal on long TR images not seen with meningiomas.

Treatment and Prognosis

Early diagnosis and surgical intervention for spinal cord meningiomas can bring about a dramatic improvement in symptomatology. A complete cure is possible if patients receive an operation before irreversible cord ischemia occurs. At 6 months after surgery, 85% of patients are found to be either neurologically intact or improved. Even paraplegic patients have a chance of returning to ambulation after surgery, given an appropriate interval of time.

The recurrence rate after surgery for meningiomas is approximately 4% on long-term follow-up, with recurrences reported up to 38 years postoperatively (200,203). Calcified meningiomas tend to have a poor neurologic outcome because of difficulty in mobilizing the tumor from surrounding tissues at surgery (200).

SECONDARY INTRADURAL EXTRAMEDULLARY TUMORS

Spinal Leptomeningeal Tumor

Both primary intracranial neoplasms and systemic tumors may spread to the CSF. Primary intracranial neoplasms are the most common, especially in the pediatric population (178,217). In 42 cases of leptomeningeal tumor due to primary intracranial neoplasms, medulloblastoma was the most frequent, representing 48% of the cases (218). Glioblastoma (grades III and IV) was next, occurring in 14%. Ependymoma was seen in 12% of the cases, oligodendroglioma 12%, astrocytoma 7%, retinoblastoma 5%, and pinealoma 3% (218). In the pediatric population, choroid plexus papilloma can also show subarachnoid spread. The importance of establishing the presence of leptomeningeal disease with an intracranial lesion is paramount because this information significantly alters therapy. If tumor is present within the spinal canal, spinal axis radiation is employed (219).

Two age peaks for leptomeningeal carcinomatosis in the pediatric population are seen, the first roughly at 6 years of age and the second at 14 to 15 years (122). The second peak occurs in patients who have had spinal axis radiation and either have delayed spread of a primary tumor into the radiated spine or have secondary recurrence intracranially with later spread through the subarachnoid space into the spinal column (122). Thirty-three percent of patients with intracranial recurrence of medulloblastoma will have leptomeningeal spread into the spine at the time of diagnosis of the recurrence (219).

Although the tumors that spread to the subarachnoid space are often primary intracranial neoplasms, tumors outside the CNS can also spread to the meninges (220). Systemic tumors may spread to the leptomeninges by many mechanisms, including direct extension into the subarachnoid space, peripheral lymphatic invasion, hematogenous dissemination, or seeding via the choroid (220).

In the spine, leptomeningeal tumor most often spreads to the lumbosacral region (73%), probably because of the effects of gravity, with most of the tumor cells settling in this area (219). However, some lesions are seen in the cervical and thoracic region. In one series, 3 of 26 patients with subarachnoid spread had lesions within the cervical region (219). Lesions in the cervical and thoracic region tend to be dorsal in location (219). Again, this distribution may reflect the natural flow of CSF because CSF travels from the brain dorsal to the cord and then returns to the brain ventral to the cord.

Frequently, subarachnoid spread of tumor can be asymptomatic (219,221). However, leptomeningeal tumor often produces a characteristic constellation of symptoms (8). Because the patients have neoplastic cells in the CSF, symptoms may be referable to any location in which the tumor cells localize. Thus, patients will often have symptoms referable to many locations in the neuraxis at the same time. For example, a patient may have headache, cranial nerve symptoms, and focal back pain at the same time. In Wasserstrom's study, 50% of 90 patients initially complained of cerebral symptoms (8). Headache was seen in 33%. Change in mental status was noted in approximately 17%. Other symptoms referable to the brain included seizures, nausea and vomiting, and polyuria, due to diabetes insipidus. Cranial nerve symptoms were seen in 38% of patients (8). Seventy percent of patients had evidence of spinal root involvement.

Of the systemic tumors, carcinoma of the breast is the most common cause, followed by carcinoma of the lung, malignant melanoma, carcinoma of the genitourinary tract, and carcinoma of the head and neck or colon.

Imaging

Contrast-enhanced MR scans, as mentioned previously, are very sensitive to the detection of subarachnoid tumor in the spine (7,16) (Fig. 20). Tumor spread can have a variety of appearances. In some cases, tumor may coat the cord or the nerve roots, resulting in a fine layer of enhancement overlying all the structures. In other cases, tumor growth may be very local, rather than diffuse, resulting in the appearance of multiple nodules in the subarachnoid space. Finally, in severe cases, enhancement of the entire thecal sac may be seen, due to tumor permeating all of the CSF space.

While the advent of gadolinium-enhanced MRI has permitted a less invasive method of the evaluation of suspected leptomeningeal tumor, large series comparing the efficacy of gadolinium-enhanced scans and the traditional modalities (myelography and postmyelography

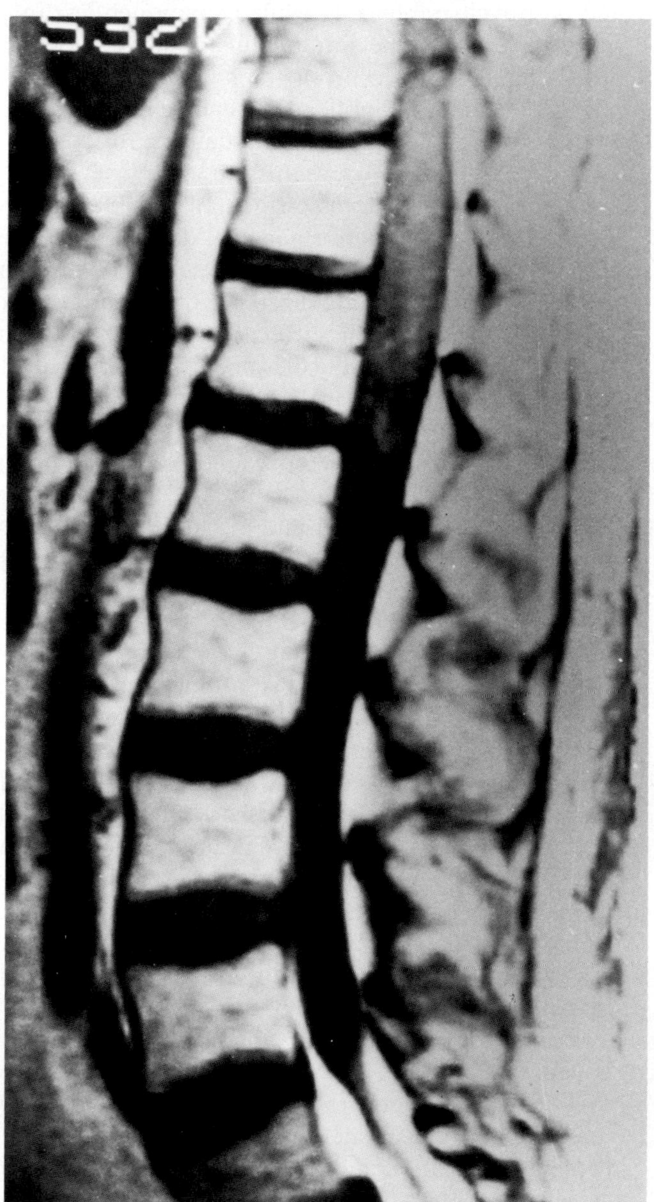

A

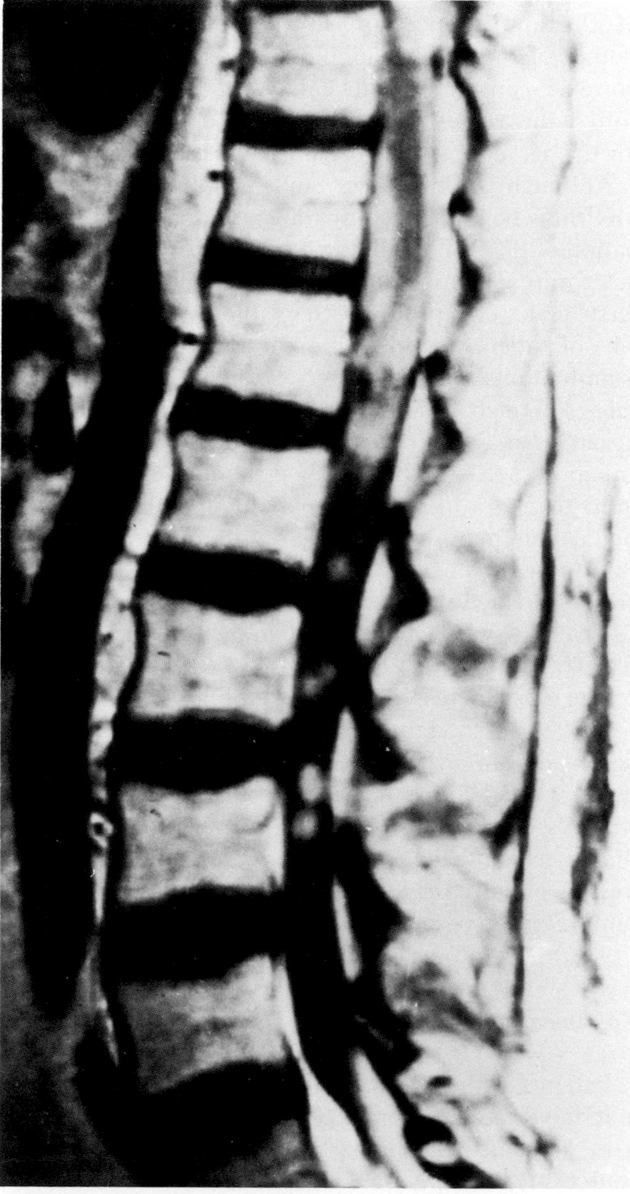

B

FIG. 20. Drop metastases from cerebral glioblastoma. **A:** Short TR (600/20) sagittal MR scan is negative except for poor definition of the conus and proximal nerve roots. On retrospect only, very vague nodules may be present in the subarachnoid space. There may be a suggestion of high intensity near the conus. **B:** Short TR (600/20) sagittal MR scan after contrast discloses enhancing subarachnoid tumor encasing the nonenhancing distal spinal cord. In addition, multiple other drop metastases are clearly visualized. (From Sze et al., ref. 7, with permission.)

CT) remain to be performed. To date, most experience is anecdotal. We have seen cases in which the myelogram and postmyelography CT suggested lesions, generally subtle, that the gadolinium-enhanced MR scans did not detect; alternatively, we have also seen cases in which the myelogram and postmyelography CT appeared normal but in which the gadolinium-enhanced MR scans proved the diagnosis. In general, if subtle irregularity of the thecal sac or minimal and localized intradural extramedullary nodules are present, the gadolinium-enhanced MRI may not be as accurate as myelography. This is particularly true if the actual pathology is so focal that it may lie in an intersection gap. However, gadolinium-enhanced MR scans appear to be superior to myelography if diffuse coating of the cord and nerve roots is suspected (222). Myelography is often insensitive to subtle changes in the caliber of the cord. Gadolinium-enhanced MR scans, however, can demonstrate enhancing tumor coating the cord in these cases. Similarly, in some cases, disease coating the nerve roots can appear as diffuse enhancement.

Although myelography and gadolinium-enhanced MRI may be roughly comparable in most cases, examination of the CSF is still the most sensitive modality for determining leptomeningeal tumor spread (8). In Wasserstrom's study, positive CSF cytology was identified in 54% of patients on initial lumbar puncture. Subsequent examinations of the CSF increase the yield of malignant cells, although CSF cytology may remain persistently negative in some patients. Findings on gadolinium-enhanced MR scan have been estimated to occur in no more than 15% to 20% in cases with proved leptomeningeal carcinomatosis. Nevertheless, the finding of the focal tumor is clinically important because these patients are best treated with radiation directed at the tumor in addition to whatever other therapy the patients may receive.

The use of increased doses of gadolinium has been suggested as a method to increase rates of detection of leptomeningeal tumor. To date, no studies of this subject have been reported. Since the primary purpose of the imaging study is often to disclose focal tumor nodules, rather than to diagnose the presence of microscopic carcinomatous meningitis, the utility of increased doses of gadolinium has yet to be demonstrated.

Treatment

Patients with primary intracranial tumors and subarachnoid spread are treated with radiation to the spinal axis. Patients with metastatic tumor from systemic sources are generally treated with intrathecal chemotherapy and radiation therapy directed at any tumor nodules that may be seen in the spine (8). The chemotherapy used in this case is nearly always methotrexate. The prognosis for patients with leptomeningeal carcinomatosis is poor. However, using aggressive therapy, a small percentage of patients may actually have tumor cells cleared from their CSF. Although they will eventually succumb to metastatic disease elsewhere, they may have their CNS cleansed of tumor.

INTRAMEDULLARY TUMORS

Technique

In the extradural space and in the intradural extramedullary space, MRI has generally proved to be equally efficacious with the traditional modalities, myelography and postmyelography CT, while being much less invasive. However, in the intramedullary space, MRI has proved far superior to myelography and postmyelography CT (1,2,223). Subtle cord enlargement is often difficult to detect with the old modalities. In fact, myelography has been shown to miss up to 50% of cord metastases. In addition, the assessment of possible cyst cavities depends on the performance of delayed CT scans, which allow iodinated contrast agents placed within the thecal sac to permeate the substance of the cord and localize in the cavities. This evaluation is time-consuming and lacks sensitivity. Furthermore, it is difficult to differentiate a benign syrinx from a tumor cyst.

The advent of MRI has tremendously increased the ability to detect and characterize lesions of the cord (Fig. 21). Short TR sagittal sequences usually demonstrate excellent morphologic detail and disclose cord widening (223). The presence and extent of any cystic cavities is generally easily assessed, although proteinaceous cysts may appear isointense (224). Long TR sagittal scans demonstrate high signal within the substance of the cord consistent with either tumor or surrounding edema (223).

Because of MRI's sensitivity to hemorrhage, areas of bleeding are easily detected. A number of different appearances may be seen. If hemorrhage into a cystic cavity occurs, fluid levels may result. Because of the evolution of hemoglobin breakdown products and other factors, the relative signal intensities of the inferior and superior components may vary. In addition, hemorrhagic cord tumors are often associated with superficial hemosiderin deposition along the surface of the cord, which appears as peripheral marked hypointensity on long TR sequences.

Although noncontrast MR scans generally detect lesions in the cord accurately, gadolinium can help in further characterization and delineation (15,225–228). Enhancement with gadolinium is most useful in cases of focal masses, especially hemangioblastomas and metastases (15,227). Both these lesions tend to be fairly well circumscribed and produce extensive surrounding edema. Because of this, cord swelling far beyond the re-

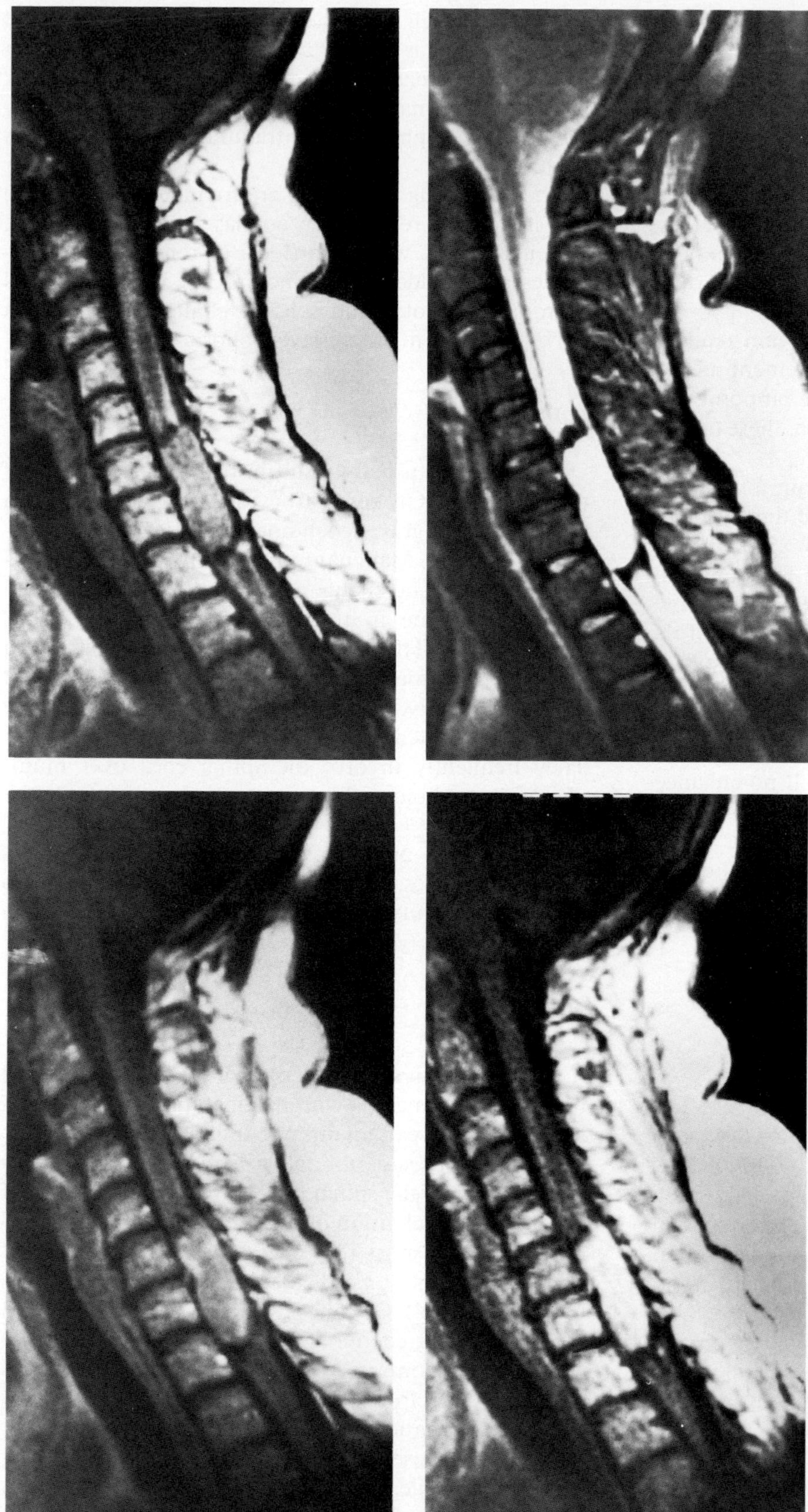

FIG. 21. Cord astrocytoma. **A,B:** Short TR (741/20) and long TR (2222/70) sagittal MRI sections disclose central nidus with superior and inferior cysts. Markedly hypointense rim was shown pathologically to be hemosiderin deposition. **C:** Enhanced short TR (741/20) sagittal MR scan 30 min after administration discloses peripheral enhancement of central lesion. **D:** One-hour delayed gadolinium-enhanced short TR (741/20) sagittal MR section shows enhancement confined to central focus. Associated cysts are not surrounded by enhancing cord parenchyma, suggesting they are benign reactive cysts, a finding confirmed at surgery, rather than tumor cysts. Necrotic nature of this tumor was shown pathologically and probably was responsible for delayed enhancement. (From Sze et al., ref. 227, with permission.)

gion of the actual tumor is often seen. The use of gadolinium can be effective in pinpointing the exact location of the lesion (215,225–228). Although the area of cord enlargement can be extensive, the actual lesion may be small, often much less than one vertebral body in height.

Results with primary cord gliomas are less dramatic. First, as in the brain, it is likely that areas of enhancement do not coincide with the actual boundaries of these infiltrative tumors. Second, unlike that seen with hemangioblastomas and metastases, enhancement is often variable.

In gliomas of the cord, enhancement again tends to be fairly focal (225–228). Areas of enhancement may be representative of more active tumor and pinpoint sites for biopsy, as is the case in the brain. Often, these tumors are associated with cysts.

Although low-grade gliomas of the brain tend not to enhance, the large majority of gliomas of the cord tend to enhance, regardless of grade (15,225–228). In fact, nonenhancing gliomas of the cord are distinctly unusual, although they have been documented. Even very low-grade tumors tend to show some enhancement. Of the 55 reported cases of cord glioma in which contrast MRI was employed, enhancement was seen in 54 (215,225–229). Because of this, the use of contrast can be helpful in differentiating suspected neoplasms from other etiology, for example, infection or benign syrinx. If no enhancement is seen the likelihood of a glioma of the cord is significantly reduced.

Because enhancement is well seen in most intramedullary tumors, no investigations of the use of increased doses of gadolinium have been reported.

PRIMARY INTRAMEDULLARY TUMORS

Astrocytoma

In reported series, gliomas constitute from 9.5% to 22.5% of all tumors of the spine, with the average being 18.7% (230–234). Approximately 36% to 54% of these are astrocytomas. Astrocytomas are especially more common in children (188,235). They represent more than 50% of intramedullary mass lesions in children, whereas ependymomas constitute approximately 24% to 38% of cases (235,236).

Overall, the peak incidence of spinal astrocytomas is in the third and fourth decade. In the Mayo Clinic series, the average age was 31 years. There is either no sexual predilection or a slight male predilection (237).

Astrocytomas are most often located in the thoracic cord. Sloof found that 17 of 86 astrocytomas were located in the cervical region, 41 were thoracic, 11 were in both the cervical and thoracic cord, 13 were in both the thoracic and lumbar cord, and 4 were lumbar (238). The prevalence of astrocytomas decreases in the lower thoracic and lumbar regions, unlike the prevalence of ependymomas, which increases in the caudal spinal canal (235). In fact, it is rare for astrocytomas to be located in the filum terminale, a common site for ependymomas. Most astrocytomas are intramedullary, although rarely they can be exophytic and intradural extramedullary in location (122).

The presenting symptoms are frequently nonspecific and ill-defined, resulting in a delay in diagnosis (237). Patients present with pain (local or remote), gait difficulties, and bladder disturbances (237,238). On physical examination motor and sensory changes can be seen (237). In children, progressive scoliosis may occur.

Pathology

These lesions usually result in fusiform expansion of the spinal cord. Grossly, astrocytomas are gray-yellow in color to reddish gray, depending on the degree of hemorrhage (185,238). Malignant tumors tend to be more vascular (239). Cystic change is present between 25% and 38% of the time in these potentially friable lesions (185,237,240). These low-grade tumors do not have a clear line of demarcation from the normal spinal cord (241). Frequently, they are eccentric in location, usually posteriorly located by the posterior columns (216,238). They frequently involve the spinal cord over multiple segments; holocord astrocytomas involve the entire cord (241).

Astrocytomas are composed of neoplastically transformed astrocytes, which vary from well differentiated to anaplastic. Seventy-five to 92% of cord astrocytomas are benign in adults (grades I and II) (239,242).

Imaging

Plain films can show widening of the spinal canal and bony erosion. Imaging with myelography and postmyelography CT reveals an intramedullary mass.

Because of its superior ability to evaluate and characterize lesions of the spinal cord, MRI is the modality of choice in the evaluation of suspected intramedullary tumors (243). On short TR images, these lesions appear of low signal intensity. Cord enlargement, often marked, is present (243,244). On long TR images, these lesions and the surrounding edema appear of high signal intensity (244). On noncontrast MRI it can be difficult to distinguish the lesion from its surrounding edema. After contrast administration these lesions almost always enhance, but because of the infiltrative nature of the tumor, without a capsule or cleavage plane between the lesion and the spinal cord, the margins of the lesion are often poorly defined and irregular (215,227). The contrast enhancement can be inhomogeneous in nature and can reveal the tumor, which might not be evident on the noncontrast portion of the exam (215,226) (Figs. 21 and 22).

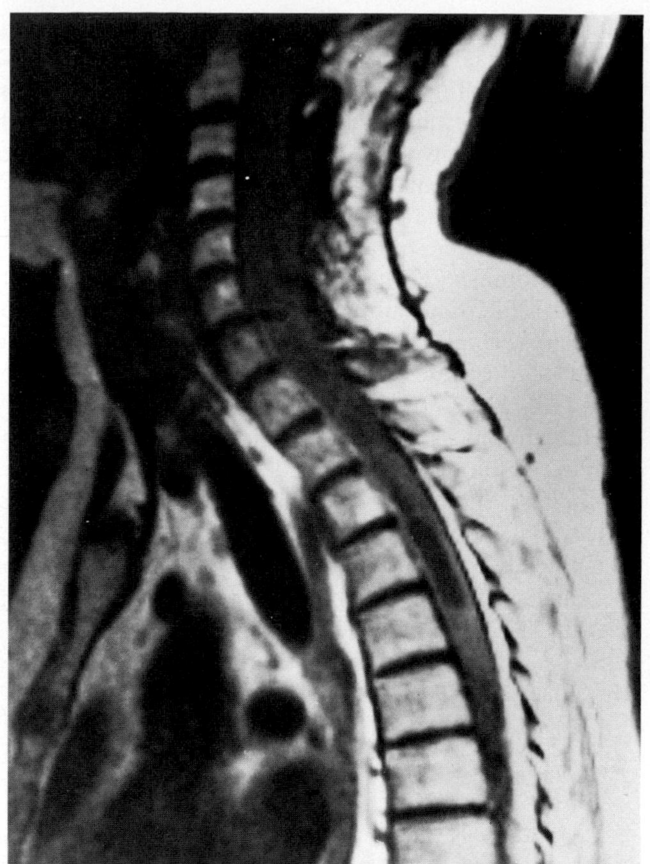

A

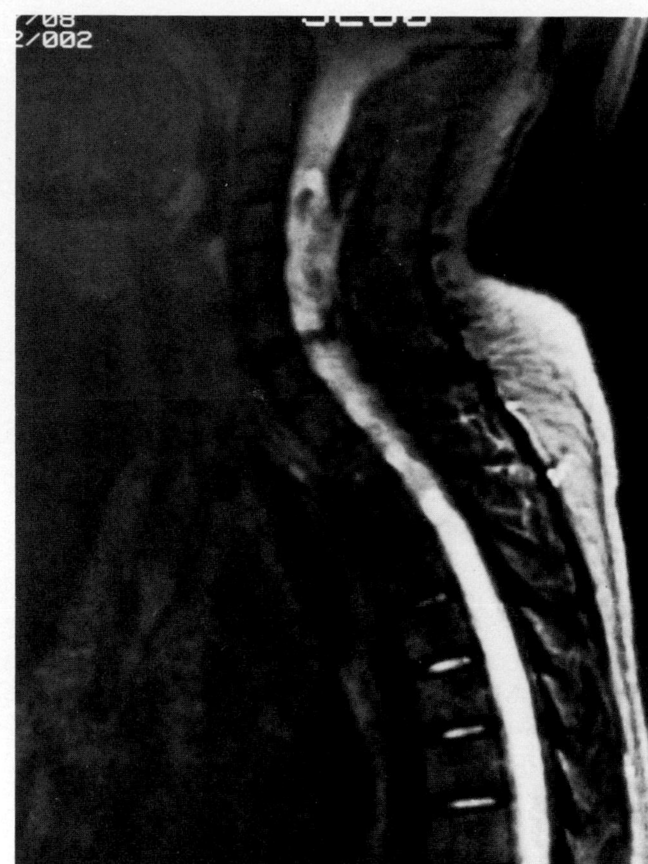

B

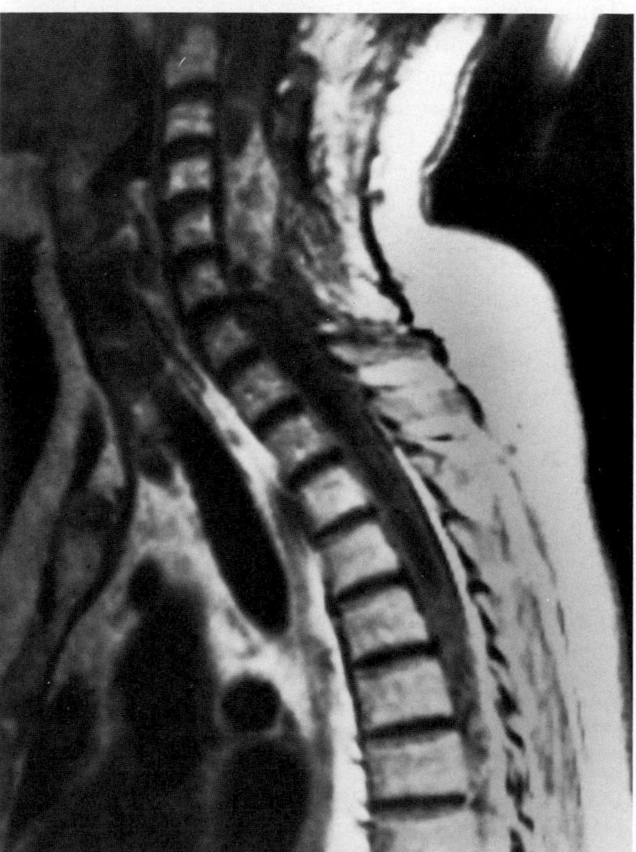

C

FIG. 22. Cord astrocytoma. A 47-year-old woman 5 years after section of cervical astrocytoma, presenting with recurrent symptoms. **A,B:** Short TR (600/20) and long TR (2118/70) sagittal MR sections disclose extensive cervical postoperative changes, with diffuse widening and some angulation of cord. Caudal cysts are noted. **C:** Gadolinium-enhanced short TR (600/20) sagittal MR section shows enhancing recurrent tumor mass confined to mid-cervical spine, distorted by postsurgical tethering and adhesion. Much of inferior cord enlargement results from combination of edema, cyst formation, and postoperative changes. (From Sze et al., ref. 227, with permission.)

Enhancement usually occurs immediately after the administration of contrast, although in necrotic tumors, delayed enhancement can be seen (181).

MRI is also advantageous in its ability to differentiate the tumor from associated cyst formation (244). Cysts can be either intratumoral or rostral and caudal (223,240). Rostral and caudal cysts tend to be benign (240). Even though the fluid within them might be proteinaceous or hemorrhagic, these cysts are usually not lined by tumor, nor do they contain tumor cells. Unlike tumor cysts, they do not require excision but are merely drained at surgery (245). Gadolinium enhancement has proved useful in identifying the nature of cysts associated with tumors (215,225–229). Tumor cysts are generally surrounded by enhancement, whereas the walls of benign cysts lack associated contrasted uptake.

Both reactive and neoplastic cysts tend to have a decreased signal intensity on T1-weighted images and an increased signal intensity on T2-weighted images in relationship to the tumor (244). However, the signal intensity can be indistinguishable from the solid tumor on noncontrast MRI, especially when the cavity is caused by necrosis within the tumor (224,245). Hemorrhage or increased protein within the cyst fluid can decrease T1 and T2 relaxation times in relation to pure CSF, making the cyst isointense with the spinal cord and tumor (244).

Complex benign syrinxes can resemble cystic astrocytomas. They have gliosis within their walls secondary to chronic CSF pulsations (236). This tissue can display increased signal intensity on long TR images and can be indistinguishable from tumor (245). On noncontrast MRI, some characteristics may favor an underlying neoplasm. These include indistinct margins to the cyst, nonuniform signal intensity of the fluid that does not parallel CSF, and the absence of pulsations (246).

Treatment

Surgery is advocated in all cases followed by radiation therapy (239,241). Histologic grade is a major facet in predicting prognosis. Low-grade tumors often have a protracted and indolent course, whereas high-grade tumors have a tendency to CSF dissemination (58%) and rapid deterioration. For all patients, the 5- and 10-year survival rates are 58% and 23%; patients with malignant tumors, however, rarely survive more than 2 years (239,247).

Ependymoma

Ependymomas are most often intracranial than intraspinal (248). Of 74 ependymomas reported by Barone, 36% were intraspinal (249). Of 62 patients with ependymoma, Rawlings found that 31% were intraspinal (250). The lesion usually presents in patients in their fourth or fifth decade of life, far older than those with intracranial ependymomas. In Barone's series, the average age was 37 years. In Rawling's series, the average age was 41 years. However, they may occur in other patients, from children to the elderly (249–251). Men predominate over women in a ratio of approximately 3:2.

Ependymoma is the most common primary cord tumor of the lower spinal cord, conus medullaris, and filum terminale (237). It represents 58% of all conus tumors (252). One subtype of ependymoma, the myxopapillary form, is particularly common in the conus and filum. It constitutes from 27% to 30% of all ependymomas (198,248,249). Of the 77 cases of myxopapillary ependymomas in the Mayo Clinic series, 65% were limited to the filum, 30% involved the filum and the conus medullaris, and only 4% were located in the cervicothoracic spinal cord (248).

Clinically, patients present most often with back or neck pain, seen in 63% of patients, or with radicular pain, seen in 89% of patients (250). Other symptoms include unsteady gait, numbness, and bowel or bladder dysfunction.

Pathology

Ependymal cells line the central spinal canal as well as the remainder of the internal surfaces of the CNS (238). Thus, ependymomas often tend to be central in location and exhibit centrifugal growth (215).

Grossly, ependymomas are cylindrical, elongated masses that cause localized fusiform expansion of the spinal cord (215). They are brownish red to blue in color, depending on their blood content. Ependymomas are soft, friable lesions that frequently have a delicate capsule forming a plane of cleavage to separate tumor from spinal cord (215,248). They can grow into the conus and adhere to the lumbar nerve roots (248). Cyst formation is seen in 50% of the cases (244). Although ependymomas in the brain frequently calcify, calcification is extremely uncommon in spinal ependymomas.

The most common histology is that of the cellular type. Well defined cuboidal or low columnar cells are arranged in a papillary fashion. However, the most common lesion of the filum terminale is the myxopapillary type, in which mucinous change is also seen. This type is especially prone to hemorrhage and can present as an unexplained subarachnoid bleed (121,248).

Imaging

Plain films are positive in 63% and show erosion of the pedicles or of the posterior surface of the vertebral bodies (197). CT and myelography disclose the typical intramedullary or conus/filum mass and can be performed to localize the lesion and show its extent and the degree of

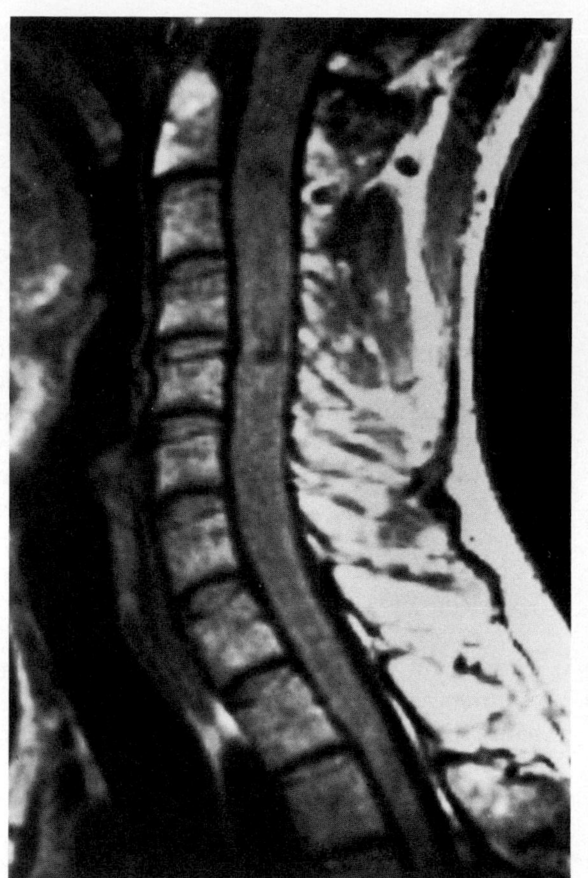

A

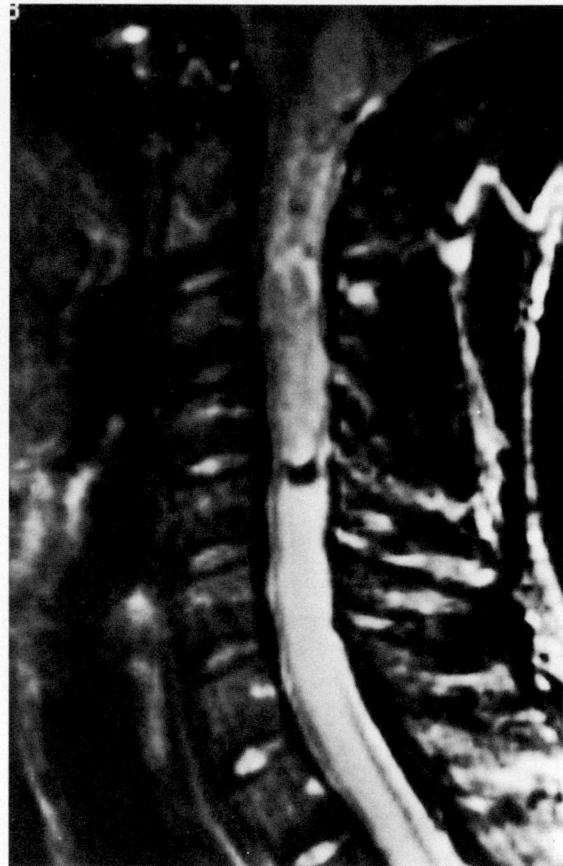

B

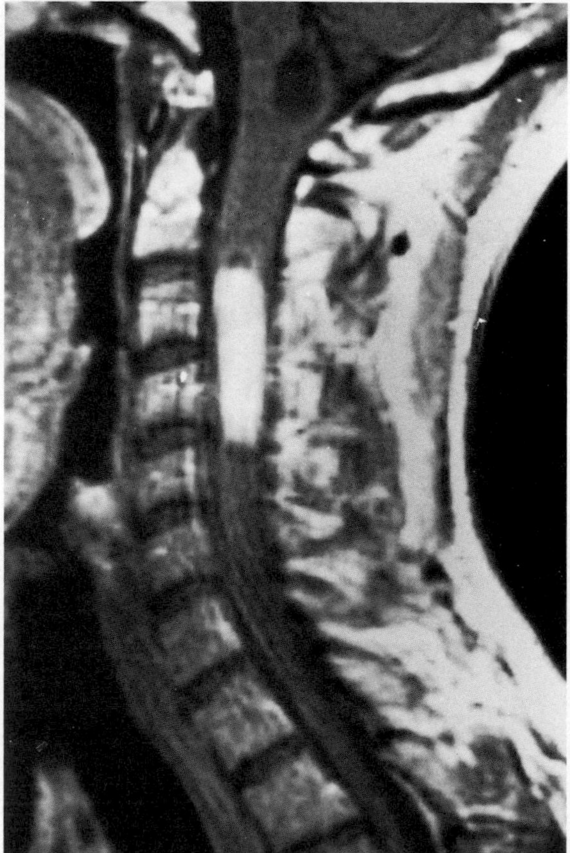

C

FIG. 23. Cord ependymoma. **A:** Short TR (600/20) sagittal MR image discloses heterogeneity and widening of the cord from the cervicomedullary junction at least to C7. **B:** Long TR (1880/70) sagittal image demonstrates heterogeneous hyperintensity of the entire cord, associated with several hypointense foci containing hemosiderin. **C:** Short TR (600/20) sagittal MR image shows focal enhancement of the tumor nidus at C3-C5. Associated benign cyst is seen at the cervicomedullary junction. (From Sze et al., ref. 270, with permission.)

spinal cord block. These modalities, however, are frequently nonspecific.

Noncontrast MRI demonstrates spinal cord widening or a mass, frequently near the conus (225–229,244) (Fig. 23). The lesion is hypointense or isointense with the cord on short TR images and hyperintense on long TR images (253). Areas of hemorrhage may appear of varying intensity on both sequences. Hemosiderin deposition is frequently encountered, particularly at the superior and inferior borders of the tumor, and appears as mildly hypointense on short TR images and markedly hypointense on long TR images. Although the tumors have a capsule and can be well delineated pathologically, it is difficult to differentiate these tumors from astrocytomas by imaging criteria.

After the administration of contrast, ependymomas tend to enhance intensely and homogeneously (215, 225,229). The lesions often have well defined borders. Gadolinium helps to better identify intratumoral and peritumoral cysts, especially those that can be isointense with the lesion and cord on noncontrast MRI (225–229,245) (Fig. 23).

The differentiation of astrocytomas and ependymomas is difficult with imaging. There are a few suggestive criteria, however. First, ependymomas occur far more often in the lower cord and conus than astrocytomas. A significant proportion, however, of ependymomas do occur in the cervical or thoracic cord. Second, astrocytomas tend to arise eccentrically within the cord, especially posteriorly. Ependymomas arise from ependymal cells in the central canal and tend to be central (Fig. 24). Third, ependymomas are more frequently hemorrhagic than astrocytomas. Hemorrhage with cord astrocytomas, however, is also not uncommon. Finally, because of the thin pseudocapsule that surrounds ependymomas, it may be possible on very thin sections to identify a plane separating the ependymoma from the cord (S. Hilal, *personal communication*), unlike astrocytomas, which tend to be infiltrative and have poorly defined borders. This plane, however, may be difficult to identify.

Treatment

Treatment is aimed at surgical removal. With complete removal of an encapsulated tumor, there is little chance for recurrence (15%) (248). However, sometimes the tumor is poorly encapsulated or cannot be removed

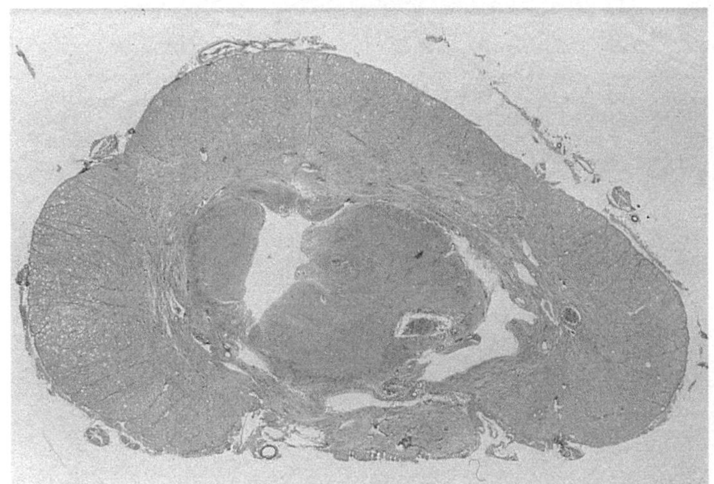

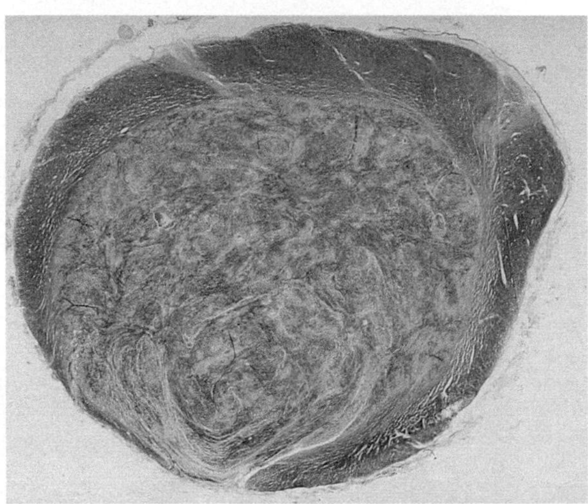

FIG. 24 Spinal cord astrocytoma vs. ependymoma. **A:** Astrocytoma. Cross-section of the upper cervical cord shows extensive replacement of spinal cord with ill-defined tumor tissue with cystic necrosis as well as syringohydromyelia. **B,C:** Ependymomas. Typical, well circumscribed, centrally located intramedullary tumor on axial section (B). Multiple well circumscribed centrally located ependymomas are also seen on longitudinal sections (C). (From Okazaki and Scheithauer, ref. 193, with permission.)

entirely (248). These tumors can metastasize via CSF dissemination or by distant metastases (248).

Hemangioblastoma

Although hemangioblastomas are the most common primary posterior fossa tumor in the adult, they rarely involve the spinal cord. They constitute 3.3% of intramedullary tumors. There is no sex predilection. These lesions usually present in the fourth decade. In a review of 85 cases in the literature, Browne et al. noted a median age of 30 years (254).

Approximately 30% of the patients with spinal cord hemangioblastomas have von Hippel-Lindau syndrome. Von Hippel-Lindau syndrome, an autosomal dominant disorder with almost 100% penetrance, is typified by cerebellar hemangioblastomas (35–60%), retinal angiomatosis (greater than 50%), renal cell carcinomas (25–38%), pheochromocytoma (greater than 10%), or spinal hemangioblastomas (less than 5%) (254–257). However, the incidence of spinal cord hemangioblastomas in von Hippel-Lindau syndrome may be underestimated because these lesions are frequently asymptomatic (256,257). An autopsy study of 10 patients with von Hippel-Lindau syndrome revealed hemangioblastomas of the cord in all (253). When patients with von Hippel-Lindau syndrome have retinal or cerebellar hemangioblastomas coexisting with spinal hemangioblastomas, they usually present with symptoms from the former le-

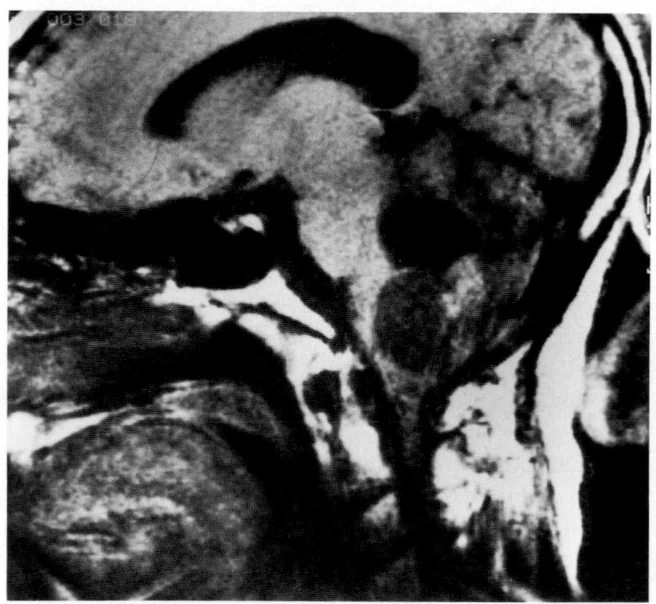

A

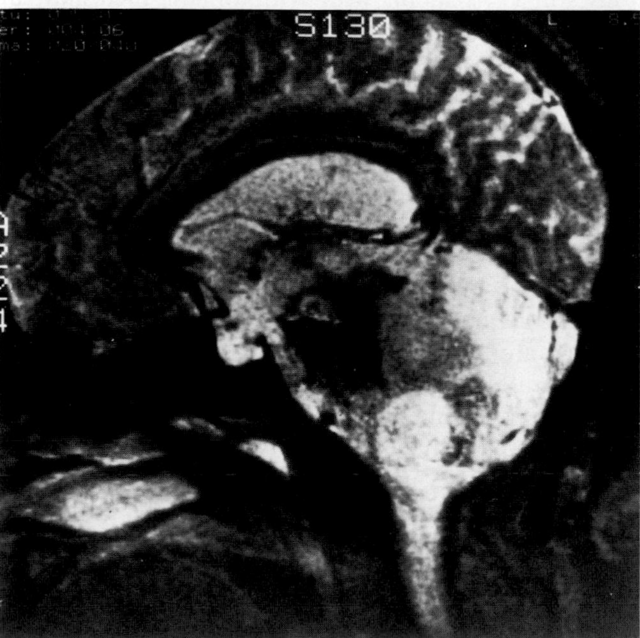

B

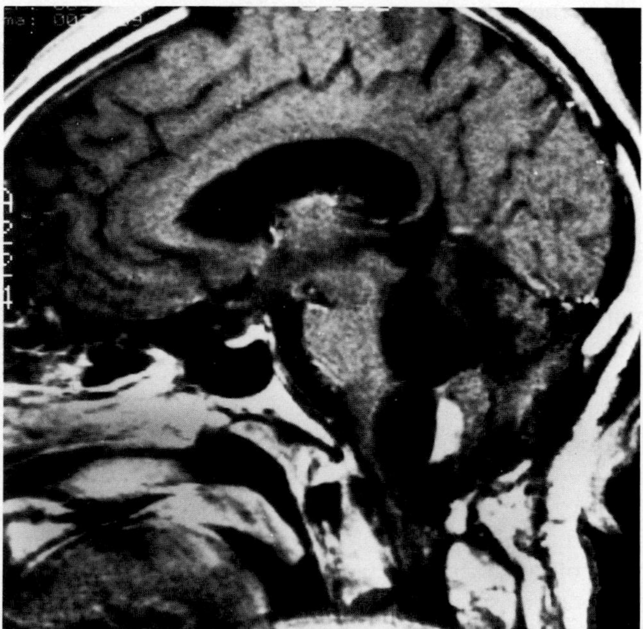

C

FIG. 25. Hemangioblastoma in a patient with von Hippel-Lindau syndrome. **A:** Short TR (600/20) sagittal MR scan of cervicomedullary region shows well circumscribed low-intensity lesion. No distinct tumor nodule is defined. **B:** Long TR (2000/70) sagittal MR scan does not provide additional information regarding nidus of lesion. High intensity in white matter of brain, especially cerebellum, is noted incidentally and probably is from postoperative and postradiation change resulting from previous resection of a cerebellar hemangioblastoma. **C:** Short TR (600/20) sagittal MR scan after administration of gadolinium reveals enhancement of nidus of cystic tumor. These findings were used to guide neurosurgeons to complete resection of nidus. (From Sze et al., ref. 227, with permission.)

sions rather than from the spinal cord lesions (255,256). In patients with a family history positive for von Hippel-Lindau syndrome, even if asymptomatic, MRI is now recommended to evaluate for cerebellar or spinal cord lesions.

Hemangioblastomas involving the spinal cord tend to be single (79%), although multiple tumors in a single patient are not unusual. In spinal hemangioblastomas, the thoracic cord is most often involved (51%), followed by the cervical cord (41%) (254,257). Most hemangioblastomas are intramedullary (60%); however, they can also be intradural extramedullary or purely extradural.

Of all spinal hemangioblastomas, 43% are associated with cysts; however, when purely intramedullary hemangioblastomas are considered, cyst formation is seen in up to 67% of the cases (254,259). The cyst fluid is often proteinaceous, either from previous hemorrhage or from transudation of fluid by the tumor. Cord hemangioblastomas are also associated with meningeal varicosities, which have been noted in 48% of cases and which usually are located on the dorsal surface of the cord.

Pathology

Histologically, hemangioblastomas are composed of endothelial cells intermixed with stromal cells containing fat and hemosiderin (254). The endothelial cells form masses, cords, and thin-walled blood vessels. It is this portion of the tumor that comprises the actual growing mass (254). Eventually the tumor consists of a compact collection of capillaries with small feeding arteries and dilated draining veins (257).

The cysts can be very large compared with the size of the tumor (255). They are lined with fibrillary neuroglia, similar to those seen with syrinxes. In three patients with cord hemangioblastomas, autopsy failed to show tumor cells in the wall of the cyst cavity (254).

Imaging

Plain films may demonstrate widening of the spinal canal. Myelography frequently shows expansion of the spinal cord and serpiginous filling defects posterior to the cord representing meningeal varicosities. CT can show widening of the cord with a hypodense tumor nidus that markedly enhances (254). Spinal angiography reveals prominent feeding arteries and draining veins and an intense blush of the tumor nidus.

Unenhanced MRI demonstrates widening of the spinal cord (259) (Fig. 25). Associated cyst formation may be noted. The cysts may vary in signal intensity, depending on their contents (259). Signal characteristics can parallel those of CSF or may be of greater intensity as a result of increased protein content (224,259). As a result of this increased signal intensity, the cyst can occasionally be indistinguishable from the tumor nidus and cord on noncontrast sequences. Cord hemangioblastomas are often associated with considerable edema, as shown by low signal on short TR and increased signal on long TR images. Adjacent serpiginous areas of signal void may be seen (257). These can represent large feeding arteries or, more commonly, draining meningeal varicosities associated with the very vascular tumor nidus (254,257).

Enhanced MRI shows a markedly enhancing tumor nidus, permitting differentiation of the often small nidus from the adjacent edematous spinal cord and the cyst (227,229). This helps to direct surgery toward accurate removal of the tumor nidus and decompression of the adjacent cyst.

Treatment

Complete surgical removal offers the only chance of cure at the present time (254). Total removal is possible in some cases because a cleavage plane often separates tumor from adjacent cord. Incomplete excision results in recurrence. The use of radiation therapy is uncertain. Possible benefits are counterbalanced by the acute risk of increased cord edema and the chronic risk of radiation myelopathy (254).

SECONDARY INTRAMEDULLARY TUMORS

Metastatic Disease to the Cord

Metastatic intramedullary tumors are rare, especially when compared with extradural metastases (260,261). The incidence of metastasis to the spinal cord in patients with systemic carcinomas has been estimated from 0.9% to 8.5% (260–262). Edelson et al. found six cord metastases in 175 patients with symptomatic metastatic disease to the spine, or 3.4% (261). However, Costigan et al., in a retrospective autopsy series, noted an incidence of 8.5% of cases of metastasis to the cord (260). This estimate is high both because of the inherent bias of retrospective autopsy series and because, in a significant number of their cases, the metastases were asymptomatic and found only as microscopic deposits.

Of all intramedullary cord metastases, carcinoma of the lung accounts for 40% to 85% of the total (260–265). Breast carcinoma, melanoma, lymphoma, colon, and kidney are other common sites (260–262).

Several routes have been suggested by which metastatic deposits may reach the cord (260,261). Because a very high percentage of patients have a primary or metastatic pulmonary neoplasm, arterial seeding is a possible mechanism because tumor must reach the lungs before disseminating through the arterial system. Tumor may also reach the cord through the vertebral venous system, known as Batson's plexus. Finally, tumor may extend to the cord by direct invasion from nerve roots or CSF. This route would explain the frequent but not inevitable association of intramedullary metastasis with leptomeningeal tumor.

Of all areas of the cord, the thoracic cord is most often involved, followed by the cervical and the lumbar cord (261). In Edelson's review of the literature combined with a contribution of nine cases, 41% occurred in the thoracic region, 29% in the cervical region, and 8% in the lumbar region (261). The remainder were at the cervicothoracic and thoracolumbar junctions. The high incidence of intramedullary metastases in the lumbar region,

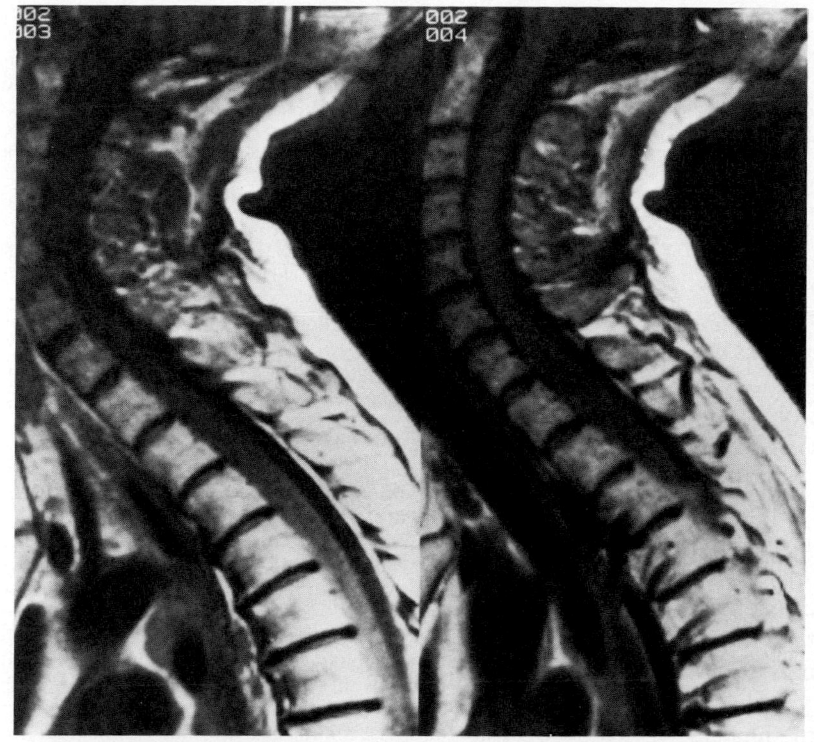

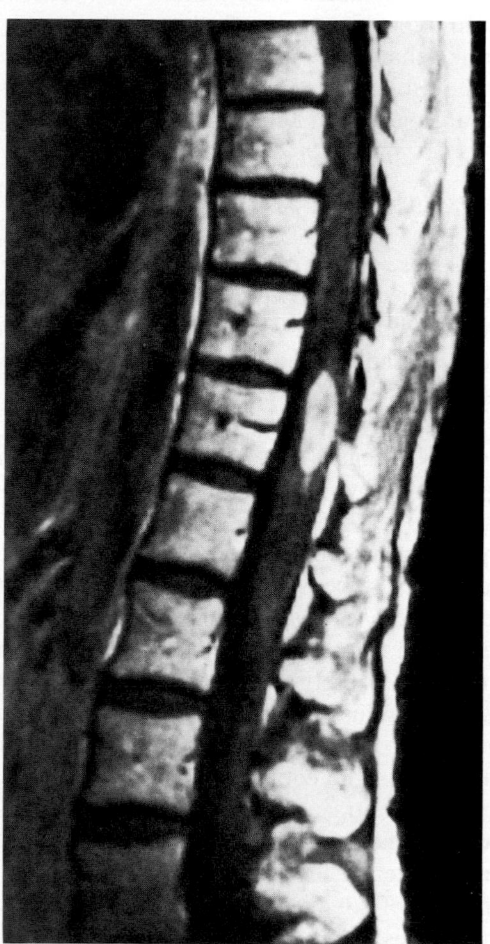

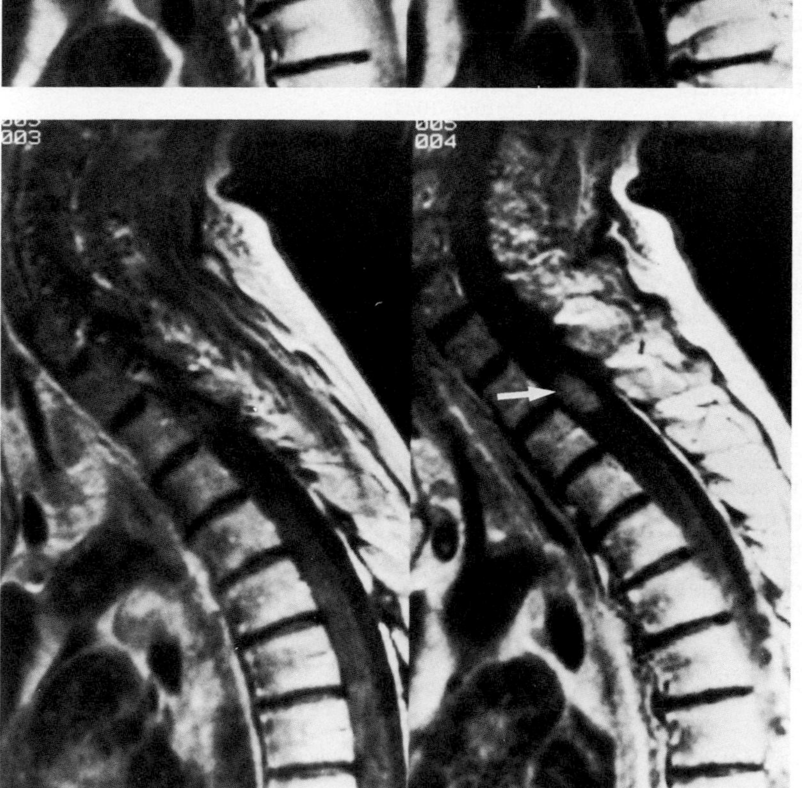

FIG. 26. Breast carcinoma metastases to the cord. **A:** Short TR (600/20) sagittal MR scan shows cord widened over considerable portion of cervical and upper thoracic spine. **B:** After administration of contrast, short TR (600/20) sagittal MR scan discloses localized region of enhancement, probably representing focal metastasis (*arrow*). Remainder of cord enlargement most likely is due to edema. **C:** Additional short TR (600/20) MR sequences after administration of gadolinium reveal second, clinically unsuspected intramedullary metastasis in distal thoracic cord. (From Sze et al., ref. 227, with permission.)

despite the disproportionately small length of the lumbar cord, may be due to the prevalence of leptomeningeal deposits in this location.

Intramedullary metastases may present with a confusing clinical picture (261–265). Pain is a common complaint (70%). Although radicular pain characterizes extradural tumors, it may also often be seen with cord metastases. Weakness (100%), paresthesias (50%), and bowel and bladder disturbances (60%) are often encountered. A striking feature is the rapid clinical progression, unlike that seen with primary cord tumors (261–265). In Edelson's series, 70% of patients exhibited complete paraplegia within 2 months (261).

Imaging

Because of the rapid progression of the syndrome, plain films are usually negative, although metastases in the vertebral bodies may be incidentally noted. Myelography is frequently normal, as noted in 13 of 30 cases by Edelson et al. (261).

MRI shows a widened cord, often extending for a considerable length (Fig. 26). On short TR scans, the cord appears of low intensity; on long TR scans, it is of high intensity (227). The low intensity on short TR images may appear to be predominantly central. This appearance can also be seen on the axial images and can lead to confusion with a syrinx. The differentiation of edematous cord from cyst is important because metastases of the cord are rarely associated with cysts. On long TR images, the nidus of the tumor can sometimes be visualized as a lower intensity structure surrounded by the higher intensity of the edematous cord. After the administration of contrast, metastases often enhance homogeneously and markedly (225,227). The size of the metastasis is often disproportionately small compared with the amount of edema. In occasional cases, intramedullary metastases may be hemorrhagic and have areas of varying signal intensity on both short TR and long TR images.

Therapy

Radiation is the therapy of choice (261–265); surgery offers little hope. However, most patients with cord metastases die soon after they present (261). Two thirds succumb within 6 months, usually because of widespread metastatic disease.

REFERENCES

1. Hans JS, Kaufman B, El Yousef SJ, et al. NMR imaging of the spine. *AJNR* 1983;4:1151–1159.
2. Norman D, Mill C, Brant-Zawadzki M, Yeates A, Crooks LE, Kaufman L. Magnetic resonance imaging of the spinal cord and canal: potential and limitations. *AJNR* 1984;5:9–14.
3. Carmody RF, Yang DJ, Seeley GW, Seeger JF, Unger EC, Johnson JF. Spinal cord compression due to metastatic disease: diagnosis with MR imaging versus myelography. *Radiology* 1989; 173:225–229.
4. Smoker WRK, Godersky JC, Nutzon RK, et al. Role of MR imaging in evaluating metastatic spinal disease. *AJNR* 1987;8:901–908.
5. Beltram J, Noto AM, Chakeres DW, Christoforidis AJ. Tumors of the osseous spine: staging with MR imaging versus CT. *Radiology* 1987;162:565–569.
6. Avrahami E, Tadmor R, Dally O, et al. Early MR demonstration of spinal metastases in patients with normal radiographs and CT and radionuclide bone scans. *J Comput Assist Tomogr* 1989;13: 598–602.
7. Sze G, Abramson A, Krol G, et al. Gadolinium-DTPA/dimeglumine in the MR evaluation of intradural extramedullary spinal disease. *AJNR* 1988;9:153-163; *AJR* 1988;150:911–921.
8. Wasserstrom WR, Glass JP, Posner JB. Diagnosis and treatment of leptomeningeal metastases from solid tumors: experience with 90 patients. *Cancer* 1982;49:759–772.
9. Daffner RH, Lupetin AR, Cash N, et al. MRI in the detection of malignant infiltration of bone marrow. *AJR* 1986;146:353–358.
10. Sze G, Krol G, Zimmerman RD, Deck MDF. Gadolinium-DTPA: malignant extradural spinal tumors. *Radiology* 1988;167: 217–233.
11. Vogler JB, Murphy WA. Bone marrow imaging. *Radiology* 1988;168:679–693.
12. Geremia GK, McCluney K, Adler S, et al. The magnetic resonance hypointense spine of AIDS. ASNR, 27th Annual Meeting, Orlando, 1989;90.
13. Stimac GK, Porter BA, Olson DO, et al. Gadolinium-DTPA-enhanced MR imaging of spinal neoplasms: preliminary investigation and comparison with unenhanced spin-echo and STIR sequences. *AJNR* 1988;9:839–846; *AJR* 1988;151:1185–1192.
14. Gusnard DA, Grossman RI, Hackney DB. The differential utility of gradient-echo and spin-echo MRI of the abnormal spine. Presented at the Twenty-Sixth Annual Meeting of ASNR, Chicago, 1988;15.
15. Yuh WTC, Zachar CK, Barloon TJ, Sato Y, Sickels WJ, Hawes DR. Vertebral compression fractures: distinction between benign and malignant causes with MR imaging. *Radiology* 1989;172: 215–218.
16. Sze G. MR of the spine: contrast agents. *Radiol Clin North Am* 1988;26:1009–1024.
17. Schmorl G, Junghanns, H. *The Human Spine in Health and Disease*, 2nd ed. New York: Grune and Stratton; 1971:325.
18. McAllister VL, Kendall BE, Bull JW. Symptomatic vertebral hemangiomas. *Brain* 1975;98:71–80.
19. Ross JS, Masaryk TJ, Modic MT. Vertebral hemangiomas: MR imaging. *Radiology* 1987;165:165–169.
20. Tekkok IH, Acikgoz B, Saglam S, Onol B. Vertebral hemangioma symptomatic during pregnancy—report of a case and review of the literature. *Neurosurgery* 1993;32(2):302–306.
21. Ghormley RK, Adson AW. Hemangioma of the vertebrae. *J Bone Joint Surg* 1941;23:887–895.
22. Krueger EG, Sobel GL, Weinstein C. Vertebral hemangioma with compression of the spinal cord. *J Neurosurg* 1961;18:331–338.
23. Laredo JD, Reizine D, Bard M, Merland JJ. Vertebral hemangiomas: radiologic evaluation. *Radiology* 1986;161:183–189.
24. Ferber L, Lampe I. Hemangioma of vertebra associated with compression of the cord. *Arch Neurol Psychiatry* 1942;47:19–29.
25. Malat J, Virapongse C, Levine A. Solitary osteochondroma of the spine. *Spine* 1986;11:625–628.
26. Karian JM, DeFilipp G, Buchheit WA, Bonakdarpour A, Eckhardt W. Vertebral osteochondroma causing spinal cord compression. *Neurosurgery* 1984;14:483–484.
27. Twersky J, Kassner EG, Tenner MS, Camera A. Vertebral and costal osteochondromas causing spinal cord compression. *AJR* 1978;124:124–128.
28. Novick GS, Pavlov H, Bullough PG. Osteochondroma of the cervical spine: report of two cases in preadolescent males. *Skeletal Radiol* 1982;8:13–15.
29. Inglis AE, Rubin RM, Lewis RJ, Villacin A. Osteochondroma of the cervical spine, case report. *Clin Ortho* 1977;126:127–129.

30. Palmer FJ, Blum PW. Osteochondroma with spinal cord compression, report of three cases. *J Neurosurg* 1980;52:842–845.
31. Cohn RS, Fielding JW. Osteochondroma of the cervical spine. *J Pediatr Surg* 1986;21:997–999.
32. Gokay H, Bucy PC. Osteochondroma of the lumbar spine, report of a case. *J Neurosurg* 1955;12:72–78.
33. Ilgenfritz HC. Vertebral osteochondroma. *Am Surg* 1951;17:917–922.
34. Fielding JW, Ratzan S. Osteochondroma of the cervical spine. *J Bone Joint Surg* 1973;55A:640–641.
35. Rose EF, Fekete A. Odontoid osteochondroma causing sudden death. *Am J Clin Pathol* 1964;42:606–609.
36. Kenney PJ, Gilula LA, Murphy WA. The use of computed tomography to distinguish osteochondroma and chondrosarcoma. *Radiology* 1981;139:129–137.
37. Dahlin DC, Unni KK. *Bone Tumors: General Aspects and Data on 8,542 Cases.* Springfield, IL: Charles C Thomas; 1986;62–69.
38. Kozlowski K, Beluffi G, Masel J, et al. Primary vertebral tumours in children. Report of 20 cases with brief review of the literature. *Pediatr Radiol* 1984;14:129–139.
39. Glass RB, Poznanski AK, Fisher MR, Shkolnik A, Dias L. Case report. MR imaging of osteoid osteoma. *J Comput Assist Tomogr* 1986;10:1065–1067.
40. Jackson RP, Reckling FW, Mantz FA. Osteoid osteoma and osteoblastoma. *Clin Orthop* 1977;128:303–313.
41. Gamba JL, Martinez S, Apple J, Harrelson JM, Nunley JA. CT of axial skeletal osteoid osteomas. *AJR* 1984;142:769–772.
42. Fountain E, Burgie C. Osteoid osteoma of the cervical spine. *J Neurosurg* 1961;18:380–383.
43. Woods ER, Martel W, Mandell SH, et al. Relative soft-tissue mass associated with osteoid osteoma: correlation of MR imaging features with pathologic findings. *Radiology* 1993;186:221–225.
44. MacLellan DI, Wilson FC. Osteoid osteoma of the spine. *J Bone Joint Surg* 1967;49:111–121.
45. Heiman ML, Cooley CJ, Bradford DS. Osteoid osteoma of a vertebral body: report of a case with extension across the intervertebral disk. *Clin Orthop* 1976;118:159–163.
46. Mustard WT, Duval FL. Osteoid osteoma of the vertebrae. *J Bone Joint Surg* 1959;41B:132–136.
47. Swee RG, McLeod RA, Beabout JW. Osteoid osteoma. *Radiology* 1979;130:117–123.
48. Freiberger RH. Osteoid osteoma of the spine. *Radiology* 1960;75:232–235.
49. Sherman MS. Osteoid osteoma. *J Bone Joint Surg* 1947;29:918–930.
50. Resjo IM, Harwood-Nash D, Fitz CR, Chuang S. CT metrizamide myelography for intraspinal and paraspinal neoplasms in infants and children. *AJR* 1979;132:367–372.
51. Balakrishnan V, Rice MS, Simpson DA. Spinal neuroblastomas diagnosis, treatment and prognosis. *J Neurosurg* 1974;40:431–438.
52. Omojola MF, Cockshott P, Beatty EG. Osteoid osteoma: an evaluation of diagnostic modalities. *Clin Radiol* 1981;32:199–204.
53. Bell RS, O'Connor GD, Waddell JP. Importance of magnetic resonance imaging in osteoid osteoma: a case report. *Can J Surg* 1989;32:276–278.
54. deSantos LA, Goldstein HM, Murray JA, Wallace S. Computed tomography in the evaluation of musculoskeletal neoplasms. *Radiology* 1978;128:89–94.
55. Doron Y, Gruszkiewicz J, Gelli B, Peyser E. Benign osteoblastoma of vertebral column and skull. *Surg Neurol* 1977;7:86–90.
56. Myles St, MacRae ME. Benign osteoblastoma of the spine in childhood. *J Neuro Surg* 1988;68:884–888.
57. Omojola MF, Fox AJ, Vinuela FV. Computed tomography metrizamide myelography in the evaluation of thoracic osteoblastoma. *AJNR* 1982;3:670–673.
58. McLeod RA, Dahlin DC, Beaubout JW. The spectrum of osteoblastoma. *AJR* 1976;126:321–335.
59. Steiner GC. Ultrastructure of osteoblastoma. *Cancer* 1977;39:2127–2136.
60. Jaffe H. Benign osteoblastoma. *Bull Hosp Joint Dis* 1956;17:141–151.
61. DeSouza L, Frost HM. Osteoblastoma of the spine, a review and report of 8 new cases. *Clin Orthop* 1973;91:144–151.
62. Dias LD, Frost HM. Osteoblastoma of the spine: a review of eight cases. *Clin Orthop* 1973;91:141–151.
63. Tonai M, Campbell CJ, Ahn GH, Schiller AL, Mankin HJ. Osteoblastoma: classification and report of 16 patients. *Clin Orthop* 1982;167:222–235.
64. Bloom MH, Bryan RS. Benign osteoblastoma of the spine, case report. *Clin Orthop* 1969;65:157–162.
65. Jackson RP, Recklin FW, Mantz FA. Osteoid osteoma and osteoblastoma. *Clin Orthop* 1977;128:303–313.
66. Omojola MJ, Fox AJ, Vinuela FV. Computed tomographic metrizamide myelography in the evaluation of thoracic spinal osteoblastoma. *AJNR* 1982;3:670–673.
67. Nguyen VD, Hersh M. A rare bone tumor in an unusual location: osteoblastoma of the vertebral body. *Comput Med Imag Graphics* 1992;16(1):11–16.
68. Tucker AS, Aramsri B, Hughes CR. Roentgenographic diagnosis of spinal tumors. *AJR* 1957;78:54–65.
69. Seki T, Fukuda H, Ishii Y, et al. Malignant transformation of a benign osteoblastoma: a case report. *J Bone Joint Surg* 1975;57:424–427.
70. Cory DA, Fritsch SA, Cohen MD, et al. Aneurysmal bone cysts: imaging findings and embolotherapy. *AJR* 1989;153:369–373.
71. Spjut HJ, Ayala AG. Skeletal tumors in childhood and adolescence. In: *Pathology of Neoplasia in Children and Adolescents.* Philadelphia: WB Saunders; 1984.
72. Dahlin DC, McLeon RA. Aneurysmal bone cyst and other nonneoplastic conditions. *Skeletal Radiol* 1982;8:243–250.
73. Biescker JL, Marcove RC, Huvos AG, Mike V. Aneurysmal bone cyst, a clinical pathologic study of 66 cases. *Cancer* 1970;26:615–625.
74. Hay MC, Paterson D, Taylor TK. Aneurysmal bone cysts of the spine. *J Bone Joint Surg* 1978;60B:406–411.
75. Gunterberg B, Kindblom LG, Laurin S. Giant cell tumor of bone and aneurysmal bone cyst. *Skeletal Radiol* 1977;2:65–74.
76. Sherman RS, Soong KY. Aneurysmal bone cyst: its roentgen diagnosis. *Radiology* 1957;68:54–64.
77. Tillman BP, Dahlin DC, Lipscomb PR, Stewart JR. Aneurysmal bone cyst: an analysis of 95 cases. *Mayo Clin Proc* 1968;43:478–495.
78. Wang A, Lipson S, Hay Kal HA, Weinberg DS, Zamanian C, Rumbaugh CL. Computed tomography of aneurysmal bone cyst of the vertebral body. *J Comput Assist Tomogr* 1984;8:1186–1189.
79. Haft H, Ransohopf J, Carter S. Spinal cord tumors in children. *Pediatrics* 1959;23:1152–1159.
80. Banna M. *Clinical Radiology of Spine and Spinal Cord.* Rockville, MD: Aspen Publishers; 1985.
81. Beltran J, Simon D, Levy M, Herman L, Weis L, Mueller CF. Aneurysmal bone cysts: MR imaging at 1.5T. *Radiology* 1986;158:689–690.
82. Munk PL, Helms CA, Holt RG, Johnston J, Steinbach L, Neuman C. MR imaging of aneurysmal bone cysts. *AJR* 1989;153:99–101.
83. Zimmer WD, Berquist TH, Sim FH, et al. Magnetic resonance imaging of aneurysmal bone cyst. *Mayo Clin Proc* 1984;59:633–636.
84. Lichtenstein L. Aneurysmal bone cyst. Further observations. *Cancer* 1953;6:1228–1273.
85. Caro PA, Mandell GA, Stanton RP. Aneurysmal bone cyst of the spine in children. MRI imaging at 0.5 tesla. *Pediatr Radiol* 1991;21:114–116.
86. McInerney DP, Middlemiss JH. Giant cell tumor of bone. *Skeletal Radiol* 1978;2:195–204.
87. Jacobs P. The diagnosis of osteoclastoma (giant cell tumours): a radiological and pathological correlation. *Br J Radiol* 1972;45:121–136.
88. Goldenberg RR, Campbell CJ, Bonfiglio M. Giant cell tumor of bone, an analysis of 218 cases. *J Bone Joint Surg* 1970;52A:619–664.
89. Williams RR, Dahlin DC, Ghormley RK. Giant cell tumor of bone. *Cancer* 1954;7:764–773.
90. Brady TJ, Gebhardt MC, Pickett IL. NMR imaging of forearms in healthy volunteers and patients with giant cell tumor. *Radiology* 1982;144:549–552.
91. Aisen AM, Martel W, Braunstein EM, McMillan KI, Phillips

WA, King TF. MRI and CT evaluation of primary bone and soft tissue tumors. *AJR* 1986;146:749–756.
92. Jaffe HL, Lichtenstein L, Portis PB. Giant-cell tumor of bone: its pathologic appearance, grading, supposed variants, and treatment. *Arch Pathol* 1940;30:993–1031.
93. Mahmood A, Caccamo DV, Morgan JK. Tenosynovial giant-cell tumor of the cervical spine. Case report. *J Neurosurg* 1992;77: 952–955.
94. Smith WL, Stokka C, Franken EA. Arteriography of sacrococcygeal teratomas. *Radiology* 1980;137:653–655.
95. Williams AO, Lagundoye SB, Bankole MA. Sacrococcygeal teratoma in Nigerian children. *Arch Dis Child* 1975;45:110–113.
96. Schey WL, Shkolnik A, White H. Clinical and radiographic considerations of sacrococcygeal teratomas: an analysis of 26 new cases and review of the literature. *Radiology* 1977;125:189–195.
97. Moazam F, Talbert JL. Congenital anorectal malformations. *Arch Surg* 1985;120:856–859.
98. Izant RJ, Filston HC. Sacrococcygeal teratomas, analysis of forty-three cases. *Am J Surg* 1975;130:617–620.
99. McDonald P. Malignant sacrococcygeal teratoma, report of 4 cases. *AJR* 1973;118:444–449.
100. Dundon CC, Williams HA, Liapply TC. Eosinophilic granuloma of bone. *Radiology* 1946;47:433–444.
101. McGavran MH, Spady HA. Eosinophilic granuloma of bone, a study of 28 cases. *J Bone Joint Surg* 1960;42A:979–992.
102. Hamilton JB, Barner JL, Kennedy PC, McCort JJ. The osseous manifestations of eosinophilic granuloma: report of nine cases. *Radiology* 1945;47:445–456.
103. Green WT, Farber S. "Eosinophilic or solitary granuloma" of bone. *J Bone Joint Surg* 1942;24:499–526.
104. Childs DS, Kennedy RL. Reticulo-endotheliosis of children: treatment with roentgen rays. *Radiology* 1951;57:653–660.
105. Oschsner SF. Eosinophilic granuloma of bone: experience with 20 cases. *AJR* 1966;97:719–726.
106. Lichtenstein L, Jaffe HL. Eosinophilic granuloma of bone. *Am J Pathol* 1940;16:595–604.
107. Arcomano JP, Barnett JC, Wunderlich WO. Histiocytosis. *AJR* 1961;85:663–679.
108. Krol G, Sundaresan N, Deck M. Computed tomography of axial chordomas. *J Comput Assist Tomogr* 1983;7:286–289.
109. Heffelfinger MJ, Dahlin DC, McCarty CS, Beabout JW. Chordomas and cartilagenous tumors at the skull base. *Cancer* 1973;32: 410–420.
110. Beaugie JM, Mann CV, Butler CB. Sacrococcygeal chordoma. *Br J Surg* 1969;56:586–588.
111. Higinbotham NL, Phillips RF, Farr HW, Hustu HO. Chordoma: thirty-five year study at Memorial Hospital. *Cancer* 1967;20: 1841–1850.
112. Firooznia H, Pinto RS, Lin JP, Zausner J. Chordoma: radiologic evaluation of 20 cases. *AJR* 1976;127:797–805.
113. Sze G, Uichanco LS, Brant-Zawadzki M, et al. Chordomas: MR imaging. *Radiology* 1988;166:187–191.
114. Winants D, Bertal A, Hennequin L, et al. Imagerie des chordomes cervicaux et thoraciques. A propos de 2 observations. *J Radiol* 1992;73(3):169–174.
115. Stowens D. Neuroblastoma and related tumors. *Arch Pathol* 1957;63:451–459.
116. Bodian M. Neuroblastoma. *Pediatr Clin North Am* 1959;6:449–472.
117. Miller JH, Sato JK. Adrenal origin tumors. In: *Imaging in Pediatric Oncology*. Baltimore, MD: Williams & Wilkins; 1985:305–339.
118. Siegel MJ, Jamroz GA, Glazer HS, Abramson CL. MR imaging of intraspinal extension of neuroblastoma. *J Comput Assist Tomogr* 1986;10:593–595.
120. Dietrich RB, Kangarloo H, Lenarsky C, Feig SA. Neuroblastoma: the role of MR imaging. *AJR* 1987;148:937–942.
120. Reed JC, Hallet KK, Feign DS. Neural tumors of the thorax: subject review from the AFIP. *Radiology* 1978;126:9–17.
121. Harwood-Nash DC, Fitz CR. *Neuroradiology in Infants and Children*. St. Louis: CV Mosby; 1976:1167–1226.
122. Punt J, Pritchard J, Pincott JR, Till K. Neuroblastoma: a review of 21 cases presenting with cord compression. *Cancer* 1980;45: 3095–3101.
123. Edeu K. The dumb-bell tumors of the spine. *Br J Surg* 1941;28: 549–569.
124. Dahlin DC, Coventry MB. Osteogenic sarcoma, a study of 600 cases. *J Bone Joint Surg* 1967;49:101–110.
125. McKenna RJ, Schwinn CP, Soong KY, Higinbotham NL. Sarcoma of the osteogenic series (osteosarcoma, fibrosarcoma, chondrosarcoma, parosteal osteogenic sarcoma, and sarcomata arising in abnormal bone). *J Bone Joint Surg* 1966;48:1–26.
126. Redmond OM, Stack JP, Dervan PA, Hurson BJ, Carney DN, Ennis JT. Osteosarcoma: use of MR imaging and MR spectroscopy in clinical decision making. *Radiology* 1989;172:811–815.
127. Marcove RC, Mike V, Hajek JV, Levin AG, Hutter RV. Osteogenic sarcoma under the age of twenty one. *J Bone Joint Surg* 1970;52:411–423.
128. Felson B, Wiot J. Osteogenic sarcoma: an update. *Semin Roentgenol* 1989;24:143–200.
129. Fielding WJ, Fietti VG, Hughes JE, Gabriellian JC. Primary osteogenic sarcoma of the cervical spine. *J Bone Joint Surg* 1976;58: 892–894.
130. Berger PE, Kuhn JP. Computed tomography of tumors of the musculoskeletal system in children. *Radiology* 1978;127:171–175.
131. Zimmer WD, Berguist TH, McLeod RA, et al. Magnetic resonance imaging of osteosarcomas, comparison with computed tomography. *Clin Orthop* 1986;208:289–299.
132. Zimmer WD, Berguist TH, McLeod RA. Bone tumors: MR imaging versus CT. *Radiology* 1985;155:709–718.
133. Sundaram M, McGuire MH, Herbold DR. Magnetic resonance imaging of osteosarcoma. *Skeletal Radiol* 1987;16:23–29.
134. Erlemann R, Reiser MF, Peters PE, Vasallo P, Nommensen B, Kusnierz-Glaz CR. Musculoskeletal neoplasms: static and dynamic GD-DTPA-enhanced MR imaging. *Radiology* 1989;171: 767–773.
135. Huvos AG, Marcove RC. Chondrosarcoma in the young. A clinicopathologic analysis of 79 patients younger than 21 years of age. *Am J Surg Pathol* 1987;11:930–942.
136. Aprin H, Riseborough EJ, Hall JE. Chondrosarcoma in children and adolescents. *Clin Orthop* 1982;166:226–232.
137. Henderson ED, Dahlin DC. Chondrosarcoma of bone. A study of 288 cases. *J Bone Joint Surg* 1963;45-A:1450–1458.
138. Blaylock RL, Kempe LG. Chondrosarcoma of the cervical spine, case report. *J Neurosurg* 1976;44:500–503.
139. Garrison RC, Unni KK, McCleod RA, Pritchard DJ, Dahlin DC. Chondrosarcoma arising in osteochondroma. *Cancer* 1982;49: 1890–1897.
140. Barnes R, Catto M. Chondrosarcoma of bone. *J Bone Joint Surg* 1966;48:729–764.
141. Marcove RC. Chondrosarcoma: diagnosis and treatment. *Orthop Clin North Am* 1977;8:811–820.
142. Wronski J, Bryc S, Kaminski J, Chibowski D. Chondrosarcoma of the cervical spine causing compression of the cord. *J Neurosurg* 1964;21:419–421.
143. Camins MB, Duncan AW, Smith J, Marcove RC. Chondrosarcoma of the spine. *Spine* 1978;3:202–209.
144. Torma T. Malignant tumors of the spine and spinal extradural space. *Acta Chir Scand (Suppl)* 1957;225:1–176.
145. Pettersson H, Gillepsy T, Hamlin D, et al. Primary musculoskeletal tumors: examination with MR imaging compared with conventional modalities. *Radiology* 1987;164:237–241.
146. Chan SL, Turner-Gomes SO, Chuang Sh, et al. A rare cause of spinal cord compression in childhood from intraspinal mesenchymal chondrosarcoma. *Neuroradiology* 1984;26:323–327.
147. Wang CC, Shulz MD. Ewing's sarcoma: a study of fifty cases treated at Massachusetts General Hospital 1930–1952 inclusive. *JAMA* 1953;248:571–576.
148. Bhansali SK, Desai PB. Ewing's sarcoma, observations of 107 cases. *J Bone Joint Surg* 1963;45A:541–553.
149. Swenson PC. The roentgenologic aspects of Ewing's tumor of bone marrow. *AJR* 1943;50:343–354.
150. Pritchard DJ, Dahlin DC, Dauphine RT, Taylor NF, Beabout JW. Ewing's sarcoma, a clinicopathological and statistical analysis of patients surviving five years or longer. *J Bone Joint Surg* 1975;57A:10–16.

151. Dahlin DC, Coventry MB, Scanlon PW. Ewing's sarcoma: a critical analysis of 165 cases. *J Bone Joint Surg* 1961;43:185–193.
152. Ginaldi S, deSantos LA. Computed tomography in the evaluation of small round cell tumors of bone. *Radiology* 1980;134:441–446.
153. Parker BR, Marglin S, Castellino RA. Skeletal manifestations of leukemia, Hodgkin disease, and non-Hodgkin lymphoma. *Semin Roentgenol* 1980;15:302–315.
154. Pinkel D. Treatment of acute leukemia. *Pediatr Clin North Am* 1976;23:117–130.
155. Pear BL. Skeletal manifestations of the lymphomas and leukemias. *Semin Roentgenol* 1974;9:229–240.
156. Murphy ML. Leukemia and lymphoma in children. *Pediatr Clin North Am* 1959;6:611–638.
157. Pierce MI, Borges WH, Heyn R, Wolff JA, Gilbert ES. Epidemiological factors and survival experience in 1770 children with acute leukemia. *Cancer* 1969;6:1296–1304.
158. Silverman FN. The skeletal lesions in leukemia clinical and roentgenographic observations in 103 infants and children with a review of the literature. *AJR* 1948;59:819–843.
159. Baty JM, Vogt EC. Bone changes of leukemia in children. *AJR* 1935;34:310–314.
160. Daffner RH, Lupetin AR, Dash N, Deeb ZL, Sefczek RJ, Shapiro RL. MRI in the detection of malignant infiltration of bone marrow. *AJR* 1986;146:353–358.
161. Moore SG, Gooding CA, Brasch RC, et al. Bone marrow in children with acute lymphocytic leukemia: MR relaxation time. *Radiology* 1986;160:237–240.
162. Young JL, Miller RW. Incidence of malignant tumor in US children. *J Pediatr* 1975;86:254–258.
163. Steinbach HL, Parker BR. Primary bone tumors. In: Parker BR, Castellino RA, eds. *Pediatric Oncologic Radiology*. St. Louis: CV Mosby; 1977;378–386.
164. Dahlin DC. Reticulum cell sarcoma of bone. *J Bone Joint Surg* 1953;35:835–842.
165. Magnus HA, Wood LC. Primary reticulosarcoma of bone. *J Bone Joint Surg* 1956;38:258–278.
166. Wilson TW, Pugh DG. Primary reticulum cell sarcoma of bone, with emphasis on roentgen aspects. *Radiology* 1955;65:343–351.
167. Sherman RS, Snyder RE. The roentgen appearance of primary reticulum cell sarcoma of bone. *AJR* 1947;58:291–306.
168. Edwards J. Primary reticulum sarcoma of the spine report of a case with autopsy. *J Bone Joint Surg* 1953;35:835–843.
169. Weaver GR, Sandler MP. Increased sensitivity of magnetic resonance imaging compared to radionuclide bone scintigraphy in the detection of lymphoma of the spine. *Clin Nucl Med* 1987;12:333–334.
170. Cohen MD, Klatte EC, Baehner R, Smith JA, Martin-Simmerman P, Carr BE. Magnetic resonance of bone marrow disease in children. *Radiology* 1984;151:715–718.
171. Kangarloo H, Dietrich RB, Taira RT, Gold RH, Lenarsky C, Boechat MI. MR imaging of bone marrow in children. *J Comput Assist Tomogr* 1986;10:205–209.
172. Gilbert RW, Kim JH, Posner JB. Epidural spinal cord compression from metastatic tumor: diagnosis and treatment. *Ann Neurol* 1978;3:40–51.
173. Berquist TH. Magnetic resonance imaging: preliminary experience in orthopedic radiology. *Magn Reson Imag* 1984;2:41–52.
174. Fornasier VL, Horne JG. Metastases to the vertebral column. *Cancer* 1975;36:590–594.
175. Livinston KE, Perrin RG. The neurosurgical managment of spinal metastases causing cord and cauda equina compression. *J Neurosurg* 1978;49:839–843.
176. Burk DL, Brunberg JA, Kanal E, Latchaw RE, Wolf GL. Spinal and paraspinal neurofibromatosis; surface coil MR imging at 1.5T. *Radiology* 1987;162:797–801.
177. Davis PC, Hoffman JC, Ball TI, et al. Spinal abnormalities in pediatric patients: MR imaging findings compared with clinical, myelographic, and surgical findings. *Radiology* 1988;166:679–685.
178. Krol G, Sze G, Malkin M, Walker R. MR of cranial and spinal meningeal carcinomatous comparison with CT and myelography. *AJNR* 1988;9:709–714.
179. Davis PC, Griedman NC, Fry SM, Malko JA, Hoffman JC, Braun IF. Leptomeningeal metastasis: MR imaging. *Radiology* 1987;163:449–454.
180. Rubin JB, Enzmann DR. Imaging of spinal CSF pulsation by 2DFT MR. *AJNR* 1987;8:297–306.
181. Sze G, Bravo S, Krol G. Spinal lesions: quantitative and qualitative temporal evolution of gadopentetate dimeglumine enhancement in MR imaging. *Radiology* 1989;170:849–856.
182. Okazaki H. *Fundamentals of Neuropathology*. New York: Igaku-Shoin; 1983:208–214.
183. Lewis TT, Kingsley DP. Magnetic resonance imaging of multiple spinal neurofibromata-neurofibromatosis. *Neuroradiology* 1987;29:562–564.
184. Brasfield RD, Das Gupta TK. Von Recklinghausen's disease: a clinical pathologic study. *Ann Surg* 1972;175:86–104.
185. Hughes JT. *Pathology of the Spinal Cord. Tumors.* London: Lloyd-Luke Ltd; 1966:160–180.
186. Rasmussen TB, Kernohan JW, Adson AW. Pathologic classification, with surgical consideration of intraspinal tumors. *Ann Surg* 1940;111:513–530.
187. Gautier-Smith PC. Clinical aspects of spinal neurofibromatosis. *Brain* 1967;90:359–393.
188. Burk DL, Brunberg JA, Kanal E, Latchaw TE, Wolf GL. Spinal and paraspinal neurofibromatosis: surface coil MR imaging at 1.5T. *Radiology* 1987;162:797–801.
189. Sordillo PP, Helson L, Hajdu SI, et al. Malignant scwannoma—clinical characteristics, survival and response to therapy. *Cancer* 1981;10:2503–2509.
190. Herman J. Sarcomatous transformation in multiple neurofibromatosis (Von Recklinghausen's disease). *Ann Surg* 1950;131:206–217.
191. Levine E, Huntrakoon M, Wetzel LH. Malignant nerve-sheath neoplasms in fibromatosis neuro: distinction from benign tumors by using imaging techniques. *AJR* 1987;149:1059–1064.
192. White HR. Survival in malignant schwannoma, an 18-year-study. *Cancer* 1971;3:720–729.
193. Okazaki H, Scheithauer B, eds. *Atlas of Neuropathology*. New York: Gower Medical Publishing; 1988.
194. Laws JW, Dallis CP. Spinal deformities in neurofibromatosis. *J Bone Joint Surg* 1963;45B:674–682.
195. Scotti G, Scialfa G, Colombo N, Landoni L. MR imaging of intradural extramedullary tumors of the cervical spine. *J Comput Assist Tomogr* 1985;9:1037–1041.
196. Augenstein H, Sze G, Becker R. Imaging of spinal meningiomas. In: Al-Mefty O, ed. *Meningiomas*. New York: Raven Press; 1991;603–613.
197. Levy WJ, Bay J, Dohn D. Spinal cord meningioma. *J Neurosurg* 1982;57:804–812.
198. Lombardi G, Passerini A. *Spinal Cord Disease: A Radiologic and Myelographic Analysis*. Baltimore, MD: Williams & Wilkins; 1964.
199. Ng THK, Chan KH, Mann KS, Fung CF. Spinal meningioma arising from a lumbar nerve root. *J Neurosurg* 1989;70:646–648.
200. Levy WJ, Bay J, Dohn D. Spinal cord meningioma. *J Neurosurg* 1982;57:804–812.
201. Zimmerman RA, Bilaniuk LT. Imaging of tumors of the spinal canal and cord. *Radiol Clin North Am* 1988;26:965–1007.
202. Nitter K. Spinal meningiomas, neurinomas and neurofibromas and hourglass tumors. In: Vinken PJ, Bruyn BW, eds. *Tumors of the Spine and Spinal Cord, Part II. Handbook of Clinical Neurology*, vol. 20. Amsterdam: North Holland; 1976;177–322.
203. Davis RA, Washburn PL. Spinal cord meningiomas. *Surg Gynecol Obstet* 1970;131:15–21.
204. Cushing H. The meningiomas (dural endotheliomas): their source, and favored seats of origin. *Brain* 1922;45:282–316.
205. Rasmussen TB, Kernohan JW, Adson AW. Pathologic classification, with surgical consideration, of intraspinal tumors. *Ann Surg* 1940;3:513–530.
206. Kaya U, Ozden B, Turantan MI, Aydin Y, Barlas O. Spinal epidural meningioma in childhood: a case report. *Neurosurgery* 1982;10:746–747.
207. Merten DF, Gooding CA, Newton TH, Malamud N. Meningiomas of childhood and adolescence. *J Pediatr* 1974;84:696–700.
208. Pitkethly DT, Hardman JM, Kempe LG, Earle KM. Angioblastic meningiomas. *J Neurosurg* 1970;32:539–544.

209. Palacios E, Azar-Kia B. Malignant metastasizing angioblastic meningiomas. *J Neurosurg* 1975;42:185–188.
210. Earle KM, Richany SF. Meningiomas: a study of the histology, incidence, and biologic behavior of 243 cases from the Frazier-Grant collection of brain tumors. *Med Ann DC* 1969;38:353–356.
211. Ibrahim AW, Satti MB, Ibrahim EM. Extraspinal meningioma. *J Neurosurg* 1986;64:328–330.
212. Singh R, Coerkamp RSG, Luyendijk W. Spinal epidural meningiomas. *Acta Neurochirurg* 1968;18:237–245.
213. Robbins SL, Cotran RS. *Pathological Basis of Disease*, 2nd ed. Philadelphia: WB Saunders; 1974.
214. Pitlyk PJ, Dockery MB, Miller RH. Hemangiopericytoma of the spinal cord. *Neurology* 1965;15:649–653.
215. Parizel PM, Baleriaux D, Rodesch G, et al. GD-DTPA enhanced MR imaging of spinal tumors. *AJNR* 1989;10:249–258.
216. Bydder GM, Kingsley PE, Brown J, Wiendorf HP, Young IR. MR imaging of meningiomas including studies with and without gadolinium-DTPA. *J Comput Assist Tomogr* 1985;9:690–697.
217. Barloon TJ, Yuh WT, Yang CJ, Schulz DH. Spinal subarachnoid tumor seeding from intracranial metastasis: MR findings. *J Comput Assist Tomogr* 1987;11:242–244.
218. Bryan P. CSF seeding of intracranial tumors: a study of 96 cases. *Clin Radiol* 1974;25:355–360.
219. Dorwart RH, Wara WM, Norman D, Levin VA. Complete myelographic evaluation of spinal metastases from medulloblastoma. *Radiology* 1981;139:403–408.
220. Kim KS, Ho SO, Weinberg PE, Lee C. Spinal leptomeningeal infiltration by systemic cancer: myelographic features. *AJNR* 1982;3:233–237.
221. Deutsch M, Reigel DH. The value of myelography in the management of childhood medulloblastoma. *Cancer* 1980;45:2194–2197.
222. Kramer ED, Raftor SE, Zimmerman RA, Packer RJ. Spinal drop metastases: comparison of myelography and enhanced MR imaging. Presented at 75th Anniversary Scientific Assembly and Annual Meeting, RSNA, Chicago, 1989, p. 404.
223. Goy AMC, Pinto RS, Raghavendra BN, et al. Intramedullary spinal cord tumors: MR imaging with emphasis on associated cysts. *Radiology* 1986;161:381–386.
224. Rubin JM, Aisen AM, DiPietro MA. Ambiguities in MR imaging of tumoral cysts in the spinal cord. *J Comput Assist Tomogr* 1986;10:395–398.
225. Bydder G, Brown J, Niendorf HP, et al. Enhancement of cervical intraspinal tumors in MR imaging with intravenous gadolinium-DTPA. *J Comput Assist Tomogr* 1985;9:847–851.
226. Dillon WP, Norman D, Newton TH, Bolla K, Mark A. Intradural spinal cord lesions: Gd-DTPA-enhanced MR imaging. *Radiology* 1989;170:229–237.
227. Sze G, Krol G, Zimmerman RD, Deck MDF. Intramedullary disease of the spine: diagnosis using gadolinium-DTPA enhanced MR imaging. *AJNR* 1988;9:847–858; *AJR* 1988;151:1193–1204.
228. Valk J. Gadolinium-DTPA in MR of spinal lesions. *AJNR* 1988;9:345–350.
229. Breger RK, Williams AL, Daniels DL, et al. Contrast enhancement in spiral MR imaging. *AJNR* 1989;10:633–637.
230. Mortara R, Parker JC, Brooks WH. Glioblastoma multiforme of the spinal cord. *Surg Neurol* 1974;2:115–119.
231. Woltman HW, Kernchan JW, Craig WM. Intramedullary tumors of the spinal cord and gliomas of the intradural portion of the filum terminate. *AMA Arch Neurol* 1951;65:378–395.
232. Wellauer J. *Die Myelographic mit Positiven Kontrastmitteln.* Stuttgart: Georg Thieme Verlag; 1961.
233. Bernasconi V, Cassinari V. Tumori e malformazioni vasali/spinali. *Acta Neurochir* [*Wien*] 1961;10:1–50.
234. Webb JH, Craig W, Kernohan JW. Intraspinal neoplasms in the cervical region. *J Neurosurg* 1952;13:348–359.
235. Farwell JR, Dohrman GJ. Intraspinal neoplasms in children. *Paraplegia* 1977;15:262–273.
236. Shenkin HA, Alpers BJ. Clinical and pathologic features of gliomas of the spinal cord. *Arch Neurol Psychiatry* 1944;52:87–105.
237. Reimer R, Onofrio BM. Astrocytomas of the spinal cord in children and adolescents. *J Neurosurg* 1985;63:669–675.
238. Sloof JL, Kernohan JW, MacCarty CS. *Primary Intramedullary Tumors of the Spinal Cord and Filum Terminale.* Philadelphia: WB Saunders; 1969.
239. Cohen AR, Wisoff JH, Allen JC, Epstein F. Malignant astrocytomas of the spinal cord. *J Neurosurg* 1989;70:50–54.
240. Poser CM. The relationship between syringomyelia and neoplasm. American Lecture Series, #262. *American Lectures in Neurology*. Springfield, IL: Charles C Thomas; 1956;28–32.
241. Epstein F, Epstein N. Surgical management of holocord spinal astrocytomas. *J Neurosurg* 1981;54:829–832.
242. Johnson DL, Schwarz S. Intracranial metastases from malignant spinal cord astrocytoma. *J Neurosurg* 1987;66:621–625.
243. Packer RJ, Zimmerman RA, Bilaniuk LT, et al. Magnetic resonance imaging of lesions of the posterior fossa and upper cervical cord in childhood. *Pediatrics* 1985;76:84–90.
244. Goy AM, Pinto RS, Raghavenda BN, Epstein FJ, Kricheff II. Intramedullary spinal cord tumors: MR imaging with emphasis on associated cysts. *Radiology* 1986;161:381–386.
245. Slasky BS, Bydder GM, Niendorf HP, Young IR. MR imaging with gadolinium-DTPA in the differentiation of tumor, syrinx and cysts of the spinal cord. *J Comput Assist Tomogr* 1987;11:845–850.
246. Williams AL, Haughton VM, Pojunas KW, Daniels DL, Kilgore DP. Differentiation by intramedullary neoplasms and cysts by MR. *AJNR* 1987;8:527–532.
247. Kopelson G, Linggood RM, Kleinman GM, Doucette J, Wang CC. Management of intramedullary spinal cord tumors. *Radiology* 1980;135:473–479.
287. Sonneland PR, Scheithauer BW, Onofrio BM. Myxopapillary ependymoma, a clinicopathologic and immunocytochemical study of 77 cases. *Cancer* 1985;56:883–893.
249. Barone BM, Elridge AR. Ependymomas, a clinical survey. *J Neurosurg* 1970;33:428–438.
250. Rawlings CE, Giangaspero F, Burger PC, Bullard DE. Ependymomas: a clinicopathologic study. *Surg Neurol* 1988;29:271–281.
251. Dohrmann GJ, Farwell JR, Flannery JT. Ependymomas and ependymoblastomas in children. *J Neurosurg* 1976;45:273–283.
252. Kernohan JW, Woltman HW, Adson AW. Gliomas arising from the region of the cauda equina. *Arch Neurol Psychiatry* 1933;29:287–307.
253. Kucharczyk W, Brant-Zawadzki M, Sobel D, et al. Central nervous system tumors in children: detection by magnetic resonance imaging. *Radiology* 1985;155:131–136.
254. Browne TR, Adams RD, Roberson GH. Hemangioblastoma of the spinal cord. Review and report of five cases. *Arch Neurol* 1976;33:435–441.
255. Kendall B, Russell J. Hemangioblastomas of the spinal cord. *Br J Radiol* 1966;39:817–823.
256. Sato Y, Wazirim, Smith W, et al. Hippel-Lindau disease: MR imaging. *Radiology* 1988;166:241–246.
257. Enomoto H, Shibata T, Ito A, Hurada T, Satake T. Multiple hemangioblastomas accompanied by syringomyelia in the cerebellum and the spinal cord. *Surg Neurol* 1984;22:197–203.
258. Levin PM. Multiple hereditary hemangioblastoma of the nervous system. *Arch Neurol Psychiatry* 1936;36:384–391.
259. Kaffenberger DA, Sah CP, Mortagh FR, Wilson C, Silbiger ML. MR imaging of spinal cord hemangioblastoma. Associated with syringomyelia. *J Comput Assist Tomogr* 1988;12:495–498.
260. Costigan DA, Winkelman MD. Intramedullary spinal cord metastasis. A clinicopathological study of 13 cases. *J Neurosurg* 1985;62:227–233.
261. Edelson RN, Deck MDF, Posner JB. Intramedullary spinal cord metastases. *Neurology* 1972;22:1222–1231.
262. Jellinger K, Kothbauer P, Sunder-Plassmann E, Weiss R. Intramedullary spinal cord metastases. *J Neurol* 1979;22:31–41.
263. Smith WT, Turner E. Solitary intramedullary carcinomatous metastasis in the spinal cord. *J Neurosurg* 1968;29:648–651.
264. Sebastian PR, Fisher M, Smith TW, Davidson RI. Intramedullary spinal cord metastasis. *Surg Neurol* 1981;16:336–339.
265. Hirose G, Shimazaki K, Takado M, Kosoegawa H, Ohya N, Mukawa A. Intramedullary spinal cord metastasis associated with pencil-shaped softening of the spinal cord. *J Neurosurg* 1980;52:718–721.

266. Sze G. Magnetic resonance imaging in the evaluation of spinal tumors. *Cancer* 1991;67(4):1229–1241.
267. Pomeranz S. *Craniospinal Magnetic Resonance*. Philadelphia: WB Saunders; 1989.
268. Twohig M, Sze G. Spinal tumors. In: Cohen MD, Edwards MK, eds. *Pediatric Magnetic Resonance Imaging*. Philadelphia: BC Decker; 1990:463–498.
269. Bronen R, Sze G. MR contrast agents: theory and application to the CNS. *J Neurosurg* 1990;73:820–839.
270. Sze G, Bartlett C, Dillon WP, et al. Multicenter study of Gd-DTPA as an MR contrast agent: evaluation in patients with spinal tumors. *AJNR* 1990;11:967–974.
271. Okazaki H. *Fundamentals of Neuropathology: Morphologic Basis of Neurologic Disorders*. New York: Igaku-Shoin; 1989.

Magnetic Resonance Imaging of the Brain and Spine, Second Edition, edited by Scott W. Atlas.
Lippincott-Raven Publishers, Philadelphia © 1996.

28

Spinal Vascular Disorders

Robert W. Hurst

Vascular disease of the spine and spinal cord comprises an important group of conditions affecting this critical portion of the central nervous system (CNS). Complete evaluation of patients with potential spinal vascular disease is a significant and often difficult task for all physicians involved in the diagnosis and treatment of disease of the spine. Magnetic resonance imaging (MRI) represents the single most important source of diagnostic information regarding spinal anatomy and pathology and is particularly important in the evaluation of the patient with possible spinal vascular disease.

A thorough familiarity with the normal vascular anatomy of the spine and spinal cord is essential for complete understanding and proper interpretation of MRI in spinal vascular disease. Just as critical is an appreciation of the varieties of vascular pathology that may afflict the spine and cord and an acquaintance with clinical situations that warrant consideration of these entities. Finally, an understanding of the strengths and limitations of MRI in spinal vascular disease will aid in formulating a diagnostic evaluation plan and assist in determining which patients will benefit from additional evaluation, including spinal angiography.

VASCULAR ANATOMY

The spinal cord receives its blood supply from the longitudinal anterior spinal artery (ASA) and the paired posterior spinal arteries (PSA). The most cranial extent of the ASA originates as separate lateralized branches from the intradural vertebral arteries at the cervicomedullary junction. A single midline ASA is formed, which courses along the ventral surface of the spinal cord adjacent to the anterior median fissure. The longest artery in the body, the ASA is usually continuous along the entire length of the spinal cord.

Predictable variations in caliber of the ASA occur along the length of the cord, reflecting variations in metabolic requirement of the various cord regions. The relatively large amounts of gray matter found within the cervical and lumbar enlargements require a larger blood supply than the white matter tracts of the cord. Consequently, the larger size of the ASA in the lower cervical and lumbosacral regions, often exceeding 1 mm in diameter, reflects this relatively large blood flow requirement. The ASA often narrows to less than 0.5 mm in diameter in the thoracic region between T2 and T9, where the cord is largely composed of white matter tracts and the metabolic demand is correspondingly low (1,2).

Each spinal nerve root receives its blood supply from a radicular artery that follows the root within the neural foramen. The radicular artery supplies the root sleeve and spinal dura and also gives supply to the vertebrae at each level (Fig. 1). Most of the radicular arteries give no supply to the spinal cord itself. At various locations along the length of the cord, however, branches from the radicular arteries contribute to both the ASA and PSA. Radicular artery branches contributing to the ASA are referred to as "radiculomedullary" arteries, whereas those giving supply to a PSA are known as "radiculopial" arteries (Fig. 2).

R. W. Hurst, M.D.: Department of Radiology, Hospital of The University of Pennsylvania, Philadelphia, PA 19104.

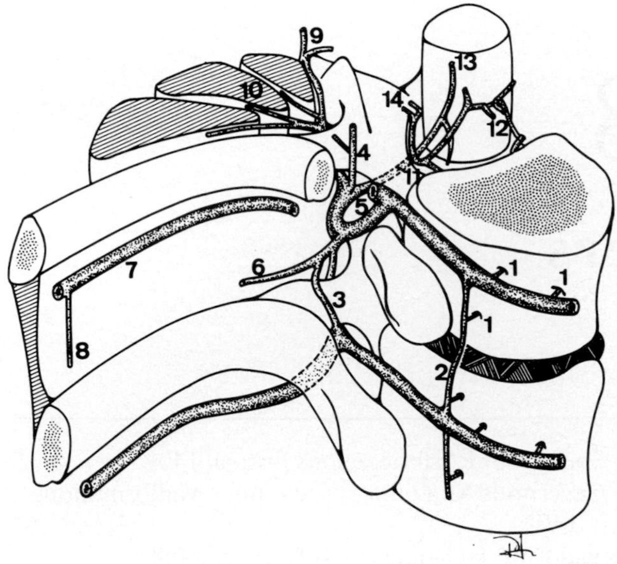

FIG. 1. Diagram of the intercostal arterial system. *1,* Arteries to the vertebral body, *2,* anterolateral anastomotic artery, *3,4,* pretransverse anastomoses, *5,* dorsospinal artery, *6,8,* ventral muscular branches, *7,* ventral branch, *9,10,* dorsal muscular branches, *11,* radicular artery, *12,14,* epidural anastomoses, *13,* dural branch. (From Lasjaunias and Berenstein, ref. 3, with permission.)

From six to eight radiculomedullary arteries arise from radicular arteries along the length of the cord. Radiculomedullary arteries follow the nerve root through the neural foramen and bifurcate on the ventral surface of the cord near the midline into ascending and descending branches, which join the ASA (3). The locations of radiculomedullary arteries along the cord follow general guidelines based on the cord blood flow requirements at various levels. Nevertheless, considerable individual variation exists in the location of radiculomedullary arteries.

Clinical consideration of the spinal cord blood supply is aided by the concept of three major regions of supply to the ASA axis (4) (Fig. 3). The three regions include the cervicothoracic, midthoracic, and thoracolumbar regions. Hemodynamic watershed areas occur at the margins of each region as flow through the ASA in one region encounters opposing ASA flow from the adjacent region. Little net flow normally occurs across the borderzone, resulting in relative hemodynamic isolation of the ASA supply of each region from its neighbor. Although the ASA is usually continuous anatomically along the length of the spinal cord, adequate collateral flow across borderzones is not always available. This is especially frequent in the midthoracic region, where the ASA may be relatively small. The spinal cord is therefore vulnerable to infarction in the event of compromise of a radiculomedullary feeding vessel or of hypotension affecting the ASA (5).

In the cervicothoracic region, radiculomedullary contributions to the ASA may originate from the vertebral artery as well as from branches of the costocervical or thyrocervical trunks. In most cases, the ASA receives a radiculomedullary branch from the vertebral artery at approximately the C3 level. In addition, a relatively constant radiculomedullary vessel, the artery of the cervical enlargement, is usually found accompanying the C6 nerve root.

The midthoracic region, consisting of the next six or seven cord segments, has a lower metabolic demand and demonstrates a correspondingly smaller blood supply. Often only one radiculomedullary artery, usually accompanying the T4 or T5 root, occurs in this region.

The thoracolumbar region, extending from the T8 segment to the conus medullaris, is provided with a relatively rich blood supply, usually originating from a single large radiculomedullary artery. This vessel, described by Adamkiewicz as the "arteria radicularis anterior magna," is also known as the artery of Adamkiewicz (Fig. 4). In 75% of cases, the artery of the lumbar enlargement enters the spinal canal at a level from T9 through T12, most commonly on the left, whereas in 10% the vessel accompanies the first or second lumbar nerves. The artery has a high origin in 15%, entering at levels

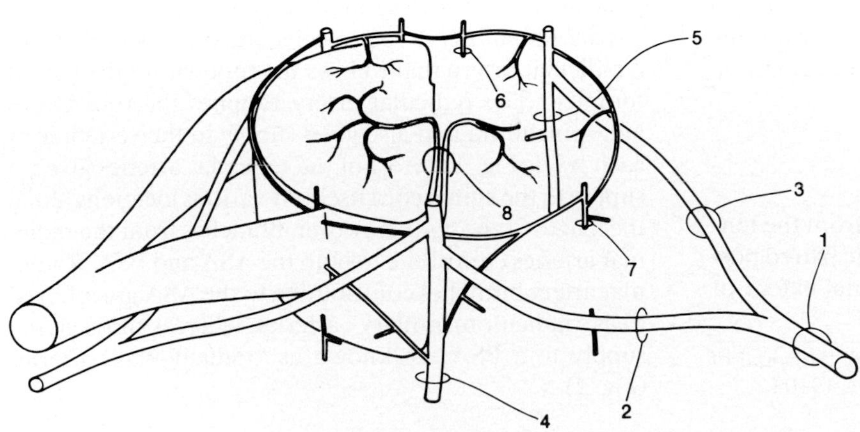

FIG. 2. Superficial arteries of the spinal cord. *1,* Radicular artery, *2,* radiculomedullary artery (to ASA), *3,* radiculopial artery (to PSA), *4,* ASA, *5,* PSA, *6,7,* circumferential pial arterial plexus, *8,* sulcocomissural arteries. (From Thron, ref. 1, with permission.)

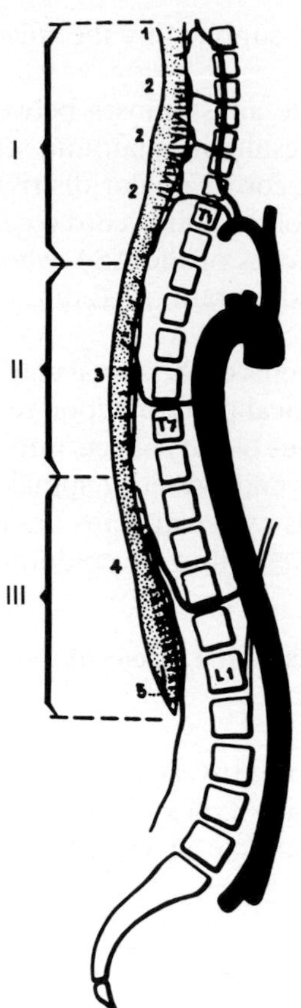

FIG. 3. Diagram of the arterial regions of the spinal cord. **I:** Superior or cervicothoracic region, **II:** intermediate or midthoracic region, **III:** lower or thoracolumbar region. *1,* ASA, *2,* artery of the spinal enlargement (variable), *3,* PSA, *4,* artery of the lumbar enlargement (artery of Adamkiewicz), *5,* anastomotic loop of the conus medullaris with continuation of the anterior spinal artery as the artery of the filum terminale. (From Lazorthes et al., ref. 4, with permission.)

from T5 through T8. Although general guidelines exist for the location of this important radiculomedullary artery, the location in a given patient is variable, ranging from the upper lumbar through midthoracic levels.

Like the ASA, the cranial extent of the paired PSAs usually originates from the intradural vertebral arteries. The PSAs, whose caliber is more uniform and usually smaller than that of the ASA, course on the dorsal surface of the cord adjacent to the dorsal roots. These features of the PSAs reflect their area of spinal cord supply, which includes mostly the dorsal white matter tracts and which demonstrates little variation in size or metabolic requirement from one cord level to another.

Frequent intercommunications connect the two PSAs across the dorsal cord surface. In contrast, collaterals around the lateral surface of the cord are infrequent and too attenuated to function reliably as anastomoses between the territories supplied by the ASA and PSAs. The absence of adequate collaterals results in functional and anatomic isolation between these two major territories of spinal cord vascular supply.

At variable locations along the length of the cord, the PSAs receive contributions from radiculopial branches of the radicular arteries. From 10 to 20 radiculopial arteries may be present, each one joining a PSA but making no contribution to the ASA.

Intrinsic Spinal Cord Supply

Two distinct groups of arteries, the sulcocommissural arteries and the rami perforantes, provide blood supply directly to the neural tissue of the cord (Fig. 5). The sulcocommissural arteries, a lateralized centrally directed system of perforating arteries, originate from the ASA. The sulcocommissural arteries course dorsally within the anterior median fissure before turning left or right to enter the cord in the region of the anterior white commissure (Fig. 6). Dense capillary networks from the sulcocommissural arteries originate within the cord substance to supply the gray matter of the anterior, intermediate, and basal dorsal horns as well as most of the white matter within the anterior and lateral funiculi.

A separate system of centripetally directed arteries known as rami perforantes receive their supply mainly via the PSAs. The rami perforantes supply the peripheral structures of the cord, including the posterior columns and the apices of the dorsal horns. A minimal amount of gray matter is supplied by the rami perforantes in com-

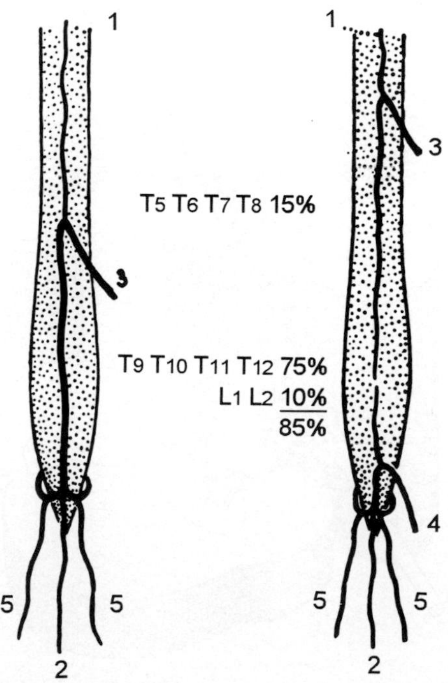

FIG. 4. Variations in the location of the artery of the lumbar enlargement. *1,* Ascending branch of the ASA, *2,* artery of the filum terminale, *3,4,* artery of the lumbar enlargement, *5,* sacral arteries. Percentages refer to the occurrence of the artery of the lumbar enlargement at specific spinal levels. (From Lazorthes et al., ref. 4, with permission.)

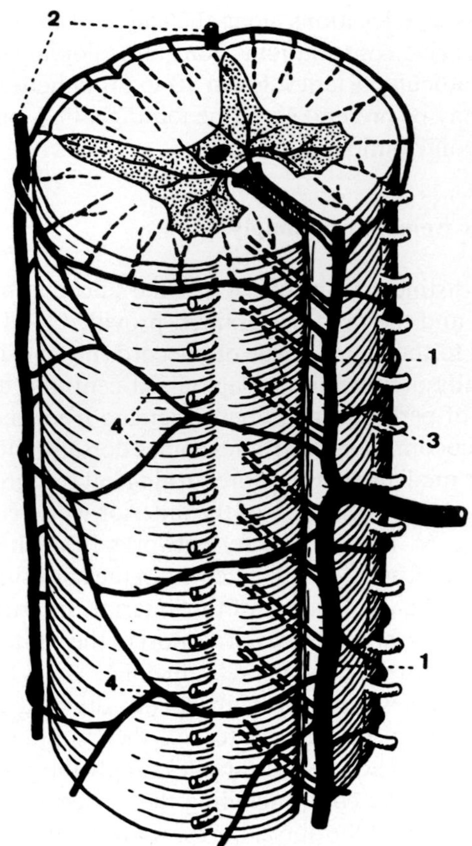

FIG. 5. Superficial and intrinsic arteries of the spinal cord. *1*, ASA, *2*, PSAs, *3*, sulcocommissural arteries, *4*, circumferential pial arterial plexus. (From Lazorthes et al., ref. 4, with permission.)

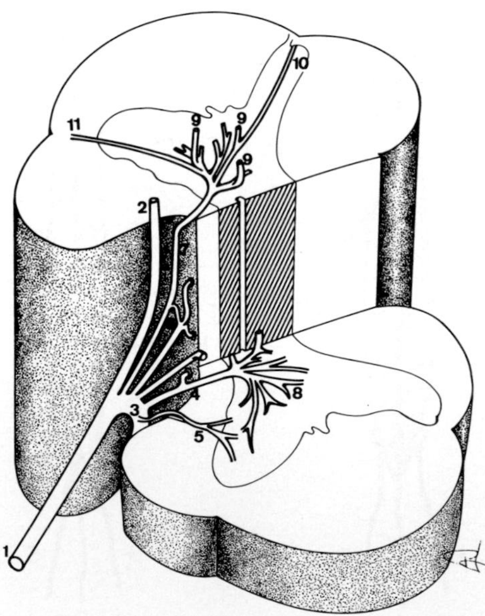

FIG. 6. Sulcocommissural branches *4, 5, 6, 7* of the descending branch of the ASA (*3*) penetrate the cord in the anterior median fissure. Both the descending and ascending (*2*) branches of the ASA are supplied by a radiculomedullary artery (*1*). The axial (*8*), (*10*), (*11*), and longitudinal (*9*) distribution of the sulcocommissural arteries is shown. (From Lasjaunias and Berenstein, ref. 3, with permission.)

parison with that supplied by the sulcocommissural arteries (Fig. 7).

The inadequate anastomoses between the ASA and PSA territories results in anatomic separation between the two intrinsic cord vascular distributions. The anterior 60% to 80% of the spinal cord receives supply exclusively from branches of the ASA whereas the posterior 20% to 30% is fed by rami perforantes originating from the PSA.

The intrinsic veins of the spinal cord collect blood in a radially symmetrical pattern. Upon reaching the surface of the cord, venous blood collects into the longitudinally directed anterior and posterior spinal veins (6) (Fig. 8). At multiple levels radicular veins drain the anterior and posterior spinal veins into the epidural venous plexus.

Evaluation of Vascular Lesions of the Spine and Spinal Cord

MRI permits noninvasive evaluation of spinal cord anatomy and many types of spine and spinal cord pathology. The complete investigation of spinal vascular

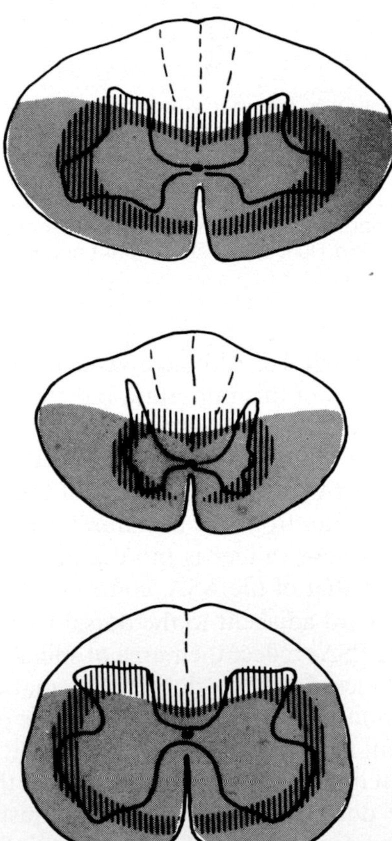

FIG. 7. Territory of the intrinsic arterial systems of the spinal cord. Cross-sections at cervical (*top*), thoracic, and lumbar (*bottom*) spinal levels. The gray zone corresponds to the area supplied by the ASA (about $\frac{2}{3}$ of the entire cross-sectional area); the dorsal white zone is supplied by branches of the PSAs. (From Thron, ref. 1, with permission.)

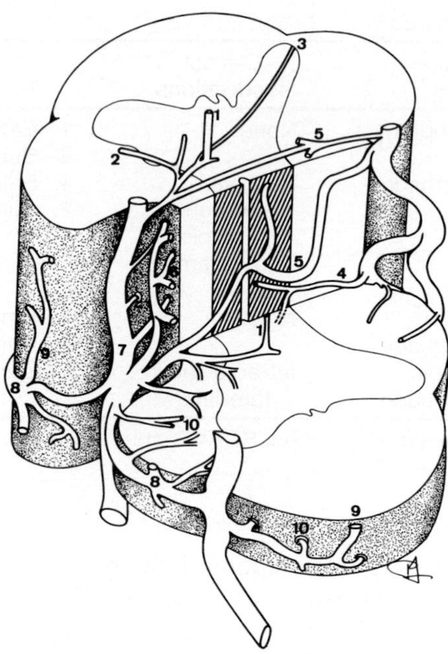

FIG. 8. Intrinsic and extrinsic veins of the cord. *1,2,3:* Intrinsic venous anastomoses, *4:* sulcal vein, *5:* transmedullary anastomoses, *7:* ventral spinal cord vein, *6,8,9:* extrinsic anastomoses, *10:* radial vein. (From Lasjaunias and Berenstein, ref. 3, with permission.)

lesions often remains difficult with MRI alone, however, and spinal angiography remains the best method for visualizing the spinal vasculature (1,2,4,7–9). Spinal MR angiography (MRA) techniques have been implemented in the diagnosis of vascular abnormalities and can be found in scattered reports in the literature (10), but at the time of this writing MRA has no significant role in these entities.

Spinal angiography is indicated when specific information regarding the vascular supply of the spine, cord, or adjacent tissue is required. Evaluation and endovascular treatment of spinal vascular malformations and some vascular tumors represent the major indications for spinal angiographic examination. In most cases, MRI findings suggestive or diagnostic of a spinal vascular malformation mandate further evaluation with spinal angiography. However, even in the face of a normal high quality MRI, catheter angiography may still be required to make the diagnosis in patients suspected of harboring these lesions. Angiographic information is particularly important in planning surgical or endovascular therapy of these lesions. In contrast, the role of angiography is limited in the evaluation of infarction or ischemia involving the spine except in cases of aortic occlusion.

SPINE AND SPINAL CORD VASCULAR MALFORMATIONS

Vascular malformations of the spine and spinal cord represent a heterogeneous group of non-neoplastic vascular abnormalities. Spinal vascular malformations are reported to make up approximately 3% to 16% of spinal mass lesions. Various classification systems and eponyms for these lesions have been used over the years with resultant confusion and difficulty in comparing and evaluating the various subgroups. The widespread use of selective angiographic examination has resulted in better delineation of the angioarchitecture and hemodynamics of the lesions, features that form the basis of the current classification. The recognition of distinct, relatively homogeneous subgroups within the spinal vascular malformations has also permitted more useful characterization of the lesions with regard to clinical behavior and therapeutic options. Major groups include spinal dural arteriovenous fistulas (SDAVF), spinal cord AVMs (SCAVM), spinal cord (perimedullary) arteriovenous fistulas (SCAVF), and cavernous malformations (11–15) (Tables 1 and 2).

Spinal Dural Arteriovenous Fistula

SDAVFs represent at least 35% of all spinal vascular malformations in large series, although some estimates range as high as 80% (16,17). The use of MRI has resulted in diagnosis of increased numbers of these lesions, which are often undetectable by other noninvasive imaging modalities. SDAVFs are believed to be acquired lesions, possibly resulting from thrombosis of the extradural venous plexus. SDAVFs are not associated with vascular malformations at other locations in the nervous system.

Anatomy and Pathophysiology

SDAVF represents an arteriovenous (AV) shunt that occurs within the dural covering of the spinal cord (Fig. 9). Usually located adjacent to the intervertebral foramen or within the dural root sleeve, the AV shunts are often tiny, with the arterial supply arising from a dural branch of the radicular artery. An intradural vein drains the shunt directly into the pial veins of the cord. The result is venous engorgement and venous hypertension involving the spinal cord. SDAVFs most commonly occur at thoracolumbar levels, usually between T5 and L3. Most often, no direct arterial supply to the spinal cord itself originates from the radicular artery feeding an SDAVF. In 10% to 15% of cases, however, the SDAVF is fed by a radicular artery that also supplies the spinal cord via a radiculomedullary or radiculopial branch (18).

TABLE 1. *Vascular malformations of the spinal cord*

Spinal dural arteriovenous fistula (SDAVF)
Spinal cord arteriovenous malformation (SCAVM)
Spinal cord (perimedullary) arteriovenous fistula (SCAVF)
Cavernous malformation (CM)

TABLE 2. *Spinal vascular malformations*

Type	Typical location	Vascular supply	Presentation & course	Clinical associations	Treatment
SDAVF	Lumbar, thoracic	Dural arteries	Chronic myelopathy	None	1. Embolization 2. Surgery
SCAVM	Cervical, thoracic, lumbar	Spinal arteries (ASA, PSA)	Acute; hemorrhage common	Vascular syndromes; paraspinal involvement rarely	1. Embolization 2. Surgery
SCAVF	Lumbar, thoracic	Spinal arteries (ASA > PSA)	Acute or chronic; may hemorrhage	None	1. Embolization 2. Surgery
CM	Cervical, thoracic, lumbar	Minimal	Acute or chronic; may hemorrhage	Intracranial or familial CM	Surgery

SDAVF, spinal dural arteriovenous fistula; SCAVM, spinal cord arteriovenous malformation; SCAVF, spinal cord arteriovenous fistula; CM, cavernous malformation.

Venous drainage from the SDAVF results in increased pressure and engorgement of the pial veins of the spinal cord. The increased venous pressure is transmitted to the intrinsic veins of the cord, reducing the intramedullary AV pressure gradient. A decrease in tissue perfusion results, with hypoxia of the neural tissue of the cord. Intramedullary vasodilation and loss of autoregulatory capacity may also occur, resulting in cord edema, stagnation of blood flow, and disruption of the blood-CNS barrier. The longitudinal extent of cord dysfunction from the venous hypertension may be very widespread and may progress over time. Poor correlation between the location of the AV shunt and the clinical level of spinal dysfunction is a frequent finding. The chronic effects of this venous hypertensive myelopathy are believed to result in a "subacute necrotizing myelopathy" identical to that described by Foix and Alajouanine in 1926 (19). SDAVF is therefore believed to represent the underlying pathology in at least some (20) of those patients with the disorder referred to as "Foix-Alajouanine syndrome" (16).

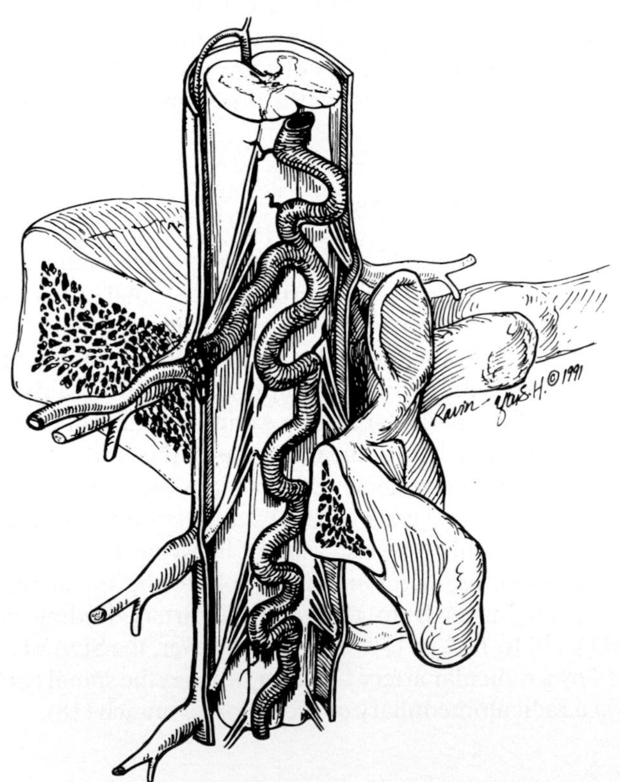

FIG. 9. Diagram of SDAVF illustrates the single dural branch of a radicular artery supplying the cluster of small vessels within the root sleeve that forms the fistula. The fistula drains into an enlarged intradural vein that communicates with and engorges the pial venous plexus of the spinal cord. (From Anson and Spetzler, ref. 14, with permission.)

The elevated pressures in spinal pial veins draining SDAVF have been found to vary in association with arterial pressure elevations, possibly accounting for the clinical worsening reported with exercise (21). The venous hypertensive myelopathy induced by SDAVF is reversible if treated early, but may become irreversible in later stages.

Clinical

SDAVF, the most common spinal vascular anomaly in the older adult, afflicts males in 80% to 90% of cases. The lesions usually present after the fourth or fifth decade; however, patients from the third through the ninth decade have been reported.

The progressive spinal venous hypertension resulting from SDAVF results in a chronic progressive myelopathy with both motor and sensory deficits (12,16,22–25). Progressive lower extremity weakness, often characterized by both upper and lower motor neuron deficits, is the most common symptom (16,25). Because of the location of the abnormal AV shunt and venous drainage, the upper extremities are not affected. Weakness is followed in frequency by localized or radicular back pain. Sensory deficits as well as bowel, bladder, and sexual dysfunction also develop in most patients before diagnosis.

Chronic progression of symptoms often exacerbated

TABLE 3. *Features of spinal dural arteriovenous fistulas (SDAVF) and spinal cord arteriovenous malformations (SCAVM)*

Feature	SDAVF	SCAVM
Age	>4th decade	2nd–3rd decade
Symptom onset	Slow progressive	Acute
Male predominance	Yes (marked)	Minimal
Hemorrhage	No	Yes (frequent)
Bruit	No	5–10%
Origin	Acquired	Congenital
Site of nidus	Dura, root sleeve	Spinal cord
Medullary arterial supply involved	10–15%	100%

Adapted from Muraszko and Oldfield, ref. 29, with permission.

by exercise characterizes the clinical course in more than 80% of SDAVF patients. The slowly progressive clinical course, often exceeding 2 to 3 years from presentation to the time of diagnosis, is unusual in most vascular diseases and often delays diagnosis. Progressive deficits with occasional remission or acute development of paraparesis or paraplegia are less frequent clinical courses. Hemorrhage has not been associated with SDAVF.

The characteristic picture of chronic myelopathy that results from SDAVF is in marked contrast to the acute onset of symptoms, often associated with hemorrhage, which frequently occurs in the presence of a SCAVM (24–29) (Table 3). The nonspecific clinical picture of chronic progressive myelopathy, usually in an older man, which characterizes SDAVF requires consideration of more common disorders in the differential diagnosis. Long-standing demyelinating disease, cervical spondylosis, and amyotrophic lateral sclerosis represent the most common causes of chronic progressive myelopathy and may often be differentiated by specific clinical features. Neoplasms, syringomyelia, degenerative processes, and infectious or inflammatory myelopathy such as that associated with acquired immunodeficiency syndrome (AIDS) are less common but may present and progress in a fashion similar to SDAVF (30). The lack of specific clinical features suggesting SDAVF means that suspicion of this entity is the most important factor in early diagnosis.

MRI

MRI findings in SDAVF include abnormal signal intensity on T1-weighted, proton-density, and T2-weighted images (Figs. 10, 11, 12, and 13). The conus and lumbar enlargement of the cord are almost uniformly affected; however, the abnormal signal may extend into upper thoracic cord levels. Diffuse enlargement of the cord may be present. These MRI findings are non-

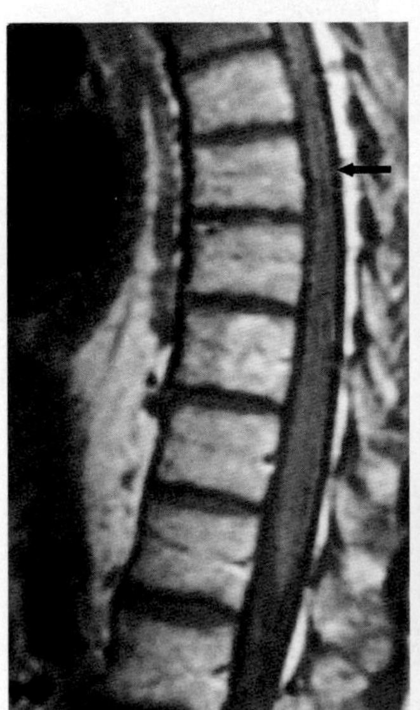
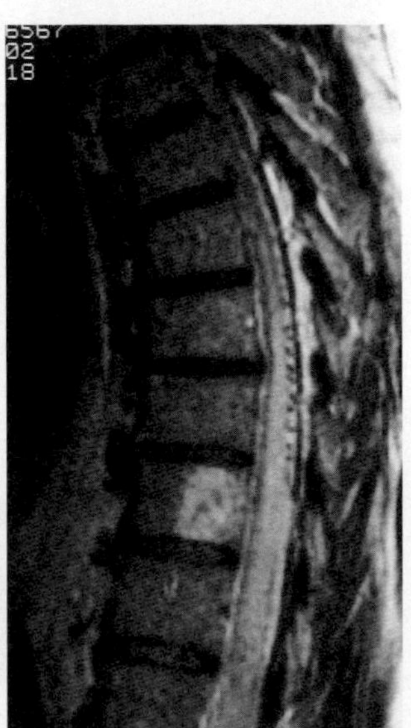
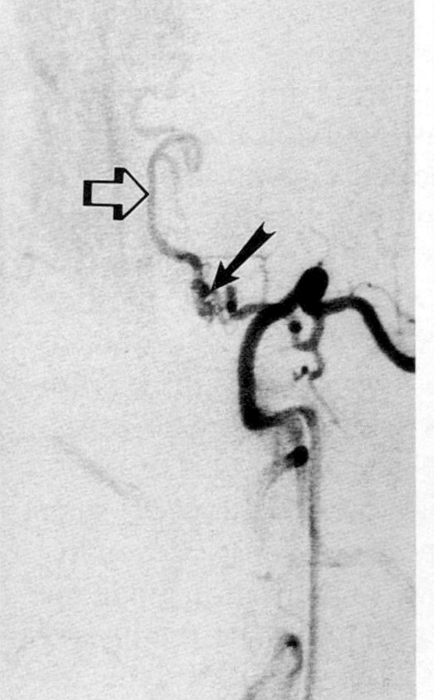
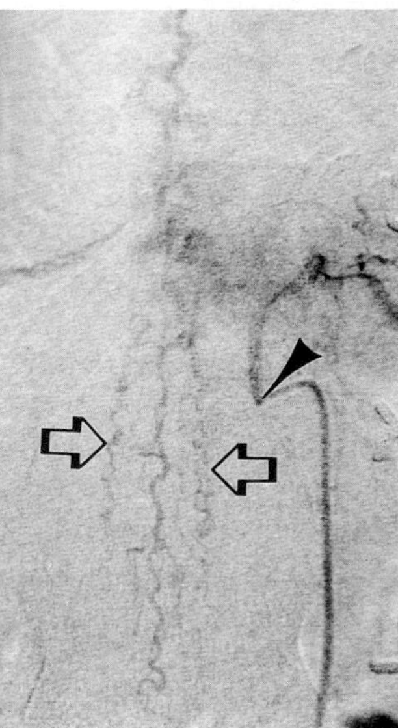

A,B C,D

FIG. 10. SDAVF. **A:** Sagittal T1- (600/10) and **B:** T2- (1800/85) weighted MR images demonstrate enlarged pial veins (*arrow*) along dorsal surface of cord. Increased intrinsic cord signal on T2-weighted images extends from conus into thoracic levels. **C:** Early phase angiographic film (AP view) of intercostal artery injection at left T10 level. SDAVF (*arrow*) fills from radicular artery with early AV shunting into pial venous system (*open arrow*). **D:** Late phase shows extensive filling of pial veins outlining cord from thoracic levels to conus (*open arrows*). *Arrowhead* at catheter tip.

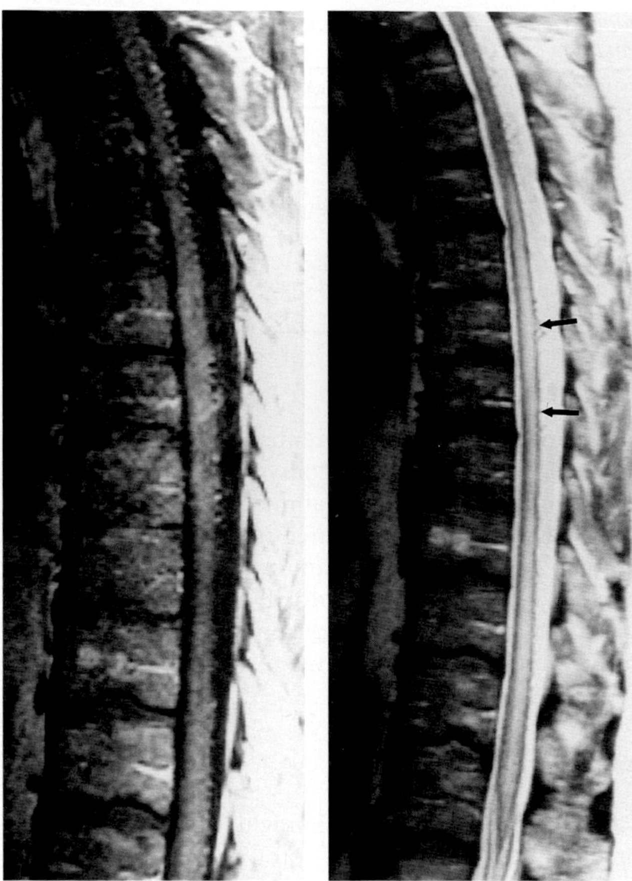

A,B

FIG. 11. SDAVF. **A:** Contrast-enhanced T1-weighted (700/11) sagittal image demonstrates flow voids along dorsal cord representing enlarged pial veins in a patient with a SDAVF. Intrinsic cord enhancement is present. **B:** Sagittal T2-weighted FSE image (4000/34) shows abnormally increased intrinsic cord signal extending from the conus to upper thoracic levels. Dorsal flow voids are visible (*arrows*).

specific and may be seen in inflammatory, demyelinating, and neoplastic conditions involving the cord. The hallmark of the diagnosis is the demonstration of dilated pial veins of the cord, most commonly along the dorsal surface. The dilated pial veins may be seen best on T2-weighted images as areas of flow void adjacent to the high signal cerebrospinal fluid (CSF). Care must be taken, however, to differentiate true flow void resulting from engorged veins from artifacts arising from CSF pulsation. This is particularly true when the veins are relatively small with slow but high pressure flow. In such cases the venous flow may appear isointense or even hyperintense if even echos or flow compensation gradients are used. Administration of gadolinium is useful and may reveal the slow flow veins as areas of high signal intensity. Intrinsic cord enhancement is frequent. The MR characteristics reflect the pathophysiologic features of SDAVF including cord edema and venous hypertension with engorgement of the pial veins. Uncommonly in patients with SDAVF, MR may be normal or demonstrate only signal abnormality within the cord without dilated pial veins. Following treatment of SDAVF with shunt occlusion, the MR abnormalities may or may not regress (31–33). Although MR may be very suggestive of the presence of SDAVF, spinal angiographic examination remains the gold standard for confirming the diagnosis, localizing the level of the abnormal AV shunt, and providing sufficient information to plan and perform therapy. MR cannot be used to exclude absolutely the presence of this lesion on the basis of absence of intradural vessels (Fig. 14).

On rare occasions, drainage from intracranial pial or dural AVMs located in the posterior fossa may engorge the pial veins of the spinal cord and result in spinal venous hypertensive myelopathy (34–36). In such cases, signal abnormalities involving the brainstem and cervical cord may be present and angiographic evaluation for intracranial lesions may reveal an otherwise occult

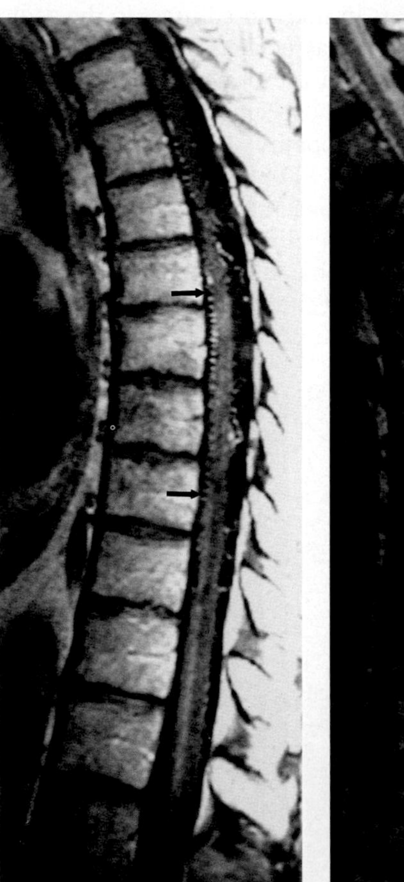

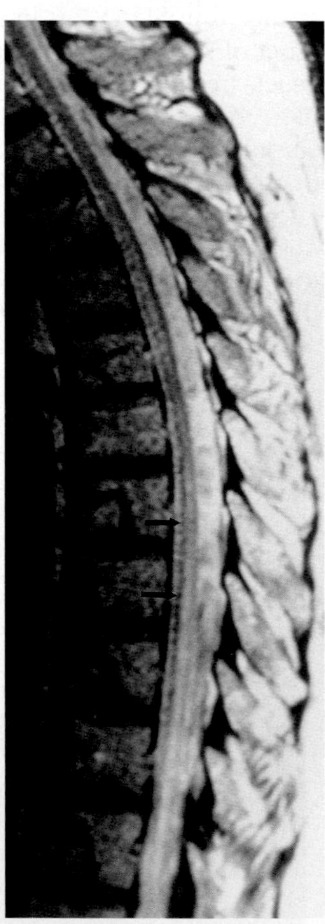

A,B

FIG. 12. SDAVF. **A:** Sagittal enhanced T1- (500/11) and (**B**) T2-weighted FSE (2700/85.2) images show enlarged pial veins as high intensity slow flow and flow voids along the ventral (*arrows*) and dorsal surfaces of the cord. Patchy intrinsic cord enhancement and T2 signal abnormality extend from thoracic levels to conus medullaris.

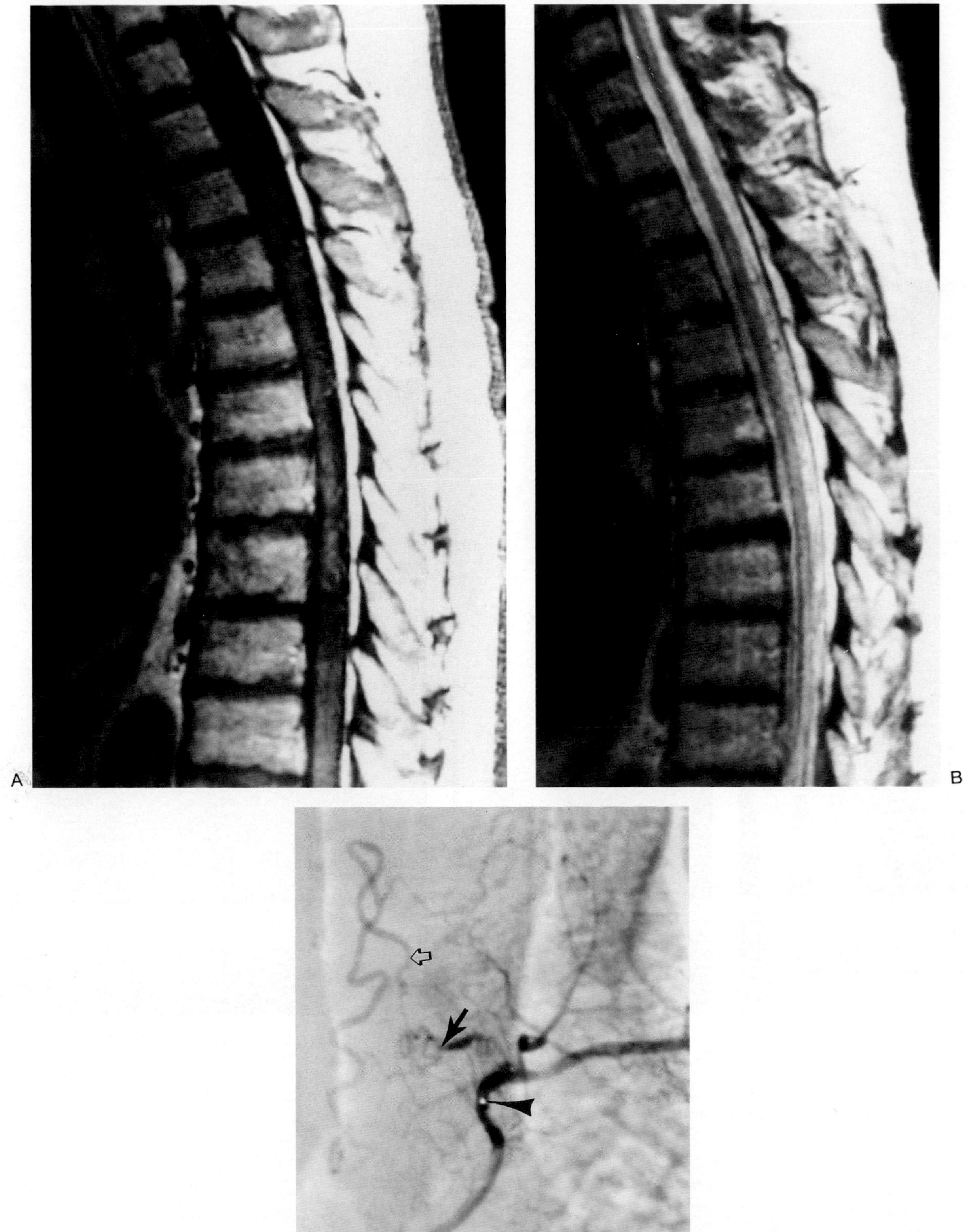

FIG. 13. SDAVF. **A:** Sagittal-enhanced T1- (600/12) and (**B**) T2- (3000/90) weighted images with dorsal flow voids on cord surface. Intrinsic cord enhancement and signal abnormality are present. **C:** AP view of angiographic injection of left T6 intercostal artery. SDAVF (*arrow*) fills from radicular artery with immediate shunting into pial veins of the cord (*open arrow*). *Arrowhead* at catheter tip.

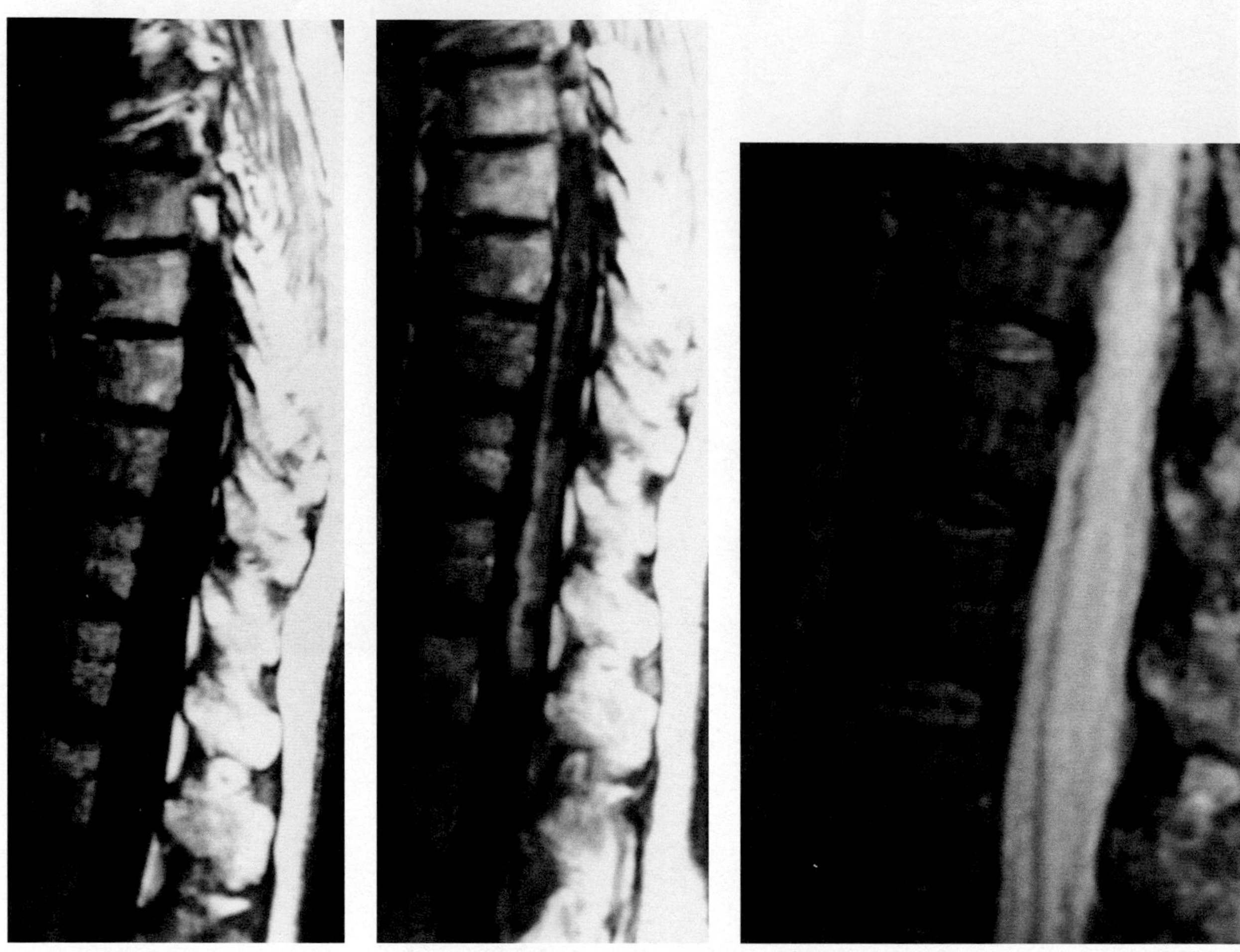

A,B

C

FIG. 14. A–M. SDAVF. A 78-year-old woman with progressive myelopathy and pathologically proven changes of Foix-Alajouanine syndrome. Sagittal unenhanced (**A**) and enhanced (**B**) T1-weighted (500/15) MRI scans demonstrate spinal cord enlargement with diffuse enhancement. No vascular flow voids are identified. **C:** Sagittal T2-weighted image shows abnormally increased intrinsic cord signal throughout the thoracic cord extending into the conus. No intradural flow voids are present.

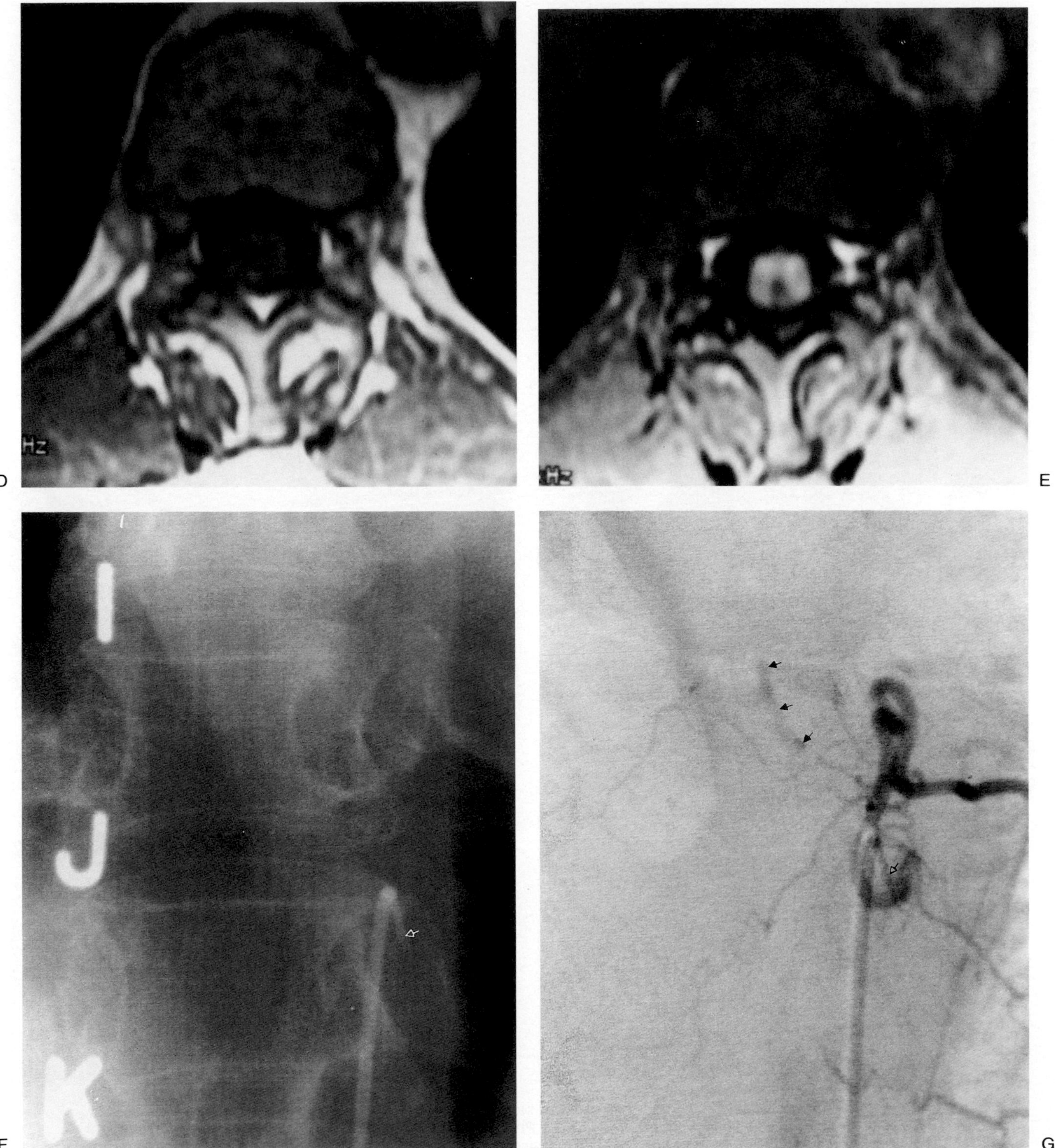

FIG. 14. (*Continued.*) Axial T1-weighted (550/16) unenhanced (**D**) and enhanced (**E**) scans at same thoracic level illustrate diffuse intramedullary enhancement. AP angiographic views unsubtracted (**F**) and subtracted (**G**) demonstrates early filling of a spinal pial vein (*arrows*) indicating the presence of a SDAVF (*open arrow* at catheter tip).

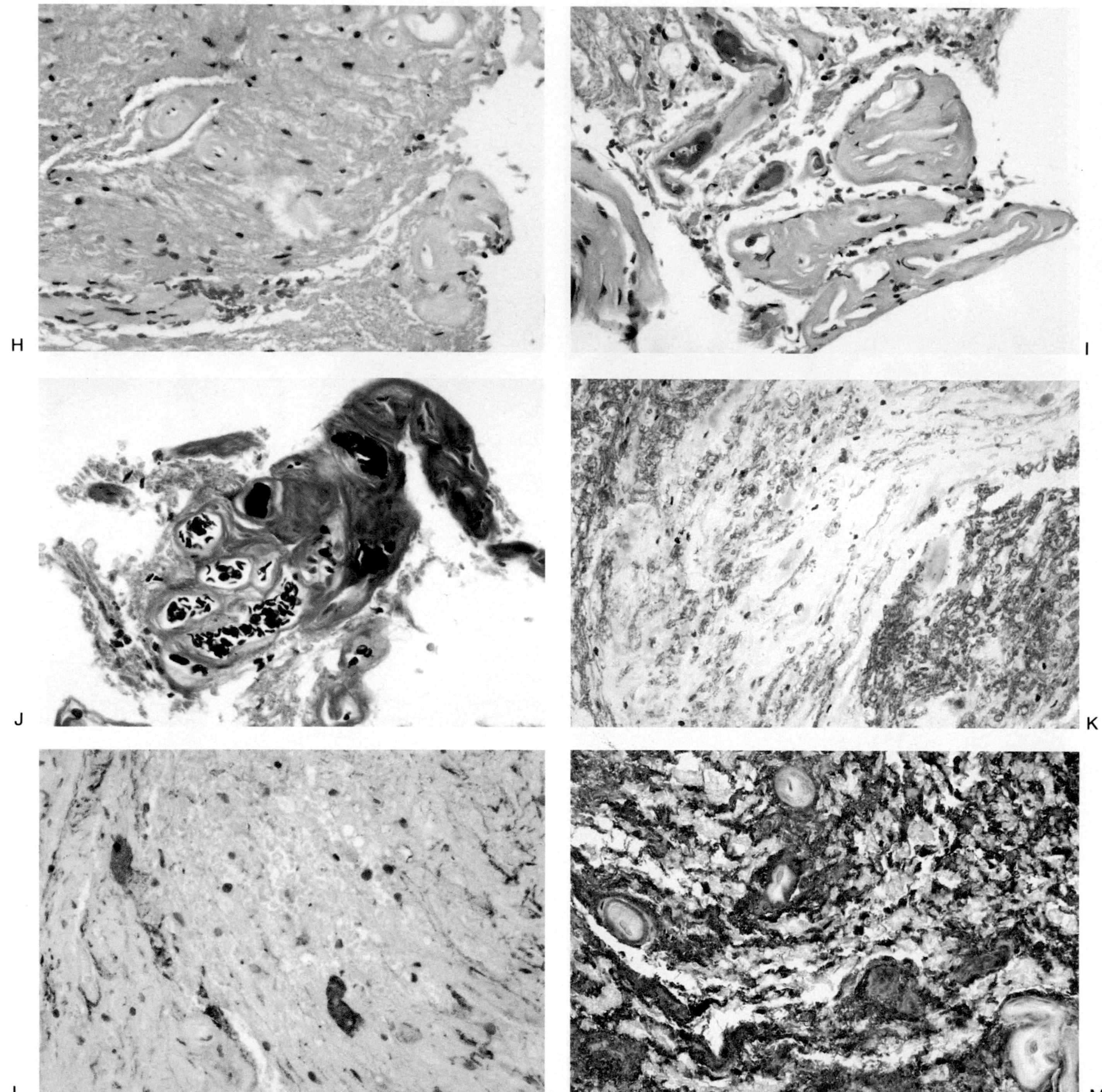

FIG. 14. (*Continued.*) Histologic sections of spinal cord biopsy showing subacute ischemic myelopathy. (Courtesy of Dr. E. Lavi, Hospital of the University of Pennsylvania, Philadelphia, PA.) **H:** Hypocellular white matter with several small hyalinized vessels. **I:** Pathologic changes in blood vessels within cord parenchyma including severe sclerosis of vessel walls and obliteration of lumen. **J:** Trichrome staining highlights collection of subpial angiomatous thickened-wall hyalinized vessels. **K:** Patchy loss of myelin within cord is shown with Luxol fast blue myelin staining. **L:** Immunohistochemical staining with antineurofilament antibodies exhibits severely decreased neurofilament expression that appears focally in clumps. **M:** Immunohistochemical staining with anti-GFAP antibodies shows severe gliosis.

source of engorgement of the spinal venous system (Fig. 15).

The presence of an SDAVF is an indication for treatment as the benefits are multiple and the risks minimal. Endovascular occlusion of SDAVF is possible in more than 80% of cases and can be accomplished at the same time as the diagnostic angiogram using permanent liquid embolic agents such as *N*-butylcyanoacrylate. In con-

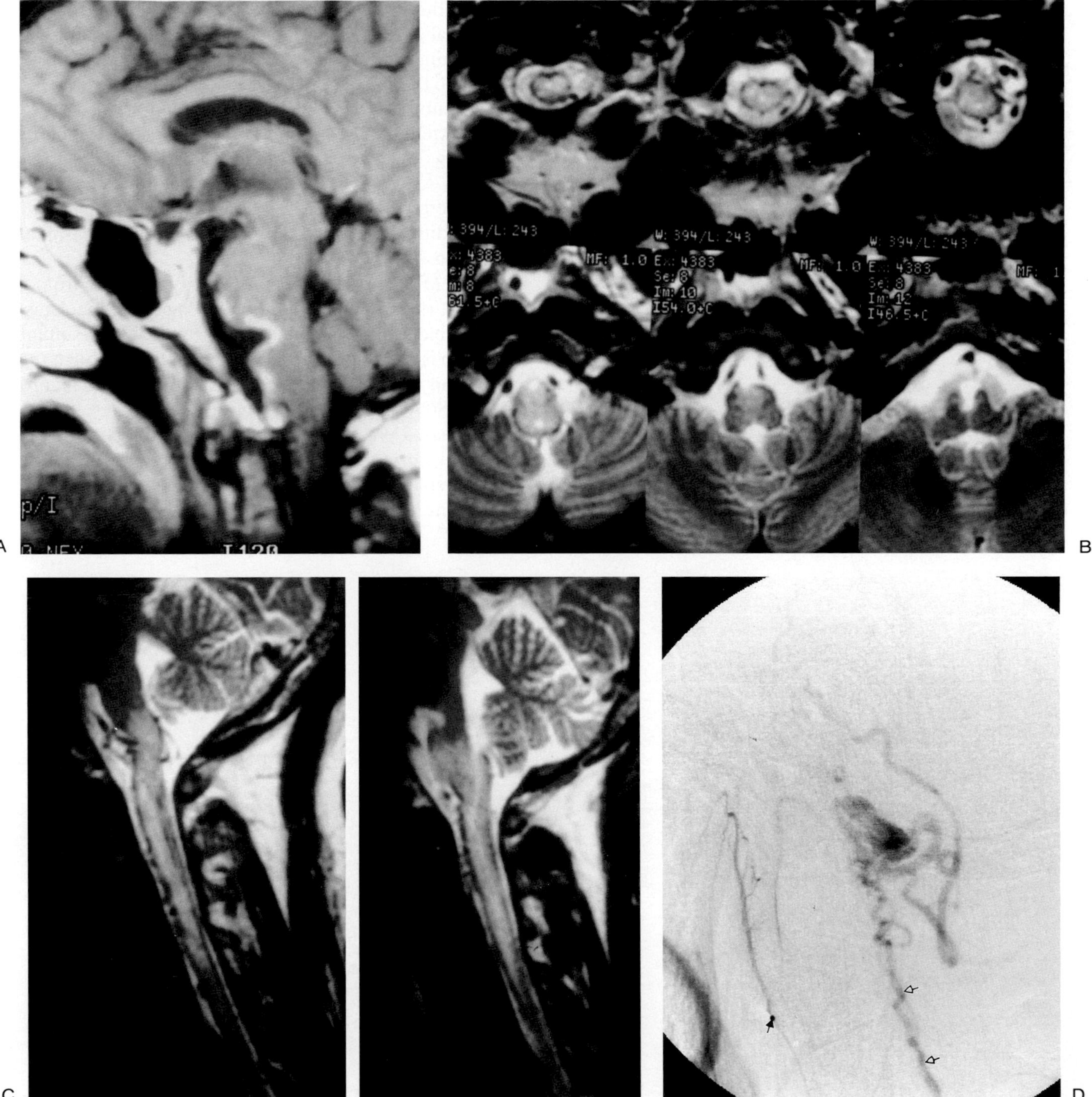

FIG. 15. Posterior fossa dural AV fistula with drainage into veins of the cervical spinal cord. A 62-year-old man with acute quadriparesis and lower cranial nerve palsies. **A:** Sagittal unenhanced T1-weighted image demonstrates high signal along the course of the thrombosed anterior median pontomesencephalic vein with extension along the ventral surface of the medulla. Sagittal (**B**) and axial (**C**) T2-weighted images showing high signal throughout the cervicomedullary junction with expansion of the upper cervical cord. **D:** Lateral view of selective injection of the right ascending pharyngeal artery (*arrow* is at catheter tip) shows dural AVM of the right jugular fossa with venous drainage inferiorly into the veins of the cervical cord.

trast, the use of nonpermanent agents such as particulate emboli for occlusion of the SDAVF results in early recanalization with progression of neurologic deficits and must be considered contraindicated (29,37,38). If endovascular therapy is unsuccessful or contraindicated, surgical coagulation or resection of the nidus and surrounding dura can be safely performed in nearly all cases (17).

Spinal Cord Arteriovenous Malformations

In contrast to SDAVF, intradural SCAVMs are congenital lesions resulting from a defect in early vascular embryogenesis. The nidus of the SCAVM is located on or within the substance of the spinal cord itself with arterial supply from vessels that also directly supply the cord (Fig. 16). The angioarchitecture of SCAVM differs significantly from SDAVF. Consequently, SCAVMs display significant differences in pathophysiology, clinical behavior, and imaging findings in comparison to SDAVF (see Table 2).

Anatomy and Pathophysiology

SCAVMs most frequently occur in the thoracolumbar region but may develop at any level of the cord, including the filum terminale.

The arterial supply to SCAVMs arises from anterior or posterior spinal arteries that also give supply to the spinal cord. The high flow through the nidus predisposes to the formation of feeding artery aneurysms, which may occur in up to 20% of cases and constitute a significant risk factor for spinal hemorrhage (17,39,40). The actual AVM nidus may be located within or on the surface of the spinal cord. Dilated ascending and descending venous drainage is usually present located both dorsal and ventral to the spinal cord.

Two subtypes of SCAVM have been described based on the extent of AVM nidus. A relatively compact nidus involving only the spinal cord characterizes the "glomus type" SCAVMs. The nidus in the much less common "juvenile type" SCAVM also involves the spinal cord with additional extramedullary and often extraspinal extension.

SCAVM may result in neurologic dysfunction from a number of potential pathophysiologic mechanisms. Steal of blood from normal neural tissue with resultant ischemia is possible because of the high flow through the nidus and the common supply to both the spinal cord and the SCAVM. Venous hypertension may result from the increased pressure in the veins draining both the lesion and normal cord tissue. Thrombosis of draining veins or enlargement with resultant mass effect may also be present. Hemorrhage, a particularly common symp-

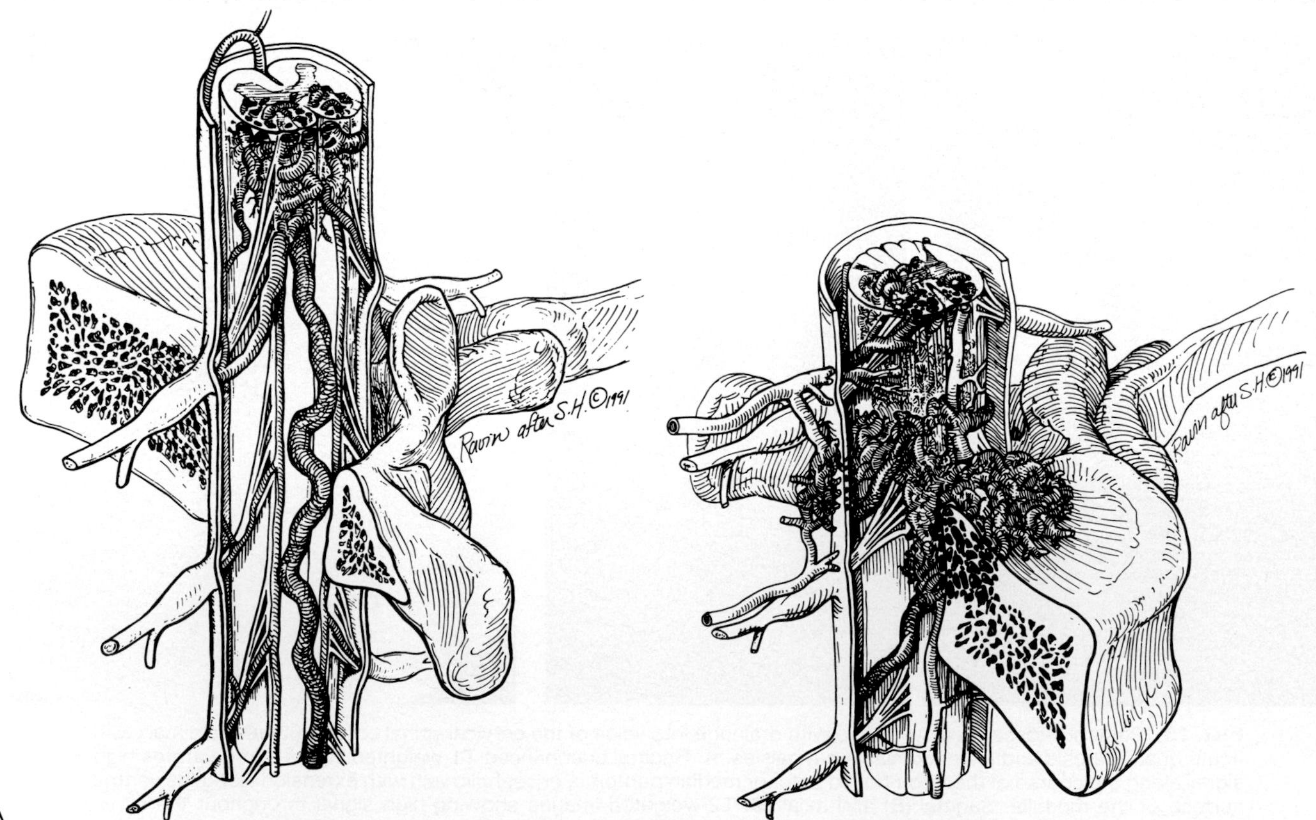

FIG. 16. SCAVM. **A:** Glomus-type SCAVM with nidus located on and within the spinal cord. **B:** Juvenile-type SCAVM with nidus involving cord as well as extending into adjacent tissue. (From Anson and Spetzler, ref. 14, with permission.)

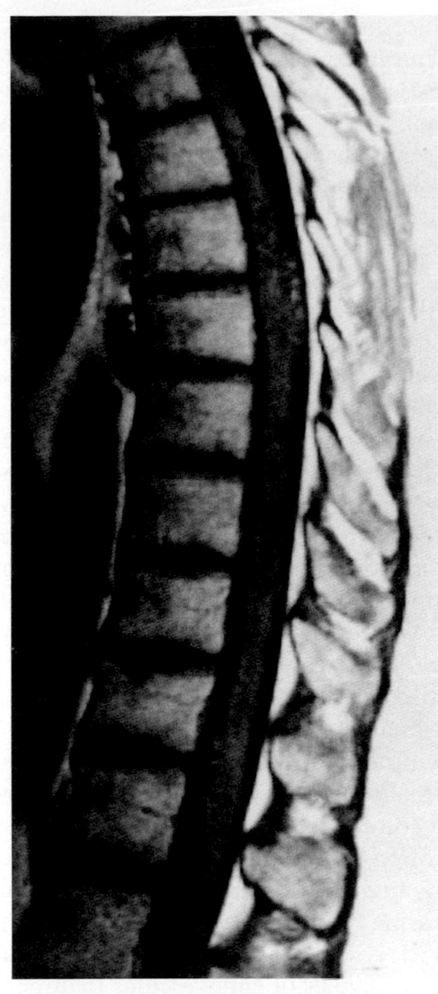

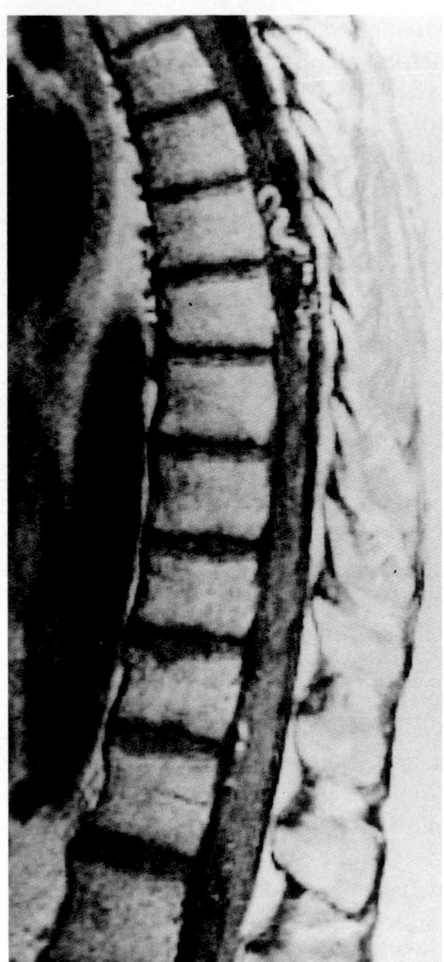

A,B

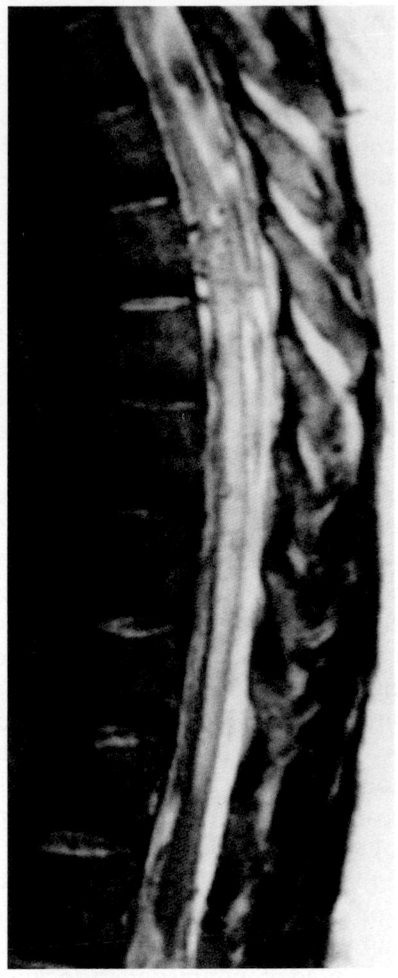

C

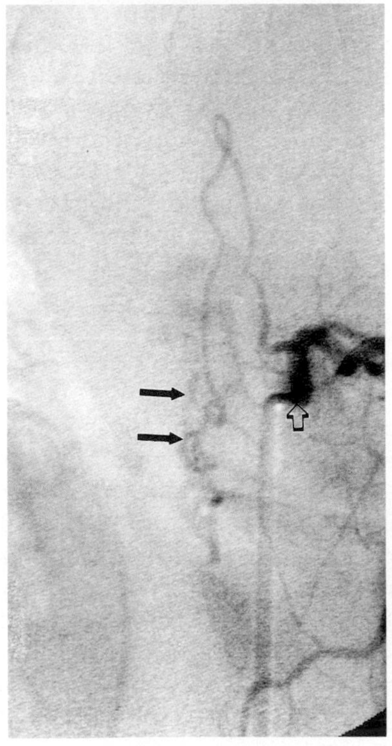

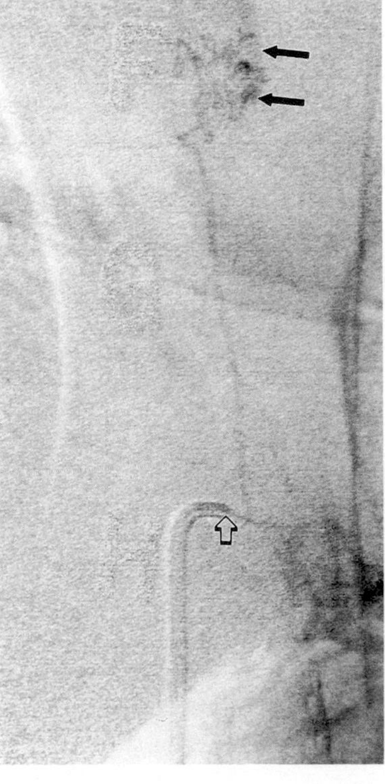

D,E

FIG. 17. SCAVM. **A:** Sagittal unenhanced T1- (400/15) weighted image shows intrinsic cord signal abnormality at T7-T8 level. High signal dorsal to cord suggests acute thrombus or hemorrhage. **B:** Enhanced T1- (400/15) weighted image reveals serpentine vascular structures within and along the surface of the cord. **C:** T2- (3500/135) weighted FSE sagittal image illustrates intrinsic cord signal abnormality with flow voids within and along surface of the cord. **D:** AP angiographic injection of left T7 and T9 (**E**) intercostal arteries shows filling of SCAVM nidus (*arrows*) via enlarged posterior spinal arteries. *Open arrow* at catheter tip.

tom in SCAVM, may arise from arterial aneurysms, the nidus itself, or the draining veins. Hematomyelia, spinal subarachnoid hemorrhage, or both may result. In most cases, a combination of pathophysiologic mechanisms probably causes the development of neurologic dysfunction with resultant deficits.

Clinical

Large series of SCAVMs have noted a slight predominance of male patients with the average age at diagnosis in the second or third decade. At the time of presentation, however, nearly half the patients are less than 16 years of age (17,24,25).

More than 30% of patients will experience weakness as the initial symptom of SCAVM; however, nearly all patients will develop some significant loss of motor function during the course. Back pain accompanies the onset in nearly one fifth of patients and actually diminishes as a significant symptom later as sensory deficits, developing in more than 70%, become more prominent. In addition, the characteristically progressive course usually involves compromise of bowel, bladder, and sexual functions. The result is confinement to bed or a wheelchair in nearly half of untreated patients within 3 years of symptom onset (41).

In contrast to SDAVF, spinal hemorrhage constitutes a prominent feature in the clinical course of more than half the patients with SCAVM. Occurring in either subarachnoid or intramedullary locations, hemorrhage is associated with both high mortality (up to 30%) and high rates of rebleeding, which may reach 40% within the first year (41,42). Less frequent features include a bruit or cutaneous angioma over the location of the nidus.

SCAVM may represent part of a more widespread systemic vascular disorder such as Rendu-Osler-Weber or Klippel-Trenauney syndrome. A complex metameric vascular malformation, Cobb's syndrome, involves all embryonic layers from the spinal cord to the skin and may be present in 5% of SCAVM patients (43,44).

Imaging

MRI provides the best noninvasive imaging information regarding spinal cord AVMs (Figs. 17, 18, and 19). Kyphosis or scoliosis may accompany SCAVM and may be so severe as to make positioning problematic. Flow voids representing enlarged arterial feeding vessels and intramedullary nidus are well seen, although flow artifact may interfere in some cases with anatomic detail. Evidence of recent or past intramedullary hemorrhage is frequently present, although determining the presence of subarachnoid hemorrhage on MRI remains difficult. Nonhemorrhagic intramedullary signal abnormality adjacent to the nidus is also frequent and most likely indicates gliosis, edema, or areas of cord infarction. Flow voids of draining veins in the subarachnoid space may show areas of ectasia, mass effect, or thrombosis. Extension of nidus into extramedullary structures, particularly vertebral bodies and paraspinal soft tissue structures, is also well seen on MR. Although MRA sequences may detect high flow, the imaging findings are usually quite characteristic of SCAVM and, at present, MRA has not developed to the point at which specific feeding and draining vessels can be reliably identified.

Angiographic evaluation of SCAVM is mandatory before planning and performance of treatment. Delineation of all feeding vessels, determining the presence of aneurysms, locating the nidus within the cord, and mapping the size and location of draining veins are important goals to be accomplished angiographically. In addition, the normal blood supply to the cord above and below the lesion must be studied. In cases of extramedullary extension, the entire extent of the nidus and its feeding vessels must be evaluated.

Treatment of symptomatic SCAVM should be aggressively pursued because of the poor outcomes in untreated patients. A combination of endovascular and surgical treatment is often appropriate and may begin at the time of diagnostic angiographic examination. In a significant and increasing number of cases, complete obliteration of SCAVM is achievable using endovascular techniques. Additional goals of endovascular treatment may include presurgical devascularization, prevention of recurrent hemorrhage, or palliation in extensive lesions (39,40,42). Surgical resection in SCAVM also aims for complete obliteration of the lesion whenever possible. In selected lesions, good outcomes have been reported in a number of series using both methods (17,24,29,45). Close coordination between the surgeon and interventional neuroradiologist is critical for proper management of these difficult lesions (46,47).

Spinal Cord Arteriovenous Fistula

SCAVFs (also known as intradural arteriovenous fistulas or perimedullary arteriovenous fistulas) consist of direct arteriovenous fistulas located on the cord and fed directly by arteries supplying the cord, most frequently the ASA. SCAVFs constitute a small homogeneous subgroup of spinal arteriovenous malformations that have been found in from 8% to 19% of patients in large series of spinal vascular malformations (13,16,24). The intradural location of the shunt, constant involvement of arteries supplying the spinal cord, and lack of intervening

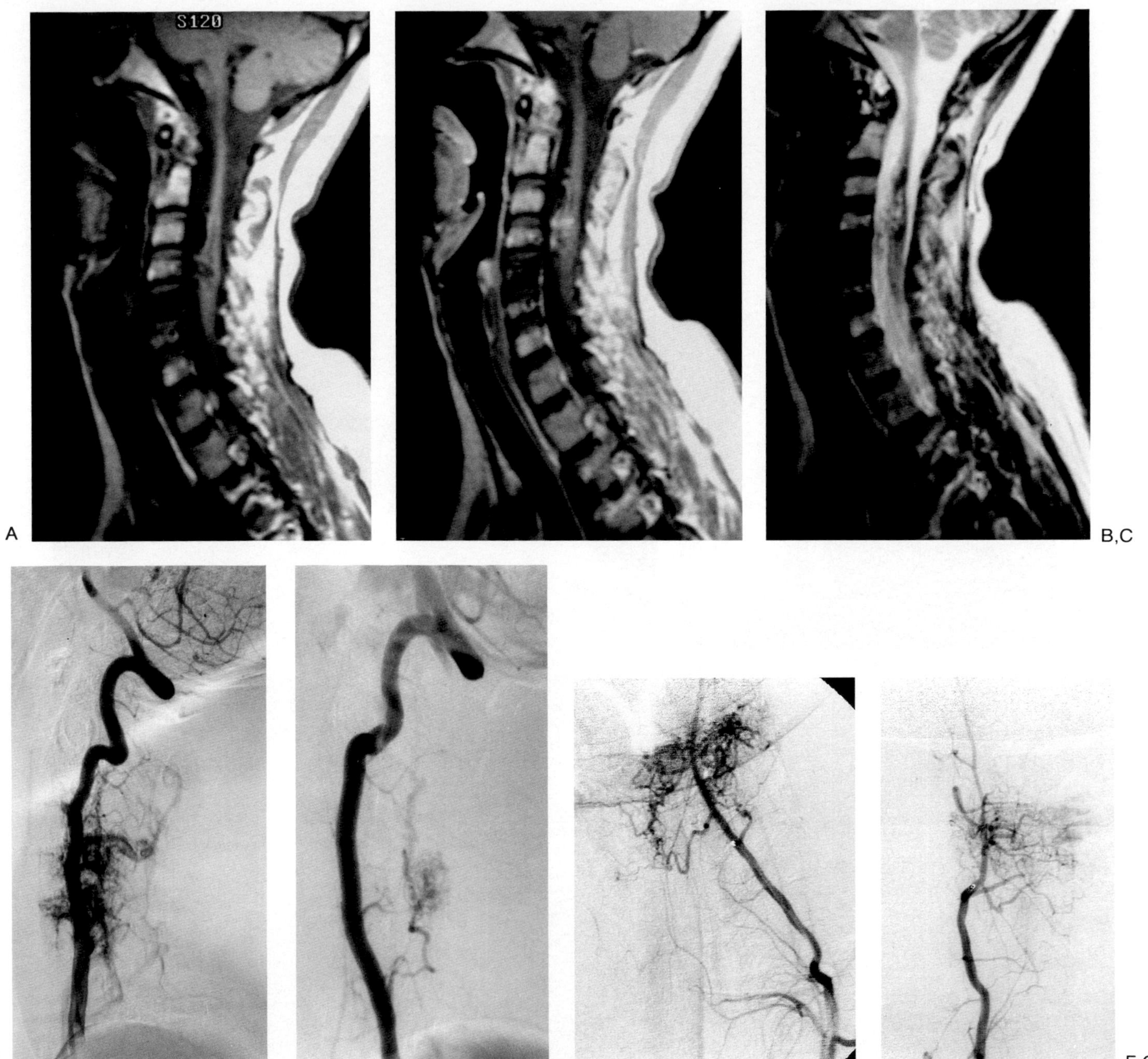

FIG. 18. SCAVM. Sagittal T1-weighted (500/17) unenhanced (**A**) and enhanced (**B**) images demonstrate intrinsic cord signal abnormality and adjacent flow void of SCAVM. Abnormal signal involving vertebral bodies indicates extensive paraspinal involvement by this juvenile-type SCAVM. **C:** T2-weighted (2700/85) FSE image demonstrates hemosiderin and blood storage products from prior hematomyelia. **D,E:** Lateral angiographic view of left and right vertebral arteries. **F,G:** AP view of left and right deep cervical arteries. Extensive supply to nidus originates from vertebral and deep cervical arteries bilaterally. Nidus involves not only spinal cord but extends into paraspinal soft tissue and vertebral bodies.

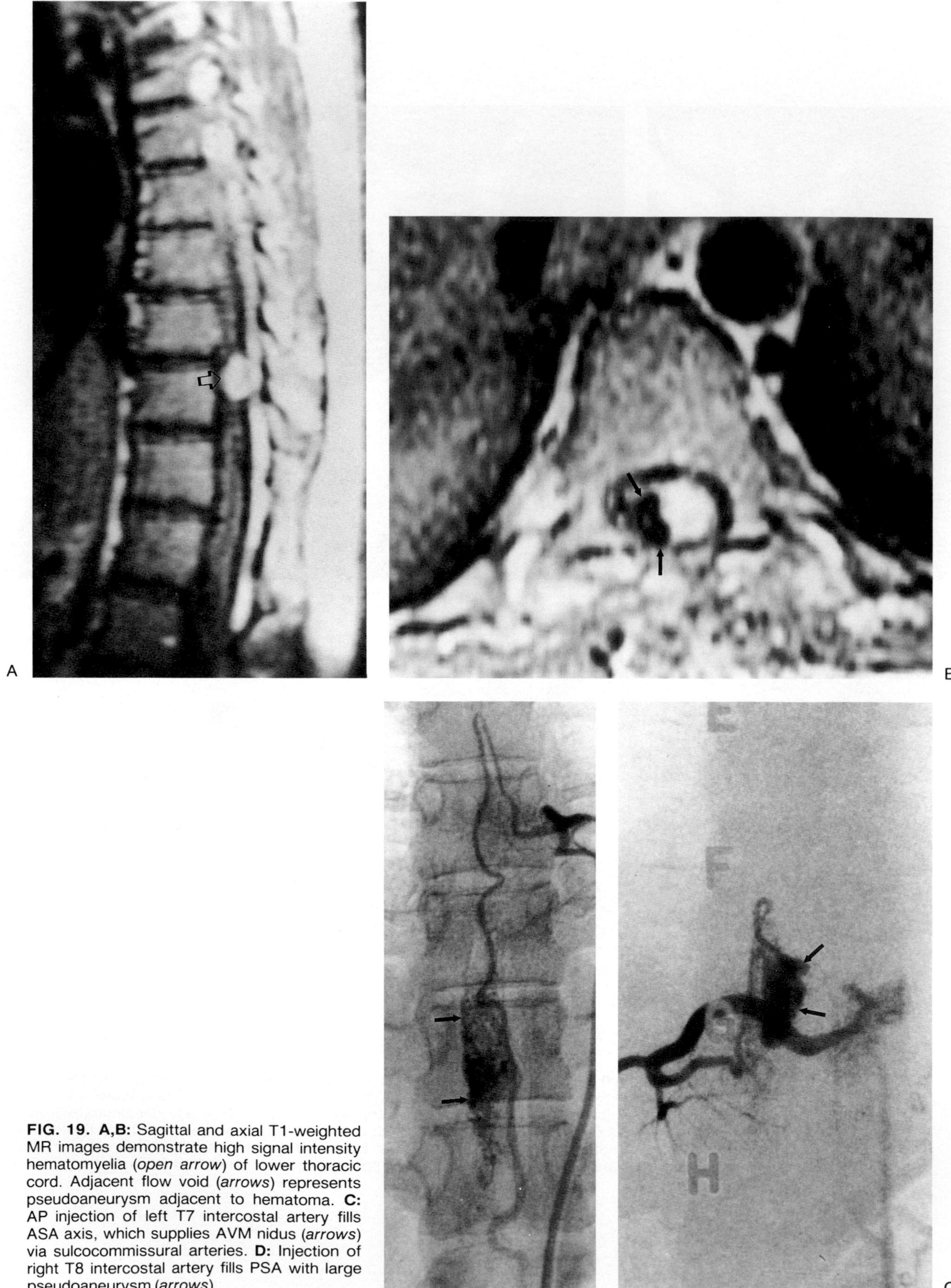

FIG. 19. A,B: Sagittal and axial T1-weighted MR images demonstrate high signal intensity hematomyelia (*open arrow*) of lower thoracic cord. Adjacent flow void (*arrows*) represents pseudoaneurysm adjacent to hematoma. **C:** AP injection of left T7 intercostal artery fills ASA axis, which supplies AVM nidus (*arrows*) via sulcocommissural arteries. **D:** Injection of right T8 intercostal artery fills PSA with large pseudoaneurysm (*arrows*).

nidus are angioarchitectural features that differentiate SCAVFs from both SDAVFs and SCAVMs (23) (Figs. 20 and 21).

Believed to be congenital lesions, SCAVFs usually present in patients in their second through fourth decade. The most common neurologic presentation is one of progressive asymmetrical radiculomedullary signs involving the lower extremities, reflecting the most common location of SCAVFs in the lower thoracic or lumbar region. Spinal subarachnoid hemorrhage is also common and has been noted in nearly one third of patients at presentation. Three subtypes of SCAVF have been identified based on the size and number of vessels involved and on the hemodynamics of the shunt (14,48).

MRI is the noninvasive imaging modality of choice. Flow voids depict the enlarged feeding and draining vessels of SCAVF. Mass effect of the enlarged vascular structures with displacement or distortion of the cord may occur. Intrinsic cord signal abnormality and evidence of hemorrhage may also be present. The small size of some lesions and lack of nidus may make differentiation from SDAVF or even detection by MRI difficult. Abnormal enhancement of the cord may be present.

Angiographic evaluation of SCAVF remains necessary for complete delineation of the angioarchitecture, particularly determining the exact location of the arteriovenous shunt. In general, smaller lesions are best treated surgically whereas larger SCAVFs are best approached by endovascular methods. The goal of endovascular treatment is occlusion of the fistula itself and the most proximal portion of the draining vein, preserving the anterior spinal artery axis. Following complete occlusion of the SCAVF, contrast enhancement and signal abnormality within the cord may persist.

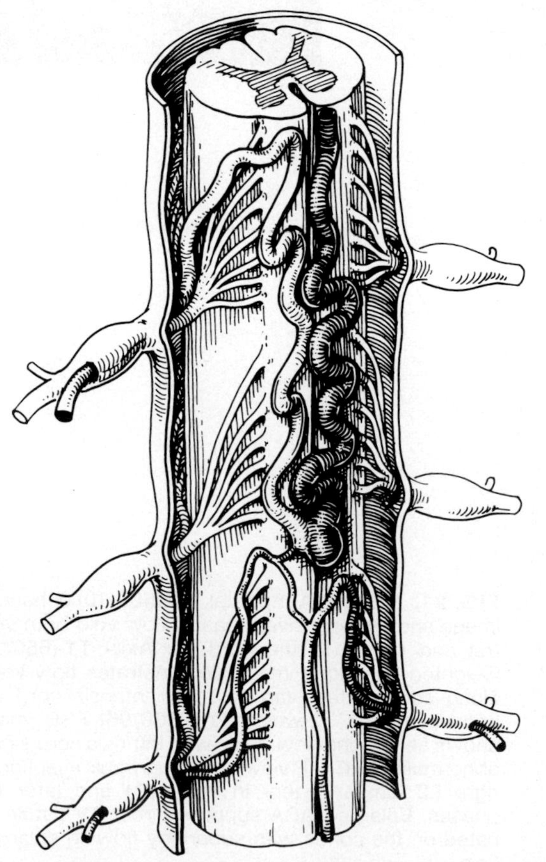

FIG. 20. Diagram of SCAVF shows the direct fistula between the ASA and an adjacent vein. (From Anson and Spetzler, ref. 14, with permission.)

Cavernous Angioma or Cavernous Malformation

Unlike the spinal AVMs previously discussed, cavernous malformations (CMs) are slow flow vascular malformations without AV shunting. The widespread use of MRI has resulted in an increase in diagnosis of CMs throughout the CNS, including lesions involving the spine. Although uncommon, the true incidence of spinal CMs is difficult to establish because most autopsy studies do not include the spinal cord. The reported incidence of CMs involving all regions of the CNS has been reported to be between 0.02% and 4%. Based on the spinal component weight and volume, it would be expected that 3% to 5% of CMs involve the spine. When the lesions do affect the spine, they are most often intramedullary and occur proportionally throughout the cord. Involvement of the cauda equina and filum terminale has also been described (49–51). In contrast to the equal male to female ratio reported in their intracranial counterparts, CMs of the spine have been noted to preferentially affect females. Kindreds have been described with multiple CMs throughout the CNS including spinal involvement (52). An autosomal dominant genetic defect with variable penetrance has been suggested as the causative factor in familial cases (53,54).

The clinical presentation of CMs involving the spinal cord is variable. Although symptoms may begin at any age, patients most often present in the fourth decade. Discrete episodic neurologic dysfunction with variable recovery between episodes has been described most commonly; however, monophasic acute or chronic deterioration of spinal cord function may also occur. The acute presentation is probably secondary to hemorrhage either within the vascular spaces of the malformation or into the surrounding parenchyma (hematomyelia). Back pain is a frequent accompaniment with the neurologic deficit beginning later and evolving over several hours to days. The pace of clinical deterioration tends to differentiate these patients from the more rapid course associated with hemorrhage from SCAVMs. Progressive myelopathy may result from growth or enlargement of the lesions by several mechanisms including vessel dilation, repeated hemorrhage, or capillary proliferation (55,56).

CMs of the spine are pathologically identical to intra-

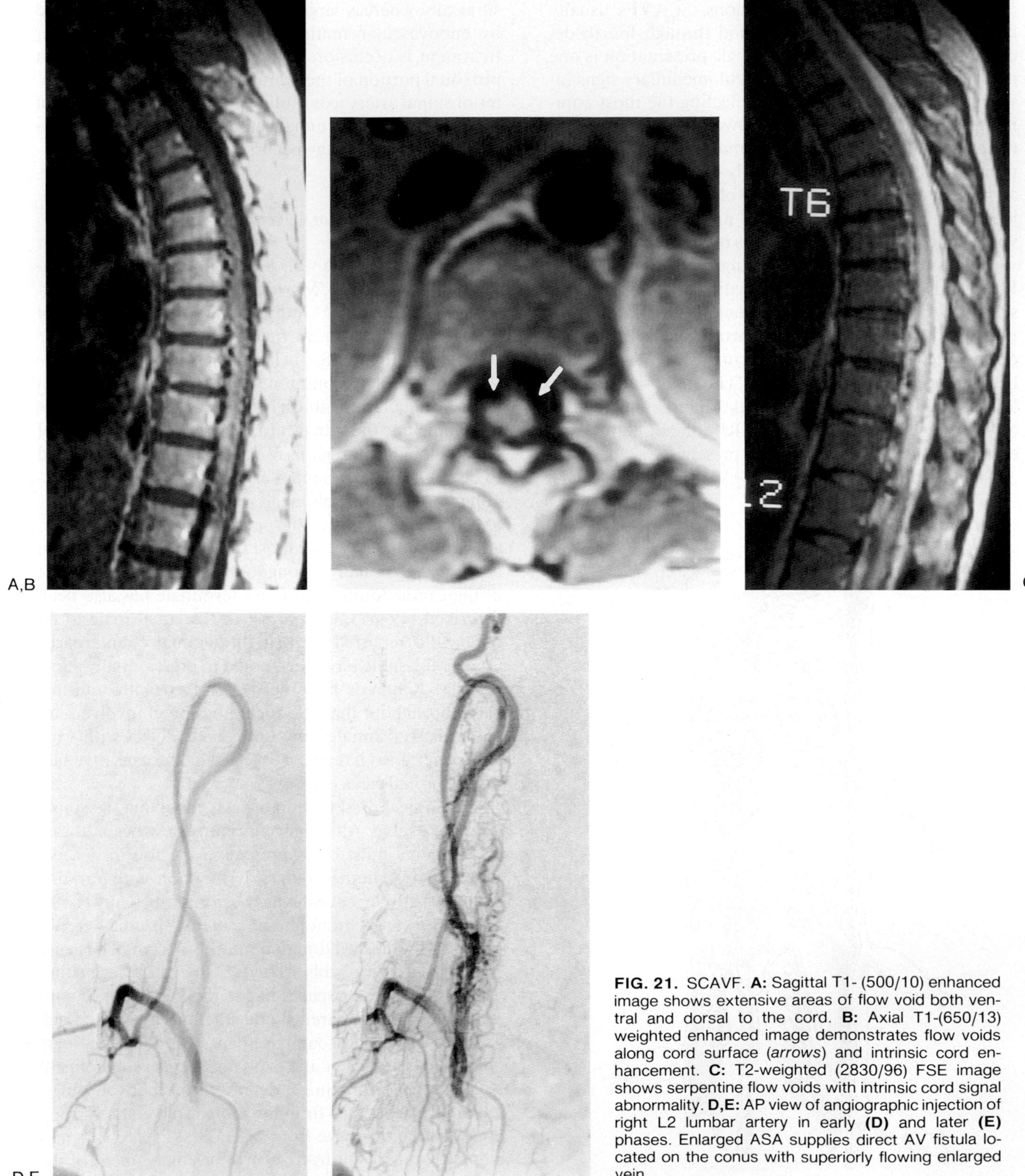

FIG. 21. SCAVF. **A:** Sagittal T1- (500/10) enhanced image shows extensive areas of flow void both ventral and dorsal to the cord. **B:** Axial T1-(650/13) weighted enhanced image demonstrates flow voids along cord surface (*arrows*) and intrinsic cord enhancement. **C:** T2-weighted (2830/96) FSE image shows serpentine flow voids with intrinsic cord signal abnormality. **D,E:** AP view of angiographic injection of right L2 lumbar artery in early **(D)** and later **(E)** phases. Enlarged ASA supplies direct AV fistula located on the conus with superiorly flowing enlarged vein.

cranial CMs and vary in size from several millimeters to more than a centimeter in diameter. Most commonly they are well-demarcated lesions surrounded by hemosiderin-stained gliotic neural tissue. The constant presence of blood storage products suggests episodic diapedesis of blood or low grade hemorrhage from the lesions. Acute hemorrhage within or adjacent to the lesions may be present in some cases. Histologically, blood-filled cysts are present, composed of closely packed sinusoidal vascular channels with very slow blood flow. The channels have variable wall thickness, ranging from a single cell layer to hyalinized thickened walls containing densely packed collagen but no elastic or smooth muscle fibers. The gliotic tissue adjacent to the CM demonstrates constant hemosiderin staining and occasional collections of inflammatory cells. Calcification, seen in up to 15% of intracranial lesions on CT scan, is rare in spinal CMs (57).

MRI findings are often characteristic and usually permit a relatively specific diagnosis. A rim of low signal intensity representing iron storage products completely surrounds the lesion. Intrinsic heterogeneous signal abnormality is present on both T1- and T2-weighted images representing blood products of various ages (Fig. 22). Gliosis, edema, or syrinx adjacent to the lesion may cause abnormal signal in the surrounding cord parenchyma. Following acute hemorrhage, the MRI appearance may be less specific and other differential considerations for hematomyelia may need to be considered (58). Although most reported cases of spinal CMs are single, multiple lesions involving the spinal cord have been reported (59). In cases with characteristic MRI features, angiographic evaluation is unnecessary.

Management of spinal CMs is dependent on the patient's age and clinical features. No treatment is currently advised for asymptomatic lesions. Surgical explo-

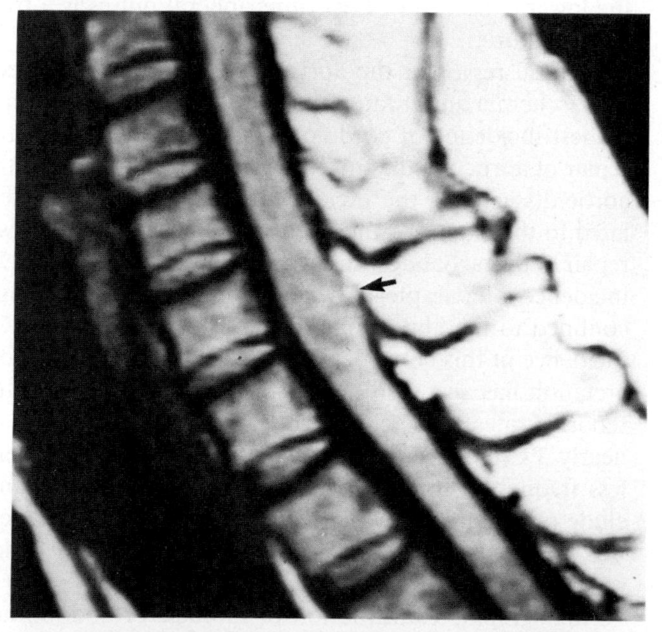

A

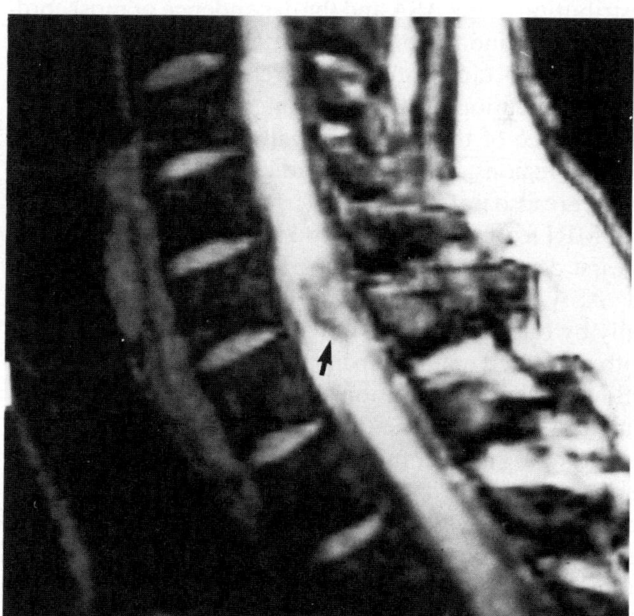

B

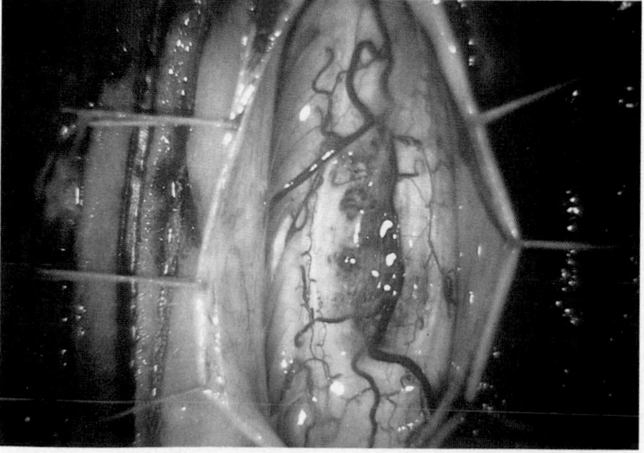

C

FIG. 22. Spinal cord CM. **A:** Sagittal T1-weighted and **B:** gradient-echo images demonstrate focal low signal intensity within the spinal cord with associated intramedullary mass. **C:** Intraoperative photograph confirms an intramedullary CM extending to the surface of the spinal cord, seen as a cluster of grapes, after exposure of the intradural space.

ration and resection is the treatment of choice for symptomatic lesions because of the potential morbidity of future neurologic deficits (56,60).

SPINAL CORD ISCHEMIA AND INFARCTION

Although frequently devastating, spinal cord ischemia is an uncommon cause of myelopathy. The exact incidence of the disorder is difficult to ascertain, however. Some studies have suggested that spinal ischemia may represent from 1% to 2% of all cases of stroke (61,62). In contrast, an autopsy study of 3,737 patients over a 50-year period found only seven incidences of nontraumatic ischemic or hemorrhagic myelopathy (63).

In cases of suspected ischemic damage to the spinal cord, MRI is the diagnostic study of choice. As is the case throughout the CNS, imaging evaluation of ischemia and infarction of the spinal cord is best approached with a thorough understanding of the vascular distributions supplying the involved region. The large intramedullary distribution of the ASA and the dependence of most cord gray matter and major white matter tracts on ASA supply are important features. The relative isolation of the ASA distribution from PSA collaterals and the frequent dependence of the ASA, especially in the thoracic and lumbar regions, on a single radiculomedullary feeding vessel are also important in determining both the clinical and MRI features of spinal cord ischemia.

First described by Spiller in 1909, ischemia involving the ASA distribution is most often characterized clinically by the abrupt onset of flaccid paralysis asssociated with decreased or absent pain and temperature sensation below the level of the lesion (64). Bowel and bladder dysfunction are also present. In contrast, posterior column functions are usually preserved because of the intact PSA supply to these cord structures. The result is a dissociated sensory deficit with loss of pain and temperature in the face of intact posterior column functions, including vibratory sensation and proprioception. The initial cord deficits are often incomplete and may be unilateral, reflecting the lateralized distribution of the sulcocommissural branches of the ASA. The sparing of posterior column function often permits clinical differentiation from a Brown-Séquard syndrome resulting from cord hemisection. Particular susceptibility of the thoracic and lumbar cord regions to ischemia results from the poor collateral flow via adjacent segments of the ASA in the event of compromise of a major radiculomedullary artery. In contrast, the multiple collateral routes to the cervical ASA seem to provide some protection from infarction at these levels, at least in cases of proximal or radiculomedullary artery obstruction. As in spinal shock associated with traumatic lesions, the initially flaccid areflexic paralysis often develops into spasticity with Babinski signs and a return of some degree of sphincter control. Although a pattern of clinical deficits referable to the ASA distribution suggests a vascular etiology, ischemia may involve both ASA and PSA distributions resulting in the less specific picture of complete loss of cord function. Ischemia confined to the PSA distribution has been described but is recognized very rarely.

Several clinical situations have been associated with infarction of the spinal cord and should prompt consideration of the diagnosis when present in the clinical history. Spontaneous aortic dissection may be the most common cause of ischemic damage to the spinal cord and has been associated with spinal infarction in nearly 2% of cases. Dissections involving the descending aorta (i.e., types I and III) are most often associated with the complication whereas those confined to the ascending aorta (type II) manifest cord ischemia only rarely. The clinical features suggest that damage to multiple radicular arteries with compromise of both ASA and PSA distributions is an important etiologic factor. Sudden onset of paraplegia and sensory loss is usually accompanied by sharp chest or abdominal pain that often radiates into the lower extremities. Loss of peripheral pulses is a frequent feature.

Surgical repair of the aorta has also been associated with ischemia and infarction of the spinal cord, with the highest incidence of cord complications resulting from repair of aortic aneurysms. Similar to the situation with aortic dissections, the incidence of cord ischemia is related to the extent of the aneurysm. In one large series, repair of thoracoabdominal aneurysms resulted in a 21% incidence of paraplegia whereas repair of aneurysms confined to the abdominal aorta resulted in only a 1% incidence of this complication (65). Repair of aortic coarctation has also resulted in spinal cord ischemia with reported rates of the complication varying from 0.4% to nearly 3% (66,67). Other surgical procedures have been less frequently implicated in cord ischemia. These include procedures in which ligation of radicular arteries was performed, such as scoliosis correction and pneumonectomy.

Angiographic examination of thoracic or abdominal branches of the aorta may rarely result in ischemic spinal cord complications. The spinal cord damage probably arises from inadvertent catheterization of branches giving rise to radiculomedullary arteries with resultant arterial spasm or accidental introduction of atheromatous emboli, blood clot, or air. Although a feared complication of spinal angiography, ischemic cord damage is uncommon with current angiographic techniques. Two recent studies evaluated the incidence of complications associated with spinal angiography in a total of 151 patients. They found that spinal angiography carries a risk of neurologic complications in the range of 2.2% to 3.6% (22,68). All complications identified in the studies were transient. Although the small numbers of patients evaluated precludes definite conclusions regarding incidence of complications, current data suggest that when performed by experienced personnel, risks of spinal angiography are similar in incidence to those associated with cerebral angiography (69).

Atherosclerotic involvement of the aorta with occlusion of radicular arteries is extremely common; nonetheless, ischemic myelopathy rarely results. The infrequency of cord ischemia may reflect the slow progression of the occlusion in atherosclerosis permitting adequate collateralization via intersegmental collaterals from adjacent levels. Similarly, thromboembolic occlusion of vessels leading to cord ischemia also appears to be a rare phenomenon. An autopsy study of 1,000 cases found only one instance of atheromatous emboli to the ASA in a patient with symptoms of cord ischemia (70). Decompression sickness has been associated with ischemic myelopathy in a number of reports (71,72). In such cases blockage of epidural veins by nitrogen bubbles appears to result in impairment of spinal cord venous return with a consequent hemorrhagic myelopathy. Cases of spinal cord ischemia have also been associated with polyarteritis, giant cell arteritis, syphilis, sickle cell anemia, and antiphospholipid antibody syndrome (73,74).

MRI findings in spinal cord ischemia are similar regardless of the etiology of the infarction (73,75,76). Areas of intrinsic cord signal abnormality are best seen on proton-density and T2-weighted images (Fig. 23). Both axial and sagittal images are useful in demonstrating the areas of abnormal signal. Signal abnormality may involve only the gray matter structures, but in more severely affected patients extends throughout the entire cross-section of the cord to affect both gray and white matter, suggesting involvement of both ASA and PSA vascular distributions. T1-weighted images are often normal or demonstrate only subtle cord enlargement in the acute stage. Following administration of gadolinium, cord enhancement may occur especially involving the gray matter. Enhancement has been noted within several days of infarction and may last as long as several months. In the chronic stages, cord atrophy may be present. MR signal abnormalities representing areas of infarction within adjacent vertebral bodies or evidence of aortic dissection may suggest the ischemic etiology of the cord signal abnormalities.

The MRI findings of cord ischemia and infarction are often nonspecific, however, and highlight the usefulness of clinical information in suggesting the diagnosis. MRI findings in patients with SDAVF may be similar and reflect venous hypertension, possibly with venous infarction of the cord. Similar MRI findings may also result from transverse myelitis, demyelinating disease, intrinsic cord tumor, or inflammatory etiologies (77–79).

HEMATOMYELIA

SCAVM is the most common cause of nontraumatic spinal hemmorhage and a finding of hematomyelia or spinal subarachnoid hemorrhage should prompt serious consideration of the diagnosis. CMs of the spinal cord,

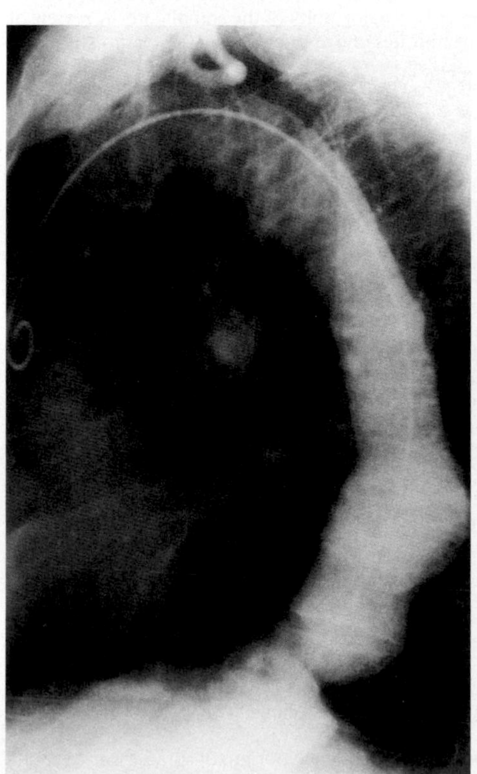

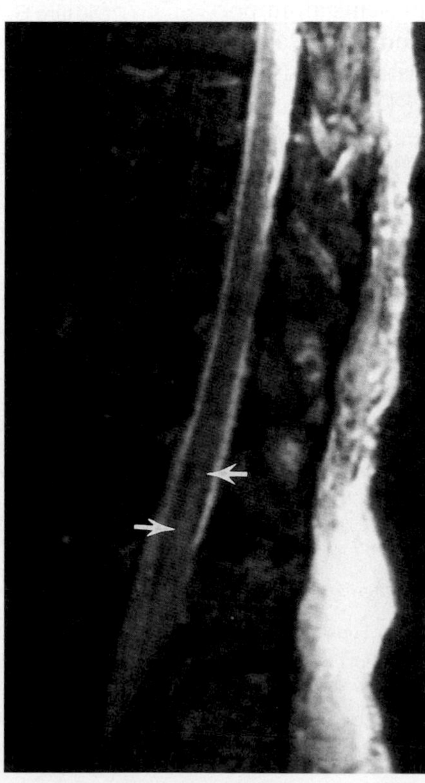

A,B

FIG. 23. A 75-year-old woman became paraplegic following resection of a thoracoabdominal aortic aneurysm shown on aortogram (**A**). **B:** Sagittal T2-weighted image (2,667/40) with increased signal intensity of cord due to infarction involving the lumbar region (*arrows*).

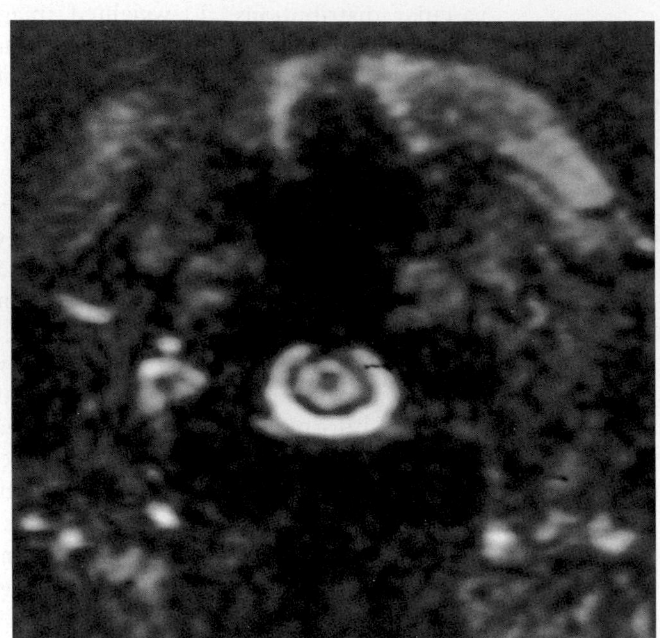

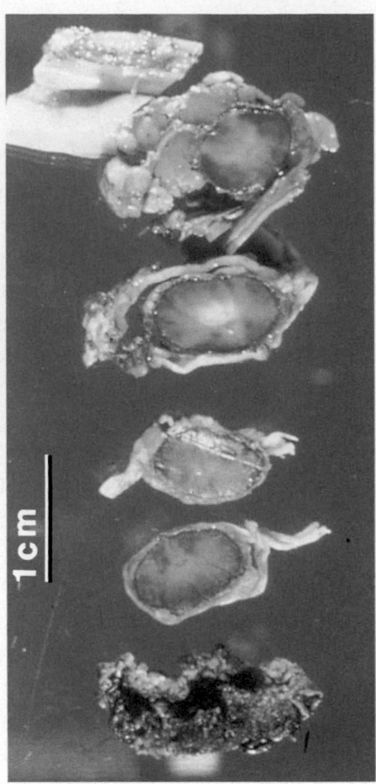

FIG. 24. Superficial hemosiderosis involving the spinal cord. **A:** T2*-weighted axial gradient-echo MRI demonstrates marked hypointensity over surface of spinal cord and within central canal. (Courtesy of Dr. S. Galetta, Hospital of the University of Pennsylvania.) **B:** Serial axial sections at post-mortem showing superficial hemosiderin deposition as depicted by positive blue Perl staining.

similar to those in the brain, may hemorrhage with resultant hematomyelia or spinal subarachnoid hemorrhage (80). Anticoagulant therapy represents an important predisposition to hematomyelia and should also be considered in any patient presenting with nontraumatic intramedullary spinal hemorrhage (81). Hemorrhage into cord tumor, syrinx, or hemorrhagic areas associated with inflammatory myelitis may also be clinically significant (82). Aside from intramedullary hematomas and their primary causative lesions, MRI may also show secondary superficial hemosiderosis from prior subarachnoid bleeding as a coat of marked hypointensity overlying the surface of the spinal cord, particularly evident on T2-weighted images (Fig. 24).

REFERENCES

1. Thron A. *Vascular Anatomy of the Spinal Cord*, 1st ed. Vienna–New York: Springer-Verlag; 1988:114.
2. Djindjian R, Hurth M, Houdart R. *Angiography of the Spinal Cord.* Baltimore: University Park Press; 1970.
3. Lasjaunias P, Berenstein A. *Surgical Neuroangiography, Vol 3: Functional Vascular Anatomy of Brain, Spinal Cord, and Spine.* Berlin–Heidelberg–New York: Springer-Verlag; 1990.
4. Lazorthes G, Gouaze A, Zadeh J, Santini J, Lazorthes Y, Burdin P. Arterial vascularization of the spinal cord. *J Neurosurg* 1971;35: 253–262.
5. Lazorthes G, ed. *Pathology, Classification, and Clinical Aspects of Vascular Diseases of the Spinal Cord.* Amsterdam–New York: Elsevier; 1972 (Vinken P and Bruyn G, eds. *Handbook of Clinical Neurology; vol 12*).
6. Gillian L. Veins of the spinal cord. *Neurology* 1970;20:860–868.
7. DiChiro G, Wener L. Angiography of the spinal cord. A review of contemporary techniques and applications. *J Neurosurg* 1973;39: 1–29.
8. Doppman J, DiChiro G, Omaya A. *Selective Arteriography of the Spinal Cord.* St. Louis: H. Green; 1969.
9. Doppman J. Spinal angiography. In: Abrams H, ed. *Abrams' Angiography*, 3rd ed. Boston: Little, Brown; 1983.
10. Gelbert F, Guichard J-P, Mourier KL, et al. Phase-contrast MR angiography of vascular malformations of the spinal cord at 0.5T. *J Magn Reson Imaging* 1992;2:631–636.
11. Kendall B, Logue L. Spinal epidural angiomatous malformation draining into intrathecal veins. *Neuroradiology* 1977;13:181–189.
12. Merland J, Riche M, Chiras J. Intraspinal extramedullary arteriovenous fistula draining into medullary veins. *J Neuroradiol* 1980;7:221–230.
13. Gueguen B, Merlane J, Reche M, Rey A. Vascular malformations of the spinal cord: intrathecal perimedullary arteriovenous fistulas fed by medullary arteries. *Neurology* 1987;37:969–979.
14. Anson J, Spetzler R. Classification of spinal arteriovenous malformations. *BNI Q* 1992;8:2–8.
15. Rodesch G, Berenstein A, Lasjaunias P. Vasculature and vascular lesions of the spine and spinal cord. In: Manelfe C, ed. *Imaging of the Spine and Spinal Cord.* New York: Raven Press; 1992:565–598.
16. Berenstein A, Lasjaunias P. *Surgical Neuroangiography, Vol 5: Endovascular Treatment of Spine and Spinal Cord Lesions.* Berlin–Heidelberg–New York: Springer-Verlag; 1992:1–109.
17. Oldfield E, DiChiro G, Quindlen E, Reith E, Doppman J. Successful treatment of a group of spinal cord arteriovenous malformations by interruption of dural fistula. *J Neurosurg* 1983;59:1019–1030.
18. Doppman J, DiChiro G, Oldfield E. Origin of spinal arteriovenous

malformation and normal cord vasculature from a commonsegmental artery: angiographic and therapeutic considerations. *Radiology* 1985;154:687–689.

19. Foix C, Alajouanine T. La myélite nécortique subaigue. Myelite centrale angio-hypertrophique à evolution progressive. Paraplégie amyotrophique lentement ascendante, d'abord spasmodique, puis flasque, s'accompagnant de dissociation albumino-cytologique. *Rev Neurol* 1926;33:1–42.
20. Burger PC, Scheithauer BW. Vascular tumors and tumor-like lesions. In: Burger PC, Scheithauer BW, eds. *Tumors of the Central Nervous System.* Washington, DC: Armed Forces Institute of Pathology; 1994:287–299.
21. Hassler W, Thron A, Grote E. Hemodynamics of spinal dural arteriovenous fistulas. *J Neurosurg* 1989;70:360–370.
22. Kendall B. Spinal angiography with Iohexol. *Neuroradiology* 1986;28:72–73.
23. Djindjian M, Djindjian R, Hurth R, Houdart R. Intradural extramedullary spinal arterio-venous malformations fed by the anterior spinal artery. *Surg Neurol* 1977;8:85–93.
24. Rosenblum B, Oldfield E, Doppman J, DiChiro G. Spinal arteriovenous malformations: a comparison of dural arteriovenous fistulas and intradural AVM's in 81 patients. *J Neurosurg* 1987;67:795–802.
25. Symon L, Kuyama H, Kendall B. Dural arteriovenous malformations of the spine. Clinical features and surgical results in 55 cases. *J Neurosurg* 1984;60:238–247.
26. Zervas N, Greenberg S, Hedley-White T, Pile-Spellman J. Case records of the Massachusettes General Hospital. *N Engl J Med* 1992;326:816–824.
27. Aminoff M, Gutin P, Norman D. Unusual type of spinal arteriovenous malformation. *Neurosurgery* 1988;22:589–591.
28. Criscuolo G, Oldfield E, Doppman J. Reversible acute and subacute myelopathy in patients with dural arteriovenous fistulas. *J Neurosurg* 1989;70:354–359.
29. Muraszko K, Oldfield E. Vascular malformations of the spinal cord and dura. *Neurosurg Clin North Am* 1990;1:631–652.
30. Adams R, Salam-Adams M. Chronic nontraumatic diseases of the spinal cord. *Neurol Clin* 1991;9:605–623.
31. Isu T, Iwasaki Y, Akino M, Koyanagi I, Abe H. Magnetic resonance imaging in cases of spinal dural arteriovenous fistula. *Neurosurgery* 1989;24:919–923.
32. Larsson E, Desai P, Hardin C, Story J, Jinkins J. Venous infarction of the spinal cord resulting from dural arteriovenous fistula: MR imaging findings. *AJNR* 1991;12:739–743.
33. Masaryk T, Ross J, Modic M, Ruff R, Selman W, Ratcheson R. Radiculomeningeal vascular malformations of the spine: MR imaging. *Radiology* 1987;164:845–849.
34. Wrobel C, Oldfield E, DiChiro G, Tarlov E, Baker R, Doppman J. Myelopathy due to dural arteriovenous fistulas draining intrathecally into spinal medullary veins. *J Neurosurg* 1988;69:934–939.
35. Dickman C, Zabramski J, Sonntag V, Coons S. Myelopathy due to epidural varicose veins of the cervicothoracic junction. *J Neurosurg* 1988;69:940–941.
36. Partington M, Rufenacht D, Marsh W, Piepgras D. Cranial and sacral dural arteriovenous fistulas as a cause of myelopathy. *J Neurosurg* 1992;76:615–622.
37. Hall W, Oldfield E, Doppman J. Recanalization of spinal arteriovenous malformations following embolization. *J Neurosurg* 1989;70:714–720.
38. Morgan M, Marsh W. Management of spinal dural arteriovenous malformations. *J Neurosurg* 1989;70:832–836.
39. Biondi A, Merland J, Hodes J, Pruvo J, Reizine D. Aneurysms of the spinal arteries associated with intramedullary arteriovenous malformations. I. Angiographic and clinical aspects. *AJNR* 1992;13:912–923.
40. Biondi A, Merland J, Hodes J, Aymard A, Reizine D. Aneurysms of the spinal arteries associated with intramedullary arteriovenous malformations. II. Results of AVM endovascular treatment and hemodynamic considerations. *AJNR* 1992;13:923–933.
41. Aminoff M, Logue V. The prognosis of patients with spinal vascular malformations. *Brain* 1974;97:211–218.
42. Casasco A, Houdart E, Gobin Y, Aymard A, Guichard J, Rufenacht D. Embolization of spinal vascular malformations. *Neuroimag Clin* 1992;2:337–358.
43. Jessen R, Thompson S, Smith E. Cobb syndrome. *Arch Dermatol* 1977;113:1587–1590.
44. Miyatake S, Kikuchi H, Koide T, et al. Cobb's syndrome and its treatment with embolization. *J Neurosurg* 1990;72:497–499.
45. Oldfield E, Doppman J. Spinal arteriovenous malformations. *Clin Neurosurg* 1979;26:543.
46. Spetzler R, Zabramski J, Flom R. Management of juvenile spinal AVM's by embolization and operative excision. *J Neurosurg* 1989;70:628–632.
47. Tuoho H, Karasawa J, Shishido H, Yamada K, Shibamoto K. Successful excision of a juvenile type spinal arteriovenous malformation following intraoperative embolization. *J Neurosurg* 1991;75:647–651.
48. Heros R, Debrun G, Ojiemann R, Lasjaunias P, Naessens P. Direct spinal arteriovenous fistula: a new type of spinal AVM. *J Neurosurg* 1986;64:134–139.
49. Golwyn D, Cardenas C, Murtagh F, Balis G, Klein J. MRI of a cervical extradural cavernous hemangioma. *Neuroradiology* 1992;34:68–69.
50. Enomoto H, Goto H. Spinal epidural cavernous angioma. *Neuroradiology* 1991;33:462–465.
51. Ramos F, de Toffol B, Aesch B, et al. Hydrocephalus and cavernoma of the cauda equina. *Neurosurgery* 1990;27:139–142.
52. Lee K, Spetzler R. Spinal cord malformation in a patient with familial intracranial cavernous malformations. *Neurosurgery* 1990;26:877–880.
53. Cosgrove R, Bertrand G, Fontaine S, Robitaille Y, Melanson D. Cavernous angiomas of the spinal cord. *J Neurosurg* 1988;68:31–36.
54. Bicknell J, Carlow T, Kornfield M, Stovring J, Turner P. Familial cavernous angiomas. *Arch Neurol* 1978;35:746–749.
55. McCormick P, Michelsen W, Post K, et al. Cavernous malformations of the spinal cord. *Neurosurgery* 1988;23:459–463.
56. McCormick P, Stein B. Spinal cavernous malformations. In: Awad A, Barrow D, eds. *Cavernous Malformations.* Park Ridge, IL: AANS; 1993.
57. Ogilvy C, Louis D, Ojemann R. Intramedullary cavernous malformations of the spine. *Neurosurgery* 1992;31:219–230.
58. Perl J, Ross J. Diagnostic imaging of cavernous malformations. In: Awad A, Barrow D, eds. *Cavernous Malformations.* Park Ridge, IL: AANS; 1993.
59. Lopate G, Black J, Grubb R. Cavernous hemangioma of the spinal cord: report of 2 unusual cases. *Neurology* 1990;40:1791–1793.
60. Barnwell S, Dowd C, Davis R, Edwards S, Gutin P, Wilson C. Cryptic vascular malformations of the spinal cord: diagnosis by magnetic resonance imaging and outcome of surgery. *J Neurosurg* 1990;72:403–407.
61. Kim S, Kim R, Choi B, et al. Nontraumatic ischemic myelopathy: a review of 25 cases. *Paraplegia* 1988;26.
62. Sandson T, Friedman J. Spinal cord infarction: report of 8 cases and a review of the literature. *Medicine* 1989;68.
63. Blackwood W. Discussion on vascular disease of the spinal cord. *Proc R Soc Med* 1958;51:543.
64. Spiller W. Thrombosis of the cervical median anterior spinal artery. *J Nerv Ment Dis* 1909;36:601.
65. Crawford E, Crawford J, et al. Thoracoabdominal aortic aneurysms: preoperative and intraoperative factors determining immediate and long term results of operation in 605 patients. *J Vasc Surg* 1986;3:389.
66. Brewer L, Fosburg R, Mulder G. Spinal cord complications following surgery for coarctation of the aorta. *J Thorac Cardiovasc Surg* 1972;64:368.
67. Costello T, Fisher A. Neurologic complications following aortic surgery. *Anaesthesia* 1983;38:230.
68. Forbes G, Nichols D, Jack C, et al. Complications of spinal cord arteriography: prospective assessment of risk for diagnostic procedures. *Radiology* 1988;169:479–484.
69. Hankey G, Warlow C, Sellar R. Cerebral angiographic risk in mild cerebrovascular disease. *Stroke* 1990;21:209–222.
70. Slavin R, Gonzalez-Vitale J, Marin O. Atheromatous emboli to the lumbosacral spinal cord. *Stroke* 1975;6:411.
71. Henson R, Persons M. Ischemic lesions to the spinal cord: an illustrated review. *Q J Med* 1967;36:205.

72. Kim S, Kim R, Choi B. Nontraumatic ischemic myelopathy: a review of 25 cases. *Paraplegia* 1988;26:262–268.
73. Hasegawa M, Yamashita J, Yamashima T, Kiyonobu I, Fujishima Y, Yamazaki M. Spinal cord infarction associated with primary antiphospholipid syndrome in a young child. *J Neurosurg* 1993;79:446–450.
74. Satran R. Spinal cord infarction. *Stroke* 1988;19:529–532.
75. Yuh W, Marsh E, Wang A, et al. MR imaging of spinal cord and vertebral body infarction. *AJNR* 1992;13:145–154.
76. Mawad M, Rivera V, Crawford S, Ramirez A, Breitbach W. Spinal cord ischemia after resection of thoracoabdominal aortic aneurysms: MR findings in 24 patients. *AJNR* 1990;11:987–991.
77. Elksnis S, Hogg J, Cunningham M. MR imaging of spontaneous cord infarction. *J Comput Assist Tomogr* 1991;15:228–232.
78. Vandertop W, Elderson A, Van Gijn J. Anterior spinal artery syndrome. *AJNR* 1991;12:505–506.
79. Friedman D, Flanders A. Enhancement of gray matter in anterior spinal artery infarction. *AJNR* 1992;13:983–985.
80. Ueda S, Saito A, Inomori S, Kim I. Cavernous angioma of the cauda equina producing subarachnoid hemorrhage. *J Neurosurg* 1987;66:134–136.
81. Constantini S, Ashkenazi E, Shoshan Y, Israel Z, Umansky F. Thoracic hematomyelia secondary to coumadin anticoagulant therapy: a case report. *Eur Neurol* 1992;32:109–111.
82. Nemoto Y, Inoue Y, Tashiro T, et al. Intramedullary spinal cord tumors: significance of associated hemorrhage at MR imaging. *Radiology* 1992;182:793–796.

Magnetic Resonance Imaging of the Brain and Spine, Second Edition, edited by Scott W. Atlas.
Lippincott-Raven Publishers, Philadelphia © 1996.

29

Fast Imaging

Principles, Techniques, and Clinical Applications

Felix W. Wehrli and Scott W. Atlas

In the early days of clinical magnetic resonance (MR) imaging, critics pointed out that MR was, and probably would remain, an intrinsically slow technique. The alleged reason for the intrinsic slowness was the acquisition rate limitation imposed by the spin-lattice relaxation times, T_1. In biological tissues, T_1 is typically on the order of hundreds of milliseconds, or even seconds (1). This, it was often contended (in spite of evidence to the contrary), would be a major physical barrier to reaching scan speeds anywhere comparable to those in computed tomography (CT). Indeed, without the advent of multiple-slice imaging (2), which somewhat mitigates the problem by making effective use of the "dead time" following data acquisition for excitation of neighboring slices, MR would probably not be clinically practical. Nevertheless, even under the best of circumstances, minimal scan times with conventional imaging remain on the order of several minutes.

The major driving forces for scan time reduction are twofold: economics (throughput) and patient comfort (for image optimization). MR is the most expensive clinical imaging modality to date. With the break-even point, depending on system and siting cost, currently ranging between 5 and 10 studies per day, the number of studies that can be performed per unit time critically affects operational economics. In a typical clinical imaging setting, the number of brain studies performed currently ranges anywhere from 1 to 3 per hour, with a significant fraction of the total study time still being scan time.

With the refinement and clinical investigation of rapid imaging techniques, it has become quite evident that speed enhancement for throughput and patient comfort is not the only basis for the utilization of these scanning techniques. Contrast characteristics of rapid scan techniques are very different from conventional spin-echo images (Fig. 1), which, when exploited, have permitted a marked increase in sensitivity for delineating certain

F. W. Wehrli, Ph.D.: Department of Radiology, Hospital of the University of Pennsylvania, Philadelphia, PA 19104.
S. W. Atlas, M.D.: Neuroradiology Division, Department of Radiology, Oregon Health Sciences University, Portland, OR 97201.

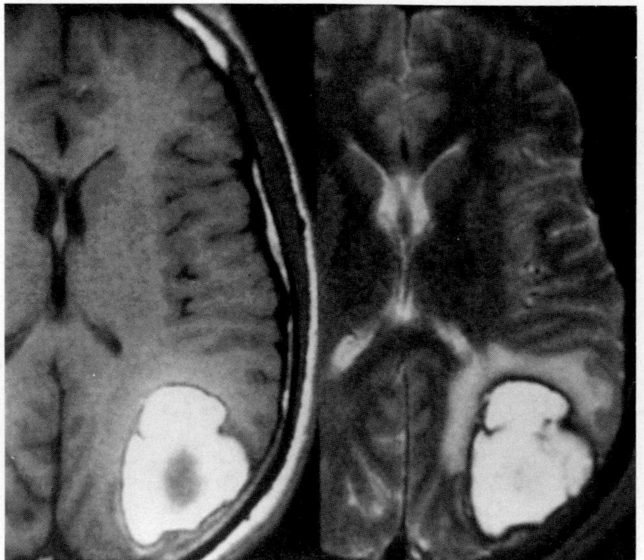

A,B

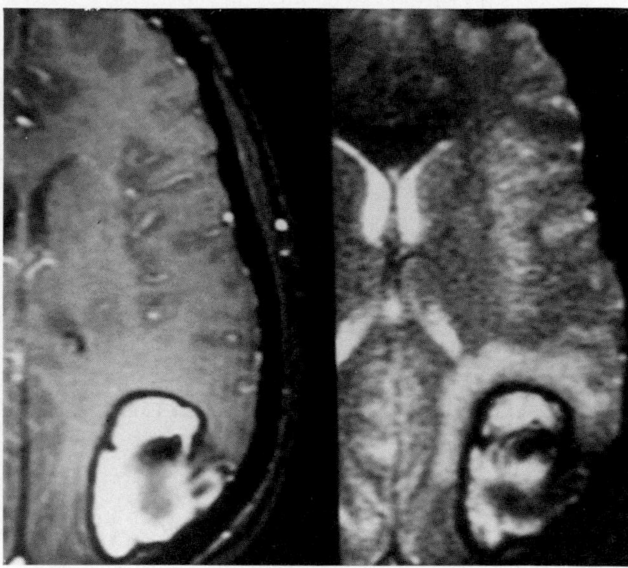

C,D

FIG. 1. Spin-echo vs. gradient-echo images, intracerebral hematoma. **A:** Conventional short TR/TE spin-echo image. **B:** Conventional long TR/TE spin-echo image. **C:** Relatively "T1-weighted" gradient-echo image (large flip angle, short TE). **D:** Relatively "T2*-weighted" gradient-echo image (small flip angle, long TE). Relatively T2*-weighted gradient-echo image (small flip angle, long TE). Gradient-echo images can be acquired to reflect contrast characteristics similar to their spin-echo counterparts, depending on specific parameters used for scanning. Although this left parietal hematoma looks similar on spin-echo images (A,B) and gradient-echo images (C,D), several differences are noted: the rim of hypointensity around the hematoma and the central hypointensity are more prominent on the gradient-echo images (C,D), and normal vessels are high intensity (C), rather than signal void (A).

pathologic conditions. In fact, rapid scan techniques have expanded the scope of possible applications into areas previously hidden from macroscopic imaging modalities. As of the writing of this text, technologies permitting shortening of MR scan times to a small fraction of a second are becoming clinically available, therefore virtually freezing physiologic motion. As these new methods evolve without excessive loss of spatial resolution and signal-to-noise compared to conventional images, MR will become an effective and elegant method of investigating physiology and function in a wide variety of areas.

Gradient-echo images can be acquired to reflect similar contrast characteristics to their spin-echo counterparts, depending on specific parameters used for scanning. Although this left parietal hematoma in Fig. 1 looks similar on spin-echo (Fig. 1A and B) and gradient-echo images (Fig. 1C and D), several differences are noted: the rim of hypointensity around the hematoma and the central hypointensity are more prominent on the gradient-echo images (C and D), and normal vessels are high intensity (C), rather than signal void (A).

BASIC PRINCIPLES OF DATA ACQUISITION AND RECONSTRUCTION

Spatial Frequency Domain

A common misconception among newcomers to MR is the notion that an image is obtained by sampling the signal emanating from the object consecutively, location by location, which then afford the individual pixel intensity values. Damadian and coworkers (3) supposedly produced images by moving the subject through a hot spot of the magnet (where the field was homogeneous) in small increments, each time recording the signal, and thus producing a pixel intensity value. Hinshaw's sensitive-point method (4), using a more elaborate approach, likewise was based on sampling the object point by point. It is easy to recognize that sensitive-point techniques are inherently inefficient since, at a given time, signal from a single location only is sampled. In all modern imaging techniques such as spin-warp imaging and its derivatives, signal is received with each data sample, from the entire imaging volume (i.e., a slice or slab of tissue). Hence, it is clear that each data sample carries information pertaining to all pixels in the image. It thus becomes obvious that we acquire data in a different domain and the question merely is how the two domains relate to one another. In other words, how do we obtain the image from the 'raw data' (spatial frequency or *k*-space domain data)? At this stage, we may rightfully ask in what way an understanding of *k*-space could further our understanding of rapid MR imaging techniques. It turns out that the *k*-space concept, described by Ljunggren (5) and Twieg (6) is an elegant and almost universally applicable way of describing the data sampling process. Further, knowledge of the basic properties of *k*-space is mandatory for understanding many of the features of such techniques as magnetization-prepared

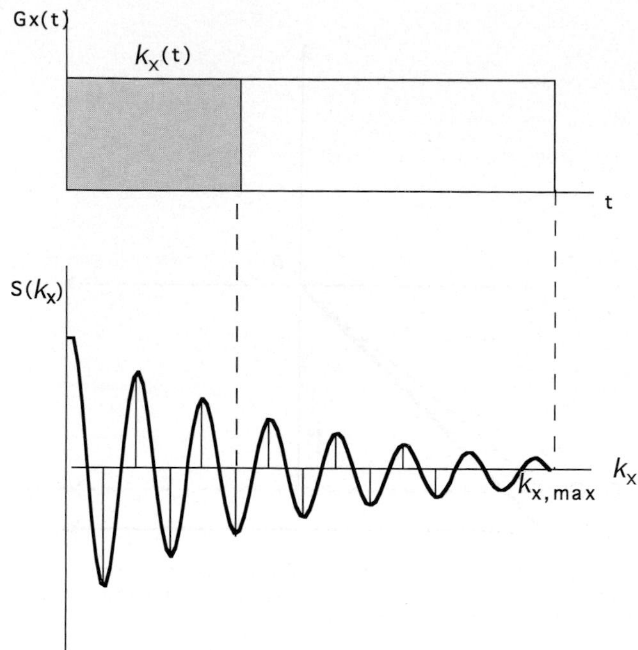

FIG. 2. The *k*-coordinate is determined by the area under the amplitude-time curve of the magnetic field gradient (*top*). The *k*-space signal arising from a single spin location is a damped cosine (*bottom*).

gradient-echo imaging, or the multi-line scanning techniques including gradient and spin-echo planar imaging, discussed later in this chapter.

The spatial frequency coordinate k expresses the phase advance of the transverse magnetization per unit length of an object when the spins are exposed to a gradient field of some amplitude G and duration t. The gradient can be the frequency-encoding gradient G_x or the phase-encoding gradient G_y or, more generally, any of the spatial-encoding gradients. In two-dimensional imaging (be this spin-warp, echo-planar, projection-reconstruction, or spiral scanning) we distinguish between the spatial frequency components k_x and k_y, defined as

$$k_x = \gamma G_x t \qquad [1a]$$

$$k_y = \gamma G_y t \qquad [1b]$$

In Equation 1 it is assumed that the gradient is constant in time, otherwise, the products have to be replaced by time integrals. If we express the gyromagnetic ratio in Hertz/Gauss (Hz/G) and the gradient strength in Gauss/centimeter (G/cm) we see that k has units of cycles/cm. Let us illustrate this concept with signal recorded from a point object at location x (e.g., a phantom one pixel wide). The phase of the transverse magnetization is given as the product $k_x \times$ x and the oscillating MR signal can be written as

$$S(k_x) = \rho(x) \cos(2\pi k_x x) \exp(-t/T_2) \qquad [2]$$

where ρ(x) is the (T1-weighted) spin density at location x and the exponential results from T2 decay. This situation is illustrated in Fig. 2. The spatial frequency at some time t is given by the area under the amplitude-time curve and thus increases from left to right. The signal is sampled at regular intervals $\Delta k_x = \gamma G_x \Delta t$ (vertical lines in bottom of Fig. 2). We shall come back later to the specific requirements for sampling. From Equation 2 we see that the k-space signal clearly contains information on the location of the spins. However, in order to determine ρ(x) a Fourier transformation has to be performed. In this simple case the Fourier transform can be done by inspection in that the location x from which the signal arises is given by the period of the oscillation.

In a more realistic situation, of course, the distribution of spin density is a continuum and the signal is a complicated sum of sinusoids which has to be unraveled in some fashion. Further, the distribution is two-dimensional and thus the spatial frequency is a vector with components k_x and k_y (Fig. 3). Also, when sampling an echo rather than an FID, sampling occurs from $-k_{max}$ to $+k_{max}$, i.e., the spatial frequency can be positive and negative.

We can scan $k_x k_y$ space in various ways. The most common sampling scheme is rectilinear whereby gradients G_x and G_y are alternately switched on. In this manner k-space is filled line by line with each step of the phase-encoding gradient advancing each k_x line by an increment Δk_y. Figure 4A shows the most fundamental spin-warp pulse sequence which samples k-space in this manner. We can easily determine the k-space location at each time point during execution of the pulse sequence, simply by taking the area under the x and y gradient at that particular time.

From Fig. 4 we see that the gradient amplitude G_x of what is commonly denoted the "frequency-encoding"

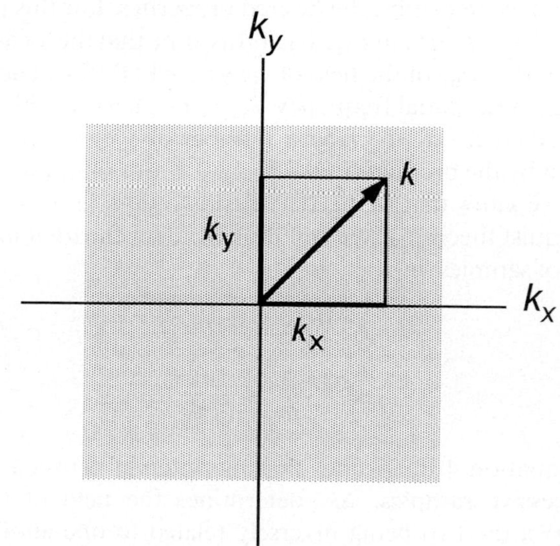

FIG. 3. In 2DFT imaging k-space is a vector whose individual components k_x and k_y represent the spatial frequencies.

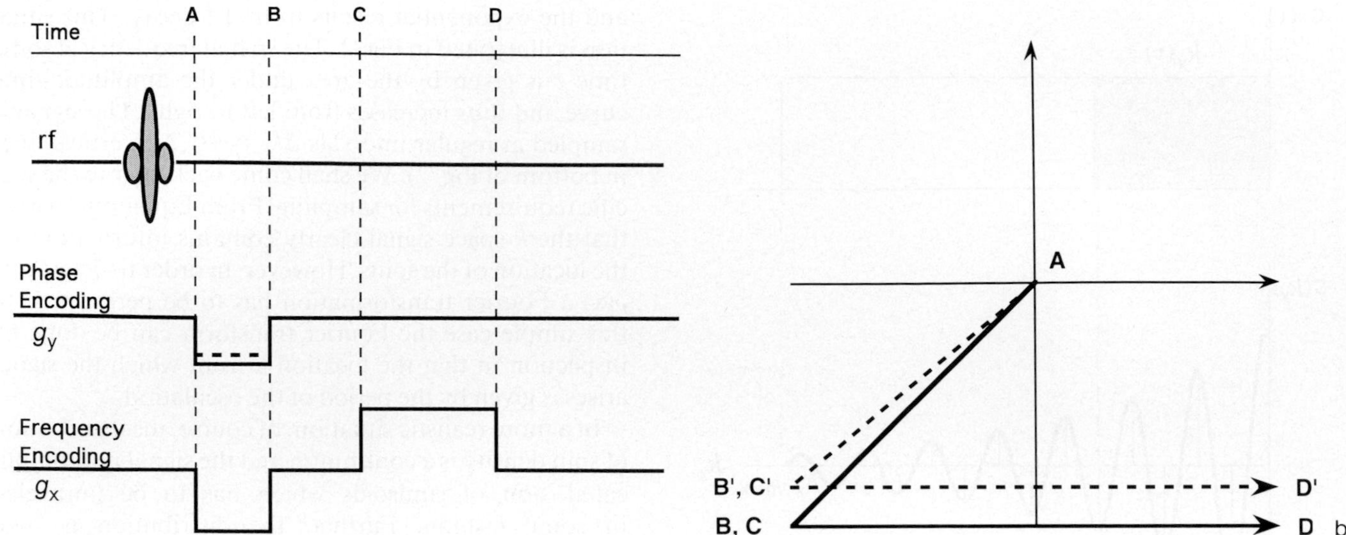

FIG. 4. Spin-warp pulse sequence (**a**) and resulting *k*-space trajectories (**b**). The time points in A correspond to the respective *k*-space locations in B. Incrementing the phase-encoding gradient (*dotted line*, A) leads to the trajectory AB′C′D′. This process is repeated N_p times, where N_p represents the number of phase encodings.

gradient, is held constant and the gradient duration is varied, whereas for phase-encoding, the duration is constant and the gradient amplitude G_y is varied. There is thus a considerable disparity in sampling time in the two spatial directions. Whereas sampling of a k_x line takes on the order of milliseconds, sampling along the phase-encoding axis is much slower, with the time interval between successive sampling points being on the order of a repetition time (TR) period. However, from the acquired *k*-space data it is no longer evident in what manner sampling had occurred. This is an important statement which conveys that it is ultimately irrelevant how a *k*-space sample S (k_{xi}, k_{xj}) was obtained.

We shall now inquire about how densely *k*-space has to be sampled and how far we have to scan in order for the image to exhibit the desired properties. For this purpose, let us return to Fig. 4A and assume that the location x is at the edge of the field of view (x = FOV/2), hence at the highest spatial frequency, k_{max}, the phase for this signal advances by the largest number of cycles, which is given by the product (FOV/2)·k_{max}. From sampling theory we know that we need at least two samples per cycle (Nyquist theorem). We can thus write for the total number of samples, n:

$$\mathrm{FOV} \cdot k_{max} = n \qquad [3]$$

$$\Delta k = \frac{k_{max}}{n} = \frac{1}{\mathrm{FOV}} \qquad [4]$$

Equation 4 thus states that the interval between two successive samples, Δk, determines the field of view (FOV), the two being inversely related to one another. Equation 4 is equally valid for k_x and k_y, i.e., for phase and frequency encoding.

Let us now examine the implications of Equation 4 in some more detail. For example, removing every other line would not lower spatial resolution, instead it would halve the FOV along that coordinate. On the other hand, doubling the size of *k*-space in both directions (by doubling the number of samples), would leave the FOV intact while increasing resolution by a factor of two in both dimensions. This brings us to a second important statement, i.e., the relationship between pixel size Δx, Δy, and *k*-space size, expressed in terms of the maximum spatial frequencies sampled in the two directions:

$$\Delta x, \Delta y = \frac{1}{k_{x,max}} \frac{1}{k_{y,max}} \qquad [5]$$

The relationship among spatial resolution, field of view, and their *k*-space counterparts is illustrated in Fig. 5.

The signal-to-noise ratio (SNR) is also related to *k*-space size, in that the noise is proportional to the square root of the *k*-space area. The following is also helpful to remember: since *k*-space and image data are the Fourier inverses of one another, each *k*-space sample contributes to the entire image. However, it is the central portions that contribute most to SNR (and therefore contrast) whereas the periphery contributes mainly to spatial resolution. The former can be conceptually understood on the basis of the circumstance that for the central rows and columns the spins have maximum phase coherence (frequency-encoding: near center of echo; phase-encoding: low amplitude of phase-encoding gradient).

Removal of high spatial frequencies thus leads to progressive image blurring. This phenomenon is illustrated with *k*-space data in Fig. 5E which was low-pass filtered by first halving k_{max} and reducing it to one quarter its

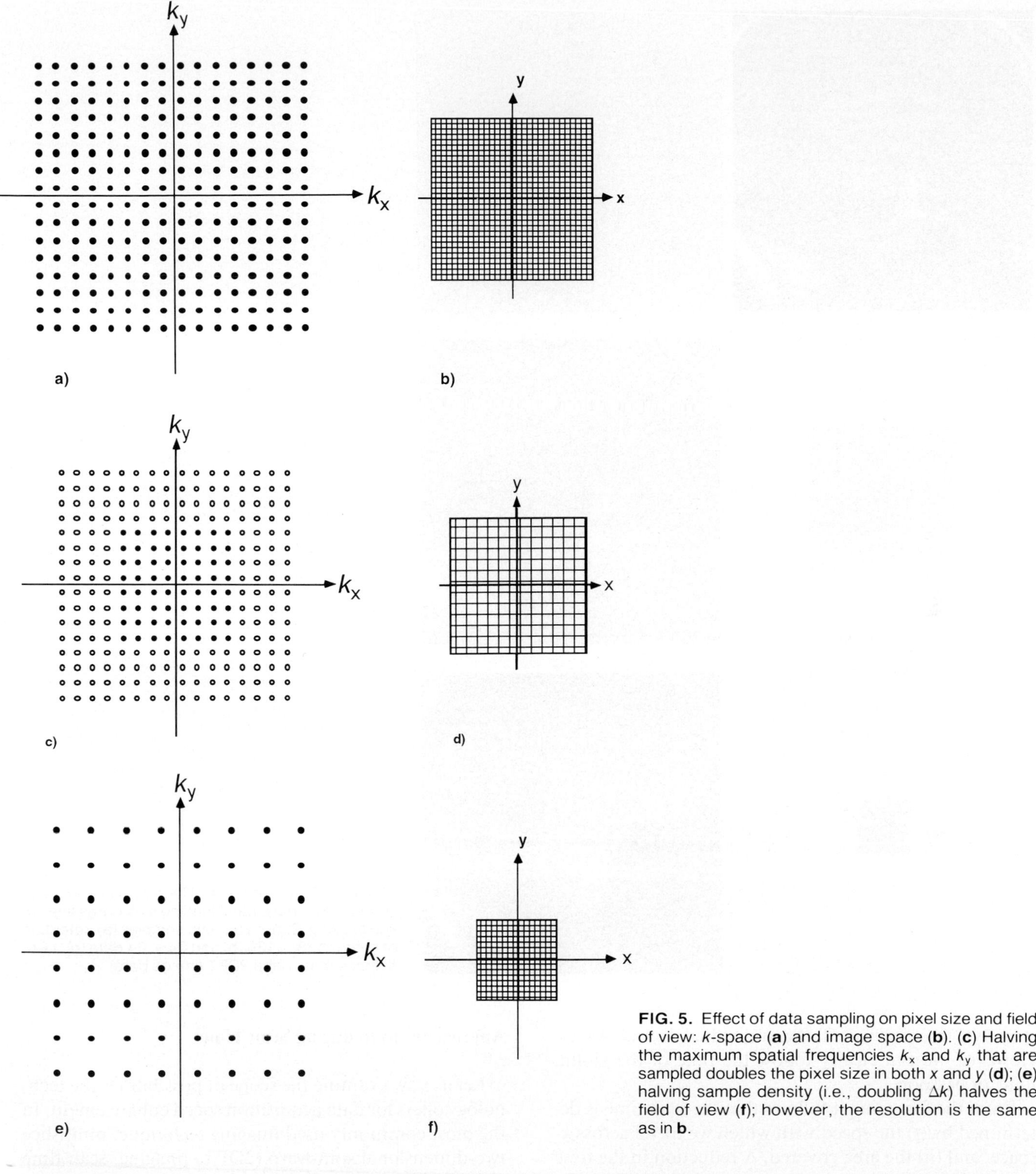

FIG. 5. Effect of data sampling on pixel size and field of view: k-space (**a**) and image space (**b**). (**c**) Halving the maximum spatial frequencies k_x and k_y that are sampled doubles the pixel size in both x and y (**d**); (**e**) halving sample density (i.e., doubling Δk) halves the field of view (**f**); however, the resolution is the same as in **b**.

original value in both the phase and frequency-encoding directions (equivalent to reducing k-space area by a factor of 4 and 16, respectively). One notices that the loss of high spatial frequency information affects mainly small structures such as the cerebral aqueduct, or the infundibulum, whereas larger structures such as the brainstem or the corpus callosum are little affected.

It is obvious from the k-space maps of Fig. 6 that this data format is not intelligible to the eye, i.e., our brain is not capable of performing a Fourier transformation of optical data into their co-domain. By contrast, our ear is an almost perfect Fourier analyzer. Listening to an orchestra concert, we hear the composite sound of the many instruments resulting from constructive and de-

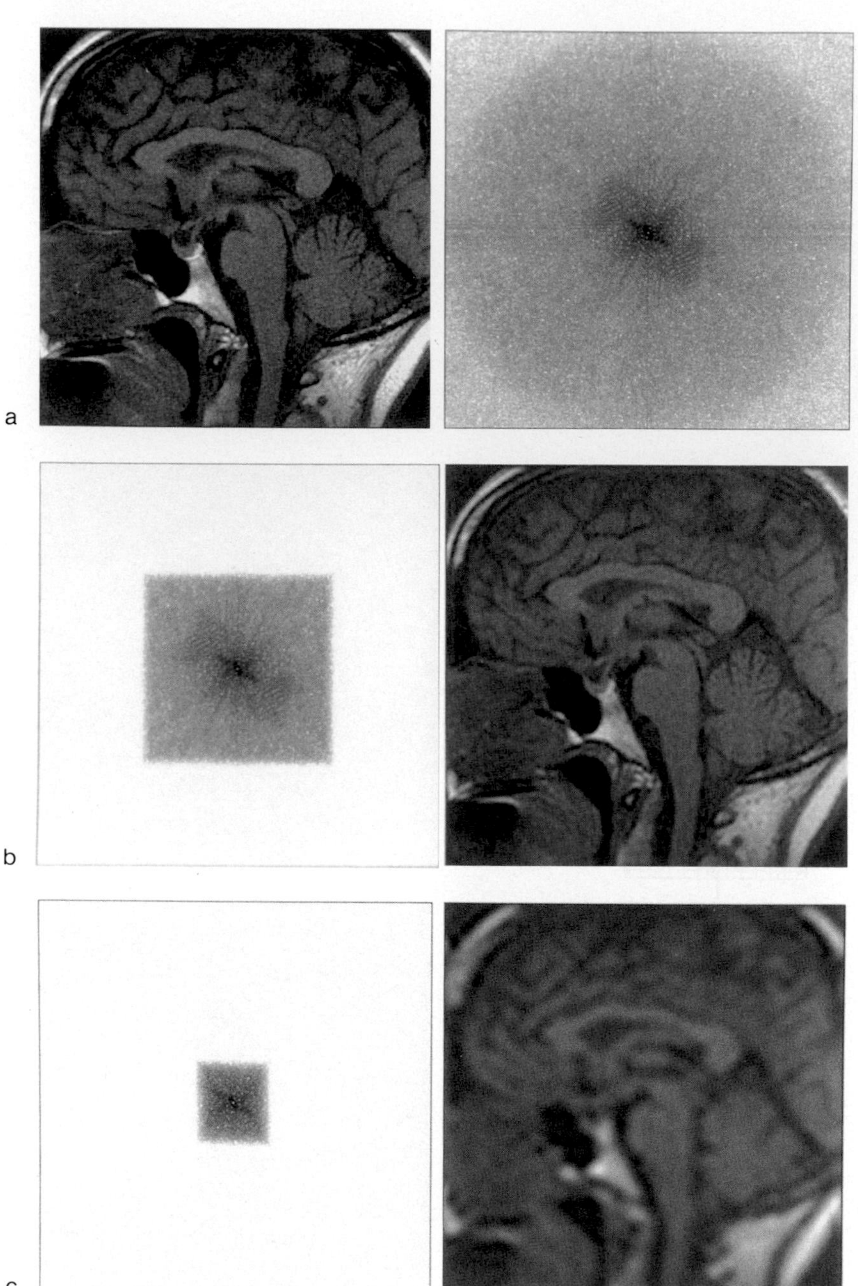

FIG. 6. Effect of removal of high spatial frequency content in *k*-space data, leading to progressive image blurring: 256 × 256 data samples (**a**); retention of center 128 × 128 (**b**) and 64 × 64 data (**c**). Left: *k*-space map, right: 2DFT (image data).

structive interference of the individual sound waves. However, we can clearly follow the tune of the violin, flute, or bassoon.

From the foregoing it follows that the scan time is determined by (i) the speed with which we travel across *k*-space, and (ii) the area covered. A reduction in the time interval between successive samples (increase in sampling rate), or a reduction in the number of data samples (reduction in FOV or pixel size) are most often invoked to reduce scan time. The latter shows that temporal and spatial resolution are often traded against one another. The third trade-off parameter is the signal-to-noise ratio (SNR) which scales as the square root of the number of data samples and inversely with voxel size.

Approaches to Reducing Scan Time

Let us now examine the scope of possibilities the technology offers for data acquisition speed enhancement. In the most commonly used imaging technique, multislice two-dimensional spin-warp (2DFT) imaging, scan time T_s is given by the following simple relationship:

$$T_s = N_y \cdot \text{TR} \cdot \text{NEX} \qquad [6]$$

where N_y is the number of phase-encoding samples, TR the pulse repetition time, and NEX the number of excitations (also termed number of acquisitions or number of averages), used for signal averaging.

The first approach that comes to mind for reducing

scan time is to minimize signal averaging, expressed in terms of the number of excitations. The obvious limit is reached once NEX = 1. Of course, as usual, we trade signal-to-noise for a reduction in scan time. It is therefore the intrinsic SNR that governs the extent to which we can reduce scan time.

Since scan time is also linearly related to the number of phase encodings, we may want to shorten data acquisition time by reducing the number of samples in the phase-encoding direction. Indeed, this is the most commonly used way of reducing scan time in conventional spin-echo imaging. Hence, often the acquisition matrix chosen is asymmetric, with fewer phase-encoding than frequency-encoding samples being collected. While the usual number of frequency encodings is 256, the number of phase-encoding samples is more often 128 or 192. Prior to Fourier transformation, the data matrix is complemented by filling in zeros for the missing views (*zero filling*). The trade-off parameter, in this case, is spatial resolution, since SNR increases as $(N_y/256)^{1/2}$ where N_y is the reduced number of phase encodings. Therefore, a 128×256 acquisition, while cutting scan time in half, also increases SNR by $\sqrt{2}$ (40%).

Partial Fourier Imaging

An elegant idea for reducing scan time exploits the symmetry of the raw data. An examination of the k-space data shows that it has *conjugate* symmetry, i.e., matrix elements k_{ij} and k_{ji} are complex conjugates ($k_{ij} = k^*_{ji}$). Therefore, instead of sampling the entire k-space, a fraction thereof can be sampled and the remainder filled in retrospectively (7,8).

It turns out that the data are conjugate only if the "real" component of the transverse magnetization is the sole contributor to the signal. This presupposes that the phase is zero at all spatial locations. In practice, spurious phase shifts occur due to a variety of reasons, including spatial nonuniformities of the magnetic field originating from imperfections in the main magnetic field or radiofrequency (rf) attenuation effects. The problem can be solved by phasing the data (9). For this purpose, slightly more than half of the k-space needs to be sampled. This technique has been termed *half-NEX imaging*, but a more appropriate term perhaps is *half Fourier imaging*. Since SNR is proportional to the square root of the total sampling time, which is halved when only half of k-space is sampled, images acquired with this technique will be penalized by a factor of $1/\sqrt{2}$ in SNR.

Gradient-Echo Imaging

The archetype of scanning techniques which shorten acquisition times is one known as *gradient-echo imaging*, a generic term which appropriately has come to represent an entire family of pulse sequences. The variety of different sequences encompassed by this title generally share two major features, which distinguish gradient-echo scanning from the more traditional counterpart of spin-echo imaging: (i) the radiofrequency (rf) excitation pulse, or flip angle, is operator-selectable, and in practice is generally less than the 90° pulse of the spin-echo sequence, and (ii) signal is acquired by virtue of reversal of the readout (frequency-encoding) gradient in the absence of the 180° refocusing rf pulse of spin-echo scanning. These two features, although quite straightforward, have profound implications with regard to image contrast and specific image characteristics found in gradient-echo images.

Reduction of Pulse Flip Angle

Since the sampling process in the phase-encoding direction is at least two orders of magnitude slower than in the frequency-encoding direction, speeding up the former promises the biggest return in terms of scan time shortening. The sampling interval in the phase-encoding direction is the product (NEX·TR). From a contrast point of view, however, shortening of TR would seem to be an undesirable approach. In addition, in multislice 2DFT imaging, it would also substantially reduce the number of sections that can be imaged.

In spin-echo imaging, the entire longitudinal magnetization at the end of the TR period is converted to transverse magnetization by means of a 90° pulse. Longitudinal magnetization then builds up in a recurrent fashion, while transverse magnetization usually decays between successive rf pulses (see Chapter 2). As TR is reduced, so is the available longitudinal magnetization, which recovers as $[1 - \exp(-TR/T_1)]$. Hence, as we shorten TR, we proceed to progressive saturation and eventual signal suppression.

One way around this problem is to operate in a regime of reduced pulse flip angles (10). In lieu of a 90° pulse, which converts the entire longitudinal magnetization to transverse magnetization, only a fraction is made transverse when using limited flip angles. Lowering the flip angle is achieved by means of either reducing the power of the B_1 field or by shortening its duration. For a rectangular rf pulse, the flip angle is given as:

$$\alpha = \gamma B_1 \tau \qquad [6a]$$

where γ is the gyromagnetic ratio, B_1 is the amplitude of the rf field (in Gauss), and τ is the pulse duration. Hence, the flip angle (expressed in radians) scales in proportion to the B_1 field amplitude and its duration τ. Since pulses typically are amplitude-modulated for slice selection (e.g., sinc modulated) in such a manner that the amplitude varies while it is played out, Equation 6a has to be modified accordingly:

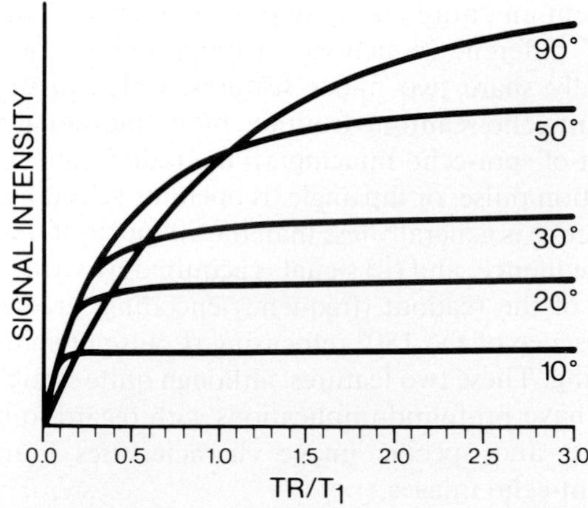

FIG. 7. MR signal as a function of the ratio TR/T_1, assuming a train of equidistant rf pulses of flip angle α and a given number of excitations. Note that, as the flip angle is lowered, the signal optimum is attained for ever smaller values of the TR/T_1 ratio. For example, at a flip angle $\alpha = 10°$ the signal is independent of T_1 at TR/$T_1 \approx 0.5$ whereas for $\alpha = 50°$, TR/$T_1 > 3$ is needed for this condition to be satisfied.

$$\alpha = \gamma \int B_1(t)dt \qquad [6b]$$

i.e., the flip angle is proportional to the integral over time of $B_1(t)$. The resultant signal then is proportional to sin α.

Assuming a train of equidistant rf pulses of flip angle α, the solution of the Bloch equation affords for the transverse magnetization:

$$M_{xy} \sim \frac{1 - \exp(-\mathrm{TR}/\mathrm{T}_1)}{1 - \cos\alpha \exp(-\mathrm{TR}/\mathrm{T}_1)} \sin\alpha \qquad [7]$$

In Fig. 7, the signal predicted by Equation 7 is plotted as a function of the ratio TR/T_1. Note that as α is reduced, the signal becomes independent of T_1, even at very short pulse intervals. Further, the absolute signal at very small TR/T_1 ratio increases as the flip angle is lowered. Hence, lowering the flip angle represents an effective means to control the degree of saturation. Indeed, at a low enough flip angle, T1-independent images

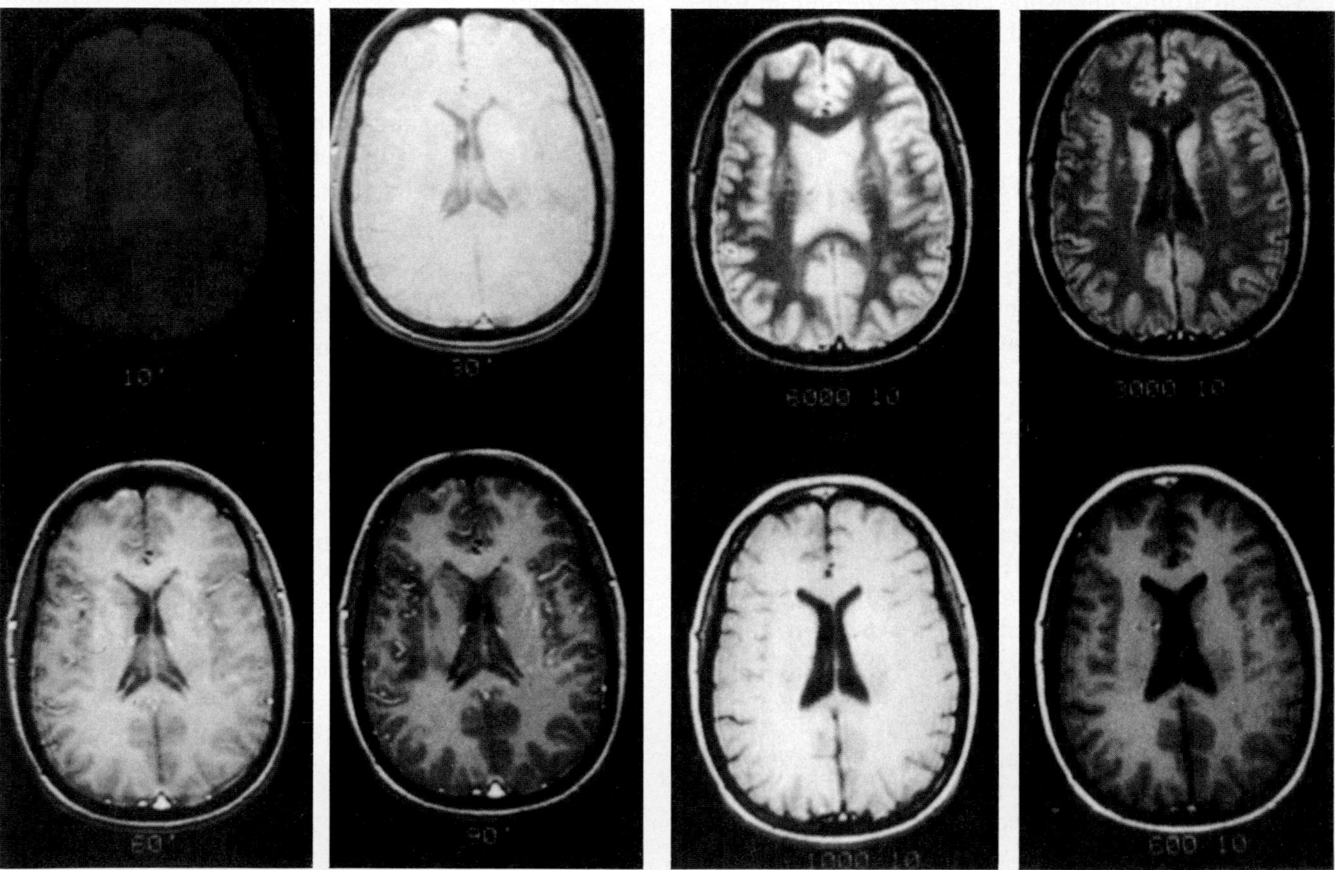

FIG. 8. Effect of flip angle on relative signal intensity in the normal brain. **A:** Gradient-echo images (TR = 200, TE = 5), varying flip angle α from 10° to 90°. **B:** Spin-echo images (TE = 10), varying TR from 6000 to 600 msec. Note that at low flip angle α, the gradient-echo image (A) has the characteristics of proton-density-weighting, with CSF being the high intensity, and white matter being low intensity. At high flip angle, T_1 is the dominant contrast parameter, so CSF has the lowest signal intensity, gray matter is intermediate, and white matter is high intensity (the overall intensity of the 30° image is highest and reflects Ernst angle effects, since all scans were obtained with identical transmit and receive attenuation factors). In an analogous situation, the introduction of T1-based contrast in spin-echo imaging (B) is imparted by virtue of shortening repetition time TR, so that at long TR, contrast is dependent mainly on spin density differences, while at short TR, T_1 differences generate most of the contrast.

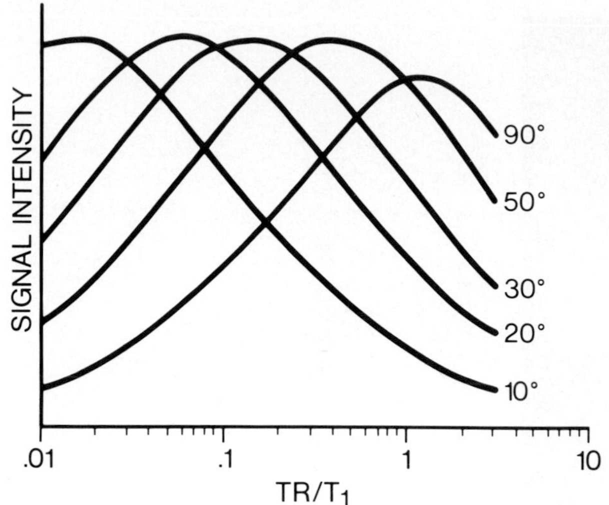

FIG. 9. Signal to noise ratio plotted as a function of the ratio TR/T_1 (assuming constant total scan time (Equation 6a) for various flip angles, showing discrete maxima). Note that the smaller the TR/T_1 ratio (short TR), the lower the flip angle needs to be chosen.

can be acquired for any given TR. It is useful to consider the pulse flip angle in partial flip angle imaging as being the counterpart of TR in conventional spin-echo imaging, in that the degree of T1-based contrast is controlled mainly by the flip angle (Fig. 8).

Another important question concerns the determination of optimum flip angle. Of course, for a fair comparison, we need to hold the total scan time constant (Fig. 9). Hence, as we shorten TR, we can increase the number of excitations (NEX). Since SNR scales as $(NEX)^{1/2}$, we need to multiply Equation 7 with $TR^{-1/2}$:

$$\mathrm{SNR} \sim \mathrm{TR}^{-1/2} \frac{1 - \exp(-\mathrm{TR}/\mathrm{T}_1)}{1 - \cos\alpha \exp(-\mathrm{TR}/\mathrm{T}_1)} \sin\alpha \quad [8]$$

The idea of shortening TR and reducing the rf flip angle has been incorporated into the original spin-warp imaging technique first conceived by Edelstein et al. (11) and by Haase et al. (12) and now forms the basis of what is commonly referred to as *partial flip angle imaging* or *FLASH* (*f*ast *l*ow-*a*ngle *sh*ot). Since this type of imaging uses a gradient echo instead of a spin echo, the term *gradient-echo imaging* is used to denote these sequences.

Gradient Echoes Versus Spin Echoes

In order to overcome the adverse effects of magnetic field inhomogeneity, we would typically utilize a 180° rf pulse and thereby generate a spin echo. Clearly, if instead of a 90° rf excitation pulse, a pulse of much lower flip angle is used ($\alpha \ll 90°$), a Hahn spin echo requiring a 180° pulse is no longer a feasible approach. It becomes apparent that the conventional phase reversal 180° rf pulse would not only generate a spin echo from the transverse magnetization produced by the initial excitation pulse of flip angle α, but it would also invert the residual longitudinal magnetization.

As a substitute for the rf-induced echo (also denoted 'Hahn' echo), the free induction decay signal (FID) is acquired. In order to sample both halves of *k*-space equally, however, we need to place the sampling window symmetrically relative to the echo time TE. Hence, the phase imparted by the readout gradient needs to be balanced, which is achieved by preceding it by a dephasing gradient, such that the spins have zero phase at the center of the sampling window. In partial flip angle imaging, this is achieved by inverting the polarity of the readout gradient. The resultant signal is also denoted as a gradient echo or field echo (11). Figure 10 shows the principle of gradient-echo formation, along with a phase map for spins located at different spatial positions on the frequency-encoding axis.

The echo illustrated in Fig. 10 clearly is not a true spin echo, in that phase shifts imparted by spurious gradients, such as those resulting from magnetic field imperfections, are not corrected. In fact, it is obvious from Fig. 10 that any static gradient superimposed on the readout gradient will cause a phase imbalance, which is not the case for a Hahn echo (13). We, therefore, must conclude that gradient echoes are intrinsically sensitive to all magnetic field inhomogeneities. The delayed readout of the signal causes a reduction in signal intensity relative to that predicted by Equation 8, by a factor $\exp(-TE/T_2^*)$ where T_2^* is the effective transverse relaxation time, i.e.,

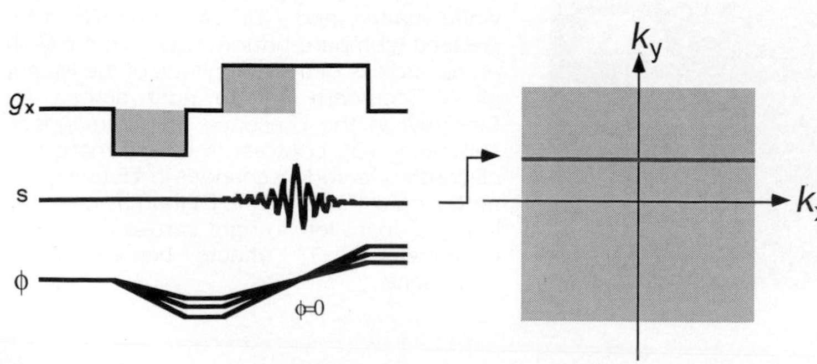

FIG. 10. Principle of gradient-echo formation. By reversing the sign of the readout gradient (G_x) the spins will rephase ($\phi = 0$) at the center of the data collection window (*left*). Note that $k_x = 0$ (echo) demands the two shaded areas of the readout gradient to be equal in magnitude. By sampling both ascending and descending portion of the echo, a full line is sampled from $k_{x,min}$ to $k_{x,max}$ (*right*).

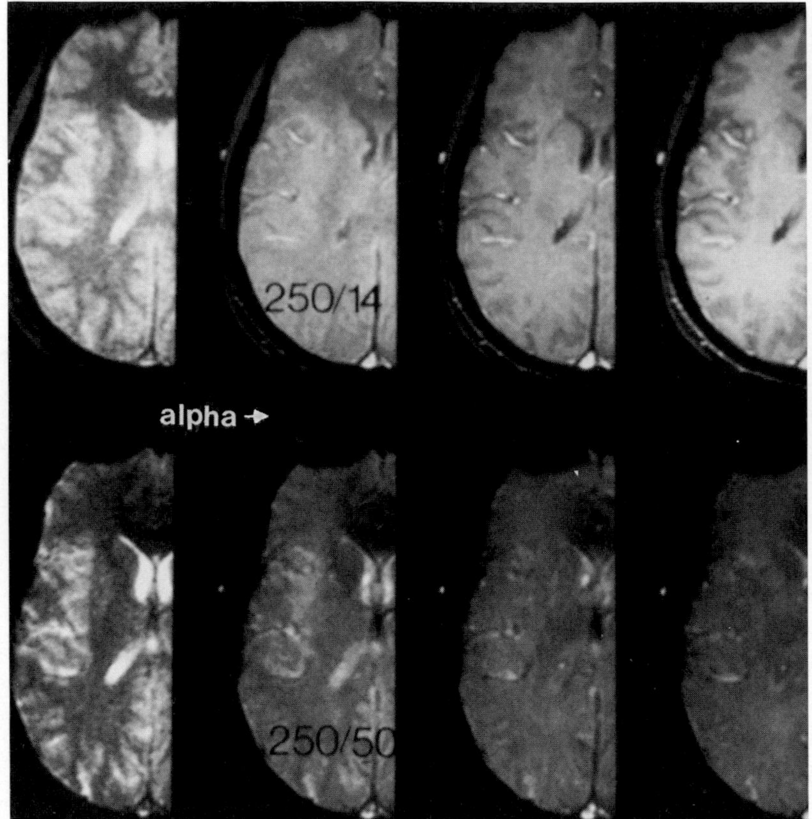

A

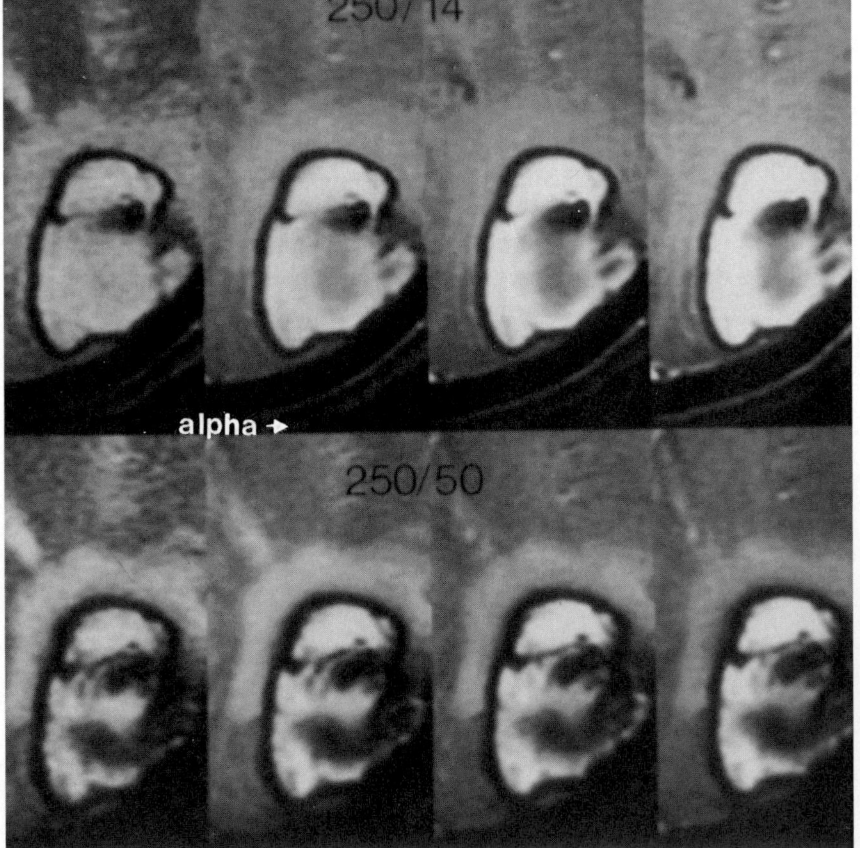

B

FIG. 11. Effect of TE on contrast in gradient-echo imaging. **A:** Normal brain, varying α from 10° to 90°. Top row: short TE (14 msec). Bottom row: long TE (50 msec). **B:** Intraparenchymal hematoma, varying α from 10° to 90°. Top row: short TE (14 msec). Bottom row: long TE (50 msec). Note significant change in contrast relationships between gray matter, white matter, and CSF (A) when TE is increased (compare bottom row to top row in A), regardless of the magnitude of the flip angle α (compare left to right across A). Similarly, in the presence of paramagnetic substance (B), contrast is clearly more significantly affected by changes in TE (compare bottom row to top row in B) than by changes in α (compare left to right across B). As TE is increased, T_2^* effects become more prominent.

the time constant for the decay of the transverse magnetization. On the assumption that no residual transverse magnetization exists at the time of the rf pulse, the gradient-echo signal, therefore, is given as:

$$S \sim M_{xy} \frac{1 - \exp(-TR/T_1)}{1 - \cos\alpha \exp(-TR/T_1)} \sin\alpha \exp(-TE/T_2^*) \quad [9]$$

From Equation 9 we see that by judiciously choosing the echo delay for the gradient-echo, images can be obtained which have contrast based on differences of T_2^* (i.e., T2*-weighted). Figure 11 shows a series of images obtained with various flip angles for both short and long echo delays, showing the effect of increased T2*-weighting as TE increases, regardless of flip angle.

The complete pulse sequence timing diagram for a generic 2DFT gradient-echo imaging pulse sequence is given in Fig. 12. Note that because of the missing 180° rf pulse, this pulse sequence permits, besides a drastic reduction in TR, also shortening of the echo delay TE, to typically less than 10 msec or, when asymmetric sampling is used, TEs of approximately 5 msec. We will see later that operation at short echo delays can be a highly desirable feature, as it minimizes artifacts from magnetic field inhomogeneity.

Contrast Implications of Varying Flip Angle

Let us now explore the effect of varying flip angle at constant pulse repetition time (TR) and echo time (TE) in some more detail. Figure 13A shows gradient-echo images acquired at TR = 300 msec with the flip angle incremented in 10° steps. Note that the image acquired with $\alpha = 10°$ has the characteristics of a proton-density-weighted image, with hyperintense CSF, followed by gray matter and white matter, i.e., contrast follows the established order of the proton densities. However, the image pertaining to a flip angle of 50° has the characteristics of a T1-weighted image, with CSF being the structure of lowest intensity, followed by gray and white matter. The relationship expressed by Equation 7 is shown quantitatively in Fig. 13B in a plot of SNR versus flip angle α for TR = 0.3 sec and T_1 relaxation times corresponding to white matter (WM), gray matter (GM), and CSF.

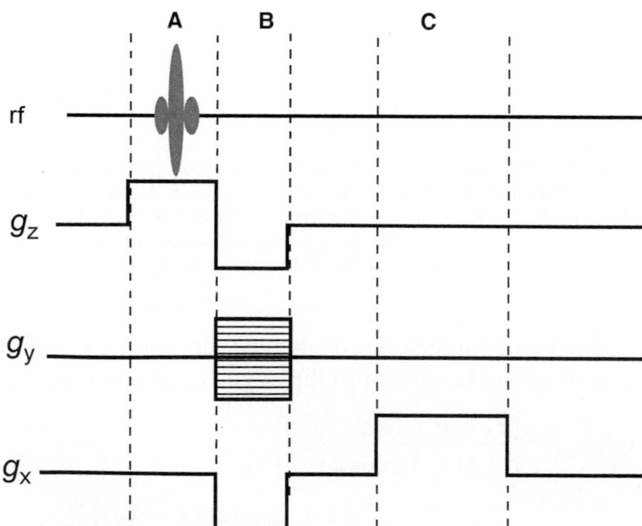

FIG. 12. Pulse sequence timing diagram of generic 2DFT gradient-echo pulse sequence showing rf, slice-selection gradient (G_z), phase-encoding gradient (G_y), and frequency-encoding gradient (G_x). The three time periods labeled *A–C* pertains to: *A:* slice selection (G_z); *B:* slice-selection rephasing gradients (G_z), phase-encoding gradient (G_y), and dephasing lobe of frequency-encoding gradient (G_x); *C:* frequency-encoding gradient (G_x).

Equation 7 assumes that the transverse magnetization has completely decayed at the time of the next echo following a pulse. We shall see that this is not necessarily the case in the very short TR regime and that refocusing effects may occur even though TR may be greater than T_2^*, the effective transverse relaxation time.

The Steady State

It is well known that any pair of rf pulses generates an echo. Furthermore, a train of rf pulses applied under the condition where TR $\ll T_2$ will generate two signals: an FID immediately following each rf pulse, and an echo-like signal from the preceding pair of rf pulses which reaches the maximum at the time of the subsequent rf pulse. This condition is called *steady state*, a dynamic equilibrium where transverse and longitudinal magnetization persist at all times. The physics of steady state has been reviewed extensively (14). An intuitive understanding of the formation of a steady state can be gained by reference to Fig. 14. Let us assume that a 90° pulse is applied, following which the spins precess by an angle $\psi = 180°$. At that time, they are subjected to another 90° rf pulse. The partially regrown longitudinal magnetization will be converted to transverse magnetization, whereas the residual transverse magnetization from the previous rf pulse will be returned to longitudinal magnetization. The forced equilibration which is a result of the condition $T_2 \gg$ TR causes the mean longitudinal magnetization to increase, relative to the one that would be present if complete decay of the transverse magnetization had already occurred. For the case of a 180° precession between successive rf pulses, the response is *maximum*, since all of the residual transverse magnetization has been converted back to longitudinal magnetization (Fig. 14B).

Let us now consider the other extreme, where the precession angle is zero (or a multiple of 2π). In this case, the next 90° rf pulse inverts the transverse magnetization, causing a net *reduction* in the mean longitudinal magnetization. It follows that the steady state signal is a function of the *precession angle* ψ (Fig. 15).

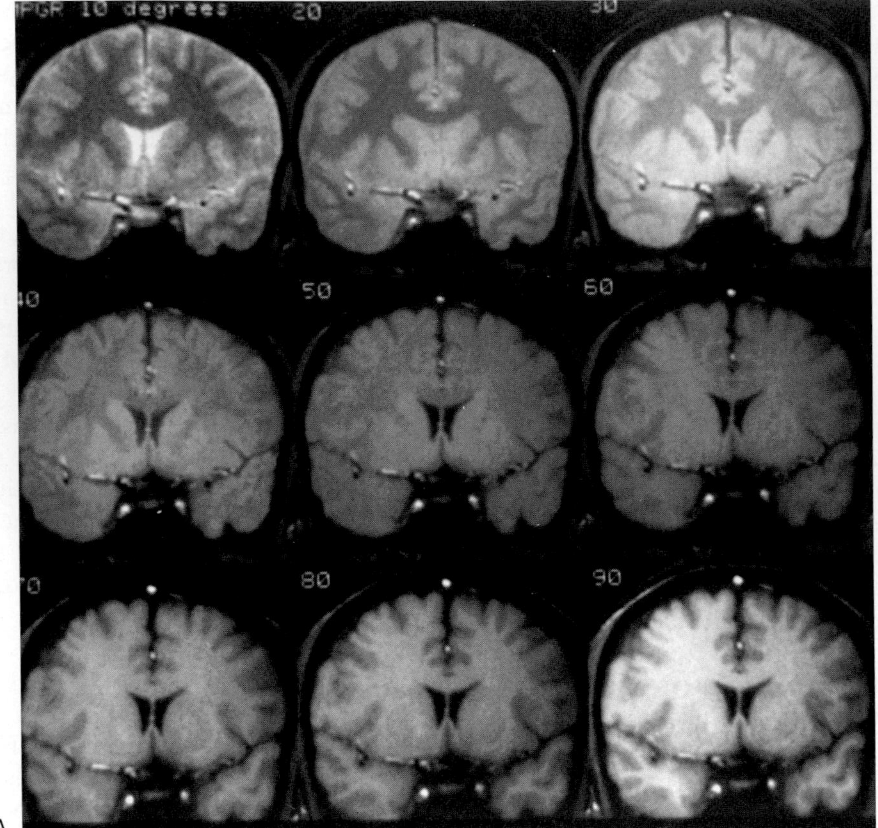

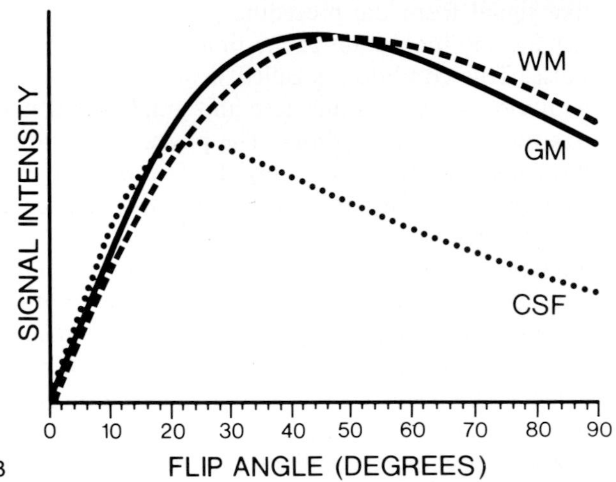

FIG. 13. A: Effect of small changes in flip angle on gradient-echo images (TR = 300 msec, short TE). Low flip angle image demonstrates expected contrast of long TR/short TE spin-echo image, while large flip angle images show contrast analogous to that of short TR/TE spin-echo images. **B:** SNR versus flip angle for a repetition time of 300 msec calculated for gray matter (GM), white matter (WM), and CSF. Note that at low flip angle the signal is determined by proton density (CSF > GM > WM) whereas at high flip angle the signal intensities follow the inverse order of T_1 (WM > GM > CSF).

The phase through which the spins precess between successive rf pulses is a function of the applied gradient. For the simplest case of a gradient G which is constant in amplitude and time, the phase advance during a pulse sequence time interval TR is:

$$\psi = \gamma \cdot G \cdot r \cdot \mathrm{TR} \qquad [10]$$

from which we can define a spatial wavelength λ, defined as the distance we have to travel from one point to the next such that the steady-state signal repeats itself in amplitude:

$$\lambda = \Delta r = 2\pi/(\gamma G \mathrm{TR}) \qquad [11]$$

Ernst and Anderson (10) showed that for a given precession angle the optimum flip angle α_{opt} is given as:

$$\cos \alpha_{\mathrm{opt}} = \left[\frac{\mathrm{E}_1 + \mathrm{E}_2(\cos \psi - \mathrm{E}_2)}{(1 - \mathrm{E}_2 \cos \psi)}\right] \times \left[\frac{1 + \mathrm{E}_1\mathrm{E}_2(\cos \psi - \mathrm{E}_2)}{(1 - \mathrm{E}_2)}\right]^{-1} \qquad [12]$$

where $\mathrm{E}_1 = \exp(-\mathrm{TR}/\mathrm{T}_1)$ and $\mathrm{E}_2 = \exp(-\mathrm{TR}/\mathrm{T}_2)$. This complicated dependence of the optimum flip angle on precession angle is found to vanish at a particular flip angle, α_{E}, called the *Ernst angle*:

$$\cos \alpha_{\mathrm{E}} = \mathrm{E}_1 \qquad [13]$$

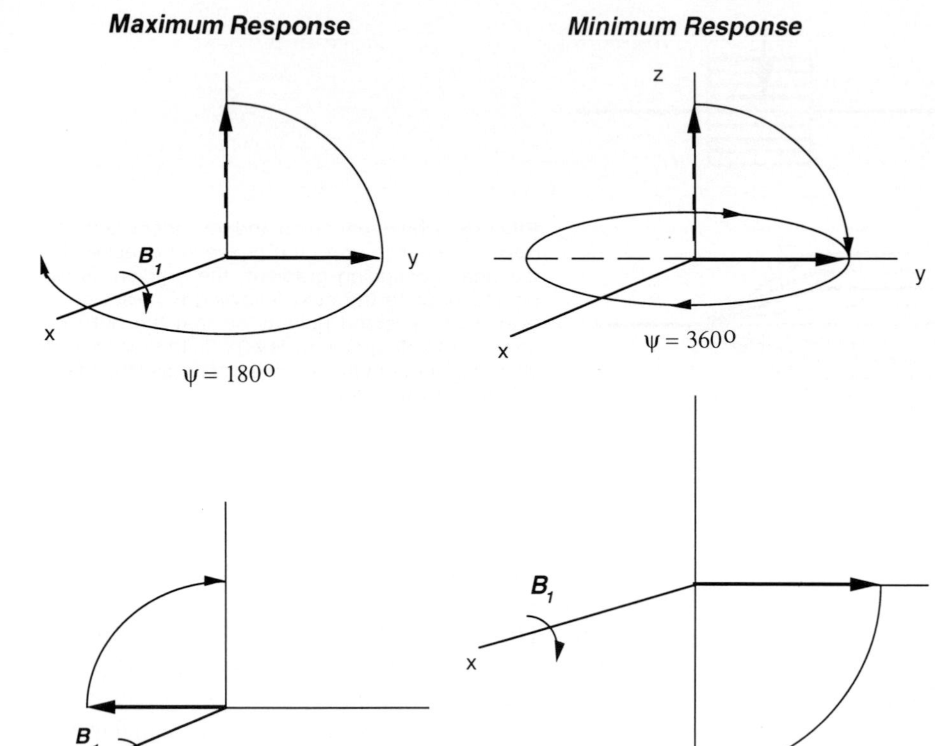

FIG. 14. Steady-state free precession: depending on the precession angle, the response may be either maximum ($\psi = 180°$) or minimum ($\psi = 360°$). In the former case (**A**), the entire residual transverse magnetization is converted to longitudinal magnetization resulting in maximum signal. In the latter situation (**B**), the signal is minimum.

We will see that in the presence of the imaging gradients the simplistic picture presented so far has to be revised since the precession angle becomes a function of spatial location. Clearly, if there were a homogeneous distribution of precession angles across the imaging voxel, the signal detected would be the mean of the one shown in Fig. 15. It is readily seen that in this case the mean signal is greater than zero, thus showing that the steady-state signal is enhanced. Sekihara et al., who carried out a detailed analysis of the steady-state signal, showed that this situation does indeed apply (15).

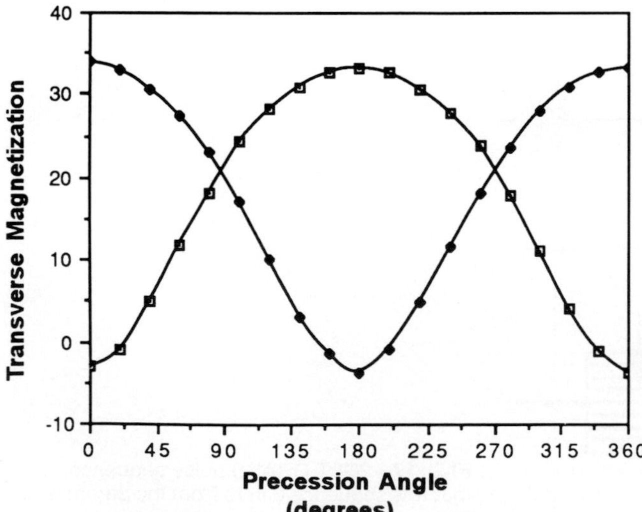

FIG. 15. The *y* component of the steady-state transverse magnetization as a function of precession angle for equally spaced rf pulses. Note that the signal is maximum when the spins precess through an angle of 180° between successive rf pulses. Curve for *filled diamonds* shows situation when the phase of the rf pulses is alternated.

GRADIENT-ECHO PULSE SEQUENCES

Gradient-Recalled Acquisition in the Steady State (GRASS)

There is one complication which requires a modification of the generic pulse sequence of Fig. 12, in that stepping of the phase-encoding gradient causes a view-dependent phase shift. Hence, whenever transverse magnetization persists between applications of the phase-encoding gradient, its phase will vary between successive phase encodes. For this reason, *phase encoding causes a view-dependent modulation of the signal intensity*, which, upon reconstruction, leads to artifacts in the images (16). This undesirable situation can be remedied by applying a gradient pulse of opposite polarity prior to the subsequent excitation. Typically, this is done by stepping the phase-encoding gradient in reverse order (17). This gradient, which removes the phase shift of the phase-encoding gradient, has also been termed "rewinder," because it rewinds the phase imparted by the phase-encoding gradient (18) (Fig. 16). Since all other gradients are view-independent, we need not be concerned with

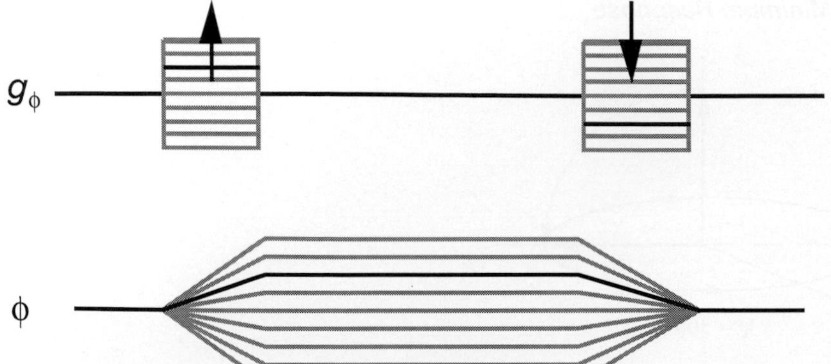

FIG. 16. Phase-encoding and rewinder gradients (**top**). In order to undo the phase shift caused by the phase-encoding gradient, the gradient is repeated prior to the next-following rf pulse, however, with reversed polarity so that the net moment from both gradients is zero. In this manner no view-dependent phase shifts occur, as the phase graph (**bottom**) shows.

them. Figure 17 shows the complete pulse sequence for what has been termed GRASS (gradient-recalled acquisition in the steady state) (19) or FISP (20).

Contrast Implications

Steady-state effects have profound implications on signal and contrast in many gradient-echo pulse sequences. Since it is the persistence of the transverse magnetization which determines the degree of signal intensity, one expects the signal for long T_2 structures to be much greater than it would in the absence of such a steady state. This is one of the manifestations of the presence of steady-state effects on clinical images: stationary fluid (e.g., CSF) is markedly hyperintense in the steady state (Fig. 18). The steady-state effect is enhanced at increased flip angle, which can readily be understood since under these conditions a greater portion of the transverse magnetization will be converted to longitudinal magnetization by the rf pulse. Note that at very low flip angle, the signal is largely independent of the relaxation times and reflects differences in proton density only. However, as the flip angle increases, the steady-state effects become more prominent. The signal intensity of CSF relative to the surrounding gray and white matter first decreases and then increases again (21–24).

Under steady-state conditions the relative signal intensity is approximately given by the ratio T_2/T_1 (for details see following section) and T_2/T_1 remains relatively invariant for most tissues, resulting from the high degree of correlation that exists between T_2 and T_1. Therefore, a characteristic feature of GRASS images is the relatively low brain parenchymal contrast. Hence, while GRASS images have been useful in the search for lesions that are associated with magnetic susceptibility differences (i.e., with T_2*-weighting) and for imaging regions of flow, they generally have not been clinically effective for evaluating brain parenchyma.

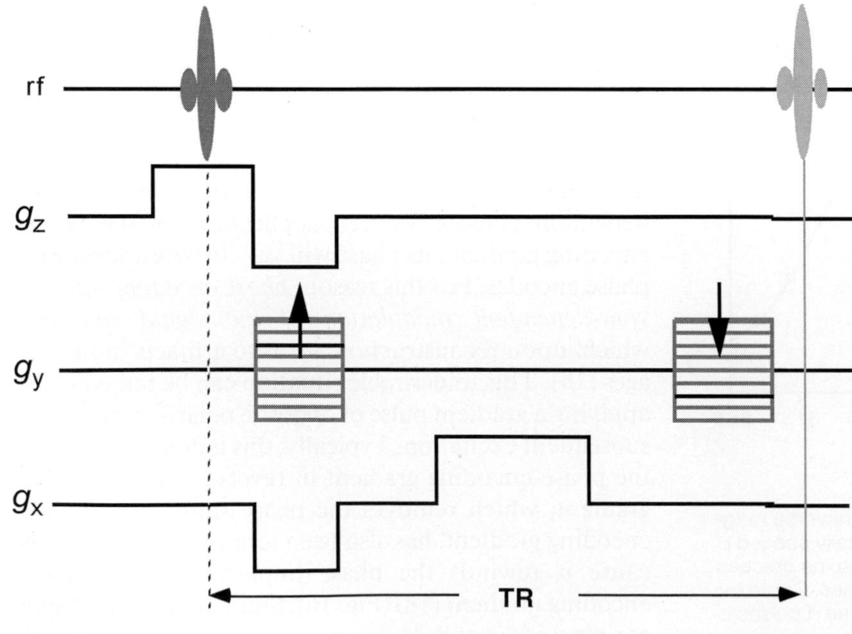

FIG. 17. 2DFT GRASS pulse sequence. Note that this sequence differs from the parent pulse sequence (Fig. 12) only in the addition of a "rewinder" gradient on the phase-encoding axis. The purpose of this rewinder gradient is to undo the phase shift induced by the initial application of phase-encoding gradient and thus prevent steady-state artifacts in the images.

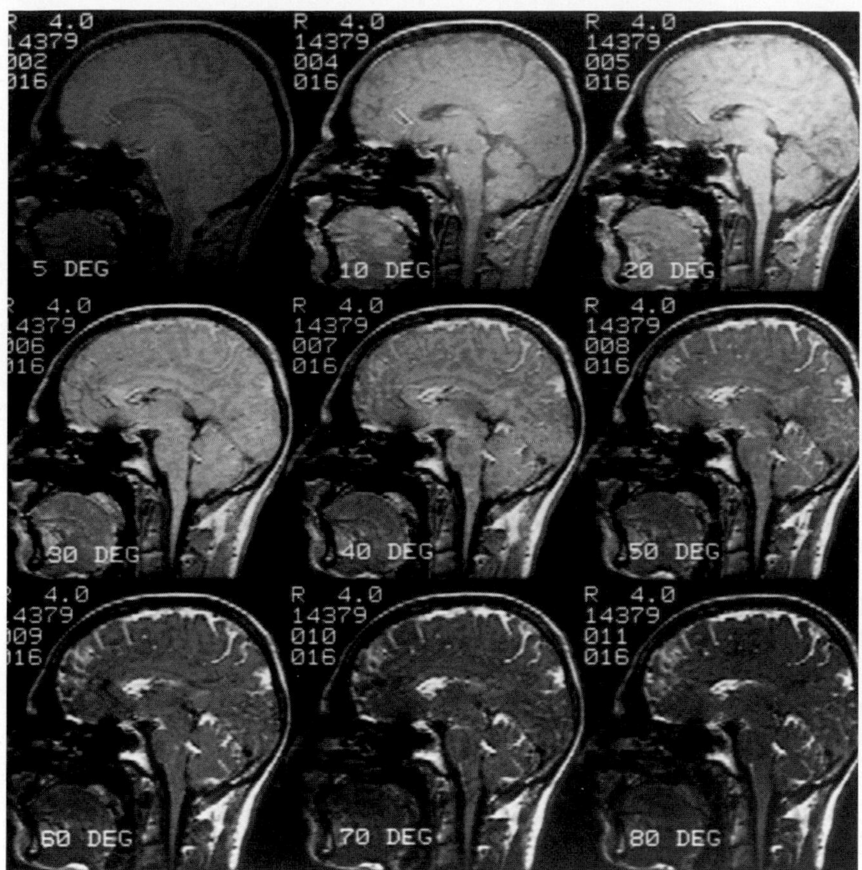

FIG. 18. Effect of motion of CSF on steady-state signal. As the flip angle α is increased, steady-state effects predominate, so CSF should become hyperintense (note high intensity of sulcal CSF at high α). However, CSF is black in areas of motion, i.e., in basal cisterns, the center of the fourth ventricle, and in the upper cervical spine.

Imaging with Fully Balanced Gradients ("True FISP")

With the gradient scheme of Fig. 17 only the phase-encoding gradient is balanced, whereas the effect of the unbalanced portions of the readout and slice selection gradient usually causes a distribution of phase angles ψ across the pixel such that $\Delta\psi \geq 360°$. However, there is no net change in phase from one pulse sequence cycle to the next, hence no artifacts should be produced. This phase distribution clearly reduces the maximum achievable signal which is now the mean of the integral over all phase angles (Fig. 15). This signal clearly is below the maximum achievable for the precession angle $\psi = 180°$ (constant rf phase) or 0° (alternating rf phase). The latter condition can easily be satisfied if all gradients are balanced, in which case $\psi = 0°$ holds (Fig. 19). This is the idea behind the original FISP pulse sequence (20) which, in order to be distinguished from the partially balanced FISP or GRASS sequence, has been termed "true FISP" (25). Unfortunately, the condition $\psi = 0°$, in practice, is difficult to achieve because of the always present static field inhomogeneities, typically arising from susceptibility effects (vide supra). These background gradients cause position-dependent phase shifts and thus local signal variations. However, at lower field strength which in the current constrained health care environment enjoy increasing popularity, these effects are minimal and true FISP thus becomes attractive.

At very short TR the FISP signal has been shown to obey the relationship (25)

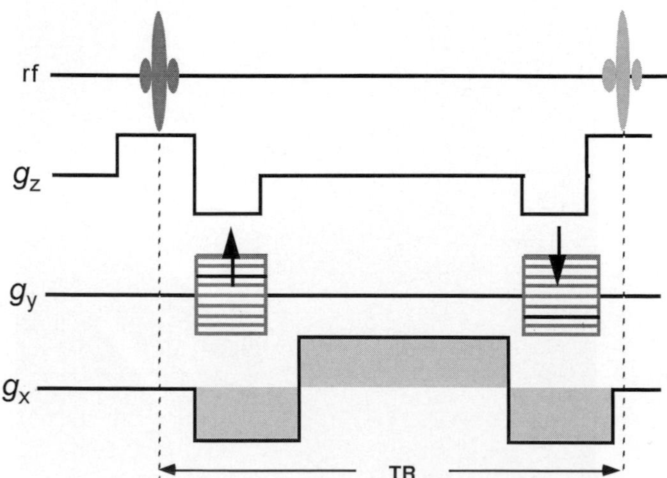

FIG. 19. True FISP pulse sequence: all gradients are balanced, i.e., the net area under the gradient-time curves, the so-called zeroth moment vanishes (*shaded area* of the frequency-encoding gradient). Under these conditions the phase angle for all spins is reset to zero at the time of the next-following rf pulse.

$$S \sim \frac{\sin \alpha}{1 + T_1/T_2 - \cos \alpha(T_1/T_2 - 1)} \quad [14]$$

which, for flip angle $\alpha = 90°$, simplifies to:

$$S \sim \frac{T_2}{(T_1 + T_2)} \quad [15a]$$

and since $T_1 \gg T_2$ usually holds,

$$S \sim \frac{T_2}{T_1} \quad [15b]$$

The above contrast behavior is illustrated by the images of Fig. 20.

It is to be noted that Equations 14 and 15 are also approximately valid for GRASS. As previously pointed out, the ratio of T_2/T_1 for most tissues is small (0.1 to 0.2), and does not vary a great deal for different tissues, so contrast among different tissues is relatively small when operating in the steady state (GRASS/FISP or "true" FISP). A noteworthy exception is CSF where $T_2/T_1 \approx 0.5$, hence the large contrast between brain tissue and CSF. In addition, while most pathologic processes cause an increase in T_1, they also cause a concomitant increase in T_2 (since the mechanisms of relaxation are similar).

A remarkable feature of the true FISP images of Fig. 20 is the retention of CSF signal, even in regions of high CSF flow (e.g., cervical spinal canal) where the signal can be markedly diminished on GRASS. This distinguishing property of true FISP is due to the fact that gradient balancing also compensates for motion at the time of the rf pulse (though not at the time of the echo). This becomes obvious when inspecting, for example, the readout gradient in Fig. 19 (shaded area) which has the 1:(−2):1 ratio needed for first moment compensation (for details of flow compensation see later in this chapter).

Spoiled Gradient-Echo Imaging

If we were to suppress steady-state coherences, we would expect contrast to be governed by the relationship expressed by Equation 9. Elimination of unwanted transverse magnetization is typically achieved with gradient pulses (spoiler gradients). While overall signal-to-noise is sacrificed in this manner, we will see that in the high flip-angle regime, parenchymal contrast can be achieved similar to or even surpassing that obtainable with spin-echo pulse sequences.

Unfortunately, effective elimination of the unwanted transverse magnetization is not straightforward. It typically does not suffice to apply a spoiler gradient of constant amplitude, because this would simply set up a new steady state based upon the spoiler gradient itself. A variety of spoiling schemes have therefore been proposed, whereby spoiler gradients are stepped in amplitude through an array of values (16) or varied in a pseudo-random fashion. None of these approaches are totally satisfactory and effective. Further, it should be noted that the phase imparted on the spins by spoiler gradients is location-dependent. Hence, at magnetic field iso-center, no phase shifts would result, since the magnetic field remains invariant there, regardless of the magnitude of applied spoiler gradients.

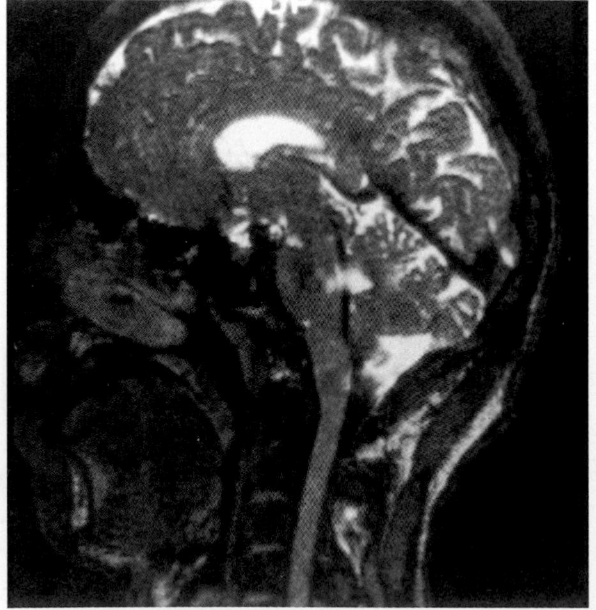
A

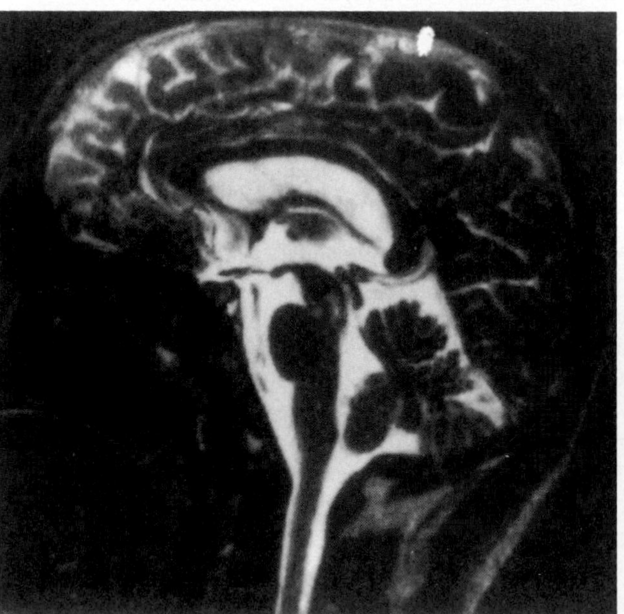
B

FIG. 20. FISP (**A**) versus true FISP (**B**): Note the loss of signal from CSF in the cisterna magna and spinal canal in image A, in contrast to the true FISP image which shows CSF uniformly bright (From Haacke et al., ref. 25, with permission.)

Phase anomalies are a well-known phenomenon in high resolution NMR spectroscopy and have been dealt with in a variety of ways. For example, it was proposed to randomize the pulse repetition time by randomly varying TR (26). Since, in this manner the precession angle is varied from pulse to pulse, the steady-state magnetization is scrambled. Alternatively, one can incrementally change the phase of the rf transmitter (and receiver) between successive views. This turns out to be a very effective approach but also instrumentally the most demanding one, as it requires excellent transmit/receive phase stability and reproducibility.

In order to understand the spoiling process, let us assume the phase to be stepped in 90° increments between views, and further, that the transverse magnetization precesses by 180° between successive views (Fig. 21). Suppose that the first rf pulse was applied along the *x* axis of the rotating frame, rotating the magnetization onto the *y* axis. Following a precession of 180° the magnetization is aligned along $-y$. The subsequent rf pulse, when applied along *x* again, restores the magnetization along *z* (maximum response, Fig. 21). However, if instead the rf pulse is applied along *y*, it will have no effect, since the magnetization is aligned along the same axis. Likewise, if the pulse is applied along $-x$, the minimum response is induced with the transverse magnetization being rotated onto the *z* axis. It is readily seen from Fig. 21 that cycling the rf phase through the four quadrants effectively eliminates the steady-state effect, thus resulting in effective spoiling. It should be noted that, in order to achieve these phase relationships, the rewinder gradient, discussed previously for the GRASS pulse sequence, needs to be applied in the RF-spoiled GRASS sequence as well.

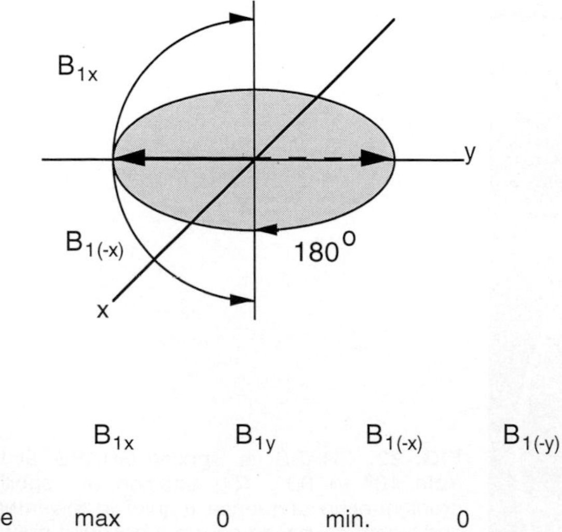

FIG. 21. Principle of rf spoiling by phase cycling: It is assumed that the transverse magnetization precesses around 180° between rf pulses and that the first rf pulse was applied along $x(B_1x)$. Note the effect of rf phase on the transverse magnetization: If the subsequent pulse has the same phase, the magnetization is returned to the $+z$ axis (maximum response) whereas a 180° phase shift ($B_{1(-x)}$) rotates it onto the $-z$ axis (minimum response).

This modification in the pulse sequence has an astounding effect on the signal characteristics as a comparison of GRASS and spoiled GRASS images (Fig. 22) demonstrates. Note that the relative signal intensities now follow the inverse of T1, with CSF exhibiting the lowest signal intensity, followed by gray matter, white matter, and subcutaneous fat, analogous to T1-weighted spin-echo images. Also note that the difference between GRASS and spoiled GRASS is not nearly as significant when one is utilizing a small flip angle, since the steady-state is not developed (Fig. 22).

Steady-State Free Precession Imaging (SSFP-Echo or CE-FAST)

A train of repetitive rf pulses applied at a rate such that $TR < T_1, T_2$ leads to two signals, an FID and an echo. The echo is formed by the two preceding rf pulses and falls on top of the next-following rf pulse[1] With the gradient-echo sequences discussed so far (e.g., GRASS, FISP, SP-GRASS), the FID is sampled and the echo is spoiled. An exception is true FISP where the balanced gradients ensure that the both FID and echo occur at the same time and thus are sampled simultaneously. It is also possible to acquire the echo and dephase the FID (28,29). In order to recover this signal, the gradients need to be balanced in such a manner that the phase is zero between the time of the echo and the next rf pulse. Further, the FID has to be destroyed which is achieved by applying the readout gradient well before sampling begins, thus dephasing the FID. A complete diagram of this pulse sequence, which is commonly referred to as CE-FAST (28) or SSFP-Echo (27), is given in Fig. 23. One notices that this pulse sequence is a time-reversed version of the GRASS/FISP pulse sequence (compare to Fig. 17). In order to understand the principle of CE-FAST, one needs to consider the phase evolution over two pulse sequence cycles. The phase trajectories for the frequency-encoding and slice-selection gradients are given in the bottom trace of Fig. 23. The phase-encoding gradient phase is nulled within each TR interval as in GRASS. Note that each rf pulse reverses the sign of the spin phase and further, that nulling of the phase from both slice-select and readout gradients is effected over the duration of two TR cycles.

The echo signal is proportional to $\exp(-2TR/T_2)$ because it can be regarded as the echo resulting from two rf pulses separated by TR milliseconds (hence causing a true spin-echo echo at time TE = 2TR). Since it is not

[1] This is a grossly simplified picture. In reality the echo at the site of the rf pulse is a superposition of a great many different echoes, both primary and stimulated.

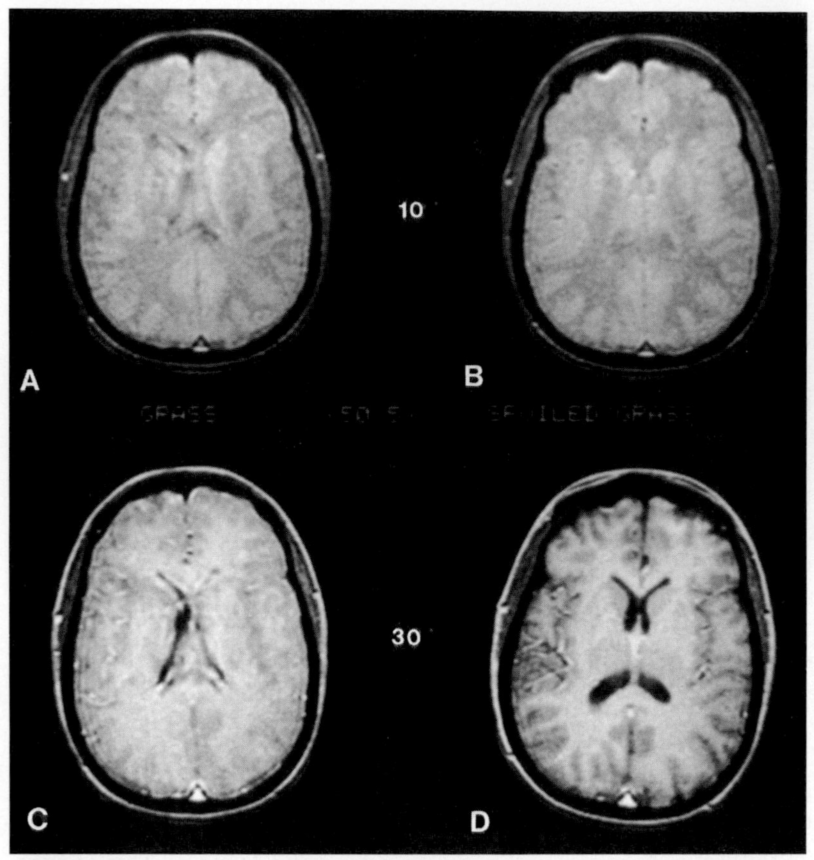

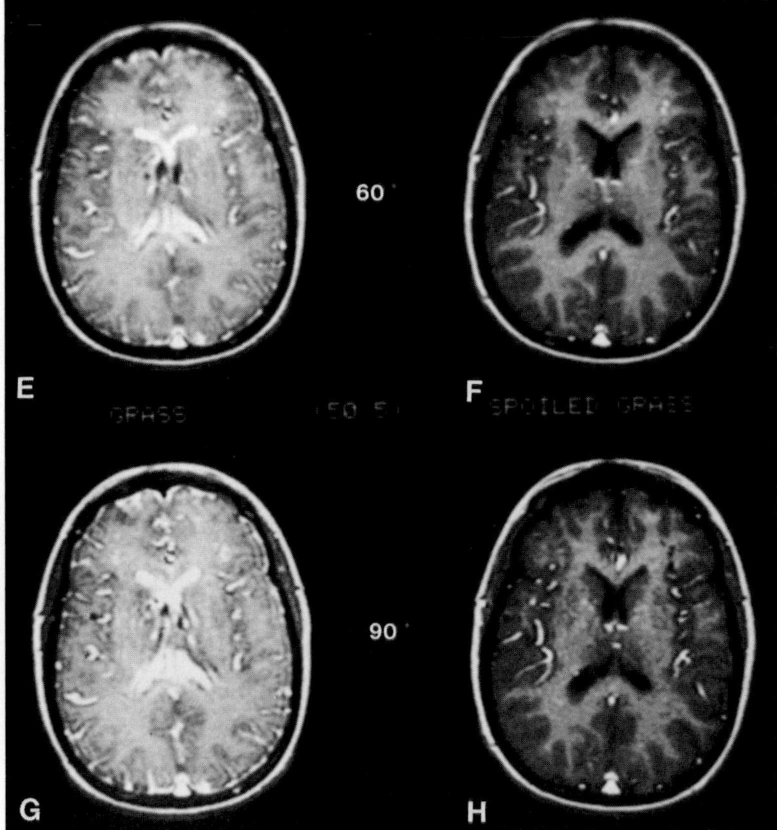

FIG. 22. GRASS vs. spoiled GRASS, at flip angles from 10° to 90°. The addition of "spoiling" to a gradient-echo sequence results in low-intensity CSF and higher T1-based contrast between gray and white matter (compare spoiled-GRASS images **B,D,F,H** to GRASS images **A,C,E,G**). Note that the effect of spoiling is more pronounced at higher flip angles (60° and 90°), since the steady state is not developed in GRASS images at lower flip angles (10° and 30°).

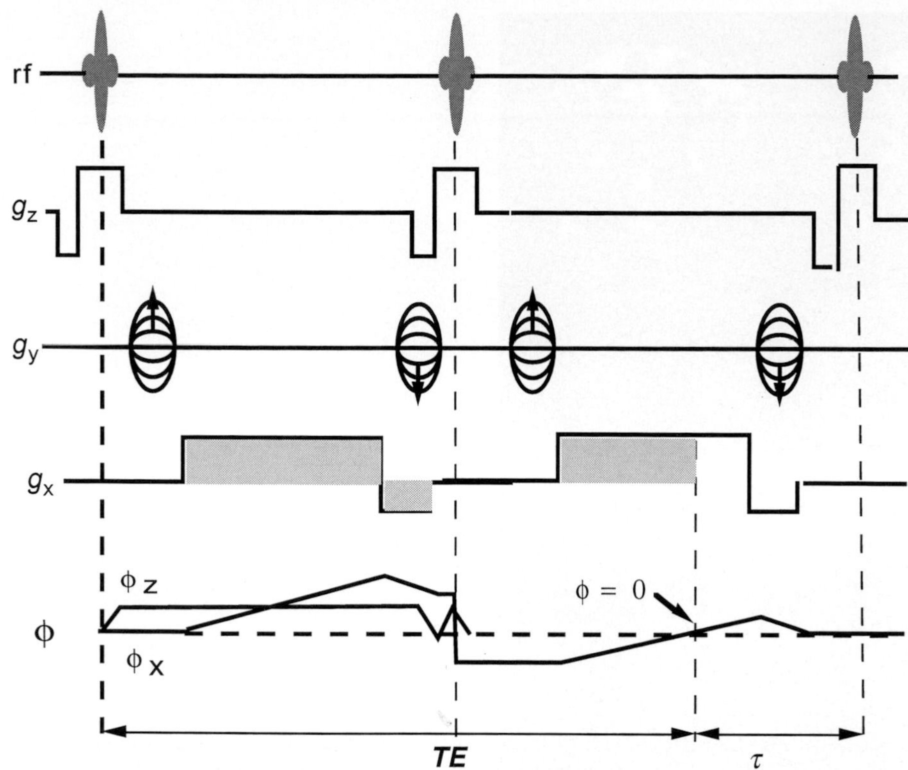

FIG. 23. Steady-state free precession echo (SSFP-echo) or CE-FAST pulse sequence. The echo, rather than the FID as in the GRASS sequence, is sampled. The readout gradient (G_x) is extended backward to spoil the FID. The time period τ represents the deviation between the rf echo which would appear at time TE = 2TR and the corresponding gradient echo which is formed at time TE = 2TR − τ. Two cycles are shown of the pulse sequence, along with phase trajectories for frequency-encoding and slice-selection gradient, showing nulling of the phase at time TE = 2TR − τ. The algebraic sum of the *shaded area* of the readout gradient is nulled (note that the rf pulse changes the sign of the gradient moment).

possible to sample the signal at the time of the rf pulse, the readout gradient is set such that refocusing occurs at time TE = 2TR − τ (Fig. 23). Thus the SSFP-echo signal is a gradient echo, like GRASS, and is sensitive to magnetic field inhomogeneity near susceptibility boundaries (vide infra). Note that the spins are only partially rephased at time t = 2TR − TE. The degree of susceptibility dephasing depends on the duration of τ. The signal is a complex function of both T_1 and T_2, but at very low flip angles the T_1 dependence vanishes (Fig. 24). One of the virtues of this pulse sequence is that it can provide T_2-weighted images at very short TR (29).

The clinical utility of such techniques is limited, however, since the recent improvement of rapid spin-echo scanning (see RARE later in this chapter) generates T_2-weighted images in short acquisition times. Therefore, although potentially generating images with relative T_2-weighting in short time frames, such sequences are probably more clinically useful for the depiction of flow (either CSF or vascular). As studied by Patz and colleagues (14), flow on steady-state images is seen as marked *hypointensity* (Fig. 25). This sequence is exquisitely sensitive to flow, on the order of millimeters per second (conventional gradient-echo imaging is sensitive to flow rates on the order of centimeters per second, and shows flow as *hyperintensity*). One cited application of the technique is in the documentation of cystic structure of mass lesions (30), where intralesional fluid motion is seen as low signal. This is used as an adjunctive pulse sequence in the clinical setting of a mass lesion when the differential diagnosis depends upon its cystic or solid structure.

High-Speed Implementations of Gradient-Echo Imaging

Reduction in Pulse Repetition and Echo Time

Until recently hardware limitations restricted the practically achievable scan times of GRASS-type pulse sequences to pulse repetition times of about 20 msec, amounting to scan times per image for a 128 × 256 data matrix of about 2.5 sec. There are several opportunities, however, for further shortening of scan time, albeit, as usual, at the expense of a further reduction in SNR or spatial resolution, or both (31,32). For more information on high-speed gradient-echo imaging the reader is referred to a review by Chien and Edelman (33).

The main target for reducing scan time is the pulse repetition time TR whose minimum is largely dictated by the time to echo and the sampling time. The echo time can be shortened by either shortening the sampling time (and thus increasing the sampling rate) or by reducing the number of samples (number of frequency-encoding steps) or both. The former entails a SNR penalty since SNR is proportional to the square root of the sampling time whereas the latter compromises spatial resolution. Another approach toward reducing echo

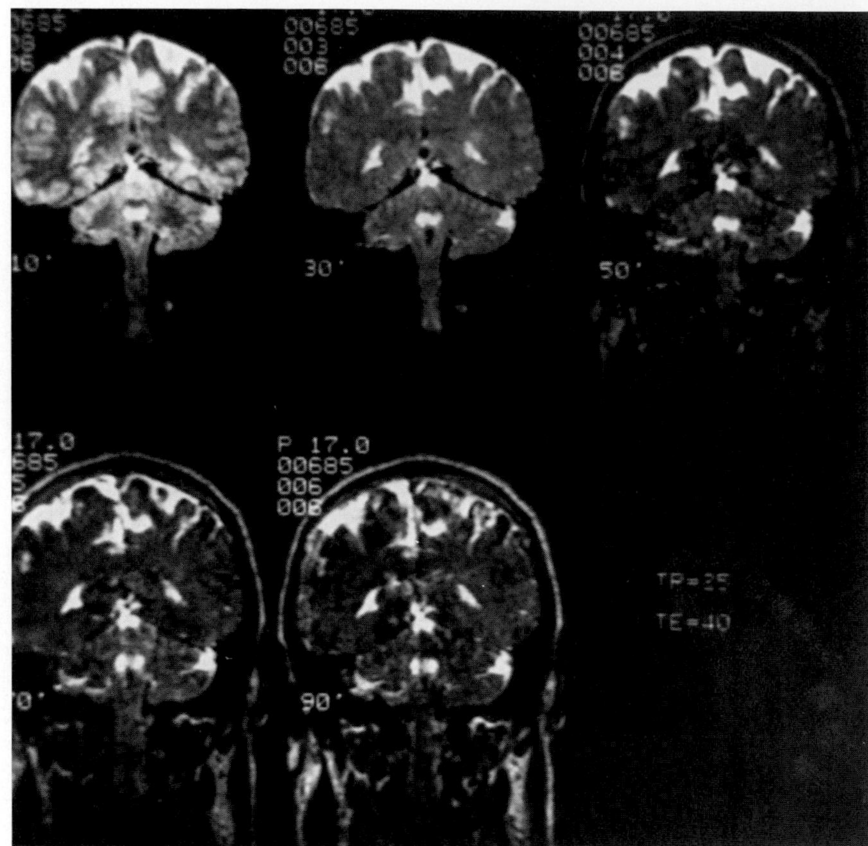

FIG. 24. Effect of flip angle on contrast in steady-state sequence (TR = 25, TE = 40 msec). Note that at low flip angle (10°), contrast is similar to that expected on long TR/TE spin-echo images.

time, previously discussed, is fractional-echo sampling (34,35). Since a reduction in sampling time requires operation at increased sampling frequency bandwidth, the gradient amplitudes need to be increased as well to maintain the field of view, thus imposing restrictions on the achievable field of view. For example, a sampling frequency bandwidth of 128 kHz, as it is required to sample 256 points in 2 msec, provides a minimum field of view of 32 cm at a gradient amplitude of 1 Gauss/cm. By acquiring only 128 frequency-encoding samples in 2 msec, the echo time can be reduced to 3 msec, permitting a TR of approximately 5 msec. Another reduction in scan time can be achieved through a reduction in the number of phase encodings. By lowering the number of phase encodings to 64, for example, scan times per image as short as 500 msec can be achieved at 1 G/cm gradient strength (31).

We will see later that increased temporal resolution exacts a price, either reduced spatial resolution, lower SNR, or both. Dynamic studies involving bolus administration of paramagnetic contrast agents (36) requires a temporal resolution of 1 to 2 images/sec, a requirement which is difficult to reconcile with gradient-echo pulse sequences except by sacrificing spatial resolution. An interesting idea which alleviates these constraints is to acquire a full k-space set only once (i.e., prior to bolus injection) and refresh only the central views during the time course to be mapped. The technique has been dubbed "keyhole" imaging[2] (37). The principle is sketched out in Fig. 26. The low-frequency data are then collected repeatedly at time intervals dictated by the time course of the physiologic process. The problems with this technique are obvious: any small detail involving the dynamic process will be lost. Nevertheless, the technique allows visualization of the temporal changes in high-resolution images. Similar view-sharing techniques have been reported earlier by Riederer et al. (38) and, more recently, by Hu et al. (39).

A potentially powerful application of high-speed gradient-echo imaging has recently been proposed as a means for monitoring interventional devices under MR fluoroscopic control (40). The idea is to track the location of an MR signal source (e.g., a small coil mounted on the tip of a catheter). In its basic implementation the method consists of sampling the signal following a nonselective rf pulse in the presence of a readout gradient. In order to obtain all three spatial coordinates, the frequency-encoding gradient is applied along x, y, and z.

[2] The term derives from the notion that by peeping through keyhole of data the entire k-space can be viewed.

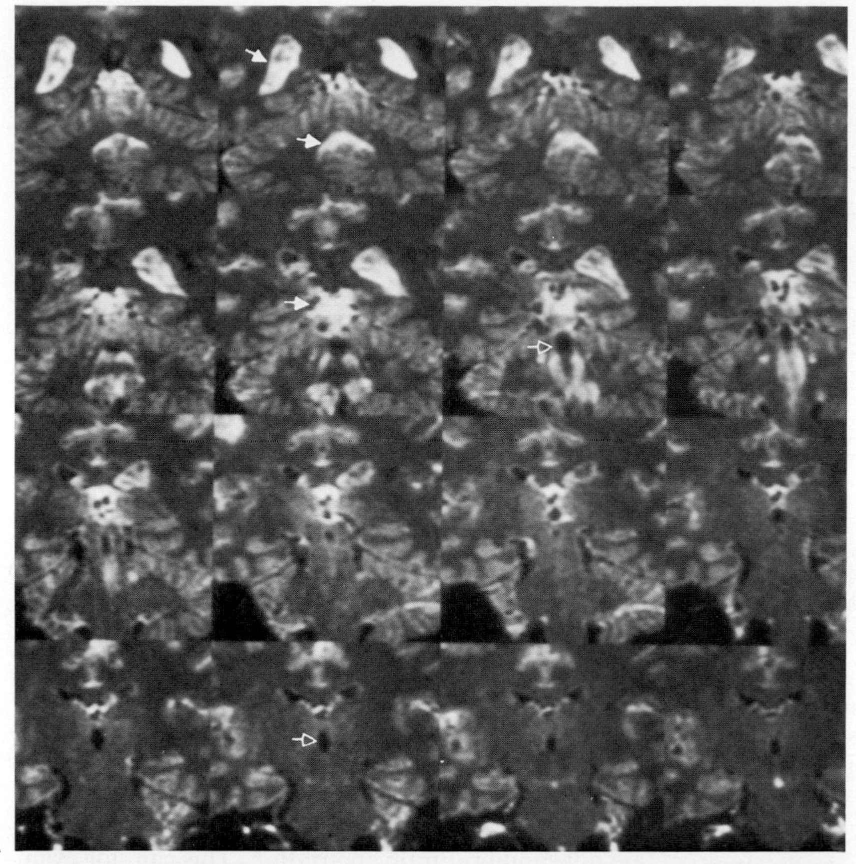

A

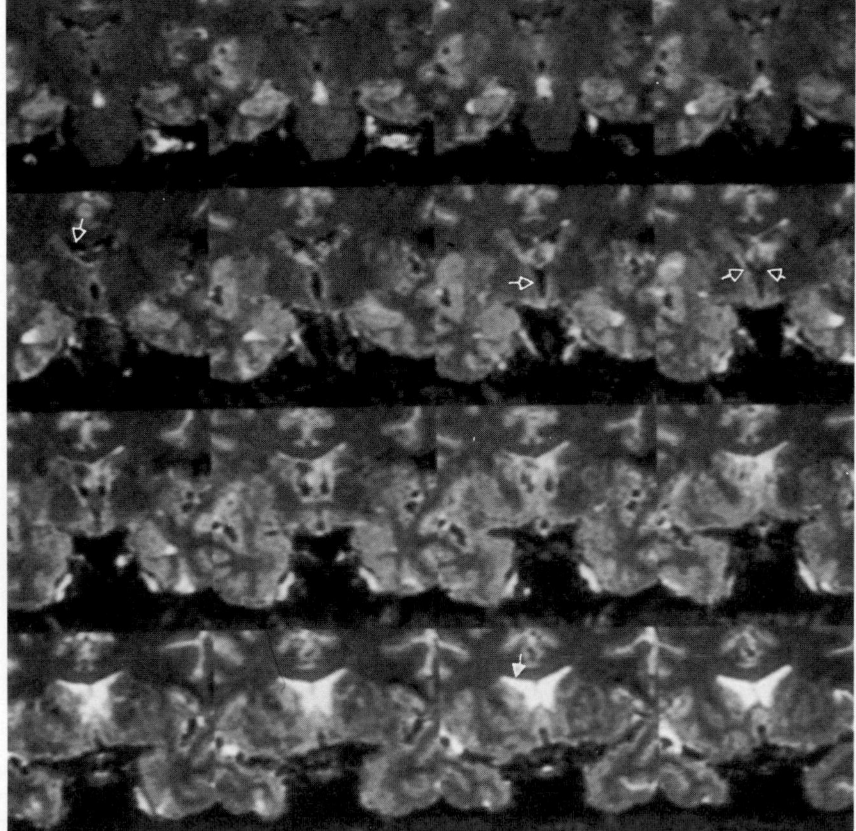

B

FIG. 25. Serial coronal 3DFT SSFP images through ventricular system (24/39/10°). Contiguous 2-mm images from posterior (**A**) to anterior (**B**) through ventricular system demonstrate that relatively stationary CSF is high intensity (i.e., atria of lateral ventricles, dorsal fourth ventricle, pineal cistern, anterior aspect of frontal horns) (*closed arrows*), while areas of flow are black (i.e., midsuperior fourth ventricle, third ventricle, foramina of Monro, and bodies of lateral ventricles) (*open arrows*).

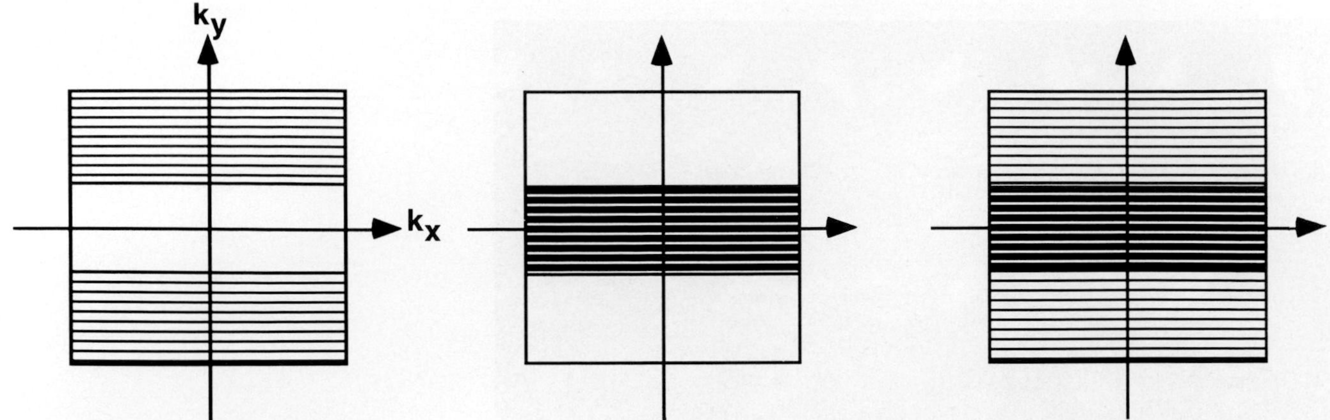

FIG. 26. Principle of keyhole imaging: the high-frequency data are derived from a reference data set (*left*) and merged with the low-frequency data acquired during the time course, to yield a composite set containing the dynamic information (*center* and *right*).

In the rotating frame the frequency of the signal ω_i ($i = x, y, z$) then is related to spatial position r_i as:

$$\omega_i = \gamma G_i r_i \qquad [16]$$

Since no phase encoding is involved, a single location measurement takes on the order 50 msec, or less, providing a frame rate of 20/sec. The basic principle is outlined in Fig. 27.

Since the signal frequency is sensitive to background gradients, more elaborate schemes are typically used whereby the polarity of the gradients is altered and gradients are applied in all three directions simultaneously (40). Figure 28 shows an image of a vascular phantom with the position of a catheter-mounted device displayed in real time.

Magnetization Preparation

Unfortunately, operation at TRs of less than 10 msec results in very low contrast, with little T_1 or proton-density discrimination, except perhaps at very low flip angles where SNR is inadequate. Signal averaging, on the other hand, would defeat the purpose of the pulse sequence, i.e., to freeze physiologic motion or to achieve sufficient temporal resolution for mapping a time-dependent physiologic process. The idea of magnetization preparation rf pulses (32,41–44) solves this dilemma.

The purpose of the preconditioning rf pulses is to create nonequilibrium magnetization. This can, for example, be achieved by inverting the equilibrium magnetization by means of an 180° rf pulse before playing out the string of low-flip-angle pulses. By appropriately delaying the acquisition by a pulse interval T1, contrast analogous to conventional inversion-recovery (45–47) can be achieved. Likewise, long-TE T2-weighted contrast can be obtained by a so-called driven-equilibrium pulse triplet in such a manner that the magnetization has decayed by a factor $\exp(-TE/T_2)$ before applying the train of low-flip-angle pulses. These two options are illustrated in Fig. 29.

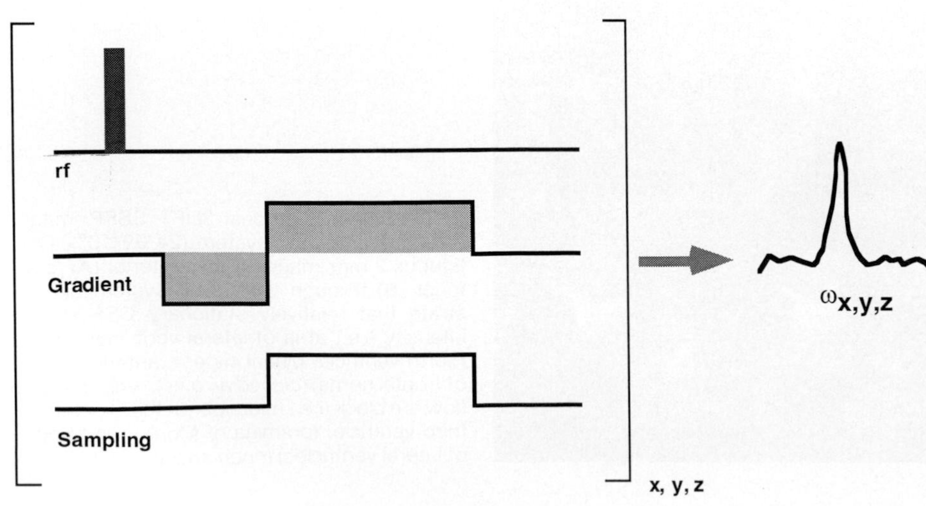

FIG. 27. Principle of determining coordinates of a signal source: a nonselective rf pulse is followed by a readout in the presence of an encoding gradient. The process is repeated for all three orthogonal orientations of the gradient. From the resulting signal frequencies the coordinates are determined from Equation 16.

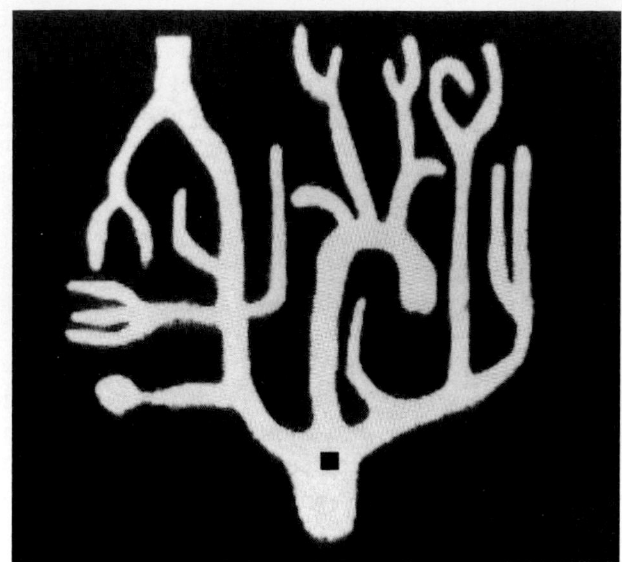

FIG. 28. Spin-echo image of vascular tree phantom. The rectangular cursor indicates the instantaneous position of a small receiver coil superimposed on the image. This position was updated at a rate of 20 locations per second (From Domoulin et al., ref. 40, with permission.)

Since most of the signal (and thus contrast) is derived from the central phase-encoded views (low spatial frequencies), it may be advantageous to ensure that these views be sampled at the appropriate time point in the pulse sequence. Hence, instead of stepping the phase-encoding gradient from its most negative to its most positive value, as it is conventionally done, a scheme, whereby the central *k*-space lines (low spatial frequencies) are sampled at the desired time point, is often employed. This view ordering may be called "centric phase encoding" (32). Alternatively, one can segment *k*-space in such a manner that the data is acquired in two or more passes. This permits better clustering of the phase-encoding views around the time point of interest (such as the T1 interval in a inversion-recovery sequence which suppresses an undesired resonance) (48). Moreover, segmented *k*-space acquisition has the advantage of providing the desired contrast for both low and high spatial frequencies. Its downside, of course, is reduced temporal resolution.

Three-Dimensional (3D) Gradient-Echo Imaging

For a large number of thin, contiguous slices, three-dimensional Fourier transformation (3DFT) imaging appears to be an extremely useful mode of data acquisition (49–51). In this acquisition mode, data are collected simultaneously from a volume, or "slab," of tissue. Partitioning into individual slices is achieved by phase encoding (also denoted "slice encoding") in a second dimension, i.e., along the slice-select axis. The timing diagram for a typical version of this pulse sequence is shown in Fig. 30. While, in principle, the z (slab-select) gradient need not be selective, a weakly selective pulse is usually chosen so as to confine excitation to a slab of tissue determining the imaging volume. In this manner, aliasing is minimized. Nevertheless, some residual aliasing is unavoidable and, in most sequences, the outer slices (e.g., slices 1, 2, 63, and 64 in a 64-slice acquisition) are automatically discarded. In practice, several additional slices at each end of the slab are impaired.

The scan time in this mode of operation scales in proportion to the number of locations scanned, analogous to the sequential mode. Unlike the 2DFT sequential

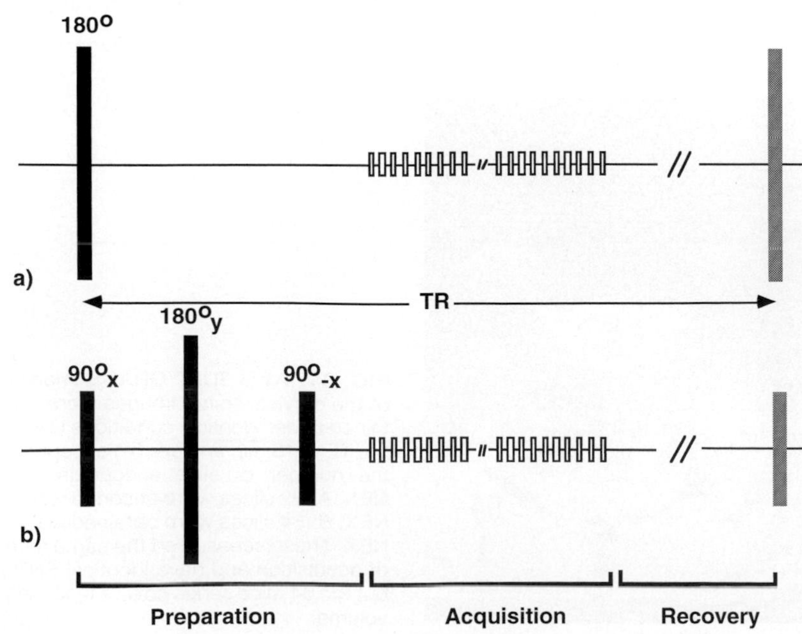

FIG. 29. Magnetization-prepared rapid gradient-echo (MP-RAGE) imaging entails one or more preparation pulses which create a nonequilibrium state of the longitudinal magnetization. **a:** Inversion-recovery for T1 weighting or selective suppression of a resonance. **b:** Driven equilibrium (DEFT) magnetization preparation; the first two pulses ($90°_x$, $180°_y$) create a spin echo, at which time a third pulse ($90°_{-x}$) restores the rephased transverse magnetization along the longitudinal axis.

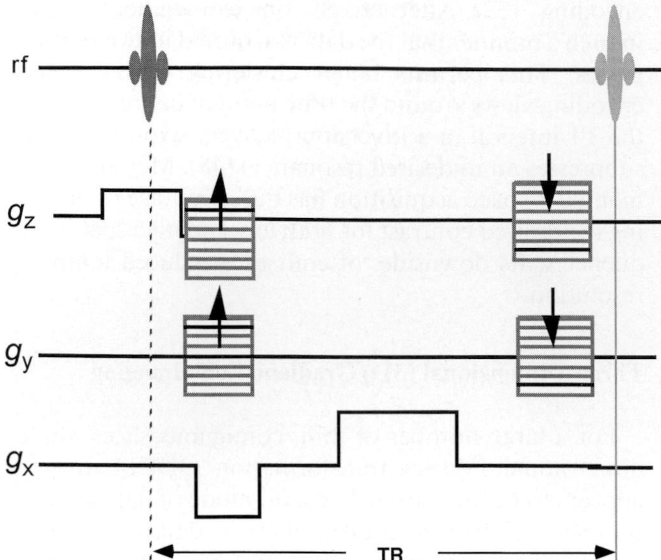

FIG. 30. Three-dimensional gradient-echo pulse sequence. Note that a slice-encoding gradient analogous to the phase-encoding gradient takes the place of the slice-selection gradient. In order to confine the 3D volume to a slab (and thus avoid aliasing in slice direction) a low-amplitude *z* gradient is typically used. The variable slice-encoding gradient is centered on the rephasing lobe of the slab-selection gradient. The version shown has rewinder gradients as they are required for GRASS/FISP.

mode, however, where any arbitrary number of slices can be acquired, a very small number of slice encodings in 3DFT causes truncation artifacts along the *z* axis. Typically, any number of locations below 32 is impractical as this is compounded with a severe degradation in image quality. Further, the fast Fourier transform algorithm demands that the number of partitions be powers of 2. The practical effect of interslice truncation artifact using 32 or 64 slices may not be significant, but this has not been fully investigated at the time of this writing.

Another distinguishing feature when compared to the 2D sequential mode relates to signal-to-noise. Whereas in the 2DFT mode, SNR is independent of the number of locations scanned, SNR in 3DFT increases as the square root of the number of slice encodings (N_{Sl}). This becomes important when designing protocols using 3DFT scanning, since SNR is proportional to both $\sqrt{N_{sl}}$ as well as to $\sqrt{\text{NEX}}$. Therefore, by halving the NEX and doubling the N_{sl}, the SNR remains unchanged, while the region of coverage has doubled at no cost in time (Fig. 31).

In 2D imaging, slice thickness is essentially limited by the available gradient power. For a typical rf pulse bandwidth of 1.25 kHz, the minimum slice thickness is 3 mm at a gradient strength of 1 G/cm, as is easily verified from Equation 17, relating rf pulse bandwidth (BW), gradient amplitude for slice selection (G_z), and slice thickness (Δ_z):

$$\gamma G_z \Delta z = 2\pi \text{BW} \quad [17]$$

By contrast, in 3D spin-warp imaging there is no slice selection, except for the application of a low-amplitude gradient for slab selection. Since partitioning of the slab is achieved analogous to in-plane phase encoding, it is subjected to the same constraints as the latter. We have seen in an earlier section of this chapter that the pixel size is given as $1/k_{max}$ (Equation 5), which in 3D imaging equally applies to the third dimension; i.e.,

$$\Delta z = \frac{1}{k_{z\max}} = \frac{1}{\gamma G_z t} \quad [18]$$

where t is the duration of the slice-encoding gradient and G_z is the maximum value of the slice-encoding gradient. Whereas the slice thickness is still inversely related to the gradient amplitude, in the event of limited gradient power the duration of the gradient can be increased. In

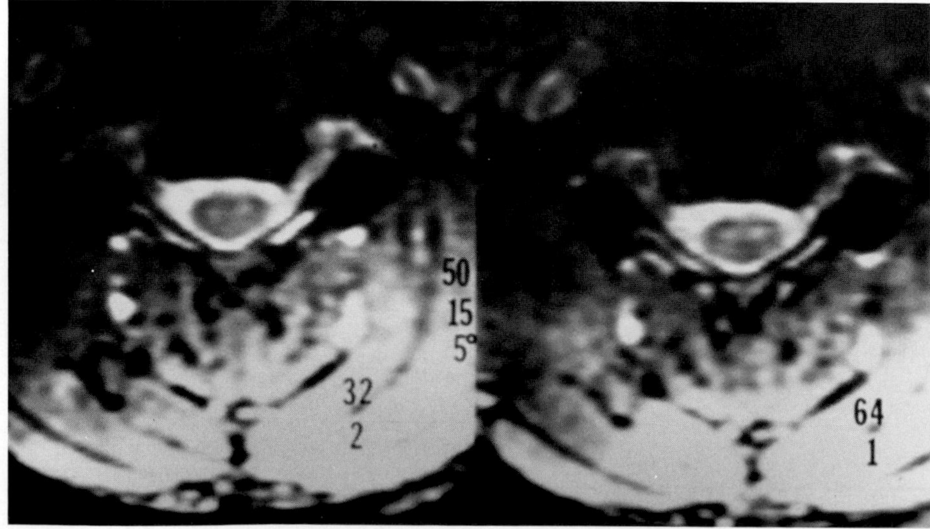

FIG. 31. Axial 3DFT GRASS images of the cervical spine. Images were obtained under identical conditions (TR = 50, TE = 15, flip angle = 5°) except for the number of slice encodings and NEX. **A:** 32 slices were encoded with 2 NEX. **B:** 64 slices were obtained with 1 NEX. These series used the same time of acquisition and have identical SNR, but the 64-slice series covers twice the volume.

3DFT imaging, in fact, the ultimate constraint to thinner slices is SNR alone. As with 2DFT imaging, SNR in 3D imaging scales proportional to voxel size, so a compromise has to be sought reconciling the spatial resolution and SNR needs when designing clinical protocols.

Among the virtues of the 3DFT mode is its capability of providing images that are contiguous but do not suffer clinically significant image degradation from interslice cross-talk, which plagues contiguous slices obtained from conventional interleaved 2DFT imaging techniques. However, it is incorrect to assume that they are totally free from cross-excitation (52). Just as the point spread function in the imaging plane causes a spread of the image intensity from individual pixels, the effect of finite sampling has similar consequences as far as slice leakage is concerned (52,53). One manifestation of 3D interslice cross-talk is the subtle superposition on the image of ghost images from adjacent slices. The effect is exacerbated for very small numbers of phase encodings (less than 32). This effect, although evident in theory, does not seem to be important clinically and, in fact, currently used clinical 3DFT protocols achieve high quality images with contiguous slices which are virtually artifact-free.

In principle, any of the pulse sequences discussed so far can be implemented in either a 2D or 3D mode. In fact, in the clinical setting where traditional anatomic information is required, high-speed gradient-echo techniques are usually applied in the 3D mode. For example, magnetization-prepared high-speed gradient-echo techniques, discussed in the previous section, can easily be extended to three spatial dimensions as shown by (43,44). In this case, following a preparation pulse, a train of low-flip-angle pulses would be administered, such that all N_z lines (number of slice encodings) are sampled and the process repeated N_y times. In this manner isotropic data sets of very good quality, covering the entire brain (128 slice encodings), can be acquired in scan times on the order of five minutes with inversion-recovery preparation (see, for example, refs. 54 and 55).

MULTI-LINE SCANNING TECHNIQUES

Fast Spin Echo and Related Techniques

Principles of RARE

The techniques described so far do not differ significantly from conventional spin-echo imaging techniques as far as the actual data acquisition process is concerned. In both techniques an echo is generated, either by reversal of the readout gradient (gradient echo) or an rf phase reversal pulse (spin echo). A characteristic trait of this mode of data acquisition is the circumstance that the signal from each excitation can generate *no more than one line* in k-space. In 1977 Mansfield first conceived the parent of a family of MR acquisition schemes known as echo-planar imaging (56,57). The underlying idea was to cover k-space by exciting the spins only once and to repeatedly recall echoes by reversing the read gradient, all while playing out a low-amplitude orthogonal gradient which, in modern parlance, takes the role of the phase-encoding gradient. Alternatively, instead of refocusing the spins by alternately reversing the polarity of the read gradient, a train of spin echoes can be generated by individually phase encoding each echo. Collecting four echoes, for example, would cover four lines of k-space, rather than one, as in conventional sampling. In this manner, the scan time can be shortened by a factor of 4 relative. Hennig first demonstrated the practicality of this approach (58,59). The images obtained in this manner, were found to exhibit a substantial degree of T_2-weighting since signals from successive k-space lines are attenuated as $\exp(-t/T_2)$. Because of its strong T_2-weighting, Hennig gave the technique the acronym RARE (*r*apid *a*cquisition with *r*elaxation *e*nhancement). The technique initially had few followers, in spite of its obvious appeal in terms of acquisition time, presumably because it was difficult to implement and because of its apparent limitations as far as contrast is concerned.

More recently, there has been a revival of the RARE technique by virtue of pulse sequence and hardware refinement (60–62). The "fast spin echo" or "turbo spin echo," as derivatives of RARE now are referred to, has had at least as significant a clinical impact as the introduction of the gradient-echo techniques had in 1986. An excellent discussion of the technique and its salient features has been published by Listerud et al. (63). Much of the renewed interest in RARE stems from advances in gradient and transceiver hardware which led to considerable improvement in image quality. For example, eddy currents sensitively affect the echo amplitude. Hence, good eddy current compensation or shielded gradients are paramount. Further, a highly stable rf system, in particular, as far as phase stability is concerned, is critical to maintaining the transverse magnetization over a period of several hundred milliseconds. One of the difficulties of generating a large number of echoes is to avoid signal loss from imperfections in the rf pulses. For example, a slight missetting of the pulse flip angle can have a cumulative effect. Such effects can be minimized if the phase of the 180° rf pulses is rotated 90° relative to the initial 90° pulse. This modification is generally referred to as "Meiboom-Gill" modification of the Carr-Purcell spin-echo train, abbreviated CPMG. Deviations of the pulse flip angle of the 180° phase reversal pulses are, of course, unavoidable for slice-selective pulses, and thus give rise to additional primary and stimulated echoes (64) which, if not properly dealt with, can give rise to artifacts (65).

Figure 32 illustrates the principle for the case of sampling of four k_y lines from the response to a single 90°

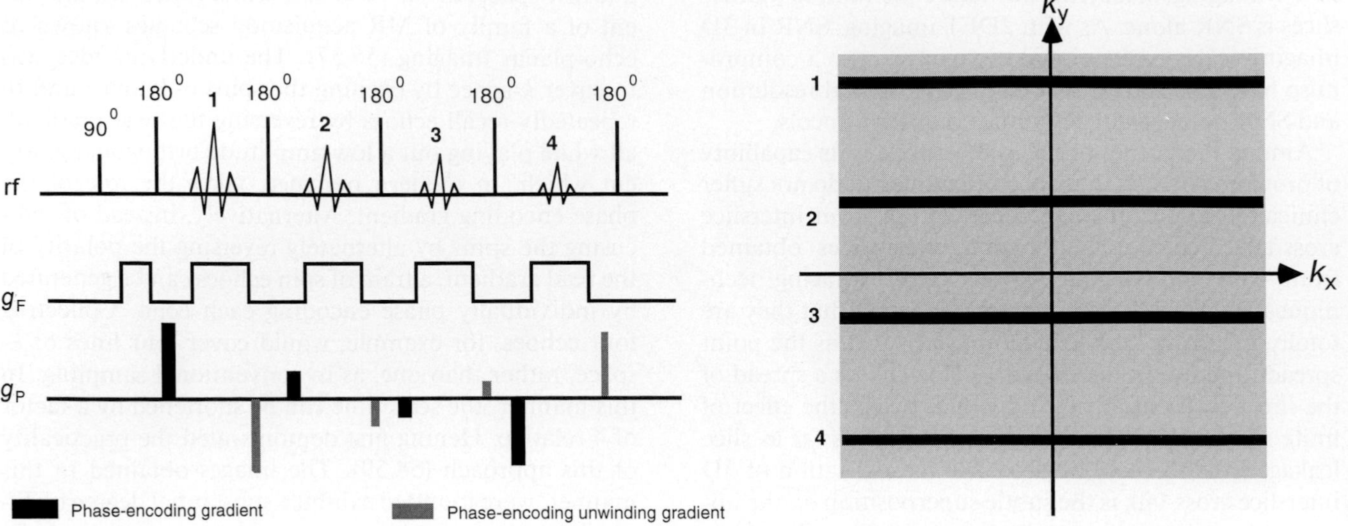

FIG. 32. Principle of fast spin echo. **A:** Multiple echoes are generated which are individually phase-encoded and frequency encoded. In this manner more than one *k*-space line can be sampled per excitation (**B**). Note in A that following echo sampling, the phase is unwound by applying the phase-encoding gradient a second time with reversed polarity.

pulse, achieved by individually encoding each of four successive echoes. An important facet in the pulse sequence of Fig. 32B is the phase unwinding gradient. One notices that after echo collection a gradient G_y of amplitude equal to the previously applied phase-encoding gradient is applied, however, with polarity opposite to the phase-encoding gradient. The purpose of this gradient is to undo the phase shift imparted by the phase-encoding gradient. We need to remember that any remaining phase would be carried over by the next-following 180° pulse since the subsequent *k*-space line is derived from the same transverse magnetization. Note also that in terms of the spatial frequency concept a 180° rf pulse brings the spatial frequency vector to its conjugate location.

The permissible length of the echo train is determined by tissue T_2. For an echo train duration of $3T_2$, for example, the last echo contributes with only about 5% of the original magnetization. We will see later, that the ratio of echo train length to T_2 is critical for minimizing artifacts.

The minimum scan time in 2D spin-warp imaging is equal to the product of the number of k_y samples, N_y, the pulse repetition time, TR, and the number of excitations. In FSE imaging each excitation (sometimes called "shot") affords *n* echoes and thus *n* lines. The scan time thus is given by the relation:

$$\text{Scan Time} = \frac{N_y \cdot \text{NEX} \cdot \text{TR}}{n} \qquad [19]$$

Since the echo train can be several hundred milliseconds long, the number of slices is reduced relative to conventional multislice spin-echo imaging. In order to account for this effect, the pulse repetition time is usually increased in FSE imaging. Hence, the scan time given by Equation 19 ought to be regarded the *minimum* scan acquisition time possible. In terms of scan time per slice the speed advantage over conventional SE imaging is less than implied by Equation 19. Nevertheless, it is clear that an enormous increase in efficiency can be achieved with this technique in that long-TR spin-echo imaging with scan times on the order of seconds, rather than minutes, becomes feasible. For example, for $n = 16$, TR = 2 sec, a scan with 128 phase encodings takes only 16 sec. This opens new avenues for imaging structures that are subjected to involuntary motion such as the globe of the orbit. Alternatively, the increased efficiency can be traded for higher resolution. A case in point is the brain image in Fig. 33, acquired with a 512 × 512 matrix, TR = 5 sec, NEX = 2, corresponding to a pixel size of $0.4 \times 0.4 \text{mm}^2$ and $n = 32$.

Contrast Manipulation by k-Space Ordering

Hennig's acronym suggests that RARE images are necessarily T_2-weighted. Naively, one would predict the contrast in these images to represent some weighted sum of the contributions from the various echoes. A longer echo train would then provide increasing T_2 weighting. Returning now briefly to the role individual spatial frequencies play in determining overall signal, it becomes immediately obvious that the above naive concept is in-

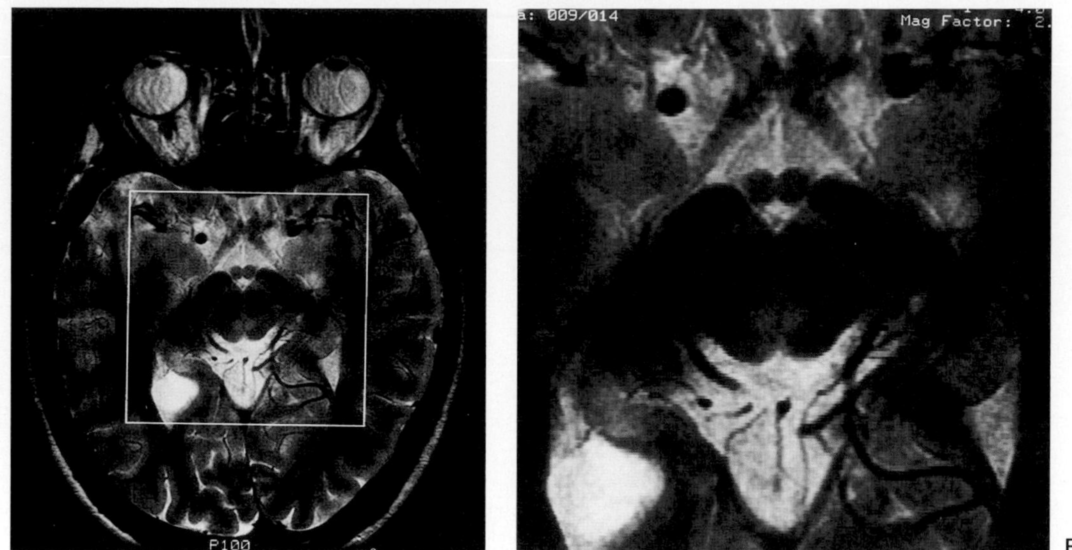

FIG. 33. A: FSE image obtained from 16-echo train (TR = 5000 ms, TE_{eff} = 80 ms, 512 × 512 matrix, 0.39 × 0.39 mm^2 pixel size), obtained in 5 minutes scan time, showing superb anatomic detail. **B:** Magnification of square region in A.

correct. If we managed to fill all lines k_y from a single echo train of duration $N_y\Delta TE$ and further, if we did so starting at $k_{y,min}$ and ending at $k_{y,max}$, by sequentially incrementing the phase-encoding gradient, we would traverse zero spatial frequency (which contributes to most of the signal and thus contrast) at time TE = $(N_y/2)\Delta TE$. In this case, the effective echo time TE_{eff} would be exactly half the echo train length.

Hennig recognized that by appropriately ordering the echoes in k-space, contrast could be altered. For example, if the central lines were acquired in such a manner that they correspond to the early echoes (i.e., by encoding with low amplitudes of the phase-encoding gradient), the resulting images would be predominantly proton-density weighted. Likewise, if the central lines were assigned to the late echoes, T_2-weighted images would be obtained. In the present case illustrating the principle, the 16 k_y lines are covered with four "shots," each generating four echoes and thus four lines. In order to achieve the least T_2-weighting (i.e., optimum proton-density weighting) one could encode the four echoes from the first shot to k_{y1}, k_{y2}, k_{y3}, and k_{y4}; the four echoes from the second shot to k_{y-1}, k_{y-2}, k_{y-3}, and k_{y-4}; the ones from the third shot to k_{y5}, k_{y6}, k_{y7}, and k_{y8}; and those from the fourth shot to k_{y-5}, k_{y-6}, k_{y-7}, and k_{y-8}; with the indices pertaining to the spatial frequencies. It turns out that such a scheme, while achieving the desired contrast, would lead to large discontinuities in the amplitude of successive spatial-frequency signals and thus artifacts. Since each line is weighted by a factor $\exp(-TE_j/T_2)$ with the index j pertaining to the jth echo, it becomes obvious that there would be a large increase in amplitude from S (k_{y4}) to S (k_{y5}). A more appropriate scheme is one in which the line-to-line variation in signal amplitude is minimized, which can be achieved by evenly distributing the echoes across one half of k-space. Hence, the four echoes from shot 1 would be assigned to spatial frequencies k_{y1}, k_{y3}, k_{y5}, and k_{y7}, the ones from shot 2 to k_{y2}, k_{y4}, k_{y6}, and k_{y8}, and likewise for the negative values of k_y. It obviously does not matter which side of k-space, $k_y > 0$ or $k_y < 0$ is filled first. Figure 34 illustrates this optimized scheme of k-space coverage for a four-echo FSE sequence with 16 k_y lines for both proton-density and T_2-weighting. The exact algorithm for assigning echoes to spatial frequency k_y for any echo train length and image matrix size to achieve a desired weighting (expressed in terms of an effective echo time, TE_{eff}), has been worked out by Melki et al. (61,62). The effective TE represents the echo time that would be required for obtaining the same contrast in a conventional spin-echo sequence. Figure 35 demonstrates the different degree of T2-weighting that can be achieved by appropriately selecting T_{eff}.

In brain imaging, we typically wish to generate two images from the same long-TR spin-echo acquisition, a first proton-density or moderately T_2-weighted image, and a second more heavily T_2-weighted image. Since in FSE imaging we use successive echoes for multi-line encoding, the reader may wonder, how more than one echo (or rather, images at two different TE_{eff}) are gathered. Because of its superior efficiency, one could simply concatenate two FSE sequences and one would still wind up with shorter scan time than in conventional spin-echo imaging. Another common approach is to split the echo train and use the early echoes for the generation of a proton-density-weighted and the later echoes for the more T_2-weighted image.

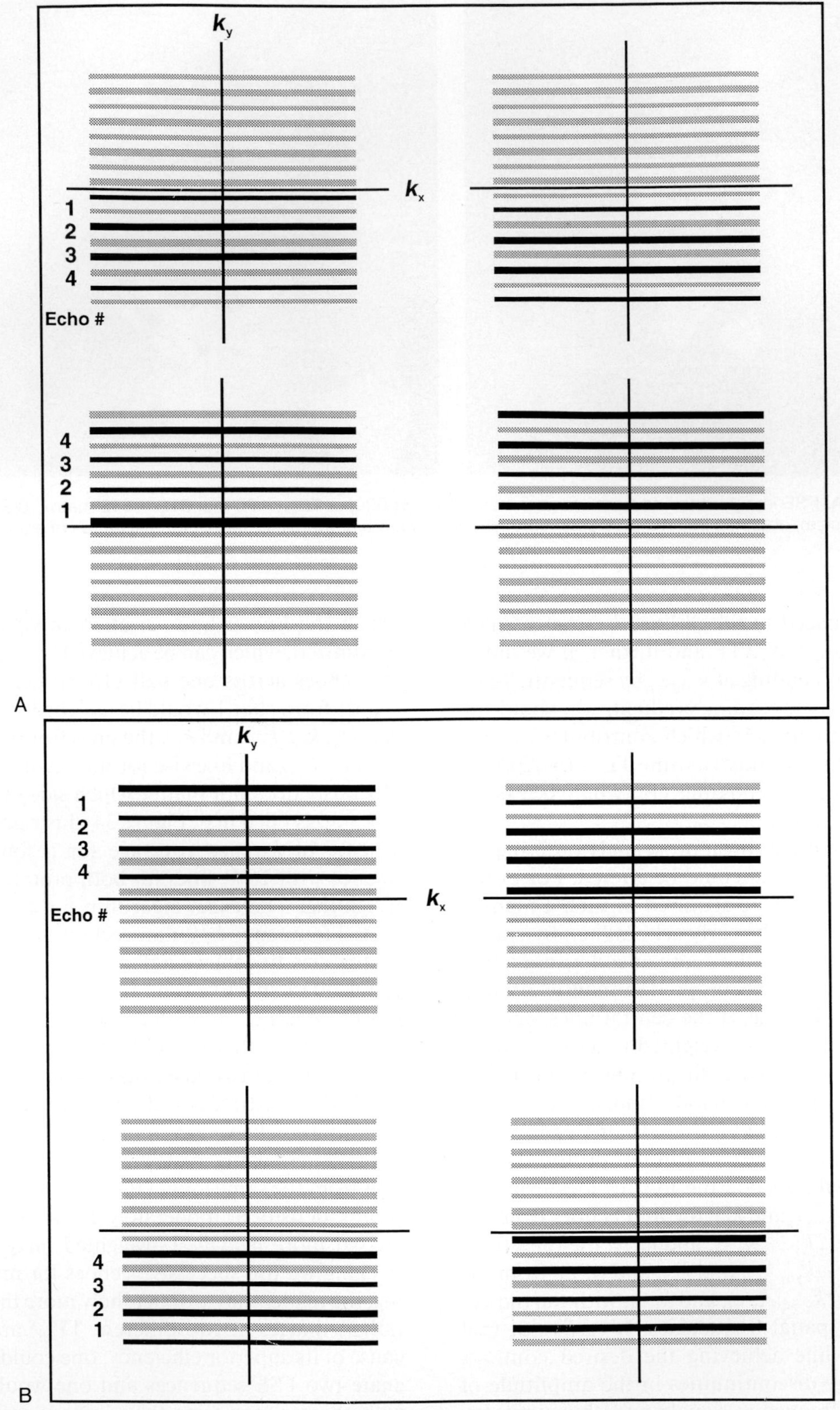

FIG. 34. Contrast in FSE imaging can be controlled by scanning the central *k*-space lines with echo times near the desired ("effective") echo time to achieve a particular contrast. The scheme shown is for a four-shot four-echo sequence, where the numbers 1, 2, 3, and 4 pertain to the four echoes. This algorithm ensures minimal signal discontinuities between successive spatial frequency signals. **A:** Encoding scheme for proton-density weighting. **B:** Encoding scheme for T_2 weighting.

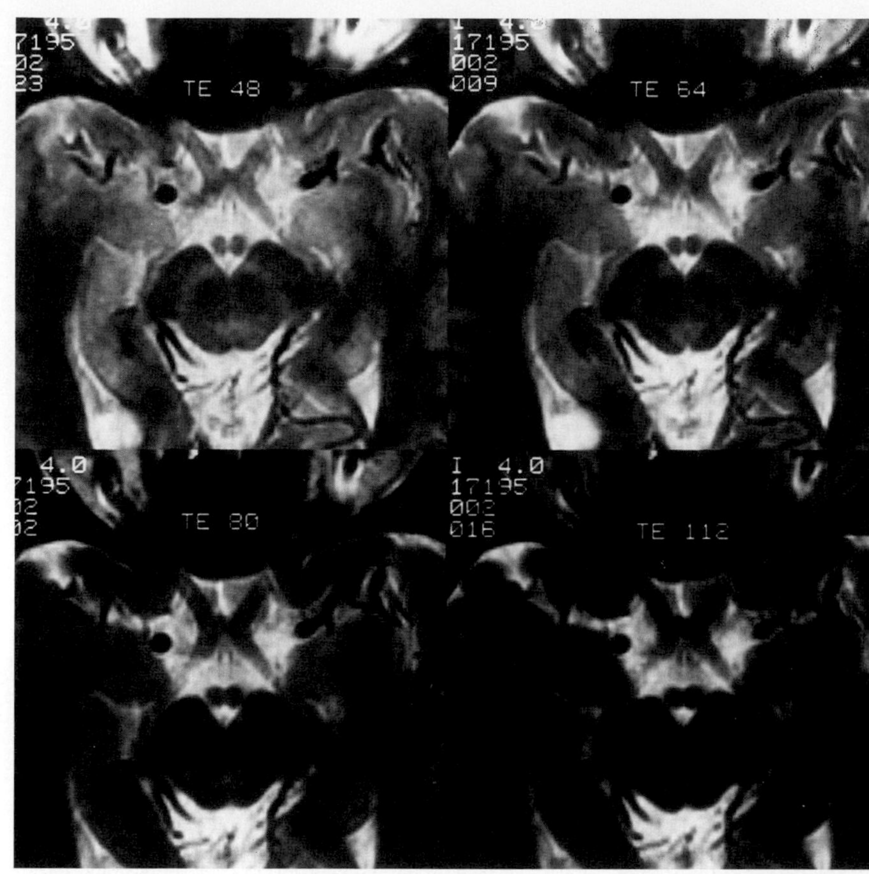

FIG. 35. The extent of T_2-weighting in FSE imaging is controlled by the effective TE, TE_{eff}. Note that the different contrasts are achieved merely by varying the order in which the spatial frequencies are assigned to the 16 echoes in the train.

Artifacts

As we have seen in the previous section, a salient feature of FSE imaging is the discrete weighting each k-space signal experiences. Notably, each signal $\rho(k_{yi})$ is weighted with a function $\exp(-TE_j/T_2)$. The discontinuous traversal of k-space can be a source of artifacts. Although the discontinuities can be minimized by adhering to Melki et al.'s scheme, they nevertheless exist and can cause a variety of artifacts. Among these are blurring, edge enhancement, ringing, and phase ghosting (61,62, 66). One of the most significant artifacts is *blurring* and *edge enhancement*. It should be realized that while edge enhancement may be referred to as artifactual, it is a clinically useful effect in certain regions, notably the lumbar spine, where nerve root morphology is clearly depicted by T_2-weighted fast spin echo but often only poorly visualized on conventional spin-echo images. In clinical practice, we routinely use fast spin echo for lumbar spine MRI for this reason.

A qualitative understanding of this effect can be obtained by considering a structure with short T_2 such as fat or cartilage. Let us first assume that we assign the early echoes to the low spatial frequencies so as to produce proton-density weighting, in which case the late echoes will correspond to the high spatial frequencies. However, since T_2 is short, there may be little signal left at the time these higher spatial frequencies are sampled (Fig. 36).

It thus becomes apparent that the spatial frequency components from the short-T_2 structure are deemphasized. Suppression of the high spatial frequencies, however, as we have seen earlier, introduces blurring. We can estimate the degree of blurring from the point spread function which determines the extent to which a point source of signal will bleed into adjacent pixels. It can readily be shown that in FSE the full width at half maximum of the point spread function is given by (63):

$$L = \frac{2\Delta y}{\pi} \frac{n \cdot \Delta TE}{T_2} \qquad [20]$$

where ΔTE is the interecho spacing and n the number of echoes in the train. Let us take fat, as an example ($T_2 \approx 60$ msec), and sampling of eight echoes, with a total echo train duration of 320 msec. Hence, according to Equation 20 this would impart a blurring of about 3.4 pixels. In other words, this particular sampling scheme is equivalent to a k-space filter. Obviously, for structures of particularly short T_2, such as articular cartilage with a T_2 of say 20 msec, blurring with a four-echo train of only 80 msec would be 3 pixels, which was found to prevent detection of small meniscal tears. Conversely, small objects may be enhanced with long effective echo times since

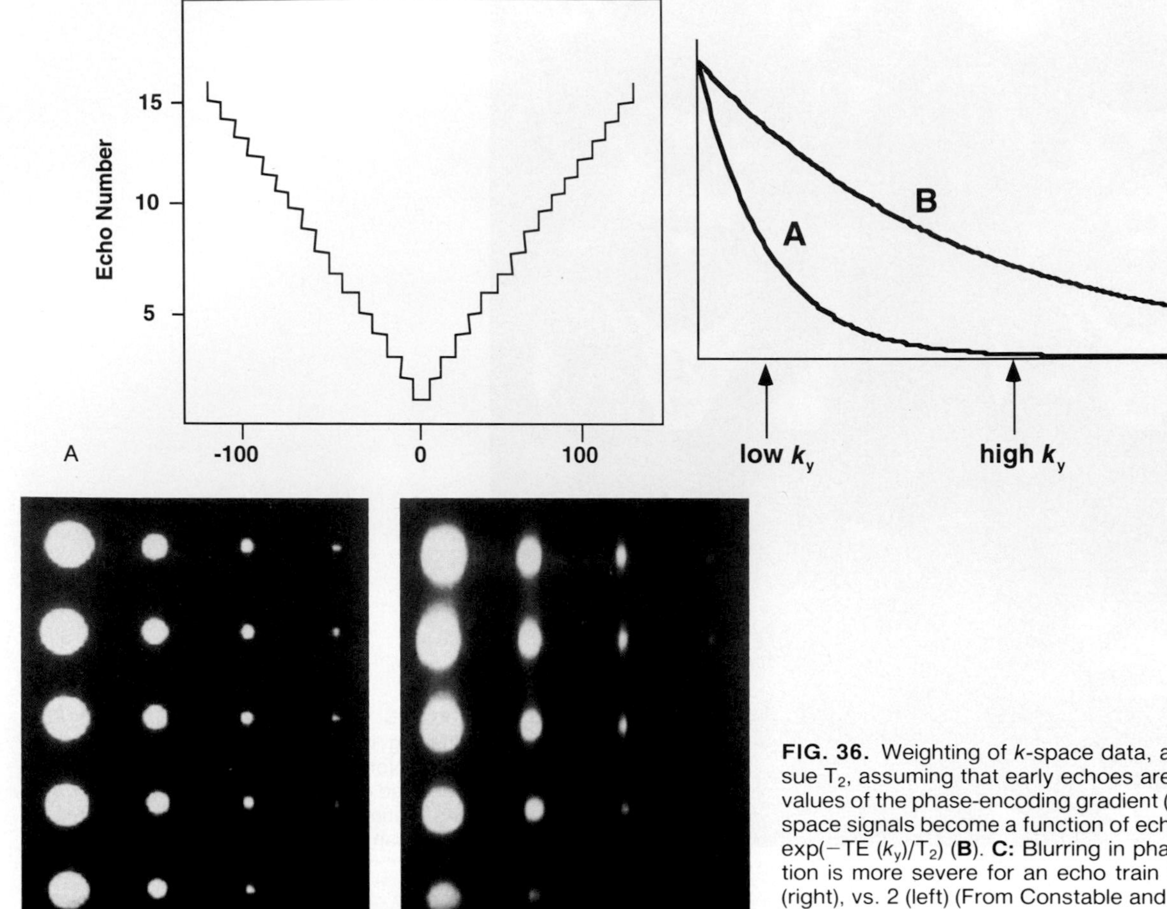

FIG. 36. Weighting of k-space data, as a function of tissue T_2, assuming that early echoes are encoded with low values of the phase-encoding gradient (**A**), showing that k-space signals become a function of echo time, i.e., S (k_y) α exp($-$TE (k_y)/T_2) (**B**). **C:** Blurring in phase-encoding direction is more severe for an echo train length (ETL) of 16 (right), vs. 2 (left) (From Constable and Gore, ref. 66, with permission).

here the spatial frequencies are collected for early echoes (having significantly more intensity). It can also be shown that large objects are not affected in their intensity by varying TE_{eff}, but significant edge enhancement occurs at long TE_{eff} (66). For a more detailed discussion of these effects in terms of the point spread function, the reader is referred to ref. 66 and ref. 63.

A different type of edge enhancement (also denoted "pseudo edge enhancement") results at the interface of structures with very different T_2 (e.g., sulci, ventricles). This effect, which can be very prominent, may be explained as resulting from blurring of the short-T_2 structure, bleeding over into the signal from the long-T_2 structure. All artifacts are alleviated by reducing echo train duration (either by lowering the number of echoes in the train or shortening interecho spacing). Figure 37A illustrates the principle along with conventional spin-echo (Fig. 37B) and FSE images of different echo train length (Fig. 37C and D).

Fast Spin Echo Versus Conventional Spin Echo

A critical issue for the clinician is the question of whether or not the contrast in FSE images is diagnostically equivalent to the one in conventional spin-echo images. While images acquired at equal "effective TE" bear close similarity to their conventional spin-echo counterparts, there are several features that are specific to FSE (61,62,64,67).

Effect of Diffusion on Brain Iron Visibility

The sensitivity to diffusion-mediated signal loss (e.g., from brain iron) is less prominent than in SE imaging. It is well known that when transverse relaxation is dominated by irreversible spin dephasing from diffusion, such as in acute hemorrhage, T_2 can be exceedingly short (68). When diffusion is operative in the presence of background gradients, the apparent T_2 is not only a function of the echo time but also of the number of echoes in the train for any given echo delay. The echo attenuation $M(\mathrm{TE})/M_o$ from diffusion is given by (69):

$$M(\mathrm{TE})/M_o = \exp(-\gamma^2 G_o^2 \mathrm{D}\ \mathrm{TE}^3/12n^2) \qquad [21]$$

where G_o is the background gradient (e.g., from intracellular deoxyhemoglobin), D is the diffusion coefficient, and n the number of echoes in the train. Figure 38 shows

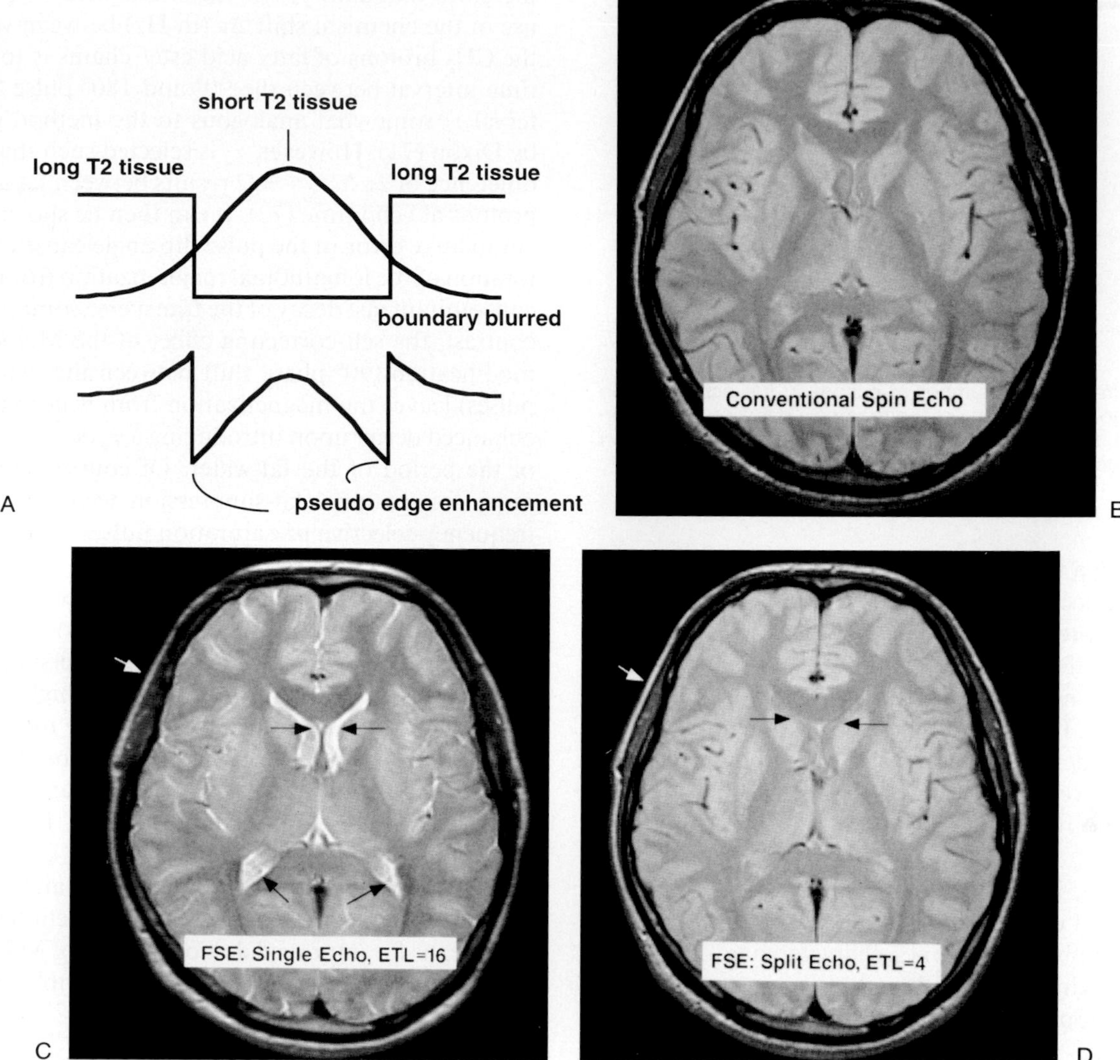

FIG. 37. A: At short effective TE the central structure of short T_2 is blurred, bleeding over into the zone pertaining to long T_2. **B–D:** Blurring and edge enhancement in proton-density-weighted FSE images; conventional spin-echo image (B); FSE image obtained with 16-echo train (echo train duration 160 ms) (C); FSE image obtained with 4-echo train (echo train duration 80 msec) (D). Note blurring of the scalp-air interface (*white arrow*) and edge enhancement at CSF–brain interface (*black arrows*). Both artifacts are greatly alleviated in D demonstrating the favorable effect of reduced echo train duration.

the dependence of the spin-echo signal on the number of echoes in the train.

Effect of J Modulation on Fat Signal

The low intensity of fat in late echoes in conventional spin-echo images has generally been ascribed to the short T_2 of fat. There is now substantial evidence that this explanation is incorrect. Contrary to this behavior FSE images exhibit anomalously intense fat signal even for effective TEs affording T_2 weighting. There has been considerable speculation about the origin of this effect and several hypotheses have been offered. There is ample evidence now that the observed effect has its origin in scalar spin-spin coupling among protons in the long-chain fatty acid protons, essentially the CH_2 protons of the aliphatic chains (see, for example, ref. 70 and references cited therein).

Spin-spin coupling is a phenomenon that is well understood and which is widely exploited in high-resolution NMR spectroscopy for the purpose of structure elucidation. In a spin-echo signal from a spin-coupling multiplet the different spectral components are phase-modulated, i.e., they get in and out of phase with each other as TE is advanced. If the multiplet components are unresolved, destructive interference and concomitant signal loss will occur when the phase shift between the various multiplet components is $\approx 180°$. This effect leads to signal loss at long echo time for single or asymmetric echoes in conventional spin-echo imaging.

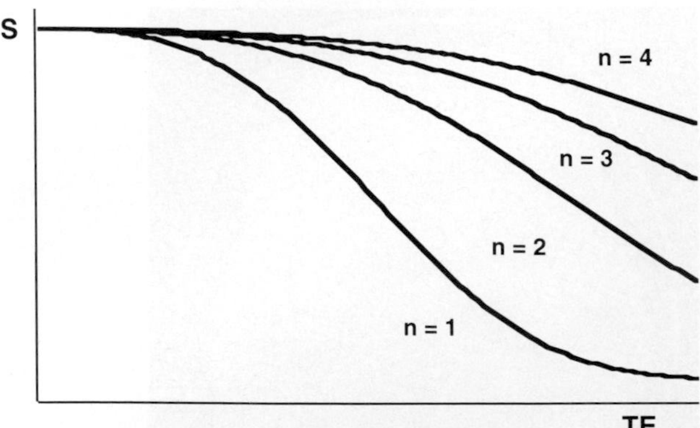

FIG. 38. Effect of the number of echoes in the echo train on the spin-echo signal in the presence of spin diffusion such as in hemorrhage. Note that as the echo number increases diffusion sensitivity decreases. Curves were computed from Equation 21.

However, in a train of closely-spaced echoes, the modulation is reduced and, in the limit of very short interecho spacing, suppressed altogether (70).

We thus infer that the retention of fat signal at long echo time is not necessarily a phenomenon unique to FSE imaging. It is generally expected to occur whenever the signal is derived from a fast CPMG spin-echo train. This may be verified by comparing a single or asymmetric dual-echo image to a CPMG multi-echo acquisition (Fig. 39).

The relative intensity of the fat in long-TE FSE images can confound clinical diagnosis in that these signals are now comparable to the ones characterizing pathologic states involving increased water concentration. For many FSE applications some form of fat suppression is therefore mandatory. An ingenious idea which makes use of the chemical shift $\Delta\nu$ (in Hz) between water and the CH_2 protons of fatty acid ester chains is to shift the time interval between the 90° and 180° pulse by an interval τ_c somewhat analogous to the method proposed by Dixon (71). However, τ_c is selected such that a phase difference of $2\pi\Delta\nu\tau_c = \pi/2$ results between fat and water protons at echo time (72). It can then be shown that the cumulative error in the pulse flip angle causes rapid restoration of the longitudinal magnetization from fat (with concomitant fast decay of the transverse component). By contrast, the self-correcting effect of the Meiboom-Gill modification (90° phase shift between the two initial rf pulses) leaves the magnetization from water intact. The enhanced decay upon introducing a τ_c delay of a quarter of the period of the fat-water. Of course, some of the more conventional fat-suppression techniques such as frequency-selective presaturation pulses (73) can readily be combined with FSE pulse sequences.

Finally, FSE imaging can be combined with magnetization preparation pulses, the most obvious one being an inversion-recovery pulse (67). Inversion-recovery (IR) images are well known to produce high gray-white matter contrast, but suffers from relative inefficiency in terms of the number of slices that can be imaged at a given TR (74). It is also useful as a means to suppress undesired signal components such as fat [short TI inversion-recovery = STIR (47)] or CSF (75). More recently, the synergistic effect prolonged T_1 and T_2 have on contrast in STIR has been used in conjunction with FSE, as a means for improved demonstration of MS lesions in the spinal cord [fast STIR, (76)], an example of which is shown in Fig. 40.

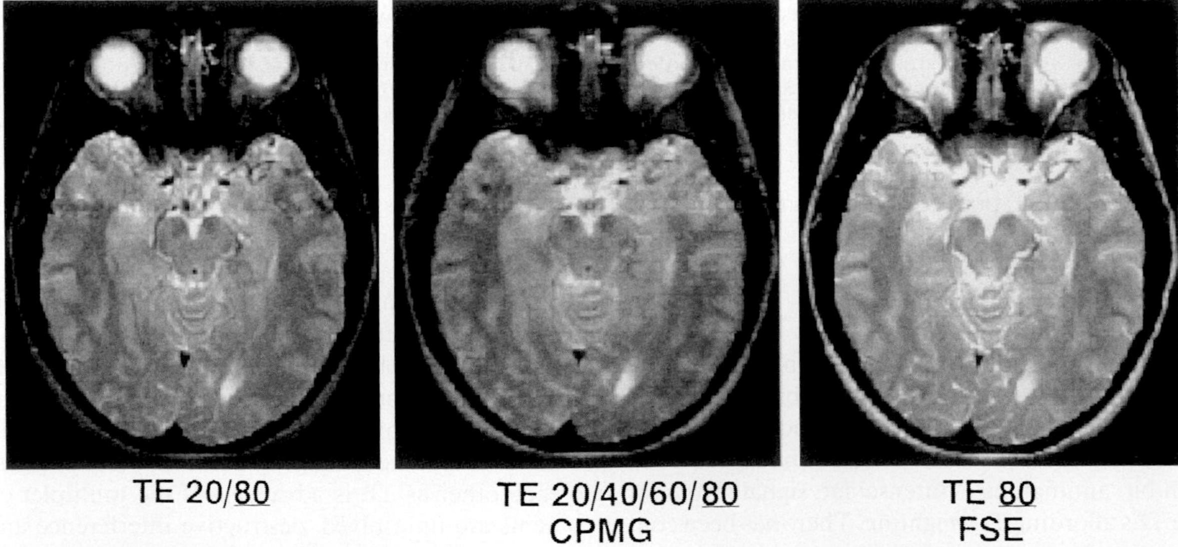

FIG. 39. Effect of echo spacing on relative fat-signal intensity for a spin-echo image obtained with an effective echo time of 80 msec. Note the increased fat intensity in the Carr-Purcell image obtained as the fourth of four equally spaced echoes, and more so, in the FSE image.

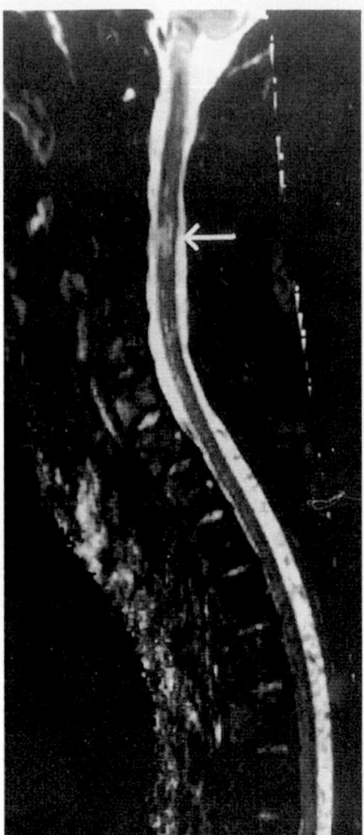
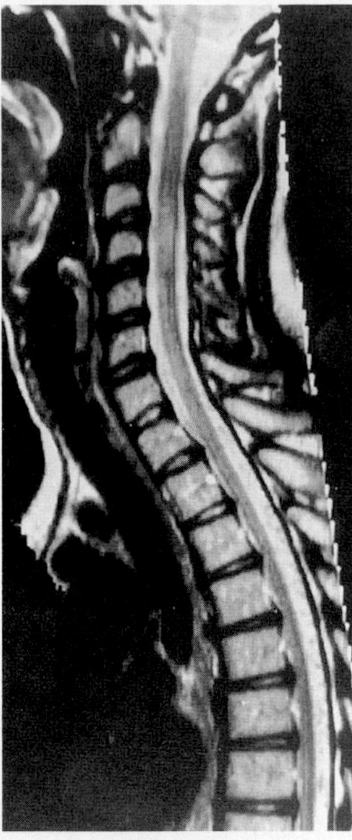

A,B

FIG. 40. MS of the cervical cord. **A:** Fast STIR. **B:** Conventional FSE. Note improved demonstration of MS lesions in A. (From Thorpe et al., ref. 76, with permission.)

Magnetization Transfer Effects

Magnetization transfer implies a process in which magnetization from a second, unobservable spin pool is transferred to the observable pool of water protons (77,78). Phenomenologically, one finds a tissue-specific decrease in signal upon irradiation off-resonance with a second radiofrequency. This effect has been ascribed to cross relaxation between the protons at the surface of macromolecules such as globular proteins and the protons in tissue water which are in contact with one another.

It is now well established that presaturation off-resonance by either a long low-amplitude pulse (77,79), or a series of short rf pulses (39), leads to tissue-specific signal attenuation. The effect has been observed in vivo (79,80) and constitutes a new type of tissue contrast. It is to be noted that the pre-irradiation need not be on-resonance (which would also saturate the observable water protons), since the linewidth of the cross-relaxing macromolecule protons is very wide. A detailed description of the mechanism will be found elsewhere in this book. While, of course, only the protons in the boundary layer (which are unobservable) are in direct contact with protein protons, the effect is transmitted to the observable tissue water protons via a phenomenon denoted "spin diffusion."

A very different and conceptually much simpler mechanism which may be operative in magnetization transfer is based on saturation transfer which would not involve cross relaxation at all. It would, in fact, simply be based on transfer of saturation of the protons in the broad resonance of hydrated water protons and the saturation would be transferred by way of chemical exchange.

However, how can this effect be present without irradiation of the protein protons? Dixon et al. (81) first analyzed what they termed "incidental magnetization transfer" effect. In order to understand this process we need to remember that the slice offset in multislice imaging is achieved by offsetting the excitation frequency in the presence of the slice-selection gradient. This is equivalent to irradiating the broad protein resonance at multiple frequencies.

While this effect is always present in 2D multislice imaging, it has been demonstrated that it is more prominent in FSE imaging (67,82). The effect was accounted to the large number of 180° pulses delivered in rapid succession at multiple offset frequencies. Particularly interesting and clinically relevant is the observation that the magnetization transfer-induced signal attenuation increases with increasing number of slices. The finding that the attenuation is greater for white matter than for gray matter further corroborates magnetization transfer as the origin of the effect. It is also noteworthy that fluids such as CSF do not exhibit attenuation with increasing number of slices thus excluding a direct interslice cross-talk effect. Also, cross talk would preferentially saturate the structures with long T_1 (i.e., CSF > GM > WM), opposite to the observed behavior. A plot of relative signal amplitude versus the number of slices imaged is shown in Fig. 41, along with FSE images acquired for different number of slices. The images in Fig. 41B clearly demonstrate increasing attenuation as the slice number is increased, as well as enhancement of gray-white matter contrast.

Flow Artifacts

We have previously seen that phase shifts experienced by moving spins from blood or CSF flow can be a significant source of artifacts, both signal loss due to intravoxel phase dispersion, and ghosting in the phase-encoding direction. The latter is a consequence of inconsistencies in phase dispersion during the cardiac cycle, leading to an amplitude modulation of the signal (vide infra for discussion of flow effects).

The phase shifts for constant velocity spins are proportional to the first moment, hence nulling of the first moment at echo time should correct the problem for flow in the frequency-encoding direction. However, in FSE imaging the echoes represent superpositions of Hahn

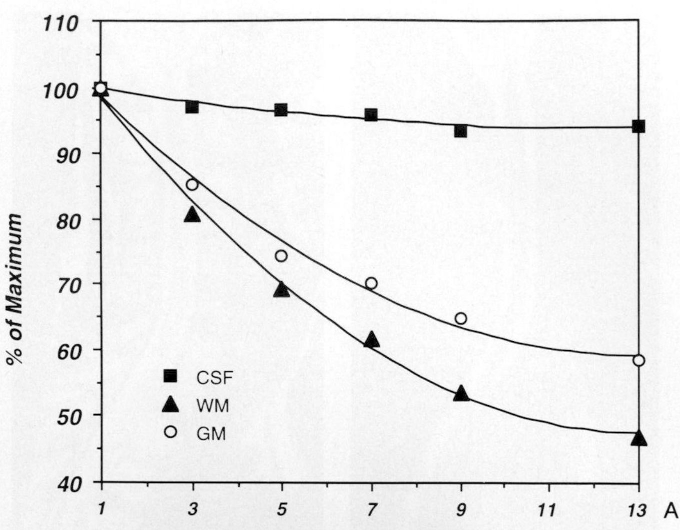

FIG. 41. Implications of the number of slices images in 2D multislice FSE imaging. **A:** Relative signal amplitude expressed as percentage of maximum versus number of slices *N* for CSF, gray matter, and white matter. (Data from Melki and Mulkern, ref. 82.) **B:** Proton-density (*top*) and T2-weighted FSE images obtained from 1, 5, and 10 slices. Images were obtained with otherwise identical parameters (B), using an interslice spacing of 100% of the slice thickness. The images have been displayed with equal display window settings. Note the marked attenuation with increasing slice number, in particular for white matter.

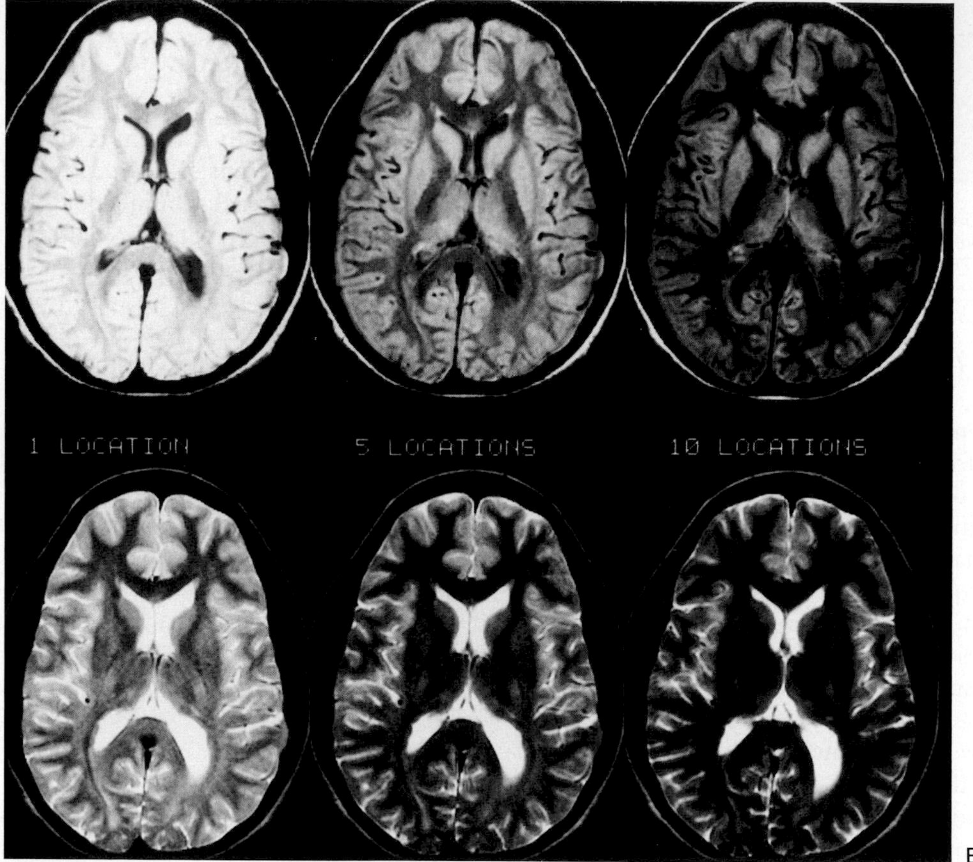

and stimulated echoes, the latter being caused by deviations in the flip angle from 180° (83). The stimulated echoes acquire phase at a different rate, leading to a phase mismatch between the two types of echoes even if the echo is first moment compensated. This problem has recently been solved by nulling the moments for both slice selection and readout gradient at the time of the refocusing pulses and preferably also at each echo (84). Figure 42 illustrates the effectiveness of FSE flow compensation.

Increased Echo Train Length

The relative efficiency of FSE imaging can be enhanced by shortening the inter-echo spacing ΔTE. The limiting factor in doing so is the time required for sampling each data line. For a given number of echoes in the train, shortened echo spacing also shortens echo train duration which, as we have seen earlier, narrows the point spread function and thus minimizes blurring

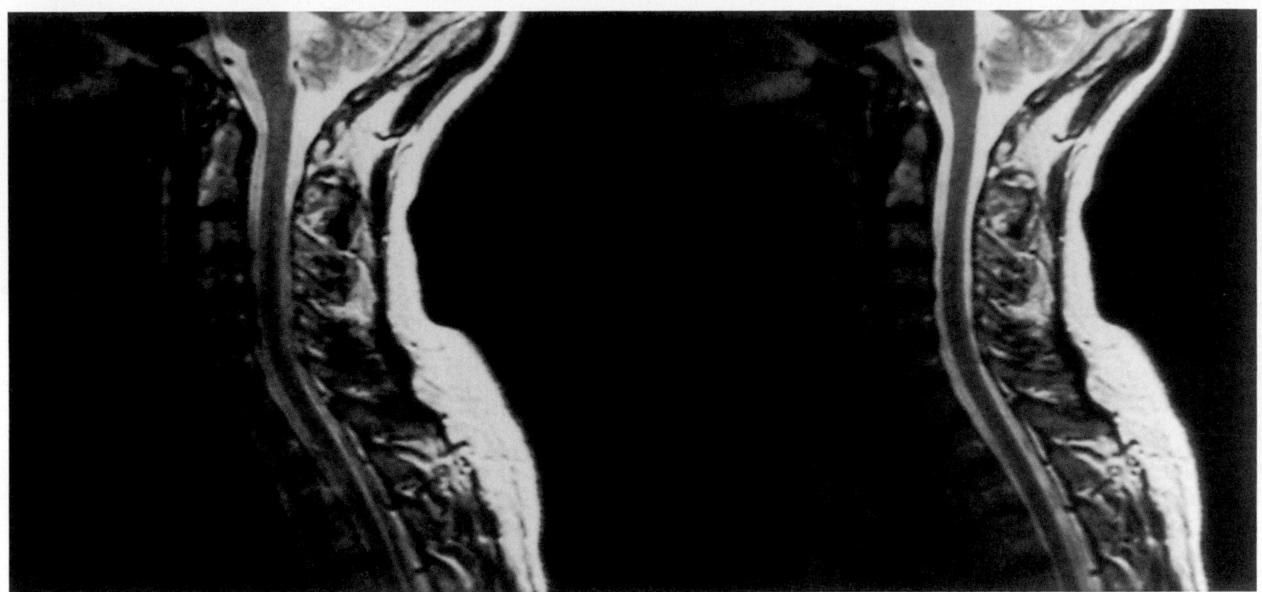

FIG. 42. FSE images of the cervical spine. **A:** Ghosting and CSF signal loss due to motion along readout gradient. **B:** Both problems are remedied by gradient moment nulling at the time of the 180° pulses (From Hinks and Constable, ref. 84, with permission.)

effects. An analysis of the time usage between successive 180° refocusing pulses shows that at least 50% is allocated to echo sampling. Shortening of the sampling period, however, requires increasing the sampling frequency bandwidth f_s, which is related to the readout gradient amplitude G_x and the field of view L by:

$$\gamma G_x L = 2\pi f_s \qquad [22]$$

From Equation 22 we recognize that increased sampling frequency bandwidth demands increased gradient amplitude which, of course, is limited by gradient hardware. This is a common limitation for many of the advanced imaging techniques and we will see in the subsequent section, on echo-planar imaging, that gradient performance, in terms of slew rate, amplitude, and permissible duty cycle, to a significant extent limit the performance of the MR imager. It has already been shown that acquisition of FSE images from a single train of 128 echoes is feasible, although $n = 32$ or 64 may be a more appropriate choice as these will allow for some contrast manipulation. Figure 43 shows a high-resolution (0.4 mm × 0.4 mm) head images obtained with a 2.2 G/cm gradient system, corresponding to $n = 32$.

It should be borne in mind that increased density of 180° pulses and the concomitant increased rf power deposition may pose some practical constraints to further enhancing efficiency in FSE imaging. Consider that the rf power deposited is proportional to $(\omega B_1)^2$, with ω being transmitter frequency and B_1 the amplitude of the rf field and further, since the flip angle α is proportional to B_1, a 180° pulse deposits four times as much power as its 90° counterpart. We also note that the problem is greatly exacerbated at high field. Hence, the specific absorption rate (SAR) essentially is determined by the number m of 180° pulses per unit time. In a typical 2D multislice pulse scan m $\approx$ 30/sec which, at 1.5-T field strength is achievable within the 2W/kg safety limit. It is readily seen that for an FSE pulse sequence with ΔTE = 15 msec, the number of 180° pulses administered is about twice this value.

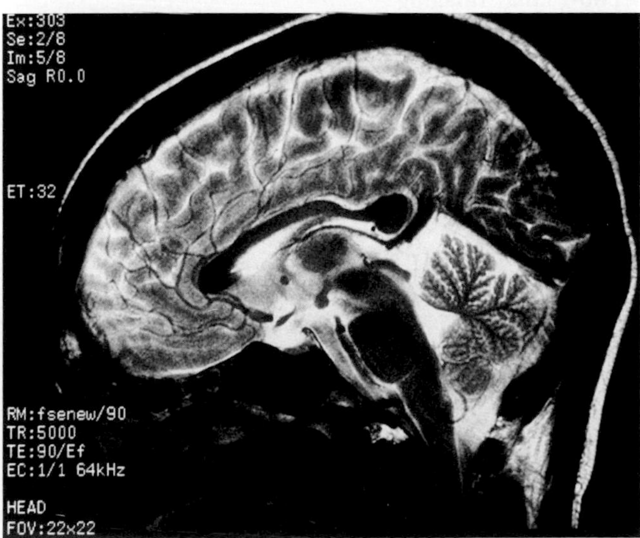

FIG. 43. High-resolution (512 × 512) FSE image obtained with echo train length $n = 32$, corresponding to inter-echo spacings of approximately 5 msec and 2 msec sampling time (±64 kHz sampling frequency bandwidth), in 5 minutes total scan time.

Three-Dimensional Fast Spin Echo

We have seen earlier that acquisition of 3D isotropic image data is a powerful means to obtain images which can be rearranged into other orthogonal or oblique planes. However, since scan time scales with the number of partitions (slice encodings), 3D spin-warp techniques demand short pulse repetition times in order to ensure tolerable scan times on the order of 10 minutes. Such a requirement is difficult to reconcile with a spin-echo technique where TR is more typically on the order of seconds, if proton-density or T2-weighting is desired. If we were able to encode 16 or 32 slices during a single-echo train, we could scan a volume in a time comparable to a 2D spin-echo acquisition. Further, since SNR scales as the square root of the number slice encodings, the improved SNR (by one order of magnitude) could then be traded for reduced slice thickness, which would obviously be needed to make multiplanar reformation practical. Recently, Yuan et al. (85) obtained 3D FSE images by stepping the slice-encoding gradient within the train of echoes, i.e., by covering k_z space, and incrementing k_y between echo trains.

The long TR required for obtaining proton-density or T2-weighted images leads to considerable dead time, which can be used by repeating the slice-encoding process on additional slabs, analogous to the multi-slab time-of-flight angiography (86). In this manner, a larger number of slices can be encoded at no additional cost in scan time. This principle is illustrated in Fig. 44.

Figure 45 shows a sagittal T_2-weighted FSE image, along with an axial image obtained by reformation of the 3D image array.

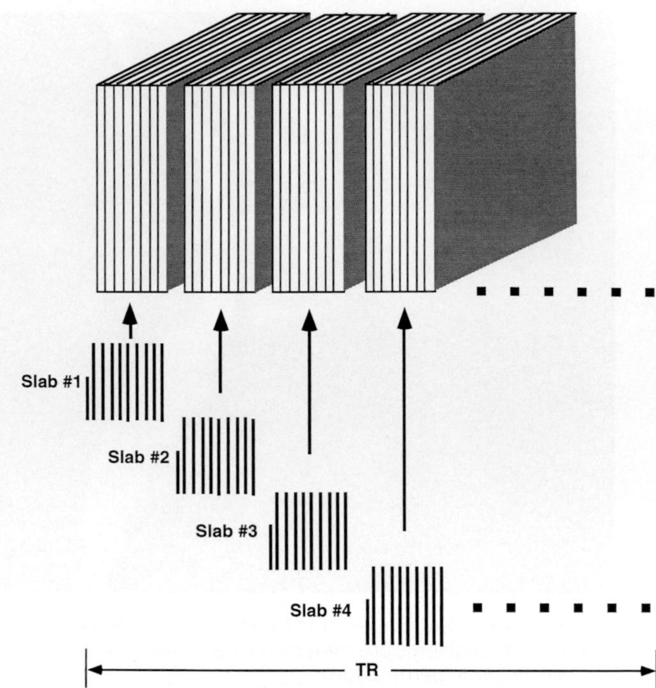

FIG. 44. Principle of multi-slab 3D FSE: each train of echoes (eight shown) partitions each of several thin slabs (four shown). In this manner, the entire TR period can be used effectively, analogous to 2D multislice imaging. In reality the slabs are placed so that they partially overlap one another and the images from border regions which are corrupted due to aliasing, are discarded.

Echo-Planar Imaging

Clearly, if we succeeded in generating as many echoes as we desire lines in k-space (number of pixels in the phase-encoding dimension), the data for an entire image could be acquired from a single excitation. The very high rf power deposition such a train of 180° pulses would entail, however, renders this proposition unrealistic. However, in lieu of 180° echoes, we can generate a series of gradient echoes, which can be acquired by means of a series of rapid reversals of the readout gradient. In addition, one needs to apply, prior to sampling of each of the echoes, a short phase-encoding gradient. This is the basis of echo-planar imaging (EPI), an experiment first reported by Mansfield more than 15 years ago (57) and first applied clinically to pediatric cardiac imaging (87). The technique was further perfected in the mid-1980s by Mansfield and coworkers (88), and, independently, Pykett and Rzedzian, who first demonstrated the feasibility of high-speed EPI at high field, using resonant gradient technology (89,90).

Single-Shot Echo-Planar Imaging

The many different approaches to single-shot EPI have been eloquently discussed in a review article by Cohen and Weisskoff (91) and some of the content of this section is excerpted from this work. It seems appropriate to begin with a brief historic overview. In Mansfield's original implementation, k-space was scanned by means of two spatial-encoding gradients: an oscillating read gradient G_x and a constant orthogonal gradient G_y (in modern parlance the "phase-encoding gradient"). The latter causes a continuous variation in k_x which, together with the oscillating read gradient leads to a zig-zag trajectory across k-space. The resulting raw data are thus not amenable to Fourier transformation without some form of pre-processing to place the data on a rectilinear grid. In Pykett and Rzedzian's approach, short phase-encoding gradients prior to each readout lead to a stepwise progression across k_y. Further, pre-encoding gradients are applied so that k_y is scanned from $-k_{y,max}$ to $+k_{y,max}$, as shown in Fig. 46. In Fig. 46A, the gradients are rectangular but for reasons discussed later, were sinusoidal. We can then, as shown earlier, construct the k-space trajectory from the gradient areas traversed at the various time points, labeled t_A through t_F (Fig. 46B). At time point t_A, before turning on any of the spatial-encoding gradients, $k_x = k_y = 0$ (center of k-space). After simultaneous appli-

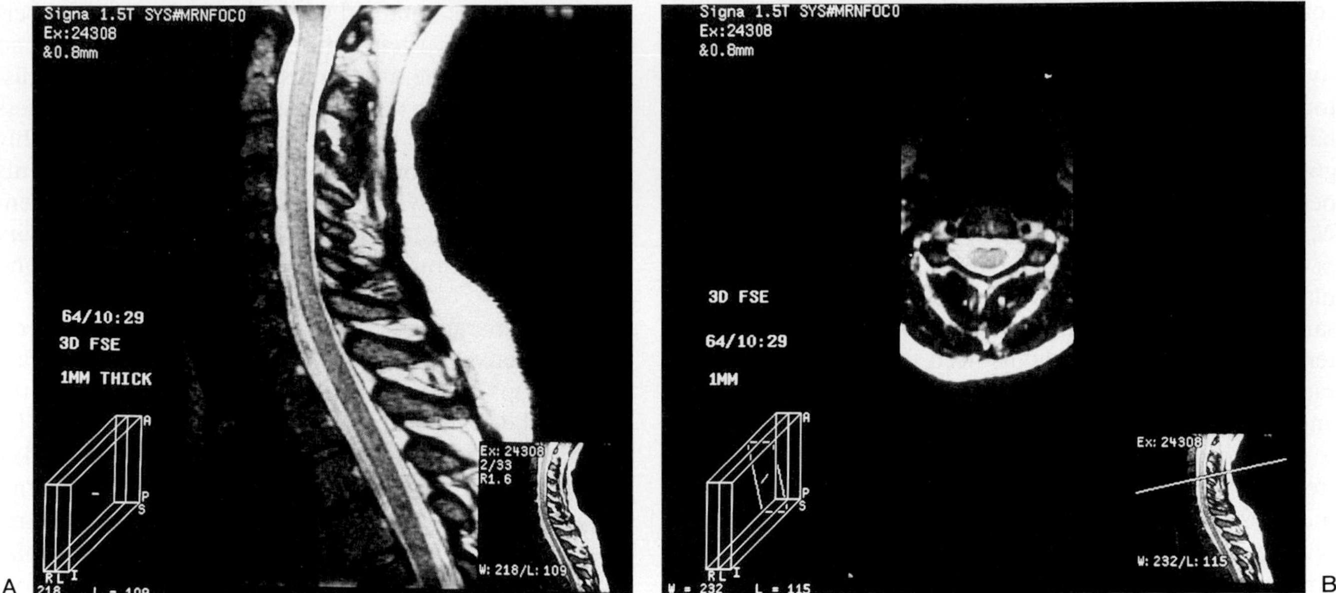

FIG. 45. A: Sagittal image (1-mm slice thickness) of C-spine, obtained from 32-slice 3D FSE series. **B:** Reformatted axial image from same data set. (Courtesy General Electric Medical Systems.)

cation of the two pre-encoding gradients, which in Fig. 46A are both positive, k_x,k_y advance to point B, the largest positive value of $k_{x,y,max}$. The subsequent 180° phase-reversal pulse leads to the corresponding conjugate location $-k_{x,y,max}$, i.e., the most negative k-value (point C). During the next-following time interval (t_C,t_D), during which only the positive read gradient is active, we sweep across k_x (with k_y constant) to end up at point D. Note that $k_x = 0$ corresponds to the center of the gradient echo which is attained when the area of the pre-encoding lobe of the frequency-encoding gradient is exactly equal to the area under the frequency-encoding gradient. Another important feature of this pulse sequence is that the center of k-space is traversed at the time of the Hahn

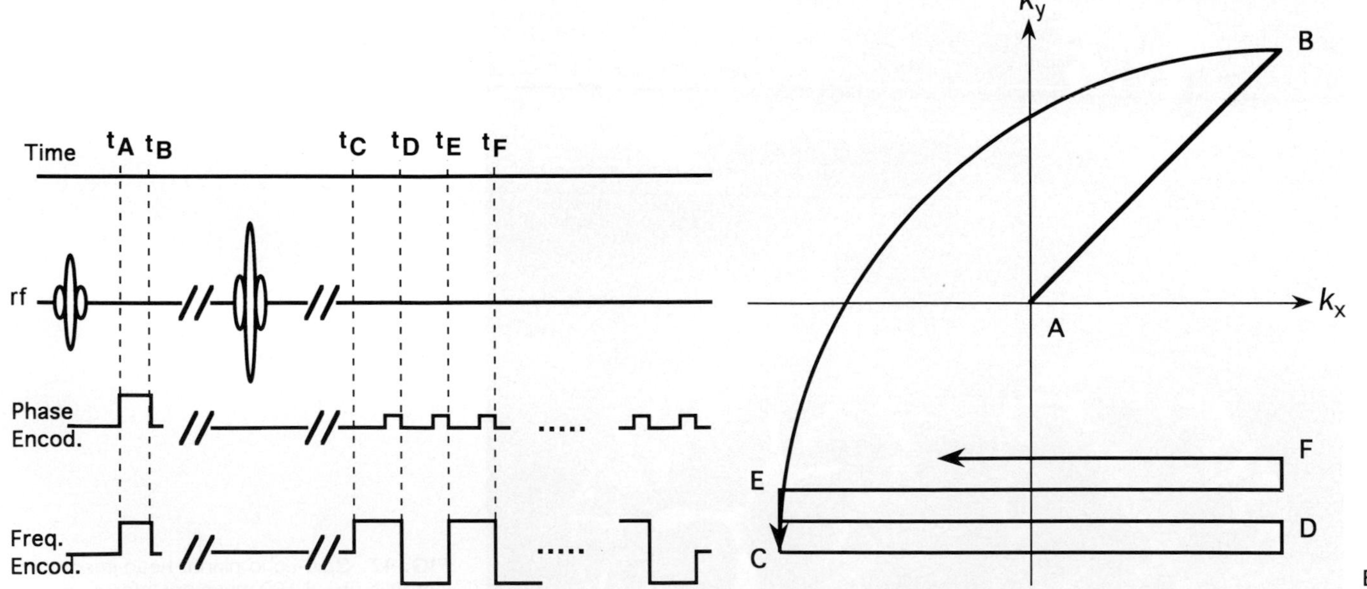

FIG. 46. A: Spin-echo EPI pulse sequence. A spin echo is produced so that $k_y = 0$ is traversed when spins are completely rephased, i.e., at echo time TE. Pre-encoding gradients ensure that both halves of k_y-space are scanned symmetrically. The time points $t_A - t_F$ correspond to locations A–F in the k-space trajectory (**B**). Note that the effect of the 180° pulse is to bring $+k_{x,y,max}$ to its conjugate $-k_{x,y,max}$. Each phase-encoding "blip" advances k_y by increment Δk_y. For simplicity, slice-selection gradients are not shown in A.

spin echo. The k trajectory in Fig. 46B scans k-space "bottom–up." It is readily seen that reversing the polarity of the y gradients would result in a top–down trajectory. The two approaches are, of course, equivalent. Perhaps the greatest technical challenge is to administer the gradient train sufficiently fast since the signal, of course, persists only for a time on the order of T_2^*. Thus the entire $N_p \times N_f$ samples have to be taken during a period comparable to T_2^*. It therefore becomes evident that an echo-planar imaging system has to operate at much higher sampling frequency than its conventional imaging counterpart. Further, the gradients need to be switched very rapidly, which requires short rise times. The phase-encoding "blip" has to be applied very rapidly as well to minimize total readout time. Since the higher spatial-frequency signals are weighted as $e^{-TE(k_y)/T_2^*}$, the technique is subjected to similar limitations as FSE, i.e., blurring in phase-encoding direction due to relative de-emphasis of high spatial frequency components may occur. In practice, however, this constraint is less severe since the resolution targeted with EPI in most instances has been lower than in FSE, with emphasis being on temporal rather than spatial resolution.

With current technology (>20 mT/m gradient amplitude and ≈200 T/m/sec slew rate), it is possible to acquire 128 × 128 echo-planar images in less than 100 msec scan time. The insensitivity to motion is exemplified with images obtained while the subject was deliberately performing a left-right tilting motion of the head (Fig. 47). While the motion resulted in gross overall displacements of the head, no effects of motion unsharpness or artifacts are seen. In neuroimaging, EPI will probably have applications for examining uncooperative patients and children who would have to be sedated for conventional imaging techniques, assuming that the sensitivity for lesion detection can approach that of fast spin-echo techniques.

When generating a train of gradient echoes under a spin-echo envelope, as shown in Fig. 46, in which case the zero spatial-frequency signals are collected at the time of the Hahn echo, the images are inherently T_2-weighted. In functional imaging (92–94) which makes use of the BOLD (blood oxygenation level dependent) contrast phenomenon (93,95,96), T_2* weighting is required. Under these constraints it is desirable to acquire the low spatial frequencies k_y data for gradient echoes with 30–50 msec echo time. For this purpose a gradient echo-planar technique is better suited. It is analogous to the pulse sequence sketched out in Fig. 46 except that the gradient-echo train begins immediately following a reduced flip-angle rf pulse (Fig. 48). Another feature of GE-EPI versus the spin-echo echo-planar (SE-EPI) variant is that the pulse sequence can be repeated more rapidly since the flip angle of the rf pulse can be adjusted.

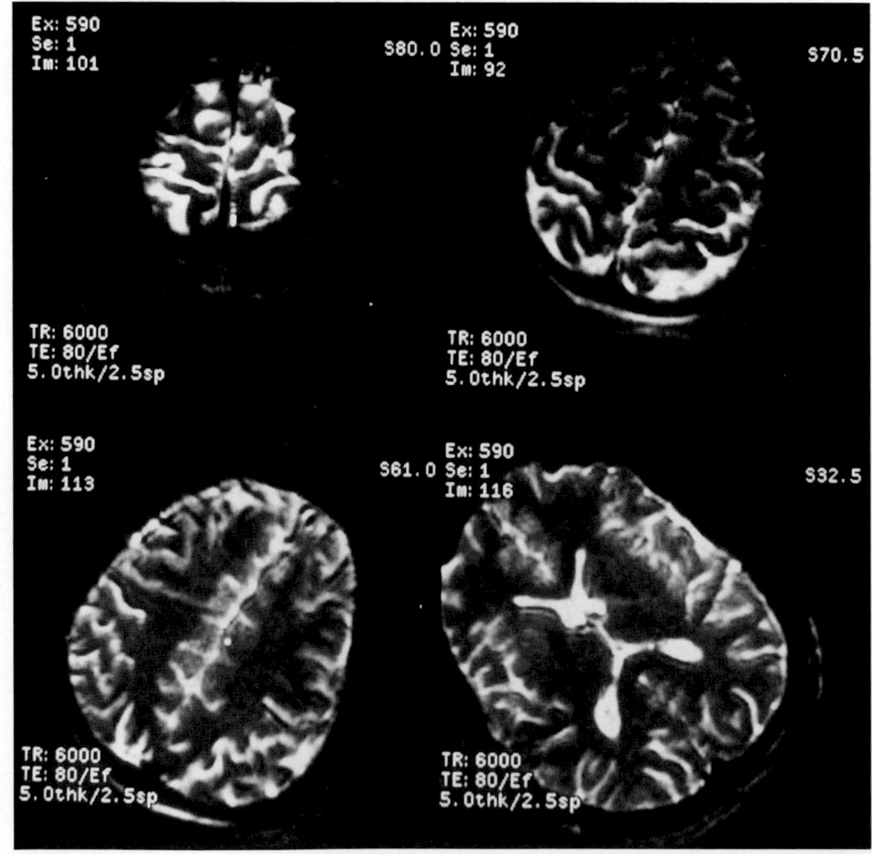

FIG. 47. Spin-echo-planar head images collected in about 100 msec per image while the subject was rocking the head sideways. Note that at this scan time motion is effectively "frozen" and the images exhibit no unsharpness or motion artifacts. (Images courtesy of General Electric Medical Systems.)

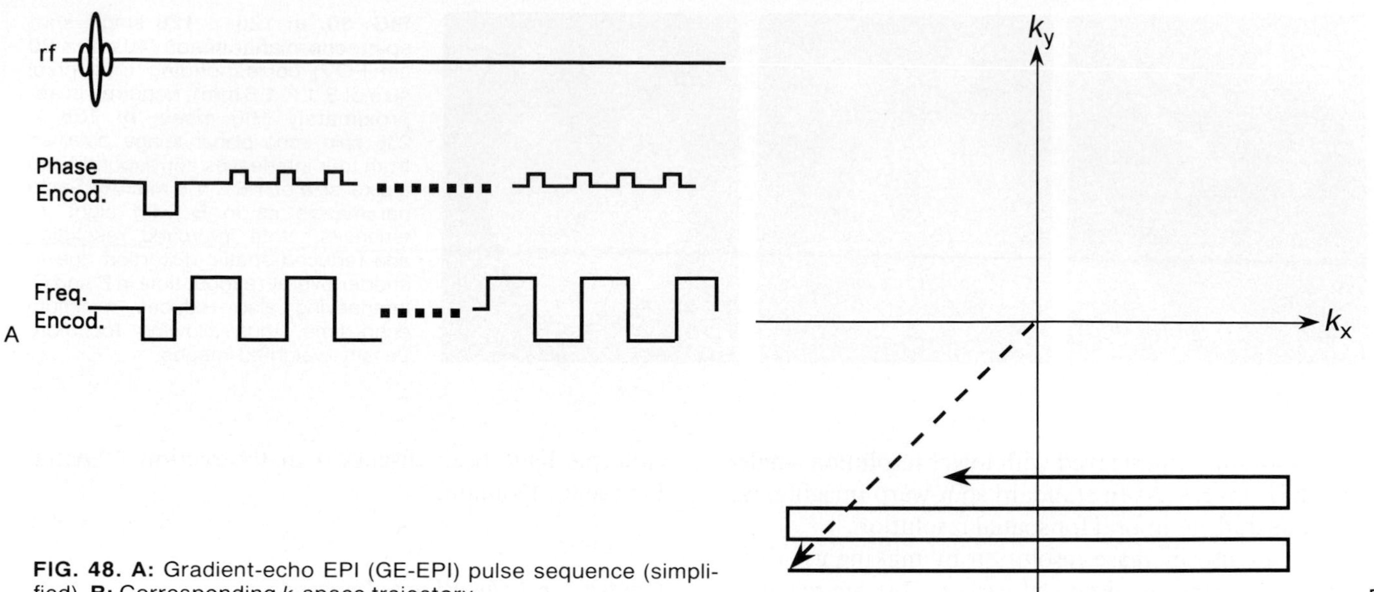

FIG. 48. A: Gradient-echo EPI (GE-EPI) pulse sequence (simplified). **B:** Corresponding *k*-space trajectory.

Hence, it entails the same advantages conventional single-line gradient-echo imaging has over spin-echo imaging. The technique is thus suited for repeated scanning, for instance for monitoring the time course of physiologic events such as following a bolus of contrast or the response to task activation (see Chapter 30).

Interleaved Echo-Planar Imaging

The hardware constraints in terms of gradient slew rates and amplitudes are relaxed if *k*-space is scanned in an interleaved manner rather than in a single traversal (97,98). In this case, it is only required that the time for an interleave be on the order of T_2^*. Since fewer lines are acquired during a single interleave, more time is available for each readout and thus the amplitude of the readout gradient can be lowered accordingly. Figure 49 shows the pulse sequence diagram for the case of two interleaves, each scanning eight lines, along with the *k*-space trajectory.

Alternatively, we can increase *y* resolution by sampling a greater number of lines without prolonging the echo train (which can cause artifacts due to phase accumulation from background gradients such as the ones arising from susceptibility effects). Figure 50 compares a

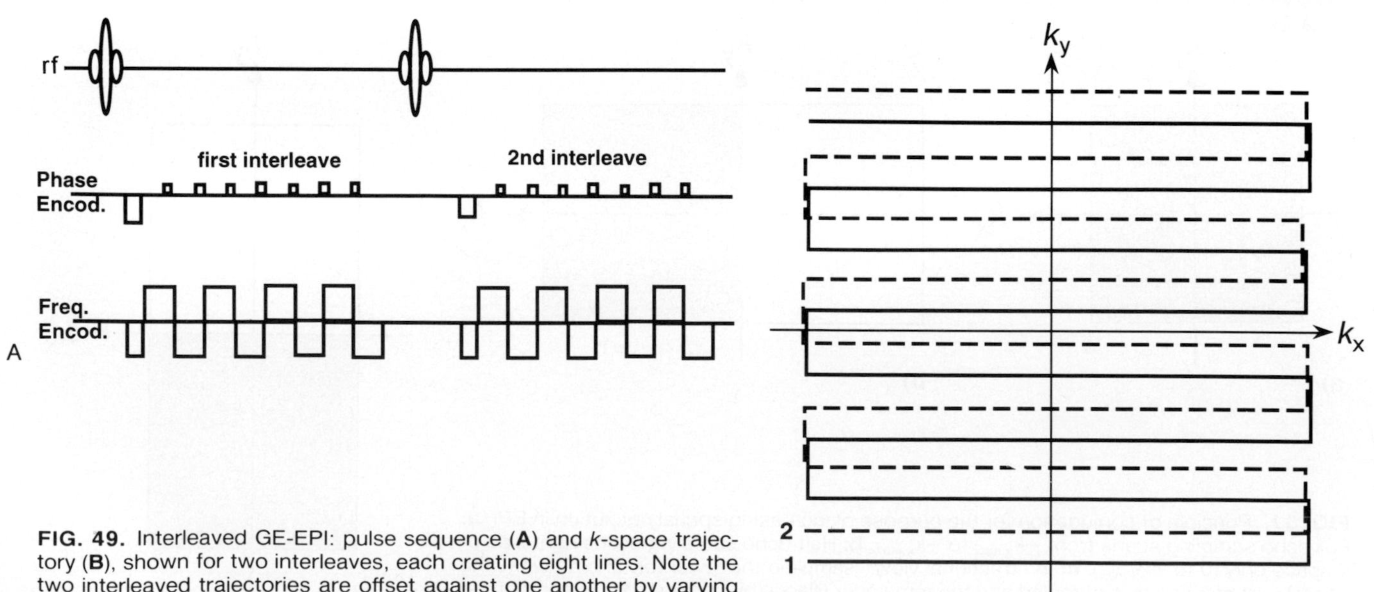

FIG. 49. Interleaved GE-EPI: pulse sequence (**A**) and *k*-space trajectory (**B**), shown for two interleaves, each creating eight lines. Note the two interleaved trajectories are offset against one another by varying the amplitude of the pre-encoding lobe of the phase-encoding gradient.

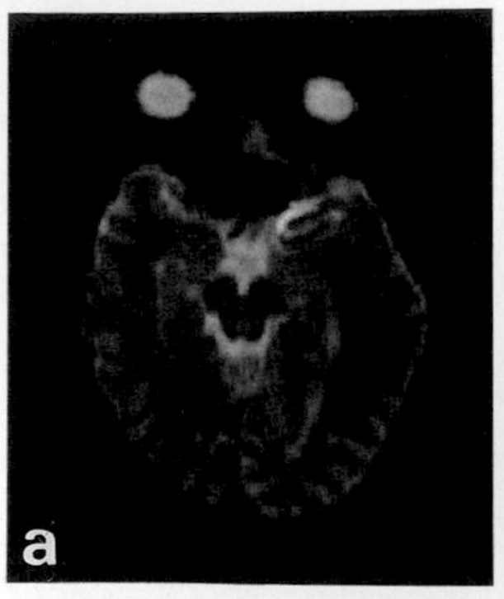

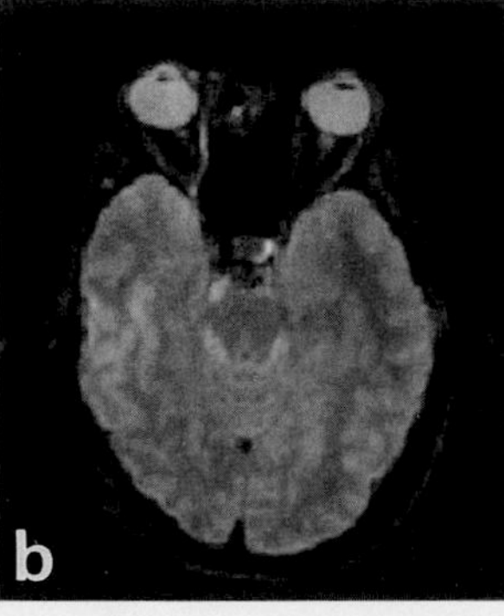

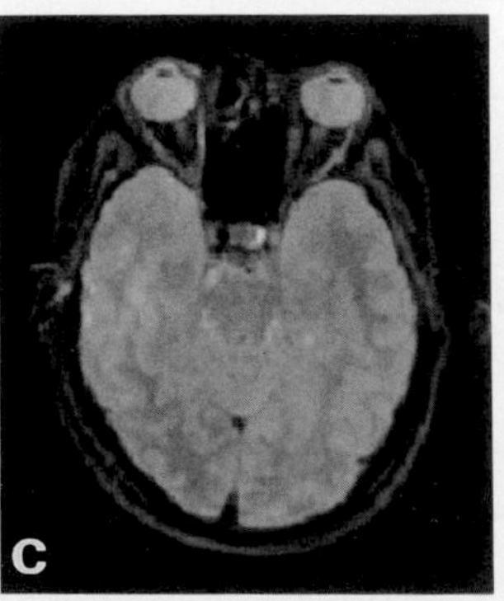

FIG. 50. a: 128 × 128 single-shot spin-echo-planar image (40 cm × 20 cm FOV) corresponding to a pixel size of 3.1 × 1.6 mm^2, acquired in approximately 100 msec. **b:** 128 × 256 spin-echo-planar image obtained from four interleaves corresponding to a pixel size of 1.6 × 1.6 mm^2. **c:** Same parameters as in B with eight interleaves. Note improved resolution and reduced spatial distortion due to shorter overall readout time in B and C. Interleaving also reduces minimum echo time, thus allowing for more density-weighted images.

high-resolution interleaved with lower resolution single-shot EPI images. As in standard spin-warp imaging, we can thus trade temporal for spatial resolution.

We can also increase resolution by making use of k-space symmetry, as discussed earlier. One approach to achieve this is to sample only a fractional echo (essentially the descending portion), rather than the full echo. The reduction in sampling time can then be used to collect the same number of samples to cover the right-hand side of k-space and fill in the left by conjugation. It is readily seen that in this manner, resolution is effectively doubled. Alternatively, the upper or lower half of data space can be sampled and the remainder again filled in retrospectively. In either case, the total readout time is essentially unaltered (which is important since any prolongation would have the usual adverse effects in terms of point spread function blurring and signal loss). Again, the constraints imposed by gradient amplitude and slew rates are relaxed if interleaved trajectories are used. The two approaches of extended sampling combined with conjugation are shown schematically in Fig. 51. These concepts have been discussed in the section, "Spatial Frequency Domain."

Contrast in Echo-Planar Imaging

Contrast in EPI is governed by the usual parameters: pulse repetition time, flip angle, and echo time at which the low spatial frequency echoes are sampled. It is readily seen, however, that in single-shot SE-EPI no TR can be defined since there is only a single pulse sequence cycle. Hence, TR = ∞ applies which, in conjunction with short effective echo time, results in heavy proton-density weighting. T_2 weighting is achieved by offsetting the 180° pulse and echo train (Fig. 48, above).

Often we wish to scan the same locations in regular time intervals, for example to follow the time course of some physiologic event, such as the passage of a bolus of contrast material or during task performance paradigms (see, for example, Chapter 30). In this case a steady state is established and gradient-echo echo-planar contrast is

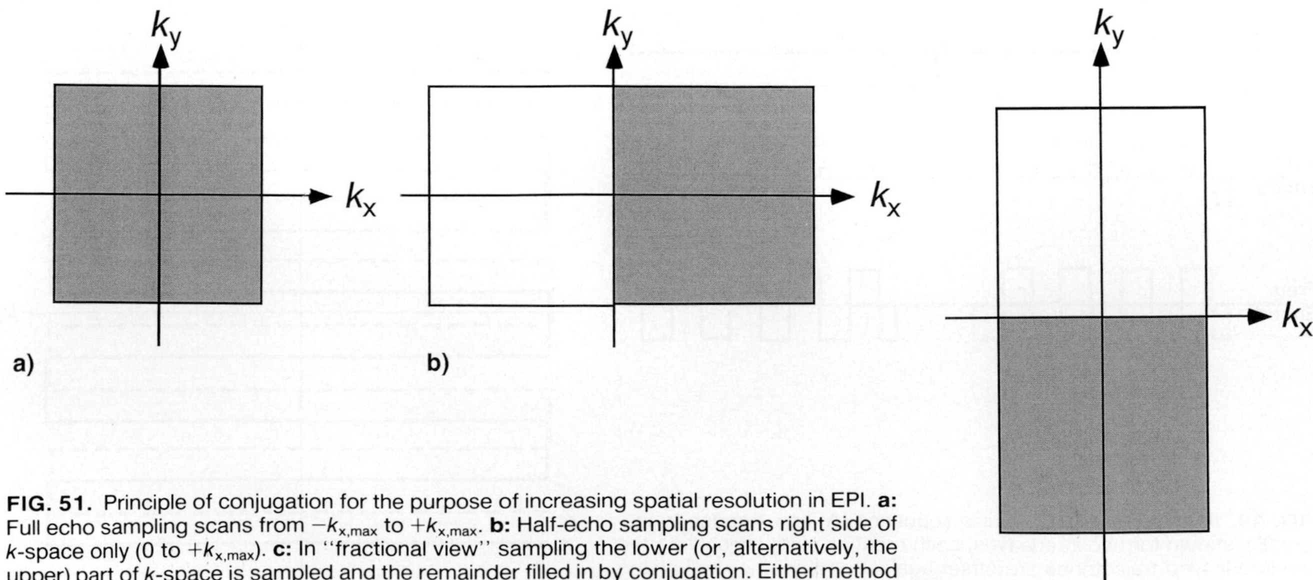

FIG. 51. Principle of conjugation for the purpose of increasing spatial resolution in EPI. **a:** Full echo sampling scans from $-k_{x,max}$ to $+k_{x,max}$. **b:** Half-echo sampling scans right side of k-space only (0 to $+k_{x,max}$). **c:** In "fractional view" sampling the lower (or, alternatively, the upper) part of k-space is sampled and the remainder filled in by conjugation. Either method allows doubling of spatial resolution in one of the in-plane spatial dimensions.

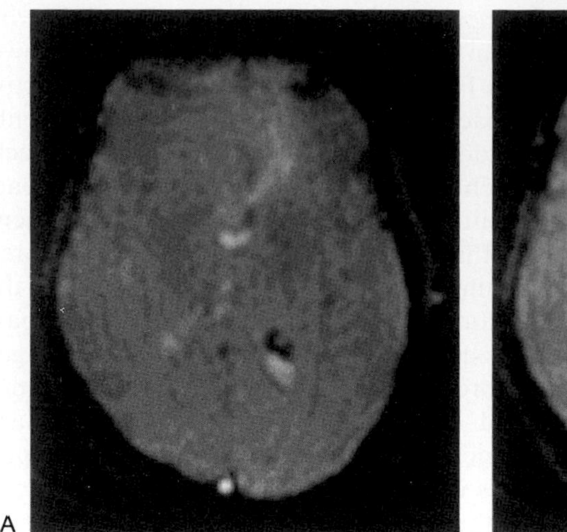
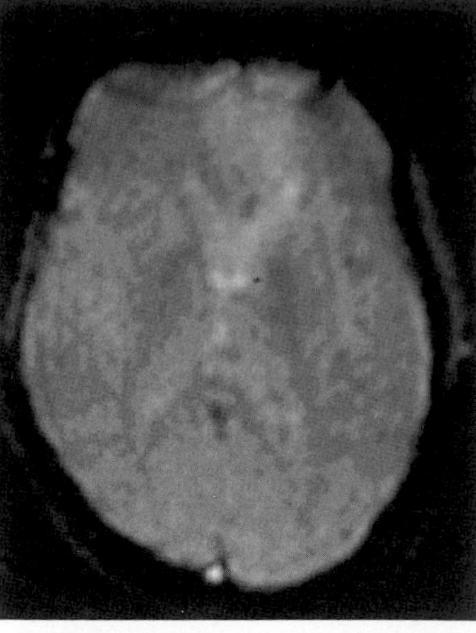
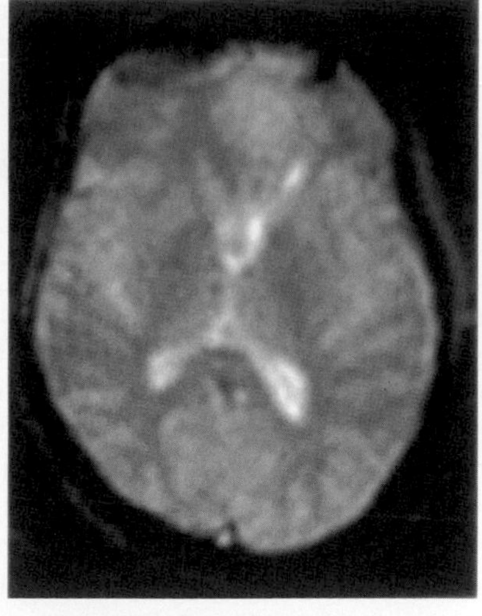

A B,C

FIG. 52. Single-shot gradient-echo-planar images obtained by repeating the scan every 500 msec, corresponding to flip angles of 90°, 55°, and 30°, respectively (**A–C**) showing the effect of decreased spin saturation as the flip angle is lowered. Images A and B are mixed weighted (T_1, T_2) whereas image C clearly exhibits the hallmarks of T2 weighting (CSF > GM > WM).

determined by TR, flip angle, and echo time obeying Equation 7 for gradient-echo imaging. Figure 52 shows the progression from T_1 to proton-density weighting.

Chemical Shift Effect

Since the sampling frequency bandwidth in EPI is very high ($\approx$500 kHz) and thus the bandwidth per pixel ($\approx$4000 Hz for 128 data samples) far exceeds the chemical shift, misregistration in frequency encoding is negligible. However, the effect is prohibitive in the phase-encoding direction. This becomes evident when we consider that 128 echoes are collected in a time on the order of 50 msec, or about 0.5 msec per sample which is equivalent to a sampling frequency of about 2000 Hz (1/0.0005). The corresponding bandwidth per pixel thus is about 15 Hz/pixel. With the chemical shift at 1.5 T being on the order of 220 Hz, the resulting pixel shift about 15 pixels or about 10% of the field of view (Fig. 53). Several schemes lend themselves to correct for this effect. The simplest approach compatible with multislice EPI is a frequency-selective presaturation pulse on-resonance with the fat signal that can be applied to eliminate the undesired resonance (99). A more elegant solution is the spatial spectral pulse, an rf pulse which is both frequency and spatially selective. Alternatively, in spin-echo EPI the 180° phase reversal pulse is made frequency-selective, by tuning it to the frequency of the water resonance (89). Other possibilities include a magnetization preparation pulse such as a 180° inversion pulse, followed by a STIR delay (74). In order to obtain images showing both water and fat, the data from two successive acquisitions (one being fat-selective, the other water-selective) could be combined.

Instrumental Requirements

We have already pointed out that a critical requirement in EPI is the condition that the echo train be played out and sampled in a time on the order of T_2^*, i.e., about 50–100 msec for most tissues. In a SE-EPI sequence of 128 data lines (phase encodings) we are thus required to read the 64 gradient echoes before and after the Hahn spin echo in about 50 msec. Hence, the echo spacing is 0.78 msec = 780 μsec. The frequency-encoding gradient

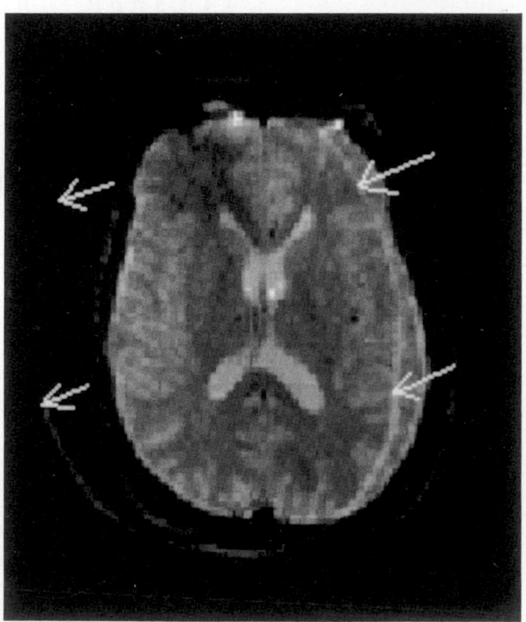

FIG. 53. Echo-planar image acquired without fat saturation, exhibiting chemical shift artifact in phase-encoding direction (*arrows*).

amplitude is dictated by the sampling rate bandwidth f_s and the FOV as usual:

$$\gamma G_x \mathrm{FOV}_x = f_s \qquad [23]$$

Further, the data sampling time is t_s given as:

$$t_s = \frac{N_x}{f_s} \qquad [24]$$

where N_x is the number of frequency encodings. Assuming a sampling frequency of 256 kHz, the sampling time, according to Equation 24 would be 0.5 msec = 500 μsec. Suppose a desired FOV in the frequency-encoding direction of 30 cm, γ = 4.25 kHz/G, Equation 23 affords for the strength of the frequency-encoding gradient G_x = 256/(4.25 × 20) = 2 G/cm. Further, since the flat top of the gradient used for sampling need at least be 500 μsec, the ramp time from 0 to 2 G/cm cannot be longer than 140 μsec, which demands a slew rate of 14.3 G/cm/msec, or 143 T/m/sec. These relationships, illustrating the critical role of gradient amplitude and slew rate in high-speed imaging, are shown graphically in Fig. 54.

Achieving rapid ramping of gradients poses significant technical challenges. An early solution to this problem is the resonant gradient technology by Rzedzian (100,101) which, in essence, is an energy recovery system allowing rapid oscillation of the gradients without excessive power requirements. The principle is to couple the inductive load to a capacitive network tuned to the gradients' switching frequency. There are two obvious drawbacks to this approach. The first is a fixed operating frequency and peak amplitude for the oscillating readout gradient. The second is that the *k*-space map obtained is not a rectilinear grid since Δk is not constant. In practice, this means that prior to Fourier reconstruction the data have to be regridded. A more recent solution which gets around these problems is the "catch and hold" technology developed by Advanced NMR Instruments and General Electric. It is based on a resonant power supply which operates in a resonant mode during the rise and fall periods of the gradient, but switches to a nonresonant mode upon reaching peak amplitude (101).

Since high-amplitude rapidly switched gradients benefit many other applications (e.g., fast spin echo with short echo spacing and flow compensation, rapid oblique imaging), a gradient system permitting generation of arbitrary waveforms would be preferable. A design overcoming the limitations of the previously mentioned approaches is based on a pulse width modulated power

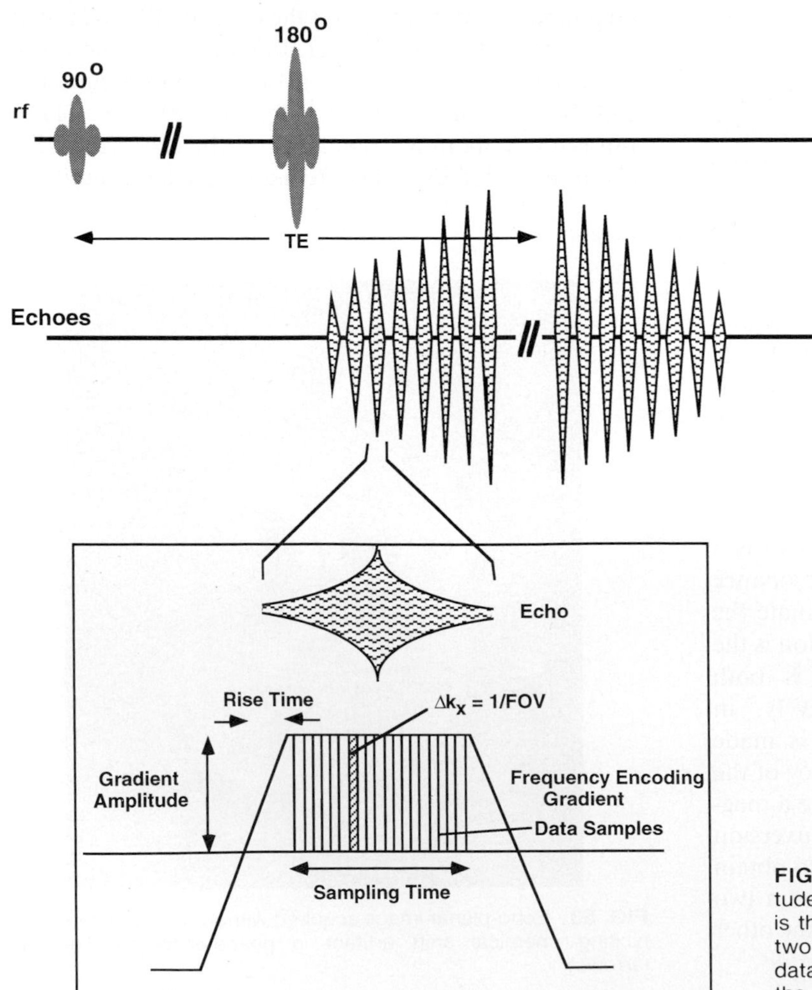

FIG. 54. Relationship between data sampling time, amplitude of the readout gradient, and FOV. Note that the FOV is the reciprocal of the area under the gradient between two successive data samples (Δk_x). The time available for data sampling is determined by the length of the flat top of the gradient which is governed by the gradients' slew rate.

supply which is capable of outputting a train of short high-amplitude pulses from which any desired gradient waveform can be synthesized (101). The three different approaches are illustrated in Fig. 55.

SNR and Spatial Resolution

Finally, one wonders what SNR penalty EPIs extraordinary scan speed exacts. At a given resolution three parameters contribute to SNR: (i) sampling time (SNR $\approx \sqrt{t_s}$), (ii) transverse relaxation losses (SNR $\approx e^{-TE/T_2}$), and (iii) the fraction of magnetization available for signal generation (determined by saturation (SNR $\approx f(TR, T_1, \alpha)$). The following comparison may be instructive. Suppose a typical tissue such as neural white matter is scanned at 1.5-T field strength ($T_1 \approx 700$ msec, $T_2 \approx 75$ msec). Then consider a high-speed gradient-echo acquisition with 128 phase encodings and 2 msec readout time, TR = 5 msec, TE $\approx$ 0, operated at the optimum flip angle, which is 6.8°, and compare it to a single-shot EPI with 50 msec total sampling time, performed such that $k_y = 0$ is sampled at TE = 30 msec. The results are summarized in Table 1. They imply a net advantage of about a factor of 5 in favor of EPI, defeating the common notion that shortened scan time inevitably exacts a SNR penalty.

Similar arguments in favor of EPI have been put forward by Cohen and Weisskoff (91). Obviously, if we were to repeat the EPI scan every 640 msec, i.e., the equivalent of the FLASH data acquisition time, this would mean that the longitudinal magnetization has only incompletely recovered, therefore requiring operation at the Ernst angle, which is 65°. Doing so reduces the transverse magnetization following the rf pulse to 0.64 (from Equation 7), thus lowering the relative SNR advantage of EPI to (a still substantial) factor of 3.

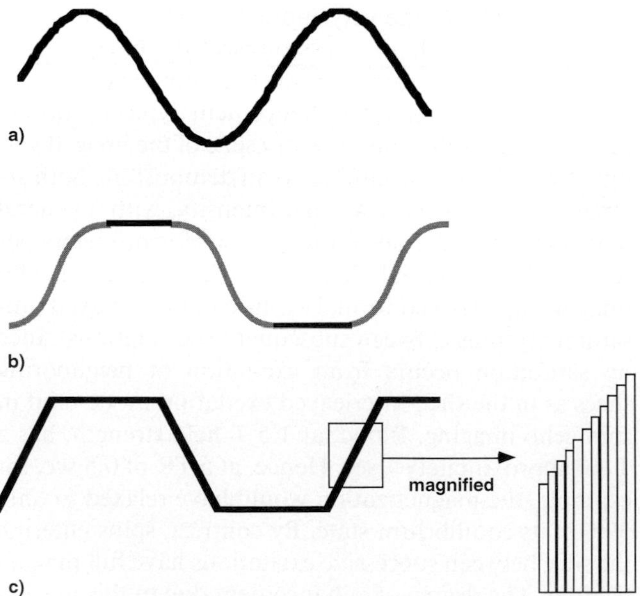

FIG. 55. Echo-planar readout gradient waveforms. **a:** sinusoidal (resonant gradients). **b:** "Catch and hold" (resonant/nonresonant). **c:** pulse width modulation technology where the gradient waveform is generated digitally from rectangular pulses of different width and amplitude.

TABLE 1. *Comparison of SNR in single-shot EPI and high-speed FLASH*[a]

	EPI	FLASH	SNR_{EPI}/SNR_{FLASH}
Sampling time (msec)	50	256	0.44
Magnetization	1	0.06	16.7
exp (−TE/T2)	0.67	1	0.67
Net gain			4.9

[a] For assumptions see text.

Figure 56A shows a series of single-shot gradient echo-planar images acquired every 500 msec (α = 30°). Multiple images are shown to demonstrate that the SNR and contrast shown is obtained in a steady-state regime, rather than with TR = ∞. Compared to the spoiled GRASS image obtained in 900 msec (TR = 7 msec, α = 5°) in Fig. 56B the echo-planar images exhibit vastly superior SNR.

CLINICAL APPLICATIONS OF FAST IMAGING IN THE CNS

At the time of this writing, many of the available fast imaging techniques have now assumed at least adjunctive roles, if not completely supplanting conventional spin-echo imaging, in routine clinical protocols for brain and spine disease. For instance, high-speed gradient-echo methods (both 2D and 3D) are the mainstay of flow imaging, most often as part of MR angiography (see Chapter 31). Gradient-echo imaging is also routinely employed in the search for intracranial hemorrhage and calcification in many clinical settings (Table 2), where it is generally used as an adjunctive scan. This clinical indication for gradient-echo imaging has become more important due to the introduction of fast spin-echo sequences, which are inherently less sensitive to susceptibility-induced signal loss than conventional spin-echo imaging. Three-dimensional volume gradient-echo acquisitions are utilized in virtually all cervical spine disc disease cases and are often the only sequence aside from an initial sagittal scan in this setting. In some centers, 3D volume methods are beginning to be used for preoperative planning in intracranial mass lesions. As already noted, steady-state gradient-echo techniques play a small part in helping to distinguish cystic from solid masses. In comparison to the somewhat limited role of gradient-echo scanning, fast spin-echo techniques have essentially replaced conventional spin-echo imaging for a wide variety of clinical indications, particularly in spinal cord evaluation (where concern for hemorrhage is less common), brain diseases not typically associated with hemorrhage, and in all cases where high resolution T_2-weighted imaging is desired (e.g., orbit, temporal

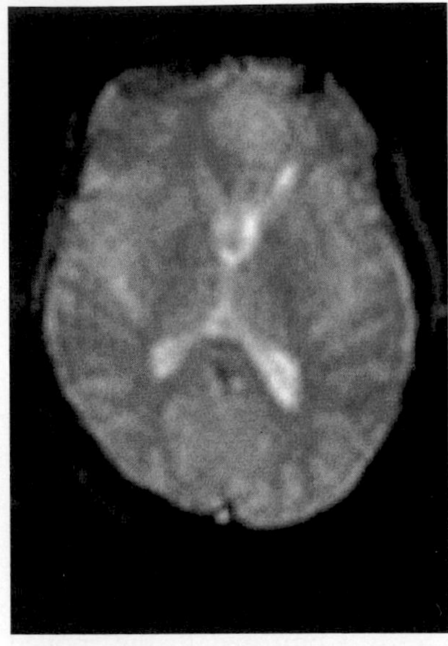
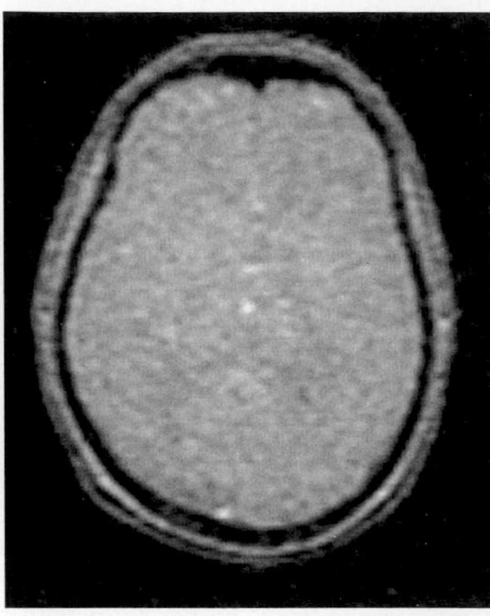

A,B

FIG. 56. A: One of a series of single-shot gradient echo-planar images acquired every 500 msec ($\alpha = 30°$) showing excellent SNR and contrast, as opposed to the spoiled GRASS image (**B**) obtained in 900 msec (TR = 7 msec, $\alpha = 5°$). The flip angles were adjusted to account for the different effective TR times.

bone). Clinical indications for ultrafast imaging methods, most commonly employing echo-planar acquisitions, are only beginning to be explored at this time (see Chapter 30). The rationale for the respective clinical roles for these fast imaging methods and principles underlying their basis will be discussed below.

Flow Imaging by Gradient-Echo Techniques

Flow often has a very characteristic appearance on gradient-echo images, and indeed the depiction of flow as high intensity is truly one of the most important and clinically useful features of these techniques, which form the basis of the vast majority of MR angiographic protocols in current use. As in spin-echo imaging, the appearance of flow is complicated by vessel orientation, flow velocity, the nature of flow (e.g., laminar versus turbulent), pulse repetition time, and the acquisition mode (2D, 3D). As a result of this, the signal emanating from flowing spins can fall virtually anywhere within the entire range of the MR grayscale (see also Chapters 4 and 31). There are three general mechanisms for the stereotypical demonstration of flowing spins as high intensity on sequentially-acquired gradient-echo scans: inflow effects from continual wash-in of unsaturated spins, lack of outflow-related signal loss because of the lack of slice-selectivity of the refocusing pulse, and the use of gradient compensation for flow-related phase-changes. This method is commonly referred to as 2D "time-of-flight" MR angiography and is probably the most commonly employed technique for extracranial carotid bifurcation evaluation, as well as having uses in the assessment of intracranial venous abnormalities.

TABLE 2. *Clinical indications for performing susceptibility-weighted gradient-echo scan*[a,b]

Hemorrhagic infarction
Occult cerebrovascular malformation (cavernous hemangioma)
Follow-up head trauma (acute or chronic)
Metastases (from tumors prone to hemorrhage, especially melanoma)
Hemorrhage from AVM
Child abuse
Seizure history

[a] Especially when the spin-echo images are normal.
[b] Using short flip angle and long TE.

Flow-Related Enhancement

A striking feature of sequential-mode gradient-echo images is the high-intensity appearance of vascular structures, especially when vessels transect the imaging slice (102–104). In contrast to multislice spin-echo imaging where such flow-related enhancement typically occurs only for venous flow on the entry slice of the imaged volume, gradient-echo techniques can demonstrate both arterial and venous flow as high intensity, with a general sensitivity to flow rates on the order of centimeters per second. In sequential 2D time-of-flight gradient-echo imaging, there is a continual wash-in of fully relaxed (unsaturated) spins between subsequent rf excitations, since no saturation occurs from excitation of neighboring slices as in the slice-interleaved excitation mode used in spin-echo imaging. Blood, at 1.5 T field strength, has a T_1 of approximately 1 sec. Hence, at a TR of 0.5 sec, for example, the magnetization would have relaxed to only 39% of its equilibrium state. By contrast, spins entering the slice between successive excitations have full magnetization. The degree of enhancement due to this mechanism is actually a function of several factors (105), including: the flow velocity v, the thickness of the imaging volume d (slice thickness in 2D techniques, slab thickness in 3D), the pulse repetition time TR, and the T_1 of the fluid. Figure 57A illustrates the degree of penetration of the fluid bolus at the end of a TR cycle for three different flow velocities labeled v_1, v_2, and v_3. Likewise, a longer TR and a thinner section will cause a higher degree of spin replacement. We, therefore, expect the degree of flow-related enhancement to be more significant in 2D GRASS than in 3D GRASS (where spins reaching the middle of the slab have already been saturated). Figure 57B shows the signal intensity plotted for a series of 90° pulses as a function of the flow velocity.

Importantly, there is a flip angle dependence of the vascular signal (105). In the non-steady-state situation, the difference in signal intensities between inflowing spins and stationary spins is, to a great extent, related to the flip angle: the larger the flip angle, the greater the difference in signal intensities. Since inflowing spins carry full magnetization, one predicts maximum signal for the condition where $\alpha = 90°$ as long as there is complete spin replacement between successive pulse sequence cycles. However, for flow this condition is usually not satisfied. Moreover, the total vascular signal (consisting of multiple fractions) may be maximal at flip angles $\alpha < 90°$ since the optimum flip angle for partially relaxed spins, as we have seen earlier, is less than 90°.

Outflow Effects

The second important difference between gradient-echo imaging and spin-echo techniques that accounts for the hyperintensity of vascular and CSF flow lies in the selectivity of the refocusing mechanism. In conventional spin-echo imaging, signal void from rapid flow can be at least partially ascribed to spins moving out of the slice between the excitation and refocusing pulses, both of which are slice-selective (106,107). To emit a signal in spin-echo imaging, both pulses must obviously be experienced by the spin. In (2DFT) gradient-echo imaging, the excitation pulse is slice-selective, just as in spin-echo imaging. However, the refocusing mechanism (in this case, reversal of the readout gradient) is not slice-selective. Therefore, spins that originally are in the appropriate slice for the application of the excitation rf pulse can still contribute signal, even if they have moved out of that plane during the "interpulse" time (TE/2), assuming that they have not left the volume subject to the application of the gradient for readout. The non-selectivity of refocusing in gradient-echo imaging does not result in absolute hyperintensity of flowing spins; it merely gives the flowing spins the same signal they would generate if they were stationary.

Phase Effects and Gradient Compensation

Let us suppose that spins residing at position r are exposed to a gradient of amplitude G. These spins resonate at frequency $\omega = \gamma G\, r$. However, spins moving in the direction of the gradient advance linearly toward higher magnetic field. As a consequence, their resonance frequency increases as $\omega = \gamma G\, r + \gamma G\, vt$ (Fig. 58). Hence they accumulate phase relative to their stationary counterparts. Since phase is the integral over time of frequency, we can write for the phase:

$$\int \omega dt = \gamma G\, r\, dt = \gamma G\, rt \qquad [25a]$$

and

$$\int \omega dt = \int (\gamma G\, r + \gamma G\, vt) dt = \gamma G\, rt + \gamma G\, r\, vt^2/2 \qquad [25b]$$

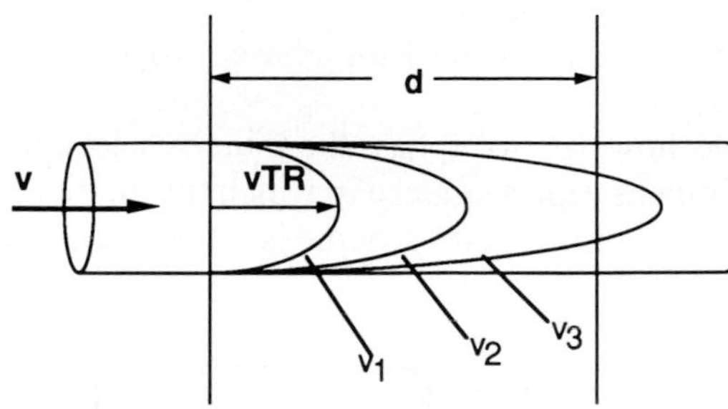

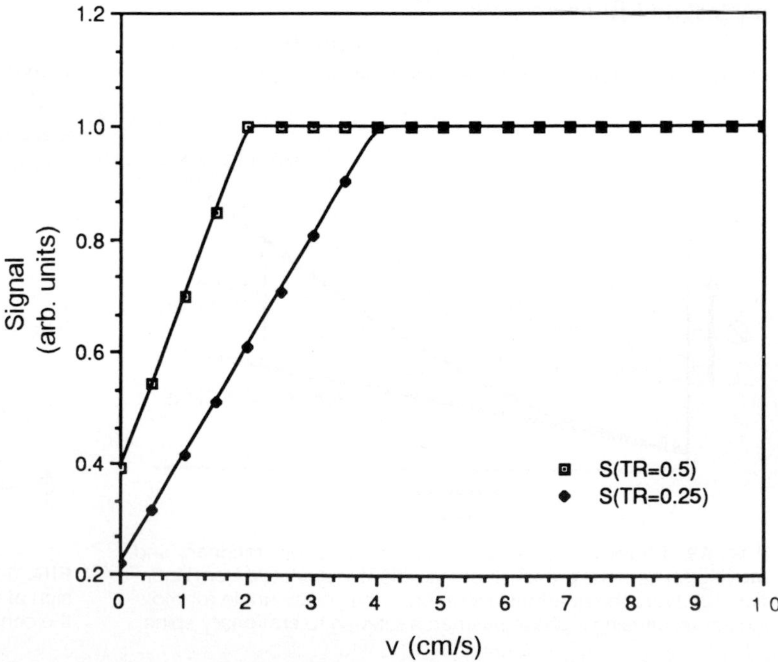

FIG. 57. Flow-related enhancement effects. **A:** Cause of flow-related enhancement: partly saturated spins are replenished due to wash-in of fully magnetized spins during the pulse recycle time TR. Note that the extent of inflow of spins without an rf history increases with increasing flow velocity ($v_3 > v_2 > v_1$). d, distance. **B:** Relative signal intensity (S) as a function of flow velocity assuming a fluid T_1 of 1 sec. The initial signal intensity is determined by partial saturation. However, as the velocity increases the fraction of unsaturated spins contributing to the signal increases until complete wash-out occurs at which point the maximum signal intensity is attained.

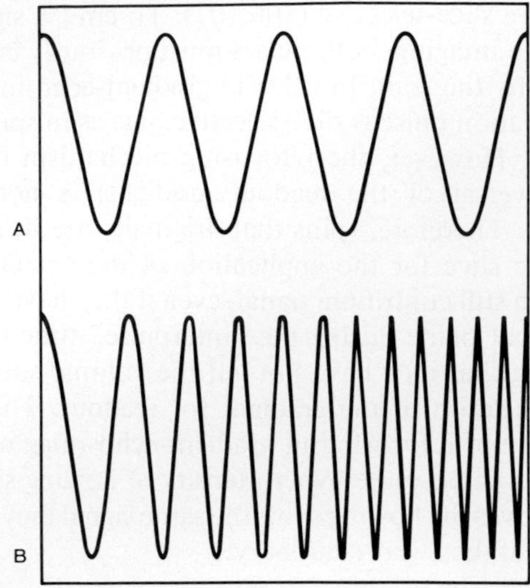

FIG. 58. Change in resonant frequency with flow. Stationary spins exposed to a magnetic field gradient resonate at constant frequency (**A**), whereas moving spins (**B**) increase in their frequency.

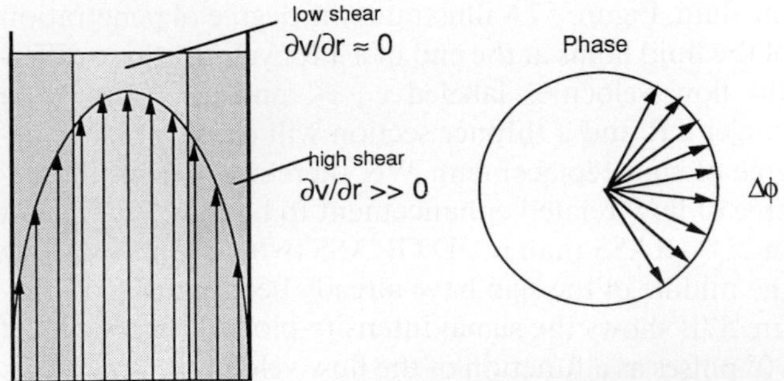

FIG. 60. Intravoxel phase dispersion. A velocity distribution such as the one caused by shear stress in laminar flow leads to phase scrambling, which, when the phase spread $\Delta\phi$ approaches 2π radians across the pixel, leads to signal attenuation.

From Equation 25b we see that in the presence of motion, the phase increases quadratically with time, as shown graphically in Fig. 59.

The phase mismatch of the moving versus stationary spins in itself is not detrimental, as long as the spins within the imaging voxel move in a coherent fashion at equal velocity (e.g., plug flow). However, if there is a distribution of velocities due to shear stress, as in laminar flow, the spin isochromats spread out (Fig. 60). Once the phase spread $\Delta\phi$ approaches 2π radians across the imaging voxel, destructive interference and thus net signal loss ensues. This type of signal loss is also denoted *intravoxel phase dispersion*. Intravoxel phase dispersion represents the single most important cause of artifactual signal loss on MR angiography.

These undesired dephasing effects can be reversed by means of rephasing gradients. In order to understand this process, let us first consider the effect of a balanced gradient on the frequency and phase of moving spins. Imaging gradients (like the slice selection and readout gradient) are balanced for stationary spins in such a manner that a phase advance is compensated by a gradient of equal area but opposite polarity (see, e.g., Fig. 61). Figure 62 shows such a gradient pair as well as a plot of frequency, in this case, however, assuming spins moving at constant velocity. During the positive portion of the gradient of duration t, frequency increases linearly. Upon reversal of the sign of the gradient, the frequency reverses sign as well (e.g., counterclockwise versus clockwise precession). The frequency then continues to increase at the same rate. The resultant phase shift is the net area under the two curves which is equal to the rectangle (the areas of the two triangles cancel). This net phase shift is equal to $\gamma G v \tau^2$. Hence, we find the same square dependence on time and linear dependence on gradient amplitude and velocity previously established for a simple gradient (Equation 25b). It thus becomes clear that a bipolar gradient (like the readout or slice-select gradient) does not cancel the phase imparted by moving spins.

It is possible, however, to rephase the spins by selecting a gradient compensation sequence in which the gradient changes its polarity twice. This scheme is called gradient

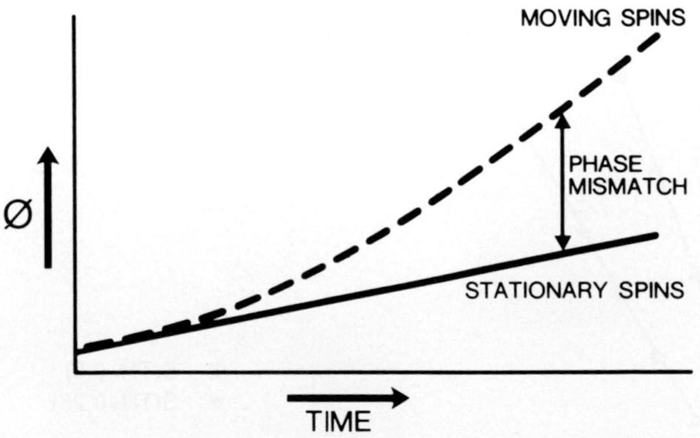

FIG. 59. Phase plotted as a function of time for stationary and moving spins in the presence of a gradient (calculated from Equation 12). Note the quadratic increase in the phase angle for moving spins, causing a phase mismatch relative to stationary spins.

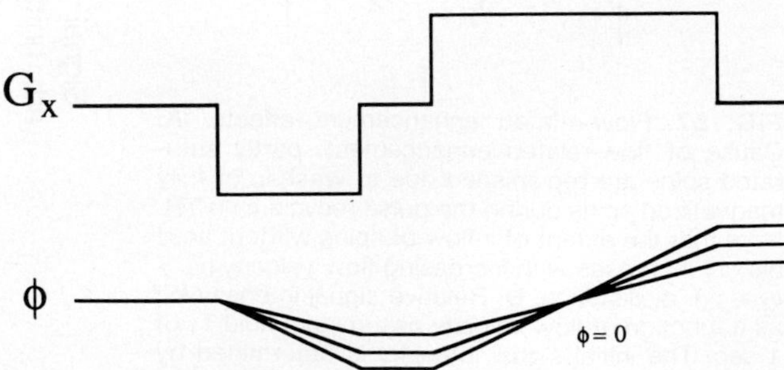

FIG. 61. Principle of gradient-echo formation. By reversing the sign of the readout gradient (G_x), the spins will rephase ($\phi = 0$) at the center of the data collection window.

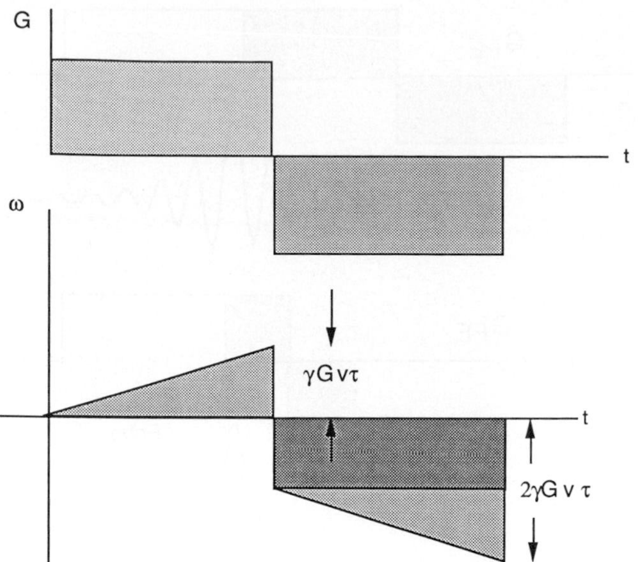

FIG. 62. Phase shifts due to flow during application of bipolar gradient. Effect of a bipolar (balanced) gradient on the frequency and phase of spins moving at constant velocity v along a gradient of amplitude G. The net phase shift is the integral over time of the frequency, which is equal to the area of the shaded rectangle: $\phi = \gamma G v \tau^2$.

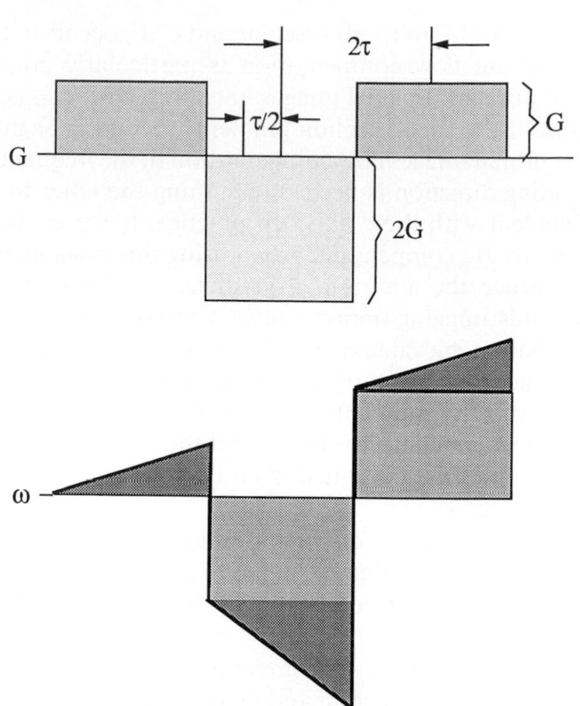

FIG. 63. Gradient (G) moment nulling. A gradient triplet of 1:(−2):1 area compensates the phase of spins moving at constant velocity. Note that the net area under the frequency curve (sum of positive and negative area) is zero.

moment nulling (108,109). Figure 63 shows such a gradient triplet and its effect on frequency and phase of the moving spins. The effect of gradient moment nulling is significant in both normal intracranial vessels (Fig. 64) and in pathology, where the use of gradient moment nulling recovers intravascular signal and makes these vessels markedly hyperintense (104). Note that rephasing induced by this method alone cannot result in higher absolute signal intensity than that of stationary fluid of the same composition, and in fact is analogous to the phenomenon of "even echo rephasing" (110).

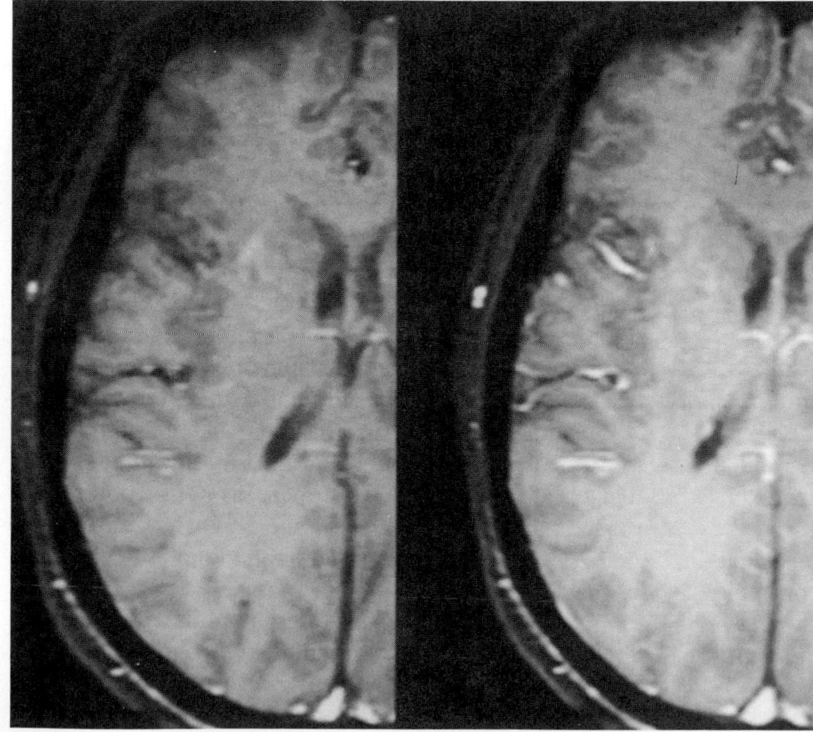

FIG. 64. Effect of gradient moment nulling on intravascular signal. **A:** Gradient-echo MR image obtained without gradient moment nulling (150/15/50°). **B:** Gradient-echo MR image obtained with first-order gradient moment nulling (150/15/50°). Although both images are from single-slice gradient-echo acquisitions, note more consistent high signal intensity from intracranial vessels when using gradient moment nulling (B).

Since most flow (both vascular and CSF) occurs in the z direction, flow compensation is particularly critical along this axis. In axial images, therefore, flow compensation of the slice-selection gradient whereas in sagittal and coronal images flow compensation in the frequency-encoding direction is needed (assuming the latter to be coincident with the z axis). In practice, however, both gradients are compensated when using this imaging option. Since the addition of gradient waveforms takes time, this imaging option causes a prolongation of the minimally achievable echo delay. It should be noted that for higher orders of motion (i.e., acceleration, jerk, etc.), their respective moments each can be nulled with further additional gradient waveforms, but the marked increase in TE from this prevents it from being clinically useful (see Chapter 4).

Intravoxel phase dispersion-induced signal losses, which can be alleviated by means of the use of rephasing gradients, as discussed above, can become particularly severe in the case of "random" motion processes such as turbulence. Gradient moment nulling, in this case, is ineffective since direction and magnitude of the velocity vector are thought to change in a more or less random manner. As noted by Listerud et al. (111), however, the degree of phase dispersion can be minimized by reducing the gradient moments with the technique of half-echo sampling, originally described as a means to minimize the echo delay (34). The underlying idea is to sample the descending part of the echo only, which results in a time savings of roughly half the sampling time and a corresponding shortening of the echo time. Figure 65 shows a comparison of the frequency-encoding gradients for full echo sampling and sampling of a fractional echo. Note the much shorter dephasing gradient needed to balance spin phase in the case of the fractional echo (Fig. 65B). Any reduction in the gradient duration, therefore, will reduce the first and subsequent moments.

The clinical impact of conventional gradient-echo imaging for the definition of vascular lesions of the CNS has been addressed by several investigations (see Chapters 12 and 31 for a more complete discussion). The value of this technique often depends on the specific lesion in question (104). Arteriovenous malformations (AVMs), for instance, are usually easily diagnosable on the basis of the spin-echo images alone (Fig. 66), since these are typically high flow abnormalities. In fact, the high intensity of CSF on T2-weighted spin-echo images is often very useful in highlighting lesions containing regions of signal void, especially when the abnormal vessels are intraventricular or over the convexities (Fig. 66) (104). On the other hand, more subtle vascular lesions, such as small venous angiomas (Fig. 67) may become more conspicuous on gradient-echo-based MR angiography images. Generally, gradient-echo-based MR angiography is utilized for these entities.

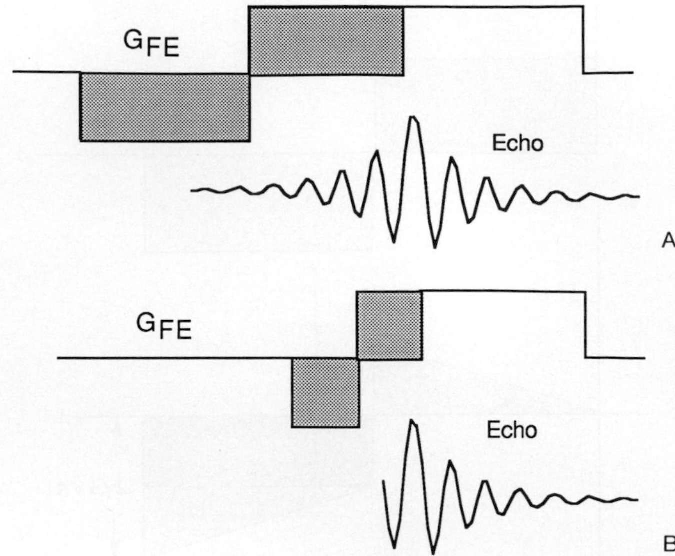

FIG. 65. The first moment ($\int G(t)tdt$) from a fractional echo (**B**) is much less than that of a full echo (**A**). For this reason, signal losses due to intravoxel phase dispersion are less severe in gradient-echo images obtained with fractional-echo B sampling.

The appearance of focal or linear regions of signal void within mass lesions can be due to multiple causes on spin-echo images, including dense calcification and flow within large tumor vessels. We do not believe that these cases necessarily require full MR angiography sequences, since in many instances single slices clarify the region in question. In these cases, the initial interpretation of hypointensity on spin-echo scans as due to vascular flow void can be rapidly verified or disproven. In partially calcified neoplasms, the absence of high intensity coupled with the heightened sensitivity of gradient-echo acquisition to magnetic susceptibility differences allows a confident diagnosis of intratumoral calcification as the etiology of spin-echo signal voids, rather than flow in vessels (Fig. 68), thereby permitting a more specific diagnosis and aiding the surgeon preoperatively. Adjunctive gradient-echo scanning of intracranial neoplasms for possible vascularity therefore is a reasonable indication for this technique, especially when one considers that the vast majority of intracranial neoplasms do not undergo catheter angiography prior to surgery. Therefore, both as a means of providing practical information that is valuable to the surgeon prior to surgery, as well as potentially a means of more complete tissue characterization (Fig. 69) (see Chapter 10), a supplemental gradient-echo scan for flow is appropriate in many cases.

Gradient-echo imaging is often helpful in ascertaining whether ambiguous intravascular spin-echo signal intensity patterns represent patent or thrombosed lumina

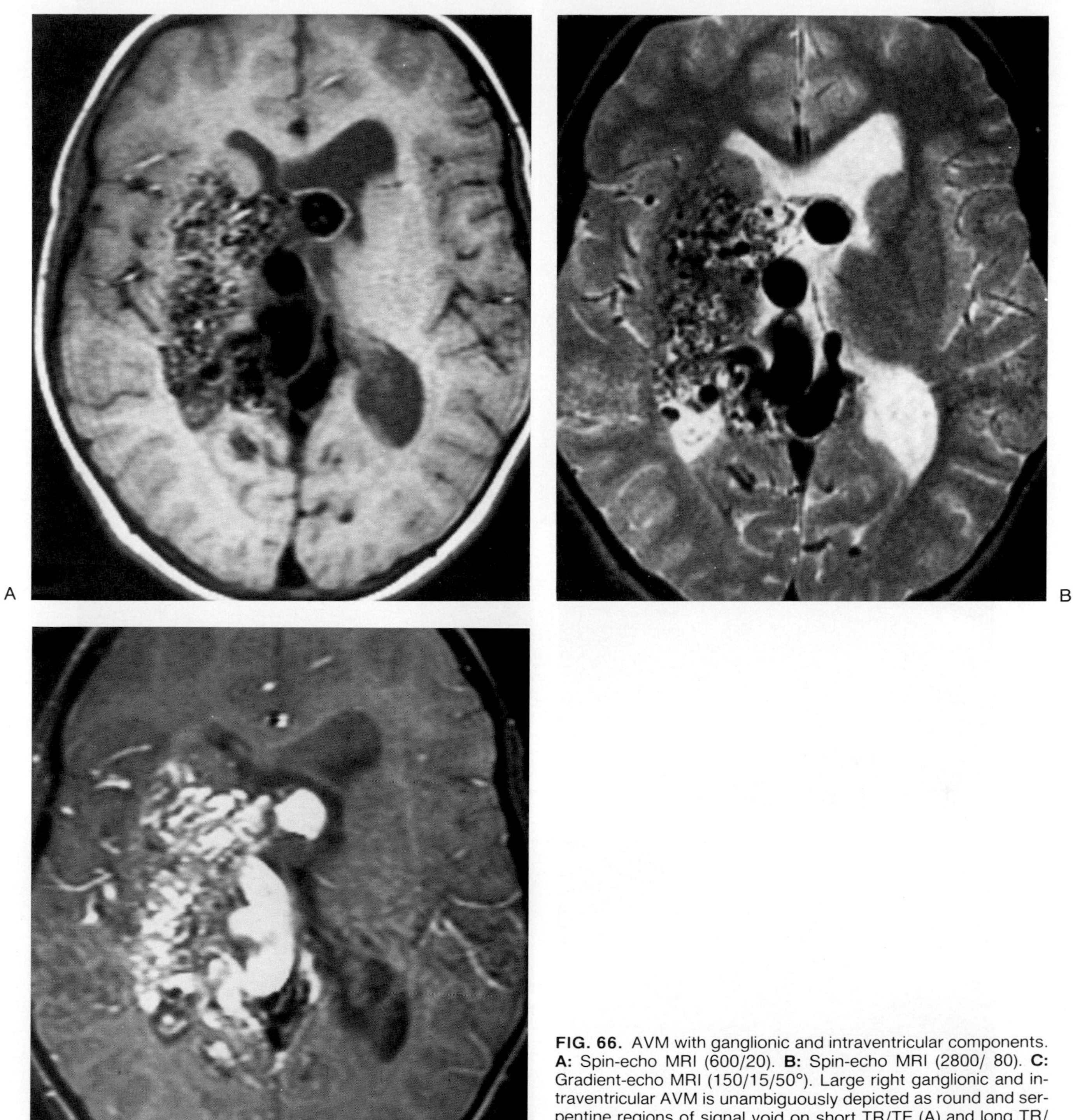

FIG. 66. AVM with ganglionic and intraventricular components. **A:** Spin-echo MRI (600/20). **B:** Spin-echo MRI (2800/ 80). **C:** Gradient-echo MRI (150/15/50°). Large right ganglionic and intraventricular AVM is unambiguously depicted as round and serpentine regions of signal void on short TR/TE (A) and long TR/TE (B) spin-echo images. Gradient-echo image (C) demonstrates high intensity in these same areas of flow. (From Atlas et al., ref. 104, with permission.)

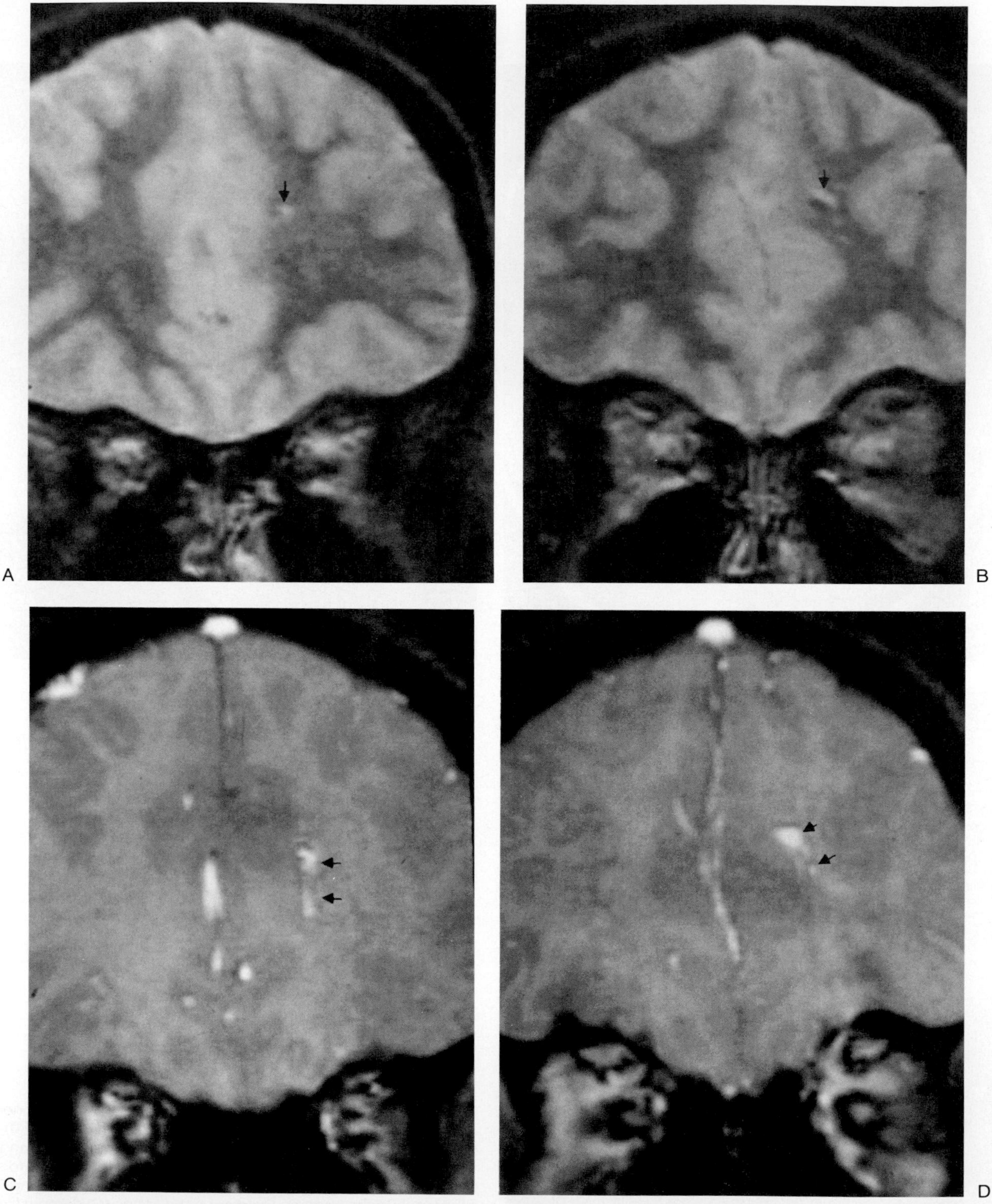

FIG. 67. Subtle venous angioma, spin-echo vs. gradient-echo MR imaging. **A,B:** Coronal long TR spin-echo MR images (2800/80). **C,D:** Coronal gradient-echo MR images (200/15/50°). On spin-echo images obtained with gradient moment nulling (A,B), lesion is seen as focal hyperintensity (*arrow*) resulting from misregistration of slow flow. Gradient-echo images (C,D) are less ambiguous and clearly show flow in venous angioma (*arrows*, C,D). (From Atlas et al., ref. 104, with permission.)

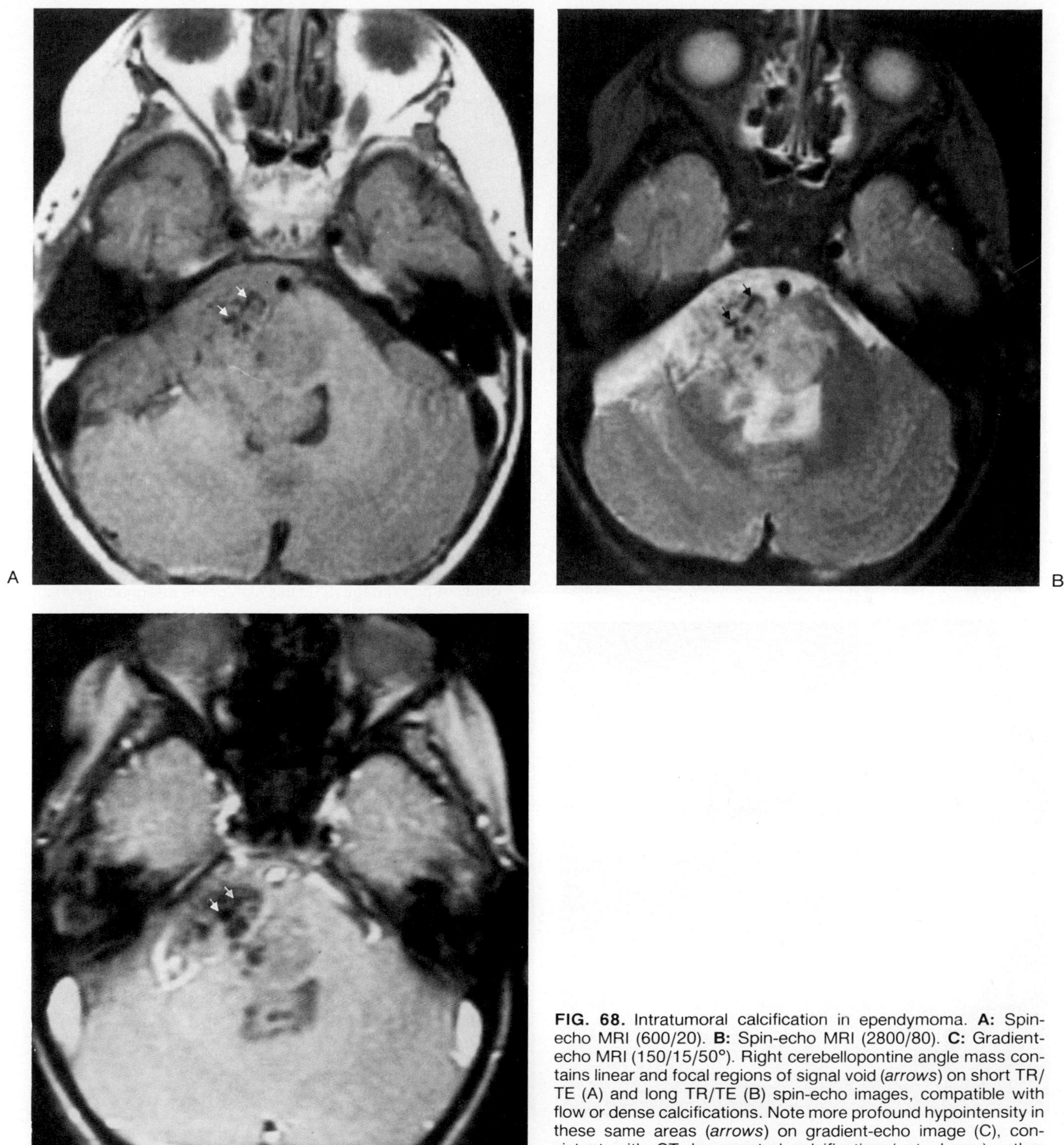

FIG. 68. Intratumoral calcification in ependymoma. **A:** Spin-echo MRI (600/20). **B:** Spin-echo MRI (2800/80). **C:** Gradient-echo MRI (150/15/50°). Right cerebellopontine angle mass contains linear and focal regions of signal void (*arrows*) on short TR/TE (A) and long TR/TE (B) spin-echo images, compatible with flow or dense calcifications. Note more profound hypointensity in these same areas (*arrows*) on gradient-echo image (C), consistent with CT-documented calcification (not shown) rather than flow in patent vessels. (From Atlas et al., ref. 104, with permission.)

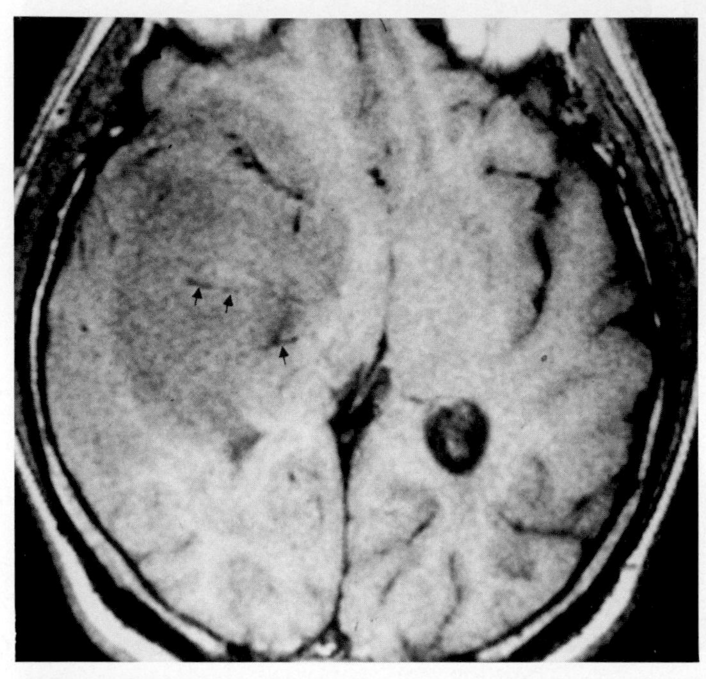

A

FIG. 69. Intratumoral vascularity suggesting high-grade glioma. **A:** Spin-echo MRI (600/20). **B:** Spin-echo MRI (2500/80). **C:** Gradient-echo MRI (150/15/50°). Large mass lesion in right hemisphere shows linear regions of low signal (*arrows*) on both short TR/TE (A) and long TR/TE (B) spin-echo images, confirmed to represent intratumoral vessels on gradient-echo image (C) in this high-grade malignant glioma.

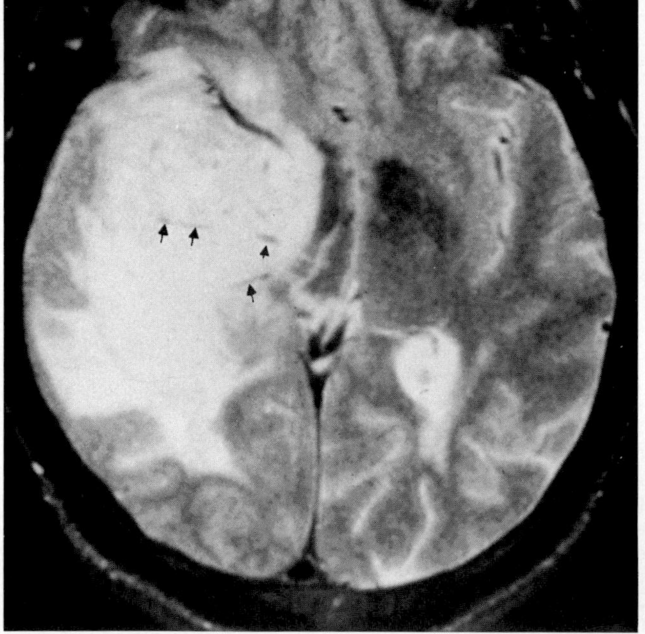

B

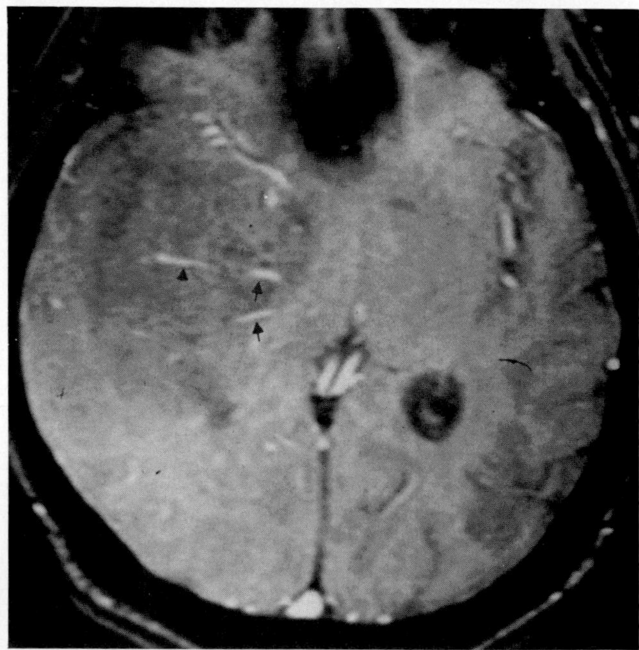

C

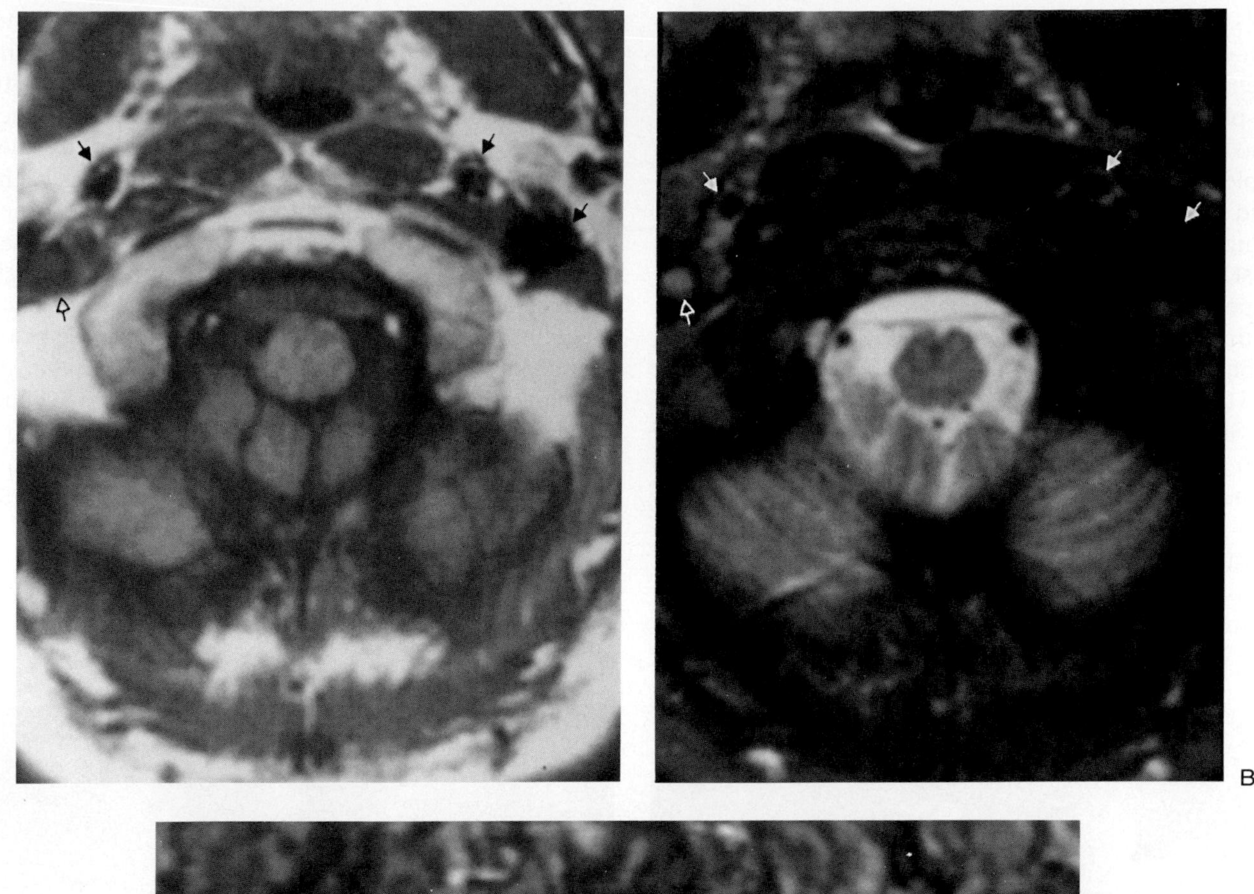

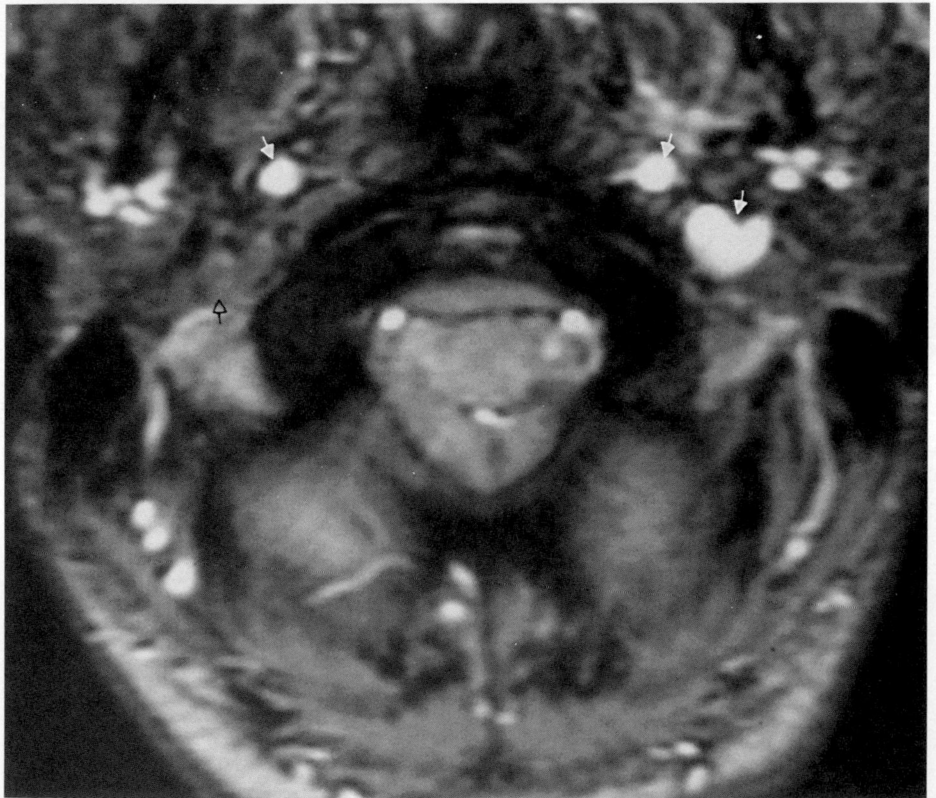

FIG. 70. Thrombosed right internal jugular vein. **A:** Spin-echo MRI (600/20). **B:** Spin-echo MRI (2800/80). **C:** Gradient-echo MRI (150/15/50°). Patent left jugular vein and left internal carotid and right internal carotid arteries (*closed arrows*) all demonstrate signal void on spin-echo images (A,B). Right internal jugular vein (*open arrow*) shows moderate intensity on short TR/TE (A) with high intensity on long TR/TE (B), indicating either slow flow or thrombosis. Gradient-echo image (C) unambiguously differentiates between high-intensity patent vessels (*closed arrows*, C) and thrombosed jugular vein (*open arrow*, C). (From Atlas et al., ref. 104, with permission.)

(Figs. 70 and 71). It has been well shown that certain spin-echo sequences may depict vascular flow as variable intensities under certain conditions, mainly based upon the phenomena of flow-related enhancement and even-echo rephasing (106,110). Furthermore, the now routine implementation of gradient moment nulling (109) in head imaging (on long TR spin-echo scans) often results in high intensity within or adjacent to patent vessels. In most of these settings, complete MR angiography should be performed. Since hyperintense clot can mimic flow on time-of-flight MR angiography, other methods, such as phase contrast techniques, can be used (see Chapter 31).

CSF flow can also be documented with the gradient-echo technique, based upon precisely the same mechanisms as defined above for intravascular flow (Fig. 72). Flow of CSF through the aqueduct, for instance, has a characteristic appearance on conventional spin-echo images, which has been ascribed to its rapid rate and bidirectional, pulsatile nature (112,113). The bidirectional jet of aqueductal CSF often results in signal void extending superiorly into the third ventricle and through the aqueduct into the superior aspect of the fourth ventricle on conventional spin-echo images. This appearance of signal loss within the aqueduct has been termed the aqueductal flow void (114), and its presence has been the sine qua non for a patent aqueduct (113–115). Concomitant with the implementation of flow compensation techniques, we and others (114,116) have noted that the aqueductal flow void sign of conventional spin-echo images has not been present in a significant proportion of patients with normal aqueductal flow [note that other factors may also be contributing to the absence of aqueductal flow void, such as diastolic pseudogating (107, 113)]. Gradient-echo imaging in conjunction with a cine mode of acquisition can be quite helpful in delineating aqueductal flow.

There are several important pitfalls in evaluating flow and vascular intracranial lesions with a gradient-echo-based flow technique (104) (for a complete discus-

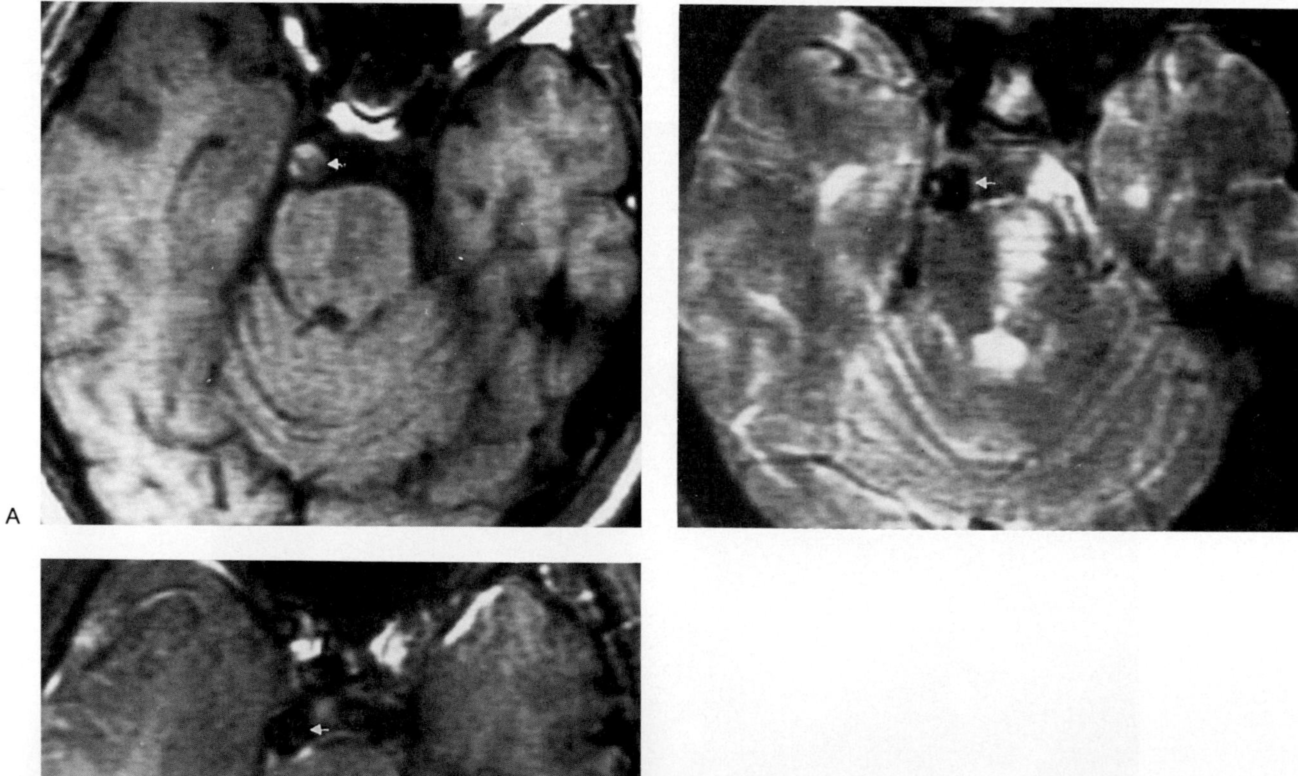

FIG. 71. Thrombosed basilar artery. **A:** Spin-echo MRI (600/20). **B:** Spin-echo MRI (2500/80). **C:** Gradient-echo MRI (150/15/50°). Mixed signal intensity pattern on spin-echo images (A,B) in basilar artery (*arrow*) could indicate either slow flow or thrombosis. Note definite low intensity in thrombosed basilar artery (*arrow*, C) on gradient-echo image (C). Left pontine infarction is clearly seen on spin-echo images (A,B). (From Atlas et al., ref. 104, with permission.)

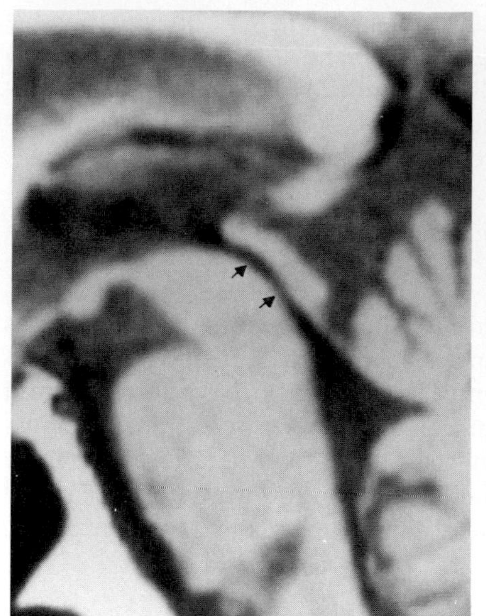
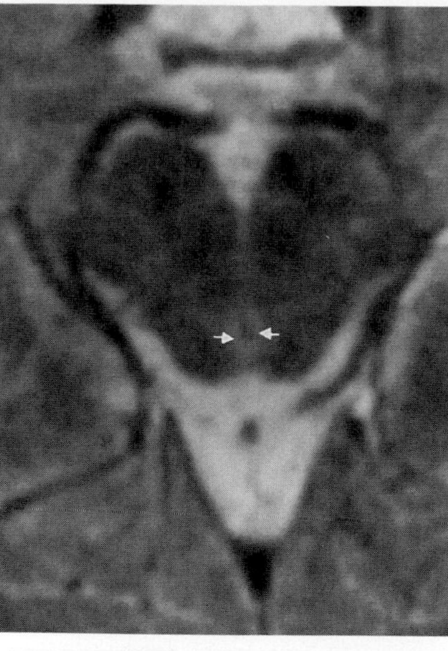
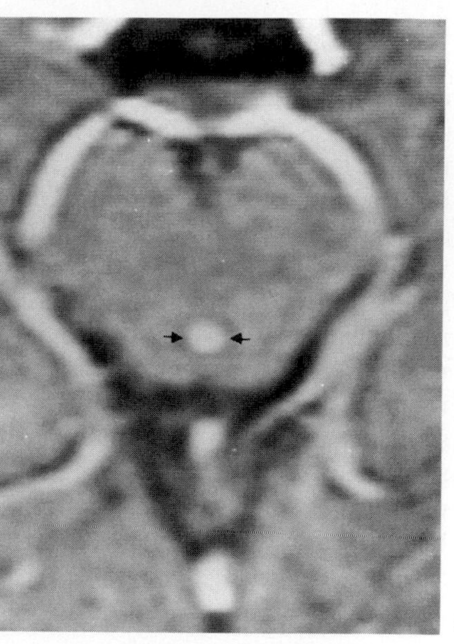

FIG. 72. Normal aqueduct using spin-echo and gradient-echo techniques. **A:** Sagittal spin-echo MRI (600/20). **B:** Axial spin-echo MRI with gradient moment nulling (2800/80). **C:** Axial gradient-echo MRI (150/15/50°). Patent aqueduct (*arrows*) shows signal void on short TR/TE image (A) and hypointensity on long TR/TE image (B). Gradient-echo image (C) depicts unambiguous high intensity in patent aqueduct (*arrows*). (From Atlas et al., ref. 104a, with permission.)

sion see Chapter 31). One major limitation lies in cases where hyperintense subacute clot (i.e., methemoglobin) is present on time-of-flight scans. In these cases, methemoglobin is also high intensity on gradient-echo images obtained to demonstrate flow as high intensity (Fig. 73), since these images are relatively T1-weighted. The location of the vascular lesion in question may be extremely problematic, particularly when section thickness is limited, as in 2D methods. For instance, in those regions of the brain in proximity to air-filled sinuses (such as the subfrontal region, inferior temporal lobes, and sella), significant hypointensity from magnetic susceptibility arti-

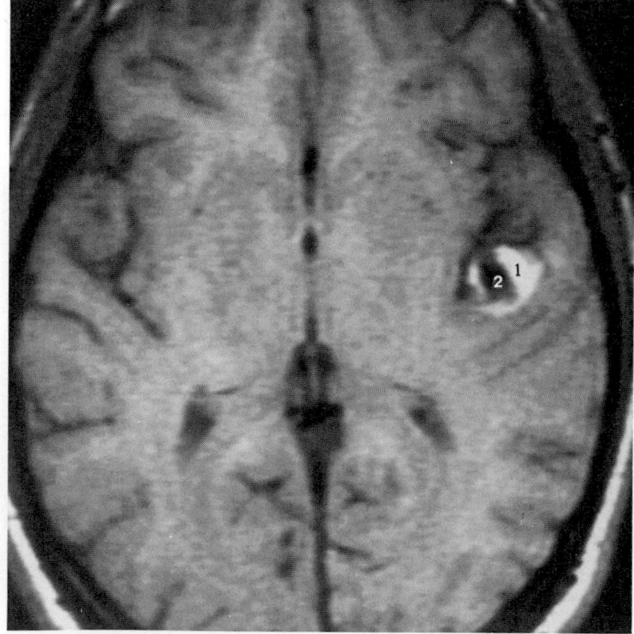

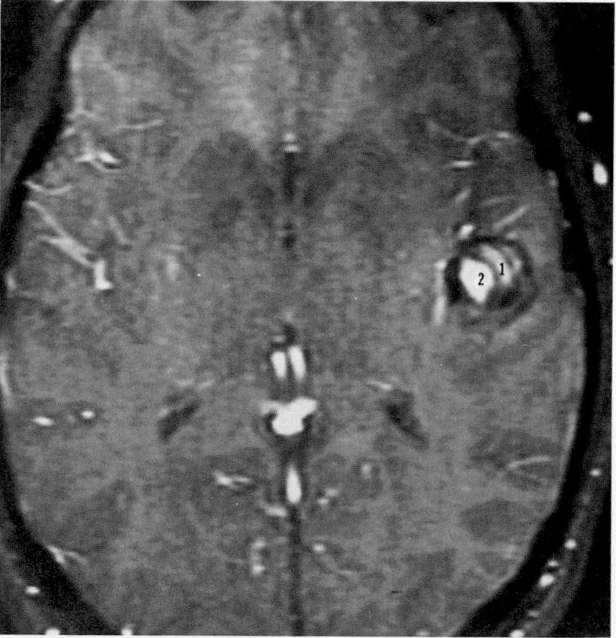

FIG. 73. Partially thrombosed left middle cerebral artery giant aneurysm. **A:** Axial spin-echo MRI (600/20). **B:** Axial gradient-echo MRI (150/15/50°). On short TR/TE spin-echo image (A), clotted portion of lumen (*1*) is high intensity and clearly distinguishable from patent portion of lumen (*2*), which demonstrates signal void. Gradient-echo technique (B) depicts both thrombosed (*1*) and patent (*2*) portions of lumen as high intensity. (From Atlas et al., ref. 104, with permission.)

fact can obscure large regions of the brain (Fig. 74) (see section on Magnetic Susceptibility Effects). Similarly, adjacent calcification or hemorrhage can mask flow. In such settings, the small voxels provided by high resolution 3D techniques minimize these artifacts. Lastly, even though flow may be present, gradient-echo-based MR angiography can still demonstrate signal void in many vascular lesions. Technical factors, such as when images are obtained without gradient moment nulling (or with inadequate compensation for higher order flow effects), results in an inconsistent demonstration of flow as high intensity (Fig. 75). Turbulent flow is seen as low intensity, since irretrievable spin dephasing occurs in this instance using conventional TEs and symmetric echo sampling (117). In one series, approximately one-third of high flow AVMs were depicted as low intensity in part, even though these regions were patent, presumably due to turbulence (Fig. 76). In-plane flow and extremely slow flow (105) can also theoretically be manifest as low intensity on gradient-echo-based MR angiography, although in practice these are not problematic.

Lesion Detection Based on Magnetic Susceptibility Effects

The 180° rf pulse of the spin-echo sequence reverses the effect of magnetic field inhomogeneities, and in fact that phenomenon was one of the driving forces behind the rapid acceptance of the sequence for clinical imaging. Gradient-echo images, on the other hand, are extremely sensitive to magnetic field nonuniformities, since signal is generated by the reversal of the readout gradient alone,

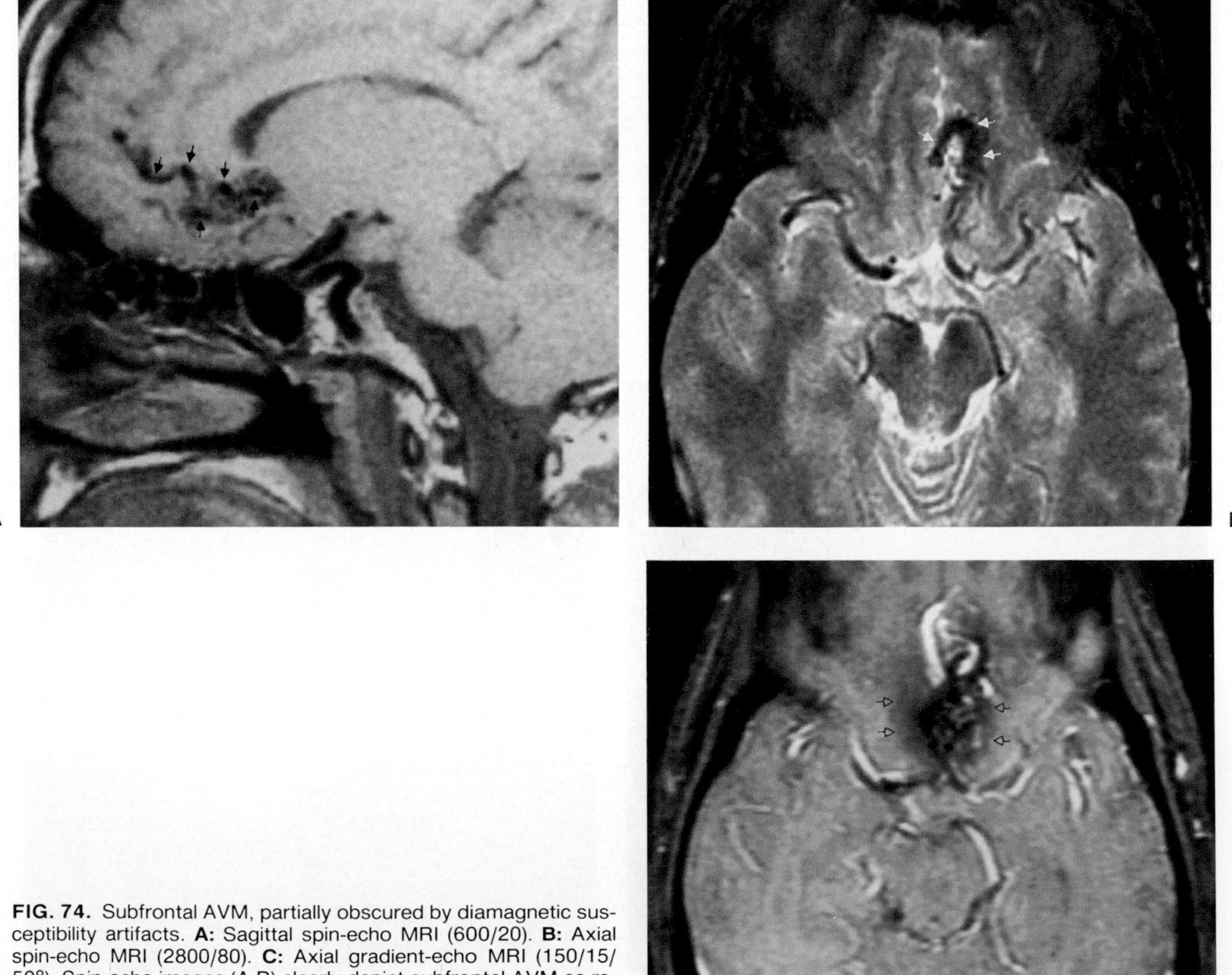

FIG. 74. Subfrontal AVM, partially obscured by diamagnetic susceptibility artifacts. **A:** Sagittal spin-echo MRI (600/20). **B:** Axial spin-echo MRI (2800/80). **C:** Axial gradient-echo MRI (150/15/50°). Spin-echo images (A,B) clearly depict subfrontal AVM as regions of signal void (*closed arrows*). Note that portions of the lesion are obscured by hypointensity (*open arrows*) on the gradient-echo image (C), due to diamagnetic susceptibility gradient-induced signal loss from nearby air-brain interface. (From Atlas et al., ref. 104, with permission.)

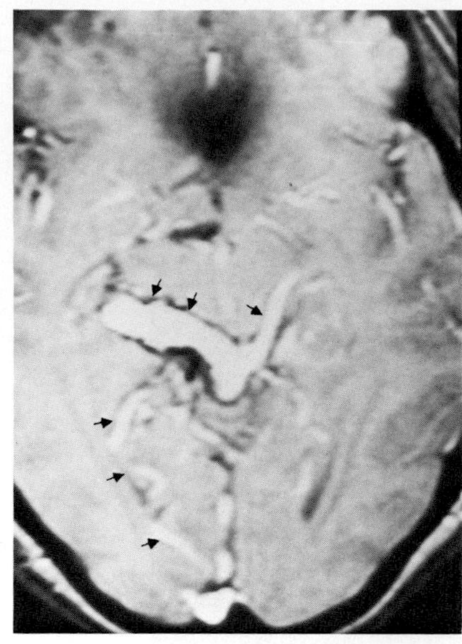
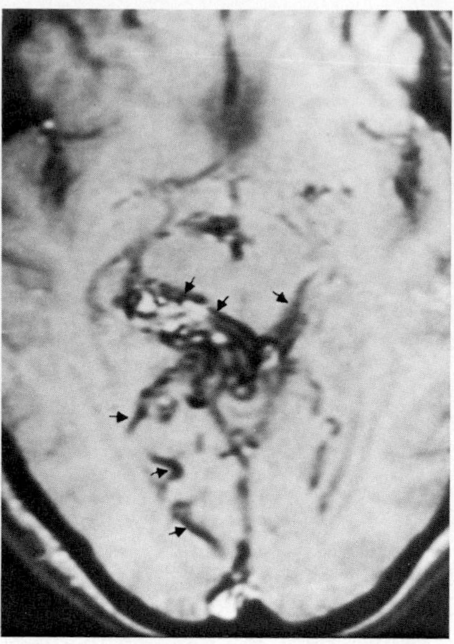

A,B

FIG. 75. Utility of gradient moment nulling in vascular pathology. **A:** Gradient-echo MRI, with gradient moment nulling (150/15/ 50°). **B:** Gradient-echo MRI, without gradient moment nulling (150/15/50°). Enlarged vessels draining AVM (*arrows*) are low intensity on gradient-echo image obtained without gradient moment nulling (B), even though sequential slice acquisition is employed. High intensity is seen within these vessels when gradient moment nulling is utilized (A). (From Atlas et al., ref. 104, with permission.)

without an accompanying 180° phase reversal pulse. The reversal of the readout gradient will rephase only what the original application of that gradient has forcibly dephased. Therefore, any magnetic field gradients that may be present will not be compensated for, and thus will attenuate the signal. Hence, whereas the spin-echo signal evolves as $\exp(-TE/T_2)$, the gradient echo is attenuated as $\exp(-TE/T_2^*)$, with T_2 and T_2^* related as:

$$1/T_2^* = 1/T_2 + 1/T_2' + 1/T_2'' \qquad [26]$$

where T_2' is the relaxation from imperfections in the main magnetic field, and T_2'' is relaxation from gradients of magnetic susceptibilities (Fig. 77). Note that $1/T_2^*$ is always greater than $1/T_2$, since there is no such thing as a perfectly homogeneous magnetic field.

One source of intrinsic magnetic field nonuniformity is the heterogeneity of the body itself. These intrinsic inhomogeneities are caused by spatial variations in the magnetic properties of human tissue. Different materials have different magnetic susceptibilities (see Chapter 9). The universal response of a material to an applied magnetic field is the generation of another magnetic field, an induced field, characteristic of the tissue involved (Table 3). According to classical electromagnetic theory, the induced magnetization M and the applied magnetic field H are related to one another as follows:

$$M = \chi \cdot H \qquad [27]$$

where χ is the *magnetic susceptibility*. Depending on the sign of χ, the induced magnetization M is parallel to (augments) the applied field ($\chi < 0$) or antiparallel (opposes) ($\chi < 0$). In air and other *diamagnetic* materials (e.g., water-containing soft tissue) $\chi < 0$. By contrast, for *paramagnetic* materials $\chi > 0$ holds. (Electronic) paramagnetism is the result of unpaired electron spins, such as occurring in transition metal ions (e.g., Fe^{2+}, Fe^{3+}, Mn^{2+}, etc.), rare earth cations (e.g., Gd^{3+}, Pr^{3+}, Dy^{3+}) or stable organic free radicals or ions (e.g., *N*-oxypyrrolidine, *N*-oxypiperidine). Molecular oxygen is a bi-radical and thus is also weakly paramagnetic. Although there are several known natural paramagnetic materials, greater than 99% of human tissue is diamagnetic. *Ferromagnetic* materials [e.g., magnetite (Fe_3O_4)] are permanently magnetic, which is the result of alignment of the electronic magnetic dipoles, caused by unpaired electron spins, arranged in domains (the so-called Weiss domains). No human tissue is ferromagnetic. If ferromagnetic particles are broken down to a size less than the that of the Weiss domains, they behave like paramagnetics, albeit exerting much enhanced paramagnetism. Such particles are called *superparamagnetic*.

Magnetic susceptibility differences between regions of tissue (e.g., tissue water and intravascular deoxygenated blood), and between tissue and adjacent structure (e.g., air, foreign body) can have profound effects on the MR signal in gradient-echo imaging. The most significant effects are those caused by local magnetic field gradients, which arise at the boundaries of zones with differing magnetic susceptibility. In this case, voxels situated near the interface of two zones are subject to spatial variations in magnetic field.

At the interface of these two regions, therefore, there is an intrinsic gradient G_i, which is proportional to $\Delta\chi$, the difference in the magnetic susceptibility of the two adjoining structures. Following excitation and generation of transverse magnetization, spins in a voxel of size Δr may thus experience a distribution of magnetic fields, causing their phases to scramble. Therefore, at echo time TE, this phase dispersion may cause a reduction in the transverse magnetization (which is the vector sum of its individual components, the spin isochromats). The

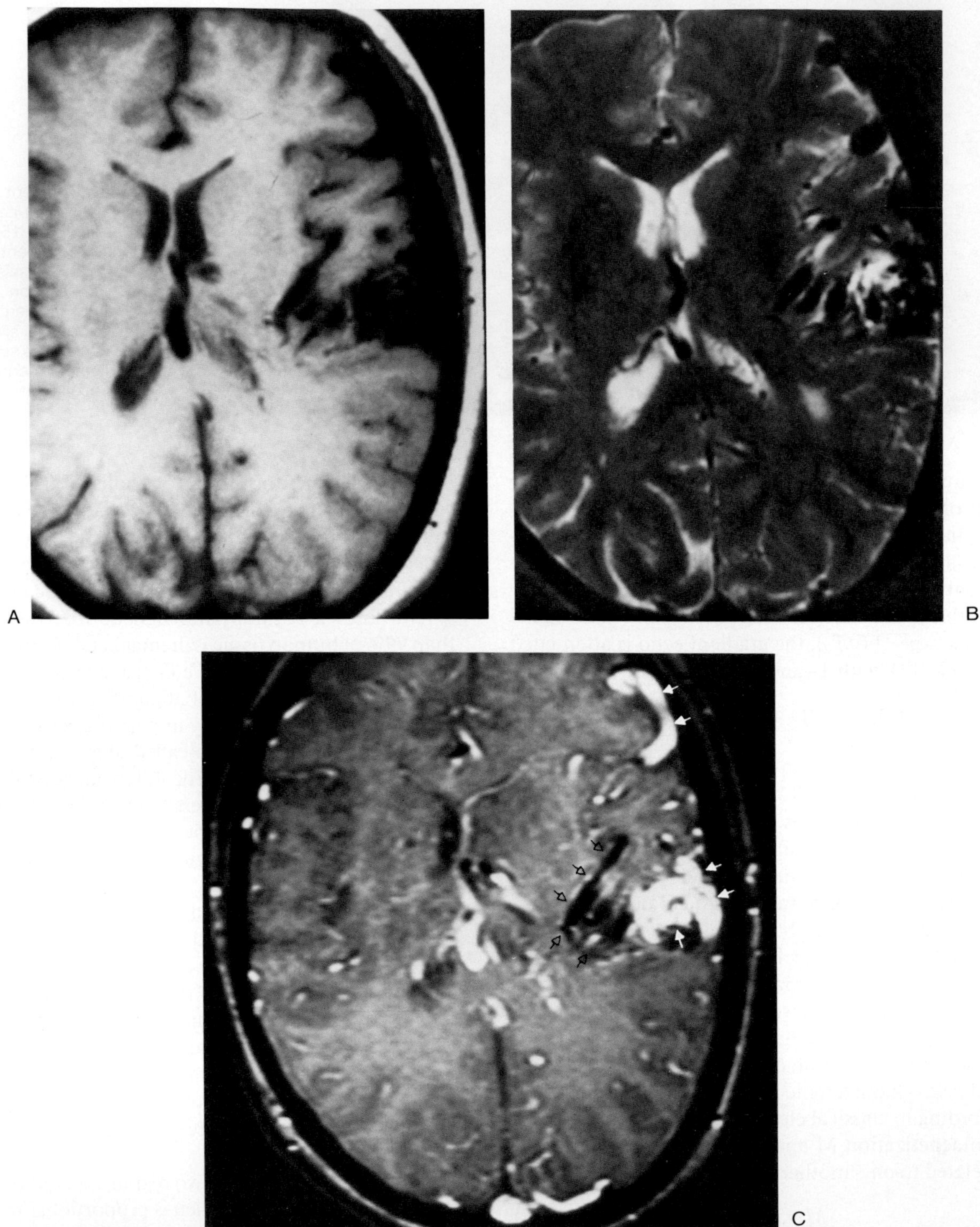

FIG. 76. Left insular AVM with turbulent flow. **A:** Spin-echo MRI (600/20). **B:** Spin-echo MRI (2800/80). **C:** Gradient-echo MRI (150/15/50°). Left insular and left frontal AVM is clearly seen as signal void on spin-echo images (A,B). Although gradient-echo image (C) depicts some areas of the lesion as high intensity (*closed arrows*, C), large regions of patency remain as signal void (*open arrows*, C), even though gradient moment nulling was employed. The persistence of signal void was presumably due to turbulence, although uncompensated higher order flow motion effects may also have been contributing to this appearance. (From Atlas et al., ref. 104, with permission.)

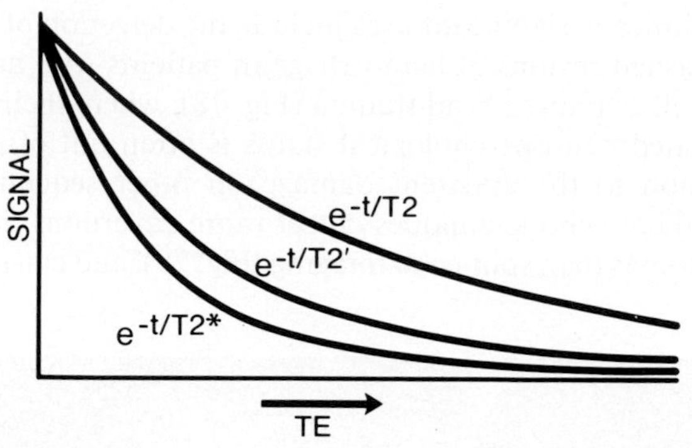

FIG. 77. Evolution of the signal intensity as a function of echo delay TE, shown for $T_2 = 2T_2'$. The time constant T_2^* for the decay of the gradient-echo signal is $[1/T_2 + 1/T_2']^{-1}$. Note that $T_2^* < T_2, T_2'$.

phase spread $\Delta\phi$ increases with increasing echo delay according to

$$\Delta\phi = \gamma \cdot G_i \cdot \Delta r \cdot \text{TE} \quad [28]$$

The clinical success of gradient-echo imaging for the detection of lesions based on susceptibility characteristics is based on the exploitation, rather than the suppression, of signal loss due to susceptibility gradients. As mentioned, the sensitivity for T2*-based signal loss is increased by lengthening the TE (118,119); T1-based contrast is reduced by decreasing the flip angle (118); imaging time is shortened by using short TR, or by implementing interleaved (multislice) acquisition or volume 3DFT scanning. Clinical protocols for this situation, therefore, generally include relatively long TE (30 to 50 msec) and relatively small flip angle (10° to 15°).

TABLE 3. *Induced magnetic fields in different forms of magnetism*

	Magnitude (vs. B_0)	Vector direction (vs. B_0)
Diamagnetic	10^{-6}	Opposed
Paramagnetic	10^{-2} or 10^{-4}	Same
Superparamagnetic	> or =	Same
Ferromagnetic	> or =	Same

It has become apparent that gradient-echo imaging is more sensitive for the detection of intracranial hemorrhage than spin-echo imaging (120,121). This phenomenon is due to the presence of paramagnetic iron associated with the various stages of the evolving hematoma (see Chapter 9). At interfaces of regions differing in magnetic susceptibility (such as in or around acute, subacute and chronic hemorrhage), *static* field inhomogeneities occur in boundary voxels which are rephased by the 180° pulse in spin-echo imaging. Diffusion of water through regions differing in susceptibility (i.e., through different

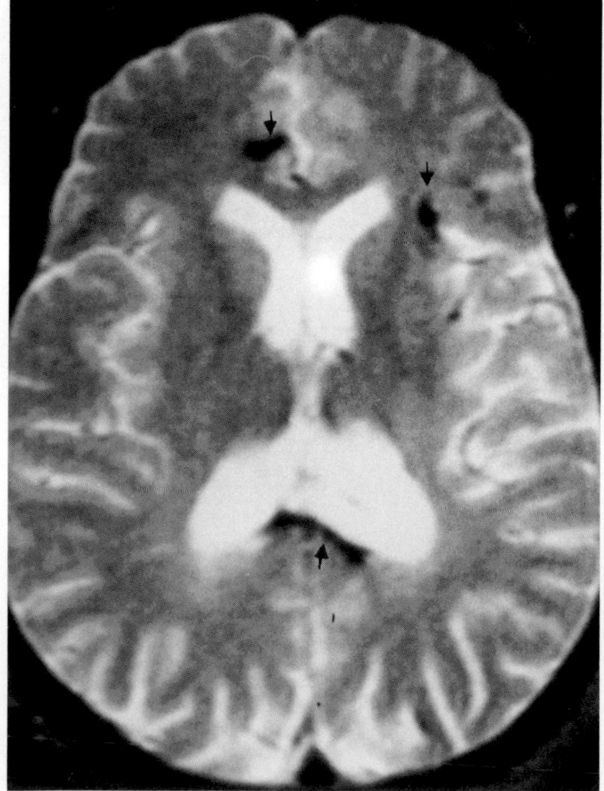

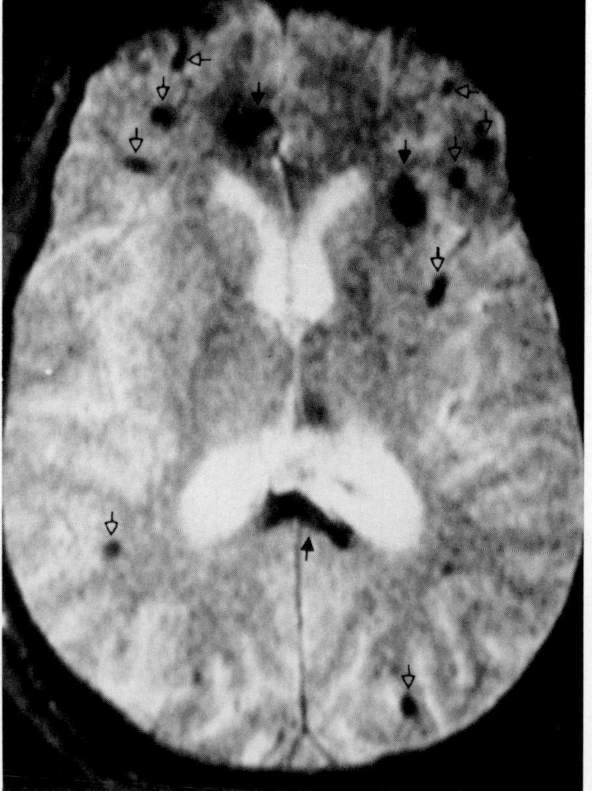

FIG. 78. Hemorrhagic shearing injuries from prior head trauma. **A:** Spin-echo MRI (2800/80). **B:** Gradient-echo MRI (180/30/15°). Foci of iron deposition at sites of shearing injuries (*closed arrows*) are seen on long TR/TE spin-echo image (A). Gradient-echo image (B) depicts numerous additional lesions scattered throughout the brain (*open arrows*), not seen on spin-echo image (A). (From Atlas et al., ref. 120, with permission.)

magnetic fields) is analogous to *time-varying* magnetic field changes, and this signal loss is not rephased by the 180° pulse. Therefore, gradient-echo imaging manifests hypointensity from *both* static field inhomogeneities (due to T_2' as well as T_2'') and diffusion-related encounters with differing fields, whereas spin-echo imaging shows signal loss only (in theory) from diffusion-related effects.

Clinically significant uses include the detection of unsuspected regions of hemorrhage in patients with acute as well as remote head trauma (Fig. 78), where their debilitated neuropsychological status is often out of proportion to the apparent damage on other sequences. Gradient-echo techniques detect more cavernous hemangiomas than spin-echo imaging (Fig. 79), and can doc-

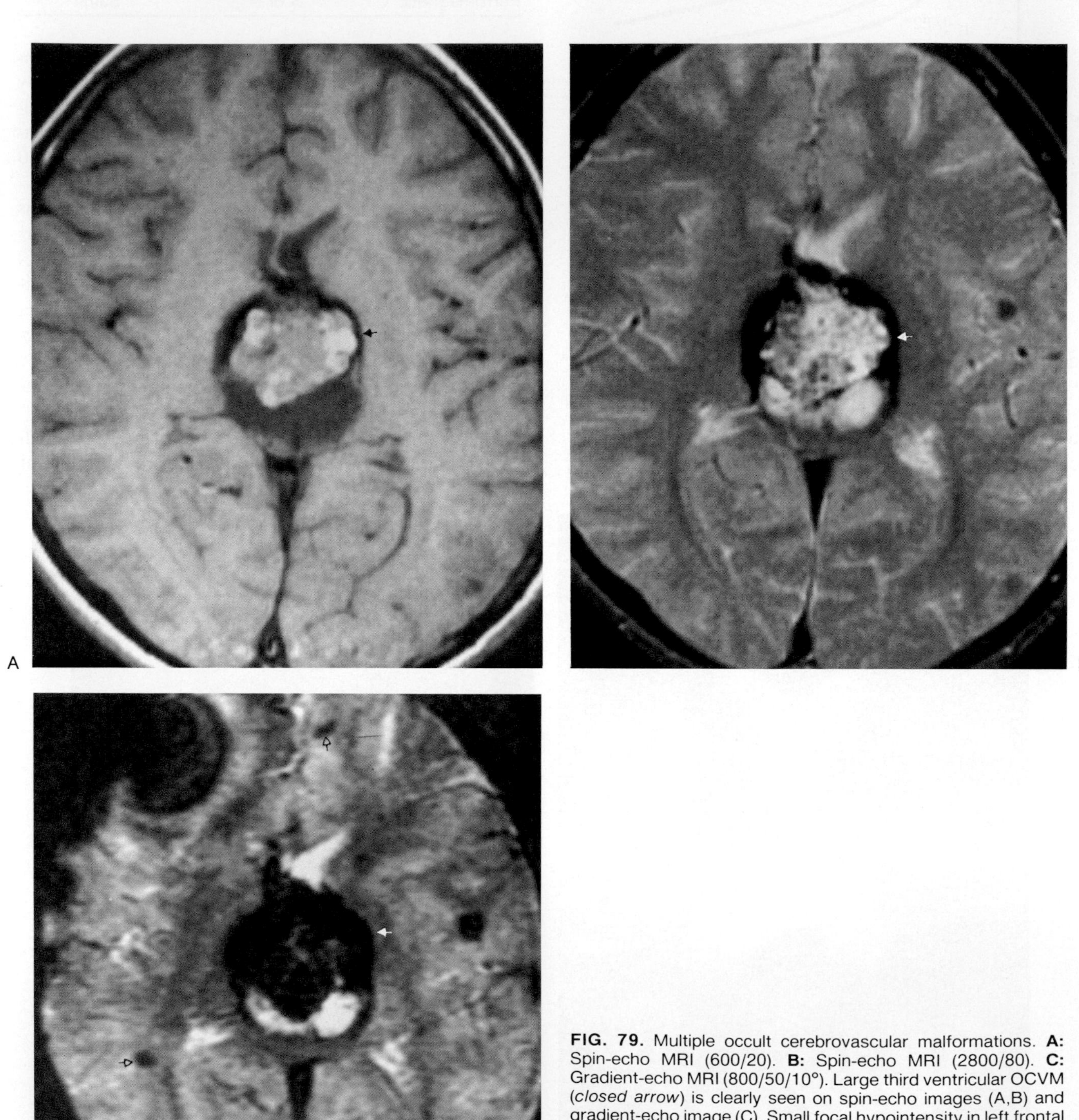

FIG. 79. Multiple occult cerebrovascular malformations. **A:** Spin-echo MRI (600/20). **B:** Spin-echo MRI (2800/80). **C:** Gradient-echo MRI (800/50/10°). Large third ventricular OCVM (*closed arrow*) is clearly seen on spin-echo images (A,B) and gradient-echo image (C). Small focal hypointensity in left frontal region, presumably representing a second OCVM, is also seen on spin-echo (B) and gradient-echo (C) images. Note additional hypointensities (*open arrows*) consistent with other OCVMS, seen only on gradient-echo image (C). (The right frontal hypointensity is from metallic residua of prior craniotomy). (From Atlas et al., ref. 120, with permission.)

ument hemorrhagic (or melanotic) metastases before they are evident on spin-echo images (Fig. 80). They are also more sensitive to the hemorrhagic sequelae of AVMs, the detection of which may offer prognostic information (see Chapter 12). Its role in patients suffering from seizures may be important: since cavernous hemangiomas most commonly present with seizures, it is a logical extension that patients with seizures who have a normal spin-echo MR should also be screened with a gradient-echo sequence (Table 2).

Calcification, which cannot be accurately identified with spin-echo imaging (122,123) can also be detected with this technique as marked hypointensity (Figs. 81 and 82) (124). The basis for the hypointensity of calcification on gradient-echo images may actually be twofold: (i) suspended particulate solids (such as diamagnetic calcium salts) alter the local magnetic field (125–128); and (ii) dystrophic calcifications are frequently found in association with paramagnetic cations (e.g., iron, copper, manganese) (129–131), which would also alter magnetic susceptibility. Perhaps most importantly, gradient-echo techniques may be most important in patients with normal spin-echo scans, in whom the search for such entities typically ends with the MRI. Moreover, since many patients now undergo fast spin echo rather than conventional spin-echo imaging, the increased sensitivity offered by gradient-echo imaging may be even more important to the ultimate diagnosis.

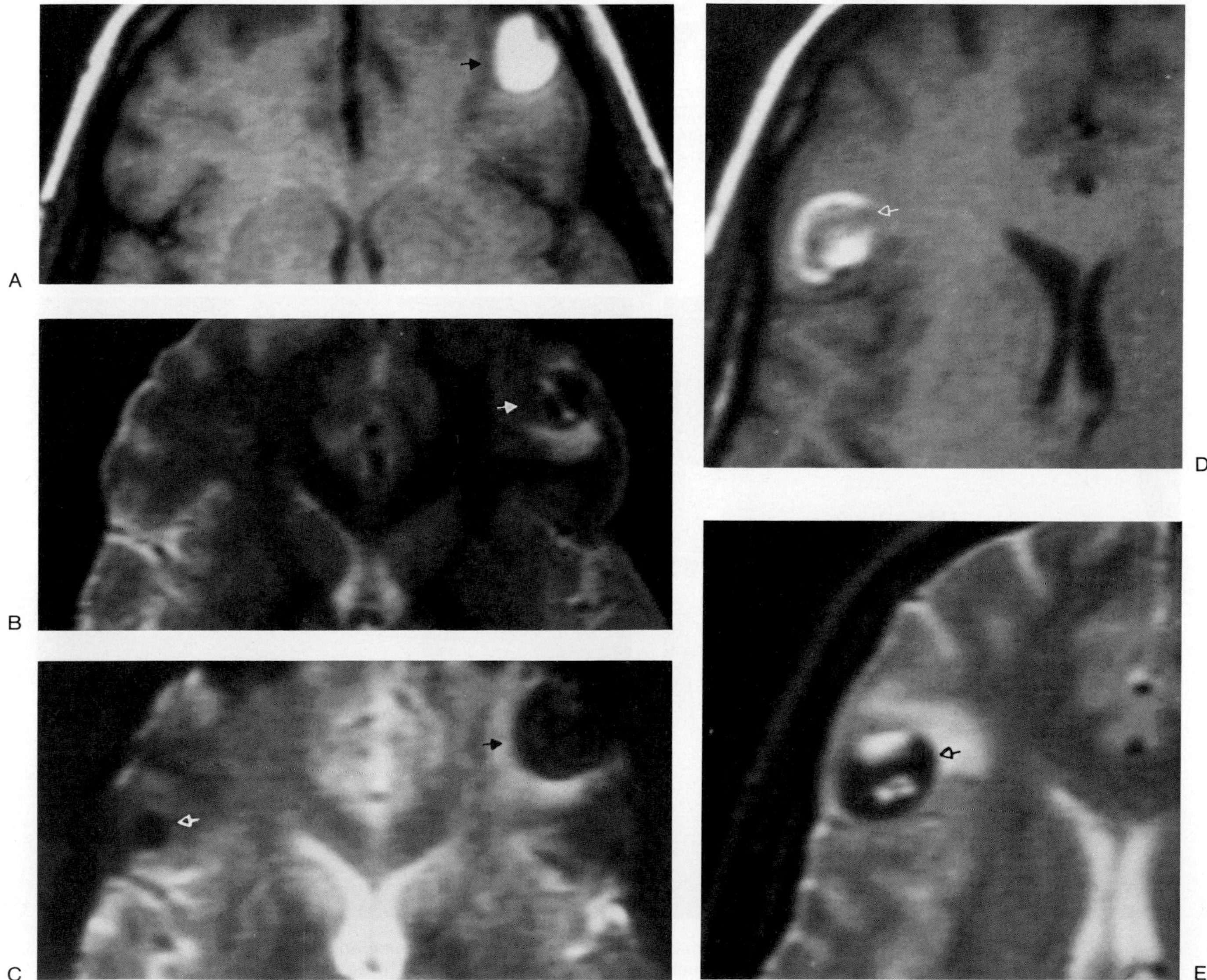

FIG. 80. Metastases from malignant melanoma. **A:** Spin-echo MRI (600/20). **B:** Spin-echo MRI (2500/80). **C:** Gradient-echo MRI (200/50/10°). **D:** Spin-echo MRI (600/20), 2 weeks later. **E:** Spin-echo MRI (2500/80), 2 weeks later. On initial scans (A–C), left frontal metastasis (*closed arrow*) was seen on spin-echo (A,B) and gradient-echo (C) images. Note additional lesion in right frontal lobe (*open arrow*, C) seen only on gradient-echo image (C). Two weeks later, intratumoral hemorrhage occurred and at that time the spin-echo images (D,E) finally showed the right frontal lesion (*open arrow*, D and E).

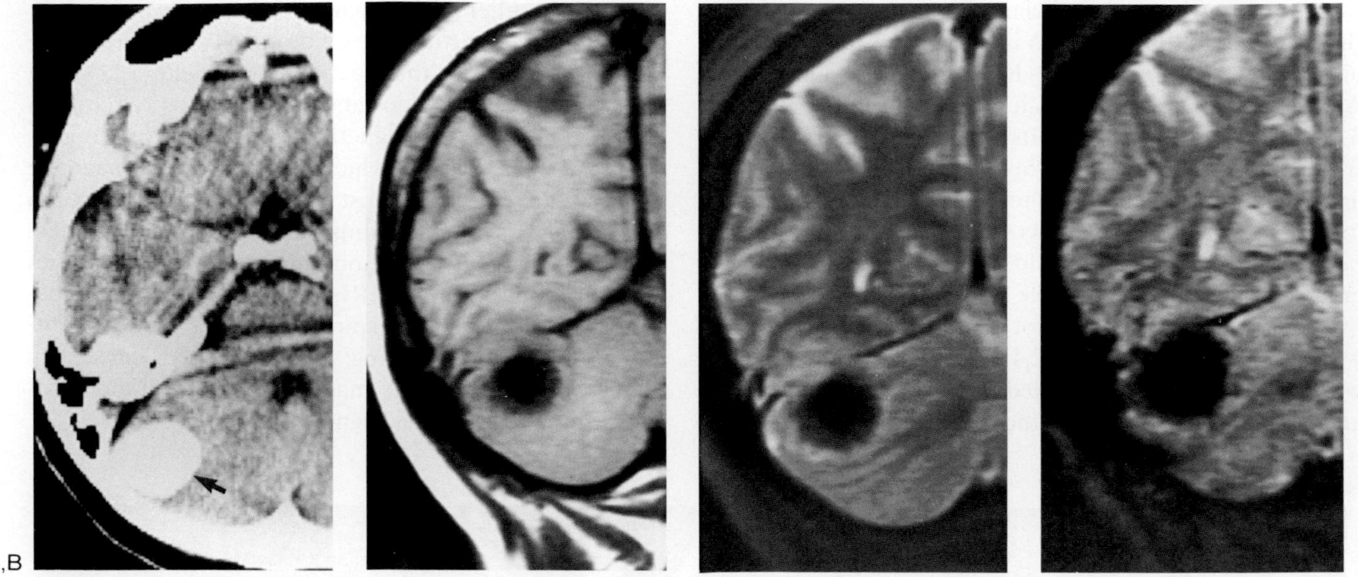

FIG. 81. Densely calcified meningioma, spin-echo vs. gradient-echo appearance. **A:** Axial CT. **B:** Coronal short TR/TE spin-echo MRI (600/20). **C:** Coronal long TR/TE spin-echo MRI (2500/80). **D:** Coronal gradient-echo MRI (750/50/10°). Densely calcified tentorial meningioma (*arrow*, A) shows central hypointensity on short (B) and long (C) TR/TE spin-echo images. More extensive hypointensity is present on gradient-echo image (D). (From Atlas et al., ref. 124, with permission.)

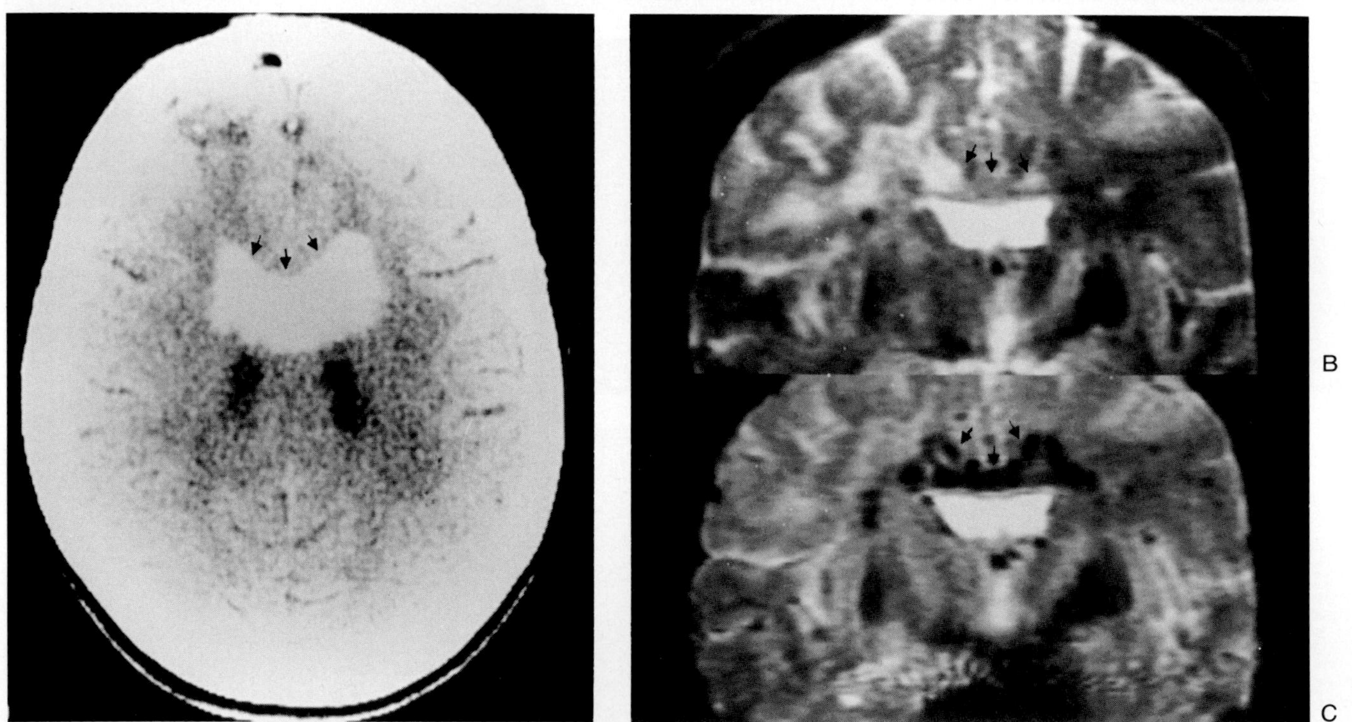

FIG. 82. Densely calcified corpus callosum glioma, spin-echo vs. gradient-echo appearance. **A:** Axial CT. **B:** Coronal long TR/TE spin-echo MRI (2500/80). **C:** Coronal gradient-echo MRI (750/50/10°). Despite dense calcification of corpus callosum glioma on CT (*arrows*, A), spin-echo image (B) shows high intensity in glioma (*arrows*, B). Gradient-echo image shows marked hypointensity throughout entire region of calcification (*arrows*, C). (From Atlas et al., ref. 124, with permission.)

The sensitivity of gradient-echo imaging for susceptibility variations has several important pitfalls. First, the heightened sensitivity of gradient-echo imaging to signal loss effects, although quite useful, is not specific (Table 4).

Second, the appearance of certain lesions on gradient-echo images is less specific than on spin-echo images, because internal signal patterns are often overwhelmed by signal loss (Fig. 83). Ironically, it has also been noted that cavernous hemangiomas can even be mimicked by an artifactual central hyperintensity within a larger hypointensity when gradient-echo images are used (see Chapter 7). The sign on spin-echo images of the *lack* of iron storage products around chronic hemorrhage (which is used

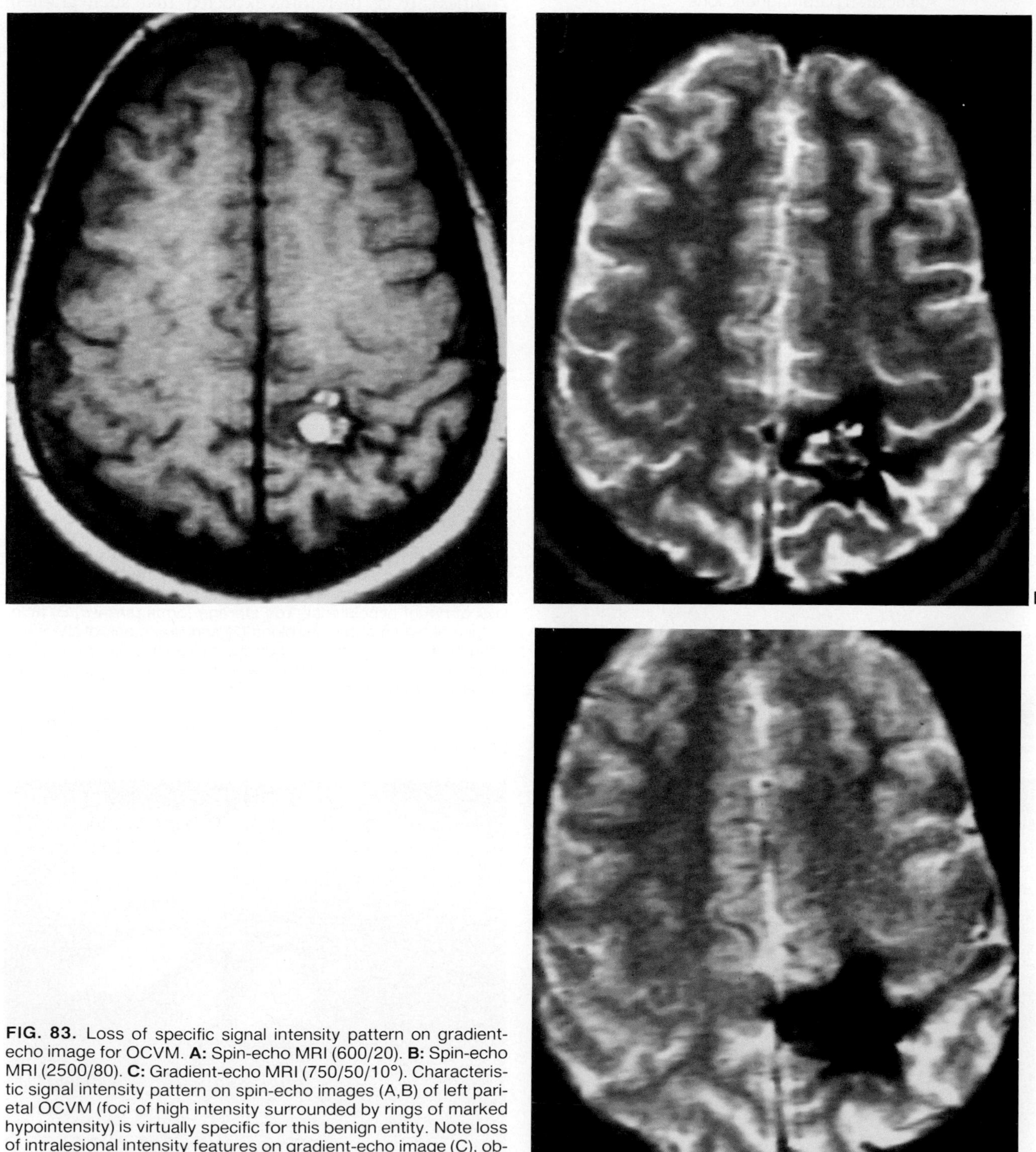

FIG. 83. Loss of specific signal intensity pattern on gradient-echo image for OCVM. **A:** Spin-echo MRI (600/20). **B:** Spin-echo MRI (2500/80). **C:** Gradient-echo MRI (750/50/10°). Characteristic signal intensity pattern on spin-echo images (A,B) of left parietal OCVM (foci of high intensity surrounded by rings of marked hypointensity) is virtually specific for this benign entity. Note loss of intralesional intensity features on gradient-echo image (C), obscuring the specific diagnosis. (From Atlas et al., ref. 120, with permission.)

TABLE 4. *Causes of hypointensity on short flip angle, long TE gradient-echo images*

Hemorrhage
Deoxyhemoglobin
Methemoglobin
Ferittin/hemosiderin
Other iron forms
Calcification
Diamagnetic calcium salts
Associated paramagnetic ions
Air-containing paranasal sinuses
Normal brain iron
Intratumoral melanin
Paramagnetic contrast agents
Ferromagnetic devices, foreign bodies
Intravascular deoxygenated blood

to suggest underlying neoplasm as the etiology for a hematoma), is lost on gradient echo MR (Fig. 84), since hypointensity will be present at the interface of paramagnetic methemoglobin and adjacent diamagnetic brain [this has been termed the "boundary effect" by Edelman et al. (119)]. Lastly, there are susceptibility-related hypointense artifacts which interfere with image interpretation by obscuring large areas of brain (Fig. 85) and, occasionally, mimicking serious intracranial pathology. The susceptibility, *c*, is larger for air than for water by about 1–2 parts per million (even though both materials are diamagnetic, there is a gradient of diamagnetic susceptibilities). It is, therefore, expected that such gradients would be manifested on images at air-tissue boundaries. In the head, for example, these occur near the posterior ethmoid and sphenoid sinuses, mastoid air cells, etc., and can obscure large portions of the subfrontal and inferior temporal lobes The dependence of the susceptibility artifact on echo delay (132,133) is demonstrated with a series of axial images slightly above the mastoid air cells, with TE increasing in 3 msec increments (Fig. 86). The presence of these artifacts precludes the use of this technique as an accurate screening tool for the detection of hemorrhagic or calcified foci.

A

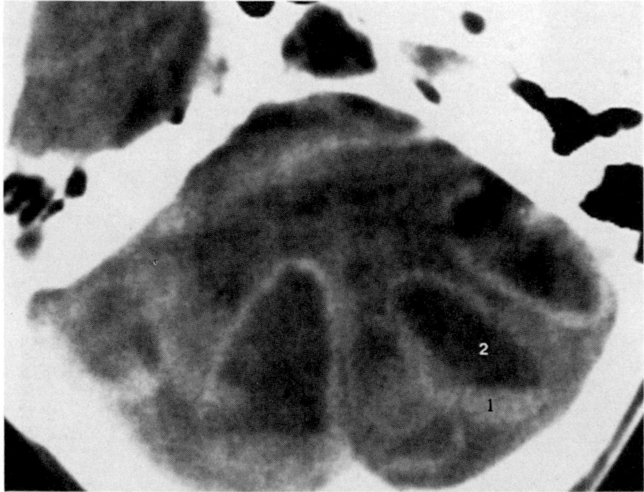

FIG. 84. Hemorrhagic metastases from lung carcinoma. **A:** CT scan. **B:** Spin-echo MRI (2500/80). **C:** Gradient-echo MRI (200/50/10°). CT (A) depicts multiple metastases with high-attenuation acute hemorrhage (*1*) layering in the dependent portions of the lesions. Long TR/TE spin-echo MRI (B) demonstrates lack of rim of hypointense iron storage forms (*arrows*, B) at interface between subacute blood (*2*) and brain, one of the signs described for suggesting underlying malignancy as the etiology of intracranial hemorrhage. Note hypointensity at this interface (*arrows*, C) on gradient-echo image, representing "boundary effect" between areas of differing magnetic susceptibility, which decreases specificity in this case. (From Atlas et al., ref. 120, with permission.)

B

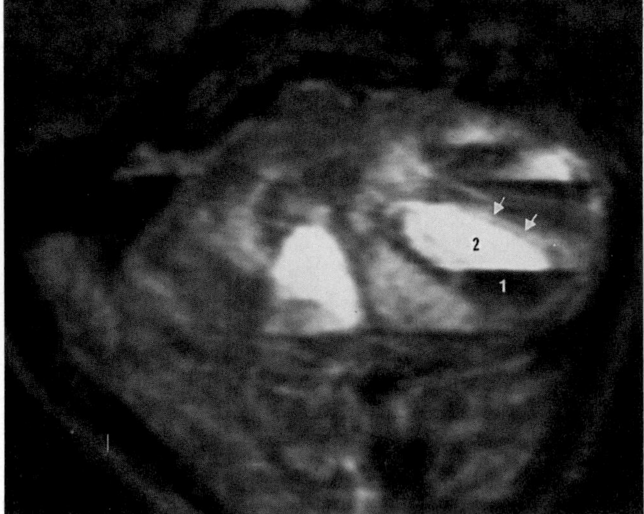

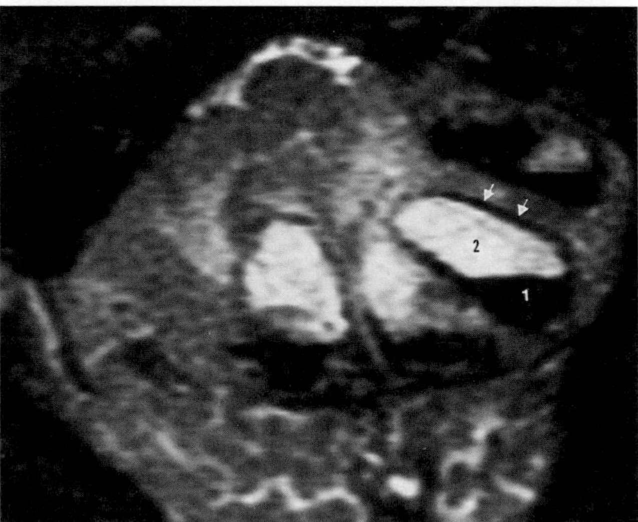

C

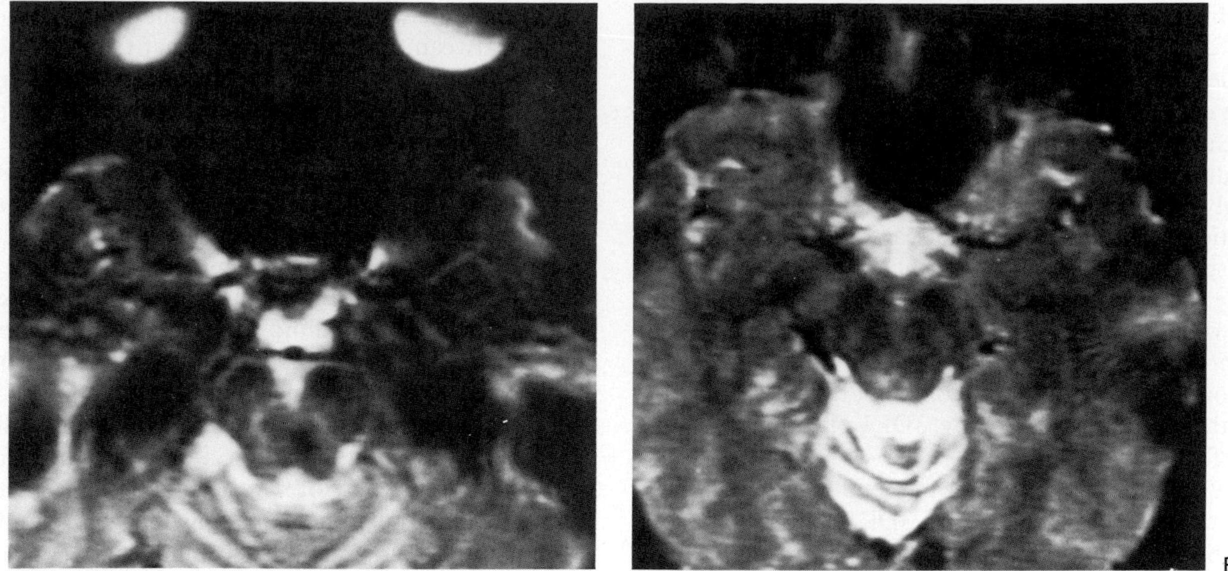

FIG. 85. Artifactual hypointensity on gradient-echo images obscuring large regions of brain (750/50/10°). Images through the base of the brain (**A,B**) are degraded by large regions of signal loss due to magnetic susceptibility differences between air-filled sinuses and mastoids and adjacent brain parenchyma. These artifacts prevent the use of this technique as a screening tool.

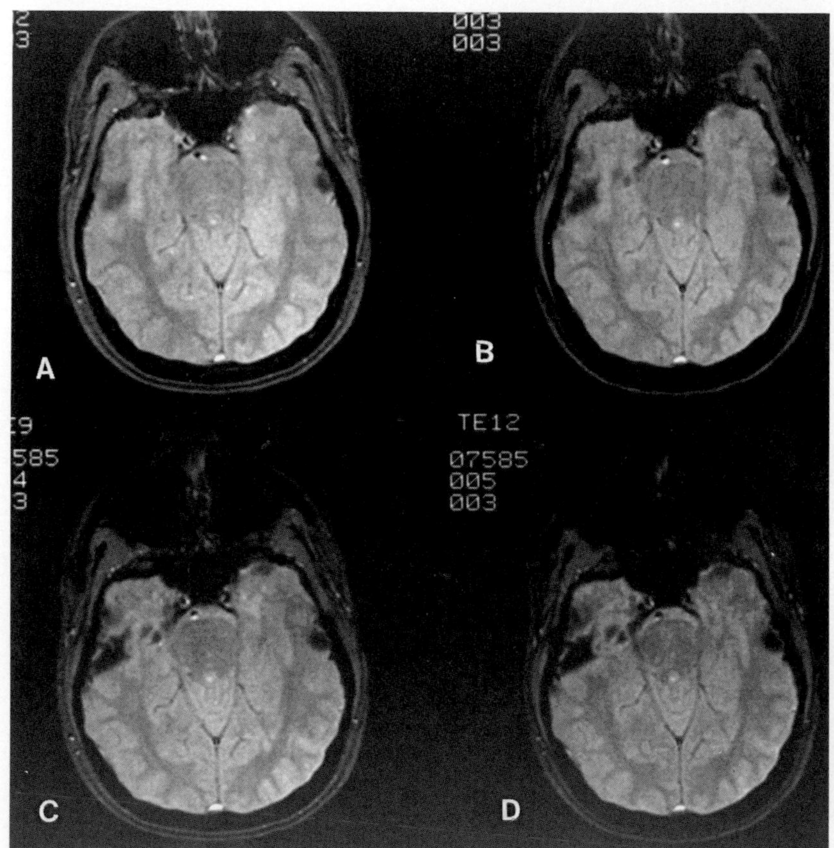

FIG. 86. Effect of small changes in TE on susceptibility artifact. Axial gradient-echo images through level just superior to mastoids at TEs of 9 (**A**), 12 (**B**), 15 (**C**), and 18 msec (**D**) show increasing degrees of signal loss in posterior temporal lobes, demonstrating that even small changes in TE can alter image quality dramatically.

3DFT Gradient-Echo Imaging

One of the major clinical applications of 3DFT imaging currently is in the evaluation of the cervical spine for extramedullary disease, specifically for degenerative disc disease. In the cervical region, the epidural space is mainly occupied by veins rather than fat, so contrast implications differ from lumbar disease. Furthermore, very thin sections are necessary for the complete evaluation of the patient with cervical radiculopathy (Fig. 87), an area where conventional 2DFT techniques are inadequate because of slice thickness limitations in comparison with the invasive "gold standard" of CT with intrathecal contrast. Therefore, 3DFT offers clear advantages for studying this region.

Importantly, contrast varies tremendously in the spine with changes in flip angle in 3DFT GRASS/spoiled GRASS (Fig. 88). Note that a high intensity CSF "myelographic" image is obtained only when the flip angle is very low, while CSF is low intensity at high flip angles. Also note that bone is always hypointense, which is a reflection of two phenomena: 1) magnetic susceptibility effects due to bony trabecular interfaces (134), and 2) chemical shift signal cancellation due to opposition of phase between marrow fat and water (see Chapter 7). The persistent hypointensity of bone at all flip angles (Fig. 88) is extremely beneficial for separating osteophyte from disc herniation (Fig. 89) since disc material is essentially virtually always hyperintense (regardless of disc dessication) on all flip angles. Note that the neural foramina are very clearly delineated with thin section 3DFT imaging, free from significant artifactual narrowing in spite of using gradient echoes (the susceptibility artifact at bone-fluid interfaces is minimized by decreasing voxel size). One randomized study (135) with blinded readings determined that the accuracy of 1.5mm contiguous sections with this technique equalled the intraobserver variability of thin section CT readings for foraminal disease (therefore, its accuracy is as high as the reproducibility of double reading the gold standard), which, until the advent of this technique, was considered to be a major weakness of MR for evaluating spinal disease. One specific limitation of the technique lies in the evaluation of the post-operative cervical spine, where ferromagnetic artifacts from metallic residua of surgical instrumentation interfere with image interpretation (Fig.

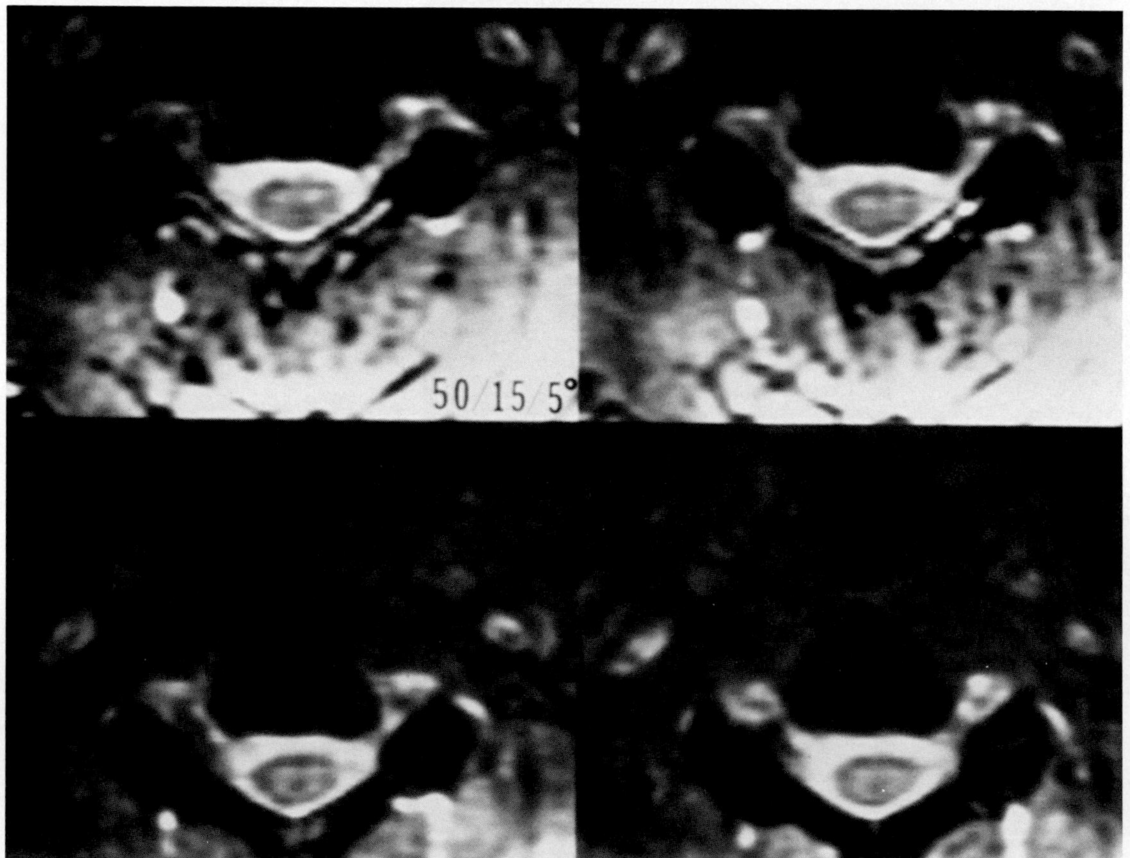

FIG. 87. Contiguous 1.5-mm slices through cervical foramina with 3DFT acquisition. Note that high-quality images can be obtained in contiguity without interference from interslice cross-talk when using 3DFT volume acquisition, clearly defining normal cervical neural foramina.

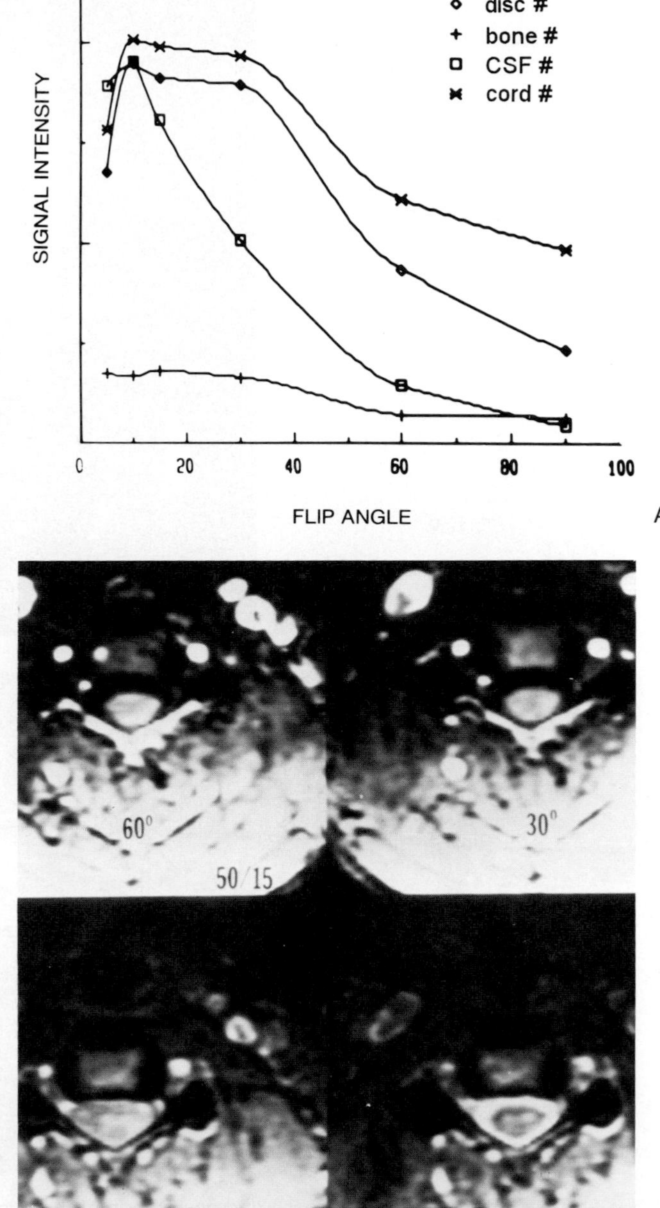

FIG. 88. Effect of flip angle on contrast in cervical spine 3DFT imaging. **A:** Graph of signal intensity vs. flip angle, axial 3DFT images of cervical spine. **B:** Axial 3DFT GRASS through vertebral body with changes in flip angle. **C:** Axial 3DFT GRASS through disc with changes in flip angle. Note from graph (A) that at very low flip angles, CSF is hyperintense to cord, and at high flip angles, CSF is hypointense to cord. Bone remains low intensity, regardless of flip angle. Also note that contrast is maintained, but overall signal drops off after flip angle exceeds 30°. Images (B,C) reflect similar contrast relationships; cord and CSF are isointense at 10°, but CSF around cord and roots is high intensity at 5° and cord is hyperintense amid low-intensity CSF at 30° and 60° flip angles. Bone is always very low intensity, while disc material (C) is hyperintense on all flip angles.

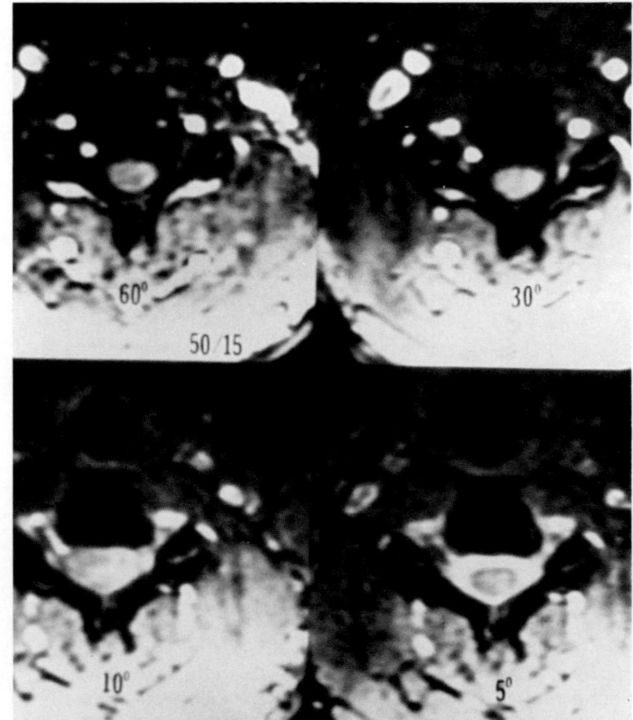

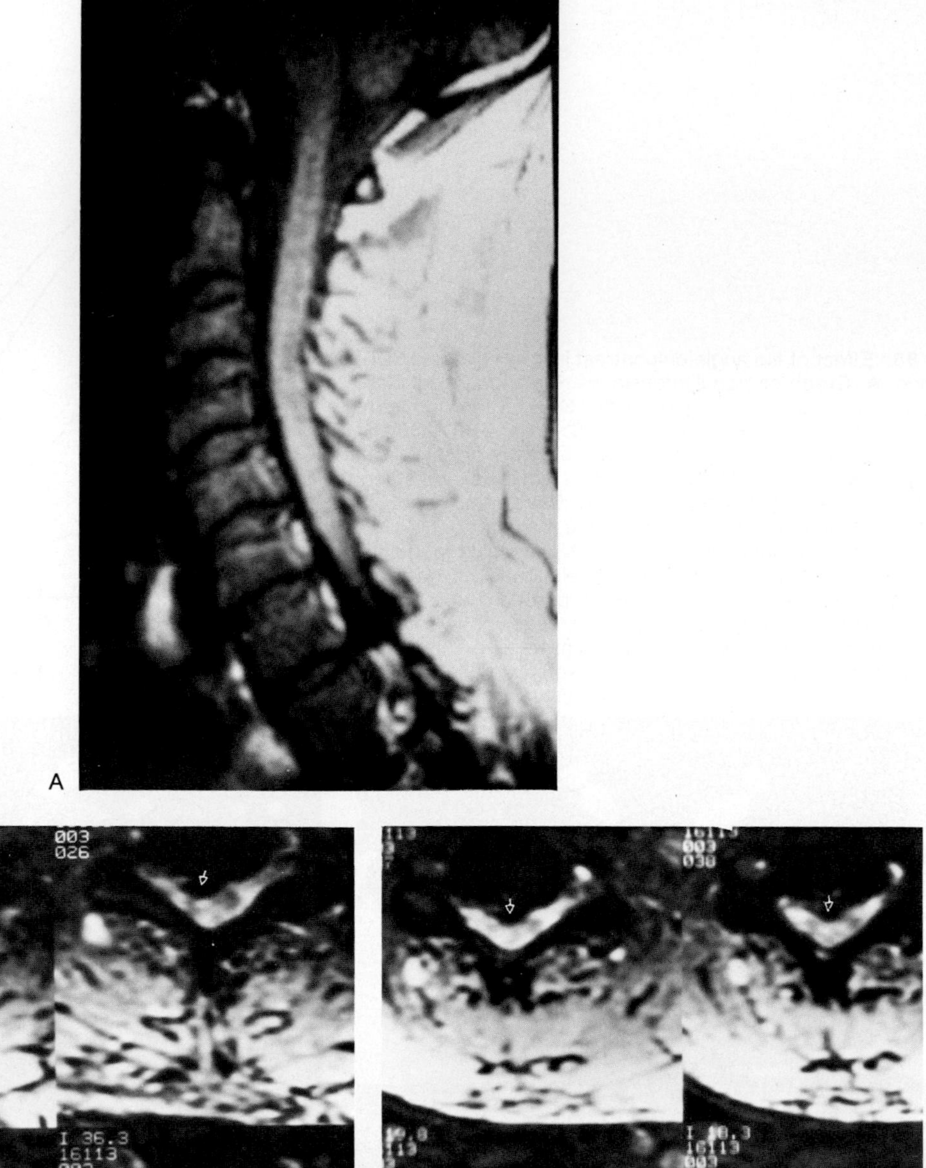

FIG. 89. Osteophytic disease and ossification of the posterior longitudinal ligament (OPLL). **A:** Sagittal spin-echo MRI (600/20). **B:** Serial axial 3DFT GRASS, 50/15/5°. **C:** Serial axial 3DFT GRASS, 50/15/5°. Midsagittal spin-echo image (A) shows mildly narrowed spinal canal. Axial gradient-echo images at two different levels in midcervical spine (B,C) clearly demonstrate OPLL and large ventral osteophyte as markedly hypointense structures (*arrows*) that compress ventrolateral cord.

90). These artifacts can be overcome by using a 3D version of fast spin-echo, rather than gradient-echo, imaging (136).

A potentially important utilization of 3DFT imaging is the capability of reformatting images in other planes after a single acquisition. The benefits of reformatting images in multiple planes from a single acquisition have been touted since the introduction of 3D scanning into the clinical setting. While the attractiveness of this idea is irrefutable, practical problems of the implementation of such a protocol have prevented its introduction at most centers. This can be traced to both the anticipated significant increase in direct physician input required for filming, as well as to the fact that at the time of this writing, no single pulse sequence seems to be optimal for both intramedullary and extramedullary disease. For instance, while 3D gradient-echo imaging has been accepted into most protocols for degenerative disc disease in the cervical spine, the vast majority of radiologists use a form of spin-echo imaging for evaluating the cervical spinal cord itself. Preliminary work on a 3DFT version of fast spin echo has been reported in an attempt to achieve this goal of a single sequence for the cervical spine with mixed results (137).

Relevant to the quality of reformatted images is the geometric characteristics of the imaging voxel. Typically, the voxel is a parallelepiped with its long side orthogonal to the slice plane. Since virtually any arbitrary slice thickness can be achieved in the 3D mode, it can be chosen such that it equals the pixel size. In this case, the voxel has a cubic shape. This acquisition mode is historically termed *isotropic* (138). Voxels from anisotropic acquisitions have unequal dimensions. The advantage of isotropic acquisition is that it permits reformation generating images in secondary display planes retrospectively with no degradation in spatial resolution than that of the original acquisition (as long as the secondary planes are orthogonal). By contrast, oblique reformations are penalized somewhat as far as spatial resolution is concerned, with a maximum degradation of $\sqrt{2}$.

3DFT imaging also shows promise in scanning intracranial regions, especially where high resolution imaging is necessary or desired, such as the temporal bone. With very thin sections (e.g., 1 mm or less) and short echo times, susceptibility artifacts which otherwise plague gradient-echo images of these areas, are minimized. For contiguous slices with T1-based contrast of brain parenchyma, spoiled gradient-echo techniques with ultra-

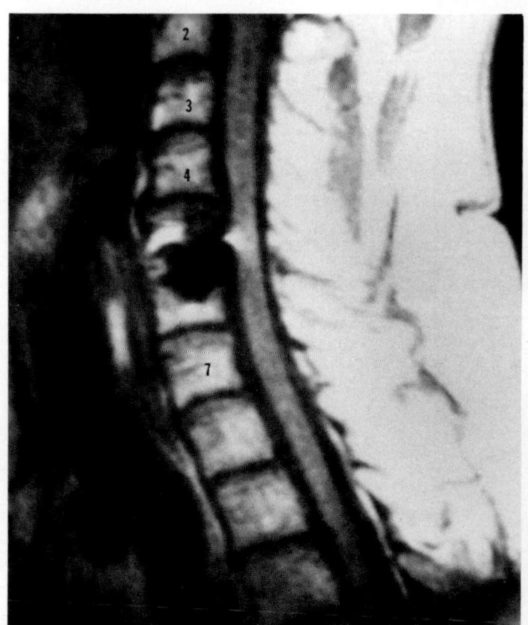

A

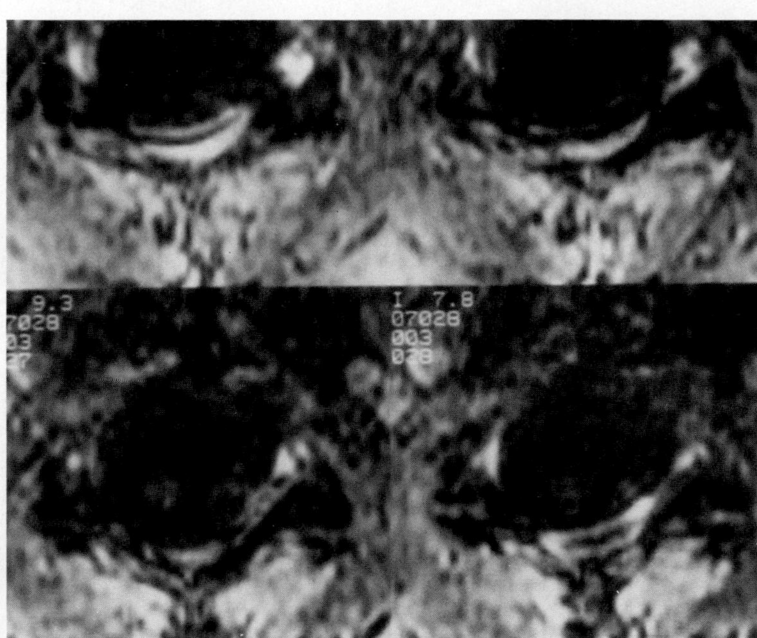

B

FIG. 90. Ferromagnetic artifact degrading 3DFT images of postoperative spine. **A:** Sagittal spin-echo MRI (600/20). **B**: Serial axis 3DFT GRASS, 50/15/5°. In this patient after C5/6 surgery, note ferromagnetic artifact obscuring C5/6 disc space on sagittal image (A). 3DFT gradient-echo images (B) are uninterpretable, due to anatomic distortions from ferromagnetic residua of surgical instrumentation.

short TE (e.g., ≤5 msec) provide superb gray-white contrast (Fig. 91) and have the potential for replacing short TR/short TE spin echo scanning. Similarly, T1-weighted images from 3D MP-RAGE with inversion preparation have been used in conjunction with 3D reformations and 3D shaded surface displays (54,55). Data from such high resolution 3D acquisitions can be combined with overlays of vascular structures for surgical planning (55) (Fig. 92).

Fast Spin-Echo Imaging

Although gradient-echo imaging and its variants have now been granted a defined, albeit limited, role in clinical imaging, the search for faster spin-echo methods (FSE) has continued. The focus on faster spin-echo techniques has been prompted by the generally accepted idea that gradient-echo imaging is less sensitive than spin-echo imaging to the vast majority of brain and spinal cord lesions, that is, those lesions that are diamagnetic and detected on the basis of altered water content, T_1, and T_2. An added advantage of the fast spin-echo technique over rapid gradient-echo imaging sequences is virtual absence of problematic magnetic susceptibility artifacts. Obvious benefits of increasing speed by the degree realized by FSE sequences are that patient throughput increases, motion artifacts due to intolerance of long scan times are reduced, and very high resolution imaging becomes feasible (139).

Overall, the major use of FSE is simply to replace conventional SE imaging, and in the spinal cord in particular, conventional spin-echo imaging is generally no longer utilized. It is clear that for large intraparenchymal lesions, the similarity of FSE to SE images is enough to obviate the latter in most instances (Fig. 93). The issue of small focal hyperintense lesions, on first consideration, may be different. This follows from the previous discussion of the point spread function, where we realize that the intensity of a small object is changed by virtue of the contribution of different lines of *k*-space to an image. In one study (140), blinded readings by several independent readers were conducted in a group of patients who had both SE and FSE sequences performed. In that study, there was a small but statistically significant increase in the number of lesions detected on SE images compared to FSE images. This difference, however, fell within the range of intra-observer variation in the interpretation of the same set of SE images twice by the same observers. The investigators concluded that, although there were

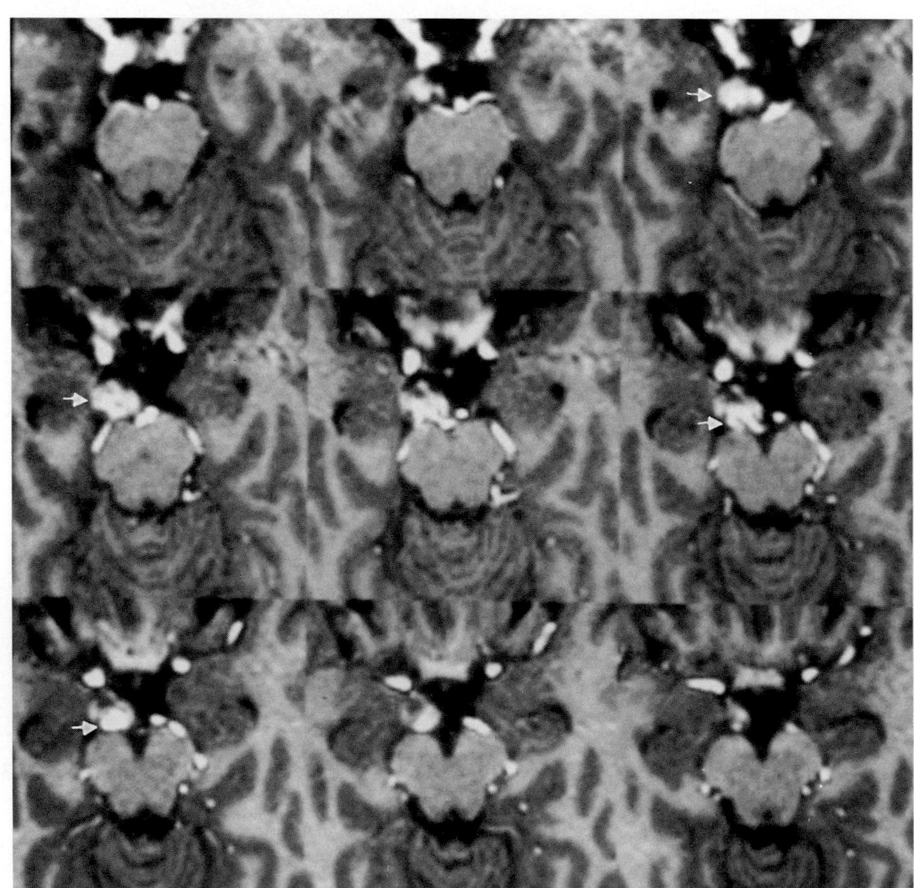

FIG. 91. Contiguous 2-mm 3DFT spoiled GRASS images at level of suprasellar cistern. Note superb contrast between gray and white matter and high intensity in circle of Willis arterial vessels, incidentally depicting small right posterior communicating artery aneurysm (*arrows*).

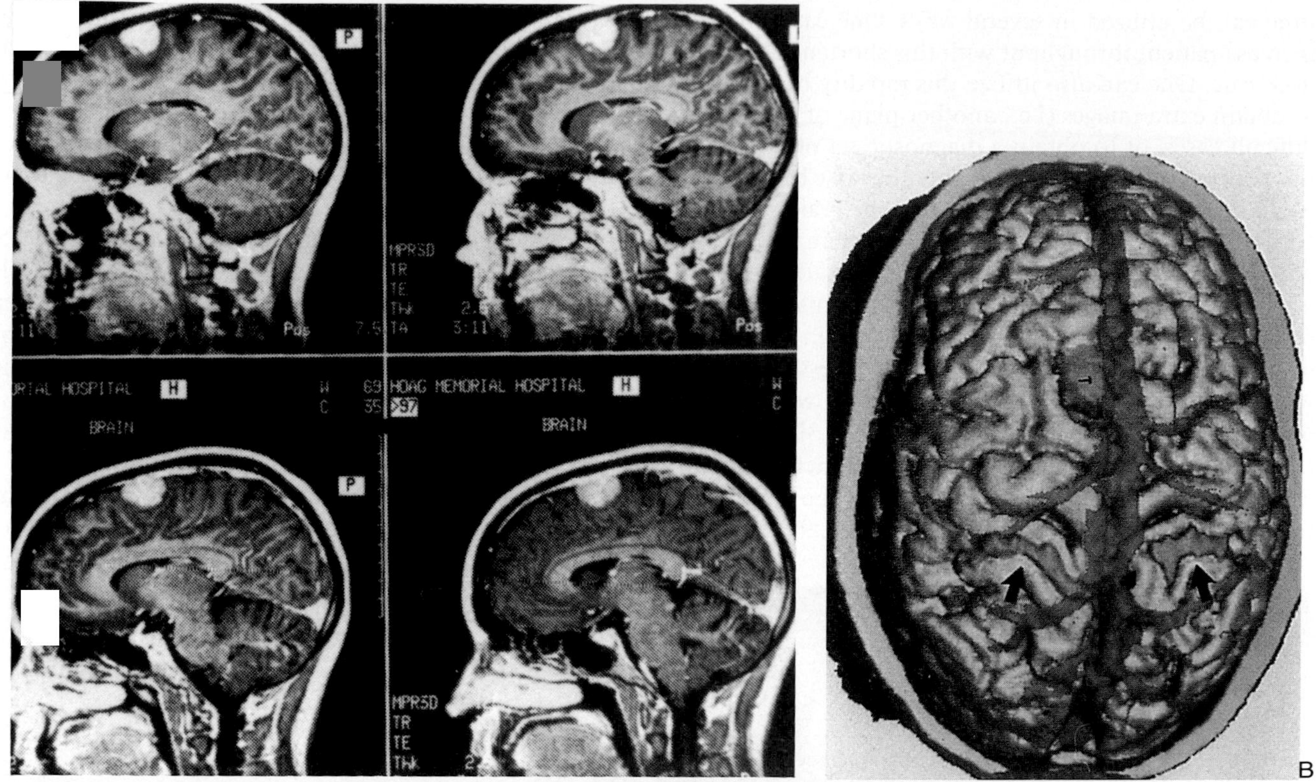

A B

FIG. 92. Post-contrast 3D MP-RAGE images (**A**) of parasagittal meningioma, along with 3D surface-rendered image (**B**), showing tumor (T) and its relationship to superior sagittal sinus. Central sulcus (*arrows*) is well posterior to the tumor (From Brant-Zawadzki et al., ref. 54, with permission.)

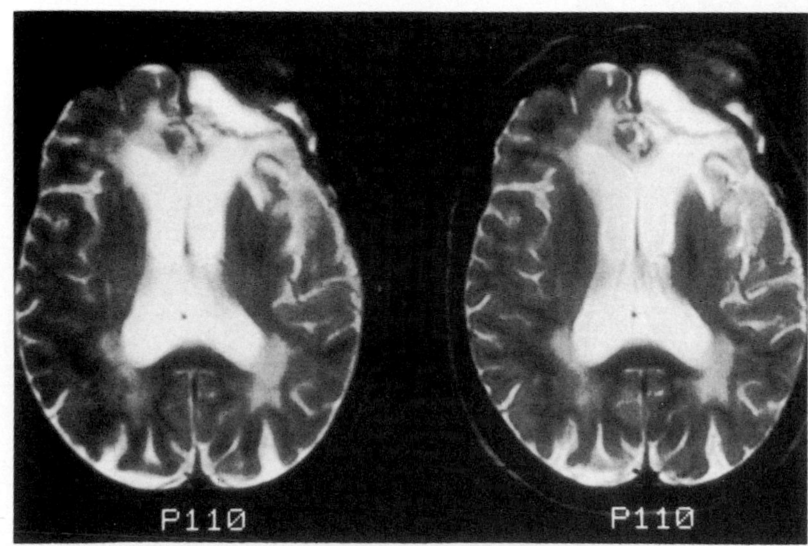

FIG. 93. Large mass lesion. SE versus FSE. On left, the conventional SE long TR/TE image shows a corpus callosum mass with postoperative changes in the left frontal lobe and high-intensity periventricular white matter. Note virtually identical appearance of abnormalities on the FSE image (right). (From Atlas et al., ref. 139, with permission.)

differences between SE and FSE images, no clinically significant difference was present (Fig. 94).

The replacement of spin echo by FSE in routine brain imaging shortens overall examination time, and this time can be utilized in several ways. One can certainly increase patient throughput with this shortened acquisition time. One can also utilize this rapidity of scanning to obtain extra images (i.e., another plane of section) in difficult cases, or to obtain a diagnostic set of images in uncooperative patients who might otherwise be impossible to image (Fig. 95). One can image the brain or spinal cord during the same setting in cases where one might otherwise only recommend this on subsequent rescanning to confirm or seek out diagnoses (e.g., multiple sclerosis). In addition, one can obtain very high resolution images in anatomic regions where it is essential and where scan times using conventional SE would have been prohibitive (Fig. 96), including in the 3DFT mode (Fig. 97). Along these lines, we now routinely generate 512 × 512 high resolution FSE images when using MR for orbital or temporal bone pathology (Fig. 98).

Another potential utilization of FSE is for the production of "black blood" MR angiograms (see Chapter 31), since FSE images show relative signal loss in the presence of intravascular flow (141). The rationale for this application lies in the well-known tendency for nearly all of the problematic artifacts of "white blood" MR angiography to appear as loss of signal, even though flow is present. The *intentional* depiction of the presence of flow as signal void, as in black blood methods (Fig. 99), would theoretically eliminate problems of signal loss due to turbulence, etc.

Practical constraints due to slice limitation of FSE have been addressed by other authors (60) and are influenced by the selection of specific technical parameters, such as the number of echoes per TR (ETL). These problems can be somewhat resolved by maneuvers like increasing the TR to allow for more slices and are of limited importance. However, there are potentially important limitations imposed by the lack of sensitivity of the FSE sequence to intracranial hemorrhage and brain iron which are inherent to the technique itself. The short

A

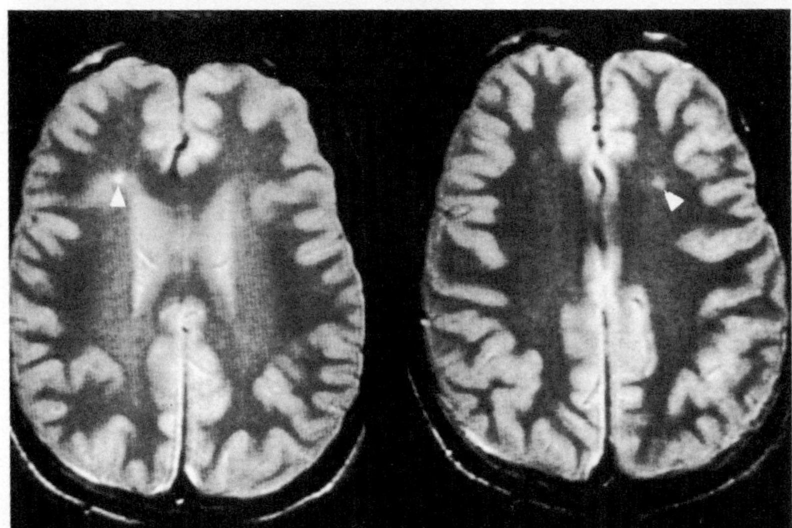

B

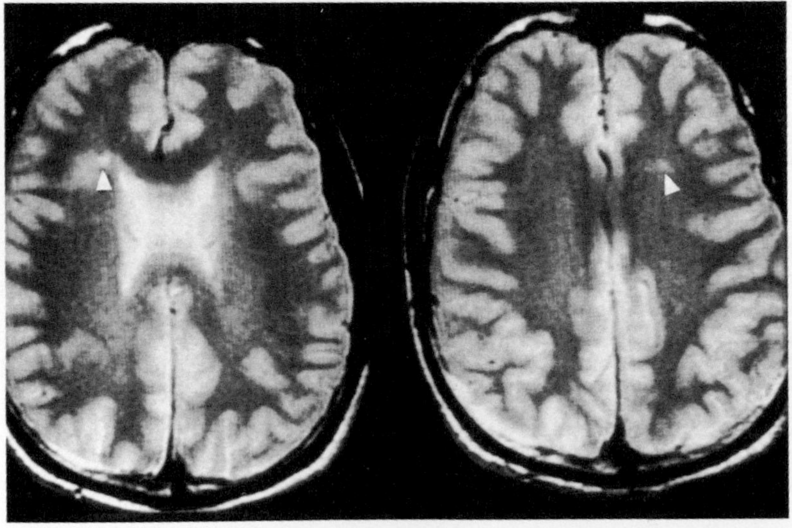

FIG. 94. Small focal white matter lesions, SE versus FSE. **A:** Conventional SE long TR/short TE images show two small focal hyperintense lesions (*arrows*). **B:** FSE long TR/short TE_{eff} shows identical appearance (*arrows*), identified correctly by blinded readers. (From Atlas et al., ref. 139, with permission.)

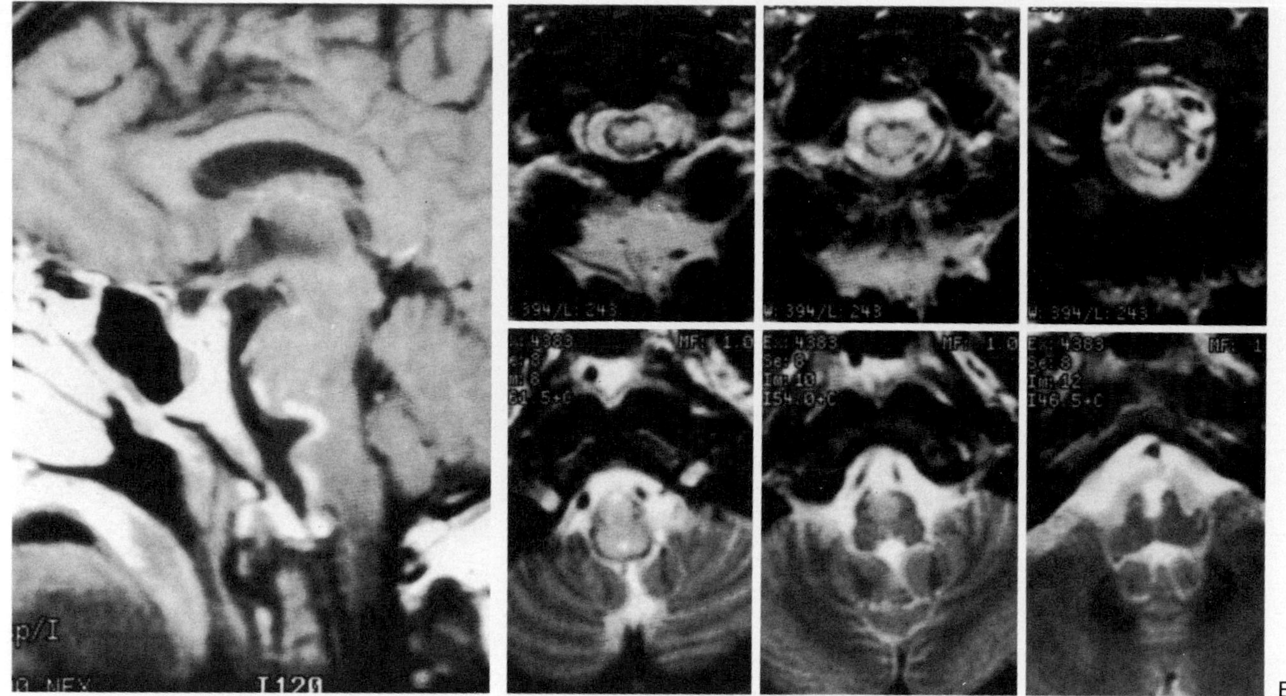

FIG. 95. Thrombosis of anterior median pontomesencephalic vein with brainstem venous infarction. **A:** Sagittal short TR/TE SE image shows hyperintense clot within midline thrombosed vein. **B:** Axial long TR FSE images obtained rapidly clearly show pathology without obscuring by motion artifact in this very ill patient unable to cooperate for long acquisition time images. (From Atlas et al., ref. 139, with permission.)

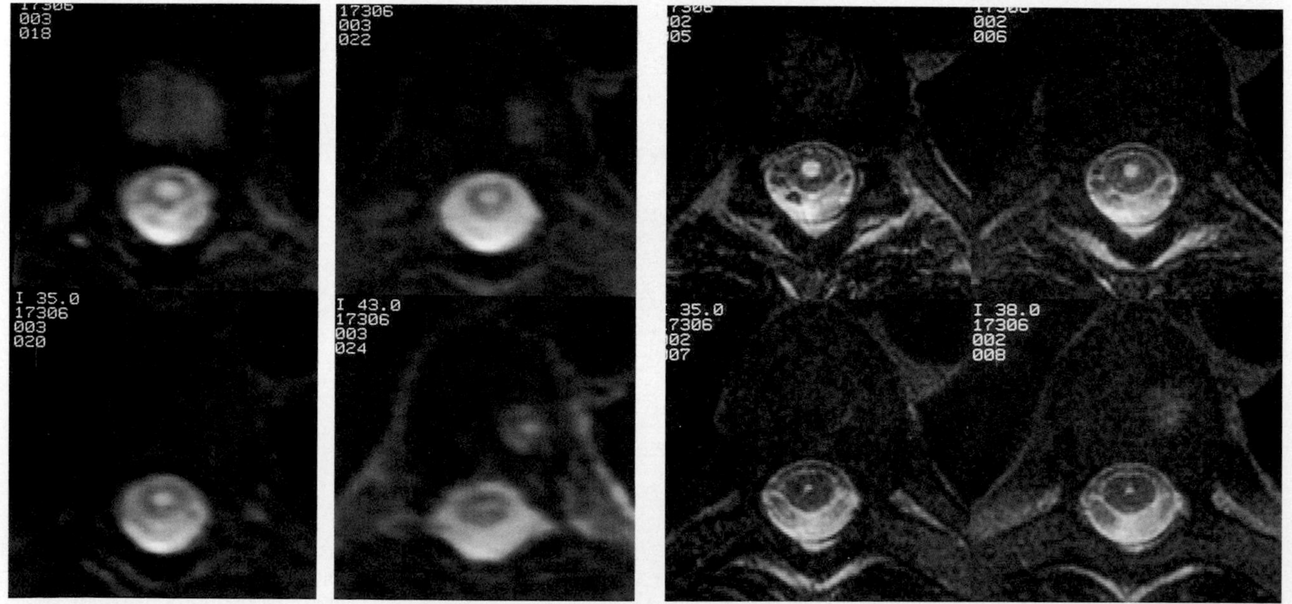

FIG. 96. High resolution T2-weighted FSE, syringomyelia. Ill-defined central hyperintensity on conventional T2-weighted spin-echo images (**A**) is clear and distinctly seen on 512 × 512 T2-weighted FSE images (**B**), which were obtained in less time.

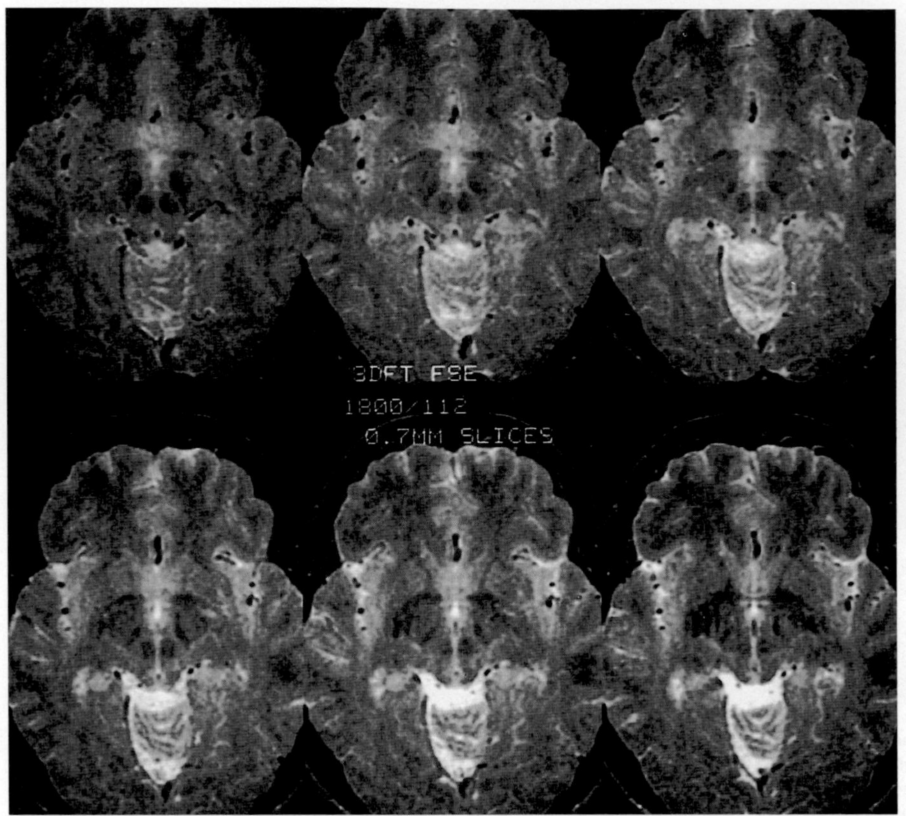

A

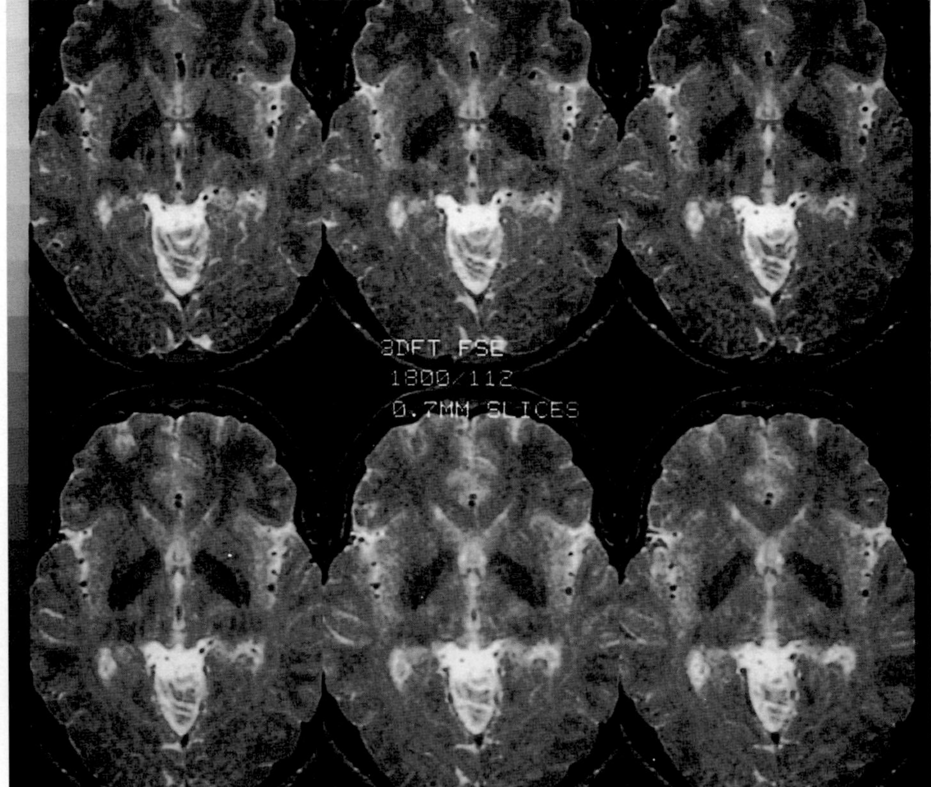

B

FIG. 97. Ultra-high resolution T2-weighted FSE using 3D volume acquisition. Contiguous 0.7-mm sections generated with 3D FSE (inferior to superior, **A–B**) show previously unobtainable high resolution T2-weighted images.

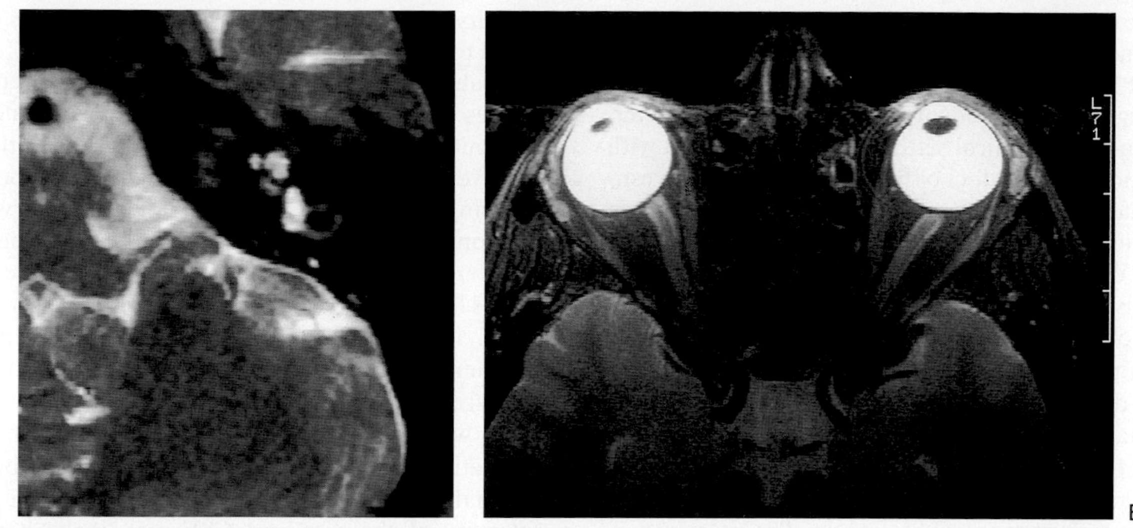

FIG. 98. A: High resolution T2-weighted FSE, temporal bone. Note clear depiction of non-bony components of normal anatomy of labyrinth on 512 × 512 FSE image. **B:** High resolution T2-weighted FSE, orbit. Rapidly acquired T2-weighted images with 512 × 512 delineate small structures of orbit, an area where conventional low resolution T2-weighted images are typically degraded by motion.

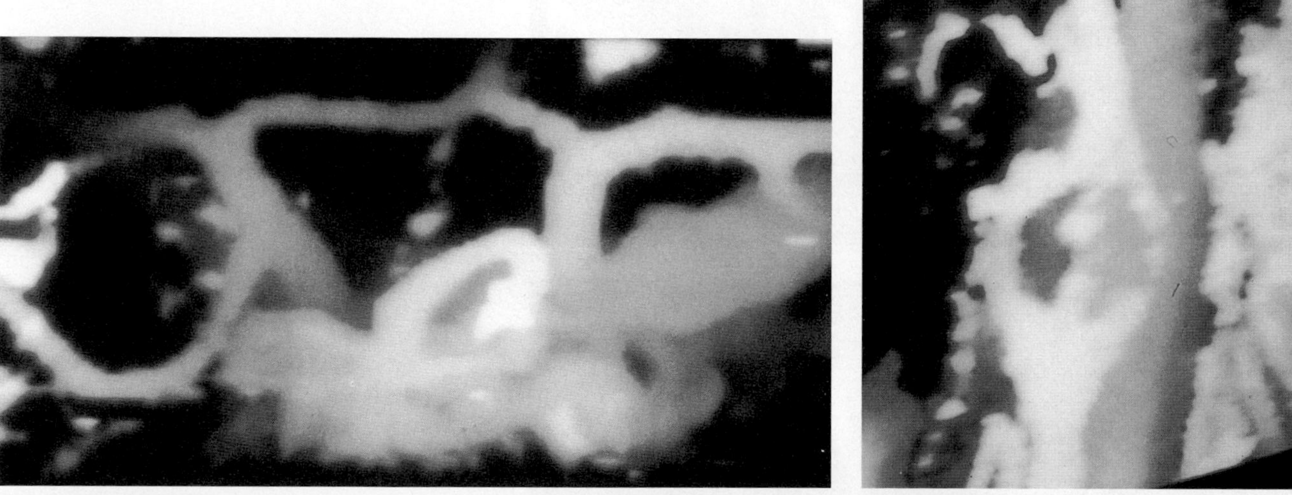

FIG. 99. Black blood MRA. (Courtesy of J. Listerud, Portland, OR.) Projection image from 3DFT FSE acquisition shows circle of willis region (**A**). Obscuring by venous system at skull base is also noted. In separate patient, projection image shows severe extracranial carotid artery bifurcation disease (**B**) which was depicted as complete signal loss on "white blood" time-of-flight image (not shown). Also note jugular vein.

interecho interval in FSE most likely accounts for the lack of signal loss in iron-containing lesions on FSE (Fig. 100).

The sensitivity for acute and remote hemorrhage, cavernous hemangiomas, hemorrhagic metastases, and hemorrhagic infarction is presumably therefore reduced (142). The clinical relevance of this reduced sensitivity to some forms of hemorrhage remains debatable, however (Figs. 101 and 102). In practice, it is likely that most hemorrhages are still evident on FSE images. Moreover, imaging in many clinical settings is not concerned with the detection of small foci of hemorrhage. Some investigators believe that supplemental gradient-echo scans in combination with FSE comprise a reasonable routine protocol. We believe that, with adequate monitoring of clinical histories, a significant proportion of brain and nearly all of spinal cord MRI can be performed with FSE rather than spin echo without a clinically relevant diminution in diagnostic sensitivity.

FSE imaging of the spine is in most ways quite similar to conventional spin-echo imaging in this region. However, several significant differences change the appearance and interpretation of FSE images. The most important differences are suppression of the cerebrospinal fluid pulsation artifact in FSE imaging and a higher fat-signal intensity on FSE than on conventional spin-echo images. There is a theoretical concern that there may be difficulties in detecting very small intramedullary lesions on the FSE images. Finally, there is an improved conspicuity of spinal nerve roots on FSE images as compared to SE images.

As already stated, the appeal of FSE is that it produces images which are very similar to those obtained using conventional spin-echo techniques. Just as in the brain, however, the great increases in imaging speed permit developing protocols which would not be feasible with conventional techniques. For example, our routine lumbar spine study for evaluating degenerative disease now includes long TR axial imaging through the entire lumbar spine. This is useful in displaying the full extent of disc fragments which have migrated away from the interspace, obtaining axial images in the upper lumbar spine where degenerative disease rarely results in disc herniations, better display of unanticipated abnormalities in the lumbar spine, and at times the change in signal intensity of the disc and CSF may make herniations

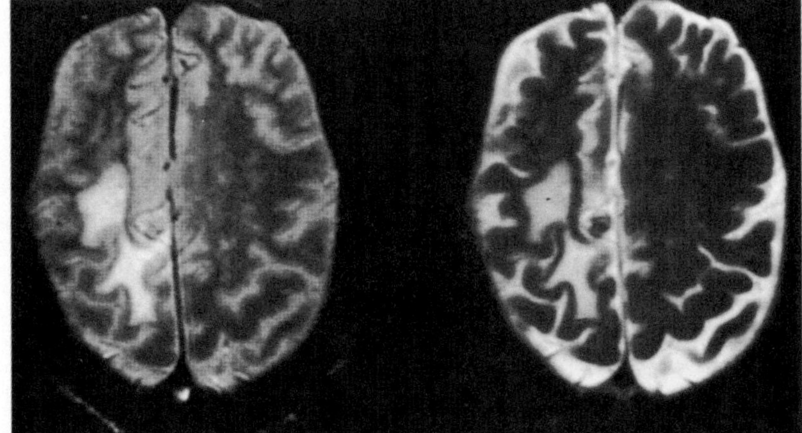

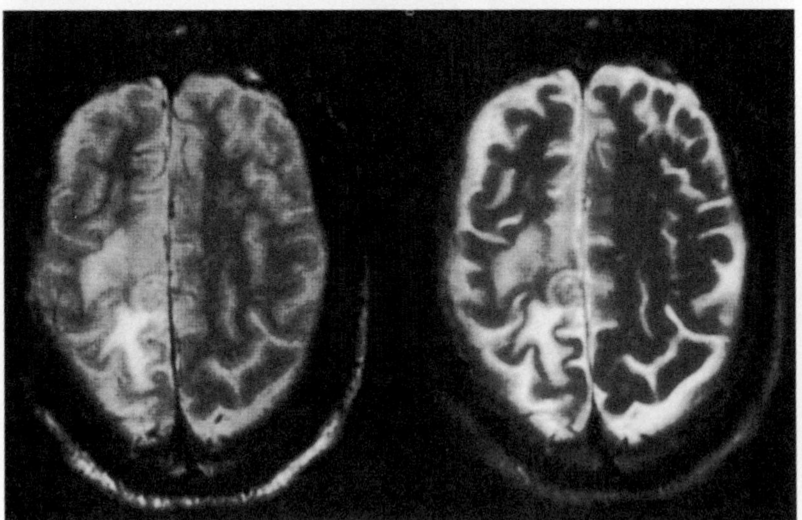

FIG. 100. Hemorrhagic metastasis, SE versus FSE. **A:** Long TR/short TE and long TR/TE SE images clearly show marked hypointensity on a long TE image, indicative of acute hemorrhage into metastasis. **B**: Long TR/short TE_{eff} and long TR/TE_{eff} show lesion but fail to demonstrate the hypointensity indicative of hemorrhage. (From Atlas et al., ref. 139, with permission.)

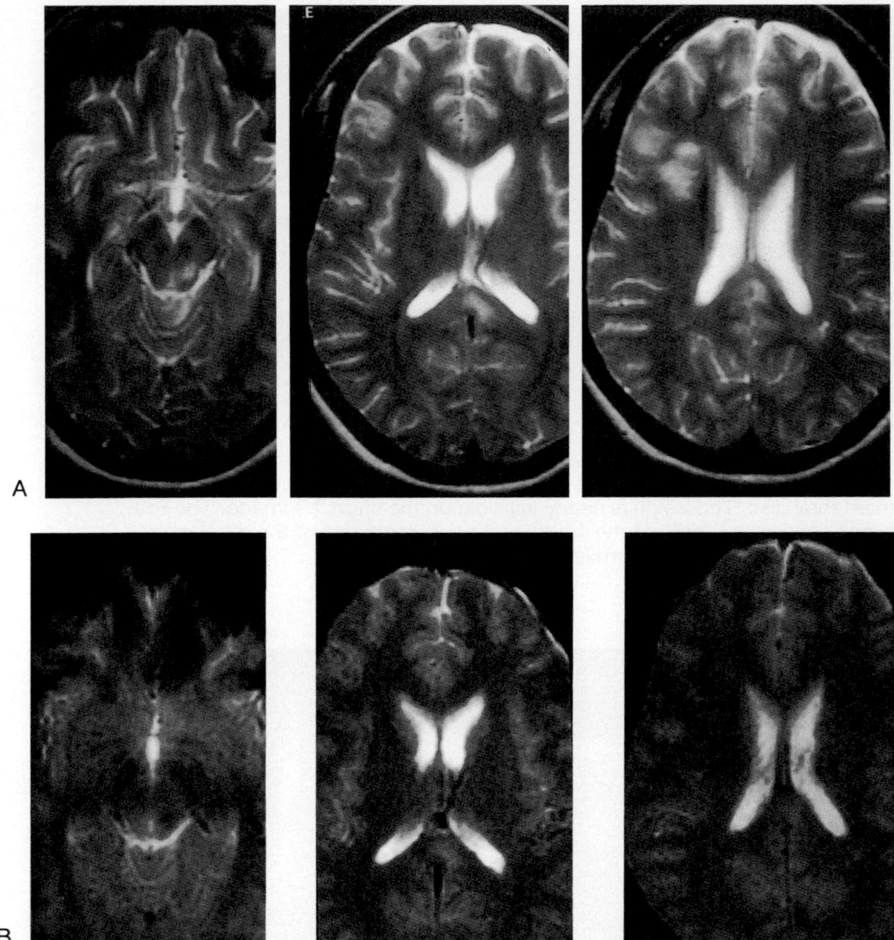

FIG. 101. Hemorrhage in diffuse axonal injury, FSE versus gradient echo. Multiple shearing injuries in dorsal midbrain, corpus callosum, and subcortical white matter on FSE (**A**) are seen as containing small hemorrhagic foci on gradient-echo scans (**B**). The significance of this finding is uncertain, but it may indicate an irreversible lesion and therefore be a clue to prognosis.

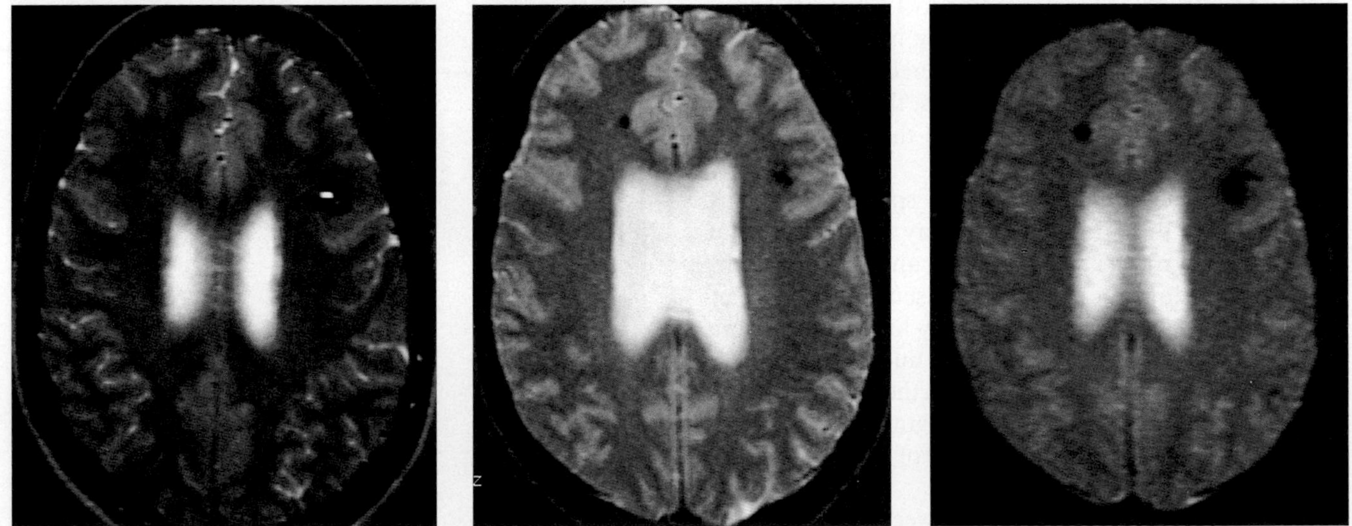

FIG. 102. Cavernous hemangiomas, FSE vs. spin echo vs. gradient echo. Two cavernous hemangiomas (right and left frontal) are identifiable on FSE (**A**), spin echo (**B**), and gradient echo (**C**), despite the differences in sensitivity to hemorrhage.

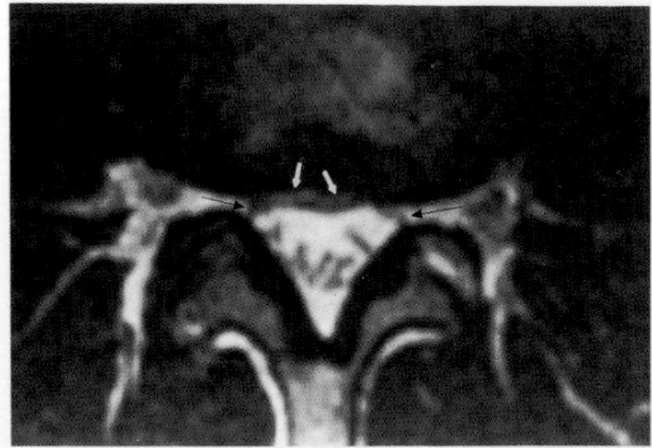
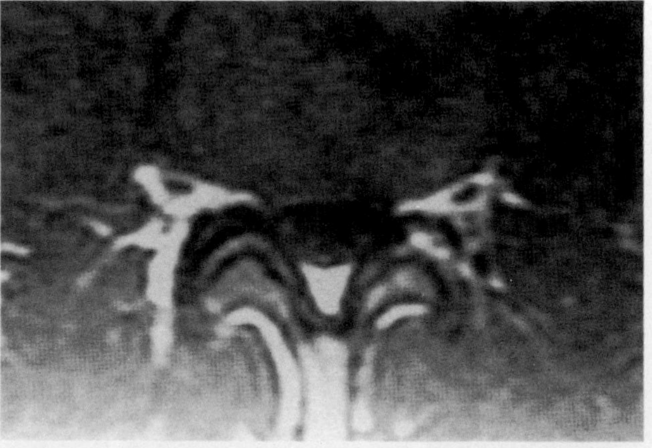

A B

FIG. 103. Axial TR = 4000, TE = 78 FSE image (**A**) showing a small L4 disc protrusion (*white arrows*). On the TR = 500, TE = 14 axial spin-echo image (**B**) at the same level there is very little contrast between the herniated fragment and the remainder of the intervertebral disc. The lesion is nearly invisible on the short TR image. The FSE image also shows striking hypointensity and conspicuousness of the intrathecal nerve roots and of the dural margin of the thecal sac (*black arrows*). (From Atlas et al., ref. 139, with permission.)

more conspicuous (Fig. 103). This study would be prohibitively time-consuming using conventional spin-echo imaging, but it is quite practical using FSE. A typical protocol would be TR = 4000, TE = 85, 256 × 256, ETL = 16. Although this may require multiple acquisitions in order to cover the entire lumbar spine, the complete examination with 4-mm sections and 1-mm gaps may be obtained in less than 6 minutes.

T2-weighted FSE images are similar to spin-echo images in that the high signal intensity of the cerebrospinal fluid produces excellent contrast between the thecal sac and epidural tissues (Fig. 103). In most cases, this produces an increase in contrast between the intervertebral disc and the thecal sac as compared to T1-weighted spin-echo images (Fig. 103). Occasionally in cases in which disc herniations, especially sequestered fragments, are hyperintense on T2-weighted images, this may result in a reduction in contrast between the thecal sac and the disc fragment.

Unlike conventional long TR/TE spin-echo imaging in which CSF pulsation artifacts may cause significant degradation of images in the cervical and thoracic spine, fast spin-echo imaging is relatively insensitive to such artifacts. Although FSE images display little artifact from CSF pulsation, gradient moment nulling techniques have been combined with FSE to further suppress these artifacts. These also require prolonging the minimum echo spacing and reduce the number of sections that can be acquired.

The most obvious difference between FSE and CSE images and the most important disadvantage of FSE imaging is the persistent high intensity of adipose tissue discussed above. In spinal imaging, the practical consequences of this fat hyperintensity are changes in the signal intensity of yellow marrow on FSE as composed to spin-echo images and a striking hyperintensity of epidural fat (Figs. 104–106). The change in marrow signal

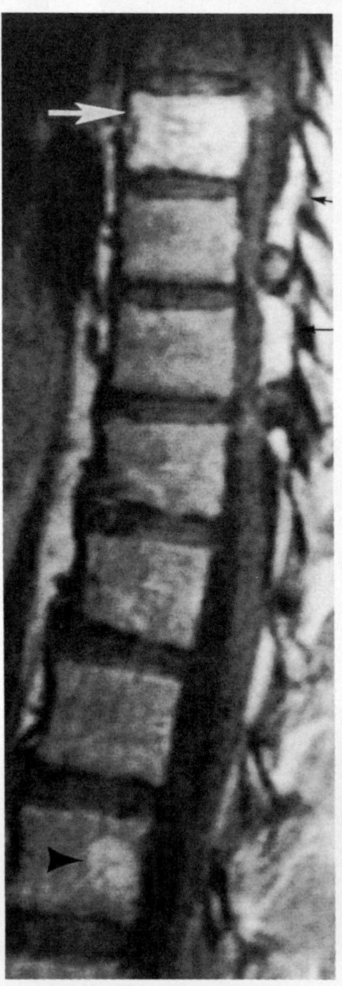
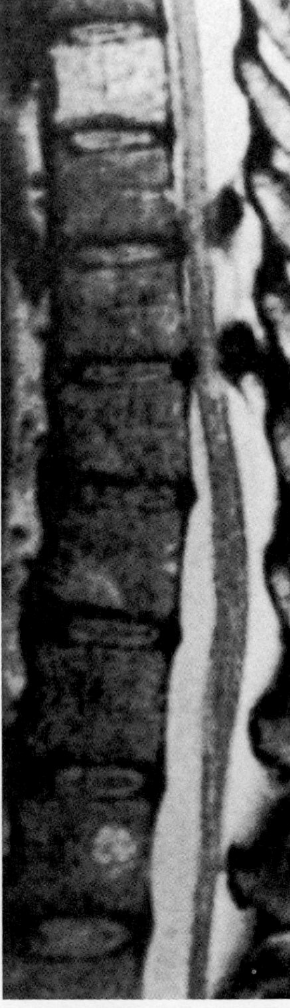

A,B

FIG. 104. Sagittal TR = 500, TE = 16 image (**A**) of a vertebral body hemangioma (*white arrow*), focal fat deposition (*arrowhead*), and calcification of the ligamentum flavum with widening of the fat-filled epidural space posteriorly (*black arrows*). On the TR = 2700, TE = 85 FSE image (**B**), both the hemangioma and the focal fat remain hyperintense. On the FSE image, the signal intensity of the epidural fat is nearly identical to that of CSF. (From Atlas et al., ref. 139, with permission.)

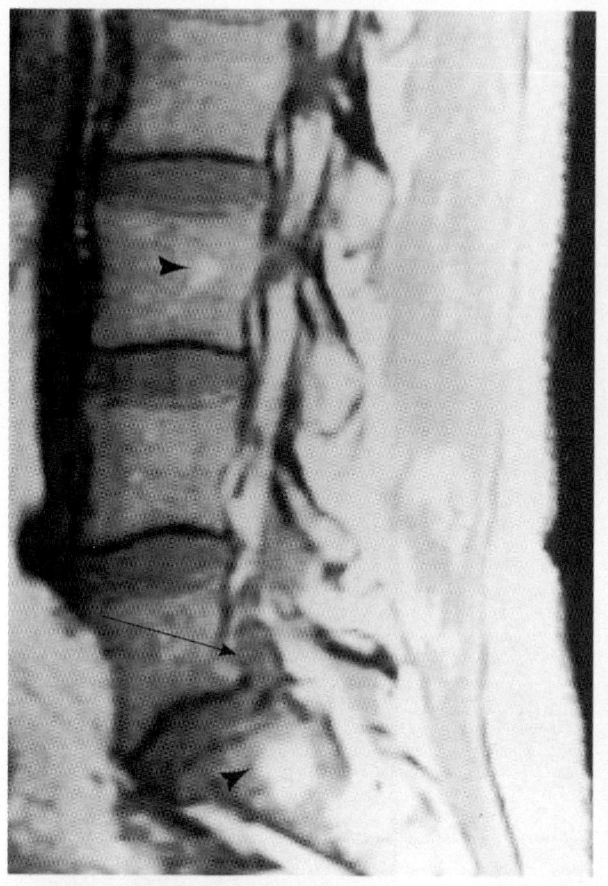

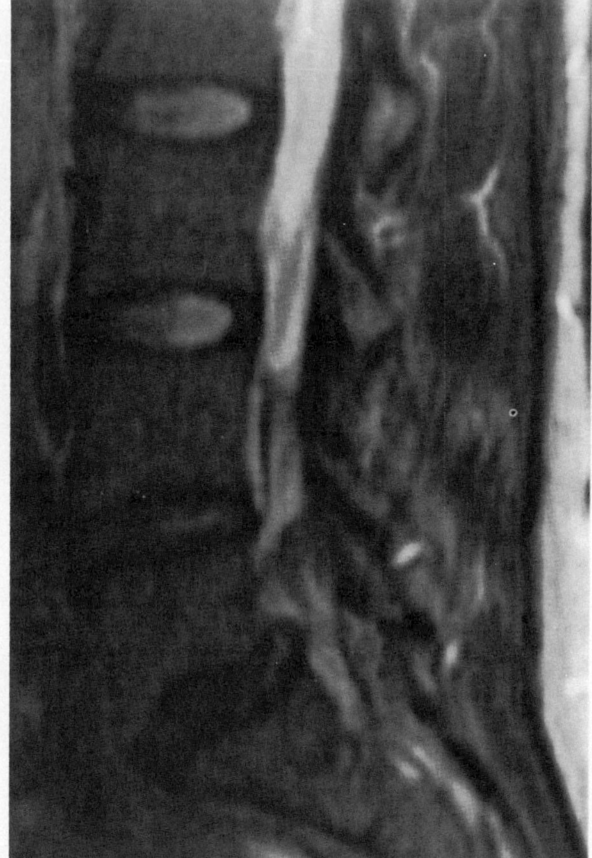

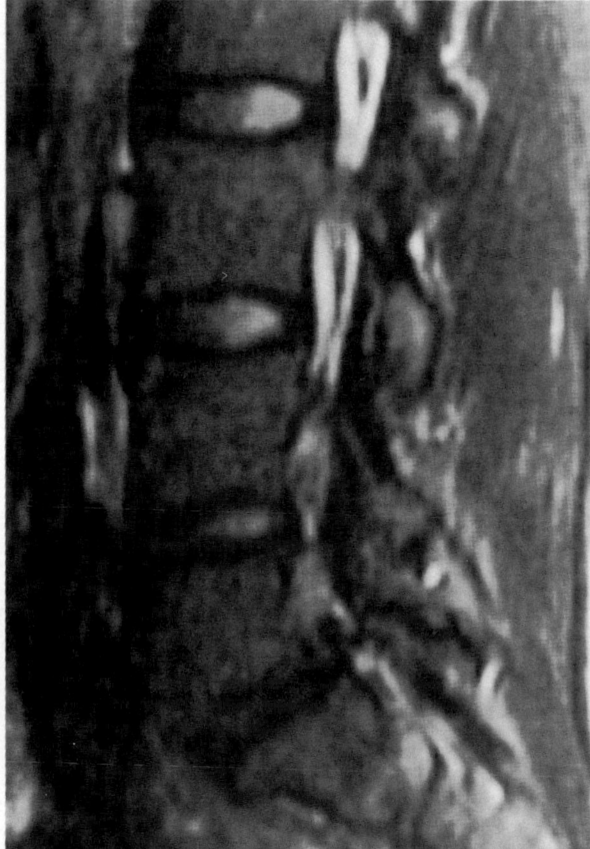

FIG. 105. TR = 600, TE = 12 sagittal spin-echo image (**A**) through the lower lumbar spine. There are areas of focal fat deposition in the sacrum and the L3 vertebral body (*arrowheads*). In addition, a large disc fragment has extended from the L5-S1 interspace into the L5 neural foramen (*arrow*). Two contiguous TR = 4000, TE = 80 FSE images with chemical shift selective fat saturation (**B** and **C**) bracket the short TR/TE image. The areas of focal fat deposition can no longer be detected. In addition, the suppression of fat-signal intensity has eliminated the tissue contrast between the disc herniation and the contents of the neural foramen. Although the L4–L5 neural foramen is normal on the short TR/TE images, the saturation has rendered the epidural fat isointense to the herniated fragment. Therefore, in this case, the use of fat saturation on the FSE images has been detrimental to detecting the disc herniation. (From Atlas et al., ref. 139, with permission.)

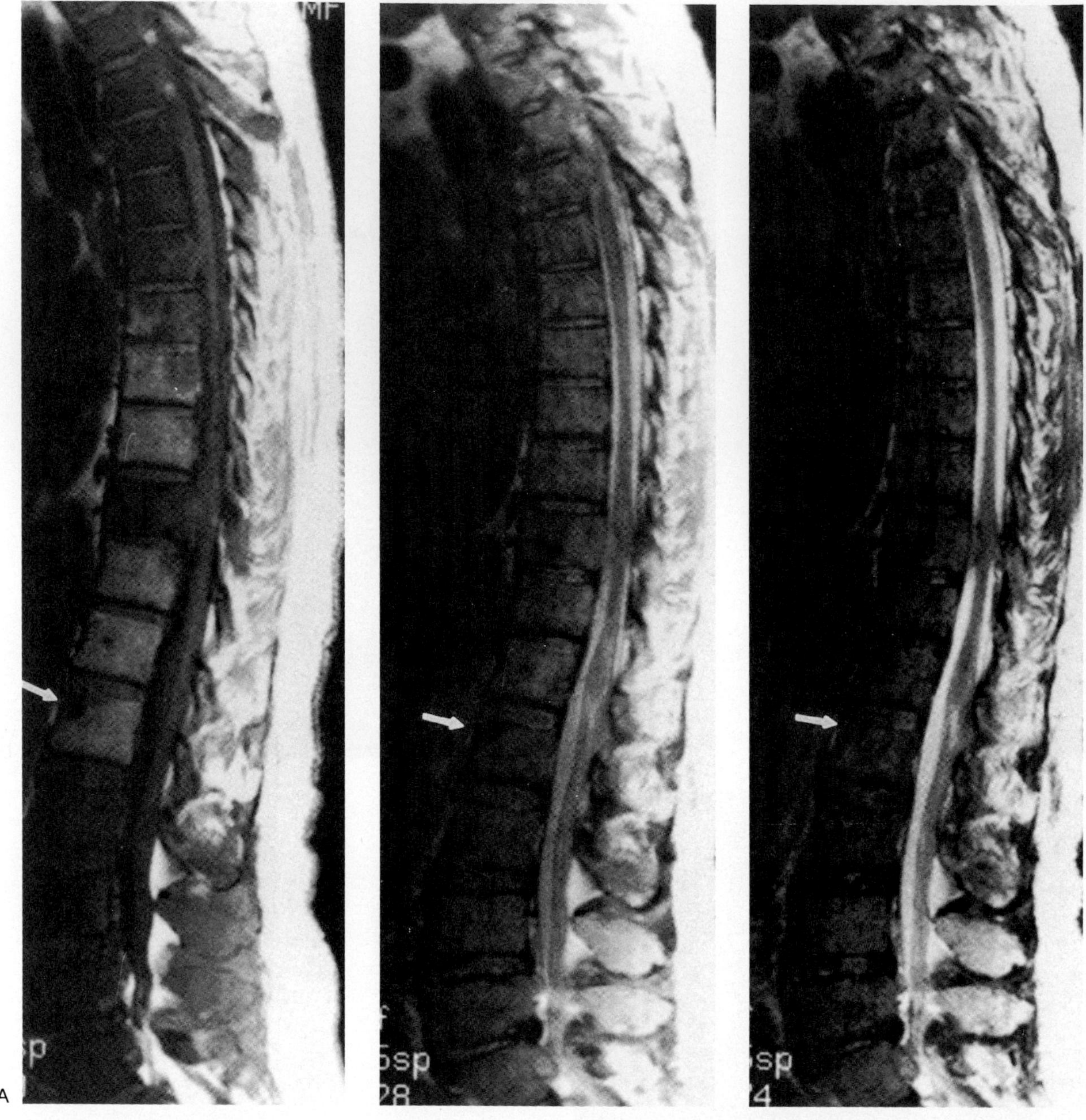

FIG. 106. Sagittal TR = 500, TE = 11 spin-echo image (**A**). The short TR/TE image shows multiple vertebral body metastases in this 68-year-old man with prostatic carcinoma. Note that the metastases appear nearly isointense to normal vertebral bodies on the TR = 4000, TE = 17 (**B**), and TR = 4000, TE = 85 (**C**) images. This persistent hyperintensity of adipose tissue on the fast spin-echo images severely reduces its sensitivity to metastases. The osteoblastic lesion is visible on all images (*arrows*).

intensity has great potential significance in image interpretation since the appearance of many abnormalities have been characterized, in part, by their signal intensity on T2-weighted images. Examples include vertebral hemangiomas (Fig. 104), focal fat deposition within vertebral bodies (Figs. 104 and 105), changes in the fat and vascular tissue content of vertebral bodies related to degenerative disease, infections of the vertebrae, metastases (Fig. 106), and compression fractures. Descriptions of the characteristic signal intensities of these abnormalities on long TR/TE images have been based upon the relative hypointensity of normal adipose tissue observed on conventional spin-echo images. The signal intensity of epidural fat also contributes to anatomic diagnoses. Figure 104 illustrates a case in which the persistent high intensity of fat makes it difficult to separate adipose tissue in an enlarged posterior epidural space from CSF on a long TR/TE FSE image. Unfortunately, chemical shift-selective fat suppression is not always desirable on FSE images. Variations in bulk susceptibility prevent uniform suppression of fat signal when large fields of view are employed—for example, when using long phased array coils. Fat suppression may also obscure lesions by removing the contrast between the abnormality and epidural adipose tissue.

On long TR images, the edge enhancement of short T_2 structures, such as nerve roots, when surrounded by long T_2 CSF, results in increased conspicuity. This feature arises as a result of the previously described point-spread function considerations. A clinical example is given in Fig. 103. Note the striking conspicuity of the roots evident on the FSE image. The same effect increases the conspicuity of the low intensity dura mater of the thecal sac and ligamentous structures against the hyperintense CSF.

This effect has made FSE the best available sequence for detecting arachnoiditis. Scarring of the pia, arachnoid, and dura produce changes which are recognized on imaging studies as arachnoiditis. When scarring of the arachnoid is present there is almost always associated pial scarring as well. The extent of dural scarring associated with pial and arachnoid inflammation appears to be more variable. The changes which may be produced by scarring of the meninges are by tradition referred to as "arachnoiditis" without distinguishing among pial, arachnoidal, or dural scarring. Three patterns of nerve root abnormality in arachnoiditis are recognized with myelographic imaging (143,144). It may be difficult to make the diagnosis of arachnoiditis on noncontrast short TR spin-echo MR studies since high spatial resolution, high contrast images are needed in order to detect abnormal arrangements of the lumbar roots (145). Although contrast-enhanced MR images may be helpful in identifying active inflammation, the pial and arachnoid scarring are diagnosed on the basis of anatomic changes. There is no apparent relationship between the presence or intensity of enhancement and the severity of anatomic abnormality or clinical findings (146).

Potential Applications of Ultrafast Imaging

The speed of echo-planar imaging is such that entire images can be acquired in less than 50 to 100 msec. Once the data sampling time has become a small fraction of the period of physiologic motion (such as respiration, peristalsis, cardiac, or CSF pulsation), such motion can no longer degrade the images. The major potential for such imaging speeds lies in the visualization of physiology and regional brain function (see Chapter 30). While many of the dynamic signal changes already described in the literature with echo-planar imaging can be noted with more conventional fast imaging methods, it is our belief that the true exploitation of this unique data in the clinical setting necessitates that the whole brain be studied. The requisite acquisition times for such imaging are achievable at present only with EPI. Patient-generated motion which typically degrades diffusion/perfusion imaging attempted in conventional time frames can be eliminated with ultrafast techniques (147).

In brain imaging, functional imaging can be performed either with or without intravenous contrast agents. One very promising application of ultrafast gradient-echo imaging exploits differentials in local magnetic susceptibility: imaging of microcirculation (perfusion) by means of intravenously administered paramagnetic (36) and superparamagnetic agents (148–150). Such methods overcome one of the major difficulties of direct imaging of tissue perfusion (151), the very small capillary volume (only a few percent of total volume which requires very high SNR to separate it from extravascular tissue). The resultant change in magnetic susceptibility by administering a paramagnetic agent intravenously causes a field gradient beyond the vascular compartment (36). Rather than signal enhancement, as it would be expected for dipole-dipole relaxation from shortening of T_1, a transient signal loss is expected due to magnetic field gradients set up in the boundary zone between capillaries, as shown schematically in Fig. 107. Villringer et al. have shown that up to 60% of the brain tissue water is within the range of these gradients. Hence, unlike conventional enhancing agents for the brain, the susceptibility effect does not reflect (nor, for that matter, does it require) alterations in blood–brain barrier permeability. Dysprosium has been reported to exert the strongest effect, consistent with its large magnetic moment, although an effect is also shown with both conventional and high dose gadolinium (36).

The decrease in intensity is more profound in gray matter, which corresponds to differences in capillary (blood) volume (Fig. 108). From integration of the concentration-time data during dynamic imaging as the agent passes through the cerebral capillaries (Fig. 109), regional cerebral blood volume can be determined and displayed in image form. This has been hypothesized as a means of assessing "tissue at risk" during an acute ischemic event. The blood volume technique is also currently being investigated as a method of discriminating recurrent tumor from radiation necrosis, based on the hypothesis that differences in metabolic rates are reflected by similar differences in blood volume (see Chapter 30).

Blood oxygen level dependent contrast (BOLD) imaging (93,95) is a noninvasive functional MRI (fMRI) technique for localizing regional brain signal intensity changes in response to task performance (94,152,153). This technique utilizes no intravenous contrast agents and depends mainly on regional changes in endogenous intravascular paramagnetic deoxyhemoglobin (154). Signal intensity changes in BOLD fMRI are attributed to the documented mismatch between increases in regional cerebral blood flow and cerebral blood volume and the

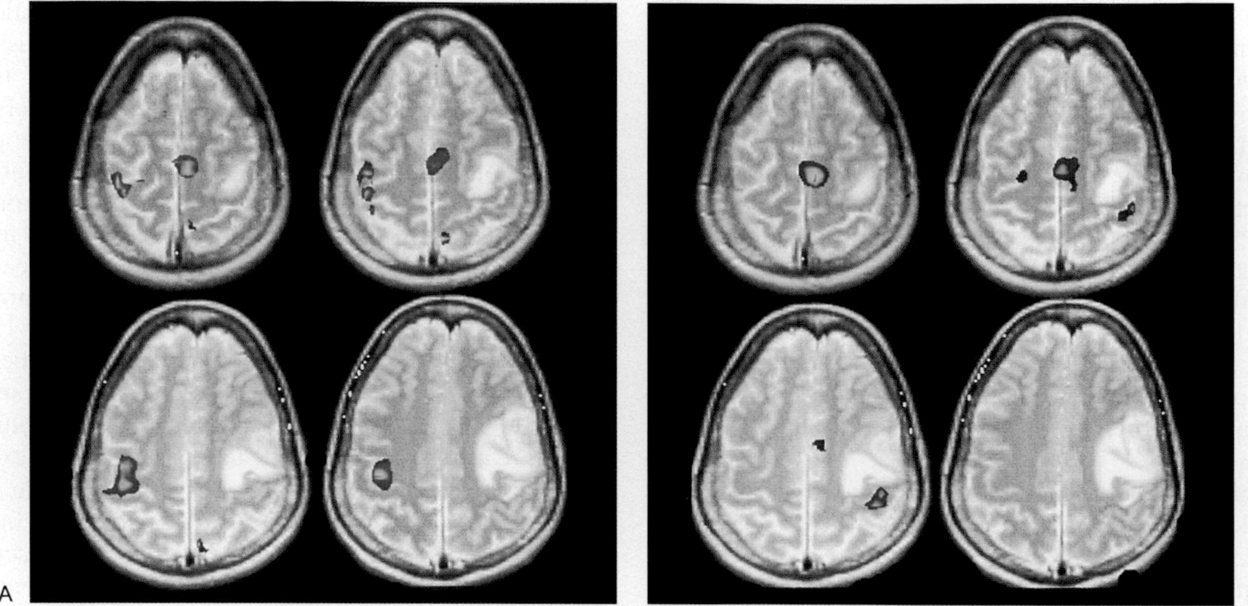

FIG. 107. BOLD task activation fMRI in infiltrative glioma. In patient harboring left posterior frontal glioma, right primary motor cortex function is noted during performance of left (normal side) hand task (**A**). Also note centrally located supplemental motor area activation. Right hand motor task (side of deficit) elicits much smaller activation in left primary motor cortex, in margin of tumor, along with supplemental motor area activation and small focus of ipsilateral primary motor cortex (**B**).

much less profound increase in oxygen utilization in response to regional activation (155,156). As opposed to contrast bolus MRI techniques (157,158) and positron emission tomography (PET), the performance of BOLD fMRI measurements are not limited by contrast agent dose or radiation limits, so several activation experiments can be performed without these considerations. Despite the fact that many questions remain regarding such fundamental concepts as the relative contributions of magnetic susceptibility versus inflow to the task-related signal changes using BOLD, and the precise anatomic sites from which these signal changes are generated (capillaries and/or post-capillary venules and/or larger veins, etc.), several recent reports illustrate the potential value of BOLD fMRI as a tool to investigate regional cerebral physiology in response to a variety of stimuli. The localization of primary sensorimotor cortex using fMRI studies has been validated with invasive cortical mapping in prior studies (159).

Using BOLD fMRI, findings supporting cortical reorganization associated with congenital lesions have been reported (160). Focal task activation within the region of

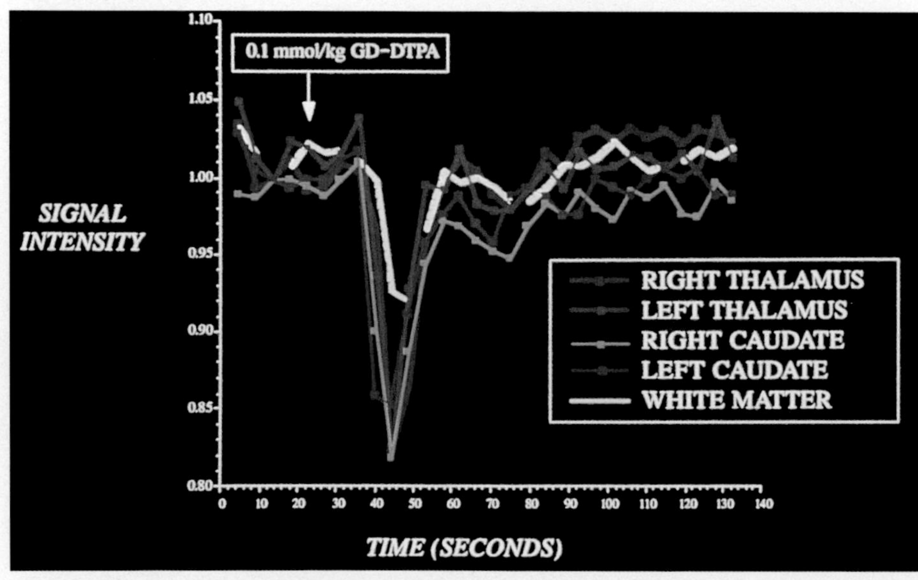

FIG. 108. Signal intensity change during passage of contrast, normal brain. Note approximately 50% difference in degree of signal intensity decrease between gray matter structures and white matter in normal brain on dynamic imaging. This difference corresponds to difference in cerebral blood volume between gray and white matter.

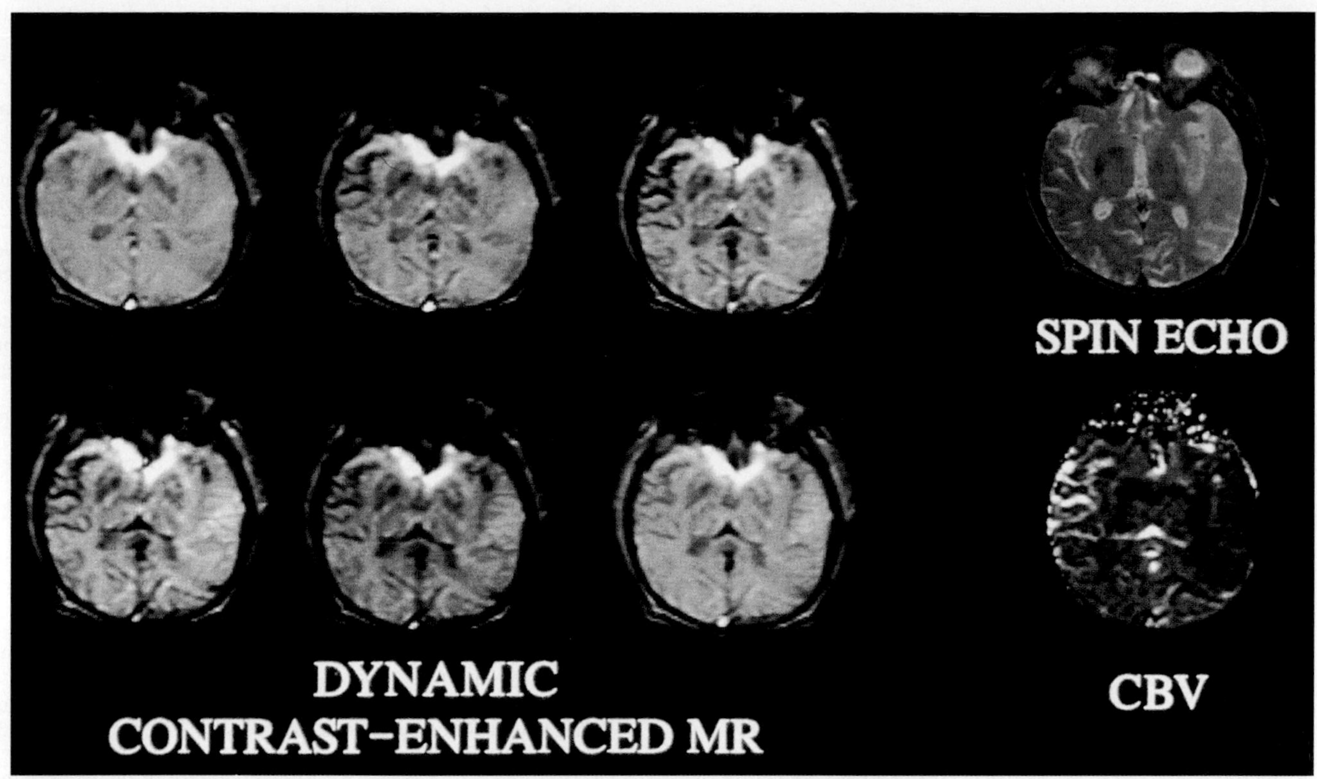

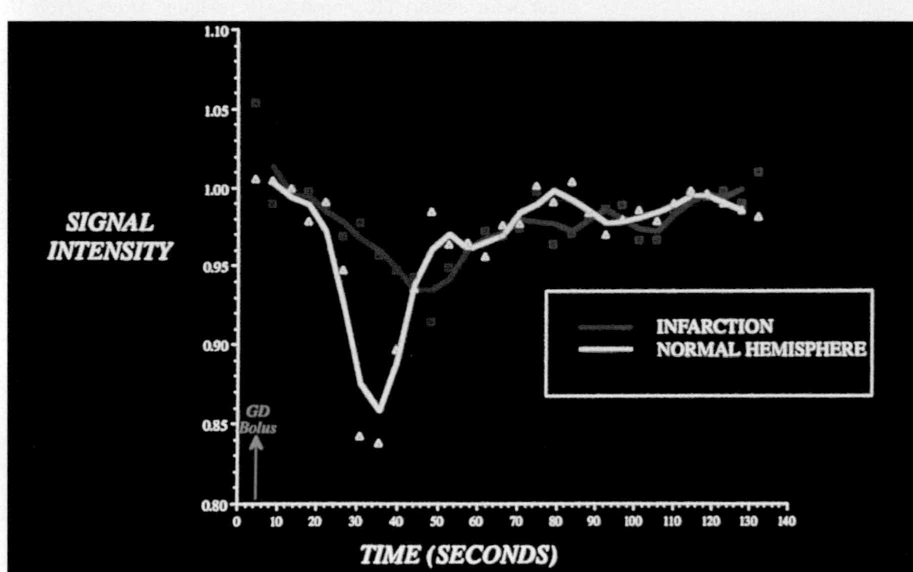

FIG. 109. Dynamic contrast bolus MRI, acute infarction. Contrast-enhanced images using gradient-echo technique show drop in signal as contrast passes through normally perfused brain. Region of infarction seen on T2-weighted spin-echo image in left middle cerebral artery distribution shows significant decrease in blood volume (CBV map). Note that CBV map is from integration of intensity-time data from region-of-interest data (see graph).

the AVM nidus has also been seen and may be a prognostic indicator for a post-therapy deficit. Preliminary data using fMRI in gliomas (161) suggest that functioning cortex within spin-echo-defined tumor margins of infiltrative gliomas can be demonstrated in patients with partially preserved clinical function (Fig. 107). Therefore, notwithstanding the many uncertainties regarding the anatomic and physical basis for signal changes on BOLD fMRI, as well as the unsettled methodology of statistical analysis for such data, we believe that patients harboring such lesions might be considered candidates for fMRI prior to surgery.

CONCLUSIONS

While conventional MRI has continued to mature and improve, a more significant advancement in fast MRI techniques has led the way to major changes in the clinical implementation of this imaging modality. These new scanning methods have dramatically improved since their initial introduction by virtue of numerous software as well as hardware innovations. At this point in time, even the most mundane clinical setting employs some type of fast MRI technique as a matter of routine. New more sophisticated methodologies have now been introduced which allow for the first time real-time high quality images of brain function to be acquired. These techniques hold promise for MR to have a much wider range of clinical applications than ever before, with potential to shed light on such poorly understood entities as mental illness and learning disabilities, as well as more basic data on the normal function involved in motor, sensory, and cognitive processes. The ultimate boundaries of its potential continue to be a matter of pure speculation.

REFERENCES

1. Bottomley PA, Foster TH, Argersinger RE, Pfeifer LM. A review of normal tissue hydrogen NMR relaxation times and relaxation mechanisms from 1 to 1000 MHz. Dependence on tissue type, NMR frequency, temperature, excision and age. *Med Phys* 1984;11:425–448.
2. Crooks LE, Ortendahl DA, Kaufman L. Clinical efficiency of nuclear magnetic resonance. *Radiology* 1983;146:123–128.
3. Damadian R, ed. *NMR in Medicine. NMR Basic Principles and Progress Series, vol 19*, New York: Springer-Verlag, 1981: chapter 1.
4. Hinshaw WS. Spin mapping the applications of moving gradients to NMR. *Phys Letters* 1974;48A:87–88.
5. Ljunggren S. A simple graphical representation of Fourier-based imaging methods. *J Magn Reson* 1983;54:338–343.
6. Twieg DB. The k-trajectory formulation of the NMR imaging process with applications in analysis and synthesis of imaging methods. *Med Phys* 1983;10:610–621.
7. Feinberg D, Hale J, Watts J, et al. Halving MR imaging time by conjugation: demonstration at 3.5 kG. *Radiology* 1986;161: 527–531.
8. Margosian P, Schmitt F, Purdy D. Faster MR imaging: imaging with half the data. *Health Care Instrum* 1986;1:195–197.
9. MacFall JR, Pelc N, Vavrek RM. Correction of spatially dependent phase shifts in partial Fourier imaging. *Magn Reson Imaging* 1988;6:143–155.
10. Ernst RR, Anderson WA. Application of Fourier transform spectroscopy to magnetic resonance. *Rev Sci Instrum* 1966;37:93–102.
11. Edelstein WA, Hutchison JMS, Johnson G, Redpath T. Spin warp imaging and applications to human whole-body imaging. *Phys Med Biol* 1980;25:756–759.
12. Haase A, Frahm J, Matthaei D, et al. FLASH Imaging: rapid NMR imaging using low flip angle pulses. *J Magn Reson* 1986;67: 258–266.
13. Hahn EL. Spin echoes. *Phys Rev* 1950;80:580–594.
14. Patz S. Steady-state free precession: an overview of basic concepts and applications. In: Feig E, ed. *Advances in Magnetic Resonance Imaging*. Norwood: Ablex Publishing; 1989:73–102.
15. Sekihara K. Steady-state magnetizations in rapid NMR imaging using small flip angles and short repetition intervals. *IEEE Trans Med Imaging* 1987;MI-6:157–164.
16. Crawley AP, Wood ML, Henkelman RM. Elimination of transverse coherences in FLASH MRI. *Magn Reson Med* 1988;8: 248–260.
17. Frahm J, Merboldt KD, Hänicke W. Transverse coherence in rapid FLASH NMR imaging. *J Magn Reson* 1987;27:307–314.
18. Glover GH, Pelc NJ. A rapid-gated cine MRI technique. In: Kressel HY, ed. *Magnetic Resonance Annual*. New York: Raven Press; 1988:299–234.
19. Wehrli FW. *Introduction to Fast-Scan Magnetic Resonance*. Milwaukee: General Electric Co; 1986.
20. Oppelt A, Graumann R, Barfuss H, et al. Fast imaging with steady state precession. *Electromedica* 1986;54:15–18.
21. Perkins TG, Wehrli FW. CSF signal enhancement in short TR gradient-echo images. *Magn Reson Imaging* 1986;4:465–467.
22. Tkach JA, Haacke EM. A comparison of fast spin echo and gradient field echo sequences. *Magn Reson Imaging* 1988;6:373–389.
23. Van Der Meulen P, Groen JP, Cuppen JJM. Very fast MR imaging by field echoes and small angle excitation. *Magn Reson Imaging* 1985;3:297–299.
24. Van der Meulen P, Groen P, Tinus AMC, Bruntink G. Fast field echo imaging: an overview and contrast calculations. *Magn Reson Imaging* 1988;6:355–368.
25. Haacke EM, Wielopolski PA, Tkach JA, Modic MT. Steady-state free precession imaging in the presence of motion: application for improved visualization of the cerebrospinal fluid. *Radiology* 1990;175:545–552.
26. Freeman R. Phase and intensity anomalies in Fourier transform NMR. *J Magn Reson* 1971;4:366–383.
27. Hawkes RC, Patz S. Rapid Fourier imaging using steady-state free precession. *Magn Reson Med* 1987;4:9–23.
28. Gyngell ML. The steady-state signals in short-repetition-time sequences. *J Magn Reson* 1988;81:474–483.
29. Gyngell ML. The application of steady-state free precession in rapid 2DFT NMR imaging: fast and CE-FAST sequences. *Magn Reson Imaging* 1988;6:415–419.
30. Menick BJ, Bobman SA, Listerud J, Atlas SW. Thin section, three dimensional Fourier transform, steady-state free precession MR imaging of the brain. *Radiology* 1992;183:369–377.
31. Frahm J, Merboldt KD, Bruhn H, Gyngell ML, et al. 0.3 second FLASH MRI of the human heart. *Magn Reson Med* 1990;13: 150–157.
32. Holsinger AE, Riederer SJ. The importance of phase-encoding order in ultra-short TR snapshot MR imaging. *Magn Reson Med* 1990;16:481–488.
33. Chien D, Edelman RR. Ultrafast imaging using gradient echoes. *Magn Reson Q* 1991;7:31–56.
34. Harms SE, Flamig DP, Fisher CF, Fulmer CM. New method for fast MR imaging of the knee. *Radiology* 1989;173:743–750.
35. Schmalbrock P, Yuan C, Chakeres DW, Kohli J, Pelc NJ. Volume MR angiography: methods to achieve very short echo times. *Radiology* 1990;175:861–865.
36. Villringer A, Rosen BR, Belliveau JW, et al. Dynamic imaging with lanthanide chelates in normal brain: contrast due to magnetic susceptibility effects. *Proceedings of the Seventh Annual Meeting of the Society of Magnetic Resonance in Medicine*. Berkeley, CA: Society of Magnetic Resonance in Medicine; 1988;6: 164–174.
37. van Vaals J, Brummer M, Dixon W, et al. "Keyhole" method for accelerating imaging of contrast agent uptake. *J Magn Reson Imaging* 1993;3:671–675.
38. Riederer SJ, Tascyan T, Farzaneh F, Lee JN, Wright RC, Herfkens RJ. MR fluoroscopy: technical feasibility. *Magn Reson Med* 1988;8:1–15.
39. Hu X, Parrish T. Reduction of field of view for dynamic imaging. *Magn Reson Med* 1994;31:691–694.
40. Dumoulin C, Souza S, Darrow R. Real-time position monitoring of invasive devices using magnetic resonance. *Magn Reson Med* 1993;29:411–415.
41. Haase A. Snapshot FLASH MRI. Applications to T1, T2 and chemical shift imaging. *Magn Reson Med* 1990;13:77–89.
42. Holsinger-Bampton A, Riederer SJ, Campeau MG, Ehman RL, Johnson CD. T1-weighted snapshot gradient-echo MR imaging of the abdomen. *Radiology* 1991;181:25–32.
43. Mugler JP 3d, Spraggins TA, Brookeman JR. T2-weighted three-dimensional MP-RAGE MR imaging. *J Magn Reson Imaging* 1991;1:731–737.
44. Mugler JP 3d, Brookeman J R. Rapid three-dimensional T1-weighted MR imaging with the MP-RAGE sequence. *J Magn Reson Imaging* 1991;1:561–567.
45. Wehrli FW, MacFall JR, Shutts D, Breger R, Herfkens RJ. Mechanisms of contrast in NMR imaging. *J Comput Assist Tomogr* 1984;8:369–380.
46. Wehrli FW, MacFall JR, Glover GH, Grigsby GN, Haughton V, Johanson J. The dependence of nuclear magnetic resonance

(NMR) image contrast on intrinsic and pulse sequence timing parameters. *Magn Reson Imaging* 1984;2:3–16.
47. Bydder GM, Young IR. Clinical use of the inversion-recovery sequence. *J Comput Assist Tomogr* 1985;9:659–675.
48. Edelman RR, Wallner B, Singer A, Atkinson DJ, Saini S. Segmented turboFLASH: method for breath-hold MR imaging of the liver with flexible contrast. *Radiology* 1990;177:515–521.
49. Frahm J, Haase A, Matthaei D. Rapid three-dimensional NMR imaging using the FLASH technique. *J Comput Assist Tomogr* 1986;10:363–368.
50. Gallimore GW Jr, Harms SE. Selective three-dimensional imaging of the spine. *J Comput Assist Tomogr* 1987;160:457.
51. Matthaei D, Frahm J, Hasse A, Hänicke W, Merboldt KD. Three-dimensional FLASH MR imaging of thorax and abdomen without triggering or gating. *Magn Reson Imaging* 1986;4:381–386.
52. Carlson J, Crooks L, Ortendahl D, et al. Signal-to-noise ratio and section thickness in two-dimensional versus three-dimensional Fourier transforms MR imaging. *Radiology* 1988;166:266–270.
53. Henkelman RM, Bronskill MJ. *Artifacts in Magnetic Resonance Imaging*. New York: Pergamon Press; 1987:126.
54. Brant-Zawadzki MN, Gillan GD, Nitz WR. MP RAGE: a three-dimensional, T1-weighted, gradient-echo sequence—initial experience in the brain. *Radiology* 1992;182:769–775.
55. Brant-Zawadzki MN, Gillan GD, Atkinson DJ, Edalatpour N, Jensen M. Three-dimensional MR imaging and display of intracranial disease: improvements with the MP-RAGE sequence and gadolinium. *J Magn Reson Imaging* 1993;3:656–662.
56. Mansfield P. Multi-planar image formation using NMR spin echoes. *J Phys Chem Solid State Phys* 1977;10:L55–L58.
57. Mansfield P, Pykett IL. Biological and medical imaging by NMR. *J Magn Reson* 1978;29:355–373.
58. Hennig J, Nauwth A, Friedburg H. RARE imaging: a fast imaging method for clinical MR. *Magn Reson Med* 1986;3:823–833.
59. Hennig J, Mueri M, Brunner P, Friedburg H. MR imaging of flow using the steady-state selective saturation method. *J Comput Assist Tomogr* 1987;11:872–877.
60. Melki PS, Mulkern RV, Panych LP, Jolesz FA. Comparing the FAISE method with conventional dual-echo sequences. *J Magn Reson Imaging* 1991;1:872–877.
61. Melki PS, Jolesz FA, Mulkern RV. Partial RF echoplanar imaging with the FAISE method. I. Experimental and theoretical assessment of artifact. *Magn Reson Med* 1992;26:328–341.
62. Melki PS, Melki PS, Jolesz FA, Mulkern RV. Partial RF echoplanar imaging with the FAISE method. II. Contrast equivalence with spin-echo sequence. *Magn Reson Med* 1992;26:342–354.
63. Listerud JL, Einstein S, Outwater E, Kressel HY. First principles of fast spin echo. *Magn Reson Q* 1992;8:199–244.
64. Constable RT, Anderson AW, Zhong J, Gore JC. Factors influencing contrast in fast spin-echo MR imaging. *Magn Reson Imaging* 1992;10:497–511.
65. Le Roux P, Hinks RS. Stabilization of echo amplitudes in FSE sequences. *Magn Reson Med* 1993;30:183–190.
66. Constable RT, Gore JC. The loss of small objects in variable TE imaging: implications for FSE, RARE, and EPI. *Magn Reson Med* 1992;28:9–24.
67. Constable RT, Smith RC, Gore JC. Signal-to-noise and contrast in fast spin echo (FSE) and inversion recovery FSE imaging. *J Comput Assist Tomogr* 1992;16:41–47.
68. Gomori JM, Grossman RI, Goldberg HI, Zimmerman RA, Bilaniuk LT. Intracranial hematomas: imaging by high-field MR. *Radiology* 1985;157:87–93.
69. Carr HY, Purcell EM. Effects of diffusion on free precession in nuclear magnetic resonance experiments. *Phys Rev* 1954;94:630.
70. Henkelman RM, Hardy PA, Bishop JE, Poon CS, Plewes DB. Why fat is bright in RARE and fast spin-echo imaging. *J Magn Reson Imaging* 1992;2:533–540.
71. Dixon WT. Simple proton spectroscopic imaging. *Radiology* 1984;153:189–194.
72. Higuchi N, Hiramatsu K, Mulkern R. A novel method for fat suppression in RARE sequences. *Magn Reson Med* 1992;27:107–117.
73. Keller PJ, Hunter WW, Schmalbrock P. Multisection fat-water imaging with chemical shift selective presaturation. *Radiology* 1987;164:539–541.
74. Bydder GM, Steiner RE, Blumgart RH, et al. MR imaging of the liver using short TI inversion recovery sequences. *J Comput Assist Tomogr* 1985;9:1084–1089.
75. Hajnal JV, Bryant DJ, Kasuboski L, et al. Use of fluid attenuated inversion recovery (FLAIR) pulse sequences in MRI of the brain. *J Comput Assist Tomogr* 1992;16:841–844.
76. Thorpe J, MacManus D, Kendall B, Tofts P, Barker G, McDonald W, Miller D. Short tau inversion-recovery fast spin-echo (fast STIR) imaging of the spinal cord in multiple sclerosis. *Magn Reson Imaging* 1994;12:983–989.
77. Wolff SD, Balaban RS. Magnetization transfer contrast (MTC) and tissue water proton relaxation in vivo. *Magn Reson Med* 1989;10:135–144.
78. Wolff SD, Eng J, Balaban RS. Magnetization transfer contrast: method for improving contrast in gradient-recalled-echo images. *Radiology* 1991;179:133–137.
79. Eng J, Ceckler TL, Balaban RS. Quantitative 1H magnetization transfer imaging *in vivo*. *Magn Reson Med* 1991;17:304–314.
80. Dousset V, Grossman RI, Ramer KN, et al. Experimental allergic encephalomyelitis and multiple sclerosis: lesion characterization with magnetization transfer imaging. *Radiology* 1992;182:483–491.
81. Dixon WT, Engels H, Sardashti M, Castillo M. Incidental magnetization transfer contrast affects ordinary multislice imaging. *Magn Reson Imaging* 1990;8:417–422.
82. Melki PS, Mulkern R. Magnetization transfer effects in Multislice RARE sequences. *Magn Reson Med* 1992;24:189–195.
83. Hennig J. Multiple sequences with low refocussing flip angles. *J Magn Res* 1988;78:397–407.
84. Hinks RS, Constable RT. Gradient moment nulling in fast spin echo. *Magn Reson Med* 1994;32:698–694.
85. Yuan C, Schmiedl UP, Weinberger E, Krueck WR, Rand SD. Three-dimensional fast spin-echo imaging: pulse sequence and in vivo image evaluation. *J Magn Reson Imaging* 1993;3:894–899.
86. Parker DL, Yuan C, Blatter DD. MR angiography by multiple thin slab 3D acquisition. *Magn Reson Med* 1991;17:434–451.
87. Rzedzian R, Mansfield P, Doyle M, et al. Real-time NMR clinical imaging in paediatrics. *Lancet* 1983;2:1281–1282.
88. Ordidge RJ, Howseman A, Coxon R, et al. Snapshot imaging at 0.5T using echo-planar techniques. *Magn Reson Med* 1989;10:227–240.
89. Pykett IL, Rzedzian RR. Instant images of the body by magnetic resonance. *Magn Reson Med* 1987;5:563–571.
90. Rzedzian RR, Pykett IL. Instant images of the human heart using a new, whole-body MR imaging system. *AJR* 1987;149:245–250.
91. Cohen MS, Weisskoff RM. Ultra-fast imaging. *Magn Reson Imaging* 1991;9:1–37.
92. Kwong KK, Belliveau JW, Chesler DA, et al. Dynamic magnetic resonance imaging of human brain activity during primary sensory stimulation. *Proc Natl Acad Sci U S A* 1992;89:5675–5679.
93. Ogawa S, Lee TM, Kay AR, Tank DW. Brain magnetic resonance imaging with contrast dependent on blood oxygenation. *Proc Natl Acad Sci U S A* 1990;87:9868–9872.
94. Ogawa S, Tank DW, Menon R, Ellerman JM, Kim S-G, Merkle HH, Ugurbil K. Intrinsic signal changes accompanying sensory stimulation: functional brain mapping with magnetic resonance imaging. *Proc Natl Acad Sci U S A* 1992;89:5951–5955.
95. Ogawa S, Lee TM, Nayak AS, Glynn P. Oxygenation-sensitive contrast in magnetic resonance imaging of rodent brain at high magnetic fields. *Magn Reson Med* 1990;14:68–78.
96. Turner R, LeBihan DL, Moonen CTW, Despres D, Frank J. Echoplanar time course MRI of cat brain oxygenation changes. *Magn Reson Med* 1991;22:159–166.
97. McKinnon G. Ultrafast interleaved gradient echo planar imaging on a standard scanner. *Magn Reson Med* 1993;30:609–616.
98. Butts K, Riederer SJ, Ehman RL, Thompson RM, Jack CR. Interleaved echo planar imaging on a standard MRI system. *Magn Reson Med* 1994;31:67–72.
99. Stehling MJ, Houseman AM, Ordidge RJ, et al. Whole-body echo-planar imaging at 0.5 T. *Radiology* 1989;170:257–263.
100. Rzedzian R. NMR gradient field modulation. U.S. Patent No. 4628264; 1986.
101. Weber D. Echoplanar imaging. General Electric Publication No. 3187; Milwaukee, WI.
102. Wehrli FW, Shimakawa A, Gullberg GT, MacFall JR. Time-of-

flight MR flow imaging: selective saturation recovery with gradient refocusing. *Radiology* 1986;160:781–785.

103. Gullberg GT, Wehrli FW, Shimakawa A, Simons MA. MR vascular imaging with a fast gradient refocusing pulse sequence and reformatted images from transaxial sections. *Radiology* 1987;165:241–246.
104. Atlas SW, Fram EK, Mark AS, Grossman RI. Vascular intracranial lesions: applications of fast scanning. *Radiology* 1988;169:455–461.
104a. Atlas SW, Mark AS, Fram EK. Aqueductal stenosis: evaluation with gradient echo imaging. *Radiology* 1988;169:449–453.
105. Fram EK, Dimick R, Hedlund LW, et al. Parameters determining the signal of flowing fluid in gradient refocused MR imaging: flow velocity, TR and flip angle. *Book of Abstracts*, SMRM Annual Meeting, Montreal: 1986:84–85.
106. Axel L. Blood flow effects in magnetic resonance imaging. *AJR* 1984;143:1157–1166.
107. Bradley WG, Waluch V. Blood flow: magnetic resonance imaging. *Radiology* 1985;154:443–450.
108. Haacke EM, Lenz GW. Improving image quality in the presence of motion by using rephasing gradients. *AJR* 1987;148:1251–1258.
109. Pattany PM, Phillips JJ, Chiu LC, et al. Motion artifact suppression technique (MAST) for MR imaging. *J Comput Assist Tomogr* 1987;11:369–377.
110. Waluch V, Bradley WG. NMR even-echo rephasing in slow laminar flow. *J Comput Assist Tomogr* 1984;4:594–598.
111. Listerud J, Chao P, Atlas S, Wehrli F, Souza S. Investigation of MR angiographic contrast in RF-spoiled GRASS (paper no. 447). Washington, DC: 1989: 29.
112. Du Boulay GH. Pulsatile movements in the CSF pathways. *Br J Radiology* 1966;39:255–262.
113. Bradley WG, Kortman KE, Burgoyne B. Flowing cerebrospinal fluid in normal and hydrocephalic states: appearance on MR images. *Radiology* 1986;159:611–616.
114. Citrin CM, Sherman JL, Gangarosa R, Scanlon D. Physiology of the CSF flow void sign: modification by cardiac gating. *AJNR* 1986;7:1021–1024.
115. Sherman JL, Citrin CM, Bowen BJ, Gangarosa RE. MR demonstration of altered cerebrospinal fluid flow by obstructive lesions. *AJNR* 1986;7:571–579.
116. Kemp SS, Zimmerman RA, Bilaniuk LT, et al. Magnetic resonance imaging of the cerebral aqueduct. *Neuroradiology* 1987;29:430–436.
117. Evans AJ, Herfkens RJ, Spritzer CE, et al. The effect of turbulent flow on MRI signal intensity using gradient refocused echoes. SMRM Annual Meeting, New York: 1987.
118. Buxton RB, Edelman RR, Rosen BR, et al. Contrast in rapid MR imaging: T1 and T2 weighted imaging. *J Comput Assist Tomogr* 1987;11:7–16.
119. Edelman RR, Johnson K, Buxton R, et al. MR of hemorrhage: a new approach. *AJNR* 1986;7:751–756.
120. Atlas SW, Mark AS, Gomori JM, Grossman RI. Intracranial hemorrhage: gradient echo imaging at 1.5T. Comparison with spin-echo imaging and clinical applications. *Radiology* 1988;168:803–807.
121. Mills TC, Ortendahl DA, Hylton NM, et al. Partial flip angle MR imaging. *Radiology* 1987;162:531–539.
122. Holland BA, Kucharcyzk W, Brant-Zawadzki M, Norman D, Haas DK, Harper PS. MR imaging of calcified intracranial lesions. *Radiology* 1985;157:353–356.
123. Oot RF, New PFJ, Pile-Spellman J, et al. The detection of intracranial calcifications by MR. *AJNR* 1986;7:801–809.
124. Atlas SW, Grossman RI, Hackney DB, et al. Calcified intracranial lesions: detection with gradient-echo-acquisition rapid MR imaging. *AJNR* 1988;9:253–259.
125. Packer KJ. The effects of diffusion through locally inhomogeneous magnetic fields on transverse nuclear spin relaxation in heterogeneous systems. Proton transverse relaxation in striated muscle tissue. *J Magn Reson* 1973;9:438–443.
126. Glasel JA, Lee KH. On the interpretation of water nuclear magnetic resonance relaxation times in heterogeneous systems. *J Am Chem Soc* 1974;96:970–978.
127. Hanus F, Gillis P. Relaxation of water adsorbed on the surface of silica powder. *J Magn Reson* 1984;59:437–445.
128. Fung BM, McGaughy TW. Magnetic relaxation in heterogeneous systems. *J Magn Reson* 1981;43:316–323.
129. Alcolada JC, Moore IE, Weller RO. Calcification in the human choroid plexus, meningiomas, and pineal gland. *Neuropathol Appl Neurobiol* 1986;12:235–250.
130. Duckett S, Galle P, Escourolle R, Poirier J, Hauw J. Presence of zinc, aluminum, magnesium in striopallidodentate (SPD) calcification (Fahr's disease): electron probe study. *Acta Neuropathol (Berl)* 1977;38:7–10.
131. Kozik M, Kulczycki L. Laser-spectroscopic analysis of the cation content in Fahr's syndrome. *Arch Psychiatr Nerv* 1978;225:135–142.
132. Wehrli FW, Chao PW, Yousem DM. Parameter dependence of susceptibility-induced signal losses in gradient-echo imaging. *Magn Reson Imaging* 1989;7(Suppl 1):139.
133. Haacke EM, Tkatch JA, Parrish TB. Reducing T2* dephasing in gradient field-echo imaging. *Radiology* 1989;170:457–462.
134. Wehrli FW, Ford JC, Gusnard DA, Listerud J. The inhomogeneity of magnetic susceptibility in vertebral body marrow. *Book of Abstracts*, SMRM Annual Meeting, Amsterdam: 1989:217.
135. Yousem DM, Atlas SW, Hackney D. Cervical spine disc herniation: comparison of CT and 3DFT gradient-echo MR scans. *J Comput Assist Tomogr* 1992;16:345–351.
136. Tartaglino L, Flanders A, Vinitski S, Friedman D. Metallic artifacts on MR images of the postoperative spine: reduction with fast spin echo techniques. *Radiology* 1994;190:565–569.
137. Howard R, Chung W, Holland G, Atlas S. 3DFT multislab fast spin echo high resolution MR imaging of cervical spine degenerative disc disease. *Abstracts of the Proceedings of the 1994 Annual Meeting of RSNA,* Chicago: 1995.
138. Buonanno FS, Pykett IL, Brady TJ, et al. Clinical relevance of two different nuclear magnetic resonance (NMR) approaches to imaging of a low-grade astrocytoma. *J Comput Assist Tomogr* 1982;6:529–535.
139. Atlas S, Hackney D, Listerud J. Fast spin echo imaging of the brain and spine. *Magn Reson Q* 1993;9:61–83.
140. Atlas SW, Hackney DB, Yousem DM, Listerud J. Fast spin echo (FSE) MR imaging: blinded comparison with conventional spin echo imaging for the detection of focal brain lesions. *Abstracts of the Proceedings of the 1991 Annual Meeting of the Society of Magnetic Resonance in Medicine*, San Francisco, CA. Berkeley, CA: Society of Magnetic Resonance in Medicine; 1991:41.
141. Listerud J, Atlas SW. The suitability of 3DFSE pulse sequences as a black blood MRA technique. *Abstracts of the Proceedings of the 1991 Annual Meeting of RSNA*, Chicago: 1991:141.
142. Norbash AM, Glover GH, Enzmann DR. Intracerebral lesion contrast with spin-echo and fast spin echo pulse sequences. *Radiology* 1992;185:661–665.
143. Jorgensen J, Hansen PH, Steenskov V, Ovesen N. A clinical and radiological study of chronic lower spinal arachnoiditis. *Neuroradiology* 1975;9:139–144.
144. Quencer R, Tenner M, Rothman L. The postoperative myelogram radiographic evaluation of arachnoiditis and dural/arachnoid tears. *Radiology* 1977;123:667–679.
145. Ross JS, Masaryk TJ, Modic MT, Delamater R, Bohlman H, Wilbur G, Kaufman B. MR imaging of lumbar arachnoiditis. *AJNR* 1987;8:885–892.
146. Johnson CE, Sze G. Benign lumbar arachnoiditis: MR imaging with gadopentetate. *AJNR* 1990;11:763–770.
147. Rosen BR, Belliveau JH, Chien D. Perfusion imaging by nuclear magnetic resonance. *Magn Reson Q* 1989;5:263–281.
148. Saini S, Stark DD, Hahn PF, et al. Ferrite particles: a superparamagnetic MR contrast agent for enhanced detection of liver carcinoma. *Radiology* 1987;162:217–222.
149. Majumdar S, Zoghbi S, Pope CF, Gore JC. Quantitation of MR relaxation effects of iron oxide particles in liver and spleen. *Radiology* 1988;169:653–655.
150. Majumdar, S, Zoghbi, SS, Gore, JC. The influence of pulse sequence on the relaxation effects of superparamagnetic iron oxide contrast agents. *Magn Reson Med* 1989;10:289–301.
151. Le Bihan D, Breton E, Lallemand D, et al. MR imaging of intra-

voxel incoherent motions: applications to diffusion and perfusion in neurologic disorders. *Radiology* 1986;161:401–407.

152. Turner R, Jezzard P, Wen H, Kwong K. Functional mapping of the human visual cortex at 4 and 1.5 tesla using deoxygenation contrast EPI. *Magn Reson Med* 1993;29:277–279.
153. Bandettini PA, Wong EC, Hinks RS, Tikofsky RS, Hyde JS. Time course EPI of human brain function during task activation. *Magn Reson Med* 1992;25:390–397.
154. Bandettini PA, Wong EC, Cox RW, Jesmanowicz A, Hinks RS, Hyde JS. Simultaneous assessment of blood oxygenation and flow contributions to activation induced signal changes in the human brain. *Abstracts of the Proceedings of the Annual Meeting of the Society of Magnetic Resonance in Medicine*. Berkeley, CA: Society of Magnetic Resonance in Medicine; 1994:621.
155. Fox PT, Raichle ME. Focal physiological uncoupling of cerebral blood flow and oxidative metabolism during somatosensory stimulation in human subjects. *Proc Natl Acad Sci U S A* 1986;83: 1140–1144.
156. Fox PT, Raichle ME, Mintun MA, Dence C. Nonoxidative glucose consumption during focal physiologic neural activity. *Science* 1988;241:462–464.
157. Belliveau JW, Rosen BR, Kantor HL, et al. Functional cerebral imaging by susceptibility-contrast NMR. *Magn Reson Med* 1990;14:538–546.
158. Belliveau J, Kennedy D, McKinstry R, et al. Functional mapping of the human visual cortex by magnetic resonance imaging. *Science* 1991;254:716–719.
159. Jack CR, Thompson RM, Butts RK, et al. Sensory motor cortex: correlation of presurgical mapping with functional MR imaging and invasive cortical mapping. *Radiology* 1994;190:85–92.
160. Maldjian J, Howard R, Alsop DA, et al. Functional MRI in AVMs prior to surgical or endovascular therapy. *Abstracts of the Proceedings of the Annual Meeting of the RSNA*; 1994.
161. Atlas SW, Howard RS, Maldjian J, et al. Functional MRI of infiltrating gliomas: findings and implications for clinical management. *Neurosurgery* 1995;[*in press*].

Magnetic Resonance Imaging of the Brain and Spine, Second Edition, edited by Scott W. Atlas. Lippincott-Raven Publishers, Philadelphia © 1996.

30

Functional MRI of the Brain

A. Gregory Sorensen and Bruce R. Rosen

DEFINITION OF FUNCTIONAL MRI

Magnetic resonance imaging (MRI) in the brain has been primarily used to evaluate neuroanatomy. Compared with previous imaging techniques, MRI is clearly superior in contrast resolution and near equivalent in spatial resolution to x-ray technologies, and has accordingly improved neuroradiologic diagnosis. This improved anatomic information has benefitted neuroscience research as well. Nevertheless, many disease processes do not have a clear anatomic correlate. Such disease entities include early ischemia, dementia, and psychiatric illnesses. In addition, many diseases may be insufficiently defined by anatomic changes alone. These include many neoplasms, particularly after treatment; epilepsy; and cerebral infarction. Finally, for preoperative planning it is frequently useful to investigate not only the location of anatomically normal brain, but also its functional activity. In each of these settings it is physiology, rather than anatomy, that is of greater interest.

Functional MRI (fMRI) of the brain is the application of MRI techniques to investigate cerebral physiology while preserving anatomic specificity. Under the umbrella term of fMRI are MRI techniques including imaging of microscopic water mobility (diffusion imaging), microvascular hemodynamics (cerebral blood flow and volume imaging), and blood oxygenation–sensitive imaging, as well as other techniques. In large measure these techniques depend on rapid acquisition of MR images (typically a complete image slice every 100 msec or so) in order to scan the entire brain with temporal resolution of a few seconds. Although these techniques are as yet unable to image neural activity directly, underlying normal or pathologic tissue function can be assessed through the use of the well established relationship between neuronal activity, cellular metabolism, and closely linked parameters of cerebral blood volume, cerebral blood flow, the oxygenation state of blood, or water diffusion (1).

To understand the potential clinical application of fMRI requires an understanding not only of the instrumentation, physics, and techniques of fMRI, but also an appreciation for underlying cerebral physiology and pathophysiology. This chapter first reviews the fundamentals of fMRI techniques and then illustrates their application in the clinical setting.

FUNCTIONAL MRI TECHNIQUES

Diffusion Imaging—Imaging of Tissue Water Mobility

Diffusion (also known as brownian motion) is the random motion of all molecules driven by thermal energy. MR imaging can be made sensitive to molecular diffusion of the primary contributor to MR signal, molecular water, through the addition of balanced gradient pulses

A. G. Sorensen, M.D., and B. R. Rosen, M.D., Ph.D.: NMR Center, Massachusetts General Hospital, Charlestown, MA 02129.

to a standard spin-echo (SE) sequence (2,3). Developed first as a quantitative tool by nuclear magnetic resonance (NMR) spectroscopists, pulse gradient diffusion MRI has provided one of the first noninvasive in vivo methods for measuring water diffusion coefficients. While diffusion and brain function may not appear to be closely linked, numerous studies have demonstrated that the apparent diffusion coefficient changes in disease states (3–10). Since diffusion in the brain has only been recently measurable in a clinical setting, its clinical utility and indications are still being investigated. Perhaps the area of diagnosis with the greatest promise is in the imaging of stroke, as is discussed below.

The physical principle behind diffusion imaging is quite analogous to that of phase contrast MR angiography (MRA). As spins (in this case water) move through magnetic field gradients, they accumulate a phase shift in their transverse magnetization relative to that of stationary spins. In phase contrast MRA, this phase shift is used to identify motion (flow) within the vessel lumen. Since the velocities of water within blood vessels is quite high (by molecular standards), only modest gradients are needed to produce significant phase shifts. In addition, since the blood is typically moving in a coherent direction, the phase shifts within the vessel are predictable, and can even be used to quantify the direction and velocity of flow. A notable exception is during turbulent flow. In this setting flow velocities are even higher than normal, and the direction of flow is no longer constant or even predictable. As MR angiographers quickly realized, under these conditions the random phase shifts imparted to the spins lead to signal dropout.

Diffusion imaging is quite analogous. Since all water in tissues is constantly in motion, water spins will naturally accumulate phase shifts if the spins move through an inhomogeneous field such as that generated by MRI gradients. As with turbulent flow, however, the diffusive motion of water is random and unpredictable, and no two water molecules take the same path. As a result, the phase shifts accumulated by the water are also random, leading to phase cancellation and hence signal loss. As with phase contrast MRA, this is enhanced by longer TE times and stronger gradients. Unlike turbulent motion in arteries, however, the motion of individual water molecules is quite small: during a typical SE sequence the water molecules in brain tissue move less than 14 μm. As a result, diffusion effects are quite subtle on conventional MR images, even at long TEs. However, by applying strong gradients for longer periods this signal loss can be enhanced, and the degree of signal loss can be directly related to the degree of random motion, measured by the diffusion coefficient D. A typical diffusion-weighted sequence therefore consists of additional gradient pulses as shown in Fig. 1. The amount of signal attenuation in a given voxel, SA, depends on the diffusion coefficient D in the voxel in an exponential fashion:

$$\text{SA} \approx e^{-b\text{D}} \quad [1]$$

The constant b depends on the duration and strength of the applied diffusion-encoding gradients, and can be calculated from the Stejskal-Tanner equation:

$$b = \gamma^2 G^2 \delta^2 (\Delta - \delta/3) \quad [2]$$

where G, δ, and Δ are defined as in Fig. 1 and γ is the standard gyromagnetic ratio. Hence, a *diffusion-weighted* image is spoken of as having a particular b value, analogous to the TE value we use to denote the degree of T2 weighting. As with TE, large b denotes greater diffusion weighting. By acquiring a series of images with different b values a map of the apparent diffusion coefficient (an *ADC map*) can be calculated. In clinical practice, both the diffusion-weighted images as well as the calculated ADC maps can be useful, because diffusion-weighted images show lesions with decreased diffusion coefficient as bright (e.g., acute stroke), whereas lesions with increased diffusion (e.g., cystic tumors) can

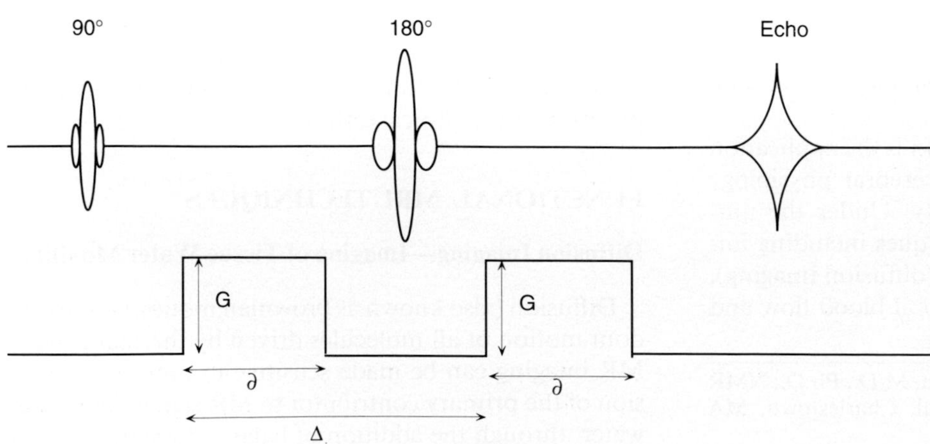

FIG. 1. In an SE experiment, the amount of signal attenuation due to diffusion experiments can be quantified by a value b, as given in Eq. 1 in the text. The values G, δ, and Δ correspond to the values of the gradient amplitude, duration, and interval, respectively, as shown in the diagram.

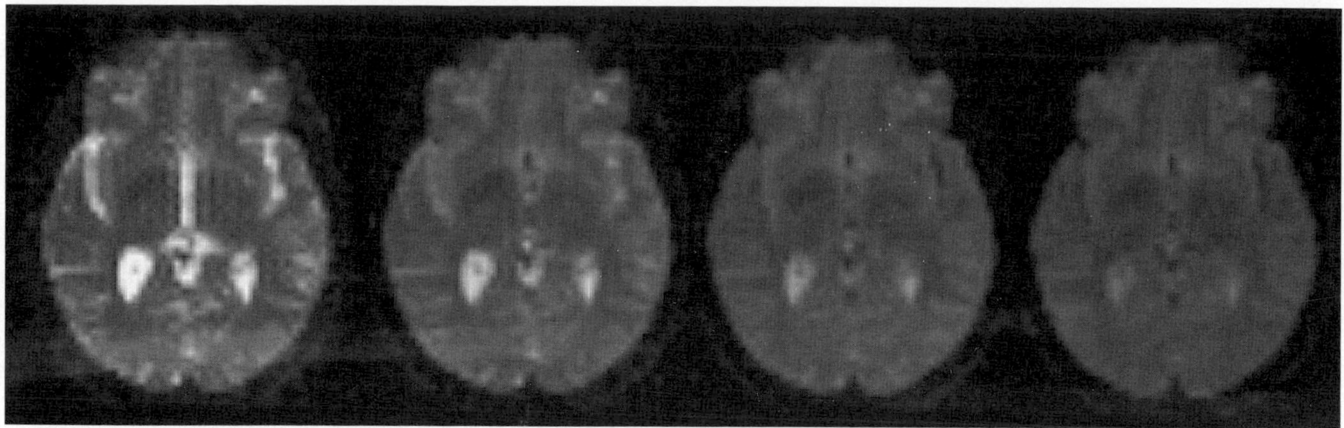

FIG. 2. Raw diffusion-weighted images in a normal subject. Four images from a set of 32 used to calculate diffusion maps. From left to right the *b* values are 0, 312, 753, and 1175 s/mm^2, in one direction. EPI single-shot SE images, TR = 8000 msec, TE = 123 msec. Note that with $b = 0$, the image is simply heavily T2-weighted, but as *b* increases the regions of lower ADC become brighter relative to CSF.

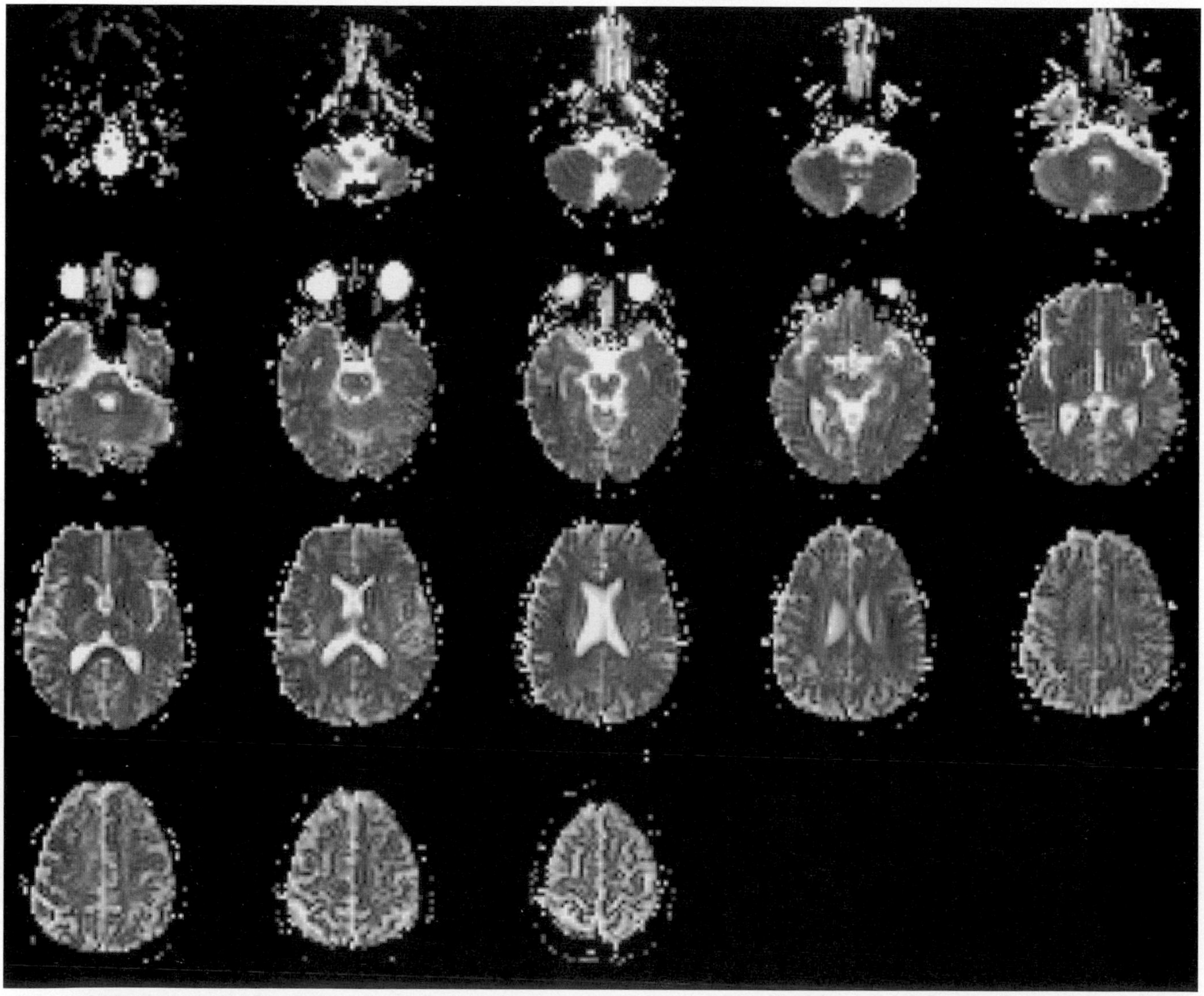

FIG. 3. Maps of ADC. These maps are calculated by applying Eq. 1 in the text to a series of images with increasing known *b* values. Note that the ADC map shows highest value in the ventricles, where there is no restriction to motion of water. 18 slices, EPI single-shot SE images, 32 *b* values/slice, TR = 8000 msec, TE = 123 msec, single direction of applied gradient.

be visualized as bright on ADC maps. Figure 2 shows normal brain imaged at increasing b values. Alternatively, one can acquire images with at least two b values (e.g., $b = 0$ and $b = 700$ sec/mm^2), solve equation 1, and create a map of the apparent diffusion coefficient (ADC). This is illustrated in Fig. 3.

Molecules can diffuse in all three dimensions. However, the local environment does influence diffusion; for example, in areas of white matter there is greater diffusion along the myelin sheaths than across them. Therefore, the diffusion of water in some tissues is anisotropic; that is, there are different apparent diffusion coefficients in each direction, whereas in other tissues it is quite isotropic. Since there is no a priori preferred direction of motion, the mathematical description of diffusion for each voxel is termed a *tensor*. Complete characterization of the molecular diffusion tensor requires at least seven measurements. For example, if diffusion gradients are applied only in a single direction, it is possible that what may appear to be abnormal diffusion because of stroke may actually be due to the local cellular alignment and environment. Figure 4 demonstrates this artifactual lowering of ADC in normal brain. In practice, two or three measurements will suffice in most clinical settings, although many investigators now recommend attempting to measure the entire tensor or some spatially invariant portion of it, such as the trace of the tensor (11–13). We favor this approach as well when practical. If one has sampled the full diffusion tensor, the tensor can be displayed graphically. This can be useful in mapping white matter tracts, as shown in Fig. 5, but has also been shown to benefit the visualization of stroke (13).

Diffusion-weighted sequences are meant to detect motion within a voxel but are exquisitely sensitive to motion of any type. Because of this, diffusion-weighted images are extremely sensitive to patient motion, and extra efforts at head restraint are required even in cooperative patients. These problems are not insurmountable with conventional MR imagers, and several important studies have been carried out with conventional equipment even at mid-field strength (e.g., ref. 5). In practical terms, the use of very high speed echo-planar imaging (EPI) or similar single-shot capabilities have made multislice diffusion imaging both rapid and robust even in noncompliant patients. As the availability of EPI systems grows, diffusion-weighted imaging will therefore become more important in clinical practice.

Imaging Cerebral Hemodynamics with Contrast Agents

MRA has demonstrated its ability to detect flow in macroscopic vasculature and is in widespread use. Hemodynamic imaging, on the other hand, is concerned with microscopic flow; that is, flow at the capillary level. Traditionally, tissue perfusion has been assessed using a variety of radiologic techniques, from conventional catheter angiography to positron emission tomography (PET) and single photon emission computed tomography (SPECT). MRI has unique features that add to its value in assessing tissue perfusion in the brain: it can be relatively sensitive to tissue microvasculature; it is minimally invasive, and has higher spatial resolution than radionuclide-based techniques. Over the past 5 years these techniques have demonstrated their utility in a wide variety of neuroradiologic applications; any disease process with microvascular alterations may potentially

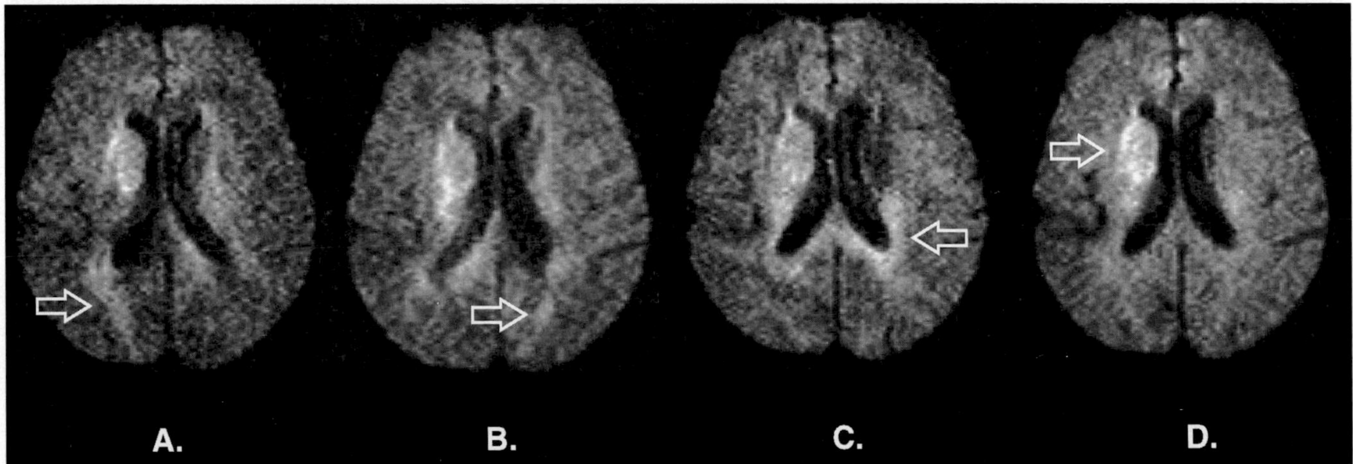

FIG. 4. The ADC is a tensor, which means it can vary directionally. Since the magnetic field used to measure the ADC is usually applied along a single axis, a low ADC may be due to pathologic lowering, or alternatively could be due to anisotropy, with a normal ADC in a direction perpendicular to the measured direction but a low ADC along the measured direction. Diffusion weighted images are shown in a patient presenting with acute stroke (same patient as in Fig. 19F), with **A**, **B**, and **C** representing three acquisitions with the diffusion measurement in orthogonal directions. From these three directions the trace of the diffusion tensor can be computed, which is spatially invariant, and an isotropic diffusion-weighted image can be computed (**D**). The *arrows* point out areas of low diffusion due to anisotropy, which is not present in all directions, while the acute stroke in the right deep gray matter is evident in all three acquisitions. A, B, C: b value of 1009 s/mm^2.

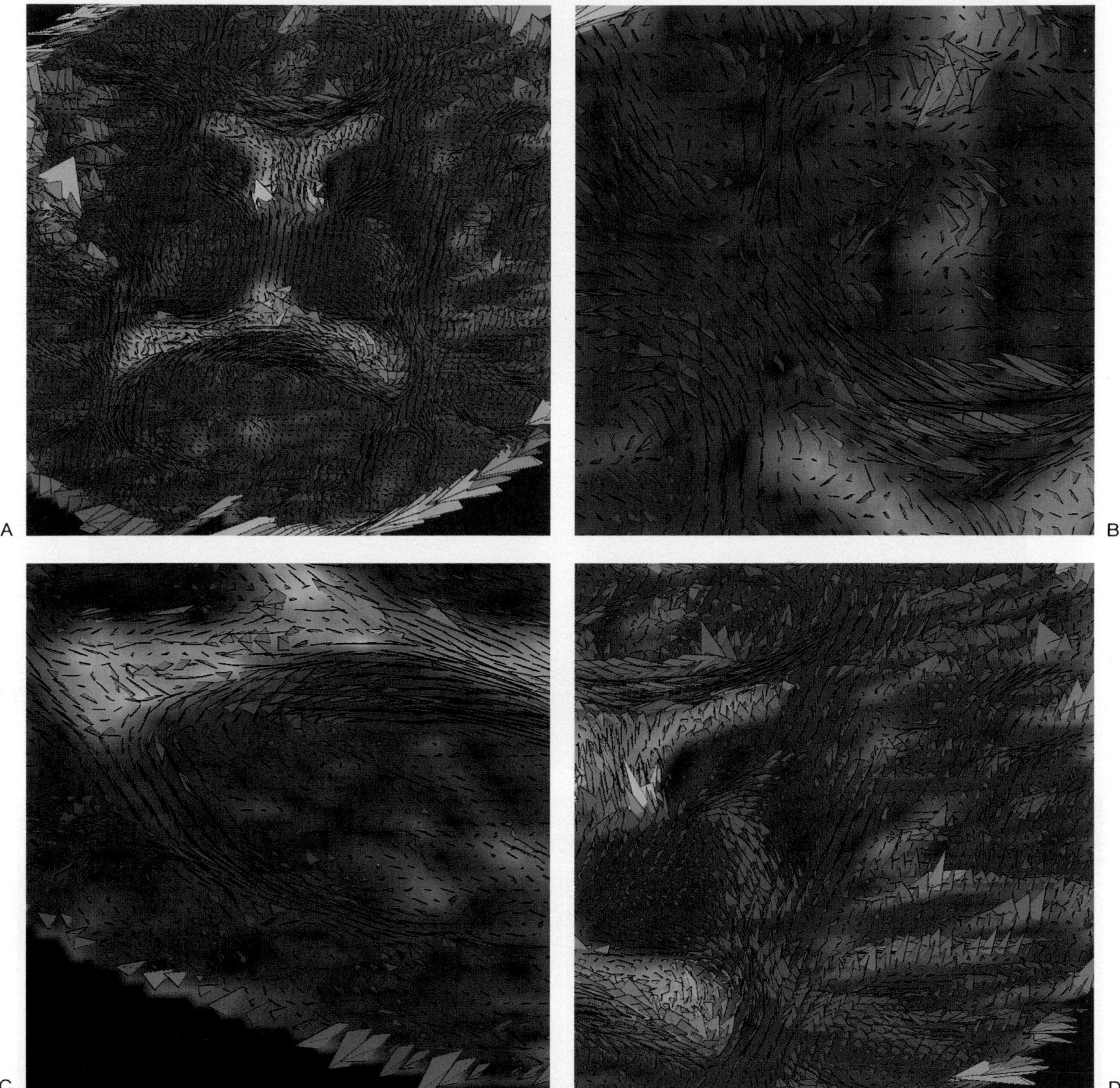

FIG. 5. Diffusion anisotropy maps. **A:** A single-slice axial anisotropy image showing, in color rhomboids, in-plane and through-plane fiber orientations over a gray-scale diffusion map. Note the three-dimensional curving of fibers in the corpus callosum, the internal capsules, and cortical radiations. (These maps are projection images; the lower right corner is tilted toward the reader.) **B:** Close-up of the genu of the corpus callosum, looking straight down onto the slice plane. The most polarized diffusion anisotropy is seen here. One can follow the fibers out into the frontal lobes. **C:** Close-up of optic radiation and splenium of corpus callosum, again in perspective, from the lower left of image A. **D:** Close-up of internal capsule, atrium of the lateral ventricle, and thalamus (on the left of the image). Multislice data allow continued tracking of the fiber orientations in three dimensions.

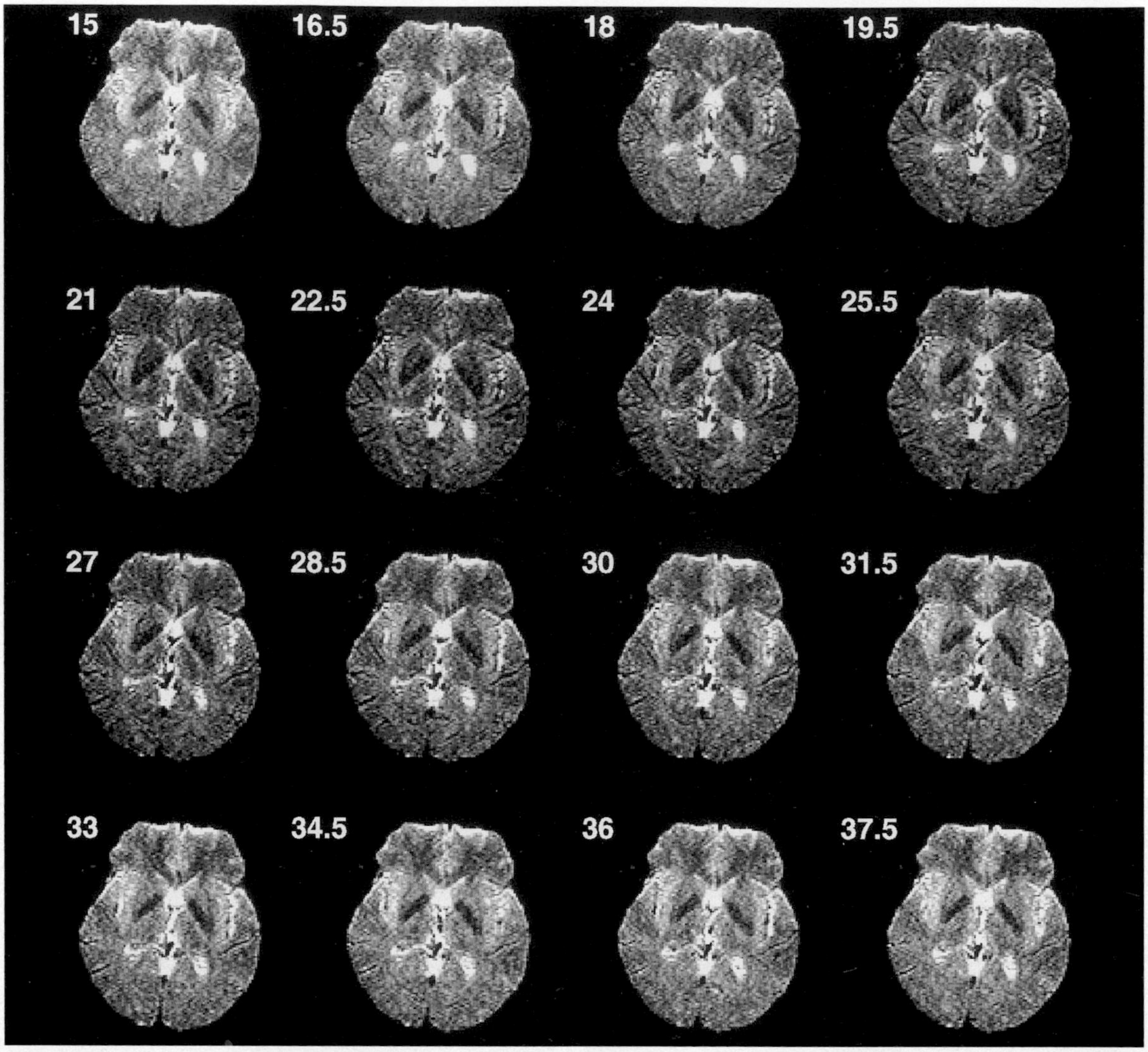

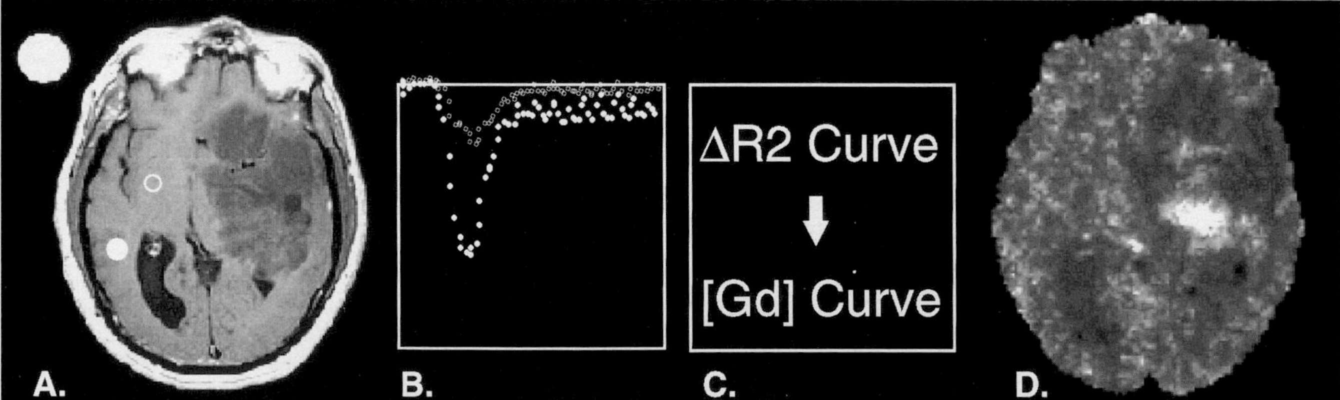

FIG. 6. 1: First pass susceptibility effect of passage of contrast through the brain. The high concentration of Gd-based contrast agent, which remains intravascular due to the BBB, causes the T2-shortening effects to overwhelm the T1-shortening effects, leading to signal loss. Loss of signal in each voxel is related to the degree of contrast medium in the voxel, or rCBV. Numbers indicate seconds from injection of bolus of gadodiamide. This and all other rCBV maps in this chapter were obtained using EPI SE imaging, typically with TR = 1500 msec, TE = 75 to 100 msec. **2:** Typical procedure for creating rCBV maps. **A:** Conventional localizing images are obtained. **B:** An MR contrast agent is injected intravenously and complete images are obtained every second or two to obtain signal versus time curves for each voxel. **C:** Using susceptibility physics and tracer kinetics principles, the signal-vs.-time curve is converted to an rCBV value for each voxel. **D:** A map of the rCBV values can be displayed for each slice.

benefit from hemodynamic imaging. First described in the brain by Villringer et al. (14), contrast-based hemodynamic imaging with MR has been applied to a variety of clinical applications including tumor characterization, stroke, and dementia, with others under active investigation (15,16).

With currently available MR contrast media, the physical basis of these techniques rests on dynamic imaging during the first passage of a contrast agent bolus. These paramagnetic chelates remain one of the most useful means of effecting tissue contrast, and their use is now routine in many clinical settings. However, the short range, dipole-dipole (relaxivity) effects conventionally used to affect T1 contrast depend on a contrast agent's direct access to water molecules to perturb the MR signal. This access is effectively limited to the intravascular space in the presence of an intact blood–brain barrier (BBB). When the BBB is intact or only minimally disrupted, the current class of contrast agents effectively become intravascular agents in the central nervous system (CNS) and hence can produce only enhancement of the blood pool itself, which in turn contributes only a small fraction of the total MRI spins from tissue (~2–4%). Susceptibility-based perfusion imaging techniques circumvent this limitation, and in fact provide their contrast only in the presence of significant compartmentalization of the contrast agent.

Magnetic susceptibility (T2 or T2*) contrast, unlike relaxivity (T1) contrast, results from microscopic variations in the magnetic field, which are caused by the heterogeneous distribution of high magnetic susceptibility contrast agents within a tissue. This microscopic heterogeneity of magnetic field leads to loss of transverse phase coherence and hence MRI signal. This mechanism is of course identical to that invoked to explain the loss of signal during hemorrhagic disease characterized by compartmentalization of iron, as either deoxygenated intact red cells acutely or as ferritin/hemosiderin clumps chronically. Image contrast in susceptibility-contrast (T2 or T2*) studies is occasioned by longer range, rather than molecular, magnetic field perturbations that the paramagnetic agents produce when compartmentalized within the vascular bed (17–19). Within this space, these magnetic susceptibility effects relax the transverse magnetization of surrounding tissue protons for a distance roughly equal to the radius of the blood vessel (14). Dynamic magnetic susceptibility contrast imaging is thus well suited to investigations of hemodynamic perturbations in the CNS, since the BBB, rather than obscuring these effects as with relaxivity (T1) contrast imaging, produces the compartmentalization needed to produce susceptibility contrast in the brain (14,20,21). An injection of any high magnetic susceptibility contrast agent (either the current class of gadolinium chelates or newer agents based on dysprosium or iron oxides) will therefore produce a significant decrease in brain signal intensity for both SE T2- and gradient-echo (GE) T2*-weighted images when present in high enough concentration, such as during the agent's first pass through the microvascular bed (14).

Magnetic susceptibility contrast phenomena can be coupled with rapid imaging to resolve the first pass tissue transit of intravenously administered contrast materials (16,22–24), thereby providing an index with which to measure cerebral blood flow (CBF) and volume. To determine quantitatively cerebral blood volume (CBV) or CBF, however, it is necessary to convert regional changes in MR signal intensity with respect to time into contrast agent tissue concentration-time curves (16,23,25). Both theoretical and empirical studies have shown that the degree of the signal drop rests on two factors: the concentration of an injected contrast agent within the blood and the fractional volume of intravascular space within the tissue (the CBV). After injection, the contrast agent's concentration varies with time, whereas blood volume may vary region by region. Both contrast agent concentration and blood volume reflect approximately linear relationships to the change observed in the T2 rate, $\Delta(1/T2) = \Delta R2$. This can be measured easily by measuring the percent-signal change from baseline (16,23). Within some limiting range, therefore, we can measure the contrast agent's concentration in tissue as a function of time (the so-called concentration-versus-time curve) by mapping tissue signal loss dynamically over time (16,23,25).

Measurement of these concentration time curves allows us to directly map important physiologic parameters in the brain. For example, integrated or summed over time, the signal changes are proportional to the blood volume in each voxel, and are similar to standard tracer experiments used in nuclear medicine. Relative microvascular CBV maps can be generated by applying susceptibility contrast physics and standard tracer kinetic principles, as illustrated in Fig. 6. Unlike conventional nuclear medicine studies, however, the principles underlying the susceptibility contrast phenomena are highly dependent on the specific acquisition technique used. Although the techniques of image acquisition and creation of the maps include many details that are beyond the scope of this chapter, a few points are worth noting. First, SE or T2-weighted imaging techniques are more sensitive to the microvasculature than are T2*-weighted GE imaging techniques. This aspect of susceptibility physics has been demonstrated using simulation studies, and is illustrated in practice in Fig. 7 (26). This provides an important advantage of the SE MRI techniques over conventional nuclear studies because the signal changes are weighted by contrast agent in the *microvasculature*, rather than in the total vascular space. This has important implications in studying neoplastic disorders, because of the role of tumor microvascular angiogenic factors in cancer pathogenesis (27). This implies that for detection of microvascular perfusion, SE tech-

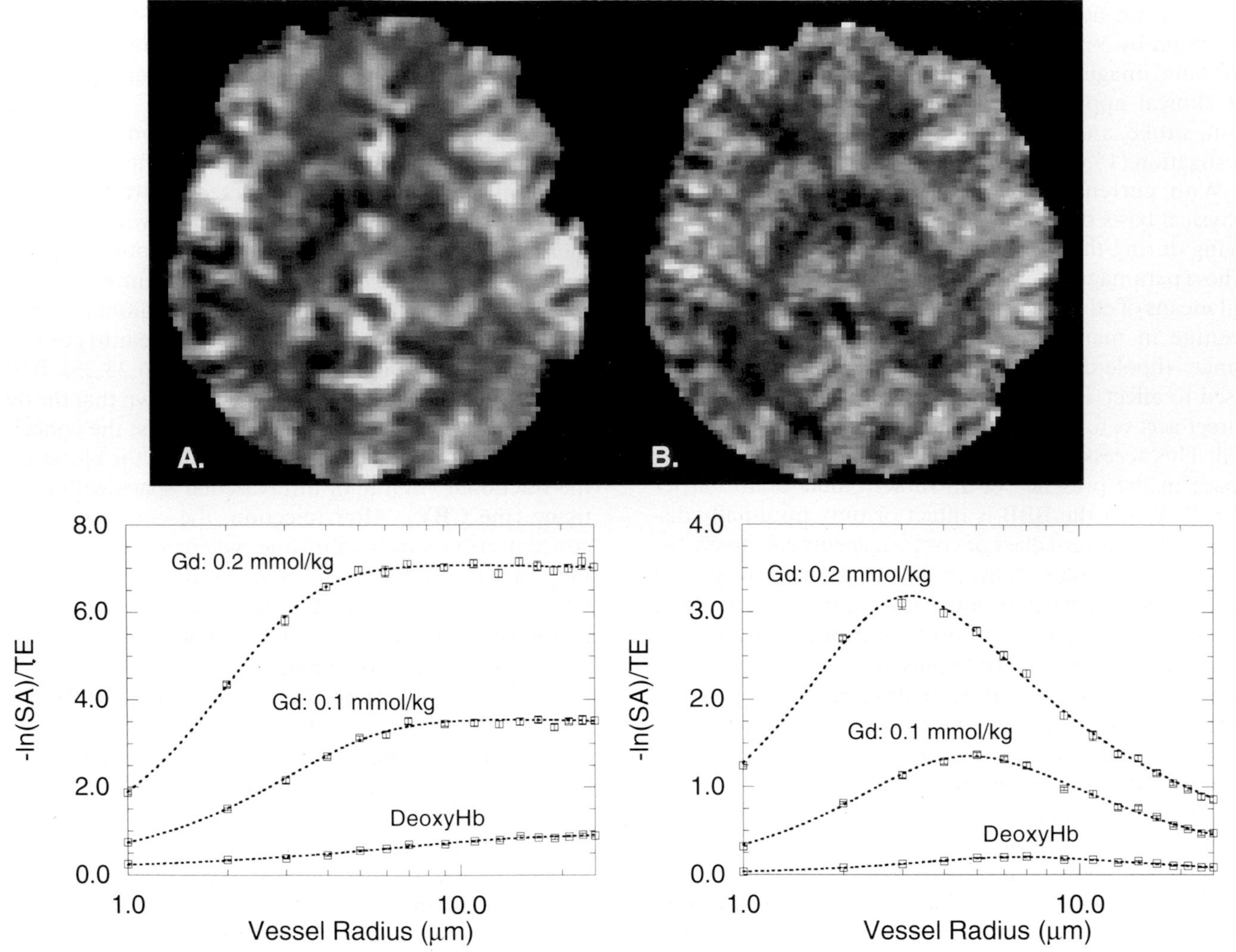

FIG. 7. GE vs. SE in rCBV maps. **A:** GE rCBV map, TE = 60, TR = 1500, injection of 0.1 mmol/Kg Gd-DTPA. **B:** SE rCBV map, TE = 100, TR = 1500, injection of 0.2 mmol/Kg of Gd-DTPA. The change in signal with injection is similar for the two studies, but the SE rCBV map is clearly superior. **C,D:** Relative sensitivity of each technique to intravascular contrast based on vessel size. These data confirm the visual impressions of the maps in A and B. For evaluation of rCBV in the microvasculature, SE techniques have a marked advantage. (Courtesy J. L. Boxerman, R. M. Weisskoff, and H. Aronen.)

niques provide an increase in specificity, although with some loss of SNR. A typical series of microvascular rCBV maps in normal subjects are shown in Figs. 8 and 9. These can be compared to a typical positron-emission study of blood volume (Fig. 10), which is dominated by the large vascular structures. Typical features of a normal SE rCBV map include a normally slightly higher rCBV in the visual cortex, and zero rCBV in the ventricles. Also note that larger vascular structures, notably cortical veins and arteries, also contribute to image contrast on these CBV maps, although much less so than on the PET map.

In clinical practice, echo-planar techniques have been predominantly used for dynamic SE acquisition, especially for multislice imaging, because conventional SE images are not fast enough to capture first-pass phenomena from multiple slices with a temporal resolution of 1 to 2 sec. Other technical issues have also been found to be of practical importance. Since blood volume is calculated on the basis of signal change from the baseline, estimating this baseline with as many images as possible improves the signal-to-noise ratio (28). As a rough rule of thumb, one should collect about as many baseline images as are acquired during the contrast passage (typically 20–40). Dose of contrast is also important. Although doses of 0.1 mmol/Kg can be used, several studies have found that higher doses than 0.2 mmol/Kg to be significantly superior, especially using gadolinium-based agents (29). For SE imaging, this produces a 20% to 30% peak signal drop in gray matter for TE = 100 msec. Finally, to produce the highest intravascular concentrations possible and to limit recirculation artifacts, contrast should be administered as a bolus injection, typically at 5 cc/sec. The use of an MR-compatible

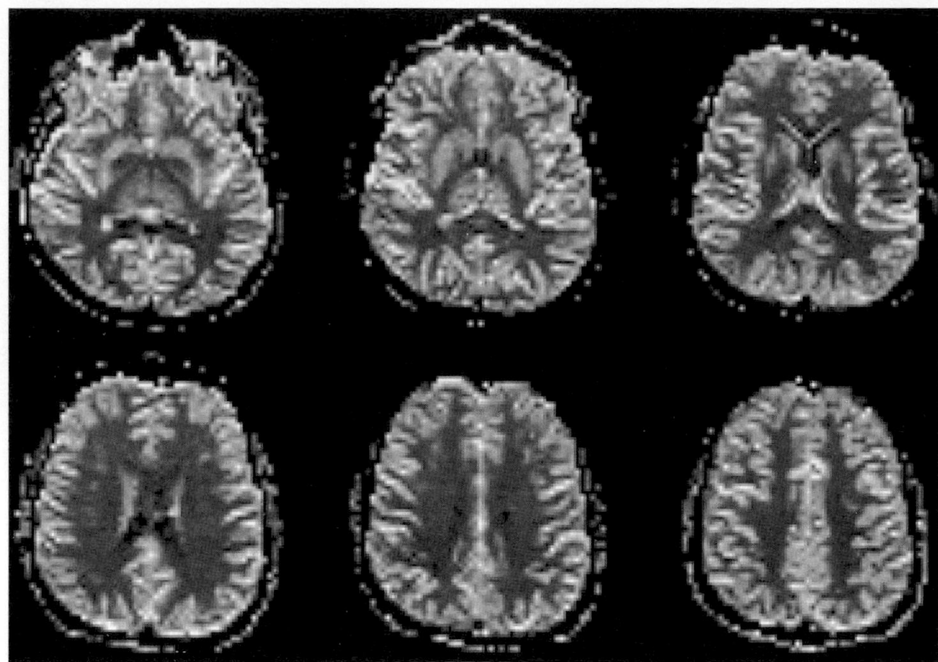

FIG. 8. Normal rCBV map using 0.2 mmol/Kg of dysprosium-DTPA-BMA. Note the excellent gray-white contrast and the relatively high signal in the normal cortical and deep veins. Acquisition parameters: TR = 1500, TE = 100, 1.5-mm × 1.5-mm × 6-mm voxels.

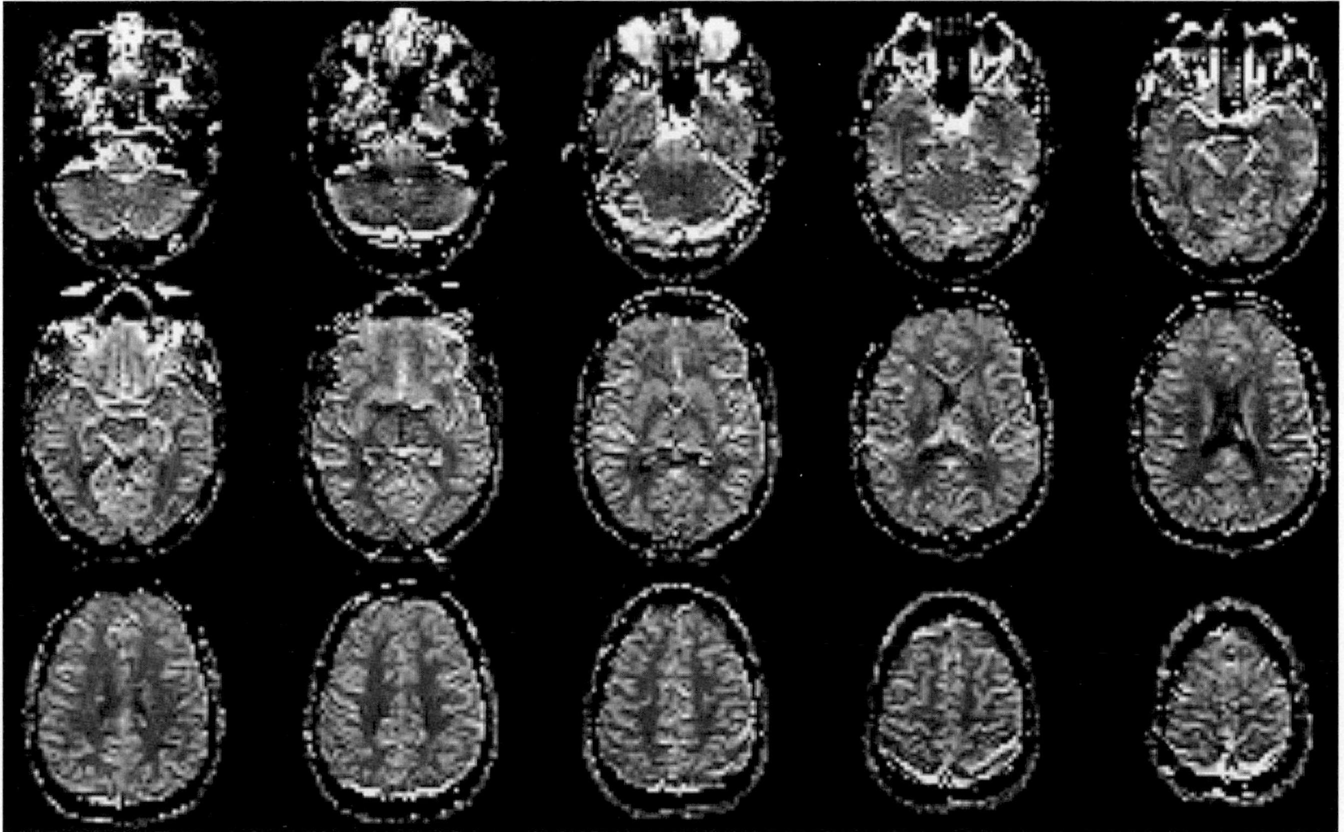

FIG. 9. Normal rCBV map using a Gd-based contrast agent (gadoteridol, 0.2 mmol/Kg). The gray-white contrast is slightly decreased when compared with the dysprosium maps, but still adequate. There is still some relatively high signal in cortical veins, which is artifactual. Note the slightly higher rCBV in the visual cortex, which is normal. There is some signal in the soft tissues as well. 15 slices, TR = 2000, TE = 100, 3-mm × 3-mm × 6-mm voxels.

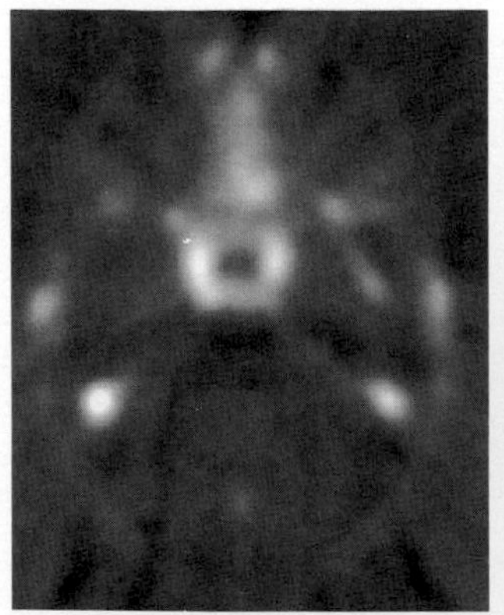
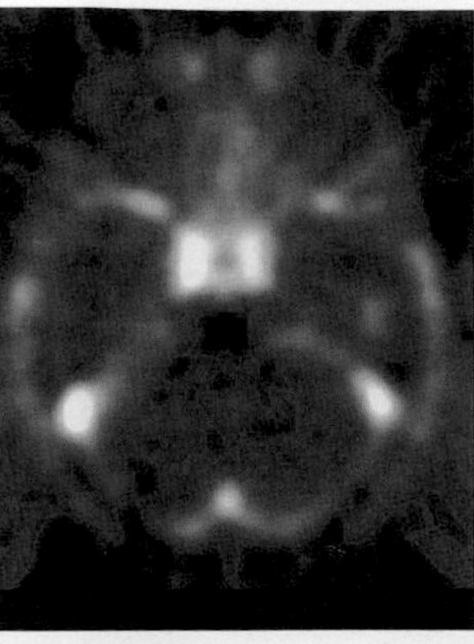
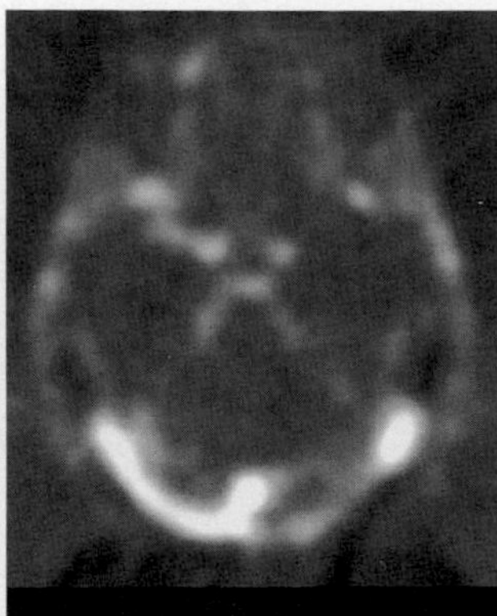
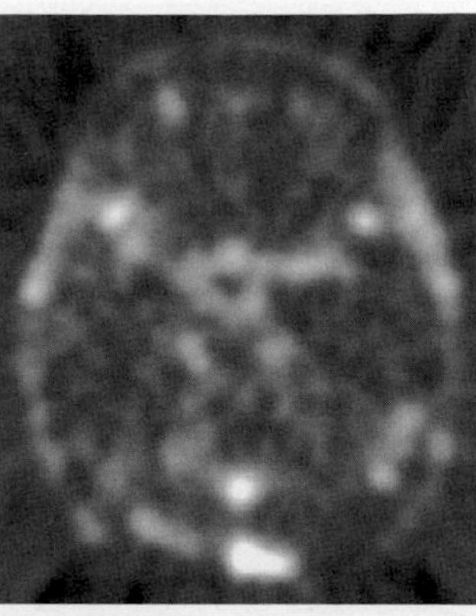

FIG. 10. Normal CO-PET study. Note that the image is dominated by the structures with highest blood volume; in particular, the venous sinuses, with 100% blood volume, have such a high signal that gray-white differences are obscured. Contrast this with fMRI rCBV maps, which emphasize the blood volume in the capillary bed.

power injector has been found to facilitate this process (30).

As with other intravascular tracer techniques, more than relative CBV can be computed from the concentration-versus-time curve. Contrast agent arrival time, time to peak change, and transit time can be calculated on a voxel-by-voxel basis, and can be used to infer information on CBF as well as CBV (31–34). Coupled with MRA, such techniques promise a complete cerebrovascular examination at the tissue as well as large vessel level.

Blood Flow/Oxygenation Imaging and Activation Mapping

As proposed as early as 1895, local cerebral hemodynamics are closely linked to local cerebral activity (1,35–37). Although fMRI is not yet sensitive to neuronal activity directly, cerebral hemodynamic changes can be used as a surrogate marker for cerebral activity (38,39). Functional MRI can detect changes in blood volume via introduction of intravenous contrast agents, as noted in the previous section. This has been used to directly observe changes in hemodynamics that accompany neuronal activation in the visual system (24). In addition, however, several more recent fMRI techniques have been developed that use intrinsic tissue contrast mechanisms.

Two basic contrast mechanisms have been elucidated that provide image contrast during changing hemodynamic state. The first of these is the so-called BOLD (for *b*lood *o*xygenation *l*evel–*d*ependent) contrast mechanism. The link between changes in deoxyhemoglobin content and MRI signal changes is founded on the observation by Linus Pauling that the magnetic properties of hemoglobin change as its oxygenation state changes. Specifically, deoxyhemoglobin is paramagnetic, whereas oxyhemoglobin loses its paramagnetism and is thus diamagnetic (40). The paramagnetic effect of deoxyhemoglobin was shown by Thulborn et al. in 1982 to shorten T2 (41). This property is familiar to neuroradiologists as the cause for the drop in T2-weighted signal seen in some stages of acute hemorrhage (42). More recently, the intrinsic contrast effects of deoxygenated paramagnetic hemoglobin with a GE technique were used by Ogawa et al. to study the influence of intravascular susceptibility perturbations on signal arising from blood vessels (43). In the last few years, several groups have demonstrated that the MR signal of brain tissue on T2, T2* and T2′-weighted images is strongly influenced by the oxygenation state of the blood (43–45).

The link between these earlier observations and changes in MR signal during neuronal activation was first established by Kwong et al. (46,47). Why does blood oxygenation state, and hence MR signal, change during conditions of increased flow seen with neuronal activation? PET and other studies have shown that oxygen delivery, CBF, and CBV all increase with activation, with the increase in CBF exceeding CBV by about a factor of 2 (48). However, there is a mismatch between oxygen delivery (governed by CBF) and oxygen utilization (the $CMRO_2$) under at least most activation paradigms, with oxygen utilization rising only slightly with cerebral activation (38,39). The combination of increased oxygen delivery without concomitant increase in oxygen extraction, coupled with a more modest increase in blood volume, leads to a decrease in the local tissue deoxyhemoglobin content during states of increased neuronal activity. This drop in paramagnetic deoxyhemoglobin leads to *increased* signal on susceptibility sensitive T2- and T2*-weighted pulse sequences. Especially when coupled with high-speed imaging, these techniques have become a powerful tool in assessing changes in regional blood, and hence tissue, oxygenation and flow (47).

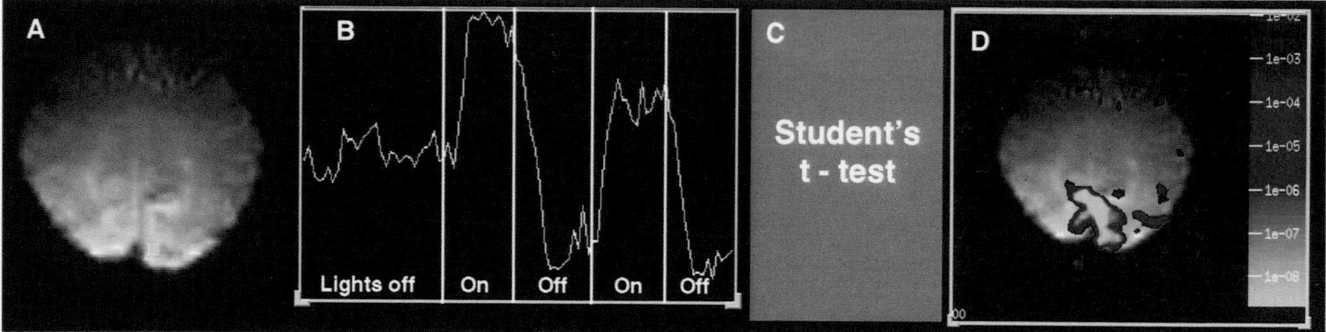

FIG. 11. Task activation fMRI. In this case the task is simply to be in the dark ("lights off") or watch LEDs flicker at 8 Hz ("lights on"). **A:** Imaging is performed, typically at one image each second or two (depending on the nature of the task), both while the control and stimulus tasks are being performed. A region of interest or the whole image can be selected for further analysis. **B:** Time course of region of interest shown in A during the task. Note the "undershoot" phenomenon and also the slight delay between onsite of task and fMRI response. Also note the possible habituation during the second stimulation, an inconstant phenomenon. **C:** Each voxel can be tested using any number of statistical tests to determine what, if any, difference in signal occurred during the stimulus condition as compared with the control condition. **D:** The probability that the differences in signal were random, or *p* value, can then be plotted over the anatomic image. The areas of brightest yellow demonstrate that the chance of the signal change observed is due to random fluctuations that have a *p* value of less than 0.00000001 ($<1 \times 10^{-8}$), before Bonferroni correction.

These allow direct visualization of brain activity using fMRI, as shown in Fig. 11.

A second technique using intrinsic tissue contrast relies on changes in the longitudinal, rather than transverse, magnetization that occurs with changing blood flow. An increase in tissue perfusion was shown by Detre et al. (49,50) to result in a drop in the apparent T1 of brain tissue. This drop in T1 leads directly to an increase in MR signal on pulse sequences sensitive to changes in T1, in a manner analogous to the increase in signal seen on T1-weighted images within flowing vessels (so-called time of flight or flow-related enhancement). Variations on this broad theme have been used to quantify absolute tissue perfusion (e.g., Detre) or map changes in tissue perfusion seen with neuronal activity either directly with T1-weighted images (e.g., Kwong) or through

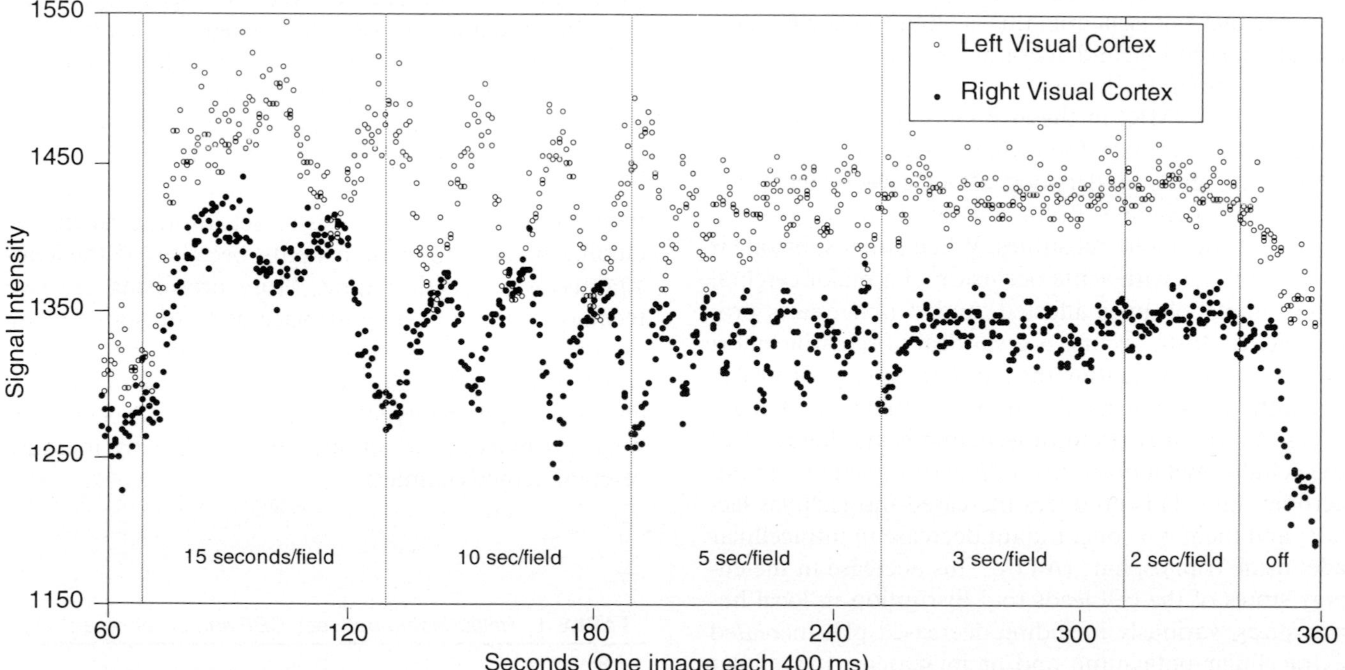

FIG. 12. Alternating hemifield stimulation. A flashing checkerboard pattern was presented first to one visual hemifield and then to the other, corresponding to excitation of one hemisphere's primary visual cortex and then the other. This stimulus was presented at increasing frequencies. Regions of interest in visual cortex (along the calcarine fissure) are then plotted, demonstrating that discrete neural events lasting as little as 3 to 5 sec can be distinguished. Acquistion parameters: EPI single-shot GE images, TR 400 msec, TE 60 msec, 3-mm × 3-mm × 7-mm voxels.

the use of modified angiographic "bolus tracking" techniques (e.g., Edelman).

By using techniques sensitive to these deoxyhemoglobin and flow changes, completely noninvasive tomographic maps of cerebral activity can be made (47). Of particular interest is the relative rapidity of the onset of the fMRI effect and its reproducibility. This is demonstrated in Fig. 12. The capability to map brain activity with MRI has already found wide application in the basic neurosciences; subsequent sections in this chapter confirm the clinical applicability of these techniques.

CLINICAL APPLICATIONS

Stroke and Cerebrovascular Disease

Acute Ischemia and Infarction

Stroke is diagnosed approximately 400,000 times per year in the United States, and contributes to approximately 150,000 deaths per year (51). In addition to the difficulty of making an accurate diagnosis clinically (estimates of false-positive rates for stroke range up to 40%), intervention may depend on a more accurate assessment than clinical evaluation. Attempts to find an effective therapy for stroke have been so far met with limited success (52), and many investigators believe that this is because of an incomplete understanding of human stroke, particularly in the acute stage. While conventional T2-weighted images are typically abnormal 12 to 24 hours after the onset of ischemia, this is often too late to allow useful intervention, and does not allow study of the early events in cerebral ischemia.

The role of fMRI in the evaluation of acute cerebral ischemia is best understood when placed in context with what is currently understood about cerebral hemodynamics and ischemia. Brain cells use both oxygen and glucose as metabolic substrates. When either substrate is unavailable, as with acute occlusion of a major cerebral artery, metabolism is affected, and if ischemia is prolonged cell death occurs. A great deal of scientific effort has gone into elucidating the pathophysiology of stroke, and although key steps remain poorly understood, it appears that the first result of ischemia is an alteration of the cellular metabolism from an aerobic state to an anaerobic state. This produces increased intracellular lactate, and there is a concomitant decrease in intracellular adenosine triphosphate (ATP). This decrease in the energy stores of the cell leads to a disruption in local homeostasis, variously including decreased pH, increased extracellular potassium, and/or increased extracellular neurotransmitters. This loss of homeostasis progresses to neuronal dysfunction, with abnormal stimulation such as spreading depression and excitotoxic activity. Neuronal dysfunction (including possibly hyperstimulation) may lead to a further loss of homeostasis, particularly increased permeability of the cell membrane to calcium. This is followed by cell death. Concomitant with this is a loss of the autoregulatory function of the brain capillary bed, such that at certain stages of ischemia, reperfusion may actually increase injury rather than reverse the cellular decline, although this is controversial (53,54).

Of course, CBF is not binary; there are degrees of ischemia. The relationship between level CBF and neuronal dysfunction is outlined in Table 1. The key finding in this table is that there is a level of CBF at which neurons stop functioning (producing observable clinical symptoms) but have not undergone cell death; therefore, the damage from this level of ischemia may be reversible. This has led to the concept of an "ischemic penumbra" (55). This penumbra has been heavily investigated in animal studies (e.g., ref. 56), and also in humans by means of nuclear medicine techniques (57,58), and currently is thought of as composed of brain tissue that is viable but ischemic. Cells in the penumbra are somewhere along the series of steps described above in the pathophysiology of stroke, but may be salvageable by intervention. Importantly, the penumbra may be as much defined by the duration of the ischemic insult as by the degree: a decrease in blood flow that does not produce cellular dysfunction acutely may do so if maintained for longer periods of time (59). Furthermore, an ischemic insult that causes no discernible injury may cause infarction if it is repeated (60).

One of the goals of fMRI in the acute setting is to visualize the ischemic penumbra, and ideally identify at an early time the difference between salvageable, nonsalvageable, and undamaged tissue. Imaging of acute stroke has been undertaken with a variety of MRI techniques, including spectroscopic, diffusion, perfusion, and conventional imaging, all with an aim to visualize one or more of the steps in the pathophysiologic process of stroke. Although spectroscopic imaging is sensitive to many of these processes, it is as yet impractical for excluding acute stroke in patients because of the constraints of acquisition time. More promising are two techniques that are now in place at some sites for use on a routine clinical basis: diffusion-weighted imaging, which is sensitive to alterations in water mobility due to changes in the energy status of the cell, and perfusion-weighted imaging, which attempts to directly measure cerebral hemodynamics.

TABLE 1. *Relationship between CBF and cerebral activity*

Blood flow (in ml/100 g/min)	Cerebral activity
50–55	Normal
18–25	EEG flat line, loss of evoked response
12	Membrane pump failure and cell death

EEG, electroencephalogram.

While the diffusion of water is not directly related to neural function, numerous studies have demonstrated that diffusion-weighted MR images can detect ischemic changes as early as 15 min after middle cerebral artery occlusion (4,5,33,34,61). Therefore, diffusion-weighted imaging has the potential to diagnose stroke in its earliest phases, before conventional MR or computed tomographic (CT) imaging techniques become sensitive. Figure 13 shows conventional and diffusion-weighted imaging in a patient approximately 10 hours after the onset of right body weakness. While T2- and postcontrast T1-weighted images were normal, the diffusion-weighted images demonstrate an area of hyperintensity. This corresponds to a decreased apparent diffusion coefficient:

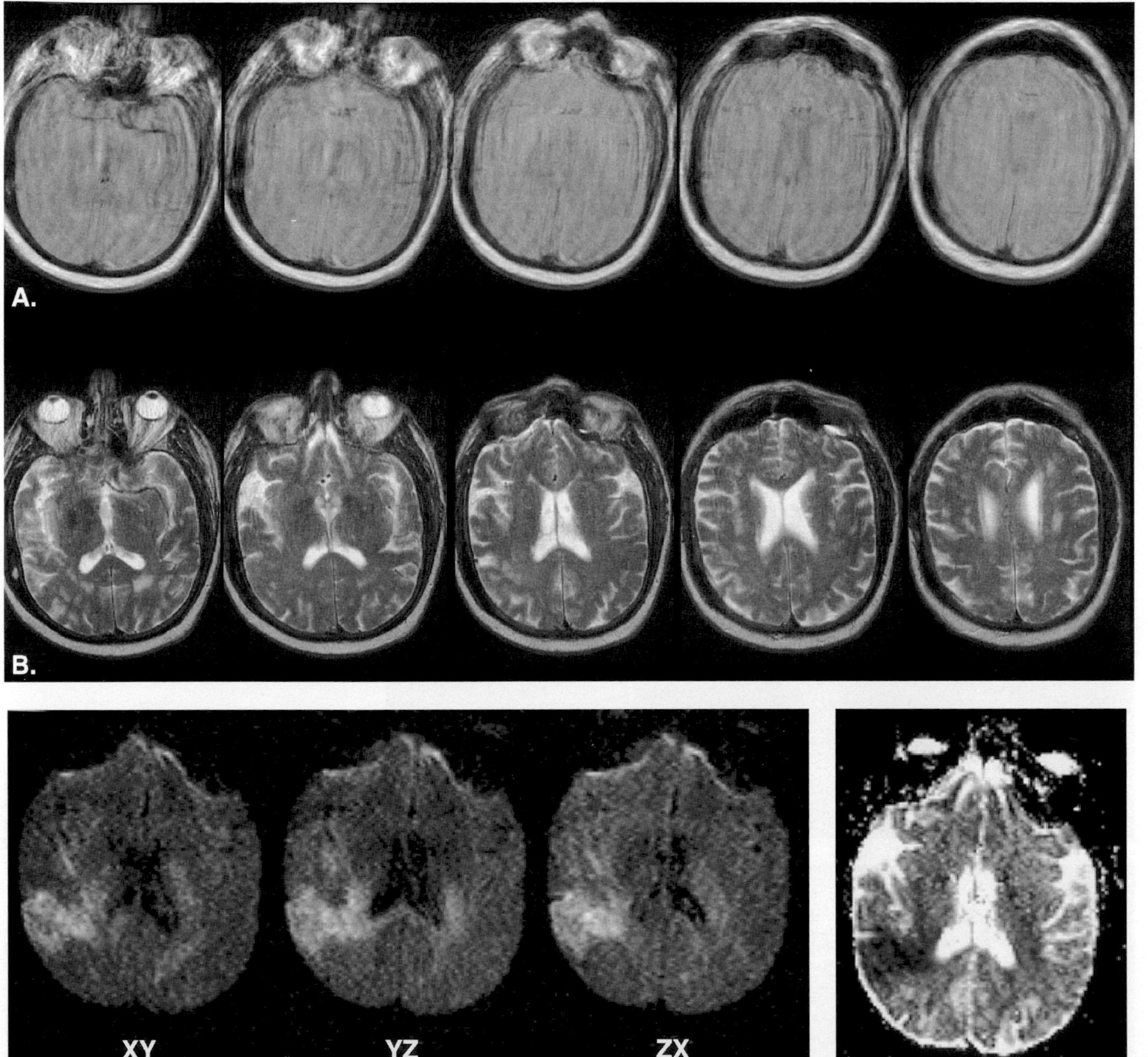

FIG. 13. Conventional and diffusion-weighted imaging in acute stroke. **A,B:** Conventional proton density-weighted and T2-weighted fast SE images demonstrate extensive patient motion, as is typical in this patient population, and no evidence of infarct. A CT before this study was also negative for infarct. **C:** Diffusion-weighted images demonstrate a large area of ischemia in the right parietal lobe. This is seen with diffusion weighting in three orthogonal directions: XY, YZ, ZX. Note the increased relative signal intensity in the corpus callosum on the YZ diffusion-weighted image; this is not present on the other images and is, therefore, due to ADC anisotropy in white matter. **D:** ADC map showing decreased ADC in the area of infarct. The ADC in the area of infarct is approximately 30% of the ADC of contralateral gray matter. Acquisition parameters: EPI SE, TR 6000, TE 151, 16 slices, 1.41 G/cm for 40 msec, 15 *b* values, total acquisition time 90 sec. Follow-up imaging confirmed the location and extent of the stroke to be similar to the initial diffusion-weighted image abnormality.

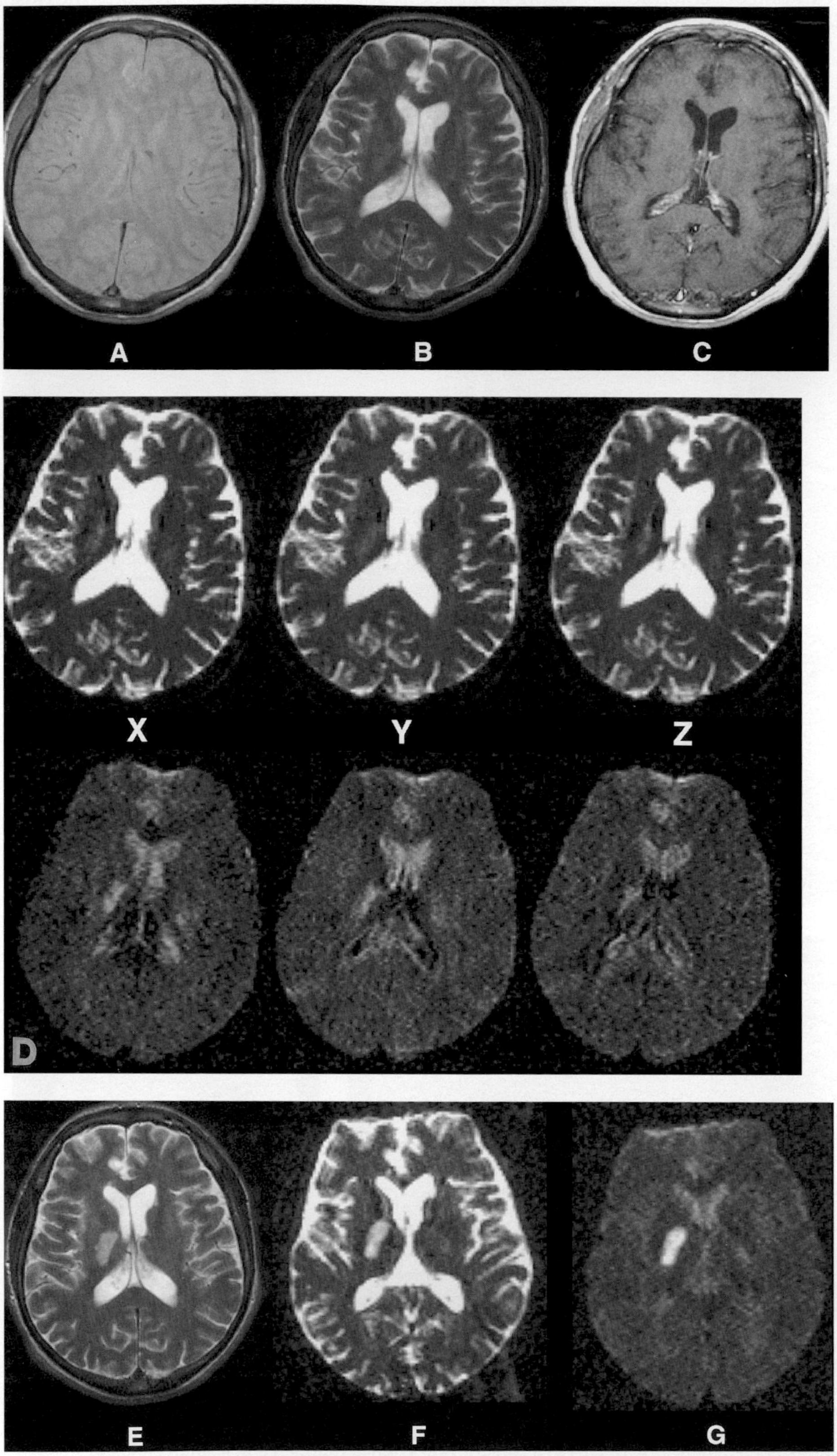

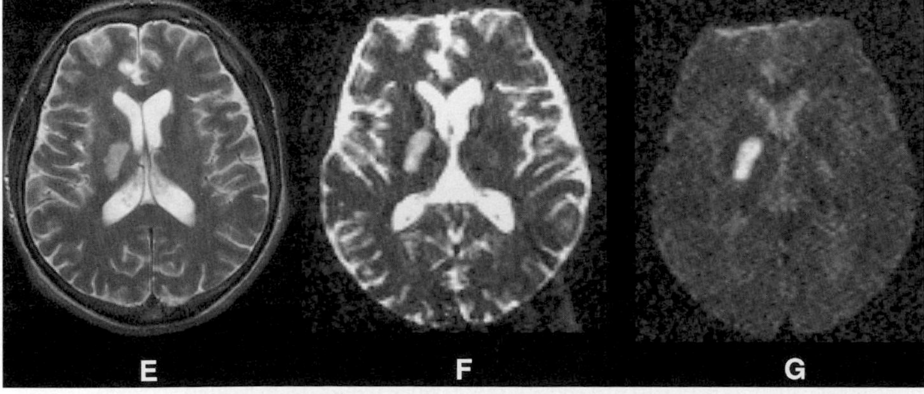

FIG. 14. Conventional and diffusion-weighted imaging in acute stroke. This patient with a known small old right frontal parasagittal stroke presented with acute left-sided weakness. **A,B,C:** Proton density-, T2-, and post-Gd T1-weighted conventional images, respectively, show no acute abnormality. **D:** Diffusion-weighted imaging shows a small focus of increased signal in the right thalamus; X, Y, and Z directions at b = 34 and b = 700 sec/mm^2 images are shown. **E,F,G:** Follow-up imaging 5 days later with T2, b = 34 sec/mm^2, and b = 700 sec/mm^2 diffusion-weighted images, respectively. These demonstrate the area of infarct, and show a slightly larger area of diffusion abnormality than the original image, perhaps indicating increase in the size of infarct.

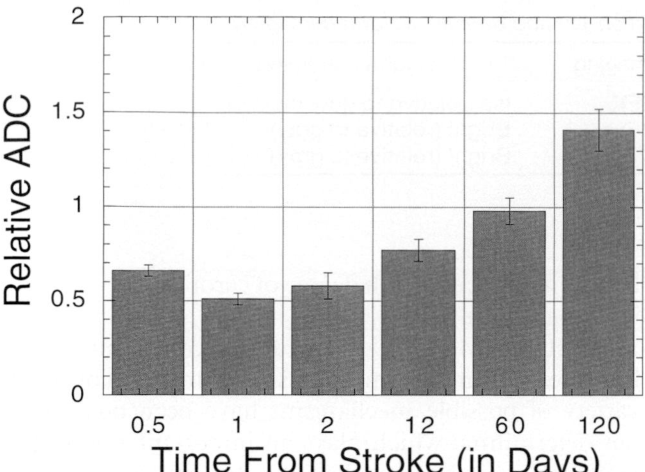

FIG. 15. Graph of relative ADC (ADC in area of abnormality divided by the ADC of the contralateral hemisphere) versus time. This demonstrates that the ADC stays depressed for days to weeks after acute ischemia. (Data from ref. 62.)

the water molecules move less, and therefore less dephasing occurs during the time the diffusion gradients are on. Figure 14 presents a second case in which follow-up imaging confirmed that this was in fact the area of infarct.

This acute decrease in water diffusion has been confirmed in animal and human studies of acute stroke. Figure 15 demonstrates that the relative ADC drops initially, remains depressed for some period of time, but then exceeds the normal diffusion coefficient of gray matter (5,62). Compare an acute infarct, as shown in Fig. 13 with a chronic infarct as shown in Fig. 16. Because of this evolution, acute, subacute, and chronic ischemia may be distinguishable on the basis of a combination of diffusion- and T2-weighted imaging, as shown in Table 2. Typical values for intracranial structures are given in Table 3.

The exact mechanism for the decrease in water diffusion in acute stroke is incompletely understood and under active investigation. Current thinking holds that a shift of water from the extravascular space, where diffusion is relatively unrestricted, to the more restricted intravascular environment, accounts for the drop in water mobility (32). This shift in water balance may reflect diminished Na/K pump activity, and hence be an indirect measure of cell ATP charge. This is supported by the close temporal correlation between diminished high energy phosphates seen on 31-P magnetic resonance spectroscopy (MRS) and ADC drop (34). Additional controversy surrounds whether or not the degree of drop in ADC corresponds to the degree of ischemia. Although some investigators have found correlations between decrease in ADC and extent of infarct (e.g., ref. 63), it is unclear whether this is simply a volume-averaging issue. It may be that quantification of ADC is similar to quantification of T1 and T2: possible, but not necessarily useful. It does appear clear that when diffusion abnormalities are present, the blood flow has dropped to the level of cell energy failure. In other words, the penumbra may well surround the area of decreased ADC, but not be included in it; for example, Roberts et al. (64) demonstrated in an animal model that the area of abnormal diffusion after middle cerebral artery (MCA) stenosis was surrounded by a larger area of abnormal perfusion. Because of this, some investigators believe that in order to visualize the ischemic penumbra a combination of diffusion and perfusion imaging will be needed. Although techniques that measure absolute CBF are not

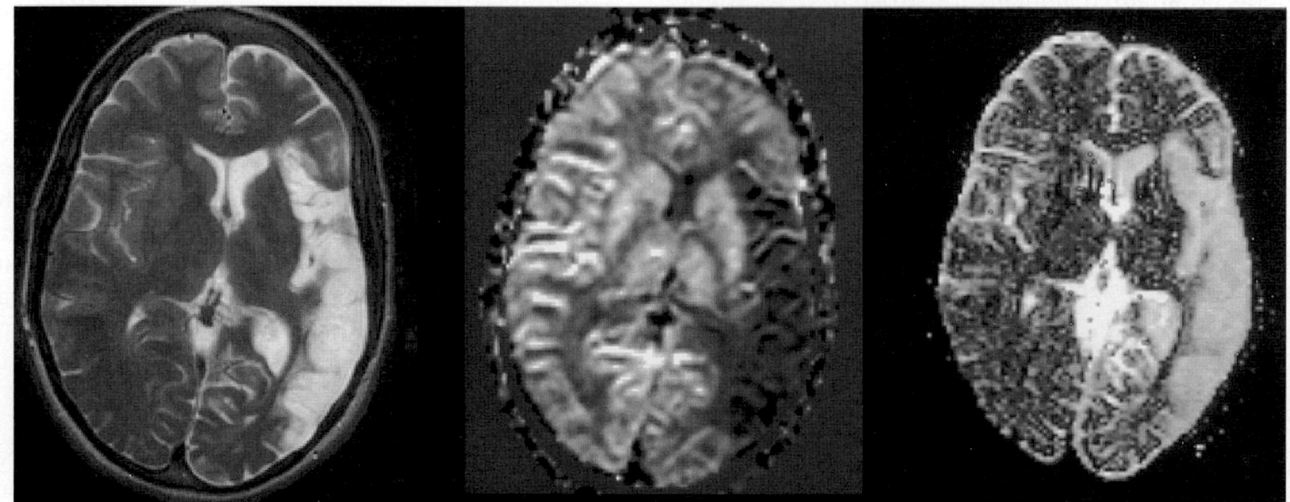

FIG. 16. Chronic stroke. These images are from a 32-year-old woman 1 year status post a large infarct. **A:** T2-weighted FSE image showing a large area of bright signal corresponding to the chronic stroke. **B:** Relative CBV map demonstrating decreased blood volume in this area. **C:** ADC map showing increase in the ADC consistent with increased free fluid due to tissue loss.

TABLE 2. *Proposed dating of ischemia based on T2- and density-weighted imaging*

	Diffusion-weighted imaging	T2-weighted imaging
Acute ischemia	Bright (relative to CSF)	Iso (relative to gray matter)
Subacute ischemia	Bright (relative to CSF)	Bright (relative to gray)
Chronic ischemia	Iso (relative to CSF)	Bright (relative to gray)

CSF, cerebrospinal fluid.

fully developed for human use (see, e.g., ref 49), useful information can be gained through the use of dynamic contrast studies. For example, Fig. 17 shows the hemodynamic maps from the acute stroke patients shown in Figs. 13 and 14, and confirms that the area of diffusion abnormality has decreased blood volume and peak contrast concentration. Figure 18 demonstrates that mapping the arrival time of the bolus of contrast agent can also be useful in determining inflow to a region; this may well be a predictor of tissue at risk, and combined with the acute diffusion imaging might predict areas corresponding to the ischemic penumbra.

Although this area of imaging is actively advancing, it seems clear that acute stroke can be imaged successfully in the clinical setting with diffusion and perfusion imaging, and with accurate identification of ischemic tissue. Characterization of the penumbra, prognostic implications, and where acute stroke imaging fits into the clinical care of the patient remain to be worked out. Figure 19 demonstrates additional application of diffusion and perfusion imaging to the diagnosis of acute stroke.

Chronic Infarction

Although assessment of acute stroke has clear clinical utility, fMRI may also be useful in the management of chronic infarction. Approximately one quarter of stroke patients hospitalized annually for stroke have recurrent disease (65). Assessment of patient pathology after stroke may help identify patients who may benefit from intervention. Figure 20 demonstrates how mapping other perfusion parameters besides relative CBV can detect differences in the passage of a bolus of contrast agent on a tomographic basis. This technique can be applied over the entire brain, providing a complete tomographic evaluation of baseline hemodynamics. For example, delay in the time to peak signal change after a bolus of contrast

TABLE 3. *Apparent diffusion coefficient values*

Tissue	ADC
Normal gray matter	1.0×10^{-3} mm^2/sec
Normal white matter	0.5×10^{-3} mm^2/sec to 0.9 mm^2/sec
Infarcted gray matter	0.4×10^{-3} to 0.7×10^{-3} mm^2/sec
CSF	3×10^{-3} mm^2/sec

CSF, cerebrospinal fluid; ADC, apparent diffusion coefficient.

has been correlated with degree of carotid artery stenosis in humans (66).

Functional MRI may also be able to contribute to clinical research into the mechanism of stroke recovery. A variety of possible mechanisms have been postulated, but determining which plays an important role in human stroke has been challenging. In 1895 and again in 1914, Von Monakow described the possible functional "shock" or dysfunction of remote intact neurons due to connectivity with neurons in the area of a stroke, which he termed "diaschisis" (67,68). Distinguishing between dysfunction due to diaschisis and dysfunction due to primary injury is not possible with conventional MRI studies because the nonfunctioning remote cortex is initially anatomically normal, until the affected neurons degenerate as in crossed-cerebellar diaschisis. However, recovery from diaschisis may play an important role in recovery from stroke, as most diaschisis is reversible (69). In a clinical setting, determining which areas of cortex are dysfunctional because of primary insult versus cortex affected by diaschisis may play a role in therapeutic choice. Functional MRI is able to map these differences, as demonstrated in Fig. 21.

Neoplasm

Diagnosis of the presence of CNS tumors has been greatly aided by the anatomic resolution of MRI. Characterization of tumor malignant potential is more difficult using conventional techniques, particularly because both the T1- and T2-relaxation times and the integrity of the BBB of neoplastic tissue has failed to be a specific indicator of malignancy. Over the last several years more physiologic parameters have been sought that may be imaged in vivo and could improve tumor characterization, including measures of tumor growth rate, metabolism, and angiogenesis. Much of this work to date has been performed using nuclear technologies, especially PET and SPECT. For example, PET studies of tumor metabolism using ^{18}FDG have shown the degree of glucose utilization to be a predictor of prognosis (70,71). However, metabolism may not be the only or the best method to evaluate cancer. To continue growth, a new tumor must induce new capillary vessels once it reaches a few millimeters in size; this is termed "angiogenesis." In 1991, Weidner et al. (72) demonstrated that, in breast carcinoma [and later lung and prostate carcinoma (27)],

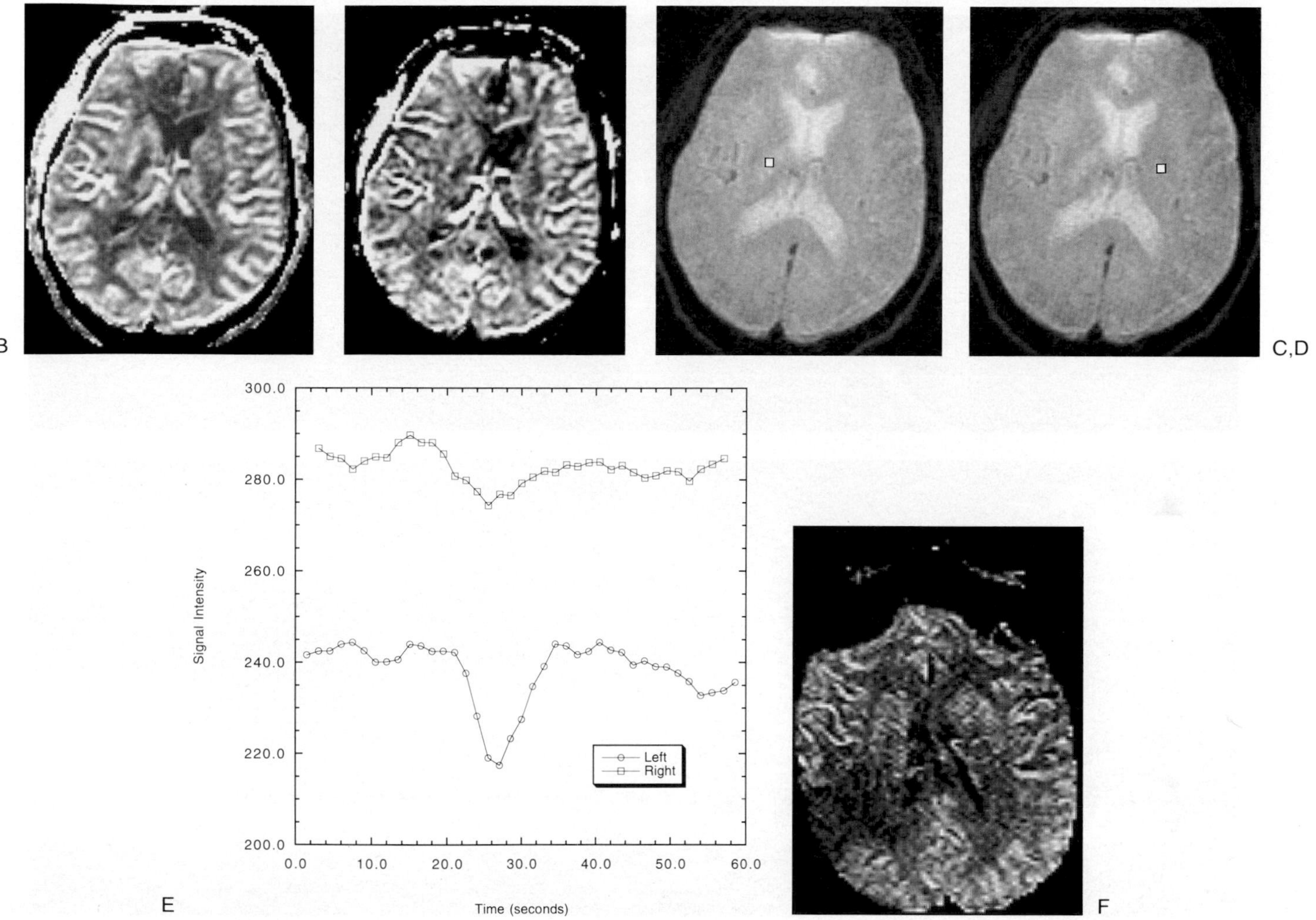

FIG. 17. Relative CBV mapping of the patients in Figs. 13 and 14. A–E, patient in Fig. 14, F, patient in Fig. 13. **A:** Map of the peak change in signal during the course of the injection (peak delta T2), showing an area of low signal intensity in the right thalamus, consistent with the diffusion and follow-up images. **B:** Same patient, map of rCBV. **C–E:** Regions of interest (ROIs) and time course for the two ROIs indicated in C and D, demonstrating the decreased change in the area of stroke, consistent with decreased delivery of gadolinium contrast agent. **F:** Relative CBV map in patient from Fig. 13. Interestingly, the rCBV defect is larger than the diffusion abnormality; their mismatch may indicate the region of the ischemic penumbra.

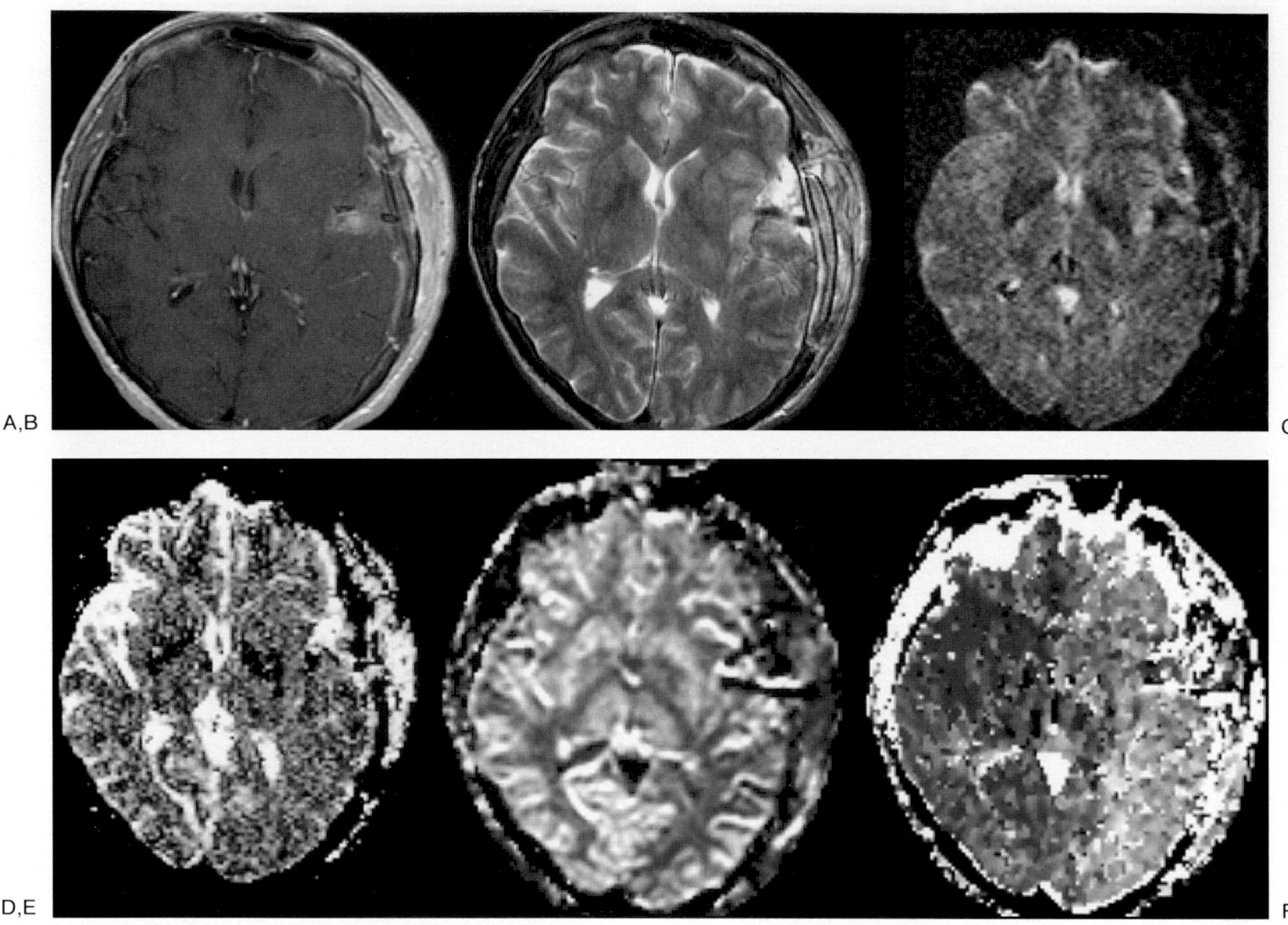

FIG. 18. A 35-year-old man status post extracranial-intracranial bypass graft for future occlusion of distal ICA to treat an aneurysm (at the time of imaging the ICA had not yet been occluded). **A:** Post-Gd T1-weighted images showing minimal enhancement in the area of surgery. **B:** T2 FSE showing again minimal local postoperative changes. **C:** Diffusion-weighted image showing no definite diffusion abnormality. **D:** ADC map confirming the findings in C. **E:** rCBV map showing no clear blood volume deficit. **F:** Image of time to peak signal change, showing a brighter left hemisphere than the right. Longer arrival times are shown as brighter signal, and region of interest analysis demonstrated that the delay in the contrast bolus between the left and right hemispheres was approximately 3 sec.

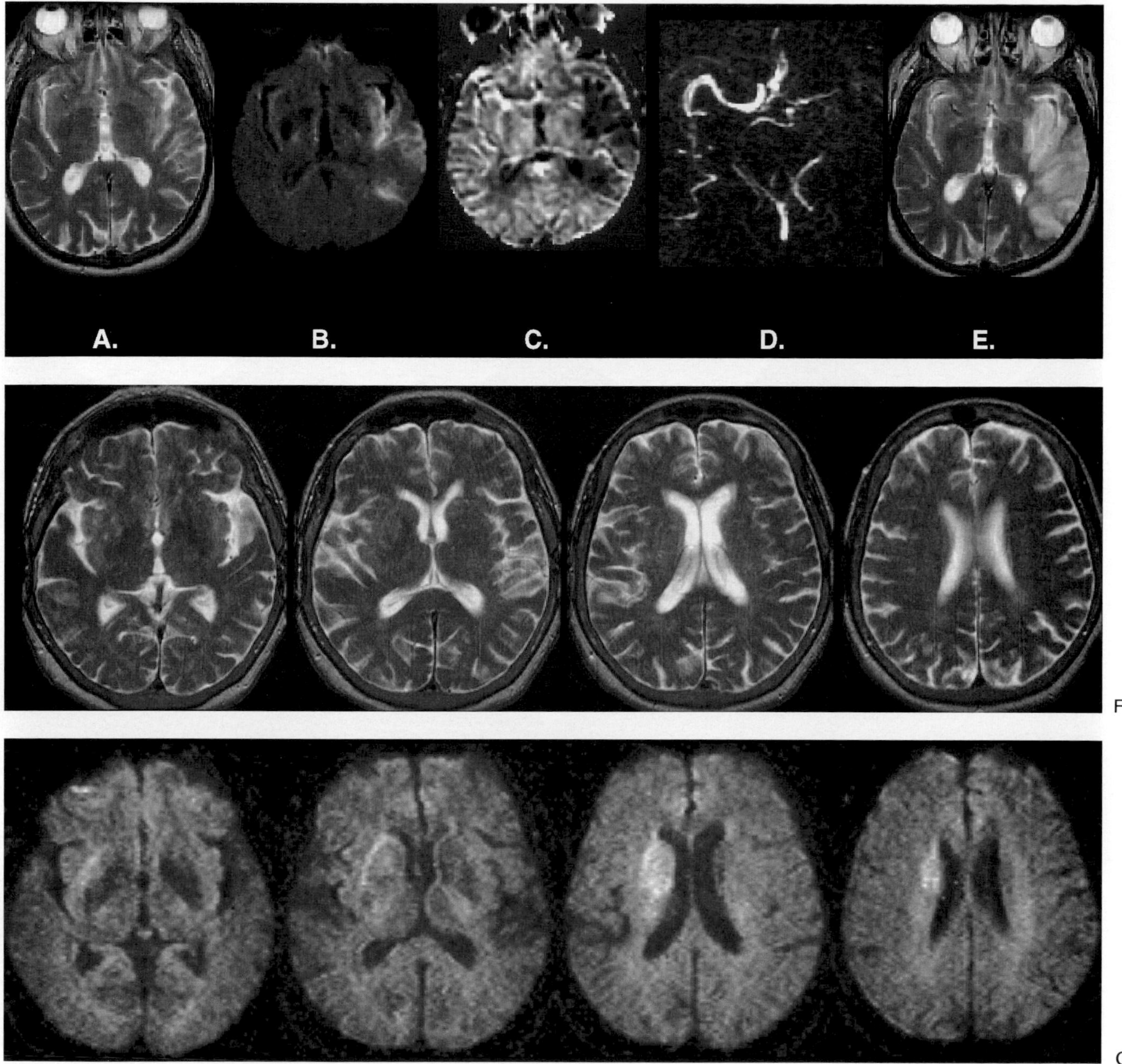

FIG. 19. Additional examples of diffusion/perfusion evaluation of acute stroke. A–E, a 62-year-old man with sudden onset dense R hemiplegia 7 hours before study. **A:** T2 FSE shows no definite abnormality. **B:** Diffusion-weighted image (b ~1000 sec/mm^2) shows diffuse cortical abnormality consistent with acute ischemia. **C:** CBV map demonstrates a large perfusion defect. **D:** 2D PC MRA shows decreased flow in the proximal MCA. **E:** Follow-up T2 FSE at 65 hours postictus demonstrates abnormal signal consistent with subacute ischemia. F–J, A 72-year-old woman with sudden onset L hemineglect, facial droop, and hemiparesis 3 hours before study. **F:** T2W FSE demonstrates no abnormal signal. Proton density-weighted images were also normal. **G:** Isotropic diffusion-weighted imaging demonstrates increased signal in the right deep gray and white matter, particularly the putamen, consistent with acute ischemic change.

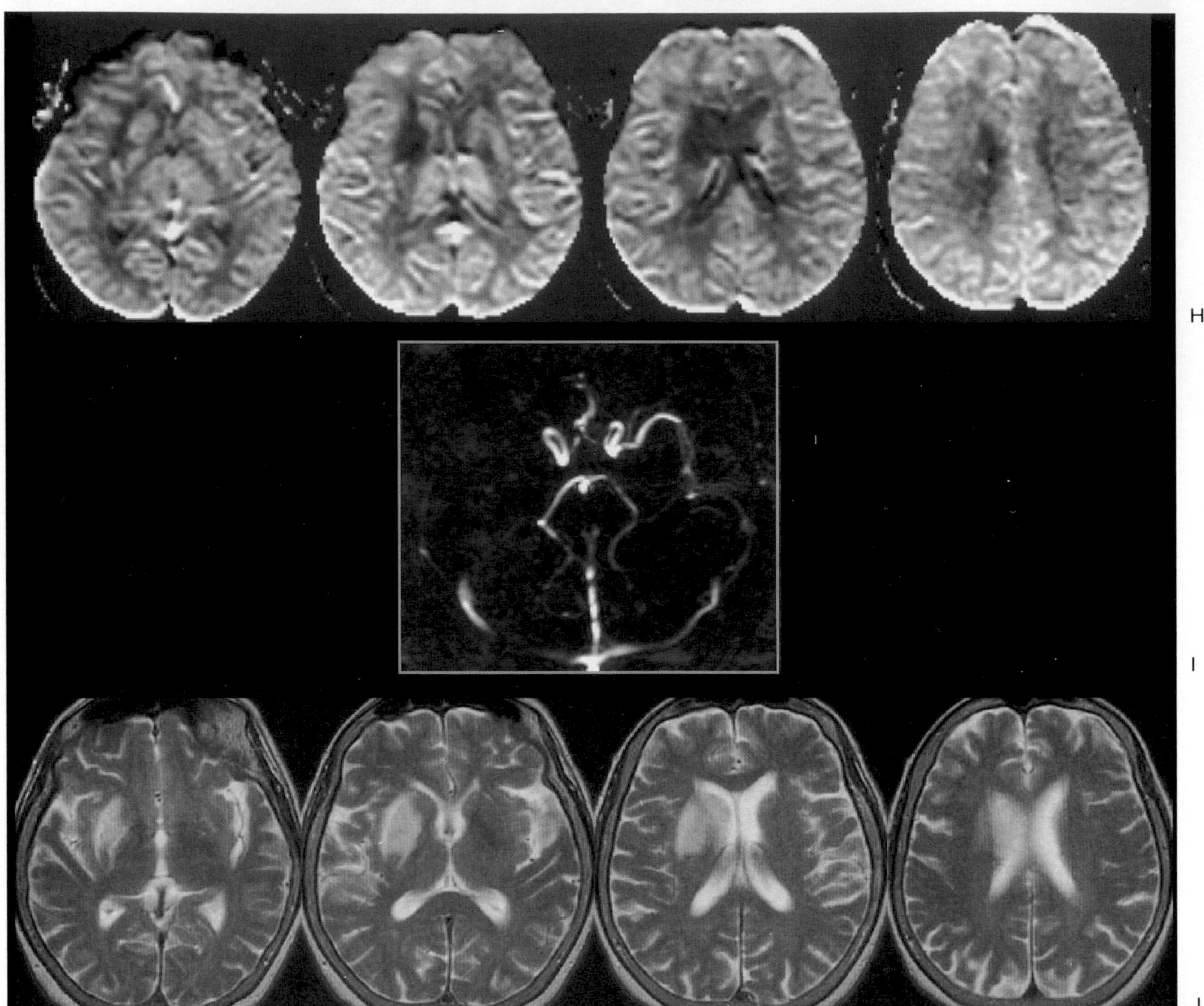

FIG. 19. (*Continued.*) **H:** rCBV maps demonstrate a perfusion defect, also consistent with acute ischemia. **I:** 2D PC MRA demonstrates no flow in the right MCA, despite a velocity encoding of 40 cm/sec. The perfusion-weighted imaging demonstrates the presence of collateral flow, however. **J:** Follow-up T2-weighted image (FSE) 5 days later confirms the infarct boundaries seen on the perfusion-weighted imaging.

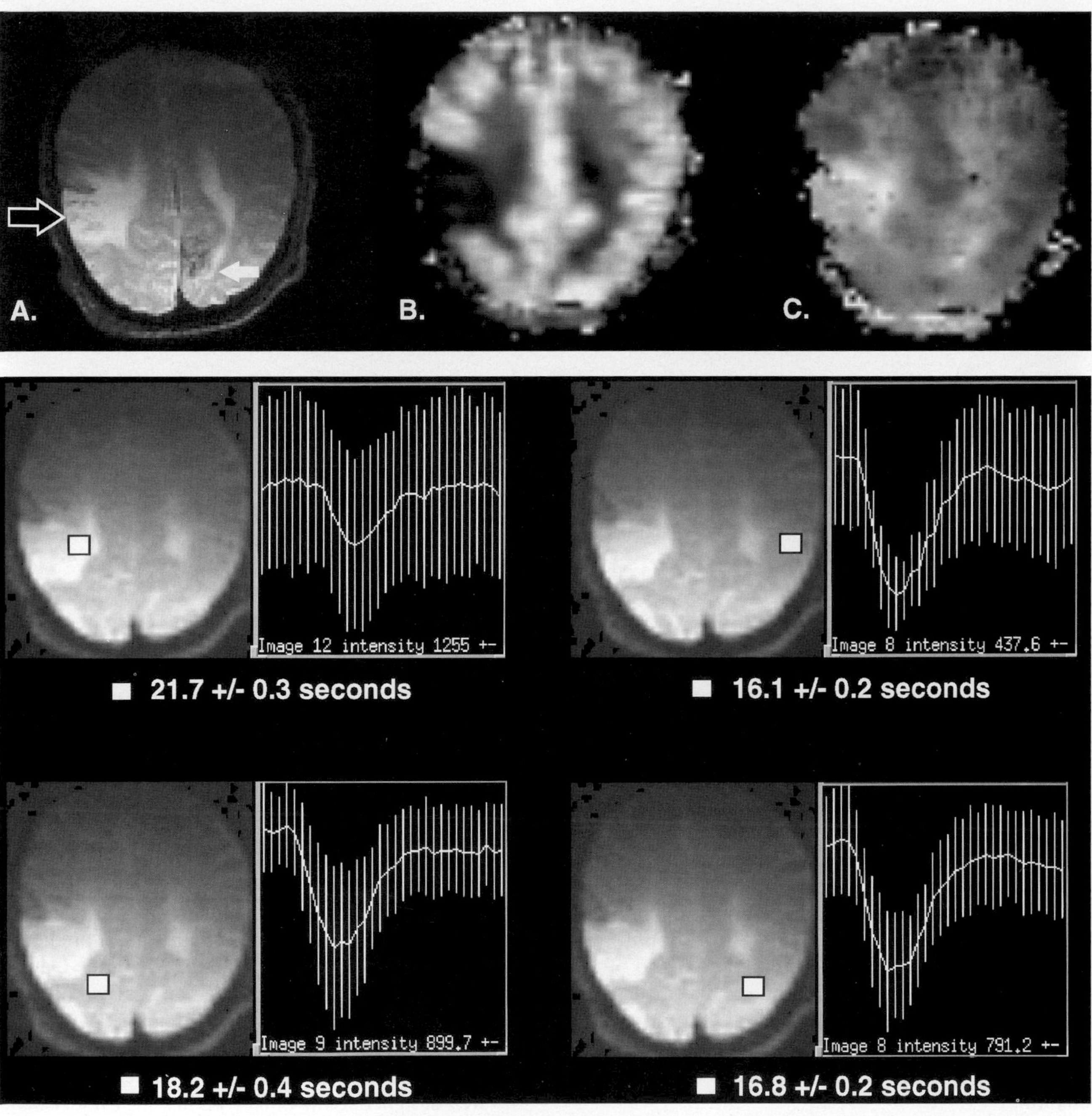

FIG. 20. Evaluation of stroke with perfusion imaging. **A:** T2-weighted image of a 74-year-old man who suffered two strokes at least 3 weeks before imaging. Abnormal signal consistent with stroke is seen in the right temporal/parietal lobe (*open arrow*) and in the left occipital lobe (*solid arrow*). **B:** rCBV map demonstrates markedly reduced rCBV in the right hemisphere lesion but only slightly reduced rCBV in the left. **C:** Map of time to peak signal change due to the contrast injection. From the time course of each voxel the time of peak $\Delta R2$ is computed. This demonstrates higher peak time (longer from time of injection in the right hemisphere, particularly in the region of stroke). **D:** Time courses for four different regions of interest. The ROIs from the map of peak $\Delta R2$ are overlaid onto a T2-weighted image. The *top left* image shows an ROI within an area of stroke, and demonstrates a delay of about 5 sec when compared with the contralateral hemisphere at the same location (shown in the *top right* image). Interestingly, in this patient there is also a delay in peak arrival time of 1.5 sec in the cortex that appears normal on conventional imaging. This delay in arrival of the bolus of contrast implies that there is some residual large vessel disease in this patient. Acquisition parameters for map: EPI SE, TR 1500, TE 100, 0.2 mmol/Kg Gd-DTPA-BMA (gadodiamide).

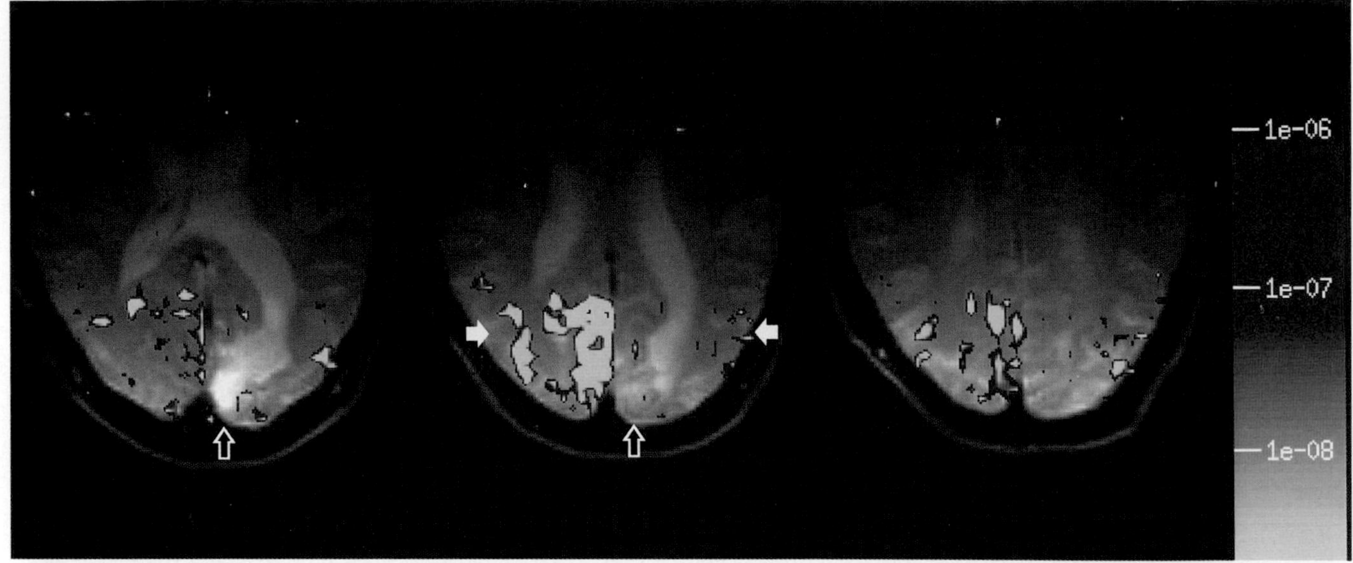

FIG. 21. Diaschisis. A small area of tissue is affected by stroke, located in the primary visual cortex (indicated by *open arrows*). Activation mapping demonstrates that in the unaffected side there is a large area of activation, consistent with both primary, secondary, and higher centers of visual processing. However, on the affected side there is absence of activation in not only the affected primary visual cortex but also in the expected areas of activation outside the primary visual cortex, in regions known to correspond to higher centers of vision (104) (indicated by *solid arrows*). Hence, a stroke in one area is demonstrated to affect distant cortex. Underlying gray-scale image: T2-weighted oblique axial SE image. Functional overlay: *t* test *p* value, ranging from $p = 1 \times 10^{-5}$ to $p = 1 \times 10^{-9}$. The test was applied to 90 images acquired during full-field stimulation with LED goggles alternating with darkness.

the number of capillaries per microscopic high power field correlated linearly with the risk of metastasis. They ascribed this to a biphasic behavior of tumors: a prevascular phase, which may last for years, during which there is limited tumor growth; and a vascular phase, in which there is bleeding, a high rate of tumor growth, and possible metastasis. Additional investigation has demonstrated that tumor angiogenesis is an independent predictor of relapse-free survival in primary breast carcinoma (73). Furthermore, in vivo animal studies demonstrate that glucose and oxygen utilization in cancer cells is limited not by the metabolic demand of the cancer cells but rather the substrate supply, that is, the capillary bed (74). These findings imply that important imaging markers of malignancy may include direct measurement of the microvasculature rather than metabolism alone.

These findings in breast and other carcinomas are relevant to understanding primary cerebral neoplasms: the degree of angiogenesis has been linked to tumor grade in human gliomas, with higher-grade lesions showing increased angiogenic factors such as renin (75) or capillary growth factors (76,77). Susceptibility contrast fMRI, with its sensitivity to the capillary bed (especially when using SE techniques), is therefore ideally suited for evaluating tumor angiogenesis in vivo. Over the past 5 years considerable clinical experience has been gained with dynamic susceptibility MRI of tumors. Functional MRI can play an important role at the major clinical decision points: diagnosis, intervention, and post-treatment monitoring.

Diagnosis

The most common primary CNS neoplasm has historically been astrocytoma, although CNS lymphoma is predicted to pass this soon (78) based on historical trends and the effects of HIV. In "ordinary" astrocytomas, histologic tumor grade at diagnosis is the major predictor of survival (79). Patients with grade I/IV (on the Daumas-Duport grading scale) have a median survival of 8 to 10 years, whereas those presenting with grade IV/IV have a median survival of less than 1 year (80). Hence, high-grade lesions warrant aggressive intervention, whereas no well designed, controlled trial has shown any benefit for any treatment of low-grade lesions (81).

Although standard radiologic criteria can provide some information as to the aggressiveness of a lesion, most treatment is based on biopsy. Increasingly, this is performed using stereotactic surgical techniques. MRI and neuroradiologists typically play a key role in guiding tumor sampling, which can be problematic. Although destruction of the BBB has typically been thought of as a correlative of high grade, other studies imply that this may not be so (82). For example, 25% of lesions are undergraded at stereotactic biopsy, most likely as a result of failure to sample the highest-grade portion of the lesion

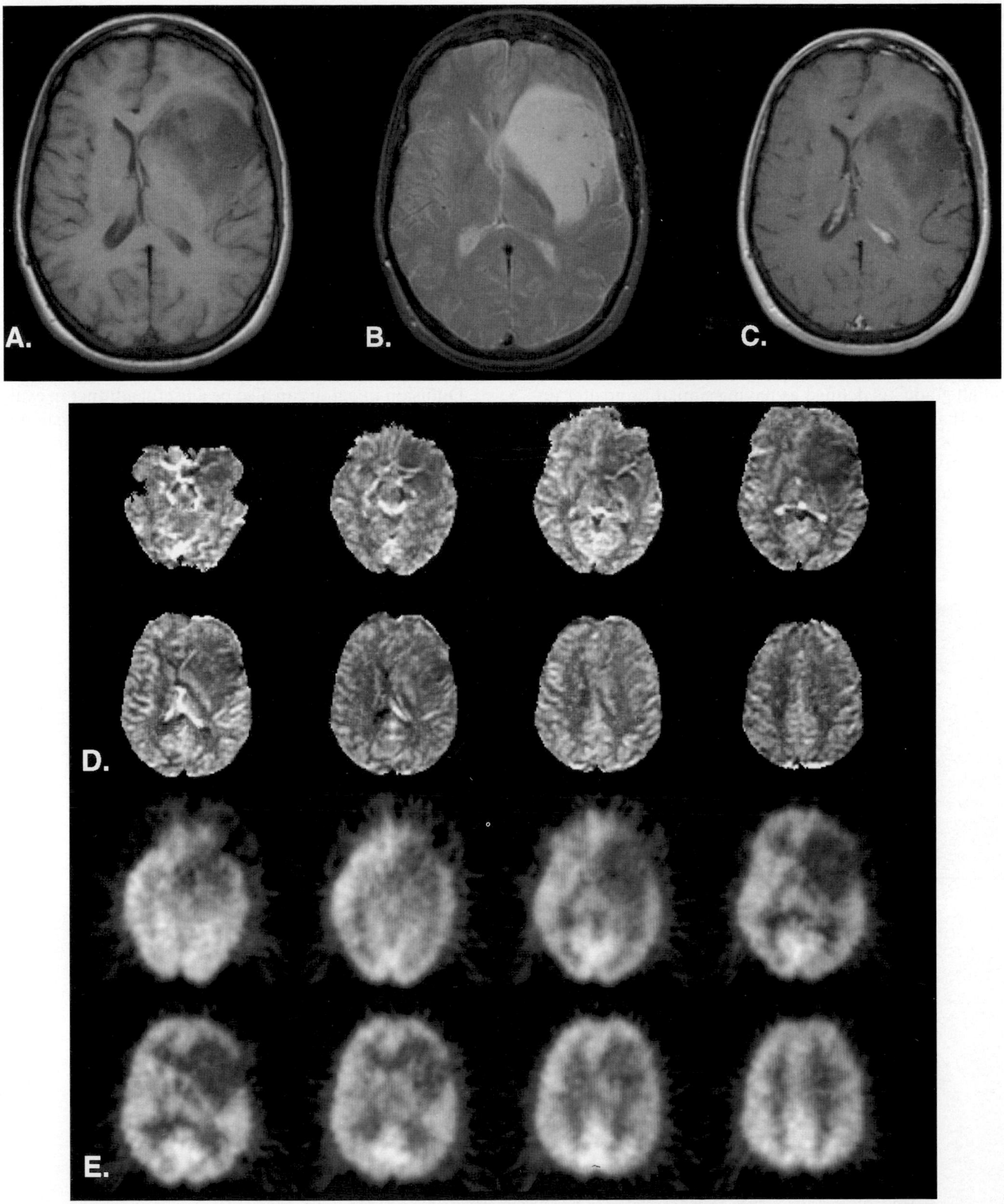

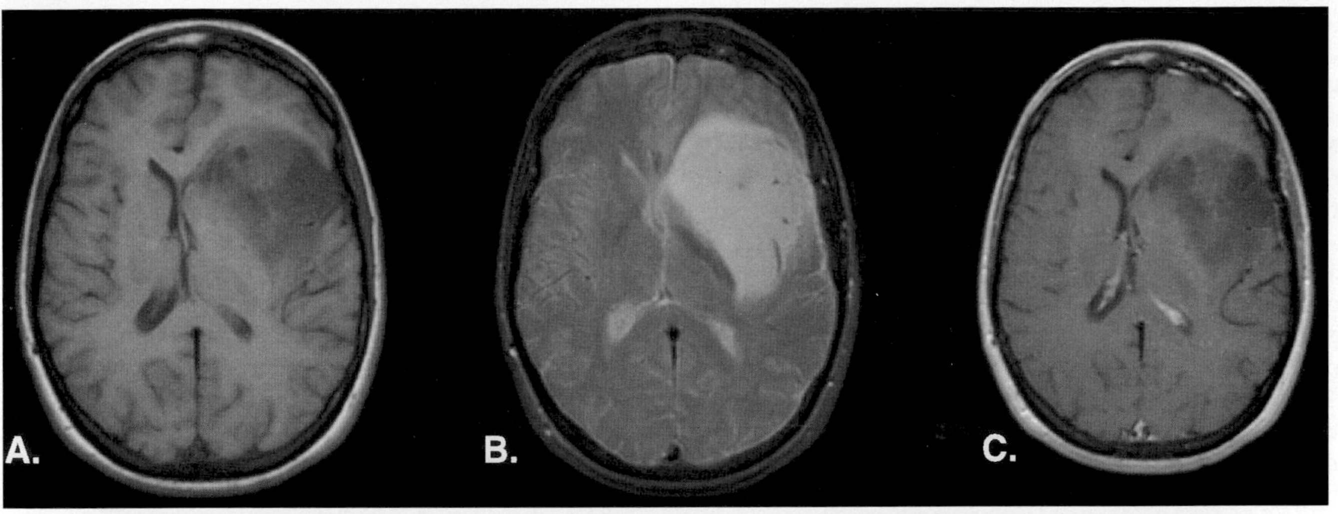

D.

E.

FIG. 22. Relative CBV map of a low-grade glioma. A 33-year-old woman presented for further evaluation of a known lesion that she had been told represented an epidermoid cyst. **A–C:** T1-weighted, T2-weighted, and post-Gd T1-weighted images, respectively, that demonstrate an extensive abnormality consistent with a low-grade intra-axial neoplasm. **D:** rCBV mapping demonstrates a large, low rCBV area consistent with a low-grade lesion. **E:** ^{18}FDG PET also demonstrates findings consistent with a low-grade lesion. Biopsy demonstrated a grade 2/4 glioma.

(83,84). A high-resolution mapping of the heterogeneity of neoplasms that could guide biopsy could reduce this undergrading.

Perfusion maps may provide such detail. Functional MR perfusion studies of lesions are typically summarized via a map of regional CBV (rCBV). As noted above, this rCBV map is mapping predominantly (but not solely) capillaries and small venules, a vessel size associated with tumor angiogenesis. In a study of 29 patients comparing fMRI rCBV with ^{18}FDG PET and pathologic grade, good correlation was found between tumor grade on biopsy, rCBV, and FDG uptake (85,86).

Interpretation of rCBV images is similar to interpretation of PET or other functional modalities. In PET scanning, the uptake of tracer in the region of a known lesion is compared with the normal gray and white matter. "High grade" is defined as having similar or greater uptake than gray matter, but usually obvious as a "hot spot" (87). A similar grading scheme has been proposed for rCBV mapping with SEs. These data have indicated that tumors with any regional rCBV value (i.e., the maximum rCBV value anywhere within the tumor) over twice that of white matter (roughly comparable to gray matter) have a high likelihood of having high-grade components (86), whereas tumors with maximum rCBV values less than 1.5 times white matter are usually low grade. Figures 22 and 23 show a typical low-grade lesions, whereas Fig. 24 shows a typical high-grade lesion. An important caveat here is the differentiation of a small focus of tumor neovascular proliferation from the high rCBV apparent from large vascular structures that may be adjacent to expansile lesions or the highly vascular choroid plexus. If questions exist, the rCBV maps should be interpreted in concert with flow-sensitive images (such as short TE GEs) and the conventional post-contrast T1-weighted studies from comparable slices to avoid these potential pitfalls.

Diffusion imaging can also be a useful adjunct in evaluating some tumors, notably in distinguishing cystic regions from solid tumors with long relaxation times, because there is a higher diffusion coefficient in fluid than in tissue even in the face of equivalent relaxation charac-

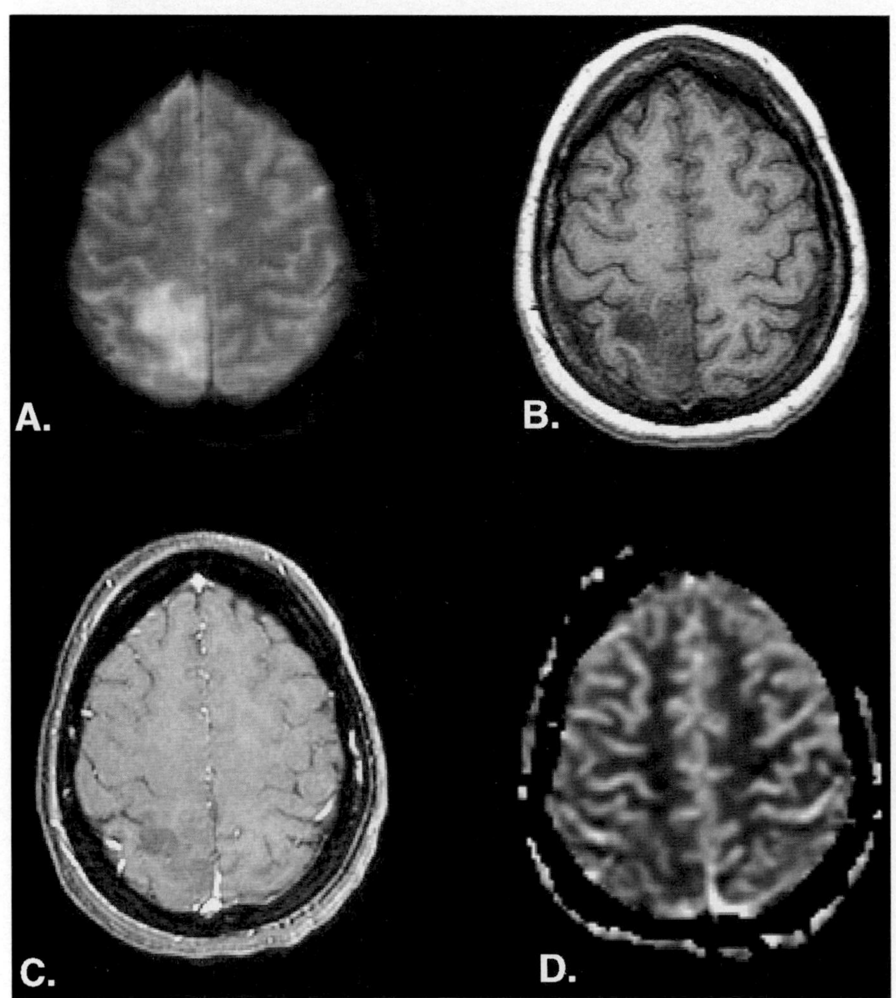

FIG. 23. Relative CBV map of a low-grade oligodendroglioma with some astrocytoma component in a 39-year-old woman. **A:** SE T2-weighted image. **B, C:** T1-weighted images pre- and postcontrast, respectively, demonstrating minimal enhancement. **D:** rCBV map demonstrating a slight decrease in rCBV compared with gray matter.

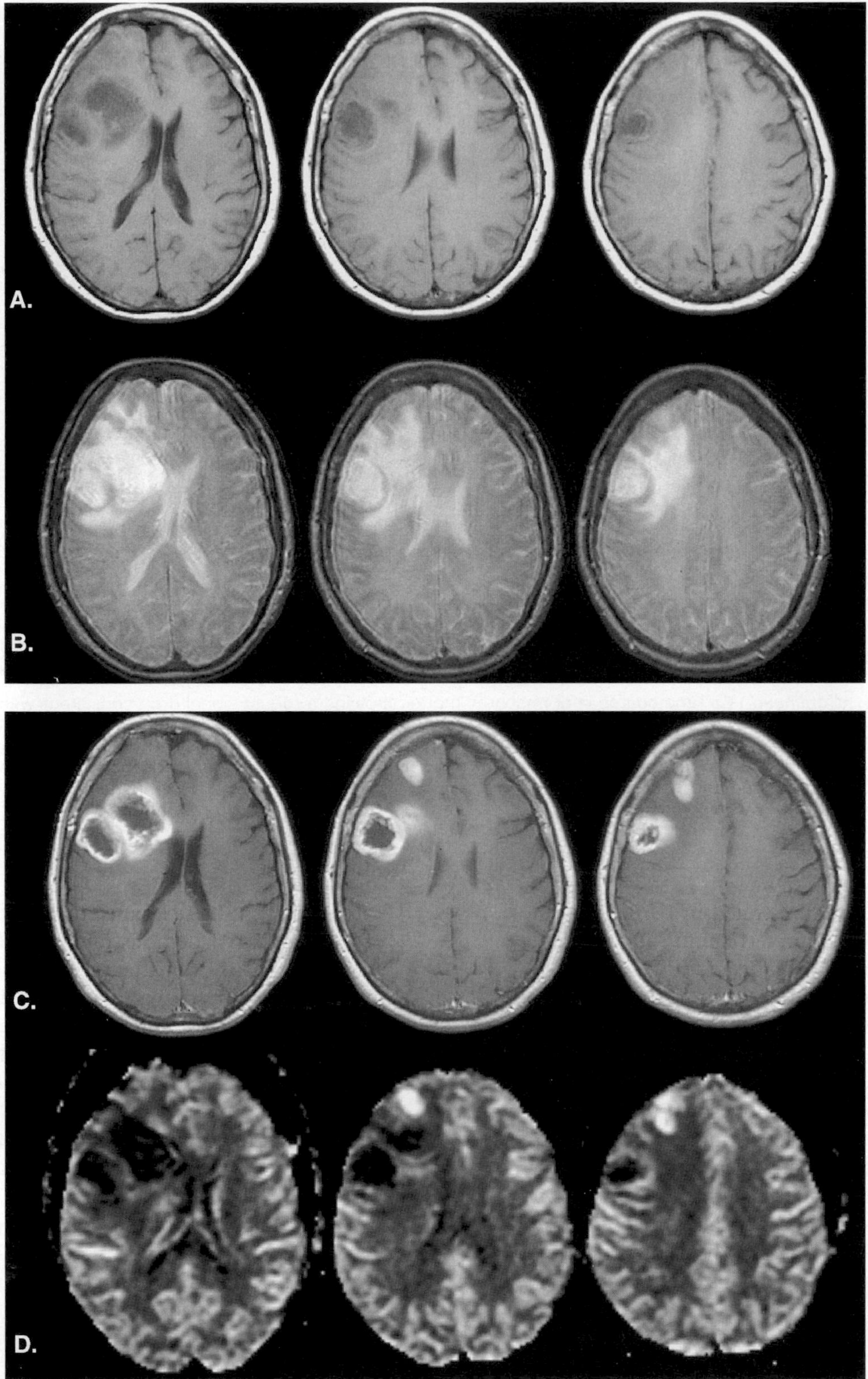

FIG. 24. Heterogeneity of high-grade lesions due to necrosis. Grade IV/IV glioma in a 65-year-old woman. **A:** Conventional T1-weighted images. **B:** Conventional T2-weighted images. **C:** Post-Gd T1-weighted images. **D:** rCBV maps using 0.2 mmol/Kg of Gd-based contrast media. The cystic regions demonstrate low CBV in the center with a question of higher CBV in the rim. The more solid lesions demonstrate clear, abnormally high rCBV. The rim of the cystic regions have somewhat heterogeneous rCBV, with possibly some high areas but also some low areas.

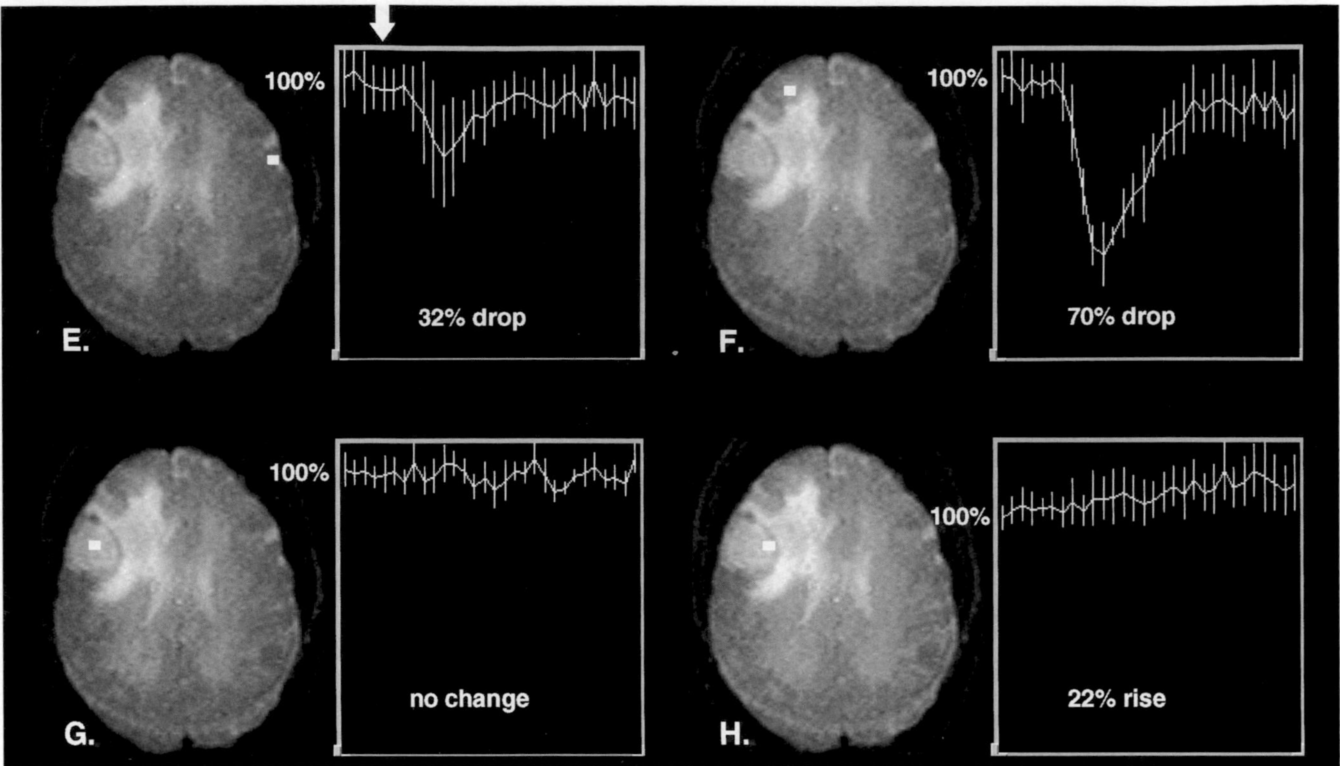

FIG. 24. (*Continued.*) **E:** Time course in normal gray matter showing a robust signal drop consistent with the first pass effect of Gd. **F:** Even greater signal drop in the area of tumor, consistent with its high blood volume. **G:** Absent signal drop in center of cyst, consistent with an area of no blood volume. **H:** Increase in signal intensity without transient signal drop in rim or cyst. The lower rCBV at the rim may be due to either the absence of viable tumor or a confounding effect from the marked disruption of the BBB. The cystic portion of the tumor contained mostly necrotic tumor cells. Tumor was also present in deep white matter, consistent with the infiltrative nature of gliomas.

teristics. This is demonstrated in Figs. 25 and 26. Data to date have not definitively demonstrated that diffusion mapping alone will provide additional diagnostic value, although early studies have demonstrated a trend toward decreased ADC in primary CNS lymphoma (88), in regions of high functional/metabolic activity (89), and during radiation treatment. Further work in this area remains to be done. Some investigators are attempting to use diffusion imaging to distinguish peritumoral edema from tumor spread; however, since a tumor often extends beyond the visualized abnormality on T2-weighted images, this technique may have inherent limitations. Relative CBV mapping may be a more relevant way to localize the aggressive portions of a tumor.

Direction of Biopsy and Surgical Debulking

Although low-grade lesions have a typical appearance on conventional MRI, on occasion lesions that appear low grade and uniform on conventional pre- and postcontrast MR studies can have focal areas of malignant dedifferentiation. Figures 27, 28, and 29 demonstrate how rCBV maps can be used to aid in determining where to biopsy or treat these lesions. In each of these cases the conventional MRI demonstrated a relatively homogeneous appearance, even after the administration of intravenous contrast. However, the rCBV and PET studies demonstrate focal areas of increased signal corresponding to higher-grade tumor. The rCBV maps cannot only be used to direct the surgical biopsy, but occasionally can directly aid the pathologist. Figure 30 demonstrates a case in which the original pathology reading was based on only some of the surgical samples (taken outside the area of high rCBV) and was reported as low-grade astrocytoma. After review of the rCBV map, which clearly showed regions of intense microvascular proliferation suggesting greater malignancy, additional tissue specimens were located from surgical samples localized to the rCBV "hot" areas. These samples subsequently documented the lesion as high grade.

In combination with rCBV mapping, activation mapping can be performed to locate a nearby eloquent cortex. As with any activation mapping techniques, this requires an "off" task (typically rest for primary somatosensory cortex) and an "on" task. For example, by using simple hand, toe, or tongue movement, centers

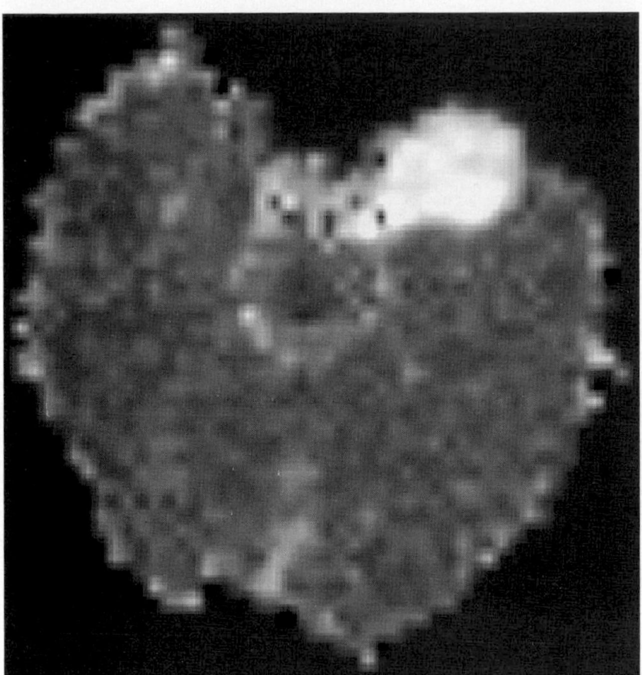

FIG. 25. Diffusion map of a temporal arachnoid cyst. The image is a map of the ADC. The water inside the cyst is less constrained than that in the brain and as a result has a higher diffusion coefficient, seen as a relatively bright area of signal on the ADC map.

along the sensorimotor cortex can be mapped using the deoxyhemoglobin-sensitive intrinsic contrast described above (90,91). This mapping is particularly useful in cases in which a tumor has displaced or destroyed normal landmarks. Figure 31 demonstrates how the displacement of normal cortex by tumor can be mapped preoperatively. Note, however, that because nearly all motor tasks have some sensory component, distinguishing between the two centers is difficult. Task activation studies can be used to demonstrate sites of residual function in patients harboring infiltrative gliomas. Atlas et al. (92) reported identification of fMRI intensity changes within margins of SE-defined tumor tissue, whereby the extent of activation correlated grossly with the degree of residual function (Fig. 32). It is presumed that fMRI will provide important information to the surgeon before debulking such lesions, so that regions with SE abnormality but intact function can be preserved.

Treatment Follow-Up

Gliomas are typically extremely infiltrative, with margins difficult to define even at pathology (93). In this setting surgical procedures are rarely curative, but rather cytoreductive, and are combined with radiation. As a re-

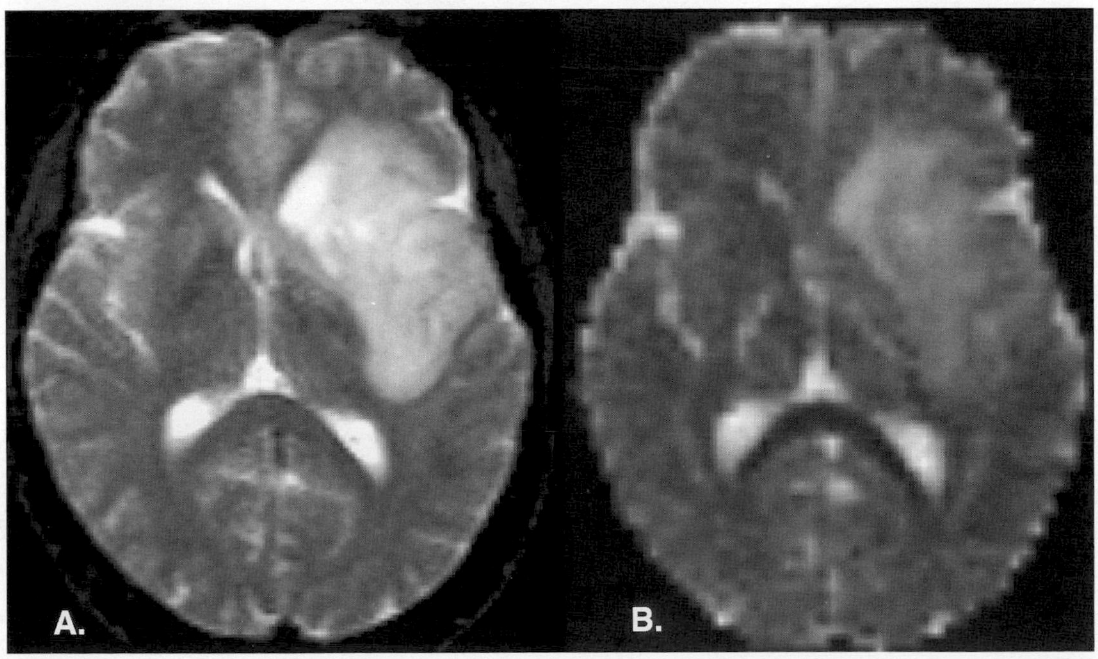

FIG. 26. Diffusion imaging of edema around tumor. **A:** T2-weighted SE image demonstrating increased signal around a poorly defined tumor. **B:** Calculated ADC map demonstrating increased diffusion in the left frontal lobe, indicating that the increased signal on the T2-weighted image was secondary to increased water from edema, which has a higher diffusion.

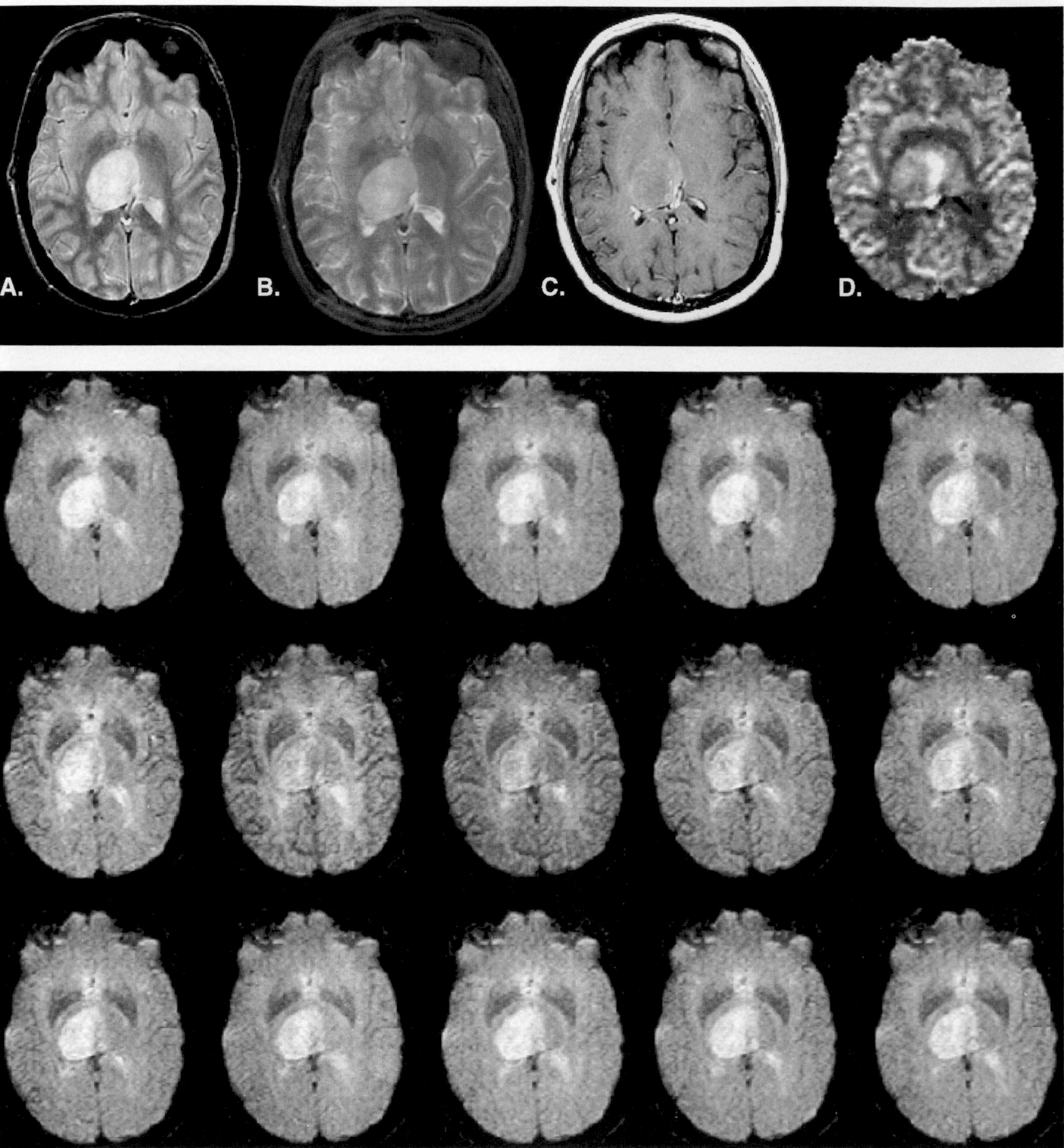

FIG. 27. Heterogeneity of glioma seen best on functional studies. A 26-year-old woman presented with headache and right-sided weakness. **A–C:** Proton density, T2-weighted, and post-Gd T1-weighted images, respectively, demonstrate minimal enhancement and fair homogeneity. **D:** fMRI rCBV mapping demonstrates an area of increased rCBV in the medial aspect of the tumor. Biopsy demonstrated grade III/IV astrocytoma. **E:** Time course images from the fMRI study demonstrate that the central, high rCBV region has a greater degree of signal loss than the peripheral portions of the tumor.

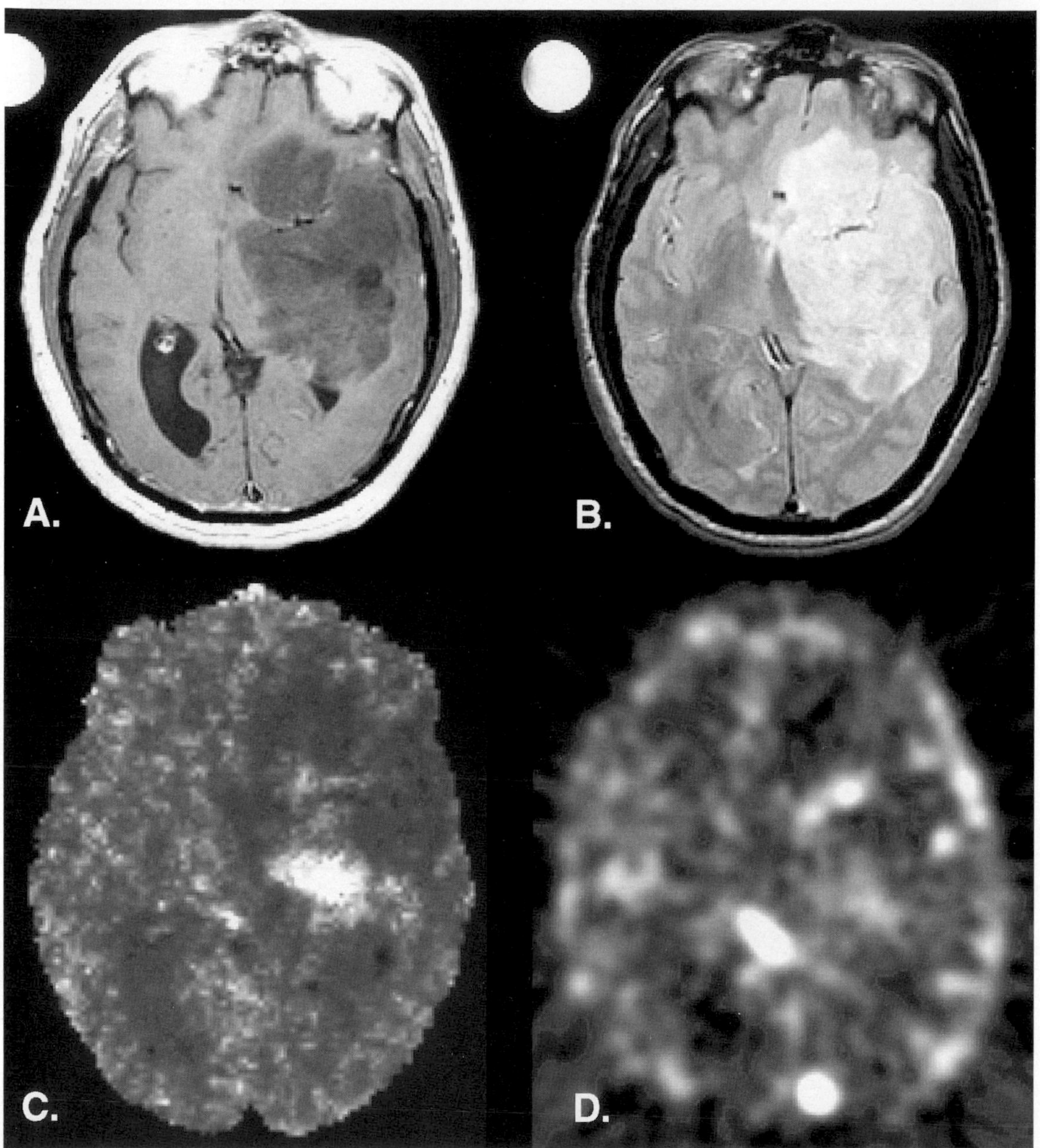

FIG. 28. Heterogeneity of glioma seen only on functional studies in a 51-year-old man. **A:** Postcontrast T1-weighted image shows marked mass effect but little enhancement. **B:** T2-weighted image shows a fairly homogeneous mass. **C:** rCBV map shows a focal area of high rCBV. **D:** PET ^{11}CO confirms the location of a more malignant focus; subsequent biopsy demonstrated that this focus indeed was malignant and eventually led to the patient's demise.

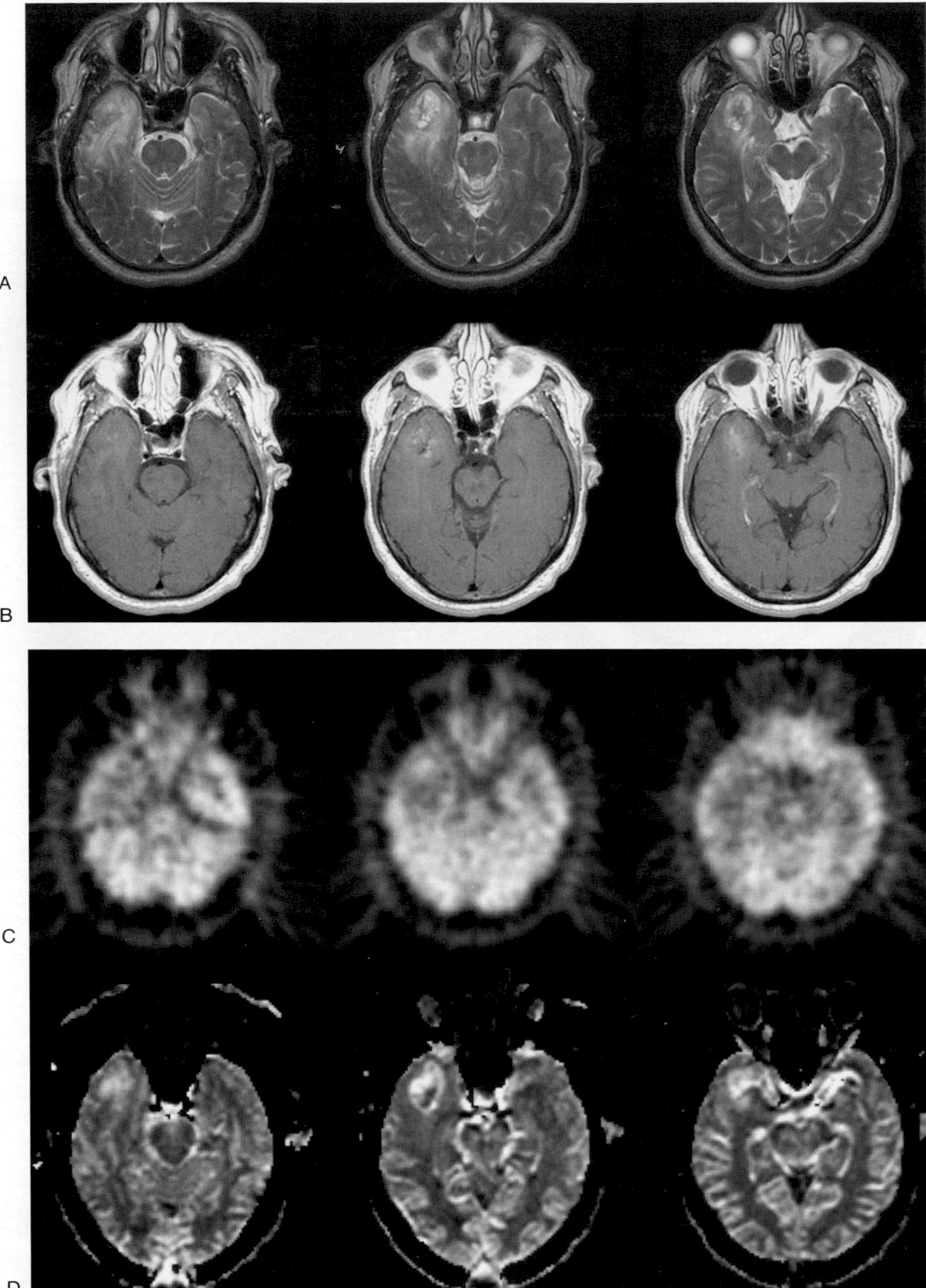

FIG. 29. PET vs. fMRI for tumor grading in a 49-year-old man with a right temporal tumor. **A:** T2-weighted FSE images demonstrate a focal lesion in the right temporal lobe. **B:** Post-Gd T1-weighted images show minimal enhancement. **C:** ^{18}FDG PET shows no clear focus of high uptake, and was interpreted as indicating the tumor was likely low grade. **D:** MRI rCBV maps show clear, high rCBV in the region of the tumor, prompting resection. Pathologic exam demonstrated a malignant mixed glioma, with 40% grade 3/4 astrocytoma and 60% oligodendroglioma.

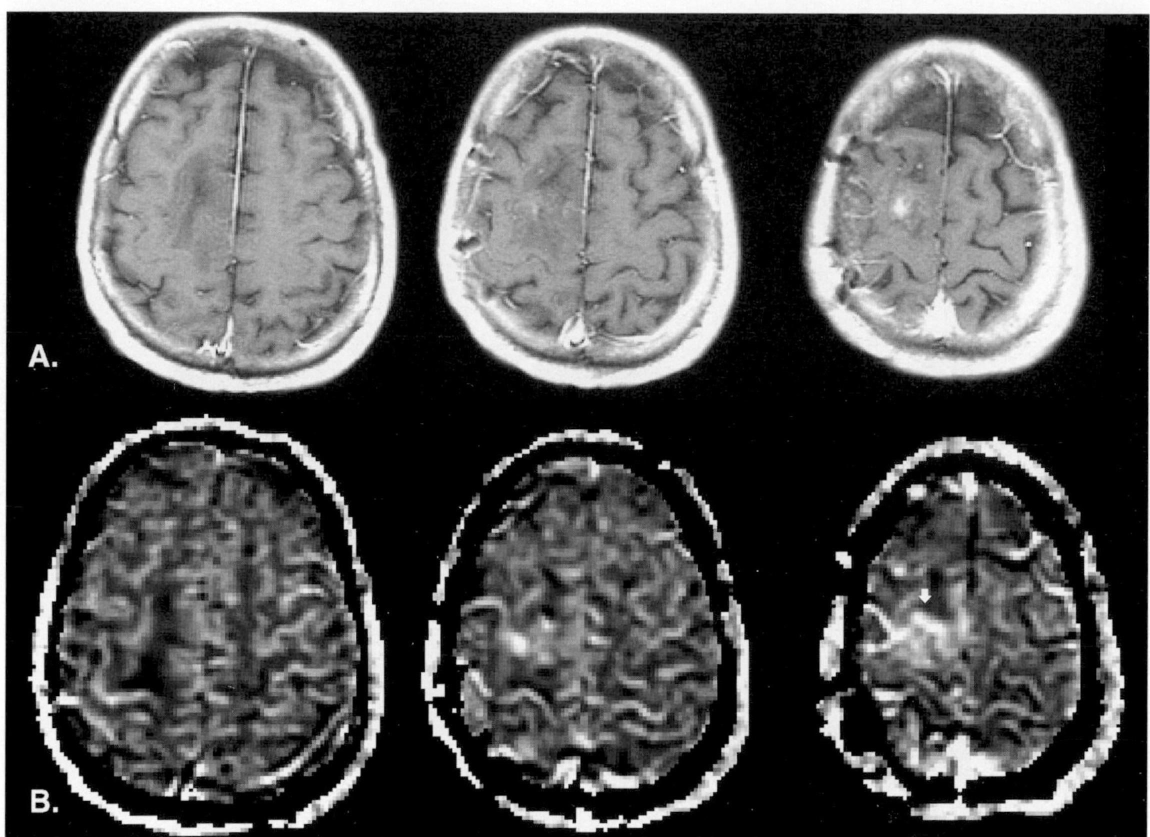

FIG. 30. Use of rCBV to direct biopsy. A 57-year-old man presented 7 years s/p resection of oligodendroglioma. **A:** Post-Gd T1-weighted images demonstrating slight enhancement in the area of prior surgery. **B:** Functional MRI rCBV mapping of the tumor demonstrates an area of increased uptake approximately 2 cm anterior to the central sulcus. Biopsies from in front and behind the area of highest rCBV demonstrated low-grade tumor, and a biopsy in the lesion in the area of highest rCBV demonstrated grade 3/4 astrocytoma.

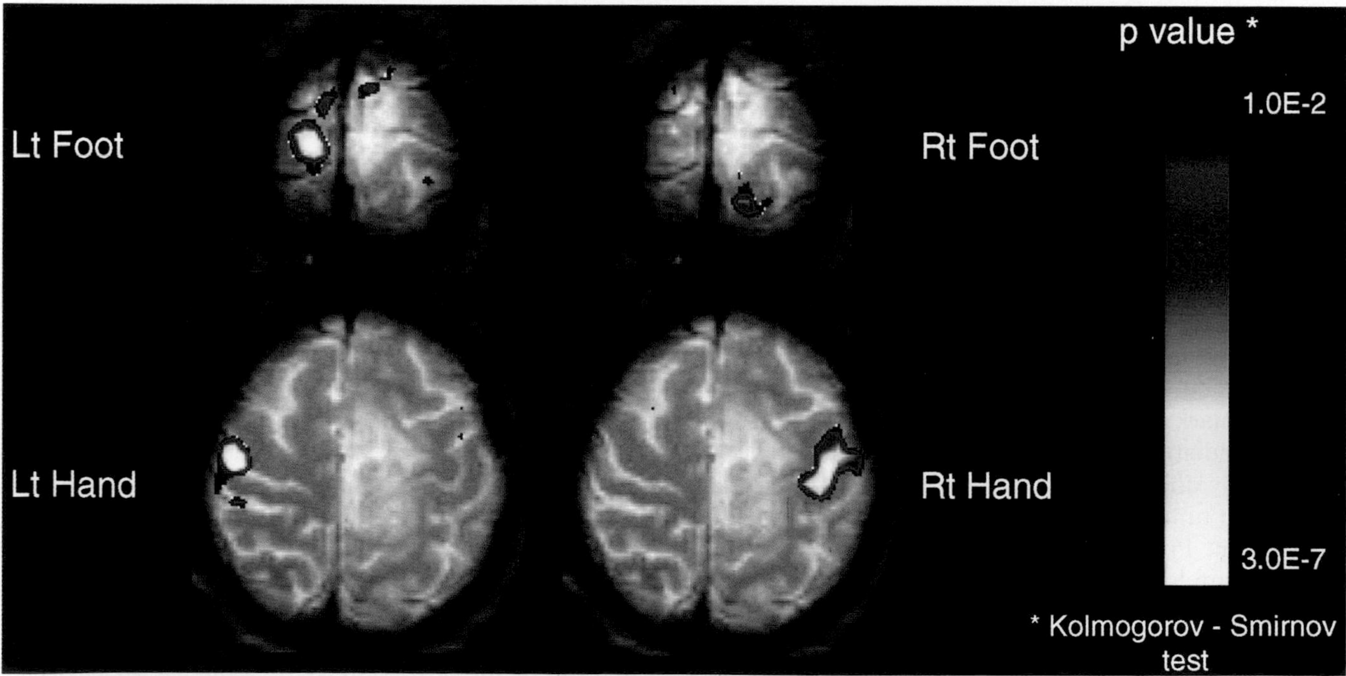

FIG. 31. Preoperative activation mapping of motor activity in a patient with an intra-axial brain tumor. Images show statistically significant changes in MRI signal as tested by the Kolmogorov-Smirnov test, a nonparametric statistical test. Note the displacement of the locus of activity of the right foot, presumably due to tumor. This was verified at surgery using intraoperative electrophysiologic cortical mapping.

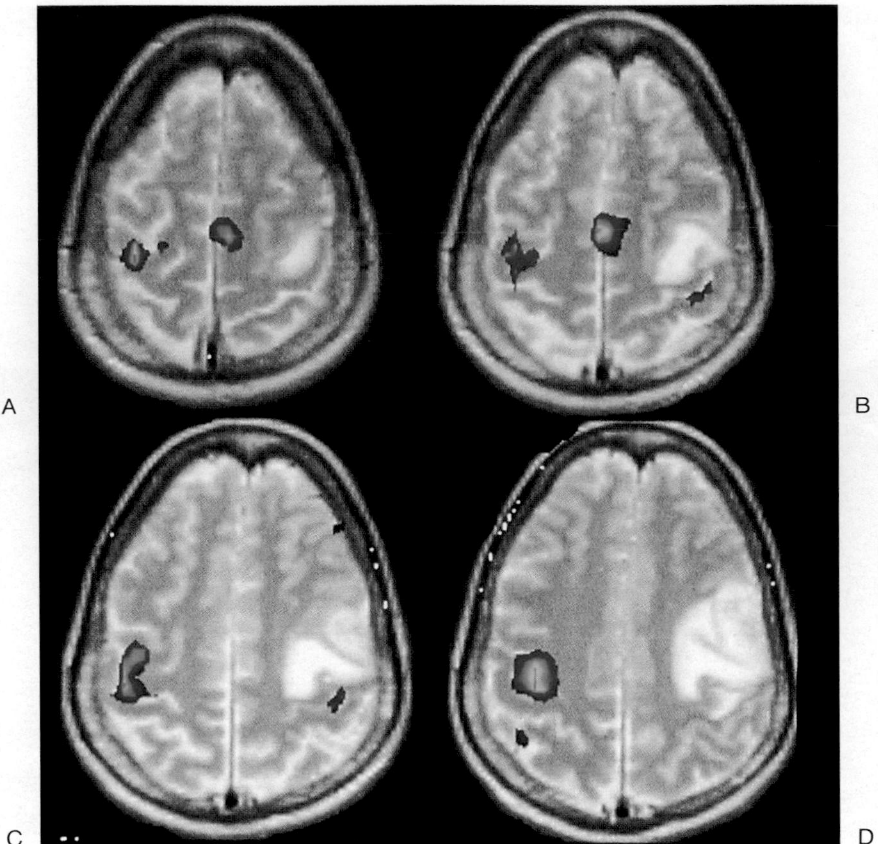

FIG. 32. A–D: Bilateral hand motor task activation map in a patient with a left posterior frontal glioma and right hemiparesis. Note significant activation in right primary sensorimotor cortex and a smaller region of left sensorimotor cortex activation in border of tumor. Significant activation is also seen midline in superior frontal gyrus, corresponding to supplemental motor area (SMA).

sult, follow-up studies are typically obtained at 3- and 6-month intervals to rule out "recurrence." Since some tumor has invariably been left behind, the questions for evaluation via follow-up imaging include the effectiveness of the radiotherapy and/or the detection of invasion or malignant degeneration in previously low-grade lesions. In particular, radiation can have a delayed effect, causing mass lesions 6 to 12 months or more after completion of therapy. While conventional MRI depends on BBB destruction and on changes in serial imaging studies, such markers are often nonspecific. The distinction between radiation necrosis and bulk tumor recurrence is particularly difficult with conventional MRI or CT because both tumor and radiation necrosis can show BBB breakdown. Previous studies using PET FDG uptake and thallium SPECT have shown promise in aiding this classification. With fMRI, perfusion imaging and rCBV mapping appear to be able to provide this same distinction, provided the rCBV maps are made with care.

Figures 33 and 34 demonstrate clinical cases of follow-up studies. Figures 35 through 38 demonstrate rCBV mapping in biopsy-proven recurrence. Figure 39 demonstrates biopsy-proven radiation necrosis. Because of the high correlation between rCBV maps, pathology, and PET studies, at our institution if the PET and fMRI rCBV maps both demonstrate the absence of a "hot" lesion the patients are not biopsied and the presumptive diagnosis of radiation effect is made. Our own experience has demonstrated that in 15 cases in which there was a clinical and radiologic question of radiation necrosis versus tumor recurrence that went to biopsy after rCBV mapping, rCBV mapping was able to predict correctly the absence or presence of tumor in 14 of 15 cases (94) Our initial experience, however, indicates that primary CNS lymphoma may often have low relative CBV, implying that MR-based rCBV mapping may not be as useful in these patients.

Interpretation of these follow-up rCBV studies is generally straightforward; however, when using gadolinium-based agents for rCBV mapping it is essential to take care to examine the post-contrast T1-weighted images. This is because of the physics of the competing effects of susceptibility and relaxivity contrast mechanisms. In lesions where the BBB is intact or only minimally disrupted, lit-

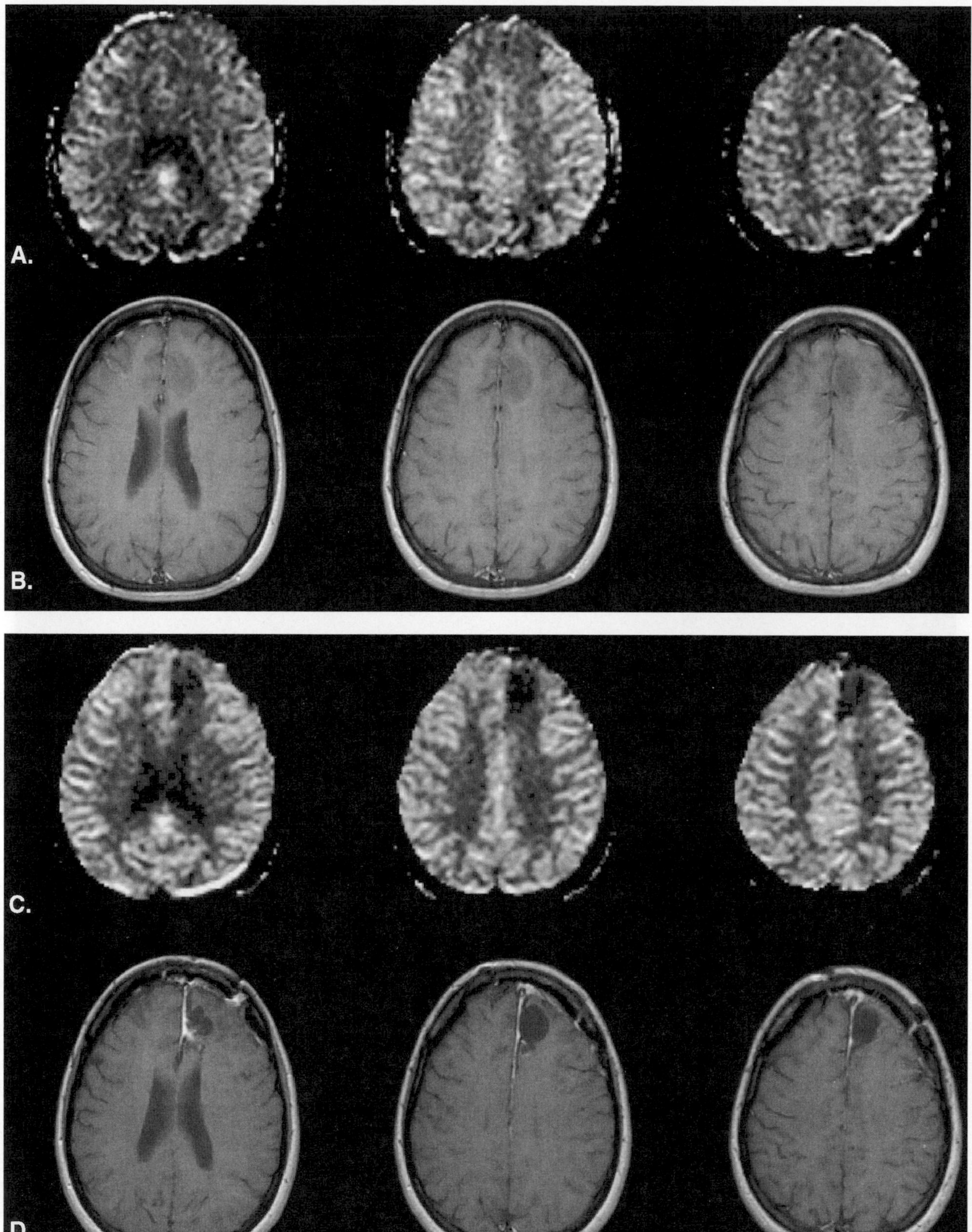

FIG. 33. Follow-up of 28-year-old woman using rCBV imaging. **A:** rCBV images preresection show no high rCBV and possibly low rCBV over the left frontal region. **B:** Post-Gd T1-weighted images indicate a nonenhancing lesion in the left frontal lobe along the midline. **C:** Postresection rCBV maps demonstrate no evidence of high rCBV to suggest malignant degeneration or recurrence. **D:** Postcontrast T1-weighted images demonstrate resection site and postsurgical enhancement. (Courtesy F. Caramia.)

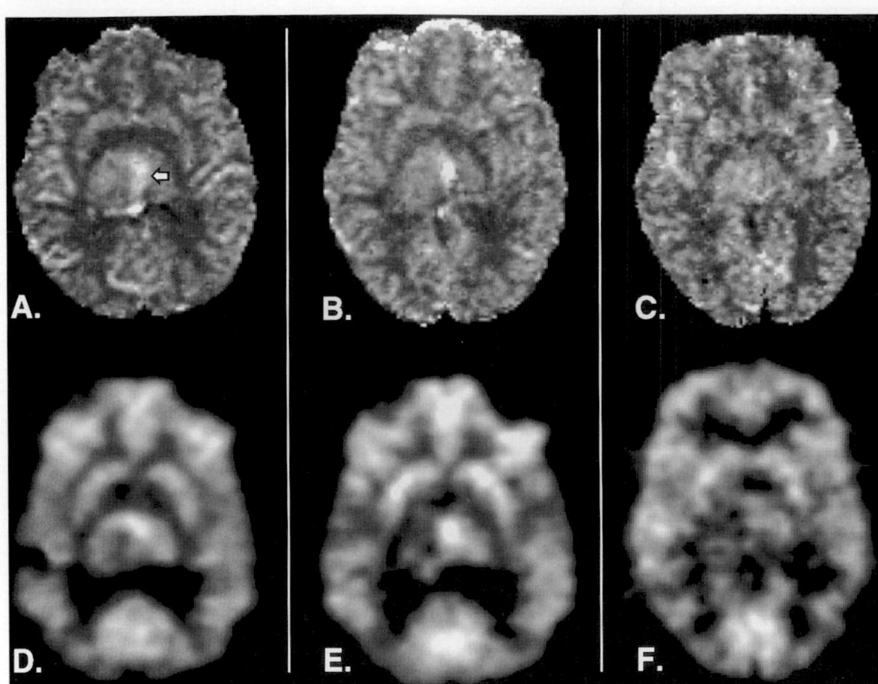

FIG. 34. Relative CBV mapping of response to therapy. Same case as in Fig. 26. Functional MRI rCBV maps and PET ^{18}FDG maps pre- and postradiation. **A–C:** rCBV maps; **D–F:** ^{18}FDG maps. A,D: preradiation; *arrow* points out region of high rCBV. B,E: 6 weeks after radiation. C,F: 5 months postradiation. (Courtesy H. Aronen.)

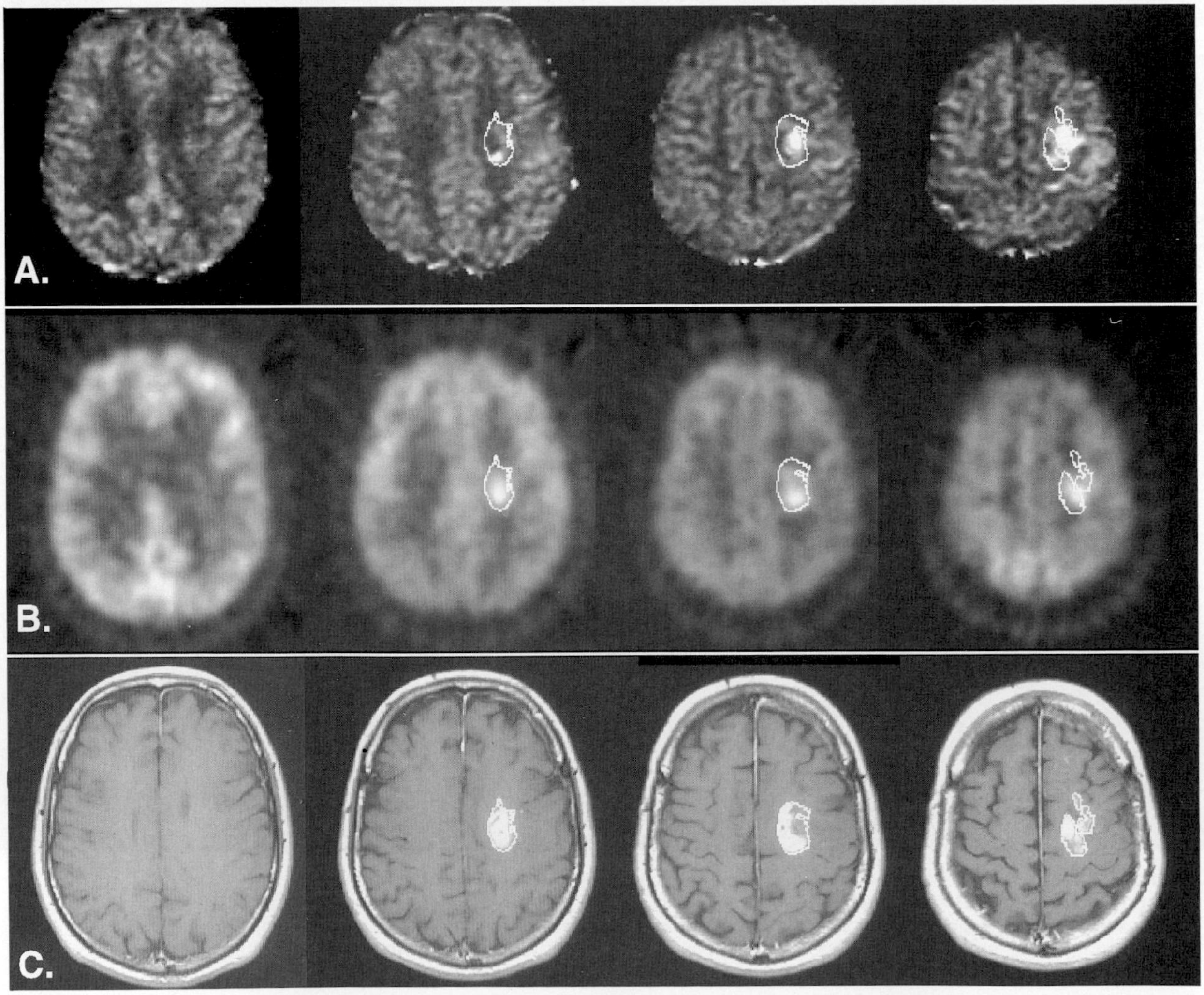

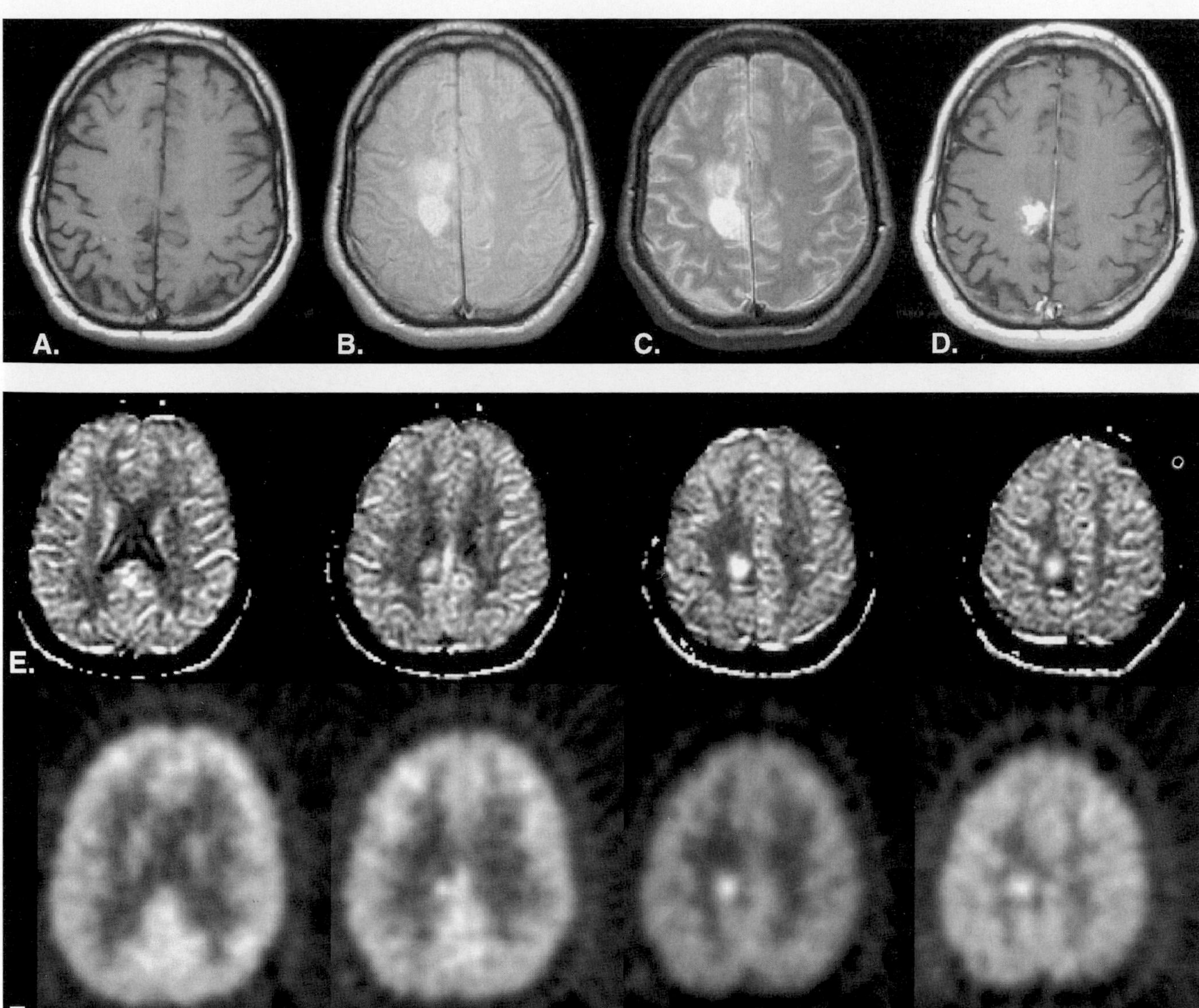

FIG. 36. rCBV mapping of high-grade lesion. A 47-year-old man with known low-grade oligodendroglioma, now with new enhancement on conventional post-Gd images. **A–D:** T1-weighted, proton density-, T2-weighted, and post-Gd T1-weighted images. **E:** rCBV mapping showing high rCBV in the area of Gd enhancement. **F:** ^{18}FDG PET demonstrating increased uptake, also consistent with high-grade lesion. Biopsy showed anaplastic astrocytoma.

FIG. 35. CBV mapping of high-grade lesion. A 47-year-old man presents with focal neurologic deficit. **A:** rCBV mapping showing a focal area of high rCBV. **B:** ^{18}FDG PET demonstrating increased uptake, also consistent with high-grade lesion. **C:** Post-Gd conventional T1-weighted images. Biopsy showed anaplastic mixed glioma/oligodendroglioma, grade III/IV. The regions of enhancement on the postcontrast T1-weighted images are outlined in white and overlaid on the PET ^{18}FDG and fMRI rCBV studies, demonstrating that the relationship between enhancement and high rCBV/FDG uptake is close but not exact. (Courtesy H. Aronen.)

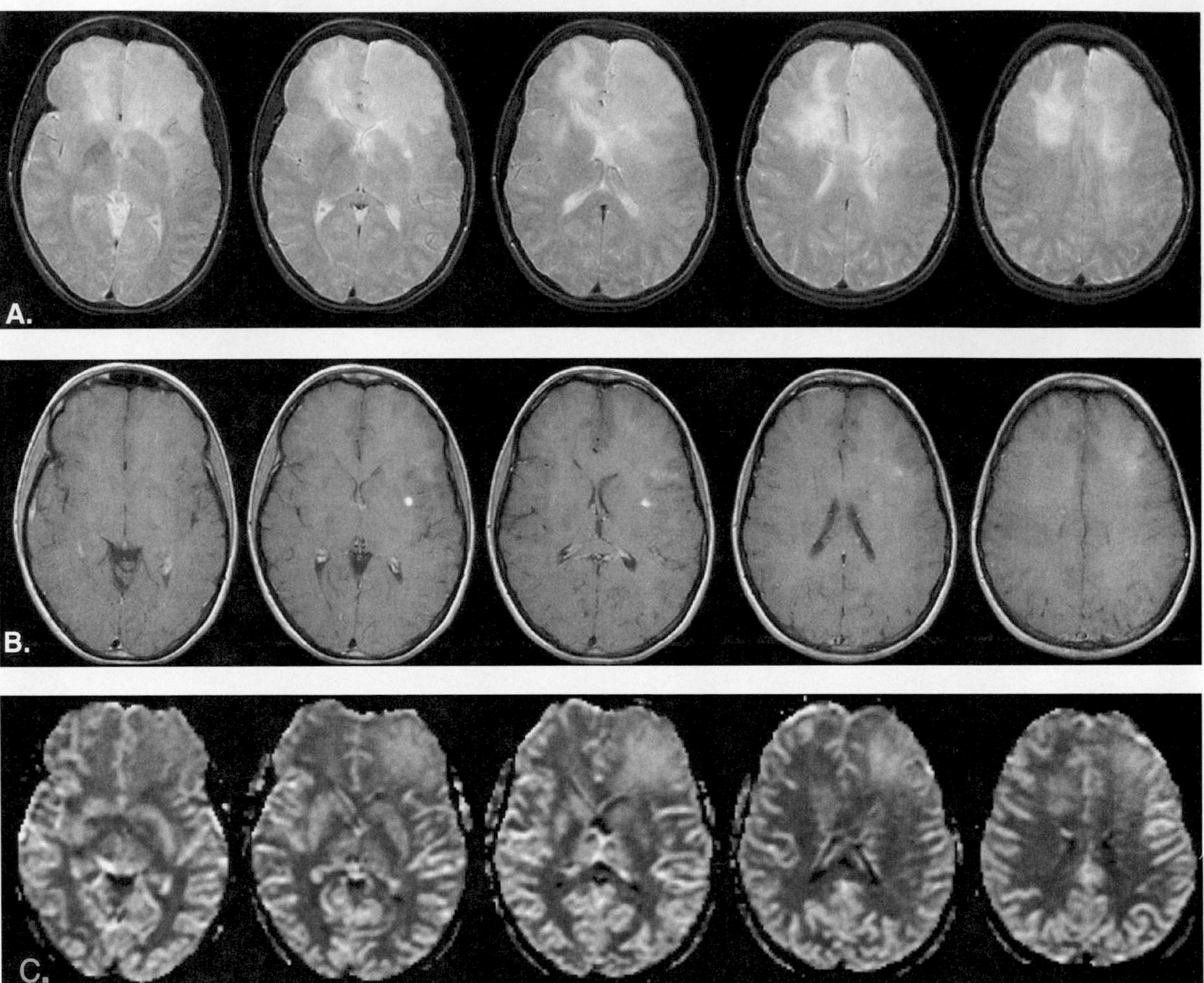

FIG. 37. Radiation effect vs. tumor degeneration. A 29-year-old woman 4 years s/p XRT for left frontal astrocytoma. **A:** Conventional T2-weighted images show diffuse increased signal intensity consistent with radiation effect or recurrent tumor. **B:** Post-Gd T1-weighted images show diffuse mild enhancement. **C:** Relative CBV maps show a large area of increased rCBV, suggesting high capillary count tissue and therefore malignancy rather than radiation effect. Biopsy showed anaplastic astrocytoma. Note the infiltrative pattern of high rCBV, consistent with the known infiltrative patterns of gliomas.

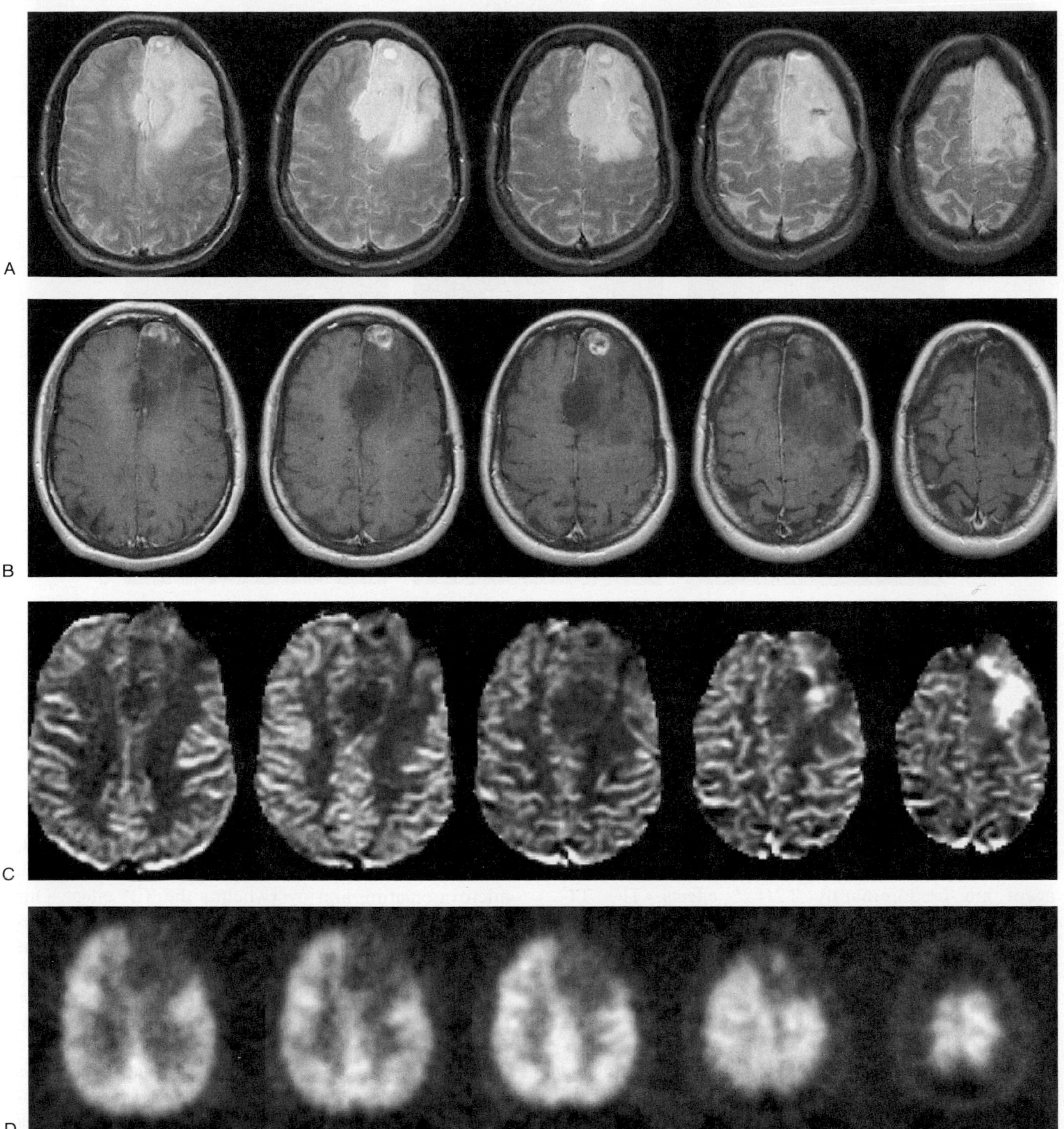

FIG. 38. Radiation necrosis versus recurrence. A 34-year-old woman 6 years s/p excision and radiation of a low-grade astrocytoma. **A:** T2-weighted images show a diffuse T2 abnormality consistent with radiation effect or tumor. **B:** Post-Gd T1-weighted images show a focus of enhancement in a ring-like fashion. This is still consistent with tumor recurrence or radiation effect. **C:** rCBV maps show that there is mildly increased rCBV in the ring-enhancing area, but that more importantly there is a large focus of high rCBV more cranially, near the vertex. Biopsy showed malignant mixed glioma. **D:** ^{18}FDG PET shows a small focus of increased glucose uptake near the vertex, and may confirm the ring-enhancing lesion, but with less confidence than the rCBV maps.

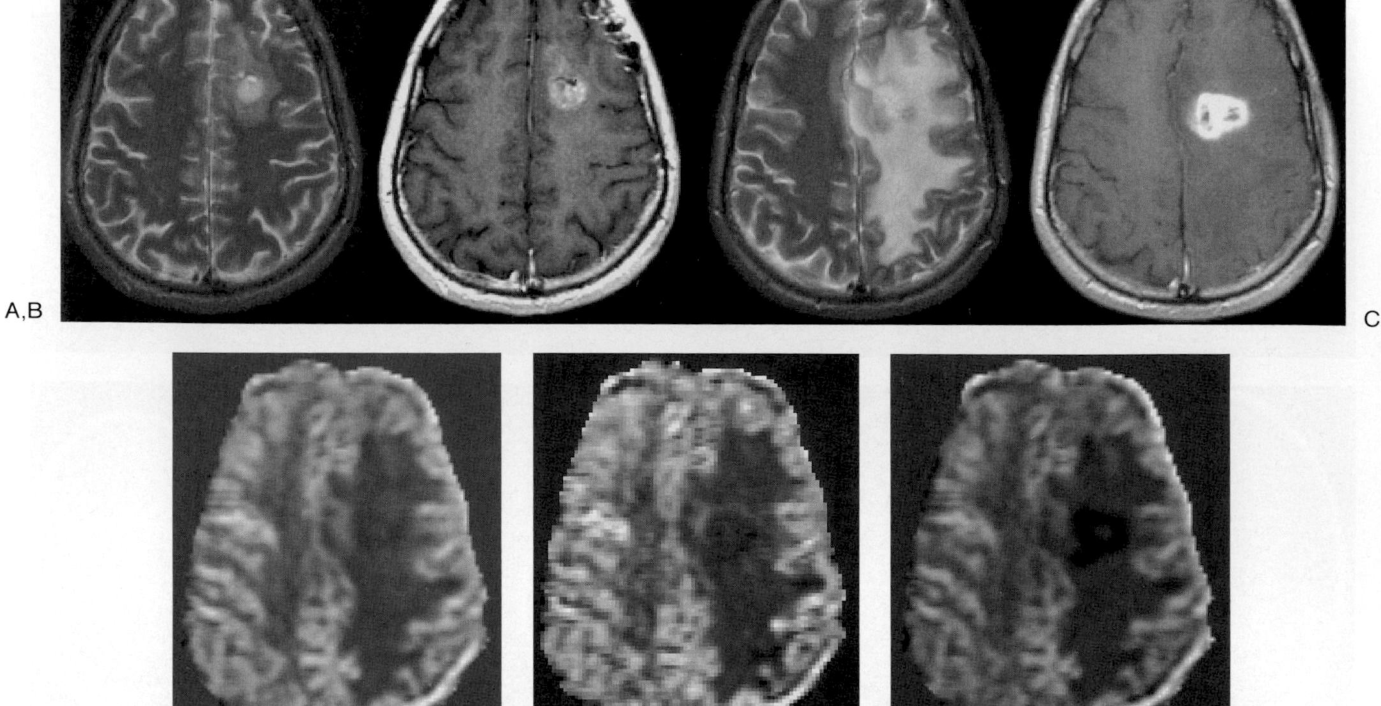

FIG. 39. Radiation necrosis vs. recurrence. A 42-year-old man 1 year s/p XRT for grade III/IV astrocytoma. **A,B:** T2-weighted images and post-Gd T1-weighted images, respectively. **C,D:** T2- and post-Gd T1-weighted images 6 months later showing increased T2 signal abnormality, increased enhancement, and greater mass effect. **E:** Gd-based rCBV map shows no areas of rCBV greater than contralateral (normal) white matter. **F:** rCBV mapping with dysprosium (Dy-DTPA-BMA, Nycomed) also demonstrates no areas of rCBV greater than contralateral (normal) white matter. (Dysprosium has essentially no T1 effect, and therefore the integrity of the BBB is less an issue than with Gd-based rCBV maps.) These images therefore suggest radiation necrosis rather than tumor. Biopsy showed radiation necrosis with no tumor. The rCBV map in E was calculated using a technique to correct for possible breakdown of the blood-brain barrier as described in (95). The uncorrected map (**G**) demonstrates artifactually low rCBV. The Dy-based map confirms the true rCBV.

tle contrast leaks out into the extravascular space during the first pass and the effects of the initial bolus of contrast agent are predominantly T2/T2* effects. The T1-relaxivity effects of gadolinium are confined to the intravascular space and are therefore dominated by the susceptibility effects, leading to transient signal loss. However, if there is significant disruption of the BBB, contrast can rapidly leak into the interstitium. In this setting the T1 enhancement that results from the gadolinium's relaxivity effect may blunt the susceptibility-related signal loss, and if severe may actually dominate and cause signal increases. Even EPI dynamic imaging is not immune to this effect because the TRs used to fully capture the first pass kinetics (typically 1–2 sec) retain a significant degree of T1 weighting. In these cases, uncorrected maps of rCBV will be spuriously low. Examination of the individual images will often allow distinction between early signal drop and later enhancement; however, if the enhancement is too prompt the rCBV maps will be nondiagnostic (see, e.g., Fig. 24H). This same effect makes rCBV mapping of extra-axial lesions difficult with gadolinium-based agents: without a BBB, the gadolinium leaks out on the first pass through the microvasculature and overwhelms the T2* effect. Our experience with meningiomas and some metastases has led us to interpret rCBV mapping of extra-axial lesions with great caution. Intra-axial metastases can be evaluated if the degree of BBB disruption is either heterogeneous enough or low enough to allow a first-pass estimation of blood volume, as shown in Fig. 40.

There are four general approaches to addressing this important problem of BBB breakdown leading to competing T1 and T2 effects. First, computer postprocessing schemes have been developed that can, at least in part, correct for the T1 enhancement by directly measuring it and subsequently removing it from the rCBV calculation algorithm (95); we now favor and use such algorithms routinely. Second, a small dose (typically 0.05 mmol/Kg) of gadolinium can be injected a few minutes before high dose rCBV mapping to effectively "presaturate" tumor regions with very high BBB permeability. This is often part of our routine protocol, especially when a leaky

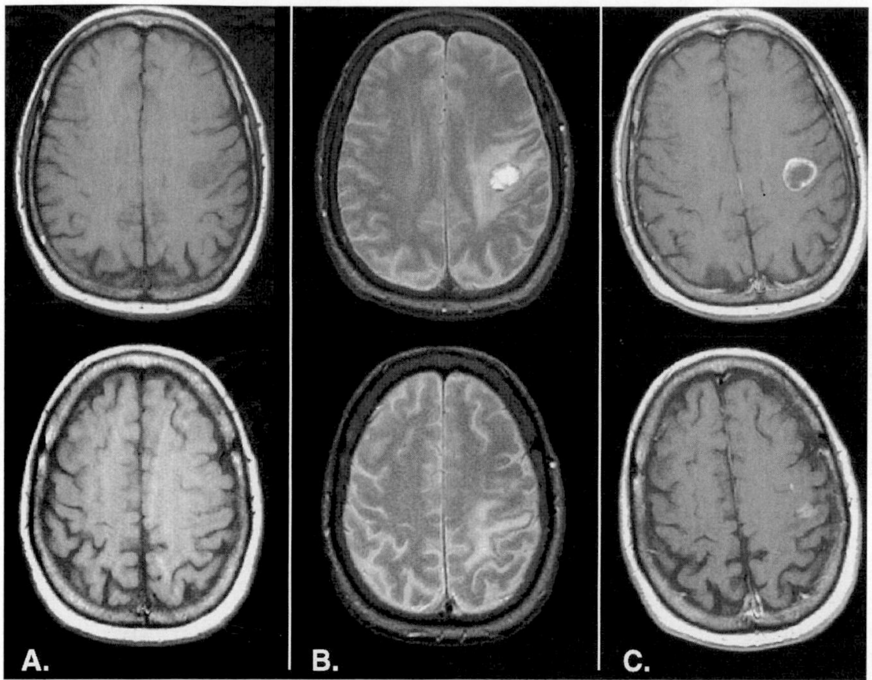

FIG. 40. CBV mapping of metastatic renal cell carcinoma in a 69-year-old man. **A–C:** T1-weighted, T2-weighted, and post-Gd T1-weighted conventional images, respectively, with two slices from each technique, demonstrating a ring-enhancing metastasis in the left frontal lobe. **D:** Functional MRI rCBV mapping just after radiation demonstrates a rim of increased signal consistent with persistent viable tumor. **E:** ^{18}FDG PET at the same time did not show any increased uptake, and was dictated as no evidence of persistent tumor. **F:** ^{18}FDG PET repeated 4 months later demonstrated the lesion, which was biopsied and shown to be persistent metastasis. This indicates that in some cases fMRI rCBV mapping can be more sensitive than PET, probably because of its higher spatial resolution.

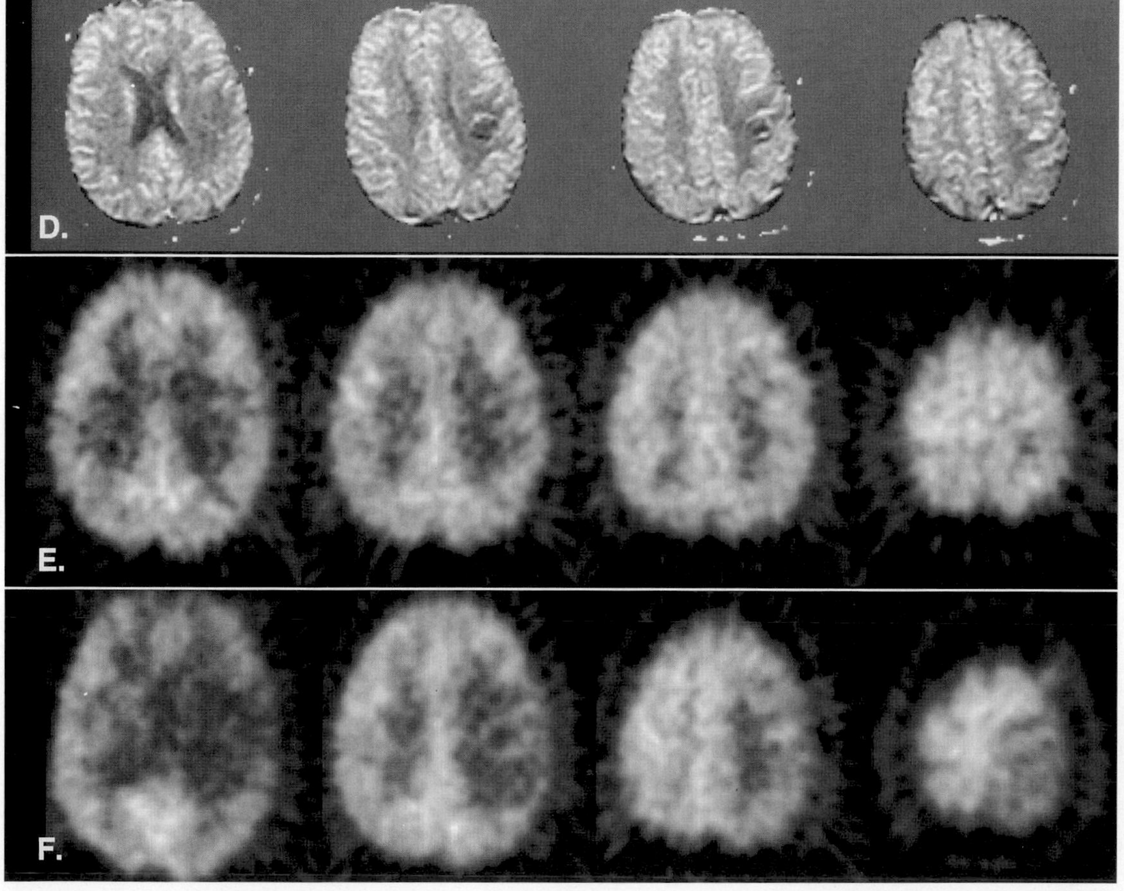

lesion is suspected as in cases of suspected recurrence. Third, the imaging sequence itself can be made less T1 sensitive, either by increasing TR or decreasing the flip angle on GE images. All these techniques can be effectively used in concert. Finally, because the problem ultimately arises from the high relaxivity effect of gadolinium, other contrast agents with high magnetic susceptibility but lower relaxivity are under development. One class of promising agents is based on dysprosium rather than gadolinium. Dysprosium has roughly one fortieth the T1 effect of gadolinium but approximately 80% greater T2 effect (14), making it a superior agent for rCBV mapping (96). Figure 39 demonstrates the difference between a gadolinium-based map and dysprosium-based map in a case of tumor recurrence versus necrosis.

In summary, perfusion mapping of tumors can greatly add to the diagnosis and management of patients with primary CNS malignancies. Because these studies can be performed as additions to conventional MR evaluations with little added time, they are a cost-effective alternative to radionuclide-based functional imaging studies. Although additional data on the ultimate clinical utility of these techniques are needed, the primary advantages of low incremental costs combined with high anatomic resolution and the ability to easily register functional with anatomic images from a single modality make it likely that these methods will find widespread use.

Nonanatomic Diseases

Conventional MRI has excelled in defining abnormal anatomy. However, there are many disease processes in which there is no reliable macroscopic anatomic abnormality. These disease processes include psychiatric disorders, some forms of epilepsy, and dementia. Functional MRI may well have a role to play in the evaluation of these patients. Although fMRI is just beginning to be applied to these patients, the initial results are encouraging and are briefly reviewed here.

Seizures

Because fMRI does not yet visualize neuronal firing, but rather the hemodynamic changes associated with neural activity, seizures are best identified ictally (97). However, this is impractical, and most imaging is done interictally. Often an anatomic abnormality can be found, such as shown in Fig. 41, in which case rCBV mapping can demonstrate the microvascularity of the tissue.

The most common cause of partial complex seizures is mesial temporal sclerosis (MTS) (98). Although PET studies in many centers have demonstrated lateralizing ability, no study comparing fMRI techniques such as rCBV mapping with PET imaging in these patients has yet been published. Because of the good correlation of PET and fMRI rCBV in tumors, similar correlation between PET and rCBV may exist in patients with MTS. This is a current area of active investigation.

In addition to mapping the primary abnormality in seizures, additional pre- and intraoperative testing commonly employed in these patients may be performed noninvasively by fMRI. Specifically, the localization of a eloquent cortex involved with motor, memory, and language currently requires the use of a battery of detailed behavioral testing pre- and intraoperative cortical mapping. Functional MRI techniques sensitive to brain activation, using either BOLD or flow contrast combined with appropriate task paradigms, may allow these studies to be performed as part of a single anatomic/functional preoperative evaluation. For example, lateralization of language may be an excellent candidate. Currently, this is typically done via the Wada test, an angiographic procedure not without some risk. Preliminary data suggest that lateralization of language function is a straightforward task with fMRI (99), and appears to be correlated with Wada results (100). Figure 42 demonstrates an illustrative case. In cases where seizure foci are near an eloquent cortex, sensorimotor cortex mapping can be performed as discussed above.

Psychiatric Disease

Numerous attempts to link structural changes with psychiatric illnesses have been made, with varied success. Functional MRI has the potential to map the abnormal function of what appears to be a structurally normal cortex. This area of exploration is still quite new, and investigators in this area face the same challenges as traditional cognitive neuroscience, including the difficulty in designing tests that are specific for a given disease. Because of the complexity of psychiatric disease, finding a simple control/stimulus paradigm that can be used in an MRI setting remains a primary challenge. Furthermore, since our knowledge of functional neuroanatomy is relatively poor, finding loci of activation does not necessarily shed light on pathophysiology. Nevertheless, these diseases will likely benefit from investigation with fMRI, particularly as fMRI expands our understanding of functional neuroanatomy.

Applications of fMRI in psychiatry so far have been limited to research investigation, similar to other functional neuroimaging techniques such as PET. Figure 43 shows activation mapping of obsessive-compulsive disorder (OCD). This disorder is amenable to fMRI activation mapping because it has definable "on" and "off" states; application of fMRI to other disease processes may require design of similar paradigms. Once such tests are demonstrated to have statistical reliability they may be applied to aid in diagnosis, intervention, and follow-up.

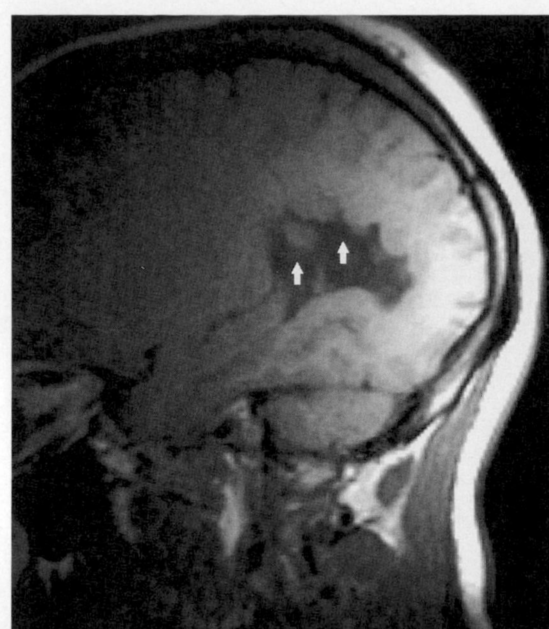

A

FIG. 41. Relative CBV mapping in a patient with seizures and known heterotopic gray matter. **A:** Conventional T1-weighted image (taken with a surface coil over the occiput) demonstrates heterotopic gray matter lining an enlarged right ventricle (*arrows*). **B:** rCBV mapping demonstrates that the blood volume in the heterotopic gray matter is similar to that in the cortical gray matter (*open arrows*). Note the normal increased rCBV in the visual cortex (*solid arrows*), the normal high rCBV in the visual cortex (*arrowheads*), and the distortion of the ventricle evident on the rCBV map.

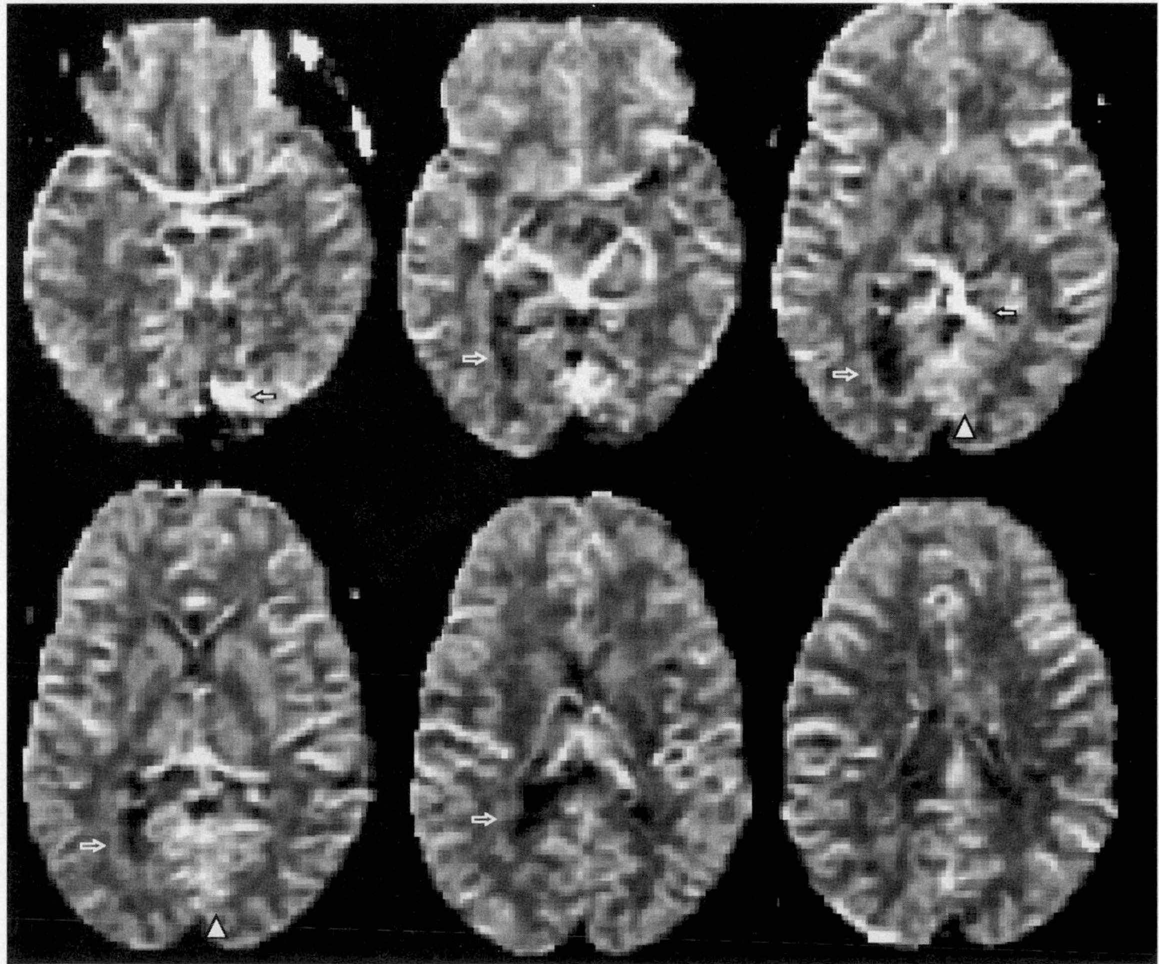

B

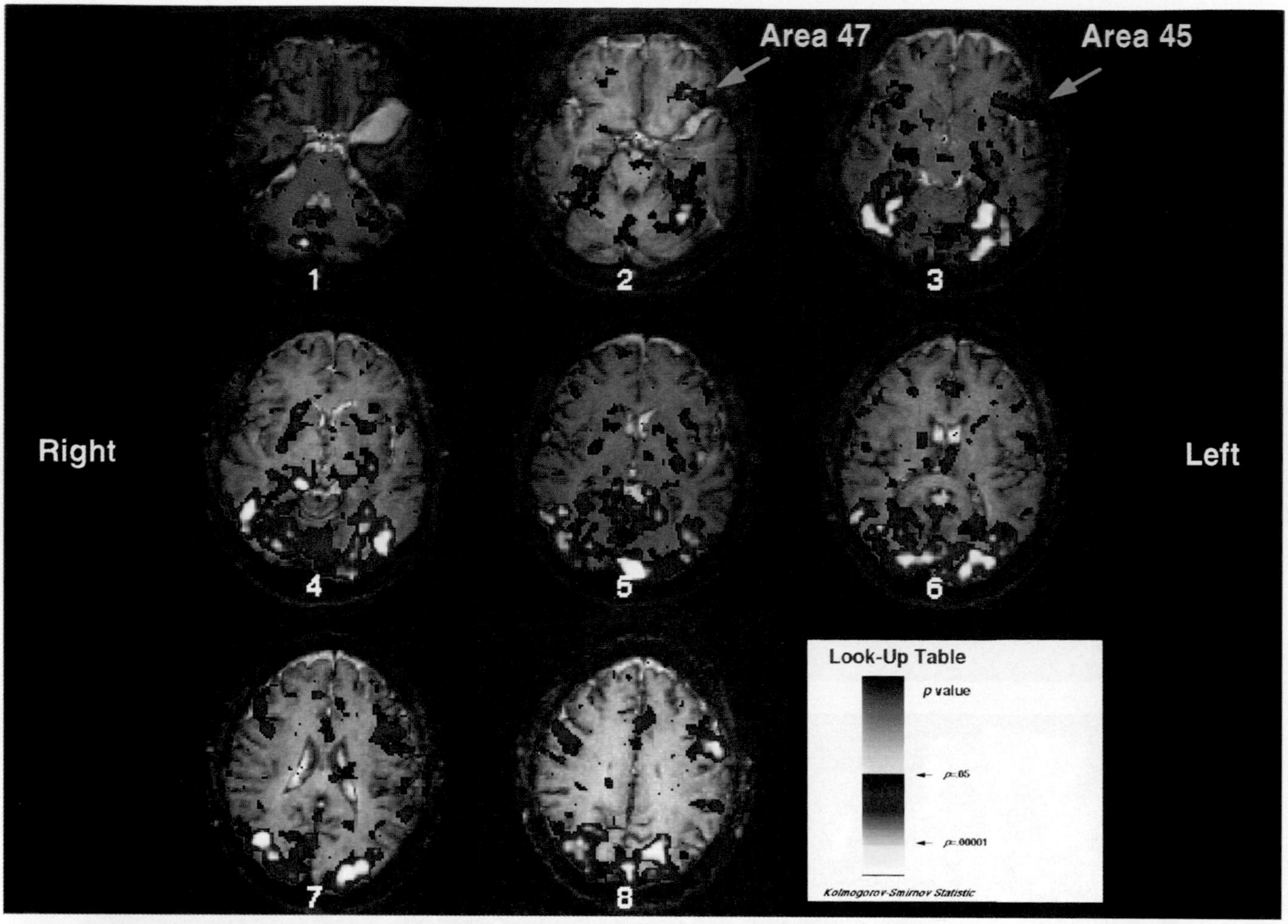

FIG. 42. Language lateralization. The stimulus task was generating verbs corresponding to objects that were projected onto a screen in the magnet during imaging. The control task was fixation on a dot. Increased activity is noted in areas 47 and 45 on this comparison, and also when comparing the verb generation to viewing the objects passively. This localizes the language activity in this subject to the left side. Of note, this patient was left handed, and also had an arachnoid cyst on the left, which gave him an increased chance of language lateralization on the right. However, Wada testing confirmed that this patient's language processing localized to the left.

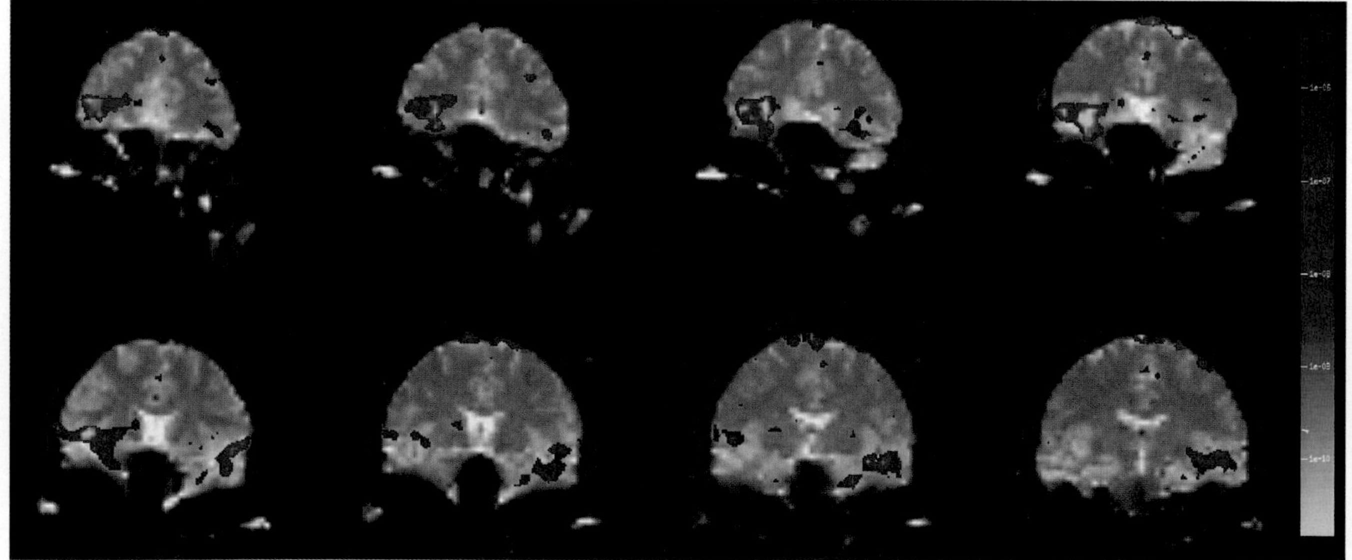

FIG. 43. Localization of obsessive-compulsive activity. The stimulus condition was a cloth on the hand in a patient known to obsess about cleanliness issues. The subject was told the cloth was dirty. The control condition was also a cloth on the hand, but the subject was told the cloth was clean. Marked activity is demonstated on these coronal images in the left frontal and temporal lobes.

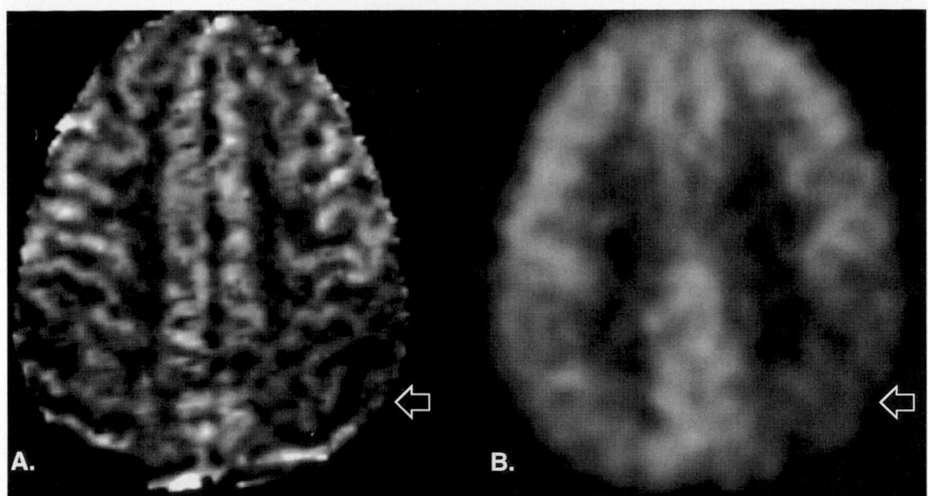

FIG. 44. Correlation of rCBV maps with PET ^{18}FDG maps in a patient with Alzheimer's disease. **A:** Functional MRI Gd-based rCBV map demonstrating a region of low blood volume (*arrow*). Decreased uptake is also seen in the contralateral hemisphere. **B:** Similar decreased uptake of tracer in the same distribution (*arrow*), in both hemispheres.

Alzheimer's/Dementia

Dementia is one of the most common diseases and yet one quite difficult to diagnose radiographically. The most common subtype, senile dementia of the Alzheimer's type (SDAT) remains particularly challenging. PET studies have shown some success in this setting (101), with characteristic decreases in ^{18}FDG uptake in moderate to severe cases of SDAT. Perfusion imaging with fMRI has been applied to this problem as well, with early studies indicating similar results to that of PET (102). These early studies indicate that fMRI rCBV mapping may have a sensitivity and specificity similar to that of PET for the diagnosis of SDAT. A typical case is illustrated in Fig. 44. Other approaches to imaging diagnosis of Alzheimer's include observing fMRI activation mapping during neuropsychiatric testing of memory formation and retrieval (104), which may be apparent earlier than the structural changes associated with changes in lobar blood volume. As in many other areas of clinical application, these works are still in progress.

CONCLUSION

Functional MRI can potentially bring a series of new patient populations and disease entities to the neuroradiologist. In addition to the clinical applications discussed above, there is a broad range of basic neuroscience questions that can be addressed by taking advantage of the high spatial and temporal resolution of fMRI techniques, and these techniques promise to expand the reach of neuroradiology. These include investigations of the human visual system, including spatial, depth, motion, and color perception, language processing; memory and cognition; and investigation into the fundamentals of the clinical problems mentioned above, including tumor biology and pathophysiology; stroke pathophysiology and recovery; epilepsy; dementia; and many others.

Understanding the technical issues of fMRI as well as the underlying cerebral physiology and pathophysiology is necessary to bring the full benefit of these techniques to patient care. Currently, fMRI can benefit patients in the evaluation of neoplasm, stroke, presurgical mapping, and epilepsy; future applications include psychiatric diseases and providing insight into the way the brain works.

ACKNOWLEDGMENTS. The authors would like to thank Drs. R. Weisskoff, K. Kwong, and J. Belliveau for many useful discussions, and T. Campbell for his expert technical assistance.

FIGURE ACKNOWLEDGMENTS. H. Aronen, data for Figs. 7, 22, 24, 27, 28, 33, 34, 36, 37, 38, 41; R. Benson, Fig. 42; J. L. Boxerman, Fig. 7; H. Breiter, Fig. 43; R. Bruening, data for Fig. 33; B. Buchbinder, Fig. 31; F. Caramia, Fig. 33; T. L. Davis, Fig. 5; G. Gonzalez, Fig. 44; S. Kulke, data for Figs. 23, 29, 30, 39; S. Warach, data for Fig. 15; R. M. Weisskoff, Fig. 7.

REFERENCES

1. Roy CS, Sherrington CS. *J Physiol* (*Lond*) 1890;11:85–108.
2. Stejskal E, Tanner J. *J Chem Physics* 1965;42:288–292.
3. Le Bihan D, Breton E, Lallemand D, Grenier P, Cabanis E, Laval-Jean M. MR imaging of intravoxel incoherent motions: application to diffusion and perfusion in neurologic disorders. *Radiology* 1986;161:401–407.
4. Chien D, Buxton RB, Kwong KK, Brady TJ, Rosen BRD. MR diffusion imaging of the human brain. *J Comput Assist Tomogr* 1990;14: 514–520.
5. Chien D, Kwong KK, Gress DR, Buonanno FS, Buxton RB, Rosen BR. MR diffusion imaging of cerebral infarction in humans. *AJNR* 1992;13:1097–1102.
6. Hajnal JV, Doran M, Hall AS, et al. MR imaging of anisotropically restricted diffusion of water in the nervous system: technical, anatomic, and pathologic considerations. *J Comput Assist Tomogr* 1991;15:1–18.
7. Hooper J, Sunder R, Rose L, Le Bihan D. *Society of Magnetic Resonance in Medicine Ninth Annual Scientific Meeting and Exhibition*. New York; 1990.
8. Larsson H, et al. *Society of Magnetic Resonance in Medicine Ninth Annual Meeting*. New York; 1991.
9. Le Bihan D, Delannoy J, Levin R. Temperature mapping with

MR imaging of molecular diffusion: application to hyperthermia. *Radiology* 1989;171:853–857.
10. Le Bihan D, Turner R, Douek P, Patronas ND. Diffusion MR imaging: clinical applications. *AJR* 1992;159:591–599.
11. Davis TL, Wedeen VJ, Weisskoff RM, Rosen BR. *Twelfth Annual Scientific Meeting of the Society of Magnetic Resonance in Medicine.* New York; 1993.
12. Moseley ME, Cohen Y, Kucharczyk J, Mintorovitch J, Asgari HS, Wendland MF. Diffusion-weighted MR imaging of anisotropic water diffusion in cat central nervous system. *Radiology* 1990;176:439–445.
13. van Gelderen P, de Vleeschouwer MH, DesPres D, Pekar J, van Zijl PC, Moonen CT. Water diffusion and acute stroke. *Magn Reson Med* 1994;31:154–163.
14. Villringer A, Rosen BR, Belliveau JW, et al. Dynamic imaging with lanthanide chelates in normal brain: contrast due to magnetic susceptibility effects. *Magn Reson Med* 1988;6:164–174.
15. Belliveau JW, et al. *Society for Magnetic Resonance in Medicine* 1987:7.
16. Belliveau JW, Rosen BR, Kantor HL, et al. Functional cerebral imaging by susceptibility-contrast NMR. *Magn Reson Med* 1990;14:538–546.
17. Henkelman RM, Hardy PA. *Seventh Annual Meeting of the Society of Magnetic Resonance Imaging.* Los Angeles; 1989.
18. Fisel CR, Ackerman JL, Buxton RB, et al. MR contrast due to microscopically heterogeneous magnetic susceptibility: numerical simulations and applications to cerebral physiology. *Magn Reson Med* 1991;17:336–347.
19. Majumdar S, Zoghbi SS, Gore JC. Regional differences in rat brain displayed by fast MRI with superparamagnetic contrast agents. *Magn Reson Imaging* 1988;6:611–615.
20. Bradbury MWB. *The Concept of a Blood-Brain Barrier.* New York: John Wiley; 1979.
21. Rapoport SI. *Blood-Brain Barrier in Physiology and Medicine.* New York: Raven Press; 1976.
22. Rosen BR, Belliveau JW, Buchbinder BR, et al. Contrast agents and cerebral hemodynamics. *Magn Reson Med* 1991;19:285–292.
23. Rosen BR, Belliveau JW, Vevea JM, Brady TJ. Perfusion imaging with NMR contrast agents. *Magn Reson Med* 1990;14:249–266.
24. Belliveau JW, Kennedy DN Jr, McKinstry RC, et al. Functional mapping of the human visual cortex by magnetic resonance imaging. *Science* 1991;254:716–719.
25. Weisskoff R, Chesler D, Boxerman J, Rosen B. Pitfalls in MR measurement of tissue blood flow with intravascular tracers: which mean transit time? *Magn Reson Med* 1993;29:553–558.
26. Boxerman JL, Weisskoff RM, Hoppel BE, Rosen BR. *Society of Magnetic Resonance in Medicine Twelfth Annual Scientific Meeting.* New York; 1993.
27. Weidner N, Carroll PR, Flax J, Blumenfeld W, Folkman J. Tumor angiogenesis correlates with metastasis in invasive prostate carcinoma. *Am J Pathol* 1993;143:401–409.
28. Boxerman J, Weisskoff R, Aronen H, Rosen B. *Society of Magnetic Resonance in Medicine Eleventh Annual Meeting.* Berlin; 1992.
29. Aronen H, et al. *Society of Magnetic Resonance in Medicine Eleventh Annual Meeting.* Berlin; 1992.
30. Saini S, Fretz CJ, Fisel CR, Rosen BR, Ferrucci J Jr. In vitro evaluation of a mechanical injector for infusion of magnetic resonance contrast media. *Invest Radiol* 1991;26:748–751.
31. Hamberg LM, Macfarlane R, Tasdemiroglu E, et al. Measurement of cerebrovascular changes in cats after transient ischemia using dynamic magnetic resonance imaging. *Stroke* 1993;24(3):444–451.
32. Moseley M, et al. Comparison of MR imaging after administration of Dysprosium-based magnetic-susceptibility contrast media with diffusion-weighted MR imaging in evaluation of regional cerebral ischemia. *Radiology* 1989;173:383.
33. Moseley ME, Kucharczyk J, Mintorovitch J, et al. Diffusion-weighted MR imaging of acute stroke: correlation with T2-weighted and magnetic susceptibility-enhanced MR imaging in cats. *AJNR* 1990;11:423–429.
34. Moseley ME, Cohen Y, Mintorovitch J, et al. Early detection of regional cerebral ischemia in cats: comparison of diffusion- and T2-weighted MRI and spectroscopy. *Magn Reson Med* 1990;14:330–346.
35. Sokoloff L, Reivich M, Kennedy C, et al. The [^{14}C]deoxyglucose method for the measurement of local cerebral glucose utilization: theory, procedure, and normal values in the conscious and anesthetized albino rat. *J Neurochem* 1977;28:897–916.
36. Posner MI, Petersen SE, Fox PT, Raichle ME. Localization of cognitive operations in the human brain. *Science* 1988;240:1627–1631.
37. Petersen SE, Fox PT, Posner MI, Mintun M, Raichle ME. Positron emission tomographic studies of the cortical anatomy of single-word processing. *Nature* 1988;331:585–589.
38. Fox PT, Raichle ME, Mintun MA, Dence C. Nonoxidative glucose consumption during focal physiologic neural activity. *Science* 1988;241:462–464.
39. Fox PT, Raichle ME. Focal physiological uncoupling of cerebral blood flow and oxidative metabolism during somatosensory stimulation in human subjects. *Proc Natl Acad Sci USA* 1986;83:1140–1144.
40. Pauling L, Coryell C. *Proceedings of the National Academy of Sciences* 1936;22:210–216.
41. Thulborn KR, Waterton JC, Matthews PM, Radda GK. Oxygenation dependence of the transverse relaxation time of water protons in whole blood at high field. *Biochim Biophys Acta* 1982;714:265–270.
42. Gomori JM, Grossman RI, Goldberg HI, Zimmerman RA, Bilaniuk LT. Intracranial hematomas: imaging by high-field MR. *Radiology* 1985;157:87–93.
43. Ogawa S, Lee TM, Nayak AS, Glynn P. Oxygenation-sensitive contrast in magnetic resonance image of rodent brain at high magnetic fields. *Magn Reson Med* 1990;14:68–78.
44. Turner R, Le Bihan D, Moonen CT, Despres D, Frank J. Echo-planar time course MRI of cat brain oxygenation changes. *Magn Reson Med* 1991;22:159–166.
45. Hoppel B, et al. *Society of Magnetic Resonance in Medicine Eleventh Annual Meeting.* Berlin; 1992.
46. Brady T. *10th Annual Meeting of the Society of Magnetic Resonance in Medicine.* San Francisco; 1991.
47. Kwong KK, Belliveau JW, Chesler DA, et al. Dynamic magnetic resonance imaging of human brain activity during primary sensory stimulation. *Proc Natl Acad Sci* 1992;89:5675–5679.
48. Grubb RL Jr, Raichle ME, Eichling JO, Ter-Pogossian MM. The effects of changes in $PaCO_2$ on cerebral blood volume, blood flow, and vascular mean transit time. *Stroke* 1974;5:630–639.
49. Williams DS, Detre JA, Leigh JS, Koretsky AP. Magnetic resonance imaging of perfusion using spin inversion of arterial water [published erratum appears in *Proc Natl Acad Sci USA* 1992 May 1,89(9):4220] *Proc Natl Acad Sci* 1992;89:212–216.
50. Detre JA, Subramanian VH, Mitchell MD, et al. Measurement of regional cerebral blood flow in cat brain using intracarotid ^2H_2O and ^2H NMR imaging. *Magn Reson Med* 1990;14:389–395.
51. American Heart Association. *1989 Stroke Facts.* Dallas: American Heart Association; 1988.
52. Wade D, Langton Hewer R. Hospital admission for acute stroke: who, for how long, and to what effect? *J Epidemiol Community Health* 1985;39:347–352.
53. Heiss WD, Graf R. The ischemic penumbra. *Curr Opin Neurol* 1994;7:11–19.
54. Davis R, Bulkley G, Traystman R. In: Tomita M, Sawada T, Naritoma H, Heiss WD, eds. *Cerebral Hyperemia and Ischemia: From the Standpoint of Cerebral Blood Volume.* Amsterdam: Excerpta Medica; 1988;151–156.
55. Symon L. The relationship between CBF, evoked potentials and the clinical features in cerebral ischaemia. *Acta Neurol Scand* 1980;62:175–190.
56. Tomlinson FH, Anderson RE, Meyer FB. Acidic foci within the ischemic penumbra of the New Zealand white rabbit. *Stroke* 1993;24:2030–2040.
57. Hakim AM, Evans AC, Berger L, et al. The effect of nimodipine on the evolution of human cerebral infarction studied by PET. *J Cereb Blood Flow Metab* 1989;9:523–534.
58. Olsen TS, Larsen B, Herning M, Skriver EB, Lassen NA. Blood

flow and vascular reactivity in collaterally perfused brain tissue. Evidence of an ischemic penumbra in patients with acute stroke. *Stroke* 1983;14:332–341.

59. Rosner G, Heiss WD. Survival of cortical neurons as a function of residual flow and duration of ischemia. *J Cereb Blood Flow Metab* 1983;3:S393–394.
60. Inoue T, Kato H, Araki T, Kogure K. Emphasized selective vulnerability after repeated nonlethal cerebral ischemic insults in rats. *Stroke* 1992;23:739–745.
61. Kucharczyk J, Mintorovitch J, Asgari HS, Moseley M. Diffusion/perfusion MR imaging of acute cerebral ischemia. *Magn Reson Med* 1991;19:311–315.
62. Warach S, Chien D, Li W, Ronthal M, Edelman RR. Fast magnetic resonance diffusion-weighted imaging of acute human stroke [published erratum appears in *Neurology* 1992;42(11): 2192]. *Neurology* 1992;42:1717–1723.
63. Hasegawa Y, Fisher M, Latour LL, Dardzinski BJ, Sotak CH. MRI diffusion mapping of reversible and irreversible ischemic injury in focal brain ischemia. *Neurology* 1994;44:1484–1490.
64. Roberts TP, Vexler Z, Derugin N, Moseley ME, Kucharczyk J. High-speed MR imaging of ischemic brain injury following stenosis of the middle cerebral artery. *J Cereb Blood Flow Metab* 1993;13:940–946.
65. Wolf PA, Belanger AJ, D'Agostino RB. Management of risk factors. *Neurol Clin* 1992;10:177–191.
66. Crosby D, et al. *Second Meeting, Society of Magnetic Resonance.* San Francisco; 1994.
67. von Monakow C. *Die Lokalistion in Grosshirn und der Abbau der Funktion durch Kortikale Herde.* Wiesbaden; J.F. Bergmann; 1914.
68. von Monakow C. *Arch Psychiatrie Nervenkrankh* 1895;27:1–128.
69. Feeney DM, Baron J-C. Diaschisis. *Stroke* 1986;17:817–830.
70. DiChiro G. Positron emission tomography [18F]fluorodeoxyglucose in brain tumors: a powerful diagnostic and prognostic tool. *Invest Radiol* 1986;22:360–371.
71. Alavi J, Alavi A, Charoluk J, et al. Positron emission tomography in patients with glioma. A predictor of prognosis. *Cancer* 1988;62:1074–1078.
72. Weidner N, Semple JP, Welch WR, Folkman J. Tumor angiogenesis and metastasis—correlation in invasive breast carcinoma. *N Engl J Med* 1991;324:1–8.
73. Toi M, Kashitani J, Tominaga T. Tumor angiogenesis is an independent prognostic indicator in primary breast carcinoma. *Int J Cancer* 1993;55:371–374.
74. Kallinowski F, Schlenger KH, Runkel S, Kloes M, Stohrer M, Okunieff P, Vaupel P. Blood flow, metabolism, cellular microenvironment, and growth rate of human tumor xenografts. *Cancer Res* 1989;49:3759–3764.
75. Ariza A, Fernandez LA, Inagami T, Kim JH, Manuelidis EE. Blood flow, metabolism, cellular microenvironment, and growth rate of human tumor xenografts. *Am J Clin Pathol* 1988;90:437–441.
76. Plate KH, Breier G, Farrell CL, Risau W. Platelet-derived growth factor receptor-beta is induced during tumor development and upregulated during tumor progression in endothelial cells in human gliomas. *Lab Invest* 1992;67:529–534.
77. Zagzag D, Miller DC, Sato Y, Rifkin DB, Burstein DE. Platelet-derived growth factor receptor-beta is induced during tumor development and upregulated during tumor progression in endothelial cells in human gliomas. *Cancer Res* 1990;50:7393–7398.
78. Eby NL, Grufferman S, Flannelly CM, Schold SC Jr, Vogel FS, Burger PC. Increasing incidence of primary brain lymphoma in the US. *Cancer* 1988;62:2461–2465.
79. Daumas-Duport C, Scheithauer B, O'Fallon J, Kelly P. Grading of astrocytomas. A simple and reproducible method. *Cancer* 1988;62:2152–2165.
80. Burger PC, Vogel FS, Green SB, Strike TA. Glioblastoma multiforme and anaplastic astrocytoma. Pathologic criteria and prognostic implications. *Cancer* 1985;56:1106–1111.
81. Morantz RA. Radiation therapy in the treatment of cerebral astrocytoma. *Neurosurgery* 1987;20:975–982.
82. Chamberlain MC, Murovic JA, Levin VA. Absence of contrast enhancement on CT brain scans of patients with supratentorial malignant gliomas [published erratum appears in *Neurology* 1988 Nov;38(11):1816]. *Neurology* 1988;38:1371–1374.
83. Coffey RJ, Lunsford LD, Taylor FH. Survival after stereotactic biopsy of malignant gliomas. *Neurosurgery* 1988;22:465–473.
84. Greenberg MS. *Handbook of Neurosurgery,* Lakeland, Fla: Greenberg Graphics; 1994.
85. Aronen H, Gazit I, Pardo F, et al. Multislice MRI CBV imaging of brain tumors: a comparison with PET studies. Presented at the *Proceedings of the Twelfth Annual Scientific Meeting,* New York, 1993.
86. Aronen H, Gazit IE, Louis DN, Buchbinder BR, Pardo FS, Weisskoff RM, Harsh GR, Cosgrove GR, Halpern EF, Hochberg FH. Cerebral blood volume maps of gliomas: comparison with tumor grade and histologic findings. *Radiology* 1994;191:41–51.
87. Di Chiro G, DeLaPaz RL, Brooks RA, Sokoloff L, Kornblith PL, Smith BH, Patronas NJ, Kufta CV, Kessler RM, Johnston GS, Manning RG, Wolf AP. Glucose utilization of cerebral gliomas measured by [18F]fluorodeoxyglucose and positron emission tomography. *Neurology* 1982;32:1323–1329.
88. DeLaPaz RL, Knott A, Rohan M, Matuzek M. *Radiological Society of North America 79th Scientific Assembly and Annual Meeting.* Chicago; 1993.
89. Gazit I, et al. *Proceedings of the 12th Annual Meeting of the Society of Magnetic Resonance in Medicine.* New York; 1993.
90. Jack C Jr, Thompson RM, Butts RK, Sharbrough FW, Kelly PJ, Hanson DP, Riederer SJ, Ehman RL, Hangiandreou NJ, Cascino GD. Sensory motor cortex: correlation of presurgical mapping with functional MR imaging and invasive cortical mapping. *Radiology* 1994;190:85–92.
91. Buchbinder BR, et al. *79th Annual Meeting of the Radiological Society of North America.* Chicago; 1993.
92. Atlas SW, Howard RS, Maldjian J, et al. Functional MRI of regional brain activity in patients with intracerebral gliomas: findings and implications for clinical management. *Neurosurgery* 1995;[*in press*].
93. Scherer HJ. The forms of growth in gliomas and their practical significance. *Brain* 1940;63:1–35.
94. Sorensen AG, Kulke S, Aronen H, Weisskoff RM, Fischman A, Hochberg FH, Pardo FS, Harsh G, Rosen, BR. Relative cerebral blood volume maps can distinguish tumor recurrence from radiation necrosis. Presented at the *Annual Meeting of the American Society of Neuroradiology,* Chicago, 1995.
95. Weisskoff R, et al. *Proceedings of the Second Meeting of the Society of Magnetic Resonance.* San Francisco; 1994.
96. Sorensen AG, et al. *American Society of Neuroradiology Annual Meeting.* Nashville; 1994.
97. Connelly A, Jackson GD, Cross JH, Gadian DG. *Society of Magnetic Resonance in Medicine Twelfth Annual Scientific Meeting.* New York; 1993.
98. Falconer MA. Mesial temporal (Ammon's horn) sclerosis as a common cause of epilepsy. Aetiology, treatment, and prevention. *Lancet* 1974;2:767–770.
99. Blamire A, et al. *Proceedings of the 11th Annual Meeting of the Society of Magnetic Resonance in Medicine.* Berlin; 1992.
100. Benson R, et al. *Proceedings of the Second Meeting of the Society of Magnetic Resonance.* San Francisco; 1994.
101. Herholz K, Perani D, Salmon E, Franck G, Fazio F, Heiss WD, Comar D. Comparability of FDG PET studies in probable Alzheimer's disease. *J Nucl Med* 1993;34:1460–1466.
102. Gonzalez R, et al. *Proceedings of the 31st Annual Meeting of the American Society of Neuroradiology.* Vancouver; 1993.
103. Stern C, et al. *Society for Neuroscience 1994 Annual Meeting.* Miami Beach; 1994.
104. Horton JC, Hoyt WF. Quadrantic visual field defects. A hallmark of lesions in extrastriate (V2/V3) cortex. *Brain* 1991;114:1703–1718.

Magnetic Resonance Imaging of the Brain and Spine, Second Edition, edited by Scott W. Atlas.
Lippincott-Raven Publishers, Philadelphia © 1996.

31

MR Angiography

Techniques and Clinical Applications

John Perl II, Patrick A. Turski, and Thomas J. Masaryk

The intrinsic sensitivity of nuclear magnetic resonance to motion was first recognized in the 1950s (1,2). From the early clinical experiences with magnetic resonance imaging (MRI) it was appreciated that moving spins exhibited signal variability. Initially this was often considered a nuisance because the signal instability produced confusing and unwanted image artifacts. Considerable effort was aimed at minimizing these troublesome manifestations (3). Subsequently, the signal alterations resulting from flowing blood have been exploited to provide vascular morphology and quantitative flow data and are the basis for magnetic resonance angiography (MRA). MRA with MRI provides additional insights into cerebrovascular diseases above that provided by either technique alone.

Conventional MRI yields parenchymal and vascular anatomic information with limited physiologic information. The addition of MRA opens the door to anatomic and physiologic vascular information often not obtainable from other diagnostic techniques. It is often tempting to assume that MRA displays the same information as conventional catheter angiography due to the similarity in the displayed information. But MRA displays the physiologic consequences of flow dynamics in blood vessels, and therefore the true anatomic lumen may not always be reflected in the MRA image. The physiologic and morphologic information that can be extracted from a particular MRA sequence varies. It is important to recognize that along with anatomic images, details of flow direction, velocity, and volume can be extracted using specific MRA techniques. Thus, MR offers the possibility of combined, noninvasive imaging of parenchymal anatomy, the vascular supply, and a quantitative measure of blood flow, in a single high-contrast, high-resolution examination. Having said this, it is still uncertain whether such information is significant in the clinical setting and in what specific circumstances should all these data be obtained.

Although extensive knowledge of MR physics is not necessary to interpret MRA images, a basic understanding is necessary to choose an appropriate MR technique for a particular clinical situation. Moreover, fundamental knowledge will allow common diagnostic pitfalls to be avoided (see also Chapter 4).

J. Perl II, M.D. and T. J. Masaryk, M.D.: Radiology, The Cleveland Clinic Foundation, Cleveland, Ohio 44195.
P. A. Turski, M.D.: Section of Neuroradiology, Department of Radiology, University of Wisconsin, Madison, WI 53792.

BASIC PRINCIPLES OF MR AND THE EFFECTS OF FLOW

The basic MR imaging experiment consists of two essential (and relatively independent) components: (a) excitation/saturation, from application of a radiofrequency pulse sequence, and (b) signal sampling/localization, forming the MR image using magnetic field gradients. Blood flow during either excitation or receiving results in two types of corresponding effects on the MR signal of moving spins: (a) the wash-in/wash-out or "flight" of spins relative to the timing and placement of a radiofrequency (rf) pulse produces so-called time-of-flight (TOF) effects, and (b) spins moving during the application, and in the direction of, an imaging gradient produce a shift in signal phase which is dependent on the type of flow (constant velocity, disturbed, etc.) and gradient in the flow direction, i.e., spin-phase phenomena (4,5). These flow-induced changes in the MR signal form the substrate for imaging and quantifying blood flow. The moving spin signal changes may be selectively displayed or enhanced as either a magnitude or phase image display.

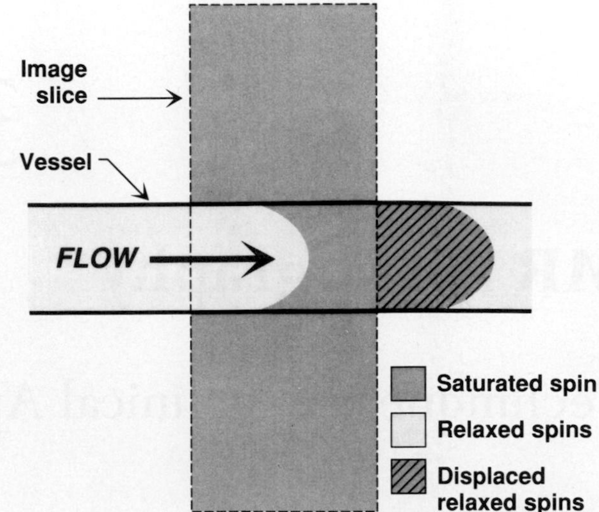

FIG. 1. Flow-related enhancement schematic of a cross-section of vessel. The relaxed spins entering the image slice result in high signal intensity because of the inflow of fully magnetized blood into the excitation volume. Signal strength is proportional to the fraction of the replacement of saturated spins within the imaging volume. Other factors that influence signal intensity include the flip angle of the radiofrequency pulse and the repetition time (TR).

TOF Effects

TOF effects influence the signal intensities of moving blood in standard imaging situations. Flow void (high velocity signal loss) and flow-related enhancement commonly seen in conventional spin-echo (SE) and gradient-echo (GE) imaging, respectively, are described in Chapter 4. TOF effects reflect the macroscopic motion of spins and their state of longitudinal magnetization. Most commonly, the magnetization of a bolus of blood is modified [with an rf pulse] at one location and detected at another. The time elapsed between the rf labeling and sampling of the flowing spin's magnetization is referred to as the TOF effect (Fig. 1).

Moving spins results in substantial alteration of both the amplitude and phase of MR signal while using conventional imaging schemes. If the direction of flow is perpendicular to the imaging slice (or volume), partially saturated spins are replaced by the inflowing unsaturated (fully relaxed and magnetized) spins during the rf repetition time (5) (Fig. 1). The displacement of partially saturated spins is directly dependent on the flow velocity and slice thickness. If the repetition time (TR) is short relative to the longitudinal relaxation time T1 of stationary tissue, the signal of the stationary material is saturated and therefore attenuated (5). Signal from the unsaturated moving blood, which entering the excitation volume between pulse sequence repetitions is not saturated (attenuated), is, consequently, high signal intensity compared to the surrounding stationary tissue ("flow-related enhancement") (Fig. 1). An important point to remember is that with conventional SE sequences, spins must receive both a 90° and 180° slice-selective rf pulses to create the echo. Hence, flow signal eventually decreases at higher flow velocities because of the outflow ("high velocity signal loss"), which occurs when the spins move outside the imaging slice before application of the 180° refocusing rf pulse (5).

Spin-Phase Phenomena

Another class of flow effects results from changes in the phase of the transverse magnetization that occur when the spins move along the magnetic field gradients used for position encoding in MRI. The phase change predicted by the Larmor equation for stationary spins is:

$$\Delta\Phi = 2\gamma \times G \times \mathrm{TE} \quad [1]$$

where $\Delta\Phi$ is the change in phase, γ is the gyromagnetic ratio, G is the magnetic field gradient, and TE is the echo time. The dephasing effect of magnetic field gradients on a sample of stationary spins is widely recognized and typically is compensated for by a second gradient (e.g., the first inverted lobe of a bipolar read gradient in a GE sequence), resulting in the complete alignment of all spins within an imaging volume element at the time the "gradient echo" is sampled.

The sequelae of motion along an imaging gradient disrupts the linear relationship predicted by the Larmor equation for stationary tissue. For moving protons, frequency and phase change exponentially with field strength as a Taylor series, which depends on the character of flow (i.e., constant velocity, accelerating, turbulent, etc.). It is important to recognize the directional nature of this phenomenon: the motion must be in the direction defined by the imaging gradient. For protons moving at constant velocity the change in phase is described as:

$$\Delta\Phi^{v} = \gamma G \times \Delta V(\mathrm{TE}/2)2 \quad [2]$$

where $\Delta\Phi^{v}$ is the velocity-induced phase difference within a given pixel resulting from the velocity distribution ΔV across the voxel with respect to the applied gradient field (G), γ is the gyromagnetic ratio, and TE the echo time (i.e., time between the centers of the rf excitation period and rf sampling or read-out interval). For example, the blood flowing in vessels (e.g., the carotid arteries in a sagittal scan of the neck) has a variety of velocities (as well as higher order motion). The spectrum of velocities and higher order motion within the voxel depicting the vascular lumen result in a variety of signal phases. In conventional SE images, this results in spatial misregistration in the phase-encode direction (i.e., ghosting) resulting from bulk phase shifts of spins flowing along the imaging gradients during the finite time required between phase-encoding and signal sampling. In addition, spin dephasing due to the range of intravoxel velocities produces a spectrum of phases within the voxel, leading to partial or complete signal loss. The phenomenon is most prominent in circumstances in which the flow has a wide variety of velocities (e.g., near vessel walls and in areas of turbulence) and when gradients are applied over a relatively long time period (of flow) with relatively large amplitude (i.e., frequency encoding). In summary, the effects of motion in the presence of conventional signal sampling gradients occur simultaneously with, but independent of, TOF effects and are known as spin-phase phenomena. These effects may be observed in conventional magnitude reconstructed images as ghosting and signal loss.

Phase shift effects are observed for flow in all directions, specifically along the slice-select, phase-encoding, and frequency-encoding gradients. The resulting phase change depends on both sequence gradient structure (timing, amplitude, etc.) and flow parameters such as velocity, acceleration, and higher order motion. The terms of Eq. 2 above can be manipulated to modify motion-induced phase changes. Reduction of echo time can result in a geometric reduction in phase change. Velocity-induced phase dispersion, present in physiologic situations, can be manipulated by employing cardiac gating. As described above, the gradient term G in Eq. 2 can be altered using additional gradients of appropriate magnitude and timing, so-called rephasing or refocusing gradients (flow compensation or gradient moment nulling) to negate flow-induced phase changes. Use of additional gradients can be employed to compensate for acceleration and other higher order motion phase changes. However, implementation of refocusing gradient pulses in a given pulse sequence prolongs the echo time, which may be counterproductive.

FLOW MEASUREMENT TECHNIQUES

Quantitative flow velocity measurements can be obtained using techniques designed to take advantage of the bulk motion of spins relative to the timing of the pulse sequence (TOF effects), and on the phase shift accrued by spins moving along a magnetic gradient of known amplitude and duration. Selection of an appropriate technique for a particular clinical application includes spatial resolution (i.e., the ability of the method to isolate flow through a particular vessel), temporal resolution (i.e., the speed of data acquisition that determines the ability to provide instantaneous measurements or mean flow rates), and dynamic range (i.e., the range of measurable flow rates).

TOF Methods

Acquisition Techniques

Several TOF velocity quantification schemes based on a variety of pulse sequences have been devised. Other monikers for these techniques include "wash-in/wash-out" or "bolus tagging." With these types of measurements, conventional imaging techniques excite a plane and create an image representing the same plane. In the first of the two bolus tracking methods to be discussed, a saturation pulse is applied orthogonal to the plane of excitation, with inflow of bright signal flowing into the saturation band of the magnitude image and progressive displacement of the saturated low signal bolus downstream. In the second technique, the imaging plane itself is applied orthogonal to the excitation plane and, hence, only excited, flowing spins (profiles) appear extending into the plane of the image.

Presaturation Bolus Tracking

This TOF method for flow measurement uses a presaturation pulse perpendicular to inplane flow with subsequent tracking of the bolus over time. Multiple images in the plane of the vessel of interest are rapidly acquired over the cardiac cycle immediately following a series of preparatory rf saturation pulses confined to a small region within the vessel (6). This is similar to the cardiac-triggered low flip-angle GE cine technique used in the heart. When the images are played back in cine fashion, the saturated (low signal) bolus is tracked visually as it flows down the vessel. A quantitative measurement is calculated based on the measured displacement over the time of image acquisition.

The accuracy of quantitative measurements is limited by several factors. Measurement of the displaced bolus may be limited by poor presaturation pulse edge definition due to an imperfect rf saturation pulse profile. Moreover, with slow flow, the dynamic range may theoretically be limited by the T1 relaxation time of the saturated bolus region. Finally, because this technique generates an actual image of in-plane vascular anatomy to follow the saturated bolus, the acquisition time is relatively long, resulting in relatively poor temporal resolution. Hence, these saturation bolus tagging methods are best suited to evaluation of relatively constant flow (i.e., venous flow) and are ill-suited to measurement of pulsatile arterial flow.

Excitation Bolus Tracking

With these methods, a plane perpendicular to flow is excited, with images acquired in the plane of the vessel. In effect, the slice-select and read gradients are in the same direction. One such excited bolus tagging technique uses SE imaging with a 90° rf excitation pulse applied at one point and a 180° rf refocusing pulse placed farther downstream in the direction of flow. The range of velocities can then be approximated by repeating the sequence with different placements of the refocusing pulse and comparing the amplitude of the resultant SEs. Variations consisting of GE sequences have been developed in which a 90° rf excitation pulse is placed perpendicular to flow and the signal is read out in the slice-select direction. The flow rate is estimated by the relative displacement of the excited bolus during the repetition time (7,8). GE techniques are significantly faster than SE methods because merely enough signal data to track the displaced bolus is collected as opposed to creation of a complete MRI. Hence, sufficient temporal resolution is achieved, allowing tracking of arterial flow over the cardiac cycle.

The accuracy of quantitative measurements may be limited, however, by poor edge definition of the tagged region due to an imperfect rf excitation slice profile and T2* decay. The potential for significant signal loss secondary to T2 or T2* effects at longer echo times presents an additional limitation of these methods. If flow is so slow that signal from the excited bolus decays (secondary to T2 relaxation) before significant flow displacement, the ability of these techniques to detect and measure flow may be limited. To overcome this limitation, the implementation of a three-pulse, stimulated-echo technique has been proposed by perpetuating the bolus signal over a longer period of time (9).

Clinical Applications

Correlation of peak flow velocity and velocity-integral measurements between the GE excitation bolus-tracking method and Doppler ultrasound (US) has been performed in the abdominal aorta in normal volunteers, revealing close agreement between the two techniques (7,8). In preliminary clinical studies, the presaturation bolus method, however, has been the more frequently applied TOF quantitative technique. This method has been used to image the slow systolic plug flow and retrograde diastolic flow in abdominal aortic aneurysms and middle cerebral arteries. Several studies have proven it to be a relatively simple method to document both flow direction and velocity in the superior sagittal sinus as well as the portal venous system, with good correlation to Doppler US (6,10–13). The feasibility of this technique is therefore already documented; the clinical applications for the central nervous system (CNS) remain to be elucidated.

Velocity and Flow Quantification from Measured Phase Shifts

Acquisition Techniques

Spins flowing along a magnetic gradient accrue a phase shift that can be employed to measure flow velocity. This is achieved by using sequences with gradient structures of specified amplitude, duration, and polarity, which in the presence of flow induce predictable phase changes (14–23).

Flow Evaluation from Two-Dimensional Phase Reconstructed Images

The implementation of the "phase-display" (phase reconstruction, or "zebra stripe") imaging concept allows velocity information to be obtained by using an uncompensated gradient structure for velocity in either the slice-select or read direction. Since the flow velocity of blood or cerebrospinal fluid (CSF) is pulsatile, cardiac gating or another form of variability suppression is applied to improve temporal resolution (e.g., systolic vs. diastolic flow). Collection of a two-dimensional (2D) image at a specified time in the cardiac cycle and reconstructing a complex image allows a phase image to be calculated at each pixel location, velocity being proportional to the phase changes (15,21,24,25). In the mid 1980s, Bryant et al. validated the accuracy of one technique of velocity-induced phase measurements based on measured phase shifts using modified standard MRI gradients and comparing flow measurements of carotid arteries to those obtained by Doppler US (14). More recently, studies have measured flow velocities and volumes in other cerebral vessels (Table 1). Similar experiments performed with conventional SE imaging sequences have been verified by in vivo electromagnetic flow meters in experimental animals with good correlation (25,26).

The practical limitations of the technique include problems relating to cardiac gating. Without gating or if frequent mistriggering occurs, pulsatility (ghosting) artifacts will be seen (27). Also, background phase errors related to radiofrequency penetration, magnetic field inhomogeneities, chemical shift, and offset (uncentered) echoes occur. Offset echoes present no major difficulties for SE techniques, but are potentially more troublesome with more commonly used GE methods. Another, more prominent, phase error results from higher order motion effects in turbulent jets, which can be reduced by the use of short echo times or higher order moment nulling (28). Moreover, each sequence gradient structure must be both optimized and calibrated to maximize the sensitivity over the desired selected velocity range. The dynamic range of the phase-sensitive flow measurement techniques is equal to a $-\pi$ to $+\pi$ ($-180°$ to $+180°$) phase difference. Flow above the selected range (based on the timing, amplitude, and duration of the gradients in the direction of flow) produces a phase difference greater than 180°, resulting in signal loss and aliasing of measured phase changes to falsely low velocity values (28,29). In this scenario, the phase difference from the rapid flow will falsely be assigned to a lower velocity value. Thus, the same technique may require several gradient structures applied over different anatomic regions and velocity ranges. Signal loss from phase dispersion due to flow in gradient directions other than the direction of interest, or from higher order motion (e.g., acceleration, jerk), can be partially suppressed by additional flow compensation with gradient moment nulling (29). This extends the dynamic range of such techniques, allowing the measurement of nonuniform flow. The sequence must also be recalibrated when the gradient strengths are changed, which occurs when the slice thickness or field of view is altered.

Flow Evaluation from 2D Gradient-Encoded Images

Using GE sequences for phase-sensitive flow measurement shortens data acquisition time, increases signal contrast between moving spins and stationary tissues, and thus facilitates quantitative measurement of rapid flow as well as time-resolved measurements throughout the cardiac cycle (19). Background phase errors are overcome by several methods. The first involves interleaving two scans, where the gradients are reversed relative to each other, generating phase changes in the regions where flow occurs (a.k.a. VIGRE for velocity imaging with gradient-recalled echoes) (30). The subtraction of the raw data of two datasets results in effectively doubling phase change due to velocity while all other spurious sources of phase are subtracted out and leads to a $\sqrt{2}$

TABLE 1. *Flow velocities in normal subjects*

Vessel (ref. #)	Volume flow (ml/min)	Mean velocity (cm/sec)	Peak velocity (cm/sec)
Artery			
Right carotid (32)	352 ± 21	46 ± 4	63 ± 4
Right carotid (393)	305 ± 31; 310 ± 34[a]		
Left carotid (32)	342 ± 15	46 ± 4	60 ± 3
Left carotid (393)	263 ± 12; 249 ± 11[a]		
Basilar (32)	164 ± 12	40 ± 3	51 ± 4
Basilar (393)	201 ± 10; 213 ± 14[a]		
Anterior cerebral (393)	(R) 49 ± 4; 49 ± 5[a]		
	(L) 41 ± 6; 38 ± 5[a]		
Middle cerebral (12)	150 ± 8.3	—	69 ± 9
Middle cerebral (393)	(R) 164 ± 34; 160 ± 35[a]		
	(L) 141 ± 12; 147 ± 20[a]		
Posterior cerebral (393)	(R) 54 ± 8; 57 ± 5[a]		
	(L) 49 ± 7; 46 ± 7[a]		
Vein			
Superior sagittal sinus (32)	435 ± 121	13 ± 1	
Superior sagittal sinus (393)	281 ± 19; 285 ± 19[a]		
Internal cerebral (393)	(R) 21 ± 1; 18 ± 1[a]		
	(L) 23 ± 1; 20 ± 2[a]		

[a] Indicates flow measurement acquired with a nongated two-dimensional phase contrast slice.

R, right; L, left.

Modified from Anderson CM, Edelman RR, Turski PA. In: *Clincal Magnetic Angiography*. New York: Raven Press; 1993; 135.

improvement in signal-to-noise. Alternatively, a corrected image can also be obtained by collecting a gated cine mode data set and subtracting the first image from all other cardiac-gated scans, providing the change in velocity and also eliminating spurious phase changes (24). The former method reveals the actual flow velocities (rather than velocity change) and improves the signal-to-noise of the measurement. If the cine data are subtracted from a control scan with full motion compensation gradients, absolute flow velocities are determined rather than velocity differences (as long as the first image is fully compensated; if not, acceleration can cause an error) (31,32). Since the gated 2D phase techniques provide both magnitude images and phase information, quantitative flow rates in ml/min can be calculated by multiplying the measured cross-sectional area of the vessel on the magnitude image by the velocities derived from the phase data (31,32).

Flow Rates from One-Dimensional Phase Measurements

One-dimensional (1D) projection techniques can also be used to extract velocity information from phase data. An advantage of this method is the high speed acquisition providing excellent temporal resolution. One such lD technique called RACE (real time acquisition and velocity evaluation) was developed to measure flow perpendicular to the slice (through plane flow) from phase data produced by motion in the slice-select direction (20). Data are generated by application of a slice-select gradient followed by a read gradient (perpendicular to the direction of flow), and with no phase-encoding gradient. The TE varies from 6 to l0 msec and TR from l0 to 40 msec (20 msec is often used to obtain sufficient sampling). The sequence is continuously repeated throughout the cardiac cycle, capturing flow information with a temporal resolution equivalent to the TR (e.g., on velocity point every 20 msec for the duration of the measurement, usually 10–20 sec). Hence, this technique sacrifices 2D spatial resolution for excellent temporal resolution, short measurement time, and no requisite gating. As with all phase methods, the sequence can be calibrated to a velocity range of interest, and echo times must be minimized to avoid higher order motion dephasing.

The measured phase difference determined by the lD methods reflects motion contributions from everything within the projection. Phase shifts from overlapping arterial, venous, CSF, and moving parenchymal structures are combined, disrupting the phase information. Overcoming motion-induced phase shifts from structures outside the region of interest, but within the projection, is achieved by several strategies, including spatial presaturation, projection dephasing (applying a gradient to suppress stationary tissue), collecting a cylinder of data (33), and using oblique measurements to project the vessel of interest free from overlap. After allowances for the phase contributions of other tissues, the velocity calculated using this method represents a projection across the vessel and, therefore, is an averaged velocity. For this reason, RACE yields peak systolic velocities lower than those determined by US, the discrepancy depending on the velocity profile across the vessel during peak flow.

Clinical Applications

Clinical implementation of these techniques in normal volunteers has been reported in the carotid, cerebral, basilar, femoral, and pulmonary arteries, as well as the heart and aorta (14,16–19,23); however, the experience in the evaluation of vascular pathology is limited. Reduction in normal velocity has been detected distal to aortic coarctation and carotid occlusion. Increases in velocity have been observed in the carotid artery of normal volunteers as well as in patients with high-flow cerebral vascular malformations (32). Characteristic velocity profiles have also been measured at sites of peripheral vascular stenosis (15,21,22). As with all quantitative methods, clinical studies proving clinical relevance are yet to be performed.

MRA TECHNIQUES

In addition to flow quantification, the signal variation from TOF and spin-phase effects can be enhanced or modified in order to derive angiographic images.

TOF Methods

TOF MRA imaging methods provide vascular contrast based on tagging of the longitudinal magnetization of spins flowing into a region of interest, typically through relaxation, inversion, or subtraction (34–47). Unique to the more common TOF approaches is the creation of vascular contrast during a single scan acquisition followed by removal of stationary tissue, not by subtraction, but by image postprocessing.

Acquisition Techniques

Adiabatic Fast Scanning Technique

The initial use exploiting TOF effects in the production of angiographic images, reported by Dixon, used a method of adiabatic fast passage that selectively tagged common carotid inflow using a separate rf coil placed low on the neck, and the carotid bifurcation image downstream using a head coil (34). Suppression of stationary tissue signal was achieved with "twister" gradient pulses. A "twister" pulse is a low-amplitude gradient pulse that causes a 360° phase wrap over a relatively large region (i.e., voxel) of soft tissue that produces signal loss secondary to phase cancellation. Vessels in this region that are significantly smaller than the voxel size reduce the phase shift and signal loss will lessen, therefore enhancing vascular contrast. Newer variations of this technique employ stationary tissue rf saturation/inversion schemes (35).

Inversion Recovery Technique

Another TOF technique developed by Nishimura and associates uses single-slice, thick-slab (i.e., "projection") images acquired with a surface coil placed at the carotid bifurcation (36). Contrary to Dixon's method mentioned above, which used an excitation coil for spin tagging low in the neck, this method employs a local receive surface coil. Vascular contrast is generated by two acquisitions by different placement (at and below the carotid bifurcation on alternate acquisitions) of a spatially selective inversion pulse (180°). The angiographic images are created by subtraction of the two data acquisitions. The vascular signal intensity from TOF effects is maximized by varying the time following the inversion pulse (TI) and cardiac gating. Signal loss from phase effects secondary to rapid flow are minimized through use of extremely short echo times and gating to diastolic signal readout. Advantages include significant background tissue suppression and the use of very short echo time (through asymmetric sampling of signal) permitting the first MRA demonstration of a significant arterial stenosis.

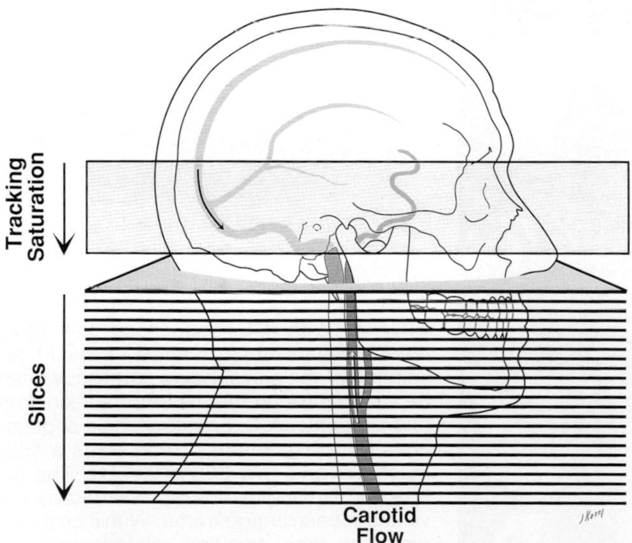

FIG. 2. Sequential 2D TOF technique schematic. Axial GE images are obtained in a craniocaudad direction with a superiorly placed tracking saturation pulse to eliminate venous signal. The direction of acquisition opposing carotid flow minimizes the saturation from a previous slice.

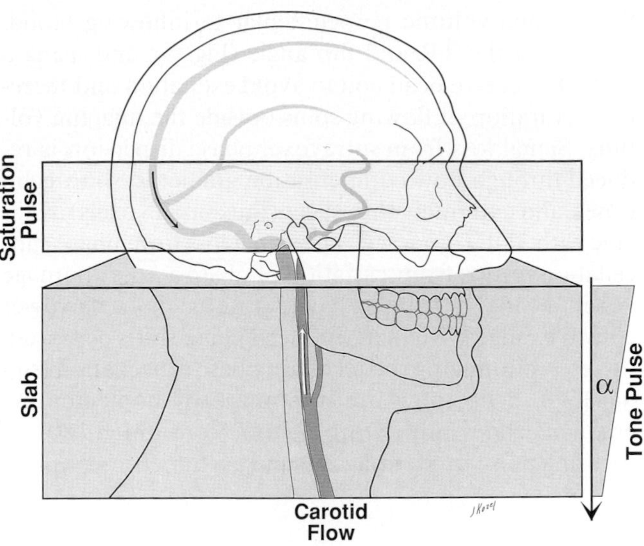

FIG. 3. 3D TOF with ramped radiofrequency pulse. The 3D volume is acquired with a ramped rf pulse to avoid progressive saturation of blood as it travels cephalad through the 3D volume. Note the amplitude of the rf excitation (α) increase across the volume. The superior saturation pulse suppresses signal from inflowing unsaturated venous blood.

2DFT Gradient-Echo TOF Technique

Inflow of unsaturated spins (flow-related enhancement) provides vascular contrast of flowing blood in vessels using sequential two-dimensional Fourier transform (2DFT) GE images oriented perpendicular to the direction of blood flow (37,38) (Figs. 1 and 2). Motion compensation gradients and relatively short echo times minimized signal loss secondary to motion-induced phase effects. The use of short repetition times allows coverage of large anatomic regions in a reasonable examination time. Initially, because the data were not displayed in a conventional angiographic format, Wehrli and Gullberg's work received little immediate attention. The potential of this technique was popularized when Keller et al. enhanced the acquisition by using thin 2DFT slices to minimize inflow saturation and displayed the data in an angiographic format using a maximum intensity projection (MIP) postprocessing algorithm (40). Sequential contiguous 2DFT TOF vascular images with selectively applied presaturation pulses have been used to produce both arteriograms and venograms in the abdomen, the carotid bifurcation, and the intracranial vessels (39,40). Acquisition and postprocessing of data is rapid and is especially useful when examining slow flow and large regions of interest.

3DFT Gradient-Echo TOF

An analogous inflow-enhancement–based TOF angiographic technique uses three-dimensional Fourier transform (3DFT) sequence acquisitions (41–43) (Fig. 3). Flow-related enhancement is maximized by orienting the imaging volume perpendicular to inflowing blood, optimizing the TR and flip angle (Fig. 4), and using a transmit/receive head coil to avoid excitation and therefore saturation of flowing spins outside the imaging volume. Signal loss from intravoxel phase dispersion is reduced through flow compensation gradients, short echo times, and extremely thin slices (thus small voxels) available with 3DFT imaging. The signal loss from phase cancellation results from variation of phase across an image voxel. Using a smaller voxel results in a narrower effective range of velocity-induced phase shifts per voxel, thereby minimizing the resultant phase cancellation (signal loss). Echo times are minimized by implementing gradient echoes (alleviating the time-consuming 180° refocusing pulse in SE imaging) and asymmetric sampling (sampling the echo earlier in the readout period). Flow compensation for acceleration or higher order motion terms is technically possible with complex gradient configurations; however, in practice using compensation gradients for first-order flow (constant velocity) alone in combination with a very short TE generally is more effective than higher order flow compensation, which slightly but detrimentally increases the echo time (42–48).

The 3D TOF MRA method excites and images a thick slab or volume of tissue. The 3DFT pulse sequence is similar to 2DFT, with the addition of an extra phase-encoding gradient along the slice-select direction to partition the thick volume into multiple, thin slices or "partitions" (usually ranging from 16 to 128 in number). The

A

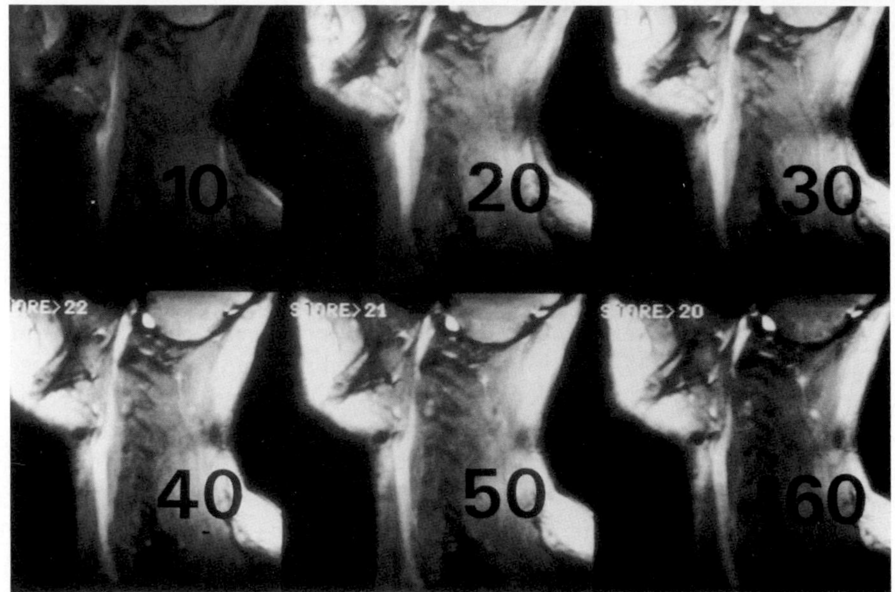

B

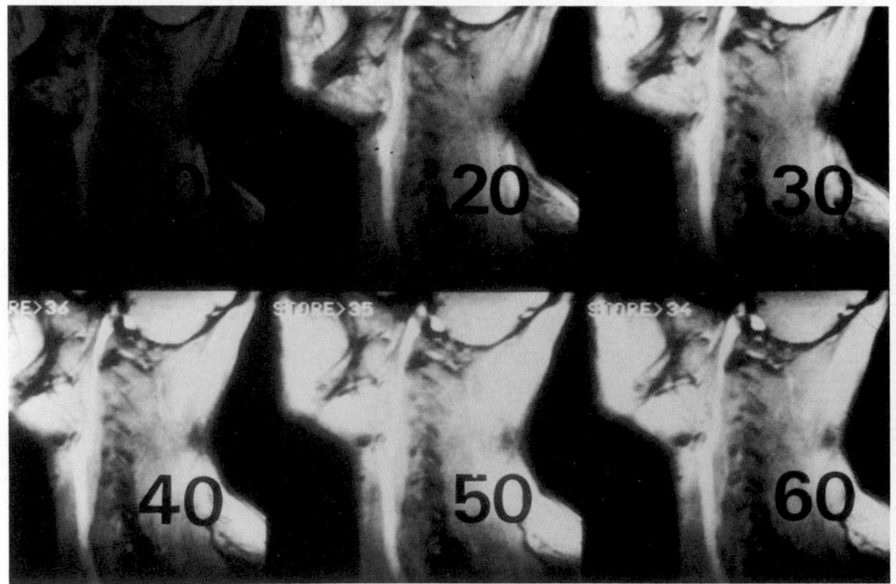

FIG. 4. With GE sequences the flow-related enhancement relative to the T1 relaxation of the surrounding soft tissues can be varied through the use of repetition time and flip angle. **A,B:** Fast low angle shot images (FLASH), where A represents a 100-msec TR and B a 200-msec TR. The respective flip angles are represented by the values in each image frame. With increasing repetition time, the flow-related enhancement extends farther along the neck, even as the echo time increases. Notice that the background also increases. (From *Top Magn Reson Imaging* 1991; 3(3):4.)

application of a 3DFT reconstructs the final image. Using this technique, production of 3D data sets with voxel dimensions of less than 0.8 × 0.8 × 0.8 mm are significantly smaller than possible with 2DFT TOF techniques (41,42). In addition, each 3DFT thin partition benefits from an increased signal-to-noise ratio (S/N × $\sqrt{n}$, where n = #3D slices), improved slice profile, and a reduction in T2* effects as compared to a 2DFT slice (44). The combination of very short echo times and first order flow compensation with the small voxel element of 3D imaging makes this technique relatively resistant to the imaging-degrading effects of disturbed flow. These advantages, in conjunction with the ability to display the vessels in multiple projections, has popularized 3DFT TOF imaging in the evaluation of the intracranial and extracranial circulation.

Using inflow of unsaturated spins (flow-related enhancement) for vascular contrast in 2DFT and 3DFT TOF methods also allows the selective imaging of vessels based on the direction of blood flow. This is accomplished by placing a presaturation 90° rf pulse adjacent to one side of the imaging slice or volume. By saturating inflowing spins before entering the imaging slice, inflow enhancement is prevented and the vessel appears iso- or hypointense compared to the stationary background tissue (47) (Figs. 2, 5, and 6). This technique allows visualization of the carotid arteries free of venous overlap, selective display of the aorta or inferior vena cava, examination of the intracranial venous system, and documentation of the direction of flow (39,40,49,50).

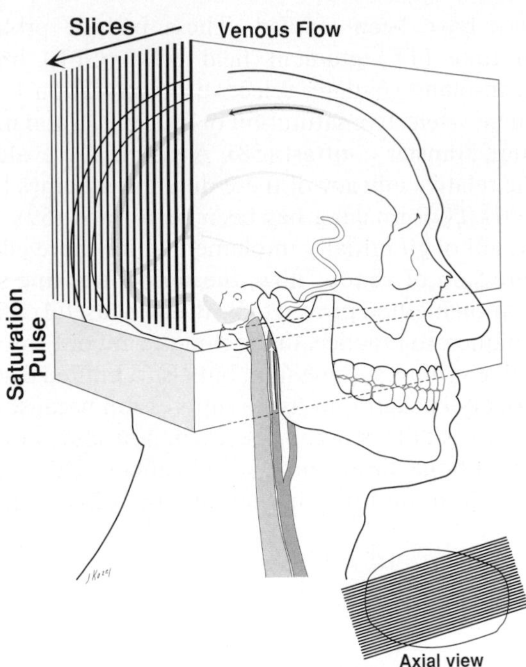

FIG. 6. Sequential 2D TOF MRV. Notice the oblique sagittal-oriented image acquisition reduces the number of slices and, thus, the acquisition time while still allowing unsaturated inflow into each slice. The inferiorly located saturation pulse saturates signal from inflowing arterial blood.

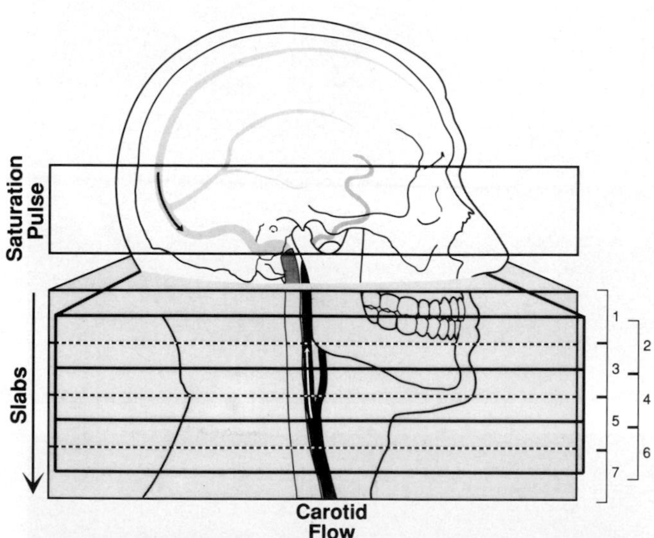

FIG. 5. Multiple overlapping 3D TOF slab technique schematic. This technique incorporates advantages of both sequential 2DFT and 3DFT exams. The axially oriented partitions maximize flow-related enhancement. The smaller 3D slabs allow thin contiguous slices to avoid flow saturation. Note the slabs are acquired in a craniocaudad direction to avoid saturation effects. With the implementation of a ramped radiofrequency pulse, larger 3D volumes are used because flow saturation is reduced with this technique. A superior saturation suppresses venous signal.

Black Blood Angiography

Despite the use of short echo times, gradient refocusing, and small voxels, the inflow or "bright blood" MRA techniques still occasionally suffer from signal loss in regions of complex flow secondary to superimposed spin-phase phenomena. This can produce signal loss leading to overestimation of stenoses or signal drop-out. One possible solution has recently been applied to the carotid bifurcation, which renders the blood "black" by presaturating inflowing arterial blood below the region of interest. Additionally, arterial spins are intentionally dephased as they flow along the imaging gradients by using relatively long echo times. Projection angiograms can be produced using a "minimum-intensity" projection method analogous to the "maximum-intensity" algorithm described for so-called bright blood methods. In this technique the presence of complex flow actually adds to vessel contrast, possibly allowing more accurate evaluation of stenoses (51,52).

Advances in TOF

Many alternative acquisition schemes to better suppress the stationary tissues and thus improve MRA images have been studied. These include prolonged echo time (TE) gradient field echo (GFE) imaging (53); in-plane spatially selective presaturation (54,55); frequency-selective saturation of fat (56,57); and magnetization transfer contrast (58). A systematic evaluation of the relative efficacy of these different schemes for 2D and 3D TOF imaging has been performed (59). Ironically, although initially implemented for more effective suppression of venous flow, the simple tracking spatial saturation method proved to be the most useful of the 2D techniques. In practice, this technique not only provided effective venous suppression, but also a limited degree of stationary background tissue suppression because of the slight cross-talk between the excitation and saturation slices without diminishing vessel caliber. This suppression is more uniform and specific than 2D frequency-selective fat saturation because the excitation produced by the higher bandwidth pulses (defining the tracking saturation pulses) is better defined and essentially insensitive to local field inhomogeneities.

Although originally viewed as a means of isolating vascular territories, work with spatially variable excitation and presaturation techniques has yielded additional improvement in image contrast, particularly at higher resolution matrices among the 3D sequences for the intracranial circulation (59–62). The most effective method of background suppression without significantly compromising vessel morphology is the combination of afrequency-selective fat saturation pulse, a superior spatial-saturation slab, and the shortest possible opposed–phase echo time (7 msec on a conventional 1.5 T imager) (Fig. 7) (Table 2) combined with magnetization transfer saturation pulses

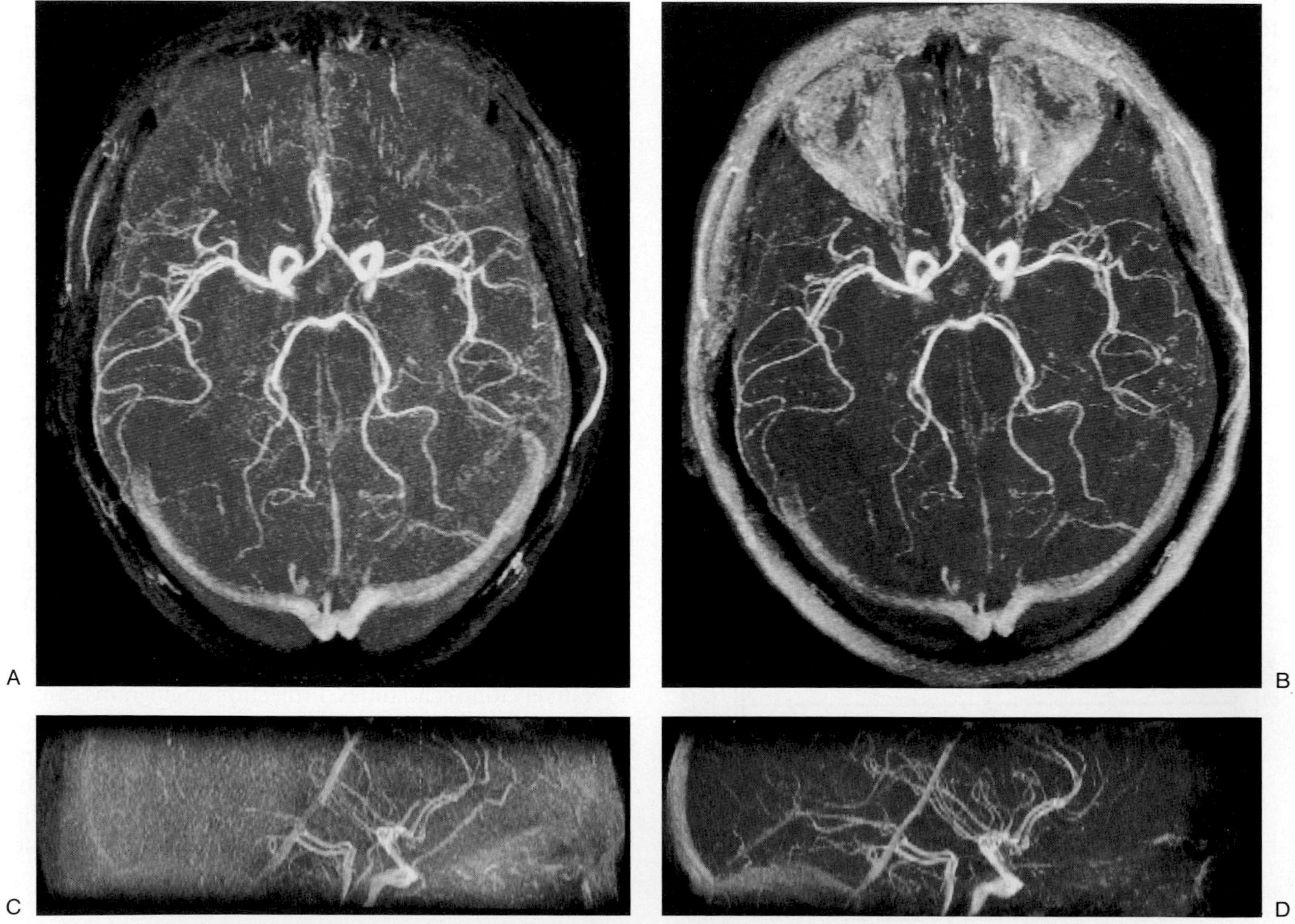

FIG. 7. Second order chemical shift artifact. Second order chemical shift artifact seen on GE images results from the transverse magnetization of both fat and water to be in phase. Because water and fat precess at slightly different rates as dictated by the main magnetic field, there are times during the decay that fat and water will be in or out of phase. **A,B:** Axial 3D TOF images at 1.5 Tesla with an echo time of 5 msec and 7.0 msec. Note the orbital and subcutaneous fat high signal intensity with the in-phase and low signal intensity with the out-of-phase acquisition with an echo time of 7.0 msec. The lateral projections (**C,D**) illustrate the image degradation by the overlapping fat.

TABLE 2. *Second order chemical shift effect*

Phase	Magnetic field strength 0.5 T (msec)	1.0 T (msec)	1.5 T (msec)
In	0	0	0
Out	6.8	3.4	2.3
In	13.6	6.8	4.5
Out	20.4	10.2	6.8
In	27.3	13.6	9.1
Out	34.1	17.0	11.4

Modified from Keller PJ, Drayer BP, Fram EK. *Neuroimag Clin North Am* 1992;2(4):643.

(Fig. 8). The background suppression is more uniform when compared to similar 2D sequences, and likely related to the larger bandwidth used in the 3D version for fat saturation and the greater number of rf pulses used to excite the 3D volume because of the second phase encoding gradient. The smaller voxels, shorter echo times, and spherical anatomy (of the head) also make it less vulnerable to T2*-related dephasing and flow-induced signal loss (59,63).

Recent interest in hybrid RARE (rapid acquisition with relaxation enhancement) sequences for conventional MRI has increased the awareness of the advantages of manipulating the way in which data are collected across *k*-space as a means to influence contrast and edge definition as displayed by MIP images (64–66). Data collected at the low spatial frequencies or central phase-encoding steps are the primary determinants of gross contrast in an image, whereas the data collected at the high spatial frequencies primarily determine edge definition and have proportionately less impact on contrast. Investigators have used these principles in MRA acquisitions to improve vessel/soft tissue contrast and reduce flow-related dephasing (67).

For example, despite the use of gradient motion refocusing, small voxels, and relatively short echo times in 3D TOF MRA sequences, there continues to be a variable degree of residual signal loss in regions of a stenosis or tortuosity. Although refocusing gradients are necessary to correct the phase errors related to first order motion (velocity), the most effective means of reducing the phase errors due to higher order motion is through the use of very short field echo times (68). With current gradient limitations in standard imaging systems, the shortest echo times achievable without gradient moment refocussing (GMR) and acceptable resolution are approximately 4.0 to 5.0 msec. At 1.5 T, this corresponds to an echo time at which the fat and water spins are in-phase such that background, stationary tissue is relatively bright and may obscure the adjacent vessels with conventional postprocessing algorithms (Fig. 7) (Table 2). The standard 3D TOF sequences can be modified to vary the echo time across *k*-space between a short in-phase (5.3 msec) and slightly longer out-of-phase (6.5 msec) echo times. As the low frequency data are the primary determinant of contrast, the signal of the orbital and subcutaneous fat can be reduced to that measured for a comparable constant TE = 6.5 msec 3D acquisition (67). The remaining phase-encoding steps are obtained with a TE of 5.3 msec because the delineation of the intracranial vessels requires sharp definition. Hence, this

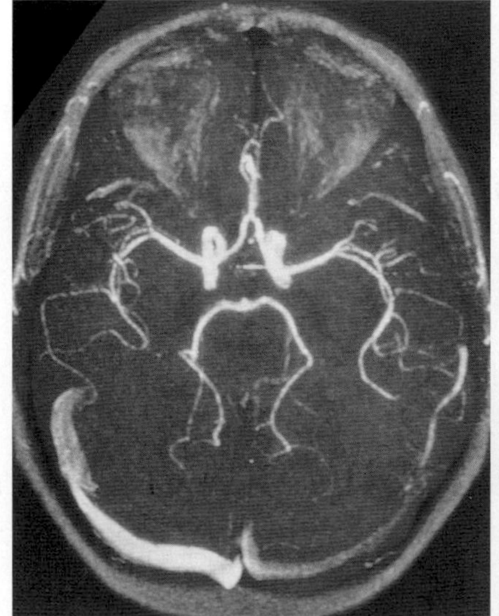
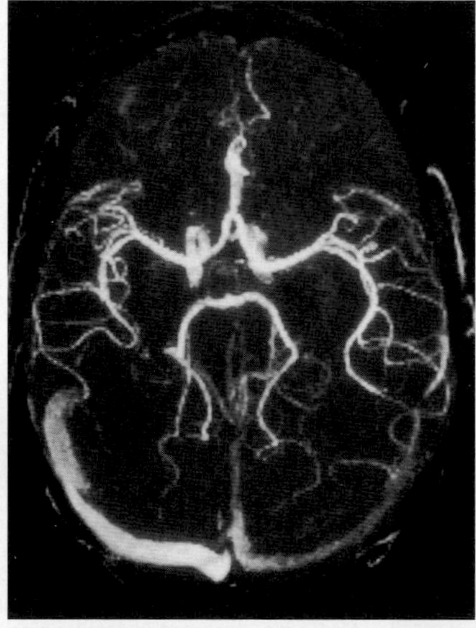
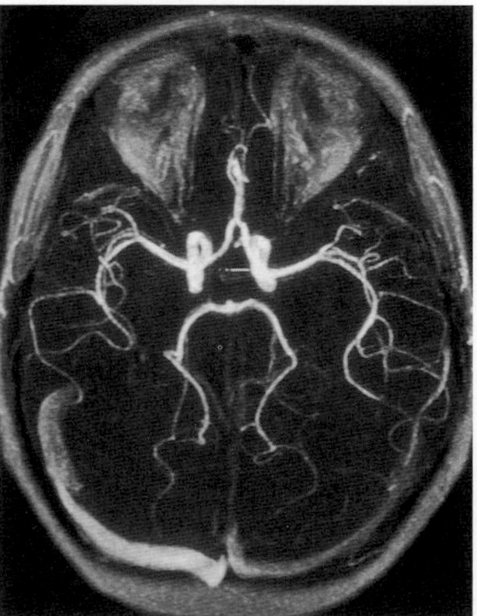

A B,C

FIG. 8. Effect of magnetization transfer. All imaging parameters were held the same. **A:** 3D TOF MRA axial image. **B:** The same image with application of magnetization transfer. Notice the superior background suppression of the brain tissue; however, the fat within the orbits and scalp is now accentuated. Note that because of the superior background suppression, the visibility of the intracranial vessels is increased. **C:** Application of magnetization transfer and fat suppression. Notice on this image the superior delineation of the vessels due to the superior background suppression from both magnetization transfer and fat suppression. (From Lin et al., ref. 60, with permission.)

technique produced effective fat suppression and, unlike the frequency selective fat saturation pulse, its performance was not compromised by static local field inhomogeneities, nor did it prolong the minimum sequence TR.

The relative speed of this method is in part due to the use of the MIP display that, in effect, replaces the acquisition of a mask image in order to produce an angiogram. This software is based on an MIP ray-tracing algorithm, projecting the 3D data set onto a 2D plane. Only the maximum voxel intensities encountered are written onto the projected plane, resulting in a single 2D projection view of all vessels within the entire 3D data set. The background signals are suppressed by nulling all pixels with signal intensities below a selected threshold. This may be performed at different angles, permitting a 360° rotational display of the data set around any axis (43,69).

Since the TOF MRA sequences are inherently T1- and spin density–weighted, any tissue with a short T1 or high spin density will appear relatively bright on the final MRA images and can lead to misrepresentation of vessel caliber and configuration on the MRA images (70). The most commonly used postprocessing (i.e., MIP) algorithm only identifies voxels of high signal intensity and cannot distinguish hyperintense tissues from bright vessels. Beyond modifications of the pulse sequence acquisition technique, other postprocessing computer algorithms have been adapted to MRA beyond the standard MIP. These include vessel tracking techniques that segment flow-enhanced vessels from stationary tissue in a 3D data set on the basis of contiguity of high signal voxels originating from an operator-selected seed point (71) (Fig. 9). This method is not exclusive of, and can be combined with, the MIP technique known as Targeted MIP (72). Atlas et al. have described another variation that uses a technique known as "soft thresholding" expanding the dynamic range of vascular information displayed in the image as well as depth cuing (Fig. 10) (73).

TOF Artifacts/Limitations

The clinical implementation of MRA has shown encouraging results in numerous applications; however, several characteristics of currently available techniques provide significant potential for misdiagnosis to the unwary, and as such merit special mention. While extremely helpful in visualizing the complex 3D nature of vascular anatomy, the MIP algorithm currently used for postprocessing results in loss of information, and may prevent the visualization of small or faint vascular structures (70,74). Since the TOF MRA sequences are inherently T1- and spin density–weighted, any tissue with a short T1 or high spin density will appear relatively bright on the final MRA images and can lead to misrepresentation of vessel caliber and configuration on the MRA

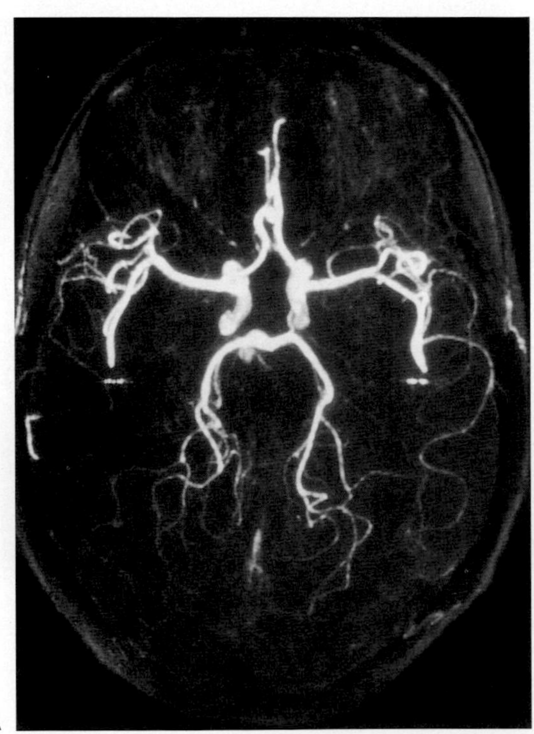

A

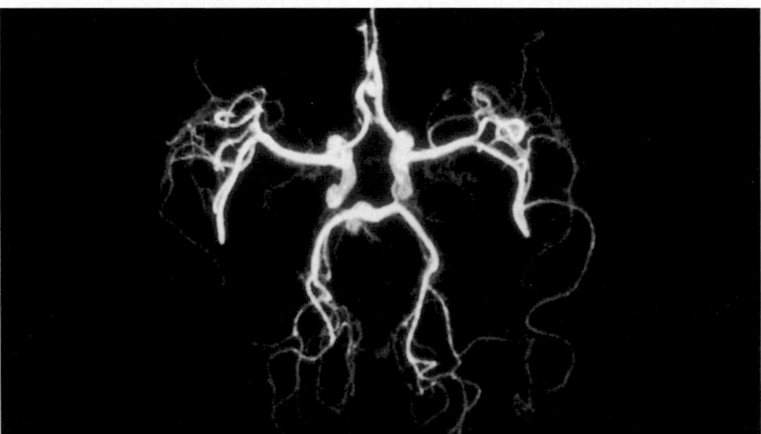

B

FIG. 9. Postprocessing algorithms. **A:** High resolution 3DFT TOF MRA of the intracranial vessels is demonstrated. The image of the data set was subjected to a maximum intensity projection postprocessing algorithm. Note the mild luminal irregularity and discontinuity of the normal vessels in the MRA image. **B:** Same data set submitted to a vessel-tracking postprocessing algorithm. Notice the vessels are more homogeneous in caliber and the background intensity dramatically suppressed. This is performed by placing a seed on the vessel of interest in the imaging volume and using localized thresholding so that the algorithm makes decisions whether the adjacent voxels represent background or are continuous with the same vessel. (From Lin et al., ref. 72, with permission.)

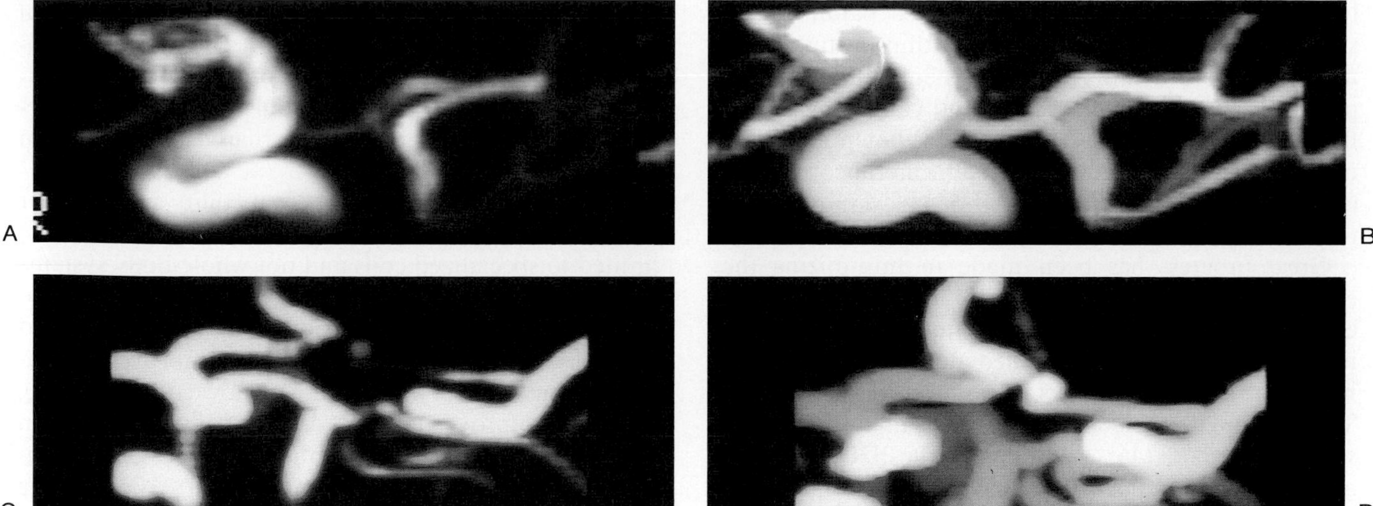

FIG. 10. Conventional MIP vs. STANDOUT postprocessing. **A,B:** Lateral view, normal circle of Willis on MIP postprocessing (A); note artifactual narrowing of cavernous carotid, areas of signal loss, and poor visualization of small vessels. Using STANDOUT (B), same data set shows better luminal definition, homogeneous intravascular signal, clear delineation of the posterior communicating artery, and depth cuing (ipsilateral carotid is higher intensity than contralateral). **C,D:** Aneurysm seen using STANDOUT, not visualized using MIP. Although no aneurysm is seen on MRA using MIP (C), clear demonstration of right basilar aneurysm and origin of right superior cerebellar artery are seen on STANDOUT (D). (From Atlas, ref. 73, with permission.)

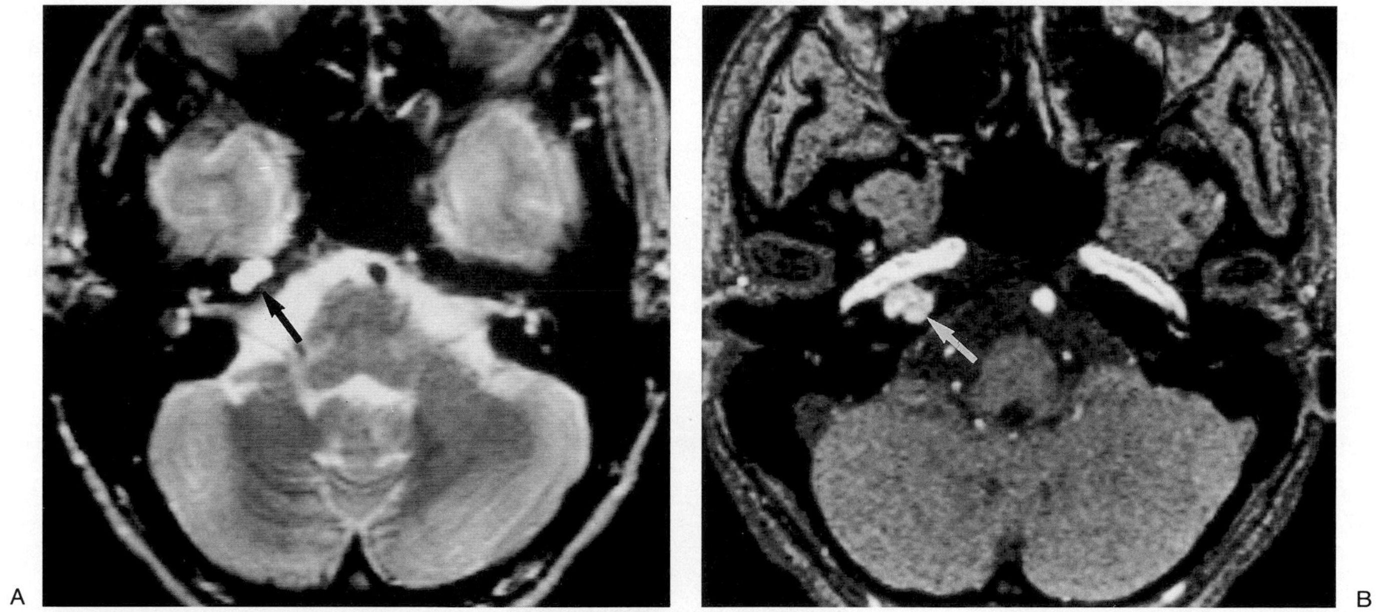

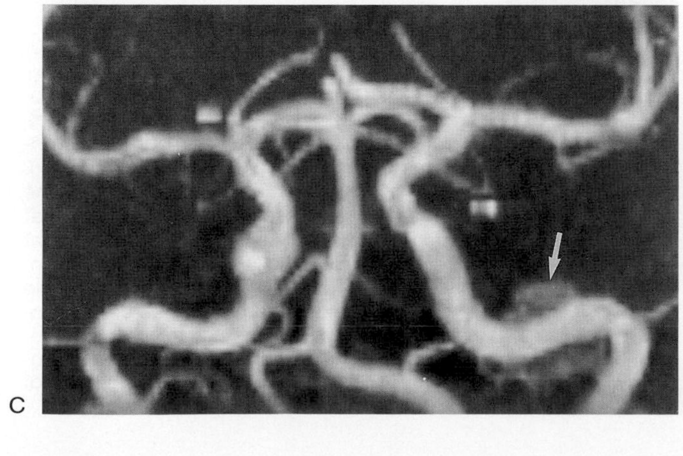

FIG. 11. Right petrous apex cholesterol cyst. **A:** Note the high signal intensity on the T2-weighted SE image just posterior to the right carotid canal (*arrow*). **B:** An axial 3DFT TOF MRA demonstrates the high signal intensity just posterior to the right petrous portion of the internal carotid artery (*arrow*). **C:** The maximum intensity imaging incorporates the high signal intensity from the cholesterol cyst into the angiogram, simulating a petrous carotid aneurysm (*arrow*).

images (59) (Fig. 11). For example, paramagnetic substances such as gadolinium within a tumor or methemoglobin within a subacute hematoma may appear bright on the TOF images, and can mimic active flow on the postprocessed images. This potential source of confusion can be avoided through careful correlation of the MRA to the standard MRI or by examination of the individual partitions or slices (Figs. 11, 12, and 13).

Great progress has been made in minimizing the effects of nonuniform or turbulent flow in MRA. However, areas of tight stenosis continue to display flow-induced signal loss at and immediately following the luminal narrowing. This effect is less pronounced with the TOF 3D and sequential 2D techniques than with phase-sensitive methods (46). Additionally, the 2DFT slices are generally thicker than the individual partitions of a 3DFT technique, resulting in a larger voxel size in the slice-select direction. Relative to the 3DFT method, this produces decreased spatial resolution in the slice-select direction and may lead to signal loss from increased intravoxel phase dispersion (discussed below). Also, the larger slice-select gradients necessary for the sequential 2DFT sequences generally prolong the minimum echo time relative to comparable 3DFT techniques. The optimization of vessel signal and reduction of flow artifact has been an area of keen interest, primarily as it relates to shortened gradient times and reduced spin dephasing (68,75–78). These efforts have been devoted both to innovations in image reconstruction as well as system hardware. The use of conventional pulse sequence design and reconstruction techniques strongly favors the use of some form of 3D TOF acquisition with first order flow compensation for delineation of the cerebral arterial tree (45,46,68,79,80). Reductions in echo time are possible in conventional systems with strategies such as truncated asymmetric rf pulses, partial Fourier reconstruction in the read direction, and alternative reconstruction methods (81).

Improved gradient hardware capability may further enhance such sequences, but until recently this has been limited to specialized coils and not whole-body systems (68). Recent technological developments that have increased the interest and diffusion of fast SE (RARE) and echo-planar imaging (EPI) should also improve the contrast and resolution of clinical MR flow studies (64,82). The same improved gradient capabilities and coil design (hardware) provide the potential for even greater improvements in routine MRA imaging (68). The absolute echo time determines signal loss due to T2* decay processes as well as to losses incurred because of motion through static local field inhomogeneities. Additional motion-induced dephasing results from motion through the applied imaging gradients, the severity of the associated signal loss depending on the gradient duration and timing (field echo) and the gradient strength (68,75). When conventional 2D and 3D TOF MRA sequences are compared to sequences incorporating the higher gradient capabilities with ultra-short echo times (but otherwise similar), the greatest single factor affecting the visualization of the simulated carotid stenoses was the field echo time (41,48,68,75). Higher order motion terms are expected within and immediately distal to a high grade stenosis. This explains the dramatic improvement in the size of the post-stenotic flow void and the visualization

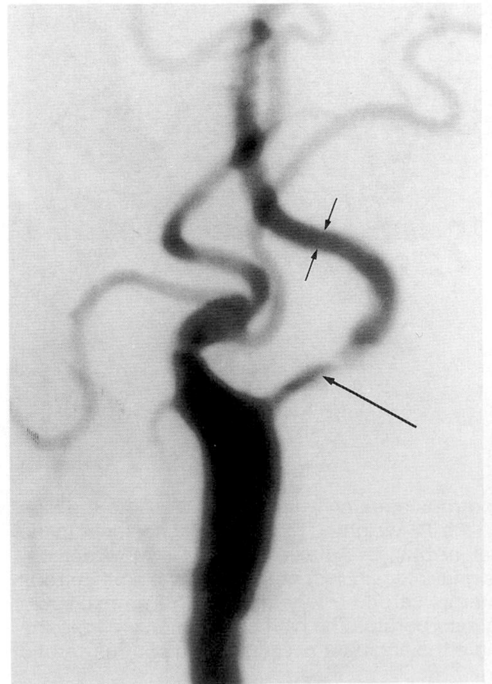

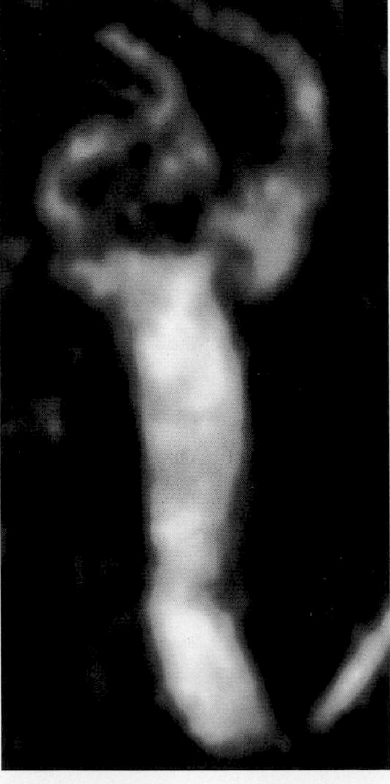

A,B

FIG. 12. Catheter digital subtraction angiogram and 3DFT TOF MRA of the carotid bifurcation. **A:** The catheter angiogram demonstrates a very severe stenosis (*long arrow*). The two facing *short arrows* demonstrate the normal arterial vessel segment diameter that would be used for calculation of the percent of stenosis using the NASCET criteria. **B:** Notice that the 3D TOF MRA does not resemble the catheter angiogram because of incorporation of high signal intensity from a mural hematoma (hemorrhagic plaque) in the angiogram. This is one of the potential pitfalls of MRA of the carotids.

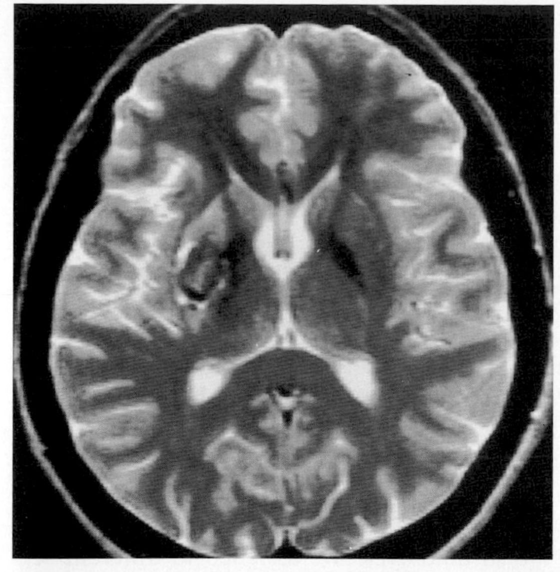

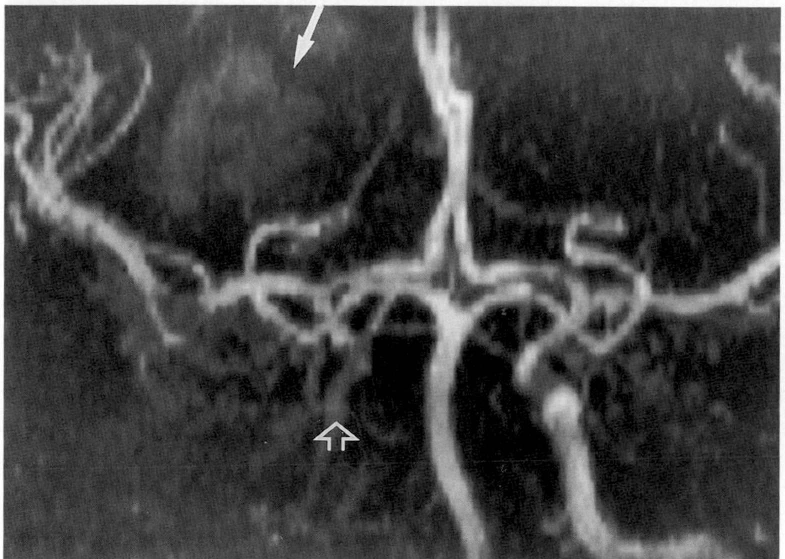

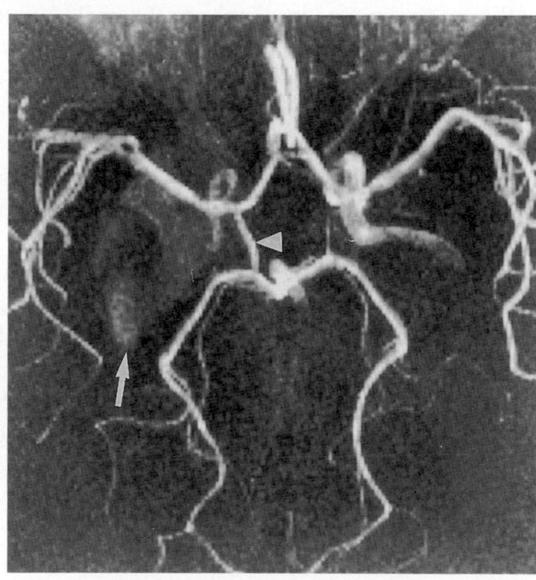

FIG. 13. Acute occlusion of the right internal carotid artery and hemorrhagic infarction of the right lentiform nucleus. **A:** The T2-weighted SE image demonstrates the hemorrhagic infarction within the lentiform nucleus. **B,C:** The 3DFT TOF MRA demonstrates minimal signal in the right carotid siphon, most likely due to retrograde flow (*open arrow*). Note the slightly diminished signal intensity in the MCA branches on the right when compared to the left due to the slower flow. In addition, there has been incorporation of the hemorrhage into the MIP algorithm (*arrow*). Notice the patent posterior communicating artery on the right side (*arrowhead*).

of the stenotic segment itself when standard sequences were replaced by the sequences designed for higher gradient capabilities. As noted by Evans et al., the field echo time should be the most important consideration and the results with longer read field echoes tended to parallel the changes seen with longer absolute TEs (75). The read field echo is affected by the receiver bandwidth, necessitating the use of longer gradients along this direction (as compared to the brief slice-select gradients applied in 3D). Consequently, with the exception of those sequences that do not employ higher than zero order GMR, the read field echo is the primary limiting factor for reducing the absolute TE. The addition of first order flow compensation in the read and slice-select directions produces a further reduction in size of post-stenotic flow void for the central and eccentric stenoses despite the longer field and absolute echo times.

The third characteristic of note reflects the physics of inflow-based TOF angiography: bright signal requires not only flow, but unsaturated spins. A disadvantage to the use of such a wide slab of excitation/saturation is that, depending on the speed of flow (i.e., residence time within the volume) and frequency of rf pulses (i.e., TR), one may lose vascular contrast deep in the volume secondary to saturation effects. It is estimated that total loss of flow-related enhancement occurs after 10 to 20 excitations (48). Although rapid arterial blood flow can retain sufficient flow-related enhancement to be successfully imaged over small regions of interest (such as the intracranial circulation or cervical carotid arteries), slowly moving venous, peripheral arterial, or pathologically slowed arterial flow may become sufficiently saturated over even small imaging volumes to prevent visualization. Thus, inflow-enhanced 3DFT methods currently appear limited to relatively small regions of rapid flow (i.e., arteries of the head and neck). Care must be taken when using the 3DFT methods to allow for adequate inflow through choice of repetition time, flip angle, and volume thickness. An inappropriate selection of parameters may result in a false appearance of vessel tapering. Such causes of signal loss, such as in-plane spin saturation, may be minimized through the administration of paramagnetic contrast material (45,83).

Spin saturation can also be circumvented without the use of contrast and without affecting examination time, by incorporating specialized radiofrequency pulses for excitation (84). These rf pulses are designed to increase linearly along the major axis of flow so a lower flip angle is applied where the flowing spins enter the volume and higher flip angles are applied distally where the vessel/soft tissue contrast would normally be limiting (79,85) (Figs. 3 and 5). Background suppression can be simultaneously performed with fat saturation and magnetization transfer pulses. Compared to the conventional MRA pulse sequences, distal small vessel visualization is improved because of the background suppression and the specialized rf pulses intracranially (Fig. 8). This is most obvious when intracranial studies are reconstructed at matrices of 512^2. In the neck, the distal cervical internal carotid arteries are well visualized despite severe stenoses at the bifurcations and slow antegrade flow distally.

The use of small, stacked 3D volumes is even more effective at reducing the problem of spin saturation (79,86). In effect, this technique combines the 2D advantages of reduced spin saturation and the short TEs and small voxels of the 3D TOF MRAs. When combined with the spatially variable rf pulses, it is possible to increase the size of the volumes, reduce the degree of overlap between the volumes, and reduce the number of volumes necessary to cover the region of interest (87) (Fig. 5).

As noted above, data collected at the low spatial frequencies or central phase-encoding steps are the primary determinants of gross contrast in an image, whereas the data collected at the high spatial frequencies primarily determine edge definition and have proportionately less impact on contrast. Investigators have used these principles in MRA acquisitions to improve vessel/soft tissue contrast and reduce flow-related dephasing (64,65,67).

Variation in the TR across *k*-space has been shown to improve vessel/soft tissue contrast and reduce acquisition time with 2D and 3D TOF acquisitions (88,89). In comparison to 2D studies, the 3D TOF MRAs are especially prone to spin saturation because the spins must flow a larger distance before exiting the imaging slab, typically residing for more than one TR interval within the imaging volume. Consequently, the moving spins experience multiple excitation pulses, and similar to the adjacent background stationary tissue, become saturated. Varying the TR across *k*-space is particularly appealing because it not only offers the possibility to limit saturation, but also potentially reduces the acquisition time. In a reverse centric acquisition (k_{max}/min to k_0), applying a longer TR interval to the lowest 22 (of 32) slice-select phase-encoding steps produced the greatest benefit in contrast and flow-related enhancement.

Although the longer TR also permits T1 relaxation of the soft tissues, it permits a longer, more effective magnetization transfer saturation pulse that improves the suppression of brain parenchyma by 10% beyond that which was possible with the constant, intermediate-length TR interval that is normally applied. The longer TR interval also allows for an additional frequency-selective fat saturation pulse to be applied immediately before the acquisition of the lower 15% of the slice-select spatial frequency information (89).

An analogous strategy can be applied in a more time-efficient manner if data acquired during different portions of the cardiac cycle are assigned to different segments of *k*-space (90). A 2D TOF sequence would seem more appropriate in this setting because of the short acquisition time relative to 3D studies, and mild improvements have been described compared to the conventional 2D sequence (90). When the lower spatial frequency data lines are acquired during systole, the rapid influx of fresh unsaturated spins provides strong flow-related enhancement in those data lines that primarily determine contrast in the image. Edge definition of the small vessels is primarily determined by the higher spatial frequency data lines that are acquired during the quiescent phase of diastole when flow artifacts should be minimized at the carotid bifurcation. Intracranially, the flow is more constant and should have less of an impact on vessel contrast and definition.

Phase-Sensitive Methods

Acquisition Techniques

Magnitude Subtraction

The use of motion-induced phase shifts, combined with subtraction, to produce projective MRAs was initially proposed in 1982 (91). The intravoxel velocity distribution may be modified by cardiac gating so that signal is alternately sampled in diastole (with a small range of intravoxel velocities/phase dispersion and high intravascular signal), or in systole (where the larger velocity distribution leads to signal loss from increased phase distribution and cancellation). The signal from stationary tissues is identical in systole and diastole, allowing subsequent magnitude subtraction of such images to yield an angiographic image (92).

Signal variability from flow-induced phase changes can be modified by several factors (see above). The simplest and possibly most effective method to limit signal loss is reduction of the echo time, which results in an exponential reduction in the motion-induced phase change. Alteration of the gradient configuration can be used to reduce signal loss from flow-induced phase shifts as well, with compensation gradients precisely designed to cancel the motion-induced phase change at the time of signal sampling (93). Images with and without these flow-compensation gradients can be obtained while maintaining other imaging parameters (TR/TE) constant in order to leave stationary tissue with the same signal allowing subsequent magnitude image subtraction to create an angiographic appearance (43,48,77,94–96).

Complex Subtraction ("Phase-Contrast")

A somewhat different use of gradient-modulated phase effects depends on detection of flow as a discrete phase shift, with subsequent complex data subtraction/phase reconstruction to produce the final angiographic image. This "phase-contrast" (PC) technique relies on paired data acquisitions with opposite bipolar flow-encoding gradient pulses, resulting in images with vascular signal approximately proportional to the velocity-induced phase shifts (97–99). As with the other phase-sensitive techniques, stationary tissue has identical signal on both acquisitions and thus subtracts out. Advantages of these phase-sensitive methods include their high sensitivity to slowly flowing protons, such as venous blood, as well as high vascular contrast resulting from excellent stationary tissue subtraction. Chung et al. compared the effect of magnetization transfer (MT) with or without ramped excitation in 3D TOF MRA to 3D PC for intravascular signal versus background (100). That study evaluated both large arteries [supraclinoid carotid and middle cerebral artery (MCA)], as well as small distal branches, and can be summarized by three findings: (a) a statistically significant improvement using MT in intracranial TOF MRA, (b) a small improvement using ramped excitation, and (c) a dramatic improvement using PC over any combination of MT +/− ramped excitation TOF. Therefore, regardless of the methods used to optimize the intravascular signal of 3D TOF intracranial MRA, there is a significant improvement from 3D PC. The gradient-sensitive techniques have the additional advantage of no requisite cardiac gating.

Phase-Sensitive Postprocessing

For sensitivity to flow along all three imaging axes, both the magnitude-subtraction (including rephase/dephase subtraction) and complex phase-subtraction techniques require three image sets, each sensitive to flow in each direction (e.g., readout, slice-select, or phase-encoding) with at least one additional reference scan to serve as the "mask" (101,102). The paired images may be integrated into a single acquisition by alternating (i.e., interleaving) phase-sensitive y-steps. This interleaved approach helps to reduce misregistration artifact secondary to motion between paired acquisitions. The three subtraction images can be analyzed separately, or combined to generate the final angiographic image. Unfortunately, the need for multiple acquisitions prolongs examination time, making such studies susceptible to gross patient motion.

Artifacts/Limitations

Implementation of flow-sensitive gradients requires additional time before signal sampling, thus prolonging TE. This is particularly disadvantageous in regions of fast nonuniform motion and in GE sequences that are sensitive to other T2* effects that may degrade image quality (99). The phase-sensitive techniques are particularly sensitive to image degradation from pulsatile flow, as well as instrument imperfections such as eddy currents (99). As with the phase-derived MR velocity measurements, signal phase aliasing is also a problem in vessels with complex or rapid flow.

It is important to appreciate that MRA is young technology; new insights into the mechanisms of flow-induced signal changes and more robust techniques with fewer artifacts (not only at the bifurcation but also at the circle of Willis) are not only on the horizon but in some instances currently available. Advanced gradient designs and more sophisticated acquisition schemes/postprocessing will continue to provide significant improvement in image quality and diagnostic accuracy over the next several years.

CLINICAL APPLICATIONS

MRA provides high-quality, reproducible images as well as flow measurements that can be applied to many types of cerebral vascular anatomy and pathology. Essential additional diagnostic information can be obtained in patients undergoing a parenchymal MRI, as well as in patient populations in whom the risk/benefit ratio of catheter arteriography is considered high. The TOF MRA-based techniques are both rapid and easily acquired as an additional pulse sequence in conjunction with a conventional parenchymal MR examination. Phase-contrast MRA studies have advantages, notably the ability to quantify flow velocities, volumes, and direction. Understanding of the relative advantages and disadvantages of the currently popular MRA methodologies (primarily TOF and PC) maximizes the diagnostic information obtained for a particular patient. Differing techniques often are complementary; combinations of techniques provide the necessary data for an accurate diagnosis and treatment planning. The relative strengths and weaknesses of the most commonly used TOF and PC techniques are presented in Table 3.

Extracranial Circulation

It is beyond the scope of this chapter for a full discussion of cerebrovascular ischemic disease; however, it is important to articulate the pathophysiology of cerebral ischemia and infarction. Several basic mechanisms have been identified resulting in ischemia and ischemic infarction, including global or local perfusion failure (as in systemic hypoperfusion) vascular occlusion from embolic events or propagation of thrombus. Clinically, characteristic signs and symptoms will often aid in differentiating the vascular territories involved and will aid in the direction of the MRA exam.

Carotid Territory Atherosclerosis

The interest in carotid imaging relates to the high incidence of thromboembolic ischemia and stroke in the United States resulting from surgically accessible lesions (103–110). Atherosclerotic carotid artery disease results in cerebral ischemia in several ways, including decreased blood flow due to stenoses, and by thrombotic or atheromatous embolization at sites of plaque ulceration that may be quite small (109–118). Thus, successful thorough evaluation of the carotid bifurcation requires both accurate depiction of the degree of luminal narrowing as well as demonstration of arterial wall irregularity.

Clinical Background

In the mid 1980s, prominent cerebrovascular experts questioned the clinical rationale justifying the increasing number of carotid endarterectomies performed in the absence of studies supporting beneficial patient outcome (119–122). Specifically, the first large randomized trial published by the Joint Study of Extracranial Arterial Occlusion revealed no difference in total number of strokes and death between the medical and surgical groups if both perioperative morbidity and mortality were included in the analysis (123). Subsequent studies failed to support conclusively benefit to patients undergoing carotid endarterectomy; however, most of the studies were not well designed. Patient selection criteria was poorly controlled and wide variation in perioperative complication rates was noted (121,122,124). Thus, a considerable amount of controversy was generated because of the numerous anecdotal cases supporting the efficacy of carotid endarterectomy.

Subsequently, efforts to define the role of endarterectomy through a carefully controlled definitive multicenter clinical trial were initiated (125). To date, the North American Carotid Endarterectomy Trial (NASCET) and the European Carotid Surgery Trial (ECST) have addressed some of the controversial issues concerning carotid endarterectomy (126–128). The NASCET objective was to determine whether carotid endarterectomy in combination with the best medical therapy was superior to the best medical treatment alone in patients with carotid stenoses and transient cerebral ischemia or partial stroke (129). The study goal was accomplished by a large, randomized, multicenter trial with strict inclusion and exclusion criteria. Multiple layers of quality control were incorporated in the study to insure proper patient selection and to minimize operative morbidity. Both randomized and nonrandomized patient data were collected and the data underwent careful statistical analysis by independent observers.

A segment of NASCET was stopped when it was recognized that patients with 70% to 99% diameter reduction of the carotid artery who had been treated with carotid endarterectomy had an absolute reduction in stroke risk of 17% at 2 years over the medically managed patient (129,130). The benefits were directly related to the severity of the stenosis, that is greater for a stenosis of 99% than 85% or even 70% stenosis. One important exclusion criterion was that of a tandem stenosis, a finding in 2% of this population. Tandem stenoses are serial stenoses involving the ipsilateral carotid bifurcation and a vessel such as the carotid siphon or MCA. Careful analysis of the data by Schuler et al. reveals that there were

TABLE 3. *Comparison of 2D and 3D TOF MRA*

	2D TOF	3D TOF	3D TOF MOTSA	2D PC[a]	3D PC[a]
Slow flow	+++	+	++	+++	+++
Fast disturbed flow	++	+++	+++	+	+
Resolution	+	+++	+++	+	+
Signed/noise	+	+++	+++		
Contrast/noise	++	+	+	+++	+++
Acquisition time	+++	+++	++	+++	+

[a] Requires a priori selection of velocity to be measured.
2D, two-dimensional; 3D, three-dimensional; TOF, time-of-flight; MOTSA, multiple overlapping thin slab acquisition; PC, phase contrast; MRA, magnetic resonance angiography.

no intra-/perioperative strokes and one death (2.1%) in patients with bifurcation disease only, whereas patients with both bifurcation and distal stenoses had 11.4% intra-/perioperative strokes and a morbidity of 9.1% (130,131). Other authors support the notion that patients with tandem stenoses are at additional risk for both types of stroke but also are more prone to significant cardiac complications (132). In addition, 2.6% of NASCET patients harbored intracranial aneurysms; 16% of these aneurysms were felt to be clinically important (133). Therefore, evaluation of both the common carotid bifurcation using the NASCET criteria in addition to the remaining extra- and intracranial circulation is not only sound medicine but probably standard of care (129,130).

The role of carotid endarterectomy in symptomatic stenoses less than 70% diameter reduction is currently not well established; however, this is currently being evaluated as NASCET continues (127,128). It is important to recognize that the severity of the stenoses were carefully calculated from the most severe stenosis demonstrated on a selective catheter angiogram. The percentage of the carotid artery narrowing was determined in a specific fashion (stenosis/normal distal lumen × 100), a standard that has been adopted by the surgical community (134,135) (see Fig. 12).

The NASCET trial has established a well-defined practice standard for preoperative evaluation of the carotid bifurcation: angiographically demonstrated and specifically measured stenosis in the absence of significant tandem lesions. Nevertheless, the authors of the NASCET report also stressed that the risk of angiography be considered when evaluating patients for endarterectomy and suggested the possible use of a noninvasive examination to screen potential catheter angiography candidates, thus sparing patients with nonsurgical disease this risk (136,137). Recently, there have been efforts to establish an entirely noninvasive approach to the preoperative imaging of patients with symptomatic carotid arterial disease through a multimodality approach using color Doppler ultrasonography and TOF MRA (138–140). A study reported by Polak et al. was designed to show that US in combination with MRA compares favorably to catheter angiography, thus fulfilling NASCET imaging standards for evaluation of bifurcation disease. Although the future of MRA supplanting catheter angiography is promising for imaging of occlusive disease of the carotid arteries, there remain unanswered questions: Does MRA/US characterize stenoses of 70% to 99% severity, distinguish complete occlusion from severe stenosis, and exclude tandem stenoses as accurately as catheter angiography (140)? These questions may also have to be evaluated for less severe stenoses depending on the outcome of the ongoing NASCET trial (133). Only a prospective study of symptomatic patients with color Doppler US, MRI/MRA, and catheter angiography will adequately address these issues and to date has not been done (130,141). Therefore, the role of MRA in symptomatic carotid occlusive disease is in flux and continues to evolve, especially as more robust MRA techniques continue to emerge (130,133,141–145).

For asymptomatic carotid artery narrowing, early work concluded that the risk of carotid endarterectomy in this patient population was greater than that of medical therapy (146). In a recent prospective trial, "The Carotid Artery Stenosis With Asymptomatic Narrowing: Operative Versus Aspirin" (CASANOVA), the authors concluded that there is no significant difference between patients medically managed with daily acetylsalicylic acid and dipyridamole versus carotid endarterectomy (147). This study is very complicated, with many variables making any solid conclusion difficult (148). The results from the VA Asymptomatic Trial revealed that carotid endarterectomy prevented transient ischemic attacks, but no statistically significant benefit was demonstrated in preventing stroke or death (148–150). However, most recently the early data from the Asymptomatic Carotid Endarterectomy Trial (151) showed that stenoses greater than or equal to 60% of luminal diameter benefit from endarterectomy. Therefore, the assessment of the degree of carotid artery bifurcation narrowing is at this point essential to patient management.

Technical Background

The anatomic representation by MRA varies widely depending on the MRA technique employed. The carotid circulation has been most extensively studied using 2DFT and 3DFT TOF techniques (42,78). The 2DFT MRA techniques provide the highest degree of flow contrast, better for slow flow (i.e., are more resistant to saturation effects) and therefore better at distinguishing severe stenosis from occlusion (Fig. 14). Alternatively, 3DFT TOF MRA techniques possess higher spatial resolution and shorter echo times, making it more resistant to signal loss due to disturbed flow, and at and distal to stenoses. (Figs. 15, 16, and 17). Clinical studies of both techniques have shown reasonably good correlation with catheter angiography; however, these studies have varied significantly in pulse sequence details of echo time and flow-compensation schemes (76). Moreover, most of these studies were conducted before the NASCET results and, thus, criteria for measurement of stenoses is not standardized.

The anatomic display that 2DFT TOF MRA displays in severe stenoses is often a "flow void" or apparent vascular interruption. Although 2DFT TOF MRA has been demonstrated to be a highly sensitive screening exam, it may not be the most appropriate technique as the definitive (i.e., final) diagnostic study before angiography and subsequent surgery. Rather, its role is most suited for determining which patients do *not* harbor significant dis-

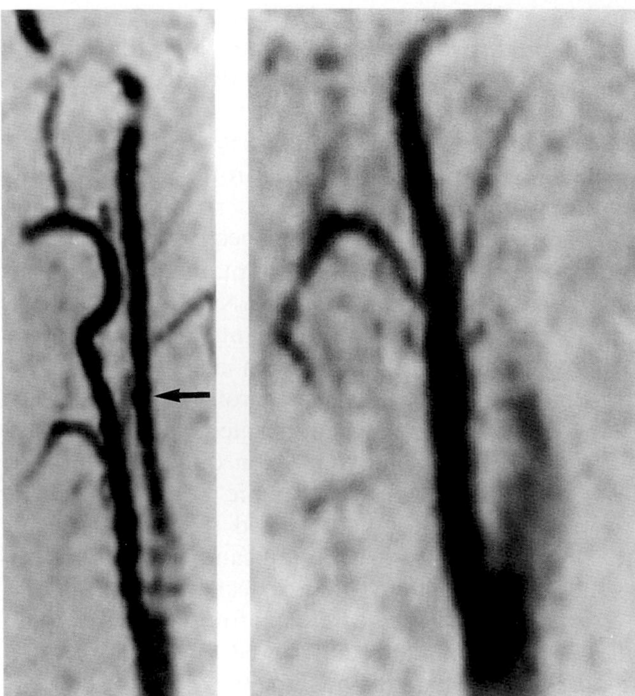

FIG. 14. Carotid artery dissection. **A:** 2D TOF of the left carotid artery demonstrating a patent internal carotid artery. Notice the size of the internal carotid artery (*arrow*) is equal to that of the external. Normally, the internal carotid artery is quite a bit larger than the external carotid artery branches. **B:** 3D TOF of the same patient. Note there is signal within the carotid bulb but, distally, the signal is not seen because of the extreme slow flow in this vessel.

ease, and hence need no further diagnostic studies. Most studies have compared 2DFT TOF MRA, or have paired US and 2DFT TOF MRA, to catheter angiography; to date there is insufficient data available that allow determination of the combined sensitivity, specificity, and accuracy for the evaluation of the carotid bifurcation and importantly distal disease (138,139,152–158). Review of the literature relevant to carotid MRA reveals several generalities: 2DFT TOF MRA overestimates stenoses with a wide variation in the correlation with catheter angiography from 35% to 79%. Most of the comparison studies had similar grading systems for stenoses, but evaluation of the percentage agreement within stenoses grades revealed some variation. In 13% to 23% of normal carotids 2DFT TOF MRA inappropriately demonstrate mild stenoses (related to the normal disturbed flow at the carotid bifurcation/bulb) (7,52,159–163). These studies indicate that the overestimation of stenoses is most problematic as the grade approaches the 70% benchmark. The significance of complete signal loss also has to be viewed with suspicion. Whereas in general complete signal loss on 2DFT TOF MRA is seen in more than 80% of stenoses greater than 70% severity, it also has been identified in stenoses of 50% (154,161,164). Alternatively, if a 2DFT TOF MRA only reveals a mild to moderate stenosis, the likelihood of the stenosis being significant by NASCET criteria is small. The technical parameters that are likely to result in overestimation in the mild to moderate severity group are longer echo times and larger voxel size (152,153,156).

Varying methods to reduce phase-shift effects have been used, including cardiac gating to diastole, flow-compensation gradients, short echo times, and small voxel size, with variable clinical success (38,42,48,77,78, 95–98,103,165,166). Current 3DFT and sequential 2DFT GE TOF methods typically include first order flow compensation, small voxel size, and the use of the shortest echo times possible (e.g., < 7 msec), resulting in successful imaging of carotid stenoses without cardiac gating (15,42,44,47,78,138,139,166,167). The dominant force in post-stenotic signal loss is related to the duration and strength of the gradient in the direction of flow; the echo time probably plays a less important role (75,168). As faster and stronger gradients become more available, these techniques will only become more powerful.

The sequential 2DFT TOF technique is typically applied in the axial plane, thus maximizing flow-related enhancement while necessitating relatively high gradient exposure in the direction of flow. The 3DFT TOF technique, alternatively, can be oriented in an axial, sagittal, or coronal orientation (42,78,169). With a sagittal or coronal approach, a local transmit-receive coil is used, limiting the region of excitation to prevent saturation of the

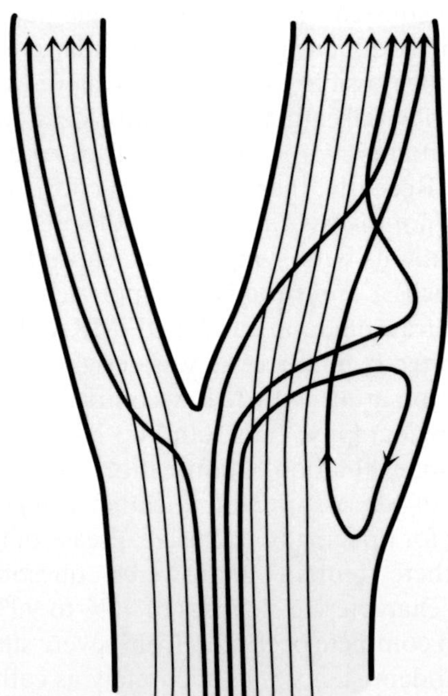

FIG. 15. Flow pattern in the normal human carotid. Note the heavy lines reflect flow resulting from the bifurcation flow divider. The blood flowing into the region of the carotid bulb is relatively stagnant, allowing progressive spin saturation. This is in part responsible for the frequent signal loss on TOF studies, especially 2DFT acquisitions. (Modified from Motomiya and Karino, ref. 162, with permission.)

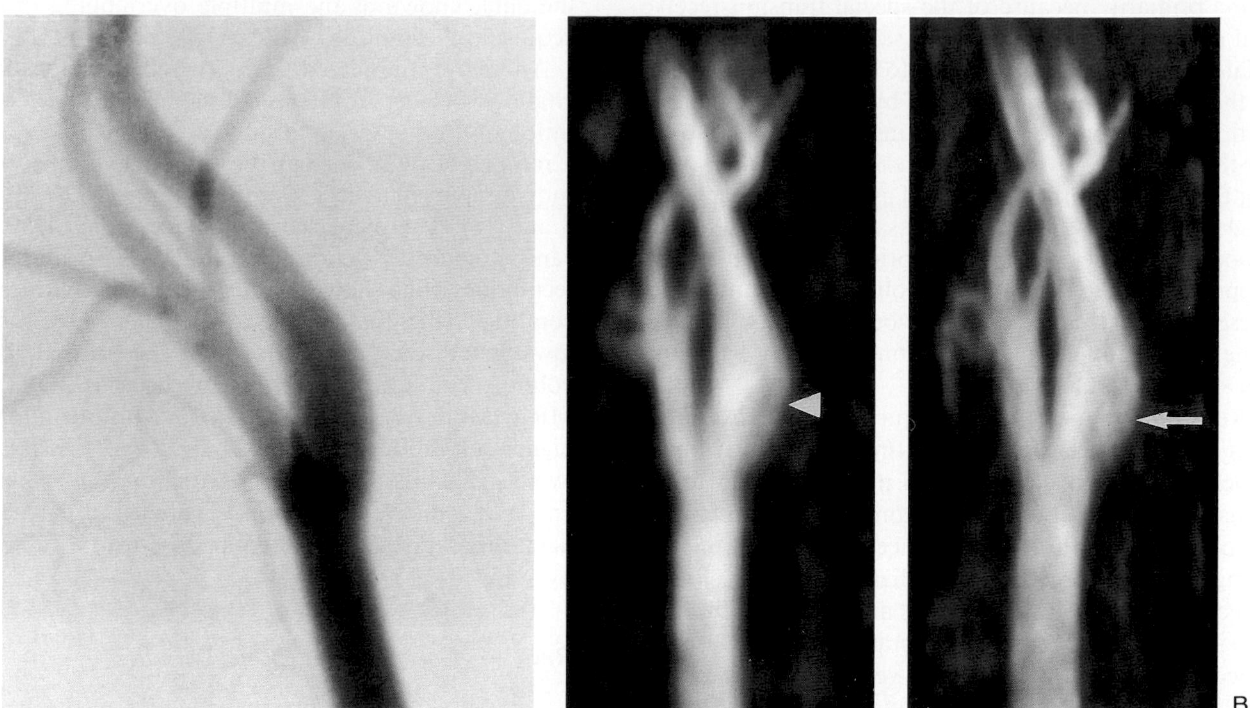

FIG. 16. Normal carotid artery bifurcation. **A:** Digital subtraction angiogram. **B:** 3D TOF MRA. **C:** 3D TOF MRA with ramped rf pulse. Notice the subtle loss of signal intensity in the carotid bulb (*white arrowhead*) resulting from the disturbed flow and recirculation due to progressive spin saturation. With the application of the ramped rf pulse, not only is there an improvement of the spin saturation in the distal internal carotid artery, but signal loss in the carotid bulb is not as striking (*arrow*).

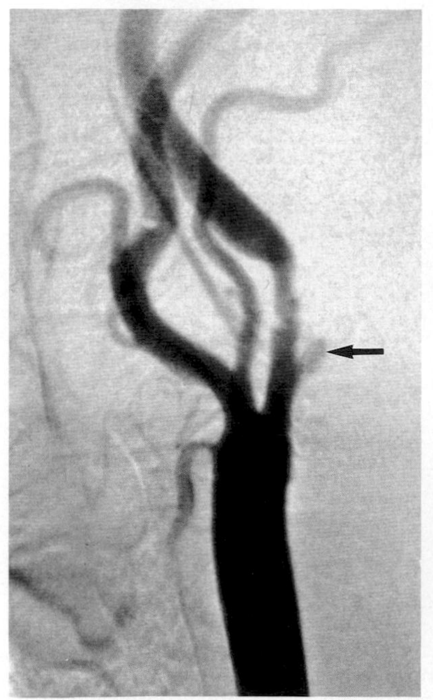

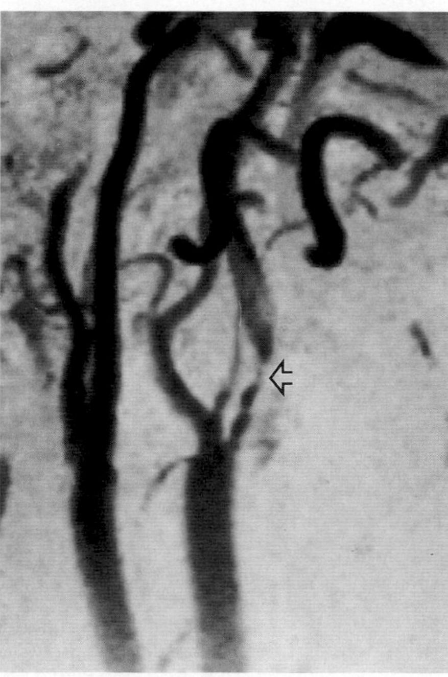

FIG. 17. A: Catheter carotid angiogram and **B,** 3DFT TOF MRA of the carotids (TE = 7.5) demonstrate a moderate long segment stenosis of the proximal internal carotid artery. Notice the outpouching along the margin of the stenosis on the conventional angiogram (*arrow*). The 3D TOF MRA accurately depicts the length of the stenosis; however, notice that the severity of the stenosis is overestimated (*open arrow*). Because of the slow flow within the outpouching, the flowing blood spins are saturated such that the outpouching is not visualized.

inflowing blood before entering the imaging volume. This approach is not used as commonly as the axial plane primarily because of the special transmit/receive coil necessary to implement the sequence. Loss of flow-related enhancement signal due to premature saturation of the inflowing blood is avoided by lengthening the repetition time (thus allowing fresh unsaturated blood to enter the imaging volume between excitations and increasing the acquisition time), as well as using a variable flip angle to decrease the progressive saturation of inflowing blood (170). The use of axially oriented, multiple overlapping thin-slab 3DFT TOF volumes also minimizes these technical considerations, but increases imaging time to cover an equivalent region of interest with similar spatial resolution.

Regardless of the TOF technique employed, examination of the cervical carotid is routinely performed with a superiorly located presaturation pulse to eliminate venous overlap. With coronal volume orientation, an additional presaturation slab is placed anterior to the imaging volume to prevent signal aliasing in the slice-select direction (169). With the sagittal and coronal 3DFT acquisition schemes, the presaturation slab is usually placed posteriorly, saturating the venous blood as it flows through the transverse and sigmoid sinuses. The axially oriented 3DFT method requires an axial presaturation volume above the imaging slab (Fig. 3), whereas the sequential 2DFT technique typically uses a traveling presaturation volume immediately cephalad to the imaging slice that shifts maintaining a constant distance above the scan plane (42,78) (Fig. 2).

Several modifications to these techniques have been proposed. First, the time of acquisition with the sequential 2DFT TOF technique can be reduced by aligning the phase-encoding gradient with the desired projection angle and reducing the number of phase-encoding steps (171,172). With this method, spatial resolution in the postprocessed angiogram at this projection angle is maintained; however, signal-to-noise is reduced, and there is potential for greater signal loss from the larger voxel size (44,45). Another modification relies on the black blood angiography techniques, which attempt to circumvent the problems of complex flow by exploiting them for the demonstration of the vessel lumen including stenoses (51,52,173). The black blood techniques are most successful in areas where the vascular anatomy is completely surrounded by higher signal soft tissue in regions with adequate anatomic separation of arteries and veins.

Recent advances in 3DFT imaging have addressed some of the issues of flow saturation and coverage. One method of decreasing flow saturation is to reduce the volume imaged; thus, the flowing blood is not exposed to as many rf excitations. This is especially important in situations of slower flow distal to severe stenoses and in small vessels. It is possible to capitalize on the advantages of 3DFT and 2DFT TOF techniques by employing multiple thin 3DFT TOF MRA volumes and combine the data, known as the multiple overlapping thin slab acquisition technique (MOTSA) (79,86,174) (Fig. 5).

Another technique, tilted optimized nonsaturating excitation (TONE), improves the signal loss due to desaturation of flowing blood through a volume by employing a ramped rf pulse so that the flip angle applied to the moving spins increases over the volume (169,170) (Figs. 3 and 18). The increased acquisition time of MOTSA can be reduced by combining the MOTSA and TONE techniques, thus allowing fewer but larger volumes to be combined (Fig. 5). The use of a smaller 3D volume allows better contrast-to-noise than the normal size 3D volume, but still not to the same level as 2DFT TOF MRA. Moreover, the 3DFT TOF technique allows for higher resolution (small voxel size) and the ability to avoid signal loss (shorter TE). To acquire MOTSA exam and avoid the venetian blind artifact (i.e., alternating light and dark bands) the volumes must be sufficiently overlapped (175) (Fig. 19).

Review of Carotid MRA Clinical Studies

In a critical evaluation by Kent et al. for the American College of Physicians, the diagnostic accuracy of nine of the more recent MRA articles addressing carotid bifur-

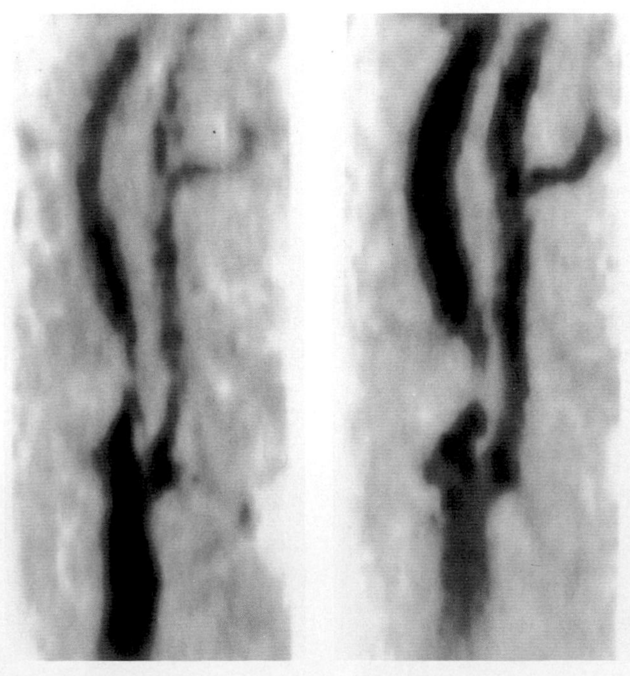

FIG. 18. The effect of a ramped rf pulse on signal saturation. Two 3D TOF MRAs of the same patient. **A:** As a normal slab and **B,** as a slab with a ramped rf pulse. Notice the progressive signal loss in the carotid arteries. This is manifested not only by diminished signal intensity but an apparent decrease in the lumen diameter.

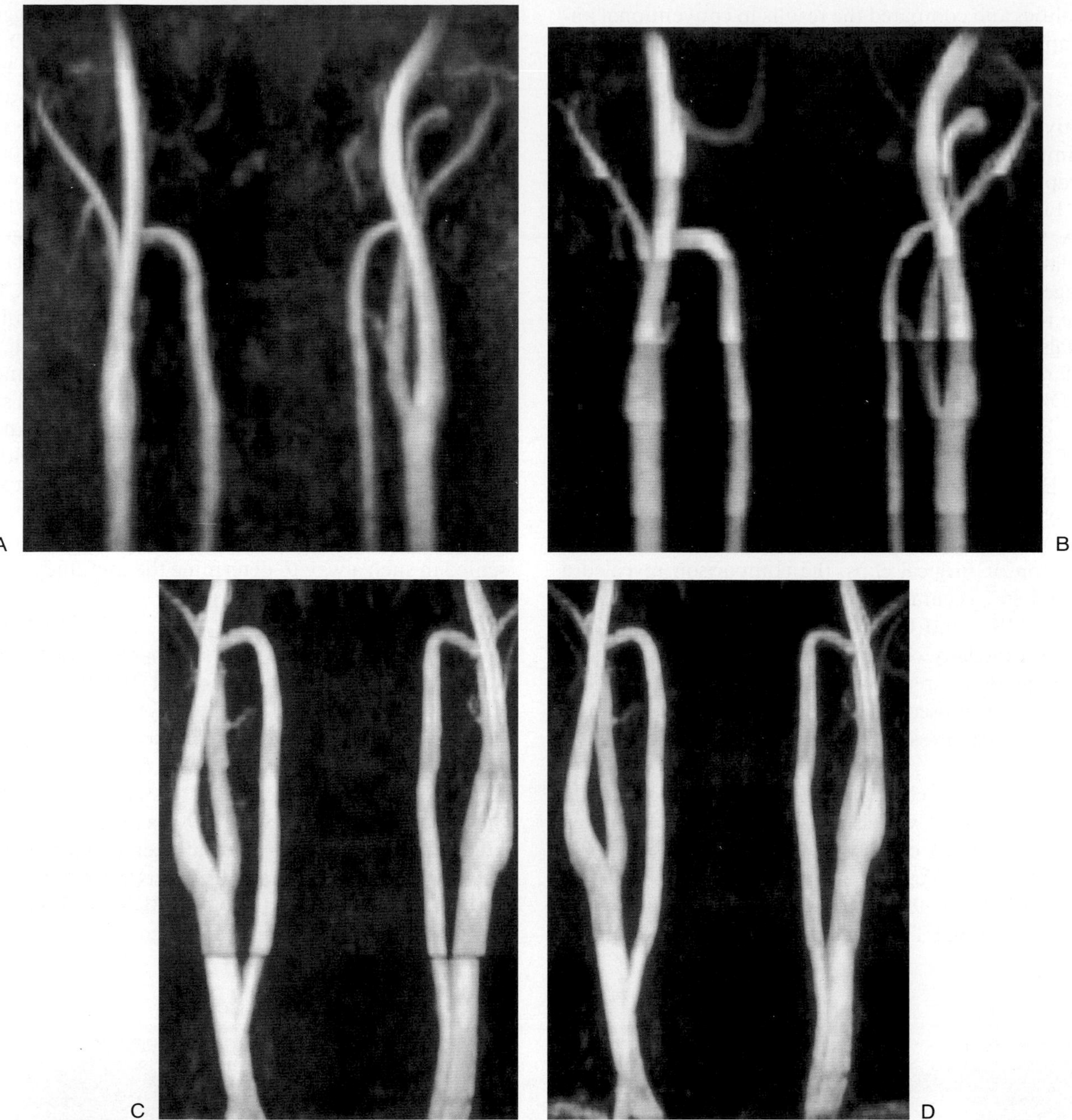

FIG. 19. Multiple overlapping slab technique. **A:** A single 3DFT TOF slab demonstrating progressive flow saturation as the image extends higher in the volume, as evidenced by the vessel tapering and the loss of signal intensity. **B:** Multiple overlapping thin slab acquisition (MOTSA) demonstrating the "venetian blind" artifact. Because of the use of the smaller imaging volumes, the effective spin saturation is not evident. **C:** Multiple overlapping thick slab acquisition with the use of a ramped rf pulse and manual integration of the slabs. Again, a "venetian blind" artifact can be seen in two locations with the integration of the three slabs. Note the uniform signal intensity and the lack of spin saturation through the use of the ramped rf pulse. **D:** Multiple overlapping thick slab acquisition with an automated algorithm integrating the three slabs. No demonstrable "venetial blind" artifact is seen. There is no loss of signal intensity due to spin saturation.

cation evaluation revealed a sensitivity of 0.86 to 1.0 and a correlation with conventional angiography in 50% to 90% of the arteries reported (145). The specificity varied from 0.60 to 0.98 (145). Polak et al. prospectively compared US and 2DFT TOF MRA in 42 bifurcations, demonstrating comparable sensitivities and specificities from both exams and correlating Doppler velocity changes with extent of MRA flow void (155). Yet, from the data presented it is not possible to determine combined sensitivity and specificity of the techniques nor how they complement one another with respect to diagnostic accuracy. Mattle et al. studied 39 vessels in 20 patients with both modalities and compared the results to conventional angiography (139). Contrary to Polak et al., they found 2DFT MRA (shorter echo times and confirmation of suspected lesions with a "black blood" technique) more sensitive and specific for stenoses greater than 70% than US. Importantly, they noted a 100% correlation with angiography when both US and MRA agreed (n = 30 vessels). Finally, Riles et al. likewise compared 2DFT TOF MRA, US, and catheter angiography and found that US correlated with catheter angiography in a greater percentage of cases (echo time not specified) (153). Notable in the reports of Riles and Mattle are both false-positive and false-negative MRA diagnoses of carotid occlusion. Similar findings were described by Buijs et al., although the 2DFT TOF MRA technique had relatively long echo times of 14 msec (163). Turnipseed et al. compared 2DFT TOF and 2DFT phase contrast MRA to duplex color Doppler and catheter angiography in 20 patients with symptomatic high grade stenoses. After excluding six carotids for technical inadequacies on MRI either due to motion or surgical clips, the comparison revealed a 91% and 86% accuracy for high grade stenoses or occlusion for MRA and US, respectively (138). Both MRA and US artificially converted two patients from a nonsurgical grade to greater than 70%. Both US and MRA accurately diagnosed carotid occlusion (138). None of these studies addressed the issue of disease distal to the bifurcation.

Mittl et al. (176) compared 2D TOF MRA to catheter angiography in 73 vessels of 38 patients in a blinded reader study. MRA demonstrated a sensitivity of 92.4%, specificity of 74.5%, and negative predictive value of 95.8% for 70% to 99% stenoses (i.e., surgical disease according to NASCET findings). Interobserver agreement was very high (κ = 0.91). The authors further suggested that combined high resolution 3D TOF with 2D TOF would obviate the overestimation of stenosis seen by 2D MRA alone (Fig. 20). In 35 of these patients, US was also compared to MRA. For the 70% to 99% stenosis cases, MRA had higher sensitivity and higher negative predictive value, but lower specificity and positive predictive value; these differences from US were not statistically significant. In that study, MRA had a clear advantage over US in the diagnosis of complete occlusion, where US had both false positives and false negatives, but MRA was 100% sensitive and specific. The issue of using combined MRA and US was also examined by Mittl et al., who found that even in those cases in which MRA and US both indicated 70% to 99% stenosis, a nonsurgical stenosis could still be found at catheter angiography. Pan et al. advocated the combined use of both 2DFT and 3DFT MRA sequences to accurately evaluate the carotid bifurcation. Their data showed a sensitivity of 0.92 and a specificity of 0.97; however, the data were not presented in such a way to determine the usefulness of each particular sequence (145,177).

Anderson et al. compared 2DFT, 3DFT TOF MRA, and color Doppler with x-ray angiography in 50 bifurcations. The findings concluded that 2DFT was complementary to 3DFT, and that 2DFT was better for slow flow and establishing vessel patency; however, 3DFT TOF MRA, because of its higher resolution, was preferred for "ulcer" detection or vessel wall irregularity. Spearman correlations were 0.94 between MRA (combined 2DFT and 3DFT) and catheter angiography, 0.85 between MRA and US, and 0.82 between US and catheter angiography. Interestingly, the 3DFT MRA detected 11 of 16 "ulcerations" and US detected none. It should

A,B

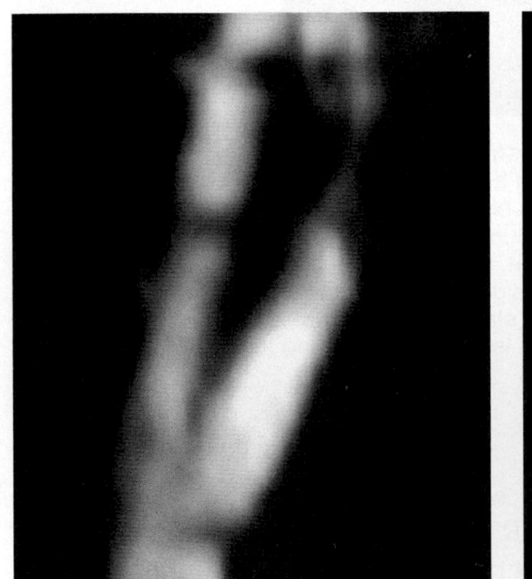

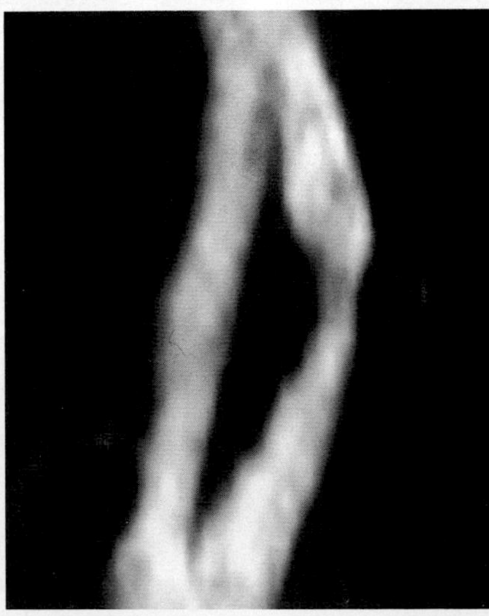

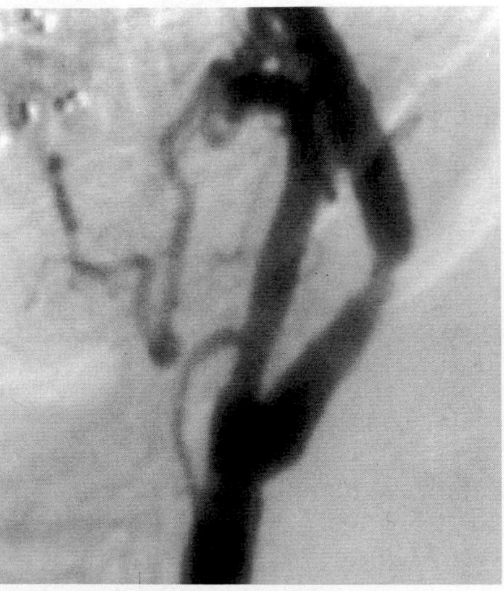

C

FIG. 20. Carotid stenosis, high resolution 3D TOF vs. 2D TOF. 2D TOF MRA (**A**) shows complete signal loss, implying tight stenosis in proximal internal carotid artery. High resolution 3D TOF (**B**) demonstrates only moderate narrowing, which matches catheter angiogram (**C**).

be noted, however, that the accuracy of the gold standard, catheter angiography, is quite low for carotid ulceration (178), so studies purporting to assess MRA or US for such pathology that are based on catheter angiography as proof should be considered with some skepticism. There were significant errors made both false positive and negative, which would alter management in five cases of US, but none involving MRA (167).

Quantification of carotid stenoses with MRA will continue to improve (38,42,78,154,155,158,162,163). From the previous discussion the largest obstacle is precise representation of stenoses in regions of disturbed flow at and immediately distal to the luminal narrowing (177) (Fig. 17). The "higher order" motion may result in significant phase dispersion, signal loss, and therefore nonvisualization of the involved arterial segment (75,77,177,179). Extensive effort has been directed at alleviating this signal loss.

Although potential solutions to the problems of imaging severe stenosis exist, the difficulties encountered in the evaluation of irregularities within atherosclerotic plaques are much more difficult to solve (Fig. 17). Not only are areas of plaque ulceration subject to disturbed flow, but clinically significant ulcerations may be below the limits of spatial resolution of MR techniques (113). Several studies have examined the appearance of atherosclerotic plaque on conventional MR, distinguishing hemorrhagic and calcific components on high resolution cross-sectional images (180,181). Occasionally, a hemorrhagic plaque may be a source of artifact, underestimating the severity of the stenosis (Fig. 12). Moreover, MRA evaluation of patients following head or neck surgery (especially carotid endarterectomy) may reveal artifactual stenoses or signal loss due local field heterogeneity from surgical hardware (Fig. 21). The comprehensive MR evaluation of carotid artery disease may require the application of multiple techniques at areas of disease in order to provide diagnostic and prognostic information unobtainable from the TOF angiogram alone.

The current role of MRA continues to be that of identifying patients *without* surgically correctable, significant stenoses at the carotid bifurcation, thus sparing these individuals an invasive study (129). Although many patients with symptoms referable to occlusive cerebrovascular will continue to be examined using MRA, we feel that MRA in this setting should be combined with MRI of the brain.

Carotid and Vertebral Artery Dissection

The etiologies of carotid and vertebral artery dissections include both intrinsic and extrinsic abnormalities of the vessel wall. The role of minor trauma in the absence of an arteriopathy has been questioned because of the difference in the clinical course of dissections resulting from severe trauma and spontaneous dissection or minor trauma (182–184). The association of intrinsic arteriopathies with dissection, including fibromuscular dysplasia, Marfans, Ehler-Danlos (IV), and cystic medial necrosis, is well known; it is estimated that 15% are related to underlying fibromuscular disease (182,184–186). Multiple cervical arteries may be involved at the time of diagnosis, although recurrent dissection is un-

A,B
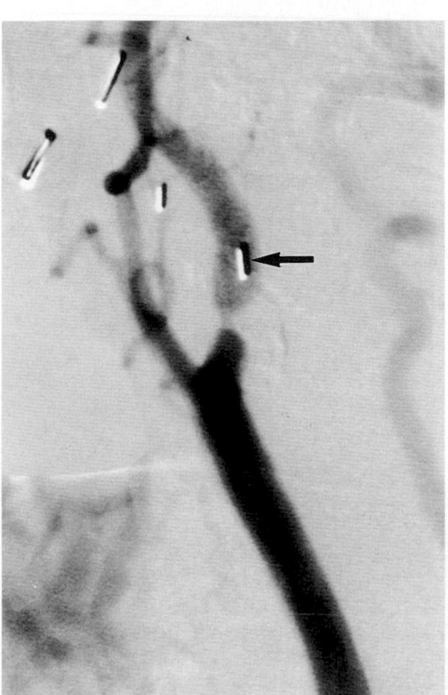
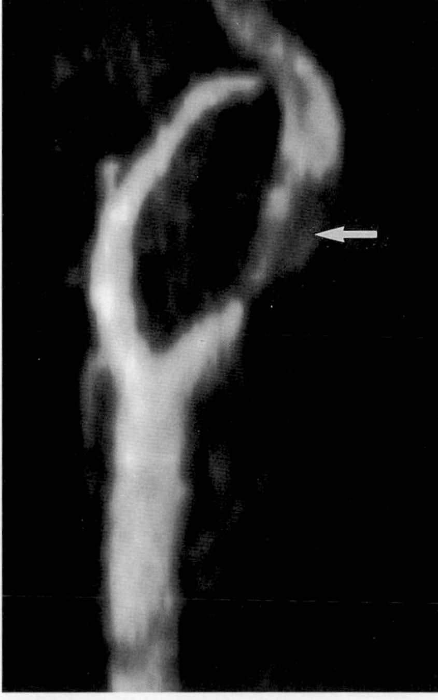

FIG. 21. A: Digital subtraction catheter angiogram and 3DFT TOF MRA of the carotid bifurcation. Notice the surgical clips overlying the carotid artery (*black arrow*) on the catheter angiogram, which results in susceptibility artifact (*white arrow*) and signal loss on the, **B,** 3D TOF angiogram, resulting in diminished signal intensity.

common and rarely involves the same vessel segment (182,184,187). When dissection recurs in the same vessel, a strong suspicion of an underlying arteriopathy such as fibromuscular disease must be considered (182). Whatever the etiology, the injury to the vessel consists of blood penetrating the intima into the vessel wall with variable (usually cephalad) extension, but rarely beyond the skull base (184–187). In contrast to extracranial dissections, dissections involving the intracranial vessels have a catastrophic clinical course (188–190). The involved vascular segment often produces a typical catheter angiographic pattern; specifically, subintimal dissections result in considerable luminal narrowing whereas subadventitial dissections often result in arterial dilatation (191).

Spontaneous Dissection

Clinical Background

Spontaneous dissection most often afflicts the cervical internal carotid artery, although common carotid artery involvement has been reported (185,192). Most often there is single vessel involvement, although additional cervical cephalic vessels are afflicted in one third of patients (185). In addition to luminal compromise and vessel thrombosis, irregularity and pseudoaneurysms may occur (183,184,192) (Fig. 22). Pathologically, the hematoma is usually between the intima and the media, but rarely is subadventitial (183). Imaging strategies for dissection have traditionally rested with catheter angiography; however, MRI with MRA probably represents the most efficacious method of evaluation of a patient with a clinical suspicion of dissection (193).

Technical Background

Levy et al., in a prospective blinded study, compared MRI to 3DFT TOF MRA to conventional angiography in a series of 19 patients with spontaneous or traumatic dissections comprising 19 carotid and 5 vertebral vessels (193). MRI and MRA demonstrated an excellent sensitivity and specificity of 84% and 99% and 95% and 99%, respectively (193). However, the vertebral arteries studied revealed a sensitivity and a specificity of 20% and 100% for MRA and 60% and 58% for MRI (193). The MRI and MRA findings consist of an "enlarged" vessel with an intramural hematoma (193–195). In addition to the enlarged vessel on MRI, there is an eccentric signal void with surrounding semilunar-shaped signal intensity

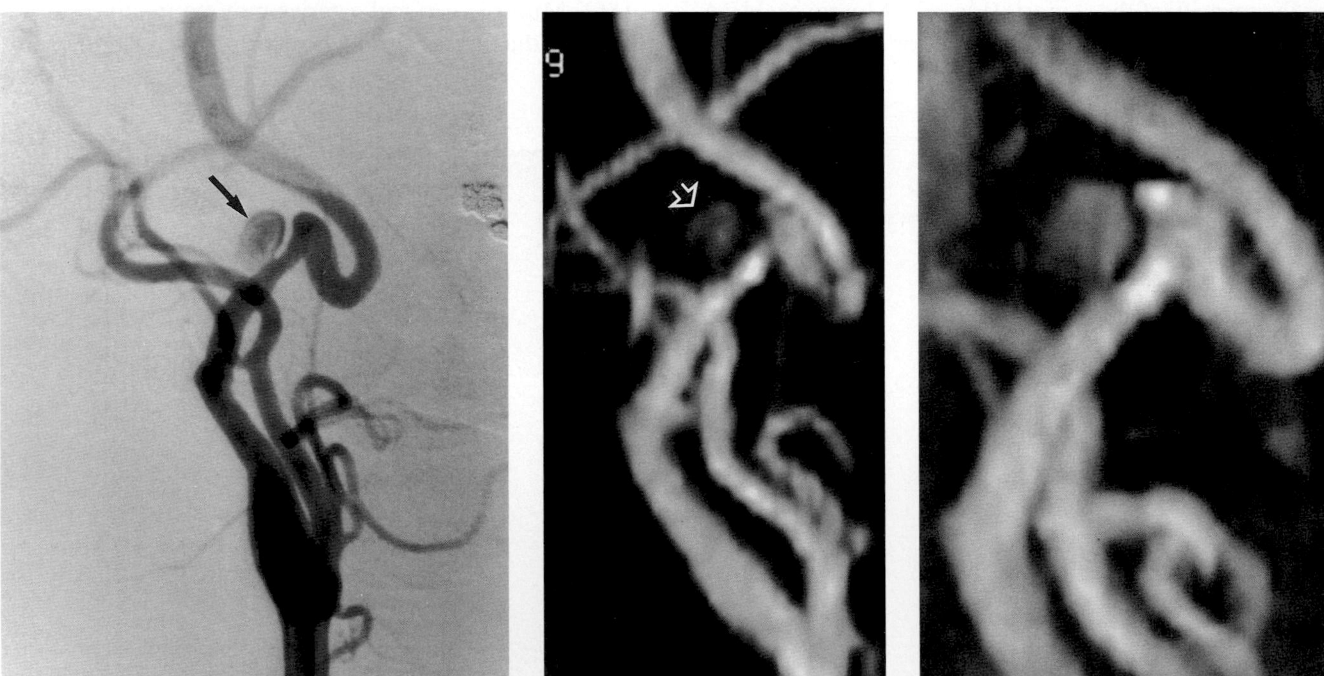

FIG. 22. Pseudoaneurysm of the internal carotid artery. **A:** Catheter angiogram. **B:** 2DFT TOF and **C:** 3DFT TOF MRAs of the carotid arteries. Notice the pseudoaneurysm in a patient who had a carotid artery dissection 1 month prior (*arrow*). The lower spatial resolution of the 2D TOF MRA image of the carotid artery pseudoaneurysm fails to reveal the neck of the aneurysm completely (*open arrow*). The 3D TOF MRA image clearly demonstrates the association of the aneurysm to the carotid artery.

representing the intramural hematoma (Fig. 23). The appearance of the hematoma varies with the state of the blood products. MRA findings of the apparent enlarged vessels occur when the mural hematoma is in the methemoglobin stage, which, because of its paramagnetic effect, is mapped into the MIP MRA as an enlarged vascular segment. The appearance of enlarged vessels as well as a slight higher signal intensity from the flowing blood (compared to the intramural hematoma) made detection of dissection by MRA reportedly easy and specific (193) (Fig. 23).

With very severe luminal compromise, where a flow through the vessel may be extremely slow, a 2DFT sequence may be helpful (Fig. 14). Phase-contrast techniques may be useful in this clinical scenario because they do not demonstrate the high signal intensity of methemoglobin and allow selection of the velocity of blood to be imaged. MRA is helpful in follow-up of patients with carotid dissections by monitoring the resolution of an intramural hematoma or the development of complications of dissection (183,192,194,195). It is important to emphasize that MRI or 3DFT TOF MRA are not nearly as helpful in the evaluation of vertebral artery dissection (193).

Fibromuscular Dysplasia

Clinical Background

Fibromuscular dysplasia is an idiopathic multifocal arteriopathy consisting of smooth muscle hyperplasia or thinning, proliferation of fibrous tissue, and elastic fiber destruction (196). It predominantly involves the renal arteries, but cephalic arteries are also commonly in-

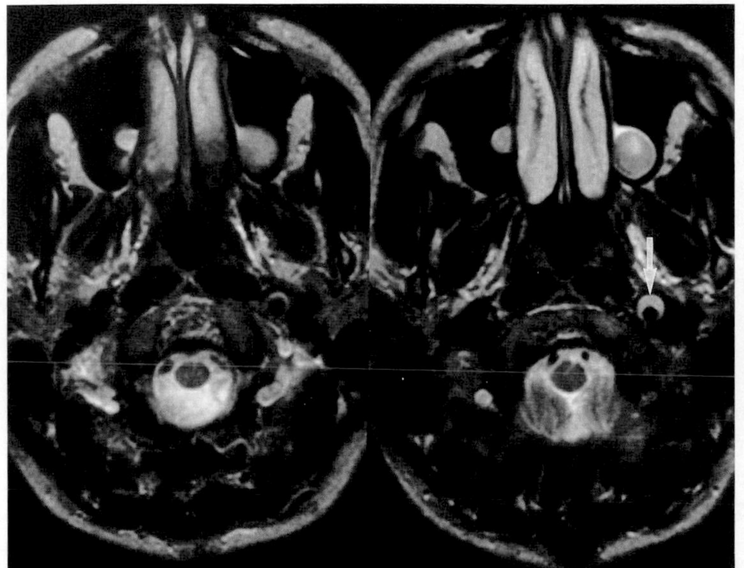

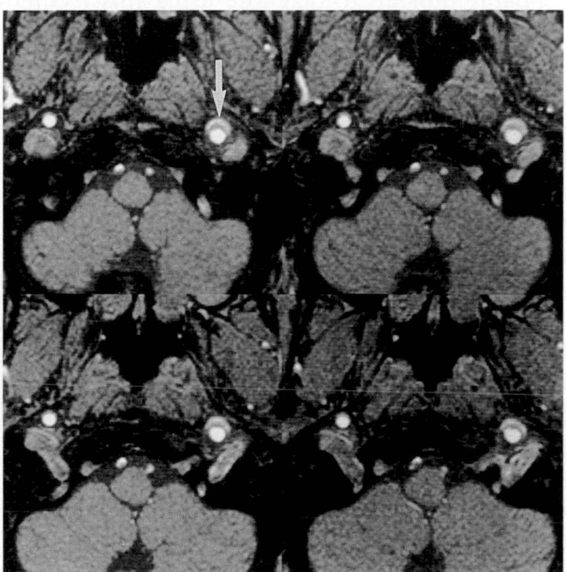

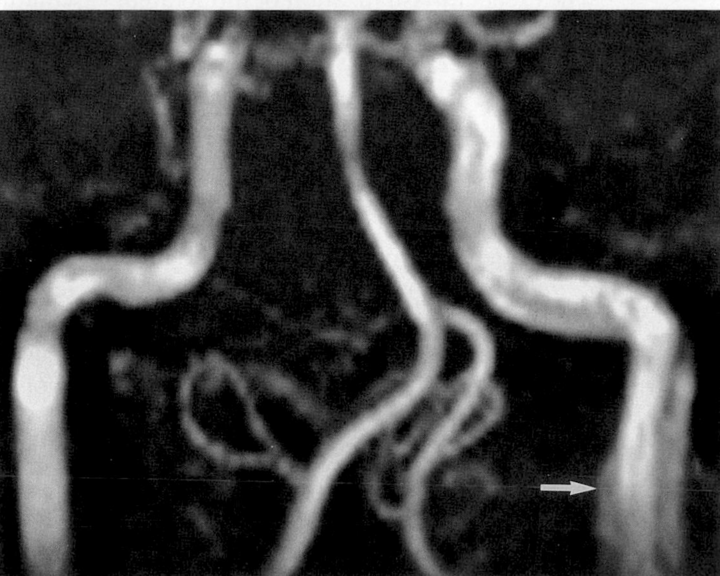

A B C

FIG. 23. Spontaneous carotid artery dissection. **A:** SE image demonstrating normal flow void in the left carotid artery and a halo of hyperintensity due to a mural hematoma (*arrow*). **B:** Individual partitions from the 3DFT TOF MRA demonstrating the normal hyperintense flow signal in the left internal carotid artery with a less hyperintense crescent-shaped rim, representing mural hematoma (*arrow*). **C:** Maximum intensity projection image of the internal carotid arteries demonstrating the surrounding slight hyperintense, but less than the flowing blood, around the left internal carotid artery (*arrow*), representing methemoglobin in the vessel wall that has been incorporated into the image by the maximum intensity projection algorithm.

volved. There are three histologic varieties of fibromuscular dysplasia: medial, intimal, and subadventitial types with the medial or muscular dysplasia occurring in 90% to 95% of cases (196,197). Multiple angiographic studies indicate that the cervical internal carotid artery is diseased in approximately 95% of cases of cephalic fibromuscular dysplasia, with bilateral involvement in 60% to 85% (196). The catheter angiogram demonstrates focal or long tubular, multifocal stenoses with adjacent dilatations, the so-called string of beads. Rarely one may appreciate an asymmetric mural septum, or outpouching (196,197).

Technical Background

An anecdotal report of imaging by 2DFT MRA of two patients with the classic alternating areas of stenosis and dilatation has been reported; however, these lesions are probably difficult to diagnose using this technique because the stenotic bands may be mistaken for a common slice misregistration artifact due to motion seen on 2DFT TOF MRA (197). In addition, because of the serrated contour, flow through the diseased segment is likely to be disturbed, resulting in dephasing artifacts. Although 3DFT TOF has greater spatial resolution than the 2D TOF technique, the disturbed flow is also likely to be problematic with this technique. No study has been performed to determine the sensitivity or specificity of MRA for this arteriopathy; however, given the known limitations of these techniques and focal multilevel stenoses, it is unlikely to be high. Alternatively, MRA is beneficial in detecting associated conditions with fibromuscular dysplasia, specifically intracranial aneurysms, a finding in approximately 21% to 51% of patients with cephalic fibromuscular dysplasia and arterial dissection (196).

Subclavian Steal Syndrome

Clinical Background

Subclavian steal syndrome results from either a very severe stenosis or occlusion of the subclavian artery proximal to the origin of the vertebral artery, resulting in blood being redirected from the contralateral vertebral artery across the vertebral basilar junction and in a retrograde direction ipsilateral to the stenosis or occlusion. The symptoms are most frequently referable to episodic ischemia of the posterior circulation, with occasional ipsilateral arm claudication (198–200).

Technical Background

As with conventional angiography and Doppler US, the findings consist of reversed flow in the vertebral artery ipsilateral to the subclavian stenosis or occlusion. The retrograde flow in the vertebral artery can be demonstrated by using TOF or PC MRA techniques (Fig. 24). Using the 2DFT TOF MRA technique requires removing the traveling or repositioning the stationary superior saturation pulse (typically employed to suppress the signal from the venous system). Because of the reverse flow in the vertebral artery, this saturation pulse has to be eliminated. In a presentation of three cases of subclavian steal, Turjman et al. employed a 2DFT TOF technique with two imaging sequences, one with the saturation superior to the image acquisition, and one inferior to the image acquisition, allowing visualization of the flow in the affected vertebral artery (201). A more elegant method of obtaining the information, which also allows quantitation of the steal, consists of a coronal 2DFT PC examination with superior to inferior flow encoding. The reverse flow in the vertebral arteries will appear as a high signal intensity, indicating flow is in the craniocaudad direction. In addition, cine phase contrast quantification of subsequent subclavian steal can be performed by measuring the flow in both vertebral arteries as well as in the basilar artery to quantify the degree of basilar artery steal. In a recent study, flow rates were quantified in the vertebral artery contralateral to the subclavian steal and within the basilar artery before and following exercise or reactive hyperemia (202). Following reactive hyperemia, flow rates ipsilateral to the subclavian steal increased by 20%, and the basilar artery flow rates decreased between 5% and 12% (202).

Intracranial Circulation

Intracranial Arterial Occlusive Disease and Stroke

Clinical Background

The excellent visualization of intracranial vasculature with current MRA techniques makes the detection of occlusive disease relatively straightforward. Strokes resulting from occlusion of the primary intracranial arteries may be classified as (a) "thrombotic," primary occlusions, (b) "embolic" strokes, or (c) infarcts due to interruption of the smaller penetrating arteries, which are called lacunes (203–205). Mohr et al. in data evaluated in 694 patients hospitalized for stroke revealed that approximately 53% were diagnosed as having large vessel thrombosis and 31% as having cerebral embolization (203). In that particular study, angiographic evidence of large vessel thrombosis was identified in all 102 of the angiographic study patients (which included internal carotid artery stenosis, note that intracranial and internal carotid artery stenosis were not separated). In patients with embolization, 73% of the catheter angiograms were positive for emboli when performed within 2 days of the stroke and only 28% were positive after the second day

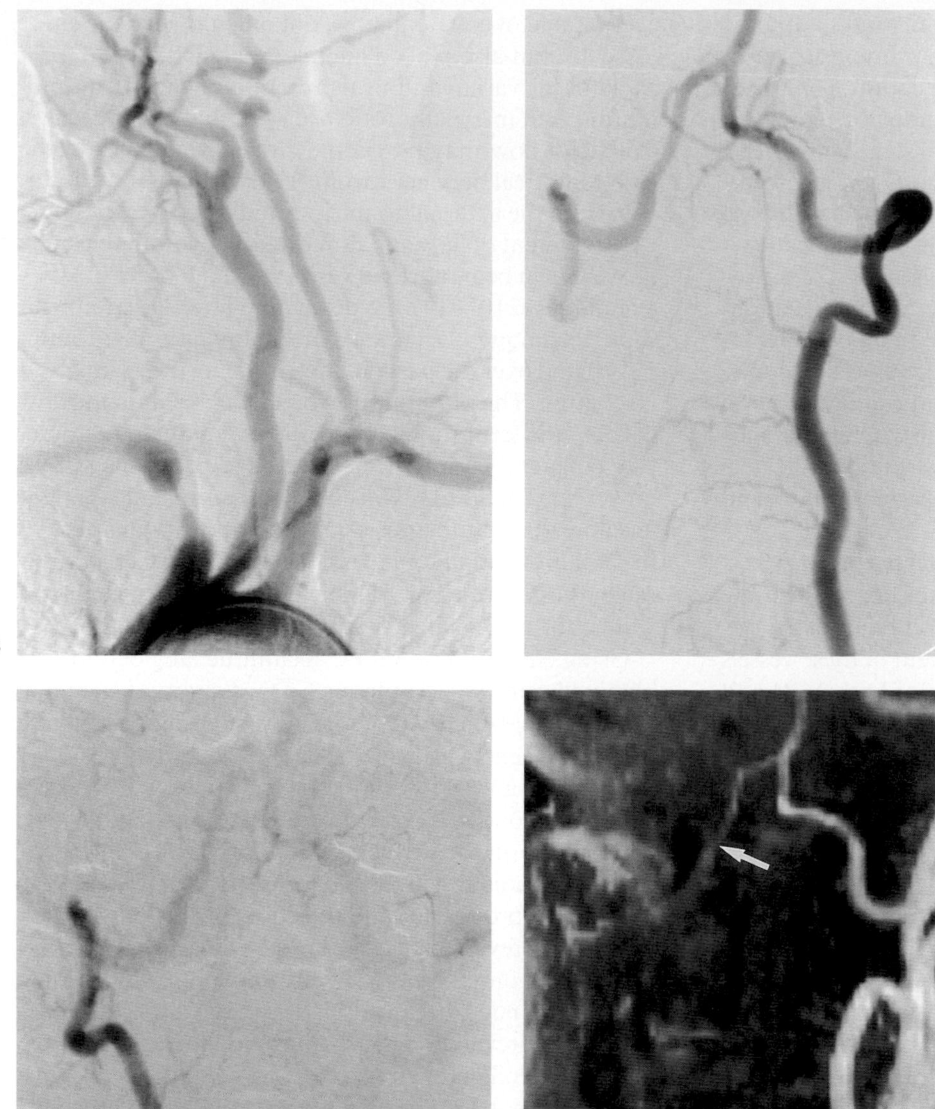

FIG. 24. Right common carotid artery occlusion, right subclavian stenosis, and subclavian steal. **A:** Catheter arch aortogram demonstrates a severe stenosis in the brachiocephalic subclavian junction and the right carotid artery is occluded. **B,C:** Two frames (early and late) from a selected left vertebral artery conventional angiogram demonstrating the retrograde flow down the right vertebral artery. **D:** A 3D TOF MRA demonstrating the retrograde flow (*arrow*) down the right vertebral artery. The signal intensity diminishes as flow extends caudad in the artery because of spin saturation. A 2D TOF sequential sequence with a tracking superior saturation pulse would saturate the entire signal of the retrograde flow in the right vertebral artery.

(203). Clearly, the temporal relationship between the frequency of a positive examination and the initial ictus of the symptoms is important.

Thrombic ischemic infarction is the result of thrombosis of a specified vessel at the level of its abnormality. This abnormality is most frequently due to atherosclerosis; however, this can occur in other diseases such as arterial dissection or vasospasm. The clinical hallmark of a thrombic stroke is that of stuttering neurologic signs and symptoms (204). The onset is progressive over time—usually minutes to hours, but occasionally as long as days. Thrombotic infarction frequently occurs during sleep, or may be preceded by transient ischemic symptoms with a stuttering onset and gradual evolution. The variation of the signs and symptoms is felt to be related to marginal tissue perfusion from inadequate collateral circulation. In patients with no vascular reserve, the signs and symptoms are influenced by systemic factors that affect cerebral perfusion pressure such as blood pressure, hydration, and cardiac output (204).

In contrast, embolic ischemic infarctions are often abruptly catastrophic, with the severity of symptoms often peaking at the ictus. The clinical signs and symptoms are referable to the vascular territory involved, most commonly the MCA (205). The most common cause of emboli is from atherosclerotic alterations of the proximal internal carotid, specifically that of stenoses or ulcerations. In approximately 25% of patients, the source of the embolus is felt to arise in patients with cardiac disease (203). It is therefore logical that evaluation of patients with cerebral infarction should have evaluation of the carotid bifurcations as well as the intracranial circulation. The intracranial abnormality detected in an embolic infarction will vary with time. In an acute phase, one may see a focal stenosis that in a subsequent examination returns to a normal-caliber vessel (Fig. 25). In the presence of massive infarction, there may be distortion in the normal course of the vessel because of the mass effect and the intracranial vessels.

MRA techniques demonstrate the larger primary vessels well; however, visualization of the lenticulostriate and thalamoperforating vessels is beyond the spatial resolution of current methods. Involvement of these vessels can be inferred with the combination of both MRI and MRA imaging.

Technical Background

The role of MRI and MRA in infarction not only displays morphologic function, but physiologic function can be appreciated. In a review of intracranial MRA in brain infarction, Johnson et al. retrospectively evaluated 78 consecutive patients with acute or subacute stroke with positive MRI findings who had undergone MRA (206). Abnormalities evaluated on MRA included stenoses and inclusion as well as collateral flow. Eighty percent of the MRA demonstrated stenoses or occlusion and abnormality was in the distribution of the infarction in 93% of cases. In the eight patients who underwent conventional angiography, there was an 87% correlation of the evaluated 90 vessels. Interestingly enough, there is no significant difference in the results of patients who were imaged acutely (less than 48 hours) and those imaged subacutely (3–14 days). In patients with the clinical event occurring 24 hours or less before the MRA examination, 54% had occlusions in the same vascular territory as the infarction versus 35% of those who presented for imaging after 24 hours. Certainly these findings are discrepant with studies that included catheter angiographic findings (203). MRA abnormalities were more commonly detected in patients with larger infarcts; however, in patients with $\leq$ 2 cm infarctions, 64% of patients had abnormalities on MRA.

The angiograms were evaluated for collateral circulation, but the role of collateral circulation in infarct size was not reported. A major consideration in the outcome of a patient undergoing a thrombic or embolic ischemic event is that of collateral flow, not only through the circle of Willis, but also pial collaterals. Collateral flow in part explains the variable clinical presentation of patients presenting with internal carotid artery occlusion (207–209). Collateral flow may be via the circle of Willis or in the case of critical cervical carotid artery stenosis or occlusion from the external to the internal carotid arteries.

Assessment of flow and flow direction within the circle of Willis can be performed with both TOF and PC MRA techniques (210–214). To determine flow direction with TOF techniques, accurate placement of presaturation pulse band over the particular vascular territory involved is required. The presaturation band will result in the flow distal to the saturation band being inapparent and therefore collateral supply from the saturated vessel will no longer be visualized (210,211). For example, if a patient has flow through the posterior communicating artery to the anterior circulation and the basilar artery is saturated, the contribution of flow to the anterior circulation will not be appreciated.

Using either 2D or 3D PC technique, angiograms are obtained using phase difference processing and encoding for velocity, which will avoid flow aliasing. The phase maps thus generated will display flow in anteroposterior (AP), right–left (RL), and superior–inferior (SI) directions. The flow toward the flow-encoding gradient will be represented on the image by white pixels and flow away from the gradient will result in dark vessels (Fig. 26). As mentioned previously, the selection of the velocity encoding to prevent phase wrap (flow aliasing) is important. Most commonly, a velocity encoding of 80 cm/sec is recommended because this is greater than velocities above the circle of Willis by transcranial Doppler in patients with collateral flow (215).

It is important to recognize that collateral flow through the circle of Willis is quite variable because of normal anatomic variability (207). Only in 21% of patients is a complete circle of Willis present (216). The presence of adequate collateral flow explains why individual patients can tolerate an internal carotid artery occlusion whereas others cannot. In a recent study by Schomer et al. using 3DFT PC MRA techniques, 29 consecutive patients were evaluated with angiographically proven internal carotid artery occlusion. The collateral pathways to the occluded vessel were evaluated including the anterior cerebral artery, the posterior communicating and the ophthalmic artery, and the leptomeningeal collaterals from the posterior cerebral artery (214). Using this technique, they demonstrated that a posterior communicating artery greater than 1 mm in diameter may protect against watershed infarctions in patients with ipsilateral occlusion of the internal carotid artery. The converse of this held true (214). The data presented support a previous study in which the size of the posterior communicating artery was a good predictor of the

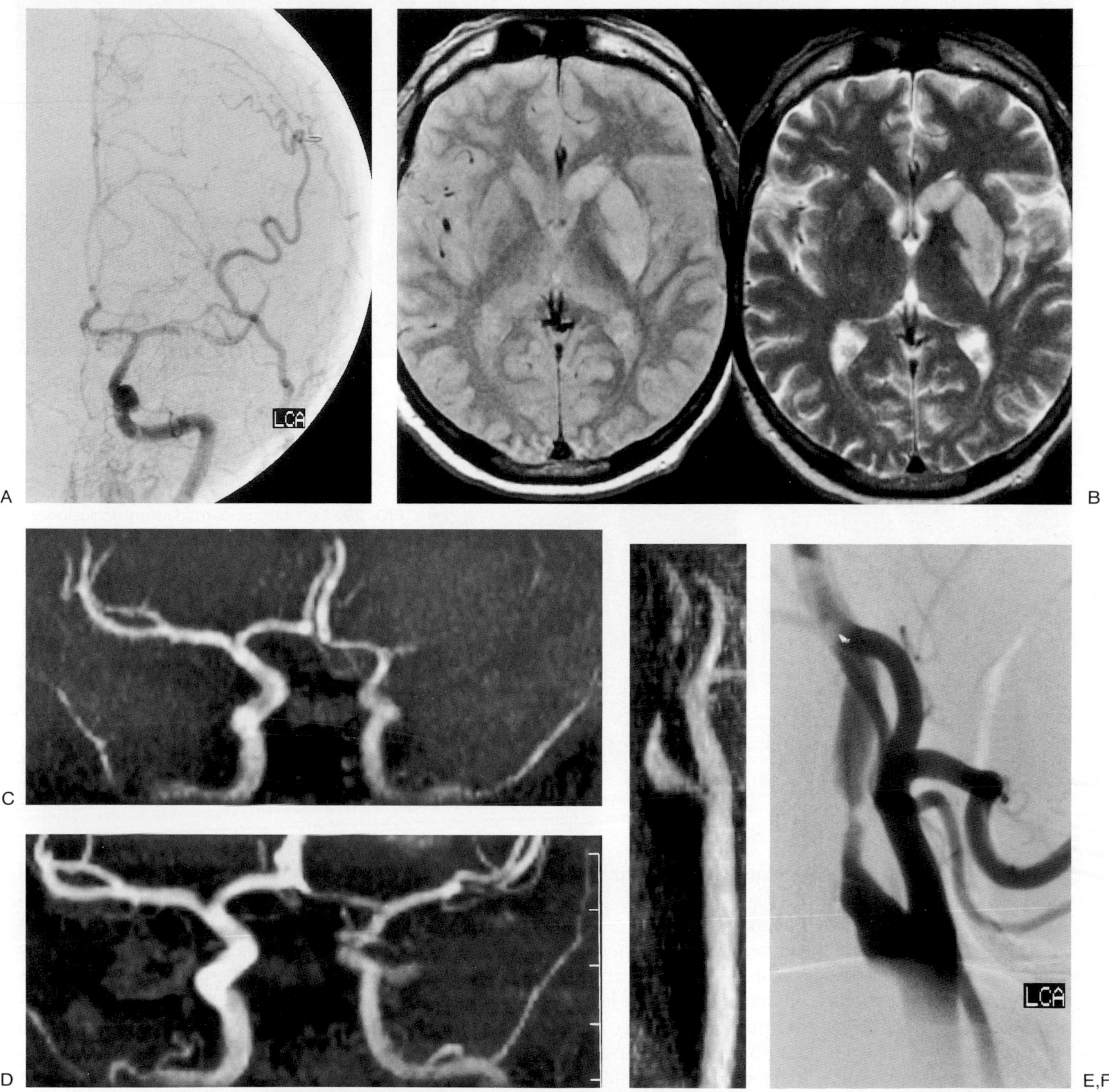

FIG. 25. MCA embolus and stroke. **A:** Digital subtraction angiogram demonstrating embolus in the left M1 segment of the MCA. **B:** SE images demonstrating the caudate head and lentiform nucleus infarction due to occlusion of the lenticulostriate arteries. **C:** 3D TOF MRA demonstrating a decreased size and signal intensity in the left internal carotid artery and in the proximal MCA. The distal MCA is not visualized. **D:** 3D TOF MRA performed a week later demonstrating decreased signal intensity within the left internal carotid artery and MCA. Note the MCA has recanalized. **E:** 3D TOF MRA of the proximal left carotid artery demonstrates a very severe stenosis with complete signal loss. **F:** Corresponding digital subtraction angiogram showing a very severe stenosis in the proximal left internal carotid artery.

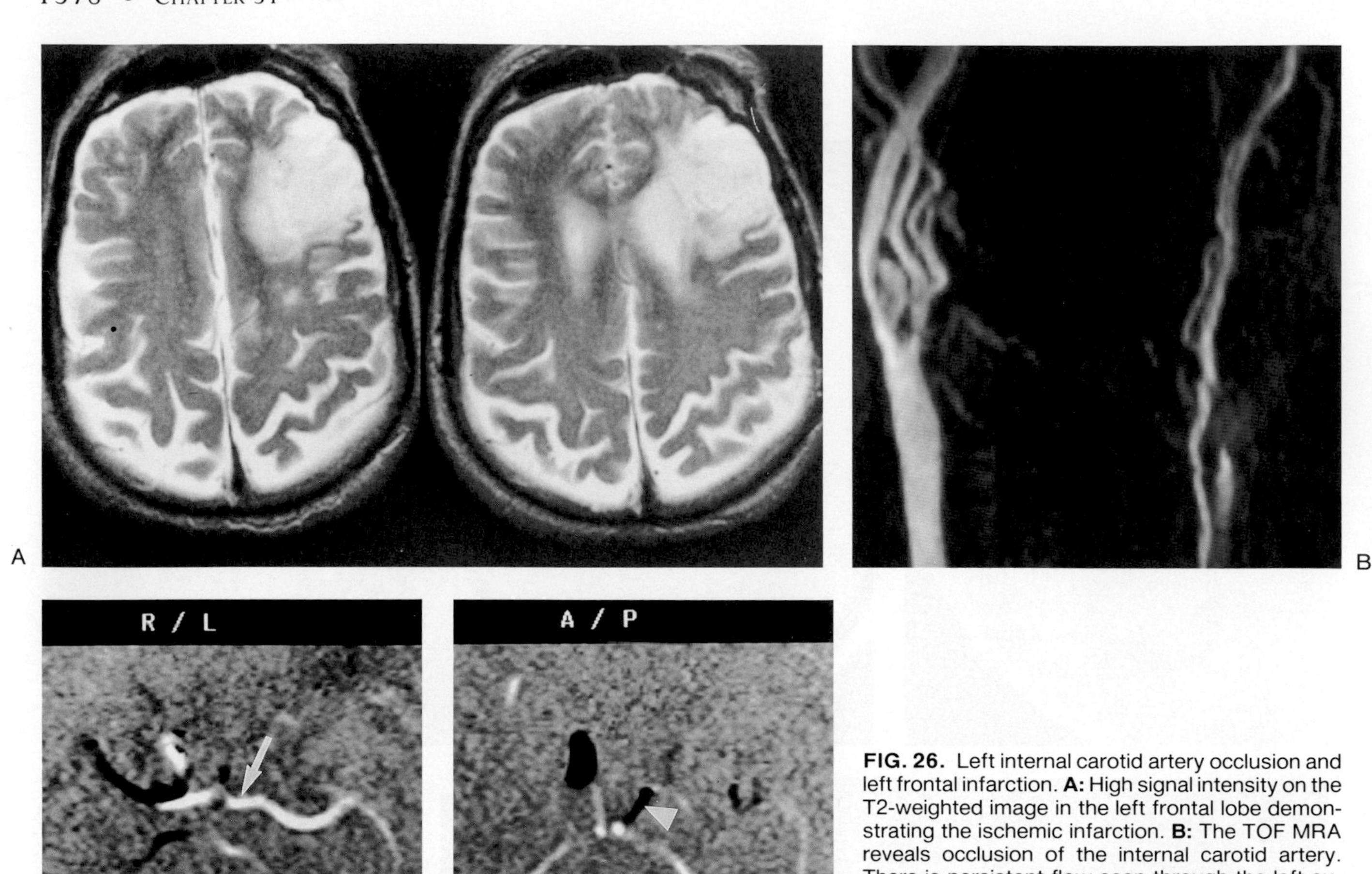

FIG. 26. Left internal carotid artery occlusion and left frontal infarction. **A:** High signal intensity on the T2-weighted image in the left frontal lobe demonstrating the ischemic infarction. **B:** The TOF MRA reveals occlusion of the internal carotid artery. There is persistent flow seen through the left external carotid artery. **C:** Phase contrast speed images in the right/left and anterior/posterior flow directions show collateral flow via the left posterior communicating artery and across the anterior communicating artery. The right to left image demonstrates reversed flow in the A1 segment (*arrow*) of the left anterior cerebral artery and posterior to the anterior flow in the left posterior communicating artery (*arrowhead*).

tolerance of ischemia after deliberate sacrifice of patients with basilar artery aneurysms (217).

In 26% of patients, the anterior communicating artery (ACOM) or A1 segment of the anterior cerebral artery is hypoplastic or absent (216). If the internal carotid artery is occluded in these patients, collateral flow may be identified through the posterior communicating artery and therefore flow will be from posterior to anterior ipsilateral to the internal carotid artery occlusion. Posterior communicating artery hypoplasia or aplasia is identified in approximately 48% of individuals (216). With an internal carotid artery occlusion, collateral flow may be identified through the ACOM, and therefore flow in the A1 segment of the anterior cerebral artery ipsilateral to the carotid artery occlusion would be reversed. The patent internal carotid artery would supply both anterior and middle cerebral arteries. In patients with an absent or inadequate circle of Willis collateral flow, the hemisphere ipsilateral to an occluded carotid artery may obtain some of its blood flow via extracranial to intracranial collateral vessels. Although there are many such collateral pathways at the skull base, the most common is through retrograde flow through the ophthalmic artery in a patient with internal carotid artery occlusion. In this scenario of internal carotid artery occlusion with no collateral vessels via the circle of Willis or from external to internal carotid artery supply, whole hemispheric infarctions involving the anterior and middle cerebral arteries may occur.

Intracranial Carotid Artery Atherosclerosis

Clinical Background

Atherosclerotic occlusive disease involving the carotid siphon is second only in location to that of the carotid bifurcation in the neck. The significance of tandem distal internal carotid artery disease is controversial, especially in light of the fact that there have been few prospective blinded studies evaluating the natural history of the disease versus that of best medical management. The incidence of an ischemic event and ischemic infarction in patients with intracranial internal carotid artery stenosis is high (132,218,219). In fact, in a retrospective review of 58 patients only 33% were alive and free from ischemic events at the end of follow-up of 30 months and 43% of patients had died during the follow-up, 36% from ischemia and 44% from cardiac disease (219). In a second retrospective study of 66 patients, the observed stroke rate was 13 times the expected infarction rate for the normal population and patients with a tandem extracranial stenosis had a greater risk of stroke than patients with isolated internal carotid artery stenosis (132). Somewhat less robust studies describe a relatively benign natural history of carotid siphon stenoses following carotid endarterectomy (132). Marzewski et al. presented the only study in which vigorous analysis of the severity of the siphon stenosis was performed; however, in no study has careful analysis of the severity and location of stenosis been performed in a fashion analogous to NASCET (132). As suggested earlier, the presence of a tandem stenosis involving the internal carotid artery, or for that matter any cerebrovascular territory with serial stenoses, may alter the benefits of endarterectomy or other therapies.

Technical Background

The complex geometric shape of the internal carotid artery as it enters the skull base, in particular the carotid siphon, present special problems when imaging with a flow modality such as MRA. The only truly successful techniques in evaluating the carotid siphon have been the 3DFT TOF methods. Despite the dramatic improvement of these techniques over the last several years, there can still be artifactual signal loss resulting from the extremely complex flow pattern in this region (Fig. 27). Not only is there disturbed flow, but the velocity profile across the vessel in a given location can be quite wide. The sharp bends cause focal areas of acceleration and deceleration of the blood. Due to secondary variations in flow velocity and disturbed flow, there may be signal loss from phase dispersion (43) (Fig. 28). Artifactual signal loss can be decreased by implementation of short gradient (echo) times, partial echo sampling, small voxel size and flow compensation (43) (Figs. 28 and 29). In addition, improvement of the display of the 3D TOF MRA can be achieved by processing the partitions to include only a single siphon.

Intracranial Carotid Artery Dissection

Contrary to extracranial carotid dissection, dissection involving intracranial vessels is commonly related to se-

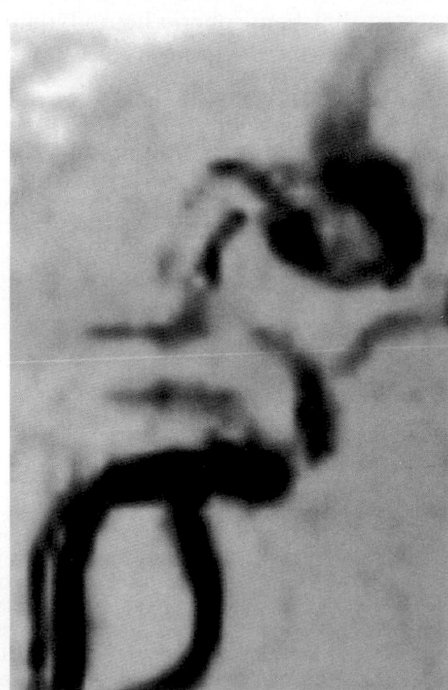

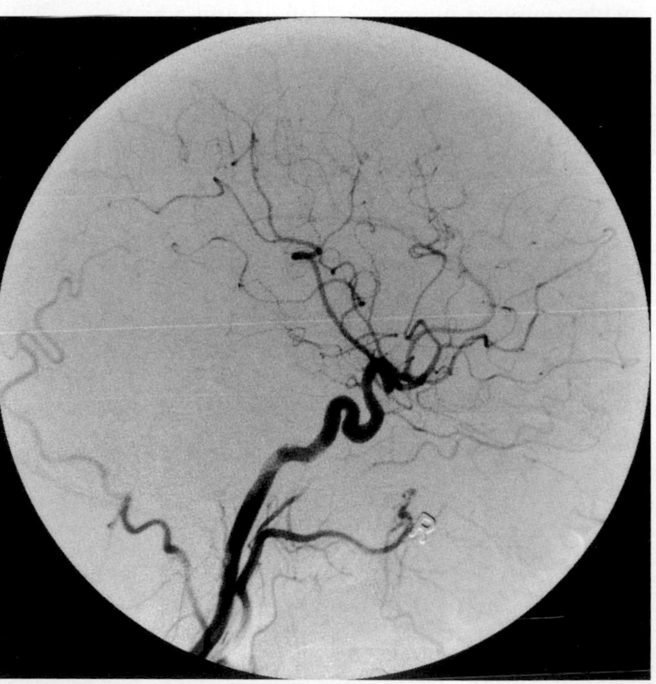

FIG. 27. A: 3DFT TOF MRA (TE = 10) of the carotid siphon demonstrating loss of signal in a tortuous carotid siphon due to acceleration and disturbed flow. **B:** The corresponding conventional angiogram demonstrates the severe tortuosity of the internal carotid artery siphon.

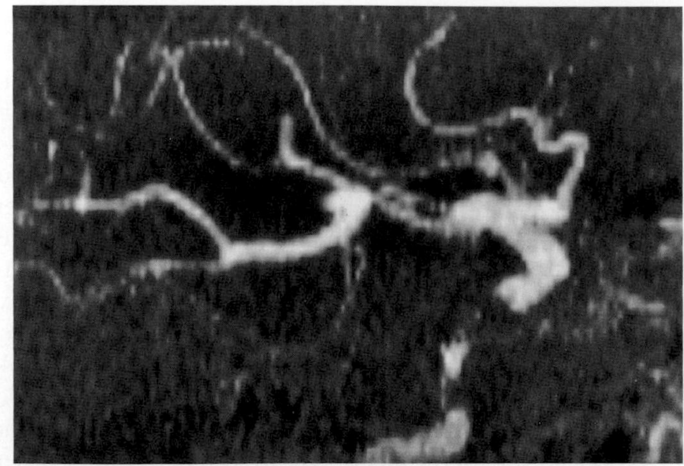

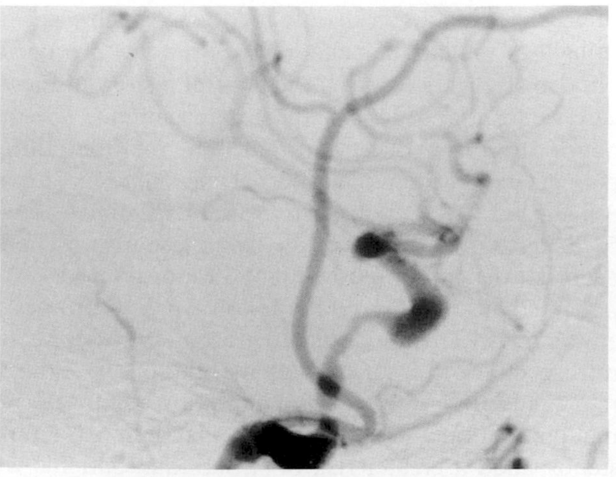

FIG. 28. Intracranial internal carotid artery stenosis. This is a patient with a severe stenosis of the carotid artery. Following carotid endarterectomy, he had persistent TIAs. **A:** Notice the severe stenosis with 3DFT TOF MRA (TE = 7). Notice the complete signal loss due to disturbed flow and acceleration through the stenoses. **B:** The corresponding conventional angiogram demonstrates the true morphology of the lesion.

vere traumatic injury (188–190,220,221). As mentioned earlier, internal carotid artery dissections are most often in the midcervical carotid artery and extend cephalad to the skull base. Intracranial artery dissections tend to occur in the supraclinoid internal carotid artery, although involvement of the anterior and middle cerebral arteries does occur (190,220,222). As with dissections elsewhere, complications such as pseudoaneurysm or extension into the anterior and middle cerebral arteries can occur (220). Unlike the cervical internal carotid arteries, dissections of the intracranial internal carotid arteries are associated with profound neurologic deficits and a high mortality rate (189,190,220). The MRA findings reveal a progressive tapering of the supraclinoid internal carotid artery and the source images may reveal an intramural hematoma.

Cerebral Artery Atherosclerosis

Clinical Background

There are few studies evaluating the clinical significance of a stenosis of the anterior middle or posterior cerebral arteries. However, it has been well documented in several studies that occasionally stenoses within the MCA can be the source of the patient's focal neurologic symptoms (223,224). Symptoms of MCA stenoses are variable, depending on the underlying etiology. Hinton et al. suggested that hemispheric hemodynamic insufficiency resulted in clinical symptoms of 13 of the 16 cases reported in their series (223). Alternatively, the symptoms may be related to embolism distal to the stenoses (224). Renewed interest in symptomatic MCA stenoses

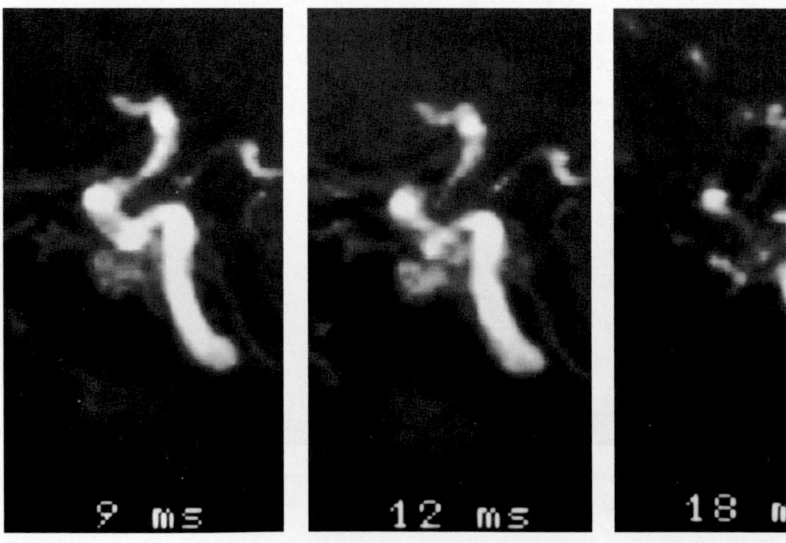

FIG. 29. The effect of echo time on reducing dephasing in regions of complex flow. TOF angiogram of the carotid siphon demonstrating the effect of prolonging the echo time from 9 msec to 18 msec. Notice the loss of signal that occurs in the carotid siphon that can result in an apparent stenosis. In addition to decreasing echo time, correlation with the SE images is important. (From Ruggieri et al., ref. 41, with permission.)

has occurred because newer treatment options consisting of intracranial angioplasty have been performed. In a recent case report this therapeutic technique improved regional cerebral blood flow and relieved the patient symptoms (225).

Technical Background

In an early study by Masaryk et al., nine patients with cerebral infarctions were studied using 3DFT TOF MRA. Artifactual signal loss in the carotid siphon, in the internal carotid bifurcation, and in the genu of the MCAs was observed (Fig. 30). This was attributed to intervoxel dephasing due to the longer gradient (echo) times in this study (226). Since that initial study there have been dramatic improvements in the spatial resolution, echo times, and techniques to reduce saturations of moving spins as well as background suppression (227). In a retrospective study, Hiserman et al. evaluated internal carotid artery and MCA stenoses with a 3DFT TOF technique and compared the MRA exams to conventional angiography (228). There were both false-positive and false-negative findings for MCA stenosis; however, occlusions were accurately identified on both studies. A similar study performed by Dagirmanjian et al. in which 3DFT MRA with magnetization transfer saturation and variable flip angle were used revealed 19 intracranial stenoses that were correctly identified on MRA and were confirmed with conventional angiography. However, eight vessels were incorrectly identified as being stenotic on MRA and were later shown to be normal on angiography and two vessels were incorrectly identified as normal on MRA and were found to be stenotic with catheter angiography (227). A recent publication by Fujita et al. discussed seven patients who were evaluated with MCA stenoses or occlusion by 2DFT and 3DFT TOF techniques. Not all the patients were evaluated with conventional angiography. In all the patients, both 2DFT and 3DFT MRA studies depicted the compromised flow in the MCA consistent with a focal discontinuity with decreased vessel caliber corresponding to the stenosis and nonvisualization of the vessels distal to the stenoses. As one would expect, the discontinuity through the area of the stenosis was more pronounced on the 2DFT MRAs; with the 3DFT techniques using the smaller voxels as well as shorter echo times with gradient echo nulling, the stenosis was less pronounced (229).

As in the anterior circulation, MRA evaluation of the posterior circulation is possible. Similar TOF techniques are used for evaluation of the distal vertebral and basilar arteries. Moreover, with the emerging techniques in treating patients with stenotic lesions of the posterior circulation, MRA can provide diagnoses and a method of noninvasive follow-up (Fig. 31).

Contrary to the anterior circulation, where the normal path of the arterial vessels is tortuous, the posterior circulation consists of relatively straight arterial segments. For this reason, as one would expect, there would be fewer problems with signal loss resulting from flow acceleration or disturbed flow. There have been few studies that have evaluated the true sensitivity and specificity of MRA in detecting lesions in the distal vertebral artery and basilar artery; however, initial studies are promising (230–232). Recently, MRA was used to assess the poste-

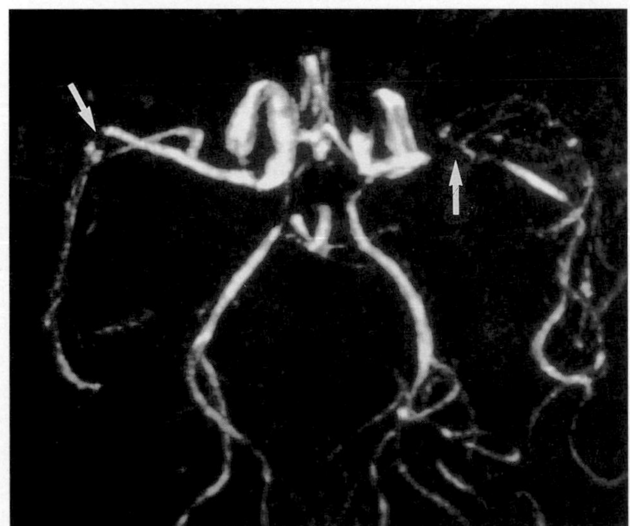

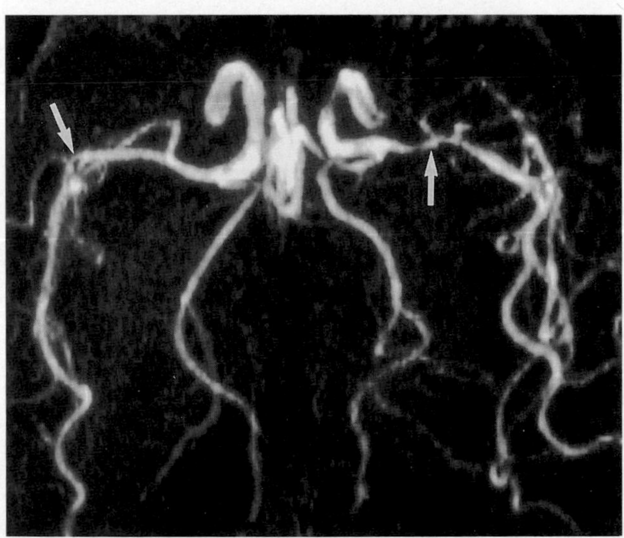

FIG. 30. Effect of echo time on stenosis. **A:** 3DFT TOF MRA of the circle of Willis with an echo time of 8.0 msec. Notice the signal loss (*arrows*) at the genu of the MCA on the right and in the horizontal segment of the left MCA on the left, as well as the poor vascular contrast seen in the distal MCAs bilaterally, worse on the right. **B:** The same patient with a shorter echo time of 6.5 msec. The genu now demonstrates near normal caliber and there is normal filling of the MCAs bilaterally; however, the serrated signal in the horizontal MCA on the left represented an MCA stenosis.

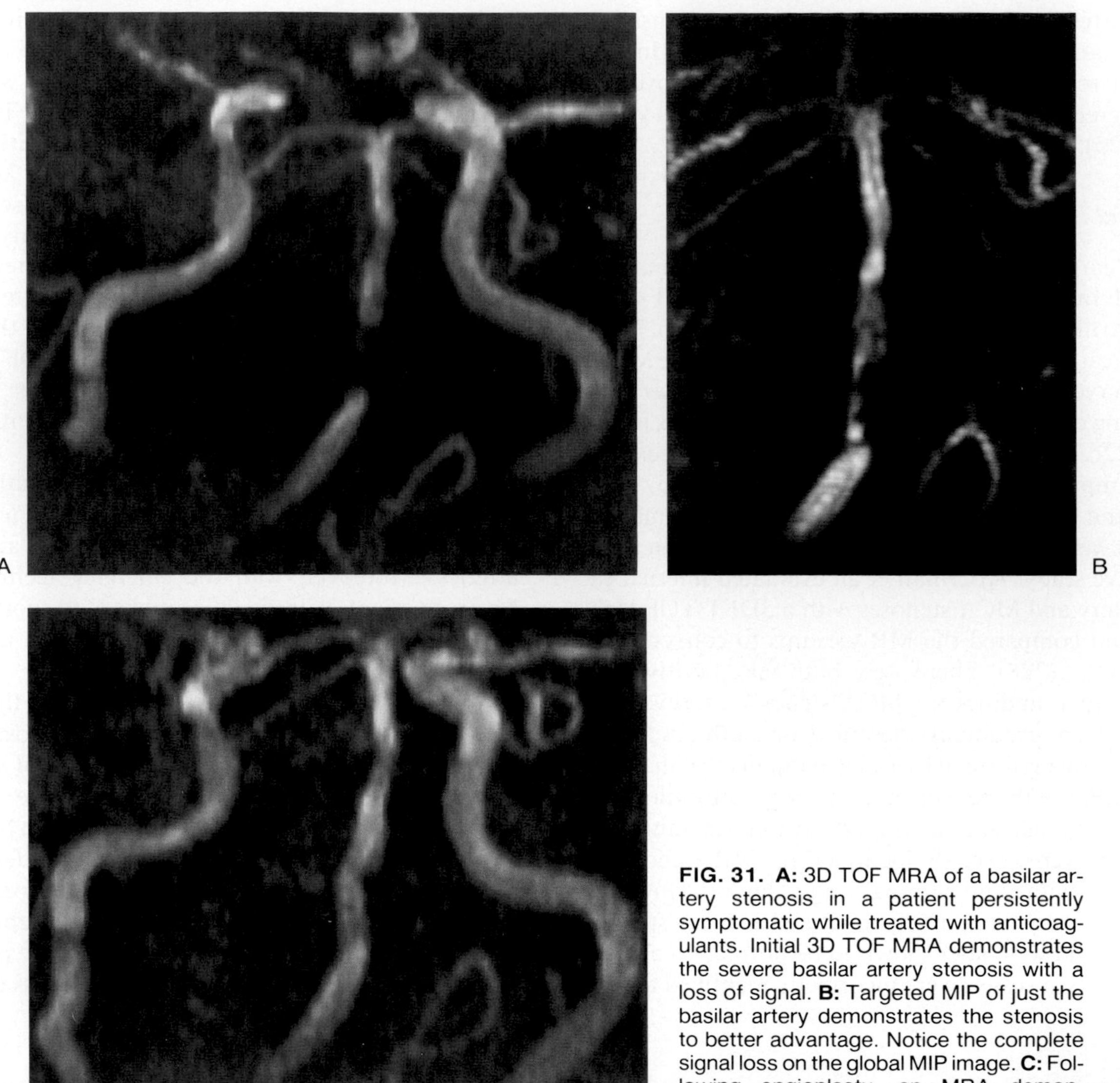

FIG. 31. A: 3D TOF MRA of a basilar artery stenosis in a patient persistently symptomatic while treated with anticoagulants. Initial 3D TOF MRA demonstrates the severe basilar artery stenosis with a loss of signal. **B:** Targeted MIP of just the basilar artery demonstrates the stenosis to better advantage. Notice the complete signal loss on the global MIP image. **C:** Following angioplasty, an MRA demonstrates the restoration of the near normal contour of the basilar artery.

rior circulation in a prospective series of 70 patients with clinical and imaging evidence of posterior circulation infarctions. Although the study was not specifically designed to verify the MRA technique, 44 of the patients had abnormalities detected on MRA. Catheter angiography was performed in 22 of the patients and accurate correlation was found in 14 patients. Three patients had distal branch occlusions that were not identified on MRA. Dolichoectatic vertebral basilar arteries were identified in 12 patients. Fifteen of the 70 patients had a potential cardiac source for embolism. Interestingly, large vessel stenoses or occlusions was seen in 46 patients. Of note is that stenosis was not declared unless the lumen diameter was reduced by at least 50% on 3DFT TOF image (230). This study excluded evaluation of the proximal vertebral arteries, which in the past have been thought to play a minimal role in posterior circulation infarction; however, a recent study by Caplan et al. strongly challenge this premise (203).

In the second prospective study of 41 patients with acute cerebellar or brainstem ischemia, MRA correctly identified the vertebral artery pathology responsible for the infarct 95% of the time, with a specificity of 99% (231). The only lesion that was missed was that of a vertebral artery dissection. In this imaging protocol, if an inconclusive finding was seen in the vertebral basilar arterial territory, additional MRA images evaluating the proximal vertebral arteries were implemented (231).

In a third study by Ruggieri et al., comparing 3DFT TOF MRA to conventional angiography of distal vertebral and basilar arteries, a sensitivity of 90% and a specificity of 75% were identified when 53 posterior circulation vessels were studied in 22 patients. Stenoses were both over- and underestimated with similar percentages; the errors occurred most frequently in the vertebral arteries (232).

Intracranial Vasculitis

Clinical Background

There is strong evidence that MRI has a close correlation with detection of intracranial vasculitis; however, no study to date has established the role of MRA. In a retrospective study of 92 patients (11 with proven vasculitis) by Harris et al., MRI was significantly abnormal in the nine patients who underwent MRI. Catheter angiography demonstrated angiographic evidence of vasculitis in 8 of 11 patients with true vasculitis (233).

Technical Background

Current MRA techniques are unlikely to detect many of the subtle small vessel contour alterations that are identified with catheter angiography in patients with vasculitis. In a study by Ruggieri et al. evaluating intracranial stenoses of the posterior circulation in 22 patients, there were three patients with large vessel vasculitis with vascular stenoses appreciated (232). Because of this preliminary work in detection of large vessel abnormalities in vasculitis, patients who are being studied for vasculitis with MRI may also gain some benefit from MRA.

Moyamoya Disease

Clinical Background

Moyamoya disease is a vasculopathy of unknown etiology; there is considerable debate as to whether the disease is actually an acquired or congenital abnormality (234). Regardless of the etiology, there is a relatively characteristic appearance identified with catheter angiography, MRI, and MRA; the exact appearance is related to the severity of the disease (211,235). The fundamental finding relates to progressive supraclinoid carotid artery narrowing that subsequently extends into the proximal segments of the anterior and middle cerebral arteries (211,234–236). As the progressive stenosis of the internal carotid artery worsens, collateral flow develops to the adjacent small perforating and leptomeningeal vessels (234,236). The angiographic pattern has been classified according to Suzuki et al., grading the severity from Stage I through Stage VI. Stage I represents narrowing of the internal carotid bifurcation, and Stage VI reflects the appearance of the classic Moyamoya pattern with extensive pial collaterals through the external carotid arteries (236) (Fig. 32). The clinical presentation tends to be related to the age when the disease develops. In the pediatric age group patients present with transient ischemic attacks and stroke, which can progress to a severe vegetative state (234,236). In the adult population, patients often present with intraventricular hemorrhage and subarachnoid hemorrhage (234).

Technical Background

Yamada et al. compared 3DFT TOF MRA with catheter angiography in 12 patients with Moyamoya disease (235). In 21 of 24 supraclinoid internal carotid stenoses, MRA accurately depicted the degree of occlusive disease; however, MRA overestimated the severity of the stenoses in three instances. Similar findings were identified with evaluation of the anterior middle and posterior cerebral arteries (MRA accurately demonstrated 61 vessels and overestimated the severity of occlusive disease in 11 arteries). As expected, when the severity of the disease worsened, the accuracy of TOF MRA diminished because of the slower flow conditions with increasing saturation of the moving spins. Identification of leptomeningeal and transdural collateral vessels were accurately identified in only 18 of 28 vessels. Given the slow flow, employing a 2DFT TOF technique in the late stage of disease may be helpful, and using a 3DFT TOF technique in the earlier stages of the disease to avoid overestimation of the severity of the stenosis. In addition, the use of intravenous contrast may be a helpful adjunct to increase intravascular contrast by shortening the T1 of blood and therefore the saturation effects (45,237,238).

Pediatric Arterial Occlusive Disease

Most MRA investigations have been directed toward two pediatric groups: patients with sickle-cell disease (SCD) complicated by strokes, and neonates following carotid cannulation for extracorporeal membrane oxygenation (ECMO) therapy.

Sickle Cell Vasculopathy

Clinical Background

Although SCD and thrombotic stroke have been known to coexist for more than 70 years, it was not until the mid 1980s that an autopsy series documented that cerebral infarction was regularly associated with carotid artery stenoses/occlusion (239–241). Infarctions occur most extensively in the territory supplied by the internal carotid artery, specifically in the region supplied by the distal watershed territories of the anterior and middle cerebral arteries (242,243). Cerebrovascular sequelae are seen in up to 17% of cases (244). Several subsequent investigations have demonstrated evidence of infarction on MRI in corresponding locations (245–248). Large

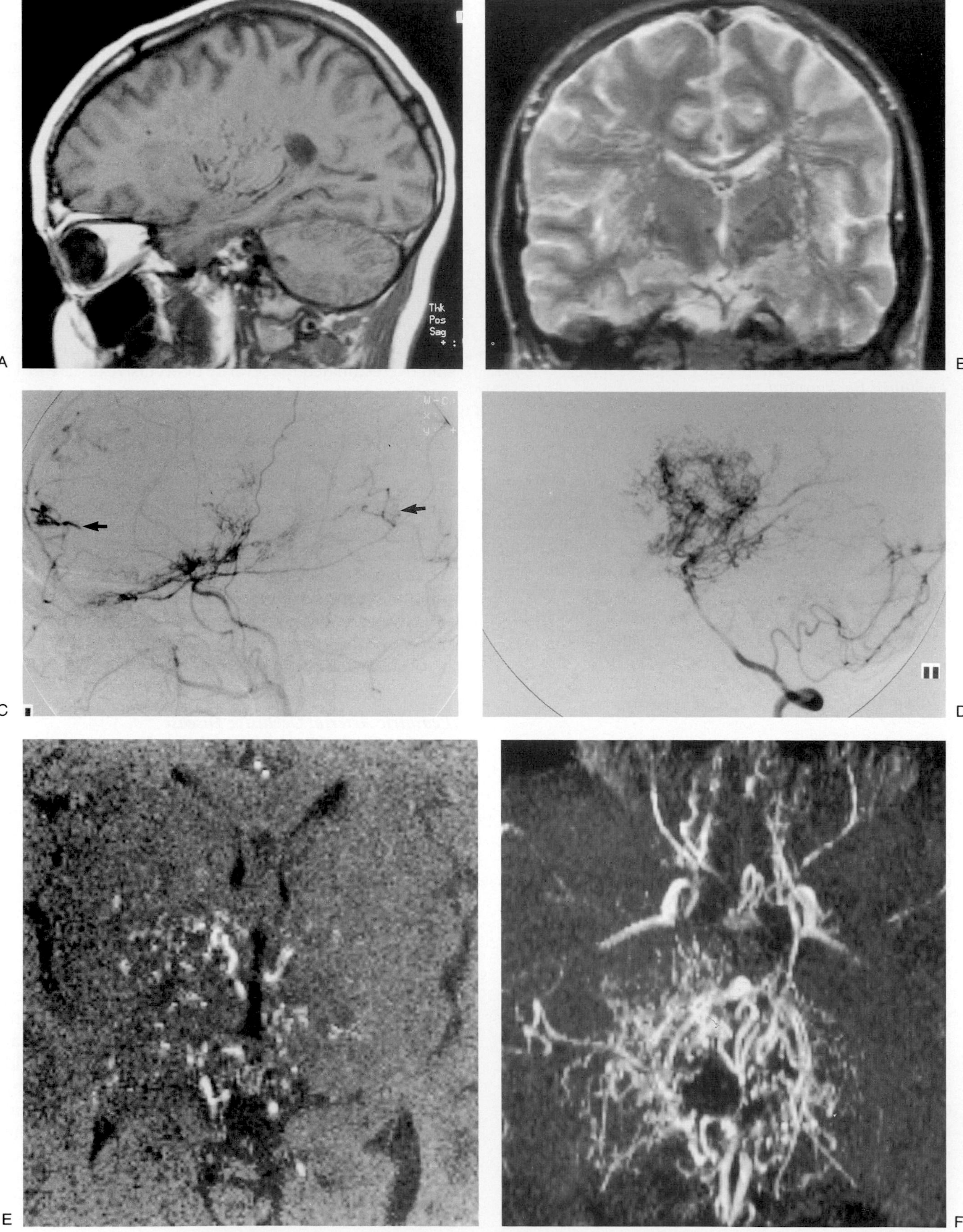
A
B
C
D
E
F
Thk
Pos
Sag

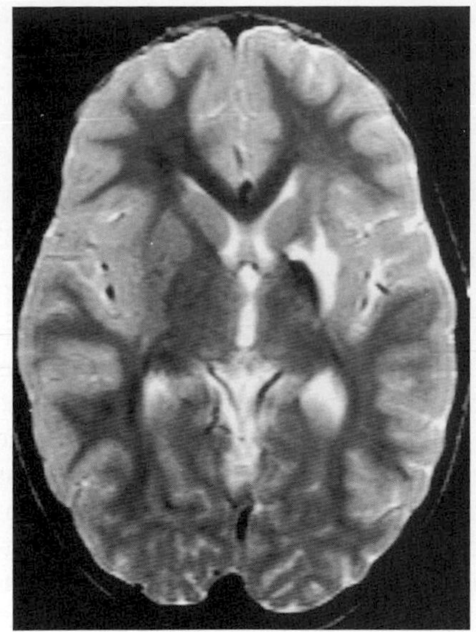

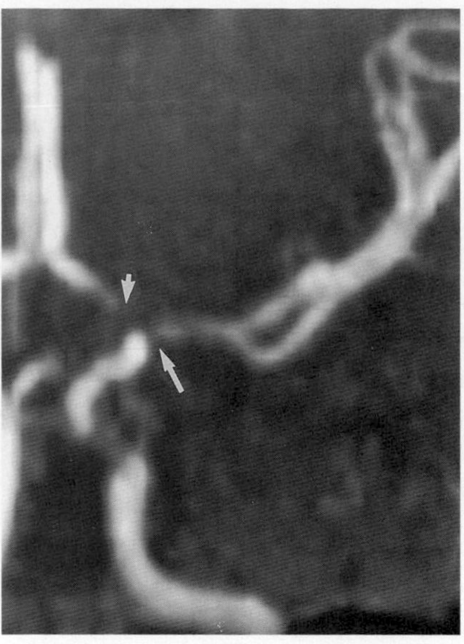

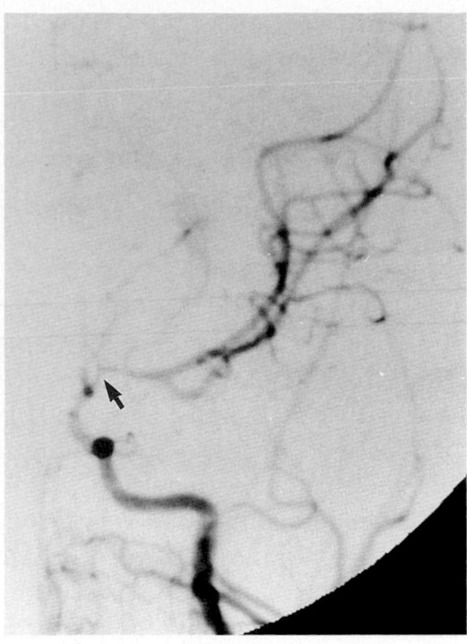

FIG. 33. A 9-year-old child with sickle cell disease. **A:** There is infarction of the left lentiform nucleus. **B:** 3D TOF MRA. There is a stenosis of the terminal portion of the internal carotid artery (*arrow*) and apparent stenosis (*short arrow*) of the proximal anterior cerebral artery as well. The digital subtraction angiogram, **C,** demonstrates the terminal internal carotid artery stenosis (*arrow*) and occlusion of the proximal anterior cerebral artery.

vessel disease, attributed to intimal proliferation, has been documented in 60% to 93% of SCD patients with stroke by catheter angiography (247–251). The theory that infarction occurs when anemia and hemodynamic insufficiency compound large vessel stenoses resulted in the institution of chronic prophylactic exchange transfusion therapy. This has been successful in preventing recurrence of clinical strokes in most SCD patients with a prior history of cerebral infarction (242,252–254). Unfortunately, the only known risk factor useful to distinguish those SCD patients at high risk of stroke, in whom prophylactic therapy would be useful, is a previous ischemic incident. This has recently been supported by MRI data in which Kugler et al. studied 16 asymptomatic patients with SCD who were imaged with MRI (255). Eight patients had no abnormalities on MRI and eight had abnormalities that were felt to be a result of ischemic infarction. They were followed longitudinally for a mean of 3.7 years and were assessed neurologically. In the group of asymptomatic patients with abnormal MRI, 38% became clinically symptomatic; however, the patients with normal MRI examinations remained normal during the study period. Interestingly, both groups of patients had a high incidence of abnormal scores in one or more areas of cognitive function (255). It has been suggested that even an asymptomatic patient with an abnormal MRI may represent a clinically silent stroke and should be started on long-term transfusion therapy to avoid a cerebrovascular catastrophe (255).

Technical Background

Catheter angiography detects the large vessel occlusions associated with infarction. It is invasive and carries an increased risk of precipitating stroke in SCD patients (256). Thus, MRA combined with parenchymal MRI appears to be well suited for the neurovascular evaluation of these patients (257). Several papers on 3DFT TOF MRA validate that it is capable of delineating vascular stenoses and occlusions in a fashion analogous to conventional angiography (217,228,229,232,235,257, 258) (Fig. 33). Additionally, normal studies may also be useful as a screening tool, thus avoiding unnecessary contrast angiography (257). There are numerous studies that have reported an increase in regional cerebral blood flow in patients with SCD (255,259,260). Attempts have been made to correlate regional blood flow using xenon CT and transcranial Doppler with varying results (260–

FIG. 32. A 10-year-old child with moyamoya disease. **A:** T1-weighted sagittal and **B:** T2-weighted coronal images demonstrate the flow voids due to the collateral flow from the enlarged perforating vessels. **C,D:** Lateral carotid and vertebral artery injections demonstrate extensive collateral flow from perforating vessels arising off the distal basilar artery and proximal posterior cerebral arteries. There is collateral dural-to-pial flow through the anterior falcine and meningeal arteries (*arrows*, C). **E:** 3D TOF MRA individual slice revealing the extensive collateral flow through perforating vessels. **F:** MIP image demonstrating the classic "puff of smoke" appearance predominantly from the thalamostriate perforators and posterior choroidal vessels seen on the vertebral artery catheter angiogram.

262). Direct flow measurements with MRA techniques may also be used at the same sitting as the conventional MRI to assess relative hemispheric blood flow.

Extracorporeal Membrane Oxygenation

Clinical Background

A second group of pediatric patients with arterial occlusion studied by MRA consists of neonates and infants following ECMO therapy, a method of partial heart-lung bypass used to treat life-threatening respiratory failure in the newborn. This therapy is performed by diverting blood from the right jugular vein through an external gas exchange membrane and returning it to the systemic circulation via the right carotid artery. Following discontinuation of ECMO therapy, the right common carotid artery and internal jugular vein are often ligated. Several studies have shown both neurologic and neurodevelopmental dysfunction following ECMO therapy, possibly due to pre-existing hypoxic damage, altered hemodynamics, ligation of the right common carotid artery or internal jugular vein, anticoagulation, or some combination thereof (263,264).

Whereas US and CT can provide important imaging information during therapy (264), MRI is primarily limited to evaluation of the infant following termination of ECMO bypass because of the adverse effects of the magnetic field on critical care instrumentation, including the bypass pump. Following completion of ECMO, MRI of the brain parenchyma is a sensitive examination for hemorrhagic and ischemic complications, in addition to the brain maturity (myelination) (265,266).

Technical Background

In a study of 23 infants, 3DFT TOF MRA evaluation of the intracranial vascular patterns following ECMO documented patency of the right internal carotid artery proximal to the ophthalmic artery in nine of 16 patients with permanent carotid ligation. The importance of the role for MRA is diminishing in this clinical scenario because of changes in therapy. Reanastomosis of the right common carotid artery following ECMO is being performed more commonly. Moreover, veno-venous ECMO is being performed to avoid the untoward side effects of arterial access. Four neonates in this study underwent reanastomosis, with patency of the carotid anastomosis documented in three patients with cervical carotid MRA (49). These findings suggest that MRA may prove to be a useful examination of the carotid arteries in infants following ECMO with surgical vascular reanastomosis. Additionally, such studies allow the natural history of cerebrovascular changes in the growing child to be followed after the anterior fontanelle has closed, a capability not shared by US. The limiting factor of spatial resolution in these small patients has been the gradient constraints of present MR systems, which, with the short TE and refocusing gradients, limit the effective field of view. As the child grows, image signal-to-noise ratio and visualization of more distal vasculature progressively improves (49).

These pediatric investigations suggest that 3DFT TOF MRA can provide good vascular detail and allow sensitive evaluation of arterial occlusive disease in the adult as well as the child. However, one basic deficiency of these preliminary MRA techniques has been their lack of the ability to demonstrate collateral flow. This drawback has been addressed in a more recent study using the sequential-2DFT TOF technique, in which pathways of collateral flow in the intracranial circulation were demonstrated by selectively placing spatial presaturation pulses at points of feeding vessels within the circle of Willis, and then imaging the flow-related enhancement through collateral vessels into these regions (267). Such studies can be implemented rapidly and can be a valuable adjunct to the angiographic examination.

Venous Occlusive Disease

Clinical Background

The wide variability and severity of the symptoms and signs of cerebral venous thrombosis (CVT) lead to difficult and often delayed diagnoses. Because of the diversity of predisposing conditions associated with dural sinus thrombosis, these often confuse the clinical presentation rather than lead toward a rapid diagnosis. Moreover, it is estimated that approximately 25% of cases are idiopathic (268–272). The most common adult conditions include local or systemic infections, intrinsic or acquired coagulopathies, trauma, pregnancy, oral contraceptive use, and collagen vascular disorders (5,268, 269,273,274). As alluded to previously, the clinical manifestation of CVT is variable; however, headache is by far the most common presenting symptom (268,271,275). Classically, additional signs and symptoms include a focal sensory or motor neurologic deficit, nausea and vomiting, seizures, and altered level of consciousness (5,268,269,272,273).

Older children have a similar presentation to adults. However, neonates tend to present with seizures (268, 272,276). Before antibiotics, most cases related to otitis or mastoiditis; however, more common associated conditions include neonatal asphyxia, severe dehydration, and congenital heart disease (268,272,276).

Classically, the mortality associated with CVT was high. Now, with the advent of angiography and newer noninvasive techniques including MRA, the diagnosis is made more frequently. Patients presenting with mild symptoms tend to have a relatively benign course with appropriate therapy (268). Because of this potentially poor outcome, rapid diagnosis is important to facilitate implementation of appropriate therapy of the predisposing condition and the use of anticoagulants (277,278) (Fig. 34).

Technical Background

CVT has traditionally been diagnosed with catheter angiography or with CT by the direct identification of thrombosed veins or the "empty delta," "sinus rectus," or "falx" signs (270,279). Several studies using MRA in the evaluation of dural sinus and deep venous thrombosis have been published (275,276,280–282) (Fig. 34). In the past, several case reports anecdotally demonstrated the utility of both TOF and PC techniques in the setting of dural sinus thrombosis (275,280). More recently, Vogl et al. analyzed 42 patients with clinical findings suggestive of dural sinus thrombosis and 10 patient control subjects were evaluated with 2DFT TOF MRAs as well as routine SE imaging. All control subjects (25 patients)

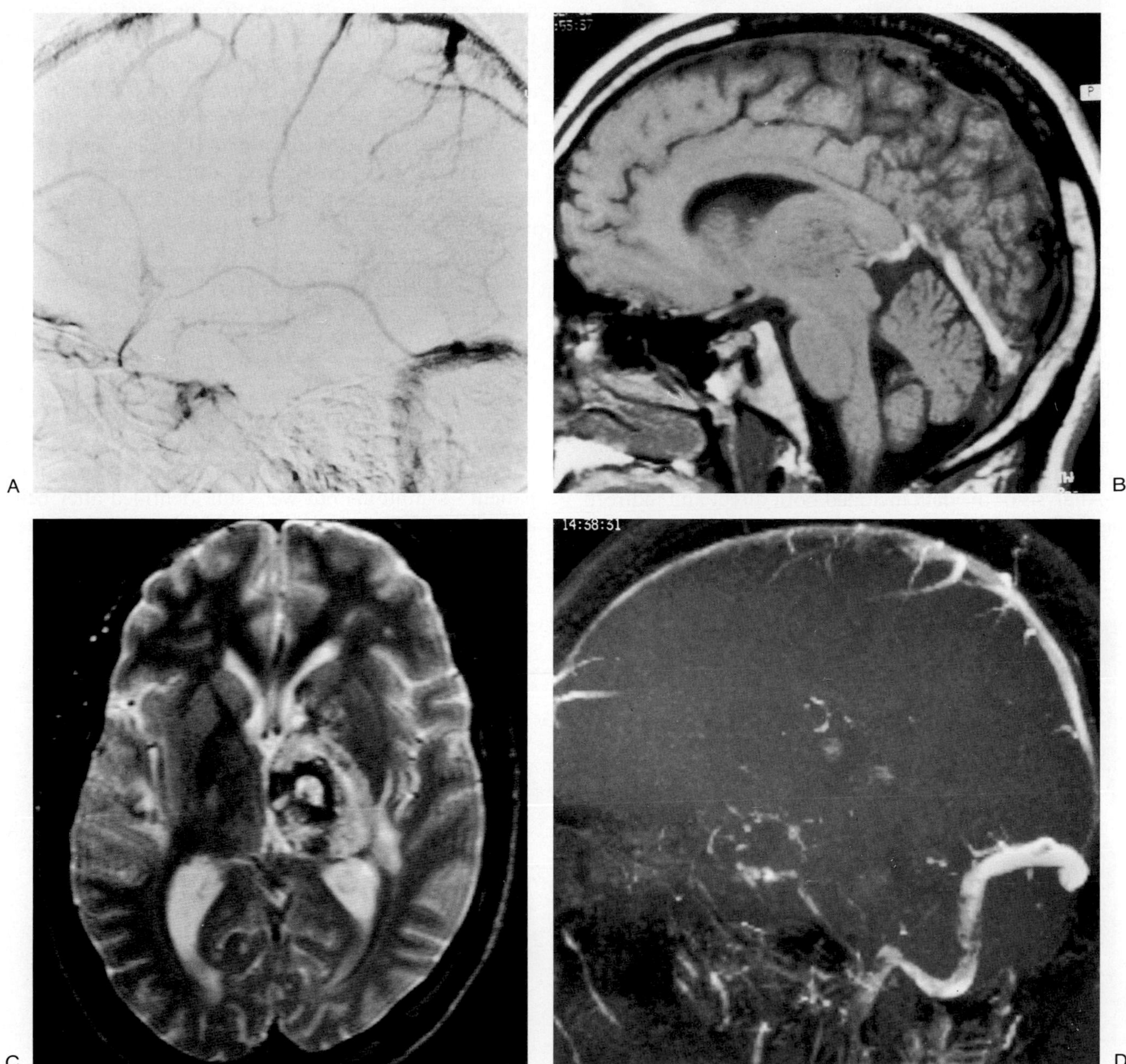

FIG. 34. Deep cerebral venous thrombosis. **A:** Venous phase of a catheter angiogram demonstrated occlusion of the deep venous system. **B:** A T1-weighted sagittal image performed the day before the angiogram demonstrates thrombosis of the internal cerebral veins, vein of Galen, and straight sinus. **C:** A T2-weighted axial image performed 10 days later shows a large hemorrhage in the thalamus and internal capsule on the left. **D:** The 2D TOF MRA 20 days after the presentation shows persistent thrombosis of the deep venous system.

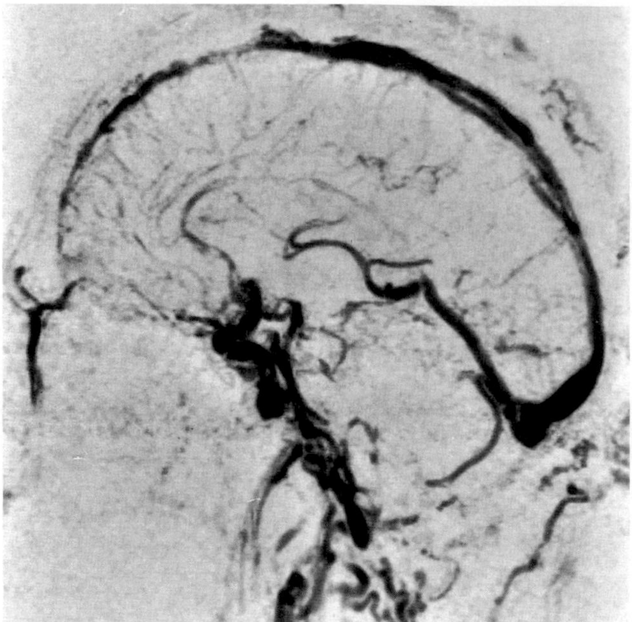

FIG. 35. 2D phase contrast MRV with a velocity encoding of 20 cm/sec in a patient with a recanalized superior sagittal sinus thrombosis. Notice the frayed appearance of the superior sagittal sinus, a common finding with recanalization.

were determined not to have dural sinus thrombosis, whereas 17 patients were felt to have dural sinus thrombosis by MRA techniques. Confirmation of the diagnosis was performed with conventional catheter angiograms in 9 of the 17 patients (282).

Analysis of the data included both direct and indirect signs of dural sinus thrombosis. Direct signs specifically included the lack of the typical high flow signal from sinuses that did not appear aplastic or hypoplastic on the individual partitions from the MRA and the frayed appearance of a thrombosed sinus that had subsequently recanalized (Fig. 35). Indirect signs of dural sinus thrombosis included unusual prominent flow signals from deep medullary veins, cerebral hemorrhage, visualization of emissary veins, and signs of increased intracranial pressure. The diagnosis was best established in the single frames from the 2DFT TOF sequences, which had characteristic appearances depending on the evolution of the blood products from the thrombus (282). Specifically, in acute cases (less than 1 week after onset of symptoms), thrombus was identified as a hypointensity approximately isointense with the surrounding brain tissue. At approximately 7 to 10 days, thrombus was identified as being homogeneous and slightly hyperintense with respect to the adjacent brain tissue (Fig. 36). In cases of nonocclusive thrombosis, a reproducible area of hypointense intraluminal signal was identified that was adherent to the venous wall and was partially surrounded by high signal from adjacent flowing blood. The maximum intensity projection reconstructions did not demonstrate the thrombus itself, and therefore were felt to be less helpful, especially in differentiating thrombotic occlusion from hypoplastic or aplastic dural sinuses (282). In seven patients in whom repeated MRA examinations were performed, progressive improvement in the MRAs was demonstrated, including the presence of intraluminal strands that were seen within 2 weeks of onset of the patient's symptoms but were still identified after being asymptomatic for months (282). In two patients, indirect

A 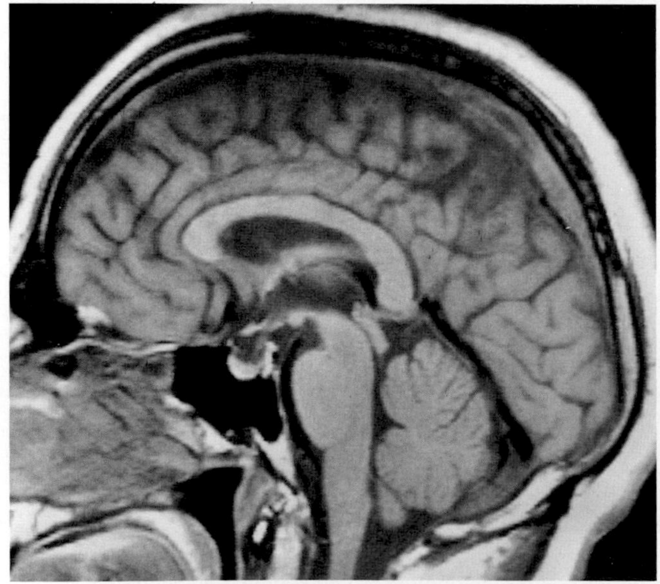

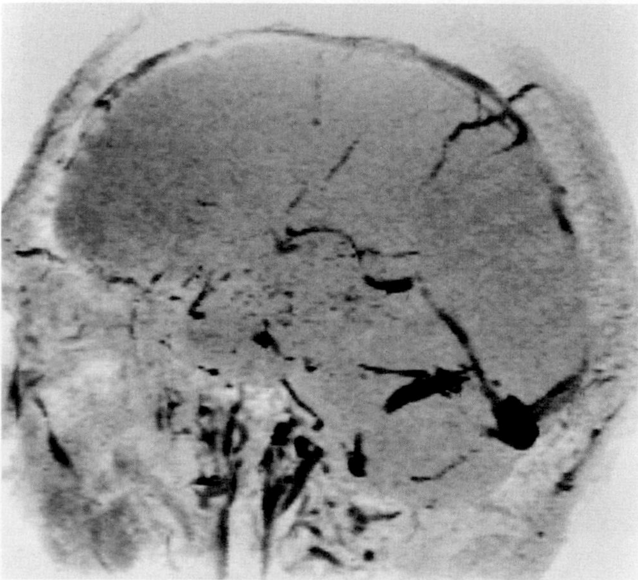 B

FIG. 36. Acute thrombosis of the superior sagittal sinus. **A:** T1-weighted sagittal image demonstrates intermediate signal intensity within the superior sagittal sinus. Note the straight sinus in the internal cerebral veins demonstrating flow void. **B:** 2D TOF MRA demonstrates thrombosis of the superior sagittal sinus.

signs such as diminished flow from inflowing arteries were conspicuous, and increased signal in collateral veins could be identified (282). In the second study, 3 of 13 patients with CVT were diagnosed with MRAs that showed similar findings consisting of stranding with recanalization of the sinus thrombosis (276).

Clearly, MRI has advanced the diagnosis of cerebral venous occlusive disease; however, SE MRI can occasionally be misleading in the presence of intravascular signal secondary to flow-related enhancement or even echo rephasing (283). In addition, depending on the stage of thrombus formation, a false impression of vessel patency on the T2-weighted images can occur if the blood is in the deoxyhemoglobin or methemoglobin stage (283). Since 2DFT TOF MRA techniques are sensitive down to the order of 3 to 4 cm/sec, this technique is especially appealing in the evaluation of the intracranial venous system (41). Initial studies evaluating the feasibility of 2DFT TOF technique revealed good correlation with the patients who had contrast angiograms (41,284). Mattle et al., in evaluation of the direct coronal, sagittal, and axial images, concluded that the direct coronal projection was the best for evaluating the intracranial venous structures (284). More recently, Lewin et al. have evaluated a sequential 2DFT TOF oblique slice technique (284) (Fig. 6). Flow-related enhancement is maximized when flow into the imaging plane is perpendicular to the imaging slice (5). The corollary is that flow-related enhancement diminishes when the plane of imaging parallels the vessel being interrogated. The above reasons make the use of direct coronal imaging attractive because it provides the greatest inflow of unsaturated spins in the midline veins but requires a large number of slices to evaluate the entire intracranial venous structures, and signal loss may be seen in the posterior aspect of the superior sagittal sinus because of in-plane spin saturation. The use of the oblique sagittal slice provides adequate flow-related enhancement, avoids spin saturation, and allows fewer slices to evaluate the intracranial venous system (283) (Fig. 6).

Limitations of the 2DFT TOF techniques include incorporation of methemoglobin within thrombus (high signal intensity), mimicking flow on the MRA (285). It is important to stress that evaluation of T1-weighted SE images should be performed to help avoid this pitfall. In addition, whereas areas of hyperintense intravascular thrombus have been detected on T1-weighted SE sequences, the signal intensity is frequently not as high as that of flowing blood and therefore may not be always incorporated into the MIP angiogram (283). In addition, signal flow voids or ghosting can be identified at junctions of complex geometry such as the sigmoid sinus and transverse sinus. Signal voids can be identified on 2DFT TOF techniques, probably arising from nonuniform flow resulting in persistent phase dispersion combined with in-plane flow from segments of the venous system within the imaging plane (283). Techniques to avoid this problem such as shortening the echo time may be helpful. In addition, it is important to recognize analysis of the MIP angiogram as well as the individual MRA slices help avoid misdiagnosing a nonocclusive thrombus (264,283).

In addition to the TOF MRA technique, PC MRA has been reported in the evaluation of dural sinus occlusion (280,286). Phase-contrast techniques have desirable features in that they are sensitive to flow in all directions, which allows imaging of regions with complex flow geometry and directions such as torcula and sigmoid sinuses (Fig. 35). In addition, PC techniques will not demonstrate the artifact from intracranial hemoglobin or other causes of high signal on T1-weighted images that can be incorporated into the TOF MRAs. In situations with an extremely slow flow, the sensitivity of PC or TOF techniques can be improved by administering a contrast agent that shortens the T1 of blood, increasing intravascular signal intensity by elevating the study state magnetization (287). The disadvantage of the PC techniques is that they require the acquisition and postprocessing manipulation of multiple views of the venous system for complete evaluation. Additionally, because of the superior background suppression and data acquisition, identification of the intraluminal thrombus is more difficult.

Technical Background

Both flow direction and flow volume analysis can be performed most easily using phase-contrast techniques. Flow direction is generated using phase-subtraction techniques. When using these techniques, the quantitative phase velocity relationships are maintained by insuring that the velocity encoding selected is higher than the greatest expected venous velocity to avoid phase wrap or aliasing (288). Flow volume measurements within the sagittal sinus can be quantitatively measured using phase-contrast techniques. The initial cine PC techniques yield a normal flow rate of approximately 285 ml/min (288). The flow values obtained both with cine PC and single-slice PC methods are lower than previously reported using bolus tracking techniques (13,288).

An alternative method to determine flow direction relies on bolus tracking technique as described previously. Mattle et al., using bolus tracking technique, measured mean flow studies in the superior sagittal sinus that equaled 420 ml/min. In addition, dynamic changes in cerebral blood flow during hyperventilation and hypercapnia were observed. Although the accuracy of these techniques needs validation, both the phase-contrast and bolus tracking techniques show promise not only to determine the degree of venous compromise but also to quantify the flow rate through a compromised vascular channel.

Vascular Compression of the Facial or Trigeminal Nerve

Clinical Background

A common etiology of trigeminal neuralgia and most cases of hemifacial spasm are felt to be caused by vascular compression of the exiting nerve root from the pons, often called the nerve root exit zone (289) (Fig. 37). Other less common etiologies include extra-axial mass lesions in the cerebellopontine angle and intraparenchymal lesions, including multiple sclerosis (290). Although some consider vascular compression of the fifth or seventh nerve root exit zone to be controversial, there is support for neurovascular compression by neuropathologic and electrophysiologic studies (291,292). Moreover, several recent MRI- and MRA-based studies have supported the notion of compression of the exiting nerve with demonstration of the compressing vascular structures preoperatively with clinical improvement following microvascular decompression (290,293–299). In an early study using MRI alone, 13 of 13 patients with clinically documented hemifacial spasm had identification of a vascular structure at the root exit zone; however, a similar finding was also found in 21% of the asymptomatic patients. In addition, identifying the specific vessel involved was not possible in this MRI-based study (297). Adler and Bernardi et al. described 37 patients with hemifacial spasm with 16 age-matched control patients in which MRI, MRA, and MR tomographic angiography were applied in the study of hemifacial spasm (299). Sixty-five percent of patients with hemifacial spasm had ipsilateral vascular compression of the seventh cranial nerve or the pons, whereas only 6.3% of control patients had similar patterns of vascular compression. The MR tomographic angiography technique was found to be more sensitive and more specific in vascular decompression.

Marked elongation and widening of the basilar artery may result in compression of the adjacent brainstem and exiting nerve roots as well as physiologic changes that are associated with slow flow due to the enlarged vessel,

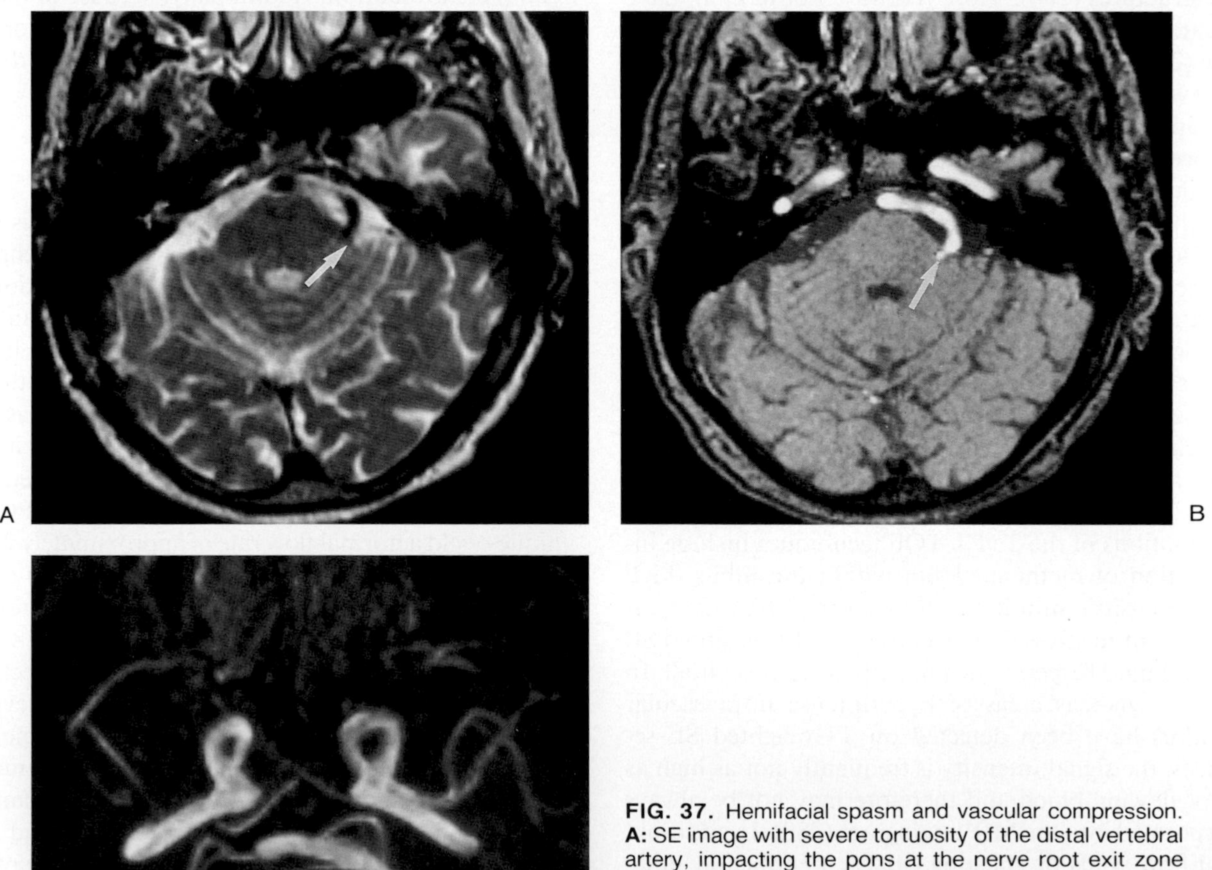

FIG. 37. Hemifacial spasm and vascular compression. **A:** SE image with severe tortuosity of the distal vertebral artery, impacting the pons at the nerve root exit zone (*arrow*). **B:** 3D TOF MRA image demonstrating flow within the vertebral artery impacting the right side of the pons at the nerve root exit zone (*arrow*). **C:** The maximum intensity projection MRA demonstrates the vascular anatomy without the benefit of having the adjacent parenchyma, making this image less helpful in the diagnosis of vascular compression.

a.k.a. basilar dolichoectasia (Fig. 38). This can result in cranial nerve palsies in up to 60% of patients with basilar dolichoectasia and symptoms of vertebral basilar insufficiency or vertebral basilar ischemic infarctions can be identified in approximately 55% of these patients. As with vascular compression in hemifacial spasm and trigeminal neuralgia, a 3DFT TOF MRA can be useful in identifying the vascular anatomy causing cranial nerve compression or compression of the midbrain itself. In patients with extremely slow flow, phase-contrast techniques employing slow velocity encoding may be helpful. In patients with vertebral basilar insufficiency or ischemic symptoms, these findings can direct therapy, which may include antiplatelet aggregating drugs.

Technical Background

MR tomographic angiography consists of using a conventional 3DFT TOF MRA technique and reformatting the original data acquisition in submillimeter coronal, sagittal, and oblique sections with the window and level adjusted to allow visualization of both vascular structures and the adjacent brainstem parenchyma as well as nerve root exit zones (290,299). The coronal reformations appear to be the most reliable for demonstrating the nerve root exit zone of the seventh cranial nerve (299). In addition, they studied gadolinium-enhanced MRI and found this to be of no additional value. Similar findings were published by Felber et al. in 14 patients with unilateral hemifacial spasm with 20 controls. MRI in combination with MRA demonstrated the neurovascular contact in 12 of 14 patients and only 4 of 20 controls. The vessels that can contribute to neurovascular compression include the vertebral artery, posterior inferior cerebellar artery, anterior inferior cerebellar artery, and less commonly the cochlear or basilar arteries (290,293,295,296). Occasionally venous structures have been implicated in the etiology of hemifacial spasm. In these particular cases, the 3DFT TOF techniques will not demonstrate the slower venous flow due to saturation effects or the presence of the venous presaturation pulse. Because of the multiple vascular structures that may be causing the vascular decompression, identifying the offending vessel has been helpful in directing the surgical approach (295,296,299).

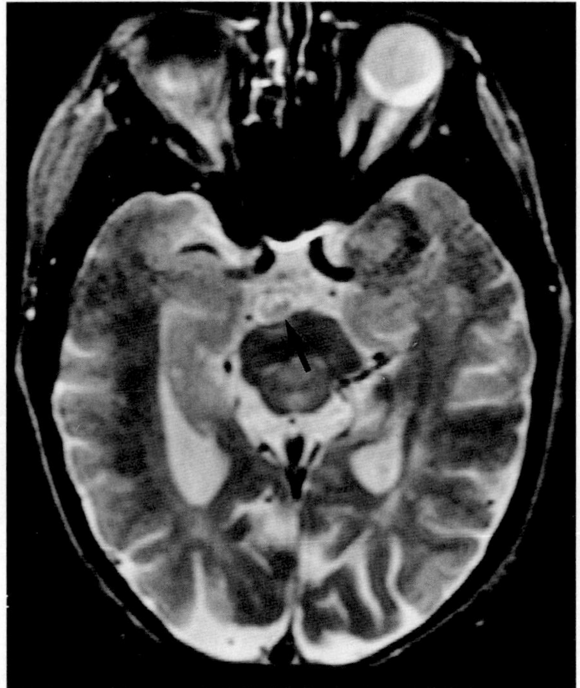
A

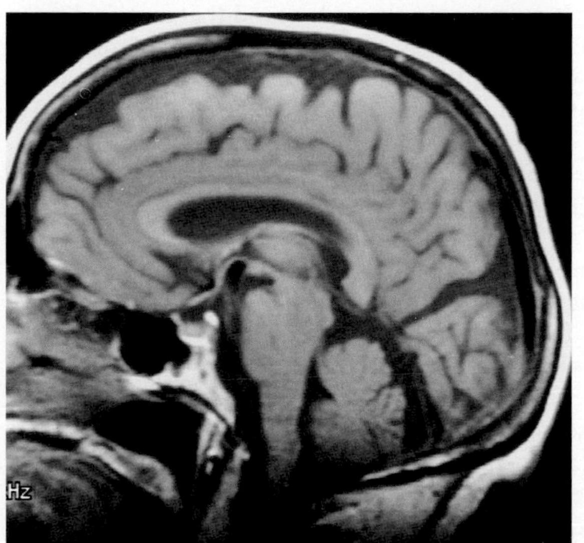

B

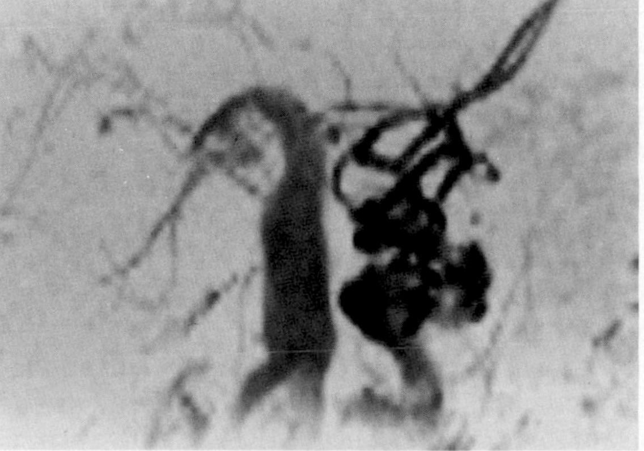
C

FIG. 38. Dolichoectasia of the basilar artery. **A:** Axial T2-weighted image demonstrates mixed signal intensity in the distal basilar artery due to slow flow. Note absence of the normal flow void (*arrow*). **B:** The sagittal T1-weighted image demonstrates the superior extent of the basilar artery with mass effect on the tuber cinereum. **C:** 3DFT TOF MRA reveals the markedly enlarged basilar artery and the signal intensity within the artery is less than that of the anterior circulation because of the slow flow within this vessel.

Intracranial Aneurysms

MRI and MRA have become more robust in the last several years. It is not only possible to establish a diagnosis of an intracranial aneurysm and to determine whether the aneurysm is solitary or multiple, but important associated characteristics may sometimes be identified, such as the size, location, relationship of the aneurysm to the apparent artery or adjacent vessels, the presence of small branches that arise off the aneurysm wall, and the demonstration of the neck of the aneurysm. All these factors may influence the surgical or endovascular approach to the treatment of these lesions. Unruptured intracranial aneurysms represent a major, growing public health problem in the United States, with a tremendous cost in terms of diagnostic work-up, hospitalization, and treatment. The value of having an imaging technique that can function reliably as a screening examination for intracranial aneurysms is irrefutable, because of the known low morbidity (4%) and mortality (0%) when an unruptured aneurysm is operated on. On the other hand, it should be stressed that any attempt to replace catheter arteriography for aneurysms with another imaging test must take into account the extremely high (60% to 70%) fatality rate in untreated ruptured aneurysms. It must be clearly understood that a missed (undetected) aneurysm is a life-threatening circumstance, because this is a treatable disease with a tragic outcome likely if left untreated.

Clinical Background

Approximately 28,000 intracranial aneurysms rupture each year in North America; 8% of these patients die before reaching the hospital and half the survivors die within the first 30 days following rupture (300,301). The prevalence of unruptured incidental aneurysms in autopsy series ranges from 1.3% to 7.9% (302,303). A more recent angiographic study by Atkinson et al. found a 1% prevalence of anterior circulation aneurysms (304). The low prevalence of incidental aneurysms suggested by this study, combined with the significant mortality and morbidity associated with ruptured aneurysms, emphasizes the need for urgent evaluation of the symptomatic patients, and also asymptomatic patients at risk (305–310).

Symptomatic patients can be divided into two groups: those who present with acute headaches/meningismus secondary to subarachnoid hemorrhage (SAH) and those who present with focal mass effect such as a cranial nerve palsy. An important limitation to the use of MRI and MRA in the detection of aneurysms is the insensitivity to subarachnoid hemorrhage (311,312). Therefore, CT and conventional intra-arterial angiography remain the most appropriate initial studies in cases of acute SAH (although in some circumstances MRI and MRA play a role). Catheter angiography as the exclusive modality of evaluation of patients with acute SAH is being challenged. In a recent case report in a patient with SAH, MRA demonstrated an anterior communicating artery aneurysm that was undetected by catheter angiography (313). Moreover, a second study comparing MRA to catheter angiography in the setting of SAH was also encouraging (314). Fourteen patients with acute SAH were evaluated with both modalities. In 3 of the 14 patients no abnormalities were detected on either diagnostic test, and two patients had two aneurysms each. MRA detected all the aneurysms with the exception of one, a 2-mm MCA aneurysm. Catheter angiography also failed to detect a 5-mm MCA aneurysm. Atlas recently reported results of a blinded reader study using a sophisticated postprocessing method and 3D TOF MRA in a large series of patients with intracranial aneurysms (315) In their study, MRA had a 96.8% sensitivity, an 86.3% specificity, a 96.9% positive predictive value, and a 91.7% negative predictive value for the presence of at least one aneurysm in patients with one or more aneurysm larger than 3 mm. They noted a very low sensitivity for aneurysms $\leq$ 3 mm in size and a low sensitivity for morphologic features suggestive of rupture. Notwithstanding these exciting preliminary reports, it still must be stated that MRA has no current role in the setting of acute SAH from a ruptured aneurysm.

The evaluation of asymptomatic cerebral aneurysms is evolving. Certain populations are at high risk for associated cerebral aneurysms and thus may be at risk for harboring nascent lesions. These include patients with polycystic kidney disease, cerebral arteriovenous malformations, fibromuscular dysplasia, coarctation of the aorta, and some connective tissue disorders (316–320). In addition, there are families with a high incidence of intracranial aneurysms (306,310,317,318,321,322). However, invasive studies are not typically performed in the asymptomatic patient unless another imaging modality is suggestive of an aneurysm. Other less invasive tests, such as CT, have significant limitations in their ability to detect small or asymptomatic aneurysms, including the requirement of intravenous, iodinated contrast agents (323,324). Indeed, MRA shows greatest promise as a screening procedure for asymptomatic aneurysms in high risk populations. The noninvasive nature and short acquisition time of 3DFT TOF MRA make the widespread screening for aneurysms possible, but also raise many questions related to patient outcome. Even though SAH associated with intracranial aneurysms is a known condition of high morbidity and mortality, there is no consensus regarding the natural history and risk of intact intracranial aneurysms (325–331). Calculating the risk of rupture, irrespective of size, is complicated by the lack of clear discrimination between symptomatic and asymptomatic aneurysms in most studies (325,328,330–333). The annual risk of rupture of an asymptomatic aneurysm has been estimated as less than 0.5% to 2% (326,327,331–334). Symptomatic intact aneurysms are associated with a significantly higher risk of hemorrhage, and these aneurysms rupture at a rate of at least 4% per year (325,329,331,332). Although the natural histories of incidental aneurysms and those discovered during the investigation of SAH from another source were not shown to be significantly different in one study (333), this point has never been properly investigated and the risk of rupture for these two groups of aneurysms may be dissimilar (334). Moreover, the prevalence of aneurysms is an important predictor of the benefit and cost effectiveness of screening, yet studies of the prevalence of aneurysms in asymptomatic subjects have been small and/or biased (317).

Three recent studies have assessed the prevalence of aneurysms in asymptomatic subjects with a history of autosomal dominant polycystic kidney disease (PKD). Chapman et al. identified two patients with aneurysms among 29 subjects with a family history of ruptured intracranial aneurysms using high resolution CT scanning; the 95% confidence interval for the prevalence of aneurysms based on this study is 0.02 to 0.23 (335). Huston et al. used MRA to identify six patients with aneurysms among 27 patients with a family history of aneurysm or SAH; the 95% confidence interval for the prevalence of aneurysms based on this study was 0.08 to 0.42 (305). Ruggieri and associates likewise used MRA to identify five patients with a saccular intracranial aneurysm among 27 patients with a family history or suspected family history of aneurysm; the 95% confidence interval for the prevalence of aneurysms based on this study was 0.09 to 0.42 (adjusted for the estimated false-negative rate of MRA) (309). In a fourth study of patients without PKD, Nakagawa and Hashi used a combination of catheter angiography and MRA to screen 400 Japanese patients with a family or clinical history of cerebrovascular disease; 26 patients (0.065) had aneurysms (307). Volunteers with a family history of SAH within the second degree of consanguinity showed a higher incidence of aneurysms (17.9%). MRI in combination with MRA holds promise for evaluation of unruptured aneurysms in asymptomatic and symptomatic patients. It was concluded by Levey et al. in a rigorous decision analysis of PKD patients that intra-arterial angiography should not be performed on a routine basis in this population because its benefit is significant only if the prevalence of aneurysms exceeds 30%, the surgical complication rate is less than 1%, and the patient is under 25 years old (317). The current data suggest that MRI with MRA can provide a noninvasive test that has the sensitivity and specificity to significantly impact high risk asymptomatic populations (308). Weibers and Torres, Ruggieri et al., and Huston and colleagues indicate that MRA may be the optimal noninvasive study to detect asymptomatic intracranial aneurysms (305,309,336). In the more recent protocol of Nakagawa and Hashi, they replaced catheter angiography with MRA as the screening method of choice (although the exact technique used is not described) (307).

Morphology and Flow

Classification of an aneurysm is often based on either the architecture or the etiology of the aneurysm. The morphologic appearance is commonly classified as saccular, or fusiform. The etiologies of aneurysms include congenital (berry), atherosclerotic, inflammatory, mycotic, dissecting, and neoplastic. The imaging evaluation of aneurysms includes demonstration of number, location, size, and morphologic appearance, as well as location of the neck in the case of saccular aneurysms (337). Intracranial aneurysms can be located intra- or extradurally. Extradural aneurysms involve the internal carotid arteries below the ophthalmic segment. Intradural aneurysms usually involve the distal internal carotid arteries, vessels of the circle of Willis, the bifurcation or trifurcation of the MCAs, and the vertebrobasilar trunk (338). Aneurysms involving more peripheral cerebral vessels are less common and are usually due to inflammatory, infectious, traumatic, or tumoral etiology (337,339–341). Posterior circulation aneurysms constitute 5% to 15% of cases. In addition, evaluation for the presence of associated vascular variants or anomalies (such as hypoplastic/aplastic segments of the circle of Willis, carotid/basilar artery anastomosis, and presence or absence of vertebral or carotid arteries) is imperative (337).

Intracranial aneurysms are most typically categorized by morphology. The subgroups include lateral saccular, bifurcation, terminal, fusiform, and giant aneurysms. The morphology results in different flow characteristics,

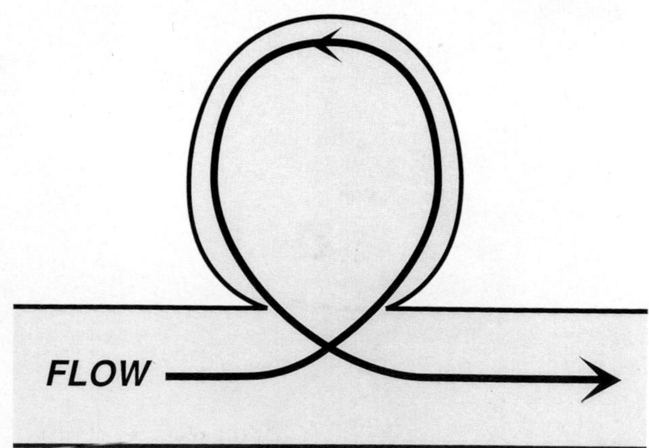

FIG. 39. Schematic of the lateral aneurysm. Notice the inflow along the distal margin of the aneurysm circulates through the dome and exits the proximal edge of the ostium of the aneurysm, a phenomenon that is not only appreciated in experimental animal aneurysms but also human aneurysms.

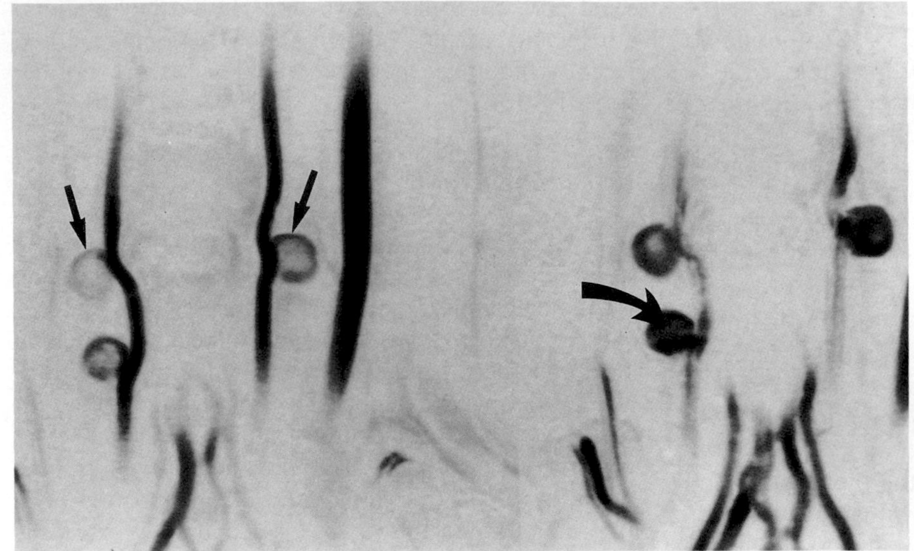

FIG. 40. Experimental lateral saccular aneurysms. **Left:** Coronal PC slab image obtained at a velocity encoding of 80 cm/sec identifies the high velocity inflow at the distal edge of the aneurysm ostium (*arrows*). **Right:** PC slab image obtained at a velocity encoding of 20 cm/sec. The central slow vortex flow within the aneurysm is better appreciated at the lower velocity encodings. Notice that the slow central flow is manifested by a lower signal intensity (*curved arrow*).

that may have implications relative to the clinical stability and growth of the lesion, and that are reflected in the appearance on MR flow images (342).

Lateral saccular aneurysms project nearly perpendicular from the side of the parent artery. The characteristic flow pattern in these aneurysms is a discrete inflow zone along the distal edge of the aneurysm ostium (Fig. 39). The blood flows in a circular fashion about the dome of the aneurysm and exits along the proximal edge of the aneurysm ostium. Centrally, recirculation of the blood results in a vortex flow pattern. These flow effects have been reported in experimental (Fig. 40) and human lateral saccular aneurysms (201,343,344) (Figs. 41 and 42). Both PC and TOF MRAs demonstrate the vortex flow as a region of central low signal intensity (201,344). The decreased signal intensity is primarily due to saturation effect rather than intravoxel dephasing. The slow central flow can be best visualized with a PC technique with a low velocity encoding (201,344).

Lateral saccular aneurysms are frequently encountered in the region of the carotid siphon. The accumulation of platelets and leukocytes along the intimal surface due to the flow stasis in lateral aneurysms reduces the oxygen diffusion and delivery of metabolites to the aneurysm wall (324). These factors have been proposed to lead to thrombus formation, thickening of the aneurysm wall, and aneurysm growth (345). Thus, the two main flow features of lateral aneurysms that impact on the MRA appearance are (a) the flow velocity is greatest within the inflow stream along the periphery of the aneurysm wall. The maximum flow velocity and shear stress is at the neck not at the dome of the aneurysm,

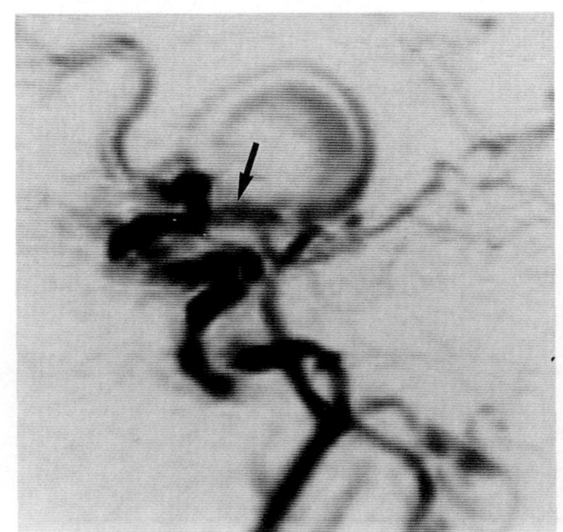

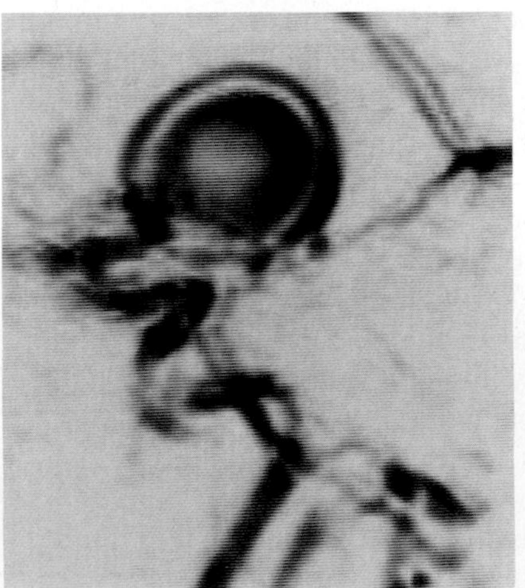

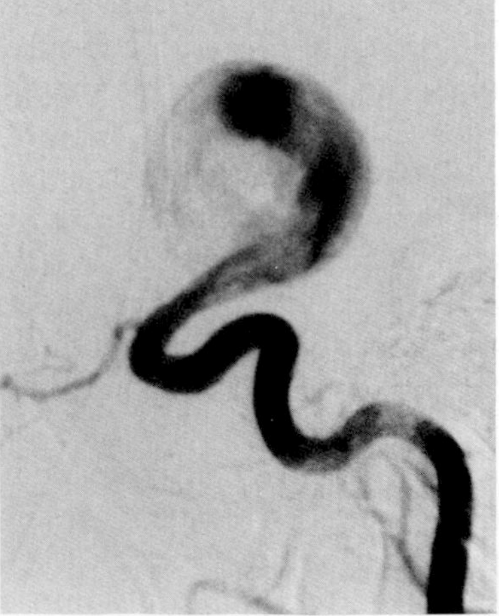

A B,C

FIG. 41. Inflow stream and vortex flow demonstrated by PC MRA on a giant internal carotid artery aneurysm. **A:** The sagittal PC slab MRA obtained at a velocity encoding of 40 cm/sec, demonstrating the relatively high inflow stream along the caudad aspect of the aneurysm (*arrow*). **B:** The second PC angiogram obtained at a velocity encoding of 10 cm/sec, revealing a slow central vortex. **C:** Catheter angiogram demonstrating the inflow jet and vortex flow. (From Anderson, Edelman and Turski, ref. 288, with permission.)

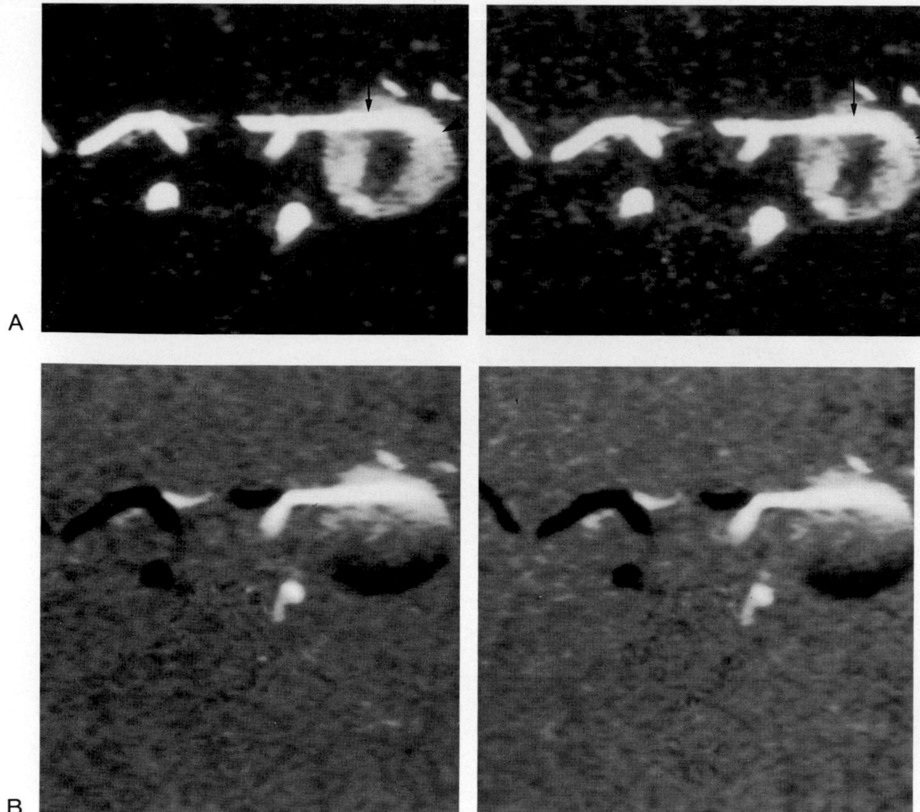

FIG. 42. Giant MCA aneurysm. **A:** cine PC speed images demonstrate a well-defined inflow stream (*arrows*) and impact zone (*arrowheads*) as well as a slow central vortex. **B:** 2D PC phase/velocity images with right to left flow encoding displayed from the systolic phase of the cardiac cycle. Again the well-defined inflow stream and impact zone can be identified.

and (b) thrombus formation within the aneurysm is a dynamic process that tends to occur in concentric layers and is related to flow. Therefore, aneurysms may appear substantially different on sequential MRI/MRA exams, even in the absence of intervening therapy.

The flow characteristics of bifurcation aneurysms have also been well documented in experimental models (343). Inflow into the aneurysm occurs at the margin of the ostium nearest to the long axis of the parent artery. Rapid helical flow is most commonly present in these aneurysms, with rotation of flow within and in the direction of the vascular outflow branch. All these flow patterns maintain a nearly laminar and relatively coherent flow profile. Since outflow is predominantly into one distal vessel, it can be difficult to visualize small branch vessels adjacent to the aneurysm. The high flow conditions within these aneurysms are sensitive to detection by 3DFT TOF MRA techniques. Loss of signal may occur from intravoxel dephasing, but the relatively high inflow into these aneurysms adequately defines the contour (Fig. 43). Bifurcation aneurysms are most often located at the MCA or internal carotid bifurcation.

The flow into terminal aneurysms is determined by a portion of the aneurysm ostium closest to a straight line drawn through the center of the stem artery (parent artery) (Fig. 44). Similar to bifurcation aneurysms, flow within terminal aneurysms is rapid and rotary in nature, with no evidence of slow central vortex patterns (346). Outflow is along the opposite edge of the aneurysm ostium and typically passes almost exclusively into the vessel nearest the outflow stream. The basilar tip aneurysm is the most common terminal aneurysm encountered clinically.

It is important to note that turbulent flow is not commonly present in any of these aneurysms. In all cases, flow within the aneurysm, although not always laminar, is seldom chaotic. Perktold and associates, using mathematical models and computer simulations to predict flow in an axisymmetric aneurysm model, noted complex consistent intra-aneurysm flow fields, with varying shear stresses in different portions of the aneurysm (347). Strother et al. have also shown that the geometric relationship between an aneurysm and its parent artery is the principal factor that determines the intra-aneurysm flow pattern (343). Flow is rather highly predictable, varying according to the geometric relationship of the aneurysm to the parent artery. Flow transitions that represent intermediate stages between laminar flow and turbulence were observed in all three aneurysm geometries. In light of the complex flow conditions, occasional difficulties may be encountered in adequately visualizing the flow within intracranial aneurysms using MRA techniques.

The predominant feature of fusiform and giant aneurysms is slow flow along the wall, often resulting in laminated mural thrombus. Because of saturation effects, the slow flow commonly makes them difficult to identify by

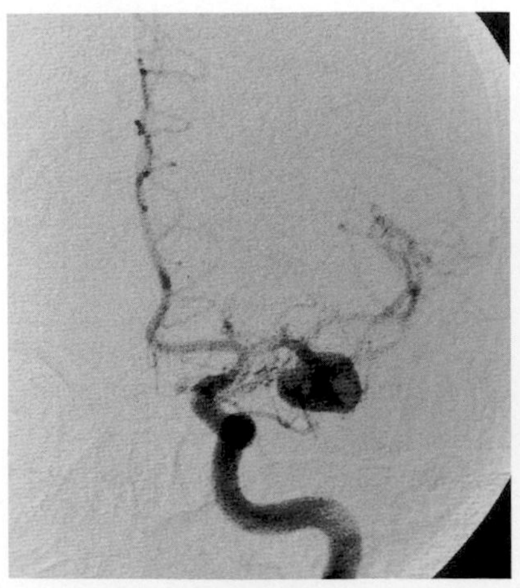

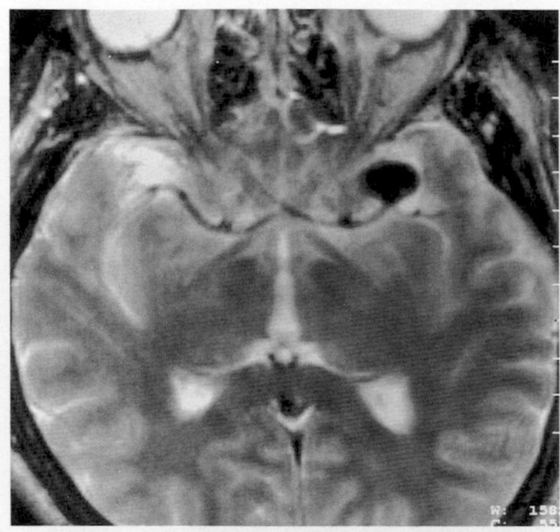

A,B

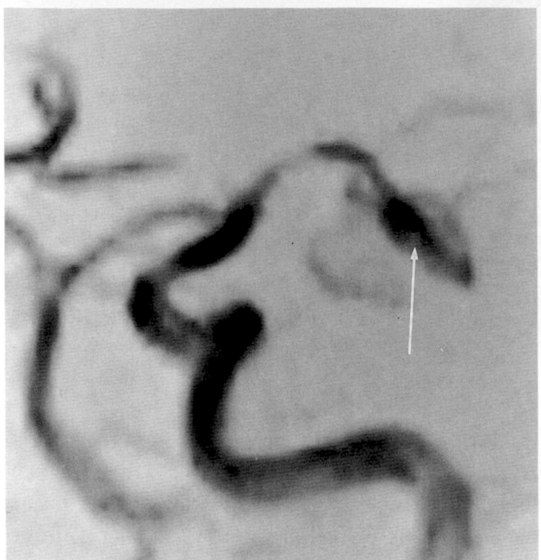

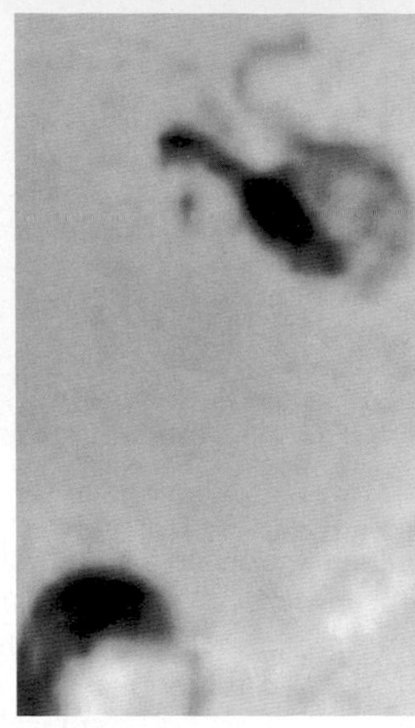

C,D

FIG. 43. Left MCA aneurysm. **A:** A 1.5-cm saccular left MCA aneurysm is demonstrated. The relationship of the neck of the aneurysm is not well appreciated and was not in any of the other catheter angiographic images. **B:** Axial SE-weighted image demonstrating the flow void within the aneurysm and the suggestion that the aneurysm arises at a bifurcation. **C:** Targeted maximum intensity projection image demonstrates the aneurysm. Note the high signal intensity of the inflow stream (*arrow*) and the lower signal intensity of the recirculating blood. On this image there is the suggestion that a branch arises from the aneurysm. **D:** Targeted MIP of the aneurysm itself demonstrates that clearly a branch arises off the aneurysm itself, requiring surgical reconstruction of the artery.

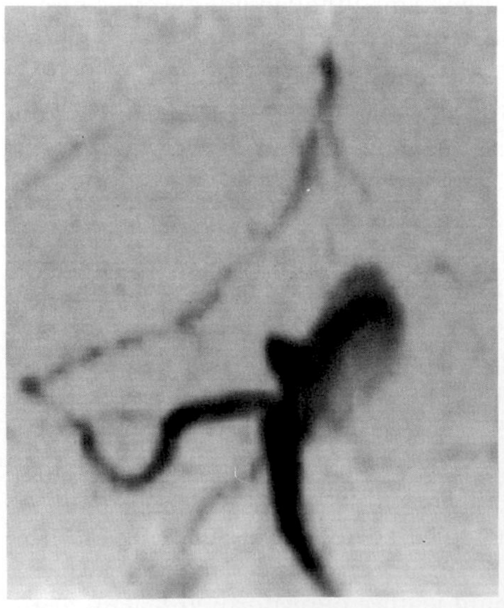

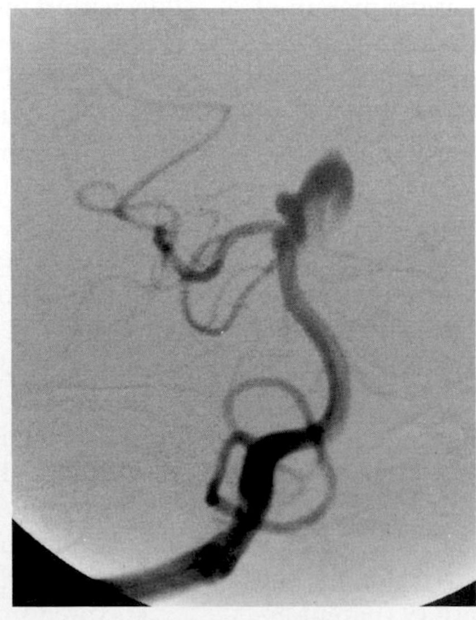

A,B

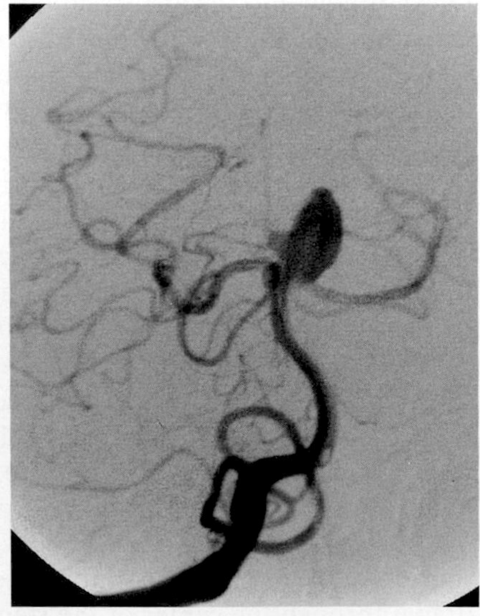

C

FIG. 44. Basilar tip aneurysm. **A:** 3D TOF MRA with a targeted MIP of a basilar tip aneurysm. Notice the outpouching along the right lateral aspect. In addition, the flow stream is identified on the right side of the aneurysm, which is oriented along the long axis of the basilar aneurysm. Notice the differential signal intensity in the left and right posterior cerebral arteries. **B,C:** Sequential frames from a catheter angiogram demonstrating the same phenomenon.

3D TOF MRA, and they may in fact appear normal in caliber on PC MRA, if the mural thrombus has sufficiently reduced the aneurysm lumen. The aneurysm size and associated thrombus can best be evaluated on SE MRI.

Technical Background

Anatomic Imaging. The spatial resolution of current 3DFT TOF angiographic methods is approximately 0.8 × 0.8 × 0.8 mm, less than catheter angiography but high enough to detect aneurysms as small as 2 to 3 mm. This has practical importance as both Loxley and McCormick et al. found no SAHs from aneurysms smaller than 3 mm (329,348). Thus, most aneurysms of clinical concern are large enough to be detected by current MRA techniques (Fig. 45).

In a small retrospective study by Ross et al., MRI and 3DFT TOF MRA were complementary, resulting in a combined sensitivity of 95% and a specificity of 100% compared to intra-arterial digital subtraction angiography (308). At least one aneurysm in each of 19 patients with saccular or giant intracranial aneurysms proven by IADSA was detected on MRA; 28 patients without a suspicion for aneurysm served as controls. These preliminary results were encouraging; however, several limitations of the study and 3DFT technique also came to light. First, the incidence of aneurysms within the study group was much higher than in the population as a whole, introducing bias into the sensitivity value. Second, vascular contrast depends on the presence of adequate inflow, with slow-flow lesions such as giant and/or fusiform intracranial aneurysms poorly visualized or underestimated in size because of saturation of the slowly moving spins. However, these were easily detected on the SE images. Finally, the aneurysm neck was often not visualized on the MRA, although the general relationship of the aneurysm to the parent vessel was appreciated. This was most commonly noted in the evaluation of internal carotid artery lesions, and less often in aneurysms at other locations (308). Although the anterior communicating artery, MCA, and basilar tip aneurysms were typically well defined, the carotid siphon proved problematic to fully characterize because of signal dropout from the uncompensated turbulent flow (Fig. 45). Potential solutions to these limitations include targeted maximum intensity projections, better flow compensation, shorter echo times, and reduced slice thickness (308). Alternative post-processing algorithms may also be of great benefit.

Giant intracranial aneurysms at any location (including the carotid siphon) present problems for MRA. These lesions are conspicuous on SE images, but may not demonstrate the same level of vascular contrast because of slow, disturbed flow with the aneurysm lumen (226,348—350) (Fig. 41). Alternatively, if an aneurysm is partially thrombosed, MRA may underestimate the true size or miss the aneurysm in a fashion analogous to catheter angiography. Additionally, most clinical TOF techniques employ an MIP algorithm to create the angiographic image from the original image data set. Although this is expeditious with respect to scan time, it does not completely exclude the angiogram signal from stationary tissue (particularly tissue with high signal such as paramagnetic blood breakdown products). This mis-

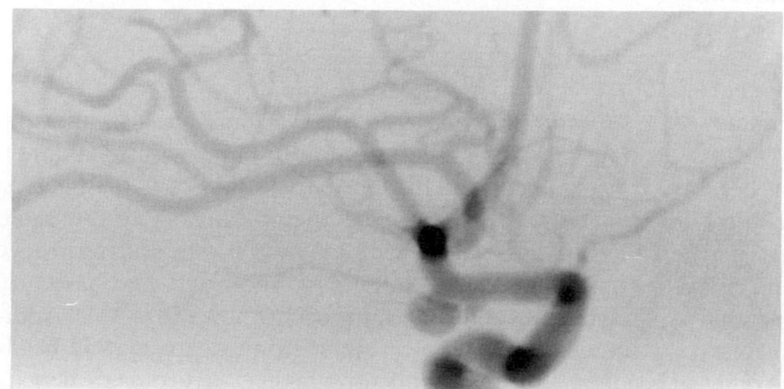
A

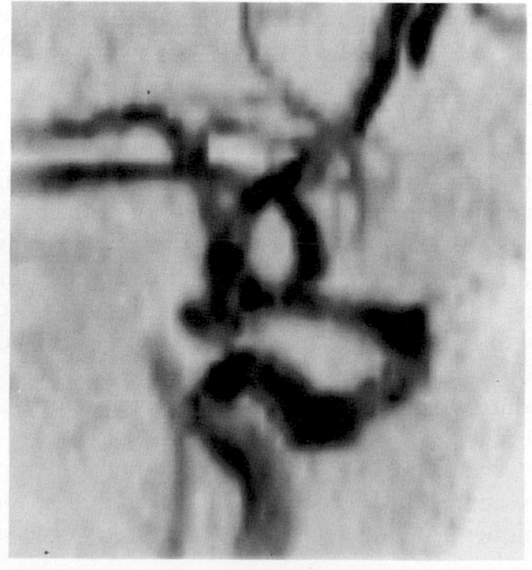
B

FIG. 45. Polycystic kidney disease and anterior choroidal aneurysm and posterior communicating artery infundibulum. **A:** The digital subtraction angiogram demonstrates the aneurysm nicely and the infundibulum well. **B:** The maximum intensity projection clearly demonstrates the aneurysm but shows the infundibulum poorly.

registration of stationary signal into the flow image may result in significant image degradation (226,348,349).

Occasionally the flexibility of postprocessing with the 3D data set of MRA images may allow visualization of certain aneurysms as well as delineating the morphology of the aneurysm (such as the neck) better than catheter angiography (350,351) (Fig. 43). A variety of pre- and postprocessing innovations have also been attempted to minimize the pitfalls of MIP rendered images. These include magnetization transfer and fat saturation pulses to minimize signal from nonvascular stationary tissue, macromolecular paramagnetic contrast agents, MOTSA 3D acquisition schemes and newer postprocessing techniques such as STANDOUT (58,72,73,352,353).

Phase-contrast MRA is not as dependent on rapid flow and hence in many cases may be better suited to giant aneurysms (see Fig. 41). This is especially true with respect to avoiding misregistration of clot into the final MIP image (225). Additional cine MR flow imaging techniques exist that can demonstrate flow and flow disturbances within aneurysms; with some it is possible to quantify blood flow and flow velocities (18,34,354). The clinical need for these images remains to be determined.

Clinical Studies in the Evaluation of Lesions Post-Therapy Evaluation

There are several studies suggesting that postoperative imaging with MRI of patients with a successfully clipped aneurysm is safe and provides more useful information than CT (355,356). Regardless of the chemical composition of the aneurysm clip, most CT images are markedly degraded by beam-hardening artifacts arising from the aneurysm clip (355,356). Often with MRI the artifacts are produced because of the magnetic properties of the alloys within the surgical clips resulting in local image distortion due to inhomogeneities produced in the magnetic field (356). The amount of artifact created on both imaging modalities relates to both the clip size and the alloy used in production of the clip (356). Nonferromagnetic aneurysm clips (not deflected in a magnetic field) have been available for several years from several manufacturers. The difficulty arises in distinguishing the ferro- from the nonferromagnetic clips once they have been placed in the patient. The safety of a magnetic clip for imaging does not imply that there will be no artifact; rather, that there will be no deflection and thus no risk of dislodging the aneurysm clip (356–358). Aneurysms wrapped with muslin gauze at surgery may be successfully evaluated with MRA techniques, as long as no other sources of artifact such as surgical clips are also present locally.

Aneurysms not amenable to surgical treatment may be approached by endovascular techniques. These techniques primarily consist of parent artery occlusion or direct aneurysm occlusion. Fox et al. successfully treated 65 of 67 patients by proximal parent artery occlusion with detachable balloons (359). Complete obliteration of the aneurysm in 65 of 84 patients by direct balloon placement into the lumen of the aneurysm was achieved by Higashida and associates (360). More recently, direct occlusion of aneurysms has been performed with Guglielmi Detachable Coils (GDC) with good success (361,362).

Identifying the location of the occluding balloon, assessing the presence of thrombus, and determining residual flow in the parent artery or aneurysm is important. Tsuruda and associates evaluated five patients treated with detachable balloons (363). Three of the five patients studied by catheter angiography had residual flow within the treated aneurysms. 3DFT TOF MRAs identified the residual aneurysm lumen in two of these patients. Methemoglobin within the thrombus obscured the flow in the third patient. Flow stasis or trapping the blood within the aneurysm results in a thrombus containing a large number of red cells and platelets and resembling venous thrombus (red thrombus) (364). Initially the thrombus is isointense on T1-weighted images, followed in 5 to 10 days by red cell lysis, oxidation to methemoglobin, and organization of the clot. After 2 to 4 weeks the predominant finding is the presence of methemoglobin (364). A second potential pitfall is slow flow within the aneurysm rest. Evaluation of patients treated with GDC with MRA has not been published to date. A canine study employing both PC and TOF techniques compared to catheter angiography revealed detection of only two of eight aneurysm rests (202). Both MRA techniques were degraded by the susceptibility artifact from the coils. Clinical implementation of both techniques has occasionally been successful (Fig. 46).

Arteriovenous Malformations

Clinical Background

Central nervous system pial arteriovenous malformations (AVMs) are less common than intracranial aneurysms, occurring in approximately 0.15% of the U.S. population (365,366). The natural history of untreated AVMs is associated with an annual rate of hemorrhage approximating 3%; subsequent morbidity and mortality related to hemorrhage approaches 50% (367–371). Additionally, patients may suffer from incapacitating headaches, seizures, and progressive neurologic deficits related to adjacent brain ischemia (367,369,370). Definitive treatment for AVMs may involve surgery, endovascular therapy, or radiation therapy. A subset of these AVMs, specifically those that are large and in deep or eloquent parts of the brain, are particularly problem-

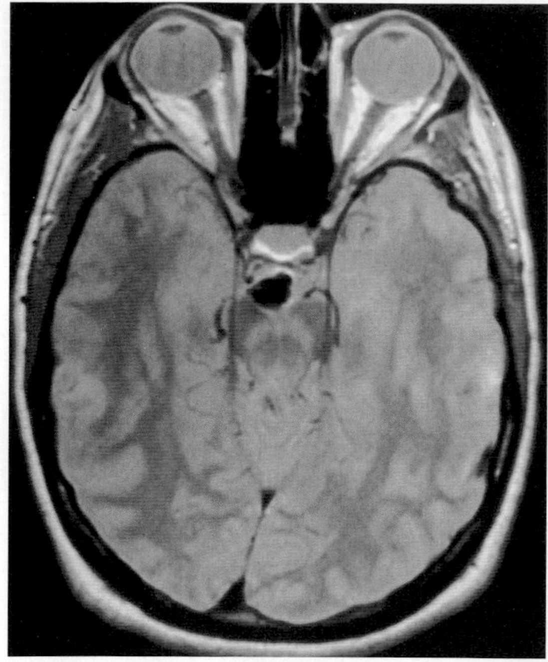

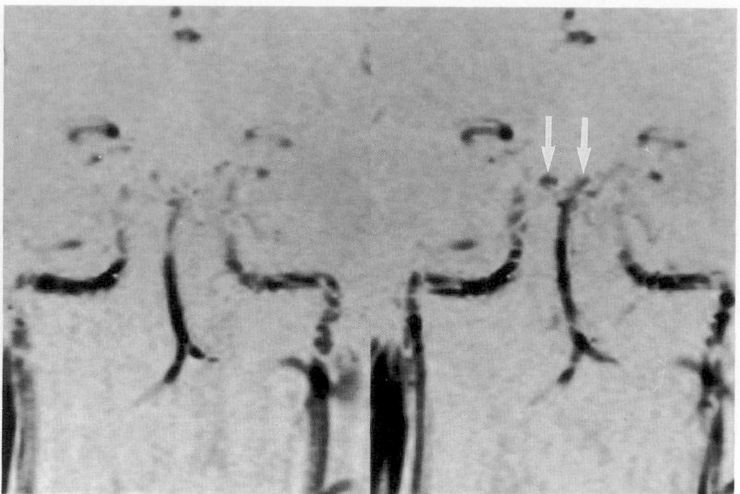

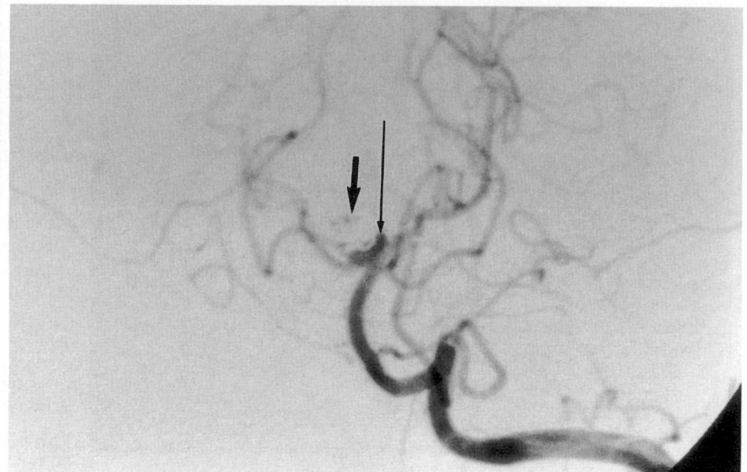

FIG. 46. Basilar tip aneurysm following treatment with GDC. **A:** An SE image demonstrating decreased signal intensity related to mild susceptibility artifact due to the GDC coils and possibly a residual aneurysm rest. **B:** A cine 2D phase-contrast MRA with a frame in diastole and systole. Note the two regions of high signal intensity adjacent to the basilar tip on the systolic frame, suggestive of residual aneurysm rest (*arrows*). **C:** Conventional angiogram demonstrating GDC coils (*thick arrow*) and aneurysm rest (*thin arrow*) that was subsequently treated with additional coils.

atic and require a coordinated, multimodality approach to their management (372).

Because of the multimodality approach of treating AVMs, it is important to establish not only the diagnosis, but the morphologic and physiologic features of the lesion that allow appropriate therapeutic decisions. To arrive at an appropriate therapeutic plan, specific features of the AVM need to be demonstrated. The afferent arterial feeding pedicles should be characterized as (a) direct terminal feeders supplying only the AVM (Fig. 47) and (b) indirect arterial pedicles supplying normal brain distal to the AVM (so-called en passage vessels). In addition, arteries providing collateral flow to ischemic brain about the AVM also exist as with secondary supply to the AVM. This supply may enlarge following incomplete treatment of the AVM (373,374). Angiomatous change or leptomeningeal collateral flow appears similar in appearance to the AVM nidus; however, distinguishing features include absence of the arteriovenous shunting and slow circulation (374). Other architectural aspects of the arterial supply that are important include the presence of arteriovenous fistulae (AVF) and flow-related saccular aneurysms seen on the supplying pedicle to the AVM (21% of cases) (375).

In addition to the afferent supply, determination of the nidus size is important. The nidus is a pathologic network of abnormal vascular channels replacing the normal arteriolar and capillary network resulting in a low resistance, arteriovenous connection. As alluded to previously, there also may be accompanying direct connections or an AVF. Nidus size varies as does its configuration; it may be compact, diffuse, and occasionally multifocal.

The efferent side of the AVM is also variable. Several large draining veins that coalesce to a single larger vein or represent several independent large veins is the most common pattern. Venous drainage is categorized as (a) superficial drainage into the sagittal, cavernous, transverse, sigmoid, and sphenoparietal sinuses (Fig. 47) and (b) the deep draining pattern that empties into the internal cerebral veins, basal vein of Rosenthal, vein of Galen, and straight sinus (Fig. 48). Besides the AVM itself, its location in the brain parenchyma is also important. Specifically, if it is located in a region controlling a

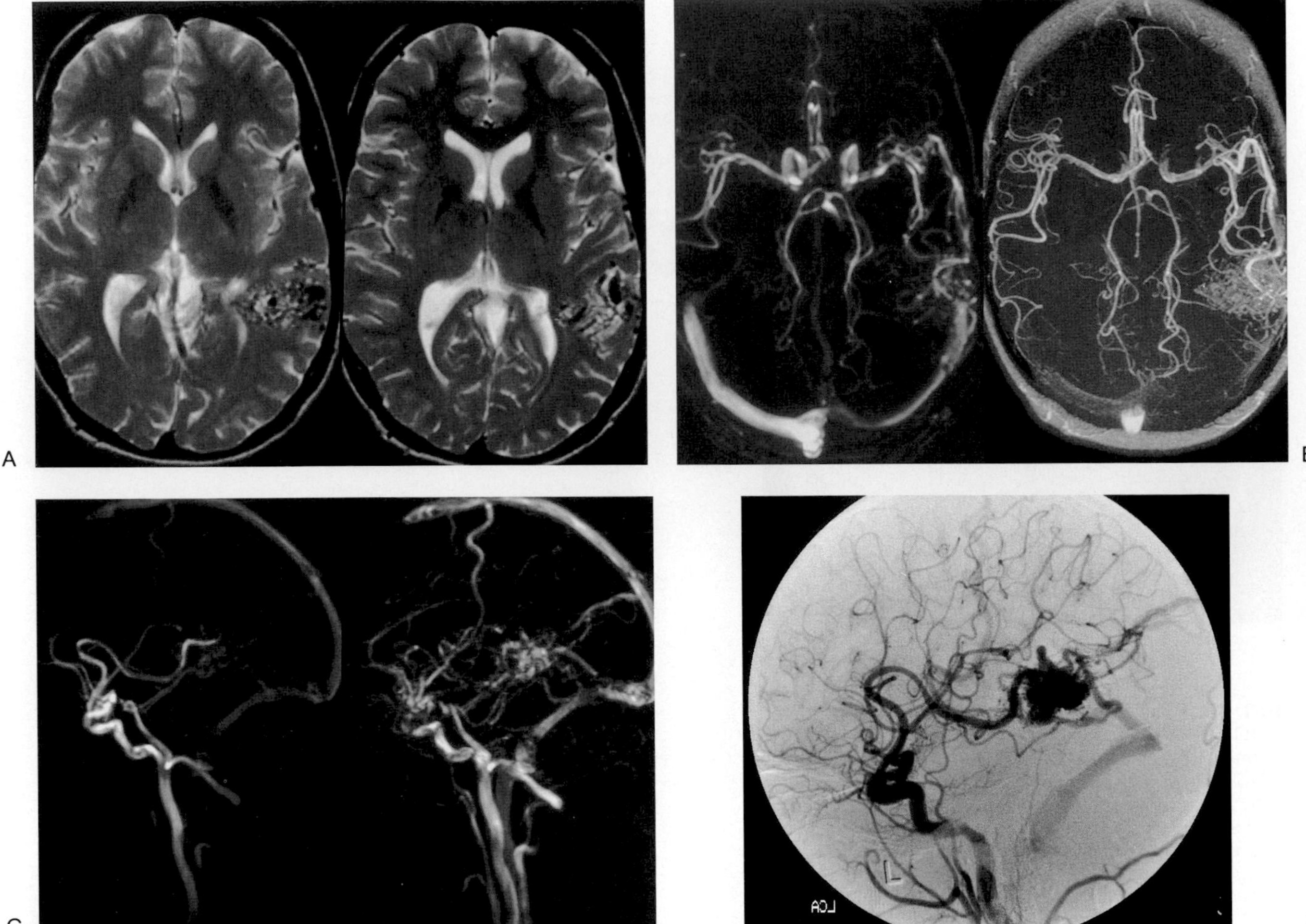

FIG. 47. Left hemisphere AVM. **A:** SE images demonstrating multiple flow voids consistent with an AVM. Note the enlarged MCA branches in the left sylvian fissure. **B:** 2D phase contrast and 3D TOF MRA. Note the conspicuity of the nidus is much better on the 3D TOF image; however, in part, this is due to high velocity encoding for the PC image (80 cm/sec). Note the delineation of the nidus is better appreciated on the TOF MRA image than on the routine SE images. **C:** 2D phase-contrast images, the left image with a velocity encoding of 80 cm/sec and the right with a velocity encoding of 30 cm/sec. Note the conspicuity of the nidus is much better on the lower velocity encoding because of the slower flow within the nidus. The arterial supply is exclusively through the MCA and venous drainage can be appreciated on the phase contrast image to the transverse sinus. Note there is no deep venous drainage and no associated aneurysm is identified on the supplying arterial pedicle. The arterial pedicle terminates in the AVM. **D:** Catheter angiogram demonstrating the AVM with the large single MCA supply that terminates in the AVM.

FIG. 48. AVM of the left frontal lobe before and after stereotactic radiosurgery. **A:** SE image demonstrating the nidus in the left frontal lobe draining centrally. **B:** The corresponding 3D TOF MRA without contrast demonstrating the AVM. Note the deep venous structures draining the AVM are not well appreciated on this sequence. **C:** SE images 14 months later demonstrating the high signal intensity in the frontal lobe corresponding to stereotactic radiation therapy changes. Note the AVM nidus is not visualized on the SE images. **D:** The 3D TOF MRA with contrast demonstrates the AVM draining into the deep venous system. Note the vein size is considerably smaller, as are the supplying MCA pedicles. **E:** SE image performed 20 months following radiation therapy demonstrating reduction in the radiation-induced high signal intensity in the left frontal lobe. **F:** The corresponding 3D TOF MRA with contrast demonstrates no AVM. Note the normal caliber of the MCA vessels.

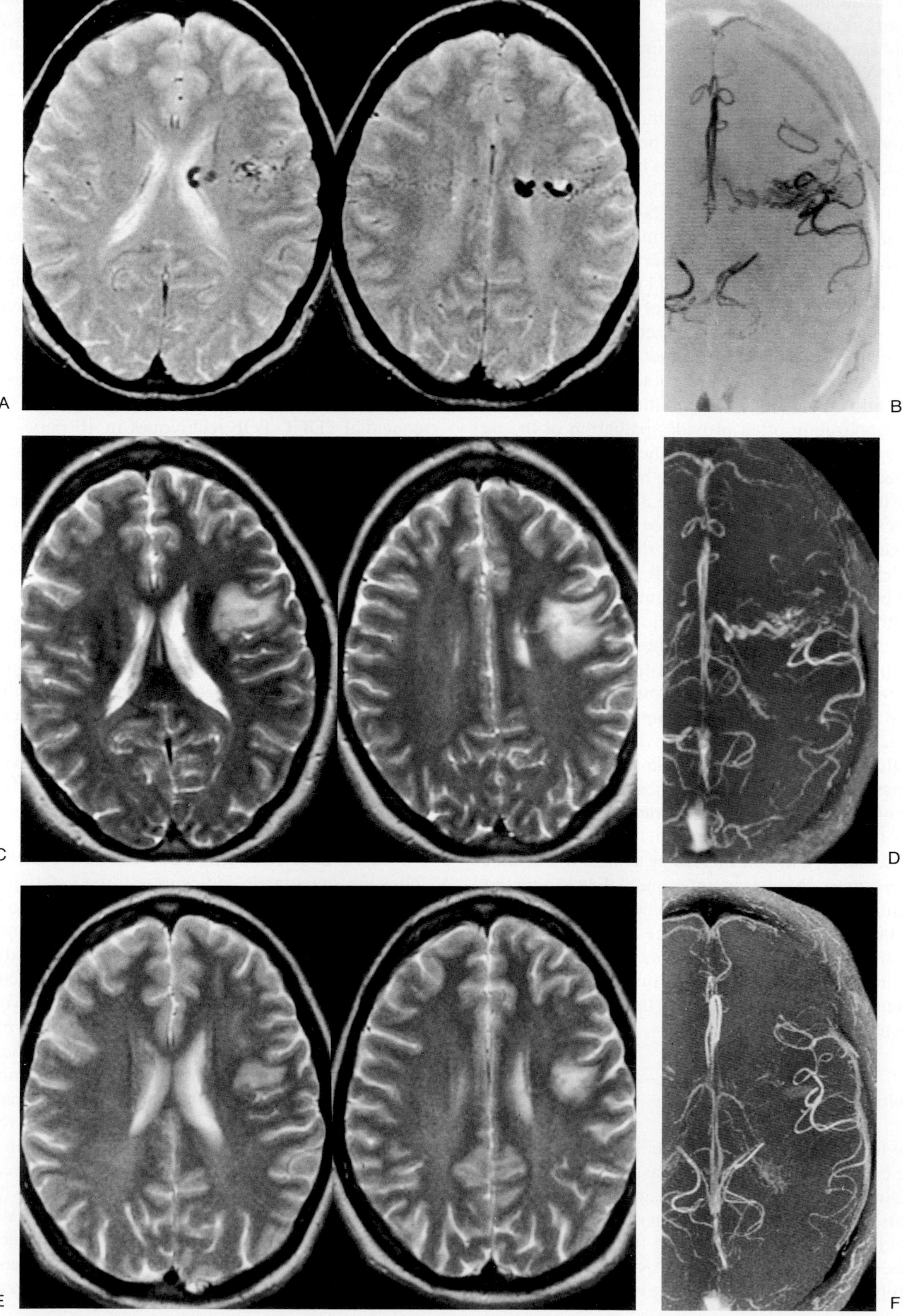
A
B
C
D
E
F

readily identifiable, focal neurologic function, this area is termed "eloquent" (376).

There are several proposed grading schemes for intracranial AVM that are formulated to predict the surgical risk of excision of an AVM (376,377). Most of these systems revolve around the issue of nidus size, location, and the pattern of venous drainage. The grading system of Spetzler and Martin and that of Shi both provide frameworks for the MRA evaluation of AVMs. The more commonly used Spetzler and Martin classification assigns a cumulative, numeric score for the nidus size, eloquence of adjacent brain, and venous pattern to arrive at a designation in ascending severity from I to VI (376). Surgery is the current treatment modality of choice for removal of lower-grade AVMs, and endovascular therapy is often recommended in patients with larger AVMs to obliterate a portion converting an AVM to a lesion that can be treated with either surgery or radiation therapy. Incomplete embolization often provides palliation of the patient's symptoms, and can arrest the neurologic decline in patients harboring large AVMs; however, it does not reduce the risk of hemorrhage (376,378). Stereotactic radiation therapy tends to be reserved for AVMs that are approximately 3 cm in size or less that are located in or near "eloquent" brain areas such that other therapy would pose a large risk to the patient. The ultimate cure rate with stereotactic radiotherapy for small AVMs without arteriovenous fistulae approaches 90% (379,380) (see Fig. 48). Both the pre- and post-treatment MRI and MRA must provide detailed information, including the afferent and efferent AVM blood supply, precise location and size of the AVM nidus, and evaluation of the flow through the nidus itself (381). The flow through the nidus becomes especially important subsequent to therapy with endovascular techniques or radiation surgery. Because of the success of treating patients with AVMs with radiation surgery and the increasing availability of radiosurgery centers, the assessment of nidal flow as a method of evaluation of AVM obliteration becomes increasingly important (381,382). However, the nonselective nature of routine MRA techniques limits the importance of MRA in AVMs, whereas in the clinical setting selective catheter angiography is essential to the diagnosis and characterization of these lesions.

Technical Background

The feasibility and utility of the 3D TOF techniques in the evaluation of pial AVMs has been demonstrated in preliminary studies in which diagnostically useful information concerning feeding arteries, draining veins, and nidus location were obtained in five patients with AVMs. However, with current MRA techniques there are problems, including areas of signal void within tortuous feeding arteries (from complex flow), inability to differentiate flow from methemoglobin within an associated, subacute hematoma, and lack of visualization of slower distal venous spins due to progressive spin saturation (226).

There have been two recent attempts to minimize this problem of spin saturation. In one approach, MRAs were obtained in 26 patients with congenital intracranial vascular lesions, with a single thick 3DFT volume in 15 cases and a technique using multiple sequentially acquired thin volumes in 11 subjects. The authors observed a significant improvement in visualization of the slowly flowing venous spins with the multiple thin-volume method as compared to the single-volume technique. A less significant improvement was noted with the single thick-volume method when intravenous gadolinium-DTPA was administered (45). The second study compared the single thick-volume 3DFT TOF and sequential 2DFT TOF techniques in 10 patients with AVMs. Similar to the findings with multiple thin 3DFT volumes, the reduction of spin saturation obtained with the sequential 2DFT technique allowed significantly improved visualization of draining veins. The single thick 3DFT technique, however, was better for the delineation of small arteries because of its higher spatial resolution and lower sensitivity to dephasing (secondary to smaller voxel size and shorter TE). An additional feature of this investigation was the application of selective spatial presaturation pulses to determine the territories supplied by a particular vessel. By selectively saturating inflowing blood from the anterior, middle, and posterior cerebral arteries while acquiring flow-compensated 2DFT images of the nidus, the authors were able to define correctly which of these arteries contributed feeding vessels to the AVM in all 10 cases, as confirmed on conventional contrast angiography (383).

Kauczor et al. evaluated the role of 3DFT TOF MRA following stereotactic radiosurgery in 18 patients prospectively (382). MRA demonstrated reduction of nidus flow in nine patients after 6 months and 15 patients after 1 year. The decreased signal was related to the reduction of the nidus in 11 of 18 patients at 1 year. This technique was more sensitive than SE imaging, which revealed a reduction of the nidus size in two patients after 6 months and eight after 1 year's follow-up. Importantly, the signal intensity of the feeding arteries was reduced in nine patients, and diminished veins were seen in six patients, implying reduced flow through to the AVM. Correlation with conventional angiography was determined in all patients. Other authors have reported excellent success using tandem 2D gradient-recalled echo images with and without gradient moment nulling to evaluate AVM following stereotactic radiosurgery (381). In a subset of patients in whom conventional angiograms were performed, there were no false positives or negatives using this MRI diagnostic algorithm (381). In addition to follow-up of radiosurgery, the use of 3DFT TOF MRA techniques as a data base for treatment planning for stereotactic radiosurgery has been reported (384–387) (Fig. 48). Advantages of using TOF MRA techniques include delineation of the stereotactic target and the adjacent normal brain parenchyma at risk for radiation injury can be performed with 3D MRA data sets with a higher reliability than with CT (384,385). Concern over the geometric distortion from magnetic field heterogeneities and gradient nonlinearities are less of a problem because of improvement in the MRI hardware, and correction algorithms that reduce distortion to 1 mm (385).

Three-dimensional PC MRA has not enjoyed the same success in evaluating the architecture of AVMs as have TOF techniques. In a small study by Nussel et al., 10 patients with AVMs were examined by PC MRA and catheter angiography (388). In 7 of 10 of the AVM patients additional data about vascular supply was obtained using this 3D phase technique complementing the MRI images. In three patients with small AVMs the abnormality could not be definitely detected. Unfortunately, the velocity-encoding values were not presented and therefore poor visualization of the AVM may be due to inappropriate application of the PC technique.

Clinical Studies of MR Flow Analysis

With phase-contrast flow analysis techniques there are opportunities for evaluation of blood flow in the vascular supply to an AVM. Marks and colleagues evaluated 16 patients with intracerebral AVMs (32). In this study, velocity and volume flow rates in both carotid arteries and the basilar artery were determined using a phase-contrast cine MRA technique. As expected, flow and velocity measurements were significantly elevated in all three arteries in patients with AVMs. The flow in the carotid artery ipsilateral to the AVM was significantly greater than the flow in the contralateral carotid artery. In four patients who underwent partial embolization corresponding decreases in flow were observed. Turski and co-workers reported preliminary data using cardiac-gated PC MRA. They demonstrated flow rates in the arterial supply in the AVMs of 200 cm/sec and venous flow rates of 20 cm/sec (354). As work in this area continues to develop, flow quantification of AVMs may allow assessment of the response therapy and quantitation of the flow of a particular arterial pedicle to guide endovascular embolization therapy.

Venous Malformations

Venous malformations (angiomas, or developmental venous anomalies) were once thought to be quite rare; however, with the advent of CT and MRI, they are known to be common vascular malformations that are most frequently incidentally discovered. Morphologically, they are characterized by mildly dilated radially oriented medullary veins that converge into a linear subcortical transcerebral vein that drains into a superficial or ependymal vein (389,390). Drainage can occur centrally toward the subependymal veins (390). Arteriovenous shunting is not identified. Approximately 50% of these lesions are identified in the frontal lobe and 25% in the cerebellar white matter (390). Pure venous malformations drain normal brains, and therefore as isolated malformations are rarely, if ever, associated with hemorrhage (390–394). Up to 33% of these malformations can be associated with a cavernous malformation (389–391). In a study by Ostertun et al., evaluation of 20 patients with 21 developmental venous malformations were studied employing a 2DFT TOF technique (391). MRA was diagnostic in 17 of the 21 developmental venous abnormalities when both the 2DFT slices (number not specified) and the maximum intensity projection images were interpreted. MRI alone frequently identified the draining of veins; however, after the administration of a Gd-DTPA, the MRI was diagnostic in 17 of 18 cases. In fact, most neuroradiologists would probably agree that MRA is not necessary for the diagnosis of these anomalies in the vast majority of cases.

The radially oriented medullary veins can be visualized on 3DFT TOF angiograms particularly the administration of intravenous contrast. The 2DFT TOF technique, because of its sensitivity to slow flow, is an ideal technique for imaging venous malformations. The typical MRA findings are similar to the catheter angiographic findings with the curvilinear venous channel coursing toward a subependymal, cortical, or dural sinus (Fig. 49). In addition, PC MRA can be employed with a selection of a low velocity encoding (10 cm/sec) to take advantage of a slow flow seen in these lesions. Intravenous contrast enhancement increases the detectability of these lesions with all MRA techniques, especially from the smaller slow flow tributaries (Fig. 49). If hemorrhage is identified on the accompanying MRI examination, a coexisting cavernous malformation should be strongly suspected (389,391).

Dural Arteriovenous Fistulae

Dural arteriovenous fistulae (DAVF) are thought to represent an acquired or developmental anomaly responsible for 15% of intracranial vascular malformations (395,396) (Figs. 50 and 51). The most common location involves the dural sinuses along the skull base, most commonly the cavernous, transverse, and sigmoid sinuses (397–399). Dural arteriovenous malformations

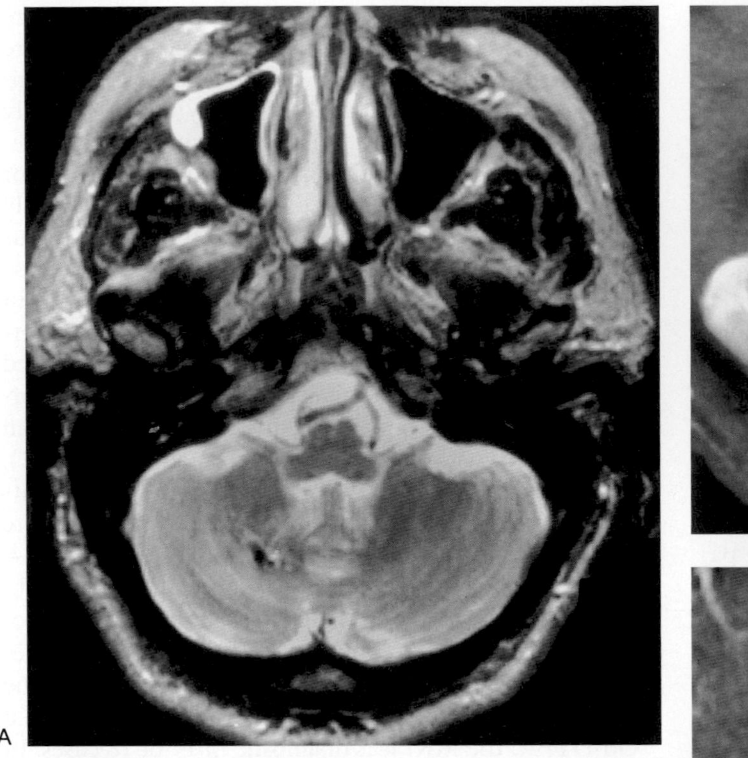

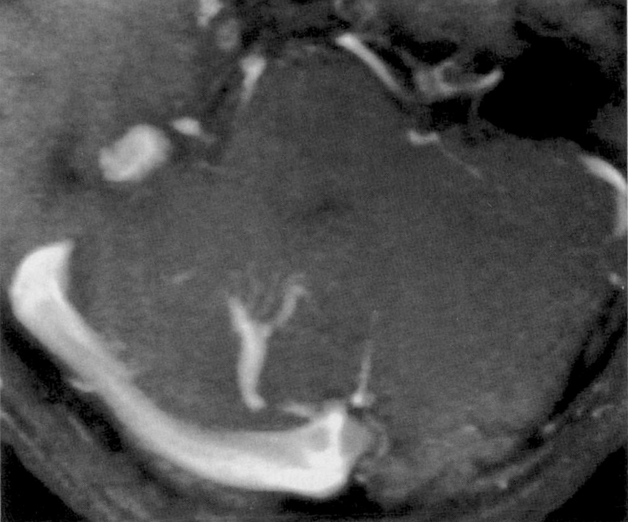

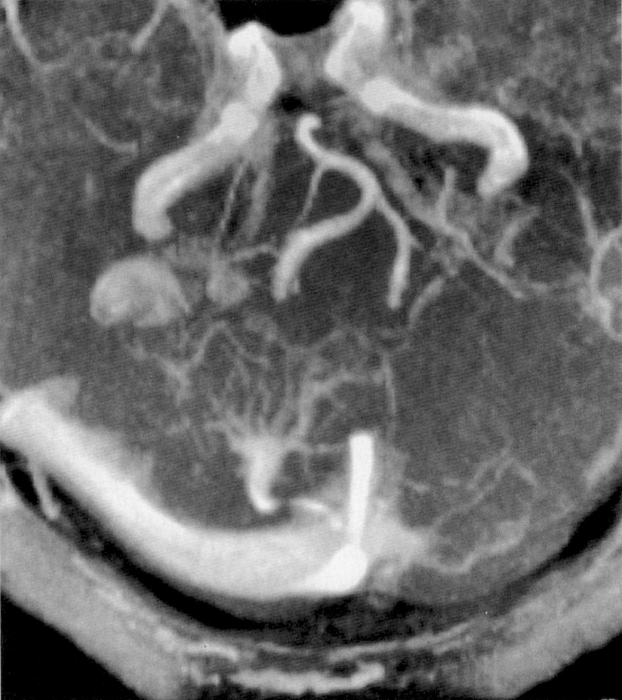

FIG. 49. Venous malformation (angioma). **A:** SE image reveals a focal area of decreased signal intensity in the right cerebellar hemisphere that could represent flow or blood by-products. **B:** A 2D TOF MRA demonstrates the venous angioma with the classic "caput medusae" draining toward the torcula. Notice the stenosis seen at the distal aspect of the venous angioma, near the junction with the dural sinus. **C:** A 3D TOF MRA after the administration of Gd-DTPA demonstrates the venous angioma to better advantage, revealing the multiple subtle radiating veins projecting toward the larger draining vein. The malformation drains normal brain parenchyma.

have a varied clinical presentation. The patient's signs and symptoms may include headaches, pulsaltic, tinnitus, otalgia, bruit, exopthalmous, chemosis, and cranial nerve palsies (397–400). The neurologic deficit apparently is related to the severity of the induced venous hypertension from the arterial to venous shunt (400,401). In addition, cortical venous involvement is associated with brain parenchymal hemorrhage. In Chen and colleagues' study, identification of DAVF proved difficult at SE MRI, confirming an earlier study performed by DeMarco et al. (397,401). In contrast, six of the seven patients in this study with DAVF were identified by MRA. In this MRA study occlusion of the dural sinus was not identified on any SE images; however, MRA also failed to diagnosis the dural sinus thrombosis in two of the three cases. This particular issue may be addressed better using techniques sensitive to slow flow.

It is important to recognize in this most recent study

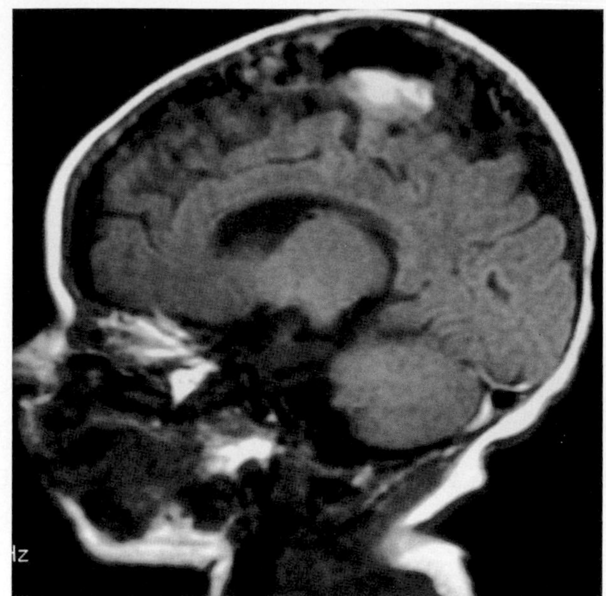

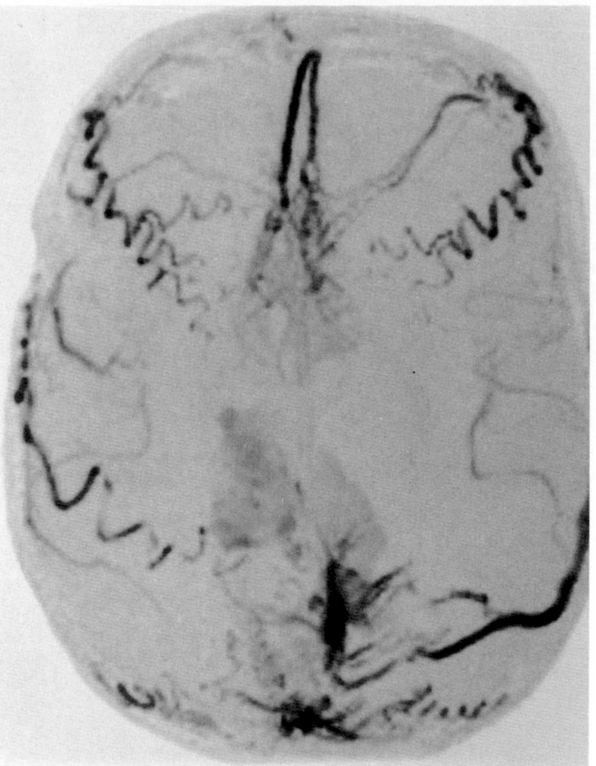

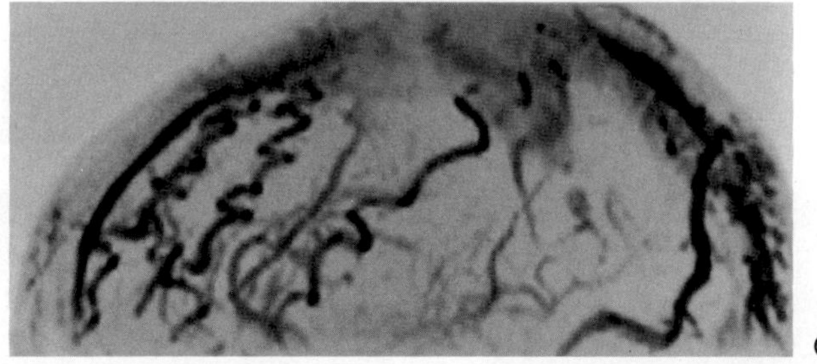

FIG. 50. A 2-week-old infant with congestive heart failure and a dural arteriovenous fistula. **A:** A markedly enlarged superior sagittal sinus is seen with multiple serpentine flow voids identified. Note the high signal intensity from thrombus within the superior sagittal sinus. **B,C:** Axial and lateral 3D TOF MRAs demonstrate the supply to this dural AVM through meningeal and scalp vessels. Note the high signal intensity from the thrombus has been incorporated into the image.

that gadopentetate dimeglumine was used in all cases except one case of cavernous sinus involvement. There was no attempt to perform 3D TOF MRA before and after the administration of the contrast agent. Although contrast was felt to improve the identification of the DAVFs, caution was expressed when imaging cavernous sinus DAVFs because flow-related enhancement cannot be well differentiated from the normal contrast enhancement pattern of a cavernous sinus (401) (Fig. 51).

In addition to the DAVFs, which consist of numerous tiny anastomoses between the branches of the dural arteries and a vein or dural sinus of the cavernous sinus, there occasionally can be a direct fistula from the carotid artery into the cavernous sinus. This finding is usually associated with trauma or secondary to a ruptured cavernous carotid aneurysm. On MRA the appearance of this should be slightly different because this is a very high flow fistula directly into the cavernous sinus in the absence of the multiple tiny dural connections (Fig. 52).

Neoplastic Disease

The role of MRA in the evaluation of neoplastic disease appears limited. Although MRA can document

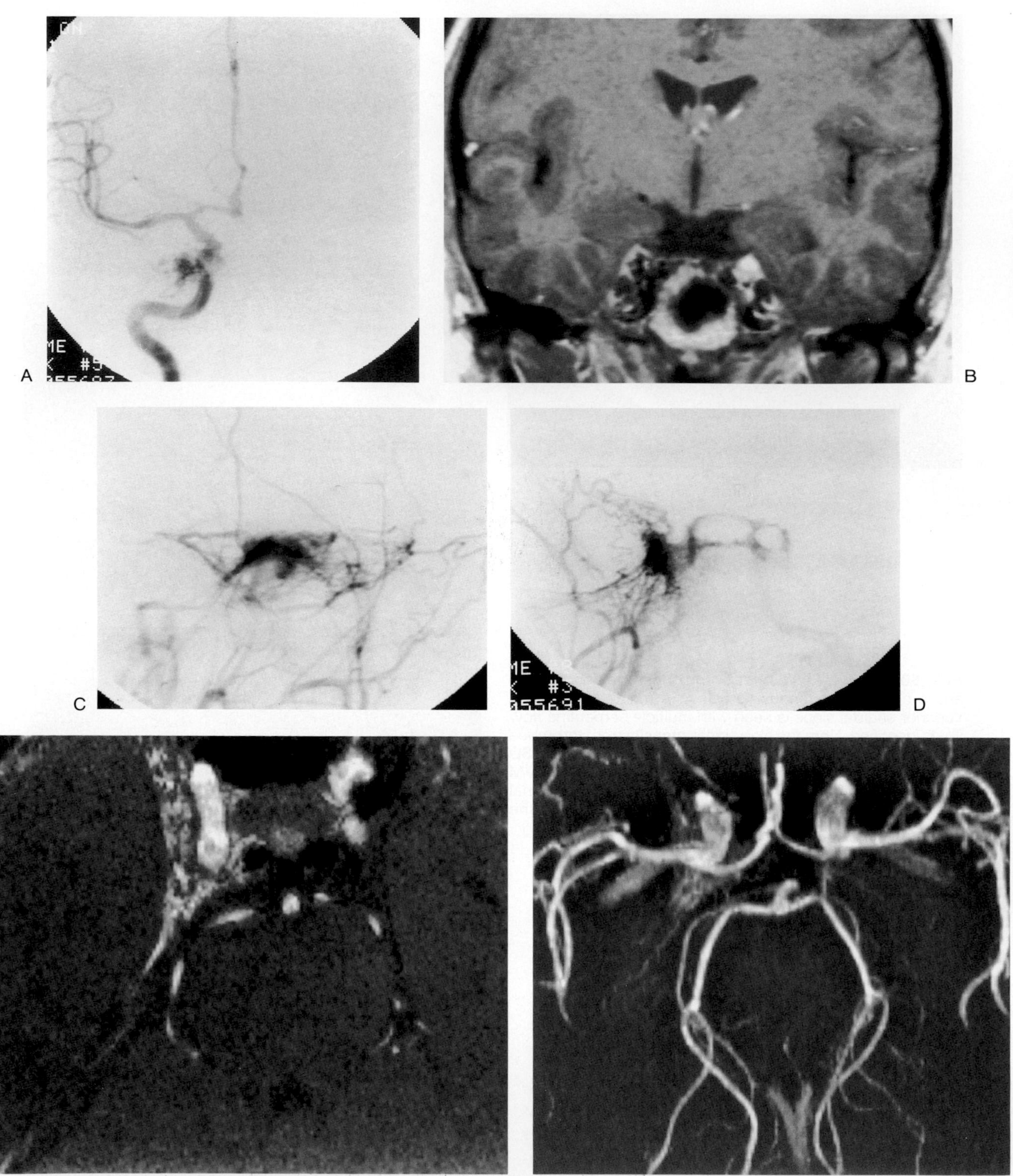

FIG. 51. Indirect dural arteriovenous fistula. **A:** A conventional common carotid artery angiogram demonstrating blush of the right cavernous sinus. **B:** The T1-weighted enhanced coronal image of the cavernous sinus demonstrates a heterogeneous area of predominantly low signal intensity in the cavernous sinus, worse on the right side. **C,D:** The selective external carotid artery angiograms show the multiple tiny vessels supplying the dural fistula. **E:** A 3D TOF image reveals a high signal intensity about the right cavernous carotid artery, due to abnormal flow in this region. **F:** A MIP 3D TOF image demonstrating the high signal intensity and the flow about the right cavernous internal carotid artery.

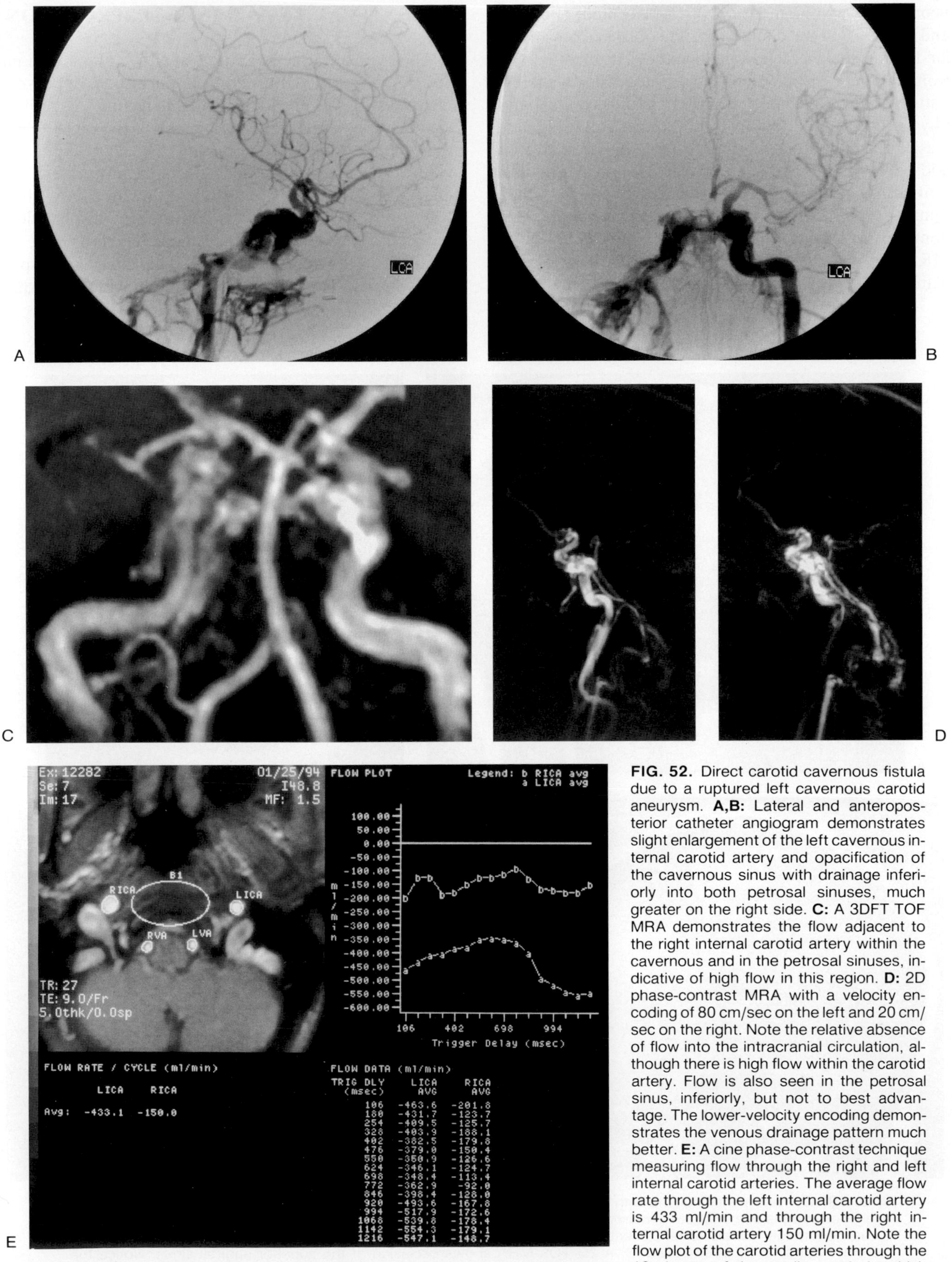

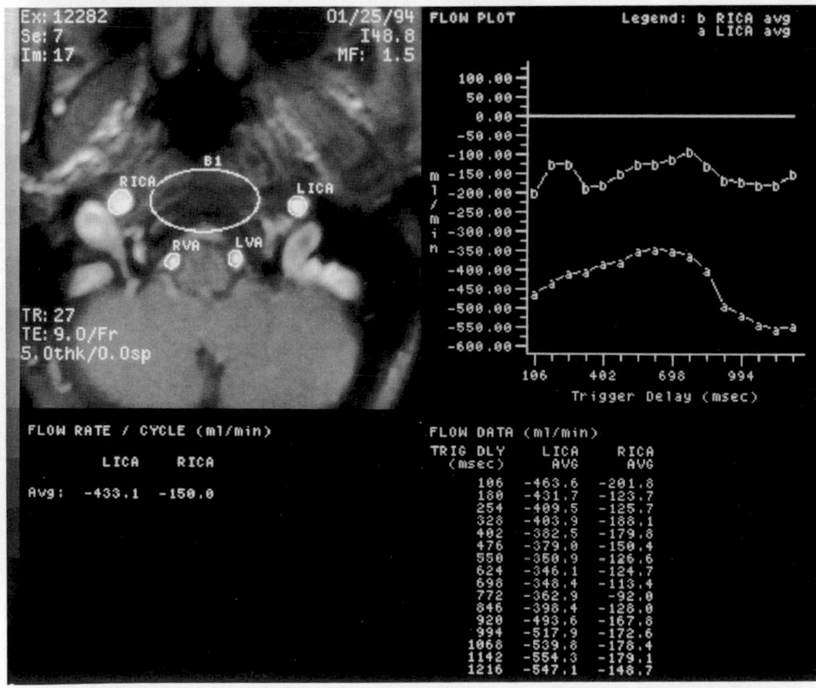

FIG. 52. Direct carotid cavernous fistula due to a ruptured left cavernous carotid aneurysm. **A,B:** Lateral and anteroposterior catheter angiogram demonstrates slight enlargement of the left cavernous internal carotid artery and opacification of the cavernous sinus with drainage inferiorly into both petrosal sinuses, much greater on the right side. **C:** A 3DFT TOF MRA demonstrates the flow adjacent to the right internal carotid artery within the cavernous and in the petrosal sinuses, indicative of high flow in this region. **D:** 2D phase-contrast MRA with a velocity encoding of 80 cm/sec on the left and 20 cm/sec on the right. Note the relative absence of flow into the intracranial circulation, although there is high flow within the carotid artery. Flow is also seen in the petrosal sinus, inferiorly, but not to best advantage. The lower-velocity encoding demonstrates the venous drainage pattern much better. **E:** A cine phase-contrast technique measuring flow through the right and left internal carotid arteries. The average flow rate through the left internal carotid artery is 433 ml/min and through the right internal carotid artery 150 ml/min. Note the flow plot of the carotid arteries through the 16 phases of the cardiac cycle in which flow data were sampled.

neoplastic vascular invasion or displacement (Fig. 53) and can assist in the distinction of neoplasm from vascular lesion (such as a calcified juxtasellar meningioma from an aneurysm), it lacks the selectivity and dynamic nature of conventional intra-arterial contrast angiography to consistently demonstrate vascular shunting, neoplastic blush, and dominant feeding vessels (Fig. 54). In addition, if a TOF MRA is performed following gadolinium administration in a case of enhancing tumor, high signal from the mass may present a "vascular pseudomass" on the postprocessed angiogram. The role of MRA for intracranial neoplastic disease is yet to be defined.

POTENTIAL PITFALLS IN INTERPRETATION

The clinical implementation of MRA has shown encouraging results in numerous applications, but several characteristics of currently available techniques provide significant potential for misdiagnosis to the unwary, and as such merit special mention.

Great progress has been made in minimizing the effects of nonuniform or turbulent flow in MRA. However, areas of tight stenosis continue to display flow-induced signal loss at and immediately following the luminal narrowing (see Fig. 17). This effect is less pronounced with the 3D TOF and sequential 2D techniques

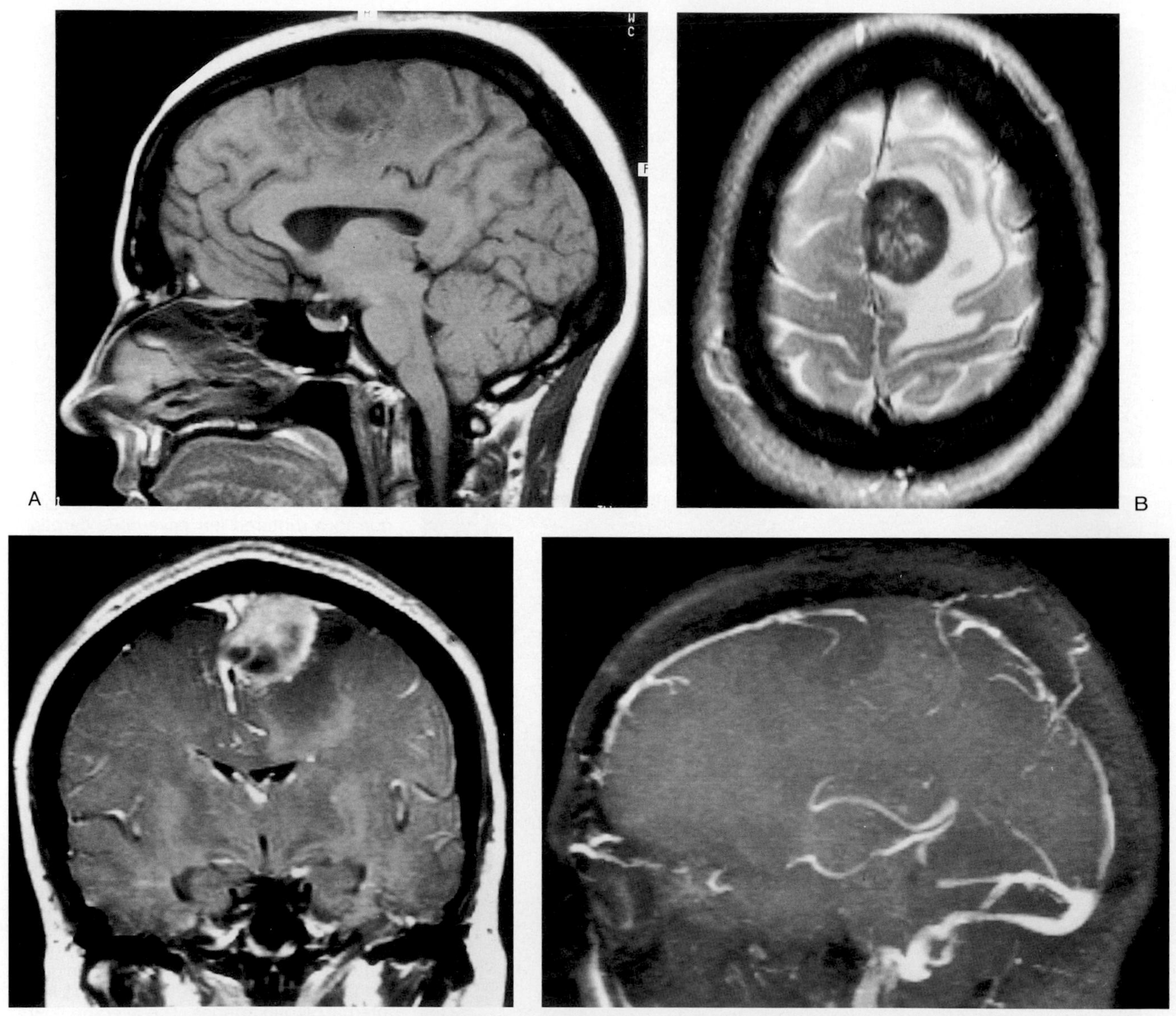

FIG. 53. Convexity meningioma with occlusion of the superior sagittal sinus. **A,B:** T1-weighted sagittal and T2-weighted images demonstrate a meningioma occluding the superior sagittal sinus. **C:** T1-weighted coronal contrast-enhanced image reveals enhancement of the meningioma as well as the adjacent dura. It is difficult to ascertain whether the sinus is thrombosed. **D:** A 2D TOF MRA shows occlusion of the superior sagittal sinus. Notice the collateral flow from the superior sagittal sinus to the superior ophthalmic vein.

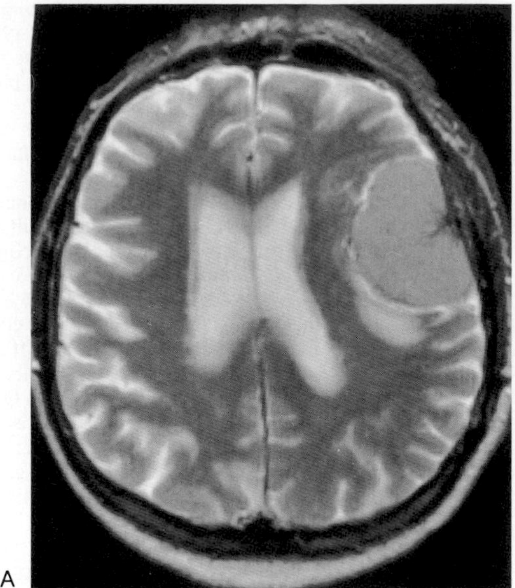

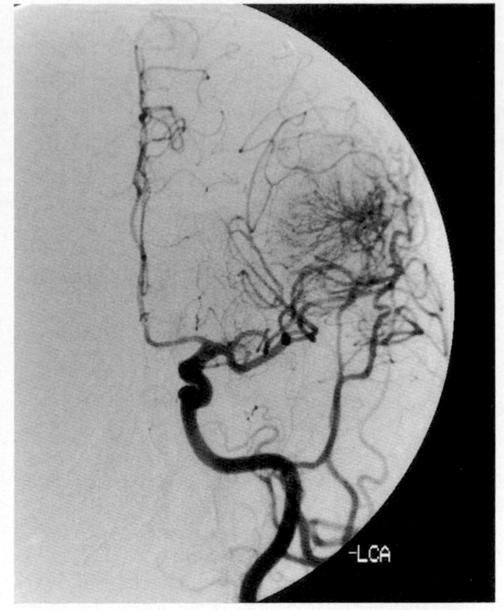

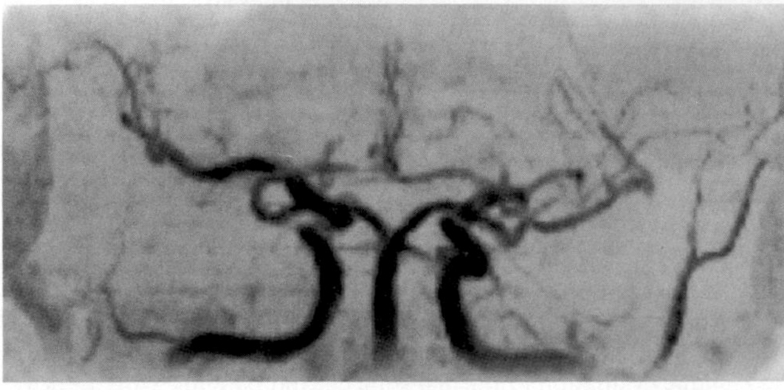

FIG. 54. Meningioma. **A:** T2-weighted axial image demonstrates a large extra-axial mass, consistent with a meningioma. **B:** Midarterial phase from a catheter angiogram demonstrating a hypervascular mass and marked enlargement of the middle meningeal artery. **C:** A 3DFT TOF MRA demonstrating marked enlargement of the middle meningeal artery; however, the vascularity of the tumor is not appreciated.

than with phase-sensitive methods (46), but must be considered when estimating the degree of tight stenoses. In addition, the diagnosis of vascular occlusion must be made with caution on MRA, as the flow void due to a tight stenosis may present with similar findings. Possible solutions to this problem include using pulse sequences with even shorter echo times through innovative design, half-Fourier reconstruction methods (402), and possibly dedicated angiographic gradient coils, as well as the use of new "black blood" techniques.

A second potential pitfall lies in the postprocessing algorithms in common use. Although extremely helpful in visualizing the complex 3D nature of vascular anatomy, the MIP algorithm currently used for postprocessing results in loss of information, and may prevent the visualization of small or faint vascular structures (70). For this reason, it may be important to examine the individual partitions or slices whenever a small abnormality or occlusion is suspected if MIP is utilized.

The third characteristic of note reflects the physics of inflow-based TOF angiography: bright signals require not only flow, but unsaturated spins. Thus, care must be taken when using the 3DFT methods to allow for adequate inflow through choice of repetition time, flip angle, and volume thickness, with the possibility of a false appearance of vessel tapering with incorrect technique (see Fig. 14). Such causes of signal loss, such as in-plane spin saturation, may be minimized through the administration of paramagnetic contrast material (45,83,287,353). In the meantime, one must be careful not to incorrectly diagnose occlusion in the presence of potentially treatable slow-flow ("string-sign") stenosis (see Fig. 14).

Also, analogous to conventional contrast angiography, both TOF and phase-sensitive techniques demonstrate only the patent portion of the vessel lumen, which may be misleading in the evaluation of aneurysms (309). Thus, examination of standard T1- or T2-weighted parenchymal images is important in addition to the MRA to exclude a partially thrombosed lesion. Finally, paramagnetic substances such as gadolinium within a tumor or methemoglobin within a subacute hematoma may appear bright on the TOF images, and can mimic active flow on the postprocessed images (see Figs. 11 and 12). This potential source of confusion can also be avoided through careful correlation of the MRA to the standard MRI.

It is important to appreciate that MRA is young technology; new insights into the mechanisms of flow-induced signal changes and more robust techniques with fewer artifacts (not only at the bifurcation but also at the circle of Willis) are not only on the horizon but in some instances currently available. Advanced gradient designs and more sophisticated acquisition schemes/postprocessing will continue to provide significant improvement in image quality and diagnostic accuracy over the next several years. In the meantime, MRA already can be an extremely valuable adjunct to the diagnosis of cerebrovascular disease with conventional MRI.

REFERENCES

1. Surjan G. Nuclear resonance in flowing liquids. *Proc Indian Acad Sci A* 1951;33:107–113.
2. Singer JR. Blood flow rates by nuclear magnetic resonance measurements. *Science* 1959;130:1652–1653.
3. Haacke EM, Patrick JL. Reducing motion artifacts in two-dimensional Fourier transform imaging. *Magn Reson Imaging* 1986;4:359–376.
4. Axel L. Blood flow effects in magnetic resonance imaging. *AJR* 1984;143:1157–1166.
5. Bradley WG, Waluch V. Blood flow magnetic resonance imaging. *Radiology* 1985;154:443–450.
6. Edelman RR, Mattle HP. Kleefield J, Silver MS. Quantification of blood flow with dynamic MR imaging and presaturation bolus tracking. *Radiology* 1989;171:551–556.
7. Matsuda T, Shimizu K, Sakurai T, et al. Measurement of aortic blood flow with MR imaging: comparative study with doppler ultrasound. *Radiology* 1987;162:857–861.
8. Shimizu K, Matsuda T, Sakurai T, et al. Visualization of moving fluid: quantitative analysis of blood flow velocity using MR imaging. *Radiology* 1986;159:195–199.
9. Finn JP, Edelman RR, Kane R, et al. MR angiography in the portal system: early clinical results. Presented at the *Eighth Annual Meeting of the Society for Magnetic Resonance Imaging*, Washington, DC, 1990.
10. Goldberg HI, Berkowitz HD, Grossman RI. Improved MR imaging of carotid artery disease. Presented at the *74th Annual RSNA Meeting*, 1988.
11. Forbes GS, Earnest F, Kispert DB, et al. Digital angiography. Introducing digital techniques to clinical cerebral angiography practice. *Mayo Clin Proc* 1982; 57:683–693.
12. Mattle H, Edelman RR, Wentz KU, et al. Middle cerebral artery: determination of flow velocities with MR angiography. *Radiology* 1991;181:527–530.
13. Mattle H, Edelman RR, Reis MA, et al. Flow quantification in the superior sagittal sinus using magnetic resonance. *Neurology* 1990;40:813–815.
14. Bryant DJ, Payne JA, Firmin DN, Longmore DB. Measurement of flow with NMR imaging using a gradient pulse and phase difference technique. *J Comput Assist Tomogr* 1984;8:588–593.
15. Underwood SR, Firmin DN, Klipstein RH, Rees RSO, Longmore DB. Magnetic velocity mapping: clinical application of a new technique. *Br Heart J* 1987;57:404–412.
16. van Dijk P. Direct cardiac NMR imaging of the heart wall and blood flow velocity. *J Comput Assist Tomogr* 1984;8(3):429–436.
17. Nayler GL, Firmin DN, Longmore DB. Blood flow imaging by cine magnetic resonance. *J Comput Assist Tomogr* 1986;10(5): 715–722.
18. Hennig J, Muri M, Brunner P, Friedburg H. Quantitative flow measurement with the fast Fourier flow technique. *Radiology* 1988;166:237–240.
19. Meir D, Maier S, Bosiger P. Quantitative flow measurements on phantoms and blood vessels with MR. *Magn Reson Med* 1988;8: 25–34.
20. Mueller E, Laub G, Graumann R, Loeffler W. RACE—Real time acquisition and evaluation of pulsatile blood flow on a whole body MRI unit. Presented at the *Seventh Annual Meeting of the Society of Magnetic Resonance in Medicine*, 1988.
21. Bendel P, Buonocore E, Bockisch A, Besozzi MC. Blood flow in the carotid arteries: quantification by using phase-sensitive MR imaging. *AJR* 1989;152:1307–1310.
22. Mohiaddin R, Sampson C, Firmin D, et al. MR anatomic and flow imaging in peripheral vascular disease. Presented at the *75th Annual RSNA Meeting*, 1989.
23. Lewin JS, Mueller E, Laub G. Magnetic resonance velocity determination in the carotid arteries with duplex ultrasonographic correlation: comparison and optimization of techniques (WIP). Presented at the *Eighth Annual Meeting of the Society for Magnetic Resonance Imaging*, Washington, DC, 1990.
24. Pelc NJ, Shimakawa A, Glover GH. Phase contrast Cine MRI. *8th Annual SMRM Book of Abstracts*, 1989:101.
25. Pettigrew RI, Dannels W, Galloway JR, Pearson T, Millikan W, Henderson JM, Peterson J, Bernadino ME. Quantitative phase-flow MR imaging by using standard sequences: Comparison with in vivo flow-meter measurements. *AJR* 1987;148:411–414.
26. Pettigrew RI, Dannels W. Use of standard gradients with compound oblique angulation for optimal MR flow imaging in oblique vessels. *AJR* 1987;148:405–409.
27. Feinberg DA, Crooks LE, Sheldon P, et al. Magnetic resonance imaging the velocity vector components of fluid flow. *Magn Reson Med* 1985;2:555–556.
28. Kilner PJ, Firmin DN, Rees RSO, et al. Valve and great vessel stenosis: assessment with MR jeg velocity mapping. *Radiology* 1991;178:229–235.
29. Moran PR, Moran RA, Karstaedt N. Verification and evaluation of internal flow and motion. *Radiology* 1985;154:433–441.
30. Spritzer CE, Pelc NJ, Lee JN, et al. Preliminary experience with rapid MR blood flow imaging using a phase sensitive limited flip angle gradient refocussed pulse sequence. *Radiology* 1990;176: 285–262.
31. Gover GH, Pelc NJ. A rapid-gated cine MRI technique. *Magn Reson Q* 1988;4:299–333.
32. Marks M, Pelc N, Ross MR, Enzmann DR. Determination of cerebral blood flow with phase contrast cine MR imaging technique evaluation of normal subjects and patients with arteriovenous malformations. *Radiology* 1992;182:467–476.
33. Hardy CJ, Pearlman JD, Moore J, et al. Continuous cardiography with a half-echo MR M-mode method. *Ninth Annual SMRM Book of Abstracts* 1990;1:280.
34. Dixon WT, Du LN, Gado M, Rossnick S. Projection angiograms of blood labeled by adiabatic fast passage. *Magn Reson Med* 1986;3:454–462.
35. Sardashti M, Schwartzberg DG, Stomp GP, Dixon WT, Philips F. Spin labeling angiography of the carotids by presaturation and adiabatic inversion. Presented at the *Eighth Annual Meeting of the Society of Magnetic Resonance in Medicine*, 1989.
36. Nishimura DG, Macovski A, Pauly JM, Conolly SM. MR angiography by selective inversion recovery. *Magn Reson Med* 1987;4:193–202.
37. Wehrli FW, Shimakawa A, Gullberg GT, MacFall JR. Time-of-flight MR flow imaging: selective saturation recovery with gradient refocusing. *Radiology* 1986;160:781.
38. Gullberg GT, Wehrli FW, Shimakawa A, Simmons MA. MR vascular imaging with fast gradient refocusing pulse sequence and reformatted images from transaxial sections. *Radiology* 1987; 165:241–246.
39. Edelman RR, Wentz KU, Mattle H, et al. Projection arteriography and venography: initial clinical results with MR. *Radiology* 1989;172:351–357.
40. Keller PJ, Drayer BP, Fram EK, Williams KD, Dumoulin CL, Souza S. MR angiography with two-dimensional acquisition and three-dimensional display. *Radiology* 1989;173:527–532.
41. Ruggieri PM, Laub GA, Masaryk TJ, Modic MT. Intracranial circulation: pulse sequence considerations in three-dimensional (volume) MR angiography. *Radiology* 1989;171:785–791.
42. Masaryk TJ, Modic MT, Ruggieri PM, et al. Three-dimensional (volume) gradient-echo imaging of the carotid bifurcation: preliminary clinical experience. *Radiology* 1989;171:801–806.
43. Laub G, Kaiser W. MR angiography with gradient motion refocusing. *J Comput Assist Tomogr* 1988;12(3):377–382.

44. Haacke EM, Tkach JA, Parrish TB. Reduction of T2* dephasing in gradient field-echo imaging. *Radiology* 1989;170:457–462 .
45. Marchal G, Bosmans H, Van fraeyenhoven L, et al. Optimization and clinical evaluation of the 3D time of flight MR—angiography sequence on intracranial vascular lesions. *Radiology* 1990;175: 443–448.
46. Lewin JS, Laub G. Comparison and optimization of three-dimensional MR angiographic techniques for evaluation of the intracranial circulation. Presented at the *75th Annual RSNA Meeting*, 1989.
47. Felmlee JP, Ehman RL. Spatial presaturation: a method for suppressing flow artifacts and improving depiction of vascular anatomy in MR imaging. *Radiology* 1987;164:559–564.
48. Lenz GW, Haacke EM, Masaryk TJ, et al. In-plane vascular imaging: pulse sequence design and strategy. *Radiology* 1988;166: 875–882.
49. Lewin JS, Masaryk TJ, Modic MT, Ross JS, Stork EK, Wiznitzer M. Extracorporeal membrane oxygenation in infants: angiographic and parenchymal evaluation of the brain with MR imaging. *Radiology* 1989;173:361–365.
50. Lewin JS, Laub G. Evaluation of the intracranial venous system with the thin-slice oblique acquisition sequential technique. Presented at the *Eighth Annual Meeting of the Society for Magnetic Resonance Imaging*, Washington, DC, 1990.
51. Wehrli FW, Hoffman E, Raya SP, et al."Black blood" MR angiography for carotid imaging. Presented at the *75th Annual RSNA Meeting*, 1989.
52. Edelman RR, Mattle H, Atkinson DJ, Kleefield J. "Black blood" angiography of the carotid bifurcation. Presented at the *Eighth Annual Meeting of the Society for Magnetic Resonance Imaging*, Washington, DC, 1990.
53. Laub G, Lewin J. T2-enhanced time-of-flight magnetic resonance angiography (abstr). Presented at the *Eighth Annual Meeting of the Society of Magnetic Resonance Imaging*, Washington, DC, 1990.
54. Norris D, Henrich D, Leibfritz D, Haase A. 3D flow imaging with snapshot FLASH (abstr). Presented at the *Eighth Annual Meeting of the Society of Magnetic Resonance Imaging*, Washington, DC, 1990.
55. Hu X, Yaun C. Technique for elimination of stationary tissue signal in 2DFT MR angiography (abstr). Presented at the *9th Annual Scientific Meeting and Exhibition of the Society of Magnetic Resonance in Medicine*, 1990.
56. Rosen BR, Wedeen VJ, Brady TJ. Selective saturation NMR imaging. *J Comput Assist Tomogr* 1984;8:813–818.
57. Keller RJ, Hunter WW, Schmalbrock P. Multisection fat-water imaging with chemical shift selective presaturation. *Radiology* 1987;164:539–541.
58. Edelman RR, et al. Improved time-of-flight MR angiography of the brain using magnetization transfer contrast. *Radiology* 1992;184:295–299.
59. Tkach JA, Ruggieri PM, Ross JS, Modic MT, Dillinger JJ, Masaryk TJ. Pulse sequence strategies for vascular contrast in time-of-flight MR angiography. *J Magn Reson Imaging* 1993;3:811–820.
60. Lin W, Tkach JA, Haacke EM, Masaryk TJ. Intracranial MR angiography: an application of magnetization transfer contrast and fat saturation to short gradient echo, velocity compensated sequences. *Radiology* 1993;186:753–761.
61. Haacke EM, Masaryk TJ, Wielopolski PA, et al. Optimizing blood vessel contrast in fast three-dimensional MRI. *Magn Reson Med* 1990;14:202–221.
62. Atkinson D, Brant-Zawadzki M, Gillan G, et al. Improved MRA: magnetization transfer suppression with variable flip angle excitation and increased resolution. *Radiology* 1994;190:890–894.
63. Ruggieri PM, Tkach JA, Modic MT, et al. High resolution, fat saturation, variable flip angle, time-of-flight MR angiography of the carotid bifurcation. Presented at the *78th Annual Meeting of the RSNA*, 1992.
64. Hennig J, Naureth A, Friedburg H, et al. RARE imaging: a fast method for clinical MR. *Magn Reson Med* 1989;3:823–833.
65. Hennig J, Friedburg H, Ott D. Fast three-dimensional imaging of cerebrospinal fluid. *Magn Reson Med* 1987;5:380–383.
66. Mulkern RV, Wong STS, Winalski C, Jolesz FA. Contrast manipulation and artifact assessment of 2D and 3D RARE sequences. *Magn Reson Imaging* 1990;8:557–566.
67. Lin W, Haacke EM, Tkach JA. Three-dimensional time-of-flight angiography with variable TE (VARIETE) for fat signal reduction. *Magn Reson Med* 1994;32:678–683.
68. Tkach JA, Ruggieri PM, Dillinger JJ, Ross JS, Modic MT, Masaryk TJ. Three-dimensional time-of-flight MR angiography with a specialized gradient head coil. *J Magn Reson Imaging* 1993;3: 365–375.
69. Rossnick S, Kennedy D, Laub G, et al. Three-dimensional display of blood vessels in MRI (*abstr*). In: *Proceedings of the IEEE Computers in Cardiology Conference.* Piscataway, NJ, 1986.
70. Anderson CM, Saloner D, Tsuruda JS, Shapeero LG, Lee RE. Artifacts in maximum–intensity–projection display of MR angiograms. *AJR* 1990;154:623–629.
71. Lin W, Masaryk TJ, Tkach JA, Haacke EM. Time-of-flight MR angiography: postprocessing with vessel track algorithms. *J Magn Reson Imaging* 1993.
72. Lin W, Haacke EM, Masaryk TJ, Smith AS. Automated local maximum-intensity projection with three-dimensional vessel tracking. *J Magn Reson Imaging* 1992;2:519–526.
73. Atlas SW, Listerud J, Chung W, et al. Intracranial aneurysms: depiction on MR angiograms with a multifeature-extraction, ray-tracing postprocessing algorithm. *Radiology* 1994;192:129–139.
74. Johnson CD, Ehman RL. MR angiography of the abdomen: clinical role of projection and tomographic formats. Presented at the *75th Annual RSNA Meeting,* 1989.
75. Evans AJ, Richardson DB, Tien R, et al. Poststenotic signal loss in MR angiography: effects of echo time, flow compensation, and fractional echo. *AJNR* 1993;14:721–729.
76. Masaryk AM, Ross JS, DiCello M, Modic MT, Paranandi L, Masaryk TJ. 3DFT magnetic resonance angiography of the cervical carotid arteries: potential and limitations as a screening exam for arteriosclerotic ischemic cerebrovascular disease. *Radiology* 1991;179:797–804.
77. Masaryk TJ, Ross JS, Modic MT, et al. Carotid bifurcation: MR imaging. *Radiology* 1988;166:461–466.
78. Masaryk TJ, Modic MT, Ruggieri PR, et al. Three-dimensional (volume) gradient echo imaging of the carotid bifurcation: preliminary experience. *Radiology* 1989;171:801–806.
79. Blatter DD, Parker DL, Robison RO. Cerebral MR angiography with multiple overlapping thin slab acquisition. Part I. Quantitative analysis of vessel visibility. *Radiology* 1991;179:805–811.
80. Wielopolski P, Zisk J, Patel M, Edelman RR. Evaluation of ultra-short echo time MR angiography with a whole body echo planar imager. Presented at the *12th Annual Scientific Meeting and Exhibition of the Society of Magnetic Resonance in Medicine*, 1994.
81. Schmalbrock P, Yuan C, Chakeres DW, et al. Volume MR angiography: methods to achieve very short echo times. *Radiology* 1990;171:801–806.
82. Oshio K, Jolesz FA, Melki PS, et al. T2 weighted thin-section imaging with the multislab three-dimensional RARE technique. *J Magn Reson Imaging* 1991;1:731–735.
83. Link KM, Margosian P, Sattin W, Souder C. Dural sinus evaluation with 3-D MRA with Gd-DTPA. Presented at the *Eighth Annual Meeting of the Society for Magnetic Resonance Imaging*, Washington, DC, 1990.
84. Laub G, Purdy DE. Variable-tip-angle slab selection for improved three-dimensional MR angiography. In: *Book of Abstracts: Society of Magnetic Resonance in Medicine 1992.* Berkeley, Calif: Society of Magnetic Resonance in Medicine, 1992.
85. Ross JS, Ruggieri PM, Tkach JA, et al. High resolution, magnetization transfer saturation, variable flip angle time-of-flight MR angiography of the intracranial vasculature. Presented at the *78th Annual Meeting of the RSNA,* 1992.
86. Blatter DD, Parker DL, Ahn SS, et al. Cerebral MR angiography with multiple overlapping thin slab acquisition. II. Early clinical experience. *Radiology* 1992;183:379–389.
87. Ding X, Tkach JA, Ruggieri PR, Masaryk TJ. Sequential 3D TOF MR angiography of the carotid arteries: value of variable excitation and postprocessing in reducing venetian blind artifact. *AJR* 1994;163:683–688.
88. Butts RK, Farzaneh F, Reiderer SJ, Rydberg JN, Grimm RC. T2 weighted spin-echo pulse sequence with variable repetition and

echo times for reduction of MR image acquisition time. *Radiology* 1991;180:551–556.
89. Tkach J, Lin W, Duda JJ Jr, et al. Optimizing three-dimensional time-of-flight MR angiography with variable TR. *Radiology* 1994.;191:805–811.
90. Daniels DL, Kneeland JB, Foley WD, Jesmanowicz A, Froncisz W, Hyde JS. Cardiac-gated local coil MR imaging of the carotid neck bifurcation. *AJNR* 1986;7:1036–1037.
91. Macovski A. Selective projection imaging: applications to radiology and NMR. *IEEE Trans Med Imag* 1982;1:42–47.
92. Wedeen VJ, Meuli RA, Edelman RR, et al. Projective imaging of pulsatile flow with magnetic resonance imaging. *Science* 1985;230:946–948.
93. Moran PR. A flow velocity zeugmatographic interlace for NMR imaging in humans. *Magn Reson Imaging* 1982;1:197–203.
94. Alfidi RJ, Masaryk TJ, Haacke EM, et al. MR angiography of peripheral, carotid, and coronary arteries. *AJR* 1987;149:1097–1109.
95. Axel L, Morton D. MR flow imaging by phase compensated/uncompensated difference images. *J Comput Assist Tomogr* 1987;11:31–34.
96. Naylor W, Firmin DN. Multislice MR angiography. *Magn Reson Imaging* 1986;4:156.
97. Pattany PM, Marino R, McNally JM. Velocity and acceleration desensitization in 2DFT MR imaging. *Magn Reson Imaging* 1986;4:154–155.
98. Dumoulin CL, Hart HR Jr. Magnetic resonance angiography. *Radiology* 1986;161:717–720.
99. Dumoulin CL, Souza SP, Walker MF, Wagle W. Three-dimensional phase contrast angiography. *Magn Reson Med* 1989;9:139–149.
100. Hiehle J, Chung W, Atlas SW, Listerud J, Goldberg HI, Schneider E. Ramped excitation magnetization transfer 3D Fourier transform time-of-flight MR angiography in the intracranial circulation: comparison with 3D Fourier transform phase contrast imaging. In*: 1993 RSNA Book of Abstracts, #14.*
101. Pelc N, Bernstein MA, Shimakawa A, Glover G. Encoding strategies for three direction phase contrast MR imaging of flow. *J Magn Reson Imaging* 1991;1:405–413.
102. Hausmann R, Lewin J, Laub G. Phase contrast MR angiography with reduced acquisition time: new concepts in sequence design. *J Magn Reson Imaging* 1991;1:415–422.
103. Haas WK, Fields WS, North RR, et al. Joint study of extracranial arterial occlusion. Organization of study and survey of patient population. *JAMA* 1968;203:961–968.
104. Hass WK, Fields WS, North RR, et al. Joint study of extracranial arterial occlusion. II. Arteriography, techniques, sites, and complications. *JAMA* 1968;203:961–968.
105. Bauer BB, et al. Progress report of controlled study of long term survival in patients with and without operation. *JAMA* 1969;208: 509–518.
106. Blaisdell WF, et al. A review of surgical considerations. *JAMA* 1969;209:1889–1895.
107. Fields WS, et al. Progress report of prognosis following surgery or non-surgical treatment for transient cerebral ischemic attacks and cervical carotid artery lesions. *JAMA* 1970;211:1993–2003.
108. Heyman A, et al. Joint study of extracranial arterial occlusion: radical differences in ischemic stroke population. *JAMA* 1972;222:285–289.
109. Kricheff II. Arteriosclerotic ischemic cerebrovascular disease. *Radiology* 1987; 162:101–109.
110. Kurtzke JF. Epidemiology of cerebrovascular disease. In: *Cerebrovascular Survey Report 1985.* Bethesda: National Institutes of Health; 1–34.
111. Kishore PRS, Chase NE, Kricheff II. Carotid stenosis and intracranial emboli. *Radiology* 1971;100:351–356.
112. Houser OW, Sundt TM, Holman CB, Sandok BA, Burton RC. Atheromatous disease of the carotid artery. *J Neurosurg* 1974;41: 321–331.
113. Hertzer NR, Beven EG, Benjamin SP. Ultramicroscopic ulcerations and thrombi of the carotid bifurcation. *Arch Surg* 1977;112:1394–1402.
114. Busuttil RW, Baker JD, Davidson RK, Machleder HI. Carotid artery stenosis: hemodynamic significance and clinical course. *JAMA* 1981;245:1438–1441.
115. Raichle ME. The pathophysiology of brain ischemia. *Ann Neurol* 1983;13:2–10.
116. Rosenorn J, Astrup J, Duel P, et al. Risiko for blodning fra ikke-rumperede intrakraniale sakkulate aneurysmer. [Risk of hemorrhage from non-ruptured intracranial sacculate aneurysms.] *Ugeskr Laeger* 1986;148:3363–3365.
117. Weinberger J, Robbins A. Neurologic symptoms associated with nonobstructive plaque at the carotid bifurcation. *Arch Neurol* 1983;40:489–492.
118. Wood EH, Correll JW. Atheromatous ulceration in major neck vessels as a cause of cerebral embolism. *Acta Radiol* 1969;9:520–536.
119. Barnett HJM, Plum F, Walton JN. Carotid endarterectomy: an expression of concern. *Stroke* 1984;15:941–943.
120. Dyken ML. Carotid endarterectomy studies: a glimmering of science. *Stroke* 1986;17:355–358.
121. Pokras R, Kyken ML. Dramatic changes in the performance of endarterectomy for diseases of the extracranial arteries of the head. *Stroke* 1988;19:1289–1290.
122. Winslow CM, Solomon DH, Chassin MR, Kosedoff J, Merrick NJ, Brook RH. The appropriateness of carotid endarterectomy. *N Engl J Med* 1988;318:721–727.
123. Fields WS, Maslenikov V, Meyer JS, Haas WK, Remington RD, MacDonald M. Joint study of extracranial arterial occlusion. V. Progress report of prognosis following surgery or nonsurgical treatment for transient cerebral ischemic attacks and cervical carotid artery lesions. *JAMA* 1970;211(12):1993–2003.
124. The Committee on Health Care Issues, American Neurological Association. Does carotid endarterectomy decrease stroke and death in patients with transient ischemic attacks? *Ann Neurol* 1987;22(1):72–76.
125. Howard VJ, Grizzle J, Diener HC, Hobson RW, Mayberg MR, Toole JF. Comparison of multicenter study designs for investigation of carotid endarterectomy efficacy. *Stroke* 1992;23(4):583–593.
126. Editorial. Operating to prevent stroke. *Lancet* 1991;337:1255–1256.
127. European Carotid Surgery Trialists' Collaborative Group. MRC European carotid surgery trial: interim results for symptomatic patients with severe (70–99%) or with mild (0–29%) carotid stenosis. *Lancet* 1991;337:1235–1243.
128. North American Symptomatic Carotid Endarterectomy Trial Investigators. Clinical alert: benefit of carotid endarterectomy for patients with high-grade stenosis of the internal carotid artery. *Stroke* 1991;22:816–817.
129. North American Symptomatic Carotid Endarterectomy Trial Collaborators. Beneficial effect of carotid endarterectomy in symptomatic patients with high grade carotid stenosis. *N Engl J Med* 1991;325:445–453
130. Masaryk TJ, Obuchowski NA. Noninvasive carotid imaging: caveat emptor. *Radiology* 1993;186:325–331.
131. Schuler JJ, Flanigan P, Lim LT, Keifer T, Williams LR, Behrend AJ. The effect of carotid siphon stenosis on stoke rate, death, and relief of symptoms following elective carotid endarterectomy. *Surgery* 1982;92:1058–1067.
132. Marzewski DJ, Furlan AJ, St Louis P, Little JR, Modic MT, Williams G. Intracranial internal carotid stenosis: long-term prognosis. *Stroke* 1982;13:821–824.
133. Barnett HJ, Barnes RW, Robertson JJ. The uncertainties surrounding carotid endarterectomy [editorial]. *JAMA* 1992;268: 3120–3121.
134. Baker JD, Rutherford RE, Bernstein EF, et al. Suggested standards for reports dealing with cerebrovascular disease. *J Vasc Surg* 1988;8:721–729
135. Fox AJ. How to measure carotid stenosis. *Radiology* 1993;186: 316–318.
136. The North American Symptomatic Carotid Endarterectomy Trial (NASCET) Steering Committee. North American symptomatic carotid endarterectomy trial: methods, patient characteristics, and progress. *Stroke* 1991;22(6):711–720.
137. Barnett HJM, Barnes RW, Robertson JT. The uncertainties sur-

rounding carotid endarterectomy [editorial]. *JAMA* 1992;268: 3120–3121.

138. Turnipseed WD, Kennell TW, Turski PA, et al. Combined use of duplex imaging and magnetic resonance angiography for evaluation of patients with symptomatic ipsilateral high-grade carotid stenosis. *J Vasc Surg* 1993;17:832–839.
139. Mattle HP, Kent KC, Edelman RR, Atkinson DJ, Skillman JJ. Evaluation of the extracranial carotid arteries: correlation of magnetic resonance angiography, duplex ultrasonography and conventional angiography. *J Vasc Surg* 1991;13:838–845.
140. Polak JF, Kalina P, Donaldson MC, O'Leary DH, Whittemore AD, Mannick JA. Carotid endarterectomy: preoperative evaluation of candidates with combined Doppler sonography and magnetic resonance angiography: work-in-progress. *Radiology* 1993;186:333–338.
141. American College of Physicians. Magnetic resonance imaging of the brain and spine: a revised statement. *Ann Intern Med* 1994;120:872–875.
142. Ackerman RH, Candia MR. Assessment of carotid artery stenosis by MR angiography. *AJNR* 1992;13:1005–1008.
143. Bowen BC, Quencer RM, Margosian P, et al. MR angiography of occlusive disease of the arteries in the neck and head: current concepts. *AJR* 1994;162:9–18.
144. Moore WS, Barnett HJM, Beebe HG, et al. Guidelines for carotid endarterectomy: A multidisciplinary consensus statement from the ad hoc committee, American Heart Association. *Stroke* 1995;26:188–201.
145. Kent DL, Haynor DR, Longstreth WT Jr, Larson EB. The clinical efficacy of magnetic resonance imaging in neuroimaging. *Ann Intern Med* 1994;120:856–871.
146. Clagett GP, Youkey JR, Brigham RA, et al. Asymptomatic cervical bruit and abnormal ocular pneumoplesysmography: a prospective study comparing two approaches to management. *Surgery* 1984;15:950–955.
147. CASANOVA Study Group. Carotid surgery versus medical therapy in asymptomatic carotid artery stenosis. *Stroke* 1991;22: 1229–1235.
148. Easton JD, Wilterdink JL. Carotid endarterectomy: Trials and tribulations. *Ann Neurol* 1994;35:5–17.
149. Veterans Administration Cooperative Study. Role of carotid endarterectomy in asymptomatic atherosclerosis. *Stroke* 1986;17: 534–539.
150. Hobson RW, Krupski WC, Weiss DG, et al. VA cooperative study group on asymptomatic carotid stenosis. Influence of aspirin in the management of asymptomatic carotid artery stenosis. *J Vasc Surg* 1993;17:257–265.
151. Moore WS, Barnett HJM, Beebe HG, et al. Guidelines for carotid endarterectomy: a multidisciplinary consensus statement from the ad hoc committee, American Heart Association. *Stroke* 1995;26;188–201.
152. Litt AW, Eidelman EM, Pinto RS, et al. Diagnosis of carotid artery stenosis: comparison of 2DFT time-of-flight MR angiography with contrast angiography in 50 patients. *AJR* 1991;156: 611–616.
153. Riles TS, Eidelman EM, Litt AW, Pinto RS, Oldford F, Schwartzenberg T. Comparison of magnetic resonance angiography, conventional angiography and duplex scanning. *Stroke* 1992;23: 341–346.
154. Wilkerson DK, Keller I, Mezrich R, et al. The comparative evaluation of three-dimensional magnetic resonance for carotid artery disease. *J Vasc Surg* 1991;14:803–811.
155. Polak JF, Bajakian RL, O'Leary DK, Anderson MR, Donaldson MC, Jolesz FA. Detection of internal carotid artery stenosis: comparative of MR angiography, color Doppler sonography and arteriography. *Radiology* 1992;182:35–40.
156. Kido DK, Barsotti JB, Rice LZ, et al. Evaluation of the carotid artery bifurcation: comparison of magnetic resonance angiography and digital subtractionarch aortography. *Neuroradiology* 1991;33:48–51.
157. Pavone P, Marsili L, Catalano C, et al. Carotid arteries: evaluation with low field strength MR angiography. *Radiology* 1992;184:401–404.
158. Laster RE JR, Acker JD, Halford HH III, et al. Assessment of MR angiography verses arteriography for the evaluation of cervical carotid bifurcation disease. *AJNR* 1993;14:681–688.
159. Listerud J, Cohen IM. Overview of flow hemodynamics. *Neuroimag Clin North Am* 1992;2(4):735–739.
160. Middleton WD, Foley WD, Lawson TL. Flow reversal in the normal carotid bifurcation: color Doppler flow imaging analysis. *Radiology* 1988;167:207–210.
161. Heiserman JE, Drayer BP, Fram EK, et al. Carotid artery stenosis: clinical efficacy of two-dimensional time-of-flight MR angiography. *Radiology* 1992;182:761–768.
162. Motomiya M, Karino T. Flow patterns in the human carotid artery bifurcation. *Stroke* 1984;15(1):50–56.
163. Buijs PC, Klop RBJ, Eikelboom BC, et al. Carotid bifurcation imaging: magnetic resonance angiography compared to conventional angiography and doppler ultrasound. *Eur J Vasc Surg* 1993;7:245–251.
164. Huston J III, Lewis BD, Wiebers DO, et al. Carotid artery: prospective blinded comparison of two-dimensional time-of-flight MR angiography with conventional angiography and duplex US. *Radiology* 1993;186:339–344.
165. Ruskowski JT, Damadian R, Giambalvo A, et al. MRI angiography of the carotid artery. *Magn Reson Imaging* 1986;4:497–502.
166. Wesbey GE, Bergan JJ, Moreland SI, et al. Cerebrovascular magnetic resonance angiography: a critical verification. *J Vasc Surg* 1992;16:619–632.
167. Anderson CM, Saloner D, Lee RE, et al. Assessment of carotid stenosis by MR angiography: comparison with x-ray angiography and color-coded Doppler ultrasound. *AJNR* 1992;13:1235–1243.
168. Urchuk SN, Plewes DB. Mechanisms of flow-induced signal loss in MR angiography. *J Magn Reson Imaging* 1992;2:453–462.
169. Masaryk TJ, Laub G, Modic MT, Ruggieri P, Ross JS. 3DFT MR angiography: a comparison of time-of-flight techniques. Presented at the *Eighth Annual Meeting of the Society of Magnetic Resonance in Medicine*, Washington, DC, 1989.
170. Atkinson D, Brant-Zawadzki M, Gillan G, Purdy D, Laub G. Improved MR angiography: magnetization transfer suppression with variable flip angle excitation and increased resolution. *Radiology* 1994;190:890–894.
171. MacFall JR, Grist TM, Spritzer CE, Evans AJ. In-plane sampling requirements of MR reprojection angiography. Presented at the *75th Annual RSNA Meeting*, 1989.
172. Brown DG, Riederer SJ, Farzaneh F, Wright RC, Ehman RL. Realtime MR angiographic line scan acquisition and reconstruction. Presented at the *Eighth Annual Meeting of the Society of Magnetic Resonance in Medicine*, 1989.
173. Napel S, Rutt BK, Dunne S. Minimum voxel and maximum gradient re-projection for MR angiography. Presented at the *Eighth Annual Meeting of the Society for Magnetic Resonance Imaging*, Washington, DC, 1990.
174. Parker DL, Yuan C, Blatter DD, et al. MR angiography by multiple thin slab 3D acquisition. *Magn Reson Med* 1991;17: 434–451.
175. Parker DL, Blatter DD. Multiple thin slab magnetic resonance angiography. *Neuroimag Clin North Am* 1992;2:677–692.
176. Mittl RL, Broderick M, Carpenter JP, et al. Blinded reader comparison of magnetic resonance angiography and duplex ultrasonography for carotid artery bifurcation stenosis. *Stroke* 1994;25: 4–10.
177. Pan XM, Anderson CM, Reilly LM, et al. Magnetic resonance angiography of the carotid artery combining two- and three-dimensional acquisitions. *J Vasc Surg* 1992;16:609–618.
178. Eikelbloom BC, Riles TR, Mintzer R, et al. Inaccuracy of angiography in the diagnosis of carotid ulceration. *Stroke* 1983;14:882–885.
179. Podolak MJ, Hedlund LW, Evans AJ, Herfkins RJ. Evaluation of flow through simulated vascular stenoses with gradient echo magnetic resonance imaging. *Invest Radiol* 1989;24(3):184–189.
180. Yuan C, Tsuruda JS, Beach KN, et al. Techniques for high resolution MR imaging of atherosclerotic plaque. *J Magn Reson Imaging* 1994;4:43–49.
181. Goldberg AL, Rosenbaum AE, Wang H, Kim WS, Lewis VL, Hanley DF. Computed tomography of dural sinus thrombosis. *J Comput Assist Tomogr* 1986;10:16–20.

182. Schievink WI, Mokri B, O'Fallon WM. Recurrent spontaneous cervical-artery dissection. *N Engl J Med* 1994;330:393–397.
183. Hart RG, Easton JD. Dissections and trauma of cervico-cerebral arteries. In: Barnett HJM, Mohr JP, Stein BM, Yatsu FM, eds. *Stroke: Pathophysiology, Diagnosis, and Management.* New York: Churchill Livingstone; 1986:775–778.
184. Mokri B, Sundt TM, Houser OW, Peipgras DG. Spontaneous dissection of the cervical internal carotid artery. *Ann Neurol* 1986;19:126–138.
185. Houser OW, Mokri B, Sundt TM Jr, et al. Spontaneous cervical cephalic arterial dissection and its residuum: angiographic spectrum. *AJNR* 1984;5:27–34.
186. O'Dwyer JA, Moscow N, Trevor R, Ehrenfeld WK, Newton TH. Spontaneous dissection of the carotid artery. *Radiology* 1980;137:379–385.
187. Pozzati E, Giuliani G, Acciarri N, Nuzzo G. Long-term follow-up of occlusive cervical carotid dissection. *Stroke* 1990;21:528–531.
188. Kitani R, Itouji T, Noda Y, Kimura M, Uchida S. Dissecting aneurysms of the anterior circle of Willis arteries. *J Neurosurg* 1987;67:296–300.
189. Morgan MK, Besser M, Johnston I, Chaseling R. Intracranial carotid artery injury in closed head trauma. *J Neurosurg* 1987;66: 192–197.
190. O'Sullivan RM, Robertson WD, Nugent RA, Berry K, Turnbull IM. Supraclinoid carotid artery dissection following unusual trauma. *AJNR* 1990;11:1150–1152.
191. Luken MG III, Ascherl GR Jr, Correll JR, et al. Spontaneous dissecting aneurysms of the extracranial internal carotid artery. *Clin Neurosurg* 1979;26:353–375.
192. Fisher CM, Ojemann RG, Roberson GH. Spontaneous dissection of cervico-cerebral arteries. *Can J Neurol Sci* 1978;5:9–19.
193. Lévy C, Laissy JP, Raveau V, et al. Carotid and vertebral artery dissections: three-dimensional time-of-flight MR angiography and MR imaging versus conventional angiography. *Radiology* 1994;190:97–103.
194. Brugières P, Castrec-Carpo A, Héran F, Coujon C, Gaston A, Marsault C. Magnetic resonance imaging in the exploration of dissection of the internal carotid artery. *J Neuroradiol* 1989;16: 1–10.
195. Gelbert F, Assouline E, Hodes JE, et al. MRI in spontaneous dissection of vertebral and carotid arteries. *Neuroradiology* 1991;33: 111–113.
196. Healton EB. Fibromuscular dysplasia. In: Barnett HJM, Mohr JP, Stein BM, Yatsu FM, eds. *Stroke: Pathophysiology, Diagnosis, and Management.* New York: Churchill Livingstone; 1986: 831–844.
197. Heiserman JE, Drayer BP, Fram EK, Keller PJ. MR angiography of cervical fibromuscular dysplasia. *AJNR* 1992;13:1454–1457.
198. Heidrich H, Bayer O. Symptomatology of the subclavian steal syndrome. *Angiography* 1969;20:406–413.
199. Killen DA, Foster JH, Gobbel WG Jr, et al. The subclavian steal syndrome. *J Thorac Cardiovasc Surg* 1965;51:539–560.
200. Santschi DR, Frahm CJ, Pascale LR, Dunamian AV. The subclavian steal syndrome. Clinical and angiographic considerations in 74 cases in adults. *J Thorac Cardiovasc Surg* 1966;51:103–112.
201. Turjman F, Tournut P, Baldy-Porcher C, Laharotte JC, Duquesnel J, Froment JC. Demonstration of subclavian steal by MR angiography. *J Comput Assist Tomogr* 1992; 16(5):756–759.
202. Perl J II, Turski PA, Kennell T, Robichaud K, Strother CM, Graves VB. Cine phase contrast quantification of subclavian steal flow rates at rest and following hand exercise or reactive hyperemia. *ASNR 32nd Annual Meeting,* Nashville, 1994.
203. Mohr JP, Caplan LR, Melski JW, et al. The Harvard cooperative stroke registry: a prospective registry. *Neurology* 1978;28:754–762.
204. Caplan LR. Diagnosis and treatment of ischemic stroke. *JAMA* 1991;266:2413–2418.
205. Adams RA, Victor M. Cerebrovascular diseases. In: *Principles of Neurology,* 4th ed. New York: McGraw-Hill; 1989:617–692.
206. Johnson BA, Heiserman JE, Drayer BP, Keller PJ. Intracranial MR angiography: its role in the integrated approach to brain infarction. *AJNR* 1994;15:901–908.
207. Battacharji SK, Hutchinson EC, McCall AJ. The circle of Willis—the incidence of developmental abnormalities in normal and infarcted brains. From the North Staffordshire Royal Infirmary. PhD Thesis entitled "The role of extracranial and intracranial arteries in cerebral infarction," accepted by the University of Birmingham, 1965.
208. Castaigne P, Lhermitte F, Gautier JC, Escourolle R, Derouesne C. Internal carotid artery occlusion. A study of 61 instances in 50 patients with post-mortem data. *Brain* 1970;93:231–258.
209. Ringelstein EB, Zeumer H, Angelou D. The pathogenesis of strokes from internal carotid artery occlusion. Diagnostic and therapeutical implications. *Stroke* 1983;14:867–875.
210. Edelman RR, Heinrich PM, O'Reilly GV, Wentz KU, Liu C, Zhao B. Magnetic resonance imaging of flow dynamics in the circle of Willis. *Stroke* 1990;21:56–65.
211. Gurst G, Steinmetz H, Fischer H, et al. Selective MR angiography and intracranial collateral blood flow. *J Comput Assist Tomogr* 1993;17:178–183.
212. Pernicone JR, Siebert JE, Laird TA, Rosenbaum TL, Potchen EJ. Determination of blood flow direction using velocity–phase image display with 3-D phase-contrast MR angiography. *AJNR* 1992;13:1435–1438.
213. Rossnick S, Kennedy D, Laub G, et al. Three-dimensional display of blood vessels in MRI (*abstr*). In: *Proceedings of the IEEE Computers in Cardiology Conference.* 1986:193–196.
214. Schomer DF, Marks MP, Steinberg GK, et al. The anatomy of the posterior communicating artery as a risk factor for ischemic cerebral infarction. *N Engl J Med* 1994;330:1565–1570.
215. Ringelstein EB, Otis SM. Physiologic testing of vasomotor reserve and collateral flow via the circle of Willis. In: Newell DN, Aasbid R, eds. *Transcranial Doppler.* New York: Raven Press; 1992;83–100.
216. Riggs HE, Rupp C. Variation in form of circle of Willis. *Arch Neurol* 1963;8:24–30.
217. Steinberg GK, Drake CG, Peerless SJ. Deliberate basilar or vertebral artery occlusion in the treatment of intracranial aneurysms: immediate results and long-term outcome in 201 patients. *J Neurosurg* 1993;79:161–173.
218. Raju S, Fredericks RK. Carotid siphon stenosis. *J Cardiovasc Surg* 1987;28:671–677.
219. Craig DR, Meguro K, Watridge C, Robertson JT, Barnett HJM, Fox AJ. Intracranial internal carotid artery stenosis. *Stroke* 1982;13:825–828.
220. Amagasa M, Sato S, Otabe K. Posttraumatic dissecting aneurysm of the anterior cerebral artery: case report. *Neurosurgery* 1988;23: 221–225.
221. Mann CI, Dietrich RB, Schrader MT, Peck WW, Demos DS, Bradley WG Jr. Posttraumatic carotid artery dissection in children: evaluation with MR angiography. *AJR* 1993;160:134–136.
222. Grosman H, Fornasier VL, Bonder D, Livingston KE, Platts MJ. Dissecting aneurysm of the cerebral arteries. *J Neurosurg* 1980; 53:693–697.
223. Hinton RC, Mohr JP, Ackerman RH, Adair LB, Fisher CM. Symptomatic middle cerebral artery stenosis. *Ann Neurol* 1979;5: 152–157.
224. Adams HP Jr, Gross CE. Embolism distal to stenosis of the middle cerebral artery. *Stroke* 1981;12:228–229.
225. Purdy PD, Devous MD Sr, Unwin DH, Giller CA, Batjer HH. Angioplasty of an atherosclerotic middle cerebral artery associated with improvement in regional cerebral blood flow. *AJNR* 1990;11:878–880.
226. Masaryk TJ, Modic MT, Ross JS, et al. Intracranial circulation: preliminary clinical results with three-dimensional (volume) MR angiography. *Radiology* 1989;171:793–799.
227. Dagirmanjian A, Ross JS, Lewin JS, Masaryk TJ, Ruggieri PM. Use of high-resolution, magnetization transfer saturation, variable flip angle, time-of-flight MR angiography in the detection of intracranial vascular stenoses. *ASNR 31st Annual Meeting,* 1993.
228. Heiserman JE, Drayer BP, Keller PJ, Fram EK. Intracranial vascular stenosis and occlusion: evaluation with three-dimensional time-of-flight MR angiography. *Radiology* 1992;185:667–673.
229. Fujita N, Hirabuki N, Fujii K, et al. MR imaging of middle cerebral artery stenosis and occlusion: value of MR angiography. *AJNR* 1994;15:335–341.
230. Bogousslavsky J, Regli F, Maeder P, Meuli R, Nader J. The etiol-

ogy of posterior circulation infarcts: a prospective study using magnetic resonance imaging and magnetic resonance angiography. *Neurology* 1993;43:1528–1533.

231. Rother J, Wentz KU, Rautenberg W, Schwartz A, Hennerici M. Magnetic resonance angiography in vertebrobasilar ischemia. *Stroke* 1993;24;1310–1315.
232. Ruggieri PM, Ross JS, Modic MT, et al. MR angiographic evaluation of symptomatic vertebrobasilar stenosis. *First Meeting of the Society of Magnetic Resonance*, 1994.
233. Harris KG, Tran DD, Sickels WJ, Cornell SH, Yuh WTC. Diagnosing intracranial vasculitis: the roles of MR and angiography. *AJNR* 1994;15:317–330.
234. Yonekawa Y, Handa H, Okuno T. Moyamoya disease: diagnosis, treatment, and recent achievement. In: Barnett HJM, Mohr JP, Stein BM, Yatsu FM, eds. *Stroke: Pathophysiology, Diagnosis and Management*. New York: Churchill Livingstone; 1986:805–830.
235. Yamada I, Matsushima Y, Suzuki S. Moyamoya disease: diagnosis with three-dimensional time-of-flight MR angiography. *Radiology* 1992;184:773–778.
236. Suzuki J, Kodama N. Moyamoya disease—a review. *Stroke* 1983;14:104–109.
237. Creasy JL, Price RR, Presbrey T, Goins D, Partain CL, Kessler RM. Gadolinium-enhanced MR angiography. *Radiology* 1990;175:280–283.
238. Marchal G, Michiels J, Bosmans H, VanHecke P. Contrast-enhanced MRA of the brain. *J Comput Assist Tomogr* 1992;16: 25–29.
239. Sydenstricker VP, Mulherin WA, Houseal RW. Sickle cell anemia. *Am J Dis Child* 1923;26:143–154.
240. Bridgers WH. Cerebrovascular disease accompanying sickle cell anemia. *Am J Pathol* 1939;15:353–361.
241. Rout D, Sharma A, Mohan PK, Rao VRK. Bacterial aneurysms of the intracavernous carotid artery. *J Neurosurg* 1984; 60:1236–1242.
242. Bogousslavsky J, Regli F. Borderzone infarctions distal to internal carotid artery disease. *Ann Neurol* 1986;20:346–350.
243. Mohr JP. Neurological complications of cardiac valvular disease and cardiac surgery. In: Vicken PJ, Bruyn GW, eds. *Handbook of Clinical Neurology*. Amsterdam: North Holland Publications; 1979:34(1);113–171.
244. Huttenlocher PR, Moohr JW, Johns L, Brown FD. Cerebral blood flow in sickle cell cerebrovascular disease. *Pediatrics* 1984;73:615–621.
245. Pavlakis SG, Bello J, Prohovnik I, et al. Brain infarction in sickle cell anemia: magnetic resonance imaging correlates. *Ann Neurol* 1988;23:125–130.
246. Adams RJ, Nichols FT, McKie V, et al. Cerebral infarction in sickle cell anemia mechanism based on CT and MRI. *Neurology* 1988;38:1012–1017.
247. Gammal T, Adams RJ, Nichols FT, et al. MR and CT investigation of cerebrovascular disease in sickle cell patients. *AJNR* 1986;7:1043–1049.
248. Zimmerman RA, Gill F, Goldberg HL, et al. MRI of sickle cell cerebral infarction. *Neuroradiology* 1987;29:232–237.
249. Stockman JA, Nigro MA, Mishkin MM, et al. Occlusion of large cerebral vessels in sickle cell anemia. *N Engl J Med* 1972;287: 846–849.
250. Adeloye A, Odeku E. Nervous system in sickle cell disease. *Afr J Med Sci* 1970;1:33.
251. Russel MO, Goldberg HI, Hodson A, et al. Effect of transfusion therapy on arteriographic abnormalities and on recurrence of stroke in sickle cell disease. *Blood* 1984;63:162–169.
252. Wilimas J, Goff JR, Anderson HR, et al. Efficacy of transfusion therapy for one to two years in patients with sickle cell disease and cerebrovascular accidents. *J Pediatr* 1980;96:205–208.
253. Lusher JM, Haghight H, Khalifa AS. A prophylactic transfusion program for children with sickle cell anemia complicated by CNS infarction. *Am J Hematol* 1976;1:265–273.
254. Schmalzer E, Chien S, Brown AK. Transfusion therapy in sickle cell disease. *Am J Pediatr Hematol Oncol* 1982;4:395–406.
255. Kugler S, Anderson B, Cross D, et al. Abnormal cranial magnetic resonance imaging scans in sickle-cell disease. *Arch Neurol* 1993;50:629–635.
256. Richards D, Nulsen FE. Angiographic media and the sickling phenomenon. *Surg Forum* 1971;22:403–404.
257. Wiznitzer M, Ruggieri PM, Masaryk TJ, Ross JS, Modic MT, Berman B. Diagnosis of cerebrovascular disease in sickle cell anemia by magnetic resonance angiography. *J Pediatr* 1990;117: 551–555.
258. Masaryk TJ, Masaryk AM, Ross JS, Modic MT, Wiznitzer M, Berman B. MR angiographic and parenchymal evaluation of cerebral infarction in sickle cell anemia. Presented at the *75th Annual RSNA Meeting*, 1989.
259. Brown MM, Marshall J. Regulation of cerebral blood flow in response to changes in blood viscosity. *Lancet* 1985;1:604–609.
260. Prohovnik I, Pavlakis SG, Piomelli S, et al. Cerebral hyperemia, stroke and transfusion in sickle cell disease. *Neurology* 1989;39: 344–348.
261. Bishop CCR, Powell S, Rutt D, Browse NL. Transcranial Doppler measurement of middle cerebral artery blood flow velocity: a validation study. *Stroke* 1986;17:913–915.
262. Sorteberg W, Lindegaard KF, Rootwelt K, et al. Blood velocity and regional blood flow in defined cerebral artery systems. *Stroke* 1989;97:47–52.
263. Towne BH, Lott IT, Hicks DA, Healey T. Long-term follow-up of infants and children treated with extracorporeal membrane oxygenation (ECMO): a preliminary report. *J Pediatr Surg* 1985;20: 410–414.
264. Schumacher RE, Barks JDE, Johnston MV, et al. Right-sided brain lesions in infants following extracorporeal membrane oxygenation. *Pediatrics* 1988;82:155–161.
265. McArdle CB, Richardson CJ, Hayden CK, Nicholas DA, Amparo EG. Abnormalities of the neonatal brain: MR imaging; Part II. Hypoxic-ischemic brain injury. *Radiology* 1987;163:395–403.
266. McArdle CB, Richardson CJ, Hayden CK, Nicholas DA, Crofford MJ, Amparo EG. Abnormalities of the neonatal brain: MR imaging; Part I. intracranial hemorrhage. *Radiology* 1987;163:387–394.
267. Mattle H, Edelman RR, O'Reilly GV, Wentz KU, Liu C, Zhao B. Evaluation of flow dynamics in the circle of Willis using magnetic resonance. Presented at the *Eighth Annual Meeting of the Society of Magnetic Resonance in Medicine*, 1989.
268. Ameri A, Bousser MG. Cerebral venous thrombosis. *Neurol Clin North Am* 1992;10:87–111.
269. Johnson BA, Fram EK. Cerebral venous occlusive disease: pathophysiology, clinical manifestations, and imaging. *Neuroimag Clin North Am* 1992;2(4):769–783.
270. Virapongse C, Cazenave C, Quisling R, Sarwar M, Hunter S. The empty delta sign: frequency and significance in 76 cases of dural sinus thrombosis. *Radiology* 1989;162:779–785.
271. Hoffmann MW, Bill PLA, Bhigjee AI, Modi G, Haribhai HC, Kelbe C. The clinicoradiological profile of cerebral venous thrombosis. *South Afr Med J* 1992;82:341–348.
272. Barron TF, Gusnard DA, Zimmerman RA, Clancy RR. Cerebral venous thrombosis in neonates and children. *Pediatr Neurol* 1992;8(2)112–116.
273. Southwick FS, Richardson EP, Swartz MN. Septic thrombosis of the dural venous sinuses. *Medicine* 1986;65(2):82–106.
274. Hesselbrock R, Sawaya R, Tomsick T, Wadhwa S. Superior sagittal sinus thrombosis after closed head injury. *Neurosurgery* 1985;16:825–828.
275. Padayachee TS, Bingham JB, Graves MJ, Colchester ACF, Cox TCS. Dural sinus thrombosis. Diagnosis and follow-up by magnetic resonance angiography and imaging. *Neuroradiology* 1991;33:165–167.
276. Medlock MD, Olivero WC, Hanigan WC, Wright RM, Winek SJ. Children with cerebral venous thrombosis diagnosed with MRI and magnetic resonance angiography. *Neurosurgery* 1992;31: 870–876.
277. Einhaupl KM, Villringer A, Meister W, et al. Heparin treatment in sinus venous thrombosis. *Lancet* 1991;338:597–600.
278. Villringer A, Garner C, Meister W, et al. High dose heparin treatment in cerebral sinus venous thrombosis. *Stroke* 1988;19:135.
279. Anderson SC, Shah CP, Murtagh FR. Congested deep cortical veins as a sign of dural venous thrombosis: MR and CT correlations. *J Comput Assist Tomogr* 1987;11:1059–1061.
280. Rippe DJ, Boyko OB, Spritzer CE, et al. Demonstration of dural

sinus occlusion by the use of MR angiography. *AJNR* 1990;11: 199–201.
281. Villringer A, Seiderer M, Bauer W, et al. Diagnosis of superior sagittal sinus thrombosis by three-dimensional magnetic resonance imaging. *Lancet* 1989;1:1086–1087.
282. Vogl TJ, Bergman C, Villringer A, Einhaupl K, Lissner J, Felix R. Dural sinus thrombosis: value of venous MR angiography for diagnosis and follow-up. *AJR* 1994;162:1191–1198.
283. Lewin JS, Masaryk TJ, Smith AS, Ruggieri PM, Ross JS. Time-of-flight intracranial MR venography: evaluation of the sequential oblique slice technique. *AJNR* 1994;15:1657–1664.
284. Mattle HP, Wentz KU, Edelman RR, et al. Cerebral venography with MR. *Radiology* 1991;178:453–458.
285. Yousem DM, Balakrishnan J, Debrun GM, Bryan RN. Hyperintense thrombus on Grass MR images: potential pitfall in flow evaluation. *AJNR* 1990;11:51–58.
286. Applegate GR, Talagala SL, Apple LJ. MR angiography of the head and neck: value of two-dimensional phase-contrast projection technique. *AJR* 1992;159:369–374.
287. Chakeres DW, Schmalbrock P, Brogan M, Yuan C, Cohen L. Normal venous anatomy of the brain: demonstration with gadopentatate dimeglumine in enhanced 3-D MR angiography. *AJNR* 1990;11:1107–1118.
288. Anderson CM, Edelman RR, Turski PA. Magnetic resonance venography and cerebral venous thrombosis. In: *Clinical Magnetic Resonance Angiography.* New York: Raven Press; 1993: 289–308.
289. Jannetta PJ, Abbasy M, Maroon JC, et al. Etiology and definitive microsurgical treatment of hemifacial spasm. Operative techniques and results in 47 patients. *J Neurosurg* 1977;47:321–328.
290. Adler CH, Zimmerman RA, Savino PJ, Bernardi B, Bosley TM, Sergott RC. Hemifacial spasm: evaluation by magnetic resonance imaging and magnetic resonance tomographic angiography. *Ann Neurol* 1992;32:502–506.
291. Coad JE, Wirtschafter JD, Haines SJ, et al. Familial hemifacial spasm associated with arterial compression of the facial nerve: case report. *J Neurosurg* 1991;74:290–296.
292. Neilsen VK, Jannetta PJ. Pathophysiology of hemifacial spasm: III. Effects of facial nerve decompression. *Neurology* 1984;34: 891–897.
293. Felber S, Birbamer G, Aichner F, Poewe W, Kampfl A. Magnetic resonance imaging and angiography in hemifacial spasm. *Neuroradiology* 1992;34:413–416.
294. Furuya Y, Ryu H, Uemura K, et al. MRI of intracranial neurovascular compression. *J Comput Assist Tomogr* 1992;16:503–505.
295. Harsh GR, Wilson CB, Hieshima GB, Dillon WP. Magnetic resonance imaging of vertebrobasilar ectasia in tic convulsif. *J Neurosurg* 1991;74:999–1003.
296. Nagaseki Y, Horikoshi T, Omata T, et al. Oblique sagittal magnetic resonance imaging visualizing vascular compression of the trigeminal or facial nerve. *J Neurosurg* 1992;77:379–386.
297. Tash R, DeMerritt J, Sze G, Leslie D. Hemifacial spasm: MR imaging features. *AJNR* 1991;12:839–842.
298. Tien RD, Wilkins RH. MRA delineation of the vertebral-basilar system in patients with hemifacial spasm and trigeminal neuralgia. *AJNR* 1993;14:34–36.
299. Bernardi B, Zimmerman RA, Savino PJ, Adler C. Magnetic resonance tomographic angiography in the investigation of hemifacial spasm. *Neuroradiology* 1993;35:606–611.
300. Drake CG. Management of cerebral aneurysm. *Stroke* 1981;12: 273–283.
301. Sypert GW. Intracranial aneurysms: natural history and surgical management. *Comprehensive Ther* 1978;4:64–73.
302. Housepian EM, Pool JL. A systematic analysis of intracranial aneurysms from the autopsy file of Presbyterian Hospital. *J Neuropathol Exp Neurology* 1958;17:409–423.
303. McCormick WF. Problems and pathogenesis of intracranial arterial aneurysms. In: Toole JF, Moosey J, Janeway R, eds. *Cerebrovascular Disorders*, 2nd ed. New York: Grune & Stratton; 1971: 219–231.
304. Atkinson JLD, Sundt TM, Houser OW, Whisnant JP. Angiographic frequency of anterior circulation intracranial aneurysms. *J Neurosurg* 1989;70:551–555.
305. Huston J III, Torres VE, Sulivan PP, Offord KP, Wiebers DO. Value of magnetic resonance angiography for the detection of intracranial aneurysms in autosomal dominant polycystic kidney disease. *J Am Soc Nephrol* 1993;3:1871–1877.
306. Leblanc R, Worsley KJ, Melanson D, Tampieri D. Angiographic screening and elective surgery of familial cerebral aneurysms: a decision analysis. *Neurosurgery* 1994;35:9–18.
307. Nakagawa T, Hashi K. The incidence and treatment of asymptomatic unruptured cerebral aneurysms. *J Neurosurg* 1994;80: 217–223.
308. Ross JS, Masaryk TJ, Modic MT, Ruggieri PM, Haacke EM, Selman W. Intracranial aneurysms: evaluation by MR angiography. *AJNR* 1990;11:449–456.
309. Ruggieri PM, Poulas N, Obuchowski N, et al. Occult intracranial aneurysms in polycystic kidney disease: screening with MR angiography. *Radiology* 1994;191:33–39.
310. ter Berg HWM, Dippel DWJ, Limburg M, Schievink WI, van Gijn J. Familial intracranial aneurysms. *Stroke* 1992;23:1024–1030.
311. DeLaPaz RL, New PFJ, Buonanno FS, et al. NMR imaging of intracranial hemorrhage. *J Comput Assist Tomogr* 1984;8:599–607.
312. Atlas SW. MR imaging is highly sensitive for acute subarachnoid hemorrhage . . . not! *Radiology* 1993;186:319–322.
313. Curnes JT, Shogry MEC, Clark DC, Elsner HJ. MR angiographic demonstration of an intracranial aneurysm not seen on conventional angiography. *AJNR* 1992;14:971–973.
314. Gouliamos A, Gotsis E, Vlahos L, et al. Magnetic resonance angiography compared to intra-arterial digital subtraction angiography in patients with subarachnoid haemorrhage. *Neuroradiology* 1992;35:46–49.
315. Sheppard L, Listerud J, Goldberg HI, Hurst RW, Flamm E, Atlas SW. MR angiography of intracranial aneurysms using a sophisticated multifeature extraction post-processing method. 1994 *RSNA Annual Meeting.*
316. Allcock JM. Aneurysms. In: Newton TH, Potts DG, eds. *Radiology of the Skull and Brain.* St. Louis: Mosby; 1974;2(4):2445–2559.
317. Levey AS, Pauker SG, Kassirer JP. Occult intracranial aneurysm in polycystic kidney disease. When is cerebral arteriography indicated? *N Engl J Med* 1983;308:986–994.
318. Perret G, Nishioka H. Report on the cooperative study of intracranial aneurysms and subarachnoid hemorrhage. Section VI. Arteriovenous malformations. An analysis of 545 cases of craniocerebral arteriovenous malformations and fistulae reported to the cooperative study. *J Neurosurg* 1966;25:467–490.
319. Steiner H, Lammer J, Kleinert R, Scheyer H. Dissecting aneurysm of cerebral arteries in congenital vascular deficiency. *Neuroradiology* 1986;28:331–334.
320. Belber CJ, Hoffman RB. The syndrome of intracranial aneurysm associated with fibromuscular hyperplasia of the renal arteries. *J Neurosurg* 1968;28:556–559.
321. Bert JWM, Overtoom TMD, Ludwig JW, et al. Detection of unruptured familial intracranial aneurysms by intravenous digital subtraction angiography. *Neuroradiology* 1987;29:272–276.
322. Schievink WI, Limburg M, Dreissen JJR, et al. Screening for unruptured familial intracranial aneurysms: subarachnoid hemorrhage 2 years after angiography negative for aneurysms. *Neurosurgery* 1991;29(3):434–438.
323. Asari S, Satoh T, Sakurai M, et al. Delineation of unruptured cerebral aneurysms by CT angiotomography. *J Neurosurg* 1982; 57:527–534.
324. Aoki S, Sasaki Y, Machida T, Ohkubo T, Minami M, Sasaki Y. Cerebral aneurysms: detection and delineation using 3-D–CT angiography. *AJNR* 1992;13:1115–1120.
325. Eskesen V, Rosenorn J, Schmidt K, et al. Clinical features and outcome in 48 patients with unruptured intracranial saccular aneurysms: a prospective consecutive study. *Br J Neurosurg* 1987;1: 47–52.
326. Graf CJ. Prognosis for patients with nonsurgically-treated aneurysms. Analysis of the cooperative study of intracranial aneurysms and subarachnoid hemorrhage. *J Neurosurg* 1971;35:438–443.
327. Heiskanen O. Risk of bleeding from unruptured aneurysms in

cases with multiple intracranial aneurysms. *J Neurosurg* 1981;55: 524–526.

328. Jane JA, Winn HR, Richardson AE. The natural history of intracranial aneurysms: rebleeding rates during the acute and long term period and implication for surgical management. *Clin Neurosurg* 1977;24:176–184.
329. Locksley HB. Report on the cooperative study of intracranial aneurysms and subarachnoid hemorrhage: Section V, Part I. Natural history of subarachnoid hemorrhage, intracranial aneurysms and arteriovenous malformations. Based on 6368 cases in the Cooperative Study. *J Neurosurg* 1966;25:219–239.
330. Rosenorn J, Eskesen V, Schmidt K. Unruptured intracranial aneurysms: an assessment of the annual risk of rupture based on epidemiological and clinical data. *Br J Neurosurg* 1988;2:369–377.
331. Wiebers DO, Whisnant JP, Sundt TM Jr, et al. The significance of unruptured intracranial saccular aneurysms. *J Neurosurg* 1987;66:23–29.
332. Wiebers DO, Whisnant JP, O'Fallon WM. The natural history of unruptured intracranial aneurysms. *N Engl J Med* 1981;304: 696–698.
333. Winn HR, Almaani WS, Berga SL, et al. The long-term outcome in patients with multiple aneurysms. Incidence of late hemorrhage and implications for treatment of incidental aneurysms. *J Neurosurg* 1983;59:642–651.
334. Wiebers DO, Whisnant JP, Sundt TM Jr, et al. Intracranial aneurysm size and potential for rupture. [Letter]. *J Neurosurg* 1987;67:476.
335. Chapman AB, Rubinstein D, Hughes R, et al. Intracranial aneurysms in autosomal dominant polycystic kidney disease. *N Engl J Med* 1992;327:916–920.
336. Weibers DO, Torres VE. Screening for unruptured intracranial aneurysms in autosomal dominant polycystic kidney disease. *N Engl J Med* 1992;327(13):953–955.
337. Fox JL. Management of aneurysms of anterior circulation of intracranial procedures. In: Youmans JR, ed. *Neurological Surgery*, 3rd ed. Philadelphia: WB Saunders; 1990:1689–1732.
338. Hacker RS, Krall SM, Fox JL. In: Fox JL, ed. *Intracranial Aneurysms*. New York: Springer-Verlag; 1983;1:19–117.
339. Hove B, Andersen BB, Christiansen TM. Intracranial oncotic aneurysms from choriocarcinoma. Case report and review of the literature. *Neuroradiology* 1990;32:526–528.
340. Nakstad P, Nornes H, Hauge HN. Traumatic aneurysms of the pericallosal arteries. *Neuroradiology* 1986;28:335–338.
341. Ruggieri PM, Laub GA, Masaryk TJ, Modic MT. Intracranial circulation: pulse sequence considerations in three-dimensional (volume) MR angiography. *Radiology* 1989;171:785–791.
342. Steiger HJ, Poll A, Liepsch DW, Reuler HJ. Basic flow structures in saccular aneurysms: a flow visualization study. *Heart Vessels* 1987;3:55–65.
343. Strother CM, Graves VB, Rappe A. Aneurysm hemodynamics: an experimental study. *AJNR* 1992;13:1089–1095.
344. Turski PA, Korosec F. Technical features and emerging clinical applications of phase contrast MRA. *Neuroimag Clin North Am* 1992;2(4):785–800.
345. Artman H, Vonofakos D, Muller H, Grau H. Neuroradiologic and neuropathologic findings with growing giant intracranial aneurysm: review of the literature. *Surg Neurol* 1984;21:391–401.
346. Steiger HJ, Liepsch DW, Poll A, Reulen JH. Hemodynamic stress in terminal saccular aneurysms—a laser Doppler study. *Heart Vessels* 1988;4:162–169.
347. Perktold K. On the path of fluid particles in an axisymmetrical aneurysm. *J Biomech* 1987;20:311–317.
348. McCormick WF, Acosta-Rua GJ. The size of intracranial saccular aneurysms. An autopsy study. *J Neurosurg* 1970;33:422–427.
349. Huston J III, Rufenacht DA, Ehman RL, Wiebers DO. Intracranial aneurysms and vascular malformations: comparison of time-of-flight and phase-contrast MR angiography. *Radiology* 1991;181:721–730.
350. Sevick RJ, Tsuruda JS, Schmalbrock P. Three-dimensional time-of-flight MR angiography in the evaluation of cerebral aneurysms. *J Comput Assist Tomogr* 1990;14:874–881.
351. Demaerel PH, Marchal G, Casteels I, et al. Intracavernous aneurysm. Superior demonstration by magnetic resonance angiography. *Neuroradiology* 1990;32:322–324.
352. Runge VM, Kirsch JE, Lee C. Contrast-enhanced MR angiography. *J Magn Reson Imaging* 1993;3:233–239.
353. Bogdanov AA Jr, Weissleder R, Frank HW, et al. A new macromolecule as a contrast agent for MR angiography: preparation, properties, and animal studies. *Radiology* 1993;187:701–706.
354. Turski PA, Korsec FR, Partington CR, Strother CM, Graves VB, Mistretta CA. Cardiac-gated and variable-velocity-phase MR angiography for evaluation of intracranial aneurysms and arteriovenous malformations (abstr). *Radiology* 1990;177(P):281.
355. Brothers MF, Fox AJ, Lee DH, et al. MR imaging after surgery for vertebrobasilar aneurysm. *AJNR* 1990;11:149–161.
356. Holtas S, Olsson M, Romner B, et al. Comparison of MR imaging and CT in patients with intracranial aneurysm clips. *AJNR* 1988;9:891–897.
357. Becker RL, Norfray JF, Teitelbaum GP, et al. MR imaging in patients with intracranial aneurysm clips. *AJNR* 1988;9:885–889.
358. Shellock FG, Morisoli S, Kanal E. MR procedures and biomedical implants, materials, and devices: 1993 update. *Radiology* 1993;189:587–599.
359. Fox AJ, Vinuela F, Pelz DM. Use of detachable balloons for proximal artery occlusion in the treatment of unclippable cerebral aneurysms. *J Neurosurg* 1987;66:40–46.
360. Higashida RT, Halbach VV, Barnwell SL. Treatment of intracranial aneurysms with preservation of the parent vessel: results of percutaneous balloon embolization in 84 patients. *AJNR* 1990;11:633–640.
361. Guglielmi G, Vinuela F, Dion J, Duckwiler G. Electrothrombosis of saccular aneurysms via endovascular approach. Part 2: preliminary clinical experience. *J Neurosurg* 1991;75(1):8–14.
362. Guglielmi G, Vinuela F, Duckwiler G, et al. Endovascular treatment of posterior circulation aneurysms by electrothrombosis using electrically detachable coils. *J Neurosurg* 1992;77(4):515–524.
363. Tsuruda JS, Sevick RJ, Halbach VV. Three-dimensional time-of-flight MR angiography in the evaluation of intracranial aneurysms treated by endovascular balloon occlusion. *AJNR* 1992;13: 1129–1136.
364. Strother CM, Eldevik P, Kikuchi Y, et al. Thrombus formation and structure and the evolution of mass effect in intracranial aneurysms treated by balloon embolization: emphasis on MR findings. *AJNR* 1989;10:787–796.
365. Jellinger K. Vascular malformation of the central nervous system: a morphological overview. *Neurosurg Rev* 1986;9:177–216.
366. Garretson HD. Intracranial arteriovenous malformations. In: Wilkins RH, Rengachary SS, eds. *Neurosurgery*. New York: McGraw–Hill; 1985:1448–1457.
367. Brown RD Jr, Wiebers DO, Forbes GS. Unruptured intracranial aneurysms and arteriovenous malformations: frequency of intracranial hemorrhage and relationship of lesions. *J Neurosurg* 1990;73:859–863.
368. Brown RD Jr, Wiebers DO, Forbes G, et al. The natural history of unruptured intracranial arteriovenous malformations. *J Neurosurg* 1988;68:352–357.
369. Crawford PM, West CR, Chadwick DW, Shaw MDM. Arteriovenous malformations of the brain: natural history in unoperated patients. *J Neurol Neurosurg Psychiatry* 1986;49:1–10.
370. Marks MP, Lane B, Steinberg GK, Chang PJ. Hemorrhage in intracerebral arteriovenous malformations: angiographic determinants. *Radiology* 1990;176:807–813.
371. Ondra SL, Troupp H, George ED, Schwab K. The natural history of symptomatic arteriovenous malformations of the brain: a 24-year follow-up assessment. *J Neurosurg* 1990;73:387–391.
372. Spetzler RF, Martin NA, Carter LP, Flom RA, Raudzens PA, Wilkinson E. Surgical management of large AVMs by staged embolization and operative excision. *J Neurosurg* 1987;67:17–28.
373. Berenstein A, Lasjaunias P. Classification of brain arteriovenous malformations. In: *Surgical Neuroangiography*. Berlin: Springer-Verlag; 1992:1–86.
374. Marks MP, Lane B, Steinberg G, Chang P. Vascular characteristics of intracerebral arteriovenous malformations in patients with clinical steal. *AJNR* 1991;12:489–496.

375. Willinsky R, Lasjaunias P, Terburgge K, et al. Brain arteriovenous malformations: analysis of the angioarchitecture in relationship to hemorrhage. *J Neuroradiol* 1988; 15:225–237.
376. Spetzler RF, Martin NA. A proposed grading system for arteriovenous malformations. *J Neurosurg* 1986;65:476–483.
377. Shi YQ, Chen XC. A proposed scheme for grading intracranial arteriovenous malformations. *J Neurosurg* 1986;65:484–489.
378. Dawson RC III, Tarr RW, Hect ST, et al. Treatment of arteriovenous malformations of the brain with combined embolization and stereotactic radiosurgery: results after one and two years. *AJNR* 1990; 11:857–864.
379. Betti OO, Munari C, Rosler R. Stereotactic radiosurgery with the linear accelerator: treatment of arteriovenous malformations. *Neurosurgery* 1989;24:311–321.
380. Winston KR, Lutz W. Linear accelerator as a neurosurgical tool for stereotactic radiosurgery. *Neurosurgery* 1988;22:454–464.
381. Quisling RG, Peters KR, Friedman WA, Tart RP. Persistent nidus blood flow in cerebral arteriovenous malformation after stereotactic radiosurgery: MR imaging assessment. *Radiology* 1991; 180:785–791.
382. Kauczor HU, Engenhart R, Layer G, et al. 3D TOF MR angiography of cerebral arteriovenous malformations after radiosurgery. *J Comput Assist Tomogr* 1993; 17:184–190.
383. Edelman RR, Wentz KU, Mattle HP, et al. Intracerebral arteriovenous malformations: evaluation with selective MR angiography and venography. *Radiology* 1989; 173:831–837.
384. Ehricke HH, Schad LR, Gademann G, Wowra B, Engenhart R, Lorenz WJ. Use of MR angiography for stereotactic planning. *J Comput Assist Tomogr* 1992; 16:35–40.
385. Mehta MP, Petereit D, Turski P, Gehring M, Levin A, Kinsella T. Magnetic resonance angiography: a three-dimensional database for assessing arteriovenous malformations. *J Neurosurg* 1993;79:289–293.
386. Phillips MH, Kessler M, Chuang FYS, et al. Image correlation of MRI and CT in treatment planning for radiosurgery of intracranial vascular malformations. *Int J Radiat Oncol Biol Phys* 1991;20:881–889.
387. Petereit D, Mehta M, Turski P, et al. Treatment of arteriovenous malformations with stereotactic radiosurgery employing both magnetic resonance angiography and standard angiography as a database. *Int J Radiat Oncol Biol Phys* 1993;25:309–313.
388. Nussel F, Wegmuller H, Huber P. Comparison of magnetic resonance angiography, magnetic resonance imaging and conventional angiography in cerebral arteriovenous malformation. *Neuroradiology* 1991;33:56–61.
389. Awad IA, Robinson JR Jr, Mohanty S, Estes M. Mixed vascular malformations of the brain: clinical and pathogenetic considerations. *Neurosurgery* 1993;33:179–188.
390. Valavanis A, Wellauer J, Yasargil MG. The radiological diagnosis of cerebral venous angioma: cerebral angiography and CT. *Neuroradiology* 1983;24:193–199.
391. Ostertun B, Solymosi L. Magnetic resonance angiography of cerebral developmental venous anomalies: its role in differential diagnosis. *Neuroradiology* 1993;35:97–104.
392. Augustyn GT, Scott JA, Olson E, et al. Cerebral venous angiomas: MR imaging. *Radiology* 1985; 156:391–395.
393. Michels LG, Bentson JR, Winter J. Computed tomography of cerebral venous angiomas. *J Comput Assist Tomogr* 1977; 1:149–154.
394. Sarwar M, McCormick WF. Intracerebral venous angioma: case report and review. *Arch Neurol* 1978;35:323–328.
395. Barnwell SL, Halbach VV, Dowd CF, Higashida RT, Hieshima GB, Wilson CB. Multiple dural arteriovenous fistulas of the cranium and spine. *AJNR* 1991; 12:441–445.
396. Houser WO, Campbell KJ, Campbell JR, Sundt TM. Arteriovenous malformation affecting the transverse dural venous sinus: an acquired lesion. *Mayo Clin Proc* 1979;54:651–661.
397. DeMarco K, Dillon WP, Halbach VV, Tsuruda JS. Dural arteriovenous fistula: evaluation with MR imaging. *Radiology* 1990; 175: 193–199.
398. Halbach VV, Higashida RT, Hieshima GB, Reicher M, Norman D, Newton TH. Dural fistulas involving the cavernous sinus: results of treatment in 30 patients. *Radiology* 1987;63:437–442.
399. Halbach VV, Higashida RT, Hieshima GB, Goto K, Norman D, Newton TH. Dural fistulas involving the transverse and sigmoid sinuses: results in 28 patients. *Radiology* 1987; 163:443–447.
400. Awad IA, Little JR, Akrawi WP, et al. Intracranial dural arteriovenous malformations: factors predisposing to an aggressive course. *J Neurosurg* 1990;72:839–850.
401. Chen JC, Tsuruda JS, Halbach VV. Suspected dural arteriovenous fistula: results with screening MR angiography in seven patients. *Radiology* 1992; 183:265–271.
402. Haacke EM, Lin W, Amartur S, Lindskog E, Masaryk TJ. Half-Fourier imaging in MR angiography. Presented at the *75th Annual RSNA Meeting,* 1989.
403. Enzmann DR, Ross MR, Marks MP, Pelk NJ. Blood flow in major cerebral arteries measured by phase-contrast cine MR. *AJNR* 1994; 15:123–129.

Magnetic Resonance Imaging of the Brain and Spine, Second Edition, edited by Scott W. Atlas. Lippincott-Raven Publishers, Philadelphia © 1996.

32

MR Spectroscopy and the Biochemical Basis of Neurological Disease

Robert E. Lenkinski and Mitchell D. Schnall

Magnetic resonance spectroscopy (MRS) provides a noninvasive, potentially risk-free method with which to monitor the biochemistry of acute and chronic stages of disease. The recent development of spatial localization methods which sample the relative levels of mobile metabolites from a volume of tissue defined from an MR image has provided a basis for integrating the biochemical information obtained by MRS with the anatomical and pathological information obtained from MRI. This combination of metabolic and anatomic information affords a new means of understanding the origins and the time course of progression in a variety of diseases.

The first discoveries of the principles of nuclear magnetic resonance (NMR) were made by Bloch and Purcell (1,2) more than 40 years ago. In 1950, Proctor (3) made the observation that the precise resonance frequency of a nucleus depended on the nature of its chemical environment leading to the definition of this phenomenon as the "chemical shift." As instrumentation has developed, NMR has become an increasingly important tool for the study of chemical structure, intra- and intermolecular exchange, and chemical dynamics. Initially, proton (^{1}H) spectra were used exclusively, although any nucleus which possesses a nuclear spin can give rise to an NMR signal. Protons were chosen initially because of their high isotopic abundance, high relative receptivity, and their relevance to organic structure determination. As more sensitive and more flexible NMR instruments became commercially available, techniques for the detection of nuclei other than ^{1}H were developed. The initial biological NMR studies focused on ^{1}H as well. In most of these studies, NMR was used to investigate aspects of cellular processes in isolation or the influences of different processes on the resonance of water in intact cells. In 1959, Odeblad reported on ^{1}H NMR studies of the chemical shift and relaxation times of water in human vaginal epithelial cells (4). As was the case in chemical applications, protons were chosen initially because of their high isoto-

R. E. Lenkinski, Ph.D., and M. D. Schnall, M.D., Ph.D.: Department of Radiology, University of Pennsylvania, Philadelphia, PA 19104.

pic abundance and high relative receptivity. Although these characteristics make detection of the NMR signal relatively easy, the complexity of the mixtures of biomolecules in intact living systems as well as the high relative concentration of water present make the proton spectra complex and therefore difficult to interpret. Phosphorus-31 is a useful nucleus for biological investigations because it is present as 100% of the naturally occurring phosphorus and is present in only a few biological molecules. Moreover, many of these phosphorus-containing compounds are involved in the processes which either produce or consume energy for the cell. Because of the large range of chemical shifts present in the different phosphorus-containing species, the ^{31}P spectra obtained from intact biological systems are relatively simple and easy to interpret. For these reasons, ^{31}P NMR spectroscopy has been widely used to study cellular metabolism, to probe the metabolic state of a variety of tissues, and to investigate the biochemical basis for diseases (5–7). The in vivo ^{31}P spectrum of a tissue generally exhibits seven distinct resonances: phosphomonoesters (PME); inorganic phosphate (Pi); phosphodiesters (PDE); phosphocreatine (PCr); and the alpha, beta, and gamma phosphorus atoms of ATP. A typical ^{31}P spectrum obtained from the brain of a normal volunteer on a 1.5T GE Signa MR scanner is shown in Fig. 1. Note that the resolution is sufficient to resolve all seven peaks. Various groups have

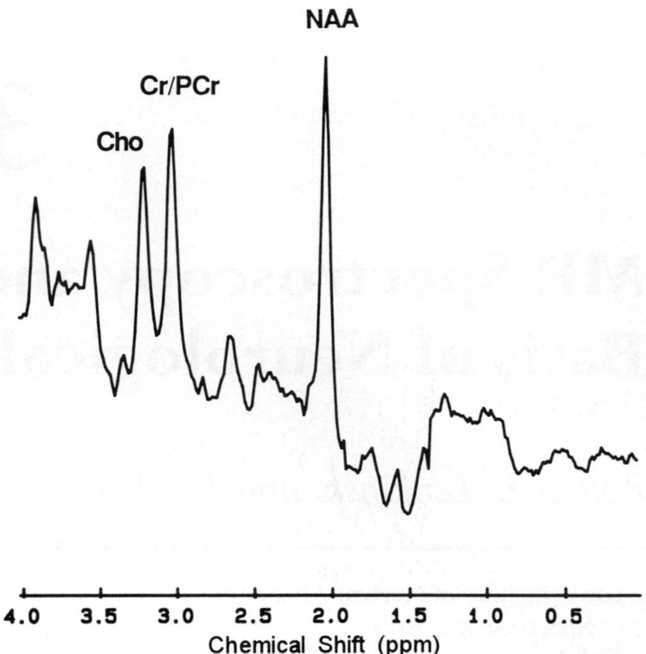

FIG. 2. A localized ^{1}H spectrum of the brain of a normal volunteer. This spectrum was obtained using the STEAM method of localization (see refs. 10 and 32) from an isotropic voxel of 2-cm linear dimension. The acquisition parameters were: 1000 Hz-sweepwidth, 2048 data points, 19-msec echo time, 8.6-msec mixing time, 2-sec repetition time, and 256 averages. The spectrum was processed with 1-Hz exponential linebroadening. No baseline correction algorithm was employed.

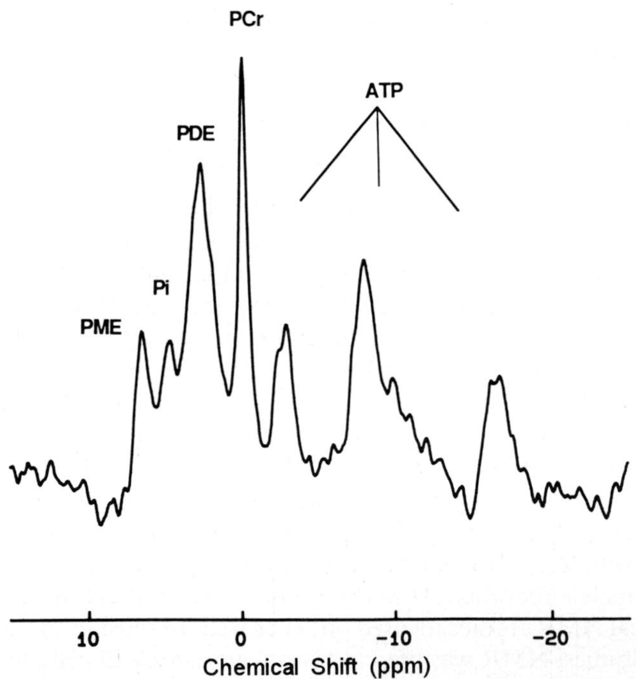

FIG. 1. A localized ^{31}P spectrum of the brain of a normal volunteer. This spectrum was obtained from a 3-cm-thick slice using the DRESS method of localization (see ref. 28) on a GE 1.5 T Signa whole body scanner. The acquisition parameters were: 2000-Hz sweepwidth, 2048 data points, 2.1-msec preacquisition delay, 4-sec repetition time, and 128 averages. The spectrum was processed with 10-Hz exponential linebroadening.

shown that, in some tissues, the intracellular pH can be determined from the separation in frequency between the Pi and PCr peaks (8,9). This separation in frequency is dependent on the pH of the solution because the Pi resonance is a population average of the various ionized species present in solution which are in rapid chemical exchange. This point will be discussed in detail in the section dealing with chemical exchange.

The application of proton MRS to the study of living tissue has in the past been hindered by the technical problems posed by the presence of 110 molar concentration of the protons of water as a background signal. The relative size of this signal can now be reduced substantially by a variety of solvent suppression schemes ranging from nonexcitation, such as 1-3-3-1 sequences, to straightforward presaturation of the water resonance (10–12). A large number of proton-containing metabolites (e.g., lactate, creatine, phosphocreatine, *N*-acetylaspartate, glutamate, and others) can be detected when these methods are employed. In addition, there have been a number of spectral editing pulse sequences reported which produce proton spectra in which only the lactate resonance is selectively inverted or detected (13). These techniques have been developed by Shulman and his group as well as in several other laboratories. A typical solvent suppressed proton spectrum obtained from the brain of a normal volunteer is shown in Fig. 2. The proton and phosphorus spectra contain different information concerning the metabolic state of the tissue being sampled. We believe that the acquisition of the spatially localized metabolic information available from either a proton, a phosphorus, or from both spectra can be correlated with the information available from MRI and other imaging methods. These correlations may lead to the development of a set of physiological, anatomical, and biochemical indices which will provide a powerful approach for investigating the underlying basis for many clinical disorders.

In this chapter, our goal is to provide the reader with an understanding of the basic principles of MRS, to review critically the spatial localization methods currently available, and to provide the basis for achieving an insight into the metabolic interpretation of spectral data. We also discuss several examples of clinical applications of magnetic resonance spectroscopy. Our emphasis in discussing the above topics is to highlight the real and potential clinical applications of the spectroscopy to the CNS.

BASIC PRINCIPLES OF NUCLEAR MAGNETIC RESONANCE SPECTROSCOPY

The ability of NMR spectroscopy to provide structural information about molecules has led to its development into perhaps the most important tool for the structure determination of organic compounds in solution. Before the development of Fourier transform methods NMR spectra were collected in the frequency domain employing methods in which the static magnetic field (B_0) of the instrument was systematically varied and an NMR absorption line was recorded. These methods are referred to as continuous wave or CW methods. The general lineshape obtained using these techniques was found to fit a lorenzian function which is the Fourier transform of a single decaying exponential function in the time domain.

Relationship Between the Free Induction Decay (FID) and the Spectrum

The behavior of the magnetization of an ensemble of nuclei detected on resonance is illustrated in Figure 3. After a 90° pulse applied along the y axis the magnetization is rotated along the x axis (Fig. 3A and B). In the rotating frame of reference we can place the detector along the x axis as well. As the magnetization returns to equilibrium its component along the x axis decreases (Fig. 3C–E) until the magnetization has returned to its initial state (Fig. 3F). The instantaneous voltage in the receiver coil at any point in time is plotted below. This variation in voltage with time is the free induction decay (FID) of the NMR signal on resonance. The Fourier transform of this FID is a single line NMR spectrum, shown in Fig. 4.

The three characteristic parameters which define this line are given in this figure. The width at half-height is related to the transverse relaxation time, T2, as follows,

$$\Delta\omega_{1/2} = 1/(\pi T2) \qquad [1]$$

where $\Delta\omega_{1/2}$ is the width at half-height of the resonance in Hz. The area under this peak can be obtained from the amplitude and linewidth directly.

The relationship between the linewidth and the T2 of the nucleus is valid only for ideal magnets where there are no contributions to the linewidths from inhomogeneities in the static magnetic field. The effects of the presence of inhomogeneity in the magnetic field increases the

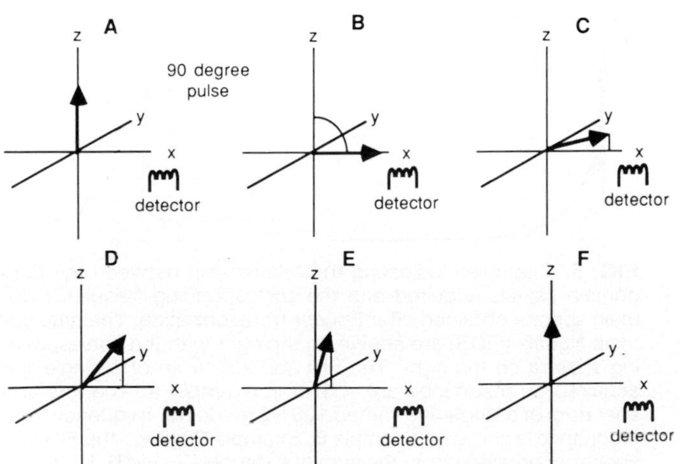

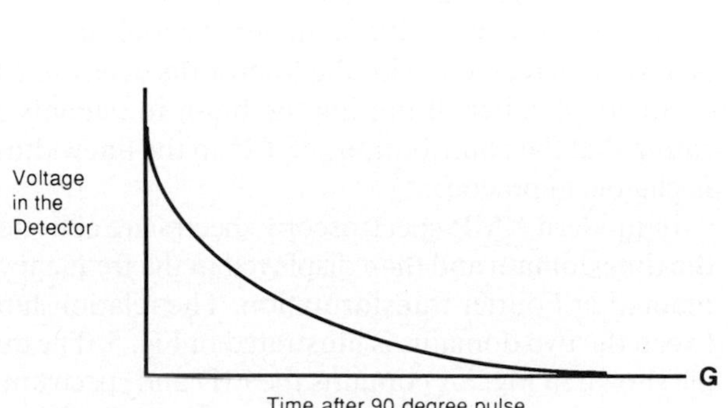

FIG. 3. A–F: A diagram of the time-dependent evolution of magnetization after a 90° rf pulse is applied along the y axis. In this diagram the receiver coil is indicated on the x axis. The magnetization after successive delays is shown in diagrams B–F. **G:** Graph showing the voltage detected in the receiver coil as a function of the delay after the 90° pulse.

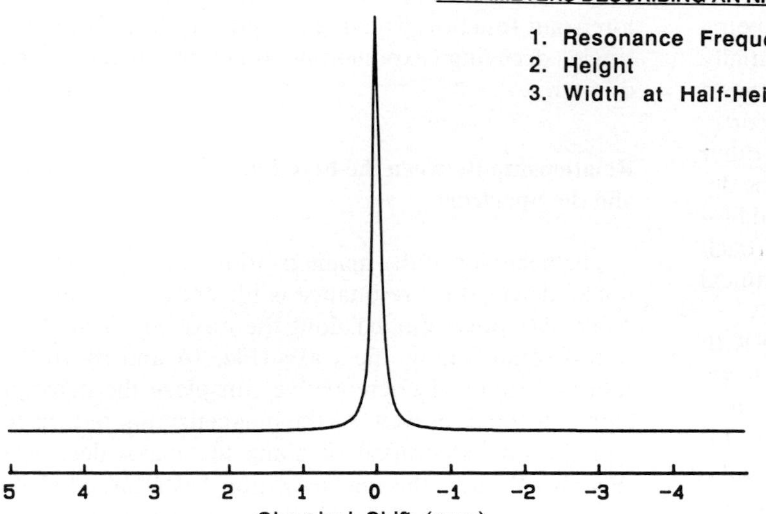

FIG. 4. The Fourier transform of the bottom graph shown in Fig. 3, which results in a lorenzian line in the frequency domain. Note that this line occurs at 0 Hz since the FID shown in Fig. 3 was obtained on resonance (see Fig. 5 for further explanation of this point). The three characteristic parameters defining this line are indicated on the figure.

linewidth beyond the natural linewidth ($1/\pi T2$). Mathematically this effect is described by the replacement of the T2 term with T2* in Equation 1. The relationship between T2 and T2* is given by,

$$1/\pi T2^* = 1/\pi T2 + 1/\pi T2\ (\text{extrinsic}) \qquad [2]$$

where $1/\pi T2^*$ is the observed linewidth in Hz, $1/\pi T2$ is the natural linewidth and $1/\pi T2$ (extrinsic) is the contribution to the linewidth arising from instrumental imperfections such as magnetic field inhomogeneities. In spectroscopy it is important to minimize the contributions of $1/\pi T2$ (extrinsic) to the linewidth, and thus make $1/\pi T2^*$ as close to $1/\pi T2$ as possible. This is usually accomplished by adjusting the homogeneity of the magnetic field over the region of interest using the linewidth of the proton resonance of water in the tissue to assess the homogeneity of the magnetic field. This procedure is known as shimming the field. As an example of the linewidths of water that can be obtained from brain tissue after shimming, consider that the T2 of water in brain tissue is about 70 msec. From Equation 1 this T2 corresponds to a width at half-height of about 4.5 Hz for the water resonance in brain. In our experience this value is in good agreement with the linewidths determined experimentally after shimming the brain in patients indicating that the contributions of T2* to the linewidths are negligible in practice.

In modern NMR spectroscopy spectra are collected in the time domain and then displayed in the frequency domain after Fourier transformation. The relationship between the two domains is illustrated in Fig. 5. The example shown in Fig. 5A contains the FID and spectrum of a single peak detected on resonance. Figure 5B shows the FID and spectrum of a peak detected 100 Hz off resonance (in this case to lower frequency). Note that the FID appears like a damped sinusoidal wave with a frequency of 100 Hz. The FID and spectrum obtained from the

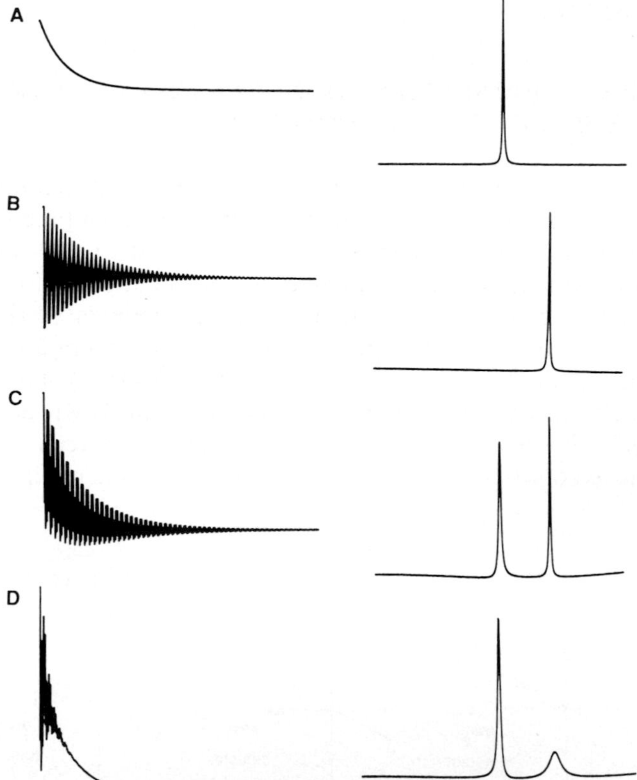

FIG. 5. Examples indicating the relationship between the time domain signals acquired and the corresponding frequency domain spectra obtained after Fourier transformation. The time domain signals (FIDS) are shown on the right with the corresponding spectra on the right. The FID and spectrum of a single line acquired on resonance are shown in example **A**. The FID and spectrum of a single line shifted 100 Hz to a lower frequency from resonance is shown in example **B**. Example **C** shows the FID and spectrum obtained from the sum of examples A and B. Note that the linewidths of the two resonances are approximately equal in this example. Example **D** illustrates the situation where the line shifted 100 Hz to a lower frequency has a shorter T2 (broader line in the spectrum) than the line on resonance. Note that the first part of the FID is similar to the one shown in example D while the later part of the FID resembles the FID shown in example A.

sum of Fig. 5A and B are shown in Fig. 5C. The effects of decreasing the T2 of the peak 100 Hz off resonance is shown in Fig. 5D. Note that the beginning of this FID appears similar to the FID shown in Fig. 5C. However, since the signal arising from the peak at 100 Hz off resonance decays more quickly, the later parts of the FID appear similar to the FID shown in Fig. 5A. The spectrum shown in Fig. 5D contains a sharp peak on resonance and a broader peak 100 Hz off resonance.

Chemical Shift

From MR imaging we are familiar with the use of external switched B_0 gradients to achieve spatial encoding. These gradients are applied at a maximum strength of around 1 gauss/cm on most commercial scanners. In the absence of these external gradients the NMR experiment is sensitive to intramolecular gradients which are caused by the distribution of the bonding electrons around the nuclei being detected. As an example we can examine the proton NMR spectrum of methanol in the presence of a small amount of water which is shown in Fig. 6. This compound which contains hydrogen atoms in two different chemical environments gives rise to two distinct NMR resonances. The ratio of the areas under the two peaks is 3:1 consistent with the fact that there are three protons in the CH_3 (methyl) group and one proton in the OH (hydroxyl) group. Also the fact that the OH resonance occurs at higher frequency than the methyl resonance can be explained as follows. The electrons associated with the carbon-hydrogen bonds in the methyl group shield the methyl hydrogens from the applied magnetic field, B_0. Thus, the field experienced by these hydrogens is slightly less than the applied field. The electronegative element oxygen causes a relative deshielding of the OH hydrogen by concentrating more of the bonding electrons around its nucleus. For this reason, the OH hydrogen experiences a net higher magnetic field than the methyl hydrogens. Although the precise magnetogyric ratios of all of these hydrogens are different it is convenient to express the differences in their Larmor frequencies with reference to a standard kind of hydrogen with a magnetogyric ratio of γS. The differences in resonant frequencies of the different hydrogens can be expressed in terms of a screening parameter, σ. These effects are summarized in the following three equations.

$$\omega_{CH_3} = \gamma_{CH_3} \cdot B_0 \quad [3]$$

$$\omega_{OH} = \gamma_{OH} \cdot B_0 \quad [4]$$

and

$$\omega_S = \gamma_S \cdot B_0(1 - \sigma) \quad [5]$$

where ωCH_3, ω_{OH}, and ω_S refer to the Larmor frequencies of the CH_3, OH, and the reference hydrogen, S, respectively. The symbols ω_{CH3}, ω_{OH}, and ω_S are the magnetogyric ratios of the methyl, hydroxyl, and reference hydrogens, respectively. The values of the screening parameters for hydrogen in different environments lie in the parts per million range of the applied magnetic field, B_0. We know from imaging that there are differences in the Larmor frequencies of fat and water. These differences are about 215 Hz at 1.5 T. These differences are expressed in terms of a dimensionless, field-independent parameter δ, given by

$$\delta_{compound} = [(\omega_{compound} - \omega_S)/(\omega_S)] \cdot 10^6 \quad [6]$$

where the ω refers to the Larmor frequency. The units of δ are given in ppm which is an abbreviation for parts per million of the applied field. This parameter is independent of the field since the distribution of the bonding electrons within a given molecule is a property of that molecule rather than the external applied field. Water resonates at 4.7 ppm and fat resonates at about 1.3 ppm on this scale. The value of δ can be characteristic of the chemical environment of the nucleus being studied. Chemists have used the chemical shift information in combination with other NMR parameters to deduce the structure of unknown compounds.

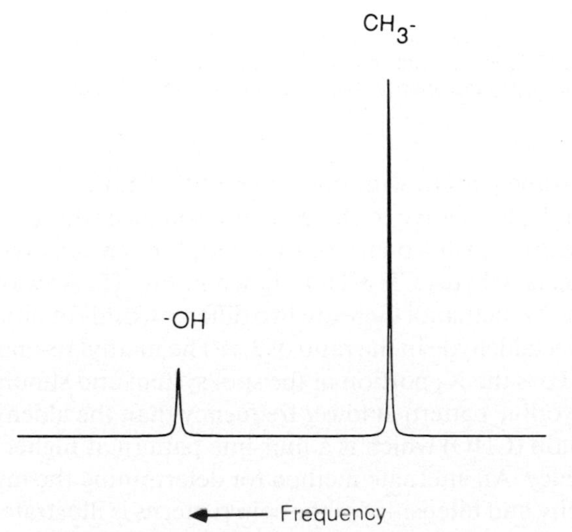

FIG. 6. A representation of the proton spectrum of methanol (CH_3OH) in the presence of a small amount of water. The area under the CH_3 resonance is three times the area under the OH resonance. Although methanol is an AX_3 spin system like acetaldehyde which is shown in Fig. 10, chemical exchange between the water and OH proton bring about collapse of the multiplet structures. This point is discussed in the text.

Spin–Spin Coupling

Another important parameter arising from interactions with the bonding electrons is the spin-spin or J coupling. An explanation for this coupling interaction was first proposed by Ramsey and Purcell in 1952 (14). There are two key features of this explanation. The first is that bonding pairs of electrons in the same molecular orbital must have antiparallel spins. This is referred to as the Pauli exclusion principle. The second point is that spins tend to align themselves in an antiparallel arrangement.

The results of these two interactions are illustrated by the example shown in Figs. 7 and 8 of two nuclear spins (normal arrows in Fig. 7) with different chemical shifts (A and X) in the presence of two bonding electrons (bold arrows in Fig. 7). The energy levels of this two-spin system in the absence of any interactions with the electrons would be:

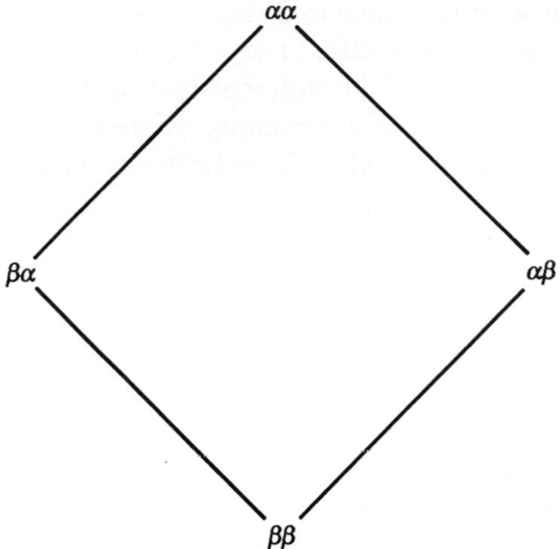

with the energies of the $\beta\alpha$ and $\alpha\beta$ states equivalent. In conventional NMR only transitions between states in which a single nucleus changes its spin are allowed. The transitions are shown in Fig. 8 and indicate that the two allowed transitions for each nucleus are equivalent. Thus, we should expect to see two resonances one at the chemical shift of the A spin and the other at the chemical shift of the X spin. The influences of the electron spins can be explained with reference to Fig. 7. In the state shown in Fig. 7C both pairs of electron nuclear spins are antiparallel while in Fig. 7B both pairs are parallel. Thus, the state illustrated in Fig. 7C should be shifted to lower energy from the case where the interactions with electronic spins were ignored and the state shown in Fig. 7B should be shifted to higher energy. The energy level diagram for this case is shown in Fig. 8. The interactions with the electrons leads to a splitting of the two resonances, so that each resonance now appears as a doublet centered at the chemical shift of the A and X resonances, respectively. The intensity of each peak in the doublet is 0.5 relative to that of the case with no coupling. The frequency separation of the doublet is referred to as J_{AX}, the spin-spin coupling constant. The magnitude of J_{AX} is independent of the applied field.

This example can be extended to AX_2 and AX_3 systems. These are illustrated in Fig. 9. In the AX_2 case the AX doublet is split again by the presence of the extra X spin. Since the magnitude of J is the same, the two central portions of the doublets overlap giving rise to a three-line pattern with intensities of 0.25, 0.5, and 0.25 relative to the unsplit case (this pattern is referred to as a triplet). The AX_3 case adds an additional splitting resulting in a four-line pattern with intensities of 0.125, 0.375, 0.375, and 0.125 relative to the unsplit resonance (this pattern is referred to as a quartet). An example of an AX_3 system is acetaldehyde, CH_3CHO, shown in Fig. 10. As was the case for methanol there are two different kinds of protons in acetaldehyde in the ratio of 3:1. The methyl resonance (CH_3) is the X_3 portion of the spin system and should be a two-line pattern at lower frequency than the aldehydic proton (CHO) which is a four-line pattern at higher frequency. An alternate method for determining the multiplicity and intensities of the spin patterns is illustrated in Fig. 10. The various combinations of spin states possible for each adjacent group are drawn below the methyl and aldehydic resonances, respectively. The aldehydic proton is split into four slightly different frequencies which depend on the orientations of the spins of the three

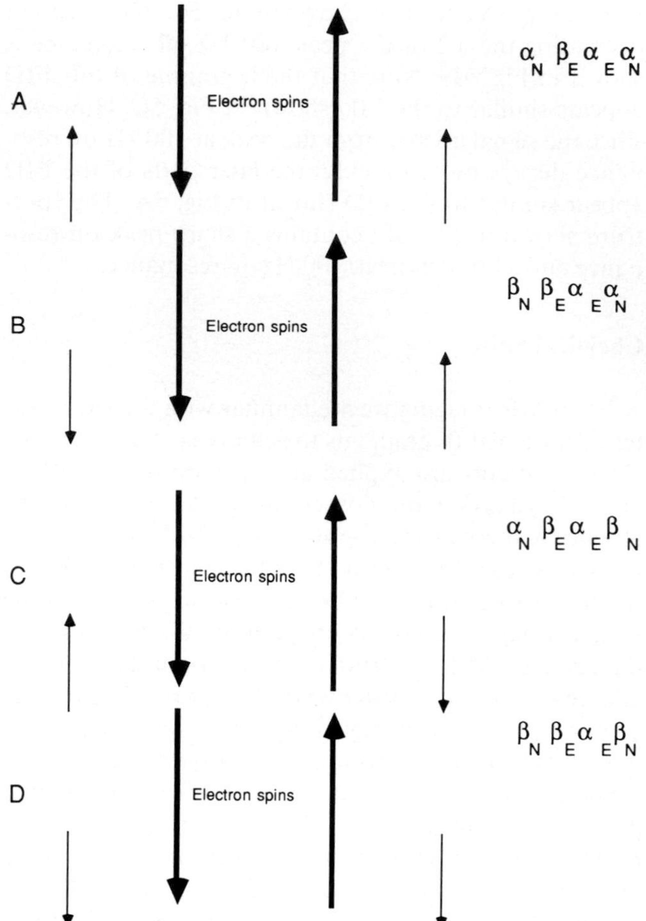

FIG. 7. A diagram illustrating the origins of electron-coupled nuclear spin-spin interactions. The electron spins are shown with *bold arrows* and are referred to by the subscript *E*. The nuclear spins are shown in regular arrows and referred to by the subscript *N*. The electron spins involved in bonding must always have an antiparallel orientation as indicated. Although the nuclear spin orientations shown in states *B* and *C* are identical, the nuclear spins are in an antiparallel orientation with respect to the electron spins in *C* and a parallel orientation in *B*. For this reason the energy of state *C* is lower than the energy of state *B*. This difference is illustrated in the energy level diagram shown in Fig. 8.

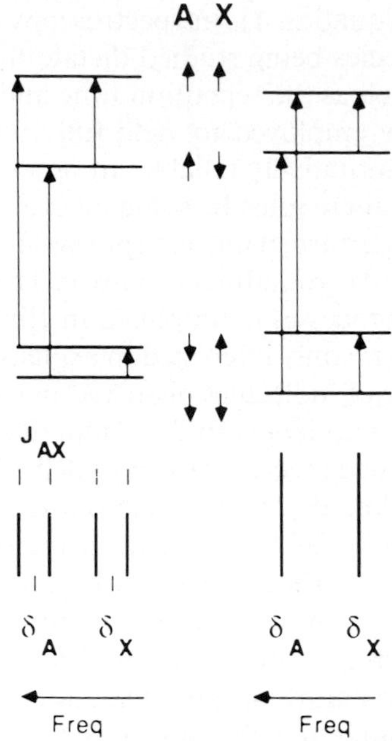

FIG. 8. The energy level diagram for an AX spin system in the absence of coupling (diagram on the right) and in the presence of spin-spin interactions (diagram on the left). The presence of coupling causes the two resonances to be split into doublets as illustrated by the simulated spectra shown below each diagram. The doublets are centered on the frequency for the A and the X spin with a splitting of J^{AX}, the value of the spin-spin coupling constant.

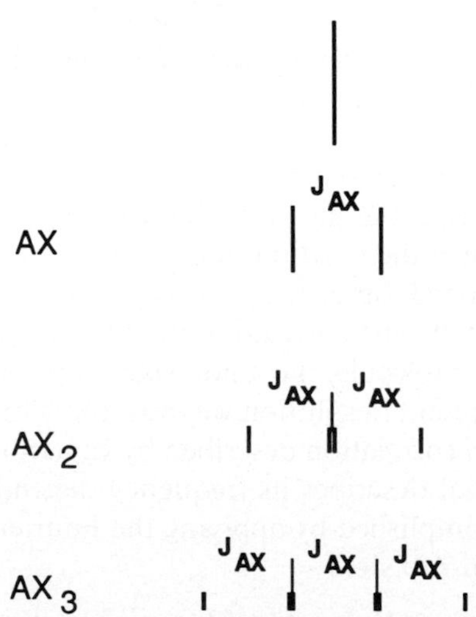

FIG. 9. A diagram illustrating the patterns observed in the A spin of AX, AX_2, and AX_3 spin systems. In the AX_2 case the presence of an additional spin-spin interaction splits the doublet into two doublets which overlap at the center of the multiplet. Note that the center line of this multiplet resonates at the frequency of the A resonance, d_A. This multiplet is a three-line pattern with intensity ratios of 1:2:1. Similarly in the AX_3 case, the presence of an additional spin-spin interaction splits each of the three lines of the AX_2 multiplet into a doublet resulting in a four-line multiplet with intensity ratios of 1:3:3:1.

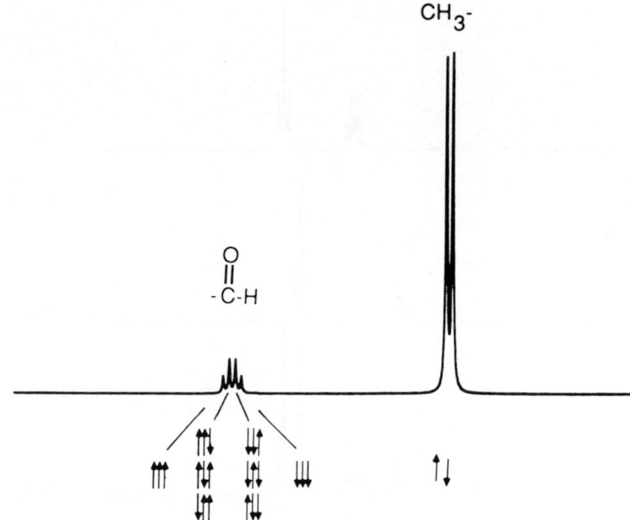

FIG. 10. A representation of the proton spectrum of acetaldehyde (CH_3CHO) which is an AX_3 spin system. The influence of the orientations of the adjacent spins is illustrated below each multiplet.

methyl protons (three up; two up and one down; two down and one up; and three down). Since there are three different ways that each of the second and third orientations can occur and only one way that the first and fourth orientations can occur, the intensities should be in the ratio of 1:3:3:1. There are only two orientations possible for the aldehydic proton, up or down with equal probability. On this basis, the methyl resonance should be split into a doublet with the relative intensity ratio of 1:1. Combining the fact that the methyl group contains three protons and the aldehydic group only one proton we can calculate the overall intensity ratios as 1.5 units for each line of the methyl doublet and 0.125, 0.375, 0.375, and 0.125 for the aldehydic quartet.

Analysis of Mixtures

An example of how NMR spectroscopy can be used to provide both qualitative and quantitative information on mixtures of compounds is shown in Fig. 11. The spectrum shown in Fig. 11C is the sum of the spectra shown in Fig. 11A and B. The chemical shift and coupling information can be used to identify the components present. The relative areas under the peaks provides an estimate of the relative concentrations of the various compounds present. The spectrum in Fig. 11A contains three different resonances: a broad resonance with relative area of one unit, a quartet with relative area of two units, and a triplet with relative area of three units. Since the triplet has an area of three units it can be identified as a CH_3 group adjacent to a CH_2 group. Similarly since the quartet has a relative intensity of two units it can be identified as a CH_2 group adjacent to a CH_3 group. The

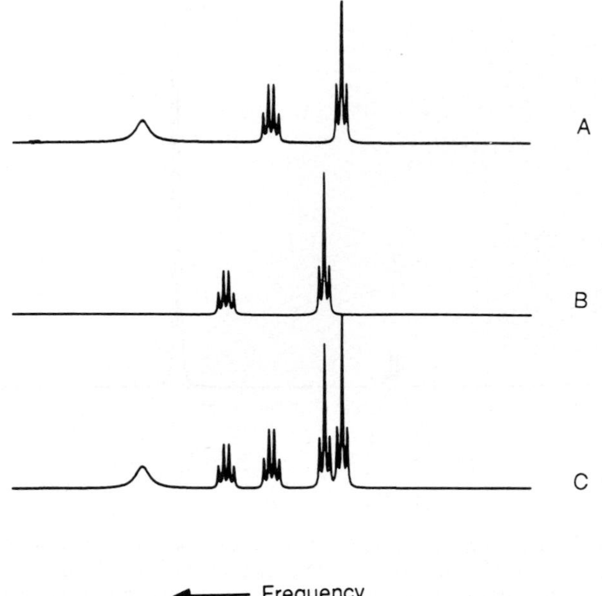

FIG. 11. An example of the analysis of mixtures by NMR spectroscopy. The spectrum shown in **A** is of ethanol. The spectrum shown in **B** is of ethylchloride. The spectrum shown in **C** is the sum of A and B.

third resonance corresponds to an OH group that is broadened due to chemical exchange with trace amounts of water present. The effects of exchange are discussed more fully in a following section. Based on these assignments we can identify the compound whose spectrum is shown in Fig. 11A as CH_3CH_2OH, or ethanol. In fact we can make the general assignment of the combination of a triplet with a quartet having the relative areas of 3:2, respectively, as a CH_3CH_2 or ethyl group. Using this assignment we can identify the compound in Figure 11B as CH_3CH_2X, where X is a substituent that contains no additional hydrogens. In fact the spectrum shown in Fig. 11B was obtained from CH_3CH_2Cl. Thus, the two compounds present can be identified as ethanol and ethylchloride. The relative areas under the triplet peaks at lower frequency indicate that there is more ethanol than ethylchloride present in this mixture.

Relaxation

In Fig. 3, we showed the behavior of the magnetization after a 90° rf pulse. From MR imaging we know that this magnetization relaxes to its equilibrium state with two characteristic time constants, T1, the spin-lattice or longitudinal relaxation time, and T2, the spin-spin or transverse relaxation time. MR imaging protocols exploit differences in the values of these relaxation times in different tissues to generate images with a high degree of contrast. In spectroscopy, we have already shown that the value of T2 is inversely related to the linewidth of the nucleus (see Equation 1). In spectroscopy the values of T1 for the species being studied dictate the acquisition parameters such as the repetition time and/or flip angle that should be employed to yield fully relaxed spectra which are quantitatively reliable. In order for T1 relaxation to occur there must be some mechanism by which the excited or perturbed nuclear spin system can transfer its energy to its surroundings or lattice. The explanation of relaxation processes is simplified in clinical spectroscopy since we are only interested in explaining the relaxation behavior of molecules dissolved in solution where these molecules undergo rapid random motion. This situation was treated theoretically in 1948 by Bloembergen, Purcell, and Pound (15) who showed that the fluctuations in magnetic fields arising from the rapid random motion of these molecules was one of the two key ingredients in the relaxation process. The timescale of these fluctuations was described in terms of a correlation time, τ_c. The precise nature of the interaction of the nucleus with its environment, referred to as the relaxation mechanism, is the second ingredient which describes the relaxation process.

The concept of a correlation time is important in MR and can be defined as the length of time a molecule can exist in a given position before its motion is changed by a collision. For relatively low molecular weight compounds in aqueous solution, this time is between 10^{-11} and 10^{-12} seconds. For larger molecules such as proteins, phospholipids, polysaccharides, and DNA this time is much longer. This concept can be described mathematically by the following equation:

$$k(\tau) = k(0)e^{-\tau/\tau_c} \quad [7]$$

where $k(\tau)$ is a correlation function which describes the position of the molecule at time τ with respect to its initial position $k(0)$ at zero τ. These two positions are related in an exponential manner. In fact the degree of correlation decays like an FID with a time constant of τ_c. After a long τ, the positions are different and are said to be uncorrelated. Since the motion of molecules in solution is random, the correlation time is an average property of the molecule. To understand the range of frequencies present in solution we must transform the time variation of correlation described by Equation 7 into an equation that describes its frequency dependence. This can be accomplished by applying the Fourier transform to Equation 7 to yield

$$J(\omega) = A[\tau_c/(1 + \omega^2\tau_c^2)] \quad [8]$$

where $J(\omega)$ is the function that describes the range of frequencies associated with τ_c, often referred to as the spectral density function, and A is a constant. From this equation it is clear that $J(\omega)$ is maximum when $\tau_c = 1/\omega$. That is, the best match between the spectral density function and τ_c occurs when $1/\tau_c$ is the Larmor frequency. Intuitively from this discussion it is clear that the most efficient T1 relaxation will occur when the frequency of molecular motion matches the Larmor frequency. A frequency of molecular motion either higher or lower than the Larmor frequency leads to less efficient relaxation.

Classically the situation where $\omega \tau_c \ll$ is called the extreme narrowing limit. When this limit is satisfied Equation 8 becomes

$$J(\omega) = A\tau_c \quad [9]$$

and $J(\omega)$ is a linear function of the correlation time. When the condition that $\omega \tau_c \gg 1$ is satisfied Equation 8 becomes

$$J(\omega) = A/\omega^2\tau_c \quad [10]$$

and $J(\omega)$ has an inverse dependence on the correlation time and also varies as the inverse of the square of the field. From Equation 9 it is clear that there should be no field dependence on the T1 in the extreme narrowing limit. Outside the extreme narrowing limit, however, the spectral density function should decrease as the inverse square of the field. Since the value of 1/T1 is proportional to the spectral density function, the value of T1 should increase as the square of the field outside of the extreme narrowing limit. This discussion has relevance toward understanding the dependence of T1 on the magnetic field employed in MRI where we are imaging primarily the water molecules in the tissue which have a fixed average τ_c.

The variation of T2 with correlation time is different from that of T1. In the extreme narrowing limit where τ_c is short T2 behaves like T1. However, outside of the extreme narrowing limit where τ_c is long, the low-frequency motions are effective in reducing T2. Thus, T2 decreases with τ_c, reaching its limiting value when the motions in solution are frozen and the solution becomes a solid.

A number of different relaxation mechanisms have been identified. These are

1. Dipole-dipole interactions (both heteronuclear and homonuclear)
2. Chemical shift anisotropy
3. Quadripolar relaxation
4. Spin-rotation
5. Scalar coupling
6. Paramagnetic relaxation.

We discuss the first two since they are the most relevant to clinical studies involving proton and ^{31}P MR spectroscopy.

Dipole–Dipole Interactions

Nuclei that are MR active produce an instantaneous magnetic field proportional to the magnetic moment of the nucleus. As the molecule containing these nuclei rotates randomly in solution, the fields produced by these nuclei oscillate. If the frequency of oscillation (which is the inverse of the correlation time for molecular rotation) is at, or near, the Larmor frequency then the nucleus being excited can experience efficient relaxation. The magnitude of the interaction which depends on both the magnetic moment of the nucleus and the distance between the interacting nuclei are also important in this mechanism. The static magnetic field produced by a nucleus j at another nucleus i is given by

$$H_{\text{local}} = \pm(\mu/r_{ij}^3)/(3\cos^2\theta_{ij} - 1) \quad [11]$$

where μ is the magnetic moment, r_{ij} is the magnitude of the vector joining the two nuclei, and θ_{ij} is the angle between this vector and the applied magnetic field. The value of this local field is about 14 Gauss for protons that are about 1 Å apart. If molecular rotation is rapid (i.e., τ_c is small) then the value of $\cos^2\theta_{ij}$ is averaged over all possible angles and the value of the local field becomes zero ($\langle\cos^2\theta_{ij}\rangle$avg $= \frac{1}{3}$). This means that there are no direct manifestations of the dipole-dipole interaction such as a shifting of the resonances in solution. However, this interaction leads to a shortening of the relaxation times. Conceptually this can be understood by considering that there can be fluctuations in the local magnetic field produced that have large amplitudes even if the average value of this interaction is zero.

The detailed treatment of this mechanism (16) shows that in the extreme narrowing limit

$$1/T1 = 1/T2 = (4\gamma_i^2\gamma_j^2 h^2 S(S+1)\tau_c)/(12\pi^2 r_{ij}^6) \quad [12]$$

where γ_i and γ_j are the magnetogyric ratios of the i and j nuclei, h is Planck's constant, S is the nuclear spin, and r_{ij} is the internuclear distance between i and j. If the two nuclei are within the same molecule (intramolecular dipole-dipole interaction) as in water then τ_c is the correlation time for molecular reorientation. If the nuclei are in different molecules (intermolecular dipole-dipole interaction), τ_c is the translational correlation time. This mechanism is important for nuclei such as protons that possess large magnetic moments. Also nuclei with smaller magnetic moments that are in molecules containing protons are relaxed efficiently through the intramolecular heteronuclear dipole-dipole interaction.

Chemical Shift Anisotropy

In Equation 5 we introduced the concept of a screening parameter, σ, in order to explain the chemical shift. The use of a single number to define the screening parameter in Equation 5 is only valid if there is rapid molecular rotation in solution leading to an averaged value of σ. This can be readily understood by remembering that σ reflects the distribution of bonding electrons around the nucleus and that at the molecular level this distribution of electrons may not be spherically symmetric. In the absence of symmetry the value of σ is said to be anisotropic and is mathematically defined as a tensor quantity which defines the values of σ along three perpendicular axes. If the signs and/or magnitudes of these three values are different then as the molecule tumbles rapidly in solution the nucleus will experience a fluctuating effective local magnetic field. If the rate of tumbling is at, or near, the Larmor frequency efficient T1 relaxation will occur. If σ is axially symmetric, that is the distribution of electrons possesses a symmetry axis, then in the extreme narrowing limit,

$$1/T1 = (2/15)\gamma^2 B_0^2(\sigma^{par} - \sigma^{perp})^2\tau_c \qquad [13]$$

where B_0 is the strength of the magnetic field, σ^{par} and σ^{perp} are the values of the shielding tensor parallel and perpendicular to the axis of symmetry. A similar relationship can be derived for T2. Equation 12 predicts that the relaxation time for a nucleus will decrease as the square of the field if the chemical shift anisotropy is the dominant relaxation mechanism. Chemical shift anisotropy may be an important relaxation mechanism in ^{31}P for some of the species being detected.

Chemical Exchange

One of the major applications of NMR has been to study the dynamics of molecules in solution (17). In organic chemistry these dynamics can be conformational interconversion such as the classic case of cyclohexane which undergoes conversion from the "boat" to the "chair" form of the cyclohexyl ring in solution. This is an example of an intramolecular exchange process. Consider the case of methanol in the presence of a small amount of water shown in Fig. 6. There is a rapid exchange between the hydroxyl proton of methanol and the protons of water,

$$CH_3O{-}H^* \leftrightarrow H{-}O{-}H. \qquad [14]$$

If the exchange is rapid on the NMR timescale an averaging of the NMR properties of the two environments occurs. In this case the chemical shift observed will be the population average chemical shift given by

$$\delta_{obs} = P_A\delta_A + P_B\delta_B \qquad [15]$$

where P_A and P_B are the fractional populations of the two sites A and B ($P_A + P_B = 1$) and δ_A and δ_B are the chemical shifts in the two sites.

pH Measurements Based on ^{31}P Spectra

As was pointed out in the introduction there have been several reports which have described a relationship between the frequency separation of the ^{31}P resonances of PCr and Pi and the pH of the solution. The position of the PCr resonance has been shown to be unaffected by both changes in pH and changes in the concentrations of the ions present in the ranges that pH and ion concentrations vary under most physiological conditions. The chemical shift of the Pi resonance is dependent on the pH. Phosphoric acid has three acid dissociation equilibria characterized by three acid dissociation constants ($pKa_1 = 2.12$; $pKa_2 = 7.21$; and $pKa_3 = 12.67$). There are four possible phosphorus-containing species present from these dissociations; H_3PO_4, $H_2PO_4^-$, HPO_4^{2-}, and PO_4^{3-}. At room temperature in aqueous solution, these four species are in fast exchange on the ^{31}P NMR chemical shift timescale and only a single resonance which is the population average of the four species is observed. Under physiological conditions (i.e, around pH 7) we can assume that the dissociation step with a pKa of 7.21 is important. This means that the predominant species present in solution are $H_2PO_4^-$ and HPO_4^{2-} and we can neglect the other two species. The chemical shifts of the two predominant species are both at higher frequency than PCr with the shift of the $H_2PO_4^-$ species closer to PCr than HPO_4^{2-}. When the pH is equal to the pKa (7.21) the concentration of the two species are equal. In Equation 13 this would mean that $P_A = P_B = 0.5$. When the solution is more acidic, there is relatively more $H_2PO_4^-$ than HPO_4^{2-} and since the Pi resonance is a population average of the two species it will shift to lower frequency (closer to the PCr resonance). Under more alkaline conditions the reverse is true. Namely there is more HPO_4^{2-} than $H_2PO_4^-$ present and the Pi resonance will shift to higher frequency (farther from the PCr resonance). Using this simple two-site exchange model for the effects of changing pH on the chemical shift of Pi we can begin to understand how we can construct a titration curve from which the precise resonance position of the Pi can be used to determine the pH.

Calculation of Free Mg^{2+} from ^{31}P Spectra

The facts that Mg^{2+} binds to ATP and that the rate of dissociation of the Mg-ATP complex is fast on the ^{31}P NMR timescale can be exploited to yield estimates of the free Mg^{2+} concentration in tissue. At neutral pH, assuming the formation of a 1:1 complex, we can write the following equilibrium

$$Mg^{2+} + ATP \leftrightarrow MgATP \qquad [16]$$

with a dissociation constant given by,

$$K_D^{MgATP} = \frac{[Mg^{2+}][ATP]}{[MgATP]} \qquad [17]$$

where [ ] denotes equilibrium concentration and [ATP] denotes all of the species of ATP not complexed to Mg^{2+}. Based on measurements made in vitro, Gupta et al. (17)

showed that the free Mg^{2+} concentration could be related to the difference in chemical shift between the α and β resonances of ATP, $\delta_{\alpha\beta}^{obs}$, by,

$$[Mg_f] = K_D^{MgATP} \frac{\delta_{\alpha\beta}^{ATP} - \delta_{\alpha\beta}^{obs}}{\delta_{\alpha\beta}^{obs} - \delta_{\alpha\beta}^{MgATP}} \quad [18]$$

where $\delta_{\alpha\beta}^{ATP}$ is the chemical shift difference observed with no Mg^{2+} present, $\delta_{\alpha\beta}^{MgATP}$ is the chemical shift difference observed when all of the ATP is bound to Mg^{2+}, and $\delta_{\alpha\beta}^{obs}$ is the observed chemical shift difference. Vink et al. (18) exploited this relationship together with the fact that the value of K_D is 50 mM (at 37°C, pH 7.2, and an ionic strength of 0.15 M) to determine the concentrations of Mg^{2+} in the brains of animals with head trauma. More recently Williams et al. (19) have described a more sophisticated method for determining the levels of Mg^{2+} present which simultaneously solves all of the equations describing the interactions of ATP both with Mg^{2+} and H^+. A computer algorithm which performs this analysis is available from these authors. Using this algorithm both the intracellular pH and Mg^{2+} concentrations can be determined simultaneously from the resonance positions of the three ^{31}P resonances of ATP.

Effects of Exchange on Relaxation Rates

Rapid exchange can lead to the collapse of expected spin multiplets. Consider the case of methanol. In the absence of exchange of the hydroxyl proton, i.e, no water present, methanol should have a spectrum with multiplets similar to that of acetaldehyde (Fig. 10); the methyl resonance should be a doublet and the hydroxyl resonance a quartet. The splitting of the methyl group arises from the fact that its Larmor frequency is affected by the orientation of the spin of the hydroxyl proton. One resonance of the doublet arises from those molecules containing the hydroxyl proton oriented with the main field. The other resonance arises from those molecules containing the hydroxyl proton in the opposite orientation. In the presence of a small amount of water, the hydroxyl proton exchanges rapidly with the water protons as indicated above. The effect of this exchange is to scramble and average the orientations of the hydroxyl protons. For example, consider the case where the hydroxyl proton is oriented parallel to the main field. As this proton exchanges with protons of water there is an almost equal probability that the proton replacing the hydroxyl proton will have a parallel or antiparallel orientation. A similar argument can be made when the hydroxyl proton is in an initial antiparallel orientation. Thus, the spectrum under conditions of fast exchange will show an unsplit resonance in the methyl region with its frequency exactly at the center of the doublet.

The presence of exchange may also affect the relaxation times. A detailed mathematical discussion of these effects has been provided in the literature (20). In general, the effects of exchange are more pronounced on T2 than T1 relaxation times. This can be understood conceptually in two ways. First the rate of exchange is usually much smaller than the Larmor frequency. As was discussed above this situation leads to inefficient interactions between the spins and the lattice. For this reason the contribution of exchange to T1 relaxation is usually small. An alternative explanation lies in the fact that exchange processes have very little effect on the longitudinal magnetization since this magnetization should be the same in all sites.

The effect on the transverse magnetization can be quite large particularly when the chemical shifts in the different sites are very different. In this case the effects of exchange modulate the transverse magnetization at a frequency that is the difference of the frequencies between the sites leading to more efficient T2 relaxation and broader lines. For the case of two-site exchange (site A and site B), under conditions of fast exchange the transverse relaxation rate is given by,

$$1/T2 = P_A/T2_A + P_B/T2_B + P_B(1 - P_B)^2[2\pi(\omega_A - \omega_B)^2]\tau_{ex} \quad [19]$$

where the symbols P, T2, and ω refer to the population, transverse relaxation time, and resonance frequency, respectively, in sites A and B and τ_{ex} is the correlation time for exchange between the two sites. The last term in Equation 19 is the mathematical representation of the effects of the modulation of the difference in chemical shift by exchange. The effects of exchange with Mg^{2+} are thought to be important in reducing the T2s of the ^{31}P resonances of ATP in vivo.

RELATIVE SENSITIVITIES OF THE VARIOUS NUCLEI

The relative sensitivities of the various nuclei routinely monitored by MRS are given in Table 1. These numbers can be used in reference with the physiological concentrations of various metabolites present to arrive at estimates of the volumes of tissue which will give rise to localized spectra with reasonable signal-to-noise (S/N). As an example we can calculate the volumes of tissue in the brain which can be currently sampled by MRS with reasonable S/N. Using the concentrations reported for *N*-acetylaspartate (NAA) and PCr measured by conventional wet chemical analysis, we can estimate the minimum voxel volumes achievable at 1.5 T by comparing the minimum volumes detectable in MRI at 1.5 T. In these estimates we are assuming that there are no S/N losses associated with the localization methods employed and that rf coils of comparable quality to the head coil employed in MRI are used in MRS. We use as our

TABLE 1. *NMR properties of select nuclei of biomedical interest*

Nucleus	Spin	Natural abundance	Frequency at 1.5 T	Physiological concentration	Relative sensitivity[b]	Receptivity at 1.5 T[c]
H-1	1/2	100	63.89	110 M	1.00	1.00
H-2	1	0.015	9.80	110 M	2.4×10^{-6}	2.4×10^{-6}
H-1		(metabolites)	63.89	1–10 mM	1.00	10^{-5}–10^{-6}
C-13	1/2	1.18	16.06	10 mM	2.5×10^{-4}	2.5×10^{-8}
F-19	1/2	100	60.08	10 mM[a]	0.85	8.5×10^{-5}
Na-23	3/2	100	16.89	80 mM	0.13	9.5×10^{-5}
P-31	1/2	100	25.85	10 mM	8.3×10^{-2}	8.3×10^{-6}
K-39	3/2	93.1	2.99	45 mM	1.0×10^{-3}	4.1×10^{-4}

[a] Introduced exogenously as a fluorinated drug like 5-fluorouracil.

[b] Relative sensitivity at 1.5 T computed by multiplying the intrinsic sensitivity at constant field by the natural abundance of the nucleus.

[c] The relative sensitivity multiplied by the physiological concentration present. For reference an entry for proton-containing metabolites such as lactate is included.

baseline MR images obtained at the highest spatial resolution possible with the head coil. In our experience these can be obtained at a field-of-view of 8 cm, slice thickness of 3 mm, and matrix size of 256 × 256, in about 13 minutes of acquisition time (TR = 2500/TE = 20). The voxel size in this protocol is (8/256) × (8/256) × (0.3) cm^3. If we wish to achieve a comparable S/N in a comparable acquisition time for MRS then we multiply this voxel volume by the appropriate sensitivity factors provided for NAA and PCr. This calculation gives a minimum voxel volume of about 2 cm^3 for the detection of NAA in the brain using solvent suppressed proton MRS. The minimum volume of brain tissue that will yield reasonable S/N for the ^{31}P resonance of PCr is about 30 cm^3. Assuming isotropic voxels, these volumes translate into linear voxel dimensions of about 1.3 cm for proton and about 3 cm for phosphorus. Although these calculations are relatively crude because they fail to take into account a number of factors such as the differences in relaxation times of the molecules being compared, we feel that they provide a realistic limit of the volumes that can be sampled by current methods. These estimates can be extended to other nuclei by scaling with the appropriate factors provided in 1. Similarly the estimates can be made for other kinds of tissue if the physiological concentrations of the metabolites of interest are known.

In all of the above estimates we have assumed that volume coils have been used both for excitation and detection. If surface coils or arrays of surface coils are employed it is possible to significantly improve the spatial resolution of the spectroscopy study. It is common to improve the S/N of MRI significantly (almost a factor of five in tissues proximal to the coil) using surface coils. This improvement would translate into a minimum voxel size of about 0.4 cm^3 for proton and about 6 cm^3 for ^{31}P. Examples of spectra obtained with this spatial resolution are given in a following section.

SPATIAL LOCALIZATION METHODS

Localization can be achieved in MRS by means of employing rf gradients, static B_0 gradients, or pulsed spatial gradients (or combinations of these). The technical details of all of these approaches have been described in detail in the literature (21–23). The latter methods are similar to those currently employed in MRI. Rather than providing details of the spin physics of the methods currently employed we feel it is important to understand the constraints placed on the choices of the various localization methods by the intrinsic properties of the molecules being monitored. For ^{31}P the relaxation times in molecules of biological interest present some important constraints. Den Hollander et al. have reported the spin-lattice relaxation times, T1s, of the phosphorus-containing metabolites observed in brain at 1.5 T (24). These values range from 3.3 sec for PCr to about 1 sec for α-ATP. Thus, for a fully relaxed spectrum one would need a recycle time, TR, of about 15 sec. The spin-spin relaxation times, T2s, of the ATP peaks have been measured in pure solution and range from 200 to 300 msec (25). In brain, however, these times are much shorter (i.e, less than 50 msec).

Any localization methods which employ spin-echo techniques must have very short TEs since long TEs will result in selective loss of ATP signal. Thus, for fully quantitative ^{31}P spectra long TRs and short TEs are required. Since achieving short TEs on conventional whole-body imaging scanners is difficult, FID-like methods which, in principle, have an almost zero TE have gained popularity. There are three classes of methods in which FID methods can be employed. The first class includes methods in which all spins except those in the location to be sampled are effectively removed. Examples are the VSE (26) and LOCUS (27) sequences. The second class includes methods in which only the desired spins are excited. These include surface coil localization and DRESS (28). The last class of methods involves the use of spatial encoding methods such as Fourier and Hadamard encoding (29). Examples include phase-encoded chemical shift imaging (CSI) (21–23), ISIS (30), and Hadamard methods (29).

Proton spectroscopy of metabolites presents a problem in that metabolites at millimolar concentrations must be detected in the presence of a background water signal that is present at about 100 molar. For this reason, solvent-suppression techniques have been combined with localization schemes to produce spatially localized solvent-suppressed spectra. The T1s of the various proton metabolites are quite long and the T2s are also quite long permitting the use of methods like the spin-echo or stimulated-echo sequences. As in the case of ^{31}P there are three classes of localization. The SPARS method (31) is an example of a localization method which preserves the magnetization of only those protons being sampled and destroys the coherence of all of the unwanted spins. When implemented as single-voxel (i.e., sampling only one region of tissue) the stimulated echo (STEAM) sequence (10,32) and PRESS (33) are examples of methods in which only those protons being sampled are excited. Both the STEAM and PRESS methods can be combined with Fourier phase-encoding methods to produce CSI sequences (21–23). The advantages of combining these spatial preselection methods with encoding schemes are that the signal from lipid arising from scalp is minimized and the volume over which the B_0 field is adjusted can be restricted to avoid air-tissue boundaries where there may be large variations in the magnetic susceptibility.

For reasons associated with instrument performance such as residual eddy current effects, many of the early reports of proton MRS employed echo delays of 135 msec or 270 msec. The choice of 135 or 270 msec is made in order to refocus the doublet resonance of the methyl resonance of lactate which has a value of about 7 Hz for the spin-spin coupling constant to its methenyl proton. As instrumental performance has improved there has been a larger emphasis placed on acquiring proton spectra at shorter echo delays (20–60 msec). One advantage of these shorter delays is the ability to detect resonances from coupled spin systems (e.g., glutamate, glutamine, inositol) whose apparent T2s are too short to permit detection at longer echo delays.

The recent development of so-called digitally-crafted or designer rf pulses (34–39) has also improved the quality of both ^{1}H and ^{31}P in vivo MRS. For example, Lim et al. (40) have recently reported a self-refocusing spin-echo CSI method for ^{31}P with an effective echo delay of 2.5 msec. The pulse sequence is shown in Fig. 12. The advantages of the shorter echo delay are shown in Fig. 13. At longer echo delays there is a selective loss in the intensity of the resonance arising from PDE. Examples of CSI

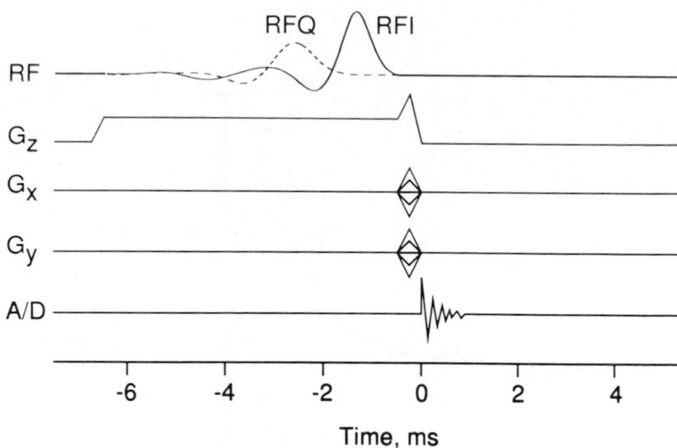

FIG. 12. The pulse sequence for 2D spectroscopic imaging using a 2.5 msec TE self-refocusing pulse. (From Lim et al., ref. 40, with permission.)

data collected at an echo delay of 2.5 msec are shown in Fig. 14. The S/N of the PCr peak obtained from one voxel ($\approx$ 40 cm^3) of the reconstructed CSI data set is about 20:1. The advantage of this method is that the spectra can be phased using zero-order phase corrections and that the signal has the characteristic advantages of a spin-echo acquisition.

We have recently assessed the precision of localization of a STEAM sequence for solvent suppressed ^{1}H spectroscopy which employs digitally-crafted excitation and solvent-suppression pulses. Consider an object of volume, V_{tot}. If we use a spatial localization method to select a smaller volume of this object V_{sel}, from which we wish to obtain a localized spectrum, then the spatial discrimination, D, of the method can be expressed as

$$D = \left[\frac{V_{tot} - V_{sel}}{V_{sel}}\right] \qquad [20]$$

Under the simplifying assumption of a uniform distribution of metabolites we can define the spatial precision required for a specified level of contamination (S_{sel}/S_{out}) of the spectrum obtained from the selected volume with signal originating from the unselected ($V_{tot} - V_{sel}$) volume as

$$SP = \left[\frac{V_{tot} - V_{sel}}{V_{sel}}\right] \times \left[\frac{S_{sel}}{S_{out}}\right] \qquad [21]$$

If we assume that the object has a total volume of 1000 cm^3 and that the selected volume is 1 cm^3, then from Equation 20 the value of D is 999. If we define 10% contamination as acceptable, then the value of SP from Equation 21 is about 10^4. From Equation 21 it is clear that as the selected volume becomes smaller the spatial precision of the method must become higher. Our results obtained on phantoms indicate that the STEAM sequence with conventional rf pulses can only achieve val-

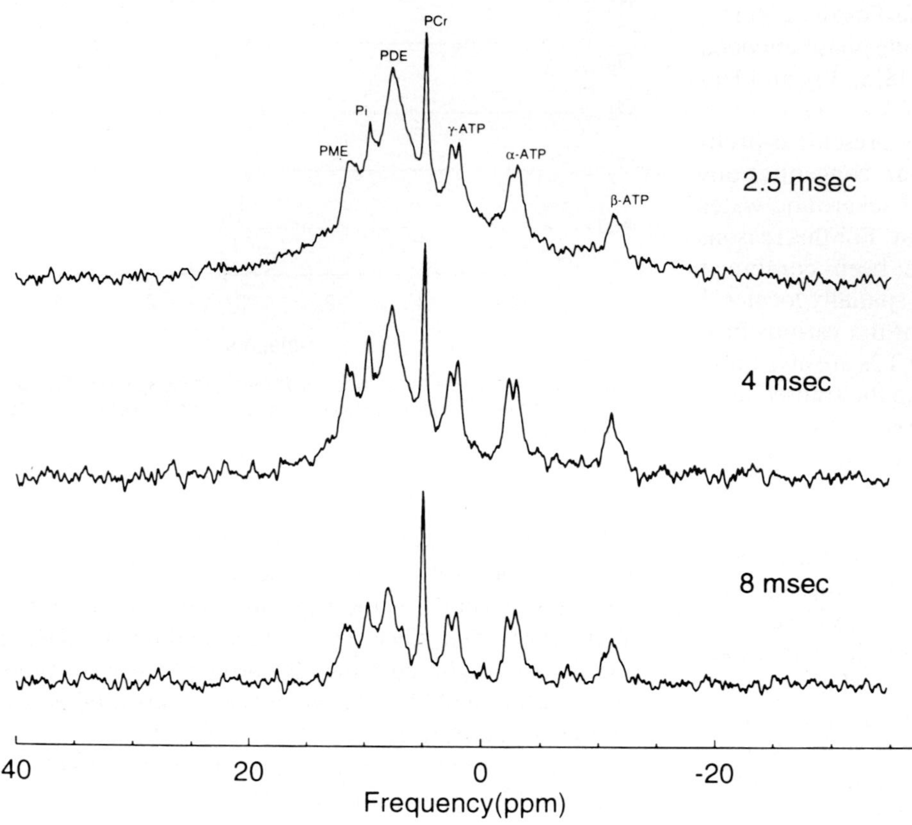

FIG. 13. Spectra obtained using the pulse sequence shown in Fig. 12 from a 33-mm slice at TR = 2000 msec and TE = 2.5, 4, and 8 msec. (From Lim et al., ref. 40, with permission.)

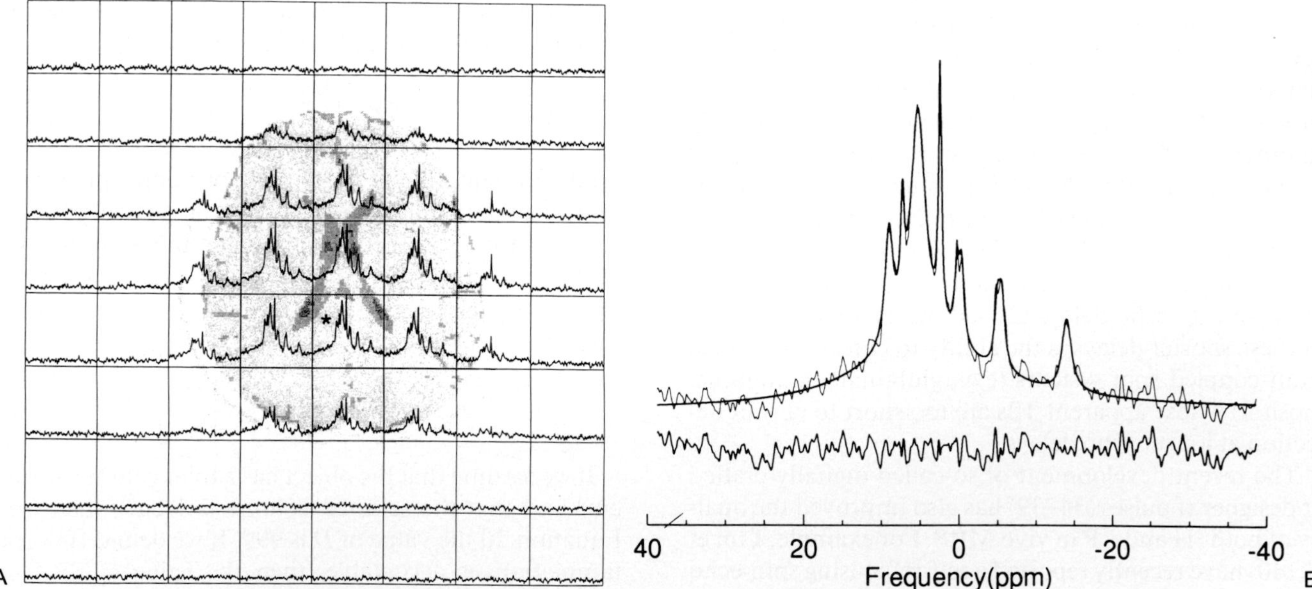

FIG. 14. A: A data set obtained using 8 × 8 phase encodes in the sequence shown in Fig. 12. The data set is superimposed over an anatomical axial MRI. The spectra were acquired from a 35-mm slice, 28-cm FOV, TR = 4 sec, TE = 2.5 sec, and total scan time of 34 min. **B:** A single spectrum obtained from the data set shown in Fig. 14A from the location indicated. (From Lim et al., ref. 40, with permission.)

ues of spatial precision of about 3000. This means that the minimum useful V_{sel} in a 1000-cm^3 object (about the size of an adult head) at a 10% level of contamination is about 2 cm^3. With rf pulses designed specifically for high spatial selectivity the spatial precision can be improved by almost an order of magnitude, making the minimum useful voxel, V_{sel}, about 0.2 cm^3. The point of the above discussion is that it may not always be S/N considerations that limit the spatial resolution achievable.

Examples of ^{1}H spectra obtained from the occipital lobes of normal volunteers from volumes of about 0.36 cm^3 are shown in Figs. 15 and 16. This level of spatial precision is necessary to obtain spectra localized to cortical gray matter since the thickness of cortical gray matter is about 3 mm in young, healthy volunteers. These spectra obtained with a surface coil indicate the potential of ^{1}H MRS for studying diseases that affect gray matter.

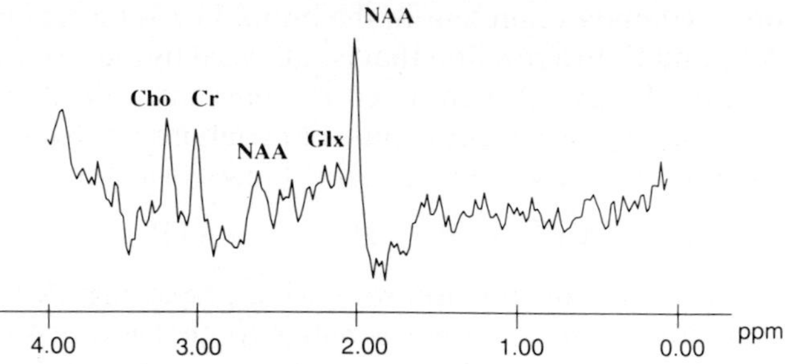

FIG. 16. A spectrum obtained from white matter in the occipital lobe. The acquisition and processing parameters are identical to those employed in Fig. 15.

METABOLIC BASIS FOR SPECTRAL INTERPRETATION

In order to appreciate the information available from MRS, it is important to review some basic concepts in brain biochemistry. Since many of the compounds measured in ^{31}P and ^{1}H MRS are key components in cellular energy metabolism, we will start by considering cellular energetics. In order to survive in a viable steady state, the rate of cellular energy production must equal the rate of energy consumption. Since ATP is the energy currency of the cell, this translates into the rate of ATP synthesis and ATP consumption being equal. Figure 17 shows a model of cellular metabolism in the brain. In this model the cycle involving ATP synthesis and consumption is the most important cycle upon which cell survival depends. Also as shown in Fig. 17, the predominant energy consuming function is the active transport of various ions that are required to maintain the proper membrane potentials. This function is performed by membrane bound ion pumps function biochemically as ATPases (ATP-splitting enzymes). The principal site of ATP synthesis is the mitochondria. The rate of mitochondrial ATP synthesis must equal the rate of consumption of ATP by ATPase conditions for steady-state survival can be maintained. It is important to understand some of the regulation that keeps this steady state viable.

The mitochondria need various substrates in order to synthesize ATP. The most important of these are ADP and Pi. In addition the mitochondria require oxygen and reducing equivalents. The reducing equivalents are supplied in the form of NADH from the Krebs cycle, as

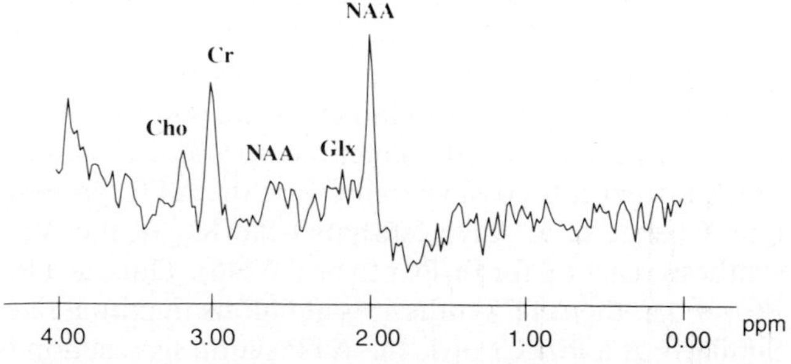

FIG. 15. Localized proton spectra obtained in cortical gray matter from an 0.6 mm × 0.6mm × 10 mm voxel using the STEAM sequence (TE = 31 msec, TM = 10.6 msec, TR = 2000 msec, 2000 Hz sweepwidth, 2048 points, and 256 acquisitions) using a 7.5-cm diameter surface coil. The spectrum was acquired with an eight-step phase-cycling scheme. The pulse sequence employed a "digitally crafted" rf pulse for slice selection and solvent suppression. No additional baseline correction was employed.

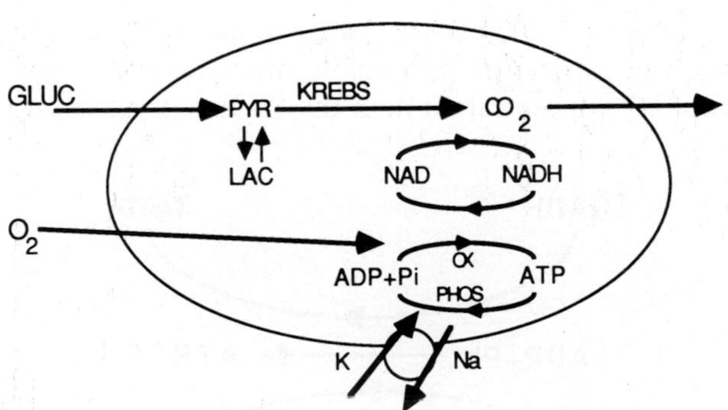

FIG. 17. Model of brain metabolism. The central cycle is the ATP-ADP cycle. ATP is consumed in the membrane bound ion pump ATPase enzymes. ATP is produced in the mitochondria. Oxygen and NADH are needed as additional substrate. The NADH is produced from NAD in the Krebs cycle.

shown in Fig. 16. Thus, the entire reaction that occurs in the mitochondria can be written, as shown in Fig. 18.

In addition to ATP, PCr is a second high-energy phosphate compound present in the brain. PCr is formed by ATP and Cr in a reaction that is catalyzed by the enzyme creatine kinase. PCr in a sense represents a dead-end compound, since its only route of metabolism is back to Cr and ATP via the same creatine kinase reaction:

$$PCr + ADP + {}^{+}H \leftrightarrow Cr + ATP \quad [22]$$

This makes its function somewhat perplexing. PCr is generally felt to represent a buffer to changes in ATP through the creatine kinase equilibrium (41). Its function as an energy reserve is often overstated. The 5 mM of PCr in the brain would only fuel the brain for 20 seconds at normal metabolic rates (42). The presence of PCr in the brain is very important to MRS, since it permits the indirect calculation of the ADP concentration. ADP is present at very small levels in the brain and cannot be detected directly by ^{31}P MRS. However, the condition of creatine kinase equilibrium requires that:

$$[ADP] = [Cr][ATP]/[PCr][H^{+}]K_{eq} \quad [23]$$

PCr and ATP can be measured directly in the ^{31}P MRS spectrum. The $^{+}$H concentration or pH can be calculated from the chemical shift of the Pi resonance. The sum of Cr and PCr is relatively constant in the brain allowing for calculation of the Cr from the PCr, and the K_{eq} is a constant that has been measured (43). In order to appreciate the importance of ADP it is useful to consider mitochondria as a single enzyme that catalyzes the ATP synthesis reaction. In this model proposed by Chance et al. (44), oxygen and reducing equivalents are considered cofactors. Since we are considering the ATP synthesis reaction as a single enzyme-mediated reaction, the rate of ATP synthesis can be expressed in terms of the concentrations of ADP and Pi according to Michaelis-Menten kinetics (45). Thus, the rate of ATP synthesis can be expressed in terms of a V_{max} and K_M and the ADP and Pi concentrations. In the brain the ADP concentration is approximately 10 μM, which is significantly lower than the 1 mM of Pi. Thus, any change in the ATP concentration will cause a proportionally much larger change in the ADP concentration than the Pi. It is possible to approximate the kinetics of ATP synthesis by considering only the ADP as the rate-controlling metabolite. Then according to simple Michaelis-Menten kinetics the rate of ATP synthesis can be expressed as

$$R = V_{max}/(1 + K_M/[ADP]) \quad [24]$$

where V_{max} is the maximal rate of mitochondrial ATP synthesis and Km is a constant (K_M represents the ADP concentration at which the V of ATP synthesis is 50% of the V_{max}). This relation can be expressed graphically as shown in Fig. 19. As the ADP concentration increases, so will the ATP synthesis rate, until it reaches V_{max}. This results in a very simple control scheme. If there is an increase in the rate of ATP consumption, the ADP concentration will increase, thus increasing the ATP synthesis rate to keep up with the increased rate of ATP consumption, and a new steady state will be established. The ADP concentration will indicate the new position on the rate curve and, thus, the reserve available. As shown by Chance et al., the Pi/PCr ratio behaves very similarly to the ADP concentration. Since this can be measured directly from the ^{31}P spectrum, this ratio becomes a convenient measure of metabolic reserve (46). The use of the Pi/PCr ratio does not account for the pH dependence of the ADP concentration (see Equation 23), and thus must be corrected for pH in order to be accurate. The Pi/PCr ratio indicates the point of operation of the system on the kinetic curve, and thus, how much further it is possible to increase the ATP synthesis rate. Chance et al. have estimated the K_M of the ATP synthesis reaction for Pi/PCr to be 0.6 (46). Thus, at a Pi/PCr of 0.6, the ATP synthesis is at half its maximal rate. Similarly at a Pi/PCr of 1, the ATP synthesis reaction is at 60% of V_{max} and on the beginning of the plateau of the kinetic curve. Thus, at a Pi/PCr of 1, the system is beginning to use up all of its reserve. In practice, it is very difficult to maintain a steady state with the Pi/PCr greater than 1. Usually, beyond this value the system can no longer maintain a steady state, and thus, there is complete metabolic collapse.

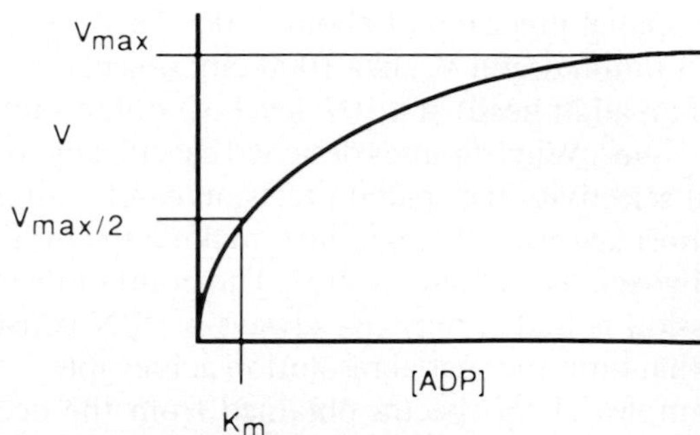

FIG. 19. Kinetics of ATP synthesis. The rate of ATP synthesis (*V*) is a function of the ADP concentration ([ADP]) according to the Michaelis-Menten kinetics. V_{max} is the maximal rate of ATP synthesis, and K_M is the concentration of ADP at which $V = \frac{1}{2} \times V_{max}$.

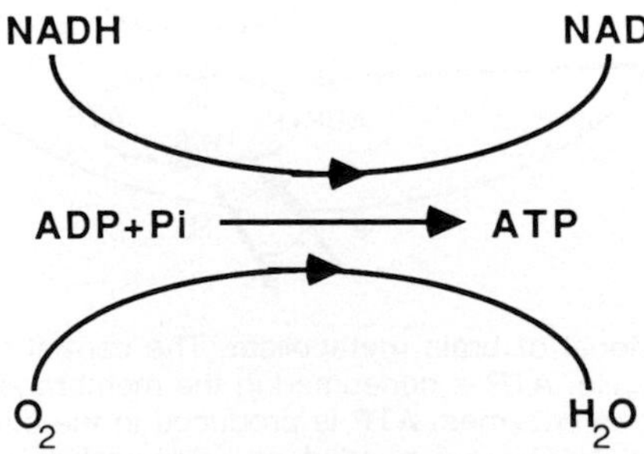

FIG. 18. The ATP synthesis reaction.

The relationship of the lactate concentration to the ATP synthesis rate is mediated by NAD/NADH ratio. This is illustrated in Fig. 18. If the rate of mitochondrial ATP synthesis decreases, there will be a decrease in the rate of turnover of NADH to NAD, and thus, the NAD concentration will decrease. Since NAD is an important substrate of the Krebs cycle, this will decrease the rate of the Krebs cycle and result in an accumulation of pyruvate (the terminal step of glycolysis) which will be converted to lactate by the lactate dehydrogenase enzyme. Thus, the accumulation of lactate is related to the disparity in rates between the Krebs cycle and glycolysis, which in the brain is almost always associated with a decrease in NADH turnover rate due to a decrease in the ATP synthesis rate.

In order to better understand the concepts discussed above we consider the effect of perturbing the normal brain metabolism on the ^{31}P and ^{1}H spectra. The perturbations we consider are hypoxia and seizure. These have been extensively studied in animal models.

The first metabolic consequence of hypoxia is a decrease in the V_{max} of mitochondrial ATP synthesis. This results in a shift to a new metabolic control curve, since as discussed above, the limitation of oxygen acts to decrease the V_{max} of the ATP synthesis in the mitochondria. This is depicted graphically in Fig. 20. In order to maintain the same ATP synthesis rate, there will be an increase in the Pi/PCr ratio, using up some of the brain's metabolic reserve. If the hypoxia is profound, the V_{max} is decreased to the point that in order to maintain a steady state, the rate of ATP consumption must decrease. This is manifested by a decrease in the electrical activity of the brain as measured by EEG. At this point, there is a net accumulation of NADH and decrease of NAD due to the reduced rate of mitochondrial ATP synthesis. This results in the accumulation of lactate. Thus, under conditions of severe hypoxia, there is a decrease in the electrical activity, increase in lactate and increase in the Pi/PCr ratio (48,49). ^{31}P and ^{1}H spectra of a cat brain

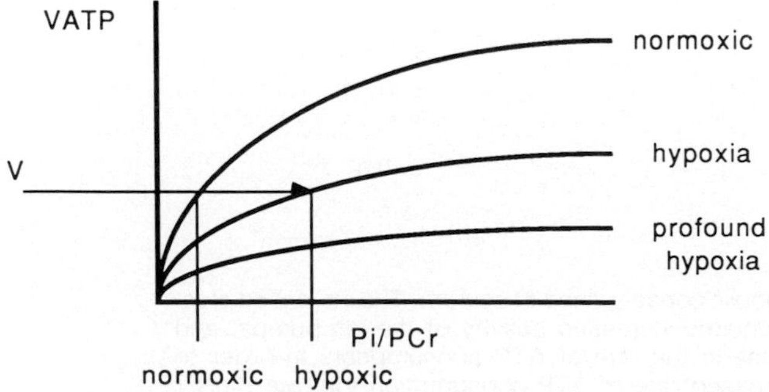

FIG. 20. Metabolic consequence of hypoxia. The decrease in O_2 causes a decrease in the V_{max} of ATP synthesis, and thus a shift to a new kinetic curve. In order to maintain the same VATP the Pi/PCr must increase as shown. If the hypoxia is profound, the decrease in V_{max} is such that no steady state can be established.

under conditions of hypoxia are shown in Fig. 21. The increased lactate production is also associated with a decrease in the intracellular pH. This is manifested by a change in the chemical shift of the Pi resonance. In cases of near anoxia, the V_{max} of ATP synthesis is nearly 0. Under these conditions no steady state is possible and there is complete metabolic collapse. If this is not reversed in approximately 5 minutes, cell death will occur. If reversed earlier, the system will return to equilibrium. It takes longer for the lactate level to return to normal values than for the PCr level to do so. The decrease in the lactate concentration is probably dominated by diffusion across the blood–brain barrier. This diffusion appears to be saturable at low concentrations of lactate, with the pseudo-zeroth order rate of lactate clearance at 0.36 mM/min (50).

In the case of grand mal seizure, the V_{max} of ATP synthesis is preserved. The increased electrical activity is manifested biochemically by an increase in ATP consumption. In order to maintain a steady state, the Pi/PCr will increase (51,52). This increases the rate of ATP synthesis to keep up with the increased ATP consumption (Fig. 22). Since there is adequate turnover of NADH into NAD within the mitochondria, there is no decrease in the rate of the Krebs cycle, and thus, unlike hypoxia, only minimal lactate accumulation. ^{1}H spectra and time course of spectra changes during seizure in the cat brain are shown in Fig. 23.

There are multiple other metabolites in the ^{31}P and ^{1}H brain spectra that are not mentioned above. The most prominent resonance in the ^{1}H spectrum is NAA, which resonates at 2.0 ppm. The function of NAA is not clear, however, it appears to be present in high levels only in neuronal tissue (53). Several functions have been proposed for NAA. These include the regulation of lipid synthesis, the regulation of protein synthesis or as a storage buffer for aspartate (54). The level of NAA is relatively constant in normal brain tissue, although it has been shown to decrease in many pathologic conditions. These decreases in NAA are detectable before any changes are observed on MRI. This has been attributed to the fact that as neurons die, the level of NAA decreases. As this occurs, the surrounding glia become hypertrophic, essentially filling the space left by neuronal loss. Conventional MRI is not sensitive to these changes. At 3.0 ppm in the ^{1}H spectrum is another prominent resonance. This resonance is from creatine from the $-CH_3$ group that is common in PCr and Cr, and thus this resonance represents the total creatine pool. This peak remains stable under many pathologic conditions in the brain, and thus is a useful reference against which the intensities of other peaks can be compared. A rough approximation is that this peak represents 11 mM total creatine (55). The resonance at 3.2 ppm is from the $N\text{-}CH_3$ group of choline. Choline (Cho) is important to cell membrane synthesis, and is often found to be elevated in malignant tumors.

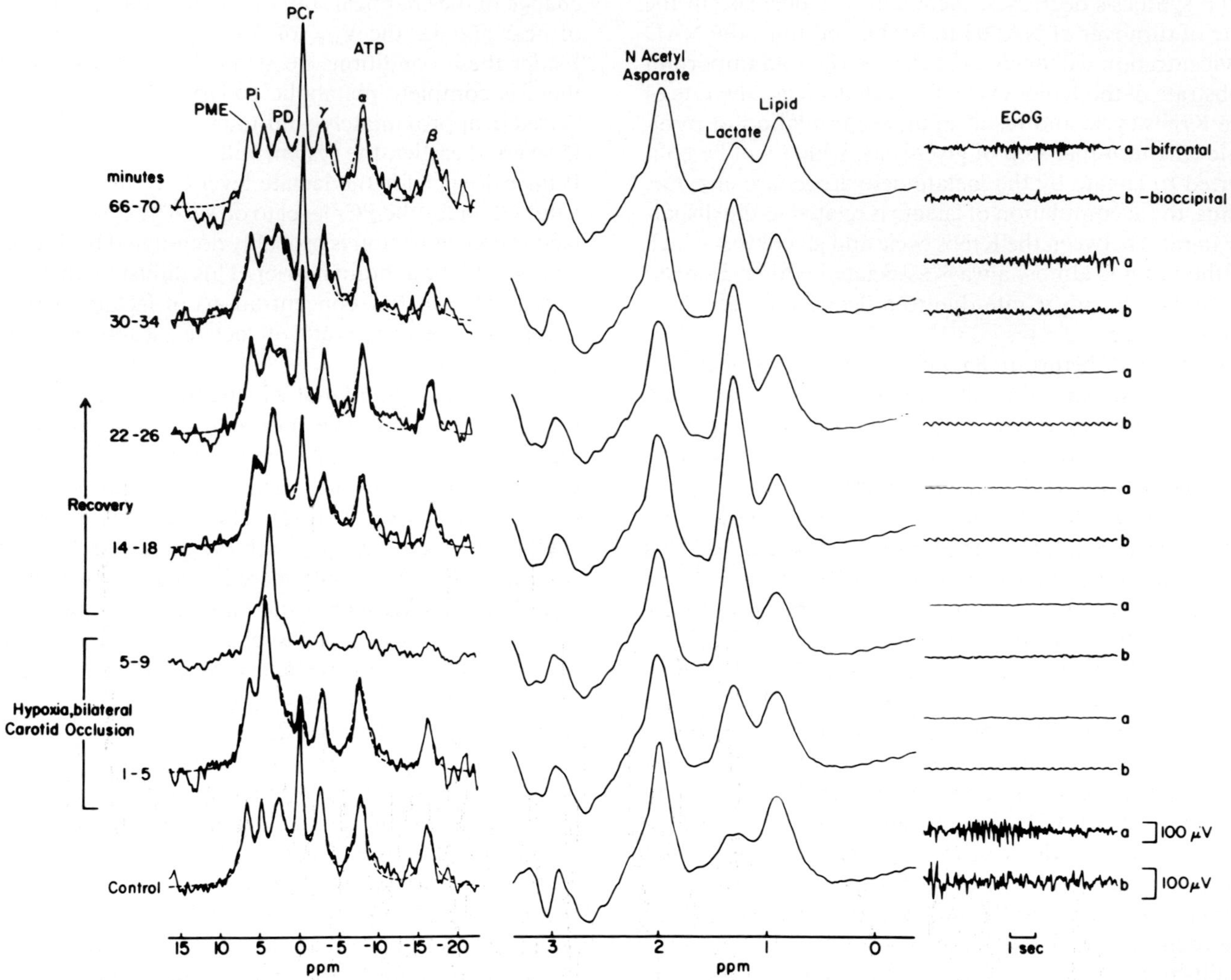

FIG. 21. ^{31}P and ^{1}H spectral changes during acute hypoxia and ischemia. The profound increase in lactate and decrease in PCr are easily observed. Note the acidic shift in the Pi resonance.

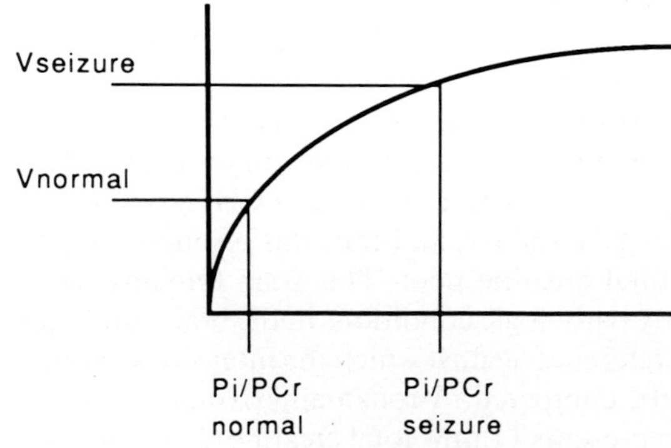

FIG. 22. Metabolic consequence of seizure. The increased electrical activity requires increased activity of the ion pumps, and thus, an increase in the rate of ATP consumption. In order to match this increased rate of ATP consumption the rate Pi/PCr increases, increasing the rate of ATP synthesis.

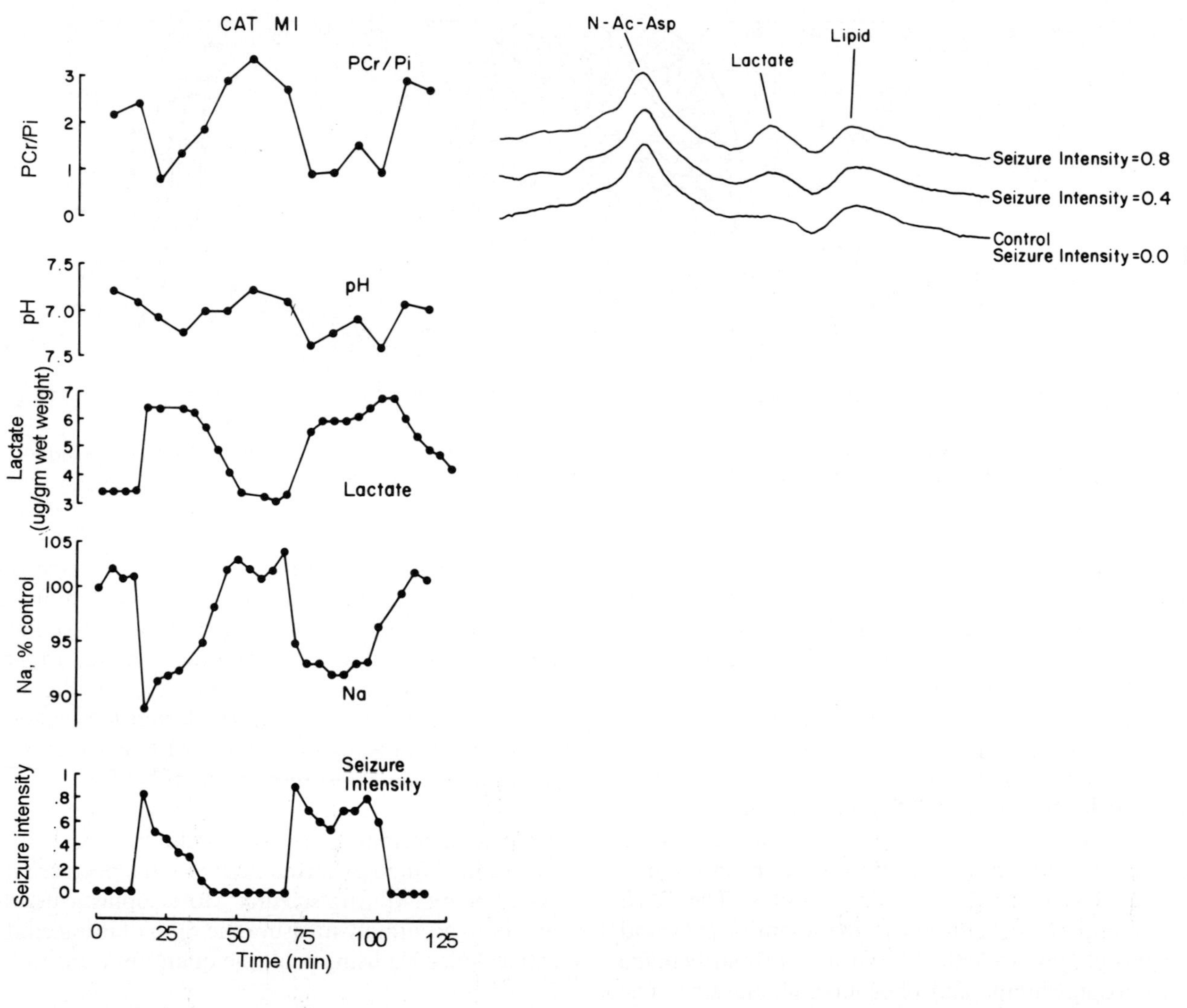

FIG. 23. Metabolic changes in a cat brain during seizure: **A:** The onset of seizure is accompanied by a decrease in the PCr/Pi (increased Pi/PCr) and only mild increase in the lactate resonance. The decrease in the ^{23}Na signal is related to Na moving from the extracellular to intracellular fluid. **B:** ^{1}H spectra of a cat brain during seizure: note when compared to Fig. 16 the increase in lactate during seizure is mild compared to that during hypoxia.

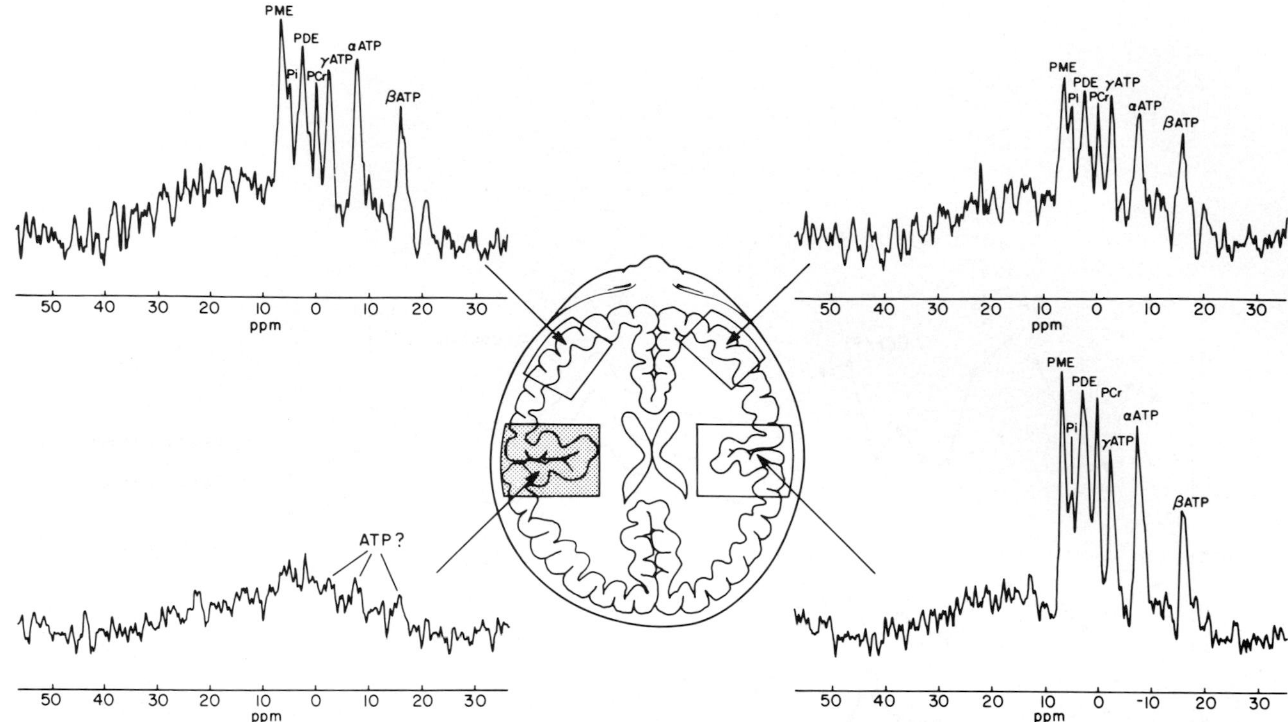

FIG. 24. Mature cerebral infarction in a neonatal human brain. Note the total absence of phosphate-containing metabolites in the infarcted region. Also note the high PME in the normal neonatal brain.

Smaller peaks from several other compounds such as the amino acids aspartate and glutamate, and the neurotransmitter GABA can also be found in the ^{1}H spectrum of the brain (56,57). In the normal brain, there is little or no signal from mobile lipids. Peaks associated with myoinositol and glucose have also been identified.

There are two prominent resonances in the ^{31}P brain spectrum that we have not yet discussed. The phosphodiester (PDE) peak at 2.5 ppm and the phosphomonoester (PME) peak at 7 ppm are composite peaks arising from compounds that are important in the metabolism of cell membrane phospholipids. The PME peak is composed of phosphorylethanolamine (58), and sugar phosphates, while the PDE peak is primarily made up of phosphocholine and phosphoethanolamine. The PME peak is interesting in that it is very elevated in the neonatal brain (Fig. 24). It is also elevated in some rapidly growing tumors (59). This suggests that the compounds that make up the PME resonance are important to rapid membrane synthesis.

In addition to ^{31}P and ^{1}H, spectra from other nuclei can also be obtained from the brain. ^{23}Na is readily detected by NMR. Most of the Na in the body is in the form of the Na^{+} ion, and therefore the ^{23}Na spectrum of the brain contains a single resonance. Although there is little interesting information available from the chemical shift of ^{23}Na, there is much interest in studying its relaxation behavior. ^{23}Na is a nucleus with a spin of 3/2. Thus, it has four possible energy states and three possible transitions (Fig. 25). The T2 relaxation of the two outside transitions, $3/2 \rightarrow 1/2$ and $-1/2 \rightarrow -3/2$, is much more sensitive to adjacent charge-carrying molecules than the central transition, $1/2 \rightarrow -1/2$. Within a cell there are more of these charge-carrying molecules, causing the outside transition to have such a short T2 that they cannot be detected. This results in a partial MR invisibility of intracellular ^{23}Na. Thus, movement of Na from the extracellular fluid into the intracellular fluid would be associated with a decrease in the size of the ^{23}Na peak (42,51). This is illustrated experimentally by the decrease in the Na resonance during seizure. More sophisticated techniques to accurately measure the ratio of intracellular to extracellular Na using multiple quantum transitions (3/

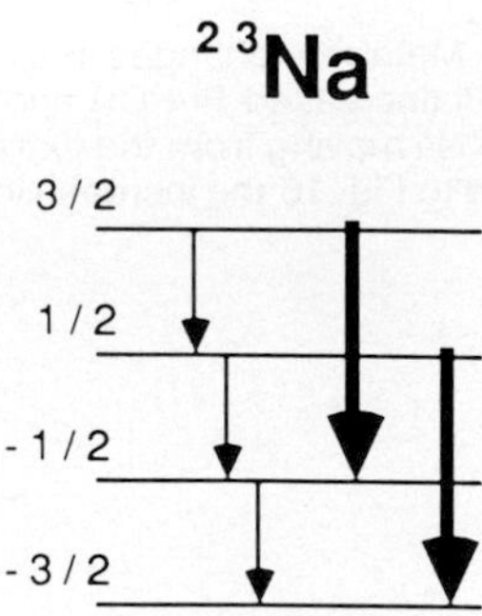

FIG. 25. ^{23}Na spin states. The *small arrows* represent single quantum transitions, the *bold arrows* represent the double quantum transitions.

2 → −1/2 and 1/2 → −3/2) have been suggested and are currently being studied.

^{13}C and ^{19}F MRS of the brain can also be performed. Although ^{13}C has only a 1% natural abundance, it can still be used to measure multiple metabolites. The real strength of ^{13}C is that the administration of ^{13}C-enriched metabolites allows one to follow the metabolite through the various metabolic pathways in vivo. Although expensive, ^{13}C-enriched compounds are not radioactive and do not appear to be harmful. Fluorine is found on many anesthetics, and thus ^{19}F MRI can be used to monitor the levels of these compounds in the brain. ^{19}F also serves as a convenient NMR visible label, to make many different molecules NMR visible (60).

Thus far we have discussed the ability of MRS to measure the concentration and relaxation of various metabolites. The ability to detect chemical exchange with MRS can also provide important information regarding reaction rates. This is most commonly achieved through the measurement of saturation transfer. Briefly, if a frequency-selective saturation is applied to one chemical species; the ^{31}P resonance of α-ATP for example, some of these saturated spins will be transferred to the PCr via the creatine kinase reaction. This results in a decrease in the amplitude of the PCr peak due to this transferred saturation. If the PCr resonance is repeatedly saturated, the PCr peak will decrease by an amount determined by the rate of chemical transfer from PCr to α-ATP. Unfortunately as these magnetically labeled (saturated) spins are transferring from α-ATP to PCr, they are also relaxing according to time T1. Thus, the actual resultant amplitude of the PCr peak is determined by the time during which the α-ATP resonance is saturated, the rate of chemical exchange and the T1 of the PCr. If the PCr amplitude is measured for two different saturation times, both the T1 and the rate of chemical exchange can be measured. Thus, this technique of saturation transfer provides the ability to measure actual reaction rates in vivo. Figure 26 shows a human muscle spectrum prior to and after the application of a frequency-selected saturation pulse to the α-ATP. Note the decrease of the intensity of the PCr peak due to transferred saturation. Although not yet applied clinically in the brain, the power of this technique for making measurements of metabolite fluxes makes it worth noting (61).

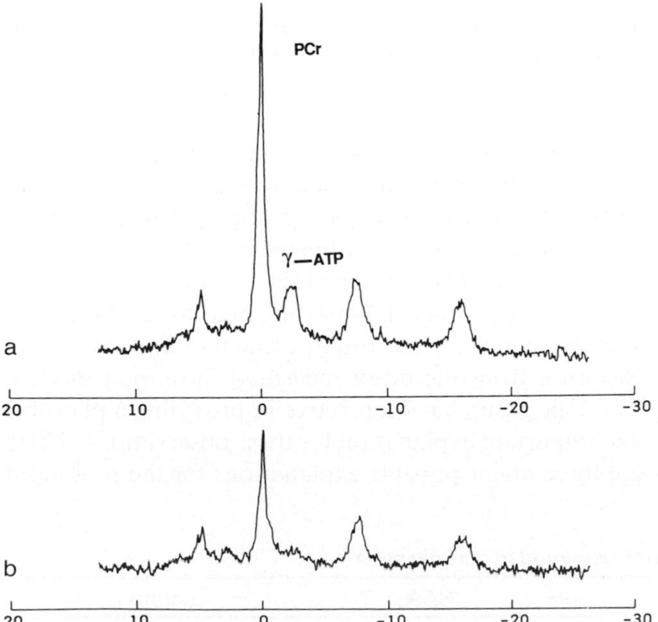

FIG. 26. Saturation transfer: **a:** Human muscle spectrum prior to the application of saturation. **b:** Spectrum after the application of a saturation pulse to γ-ATP. Note the decrease in the PCr peak from the transferred saturation.

CLINICAL MRS

When this chapter first appeared in 1991, it was our opinion that the clinical applications of MRS were in a very early stage of development. In the intervening five years there have been advances made in the technique and the number of clinical cases examined has increased to the point where interpretations of spectral data can be made in terms of the pathophysiology and biochemistry of the diseases being studied. The number of institutions performing localized MRS in a clinical setting has increased dramatically. Most of these institutions employ localized ^{1}H spectroscopy on a routine basis with a smaller number using ^{31}P. The emphasis on ^{1}H MRS in the brain has occurred for a number of reasons. First these studies can be performed on clinical MRI scanners with no additional hardware requirements. For these reasons ^{1}H MRS can be implemented on most commercial scanners operating at 1.5 T. There have been several localization methods developed for protons that are robust and easy to implement. In fact parts, if not all, of the MRS examination have been automated (62). These developments have led to the firm establishment of normal spectral parameters for ^{1}H with statistically tight standard deviations. This has led to a general consensus regarding the definition of what constitutes an abnormal spectral result. Finally and perhaps most important, there is agreement that there is information available from the localized spectra that cannot be obtained from conventional MRI. An example of this kind of information was discussed earlier. That is, changes in the level of NAA will occur earlier in the course of neuronal damage than can be detected by conventional MRI.

As might be expected from this discussion there has been a dramatic increase in the number of reports dealing with clinical studies of MRS. Rather than review all of these exhaustively, we will focus on several diseases in which there are indications that MRS has made an impact or shows the promise of affecting clinical decisions. These include stroke, birth asphyxia, epilepsy, HIV infection, dementias, and brain tumors.

Stroke

In stroke the supply of blood to a particular region of the brain is markedly reduced for a period of time. Based on the example of hypoxia/ischemia shown in Figs. 21 and 22, we can predict that acutely, the level of PCr/Pi should fall and the level of lactate should increase. After 10 minutes all of the PCr will disappear followed by a decrease in the level of ATP. Although it is easy to predict the acute changes that occur in stroke, it is almost impossible to study patients in this time interval. After this acute phase the progression of the infarcted region is highly complex and variable. If reperfusion occurs over the appropriate time period, there is a possibility of recovery of full metabolic function. If on the other hand there are parts of the infarcted region in which reperfusion does not occur (or occurs too late to reverse the metabolic state) the tissue in these regions will die. This damaged tissue is replaced by activated leukocytes, reactive astrocytes, and glia. Since it is unlikely that all of the regions of the infarct will behave identically, there has been a hypothesis made for the existence of a "reversible" ischemic transition zone of tissue which can exist over prolonged periods of time. Based on this discussion we can predict the alterations in the MRS spectra which should occur in each state. Note that under ischemic conditions the entire phosphate pool is converted to Pi in approximately 5–10 minutes. With subsequent cell death and lysis, there is diffusion of the Pi into the interstitial space. This results in the infarcted area being completely devoid of phosphate. In the absence of oxygen, the only source of ATP is through the conversion of glucose to lactate (glycolysis). If this is the only source of ATP production the concentration of lactate should increase acutely (to a maximum of about 10 mM) and then decrease since glucose can no longer be delivered to the cell. As pointed out earlier, the decrease in the lactate concentration is probably dominated by diffusion across the blood–brain barrier. This diffusion appears to be saturable at low concentrations of lactate, with the pseudo-zeroth order rate of lactate clearance at 0.36 mM/min (50). If no additional lactate is being produced or lactate is not "trapped" in some non-diffusible pool, all of the lactate should be cleared in less than 2 hours. Chronically, since neuronal death should occur in the regions with irreversible damage, the levels of NAA should be decreased. Because most patients will not be available for MRS studies in the acute or sub-acute stage of their stroke we have listed the spectral alterations expected in the chronic phase for each of the three states described above, namely reperfusion, reversible ischemia, and irreversible ischemia, in Table 2.

There have been several reports in the literature of localized ^{31}P MRS of stroke patients (63). Studies of patients with mature cerebral infarction failed to show any significant difference in the ratios of the various metabolites as compared to controls. There were early data suggesting that the pH in the infarcted regions was actually higher than that in normal areas of the brain (64). These findings were supported by the more recent spectroscopic imaging studies (^{1}H and ^{31}P) of stroke reported by Hugg et al. (65). Paradoxically, the regions with highest lactate showed alkaline pHs. Alkaline pHs have also been reported in a ^{31}P MRS study of head injury (66).

In regions of mature irreversible damage there should be no ^{31}P signals. The spectrum from the infarcted area will only have contributions from those residual areas of viable tissue. The resultant ^{31}P spectrum may be expected to show an overall decrease in spectral amplitude, but normal ratios of metabolites in the remaining viable tissue. Information about the absolute levels of the metabolites is necessary in order to detect this state. A report on the use of a quantitative technique to study the ^{31}P spectrum of patients with mature cerebral infarcts does indeed indicate that the overall concentration of the various metabolites are decreased despite normal relative concentrations (67).

There have been several studies using ^{1}H MRS to examine patients with stroke. An early report of ^{1}H MRS on patients with known cerebral vascular disease followed serially at various times after an acute stroke showed a marked decrease in the NAA resonance and persistently elevated lactate levels (32). In one case there was a suggestion that the lactate concentration actually decreased following bypass surgery (68). These early reports have been confirmed by other groups (65,69–74) who have shown elevated lactate levels many days after stroke. These spectroscopic findings are in agreement with reports (75,76) of prolonged elevated lactate levels in CSF several days after the infarct occurred. These observations are somewhat puzzling in terms of the discussion presented on the origin of lactate and its rate of clearance from the brain measured in animal models. The Yale group has been active in providing a plausible and important explanation for these observations. There are three major possible explanations for the prolonged

TABLE 2. *Predicted MRS alterations observed in chronic stroke*

State	PCr/Pi	ATP	pH	NAA	Lactate
Reperfused	Normal	Normal	Normal	Normal	Normal
Reversible ischemia	Low	Normal–low	Acidic	Normal?	High
Irreversible ischemia	No ^{31}P metabolites from resident tissue		?	Low	Low unless produced by WBC, activated astrocytes

lactate levels: a trapped pool of lactate which is not turning over metabolically; an ischemic penumbra that continues to produce lactate by glycolysis; and lactate production by the cellular infiltrates (activated macrophages, reactive astrocytes, etc).

There are two reports of the Yale group that indicate that the third explanation is important (77,78). In a patient with a 16-day-old infarct, Petroff et al. (77) found that the regions of the brain that showed elevated levels of lactate on MRS had the highest density of macrophages on histopathology. Rothman et al. (78) used an infusion of ^{13}C-labeled glucose in a patient with a 32-day-old infarct to show that all of the lactate was metabolically turning over, and thus being labeled. These two observations clearly show that the lactate is not "trapped" and may be produced by activated macrophages.

The discussion presented above should serve to reinforce two points concerning the value of clinical MRS. It is clear that the metabolic information contained in the large body of MRS data collected in animal models of cerebral ischemia is critically important in the interpretation of the MRS results found in patients with stroke. Also it is important to consider metabolic manipulations of patients performed in order to test physiological hypotheses in order to augment the understanding of the underlying basis for spectral interpretations.

Birth Asphyxia

^{31}P MRS has been used to study brain metabolism in neonates who have had a suspected hypoxic or ischemic insult, including birth asphyxia, periventricular hemorrhage, and infarction. Results show a definite decrease in the PCr/Pi ratio in areas felt to be affected by the injury (79) (Fig. 27). This has important implications for the prognosis of these patients. Hamilton et al. reported that in a study of 27 infants with ultrasound evidence of hypoxic/ischemic brain injury (hyperechoic area), the patients with PCr/Pi below the 95% confidence limits for normal had a significantly worse outcome than those with PCr/Pi within the normal limits. Nine of 15 patients with abnormal PCr/Pi died and the remaining six had significant areas of brain atrophy. In patients with normal PCr/Pi, none died and three had small areas of atrophy (80). This same group confirmed these results in a larger study of 61 newborn infants with suspected hypoxic/ischemic insults (81). Based on a statistical analysis of the ^{31}P spectra (employing 95% confidence limits for normal as cutoff points) correlated with outcome, these authors concluded that when reduced values for PCr/Pi are found in the brains of infants suspected of hypoxic-ischemic injury, the prognosis for survival without serious neurological impairments is very poor, and that when ATP/total phosphorus ratio is reduced, death is almost inevitable. Thus, ^{31}P MRS appears to be very important in assessing the extent of suspected brain injury in neonates and their long-term prognosis.

Epilepsy

As indicated in Fig. 22, the metabolic consequences of seizure should be an increase in the rate of turnover of ATP manifested by a decrease in the PCr/Pi ratio. If all of the ATP can be produced by oxidative metabolism, there should be no increase in the production of lactate or drop in pH. Prichard has recently presented an overview of the results obtained in animals and patients (82). During seizure discharge, acidosis, reduction of phosphocreatine, and elevation of lactate have all been demonstrated in the human brain (82). These results indicate that the energy demand placed on the region undergoing seizure exceeds the energy available through oxidative metabolism. Since lactate is detected some of the energy demand is being met by glycolysis. Prichard also reported chronic reductions of *N*-acetylaspartate in limbic

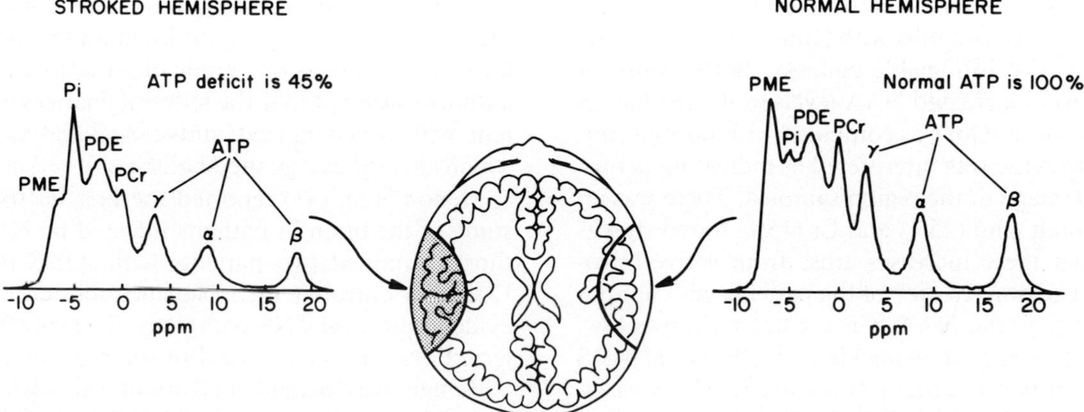

FIG. 27. Acute respiratory distress in a neonate. Note the increased Pi and decreased PCr in the affected area.

regions probably reflecting neuronal loss which may correlate with mesial temporal sclerosis (82).

Weiner and coworkers have employed MR spectroscopic imaging (both ^{1}H and ^{31}P) to determine the focus of seizure (in both temporal and frontal lobe epilepsy) (83–85). The ^{31}P spectra showed reported decreased levels of Pi, decreased levels of PME, and alkalosis in the seizure focus. On ^{1}H MRS, the levels of NAA were reduced substantially and no signals arising from lactate were observed. Rather than employing a statistical analysis of these results based on comparisons made from single peaks, this group proposed the use of a combined spectral parameter which reflected all of the spectral abnormalities observed. Using this approach, this group could correctly identify the focus of seizure in virtually all of the cases studied.

Kuzniecky et al. (86) employed ^{31}P MRS to study patients with temporal lobe epilepsy. In contrast to the findings of Weiner and coworkers, this group found that the values obtained for pH and PME were the same as found in normal controls. The levels of PCr/Pi were reduced by 50% in the affected region as compared with normal controls. This difference was found to be highly statistically significant ($p > 0.005$). The PCr/Pi ratio was reduced by 35% in the affected region when compared with the contralateral region ($p > 0.05$).

Cendes et al. (87) employed ^{1}H MR spectroscopic imaging to study ten patients with temporal lobe epilepsy. Decreased levels of NAA were found in these patients. Although two patients showed NAA levels lower than normal in both temporal lobes, the region showing the lowest levels of NAA always corresponded to the lobe identified by clinical electroencephalography. Eight of these ten patients demonstrated atrophy of their amygdala and hippocampus on MRI. The authors concluded that the spectroscopic imaging approach had advantages over single voxel methods since the site of the lesion was not always known a priori. They also suggested that the ability to identify a region of "maximum metabolic abnormality" should provide a very sensitive method for the identification of the affected site.

Gadian and coworkers (88,89) have employed ^{1}H MR spectroscopy to study adults with temporal lobe epilepsy and children with intractable epilepsy. Both groups of patients showed decreased NAA levels in the medial region of the temporal lobe as compared with normal controls. This decrease was interpreted as indicating neuronal loss or damage in the region sampled. There was an increase in both Cho (25%) and Cr (15%) found. It was suggested that these increases arose from active astrocytosis in the region. In 88% of the patients with temporal lobe epilepsy, the NAA/[Cr + Cho] ratio was low, with 40% of the cases showing bilateral effects. ^{1}H MRS correctly identified the focus of seizure in 15/18 cases. The three incorrect cases had marked evidence for bilateral disease. The authors concluded that ^{1}H MRS could be useful in guiding operative procedures and detecting bilateral abnormalities.

The results discussed above show that there is a consensus regarding the clinical utility of MRS in temporal lobe epilepsy. While there may still be slight disagreements concerning the spectral abnormalities observable in this disease, it is clear that several independent groups have had success in employing MRS to determine the laterality of the focus of seizure. There are indications that this distinction can be made based on decreases in NAA observed by ^{1}H MRS. However, the statistical certainty with which this distinction can be made is probably improved with the use of aggregate spectral parameters of the kind reported by Weiner and coworkers (83–85).

HIV Infection of the CNS

There is a clear rationale for employing MRS in studies of HIV migration to the CNS. It is generally recognized that conventional MRI is not sensitive to the detection of the earliest stages of HIV infection of the brain. The currently accepted "gold standard" for the early detection is based on cognitive dysfunction as assessed by neuropsychological tests. Although HIV infection of the brain is not considered to be a disease which affects neurons in its early stages, there is histopathological evidence suggesting that early in the disease process microglia become infected with the virus. Based on the discussion presented in the previous sections there are suggestions that MRS may be able to detect the metabolic products of activated immune cells. In the intermediate stages of disease there is evidence for neuronal loss which should be reflected in reductions in NAA levels.

Bottomley et al. (90) employed localized ^{31}P MRS to examine 12 patients with mild to moderate AIDS. The absolute concentrations of PCr and NTP were significantly reduced in the centrum semiovale when compared to normal controls (n = 29). It is important to note that the ratios of metabolites were not significantly different between the two groups. The regions in which there were reduced levels of metabolites did not show focal abnormalities or significant atrophy on MRI. The authors suggested that the spectral changes were consistent with a generalized virus-associated toxic process which affected energy metabolism.

Menon et al. (91) reported the first ^{1}H spectroscopic study of the brain in patients infected by HIV. The authors examined two patients with AIDS (Centers for Disease Control (CDC) classification group IV) and evidence of focal CNS pathology. The spectra were collected from a 64-cm^3 voxel in the right parietal region. Although these patients had abnormal MRI, the spectra were taken in areas of normal-appearing white matter. In both cases the spectra showed a marked reduction in the ratio of NAA/Cho and NAA/creatine (NAA/Cr) when compared with control subjects. The authors proposed that the spectral changes in these regions which appear as normal brain on MRI may be attributed to other causes but is most likely to be due to primary HIV infection. The authors first demonstrated the ability of proton MRS to detect brain abnormalities in HIV-infected patients at a stage when it is undetectable by imaging and proposed a possible role for the early selection of patients for treatment with antiviral drugs.

The same group examined 11 patients with HIV infection and varying stages of AIDS dementia complex (ADC) (actually known as HIV-1-associated cognitive/motor complex) (92). In this study, patients with pathology seen on MR imaging that could not be directly attributed to HIV infection of the brain, were excluded from the study. Spectra were obtained from 27 to 64 cm^3 voxels in parieto-temporal regions. Spectra from patients with moderate (stage 2) to severe ADC (stage 3), when compared with spectra from normal volunteers, exhibited significant reductions in NAA/Cr ratio and a tendency toward increased Cho/Cr ratio, although this last trend did not reach statistical significance. Spectra from patients with no ADC (stage 0) or early ADC (stage 1) were not significantly different from normal volunteers.

Many of the patients in this study exhibited abnormalities on MRI, but apart from the presence of atrophy, which was seen in all of the patients with moderate to severe ADC, MRI did not seem to discriminate between patients with and without ADC. The authors concluded that although the NAA/Cr ratio may not be an early or sensitive marker of ADC it may be relatively specific, since all of the patients with significantly low values of this ratio had a clinical diagnosis of ADC.

Meyerhoff et al. (93) examined 14 HIV-seropositive patients, 10 with varying degrees of cognitive impairment and 4 who were cognitively asymptomatic. Spectra were obtained from nine 2.5-cm^3 volumes in the centrum semiovale and the mesial cortex in each patient. Significantly reduced NAA/Cho and NAA/Cr ratios were observed in cognitively impaired subjects versus normal controls, without significant regional differences between the voxels studied. No significant differences were found between groups with cognitive impairment and asymptomatic groups or between asymptomatic and control groups. This study reported diffuse reductions in NAA in individuals with cognitive impairment due to HIV. Most of the patients in this study had normal appearing MRI (80%), suggesting that proton MRS is more sensitive than imaging in assessing the effects of HIV infection on the brain.

This same group followed up the previous study with a report of an additional 13 patients who were cognitively impaired (94). Ten high-risk seronegative homosexual males were used as controls. The levels of NAA/Cr and NAA/Cho were found to be lower in the patients, while the Cho/Cr ratio was the same in the two groups. Six cognitively normal patients had NAA/Cho and NAA/Cr ratios that were similar to those of the controls. The metabolite ratios of the high-risk control group were similar to those found in a heterosexual seronegative low-risk group.

Jarvik et al. (95) examined 11 HIV-seropositive patients without clinical, radiological, or laboratory evidence of CNS infections other than HIV. Voxels of 3.4 to 8 cm^3 were chosen to cover areas of abnormal white matter signal intensity if present or centrum semiovale if the white matter appeared normal at imaging. The analysis of the images showed that there was a significant difference between the patients and control subjects with respect to atrophy, although no significant difference was found between the appearance of the white matter in patients and control subjects. The analysis of the spectra showed that the NAA/Cr ratio was significantly lower and that Cho/Cr and marker peak/Cr (marker peak was defined as the resonances between 2.1 to 2.6 ppm) ratios were significantly higher in patients as compared with control subjects. The authors calculated an aggregate score that combined these three ratios. This aggregate score proved to be a good discriminator between the patient and control populations ($p = 0.001$).

The aggregate scores were abnormal (< 2 SDs from the mean of the control subjects) in 13 of 15 patients' spectra (87%), while 8 of 11 patients (73%) had abnormal MR images. Moreover, only 1 of 10 control spectra (10%) was abnormal while 4 of 11 controls (36%) had abnormal imaging. These results suggested that MRS may be more sensitive and specific than MR imaging in detecting CNS involvement in HIV-infected patients.

Chong et al. (96) reported the largest study in which proton MRS was performed in 103 HIV-seropositive patients and 23 control subjects. Spectra were collected from an 8-cm^3 voxel placed in a normal parieto-occipital region of the brain using a spin-echo sequence (PRESS), TR of 1600 msec, and TE of 135 msec. In the first part of the study, the spectra of HIV-seropositive patients were compared and correlated with clinical, immunologic, and radiologic measures of HIV infection. A significant reduction in the NAA/Cr ratio was seen in patients with late-stage disease (CDC group IV). The NAA/Cr and NAA/Cho ratios were also reduced in patients with CD4 counts < 200/mm^3 and in patients with neurologic signs. Significant increases in Cho/Cr ratios were seen in patients with low CD4 counts and abnormal MR images. Reduced NAA ratios correlated with diffuse but not focal MR imaging abnormalities. In the second part of the study the authors evaluated the utility of combining the results of MR imaging and spectroscopy, finding that the combination of both modalities provides closer relationships to clinical and immunologic measures of disease than either modality alone. Moreover, abnormal spectra correlated more with abnormal neurologic findings than did abnormal MR images suggesting that spectroscopy may be sensitive to changes in cerebral chemistry that are clinically relevant and are not apparent on MR images.

The same authors (97) studied 43 HIV-seropositive patients, including 26 who had clinical or radiologic evidence of late-stage disease (CDC group IV) and 17 in the early stages of infection (CDC groups II and III). Using the same sequence described above, spectra were obtained from an 8-cm^3 voxel placed in a normal parieto-occipital region of the brain. When patients grouped by different criteria were compared, a significant reduction in the NAA/(NAA + Cho + Cr) ratio was found in patients in the late stage of the disease as compared with those in early-stage disease. This ratio was lower in patients with HIV-1-associated cognitive/motor complex as compared with patients who were neurologically healthy. Also this ratio was decreased in patients with abnormal MR images (diffuse white matter abnormalities) as compared with those with normal-appearing white matter. When patients were compared with healthy control subjects, the NAA/(NAA + Cho + Cr) ratios were significantly higher in control subjects than in CDC group II and III patients and also significantly higher than in all seropositive patients with normal MR imaging. The authors noted, however, that the control group was younger and so these last results may be influenced by the expected decrease in NAA levels which parallel neuronal loss with age. The authors reported the first follow-up spectroscopic study performed in 15 patients between 3 and 8 months after their initial studies. A significant reduction in NAA/(NAA + Cho + Cr) ratio was observed at follow-up study when compared with the initial examinations.

The results of all of the studies of HIV are summarized in Table 3. A common finding in all of the studies on HIV infection of the brain is the reduced level of NAA. This finding is consistent with the pathologic evidence of neuronal loss reported in HIV-1-infected patients. Another common finding, although not present in all of the studies, is the increase in Cho/Cr ratio. Choline, which resonates at 3.2 ppm, is an important precursor of cell membrane synthesis and is often found to be elevated in tissues that are rapidly regenerating or undergoing membrane disruption. The significance of the elevation in Cho/Cr ratio remains uncertain. A possible interpretation for this increase in HIV-1-infected patients is that the increased Cho may not directly arise from changes in neurons but may result from metabolic alterations in glial or inflammatory cells. An alternate interpretation is that the increase in Cho/Cr ratio combined with the increase in marker/Cr ratio, also observed in these patients, may reflect myelin damage. Choline phosphoglycerides contribute 11.2% of myelin lipids with phosphatidylcholine being the most abundant. Therefore, as myelin damage occurs free choline may be released increasing the choline resonance detected by MRS. The "marker peak," region between 2.1 and 2.6 ppm, may be a combination of nonspecific amino acids and possibly myelin catabolites which may increase with myelin breakdown. Both explanations for the increase in Cho/Cr ratio are consistent with the neuropathologic finding of inflammatory infiltrates and white matter abnormalities in the brain of HIV-1-infected patients. An alternative explanation proposed for the increase in this ratio is the decrease in Cr resonance. The decrease in creatine pool may indicate impairment of cellular metabolism in the brain of these patients and is supported by the decrease in PCr peak observed in phosphorus MRS studies.

Abnormal proton spectra may be found in normal-appearing white matter on imaging suggesting that MRS may be more sensitive than MRI in detecting CNS involvement in HIV-1-infected patients. Moreover, MRS seems to be a better discriminator between the patient and control populations than MRI suggesting that MRS may be also more specific. When individuals displaying different manifestations of illness were compared, the abnormalities in the spectra correlated with the presence and the severity of the cognitive impairment and with clinical and immunologic measures of late-stage disease. These findings suggest that MRS may serve as an indicator of the degree of CNS involvement. MRS may serve to monitor the course of disease progression and may have a prognostic role regarding CNS involvement. This modality may provide a sensitive method for the early detection of HIV migration to the CNS. Finally, MRS can be employed in longitudinal studies to monitor the response to therapy, and thus may lead to individual optimized treatment effectiveness.

Dementias

The rationale for employing MRS to study dementias is based on the ability of proton MRS to detect neuronal loss and on the fact that the precise differential diagnosis of these conditions remains a clinical challenge. It is also important to note that some of the genetic markers which define high-risk populations for these diseases have been identified. This places an enormous stress on the development of methods with which to identify the earliest signs of the disease and monitor response to therapy.

Alzheimer's Dementia

Pettegrew and coworkers have reported the results of several studies using localized ^{31}P MRS to investigate patients with Alzheimer's dementia (AD) (98–102). Patients with AD exhibited increased levels of PME and decreased levels of PCr compared to normal controls. The increase in PME has been interpreted in terms of

TABLE 3. *A summary of the proton MRS findings in HIV*

Study	Patients(p)/ Controls(c)	Stage[a]	Clinical evidence of[b] CNS involvement	MRI findings[c]	MRS sequence and parameters	MRS findings	Groups statistically distinguished by MRS
Menon et al., 1990	2p/6c	Late-stage 2	Cogn. imp. + focal signs 1 Focal signs 1	Focals lesions not attributed to HIV 2	MESA TR-2000/TE-270 V = 64 cm^3 normal parietal region	↓ NAA/Cho ↓ NAA/Cr	Patients/controls
Menon et al., 1992	11p/8c	Late stage 10 Early-stage 1	Cogn. imp. (ADC) 7 No cogn. imp. 4	Abnormal 9 Normal 2	MESA TR-2000/TE-270 V = 27–64 cm^3 parieto-temporal region	↓ NAA/Cr ↑ Cho/Cr (NS)	ADC stage 2/3/ controls
Meyerhoff et al., 1993	14p/7c	Late-stage 4 Early-stage 10	Cogn. imp. 10 No cogn. imp. 4	Abnormal 3 Normal 11	CSI V = 2.5 cm^3 centrum semiovale and mesial cortex	↓ NAA/Cr ↓ NAA/Cho	Cogn. imp./controls
Jarvik et al., 1993	11p/8c	Late-stage 4 Early-stage 7	Cogn. imp. 9 No cogn. imp. 2	Abnormal 8 Normal 3	STEAM TR-2000/TE-19/ TM-10.6 V = 3.4–8 cm^3 abnormal white matter or centrum semiovale	↓ NAA/Cr ↑ Cho/Cr ↑ Marker peak/Cr	Patients/controls
Chong et al., 1993[d]	103p/23c	Late-stage 70 Early-stage 22	Neurlogic signs 19 No neurologic signs 31	Abnormal 34[e] Normal 36	PRESS TR-1600/TE-135 V = 8 cm^3 normal parieto-occipital region	↓ NAA/Cr ↓ NAA/Cho ↑ Cho/CR	Late-stage/early-stage <CD4 count/>CD4 count Neurologic signs/no neurologic signs Abnormal MRI/normal MRI
Chong et al., 1994[d]	43p/8c	Late-stage 26 Early-stage 17	Cogn. imp. (HIV-1-associated cognitive/ motor complex) 6 No cogn. imp. 14	Abnormal 9 Normal 34	PRESS TR-1600/TE-135 V = 8 cm^3 normal parieto-occipital region	↓ NAA/NAA + Cho + Cr	Late stage/early stage Cogn. imp./no cogn. imp. Abnormal MRI/normal MRI Early-stage/controls Normal MRI patients/ controls

[a] Stage: late stage refers to CDC group IV, early stage to CDC groups II and III.

[b] ADC, AIDS dementia complex, actually known as HIV-1-associated cognitive/motor complex; Cogn. imp., cognitive impairment.

[c] Abnormal MRI: abnormalities were either gray matter atrophy or white matter signal changes.

[d] Not all of the subjects had complete neurological examinations.

[e] Some of the patients (33) were excluded because they exhibited focal lesions on MRI.

defects in membrane metabolism in these patients. As the dementia worsens, the level of PME decreases and the level of PCr increases. The authors suggested that the changes in energy metabolites with increasing dementia could be a consequence of nerve terminal degeneration and pointed out that these results are consistent with previous PET findings.

The same group employed ^{31}P MRS to successfully distinguish patients with AD from patients with multiple subcortical infarctions (MSID) based on spectral profiles. The MSID patients demonstrated elevations in the PCr/Pi ratio in both the temporoparietal and frontal regions. PME and the ratio of PME to PDE were elevated in the temporoparietal region of AD. Pi was also elevated in the frontal and temporoparietal regions of AD. These ^{31}P MR spectral profiles were accurate in distinguishing MSID from AD. Values of PCr/Pi accurately classified 100% of the MSID patients and 92% of the AD patients. When Pi and PME were considered jointly, MRS also accurately classified all of the MSID group and all but one of the AD group.

Bottomley et al. (103) also employed ^{31}P to study patients with AD. In contrast to the previous discussion, these authors found no differences in metabolite ratios between patients and normal controls.

Pettegrew and coworkers (104) have also used high resolution ^{1}H NMR on extracts of samples of brain tissue in patients with AD to identify the metabolites present. The analysis of perchloric acid extracts of 12 AD and 5 control brain samples indicated no significant changes in taurine, aspartate, or glutamine. The level of NAA was lower in AD samples than controls, and this decrease correlated with the number of senile plaques and neurofibrillary tangles in adjacent tissue sections. Glutamate levels were higher in AD patients, and showed an inverse correlation with NAA levels. The levels of GABA were lower in the AD samples. The authors suggested that the lower levels of NAA were indicative of neuronal loss. If the remaining neurons were exposed to the imbalance of glutamate and GABA this might result in further neuronal damage.

Miller et al. (105) used the STEAM sequence to acquire proton spectra from 10–15-ml voxels in white matter located in the parietal area (WM) and gray matter (GM) in the occipital cortex of patients with AD. Summed spectra are shown in Fig. 28. They reported an increased myo-inositol/creatine (MI/Cr) ratio, which suggested abnormalities in the inositol polyphosphate messenger pathway, and reduced NAA/Cr in AD compared to controls. The difference in NAA/Cr level was small but statistically significant in both WM and GM voxels. The increase in MI/Cr was more prominent especially in GM. However, there was no correlation between the severity of the disease and spectroscopic findings.

This same group has carried out a thorough investigation of the relaxation times and concentrations (both relative and absolute) in ten patients with probable AD (106). There was a 50% increase observed in myo-inositol in the AD patients. In these patients, the levels of NAA were lower in occipital GM. There was also a decrease observed in the manifold of glutamate/glutamine resonances. The levels of glucose were found to be increased. The level of choline was found to be about the same as for age-matched controls.

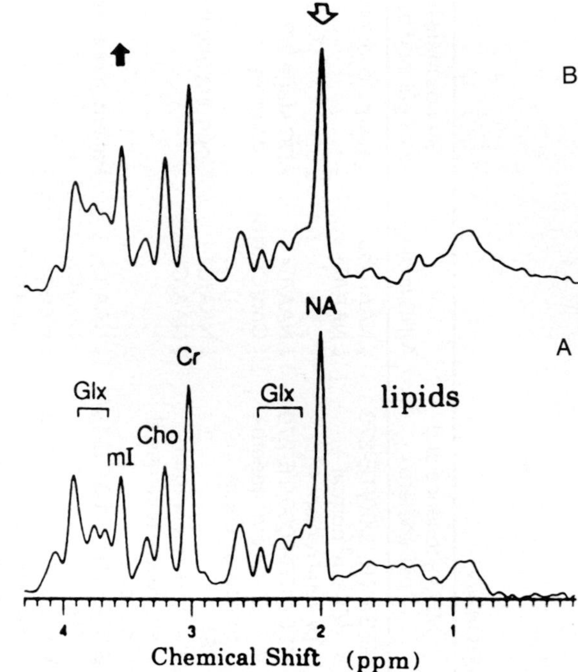

FIG. 28. Representative summed solvent-suppressed proton spectra obtained using the STEAM sequence (TR = 1500, TE = 30) from normal volunteers (n = 8) (**A**) and patients with AD (n = 8) (**B**). (From Miller et al., ref. 105, with permission.)

Schiino et al. (107) studied a patient group (n = 9) with primary degenerative dementia (PDD) that included 7 patients with probable AD, 3 normal pressure hydrocephalus (NPH), and healthy controls. The DRY STEAM technique was applied with a TR of 2500 msec, TE of 19, and TM of 5.7 msec. The ratio of NAA/Cr was significantly reduced in patients with PDD with no significant brain atrophy or reduction in regional blood flow detected by SPECT. There was no reduction of NAA/Cr in NPH. These authors concluded that, in the appropriate clinical setting, proton MRS was a useful measure for the early detection and study of PDD.

Meyerhoff et al. (108) used ^{1}H spectroscopic imaging to study 8 patients with probable AD. A group of 10 age-matched controls was used for comparison. Since the spectra were obtained over the whole brain, the authors could compare the regional distributions of metabolites. Under the acquisition conditions employed, the method detected three major resonances: NAA, Cho, and Cr. The NAA/Cr ratio was found to be lower in the white matter of the patients. In these regions the Cho/Cr ratio was normal. In mesial GM regions the NAA/Cho ratio was lower than normal and the Cho/Cr ratio was elevated. Similar observations were made in the posterior regions of the centrum semiovale. In these regions the level of NAA was normal suggesting that the level of Cho was elevated. This observation is in contrast with the results obtained by Ross and coworkers (see above). The elevated Cho levels were interpreted in terms of membrane alterations in both gray and white matter in the patients with AD.

Parkinson's Disease

Shiino et al. (107) examined two patients with Parkinson's disease (PD) using proton MRS. Spectra were acquired from a 27-cm^3 voxel located in the insular area of the brain. A decrease in the NAA/Cr ratio was observed in the two patients with PD when compared with control subjects. Even though the mean age in the control group was lower, the authors observed that there were no age-related changes in the mean area ratio of NAA/Cr in this group. Both PD patients exhibited marked atrophy on MRI and since the spectra were obtained from voxels placed in the insular area, these results should be interpreted with caution.

Huntington's Disease

Jenkins et al. (109) reported the results of a proton MRS study in a series of Huntington's disease (HD) patients. Sixteen patients with clinical signs of definite HD and confirmed family history and two individuals without neurologic affectation but with linked DNA markers indicating a high probability to have inherited the HD gene were examined. Proton spectroscopy was performed using a STEAM sequence with TR of 2000 msec, TE of 272 msec, and TM of 10 msec. Spectra were collected from a 15.6-cm^3 voxel placed over the visual cortex and from a 5.4- to 20-cm^3 voxel placed in basal ganglia. A 5-inch surface coil was used to study the occipital cortex and the quadrature head coil was used for studies of the basal ganglia. Elevated lactate levels were observed in the occipital cortex in all of the symptomatic patients when compared with normal controls. The lactate level correlated with the duration of illness. Lactate levels were normal in the two asymptomatic subjects. In the basal ganglia the levels of NAA were decreased and the levels of Cho elevated, relative to creatine. Several patients also showed elevated lactate levels in the basal ganglia. The authors suggested that the increase in lactate may be explained by a defect in oxidative phosphorylation in HD. This possibility is supported by biochemical studies that have reported reduced mitochondrial enzyme activity in HD patients, and ultrastructural studies that have shown abnormalities in the mitochondria of these patients. The reduced NAA and increased Cho were interpreted in these patients to result from neuronal loss and gliosis. The authors suggested that lactate likely precedes neuronal death and that this may be the explanation for the more variable lactate elevation in the basal ganglia where evidence of more neuronal loss and gliosis was found. On this basis, they proposed that the elevated lactate may provide a simple marker to monitor the progression of the disease and possible therapies for HD patients.

High resolution proton MRS was employed by Nicoli et al. (110) to study CSF and serum metabolic samples obtained from patients with HD. Serum and CSF samples were collected from 11 patients suffering from HD and 12 reference patients suffering from miscellaneous neurological diseases. A significant increase in the pyruvate concentration in CSF was found in patients with HD. This finding may be explained by the decrease of pyruvate-dehydrogenase and Krebs cycle enzyme activity observed in HD patients. This observation is consistent, as was the finding of elevated lactate reported by Jenkins et al. (109), with the hypothesis of the existence of a defect in oxidative phosphorylation present in this disease.

Brain Tumors

Another clinical area in which MRS has been applied is the study of brain tumors. This field has been recently reviewed by Negendank (111). An early study of ^{31}P MRS of human neuroblastoma had suggested that there was a significant increase in the PME peak associated with malignant as opposed to benign tumors (59). This finding raised speculation that this elevated PME may be a general fingerprint of malignant tumors. ^{31}P MRS studies since that time have shown that this is not the case. There does not appear to be a specific ^{31}P MRS fingerprint of brain tumors (111). A summary of the results as reviewed by Negendank (111) is given in Table 4. An alkaline shift in the pH does appear to be a consistent finding. Often, there is a decrease in the PCr/Pi ratio. One rationale for using ^{31}P MRS is to determine whether a tumor is hypoxic since it is believed that hypoxic tumors are less responsive to radiation treatment. These tumors might be candidates for radiation-sensitizing agents. Thus, although ^{31}P MRS has not yet been shown to provide information that will help make a specific diagnosis of brain tumors, it does provide some metabolic data that may help in planning therapy.

^{1}H MRS has also been applied to the study of brain tumors. This technique is very appealing since it does not require a change in the resonant frequency of the rf coil when switching from MRI, and the increased sensitivity

TABLE 4. *A summary of the ^{31}P MRS profiles of primary brain tumors*

Tumor	High PME	Low PDE	Low Pi	Low PCr
Low-grade glial	0.10 (31)	0.26 (27)	0.0 (22)	0.21 (29)
High-grade glial	0.29 (48)	0.81 (41)	0.07 (30)	0.47 (045)
Meningiomas	0.55 (22)	0.96 (29)	0.40 (10)	0.96 (29)
Pituitary adenomas	1.00 (4)	0.75 (4)	0.75 (4)	1.00 (4)

From Negendank, ref. 111.
The number given is the fraction of total cases with the profile described in each category. The value in parentheses is the total number of cases analyzed.

enables spectra from smaller voxels to be measured in shorter periods of time. The ^{1}H spectra from most tumors are very different from those in normal brain. A summary of the results obtained by ^{1}H as reviewed by Negendank is presented in Table 5. One feature of most brain tumor spectra is a decrease in the NAA signal relative to normal brain. As previously discussed, NAA is found primarily in the neuronal cells, and any tumor that replaces the normal neurons can be expected to reduce the NAA level. Unfortunately, this is not a specific feature of neoplasia since any pathologic condition that causes neuronal loss will cause this same spectroscopic finding. Other spectral abnormalities have been reported in various types of brain tumors. Meningiomas, in addition to lowered NAA, are reported to have lowered Cr, only a mild elevation of lactate, and a prominent choline peak. The ^{1}H spectrum of gliomas tends to be dependent on the grade of the tumor. Low-grade gliomas are reported to have decreased, but detectable, NAA and Cr with a moderate increase in lactate. Higher-grade gliomas tend to have decreased NAA, lower Cr, increased Cho, and more significant elevations of the lactate peak.

Multiple Sclerosis

There have been several studies which have employed proton MRS to study MS plaques. This is potentially an important area for MRS since MRS can in principle provide a biochemical basis for plaque characterization and evolution. At this time, however, although the data reported in the literature have shown a variety of interesting results it may be premature to arrive at a consensus regarding the ultimate role of MRS. This may be a result of the heterogeneous nature of the disease or the fact that the spectral data have been acquired with different pulse sequences, localization methods, and echo delays.

Wolinski et al. (112) monitored 28 plaques in 13 patients with MS. Resonances consistent with the presence of cholesterol and/or fatty acids were observed in 5 of 21 interpretable spectra. In one of the patients who was followed serially, these additional resonances disappeared after 2 weeks. The authors concluded that demyelination was a dynamic process based on the changing level of cholesterol and/or fatty acids and suggested serial monitoring of plaques in patients with MS. Gd-DTPA was not utilized in this imaging protocol. Narayana et al. (113) later studied patients with lesions that enhanced after injection of Gd-DTPA. This group observed prominent resonances in the 0.5–2.0 ppm region in six of nine enhancing lesions. They speculated that these resonances arose in lipids and other myelin breakdown products. In their cohort of enhancing lesions, there was no significant decrease in NAA.

Matthews et al. (114) examined seven patients with MS. In three patients with moderate to severe chronic disability, the NAA/creatine ratio was lower (1.6–2.0) than observed in normals (2.4–2.9). In three of four patients with minimal or no disability, the NAA/creatine ratio was normal. No lipid resonances were observed in any of the patients studied. The authors attributed the decrease in the NAA/creatine ratio to cumulative irreversible tissue damage rather than a response to acute inflammation. Based on these results, the authors suggested that: (i) in hyperacute plaques, the metabolite ratios would be unchanged; (ii) demyelinating plaques would exhibit increased choline/creatine; and (iii) subacute to chronic plaques would have decreased NAA/creatine ratios. Gd-DTPA was not utilized in this protocol. The same authors employed MRS in a longitudinal study of 7 patients with MS (4 with recurrent relapses and 3 with a secondary progressive course) (115). MRS

TABLE 5. *A summary of the profiles of metabolites of brain tumors on ^{1}H MRS*

Tumor	High Cho	Low Cr	Low NAA	High Lac
Low-grade glial	0.70 (40)	0.50 (16)	0.78 (40)	0.65 (40)
High-grade glial	0.71 (55)	0.79 (29)	0.96 (55)	0.80 (55)
Meningiomas	0.95 (19)	0.76 (17)	0.89 (19)	0.12 (17)
Neurinomas	1.00 (3)	1.00 (3)	1.00 (3)	1.00 (3)
Lymphomas	0.50 (2)	0.00 (2)	1.00 (2)	0.00 (2)
Metastases	0.60 (10)	0.83 (6)	0.80 (10)	0.90 (6)

From Negendank, ref. 111.
The number given is the fraction of total cases with the profile described in each category. The value in parentheses is the total number of cases analyzed.

examinations were performed every six months. Initially the NAA/Cr ratio was lower than normal in the patients compared to normal controls. This ratio decreased in subsequent studies while the lesion volumes determined from MRI and disability scores did not change significantly. The changes in NAA/Cr between successive 6-month intervals showed a significant correlation with lesion volume in the relapsing patients.

Van Hecke et al. studied 18 patients with MS (116). These patients showed a significant reduction in NAA relative to normals. These investigators did not employ Gd-DTPA to separate the enhancing from the unenhancing lesions.

Larsson et al. (117) employed proton MRS to study 15 patients with acute or chronic multiple sclerosis. Some of the patients were investigated serially, being given a total of 22 spectroscopic investigations. Resonances corresponding to free lipids were observed in six plaques. This was distinctly seen in two plaques at 70 and 85 days after the occurrence of the plaques. A lower content of lipids in plaques was observed as early as day 10 and as late as nearly 1 year after occurrence. The relative concentration of NAA was significantly lower in patients than in controls, and the relative concentration of choline was significantly higher in patients than in controls. The authors suggested that these differences were most pronounced in older plaques. MR spectroscopic demonstration of lipids in an MS plaque probably reflects disintegration of myelin, and a decreased NAA/Cho ratio may be related either to gliosis or to axonal degeneration, which sometimes occurs in longstanding MS.

Husted et al. (118,119) studied 13 subjects with clinically definite MS with both ^{1}H and ^{31}P CSI, and 19 controls were studied with either ^{1}H, ^{31}P MRS, or both. MS lesion, MS normal-appearing white matter, and region-matched control spectra from the centrum semiovale were analyzed. The major findings of this study were that in both white matter lesions and normal-appearing white matter in patients with MS, the metabolite ratio NAA/creatine and the total ^{31}P-peak integrals were significantly reduced compared with controls. In addition, in MS lesions NAA/Cho and phosphodiesters/total ^{31}P were significantly reduced compared with controls, and in MS normal-appearing white matter there was a trend for NAA/Cho to be reduced compared with controls. In normal-appearing white matter in patients with MS, total creatine and phosphocreatine were significantly increased compared to controls, as detected with both ^{1}H (total creatine peak integrals) and ^{31}P (phosphocreatine/total ^{31}P) CSI techniques. These results suggest reduced neuronal density and altered phospholipid metabolites in white matter lesions in patients with MS.

Grossman et al. (120) examined 16 patients with a total of 21 lesions. They demonstrated decreased levels of NAA in 17 of the 21 lesions. No correlation was found between NAA concentration and degree of enhancement with Gd-DTPA. Extra peaks were observed between 2.1 and 2.6 ppm ranging in concentration from 10–50 mM protons. This region corresponds to areas of known amino acid resonance including GABA and glutamate. As these peaks were observed in 5 of 7 enhancing lesions and enhancement is thought to correlate with lesion activity, these authors termed these peaks, "marker peaks," representing markers of demyelination.

Hiehle et al. (121) took the analysis of these marker peaks a step further. Eleven patients with clinically diagnosed MS were independently evaluated with both MRS and magnetization transfer (MT). Only two of the eleven lesions enhanced. The MT ratio of white matter lesions in MS was markedly decreased with the lowest values seen in lesions that enhance. A linear inverse relationship was seen between the degree of MT ratio and concentration of the marker peaks. There was no correlation between MT ratio and the concentration of NAA.

CONCLUSIONS AND FUTURE DIRECTIONS

There has been a dramatic increase in the number of studies reported which have employed MRS in the clinical setting. This increase has primarily involved reports which have employed ^{1}H MRS in the brain. A major reason for the increased emphasis on ^{1}H MRS is the fact that there have been major technical improvements made by all commercial manufacturers in terms of the acquisition of high-quality ^{1}H MR spectra of the brain. These improvements have made ^{1}H MRS almost as routine as many MRI studies. There are still efforts underway to further improve and automate these spectral methods. One area of intense investigation is the development of robust CSI methods for ^{1}H which can be performed at both long and short echo delays. There are efforts underway to provide automated methods for data analysis. These methods are necessary for two reasons: to remove operator bias and to analyze the large volume of data generated by CSI studies. Methods to analyze spectra in terms of absolute as well as relative concentrations are being developed. We expect that all of these developments will continue to improve the quality of the MRS study.

As was implied in many of the discussions of disease, MRS provides a bridge between imaging and metabolism. In the case of ^{1}H this bridge is not completed leaving several important scientific challenges. The precise biochemical role(s) of many of the compounds detected by ^{1}H remains unclear. Although there is a consensus that NAA is a marker for neuronal integrity, its biochemical function is unknown. In fact it is possible that it may have a different role in gray matter than in white matter. The rate of turnover of NAA is still unknown. As a result, we cannot rule out the possibility that there may be conditions under which transient changes in NAA occur. For these reasons as we focus our efforts on improving the acquisition of the spectral data we must also strengthen our efforts in providing a better biochemical interpretation of the spectral alterations observed. There have been significant improvements made in ^{31}P MRS. The examples provided in Figs. 12–14 demonstrate the improvements possible through the use of "digitally crafted" rf pulses. We previously highlighted the results reported by den Hollander and Luytens and coworkers (122) as clearly indicating the potential improvements possible for ^{31}P available through proton decoupling of the ^{31}P spectrum. These improvements have been implemented in conjunction with CSI methods by Murphy-Boesch et al. (123).

There has been an increased interest in employing higher field 3–4 T whole-body scanners in MRS studies. It is clear that the increased S/N available at higher field is of benefit to MRS. The increased chemical shift dispersion available at higher field has resulted in the better interpretation of solvent-suppressed proton spectroscopy. Increasing the field strength alone, however, may result in minimal reductions in the linear dimensions of these voxels since the S/N scales almost linearly with the field and the linear dimensions will be reduced by a factor proportional to the cube root of the S/N increase.

We have presented several examples of diseases in which MRS plays an important role. The ability of MRS to provide biochemical information from specific regions of tissue guarantees its potential in the clinical setting. As indicated by some of the diseases discussed, there are already applications in which there is clinically relevant information provided by MRS that cannot be obtained by any other modality.

It is clear that over the past five years there has been a great deal of progress. Over the next five years it is almost certain that MRS will become increasingly important in diagnosing and treating diseases of the CNS.

REFERENCES

1. Purcell EM, Torrey HC, Pound RV. Resonance absorption by nuclear magnetic moments in solids. *Phys Rev* 1946;69:37–38.
2. Bloch R, Hansen WW, Packard M. Nuclear induction. *Phys Rev* 1946;69:127.
3. Proctor WG, Yu FC. The dependence of nuclear magnetic resonance frequency upon chemical compound. *Phys Rev* 1950;70: 717.
4. Odeblad E, Lindstrom G. Some preliminary observations on the proton magnetic resonance in biologic samples. *Acta Radiol* 1966;43:469–476.
5. Weiner MW. The promise of magnetic resonance spectroscopy for medical diagnosis. *Invest Radiol* 1988;23:253–261.
6. Bottomley PA. Human in vivo NMR spectroscopy in diagnostic medicine: clinical tool or research probe? *Radiology* 1989;170:1–15.
7. Radda GK, Rajagopalan B, Taylor DJ. Biochemistry in vivo: an appraisal of clinical magnetic resonance spectroscopy. *Magn Reson Q* 1989;5:122–151.
8. Burt CT, Glonek T, Barney M. Analysis of phosphate metabolites, the intracellular ph, and the state of adenosine triphosphate in intact muscle by phosphorus nuclear magnetic resonance. *J Biol Chem* 1976;252:2584–2591.
9. Pettegrew JW, Withers G, Panchalingam K, et al. Considerations for brain pH assessment by ^{31}P NMR. *Magn Reson Imaging* 1988; 6:135–142.
10. Frahm J, Bruhn H, Gyngell ML, et al. Localized high resolution proton NMR spectroscopy using stimulated echos: initial applications to human brain in vivo. *Magn Reson Med* 1989;9:79–93.
11. Bottomley PA. Spatial localization in NMR spectroscopy in vivo. In: Cohen SM, ed. *Physiological NMR Spectroscopy: From Isolated Cells to Man*, vol 508. New York: Annals New York Academy of Science; 1987;333–348.
12. den Hollander JA, Luyten PR. Image-guided ^{1}H and ^{31}P NMR spectroscopy of humans. In: Cohen SM, ed. *Physiological NMR Spectroscopy: From Isolated Cells to Man*, vol 508. New York: Annals New York Academy of Science; 1987;386–397.
13. Rothman DL, Behar KL, Hetherington HP, et al. ^{1}H-observe/^{13}C-decouple spectroscopic measurements of lactate and glutamate in the rat brain in vivo. *Proc Natl Acad Sci U S A* 1985;82: 1633–1637.
14. Ramsey NF, Purcell. Interactions between nuclear spins in molecules. *Phys Rev* 1952;85:143–144.
15. Bloembergen N, Purcell EM, Pound RV. Relaxation effects in nuclear magnetic resonance absorption. *Phys Rev* 1948;73:679–713.
16. Abragam A. *The Principles of Nuclear Magnetism*. New York: Oxford University Press; 1961.
17. Gupta RK, Benovic JL, Rose BZ. The determination of free magnesium level in the human red blood cell by ^{31}P NMR. *J Biol Chem* 1978;253:6172–6176.
18. Vink R, McIntosh TK, Demediuk P, Weiner MW, Faden AI. Decline in intracellular free Mg^{2+} is associated with irreversible tissue injury after brain trauma. *J Biol Chem* 1988;263:757–761.
19. Williams GD, Mosher TJ, Smith MB. Simultaneous determination of intracellular magnesium and pH from the three ^{31}P NMR chemical shifts of ATP. *Anal Biochem* 1993;214:458–467.
20. Sandstrom J. *Dynamic NMR Spectroscopy*. New York: Academic Press; 1982.
21. Aue WP. Localization methods for in vivo nuclear magnetic resonance spectroscopy. *Rev Magn Reson Med* 1986;1:21–72.
22. Narayana PA, DeLayre JL. In: Partain CL, Price RR, Patton JA, Kulkarni MV, James AE Jr, eds. *Magnetic Resonance Imaging, 2nd ed. vol II. Physical Principles and Instrumentation*. Philadelphia: WB Saunders; 1988:1609.
23. Bollinger L, Lenkinski RE. Localization in clinical MR spectroscopy. In: Berliner LJ, Reuben J, eds. *Biological Magnetic Resonance*, vol 11. New York: Plenum Press; 1992.
24. den Hollander JA, Luyten PR, Marien AJH, et al. Potentials of quantitative image-localized human ^{31}P nuclear magnetic resonance spectroscopy in the clinical evaluation of intracranial tumors. *Magn Reson Q* 1989;5:152–168.
25. Albrand JP, Foray MF, Decorps M. ^{31}P NMR measurements of T2 relaxation times of ATP with surface coils: suppression of j modulation. *Magn Reson Med* 1986;3:941–945.
26. Aue WP, Mueller S, Cross TA, et al. Volume selective excitation. A novel approach to topical NMR. *J Magn Reson* 1984;56:350–354.
27. Haase A. Localization of unaffected spins in NMR imaging and spectroscopy (LOCUS spectroscopy). *Magn Reson Med* 1986;3: 963–969.
28. Bottomley PA, Foster TB, Darrow RB. Depth-resolved surface-coil spectroscopy (DRESS) for in vivo H-1, P-31 and C-13 NMR. *J Magn Reson* 1984;59:338–342.
29. Leigh JS, Haselgrove JC. Chemical shift imaging using Hadamard encoding. *Abstracts of the Proceedings of the Fourth Annual Meeting of the Society of Magnetic Resonance in Medicine*, August 1985. Berkeley, CA: Society of Magnetic Resonance in Medicine; 1986:164.
30. Ordridge RJ, Connelly A, Lohman JAB. Image-selected in vivo

spectroscopy (ISIS). A new technique for spatially selective NMR spectroscopy. *J Magn Reson* 1986;66:283–294.

31. Luyten PR, Marien AJH, Systma B, et al. Solvent suppressed spatially resolved spectroscopy: an approach to high resolution NMR on a whole body MR system. *J Magn Reson* 1986;67:148–155.
32. Bruhn H, Frahm J, Gyngell ML, et al. Cerebral metabolism in man after acute stroke: new observations using localized proton NMR spectroscopy. *Magn Reson Med* 1989;9:126–131.
33. Bottomley PA. Selective Volume Method for Performing Localized NMR Spectroscopy. U.S. Patent 4 480 228; 1984.
34. Shinnar M, Bolinger L, Leigh JS. The use of finite impulse response filters in pulse design. *Magn Reson Med* 1989;12:81–87.
35. Shinnar M, Bolinger L, Leigh JS. The synthesis of soft pulses with a specified frequency response. *Magn Reson Med* 1989;12:88–92.
36. Shinnar M, Leigh JS. The application of spinors to pulse synthesis and analysis. *Magn Reson Med* 1989;12:93–98.
37. Pauly J, Le Roux P, Nishimura D, Macovski A. Parameter selection for the Shinnar-Le Roux excitation pulse design algorithm. *IEEE Trans Med Imaging* 1991;10:53–65.
38. Spielman D, Pauly J, Macovski A, Enzmann D. Spectroscopic imaging with multidimensional pulses for excitation: SIMPLE. *Magn Reson Med* 1991;19:67–84.
39. Conolly S, Pauly J, Nishimura D, Macovski A. Two-dimensional selective adiabatic pulses. *Magn Reson Med* 1992;24:302–313.
40. Lim KO, Pauly J, Webb P, Hurd R, Macovski A. Short TE phosphorus spectroscopy using a spin-echo pulse. *Magn Reson Med* 1994;32:98–103.
41. Meyer RA, Sweeney AH, Kushmerick MJ. A simple analysis of the 'phosphocreatine shuttle.' *Am J Physiol* 1984;246:365
42. Schnall MD. *Multinuclear NMR Studies of Cat Brain Metabolism* [Thesis, 1986]. Philadelphia, PA: University of Pennsylvania.
43. Veech RL, Lawson RL, Cornell NW, Krebs HA. Cytosolic phosphorylation potential. *J Biol Chem* 1979;254:6538.
44. Chance B, Leigh JS Jr, Clark BJ, et al.. Control of oxidative metabolism and oxygen delivery in human skeletal muscle: a steady state analysis of the work/energy cost transfer function. *Proc Natl Acad Sci USA* 1985;82:8384.
45. Michaelis L, Menten M. Die kinetic der intervertasewirkung. *Biochem Z* 1913;49:333.
46. Chance B, Leigh JS, Kent J, et al. Multiple controls of oxidative metabolism in living tissues as studied by phosphorus magnetic resonance. *Proc Natl Acad Sci U S A* 1986;83:9458.
47. Chance B, Smith D, Nioka S, et al. Nature of ischemic injury. In: Cerra F, Shoemaker WC, eds. *Critical Care: State of the Art*, vol 8. Fullerton, CA: Society of Critical Care Medicine; 1987:1–11.
48. Hilberman M, Subramanian VH, Hazelgrove J. In vivo time resolved brain phosphorus nuclear magnetic resonance. *J Cereb Blood Flow Metab* 1984;4:334.
49. Behar K, den Hollander JA, Stromski ME, et al. High resolution ^{1}H nuclear magnetic resonance study of cerebral hypoxia in vivo. *Proc Natl Acad Sci U S A* 1983;80:4945–4948.
50. Gyulai L, Schnall MD, McLaughlin AC, et al. Simultaneous ^{31}P and ^{1}H nuclear magnetic resonance studies of hypoxia and ischemia in the cat brain. *J Cereb Blood Flow Metab* 1987;7:543–551.
51. Schnall MD, Yoshizaki K, Leigh JS. Triple nuclear NMR studies of cat brain metabolism during seizure. *Magn Reson Med* 1988;6:15–23.
52. Petroff OAC, Prichard JW, Behar KL, et al. In-vivo phosphorus nuclear magnetic resonance spectroscopy in status epilepticus. *Ann Neurol* 1985;16:169–177.
53. Nadler JV, Cooper JR. N-Acetyl-L-Aspartic acid content of human neural tumors and bovine peripheral nervous tissues. *J Neurochem* 1972;19:313–319.
54. Birken D, Oldendorf WH. N-Acetyl-L-Aspartic acid: review of a compound prominent in the ^{1}H NMR spectroscopic studies of brain. *Neurosc Behav Rev* 1989;13:23–30.
55. Ljunggren R, Ratcheson A, Seisjo BK. Cerebral metobolic state following complete compression ischemia. *Brain Reson* 1974;73:291.
56. Frahm J, Michaelis T, Merboldt KM, et al. Localized NMR spectroscopy in vivo. *NMR Biomed* 1989;2:188–195.
57. Hanstock CL, Rothman DL, Prichard JW, et al. Spatially localized 1H NMR spectra of metabolites in the human brain. *Proc Natl Acad Sci U S A* 1988;85:1821.
58. Gyulai L, Bolinger L, Leigh JS Jr. Phosphorylethanolamine—the major constituent of the phosphomonoester peak observed by ^{31}P NMR on the developing dog brain. *FEBS Lett* 1984;178:137.
59. Marris JM, Evans AE, McLaughlin AC, et al. ^{31}P nuclear magnetic resonance spectroscopic investigation of human neuroblastoma in situ. *N Engl J Med* 1985;312:1500.
60. Nakeda T, Kwee I, Card P, et al. ^{19}F NMR imaging of glucose metabolism. *Magn Reson Med* 1988;6:307–313.
61. Bittl J, Ingwall J. Comparative analysis of creatine kinase flux and enzyme content in the heart, brain and skeletal muscle of rat. *Abstracts of the Proceedings of the Society of Magnetic Resonance in Medicine.* Berkeley, CA: Society of Magnetic Resonance in Medicine; 1985:1:445.
62. Webb PG, Sailasuta P, Kohler SJ, Raidy T, Moats, RA, Hurd RE. Automated single-voxel proton MRS: technical development and multisite verification. *Magn Reson Med* 1994;31:365–373.
63. Bottomley PA, Drayer BP, Smith LS. Chronic adult cerebral infarction studied by phosphorus NMR spectroscopy. *Radiology* 1986;160:763–766.
64. Levine S, Welch K, Gdowski J, et al. The relationship of brain pH to energy metabolism and clinical outcome in acute human cerebral ischemia. *J Cereb Blood Flow Metab* 1989;9(Suppl 1):357.
65. Hugg JW, Duijn JH, Matson JB, Maudsley AA, Tsuruda JS, Gelinas DF, Weiner MW. Elevated lactate and alkalosis in chronic human brain infarction oberved by ^{1}H and ^{31}P MR spectroscopic imaging. *J Cereb Blood Flow Metab* 1992;12:734–744.
66. Rango M, Lenkinski RE, Alves W, Gennarelli TA. Brain pH in head injury. An image guided ^{31}P magnetic resonance spectroscopy study. *Ann Neurol* 1990;28:661–667.
67. Weiner MW, Hetherington H, Hubesch B, et al. Clinical magnetic resonance spectroscopy of brain, heart, liver, kidney and cancer: a quantitative approach. *NMR Biomed* 1989;2:290–297.
68. Berkelbach van der Sprenkel JW, Luyten PR, van Rijen PC, Tulleken CAF, den Hollander JA. Cerebral lactate detected by proton magnetic resonance spectroscopy in a patient with cerebral infarction. *Stroke* 1988;19:1556–1560.
69. Fenstermacher MJ, Narayana PA. Serial proton magnetic resonance spectroscopy of ischemic brain injury in humans. *Invest Radiol* 1990;25:1034–1039.
70. Ford CC, Griffey RH, Matwiyoff NA, Rosenberg GA. Multivoxel ^{1}H-MRS of stroke. *Neurology* 1992;42:1408–1412.
71. Felber SR, Aichner FT, Sauter R, Gerstenbraind F. Combined magnetic resonance imaging and proton magnetic resonance spectroscopy of patients with acute stroke. *Stroke* 1992;23:1106–1110.
72. Duijn JH, Matson GB, Maudsley AA, Hugg JW, Weiner MW. Proton spectroscopic imaging of human brain infarction. *Radiology* 1992;183:711–718.
73. Graham GD, Blamire AM, Howseman AM, Rothman DL, Fayad PB, Brass LM, Petroff OAC, Shulman RG, Prichard JW. Proton magnetic resonance spectroscopy of cerebral lactate and other metabolites in stroke patients. *Stroke* 1992;23:333–340.
74. Gideon P, Henriksen O, Sperlin B, Christiansen P, Olsen TS, Jorgensen HS, Arlien-Soborg P. Early time course of N-acetyl aspartate, creatine plus phosphocreatine and choline containing compounds in the brain after acute stroke: a proton magnetic resonance spectroscopy study. *Stroke* 1992;23:1566–1572.
75. Posner JB, Plum F. Independence of blood and cerebrospinal fluid lactate. *Arch Neurol* 1967;16:492–496.
76. Zupping R, Kaasik AE, Raudam E. Cerebrospinal fluid metabolic acidosis and brain oxygen supply. *Arch Neurol* 1971;23:33–38.
77. Petroff OAC, Graham GD, Blamire AM, Al-Rayes M, Rothman DL, Fayad PB, Brass LM, Shulman RG, Prichard JW. Spectroscopic imaging of stroke in man: histopathological correlates of spectral changes. *Neurology* 1992;42:1349–1354.
78. Rothman DL, Howseman AM, Graham GD, Petroff OAC,

Lantos G, Fayad PB, Brass LM, Shulman GI, Shulman RG, Prichard JW. Localized proton NMR observation of [3–^{13}C] lactate in stroke after [1–^{13}C] glucose infusion. *Magn Reson Med* 1991;21:302–307.

79. Chance B, Smith D, Delvoria-Papadopoulos M, Younkin D. New techniques for evaluating metabolic brain injury in newborn infants. *Basic Science Applications to Critical Care.* 1989;17: 405–409.
80. Hamilton PA, Hope PL, Cady EB, et al. Impaired energy metabolism in brains of newborn infants with increased crebral echodensities. *Lancet* 1986;1:1242–1246.
81. Azzopardi D, Wyatt JS, Cady EB, Delpy DT, Baudin J, Stewart AL, Hope PL, Hamilton PA, Reynolds EO. Prognosis of newborn infants with hypoxic-ischemic brain injury assessed by phosphorus magnetic resonance spectroscopy. *Pediatr Res* 1989;25:445–451.
82. Prichard JW. Nuclear magnetic resonance studies of seizure states. *Epilepsia* 1994;35(Suppl 6):S14–20.
83. Hugg JW, Laxer KD, Matson GB, Maudsley AA, Husted CA, Weiner MW. Lateralization of human focal epilepsy by ^{31}P magnetic resonance spectroscopic imaging. *Neurology* 1992;42: 2011–2018.
84. Hugg JW, Laxer KD, Matson GB, Maudsley AA, Weiner MW. Neuron loss localizes human temporal lobe epilepsy by in vivo magnetic resonance spectroscopic imaging. *Ann Neurol* 1993;34: 788–794.
85. Garcia PA, Laxer KD, van der Grond J, Hugg JW, Matson GB, Weiner MW. Phosphorus magnetic resonance spectroscopic imaging in patients with frontal lobe epilepsy. *Ann Neurol* 1994;35: 217–221.
86. Kuzniecky R, Elgavish GA, Hetherington HP, Evanochko WT, Pohost GM. In vivo ^{31}P nuclear magnetic resonance spectroscopy of human temporal lobe epilepsy. *Neurology* 1992;42:1586–1590.
87. Cendes F, Andermann F, Preul MC, Arnold DL. Lateralization of temporal lobe epilepsy based on regional metabolic abnormalities in proton magnetic resonance spectroscopic images. *Ann Neurol* 1994;35:211–216.
88. Connelly A, Jackson GD, Duncan JS, King MD, Gadian DG. Magnetic resonance spectroscopy in temporal lobe epilepsy. *Neurology* 1994; 44:1411–1417.
89. Gadian DG, Connelly A, Duncan JS, Cross JH, Kirkham FJ, Johnson CL, Vargha-Khadem F, Nevile BG, Jackson GD. ^{1}H magnetic resonance spectroscopy in the investigation of intractable epilepsy. *Acta Neurol Scand Suppl* 1994;152:116–121.
90. Bottomley PA, Hardy CJ, Cousins JP, Armstrong M, Wagle WA. AIDS dementia complex: brain high-energy phosphate metabolite deficits. *Radiology* 1990;176:407–411.
91. Menon DK, Baudouin CJ, Tomlinson D, Hoyle C. Proton MR spectroscopy and imaging of the brain in AIDS: evidence of neuronal loss in regions that appear normal with imaging. *J Comput Assist Tomogr* 1990;14:882–885.
92. Menon DK, Ainsworth JG, Cox IJ, Coker RC, Sargentoni J, Coutts GA, Baudouin CJ, Kocsis EA, Harris JRW. Proton MR spectroscopy of the brain in AIDS dementia complex. *J Comput Assist Tomogr* 1992;16:538–542.
93. Meyerhoff DJ, Mackay S, Bachman L, Poole N, Dillon WP, Weiner MW, Fein G. Reduced brain N-acetylaspartate suggests neuronal loss in cognitively impaired human immunodeficiency virus-seropositive individuals: in vivo ^{1}H magnetic resonance spectroscopic imaging. *Neurology* 1993;43:509–515.
94. Meyerhoff DJ, MacKay S, Poole N, Dillon WP, Weiner MW, Fein G. N-acetylaspartate reductions measured by ^{1}H MRSI in cognitively impaired HIV-seropositive individuals. *Magn Reson Imaging* 1994;12:653–659.
95. Jarvik JG, Lenkinski RE, Grossman RI, Gomori JM, Schnall MD, Frank I. Proton MR spectroscopy of HIV-infected patients: characterization of abnormalities with imaging and clinical correlation. *Radiology* 1993;186:739–744.
96. Chong WK, Sweeney B, Wilkinson ID, Paley M, Hall-Craggs MA, Kendall BE, Shepard JK, Beecham M, Miller RF, Weller IVD, Newman SP, Harrison MJG. Proton spectroscopy of the brain in HIV infection: correlation with clinical, immunologic, and MR imaging findings. *Radiology* 1993;188:119–124.
97. Chong WK, Paley M, Wilkinson ID, Hall-Craggs MA, Sweeney B, Harrison MJG, Miller RF, Kendall BE. Localized cerebral proton MR spectroscopy in HIV infection and AIDS. *AJNR* 1994;15:21–25.
98. Pettegrew JW, Withers G, Panchalingam K, Post JF. ^{31}P nuclear magnetic resonance (NMR) spectroscopy of brain in aging and Alzheimer's disease. *J Neural Transmission* [*Suppl*] 1987;24: 261–268.
99. Pettegrew JW, Panchalingam K, Moossy J, Martinez J, Rao G, Boller F. Correlation of phosphorus-31 magnetic resonance spectroscopy and morphologic findings in Alzheimer's disease. *Arch Neurol* 1988;45:1093–1096.
100. Pettegrew JW, Moossy J, Withers G, McKeag D, Panchalingam K. ^{31}P nuclear magnetic resonance study of the brain in Alzheimer's disease. *J Neuropathol Exp Neurol* 1988;47:235–248.
101. Pettegrew JW. Molecular insights into Alzheimer's disease. *Ann N Y Acad Sci* 1989;568:5–28.
102. Pettegrew JW, Panchalingam K, Klunk WE, McClure RJ, Muenz LR. Alterations of cerebral metabolism in probable Alzheimer's disease: a preliminary study. *Neurobiol Aging* 1994;15:117–132.
103. Bottomley PA, Cousins JP, Pendrey DL, Wagle WA, Hardy CJ, Eames FA, McCaffrey RJ, Thompson DA. Alzheimer dementia: quantification of energy metabolism and mobile phosphoesters with P-31 NMR spectroscopy. *Radiology* 1992;183:695–699.
104. Klunk WE, Panchalingam K, Moossy J, McClure RJ, Pettegrew JW. N-acetyl-L-aspartate and other amino acid metabolites in Alzheimer's disease brain: a preliminary proton nuclear magnetic resonance study. *Neurology* 1992;42:1578–1585.
105. Miller BL, Moats RA, Shonk T, Ernst T, Woolley S, Ross BD. Alzheimer disease: depiction of increased cerebral myo-inositol with proton MR spectroscopy. *Radiology* 1993;187:433–437.
106. Moats RA, Ernst T, Shonk TK, Ross BD. Abnormal cerebral metabolite concentrations in patients with probable Alzheimer's disease. *Magn Reson Med* 1994;32:110–115.
107. Shiino A, Matsuda M, Morikawa S, Inubushi T, Akiguchi I, Handa J. Proton magnetic resonance spectroscopy with dementia. *Surg Neurol* 1993;39:143–147.
108. Meyerhoff DJ, MacKay S, Constans JM, Norman D, Van Dyke C, Fein G, Weiner MW. Axonal injury and membrane alterations in Alzheimer's disease suggested by in vivo proton magnetic resonance spectroscopic imaging. *Ann Neurol* 1994;36:40–47.
109. Jenkins BG, Koroshetz WJ, Beal MF, Rosen BR. Evidence for impairment of energy metabolism in vivo in Huntington's disease using localized ^{1}H NMR spectroscopy. *Neurology* 1993;43:2689–2695.
110. Nicoli F, Vion-Dury J, Maloteaux JM, Delwaide C, Confort-Gouny S, Sciaky M, Cozzone P. CSF and serum metabolic profile of patients with Huntington's chorea: a study by high resolution proton NMR spectroscopy and HPLC. *Neurosci Lett* 1993;154: 47–51.
111. Negendank W. Studies of human tumors by MRS: a review. *NMR Biomed* 1992;5:303–324.
112. Wolinsky JS, Narayana PA, Fenstermacher MJ. Proton magnetic resonance spectroscopy in multiple sclerosis. *Neurology* 1990; 40(11):1764–1769.
113. Narayana PA, Wolinsky JS, Jackson EF, McCarthy M. Proton MR spectroscopy of gadolinium-enhanced multiple sclerosis plaques. *J Magn Reson Imaging* 1992;2(3):263–270.
114. Matthews PM, Francis G, Antel J, Arnold DL. Proton magnetic resonance spectroscopy for metabolic characterization of plaques in multiple sclerosis [published erratum appears in *Neurology* 1991;41(11):1828]. *Neurology* 1991;41(8):1251–1256.
115. Arnold DL, Riess GT, Matthews PM, Francis GS, Collins DL, Wolfson C, Antel JP. Use of proton magnetic resonance spectroscopy for monitoring disease progression in multiple sclerosis. *Ann Neurol* 1994;36(1):76–82.
116. Van Hecke P, Marchal G, Johannik K, Demaerel P, Wilms G, Carton H, Baert AL. Human brain proton localized NMR spectroscopy in multiple sclerosis. *Magn Reson Med* 1991;18(1):199–206.
117. Larsson HB, Christiansen P, Jensen M, Frederiksen J, Heltberg A, Olesen J, Henriksen O. Localized in vivo proton spectroscopy in the brain of patients with multiple sclerosis. *Magn Reson Med* 1991;22(1):23–31.

118. Husted CA, Matson GB, Adams DA, Goodin DS, Weiner MW. In vivo detection of myelin phospholipids in multiple sclerosis with phosphorus magnetic resonance spectroscopic imaging. *Ann Neurol* 1994;36(2):239–241.
119. Husted CA, Goodin DS, Hugg JW, Maudsley AA, Tsuruda JS, de Bie SH, Fein G, Matson GB, Weiner MW. Biochemical alterations in multiple sclerosis lesions and normal-appearing white matter detected by in vivo 31P and 1H spectroscopic imaging. *Ann Neurol* 1994;36(2):157–165.
120. Grossman RI, Lenkinski RE, Ramer KN, Gonzalez-Scarano F, Cohen JA. MR proton spectroscopy in multiple sclerosis. *AJNR* 1992;13(6):1535–1543.
121. Hiehle JF, Lenkinski RE, Grossman RI, Dousset V, Ramer KN, Schnall MD, Cohen JA, Gonzalez-Scarano F. Correlation of spectroscopy and magnetization transfer imaging in the evaluation of demyelinating lesions and normal appearing white matter in multiple sclerosis. *Magn Reson Med* 1994;32(3):285–293.
122. Luyten PR, Brutink G, Sloff FM, et al. Broadband proton decoupling in human ^{31}P NMR spectroscopy. *NMR Biomed* 1989;1: 177–183.
123. Murphy-Boesch J, Stoyanova R, Srinivasan R, Willard T, Vignernon D, Nelson S, Taylor JS, Brown TR. Proton-decoupled ^{31}P chemical shift imaging of human brain in normal volunteers. *NMR Biomed* 1993;6:173–180.

Subject Index

J

K

L

T

U

V

ISBN 0-7817-0282-8

9 780781 702829